WebMD

SCIENTIFIC AMERICAN®
MEDICINE

2003 Edition

WebMD

SCIENTIFIC AMERICAN®
MEDICINE

2003 Edition

Volume 1

David C. Dale, M.D., F.A.C.P.

Professor of Medicine
University of Washington Medical Center

EDITOR-IN-CHIEF

Daniel D. Federman, M.D., M.A.C.P.

The Carl W. Walter Distinguished Professor of Medicine and Medical Education
and Senior Dean for Alumni Relations and Clinical Teaching
Harvard Medical School

FOUNDING EDITOR

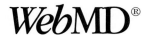

ISBN: 0-9703902-5-4

Vice President and Publisher	Nancy E. Chorpenning
Director, Electronic Publishing	Liz Pope
Managing Editor	Nancy Terry
Development Editor	John Heinegg
Senior Copy Editor	John J. Anello
Copy Editor	Dave Terry
Art and Design Editor	Elizabeth Klarfeld
Electronic Composition	Diane Joiner, Jennifer Smith
Manufacturing Producer	Kelly Mercado
Indexer	Julia Brooks Figures

Printed in the United States of America

Published by WebMD Inc.

WebMD Scientific American® Medicine
WebMD Professional Publishing
224 West 30th Street
Fourth Floor
New York, NY 10001-4905

The authors, editors, and publisher have conscientiously and carefully tried to ensure that recommended measures and drug dosages in these pages are accurate and conform to the standards that prevailed at the time of publication. The reader is advised, however, to check the product information sheet accompanying each drug to be familiar with any changes in the dosage schedule or in the contraindications. This advice should be taken with particular seriousness if the agent to be administered is a new one or one that is infrequently used. *WebMD Scientific American® Medicine* describes basic principles of diagnosis and therapy. Because of the uniqueness of each patient and the need to take into account a number of concurrent considerations, however, this information should be used by physicians only as a general guide to clinical decision making.

Editorial Board

Contributors

Elizabeth A. Abel, M.D.   Clinical Professor of Dermatology, Stanford University School of Medicine

W. Stewart Agras, M.D.   Professor of Psychiatry (Emeritus), Department of Psychiatry and Behavioral Sciences, Stanford University School of Medicine

Aijaz Ahmed, M.D.   Assistant Professor of Medicine, Stanford University School of Medicine

Joseph Alpert, M.D.   Robert S. and Irene P. Flinn Professor of Medicine and Head, Department of Medicine, University of Arizona College of Medicine

Nancy A. Alvarez, Pharm.D.   Product Information Manager, Medical Affairs, Endo Pharmaceuticals, Inc.

Michael J. Aminoff, M.D., D.Sc.   Professor of Neurology, University of California, San Francisco, School of Medicine

Paul Anderson, M.D., Ph.D.   Associate Professor of Medicine, Harvard Medical School, and Rheumatologist, Division of Rheumatology and Immunology, Brigham and Women's Hospital

Gerald B. Appel, M.D.   Professor of Clinical Medicine, Columbia University College of Physicians and Surgeons, and Director of Clinical Nephrology, New York Presbyterian Hospital

Frederick R. Appelbaum, M.D.   Professor and Head, Division of Medical Oncology, University of Washington School of Medicine, and Member and Director, Clinical Research Division, Fred Hutchinson Cancer Research Center

William F. Armstrong, M.D.   Professor of Internal Medicine, Associate Clinical Chief of Cardiology, and Director of the Echocardiography Laboratory, University of Michigan Health System

Frank C. Arnett, M.D.   Chairman, Department of Internal Medicine, and Professor of Internal Medicine and of Pathology and Laboratory Medicine and Elizabeth Bidgood Chair in Rheumatology, University of Texas Health Science Center at Houston

Bimal H. Ashar, M.D.   Assistant Professor of Medicine, Johns Hopkins University School of Medicine

Michael Augenbraun, M.D.   Associate Professor of Medicine, State University of New York Downstate Medical Center

Robert L. Barbieri, M.D.   Kate Macy Ladd Professor of Obstetrics, Gynecology, and Reproductive Biology, Harvard Medical School, and Head, Department of Obstetrics, Gynecology, and Reproductive Biology, Brigham and Women's Hospital

Michael J. Barry, M.D.   Associate Professor of Medicine, Harvard Medical School, and Chief, General Medical Unit, Massachusetts General Hospital

Dennis J. Beer, M.D.   Chief of Pulmonary Medicine and Director, Critical Care Unit, Newton-Wellesley Hospital

Vincent S. Beltrani, M.D.   Visiting Professor of Medicine, University of Medicine and Dentistry of New Jersey/Robert Wood Johnson Medical School

Sarah L. Berga, M.D.   Professor of Obstetrics, Gynecology, and Reproductive Sciences and Professor of Psychiatry, University of Pittsburgh School of Medicine, and Director, Division of Reproductive Endocrinology and Infertility, Magee-Women's Hospital

Peter B. Berger, M.D.   Professor of Medicine, Mayo Medical School, and Consultant, Cardiac Catheterization Laboratory and Coronary Care Unit, Mayo Clinic

Robert M. Black, M.D.   Associate Professor of Medicine, University of Massachusetts Medical School, and Director, Division of Renal Medicine, Worcester Medical Center

Gary M. Brittenham, M.D.   Professor of Pediatrics and Medicine, Columbia University College of Physicians and Surgeons

Beth L. Brogan, M.D.   Department of Medicine, Vanderbilt University School of Medicine

Virginia C. Broudy, M.D.   Professor of Medicine, Division of Hematology, University of Washington School of Medicine, and Chief, Section of Hematology, Harborview Medical Center

J. Steven Burdick, M.D.   Associate Professor of Medicine, University of Texas Southwestern Medical Center at Dallas, and Medical Director, Gastroenterology and Endoscopy, Parkland Health and Hospital System

Jean-Claude Bystryn, M.D.   Professor of Dermatology, New York University School of Medicine, and Director, Melanoma Immunotherapy Clinic, NYU Kaplan Comprehensive Cancer Center

David A. Calhoun, M.D.   Assistant Professor of Medicine, Division of Cardiovascular Disease, and Medical Director, Vascular Biology and Hypertension Program, University of Alabama at Birmingham School of Medicine

Michael Camilleri, M.D.   Professor of Medicine and Physiology, Mayo Medical School, and Consultant, Internal Medicine and Gastroenterology, Mayo Clinic

Stephen A. Cannistra, M.D.   Associate Professor of Medicine, Harvard Medical School, and Director, Gynecologic Medical Oncology, Beth Israel Deaconess Medical Center

Robert L. Carithers, Jr., M.D. Professor of Medicine and Director, Hepatology Section, Division of Gastroenterology, Department of Medicine, and Medical Director, Liver Transplantation Program, University of Washington School of Medicine

Robert W. Carlson, M.D. Professor of Medicine, Division of Oncology, Stanford University School of Medicine

Maria Torroella Carney, M.D. Geriatrics and Adult Development, Mount Sinai School of Medicine

Charles B. Carpenter, M.D. Professor of Medicine, Harvard Medical School, and Senior Physician, Brigham and Women's Hospital

Christine K. Cassel, M.D. Dean and Vice President for Medical Affairs, Oregon Health Sciences University School of Medicine

Ned H. Cassem, M.D. Professor of Psychiatry, Harvard Medical School, and Psychiatrist, Massachusetts General Hospital

Colin H. Chalk, M.D., C.M. Associate Professor, Department of Neurology and Neurosurgery, McGill University Faculty of Medicine, and Associate Physician, Division of Neurology, Montreal General Hospital

Bruce D. Cheson, M.D. Head, Medicine Section, Clinical Investigations Branch, Cancer Therapy Evaluation Program, National Cancer Institute

Sudhansu Chokroverty, M.D. Professor of Neurology, New York Medical College; Clinical Professor of Neurology, University of Medicine and Dentistry of New Jersey/Robert Wood Johnson Medical School; and Associate Chairman and Program Director, Department of Neurology, Chairman, Division of Clinical Neurophysiology, and Director, Center of Sleep Medicine, St. Vincent's Hospital and Medical Center

Mina Chung, M.D. Electrophysiologist, Department of Cardiovascular Medicine, Cleveland Clinic Foundation

W. Hallowell Churchill, M.D. Associate Professor of Medicine, Harvard Medical School, and Medical Director, Therapeutic Services, Brigham and Women's Hospital

Eric P. Cohen, M.D. Professor of Medicine, Division of Nephrology, Department of Medicine, Medical College of Wisconsin

Robert W. Coombs, M.D., Ph.D. Associate Professor, Department of Laboratory Medicine, University of Washington School of Medicine

Kevin D. Cooper, M.D. Professor and Chair, Department of Dermatology, Case Western Reserve University School of Medicine; Director, Department of Dermatology, University Hospitals of Cleveland; and Director, NIAMS Skin Disease Research Center

Mark A. Creager, M.D. Associate Professor of Medicine, Harvard Medical School; and Director, Vascular Center, and Member, Vascular Medicine Section, Cardiovascular Division, Brigham and Women's Hospital

Mark R. Cullen, M.D. Professor of Medicine and Public Health and Director, Occupational and Environmental Medicine Program, Yale University School of Medicine

Pamela J. Daffern, M.D. Assistant Professor of Internal Medicine, Division of Rheumatology, Allergy, and Immunology, Medical College of Virginia at Virginia Commonwealth University

Marinos C. Dalakas, M.D. Chief, Neuromuscular Diseases Section, National Institute of Neurological Disorders and Stroke, National Institutes of Health

David C. Dale, M.D. Professor of Medicine, University of Washington Medical Center

C. Ralph Daniel III, M.D. Clinical Professor of Medicine (Dermatology), University of Mississippi Medical Center

John R. David, M.D. Richard Pearson Strong Professor, Department of Immunology and Infectious Diseases, Harvard School of Public Health, and Professor of Medicine, Harvard Medical School

Nancy E. Davidson, M.D. Professor of Oncology and Breast Cancer Research Chair in Oncology, Johns Hopkins University School of Medicine, and Director, Breast Cancer Program, Johns Hopkins Oncology Center

G. William Dec, M.D. Associate Professor of Medicine, Harvard Medical School; and Medical Director, Cardiac Transplantation Program, and Director, Clinical Cardiology, Massachusetts General Hospital

Alan H. DeCherney, M.D. Professor of Obstetrics and Gynecology, UCLA School of Medicine

Mahlon R. DeLong, M.D. Professor and Chairman, Department of Neurology, Emory University School of Medicine

James Q. Del Rosso, D.O. Clinical Assistant Professor, Department of Dermatology, University of Nevada School of Medicine

David B. DeLurgio, M.D. Assistant Professor of Cardiac Electrophysiology, Emory University School of Medicine, and Electrophysiologist, Emory Crawford Long Hospital

Roman W. DeSanctis, M.D. Evelyn and James Jenks/Paul Dudley White Professor of Medicine, Harvard Medical School, and Physician and Director (Emeritus) of Clinical Cardiology, Massachusetts General Hospital

Adrian S. Dobs, M.D., M.H.S. Professor of Medicine and Oncology and Director, Clinical Trials Unit, Johns Hopkins University School of Medicine

Michael S. Donnenberg, M.D. Professor of Medicine, Professor of Microbiology and Immunology, and Head, Division of Infectious Diseases, University of Maryland School of Medicine

William H. Dribben, M.D. Assistant Professor of Medicine, Washington University School of Medicine, St. Louis

Jeffrey Duchin, M.D. Assistant Professor of Medicine, Division of Allergy and Infectious Disease, University of Washington School of Medicine, and Chief, Communicable Disease Control, Department of Public Health, Seattle and King County, Washington

Pamela Woods Duncan, Ph.D., P.T. Professor, Health Services Administration and Physical Therapy, Director, Brooks Center for Rehabilitation Studies, and Director, Department of Veterans Affairs Rehabilitation Outcomes Research Center, University of Florida College of Medicine

Peter James Dyck, M.D. Professor of Neurology, Mayo Medical School, and Consultant, Department of Neurology, Mayo Clinic

Kim A. Eagle, M.D. Albion Walter Hewlett Professor of Internal Medicine and Chief of Clinical Cardiology, University of Michigan Health System

Helen K. Edelberg, M.D. Assistant Professor, Department of Geriatrics, Mount Sinai School of Medicine

Randolph W. Evans, M.D. Clinical Associate Professor of Medicine, Department of Neurology, University of Texas at Houston Medical School

Stefan Faderl, M.D. Assistant Professor, Department of Leukemia, University of Texas M.D. Anderson Cancer Center

Douglas Fearon, M.D. Wellcome Trust Professor of Medicine, Wellcome Trust Immunology Unit, University of Cambridge School of Clinical Medicine, England

Daniel D. Federman, M.D. The Carl W. Walter Distinguished Professor of Medicine and Medical Education and Senior Dean for Alumni Relations and Clinical Teaching, Harvard Medical School

Mark Feldman, M.D. William O. Tschumy, Jr., M.D. , Chair of Internal Medicine and Clinical Professor of Internal Medicine, University of Texas Southwestern Medical School at Dallas, and Director, Internal Medicine Residency Program, Presbyterian Hospital of Dallas

Paul E. Fenster, M.D. Associate Professor of Medicine, University of Arizona College of Medicine

Gary S. Firestein, M.D. Professor of Medicine and Chief, Division of Rheumatology, Allergy and Immunology, University of California, San Diego, School of Medicine

Stephen P. Fortmann, M.D. C. F. Rehnborg Professor of Preventive Medicine and Director, Stanford Center for Research in Disease Prevention, Stanford University School of Medicine

Elliot M. Frohman, M.D., Ph.D. Director of the Multiple Sclerosis Program and Associate Professor of Neurology, University of Texas Southwestern Medical School

Bradley Galer, M.D. Vice President, Scientific Affairs, Endo Pharmaceuticals, Inc., and Director of Clinical Studies, Institute for Education and Research in Pain, Beth Israel Medical Center

Arnold Gammaitoni, Pharm.D. Manager, Medical Affairs, Endo Pharmaceuticals, Inc.

Marc B. Garnick, M.D. Clinical Professor of Medicine, Harvard Medical School; Physician, Hematology and Oncology Division, Beth Israel Deaconess Medical Center; and Chief Medical Officer, Praecis Pharmaceuticals, Inc.

Layne O. Gentry, M.D. Clinical Professor of Medicine, Baylor College of Medicine; and Chief, Infectious Disease Section, and Medical Director, Infection Control, St. Luke's Episcopal Hospital

Saul Genuth, M.D. Professor of Medicine, Division of Clinical and Molecular Endocrinology, Case Western Reserve University School of Medicine

Donald H. Gilden, M.D. Professor and Chairman, Department of Neurology, University of Colorado Health Sciences Center

Marcia B. Goldberg, M.D. Associate Physician, Division of Infectious Disease, Massachusetts General Hospital, and Associate Professor of Medicine (Microbiology and Molecular Genetics), Harvard Medical School

David B. K. Golden, M.D. Associate Professor of Medicine, Johns Hopkins University School of Medicine

Matthew R. Golden, M.D., M.P.H. Assistant Professor of Medicine, University of Washington School of Medicine

Stanley Goldfarb, M.D. Professor of Medicine and Interim Chair, Department of Medicine, University of Pennsylvania School of Medicine

Francisco González-Scarano, M.D. Professor of Neurology and Microbiology, Department of Neurology, University of Pennsylvania School of Medicine

Mitchell H. Grayson, M.D. Instructor, Department of Medicine, Division of Allergy/Immunology, Washington University School of Medicine, St. Louis

Brian P. Griffin, M.D. Staff Cardiologist, Section of Imaging, and Director, Cardiovascular Training Program, Department of Cardiology, Cleveland Clinic Foundation

Pearl E. Grimes, M.D. Clinical Associate Professor of Dermatology, Division of Dermatology, University of California, Los Angeles, School of Medicine, and Director, Vitiligo and Pigmentation Institute of Southern California

Duane J. Gubler, Sc.D. Adjunct Professor, Department of Microbiology, Colorado State University; Adjunct Professor, Department of International Health, Johns Hopkins University School of Public Health; and Director, Division of Vector-Borne Infectious Diseases, National Center for Infectious Diseases, Centers for Disease Control and Prevention

Kalpana Gupta, M.D., M.P.H. Acting Assistant Professor of Medicine, Division of Infectious Diseases, Department of Medicine, University of Washington School of Medicine

Daniel A. Haber, M.D., Ph.D. Professor of Medicine, Harvard Medical School, and Director, Center for Cancer Risk Analysis, Massachusetts General Hospital Cancer Center

William N. Hait, M.D., Ph.D. Professor of Medicine and Pharmacology and Associate Dean, Oncology Program, University of Medicine and Dentistry of New Jersey/Robert Wood Johnson Medical School, and Director, Cancer Institute of New Jersey

Allan C. Halpern, M.D. Associate Professor of Dermatology, Joan and Sanford I. Weill Medical College of Cornell University, and Chief, Dermatology Service, Memorial Sloan-Kettering Cancer Center

Stephen B. Hanauer, M.D. Professor of Medicine and Clinical Pharmacology, University of Chicago Pritzker School of Medicine, and Director, Section of Gastroenterology/Nutrition, University of Chicago Hospital

E. William Hancock, M.D. Professor of Medicine Emeritus (Cardiovascular Medicine), Stanford University School of Medicine

William V. Harford, Jr., M.D. Professor of Medicine, Department of Medicine, University of Texas Southwestern Medical School at Dallas, and Director, Clinical Gastroenterology Laboratory, Dallas Veterans Affairs Medical Center

Frederick G. Hayden, M.D., Ph.D. Stuart S. Richardson Professor of Clinical Virology and Professor of Medicine and Pathology, Departments of Internal Medicine and Pathology, University of Virginia School of Medicine

Brian Haynes, M.D., Ph.D. Professor of Clinical Epidemiology and Medicine and Chair, Department of Clinical Epidemiology and Biostatistics, McMaster University Health Sciences Centre

Martin S. Hirsch, M.D. Professor of Medicine, Harvard Medical School, and Physician, Massachusetts General Hospital

Jan V. Hirschmann, M.D. Professor of Medicine, University of Washington School of Medicine, and Assistant Chief, Medical Service, Puget Sound Veterans Affairs Medical Center

Jack Hirsh, M.D. Professor Emeritus, McMaster University, and Director, Hamilton Civic Hospitals Research Centre

Michael K. Hise, M.D. Associate Professor of Medicine, University of Maryland School of Medicine

Eric G. Honig, M.D. Professor of Medicine, Emory University School of Medicine

Sandra J. Horning, M.D. Professor of Medicine, Stanford University School of Medicine

Christian E. Huber, M.D. Postdoctoral Research Fellow, Infectious Disease Division, Brown University School of Medicine

Adolph M. Hutter, Jr., M.D. Professor of Medicine, Harvard Medical School, and Physician, Massachusetts General Hospital

Steven E. Hyman, M.D. Provost, Harvard University, and past Director, National Institute of Mental Health

Conrad Iber, M.D.   Associate Professor of Medicine, Department of Medicine, University of Minnesota Medical School, and Pulmonologist, Division of Pulmonary and Critical Care Medicine, Hennepin County Medical Center

Roland H. Ingram, Jr., M.D.   Martha West Looney Professor of Medicine (Emeritus), Emory University School of Medicine

Silvio E. Inzucchi, M.D.   Associate Professor of Medicine, Section of Endocrinology, Yale University School of Medicine

Michael G. Ison, M.D.   Fellow, Division of Infectious Diseases, University of Virginia School of Medicine

Khursheed N. Jeejeebhoy, M.B.B.S., Ph.D.   Professor of Medicine, Nutrition and Physiology, University of Toronto

Jorge L. Juncos, M.D.   Associate Professor, Department of Neurology, Emory University School of Medicine, Wesley Woods Geriatric Center

Kefei Kang, M.D.   Associate Professor of Dermatology, Case Western Reserve University School of Medicine

Hagop M. Kantarjian, M.D.   Professor of Medicine and Chairman, Department of Leukemia, University of Texas M. D. Anderson Cancer Center

Philip W. Kantoff, M.D.   Associate Professor of Medicine, Harvard Medical School, and Director, Lank Center for Genitourinary Oncology, Dana-Farber Cancer Institute

Adolf W. Karchmer, M.D.   Professor of Medicine, Harvard Medical School, and Chief, Division of Infectious Diseases, Beth Israel Deaconess Medical Center

Scott E. Kasner, M.D.   Assistant Professor, Department of Neurology, University of Pennsylvania School of Medicine, and Director, Comprehensive Stroke Center, University of Pennsylvania Medical Center

Carol A. Kauffman, M.D.   Professor of Medicine, Department of Internal Medicine, University of Michigan Medical School

Clive Kearon, M.B., Ph.D.   Associate Professor of Medicine, McMaster University, and Head of the Thrombosis Service, Henderson General Hospital, Hamilton Health Sciences

Emmet B. Keeffe, M.D.   Professor of Medicine, Stanford University School of Medicine; and Co-Director, Liver Transplant Program, and Chief of Hepatology, Stanford University Medical Center

Nino Khetsuriani, M.D., Ph.D.   Medical Epidemiologist, Respiratory and Enteric Viruses Branch, Centers for Disease Control and Prevention

David K. Klassen, M.D.   Professor of Medicine, University of Maryland School of Medicine

Allan Klein, M.D.   Professor of Medicine and Director, Cardiovascular Imaging Research, Department of Cardiovascular Medicine, Cleveland Clinic Foundation

Sandra Knowles, B.Sc.Pharm.   Pharmacist, Drug Safety Clinic, Sunnybrook and Women's College Health Science Centre

Phillip Korenblat, M.D.   Professor of Clinical Medicine, Washington University School of Medicine, St. Louis

Stephen M. Krane, M.D.   Persis, Cyrus, and Marlow B. Harrison Professor of Medicine, Harvard Medical School, and Physician, Medical Services, Massachusetts General Hospital

Jonathan J. Langberg, M.D.   Professor of Medicine, Cardiology Division, Emory University School of Medicine, and Director, Cardiac Electrophysiology Laboratory, Emory University Hospital

Richard A. Larson, M.D.   Professor of Medicine, University of Chicago Pritzker School of Medicine

Mark Lebwohl, M.D.   Sol and Clara Kest Professor and Chairman, Department of Dermatology, Mount Sinai School of Medicine

Lawrence L. K. Leung, M.D.   Professor of Medicine and Chief, Division of Hematology, Department of Medicine, Stanford University School of Medicine

Mark D. Levine, M.D.   Clinical Instructor in Emergency Medicine, Washington University School of Medicine, St. Louis

Lawrence M. Lewis, M.D.   Associate Professor of Medicine and Chief, Division of Emergency Medicine, Washington University School of Medicine, St. Louis

Frederick P. Li, M.D.   Professor of Clinical Cancer Epidemiology, Harvard School of Public Health; Professor of Medicine, Harvard Medical School; and Harry and Elsa Jiler American Cancer Society Clinical Research Professor

W. Conrad Liles, M.D., Ph.D.   Associate Professor of Medicine, University of Washington School of Medicine

J. William Lindsey, M.D.   Assistant Professor of Neurology, University of Texas Health Science Center at Houston

Michael D. Lockshin, M.D.   Director, Barbara Volcker Center for Women and Rheumatic Disease, Hospital for Special Surgery, New York

Brian F. Mandell, M.D., Ph.D.   Education Program Director, Department of Rheumatic and Immunologic Diseases, and Senior Associate Program Director, Internal Medicine Residency Program, Cleveland Clinic Foundation

Charles M. Mansbach II, M.D.   Professor of Medicine and Physiology and Chief, Division of Gastroenterology, Department of Medicine, University of Tennessee, Memphis, College of Medicine

David J. Maron, M.D.   Associate Professor of Medicine and Director, Preventive Cardiology, Division of Cardiovascular Medicine, Vanderbilt University School of Medicine

Jeanne M. Marrazzo, M.D., M.P.H.   Assistant Professor of Medicine, University of Washington School of Medicine

Robert J. Mayer, M.D.   Professor of Medicine, Harvard Medical School, and Vice Chair for Academic Affairs, Department of Adult Oncology, Dana-Farber Cancer Institute

Elaine T. McParland, M.D., J.D.   Research Associate, Department of Geriatrics, Mount Sinai School of Medicine

Terry J. Mengert, M.D.   Associate Professor of Medicine, University of Washington School of Medicine

Edgar L. Milford, M.D.   Associate Professor of Medicine, Harvard Medical School

Lewis B. Morgenstern, M.D.   Associate Professor of Neurology and Epidemiology and Co-Director, Stroke Program, University of Texas–Houston Medical School

Robb Moses, M.D.   Professor and Chair, Department of Molecular and Medical Genetics, Oregon Health Sciences University School of Medicine

Marc Moss, M.D.   Associate Professor of Medicine, Emory University School of Medicine, and Director, Medical Intensive Care Unit, Grady Memorial Hospital

George Moxley, M.D.   Associate Professor, Division of Rheumatology, Allergy and Immunology, Medical College of Virginia at Virginia Commonwealth University, and Chief, Rheumatology Section, McGuire Veterans Affairs Medical Center

Mary P. Mullen, M.D., Ph.D.   Instructor in Pediatrics, Harvard Medical School, and Assistant in Cardiology, Children's Hospital, Boston

Patricia L. Myskowski, M.D. Associate Professor of Dermatology, Joan and Sanford I. Weill Medical College of Cornell University, and Associate Attending Physician, Dermatology Service, Memorial Sloan-Kettering Cancer Center

Patrick G. O'Connor, M.D., M.P.H. Professor of Medicine and Chief, Program in Primary Care Medicine, Yale University School of Medicine, and Director, Primary Care, Yale-New Haven Hospital

Nancy J. Olsen, M.D. Professor of Medicine, Vanderbilt University School of Medicine

Kent R. Olson, M.D. Clinical Professor of Medicine, Pediatrics and Pharmacy, University of California, San Francisco, Schools of Medicine and Pharmacy, and Medical Director, San Francisco Division, California Poison Control System

Steven M. Opal, M.D. Professor of Medicine, Department of Medicine, Brown University School of Medicine

Suzanne Oparil, M.D. Professor of Medicine, Professor of Physiology and Biophysics, and Director of the Vascular Biology and Hypertension Program of the Division of Cardiovascular Disease, University of Alabama at Birmingham School of Medicine

Catherine M. Otto, M.D. Professor of Medicine and Acting Director, Division of Cardiology, and Director, Cardiology Fellowship Program, University of Washington School of Medicine

Roberta A. Pagon, M.D. Professor of Pediatrics, University of Washington School of Medicine; Medical Director, GeneTests Genetic Testing Resource, Children's Hospital and Regional Medical Center; and Editor-in-Chief, GeneClinics: Medical Genetics Knowledge Base, University of Washington

Biff P. Palmer, M.D. Professor of Medicine, University of Texas Southwestern Medical Center at Dallas

Robert M. Palmer, M.D. Head, Section of Geriatric Medicine, Cleveland Clinic Foundation

Umesh D. Parashar M.D., M.P.H. Medical Epidemiologist, Centers for Disease Control and Prevention

Manish M. Patel, M.D. Assistant Professor, Department of Emergency Medicine, Emory University School of Medicine

James D. Perkins, M.D. Professor of Surgery, and Chief, Division of Transplantation, University of Washington Medical Center

Mark G. Perlroth, M.D. Professor of Medicine, Division of Cardiovascular Medicine, Stanford University School of Medicine

Lyle R. Petersen, M.D., M.P.H. Deputy Director for Science, Division of Vector-Borne Infectious Diseases, Centers for Disease Control and Prevention

Jerome B. Posner, M.D. George C. Cotzias Chair in Neuro-Oncology and Member, Memorial Sloan-Kettering Cancer Center

Ruth B. Purtilo, Ph.D. Director and Dr. C. C. and Mabel Criss Professor of Clinical Ethics, Creighton University Center for Health Policy and Ethics

Bruce G. Redman, D.O. Associate Professor of Internal Medicine, Division of Hematology/Oncology, University of Michigan Medical School

David A. Relman, M.D. Associate Professor, Department of Medicine (Infectious Diseases) and Department of Microbiology and Immunology, Stanford University School of Medicine, and Staff Physician, Veterans Affairs Palo Alto Health Care System

John T. Repke, M.D. The Chris J. and Marie A. Olson Distinguished Professor of Obstetrics and Gynecology, University of Nebraska Medical Center

Jennifer Rhodes-Kropf, M.D. Geriatrics and Adult Development, Mount Sinai School of Medicine

Ross E. Rocklin, M.D. Senior Director, Clinical Research, and Senior Scientist, Astra U.S.A.

Fred S. Rosen, M.D. James L. Gamble Professor of Pediatrics, Harvard Medical School, and President, Center for Blood Research, Boston

Linda Rosenstock, M.D., M.P.H. Dean, University of California, Los Angeles, School of Public Health

Allen D. Roses, M.D. Senior Vice President, Genetics Research, GlaxoSmithKline

Eric H. Rubin, M.D. Associate Professor of Medicine and Pharmacology, University of Medicine and Dentistry of New Jersey/Robert Wood Johnson Medical School, and Director of Clinical Pharmacology, Cancer Institute of New Jersey

Shaun Ruddy, M.D. Elam C. Toone Professor of Internal Medicine, Microbiology and Immunology, and Professor (Emeritus), Division of Rheumatology, Allergy and Immunology, Medical College of Virginia at Virginia Commonwealth University

Matthew V. Rudorfer, M.D. Assistant Chief for Adult and Geriatric Treatment and Preventive Intervention, Division of Services and Intervention Research, National Institute of Mental Health

Andres M. Salazar, M.D. Professor of Neurology, Uniformed Services University of the Health Sciences

Jone E. Sampson, M.D. Assistant Professor, Department of Molecular and Medical Genetics, Oregon Health Sciences University School of Medicine

Ann M. Saunders, Ph.D. Associate Research Professor, Department of Medicine, Duke University Medical Center

Lawrence R. Schiller, M.D. Program Director, Gastroenterology Fellowship, Baylor University Medical Center, and Clinical Professor of Internal Medicine, University of Texas Southwestern Medical Center

Stanley L. Schrier, M.D. Professor of Medicine (Active Emeritus), Division of Hematology, Stanford University School of Medicine

Lawrence B. Schwartz, M.D., Ph.D. Professor of Internal Medicine, Division of Rheumatology, Allergy, and Immunology, Medical College of Virginia, Virginia Commonwealth University School of Medicine

F. John Service, M.D., Ph.D. Earl and Annette R. McDonough Professor of Medicine, Mayo Medical School

Sudhir V. Shah, M.D. Professor, Department of Medicine, and Director, Division of Nephrology, University of Arkansas for Medical Sciences

Stuart J. Shankland, M.D. Associate Professor of Medicine and Director, Nephrology Fellowship Program, Division of Nephrology, University of Washington School of Medicine

Lori Shapiro, M.D. Assistant Professor, Department of Medicine, University of Toronto Faculty of Medicine, and Physician, Drug Safety Clinic, Sunnybrook and Women's College Health Science Centre

David M. Shavelle, M.D. Interventional Fellow, Good Samaritan Hospital, Los Angeles

Mary Jo Shaver, M.D. Assistant Professor, Department of Medicine, Division of Nephrology, University of Arkansas for Medical Sciences

Neil H. Shear, M.D.   Professor of Medicine, Pharmacology, Pediatrics, and Pharmacy, University Director of Dermatology, and Director of the Drug Safety Research Group, University of Toronto Faculty of Medicine; and Director of Dermatology, Sunnybrook and Women's College Health Science Centre

Harvey B. Simon, M.D.   Associate Professor of Medicine, Harvard Medical School; Health Sciences and Technology Faculty, Massachusetts Institute of Technology; and Physician, Massachusetts General Hospital

Lee Simon, M.D.   Associate Professor of Medicine, Harvard Medical School; and Associate Chief of Medicine for External Affairs and Director, Graduate Medical Education, Beth Israel Deaconess Medical Center

Arthur T. Skarin, M.D.   Associate Professor of Medicine, Harvard Medical School; and Medical Director, Thoracic Oncology Program, Consultant, Hematology Laboratory, and Associate Physician in Medicine, Dana-Farber Cancer Institute

Shawn J. Skerrett, M.D.   Associate Professor of Medicine, University of Washington School of Medicine

Raymond G. Slavin, M.D.   Professor of Internal Medicine and Microbiology and Director, Division of Allergy and Immunology, Saint Louis University School of Medicine

Christopher F. Snow, M.D.   Clinical Professor of Medicine, Stanford University School of Medicine

Frederick S. Southwick, M.D.   Professor and Chief, Division of Infectious Diseases, and Associate Chairman, Department of Medicine, University of Florida College of Medicine

Harold C. Sox, Jr., M.D.   Editor, *Annals of Internal Medicine*

David H. Spach, M.D.   Associate Professor of Medicine, Division of Allergy and Infectious Diseases, University of Washington School of Medicine

Walter E. Stamm, M.D.   Professor of Medicine and Head, Division of Allergy and Infectious Disease, University of Washington School of Medicine

Gerald W. Staton, Jr., M.D.   Professor of Medicine, Emory University School of Medicine, and Chief of Pulmonary and Critical Care Medicine, Crawford Long Hospital

Richard H. Sterns, M.D.   Professor of Medicine, University of Rochester School of Medicine and Dentistry, and Chief of Medicine, Rochester General Hospital and the Genesee Hospital

Seth R. Stevens, M.D.   Assistant Professor of Dermatology, Case Western Reserve University School of Medicine/University Hospitals of Cleveland, and Acting Chief of Dermatology, Cleveland Louis Stokes Veterans Affairs Medical Center

Stephanie Studenski, M.D., M.P.H.   Professor of Medicine, University of Kansas Medical Center

S. H. Subramony, M.D.   Professor of Neurology and Vice Chairman, Department of Neurology, University of Mississippi Medical Center

Suzanne K. Swan, M.D.   Associate Professor of Medicine, Division of Nephrology, Hennepin County Medical Center, University of Minnesota Medical School

Morton N. Swartz, M.D.   Professor of Medicine, Harvard Medical School; and Chief, James Jackson Firm, Medical Services, and Chief (Emeritus), Infectious Disease Unit, Massachusetts General Hospital

James S. Taylor, M.D.   Head, Section of Industrial Dermatology, Department of Dermatology, Cleveland Clinic Foundation

Patrick J. Tchou, M.D.   Section Head, Electrophysiology and Pacing, Department of Cardiology, Cleveland Clinic Foundation

Cox Terhorst, Ph.D.   Professor of Medicine, Harvard Medical School, and Chief, Division of Immunology, Beth Israel Deaconess Medical Center

Robert F. Todd III, M.D., Ph.D.   Frances and Victor Ginsberg Professor of Hematology/Oncology, Professor of Internal Medicine, and Chief, Division of Hematology/ Oncology, University of Michigan Medical School; and Associate Vice President for Research, Health Affairs, University of Michigan

Richard G. Trohman, M.D.   Professor of Medicine, Rush Medical College of Rush University; and Director, Heart Station, Rush Heart Institute, and Director, Electrophysiology, Arrhythmia and Pacemaker Services, Rush-Presbyterian–St. Luke's Medical Center

Jo-Anne van Burik, M.D.   Assistant Professor, University of Minnesota Medical School

Everett E. Vokes, M.D.   John E. Ultmann Professor of Medicine and Radiation Oncology and Director, Section of Hematology/Oncology, University of Chicago Pritzker School of Medicine

Deborah L. Warden, M.D.   Associate Professor of Neurology and Psychiatry and Director, Clinical Research Division, Department of Neurology, Uniformed Services University of the Health Sciences; and Director, Defense and Veterans Head Injury Program, Walter Reed Army Medical Center

Matthew R. Weir, M.D.   Professor of Medicine, University of Maryland School of Medicine

Peter F. Weller, M.D.   Professor of Medicine, Harvard Medical School; and Co-Chief, Infectious Diseases Division, and Chief, Allergy and Inflammation Division, Beth Israel Deaconess Medical Center

James W. Wheless, M.D.   Professor of Neurology and Pediatrics, University of Texas Health Science Center at Houston Medical School; and Medical Director, Epilepsy Monitoring Unit, Director of Clinical Electroencephalography, and Director, Texas Comprehensive Epilepsy Program, Hermann Hospital

David A. Whiting, M.D.   Associate Professor of Dermatology, University of Texas Southwestern Medical Center at Dallas, and Medical Director, Baylor Hair Research and Treatment Center

Christopher Wise, M.D.   W. Robert Irby Associate Professor of Internal Medicine, Division of Rheumatology, Allergy and Immunology, Medical College of Virginia at Virginia Commonwealth University

Jerry S. Wolinsky, M.D.   The Bartels Family Professor of Neurology, University of Texas Health Science Center at Houston Medical School, and Attending Neurologist, Hermann Hospital

Harvey S. Young, M.D.   Clinical Associate Professor of Medicine, Department of Gastroenterology and Hepatology, Stanford University School of Medicine

Fuad N. Ziyadeh, M.D.   Professor of Medicine, Division of Renal-Electrolyte and Hypertension, University of Pennsylvania School of Medicine

Contents

Volume 1

CARDIOVASCULAR MEDICINE

DERMATOLOGY

Volume 2

INFECTIOUS DISEASE

About WebMD Scientific American® Medicine

While you may not realize it, you are holding part of an electronic medical database in your hands. This annually-published, bound two-volume edition of *WebMD Scientific American® Medicine* constitutes just one component of a larger network providing continually updated medical information for practicing physicians and other health care professionals. The heart of this network is an electronic database. Spreading out from this database like spokes of a wheel are the various methods that we have developed to provide current medical information the way our readers need it.

In addition to these volumes, *WebMD Scientific American® Medicine* also exists online at www.samed.com, a continually updated, rapidly searchable Web site with links to the broad resources of the Internet. A free email service alerts you to new information on our Web site. To present the key recommendations from new chapters, the email alert links directly to our online monthly newsletter, *What's New in Medicine.*

Also online, we offer a CME center, where you can earn up to 120 credits of category 1 CME (AMA and AAFP) a year. This CME program features a CME tracker that monitors your credits as you earn them and lets you print out your certificates whenever you need them. We also invite you to try our online service at www.samed.com for yourself, using the free three-month trial that we are offering with the purchase of this edition. Please turn to the inside front cover of this volume for more information on the features of *WebMD Scientific American® Medicine Online.*

As was true with each of these resources, we developed this edition by first asking our loyal readership how they would prefer to receive updated medical information. And as anyone who knows physicians could have predicted, when the answers rolled in, it was not as with one voice but with many. Some wanted updates each month; some every six months; some every year. Many told us that it is too time-consuming to swap new chapters into the loose-leaf binders that were the precursors to this edition.

Thus, we took physicians' needs into account and created an annual bound edition of *WebMD Scientific American® Medicine*, using the continually updated information from our electronic database, including information as recent as the beginning of 2003. We then included the free access to the Web site mentioned above, so that readers can determine how frequently they would like to receive updates. As we hear from you in the future, we will continue to expand the number of ways you can find the current medical information you need in a format that best serves your needs.

Nancy E. Chorpenning
Publisher
publisher@webmd.net

Preface

WebMD Scientific American® Medicine is intended to answer particular needs and work habits of practicing physicians. Issued annually and based on our continually updated electronic database, it provides a "snapshot" of the current state of medical knowledge. Its coverage spans the subspecialties of internal medicine, women's health, geriatrics, palliative medicine, psychology, dermatology, and neurology. Special attention has been given to topics of emerging interest to practitioners, such as bioterrorism, complementary/alternative medicine, and ethical choices in medical care. While the information is written by the world's leading specialists, we have taken pains to make their recommendations accessible for clinicians practicing outside the subspecialty.

The most common and clinically significant patient presentations are represented in these pages. Each chapter is organized consistently to allow readers to easily locate the information they require. If a physician has a pressing clinical question, he or she can go directly to the sections on diagnostic workup and recommendations for management. Epidemiologic data, risk factors, pathogenic processes, and differential diagnoses are covered in the early sections of each chapter and are designed to give current overviews of diseases most frequently encountered in practice.

Key recommendations are readily accessible in the over 700 tables on drug regimens, differential diagnoses, common presenting symptoms, and risk factors. *WebMD Scientific American® Medicine* is renowned for its rich illustrations, which enhance learning by distilling text into lucid visual explanations. The over 1,000 figures include diagrams depicting disease processes, algorithms outlining best diagnostic and management strategies, four-color images of dermatologic presentations and histologic findings, and radiographs, CT scans, MRIs, and ECG findings—all of which have been carefully selected to aid in sharpening the practitioner's diagnostic skills.

We hope that you find this book helpful in your daily practice of medicine and that it contains the information necessary for you to provide excellent care of your patients.

David C. Dale, M.D.
Editor-in-Chief
daviddalemd@webmd.net

Dedication

This new edition of *WebMD Scientific American® Medicine* is dedicated to our Founding Editors, Edward Rubenstein, M.D., and Daniel D. Federman, M.D., whose foresight created the first edition of this text over 25 years ago. We recognize Nancy Terry, our Managing Editor, and the scores of devoted authors and staff members whose writing, editing, and illustrations have given *WebMD Scientific American® Medicine* its unique standing as a resource for reliable and current medical information. We thank Nancy Chorpenning, our Publisher, for her exceptional leadership in completing this edition, and Rose Marie Dale for her patience with the Editor-in-Chief.

David C. Dale, M.D. (on behalf of the editors)
Editor-in-Chief

On Being a Physician

David C. Dale, M.D., and Daniel D. Federman, M.D.

Looking back over the past hundred years, it is easy to see that the scientific basis for medical practice and the organization of hospitals and clinics have changed dramatically. The future will bring even more changes. Population growth, environmental pollution, emerging infectious diseases, and global warming, for example, are worldwide problems that have immense medical implications. But on the positive side, the human genome project and the imminent development of new drugs and vaccines hold great promise.

Other aspects of medicine, however, have not changed so rapidly. In the community and in the patient-doctor relationship, physicians are still seen as persons skilled in the art of healing and in teaching others about health and disease. Physicians are still the ones who receive the extensive training, the licensure by the state, and the approval of society to provide all levels of care: to give advice for a healthy life, to examine and diagnose illness, to prescribe drugs to relieve suffering, and to care for those who are seriously ill and dying. Although physicians now share the many responsibilities involved in patient care and work closely with nurses, physician assistants, pharmacists, technicians, therapists, and family members of patients, it is still the physician who bears most of the responsibility for the care of the patient.

Being a patient's physician carries many responsibilities and requires at least three attributes. First, knowledge of applicable biomedical science and clinical medicine is necessary to understand a patient's problem. There is no limit to the knowledge that may be needed, but it is important to be able to answer correctly the patient's questions, such as "How did this happen to me?" and "Will I be better soon?" The physician needs to understand disease processes well enough to identify and categorize a patient's problem quickly. It is important, and sometimes critical, to know whether the problem will resolve spontaneously or whether detailed investigations, consultations, or hospitalization is needed. A thorough and up-to-date understanding of pathophysiology, diagnosis, and treatment is essential for the day-to-day exchange of information that occurs between physicians as they solve the problems of individual patients and work together to organize systems to improve patient care.

The physical examination remains a fundamental skill; the ability to recognize the difference between normal and abnormal findings, adjusting for age, sex, ethnicity, and other factors, is crucial. Good record keeping is essential—with regard to both a written record and a mental record—so that the circumstances of visits are remembered and changes in a patient's appearance or other characteristics that may not have been recorded can be recognized. With practice and attention, these skills—history taking, physical examination, and record keeping—can grow throughout a professional lifetime. Other aspects of care, such as selecting and performing diagnostic tests, procedures, and treatments, require evolving expertise. For all physicians, it is necessary both to practice medicine and to study regularly to maintain all of these essential skills.

In addition to having the specific skills necessary to diagnose and treat a patient, a good physician must recognize the role personal skills play in medical practice. The ability to communicate—both to speak and to listen—remains essential, especially for physicians providing primary care. Effective and sensitive communication can be challenging in communities characterized by diverse cultures and languages. At times, the physician must be, in part, an anthropologist to grasp the patient's understanding of illness and of the roles of patient and doctor. Knowing how to communicate empathically is invaluable: it is important to welcome each patient at every visit, to reach out and hold the hand of a troubled person, and to express understanding and concern.

The third, but by no means least important, attribute is the physician's responsibility to the patient and the medical community to conform to appropriate professional and ethical conduct. The first principle of the doctor-patient relationship is that the patient's welfare is paramount. Putting the patient first necessitates understanding the patient and the patient's values. It often means spending precious personal time explaining illness, determining the best method of treatment, or dealing with emergencies. It places the physician in service to the patient. Ethical conduct includes seeing clearly and acknowledging situations in which the physician's interest may conflict with the interest of the patient. Finally, personal exploitation of the intimacy and privacy of the doctor-patient relationship is never allowed.

Thus, the physician's work—recognizing illness, providing advice and comfort, relieving pain and suffering, and dealing with illness and death—has not changed much even since ancient times. On another level, however, the work has changed greatly. Better medical record keeping, quantitative observation, meticulous experimentation, and carefully conducted clinical trials have contributed to the rapid evolution of medical practice over the past hundred years. Simultaneously, medical education at the undergraduate, graduate, and postgraduate levels has been dedicated to the organization of a truly scientific knowledge base and its translation into intellectually cohesive approaches to understanding disease. Extraordinary advances in the biologic sciences, the development of medical and surgical specialties, and the explosion of medical information have brought with them great benefits. They have also added to the costs and the potential costs of almost every aspect of health care.

Efficiency and cost containment are now watchwords of the payers for health service. Practice guidelines, hospital care pathways, and other efforts to codify the practice of medicine are receiving much attention. When based on good evidence, these efforts are beneficial; they save precious resources—time and money—for both patients and physicians. The development of managed care in the United States has created a new challenge for physicians: to serve as advocates for their patients. In this role, physicians are responsible for overcoming organizational, geographic, and financial barriers to the provision of services that are important for their patients. In organizations in which guidelines for care have been established, it may be necessary for a physician to explain to administrators the specific needs and problems of individual patients—sometimes over and over again, because laypersons may be less apt to recognize that guidelines for clinical practice must remain just guidelines. Because more and more physicians are salaried and thus bound to the needs of populations of patients, physicians face the problem of balancing the needs of individual patients with the expectations of the employer. This is a delicate and, in some places, even fragile balance. To serve both patients and the employer well, a physician must develop good judgment in managing patient care under conditions in which the allocation of resources is conservative.

The increasing organization of health care on a for-profit basis has raised new issues. The physician's obligation to put the patient first, the thoroughness inculcated in physicians throughout their training, and the increasing costs of diagnostic tests and therapies can collide head-on with health care management's attempts to protect earnings for investors. Professional responsibility to patients and the public good is clear and at times poses difficult challenges for the physician.

A profession is defined by a specialized body of knowledge requiring advanced training and by the dedication of its practitioners to the public good over their own enrichment. In exchange, professionals are granted considerable autonomy in setting standards and in the conduct of their work. Circumstances within the medical profession have changed. The public in general and patients in particular have much more knowledge of medicine than at any time in the past, and the modern organization of medicine has severely restricted the autonomy of physicians. But delivery of expert medical care and the welfare of the patient remain central to the physician's professional responsibility. Maintaining professionalism as the ground moves under us is more important than ever.

The weight of all these responsibilities may suggest that it is impossible, or nearly impossible, to be a good physician. Quite the contrary, persons with vastly different personalities, interests, and intellects have become and are becoming good physicians and are deeply satisfied in this role. The information necessary for practicing medicine is now more accessible than ever before. The skills the physician needs can be learned through experience, sharpened through practice, and focused through specialization. The ethical requirements of physicians are not onerous. They are, in fact, expectations of all good citizens, regardless of their careers. Being a physician is both exciting and satisfying; it provides a unique opportunity to combine modern scientific knowledge with the traditions of an ancient and honored profession in serving and helping one's fellow man.

WebMD Scientific American® Medicine is written and edited by physicians to help other physicians meet the ideals enunciated in this introduction. A principal goal of *WebMD Scientific American® Medicine* is to be the most up-to-date textbook of medicine available. The contents summarize the most important information from general and specialty journals, as interpreted by experienced clinicians. The material is evidence-based, with extensive bibliographic citations that are updated regularly. Authors are selected who understand both the constraints of managed care and the quality of care that is possible with scientific advances. In short, *WebMD Scientific American® Medicine* is committed to conveying the information necessary for physicians to provide excellent care to their patients.

CLINICAL ESSENTIALS

1 Contemporary Ethical and Social Issues in Medicine

Christine K. Cassel, M.D., *Ruth B. Purtilo,* Ph.D., *and Elaine T. McParland,* M.D., J.D.

At one time, medical ethics was thought to refer solely to proscriptions against physicians advertising their services and fees or engaging in questionable economic arrangements such as fee-splitting. Within the past 20 years, however, medical ethics has evolved into a discipline of clinicians (physicians, nurses, and other health professionals), philosophers, theologians, and social scientists who have become familiar enough with clinical matters to speak knowledgeably about value conflicts that arise in the practice of medicine. Advances in biomedical science and technology, changes in the delivery of health care, changing worldwide demographic trends, AIDS, and a growing understanding of the interconnectedness of individual and public health concerns are just some of the reasons why physicians have recognized the need to be knowledgeable about complex and wide-ranging moral issues.

The rapid advance of medical technology has raised a host of new moral issues around such fundamental questions as when does life begin, when and how does life end, which services can patients require of physicians, and which requests can physicians legitimately refuse. These questions become even more complex in a society as diverse and multicultural as our own, where moral norms may conflict. Such conflicts can be analyzed as ethical dilemmas. Consider the following ethical dilemmas and the questions that each one raises for physicians today:

• A 90-year-old Auschwitz survivor, totally disabled from several strokes, lives at home with 24-hour care. Her strokes have left her cognitively impaired and unable to communicate. Her husband is her designated health care proxy. She was hospitalized because she had stopped eating and later developed aspiration pneumonia. Four days into her hospitalization, she developed a bleeding ulcer and hemorrhaged several units of blood. She had a cardiac arrest, was resuscitated after 45 minutes of asystole, and is now unresponsive and ventilator dependent. Her husband insists she should be kept alive by whatever means possible. The hospital team is strongly divided about the morally appropriate course of action. Some agree with the patient's husband: she should receive life-sustaining treatment even though she has virtually no chance of recovery. Others argue that it would be more respectful to discontinue intrusive medical care and allow her to die. What clinical and moral value considerations should finally govern their decision?

• A 58-year-old man living in Oregon is suffering from end-stage AIDS with lymphopenia, multiple refractory fungal infections, and Kaposi sarcoma. He has significant pain from mucosal lesions and skin breakdown and has sustained fractures, including one from a spinal metastasis that has led to paraplegia and urinary and fecal incontinence. He is cognitively intact and has given oral and written directives that he does not want to be kept alive any longer. He has repeatedly asked his physician to give him an overdose of sedative so that he will die and be released from his intractable suffering. The physician is convinced that this patient is competent and that his wish is well informed and made in good faith. His companion of 15 years agrees with his decision. Both have known the physician for a long time and trust her judgment. Physician-assisted suicide is currently legal in Oregon. Should the physician comply with this patient's wishes? If she cannot do so in good conscience, must she refer her patient to a physician who can? Why or why not?

• Science allows physicians to transplant hearts, livers, kidneys, and other living organs, tissues, and cells. Overall, there are drastic shortages of donors. Hundreds, sometimes thousands, of people die each year before a match becomes available. Currently in the United States, people who wish to donate organs are encouraged to indicate that wish on their driver's licenses. In the absence of such clear evidence of consent, physicians and other hospital staff are often reluctant to ask bereaved family members for donations because many people, understandably, cannot deal with such a request in a time of crisis. Should the United States adopt a policy—already practiced in other countries—allowing hospitals to harvest organs upon the death of a patient unless that person has specified otherwise? Could one policy ever work to everyone's benefit in a diverse society where there may be differing attitudes about treatment of the dead, the moral use of animals, and other culturally derived considerations? Would cloning or xenotransplantation provide ethically preferable alternatives?

• Health plans and health care providers should be accountable for the quality of care they provide. Better information about health care outcomes is needed to monitor care, which is possible with electronic information systems. Such monitoring requires that information from patient encounters (e.g., diagnosis, medications and other treatments, and outcomes) be recorded in clinical databases. Some critics are concerned that this practice threatens the privacy of clinical information and breaches physician-patient confidentiality. Are the concerns about accountability and quality of care afforded by clinical databases overriding values? Are there any ethically preferable alternatives?

These examples highlight the complexity of ethical dilemmas and the need for a common language by which clinicians and society can openly deliberate about ethical issues. Often, there is not a single right answer to an ethical dilemma; in almost all cases, there are competing values that need to be weighed against each other before a decision is made that most fully upholds the moral values by which physicians must guide their practice. As in many other areas of medicine, there may be a high degree of uncertainty. For that reason alone, it is useful to have a framework for ethical decision making.

A Context and Process for Ethical Decision Making

A conflict of values lies at the center of each ethical dilemma. Most medical ethicists agree that several fundamental ethical norms can be drawn from the overarching principle to treat the patient with respect. These ethical norms include the responsibility to act in a way that benefits the patient (beneficence); the responsibility, whenever possible, to do no harm (nonmaleficence); the responsibility to acknowledge the autonomy of the patient and his or her right to self-determination; and, finally, the responsibility to treat people fairly and equitably. Although it would be hard to argue with any of these values taken individually, they come into conflict with one another every day in medical practice. Three steps are useful tools for decision making when conflicts arise.

First, the clinician needs to gather all available relevant information regarding the patient; inadequate information can result in decisions that do not reflect the interests and desires of the patient. Key information includes not only the medical condition of the patient but also the patient's values and preferences, the family and social situation, and the realities of the options open to her or him.

Second, ethical dilemmas must be clarified and presented clearly to all those involved in the decision-making process. For example, a spouse of an incompetent patient arguing for aggressive, clinically futile treatment in the face of an imminently terminal and untreatable illness can present the physician with a conflict between respecting the considered wishes of family members and doing what the physician judges is best for the patient. Sometimes, enhanced communication between physician, patient, and family helps bring the matter to resolution. For example, having a discussion with the family that is focused on the likelihood that aggressive measures would only prolong the suffering of the patient may convince them to end life-prolonging interventions. In other circumstances, however, the patient's and family's beliefs may necessitate that the physician take aggressive measures to preserve life at all costs. It may be important to discuss the spiritual and moral dimensions of the impending decision explicitly. The involvement of other physicians or nonphysician mediators, such as the hospital ethicists, patient advocates, social workers, and clergy members, in the decision-making process is often helpful. Once values are explicitly discussed and differences clarified, a plan may be agreed upon by which all parties can abide.

Third, once a decision has been made, it is essential that the decision be carried out effectively, compassionately, and with continuing respect for the patient's needs and wishes. For example, if genetic testing is indicated and there are potential consequences regarding the patient's future eligibility for health insurance, the physician must ensure the confidentiality of information about the tests. If complete confidentiality is not possible, the physician should be sure that the patient understands and accepts the risks. Whatever the topic at hand, the physician must employ the clinical and interpersonal skills necessary to carry out the patient's wishes respectfully and compassionately.

Areas of Current Ethical Debate

Three broad societal concerns that have important implications for clinical practice lie at the center of many current ethical dilemmas.

DIFFERENCES OF OPINION ABOUT THE MORAL LIMITS OF MEDICAL INTERVENTION IN AN ERA OF TECHNOLOGICAL IMPERATIVES

Modern medicine has been criticized for generating an ethos in which clinicians assume that if an intervention is available, it should always be used. A physician might offer a new intervention as a way of either sustaining hope for the patient and family or avoiding the reality of a poor prognostic situation. In these circumstances, the chances of success can sometimes be overestimated. There are times when the better course is to help patients and families deal realistically with their losses. Physicians' ethics should allow them to consider each medical intervention in the light of their patient's values and wishes and with due regard for the appropriateness of the treatment in that particular setting. Several questions frame the current debate about the appropriate use of medical technology, among them issues related to life span, quality of life, and medical futility.

THE ENIGMA OF WHAT CONSTITUTES A PERSON AND WHEN LIFE BEGINS AND ENDS

Physicians sometimes face extreme and unfamiliar situations in discharging their duty to respect a patient's autonomy. Current research in genetics, for example, challenges traditional assumptions of the uniqueness of individual identity and the acceptability of genetic interventions. Germline interventions were considered completely ethically unacceptable just a few years ago because of the reluctance on the part of geneticists to create changes that would persist through subsequent generations. However, research has now progressed to the point of growing human stem cells under laboratory conditions, and stem cell research is thought to be one of the most promising new areas for clinical interventions. The ethical debate has shifted somewhat, as many in the scientific community are now actively supporting stem cell research and taking steps to address some of the ethical concerns raised by the use of these cells. This shift has occurred in part because stem cell techniques do not create permanent germline changes. Also, attempts to promulgate practice guidelines governing the conduct of such research are being extensively debated in some segments of the United States society and continue to generate rich ethical discourse that addresses the very essence of personhood. Reproductive technologies, including the potential for cloning, have an impact on this issue as well and have spurred new questions about the ethical limits of medical intervention in human reproduction. The debate about abortion in the United States continues to encompass many points of controversy that directly affect the practice of medicine, sometimes violently.

At the other end of the continuum of care, the question of when life ends is brought into sharp focus by dramatic life-extending technologies. For example, although there have been rational criteria for brain death that have guided organ transplantation, the extreme shortage of donor organs and evolving technological capabilities have prompted new ethical considerations regarding organ recovery. As utilization of organ donations from non–brain-dead but irreversibly comatose persons has become an increasingly common practice, commitment to clarifying and addressing the ethical dilemmas associated with the use of such donors remains warranted. Finally, the debate about assisted suicide raises profound questions of quality of life and the limits of personal choice [see Chapters 10 and 84].

APPROPRIATE APPROACHES TO ASSESSING QUALITY OF LIFE

Discussions of quality of life gain broader clinical relevance as technical advances make it easier to extend life beyond a point when many people would consider it meaningful. When a patient or family member raises the issue, it is important for

Biomedical Ethics Information on the Internet

Federal Government

Bioethicsline

http://www.nih.gov/sigs/bioethics

The National Library of Medicine's database of peer-reviewed bioethics literature.

National Bioethics Advisory Commission

http://bioethics.gov

Agendas and transcripts of meetings, online publications, and other information primarily regarding genetics research and research involving humans.

Ethical, Legal and Social Implications Program, National Human Genome Research Institute

http://www.nhgri.nih.gov/ELSI

Information on policy and legislation, research opportunities, grant products and publications, education and training activities.

Professional Societies

American College of Physicians Center for Ethics and Professionalism

http://www.acponline.org/ethics

Position papers, educational programs, and other resources on end-of-life care, managed care, and other issues related to medical ethics.

American Medical Association Institute for Ethics

http://www.ama-assn.org/ama/pub/category/2558.html

Educational and outreach programs for physicians, including the Education for Physicians on End-of-life Care Project.

American Society for Bioethics and Humanities

http://www.asbh.org

Consolidation of the Society for Health and Human Values, the Society for Bioethics Consultation, and the American Association of Bioethics; meeting agendas, position papers.

American Society of Law, Medicine & Ethics

http://www.aslme.org

Conference agendas, publications, online forum.

International Association of Bioethics

http://www.uclan.ac.uk/facs/ethics/iab.htm

Congress and conference agendas, online newsletter, discussion networks.

Institutes and Centers

Case Western Reserve University Center for Biomedical Ethics

http://www.cwru.edu/med/bioethics/bioethics.html

Program news, events, online newsletter.

Georgetown University Kennedy Institute of Ethics

http://www.georgetown.edu/kie

Information on symposia, publications, and services, including the National Reference Center for Bioethics Literature. (**http://www.georgetown.edu/nrcbl**)

The Hastings Center

http://www.thehastingscenter.org

Research and educational programs on ethical issues in medicine, the life sciences, and the environment.

University of Chicago MacLean Center for Clinical Medical Ethics

http://ethics.bsd.uchicago.edu/home.html

Comprehensive guide to online resources in biomedical ethics; online newsletter.

University of Pennsylvania Center for Bioethics

http://www.med.upenn.edu/bioethic

Online bioethics tutorial, publications, discussion groups; special sections on genetics, cloning, and physician-assisted suicide.

---

the physician to learn more about what that person means by "quality of life." Physicians, family members, and patients may disagree about what constitutes an acceptable quality of life. Often, the phrase is used in the context of how long clinicians should continue attempts to extend life. The ideal setting for gathering this key information is in an ongoing caregiving relationship that allows the patient time to think about the issues, discuss them with those close to him or her, and come back to the physician for a fuller discussion. Unfortunately, this ideal relationship is increasingly rare. Crucial decisions must often be made among relative strangers in times of great stress (for example, in an ICU or on the brink of a cardiac arrest precipitated by critical illness).

For that reason, physicians should try to open the door to these discussions with patients ahead of time whenever appropriate. Increasingly frequent discussions of death and dying in the popular media have set the stage for patients and families to be receptive to such discussions and to be better informed about the facts and issues involved.

In general, questions related to acceptable quality of life should be answered by the patient. Often, however, the patient is unable to speak for himself or herself when the answer is needed. A proxy decision maker, usually a family member or a friend, should be asked about the patient's likely wishes in such a situation. It is crucial to emphasize to a proxy that it is the patient's values, not his or her own own, that should be conveyed in these situations. In addition to providing clear information about prognosis and likely outcomes, it is important

for the clinician to recognize that a proxy is in a very difficult position—often in the midst of acute grief or anxiety—and should be provided a comforting context in which to make a decision. A proxy should not be made to feel that he or she is alone in making this decision, especially in the common situation in which the patient is likely to die in any case. Written advance directives—so-called living wills—can be helpful in this regard, mostly as adjuncts to discussions between patient and physician. Assigning a trusted proxy is still recommended, however, because situations are often more complex than can be adequately addressed in a written document.

Traditional Medical Ethics and the Changing World of Medicine

One of the reasons the medical profession has been able to maintain a strong ethical standard for more than 2,000 years is that the standard has been so simple. From the Hippocratic oath to the prayer of Moses Maimonides, statements of medical ethics have required the physician to do what is best for the patient, putting the patient's interest before his or her own. Admittedly, there have been breaches of the standard. Many physicians became rich selling unproven patent medicines before the advent of scientific medicine. More recently, some have overcharged patients or ordered unnecessary tests and procedures to further their own financial interests. In the past, however, the accountability structure was clearly delineated between physician and patient. Today, changes in the economics and delivery systems of health care have so affected this classic ethical construct of undivided loyalty to the patient that even previously inviolable ethical relationships are being challenged. Currently, for example, many physicians are concerned about pressure to reduce health care expenditures by withholding needed care. Recent United States Supreme Court decisions have suggested that a health care provider's fiduciary duty to the patient does not preclude financial incentives to physicians to withhold treatment. Such incentives, challenged by a patient in a Texas court, were upheld by the Supreme Court as a legitimate business practice. Pressures on physicians to depart from traditional ethical standards are increasing, as has been illustrated by judicial endorsement of such incentives. Understanding the fundamental responsibility of the profession to the welfare of the patient is an important beginning for dealing with any ethical problems presented by social change, technological innovation, and changes in the delivery and financing of health care.

POPULATION-BASED MEDICINE AND THE RIGHTS OF THE INDIVIDUAL

Although simple in the abstract, the physician's responsibility to the patient is not always clear in actual practice. For example, the traditional standard requires a physician to do everything possible for patients directly in his or her care. Arguing that a more utilitarian standard is needed, some theorists have suggested changes to meet the requirements of population-based medicine, in which some treatments that are potentially beneficial to the individual patient are forgone to benefit larger numbers of patients with the resources thus recovered.

Utilitarian considerations are sometimes discussed in the context of a communitarian philosophy, which holds that all members of the society are better off if standards are based on the benefit to communities rather than to individuals exclusively. Many European governments base policies on communitarian premises, whereas in the United States, policy makers have traditionally focused more sharply on the rights of the individual. However, it may be that the rights of a far greater number of individuals would be better served with a health care structure that emphasizes more collective responsibility and resolution.

One area where this tension can be seen is in end-of-life care. In recent decades, there has been a presumption and a legal standard in the United States that patients may make their own decisions about the care they receive at the end of life and, in particular, that every person has the right to refuse life-sustaining treatment. This freedom of choice is the thrust of the Patient Self-Determination Act of 1990, which requires hospitals and nursing homes to inform patients of local laws regarding advance directives and to help them prepare advance directives if they choose to do so. Before 1990, in several well-publicized cases (e.g., the Quinlan case and the Cruzan case), courts supported families or patients who wished to end life-sustaining treatment. However, attention is now being drawn to instances in which patients or their proxies are asking for life-sustaining treatment over objections from health care payors and, sometimes, providers. In the relatively few cases in which such conflicts have been brought to litigation, courts, again, have been generally supportive of patients' and families' desires. Interestingly, these cases conflict with the recent judgments that financial incentives to restrict care are acceptable in the context of insurance law.

In recent years, some ethicists have worked to define a standard of medical futility that would give physicians the right to withhold treatment in specific cases. There is profound disagreement, however, about the definition of futility and its statistical basis. For example, the chances of success with cardiopulmonary resuscitation are remarkably small in patients of very advanced age, debilitating illness, and poor functional status, particularly in cases of an unwitnessed cardiac arrest; however, many physicians would be uncomfortable making the decision to withhold CPR without consulting the patient's family. From one perspective, this instinct to involve and communicate with patient and family is a sound one, motivated by respect and caring. In other cases, however, an insistence on family permission in an essentially medical context of futility is a misguided gesture, perhaps driven by liability concerns. Ethicists have asserted the physician's duty to regain the responsibility of prognostication and decision making inherent in the older paternalistic model of medical practice. This belief can be supported by two arguments: (1) there is a responsibility to avoid wasteful use of scarce resources and (2) the attitude of caring supports not inflicting unrealistic choices on grieving families but, rather, offering reassurances of aggressive palliative care and relief from suffering for patients who are dying.

A BROADER CONTEXT FOR CLINICAL DECISION MAKING

The role of the physician and the nature of the doctor-patient relationship may be challenged, not only by changes in the practice of medicine but also by the increasing interconnectedness of communities and societies and the emergence of public health as a global concern. Regional and national health care systems are commonplace; epidemics can occur worldwide because of widespread international travel, immigration, and dislocation caused by war and civil strife.

The global, multicultural aspect of modern medicine will have increasingly significant implications for ethical decision making in clinical practice in coming years. For example, in seeking to honor a patient's right to autonomy, a physician may have to balance the traditional standard of care with a patient's desire to choose an alternative or complementary therapy. Or following the traditional Hippocratic model, a physician may feel justified in using the most powerful antibiotic available to treat a patient's infection, even as the widespread use of powerful antibiotics leads to the emergence of new and more resistant organisms throughout the world.

Caring for patients in this new environment raises challenges for physicians that their predecessors never faced. Physicians must now analyze ethical issues systematically, understand the conflicts modern medicine poses for some traditional Hippocratic precepts, and come to terms with a combined responsibility to their patients and to the consequences of individual clinical decisions for the broader population. Even as electronic communication systems evolve to keep physicians abreast of new global realities, the moral and ethical framework of clinical decision making must begin to encompass those realities [see Sidebar Biomedical Ethics Information on the Internet]. It is critical that physicians learn the language of medical ethics and follow its literature closely so that their voices will help shape the future of basic medical values, even as they cope with complex ethical challenges in their daily practice.

Selected Readings

Bloche MG, Jacobson PD: The Supreme Court and bedside rationing. JAMA 284:2776, 2000

Cantor NL: Can healthcare providers obtain judicial intervention against surrogates who demand "medically inappropriate" life support for incompetent patients? Crit Care Med 24:883, 1996

Cranford RE: The vegetative and minimally conscious states: ethical implications. Geriatrics 53(suppl 1):S70, 1998

DeVita MA, Snyder JV, Arnold RM, et al: Observations of withdrawal of life-sustaining treatment from patients who became non-heart-beating organ donors. Crit Care Med 28:1709, 2000

Doukas DJ, McCullough LB: A preventive ethics approach to counseling patients about clinical futility in the primary care setting. Arch Fam Med 5:589, 1996

Drickamer MA, Lee MA, Ganzini L: Practical issues in physician-assisted suicide. Ann Intern Med 126:146, 1997

Dunn PM, Gallagher TH, Hodges MO, et al: Medical ethics: an annotated bibliography. Ann Intern Med 121:627, 1994

Edwards SJL, Lilford RJ, Hewison J: The ethics of randomised controlled trials from the perspectives of patients, the public, and healthcare professionals. BMJ 317:1209, 1998

Hall MA, Berenson RA: Ethical practice in managed care: a dose of realism. Ann Intern Med 128:395, 1998

Herdman R, Beauchamp TL, Potts JT: The Institute of Medicine's report on non-heart-beating organ transplantation. Ken Inst Ethics J 8:83, 1998

Kassirer JP: Managed care and the morality of the marketplace. N Engl J Med 333:50, 1995

Lee S: Human stem cell research: NIH releases draft guidelines for comment. J Law Med Ethics 28:81, 2000

Meier DE, Morrison RS, Cassel CK: Improving palliative care. Ann Intern Med 127:225, 1997

Meisel A, Kuczewski M: Legal and ethical myths about informed consent. Arch Intern Med 156:2521, 1996

Muskin PR: The request to die: role for a psychodynamic perspective on physician-assisted suicide. JAMA 279:323, 1998

Pellegrino ED: Ethics. JAMA 275:1807,1996

Pellegrino ED: The metamorphosis of medical ethics: a 30-year retrospective. JAMA 269:1158, 1993

Post LF, Blustein J, Gordon E, et al: Pain: ethics, culture, and informed consent to relief. J Law Med Ethics 24:348, 1996

Post SG, Whitehouse PJ, Binstock RH, et al: The clinical introduction of genetic testing for Alzheimer disease: an ethical perspective. JAMA 277:832, 1997

Quill TE, Brody H: Physician recommendations and patient autonomy: finding a balance between physician power and patient choice. Ann Intern Med 125:763, 1996

Quill TE, Cassel CK: Nonabandonment: a central obligation for physicians. Ann Intern Med 122:368, 1995

Roter DL, Stewart M, Putnam SM, et al: Communication patterns of primary care physicians. JAMA 277:350, 1997

Schneiderman LJ, Jecker NS, Jonsen AR: Medical futility: response to critiques. Ann Intern Med 125:669, 1996

Sharpe VA, Faden AI: Appropriateness in patient care: a new conceptual framework. Milbank Q 74:115, 1996

Snyder L: Ethical choices: case studies for medical practice. American College of Physicians, Philadelphia, 1996

Whittaker L: Clinical applications of genetic testing: implications for the family physician. Am Fam Physician 53:2077, 1996

Practice Guidelines and Consensus Statements

American College of Physicians: Ethics manual: fourth edition. Ann Intern Med 128:576, 1998

Consensus statement of the Society of Critical Care Medicine's Ethics Committee regarding futile and other possibly inadvisable treatments. Crit Care Med 25:887, 1997

Council on Ethical and Judicial Affairs, American Medical Association: Ethical considerations in the allocation of organs and other scarce medical resources among patients. Arch Intern Med 155:29, 1995

Emanuel LL: A professional response to demands for accountability: practical recommendations regarding ethical aspects of patient care. Working Group on Accountability. Ann Intern Med 124:240, 1996

Fletcher JC, Siegler M: What are the goals of ethics consultation? A consensus statement. J Clin Ethics 7:122, 1996

2 Quantitative Aspects of Clinical Decision Making

Brian Haynes, M.D., Ph.D, and Harold C. Sox, Jr., M.D.

An increasing amount of very useful quantitative evidence from health care research has become available to practitioners. This information addresses issues related to such important clinical topics as screening and diagnostic tests, preventive and therapeutic interventions, prognosis, risk of adverse outcomes, improvement in quality of care, and cost-effectiveness. Clinical application of this evidence, however, has lagged, not only because clinicians are often slow to adopt new research findings[1] but also because many clinicians are unfamiliar with the concepts that lie behind the application of quantitative reasoning to clinical care.

This lack of precision in clinical thinking is beginning to yield to several encouraging developments. The most important developments include the application of principles of critical appraisal to evidence in the medical literature; the formulation of methods for medical decision analysis; the introduction of terms such as sensitivity, specificity, likelihood ratio, number needed to treat, and confidence interval; and the creation of print and electronic resources that greatly reduce the amount of time and effort required to find and interpret valid quantitative evidence. These developments notwithstanding, the possibility of miscommunication still exists. A 1992 study[2] showed that clinicians had widely differing interpretations of the impact of an intervention, depending on how the figures were presented. For example, when the authors described a therapeutic effect as a reduction in relative risk, the clinicians believed the effect to be larger than when the authors described the same results as a reduction in absolute risk or as the number needed to treat. Patients are entitled to expect clearer thinking from their physicians. Moreover, the current health care environment increasingly demands that physicians be able to justify clinical policies and decisions with an evidence-based, quantitative approach.

We have two principal goals in this subsection. The first is to provide a basic explanation of the measurements used in critical appraisal of the literature and the ways in which physicians interpret these measurements in evidence-based clinical decision making. With the advent of electronic access to MEDLINE and its clinical subsets, specialized compendia of studies (e.g., *Best Evidence*[3] and *Clinical Evidence*[4]), and systematic reviews of studies (e.g., *The Cochrane Library*[5]), the current best evidence for clinical practice is becoming more and more accessible to clinicians.

The second goal is to introduce the topic of medical decision analysis. Clinicians use decision analysis in two ways: indirect and direct. The indirect method involves reliance on products of decision analyses conducted by others. For example, practice guidelines increasingly influence many of the quick, straightforward decisions that occur in daily practice. Many of these guidelines are based on formal decision analyses. The direct method is the use of decision analysis tools to assist in making major decisions about the care of an individual patient. It is not necessary for physicians to spend hours conducting formal decision analyses from scratch. Many of the tools of decision analysis (e.g., likelihood ratios of test results) are easy to apply, and some decision analyses themselves are accessible by desktop or handheld computer and require only that the clinician enter the clinical findings.

This effort to achieve precision and quantitation in measurement and decision making has an important goal: to enhance the quality of patient care by making it more specific to the individual. Anything that can be measured, even if only qualitatively, can be counted and expressed as a clinically useful quantitative measure. For example, a study might classify clinical outcomes qualitatively as satisfactory or unsatisfactory, but if the participants in the study who fall into various categories are counted, the result is quantitative. If physicians can define individual states and measure them quantitatively by using a continuous scale to assess functional status, they can describe individual patient status more precisely and therefore can make finer distinctions between groups of patients. By placing patients in distinctive groups, physicians can help patients make the choice between alternative treatments on the basis of the predicted response to one treatment or the other.

What is the role of the individual practitioner in retrieving and evaluating evidence from research and incorporating it into individual clinical decisions? The answer to this innocuous question distills the angst associated with contemporary health care. In some settings, the practitioner has the freedom to act as circumstances dictate, whereas in others (e.g., some managed-care settings), someone else dictates how to translate research results into patient care. We believe that practitioners cede their responsibility for clinical decision making to others at great risk to themselves and their patients, because any clinical decisions must take into account not only the evidence available and the guidelines in force but also the patient's unique circumstances and individual wishes. In today's world, the freedom to determine the content of one's practice is an increasingly precious opportunity. To use this opportunity responsibly, practitioners must have ready access to information that is based on current evidence, must understand the basic principles of quantitative decision making and decision analysis, must be able to determine whether others have applied these principles appropriately in published works or in practice, and must be able to understand how to use evidence from research to make decisions in clinical practice.

Measurements Used in Critical Appraisal of the Literature

HOW TO CRITICALLY EVALUATE RESEARCH REPORTS

To use numbers wisely in making decisions about patients, a physician must have some way of determining whether the numbers are derived from sound research. Detailed users' guides for interpreting the medical literature are available.[6] In an effort to simplify this issue, we have provided an abbreviated set of such guides [see Table 1].[7] These guides are especially useful for physicians who read research reports in the primary literature. However, physicians who are willing to cede the responsibility for getting and interpreting evidence to the authors of review articles, textbook chapters, and practice guidelines must also remember that not all quantitative findings are equally valid or significant. The value of a numerical result depends on the soundness of the methods used to obtain it.

Table 1   Abbreviated Users' Guides for Appraisal of Medical Journal Articles

Purpose of Study	Source of Data	Method of Arriving at Findings	Method of Reducing Bias of Findings
Diagnosis	Clearly identified comparison groups, all suspected of having the disorder, but one of which is free of the disorder	Objective or reproducible diagnostic standard applied to all participants	Blinded assessment of test and diagnostic standard
Therapy	Random allocation of patients to comparison groups	Outcome measure of known or probable clinical importance	Follow-up of ≥ 80% of subjects
Prognosis	Inception cohort, early in the course of the disorder and initially free of the outcome of interest	Objective or reproducible assessment of clinically important outcomes	Follow-up of ≥ 80% of subjects
Causation	Clearly identified comparison group for those who are at risk for, or for those having, the outcome of interest	Blinding of observers of outcome to exposure; blinding of observers of exposure to outcome	—
Review	Comprehensive search for relevant articles	Explicit criteria for rating relevance and merit of studies	Inclusion of all relevant studies

HOW TO APPLY RESEARCH RESULTS TO PATIENT CARE

Once a physician is satisfied that the quantitative results of research were derived from sound methods, he or she can interpret them in light of the patient's circumstances and use them to help determine the best course of treatment. The interpretation of research results takes five main forms: (1) measures of disease frequency, (2) measures of diagnostic certainty, (3) measures of diagnostic test performance and interpretation, (4) measures of the effects of treatment, and (5) measures of treatment outcomes adjusted for quality of life.

Measures of Disease Frequency

Clinically useful measures of disease frequency include incidence, prevalence, the case-fatality rate, the *P* value, and the confidence interval (CI) [*see Table 2*].

Measures of Diagnostic Certainty: Use of Probabilities

When asked how sure they are of their diagnoses, most physicians express their degree of certainty in words rather than numbers. A classic study illustrates the difficulty of this approach.[8] The authors examined pathology and radiology reports and recorded various terms expressive of the probability of a disorder, such as "compatible with," "consistent with," "likely," "probably," and "pathognomonic." They then asked a group of clinicians to assign numerical probabilities to all of these terms. For each term (even "pathognomonic"), the range of probabilities stretched over half the scale. For example, to one physician, "likely" meant there was a 45% chance that the disease in question was present, whereas to another, "likely" meant the probability was higher than 90%. When diagnostic-test specialists were asked on two occasions what they meant by these terms, the earlier and later answers were highly consistent for each individual specialist but highly inconsistent from one specialist to the next.

An alternative to using words to express the degree of diagnostic certainty is to use a number—namely, the probability that the diagnosis is present. A probability is a number between 0 and 1, expressing the likelihood that an event will occur; 0 represents certainty that it will not occur, and 1 represents certainty that it will. Using probability to express diagnostic certainty has two key advantages. First, it facilitates precise communication. Comparison of probability estimates is a far more precise method of comparing degrees of diagnostic certainty than exchanging verbal assessments. Second, there exists an ac-

curate method of calculating changes in the likelihood of disease as new information (e.g., a test result) becomes available. This method, the Bayes theorem, should be one of the central principles that underlie medical practice.

The probability of an event is not precisely the same thing as the odds of an event, even though the two are equivalent ways of expressing diagnostic uncertainty. Habitués of the racetrack are reputed to use odds directly, but most clinicians are likely to find probabilities easier to use. Each of these measures can be readily converted to the other, as follows:

$$\text{Odds} = \frac{\text{probability}}{1 - \text{probability}}$$

$$\text{Probability} = \frac{\text{odds}}{1 + \text{odds}}$$

To use a test result quantitatively, a physician must first estimate the pretest probability of the disease. Unaided, physicians are not particularly good at this task. In a 1982 study, when primary care physicians were given clinical scenarios and asked for

---

Table 2   Clinically Useful Measures of Disease Frequency

- Incidence: the proportion of new cases of a disorder occurring in a defined population during a specified period of time, typically 1 year.
- Prevalence: the proportion of cases of a disorder at a designated point in time in a specified population.
- Case-fatality rate: the proportion of cases of a specified disorder that are fatal during a specified period of follow-up (typically 1 yr) from the onset of the disorder.
- Quality-adjusted life year (QALY): a measure of survival in which each year of a patient's survival is discounted according to a measure (usually an index) of the patient's quality of life.
- *P* value: the probability of obtaining the observed data, or more unlikely data, when the null hypothesis is true. The *P* value does not indicate the magnitude of the effect of interest, or even its direction, nor does it indicate how much uncertainty is associated with the results.
- Confidence interval (CI): the range of values of a true effect that is consistent with the data observed in a study. A common (although not entirely correct) interpretation of a 95% confidence interval is that 95% of the time, the true value lies within the stated range of values.

Table 3 Definitions of Clinically Useful Measures of Diagnostic Test Performance and Interpretation

The typical approach to evaluation of most diagnostic tests, particularly those with so-called binary outcomes (e.g., a positive or a negative test result, with no other categories), makes use of a 2 × 2 table, as follows:

Diagnostic Test Result	Presence or Absence of Disease on a Reference Test (Gold Standard)		No. of Patients with Given Test Result
	Present	Absent	
Positive	a	b	a + b
Negative	c	d	c + d
Total	a + c	b + d	

Measures of diagnostic test performance, defined below, are calculated from this table.

- Sensitivity: the proportion of people with a disease of interest who are detected by a diagnostic test; calculated as $a/(a+c)$.
- Specificity: the proportion of people who do not have a disease who are correctly identified by a diagnostic test; calculated as $d/(b+d)$.
- Likelihood ratio: the odds that a given test result comes from a person who has the disease for which the test was ordered, compared with the odds that the result came from someone who does not have the disease; calculated as $[a/(a+c)]/[b/(b+d)]$ for a positive test result and as $[c/(a+c)]/[d/(b+d)]$ for a negative test result. According to an alternative, more useful definition, the likelihood ratio is the amount by which the odds of disease change after a test result.
- Pretest probability: the proportion of people with the disorder of interest in a group suspected of having the disorder; calculated as $(a+c)/(a+b+c+d)$.
- Odds: calculated as probability/(1 – probability).
- Probability: calculated as odds/(1+ odds).
- Posttest odds: calculated as pretest odds × likelihood ratio.
- Probability after a positive test: the proportion of people with a positive test result who have the disease of interest; calculated as $a/(a+b)$.
- Probability after a negative test: the proportion of people with a negative test result who have the disease of interest; calculated as $c/(c+d)$.

their estimates of the probabilities of given disorders, they provided estimates—quite confident ones—but their estimates did not agree with those of their fellow clinicians.[9] Indeed, when individual physicians were tested subsequently with the same scenarios, their later estimates did not agree with their initial ones.

How does a physician estimate the probability that a patient's chief complaint is a symptom of a particular disease? The first step is to take a careful history and perform a physical examination. From this point, the physician may take any of three basic approaches to estimating the probability of a disease[10]: (1) subjective estimation, (2) estimation based on the prevalence of disease in other patients with the same syndrome, or (3) application of clinical prediction rules.

Subjective estimation   In principle, the physician can draw on personal experience with similar patients and use the estimated frequency of the disease in those patients. In practice, this approach is little more than a semiquantitative guess and is prone to error because of defective recall as well as to bias in the application of the heuristics (i.e., the rules of thumb) for estimating probability. Examples of such heuristics are representativeness, by which one estimates a probability on the basis of

the similarity of the patient's signs and symptoms to the features of the classic description of the disease, and availability, by which one estimates a probability partly on the basis of how easy it is to recall similar cases. One very useful heuristic is anchoring and adjustment, by which one establishes an initial estimate (e.g., the prevalence of pulmonary embolism in 100 patients presenting to the emergency department with pleuritic chest pain) and then adjusts the estimate upward or downward by taking into account the patient's findings (e.g., hypoxemia, unilateral leg swelling, or a history of cancer). Physicians can, in principle, calculate the extent of such adjustments by using the Bayes theorem.

Estimation based on the prevalence of disease in other patients with the same syndrome   One antidote to the failures of subjective probability estimation is to base the estimate on accurate diagnoses established in a series of patients with the same clinical syndrome as the patient under consideration. The best example is the diagnosis of suspected coronary artery disease in patients with chronic chest pain. On the basis of the clinical history, the physician can place the patient in one of three categories: typical angina pectoris, atypical angina, or nonanginal chest pain. Many published studies have measured the frequency of angiographically proven coronary disease in patients with these syndromes. These studies have shown, for example, that in an adult male patient with atypical angina, the probability of significant coronary artery disease is approximately 0.70.

Application of clinical prediction rules   Clinical prediction rules describe the key clinical findings that predict a disease and show how to use these findings to estimate the probability of disease in a patient. Such rules are based on analysis of a standardized set of data, including clinical findings and the final diagnosis, for each of many patients with a diagnostic problem. One type of clinical prediction rule uses regression analysis to identify the best clinical predictors and their diagnostic weights. The sum of the diagnostic weights corresponding to a patient's findings is a score, and the probability of disease for each patient is equivalent to the prevalence of disease among patients with similar scores. A well-known example of this approach is the rule for estimating the probability of cardiac complications from noncardiac surgery.[11] Another interesting example showed that the prevalence of coronary artery disease in patients with similar chest pain scores varied systematically according to the overall prevalence of coronary artery disease in several study populations.[12] This study suggested that the probability of disease corresponding to a patient's clinical history will vary depending on whether the setting of care is a primary care practice or a referral practice. The book *Diagnostic Strategies for Common Medical Problems*[13] is an excellent source of pretest probabilities, as is the electronic publication *Best Evidence*.[3]

Measures of Diagnostic Test Performance and Interpretation

Clinically useful measures of diagnostic test performance include sensitivity, specificity, and the likelihood ratio. Clinically useful measures of test interpretation include pretest odds, pretest probability, probability after a positive test result, and probability after a negative test result [*see Table 3*]. Physicians should memorize and internalize the definitions of these terms to avoid becoming muddled when attempting to use information from diagnostic tests in decision making.

Table 4 Performance of Ventilation-Perfusion Scanning Compared with Angiography in the PIOPED Study

| Ventilation-Perfusion Scan Result | Pulmonary Embolism | | | | Likelihood Ratio for Scan Results |
| | Present | | Absent | | |
	No.	Proportion	No.	Proportion	
High probability of PE	102	102/251 = 0.41	14	14/630 = 0.02	0.41/0.02 = 20.5
Intermediate probability of PE	105	105/251 = 0.42	217	217/630 = 0.34	0.42/0.34 = 1.24
Low probability of PE	39	39/251 = 0.16	273	273/630 = 0.43	0.16/0.43 = 0.37
Normal or near normal	5	5/251 = 0.02	126	126/630 = 0.20	0.02/0.20 = 0.10
Total	251	—	630	—	—

PE—pulmonary embolism   PIOPED—Prospective Investigation of Pulmonary Embolism Diagnosis

Until recently, articles usually described the performance of a diagnostic test only in terms of sensitivity and specificity. These familiar terms do not directly describe the effect of a test result on the probability of disease. To correct this shortcoming, many articles now use the likelihood ratio (LR), which is the amount by which the odds of a disease change with new information. This value is calculated as follows:

$$\text{Likelihood ratio} = \frac{p \text{ [test result if disease present]}}{p \text{ [test result if disease absent]}}$$

Because physicians often express test results as either positive or negative, there is a likelihood ratio for a positive test result (LR$^+$) and a likelihood ratio for a negative test result (LR$^-$). The formula for the likelihood ratio for a positive test result is

$$LR^+ = \frac{\text{sensitivity}}{1 - \text{specificity}}$$

The formula for the likelihood ratio for a negative test result is

$$LR^- = \frac{1 - \text{sensitivity}}{\text{specificity}}$$

The likelihood ratio is generally a better descriptor than sensitivity or specificity because it more directly describes the effect of a test result on the odds of disease. The probability after obtaining new information is an application of the Bayes theorem. The most useful form of the Bayes theorem for this purpose is the odds ratio format:

$$\text{Posttest odds} = \text{pretest odds} \times \text{likelihood ratio}$$

This form of the Bayes theorem illustrates a very powerful concept that clinicians often overlook: new information has meaning only in context. Operationally, the statement means that a test result should never be interpreted in isolation; the individual's pretest probability should also be taken into account. It is not necessary to use the Bayes theorem to apply this principle, however. A physician can simply recall that after a positive test result, the posttest probability will be greater for a high pretest index of suspicion than for a low pretest index of suspicion. The most important practical application of this reasoning is to be suspicious when a test result is negative in a patient whose clinical findings strongly point toward a disease.

The evaluation of suspected pulmonary embolism is a good example of the practical use of these statistical terms and methods. A 37-year-old woman presents to the emergency department (ED) with pleuritic chest pain and new dyspnea. She has a low-grade fever and has no cough or hemoptysis, but the ED physician believes it necessary to rule out pulmonary embolism (PE). The patient has none of the other known risk factors for PE (e.g., recent surgery, prolonged bed rest, previous deep vein thrombosis [DVT], coagulopathy, malignancy, pregnancy, and use of oral contraceptives), and physical examination reveals no evidence of DVT. The arterial oxygen tension (P_aO_2) is 92 mm Hg with the patient on room air. The patient is quite distressed. The ED physician orders a chest x-ray and a ventilation-perfusion scan. The scan is interpreted as indicating an intermediate probability of PE. The resident wishes to explain this result to the patient and then to take the appropriate next steps.

A useful flowchart for working up patients with suspected PE is provided elsewhere [*see Chapter 29*]; however, this chart provides no guidance on how to estimate the clinical probability of PE. It is instructive to examine how the results of a quantitative, evidence-based approach to this patient's case relate to the recommendations outlined in the flowchart.

The first step is to estimate the pretest probability of PE by one of two approaches. The first approach is to use the anchoring and adjustment heuristic. The anchor, or starting point, is the prevalence of PE in adults who present to the ED with pleuritic chest pain. One very carefully done study found that 21% of such patients (36 of 173) had a positive pulmonary angiogram.[14] The physicians should use this 21% initial probability as the starting point (the anchor) for the patient under discussion and adjust it on the basis of the history and the physical examination. As noted, this patient has no predisposing factors for PE and no evidence of DVT, and her P_aO_2 is greater than 90 mm Hg. Using this approach, the ED physician concludes that the probability of PE before ventilation-perfusion scanning is quite low, perhaps 10%.[15]

The second approach is to use a newly developed clinical prediction rule.[16] This model places patients into three categories based on the clinical findings (typical for PE, atypical for PE, severe PE), the likelihood of alternative diagnoses, and the presence of risk factors for deep vein thrombosis. The prevalences of PE in the three categories are 3.4%, 27.8%, and 78.4%, respectively. The algorithm for placing patients into one of the three categories is somewhat complex but is easy to use when represented on the screen of a handheld computer. Assuming that the ED physician did not identify an alternative diagnosis that he thought was more likely than PE, the patient's pretest probability of PE was 28%, considerably higher than the ED physician's subjective probability.

With an estimate for the pretest probability of PE, the next step is to obtain the likelihood ratio for an intermediate-probability ventilation-perfusion scan. A good source for the data needed to calculate this number is the Prospective Investigation of Pulmonary Embolism Diagnosis (PIOPED) study,[17] which compared ventilation-perfusion scanning with pulmonary angiography or follow-up in a large series of patients with suspected PE [*see Table 4*]. This study met the criteria for diagnostic test evaluations mentioned earlier [*see Table 1*]: it provided independent (i.e., blinded or masked) comparisons of ventilation-perfusion scanning with a reproducible diagnostic standard in patients suspected of having the disorder, of whom some were ultimately found to have PE and others were found to be free of PE. Thus, the findings of the PIOPED study are likely to be valid for guiding the interpretation of this patient's problem.

To calculate the posttest odds of PE, the ED physician must combine the patient's pretest odds with the test's likelihood ratio by means of the odds-ratio format of the Bayes theorem mentioned earlier (posttest odds = pretest odds × likelihood ratio). An alternative to converting the pretest probability to odds and doing the calculation of posttest odds is to use a nomogram [*see Figure 1*]. To estimate posttest probability, anchor a straight edge at a pretest probability of 10% (corresponding to the ED physician's subjective estimate of pretest probability) in the left-hand column; then pass the straight edge through a likelihood ratio for an intermediate-probability scan, 1.21, in the middle column. Read the posttest probability, about 12%, from the right-hand column. The math for the ED clinician's estimate is as follows:

First, the 0.10 pretest probability of PE must be converted to pretest odds:

$$
\begin{aligned}
\text{Pretest odds} &= \text{pretest probability}/(1 - \text{pretest probability}) \\
&= 0.1/0.9 \\
&= 0.11
\end{aligned}
$$

Now determine the post–ventilation-perfusion scan odds of PE for this patient by multiplying the pretest odds of PE, 0.11, by the likelihood ratio for an intermediate-probability scan, 1.21 [*see Table 4*]:

$$
\begin{aligned}
\text{Posttest odds} &= \text{pretest odds} \times \text{likelihood ratio} \\
&= 0.11 \times 1.21 \\
&= 0.13
\end{aligned}
$$

Convert the posttest odds to the posttest probability, as follows:

$$
\begin{aligned}
\text{Posttest probability} &= \text{posttest odds}/(1 + \text{posttest odds}) \\
&= 0.13/(1 + 0.13) \\
&= 0.12
\end{aligned}
$$

Using the clinical prediction rule of Wells and colleagues,[16] the corresponding result would be a change from a pretest estimate of 28% to a posttest estimate of about 32%. Thus, the intermediate-probability scan provides almost no useful information and leaves the patient with about the same probability of PE as before the test. The recommended approach for this situation [*see Chapter 29*] is to assess the patient further for DVT; if, as in this case, the physical findings of DVT are absent, the next step is to perform compression ultrasonography on days 1, 3, 7, and 14 to rule out an evolving clot.

Measures of Treatment Effects

One of the most important tasks of clinicians is to advise patients about the current best treatment for their condition. Such advice is based on the best evidence available. Clinically useful measures of treatment effects reported in clinical trials include the experimental event rate (EER), the control event rate (CER), relative risk reduction (RRR), absolute risk reduction (ARR), and the number needed to treat (NNT) [*see Table 5*]. These measures can be effective tools for quantifying the magnitude of treatment benefits, provided that there is a statistically significant difference in the clinical event rate between experimental subjects and control subjects (i.e., between the EER and the CER).

Again, we illustrate the practical application of these terms with a specific example. A 69-year-old hypertensive male smoker has experienced a partial left hemispheric stroke, with good recovery of function, and has ipsilateral 75% internal carotid artery stenosis. One option would be to give this patient aspirin or clopidogrel and manage his risk factors for cerebrovascular disease; another would be to offer him carotid endarterectomy in addition to medical treatment. The question is, how and on what evidentiary basis does the clinician choose one treatment over another? It is tempting to think of treatments in black-and-white terms, as either working or not working, but the reality is rarely so absolute; often, the choice is between two or more treatments, each of which works after a fashion in certain situations. To apply the available evidence to the decision-making process in the most effective manner, the clinician must interpret it quantitatively, offering accurate, relevant figures instead of gut feelings when the patient asks what his chances are with each therapeutic approach.

Elsewhere [*see Chapter 179*], three randomized controlled trials of carotid endarterectomy for symptomatic carotid artery stenosis[18-20]

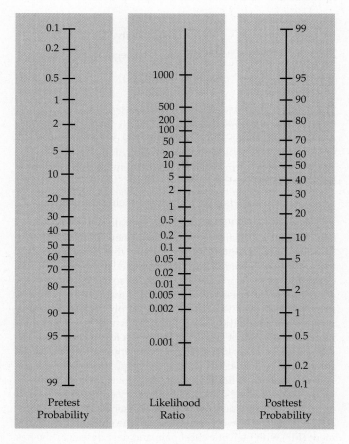

Figure 1 **Nomogram for converting pretest probabilities to posttest probabilities when test results are presented as likelihood ratios.**

Table 5 Definitions of Clinically Useful Measures of Treatment Effects from Clinical Trials

Like evaluation of diagnostic tests, evaluation of treatment effects often makes use of a 2×2 table, as follows:

Treatment Group	Treatment Outcome		No. of Patients in Treatment Group
	Bad	Good	
Experimental	a	b	a + b
Control	c	d	c + d
Total	a + c	b + d	

Measures of treatment effects when treatment reduces the risk of bad outcomes are calculated from this table.

- Experimental event rate (EER): the rate of an adverse clinical outcome in the experimental group; calculated as $a/(a+b)$.
- Control event rate (CER): the rate of an adverse clinical outcome in the control group; calculated as $c/(c+d)$.
- Absolute risk reduction (ARR): the absolute arithmetic difference in outcome rates between control and experimental groups in a trial; calculated as CER – EER, or $[c/(c+d)] – [a/(a+b)]$.
- Relative risk reduction (RRR): the proportional reduction in the rate of an adverse clinical outcome in the experimental group in comparison with the control group in a trial; calculated as ARR/CER, or (CER – EER)/CER, or $\{[c/(c+d)] – [a/(a+b)]\}/[c/(c+d)]$.
- Number needed to treat (NNT): the number of patients to whom one would have to give the experimental treatment to prevent one adverse clinical outcome; calculated as 1/ARR, or $1/\{[c/(c+d)] – [a/(a+b)]\}$, and reported as a whole number rounded to the next highest integer.
- Odds ratio: the odds that an experimental patient will experience an adverse event relative to the odds that a control subject will experience such an event; calculated as $(a/b)/(c/d)$.

are discussed in some detail. Examination of the North American Symptomatic Carotid Endarterectomy Trial (NASCET)[14] in the light of the users' guides discussed earlier [see Table 1] reveals that it meets the three criteria for a study focusing on therapy. First, patients with symptomatic hemispheric transient ischemic attacks or partial strokes and ipsilateral 70% to 99% carotid stenosis were randomly assigned to either an experimental group that underwent carotid endarterectomy or a control group that did not, and all patients received continuing medical care with special attention to risk factors for cerebrovascular disease. Second, the study assessed the effect of carotid endarterectomy on important clinical events—namely, recurrence of stroke or perioperative stroke or death. Third, none of the patients were lost to follow-up. Consequently, the data from the study are likely to be valid guides in determining which treatment is best for this patient.

In the NASCET report, the risk of major or fatal ipsilateral stroke within a 2-year follow-up period was 2.5% in the group that underwent carotid endarterectomy and 13.1% in the control group. The absolute risk reduction, therefore, was 13.1% – 2.5%, or 10.6% ($P < 0.001$; CI, 5.5% to 15.7%), and the relative risk reduction was 10.6%/13.1%, or 81%. The number needed to treat was 10 (1/10.6); that is, 10 patients (CI, 7 to 18) would have to be treated with carotid endarterectomy (rather than medical treatment alone) to ensure that one major or fatal ipsilateral stroke would be prevented. The NASCET report indicates that this benefit is somewhat lower for patients with less severe stenosis (70% to 79%) and somewhat higher for patients with multiple risk factors for cerebrovascular disease, circum-

stances that offset one another in the case of the patient under consideration here.

The NNT having been determined, the next question is whether an NNT of 10 for major or fatal stroke over a 2-year period is a small benefit or a large one. By contrast, treatment of elevated diastolic blood pressures that do not exceed 115 mm Hg is associated with an NNT of 167 to prevent one stroke over a 5-year period.[18] Thus, for patients who have symptomatic, severe carotid artery stenosis, carotid endarterectomy is highly beneficial.

Given this conclusion, the next question is whether these research results apply to a specific patient, hospital, and surgeon. For example, the NASCET data reflect operative procedures performed by highly competent surgeons in specialized centers. A physician would have to know the perioperative complication rates for local surgeons to be able to assess a patient's chances if referred to them. If the local perioperative complication rates for carotid endarterectomy are lower than 7%, the results will be comparable to the NASCET results. On the other hand, patients with less than 70% stenosis are at substantially less risk for subsequent stroke to begin with. Potential benefit is similar to potential harm for patients with 50% to 70% stenosis; for patients with less than 50% stenosis, current evidence indicates that carotid endarterectomy would not yield any net reduction of this risk, even when the procedure is done by a highly skilled surgeon.[21]

Measures of Treatment Outcome Adjusted for Quality of Life

Measures of treatment outcome, such as reduction in mortality, are important in helping to determine whether a medication should be started or an operation should be performed. However, these measures do not answer a question that is important to many patients: How much longer can the patient expect to live if treatment is started? One way of responding is to frame the answer in terms of life expectancy, the average length of life after starting treatment, which has a simple relation to the annual mortality in patients undergoing treatment.[9]

Life expectancy is a useful measure of treatment outcome, but it places the same value on years in perfect health as on years in poor health. Many clinicians would argue that a year with partially treated chronic disease is not equivalent to a year in perfect health. The solution to this problem is to adjust life expectancy for the quality of life that the patient experiences during a year in poor health by multiplying life expectancy by a number, on a scale of 0 to 1, that reflects how the patient feels about the quality of life experienced during an illness. This number is usually called a utility. When life expectancy, expressed in years, is multiplied by a utility, the result is a quality-adjusted life year (QALY). One QALY is equivalent to a year in perfect health.

Medical Decision Analysis

Clearly, there is more to clinical decision making than simply collecting numbers that measure treatment effects. Reports of treatment effects in randomized, controlled trials are important starting points that help determine whether a treatment has merit in its own right, but the actual decision whether to offer a given patient a particular treatment is complex and must take into account each patient's specific clinical circumstances and individual wishes. For example, if a patient has significant comorbidity that would result in an especially high risk of perioperative complications, surgical therapy may not be the best choice. Even if the patient is well enough to undergo an operation, individual

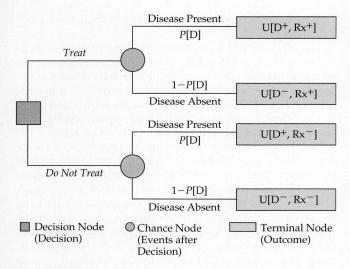

Disease Present
$P[D]$ $U[D^+, Rx^+]$

Treat

$1 - P[D]$
Disease Absent $U[D^-, Rx^+]$

Disease Present
$P[D]$ $U[D^+, Rx^-]$

Do Not Treat

$1 - P[D]$
Disease Absent $U[D^-, Rx^-]$

▪ Decision Node   ● Chance Node   ▭ Terminal Node
(Decision)   (Events after   (Outcome)
             Decision)

Figure 2   **Shown is a decision tree for calculating the treatment threshold probability in a patient who is a possible candidate for carotid endarterectomy. (U—utility; D—disease)**

preferences and values must be taken into account: the patient may be strongly averse to the immediate risks posed by surgery or may lack the resources to pay for the procedure.

THE THRESHOLD MODEL OF DECISION MAKING

At the conclusion of every history and physical examination, the clinician must choose one of three options: to treat, to observe, or to obtain more information. The optimal approach to making this decision starts with the assumption that the physician will seek more information (i.e., order diagnostic tests) only if the results may alter the treatment decision. Although occasional exceptions can be easily justified, this rule is a good guiding principle for a lean style of practice. It is also the central assumption behind the threshold model of decision making.

When a diagnosis is uncertain, the decision to start treatment depends on the probability of the diagnosis. If the probability is 0, no one would start treatment; if the probability is 1, everyone would start treatment. Therefore, there must be a probability between 0 and 1 at which a physician would have no preference between treating and not treating. This probability is called the treatment threshold probability.

The treatment threshold probability is a key to solving the important decision-making problem of whether to treat, to observe, or to obtain more information. The most elegant way of obtaining the treatment threshold probability is to construct a decision tree that represents the choice between starting treatment and withholding treatment [*see Figure 2*]. In a decision tree, decisions are represented by squares (decision nodes), and the chance events that follow a decision are represented by circles (chance nodes). The probabilities of the events after a chance node must total 1.0. A terminal node (represented by a rectangle enclosing the name of the state) represents a state in which there are no subsequent chance events. Each terminal node has a value, which is a measure of the outcome associated with the event.

In a decision tree for starting or withholding treatment, each branch of the two chance nodes ends in a terminal node whose value is the utility (U) for being in the state specified. For example, U[D⁺, Rx⁺] is the utility for having the disease (D) and being

treated for it, which one could calculate by representing that state as a tree with chance nodes and terminal nodes. To obtain the treatment threshold probability, one sets the expected utility of treatment at a value equal to the value for the expected utility of no treatment and then solves for the probability of disease. The general solution to the equation is as follows:

$$\text{Treatment threshold probability} = \frac{\text{harm}}{\text{harm} + \text{benefit}}$$

where harm is the net utility of being treated when disease is absent (U[D⁻, Rx⁺] – U[D⁻, Rx⁻]) and benefit is the net utility of being treated when disease is present (U[D⁺, Rx⁺] – U[D⁺, Rx⁻]). This relation between benefits and harms of treatment is fundamental to solving the problem of making decisions about treatment when the diagnosis is not known with certainty. Because the treatment threshold depends on the benefits and harms of the treatment, it will vary from treatment to treatment. When the benefit of a treatment exceeds harm, which is usually the case, the treatment threshold probability must be less than 0.50.

To make the choice between treating, not treating, and ordering tests to obtain additional information, the physician needs to know the range of probabilities of disease within which testing is the preferred action. The probability scale can be divided into three ranges [*see Figure 3*], one of which is the test range. The first step in defining the test range is to establish the treatment threshold probability. For the next step, we must invoke the principle that the physician should seek more information only if the results might alter the treatment decision. Translated to the threshold model, this principle takes the following form: testing is indicated only if the result of the test might move the probability of disease from one side of the treatment threshold (the do-not-treat side) to the other (the treat side). A physician can use this principle to decide whether to obtain a test in an individual patient. If the patient's pretest probability is below the treatment threshold and therefore in the do-not-treat zone, the physician should order the test only if the posttest probability of disease after a positive test result would be higher than the treatment threshold probability.

To obtain the test range, we must extend this example to a more general solution, which is to use the test's likelihood ratio and the Bayes theorem to calculate the pretest probability at which the posttest probability is exactly equal to the treatment threshold probability [*see Figure 3*]. This probability is called the no treat–test threshold probability. Clearly, if the pretest probability is lower than the no treat–test threshold probability, the test should not be done, because the posttest probability will be lower than the treatment threshold probability (i.e., a positive

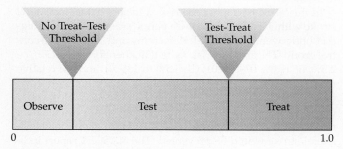

Figure 3   **Probability scale showing the ranges of probability corresponding to different actions after the initial history and physical examination.**

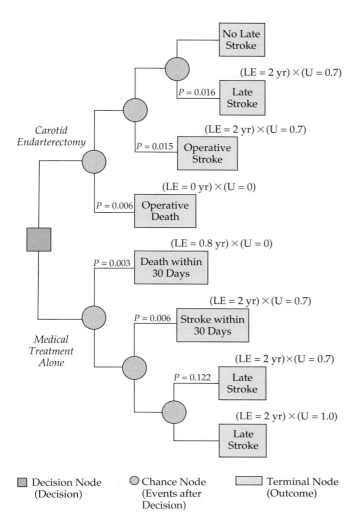

Figure 4 **Shown is a decision tree depicting the application of expected-outcome decision analysis to the same patient referred to in Figure 2. (LE—life expectancy; U—utility)**

result will not change the management decision); conversely, if the pretest probability is higher than the no treat–test threshold probability, the test should be done, because the posttest probability will be higher than the treatment threshold probability (i.e., a positive test result would change the management decision from do not treat to treat).

The size of the test range depends on the likelihood ratios reported for the test. If LR⁻ is close to zero and LR⁺ is much greater than 1.0, the test range will be very wide. In general, the better the test, the larger the test range. If the posttest probability falls within the treat zone, the physician must then decide which treatment to offer. The choice among treatments offers a good opportunity to explore the principles of decision making under conditions of uncertainty.

MEASURES OF EXPECTED-OUTCOME DECISION MAKING: THE TREATMENT DECISION

The purpose of decision analysis is to help with those decisions for which the outcome cannot be foretold (e.g., the decision whether to treat carotid artery stenosis surgically). Even when randomized trial results indicate that one treatment generally gives better results than another, some degree of uncertainty re-

mains: individual patients may still exhibit idiosyncratic outcomes or may experience unusual but serious side effects of treatment. Faced with this uncertainty, most physicians choose the treatment that gives the best results averaged over a large number of patients. In so doing, they become, perhaps unwittingly, what are known as expected-value decision makers. Expected value is the value of an intervention when the outcomes of that intervention are averaged over many patients. A more general term might be expected-outcome decision maker, which would denote a physician who chooses the treatment that gives the best outcome when averaged over many patients. This concept is the basis of expected-outcome decision analysis, which is a method of framing a decision problem in terms of the expected outcome of each decision alternative. Thus, one would decide between medical management of stable angina, coronary angioplasty, or coronary artery bypass surgery by calculating a patient's life expectancy, expressed in years in good health, after undergoing each of these treatment options.

We can illustrate the application of expected-outcome decision making by returning to the example of the 69-year-old male patient who has recovered from a hemispheric stroke and has 75% carotid stenosis. The question to be answered is the same: Should the patient be offered carotid endarterectomy in addition to best medical treatment? The first step is to represent the problem by a decision tree [*see Figure 4*]. Each of the terminal nodes in this decision tree is associated with a life expectancy as well as a utility representing the value of life in the outcome state represented by the terminal node. As noted earlier [*see* Measurements Used in Critical Appraisal of the Literature, Measures of Treatment Outcome Adjusted for Quality of Life, *above*], life expectancy by itself is not a sufficiently precise measure. Clearly, 2 years of life after a major stroke is not equivalent to 2 years in perfect health. The decision maker needs a quantitative measure of the patient's feelings about being in an outcome state. The physician can obtain the patient's utility for that state by asking the patient to indicate the length of time in perfect health that he or she would consider equivalent to his or her life expectancy in a disabled state (e.g., after a major stroke). This technique is called time trade-off. Other techniques used to obtain this utility include linear scaling and the standard reference gamble.[10]

To calculate the expected value of surgical management, the decision maker starts at the chance nodes that are farthest from the decision node (the tips of the branches of the decision tree), multiplies the probability of each event at each chance node by the value of the event, and sums these products over all the events at the chance node. This calculation is known as averaging out at a chance node [*see Figure 5*]. The value obtained for each chance node by means of this process becomes the outcome measure for the next step, which is to repeat the averaging-out process at the next chance node to the left.

With either therapeutic option—aspirin combined with carotid endarterectomy or continued management with aspirin alone—there is a chance of death within 30 days or a chance of stroke within 30 days to 2 years [*see Figure 4*]. As demonstrated [*see* Measures of Treatment Effects, *above*], reliable data on the probabilities of these adverse events are available in the NASCET report.[18] To simplify the presentation of the decision analysis, we measure survival only within the 2-year time frame addressed in the NASCET report, and we assume that all late strokes occur at the start of this 2-year period. Further, we assume that a patient would value 2 years of disability resulting from a stroke as equivalent to 17.5 months of healthy life, which means that the

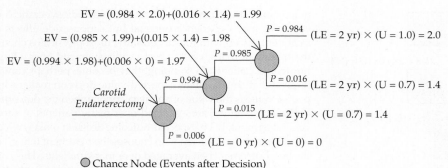

EV = (0.984 × 2.0)+(0.016 × 1.4) = 1.99

EV = (0.985 × 1.99)+(0.015 × 1.4) = 1.98

EV = (0.994 × 1.98)+(0.006 × 0) = 1.97

P = 0.984 (LE = 2 yr) × (U = 1.0) = 2.0

P = 0.985

Carotid Endarterectomy

P = 0.994

P = 0.016 (LE = 2 yr) × (U = 0.7) = 1.4

P = 0.015 (LE = 2 yr) × (U = 0.7) = 1.4

P = 0.006 (LE = 0 yr) × (U = 0) = 0

◯ Chance Node (Events after Decision)

Figure 5 **Illustrated is the process of averaging out at a chance node, as applied to the upper (carotid endarterectomy) portion of the decision tree depicted in Figure 2. (EV—expected value; LE—life expectancy; U—utility)**

utility representing the state of having experienced a major stroke is 0.70.

The decision analysis indicates that the decision maker should prefer surgical treatment to medical treatment. The expected value of carotid endarterectomy for this patient is 1.96 quality-adjusted life years, whereas the expected value of medical treatment is 1.91 quality-adjusted life years. Admittedly, this difference is not very large, indicating a close call, and it is reasonable to ask how high the operative mortality would have to be to make medical treatment the favored approach. Sensitivity analysis, one of the most powerful features of decision analysis, shows that the operative mortality would have to increase considerably before medical treatment would become preferable. The baseline figure for operative mortality in the NASCET report was 0.6%. The sensitivity analysis indicates that medical treatment would have a higher expected value than surgical treatment only if the operative mortality were 3.2% or higher, which might be the case if considerable comorbidity were present or if the surgeon seldom performed carotid endarterectomy. Although most physicians would not have the time or expertise to carry out this decision analysis, storing the appropriate decision tree in a handheld computer would make it possible to do the decision analysis easily in the office setting, using values specific to the clinical setting and the patient.

COST-EFFECTIVENESS ANALYSIS

Cost-effectiveness analysis is a method for comparing the impact of expenditures on different health outcomes. Cost-effectiveness analysis assesses the trade-off between added benefit and added cost by examining costs and benefits at the margin (i.e., comparing one intervention with another or with no intervention). The cost-effectiveness of one intervention (A) versus another (B) is calculated as follows:

$$\text{Cost-effectiveness (A vs. B)} = \frac{\text{cost A} - \text{cost B}}{\text{effectiveness A} - \text{effectiveness B}}$$

In the carotid endarterectomy example, the costs would include all costs associated with a subsequent stroke. If we assume that the average lifetime cost associated with carotid endarterectomy is $10,000 and the average lifetime cost associated with medical treatment is $8,000, then the cost-effectiveness of surgical treatment, as compared with medical treatment, would be

Cost-effectiveness (surgery vs. no surgery)
= ($10,000 – $8,000)/(1.96 –1.91 QALY)
= $2,000/0.05 QALY
= $40,000/QALY

The following question may arise: Is a decision that costs $40,000 for each extra QALY cost-effective? There is no absolute answer to this question. In practice, a physician compares the cost-effectiveness of carotid endarterectomy with that of other interventions. How this information should affect the decision regarding whether to offer surgical treatment to any given patient is an even more difficult question. Indeed, most experts would say that cost-effectiveness is a technique for deciding policies that would apply to many patients. An organization with limited resources would apply them to interventions with the lowest cost per added QALY. The organization would not offer interventions that cost much relative to the magnitude of the anticipated benefit.

Conclusion

Quantitative approaches to clinical reasoning are still evolving. By combining better evidence from health care research with today's burgeoning information technology, physicians can apply evidence effectively to real-time individual patient care. Managed care, with its ever-increasing demands for efficiency and accountability, is placing more and more pressure on physicians to adopt a quantitative, evidence-based approach to patient care. Physicians who can back up their decisions with sound research and sound reasoning will be in a better position to provide their patients with optimal care.

References

1. Antman EM, Lau J, Kupelnick B, et al: A comparison of results of meta-analyses of randomized control trials and recommendations of experts. JAMA 268:240, 1992

2. Naylor CD, Chen E, Strauss B: Measured enthusiasm: does the method of reporting trial results alter perceptions of therapeutic effectiveness. Ann Intern Med 117:916, 1992

3. Best Evidence 2: Linking Medical Research to Practice (CD-ROM). Haynes RB, Ed. American College of Physicians, Electronic Products, Philadelphia, 1998

4. Clinical Evidence: A compendium of the best available evidence for effective health care. BMJ Publishing Group, Serial Electronic Publication, London, 1999 (www. clinicalevidence.org)

5. The Cochrane Library. Serial Electronic Publication, Oxford, 2000 (www.update-software.com/cochrane)

6. Sackett DL, Straus S, Richardson SR, et al: Evidence-Based Medicine: How to Practice and Teach EBM, 2nd ed. Churchill Livingstone, London, 2000

7. Haynes RB, Sackett DL, Cook DJ, et al: Transferring evidence from health care research into medical practice: II. Getting the evidence straight. ACP J Club 126:A-14, 1997

8. Bryant G, Norman G: Expression of probability: words and numbers (letter). N Engl J Med 302:411, 1980

9. Feightner JW, Norman GR, Haynes RB: The reliability of likelihood estimates by physicians. Clin Res 30:298A, 1982

10. Sox HC, Blatt M, Marton KI, et al: Medical Decision Making. Butterworths, Stoneham, Massachusetts, 1988

11. Goldman L, Caldera DL, Nussbaum SR, et al: Multifactorial index of cardiac risk in noncardiac surgical procedures. N Engl J Med 297:845, 1977

12. Sox HC, Hickam DH, Marton KI, et al: Using the patient's history to estimate the probability of coronary artery disease: a comparison of referral and primary care practice. Am J Med 89:7, 1990

13. Black E, Bordley DR, Tape TG, et al: Diagnostic Strategies for Common Medical Problems, 2nd ed. ACP Publications, Philadelphia,1999

14. Hull RD, Raskob GE, Carter CJ, et al: Pulmonary embolism in outpatients with pleuritic chest pain. Arch Intern Med 148:838, 1988

15. Mayewski RJ: Respiratory problems: pulmonary embolism. Diagnostic Strategies for Common Medical Problems. Panzer R, Black E, Griner P, Eds. ACP Library on Disk (CD-ROM publication). American College of Physicians, Philadelphia, 1996

16. Wells PS, Ginsberg JS, Anderson DR, et al: Use of a clinical model for safe management of patients with suspected pulmonary embolism. Ann Intern Med 129:997, 1998

17. Value of ventilation/perfusion scan in acute pulmonary embolism: results of the Prospective Investigation of Pulmonary Embolism Diagnosis (PIOPED). The PIOPED Investigators. JAMA 263:2753, 1990

18. Beneficial effect of carotid endarterectomy in symptomatic patients with high-grade carotid stenosis. North American Symptomatic Carotid Endarterectomy Trial collaborators. N Engl J Med 325:445, 1991

19. Cook RJ, Sackett DL: The number needed to treat: a clinically useful measure of treatment effect. BMJ 310:452, 1995

20. Endarterectomy for moderate symptomatic carotid stenosis: interim results from the MRC European Carotid Surgery Trial. European Carotid Surgery Trialists' Collaborative Group. Lancet 347:1591, 1996

21. Cina CS, Clase CM, Haynes RB: Carotid endarterectomy for symptomatic carotid stenosis (Cochrane Review). The Cochrane Library, Issue 2, Oxford, England, 2000

3 Reducing Risk of Injury and Disease

Harold C. Sox, Jr., M.D.

Prevention: A Brief Overview

During the past 2 decades, disease and injury prevention has occupied an expanding share of medical practice. Public interest in prevention is very high, driven by a steady accumulation of high-quality evidence that preventive interventions do reduce cause-specific death rates. The purpose of these interventions is to eliminate the root causes of diseases that precede death (e.g., heart disease, cancer, and stroke), which in the United States in 1990 were tobacco use (400,000 deaths), poor diet and inadequate physical activity (300,000 deaths), alcohol consumption (100,000 deaths), microbial agents (90,000 deaths), toxic agents (60,000 deaths), firearms (35,000 deaths), unprotected sexual intercourse (30,000 deaths), motor vehicle accidents (25,000 deaths), and use of illicit drugs (20,000 deaths).[1] These causes of death are the targets of disease and injury prevention. They contribute to 50% of the deaths in the United States. Most are simply bad habits, and changing those habits reduces the risk of dying.

Physicians have two principal roles in prevention: they identify risk factors for disease and injury, and they act as teachers and counselors. Physicians must expand their routine questioning beyond diet, exercise, and substance abuse to include recreational activities that increase the risk of death (e.g., boating, bicycling, and riding motorcycles), gun ownership, use of swimming pools, smoke detectors in the home, and domestic violence. In counseling patients about a healthy diet (including vitamin supplements), exercise, and other elements of a healthy lifestyle, physicians must often help patients adopt healthy living habits. Some patients simply require reinforcement of a chosen lifestyle. Others need help in changing harmful habitual behaviors to healthy behaviors.

The report of the United States Preventive Services Task Force (USPSTF)[2] contains evidence-based guidelines on 70 prevention topics [*see Table 1*]. Other literature is also helpful [*see Chapters 4, 5, 206, and 207*].

CAVEATS IN DISEASE AND INJURY PREVENTION

Although disease and injury prevention can have a significant effect on the health of the public, physicians should observe several caveats. First, the baseline risk of most diseases is very low in the average person. Each year, colon cancer will occur in 165 men in a cohort of 100,000 men 60 to 64 years of age. The low baseline risk means that the number needed to screen or treat to prevent one death is often very high. Annual fecal occult blood testing must be performed on more than 300 people for 12 years to prevent one death from colon cancer. Whether this inefficiency is important depends partly on the cost of the intervention. Fecal occult blood testing can be costly because it must be performed annually and because abnormal results trigger costly diagnostic tests. Seat belts and smoke alarms are very cost-effective because they incur a onetime cost.

Second, disease prevention does not prevent death. At best, it postpones death by shifting the cause of death from the targeted disease to another disease that strikes later in life. In the Minnesota Colon Cancer Control Study, a randomized trial of fecal occult

blood testing, annual testing reduced deaths from colon cancer during 13 years of surveillance. However, the total mortality was the same in the control group and the intervention groups. Our preventive efforts may reduce the likelihood of death from the target disease, whose identity and natural history we know. Inevitably, we raise the lifetime probability of dying from another disease, whose identity and natural course are unknown to us.

Third, we know little about the age at which we should stop our efforts to prevent disease. Our studies provide good informa-

---

Table 1 Recommendations of the United States Preventive Services Task Force[2]

Tobacco Use
Provide tobacco cessation counseling to patients who use tobacco products. Counsel pregnant women and parents about the potentially harmful effects of smoking on fetal and child health. Prescribe nicotine patches or gum to selected patients as an adjunct to counseling. Give antitobacco messages to young people as part of health promotion counseling.

Alcohol Abuse
Screen all adults and adolescents for problem drinking, using a careful history or a standardized screening questionnaire. Advise pregnant women to limit or abstain from drinking. Counsel all persons who use alcohol about the dangers of operating a motor vehicle or engaging in other potentially dangerous activities while drinking.

Drug Abuse*
Although the evidence is insufficient for a strong recommendation to be made, it is reasonable to ask adolescents and adults about drug use and drug-related problems. All pregnant women should be advised of the potential adverse effects of drug use on fetal development. Refer drug-abusing patients to specialized treatment facilities where available.

Preventing Motor Vehicle Injuries†
Counsel all patients and the parents of young people to use occupant restraints (lab/shoulder safety belts and child safety seats), to wear helmets when riding motorcycles, and to refrain from driving while under the influence of alcohol or other drugs.

Preventing Falls†
Counsel elderly patients on specific measures to reduce the risk of falls. Effective measures include exercise, balance training, environmental hazard reduction, and monitoring and adjusting medications. Provide multifactorial individualized interventions to elderly patients at especially high risk for falls.

Fires
Advise homeowners to install smoke detection devices and test them periodically. Infants and children should wear flame-resistant nightclothes. Smokers should cease or reduce smoking.

Drowning
Families with swimming pools should install four-sided 4-ft isolation fences with self-latching gates.

Firearm Injuries
Remove firearms from the home or store them unloaded in a locked compartment.

---

*There is insufficient evidence to recommend routine screening for drug abuse with standardized questionnaires or biologic assays.
†There is insufficient evidence to recommend for or against counseling patients to avoid pedestrian injuries.
‡There is insufficient evidence of effectiveness of external hip protectors.

tion on effectiveness in the study population, which is usually in middle age, but we do not know how the results apply to older people, whose care will occupy an increasing amount of the primary care physician's time.[3] Interventions that take years to show their impact may be ill suited to people whose life expectancy is measured in years rather than decades.

The decision to do a screening test on an older person should depend on the person's general health, which may be quantified as the person's physiologic age. The physician can determine a patient's physiologic age by asking the patient to rate his or her health as excellent, good, fair, or poor. The most likely age at death is the sum of the patient's actual age and the life expectancy that corresponds to the patient's physiologic age. A 75-year-old man in excellent health has a physiologic age of 67 years, which corresponds to a 12.9-year life expectancy [see Figure 1]. The most likely age at death is 75 years plus 12.9 years, or 88 years. This information can be very helpful in deciding how hard to press preventive efforts. With a 13-year life expectancy, a 75-year-old man has plenty of time in which to experience gains from preventive efforts.

CHANGING BEHAVIOR

Many interventions of proven efficacy are not completely effective because patients are reluctant to change long-established risky behaviors. The United States Preventive Services Task Force recommends the following steps for helping patients use their ability to change (self-efficacy)[4]:

1. Match teaching to the patient. Identify a patient's beliefs about a behavior, and adjust advice to the patient's lifestyle. Building the patient's confidence in his or her ability to change requires recognizable successes; define success in terms of goals the patient can achieve.

2. Tell why, what, and when. Patients need to know the reason for a recommendation and the results of following the recommendation. They must also know the time scale for the results, so they do not become discouraged when results do not occur immediately.

3. Small changes succeed. As the patient achieves small successes, propose larger but achievable goals.

4. Be specific. Couch suggestions in terms of current behavior, and give precise instructions in writing.

5. Add new behaviors. Adopting good habits is often easier than discarding bad ones.

6. Link positive behaviors with the daily routine. For example, patients can be encouraged to exercise before lunch or to take medication immediately after brushing teeth.

7. Do not mince words. Tell the patient directly, simply, and specifically what you want and why.

8. Extract promises. Get explicit commitments from the patient. Have the patient tell you exactly how he or she will achieve a goal. Assess the patient's self-confidence and address concerns about succeeding.

9. Use combination strategies. An approach that combines several strategies is more likely to succeed than a single strategy.

10. Involve others. Members of the physician's office staff can become educators. Anyone can offer encouragement to patients.

11. Refer. Subspecialists in many chronic diseases have trained teams that can educate patients far more effectively than individual physicians can. Another form of referral is sending novice patients to talk with successful patients.

12. Stay interested. According to research findings, a call from a health professional to inquire about progress is very effective in changing a behavior. A well-organized office will have a protocol for making these calls a matter of routine.

Health Risks from Substance Abuse

Substance abuse exacts a large toll on the health of the American people, accounting for at least 520,000 deaths in 1990, 24% of all deaths.[1] Unfortunately, many physicians do not place diseases resulting from self-abuse in the same category as diseases that strike seemingly by chance. Two factors make helping patients shed their habitual use of tobacco, alcohol, and illicit drugs a very efficient way for physicians to add healthy years to patients' lives. First, there is a high baseline risk that substance abuse will lead to serious disease. Therefore, the absolute reduction in risk from a successful intervention is high. This principle is especially true of substance abuse during pregnancy. Second, substance abuse is primarily a problem of youth and middle age, so a successful intervention can add many years of healthy life.

TOBACCO USE

Tobacco contains an addictive drug, nicotine, as well as other substances that contribute to death from cardiovascular disease, cancer, and chronic lung disease. Smoking also contributes to 10% of infant deaths and 20% to 30% of low-birth-weight infants.[5] Tobacco use contributed to one in every five deaths in the United States in 1990 (420,000 deaths a year). In one 40-year cohort study of male physicians in the United Kingdom, half of the deaths after age 35 were smoking related, and smoking caused 25% of the residential fires that resulted in death.[5] Tobacco use is less common than it was several decades ago, but 25% of adults smoke, and an increasing number of smokers are women. Women are starting to smoke earlier—many as high-school students—and they are heavier smokers; nearly twice as many women smoked at least 25 cigarettes a day in 1985 as in 1965.[6]

Cigarettes are highly addictive. Fewer than 10% of people who

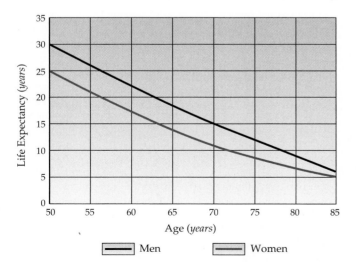

Figure 1 **Life expectancy of men and women in the United States. Source: Life table from the *Vital Statistics of the United States, 1980.***

quit smoking for a day are still abstinent 1 year later. Nicotine, like other highly addictive substances, acts on the dopaminergic mesolimbic pathway, the brain reward pathway that controls motivated behaviors [see Chapter 207]. The use of nicotine is self-reinforcing, leading to compulsive use. Nicotine produces a withdrawal syndrome that begins within a few hours of abstinence, peaks within the first week, and continues for several weeks. The withdrawal syndrome includes dysphoria, insomnia, irritability, anxiety, difficulty in concentrating, restlessness, slowed heart rate, and increased appetite.[7]

Detection of cigarette smoking is easy; most smokers are truthful when asked about their habit and its extent.

Smoking cessation reduces mortality dramatically. The risk of some diseases (e.g., myocardial infarction and stroke) declines rapidly within a few years of quitting [see Table 2].[8] This information is important when one is trying to convince long-term smokers to quit.

Research has shown that a strong message from a personal physician is the most important factor in successful quitting. The elements of successful quitting are consistent, repeated, and strong advice to stop smoking; setting a specific quit date; and follow-up visits to reinforce behavior [see Table 3]. However, not all physicians counsel smokers to quit. In one study, only 78% of cigarette smokers reported that their physician had advised them to quit.[9]

School-based prevention has received extensive study, and it is effective for at least 2 to 4 years. Clinicians, especially those caring for adolescents, must reinforce the messages of school-based programs.

Nicotine products are an important adjunct to counseling.[10] Drugs are most reinforcing when the level in the brain rises very rapidly, as with inhaled nicotine. Nicotine in medication form, especially transdermal products, appears in the blood much more slowly than inhaled nicotine and produces much less of the reinforcing effect that leads to craving for cigarettes. Plasma nicotine concentrations after transdermal administration reach stable levels in 2 to 3 days. Nicotine medications reduce the symptoms of withdrawal, so that symptoms in the first week are reduced to the level of symptoms at 5 to 10 weeks. Nicotine medications may also provide some nicotinelike effects, such as helping patients to sustain concentration and deal with stress.

Nicotine medications improve abstinence rates, but abstinence at 1 year is still the exception. A meta-analysis summarized the results of 46 trials of nicotine gum and 20 trials of nicotine patches.[11] At 12 months, 19% of patients who received nicotine gum were abstinent, as compared with 11% of patients who did not receive gum. The number needed to treat to achieve one success at 1 year (NNT) was 17 (P < 0.001). Transdermal nicotine led to sim-

Table 3 Elements of a Successful Smoking Cessation Strategy

Direct, face-to-face advice and suggestions
Reinforcement, especially in first 2 weeks
Office reminders: a sticker on chart of smokers may stimulate physician to deliver antitobacco message at each visit
Self-help materials
Community programs for additional help
Drug therapy

ilar rates. At 12 months, 16% of patients who received a transdermal nicotine patch had quit smoking, as compared with 9% who did not receive the patch (NNT 16). Clonidine also increases the rate of abstinence at 12 months. Weight gain is a common occurrence in patients who have stopped smoking. The average gain in a national sample of adults who had stopped smoking was 4.4 kg for men and 5.0 kg for women.[12]

The dose of nicotine medications should depend on the degree of nicotine dependence.[10] The score on the Fagerstrom questionnaire[13] and the number of cigarettes a day are measures of dependence. Follow-up calls at prearranged times will help the patient to maintain abstinence. It is best to designate a specific member of the physician's office staff to be the smoking-cessation coordinator.

The starting dose of nicotine gum (nicotine polacrilex) is 2 mg per two cigarettes; in patients who smoke more than 20 cigarettes a day, the dose should be 4 mg per three or four cigarettes. Patients may take additional unit doses if their withdrawal symptoms are unpleasant. The medication should be taken at regular intervals throughout the waking hours. The patient should compress the gum a few times with the teeth and then hold it in the mouth, repeating the cycle every minute or so for 15 to 30 minutes for each dose. After 1 to 2 months, weaning can begin with a reduction of 1 unit dose a week.

With transdermal nicotine, patients who smoke more than 10 cigarettes a day should use the largest patch (21 mg). After 1 to 2 months, weaning can begin with each of the lower doses (usually 14 mg and 7 mg, respectively), prescribed for 2 to 4 weeks. Patients who smoke fewer than 10 cigarettes a day can start with the 14 mg dose. A hairless site allows the best absorption. The patient should rotate sites to avoid skin irritation.

Nicotine medications are quite safe[10]—certainly safer than cigarette smoking—even for patients with cardiovascular disease. The only contraindication is hypersensitivity to nicotine or to a component of the delivery system. Twenty-four-hour application of transdermal medication can result in sleep disturbance, which subsides if the medication is removed before sleep. Nicotine medication during pregnancy is of concern but probably of less concern than heavy smoking during pregnancy. Medication during pregnancy should be reserved for women who have failed to quit without medication and who smoke more than 10 to 15 cigarettes a day. Dependence on nicotine medications is most likely with delivery systems such as a nasal spray, which causes a rapid rise in the plasma nicotine concentration, and a small number of patients will still be using nicotine medication 1 year after starting treatment.

Nicotine therapy is not the only pharmacologic approach to smoking cessation. Another approach focuses on dopamine. Nicotine releases norepinephrine in the brain and increases dopamine in areas of the brain associated with reinforcing the effects of addictive substances, such as opioids. Bupropion potentiates the effect of norepinephrine and dopamine by acting as a weak

Table 2 Years of Smoking Abstinence Needed to Reduce Risk of Disease[2,8]

Disease	Years until Risk Is Half of a Nonsmoker's Risk	Years until Risk Is Equal to a Nonsmoker's Risk
Recurrent myocardial infarction or death from coronary artery disease	1	15
Stroke	2–4	5–15
Oral and esophageal cancer	5	
Lung cancer	10	20

Table 4 Test Performance of Screening Questionnaires for Alcohol Abuse[2]

Screening Instrument	Number of Items	Sensitivity (%)	Specificity (%)	Likelihood Ratio Positive	Likelihood Ratio Negative
MAST	25	84–100	87–95	10.2	0.10
CAGE	4	74–89	79–95	6.3	0.21
AUDIT*	10	96	96	24	0.04
AUDIT†	10	61	90	6.1	0.43

*In inner-city clinic population.
†In rural clinic.
AUDIT—Alcoholism Use Disorders Identification Test   CAGE—see Table 5   MAST—Michigan Alcoholism Screening Test

inhibitor of their neuronal uptake. Thus, bupropion can mimic some of the central nervous system effects of nicotine and act as a substitute for nicotine in people who are trying to quit cigarettes. A recent double-blind, placebo-controlled, randomized clinical trial suggests that bupropion has a role in smoking cessation.[14] The study subjects averaged just over one pack a day of cigarettes and were moderately addicted to nicotine. Forty percent had used nicotine products, but no one was using them at the time of the trial. The proportions of subjects not smoking after 7 weeks of active treatment were 19%, 29%, 39%, and 44% in the groups on placebo, 100 mg bupropion, 150 mg bupropion, and 300 mg bupropion, respectively. (*P* values for comparing active treatment with placebo were less than 0.001 for 150 mg and 300 mg of active drug.) No one took bupropion after the seventh week. At 1 year, the rates of abstinence from tobacco were 12%, 20%, 23%, and 23% for those taking placebo, 100 mg bupropion, 150 mg bupropion, and 300 mg bupropion, respectively.

Side effects of bupropion include agitation and insomnia. Seizures are very uncommon when the daily dose of bupropion is 300 mg or less, and seizures did not occur in the trial. Patients on placebo were as likely to discontinue medication as those on active drug.

The recommended dose of bupropion is 150 mg/day for the first 3 days and then 150 mg twice daily. The patient should wait to stop smoking until he or she has been on bupropion for 1 week. There are no peer-reviewed reports comparing nicotine-replacement products with bupropion or detailing possible synergy between the two drugs.

ALCOHOL ABUSE

Habitual excessive alcohol consumption causes 100,000 deaths annually in the United States.[1] Although more than one million adults are under treatment for alcoholism, a far greater number engage in drinking that injures their health or has social consequences. The Institute of Medicine estimates that 20% of the population of the United States are problem drinkers, but only 5% are alcohol dependent.[15] Therefore, it is important to distinguish alcohol dependence from problem drinking. Alcohol dependence is associated with major withdrawal symptoms, tolerance, complete loss of self-control, and preoccupation with drinking. Problem drinking, on the other hand, is a less severe condition. Problem drinkers are younger, have a shorter drinking history, have fewer alcohol-related job problems, and have better social resources. In community surveys, the prevalence of problem drinking has been shown to be highest in young men (17% to 24% in 18- to 29-year-olds) and lowest in men and women over age 65 (1% to 3% and less than 1%, respectively). Women are more frequently problem drinkers than alcohol dependent.

Problem drinking has consequences that affect others, such as motor vehicle accidents, fetal-alcohol syndrome, unsafe sex, domestic violence, and psychological damage to children of problem drinkers. Binge drinking, which is especially prevalent in young adults, leads to violence, unsafe sex, and drunk driving.

Screening for problem drinking and alcohol dependence can be time consuming, and most methods are inaccurate. The gold standard test for alcoholism is the *Diagnostic and Statistical Manual of Mental Disorders* (DSM-IV) criteria, which require a detailed interview and do not constitute a suitable screening instrument. Results of physical examination and laboratory tests are often normal in problem drinkers. Screening questionnaires such as the modified Michigan Alcoholism Screening Test (MAST), the Alcohol Use Disorders Identification Test (AUDIT), and the CAGE test are the most accurate instruments for detecting problem drinking[2] [*see Tables 4 and 5 and Chapter 206*]. The questions in the MAST and CAGE instruments focus on alcohol dependence and are much less sensitive or specific for binge drinking. The AUDIT screening instrument[2] may be more generally useful because it also asks about quantity of alcohol imbibed, frequency of drinking, and binge behavior. The CAGE and MAST questionnaires may also fail to detect a level of alcohol use that is dangerous during pregnancy.

The treatment of problem drinking depends on the severity of the problem. Problem drinkers often respond to brief office interventions (as short as 10 or 15 minutes), which use motivational techniques such as goal setting, contracts, and enhancing self-efficacy. In most instances, the goal is usually controlled moderate drinking rather than abstinence. The first step toward successful counseling is to get the patient to recognize that there is a problem. It is important to help the patient see a relationship between drinking and current medical or psychosocial problems. Strong advice to reduce consumption is also important. Regular follow-up visits to monitor progress are just as important for problem drinkers as they are for patients with high blood pressure.[16] One meta-analysis of brief intervention trials for nondependent problem drinkers showed a reduction of 24% in average alcohol consumption.[17] Another meta-analysis of nine studies showed some-

---

Table 5 The CAGE Questionnaire

C: Have you ever felt you ought to **C**ut down on drinking?

A: Have people **A**nnoyed you by criticizing your drinking?

G: Have you ever felt bad or **G**uilty about your drinking?

E: Have you ever had a drink in the morning to steady your nerves or get rid of a hangover (**E**ye-opener)?

what smaller effects. In five of nine studies in men, the number of drinks a week decreased (range of decrease, five to 20 a week). The effects in women were smaller.[18] A third meta-analysis of nine randomized trials found that brief interventions were associated with alcohol moderation 6 to 12 months later (pooled odds ratio, 1.91; 95% confidence interval = 1.61 to 2.27).[19] An excellent guide to managing problem drinking is available from the National Institute on Alcohol Abuse and Alcoholism.

In contrast to the success of brief office-based interventions for problem drinking, successful treatment of alcohol dependence requires intensive therapy from specialists in substance abuse. A randomized trial of employees with alcohol dependence showed the importance of intervening intensively. Participants were randomly allocated to compulsory 3-week hospitalization followed by 1 year of attendance at Alcoholics Anonymous (AA) meetings, mandatory attendance at AA meetings at least three times a week, or a choice of treatment. Rates of being fired from work were similar in all groups, but rates for hospitalization for additional alcohol treatment were much lower in the mandatory-hospitalization group.[20]

The personal physician does have an important role to play in the management of patients with alcohol dependence. In addition to managing medical complications of alcoholism, physicians should be able to use adjunctive therapy for alcohol dependence, such as naltrexone. Another key role for the personal physician is encouragement. Patients need to know that the abstinence rate can be as high as 60% at 10 years after intensive treatment. Finally, the personal physician can lead efforts to help patients solve life problems that are contributing to alcohol dependence.

DRUG ABUSE

The abuse of illicit and legal drugs is a large problem in the United States. A household survey showed that 14% of adults between 18 and 25 years of age and 3% of those older than 35 years reported having used illicit drugs within the previous month. Casual use of marijuana accounts for most of these reports, but as many as 500,000 Americans use cocaine weekly and 500,000 use heroin or another injectable drug. The drug abuser is at risk for many medical complications, but the social cost of drug abuse far outweighs the personal costs. Illicit drug use plays a major role in spreading HIV infection and in homicide, suicide, and motor vehicle accidents. The health care costs of drug abuse are estimated to be $3.2 billion annually, and the cost of federal and state government efforts to stem the flow of illicit drugs is several times higher [see Chapter 207].

Many professional organizations recommend that physicians ask about drug abuse as part of a periodic health examination of a well person. However, learning about drug abuse may be difficult in the office setting. Patients may be unwilling to acknowledge drug abuse until presented with incontrovertible evidence or after persistent questioning by an alerted physician. There is little information about the accuracy of the history or questionnaires in detecting drug abuse.

Toxicologic testing is the best way to detect illicit drug use. Current tests can detect drugs in the urine with 99% sensitivity compared with reference tests. However, detection depends on when the patient supplies the specimen relative to the last drug exposure. Marijuana is detectable up to 14 days after use, whereas cocaine, opiates, amphetamines, and barbiturates are present for only 2 to 4 days after use.

Although physicians sometimes test for illicit drugs without obtaining the patient's consent, they do so in the context of trying to determine the cause of a clinical problem that could be caused by an illicit drug. Whether it is ethical to test for illicit drugs in an apparently healthy person who is at high risk for drug abuse is an open question. Regardless of the circumstances leading to testing, abnormal results deserve the physician's best efforts to maintain confidentiality, because they may affect the patient's employability, insurability, and personal relationships. At present, no professional organization recommends drug testing in apparently healthy people.

Physicians must learn to think of drug abuse as a chronic disease. Recidivism after intensive treatment programs is very common, no doubt in part because psychiatric disorders, unemployment, and homelessness often coexist with drug abuse. On the other hand, treating heroin abuse with maintenance methadone, an opioid agonist, can dramatically reduce the social effects of abusing the drug. Heroin addicts in methadone maintenance programs report less use of heroin and reduced rates of HIV infection, criminal behavior, and unemployment. There is no similarly effective treatment for cocaine addiction.

Health Risks from Accidents and Violence

A person's environment contains many threats to health: motor vehicle accidents, accidents in the home, recreation-related accidents, and domestic violence. Passive strategies, which change the environment in which accidents can occur, are generally more successful at accident prevention than active strategies, which require people to change their behavior. Improving roads saves more lives than exhorting people to drive carefully. For a fuller account, refer to the report of the USPSTF[2] and to a comprehensive review published in 1997.[21]

MOTOR VEHICLE INJURIES

Motor vehicle accidents are the leading cause of loss of potential years of life before age 65. Alcohol-related accidents account for 44% of all motor vehicle deaths. One can experience a motor vehicle accident as an occupant, as a pedestrian, or as a bicycle or motorcycle rider.

Injuries to Motor Vehicle Occupants

In 1994, 33,861 people died of injuries sustained in motor vehicle accidents in the United States.[21] The two greatest risk factors for death while one is driving a motor vehicle are driving while intoxicated and failing to use a seat belt. The physician's role is to identify patients with alcoholism [see Alcohol Abuse, above], to inquire about seat-belt use, and to counsel people to use seat belts and child car seats routinely. In one study, 53.5% of patients in a university internal medicine practice did not use seat belts. Problem drinking, physical inactivity, obesity, and low income were indicators of nonuse. The prevalence of nonuse was 91% in people with all four indicators and only 25% in those with no indicators.[22] Seat belts confer considerable protection, yet in one survey, only 3.9% of university clinic patients reported that a physician had counseled them about using seat belts.[22]

Three-point restraints reduce the risk of death or serious injury by 45%.[23] Air bags reduce the risk of death by an additional 9% in drivers using seat belts.[24] Because air bags reduce the risk of death by only 20% in unbelted drivers,[24] physicians must tell their patients not to rely on air bags.

Injuries to Motorcyclists

There were 1,775 motorcycle deaths in the United States in 1994.[21] The chance of death per mile when one is riding a motorcycle is 35 times higher than when one is riding in an automobile. Most deaths are caused by head injuries. Helmets reduce the risk of a fatal head injury by 27%, but only 50% of riders use helmets. Laws mandating helmet use are quite effective; the rate of helmet use rose to 95% in California after passage of a law, and the rate of head injuries dropped by 34%. Substance abuse is very common among injured motorcyclists.

Physicians should inquire about motorcycle use. They should redouble their efforts to screen for substance abuse in motorcyclists and should recommend using helmets.

Injuries to Pedestrians

Pedestrian injuries caused by motor vehicles accounted for 6,221 deaths in 1994. Children are at greatest risk for injury. Among adults, the elderly are at greatest risk, principally because of sensory deficits, locomotor disability, and inability to process simultaneous stimuli.

Injuries to Cyclists

There were 800 deaths from bicycle injuries in 1994.[21] Children are at greatest risk. Head injuries account for two thirds of hospitalizations and three quarters of deaths related to bicycling. A population-based case-control study showed that children's use of safety helmets was associated with a much reduced risk of head injuries (15% of that of unhelmeted riders).[25] Helmets are effective for all ages and protect even in collisions with motor vehicles. Community-based education efforts have raised the rate of helmet use to 50%. Physicians should ask about bicycle use and counsel riders to use safety helmets.

INJURIES FROM FALLING

Falling is a serious health risk for older persons [see Table 6]. The lifetime risk of hip fracture, perhaps the most important consequence of a fall, is 40% for a 50-year-old woman. One approach to reducing the risk of hip fracture is to prevent osteoporosis. Strategies for prevention of osteoporosis include vitamin D and supplementation of dietary calcium intake, estrogen replacement after menopause, and drugs that increase bone mass, such as etidronate and alendronate. In a cohort study, weight-bearing exercise, such as walking, was associated with a 40% lower risk of hip fracture in women and a 50% lower risk in men.[26] Exercise works in part by increasing bone mass and in part by reducing the likelihood of a fall. Combined interventions that included home visits, modifying home hazards, and exercise and gait programs reduced the risk of falls by 31% in a randomized clinical trial.[27] Physicians should identify patients who are at greatest risk for falling [see Table 6], treat osteoporosis, and link the patient to community-based programs for improving mobility and reducing hazards in the home.

INJURIES FROM FIRE

Prevention of death from fires is an example of a successful passive strategy. Smoke detectors prevent fire injury. A study in Oklahoma City measured the effects of door-to-door distribution of smoke detectors to residents of an area that had much higher rates of burn injuries than the rest of the city. The fire-injury rate declined 80%, to the same level as that in the rest of the city. The injury rate per fire also declined dramatically.[28] Physicians should inquire about smoke detectors in the home and recommend them to people who don't have them. Persons who are alcohol dependent or who smoke in bed are at high risk and need special effort.

Table 6 Risk Factors for Falls among the Elderly[27]	
Prior falls	Low body mass index
Cognitive impairment	Female sex
Chronic illness	General frailty
Balance and gait impairment	Hazards in the home

DROWNING

In most instances of witnessed drowning, bystanders report that the victim becomes motionless while swimming or simply fails to surface after a dive. Struggle is unusual. This observation raises the possibility that many cases of drowning occur when something such as a seizure, an arrhythmia, or an injury occurs.[29]

All victims of immersion have hypoxemia. Aspirated freshwater is hypotonic and therefore rapidly absorbed by the pulmonary circulation and distributed throughout the body water compartment. Freshwater alters pulmonary surfactant and causes alveolar collapse and atelectasis. Saltwater is hypertonic and draws water into the alveoli, causing perfused but poorly ventilated alveoli and hypovolemia with concentration of electrolytes. The end result with both types of water is venous admixture and hypoxemia, often resulting in metabolic acidosis. Saltwater drowning often leads to hypovolemia as well.

The main goal of treatment is to prevent brain injury.[29] The first step is to initiate cardiopulmonary resuscitation if the victim is apneic and pulseless. The American Heart Association recommends abdominal thrusts only to clear the airway in case of suspected foreign-body aspiration or failure to respond to artificial ventilation. Supplemental oxygen is indicated as long as the patient is hypoxemic. The most effective single treatment of hypoxemia is continuous positive airway pressure (CPAP), using mechanical ventilation to expand collapsed alveoli caused by freshwater immersion.[29] Hypothermia, which often accompanies near-drowning, can protect the brain from injury by reducing its metabolic requirements when the patient is hypoxemic.

Most efforts to prevent drowning focus on children, for whom the passive strategy of requiring fencing around swimming pools is associated with reduced drowning rates. In adults, alcohol ingestion is a risk factor for drowning. The efficacy of personal flotation devices is not known. Relatively few boaters (14%) wear personal flotation devices, but this rate is similar to that of drowning victims. Physicians should ask patients whether they use boats recreationally and advise avoiding alcohol and using a personal flotation device while boating.

Domestic Violence Information on the Internet

Medical Resources
  Family Peace Project
  http://www.family.mcw.edu/ahec/ec/medviol.html
  Domestic Violence: A Practical Approach for Clinicians
  http://www.sfms.org/domestic.html

Legal Resources
  Nashville, Tennessee, Police Department
  http://www.telalink.net/~police/abuse/index.html
  American Bar Association Commission on Domestic Violence
  http://www.abanet.org/domviol/home.html

DOMESTIC VIOLENCE

For women especially, the home is the most dangerous place. In one large study of women in a primary care clinic, one in 20 had experienced domestic violence in the previous year, one in four had experienced it as adults, and one in three had experienced it in their lifetime.[30,31] A condition so prevalent in primary care practice demands the attention of the physician.

Among those abused in the previous year, approximately equal numbers had been abused once, two or three times, or four or more times. In this study, the definition of domestic violence was an affirmative answer to the question "Have you been hit, slapped, kicked, or otherwise physically hurt by someone?" or "Has anyone forced you to have sexual activities?" Generally, a husband, exhusband, boyfriend, or relative is the abuser in domestic violence.

Most of the rapidly developing literature on domestic violence focuses on screening, diagnosis, and management, and there is little on preventing the first episode. Screening for domestic violence typically occurs in the office setting. Many authorities recommend that physicians routinely ask about domestic violence as part of the screening history.[31,32] Domestic violence occurs in homosexual relationships as well, so it is best to ask both men and women. Some physicians introduce the question by saying that they are now asking all their patients about domestic abuse, in view of the growing awareness of the problem. Then they ask, "At any time [or since I last saw you] has your husband [lover, partner, boyfriend] hit, kicked, threatened, or otherwise frightened you?" If the patient replies in the affirmative, the physician should gather more information, including the name of the abuser, and record it. Because many people are ashamed of their situation and their inability to break out of it, the physician should avoid any judgmental statements other than to confirm that what is being done to the patient is wrong.

In many cases, patients will not disclose an abusive relationship but their medical and social history contains clues to the true situation. Somatic symptoms that are particularly indicative (prevalence ratio > 2.5) of an abusive relationship include multiple symptoms (especially with no apparent physical cause), poor appetite, nightmares, eating binges, pain in the pelvic region, vaginal discharge, musculoskeletal injuries, and diarrhea.[30] Even more indicative are emotional symptoms such as high anxiety, severe depression, a high level of somatization, and low self-esteem; current or past use of street drugs; positive items on the CAGE questionnaire for alcohol abuse; a current or past drinking problem; a husband or partner who abuses alcohol or uses street drugs; a history of suicide attempt; and abuse as a child (prevalence ratio > 10.0 for all of these).[30,33] Pregnancy is often associated with an escalation of violence.

Some abused patients will disclose a history of abuse, but many will not. Therefore, during the physical examination, the physician should be alert to signs of injury. One expert states that a woman who presents with any injury should be considered a victim of domestic abuse until proved otherwise.[32] Trauma to the face, abdomen, breasts, or genitals is especially likely to be from domestic abuse, as are bilateral or multiple injuries, injuries in different stages of healing, and injuries that occurred well before the patient sought help. Injuries to the ulnar aspect of the elbows may occur as a woman raises her hands to protect herself during an assault.

The physician should communicate concern and validate the patient's belief that domestic abuse is wrong. The physician should not only provide medical treatment of injuries but also talk with the patient about how to avoid serious injury during an assault, review the patient's options, and facilitate referral to community and other resources for abused partners [see Sidebar Domestic Violence Information on the Internet].

INJURIES FROM FIREARMS

The rate of death by firearms in the United States has risen at an alarming rate, from 23,875 in 1968 to 39,720 in 1994.[34] Firearms accounted for 1,356 accidental deaths, 17,886 homicides, and 18,765 suicides in 1994. In two large communities, 58% of suicide victims used a firearm. Seventy percent of the suicides occurred at home. Firearms kill more teenagers than all natural causes of death combined. The Bureau of Alcohol, Tobacco and Firearms estimates that there are 192 million firearms in private hands. Firearms, often bought for protection in the home, are far more dangerous to the occupants than to an intruder. After controlling for other suicide risk factors, the odds of suicide were 1.9 times greater in homes in which there was at least one gun.[35,36] The odds of homicide increase by 2.2 in homes in which there is a firearm.[37]

Physicians strongly support regulation of firearms and community efforts to restrict ownership.[38] Physicians also have a role to play in preventing injury from firearms.[34] They should inquire about firearms in the home and counsel owners about storing their firearms in a safe place. With the increased number of teenagers who own guns and commit homicide with guns, the need to educate parents is urgent. The American Academy of Pediatrics has developed an information kit for physicians to use in counseling parents and children. Kits are available without charge from the Center to Prevent Handgun Violence, 1225 "I" Street NW, Suite 1100, Washington, DC 20005.

References

1. McGinnis JM, Foege WH: Actual causes of death in the United States. JAMA 270: 2207, 1993

2. United States Preventive Services Task Force: Guide to Clinical Preventive Services. Williams & Wilkins, Baltimore, 1996

3. Welch HG, Albertsen PC, Nease RF, et al: Estimating treatment benefits for the elderly: the effect of competing risks. Ann Intern Med 124:577, 1996

4. Lorig K: Patient Education and Counseling. United States Preventive Services Task Force. Williams & Wilkins, Baltimore, 1996

5. Doll R, Peto R, Wheatley K, et al: Mortality in relation to smoking: 40 years' observations on male British doctors. BMJ 309:901, 1994

6. Bartecchi CE, MacKenzie TD, Schrier RW: The human costs of tobacco use. N Engl J Med 330:907, 1994

7. Diagnostic and Statistical Manual of Mental Disorders, 4th ed.: DSM-IV. American Psychiatric Association, Washington, DC, 1994

8. Kawachi I, Colditz GA, Stampfer MJ, et al: Smoking cessation and decreased risk of stroke in women. JAMA 269:232, 1993

9. Dietrich AJ, O'Connor GT, Keller A, et al: Cancer: improving early detection and prevention: a community practice randomised trial. BMJ 304:687, 1992

10. Henningfield JE: Nicotine medications for smoking cessation. N Engl J Med 333:1196, 1995

11. Silagy C, Mant D, Fowler G, et al: The effect of nicotine replacement therapy on smoking cessation. Tobacco Addiction Module of the Cochrane Database of Systematic Reviews, Issue 2. Cochrane Library, Oxford: Update Software, 1996

12. Flegal KM, Troiano RP, Pamuk ER, et al: The influence of smoking cessation on the prevalence of overweight in the United States. N Engl J Med 333:1165, 1995

13. Heatherton TF, Kozlowski LT, Frecker RC, et al: The Fagerstrom test for nicotine dependence: a revision of the Fagerstrom Tolerance Questionnaire. Br J Addict 86:1119, 1991

14. Hurt RD, Sachs DPL, Glover ED, et al: A comparison of sustained-release bupropion and placebo for smoking cessation. N Engl J Med 337:1195, 1997

15. Institute of Medicine. Broadening the base of treatment for alcohol problems. National Academy Press, Washington, DC, 1990

16. Bien TH, Miller WR, Tonigan JS: Brief interventions for alcohol problems: a review. Addiction 88:315, 1993

17. Brief interventions and alcohol use. Effective Health Care, Bulletin No. 7. Nuffield Institute for Health Care, University of Leeds, Leeds, England, 1993

18. Kahan M, Wilson L, Becker L: Effectiveness of physician-based interventions with problem drinkers: a review. Can Med Assoc J 152:851, 1995

19. Wilk AI, Jensen NM, Havighurst TC: Meta-analysis of randomized control trials addressing brief interventions in heavy alcohol drinkers. J Gen Intern Med 12:274, 1997

20. Walsh DC, Hingson RW, Merrigan DM, et al: A randomized trial of treatment options for alcohol-abusing workers. N Engl J Med 325:775, 1991

21. Rivara FP, Grossman DC, Cummins P: Medical progress: injury prevention. N Engl J Med 337: 536, 1997

22. Hunt DR, Lowenstein SR, Badgett RG, et al: Safety belt nonuse by internal medicine patients: a missed opportunity in preventive medicine. Am J Med 98:343, 1995

23. Effectiveness of occupant protection systems and their use: third report to Congress. National Highway Traffic Safety Administration, Washington, DC, 1996

24. Kahane CJ: Fatality reduction by airbags: analyses of accident data through early 1996. National Highway Traffic Safety Administration, Washington, DC, 1996 (Report No. DOT HS 808 470)

25. Thompson RS, Rivara FP, Thompson DC: A case-control study of the effectiveness of bicycle safety helmets. N Engl J Med 320:1361, 1989

26. Paganini-Hill A, Chao A, Ross RK, et al: Exercise and other risk factors in the prevention of hip fracture: the Leisure World Study. Epidemiology 2:16, 1991

27. Tinetti ME, Baker DI, McAvay G, et al: A multi-factorial intervention to reduce the risk of falling among elderly people living in the community. N Engl J Med 331:821, 1994

28. Mallonee S, Istre GR, Rosenberg M, et al: Surveillance and prevention of residential-fire injuries. N Engl J Med 335:27, 1996

29. Modell JH: Drowning. N Engl J Med 328:253, 1993

30. McCauley J, Kern DE, Kolodner K, et al: The "battering syndrome": prevalence and clinical characteristics of domestic violence in primary care internal medicine practices. Ann Intern Med 123:737, 1995

31. Barrier PA: Domestic violence. Mayo Clin Proc 73:271, 1998

32. Alpert EJ: Violence in intimate relationships and the practicing internist: new "disease" or new agenda? Ann Intern Med 123:774, 1995

33. Kyriacou DN, McCabe F, Anglin D, et al: Emergency department–based study of risk factors for acute injury from domestic violence against women. Ann Emerg Med 31:502, 1998

34. American College of Physicians: Firearm injury prevention. Ann Intern Med 128:236, 1998

35. Kellerman AL, River FP, Somes G, et al: Suicide in the home in relation to gun ownership. N Engl J Med 327:467, 1992

36. Cummings P, Koepsell TD: Does owning a firearm increase or decrease risk of death? JAMA 280:471, 1998

37. Kellerman AL, River FP, Rushforth NB, et al: Gun ownership as a risk factor for homicide in the home. N Engl J Med 329:1084, 1993

38. Cassel CK, Nelson EA, Smith TW, et al: Internists' and surgeons' attitudes toward guns and firearm injury prevention. Ann Intern Med 128:224, 1998

Acknowledgment

Figure 1   Marcia Kammerer.

4 Diet and Exercise

Harvey B. Simon, M.D.

Many chronic diseases result from unhealthful eating and a sedentary lifestyle. Poor nutrition and inadequate exercise substantially increase the risk of such maladies as coronary artery disease, hypertension, stroke, diabetes, obesity, osteoporosis, and certain cancers and account for about 300,000 deaths in the United States each year.[1] Dietary factors also contribute to cholelithiasis, hemorrhoids, hernias, constipation, irritable bowel syndrome, and diverticulosis.

Diet

In the 20th century, the average American diet shifted from one based on fresh, minimally processed vegetable foods to one based on animal products and highly refined, processed foods. As a result, Americans now consume far more calories, fat, cholesterol, refined sugar, animal protein, sodium, and alcohol and far less fiber and starch than is healthful.

In the United States, 42% of men and 28% of women are overweight (body mass index [BMI] of 25 to 30) and an additional 21% of men and 28% of women are obese (BMI > 30)[2]; the health burden is substantial.[3]

Obesity is a complex, multifactorial disorder, but an element common to all cases is a positive energy balance in which more calories are consumed than expended. Excess calories are stored in body fat; each pound of adipose tissue contains 3,500 calories. Weight loss is accomplished only by achieving a negative energy balance.

ENERGY

Genetic, metabolic, and behavioral variables make it difficult to predict an individual's caloric requirements with precision. However, physicians can provide estimates: sedentary adults require about 30 cal/kg/day to maintain body weight; moderately active adults require 35 cal/kg/day; and very active adults require 40 cal/kg/day. On average, therefore, a 70 kg (154 lb) person can expect to maintain body weight by consuming 2,100 to 2,800 calories daily.

Although any source of dietary energy, including carbohydrate, protein, and alcohol, can be converted in the body to fatty acids and cholesterol, the caloric value of foods varies considerably; for example, fat provides 9 cal/g and alcohol provides 7 cal/g, but protein and carbohydrates each provide only 4 cal/g. Patients with excess body fat should be encouraged to shift from high-fat, calorie-dense foods to low-fat, less-caloric foods. To lose 1 lb a week, patients must consume 500 fewer calories than they expend each day; in almost all cases, sustained weight loss requires both a low-fat, high-fiber diet and regular vigorous exercise.

FAT AND CHOLESTEROL

Structure

Most dietary lipids are triglycerides, in which three fatty acids are joined to one glycerol molecule. At the core of every fatty acid is a chain of carbon atoms with a methyl group at one end and a carboxyl group at the other [*see Figure 1*]. The biologic properties of fatty acids are determined by the presence or absence of double bonds between carbon atoms, the number and location of the double bonds, and the configuration of the molecules.

Most of the fatty acids in foods are composed of an even number of carbon atoms, generally in chains of 12 to 22 atoms. The number of double bonds between carbon atoms determines the saturation of fats. Fatty acids with no double bonds are fully saturated; they have no room for additional hydrogen atoms. Fatty acids with one double bond are monounsaturated, and those with two or more double bonds are polyunsaturated.

Fatty acids contain zero to six double bonds, where additional hydrogen atoms can be attached. The location of the double bonds is of great physiologic importance; an unsaturated fatty acid's group (i.e., omega-3, omega-6, or omega-9) is determined by the position of the double bond closest to the methyl group. In omega-3 fatty acids, for example, three carbon atoms lie between the methyl end of the chain and the first double bond.

Most of the fatty acids in natural foods are in the curved, or *cis*, configuration. When hydrogen is added back to unsaturated fats during food manufacturing, however, the molecules assume a straightened, or *trans*, configuration [*see Figure 1*].

Cholesterol is a waxy, fatlike molecule that is present in the membranes of all animal cells but is absent from plant cells. Although cholesterol is a sterol rather than a true fat, its metabolism is intimately linked to the dietary intake of fatty acids.

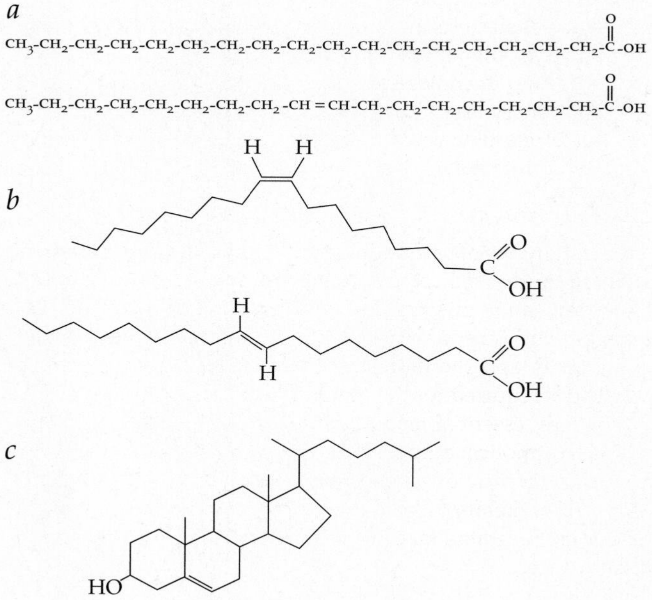

Figure 1 The structure of fat and cholesterol is shown. (*a*) Stearic acid (top) is a saturated fatty acid. Oleic acid (bottom) is a monounsaturated omega-9 fatty acid. (*b*) Oleic acid (top) displays a *cis* double bond. Elaidic acid (bottom) displays a *trans* double bond. (c) Cholesterol has a structure similar to that of fatty acids.

Effects on Blood Lipids and Cardiovascular Risk

Although all fats have the same caloric value (9 cal/g), their effects on human health vary greatly, largely because of their disparate effects on blood cholesterol levels. Saturated fats stimulate hepatic cholesterol production, thus increasing blood cholesterol levels. Of the four saturated fatty acids that predominate in the American diet, myristic acid (14 carbons) has the most potent hypercholesterolemic effect, followed by palmitic acid (16 carbons) and lauric acid (12 carbons). Stearic acid (18 carbons) has little effect on blood cholesterol levels.

Unsaturated fatty acids generally derive from vegetable and marine sources; they are often called oils rather than fats because they are liquid at room temperature. When monounsaturated or polyunsaturated fatty acids are substituted for saturated fats, blood cholesterol levels fall. Neither type of unsaturated fat, however, has a direct ability to lower low-density lipoprotein (LDL) or raise high-density lipoprotein (HDL) cholesterol levels. Although monounsaturated and polyunsaturated fats have a similar, generally neutral, effect on blood cholesterol levels, monounsaturated fats are less susceptible to oxidation and may therefore be less atherogenic.

Consumption of the omega-3 fatty acids is inversely related to the incidence of atherosclerosis and the risk of sudden death.[4] In high doses, omega-3 fatty acids may reduce blood triglyceride levels, but in dietary amounts, they have little effect on blood lipids. Even in modest amounts, however, omega-3 fatty acids reduce platelet aggregation, impairing thrombogenesis; they may also have antiarrhythmic properties.[5] Diets high in α-linolenic acid appear to reduce the risk of coronary artery diseases[6,7] and stroke.

Like saturated fats, *trans* fatty acids increase blood LDL cholesterol levels; unlike saturated fats, *trans* fatty acids reduce HDL cholesterol levels, making *trans* fatty acids even more detrimental.[8] Diets high in *trans* fatty acids have been associated with an increased risk of atherosclerosis and coronary events.

Dietary cholesterol increases blood LDL cholesterol levels but has a less potent hypercholesterolemic effect than saturated fat. Diets high in cholesterol are associated with an increased risk of coronary artery disease independent of their effects on blood cholesterol levels,[6] reinforcing the importance of reducing cholesterol intake.

Fat and Health

A high intake of saturated fat from animal sources appears to increase the risk of colon cancer[9] and prostate cancer.[10] However, some dietary fat is essential. For example, the omega-3 and omega-6 fatty acids cannot be synthesized endogenously and therefore must be obtained from food. Dietary fat is required for the absorption of fat-soluble vitamins. Lipids are essential components of cell membranes and steroid hormones; adipose tissue is the body's major energy depot, and it provides insulation against heat loss. As little as 15 to 25 g of dietary fat a day can provide essential physiologic functions. Saturated fat does not appear to increase the risk of breast cancer.[11]

Dietary Recommendations

The American Heart Association (AHA) dietary guidelines[12] for healthy adults suggest that no more than 30% of calories should come from fat, with less than 10% coming from saturated fat and the remainder coming from unsaturated fat in vegetables, fish, legumes, and nuts. The AHA guidelines also spec-

ify consumption of less than 300 mg of cholesterol a day. Patients with atherosclerosis or diabetes and persons who are hyperlipidemic or obese should follow more stringent limits, such as a saturated-fat intake of no more than 7% of daily calories, with a corresponding decrease in cholesterol consumption to less than 200 mg a day. In some persons, very low fat diets providing 15% to 22% of calories from fat can reduce blood HDL levels and produce other adverse effects,[13,14] but in carefully monitored high-risk persons, diets with about 10% fat and virtually no cholesterol have been beneficial.[15] Although reductions in total fat intake can help reduce body fat and serum cholesterol levels [see Table 1], the risk of coronary artery disease may depend more on the type of fat in the diet; saturated fats and *trans* fatty acids are the most atherogenic, whereas monounsaturated and omega-3 fatty acids are the most desirable.[4,6-8,12,16]

Food labels list the fat, saturated fat, and cholesterol contents of packaged foods. They are not required to list *trans* fatty acids, so patients should be advised to check the ingredients list at the bottom of the label for the presence of partially hydrogenated vegetable oils.

CARBOHYDRATES

Carbohydrates are a vital source of energy for metabolic processes. They are also vital constituents of nucleic acids, glycoproteins, and cell membranes.

Plants are the principal dietary sources of carbohydrates. The only important carbohydrates that originate from animal sources are the lactose in milk and the glycogen in muscle and liver. Carbohydrate-rich foods contain varying amounts of simple and complex carbohydrates. Simple carbohydrates include monosaccharides such as glucose, fructose, and galac-

Table 1 Suggested Fat-Intake Target Values

Calories/Day	Calories from Fat (%)	Fat Allowed (g)
1,200	15	20
	20	27
	25	33
	30	40
1,500	15	25
	20	33
	25	42
	30	50
1,800	15	30
	20	40
	25	50
	30	60
2,000	15	33
	20	44
	25	56
	30	66
2,500	15	42
	20	56
	25	70
	30	84
3,000	15	50
	20	66
	25	84
	30	100

tose and disaccharides such as sucrose (table sugar), maltose, and lactose. Complex carbohydrates include polysaccharides (e.g., starch and glycogen that can be digested into sugars by intestinal enzymes) and fiber (i.e., high-molecular-weight carbohydrates that cannot be split into sugars by human intestinal enzymes). Sugars, starches, and glycogen provide 4 cal/g; because fiber is indigestible, it has no caloric value.

Carbohydrates contribute about 50% of the calories in the average American diet—half from sugar and half from complex carbohydrates. Because sugars are more rapidly absorbed, they have a higher glycemic index than starches. In addition to provoking higher insulin levels, carbohydrates with a high glycemic index appear to reduce HDL cholesterol levels and may increase the risk of coronary artery disease.[17] Processed foods containing simple sugars are often calorie dense, whereas foods that are rich in complex carbohydrates provide vitamins, trace minerals, and other valuable nutrients. A healthful diet should provide 55% to 65% of calories from complex carbohydrates found in fresh fruits and vegetables, legumes, and whole grains.[12]

DIETARY FIBER

Dietary fiber is a heterogeneous mix of very long chain branched carbohydrates that resist digestion by human intestinal enzymes because of the ways their monosaccharide components are linked to one another. Fiber is found only in plants, particularly in the bran of whole grains, in the stems and leaves of vegetables, and in fruits, seeds, and nuts. The two general categories of dietary fiber are soluble and insoluble.

Soluble fiber delays gastric emptying, which produces a sensation of satiety, and slows the absorption of digestible carbohydrates, which reduces insulin levels. Soluble fiber also lowers blood cholesterol levels, probably by inhibiting bile acid and nutrient absorption in the small intestine and by promoting bile acid sequestration by colonic bacteria.[18] Because soluble fiber is metabolized by these bacteria, it has little effect on fecal bulk. In contrast, insoluble fiber increases the water content and bulk of feces and shortens intestinal transit time [see Table 2].

Diets that are high in fiber also tend to be low in fat. Such diets have been associated with a reduced risk of intestinal disorders, including constipation, irritable bowel syndrome, cholelithiasis, hemorrhoids, and diverticulosis but not colon cancer.[19] A high intake of fiber is associated with a reduced risk of diabetes[20] and, in patients with diabetes, improved glycemic control and decreased blood lipids[21]; it is also associated with a reduced risk of obesity[22] and coronary artery disease[23,24] and a lower all-cause mortality. A healthful diet should contain at least 25 to 30 g of fiber a day, including substantial amounts of soluble fiber.

PROTEINS

Unlike reserves of fat (which is stored in large amounts as triglyceride in adipose tissue) and reserves of carbohydrate (which is stored in small amounts as glycogen in liver and muscle), there are no endogenous reserves of amino acids or protein; all the proteins in the body are serving a structural or metabolic function. As a result, bodily function can be impaired if proteins are catabolized because of energy deficiency, wasting diseases, or dietary protein intake that is not sufficient to replace protein losses.

All proteins in human cells are continuously catabolized and

Table 2 Types of Dietary Fiber and Representative Food Sources

Fiber Type	Food Sources
Gums*	Oats, beans, legumes, guar
Pectin*	Apples, citrus fruits, soybeans, cauliflower, squash, cabbage, carrots, green beans, potatoes
Mucilage*	Psyllium
Hemicellulose*†	Barley, wheat bran and whole grains, brussels sprouts, beet roots
Lignin†	Green beans, strawberries, peaches, pears, radishes
Cellulose†	Root vegetables, cabbage, wheat and corn, peas, beans, broccoli, peppers, apples

*Soluble fiber   †Insoluble fiber

resynthesized. In a healthy 70 kg adult, about 280 g of protein is degraded and replaced daily. In addition, about 30 g of protein is lost externally through the urine (urea), feces, and skin.

In healthy adults, daily protein losses can be fully replaced by as little as 0.4 g/kg. Because not all dietary proteins are fully digestible, the recommended dietary allowance (RDA) of protein for healthy adults is 0.8 g/kg. People who exercise strenuously on a regular basis may benefit from extra protein to maintain muscle mass; a daily intake of about 1 g/kg has been recommended for athletes. Women who are pregnant or lactating require up to 30 g/day in addition to their basal requirements. To support growth, children should consume 2 g/kg/day.

A healthful diet should provide 10% to 15% of its calories from protein. For healthy, nonpregnant women, an intake of 44 to 50 g/day of protein is required, and for men, an intake of 45 to 63 g/day of protein is needed. Although excessive protein intake has not been proved to be harmful, there are several potential disadvantages to a very high protein intake. The protein in foods derived from animals is often accompanied by large amounts of fat. In the body, excessive protein can be transaminated to carbohydrate, adding to the energy surplus responsible for obesity. When excess protein is eliminated from the body as urinary nitrogen, it is often accompanied by increased urinary calcium, perhaps increasing the risk of nephrolithiasis and osteoporosis. Because nitrogen is excreted in the urine, an increased protein intake is associated with an increase in renal plasma flow and glomerular filtration rates and, eventually, with increased renal size. In some animal models, increased dietary protein is associated with accelerated renal aging, and in humans with kidney disease, high dietary protein intake is associated with more rapid disease progression.[25] On the other hand, high dietary protein appears linked to somewhat reduced blood pressure readings,[26] possibly because of increased urinary sodium losses, and protein supplements may be beneficial for patients with acute or chronic illnesses.[27]

The thousands of proteins in the human body are synthesized from just 21 amino acids. Most amino acids can be synthesized endogenously, but nine cannot. Not all dietary proteins contain all nine essential amino acids; in particular, vegetable proteins may be incomplete. However, by eating a varied diet with foods that contain a mix of proteins, even strict vegetarians can obtain all the amino acids they need.

VITAMIN AND MINERAL CONSUMPTION

Vitamins

Vitamins are either fat soluble or water soluble. Vitamins A, D, E, and K are fat soluble. They are found in fatty foods and are absorbed, transported, and stored with fat. Because excretion is minimal and storage in fat is abundant, deficiencies of fat-soluble vitamins are rare, but toxic amounts can accumulate if intake is excessive. Vitamin C and the B-complex group are water soluble; they are absorbed in the intestine, bound to transport proteins, and excreted in the urine. Because storage is minimal, water-soluble vitamins should be ingested regularly, and except for large doses of B_3 and B_6, toxicity is rare [see Table 3].

Although there is great disparity between popular beliefs about vitamins and their known physiologic effects, new medical information may narrow the gap. First, it is becoming clear that many Americans, particularly the elderly and the poor, do not consume adequate amounts of vitamin-rich foods. Second, laboratory and animal experiments demonstrate that antioxidant vitamins can retard atherogenesis and suggest that antioxidants may lower the risk of carcinogenesis. Indeed, many epidemiologic and observational studies have demonstrated an association between a low dietary intake or low plasma levels of antioxidants and an increased risk of atherosclerosis and certain cancers. Similarly, studies have linked low levels of folic acid, vitamin B_6, and vitamin B_{12} with elevated blood homocysteine levels and increased cardiovascular risks.[28] People who consume multivitamins appear to have a reduced risk of coro-

Table 3 The Vitamins

Vitamin	Functions	Deficiency Effects	Toxic Effects	Sources	RDA for Adults
A (retinol, retinoic acid)	Vision, epithelial integrity; possible protection against epithelial cancers and atherosclerosis	Night blindness; increased susceptibility to infection	Teratogenicity, hepatotoxicity, cerebral edema, desquamation; yellowish skin discoloration by carotenoids	Liver, dairy products, eggs; dark-green and yellow-orange vegetables (carotenoids)	Men, 5,000 IU or 1,000 RE; women, 4,000 IU or 800 RE
B_1 (thiamine)	Metabolism of carbohydrates, alcohol, and branched-chain amino acids	Beriberi, Wernicke-Korsakoff syndrome	None	Grains, legumes, nuts, poultry, meat	Men 19–50 yr: 1.5 mg; men > 50 yr: 1.2 mg; women 19–50 yr: 1.1 mg; women > 50 yr: 1.0 mg
B_2 (riboflavin)	Cellular oxidation-reduction reactions	Stomatitis, dermatitis, anemia	None	Grains, dairy products, meat, eggs, dark-green vegetables	Men 19–50 yr: 1.7 mg; men > 50 yr: 1.4 mg; women 19–50 yr: 1.3 mg; women > 50 yr: 1.2 mg
B_3 (niacin, nicotinic acid)	Oxidative metabolism; reduces LDL cholesterol; increases HDL cholesterol	Pellagra	Flushing, headaches, pruritus, hyperglycemia, hyperuricemia, hepatotoxicity	Meat, poultry, fish, grains, peanuts; synthesized from tryptophan in foods	Men 19–50 yr: 19 mg; men > 50 yr: 15 mg; women 19–50 yr: 15 mg; women > 50 yr: 13 mg
B_6 (pyridoxine)	Amino acid metabolism and heme synthesis; neuronal excitability; reduces blood homocysteine levels	Anemia, cheilosis, dermatitis	Neurotoxicity	Meat, poultry, fish, grains, soybeans, bananas, nuts	2 mg
B_{12} (cobalamin)	DNA synthesis (with folate); myelin synthesis (without folate); reduces blood homocysteine levels	Megaloblastic anemia, neuropathies	None	Meat (especially liver), poultry, fish, dairy products	2–4 μg
Folic acid	DNA synthesis (with B_{12}); reduces blood homocysteine levels	Megaloblastic anemia, birth defects	None	Vegetables, legumes, grains, fruit, poultry, meat	400 μg
Biotin	Metabolic processes	Rare	None	Many foods	30–100 μg
Pantothenic acid	Metabolic processes	Rare	None	Many foods	4–7 mg
C (ascorbic acid)	Collagen synthesis; possible protection against certain neoplasms	Scurvy	Nephrolithiasis, diarrhea	Fruits, green vegetables, potatoes, cereals	Men, 90 mg; women, 75 mg
D (calciferol)	Intestinal calcium absorption	Osteomalacia and rickets	Hypercalcemia	Fortified dairy products, fatty fish, egg yolks, liver	< 50 yr, 200 IU; 50–70 yr, 400 IU; > 70 yr, 600 IU
E (α-tocopherol)	Reduces peroxidation of fatty acids: possible protection against atherosclerosis	Rare	Antagonism of vitamin K, possible headaches	Vegetable oils, wheat germ, nuts, broccoli	15 mg
K	Synthesis of clotting factors VII, IX, X, and possibly V	Hemorrhagic diathesis	None	Leafy green vegetables (K_1), intestinal bacteria (K_2)	Men, 120 μg; women, 90 μg

HDL—high-density lipoprotein   IU—international units   LDL—low-density lipoprotein   RDA—recommended dietary allowance   RE—retinol equivalents

nary artery disease[29] and colon cancer[30]; protection may be attributed principally to folic acid. However, with the exception of the Cambridge Heart Antioxidant Study, which demonstrated the efficacy of vitamin E in reducing the risk of myocardial infarction in patients with coronary artery disease, randomized trials have not demonstrated benefit from vitamin supplements,[31] and β-carotene supplements actually appear to increase the risk of lung cancer in smokers.[32] It is clear that additional studies are required to clarify the impact of vitamins on health.

Women of childbearing age, the elderly, and people with suboptimal nutrition should take a single multivitamin tablet daily; others may benefit as well.[33] Strict vegetarians should take vitamin B_{12} in the recommended daily amount (2.4 mg); because many people older than 60 years have atrophic gastritis and cannot absorb B_{12} bound to food protein, they may also benefit from supplementary B_{12}. Multivitamin supplements may also be necessary to avert vitamin D deficiencies, particularly in the elderly.[34] Although higher doses of vitamins have no proven health benefits, some people may reasonably choose to take higher doses of vitamin E (100 to 400 U/day) or vitamin C (250 to 500 mg/day), particularly if they are at increased risk for cardiovascular disease.

Use of so-called megadose vitamins should be discouraged. Expensive brand-name and so-called all-natural preparations are no more effective than reputable generic preparations. In any case, vitamin supplements should never be used as a substitute for a balanced healthful diet that provides abundant amounts of vitamin-rich foods.

Minerals

Although minerals are chemically the simplest of nutrients, their roles in metabolism and health are complex. At least 16 minerals are essential for health [see Table 4]; 10 are classified as trace elements because only small amounts are required. Other minerals, such as boron, nickel, vanadium, and silicon, have been shown to be essential in various animal studies but have not been found to be necessary for humans. Many Americans consume too little of some minerals (e.g., calcium and iron) or too much of others (e.g., sodium).

Sodium   The body can conserve sodium so effectively that only small amounts are required in the diet. The Food and Nutrition Board of the National Academy of Science estimates that an intake of no more than 500 mg of sodium a day is needed for health; the average American diet contains more than 4,000 mg a day.

Population studies demonstrate conclusively that a high sodium intake increases blood pressure, especially in older people.[35] The Dietary Approaches to Stop Hypertension (DASH) trial demonstrated that reduction of sodium intake from high amounts to moderate amounts will result in lower blood pressures and that further reductions in sodium intake will produce additional benefits.[36] When combined with other elements of the DASH diet (increased consumption of fruits, vegetables, whole grains, and low-fat dairy products, along with decreased consumption of saturated fat and sugar), sodium restriction can lower systolic blood pressure by an average of 7.1 mm Hg in normotensive persons and 11.5 mm Hg in patients with hypertension. Hence, reductions in dietary sodium could substantially reduce the risk of stroke and coronary artery disease. A high sodium intake also increases urinary cal-

Table 4   Essential Minerals and Trace Elements

Minerals and Elements	RDA/ESADDI for Healthy Individuals
Macrominerals	
Calcium	1,000 mg before age 50; 1,200 mg after age 50
Phosphorus	800 mg
Magnesium	Women, 280 mg; men, 350 mg
Sodium	1,100–3,300 mg
Potassium	1,875–5,625 mg
Chloride	1,700–5,100 mg
Trace elements	
Iron	Men and postmenopausal women, 8 mg; premenopausal women, 18 mg; pregnant women, 27 mg
Zinc	Women, 12 mg; men, 15 mg
Iodine	150 µg
Copper	1.5–3.0 mg
Manganese	2–5 mg
Fluoride	1.5–4.0 mg
Chromium	Women, 25 µg; men, 35 µg
Molybdenum	75–250 µg
Selenium	55 µg
Cobalt	Required in small amount as a component of vitamin B_{12}

ESADDI—estimated safe and adequate daily dietary intake   RDA—recommended dietary allowance

cium excretion, which increases the risk of osteoporosis.

There is no RDA for sodium, and additional controlled clinical trials will be needed to provide conclusive evidence that sodium restriction is beneficial to normotensive persons. Pending such information, the AHA recommends that daily consumption of sodium not exceed 2,400 mg,[12] and the National Academy of Science proposes a 2,000 mg maximum. Patients with illnesses such as hypertension, congestive heart failure, cirrhosis, and nephrotic syndrome may benefit from substantially lower sodium intakes.

About 80% of dietary sodium comes from processed foods. Physicians should review these hidden sources of salt with patients who would benefit from sodium restriction.

Calcium   A high intake of calcium, either from dairy products or supplements,[37] improves bone density. Dietary calcium intake is inversely related to blood pressure[38] and to the risk of stroke[38,39]; however, calcium supplements produce only small reductions in systolic blood pressure.[40] Calcium supplements appear to reduce the risk of colorectal adenomas[41] but may increase the risk of prostate cancer.[42]

At present, fewer than 50% of Americans consume the RDA of calcium [see Table 4]. Persons who do not consume enough calcium from foods should consider a supplement such as calcium carbonate or calcium citrate. High-calcium diets do not increase the risk of nephrolithiasis,[43] but prolonged overdoses of supplements may produce hypercalcemia (milk-alkali syndrome) or nephrolithiasis.

Iron   Iron deficiency is the most common cause of anemia. In the United States, 9% to 11% of women of childbearing age are iron deficient and 2% to 5% have iron deficiency anemia, but only 1% of men are iron deficient. Routine administration of iron supplements is recommended only for infants and pregnant women[44]; dietary sources should provide adequate amounts of iron for other healthy people.

A high intake of iron is harmful for patients with hemochromatosis and for others at risk for iron overload. A Finnish study linked high iron levels to cardiac risk.[45] However, American studies have not confirmed these observations, and one study indicated a possible inverse association between iron stores and mortality from cardiovascular disease and other causes.[45]

Potassium   Dietary potassium is inversely related to blood pressure and to stroke mortality in hypertensive men.[46] Although potassium supplements may assist in the treatment of hypertension,[47] current data do not justify the routine use of potassium supplements. Physicians should encourage a high dietary potassium intake in most individuals,[12,36] but low potassium diets may be necessary for patients with renal disease or other conditions that cause hyperkalemia.

Selenium   Selenium is a cofactor of the free radical scavenger enzyme glutathione peroxidase. A randomized clinical trial reported that selenium supplements of 200 μg/day appear to reduce mortality from various cancers.[48] Selenium levels have been inversely associated with mortality from prostate cancer[49] and gastroesophageal maligancies.[50] These data, however, do not yet support the routine use of selenium supplements, which can be toxic in high doses. Selenium is present in many foods, including tomatoes, poultry, shellfish, garlic, meat, egg yolks, and grains grown in selenium-rich soil.

Chromium   Although chromium plays a role in glucose metabolism, there is no scientific basis for the claims that chromium supplements contribute to weight loss or increased energy. Chromium supplements may be beneficial for persons with low HDL cholesterol levels, but more study is needed. Dietary sources of chromium include brewer's yeast, whole grains, legumes, peanuts, and meats.

Magnesium   Magnesium deficiency is common in diabetics, alcoholics, patients who take diuretics, and hospitalized patients. Persons with hypomagnesemia may require magnesium supplements, but others can rely on foods such as green vegetables, whole grains, bananas, apricots, legumes, nuts, soybeans, and seafood to provide magnesium.

WATER AND FOOD CONSUMPTION

Water

On average, adults consume about 2 L/day of water, with two thirds coming from beverages and the remainder coming from food. Healthy people have no need to track their water intake. Patients with conditions such as nephrolithiasis and urinary tract infections may benefit from consciously increasing their fluid intake; patients who are at risk for hyponatremia should restrict their water consumption.

Foods

Fruits and vegetables   Fruits and vegetables provide many desirable nutrients, including complex carbohydrates, fiber, vitamins, and minerals. Deep-green and yellow-orange vegetables may be particularly beneficial because of their carotenoids, and citrus fruits may be valuable because of their vitamin C, soluble fiber, and potassium. Cruciferous vegetables, such as cabbage, may reduce the risk of certain cancers.

Vegetables and fruits are low in sodium and calories; none contain cholesterol, and only coconut, palm oil, and cocoa butter contain saturated fat.

The findings of case-control and cohort studies strongly suggest that the consumption of fruits and vegetables is inversely related to the risk of coronary artery disease,[51] stroke,[52] malignancies of the respiratory and digestive tracts, and all-cause mortality.[53] A dietary-intervention trial demonstrated that a diet rich in vegetables, fruits, and low-fat dairy products can substantially reduce blood pressure.[36] The United States Department of Agriculture's Dietary Guidelines for Americans recommends eating two to four servings of fruit and three to five servings of vegetables a day; at present, only 32% of Americans meet these standards.

Legumes   Often neglected in the Western diet, legumes (beans, peas, and lentils) are rich in complex carbohydrates with low glycemic indices, iron, and B vitamins. Legumes are an excellent source of dietary fiber, including soluble fiber that can reduce blood cholesterol levels. Because of their high protein content, legumes are an excellent meat substitute. Soy protein can reduce blood cholesterol levels, and soy intake is inversely related to the risk of prostate and breast cancers.

Legumes can increase intestinal gas, causing bloating, flatulence, and cramps. Distress can be minimized by use of the nonprescription α-galactosidase preparation Beano.

Grains   The seed-bearing fruits of grains, called kernels, consist of three layers: the inner germ, which contains vitamins and polyunsaturated fats; the middle endosperm, which contains complex carbohydrates; and the outer bran, which contains dietary fiber. Because milling removes the bran and endosperm, whole grains are nutritionally superior to refined grain; whole-grain consumption is inversely related to the risk of coronary artery disease[54] and stroke.[55] Whole-grain flour can be used to make cereals, baked goods, and even pasta. Whole grains such as brown rice, couscous, and yellow cornmeal (polenta) are easily prepared and healthful side dishes. Oats and barley contain soluble fiber that can lower blood cholesterol levels.

Meat and poultry   Although meat is a source of protein, vitamins, and iron and other minerals, its high content of saturated fat, cholesterol, and calories makes it a potentially unhealthy food. Patients who eat meat should be encouraged to select lean cuts, trim away visible fat, and use cooking methods that remove, rather than add, fat. It is even more beneficial to reduce the amount of meat consumed by reducing portion size and frequency; a reasonable goal is to eat about 4 oz one to three times a week.

Poultry is a more healthful source of protein and other nutrients. Chicken and turkey are best, but the skin should be removed before cooking to reduce the fat content.

Dairy products and eggs   To reduce intake of saturated fat and cholesterol, nonfat or low-fat dairy products can be substituted for whole-milk products. The use of nondairy creamers, imitation cheese, margarine, and other products that contain *trans* fatty acids in partially hydrogenated vegetable oils should be limited. The consumption of up to one egg a day does not appear to increase the risk of cardiovascular disease in healthy, nondiabetic people,[56] but additional egg-yolk consumption should be limited. One egg yolk contains about two thirds of the total amount of cholesterol that is recommended for an entire day. Egg whites and egg substitutes are good alternatives to egg yolks.

Fish   A 1997 study reported that participants who consumed 245 g or more of fish a week enjoyed a 38% reduction in fatal myocardial infarctions over a 30-year period.[57] Although at least three other observational studies did not find that fish consumption was protective, a 1989 intervention trial that randomized 2,033 myocardial infarction survivors to usual care or usual care plus fish consumption found that eating two or three fish meals a week reduced 7-year mortality by 29%.[58] Fish consumption has also been associated with a reduced risk of primary cardiac arrest,[59] hypertension, and stroke.

As little as 4 oz of fish twice a week may provide protection.[12] Fish should be baked, broiled, grilled, steamed, or poached rather than fried, and high-fat sauces should be avoided. Because of their higher content of omega-3 fatty acids, oily, deep-water fish may be best. Despite the apparent benefit of eating fish, fish oil supplements have only a modest ability to retard atherosclerosis.[60] More study is required to confirm the value of eating fish and to define the optimal types and amounts of fish.

Cooking oils   Canola oil contains an omega-3 fatty acid, α-linolenic acid. High serum levels of α-linolenic acid have been associated with a decreased risk of stroke, and consumption of canola oil is inversely related to the risk of myocardial infarction.[6] Canola oil and olive oil have a high content of oxidation-resistant monounsaturated fatty acids. Olive oil may be a cardioprotective element in the Mediterranean diet and may also reduce the risk of breast cancer. Although more study is

needed, canola and olive oils appear to be the most beneficial oils for food preparation.

Nuts   Nuts are high in monounsaturated and polyunsaturated fatty acids and fiber. Nut consumption appears to be inversely related to the risk of coronary artery disease.[61]

Garlic   Medical studies of garlic have shown mixed results. Some meta-analyses suggest that garlic extracts can improve blood cholesterol levels, but others do not.[62] The putative benefits of garlic on blood pressure and coagulation are even less clear.

Flavonoid-rich foods   Flavonoids are polyphenolic antioxidants that are found in a variety of vegetable foods, including apples, onions, tea, and red wine. Although not all studies agree, consumption of these foods has been inversely related to the risk of coronary artery disease and stroke.[63]

Alcohol   Rarely regarded as a nutrient, alcohol should be considered when dietary recommendations are formulated. Containing 7 cal/g, alcohol is a calorie-dense food. Numerous studies demonstrate that low to moderate alcohol consumption substantially reduces the risk of coronary artery disease, peripheral vascular disease, and all-cause mortality.[64] The major mechanism of protection is alcohol's ability to increase HDL cholesterol levels; favorable effects on blood coagulation mechanisms may also contribute. Protective doses of alcohol can be obtained from one to two drinks a day; 5 oz of wine, 12 oz of beer, or 1.5 oz of spirits is counted as one drink. Despite its antioxidant content, red wine is no more protective than other alcoholic beverages.

Coffee   Studies have failed to confirm putative links between caffeine and peptic ulcers, hypertension, coronary artery disease, breast disease, or cancer. Caffeine can trigger migraines in sensitive individuals, and caffeine withdrawal can precipitate headaches or depression in habitual consumers. Caffeine can cause anxiety, insomnia, and gastroesophageal reflux. Brewed coffee can increase blood cholesterol levels, but filtered coffee does not. The effects of caffeine on pregnancy are not fully understood, but it is reasonable to discourage consumption of large amounts.[65] Caffeine restriction does not reduce palpitations in patients with idiopathic premature ventricular contractions.[66]

DIET AND HEALTH

Much remains to be learned about the complex relation between nutrition, health, and disease. Dietary preferences are no less complex and individual. Despite these uncertainties, a dietary pattern characterized by a high intake of vegetables, fruits, legumes, whole grains, fish, and poultry is associated with major health benefits for men [67] and women.[68] Physicians have an important role in educating patients about healthful nutrition and providing dietary guidelines [*see Table 5*].

Exercise

Numerous observational studies have demonstrated a dose-related inverse relation between habitual physical activity and the risk for many of the chronic illnesses that afflict people in industrialized societies. The protective effect of exercise is

---

Table 5   **Dietary Guidelines for Healthy People**

Eat more vegetable products than animal products

Eat more fresh and homemade foods than processed foods

Less than 30% of calories should come from fat

Limit cholesterol to less than 300 g a day

Eat at least 25 g of fiber a day

55%–65% of calories should come from complex carbohydrates

10%–15% of calories should come from protein

Limit sodium to less than 2,400 mg a day

Obtain 1,200–1,500 mg of calcium a day from food or supplement

Eat 6 or more servings of grain products a day

Eat 3–5 servings of vegetables and legumes a day

Eat 2–4 servings of fruit a day

Eat two 4 oz servings of fish a week

Eat no more than two 4 oz servings of red meat a week

Chicken and turkey should be eaten in moderation with skin removed

Eat no more than one egg yolk a day, including those used in cooking and baking

Use vegetable oils, preferably olive and canola oils, in moderation

Have no more than two alcoholic drinks a day

Adjust caloric intake and exercise level to maintain a desirable body weight

Avoid fad diets and extreme or unconventional nutrition schemes

Avoid untested nutritional supplements, including megavitamins, herbs, food extracts, and amino acids

strongest against coronary artery disease but is also significant against hypertension, stroke, type 2 (non–insulin-dependent) diabetes mellitus, obesity, anxiety, depression, osteoporosis, and cancers of the colon, breast, and female reproductive tract. Despite these proven benefits, only 22% of people in the United States exercise at recommended levels. Of all deaths in the United States, as many as 12%, or about 250,000 annually, can be attributed to a sedentary lifestyle.[69]

EXERCISE PHYSIOLOGY

The physiologic effects of exercise depend on the type of exercise, its intensity, its duration, and its frequency.[70] Exercise is either isometric or isotonic. Isometric contraction of muscle is characterized by an increase in muscle tension without a significant change in fiber length. No external work is accomplished, but substantial energy is expended. Examples of isometric work include handgrip exercises, pushing or pulling against a fixed resistance, and holding a heavy weight. In contrast, isotonic work involves a shortening of muscle fibers with little increase in tension; examples include swimming, bicycling, and running. Most exercise includes both isometric and isotonic elements.

Isometric and isotonic exercises differ substantially in their physiologic effects. Isometric work increases total peripheral resistance; both systolic blood pressure and diastolic blood pressure rise substantially, with relatively little increase in stroke volume or cardiac output. Isotonic work lowers total peripheral resistance, but heart rate and cardiac output rise. Systolic blood pressure rises substantially, but diastolic pressure changes little, resulting in a small increase in mean arterial pressure. Isometric work places a pressure load on the heart, whereas isotonic work imposes a volume load.

Isometric exercise increases muscle strength and bulk, which is desirable for competitive athletes, for patients recovering from musculoskeletal injuries, and for individuals who wish to attenuate the loss of muscle mass and bone strength that accompanies sedentary aging. However, static exercises produce minimal cardiovascular conditioning, and the circulatory demands of intense isometric work can be hazardous to patients with heart disease. In contrast, dynamic exercises enhance endurance and can produce adaptive cardiovascular changes in healthy individuals and cardiac patients.

Cardiovascular Response to Dynamic Exercise

The acute circulatory response to maximal dynamic exercise is a dramatic rise in cardiac output, from about 5 L/min to 20 L/min in healthy young men. The increased cardiac output results from a 300% increase in heart rate. This increased transport of oxygen is matched by a threefold increase in peripheral oxygen extraction. Total peripheral resistance falls, and blood is shunted away from nonworking muscles and the viscera toward exercising muscles and the coronary circulation, where blood flow increases fourfold.

The physiologic adaptations produced by repetitive dynamic exercise are known collectively as the training effect. The magnitude of the training effect depends on the intensity, duration, and frequency of exercise. Training requires rhythmic, repetitive use of large muscle groups for prolonged periods. Fitness can be developed and maintained in healthy adults with three to five exercise sessions a week. Each day's exercise should involve isotonic work at 60% to 90% of maximal heart rate for 20 to 60 minutes, either continuously or in increments

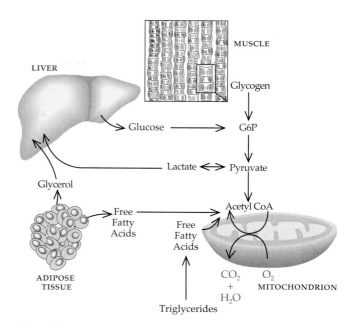

Figure 2   During exercise, catecholamine stimulation of adipose tissue rapidly mobilizes free fatty acids to achieve blood levels that are six times the normal level, which are far higher than the muscle can use. Glucose derived from the liver and muscle glycogen are initially phosphorylated to yield glucose-6-phosphate (G6P). The G6P, the free fatty acids fom adipose tissue, and the muscle's own triglycerides are metabolized to acetyl coenzyme A (acetyl CoA). This compound then undergoes oxidative metabolism in the mitochondrial Krebs cycle (blue), thus providing energy for exercising muscle.

of 10 minutes or longer.[71] Obviously, sedentary persons and patients with cardiopulmonary disease must initiate training at lower intensities and shorter durations and build up gradually.

Perhaps the most obvious training effect is resting bradycardia; heart rates of 40 to 50 beats/min are common in highly trained endurance athletes. The mechanisms responsible are not fully understood but probably involve increased vagal tone, decreased sympathetic activity, and increased stroke volume. The best overall measurement of the training effect and of physical fitness is the maximal oxygen uptake ($\dot{V}O_{2MAX}$).

Oxygen consumption relates directly to the amount of muscular work; maximal oxygen uptake therefore reflects maximal work capacity. Many factors determine an individual's $\dot{V}O_{2MAX}$, including age, gender, lean body mass, genetics, and, most important, the level of habitual exercise. Just 3 weeks of bed rest will cause a 20% to 25% decline in $\dot{V}O_{2MAX}$. It is no wonder that patients are debilitated after being confined to bed by illness or treatment regimens. In contrast, regular training lasting weeks or months will increase $\dot{V}O_{2MAX}$, typically by 30% to 40%.

Both central (cardiac) and peripheral (muscular) adaptations are involved in the training effect. In healthy individuals, training produces dramatic changes in cardiac structure. The dimensions of all cardiac chambers increase by up to 20%, and myocardial mass may increase as much as 70%.[72] Although increased coronary flow and collateralization have not been demonstrated directly in humans, echocardiographic studies show that elite athletes have increased proximal coronary artery size, which is proportional to their increased left ventricular mass. Cardiac function is also enhanced by training; left ventricular contractility and stroke volume increase, and angiographic studies have demonstrated increased dilating capacity in the coronary arteries of endurance athletes. Exercise training also improves endothelial function in patients with coronary artery disease and in elderly persons.[73,74]

In addition to these cardiac changes that allow enhanced oxygen delivery, there is improvement in peripheral oxygen extraction caused by enhanced O_2 extraction by the skeletal muscles themselves. This effect on skeletal muscle is specific for the muscles that have been trained; if only leg muscles are trained, the circulatory response to strenuous leg exercise will improve, but the response to vigorous arm exercise will not change.

Exercise training decreases the risk of hypertension. A meta-analysis of 36 controlled intervention studies concluded that isotonic exercise training lowers both systolic and diastolic blood pressure levels by about 5 mm Hg.[75] Regular exercise can even reduce left ventricular hypertrophy and blood pressure in patients with severe hypertension.[76] Regular exercise also lowers catecholamine levels, which may protect against arrhythmias, and it reduces myocardial oxygen demands.

Although isotonic exercise reduces resting blood pressure, isometric exercise increases total peripheral resistance and acutely elevates blood pressure. However, sustained hypertension is not a complication of resistance training, which may even reduce resting blood pressure.[77] Unsupervised isometric exercising should be avoided by patients with cardiovascular disease; with appropriate precautions, however, it can be safe for selected cardiac patients and can produce favorable effects on muscular function.[78]

Pulmonary Response

Except in people with intrinsic lung disease, the pulmonary diffusion capacity does not limit exercise. At heavy work loads, however, skeletal muscle oxygen demands exceed oxygen delivery. As a result, muscle metabolism becomes anaerobic; the lactic acid that accumulates is buffered by bicarbonate, so that the pH remains nearly normal. The CO_2 that is liberated by the buffering reaction produces an increased ventilatory drive and tachypnea. Athletes know when they have crossed the anaerobic threshold by a markedly increased respiratory rate and a sensation of dyspnea. Habitual exercise does not improve pulmonary function in healthy people, but exercise training may be helpful in patients with chronic lung disease as a result of adaptations in muscles rather than in the lungs.

Musculoskeletal Response

Isotonic exercises increase muscle endurance. Training increases capillary density, and it can increase muscle mitochondria and oxidative capacity more than twofold. These changes account for the greater oxygen extraction that is an important element of the training effect. Isometric training builds muscle mass, which improves performance and may decrease injuries. Isometric exercises involving slow repetitions of work against high resistance produce fiber hypertrophy and strength but do not alter muscle enzyme content.

Exercise training affects tissues in addition to muscles. Of great importance, weight-bearing exercises increase bone mineral density, reducing the risk of osteoporosis. Repetitive performance of athletic tasks improves coordination and efficiency; changes in neuromuscular recruitment may be partially responsible. Tendon strength and bone density increase as a result of repetitive use. Joint wear and tear remains a concern,

but as long as there is no trauma, habitual exercise probably does not produce degenerative joint disease.

Metabolic Effects

Skeletal muscle contains only very limited energy stores; preformed adenosine triphosphate (ATP) and creatine phosphate (CP) can supply less energy than is consumed in a 100-yard dash. Clearly, ATP and CP must be generated during exercise. Only three sources of fuel are available to skeletal muscle for this purpose: endogenous muscle glycogen, blood glucose, and free fatty acids (FFAs) derived either from muscle triglyceride or from adipose tissue. Normally, the body's skeletal muscle contains only 120 g of glycogen and the liver only 70 g. The 600 kcal of energy available from these two sources could sustain running for only 6 miles. The blood glucose provides only 40 kcal more. In contrast, the average person's 15,000 g of adipose tissue provides 100,000 kcal of energy, theoretically enough to fuel a run from Boston to Atlanta.

At rest and during low-intensity exercise, both FFAs and muscle glycogen provide energy. As exercise begins, catecholamines stimulate adipose lipase, which cleaves triglyceride into glycerol and three FFA molecules [see Figure 2]. In muscle cells, FFAs are metabolized to acetyl coenzyme A (acetyl CoA); in the presence of oxygen, acetyl CoA undergoes oxidative metabolism by enzymes of the citric acid (Krebs) cycle in mitochondria.

As the intensity of exercise increases, the relative contribution of FFAs decreases and glycogen becomes more important, and at maximum work, muscle depends entirely on glycogen. When oxygen is available, glycogen is metabolized in the cytoplasm to pyruvate, which then undergoes oxidation in the mitochondria via the citric acid cycle to water and CO_2. However, when the demands of muscle outstrip the availability of oxygen, energy can be generated only anaerobically via glycolysis. Anaerobic metabolism is much less efficient: from a gram of glycogen, anaerobic metabolism generates only 5% of the energy that aerobic metabolism generates. In addition, pyruvate cannot be converted to acetyl CoA. Instead, pyruvate is reduced to lactate. Acidosis limits muscular performance, and buffering by the bicarbonate system generates CO_2, causing tachypnea.

Although the blood glucose itself constitutes only a modest caloric reserve, glucose turnover is greatly accelerated by exercise. During exercise, the liver releases glucose by both glycogenolysis and gluconeogenesis. Simultaneously, peripheral glucose uptake is enhanced. As a result of these metabolic events, blood glucose can account for 10% to 30% of exercising muscle's metabolic needs. The blood glucose level remains normal and may even rise during modest exertion. However, hypoglycemia can occur if hepatic glycogen stores are depleted and high-intensity exercise continues to consume blood glucose and muscle glycogen.

These changes in glucose metabolism are moderated by a number of hormonal alterations. Circulating catecholamines, growth hormone, cortisol, and glucagon levels rise. Insulin levels fall. All of these factors tend to elevate blood glucose levels. Glucose that is ingested during exercise will also tend to maintain blood glucose levels, but ingestion of glucose before exercise may actually raise insulin levels, thus impeding energy mobilization. Contrary to popular so-called instant-energy theories, preexercise meals should not contain concentrated sweets. Indeed, preexercise meals should be sparse, and people should probably ingest little other than water during the 2 hours before exercise.

Exercise increases the insulin sensitivity of muscle, thereby increasing glucose transport and muscle glycogen synthesis. Even moderate physical activity such as walking can help prevent the development of type 2 diabetes mellitus.[79] Because exercise improves glucose tolerance in diabetic patients, patients taking insulin may require special precautions to exercise safely [see Medical Complications of Exercise, below].

During exercise, the rate of protein synthesis is depressed. As a result, amino acids are available for anabolic processes, including hepatic gluconeogenesis. Amino acids also may directly provide a small fraction of the energy needed for muscle contraction. It is not clear whether athletes have higher nutritional protein requirements than sedentary persons; the ingestion of protein and amino acid supplements does not enhance athletic performance.

Regular aerobic exercise also alters body weight and body composition. If dietary caloric intake remains constant, exercise will produce slow weight loss. It takes 35 miles of walking or jogging to consume the calories present in 1 lb of adipose tissue. Intense exercise also stimulates both energy expenditure and lipid oxidation for up to 17 hours after exercise itself, thus further contributing to a reduction in body fat. Even as body fat declines, muscle mass increases; because muscle is denser than fat, net weight loss may be slight. Swimming appears to be less effective than land exercise for reducing body fat and increasing bone mineral content.

Effects on Blood Lipids

Exercise increases serum levels of HDL-associated cholesterol (HDL-C), probably by delaying hepatic HDL-C catabolism. The amount of exercise appears to be the major determinant of the magnitude of the increase in HDL-C. As little as 5 to 10 miles of jogging a week will elevate HDL-C levels, which rise with increasing exercise in a dose-response fashion; beyond about 35 miles a week, however, additional training does not produce a further increase in HDL-C levels.[80] Similar changes in HDL levels have also been demonstrated in walkers, cross-country skiers, tennis players, bicyclists, and other endurance athletes. The effects of exercise are independent of other factors known to alter HDL-C levels, such as diet, body weight, smoking, and alcohol consumption. Exercise must be sustained to maintain high HDL-C levels.

The effects of exercise on HDL-C levels are observed consistently, but changes in the other blood lipid levels have varied. In general, exercise produces a fall in triglyceride and chylomicron levels. Total cholesterol and LDL cholesterol levels also tend to decline.

Hematologic Effects

A mild decrease in hematocrit is commonly observed in endurance athletes. This so-called sports anemia is usually a pseudoanemia, because red blood cell mass is normal but plasma volume is increased; decreased viscosity has also been observed. Exercise-related hemolysis or gastrointestinal blood loss may be an additional factor in some cases of anemia in athletes. No consistent long-term changes in polymorphonuclear leukocytes, lymphocytes, or immunoglobulins have been noted.

Hemostatic mechanisms are influenced by exercise. Endurance exercise acutely increases fibrinolytic activity, and repetitive exercise is associated with reduced fibrinogen levels.

In contrast, intense exercise can activate platelets,[81] perhaps contributing to a prothrombotic state that may contribute to exertion-induced cardiac events[82] [see Medical Complications of Exercise, below]. The effects of exercise on platelet function require further study.

Effects on Body Fluids

During exercise, skeletal muscle generates a tremendous amount of heat. Sweating is necessary to dissipate this heat. During strenuous exercise in a warm environment, up to 2 L can be lost each hour. Because sweat is hypotonic, the serum sodium concentration rises. Even in the absence of systemic acidosis, serum potassium levels may rise because of an efflux of potassium from muscle cells, but potassium levels normalize within minutes after exertion ceases.

The decline in blood volume, together with a shift in blood flow from the kidneys to skeletal muscle, produces a sharp decline in urine volume during exercise. The rise in plasma osmolarity increases thirst. However, thirst lags behind volume requirements, and fluid intake is often inadequate during athletic events. Volume depletion impairs athletic performance and can contribute to renal dysfunction or heatstroke. Unfortunately, coaching lore often limits fluid intake for fear of cramps, when, in fact, athletes can tolerate large volumes of water during brief pauses in exercise. Athletes do not require supplemental potassium or salt, so popular glucose-sodium-potassium solutions make little sense physiologically.

Psychological Effects

Endurance exercise produces improvements in mood, self-esteem, and work behavior both in healthy people and in patients undertaking cardiac rehabilitation; exercise training can help treat depression.[83] Several mechanisms have been suggested to explain the psychological effects of exercise. Purely psychological factors, such as distraction, may be involved. The serum levels of β-endorphin, monoamines, and other neuropeptides are affected by exercise in direct relation to the intensity and duration of exercise. Changes in endogenous opioid peptides may mediate the subjective effects of exercise (so-called runner's high).

EXERCISE AND AGING

Many physiologic changes attributed to aging closely resemble those that result from inactivity. In both circumstances, bone calcium wastage occurs, and there are decreases in $\dot{V}O_{2MAX}$, cardiac output, red blood cell mass, glucose tolerance, and muscle mass; total peripheral resistance and systolic blood pressure are increased, as are body fat and serum cholesterol levels. Regular exercise appears to retard these age-related maladies. Exercise training improves left ventricular systolic function and increases stroke volume to maintain exercise cardiac output in healthy, active older people. The age-related decline in $\dot{V}O_{2MAX}$ has been found to be twice as great for sedentary men as for active men, and even low-intensity training can improve $\dot{V}O_{2MAX}$ in the elderly. Exercise training also helps blunt the age-related decline in peripheral vascular function experienced by sedentary people. Endurance training improves glucose tolerance and serum lipid levels in older men and women, and regular exercise appears to blunt the age-related decline in resting metabolic rate. Physical activity in the elderly is associated with increased functional status and decreased mortality. Exercise is safe in the elderly if simple precautions are observed [see Prescribing Exercise, below]. Walking programs increase aerobic capacity in persons 70 to 79 years of age, with few injuries; healthy elderly persons who are randomly assigned to aerobic exercise acquire fewer new cardiovascular disorders than control subjects. Appropriate resistance weight programs are not hemodynamically stressful in the elderly and produce increases in muscle strength, functional mobility, and walking endurance. Even frail nursing home residents (mean age, 87 years) responded to resistance training with an increase in muscle mass and strength, as well as improved gait velocity, stair-climbing power, and spontaneous activity. Although more studies are needed to clarify correlations between aging, inactivity, and exercise, enough information is available to warrant a recommendation of carefully planned exercise programs for the elderly.

EXERCISE AND LONGEVITY

Primary Prevention of Atherosclerosis

Exercise training can favorably modify many of the conditions associated with an increased risk of coronary artery disease, including hypercholesterolemia, elevated blood pressure, glucose intolerance, obesity, and the less firmly incriminated traits of hypertriglyceridemia, hyperinsulinemia, hyperfibrinogenemia, and psychological stress. Studies conducted in men, women, and children demonstrated a consistent inverse relation between physical fitness and body weight, percent body fat, systolic blood pressure, and serum levels of cholesterol, triglycerides, and glucose.[84]

Is a sedentary way of life itself a risk factor independent of these other traits? Investigators at the Centers for Disease Control and Prevention (CDC) reviewed 43 methodologically sound studies of exercise and coronary artery disease.[85] Collectively, these studies showed that sedentary living increases coronary risk by 1.9 times. An independent meta-analysis derived the same relative risk.[86] The magnitude of this excess risk is similar to that conferred by other risk factors: hypertension, 2.1 times; hypercholesterolemia, 2.4 times; and cigarette smoking, 2.5 times.[85] Because sedentary living is at least two to three times more prevalent than any of these other risk factors, it can be argued that physical inactivity makes the most significant contribution to the epidemic of coronary artery disease in the United States. Maintaining a physically active way of life can be expected to reduce the risk of myocardial infarction by 35% to 70%.

Although reductions in coronary artery disease account for the great majority of the improvements in survival conferred by exercise, other factors may play a role. Physical activity protects against stroke[87] and reduces the risk of colon cancer.[88] Exercise also reduces the risk of breast cancer[89] and cancer of the reproductive organs in women, and very intensive exercise may reduce the risk of prostate cancer. Current studies continue to confirm observations that have occurred over the past 50 years, demonstrating that there is a graded, inverse association between activity and mortality.[90,91]

Secondary Prevention of Ischemic Heart Disease

Since the 1970s, interest in the potential role of exercise in the rehabilitation of patients after myocardial infarction and in the prevention of recurrent cardiac events has grown. Certain benefits of supervised exercise programs have been clearly established, including physiologic and symptomatic improvements and the reduction of risk factors. Patients completing exercise programs demonstrate the training effect, including a lower heart rate at rest and both a lower heart rate and a lower systolic blood pressure at submaximal work loads. These changes reduce myocardial oxygen demands, thereby increasing the angina threshold. Significant improvements in maximal oxygen uptake and work capacity can also be demonstrated. Exercise can be useful even for patients with severe ischemic left ventricular dysfunction and chronic congestive heart failure, although extra precautions should be taken in these patients. In addition, cardiac exercise programs are safe.[92] Most centers note a substantial improvement in mental attitudes, a decrease in the use of medications, and widespread patient satisfaction. Most important, randomized trials demonstrate that cardiac exercise programs reduce mortality by 20% to 25%.[92,93]

PRESCRIBING EXERCISE

Physicians can provide important incentives for their patients by educating them about the benefits, as well as the risks, of habitual exercise. Healthy, sedentary individuals are the largest group in need of such advice. In addition, physicians may be responsible for the medical screening of competitive athletes or for prescribing exercise for patients with chronic illnesses.

A careful history and physical examination are central to the medical evaluation of all potential exercisers. Particular attention should be given to a family history of coronary disease, hypertension, stroke, or sudden death and to symptoms suggestive of cardiovascular disease. Cigarette smoking, sedentary living, hypertension, diabetes, and obesity all increase the risks of exercise and may indicate the need for further testing. Physical findings suggestive of pulmonary, cardiac, or peripheral vascular disease are obvious causes for concern. A musculoskeletal evaluation is also important.

The choice of screening tests for apparently healthy individuals is controversial. A complete blood count and urinalysis are reasonable in all cases. Determination of blood glucose, serum cholesterol, and creatinine levels may also be useful in screening for risk factors or occult disease. The Valsalva maneuver and the isometric handgrip may be useful additions to the workup.

Young adults who are free of risk factors, symptoms, and abnormal physical findings do not require further evaluation. It is not at all clear that more aggressive medical screening can prevent sudden cardiac death. Although echocardiography and electrocardiography might reveal asymptomatic hypertrophic cardiomyopathy in some patients, the infrequency of this problem makes routine screening impractical.

The role of exercise electrocardiography as a screening test before an individual begins an exercise program is controversial. The American Heart Association recommends exercise testing before the start of a vigorous exercise program for all individuals older than 40 years, even if they are asymptomatic and free of cardiac risk factors.[94] However, a study of 3,617 asymptomatic men 35 to 59 years of age casts doubt on the value of exercise electrocardiography for routine preexercise screening.[95] None of the men had known coronary artery disease on entry into the study, but all were at increased risk because of hypercholesterolemia. Each subject had an exercise test on entry; the tests were repeated annually over a mean follow-up period of 7.4 years. Exercise proved safe in this group, with approximately 2% experiencing exercise-related cardiac events. Only 11 of the 62 men who experienced such events had abnormal exercise tests on entry, a sensitivity of only 18%. The cumulative sensitivity of annual tests was also low (24%). Even in elderly people, routine exercise testing before starting a moderate exercise program may not be necessary.[96]

Despite its limitations as a screening test for silent coronary artery disease, exercise testing can be useful for detecting exercise-induced arrhythmias, establishing a maximal heart rate for the exercise prescription, and determining work capacity. Serial testing may help motivate a patient by demonstrating increased work capacity. Specialized tests such as pulmonary function tests and exercise ergometry, Holter or telemetric monitoring during exercise, and echocardiography may be very useful in the evaluation of patients who have known or suspected cardiovascular abnormalities.

Screened patients will fall into one of three groups:

1. Healthy persons who can exercise without supervision. (Medical guidelines, as discussed below, may still be helpful.)
2. Patients with ischemic heart disease or other significant cardiovascular abnormalities who should have medically supervised, graded exercise programs. (If structured programs are not available, such patients should engage in milder forms of exercise, such as walking or bicycling, with appropriate precautions.)
3. Patients for whom physical exertion is contraindicated because of decompensated congestive heart failure, complex ventricular irritability, unstable angina, significant aortic valve disease, aortic aneurysm, uncontrolled diabetes, or uncontrolled seizure disorders.

People can exercise in the course of daily life or in formal exercise programs. Although most physicians have recommended structured exercise, recent studies demonstrate that even modest levels of physical activity are beneficial.[97] Walking and gardening are good examples[91,97,98]; such activities are protective even if they are not started until midlife or late in life.[99,100] In one study, for example, elderly men who walked less than 1 mile a day had nearly twice the mortality of men who walked more than 2 miles a day. Compliance with walking is good,[101] and lifestyle interventions appear to be as effective as formal exercise programs of similar intensity in improving cardiopulmonary fitness, blood pressure, and body composition.[102,103]

People should be encouraged to exercise nearly every day. Formal, intense exercise is not necessary; even moderate exercise that consumes about 150 kcal/day or 1,000 kcal/wk is very beneficial to health. Warm-ups, stretches, and a graded increase in exercise intensity can help prevent musculoskeletal problems.

Whereas all people can benefit from moderate daily activity, additional benefit can be obtained from more intense exercise; people who consume about 2,000 kcal in exercise a week obtain the greatest reduction of cardiovascular risk and mortality [see Table 6].[90,104] On average, people can obtain optimal health benefits from about 30 minutes of intense exercise or 45 to 60 minutes of mild to moderate exercise a day.

Physicians who provide specific practical advice are most likely to motivate their patients to adopt better health habits, including diet and exercise [see Table 7].

The success of a structured fitness program depends on the frequency, duration, and intensity of exercise. At least three sessions a week are needed. An alternate-day schedule will help prevent muscle soreness, but as fitness improves, individuals

Table 6 Exercise Time Required to Consume 2,000 kcal

Activity	Time (hr)
Strolling	10
Bowling	8.5
Golf	8
Raking leaves	7
Doubles tennis	6
Brisk walking	5.5
Biking (leisurely)	5.5
Ballet	4.5
Singles tennis	4.5
Racquetball, squash	4
Biking (hard)	4
Jogging	4
Downhill skiing	4
Calisthenics, brisk aerobics	3.3
Running	3
Cross-country skiing	3

should be encouraged to increase exercise sessions to five or even seven times a week. Each session consists of 15 to 60 minutes of continuous aerobic activity. Untrained individuals may not be able to sustain even 15 minutes at first, but they should be encouraged to progress slowly as they improve. Each exercise session should be preceded by a 5- to 10-minute warm-up period and followed by a 5- to 10-minute cool-down period; stretching, gentle calisthenics, and walking are ideally suited for this purpose. These same exercises are excellent for a 5- to 10-minute cool-down period.

The intensity of exercise can best be judged by the target heart rate. A heart rate of 60% to 85% of maximum is considered optimal for training. If an exercise test has not been performed, a maximal heart rate can be calculated by subtracting the patient's age from 220. Unfit people should start at the lower end of the target heart rate range. Healthy people need not monitor pulse rate. Instead, they can adjust the intensity of effort to a talking pace: they are working hard but still able to talk to a companion without a sensation of dyspnea.

Many kinds of exercise can be used to attain fitness. Dynamic (i.e., isotonic or aerobic) exercises in which large muscle groups are used continuously in a rhythmic, repetitive fashion for prolonged periods are ideal. The energy requirements of various activities have been measured. An energy expenditure of 5 to 6 METs (metabolic equivalents) or more is desirable for exercise training (1 MET is equal to the energy expenditure at rest or equivalent to approximately 3.5 ml O_2/kg body weight/min). Brisk walking, jogging, swimming, cross-country skiing, skating, bicycling, and vigorous singles racket sports all provide good conditioning. Sports that allow prolonged periods of inactivity, such as doubles tennis, golf, bowling, and baseball, are much less desirable for fitness.[90] Activities requiring sudden bursts of intense isometric activity, such as weight lifting, provide little cardiovascular conditioning and are contraindicated for patients with hypertension or heart disease. Contact sports cannot be recommended for health.

Although physicians should encourage patients to choose the sports that appeal most to them, medical considerations may also be important. For example, swimming is particularly desirable for individuals who have various musculoskeletal problems, and it is also ideal for people who experience exercise-induced asthma (EIA). Walking and bicycling are ideal for older individuals or for anyone who is starting from a low level of fitness. Jogging can be recommended because it is convenient and because the participants can easily adjust intensity and duration upward as fitness develops. Most desirable of all is a balanced program containing a variety of activities that exercise different muscle groups. People who have several activities at their command find it easier to remain active despite constraints of climate, schedules, and minor injuries. Although aerobic exercise is most important for metabolic improvement and cardiovascular health, exercises for flexibility and strength should be part of a balanced fitness program.[71] Stretching exercises promote flexibility and help prevent injuries. A stretching routine should be performed at least two to three times a week, but it is best when incorporated in the warm-up and cool-down periods that should surround aerobic exercise. Low-resistance strength training is important to preserve muscle mass and power in the face of the aging process; two to three sessions a week are ideal.

PREVENTING COMPLICATIONS

Physicians can minimize complications by educating patients about potential problems. Physicians should stress the need for such safety devices as helmets for biking, eye guards for squash and racquetball, and elbow and knee pads for roller-skating. Diet, weight control, stress management, smoking cessation, and other preventive health measures should be discussed, as should the warning signs of cardiac disease and the precautions for exercising in cold or hot climates.

MEDICAL COMPLICATIONS OF EXERCISE

Exercise promotes health, but it can also have adverse consequences. In some cases, the physiologic adaptations to exercise produce changes that may be misinterpreted as pathologic; athlete's heart is one example. In other cases, however, exercise can precipitate clinically important problems.

The cardiac complications of exercise include ischemia, infarction, and sudden death, often caused by rupture of an atherosclerotic plaque.[105] These dire events are infrequent and can be minimized by proper patient screening and instruction [see Prescribing Exercise, above]. Exercise-induced cardiac events are less common in people who exercise regularly than in sedentary individuals.[106] On balance, exercise is clearly beneficial for the heart.

The most common pulmonary complication of exercise is exercise-induced asthma, which usually responds well to treatment.[107] A much less common problem that can mimic hypersensitivity disorders is exercise-induced anaphylaxis.

The gastrointestinal response to exercise may produce reflux, diarrhea, or bleeding, which is usually occult and transient. Women who exercise very strenuously may experience oligomenorrhea or amenorrhea; the menstrual dysfunction is reversible but may be accompanied by osteoporosis. With appropriate precautions, exercise is safe during pregnancy. Precautions are also in order for prevention of hypoglycemia in diabetics who exercise.

People who exercise regularly can experience increased plasma volume that produces hemodilution or pseudoanemia. True anemia is less common but may result from shortened red cell life span caused by vascular trauma or iron deficiency. Exercise can produce proteinuria or hematuria; both are benign but are indications for studies to rule out renal disease. In warm, humid weather, exercise can produce heat cramps, hyperthermia, or heatstroke, all of which are preventable.

Exercise does not appear to cause or accelerate osteoarthritis. Acute muscle injury, manifested by transient elevation of creatine phosphokinase levels, is common, but exertional rhabdomyolysis is rare. Musculoskeletal problems, however, are the most frequent side effects of exercise. Overstress, overuse, or trauma is usually responsible. Poor technique, faulty equipment, or fatigue often contributes to injury. Soft tissue injuries such as sprains, strains, and tendinitis usually respond well to simple treatment regimens. The same is true of stress fractures. Primary care physicians can manage many of these problems, but more serious injuries may merit referral to a sports medicine facility.

Table 7 Exercise Advice for Patients

Get a medical check-up before beginning a formal exercise program

Warm up before each exercise session, and cool down afterward with 10 minutes of stretching and light calisthenics

Start slowly and build up to 30 minutes of moderate to intense exercise or 45–60 minutes of mild to moderate exercise

Begin with aerobic-type exercise, and later add stretching exercises for flexibility and low-resistance weight training for strength

Exercise daily if possible, and alternate harder workouts with easier ones

Dress comfortably

Use good equipment, especially good shoes

Do not eat during the 2 hr before you exercise, but drink plenty of water before, during, and after exercise, particularly in warmer weather

Do not ignore aches and pains that may signify injury

Do not exercise if you are feverish or ill

Learn warning signals of heart disease, including chest pain or pressure, disproportionate shortness of breath, fatigue, sweating, erratic pulse, light-headedness, or even indigestion

Consider getting instruction or joining a health club

References

1. McGinnis JM, Foege WH: Actual causes of death in the United States. JAMA 270:2207, 1993

2. Must A, Spandano J, Coakley EH, et al: The disease burden associated with overweight and obesity. JAMA 282:1523, 1999

3. Calle EE, Thun MJ, Petrelli JM, et al: Body-mass index and mortality in a prospective cohort of U.S. adults. N Engl J Med 341:1097, 1999

4. Rissanen T, Voutilainen S, Nyyssonen K, et al: Fish oil–derived fatty acids, docasahexaenoic acid and docosaentaenoic acid, and the risk of acute coronary events. The Kuopio Ischaemic Heart Disease Risk Factor Study. Circulation 102:2677, 2000

5. Kang JX, Leaf A: The cardiac antiarrhythmic effects of polyunsaturated fatty acid. Lipids 31:S-41, 1996

6. de Lorgeril M, Salen P, Martin J-L, et al: Mediterranean diet, traditional risk factors, and the rate of cardiovascular complications after myocardial infarction. Final report of the Lyon Diet Heart Study. Circulation 99:779, 1999

7. Hu FB, Stampfer MJ, Manson JE, et al: Dietary intake of α-linolenic acid and risk of fatal ischemic heart disease among women. Am J Clin Nutr 69:890, 1999

8. Lichtenstein AH, Ausman LM, Jalbert SM, et al: Effects of different forms of dietary hydrogenated fats on serum lipoprotein cholesterol levels. N Engl J Med 340:1933, 1999

9. Cummings JH, Bingham SA: Diet and the prevention of cancer. BMJ 317:1636,1998

10. Kolonel LN, Nomura AMY, Cooney RV: Dietary fat and prostate cancer: current status. J Natl Cancer Inst 91:414, 1999

11. Velie E, Kulldorff M, Schairer C, et al: Dietary fat, fat subtypes, and breast cancer in postmenopausal women: a prospective cohort study. J Natl Cancer Inst 92:833, 2000

12. Krauss RM, Eckel RH, Howard B, et al: AHA dietary guidelines. Revisions 2000: a statement for healthcare professionals from the nutritional committee of the American Heart Association. Circulation 102:2284, 2000

13. Knopp RH, Walden CE, Retzlaff BM, et al: Long-term cholesterol-lowering effects of 4 fat-restricted diets in hypercholesterolemic and combined hyperlipidemic men. The Dietary Alternatives Study. JAMA 278:1509, 1997

14. Barnard ND, Scialli AR, Berton R, et al: Effectiveness of a low-fat vegetarian diet in altering serum lipids in healthy premenopausal women. Am J Cardiol 85:969, 2000

15. Ornish D, Scherwitz LW, Billings JH, et al: Intensive lifestyle changes for reversal of coronary heart disease. JAMA 280:2001, 1998

16. Hu FB, Stampfer MJ, Manson JE, et al: Dietary fat intake and the risk of coronary heart disease in women. N Engl J Med 337:1491, 1997

17. Frost G, Leeds AA, Madeiros DS, et al: Glycaemic index as a determinant of serum HDL-cholesterol concentration. Lancet 353:1045, 1999

18. Spiller RC: Cholesterol, fibre, and bile acids. Lancet 347:415, 1996

19. Fuchs CS, Giovannucci EL, Colditz GA, et al: Dietary fiber and the risk of colorectal cancer and adenoma in women. N Engl J Med 340:169, 1999

20. Salmeròn J, Manson JE, Stampfer MJ, et al: Dietary fiber, glycemic load, and risk of non-insulin-dependent diabetes mellitus in women. JAMA 277:472, 1997

21. Chandalia M, Garg A, Lutjohann D, et al: Beneficial effects of high dietary fiber intake in patients with type 2 diabetes mellitus. N Engl J Med 342:1391, 2000

22. Ludwig DS, Pereira MA, Kroenke CH, et al: Dietary fiber, weight gain, and cardiovascular disease risk factors in young adults. JAMA 282:1539, 1999

23. Rimm EB, Ascherio A, Giovannucci E, et al: Vegetable, fruit, and cereal fiber intake and risk of coronary heart disease among men. JAMA 275:447, 1996

24. Wolk A, Manson JE, Stampfer ME, et al: Long-term intake of dietary fiber and decreased risk of coronary heart disease among women. JAMA 281:1998, 1999

25. Pedrini MT, Levey AS, Lau J, et al: The effect of dietary protein restriction on the progression of diabetic and nondiabetic renal diseases: a meta-analysis. Ann Intern Med 124:627, 1996

26. Stamler J, Elliott P, Kesteloot H, et al: Inverse relation of dietary protein markers with blood pressure: findings for 10,020 men and women in the INTERSALT study. Circulation 94:1629, 1996

27. Potter J, Langhorne P, Roberts M: Routine protein energy supplementation in adults: systemic review. BMJ 317:495, 1998

28. Robinson K, Arheart K, Refsum H, et al: Low circulating folate and vitamin B$_6$ concentrations risk factors for stroke, peripheral vascular disease, and coronary artery disease. Circulation 97:437, 1998

29. Rimm EB, Willett WC, Hu FB, et al: Folate and vitamin B$_6$ from diet and supplements in relation to risk of coronary heart disease among women. JAMA 279:359, 1998

30. Giovannucci E, Stampfer MJ, Colditz GA, et al: Multivitamin use, folate, and colon cancer in women in the Nurses' Health Study. Ann Intern Med 129:517, 1998

31. Low-dose aspirin and vitamin E in people at cardiovascular risk: a randomized trial in general practice. Collaborative Group of the Primary Projection (PPP). Lancet 357:89, 2001

32. Omenn GS, Goodman GE, Thornquist MD, et al: Effects of a combination of beta carotene and vitamin A on lung cancer and cardiovascular disease. N Engl J Med 334:1150, 1996

33. Vitamin supplements. The Medical Letter 40:75, 1998

34. Utiger RD: The need for more vitamin D. N Engl J Med 338:828, 1998

35. Elliott P, Stamler J, Nichols R, et al: INTERSALT revisited: further analyses of 24 hour sodium excretion and blood pressure within and across populations. BMJ 312:1249, 1996

36. Sacks FM, Svetkey LP, Vollmer WM, et al: Effects on blood pressure of reduced dietary sodium and the dietary approaches to stop hypertension (DASH) diet. N Engl J Med 344:3, 2001

37. Dawson-Hughes B, Harris SS, Krall EA, et al. Effect of calcium and vitamin D supplementation on bone density in men and women 65 years of age or older. N Engl J Med 337:670, 1997

38. Iso H, Stampfer MJ, Manson JE, et al: Prospective study of calcium, potassium, and magnesium intake and risk of stroke in women. Stroke 30:1772, 1999

39. Abbott RD, Curb JD, Rodriguez BL, et al: Effect of dietary calcium and milk consumption on risk of thromboembolic stroke in older middle-aged men: the Honolulu Heart Program. Stroke 27:813, 1996

40. Allender PS, Cutler JA, Follmann D, et al: Dietary calcium and blood pressure: a meta-analysis of randomized clinical trials. Ann Intern Med 124:825, 1996

41. Baron JA, Beach M, Mandel JS, et al: Calcium supplements for the prevention of colorectal adenomas. N Engl J Med 340:101, 1999

42. Giovannucci E, Rimm EB, Wolk A, et al: Calcium and fructose intake in relation to risk of prostate cancer. Cancer Res 58:442, 1998

43. Curhan GC, Willett WC, Speizer FE, et al: Comparison of dietary calcium with supplemental calcium and other nutrients as factors affecting the risk for kidney stones in women. Ann Intern Med 126:497,1997

44. U.S. Department of Health and Human Services: Recommendations to prevent and control iron deficiency in the United States. MMWR Morb Mortal Wkly Rep 47:1, 1998

45. Danesh J, Appleby P: Coronary heart disease and iron status: meta-analyses of prospective studies. Circulation 99:852, 1999

46. Fang I, Madhavan S, Alderman MH: Dietary potassium intake and stroke mortality. Stroke 31:1532, 2000

47. Whelton PK, He J, Cutler JA, et al: Effects of oral potassium on blood pressure: meta-analysis of randomized controlled clinical trials. JAMA 277:1624, 1997

48. Clark LC, Combs GF, Turnbull BW, et al: Effects of selenium supplementation for cancer prevention in patients with carcinoma of the skin: a randomized controlled trial. JAMA 276:1957, 1996

49. Yoshizawa K, Willett WC, Morris SJ, et al: Study of prediagnostic selenium level in toenails and the risk of advanced prostate cancer. J Natl Cancer Inst 90:1219, 1998

50. Mark SD, Qiao Y-L, Dawsey SM, et al: Prospective study of serum selenium levels and incident esophageal and gastric cancers. J Natl Cancer Inst 92:1753, 2000

51. Liu S, Manson JE, Lee I-M, et al: Fruit and vegetable intake and risk of cardiovascular disease: the Women's Health Study. Am J Clin Nutr 72:922, 2000

52. Joshipura KJ, Ascherio A, Manson JE, et al: Fruit and vegetable intake in relation to risk of ischemic stroke. JAMA 282:1233, 1999

53. Gillman MW: Enjoy your fruits and vegetables: eating fruits and vegetables protects against the common chronic diseases of adulthood (editorial). BMJ 313:765, 1996

54. Liu S, Stampfer MJ, Hu FB, et al: Whole-grain consumption and risk of coronary heart disease: results from the Nurses' Health Study. Am J Clin Nutr 70:412, 1999

55. Liu S, Manson JE, Stampfer MJ, et al: Whole grain consumption and risk of ischemic stroke in women: a prospective study. JAMA 284:1534, 2000

56. Hu FB, Stampfer MJ, Rimm EB, et al: A prospective study of egg consumption and risk of cardiovascular disease in men and women. JAMA 281:1387, 1999

57. Daviglus ML, Stamler J, Orencia AJ, et al: Fish consumption and the 30-year risk of fatal myocardial infarction. N Engl J Med 336:1046, 1997

58. Burr MK, Fehily MA, Gilbert JF, et al: Effects of changes in fat, fish, and fibre intakes on death and myocardial reinfarctions: diet and reinfarction trial (DART). Lancet 2:757, 1989

59. Albert CM, Hennekens CH, O'Donnell CJ, et al: Fish consumption and risk of sudden cardiac death. JAMA 279:4, 1998

60. von Schacky C, Angerer P, Kothny W, et al: The effect of dietary omega-3 fatty acids on coronary atherosclerosis: a randomized, double-blind, placebo-controlled trial. Ann Intern Med 130:554, 1999

61. Tunstall-Pedoe H: Nuts to you (...and you, and you): eating nuts may be beneficial—though it's unclear why. BMJ 317:1332, 1998

62. Neil HAW, Silagy CA, Lancaster T, et al: Garlic powder in the treatment of moderate hyperlipidaemia: a controlled trial and meta-analysis. J R Coll Physicians Lond 30:329, 1996

63. Keli SO, Hertog MGL, Feskens EJM, et al: Dietary flavonoids, antioxidant vitamins, and incidence of stroke: the Zutphen Study. Arch Intern Med 154:637, 1996

64. Camargo CA, Hennekens CH, Gaziano JM, et al: Prospective study of moderate alcohol consumption and mortality in US male physicians. Arch Intern Med 157:79, 1997

65. Hinds TS, West WL, Knight EM, et al: The effect of caffeine on pregnancy outcome variables. Nutr Rev 54:203, 1996

66. Newby DE, Neilson JMM, Jarvie DR, et al: Caffeine restrictions has no role in the management of patients with symptomatic idiopathic ventricular premature beats. Heart 76:355, 1996

67. Hu FB, Rimm EB, Stampfer MJ, et al: Prospective study of major dietary patterns and risk of coronary heart disease in men. Am J Clin Nutr 72:912, 2000

68. Kant AK, Schatzkin A, Graubard BI, et al: A prospective study of diet quality and mortality in women. JAMA 283:2109, 2000

69. Pate RR, Pratt M, Blair SN, et al: Physical activity and public health: a recommendation from the Centers for Disease Control and Prevention and the American College of Sports Medicine. JAMA 273:402,1995

70. Jones NL, Killian KJ: Exercise limitations in health and disease. N Engl J Med 343:632, 2000

71. Pollock ML, Gaessar GA, Butcher JD, et al: The recommended quantity and quality of exercise for developing and maintaining cardiorespiratory and muscular fitness, and flexibility in healthy adults. Med Sci Sports 30:975, 1998

72. Huonker M, Halle M, Keul J: Structural and functional adaptations of the cardiovascular system by training. Int J Sports Med 17:S164, 1996

73. Hambrecht R, Wolf A, Gielen S, et al: Effect of exercise on coronary endothelial function in patients with coronary artery disease. N Engl J Med 342:454, 2000

74. Taddei S, Galetta F, Virdis A, et al: Physical activity prevents age-related impairment in nitric oxide availability in elderly athletes. Circulation 101:2896, 2000

75. Fagard RH: Physical fitness and blood pressure. J Hypertens 11(suppl 5):S47, 1993

76. Kokkinos PF, Narayan P, Colleran JA, et al: Effects of regular exercise on blood pressure and left ventricular hypertrophy in African-American men with severe hypertension. N Engl J Med 333:1462, 1995

77. Kelley GA, Kelley KS: Progressive resistance exercise and resting blood pressure: a meta-analysis of randomized controlled trials. Hypertension 35:838, 2000

78. Pollock MK, Franklin BA, Balady GJ, et al: Resistance exercise in individuals with and without cardiovascular disease: an advisory from the committee on exercise, rehabilitation, and prevention, Council on Cardiology, American Heart Association (AHA Science Advisory). Circulation 101:828, 2000

79. Hu FB, Sigal RJ, Rich-Edwards JW, et al: Walking compared with vigorous physical activity and risk of type 2 diabetes in women: a prospective study. JAMA 282,1433, 1999

80. Williams PT: Relationship of distance run per week to coronary heart disease risk factors in 8,283 male runners: the National Runners' Health Study. Arch Intern Med 157:191, 1997

81. Li N, Wallen NH, Hjemdahl P: Evidence for prothrombotic effects of exercise and limited protection by aspirin. Circulation 100:1374, 1999

82. Bartsch P: Platelet activation with exercise and risk of cardiac events. Lancet 354:1747, 1999

83. Blumenthal JA, Babyak MA, Moore KA, et al: Effects of exercise training on older patients with major depression. Arch Intern Med 159:2349, 1999

84. LaMonte MJ, Eisenman PA, Adams TD, et al: Cardiorespiratory fitness and coronary heart disease risk factors. The LDS Hospital Fitness Institute Cohort. Circulation 102:1623, 2000

85. Protective effect of physical activity on coronary heart disease. MMWR Morb Mortal Wkly Rep 36:426, 1987

86. Berlin JA, Colditz GA: A meta-analysis of physical activity in the prevention of coronary heart disease. Am J Epidemiol 132:612, 1990

87. Hu FB, Stampfer MJ, Colditz GA, et al: Physical activity and risk of stroke in women. JAMA 283:2961, 2000

88. Batty D, Thune I: Does physical activity prevent cancer? Evidence suggests protection against colon cancer and probably breast cancer. BMJ 321:1424, 2000

89. Verloop J, Rookus MA, van der Kooy K, et al: Physical activity and breast cancer risk in women aged 20-54 years. J Natl Cancer Inst 92:128, 2000

90. Lee I-M, Paffenbarger RS Jr: Association of light, moderate and vigorous intensity physical activity with longevity. The Harvard Alumni Health Study. Am J Epidemiol 151:293, 2000

91. Anderson LB, Schnohr P, Schroll M, et al: All-cause mortality associated with physical activity during leisure time, work, sports, and cycling to work. Arch Intern Med 160:1621, 2000

92. Frankin BA, Bonzheim K, Gordon S, et al: Safety of medically supervised outpatient cardiac rehabilitation exercise therapy: a 16-year follow-up. Chest 114:902, 1998

93. Ades PA, Coello CE: Effects of exercise and cardiac rehabilitation on cardiovascular outcomes. Med Clin North Am 84:251, 2000

94. Maron BJ: Cardiovascular risks to young persons on the athletic field. Ann Intern Med 129:379, 1998

95. Siscovick DS, Ekelund LG, Johnson JL, et al: Sensitivity of exercise electrocardiography for acute cardiac events during moderate and strenuous physical activity. Arch Intern Med 151:325, 1991

96. Gill TM, DiPietro L, Krumholz HM: Role of exercise stress testing and safety monitoring for older persons starting an exercise program. JAMA 284:342, 2000

97. Lemaitre RN, Siscovic DS, Raghunathan TE, et al: Leisure-time physical activity and the risk of primary cardiac arrest. Arch Intern Med 159:686, 1999

98. Manson JE, Hu FB, Rich-Edwards JW, et al: A prospective study of walking as compared with vigorous exercise in the prevention of coronary heart disease in women. N Engl J Med 341:650, 1999

99. Wannamethee SG, Shaper AG, Walker M: Changes in physical activity, mortality, and incidence of coronary heart disease in older men. Lancet 351:1603, 1998

100. Hakim AA, Petrovitch H, Burchfiel CM, et al: Effects of walking on mortality among nonsmoking retired men. N Engl J Med 338:94, 1998

101. Pereira MA, Kriska AM, Day RD, et al: A randomized walking trial in postmenopausal women: effects of physical activity and health 10 years later. Arch Intern Med 158:1695, 1998

102. Andersen RE, Wadden TA, Bartlett SJ, et al: Effects of lifestyle activity vs structured aerobic exercise in obese women: a randomized trial. JAMA 281:335, 1999

103. Dunn AL, Marcus BH, Kampert JB, et al: Comparison of lifestyle and structured interventions to increase physical activity and cardiorespiratory fitness: a randomized trial. JAMA 281:327, 1999

104. Sesso HD, Paffenbarger RS, Lee I-M: Physical activity and coronary heart disease in men. The Harvard Alumni Health Study. Circulation 102:975, 2000

105. Burke AP, Farb A, Malcom GT, et al: Plaque rupture and sudden death related to exertion in men with coronary artery disease. JAMA 281:921, 1999

106. Albert CM, Mittleman MA, Chae CU, et al: Triggering of sudden death from cardiac causes by vigorous exertion. N Engl J Med 343:1355, 2000

107. Leff JA, Busse WW, Pearlman D, et al: Montelukast, a leukotriene receptor antagonist, for the treatment of mild asthma and exercise-induced bronchoconstriction. N Engl J Med 339:147,1998

Acknowledgments

Figure 1   Marcia Kammerer.

Figure 2   Talar Agasyan.

5   Adult Preventive Health Care

Christopher F. Snow, M.D.

The Evolution of Preventive Care Guidelines

In the United States, the idea that detection of disease in asymptomatic persons may prevent morbidity and prolong life has gained an increasing foothold since World War II. The concept was initially embodied in recommendations that adults receive a complete annual physical examination. In 1975, Frame and Carlson published a series of articles that challenged the scientific basis for the routine physical.[1] In the subsequent 25 years, many groups have published preventive care guidelines tailored to the age, sex, and risk factors of individual patients. Among these guidelines, recommendations of the Canadian Task Force (CTF),[2] the United States Preventive Services Task Force (USPSTF),[3] and the American College of Physicians (ACP) are notable for the quality of their evidence-based approach.[4] Updated recommendations of these groups and others have been summarized and discussed in a U.S. Government handbook.[5]

The emergence of a burgeoning preventive medicine literature has, in some areas, eased the task of planning and implementing preventive care for individual patients. However, for many preventive interventions, disparities in published recommendations have caused uncertainty. For example, the American Cancer Society recommends that annual screening for prostate cancer be offered to men beginning at age 50,[6] whereas the USPSTF recommends against such screening.[3] One reason for differing recommendations is the relative paucity of randomized controlled trials for preventive maneuvers; such trials are inherently difficult and expensive to perform because of the large number of subjects who must be enrolled and followed for many years in order to demonstrate statistical differences in end points.

Ideally, any condition for which a preventive measure is recommended should meet the following criteria: (1) The burden of illness caused by the condition must be sufficient to justify the costs of the preventive measure; (2) detection and treatment of the condition before symptoms occur, compared with detection and treatment after onset of symptoms, must reduce morbidity and mortality; and (3) the benefits of the proposed preventive measure must outweigh any harm, including discomfort and anxiety, engendered by it.

These principles seem straightforward, but to apply them requires what must ultimately be a subjective process: the balancing of benefits and risks, involving such disparate factors as mortality reduction and costs or burden of illness and patient discomfort.

The emergence of managed care in the United States may influence the practice of preventive health care. In managed care organizations, the use of such preventive interventions as mammography screening and influenza vaccination is often audited. Compliance rates are used by watchdog agencies and public interest groups as one way of comparing the quality of care offered by different managed care organizations. There is concern, however, that managed care organizations may attempt to influence affiliated practitioners to perform preventive maneuvers of questionable value, including the complete annual physical examination.[7] The provision of comprehensive preventive health care is a major advertising focus of managed care organizations, and in capitated systems, the cost of prevention is borne by the primary provider groups.

Counseling and Education of Patients

Numerous interventions involving counseling and education of patients have been proposed, especially by the CTF and the USPSTF [see Table 1]. For some health-related behaviors, such as smoking, there is good evidence that counseling by clinicians can help change patient behavior.[8] For many other behaviors, the effects of counseling, in the office setting, on patient behavior and on the reduction of morbidity have never been rigorously examined. In general, preventive interventions involving counseling and patient education are safe, inexpensive, and unlikely to cause discomfort or anxiety. However, some types of counseling are potentially harmful and costly. For example, there is evidence that breast self-examination leads to an increase in biopsies of benign lesions.[9] Patient education is time-consuming for the busy practitioner; counseling by nonphysicians may be more cost-effective.

Table 1   Selected Recommendations for Counseling and Patient Education

Type of Counseling	CTF	USPSTF
Inquire and counsel about the following risks:		
Tobacco use	Yes	Yes
Alcohol use/driving after drinking	Yes	Yes
Unsafe sexual practices	Yes	Yes
Water-heater temperature > 120°–130° F	NR	Yes
Smoking near bedding and upholstery	NR	Yes
Illicit drug use	I	Yes
Unsafe storage of firearms	I	Yes
Counsel about the benefits of the following:		
Good nutrition	Yes	Yes
Exercise	Yes	Yes
Use of seat belts	Yes	Yes
Regular dental care	Yes	Yes
Avoidance of sun exposure/use of protective clothing	Yes	Yes
Adequate calcium intake (women)	NR	Yes
Use of smoke detectors	NR	Yes
Use of bicycle helmets	I	Yes
Use of motorcycle/all-terrain-vehicle helmets	I	Yes
Use of sunscreens	I	I
Inquire about the following:		
Functional status at home (elderly)	Yes	Yes
Contraceptive practices	Yes*	Yes
Family violence or abuse	NR	Yes
Educate patients about the following:		
Benefits/risks of estrogen replacement (perimenopausal women)	Yes	Yes
CPR training (household members of elderly patients)	NR	Yes
Prevention of falls (elderly persons)	I	Yes
Heimlich maneuver for accidental choking	I	NR
Self-examination of testes	I	I
Self-examination of skin	I	I
Self-examination of breasts	I	I

*Reviewed only for adolescents.
CPR—cardiopulmonary resuscitation   CTF—Canadian Task Force on the Periodic Health Examination   I—insufficient evidence to recommend for or against use of this preventive measure   NR—not reviewed or specifically discussed   USPSTF—United States Preventive Services Task Force

Table 2   Expert Panel Recommendations for Cancer Screening

Condition/Intervention	CTF	USPSTF	ACP
Bladder cancer Urine dipstick for hematuria Urine cytology	Screening of general population not recommended; insufficient evidence to recommend for or against screening in men older than 60 yr who have smoked or who have had industrial exposure to aromatic amines	Screening of general population not recommended	Not reviewed
Breast cancer Clinical breast examination Mammography Teaching of breast self-examination	Annual clinical breast examination and mammography in women 50 to 69 yr of age; insufficient evidence to recommend for or against the teaching of breast self-examination	Mammography every 1 to 2 yr with or without annual clinical breast examination for women 50 to 69 yr of age, for high-risk women 40 to 49 yr of age, and for women 70 yr of age and older with a reasonable life expectancy; insufficient evidence to recommend for or against the teaching of breast self-examination	Under review
Cervical cancer Papanicolaou smear	Starting at the onset of sexual activity or at 18 yr of age, two smears 1 year apart, then every 3 years until 69 yr of age; consider more frequent screening in high-risk women	Starting at the onset of sexual activity, at least every 3 yr; women with consistently normal smears may discontinue screening after age 65; consider more frequent screening in high-risk women	In sexually active women 20 to 65 yr of age, two or three smears 1 yr apart, then every 3 years; screen women 66 to 75 yr of age who have not been screened within the 10 yr before age 66; screen every 2 yr in high-risk women
Colorectal cancer Digital rectal examination Fecal occult blood testing Barium enema Sigmoidoscopy Colonoscopy	Insufficient evidence to recommend for or against the use of fecal occult blood testing, sigmoidoscopy, or colonoscopy in screening persons older than 40 yr	Screening recommended starting at age 50 using either annual fecal occult blood testing, sigmoidoscopy (periodicity unspecified), or both; use of digital rectal examination, barium enema, or colonoscopy not recommended	Under review
Lung cancer Chest radiography Sputum cytology	Screening not recommended	Screening not recommended	Screening not recommended
Oral cancer Examination of the oral cavity	Annual oral examination by a physician or dentist should be considered for persons older than 60 yr who use tobacco in any form or who use alcohol on a regular basis; insufficient evidence to recommend for or against screening average-risk persons	Insufficient evidence to recommend for or against screening; clinicians may wish to screen tobacco users or older persons who drink regularly; all patients, especially those at increased risk, should be advised to receive a complete dental examination on a regular basis	Not reviewed

ACP—American College of Physicians   CTF—Canadian Task Force on the Periodic Health Examination   USPSTF—United States Preventive Services Task Force

Cancer Screening

The CTF, the USPSTF, and the ACP have issued recommendations for cancer screening in average and high-risk individuals [*see Table 2*].[10,11] At present, most cancer screening interventions involve breast, cervical, colorectal, and prostate cancers. In the future, technological innovations, such as the use of helical low-dose computed tomography for early detection of lung cancer,[12] may cause this list of recommendations to grow.

BREAST CANCER

Modalities for breast cancer screening include mammography, clinical breast examination, and breast self-examination. In women 50 to 69 years of age, mammography has been shown to reduce mortality from breast cancer by about 30%.[13] Although biennial screening appears to be about as effective as annual screening,[14] screening every 3 years may be less effective.[15] Whether to extend mammographic screening to younger and older women has been controversial. In the Gothenburg trial,[16] Swedish women ranging from 39 to 49 years of age were randomized to two groups: the study group was offered mammography every 18 months, but the control group was not invited to undergo mammographic screening until 6 to 7 years after randomization. Although a significant reduction in breast cancer mortality was observed in the study group, the absolute risk reduction was small, with about one breast cancer death being prevented for each 1,000 women screened. By comparison, six breast cancer deaths would be prevented by mammographic screening of 1,000 women 60 to 69 years of age.[17] Also, the false positive rate is higher in younger women[18]; the cumulative risk of a false positive test after five mammograms in women 40 to 49 years of age is 30%.

For women 70 years of age and older, there are insufficient data to draw firm conclusions about the utility of mammographic screening. On the one hand, screening in older women detects substantially more cancers than does screening in younger women, because older women have a higher incidence of such cancers and because test performance is better in this age group. Also, cancers detected in elderly women are usually less advanced.[19] On the other hand, older women who develop breast cancer are more likely than younger women to die of unrelated conditions. Thus, the physician who considers screening a woman older than 69 years must take her life expectancy and

Table 2   (*continued*)

Condition/Intervention	CTF	USPSTF	ACP

Ovarian cancer
  Pelvic examination
  Abdominal or transvaginal ultrasonography
  Serum CA-125
	Screening not recommended for women at average risk; insufficient evidence to recommend for or against screening women with one or more first-degree relatives with ovarian cancer; examination of the adnexae is reasonable if a pelvic examination is being done for another reason	Screening for average-risk women is not recommended; insufficient evidence to recommend for or against screening women at increased risk	Adnexal examination is reasonable when pelvic examination is done for other clinical reasons; screening with ultrasonography or CA-125 levels not recommended for either average-risk or high-risk women; however, women with the hereditary ovarian cancer syndrome should be referred for specialist care[10]

Pancreatic cancer
  Abdominal examination
  Ultrasonography
  Serologic markers
	Screening not recommended	Screening not recommended	Not reviewed

Prostate cancer
  Digital rectal examination
  Serum prostate-specific antigen
  Transrectal ultrasonography
	Insufficient evidence to recommend for or against use of digital rectal examination for men older than 50 yr; use of prostate-specific antigen levels and transrectal ultrasonography in screening not recommended	Screening not recommended; patients who request screening should be given information about the potential benefits and harms of early detection and treatment; if screening is performed, digital rectal examination and prostate-specific antigen levels should be used and screening should be limited to men with a life expectancy > 10 yr	Physicians should discuss the potential benefits and known harmful effects of screening, diagnosis, and treatment; listen to the patient's concerns; then individualize the decision to screen. Available evidence does not suggest that high-risk men should be cared for differently from men at average risk; if screening is elected, men between 50 and 69 yr of age are most likely to benefit, using one-time or repeated screening with digital rectal examination, prostate-specific antigen levels, or both; transrectal ultrasonography not recommended for use in screening[11]

Skin cancer
  Clinical skin examination
  Counseling to perform skin self-examination
	Screening by clinical examination not recommended for average-risk persons; for persons with a family history of malignant melanoma, periodic clinical examination may be prudent; insufficient evidence to recommend for or against counseling patients to perform skin self-examination	Insufficient evidence to recommend for or against screening for average-risk men; persons at increased risk for malignant melanoma because of family history or precursor lesions should be referred to skin cancer specialists for surveillance	Not reviewed

Testicular cancer
  Testicular examination
  Teaching of testicular self-examination
	Insufficient evidence to recommend for or against screening for average-risk men; regular screening in persons with a history of cryptorchidism, testicular atrophy, or ambiguous genitalia may be prudent	Insufficient evidence to recommend for or against screening for average-risk men; men with a history of cryptorchidism or atrophic testes should be informed of their increased risk and counseled about the options for screening	Not reviewed

Thyroid cancer Thyroid examination	Insufficient evidence to recommend for or against screening	Screening not recommended for persons at average risk; periodic screening recommended in persons with a history of external upper body irradiation in infancy or childhood	Not reviewed

comorbid conditions into account. The incremental value of clinical breast examination in women who undergo regular mammography is another area of controversy. In the Ontario Breast Screening Program, women 50 to 69 years of age received nurse-examiner clinical breast examination and mammography every 2 years. Only 5% of cancers were detected by clinical breast examination but not by mammography, whereas almost half of cancers were detected by mammography but not by clinical breast examination.[20] This small incremental value of clinical breast examination is borne out by a meta-analysis, which concluded that clinical breast examination does not reduce breast cancer mortality beyond the reduction provided by screening mammography.[14] The use of clinical breast examina-

tion in younger women is often advocated; for example, the American Cancer Society recommends regular clinical breast examination for women starting at age 20.[21] However, the false positive rate of clinical breast examination in younger women is much higher than that in older women.[18]

Ongoing randomized trials of breast self-examination training from China[9] and Russia[22] have as yet failed to show a reduction in breast cancer mortality or an improvement in tumor stage among women receiving instruction in breast self-examination. In both trials, women who had been instructed in breast self-examination were more likely to seek medical advice for benign breast lesions.

The Breast Cancer Prevention Trial studied the use of tamoxifen to prevent breast cancer in women at increased risk.[23] Over-

Table 3 Other Preventive Interventions to Be Considered for Persons at Average Risk

Condition	Preventive Measure	CTF	USPSTF	ACP	Comments
Abdominal aortic aneurysm in elderly males	Abdominal palpation, ultrasonography	I	I	NR	Males older than 60 yr who smoke, are hypertensive, or have vascular disease or a family history of abdominal aortic aneurysm are at increased risk; screening with abdominal palpation is less expensive than screening with ultrasonography but is less sensitive; a single screening test for abdominal aortic aneurysm in males aged 60 to 80 yr of age may be cost-effective but repeat screening is not[64]
Bacteriuria in elderly women	Dipstick testing for leukocyte esterase or nitrite	I	No	No	Treatment of asymptomatic bacteriuria has not been shown to reduce mortality,[65] and relapse rates are high
Carotid artery stenosis	Neck auscultation, carotid ultrasonography	No	I	No[66]	Although the Asymptomatic Carotid Artery Stenosis study showed a benefit to carotid endarterectomy in highly selected persons with asymptomatic carotid stenoses of greater than 60% reduction in diameter,[67] a consensus conference of Canadian neurologists using CTF guidelines for evidence-based medicine concluded that there is insufficient evidence to recommend screening for asymptomatic carotid disease even in high-risk groups[68]
Dementia in elderly persons	Standardized mental status instruments	I	I	NR	Although some causes of cognitive impairment, including drug toxicity and depression, are reversible, there is no evidence to indicate that early diagnosis of the most common causes of dementia is beneficial; the CTF, USPSTF, and ACP all recommend functional status assessment of the elderly
Depression	Standardized questionnaires	No	I	NR	Although there is no consensus that the use of questionnaires in the diagnosis of depression is helpful, the expert panels recommend that clinicians maintain a high level of clinical sensitivity to the presence of this treatable disorder
Glaucoma	Funduscopy, tonometry, automated perimetry	I[69]	I	NR	Referral of high-risk patients to an eye specialist is considered prudent by both the CTF and the USPSTF; persons at increased risk include African Americans older than 40 yr and persons with severe myopia, diabetes, or a family history of glaucoma
Hearing impairment in elderly persons	Directed questioning, the whispered-voice test, or audiometry	Yes	Yes	NR	Hearing loss is prevalent in the elderly and may lead to social isolation, depression, and exacerbation of coexisting psychiatric conditions; the USPSTF recommends directed questioning but neither endorses nor discourages the use of audiometry, a more costly means of screening [*see Chapter 74*]

ACP—American College of Physicians CTF—Canadian Task Force on the Periodic Health Examination I—insufficient evidence to recommend for or against use of this preventive measure NR—not reviewed or specifically discussed USPSTF—United States Preventive Services Task Force

all, women who received tamoxifen daily for an average of more than 4 years had a 49% reduction in the risk of invasive breast cancer compared with a control group taking placebo (22 versus 43.4 cases per 1,000 women). Women receiving tamoxifen—especially those 50 years of age or older—had an increased risk of stage I endometrial cancer, stroke, pulmonary embolism, and deep vein thrombosis. Another controlled trial, designed to study the effectiveness of raloxifene (a selective estrogen receptor modulator) in the prevention of osteoporotic fractures, found a 76% reduction in the risk of invasive breast cancer in women who had been receiving raloxifene for 3 years.[24] As would be predicted by its antiestrogenic effects on endometrial receptors, raloxifene did not increase the risk of endometrial cancer. However, women who received raloxifene had a threefold increase in the incidence of thromboembolic disease, as well as significant increases in side effects, including hot flashes and leg cramps.

CERVICAL CANCER

Although there are no data from randomized controlled trials to support the value of the Papanicolaou (Pap) smear in reducing mortality from cervical cancer, indirect evidence suggests that this inexpensive test may be among the most effective cancer screening techniques.[25] Screening is recommended at the onset of sexual activity, because it appears that women who have never been sexually active are not at risk for cervical neoplasia. Although many practitioners advise their patients to undergo annual screening, it is rational and cost-effective to screen less frequently,[26] because cervical dysplasia is slow to progress to invasive carcinoma. Although the exact sensitivity of the Pap test in detecting dysplasia and cancer is unknown, false negative results are sufficiently common that the ACP-ASIM and the CTF recommend that the first two or three smears be obtained at 1-year intervals. Screening may be discontinued in older women who have been screened regularly and have had normal results.[27] Women who have had a hysterectomy for benign disease are unlikely to benefit from cytologic sampling of the vaginal wall.[28]

The greatest obstacle to early detection of cervical neoplasia by use of the Pap smear is the failure to enroll and maintain women in screening programs. Women of low socioeconomic status are at increased risk for development of cervical cancer and are also less likely to be screened regularly. Other risk factors include smoking, onset of sexual activity at an early age, a history of multiple sexual partners, and a history of sexually transmitted diseases, especially human papillomavirus (HPV) or HIV. Efforts to screen women for HPV infection and to use HPV typing to identify the serotypes most closely associated with cervical neoplasia have not yet been proved to be useful adjuncts to the Pap smear.[29]

Table 3   *(continued)*

Condition	Preventive Measure	CTF	USPSTF	ACP	Comments
Hyperlipidemia	Measurement of serum cholesterol with or without lipoprotein	I	Yes	Yes[70]	Randomized controlled trials using statin drugs have shown reductions in mortality from coronary heart disease[71] and stroke[72]; the CTF endorses case findings in men 30 to 59 yr of age; the other expert panels target men 35 to 65 yr of age and women 45 to 65 yr of age; repeated screening is most appropriate in patients whose initial result is near a treatment threshold [*see Chapter 54*]
Hypertension	Measurement of blood pressure	Yes	Yes	Yes[73]	The benefits of treatment for systolic and diastolic hypertension are well documented, and most persons have their blood pressure measured periodically without the need for community screening programs or scheduled screening visits; it is important to confirm elevated readings on several occasions, as misclassifying normotensive persons as hypertensive may have adverse consequences[74]; in uncertain cases, self-measurement of blood pressure and use of automated ambulatory monitoring devices may provide useful information[75,76] [*see Chapter 16*]
Obesity	Measurement of weight or body mass index	I[77]	Yes	NR	The CTF makes no recommendation for or against screening average-risk persons but recommends body mass index measurement for people with obesity-related diseases (diabetes, hypertension, coronary artery disease, hyperlipidemia, or obstructive sleep apnea), with weight reduction attempts recommended for consideration in patients with a body mass index of more than 27 [*see Chapter 53*]
Thyroid dysfunction in women older than 50 yr	Serum thyroid-stimulating hormone	I	I	Yes[78]	Older women have a high prevalence of thyroid dysfunction; although screening, by definition, is normally targeted at asymptomatic persons, the principal benefit of screening for thyroid dysfunction using the serum thyroid-stimulating hormone may be the detection of treatable symptoms that would otherwise go unnoticed[78]; other potential benefits include the prevention of osteoporosis and atrial fibrillation in hyperthyroid patients and the ability to lower lipid levels by treatment of hypothyroid patients; the ACP recommends follow-up screening every 2–5 yr[79]
Visual impairment in elderly persons	Use of the Snellen eye chart	Yes[69]	Yes	NR	Visual loss may be insidious, especially in elderly persons, and may increase the risk of various traumatic injuries, including hip fractures [*see Chapter 74*]

Other obstacles to effective screening by use of the Pap smear are errors in sampling, preparation, and interpretation. Women should not be screened during menses or when evidence of cervical or vaginal infection is present. No lubricants other than water should be used before obtaining the specimen. The best sensitivity (defined by the presence of endocervical cells) is achieved by sampling with both a spatula and an endocervical brush. However, the importance of obtaining endocervical cells and the need to repeat a Pap smear if no endocervical cells are obtained has been questioned.[29] According to federal guidelines, laboratories must rescreen at least 10% of smears initially classified as negative. Use of automated rescreening technologies has been approved by the United States Food and Drug Administration. Use of another technique, in which the sampling device is rinsed in a preservative solution, followed by filtration of the cells and preparation of a thin-layer slide sample, may result in a higher proportion of satisfactory slides and a higher detection rate for abnormal cells.[30] Use of these newer methods adds to the expense of screening programs; whether this expense can be justified by improvements in test sensitivity is uncertain.[29,31]

The specificity of Pap smears for detection of dysplasia and cancer is also uncertain. False positive results occur infrequently, but Pap smears may correctly detect a large number of low-grade lesions that, without treatment, would remain stable or regress.[32] As a consequence, many women who would never develop invasive cervical cancer are subjected to anxiety and to colposcopy and biopsy.

COLORECTAL CANCER

Potential screening modalities for colorectal cancer include digital rectal examination (DRE), fecal occult blood testing (FOBT), sigmoidoscopy, double-contrast barium enema, colonoscopy, and computed tomography colonography.

It has been estimated that fewer than 10% of colorectal cancers can be reached by the finger of an examiner performing DRE. Most of these cancers would be detected by the use of other screening modalities. FOBT is the only screening modality that has been shown in randomized controlled trials to reduce colorectal cancer mortality. In the Minnesota Colon Cancer Control Study,[33] volunteers 50 to 80 years of age were randomized to annual FOBT, biennial FOBT, or a control group. After 18 years of follow-up, colorectal cancer mortality was 33% less in the annual group and 21% less in the biennial group than in the control group.[34] In this study, the slides were rehydrated, a technique that increases sensitivity but reduces specificity; during the trial, 38% of patients in the annual group underwent colonoscopy because of a positive test result. Two randomized controlled trials from Europe have demonstrated 16% and 18% reductions in colorectal cancer mortality using FOBT.[35,36] In contrast to the Minnesota study, in the European trials, patients were drawn from the general population, the slides were not rehydrated, and all testing was biennial.

The 60 cm flexible sigmoidoscope can detect more than 50% of colorectal cancers, and approximately 25% of cancers beyond the reach of the scope will be associated with a so-called

Table 4 Preventive Interventions to Be Considered for Persons at Increased Risk*

Condition	Persons at Increased Risk[†]	Preventive Measure	CTF	USPSTF	ACP	Comments
Anemia, iron deficiency	Recent immigrants from developing countries, institutionalized elderly persons[80]	Hemoglobin measurement	NR	No	I[80]	In recommending against screening, the USPSTF cites the low prevalence of iron deficiency anemia, the cost of screening, and the potential adverse effects of iron therapy
Chlamydial infection	Sexually active women who are younger than 25 yr, who have had new or multiple partners in the past year, or who use nonbarrier contraception[2]	Cervical culture or nonculture testing	Yes[81]	Yes	NR	The USPSTF also recommends screening high-risk young men, although it concedes that there is a lack of evidence to support the practice [*see Chapter 129*]
Coronary artery disease	Older males with at least one additional risk factor for coronary artery disease[4]	Exercise ECG	NR	I	I	The USPSTF recommends screening persons in occupations that involve public safety (e.g., pilots, truck drivers) and states that screening other persons with multiple coronary artery disease risk factors may be indicated if the results will alter treatment decisions
Type 2 (non–insulin-dependent) diabetes mellitus	Obese persons older than 40 yr, persons with a strong family history of diabetes mellitus, and members of certain ethnic groups[3]	Fasting blood glucose measurement	I	I	Yes	The main rationale for screening is that long-term glycemic control may reduce complications in patients with type 2 diabetes mellitus[82] [*see Chapter 48*]
Gonorrhea	Persons younger than 30 yr who have had at least two sexual partners in the past year or who first had intercourse at a young age; prostitutes; sexual contacts of individuals known to have a sexually transmitted disease[2]	Gram stain and culture of cervical or urethral smear	Yes	Yes	NR	Both the CTF and the USPSTF recommend against screening the general population; the USPSTF states that the evidence for screening high-risk women is stronger than that for screening high-risk men
Hemoglobin-opathies	Persons of reproductive age who are at increased risk because of family history or ethnic or racial background[2]	Complete blood count, hemoglobin electrophoresis, or both	I	Yes	NR	Although the USPSTF concedes that there is a lack of evidence to support screening, it recommends that it be offered on other grounds, including patient preference and burden of suffering
HIV infection	Persons with sexually transmitted diseases, injection drug users, homosexual and bisexual men, persons who received blood transfusions between 1978 and 1985, sexual contacts of persons at risk, and persons who identify themselves as at risk[83]	Serum antibody testing	Yes	Yes	Yes[83]	The CTF and the USPSTF state that there is insufficient evidence to recommend for or against screening persons without identified risk factors [*see Chapter 133*]
Influenza	Nonimmunized persons exposed to influenza A virus during an outbreak, especially if they are at high risk for complications[2] [*see Table 5*]	Administration of amantadine or rimantadine	Yes	Yes	NR	The USPSTF suggests prophylaxis to supplement the vaccine in persons expected to have a poor antibody response or when the vaccine may be ineffective because of major antigenic changes in the virus, or to substitute for the vaccine in high-risk persons for whom it is contraindicated [*see Chapter 150*]
Myocardial infarction	Males 40 yr of age and older with risk factors such as high cholesterol levels, smoking, diabetes, and family history of early onset coronary artery disease[3]	Administration of aspirin	I	I	NR	The USPSTF states that if relative contraindications to aspirin use are present, the risk of use may outweigh the benefits
Osteoporosis	Postmenopausal women who are white or have low body weight; women who have undergone oophorectomy before menopause[3]	Bone densitometry	I	I	I	All three expert panels recommend against routine screening but state that screening may be appropriate in selected women to aid decisions about estrogen replacement therapy
Renal failure, chronic	Patients with insulin-dependent diabetes mellitus[2]	Dipstick urinalysis for protein measurement	Yes	NR	NR	The CTF states that screening for microalbuminuria in patients with insulin-dependent diabetes mellitus who are dipstick negative may also be useful [*see Chapter 48*]

*This table excludes recommendations for pregnant women.

[†]Each expert panel has its own definition of high-risk subsets for a given disorder. Only one representative example has been chosen for use in this table.

ACP—American College of Physicians   CTF—Canadian Task Force on the Periodic Health Examination   I—insufficient evidence to recommend for or against use of this preventive measure   NR—not reviewed or specifically discussed   USPSTF—United States Preventive Services Task Force

Table 4   (continued)

Condition	Persons at Increased Risk[†]	Preventive Measure	CTF	USPSTF	ACP	Comments
Retinopathy	Patients with diabetes[2]	Funduscopy or retinal photography	Yes[69]	NR	Yes[84]	For type 1 diabetics, the ACP recommends annual screening beginning 5 yr after onset; for type 2 diabetics, screening at the time of diagnosis is recommended; if screening is negative, further screening may be delayed for 4 yr, with annual screening thereafter [see Chapter 48]
Syphilis	Prostitutes; persons with other sexually transmitted diseases; sexual contacts of patients with active syphilis[3]	Serologic testing	Yes	Yes	Yes	Nontreponemal tests (e.g., the rapid plasma reagin test) are recommended for initial screening [see Chapter 143]
Tuberculosis	Persons infected with HIV; close contacts of persons with known or suspected tuberculosis; persons with medical risk factors associated with tuberculosis (see comments); immigrants from endemic areas; medically underserved populations; alcoholics; injection drug users; residents of long-term care facilities[3]	Tuberculin skin testing, with selective use of isoniazid prophylaxis for positive reactors	Yes	Yes	NR	In most high-risk persons, 10 mm or more of induration is considered a positive reaction; however the USPSTF suggests that 5 mm of induration should be used as the cutoff for persons with HIV infection, with an abnormal chest x-ray, or with recent exposure to an active case. Prior vaccination with bacillus Calmette-Guérin is not considered a valid basis for dismissing positive test results

distal sentinel polyp. Randomized controlled trials of sigmoidoscopy in colorectal cancer screening are under way in the United States and Europe. Current evidence for the efficacy of sigmoidoscopy comes from case-control studies,[37,38] which suggest that the protective effect of a single sigmoidoscopy lasts at least 6 years. Although the risks of sigmoidoscopy are small, many patients find the procedure uncomfortable and embarrassing.

A Veterans Affairs cooperative study, using colonoscopy as the reference standard, examined the sensitivity of FOBT and sig-

moidoscopy for the detection of advanced neoplasia (defined as including tubular adenomas 10 mm or more in diameter or with high-grade dysplasia, villous adenomas, or invasive cancer). Asymptomatic persons 50 to 75 years of age provided three FOBT specimens, which were rehydrated before testing, and underwent colonoscopy. Examination of the rectum and sigmoid colon during colonoscopy was defined as a surrogate for sigmoidoscopy. The sensitivity of sigmoidoscopy was estimated by determining how many patients with advanced neoplasia had an

Selected Internet Resources for Preventive Health Care

Resources for Practitioners

U.S. Department of Health and Human Services
http://www.ahrq.gov/clinic/ppipix.htm
Includes full text of *Clinician's Handbook of Preventive Services,*[5] flowcharts for preventive care, and other useful materials

Agency for Health Care Policy and Research: National Guideline Clearinghouse
http://www.guideline.gov/index.asp
A searchable index for evidence-based practice guidelines; includes more than 100 preventive medicine topics, often abstracted from the U.S. Preventive Services Task Force report[3]

Immunization Action Coalition
http://www.immunize.org
A nonprofit group collaborating with the Centers for Disease Control and Prevention (CDC); includes downloadable vaccine information statements in many languages

CDC Recommends: The Prevention Guidelines System
http://www.phppo.cdc.gov/cdcRecommends/AdvSearchV.asp
Contains CDC-approved preventive guidelines and recommendations

National Cancer Institute (NCI) Physicians Data Query
http://cancernet.nci.nih.gov/index.html
Referenced recommendations for cancer screening from the NCI

Resources for Patients

National Institutes of Health Consumer Health Information
http://www.nih.gov/health/consumer/conkey.htm
A large index of articles for patients on a variety of health topics

National Heart, Lung, and Blood Institute
http://www.nhlbi.nih.gov
Information for patients and clinicians on obesity, hypertension, and hyperlipidemia

CDC Guide to Smoking Cessation
http://www.cdc.gov/tobacco/how2quit.htm
A booklet for patients on smoking cessation

National Institute on Aging
http://www.nia.nih.gov/health/agepages/osteo.htm
Patient information on osteoporosis

American Academy of Family Physicians Colorectal Cancer Screening Information
http://familydoctor.org/handouts/556.html
A patient information sheet on colorectal cancer screening

American Academy of Family Physicians: The Slightly Abnormal Pap Smear
http://www.familydoctor.org/handouts/223.html
A patient information sheet regarding mildly abnormal Pap smears

Table 5 Summary of Recommendations for Adult Immunization

Vaccine	CTF	USPSTF	ACP	Comments
Hepatitis A vaccine	Not reviewed	Recommended for adults at high risk; may also be considered for institutionalized persons, and workers in those institutions and in day care centers	Not reviewed	High-risk groups include persons living in or traveling to endemic areas, homosexual and bisexual men, injection and other street-drug users, military personnel, and certain hospital and laboratory workers; the ACIP also recommends vaccination of patients with chronic liver disease (including hepatitis B and C) and patients with clotting disorders; prevaccination serologic testing is likely to be cost-effective in persons older than 40 yr and in younger persons with a high probability of prior infection; the vaccine is given in two doses, with the second given at least 6 mo after the first [*see Chapter 64*]
Hepatitis B vaccine	Use in adults not reviewed	Recommended for young adults who were not previously immunized and for older adults at high risk	Same as USPSTF recommendation	High-risk groups include injection drug users, homosexual and bisexual males, heterosexuals with multiple sex partners, patients with other sexually transmitted diseases, household and sexual contacts of HbsAg-positive persons, hemodialysis and predialysis patients, and recipients of certain blood products; vaccination is also recommended for health care workers, clients and staff of institutions for the developmentally disabled, inmates of long-term correctional facilities, patients with hepatitis C, and certain international travelers; the vaccine is given in three doses at 0, 1, and 6 mo; prevaccination and serologic testing may be cost-effective if the probability of prior infection is deemed to be high; for selected persons, postvaccination serologic testing 1–6 mo after completion of the series is recommended[85] [*see Chapter 64*]
Influenza vaccine	Annually for persons 65 yr of age and older and for younger persons at increased risk; insufficient evidence to recommend for or against use in healthy younger persons	Annually for persons 65 yr of age and older and for younger persons at increased risk	Same as USPSTF recommendation	Persons of any age at increased risk include those with cardiopulmonary disease, diabetes mellitus, renal insufficiency, hemoglobinopathies, and other conditions causing immunosuppression; influenza vaccine is also recommended for health care workers, for residents of long-term care facilities and their caregivers, for women who will be in the second or third trimester of pregnancy during influenza season, and for anyone else who desires it; protective antibodies develop 2 wk after immunization, peak at 4 to 6 wk, and wane after 6 mo; optimal time for immunization is October to mid-November, but the vaccine may be beneficial even if given as late as March or April; see Table 4 for information about amantadine and rimantadine use in influenza prophylaxis
Measles-mumps-rubella (MMR) vaccine	Recommended for susceptible nonpregnant women of childbearing age; not reviewed for prevention of measles or mumps in adults	Recommended for adults at high risk; may also be considered for institutionalized persons, and workers in those institutions and in day care centers	Same as USPSTF recommendation	Adults born before 1957 are likely to be immune because of natural infection; in younger persons, documentation of immunity requires serologic testing or physician records documenting live virus vaccine after the first birthday or natural infection; although children receive two doses of MMR vaccine, a single dose is considered sufficient for unimmunized adults; however, for health care workers, students entering postsecondary educational institutions, and persons traveling to an area where measles is endemic, a second dose, given no sooner than 4 wk after the first dose, is recommended.[85] Physicians must be aware of contraindications to the use of this vaccine within 3 mo of pregnancy and in some immunocompromised patients [*see Chapter 149*]

ACIP—Advisory Committee on Immunization Practices, Centers for Disease Control and Prevention   ACP—American College of Physicians   CTF—Canadian Task Force on the Periodic Health Examination   USPSTF—United States Preventive Services Task Force

adenoma of any size in the distal colon. The sensitivities of FOBT and sigmoidoscopy for the detection of advanced neoplasia were 24% and 70%, respectively, and the sensitivity of combined screening was 76%.[39]

Because of the imperfect sensitivity of FOBT and sigmoidoscopy and because many patients who undergo these procedures end up requiring colonoscopy anyway, many clinicians are advising their average-risk patients to undergo colonoscopy as a screening test, either as a one-time procedure or periodically (e.g., every 10 years) beginning at age 50. The expert panels have yet to endorse this approach to screening [*see Table 2*], presumably because of concerns about the lack of randomized trial data supporting screening colonoscopy, issues of cost-effectiveness, the risks of the procedure itself, and the availability of skilled colonoscopists for widespread population screening.

Radiologic procedures may provide an alternative to colonoscopy for full colon screening. The Agency for Healthcare Policy and Research has endorsed the use of the double-contrast barium enema, performed every 5 to 10 years, as an alternative screening modality.[40] However, no direct evidence supports this approach, and there are concerns about the sensitivity of the test.[41] A new procedure, CT colonography, may prove to be more sensitive and better tolerated than double-contrast barium enema and provide greater safety and generate less expense than colonoscopy.[42]

PROSTATE CANCER

The topic of prostate cancer screening is highly controversial for many reasons, including the following: (1) there are no completed randomized controlled trials of screening, although studies are ongoing in the United States[43] and in Europe[44]; (2) although prostate cancer is a major cause of death from cancer in men, many cases are clinically indolent (in autopsy studies, the prevalence of histologic prostate cancer in men older than 50 years is about 30%, but only 3% of men die of prostate cancer)[45]; (3) the value of treatment for the localized cancers targeted by screening is unknown; the one randomized controlled trial of radical prostatectomy, which found no improvement in the 15-year survival rates of patients undergoing surgery, has

Table 5 *(continued)*

Vaccine	CTF	USPSTF	ACP	Comments
Pneumo-coccal vaccine	Once for older adults who live in an institution or live or work under crowded conditions, who have sickle cell anemia, or who have undergone splenectomy; insufficient evidence to recommend for or against use in immunocompetent adults 55 yr of age and older; not recommended for immunocompromised patients	Once for adults 65 yr of age and older and for younger adults at high risk; periodic revaccination should be considered for selected persons at high risk	Once for adults 65 yr of age and older and for younger adults at high risk; revaccination recommended at 65 yr of age if 6 yr or more have passed since initial vaccination	High-risk groups for pneumococcal infection include patients with cardiopulmonary disease, diabetes mellitus, alcoholism, cirrhosis, chronic renal failure, nephrotic syndrome, cerebrospinal fluid leaks, anatomic or functional asplenia, and other conditions causing immunosuppression; the controversy among the expert panels regarding vaccination recommendations relates to the fact that vaccine efficacy is best documented in immunocompetent adults at low risk; the ACIP has recommended a single vaccination after 5 yr or more for persons 65 yr of age or over who receive the initial vaccine before 65 yr of age, and for younger patients who are immunocompromised[86]; revaccination increases the risk of local injection site reactions[87] [see *Chapter 134*]
Tetanus-diphtheria vaccine	Every 10 yr after primary immunization series	Periodically after primary immunization series	After primary immunization series, either every 10 yr or once at 50 yr of age (assuming teenage or young adult booster was received)	Although antibody levels decline 10 yr after tetanus immunization, tetanus is unlikely to occur in persons who have received a primary immunization series; although booster immunizations every 10 yr have been recommended for adults, the focus in prevention should be to ensure that unimmunized persons are vaccinated and that wound management guidelines are followed; a primary immunization series for adults consists of a second dose 4–8 wk after the first and a third dose 6–12 months later; use of the combined adsorbed toxoid vaccine for adults is recommended [*see Chapter 136*]
Varicella vaccine	Not reviewed	Recommended for healthy adults with no history of varicella or previous vaccination; strongly recommended for susceptible health care workers, family contacts of immunocompromised patients, and workers in day care centers and other sites in which transmission is likely to occur	Not reviewed	Adults with reliable histories of chickenpox can be assumed to be immune; in others, serologic testing may be cost-effective because most adults with a negative or uncertain history of chickenpox are immune; the vaccine is administered in two doses, with the second given 4–8 wk after the first; physicians must be aware of contraindications to the use of this live attenuated virus vaccine within 1 mo of pregnancy and in immunocompromised patients

been criticized for methodologic problems[46] (another randomized controlled trial comparing expectant management with radical prostatectomy for the treatment of localized cancer is under way)[47]; (4) aggressive treatments for localized disease are associated with significant morbidity; and (5) as with colorectal cancer screening, serendipity may play a role in the discovery of many cancers ostensibly detected by screening,[48] making the value of screening harder to ascertain.

Available modalities for prostate cancer screening include DRE, measurement of serum prostate-specific antigen (PSA), and transrectal ultrasonography (TRUS). TRUS is used primarily as a follow-up study for men with abnormal findings after screening with DRE or PSA measurement; none of the expert panels advocate the use of TRUS in screening [*see Table 2*].

DRE is an inexpensive screening technique, but because up to 15% of men older than 50 years who undergo this examination have suspicious findings, the costs of follow-up testing and treatment are considerable. Even among urologists, the interobserver variability of DRE is substantial.[49] In a report from the European Randomized Study of Screening for Prostate Cancer, in which DRE, PSA measurement, and TRUS were used, the overall sensitivity of DRE was 37%, and its overall specificity was 91%.[50]

Of 473 cancers detected, 44 were found only by DRE and 125 were found only by measurement of PSA. In this study, the positive predictive value (PPV) of DRE in men with a PSA of 0 to 2.9 ng/ml was low (4% to 11%); for men with a PSA of 3 to 3.9 ng/ml, the PPV of DRE rose to 33%. Because most men with a PSA of 4 ng/ml or greater will undergo further evaluation, this increase in the PPV suggests that in screening programs where both modalities are used, DRE may be most helpful in men with a PSA of 3 to 3.9 ng/ml. Case-control studies of the value of DRE in screening have provided conflicting results.[51,52]

PSA is a serine protease that is secreted exclusively by prostatic epithelial cells. The true sensitivity and specificity of PSA measurement for the detection of prostate cancer are unknown. In one study in which men were screened using DRE, PSA measurement, and TRUS, 74% of cancers detected were associated with a PSA level above the usual cutoff of 4 ng/ml.[50] Of the men in this study with an elevated PSA who underwent biopsy, 24% of those with a PSA of 4.0 to 9.9 ng/ml had cancer, and 58% of men with a PSA of 10 ng/ml or greater had cancer. Although the PPV of PSA increases as the level rises, cancers in men with levels of 10 ng/ml or greater are less likely to be curable. Because PSA levels increase in men with benign prostatic hyperplasia, the specificity of PSA measurement declines with increasing age; however, presumably because this loss of specificity is counterbalanced by increased disease prevalence, the PPV of the test appears to vary little with age.[53]

Pending the results of ongoing trials, the expert panels [*see Table 2*] have been reluctant to endorse the use of PSA measurement in prostate cancer screening. The ACP recommends the use of informed consent regarding the potential risks and benefits of screening by use of PSA measurement. When such informed consent is given, patient interest in screening diminishes.[54] If screening is undertaken, several caveats should be noted. Many factors other than the presence of cancer or benign prostatic hyperplasia can affect PSA levels.[55] Acute prostatitis, urinary retention, and prostatic biopsy can all cause significant and prolonged elevations of serum PSA levels. It is recommended that men abstain from ejaculation for 48 hours before the PSA is drawn. PSA levels are higher in hospitalized men than in ambulatory men, perhaps because of the physiologic stress of hospitalization. However, DRE, prostatic massage, urethral catheterization, TRUS, the presence of end-stage renal disease, and hemodialysis do not appear to cause significant alterations in serum PSA. Men of African descent with and without prostate cancer have higher PSA levels than men of European descent.[56] PSA may be an insensitive indicator of prostate cancer in men with low serum testosterone levels.[57] Treatment with finasteride but not with terazosin causes PSA levels to fall.[58]

Several refinements of PSA measurement may prove to be useful. Age-specific reference ranges may be used to increase sensitivity in younger men and to increase specificity in older men who are more likely to have benign prostatic hyperplasia.[59] However, because this strategy reduces specificity in younger men and sensitivity in older men, it has not been universally embraced. A PSA velocity (the rate of change of the PSA level over time) of 0.75 ng/ml/year or greater may identify men at increased risk for prostate cancer.[60] However, individual fluctuations in PSA levels, which increase as mean PSA increases, are a confounding factor.[61] PSA density adjusts raw PSA value according to the volume of the gland or the transition zone of the gland,[62] on the basis of the concept that the PSA content of a given volume of cancerous tissue is higher than that of benign tissue. Because measurement of PSA density requires TRUS, it is expensive and impractical for use in primary care settings. Men with prostate cancer appear to have a lower ratio of free PSA to total PSA in serum than do men with benign prostatic hyperplasia. The authors of one prospective trial have suggested that for men with a PSA value between 4 and 10 ng/ml and a palpably benign gland, biopsy should be performed only for those with a free PSA of 25% or less.[63]

Other Screening and Preventive Measures

The CTF, USPSTF, and ACP-ASIM have also examined the use of preventive interventions and immunizations for conditions other than cancer in average-risk and high-risk patients [*see Tables 3, 4, and 5*]. A variety of Internet sites provide useful information on preventive health care, for both practitioners and patients [*see Sidebar*, Selected Internet Resources for Preventive Health Care].

References

1. Frame CS, Carlson SJ: A critical review of periodic health screening using specific screening criteria. J Fam Pract 2:29, 1975

2. Canadian Task Force on the Periodic Health Examination: The Canadian Guide to Clinical Preventive Health Care. Canada Communication Group, Publishing, Ottawa, Canada, 1994

3. US Preventive Services Task Force: Guide to Clinical Preventive Services: Report of the US Preventive Services Task Force, 2nd ed. Williams & Wilkins, Baltimore, 1996

4. Common Screening Tests. Eddy DM, Ed. American College of Physicians, Philadelphia, 1991

5. Put Prevention into Practice: Clinician's Handbook of Preventive Services, 2nd ed. U.S. Government Printing Office, Washington, DC, 1998

6. von Eschenbach A, Ho R, Murphy GP, et al: American Cancer Society guideline for the early detection of prostate cancer: update 1997. CA Cancer J Clin 47:261, 1997

7. Gordon PR, Senf J, Campos-Outcalt D: Is the annual complete physical examination necessary? Arch Intern Med 159:909, 1999

8. Kottke TE, Battista RN, DeFriese GH, et al: Attributes of successful smoking cessation interventions in medical practice: a meta-analysis of 39 controlled trials. JAMA 259:2882, 1988

9. Thomas DB, Gao DL, Self SG, et al: Randomized trial of breast self-examination in Shanghai: methodology and preliminary results. J Natl Cancer Inst 89:355, 1997

10. American College of Physicians: Screening for ovarian cancer: recommendations and rationale. Ann Intern Med 121:141, 1994

11. American College of Physicians: Screening for prostate cancer. Ann Intern Med 126:480, 1997

12. Henschke CI, McCauley DI, Yankelevitz DF: Early lung cancer action project: overall design and findings from baseline screening. Lancet 354:99, 1999

13. Nystrom L, Rutqvist LE, Wall S, et al: Breast cancer screening with mammography: overview of Swedish randomised trials. Lancet 341:973, 1993

14. Kerlikowske K, Grady D, Rubin SM, et al: Efficacy of screening mammography: a meta-analysis. JAMA 273:149, 1995

15. Woodman CBJ, Threlfall AG, Boggis CRM, et al: Is the three year breast screening interval too long? Occurrence of interval cancers in NHS breast screening programme's north western region. BMJ 310:224, 1995.

16. Bjurstam N, Björneld L, Duffy SW, et al: The Gothenburg breast screening trial: first results on mortality, incidence, and mode of detection for women ages 39-49. Cancer 80:2091, 1997.

17. Antman K, Shea S: Screening mammography under age 50. JAMA 281:1470, 1999

18. Elmore JG, Barton MB, Moceri VM, et al: Ten-year risk of false positive screening mammograms and clinical breast examinations. N Engl J Med 338:1089, 1998

19. Faulk RM, Sickles EA, Sollitto RA, et al: Clinical efficacy of mammographic screening in the elderly. Radiology 194:193, 1995

20. Knight JA, Libstug AR, Moravan V, et al: An assessment of the influence of clinical breast examination reports on the interpretation of mammograms in a breast screening program. Breast Cancer Res Treat 48:65, 1998

21. Mettlin C, Smart CR: Breast cancer detection guidelines for women aged 40 to 49 years: rationale for the American Cancer Society reaffirmation of recommendations. CA Cancer J Clin 44:248, 1994

22. Semiglazov VF, Moiseenko VM, Manikhas AG, et al: Interim results of a prospective randomized study of self-examination for early detection of breast cancer. Vopr Onkol 45:265, 1999

23. Fisher B, Costantino JP, Wickerham DL, et al: Tamoxifen for prevention of breast cancer: report of the National Surgical Adjuvant Breast and Bowel Project P-1 Study. J Natl Cancer Inst 90:1371, 1998

24. Cummings SR, Eckert S, Krueger KA, et al: The effect of raloxifene on risk of breast cancer in postmenopausal women. JAMA 281:2189, 1999

25. Guzick DS: Efficacy of screening for cervical cancer: a review. Am J Public Health 68:125, 1978

26. Eddy DM: Screening for cervical cancer. Ann Intern Med 113:214, 1990

27. Fahs MC, Mandelblatt J, Schechter C, et al: Cost effectiveness of cervical cancer screening for the elderly. Ann Intern Med 117:520, 1992

28. Piscitelli JT, Bastian LA, Wilkes A, et al: Cytologic screening after hysterectomy for benign disease. Am J Obstet Gynecol 173:424, 1995

29. Walsh JME: Cervical cancer: developments in screening and evaluation of the abnormal Pap smear. West J Med 169:304, 1998

30. Diaz-Rosario LA, Kabawat SE: Performance of a fluid-based, thin-layer Papanicolaou smear method in the clinical setting of an independent laboratory and an outpatient screening population in New England. Arch Pathol Lab Med 123:817, 1999

31. O'Leary TJ, Tellado M, Buckner S, et al: PAPNET-assisted rescreening of cervical smears: cost and accuracy compared with a 100% manual rescreening strategy. JAMA 279:235, 1998

32. Östör AG: Review. Natural history of cervical intraepithelial neoplasia: a critical review. Int J Gynecol Pathol 12:186, 1993

33. Mandel JS, Bond JH, Church TR, et al: Reducing mortality from colorectal cancer by screening for fecal occult blood. N Engl J Med 328:1365, 1993

34. Mandel JS, Church TR, Ederer F, et al: Colorectal cancer mortality: effectiveness of biennial screening for fecal occult blood. J Natl Cancer Inst 91:434, 1999

35. Hardcastle JD, Chamberlain JO, Robinson MHE, et al: Randomised controlled trial of faecal-occult-blood screening for colorectal cancer. Lancet 348:1472, 1996

36. Kronborg O, Fenger C, Olsen J, et al: Randomised study of screening for colorectal cancer with faecal-occult-blood test. Lancet 348:1467, 1996

37. Selby JV, Friedman GD, Quesenberry CP Jr, et al: A case-control study of screening sigmoidoscopy and mortality from colorectal cancer. N Engl J Med 333:1301, 1995

38. Muller AD, Sonnenberg A: Prevention of colorectal cancer by flexible endoscopy

and polypectomy: a case-control study of 32,702 veterans. Ann Intern Med 123:904, 1995

39. One-time screening for colorectal cancer with combined fecal occult-blood testing and examination of the distal colon. Veterans Affairs Cooperative Study Group 380. N Engl J Med 345:555, 2001

40. Winawer SJ, Fletcher RH, Miller L, et al: Colorectal cancer screening: clinical guidelines and rationale. Gastroenterology 112:594, 1997

41. Rex D: Barium enema: detection of colonic lesions in a community population. Am J Gastroenterol 92:1570, 1997

42. Johnson CD, Ahlquist DA: Computed tomography colonography (virtual colonoscopy): a new method for colorectal screening. Gut 44:301, 1999

43. Gohagan JK, Prorok PC, Kramer BS, et al: Prostate cancer screening in the Prostate, Lung, Colorectal and Ovarian Cancer Screening Trial of the National Cancer Institute. J Urol 151:1283, 1994

44. Schroder FH, Kranse R, Rietbergen J, et al: The European randomized study of screening for prostate cancer (ERSPC): an update. Eur Urol 35:539, 1999

45. Coley CM, Barry MJ, Fleming C, et al: Early detection of prostate cancer: part I: prior probability and effectiveness of tests. Ann Intern Med 126:394, 1997

46. Graversen PH, Corle DK, Nielsen KT, et al: Radical prostatectomy versus expectant primary treatment in stages I and II prostatic cancer: a fifteen-year follow-up. Urology 36:493, 1990

47. Wilt TJ, Brawer MK: The prostate cancer intervention versus observation trial (PIVOT). Oncology 8:1133, 1997

48. Collins MM, Ransohoff, DF, Barry MJ: Early detection of prostate cancer: serendipity strikes again. JAMA 278:1516, 1997

49. Smith DS, Catalona WJ: Interexaminer variability of digital rectal examination in detecting prostate cancer. Urology 45:70, 1995

50. Schröder FH, van der Maas P, Beemsterboer P, et al: Evaluation of the digital rectal examination as a screening test for prostate cancer. J Natl Cancer Inst 90:1817, 1998

51. Friedman GD, Hiatt RA, Quesenberry CP Jr, et al: Case-control study of screening for prostatic cancer by digital rectal examinations. Lancet 337:1526, 1991

52. Jacobsen SJ, Bergstralh EJ, Katusic SK, et al: Screening digital rectal examination and prostate cancer mortality: a population-based case-control study. Urology 52:173, 1998

53. Richie JP, Catalona WJ, Ahmann FR, et al: Effect of patient age on early detection of prostate cancer with serum prostate-specific antigen and digital rectal examination. Urology 42:365, 1993

54. Wolf AMD, Nasser JF, Wolf AM, et al: The impact of informed consent on patient interest in prostate-specific antigen screening. Arch Intern Med 156:1333, 1996

55. Tchetgen MN, Oesterling JE: The effect of prostatitis, urinary retention, ejaculation, and ambulation of the serum prostate-specific antigen concentration. Urol Clin North Am 24:283, 1997

56. Morgan TO, Jacobsen SJ, McCarthy WF, et al: Age-specific reference ranges for serum prostate-specific antigen in black men. N Engl J Med 335:304, 1996

57. Morgentaler A, Bruning CO, DeWolf WC: Occult prostate cancer in men with low serum testosterone levels. JAMA 276:1904, 1996

58. Brawer MK, Lin DW, Williford WO, et al: Effect of finasteride and/or terazosin on serum PSA: results of VA Cooperative Study #359. Prostate 39:234, 1999

59. Oesterling JE, Jacobsen SJ, Chute CG, et al: Serum prostate-specific antigen in a community-based population of healthy men: establishment of age-specific reference ranges. JAMA 270:860, 1993

60. Carter HB, Pearson JD, Metter EJ, et al: Longitudinal evaluation of prostate-specific antigen levels in men with and without prostate disease. JAMA 267:2215, 1992

61. Kadmon D, Weinberg AD, Williams RH, et al: Pitfalls in interpreting prostate specific antigen velocity. Urology 155:1655, 1996

62. Djavan B, Zlotta A, Kratzik C, et al: PSA, PSA density, PSA density of transition zone, free/total PSA ratio, and PSA velocity for early detection of prostate cancer in men with serum PSA 2.5 to 4.0 ng/mL. Urology 54:517, 1999

63. Catalona WJ, Partin AW, Slawin KM, et al: Use of the percentage of free prostate-specific antigen to enhance differentiation of prostate cancer from benign prostatic disease: a prospective multicenter clinical trial. JAMA 279:1542, 1998

64. Frame PS, Fryback DG, Patterson C: Screening for abdominal aortic aneurysm in men ages 60 to 80 years. A cost-effectiveness analysis. Ann Intern Med 119:411, 1993

65. Abrutyn E, Mossey J, Berlin J, et al: Does asymptomatic bacteriuria predict mortality and does antimicrobial treatment reduce mortality in elderly ambulatory women? Ann Intern Med 120:827, 1994

66. American College of Physicians: Diagnostic evaluation of the carotid arteries. Ann Intern Med 109:835, 1988

67. Executive Committee for the Asymptomatic Carotid Atherosclerosis Study: Endarterectomy for asymptomatic carotid artery stenosis. JAMA 273:1421, 1995

68. Perry JR, Szalai JP, Norris JW: Consensus against both endarterectomy and routine screening for asymptomatic carotid artery stenosis. Arch Neurol 54:25, 1997

69. Canadian Task Force on the Periodic Health Examination: Periodic health examination, 1995 update: 3. Screening for visual problems among elderly patients. Can Med Assoc J 152:1211, 1995

70. American College of Physicians: Clinical guideline: guidelines for using serum cholesterol, high-density lipoprotein cholesterol, and triglyceride levels as screening tests for preventing coronary heart disease in adults (pt 1). Ann Intern Med 124:515, 1996

71. Shepherd J, Cobbe SM, Ford I, et al: Prevention of coronary heart disease with pravastatin in men with hypercholesterolemia. N Engl J Med 333:1301, 1995

72. Hebert PR, Gaziano JM, Chan KS, et al: Cholesterol lowering with statin drugs, risk of stroke, and total mortality: an overview of randomized trials. JAMA 278:313, 1997

73. Littenberg B: A practice guideline revisited: screening for hypertension. Ann Intern Med 122:937, 1995

74. MacDonald LA, Sackett DL, Haynes RB, et al: Labelling in hypertension: a review of the behavioural and psychological consequences. J Chronic Dis 37:933, 1984

75. American College of Physicians: Automated ambulatory blood pressure and self-measured blood pressure monitoring devices: their role in the diagnosis and management of hypertension. Ann Intern Med 118:889, 1993

76. Sixth Report of the Joint National Committee on Prevention, Detection, Evaluation, and Treatment of High Blood Pressure. Arch Intern Med 157:2413, 1997

77. Douketis JD, Feightner JW, Attia J, et al: Periodic health examination, 1999 update: 1. Detection, prevention and treatment of obesity. CMAJ 160:513, 1999

78. American College of Physicians: Screening for thyroid disease. Ann Intern Med 129:141, 1998

79. Helfand M, Redfern CC: Screening for thyroid disease: an update. Ann Intern Med 129:144, 1998

80. Common diagnostic tests: use and interpretation, 2nd ed. Sox HC Jr, Ed. American College of Physicians, Philadelphia, 1990

81. Davies HD, Wang EEL: Periodic health examination, 1996 update: 2. Screening for chlamydial infections. CMAJ 154:1631, 1996

82. UK Prospective Diabetes Study (UKPDS) Group: Intensive blood-glucose control with sulphonylureas or insulin compared with conventional treatment and risk of complications in patients with type 2 diabetes (UKPDS 33). Lancet 352:837, 1998

83. American College of Physicians, Infectious Diseases Society of America: Human immunodeficiency virus (HIV) infection. Ann Intern Med 120:310, 1994

84. American College of Physicians, American Diabetes Association, American Academy of Ophthalmology: Screening guidelines for diabetic retinopathy. Ann Intern Med 116:683, 1992

85. American College of Physicians Task Force on Adult Immunization, Infectious Diseases Society of America: Guide for Adult Immunization, 3rd ed. American College of Physicians, Philadelphia, 1994

86. Prevention of pneumococcal disease. Recommendations of the Advisory Committee on Immunization Practices (ACIP). MMWR Morb Mortal Wkly Rep 46:RR-8:1, 1997

87. Jackson LA, Benson P, Sneller V, et al: Safety of revaccination with pneumococcal polysaccharide vaccine. JAMA 281:243, 1999

6 Occupational Safety and Health

Mark R. Cullen, M.D., and Linda Rosenstock, M.D., M.P.H.

Awareness of the impact of the work environment on health has increased dramatically in the past two decades. Common clinical problems, such as carpal tunnel syndrome and respiratory irritation and allergy, are increasingly being related to physical, chemical, and biologic hazards at work.[1] In this chapter, we cover some of the most common occupational disorders diagnosed in industrialized countries and present examples of known or suspected causes [*see Table 1*]. More extensive descriptions of specific disorders are presented in other sections of *WebMD Scientific American® Medicine* and in textbooks of occupational medicine.[2-9]

Data on the frequency of occurrence of most occupational disorders are limited; however, general figures illustrating the extent of the problem are available. For example, in 1998, private employers in the United States reported 5.5 million nonfatal work injuries and 390,000 cases of occupational illness.[10] The National Safety Council estimates the total cost of occupational deaths and injuries at $125 billion in medical expenses, wage and productivity losses, and other associated expenses.[11] Illness from the workplace occurs frequently and has substantial clinical ramifications.

Basic Principles of Occupational Disease

It is important to debunk the widespread and erroneous perception that most occupational disorders are pathologically unique. Although some disorders, such as silicosis, do have distinguishing pathologic characteristics, the majority do not. Most—such as lung cancer induced by ionizing radiation, bladder cancer caused by fumes from coke ovens, asthma triggered by inhalation of platinum salts, and fatty liver resulting from the absorption of the solvent dimethylformamide through the skin—are pathologically indistinguishable from disorders with more familiar causes. However, it is virtually always possible to differentiate occupational diseases from their nonoccupational counterparts. Laboratory testing and data gathering provide the best clues for the diagnosis of occupational disease, but to recognize these disorders, it is critical to ask appropriate questions when taking the medical history [*see* Clinical Evaluation, *below*].

Workplace toxins and hazards, when adequately studied, have predictable and discrete pathologic consequences. Although other diseases share common final pathways, the initial mechanisms of injury are generally highly specific for each agent. Aside from the possibility of idiosyncratic responses, as with pharmacologic agents, the actual potential effects of most toxins are few. For example, beryllium may cause an acute inflammatory pneumonia (acute beryllium disease) within hours after intense exposure, or it may cause a delayed hypersensitivity response with granulomatous lung disease (chronic beryllium disease [CBD]) in persons with recurrent or chronic exposures; no other form of nonmalignant lung disease is known to be caused by this metal or its salts.

Both the likelihood that workplace hazards will produce effects and the severity of those effects are determined by the dose of exposure. The nature of the relation between dose and response depends on the mechanism of action of the agent. For direct-acting toxins, which cause effects by directly disrupting cellular function or cell death at the target-organ level, there is usually a dose beneath which no biologic effects are observed, a

so-called threshold level. Above this level, there is typically a sigma-shaped dose-response correlation as dose rises, until a lethal dose is reached. Similarly, a rising fraction of the exposed population is affected as dose rises; eventually, everyone is affected. This is characteristic of heavy metals, organic solvents, and pesticides. For agents that cause allergic-type or idiosyncratic responses, such as latex and epoxy resins, which affect only susceptible people, dose contributes to the likelihood of sensitization, though not necessarily to the severity of the reaction. Further, once a worker has become sensitized, a very low dose may be sufficient to induce a full-blown clinical response. For mutagens and carcinogens, current knowledge presumes a linear dose-response model, with each increment in cumulative dose resulting in a proportional increase in the risk of cancer. The severity of the resultant cancer bears no predictable relation to the induction dose, though the time from exposure to onset generally is shorter when doses are higher.

The temporal relation between exposure and effect is highly predictable for each agent and each effect. For many direct toxins, effects occur within minutes or hours of exposure to an appropriate dose, such as the syndrome of cholinergic storm after organophosphate pesticide poisoning. Similarly, immunologically mediated responses, such as asthma and dermatitis, will occur within minutes or hours after exposure. Conversely, other effects are predictably delayed. Asbestos and silica rarely cause pneumoconiosis in less than 10 years after first exposure, except after very high exposure levels. Solid tumors, such as lung cancer associated with these same dusts, emerge, on average, 20 to 30 years after first exposure. Other effects occur in an intermediate time frame: some organophosphates cause a paralysis delayed in onset by weeks to months after an intense overexposure. The presentations of acute lead, mercury, or arsenic poisoning are insidious, coming after the poison accumulates to a dangerous level, usually after weeks or months of exposure.

From the clinician's perspective, an approach to patients with new medical problems should take into consideration occupational causes. If the problem is acute, such as the relatively sudden onset of a rash or of liver function abnormalities or hemolysis, the search for a possible occupational cause should focus on recent events: Has there been a new or increased exposure to an agent that can cause such toxicity in the hours, days, or, at most, weeks before onset? On the other hand, for chronic disorders, such as pulmonary fibrosis and cancer, the search for causes should begin with a work history that goes back years.

With regard to work histories, it is important to note that host factors may modify temporal and dose-response correlations; all workers do not react alike to comparable exposures. Every workplace has some people who appear to be immune to the effects of even the most toxic agents and others who seem to react to low doses, often lower than the threshold deemed toxic by regulatory authorities. These differences may be caused by genetic, dietary, or constitutional factors or by the preexistence of other illnesses.

In addition, many workplace hazards and toxins interact with one another and with nonoccupational factors in the induction of disease. Dose-response correlations for industrial hazards may be markedly shifted in the presence of other hazards,

Table 1 Common Occupational Disorders

Disorders	Examples of Causal Factors
Respiratory tract	
Pneumoconiosis	Coal, silica, asbestos
Asthma	Latex, polyurethane
Allergic alveolitis	Vegetable matter, machining fluids
Metal fume fever	Metal fumes
Skin	
Contact dermatitis	Oils, rubber, metals
Acne	Herbicides, oils, friction
Urticaria	Latex
Urinary tract	
Glomerular disease	Organic solvents, mercury
Tubulointerstitial disease	Cadmium, lead
Liver	
Acute or subacute necrosis	Organic solvents, TNT, 2-nitropropane
Cholestatic hepatitis	Methylene dianiline
Acute and chronic hepatitis	Viruses (hepatitis B, C)
Steatosis	Organic solvents
Hepatoportal sclerosis	Vinyl chloride, arsenical compounds
Hepatocellular injury	Lead, arsenic, phosphorus, dioxin
Musculoskeletal	
Carpal tunnel syndrome	Repetitive trauma
Raynaud phenomenon	Repetitive vibrations, vinyl chloride
Scleroderma	Coal mining
Nervous system	
Parkinsonism	Manganese
Peripheral neuropathy	Solvents, lead, acrylamide, arsenic
Acute encephalopathy	Organic solvents, asphyxiants
Acute or subacute cholinergic crisis	Organophosphate and carbamate pesticides
Subacute encephalopathy	Mercury, lead, arsenic, manganese, carbon disulfide
Subacute peripheral neuropathy	Organophosphates
Chronic basal gangliar disorder	Manganese, carbon monoxide (postasphyxiation)
Chronic encephalopathy	Recurrent organic solvent exposures
Hematologic conditions	
Hemolysis	Lead, organic nitrites
Accelerated red cell destruction	
Acute hemolysis	Nitro and amine compounds
Subacute hemolysis	Lead
Disorders of oxygen transport	
Methemoglobinemia	Nitro and amine compounds
Carboxyhemoglobinemia	Carbon monoxide
Disorders of red cell production	
Hyperplastic anemia	Lead
Aplastic anemia, hypoplastic anemia	Ethylene glycol ethers, benzene, arsenic, ionizing radiation
Myelodysplasia	Benzene, ionizing radiation
Polycythemia	Cobalt
Endocrine and reproductive	
Hypogonadism	Lead
Azoospermia, oligospermia	DBCP, ionizing radiation
Teratogenesis	Organic mercury, PCBs

DBCP—1,2-dibromo-3-chloropropane (pesticide) PCBs—polychlorinated biphenyls

habits, or medications. An important example is the likelihood of disease resulting from thermal stress (i.e., heat or cold) in the presence of hemodynamically active agents, such as calcium channel blockers, autonomic agents, and diuretics.[12] Likewise, the effects of vibration trauma on wrists and digits may be amplified by nicotine.[13] The effects of one hazard may be significantly altered in the presence of another; for example, the combined effect of noise and solvents on hearing loss[14] and of asbestos and smoking on lung cancer[15] are greater than the effect of exposure to each hazard alone.

Clinical Evaluation

DEFINING THE PATHOPHYSIOLOGIC BASIS OF THE PATIENT'S COMPLAINTS

When searching for the pathophysiologic basis of a patient's complaints, it is important to ascertain the following: Is the process an acute or relapsing process, with precipitous changes in physiologic status, reflecting a recent or ongoing exposure? Or is it a chronic process, more likely to have resulted from noxious exposure in the distant past? Dysfunction of what organ or organs best explains symptoms? Is there evidence of physiologic disruption, or is the disorder predominantly one of subjective difficulties?

TAKING THE OCCUPATIONAL HISTORY

Every patient should be questioned regarding the essentials of occupation, including current and past workplaces, job type, and materials used. Open-ended questions are always appropriate (e.g., "Are there dangerous materials or hazards in your workplace?" and "Do you believe that your work is causing you any health problems?").[16] The exploration of work as the basis for a complaint or medical problem entails an incisive approach and depends on the nature of the clinical problem being investigated.

Approach to the Patient with an Acute Disorder

The emphasis should be on new exposures, increased exposures, and accidental exposures. Has the patient recently begun a new job or task involving hazards? Were new materials recently introduced at work? Has there been a change in working conditions, such as a failure of the ventilation system? Has there been a leak, spill, or accident? If the answer to all of these questions is no, the likelihood is low that the acute illness is related to work processes or chemicals.

Other than acute effects that are immunologically mediated, most are not idiosyncratic and will follow a sigma-shaped dose-response correlation like that discussed for direct-acting toxins (see above). In such circumstances, a high proportion of exposed persons are expected to be affected, although individual thresholds and dose responses may differ. Questions probing effects in other exposed persons are extremely helpful, as in the investigation of food poisoning or respiratory infections. Although a negative answer does not exclude a work-related effect, suggestion of an outbreak or cluster makes the probability of an association high and increases the urgency of a prompt, correct diagnosis.

Approach to the Patient with Recurrent Manifestations

A patient may have repeated or recurring manifestations, such as intermittent cough, rash, or nausea. Although the cause may be difficult to establish in some situations, especially when symptoms have been very persistent or chronic, the time course,

Table 2 Common Occupational Hazards for Which There Are Widely Available Biologic Tests of Exposure

Hazard	Comments
Metals	
Arsenic	Hair sampling can detect historic exposures
Cadmium	Detectable in urine for many years if there is renal injury
Fluorides	Transient in urine
Lead	Half-life 40 days in blood
Mercury	Detectable in urine for days to weeks
Asphyxiants	
Carbon monoxide	Half-life 4 hr in blood
Pesticides	
Organophosphates	Detectable indirectly, by measurement of cholinesterase, which may be depressed for days to months
Organochlorines (e.g., DDT, chlordane, dieldrin)	Persists in blood
Organic solvents	
Benzene and toluene	Metabolites transiently in urine
Antigens	IgE antibodies measurable by RAST
Miscellaneous	
PCBs	Persists in blood

PCBs—polychlorinated biphenyls   RAST—radioallergosorbent test

particularly at the onset of recurring manifestations, is often extremely revealing. For example, a new asthma patient whose symptoms occur on vacations and weekends is unlikely to have an occupationally related disorder.

Approach to the Patient with Chronic Disease

When patients present with evidence of irreversible organ damage or malignancy, the approach is altogether different. Although the longer latency between initial exposure and disease onset will be useful in determining whether occupational exposures have played an important role, questions directed at temporal associations between symptoms and exposures are not helpful. Rather, the first step is to establish a clear pathophysiologic picture of the disease process itself. Sometimes, knowledge of past exposures may assist in directing this evaluation. For example, a malignant pleural effusion in a worker exposed to asbestos should be carefully evaluated for the possibility of mesothelioma, which is otherwise an uncommon disorder.

Once the disease process is characterized, a role for occupational factors can be more seriously considered by obtaining a more detailed history of exposures. Because only a handful of agents are suspected of causing or have been proved to cause any single chronic disease, the goal of this history is to determine whether exposure to any of those agents has occurred and whether the exposure occurred at a time and dose that suggest a causal connection to the disease.

Approach to Subacute and Insidious Disease

The greatest challenge in clinical occupational medicine is the clinical disorder of gradual onset over days to weeks that meets none of the above approaches. Examples include peripheral neuropathies, anemia, and change in bowel habit without evidence of malignant or irreversible organ system damage. Often, in such cases, the search for the underlying pathophysiologic process and the search for its cause seem intricately related and must proceed simultaneously. Lessons from these paradigms may be helpful. If indeed the subacute process is toxic, it most likely reflects effects of a recent exposure, typically of an agent that is accumulating slowly. Heavy metals, pesticides, and various toxic organic chemicals often behave in this fashion, taking weeks or months for levels of pathogenic significance to accrue under typical conditions of exposure. Although it is unnecessary to identify an accidental leak or spill, it is key to note an enhanced opportunity for exposure or a novel exposure over a relatively short time frame. The distant exposure history is not likely to be helpful, because the subacute disorders almost always present at the point of maximal accumulation; once the worker is removed from exposure, latency or delay in onset is unusual.

CONFIRMING AND QUANTIFYING EXPOSURE

There are two basic approaches to obtaining additional exposure information. The first involves collection of independent information about present or former work (depending on which is relevant). After the physician obtains consent from the patient (to ensure that the patient is protected from unwanted consequences), information about exposures is requested from the employer, a trade union, or a regulatory agency. The usual form of such information is a material safety data sheet (MSDS). The MSDS provides generic chemical names, compositions, and basic toxicity information of all materials used. In addition, employers may be able to provide evidence of objective sampling that may have been done to test air levels of hazardous substances. Job descriptions, results of medical tests performed at work, information about other workers with health problems, and use of protective equipment or other methods to limit exposure may all be of value in assessing workplace exposures.

The second potential source of dose information is biologic testing. For a few hazards, urine, blood, or hair testing may enable the physician to determine body burden of the agent, which correlates with current or recent levels, or both, and less commonly with remote exposures [*see Table 2*]. Most of these tests cannot detect chemicals that have been cleared from the body or deposited in body organs; this substantially limits their usefulness for diagnostic decision making. Of course, there are no simple tests for chemicals that cause topical injury to skin or respiratory mucosa but are not absorbed. For agents that act by immune sensitization, radioallergosorbent testing or skin-patch testing may be useful both for documenting exposure and for subsequent elicitation of an immune response.

Most important of all is to remember that a test for exposure can be interpreted only in the context of the history and clinical problem. It should not be directly interpreted as a test for disease, regardless of how the laboratory reports the data. For example, a whole blood lead level of 25 mg/dl is clear evidence of excess lead exposure. If the history indicated that the patient had recently been exposed for the first time, this level would suggest a modest, generally subtoxic dose of exposure. If, however, the patient had worked around lead for many years and quit a year before the test was performed, this same value would suggest a very high previous exposure and might well be associated with health effects caused by high chronic exposure. Similarly, a large proportion of bakers working around flour dust may have IgE antibodies to wheat, rye, or other grain antigens, even though the vast majority of those bakers are symptom free and will most likely remain so. Given all these limitations, biologic testing plays only a limited role in occupational medicine and can never substitute for the occupational history.

DIAGNOSTIC DECISION MAKING

The determination that a patient's symptoms are work related often entails extensive ramifications for the patient's employer, as well as potentially serious public health and medicolegal implications. These may present a significant challenge to the clinician, because for many occupational disorders, there is no gold standard for diagnosis.

The decision-making process should address the following questions:

1. Is the clinical illness, including the history, physical examination, and laboratory findings, consistent with other case descriptions?
2. Is the timing between exposure and clinical onset compatible with the known biologic facts about the hazard?
3. Is the exposure dose within the range of doses believed to cause such effects?
4. Are there special attributes of the particular patient that make it more or less likely that he or she would be so affected?
5. Are there alternative ways of constructing the case that better fit the available facts?
6. Where there remains significant uncertainty about the cause, how important is it to be certain?

Regarding the certainty of identifying the cause, the general legal standard for workers' compensation purposes is "more likely than not," which is a relatively low hurdle of certainty (i.e., at least 50% certain). However, there may be other situations that demand a higher level of confidence, irrespective of the standard for obtaining compensation benefits. In general, problems involving current working conditions demand a far greater level of certainty than historical ones. For example, a diagnosis of occupational asthma in a spray painter would likely dictate removing the patient completely from exposure to the offending paint or constituent; correct identification of that agent might be crucial to save his or her career. Similarly, if a surgeon presented with recurrent anaphylactic reactions, it would be very important to determine whether the reactions were to latex, an anesthetic agent, or some extrinsic factor.

In situations where a high level of certainty is needed, it is often worth the effort to refine the diagnostic impression by serial observations, usually while the patient remains exposed, or by utilizing diagnostic challenges of removal followed by reexposure. Using serial functional measurements, such as peak expiratory flow records or serial blood tests, a more certain judgment can be made. This may also be an appropriate circumstance for referral to occupational physicians who specialize in evaluating challenging cases.

Major Occupational Disorders in Developed Countries

The spectrum of occupational disorders of clinical importance is rapidly shifting as a result of several factors: they include changes in the economy, which have brought about a decline in traditional manufacturing and a rise in service-sector activities; better control of many hazards, such as mineral dusts (asbestos, silica, coal), heavy metals (lead, arsenic, mercury), and the most toxic solvents (e.g., benzene); rapid introduction of many new technologies whose health risks remain inadequately characterized; and changing demographics in the workplace, with an in-

creasing proportion of women, minority, and older workers. In the sections that follow, the disorders that are most important in clinical practice in developed countries are briefly discussed by organ system.

OCCUPATIONAL CANCER

Only a small fraction of known chemical agents and a handful of physical and biologic hazards appear capable of inducing neoplastic change in mammalian tissues. In general, the risk of cancer being induced increases in direct proportion to total dose of exposure. Typically, the target organ is relatively specific, based on the metabolism and transport of the agent. However, a few agents, including ionizing radiation and asbestos, appear to have potential to cause malignancy at more than one human site. There is invariably a long lag time between initial exposure and onset of clinical disease. Only a small number of hazards found in the workplace have been clearly established as carrying substantive cancer risk for workers. An additional group of hazards are suspected, but additional studies are needed. The list of potential carcinogens is expanding; for example, recent evidence suggests that exposure to cadmium may play a role in the development of prostate cancer.[17] In a recent study, there was some indication that workers in print shops, workers in gardening nurseries, horticulturists, farmers, and aircraft mechanics were at excess risk for renal cell carcinoma[18] [see Table 3].

RESPIRATORY TRACT DISORDERS

The respiratory tract is a frequent target of toxic effects. Complaints referable to the lungs or upper respiratory tract often require a careful evaluation for occupational causes. The presence of other possible causal factors, such as common allergy and smoking, does not exclude the possibility of an occupational cause and may, in fact, increase the likelihood of one.

Acute Disorders and Recurrent Disorders

The most prevalent acute effects—inflammatory reactions of the mucosae of the upper or lower airway systems—are caused by environmental irritants.[19] An extraordinary array of agents are irritating, including simple inorganic gases (e.g., ammonia and chlorine), organic solvents, acid and alkaline mists, metal fumes (tiny particles of metal and metal oxide that occur when vaporized metals hit cool air), mineral dusts (e.g., fibrous glass and coal), and almost all the pyrolytic products of combustion. The anatomic site of irritation for dusts, mists, and fumes depends on the deposition of particles; for gases, it depends on water solubility (i.e., the more water soluble the gas, the more it will dissolve in the upper respiratory tract). Expression of symptoms, from mild burning of eyes, nose, and throat to small airway and alveolar injury with the acute respiratory distress syndrome, depends on dose, duration of exposure, and the potency and composition of the irritant; there is also substantial host variability. Delay from the time of exposure to onset of symptoms is very brief for the upper respiratory structures and can be from minutes to hours for lower structures.

Most of the consequences of acute irritation are self-limited; the upper respiratory tract is particularly resilient, although patients who work in areas of poor air quality will experience frequent recurrences, punctuated by commonplace complications such as sinusitis. Such cases require steps to modify exposure. More severe insults may result in fixed scarring of airways or lung parenchyma; late inflammatory sequelae such as bronchiolitis obliterans are occasionally reported. A newly recognized

Table 3 Established Occupational Carcinogens

Cancer Site	Hazard	Setting
Lung	Asbestos	Insulation, textiles
	Ionizing radiation	Uranium mining
	Arsenic	Refining
	Polyaromatic hydrocarbons	Coke ovens
	Nickel	Nickel refining
	Chromium	Tanning, pigments
	Alkylating agents	Chemical industry
	Silica	Mining, stonecutting
	Ceramic fibers	Insulation
	Formaldehyde	Chemicals, plastics
	Beryllium	Nuclear weapons, aerospace industry
	Cadmium	Batteries
	Acrylonitrile	Plastics
	1,3-Butadiene	Rubber, plastics
Pleura and peritoneum	Asbestos	Construction materials
Upper respiratory tract	Wood dust	Carpentry
	Nickel	Refining
	Chromium	Plating
	Asbestos	Friction products
	Formaldehyde	Chemicals, plastics
Urinary bladder	Benzidine and related amines	Dyes, chemicals
	Polyaromatic hydrocarbons	Aluminum reduction
Liver	Vinyl chloride monomer	Plastics
	Arsenic	Pesticides
Upper GI tract	Asbestos	Shipbuilding
	Coal dust	Mining
	Acrylonitrile	Plastics
Hematologic system	Benzene	Chemicals, rubber
	Ionizing radiation	Defense industry
	Ethylene oxide	Chemicals, sterilizers
Soft tissue	Dioxin	Chemical industry

and probably common outcome of significant lower airway injuries is the occurrence of persistent mucosal irritation and bronchospasm, a variant of asthma induced by a single exposure or repeated exposures to irritants. Initially dubbed reactive airways dysfunction syndrome,[20] this disorder is best classified as nonimmune occupational asthma or simply asthma without latency. Unfortunately, the condition tends to be highly resistant to therapy, and patients are only modestly benefited from inhaled steroids or other bronchodilators. Typically, cough with some phlegm, chest discomfort, and occasionally even dyspnea persist despite early and intensive therapy. Reassurance and reduction of further exposures to irritants are the mainstays of treatment.

Occupational asthma, including the nonimmune- and the immune-mediated varieties, is prevalent.[21] There are now over 200 established causes of presumed immune-mediated asthma,[22] usually separated into proteins and other high-molecular-weight antigens (e.g., animal danders, latex antigens, and grains) and small molecules such as the isocyanates—the ubiquitous chemicals used in polyurethane products. Typically, the classic antigens differentially affect those with atopy and are associated with identifiable IgE antibody responses to the sensitizer.[23] In such cases, the greatest diagnostic dilemma is distinguishing occupational sources from other causes of asthma, though the peri-

odicity as documented by history or peak expiratory flow records (PEFR) aid in identifying a relation to work. Latex has become a particularly important cause, especially when rendered airborne in association with the use of powdered gloves.[24,25] More troublesome are the low-molecular-weight agents such as toluene-2,4-diisocyanate (TDI) and other isocyanates, for which atopy is not a risk factor.[22,26] Onset is often insidious, with cough and chest discomfort relatively more common than in asthma of other causes. Far more often than with the IgE-mediated agents, symptoms may be delayed some hours after exposure, so patterns may include nocturnal complaints. Once the physiologic hallmarks of asthma are established, the history and PEFR are the keys to specific diagnosis. Studies have shown that detailed histories can be inconclusive[27]; in some cases, objective measurements can establish the diagnosis of occupational asthma.[27,28] Specific inhalation tests may be valuable, but they should be performed only under medical supervision.[27]

Current evidence suggests that correct diagnosis of occupational asthma makes a difference. People who are removed early from further contact have a better likelihood of reducing their dependence on medication; many will become nonasthmatic over time.[22,23] Most who remain exposed will develop persistent nonspecific bronchial hyperreactivity, as well as possible fixed obstructive changes. These patients will typically fail to recover after they are removed from contact with the agent, and their conditions may even worsen; this is the basis for an aggressive posture toward early evaluation and management.

Allergic alveolitis, with its more benign variants, such as humidifier fever, continues to occur sporadically in a wide range of settings.[29] This disorder was traditionally associated with agricultural exposures to molds and bacilli. Cases are now reported to occur in manufacturing and other industrial settings because of the appearance of a few chemicals that appear capable of inducing the immune response (e.g., plastic resin constituents) and because of the contamination of many industrial processes with microorganisms.[30] The office environment continues to be an occasional source of this condition as well, though the reservoir of causal microbes may be obscure; such organisms may potentially reside in heating and air-conditioning systems remote from the patient's work area.[31]

Chronic Conditions

The pneumoconioses continue to occur, in part because of their very long latency from first exposure and because pockets of very poor industrial conditions continue to exist even in developed countries. Construction activities have been particularly problematic. In general, asbestosis, silicosis, and coal workers' pneumoconiosis are diseases that occur after extensive work exposures. The diagnosis can usually be made on the basis of clinical findings and the history of exposure, once the patient's lifetime job history is obtained.

The granulomatous diseases, including chronic beryllium disease, or CBD, and so-called hard metal disease, are less common but important and increasingly recognized disorders of sensitization. CBD is clinically almost identical to idiopathic sarcoidosis except that all cases involve the lung and that the prognosis— even after the patient is removed from exposure to beryllium metal, compound, or fumes—is generally unfavorable. All patients with sarcoidosis should be asked if they work with metals, and the least suspicion should prompt specific testing; there is a highly sensitive test that can distinguish sarcoidosis from CBD on blood or bronchoalveolar lavage (BAL) fluid.[32] Hard metal disease is a giant cell alveolitis induced via an idiosyncratic reaction in workers exposed to the metal cobalt.[33] Most often, it occurs in workers making or using tungsten carbide, the very hard metal used for machine tools. Onset may be insidious and may include asthmatic symptoms, because cobalt is asthmogenic as well. Recognition of the parenchymal process by BAL or biopsy is crucial because hard metal disease is progressive, often refractory to treatment with steroids, and often lethal; there is anecdotal evidence favoring the use of cytotoxic drugs. Once hard metal disease is diagnosed, the patient should be promptly removed from any further exposure.

In 1998, a novel form of interstitial fibrosis related to an industrial exposure was reported: flock worker's lung, named after the nylon flocking used for making feltlike textiles.[34] Cases of flock worker's lung are distinctive, with pathologic evidence of both parenchymal fibrosis and lymphocytic bronchiolitis. This report underscores a key principle of occupational medicine: that new occupational diseases and other clinical consequences of work continue to be uncovered.[35]

DERMATOLOGIC DISORDERS

Despite increased recognition of the need to reduce contact between the skin and the chemical and physical environment, dermal conditions remain responsible for significant morbidity in the workplace. Most disorders are caused by direct exposure of the skin to workplace irritants, sensitizers, pigments, carcinogens, and materials that interfere with normal dermal function by disrupting sebaceous and follicular secretions (e.g., oils that cause acne) or solvents that erode protective lipids. Trauma, foreign bodies, ionizing and nonionizing radiation, and extremes of temperature may modify or disrupt skin growth, vascular integrity, or both. On occasion, systemic exposure may have a dermal consequence, as in urticarial responses to inhaled antigens, pigmentary alterations from deposition of metals (e.g., silver), and the much-described though rarely seen chloracne, a variant of acne induced by dioxins and related chemicals. Workers who are at increased risk for allergic contact dermatitis include tanners, cast concrete product workers, leather goods workers, footwear workers, machine and metal product assemblers, electrical and telecommunications equipment assemblers, printshop workers, and machine and engine mechanics.[36] There are several excellent texts of occupational skin disease available.[37-39]

Overwhelmingly, the major skin problem in the workplace remains dermatitis, either irritant induced or caused by allergy. Many agents may be responsible, including organic and inorganic chemicals, plastics and rubber, oils and lubricants, metals and construction materials, paints, and coatings. Both allergic dermatitis and irritant-induced dermatitis are more likely to affect persons with atopic conditions, dry skin, or other dermal risk factors. Distinguishing between the two is less important than recognizing occupational precipitants in the first place; both are difficult to differentiate from other commonplace skin disorders, such as eczema. The key to correct diagnosis is the history of skin contact and the temporal relation between contact and manifestations. Unfortunately, there is seldom a perfect or obvious correlation between the two, and some sleuthing is necessary, especially to discern the extent to which chemical contact may spread to places like the groin or areas where hand contact occurs. Airborne exposure may cause lesions in apparently untouched areas, such as the face, a sign of likely hypersensitivity. Vexingly, symptoms do not always abate dramatically over weekends or short periods in which exposure is avoided, so that removing the patient from the toxin for a week or two may be necessary to observe response; combined with observation of the patient during reexposure, this is often the most valuable diagnostic test. Patch testing, performed by an experienced clinician aware of the exposures of concern, may be useful in difficult cases, though the clinician should keep in mind that irritants may yield false negative results and that even many healthy atopic persons will react to common contactants, such as nickel. Often, complete isolation from offending agents is economically infeasible, and materials that previously were well tolerated become sources of irritation and exacerbation. Combinations of work modification, aggressive treatment of flares and complications, and careful attention to routine skin care are necessary to control disease.

DISORDERS OF THE URINARY TRACT

Although there are innumerable toxins known to cause acute injury to the kidney, exposures to chemical and physical agents at concentrations extant in the workplace rarely cause such effects (exceptions include cases involving overwhelming accidental overexposure or ingestion). Of far greater concern are recurring exposures to agents at more typical workplace dose levels that have subclinical effects but can lead to late nephropathy. Although there remains a vast burden of unexplained nephropathology in the population and despite epidemiologic data suggesting an occupational cause,[40,41] chronic renal injury resulting from workplace exposures remains poorly characterized.

The best-established effects on the urinary tract are those caused by exposure to heavy metals, especially lead, mercury, and cadmium; each of these metals is associated with a unique pattern of effects. Workers whose jobs entail exposure to lead include traffic police, hazardous-waste incineration workers, industrial workers, and furniture strippers; workers at risk for exposure to mercury include goldmine workers, workers at chlor-alkali plants, workers exposed to hazardous waste, and construction workers; workers at risk for exposure to cadmium include those involved in the manufacture of batteries. Long-standing heavy lead exposure results in a pattern of injury difficult to distinguish pathologically and clinically from the effects of hypertension; signs and symptoms include nephrosclerosis and evidence of both glomerular and tubular defects. The ability to clear urate is impaired early in the course and may be a clue; saturnine gout may occur a decade later. There is debate about the possibility that low-level or brief exposures to lead may predispose to hypertension or that such exposures may enhance the degree of renal injury associated with essential hypertension or gout.[42,43] Proponents of this view stress the importance of assessment of lead exposure in patients with mild chronic renal insufficiency.[44]

Chronic occupational exposure to inorganic mercury—principally through exposure to mercury vapor—may result in renal alterations involving the tubules and glomeruli. The monitoring of urinary mercury is useful for controlling such risk.[45]

Cadmium exposure in jewelry making, battery production, and other metal-processing operations leads to bioaccumulation of cadmium in the kidney, which results in proximal tubular injury with excessive excretion of β_2-microglobulin and other tubular proteins. Later, a pattern of renal tubular acidosis may occur, with renal insufficiency developing late. Since the condition is only partially reversible,[46] the key is to carefully monitor cadmium exposure, which is best done with regular blood and urine cadmium testing.[47] Renal damage can occur at relatively low levels of cadmium exposure.[48]

The role of organic solvents in renal tubular and renal parenchymal injury remains uncertain.[49] The growing evidence, however, suggests evaluation of all new cases of unexplained nephropathy.

LIVER DISEASE

The liver is highly sensitive to effects of numerous organic and inorganic substances used in the workplace [see Table 1]. Despite the impressive potential for harm, often at exposure levels not uncommon in the workplace, occupational liver diseases are rarely recognized except during outbreaks. This is almost certainly because the clinical presentation is nonspecific, most often consisting of unsuspected elevations of hepatocellular enzymes occasionally associated with mild gastrointestinal symptoms. The single exception to this is the now extremely rare vascular disorder resembling veno-occlusive disease caused by vinyl chloride.

The more common hepatic effects of occupational hazards—steatosis and nonspecific hepatocellular injury—have numerous causes and are prevalent in the general population; a given case may be readily attributed to infection, alcohol use, drug toxicity, biliary tract disease, diabetes, obesity, or weight change. When persistent elevations of hepatic enzymes prompt more extensive workup with radiographic studies and biopsy, results rarely provide specific evidence of an occupational cause. Only high suspicion of a workplace culprit, combined with evidence of exposure to a suspect agent, serves to distinguish etiology.

CENTRAL AND PERIPHERAL NERVOUS SYSTEMS

Most pesticides,[50,51] organic solvents,[52] and many metals[53] are neurotoxic at doses that may be seen in the workplace [see Table 1]. A handful of other chemicals used in plastics, lubricating fluids, and chemical operations also have neurotoxicity, most usually relevant after accidental or unusual exposures. In addition, persons exposed to asphyxiants, such as carbon monoxide and cyanide, may present with acute or recurring central nervous system symptoms. Both acute and late effects may occur—the former typically occurring immediately after an intense exposure, the latter often after prolonged periods of exposure. Importantly, the late or chronic effects usually result from prolonged periods of bioaccumulation or recurrent mild or subclinical acute exposures or as sequelae of acute intoxication. A direct consequence of this toxicologic fact is that neurotoxicity almost invariably presents during the time of occupational exposure to the offending agent and not long afterward, as may occur with carcinogenic substances or dusts causing pneumoconiosis.

Because of the extraordinarily diverse range of clinical symptoms that may herald CNS toxicity, including subtle changes in cognitive and affective function, the evaluation of suspected cases follows the general principles for all occupational disease, with increased attention given to recent exposures. The acute disorders usually occur as mild alterations of CNS function, often with associated GI or other systemic effects; they are often recurrent, cycling with periods of work exposure, as might be seen in a painter (through exposure to solvents) or pest-control operator. The key to recognition is the temporal pattern, with remission of symptoms occurring over a course of time consistent with the metabolism of the toxin. There may also be evidence of symptoms associated with withdrawal, similar to the effects associated with ethyl alcohol. For the subacute and chronic effects, the key to diagnosis is identification of evidence of substantial exposure occurring over a course of time consistent with an evolving neurotoxic picture. None of the neurologic disorders appear to involve allergy or idiosyncrasy; thus, the doses of exposure involved must be substantive.

In many cases, the exposure to the agent can be biologically confirmed with measurement of urine or blood metal levels, measurement of cholinesterase levels, or identification of a metabolite of an organic chemical in urine. There may also be some clinical or pathophysiologic clues. For example, the constellation of cerebellar ataxia, personality change, and salivary gland hypersecretion should prompt consideration of inorganic mercurialism, possibly with associated renal effects. An asymmetrical motor neuropathy should always raise the specter of lead poisoning. Insidious symmetrical distal sensory neuropathies, on the other hand, are far more common with solvents and acrylamide; electrophysiologic or pathologic evaluation reveals almost pure axonal degeneration, with minimal secondary demyelination, an important differential feature. Highly localized neuropathies, either unilateral or bilateral, should raise the possibility of a compressive etiology, not uncommon with repetitive work activities [see Musculoskeletal Disorders, below].

Although diagnosis may be straightforward once the possibility of a workplace agent is considered, management remains challenging. Treatment of acute disorders involves ending the exposure and providing support where clinically necessary. Several hazards, such as certain cholinesterase inhibitors and cyanide, have specific antidotes that should be administered under medical supervision. The subacute and chronic conditions all require removal from further exposure. In addition, patients with heavy metal exposure may be given chelation therapy when signs and symptoms of severe intoxication are evident; this, too, must be done under very close supervision in view of the risk of enhancing CNS effects early in treatment. Moreover, the possibility of rebound effects from reequilibration of metal into the nervous system must be anticipated when chelation is stopped. Most important, whatever strategy is chosen, physician and patient must be aware that the prognosis for full recovery from all but the most acute effects is somewhat guarded. Axons regrow very slowly, and higher integrative functions, such as affective or cognitive functions of the CNS, resolve even more slowly or not completely. Early efforts at functional rehabilitation, as may be used for trauma or stroke patients, are indicated when impairments limit work or other major life activities.

Possibly the most challenging situation in occupational neurology is the worker who presents with CNS-related complaints that exhibit a temporal pattern consistent with a workplace origin but who does not have substantial exposure to neurotoxic agents. Such symptoms are a common part of the so-called sick-building syndrome, now referred to as nonspecific building-related illness, and are universal among persons who have acquired intolerance to low levels of chemicals (multiple chemical sensitivities).[54] It is important to recognize early that these syndromes are different from the neurotoxic disorders discussed above in approach to evaluation, in prognosis, and in treatment. They are discussed more fully later in this chapter [see Clinical Problems Associated with Low-Level Environmental Exposures, below].

MUSCULOSKELETAL DISORDERS

There has been a marked increase in the awareness of the role that work factors play in musculoskeletal disorders, ranging from such well-defined clinical problems as arthropathies and nerve compression syndromes to the less well characterized ailments causing pain of the trunk and extremities.[55,56] In developed countries, such disorders account for billions of dollars of costs in medical care and lost productivity. The overwhelming bulk of this epidemic relates to suspected consequences of physical stressors and trauma that occur at work. The reader should be reminded, though, that a number of systemic occupational disorders may also have expression in the muscles, bones, joints, and connective tissues; important examples of such disorders are the arthralgias and gouty consequences of lead intoxication, bony pain in association with systemic fluorosis, and the apparent increased risk of scleroderma in miners.[57]

It is clinically useful to divide potential occupational musculoskeletal disorders into those that have a well-defined anatomic structure of involvement, such as carpal tunnel syndrome, and those that lack such a clear-cut pattern, such as low back pain.[58-60] Although there are extensive data suggesting that physical aspects of work, such as overall force, repetition, awkward posture, and vibration, contribute in a cumulative fashion to the development of both localizable and nonspecific symptomatology, the approach to diagnosis and treatment is somewhat different for each. There is also evidence that factors other than physical strain, such as work stress, work fatigue, and adverse relationships in the workplace, may be important contributory factors, partially explaining high rates of musculoskeletal disorders among certain white-collar workers.[61,62]

For the new onset of disorders involving the trunk or extremities, or for such disorders that are clinically mild, the initial approach should be short-term palliation with minimal workup. Rest from physically demanding tasks, use of nonsteroidal anti-inflammatory drugs (NSAIDs) or other nonnarcotic pain relievers, reassurance, and follow-up in a few days are suggested; further evaluation is indicated only if suggested by physical findings. If conservative steps fail to alleviate symptoms rapidly, additional examination and laboratory evaluation may be appropriate to rule out an anatomically discrete lesion that could be amenable to treatment. Where specific lesions are identified, such as compression of a nerve or disk or tenosynovial inflammation, longer-term efforts at elimination of strain in the affected region combined with anti-inflammatory drugs or other therapies are appropriate, followed by surgical intervention should these fail. In such cases, it is crucial to remember that the work-related stressors that caused the problem will complicate recovery unless they are modified.[63-65]

The most perplexing problem is management of patients whose complaints cannot be specifically localized by physical examination or, when necessary, electrophysiologic or radiologic evaluation. Such complaints are no less real than those that are more readily understood and treated. Modification of work activities is often necessary but rarely sufficient to resolve the problem. Pain may be persistent and refractory to treatment, and the value of physical therapy or pain medications is questionable. Rather, it is important for the treating physician to establish early that the symptoms are troublesome but not the result of a progressive process and that the patient may have to adapt to them despite discomfort. Expectation of cure often leads to unnecessary treatment, prolonged (and clinically unhelpful) loss of work time, and, ultimately, frustration on the part of the employer, insurance company, patient, and physician.

HEMATOLOGIC DISORDERS

A host of disturbances of red cell function, survival, and production have been attributed to workplace exposures, including acute, subacute, and chronic processes [see Table 1]. Effects involving other cell lines have seldom been reported and will not be discussed. In clinical practice, the biggest concerns are the risk of acute hemolysis in workers exposed to nitrogen-containing oxidant chemicals in pharmaceutical, chemical, and explosives manufacture; the effects of lead, which remains ubiquitous in the work environment; and the potential for solvent-induced marrow injury. The problem of oxidant stressors is somewhat difficult. Although workers with marked deficiency of glucose-6-phosphate dehydrogenase (G6PD) should probably be excluded from significant contact with such chemicals, there is not a clear relation between any of the measurable enzyme levels and risk. It is prudent to periodically screen all exposed workers for subclinical evidence of hemolysis, as well as for subclinical accumulation of methemoglobin, which is often induced by the same agents; workers who show evidence of early effects should probably be removed from harm's way, irrespective of identifiable factors.[66]

The hematologic effects of lead are widely misunderstood.[67,68] Although there is a dose-related inhibition of heme synthetase by lead that can be readily quantified by determining the accumulation of the precursor protoporphyrin (usually measured as whole blood zinc protoporphyrin), this biochemical effect of lead on blood hemoglobin or hematocrit is minimal until very high levels are reached, and there is almost no impact on red cell volume. In other words, anemia based on hypoproliferation of red cells is very rare, and the absence of anemia should never be used to exclude a role for lead in causing toxicity to organs and systems that are far more sensitive, such as the nervous system and renal tubules. Furthermore, microcytosis can only occasionally be attributed to lead alone; when it is seen, especially in children, it most often signifies coincident iron deficiency. On the other hand, rapid accumulation of lead in acute lead poisoning, typically heralded clinically by the onset of abdominal pain, is almost always associated with evidence of rapid hemolysis; reticulocyte counts are in the range of 5% to 20%. In this setting, the notorious basophilic stipples are frequently seen as well, though they are by no means pathognomonic for lead toxicity. In general, this syndrome will occur only after lead levels have exceeded 60 mg/dl in whole blood. The hemolysis tends to abruptly stop after effective chelation therapy, which is usually indicated in this acute symptomatic form of lead poisoning.

The bone marrow effects of workplace chemicals are only slowly being unraveled, but certain conclusions seem warranted. Benzene, the aromatic constituent of petroleum products, was once widely prevalent in the work environment as a solvent and gasoline component. It can cause hypoplastic injury to the marrow, which may directly progress to a chronic blood dyscrasia (i.e., myelodysplasia or leukemia), or dyscrasia may occur after apparent recovery.[69] In other words, an exposed worker may show depressed cell counts, be removed from the source of toxicity, improve, and years later (possibly long after exposure ceases) develop myelodysplasia or a myeloproliferative syndrome. It is likely that some workers will develop the obviously more serious dyscrasias without direct marrow injury having been recognized while exposure was ongoing. There are no hallmark features of either the hypoplastic state (occurring during ongoing exposure) or the myelodysplastic one (occurring later) that distinguish benzene toxicity from other causes of such disorders; this differentiation depends on the history of substantial benzene exposure, because the disorders are not believed to be idiosyncratic but dose related. Although there is some evidence that a few other solvents, such as the glycol ethers that are widely used in paints and coatings,[70] may cause such injury, the vast majority of solvents, including many benzene congeners such as toluene and xylene, do not appear to have potential for marrow injury. For this reason, most products that formerly contained benzene that are used in developed countries have been modified, and benzene is not used directly except for specific purposes in the manufacture of chemicals and pharmaceuticals. Obviously, exposed persons should be carefully monitored for hematologic effects, which would be clear evidence of overexposure.

ENDOCRINE AND REPRODUCTIVE EFFECTS

Despite an exceptional upsurge in interest in the endocrine-disrupting effects of environmental contaminants, there is little evidence that occupational exposures to chemical hazards cause clinically relevant endocrinopathies in adults.[71] Lead has been shown to impair hypothalamic-pituitary axis secretions and probably testosterone regulation in men heavily exposed, but the clinical relevance of these observations is unclear. Several compounds used in the pharmaceutical industry and other industries have been shown to have estrogenic activity, with predictable clinical consequences in both men and women.

The effects of work on male and female reproduction are a more formidable concern.[5,8] Although data are far from complete because so many chemicals have never been studied adequately, several substances at occupational levels of exposure have been proved to cause decreased sperm counts and infertility, including lead, the pesticides DBCP (1,2-dibromo-3-chloropropane) and ethylene dibromide (EDB), ethylene glycol ethers, and carbon disulfide, as well as heat and ionizing radiation. In addition, a host of other metals, anesthetic agents, and plastic reagents have been shown to cause worrisome gonadal effects in toxicologic experiments on male animals. For this reason, infertile men should be carefully questioned about work exposures and should be observed for signs of improvement for about 9 months (which equals four cycles of spermatogenesis) should suspicion of an occupational cause be entertained.

Female reproduction is harder to study for lack of a single body fluid to analyze and because of the absence of a simple animal model. There is evidence that several common exposures, including waste anesthetic gases, lead, glycol ethers, ethylene oxide, and antineoplastic drugs, have the potential to increase the risk of miscarriage. Lead, organic mercury, polychlorinated biphenyls (PCBs), heat, and ionizing radiation are established teratogens; organic solvents are also suspect, based on animal studies and new epidemiologic reports.[72] Most of the agents that cause human cancer [see Table 3] are considered likely fetal hazards as well. In most cases, there is risk of adverse effects at doses considered acceptable in the workplace, because regulations have not traditionally been developed on the basis of reproductive concern. To a disturbing degree, knowledge of reproductive effects of thousands of additional chemicals is frankly unknown. Even the effects of hard physical work during pregnancy remain unclear, though there is evidence that excessive lifting and standing late in the third trimester may induce prematurity.

With the majority of women of reproductive age now in the workforce, many are questioning the safety of work during pregnancy, and clinicians are being confronted with trade-offs between the fetal risks and the worker's economic security. Although each case must be studied individually, a reasonable guideline is to rigorously protect patients from the established teratogens or ensure the levels of exposure below those established for pregnancy. For others, reasonable steps can be taken to minimize exposure, including job transfer if the patient prefers and the employer has alternative work. For the patient for whom any risk represents an unacceptable psychological impediment, transfer or removal is probably in the best interest of all parties.

CLINICAL PROBLEMS ASSOCIATED WITH LOW-LEVEL ENVIRONMENTAL EXPOSURES

One of the most common problems emerging in developed countries is the constellation of respiratory and systemic complaints that are appearing with increasing frequency in office workers and others in what are traditionally considered safe jobs.[73,74] Typical symptoms of sick-building syndrome, or nonspecific building-related illness, include upper and lower respiratory symptoms, often combined with neurologic problems, such as fatigue, headache, and cognitive deficits, as well as rashes and other nonspecific complaints.[74] Usually, the patient will relate that others in the environment are experiencing similar difficulties and that the symptoms improve when the patient is away from work and return upon reexposure. Although in a minority of cases, investigation may reveal a specific allergy (with asthma, rhinitis, or allergic alveolitis) or a specific hazard (e.g., fibrous glass released from a renovation or ventilation duct, causing pruritus), in the majority of cases, the environment is usually best described as poorly ventilated.[74] At present, there is no specific treatment for this syndrome other than palliative care and reassurance that it is neither progressive nor life threatening.[75,76] Expensive testing of either the patient or the work environment is rarely necessary or beneficial.[74] Ideally, remediation of both should be undertaken as soon as more dire possibilities are excluded by history and a walk-through of the workplace by an industrial hygienist or comparable environmental professional. In the vast majority of cases, improvement of ventilation will result in symptomatic improvement for most workers.[74]

On occasion, a patient in an affected building will start to experience similar discomfort in other situations, such as driving behind a bus, being in a store, or using a perfume or detergent.[54] The net impression is that the patient has become reactive to everything that has an odor. Many also have fatigue or other asthenic symptoms between exposures. Symptoms reminiscent of those in panic disorder may also occur. Dubbed multiple chemical sensitivities (MCS), this disorder is not associated with measurable abnormalities of organ system function but may be highly disabling.[54] Although there are many physical and psychological theories regarding the origin of MCS, present knowledge is limited. Patients do not easily tolerate pharmacologic agents and usually do not respond to treatment for anxiety or depression. Avoidance is equally fruitless, with shorter and more trivial exposures causing problems in those who quit work and minimize human contact. At present, the recommended treatment is supportive care coupled with moderate life modifications to avoid the most provocative exposures while preserving everyday functioning, including work if possible. Unrealistic expectations of cure or remission are as harmful as unwarranted fears of deterioration; neither outcome appears common among patients followed for many years.

Additional Information

An increasing amount of information about occupational safety and health is available on the Internet from the National Institute for Occupational Safety and Health (http://www.cdc.gov/niosh) and the Occupational Safety and Health Administration (http://www.osha.gov). In 1999, NIOSH issued guidelines to reduce the incidence of needle-stick injuries in health care workers[77] and OSHA published a proposed ergonomics standard to help prevent work-related musculoskeletal disorders,[78] among other resources.

References

1. Palmer K, Coggon D: ABC of work related disorders: investigating suspected occupational illness and evaluating the workplace. BMJ 313:809, 1996

2. Encyclopedia of Occupational Health and Safety, 4th ed. Stellman JM, Ed. International Labor Office, Geneva, Switzerland, 1988

3. Maxcy Rosenau Textbook of Public Health and Preventive Medicine, 14th ed. Last WB, Ed. Appleton & Lange, Norwalk, Connecticut, 1998

4. Levy B, Wegman D: Occupational Health: Recognizing and Preventing Work-Related Disease, 4th ed. Lippincott Williams & Wilkins, New York, 1999

5. Occupational and Environmental Reproductive Hazards: A Guide for Clinicians. Paul M, Ed. Williams & Wilkins, Baltimore, 1993

6. Environmental and Occupational Medicine, 2nd ed. Rom WN, Ed. Little, Brown & Co, Boston, 1992

7. Textbook of Clinical Occupational and Environmental Medicine. Rosenstock L, Cullen M, Eds. WB Saunders Co, Philadelphia, 1994

8. Reproductive Hazards of the Workplace. Frazier LM, Hage ML, Eds. John Wiley & Sons, New York, 1998

9. Occupational and Environmental Respiratory Disease. Haber P, Schenker MB, Balmes JR, Eds. Mosby, St. Louis, 1996

10. Workplace injuries and illnesses in 1998. Bureau of Labor Statistics News. USDL 99-358. Washington, DC, 1999

11. Injury Facts, 1999. National Safety Council. Itasca, Illinois, 1999

12. Epstein Y, Albukrek D, Kalmovitc B, et al: Heat intolerance induced by antidepressants. Ann NY Acad Sci 813:553, 1997

13. Tanaka S, Wild DK, Cameron LL, et al: Association of occupational and non-occupational risk factors with the prevalence of self-reported carpal tunnel syndrome in a national survey of the working population. Am J Ind Med 32:550, 1997

14. Lataye R, Campo P: Combined effects of a simultaneous exposure to noise and toluene on hearing function. Neurotoxicol Teratol 19:373, 1997

15. Erren TC, Jacobssen M, Piekarski C: Synergy between asbestos and smoking on lung cancer. Epidemiology 10:405, 1999

16. Lax MB, Grant WD, Manetti FA, et al: Recognizing occupational disease: taking an effective occupational history. Am Fam Physician 58:935, 1998

17. Achanzar WE, Diwan BA, Liu J, et al: Cadmium-induced malignant transformation of human prostate epithelial cells. Cancer Res 61:455, 2001

18. Parent ME, Hua Y, Siemiatycki J: Occupational risk factors for renal cell carcinoma in Montreal. Am J Ind Med 38:609, 2000

19. Baur X, Chen Z, Liebers V: Exposure-response relationships of occupational inhalative allergens. Clin Exp Allergy 28:537, 1998

20. Brooks SM, Bernstein IL: Reactive airways dysfunction syndrome or irritant induced asthma. Asthma in the Workplace. Bernstein IL, Chan-Yeung M, Malo JL, et al, Eds. Marcel Dekker, New York, 1993, p 533

21. Rabatin JT, Cowl CT: A guide to the diagnosis and treatment of occupational asthma. Mayo Clin Proc 76:633, 2001

22. Chan-Yeung M, Malo JL: Occupational asthma. N Engl J Med 333:107, 1995

23. Bernstein DI, Malo JL: High molecular weight agents. Asthma in the Workplace. Bernstein IL, Chan Yeung M, Malo JL, et al, Eds. Marcel Dekker, New York, 1993, p 573

24. Liss GM, Sussman GL: Latex sensitization: occupational versus general population prevalence rates. Am J Ind Med 35:196, 1999

25. Wooding LG, Teuber SS, Gershwin ME: Latex allergy. Compr Ther 22:384, 1996

26. Meredith SK, Bugler J, Clark RL: Isocyanate exposure and occupational asthma: a case-referent study. Occup Environ Med 57:830, 2000

27. Dykewicz MS: Occupational asthma: a practical approach. Allergy Asthma Proc 22:225, 2001

28. Malo JL, Chan-Yeung M: Occupational asthma. J Allergy Clin Immunol 108:317, 2001

29. Grammer LC: Occupational allergic alveolitis. Ann Allergy Asthma Immunol 83:602, 1999

30. Fox J, Anderson H, Moen T, et al: Metal working fluid-associated hypersensitivity pneumonitis: an outbreak investigation and case-control study. Am J Ind Med 35:58, 1999

31. Hoffman RE, Wood RC, Kreiss K: Building-related asthma in Denver office workers. Am J Public Health 83:89, 1993

32. Middleton DC: Chronic beryllium disease: uncommon disease, less common diagnosis. Environ Health Perspect 106:765, 1998

33. Cugell DW: The hard metal diseases. Clin Chest Med 13:269, 1992

34. Kern DG, Crausman RS, Durand KT, et al: Flock worker's lung: chronic interstitial lung disease in the nylon flocking industry. Ann Intern Med 129:261, 1998

35. Davidoff F: New disease, old story. Ann Intern Med 129:327, 1998

36. Kanerva L, Jolanki R, Estlander T, et al: Incidence rates of occupational allergic contact dermatitis caused by metals. Am J Contact Dermat 11:155, 2000

37. Hogan DJ: Occupational Skin Disorders. Igaku-Shoin, New York, 1994

38. Adams R: Occupational Skin Disease, 3rd ed. WB Saunders Co, Philadelphia, 1999

39. Marks JG, DeLeo VA: Contact and Occupational Dermatology, 2nd ed. Mosby, St. Louis, 1997

40. de Broe ME, D'Haese PC, Nuyts GD, et al: Occupational renal diseases. Curr Opin Nephrol Hypertens 5:114, 1996

41. Wedeen RP: Occupational and environmental renal disease. Semin Nephrol 17:46, 1997

42. Batuman V, Landy E, Maesaka JK, et al: Contribution of lead to hypertension with renal impairment. N Engl J Med 309:17, 1983

43. Batuman V, Maesaka JK, Haddad B, et al: The role of lead in gouty nephropathy. N Engl J Med 304:520, 1981

44. Erhlich R, Robins T, Jordaan E, et al: Lead absorption and renal dysfunction in a South African battery factory. Occup Environ Med 55:453, 1998

45. Roels HA, Hoet P, Lison D: Usefulness of biomarkers of exposure to inorganic mercury, lead, or cadmium in controlling occupational and environmental risks of nephrotoxicity. Ren Fail 21:251, 1999

46. Roels HA, Van Assche FJ, Overstseyns M, et al: Reversibility of microproteinuria in cadmium workers with incipient tubular dysfunction after reduction of exposure. Am J Ind Med 31:645, 1997

47. Jarup L, Persson B, Elinder CG: Blood cadmium as an indicator of dose in a long-term follow-up of workers previously exposed to cadmium. Scand J Work Environ Health 23:31, 1997

48. Jarup L, Hellstrom L, Alfven T, et al: Low level exposure to cadmium and early kidney damage: the OSCAR study. Occup Environ Med 57:668, 2000

49. Pai P, Stevenson A, Mason H, et al: Occupational hydrocarbon exposure and nephrotoxicity: a cohort study and literature review. Postgrad Med J 75:225, 1998

50. Jamal GA: Neurological syndromes of organophosphorus compounds. Adverse Drug React Toxicol Rev 16:133, 1997

51. Keifer MC, Mahurin RK: Chronic neurologic effects of pesticide overexposure. Occup Med 12:291, 1997

52. White RF, Proctor SP: Solvents and neurotoxicity. Lancet 349:1239, 1997

53. Manzo L, Artigas F, Martinez E, et al: Biochemical markers of neurotoxicity: a review of mechanistic studies and applications. Hum Exp Toxicol 15(suppl):S20, 1996

54. Cullen MR: Low-level environmental exposures. Textbook of Clinical Occupational and Environmental Medicine. Rosenstock L, Cullen M, Eds. WB Saunders Co, Philadelphia, 1994, p 667

55. Rheumatologic Diseases and the Environment. Kaufman CD, Varga J, Eds. Chapman & Hall, New York, 1996

56. Tanaka S, Petersen M, Cameron L: Prevalence and risk factors of tendinitis and related disorders of the distal upper extremity among U.S. workers: comparison to carpal tunnel syndrome. Am J Ind Med 39:328, 2001

57. Katz JN, Brissot R, Liang MH: Systemic rheumatologic disorders. Textbook of Clinical Occupational and Environmental Medicine. Rosenstock L, Cullen M, Eds. WB Saunders Co, Philadelphia, 1994, p 376

58. Cherniack M: Upper extremity disorders. Textbook of Clinical Occupational and Environmental Medicine. Rosenstock L, Cullen M, Eds. WB Saunders Co, Philadelphia, 1994, p 344

59. Pascarelli EF, Hsu YP: Understanding work-related upper extremity disorders: clinical findings in 485 computer users, musicians, and others. J Occup Rehabil 11:1, 2001

60. Hoogendoorn WE, Bongers PM, de Vet HC, et al: Flexion and rotation of the trunk and lifting at work are risk factors for low back pain: results of a prospective cohort study. Spine 25:3087, 2000

61. Macfarlane GJ, Hunt IM, Silman AJ: Role of mechanical and psychosocial factors in the onset of forearm pain: prospective population based study. BMJ 321:676, 2000

62. Haufler AJ, Feuerstein M, Huang GD: Job stress, upper extremity pain and functional limitations in symptomatic computer users. Am J Ind Med 38:507, 2000

63. Jayson MI: ABC of work related disorders: back pain. BMJ 313:355, 1996

64. Hagberg M: ABC of work related disorders: neck and arm disorders. BMJ 313:419, 1996

65. Buckle PW: Work factors and upper limb disorders. BMJ 315:1360, 1997

66. Luster MI, Wierda D, Rosenthal GJ: Environmentally related disorders of the hematologic and immune systems. Med Clin North Am 74:425, 1990

67. Nelson JC, Westwood M, Allen KR, et al: The ratio of erythrocyte zinc-protoporphyrin to protoporphyrin IX in disease and its significance in the mechanism of lead toxicity on haem synthesis (pt 3). Ann Clin Biochem 35:422, 1998

68. Solliway BM, Schaffer A, Pratt H, et al: Effects of exposure to lead on selected biochemical and haematological variables. Pharmacol Toxicol 78:18, 1996

69. Smith MT: Overview of benzene-induced aplastic anaemia. Eur J Haematol 57:107, 1996

70. Cullen MR, Solomon L, Pace PE, et al: Morphologic, biochemical and cytogenetic studies of bone marrow and circulating blood cells in painters exposed to ethylene glycol ethers. Environ Res 59:250, 1992

71. Cullen MR: Endocrine disorders. Textbook of Clinical Occupational and Environmental Medicine. Rosenstock L, Cullen M, Eds. WB Saunders Co, Philadelphia, 1994, p 442

72. Khattak S, Moghtader GK, McMartin K, et al: Pregnancy outcome following gestational exposure to organic solvents. JAMA 281:12, 1999

73. Seltzer JM: Effects of the indoor environment on health. Occupational Medicine: State of the Art Reviews 10:1, 1995

74. Redlich CA, Sparer JS, Cullen MR: Sick building syndrome. Lancet 349:1013, 1997

75. Husman T: Health effects of indoor-air microorganisms. Scand J Work Environ Health 22:5, 1996

76. Bascom R, Kesavanathan J, Swift DL: Human susceptibility to indoor contaminants. Occup Med 10:119, 1995

77. Preventing needlestick injuries in health care settings. NIOSH Alert. DHHS (NIOSH) Publication 2000-108. Cincinnati, Ohio, 1999

78. Ergonomics Program, Proposed Rule. 64(225) Federal Register 65767-66078 (Nov 23, 1999)

7 Health Advice for International Travelers

Peter F. Weller, M.D.

Pretravel Evaluation and Immunizations

The provision of health advice and the administration of prophylactic measures can help reduce the morbid and, at times, mortal risks of infectious illnesses that may be acquired during international travel. The Centers for Disease Control and Prevention (CDC) annually publishes Health Information for International Travel—available from the United States Government Printing Office, Washington, DC 20402 (202-512-1800)—that provides information on required and recommended vaccinations and malaria prophylaxis as well as general advice.[1] Updated information may be obtained from state public health departments, from local physicians or clinics catering to travelers, from the embassies of individual countries, and from Internet-based advisory services. The CDC has made information readily available on the Internet (http://www.cdc.gov). The Travelers' Health page provides online access to a variety of information sources, including Health Information for International Travel 2000–2001; the weekly Blue Sheet, which updates lists of countries with known cases of cholera and yellow fever; the Green Sheet, which provides reports of cruise-ship sanitation inspections; detailed guidelines on the need for yellow fever immunizations; guidelines on international health issues for travelers by country; recently recognized disease outbreaks; and general guidelines on immunizations and other medical issues for travelers. Even the most up-to-date information sources, however, may not be able to provide precise information on specific diseases prevalent in specific locales, because mechanisms for recognizing and reporting diseases are often lacking in developing areas.

Medical consultation should be obtained at least 1 month before travel to allow time for immunizations [*see Table 1*]. A general medical history should be obtained to define pertinent underlying medical conditions. For instance, splenectomy predisposes a person to more severe malaria, babesiosis, and infections with encapsulated bacteria, including meningococcal infections. A history of allergies to antimicrobial agents or to other components of vaccines should be determined. Knowledge of the duration and purpose of a trip, as well as of the countries and locales to be visited, can help in estimating the risks of exposure to endemic diseases.

REQUIRED IMMUNIZATIONS

The only immunization legally required for entrance into specific countries is that for yellow fever. Although cholera immunization is not officially required for entrance into any country, some local authorities may still require proof of cholera immunization.

Yellow Fever

Yellow fever is endemic and resurgent in equatorial Africa and in areas of South America [*see Figure 1*].[1,2] Persons older than

Table 1   Guidelines for Immunizations for Travelers

	Asia	Eastern Mediterranean, North Africa	Middle East	Sub-Saharan Africa	Pacific Islands	Caribbean, Mexico, Central and South America	North America, Northern and Western Europe, Japan, Australia, New Zealand
Yellow fever				X (some countries)		X (some South American countries)	
Cholera*							
Polio	X	X	X	X	X		
Tetanus/diphtheria	X	X	X	X	X	X	X
Measles (if born after 1957 and not recipient of 2 doses of vaccine)	X	X	X	X	X	X	X
Typhoid	X	X	X	X	X	X	
Rabies (for prolonged visits)	X	X	X	X		X	
Hepatitis A	X	X	X	X	X	X	
Hepatitis B (especially for prolonged visits)	X	X	X	X	X	X	
Meningococci	X (especially Nepal and parts of India)	X (especially North Africa)	X (especially Mecca)	X		X (during outbreaks)	
Japanese encephalitis	X[†]						

*Only if required by a country.
[†]Prolonged visits to some regions.

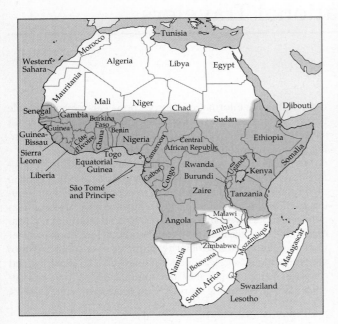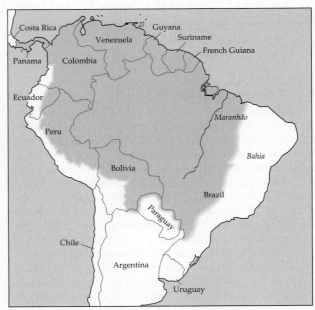

Figure 1   Yellow fever (gray areas) is endemic in parts of Africa (left) and South America (right). Several countries consider these zones infected areas and require an International Certificate of Vaccination against yellow fever from travelers from these zones. The country formerly called Zaire is now the Democratic Republic of Congo.

6 months visiting countries where yellow fever is known to exist should be immunized. In addition, those traveling outside of urban areas in countries that are in the yellow fever endemic zones but are not officially reporting the infection should be immunized because the disease may be underrecognized. Some countries require yellow fever immunizations for entry, especially for persons who have traveled in potentially endemic countries.[1] Yellow fever vaccine, a live virus vaccine grown in chick embryos, is safe and effective. Initially, a single subcutaneous dose of 0.5 ml is given. A booster dose is required every 10 years. Immunizations are available only from designated centers. For those persons allergic to egg proteins, skin testing with yellow fever vaccine may help ascertain whether vaccine can be given safely.[3]

Cholera

Cholera is caused by toxigenic *Vibrio cholerae* groups 01 and 0139. Although the number of cases of cholera seen in the United States has increased in recent years, many of those cases were the result of the illness being imported into the United States by travelers from other countries; tourists from the United States visiting other countries were only rarely infected.[4] In the United States, the only currently available cholera vaccine, prepared from killed bacteria, is only about 50% effective in preventing group 01 cholera for 3 to 6 months and is likely to be ineffective against group 0139 cholera. This parenteral vaccine frequently causes inflammation at the injection site, possibly accompanied by malaise, fever, or headache.[1]

Cholera is acquired by ingestion of contaminated water, ice, or food, including raw or undercooked fish and shellfish. Travelers in endemic regions should be advised of the precautions that minimize risks of acquiring cholera and other enteric infections [*see* Travel-Related Illness, *below*] and of the importance of rehydration in treating cholera. In addition to consuming only boiled or treated water and eating thoroughly cooked food and only fruit they have peeled themselves, travelers should avoid undercooked or raw fish or shellfish, including seviche.

Routine immunization is not recommended for travelers,[1] and cholera vaccination is not required for entry into or exit from any Latin American country or the United States. Currently, no country requires proof of cholera immunization as a condition for entry, and the World Health Organization recommends against such a requirement. Some local authorities, however, may require immunization (to determine local requirements, travelers may consult the embassies of the countries to which they will be traveling); a single 0.5 ml dose administered no more than 6 months before entry satisfies this requirement. Booster doses are needed after 6 months. Full primary immunization, however, requires two doses, 0.5 ml each, administered subcutaneously or intramuscularly at least 1 week apart and is reserved for persons at special risk, such as individuals who have achlorhydria—including those on antacid therapy and those who have had ulcer surgery—or individuals visiting highly endemic areas where sanitation is poor [*see* Chapter 135].

Cholera vaccine is not recommended for children younger than 6 months. Primary and booster doses are 0.2 ml each for children 6 months to 4 years of age, 0.3 ml each for children 5 to 10 years of age, and 0.5 ml each for children older than 10 years; all doses should be administered subcutaneously or intramuscularly. Cholera vaccine and yellow fever vaccine should be administered at least 3 weeks apart, if possible, because there are suggestions that simultaneous administration of cholera and yellow fever vaccines impairs responses to both vaccines. If a 3-week interval is not possible, administration within the time available before travel is advised.[1] Travelers who may be at risk for cholera and who may be in areas far removed from medical care should take with them packets of oral rehydration salts. Antimicrobial agents often employed for therapy for traveler's diarrhea, such as ciprofloxacin, are usually very effective in helping terminate cholera infections.[5]

Poliomyelitis

Travelers to countries in which polio is endemic or in which there is a current epidemic are at risk for the disease and should

be immunized. Countries considered to be free of wild poliovirus are all countries in the Americas, Australia, New
Zealand, Japan, and most European countries.[1,6] Polio transmission continues in developing countries of Asia, Africa, Eastern
Europe, and the Middle East, although efforts are ongoing in all
regions to achieve the global eradication of polio. Travelers who
have been immunized previously should receive one booster
dose of polio vaccine. Patients with an altered immune status
should receive inactivated vaccine. Oral live virus vaccine
should be avoided in those with altered immune status, and oral
live virus vaccine is no longer recommended for immunizations
in the United States.[7] Children who have not been immunized
should receive a full series of immunizations with inactivated
polio vaccine. Adults who have not been immunized should receive a series of three doses of enhanced-potency inactivated
vaccine.[1] The inactivated vaccine is preferred to avoid the small
risk of paralytic disease from the oral vaccine. If there is insufficient time before travel for at least three doses of inactivated vaccine to be given at intervals of 1 to 2 months, the following alternatives are recommended.[1] If less than 1 month is available before travel, a single dose of inactivated vaccine is given. If
between 1 and 2 months is available before travel, two doses of
inactivated vaccine are administered 4 weeks apart. Travelers
who were incompletely immunized previously should receive
the remaining required doses of vaccine.

Tetanus and Diphtheria

A tetanus-diphtheria booster should be administered every 10
years [see Chapter 136].[1] Older persons and women are more likely to lack the tetanus and diphtheria antibodies and thus are
more likely to require boosters.[8,9]

Measles

Because of the declining prevalence of measles in the United
States, disease imported by immigrants and by returning residents accounts for an increasing proportion of cases in this country. Measles may be acquired during travel in developed countries, including those in Europe, as well as in less developed
countries.[10] Most persons who were born before 1957 are immune
because of natural exposure and do not require vaccination. Persons who were born after 1956 who either have not been immunized or were immunized before 1980 and who have neither serologic evidence of infection nor a history of physician-diagnosed
measles should be immunized with a single subcutaneous dose
of measles vaccine before travel. Measles vaccine is contraindicated for both pregnant and immunodeficient patients. HIV-infected
patients, unless they are severely immunocompromised, should
be immunized before travel because measles can be severe and
even fatal in persons with HIV infection.[1,11]

Typhoid

Salmonella typhi infection is prevalent in many areas of Asia,
Africa, and Latin America. Although foreign travel has accounted for an increasing proportion of typhoid cases in the United
States, the risk of acquiring typhoid during travel remains low
(2.3 cases per million travelers).[12]

The risk has been greater for those traveling to the Indian subcontinent (812 cases per million travelers) but has not been
markedly elevated for travelers to Southeast Asia or sub-Saharan
Africa. Because infection is acquired from contaminated food or
water, typhoid vaccine is recommended for persons traveling to
areas off the usual tourist itinerary and to areas that have typhoid

epidemics. Three vaccines are available for typhoid. The oldest
vaccine, Typhoid Vaccine USP, Wyeth (Wyeth-Ayerst), is a parenteral vaccine prepared from heat-killed and phenol-killed bacteria. With this parenteral vaccine, primary immunization consists of two subcutaneous doses, 0.5 ml each, given 4 or more
weeks apart; for children younger than 10 years, two doses of
0.25 ml each are given. If there is insufficient time for the two doses to be administered 4 or more weeks apart, three doses of vaccine in the same recommended volume can be given at weekly
intervals. Booster doses are required every 3 years. This parenteral vaccine does not offer complete protection and often causes
discomfort at the injection site and febrile reactions.

The second typhoid vaccine, an oral vaccine (Vivotif Berna),
uses the attenuated Ty21a strain of S. typhi and is at least as effective as the parenteral vaccine but does not cause the local and systemic side effects frequently produced by the older, parenteral
vaccine.[13,14] The oral vaccine is supplied as a packet of four enteric-
coated capsules that must be refrigerated. Patients need explicit
guidance on refrigerating the vaccine because failure to do so
might compromise its efficacy.[14,15] At least 2 weeks before departure, the traveler takes one capsule every other day until all four
capsules have been taken. Because mefloquine and antibiotics inhibit the growth in vitro of S. typhi strains, including Ty21a, it is
prudent to separate the oral administrations of mefloquine and
antibiotics and of Ty21a vaccine by 24 hours.[1] It is recommended
that a booster dose of Ty21a vaccine, consisting of four capsules
taken on alternate days, be given every 5 years to persons who
continue to be at risk for exposure to typhoid. The safety of the
oral vaccine has not been established for patients with deficient
humoral or cell-mediated immunity, and thus, patients with congenital or acquired immunodeficiencies should not receive it.

The most recent typhoid vaccine is a capsular polysaccharide vaccine for parenteral use (Typhim Vi, Pasteur
Mérieux/Connaught). Primary vaccination consists of one I.M.
dose of 0.5 ml. The vaccine is well tolerated and, like the other
two vaccines, protects 50% to 80% of recipients.[1,16] This vaccine
is safe for immunocompromised persons, including HIV-infected patients.[1] The only contraindication is a history of serious reactions to the vaccine. It may be given to children 2 years
of age and older.

Rabies

Rabies vaccine, either human diploid cell rabies vaccine
(HDCV) or rabies vaccine adsorbed (RVA), is an inactivated viral preparation. Preexposure vaccination with rabies vaccine is
not indicated for most travelers but should be considered for
persons who anticipate contact with wild animals or who are
living for a month or more where rabies is endemic. Dog rabies
is present in most countries of Asia, Africa, and Central and
South America and is prevalent in parts of Mexico, El Salvador,
Guatemala, Colombia, Ecuador, Peru, India, Nepal, the Philippines, Sri Lanka, Thailand, and Vietnam.[1] Preexposure immunization does not eliminate the need for postexposure treatment
but abbreviates its course and eliminates the need to administer
rabies immune globulin. Only HDCV may be administered intradermally, but chloroquine phosphate and, possibly, mefloquine may interfere with the antibody response to the intradermally administered vaccine.[1] Intradermal administration of
0.1 ml of vaccine on days 0, 7, and 21 or 28 should be completed
1 month before initiation of chloroquine phosphate or mefloquine. Alternatively, three I.M. doses, 1 ml each, of either
HDCV or RVA vaccine may be administered on days 0, 7, and

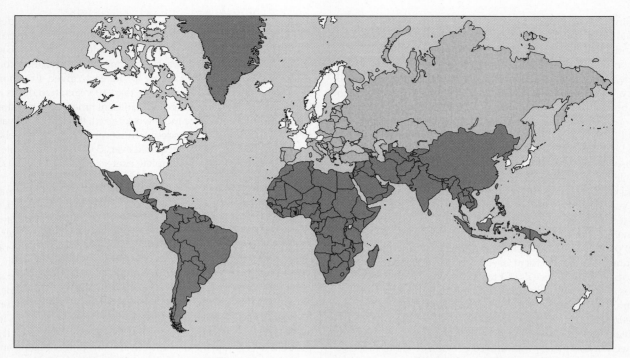

Figure 2   **The prevalence of hepatitis A is high in those countries shaded blue, intermediate in those shaded gray, and low in the white areas of the map.**

21 or 28; chloroquine phosphate does not interfere with the antibody response to vaccine given by this route.[1]

Plague

Vaccination against plague is not indicated for most travelers.[1] Vaccination is reserved for those with a high probability of exposure in rural upland areas of South America, Africa, and Asia, including persons who will have direct contact with rodents or rabbits and those who will live in these areas.

Typhus

Typhus vaccine is no longer made in the United States and is not indicated for most travelers.[1]

Hepatitis A

Immunization for hepatitis A has usually been recommended for travelers to developing countries who are going outside the usual tourist routes or who are planning to stay for longer than 3 months.[1] Hepatitis A is prevalent in many less-developed countries [*see Figure 2*] and is the most common preventable infection acquired by travelers. In visitors to developing countries, even those staying in luxury hotels, the incidence of hepatitis A in unprotected travelers is about 3 per 1,000 travelers per month of stay, and this rate rises to 20 per 1,000 travelers per month for those eating or drinking under poor hygienic conditions.[17] Although hepatitis A has previously been prevented solely by the administration of immune globulin, two inactivated vaccines have been introduced for hepatitis A. Havrix (SmithKline Beecham) and VAQTA (Merck) have proved safe and highly effective.[18,19] For adults, two I.M. 1.0 ml doses should be administered in the deltoid muscle at 0 and 6 to 12 months. For persons between 2 and 18 years of age, two doses, 0.5 ml each, should be administered at 0 and 6 to 12 months. For travelers allergic to vaccine components or who opt not to receive the vaccine, immune globulin should be administered. Administration of immune globulin should begin

shortly before departure in a dose of 2.0 ml I.M. for adults (1.0 ml for patients weighing 23 to 45 kg; 0.5 ml for those weighing less than 23 kg). If the stay is to be longer than 3 months, the adult dose is 5.0 ml (2.5 ml for patients weighing 23 to 45 kg; 1.0 ml for those weighing less than 23 kg). If the duration of stay is prolonged, the latter dosage schedule should be repeated every 4 to 6 months. Immune globulin should be given at least 2 weeks after measles, mumps, or rubella live virus vaccines. Conversely, these vaccines should be given at least 3 months after immune globulin. Immune globulin does not interfere with the immune response to killed virus vaccines or to yellow fever or live polio vaccines.

Because immune globulin has been in limited supply and because the hepatitis A vaccine has proved highly effective against hepatitis A infection, which is frequent in travelers, immunization with hepatitis A vaccine has become the principal approach for preventing hepatitis A infection in travelers.

Hepatitis B

The risk to travelers of acquiring hepatitis B is generally low, compared with the risk of acquiring hepatitis A. The risk increases, however, in regions where hepatitis B is highly prevalent [*see Figure 3*], if there is contact with blood or bodily secretions, if sexual contact with infected persons occurs, or if travel is prolonged.[1] Immunization for hepatitis B, recommended for all persons who work in health care fields with potential exposure to human blood, is especially important for traveling medical workers in countries with high or intermediate hepatitis B endemicity. Hepatitis B immunization should be considered for those residing for more than 6 months in regions where hepatitis B is endemic and for those with potential contact with blood, with potential sexual contact, or with potential need for medical or dental procedures. The available recombinant hepatitis B vaccines are safe and efficacious, and there are no contraindications, including pregnancy and immunosuppression, for administration of these vaccines. The two vaccines, Recombivax HB (Merck) and

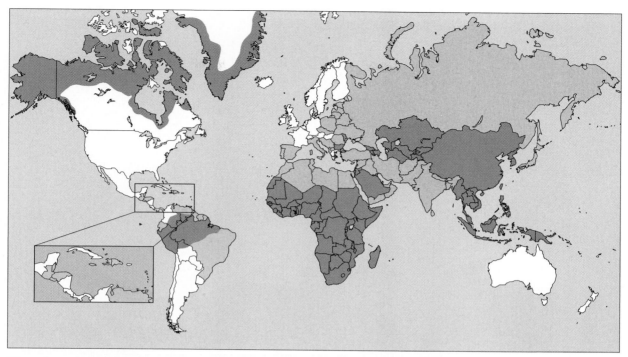

Figure 3 **Hepatitis B is highly endemic in those countries shaded blue (prevalence > 8%). Those regions shaded gray, where the prevalence is 2% to 7%, are considered to be of intermediate endemicity. The prevalence of hepatitis is less than 2% in the white areas of the map.**

Engerix-B (SmithKline Beecham), are administered in three I.M. doses: initially and 1 month and 6 months after the first dose. Engerix-B may also be given in four doses: initially and 1 month, 2 months, and 12 months after the first dose. Immunization should start 6 months before travel, but if this schedule is not feasible, some protection is afforded by one or two doses administered before travel. Full protection will be achieved by completion of the three-dose or four-dose schedule.[1]

Meningococcal Disease

Although acquisition of meningococcal disease is uncommon in travelers from the United States, immunization should be considered for travelers to areas with recognized epidemics or to regions where such disease is hyperendemic, especially if prolonged contact with the local populace is anticipated. Epidemics of meningococcal disease are frequent in the area of sub-Saharan Africa extending from Guinea in the west to Ethiopia in the east [*see Figure 4*]. Vaccination against meningococcal disease is legally required only for pilgrims who make the hajj to Mecca, Saudi Arabia. Routine immunization is also indicated for those who have either deficiencies of terminal complement components or functional or anatomic asplenia. The currently available quadrivalent vaccine is composed of meningococcal polysaccharides from *Neisseria meningitidis* serogroups A, C, Y, and W-135. A single 0.5 ml subcutaneous dose of vaccine is administered to both adults and children and will induce an antibody response in 10 to 14 days.[1]

Japanese Encephalitis

Japanese encephalitis, an arboviral infection transmitted by mosquitoes, may occur in epidemics during the late summer and autumn in northern tropical areas and temperate regions of Bangladesh, Cambodia, China, India, Korea, Laos, Myanmar (Burma), Nepal, Thailand, Vietnam, and the eastern areas of the former Soviet Union. The risk of acquiring infection is lower in endemic regions, including tropical areas of Indonesia, Malaysia, the Philippines, Singapore, Sri Lanka, Taiwan, southern India, and Thailand, where transmission occurs year-round. The disease rarely occurs in Hong Kong or Japan. Persons at highest risk are those who live for extended periods in endemic or epidemic areas. The risk for short-term travelers to urban centers is low, and in temperate countries, the risk for travelers to either an urban or a rural area is negligible during the winter.

Although Japanese encephalitis is highly uncommon, prevention is important for those traveling specifically to epidemic or endemic areas [*see Table 2*] because the risk of serious neurologic sequelae is high. Exposure to mosquitoes should be minimized by the use of insect repellents, protective clothing, and mosquito screens. Also, vaccination should be considered for persons traveling during summer monsoon months, for those visiting rural areas, and for those planning to stay more than 1 month in urban or rural areas.

Vaccination is not usually recommended for travelers to Singapore or Hong Kong, urban Japan or China, or high-altitude regions in Nepal. An effective formalin inactivated vaccine (JE-Vax, Connaught) has been licensed by the Food and Drug Administration. Primary immunization for persons older than 3 years consists of three doses, 1 ml each, administered subcutaneously on days 0, 7, and 30. A booster dose of 1 ml may be administered after 3 years. Allergic reactions, including urticaria, angioedema, and anaphylaxis, have developed in about 1 in every 1,000 recipients; at times, the onset of allergic reaction is delayed for hours or even days after vaccine administration.[1,20,21]

VACCINE CONTRAINDICATIONS

Vaccines that contain live attenuated viruses (i.e., oral polio, measles, mumps, rubella, or yellow fever vaccines) should not

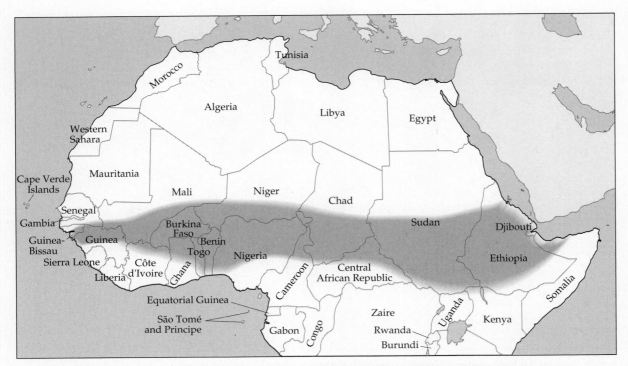

Figure 4 Epidemics of meningococcal disease are frequent in the area of sub-Saharan Africa that extends from Guinea in the west to Ethiopia in the east. The country formerly called Zaire is now the Democratic Republic of Congo.

be given to pregnant women or to persons who have known or potential immunodeficiencies—including leukemia, lymphoma, or a generalized malignant disorder—and those receiving corticosteroids, alkylating agents, antimetabolites, or irradiation. Oral polio vaccine should not be given to a patient if an immunodeficient person resides in the same household.[22] If a pregnant woman cannot defer travel to areas of high risk for yellow fever, yellow fever vaccine may be given.[23] For travelers infected with HIV, immunization with live oral polio and attenuated oral typhoid vaccines should be avoided in favor of killed parenteral vaccines. The risks of live yellow fever vaccine have not been defined for HIV-infected persons, but persons with asymptomatic HIV infection who cannot avoid exposure in areas endemic for yellow fever should be offered the choice of immunization.[1] Because measles can be severe in patients with HIV, measles immunization should be provided, unless the patient is severely immunocompromised.[11]

Contraindications to vaccination also include hypersensitivity to components of the vaccine. Neomycin is present in some vaccines. Persons who have immediate hypersensitivity reactions to neomycin or to preservative agents should avoid vaccines containing these substances. Yellow fever vaccine, which contains significant amounts of egg antigens, may be contraindicated in patients who have allergic reactions to egg proteins. In general, there is a poor correlation between a history of egg sensitivity and skin-test reactivity to egg antigen. The most reliable predictor of reactions to egg-containing vaccines is skin testing with the vaccine itself.[3] If travel plans cannot be changed, persons who have positive skin tests or known egg hypersensitivity (i.e., urticaria, oropharyngeal swelling, bronchospasm, or hypotension) should be given a letter documenting the contraindication to immunization and obtain a waiver from the embassy of any country requiring yellow fever immunization.

Malaria Chemoprophylaxis

The provision of appropriate malaria chemoprophylaxis is the most important preventive measure for travelers to malarious areas. Several hundred United States civilians contract malaria each year,[1] and infections from *Plasmodium falciparum* are potentially lethal and do cause deaths in travelers [*see Chapter 156*].[24] Morbidity and mortality are largely avoidable with chemoprophylaxis. Malaria is prevalent in parts of Mexico, Haiti, Central and South America, Africa, the Middle East, Turkey, the Indian subcontinent, Southeast Asia, China, the Malay archipelago, and Oceania. Chloroquine-resistant *P. falciparum* (CRPF) malaria occurs in many areas [*see Table 3*] and is becoming more prevalent [*see Figure 5*]. Details on prevalence by country of both malaria and CRPF malaria are reported annually.[1] Because even brief exposure to infected mosquitoes can produce malaria, travel in malarious regions, no matter how brief, mandates the use of chemoprophylaxis. When uncertainty exists over the need for chemoprophylaxis, it should be initiated. If a traveler can ascertain that malaria is not a risk after arriving in an area, prophylaxis can be terminated as long as further travel into malarious areas is not planned.

Travelers should be advised that it is possible to acquire malaria despite prophylaxis and regardless of the prophylactic regimen used. Symptoms can begin as early as 8 days after infection or as late as several months after departure from a malarious area. Travelers should be cautioned to seek medical attention promptly for any febrile illness and to inform the physician of their itinerary. The wisdom of general protective measures against mosquito bites should also be stressed, particularly for travelers to Africa. Because the vector mosquitoes usually feed at night, it is advisable to diminish exposure between dusk and dawn by remaining in screened areas; using mosquito netting, ideally treated with permethrin; covering exposed skin with clothing; and using insect repellent.

The most effective insect repellents contain *N,N*-diethyl-*m*-toluamide (DEET). DEET is available in many products in concentrations ranging from 25% to more than 75% and repels mosquitoes, ticks, fleas, and biting flies. Protection lasts for several hours but is shortened by losses from swimming, washing, rainfall, sweating, and wiping. Long-acting formulations, which contain polymer to limit the losses of DEET that result from dermal absorption and evaporation, are being used in the military. The absorption of DEET through the skin can cause such adverse reactions as dermatitis, allergic reactions, and neurotoxicity. Several precautions should be taken to minimize the potential for such adverse reactions: the repellent should be applied sparingly to clothing and exposed skin only; products with a high concentration of DEET should not be applied to the skin, especially of children; the repellent should not contact wounds or irritated skin, which could enhance absorption; and the product should be ap-

plied carefully to avoid introducing it into the eyes and to prevent inhalation or ingestion. Clothing and bed netting can also be treated with permethrin for protection against mosquitoes and ticks.[25] Treated clothing will effectively repel mosquitoes for more than 1 week even with washing and field use. Permethrin is available, often in outdoor supply stores, as a nonstaining aerosol clothing spray (Permanone Tick Repellent).

CHEMOPROPHYLACTIC AGENTS

Chloroquine

The first-line chemoprophylactic agent for malaria is chloroquine, given as either chloroquine phosphate (Aralen) or hydroxychloroquine sulfate (Plaquenil).[1] Chloroquine phosphate, 500 mg (300 mg of chloroquine base), or hydroxychloroquine sulfate, 400 mg (310 mg of hydroxychloroquine base), should be

Table 2 Risk of Japanese Encephalitis by Country, Region, and Season

Country	Affected Areas	Transmission Season
Australia	Islands of Torres Strait	Probably year-round transmission
Bangladesh	Few data, probably widespread	Possibly July through December
Bhutan	No data	No data
Brunei	Presumed to be sporadic; endemic, as in Malaysia	Presumed year-round transmission
Myanmar (Burma)	Presumed to be endemic; hyperendemic countrywide	Presumed to be May through October
Cambodia	Presumed to be endemic; hyperendemic countrywide	Presumed to be May through October
Hong Kong	Rare cases in new territories	April through October
India	Reported cases from many states	South India: May through October in Goa, October through January in Tamil Nadu, and August through December in Karnataka Andhra Pradesh: September through December North India: July through December
Indonesia	Kalimantan, Bali, Nusa Tenggara, Sulawesi, Mollucas, West Irian, Java, and Lombok	Probably year-round risk (varies by island); peak risks associated with rainfall, rice cultivation, and presence of pigs Peak periods of risk are November through March and, in some years, June through July
Japan	Rare, sporadic cases on all islands, except Hokkaido	June through September; Ryukyu Islands (Okinawa), April through October
Korea	Sporadic in South Korea; endemic with occasional outbreaks	July through October
Laos	Presumed to be endemic; hyperendemic countrywide	Presumed to be May through October
Malaysia	Sporadic; endemic in all states of Malay Peninsula, Sarawak, and probably Sabah	No seasonal pattern; year-round transmission
Nepal	Hyperendemic in southern lowlands	July through December
People's Republic of China	Hyperendemic in southern China; periodically epidemic in temperate areas	Northern China: May through September Southern China: April through October
Pakistan	May be transmitted in central deltas	Presumed to be June through January
Philippines	Presumed to be endemic on all islands	Uncertain
Russia	Far eastern maritime areas south of Khabarovsk	Peak period July through September
Singapore	Rare cases	Year-round transmission; April peak
Sri Lanka	Endemic in all but mountainous areas; periodically epidemic in northern and central provinces	October through January; secondary peak of enzootic transmission May through June
Taiwan	Endemic, sporadic cases island-wide	April through October; June peak
Thailand	Hyperendemic in north; sporadic, endemic in south	May through October
Vietnam	Endemic, hyperendemic in all provinces	May through October

taken once weekly beginning 1 to 2 weeks before travel and continuing during the stay and for 4 weeks after departure from malarious areas. Minor side effects, including gastrointestinal disturbances, dizziness, blurred vision, and headache, may be alleviated by taking the drug after meals. Serious side effects are rare. Specifically, retinal injury, which can occur when high doses of chloroquine are used to treat rheumatoid arthritis, does not occur with the weekly dosages used for malaria prevention, even when such a regimen is continued for 5 years. However, deaths from malaria have occurred among tourists from the United States who avoided chloroquine prophylaxis out of a misguided concern for ocular toxicity.

Mefloquine

Mefloquine (Lariam) is active against CRPF and against *P. falciparum* that is resistant to sulfadoxine with pyrimethamine (Fansidar). With the now-widespread geographic prevalence of CRPF [*see Figure 5*], mefloquine is for many travelers the mainstay of malarial chemoprophylaxis. Strains of *P. falciparum* that are resistant to mefloquine, however, have been recognized in Africa and along the border between Thailand and Cambodia. Mefloquine is used in place of chloroquine and should be used by travelers to areas with CRPF malaria. Mefloquine (250 mg) is taken once a week, beginning 1 to 2 weeks before travel and continuing during the stay and for 4 weeks after departure from a malarious area.[1] (This schedule is similar to that for chloroquine.) For travelers who will be immediately arriving in malarious areas, a loading dose of mefloquine (250 mg daily for the first 3 days) is advisable.

Despite the benefits of mefloquine to travelers in regions with CRPF malaria, mefloquine has acquired an unsalutary reputation for two reasons: First, British malariologists and travel medicine physicians preferred a combination of chloroquine and chloroguanide (the latter is called proguanil in Europe) for prophylaxis. This combination has now, however, proved inadequate for protection in regions with CRPF malaria.[26,27] Second, mefloquine causes side effects, including nausea, dizziness, vertigo, light-headedness (described as an inability to concentrate), bad dreams, seizures, and psychosis. These reactions occur principally when the drug is given at therapeutic doses, which are higher than those given for prophylaxis. The incidence of psychosis or seizures has been about 1 in every 10,000 travelers treated with chemoprophylactic mefloquine, which is comparable to the incidence associated with chloroquine use.[28] Other controlled trials have demonstrated that mefloquine is reasonably well tolerated in groups receiving this agent.[29-31] Thus, the uncommon and self-limited, but bothersome, side effects of mefloquine are to be weighed against the very real risks of serious and fatal malaria in many nonimmune travelers.

Mefloquine use has also been associated with sinus bradycardia and prolongation of the QT interval. Therefore, mefloquine probably should not be used by persons with cardiac conduction abnormalities but may be used by patients without arrhythmias who are taking beta blockers.[1] Other contraindications to mefloquine include a history of serious neuropsychiatric disorders or seizures. Despite recommendations to the contrary, mefloquine appears to be safe and effective for young children[32] and for use during pregnancy[33-35]; it has no deleterious effects on fine motor skills, such as those required by airplane pilots.[36]

Atovaquone-Proguanil

Atovaquone/proguanil (Malarone), which is available in many countries, has been approved for use in the United States for the

---

Table 3   Areas with Reported CRPF Malaria

Africa[*]

Angola, Benin, Botswana, Burkina Faso, Burundi, Cameroon, Central African Republic, Chad, Comoros, Congo, Côte d'Ivoire, Democratic Republic of Congo (formerly Zaire), Djibouti, Equatorial Guinea, Eritrea, Ethiopia, Gabon, Gambia, Ghana, Guinea, Guinea-Bissau, Kenya, Liberia, Madagascar, Malawi, Mali, Mauritania, Mayotte, Mozambique, Namibia, Niger, Nigeria, Rwanda, São Tomé and Principe, Senegal, Sierra Leone, Somalia, South Africa, Sudan, Swaziland, Tanzania, Togo, Uganda, Zambia, Zimbabwe

Oceania[*]

Papua New Guinea, Solomon Islands, Vanuatu

Asia

Afghanistan, Cambodia,[*] China (Hainan and southern provinces), Indonesia,[†] Iran, Laos,[‡] Malaysia, Myanmar (Burma), Nepal,[§] Oman, the Philippines (Basilan, Luzon, Mindanao, Mindoro, and Palawan; Sulu archipelago), Saudi Arabia, Sri Lanka,[ǁ] Thailand,[¶] United Arab Emirates, Vietnam, Yemen

Central and South America

Bolivia, Brazil,[**] Colombia, Ecuador,[††] French Guiana, Guyana, Panama (east of the Canal Zone, including the San Blas Islands), Peru (provinces bordering Brazil and Ecuador), Suriname, Venezuela

Indian Subcontinent

Bangladesh, Bhutan (near India), India, Pakistan

Note: see reference 1. There is no malaria risk in urban areas unless otherwise indicated. See text for recommended prophylaxis.
[*]Malaria risk exists in urban areas except Phnom Penh.
[†]Malaria risk exists mostly in rural areas, except all of West Irian.
[‡]Malaria risk exists in all urban areas except city of Vientiane.
[§]No malaria risk in Katmandu.
[ǁ]Malaria risk in all areas except Colombo, Kalutara, and Nuwara Eliya.
[¶]Malaria risk mostly in rural areas.
[**]Malaria risk exists in urban areas of interior Amazon River region.
[††]Malaria risk exists in urban areas of Cañar Cotopasi, El Oro, Esmeraldas, Guayas (including city of Guayaquil), Los Ríos, Manabi, Morona-Santiago, Napo, Pastaza, Pichincha, Sucumbios, and Zamora-Chinchipe provinces. Malaria risk does not exist in Quito, the central highland tourist area, or the Galapagos Islands.

---

chemoprophylaxis of malaria. Atovaquone-proguanil is available as a fixed-dose tablet in adult strength (250 mg atovaquone/100 mg proguanil) and in pediatric strength (62.5 mg atovaquone/25 mg proguanil). For prophylaxis, one tablet is taken daily, beginning 1 to 2 days before travel and continuing for the duration of travel and for 1 week after departure from malarious areas. One, two, or three pediatric-strength tablets are taken by children weighing 11 to 20 kg, 21 to 30 kg, or 31 to 40 kg, respectively. Atovaquone-proguanil is well tolerated; side effects, which are uncommon, are abdominal pain, nausea, vomiting, headache, and rash. Atovaquone-proguanil is safe and efficacious for prophylaxis of *P. vivax* and *P. falciparum* malaria, including CRPF.[37,38] For *P. vivax* and *P. ovale* malaria, malarone does not prevent development of hepatic hypnozoite stages, so terminal prophylaxis with primaquine may be necessary to prevent relapses with these species. Atovaquone-proguanil, therefore, is an alternative to mefloquine for malaria chemoprophylaxis.[37]

Doxycycline

Doxycycline, taken alone, is an alternative chemoprophylactic agent.[1] It should be taken in a dosage of 100 mg daily, beginning 1 to 2 days before travel and continuing for 4 weeks after departure from malarious areas. The use of doxycycline is appropriate for persons who are intolerant of sulfonamides, pyrimethamine, chloroquine, or mefloquine and for persons who are planning

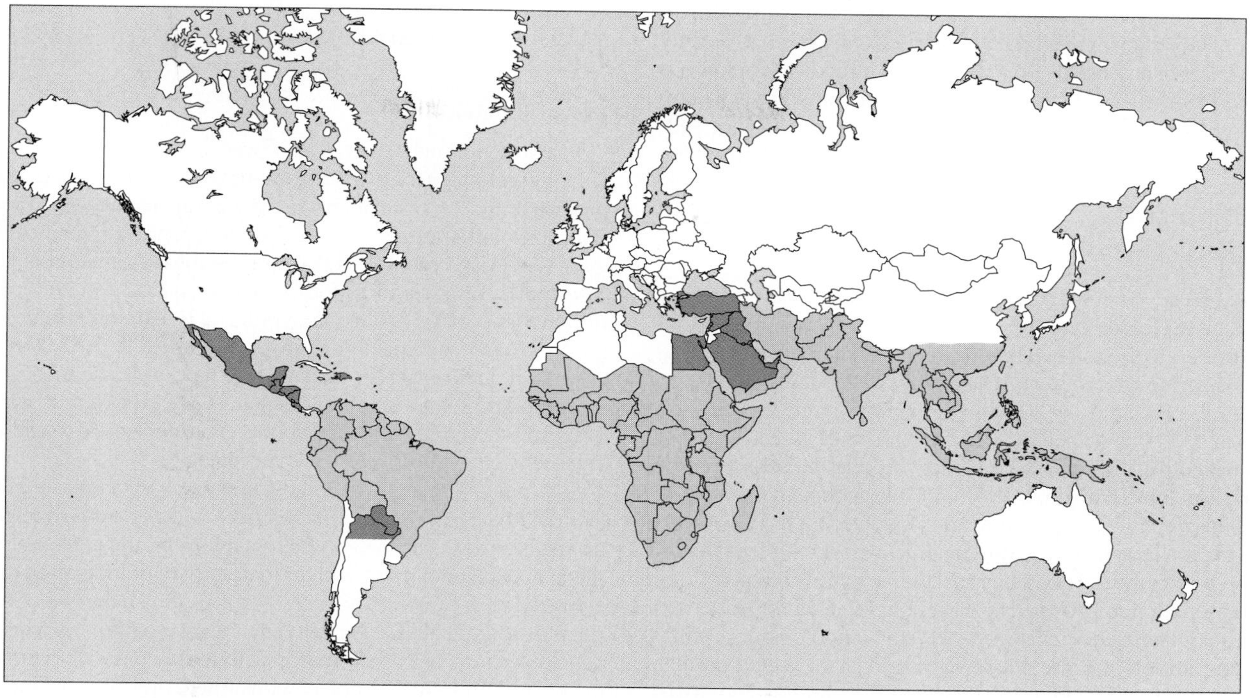

Figure 5   **This map displays the distribution of the chloroquine-resistant *Plasmodium falciparum* malaria (gray areas) and chloroquine-sensitive malaria (blue areas).**

short-term visits in forested areas of Thailand, Myanmar (Burma), or Cambodia, where strains of malaria that are resistant to chloroquine, mefloquine, and Fansidar are present.[1] Doxycycline may cause photosensitivity skin reactions and is contraindicated in pregnant women and in children younger than 8 years.

Proguanil

Proguanil (Paludrine) is not available in the United States but is available in Canada, Europe, and much of Africa. This agent, like pyrimethamine, is a dehydrofolate reductase inhibitor, and some strains of malaria are resistant to it. Proguanil (200 mg) should be taken daily in combination with a weekly dose of chloroquine. The combination of proguanil and chloroquine is less effective than mefloquine or malarone against resistant falciparum malaria and hence is not recommended.

Primaquine

Primaquine may be used either as a single agent taken daily for chemoprophylaxis against all species of malaria or as an agent to eradicate residual intrahepatic stages of *P. vivax* and *P. ovale*. For the latter purpose, primaquine is administered during the last weeks of or just after a course of prophylaxis with either chloroquine or mefloquine. Primaquine may be administered as 15 mg of the base daily for 14 days or as 45 mg of the base once a week for 8 weeks. Such terminal prophylaxis is generally reserved for persons who have had more than a casual potential exposure to *P. vivax* or *P. ovale*; other persons may be followed clinically and evaluated if they become symptomatic. For use as a primary chemoprophylactic agent, 30 mg of primaquine base is taken daily starting 1 day before travels and continuing for 2 days after departure from a malarious area.[25,39] Because primaquine can cause severe hemolysis in patients who have glucose-6-phosphate dehydrogenase (G6PD) deficiency, this disorder should be excluded before the drug is administered.

Fansidar

For chemoprophylaxis in areas where CRPF malaria occurs, it was formerly recommended that a single tablet of Fansidar, which contains 500 mg of long-acting sulfadoxine and 25 mg of pyrimethamine, be taken once a week along with chloroquine beginning 1 to 2 weeks before arrival in an endemic area and continuing for 4 weeks after departure from such an area. However, severe mucocutaneous reactions, including erythema multiforme, Stevens-Johnson syndrome, and toxic epidermal necrolysis, have developed after the use of two or more doses of Fansidar. These reactions produced fatalities with an incidence of about 1 in 11,000 to 20,000 travelers from the United States. Consequently, Fansidar is not recommended for routine chemoprophylactic use.

PROPHYLAXIS IN REGIONS WITH CRPF MALARIA

Africa

About 80% of recent cases of malaria in civilian travelers from the United States were acquired in sub-Saharan Africa; the risk of malaria infection among travelers in this area is 0.5% to 2.5%, and the case-fatality rate is 1% to 2%.[1] Except in the city of Nairobi, where the risk is low, there is a particularly high risk of acquiring CRPF malaria in the areas of East Africa that tourists often visit. The most effective chemoprophylactic regimen is either mefloquine (taken weekly starting 1 to 2 weeks before travel, during travel, and for 4 weeks after departure from malarious areas) or malarone (taken daily starting 1 to 2 days before travel, during travel, and for 1 week after departure from malarious areas). Alternatives to mefloquine or malarone include the daily use of doxycycline or primaquine. For travelers unable to take mefloquine, malarone, doxycycline, or primaquine, weekly chloroquine is the next, but least effective, alternative. Those who use chloroquine prophylaxis (with or without proguanil) and who are not intolerant of sulfonamides or pyrimethamine should carry a single-treatment dose of Fansidar (three tablets for adults), to be taken promptly at the onset of any febrile or flulike illness if medical attention is not readily available.[1] On rare occasions, Stevens-Johnson syndrome has developed in persons who used Fansidar for self-treatment of suspected malaria. Furthermore, cases in which self-treatment of CRPF malaria with Fansidar failed have been reported in travelers returning from East Africa.

Oceania

Because of intense malaria transmission in many areas of Papua New Guinea, West Irian, the Solomon Islands, and Vanuatu, travelers to these areas should use the chemoprophylactic regimens described for areas of Africa where CRPF malaria occurs.

China and Southeast Asia

Travelers to most parts of China, Indonesia, Malaysia, the Philippines, and Thailand do not frequently acquire malaria. Thus, no chemoprophylaxis is recommended for persons who visit urban areas of Asia or who have only daytime exposure in rural areas. For those who diverge from the usual tourist routes and spend time outdoors in rural areas during evening hours, the recommendations for CRPF malaria-endemic regions of Africa should be applied. In Thailand, strains of *P. falciparum* that are resistant to chloroquine, mefloquine, and Fansidar are prevalent in rural forested areas, and travelers with evening and nighttime exposures in rural areas should be given malarone or doxycycline prophylaxis.

South America

In South America, malaria is transmitted primarily in rural areas. Transmission also occurs in certain urban areas of the interior Amazon River basin and on the coast of Ecuador. Chemoprophylaxis is usually reserved for persons who visit malarious areas at night. Chemoprophylactic regimens for CRPF malaria are identical to those suggested for Africa.

The Indian Subcontinent

Malaria transmission occurs in both urban and rural areas of India, Pakistan, and Bangladesh, and CRPF malaria is present in these countries. Chemoprophylactic regimens for CRPF malaria are identical to those suggested for travelers to Africa.

PROPHYLAXIS DURING PREGNANCY

Malaria infections represent a major health hazard to the mother and fetus.[40,41] Infections are potentially more serious during pregnancy and increase the risks of stillbirths, abortions, and other adverse pregnancy outcomes. For pregnant women who cannot defer travel or residence in malarious areas, chloroquine, which is without established teratogenicity, may be used.[1] Although complete information is not yet available, mefloquine appears to be safe in pregnancy.[34,35] For the pregnant traveler in regions with CRPF malaria, the benefits of effective mefloquine chemoprophylaxis need to be balanced with any potential, but as yet not recognized, adverse effects of mefloquine in pregnancy. Sulfadoxine should be avoided before delivery because of the risk of neonatal jaundice. Pyrimethamine, which is teratogenic in animals because it interferes with folate metabolism, is generally avoided but probably could be used. Doxycycline should not be used during pregnancy because of the effects of tetracyclines on the fetus, which include dental discoloration and dysplasia and inhibition of bone growth. To avoid the risk of inducing hemolytic anemia in utero in a G6PD-deficient fetus, primaquine should

not be taken during pregnancy. The safety of malarone in pregnancy has not been established.

Travel-Related Illness

In a study of more than 10,000 Swiss who had traveled in developing countries for less than 3 months, 15% experienced health problems, and 3% were unable to work for an average of 15 days.[42] Infections with the greatest incidence per month abroad included giardiasis (seven cases per 1,000 months abroad), amebiasis (four cases per 1,000), hepatitis (four cases per 1,000), and gonorrhea (three cases per 1,000). Malaria, syphilis, and helminthic infections occurred at a lower incidence (fewer than one case per 1,000). No cases of typhoid fever or cholera were reported. The most common modes of acquisition of infection were enteral and sexual. Travelers should be cautioned about sexual contacts, especially in areas where hepatitis B or HIV is prevalent.

Stays at major resorts and first-class hotels are associated with less risk than stays at less established locales or rural dwellings or encampments. In areas where sanitation and personal hygiene may be poor, it is prudent to be careful of food and water, although such care does not necessarily diminish the risk of diarrheal disease. Fruit that is peeled by the traveler is safe, whereas vegetables may be contaminated with fecally passed organisms in the soil and should not be consumed raw. Unpasteurized dairy products should be avoided, as should inadequately cooked fish or meat. If water is of uncertain quality, travelers should avoid drinking it or using ice made from it. Boiling will render water safe. Chlorination will kill most bacterial and viral pathogens, but protozoal cysts of *Giardia lamblia* and *Entamoeba histolytica* may survive. Carbonated beverages, beer, wine, and drinks made from boiled water are safe.

In areas where schistosomiasis is prevalent, swimming in freshwater should be avoided, although swimming in chlorinated or saltwater is safe. Even short exposures to infested water during rafting or swimming have caused the onset of acute schistosomiasis.

Most infections acquired during travels will present within weeks of travel, but some may not manifest themselves until much later; hence, knowledge of a patient's travel history is important.

TRAVELER'S DIARRHEA

Diarrhea is the most common illness of travelers.[43] Infectious agents, primarily bacterial but also viral and parasitic pathogens, are responsible for traveler's diarrhea. Over three fourths of cases of traveler's diarrhea are caused by bacteria, with enterotoxigenic *Escherichia coli* being the most frequent cause. Other common bacterial causes of traveler's diarrhea include *Shigella* species, *Campylobacter jejuni*, *Aeromonas* species, *Plesiomonas shigelloides*, *Salmonella* species, and noncholera *Vibrio* species.[44] Rotavirus and Norwalk agent are the most common viral causes; *Giardia*, *Cryptosporidium*, *Cyclospora*, and, less commonly, *Dientamoeba fragilis*, *Isospora belli*, *Balantidium coli*, *Strongyloides stercoralis*, and *E. histolytica* are parasitic causes.

In addition to exercising caution about food and water,[45] travelers may take either of two approaches: chemoprophylaxis and postonset treatment.[44] The benefits of chemoprophylaxis may be offset by the risks of taking chemoprophylactic agents. Side effects of short-term prophylactic doses of bismuth subsalicylate may include tinnitus, blackening of the stool and tongue, and impaired absorption of doxycycline, which is important if doxycycline is used as daily antimalarial chemoprophylaxis. Side effects of antibiotics may include skin rashes and vaginal candidiasis,

Table 4 Chemoprophylaxis and
Treatment of Traveler's Diarrhea

Drug	Dose
Prophylaxis	
Bismuth subsalicylate	Two 262 mg tablets chewed q.i.d. with meals and at bedtime
Quinolone antibiotics	
Norfloxacin	400 mg/day
Ciprofloxacin	500 mg/day
Ofloxacin	300 mg/day
Trimethoprim-sulfamethoxazole	160 mg:800 mg/day
Doxycycline	100 mg/day
Treatment	
Loperamide	4 mg loading dose, then 2 mg after each loose stool, to a maximum of 16 mg/day
Quinolone antibiotics	
Norfloxacin	400 mg b.i.d. for up to 3 days
Ciprofloxacin	500 mg b.i.d. for up to 3 days
Ofloxacin	300 mg b.i.d. for up to 3 days
Trimethoprim-sulfamethoxazole	160 mg:800 mg b.i.d. for up to 3 days

photosensitivity skin eruptions (especially with doxycycline), and, in rare instances, potentially life-threatening bone marrow suppression, mucocutaneous reactions, or anaphylaxis. Although these potential side effects temper the routine use of chemoprophylaxis, specific needs or wishes of travelers may dictate its use. Patients with underlying medical conditions that may be aggravated by a serious diarrheal illness, including active inflammatory bowel disease, type 1 (insulin-dependent) diabetes mellitus, and heart disease in the elderly, as well as patients whose activities during travel cannot tolerate interruption by an episode of diarrheal illness, should consider chemoprophylaxis. Several regimens are available [*see Table 4*].[44] Bismuth subsalicylate, which should not be taken by persons with peptic ulcer disease, coagulopathies, or allergies to salicylates, is not as completely effective as quinolone antibiotics but has fewer side effects and enables the use of quinolone antibiotics, if they are needed for therapy. Resistance among bacterial causes of traveler's diarrhea is rare at present for the quinolone antibiotics but is quite common for trimethoprim-sulfamethoxazole and doxycycline, limiting their efficacy.[44] Chemoprophylactic medications should be started on the first day of arrival and continued for 1 to 2 days after returning home but not for more than 3 weeks' duration.

A generally preferable alternative to chemoprophylaxis is early therapy for traveler's diarrhea [*see Table 3*]. Because of the likelihood of bacterial resistance, trimethoprim-sulfamethoxazole is less effective than regimens employing quinolone antibiotics. Antibiotics will shorten the duration of traveler's diarrhea to a range of 16 to 30 hours from a range of 59 to 93 hours in those not receiving antibiotics.[44] The use of loperamide, which diminishes intestinal motility and fluid and electrolyte losses, together with antibiotics can further abbreviate symptoms. In a study of patients with dysentery caused by *Shigella* or enteroinvasive *E. coli*, the use of loperamide with ciprofloxacin, in comparison with ciprofloxacin alone, led to briefer (median, 19 hours versus 42 hours) and milder (median, two stools versus 6.5 stools) diarrheal illness, without untoward effects.[46] Loperamide has not been studied in children, and adults with prolonged fever or bloody stools should be advised to cease loperamide use and seek medical attention.

For any diarrheal illness, maintenance of hydration is of cardinal importance and can often be achieved by oral replacement of lost fluid and electrolytes. Convenient and inexpensive packets of oral rehydration salts formulated according to World Health Organization recommendations (i.e., 3.5 g of sodium chloride, 1.5 g of potassium chloride, 20 g of glucose, and 2.9 g of trisodium citrate in each packet) are available in developed as well as in developing countries. Each packet of oral rehydration salts is added to a liter of boiled or treated water and should be consumed or discarded within 12 hours (if kept at ambient temperature) or 24 hours (if kept refrigerated).

MEDICAL ISSUES DURING TRANSIT

Cruise ships that dock at ports in the United States are inspected for sanitation by officials from the CDC. Inspections are aimed at minimizing the potential for outbreaks of gastrointestinal disease on board. Travelers may obtain information on whether specific cruise ships meet sanitation standards from travel agents, state health departments, or the CDC.[44] Outbreaks of influenza have occurred aboard cruise ships in recent years in various regions, including Alaska and the Yukon Territory.[47] Travelers older than 50 years should consider influenza vaccination.

Because jet aircraft are not pressurized to sea level, passengers will be exposed to high-altitude environments. The atmospheric pressure maintained within the cabin of an airplane flying at 27,000 to 42,000 ft is equivalent to the pressure at an altitude of 3,000 to 8,000 ft, so that at a cruising altitude of 35,000 ft, the cabin pressure is about 600 mm Hg. Because of the decreased pressure, the arterial oxygen tension (P_aO_2) of normal persons will fall to about 68 mm Hg. In patients with chronic obstructive lung disease, the P_aO_2 will fall even lower. However, despite a fall in P_aO_2, patients may not show symptoms of hypoxia. Although hypoxia occurs in pregnant women, jet air travel has no deleterious effects on them or their fetuses. It is difficult to establish precise criteria for the use of supplemental oxygen for air travelers. Caution is indicated, however, for patients with impaired cardiopulmonary function: supplemental oxygen may be administered during flights at altitudes higher than 22,500 ft.

Scuba divers should wait 12 to 48 hours, depending on the length of their diving exposures, before boarding a commercial aircraft. This measure is important for avoiding the occurrence of aeroembolism, commonly known as the bends, which could develop in an underpressurized cabin if nitrogen gas dissolved in the person's fat cells is mobilized.

In patients with upper respiratory tract infections, differential air pressures between blocked eustachian tubes or sinuses and the cabin may develop on ascent or descent and impair hearing or cause pain in the ears or sinuses; symptoms can be relieved by the use of decongestants. Persons prone to motion sickness should take a prophylactic medication. Prolonged immobilization during flight may cause venous thrombosis in individuals with preexisting thrombotic or venous disease.

References

1. Centers for Disease Control and Prevention: Health information for international travel 1999-2000. US Department of Health and Human Services, Atlanta, 2000
2. Robertson SE, Hull BP, Tomori O, et al: Yellow fever: a decade of reemergence. JAMA 276:1157, 1996
3. Mosimann B, Stoll B, Francillon C, et al: Yellow fever vaccine and egg allergy (letter). J Allergy Clin Immunol 95:1064, 1995
4. Mahon BE, Mintz ED, Greene KD, et al: Reported cholera in the United States, 1992–1994: a reflection of global changes in cholera epidemiology. JAMA 276:307, 1996

5. Khan WA, Bennish ML, Seas C, et al: Randomised controlled comparison of single-dose ciprofloxacin and doxycycline for cholera caused by *Vibrio cholerae* 01 or 0139. Lancet 348:296, 1996

6. Apparent global interruption of wild poliovirus type 2 transmission. MMWR Morb Mortal Wkly Rep 50:222, 2001

7. Poliomyelitis prevention in the United States. Updated recommendation of the Advisory Committee on Immunization Practices (ACIP). MMWR Morb Mortal Wkly Rep 49(RR-5):1, 2000

8. Maple PA, Jones CS, Wall EC, et al: Immunity to diptheria and tetanus in England and Wales. Vaccine 19:167, 2000.

9. Gergen PJ, McQuillan GM, Kiely M, et al: A population-based serologic survey of immunity to tetanus in the United States. N Engl J Med 332:761, 1995

10. Vitek CR, Redd SC, Redd SB, et al: Trends in importation of measles to the United States, 1986–1994. JAMA 277:1952, 1997

11. Measles immunization in HIV-infected children. American Academy of Pediatrics. Committee on Infectious Diseases and Committee on Pediatric AIDS. Pediatrics 103:1057, 1999

12. Mermin JH, Townes JM, Gerber M, et al: Typhoid fever in the United States, 1985–1995: changing risks of international travel and antimicrobial resistance. Arch Intern Med 158:633, 1998

13. Engels EA, Falagas ME, Lau S, et al: Typhoid fever vaccines: a meta-analysis of studies on efficacy and toxicity. BMJ 316:110, 1998

14. Rahman S, Barr W, Hilton E: Use of oral typhoid vaccine strain Ty21a in a New York State travel immunization facility. Am J Trop Med Hyg 48:823, 1993

15. Stubi CL, Landry PR, Petignat C, et al: Compliance to live oral Ty21a typhoid vaccine, and its effect on viability. J Travel Med 7:133, 2000

16. Plotkin SA, Bouveret-Le Cam N: A new typhoid vaccine composed of the Vi capsular polysaccharide. Arch Intern Med 155:2293, 1995

17. Steffen R, Kane MA, Shapiro CN, et al: Epidemiology and prevention of hepatitis A in travelers. JAMA 272:885, 1994

18. Prevention of hepatitis A through active or passive immunization: recommendations of the Advisory Committee on Immunization Practices (ACIP). MMWR Morb Mortal Wkly Rep 48(RR-12):1, 1999

19. Bader TF: Hepatitis A vaccine. Am J Gastroenterol 91:217, 1996

20. Nothdurft HD, Jelinek T, Marschang A, et al: Adverse reactions to Japanese encephalitis vaccine in travellers. J Infect 32:119, 1996

21. Plesner A, Ronne T, Wachmann H: Case-control study of allergic reactions to Japanese encephalitis vaccine. Vaccine 18:1830, 2000

22. Sutter RW, Prevots DR: Vaccine-associated paralytic poliomyelitis among immunodeficient persons. Infect Med 11:426, 1994

23. Nasidi A, Monath TP, Vandenberg J, et al: Yellow fever vaccination and pregnancy: a 4-year prospective study. Trans R Soc Trop Med Hyg 87:337, 1993

24. Humar A, Sharma S, Zoutman D, et al: Fatal falciparum malaria in Canadian travellers. CMAJ 156:1165, 1997

25. D'Allessandro V: Insecticide treated bed nets to prevent malaria BMJ 322:249, 2001

26. Barnes AJ, Ong EL, Dunbar EM, et al: Failure of chloroquine and proguanil prophylaxis in travellers to Kenya (letter). Lancet 338:1338, 1991

27. Weiss WR, Oloo AJ, Johnson A, et al: Daily primaquine is effective for prophylaxis against falciparum malaria in Kenya: comparison with mefloquine, doxycycline, and chloroquine plus proguanil. J Infect Dis 171:1569, 1995

28. Steffen R, Fuchs E, Schildknecht J, et al: Mefloquine compared with other chemoprophylactic regimens in tourists visiting East Africa. Lancet 341:1299, 1993

29. Jaspers CA, Hopperus Buma AP, van Thiel PP, et al: Tolerance of mefloquine chemoprophylaxis in Dutch military personnel. Am J Trop Med Hyg 55:230, 1996

30. Davis TM, Dembo LG, Kaye-Eddie SA, et al: Neurological, cardiovascular and metabolic effects of mefloquine in healthy volunteers: a double-blind, placebo-controlled trial. Br J Clin Pharmacol 42:415, 1996

31. Croft AM, Clayton TC, World MJ: Side effects of mefloquine prophylaxis for malaria: an independent randomized controlled trial. Trans R Soc Trop Med Hyg 91:199, 1997

32. Luxemburger C, Price RN, Nosten F, et al: Mefloquine in infants and young children. Ann Trop Paediatr 16:281, 1996

33. Smoak BL, Writer JV, Keep LW, et al: The effects of inadvertent exposure of mefloquine chemoprophylaxis on pregnancy outcomes and infants of US Army servicewomen. J Infect Dis 176:831, 1997

34. Steketee RW, Wirima JJ, Slutsker L, et al: Malaria treatment and prevention in pregnancy: indications for use and adverse events associated with use of chloroquine or mefloquine. Am J Trop Med Hyg 55(suppl 1):50, 1996

35. Schlagenhauf P: Mefloquine for malaria chemoprophylaxis 1992–1998: a review. J Travel Med 6:122, 1999

36. Schlagenhauf P, Lobel H, Steffen R, et al: Tolerance of mefloquine by SwissAir trainee pilots. Am J Trop Med Hyg 56:235, 1997

37. Hogh B, Clarke PD, Camus D, et al: Atovaquone-proguanil versus chloroquine-proguanil for malaria prophylaxis in non-immune travellers: a randomised, double-blind study. Malarone International Study Team. Lancet 356:1888, 2000

38. Shanks GD, Gordon DM, Klotz FW, et al: Efficacy and safety of atovaquone/proguanil as suppressive prophylaxis for *Plasmodium falciparum* malaria. Clin Infect Dis 27:494, 1998

39. Schwartz E, Rgev-Yochay G: Primaquine as prophylaxis for malaria for nonimmune travelers: a comparison with mefloquine and doxycycline. Clin Infect Dis 29:1502, 1999

40. Steketee RW, Wirima JJ, Hightower AW, et al: The effect of malaria and malaria prevention in pregnancy on offspring birthweight, prematurity, and intrauterine growth retardation in rural Malawi. Am J Trop Med Hyg 55(suppl):33, 1996

41. Steketee RW, Wirima JJ, Slutsker L, et al: Malaria parasite infection during pregnancy and at delivery in mother, placenta, and newborn: efficacy of chloroquine and mefloquine in rural Malawi. Am J Trop Med Hyg 55(suppl 1):24, 1996

42. Steffen R, Rickenbach M, Wilhelm U, et al: Health problems after travel to developing countries. J Infect Dis 156:84, 1987

43. Ryan ET, Kain KC: Health advice and immunizations for travelers. N Engl J Med 342:1716, 2000

44. DuPont HL, Ericsson CD: Prevention and treatment of traveler's diarrhea. N Engl J Med 328:1821, 1993

45. Herwaldt BL, de Arroyave KR, Roberts JM, et al: A multiyear prospective study of the risk factors for and incidence of diarrheal illness in a cohort of Peace Corps volunteers in Guatemala. Ann Intern Med 132:982, 2000

46. Murphy GS, Bodhidatta L, Echeverria P, et al: Ciprofloxacin and loperamide in the treatment of bacillary dysentery. Ann Intern Med 118:582, 1993

47. Update: Influenza activity—United States and worldwide, 1999–2000 season, and composition of the 2000-01 influenza vaccine. MMWR Morb Mortal Wkly Rep 49:375, 2000

Acknowledgment

Figures 1 through 5   Tom Moore.

8 Complementary and Alternative Medicine

Adrian S. Dobs, M.D., M.H.S., and Bimal H. Ashar, M.D.

Definitions

Alternative medicine is an umbrella term that encompasses a spectrum of approaches to medical conditions not routinely used by conventional practitioners. Historically, the term has been used to convey negative conceptions about medical practices that did not conform to accepted standards of care. The term complementary medicine has since evolved to describe a more positive, symbiotic relationship between unconventional medicine and conventional medicine. The field of complementary and alternative medicine (CAM) now encompasses a multitude of different approaches and beliefs that are generally linked by their emphasis on so-called natural modalities of healing and wellness.

Classification

Patient demand, media attention, and the growth of an almost $30 billion industry[1] have stimulated leaders in governmental agencies and academic medicine to recognize and categorize CAM and to direct research initiatives on the subject. Although there is currently no universally accepted classification of CAM modalities, the National Center for Complementary and Alternative Medicine (NCCAM) has grouped CAM practices into five domains [see Table 1]. It should be recognized that these categories are not mutually exclusive. Certain practices will overlap (e.g., qigong is considered an energy therapy but is part of Chinese medicine, which is an alternative medical system). Also, as evidence emerges regarding mechanisms of action, safety, and efficacy, certain modalities will naturally move beyond the CAM label and become part of mainstream medicine.

Use of CAM

PREVALENCE AND DEMOGRAPHICS

The widespread use of CAM by the public has been well documented. In 1997, approximately 42% of people in the United States reported using at least one form of alternative medicine within the previous year.[1] It has been estimated that nearly 70% of people in the United States have used at least one CAM therapy over their lifetime.[2] Public opinion surveys have suggested similar overall patterns of use in European countries, although the popularity of specific CAM modalities varies greatly from country to country.[3] Patients across all demographic groups use alternative medicine. However, some surveys have noted that predictors of CAM use may include female gender, white race (as opposed to African American or Hispanic), higher socioeconomic status, and higher levels of education.[4,5] Many CAM users have chronic, non–life-threatening medical conditions[4,6] and may have an interest in spirituality.[7] A number of diagnosis-based surveys have suggested exceptionally high usage of alternative medicine among patients with cancer,[8] HIV infection,[9] fibromyalgia,[10] and inflammatory bowel disease.[11]

PUBLIC PERCEPTION

The alternative-medicine movement has clearly been a public-driven process that has spanned decades. It was initially thought that this movement was primarily the result of dissatisfaction with conventional medicine.[12] Recent studies, however, have shown that this is not the case.[7,13] Patients continue to see their conventional practitioners while using CAM therapies. Two disturbing observations are that most patients do not disclose their use of alternative therapies to their physicians and that such patients are never asked about CAM use by their physicians.[1] Furthermore, many patients feel no need to communicate their CAM use to their physicians because they believe that their physicians would be unable to understand and incorporate that information into their treatment plan.[13,14]

A number of other factors have stimulated public use of alternative medical therapies. The fact that many CAM modalities emphasize natural forms of healing seems to form the fundamental basis for its use. Many patients desire a more holistic approach to their medical care.[7] They may feel that conventional medicine focuses excessively on suppression of symptoms (e.g., pharmacologic lowering of elevated blood pressure) rather than addressing the root cause of symptoms. They believe that so-called natural products are better and safer than synthetic medications. In many cases, they may turn to alternative medical practices to get relief from chronic conditions that have not responded to conventional symptomatic therapy. Additionally, media hype, direct-to-consumer advertising, and the widespread availability of information over the Internet have all played a role in the popularity of CAM and have served to expand the public's health care choices. Of concern to many physicians is that these choices are frequently based on insufficient basic science or clinical evidence.

Table 1 NIH/NCCAM Classification of Complementary and Alternative Medicine Practices

Category	Examples
Alternative medical systems	Ayurveda (traditional Indian medicine), traditional Chinese medicine, homeopathy
Mind-body interventions	Biofeedback, hypnosis, meditation, prayer
Biologic-based therapies	Dietary therapy, herbal medicine, megavitamins, shark cartilage
Manipulative and body-based methods	Chiropractic, massage therapy
Energy therapies	Therapeutic touch, qigong, bioelectric field manipulation, reiki

NIH/NCCAM—National Institutes of Health/National Center for Complementary and Alternative Medicine

Research Concerns

Scientific Issues

One of the defining characteristics of alternative medicine is the paucity of definitive evidence supporting mechanism of action, efficacy, and safety. Although a number of clinical trials on CAM have been published, the overall quality is quite poor, primarily because of inadequate sample size, randomization, and blinding.[15,16] Additionally, publication bias may be common in the international literature. Critical reviews of published studies on CAM therapies from a number of countries have shown that the studies report almost universally positive findings pertaining to CAM. This suggests that studies reporting negative findings may never make it to press.[17,18]

There are a number of barriers to the proper evaluation of CAM studies. First, the establishment of adequate control groups is frequently very difficult. Studies on acupuncture, for example, have attempted to incorporate a placebo control by stimulating nonacupuncture points, stimulating actual points unrelated to the treated condition, or applying pressure instead of inserting needles. Some critics argue that so-called sham acupuncture is an inadequate placebo that does not preserve subject blinding. Proponents of acupuncture may argue that such control methods are still potentially therapeutic because of their possible positive effect on the flow of subtle energy through the body. Similar pitfalls are inherent in mind-body research. In the study of personal prayer, prayer groups, or intercessory prayer in the presence of the patient, the intervention group can be compared with those who do not partake in organized prayer. Such a design clearly does not lend itself to adequate blinding. Additionally, any positive results could result from aspects of prayer not related to its spiritual qualities (e.g., relaxation), making definitive conclusions difficult.

Another major problem with interpreting CAM research stems from inconsistencies in the intervention groups. Drawing meaningful conclusions from herbal-medication studies is difficult because extracts are not standardized. For example, although positive effects have been seen in a number of published clinical trials on the plant genus *Echinacea* for treatment of upper respiratory tract infections, definitive conclusions cannot be drawn because of variation in the species of plant studied, the part of the plant utilized (root, leaf, or flower), and extraction methods.[19] Lack of standardization is also a flaw in acupuncture research. Many different types of acupuncture are practiced around the world. Each form of acupuncture may utilize a completely different set of points for the same condition. Even among providers who practice the same type of acupuncture, variation in point selection is common because of different approaches based on the patient's history and physical examination and on the acupuncturist's personal style. This individualization of therapy is alluring to patients, but the unwillingness of practitioners to agree on what constitutes acceptable technique challenges conventional study methodology.

Financial Issues

Unlike conventional pharmaceutical and medical-device research, large-scale studies in CAM derive their funding almost exclusively from government resources. Modalities such as prayer, acupuncture, and massage therapy are not lucrative enough endeavors to support large privately funded trials. Dietary supplements, such as herbs, may have a significant profit potential, but the incentive for research is weakened by the fact that herbs, like other natural substances, cannot be patented. In addition, foods and natural products are regulated under rules different from those for pharmaceuticals, which must meet stringent standards of efficacy and safety. Nevertheless, many CAM treatments are profitable enough that legislation could require testing, at least of products not currently on the market or of any new claims that are made about existing products. For example, new regulations are under consideration in Canada that would require manufacturers to declare natural products as either foods (in which case no health claims can be made) or medicinals, in which case health claims can be made—but such claims must be supported by evidence.

In an effort to boost CAM research, the United States Government has set up the NCCAM (http://nccam.nih.gov) under the National Institutes of Health (NIH). With an annual working budget of about $70 million, NCCAM has funded a number of individual projects, as well as specialty centers around the country [see Table 2].

Table 2 Government-Funded Specialty Centers for Research into Complementary and Alternative Medicine

Specialty	Center and Location
Addictions	Minneapolis Medical Research Foundation, Minneapolis
Aging and women's health	Columbia University, New York
Arthritis	University of Maryland, Baltimore
Botanical treatment of age-related diseases	Purdue University, West Lafayette, Indiana
Botanical dietary supplements for women's health	University of Illinois, Chicago
Botanical dietary supplements	UCLA, Los Angeles
Cancer	Johns Hopkins University, Baltimore
Cancer and hyperbaric oxygen	University of Pennsylvania, Philadelphia
Cardiovascular diseases	University of Michigan, Ann Arbor
Cardiovascular disease and aging in African Americans	Maharishi University of Management, Fairfield, Iowa
Chiropractic	Palmer Center for Chiropractic Research, Davenport, Iowa
Craniofacial disorders	Kaiser Foundation Hospitals, Portland, Oregon
Neurodegenerative diseases	Emory University School of Medicine, Atlanta
Neurologic disorders	Oregon Health Sciences University, Portland
Pediatrics	University of Arizona Health Sciences Center, Tucson
Phytomedicine	University of Arizona, Tucson

Specific CAM Modalities

ALTERNATIVE MEDICAL SYSTEMS

Acupuncture

Acupuncture has been used for centuries as a component of traditional Chinese medicine (TCM). It involves the insertion of thin needles into specific points on the skin to facilitate the movement of energy (qi). Chinese medicine posits that qi (pronounced *chee*) flows along distinct channels (called meridians) in the body and that balanced circulation of qi is a prerequisite for good health. A block in the flow of qi can result in a deficiency or excess of qi along a meridian, and those imbalances can be corrected by accurate needle placement (or pressure, in the case of acupressure) at specific points on the body. Acupuncture practitioners often enhance the effect of the needles by electrical stimulation; manual manipulation (e.g., twirling); or moxibustion, which involves burning mugwort (*Artemisia vulgaris*) on the acupuncture point or the end of the needle. Practitioners of TCM frequently combine acupuncture with other modalities, including herbal remedies, to achieve the desired physiologic response. Each treatment is individualized on the basis of the patient's history and physical examination, including pulse and tongue examinations. Many types of acupuncture are practiced today; a few examples are traditional Chinese acupuncture, five-elements acupuncture, and auricular acupuncture.

To date, no clear physical mechanism of action has emerged to explain the potential therapeutic response to acupuncture. Changes in blood flow and biologic mediators (hormones, neurotransmitters, and endorphins) have been shown to occur with needle manipulation.[20, 21] There are numerous published clinical studies on acupuncture treatment for a variety of ailments. Most are small in size and have methodologic flaws that make consensus difficult. Nevertheless, in 1997 an NIH consensus panel concluded that there is clear evidence to support the use of acupuncture for postoperative, chemotherapy-induced, and probably pregnancy-associated nausea and vomiting.[21] Although the data are less compelling, evidence also suggests a positive effect of acupuncture on idiopathic headache,[22] fibromyalgia,[23] and osteoarthritis of the knee.[24] Current evidence does not support its use for smoking cessation.[25]

Done correctly, acupuncture is quite safe. Rare case reports of serious adverse events, including skin infections, hepatitis, pneumothorax, and cardiac tamponade, seem to stem from inadequate sterilization of needles and practitioner negligence.[26,27] To prevent transmission of infection, some practitioners now use disposable needles. Minor side effects, including insertion site pain or bleeding, fatigue, and vasovagal syncope, are probably more common.[28]

Homeopathy

Homeopathy is one of the most controversial modalities in CAM, primarily because of its theoretical implausibility. The roots of homeopathy trace back to the 1700s, when it was first described by Samuel Hahnemann. Homeopathic principles revolve around two basic tenets: the law of similars and serial dilutions. According to the law of similars, substances that cause symptoms in healthy people can cure those same symptoms in people who are sick. A number of examples of this principle exist in conventional medicine. Digoxin is used to treat the same arrhythmias that it is capable of inducing. Similarly, methyl-

phenidate, which is a stimulant, has been used to treat attention-deficit/hyperactivity disorder.[29]

The principle of serial dilutions (or the minute dose) is another controversial aspect of homeopathy. It suggests that medications can have a biologic effect even if diluted to levels at which the original substance is undetectable (a so-called homeopathic dose).

A homeopath's approach to patients differs from that of the conventional physician. Homeopaths concentrate almost exclusively on subjective symptoms and sensations. They choose medications on the basis of the patient's symptomatology rather than on the objective medical diagnosis. This results in a wide array of different medications being used for any one conventionally diagnosed condition. A number of homeopathic encyclopedias (*materia medica*) are available that describe symptoms induced by different remedies when given to healthy individuals (provings). These provings are matched to a patient's symptoms to determine the therapeutic regimen. Patients are typically followed closely so that the homeopath can titrate dosing schedules.

Meta-analyses of a number of trials of homeopathic remedies have suggested an effect superior to placebo.[30,31] However, many studies and reviews on specific medications have shown negative or inconclusive results.[31-34] Given the conflicting clinical data and the lack of evidence regarding mechanism of action, it is difficult to support general use of homeopathy.

Because homeopathic remedies typically contain little or no detectable active ingredients, serious side effects are rare. Homeopathic preparations are generally marketed as over-the-counter remedies and are usually exempt from government requirements for finished product testing or expiration dating. It should also be noted that these remedies are not restricted to the 10% alcohol limit of conventional drugs.[35]

Mind-Body Interventions

The relationship between psychological stress and physical health has been studied extensively over the past 30 years. Despite positive results from some trials, interventions designed to alter the stress response have not become part of mainstream medical practice. The reluctance of physicians to incorporate mind-body strategies into their therapeutic armamentarium likely stems from their unfamiliarity with such interventions, time constraints, and the lack of a clear mechanistic pathway to disease. Furthermore, many physicians may feel that these therapies need to be patient driven rather than physician driven, because they require significant changes in self-care.

The proposed theory of mind-body medicine stems from work done in the 1900s. The fight-or-flight response was described as physiologic preparation for combating or fleeing an external threat.[36] Stimulation of the hypothalamus and increased sympathetic nervous system activity leads to neurohormonal stimulation and increases in blood pressure, heart rate, respiratory rate, and muscle tension. This response has historically been protective, ensuring survival in the face of physical danger. In today's society, however, we are faced with innumerable stressors that can chronically elicit the fight-or-flight response, yet fighting or running away is inappropriate or impossible. The body is primed for action but can take none. This chronic physiologic stimulation is thought to increase the likelihood of disease. Furthermore, the development of a chronic disease may feed back and stimulate the response, potentially worsening the condition. The effect of the chronic

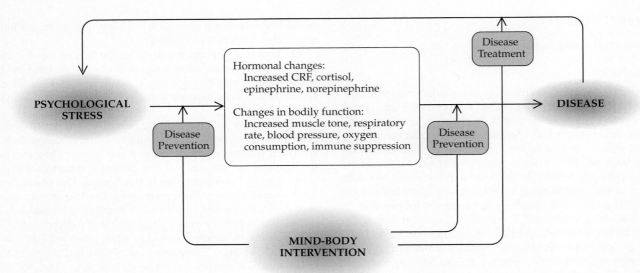

Figure 1   **Possible mechanism of mind-body interventions. (CRF—corticotropin-releasing factor)**

fight-or-flight response on immunosuppression and cytokine and hormone production needs greater elucidation.

Mind-body interventions can elicit a relaxation response that may prevent or aid in the treatment of a number of medical ailments[37] [*see Figure 1*]. A number of modalities can be used for this purpose. Many people have incorporated yoga, meditation, or self-hypnosis into their daily self-care regimen. Several clinical studies have suggested that there are positive results from mind-body modalities for many conditions [*see Table 3*]. As with other CAM interventions, however, limitations in study methodology and sample size, as well as lack of an adequate control, make definitive conclusions difficult.

The mind-body category also encompasses techniques for which a mechanism is not even remotely understood. No physical explanation for distant healing modalities—such as intercessory prayer, spiritual healing, and mental healing—is currently accepted, despite some evidence for positive treatment effects.[38] No harmful effects are seen when most mind-body interventions are used as an adjunct to conventional care. However, there is concern that patients might choose exclusive use of one or more of these methods in lieu of appropriate diagnosis and therapy.

Biologic-Based Therapies

Biologic therapy is the most popular of all fields of CAM. Its popularity stems from its similarity to the process of using conventional medications. Some persons consider biologics to be a possible quick fix for their ailments, without the need for physician visits or potentially harmful prescription medications. Others turn to biologics in the hope of preventing potentially serious diseases through the use of so-called natural substances.

Dietary supplements, including herbal and nonherbal products, make up the preponderance of medications in this category. The supplement industry has become a billion-dollar business, largely as a result of loosening of federal regulations. The Dietary Supplement Health and Education Act (DSHEA) of 1994 expanded the definition of dietary supplements to include vitamins, amino acids, herbs, and other botanicals. Furthermore, under DSHEA, supplements no longer require premar-

ket testing for safety and efficacy. Supplements are assumed to be safe unless proven otherwise by the Food and Drug Administration. Given the number and variety of products currently available, the FDA's ability to effectively regulate all products after they have been marketed is limited. The potential for harm from the lack of regulation can be seen from examples of misidentification of plant species,[39] contamination with heavy metals, and addition of pharmaceutical agents.[40,41]

Overall, there is only limited evidence supporting the use of most dietary supplements. Most clinical trials have been small, nonrandomized, or unblinded. In general, physicians and patients should view these products as medications. Physicians should advise patients to be wary of products for which grandiose claims are made. The potential for significant toxicity and drug interactions does exist. The list of currently used supplements is immense, and this chapter can touch on only the most popular [*see Tables 4 through 6*]. More comprehensive resources are available, however. James A. Duke, an ethnobotanist with the United States Department of Agriculture, has compiled a phytochemical and ethnobotanical database that can be accessed via the Internet (http://www.ars-grin.gov/duke/index.html). In 1978, the German government established an expert committee, the Commission E, to evaluate the safety and efficacy of herbs and herb combinations sold in Germany. Commission E published official monographs that give the approved uses, contraindications, side effects, dosages, drug interactions, and other therapeutic information regarding the use of 300 herbs and phytomedicines. These monographs have now been translated into English and total 8,500 pages.[42]

MANIPULATIVE AND BODY-BASED THERAPIES

Chiropractic

Many would argue that chiropractic medicine should not be considered alternative therapy. Patients, physicians, and insurance companies have all shown some degree of support for chiropractic care in recent years. Between 10% and 20% of the population use chiropractors.[17] Health care insurance plans, including Medicare, cover many of the services performed during chiropractic visits. In 1994, the Agency for Health Care Policy and Research (now the Agency for Healthcare Research and Quality) included spinal manipulation as part of its clinical practice guideline for acute low back pain.[43] This guideline is now outdated; however, chiropractic use continues to soar.

The tenets of chiropractic medicine place the spinal cord and nervous system at the center of a person's well-being. The nervous system is thought to control and influence all other body systems. Malalignments (subluxations) of the vertebrae are thought to cause or perpetuate disease. Once these subluxations are identified and corrected (via manipulation), the body uses its natural healing abilities to restore physiologic balance and health. Chiropractors typically look for spinal pain, asymmetry, impaired range of motion, or abnormalities in tone, texture, and temperature when evaluating patients.[44] Diagnostic testing, including x-rays, electromyography (EMG), and ultrasonography may be used to aid in diagnosis. Actual spinal manipulation is performed by direct or indirect delivery of thrusts to the spine. Frequently, the patient will experience a cracking noise. Some chiropractors may use adjunctive therapies, including massage, heat, and trigger-point injections.[44]

Chiropractic manipulation has been touted as treatment for a number of conditions, including hypertension, asthma, menstrual pain, and fibromyalgia. Very few data exist to support its use for these conditions, however. Use of chiropractic therapy for neck pain and headaches is also weakly supported. Much of the current use of chiropractic care stems from its utility in cases of low back pain. A number of controlled trials on chiropractic treatment for low back pain have been done, with conflicting results. A meta-analysis suggested that research was insufficient to prove a benefit for acute or chronic low back pain.[45] However, patient satisfaction seems to be high with such therapy.[46]

Serious complications from lumbar spinal manipulation seem to be uncommon, although there are reports of cauda equina syndrome.[47] Brain stem or cerebellar infarction, vertebral fracture, tracheal rupture, internal carotid artery dissection, and diaphragmatic paralysis have all been reported with cervical manipulation.[48] For that reason, it is difficult to advocate routine use of this technique for treatment of neck or headache disorders. Physicians should also recognize potential contraindications to chiropractic therapy. Patients with coagulopathy, osteoporosis, rheumatoid arthritis, spinal neoplasms, or spinal infections should be advised against such treatments.[49]

Massage Therapy

A number of different types of massage are in practice today. Many therapists combine aspects of Swedish massage (stroking and kneading), shiatsu (pressure-point manipulation), and neuromuscular massage (total body, deeper therapy) to relieve stress, anxiety, and muscle tension, as well as im-

Table 3   Selected Mind-Body Interventions

Modality	Description	Potential Applications	Comments
Aromatherapy	The use of essential oils (e.g., jasmine, chamomile, lavender) to enhance physical or psychological well-being	Anxiety	Long-term efficacy data are lacking[60]
Biofeedback	Voluntary control of physiologic processes—e.g., brainwaves, smooth muscle contraction, vasodilation—learned and reinforced with the aid of instrumentation (EEG, EMG, skin temperature/sweat monitors)	Asthma, ADHD, back pain, fibromyalgia, headache, hypertension, incontinence, neuromuscular disorders, Raynaud disease	Techniques utilized may vary between patients and practitioners; learning process can be slow, requiring multiple sessions with therapist and regular practice by patient
Guided imagery	Use of the imagination to positively stimulate the senses to bring about emotional and physiologic change	Chronic pain, headaches, nausea, post-traumatic stress disorder	Some studies suggest a positive impact on quality of life
Hypnotherapy	The induction of a trancelike state to induce relaxation and susceptibility to positive suggestion; used as a diagnostic and therapeutic tool	Anesthesia, headache, irritable bowel syndrome, smoking cessation	Success of therapy may depend on patient susceptibility and attitude toward hypnosis; no conclusive data on most conditions
Intercessory prayer	Request to God (or other spiritual beings) for the benefit of others; can take place in the presence of the patient or at a distance	Cardiac disease, HIV infection, RA	Studies are conflicting and inconclusive; mechanism is unclear
Meditation	Release of the mind from attachment to discursive thought, typically aided by focusing on the breath or a mantra	Anxiety, chronic pain, hypertension, substance abuse	Many types of meditation exist; large-scale studies are needed to prove the absolute impact of this simple intervention on health
Music therapy	Use of music to improve psychological, physical, cognitive, or social functioning	Anxiety, dementia, chronic pain, Parkinson disease	Treatment is guided by a trained music therapist; data lacking to draw conclusions regarding specific indications
Writing therapy	Creative writing exercise about an emotionally traumatic event	General emotional health, asthma, RA	Only one study, on asthma and RA, with 4-month follow-up[61]
Yoga	An Indian practice that involves specific postures; gentle, slow stretching; breathing exercises; and meditation to achieve self-guided relaxation	Asthma, cardiovascular disease, carpal tunnel syndrome, epilepsy, osteoarthritis	Most studies are short-term, with small sample sizes

ADHD—attention-deficit/hyperactivity disorder   EEG—electroencephalography   EMG—electromyography   RA—rheumatoid arthritis

Table 4   Commonly Used Herbal Dietary Supplements

Herb	Suggested Uses	Potential Toxicity	Potential Drug Interactions	Comments
Black cohosh (*Cimicifuga racemosa*)	Menopausal symptoms	Gastrointestinal discomfort	None known	No long-term studies showing efficacy or safety
Chaste tree berries (*Vitex agnus-castus*)	Premenstrual syndrome, mastodynia	Pruritus	May have dopaminergic activity; therefore, avoid with use of dopamine-receptor antagonists (e.g., neuroleptics)	Small, short-term studies suggest efficacy
Cranberry (*Vaccinium macrocarpon*)	Urinary tract infections	Nephrolithiasis (with cranberry concentrate tablets)[62]	None known	Treatment efficacy not proven; small studies show possible efficacy for prevention[63,64]
Dong quai (*Angelica sinensis*)	Menopausal symptoms	Rash	Increased international normalized ratio in patients taking warfarin	No clinical evidence of efficacy
Echinacea (*E. purpurea, E. pallida, E. angustifolia*)	Upper respiratory infections	Hypersensitivity reactions	Theoretically, may antagonize the effect of immunosuppressive medications	Variations in plant species studied, part of plant used, and extraction methods make conclusions regarding efficacy difficult
Ephedra (*E. sinica,* mahuang)	Asthma, congestion, weight loss	Hypertension, arrhythmia, myocardial infarction, stroke	Avoid use with monoamine oxidase inhibitors and cardiac glycosides; potential for serious toxicity when combined with other stimulants	Probably effective for short-term weight loss when combined with caffeine; long-term data lacking
Evening primrose (*Oenothera biennis*)	Eczema, irritable bowel syndrome, mastalgia, premenstrual syndrome, rheumatoid arthritis	Nausea, vomiting, diarrhea, flatulence	Possible lowering of seizure threshold in patients taking antiepileptic medications[65]	Conflicting efficacy data for a number of conditions
Feverfew (*Tanacetum parthenium*)	Migraine prophylaxis	Hypersensitivity reactions	Theoretical risk of increased bleeding when combined with anticoagulants	Few studies support efficacy[66]
Garlic (*Allium sativum*)	Cardiovascular protection	Gastrointestinal upset, bleeding	Theoretical risk of increased bleeding when combined with anticoagulants	Beneficial effects unproven
Ginger (*Zingiberis rhizoma*)	Motion sickness, dyspepsia	None known	Theoretical risk of increased bleeding when combined with anticoagulants	Has also been used for nausea and vomiting of pregnancy[67] and osteoarthritis[68]

prove circulation. Frequently, aromatic oils are employed to enhance the relaxation response. Many small studies support the use of massage for low back pain, fibromyalgia, chronic fatigue, anxiety, and depression.[50] No significant adverse effects are seen with massage, although caution must be advised for patients with coagulation disorders.

Structural integration (rolfing) is a system of deep-tissue manipulation that involves stretching of the fascial planes. In this system, the fascia is thought to be the key supporting structure for bones and muscles. When injury or stress occurs, the fascia tends to become shorter and thicker. Manipulation of the fascia with fingers, thumbs, and elbows is supposed to relieve tension, restore structural integrity, and improve physiologic and psychological function.[50] Limited data exist to support the efficacy of rolfing for any particular condition.

ENERGY THERAPIES

Many traditional cultures describe the physical body as existing within a field of energy. This energy is called prana by Indians and qi by the Chinese; English terms include subtle energy, vital energy, and life energy. Many ancient and modern CAM techniques involve the manipulation of this energy or the transfer of additional energy into the patient's field. Because the field extends beyond the body, energy therapies do not always involve physical contact between practitioner and patient. Further, the presumed connection of these individual fields via immersion in a universal field is believed to permit the use of some of these therapies at a distance.

Qigong

Qigong is a branch of traditional Chinese medicine designed to affect the flow of energy (qi) to preserve health. This system combines relaxation techniques with movement to achieve a meditative state designed to ensure mental and physical health. Tai chi (tai chi chuan) is a type of movement-oriented qigong that utilizes a sequence of slow, dancelike maneuvers to enhance the flow of qi through the body. In the course of a tai chi session, the person shifts body weight constantly from one foot to the other. Studies of tai chi in elderly persons have shown that long-term regular practice improves balance and cardiovascular fitness and reduces the risk of multiple falls.[51,52]

Meditative qigong is accomplished without movement and is intended to establish inner harmony. Breathing exercises can

Table 4   (*continued*)

Herb	Suggested Uses	Potential Toxicity	Potential Drug Interactions	Comments
Ginkgo biloba	Dementia, claudication, tinnitus	Gastrointestinal upset, headache, dizziness, bleeding, seizure	Theoretical risk of increased bleeding when combined with anticoagulants	May have modest effects on cognitive performance and functioning in patients with Alzheimer disease or multi-infarct dementia[69]; no evidence to support prevention of memory loss or dementia
Ginseng (*Panax* species; Asian ginseng, Korean ginseng, American ginseng)	Fatigue, diabetes	Generally considered safe; rare reports of hypertension, insomnia, headache, and mastalgia	May interact with monoamine oxidase inhibitors and warfarin (decreased prothrombin time)	Currently, little data to support its use[70]
Kava kava (*Piper methysticum*)	Anxiety	Rash, sedation, liver toxicity	May potentiate effects of benzodiazepines; best to avoid with other anxiolytics or alcohol because of risk of excess sedation	Studies suggest efficacy[71]; no data on addiction potential
Kola nut (*Cola nitida*)	Fatigue	Irritability, insomnia	Caution when used with other stimulants	Contains caffeine
Saw palmetto (*Serenoa repens*)	Prostatic hyperplasia	Mild gastrointestinal effects	None known	Short-term studies show improvement in symptoms[72]; no evidence for prevention of BPH or prostate cancer
St. John's wort (*Hypericum perforatum*)	Depression, anxiety	Headache, insomnia, dizziness, gastrointestinal irritation	Can decrease levels of cyclosporine, digoxin, oral contraceptives, theophylline, and indinavir; serotonin syndrome can occur when combined with prescription SSRIs	May be effective for mild to moderate depression[73,74]
Valerian (*Valeriana officinalis*)	Insomnia	Headaches	Avoid use with benzodiazepines because of sedation	Theoretical risk of addiction with prolonged use

BPH—benign prostatic hyperplasia SSRI—selective serotonin reuptake inhibitor

also be part of qigong. They are designed to enhance circulation of qi and expel negative energy.

Qigong has been used extensively in China for a number of conditions, including hypertension, anxiety, asthma, and nausea and vomiting.[53] Although the principles of qigong seem simple, it involves a complex set of processes that are not clearly understood. Inappropriate training has reportedly been associated with physical and mental disturbances.[54,55]

Therapeutic Touch

Therapeutic touch is the use of the hands, without actual physical touching, to influence or direct life energy throughout the body in an effort to promote healing. Therapeutic touch was codeveloped by a nurse, Dolores Krieger,[56] and many of its practitioners are nurses who use the technique for hospital inpatients.

In a therapeutic-touch session, which generally lasts 20 to 30

Table 5   Commonly Used Nonherbal Dietary Supplements

Herb	Suggested Uses	Potential Toxicity	Potential Drug Interactions	Comments
Coenzyme Q10	CHF, hypertension, angina	Nausea, heartburn, diarrhea	Decreased INR in patients on warfarin	No data to support use for angina, hypertension, or prevention of cardiovascular disease; no evidence of improved mortality in patients with CHF
Glucosamine sulfate/chondroitin sulfate	OA	Gastrointestinal side effects	Theoretical risk of increased bleeding in patients taking chondroitin sulfate and anticoagulants	Current data suggest symptomatic improvement for OA of the hips and knees[75]
Melatonin	Jet lag, insomnia	Fatigue, drowsiness	None known	Studies show efficacy at doses ≤ 1 mg,[76] but larger doses often sold; no data on long-term use
SAMe (S-adenosylmethionine)	OA, depression	Nausea, abdominal discomfort	Can increase toxicity of tricyclic antidepressants	Efficacy data lacking

CHF—congestive heart failure INR—international normalized ratio MAO—monoamine oxidase OA—osteoarthritis

Table 6   Popular Uses for Common Dietary Supplements*

Use	Supplement
Anxiety	Kava kava, St. John's wort
Asthma	Ephedra
Cardiovascular protection	Garlic
Claudication	*Ginkgo biloba*
Dementia	*Ginkgo biloba*
Depression	SAMe, St. John's wort
Dyspepsia	Ginger
Fatigue	Ginseng
Hypertension	Coenzyme Q10, garlic
Insomnia	Melatonin, valerian
Irritable bowel syndrome	Evening primrose
Jet lag	Melatonin
Menopausal symptoms	Black cohosh, Dong quai
Migraine prophylaxis	Feverfew
Motion sickness	Ginger
Osteoarthritis	Glucosamine sulfate–chondroitin sulfate
Premenstrual syndrome	Chaste tree berries, evening primrose
Prostatic hyperplasia	Saw palmetto
Tinnitus	*Ginkgo biloba*
Upper respiratory infections	Echinacea
Urinary tract infections	Cranberry
Weight loss	Ephedra

*See Tables 4 and 5 for potential toxicity, drug interactions, and comments.

minutes, the practitioner enters a meditative state (centering) and then assesses the patient's energy field. To do so, the practitioner holds his or her hands a few inches from the patient's body and moves from head to foot. Downward sweeping movements are then used to remove any blockages of energy and correct any energy-field imbalances. The practitioner then transfers energy to the patient's field and finishes the session by smoothing the field.

A small study of therapeutic touch, done as part of a fourth-grade science project, suggested that there was no basis to support practitioners' abilities to manipulate or detect human energy fields,[57] but this study was criticized as "simpleminded, methodologically flawed, and irrelevant."[58] In contrast, a number of clinical studies have suggested that there is a positive effect of therapeutic touch on wound healing, osteoarthritis, anxiety, and tension headache.[38] More vigorous trials need to be performed to determine the true efficacy of this technique.

CAM and the Practicing Physician

The field of research in complementary and alternative medicine is in its infancy. Current levels of evidence are insufficient to support or disprove a majority of CAM modalities. Despite these limitations, the public continues to embrace CAM therapies as alternatives or adjuncts to conventional care. Given that most patients currently do not inform their physicians of their CAM use, it is imperative that physicians take the lead in inquiring about such therapies. Open dialogue needs to be established to uncover the types of modalities being utilized, reasons for pursuing such therapy, and patient experiences. From there, a discussion of the current data on level of efficacy and toxicity can follow. Ultimately, primary care physicians may need to develop referral networks of trusted CAM practitioners who are open to reciprocal communication. These steps should serve to strengthen the physician-patient relationship while limiting the potential for adverse outcomes.

Specific emphasis should be placed on the role of dietary supplements, which pose a risk of significant toxicity and drug interactions. To ensure patient safety, the medication history should include specific questioning about what vitamins, herbs, or other supplements the person is taking. Unfortunately, supplements are often sold as combination products that are identified only by their catchy trade names. Patients should be encouraged to bring in all new medications and supplements at each visit. Depending on their side effect profile or potential for drug interactions, certain supplements should be discontinued in the perioperative period.[59] Finally, any suspected adverse reactions or drug-supplement reactions should be reported to the FDA's MedWatch program (http://www.fda.gov/medwatch or 1-800-FDA-1088).

References

1. Eisenberg DM, Davis RB, Ettner SL, et al: Trends in alternative medicine use in the United States, 1990-1997. JAMA 280:1569, 1998
2. Kessler RC, Davis RB, Foster DF, et al: Long-term trends in the use of complementary and alternative medical therapies in the United States. Ann Intern Med 135:262, 2001
3. Fisher P, Ward A: Medicine in Europe: complementary medicine in Europe. BMJ 309:107, 1994
4. Bausell RB, Lee WL, Berman BM: Demographic and health-related correlates of visits to complementary and alternative medical providers. Med Care 39:190, 2001
5. Population-based survey of complementary and alternative medicine usage, patient satisfaction, and physician involvement. South Carolina Complementary Medicine Program Baseline Research Team. South Med J 93:375, 2000
6. Eisenberg DM, Kessler RC, Foster C, et al: Unconventional medicine in the United States. N Engl J Med 328:246, 1993
7. Astin JA: Why patients use alternative medicine. JAMA 279:1548, 1998
8. Bernstein BJ, Grasso J: Prevalence of complementary and alternative medicine use in cancer patients. Oncology 15:1267, 2001
9. Sparber A, Wootton JC, Bauer L, et al: Use of complementary medicine by adult patients participating in HIV/AIDS clinical trials. J Altern Complement Med 6:415, 2000
10. Pioro-Boisset M, Esdaile JM, Fitzcharles MA: Alternative medicine use in fibromyalgia syndrome. Arthritis Care Res 9:13, 1996
11. Rawsthorne P, Shanahan F, Cronin NC, et al: An international survey of the use and attitudes regarding alternative medicine by patients with inflammatory bowel disease. Am J Gastroenterol 94:1298, 1999
12. Campion EW: Why unconventional medicine? N Engl J Med 328:282, 1993
13. Eisenberg DM, Kessler RC, Van Rompay MI, et al: Perceptions about complementary therapies relative to conventional therapies among adults who use both: results from a national survey. Ann Intern Med 135:344, 2001
14. Blendon RJ, DesRoches CM, Benson JM, et al: Americans' views on the use and regulation of dietary supplements. Arch Intern Med 161:805, 2001
15. Bloom BS, Retbi A, Dahan S, et al: Evaluation of randomized controlled trials on complementary and alternative medicine. Int J Technol Assess Health Care 16:13, 2000
16. Linde K, Jonas WB, Melchart D, et al: The methodological quality of randomized controlled trials of homeopathy, herbal medicines and acupuncture. Int J Epidemiol 30:526, 2001
17. Vickers A, Goyal N, Harland R, et al: Do certain countries produce only positive results? A systematic review of controlled trials. Control Clin Trials 19:159, 1998
18. Tang JL, Zhan SY, Ernst E: Review of randomized controlled trials of traditional Chinese medicine. BMJ 319:160, 1999

19. Melchart D, Linde K, Fischer P, et al: Echinacea for preventing and treating the common cold (review). Cochrane Database Syst Rev (2):CD000530, 2000

20. Yuan X, Hao X, Lai Z, et al: Effects of acupuncture at fengchi point (GB 20) on cerebral blood flow. J Tradit Chin Med 18:102, 1998

21. Acupuncture. NIH Consensus Statement 15(5):1, 1997

22. Linde K, Melchart D, Fischer P, et al: Acupuncture for idiopathic headache (review). Cochrane Database Syst Rev (1):CD001218, 2001

23. Berman BM, Ezzo J, Hadhazy V, et al: Is acupuncture effective in the treatment of fibromyalgia? J Fam Pract 48:213, 1999

24. Ezzo J, Hadhazy V, Birch S, et al: Acupuncture for osteoarthritis of the knee: a systematic review. Arthritis Rheum 44:819, 2001

25. White AR, Rampes H, Ernst E: Acupuncture for smoking cessation (review). Cochrane Database Syst Rev (2):CD000009, 2000

26. Ernst E, White A: Life-threatening adverse reactions after acupuncture? A systematic review. Pain 71:123, 1997

27. Yamashita H, Tsukayama H, Tanno Y, et al: Adverse events related to acupuncture. JAMA 280:1563, 1998

28. Ernst E, White AR: Prospective studies of the safety of acupuncture: a systematic review. Am J Med 110:481, 2001

29. Chapman EH: Homeopathy. Essentials of Complementary and Alternative Medicine. Jonas W, Levin JS, Eds. Lippincott Williams & Wilkins, Philadelphia, 1999, p 472

30. Kleijnen J, Knipschild P, ter Riet G: Clinical trials of homeopathy. BMJ 302:316, 1991

31. Linde K, Clausius N, Ramirez G, et al: Are the clinical effects of homoeopathy placebo effects? A meta-analysis of placebo-controlled trials. Lancet 350:834, 1997

32. Long L, Ernst E: Homeopathic remedies for the treatment of osteoarthritis: a systematic review. Br Homeopath J 90:37, 2001

33. Ernst E, Pittler MH: Efficacy of homeopathic arnica: a systematic review of placebo-controlled clinical trials. Arch Surg 133:1187, 1998

34. Linde K, Jobst KA: Homeopathy for chronic asthma (review). Cochrane Database Syst Rev (2):CD000353, 2000

35. Stehlin I: Homeopathy: real medicine or empty promises? FDA Consumer 30, 1996 http://www.fda.gov/fdac/096_toc.html

36. Cannon WB: The emergency function of the adrenal medulla in pain and the major emotions. Am J Physiol 33:356, 1914

37. Benson H: The Relaxation Response. William Morrow, New York, 1975

38. Astin JA, Harkness E, Ernst E: The efficacy of "distant healing": a systematic review of randomized trials. Ann Intern Med 132:903, 2000

39. Nortier JL, Martinez MC, Schmeiser HH, et al: Urothelial carcinoma associated with the use of a Chinese herb (*Aristolochia fangchi*). N Engl J Med 342:1686, 2000

40. Ko RJ: Adulterants in Asian patent medicines. N Engl J Med 339:847, 1998

41. Fugh-Berman A: Herb-drug interactions. Lancet 355:134, 2000

42. Complete German Commission E Monographs: Therapeutic Guide To Herbal Medicines. Blumenthal M, Ed. American Botanical Council, Texas, 1998

43. Bigos S, Bowyer O, Braen B, et al: Acute Low Back Problems in Adults. Clinical Practice Guideline, No. 14. US Dept of Heath and Human Services (AHCPR Publication No. 95-0642), Rockville, Maryland, 1994

44. Lawrence DJ: Chiropractic medicine. Essentials of Alternative and Complementary Medicine. Jonas WB, Levin JS, Eds. Lippincott Williams & Wilkins, Philadelphia, 1999, p 275

45. Koes BW, Assendelft WJ, van der Heijden GJ, et al: Spinal manipulation for low back pain: an updated systematic review of randomized clinical trials. Spine 21:2860, 1996

46. Cherkin DC, Deyo RA, Battie M, et al: A comparison of physical therapy, chiropractic manipulation, and provision of an educational booklet for the treatment of patients with low back pain. N Engl J Med 339:1021, 1998

47. Kaptchuk TJ, Eisenberg DM: Chiropractic: origins, controversies, and contributions. Arch Intern Med 158:2215, 1998

48. Ernst E: Adverse effects of spinal manipulation. Essentials of Complementary and Alternative Medicine. Jonas WB, Levin JS, Eds. Lippincott Williams & Wilkins,

Philadelphia, 1999, p 176

49. Field T: Massage therapy. Essentials of Complementary and Alternative Medicine. Jonas W, Levin JS, Eds. Lippincott Williams & Wilkins, Philadelphia, 1999, p 383

50. Rubik B, Pavek R, Greene E, et al: Manual healing methods. Alternative medicine: expanding medical horizons: a report to the National Institutes of Health on alternative medical systems and practices in the United States, prepared under the auspices of the Workshop on Alternative Medicine. NIH publication (No. 94-066). Washington, D.C., 1994, p 132

51. Lin YC, Wong AM, Chou SW, et al: The effects of Tai Chi Chuan on postural stability in the elderly: preliminary report. Changgeng Yi Xue Za Zhi 23:197, 2000

52. Hong Y, Li JX, Robinson PD: Balance control, flexibility, and cardiorespiratory fitness among older Tai Chi practitioners. Br J Sports Med 34:29, 2000

53. Lee CT, Lei T: Qigong. Essentials of Complementary and Alternative Medicine. Jonas W, Levin JS, Eds. Lippincott Williams & Wilkins, Philadelphia, 1999, p 392

54. Shan HH, Yan HQ, Xu SH, et al: Clinical phenomenology of mental disorders caused by Qigong exercise. Chin Med J (Engl) 102:445, 1989

55. Xu SH: Psychophysiological reactions associated with qigong therapy. Chin Med J (Engl) 107:230, 1994

56. Krieger D: Accepting Your Power to Heal: The Personal Practice of Therapeutic Touch. Bear & Company, Rochester, Vermont, 1993

57. Rosa L, Rosa E, Sarner L, et al: A close look at therapeutic touch. JAMA 279:1005, 1998

58. Freinkel A: An even closer look at therapeutic touch. JAMA 280:1905, 1998

59. Ang-Lee MK, Moss J, Yuan CS: Herbal medicines and perioperative care. JAMA 286:208, 2001

60. Cooke B, Ernst E: Aromatherapy: a systematic review. Br J Gen Pract 50:493, 2000

61. Smyth JM, Stone AA, Hurewitz A, et al: Effects of writing about stressful experiences on symptom reduction in patients with asthma or rheumatoid arthritis. JAMA 281:1304, 1999

62. Terris MK, Issa MM, Tacker JR: Dietary supplementation with cranberry concentrate tablets may increase the risk of nephrolithiasis. Urology 57:26, 2001

63. Avorn J, Monane M, Gurwitz JH, et al: Reduction of bacteriuria and pyuria after ingestion of cranberry juice. JAMA 271:751, 1994

64. Jepson RG, Mihaljevic L, Craig J: Cranberries for preventing urinary tract infections (review.) Cochrane Database Syst Rev (3):CD001321, 2001

65. Miller LG: Herbal medicinals: selected clinical considerations focusing on known or potential drug-herb interactions. Arch Intern Med 158:2200, 1998

66. Ernst E, Pittler MH: The efficacy and safety of feverfew (*Tanacetum parthenium L.*): an update of a systematic review. Public Health Nutr 3:509, 2000

67. Vutyavanich T, Draisarin T, Ruangsri R: Ginger for nausea and vomiting in pregnancy: randomized, double-masked, placebo-controlled trial. Obstet Gynecol 97:577, 2001

68. Altman RD, Marcussen KC: Effects of ginger extract on knee pain in patients with osteoarthritis. Arthritis Rheum 44:2531, 2001

69. LeBars PL, Katz MM, Berman N, et al: A placebo-controlled, double-blind, randomized trial of an extract of *Ginkgo biloba* for dementia. JAMA 278:1327, 1997

70. Vogler BK, Pittler MH, Ernst E: The efficacy of ginseng: a systematic review of randomized clinical trials. Eur J Clin Pharmacol 55:567, 1999

71. Pittler MH, Ernst E: Efficacy of kava extract for treating anxiety: systematic review and meta-analysis. J Clin Psychopharmacol 20:84, 2000

72. Wilt TJ, Ishani A, Stark G, et al: Saw palmetto extracts for the treatment of benign prostatic hyperplasia: a systematic review. JAMA 280:1604, 1999

73. Linde K, Mulrow CD: St. John's wort for depression (review). Cochrane Database Syst Rev (2):CD000448, 2000

74. Gaster B, Holroyd J: St John's wort for depression: a systematic review. Arch Intern Med 160:152, 2000

75. McAlindon TE, LaValley MP, Gulin JP, et al: Glucosamine and chondroitin for treatment of osteoarthritis. JAMA 283:1469, 2000

76. Zhdanova IV, Lynch HJ, Wurtman RJ: Melatonin: a sleep-promoting hormone. Sleep 20:899, 1997

9 Symptom Management in Palliative Medicine

Maria Torroella Carney, M.D., and Jennifer Rhodes-Kropf, M.D.

The goal of palliative care is to provide comfort and support for both patient and family through the course of a life-threatening illness. Symptom control is essential to meeting that goal. This chapter discusses symptoms that commonly contribute to patients' suffering in terminal illness: pain; respiratory, gastrointestinal, mouth, and skin problems; and delirium.

Although this chapter focuses on physical and psychological symptoms, achieving symptom control requires the physician to address the patient's suffering in all its aspects: physical, psychological, social, and spiritual. Physical distress cannot be effectively treated in isolation from the emotional and spiritual components that contribute to it, nor can these sources of suffering be addressed adequately when patients are in physical distress. The various components of suffering must be addressed simultaneously [*see Chapter 10*].

Symptom Assessment

A full and formal symptom assessment is necessary before effective treatment can be instituted.[1] Symptoms are inherently subjective[2]; therefore, patient self-reporting must be the primary source of information, and the clinician must believe what the patient says. If the patient is unable to report, a family member or professional can provide a surrogate assessment. However, several studies have demonstrated that observer and patient assessments are not well correlated.[3,4]

To compensate for this inherent subjectivity, researchers have developed symptom measurement systems that are intended to quantify patients' perceptions in a manner that is valid and reliable. Often, these measurement systems have taken the form of symptom checklists.[5,6] For example, the Edmonton Symptom Assessment Scale[5] comprises 14 questions that evaluate eight physical and psychological symptoms [*see Table 1*]. This scale has been extensively employed in palliative care research, in part because of its ease of use. Although the scale yields a numeric score (the higher the score, the more severe the patient's condition), the formal scoring mechanism is used only in research. In clinical practice, the scale can be used informally to evaluate a patient's status and follow it over time.

The Memorial Symptom Assessment Scale[7] characterizes 32 physical and psychological symptoms in terms of intensity and frequency, as well as the level of distress from the symptoms [*see Table 2*]. Although the Memorial Symptom Assessment Scale provides a greater range of information than the Edmonton Symptom Assessment Scale, the former is correspondingly more time consuming to use.

Physical Symptoms

PAIN

Diagnosis

Management of pain begins with a careful and detailed assessment [*see Chapter 173*]. The goal of this assessment is to determine the location and character of the pain, define its cause (or causes), and develop a plan of care.

Pain cannot be measured objectively, and several studies have shown that medical care providers' estimates of patients' pain severity are significantly lower than the patients' self-reports.[8,9] Pain is independent of age, gender, marital status, physical function, and cognitive function.[10] Therefore, the central guiding principle of pain assessment is to ask the patient and believe the patient's description of pain.

Pain assessment in the elderly is often complicated by coexistent cognitive impairment. The cognitively impaired patient may be unable to express pain adequately or request analgesics and, therefore, is at increased risk for undertreatment of pain.[11,12] As with cognitively intact patients, the first step in the assessment of pain in demented patients is to ask them about their pain. Although patients with severe dementia may be incapable of communicating, many patients with mild or moderate impairment can accurately localize and grade the severity of their pain,[13] and these self-reports should be regarded as valid.

Untreated pain can result in agitation and disruptive behavior, and it may worsen or precipitate delirium, particularly in cognitively impaired patients.[14,15] When delirium prevents communication with the patient, the physician may have to infer that pain is present and proceed with treatment.

Treatment

Opioids are the standard choice for treating pain in terminally ill patients. The physician who provides palliative care needs to have the confidence and competence to prescribe opioids at whatever dose is needed to control pain, as well as the skill to determine when adjuvant analgesics (e.g., antidepressant or antiseizure medication) are needed to manage certain types of pain.[16,17] Terminally ill patients are a special population, often suffering chronic pain and taking pain medications over longer periods of time and at higher dosages.[18] Indeed, tolerance to opioids may require that they be used in amounts that would be fatal to the opioid-naive patient.

In a multisite study of terminally ill patients in the United States, Weiss and colleagues[19] found that half of terminally ill patients experienced moderate to severe pain but that less than one third wanted additional pain treatment from their primary care physician. Reasons for not wanting additional therapy included dislike of analgesic side effects and not wanting to take more pills or injections. Some patients, however, mentioned fear of addiction. This is a common—and unwarranted—concern not only of patients but of some medical personnel, as well.

As the goals of care change in the course of a life-threatening illness, higher dosages of pain medication may be needed to achieve comfort. In the last days of life, relief of suffering may require sedation to the point of unconsciousness, a technique referred to as palliative sedation (see below).

RESPIRATORY SYMPTOMS

Dyspnea

Shortness of breath has been described in 70% of cancer patients during the last 6 weeks of life[20] and in 50% to 70% of patients dying

Table 1 Modified Edmonton Symptom Assessment Scale[5]

1a. Please rate your *pain* now.
1. ☐ No pain
2. ☐ Mild pain
3. ☐ Moderate pain
4. ☐ Severe pain

1b. Please rate your *pain* over the past 3 days.
1. ☐ No pain
2. ☐ Mild pain
3. ☐ Moderate pain
4. ☐ Severe pain

1c. Is your *pain control* acceptable to you?
1. ☐ Very acceptable
2. ☐ Acceptable
3. ☐ Not acceptable

2. How would you describe your *activity level* over the past 3 days?
1. ☐ Very active
2. ☐ Somewhat active
3. ☐ Minimally active
4. ☐ Not active

3. How would you describe your amount of *nausea* over the past 3 days?
1. ☐ Not nauseated
2. ☐ Mildly nauseated
3. ☐ Moderately nauseated
4. ☐ Very nauseated

4a. How would you describe your level of *constipation* over the past 3 days?
1. ☐ No constipation
2. ☐ Mild constipation
3. ☐ Moderate constipation
4. ☐ Severe constipation

4b. When was your *last bowel movement*?
1. ☐ Today
2. ☐ Yesterday
3. ☐ 2–3 days ago
4. ☐ More than 4 days ago

5. How would you describe your feelings of *depression* over the past 3 days?
1. ☐ Not depressed
2. ☐ Mildly depressed
3. ☐ Moderately depressed
4. ☐ Very depressed

6. How would you describe your feelings of *anxiety* over the past 3 days?
1. ☐ Not anxious
2. ☐ Mildly anxious
3. ☐ Moderately anxious
4. ☐ Very anxious

7. How would you describe your level of *fatigue* over the past 3 days?
1. ☐ Not fatigued
2. ☐ Mildly fatigued
3. ☐ Moderately fatigued
4. ☐ Very fatigued

8. How has your *appetite* been over the past 3 days?
1. ☐ Very good appetite
2. ☐ Moderate appetite
3. ☐ Poor appetite
4. ☐ No appetite

9. How would you describe your sensation of *well-being* over the past 3 days?
1. ☐ Very good sensation of well-being
2. ☐ Moderately good sensation of well-being
3. ☐ Not very good sensation of well-being
4. ☐ Poor sensation of well-being

10. How *short of breath* have you been over the past 3 days?
1. ☐ No shortness of breath
2. ☐ Mild shortness of breath
3. ☐ Moderate shortness of breath
4. ☐ Very short of breath

11. How has your *physical discomfort* been over the past 3 days?
1. ☐ No physical discomfort
2. ☐ Mild physical discomfort
3. ☐ Moderate physical discomfort
4. ☐ Severe physical discomfort

of other illnesses.[21] Ventafridda and colleagues[22] observed "horrible and unpleasant" dyspnea in 10% of cancer patients dying in a palliative care unit. Like pain, dyspnea is a subjective symptom that may not correlate with any objective signs of respiratory compromise,[23] and hence, its management can be challenging.

It is important to diagnose and treat any underlying reversible causes of dyspnea. For example, dyspnea caused by congestive heart failure will require diuretics and inotropic support [*see Chapter 22*].

When therapy specific to the underlying cause is unavailable or ineffective, several techniques may alleviate breathlessness. Simple measures include pursed-lip breathing and diaphragmatic breathing, leaning forward with arms on a table, cool-air ventilation (from a fan or an open window), and nasal oxygen. Opioids have been shown in numerous studies to be highly effective in the amelioration of dyspnea.[24,25] In one study,[24] morphine in doses sufficient to relieve dyspnea had no measurable adverse effect on respiratory rate or effort, oxygen saturation, and carbon dioxide concentration. Therefore, morphine is the drug of choice for treating otherwise refractory dyspnea in terminal illness.

Lorazepam and other benzodiazepines are also widely used, especially in terminally ill patients whose dyspnea has an anxiety component, although evidence to support this practice is limited.[26] In addition, steroids and oxygen therapy may be of benefit [*see Table 3*].

Cough

Cough can be an annoyance or can develop into a major source of suffering by causing muscle strain, increasing fatigue, and interrupting sleep. In one study of lung cancer patients, cough was the most common symptom, affecting 80% of patients until just before death.[27] Because the causes of cough are varied, the optimal treatment is treatment of the underlying problem, if possible. When such treatment is not possible, management depends on whether the cough is productive [*see Figure 1*].[28] A productive cough may improve with chest physiotherapy, oxygen, humidity, and suctioning. Antibiotics for infection, *N*-acetylcysteine, bronchodilators, and guaifenesin are also effective.[29,30] Opioids, antihistamines, and anticholinergics decrease mucus production, which can decrease the stimulus for cough. Cough suppressants can be harmful if used in patients with productive coughs by causing mucus retention,[29,30] which may lead to the formation of mucous plugs and airway obstruction. A patient with a nonproductive cough may benefit from a cough-suppressing agent such as a local anesthetic (e.g., nebulized bupivacaine), bronchodilators, opioids, or a soothing agent such as a lozenge. Benzonatate, steroids, and opiates are effective treatments. Opioids act centrally and are one of the most effective agents against cough. Nonopioid antitussives, such as dextromethorphan, may work synergistically with opiates.[30]

GASTROINTESTINAL SYMPTOMS

Anorexia, nausea and vomiting, constipation, bowel obstruction, and diarrhea are common and potentially devastating in terminal illness.

Anorexia

Anorexia is nearly universal in patients with a terminal illness.[31] Evaluation of anorexia should be concentrated on finding a reversible or treatable cause. It is important to note that cognitive impairment, which is also highly prevalent in advanced disease, may cause a person to be misdiagnosed as anorexic, because the person may be unable to obtain, prepare, or eat meals.[32] Often in terminal disease, however, the patient simply loses the desire to eat.

Patients themselves may complain of anorexia, in some cases because they find the resulting cachexia unacceptable. In those cases, the decision to treat is straightforward. However, anorexia can often be of more concern to family, friends, and medical staff than to patients themselves. The family may be concerned because loss of appetite is seen as a certain sign of impending death.[33] Concern about anorexia may also be rooted in the emotional and psychological meanings that surround food and its consumption: not feeding the patient may be considered equivalent to not caring about the patient. The family should be reassured that anorexia in terminal disease is usually not associated with suffering; especially at the end of life, patients rarely feel hunger or thirst, and many patients who stop eating experience analgesia and even euphoria. Excessive proteins and lipids can induce nausea and vomiting in such cases, and excessive hydration can result in edema and dyspnea.[34]

In the early stages of terminal illness, however, studies have shown that the treatment of anorexia with appetite stimulants may improve patients' quality of life.[35,36] Treatment can begin with simple measures. The patient should be encouraged to eat without any restrictions on sugar, salt, or fats, when possible. Alcohol has appetite-stimulating properties, so patients may wish to consider a cocktail or glass of wine before the evening meal.[37]

Appetite stimulants with proven efficacy in palliative care include dexamethasone, in dosages of 2 to 20 mg/day (recommended because its long half-life permits once-daily dosing and because it has minimal mineralocorticoid effects); megestrol acetate (beginning with 200 mg every 8 hours and titrating to 800 mg/day); and cannabinoids (e.g., tetrahydrocannabinol [THC]), starting with a small dose and titrating to effect and tolerability. Dexamethasone and megestrol tend to be used more often than cannabinoids because of the restricted availability of cannabinoids.

Anorexia in patients with dementia Because Alzheimer disease destroys higher brain function while sparing the other major organ systems, many patients with Alzheimer disease progress to a stage at which they are unable to eat on their own or even chew and swallow reliably but may survive for years if artificial hydration and nutrition are provided. Deciding whether to insert a gastrostomy tube in such patients can be challenging. Complications of tube feeding are common and include repeated infections, whose treatment may require needle sticks, transfer to a hospital, and restraints; these are especially burdensome for a confused patient who cannot understand the reason for such interventions.[38] In addition, patients with advanced neurologic impairment are at high risk for pneumonia from a variety of causes, including but not limited to aspiration. There is no evidence that tube feeding reduces the risk of pneumonia in such patients; it may even increase the risk.[39] One may ask what is to be gained with artificial nutrition and hydration in such cases.

Because of the terminal and irreversible nature of end-stage dementia and the substantial burden that continued life-prolonging care may pose for these patients, they may be better served by palliative care that focuses predominantly on their comfort. Comfort care is viewed as preferable to life-prolonging

---

Table 2 Memorial Symptom Assessment Scale[14]

For physical symptoms, patients are instructed to check off all symptoms experienced during the past week and the degree to which the symptom bothered or distressed them. Categories and scores are as follows: Not at all (0), A little bit (1), Somewhat (2), Quite a bit (3), and Very much (4). Patients may also add symptoms not listed and rate them on the same scale. For psychological symptoms, patients are instructed to check off all symptoms experienced during the past week and how often each occurred. Categories and scores are as follows: Rarely (1), Occasionally (2), Frequently (3), and Almost constantly (4). Patients may also add symptoms not listed and rate them on the same scale.

Physical Symptom	Severity				
	0	1	2	3	4
Difficulty concentrating					
Pain					
Lack of energy					
Cough					
Changes in skin					
Dry mouth					
Nausea					
Feeling drowsy					
Numbness or tingling in hands and feet					
Hair loss					
Constipation					
Swelling of arms or legs					

Psychological Symptom	Frequency				
	0	1	2	3	4
Feeling sad					
Worrying					
Feeling irritable					
Feeling nervous					

Table 3   Drug Treatment for Dyspnea[33]

Drug (Trade Name)	Dosage	Comment
Oral morphine	2.5–5 mg p.o., q. 4 hr while awake	Doses for opiate-naive patients
I.V. morphine	0.5 mg/hr; titrate to relief	Once dose requirement established, switch to long-acting oral opiate or fentanyl patch
Nebulized morphine	2.5–10 mg injectable in 2 ml NS	—
Nebulized hydromorphone	0.25–1 mg injectable in 2 ml NS	—
Nebulized albuterol	0.083% (3 ml)	Possible adjunct to opioid
Nebulized methylprednisolone (Solu-Medrol)	10 mg	Possible adjunct to opioid
Dexamethasone	Day 1: 16 mg p.o.; days 2–3: 8 mg b.i.d.; days 3–4: 4 mg b.i.d.; subsequent: 2 mg b.i.d.	Possible adjunct to opioid
Prednisone	40 mg b.i.d. for 5–7 days	Possible adjunct to opioid
Lorazepam (Ativan)	1–10 mg/day in two or three divided doses; usual dose, 2–6 mg/day in divided doses. Elderly: 0.5–4 mg/day	For patients whose dyspnea has an anxiety component
Oxygen	2 L/min by nasal cannula; titrate to relief	—

NS—normal saline

measures by a substantial proportion of nursing home patients and family members.[40] Families should be reassured that it is never unethical to withhold nutrition and hydration if they are not helping the patient.

Nausea and Vomiting

Nausea and vomiting occur in up to 62% of patients with terminal cancer[41] and 27% of patients dying of other causes. There are multiple potential causes for both nausea and vomiting [see Table 4].[37] Once the cause has been determined, symptomatic relief is relatively easy to achieve with the appropriate medications [see Table 5].[28] Without an understanding of the underlying etiology, it may be impossible to find the most beneficial form of treatment.

The central nervous system and the gastrointestinal tract are particularly important in nausea and vomiting.[42] The gastric lining, the chemoreceptor trigger zone in the base of the fourth ventricle, the vestibular apparatus, and the cortex are all involved in the physiology of nausea. Stimulation of the vomiting center in the brain from one or more of these areas is mediated through the neurotransmitters serotonin, dopamine, acetylcholine, and histamine. Serotonin seems to be important in the gastric lining and the CNS, whereas acetylcholine and histamine are important in the vestibular apparatus. Cortical responses are mediated via both neurotransmitters and learned responses (e.g., nausea related to anxiety or anticipatory nausea with chemotherapy).

The major causes of nausea and vomiting can be classified by the mechanisms' principal site of action. Dopamine-mediated nausea is probably the most common form of nausea and the most frequently targeted one for initial symptom management. Antidopamine medications are phenothiazines and butyrophenone neuroleptics (metoclopramide and prochlorperazine). They may cause drowsiness and extrapyramidal symptoms. Haloperidol is a highly effective antinausea agent and may be less sedating. Antihistamines such as diphenhydramine can be used to control nausea, but they may cause sedation. Antihistamines also have anticholinergic

properties. Serotonin has been implicated in chemotherapy-associated nausea. Antiserotonin medications (e.g., odansetron) can be effective, but they are expensive.

Nausea can also result from slow gastric and intestinal motility, so-called squashed stomach syndrome from mechanical compression of the stomach, and constipation. Hence, prokinetic agents (e.g., metoclopramide) and aggressive fecal disimpaction and institution of a bowel regimen (see below) should be considered as therapeutic modalities. In some patients, hyperacidity and mucosal erosion may be associated with significant nausea. In these patients, consider the use of antacids, histamine$_2$ blockers, proton-pump inhibitors, and misoprostol [see Chapter 62].

Constipation

Constipation can lead to serious complications, such as bowel obstruction, ulceration, or perforation, as well as delirium. Because constipation is so common in terminal illness, appropriate management includes the institution of preventive measures in patients at high risk for this complication.

Diagnosis   Assessment of constipation begins with inquiry about the frequency and consistency of stools; possible contributing factors, such as medications, reduced mobility, and a low-fiber diet; and any accompanying symptoms that suggest complications, such as nausea, vomiting, abdominal pain, distention, and discomfort.[43] As with any symptom, the search for a reversible cause is primary. A plain x-ray can be useful to evaluate for ileus or bowel obstruction. Invasive evaluation with colonoscopy should be considered in difficult, refractory, or complicated cases.

Many medications can contribute to constipation. These include beta blockers, calcium channel blockers, anticholinergic agents, and diuretics.[43,44] First and foremost, however, are opioid analgesics: constipation is a universal side effect of opioid therapy, especially in the terminally ill. For that reason, every terminally ill patient who is placed on opioids should also be started on a preventive regimen for constipation. The bowel regimen in these patients starts with stool softeners and stimulant laxatives and progresses through hyperosmotic agents and enemas, as necessary [*see Table 6*].[45] This regimen can also be utilized for treatment of constipation from other causes, once intestinal obstruction is ruled out.

Treatment Treatment of constipation is with oral agents, rectal suppositories, or enemas and can focus on softening the stool, enlarging stool volume, or promoting bowel peristalsis. Laxative categories include detergents, stimulants, osmotic agents, prokinetic agents, lubricant stimulants, and large-volume enemas [*see Table 7*]. Polyethylene glycol solution (GoLYTELY) or powder (MiraLax) is an osmotic agent that is marketed as a bowel cleanser to prepare patients for colonoscopy, but it is often effective in relieving constipation and may cause less cramping than other laxatives. Whichever laxative is chosen, the clinician should prescribe the maximum therapeutic dose of the agent before switching to another one.

Fecal impaction Although impaction of stool in the rectum is a complication of constipation, the typical clinical manifestation is so-called overflow diarrhea from leakage of unformed stool around the obstruction. A digital rectal examination may confirm fecal impaction in the distal rectum, but abdominal x-rays may be required for the diagnosis of more proximal impaction. Treatment of fecal impaction is from below, utilizing digital disimpaction and rectal laxatives (suppositories, enemas, or both); only if those fail should oral treatment be attempted.[43]

Bowel Obstruction

The prevalence of bowel obstruction is as high as 40% in bowel and pelvic cancers.[46] Constipation and fecal impaction are the most common causes of bowel obstruction in terminal illness. Symptoms of bowel obstruction include anorexia, confusion, nausea and vomiting, constipation, and pain. Diagnosis is made on the basis of the clinical presentation and abdominal x-rays.

Consultation with a surgeon is advisable to establish a treatment plan. In addition to aggressive measures to prevent or treat constipation and fecal impaction (see above), treatment of bowel obstruction may involve surgical relief of obstruction, nasogastric suction, and pharmacologic measures. Colicky or cramping pain may respond to dicyclomine, opioids (parenteral or rectal), and warm soaks to the abdomen. The obstruction and associated nausea and vomiting may respond to metoclopramide, haloperidol, or dexamethasone. Parenteral octreotide is also useful in this setting to decrease the volume of bowel secretions.

Diarrhea

Diarrhea, which is often secondary to fecal impaction or antibiotic-associated colitis, is a particularly distressing and exhausting symptom in the terminally ill patient.[43] Once impaction, overgrowth, and other causes (e.g., gastrointestinal bleeding, malabsorption, and medications) have been ruled out, kaolinpectin, psyllium, loperamide, or tincture of opium may be tried.

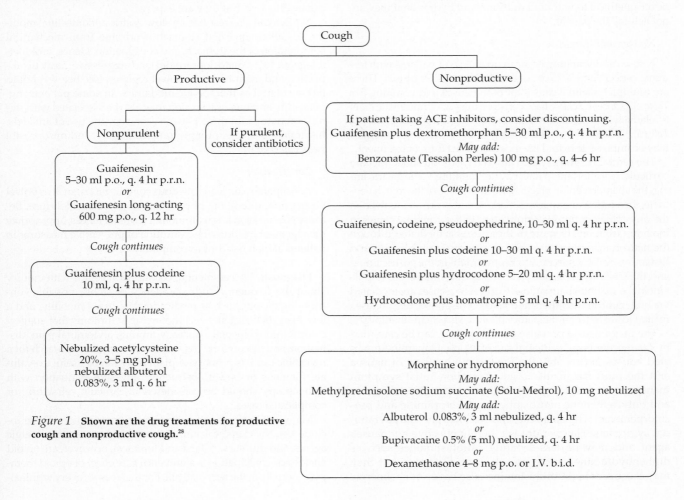

Figure 1 **Shown are the drug treatments for productive cough and nonproductive cough.**[28]

Table 4   Management of Nausea and Vomiting[37]

Etiology	Pathophysiology	Therapy
Mechanical obstruction—intraluminal	Constipation, obstipation	Laxatives; disimpaction
Mechanical obstruction—extraluminal	Tumor, fibrotic stricture	Surgery, fluid management, steroids, octreotide, scopolamine
Medications—chemotherapy	Chemoreceptor trigger zone, GI tract	Antiserotonin, antidopamine, steroids
Medications—NSAIDs	GI tract irritation	Cytoprotective agents, antacids
Medications—opioids	Chemoreceptor trigger zone, vestibular effect, GI tract	Antidopamine, anticholinergic, prokinetic agents, stimulant cathartics
Medications—other	Chemoreceptors	Antidopamine, antihistamine
Meningeal irritation	Increased intracranial pressure	Steroids
Mentation (e.g., anxiety)	Cortical	Anxiolytics
Metabolic—hypercalcemia	Chemoreceptor trigger zone	Antidopamine, antihistamine
Metabolic—hyponatremia	Chemoreceptor trigger zone	Antidopamine, antihistamine
Metabolic—hepatic/renal failure	Chemoreceptor trigger zone	Rehydration, steroids
Metastases—cerebral	Increased intracranial pressure	Steroids, mannitol
	Chemoreceptor trigger zone	Antidopamine, antihistamine
Metastases—liver	Toxin buildup	Antidopamine, antihistamine
Microbes—gastroenteritis	GI tract	Anti-infectives, antacids
Microbes—sepsis	Chemoreceptor trigger zone	Antidopamine, antihistamine, anti-infectives
Movement	Vestibular stimulation	Anticholinergic
Mucosal irritation	GI hyperacidity, GERD	Cytoprotective agents, antacids
Myocardial—ischemia, CHF	Vagal stimulation, cortical, chemoreceptor trigger zone	Oxygen, opioids, antidopamine, antihistamine, anxiolytics

CHF—congestive heart failure   GERD—gastroesophageal reflux disease   NSAIDs—nonsteroidal anti-inflammatory drugs

Octreotide (see above) is an effective means of reducing gastrointestinal secretions.

MOUTH SYMPTOMS

Oral problems can cause altered taste, pain, and difficulty swallowing, which may lead to reduced food and fluid intake. Good hydration, hygiene, and regular observation can keep oral problems to a minimum. The patient's teeth should be brushed twice daily with toothpaste. Daily observation of the oral mucosa is recommended.

Dentures also require regular cleansing. Dentures may cease to fit properly in patients who lose a significant amount of weight. Some of those patients may wish to have their dentures refitted; others (especially those nearing death) will choose to forgo this arduous process.

Key questions to ask regarding the mouth include the following: Is the mouth dry? Is infection present? Is the mouth dirty? Is the mouth painful? Are oral ulcerations present? [*see Table 8*][47]

Dry Mouth

The presence of saliva is usually taken for granted, but the lack of it can seriously damage the quality of life. Xerostomia (the subjective sensation of dry mouth) may result from salivary gland disease or systemic conditions such as Sjögren syndrome, Parkinson disease, AIDS, or diabetes[48]; it may also be a side effect of medications, including those with anticholinergic action, benzodiazepines, diuretics, and interleukin-2.[49] Regardless of the cause, xerostomia almost always requires symptomatic treatment. The goal of therapy is to moisten the oral mucosa, and the best, simplest way is for the patient to sip water frequently. However, mouth moisteners and artificial salivas exist and may be preferred by some patients.[47,49] Pilocarpine tablets may be used, at a dosage of 5 to 10 mg every 8 hours, if the above measures fail. Side effects may include nausea, diarrhea, urinary frequency, and dizziness. Other nonpharmacologic treatments include eating ice chips and sucking on hard candy.

Oral Ulcers/Mucositis

Oral infection can have multiple causes. Aphthous ulcers are common and can be eased by topical corticosteroids, tetracycline mouthwash, or thalidomide. Oral candidiasis usually presents as adherent white plaques but can also present as erythema or angular cheilitis. Nystatin suspension is the usual treatment, but a 5-day course of oral ketoconazole, 200 mg daily, can also be used. Severe viral infection (herpes simplex or zoster) requires treatment with acyclovir, 200 mg every 4 hours for 5 days. Malignant ulcers are often associated with anaerobic bacteria and may respond to metronidazole, 400 to 500 mg orally or rectally every 12 hours or as a topical gel.[47]

SKIN SYMPTOMS

Pressure Ulcers

Pressure ulcers typically result from both intrinsic and extrinsic factors [*see Table 9*]. Major sites of pressure ulcers in terminally ill patients include the ear and the skin overlying the spine (apex of kyphosis), sacrum, greater femoral trochanter, head of the fibula, and malleolus. Prevention should emphasize these sites and should include daily visual inspection of them in patients at risk for pressure sores.

Prevention and treatment of pressure sores require targeting risk factors and minimizing them. Caregivers need to minimize pressure by turning and repositioning the patient frequently and avoiding shear (sliding movement) and friction. They should be

Table 5 Medications for Nausea and Vomiting[28]

Administration	Category	Drug (Trade Name)	Dosage
Oral	Corticosteroid	Dexamethasone	2–8 mg q. 6–12 hr
	Antidopamine	Haloperidol (Haldol)	0.5–5 mg q. 6–8 hr
		Prochlorperazine (Compazine)	5–10 mg q. 4–6 hr
		Prochlorperazine SR	10–15 mg b.i.d.
	Antihistamine	Diphenhydramine (Benadryl)	25–50 mg q. 4–6 hr
		Hydroxyzine (Atarax)	25–50 mg t.i.d.–q.i.d.
		Promethazine (Phenergan)	12.5–25 mg t.i.d.–q.i.d.
	Anticholinergic	Hyoscyamine (Levsin)	0.125–0.25 S.L. q. 4 hr
		Meclizine (Antivert)	12.5–25 mg b.i.d.–q.i.d.
	Anxiolytic	Lorazepam (Ativan)	1–2 mg q. 2–4 hr
	Prokinetic	Metoclopramide (Reglan)	10–40 mg q.i.d.
	Antiserotonin	Ondansetron (Zofran)	8 mg p.o., t.i.d.–q.i.d.
	Other	Dronabinol (Marinol)	2.5–10 mg b.i.d., t.i.d.
		Thiethylperazine (Torecan)	10 mg q.d.–t.i.d.
		Trimethobenzamide (Tigan)	250 mg t.i.d.–q.i.d.
Rectal suppositories	Antidopamine	Prochlorperazine (Compazine)	25 mg q. 6 hr
	Antihistamine	Promethazine (Phenergan)	12.5, 25, 50 mg t.i.d.–q.i.d.
	Other	Trimethobenzamide (Tigan)	200 mg t.i.d.–q.i.d.
Continuous intravenous infusion	Corticosteroids	Dexamethasone	8–100 mg/24 hr
	Antidopamine	Haloperidol (Haldol)	2.5–10 mg/24 hr
	Anticholinergic	Hyoscyamine (Levsin)	1–2 mg/24 hr
		Scopolamine	0.8–20 mg/24 hr
	Antiserotonin	Odansetron (Zofran)	0.45 mg/kg/24 hr
	Prokinetic	Metoclopramide (Reglan)	20–80 mg/24 hr
Intermittent intravenous infusion	Corticosteroids	Dexamethasone	2–8 mg q. 4–6 hr
	Antidopamine	Haloperidol (Haldol)	0.5–2 mg q. 4–6 hr
		Prochlorperazine (Compazine)	5–10 mg q. 4–6 hr
	Antihistamine	Diphenydramine (Benadryl)	25–50 mg q. 6 hr
	Anxiolytic	Lorazepam (Ativan)	1–2 mg q. 6–8 hr
	Prokinetic	Metoclopramide (Reglan)	10–20 mg q. 6 hr
	Antiserotonin	Ondansetron (Zofran)	4–8 mg q. 8 hr
		Granisetron (Kytril)	10 µg/kg q.d.
	Other	Dronabinol (Marinol)	5 mg/m² q. 4 hr (maximum, six doses/day)

aware that even crumpled bedclothes can impair circulation. How a patient moves or is moved by caregivers needs to be assessed and monitored. Even with regular turning and careful lifting and positioning, special pressure surfaces or mattresses are sometimes needed.[47] Fragile skin that is at risk for breakdown should be covered with clear, occlusive dressings; pressure points should be covered with thin, hydrocolloid dressings.

Caregivers must keep the patient's skin clean and dry. Absorbent surfaces, urinary catheters, and rectal tubes may be helpful, but they must be used carefully because of their attendant complications.[37]

Nutrition is an important factor in both prevention and treatment. Good hydration, a diet that is high in protein and carbohydrates, and vitamin C supplements help maintain skin integrity and encourage healing.

If pressure ulcers develop, they should be covered with gel or colloid dressings, which keep the area moist, reduce pain, and can be left in place for several days. The pain of dressing changes can be eased by extra analgesia before each change.[47] The clinician should instruct caretakers to give oral pain medication one-half hour before the dressing change. The dose is determined by whether or not the patient is on regular opioid medications. If the patient is not on regular pain medications, start with 15 mg of immediate-release morphine. If the patient is on a regular opioid regimen, the predressing dose should be the same as the rescue dose.

Pressure ulcer management needs to be consistent with the overall goals of care. If maintenance or improvement of function is the goal and the patient's life expectancy is weeks to months, the ulcer should be treated according to the usual management guidelines. If life expectancy is very limited (e.g., days), the intent should be to optimize quality of life and minimize pain and discomfort (such as from excessive dressing changes or debridement).

Malignant Ulcers

For uncomplicated malignant ulcers, pain relief and wound care are managed in the same way as pressure ulcers. Malignant wounds can present special problems, however, which may include bleeding, exudate, infection, odor, and disfigurement. A bleeding malignant ulcer should be treated with radiation therapy, topical sucralfate, or topical tranexamic acid. Dirty ulcers should be debrided, which can be accomplished chemically. Altered body image from disfiguring wounds can be lessened with cavity foam dressings. Furthermore, empathetic listening is often therapeutic in itself. Anxiety, anger, or depression needs specific support, however[47] [see Chapter 10].

Foul-Smelling Wounds

Odors may be very distressing to patients, families, and caregivers and may lead to poor quality of care, as even professional caregivers tend to avoid sickening smells. Odors are usually due to anaerobic infections or poor hygiene. Treat superficial infections with topical metronidazole or silver sulfadiazine. These agents are expensive, however; and if a less costly alternative is required, a diluted hydrogen peroxide solution can be used.[37] For soft tissue infections, add systemic metronidazole to topical management.

To control odors, place a pan containing kitty litter or activated charcoal under the patient's bed, provide adequate room ventilation, place an open cup of vinegar in the room, or burn a can-

dle. Special charcoal-impregnated dressings placed over the odorous wound may also be helpful.[37]

Psychiatric Symptoms

Adjustment disorders, depression, anxiety, dementia, and delirium are the most common psychiatric problems encountered in dying patients.[50,51] Depending on their severity, management of these psychiatric problems may be within the capacity of the primary care physician or may require referral [see Chapter 10].

DELIRIUM

Delirium occurs in roughly 75% of terminally ill patients.[52,53] Symptoms of delirium include inability to maintain attention, waxing and waning of consciousness, psychomotor changes, disturbance of sleep-wake cycle, disorientation, visual or auditory hallucinations, and problems with memory and language.[54] Other terms often used synonymously with delirium include acute confusional state, metabolic encephalopathy, and sundowning. In contrast to dementia, delirium is more rapid in onset (developing over hours to days), fluctuates in severity, is potentially reversible, and is associated with a lesser degree of memory impairment.

Table 6   A Progressive Bowel Regimen for Patients Receiving Opioid Therapy[45]*

Step 1
    Docusate, 100 mg b.i.d.
    Senna, 1 tablet q.d. or b.i.d.
Step 2
    Docusate, 100 mg b.i.d.
    Senna, 2 tablets b.i.d.
    Bisacodyl rectal suppositories, 1–2 after breakfast
Step 3
    Docusate, 100 mg b.i.d.
    Senna, 3 tablets b.i.d.
    Bisacodyl rectal suppositories, 3–4 after breakfast
Step 4
    Docusate, 100 mg b.i.d.
    Senna, 4 tablets b.i.d.
    Lactulose or sorbitol, 15 ml b.i.d.
    Bisacodyl suppositories, 3–4 after breakfast
Step 5
    Sodium phosphate or oil-retention enema; if no results, add
        a high-colonic tap-water enema
Step 6
    Docusate, 100 mg b.i.d.
    Senna, 4 tablets b.i.d.
    Lactulose or sorbitol, 30 ml b.i.d.
    Bisacodyl rectal suppositories, 3–4 after breakfast
Step 7
    Docusate, 100 mg b.i.d.
    Senna, 4 tablets b.i.d.
    Lactulose or sorbitol, 30 ml q.i.d.
    Bisacodyl rectal suppositories, 3-4 after breakfast

*The bowel regimen is started at the time of or before the initiation of opioid therapy, and it should be continued for the duration of opioid therapy. The clinician should start with step 1 and progress through higher steps until an effective regimen is found.

Table 7   Treatments for Constipation

Laxative type	Mechanism	Agent	Dosage	Comment
Stimulant	Irritate the bowel and increase peristaltic activity	Prune juice	120-240 ml q.d. or b.i.d.	
		Senna	1–2 tablets p.o., q.h.s.	Titrate to effect; ≤ 8 tablets b.i.d.
		Bisacodyl	10–15 mg p.o., h.s.; or 10 mg p.r., after breakfast	Titrate to effect
Osmotic	Draw water into the bowel lumen, increase overall stool volume	Lactulose	30 ml p.o., q. 4–6 hr	Titrate to effect
		Sorbitol, 70% solution	2 ml/kg, up to 50 ml p.o., q.d.–t.i.d.	
		Milk of magnesia	1–2 tbsp, q.d.–t.i.d.	
		Magnesium citrate	1–2 bottles p.r.n.	
		Polyethylene glycol solution	1–4 L p.o.	Drink 8 oz q. 10 min until consumed
		Polyethylene glycol powder	17 g (1 tbsp) powder in 8 oz water, q.d.	2–4 days may be required to produce a bowel movement; increase dose as needed
Detergent (stool softeners)	Increase water content in stool by facilitating the dissolution of fat	Docusate sodium	1–2 capsules p.o., q.d.–b.i.d.	Titrate to effect
		Docusate calcium*	1–2 capsules p.o., q.d.–b.i.d.	Titrate to effect
Prokinetic agents	Stimulate the bowel's myenteric plexus, and increase peristaltic activity and stool movement	Metoclopramide	10–20 mg p.o., q. 6 hr	
Lubricant stimulants	Lubricate the stool and irritate the bowel, increasing peristaltic activity and stool movement	Glycerin suppositories	Daily	
		Mineral oil or peanut oil enema	Daily	
Large-volume enemas	Soften stool by increasing its water content; distend the colon and induce peristalsis	Warm-water enema	Daily	Addition of soapsuds irritates bowel wall to induce peristalsis
High-colonic enemas	Utilize gravity to bring fluid to more proximal parts of bowel	2 L of water or saline warmed to body temperature, hung on I.V. pole at ceiling level	Run in over 30 min, repeat q. 1 hr	

*Not available in the United States.

Delirium is a multifactorial syndrome, involving preexisting risk factors and precipitating factors that occur during hospitalization. Factors that predispose a patient to delirium include vision impairment, severe illness, cognitive impairment, and dehydration.[55] In older patients, cognitive impairment that is so mild as to be inapparent when they are well may nevertheless increase the risk of delirium. Precipitating factors include the use of physical restraints, malnutrition, taking more than three drugs, bladder catheter use, and any iatrogenic event.[55] Prevention of delirium can be accomplished by targeting risk factors.[55]

Management of delirium in the terminally ill patient includes correction of the cause and provision of symptomatic relief. Identification and treatment of underlying diseases or conditions is paramount—for example, give antibiotics for sepsis or oxygen for shortness of breath. In patients with underlying dementia, the possibility of untreated pain deserves special consideration. In the past, physicians were taught that the use of narcotic analgesics is dangerous in patients with dementia because those agents cause delirium. That is not true of a demented patient who becomes agitated or belligerent because of pain, however; in those cases, a dose of a narcotic analgesic may calm the patient within an hour or so. The risk of undertreating severe pain should be of greater concern, both medically and ethically, than the risk of worsening delirium with analgesic medications.

Additional means of treating delirium include minimizing any sensory impairments by providing appropriate eyeglasses or hearing aids and maintaining a quiet, familiar, and reassuring

Table 8   Local Measures for Oral Problems[47]

Dry mouth
    Semifrozen fruit juice
    Frequent sips of cold water or water sprays
    Petroleum jelly rubbed on lips
Dirty mouth
    Regular brushing with soft toothbrush and toothpaste
    Pineapple chunks
    Cider and soda mouthwash
Infected mouth
    Tetracycline mouthwash, 250 mg every 8 hr (one capsule dissolved in 5 ml water)
Painful mouth
    Topical corticosteroids: betamethasone, 0.5 mg in 5 ml water, as mouthwash; or triamcinolone in carmellose paste
    Coating agents: sucralfate suspension as mouthwash, carmellose paste, carbenoxolone
    Topical anesthesia: benzocaine or lozenges containing local anesthetics

setting. It is important to maintain communication with the patient, using frequent reorientation; familiar objects, places, and people; and avoidance of stimulus overload or deprivation.[56]

Pharmacologic symptom relief is best achieved with the use of an antipsychotic agent such as haloperidol or risperidone [see Table 10]. Benzodiazepines or sedatives should be used only if antipsychotic agents fail.[57]

Terminal Delirium

Delirium may be an irreversible part of the dying process. Many terminally ill patients have escalating restlessness, agitation, or hallucinations that can be relieved only with sedation.[58] When death is imminent, reversing the underlying causes of delirium is not possible. Instead, the clinician should focus on the management of the symptoms associated with the terminal delirium and bring comfort to the patient and family.

Benzodiazepines are widely used in the management of terminal delirium because they are anxiolytics, amnestics, skeletal muscle relaxants, and antiepileptics. Oral lorazepam (1 to 2 mg as an elixir, or the tablet predissolved in 0.5 to 1.0 ml of water and administered against the buccal mucosa) should be given every hour as needed; it will settle most patients at a daily dose of 2 to 10 mg. The lorazepam can then be given in divided doses, every 3 to 4 hours, to keep the patient settled. For a few extremely agitated patients, high doses of lorazepam—20 to 50 mg or more per 24 hours—may be required. A midazolam infusion (1 to 5 mg S.C. or I.V. every 1 hour, preceded by repeated loading boluses of 0.5 mg every 15 minutes to effect) may be a rapidly effective alternative.[37]

Palliative sedation When terminal delirium cannot be adequately controlled despite aggressive efforts to identify a tolerable therapy that does not compromise consciousness, it may be necessary to resort to palliative sedation. Most physicians define palliative sedation as the act of purposely inducing and maintaining a pharmacologically sedated and unconscious state, without the intent to cause death.

Once palliative sedation is initiated, the dosage of the sedative agent should not be increased unless the patient awakens or becomes restless, tachypneic, or tachycardic. Increasing the

Table 9 Risk Factors for Pressure Ulcers

Intrinsic	Extrinsic
Malnutrition	Pressure
Protein	Shear
Vitamin C	Trauma
Zinc	Friction
Diminished mobility	Crumpled bedclothes
Tissue fragility	Restraints
Anemia	Bed rails
Dehydration	Poor hygiene
Hypotension	Hospital equipment
Poor peripheral perfusion	Oxygen tubing
Incontinence	Heart monitor wires
Neurologic deficit	
Sensory	
Motor	
Older age	
Coma	
Moribund state	

Table 10 Drug Treatment for Agitation or Delirium[28]

Acute	Haloperidol, 0.5–5 mg p.o., p.r., I.M., I.V., or S.C.; titrate until calm
	Chlorpromazine, 1 mg I.V. q. 2 min until calm
Chronic	Haloperidol, 0.5–5 mg p.o. or p.r., b.i.d. (maximum dose, 100 mg/day)
	Thioridazine, 10–25 mg p.o., b.i.d. (maximum dose, 800 mg/day)
	Risperidone, 0.5 mg p.o., b.i.d.; increase by 0.5 mg b.i.d. q. 24 hr (maximum dose, 6 mg/day)
	Chlorpromazine, 10–50 mg p.o. or p.r., b.i.d. (maximum dose, 500 mg/day)
	Olanzepine, 2.5–15 mg p.o., q.d.

level of sedation in the absence of a clinical indication might imply that the physician is intending to hasten death, which if true would cross the line between palliative sedation and physician-assisted suicide or euthanasia.[59]

Terminal Wean

Mechanical ventilation is often tried in patients with respiratory distress, when there is hope that their condition will improve. This is best referred to as a time-limited trial. If reversal of the acute medical condition proves unsuccessful, the physician needs to discuss discontinuance of ventilation with the family.

Terminal ventilation withdrawal should be approached with attention to ensuring the patient's comfort and to enhancing the family's access to the bedside. Miles[60] recommends a 10-step protocol, which applies to unconscious patients dependent on a ventilator:

1. Shut off and remove all monitors and alarms from the patient's room.
2. Remove equipment that impedes access to the patient's hands (e.g., intravenous lines, pulse oximeter, restraints). Hands are for holding.
3. Remove encumbering or disfiguring devices from the bedside.
4. Invite the family to be with the patient.
5. Quietly and personally request that pressors be turned off and that intravenous infusions be set to keep veins open.
6. Watch for distressing symptoms, such as agitation, tachypnea, or seizures; treat appropriately (e.g., with diazepam) if they appear.
7. Turn the fraction of inspired oxygen (F_IO_2) down to 20% and observe the patient for respiratory distress.
8. If the patient appears comfortable, remove the endotracheal tube with a clean towel in hand.
9. Educate and debrief the house staff and nursing staff about the process.
10. Consider contacting the family during the bereavement period, whether by letter or visit.

The goal is for a peaceful, pain-free death for the patient and a supportive, comfortable environment for the family and friends. It is important to warn family that a patient removed from the ventilator may live for hours to days afterward and to reassure them that all measures necessary to ensure comfort during the dying process will be used.

Symptom Management in the Last Hours of Life

The final hours of living can be some of the most important ones for the patient and for family. Managed well, they can lead to a peaceful death and healthy grief and bereavement.[37]

During the final hours, patients usually need skilled care around the clock. Ideally, the environment will allow family and friends both easy access to their loved one and privacy. All who are present should presume that the unconscious patient hears everything.[37]

It is important to be knowledgeable about the normal physiologic changes that occur in the last hours and to educate the patient's family about them. Reassure the family that dehydration in the final hours of living does not cause distress and may stimulate endorphin release that adds to the patient's sense of well-being. Moaning and groaning, although frequently misinterpreted as pain, is often terminal delirium (see above). Decreased hepatic and renal function lead to the accumulation of metabolites, which may cause terminal delirium. Use only essential medications and dose them accordingly.[37]

In the final hours of life, many persons in semiconscious or unconscious states are unable to swallow saliva reflexively or to cough up mucus. This inability to clear secretions from the oropharynx and trachea results in the so-called death rattle—noisy respiration as the secretions move up and down with expiration and inspiration. Explain the reason for the death rattle to the family and administer an anticholinergic drug to reduce pharyngeal secretions (e.g., hyoscine, as a single parenteral dose or by continuous infusion, or scopolamine by patch).[61] At times, it may be necessary to reposition the patient or to suction the airway gently with a soft catheter. Reassure the family that despite the way the breathing sounds, the patient is not uncomfortable.

The removal of the body too soon after death can be even more upsetting to the family than the moment of death, so give the family time with the body.[37] After the patient has died, follow-up with the family is important to ensure that grief and bereavement are progressing normally [see Chapter 10].

References

1. O'Neill B, Fallon M: Principles of palliative care. BMJ 315:801, 1997

2. Ingham J, Portenoy RK: The measurement of pain and other symptoms. Oxford Textbook of Palliative Medicine. Doyle D, Hanks GW, MacDonald N, Eds. Oxford University Press, Oxford, England, 1993, p 202

3. Grossman SA, Sheidler VR, Swedeen K, et al: Correlation of patient and caregiver ratings of cancer pain. J Pain Symptom Manage 6:53, 1991

4. Clipp EC, George LK: Patients with cancer and their spouse caregivers: perceptions of the illness experience. Cancer 69:1074, 1992

5. Bruera E, Kuehn N, Miller M, et al: Symptom Assessment System: a simple method for the assessment of palliative care patients. J Palliative Care 7:6, 1991

6. Donnelly S, Walsh D: The symptoms of advanced cancer. Semin Oncol 22 (suppl 3):67, 1995

7. Portenoy RK , Thaler HT, Kornblith AB, et al: The Memorial Symptom Assessment Scale: an instrument for the evaluation of symptom prevalence, characteristics and distress. Eur J Cancer 30A:1326, 1994

8. Camp L: A comparison of nurses' record assessment of pain with perceptions of pain as described by cancer patients. Cancer Nurs 11:237, 1988

9. Teske K, Daut R, Cleeland C: Relationships between nurses' observations and patients' self-reports of pain. Pain 16:289, 1983

10. Bernabei R, Gambassi G, Lapane K, et al: Management of pain in elderly patients with cancer. SAGE Study Group. Systematic Assessment of Geriatric Drug Use via Epidemiology. JAMA 279:1877, 1998

11. Feldts KS, Ryder MB, Miles S: Treatment of pain in cognitively impaired compared with cognitively intact older patients with hip fracture. J Am Geriatr Soc 46:1069, 1998

12. Morrison RS, Siu AL: A comparison of pain and its treatment in advanced dementia and cognitively intact patients with hip fracture. J Pain Symptom Manage 19:240, 2000

13. Ferrell B, Ferrell B, Rivera L: Pain in cognitively impaired nursing home patients. J Pain Symptom Manage 10:591, 1995

14. Duggleby W, Lander J. Cognitive status and postoperative pain: older adults. J Pain Symptom Manage 9:19, 1994

15. Lynch EP, Lazor MA, Gellis JE, et al: The impact of postoperative pain on the development of postoperative delirium. Anesth Analg 86:781, 1998

16. Super A: Going one step further: skilled pain assessment and the art of adjuvant analgesia. Am J Hosp Palliat Care 14:279, 1997

17. Ahmedzai S: Current Strategies for Pain Control. Ann Oncol 8 (suppl 3):521, 1997

18. Sallerin-Caute B, Lazorthes Y, Deguine O, et al: Does intrathecal morphine in the treatment of cancer pain induce the development of tolerance? Neurosurgery 42:44, 1998

19. Weiss SC, Emanuel LL, Fairclough DL, et al: Understanding the experience of pain in terminally ill patients. Lancet 357:1311, 2001

20. Reuben DB, Mor V: Dyspnea in terminally ill cancer patients. Chest 89:234, 1986

21. Hockely JM, Dunlop R, Davies RJ: Survey of distressing symptoms in dying patients and their families in hospital and their response to a symptom control team. BMJ 296:1715, 1988

22. Ventafridda V, De Conno F, Ripamonti C, et al: Quality-of-life assessment during a palliative care programme. Ann Oncol 1: 415, 1990

23. Carrieri VK, Janson-Bjerklie S: The sensation of dyspnea: a review. Heart Lung 13:436, 1984

24. Bruera E, Macmillan K, Pither J, et al: Effects of morphine on the dyspnea of terminal cancer patients. J Pain Symptom Manage 5:341, 1990

25. Cohen MH, Anderson AJ, Krasnow SH, et al: Continuous intravenous infusion of morphine for severe dyspnea. South Med J 84:229, 1991

26. Bruera E, Neumann CM: Management of specific symptom complexes in patients receiving palliative care. CMAJ 159:1242, 1998

27. Muers MF, Round CE: Palliation of symptoms in non-small cell lung cancer: a study by the Yorkshire Regional Cancer Organization Thoracic Group. Thorax 48:339, 1993

28. Stegman MB: Non-pain symptoms. Pain and Symptom Control in Palliative Medicine. Stegman MB, Ed. Hospice Resources, Fort Myers, Florida, 1997, p 6.1

29. Fuller RW, Jackson DM: Physiology and treatment of cough. Thorax 45:425, 1990

30. Hagen NA: An approach to cough in cancer patients. J Pain Symptom Manage 6:257, 1991

31. Bruera E: ABC of palliative care: anorexia, cachexia, and nutrition. BMJ 315:1219, 1997

32. Bruera E, Miller L, MacCallion J, et al: Cognitive failure in patients with terminal cancer: a prospective study. Proc Am Soc Clin Oncol 9:308, 1990

33. Holden CM: Anorexia in the terminally ill cancer patient: the emotional impact on the patient and the family. Hosp J 7:73, 1991

34. Strang P: Quality of life is the most important goal in nutritional support of the dying. Lakartidningen 97:1141, 2000

35. Bruera E, Macmillan K, Hanson J, et al: A controlled trial of megestrol acetate on appetite, caloric intake, nutritional status, and other symptoms in patients with advanced cancer. Cancer 66:1279, 1990

36. Tchekmedyian NS, Hariri L, Siau J, et al: Megestrol acetate in cancer anorexia and weight loss. Proc Am Soc Clin Oncol 9:336, 1990

37. Emanuel LL, von Gunten CF, Ferris FD: The Education for Physicians on End-of-Life Care (EPEC) Curriculum, Institute for Ethics at the American Medical Association, 1999, p 14

38. Volicer L, et al: Ethical issues in the treatment of advanced Alzheimer dementia: hospice approach. Clinical Management of Alzheimer Disease. Aspen Publishers, Rockville, Maryland, 1988, p 167

39. Finucane TE, Christmas C, Travis K: Tube feedings in patients with advanced dementia: a review of the evidence. JAMA 284:1365, 1999

40. Luchins DJ, Hanrahan P: What is appropriate health care for end-stage dementia? J Am Geriatr Soc 41:25, 1993

41. Reuben DB, Mor V: Nausea and vomiting in terminally ill cancer patients. Arch Intern Med 146:2021,1986

42. Baines MJ: ABC of palliative care: Nausea, vomiting and intestinal obstruction. BMJ 315:1148, 1997

43. Fallon M, O'Neill B: ABC of palliative care: constipation and diarrhea. BMJ 315:1293, 1997

44. Meiring PJ, Joubert G: Constipation in elderly patients attending a polyclinic. S Afr Med J 88:888, 1998

45. Carney MT, Meier DE: Palliative care and end-of-life issues. Anaesthesiol Clin North America 18:183, 2000

46. Ripamonti C: Malignant bowel obstruction in advanced and terminal cancer patients. European Journal of Palliative Care 1:23, 1994

47. Regnard C, Allport S, Stephenson L: ABC of palliative care: mouth care, skin care, and lymphoedema. BMJ 315:1002, 1997

48. Fox PC, Van der Ven PF, Sonies BC, et al: Xerostomia: evaluation of a symptom with increasing significance. J Am Dent Assoc 110:519, 1985

49. Narhi TO, Meurman JH, Ainamo A: Xerostomia and hyposalivation: causes, consequences and treatment in the elderly. Drugs and Aging 15:103,1999

50. Breitbart W, Passik SD: Psychiatric aspects of palliative care. Oxford Textbook of Palliative Medicine. Doyle D, Hanks GW, MacDonald N, Eds. Oxford University Press, Oxford, England, 1993, p 609

51. Barraclough J: ABC of palliative care: depression, anxiety, and confusion. BMJ 315:1365, 1997

52. Massie MJ, Holland J, Glass E: Delirium in terminally ill cancer patients. Am J Psychiatry 140:1048, 1983

53. Leipzig RM, Goodman H, Gray G, et al: Reversible, narcotic-associated mental status impairment in patients with metastatic cancer. Pharmacology 35:47, 1987

54. Lipowski ZJ: Delirium. Acute Confusional States. Oxford University Press, New York, 1990

55. Inouye SK: Prevention of delirium in hospitalized older patients: risk factors and targeted intervention strategies. Ann Med 32:257, 2000

56. Rummans TA, Evans JM, Krahn LE, et al: Delirium in elderly patients: evaluation and management. Mayo Clin Proc 70:989, 1995

57. Pan CX, Meier DE: Clinical aspects of end-of-life care. Annual Review of Gerontology and Geriatrics, Year 2000: Focus on the End-of-life: Scientific and Social Issues, Lawton P, Ed. Springer-Verlag, New York, 2000, p 273

58. Fainsinger RL, Waller A, Bercovici M, et al: A multicentre international study of sedation for uncontrolled symptoms in terminally ill patients. Palliat Med 14:257, 2000

59. Rousseau P: Existential suffering and palliative sedation: a brief commentary with a proposal for clinical guidelines. Am J Hospice Palliat Care 18:299, 2001

60. Miles S: Protocol for rapid withdrawal of ventilator support in anticipation of death. Ethical Currents 45(Spring), 1996

61. Doyle D: Domiciliary Terminal Care. Churchill Livingstone, Edinburgh, Scotland, 1987

10 Management of Psychosocial Issues in Terminal Illness

Jennifer Rhodes-Kropf, M.D., and Ned H. Cassem, M.D.

Like all good medical care, palliative care addresses patients' needs at many levels. The physical deterioration as death approaches can challenge the ingenuity and equanimity of health care professionals [*see Chapter 9*]. Yet symptom management is only one aspect of the care that these patients need; the psychosocial and spiritual problems that arise at the end of life also require attention.

A fatal illness—such as untreatable heart disease, terminal cancer, or AIDS—brings with it not only physical pain but also emotional suffering. Fear is prominent. The body, once regarded as a friend, may seem more like a dormant adversary programmed for betrayal. Even innocuous bodily changes may be interpreted as ominous. Patients become fearful before disease symptoms occur. Cancer patients, for example, fear pain, shortness of breath, nausea and vomiting, anorexia, dyspnea, and isolation.[1] Well before the terminal stages of an illness, patients fear the unknown, losing autonomy, disfigurement, dementia, and, last but not least, becoming a burden to their families.

The stress of terminal illness may manifest itself in many ways. Patients may deny or be unable to accept diagnosis or treatment; they may have unrealistic hopes of being cured, and they may persistently ask why there is no improvement. They may express anxiety, often extreme, with near panic and unspecifiable fears about dying. They may experience intense feelings of ambivalence and guilt regarding their personal relationships.

Considering the severe distress that is frequently involved, it is remarkable how well most patients do cope with a terminal illness and its treatments. The unique set of coping mechanisms that they have used to maintain self-esteem and stability in the past plays a vital role in this process. Religion and spirituality may be most helpful to patients and families at the end of a patient's life and should therefore be recognized and encouraged.

When a patient is dying, the entire family is the appropriate focus of treatment. A family member may be the first to notice a symptom, such as a personality change, in the patient or in another family member and can thus serve as an indispensable historian. The physician must also contend with the psychosocial forces that can lead to family fragmentation and interfere with care. A family member may have more difficulty than the patient in coping with the illness; this may irritate and distract caregivers and ultimately disrupt the relationship between the physician and the family. For example, the physician may be inclined to schedule visits to the patient so as to avoid encounters with the family. This could seriously jeopardize the patient's treatment and the chance to make the patient's death meaningful and dignified. After the patient's death, the survivors may experience abnormal grieving patterns that deserve medical attention.

Most of the psychosocial aspects of palliative care are within the capability of the primary care physician. In some cases, however, psychiatric consultation may be necessary to help the dying patient cope with major depression, personality disorders, continuous treatment-resistant pain, substance abuse, or grieving.

Preliminary Considerations

BREAKING BAD NEWS

Psychosocial care of the patient with terminal illness begins with delivery of the diagnosis. Because there are so many possible reactions a patient may have when informed of the diagnosis, it is helpful to have some plan of action in mind that will permit the greatest range and freedom of response by the patient. When the diagnosis is made and it is time to inform the patient, the physician should meet with the patient in a private place. The spouse (and sometimes the family) should be included in the discussion, unless there is a good reason not to do so. If possible, the patient should be informed ahead of time that after all the tests are completed the physician will review the results and discuss treatment plans in detail. With inpatients, the physician should sit down at the bedside to deliver bad news. Standing while conveying bad news may be regarded by a patient as unkind and expressive of wanting to leave as quickly as possible. If the patient is tested as an outpatient and returns home before the results are known, he or she should be told that the diagnostic information is too important to convey by phone, and a meeting to discuss the results should be arranged. Relaying bad news by phone may be perceived by patients as thoughtless, even though they may have asked for information. A physician must also be prepared to respond to a patient who wishes no or minimal information about the diagnosis.

When the findings are life threatening (e.g., a biopsy positive for malignancy), how can the news best be conveyed? A good opening statement is one that is (1) rehearsed so that it can be delivered calmly, (2) brief (three sentences or less), (3) designed to encourage further dialogue, and (4) reassuring of continued attention and care. A typical delivery might go as follows: "The tests confirmed that your tumor is malignant. I have therefore asked the surgeon (or radiotherapist or oncologist) to speak with you, examine you, and make recommendations for treatment. After this, we can discuss how we should proceed." Silence and quiet observation at this point will yield more valuable information about the patient than any other part of the exchange. What are the emotional reactions? What sort of coping is seen at the very start? While observing, one can decide how best to continue with the discussion. Just sitting with the patient for a period of time, however, is the most important part of this initial encounter with a grim reality that both patient and physician will continue to confront together, possibly for a long time.

TELLING THE TRUTH

Given the difficulties that can follow the disclosure of a life-threatening illness, it may be tempting to avoid telling the patient the diagnosis. This tactic has ancient roots: Hippocrates himself recommended concealing bad news from patients, lest they become discouraged.[2] Nevertheless, most empirical studies in which patients were asked whether they wanted to be told the truth about malignancy have indicated an overwhelming desire in the affirmative. Of 740 patients in a cancer-detection clinic who were asked before diagnosis whether they wanted to be told their diagnosis, 99% said that they did.[3] Another group of patients in this clinic were asked the same question after the diagnosis was established, and 89% of them replied affirmatively, as did 82% of patients in still another group who had been examined and found to be free of malignancy.

The desire for truth telling may vary among different ethnic groups. In a study of elderly persons in the United States, Korean Americans and Mexican Americans were less likely than African Americans and European Americans to believe that a patient should be told the diagnosis of metastatic cancer.[4] Socioeconomic factors may also be involved: younger age and higher income and education make patients more likely to want detailed diagnostic information.[5]

Is the truth harmful? Gerle and colleagues[6] studied 101 patients who were divided into two groups, with one group, along with their families, being told the frank truth of their diagnoses and the other group being excluded from discussion of the diagnosis (although the patients' families were informed). Initially, there appeared to be greater emotional upset in the group of patients and families who were informed together. The investigators observed in follow-up, however, that the emotional difficulties of the families of the patients who were shielded from the truth far outweighed those of the patients and families that were told the diagnosis simultaneously. In general, empirical studies support the idea that the truth about the diagnosis is desired by terminally ill patients and does not harm those to whom it is told. Honesty sustains the relationship with a dying person rather than jeopardizes it.

Individual variations in willingness to hear the initial diagnosis are extreme, however, and diagnosis is entirely different from prognosis. Many patients have said that they were grateful to their physician for telling them they had a malignancy. Very few, however, reacted positively to being told that they were dying. In our experience, "Do I have cancer?" is a common question, whereas "Am I dying?" is a rare one. The question about dying is more commonly heard from patients who are dying rapidly, such as those in cardiogenic shock.

Honest communication of the diagnosis by no means precludes later avoidance or even denial of the truth of the diagnosis. In two studies, patients who had been explicitly told their diagnosis (using the words cancer or malignancy) were asked 3 weeks later what they had been told: in both studies, about 20% of the patients sampled denied that their condition was cancerous or malignant.[7,8] Croog and colleagues[9] interviewed 345 men 3 weeks after myocardial infarction; 20% of those patients said they had not had a heart attack. All had been explicitly told their diagnosis. For a person to function effectively, truth's piercing voice may be muted or even excluded from awareness. Denial can reduce psychological distress, and preliminary evidence suggests that in women with nonmetastatic breast cancer, it may be associated with prolonged survival.[10]

Communicating a diagnosis honestly, though difficult, is easier than the labors that lie ahead. Telling the truth is merely a way to begin, but it provides a firm basis on which to build a relationship of trust.

COMMUNICATING WITH THE PATIENT

The most important component of communication is listening. The real issue is not what you tell your patients but, rather, what you let your patients tell you.[1] Most people are afraid to let dying patients say what is on their minds. If a patient who is presumed to be 3 months from death says, "My plan was to buy a new car in 6 months, but I guess I won't have to worry about that now," a poor listener might say nothing or, "Right. Don't worry about it." A better listener might ask, "What kind of car were you thinking about?"

It is essential to get to know the patient as a person. The best way to recognize and acknowledge the person's worth is to learn those features of his or her history and nature that make him or her unique. Encourage dying persons to tell their stories. Learn about significant areas of the patient's life—such as family, work, or school—and chat about common interests. This is the most natural way to give the patient the sense that she or he is known and appreciated.

Patients occasionally complain about professionals and visitors who regard them as "the dying patient," not as a unique person. The physician can help dissolve communication barriers for staff members by showing them the remarkable qualities of each patient. Comments such as, "She has 34 grandchildren," or, "This woman was an Olympic sprinter," convey information that helps other members of the health care team appreciate their patient and to find something to talk about with them. Listen for the patient's own conversational cues whenever possible. Awkwardness subsides when a patient is appreciated as a real person and not merely "a breast cancer patient." This rescue from anonymity is essential to prevent a sense of isolation.

The most important communication is often not verbal. A pat on the arm, a wave, a wink, or a grin communicates important reassurances. Back rubs and physical examinations can also be an opportunity to convey reassurance.

Psychosocial Support during Terminal Illness

The diagnosis of a terminal illness impacts the patient's relationships with family, friends, and coworkers and can thus undermine the patient's sense of self. Although death is a natural part of life, the adjustment to diminished function and role in relationships can be stressful, both for the patient and the patient's family.

FAMILY AND FRIENDS

Family members and friends must be helped to support the patient and one another. To provide this help, the physician must get to know both the patient and family members. When patients are permitted to give support to their families, they often feel they are less of a burden.

One must appreciate the fact that for family and close friends, a fatal illness of a loved one may be the only event important enough to resolve long-standing conflicts. Peacemaking should be a priority. Specific plans for the family are important. The writing of wills, the clarification of family history, the review of memorable family gatherings and achievements, the carrying out of such family projects as trips or photo-album reviews, and planning a funeral or memorial service are all important activities.

The care of a dying person can be a process of mutual growth for the patient and the family. Just as the deterioration of a person with a fatal disease can be threatening (loved ones feel both horrified at the prospect of the same thing happening to them and helpless to assist), the response of the dying person to the challenge may be not only edifying but also an invaluable lesson in coping. Indeed, family members who act as caregivers report strong positive emotions regarding the opportunity to express their love through care. Those caregivers may experience extreme grief after the patient's death, however, and may require special support and attention from health care providers at that time.[11]

Near the end of life, a patient may be too weak to communicate by speech, and sometimes consciousness itself may be difficult to assess. Most patients who have lost the ability to communicate have a period when they can still hear or perceive those in attendance. Family feelings of helplessness can be minimized by reading especially meaningful passages to the dying person (e.g., the daily headlines, articles by favorite authors or columnists, poetry, passages from the Bible, the Dow-Jones average, sports scores, and letters new and old). Conversations should make natural reference to the person as though hearing and understanding were intact. Singing favorite songs, playing favorite music, or praying aloud may increase the sense of unity and purpose for the family. Although the patient may never be able to tell us how important that time is, an occasional incident will do so dramatically, as when a supposedly unconscious person suddenly smiles appropriately, gestures, or even speaks. Often, this conveys gratitude for the attention given to him or her, which is very rewarding for the loved ones in attendance.

The end of life is an opportunity to educate the younger generation. Whenever possible, children should be included in all the planning, meetings, discussions, activities, and care, as well as the final attendance at death. Children can learn that death need not be violent or terrifying and that we face our losses best when we face them together.

Investigators have consistently learned that the visits of children are as likely as any other intervention to bring consolation and relief to the terminally ill patient. How can one determine whether a particular child should visit a dying patient? No better approach has been found than asking the child directly whether he or she wants to visit.

Ideally, this mutual work at the end of life will confirm the dying person's sense of self. It also can give family, friends, and caregivers the wonderful feeling that they have provided good care and safe passage.

OCCUPATION AND WORK

Work is critical for the self-esteem of many people. Many people begin to feel less valuable when work ceases or they retire, and the approaching end of life may intensify a sense of failure. The continuation of work for as long as feasible, as well as continued contact with work colleagues, can remind the dying of who they are and what they have accomplished. It encourages the belief that they are remembered and respected, regardless of their illness. Similarly, continued involvement in recreational activities can be very satisfying.

Near the end of life, a person is often too disabled to get around or to contact colleagues and friends. Wherever possible, such contact should be arranged for and encouraged.

RELIGION AND SPIRITUALITY

Studies find that people who have a strong internalized faith possess a resource that helps significantly in coping with a fatal illness.[1, 12-16] It is a well-documented finding that religious persons usually belong to a community that can be unusually thoughtful and generous in providing support. However, the community may not know of the patient's plight and may need to be contacted. Thus, the appreciation of a person's religion or spirituality is extremely important.

The Physician's Psychological Role in Patient Care

The first responsibility of the caregiver, as Saunders[17] points out, is "above all to listen." A suffering person often wants to communicate just how awful a fatal illness is. Words from the caregiver may be irrelevant: "When no answers exist," says Saunders, "one can offer silent attention."

It is important to be aware of the impact that patients' feelings can have on one's own mood and the amount of time spent with the patient. The relentless approach of death from cancer or AIDS may leave a patient with feelings of terror, hopelessness, and despair. Those feelings tend to be contagious, intensifying our feelings of impotence. A caregiver's own helplessness and despair may result in neglect or avoidance of the patient or feelings that the patient would be better off dead. Sensing that a patient is burdensome to caregivers can be devastating to the patient who looks to a doctor or nurse for some sense of hope. Thus, it is of the utmost importance that caregivers reassure patients that they will continue to be there for them at all stages of their illness and that caregivers learn to live with these negative feelings and resist the urge to avoid certain patients—attitudes that could convey that care of a patient is difficult for us or that the patient no longer matters to us.

COMPASSION

Of all attributes in physicians and nurses, none is more highly valued by terminally ill patients than compassion. Although they may never convey it precisely by words, some physicians and nurses are able to tell the patient that they are genuinely touched by his or her predicament. Although universally praised as a quality for a health professional, compassion exacts a cost that is usually overlooked in professional training. This cost is conveyed by its two Latin roots: *com*, meaning with, and *passio*, from *pati*, meaning to suffer—that is, to suffer with another person. It is important for caregivers to have a source of support for themselves—such as colleagues, friends, and family—so that they can continue to be there for their patients.

CHEERFULNESS

The possessor of a gentle and appropriate sense of humor can bring relief to all parties involved. Often patients provide this, and their wit may soften many a difficult incident. Humor needs to be used sensitively, however: forced or inappropriate mirth with a sick person can increase feelings of distance and isolation.

CONSISTENCY AND PERSEVERANCE

Dying patients have a realistic fear of progressive isolation. The physician or nurse who regularly visits the sickroom provides tangible proof of continued support and concern. A brief visit is far better than no visit at all; the patient may not even be able to tolerate a prolonged visit. Do continue to visit: patients are quick to identify those who show interest at first but gradually disappear from the scene. Stay the course even if this means that you must listen to repeated or irrelevant complaints.

The Patient's Psychological Response to Terminal Illness

Any serious illness inflicts some loss on the patient. A diagnosis itself, with no change in subjective symptoms, can cause a feeling of loss, as concepts of self and plans for the future are swept away.

The emotional reactions to a myocardial infarction serve as a model for the reactions of a person who has experienced physical loss. In a series of 149 coronary patients whose emotional difficulties were severe enough to warrant psychiatric consultation, the majority of problems during the first 2 days stemmed from fear and anxiety. These patients generally showed a sequence of emotions beginning with anxiety, followed shortly thereafter by denial (at this stage, a few wanted to sign out of the hospital) and then by despondency, which sometimes persisted. A final group of management problems, related mostly to dependency or personality disorders, rounded out the sequence.[18]

In essence, this reaction pattern suggests that the most common difficulty for a patient immediately after admission is fear. The patient fears imminent death, the presence or return of pain or breathlessness, or some vague but ominous threat to well-being. As symptoms stabilize or subside, the patient is likely to imagine that admission symptoms were false alarms and, in some cases, to insist on signing out of the hospital. When the diagnostic tests confirm the presence of myocardial infarction, however, the patient is confronted with the reality of the illness and feels demoralized. As hospitalization continues, any personality flaws (e.g., passive aggression) further complicate interactions between the patient and the hospital personnel. The sequence of acute onset of illness, fear, stabilization, denial, confirmation of illness, and depression provides a convenient framework for assessing the mental state of an individual hospitalized for any serious illness.

FEAR

Anxiety and despondency are the most common emotional reactions to illness. Panic distorts personality as nothing else does. Yet fear assumes many guises. If a patient seems impossible to deal with on the first day of hospitalization, the reason very likely is underlying fright. However, if difficult behavior continues after 4 or 5 days in the absence of new events that are frightening, it is probably because of the patient's personal style. Excessive talkativeness or mute withdrawal is a typical sign of fear in the acute phase.

Medication, quiet reassurance, or both can relieve a patient's fear and anxiety. Minor tranquilizers are the agents most commonly employed, but explanation and reassurance can be even more effective than medication.

When the physician senses that the patient is afraid, it is safe to assume that the patient regards the illness as an overwhelming threat to well-being. This threat is based on what the patient already knows or presumes about the disease. The physician, therefore, may ask questions designed to uncover erroneous concepts about their condition, such as, "Have you ever known anyone with this disease?" or, "What is your notion of this disease?" If any family member has died of the disease, his or her age at death may also contribute heavily to the patient's fear of the same fate.

After false notions have been corrected, it is important to emphasize the positive aspects of the treatment plan. Even when the prognosis is grave, a calm statement of the treatments planned to counteract and contain the disorder is of val-

ue to the anxious patient. The more ominous the prognosis, the more important it is to encourage the patient to specify the fear, so that correspondingly true reassurances (e.g., "the medication can control pain") can be given. False comfort is not recommended. It robs the physician of credibility and, therefore, of the ability to reassure the patient as the illness progresses.

DENIAL AND PANIC

Denial is a common defense mechanism in the initial stage of life-threatening illness. The ability to minimize or to completely deny the threatening implications of the disease ("There's nothing to worry about; I'll be all right.") is essential for controlling panic. When panic sets in, denial fails and people want to flee. Panic is the most common reason why acutely sick patients sign out of a hospital. Although it may simply mean that the patient does not take his or her illness seriously enough, the threat to sign out should be considered a panic reaction. The patient's panic conviction is, "I'll die if I don't get out of here."

Because patients who are experiencing a panic reaction are feeling desperate, they may become antagonistic to efforts to detain them. A gentle approach is essential. For example, the doctor, seated if possible, may begin with "Mr. Jordan, I'm not here to force you to do anything; I just ask that you hear me out." Then the patient needs to hear the truth—that he is seriously ill—expressed in direct but reassuring terms. To quiet the panic, it is most important to explain that the illness is manageable. As the patient calms down, other questions designed to reduce fear can be asked. Even if calmed, however, an anxious patient will not remain calm for long and should be promptly medicated. Family members should also be mobilized and informed.

ANXIETY

Anxiety disorders may or may not intensify during a terminal illness, but they clearly require psychiatric attention when they do. The four most common anxiety-provoking fears associated with death are (1) helplessness or loss of control, (2) being considered bad (guilt and punishment), (3) physical injury or symbolic injury (castration), and (4) abandonment.[19]

In the clinical examination, a severely anxious patient usually does not know what it is about death that is so frightening. Increased anxiety may result from specific memories and associations related to the death of parents or others with whom one identifies; patients may picture the same fate for themselves (e.g., agonizing pain or excessive use of technology). Memories of someone who died of the same illness (e.g., a woman with breast cancer who had relatives who died of breast cancer or a patient with AIDS who tended to a lover dying of AIDS) or particular associations with the illness may produce specific reasons for anxiety (e.g., the disease will be disfiguring). For the sake of the patient's mental health, it is important to explore these issues.

DESPONDENCY

Despondency—a mixture of dread, bitterness, and despair—is the result of an attack on the patient's self image. The patient feels broken, scarred, and ruined. Work and personal relationships appear jeopardized. It may seem too late to realize cherished goals. The patient is haunted by disappointment with both what has been done and what has been missed. He or she may feel old and that life has been a failure.

Despondency is a contagious feeling, and in most cases the physician can sense that the patient is depressed. Simply ask-

Table 1 Antidepressant Medications Used in Patients with Advanced Disease[22,24,40-44]

Class	Agent (Trade Name)	Dosage
Tricyclic antidepressants	Amitriptyline (Elavil)	10–150 mg p.o./I.M./p.r., q.d.
	Clomipramine (Anafranil)	10–150 mg p.o., q.d.
	Desipramine (Norpramin)	12.5–150 mg p.o./I.M. q.d.
	Doxepin (Sinequan)	12.5–150 mg p.o./I.M. q.d.
	Imipramine (Tofranil)	12.5–150 mg p.o./I.M. q.d.
	Nortriptyline (Pamelor)	10–125 mg p.o., q.d.
Second-generation antidepressants	Bupropion (Wellbutrin)	200–450 mg p.o., q.d.
	Fluoxetine (Prozac)	10–60 mg p.o., q.d.
	Fluvoxamine (Luvox)	50–300 mg p.o., q.d.
	Paroxetine (Paxil)	10–60 mg p.o., q.d.
	Sertraline (Zoloft)	25–200 mg p.o., q.d.
	Trazodone (Desyrel)	25–300 mg p.o., q.d.
	Venlafaxine (Effexor)	37.5–225 mg p.o., q.d.
Psychostimulants	Dextroamphetamine (Dexedrine)	2.5–20 mg p.o. in the morning and at noon*
	Lithium carbonate	600–1,200 mg p.o., q.d.
	Methylphenidate (Ritalin)	2.5–20 mg p.o. in the morning and at noon*
	Pemoline (Cylert)	37.5–75 mg p.o. in the morning and at noon*

*Give last dose at noon to avoid insomnia at night.

ing about the depression is helpful: "You look a bit blue today. What's on your mind?" The patient is likely to respond with the feelings already described. The patient should be told that such feelings are a normal part of any serious illness. It is important to remind even those who deny despondency that there is nothing unusual about feeling low from time to time in the struggle with any illness and that these feelings are time-limited. When the patient has acknowledged feelings of depression, even in the first few days of illness, it is very helpful if the physician describes future plans for medical treatment.

DEPRESSION

The more seriously ill a patient becomes, the more likely it is that a major depression will develop.[20] Researchers identified depression in 62% of patients in a palliative care unit in Winnipeg, Canada.[21] Standard depression inventories (e.g., Beck) are not as useful for diagnosing depression in terminal patients, because some of the physical symptoms of depression that these inventories target can occur in terminal illness without depression. At present, there is no validated instrument to assess depression in patients with terminal illness, although research is under way. Emotional symptoms remain helpful, however. These include anhedonia, depressed mood, suicidal thoughts, and guilt.

Patients in pain have a significantly higher rate of depression than comparable patients without pain.[22] Extreme depres-

sion and hopelessness are the strongest predictors that patients may develop a desire for hastened death.[23] Ganzini and colleagues documented that severely depressed patients make more restricted advance directives when depressed and change them when the depression is in remission.[24]

Pharmacologic options for depression in palliative care extend beyond the traditional agents [*see Table 1*]. Because standard antidepressant medications typically require several weeks to take effect, psychostimulants such as methylphenidate (Ritalin) and pemolin (Cylert) are increasingly being used for short-term treatment of depression for terminally ill patients in pain. They may be used instead of traditional antidepressants, in patients whose life expectancy is less than 3 weeks, or as an interim measure until traditional antidepressants take effect. They are also useful to counteract opiate-induced sedation and may potentiate opiate analgesia.

Of the antidepressant agents, the selective serotonin reuptake inhibitors (SSRIs) are associated with fewer side effects than traditional tricyclic agents, which have a high incidence of anticholinergic toxicity, including constipation, urinary retention, confusion, and altered cardiac conduction. The SSRIs (fluoxetine, sertraline, and paroxetine) are effective antidepressants and are generally well tolerated. Major side effects include anorexia, nausea, restlessness, and insomnia. Antidepressants with demonstrated efficacy as adjuvant therapy for treatment of pain include the tricyclic antidepressants and paroxetine.

PERSONALITY DISORDERS

Seriously ill people share common objectives with their physician: the relief of suffering and, as far as possible, the restoration of health. Dysfunctional personality traits (e.g., passive, hysterical, obsessive, dependent) that are the residue of past problems, such as parental conflicts, can distract both patient and doctor from those shared objectives. The doctor has enough to do to care for the physical illness and its normal emotional consequences to the patient (fear, anger, or despondency) without trying to alter personality traits. If reasonable efforts do not suffice, further intervention is best left to a consulting psychiatrist.

Preparation for the End of Life

THE CHOICE OF WHERE TO DIE

Where a person wishes to spend the end of his or her life is a very personal decision. The options are to remain at home, to move to an inpatient hospice [*see Chapter 10*], or to die in the hospital. Factors that influence this decision include the amount of support at home to care for the patient (emotional and physical), how comfortable the caretakers are with the care of a person who is dying, financial resources, and the technical support needed to keep the patient comfortable. In most cases, special equipment and services can be set up in the home, but this can be prohibitively expensive.

If it is anticipated that the patient has less than 6 months before death, this is an appropriate time to discuss hospice, whether inpatient or at home [*see Chapter 10*].

Health care providers frequently overlook the financial burden for patients and families resulting from terminal illness. Financial costs can be devastating. It is important to address this issue with patients and families and to refer them to appropriate financial counseling. Social workers can provide invaluable assistance in facilitating the provision of the home services to which patients are entitled under Medicare or Medicaid, and they can usually tell the patient and family what services will have to be paid for out of pocket.

Remember that while patients are in the hospital, caregivers surround them. When they return home, they often feel isolated and abandoned. Every effort should be made to maintain channels of communication among patients, family, and home health care workers.

ADVANCE DIRECTIVES

It is a mistake to delay the discussion of advance directives until the patient is in the terminal stages of illness. Rather, this issue should be dealt with soon after the diagnosis of terminal illness [*see Chapter 10*].

FINAL CLOSURE

The end of life is the opportunity for closure in relationships with loved ones. Relationship completion comprises five types of communications: I forgive you; forgive me; thank you; I love you; and goodbye.[25] These messages are vital to the peace of mind of the patient and the patient's family and should be encouraged by the physician as an aspect of standard palliative care.

Other actions that help with life's closure are a discussion of personal preferences for a memorial service, the settlement of financial affairs, and, if applicable, the completion of a plan for care of the children.

The physician should instruct the family in practical considerations concerning their loved one's death. For instance, the family should be told that there is no need to call 911 when the patient dies; instead, they should contact the funeral director. If a patient is dying at home and the family panics and calls 911, it is important that they have a "Do Not Resuscitate (DNR)" form in the home. Otherwise, the emergency medical services in some states are required to automatically intubate the patient.

Grief and Bereavement

In one respect, life can be described as one loss after another. The degree of recovery from each loss determines whether an individual regains a stable life or remains disabled. When losses occur, the resulting sadness can eventually give way to a process of reorganization that restores the person's ability to function normally. For example, the death of a parent can cause a child to become self-reliant. Some persons maintain a satisfying, productive life despite seemingly overwhelming losses, whereas others never recover from less severe losses. What makes the difference?

NORMAL GRIEVING

Grief is the psychological process by which an individual copes with loss, struggles to understand it, regains perspective, and goes on with life. Causes of grief include not only the loss of a loved one, of valued possessions, or of employment but also the loss of good health that occurs with major illness or injury. Serious illness or injury challenges personal integrity; it could be said, for example, that every myocardial infarction causes an ego infarction. Therefore, recovery from major illness is not complete until the patient has also recovered from the accompanying emotional damage to the self.

Surrounded daily by the sick and injured, physicians see grief work in process. It is important for the physician to realize that grief is a normal reaction serving an important restitutive function, that it follows a typical pattern, and that marked deviation from this pattern may be a sign that psychological intervention is required.

The normal grieving process follows a similar course in individuals suffering from any serious loss. Several prominent features of normal grieving have been identified.[26,27] Because these features are often mistakenly labeled as pathologic, familiarity with their correlation to grief can prevent well-meaning but misguided efforts to intervene in a necessary process.

Somatic symptoms of grieving may be prominent, including sighing respirations, exhaustion, gastrointestinal symptoms of all kinds, restlessness, yawning, and choking. Feelings of guilt, especially early in the wake of loss, seem to be universal. "What more could I have done?" or other references to unresolved emotional conflicts are common expressions of these feelings.

Preoccupation with the image of the deceased person, often seeming bizarre even to the griever, is a sure sign that normal mourning is under way. The intense focus on the deceased may be manifested in several ways: by continual mental conversations with the dead person; by a sense of the dead person's presence so vivid, especially at night, that the griever hears, sees, or is touched by the person; or by the simultaneous feeling that all other persons are emotionally distant.

Hostile reactions and irritability also seem to be the rule, combined with a disconcerting loss of warm feelings toward others. Some disruption of normal patterns of conduct is present, such as a desire to be alone, uncharacteristic procrastination, and indecisiveness toward others. The style, traits, mannerisms, or even the physical symptoms of the dead person may alarmingly appear in the mourner; such identification phenomena signify only that grief is in process. Finally, it is routine for the griever to feel that part of the self has been destroyed or mutilated.

How long will it take for the acute symptomatology of grieving to subside? Although the usual estimate is 1 to 3 months, many factors affect the actual time required. They include the number of strong remaining relationships, the intensity and duration of the bond with the lost person, the number and severity of any unresolved conflicts, the degree of dependence on the lost person, and how much of the survivor's mental life habitually assumed the dead person's physical or emotional presence. The main signs of resolution of acute grief are the reappearance of normal functioning, the capacity to experience pleasure, and the ability to enter new relationships.

The acute phase is followed by the disorganization phase. In this phase, the pain of the experience becomes foremost in the person's consciousness. Turmoil, emptiness, despair, and thoughts about the pointlessness of life and the reasonableness of suicide are common. Social interaction seems impossible and is avoided, even though solitude itself is dreaded and intolerable.

Finally, there is reorganization, characterized by a return of normal functioning and behavior. Reversals during this time are the rule, and reappearance of the earlier two phases should be expected. The bereaved person is caught off guard by sudden reminders of the lost person (e.g., a special coat discovered in storage) or by new and painful realizations (e.g., no more shared holidays) that reopen the wound of loss.

The grieving process is often delayed when death follows a prolonged and difficult illness. In such circumstances, death is entirely acceptable, even welcomed as the end of suffering. Later, especially when returning to a scene that sharply evokes the memory of the dead person when healthy, death becomes unacceptable, and feelings of protest or resentment spontaneously emerge.

ABNORMAL GRIEVING

Preexisting personality traits in survivors can interfere with the normal grief process. Additionally, survivors are at heightened risk of abnormal or complicated bereavement if the loved one died suddenly or unexpectedly, if the death was violent, or if no bodily remains were found. Because grief serves an important restitutive function, failure to grieve normally may result in serious psychological symptoms.

Some markers of abnormal grief are evident immediately; others do not appear for 3 months or longer after the loss. An inability to grieve immediately after the loss, typically manifested by absence of weeping, is the best predictor of later problems. Prolonged hysterical grieving that is defined as excessive by the individual's own subcultural norms (not those of the physician) is an equally ominous prognostic sign. Overactivity without a sense of loss is an early sign of distorted grieving. Furious hostility against specific persons—for example, the doctor or hospital staff—which may assume true paranoid proportions, can be regarded as a sign of abnormality when the individual dwells on it to the exclusion of the other concerns of normal grief. A suppression of hostility to the degree that the person's affect and conduct appear frozen (masklike appearance, stilted robotlike movements, and no emotional expressiveness) and self-destructive behavior (giving away belongings, foolish business deals, or other self-punitive actions with no attendant guilt feelings) are also early indicators of abnormal grieving.

Ultimately, it may become apparent that social isolation has become progressive, with a lasting loss of interpersonal initiative. When symptoms of the deceased person appear in the survivor as conversion symptoms or have become the focus of hypochondriacal complaints overshadowing all other manifestations of grief, pathologic grief is likely. Unresolved grief can also be suspected when the dead person is portrayed either as a saint who had no shortcomings or as one who never occasioned the least feeling of anger, burden, or disagreement in the survivor. In such cases, the mourner usually harbors intense feelings that are in conflict with those feelings outwardly expressed, and fear that these feelings will be discovered immobilizes the grieving process.

The result of prolonged grieving may be prolonged sadness, social isolation, somatic complaints, or loss of ability to function. A few sessions with a psychiatrist, aimed at helping the patient bring his or her own feelings into the open so that the process of grieving can be completed, often provide great relief.

Helping the Bereaved

Mourners tend to be outcasts from society. Their presence is painful to many around them, and efforts to silence, impede, or stop the manifestations of their grief are common. Allowing the grieving person to express feelings is essential, however. Most important is avoidance of maneuvers that negate grieving, such as clichés ("It's God's will"), efforts to distract ("After all, you've got three other children"), and outright exhortations to stop grieving ("Cheer up, life must go on").

Seeing the body of the deceased facilitates grieving, probably by establishing the irrevocable fact of death.[26] Permitting survivors to express their feelings and reminders that grief is a normal process are helpful. Gentle review of the deceased person's last days of life, last conversations, and final exchange of words, as well as talking about the deceased's general lifestyle, help initiate grieving. The memories most obstructive of grieving are those of hostile interactions with the deceased and any other interactions that leave the survivor feeling guilty. The more negative these interactions were, the longer it takes to begin recalling and discussing them.

In helping the bereaved, presence means more than words. Someone who can remain calm and accepting in the presence of a weeping, angry, or bitter mourner is highly valued. A hand on the shoulder can be just what is needed. Over time, helping the griever complete memories of the deceased also facilitates mourning. Old photograph albums and letters can be helpful in this regard. Anniversaries are key points in the grieving process, and special attention to the bereaved on these days is a basic element in the care of mourners.

A return to a job is an essential feature of the recovery process because it brings the mourner back into contact with concerned fellow workers. In addition, the therapeutic effects of work on self-esteem play an important part in alleviating the narcissistic component of the response to the loss. Most bereaved persons benefit from returning to work within 2 to 4 weeks after the death of a loved one.

Self-help groups can be extremely effective for permitting expression of emotion, showing that grief is universal, and supplying the compassion and respect necessary for rebuilding self-esteem. Books that recount events such as losing a spouse or that give instructions for the surviving spouse and children may be helpful.

SPECIFIC TYPES OF LOSS

Each type of loss carries specific challenges to mourners, and each type has a specific literature that can be helpful.[28] Loss of a parent by an adult, although a nearly universal occurrence, is not trivial, and loss of the second parent may leave the bereaved feeling particularly alone and vulnerable. Loss of a parent by a child invariably worries the adult survivors responsible for the child's care because successful mourning in a child is a more complex process than in an adult.[29] For example, the child may face adjustment to parental surrogates, to a parent stressed by the responsibility of raising the child alone, to the loss of a gender role model, or, eventually, to the replacement of the deceased parent by remarriage and competition for the affection of the surviving parent. However, studies of bereaved children from stable families have shown optimistic results: 8 weeks after the death of a parent, children 5 to 12 years of age were similar to nonbereaved children in school behavior, interest in school, peer involvement, peer enjoyment, and self-esteem.[30]

Research on loss of a sibling appears to be lacking, but the available data indicate that death of a sibling forces surviving siblings to reorganize their roles and relationships with their parents and with one another.[28]

Loss of a spouse, ranked on life-event scales as the most stressful of all possible losses,[31] is more detrimental for men than for women and leads to increased morbidity and mortality in elderly men.[32] The bereaved spouse is left with sole responsibility for children, finances, management, and planning;

faced with possible loss of income; and forced to cope with a changed social role in the community.

Each year, about 800,000 parents lose a child younger than 25 years. This loss is particularly traumatic because it is so contrary to life-cycle expectancies.[33]

Sudden death, such as death in an emergency ward, stillbirth, sudden infant death, accidental or traumatic death, cardiac arrest, or death during or after surgery, inflicts a uniquely intense trauma on the survivors. Shock is dramatically intensified. Guilt is likely to be a much more serious problem than it is with nonsudden death because of the total absence of preparation. Violence or disfigurement further intensifies the survivor's feelings.

General rules for dealing with the bereaved also apply here, with certain specific emphases. The chance to view the body, even when mutilated, should be offered to the family members. If there is severe mutilation, the family should be warned. The need to view the body, an aid to normal mourning, is greater when death is sudden.

Suicide is an especially difficult way to lose a loved one. Feeling abandoned and rejected, the survivor often experiences unsettling anger or, if the relationship had been hostile and stormy, equally unsettling relief. The bereaved scours through memories for an action that might have caused or prevented the suicide. Guilt is such an inevitable consequence of suicide that even casual acquaintances wonder what they might have done that contributed to the death. Shame can cause avoidance of others, falsification of the event as an accident, or unwillingness even to let others know that a family member has died. A scapegoat may be sought, such as the deceased's therapist, spouse, or boss or the medical examiner who labeled the death a suicide.[34]

Loss by homicide also produces especially intense grief reactions.[35] Flashbacks of the violent death are unavoidable. Survivors tend to avoid locations associated with the death and to stop watching television news because of possible reports of violence. Rage and desire for proportional revenge may cause intense discomfort for the bereaved, if suppressed, or for those around the bereaved, if excessively expressed. Children who witness the murder of one parent by another are afflicted with traumatic intrusive memories of the parents, massive conflicts of loyalty, and the intense need for secrecy because of the stigmatizing nature of their loss. They may inadvertently become so-called neglected victims and are at risk for perpetuating an intergenerational cycle of violence.[36,37]

Patience and gentleness with the family's prolonged numbness and shock are essential features of caring for bereaved family members. Physical acts of kindness may be the only avenue of communication at first. Leading the family to a quiet room, providing comfortable seats, bringing beverages, and making sure that all possible members are included are all helpful and may lay the groundwork for dialogue.

Immediately after imparting the news of death, the physician may be able to bring the family together and start a dialogue by offering to give them as detailed an account as possible. Teamwork is usually required to get everyone present and seated with beverages, ashtrays, and any other comforts that seem appropriate. Survivors may benefit from very gentle questions about the last hours of the deceased: Were there any prodromal syndromes? Any premonitions? Who saw the deceased last? Families who do not wish to explore these crucial questions at this time should not be pushed, however.

A chaplain, nurse, or other team member with counseling skills, present from the time the physician begins communicating the bad news, may be able to address sensitive issues that arise. Family members or other supportive figures (e.g., family doctor or clergyman) who are absent should be notified and asked to come to the hospital when appropriate. When the family members are too shaken to sit down or participate in any dialogue, it is important to leave them a telephone contact at the hospital should any questions arise.

MEDICATIONS AND BEREAVEMENT

Treatment of bereavement-related major depressive episodes has recently been shown to be beneficial. In one trial, persons who had lost their spouses within 6 to 8 weeks and met the Diagnostic and Statistical Manual of Mental Disorders, fourth edition (DSM IV), criteria for a major depressive episode were treated with sustained-release bupropion. Improvement was noted in both depression and grief intensity.[38] In another study, persons with major depressive episodes that began within 6 months before or 12 months after the loss of a spouse were randomly assigned to a 16-week double-blind trial of one of four treatments: nortriptyline plus interpersonal psychotherapy, nortriptyline alone in a medication clinic, placebo plus interpersonal psychotherapy, or placebo alone in a medication clinic. Nortriptyline proved superior to placebo in achieving remission of bereavement-related major depressive episodes, but the combination of medication and psychotherapy was associated with the highest rate of treatment completion. The investigators concluded that the results support the use of pharmacologic treatment of major depressive episodes in the wake of a serious life stressor such as bereavement.[39]

References

1. Magni KG: The fear of death. Death and Presence. Godin A, Ed. Lumen Vitae, Brussels, Belgium, 1972, p 125

2. Hippocrates: Decorum, XVI. Hippocrates with an English Translation, Vol 2. Jones WH, Ed. Heinemann, London, England, 1923

3. Kelly WD, Friesen SR: Do cancer patients want to be told? Surgery 27:822, 1950

4. Blackhall LJ, Murphy ST, Frank G, et al: Ethnicity and attitudes toward patient autonomy. JAMA 274:820, 1995

5. Sullivan RJ, Menapace LW, White RM: Truth-telling and patient diagnoses. J Med Ethics 27:192, 2001

6. Gerle B, Lunden G, Sandblom P: The patient with inoperable cancer from the psychiatric and social standpoints. Cancer 13:1206, 1960

7. Aitken-Swan J, Easson EC: Reactions of cancer patients on being told their diagnosis. Br Med J 1:779, 1959

8. Gilbertsen VA, Wangensteen OH: Should the doctor tell the patient that the disease is cancer? Surgeon's recommendation. The Physician and the Total Care of the Cancer Patient. American Cancer Society, New York, 1962, p 80

9. Croog SH, Shapiro SD, Levine S: Denial among male heart patients. Psychosom Med 33:385, 1971

10. Greer S: The management of denial in cancer patients. Oncology (Huntingt) 6:33, 1992

11. Grbich C, Parker D, Maddocks I: The emotions and coping strategies of caregivers of family members with a terminal cancer. J Palliat Care 17:30, 2001

12. Koenig HG, Idler E, Kasi S, et al: Religion, spirituality, and medicine: a rebuttal to skeptics. Int J Psychiatry Med 29:123, 1999

13. Larson DB, Swyers JP, McCullough ME: Scientific research on spirituality and health: a consensus report. National Institute for Healthcare Research, Rockville, Maryland, 1998

14. Mueller PS, Plevak DJ, Rummans TA: Religious involvement, spirituality and medicine: implications for clinical practice. Mayo Clin Proc 76:1225, 2001

15. Sloane RP, Bagiella E, Powell T. Religion, spirituality, and medicine. Lancet 353:664, 1999

16. Post SG, Puchalski CM, Larson DB: Physicians and patient spirituality: professional boundaries, competency, and ethics. Ann Intern Med 132:578, 2000

17. Saunders C: Foreword. Mortally Wounded. Kearney M, Ed. Marino Books, Dublin, Ireland, 1996, p 11

18. Cassem NH, Hackett TP: Psychiatric consultation in a coronary care unit. Ann Intern Med 75:9, 1971

19. Reiss D, Gonzalez S, Kramer N: Family process, chronic illness, and death. Arch Gen Psychiatry 43:795, 1986

20. Cassem NH: Depression and anxiety secondary to medical illness. Psychiatry Clin North Am 13:597, 1990

21. Chochinov HM: Management of grief in the cancer setting. Psychiatric Aspects of Symptom Management in Cancer Patients. Breitbart W, Holland JC, Eds. American Psychiatric Press, Washington, DC, 1993, p 231

22. Plumb MM, Holland JC: Comparative studies of psychological function in patients with advanced cancer. Psychosom Med 39:264, 1977

23. Breitbart W, Rosenfeld B, Pessin H, et al: Depression, hopelessness, and desire for hastened death in terminally ill patients with cancer. JAMA 284:2907, 2000

24. Ganzini L, Lee MA, Heintz RT, et al: The effect of depression treatment on elderly patients' preferences for life-sustaining medical therapy. Am J Psychiatry 151:1631, 1994

25. Byock I. Dying Well. Riverhead Books, The Berkley Publishing Group, New York, 1997, p 140

26. Parkes CM, Weiss RS: Recovery from Bereavement. Basic Books Inc, New York, 1983

27. Lindemann E: Symptomatology and management of acute grief. Am J Psychiatry 101:141, 1944

28. Bereavement: Reactions, Consequences, and Care. Osterweis M, Solomon F, Green M, Eds. National Academy Press, Washington, DC, 1984

29. Furman E: A Child's Parent Dies: Studies in Childhood Bereavement. Yale University Press, New Haven, Connecticut, 1974

30. Fristad MA, Jedel R, Weller RA, et al: Psychosocial functioning in children after the death of a parent. Am J Psychiatry 150:511, 1993

31. Holmes TH, Rahe RH: The social readjustment rating scale. J Psychosomatic Res 11:213, 1967

32. Rogers MP, Reich P: On the health consequences of bereavement (editorial). N Engl J Med 319:510, 1988

33. Cassem EH: The person confronting death. The New Harvard Guide to Psychiatry. Nicholi AM, Ed. Harvard University Press, Cambridge, Massachusetts, 1988, p 728

34. Ness DE, Pfeffer CR: Sequelae of bereavement resulting from suicide. Am J Psychiatry 147:279, 1990

35. Rynearson EK, McCreery JM: Bereavement after homicide: a synergism of trauma and loss. Am J Psychiatry 150:258, 1993

36. Black D, Kaplan T: Father kills mother: issues and problems encountered by a child psychiatric team. Br J Psychiatry 153:624, 1989

37. McCune N, Donnelly P: Child surviving parental murder (letter). Br J Psychiatry 154:889, 1989

38. Zisook S, Shucter SR, Pedrelli P, et al: Buproprion sustained release for bereavement: results of an open trial. J Clin Psychiatry 62:227, 2001

39. Reynolds CF 3rd, Miller MD, Pasternak RE, et al: Treatment of bereavement-related major depressive episodes in later life: a controlled study of acute and continuation treatment with nortriptyline and interpersonal psychotherapy. Am J Psychiatry 156:202, 1999

40. Stegman MB: Non-pain symptoms. Hope Hospice Pain and Symptom Control in Palliative Medicine. Stegman MB, Ed Part Six.

41. Breitbart W, Passik SD: Psychiatric aspects of palliative care. Oxford Textbook of Palliative Medicine. Doyle D, Hanks GW, MacDonald N, Eds. Oxford University Press, Oxford, England,1993, p 609.

42. Barraclough J: ABC of palliative care: depression, anxiety, and confusion. BMJ 315:1365, 1997

43. Massie MJ: Depression. Handbook of Psycho-oncology. Holland JC, Rowland JH, Eds. Oxford University Press, New York, 1989, p 283

44. Massie MJ, Holland JC: Depression and the cancer patient. J Clin Psychiatry 51: 12, 1990

BIOTERRORISM AND MEDICAL EMERGENCIES

11 Bioterrorism

Jeffrey Duchin, M.D.

Well before the 2001 anthrax outbreak, public health and government leaders in the United States recognized the need for increased preparedness to detect and respond to acts of biologic terrorism. Concern about the vulnerability of the United States to a biologic attack grew with revelations about the offensive biologic weapons programs of the former Soviet Union and Iraq, as well as uncertainty about the whereabouts of and accountability for biologic agents produced through those programs; the successful chemical attack on the Tokyo subway system by the Aum Shinrikyo cult, coupled with information that the cult was actively experimenting with biologic agents; and information about the potential for domestic bioterrorism.[1-5]

In April 2000, the Centers for Disease Control and Prevention (CDC) published a strategic plan for preparedness and response to biologic and chemical terrorism.[6] This chapter describes the clinician's role in recognizing and responding to biologic terrorism, as presented in the CDC plan; summarizes current information on the diagnosis and management of the most likely agents of bioterrorism; and describes current resources for authoritative information and guidelines related to bioterrorism.

The Clinician's Role in Bioterrorism Preparedness and Response

For clinicians, the response to a bioterrorism attack is in many ways the same as the response to naturally occurring outbreaks of communicable disease.[7,8] Both situations typically require early identification of ill or exposed persons, rapid implementation of preventive therapy, special infection control considerations, and collaboration or communication with the public health system. Examples of naturally occurring communicable diseases that require such a response include meningococcal disease[9]; enteric infection with *Escherichia coli* 0157:H7, *Salmonella*, or *Shigella*[10]; pertussis, rubella, measles, or chickenpox occurring in health care facilities and clinics[11-14]; unusual or newly emerging infections such as West Nile virus and hantavirus pulmonary syndrome[15-17]; and the inevitable reappearance of pandemic influenza.[18]

The first indication of an unannounced biologic attack will likely be an increase in the number of persons seeking care from primary care physicians. In the 2001 anthrax outbreak, as well as in the outbreaks of *E. coli* 0157:H7 disease and hantavirus pulmonary syndrome in 1993 and West Nile virus in 1999, alert clinicians initiated the public health response by recognizing an unusual clinical syndrome, ordering appropriate laboratory tests, and notifying public health officials.[10,16,17] Similarly, primary care physicians and subspecialists alike must be familiar with both the specific clinical syndromes associated with agents of bioterrorism and the ways to rapidly notify public health authorities. In addition to identifying cases and treating ill patients, clinicians also play a critical role in managing postexposure prophylaxis and its complications, as well as psychological and mental health problems brought on by the event.

During both bioterrorism attacks and naturally occurring outbreaks, clinicians are faced with the challenge of excluding the outbreak disease in persons who are worried about potential exposure or who are ill with signs and symptoms similar to those of the outbreak disease. The clinician must have knowledge of the modes of transmission, incubation periods, and communicable periods of these diseases, as well as skill in both clinical evaluation and eliciting an appropriate and thorough history, including relevant occupational, social, and travel information. In the 2001 anthrax outbreak, for example, the epidemiologic setting of cases played an important role in guiding diagnostic tests and treatment.[19] The primary care clinician has the best opportunity to obtain relevant information early in the evaluation; this is important because such information may be more difficult to obtain as time goes on, particularly if the patient's condition deteriorates.

Physicians and other health care providers should have a working knowledge of the basic classes of isolation and infection control measures recommended for patients exposed to agents of potential bioterrorism. Again, these measures are also used in the management of common communicable diseases.[14,20-22]

Recognition of Potential Bioterrorism Agents

The CDC has developed a list of bacteria, viruses, and toxins thought to pose the greatest risk for use in a bioterrorist attack [*see Table 1*].[23] Agents were included in the list on the basis of their ability to cause disease that (1) is easily disseminated or transmitted from person to person; (2) has high mortality, with potential for major public health impact; (3) may result in panic and social disruption; and (4) requires special action for public health preparedness. Category A agents are thought to pose the highest immediate risk for use as biologic weapons; and category B agents, the next highest risk. Category C agents are thought to pose a potential, but not immediate, risk for use as biologic weapons.

As in naturally occurring outbreaks, early recognition of a bioterrorist attack is critical for rapid implementation of preventive measures and treatment. Early recognition can be challenging, however, because patients presenting for medical care after exposure to a biologic agent may initially exhibit nonspecific symptoms, and pathogens that ordinarily occur in the community, particularly enteric organisms, may be used in a biologic attack.[24,25] A heightened level of suspicion, plus knowledge of the relevant epidemiologic clues, should help physicians recognize changes in illness patterns, including clusters and increases in observed cases over the number expected [*see Table 2*].[26] Physicians should also be able to recognize diagnostic clues in single cases of a syndrome of concern (e.g., inhalational anthrax, plague and tularemia, botulismlike illness, and possible smallpox).[27] Familiarity with the clinical features of diseases from potential bioterrorist agents and diseases prevalent in the community will allow recognition of potentially significant differences from naturally occurring cases. One of the most important lessons learned from the 2001 anthrax attack was that clinical illness caused by agents prepared as biologic weapons may differ from typical natural infections.

The identification of a bioterrorist attack requires clinicians to be prepared, alert, and open-minded [*see Sidebar* Internet Resources on Bioterrorism]. Many local and state health departments post current information about communicable diseases

Table 1 Critical Biologic Agent Categories for Public Health Preparedness

Category	Biologic Agent	Disease
A (highest immediate risk)	Variola major *Bacillus anthracis* *Yersinia pestis* *Clostridium botulinum* (botulinum toxins) *Francisella tularensis* Filoviruses and arenaviruses (e.g., Ebola virus, Lassa virus)	Smallpox Anthrax Plague Botulism Tularemia Viral hemorrhagic fevers
B (next highest risk)	*Coxiella burnetii* *Brucella* species *Burkholderia mallei* *Burkholderia pseudomallei* Alphaviruses (VEE, EEE, WEE) *Rickettsia prowazekii* Toxins (e.g., ricin, staphylococcal enterotoxin B) *Chlamydia psittaci* Food-safety threats (e.g., *Salmonella* species, *E. coli* 0157:H7) Water-safety threats (e.g., *Vibrio cholerae*, *Cryptosporidium parvum*)	Q fever Brucellosis Glanders Melioidosis Encephalitis Typhus fever Toxic syndromes Psittacosis
C (potential, but not immediate, risk)	Emerging-threat agents (e.g., Nipah virus, hantavirus)	

EEE—eastern equine encephalitis   VEE—Venezuelan equine encephalitis   WEE—western equine encephalitis

on their Web sites and distribute informational newsletters with relevant data. The CDC's weekly bulletin, *Morbidity and Mortality Weekly Report* (*MMWR*), contains current information on medical conditions of public health importance in the United States. Subscriptions to *MMWR* are available online at http://www.cdc.gov/mmwr/mmwrsubscribe.html.

Communication with Authorities

Once a potential outbreak or significant cluster or event has been detected, prompt consultation with appropriate medical specialists and public health authorities is indicated. Clinicians must have reliable, around-the-clock contact information for emergency resources in the geographic area where they practice; these resources include specialist consultants (e.g., consultants in infectious disease, dermatology, or pulmonary medicine) and infection control professionals or hospital epidemiologists. All clinicians should know how to contact their local or state public health department 24 hours a day to report suspicious or otherwise immediately notifiable cases or for consultation. Many local and state health departments have such contact numbers on their Web sites. Clinicians should have these numbers readily accessible and keep them current.

Clinicians must also ensure that they have a reliable way to promptly receive urgent communications from public health authorities, both for naturally occurring outbreaks of local significance and for a bioterrorist event or outbreak. Increasingly, public health authorities are disseminating health alerts over the Internet, through Web sites and e-mail listserves.

Smallpox

Smallpox is caused by variola virus, an orthopox virus unique to humans. No known animal or insect reservoirs or vectors exist.[28] Related orthopox viruses infecting humans in-

clude vaccinia (smallpox vaccine), monkeypox, and cowpox. Smallpox existed in two forms: variola major, which accounted for most morbidity and mortality, and a milder form, variola minor. Variola major is the type of concern in the context of biologic terrorism.

Smallpox was declared eradicated in 1980, 3 years after the last naturally occurring case was reported from Somalia. Stocks of smallpox virus were retained, however, by World Health Organization (WHO) reference laboratories at the Institute of Virus Preparations in Moscow, Russia, and at the CDC in Atlanta, Georgia. In the late 1990s, allegations were published describing the production of large quantities of smallpox virus by the former Soviet Union. These stores, which may have become disseminated after the breakup of the Soviet Union, would presumably be the source for a bioterrorist attack involving smallpox.

Smallpox is stable and highly infectious in the aerosol form. The risk for a smallpox attack currently is considered low but not zero.[1,4,29,30]

Table 2 Epidemiologic Clues of a Biologic Attack

Presence of a large epidemic
Unusually severe disease or unusual routes of exposure
Unusual geographic area, unusual season, or absence of normal vector
Multiple simultaneous epidemics of different diseases
Outbreak of zoonotic disease
Unusual strains of organisms or antimicrobial-resistance patterns
Higher attack rates in persons with common exposures
Credible threat, as determined by authorities, of biologic attack
Direct evidence of biologic attack

Internet Resources on Bioterrorism

General

CDC portal to information for laboratory and health professionals
http://www.bt.cdc.gov/healthprofessionals/index.asp

Contact information for U.S. state and local health departments
http://www.cdc.gov/other.htm#states

CDC Emergency Response Hotline (24 hours): 770-488-7100
Program questions: 404-639-0385

American College of Physicians–American Society of Internal Medicine (ACP-ASIM) bioterrorism resources
http://www.acponline.org/bioterro/?hp

Association for Professionals in Infection Control and Epidemiology, Inc.
http://www.apic.org/bioterror/

Bioterrorism Preparedness and Response Program, National Center for Infectious Diseases, Centers for Disease Control and Prevention—information for laboratory and health professionals
http://www.bt.cdc.gov/healthprofessionals/index.asp

Center for Infectious Disease Research & Policy (CIDRAP), University of Minnesota
http://www1.umn.edu/cidrap/content/bt/bioprep

FDA bioterrorism site
http://www.fda.gov/oc/opacom/hottopics/bioterrorism.html

Department of Health and Human Services Preparedness and Response
http://www.hhs.gov/hottopics/healing/biological.html

Infectious Diseases Society of America
bioterrorism: **http://www.idsociety.org/BT/ToC.htm**
practice guidelines: **http://www.idsociety.org/PG/toc.htm**

Johns Hopkins University Center for Civilian Biodefense Strategies
http://www.hopkins-biodefense.org

National Academies' Expert-selected Web Resources for "First Responders" on Bioterrorism
http://www.nap.edu/shelves/first

National Institute of Allergy and Infectious Diseases
http://www.niaid.nih.gov/publications/bioterrorism.htm

National Library of Medicine Specialized Information Services
http://www.sis.nlm.nih.gov/Tox/biologicalwarfare.htm

St. Louis University Center for Study of Bioterrorism
http://bioterrorism.slu.edu

Treatment of Biological Warfare Agent Casualties (July 17, 2000), U.S. Army Field Manual on Treatment of Biological Warfare Casualties
http://www.nbc-med.org/SiteContent/MedRef/OnlineRef/FieldManuals/Fm8_284/fm8_284.pdf

USAMRIID's Medical Management of Biological Casualties Handbook (Blue Book)
http://www.usamriid.army.mil/education/bluebook.html
word format: **http://www.nbc-med.org/SiteContent/HomePage/WhatsNew/MedManual/Feb01/handbook.htm**

JAMA consensus statement series
http://pubs.ama-assn.org/bioterr.html

Specific Agents

Anthrax as a Biological Weapon, 2002. Updated Recommendations for Management
http://jama.ama-assn.org/issues/v287n17/ffull/jst20007.html

Armed Forces Institute of Pathology site on inhalational anthrax, including slides
http://anthrax.radpath.org

Botulinum Toxin as a Biological Weapon. Medical and Public Health Management
http://jama.ama-assn.org/issues/v285n8/ffull/jst00017.html

Hemorrhagic Fever Viruses as Biological Weapons. Medical and Public Health Management
http://jama.ama-assn.org/issues/v287n18/ffull/jst20006.html

Plague as a Biological Weapon. Medical and Public Health Management
http://jama.ama-assn.org/issues/v283n17/ffull/jst90013.html

Smallpox as a Biological Weapon. Medical and Public Health Management
http://jama.ama-assn.org/issues/v281n22/ffull/jst90000.html

Tularemia as a Biological Weapon. Medical and Public Health Management
http://jama.ama-assn.org/issues/v285n21/ffull/jst10001.html

CLASSIFICATION

On the basis of a study from India, the WHO has classified smallpox into five clinical forms: ordinary, flat-type, hemorrhagic, modified, and sine eruptione.[31] These forms reflect different host reactions to the same strain of virus.

Ordinary Smallpox

Ordinary smallpox is the most common form seen in nonimmune persons; it accounted for 90% of cases in the WHO study and had an average case-fatality rate of 30%. The incubation period is 7 to 17 days (mean, 10 to 12 days). Symptoms of the prodromal phase include the acute onset of high fever, malaise, headache, backache, and prostration. Other prominent symptoms include vomiting and abdominal pain.

The characteristic rash occurs 2 to 3 days later, appearing first on the face and forearms. An enanthem involving the oropharyngeal mucosa precedes the rash by a day. The rash progresses slowly, from macules to papules to vesicles and pustules and finally to scabs, with each stage lasting 1 to 2 days. The lesions are firm, discrete vesicles or pustules (4 to 6 mm in diameter) deeply embedded in the dermis; they may become umbilicated or confluent as they evolve [*see Figure 1*]. The patient remains febrile throughout the evolution of the rash, which may become painful as pustules enlarge. A second fever spike 5 to 8 days after onset of the rash may signify a secondary bacterial infection. Pustules remain for 5 to 8 days, after which umbilication and crusting occur. Lesions are in the same stage of development on any given part of the body. They are peripherally distributed, more concentrated on the face and distal extremities than on the trunk, and may involve the palms and soles. Scarring occurs with scab separation from destruction of sebaceous glands.

Experience during the global smallpox eradication program suggests that the onset of communicability coincides with the development of rash, approximately 2 days after the onset of the acute febrile prodrome. However, because the oropharyngeal enanthem and associated release of virus into oral secretions may precede rash onset, it is recommended that for the purposes of postexposure management, anyone who has contact with smallpox patients from the time of onset of fever should be considered potentially exposed [*see Infection Control, below*].[32]

Complications of smallpox include fluid and electrolyte disturbances; extensive desquamation that clinically resembles

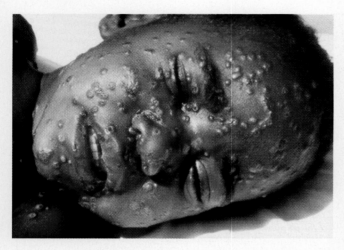

Figure 1 **Smallpox lesions.**

burns; bronchitis and pneumonitis; panophthalmitis and blindness from viral keratitis or secondary infection of the eye; arthritis (developing in up to 2% of children); and encephalitis (less than 1% of cases). Death results from toxemia associated with circulating immune complexes and variola antigens.[33]

Other Forms of Smallpox

Flat-type (or malignant) smallpox occurs in 5% to 10% of cases and is severe, with a 97% case-fatality rate among unvaccinated persons. In this form, lesions are flat and become densely confluent, evolving slowly and coalescing with a soft, velvety texture. Hemorrhagic smallpox was reported in less than 3% of cases, occurring particularly in pregnant women. It is a severe, rapidly progressive, uniformly fatal illness. A dusky erythema develops, followed by hemorrhages into the skin and mucous membranes. Both hemorrhagic and flat-type smallpox have an accelerated and more severe prodromal phase and are thought to be associated with underlying immune dysfunction.

Modified smallpox is a mild form that accounted for 2% of cases in unvaccinated patients and 25% in previously vaccinated patients. This form rarely resulted in death, and these patients had fewer, smaller, more superficial, and more rapidly evolving lesions. Smallpox sine eruptione (without rash) occurs in previously vaccinated persons or children with maternal antibodies to smallpox. It is a mild or asymptomatic illness that has not been documented to be transmissible.[31,33-35]

DIAGNOSIS

A suspected case of smallpox is a public health emergency. Local and state health authorities, the hospital epidemiologist, and other members of a hospital response team for biologic emergencies should be notified immediately (see the CDC Interim Smallpox Response Plan and Guidelines at http://www.bt.cdc.gov/documentsapp/SmallPox/RPG/ContactInfo.asp).

The differential diagnosis of smallpox includes other illnesses that can cause fever and a rash [*see Table 3*]. Severe varicella is the disease most likely to be confused with smallpox. However, familiarity with the clinical features of the two diseases, particularly the rash, should help differentiate them [*see Table 4*]. Additional information that may be useful in differentiating smallpox from chickenpox includes a history of exposure to persons with chickenpox, a personal history of chickenpox, a history of vaccination against varicella or smallpox, and the clinical course of illness.

If shingles or disseminated herpes infection is a consideration, direct fluorescent antibody testing for varicella-zoster virus can rapidly confirm varicella-zoster virus and herpes simplex virus infection in patients not considered at high risk for smallpox. Such testing should not be done in patients who are considered at high risk, to avoid exposing laboratory workers to smallpox virus. Certain laboratories can also perform

Table 3 Diagnosis of Smallpox

Incubation Period	Clinical Presentation	Differential Diagnosis	Diagnostic Testing
7–17 days; mean, 10–12 days	Severe, acute febrile prodrome 1–4 days before rash onset, with temperature ≥ 101° F (38.3° C), headache, backache, chills, vomiting, abdominal pain, prostration Enanthem on oropharyngeal mucosa, followed by rash on face, forearms, distal extremities, then trunk; lesions most concentrated on face and distal extremities Lesions evolve slowly from macules to papules to deep-seated, firm, nodular, round, well-circumscribed vesicles or pustules to scabs over 1–2 days per stage; are in same stage of evolution on a given area of the body; may become umbilicated or confluent Hemorrhagic smallpox: bleeding into skin and mucous membranes Flat-type/malignant smallpox: lesions remain soft and flattened, coalesce Modified smallpox: less severe with fewer, more superficial and rapidly evolving lesions	Varicella (chickenpox); disseminated herpes zoster and simplex; drug eruptions; erythema multiforme; enteroviral infections; secondary syphilis; contact dermatitis; impetigo; scabies; molluscum contagiosum Hemorrhagic smallpox: meningococcemia, Rocky Mountain spotted fever, ehrlichiosis, gram-negative bacterial sepsis, severe acute leukemia Malignant smallpox: hemorrhagic chickenpox	Diagnostic testing at BSL-4 laboratory, including skin biopsy, electron microscopic examination of vesicular and pustular fluid, culture, PCR; serology Appropriate infection control precautions

Note: The clinical manifestations of infections acquired during a biologic attack may differ from those of naturally occurring infections. Clinicians should remain alert for compatible syndromes that vary from the descriptions given.
BSL-4—biosafety level 4   PCR—polymerase chain reaction

Table 4 Differentiating Features of Smallpox and Chickenpox

Clinical Feature	Smallpox	Chickenpox
Prodromal illness	Febrile prodrome lasting 1–4 days; patient appears ill or toxic	No or mild prodrome; patients typically do not appear ill
Appearance of lesions	Firm, round, well-circumscribed, deep-seated lesions; may be umbilicated	Superficial lesions
Stage of lesions on any one part of the body	Lesions are all at the same stage of development on a given area of the body	Lesions occur in crops with various stages of development evident on a given area of the body
Initial lesions	Oral mucosa, face, or forearms	Face, then trunk
Oral lesions	Early; may not be evident	May occur
Severity of illness	Typically severe	Typically not severe
Distribution of rash	Centrifugal: lesions concentrated on the face and extremities, with relative sparing of the trunk	Centripetal: lesions concentrated on the trunk with relative sparing of the face and extremities
Lesions on palms or soles	Lesions on palms and soles in majority of cases	Lesions on palms and soles uncommon
Rate of evolution of rash	Slow evolution of lesions from macules to papules to pustules over days	Rapid evolution from macules to papules to crusted lesions within 24 hours
Presence of pruritus	Lesions may be painful and are not usually pruritic until scabbing occurs	Often pruritic, typically not painful in the absence of secondary infection
Hemorrhagic lesions	Can occur	Can occur

polymerase chain reaction (PCR) testing for herpes simplex virus and varicella-zoster virus. Consultation with an infectious disease specialist, a dermatology specialist, or both is recommended.

Flat-type and hemorrhagic smallpox may be difficult to recognize because of the absence of the characteristic rash of ordinary smallpox, yet these cases are highly infectious. Hemorrhagic smallpox cases may be mistaken for meningococcemia or acute leukemia. All patients with potential smallpox should be asked about their travel history, level of immunocompetence, and current medications.

The local or state health department should be contacted to facilitate specimen collection for smallpox testing (http://www.statepublichealth.org). Protocols for specimen collection for smallpox testing have been published by the CDC and are available at the following Internet address: http://www.bt.cdc.gov/documentsapp/SmallPox/RPG/GuideD/Guide-D.pdf. These protocols are also available through the CDC's smallpox information Web page: http://www.bt.cdc.gov/Agent/Smallpox/SmallpoxGen.asp.

Diagnostic testing is available at designated biosafety level 4 (BSL-4) laboratories and includes electron microscopy, immunohistohemical tests, and viral culture with PCR and restriction fragment length polymorphism (RFLP) testing. Only personnel who have undergone successful smallpox vaccination recently (within 3 years) and who are wearing appropriate barrier protection (gloves, gown, and shoe covers) should be involved in specimen collection for suspected cases of smallpox. Respiratory protection is not needed for personnel with recent, successful vaccination. Masks and eyewear or face shields should be used if splashing is anticipated. If unvaccinated personnel must collect specimens, only those who are without contraindications to vaccination should do so, because they would require immediate vaccination if the diagnosis of smallpox were confirmed. Vesicular or pustular fluid, scabs, punch biopsies of skin lesions, blood, and tissue from autopsy specimens should

be obtained, packaged, and transported according to CDC protocol (http://www.bt.cdc.gov/labissues/PackagingInfo.pdf; http://www.bt.cdc.gov/documentsapp/SmallPox/RPG/index.asp).[32,35]

The CDC has developed a protocol in poster format for evaluating patients with an acute vesicular or pustular rash illness and for determining the risk of smallpox. The protocol, including color pictures of smallpox lesions, is available on the Internet at the following address: http://www.bt.cdc.gov/agent/smallpox/index.asp.

INFECTION CONTROL AND POSTEXPOSURE ISOLATION

In the event of a limited outbreak, patients should be admitted to the hospital and confined to rooms that are under negative atmospheric pressure and equipped with high-efficiency particulate air (HEPA) filtration. Standard, contact, and airborne precautions, including use of gloves, gowns, and masks, should be strictly observed. Unvaccinated personnel caring for patients suspected of having smallpox should wear fit-tested N95 or higher-quality respirators. Once successful vaccination is confirmed, care providers are no longer required to wear an N95 mask.[35] Patients should wear a surgical mask and be wrapped in a gown or sheet to cover the rash when they are not in a negative-airflow room. All laundry and waste should be placed in biohazard bags and autoclaved before being laundered or incinerated. Surfaces that may be contaminated with smallpox virus can be decontaminated with disinfectants that are used for standard hospital infection control, such as hypochlorite and quaternary ammonia.

Persons suspected of being infected with smallpox should be immediately isolated, and all their household members and others who have had face-to-face contact with the infected patient after the onset of fever should be vaccinated and placed under surveillance. Because persons who have had contact with an infected patient would not be contagious until the onset of rash, they should take their temperatures at least once daily, preferably in the evening. Any temperature higher than 101° F (38.3° C) during the 17-day period after the last exposure to the infected patient would suggest the possibility of the development of smallpox. This would be cause for immediate isolation until the diagnosis can be determined clinically, by laboratory examination, or both.

In the event of an outbreak, the following high-risk groups should be given priority for vaccination: (1) persons exposed to the initial release of the virus; (2) contacts of suspected or confirmed smallpox patients; (3) personnel who are directly involved in medical or public health evaluation of suspected or confirmed smallpox patients, as well as the care or transportation of such patients; (4) laboratory workers involved in the collection or processing of possible smallpox specimens; (5) other persons who may be in contact with infectious material, such as hospital laundry, medical waste, and mortuary workers; (6) other groups essential to response activities, such as law enforcement, emergency response, or military personnel; and (7) all persons in a hospital where there is a smallpox patient who is not isolated appropriately. Employees for whom vaccination would be contraindicated (see below) should be furloughed.[32,35]

Smallpox Vaccine

Vaccinia vaccine does not contain smallpox (variola) virus. Currently, there are no commercially available (i.e., licensed) smallpox vaccines, and existing supplies of vaccine are available only under Investigational New Drug (IND) protocols held by the CDC. Existing vaccines were prepared from calf lymph with a seed virus derived from the New York City Board of Health strain of vaccinia virus. A reformulated vaccine, produced by using cell-culture techniques, is now being developed.

The immune status of those vaccinated more than 27 years ago is not clear. Studies have demonstrated persistence of T cell and humoral responses, but absolute levels of neutralizing antibodies decline substantially during the first 5 to 10 years after vaccination. Epidemiologic studies conducted during endemic smallpox outbreaks suggested that remote vaccination can ameliorate disease but does not prevent disease in most persons with high-risk exposures.[30]

Complications of smallpox vaccination Current data on complication rates after primary vaccination are derived from observations made when smallpox vaccine was in routine use in the United States, over 30 years ago.[28] Higher rates of vaccine complications would likely occur today, given the increased number of persons with medical conditions or medications that compromise the immune system. Moderate and severe complications of vaccinia vaccination include eczema vaccinatum, generalized vaccinia, progressive vaccinia, and postvaccinial encephalitis. These complications are rare but are at least 10 times more common after primary vaccination than after revaccination; they occur more frequently in infants than in older children and adults.

The most common complication of smallpox vaccination, occurring in 529.2 cases per million doses, is localized vaccinia infection resulting from inadvertent transfer (autoinoculation) of vaccinia from the vaccination site to other parts of the body. In addition, transmission of vaccinia virus can occur when a recently vaccinated person has contact with a susceptible person; in one study, 30% of smallpox patients were persons who had had such contact.[28,36] Inadvertent transfer of vaccinia from the

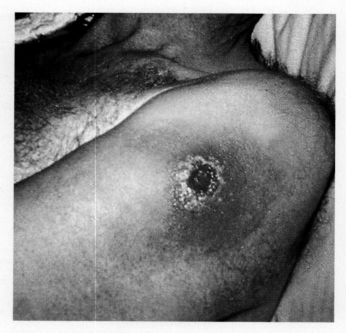

Figure 2 **Progressive vaccinia (vaccinia necrosum) at the site of smallpox vaccination in a 64-year-old man.**

vaccination site to other parts of the body can be prevented by careful hand washing after touching the vaccination site and by keeping the site covered.

Eczema vaccinatum (38.5/million doses) is a localized or systemic dissemination of vaccinia virus that occurs in persons who have eczema or a history of eczema or other chronic or exfoliative skin conditions (e.g., atopic dermatitis). Illness is usually mild and self-limited but can be severe or fatal. Severe cases have also been observed in persons with active eczema or a history of eczema, after contact with recently vaccinated persons.

Generalized vaccinia (241.5/million doses) is characterized by a vesicular rash of varying extent that can occur in persons without underlying illness. The rash is generally self-limited and requires minor or no therapy except in patients whose condition might be toxic or who have serious underlying immunosuppressive illnesses.

Progressive vaccinia (vaccinia necrosum, 1.5/million doses) is a severe, potentially fatal illness characterized by progressive necrosis in the area of vaccination, often with metastatic lesions [*see Figure 2*]. It has occurred almost exclusively in persons with cellular immunodeficiency.

The most common serious complication is postvaccinial encephalitis (12.3/million doses). It occurs mostly in infants younger than 1 year and, less often, in adolescents and adults receiving a primary vaccination. Rates of this complication were influenced by the strain of virus used in the vaccine and were higher in Europe than in the United States. The principal strain of vaccinia virus used in the United States—the New York City Board of Health (NYCBOH) strain—was associated with the lowest incidence of postvaccinial encephalitis. Approximately 15% to 25% of affected vaccinees with this complication die, and 25% have permanent neurologic sequelae.

Fatal complications caused by vaccinia vaccination are rare, with approximately one death per million primary vaccinations and 0.25 deaths per million revaccinations. Death is most often the result of postvaccinial encephalitis or progressive vaccinia.

Contraindications Groups at special risk for complications include persons with eczema or other significant exfoliative conditions; patients with leukemia, lymphoma, or generalized malignancy who are receiving therapy with alkylating agents, antimetabolites, radiation, or large doses of corticosteroids; patients with HIV infection; persons with hereditary immune disorders; and pregnant women. In persons with contraindications who require vaccination because of exposure to smallpox virus from a bioterrorist attack, the risk of complications can be reduced by giving vaccinia immune globulin (VIG; see below) simultaneously with vaccination. However, current stores of VIG are insufficient to allow its prophylactic use. Even if VIG is not available, vaccination may still be warranted, given the far higher risk of an adverse outcome from smallpox than from vaccination.

Vaccinia immune globulin Complications of vaccinia vaccination can be prevented or treated with VIG, which is an isotonic sterile solution of the immunoglobulin fraction of plasma from persons vaccinated with vaccinia vaccine. For prophylactic use, in persons with contraindications who require vaccination, VIG is given along with vaccinia vaccine.[28] Very large amounts are required: VIG is administered intramuscularly in a dose of 0.3 ml/kg (e.g., 22.5 ml I.M. for a 75 kg patient) At present, however, supplies of VIG are so limited that its use should be reserved for treatment of patients with the most serious vaccine complications.

For treatment of vaccinia vaccination complications, VIG is administered intramuscularly; 0.6 ml/kg is given in divided doses over a 24- to 36-hour period. A repeat dose may be given 2 to 3 days later if improvement does not occur. VIG is effective for treatment of eczema vaccinatum and certain cases of progressive vaccinia; it might be useful also in the treatment of ocular vaccinia resulting from inadvertent implantation. VIG is contraindicated for the treatment of vaccinial keratitis. VIG is recommended for severe generalized vaccinia if the patient is extremely ill or has a serious underlying disease. VIG provides no benefit in the treatment of postvaccinial encephalitis and has no role in the treatment of smallpox.[28,32]

Anthrax

Anthrax is a zoonotic disease caused by the spore-forming bacterium *Bacillus anthracis*, a large, nonmotile, nonhemolytic, gram-positive rod [see Chapter 135]. The organism is distributed worldwide in soil. Animals, primarily herbivores, become infected through grazing in contaminated areas. Under natural conditions, humans contract the disease after close contact with infected animals or contaminated animal products such as hides, wool, or meat.[37] Hardy spores resistant to heat and environmental degradation are the usual infective form. The spores develop in response to exposure to ambient air. On exposure to favorable, nutrient-rich environmental conditions such as tissues or blood of an animal or human host, the spores germinate, producing vegetative cells.[38]

CLASSIFICATION AND EPIDEMIOLOGY

Anthrax occurs in three clinical forms in humans: inhalational, cutaneous, and gastrointestinal. In a biologic attack, aerosol exposure to anthrax spores would be most likely.[29] Only 18 cases of inhalational anthrax were reported in the United States in the 20th century, none of them after 1976. Sixteen of these cases

were attributable to an industrial source of infection, and two cases were laboratory associated.[39] Before 2001, exposure to powdered anthrax spores in an envelope or package was not thought to be an efficient means of causing inhalational disease. However, exposure to anthrax spores sent through the United States mail in the 2001 anthrax attack resulted in 11 cases of inhalational anthrax and 11 cases of cutaneous disease.[19,40,41] Recent research has demonstrated the unanticipated potential for significant dispersion of respirable aerosol particles of spores through opening of a contaminated envelope.[42] In addition, expected clinical findings based on previous experience with naturally occurring anthrax infections did not entirely correspond to the clinical presentation in persons exposed to anthrax in the context of a biologic attack, although there was considerable overlap between the two.

Cutaneous anthrax accounts for the majority of naturally occurring anthrax cases worldwide. It results from inoculation of spores subcutaneously through a cut or abrasion.[43] Given that cutaneous anthrax cases occurred during the 2001 anthrax outbreak, it is possible that a bioterrorist attack could be detected through recognition of cutaneous anthrax cases.[19] Gastrointestinal and oropharyngeal anthrax occur in rural parts of the world where anthrax is endemic. They result from ingestion of meat contaminated with spores or large numbers of vegetative cells.[44] No cases of gastrointestinal anthrax occurred during the 1979 accidental release of anthrax from a military facility in Sverdlovsk, Russia, in which 77 inhalational cases occurred, or during the 2001 outbreak in the United States. Because of the logistic difficulty of effectively contaminating food and water supplies, it is thought that this form of anthrax would be less likely to occur as a result of a biologic attack.[29]

PATHOPHYSIOLOGY

Anthrax is a toxin-mediated disease. In inhalational anthrax, 1 to 5 μm particle–bearing spores are deposited in the terminal airways or alveoli, phagocytized by alveolar macrophages, and transported to mediastinal and peribronchial lymph nodes. Spores may stay in the mediastinal lymph nodes for extended periods and can germinate for up to 60 days or longer.[45] Cases of inhalational anthrax occurred up to 43 days after exposure in the Sverdlovsk outbreak.[46] Spores germinate into vegetative cells, which escape from the macrophages, multiply in the lymphatics, and ultimately gain access to the bloodstream, where they can reach high concentrations (107 to 108 organisms per milliliter of blood). Hemorrhagic meningitis is a complication of bacteremic spread; it develops in up to one half of cases.

In anthrax, tissue damage is mediated by two toxins: edema toxin and lethal toxin. These two toxins are composed of edema factor, lethal factor, and protective antigen. These three components of edema toxin and lethal toxin are produced by vegetative cells. Vegetative cells also produce an antiphagocytic capsule that is necessary for virulence.[47] Lethal toxin is a combination of lethal factor and protective antigen that interferes with cellular protein synthesis; it causes macrophages to release tumor necrosis factor and interleukin-1. In severe cases, it contributes to sudden death from toxemia. Edema toxin is a combination of edema factor and protective antigen that causes increased cellular levels of cyclic adenosine monophosphate (cAMP) and altered water homeostasis, resulting in massive edema. Together, edema toxin and lethal toxin cause edema, hemorrhage, necrosis, and shock. In cutaneous and gastrointestinal anthrax, toxin production results in a similar patho-physiologic process that causes edema and hemorrhagic necrosis in the skin and gastrointestinal mucosa, respectively.

INHALATIONAL ANTHRAX

Clinical Presentation and Diagnosis

Recent information on the clinical manifestations of inhalational anthrax from the 2001 anthrax outbreak both confirms many of the features reported in naturally occurring anthrax cases and reveals unanticipated differences.[39,45,48] The infectious dose of anthrax is not known with certainty. Animal data suggest that the median lethal dose (LD_{50}, which is the dose sufficient to kill 50% of exposed subjects) is 2,500 to 55,000 inhaled spores. Data from naturally occurring cases and from two cases in the 2001 outbreak suggest that the infectious dose may be very low in some persons, particularly those with underlying pulmonary disease.[45,49]

Clinical symptoms develop rapidly after germination of anthrax spores. The incubation period for inhalational disease is most commonly reported as 1 to 6 days but may be prolonged by antibiotic administration or, presumably, a low infectious dose.[50,51] In the 2001 anthrax outbreak, the median incubation period was 4 days (range, 4 to 6 days) for the six cases in which it could be calculated.

Inhalational anthrax has been described as a two-stage disease. The initial stage is a nonspecific, flulike illness lasting from several hours to a few days. In the 2001 bioterrorism-associated anthrax cases, this early clinical presentation included some combination of fever, myalgia, headache, cough, mild chest discomfort, weakness, abdominal pain, and chest pain. Profound malaise, fever, and drenching sweats were prominent symptoms, and nausea and vomiting were frequent. Classically, the initial stage is followed 1 to 3 days later, sometimes after brief improvement, by the rapidly progressive second stage, characterized by fever, dyspnea, diaphoresis, cyanosis, and shock. In the 2001 cases, no brief improvement between stages was observed.

Laboratory studies are nonspecific or unremarkable during the early stage of disease.[48] Chest x-rays were abnormal on initial presentation in all 10 recent cases, although only seven patients had the classic finding of mediastinal widening [see Figure 3]. Pleural effusions were present in all cases. These effusions were often small on presentation and were progressive, requiring drainage in the majority of patients. In contrast to previous descriptions, seven patients had pulmonary infiltrates consistent with pneumonia at presentation, and one patient was thought to have heart failure with pulmonary congestion. Other abnormalities included paratracheal and hilar fullness. The CT scan was valuable in further characterizing abnormalities in the lungs and mediastinum and was more sensitive than the chest x-ray in revealing mediastinal changes. Blood cultures can be diagnostic, although appropriate antibiotic therapy rapidly reduces the likelihood of isolating the organism. In the 2001 cases, B. anthracis was isolated from blood cultures obtained before antibiotic therapy was given, but not from those obtained afterward.

The initial manifestations of inhalational anthrax are nonspecific and are consistent with flulike illnesses caused by a variety of respiratory viruses, as well as with community-acquired bacterial infections. Adults can average one to three episodes of flulike illness a year, and millions of cases occur

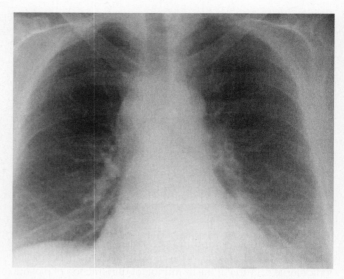

Figure 3 **Chest x-ray of a patient with inhalational anthrax showing mediastinal widening and a small left pleural effusion.**

throughout the United States.[52] Because of the high frequency of flulike illnesses and the low likelihood of inhalational anthrax in a given patient, a combination of epidemiologic, clinical, and (if indicated) laboratory testing should be used to evaluate potential cases of inhalational anthrax [see Figure 4]. According to CDC guidelines, consideration of inhalational anthrax hinges on a history of exposure or occupational/environmental risk within 2 to 5 days before illness onset.[19] Whenever possible, exposure and risk determinations should be made in consultation with public health authorities before initiating treatment or preventive therapy.

Diagnostic testing for anthrax should be done in patients whose signs and symptoms are consistent with anthrax and when one or more of the following conditions are present: a history of a recent anthrax case or outbreak in the community; a credible threat of anthrax exposure, as determined by law enforcement and public health authorities; a cluster of anthraxlike cases characterized by rapid deterioration. Anthrax should also be considered in any patient with compatible symptoms and rapid deterioration. All cases of suspected anthrax should be reported immediately to local or state public health authorities and the hospital epidemiologist (http://www.statepublic health.org). The clinical laboratory should also be alerted when diagnostic specimens of suspected anthrax are submitted to ensure that appropriate precautions are taken to protect laboratory staff, facilitate proper evaluation of the isolate, and expedite confirmatory testing at the nearest laboratory that belongs to the public health Laboratory Response Network.[6]

There is no rapid screening test to diagnose inhalational anthrax in its early stages. In persons with a compatible clinical illness for whom there is a heightened suspicion of anthrax based on clinical and epidemiologic data, the appropriate initial diagnostic tests are a chest x-ray or chest CT scan, or both, and culture and smear of peripheral blood. On chest x-rays, the posteroanterior and lateral view may be more sensitive than the anteroposterior (portable) view in detecting pulmonary abnormalities. Mediastinal widening or hyperdense mediastinal lymphadenopathy (secondary to hemorrhagic lymph nodes) on a nonenhanced CT scan should raise the suspicion of pul-

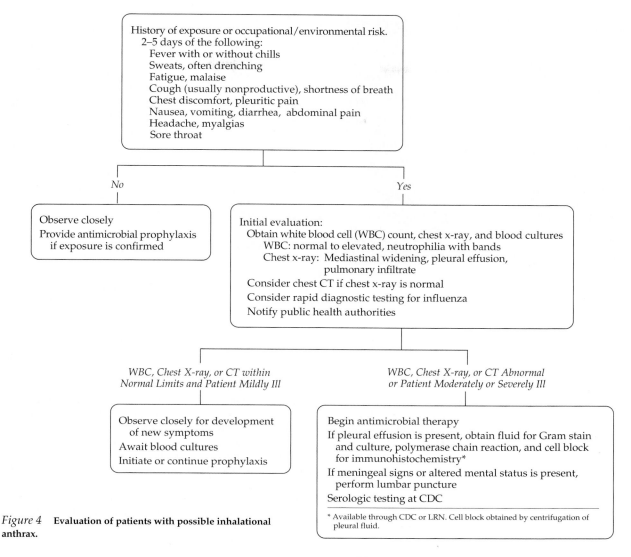

Figure 4 **Evaluation of patients with possible inhalational anthrax.**

monary anthrax [*see Figure 5*]. Most persons with flulike illnesses do not have radiologic findings of pneumonia; such findings occur most often in the very young, the elderly, and persons with chronic lung disease.

Pleural fluid and cerebrospinal fluid, as well as biopsy specimens taken from the pleura and lung, are also potentially useful for culture and other testing when disease is present in these sites, whereas sputum culture and Gram stain are unlikely to be useful. In highly suspicious cases, local or state health departments can arrange for additional diagnostic testing, including immunohistochemical staining and PCR at the CDC. Serologic testing is not useful in clinical management but may be used in epidemiologic investigations. Similarly, nasal swabs are of potential value in epidemiologic investigations for determining the route and extent of spread of anthrax in a population, but they have no role in clinical management.

A rapid influenza test can be used when influenza itself is a consideration in a patient with flulike illness, but these kits have limited value because their sensitivity can be relatively low (45% to 90%). However, rapid influenza testing with viral culture can help indicate whether influenza viruses are circulating among certain populations, and this epidemiologic information can be useful in diagnosing flulike illnesses.[52]

Treatment

Early intravenous antibiotic treatment may improve survival in inhalational anthrax.[53] In contrast to the reported case-fatality rate of 85% for 20th-century inhalational anthrax cases, 6 of 11 patients in the 2001 outbreak survived; all the survivors presented during the initial phase of the illness and received treatment the same day with antibiotics active against *B. anthracis*. Fatal cases occurred in patients who had severe disease by the time they first received antibiotics with activity against *B. anthracis*. Aggressive supportive care—including attention to fluid, electrolyte, and acid-base disturbances and drainage of pleural effusions—also played an important role in treatment.[48]

Current CDC treatment recommendations and related guidelines and information can be obtained at http://www.bt.cdc.gov/HealthProfessionals/index.asp. Before initiating treatment, clinicians should review this site to stay informed of revisions and updates. The Working Group on Civilian Biodefense has published similar recommendations with a detailed accompanying text.[45]

At present, intravenous ciprofloxacin or doxycycline plus one or two additional antimicrobials with in vitro activity against *B. anthracis* are recommended for initial empirical treatment [*see Table 5*]. Antibiotic therapy should be modified ac-

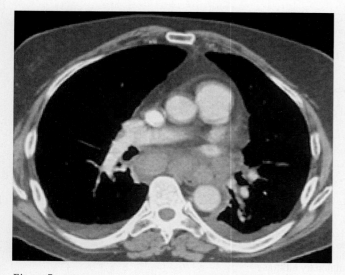

Figure 5 **CT scan of the chest of a patient with inhalational anthrax showing mediastinal lymphadenopathy and small bilateral pleural effusions.**

cording to the results of antimicrobial susceptibility testing to ensure that the most effective and least toxic regimen is used. The duration of antimicrobial therapy should be at least 60 days. Once clinical improvement occurs, it may be possible to complete the course of treatment with one or two agents given orally. Corticosteroid therapy has been suggested as adjunct therapy for inhalational anthrax associated with extensive edema, respiratory compromise, and meningitis.[19,43,45]

Prevention

Ciprofloxacin and doxycycline are recommended first-line agents for prophylaxis in persons exposed to inhalational anthrax. In vivo data suggest that other fluoroquinolone antibiotics would have efficacy equivalent to that of ciprofloxacin.[45] High-dose amoxicillin is an option when ciprofloxacin or doxy-

cycline is contraindicated [*see Table 6*]. Postexposure prophylaxis should continue for at least 60 days.[54] Given the uncertainty about the length of time viable spores can persist in the lungs, patients should be instructed to seek prompt medical evaluation if symptoms compatible with anthrax develop after discontinuance of postexposure prophylaxis. Because of uncertainty about the length of time that anthrax spores can remain viable in the lungs, the United States Department of Health and Human Services made two additional options available for preventive treatment for persons exposed to inhalational anthrax in the 2001 outbreak. These options were to follow a 60-day course of antibiotic treatment with either (1) an additional 40 days of antibiotic treatment or (2) an additional 40 days of antibiotic treatment plus three doses of anthrax vaccine over a 4-week period.[55]

Anthrax vaccine   The only licensed human anthrax vaccine available in the United States is anthrax vaccine adsorbed (AVA). This is an inactivated, cell-free filtrate of a nonencapsulated attenuated strain of *B. anthracis* (BioPort Corporation, Lansing, Michigan).[51] Primary vaccination consists of three subcutaneous injections at 0, 2, and 4 weeks and three booster vaccinations at 6, 12, and 18 months. To maintain immunity, the manufacturer recommends an annual booster injection. The basis for this recommended schedule of vaccination is not well defined.

Vaccination of adults with the licensed vaccine induced an immune response, as measured by indirect hemagglutination, in 83% of vaccinees 2 weeks after the first dose and in 91% of vaccinees who received two or more doses. Approximately 95% of vaccinees undergo seroconversion after three doses, with a fourfold rise in titers of IgG against protective antigen (the principal antigen responsible for inducing immunity). However, the precise correlation between antibody titer (or concentration) and protection against infection is not defined. The vaccine has shown efficacy in experiments involving animal models of inhalational anthrax in preexposure settings and, in combination with antibiotics, in postexposure settings.[45,52]

Table 5 Treatment of Inhalational Anthrax

Patients	Medication and Dosage	Comments
Adults, including pregnant women and immunocompromised persons	Ciprofloxacin, 400 mg I.V., q. 12 hr *or* Doxycycline, 100 mg I.V. , q. 12 hr *and* One or two additional antimicrobials*	If meningitis is suspected, doxycycline may be less optimal because of poor central nervous system penetration Modify regimen on the basis of susceptibility testing of isolate; can switch to p.o. after patient is clinically stable; continue treatment for at least 60 days Consider corticosteroids for meningitis, severe edema, or respiratory compromise
Children, including those who are immunocompromised	Ciprofloxacin, 10–15 mg/kg I.V., q. 12 hr, not to exceed 1 g/day *or* Doxycycline If > 8 yr and > 45 kg, give adult dosage If ≤ 8 yr or if > 8 yr but ≤ 45 kg, give 2.2 mg/kg q. 12 hr (maximum, 200 mg/day) *and* One or two additional antimicrobials*	If meningitis is suspected, doxycycline may be less optimal because of poor central nervous system penetration Modify regimen on the basis of susceptibility testing of isolate; can switch to p.o. after patient is clinically stable; continue treatment for at least 60 days Consider corticosteroids for meningitis, severe edema, or respiratory compromise

Note: Treatment recommendations may change over time and according to antimicrobial susceptibility test results during a biologic attack and to availability of selected antimicrobial agents. Before initiating treatment, clinicians should consult with an infectious disease specialist and public health authorities and should check for revisions and updates at http://www.bt.cdc.gov/HealthProfessionals/index.asp. This information is adapted from CDC and Working Group on Civilian Biodefense recommendations and may not represent FDA-approved uses.

*Other agents with in vitro activity against anthrax include rifampin, vancomycin, penicillin, ampicillin, chloramphenicol, imipenem, clindamycin, and clarithromycin.

Table 6   Postexposure Prophylaxis for Anthrax in the Setting of a Bioterrorist Attack

Patients	Medication	Comments
Adults, including immuno-compromised persons	Ciprofloxacin, 500 mg p.o., q. 12 hr *or* Doxycycline, 100 mg p.o., q. 12 hr *or, if strain proved susceptible,* Amoxicillin, 500 mg p.o., q. 8 hr	Give prophylaxis for at least 60 days
Pregnant women	Ciprofloxacin, 500 mg p.o., q. 12 hr *or, if strain proved susceptible,* Amoxicillin, 500 mg p.o., q. 8 hr	Give prophylaxis for at least 60 days
Children, including those who are immunocom-promised	Ciprofloxacin, 10–15 mg/kg p.o., b.i.d., not to exceed 1g/day *or, if strain proved susceptible,* Amoxicillin If ≥ 20 kg: 500 mg p.o., q. 8 hr If < 20 kg: 80 mg/kg/day p.o., in divided doses q. 8 hr (maximum, 500 mg/dose)	Give prophylaxis for at least 60 days

Note: Prophylaxis recommendations may change over time and according to antimicrobial susceptibility test results during a biologic attack and to availability of selected antimicrobial agents. Before initiating prophylaxis, clinicians should consult with an infectious disease specialist and public health authorities and should check for revisions and updates at http://www.bt.cdc.gov/HealthProfessionals/index.asp. This information is adapted from CDC and Working Group on Civilian Biodefense recommendations and may not represent FDA-approved uses.

Anthrax vaccine is considered acceptably safe by the Advisory Committee on Immunization Practices and the Institute of Medicine.[51,56] Supplies of anthrax vaccine are limited and are held by the United States Department of Defense. A combination of antibiotics and anthrax vaccine, if available, is recommended for exposed persons after a biologic attack.[45,57] At this time, preexposure use of anthrax vaccine is not recommended.

CUTANEOUS ANTHRAX

After an incubation period of approximately 7 days (range, 1 to 12 days), the primary lesion of cutaneous anthrax appears as a nondescript, painless, pruritic papule, usually on an exposed area such as the face, head, neck, or upper extremity. The papule enlarges and develops a central vesicle or bullae with surrounding brawny, nonpitting edema. The central vesicle enlarges and ulcerates over 1 to 2 days, becoming hemorrhagic, depressed, and necrotic and leading to a central black eschar [*see Figure 6*]. Satellite vesicles may be present. The eschar dries and falls off over the next 1 to 2 weeks. The findings of a painless lesion and edema out of proportion to the size of the lesion and the fact that pustules are rarely present in cutaneous anthrax are clinically useful. Tender regional lymphadenopathy, fever, chills, and fatigue may occur. Systemic disease has been reported to have a mortality of 20% if untreated. Cutaneous anthrax of the face or neck may lead to respiratory compromise from massive edema.[43,45,47,58]

The differential diagnosis of cutaneous anthrax includes other causes of eschar and ulceration and the ulceroglandular syndrome.[57] Guidelines for the diagnosis of cutaneous anthrax have been published by the American Academy of Dermatology (http://www.aad.org/BioInfo/anthrax.html).

For patients with the typical appearance and progression of cutaneous anthrax, a Gram stain and culture of the skin lesion should be obtained using a dry swab for unroofed vesicle fluid and a moist swab for the base of the ulcer and edges underneath the eschar. Blood cultures are also recommended. If the patient is taking antimicrobial drugs or if the Gram stain and culture are negative for *B. anthracis* or clinical suspicion remains high, two punch biopsies for culture (with the specimen placed in saline) and immunohistochemical staining should be per-

formed; PCR (with the specimen placed in formalin) should be performed, or both should be considered [*see Figure 7*]. Immunohistochemical staining and PCR testing at the CDC should be arranged through local public health authorities.[19,45]

Management

Antibiotic treatment is curative in cutaneous anthrax and can be initiated pending confirmation of anthrax infection. Ciprofloxicin and doxycycline are first-line agents for the empirical treatment of cutaneous anthrax and may be administered orally. Intravenous therapy with multiple drugs, as for inhalational anthrax (see above), is recommended for patients with signs of systemic involvement, extensive edema, or lesions of the face and neck.[53]

GASTROINTESTINAL AND OROPHARYNGEAL ANTHRAX

Symptoms appear 2 to 5 days after ingestion of contaminated food and include nausea, vomiting, fever, malaise, and abdominal pain. Severe bloody diarrhea with rebound abdominal tenderness develops. Ulcerative lesions occur primarily in the terminal ileum and cecum. Gastric ulcers with hemateme-

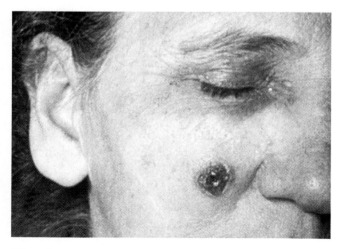

Figure 6   **Cutaneous anthrax lesion, 11 days old.**

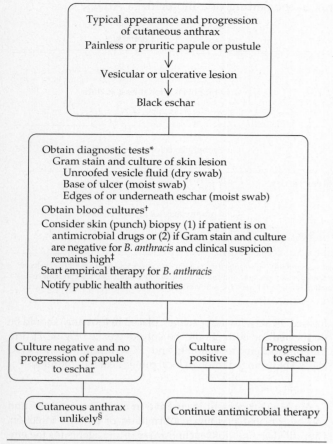

Typical appearance and progression
of cutaneous anthrax
Painless or pruritic papule or pustule

↓

Vesicular or ulcerative lesion

↓

Black eschar

Obtain diagnostic tests*
    Gram stain and culture of skin lesion
        Unroofed vesicle fluid (dry swab)
        Base of ulcer (moist swab)
        Edges of or underneath eschar (moist swab)
Obtain blood cultures†
Consider skin (punch) biopsy (1) if patient is on
    antimicrobial drugs or (2) if Gram stain and culture
    are negative for *B. anthracis* and clinical suspicion
    remains high‡
Start empirical therapy for *B. anthracis*
Notify public health authorities

Culture negative and no progression of papule to eschar

Culture positive

Progression to eschar

Cutaneous anthrax unlikely§

Continue antimicrobial therapy

* Serologic testing available at CDC may be an additional diagnostic technique for confirmation of cases of cutaneous anthrax.

† If blood cultures are positive for *B. anthracis*, treat with antimicrobials as for inhalational anthrax.

‡ Punch biopsy should be submitted in formalin to CDC. Polymerase chain reaction can also be done on formalin-fixed specimen. Gram stain and culture are frequently negative for *B. anthracis* after initiation of antimicrobials.

§ Continue antimicrobial prophylaxis for inhalational anthrax for 60 days if aerosol exposure to *B. anthracis* is known or suspected.

Figure 7   **Evaluation of patients with possible cutaneous anthrax.**

sis, hemorrhagic mesenteric lymphadenitis, and marked ascites may occur. Mediastinal widening has also been reported with gastrointestinal anthrax. Morbidity results from blood loss, fluid and electrolyte imbalances, and shock. The case-fatality rate is reportedly greater than 50%; death results from toxemia or intestinal perforation.[29,44,45]

Oropharyngeal anthrax is characterized by sore throat, fever, dysphagia, and marked edema and lymphadenitis. Ulcerative lesions may have an associated pseudomembrane. Specimens for diagnosis of gastrointestinal anthrax may include ascitic fluid for Gram stain and culture, blood cultures, and tissue samples from affected mucosal sites.

Treatment for gastrointestinal anthrax and oropharyngeal anthrax is the same as that for inhalational anthrax (see above).

INFECTION CONTROL

Person-to-person transmission of anthrax is not known to occur. Patients may be hospitalized in a standard hospital room with standard barrier isolation precautions. No treatment is necessary for contacts of cases.

The microbiology laboratory should be notified upon suspi-

cion of anthrax to ensure that appropriate precautions are taken under BSL-2 conditions when specimens are processed for culture.[59] Sporicidal solutions approved for use in hospitals and commercially available bleach or a 0.5% hypochlorite solution (1:10 dilution of household bleach) are effective for decontamination of contaminated areas. Precautions should be taken during autopsies, and cremation of human remains should be considered to prevent further transmission of disease.[20]

Plague

Plague is caused by the gram-negative coccobacillus *Yersinia pestis*, of the family Enterobacteriaceae. Wild rodents are the animal reservoir for the disease. Under natural conditions, plague is transmitted to humans by the bite of an infectious flea and, less frequently, by direct contact with infectious body fluids or tissues of an infected animal or by inhaling infectious droplets.[60] Plague has a long history of use and development as a biologic weapon, including the catapulting of plague victims' corpses over the walls of a besieged city in the 14th century. The most likely presentation after a biologic attack is primary pneumonic plague.[29] Additional information on plague, including the nonpneumonic forms (bubonic and septicemic plague), microbiology, and pathogenesis, is available elsewhere [*see Chapter 141*].

CLINICAL PRESENTATION

Plague is a severe febrile illness. Pneumonic plague, the most fatal form of the infection, can develop from inhalation of plague bacilli (primary pneumonic plague) or from hematogenous spread secondary to septicemic plague. Approximately 12% of cases of bubonic and primary septicemic plague develop into secondary pneumonic plague. Conversely, septicemic plague can be secondary to primary pneumonic plague.

The incubation period for pneumonic plague is typically 2 to 4 days (range, 1 to 6 days). Presenting symptoms typically include the acute onset of malaise, high fever, chills, headache, chest discomfort, dyspnea, and cough concomitant with or followed rapidly by clinical sepsis. Hemoptysis is a classic sign that should suggest plague in the appropriate clinical context, but sputum may be watery or purulent. Gastrointestinal symptoms may be prominent with pneumonic plague; these include nausea, vomiting, diarrhea, and abdominal pain. A cervical bubo is infrequently present.

The disease is rapidly progressive, with increasing dyspnea, stridor, and cyanosis. Rapidly progressive respiratory failure and sepsis within 2 to 4 days of onset of illness is typical of pneumonic plague. Abnormalities on chest x-ray are variable but frequently show bilateral patchy infiltrates or consolidation. The mortality for pneumonic plague is reported to be 57% and is extremely high when initiation of treatment is delayed beyond 24 hours after symptom onset.[61] Complications of septicemic plague include disseminated intravascular coagulation (DIC), purpuric skin lesions and gangrene of extremities (so-called black death), acute respiratory distress syndrome (ARDS), meningitis, and multiorgan failure with shock.[29,62-64]

DIAGNOSIS

During a confirmed outbreak of pneumonic plague after a biologic attack, a presumptive diagnosis can be made on the basis of symptoms, especially if there is a high index of suspicion. However, other causes of severe pneumonia or rapidly

Table 7 Antimicrobial Treatment of Pneumonic Plague

Patients	Drug	Comments
Adults	Streptomycin, 1 g I.M., b.i.d. *or* Gentamicin, 5 mg/kg I.M. or I.V., q.d., or 2 mg/kg loading dose followed by 1.7 mg/kg I.M. or I.V., t.i.d. *Alternative choices:* Doxycycline, 100 mg I.V., b.i.d., or 200 mg I.V., q.d. Ciprofloxacin, 400 mg I.V., b.i.d. Chloramphenicol, 25 mg/kg I.V., q.i.d.	Treat for 10 days; during a community outbreak of pneumonic plague, all persons developing a temperature ≥ 101.3° F (38.5° C) or greater or a new cough should begin parenteral antibiotic treatment; oral treatment may be given when resources for parenteral treatment are limited; pregnant women should not receive streptomycin or chloramphenicol; tetracycline may be substituted for doxycycline
Children	Streptomycin, 15 mg/kg I.M., b.i.d. (maximum, 2 g/day) *or* Gentamicin, 2.5 mg/kg I.M. or I.V., t.i.d. *Alternative choices:* Doxycycline: if ≥ 45 kg, adult dosage; if < 45 kg, 2.2 mg/kg b.i.d. (maximum, 200 mg/day) Ciprofloxacin, 15 mg/kg I.V., b.i.d. Chloramphenicol, 25 mg/kg I.V., q.i.d.; maintain serum concentration between 5 and 20 µg/ml	Use chloramphenicol in plague meningitis

Note: Treatment recommendations may change over time and according to antimicrobial susceptibility test results during a biologic attack and to availability of selected antimicrobial agents. Before initiating treatment, clinicians should consult with an infectious disease specialist and public health authorities and should check for revisions and updates at http://www.bt.cdc.gov/HealthProfessionals/index.asp. This information is adapted from CDC and Working Group on Civilian Biodefense recommendations and may not represent FDA-approved uses.

progressive respiratory infection with or without sepsis should be considered. Suspected cases of plague should be immediately reported to the local public health department and the hospital epidemiologist.

There are no widely available, rapid confirmatory tests for *Y. pestis*. Specimens for bacteriologic and serologic testing should be collected before initiating therapy. Sputum, blood, and lymph node aspirate should be submitted for Gram stain and culture. Microscopic examination of clinical specimens or buffy coat may show a gram-negative coccobacillus; Wright, Giemsa, or Wayson stains may show bipolar (safety pin) staining. Sera for acute and convalescent antibody detection should be obtained, but findings are primarily of epidemiologic value. Additional diagnostic testing, including antigen detection, IgM immunoassay, immunostaining, PCR testing, and antimicrobial susceptibility testing, is available through the CDC and designated public health laboratories (http://www.state publichealth.org). Specimen submission should be arranged through local public health authorities. The laboratory should be notified whenever plague is suspected, to help prevent exposures to staff and to facilitate appropriate testing.[29,61,64]

Laboratory findings are consistent with the systemic inflammatory response syndrome. The leukocyte count is elevated and the differential shows a neutrophil predominance, including immature forms. Platelets may be normal or low. Coagulation abnormalities include increased fibrin degradation products, hypofibrinogenemia, and prolongation of the prothrombin time (PT) and partial thromboplastin time (PTT). Elevated liver function tests and abnormal renal function tests are seen with systemic disease.

TREATMENT

When plague is suspected, antibiotic treatment should begin before laboratory confirmation of the diagnosis [see Table 7]. Whenever possible, specimens should be collected for bacteriologic and serologic testing before the start of therapy. Antibiot-

ic resistance is rare with naturally occurring *Y. pestis* but may be present in strains used as biologic weapons. Treatment should be continued for 10 days or for 3 days after defervescence and improvement in symptoms. The route of administration can be changed from intravenous to oral after the patient is clinically stable. The choice of antibiotic may be modified after microbial sensitivity testing is completed. The CDC bioterrorism Web site or local public health authorities should be consulted for updated treatment recommendations.[29,61,64]

Postexposure Prophylaxis for Pneumonic Plague

All persons potentially exposed to aerosolized *Y. pestis* and all persons in close contact with pneumonic plague patients (close contact is defined as exposure within 2 m [6.5 ft]) should be treated for 7 days after the last exposure [see Table 8]. Persons receiving prophylactic antibiotic treatment should seek medical evaluation immediately if fever or illness with cough develops.

There is no currently available vaccine for pneumonic plague. The previously available licensed plague vaccine in the United States was discontinued in 1999. That vaccine was demonstrated to reduce the severity of illness with bubonic plague but not pneumonic plague.[62]

Communicability and Infection Control Considerations

Pneumonic plague is transmitted person to person through respiratory droplets. Aerosol transmission has not been demonstrated. For patients with pneumonic plague, respiratory droplet precautions as well as standard precautions are recommended, including the use of gowns, gloves, eye protection, and surgical masks for the first 48 hours of antimicrobial therapy and until clinical improvement occurs. Hospitalized patients should remain in isolation for the first 48 hours of antimicrobial therapy and until clinical improvement occurs. Hospitalized patients should wear a mask during transport.

Y. pestis is rapidly destroyed by sunlight and drying. Environmental surfaces can be decontaminated with a standard dis-

Table 8 Postexposure Prophylaxis of Pneumonic Plague

Patients	Drug	Comments
Adults, including pregnant women	Doxycycline, 100 mg p.o., b.i.d. Ciprofloxacin, 500 mg p.o., b.i.d. *Alternative:* Chloramphenicol, 25 mg/kg p.o., q.i.d.	Asymptomatic household contacts, hospital contacts, or other close contacts should receive postexposure prophylaxis for 7 days; contacts who develop fever or cough while receiving prophylaxis should begin antibiotic treatment for plague.
Children	Doxycycline: if ≥ 45 kg, adult dosage; if < 45 kg, 2.2 mg/kg p.o., b.i.d. (maximum, 200 mg/day) Ciprofloxacin, 20 mg/kg p.o., b.i.d. *Alternative:* Chloramphenicol, 25 mg/kg p.o., q.i.d.	Asymptomatic household contacts, hospital contacts, or other close contacts should receive postexposure prophylaxis for 7 days; contacts who develop fever or cough while receiving prophylaxis should begin antibiotic treatment for plague.

Note: Prophylaxis recommendations may change over time and according to antimicrobial susceptibility test results during a biologic attack and to availability of selected antimicrobial agents. Before initiating prophylaxis, clinicians should consult with an infectious disease specialist and public health authorities and should check for revisions and updates at http://www.bt.cdc.gov/HealthProfessionals/index.asp. This information is adapted from CDC and Working Group on Civilian Biodefense recommendations and may not represent FDA-approved uses.

infectant. Persons exposed to aerosolized plague bacilli during a biologic attack should shower with warm water and soap. Clothing of persons exposed to an aerosol of *Y. pestis* and linens of plague patients should be washed in hot water.[20,62,63]

Botulism

Botulism is a paralytic illness caused by a potent neurotoxin produced by *Clostridium botulinum*, an anaerobic, spore-forming bacterium. Natural forms of the disease are foodborne botulism, wound botulism, and infant botulism. Foodborne botulism results from ingestion of improperly processed foodstuffs containing preformed toxin produced by *C. botulinum*. Wound botulism results from production of botulinum toxin by *C. botulinum* organisms that contaminate wounds. Infant botulism results from the colonization of the intestinal tract of infants after ingestion of spores. Botulinum toxin has been developed as a biologic weapon. An aerosol attack is considered the most likely use of botulinum toxin for bioterrorism, although intentional contamination of food supplies is possible.[29,65] Additional information about the pathogenesis and epidemiology of noninhalational forms of botulism is available elsewhere [*see Chapter 136*].

Botulinum toxin is the most potent lethal toxin known. The estimated toxic dose of type A botulinum toxin is 0.001 μg/kg of body weight. There are seven distinct antigenic types of botulinum neurotoxins—types A through G—produced by different strains of *C. botulinum*. Human botulism is caused primarily by toxin types A, B, and E. Botulinum toxin acts to block neurotransmission by binding irreversibly to the presynaptic nerve terminal at the neuromuscular junction and preventing the release of acetylcholine, resulting in bulbar palsies and skeletal muscle weakness. The toxin is colorless, odorless, and presumably tasteless.[29,66,67]

CLINICAL PRESENTATION

The incubation period for foodborne botulism is 2 hours to 8 days; the typical incubation period is 12 to 72 hours. The incubation period for inhalational botulism is not established. Aerosol exposures of monkeys and accidental aerosol exposure of humans have resulted in clinical illness developing 12 to 80 hours after exposure. Type A toxin is associated with more severe disease and a higher fatality rate than type B or E. The neurologic features of all forms of botulism are similar.[29,66,67] Although initial symptoms in foodborne botulism may include nausea, vomiting, abdominal cramps, and diarrhea, these symptoms are thought to result from other bacterial metabolites in contaminated food and may not occur in inhalational botulism.

The so-called classic triad of botulism summarizes the clinical presentation: an afebrile patient, symmetrical descending flaccid paralysis with prominent bulbar palsies, and a clear sensorium.[66-68] Symptoms of cranial nerve abnormalities nearly always begin in the bulbar musculature; patients typically present with difficulty seeing, speaking, or swallowing. Clinical hallmarks include ptosis, blurred vision, and the so-called four Ds: diplopia, dysarthria, dysphonia, and dysphagia. Cranial nerve abnormalities and bulbar weakness are followed by symmetrical descending weakness and paralysis with progression from the head to the arms, thorax, and legs. The extent of paralysis and rapidity of onset of symptoms are proportional to the dose of toxin absorbed into the circulation. Recovery depends on the regeneration of new motor axon twigs to reinnervate paralyzed muscle fibers; recovery may take weeks to months.

Anticholinergic symptoms are common, including dry mouth, ileus, constipation, nausea and vomiting, urinary retention, and mydriasis. Other symptoms include dizziness and sore throat. Sensory findings are not present, with the exception of circumoral and peripheral paresthesias secondary to hyperventilation resulting from anxiety. Botulinum toxin does not cross the blood-brain barrier. Cranial nerve dysfunction and facial nerve weakness may make communication difficult; these symptoms may be mistaken for lethargy and signs of central nervous system involvement.

DIAGNOSIS

Initiation of treatment with botulinum antitoxin should be based on the clinical diagnosis and should not await laboratory confirmation. A clinician who suspects botulism should immediately contact the local or state health department to facilitate procurement of antitoxin for treatment; arrangements should be made for confirmatory diagnostic testing and initiation of an epidemiologic investigation to identify the source of infection. In cases of potential foodborne botulism, any leftover foodstuffs or containers should be held for testing by the public health laboratory.

Demonstration of botulinum toxin in serum samples by mouse bioassay is diagnostic. Samples of serum (in adults, > 30 ml blood in a tiger-top or red-top tube) obtained before administration of botulinum antitoxin should be submitted for testing. For potential foodborne botulism, samples of stool, gastric aspirate, emesis, and suspect foods should also be submitted.[67] The likelihood of finding toxin in the sera of affected patients decreases with time; it is detectable in only 13% to 28% of patients more than 2 days after ingestion.[69]

The possibility of a bioterrorist attack should be considered in any outbreak of botulism. A bioterrorist attack should especially be considered when a cluster of cases occurs; when an outbreak has a common geographic location but there is no common dietary exposure (suggestive of possible aerosol exposure); when there is an outbreak of an unusual botulinum toxin type; or when multiple simultaneous outbreaks occur. A careful dietary and travel history must be taken to help identify the source. Patients should be asked if they know of others with similar symptoms.

The differential diagnosis of botulism includes stroke and other neuromuscular disorders.[66,67] A CT scan of the head may be used to exclude cerebrovascular accident, although it is relatively insensitive in early ischemic stroke [see Chapter 174]. Patients with myasthenia gravis will often have characteristic electromyographic findings and serum antibody tests. A test dose of edrophonium (Tensilon) may briefly reverse paralysis in patients with myasthenia gravis but also, reportedly, in some cases of botulism. Guillain-Barré syndrome typically results in ascending paralysis and sensory abnormalities. Cerebrospinal fluid protein is normal in patients with botulism and is normal or elevated in patients with Guillain-Barré syndrome. The rare Miller-Fisher variant of Guillain-Barré syndrome is characterized by descending paralysis and may be confused with botulism. Other conditions that mimic botulism include tick paralysis; poliomyelitis; Eaton-Lambert syndrome; paralytic shellfish poisoning; pufferfish ingestion; and anticholinesterase intoxication with organophosphates, atropine, carbon monoxide, or aminoglycosides.

The electromyogram (EMG) can help distinguish different causes of paralysis. The EMG in botulism demonstrates normal nerve conduction velocity, normal sensory nerve function, and small amplitude motor potentials with facilitation to repetitive stimulation at 50 Hz.[70]

TREATMENT

The mainstay of treatment for botulism is supportive care, including intensive care, mechanical ventilation, and parenteral nutrition. Morbidity and mortality are usually from pulmonary aspiration secondary to loss of the gag reflex and dysphagia leading to inability to control secretions, respiratory failure secondary to inadequate tidal volume from diaphragmatic and accessory respiratory muscle paralysis, and airway obstruction from pharyngeal and upper airway muscle paralysis. Careful and frequent monitoring of the gag and cough reflexes, swallowing, oxygen saturation, vital capacity, and inspiratory force are critical. Airway intubation is indicated for inability to control secretions and impending respiratory failure. Secondary infections are common and should be sought in patients who develop fever.

Trivalent (ABE) equine antitoxin is available from the CDC through state and local health departments and should be administered as soon as possible after clinical diagnosis. Antitoxin can prevent progression of disease caused by subsequent binding of toxin but does not reverse the effects of already bound toxin. For this reason, antitoxin is not useful if the patient is no longer showing progression of disease or is improving from maximum paralysis. The amount of neutralizing antibody present in the standard treatment dose of antitoxin far exceeds maximum serum toxin concentrations in foodborne botulism patients, and repeat doses are usually not required. In a biologic attack, however, patients may be exposed to unusually high concentrations of toxin, so serum toxin levels should be assessed after initiation of treatment in such cases to determine the need for repeat doses. Botulism caused by toxin types other than A, B, or E would not respond to the trivalent antitoxin. Limited quantities of an investigational heptavalent (A-G) antitoxin are held by the United States Army. However, because of the time delay involved in typing the toxin, the utility of this product in a biologic attack is probably minimal.[66,68]

Hypersensitivity reactions, including anaphylaxis, have occurred after administration of botulism antitoxin. For that reason, all patients should undergo a skin test before receiving the antitoxin, and resuscitation equipment should be immediately available. Patients showing a positive hypersensitivity reaction on the skin test can be desensitized over several hours.[71,72]

Before administering antitoxin, physicians should carefully review the package insert for dosage and adverse effects. Standard regimens can be used in children, pregnant women, and immunocompromised persons with botulism. Botulism immune globulin intravenous is an investigational human-derived neutralizing antibody that is available only for treatment of infant botulism from the California Department of Health Services, Berkeley. The CDC bioterrorism Web site or local public health authorities should be consulted for updated treatment recommendations.[29,66,67]

Transmissibility and Infection Control

Botulism is an intoxication, not an infection, and thus is not transmitted from person to person. Botulinum toxin does not penetrate intact skin. Standard infection-control precautions are adequate unless meningitis is suspected, in which case droplet precautions are indicated. Clothes of persons exposed to an aerosol release of botulinum toxin should be removed and washed. Exposed persons should shower with soap and hot water. Exposed environmental surfaces can be decontaminated with 0.1% hypochlorite bleach solution.[67]

Tularemia

Tularemia is a zoonotic infection caused by *Francisella tularensis*, a small, nonmotile, gram-negative, pleomorphic coccobacillus. The disease is typically acquired through contact with blood or tissue fluids of infected animals or through the bite of an infected deerfly, tick, or mosquito.[73] Inhalation of organisms aerosolized from the environment and the drinking of contaminated water can also result in human infection.[74] *F. tularensis* was developed for use as a biologic weapon by the United States (before its offensive biologic weapons program was terminated) and other countries.[29] The epidemiology, pathogenesis, and clinical manifestations of the naturally occurring forms of tularemia are discussed in more detail elsewhere [see Chapter 141].

CLINICAL PRESENTATION

Tularemia can take several forms in humans, depending on the route of infection. Ulceroglandular, oculoglandular, glandular, typhoidal, and pharyngeal tularemia are discussed elsewhere [*see Chapter 141*]. Inhalational tularemia is a term used to describe infection resulting from an aerosol release of *F. tularensis*.[75] Most patients with inhalational tularemia develop pleuropulmonary tularemia (tularemia pneumonia), but many patients may present with an undifferentiated febrile illness. The infectious dose is as low as one to 50 organisms, and the incubation period is typically 3 to 5 days (range, 1 to 14 days).[29]

The clinical course of inhalational tularemia is less rapidly progressive than that of pulmonary anthrax or plague. Illness onset is acute, with some combination of fever, chills, sweats, myalgias, headache, coryza, and sore throat. Nausea, vomiting, diarrhea, and abdominal pain are common. Anorexia and weight loss may occur as the illness continues. Cough may be dry or mildly productive. Hemoptysis is uncommon. Pleuritic chest pain, substernal chest discomfort, and dyspnea may be present. Chest x-rays may be normal or minimally abnormal or show a variety of abnormalities, including peribronchial patchy infiltrates, effusions, and hilar adenopathy.[76]

F. tularensis infection may be mild and nonspecific or rapidly progressive. Any form of tularemia may result in hematogenous spread with secondary pleuropneumonia, sepsis, and, rarely, meningitis. If left untreated, tularemia can progress to respiratory failure; liver, kidney, and splenic involvement; meningitis; sepsis; shock; and death. There is usually complete recovery with early diagnosis and treatment. Mortality is less than 2% if the patient is treated; it can be as high as 60% for untreated severe disease and pneumonia.[75,77,78]

DIAGNOSIS

A clustering of sudden, severe pneumonias in previously healthy patients should raise the possibility of an intentional aerosolized release of tularemia. Clusters of patients with tularemia and cases in which there is no natural explanation for the disease should be reported immediately to the local or state health department (http://www.statepublichealth.org). There are no rapid confirmatory tests for *F. tularensis*. Gram stain of sputum is not diagnostic but may identify other potential etiologies.[78,79] In the context of a known or suspected outbreak, a presumptive diagnosis can be made on the basis of symptoms. A chest x-ray should be obtained for patients with suspected pleuropulmonary tularemia. The x-ray may show infiltrates, effusion, hilar adenopathy, or subtle abnormalities, or it may be normal. Recent experience with inhalational anthrax suggests that chest CT scans of patients with tularemia may show pulmonary abnormalities, including infiltrates, effusions, and adenopathy, before they are evident on x-ray.[48]

Specimens of respiratory secretions and blood for bacteriologic and serologic testing should be collected before initiating therapy. Pharyngeal washings, sputum specimens, fasting gastric aspirates, and blood can be cultured for *F. tularensis*. Growth may be slow, so cultures should be held for 10 days. Cysteine-enriched culture media should be used to improve yield. Direct examination (by direct fluorescent antibody staining or immunohistochemical testing, antigen detection, microagglutination antibody testing, PCR, and other research tests) is available through designated public health laboratories. Acute and convalescent serologies are valuable for epidemiologic purposes.[75,79]

TREATMENT AND POSTEXPOSURE PROPHYLAXIS

When the index of suspicion is high, antibiotic treatment should be started before diagnosis is confirmed. Streptomycin or gentamicin is the preferred agent. All persons potentially exposed to aerosolized *F. tularensis* should be treated with doxycycline or ciprofloxacin. Close contacts of patients with tularemia pneumonia do not need prophylactic antibiotics. No vaccine for tularemia is currently available. The CDC bioterrorism Web site, local public health authorities, or both should be consulted for updated treatment recommendations.[29,75,80]

Transmissibility and Infection Control

Tularemia is not transmitted from person to person, and isolation of patients with tularemia is not necessary. Standard precautions are recommended for all patients with tularemia. Microbiology staff must be alerted when tularemia is suspected, so they can take precautions to prevent laboratory-acquired infection from culture plates and other infectious materials. Contaminated environmental surfaces can be disinfected with a 10% bleach solution followed by cleansing with 70% alcohol.[75]

Hemorrhagic Fever Viruses

Hemorrhagic fever viruses (HFVs) are RNA viruses classified in several taxonomic families. HFVs cause a variety of disease syndromes with similar clinical characteristics, referred to as acute hemorrhagic fever syndromes [*see Chapter 153*]. The pathophysiologic hallmarks of HFV infection are microvascular damage and increased vascular permeability. HFVs that are of concern as potential biologic weapons include Arenaviridae (Lassa, Junin, Machupo, Guanarito, and Sabia viruses, which are the causative agents of Lassa fever and Argentine, Bolivian, Venezuelan, and Brazilian hemorrhagic fevers, respectively); Filoviridae (Ebola and Marburg viruses); Flaviviridae (yellow fever, Omsk hemorrhagic fever, and Kyasanur Forest disease viruses); and Bunyaviridae (Rift Valley fever [RVF]). Under natural conditions, humans are infected through the bite of an infected arthropod or through contact with infected animal reservoirs. Hemorrhagic fever viruses are highly infectious by aerosol; are associated with high morbidity and, in some cases, high mortality; and are thought to pose a serious risk as biologic weapons.[29] All suspected cases of HFV infection should be reported immediately to the local or state health department and the hospital epidemiologist.

PATHOPHYSIOLOGY

The exact pathogenesis for HFVs varies according to the etiologic agent. The major target organ is the vascular endothelium. Immunologic and inflammatory mediators are thought to play an important role in the pathogenesis of HFVs. All HFVs can produce thrombocytopenia, and some also cause platelet dysfunction. Infection with Ebola and Marburg viruses, Rift Valley fever virus, and yellow fever virus causes destruction of infected cells. DIC is characteristic of infection with Filoviridae. Ebola and Marburg viruses may cause a hemorrhagic diathesis and tissue necrosis through direct damage to vascular endothelial cells and platelets with impairment of the microcirculation, as well as cytopathic effects on parenchymal cells, with release of immunologic and inflammatory mediators. Arenaviridae, on the other hand, appear to mediate hemorrhage via the stimulation of inflammatory mediators by macrophages, thrombocytopenia, and the inhibition of platelet aggregation. DIC is not a major pathophysiologic mechanism in arenavirus infections.[81,82]

CLINICAL PRESENTATION

The incubation period of HFVs ranges from 2 to 21 days. The clinical presentations of these diseases are nonspecific and variable, making diagnosis difficult. It is noteworthy that not all patients will develop hemorrhagic manifestations. Even a significant proportion of patients with Ebola virus infections may not demonstrate clinical signs of hemorrhage.[83]

Initial symptoms of the acute HFV syndrome may include fever, headache, myalgia, rash, nausea, vomiting, diarrhea, abdominal pain, arthralgias, myalgias, and malaise. Illness caused by Ebola, Marburg, Rift Valley fever virus, yellow fever virus, Omsk hemorrhagic fever virus, and Kyasanur Forest disease virus are characterized by an abrupt onset, whereas Lassa fever and the diseases caused by the Machupo, Junin, Guarinito, and Sabia viruses have a more insidious onset. Initial signs may include fever, tachypnea, relative bradycardia, hypotension (which may progress to circulatory shock), conjunctival injection, pharyngitis, and lymphadenopathy. Encephalitis may occur, with delirium, seizures, cerebellar signs, and coma. Most HFVs cause cutaneous flushing or a macular skin rash, although the rash may be difficult to appreciate in dark-skinned persons and varies according to the causative virus. Hemorrhagic symptoms, when they occur, develop later in the course of illness and include petechiae, purpura, bleeding into mucous membranes and conjunctiva, hematuria, hematemesis, and melena. Hepatic involvement is common, and renal involvement is proportional to cardiovascular compromise.[29,81,83,84]

Laboratory abnormalities include leukopenia (except in some cases of Lassa fever), anemia or hemoconcentration, and elevated liver enzymes; DIC with associated coagulation abnormalities and thrombocytopenia are common. Mortality ranges from less than 1% for Rift Valley fever to 70% to 90% for Ebola and Marburg virus infections.[29,81,83-85]

DIAGNOSIS

The nonspecific and variable clinical presentation of the HFVs presents a considerable diagnostic challenge. Clinical diagnostic criteria based on WHO surveillance standards for acute hemorrhagic fever syndrome include temperature greater than 101° F (38.3° C) of less than 3 weeks' duration; severe illness and no predisposing factors for hemorrhagic manifestations; and at least two of the following hemorrhagic symptoms: hemorrhagic or purple rash, epistaxis, hematemesis, hematuria, hemoptysis, blood in stools, or other hemorrhagic symptom with no established alternative diagnosis. Any suspected case of HFV should result in immediate notification of the hospital epidemiologist, local public health department, and clinical laboratory personnel.[82,86] Laboratory testing is currently available only at the CDC and the United States Army Medical Research Institute for Infectious Diseases. Laboratory techniques for the diagnosis of HFVs include antigen detection, IgM antibody detection, isolation in cell culture, visualization by electron microscopy, immunohistochemical techniques, and reverse transcriptase–polymerase chain reaction. Submission of clinical specimens, including processing and transport, should be arranged through consultation with local public health authorities. The CDC's Packaging Protocols for Biologic Agents/Diseases are available at (http://www.bt.cdc.gov/agent/vhf/index.asp).

TREATMENT

Therapy for HFVs is largely supportive. Treatment of other suspected causes of infection should be administered pending confirmation of HFV infection. Hypotension and shock may require early administration of vasopressors and hemodynamic monitoring with attention to fluid and electrolyte balance, circulatory volume, and blood pressure. HFV patients tend to respond poorly to fluid infusions and rapidly develop pulmonary edema.

Secondary infections may occur and should be diagnosed and treated. Intravenous lines, catheters, and other invasive procedures should be avoided unless they are clearly indicated. The management of bleeding is controversial. Recent recommendations include not treating mild bleeding and use of replacement therapy and heparin for severe bleeding with DIC.[29] Intramuscular injections and medications that interfere with platelet function or coagulation should be avoided.

No treatments of HFVs have been approved by the Food and Drug Administration. Ribavirin is a nucleoside analogue with activity against some Arenaviridae and Bunyaviridae (including the viruses that cause Lassa fever, Argentine hemorrhagic fever, and Crimean-Congo hemorrhagic fever) but not against Filoviridae or Flaviviridae. Ribavirin may be used under an IND protocol for the empirical treatment of HFV patients while awaiting identification of the etiologic agent. Current treatment protocols and dosing recommendations for ribavirin should be obtained through local public health authorities or the CDC's bioterrorism Web site.

Postexposure Prophylaxis

Postexposure prophylaxis is currently recommended only for persons potentially exposed to HFV and for known high-risk contacts or close contacts of HFV patients who develop fever or other clinical criteria of HFV infection with no alternative diagnosis, unless the etiologic agent is known to be a filovirus or a flavivirus.[81]

Infection Control Considerations

Ebola virus, Marburg virus, Lassa fever virus, and the New World arenaviruses are transmissible from person to person through direct contact with blood and body fluids. Airborne transmission of HFVs is unlikely but cannot be completely ruled out. The risk of person-to-person transmission is highest during the latter stages of illness, which are characterized by vomiting, diarrhea, shock, and, often, hemorrhage. The most important step in preventing transmission of HFVs is strict attention to implementation of appropriate barrier infection control measures, including double gloves, impermeable gowns, face shields, eye protection, and leg and shoe coverings.

Airborne precautions are recommended during care of patients with possible HFV infections. Airborne precautions include high-efficiency particulate respirators such as N-95 masks or powered air-purifying respirators (PAPRs) for all persons entering the patient's room. Patients should be placed in a negative-pressure isolation room with 6 to 12 air changes per hour.[82,87]

High-risk contacts of HFV patients include persons having contact with mucous membranes (e.g., through kissing or sexual intercourse) or with secretions, excretions, or blood (through percutaneous injury) of the infected person. Close contacts are persons who have other direct contact with the patient (e.g., shaking hands or hugging), provide medical care to the patient, or process laboratory specimens from a patient with HFV before initiation of infection-control precautions.

Persons potentially exposed to HFVs in a bioterrorist attack and their close and high-risk contacts should be placed under medical surveillance for 21 days from the day of exposure. Temperatures should be recorded twice daily, and any temperature of 101° F (38.3° C) or higher should be reported to the designated clinical or public health authority. Therapy with ribavirin should be initiated promptly unless an alternative diagnosis is established or the etiologic agent is known to be a filovirus or a flavivirus [see Treatment, above].[81]

HFVs are highly infectious in the laboratory setting through small-particle aerosols generated through procedures such as centrifugation. Laboratory personnel should be alerted when HFV infections are suspected, and appropriate personal-protection precautions and laboratory biosafety procedures should be implemented.

References

1. Davis CJ: Nuclear blindness: an overview of the biological weapons programs of the former Soviet Union and Iraq. Emerg Infect Dis 5:509, 1999

2. Stern J: The prospect of domestic bioterrorism. Emerg Infect Dis 5:517, 1999

3. Kortepeter MG, Parker GW: Potential biological weapons threats. Emerg Infect Dis 5:523, 1999

4. Alibek K: Biohazard. Random House, Inc. New York, 1999

5. Henderson DA: The looming threat of bioterrorism. Science 283:1279, 1999

6. Biological and chemical terrorism: strategic plan for preparedness and response. Recommendations of the CDC Strategic Planning Workgroup. MMWR Morb Mortal Wkly Rep 49:1, 2000

7. Gerberding JL, Hughes JM, Koplan JP: Bioterrorism preparedness and response: clinicians and public health agencies as essential partners. JAMA 287:898, 2002

8. Lane HC, Fauci AS: Bioterrorism on the home front: a new challenge for American medicine. JAMA 286:2595, 2001

9. Meningococcal disease and college students. Recommendations of the Advisory Committee on Immunization Practices (ACIP). MMWR Morb Mortal Wkly Rep 49:13, 2000

10. Bell BP, Goldoft M, Griffin PM, et al: A multistate outbreak of Escherichia coli 0157:H7-associated bloody diarrhea and hemolytic uremic syndrome from hamburgers: the Washington experience. JAMA 272:1349, 1994

11. Weber DJ, Rutala WA: Pertussis: a continuing hazard for healthcare facilities. Infect Control Hosp Epidemiol 22:736, 2001

12. Measles, mumps, and rubella: vaccine use and strategies for elimination of measles, rubella, and congenital rubella syndrome and control of mumps. Recommendations of the Advisory Committee on Immunization Practices (ACIP). MMWR Morb Mortal Wkly Rep 47:1, 1998

13. Prevention of varicella. Updated Recommendations of the Advisory Committee on Immunization Practices (ACIP). MMWR Morb Mortal Wkly Rep 48:1, 1999

14. Bolyard EA, Tablan OC, Williams WW, et al: Guideline for infection control in healthcare personnel, 1998. Hospital Infection Control Practices Advisory Committee. Infect Control Hosp Epidemiol 19:386, 1998

15. Suspected brucellosis case prompts investigation of possible bioterrorism-related activity–New Hampshire and Massachusetts, 1999. MMWR Morb Mortal Wkly Rep 49:509, 2000

16. Duchin JS, Koster FT, Peters CJ, et al: Hantavirus pulmonary syndrome: a clinical description of 17 patients with a newly recognized disease. The Hantavirus Study Group. N Engl J Med 330:949, 1994

17. Fine A, Layton M: Lessons from the West Nile viral encephalitis outbreak in New York City, 1999: implications for bioterrorism preparedness. Clin Infect Dis 32:277, 2001

18. Pandemic influenza: confronting a re-emergent threat. Proceedings of a meeting. Bethesda, Maryland, 11-13 December 1995. J Infect Dis 176:S1, 1997

19. Update: investigation of bioterrorism-related anthrax and interim guidelines for clinical evaluation of persons with possible anthrax. MMWR Morb Mortal Wkly Rep 50:941, 2001

20. Control of Communicable Diseases Manual, 17th ed. Chin JE, Ed. American Public Health Association, Washington DC, 2000

21. Garner JS: Guideline for isolation precautions in hospitals. Infect Control Hosp Epidemiol 17:53, 1996

22. Immunization of health-care workers. Recommendations of the Advisory Committee on Immunization Practices and the Hospital Infection Control Practices Advisory Committee. MMWR Morb Mortal Wkly Rep 46:1, 1997

23. Rotz LD, Khan AS, Lillibridge SR, et al: Public health assessment of potential bioterrorism agents. Emerg Infect Dis 8:225, 2002

24. Torok TJ, Tauxe RV, Wise RP, et al: A large community outbreak of salmonellosis caused by intentional contamination of restaurant salad bars. JAMA 278:389, 1997

25. Kolavic SA, Kimura A, Simons SL, et al: An outbreak of Shigella dysenteriae type 2 among laboratory workers due to intentional food contamination. JAMA 278:396, 1997

26. Pavlin JA: Epidemiology of bioterrorism. Emerg Infect Dis 5:528, 1999

27. Recognition of illness associated with the intentional release of a biologic agent. MMWR Morb Mortal Wkly Rep 50:893, 2001

28. Vaccinia (smallpox) vaccine. Recommendations of the Advisory Committee on Immunization Practices (ACIP), 2001. MMWR Morb Mortal Wkly Rep 50:1, 2001

29. Franz DR, Jahrling PB, Friedlander AM, et al: Clinical recognition and management of patients exposed to biological warfare agents. JAMA 278:399, 1997

30. Draft Supplemental Recommendation of the ACIP. Use of Smallpox (Vaccinia) Vaccine, June 2002.
http://www.cdc.gov/nip/smallpox/supp_recs.htm

31. Fenner F, Henderson DA, Arita I, et al: Smallpox and its eradication. World Health Organization, Geneva.
http://www.who.int/emc/diseases/smallpox/Smallpoxeradication.html

32. Smallpox as a biological weapon: medical and public health management. Working Group on Civilian Biodefense. JAMA 281:2127, 1999

33. Breman, JG, Henderson DA: Diagnosis and management of smallpox. N Engl J Med 346:1300, 2002

34. Henderson DA: Smallpox: clinical and epidemiologic features. Emerging Infect Dis 5:537, 1999

35. CDC Interim smallpox response plan and guidelines.
http://www.bt.cdc.gov/agent/smallpox/response-plan/index.asp

36. Lane JM, Ruben FL, Neff JM, et al: Complications of smallpox vaccination, 1968: results of ten statewide surveys. J Infect Dis 122:303, 1970

37. Acha PN, Szyfres B: Zoonoses and Communicable Disease Common to Man and Animals, 3rd ed. Vol I. Pan American Health Organization, Washington, DC, 2001

38. Swartz MN: Recognition and management of anthrax: an update. N Engl J Med 345:1621, 2001

39. Brachman PS: Bioterrorism: an update with a focus on anthrax. Am J Epidemiol 155:981, 2002

40. Update: investigation of bioterrorism-related anthrax and adverse events from antimicrobial prophylaxis. MMWR Morb Mortal Wkly Rep 50:973, 2001

41. Cieslak TJ, Eitzen HM Jr: Bioterrorism: agents of concern. J Public Health Manag Pract 6:19, 2000

42. Kournikakis B, Armour SJ, Boulet CA, et al: Risk assessment of anthrax threat letters. Technical Report 2001-048. Defense Research Establishment, Suffield, Canada, 2001

43. Dixon TC, Meselson M, Guillemin J, et al: Anthrax. N Engl J Med 341:815, 1999

44. Sirisanthana T, Brown AE: Anthrax of the gastrointestinal tract. Emerg Infect Dis 8:649, 2002

45. Inglesby TV, O'Toole T, Henderson DA, et al: Anthrax as a biological weapon, 2002: updated recommendations for management. JAMA 287:2236, 2002

46. Meselson M, Guillemin J, Hugh-Jones M, et al: The Sverdlovsk anthrax outbreak of 1979. Science 266:1202, 1994

47. LaForce FM. Anthrax. Clin Infect Dis 19:1009, 1994

48. Jernigan JA, Stephens DS, Ashford DA, et al: Bioterrorism-related inhalational anthrax: the first 10 cases reported in the United States. Emerg Infect Dis 7:933, 2001

49. Brachman PS: Inhalation anthrax. Ann NY Acad Sci 353:83, 1980

50. USAMRIID's Medical Management of Biological Casualties Handbook (USAMRIID Blue Book), 4th ed. United States Army Medical Research Institute of Infectious Diseases, Fort Detrick, Maryland, February, 2001
http://www.usamriid.army.mil/education/bluebook.html

51. Use of anthrax vaccine in the United States. Recommendations of the Advisory Committee on Immunization Practices. MMWR Morb Mortal Wkly Rep 49:1, 2000

52. Considerations for distinguishing influenza-like illness from inhalational anthrax. MMWR Morb Mortal Wkly Rep 50:984, 2001

53. Update: investigation of bioterrorism-related anthrax and interim guidelines for exposure management and antimicrobial therapy, October 2001. MMWR Morb Mortal Wkly Rep 50:909, 2001

54. Update: investigation of anthrax associated with intentional exposure and interim public health guidelines, October 2001. MMWR Morb Mortal Wkly Rep 50:889, 2001

55. Statement by the Department of Health and Human Services regarding additional options for preventive treatment for those exposed to inhalational anthrax. Dec. 18, 2001.
http://www.hhs.gov/news/press/2001pres/20011218.html

56. Committee to Assess the Safety and Efficacy of the Anthrax Vaccine. Medical Follow-Up Agency: The Anthrax Vaccine: Is It Safe? Does It Work? Joellenbeck LM, Zwanziger LL, Durch JS, et al, Eds: Institute of Medicine, National Academy Press, Washington, DC, 2002
http://www.iom.edu/iom/iomhome.nsf/Wfiles/Anthrax-8-pager1FINAL/$file/Anthrax-8-pager1FINAL.pdf

57. Additional options for preventive treatment for persons exposed to inhalational anthrax. MMWR Morb Mortal Wkly Rep 50:1142, 2001

58. Carucci JA, McGovern TW, Norton SA, et al: Cutaneous anthrax management algorithm. J Am Acad Dermatol (online), November 21, 2001
http://www.aad.org/BioInfo/Biomessage2.html

59. Biosafety in Microbiological and Biomedical Laboratories (BMBL) 4th Edition. U.S. Department of Health and Human Services Centers for Disease Control and Prevention and National Institutes of Health, May 1999. US Government Printing Office, Washington, DC, 1999
http://www.cdc.gov/od/ohs/biosfty/bmbl4/bmbl4toc.htm

60. Perry RD, Fetherston JD: Yersinia pestis—etiologic agent of plague. Clin Microbiol Rev 10:35, 1997

61. Gage KL, Dennis DT, Orloski KA, et al: Cases of cat-associated human plague in the

western U.S., 1977–1998. Clin Infect Dis 30:893, 2000

62. Inglesby TV, Dennis DT, Henderson DA, et al: Plague as a biological weapon: medical and public health management. Working Group on Civilian Biodefense. JAMA 283:2281, 2000

63. Prevention of plague. Recommendations of the Advisory Committee on Immunization Practice. MMWR Morb Mortal Wkly Rep 45:1 1996

64. McGovern TW, Friedlander AM: Plague. Medical Aspects of Chemical and Biological Warfare. Textbook of Military Medicine Series. Part I, Warfare, Weaponry and the Casualty. Sidell FR, Takafuji ET, Franz DR, Eds. TMM Publications, Washington, DC, 1997

65. Shapiro RL, Hatheway C, Becher J, et al: Botulism surveillance and emergency response: a public health strategy for a global challenge. JAMA 278:433, 1997

66. Shapiro RL, Hatheway C, Swerdlow DL: Botulism in the United States: a clinical and epidemiologic review. Ann Intern Med 129:221, 1998

67. Arnon SS, Schechter R, Inglesby TV, et al: Botulinum toxin as a biological weapon: medical and public health management. JAMA 285:1059, 2001

68. Cherington M: Clinical spectrum of botulism. Muscle Nerve 21:701, 1998

69. Woodruff BA, Griffin PM, McCroskey LM, et al: Clinical and laboratory comparison of botulism toxin types A, B and E in the United States, 1975–1988. J Infect Dis 166:1281, 1992

70. Angulo FJ, Getz J, Taylor JP, et al: A large outbreak of botulism: the hazardous baked potato. J Infect Dis 178:172, 1998

71. Eitzen E: Medical management of biological casualties, 3rd ed. U.S. Army Medical Research Institute of Infectious Diseases, Fort Detrick, Frederick, Maryland, 1998

72. Black RE, Gunn RA: Hypersensitivity reactions associated with botulinal antitoxin. Am J Med 69:567, 1980

73. Tularemia—United States, 1999–2000. MMWR Morb Mortal Wkly Rep 51:181, 2002

74. Feldman KA, Enscore RE, Lathrop SL, et al: An outbreak of primary pneumonic tularemia on Martha's Vineyard. N Engl J Med 345:1601, 2001

75. Dennis DT, Inglesby TV, Henderson DA, et al: Tularemia as a biological weapon: medical and public health management. JAMA 285:2763, 2001

76. Choi E: Tularemia and Q fever. Med Clinics North Am 86:393, 2002

77. Evans ME, Gregory DW, Schaffner W, et al: Tularemia: a 30-year experience with 88 cases. Medicine (Baltimore) 64:251, 1985

78. Gill V, Cunha BA: Tularemia pneumonia. Semin Respir Infect 12:61, 1997

79. Evans ME, Friedlander AM: Tularemia. Medical Aspects of Chemical and Biological Warfare. Textbook of Military Medicine Series. Part I, Warfare, Weaponry and the Casualty. Sidell FR, Takafuji ET, Franz DR, Eds. TMM Publications, Washington, DC, 1997

80. Limaye AP, Hooper CJ: Treatment of tularemia with fluoroquinolones: two cases and review. Clin Infect Dis 29:922, 1999

81. Borio L, Inglesby T, Peters CJ, et al: Hemorrhagic fever viruses as biological weapons: medical and public health management. JAMA 287:2391, 2002

82. Khan AS, Sanchez A, Pflieger AK: Filoviral hemorrhagic fevers. Br Med Bull 54:675, 1998

83. Bwaka MA, Bonnet MJ, Calain P, et al: Ebola hemorrhagic fever in Kikwit, Democratic Republic of the Congo: clinical observations in 103 patients. J Infect Dis 179:S1, 1999

84. Jahrling PB: Viral hemorrhagic fevers. Textbook of Military Medicine Series. Part I, Warfare, Weaponry and the Casualty. Sidell FR, Takafuji ET, Franz DR, Eds. TMM Publications, Washington, DC, 1997

85. Isaacson M: Viral hemorrhagic fever hazards for travelers in Africa. Clin Infect Dis 33:1707, 2001

86. Acute hemorrhagic fever syndrome. World Health Organization. http://www.who.int/emcdocuments/surveillance/docs/whocdscsrisr992.html/41Acute%20haemorrhagic%20fever%20syndrome.htm

87. Update: management of patients with suspected viral hemorrhagic fever—United States. MMWR Morb Mortal Wkly Rep 44:475, 1995

Acknowledgments

Figures 1, 3, 4, and 5   Centers for Disease Control and Prevention Public Health Image Library.

Figure 2   Centers for Disease Control and Prevention Public Health Image Library (Dr Duma).

12 Cardiac Resuscitation

Terry J. Mengert, M.D.

Sudden cardiac arrest outside the hospital is expected to claim the lives of at least 300,000 persons in the United States in 2003, making it the single leading cause of death.[1-4] In fact, approximately 50% of all cardiac deaths are sudden deaths. In hospitals, a minimum of 370,000 patients will also suffer a cardiac arrest, followed by an attempted, but only sometimes successful, resuscitation.[5] Although most victims of sudden death have underlying coronary artery disease (70% to 80%), sudden death is the first manifestation of the disease in half of these persons.[2] Other causes and contributing factors to sudden death include abnormalities of the myocardium (i.e., chronic heart failure or hypertrophy from any other cause), electrophysiologic abnormalities, valvular heart disease, congenital heart disease, and miscellaneous inflammatory and infiltrative disease processes (e.g., myocarditis, sarcoidosis, and hemochromatosis).[6,7]

The pathophysiology that culminates in a sudden cardiac death is complex and poorly understood. It likely represents a mix of electrical abnormalities combined with acute functional triggers, such as myocardial ischemia, central and autonomic nervous system effects, electrolyte abnormalities, and even pharmacologic influences.[1] Classically, most sudden deaths that occur in adults in the community are thought to be secondary to ventricular tachycardia (VT) that degenerates into ventricular fibrillation (VF). During the past 10 years in the Seattle area, the different arrhythmias found in prehospital cardiac arrest patients presumed to have underlying cardiovascular disease were VF (45%), asystole (31%), pulseless electrical activity (PEA; 10%), VT (1%), and other miscellaneous arrhythmias (14%).[3]

The Chain of Survival

The resuscitation of an adult victim of sudden cardiac arrest should follow an orderly sequence, no matter where the patient's collapse occurs. This sequence is called the chain of survival.[8] It comprises four elements, all of which must be instituted as rapidly as possible: activation of the emergency medical service network, cardiopulmonary resuscitation (CPR), defibrillation, and provision of advanced care.

ACTIVATION OF EMERGENCY MEDICAL SERVICES

A person in cardiac arrest will be unresponsive and pulseless, but agonal respirations may last for minutes. Unresponsiveness should be confirmed by speaking loudly to and shaking the patient. If the patient is unresponsive, help should immediately be sought through activation of the emergency medical service in the community (in most locales, this means calling 911); if the patient is already in the hospital, a code should be called (e.g., code blue, code 199). If an automated external defibrillator (AED) is available, it should be brought to the resuscitation scene; AEDs are easily used and can be lifesaving.[9-12]

INITIATION OF CPR

While awaiting the arrival of a defibrillator and advanced help, the rescuer should assess the patient's airway, breathing, and circulation [see The Primary Survey, *below*], and CPR should be initiated [see Table 1]. When CPR is started within 4 minutes of collapse, the likelihood of patient survival at least doubles.[13,14]

INITIATION OF DEFIBRILLATION

When the AED or monitor-defibrillator arrives, the device should be appropriately attached to the patient and the rhythm should be analyzed; if the patient is in pulseless VT or VF, a defibrillatory shock should be rapidly applied [see Tables 2 and 3]. If required, two additional shocks may be administered sequentially. The importance of rapid access to defibrillation cannot be overemphasized. In a patient who is dying from a shockable rhythm, the chance of survival declines by 7% to 10% for every minute that defibrillation is delayed.[15]

INITIATION OF ADVANCED CARE

If the patient remains pulseless despite the steps described above, CPR should be continued; a definitive airway should be secured; intravenous access should be established; and appropriate medications should be administered, as determined by the rhythm and the arrest circumstances. If the patient is in pulseless VT or VF, repeated attempts at defibrillation are interspersed with delivery of vasoactive and antiarrhythmic medication [see Table 4].

RESUSCITATION OUTCOME

When every link in this described chain is quickly and sequentially available, the patient is provided an optimal opportunity for return of spontaneous circulation.[15-18] In the United States, individual communities report survival rates of 4% to 33% or more in cases of sudden cardiac death.[19-22] Prehospital victims of VF have had survival rates to hospital discharge of greater than 50% when an AED was expeditiously used.[23] Many other factors

---

Table 1 **Initial Resuscitation Steps in the Unresponsive Patient**

Confirm unresponsiveness
Activate the emergency medical system
   In the community, call 911 in most locales
   In the hospital, activate the appropriate code response
Call for an automatic external defibrillator (AED)
Begin basic life support (CPR)
   Open airway
   Check breathing; if not breathing, deliver two initial breaths
   Check for a carotid pulse; if pulseless, do the following:
      Begin chest compressions at the rate of 100 compressions/min, depressing the sternum 1.5–2 in. per compression in patients older than 8 yr
      Intersperse ventilations with chest compressions: in nonintubated patients, deliver 15 compressions, pause for two breaths, then repeat; in intubated patients, deliver one breath every 5 sec, with no pause in compressions
Reassess for return of spontaneous circulation every 1–3 min
When defibrillator arrives, immediately analyze and treat arrhythmia
   Attach patient to AED [see Table 2] or the monitor-defibrillator [see Table 3]
   Analyze arrhythmia and treat as appropriate [see Figure 2]

Table 2 Using an Automatic External Defibrillator

Automatic external defibrillator (AED) arrives (CPR is in progress)
  Place AED beside patient.
  Turn on the AED.
  Attach the electrodes to the AED (they may be preattached).
  Attach the electrode pads to the patient (as diagrammed on the pads).
AED analyzes patient's rhythm
  Stop CPR (and ensure no one is touching the patient).
  Press the Analyze button on the AED (some devices analyze the rhythm automatically as soon as the pads are placed on the patient).
AED instructs rescuers (via an audible voice prompt and/or on-screen instructions)
  Shock is indicated: clear the patient (ensure no one is touching the patient) and push the Shock button.
  After delivering shock, press the Analyze button again; the sequence of analysis followed by shock (if so indicated) may be performed a total of three times.

or

  Shock not indicated: reassess the patient for signs of circulation; if present, assess the adequacy of breathing; if there are no signs of circulation, resume CPR for 1–2 min. After 1 min of CPR, assess the patient again for signs of circulation; if present, assess the adequacy of breathing. If the patient is still pulseless, repeat analysis, followed (if indicated) by shock steps.

---

also influence patient survival, however; these include whether the patient's collapse was witnessed, the rhythm associated with the cardiac arrest, and underlying comorbidities.[24,25] With inpatient cardiac arrest, for example, overall survival rates vary from 9% to 32%,[26-32] but in one study, survival to hospital discharge was 30% for patients with primary heart disease, 15% for patients with infectious diseases, and only 8% for patients with other end-stage diseases (e.g., cancer, lung disease, liver failure, or renal failure).[33]

Such statistics underline the importance of using cardiac resuscitation appropriately and with discrimination. Cardiac resuscitation provides rescuers with powerful tools that save the lives of thousands of people every year. These techniques are capable of returning patients who would otherwise die to productive and meaningful lives. However, cardiac resuscitation should not be employed to reverse timely and natural death. Under those circumstances, it has the potential to lengthen the dying process and to increase human suffering. All practitioners are well advised to remember that "death is not the opposite of life, death is the opposite of birth. Both are aspects of life."[34] It is untimely death that requires immediate intervention and a well-conducted cardiac resuscitation.

The Primary and Secondary Surveys of Cardiac Resuscitation

A cardiac resuscitation is a stressful event for everyone involved. Too often, clinic and inpatient cardiac arrests and their management are episodes of chaos in the busy lives of resident and attending physicians. Yet, it has been eloquently stated that a good resuscitation team should function like a fine symphony orchestra.[35] Such skill levels require dedicated individual and team practice and careful code team organization. Mastery in cardiac resuscitation is in fact a lifelong pursuit that requires

training and retraining in advanced cardiac life support (ACLS); regular practice and review; and leadership and team skill development. Its key elements include not only the resuscitation itself but the response to the announcement of a code, postresuscitation stabilization of the patient, notification of the family and primary care provider, and code critique and debriefing. To help practitioners learn and apply some of the most essential techniques used in cardiac resuscitation more easily and effectively, the American Heart Association (AHA) has developed the concepts of primary and secondary surveys of a patient in atraumatic cardiac arrest.[36]

THE PRIMARY SURVEY

The primary survey for the victim of sudden cardiac arrest consists of the appropriate assessment of the patient's airway (A), breathing (B), and circulation (C) and the simultaneous ap-

---

Table 3 Using a Manual Defibrillator[45,71]

Defibrillator arrives (CPR is in progress)
  Place defibrillator beside patient.
  Turn defibrillator on (initial energy level setting is typically 200 J).*
  Set Lead Select switch to Paddles. Alternatively, if patient is already attached to monitor leads, set Lead Select switch to lead I, II, or III; ensure all three leads are correctly attached to the patient and the defibrillator: white to right shoulder, black to left shoulder, red to ribs on left side.
  Apply gel to paddles or place conductor pads on patient's chest. Some devices use disposable electrode patches that are prepasted with a conducting gel. In either case, the appropriate positions of the paddles with applied gel, conductor pads, or disposable paddles are as follows: sternal paddle is placed to the right of the sternum, just below the right clavicle; apex paddle is placed to the left of the left breast, centered in the left midaxillary line at the fifth intercostal space.
Analyze rhythm
Briefly withhold CPR
  If using paddles to assess rhythm, apply paddles as described with firm pressure (25 lb of pressure to each paddle) and visually assess rhythm on monitor (if using leads, briefly withhold CPR and assess rhythm in leads I, II, or III). If rhythm is either pulseless VT or VF, proceed as follows:
Defibrillate, then reassess
  Announce to resuscitation team, "Charging defibrillator, stand clear!" and press Charge button on either paddles or defibrillator (initial energy, 200 J, not synchronized).*
  Warn resuscitation team that a defibrillatory shock is coming: "I am going to shock on three! ONE, I'm clear; TWO, you're clear, THREE, everybody's CLEAR!" Simultaneously with these statements, visually ensure that no resuscitation team member is in contact with patient.
  Press the Discharge buttons on both paddles simultaneously to deliver a defibrillatory shock.
  Reassess rhythm on monitor; if patient is still in VT or VF, recharge defibrillator (now 300 J)* and repeat process of loudly informing team members by giving the warning statements as above, and then apply defibrillatory shock.
  Reassess rhythm on monitor; if patient is still in VT or VF, recharge defibrillator (now 360 J)* and repeat process of loudly informing team members by giving the warning statements as above, and then apply defibrillatory shock.
  Reassess rhythm on monitor; if patient is still in VT or VF, resume CPR and continue with resuscitation sequence [*see Figure 2*].

---

*Note: if using a biphasic defibrillator, a lower initial defibrillatory energy level (< 200 J) without energy escalation on subsequent shocks is acceptable.
VF—ventricular fibrillation   VT—ventricular tachycardia

Table 4   Drugs Useful in Cardiac Arrest[3,72]

Category	Drug and Doses Supplied	Indications in Cardiac Arrest	Adult Dosage	Comments
Vasopressors	Epinephrine, 1 mg in 10 ml emergency syringe; 1 mg/ml (1 ml and 30 ml vials)	Pulseless VT or VF unresponsive to initial defibrillatory shocks; PEA; asystole	1 mg I.V. push; may repeat every 3–5 min for as long as patient is pulseless; can also be given via the endotracheal route: 2–2.5 mg diluted with normal saline (NS) to 10 ml total volume	I.V. boluses of epinephrine (1 mg) are appropriate only in pulseless cardiac arrest patients; if continued epinephrine is required postresuscitation, a continuous infusion should be started (1–10 μg/min). High-dose epinephrine (up to 0.2 mg/kg IV per dose) does not improve survival to hospital discharge in cardiac arrest patients and is no longer recommended in adults.
	Vasopressin, 20 IU/ml (1 ml vial)	Pulseless VT or VF unresponsive to initial defibrillatory shocks	40 IU I.V. push, single dose only; can also be given via endotracheal tube: same dose, diluted with NS to 10 ml total volume	If no response after 10 min of continued resuscitation, administer epinephrine, as above.
Antiarrhythmics	Amiodarone, 50 mg/ml (3 ml vial)	Pulseless VT or VF unresponsive to initial defibrillatory shocks and epinephrine plus shock(s)	VT/VF: 300 mg diluted in 20–30 ml; NS or D5W rapid I.V. push; a repeat dose of 150 mg may be given if required in 5 min; maximum dose in 24 hr should not exceed 2,200 mg	Side effects may include hypotension and bradycardia in the postresuscitation phase.
	Lidocaine, 50 mg or 100 mg in 5 ml emergency syringes; premixed bag, 1 g/250 ml or 2 g/250 ml	Pulseless VT or VF unresponsive to initial defibrillatory shocks and epinephrine plus shock(s)	Initial dose: 1–1.5 mg/kg I.V.; for refractory VF or unstable VT, may repeat 1–1.5 mg/kg I.V. in 3–5 min; maximum dose, 3 mg/kg. May also be given endotracheally: 2–4 mg/kg diluted with normal saline to 10 ml total volume	If lidocaine is effective, initiate continuous I.V. infusion at 2–4 mg/min when patient has return of a perfusing rhythm (but do not use if this rhythm is an idioventricular rhythm or third-degree heart block with an idioventricular escape rhythm). Continuous infusion should begin at 1 mg/min in congestive heart failure or chronic liver disease or in elderly patients.
	Magnesium sulfate, 500 mg/ml (2 ml and 10 ml vials), or 10 ml emergency syringe	Pulseless VT or VF unresponsive to initial defibrillatory shocks and epinephrine plus shock(s) if suspected hypomagnesemic state	Administer 1–2 g diluted in 100 ml D5W I.V. over 1–2 min. Total body magnesium deficits should be replaced gradually after initial therapy has stabilized the emergency: administer 0.5–1 g/hr for 3–6 hr, then reassess continued need	Measured magnesium levels correlate only approximately with the actual level of deficiency. Patients with renal insufficiency are at risk for dangerous hypermagnesemia; use appropriate caution. Side effects may include bradycardia, hypotension, generalized weakness, and temporary loss of reflexes.
	Procainamide, 100 mg/ml (10 ml injection); 500 mg/ml (2 ml vial)	Recurrent or intermittent pulseless VT or VF	20–30 mg/min I.V. (up to 50 mg/min if situation is critical); maximum dose is 17 mg/kg over time (but maximum dose is reduced to 12 mg/kg in setting of cardiac or renal dysfunction). Maintenance infusion is 1–4 mg/min	Administer procainamide during a perfusing rhythm. Stop procainamide administration when arrhythmia is adequately suppressed, hypotension occurs, QRS widens to > 50% of original duration, or maximum dose is administered.
Anticholinergic	Atropine, 1 mg in 10 ml emergency syringe	Asystole or PEA (if rate of rhythm is slow)	For asystole or PEA: 1 mg I.V. every 3–5 min up to 3 mg. May be given via ET tube: 2–3 mg diluted with normal saline to 10 ml	Minimal adult dose is 0.5 mg. Avoid use in type II second-degree heart block or third-degree heart block.
Miscellaneous	Bicarbonate, 50 mEq in 50 ml emergency syringe	Significant hyperkalemia. Significant metabolic acidosis unresponsive to optimal CPR, oxygenation, and ventilation. Certain drug overdoses, including tricyclic antidepressants and aspirin	Hyperkalemia therapy: 50 mEq I.V. Metabolic acidosis: 1 mEq/kg slow I.V. push; may repeat half initial dose in 10 min; ideally, ABGs should help guide further therapy. Use in overdose: discuss with toxicologist	In non–dialysis-dependent hyperkalemic patients, bicarbonate is most useful if metabolic acidosis is also present; bicarbonate is less effective in dialysis dependent renal failure patients. The use of bicarbonate in metabolic acidosis management in cardiac arrest patients is controversial. Side effects may include sodium overload, hypokalemia, and metabolic alkalosis.
	Calcium chloride, 100 mg/ml in 10 ml prefilled syringe	Significant hyperkalemia. Calcium channel blocker drug overdose. Profound hypocalcemia of other causes	In hyperkalemia: 5–10 ml slow I.V. push; may repeat if required. In calcium channel blocker overdose: discuss with toxicologist	Do not use if cause of hyperkalemia is suspected acute digoxin poisoning. Do not combine in same I.V. with sodium bicarbonate. Calcium chloride is not a routine medication in cardiac arrest.

Note: All medications used during cardiac arrest, when given via a peripheral venous site in an extremity, should be followed by a 20 ml I.V. saline bolus and elevation of the extremity for 10 to 20 sec.

ABG—arterial blood gases   D5W—5% dextrose in water   ET—endotracheal   PEA—pulseless electrical activity   VF—ventricular fibrillation   VT—ventricular tachycardia

plication of expert CPR until defibrillation (D) becomes possible (assuming the patient is in pulseless VT or VF). Thus, the primary survey includes the second and third links in the chain of survival (see above). In 1958, Kouwenhoven noted that when his research fellow forcefully applied external defibrillating electrodes on a dog's chest in the laboratory, an arterial pressure wave occurred.[37] Further study and refinements led to the technique of closed chest CPR, the careful description of which was published in 1960.[38] The first report of the use of this technique in patients was in 1961.[39] Since those early days, the fundamentals of closed-chest CPR have remained relatively unchanged. Mouth-to-mouth, mouth-to-mask, or bag-valve-mask ventilation oxygenates the blood. Chest compressions produce forward blood flow. This flow appears to result from a combination of direct compression of the heart and intrathoracic pressure changes.[40,41]

CPR in isolation does not defibrillate the heart. Its main benefit is to extend patient viability until a defibrillator and advanced interventions become available and, one hopes, succeed in restoring spontaneous circulation in the patient. CPR is not nearly as effective as a contracting heart; systolic arterial pressure peaks of 60 to 80 mm Hg may be generated, but diastolic blood pressure remains low, and a cardiac output of only 25% to 30% of normal can be achieved.[42] Still, effective CPR is critical to keeping the patient alive. It is worth remembering that the most important rescuers at a cardiac resuscitation are those who are performing expert CPR, because it is only through their efforts that the patient's heart and brain are kept viable until defibrillation and other advanced interventions can restore spontaneous circulation.

After unresponsiveness is confirmed, the emergency medical system is activated, and an AED is called for, the primary survey (A, B, C, and D) proceeds as described below.

Optimization of the Airway

The patient's mouth should be opened and the airway optimized by use of the head-tilt and chin-lift maneuver. A jaw-thrust maneuver should be used instead of the head-tilt technique if cervical spine injury is suspected. It should be remembered that in patients with suspected spine injury, proper spine alignment must be maintained throughout all phases of the resuscitation. In such circumstances, as equipment becomes available, the patient's spine should be immobilized with a padded backboard, hard cervical collar, appropriate bolstering around the patient's head to prevent movement, and strapping of the patient to the backboard.[43]

Assessment of Breathing

To assess breathing, the rescuer should place his or her cheek close to the patient's mouth and look, listen, and feel for the patient's breath. If the respirations are agonal or the patient is apneic, the rescuer should deliver two initial breaths. Each breath should be delivered over 1.5 to 2.0 seconds. The patient's chest should rise with each delivered breath, and exhalation should be allowed for between breaths. Breaths may be delivered using mouth-to-mouth technique with appropriate barrier precautions (the patient's nose should be pinched if the mouth-to-mouth technique is used) or mouth-to-mask technique. The ideal device, if available, is a bag-valve mask device attached to high-flow oxygen; this allows the delivery of a substantially higher oxygen concentration to the patient. If the patient cannot be ventilated, the airway should be repositioned and the technique attempted again. If the airway is still obstructed, up to five abdom-

inal thrusts should be delivered, followed by a finger sweep of the oropharynx, then ventilation attempts repeated. Definitive intervention for an obstructed airway in the hospital setting may involve laryngoscopic visualization of the cause of obstruction and foreign-body removal. If an adequate airway cannot be established by less-invasive means, cricothyrotomy may be required.

Initiation of CPR

A check should be made for the carotid pulse, but no more than 10 seconds should be spent doing this. (The AHA no longer recommends pulse checks for rescuers who are not health care providers.[44] Instead, lay rescuers should initiate chest compressions if the patient is not breathing, coughing, or moving after the initial two breaths.) If the patient has no carotid pulse, chest compressions should be initiated. The patient should be on a firm surface, and the heel of the rescuer's hand should be in the center of the inferior half of the patient's sternum (but cephalad to the xiphoid process). The rescuer's other hand is placed on top of the lower hand, with the fingers interlocked.

The rescuer's arms should be straight, and the force of each compression should come from the rescuer's trunk. In patients older than 8 years, the sternum should be smoothly compressed by 1.5 to 2.0 inches, then released. The duration of the compression-release cycle should be divided equally between compression and release. The rate of chest compression should be 100 compressions/min. The chest should be allowed to rebound to its precompression dimensions between compressions, but the resuscitator's palm closest to the patient should remain in contact with the sternum.

In nonintubated patients, chest compressions are regularly interrupted for the delivery of ventilations. The sequence is the same, regardless of whether one-rescuer or two-rescuer CPR is being performed: the rescuer delivers 15 compressions, pauses for two breaths (each given over 1.5 to 2 seconds), then resumes compressions. In endotracheally intubated patients, chest compression and ventilation are not synchronized; every 5 seconds, one ventilation is delivered over a period of 2 seconds, while compressions continue without pause.[14]

Good technique is critical throughout CPR delivery. There should be carotid pulses with chest compressions and appropriate breath sounds and chest movement with ventilations. Interestingly, femoral pulsations with CPR do not necessarily indicate effective CPR; frequently, these pulsations are venous rather than arterial. Quantitative end-tidal carbon dioxide levels can be monitored, if practicable. Higher levels correlate with more effective CPR and improved survival of cardiac arrest.[45] The patient should be reassessed for return of spontaneous circulation every 1 to 3 minutes [see Table 1].

Initiation of Defibrillation

When the monitor-defibrillator or AED arrives, it should be attached to the patient; the rhythm should be analyzed, and, if the patient is in pulseless VT or VF, defibrillation should be given [see Tables 2 and 3].

Defibrillation works by simultaneously depolarizing a sufficient mass of cardiac myocytes to make the cardiac tissue ahead of the VT or VF wave fronts refractory to electrical conduction. Subsequently, the sinus node or another appropriate pacemaker region of the heart with inherent automaticity can resume orderly depolarization-repolarization, with return of a perfusing rhythm.[12,46] The sooner defibrillation occurs, the higher the likelihood of resuscitation. When provided immediately after the onset of VF, the success of defibrillation is extremely high.[47] In a study of sudden cardiac arrest patients in Nevada gambling casinos, the survival rate to hospital discharge was 74% for patients who received their first defibrillation no later than 3 minutes after a witnessed collapse.[23] In this study, defibrillation was delivered via an AED operated by casino security officers.

Early defibrillation is so critical that if a defibrillator is immediately available, its use takes precedence over CPR for patients in pulseless VT or VF. If CPR is already in progress, it should of course halt while defibrillation takes place. Newer defibrillators can compensate for thoracic impedance, ensuring that the selected energy level is in fact the energy that is delivered to the myocardial tissue. In addition, defibrillators that deliver biphasic defibrillation waveforms instead of the standard monophasic damped sinusoidal waveforms allow effective defibrillation at lower energy levels (< 200 joules) and without the need for escalating energy levels during subsequent shocks.[12,48-51] In the Optimized Response to Cardiac Arrest (ORCA) study, which involved 115 patients with prehospital VF, the 150-joule biphasic-shock AED was more effective than the traditional high-energy monophasic-shock AED in four respects: it produced successful defibrillation with the first shock (96% versus 59%); it led to a higher rate of ultimate success with defibrillation (100% versus 84%); it had a better rate of return of spontaneous circulation (76% versus 54%); and its use was associated with a higher rate of ultimate good cerebral performance in the survivors (87% versus 53%).[52] There were no differences, however, in terms of survival to hospital admission or discharge. Current AHA guidelines state that lower energy biphasic waveform defibrillators are safe and have equivalent or higher efficacy for termination of VF, as compared with the standard monophasic wave-form defibrillator.[12,44]

THE SECONDARY SURVEY

The secondary survey for a victim of persistent cardiac arrest takes place after completion of the primary survey. Like the primary survey, the secondary survey follows an ABCD format, which in this case consists of advanced airway interventions (A); optimized oxygenation and ventilation by confirmation of endotracheal (ET) tube placement and repeated reassessment of the adequacy of delivered breaths (B); intravenous access and appropriate medication delivery to the patient's circulation (C); and definitive therapy (D), based on a differential diagnosis that considers the specific disease processes thought to be responsible for, or contributing to, the cardiac arrest. The secondary survey includes the fourth link in the chain of survival, rapid advanced care (see above).

Placement of an Advanced Airway

Patients who remain in cardiac arrest after completion of the primary survey require placement of an advanced airway. Depending on the setting and the experience of the rescuers, this advanced airway may be a laryngeal mask airway, an esophageal-tracheal Combitube (a tracheal tube bonded side by side with an esophageal obturator), or an ET tube.[36,53,54] The laryngeal mask airway and the Combitube can be placed by personnel with less training than that required for endotracheal intubation, and they do not require special equipment or visualization of the vocal cords. Nevertheless, endotracheal intubation is generally the preferred advanced airway technique for cardiac resuscitation, both in the hospital setting and in many paramedic systems throughout the United States. Endotracheal intubation

isolates the airway, maintains airway patency, helps protect the trachea from the ever-present risk of aspiration, helps permit optimal oxygenation and ventilation of the patient, allows for tracheal suctioning, and even provides a route for delivery of some medications to the systemic circulation (via the pulmonary circulation) if intravenous access is unobtainable or lost.[53]

Optimization of Breathing and Ventilation

When a cardiac arrest patient undergoes endotracheal intubation, correct positioning of the tube must be immediately confirmed and regularly reconfirmed during and after the resuscitation [see Table 5]. Routine use of an esophageal detector device or end-tidal CO_2 detector is recommended, along with careful patient examination. Caution is necessary with qualitative colorimetric end-tidal CO_2 detectors, because both false positive and false negative results have been documented during cardiac arrests.[55] Breath sounds should be present during auscultation over the anterior and lateral chest walls, and the patient's chest should rise and fall with delivered ventilations. No gurgling should be heard when the epigastrium is auscultated. The ET tube should be inserted to the appropriate depth marking: 21 cm at the corner of the mouth in the average adult woman, 23 cm in the average adult man. The patient's skin color should be reasonable (i.e., not dusky or cyanotic), provided the patient's pigmentation allows such assessment.

Once correct positioning is confirmed, the ET tube should be appropriately secured to prevent its dislodgment. When feasible, an arterial blood gas (ABG) measurement should be obtained to confirm the adequacy of oxygenation and ventilation as the resuscitation proceeds.

Establishment of Circulation Access

Access to the patient's venous circulation is mandatory; such access may be achieved by a code team member or members simultaneously while other resuscitators pursue steps A and B of the secondary survey. Ideally, a large intravenous cannula should be placed in a prominent upper-extremity vein or exter-

---

Table 5   Confirmation of Endotracheal
Tube Placement

Intubation process
  Vocal cords are visualized by intubator
  Tip of ET tube is seen passing between the cords
  Cuff of ET tube also passes cords by 1 cm
Postintubation checks
  Esophageal detector device or end-tidal CO_2 detector confirms
    ET tube placement in trachea
  Breath sounds are symmetrical (auscultate over lateral anterior
    chest and in midaxillary line bilaterally)
  No gurgling with auscultation over epigastrium
  Patient's chest rises and falls appropriately with ventilation
  ET tube depth is appropriate: 21 cm at the corner of the mouth
    in adult women, 23 cm in adult men
Secure the ET tube to prevent dislodgment
Reassess the adequacy of oxygenation and ventilation throughout
  the resuscitation (bedside patient assessment; also obtain ABGs
  when feasible)
Postresuscitation, obtain a portable chest radiograph

ABG—arterial blood gas   ET—endotracheal

nal jugular vein to optimize delivery of needed medications. If a peripheral line is not achievable, additional possibilities include central line placement via the internal jugular, subclavian (via the supraclavicular approach) or, less ideally, femoral vein; even intraosseous access is possible (intraosseous access is a common emergency vascular access site in pediatric patients, but it is an unusual route of access in adults). It is useful to remember, as already noted, that some important resuscitation medications can be delivered via the ET tube in cases of failed intravenous access; such medications include naloxone, atropine, vasopressin, epinephrine, and lidocaine (a mnemonic for these agents is NAVEL).

The commonly used medications in cardiac resuscitation may be grouped into the following general categories: vasopressors (epinephrine or vasopressin), antiarrhythmics (amiodarone, lidocaine, magnesium, and procainamide), anticholinergic agents (atropine, if the arrest arrhythmia is asystole or PEA is slow), and miscellaneous drugs used to treat specific problems contributing to the arrest state, such as sodium bicarbonate (for severe metabolic acidosis, hyperkalemia, and certain drug overdoses), and calcium chloride (for hyperkalemia, calcium channel blocker drug overdose, or severe hypocalcemia) [see Table 4].

Persons in cardiac arrest (which can result from pulseless VT or VF, PEA, or asystole) should receive 1 mg of epinephrine intravenously every 3 to 5 minutes for as long as they are pulseless. Epinephrine stimulates adrenergic receptors, which leads to vasoconstriction and optimization of CPR-generated blood flow to the heart and brain. In patients with pulseless VT or VF, vasopressin (40 units I.V. once only) is a reasonable alternative to epinephrine, at least initially. Vasopressin in the recommended dose is a potent vasoconstrictor. It also has the theoretical advantage over epinephrine of not increasing myocardial oxygen consumption or lactate production in the arrested heart.[56] Despite its potential advantages, however, a recent study of 200 inpatient cardiac arrest patients found no differences in survival between those given vasopressin and those given epinephrine.[57]

During resuscitation with ongoing CPR, medication delivery through an intravenous cannula should be followed by a 20 ml saline bolus; if the cannula is in a peripheral vein, the extremity containing the cannula should then be elevated for 10 to15 seconds to augment delivery of the medication to the central circulation. This is especially important because of the low-flow circulatory state with closed-chest CPR.

Differential Diagnosis and Definitive Care

The most challenging part of the secondary survey, and of cardiac resuscitation management in general, is the problem-solving required when spontaneous circulation does not return despite appropriate interventions. This situation poses a critical question to the resuscitators: Why is this patient dying right now? The intellectual challenge of that question, which the resuscitators must try to answer expeditiously and at the bedside, is compounded by the emotional intensity that pervades most cardiac resuscitations.

The solvable problems that can interfere with resuscitation can be grouped into three broad categories: technical [see Table 6], physiologic, and anatomic [see Table 7]. Technical problems consist of difficulties with the resuscitators' equipment or skills; such difficulties include ineffective CPR, inadequate oxygenation and ventilation, ET tube complications, intravenous access difficulties, and monitor-defibrillator malfunction or misuse. The physiologic and anatomic problems consist of life-threatening but poten-

tially treatable conditions that may have led to the cardiac arrest in the first place. This differentiation between physiology and anatomy is admittedly artificial, given that physiology is always involved in a cardiac arrest, but it has some usefulness as a teaching and problem-solving tool. Physiologic problems classically include hypoxia, acidosis, hyperkalemia, severe hypokalemia, hypothermia, and drug overdose. Anatomic problems are hypovolemia/hemorrhage, tension pneumothorax, cardiac tamponade, myocardial infarction, and pulmonary embolism.[36]

Whenever possible, the patient's medical and surgical history and the circumstances and symptoms immediately before the cardiac arrest should be sought from family members, bystanders, or hospital staff as the resuscitation proceeds. This information may contain important clues to the principal arrest problem and how it may be expeditiously treated. For example, a patient who presents to an emergency department with chest pain and then suffers a VF cardiac arrest is probably dying of a massive myocardial infarction, pulmonary embolism, or aortic dissection. A tension pneumothorax or cardiac tamponade is also a possibility.

Specific questions to consider include the following: Does the patient have risk factors for heart disease, pulmonary embolism, or aortic disease? What was the quality of the patient's pain and its radiation before the cardiac arrest? What were the prearrest vital signs and physical examination findings? What did the prearrest ECG show (if available)? Can any of this information be used now, at the bedside, to dictate the needed resuscitation interventions during the D phase of the secondary survey? For example, if the prearrest ECG showed prominent ST-segment elevation in leads V1 through V4 consistent with a large anterior myocardial infarction, if the patient's resuscitation is failing despite appropriate interventions, and if there appear to be no technical problems hampering the resuscitation, then a working diagnosis of massive myocardial infarction can be made; intravenous thrombolytic therapy may be a reasonable part of the resuscitation in such a setting.[58]

Thoughtful consideration of the possible reasons that resuscitation is failing will regularly push the code captain's and the resuscitation team's expertise and clinical skills to the limits. Nevertheless, the failure to consider these formidable issues will deprive the patient of an optimal opportunity to survive the cardiac arrest.

Cardiac Resuscitation Based on Rhythm Findings

When a monitor-defibrillator arrives at the scene of a cardiac arrest, the patient's rhythm is immediately analyzed (the beginning part of step D in the primary survey). There are four rhythm possibilities [see Figure 1]: (1) pulseless VT, (2) pulseless VF, (3) organized or semiorganized electrical activity despite the absence of a palpable carotid pulse, which defines PEA, and (4) asystole. The detailed management of these different cardiac resuscitation scenarios is based on the recommendations of the AHA[44] and the International Liaison Committee on Resuscitation.[59]

PULSELESS VENTRICULAR TACHYCARDIA OR VENTRICULAR FIBRILLATION

The appearance of either pulseless VT or VF on the rhythm monitor in a patient with ongoing CPR is a relatively favorable finding, because there is reasonable hope for a successful outcome with these rhythms. In addition, the interventions and medications sequentially used in the resuscitation are plainly de-

Table 6   Technical Problems That May Prevent a Successful Resuscitation

Problem	Patients at Risk	Recommendations
Ineffective CPR	All cardiac arrest patients	Ensure technically perfect CPR. Confirm carotid pulses with CPR. If arterial line was in place before cardiac arrest, confirm adequate arterial waveform with CPR on arterial line monitor. Monitor end-tidal CO_2 if available (higher levels correlate with better CPR and improved patient survival). Confirm adequate oxygenation with an ABG when feasible.
Inadequate oxygenation and ventilation	All cardiac arrest patients	Ensure optimal airway positioning and control. Have suction immediately available to manage pharyngeal and airway secretions. Ensure use of properly fitting, tightly sealed face mask for bag-valve mask (BVM) ventilation until a definitive airway is established. Apply cricoid pressure to prevent gastric distention during BVM ventilation until a definitive airway is established. Ensure that supplemental oxygen is flowing to BVM at 15 L/min. Deliver an appropriate tidal volume per breath (6–7 ml/kg if oxygen is available) at the rate of 12–15 breaths/min. Confirm bilateral and equal breath sounds with ventilation. Confirm that patient's chest rises with each ventilation. Allow adequate time for exhalation between breaths. Confirm optimal oxygenation and ventilation with an ABG when feasible.
ET tube difficulties	All patients intubated with ET tube	Allow ≤ 20–30 sec/intubation attempt. Intubator should see tip of ET tube and cuff pass between vocal cords at time of intubation. After intubation, immediately confirm correct ET tube placement; regularly reconfirm ET tube placement throughout resuscitation. Confirm adequacy of oxygenation and ventilation with an ABG. After intubation, consider nasogastric tube placement to decompress stomach and optimize diaphragmatic excursions with ventilation.
Intravenous line difficulties	All cardiac arrest patients	Place one or more 18-gauge or larger I.V. cannulas in an antecubital or external jugular vein site. Check for I.V. infiltration regularly throughout the resuscitation. Follow all medications administered through a peripheral I.V. site with a 20 ml saline bolus and elevation of the extremity containing the I.V. for 10–15 sec (if possible). Consider central line placement if the resuscitation is prolonged. Be aware of all I.V. infusions the patient is receiving. Stop all nonessential medications that had been started before the cardiac arrest. During the resuscitation, the only infusions the patient should receive are normal saline, blood products (if clinically indicated), and pertinent medications necessary to assist with return of spontaneous circulation. Pulmonary artery catheters and central lines occasionally act as an arrhythmogenic focus within the right ventricle. If applicable, deflate all relevant balloons on the catheter and withdraw the catheter to a superior vena cava position. Make sure Synchronization Mode button is in the off position when defibrillating patients in pulseless VT or VF. Make sure electricity is not arcing over the patient's chest because of perspiration or smeared conducting gel; dry patient's chest with a towel except for areas directly beneath pads or paddles. Do not administer shock through nitroglycerin paste or patches. If the patient has an internal cardioverter-defibrillator (ICD) or a pacemaker, the patient may still be manually defibrillated, but do not shock directly over the internal device. Under these circumstances, place the pads or paddles at least 1 in. away from the patient's internal device. If the ICD is intermittently firing but not defibrillating the patient and if the ICD is thought to be compromising the resuscitation, turn the device off with a magnet so that manual defibrillation may take place without interference. Maximize the gain or electrocardiography "size" and check the rhythm in several leads (or change the axes of the paddles if reading the rhythm in Paddles mode) to confirm asystole when the initial rhythm appears to be asystole.

ABG—arterial blood gas   ET—endotracheal   VF—ventricular fibrillation   VT—ventricular tachycardia

lineated, and the initial course of action is clear. Pulseless VT or VF is managed identically.

Initiation of Defibrillation

Defibrillation with 200 joules should be attempted immediately; if the VT or VF persists, subsequent attempts should be made with 200 to 300 joules and then 360 joules, successively [*see Figure 2*]. A lower, nonescalating equivalent biphasic ener-gy level is acceptable, if the defibrillator offers this option. It is no longer recommended that the patient's carotid pulse be manually checked between shocks, but the displayed rhythm on the monitor must be carefully assessed after each defibrillation attempt. If there are any doubts concerning the rhythm or if there is suspicion of a dysfunctional lead or paddle cable, then a manual pulse check would be appropriate. If pulseless VT or VF persists, CPR should be resumed, the patient should

Table 7 Potentially Treatable Conditions That May Cause or Contribute to Cardiac Arrest[3]

Condition	Clinical Setting	Diagnostic and Corrective Actions
Acidosis	Preexisting acidosis, diabetes, diarrhea, drugs, toxins, prolonged resuscitation, renal disease, shock	Obtain stat ABG. Reassess technical quality of CPR, oxygenation, and ventilation. Confirm correct endotracheal tube placement. Hyperventilate patient (P_aCO_2 of 30–35 mm Hg) to partially compensate for metabolic acidosis. If pH < 7.20 despite above interventions, consider I.V. sodium bicarbonate, 1 mEq/kg I.V. slow push.
Cardiac tamponade	Hemorrhagic diathesis, malignancy, pericarditis, postcardiac surgery, postmyocardial infarction, trauma	Initiate large-volume I.V. crystalloid resuscitation. Confirm diagnosis with emergent bedside echocardiogram, if available. Perform pericardiocentesis. Immediate surgical intervention is appropriate if pericardiocentesis is unhelpful but cardiac tamponade is known or highly suspected clinically.
Hypoglycemia	Adrenal insufficiency, alcohol abuse, aspirin overdose, diabetes, drugs, toxins, liver disease, renal disease, sepsis, certain tumors	Consider clinical setting and obtain finger-stick glucose or stat blood glucose measurements (may be obtained on ABG specimen). If glucose < 60 mg/dl, treat: 50 ml = 25 g of D50W I.V. Follow glucose levels closely posttreatment.*
Hypomagnesemia	Alcohol abuse, burns, diabetic ketoacidosis, severe diarrhea, diuretics, drugs (e.g., cisplatin, cyclosporine, pentamidine), malabsorption, poor intake, thyrotoxicosis	Obtain stat serum magnesium level. Treat: 1–2 g magnesium sulfate I.V. over 2 min. Follow magnesium levels over time, because blood levels correlate poorly with total body deficit.
Hypothermia	Alcohol abuse, burns, central nervous system disease, debilitated and elderly patients, drowning, drugs, toxins, endocrine disease, exposure history, homelessness, poverty, extensive skin disease, spinal cord disease, trauma	Obtain core body temperature. If severe hypothermia (< 30° C), limit initial shocks for pulseless VT/VF to three, initiate active internal rewarming and cardiopulmonary support, and hold further resuscitation medications or shocks until core temperature > 30° C.† If moderate hypothermia (30°–34° C), proceed with resuscitation (space medications at intervals greater than usual), passively rewarm, and actively rewarm truncal body areas.
Hypovolemia, hemorrhage, anemia	Major burns, diabetes, gastrointestinal losses, hemorrhage, hemorrhagic diathesis, malignancy, pregnancy, shock, trauma	Initiate large-volume I.V. crystalloid resuscitation. Obtain stat hemoglobin level on ABG specimen. Emergently transfuse packed red blood cells (O negative if type-specific blood not available) if hemorrhage or profound anemia is contributing to arrest. Emergently consult necessary specialty for definitive care. Emergent thoracotomy with open cardiac massage is a consideration if experienced providers are available for the patient with penetrating trauma and cardiac arrest.
Hypoxia	All cardiac arrest patients are at risk	Reassess technical quality of CPR, oxygenation, and ventilation. Confirm correct ET tube placement. Obtain stat ABG to confirm adequate oxygenation and ventilation.
Myocardial infarction	Consider in all cardiac arrest patients, especially those with risk factors for coronary artery disease, a history of ischemic heart disease, or prearrest picture consistent with an acute coronary syndrome	Review prearrest clinical presentation and ECG. Continue resuscitation algorithm; proceed with definitive care as appropriate for the immediate circumstances (e.g., thrombolytic therapy, cardiac catheterization/coronary artery reperfusion, circulatory assist device, emergent cardiopulmonary bypass).

(continued)

be intubated, correct ET tube placement should be confirmed, and the tube should be secured. Simultaneously, intravenous access should be established.

Initiation of Drug Therapy

A parenteral drug should then be administered, after which further attempts at defibrillation should be made. The first medication given is a vasoconstrictor (either epinephrine or vasopressin) [*see* Table 4]. If there is no intravenous access, this drug can be given endotracheally. After each intravenous dose, a 20 ml saline bolus should be administered, and the extremity that contains the intravenous line should be elevated. The rescuers should continue CPR for 30 to 60 seconds to allow the drug to reach the heart, after which defibrillation should again be attempted with one to three shocks at 360 joules each. As long as the patient remains pulseless, epinephrine should be repeatedly administered every 3 to 5 minutes, with each dose followed by

one to three attempts at defibrillation. When vasopressin is the chosen initial drug, only a single dose is given; if the resuscitation continues 10 minutes or longer after vasopressin is administered, epinephrine should be substituted for vasopressin for the remainder of the code. If pulseless VT or VF persists despite the initial administration of a vasoconstrictor and repeated defibrillation attempts, antiarrhythmic drug therapy is added; amiodarone or lidocaine is an appropriate agent [*see* Choice of Antiarrhythmic Drugs, *below*]. Throughout all of these steps, the code team leader should actively look for technical and physiologic/anatomic problems that may be preventing a successful resuscitation and should correct any problems that are found [*see* Table 6].

Emergency Laboratory Tests

If spontaneous circulation does not return after the first round of antiarrhythmic drug therapy, the resuscitation team must also

Table 7   (continued)

Condition	Clinical Setting	Diagnostic and Corrective Actions
Poisoning	Alcohol abuse, bizarre or puzzling behavioral or metabolic presentation, classic toxic syndrome, occupational or industrial exposures, history of ingestion, polysubstance abuse, psychiatric disease	Consider clinical setting and presentation; provide meticulous supportive care. Emergently consult toxicologist (through regional poison center) for resuscitative and definitive care advice, including appropriate antidote use. Prolonged resuscitation efforts are appropriate. If available, immediate cardiopulmonary bypass should be considered.
Hyperkalemia	Metabolic acidosis, excessive administration, drugs and toxins, vigorous exercise, hemolysis, renal disease, rhabdomyolysis, tumor lysis syndrome, significant tissue injury	Obtain stat serum potassium level on ABG specimen. Treatment: calcium chloride 10% (5–10 ml I.V. slow push [do not use if hyperkalemia is secondary to digitalis poisoning]), followed by glucose and insulin (50 ml of D50W and 10 U regular insulin I.V.); sodium bicarbonate (50 mEq I.V.); albuterol (15–20 mg nebulized or 0.5 mg I.V. infusion).[‡]
Hypokalemia	Alcohol abuse, diabetes, diuretic use, drugs and toxins, profound gastrointestinal losses, hypomagnesemia, excess mineralocorticoid states, metabolic alkalosis	Obtain stat serum potassium level on ABG specimen. If profound hypokalemia (K[+] < 2–2.5 mEq/L) is contributing to cardiac arrest, initiate urgent I.V. replacement (2 mEq/min I.V. for 10–15 mEq) then reassess.[§]
Pulmonary embolism	Hospitalized patients, recent surgical procedure, peripartum, known risk factors for venous thromboembolism (VTE), history of VTE, prearrest presentation consistent with acute pulmonary embolism	Review prearrest clinical presentation; initiate appropriate volume resuscitation with I.V. crystalloid and augment with vasopressors as necessary. Attempt emergent confirmation of diagnosis, depending on availability and clinical circumstances; consider emergent cardiopulmonary bypass to maintain patient viability. Continue resuscitation algorithm; proceed with definitive care (thrombolytic therapy, embolectomy via interventional radiology, or surgical thrombectomy) as appropriate for immediate circumstances and availability.
Tension pneumothorax	Postcentral line placement, mechanical ventilation, pulmonary disease (including asthma, COPD, necrotizing pneumonia), postthoracentesis, trauma	Consider risks and clinical presentation (prearrest history, breath sounds, neck veins, tracheal deviation). Proceed with emergent needle decompression, followed by chest tube insertion.

*Unrecognized hypoglycemia can cause significant neurologic injury and can be life threatening, but caution with I.V. glucose is appropriate in the setting of cardiac arrest. Available evidence indicates that hyperglycemia may contribute to impaired neurologic recovery in cardiac arrest survivors.

†Active internal or core rewarming includes warm (42°–46° C) humidified oxygen delivered through the endotracheal tube; warm I.V. fluids; peritoneal lavage; esophageal rewarming tubes; bladder lavage; and extracorporeal rewarming if immediately available. Active external rewarming includes warming beds, hot-water bottles, heating pads, and radiant heat sources applied externally to the patient.

‡Glucose is not necessary initially if patient is already hyperglycemic, but glucose levels should be followed closely after administration of I.V. insulin because of the risk of hypoglycemia (especially in patients with renal failure, because of the long duration of action of I.V. insulin in such patients). Sodium bicarbonate is most helpful in patients with concomitant metabolic acidosis; it is less effective in lowering serum potassium in dialysis-dependent renal failure patients. High-dose nebulized albuterol should lower serum potassium by 0.5 to 1.5 mEq/L within 30 to 60 min, but administration during cardiac arrest may be difficult.

§In a non–cardiac arrest situation, usual I.V. potassium replacement guidelines for patients requiring parenteral therapy are generally 10 to 20 mEq/hr with continuous electrocardiographic monitoring. If profound hypokalemia is contributing to cardiac arrest, however, these usual replacement rates are not timely enough, given the critical nature of the situation. Under these circumstances, potassium chloride, 2 mEq/min I.V. for 10 to 15 mEq, is reasonable, but reassessment and careful attention to changing levels, redistribution, and ongoing clinical circumstances are essential to prevent life-threatening hyperkalemia from developing.

ABG—arterial blood gas   COPD—chronic obstructive pulmonary disease   D50W—50% dextrose in water   ET—endotracheal   VF—ventricular fibrillation
VT—ventricular tachycardia

endeavor to identify and treat the clinically relevant conditions causing or contributing to the cardiac arrest [*see Table 7*]. In theory, the interventions conducted to this point should have resulted in a perfusing rhythm. The code team must ask why this has not occurred, and it must attempt to answer this question as the resuscitation continues. Emergency laboratory studies that may prove helpful include a stat ABG measurement and measurements of hemoglobin, potassium, magnesium, and blood glucose levels (most of which can be obtained from the ABG specimen).

Choice of Antiarrhythmic Drugs

There are four antiarrhythmic drugs used in cardiac resuscitation: amiodarone, lidocaine, magnesium (if the patient is thought or proven to be hypomagnesemic), and procainamide (for intermittent or recurrent VT or VF that initially responds to defibrillation).[60] It is not known which one of these drugs or which combination of them will optimize the chances of patient survival to hospital discharge. Despite many years of routine use, there are no controlled studies demonstrating a survival benefit from lidocaine versus placebo in the management of pulseless VT or VF. Two recent studies in patients with shock-refractory prehospital

VF showed that survival to hospital admission was better with amiodarone than with placebo (44% versus 34%; *P* = 0.03)[61] or with lidocaine (22.8% versus 12.0%; *P* = 0.009).[62] Neither of these studies demonstrated an improved survival to hospital discharge in the amiodarone groups, but neither study had the statistical power to demonstrate such a difference. The optimal role and exact benefit of antiarrhythmic medications in cardiac resuscitation has yet to be fully elucidated. According to AHA guidelines, either amiodarone or lidocaine is an acceptable initial antiarrhythmic drug for the treatment of patients with pulseless VT or VF that is unresponsive to initial shocks, CPR, airway management, and administration of epinephrine or vasopressin plus shocks. On the basis of available evidence, however, amiodarone appears to be the antiarrhythmic agent of first choice in the setting of prehospital refractory VF.[60-62]

PULSELESS ELECTRICAL ACTIVITY

Community ACLS providers are encountering nonventricular arrhythmias (i.e., PEA and asystole) with increasing frequency. Classically, the prognosis for PEA has been poor, with outpatient survival rates generally reported as 0% to 7%.[63,64] The sequence of resuscitation steps in the management of PEA is as follows: activation of the emergency medical or code response, primary survey (CPR and rhythm evaluation), and secondary survey (intubation and confirmation of correct ET tube placement, optimal oxygenation and ventilation, establishment of I.V. access, epinephrine administration, and, finally, problem solving for technical difficulties and establishment of cause of cardiac arrest) [see Figure 2]. The two core drugs for PEA management are epinephrine (repeated every 3 to 5 minutes for as long as the patient is pulseless) and atropine (up to 3 mg over time if the PEA rhythm on the monitor is inappropriately slow). The best hope for a successful resuscitation is to find and treat the cause of PEA; therein lies the exceptionally challenging aspect of PEA resuscitation management [see Tables 6 and 7]. Because coronary artery thrombosis and pulmonary thromboembolism are common causes of cardiac arrest, a recent trial evaluated the efficacy of tissue plasminogen activator (t-PA) in the setting of PEA of unknown or presumed cardiovascular cause in 233 patients in prehospital and emergency department settings.[65] No benefit was found with thrombolytic therapy for PEA in this study; the proportion of patients with return of spontaneous circulation was 21.4% in the t-PA group and 23.3% in the placebo group.

ASYSTOLE

The prognosis for asystole is generally regarded as dismal unless the patient is hypothermic or there are other extenuating but treatable circumstances. The sequence of resuscitation steps in the management of asystole is as follows: activation of the emergency medical or code response, primary survey (CPR, rhythm evaluation, and asystole confirmation), and secondary survey (intubation and confirmation of correct ET tube placement, optimal oxygenation and ventilation, I.V. access with epinephrine and atropine administration, immediate transcutaneous pacing if available, and problem solving for technical difficulties and establishment of cause of cardiac arrest) [see Figure 2]. The two core drugs for asystole management are epinephrine (repeated every 3 to 5 minutes for as long as the patient is pulseless) and atropine (up to 3 mg over time). Potentially treatable causes of asystole have traditionally included hypoxia, acidosis, hypothermia, hypokalemia, hyperkalemia, and drug overdose. Resuscitation efforts should stop if asystole persists for longer than 10 minutes despite optimal CPR, oxygenation and ventilation, and epinephrine/atropine administration; if extenuating circumstances (e.g., hypothermia, cold-water submersion, or drug overdose) are not present; and if no other readily treatable condition is identified.

Immediate Postresuscitation Care

Even when the resuscitation is successful, the patient's situation remains tenuous and continued meticulous patient care is essential. When the cardiac monitor indicates what should be a perfusing rhythm, one should immediately confirm the presence of a palpable pulse in the patient. If there is a pulse, the patient's blood pressure should be obtained. Simultaneously, resuscitation team members should quickly reassess the adequacy of the patient's airway, the ET tube position, oxygenation and ventilation, and the patient's level of consciousness.

If the patient is hypotensive, appropriate blood pressure management depends on the presence or absence of fluid overload, as judged at the bedside. If the patient is clinically volume overloaded or in frank pulmonary edema, dopamine should be started at inotropic doses (5 μg/kg/min I.V.) and titrated to a target

systolic blood pressure of 90 to 100 mm Hg. If the patient's clinical status suggests normovolemia or hypovolemia, intravenous crystalloid boluses (in 250 to 500 ml increments) should be administered instead of dopamine to support adequate tissue perfusion. If the patient is regaining consciousness, the level of com-

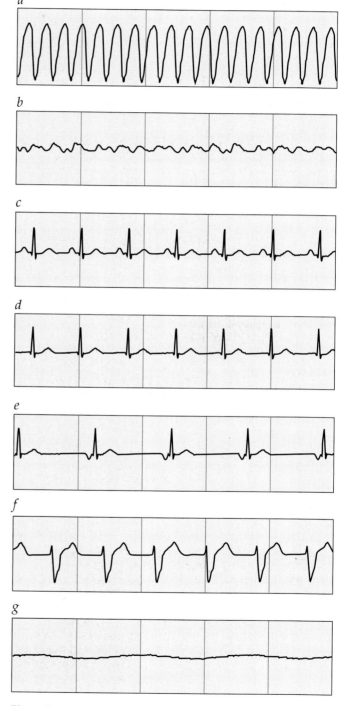

Figure 1 The sudden cardiac arrest arrhythmias. (a) Ventricular tachycardia. (b) Ventricular fibrillation. Pulseless electrical activity encompasses any of several forms of organized electrical activity in the pulseless patient; these include (c) normal sinus rhythm, (d) junctional rhythm, (e) bradycardic junctional rhythm, and (f) idioventricular rhythm. (g) Asystole.

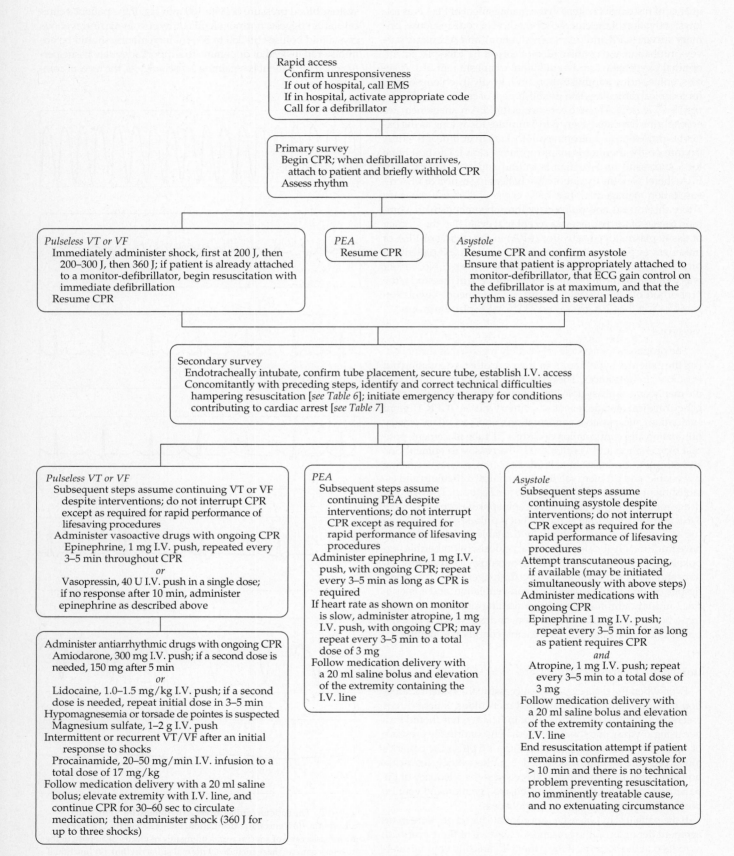

Figure 2 Treatment algorithm for patients with VT, VF, PEA, or asystole. (PEA—pulseless electrical activity;
VF—ventricular fibrillation; VT—ventricular tachycardia)

fort should be carefully assessed and analgesia and sedation administered, as indicated.

If the arrest rhythm was either VT or VF, the parenteral antiarrhythmic drug used immediately before the return of spontaneous circulation is continued as a maintenance infusion (amiodarone, 1 mg/min for 6 hr, then 0.5 mg/min for 18 hr as blood pressure allows; lidocaine, 2 to 4 mg/min). If an antiarrhythmic drug has not yet been administered, it is usually started at this point to prevent the recurrence of pulseless VT or VF. There are important exceptions to this guideline, however. If the perfusing postarrest arrhythmia is an idioventricular rhythm or third-degree heart block accompanied by an idioventricular escape rhythm, an antiarrhythmic medication should not be started at this time, because the antiarrhythmic agent could eliminate the ventricular perfusing focus and return the patient to pulselessness.

Initial postresuscitation studies usually include ECG, portable chest radiography, ABG measurement, serum electrolyte panel, fingerstick or blood glucose measurement, measurement of serum magnesium and cardiac enzyme levels, and measurement of hemoglobin and hematocrit. The resuscitated patient requires urgent transfer to the optimal site for continued definitive care. Depending on the circumstances, this may be either the cardiac catheterization laboratory or the intensive care unit.

Ending a Resuscitation Attempt

Throughout the resuscitation, the team leader should speak with calmness and authority; the leader should orchestrate the resuscitation with clarity and finesse and should make clinical decisions without directly performing specific procedures (if that is possible). All cardiac arrests are emotionally charged, but the leader must insist on a composed, orderly, and technically sound resuscitation. It is appropriate to invite suggestions from team members and to ensure that all members are comfortable with the decision to stop the resuscitation, should that time arrive.

The decision to stop a cardiac resuscitation is burdensome. Clearly, the circumstances of the event, patient comorbidities, the nature of the lethal arrhythmia, and the resuscitation team's ability to correctly identify and treat potential contributing causes to the arrest are all important considerations. Resuscitation efforts beyond 30 minutes without a return of spontaneous circulation are usually futile unless the cardiac arrest is confounded by intermittent or recurrent VT or VF, hypothermia, cold-water submersion, drug overdose, or other identified and readily treated conditions.[66,67]

In the prehospital setting (assuming proper equipment and medications are available and no extenuating circumstances suggest otherwise), full resuscitation efforts should take place at the scene of a nontraumatic cardiac arrest in preference to rapid transport to an emergency department. A prehospital resuscitation that has been appropriately conducted but has not resulted in at least temporary return of spontaneous circulation to the patient may be discontinued. It is important that certain criteria are adhered to, however, including the following: high-quality CPR was provided, an adequate airway was successfully placed, appropriate oxygenation and ventilation occurred, intravenous access was established, appropriate medications specific to the arrest scenario were administered, resuscitation was attempted for at least 10 minutes, the patient is not in persistent VF, and there are no extenuating circumstances that mandate in-hospital continuation of the resuscitation (e.g., hy-

pothermia, drug overdose). The decision to cease resuscitation efforts in the field is enhanced by direct discussion with EMS physicians. It is also essential that services be available to provide immediate assistance and support to the family and loved ones of the patient who has now died.

Discontinuing in-hospital resuscitations is advisable if the arrest was unwitnessed, the initial rhythm was other than VT or VF, and spontaneous circulation does not return after 10 minutes of ongoing resuscitation.[68] In a study of this decision rule, only 1.1% of patients (3 out of 269) who met these three parameters survived to hospital discharge, and none of these survivors were capable of independent living.[69] In a recent study of 445 prospectively recorded resuscitation attempts in hospitalized patients, no patient survived who suffered a cardiac arrest between 12 A.M. and 6 A.M. if the arrest was unwitnessed and if it occurred in an unmonitored bed.[33]

A resuscitation attempt in a persistently asystolic patient should not last longer than 10 minutes, assuming all of the following conditions apply: asystole is confirmed through proper rhythm monitoring and assessment, high-quality CPR is taking place, ET intubation was correctly performed and confirmed, adequate oxygenation and ventilation have occurred, intravenous access is present, appropriate medications (epinephrine and atropine) have been administered, and the patient is not the victim of hypothermia, cold-water submersion, drug overdose, or other readily identified and reversible cause.

After all resuscitation attempts, the code leader should debrief the team so that all may learn from the experience. Finally, marked empathy and skill are needed to carefully and compassionately inform family members about the outcome of the resuscitation.[70]

References

1. Callans DJ: Management of the patient who has been resuscitated from sudden cardiac death. Circulation 105:2704, 2002

2. Zipes DP, Wellens HJ: Sudden cardiac death. Circulation 98:2334, 1998

3. Eisenberg MS, Mengert TJ: Cardiac resuscitation. N Engl J Med 344:1304, 2001

4. 1999 Heart and Stroke Statistical Update. American Heart Association, Dallas, 1998

5. Ballew KA, Philbrick JT: Causes of variation in reported in-hospital CPR survival: a critical review. Resuscitation 30:203, 1995

6. Myerburg RJ, Castellanos A: Cardiac arrest and sudden cardiac death. Heart Disease: A Textbook of Cardiovascular Medicine. Braunwald E, Ed. WB Saunders Co, Philadelphia, 1997, p 742

7. Osborn LA: Etiology of sudden death. Cardiac Arrest: The Science and Practice of Resuscitation Medicine. Paradis NA, Halperin HR, Nowak RM, Eds. Williams & Wilkins, Philadelphia, 1996, p 243

8. Cummins RO, Ornato JP, Thies W, et al: Improving survival from cardiac arrest: the chain of survival concept: a statement for health professionals from the Advanced Cardiac Life Support Subcommittee and the Emergency Cardiac Care Committee, American Heart Association. Circulation 83:1832, 1991

9. Capussi A, Aschieri D, Piepoli MF, et al: Tripling survival from sudden cardiac arrest via early defibrillation without traditional education in cardiopulmonary resuscitation. Circulation 106:1065, 2002

10. Callaham M, Madsen CD: Relationship of timeliness of paramedic advanced life support interventions to outcome in out-of-hospital cardiac arrest treated by first responders with defibrillators. Ann Emerg Med 27:638, 1996

11. Marenco JP, Wang PJ, Link MS, et al: Improving survival from sudden cardiac arrest: the role of the automated external defibrillator. JAMA 285:1193, 2001

12. Peberdy MA: Defibrillation. Cardiol Clin 20:13, 2002

13. Cummins RO, Eisenberg MS: Prehospital cardiopulmonary resuscitation: is it effective? JAMA 253:2408, 1985

14. Stapleton ER: Basic life support cardiopulmonary resuscitation. Cardiol Clin 20:12, 2002

15. Valenzuela TD, Roe DJ, Cretin S, et al: Estimating effectiveness of cardiac arrest interventions: a logistic regression survival model. Circulation 96:3308, 1997

16. Eisenberg MS, Bergner L, Hallstrom A: Cardiac resuscitation in the community: the importance of rapid delivery of care and implications for program planning. JAMA 241:1905, 1979

17. Weaver WD, Cobb LA, Hallstrom AP, et al: Considerations for improving survival from out-of-hospital cardiac arrest. Ann Emerg Med 15:1181, 1986

18. Larsen MP, Eisenberg MS, Cummins RO, et al: Predicting survival from out-of-hospital cardiac arrest: a graphic model. Ann Emerg Med 270:1211, 1993

19. Eisenberg MS, Horwood BT, Cummins RO, et al: Cardiac arrest and resuscitation: a tale of 29 cities. Ann Emerg Med 19:179, 1990

20. Lombardi G, Gallagher J, Gennis P: Outcome of out-of-hospital cardiac arrest in New York City: The Pre-Hospital Arrest Survival Evaluation (PHASE) study. JAMA 271:678, 1994

21. Becker LB, Ostrander MP, Barrett J, et al: Outcome of CPR in a large metropolitan area: where are the survivors? Ann Emerg Med 20:355, 1991

22. Killien SY, Geyman JP, Gossom JB, et al: Out-of-hospital cardiac arrest in a rural area: a 16-year experience with lessons learned and national comparisons. Ann Emerg Med 28:294, 1996

23. Valenzuela TD, Roe DJ, Nichol G, et al: Outcomes of rapid defibrillation by security officers after cardiac arrest in casinos. N Engl J Med 343:1206, 2000

24. Eisenberg M, Bergner L, Hallstrom A: Sudden Cardiac Death in the Community. Praeger, Philadelphia, 1984

25. Becker L: The epidemiology of sudden death. Cardiac Arrest: The Science and Practice of Resuscitation Medicine. Paradis NA, Halperin HR, Nowak RM, Eds. Williams & Wilkins, Philadelphia, 1996, p 28

26. Jastremski MS: In-hospital cardiac arrest. Ann Emerg Med 22:113, 1993

27. Rosenberg M, Wang C, Hoffman-Wilde S, et al: Results of cardiopulmonary resuscitation failure to predict survival in two community hospitals. Arch Intern Med 153:1370, 1993

28. Ballew KA, Philbrick JT, Caven DE, et al: Predictors of survival following in-hospital cardiopulmonary resuscitation: a moving target. Arch Intern Med 154:2426, 1994

29. De Vos R, Koster RW, deHaan RJ, et al: In-hospital cardiopulmonary resuscitation: prearrest morbidity and outcome. Arch Intern Med 159:845, 1999

30. Goodlin SJ, Zhong Z, Lynn J, et al: Factors associated with use of cardiopulmonary resuscitation in seriously ill hospitalized adults. JAMA 282:2333, 1999

31. Van Walraven C, Forster AJ, Stiell IG: Derivation of a clinical decision rule for the discontinuation of in-hospital cardiac arrest resuscitations. Arch Intern Med 159:129, 1999

32. Zoch TW, Desbiens NA, DeStefano F, et al: Short- and long-term survival after cardiopulmonary resuscitation. Arch Intern Med 160:1969, 2000

33. Dumot JA, Burval DJ, Sprung J, et al: Outcome of adult cardiopulmonary resuscitations at a tertiary referral center including results of "limited" resuscitations. Arch Intern Med 161:1751, 2001

34. Meade M: Men and the Water of Life. Harper, San Francisco, 1993, p 442

35. Burkle FM Jr, Rice MM: Code organization. Am J Emerg Med 5:235, 1987

36. ACLS Provider Manual. American Heart Association, Dallas, 2001

37. Safar P: On the history of modern resuscitation. Anesthesiol Clin North Am 13:751, 1995

38. Kouwenhoven WB, Jude JR, Knickerbocker GG: Closed-chest cardiac massage. JAMA 173:1064, 1960

39. Jude JR, Kouwenhoven WB, Knickerbocker GG: Cardiac arrest: report of application of external cardiac massage on 118 patients. JAMA 178:1063, 1961

40. Halperin HR: Mechanisms of forward flow during external chest compression. Cardiac Arrest: The Science and Practice of Resuscitation Medicine. Paradis NA, Halperin HR, Nowak RM, Eds. Williams & Wilkins, Philadelphia, 1996, p 252

41. Ornato JP, Peberdy MA: Cardiopulmonary resuscitation. Textbook of Cardiovascular Medicine. Topol EJ, Ed. Lippincott-Raven, Philadelphia, 1998, p 1779

42. Paradis NA, Martin GB, Goetting MG, et al: Simultaneous aortic, jugular bulb, and right atrial pressures during cardiopulmonary resuscitation in humans: insights into mechanisms. Circulation 80:361, 1989

43. Daya MR, Mariani RJ: Out-of-hospital splinting. Clinical Procedures in Emergency Medicine, 3rd ed. Roberts JR, Hedges JR, Eds. WB Saunders Co, Philadelphia 1998, p 1297

44. Guidelines 2000 for cardiopulmonary resuscitation and emergency cardiovascular care: international consensus on science. Circulation 102(suppl I):1, 2000

45. Levine RL, Wayne MA, Miller CC: End-tidal carbon dioxide and outcome of out-of-hospital cardiac arrest. N Engl J Med 337:301, 1997

46. Hedges JR, Greenberg MI: Defibrillation. Clinical Procedures in Emergency Medicine, 3rd ed. Roberts JR, Hedges JR, Eds. WB Saunders Co, Philadelphia, 1998, p 1297

47. Hossack KF, Hartwig R: Cardiac arrest associated with supervised cardiac rehabilitation. J Cardiac Rehab 2:402, 1982

48. Bardy GH, Marchlinski FE, Sharma AD, et al: Multicenter comparison of truncated biphasic shocks and standard damped sine wave monophasic shocks for transthoracic ventricular defibrillation. Circulation 94:2507, 1996

49. Gliner BE, White RD: Electrocardiographic evaluation of defibrillation shocks delivered to out-of-hospital sudden cardiac arrest patients. Resuscitation 41:129, 1999

50. Gliner BE, Jorgenson DB, Poole JE, et al: Treatment of out-of-hospital cardiac arrest with a low-energy impedance-compensating biphasic waveform automatic external defibrillator. Biomed Instrum Technol 32:631, 1998

51. Poole JE, White RD, Kanz KG, et al: Low-energy impedance-compensating biphasic waveforms terminate ventricular fibrillation at high rates in victims of out-of-hospital cardiac arrest. J Cardiovasc Electrophysiol 8:1373, 1997

52. Schneider T, Martens PR, Paschen H, et al: Multicenter, randominzed, controlled trial of 150-J biphasic shocks compared with 200- to 360-J monophasic shocks in the resuscitation of out-of-hospital cardiac arrest victims. Circulation 102:1780, 2000

53. Aehlert B: ACLS: Quick Review Study Guide, 2nd ed. CV Mosby, St Louis, 2001

54. Rumball CJ, MacDonald D: The PTL, Combitube, laryngeal mask, and oral airway: a randomized prehospital comparative study of ventilatory device effectiveness and cost-effectiveness in 470 cases of cardiorespiratory arrest. Prehosp Emerg Care 1:1, 1997

55. Garnett AR, Ornato JP, Gonzales ER, et al: End-tidal carbon dioxide monitoring during cardiopulmonary resuscitation. JAMA 257:512, 1987

56. Paradis NA, Wenzel V, Southall J: Pressor drugs in the treatment of cardiac arrest. Cardiol Clin 20:61, 2002

57. Stiell IG, Hebert PC, Wells GA, et al: Vasopressin versus epinephrine for inhospital cardiac arrest: a randomized controlled trial. Lancet 358:105, 2001

58. Tiffany PA, Schultz M, Stueven H: Bolus thrombolytic infusions during CPR for patients with refractory arrest rhythms: outcome of a case series. Ann Emerg Med 31:124, 1998

59. Cummins RO, Chamberlain DA: Advisory statements of the International Liaison Committee on Resuscitation. Circulation 95:2172, 1997

60. Kudenchuk PJ: Advanced cardiac life support antiarrhythmic drugs. Cardiol Clin 20:79, 2002

61. Kudenchuk PJ, Cobb LA, Copass MK, et al: Amiodarone for resuscitation after out-of-hospital cardiac arrest due to ventricular fibrillation. N Engl J Med 341:871, 1999

62. Dorian P, Cass D, Schwartz B, et al: Amiodarone as compared with lidocaine for shock-resistant ventricular fibrillation. N Engl J Med 346:884, 2002

63. Myerburg RJ, Conde CA, Sung RJ, et al: Clinical, electrophysiologic, and hemodynamic profile of patients resuscitated from prehospital cardiac arrest. Am J Med 68:568, 1980

64. Stratton SJ, Niemann JT: Outcome from out-of-hospital cardiac arrest caused by nonventricular arrhythmias: contribution of successful resuscitation to overall survivorship supports the current practice of initiating out-of-hospital ACLS. Ann Emerg Med 32:448, 1998

65. Abu-Laban RB, Christenson JM, Innes GD, et al: Tissue plasminogen activator in cardiac arrest with pulseless electrical activity. N Engl J Med 346:1522, 2002

66. Bonnin MJ, Pepe PE, Kimball KT, et al: Distinct criteria for termination of resuscitation in the out-of-hospital setting. JAMA 270:1457, 1993

67. Kellermann AL, Hackman BB, Somes G: Predicting the outcome of unsuccessful prehospital advanced cardiac life support. JAMA 270:1433, 1993

68. Van Walraven C, Forster AJ, Stiell IG: Derivation of a clinical decision rule for the discontinuation of in-hospital cardiac arrest resuscitations. Arch Intern Med 159:129, 1999

69. Van Walraven C, Forster AJ, Parish DC, et al: Validation of a clinical decision aid to discontinue in-hospital cardiac arrest resuscitations. JAMA 285:1602, 2001

70. Iserson K: Grave Words: Notifying Survivors about Sudden, Unexpected Deaths. Galen Press, Tucson, Arizona, 1999

71. Cummins RO, Field JM, Hazinski MF, et al: ACLS Provider Manual. American Heart Association, Dallas, 2001, p 36

72. Part 1: introduction to the international guidelines 2000 for CPR and ECC: a consensus on science. Circulation 102(8 suppl):I1, 2000

13 Management of Poisoning and Drug Overdose

Kent R. Olson, M.D., and Manish M. Patel, M.D.

Drug overdose and poisoning are leading causes of emergency department visits and hospital admissions in the United States, accounting for more than 250,000 emergency department visits[1] and 7,000 deaths[2] each year. Exposure to poison can occur in several ways. The patient may have ingested it accidentally or for the purpose of committing suicide, may be a victim of accidental intoxication from acute or chronic exposure in the workplace, may be suffering from unexpected complications or overdose after intentional drug abuse, or may be a victim of an assault or terrorist attack. Poisons can include drugs; chemicals; biotoxins in plants, mushrooms, or foods; and toxic gases. In all cases of poisoning, the clinician has several priorities: (1) immediately stabilize the patient and manage life-threatening complications; (2) perform a careful diagnostic evaluation, which includes obtaining a directed history, performing a physical examination, and ordering appropriate laboratory tests; (3) prevent further absorption of the drug or poison by decontaminating the skin or gastrointestinal tract; and (4) consider administering antidotes and performing other measures that enhance elimination of the drug from the body. For expert assistance with identification of poisons, diagnosis and treatment, and referral to a medical toxicologist, the clinician should consider consulting with a regional poison-control center.

Initial Stabilization

In many cases of poisoning, the patient is awake and has stable vital signs, which allows the clinician to proceed in a stepwise fashion to obtain a history and to perform a physical examination. In other cases, however, the patient is unconscious, is experiencing convulsions, or has unstable blood pressure or cardiac rhythm, thus requiring immediate stabilization [*see Table 1*].

The first priority is the airway. The airway's reflex protective mechanisms may be impaired because of drug-induced central nervous system depression (e.g., from opioids or sedative-hypnotic agents), excessive bronchial and oral secretions (e.g., from organophosphate insecticides), or swelling or burns (e.g., from corrosive agents or irritant gases). The airway should be cleared by the use of suction and by repositioning the patient; if the patient has an impaired gag reflex or other evidence of airway compromise, a cuffed endotracheal tube should be inserted. The adequacy of ventilation and oxygenation should be determined by clinical assessment, pulse oximetry, measurement of arterial blood gases, or a combination of these techniques. Supplemental oxygen should be administered, and if necessary, ventilation should be assisted with a bag/valve/mask device or a ventilator.[3] Even if the patient is not unconscious or hemodynamically compromised on arrival in the emergency department, continued absorption of the ingested drug or poison may lead to more serious intoxication during the next several hours. Therefore, it is prudent to keep the patient under close observation, with continuous or frequent monitoring of alertness, vital signs, the electrocardiogram, and pulse oximetry.

Management of Common Complications

COMA

Poisoning or drug overdose depresses the sensorium, the symptoms of which may range from stupor or obtundation to unresponsive coma. Deeply unconscious patients may appear to be dead because they may have nonreactive pupils, absent reflexes, and flat electroencephalographic tracings; however, such patients may have a complete recovery without neurologic sequelae as long as they receive adequate supportive care, including airway protection, oxygenation, and assisted ventilation.[4]

All patients with a depressed sensorium should be evaluated for hypoglycemia because many drugs and poisons can directly reduce or contribute to the reduction of blood glucose levels. A finger-stick blood glucose test and bedside assessment should be performed immediately; if such testing and assessment are impractical, an intravenous bolus of 25 g of 50% dextrose in water should be administered empirically before the laboratory report arrives.[5] For alcoholic or malnourished persons, who may have vitamin deficiencies, 50 to 100 mg of vitamin B_1 (thiamine) should be administered I.V. or I.M. to prevent the development of Wernicke syndrome.[5] If signs of recent opioid use (e.g., suspicious-looking pill bottles or I.V. drug paraphernalia) are in evidence or if the patient has clinical manifestations of excessive opioid effect (e.g., miosis or respiratory depression), the administration of naloxone may have both therapeutic and diagnostic value. Naloxone is a specific opioid antagonist with no intrinsic opioid-agonist effects.[6,7] Initially, a dose of 0.2 to 0.4 mg I.V. should be administered, and if there is no response, repeated doses of up to 4 to 5 mg should be given; doses as high as 15 to 20 mg may be administered if overdose with a resistant opioid (e.g., propoxyphene, codeine, or some fentanyl derivatives) is suspected.[6,7] Patients with opioid intoxication usually become fully awake within 2 to 3 minutes after naloxone administration. Failure to respond to naloxone suggests that (1) the diagnosis is

---

Table 1 The ABCDs of Initial
Stabilization of the Poisoned Patient

Airway
Position the patient to open the airway; suction any secretions or vomitus; evaluate airway protective reflexes; consider endotracheal intubation

Breathing
Determine adequacy of ventilation; assist ventilation, if necessary; administer supplemental oxygen

Circulation
Evaluate perfusion, blood pressure, and cardiac rhythm; determine QRS complex; attach continuous cardiac monitor

Dextrose
Quickly determine blood glucose by finger-stick test; give dextrose if patient is suspected of having hypoglycemia

Decontamination
Perform surface and gastric decontamination to limit absorption of poisons

---

Table 2 Mechanisms of Drug-Induced Hypotension

Mechanism	Selected Causes
Hypovolemia	
Vomiting and diarrhea	Iron; arsenic; food poisoning; organophosphates and carbamates; mushroom poisoning; thallium
Sweating	Organophosphates and carbamates
Venodilatations	Barbiturates; other sedative-hypnotic agents
Depressed cardiac contractility	Tricyclic antidepressants; beta blockers; calcium antagonists; class IA and class IC antiarrhythmic agents; sedative-hypnotic agents
Reduced peripheral vascular resistance	Theophylline; beta$_2$-adrenergic stimulants; phenothiazines; tricyclic antidepressants; hydralazine

incorrect [see Factors to Be Excluded in Diagnosis, *below*]; (2) other, nonopioid drugs may have been ingested; (3) a hypoxic insult may have occurred before the victim was found and resuscitated; or (4) an inadequate dose of naloxone was given.

Flumazenil, a short-acting, specific benzodiazepine antagonist with no intrinsic agonist effects, can rapidly reverse coma caused by diazepam and other benzodiazepines.[5,7] However, it has not found a place in the routine management of unconscious patients with drug overdose, because it has the potential to cause seizures in patients who are chronically consuming large quantities of benzodiazepines or who have ingested an acute overdose of benzodiazepines and a tricyclic antidepressant or other potentially convulsant drug [see Sedative-Hypnotic Agents, *below*]. [5,7]

HYPOTENSION AND CARDIAC DYSRHYTHMIAS

The hypotension that commonly complicates drug intoxication has many possible causes [see *Table 2*].[8,9] Hypotension may result from volume depletion caused by severe drug-induced vomiting or diarrhea. In addition, relative hypovolemia may be caused by the venodilating effects of many drugs. Certain drugs or poisons can have direct negative inotropic or chronotropic effects on the heart, reducing cardiac output. Others can cause a severe reduction in peripheral vascular resistance. Some drugs or poisons can cause shock by a combination of these mechanisms.

Treatment of drug-induced shock includes rapid assessment of the likely cause, which is suggested by the history of exposure and the clinical findings. Hypotension with tachycardia suggests that the cause is volume depletion or reduced peripheral vascular resistance, whereas hypotension with bradycardia suggests that the cause is disturbance of cardiac rhythm or generalized cardiodepressant effects of the drug. Regardless of the etiology, most patients benefit from an I.V. bolus of fluid (e.g., 0.5 to 1 L of normal saline) and empirical pressor therapy with dopamine or norepinephrine.[10] However, if hypoperfusion persists, it may be necessary to insert a pulmonary arterial catheter to obtain more specific information about volume and hemodynamic status.

A variety of cardiac dysrhythmias may occur as a result of drug intoxication or poisoning [see *Table 3*]. In addition to the direct pharmacologic actions of the drug or poison, impaired ventilation and oxygenation may trigger disturbances of cardiac rhythm.[10]

Treatment of a cardiac dysrhythmia depends on its etiology. Because conventional advanced cardiac life support (ACLS) protocols were not designed with poisoning in mind, use of these guidelines may have inappropriate or dangerous effects. For ex-

ample, a patient with tricyclic antidepressant intoxication (see below) may have wide-complex tachycardia resulting from severe depression of sodium-dependent channels in the myocardial cell membrane. However, use of the ACLS protocols for wide-complex tachycardia or possible ventricular tachycardia may lead the treating physician to administer procainamide, a class IA antiarrhythmic agent with cardiodepressant effects that are additive to those of the tricyclic antidepressants.[10] A patient with multiple premature ventricular contractions or runs of ventricular tachycardia after intoxication with chloral hydrate or inhalation of a chlorinated solvent would respond more readily to a beta blocker than to lidocaine, the drug recommended by the ACLS protocols.[11] Finally, cardiac dysrhythmias from digitalis intoxication are most appropriately treated with digoxin-specific antibodies (see below).

HYPERTENSION

Although hypertension is not commonly recognized as a serious pharmacologic effect of drug intoxication, it may have life-threatening consequences and requires aggressive treatment. Hypertension may result from generalized CNS and sympathetic stimulation (e.g., by amphetamines or cocaine) or from the peripheral actions of drugs such as phenylpropanolamine, a potent alpha-adrenergic agonist.[12] (Although the Food and Drug Administration removed phenylpropanolamine from the market in the United States in November 2000, patients may have access to phenylpropanolamine purchased before then; also, phenylpropanolamine is still available in other countries.) In addition, hypertension may result from the pharmacologic interaction of two agents, such as in the use of a stimulant or the ingestion of an inappropriate food by a person taking monoamine oxidase (MAO) inhibitors.[13] Severe hypertension can lead to intracranial hemorrhage, aortic dissection, or other catastrophic complications.[14,15]

Hypertension may be accompanied by tachycardia, as commonly occurs in cases of intoxication with generalized stimulants such as cocaine and amphetamine derivatives. Hypertension may also be accompanied by bradycardia or even atrioventricu-

Table 3 Causes of Cardiac Disturbances

Type of Disturbance	Selected Causes
Sinus tachycardia	Anticholinergic agents (e.g., diphenhydramine, atropine, tricyclic antidepressants); theophylline and caffeine; cocaine and amphetamines; volume depletion
Bradycardia or atrioventricular block	Beta blockers; calcium antagonists; tricyclic antidepressants; class IA and class IC antiarrhythmic agents; organophosphate and carbamate insecticides; digitalis glycosides; phenylpropanolamine (hypertension with reflex bradycardia)
Widening of the QRS complex	Tricyclic antidepressants; class IA and class IC antiarrhythmic agents; diphenhydramine; thioridazine; propoxyphene; hyperkalemia; hypothermia
Ventricular tachycardia or ventricular fibrillation	Tricyclic antidepressants; cocaine and amphetamines; theophylline; digitalis glycosides; fluoride or hydrofluoric acid burns (hypocalcemia); trichloroethane and numerous other chlorinated, fluorinated, and aromatic solvents; chloral hydrate; agents that cause prolongation of the QT interval (e.g., quinidine, sotalol)

lar (AV) block, which may occur after phenylpropanolamine overdose because of the reflex baroreceptor response.

Treatment is directed at the cause of the hypertension. In patients who have taken cocaine, amphetamines, or other generalized stimulants, mild or moderate increases in blood pressure may be reduced simply by providing a quiet environment and administering a sedative agent such as diazepam. In persons who have taken an overdose of phenylpropanolamine, administration of a specific alpha-adrenergic antagonist, such as phentolamine (2 to 5 mg I.V.), is extremely effective and usually leads to normalization of the slow heart rate or reversal of the AV block.[12] In general, beta blockers should not be used as single agents in the treatment of drug-induced hypertension, because their use may lead to unopposed alpha-adrenergic activity with paradoxically worsened hypertension.[16]

SEIZURES

Seizures may result from a number of factors, including a variety of drugs and poisons. The drugs that most commonly induce seizures are tricyclic antidepressants, cocaine and related stimulants, antihistamines, and isoniazid [see Table 4].[17] Prolonged or repeated convulsions can lead to serious complications, including hyperthermia, rhabdomyolysis, brain damage, and death. In addition, seizure activity causes metabolic acidosis, which may worsen cardiotoxicity in patients who have taken an overdose of a tricyclic antidepressant.[10,17] Seizures can also result from hypoxia, hypoglycemia, head trauma, stroke, or serious CNS infections [see Factors to Be Excluded in Diagnosis, below].

Treatment of seizures includes taking immediate steps to protect the airway and provide oxygen while administering anticonvulsant drugs. The blood glucose level should be determined and dextrose administered if needed [see Coma, above]. Initial anticonvulsant therapy consists of diazepam (5 to 10 mg I.V.), lorazepam (1 to 2 mg I.V.), or midazolam (3 to 5 mg I.V. or, if I.V.

access is not immediately available, 5 to 10 mg I.M.). Repeated doses are given if the initial therapy is ineffective. If convulsions persist, administer phenobarbital at a dosage of 15 to 20 mg/kg (1 to 1.5 g) I.V. over 20 to 30 minutes.[18] Phenytoin is not a first-line anticonvulsant agent for drug- or toxin-induced seizures. If seizure activity continues, the physician should consult with a neurologist and consider administering pentobarbital, another short-acting barbiturate, or propofol.[18] In addition, inducing neuromuscular paralysis (e.g., with pancuronium) should be considered to control the muscle hyperactivity, which may be necessary to control the hyperthermia, rhabdomyolysis, or metabolic acidosis. If neuromuscular paralysis is induced, however, the physician should be aware that seizure activity in the brain may persist but may not be apparent.[18] If isoniazid poisoning is suspected, administer pyridoxine (vitamin B_6), 5 g intravenously; or if more than 5 g of isoniazid was ingested, administer B_6 in an amount (in grams) equal to that of the isoniazid overdose.

HYPERTHERMIA

Hyperthermia is an underrecognized complication of poisoning and drug overdose that is associated with high morbidity and mortality.[19] It may result from the pharmacologic effects of the agent or as a consequence of prolonged muscle hyperactivity or seizures [see Table 5]. Severe hyperthermia (rectal temperature > 104° F [40° C]) that goes untreated may lead to brain damage, coagulopathy, rhabdomyolysis, hypotension, and, ultimately, death.[19]

Because it is immediately life threatening, hyperthermia warrants immediate and aggressive treatment.[19] Therapy is directed at the underlying cause, which is usually excessive muscle activity or rigidity. For mild or moderate cases, the physician should use appropriate pharmacologic agents (e.g., sedatives for cases of stimulant-induced psychosis and hyperactivity and anticonvulsants for cases of seizure), remove the patient's clothing, and maximize evaporative cooling by spraying the exposed skin with tepid water and fanning the patient. For severe cases, the most rapidly effective treatment is neuromuscular paralysis accompanied by maximal evaporative cooling.[19] In some cases, a specific antidote or therapeutic agent may be available [see Table 5].

HYPOTHERMIA

Hypothermia may accompany drug overdose and is usually caused by environmental exposure combined with inadequacy of the patient's response mechanisms. These inadequate mechanisms may include impaired judgment (in patients who have taken opioids, sedative-hypnotic agents, or phenothiazines or who have underlying mental disorders), a reduced shivering response (in those who have taken phenothiazines or sedative-hypnotic agents), and peripheral vasodilatation (in those who have taken phenothiazines or vasodilators).[20] Severe hypothermia (core temperature < 82° F [28° C]) may cause the patient to appear to be dead and may be associated with barely perceptible blood pressure, heart rate, or neurologic reflexes. Hypotension, bradycardia, and ventricular arrhythmias may fail to respond to pharmacologic treatment until the patient is warmed.[20,21] Because no controlled trials comparing rewarming methods exist, management protocols vary institutionally and are often controversial.[20] Treatment of hypothermia is generally administered gradually because more aggressive management may precipitate cardiac dysrhythmias. Passive external rewarming is an acceptable treatment if the patient's condition is stable. Administration of a warmed mist inhalation or warmed I.V. fluids may be helpful, as

Table 4 **Drug-Induced Seizures**

Common Causes	Comments
Tricyclic antidepressants	Seizure activity and resulting metabolic acidosis often aggravate cardiotoxicity; protracted seizures with absent sweating may lead to hyperthermia; phenytoin worsens cardiotoxicity in animal models; treat with benzodiazepines or phenobarbital
Cocaine and amphetamines	Seizures are usually brief and self-limited; prolonged seizures suggest an alternative diagnosis or complication (e.g., hyperthermia or intracranial hemorrhage)
Theophylline	Seizures are often prolonged, recurrent, and refractory to anticonvulsant therapy; phenytoin is ineffective in animal models; administer high-dose phenobarbital (at least 15–20 mg/kg I.V.); for patients with serum theophylline levels > 100 mg/L or status epilepticus, consider hemoperfusion or hemodialysis
Diphenhydramine	Seizures are usually brief and self-limited; in patients with massive intoxication (e.g., > 4–5 g), tricycliclike cardiotoxicity may also occur
Isoniazid	Seizures are often accompanied by severe lactic acidosis; the specific antidote for seizures and coma is vitamin B_6 (pyridoxine), 5–10 g I.V., or, if the amount of ingested isoniazid is known, the equivalent gram-for-gram amount of vitamin B_6

Table 5 Drug-Induced Hyperthermia

Mechanisms	Selected Causes and Comments
Increased metabolic activity	Causes include salicylates, dinitrophenol, and cocaine and amphetamines
Reduced sweating	Causes include anticholinergic agents (e.g., tricyclic antidepressants, antihistamines, many plants, and some mushrooms)
Increased muscle activity or exertion	Causes include cocaine and amphetamines, phencyclidine, and exertional heatstroke
Neuroleptic malignant syndrome	Causes include haloperidol, related antipsychotic agents, and lithium; patients have lead-pipe rigidity, acidosis, and an elevated creatine kinase level that are caused by CNS dopamine blockade; specific treatment is bromocriptine (2.5–10.0 mg by nasogastric tube two to six times daily)[146]; treat severe hyperthermia with neuromuscular paralysis
Malignant hyperthermia	An inherited disorder of muscle cell function, commonly triggered by certain anesthetic agents (e.g., succinylcholine or halothane); causes severe muscle rigidity and acidosis not responsive to neuromuscular paralysis; treatment is dantrolene (2–5 mg/kg I.V.)[147]
Serotonin syndrome	Associated with the use of serotonin-enhancing agents (e.g., meperidine, dextromethorphan, fluoxetine, paroxetine, sertraline, L-tryptophan, or trazodone), especially in patients taking monoamine oxidase inhibitors; causes muscle rigidity, acidosis, and hyperthermia; treatment is neuromuscular paralysis; for mild cases, consider cyproheptadine (4 mg p.o. every hour for three or four dosages)[148] or methysergide (2 mg p.o. every 6 hr for three or four dosages)[149]

may gastric or peritoneal lavage with warmed fluids, although the heat transfer involved in these measures is variable. For profound hypothermia accompanied by evidence of severe hypoperfusion (e.g., cardiac arrest or ventricular fibrillation), more aggressive measures, such as partial cardiopulmonary or femorofemoral bypass, may be required.[20,21] Of note is that patients with severe hypothermia can withstand cardiorespiratory arrest longer than a normothermic patient—hence the old adage, "No one is dead until warm and dead."[21]

RHABDOMYOLYSIS

Rhabdomyolysis, a common complication of severe poisoning or drug overdose, may result from direct myotoxic effects of the agent, from prolonged or recurrent muscle hyperactivity or rigidity, or from prolonged immobility with mechanical compression of muscle groups.[22] Severe rhabdomyolysis (usually associated with markedly elevated serum creatine kinase levels) may cause massive myoglobinuria that results in acute tubular necrosis and renal failure. Myoglobinuria is usually recognized by the pink or reddish hue of spun serum or by a positive dipstick test for hemoglobin in the urine, with few or no red blood cells seen on microscopic examination. Severe rhabdomyolysis may also cause hyperkalemia, which results from loss of potassium from dead or injured cells.

Treatment of rhabdomyolysis includes measures to prevent further muscle breakdown (e.g., control of muscle hyperactivity and treatment of hyperthermia) and to prevent deposition of toxic myoglobin in the renal tubules. Unequivocally, the mainstay of treatment in rhabdomyolysis is aggressive volume expansion with normal saline early in the disease to maintain urine output of 200 to 300 ml/hr in those who can tolerate the fluid load.[22] Nonrandomized trials have also shown alkalinization of urine to be beneficial, but the role of mannitol and furosemide in rhabdomyolysis is less clear.[22]

Clinical Evaluation

Although the history recounted by patients who have intentionally taken a drug overdose may be unreliable, it should not be overlooked as a valuable source of information. If the patient is unwilling or unable to specify which drugs were taken and when they were ingested or to provide a pertinent medical history, family and friends may be able to do so. Family members should be asked about other medications available in the household and about exposure in the workplace and through hobbies. In addition, paramedics should be asked for any pill bottles or drug paraphernalia that they may have obtained at the scene.

A directed toxicologic physical examination may yield important clues about the drugs or poisons taken. Pertinent variables include the patient's vital signs, pupil size, lung sounds, peristaltic activity, skin moisture and color, and muscle activity; the presence or absence of unusual odors; and the presence or absence of track marks associated with I.V. drug abuse. Signs of one of the so-called autonomic syndromes [*see Table 6*] may suggest diagnostic possibilities and potential empirical interventions.[9]

The clinical laboratory may provide useful information that obviates an expensive and time-consuming toxicology screen. Recommended laboratory tests in the patient with an overdose of unknown cause include a complete blood count; measure-

Table 6 Autonomic Syndromes Induced by Drugs or Poisons

Autonomic Syndrome	Selected Causes	Empirical Interventions
Sympathomimetic (agitation; dilated pupils; elevated BP and HR; sweaty skin; hyperthermia)	Cocaine; amphetamines; pseudoephedrine	Induce sedation; initiate aggressive cooling; treat hypertension with phentolamine; treat tachycardia with beta blockers
Sympatholytic (lethargy or coma; small pupils; normal or low BP and HR; low temperature)	Barbiturates; opioids; clonidine; benzodiazepines	Give naloxone for suspected opioid overdose; consider flumazenil for benzodiazepine overdose
Cholinergic (pinpoint pupils; variable HR; sweaty skin; abdominal cramps and diarrhea)	Organophosphate and carbamate insecticides; chemical warfare nerve agents	Give atropine and pralidoxime; obtain measurements of serum and RBC cholinesterase activity
Anticholinergic (agitation; delirium; dilated pupils; tachycardia; decreased peristalsis; dry, flushed skin)	Atropine and related drugs; antihistamines; phenothiazines; tricyclic antidepressants	Obtain immediate ECG tracing to evaluate for poisoning with tricyclic antidepressants; consider physostigmine only if tricyclics are not involved

Table 7   Use of the Clinical Laboratory in the Initial Diagnosis of Poisoning

Test	Finding	Selected Causes
Arterial blood gases	Hypoventilation (elevated P_{CO_2})	CNS depressants (e.g., opioids, sedative-hypnotic agents, phenothiazines, and ethanol)
	Hyperventilation	Salicylates; carbon monoxide; other asphyxiants
Electrolytes	Anion-gap metabolic acidosis	Salicylates; methanol; ethylene glycol; carbon monoxide; cyanide; iron; isoniazid; theophylline
	Hyperkalemia	Digitalis glycosides; fluoride; potassium
	Hypokalemia	Theophylline; caffeine; beta-adrenergic agents (e.g., albuterol); soluble barium salts
Glucose	Hypoglycemia	Oral hypoglycemic agents; insulin; ethanol
Osmolality and osmolar gap	Elevated osmolar gap*	Ethanol; methanol; ethylene glycol; isopropyl alcohol; acetone
ECG	Wide QRS complex	Tricyclic antidepressants; quinidine and other class IA and class IC antiarrhythmic agents
	Prolongation of the QT interval	Quinidine and related antiarrhythmic agents
	Atrioventricular block	Calcium antagonists; digitalis glycosides
Plain abdominal x-ray	Radiopaque pills or objects	Iron; lead; potassium; calcium; chloral hydrate; some foreign bodies
Serum acetaminophen	Elevated level (> 140 mg/L 4 hr after ingestion)	Acetaminophen (may be the only clue to a recent ingestion)

*Osmolar gap = measured osmolality – calculated osmolality. Measured osmolality is performed in the laboratory using a freezing-point-depression device (do not use the vaporization method). Calculated osmolality = 2(Na) + [BUN/2.8] + [glucose/18]. The normal osmolar gap is 0 ± 5 mOsm/L.
BUN—blood urea nitrogen P_{CO_2}—carbon dioxide tension

ments of glucose, electrolytes, blood urea nitrogen, creatinine, aspartate aminotransferase (AST), and serum osmolality (both measured and calculated); ECG; and plain abdominal x-ray (KUB [kidneys, ureters, and bladder] view) [*see Table 7*]. A quantitative serum acetaminophen level should be obtained immediately because acetaminophen overdose may be difficult to diagnose in the absence of a complete and reliable history, does not produce suggestive clinical or laboratory findings, and requires prompt administration of an antidote in patients with a serious acute ingestion if hepatic injury is to be prevented.[9,23,24]

Obtaining a thorough history, performing a careful physical examination, and using the clinical laboratory in a logical manner can often enable the physician to make a tentative diagnosis and to order specific quantitative measurements of certain drugs (e.g., salicylates, valproic acid, or digoxin) when the results of such tests may alter therapy. It is rarely useful, especially in the emergency management of a poisoning victim, to order a comprehensive toxicology screen. Generally, this test is performed at an outside reference laboratory at considerable expense, and patients often awaken and confirm the tentative diagnosis before results are available (usually 1 to 2 days after testing). In addition, many common dangerous drugs and poisons (e.g., isoniazid, digitalis glycosides, calcium antagonists, beta blockers, metals, and pesticides) are not included in the screening procedure; thus, a negative toxicology screen does not rule out the possibility of poisoning.[25] So-called drugs of abuse screens for opioids, amphetamines, and cocaine are commonly performed by hospital laboratories and are useful in identifying intoxication by these substances, but should not be mistaken for a comprehensive toxicologic screening test.

FACTORS TO BE EXCLUDED IN DIAGNOSIS

Whenever a patient with suspected poisoning or drug overdose is evaluated, the possibility that other illnesses are mimicking or complicating the presentation should always be considered. These illnesses include head trauma (e.g., in the ethanol-intoxicated patient, who often falls); cerebrovascular accident; meningitis; metabolic abnormalities, such as hypoglycemia, hyponatremia, and hypoxemia; underlying liver disease; and the postictal state. In any patient with altered mental status, computed tomography of the head and lumbar puncture should be considered.

Management Issues

DECONTAMINATION AFTER ACUTE INGESTION

Nowhere in the field of toxicology is there more controversy than in the debate about gastrointestinal decontamination.[26-29] Techniques for gut decontamination include emesis, gastric lavage, administration of activated charcoal, and whole bowel irrigation [*see Table 8*].

Ipecac-induced emesis, which as recently as a decade ago was the preferred technique for gut emptying, has been almost completely abandoned. One reason it has fallen out of favor is that treated patients run the risks of sudden, unexpected deterioration from the effects of the overdose and subsequent pulmonary aspiration; more important, however, is the lack of evidence of the efficacy of ipecac-induced emesis, especially when emesis is induced more than 1 hour after the ingestion.[26,30]

Gastric lavage is still an accepted method for gut decontamination in hospitalized patients who are obtunded or comatose, but several prospective, randomized, controlled trials have failed to show that emesis or lavage plus charcoal provides better clinical results than administration of activated charcoal alone. In one study,[30] patients given a regimen of activated charcoal and patients given a combination regimen of gastric lavage and charcoal showed no significant differences in all outcome parameters, including clinical deterioration, length of hospital stay, complications, and mortality. Studies of volunteers have shown that the amount of ingested material returned with gastric lavage is only about 30%.[26,29] However, many authors agree that it may still provide results if the ingested material has caused slowing of peristalsis (e.g., in the case of anticholinergic agents or opioids) or pyloric spasm (e.g., in the case of salicylates) or is a potentially life-threatening amount of poison (e.g., 5 g of a tricyclic antidepressant).[26,27] Some investigators have suggested that gastric lavage is associated with an increased rate of complications, although adverse events are rare in clinical practice.[29]

Activated charcoal, a finely divided product of the distillation of various organic materials, has a large surface area that is capable of adsorbing many drugs and poisons.[27,29] Studies of volunteers and clinical trials have suggested that administration of activated charcoal without gastric lavage may be as effective as, or superior to, its administration after gut emptying.[26,29,30] Although it seems logical that gastric lavage in combination with the use of activated charcoal would be more effective than the use of activated charcoal alone, this hypothesis has not been proved. Most clinicians now employ oral activated charcoal without prior gut emptying in the awake patient who has taken a moderate overdose of a drug or poison; some clinicians still recommend lavage after a massive ingestion of a highly toxic drug.

There is no consensus about the use of cathartic agents with activated charcoal, although it seems logical to hasten passage of the charcoal-drug material from the intestinal tract. If cathartic agents are used, their potential adverse effects should be taken into account, especially in the very young or old (who may not be able to tolerate fluid shifts associated with osmotic cathartics such as sorbitol) or in patients with renal insufficiency (who may not be able to tolerate large doses of magnesium or sodium).

Whole bowel irrigation is a technique that was introduced for gut cleansing before surgical or endoscopic procedures and that has recently been adopted for gut decontamination after certain ingestions.[29] It involves the use of a large volume of an osmotically balanced electrolyte solution, such as Colyte or GoLYTELY, that contains nonabsorbable polyethylene glycol and that cleans the gut by mechanical action without net gain or loss of fluids or electrolytes. Whole bowel irrigation is well tolerated by most awake patients. Although no controlled clinical trials to date have demonstrated improved outcome, it is recommended for those who have ingested large doses of poisons that are not well adsorbed to charcoal (e.g., iron or lithium), for those who have ingested sustained-release or enteric-coated products, and for those who have ingested drug packets or other potentially toxic foreign bodies.[29,31]

ENHANCED ELIMINATION

Measures to enhance elimination of drugs and poisons are less popular than they were 20 years ago, primarily because it has since been recognized that the available techniques do not have a significant effect on total drug elimination of many of the most commonly ingested products and that they have little effect on the clinical course of intoxication.[8] In addition, hemodialysis and hemoperfusion are invasive procedures that require systemic anticoagulation and that are associated with potential morbidity. For a drug or poison to be considered for removal by hemodialysis or another procedure, it should have a relatively small volume of distribution, have a slow intrinsic rate of removal (clearance), and cause life-threatening intoxication that is poorly responsive to supportive measures.[8] Only a few drugs and poisons meet these criteria and are therefore efficiently removed by hemodialysis or hemoperfusion [see Table 9].

Repeated oral doses of activated charcoal can reduce the elimination half-life of some drugs and poisons by interrupting enterohepatic or enteroenteric recirculation.[26,32] This technique was introduced in the late 1970s, after studies reported its efficacy in volunteers, and it was considered a benign, noninvasive treatment. However, reports of fluid depletion and shock caused by excessive coadministration of sorbitol, as well as the paucity of evidence of clinical benefit, have reduced the initial optimism about this treatment.[26,32]

Specific Drugs and Poisons

ACETAMINOPHEN

Acetaminophen is a widely used analgesic and antipyretic drug that is found in a number of over-the-counter and prescription products. When it is taken in combination with another drug that has acute toxic effects (e.g., an opioid), the more obvious and more rapidly apparent manifestations of the second drug may cause the clinician to overlook the subtle and nonspecific symptoms of acetaminophen poisoning. As a result, the op-

Table 8 Methods of Gastrointestinal Decontamination

Method and Technique	Useful Situations	Comments
Emesis: give syrup of ipecac, 30 ml p.o. in adults (15 ml in children), along with one to two glasses of water; may repeat after 30 min if no emesis occurs; alternatively, give 1–2 tbsp of liquid handwashing or dishwashing soap	Most useful in the home for children with recent ingestions; possibly useful for ingestion of sustained-release or enteric-coated pills	Contraindicated in ingestions of corrosive agents and most hydrocarbons, when the patient is lethargic, or when the ingested substance is likely to cause abrupt onset of coma or seizures
Gastric lavage: insert large-bore nasogastric or orogastric tube, empty stomach contents, and lavage with 100–200 ml aliquots of water or saline until clear	Useful in obtunded or comatose patients, in recent ingestions (< 1 hr), or in ingestion of anticholinergic agents or salicylates (delayed gut emptying)	Obtunded patient should have prior endotracheal intubation to protect airway; best position is left lateral decubitus to reduce movement of poison into small intestine
Activated charcoal: give 50–60 g of charcoal slurry p.o. or by gastric tube; goal is approximately 10:1 ratio of charcoal to ingested poison; usually given with one dose of a cathartic agent	Often useful because it adsorbs most drugs and poisons; may be equally effective when given alone as when given after emesis or lavage	Not effective for ingestions of iron, lithium, potassium, sodium, or alcohols; may need to repeat two or three times or more for large ingestions; repeated dosing may also enhance elimination of some drugs
Whole bowel irrigation: give Colyte or GoLYTELY, 1–2 L/hr p.o. or by gastric tube, until rectal effluent is clear or x-ray is negative for radiopaque materials	Useful in ingestions of iron, lithium, sustained-release or enteric-coated pills, and drug packets or other foreign bodies	Generally well tolerated; no significant fluid or electrolyte gain or loss occurs; most useful in awake, ambulatory patients; may reduce effectiveness of activated charcoal

Table 9 Methods of and Indications for Enhanced Drug Removal

Drug or Poison	Preferred Elimination Method and Indications
Carbamazepine	Hemoperfusion is indicated for severe poisoning with status epilepticus or cardiotoxicity; repeated doses of charcoal are of possible benefit for mild to moderate poisoning and for gut decontamination
Ethanol, isopropyl alcohol	Hemodialysis is rarely indicated because supportive care is generally successful; consider hemodialysis for deep coma with refractory hypotension
Lithium	Hemodialysis is indicated for severe neurologic manifestations (deep coma or seizures); I.V. saline is fairly effective for mild to moderate intoxication
Methanol, ethylene glycol	Hemodialysis is indicated for severe acidosis or for estimated or measured drug levels > 20–50 mg/dl
Phenobarbital	Hemoperfusion is indicated for refractory shock and drug levels > 200 mg/L; repeated doses of charcoal are of questionable clinical benefit
Salicylates	Hemodialysis is indicated for severe acidosis and drug levels > 100 mg/dl; consider hemodialysis at lower salicylate levels (> 60 mg/dl) in elderly patients with chronic, accidental intoxication
Theophylline	Hemoperfusion or hemodialysis is indicated for drug levels > 100 mg/L or status epilepticus; repeated doses of charcoal are indicated for less severe cases
Valproic acid	Hemodialysis or hemoperfusion is indicated for severe cases (coma, acidosis, and drug levels > 1,000 mg/L); repeated doses of charcoal are of theoretical benefit

portunity to administer the highly effective prophylactic antidote acetylcysteine may be missed.

Acetaminophen is metabolized by various processes in the liver and, to a lesser extent, in the kidneys. One of the minor pathways of acetaminophen metabolism in the liver involves the cytochrome P-450 system, which generates a highly reactive intermediate metabolite. Normally, this toxic intermediate metabolite is readily scavenged by the intracellular antioxidant glutathione. In overdose, however, exhaustion of glutathione stores by production of the toxic intermediate metabolite allows the metabolite to react with cellular macromolecules, leading to cell injury and death. A similar process occurs in kidney cells.

The minimum acutely toxic single dose of acetaminophen is approximately 150 to 200 mg/kg, or about 7 to 10 g in adults.[33] Alcoholics are at risk for toxicity at lower doses, particularly when the drug is taken for several days, presumably because they have increased cytochrome P-450 metabolic activity and reduced glutathione stores.[34] Enhanced susceptibility to toxic effects has also been reported in persons who are fasting and in patients receiving long-term anticonvulsant therapy[35] or taking isoniazid.[34] Severe toxicity may result in fulminant hepatic and renal failure.[33]

Diagnosis

Early after acute ingestion of acetaminophen, the patient may have few or no symptoms.[36] Vomiting is not uncommon in those who have taken large doses. Other than what can be found in the patient's history, the only reliable early diagnostic clue is provided by a quantitative measurement of the serum acetaminophen level, which can be provided immediately by most hospital laboratories. Clinical evidence of liver and kidney damage is usually delayed for 24 hours or more after ingestion. The earliest evidence of toxicity is elevated levels of hepatic aminotransferases (AST and alanine aminotransferase [ALT]), followed by a rising prothrombin time (PT) and bilirubin level. Hypoglycemia, metabolic acidosis, and encephalopathy are signs of a poor prognosis.[33]

Treatment

Oral activated charcoal should be administered. Ipecac-induced emesis is not recommended, because it often leads to protracted vomiting, which makes administration of the oral antidote difficult. A serum acetaminophen level should be obtained approximately 4 hours after ingestion, and the result should be plotted on the Rumack-Matthew nomogram [see Figure 1]. Ingestion of massive quantities of acetaminophen or a modified-release preparation or the coingestion of a drug that slows gastric emptying may result in delayed peak serum acetaminophen levels; in such cases, repeated measurements of serum concentrations should be obtained. If the acetaminophen level is above the probable toxicity line (many clinicians use the possible toxicity line instead), treatment should be initiated with acetylcysteine, 140 mg/kg orally as a loading dose followed by 70 mg/kg orally every 4 hours. If the patient has additional risk factors for hepatotoxicity (e.g., chronic alcohol abuse, chronic use of anticonvulsants or isoniazid, or unreliable history of time of ingestion), it is prudent to treat for toxicity even with levels below the lower possible toxicity line. Acetylcysteine, an antioxidant that substitutes for glutathione as a scavenger, is highly effective in preventing liver damage from acetaminophen toxicity,

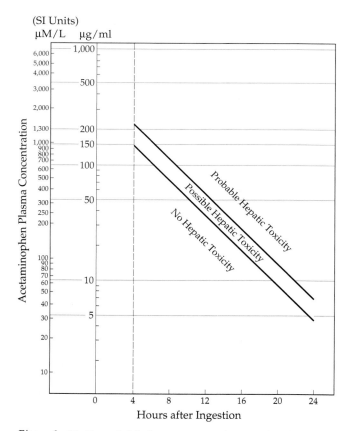

Figure 1 **The Rumack-Matthew nomogram for acetaminophen poisoning.**

especially if therapy is initiated within 8 to 10 hours after the ingestion of acetaminophen.[36] It is less effective when initiated after 12 to 16 hours after acetaminophen ingestion; but it should be given in such cases anyway because it still has beneficial effects, presumably owing to its antioxidant and anti-inflammatory properties, and increases survival in patients with hepatic failure.[36] The treatment protocol approved by the FDA for the oral administration of acetylcysteine stipulates that 17 doses (approximately 3 days of therapy) be administered; however, shorter courses (20 hours of I.V. therapy, as is given in the United Kingdom and Canada, and 48 hours of I.V. therapy, as was given in one study) have been shown to be equally effective in patients who were treated within 8 to 10 hours after ingestion of acetaminophen.[36,37] At our institution, we usually administer oral acetylcysteine until 36 hours after the ingestion and then stop its administration if the liver enzymes (e.g., AST and ALT) reach normal levels. A retrospective study showed that the 36-hour regimen has a safety and efficacy profile similar to that of the traditional 72-hour protocol.[38] A longer course may be given to high-risk patients (e.g., patients who arrive in the emergency department late in the course of overdose or who have evidence of liver injury).[36]

Aggressive intervention is recommended to ensure that the loading dose is given within the first 8 hours of overdose. Occasionally, however, patients cannot tolerate oral acetylcysteine because the drug has a disagreeable odor and they are already vomiting. In such cases, it is advisable to administer a strong antiemetic (e.g., metoclopramide, 60 to 70 mg I.V. over 1 to 2 minutes) and to give the acetylcysteine through a gastric tube. Rarely, recalcitrant vomiting indicates the need to administer the drug by the I.V. route. Because the preparation is not approved for I.V. administration and may not be free of pyrogens, it should be administered slowly through a micropore filter. A slow I.V. infusion rate is also recommended because rapid administration can cause an anaphylactoid reaction (skin flushing and hypotension).[39,40]

ANTICHOLINERGIC AGENTS AND ANTIHISTAMINES

Intoxication with anticholinergic agents can involve a variety of over-the-counter and prescription products, including antihistamines, antispasmodic agents, antipsychotic drugs, and antidepressants. In addition, several plants and mushrooms (e.g., *Datura stramonium* [angel's trumpet],[41] *Atropa belladonna*, and *Amanita phalloides*) contain potent anticholinergic alkaloids [see *Amanita phalloides* Mushrooms, *below*]. Anticholinergic agents competitively inhibit the action of acetylcholine at muscarinic receptors. Antihistamines are commonly found in a variety of over-the-counter and prescription medications for the treatment of cough and cold symptoms, itching, dizziness, nausea, and insomnia. The most commonly used nonprescription antihistamine is diphenhydramine.

Diagnosis

Clinical manifestations of intoxication with anticholinergic agents include delirium, flushed skin, dilated pupils, tachycardia, ileus, urinary retention, jerky muscle movements, and occasionally hyperthermia. Coma and respiratory arrest may occur. Tricyclic antidepressants (see below) and phenothiazines may also cause seizures and quinidinelike cardiac conduction abnormalities. Therefore, an ECG should be obtained and the QRS complex and cardiac rhythm monitored in any patient who displays anticholinergic manifestations of intoxication.

Antihistamine intoxication is similar to anticholinergic poisoning and may also be associated with seizures[17] and tricyclic-like cardiac conduction abnormalities.[42] The older nonsedating antihistamines terfenadine and astemizole were associated with prolongation of the QT interval and the occurrence of atypical (torsade de pointes) ventricular tachycardia both after overdose and after coadministration of macrolide antibiotics or other drugs that interfere with their elimination.[43] Because safer agents are available, both of these drugs were removed from the United States market by the manufacturers in 1999; however, the drugs are still commonly used in other countries.[44]

Treatment

Activated charcoal and a cathartic agent should be administered to patients with anticholinergic or antihistamine intoxication. Gastric lavage should be considered in cases of a large ingestion; this measure may be appropriate even if some time has passed, because ileus may delay gastric emptying. Coma and respiratory depression should be treated with the usual supportive measures. The physician should consider administering physostigmine, 0.5 to 2.0 mg in a slow I.V. infusion, in patients with pure anticholinergic intoxication (i.e., intoxication with agents other than tricyclic antidepressants or antihistamines) and severe delirium.[45] Drowsiness, confusion, and sinus tachycardia usually resolve without aggressive intervention. Prolongation of the QT interval and atypical ventricular tachycardia can be treated with magnesium, 1 to 2 g I.V., or overdrive pacing.

ANTICOAGULANTS

The anticoagulants include warfarin and the so-called super-warfarin rodenticides. Accidental intoxication with warfarin may result from long-term therapeutic overmedication or from the addition of a drug that interacts with it (e.g., allopurinol, cimetidine, nonsteroidal anti-inflammatory drugs, quinidine, salicylates, or sulfonamides). Acute ingestion of a single dose of warfarin rarely causes significant anticoagulation. However, a single dose of brodifacoum or one of the other superwarfarins can cause severe and prolonged anticoagulation that lasts for weeks to months.[46]

Diagnosis

All anticoagulants inhibit the hepatic production of clotting factors II, VII, IX, and X and prolong the PT. Circulating factors are not affected; the peak effect of anticoagulants on the PT is not seen until 36 to 48 hours after administration, when circulating factors are degraded. Severe anticoagulation can result in hemorrhage, which may be fatal.[46]

Treatment

Acute superwarfarin overdose should be treated with oral activated charcoal and a cathartic agent. A baseline PT should be obtained on presentation and 24 and 48 hours later. If prolongation of the PT occurs, the physician should administer oral vitamin K_1 (phytonadione), 25 to 50 mg/day, and monitor the PT; in rare instances, as much as 150 to 200 mg/day may be necessary to correct the PT. It may also be necessary to continue treatment for several weeks or even months.[47] Patients should not be treated prophylactically with vitamin K_1 after an acute ingestion, because such treatment would mask the rise in PT for about 3 to 5 days or more, preventing early diagnosis. As a result, the patient would require prolonged follow-up even in the case of a subtoxic ingestion.

Vitamin K_1 may be given subcutaneously or, cautiously, by the I.V. route to patients with severe prolongation of the PT.

However, because vitamin K_1 does not restore clotting factors immediately, patients who have active bleeding may require fresh frozen plasma or whole blood. Because coagulopathy after a superwarfarin overdose may last for weeks to months, high-dose oral vitamin K_1 therapy (5 mg/kg over 24 hours) may be necessary for outpatient therapy.[48]

BETA BLOCKERS

Beta blockers are used for the treatment of hypertension, angina pectoris, migraine, and cardiac arrhythmias. Propranolol is the prototypical beta blocker but is also the most toxic [see Table 10].[49] All of these agents act competitively at beta-adrenergic receptors; at therapeutic doses, some have a degree of selectivity for beta$_1$- or beta$_2$-adrenergic receptors that is not apparent at high doses. Propranolol and a few of the other agents also have depressant effects on the myocardial cell membrane that are similar to those of quinidine and the tricyclic antidepressants.[50]

Diagnosis

Beta blockade typically causes hypotension and bradycardia. Severe overdose may cause cardiogenic shock and asystole. Bronchospasm and hypoglycemia may also occur. In addition, propranolol overdose may cause widening of the QRS complex and CNS intoxication, including seizures and coma.[50] Most patients with beta-blocker poisoning manifest symptoms within 6 hours after an acute ingestion.[51]

Treatment

Treatment of overdose with a beta blocker includes aggressive gut decontamination. In cases of a large or recent ingestion, gastric lavage and the administration of activated charcoal and a cathartic agent should be initiated.

Hypotension and bradycardia are unlikely to respond to beta-adrenergic–mediated agents such as dopamine and isoproterenol; instead, the patient should receive high dosages of glucagon (5 to 10 mg I.V. followed by 5 to 10 mg/hr). Glucagon is a potent inotropic agent that does not require beta-adrenergic receptors to activate cells.[50,52] When glucagon fails, an epinephrine drip may be more beneficial in increasing heart rate and contractility than isoproterenol or dopamine. If pharmacologic therapy is unsuccessful, transvenous or external pacing should be used to maintain heart rate.[50,52] Use of hemodialysis in atenolol poisoning has been reported.[50]

CALCIUM ANTAGONISTS

Calcium channel blockers are used for the treatment of angina pectoris, hypertension, hypertrophic cardiomyopathy, migraine, and supraventricular tachycardia. These agents have a relatively low toxic-to-therapeutic ratio, and life-threatening toxicity can occur after accidental or intentional overdose. Calcium antagonists block the influx of calcium through calcium channels and act mainly on vascular smooth muscle, resulting in vasodilatation, reduced cardiac contractility, and slowed AV nodal conduction and sinus node activity. The most commonly used calcium antagonists in the United States are nifedipine, verapamil, and diltiazem. Although each of these agents has a different spectrum of activity, this selectivity is usually lost in overdose.[50]

Diagnosis

Manifestations of intoxication with a calcium antagonist include hypotension and bradycardia. Bradycardia may result from AV block or sinus arrest with a junctional escape rhythm.

The QRS complex is usually normal. Severe poisoning may cause profound shock followed by asystole. Overdose with sustained-release forms of nifedipine and verapamil, which are very popular, may be associated with delayed onset of toxicity.[53]

Treatment

Treatment of overdose of an orally administered calcium antagonist includes aggressive gut decontamination. Gastric lavage and administration of activated charcoal are recommended. For patients who have ingested a large dose of a sustained-release preparation, the physician should consider whole bowel irrigation[53] in combination with administration of repeated doses of activated charcoal; in such cases, the patient should be observed closely for possible delayed-onset effects.

Hypotension should be initially treated with boluses of fluid, vasopressors, and I.V. calcium chloride (10 ml of a 10% solution) or calcium gluconate (20 ml of a 10% solution).[54] Doses of calcium should be repeated as needed; in some case reports, as much as 5 to 10 g of calcium has been given.[55] Calcium administration may improve cardiac contractility but has less effect on AV nodal conduction or peripheral vasodilatation. Infusion of glucagon (5 to 10 mg I.V.) or epinephrine has been recommended for patients with unresponsive hypotension; in one reported case, cardiopulmonary bypass was also shown to be effective. In a verapamil-toxic canine model, the survival rate was higher with high-dose insulin therapy (insulin-dextrose infusion) than with high doses of epinephrine, calcium chloride, or glucagon. A small, uncontrolled case series of patients with calcium channel blocker poisoning showed improvement with high-dose insulin therapy, but a prospective, controlled trial is still pending.[56] Hemodialysis and hemoperfusion are not effective.[50]

CARBON MONOXIDE

Carbon monoxide is a colorless, odorless, nonirritating gas that is produced by the combustion of organic material. It is responsible for more than 5,000 deaths in the United States each year, most occurring from suicidal inhalation. Sources of carbon monoxide include motor vehicle exhaust, improperly vented gas or wood stoves and ovens, and smoke generated by fire. Children riding under closed canopies in the backs of pickup trucks have been poisoned from the exhaust, and campers have been poisoned by using propane stoves or charcoal grills inside their tents.[57] The blizzards that hit the eastern United States in the winter of 1996 produced reports of carbon monoxide poisoning associated with snow-obstructed vehicle exhaust systems.[58]

Tissue hypoxia, which occurs as a consequence of the high affinity of carbon monoxide for hemoglobin, is the major pathophysiologic disturbance in carbon monoxide poisoning: at a carbon monoxide concentration of only 0.1%, as many as 50% of hemoglobin binding sites may be occupied by carbon monoxide. In addition to reducing the oxygen-carrying capacity of the blood, carbon monoxide interferes with release of oxygen to the tissues. Carbon monoxide may also inhibit intracellular oxygen utilization by binding to myoglobin and cytochromes.[59]

Diagnosis

Carbon monoxide poisoning produces the symptoms and signs commonly associated with hypoxia, such as headache, confusion, tachycardia, tachypnea, syncope, hypotension, seizures, and coma. Clinical manifestations depend on the duration and intensity of exposure: an acute, sizable exposure may produce rapid unconsciousness, seizures, and death, whereas prolonged,

Table 10 Toxicity of Common Beta Blockers[150]

Drug	Usual Daily Dose (mg)	Cardioselective	Myocardial Cell Membrane Depression
Acebutolol	400–800	+	+
Atenolol	50–100	+	–
Labetalol	200–800	–	+
Metoprolol	100–450	+	Variable
Nadolol	40–240	–	–
Propranolol	40–360	–	++

low-level exposure may cause vague and nonspecific symptoms such as headache, dizziness, nausea, and weakness. Mild cases may be mistakenly diagnosed as influenza or migraine headache. So-called classic features of carbon monoxide poisoning, such as cherry-red skin coloring and bullous skin lesions, are not always present. Survivors of severe carbon monoxide poisoning may be left with permanent neurologic sequelae. These sequelae can include gross deficits, such as a permanent vegetative state or parkinsonism, or more subtle deficits, such as memory loss, depression, and irritability. In some cases, delayed neurologic deterioration may occur after 1 to 2 weeks.[59,60]

Laboratory findings may include metabolic acidosis and cardiac ischemia on ECG. The oxygen tension is usually normal because carbon monoxide binds to hemoglobin but does not disturb levels of dissolved oxygen; therefore, the calculated oxygen saturation is falsely normal. Furthermore, indirect measurement of oxygen saturation by pulse oximetry is inaccurate because of the similar absorption characteristics of oxyhemoglobin and carboxyhemoglobin.[61] Thus, correct diagnosis depends on direct spectrophotometric measurement of oxyhemoglobin and carboxyhemoglobin in a blood sample or direct measurement of exhaled carbon monoxide. Carboxyhemoglobin levels greater than 20% to 30% are usually associated with moderate symptoms of intoxication, and levels greater than 50% to 60% are associated with a serious or fatal outcome. There is considerable variability, however, and levels do not always correlate with symptoms.[59]

Treatment

The victim of carbon monoxide poisoning should immediately be removed from the site of exposure and given supplemental oxygen in the highest available concentration. Oxygen competes with carbon monoxide for hemoglobin binding sites, and administration of 100% oxygen can reduce the half-life of carboxyhemoglobin to approximately 40 to 60 minutes, thereby restoring normal oxygen saturation within about 2 to 3 hours. It should be noted that it is difficult to deliver 100% oxygen unless the patient is endotracheally intubated. Hyperbaric oxygen (HBO) administered in a sealed chamber can deliver oxygen at a pressure of 2.5 to 3.0 atm and has been reported to speed recovery and reduce neurologic sequelae.[59,62] Proponents of hyperbaric oxygen therapy assert that this treatment can reduce cerebral edema and quell lipid peroxidation and other postinjury mechanisms of cellular destruction.[59,63] However, hyperbaric chambers are not readily available, and until recently, the few clinical studies to have compared HBO therapy with 100% oxygen at ambient pressure produced conflicting or inconclusive results or were otherwise unsatisfactory.[64,65]

A recent report from Australia describes a randomized, double-blind, placebo-controlled (with sham HBO treatments) study of hyperbaric versus normobaric oxygen in a large number of patients with significant carbon monoxide poisoning; the authors found that HBO provided no greater benefit than normobaric oxygen.[66] Although the role of HBO in carbon monoxide poisoning is questionable, proponents of HBO generally advise its use for patients who have a history of unconsciousness, a detectable neuropsychiatric abnormality on bedside testing, or a carboxyhemoglobin level greater than 25%.[59] Because of concerns about the higher affinity of carbon monoxide for fetal hemoglobin, the recommended threshold for treatment of young infants and pregnant women is usually lower.[67] However, there are no controlled studies evaluating HBO therapy in pregnancy.

In patients with carbon monoxide poisoning associated with smoke inhalation, the physician must also consider the potential role of other toxic gases produced during combustion, such as cyanide, phosgene, nitrogen oxides, and hydrogen chloride, as well as the possibility that direct thermal injury to the airway and respiratory tract has been caused by inhaled soot or steam.

COCAINE, AMPHETAMINES, AND OTHER STIMULANTS

Cocaine is now used by as many as six million persons in the United States.[68] In 1991, acute cocaine-related emergencies accounted for more than 100,000 hospital visits; in 1997, cocaine abuse was the leading cause of drug-related deaths (3,465 mentions by medical examiners).[1] Cocaine and the amphetamines [*see Table 11*] stimulate the CNS and the sympathetic nervous system and may act directly on peripheral adrenergic receptors.[68,69] Although cocaine also has local anesthetic properties and may cause sodium channel blockade in high doses, the clinical manifestations and treatment of cocaine overdose are essentially the same as those of amphetamine overdose. These drugs can be taken orally or can be snorted, smoked, or injected. So-called crack cocaine is a crudely prepared nonpolar derivative of the hydrochloride salt that is more easily volatilized and is thus the preferred form for smoking. The combined use of ethanol and cocaine may create the highly potent metabolite cocaethylene, which has a longer half-life than does cocaine and may contribute to the development of delayed toxic effects.[69,70]

Another common drug of abuse, particularly among teenagers and young adults, is methylenedioxymethamphetamine (MDMA), or ecstasy. National surveys suggest a marked increase in the prevalence of MDMA use in the United States. A survey of 14,000 college students reported a 69% increase in the use of MDMA between the years 1997 and 1999.[71] Additionally, the number of emergency room visits in which MDMA was involved soared by over 1,600%, from 253 in 1994 to 4,500 in 2001.[72] Although MDMA is an amphetamine derivative

Table 11 Common Stimulant Drugs

Drug	Street Names
Cocaine	Coke, crack (free-base cocaine)
Methamphetamine	Speed, crystal, ice
3,4-Methylenedioxymethamphetamine (MDMA)	Ecstasy
Methylphenidate	Ritalin*
Methcathinone†	Cat

*Ritalin is the trade name, not the street name.
†An illegally synthesized ephedrine derivative.

with psychoactive properties similar to the hallucinogen mescaline, MDMA toxicity appears to be related to its stimulant properties. The subjective effects of MDMA include euphoria, sexual arousal, enhanced sensory perception, increased endurance, and greater sociability.[73] Adverse reactions from MDMA abuse reported in the literature include hyperthermia, hyponatremia, seizures, hepatitis, cerebrovascular accidents, and cardiac arrhythmias.[73] As MDMA use rises, health care providers are likely to see more patients with adverse reactions from this drug.

Methylphenidate (Ritalin) toxicity may be an increasing cause of sympathomimetic toxicity in children. Between 1990 and 1995, the prevalence of methylphenidate treatment in the United States increased 2.5-fold; by mid-1995, approximately 2.8% of youths 5 to 18 years of age were receiving methylphenidate for attention deficit disorders.[74] Methylphenidate toxicity is most commonly the result of therapeutic error in children treated with the drug.[75] Abuse of methylphenidate has been reported, but its prevalence remains uncertain.[76]

Diagnosis

Clinical manifestations of mild stimulation include euphoria, alertness, and anorexia. More severe intoxication causes agitation, psychosis, tachycardia, hypertension, and diaphoresis. The pupils are usually dilated. Severe poisoning may result in convulsions, hypertensive crisis (e.g., intracerebral hemorrhage or aortic dissection), and hyperthermia.[15,16] Consequences of severe hyperthermia include shock, brain damage, coagulopathy, and hepatic and renal failure.[19]

The differential diagnosis includes acute functional psychosis, acute exertional heatstroke, and intoxication with other drugs. Phencyclidine, a ketaminelike dissociative anesthetic, may produce stimulant effects, but victims of overdose often have a waxing-and-waning encephalopathy with periods of flaccid stupor or coma.[15] Anticholinergic agents (see above) may also cause dilated pupils, tachycardia, and agitation, but these toxins usually cause the skin to be dry and flushed; stimulants generally cause the skin to be pale, clammy, and diaphoretic.

Treatment

Mild or moderate intoxication with a stimulant can often be successfully managed by administering a sedative agent, such as diazepam or lorazepam, and by providing the patient with a quiet room. If hypertension is severe and does not improve after sedation, phentolamine (2 to 5 mg I.V. at 5- to 10-minute intervals) or nitroprusside (0.5 to 10 mg/kg/min) should be administered. For patients with tachycardia or ventricular arrhythmias, a short-acting beta blocker such as esmolol (50 to 100 mg/kg/min) is recommended, although it should be cautioned that beta blockers may worsen hypertension because of unopposed alpha-adrenergic effects of the stimulant drug.[16] Wide-complex dysrhythmias in cocaine overdose should be treated with sodium bicarbonate.[68] Severe hyperthermia should be treated aggressively to prevent brain damage and multiorgan complications [see Hyperthermia, above].

Because acute myocardial infarction may occur even in young persons with normal coronary arteries, all patients with chest pain should be evaluated carefully for evidence of ischemia.[16] Other causes of chest pain in these patients may include mechanical trauma to the chest wall, pneumomediastinum from hard coughing or the Valsalva maneuver, or pectoral muscle ischemia.[16]

CORROSIVE AGENTS

A number of agents with caustic or corrosive properties [see Table 12] are used for a variety of purposes in industry, as cleaning agents in the home, and in hobbies. Exposure to these agents may occur accidentally or as a result of suicidal ingestion. In some cases, the corrosive effect of these agents is a direct result of the high concentration of hydrogen (H^+) or hydroxyl (OH^-) ions and can be predicted from the very low or very high pH of the product. In other cases, toxicity may result from the product's oxidizing, alkylating, or other cytotoxic effects. Systemic toxicity can occur as a result of absorption across burned skin or after ingestion (e.g., in the case of hydrofluoric acid, phenol, or paraquat) [see Table 12].[77]

Diagnosis

Manifestations of toxicity usually occur immediately after exposure to the corrosive or caustic agent and include burning pain and erythema at the site of exposure. Immediate effects occur most commonly with acids. Injury caused by alkali burns can evolve over several hours and takes the form of a penetrating liquefaction necrosis. Burns may also be delayed in cases of exposure to hydrofluoric acid (hydrogen fluoride in aqueous solution); the toxicity of this agent is mediated through its fluoride component, which combines with calcium and magnesium ions. With hydrofluoric acid burns, pain and swelling may not be apparent until several hours after exposure, especially after exposure to relatively dilute solutions.

Treatment

Treatment of toxicity from corrosive or caustic agents must be initiated rapidly to reduce injury. Exposed areas should be flushed with copious amounts of plain water and any contaminated clothing removed (health providers must be careful not to become exposed while assisting victims). For patients whose eyes have been exposed to the agent, the physician should use an eyewash fountain or should splash water into the face, then pour water directly over the eyes from a pitcher or glass. Patients who have ingested a corrosive agent should drink one to two glasses of water. Although use of gastric lavage is controversial because of concerns about possible mechanical damage to the esophagus, our gastrointestinal consultants recommend gastric intubation with a small flexible tube as soon as possible after corrosive-liquid ingestion, to remove as much of the injurious material as possible. Neutralizing agents should not be administered in an attempt to normalize the pH; they may modify the pH too far in the opposite direction, and the heat of neutralization may cause thermal injury. There are a few exceptions to this rule; for example, after exposure to hydrofluoric acid, soaking the skin in a solution or gel that contains calcium (e.g., 2.5% calcium gluconate gel) or magnesium or in benzalkonium chloride may bind the toxic fluoride ion before it can be absorbed[78]; calcium is sometimes injected subcutaneously or by the intra-arterial route for deeper burns. For management of exposure to hydrofluoric acid, the physician should consult a regional poison-control center, a medical toxicologist, or a plastic or hand surgeon.

CYANIDE

Cyanide (the CN^- anion or a salt that contains this ion) is a highly toxic chemical that is used in a variety of industries, including electroplating, chemical synthesis, and laboratory analysis.[79] Cyanide is also released in the I.V. administration of nitroprusside. Acetonitrile, which is found in some glue removers for

Table 12 Corrosive Agents

Corrosive or Caustic Agent	Comments
Mineral acids (e.g., hydrochloric, sulfuric, nitric, and phosphoric acids)	Produce rapidly painful coagulation necrosis of skin and eyes; inhalation of mists or vapors can cause irritation, bronchospasm, and chemical pneumonitis
Hydrofluoric acid	Highly electronegative fluoride ion causes deep tissue injury, which may have a delayed onset; systemic absorption from the skin or after ingestion may cause fatal hypocalcemia or hyperkalemia[151,152]
Caustic alkalis (e.g., sodium, potassium, calcium, and ammonium hydroxides)	Injury is often progressive and deep because of tissue saponification and resulting liquefaction necrosis
Phenol (carbolic acid)	Liquid and vapor are rapidly absorbed across the skin, causing severe systemic toxicity (shock, convulsions, and coma)[153]; isopropyl alcohol may speed its removal from skin[154]
Paraquat	Ingestion causes severe corrosive injury; systemic absorption leads to progressive and ultimately fatal pulmonary fibrosis[155]

artificial fingernails, is metabolized to cyanide and has caused death in children.[79] Natural sources of cyanide (cyanogenic glycosides) include cassava, apricot pits, and several other plants and seeds. Hydrogen cyanide gas is generated from the combustion of many natural and synthetic materials that contain nitrogen and is a common component of the smoke generated by fire [*see* Smoke Inhalation, *below*].[80]

Cyanide is a highly reactive chemical that binds to intracellular cytochrome, blocking the utilization of oxygen. The resulting cellular asphyxia leads to headache, confusion, dyspnea, syncope, collapse, and death.[79,81] Although these effects occur rapidly after inhalation of hydrogen cyanide gas, symptoms of intoxication may be delayed for minutes after the ingestion of cyanide salts or even for hours after the ingestion of cyanogenic glycosides or acetonitrile.[79]

Diagnosis

Diagnosis of cyanide poisoning is based on a history of possible exposure (e.g., in a laboratory worker who attempts to commit suicide; in a person who has ingested laetrile, a cyanogenic glycoside; in a victim of smoke inhalation; or in a patient who has received a rapid high-dose infusion of nitroprusside) and the presence of characteristic symptoms. Any victim of smoke inhalation who has altered mental status should be suspected of having been poisoned with cyanide as well as with carbon monoxide. The so-called smell of bitter almonds may be present after cyanide ingestion, but only about 50% of the general population has the ability to perceive this odor. Severe lactic acidosis is usually present. Because cyanide blocks the cellular utilization of oxygen, venous blood may have an elevated oxygen content; a venous oxygen saturation of greater than 90% suggests the diagnosis.

Treatment

Once cyanide poisoning is suspected, immediate measures must be taken to prevent further exposure and to provide an antidote. For an ingestion, oral activated charcoal should be imme-

diately administered; although the adsorption of cyanide to charcoal is relatively low, a standard dose of charcoal (e.g., 50 to 60 g) is sufficient to adsorb several hundred milligrams of cyanide salts. If charcoal is not available and there will be a delay before the patient reaches the hospital, emesis should be induced with ipecac. If ipecac is not available, emesis should be induced by mechanical gagging.

The antidotes for cyanide poisoning consist of nitrites, which oxidize hemoglobin to methemoglobin; in turn, methemoglobin binds free cyanide ions. If I.V. access is not immediately available, break a pearl of amyl nitrite and have the victim inhale the contents. As soon as possible, administer sodium nitrite, 300 mg I.V. The other antidote is sodium thiosulfate (12.5 g I.V.), which enhances the conversion of cyanide to the less toxic thiocyanate by the endogenous enzyme rhodanese. Although nitrites produce serious side effects (methemoglobinemia reduces the oxygen-carrying capacity, and vasodilatation may cause hypotension), sodium thiosulfate is relatively benign and can be used empirically as a single agent when the diagnosis is uncertain. Other potential antidotes include cobalt ethylenediaminetetraacetic acid (cobalt EDTA) and vitamin B_{12a} (hydroxocobalamin), but these agents have not been approved for use in the United States, and hydroxocobalamin, although used in the United States for treatment of pernicious anemia, is not available in a concentrated high-strength form needed for antidotal treatment of cyanide poisoning.[79]

DIGITALIS GLYCOSIDES

Digitalis glycosides are found in a variety of plants, including foxglove, oleander, and rhododendron,[82] and have been used for centuries to treat heart failure. Digoxin is the most commonly prescribed digitalis glycoside. Digitalis poisoning may occur after accidental or suicidal acute overdose, as a result of chronic accumulation (usually because of renal insufficiency or overmedication), or as a drug interaction. There have been many reports of elevated digoxin levels resulting from the interaction of digoxin with commonly used drugs, such as quinidine, amiodarone, and macrolide antibiotics.[83] Digitalis glycosides inhibit the Na^+,K^+-ATPase pump, which returns potassium to cells and increases the intracellular calcium concentration.[84]

Diagnosis

After an acute overdose, serum potassium levels are often elevated and AV nodal conduction is impaired, leading to varying degrees of AV block. Additionally, gastrointestinal symptoms of nausea, vomiting, and anorexia are often described after acute digitalis poisoning. With chronic poisoning, in contrast, ventricular dysrhythmias (e.g., ventricular ectopic beats or bidirectional ventricular tachycardia) predominate, and the potassium level is often normal or low, perhaps in part because of long-term coadministration of diuretic agents. The digitalis level is usually markedly elevated; however, if the sample is drawn within a few hours of overdose or the last therapeutic dose, the result may be misleading because the drug has not been fully distributed to tissues.[85]

Treatment

Management of acute digitalis poisoning includes gut decontamination with the oral administration of activated charcoal and, if the ingestion was large and occurred shortly before presentation, gastric lavage. Ipecac is not recommended, because it may enhance the vagotonic effects of the digitalis. Initially, sinus bradycardia or uncomplicated AV block should be treated with atropine (0.5 to 2 mg I.V.). A temporary pacemaker may be needed in patients with persistent symptomatic bradycardia; however, such patients should also receive digoxin-specific antibodies.

Digoxin-specific antibodies (e.g., Digibind) are indicated for patients with manifestations of severe intoxication (marked hyperkalemia and symptomatic dysrhythmias). These antibodies are derived from sheep and then cleaved to leave only the Fab fragment, which is small enough to be filtered and eliminated by the kidney after binding to digoxin. Extensive clinical experience with dixogin-specific antibodies has shown that they are safe and highly effective, with peak activity occurring within 20 to 30 minutes after administration.[7] The dose of digoxin-specific antibodies depends on the type of intoxication [see Table 13]. After acute ingestion, the serum level of drug does not predict the body burden because of ongoing tissue distribution[85]; therefore, the dose of digoxin-specific antibodies is calculated by estimating the amount of drug ingested. In patients with chronic poisoning in whom a steady-state digoxin level can be obtained, the body burden can be estimated on the basis of the serum level and the average apparent volume of distribution. When the ingested dose is not known or a steady-state level cannot be obtained, patients should be treated empirically: initially, one to five vials should be administered, depending on the severity of toxicity. It may also be appropriate to start with small doses and to titrate them to clinical effect in patients who have preexisting disease that requires residual digitalis effect (e.g., those with congestive heart failure or atrial fibrillation).

ETHANOL, METHANOL, AND ETHYLENE GLYCOL

Ethanol (grain alcohol) is probably the most widely used drug in the United States, and complications related to acute intoxication, as well as related medical illness and trauma, are commonly encountered. Ethanol-related illnesses account for nearly 20% of the national expenditure for hospital care, and ethanol is involved in about 50% of all fatal motor vehicle accidents.[86] Ethanol is frequently ingested with other drugs, both in suicide attempts and in recreational drug abuse. Ethylene glycol (antifreeze) and methanol (wood alcohol) are other alcohols that cause profound and often fatal poisoning when mistakenly ingested as substitutes for ethanol.

Ethanol

Diagnosis Acute ethanol intoxication produces an easily recognized state of inebriation that includes disinhibition,

Table 13 Dosing of Digoxin-Specific Antibodies

Type of Intoxication	Dose Needed to Provide Complete Binding of Digoxin
Acute ingestion*	Administer one vial (40 mg) for each 0.5 mg of digoxin expected to be absorbed (because bioavailability is 80%, multiply ingested dose by 0.8 to estimate absorbed dose)
Chronic intoxication†	Use the following formula to calculate the number of vials needed: $\dfrac{\text{Serum digoxin level (ng/ml)} \times \text{body weight (kg)}}{100}$

*Dose of digoxin-specific antibodies is based on the estimated amount of digoxin ingested.
†Dose of digoxin-specific antibodies is based on the steady-state serum digoxin level.

slurred speech, ataxia, stupor, and coma.[15] Loss of protective reflexes in the airway may permit pulmonary aspiration of gastric contents, possibly causing respiratory arrest in those who are in a deep coma. In most states, a blood ethanol level above 80 to 100 mg/dl is considered sufficient evidence to charge a driver with the crime of driving while intoxicated. A level above 300 mg/dl is generally considered sufficient to cause deep coma and respiratory arrest; however, because tolerance to ethanol develops, chronic drinkers with these levels are often awake and even able to ambulate.[15] Acute ethanol ingestion can also cause hypoglycemia because of the inhibitory effect of ethanol on gluconeogenesis.

Treatment Treatment of ethanol intoxication usually consists of supportive care. The blood ethanol level decreases at an average (but variable) rate of about 20 mg/dl/hr,[15] and most patients are awake and ambulatory within 6 to 12 hours or less. The physician should protect the airway and, if necessary, intubate the trachea and assist ventilation. The patient should be evaluated for hypoglycemia, and glucose-containing fluids should be given as necessary; vitamin B_1, 100 mg I.V. or I.M., should be administered to malnourished or chronic alcoholic patients. Hypotension, although uncommon, may result from vasodilatation and dehydration and usually responds to an I.V. bolus of fluid. Although such patients often come to medical attention because of falls, even those without a history of trauma should be examined for occult injuries (especially to the head, neck, and abdomen) because inebriated patients often have such injuries. In addition, serious infections, vitamin deficiencies (especially of vitamin B_1 and folic acid), and metabolic abnormalities also occur frequently in chronic alcoholic patients[16]; if any of these are present, they should be treated.

Methanol and Ethylene Glycol

Diagnosis Methanol or ethylene glycol poisoning produces an initial clinical picture that is similar to that of ethanol intoxication. However, these alcohols are gradually metabolized to highly toxic organic acids that can have disastrous effects [see Table 14]. After a delay of up to several hours, the patient develops severe metabolic acidosis and evidence of endorgan injury from the accumulation of the toxic acid metabolites. Diagnosis of methanol or ethylene glycol poisoning is based on the patient's history of exposure and the presence of severe metabolic acidosis. The osmolar gap is usually elevated, especially early after ingestion when the parent compounds are present, but toxic products can be present with a seemingly normal osmolar gap.[87] The serum lactate level is relatively low despite a large anion gap.[88]

Treatment If methanol or ethylene glycol poisoning is suspected, immediate measures should be instituted to reduce absorption, prevent metabolism, and remove the toxic acid metabolites.[88] If the ingestion occurred shortly before presentation (i.e., less than an hour), gastric lavage should be performed; activated charcoal does not efficiently adsorb the alcohols. Metabolism of the alcohols can be prevented by giving ethanol or fomepizole (4-methylpyrazole), which competitively inhibit the enzyme alcohol dehydrogenase. If ethanol is used, a loading dose of approximately 750 mg/kg orally or I.V. usually produces an ethanol level of about 100 mg/dl[88]; an infusion of 100 to 150 mg/kg/hr is given to maintain this level. An ethanol drip is difficult to manage, and the ethanol may contribute to obtunda-

Table 14   Poisoning with Ethylene Glycol, Isopropyl Alcohol, or Methanol

Alcohol	Metabolic Products	Treatment
Ethylene glycol	Oxalic, hippuric, and glycolic acids cause severe anion-gap metabolic acidosis; calcium oxalate crystals precipitate in tissues and kidneys[156]	Fomepizole or ethanol infusion; perform hemodialysis if there is severe acidosis, if serum level > 20–50 mg/dl, or if osmolar gap > 10 mOsm/L
Isopropyl alcohol	Acetone causes characteristic odor; toxicity includes CNS depression, but there are no toxic acid by-products[157]	Isopropyl alcohol is a potent CNS depressant and gastric irritant, but its toxicity is usually managed supportively
Methanol	Formic acid causes severe anion-gap metabolic acidosis and visual disturbances that can lead to blindness and death[158]	Fomepizole or ethanol infusion; perform hemodialysis if there is severe acidosis, if serum level > 20–50 mg/dl, or if osmolar gap > 10 mOsm/L

tion. Fomepizole is easier to administer, has few side effects, and, if initiated early after ethylene glycol ingestion, may eliminate the need for dialysis (this is not the case for methanol). Although costly, fomepizole therapy may be less expensive than the combined costs of hemodialysis, intensive care, and serial blood work during an ethanol drip.[88] Administration of folic acid (50 mg I.V. every 4 hours), vitamin B_1 (100 mg I.M. or I.V. every 6 hours), and vitamin B_6 (pyridoxine; 50 mg I.V. every 6 hours) is also recommended to enhance the metabolism of the toxic organic acids, and sodium bicarbonate should be given as needed to restore normal serum pH and enhance renal elimination of the toxic acid metabolites.

If the measured or estimated serum level of the toxic alcohol is greater than 50 mg/dl or if severe metabolic acidosis is present, hemodialysis is indicated to remove the parent compounds and their metabolites. During hemodialysis, the ethanol infusion is usually increased twofold, and fomepizole is administered every 4 hours to replace the respective drugs that are lost during the procedure.[88]

γ-HYDROXYBUTYRIC ACID (GHB)

γ-Hydroxybutyric acid (GHB) is a naturally occurring four-carbon compound that was first synthesized in 1960. Since then, the drug has been used for various clinical purposes, including induction of general anesthesia, treatment of alcohol withdrawal and narcolepsy, and even as a protective agent during tissue ischemia.[89] In the United States, it has been available only under an FDA investigational new drug (IND) exemption for the treatment of narcolepsy. However, in the late 1980s, GHB gained popularity among some bodybuilders who believed it could enhance muscle mass through stimulation of growth hormone release. It is now promoted popularly as a sleep aid, a diet agent, and a euphorigenic drug. Its increasing use has been accompanied by a number of reports of severe and fatal effects. Its illegal recreational abuse has become a part of the underground drug culture (e.g., at rave parties and dance clubs). It has also been used to facilitate rape and assault because it produces rapid loss of consciousness. Innovative ways to continue GHB use despite FDA and Drug Enforcement Administration (DEA) restrictions have included the sale of precursors of the drug such as γ-butyrolactone (GBL) and 1,4-butanediol, marketed as dietary supplements at health food stores and on the Internet under several trade names (e.g., Renew Trient and Revivarant). These precursors are metabolized to GHB in the body, and toxic effects are similar or identical to those of GHB.[90] After numerous reports of adverse reactions to these agents, including one death, the FDA asked manufacturers on January 21, 1999, to recall their GBL-containing products and warned consumers to avoid taking these products.[90]

Diagnosis

Clinically, patients poisoned by GHB or analogues usually present with profound CNS and respiratory depression, with possible loss of laryngeal reflexes and apnea. Symptoms usually last less than 4 to 6 hours, and patients often have sudden awakening and agitation, particularly in response to painful stimuli (e.g., intubation).[91] Concurrent sinus bradycardia, myoclonic movements, and vomiting are common. Delirium and tonic-clonic seizures have been reported. There is an additive effect of GHB when it is taken in conjunction with sedative agents or alcohol. GHB is absorbed within 10 to 15 minutes, and because of its short half-life of 27 minutes, plasma blood levels are undetectable within 4 to 6 hours of therapeutic ingestion.[89] A recent report suggests that GHB dependence may lead to severe withdrawal after sudden discontinuance. Symptoms are similar to alcohol withdrawal but may last 7 to 14 days; these patients often require very large doses of benzodiazepines and barbiturates to control agitation.[92]

Treatment

There is no specific antidote for GHB. Therapy consists of airway protection, with rapid-sequence intubation if needed [*see* Initial Stabilization, *above*]. Because of the short half-life of GHB, patients without complications from GHB (e.g., prolonged hypoxia, aspiration, or untoward effects of mechanical ventilation) are often extubated and discharged from the emergency room within 3 to 7 hours.[91] Symptomatic bradycardia can be successfully treated with atropine.[91] Decontamination measures, such as gastric lavage and activated charcoal, are of little benefit because of GHB's rapid absorption, although it should be considered for large overdoses or if a coingestion is suspected. GHB withdrawal can be treated in the same manner as alcohol withdrawal, although physicians should recognize the potential need for a longer treatment period.[93]

IRON

Iron poisoning is typically seen in children who accidentally ingest their parents' iron supplements, but intentional overdose occasionally occurs in adults.[94] Iron in large quantities is corrosive to the gastrointestinal tract, causes nausea and vomiting, and sometimes causes bloody emesis and diarrhea. Intestinal perforation occasionally occurs. Shock may result from volume loss and fluid shifts, as well as from iron-induced peripheral vasodilatation. In addition, free iron is cytotoxic, and coma, metabolic acidosis, and liver failure may develop from excessive, acute systemic absorption.[94]

Diagnosis

Diagnosis of acute iron poisoning may be based on a history of exposure or may be suspected in a patient with severe gastroenteritis and hypotension, especially if such a patient also has metabolic acidosis, hyperglycemia, and leukocytosis.[94] A plain x-ray of the abdomen (KUB view) may reveal radiopaque iron tablets. Serum iron levels in patients with severe poisoning are usually higher than 600 to 1,000 mg/dl, although lower levels may be seen if the sample is drawn late in the course of intoxication. In the past, it was common to estimate the quantity of free iron by subtracting the total iron-binding capacity (TIBC) from the serum iron level. However, it has since been shown that the TIBC is falsely elevated during iron poisoning, and this value is no longer considered useful for the purpose.[95]

Treatment

Treatment of acute iron overdose includes gut decontamination, I.V. administration of fluids, and, possibly, chelation with deferoxamine. Patients who are in shock should receive vigorous I.V. fluid replacement. Because activated charcoal does not bind iron, it should not be given unless overdose of other drugs is also suspected. Gastric lavage may be useful in patients who have taken liquid iron preparations or chewable products; however, if intact tablets are seen on x-ray, it is unlikely that they can be removed through even the largest-bore gastric hose. Attempts to render the iron insoluble by gastric lavage with bicarbonate- or phosphate-containing solutions have proved ineffective or dangerous. Currently, the recommended method of gut decontamination in patients with large ingestions is whole bowel irrigation,[23,29] which is achieved by administering polyethylene glycol–electrolyte solution (e.g., GoLYTELY or Colyte), 1 to 2 L/hr by nasogastric tube for several hours, until the rectal effluent is clear and the x-ray shows no radiopacities.

Therapy with deferoxamine, a specific chelator of iron, is indicated in patients who have evidence of severe poisoning, but such therapy should not replace thorough gut decontamination and aggressive volume replacement.[94] The I.V. route is preferred, and an initial dosage of 10 to 15 mg/kg/hr should be given. Dosages as high as 40 to 50 mg/kg/hr may be given in particularly severe cases of poisoning. The iron-deferoxamine complex imparts an orange or vin rosé color to the urine that is sometimes used as evidence of the continued presence of chelatable (free) iron. Inasmuch as serum iron levels are readily available in most hospitals, the so-called vin rosé test is seldom used as an indication to continue therapy. Many clinicians stop administering deferoxamine as soon as the serum iron level is lower than 350 mg/dl, because prolonged infusions have been associated with acute respiratory distress syndrome (ARDS).[7]

ISONIAZID

Isoniazid is widely used in the treatment of tuberculosis. Long-term use of isoniazid has been associated with hepatitis and peripheral neuropathy [see Chapters 65 and 122]. Acute overdose of isoniazid is a well-known cause of seizures and metabolic acidosis.[96,97] Isoniazid causes acute toxicity by competing with pyridoxal 5′-phosphate (the active form of vitamin B_6), resulting in lowered γ-aminobutyric acid (GABA) levels in the brain. It also inhibits the hepatic metabolism of lactate to pyruvate. As little as 1.5 g of isoniazid may cause toxicity, with severe toxicity likely to occur after administration of 5 to 10 g.

Diagnosis

Acute overdose of isoniazid causes confusion, seizures, and coma; the onset is abrupt, often occurring within 30 to 60 min-utes of ingestion. Lactic acidosis is often severe, and its severity is disproportional to the duration or intensity of seizure activity. Diagnosis is based on a history of isoniazid ingestion and should be suspected in any person who experiences the acute onset of seizures and who may be taking the drug (e.g., persons who have tuberculosis or AIDS and recent immigrants who test positive on the purified protein derivative [PPD] skin test). Results of testing for serum isoniazid levels are not generally available immediately, and routine toxicology screens do not ordinarily test for the drug.

Treatment

Activated charcoal should be administered to any person who is suspected of having isoniazid intoxication. Emesis should not be induced because of the risk of abrupt onset of seizures and coma. Gastric lavage is appropriate in cases of large, recent ingestion. Seizures should be treated initially with diazepam, 5 to 10 mg I.V., or with lorazepam, 1 to 2 mg I.V. Vitamin B_6 is a specific antidote and should be given to all patients who have taken more than 3 to 5 g of isoniazid. In cases in which the amount of isoniazid ingested is unknown, the dose is 5 to 10 g I.V.; if the amount is known, an equivalent gram-for-gram amount of vitamin B_6 should be given.[96] Administration of vitamin B_6 effectively stops resistant seizures and improves metabolic acidosis. It has also reportedly reversed isoniazid-induced coma.[98]

LEAD

Lead poisoning primarily occurs in the occupational setting, with exposure occurring over a period of months or years. However, lead is a ubiquitous metal found in the paint of older houses, car batteries and radiators, some pottery glazes and solders, and some folk medicines[99]; thus, it may be encountered by hobbyists, home-repair buffs, and those who use ceramic cookware.

Diagnosis

The clinical manifestations of lead poisoning are sufficiently variable and nonspecific that lead poisoning should be suspected in any patient who has multisystem illness, especially if the illness involves the neurologic, hematopoietic, and gastrointestinal systems.[99] Lead poisoning rarely results from a single ingestion, although such occurrences have been reported.[31] More commonly, exposure occurs repeatedly and gradually. Patients typically have cramplike abdominal pain or nausea and may have chronic systemic symptoms such as irritability, malaise, and weight loss. Other manifestations of lead poisoning include peripheral motor neuropathy (wristdrop) and anemia, which is often microcytic and accompanied by basophilic stippling. Lead encephalopathy, manifested by coma and seizures, is rare.

Chronic lead poisoning has been misdiagnosed as porphyria, in part because they both involve alteration of heme metabolism.[100] Diagnosis of lead poisoning is usually based on the lead level in whole blood. Symptoms generally occur in patients with lead levels above 25 to 40 mg/dl, but lower levels have been associated with impaired neurobehavioral development in children.[101] Lead levels above 80 mg/dl are often associated with severe overt toxicity. The free erythrocyte protoporphyrin (FEP) concentration, which is elevated (> 35 mg/dl) in persons with chronic intoxication, has been used to screen large populations for lead poisoning but is not sufficiently sensitive for the identification of low blood lead levels (< 30 mg/dl) in children.

Treatment

For patients with an acute ingestion of lead (e.g., a fishing weight, bullet, or curtain weight), a plain x-ray of the abdomen should be obtained. If the object is in the stomach, there is a risk that the action of stomach acid may create enough absorbable lead to cause systemic toxicity; therefore, the object should be removed by the use of cathartic agents, whole bowel irrigation, or endoscopy. Objects that clearly lie beyond the pylorus are likely to pass uneventfully into the stool, but confirmation of this supposition should be obtained by close follow-up with repeated x-rays and measurement of blood lead levels.[31]

Several chelating agents are available for the treatment of patients with acute or chronic intoxication who are symptomatic and have elevated blood lead levels.[101,102] The oldest chelating agent, dimercaprol, is reserved for patients with lead encephalopathy (but even this use is controversial). For less severe intoxication, the physician should administer I.V. calcium EDTA or oral succimer (meso-2,3-dimercaptosuccinic acid, or DMSA). Triple-chelation therapy with dimercaprol, EDTA, and oral succimer has been used in conjunction with whole bowel irrigation following an extremely high lead level in a 3-year-old child with encephalopathy.[102] A recent trial suggests that succimer does not provide any benefit in children with chronically elevated blood lead levels between 20 and 44 µg/dl.[103] However, the findings of this study, the indications for treatment, and the recommended agents and doses are controversial; the physician should consult with a specialist in occupational medicine or toxicology or contact a regional poison-control center for specific advice about the doses and side effects of these drugs.

Health care providers should be aware that the Occupational Safety and Health Administration (OSHA) has provided specific guidelines for monitoring and managing workers who have been exposed to lead [see Chapter 6]; these guidelines stipulate that such workers be removed from exposure if a single blood lead level exceeds 60 µg/dl or if the average of a series of three successive periodic screening levels exceeds 50 µg/dl.[104] For further information, a regional OSHA office or an occupational medicine specialist should be consulted. (A directory of regional offices is available at the OSHA Web site, at http://www.osha.gov.) Finally, because household members of persons who have been occupationally exposed to lead may be contaminated by the poisoned individual, household members should also be evaluated for lead poisoning even if they are apparently asymptomatic, and measures should be taken to reduce or prevent further exposure.

LITHIUM

Lithium is a simple cation that is widely used for the treatment of manic-depressive illness and other psychiatric disorders. It is also used to elevate the white blood cell count in patients with severe leukopenia. Lithium is excreted renally, and severe intoxication usually results from drug accumulation caused by renal impairment or excessive overmedication. An acute single overdose, however, is less likely to result in severe poisoning.

Diagnosis

The usual therapeutic level of lithium is 0.6 to 1.2 mEq/L. Chronic intoxication can occur with levels only slightly above 1.2 mEq/L, but patients with acute overdose may remain asymptomatic despite having much higher levels early after ingestion of the drug.[105] Manifestations of lithium intoxication include confusion, lethargy, tremors, and muscle twitching. The ECG may show flattening of T waves, the presence of U waves, and prolongation of the QT interval. In severe cases, coma and convulsions may occur.[105] Symptoms may take several days to weeks to resolve, and some patients are left with permanent neurologic impairment.[106] Other toxic effects of lithium intoxication are nephrogenic diabetes insipidus and neuroleptic malignant syndrome [see Table 5]. These effects can occur at therapeutic levels of the drug.

Treatment

Treatment of acute lithium overdose consists mainly of gut decontamination and fluid therapy. Because lithium is poorly adsorbed to activated charcoal, administration of this agent is not necessary unless the physician suspects that another drug has also been ingested. Gastric lavage or ipecac-induced emesis may reduce the gastric burden of lithium. Whole bowel irrigation should be considered, especially if the patient has ingested a sustained-release form of the drug.[105] Limited experimental and anecdotal evidence suggests that administration of sodium polystyrene sulfonate reduces absorption and enhances elimination of lithium, although its role in acute lithium overdose remains to be established.[107]

Fluid therapy is an essential part of treatment of lithium intoxication. The physician should restore volume with 1 to 2 L of normal saline, then continue the I.V. administration of fluids at a rate sufficient to produce urine at a rate of about 100 ml/hr. The indications for hemodialysis in the setting of lithium toxicity are controversial. A recent review article recommends the following guidelines for hemodialysis: a lithium level greater than 6 mEq/L in any patient; a lithium level greater than 4 mEq/L in any patient on long-term lithium therapy (in contrast to an acute overdose); or a lithium level of 2.5 to 4.0 mEq/L in any patient with severe neurologic symptoms, renal insufficiency, hemodynamic instability, or neurologic instability.[105] One poison-control center–based study did not observe any significant difference in lithium toxic patients in whom hemodialysis was recommended by the poison-control center but not performed and in whom hemodialysis was performed.[108] These authors recommend reserving hemodialysis for severe cases of lithium toxicity. Blood should be drawn at least 8 to 12 hours after the last dose of lithium is given to prevent misinterpretation caused by falsely high levels before drug distribution in tissues. Serial lithium measurements should be obtained until the level clearly drops, to exclude ongoing absorption or rebound after hemodialysis. Consultation with a regional poison-control center, medical toxicologist, and nephrologist should be obtained early to help manage a lithium-toxic patient.

METHEMOGLOBINEMIA-INDUCING AGENTS

Methemoglobin is an oxidized form of hemoglobin that is incapable of carrying and delivering oxygen normally. A number of oxidant drugs and chemicals can convert hemoglobin to its oxidized form, causing methemoglobinemia.[109] These agents include local anesthetics (e.g., benzocaine and lidocaine), antimicrobial agents (e.g., chloroquine, dapsone, primaquine, and sulfonamides), analgesics (e.g., phenazopyridine and phenacetin), nitrites and nitrates (e.g., amyl nitrite, butyl nitrite, isobutyl nitrite, and sodium nitrite), and several miscellaneous drugs and chemicals (e.g., aminophenol, aniline dyes, bromates, chlorates, metoclopramide, nitrobenzene, nitrogen oxides, and nitroglycerin). Persons with glucose-6-phosphate dehydrogenase (G6PD) deficiency and congenital methemoglobin reductase deficiency are more likely than persons without these conditions to accumulate methemoglobin after exposure to an oxidant.

Diagnosis

Methemoglobinemia causes cellular asphyxia. Symptoms of mild to moderate methemoglobinemia include headache, nausea, dizziness, and dyspnea. Methemoglobin levels as low as 15% can cause the patient to appear cyanotic despite having a normal oxygen tension. The blood usually has a dark or chocolate-brown appearance. Although pulse oximetry is abnormal, the reported drop in oxygen saturation does not correlate with the actual reduction in oxyhemoglobin saturation, and specific testing for methemoglobinemia should be performed.[110]

Treatment

Mild methemoglobinemia (methemoglobin levels < 15% to 20%) usually resolves spontaneously, requiring no treatment. Patients who have more severe intoxication should be given the antidote methylene blue (1 to 2 mg/kg I.V. [0.1 to 0.2 ml/kg of a 1% solution] over several minutes).[109] The dosage may be repeated once. Although symptoms and signs usually resolve quickly, methemoglobinemia may recur with the administration of long-acting oxidants such as dapsone [see Chapter 89].[109]

OPIOIDS

The opioids and opiates include several synthetic and naturally occurring compounds that are widely used for their analgesic properties. Common opium derivatives include morphine, heroin, hydrocodone, and codeine. Synthetic opioids include fentanyl, methadone, and butorphanol. Preparations of hydrocodone or codeine for oral use commonly contain aspirin or acetaminophen, which may themselves be responsible for serious toxicity in an overdose. Opioids stimulate several receptors in the CNS, resulting in sedation and reduced sympathetic outflow.[6,7] Excessive opioid effect may cause coma and blunting of the respiratory response to hypercapnia. The opioids meperidine and dextromethorphan may cause serious rigidity and hyperthermia in persons who are taking MAO inhibitors or other serotoninergic drugs (e.g., selective serotonin reuptake inhibitors [SSRIs]).[111]

Diagnosis

Patients may have opioid intoxication as a result of unintentional overdose or attempted suicide. Signs of intoxication include lethargy or coma, pinpoint pupils, and respiratory depression. Acute noncardiogenic pulmonary edema may occur.[6] Seizures are not typical but may occur with acute propoxyphene overdose; repeated therapeutic doses of meperidine can also cause seizures, especially in persons with renal failure because of accumulation of the metabolite normeperidine.

Diagnosis of opioid intoxication is usually not difficult in a person who is in a coma and has pinpoint pupils and apnea.[5,6] Paramedics may discover I.V. drug paraphernalia or empty prescription bottles at the scene. Exposure to other drugs, however, may complicate the clinical picture.

Treatment

The physician should immediately establish that the airway is not obstructed and that ventilation is adequate and then administer supplemental oxygen as necessary. After these initial measures, the specific opioid antagonist naloxone should be given (0.2 to 2 mg I.V. or S.C.). A recent trial has shown similar results with subcutaneous and intravenous naloxone.[112] Persons who are suspected of chronic narcotic abuse should be started with smaller doses of naloxone to minimize the severity of an acute withdrawal reaction. Patients usually become fully awake within a few minutes after administration. If the initial dose is not effective, additional doses (up to 15 to 20 mg if opioid intoxication is strongly suspected) should be given until a satisfactory response is achieved. The plasma half-life of naloxone is about 60 minutes, which is shorter than that of most of the opioids whose actions it reverses; therefore, patients who respond to the antidote should be observed for at least 3 hours after the last dose for the recurrence of sedation. Traditionally thought to be an innocuous drug, naloxone has been associated with an approximately 1.6% complication rate. Complications include asystole, seizures, pulmonary edema, and severe agitation.[6]

Oral ingestion of an opioid should be treated with activated charcoal. Gastric lavage should be considered in cases of large or recent overdose. There is no role for hemodialysis or other enhanced removal procedures in the treatment of opioid overdose.

ORGANOPHOSPHATES AND RELATED AGENTS

Organophosphates and carbamates are widely used as pesticides,[113] and several of the nerve agents developed for chemical warfare[114] are rapidly acting and potent organophosphates. All of these poisons inhibit the enzyme acetylcholinesterase, preventing the breakdown of acetylcholine at cholinergic synapses. Whereas the organophosphates may cause permanent damage to the enzyme, carbamates have a transient and reversible effect. Many of these agents are well absorbed through intact skin. Persons may be exposed accidentally while working with or transporting the chemicals or as a result of accidental or suicidal ingestion.

Diagnosis

Excessive activity of acetylcholine may occur at nicotinic, muscarinic, and CNS cholinergic receptors. The most common presenting symptoms of poisoning are abdominal cramps and vomiting accompanied by sweating and hypersalivation [see Table 15]. The patient usually has small or pinpoint pupils. Because of the mixed effects of poisoning on sympathetic ganglia and parasympathetic synapses, the heart rate may be either slow or fast. Life-threatening manifestations of acetylcholinesterase inhibition include muscle weakness with respiratory arrest, as well as severe bronchospasm. Significant volume loss may result from excessive sweating, salivation, vomiting, and diarrhea.[113]

Treatment

Contaminated clothing should be removed immediately and all exposed areas washed thoroughly with soap and water. Rescue personnel should take precautions to avoid secondary contamination from direct contact with the victim's skin, clothing, or vomitus. Xylene or other solvent vapors emanating from the victim are not life threatening to medical personnel but may cause dizziness, nausea, and headache. In patients who have ingested an organophosphate or a carbamate, gastric lavage should be performed with the use of a closed-container unit and activated charcoal should be administered.

Specific therapy includes administration of atropine and pralidoxime (2-PAM). Atropine is not a physiologic antidote but can reverse excessive muscarinic stimulation, thereby alleviating abdominal cramps, bronchospasm, and hypersalivation. It does not reverse muscle weakness. All patients with organophosphate poisoning should also be given 2-PAM because it can

Table 15 Manifestations of Excessive
Activity of Acetylcholine

Site of Activity	Clinical Manifestations
Postganglionic muscarinic receptors	Bradycardia; miosis; salivation; lacrimation; bronchorrhea; increased peristalsis; sweating
Autonomic ganglia	Tachycardia; hypertension
Skeletal muscle nicotinic receptors	Muscle fasciculations followed by weakness; neuromuscular paralysis
CNS cholinergic receptors	Agitation; seizures

chemically restore the enzyme acetylcholinesterase; in persons who go untreated, the organophosphate's binding to acetylcholinesterase may become permanent (the so-called aging effect). Because carbamates have a transient effect, 2-PAM therapy is not needed in patients who have been poisoned with these agents. However, because the exact product causing cholinergic excess is often not known initially or because it may be a mix of organophosphate and carbamate, 2-PAM may be initiated empirically. Additionally, several case reports suggest that 2-PAM may be useful in carbamate poisoning.[115]

The dosage of 2-PAM is 1 to 2 g I.V. initially, followed by a continuous infusion of 200 to 500 mg/hr, depending on the patient's response. The infusion should be continued until the patient can be weaned from the drug without experiencing recurrence of weakness or muscarinic manifestations. This process may take several days in persons who have been exposed to highly lipid-soluble agents such as fenthion or dichlorvos.[7] A so-called intermediate syndrome has been described in which some patients experience recurrent muscle weakness several days after initially successful treatment[116]; this syndrome may be caused by neurotoxic components of the agent, continued toxicity from a lipid-soluble product, or inadequate 2-PAM therapy.

SALICYLATES

Aspirin (acetylsalicylic acid) and other salicylates are widely used for their antipyretic, anti-inflammatory, and analgesic effects and can be found alone or in combination in a number of prescription and over-the-counter products (e.g., oil of wintergreen, Pepto-Bismol). Salicylates interfere with the metabolism of glucose and fatty acids; they also uncouple oxidative phosphorylation, leading to inefficient production of adenosine triphosphate, accumulation of lactic acid, and production of heat. Poisoning may result from an acute single ingestion (usually in a dose > 200 mg/kg) or from chronic overmedication.[117] Chronic poisoning occurs most commonly in elderly persons who regularly take large doses of aspirin (e.g., for osteoarthritis) and who gradually begin to take larger doses or in whom renal insufficiency develops. In such cases, the diagnosis of salicylism is often overlooked, and patients may be assumed to have sepsis, gastroenteritis, or pneumonia on admission to the hospital.[117]

Diagnosis

The most common initial manifestation of salicylate poisoning is hyperventilation, which occurs largely as a result of central stimulation of respiratory drive and partly in response to metabolic acidosis. Measurement of arterial blood gases usually reveals respiratory alkalosis with predominant alkalemia and underlying metabolic acidosis. Other findings include tinnitus, confusion, and lethargy. Patients with severe intoxication may experience coma, seizures, hyperthermia, noncardiogenic pulmonary edema, and circulatory collapse. The serum salicylate level in such cases usually exceeds 100 mg/dl (1,000 mg/L), although patients with chronic intoxication may experience severe effects with much lower serum levels.[118]

Treatment

For patients with an acute ingestion, activated charcoal should be administered and gastric lavage considered if the ingestion was large (e.g., > 10 to 15 g). Because salicylates cause pylorospasm and delay gastric emptying, lavage may be successful even after a delay of several hours. For a patient who has taken a massive ingestion, extra dosages of activated charcoal (50 to 60 g every 4 to 6 hours for the first 1 to 2 days) may be needed to achieve the desired 10-to-1 ratio of charcoal to drug. Massive ingestions, as well as those involving enteric-coated aspirin, may lead to prolonged or delayed absorption and the potential for catastrophic worsening after 1 to 2 days.[117] In such cases, close observation of the patient should be maintained, and measurement of the serum salicylate level should frequently be performed until the level clearly drops into the therapeutic range (10 to 20 mg/dl).

Enhanced elimination procedures can effectively reduce elevated salicylate levels. Alkalinization of the urine traps the ionized form of salicylate in the kidney tubules, increasing renal elimination.[110] To initiate alkalinization, the physician should add 100 mEq of sodium bicarbonate to 1 L of 5% dextrose in quarter-normal (0.225%) saline, then infuse the solution at 200 ml/hr while monitoring the pH of the urine (the goal is to achieve a pH of 7 to 8). It may be difficult to perform alkalinization in patients with volume and potassium deficits without first replacing these losses. Hemodialysis rapidly lowers serum salicylate levels and can restore fluid and electrolyte balances. Hemodialysis is recommended for patients who are unable to tolerate fluid challenges (e.g., as in cerebral edema or pulmonary edema) and those who have worsening renal insufficiency, severe metabolic acidosis, or a serum salicylate level greater than 100 mg/dl (1,000 mg/L).

SEDATIVE-HYPNOTIC AGENTS

The sedative-hypnotic agents include the barbiturates (e.g., phenobarbital, pentobarbital, butalbital, and amobarbital) and the benzodiazepines (e.g., alprazolam, diazepam, lorazepam, and triazolam), as well as several other drugs, such as meprobamate, glutethimide, ethchlorvynol, chloral hydrate, zolpidem, and buspirone. These drugs cause generalized depression of CNS activity and are commonly used to alleviate anxiety or to induce sleep. The mechanisms of action and pharmacokinetics are different for each drug group.[11,119,120]

Diagnosis

Overdose of a sedative-hypnotic drug causes lethargy, ataxia, and slurred speech. In patients with severe poisoning, coma and respiratory arrest may occur, especially when sedative-hypnotic drugs are combined with other depressants, such as ethanol. The blood pressure and pulse rate are usually decreased, the temperature may be low because of exposure and venodilatation, and the pupils are usually small (although they may be dilated in patients with glutethimide overdose). Patients who are in a deep coma may appear to be dead because they may have absent reflexes, fixed pupils, and even flat EEG tracings.[121] In patients with chloral hydrate overdose, ventricular ectopy and ventricular tachycardia may develop; these effects are caused by generation of the metabolite trichloroethanol, which, like other chlorinated hydrocarbons, can sensitize the myocardium to the effects of epinephrine.[122] In cases of phenobarbital overdose, blood levels of the drug can be obtained in most hospital laboratories, but in cases of overdose of most of the other sedative-hypnotic agents, blood levels are neither clinically useful nor readily available.

Treatment

The physician should maintain an unobstructed airway and administer supplemental oxygen, then intubate the trachea and assist ventilation, if necessary. Uncomplicated hypothermia should be treated with gradual passive external rewarming. I.V. crystalloids should be administered to patients with low blood pressure; if necessary, dopamine and other pressor agents should be given. For patients with ventricular arrhythmias caused by chloral hydrate overdose, propranolol (1 to 5 mg I.V.) or esmolol (25 to 100 mg/kg/min) should be given.[122] Activated charcoal should be administered. For cases of massive ingestion, gastric lavage should be considered.

Flumazenil is a specific benzodiazepine antagonist that has been proved effective in reversing the coma caused by benzodiazepine overdose. It has a rapid onset of action after I.V. administration (0.5 to 3.0 mg); because its effects last for only about 2 to 3 hours, resedation may occur. Flumazenil is contraindicated in patients with a known or suspected overdose of a tricyclic antidepressant and in patients who have been given a benzodiazepine for control of status epilepticus, because flumazenil may induce seizures in these patients. It should also not be used in patients who have increased intracranial pressure and who are receiving benzodiazepines for sedation. The use of flumazenil in persons who have been taking large quantities of benzodiazepines for long periods may provoke an acute withdrawal syndrome.[5,7]

Enhanced removal procedures are rarely needed in patients with sedative-hypnotic overdose because most will recover with airway management, assisted ventilation, and other supportive measures. When supportive measures fail, hemoperfusion can effectively reduce blood concentrations of phenobarbital, pentobarbital, meprobamate, glutethimide, and ethchlorvynol.[123]

THEOPHYLLINE

Although no longer a first-line drug, theophylline is still used for the treatment of asthma and other bronchospastic disorders, congestive heart failure, and neonatal apnea. It is available in regular and sustained-release formulations for oral use. Aminophylline, the ethylenediamine salt of theophylline, is used for I.V. infusions. Theophylline intoxication may occur after an acute single overdose or as a result of chronic overmedication.[124] Chronic intoxication may also be caused by reduced theophylline metabolism resulting from the addition of an interfering drug (e.g., cimetidine or erythromycin) or from an intercurrent illness (e.g., congestive heart failure or liver failure). The normal elimination half-life, 4 to 6 hours, may be prolonged to more than 20 hours in theophylline overdose.

Diagnosis

Acute theophylline overdose causes vomiting, tremors, and tachycardia. Laboratory findings include hypokalemia, hypophosphatemia, and hyperglycemia. These metabolic effects, as well as tachycardia and vasodilatation, are thought to be mediated through excessive beta$_2$-adrenergic stimulation. If serum theophylline levels exceed 100 mg/L, seizures, hypotension, and

ventricular arrhythmias are likely to develop.[124] The seizures are often refractory to anticonvulsant therapy. Serum drug levels may not peak for 16 to 24 hours after theophylline ingestion, especially if the drug was in a sustained-release formulation.

Chronic intoxication may develop gradually, with toxicity possibly occurring at serum drug levels that are much lower than those associated with acute overdose: seizures have been reported to occur at levels as low as 14 to 35 mg/L.[124] Unlike the findings in acute overdose, hypokalemia and hypotension are not common.

Treatment

In cases of acute ingestion of theophylline, activated charcoal should be given. Gastric lavage should be considered for large ingestions (more than 15 to 20 tablets). However, it is unlikely that lavage will remove intact sustained-release tablets, and severe or fatal intoxication may ensue despite aggressive attempts at decontamination.[125] Although some toxicologists have suggested administering repeated doses of activated charcoal in combination with whole bowel irrigation for massive ingestions of sustained-release medications, this approach remains controversial.[125]

Hypotension should be treated with esmolol (25 to 100 mg/kg/min) rather than a beta-adrenergic agonist because the hypotension is probably caused by beta$_2$-adrenergic–mediated vasodilatation.[126] Seizures should be treated with phenobarbital (15 to 20 mg/kg I.V.) rather than with phenytoin, which is ineffective.[125] For patients with recurrent seizures and for those with serum theophylline levels of around 100 mg/L or greater, excess theophylline should be removed as quickly as possible by hemodialysis or hemoperfusion.[127] Administration of multiple repeated doses of activated charcoal [see Enhanced Elimination, above] can effectively shorten the elimination half-life of theophylline, but such administration is often not practical in the critically ill patient.

TRICYCLIC ANTIDEPRESSANTS AND RELATED COMPOUNDS

Tricyclic antidepressants, also known as cyclic antidepressants, were once a leading cause of seizures and death from acute drug overdose.[123] Although most of the newer SSRI antidepressants are much less toxic [see Table 16], tricyclic antidepressants are still commonly used for the treatment of depression, enuresis, and other disorders.

The toxicity of the tricyclic antidepressants is caused by various pharmacologic properties of this class of agents, including anticholinergic activity, inhibition of norepinephrine reuptake, alpha-adrenergic blockade, and, most important, depression of the fast sodium channel in cardiac cells (the so-called quinidine-like or membrane-depressant effect). This last property is responsible for prolongation of conduction and depressed cardiac contractility.[128] Ingestion of approximately 1 g of a tricyclic antidepressant is likely to produce severe toxicity.

Diagnosis

Initially, persons with tricyclic antidepressant overdose have anticholinergic signs, including tachycardia; dilated pupils; reduced peristalsis; muscle twitching; and dry, flushed skin. Lethargy and slurred speech are common. The abrupt onset of seizures, coma, and hypotension signals severe toxicity, which may occur within 30 to 60 minutes of ingestion or may be delayed because of slowed gut absorption. In patients with severe intoxication, the ECG shows a QRS complex that is usually

Table 16   Common Tricyclic and Other Antidepressants

Tricyclic antidepressants and related agents (may induce cardiotoxicity, including widening of the QRS complex)
  Amitriptyline
  Desipramine
  Doxepin
  Imipramine
  Maprotiline
  Nortriptyline

Newer-generation antidepressants (cardiotoxicity is unlikely but seizures may occur)
  Amoxapine
  Bupropion
  Fluoxetine
  Paroxetine
  Sertraline
  Trazodone
  Venlafaxine

wider than 0.12 second[128,129]; however, this finding may initially be absent if the drug has not been absorbed or in cases of overdose with amoxapine or another noncardiotoxic drug. In some patients, right-axis deviation of the terminal 40 msec of the QRS complex may represent early evidence of a conduction disturbance.[129] Death may result from profound depression of cardiac conduction and contractility; respiratory arrest; or complications of pulmonary aspiration, aspiration pneumonia, or hyperthermia (caused by muscle twitching and seizures coupled with the absence of sweating).

Treatment

The physician should administer activated charcoal. Gastric lavage should be considered for patients with massive ingestions (e.g., > 4 to 5 g), especially if less than 1 hour has elapsed since the overdose. All patients should be monitored closely for at least 6 hours; any person with altered mental status, evidence of anticholinergic toxicity, or cardiac conduction abnormalities should be admitted to the hospital and monitored closely. The physician should maintain an unobstructed airway, intubate the trachea, and assist ventilation if needed.

Seizures should be treated with benzodiazepines and pheno-barbital (see above). Physostigmine should not be administered, because it may cause seizures and can worsen cardiac conduction disturbances. Initially, hypotension should be treated with I.V. boluses of normal saline. If there is evidence of depression of the sodium channel (i.e., a wide QRS complex), sodium bicarbonate should be administered at a dosage of 50 to 100 mEq I.V.[10,128] Repeated doses may be given as needed, although the serum pH should be monitored for excessive alkalemia. If hypotension does not respond to administration of fluids and sodium bicarbonate, dopamine or norepinephrine should be given. Norepinephrine may be more effective than dopamine in some patients, possibly because of tricyclic antidepressant–induced depletion of norepinephrine, but in one study, no difference between these agents was found.[128] Partial cardiopulmonary bypass has been suggested for patients with refractory hypotension and agonal cardiac rhythm, although there is little likelihood of survival.[54] There is no known role for hemodialysis or hemoperfusion in this setting.

Food Poisoning

A variety of toxins may produce illness after consumption of fish, shellfish, or mushrooms. Illness caused by bacterial or viral contamination of food, including botulism, is discussed elsewhere [see Chapter 136].

SEAFOOD

The mechanism of toxicity varies with each toxin [see Table 17]. In general, the seafood-associated toxins are heat stable; therefore, cooking does not render the food safe to eat. In some cases (e.g., ciguatera and paralytic shellfish poisoning [PSP]), the poisons are highly potent neurotoxins elaborated by dinoflagellates, which are then consumed by fish or concentrated by filter-feeding clams and mussels. Scombroid poisoning results from bacterial overgrowth in inadequately refrigerated fish (although the fish may look and smell fresh); scombrotoxin is a mixture of histamine and histaminelike compounds produced by the breakdown of histidine in the fish flesh. Tetrodotoxin is produced by microorganisms associated with the puffer fish (as well as the California newt and some species of South American frogs) and concentrated in various internal organs. Although the fish is deadly and ranks as the leading cause of fatal food poisoning in Japan, it is also considered a delicacy; extreme care is required in preparation of this fish by specially trained chefs to separate the edible muscle from

Table 17   Seafood Poisonings[159]

Type	Onset	Common Sources	Syndrome	Treatment
Ciguatera	1–6 hr	Barracuda, red snapper, grouper	Gastrointestinal upset, paresthesias, sensation of hot and cold reversal, itching, weakness, myalgias, orthostatic hypotension	Supportive; ?mannitol
Paralytic shellfish poisoning	30 min	Bivalve mollusks (mussels, clams), associated with algae bloom (red tide)	Gastrointestinal upset, paresthesias, ataxia, weakness, respiratory muscle paralysis, respiratory arrest	Supportive
Scombroid	Minutes to hours	Tuna, mahi-mahi, bonito, mackerel	Gastrointestinal upset, flushed skin, urticaria, wheezing	Antihistamines
Tetrodotoxin	30 min	Puffer fish (fugu), sunfish, porcupine fish	Vomiting, paresthesias, perioral tingling, muscle weakness, respiratory paralysis, respiratory arrest	Supportive

the toxin-containing organs. Poisoning from saxitoxin (the culprit in PSP) has recently been reported in persons who ate puffer fish caught in waters near Titusville, Florida.[130]

Diagnosis

Signs and symptoms of seafood poisoning vary with the toxin [see Table 17]. Diagnosis is based on the clinical presentation and history of ingested seafood. In some cases, laboratory confirmation can be carried out with the assistance of the regional or state health department.

Treatment

In general, treatment is supportive. For neurotoxic poisonings such as PSP and tetrodotoxin, prompt medical attention may be required to prevent death from sudden respiratory arrest. Scombroid poisoning is often treated with H_1 and H_2 histamine blockers (e.g., diphenhydramine and cimetidine). For ciguatera poisoning, previous anecdotal reports have suggested benefit from mannitol, but a recent randomized, controlled blinded trial showed that mannitol did not relieve symptoms of ciguatera poisoning and resulted in more side effects than normal saline.[131] Ciguatera poisoning can produce chronic symptoms, which may resemble multiple sclerosis or chronic fatigue syndrome.[132] Improvement in chronic symptoms has been reported in patients treated with amitriptyline or fluoxetine[133,134]; polyneuropathy has responded to gabapentin.[135] Recurrence of symptoms, which may be worse than the initial attack, can be triggered by ingestion of fish or alcohol.

AMANITA PHALLOIDES MUSHROOMS

The *A. phalloides* mushroom ("death cap") has been known and feared for at least two millennia and continues to cause serious illness and death, although in recent years, mortality has declined because of the availability of orthotopic liver transplantation for patients with fulminant liver failure. This mushroom, as well as several others that contain the cellular toxin amanitin (also known as amatoxin), are found throughout Europe and the United States. Most victims are amateur or novice mushroom hunters who mistake this mushroom for another, edible species. The toxin is heat stable and is not destroyed by cooking. Once absorbed, it binds to RNA polymerase and inhibits cellular protein synthesis. Hepatocytes and rapidly dividing cells are most sensitive.

Diagnosis

Severe abdominal cramps, vomiting, and diarrhea begin about 8 to 12 hours or longer after a meal. Diarrhea can be so severe that it results in severe volume depletion and cardiovascular collapse. After apparent recovery from the gastrointestinal syndrome, patients can develop rapidly progressive hepatic failure.

Treatment

Treatment of suspected amatoxin poisoning includes aggressive fluid replacement and administration of activated charcoal by mouth to bind any unabsorbed toxin in the gut and to prevent enterohepatic reabsorption, which can be significant.[136] Patients who develop severe liver injury with encephalopathy are candidates for emergency liver transplantation. Various antidotes have been described over the years, including high-dose intravenous penicillin G, corticosteroids, thioctic acid, and silibinin (an extract of the milk thistle plant), but none have proved to be effective in controlled studies, and neither thioctic acid nor

silibinin is available in the United States.[136] (Milk thistle extract can be found in some stores selling dietary and nutritional supplements, however.)

MONOSODIUM GLUTAMATE

Monosodium glutamate (MSG) is a food additive used to enhance flavor and add body to prepared foods. It is also found as a component of hydrolyzed vegetable protein. Consumption of MSG can invoke, in susceptible persons, a syndrome originally coined the Chinese-restaurant syndrome and now known as the MSG symptom complex. The syndrome, which begins about 15 to 30 minutes after ingestion, includes a burning sensation or pressure in the face, behind the eyes, and in the chest, neck, shoulders, forearms, and abdomen. Headache, syncope, and, rarely, cardiac arrhythmias have been described. Not everyone who ingests MSG experiences the reaction. The etiology of the syndrome is not clearly understood. Symptoms usually last no more than 2 to 3 hours, and there is no specific treatment.[137-139]

HERBAL REMEDIES AND DIETARY SUPPLEMENTS

Approximately 25% of patients use alternative therapies, such as herbal products, for a health problem[140] [see Chapter 8]. Herbal products are not subject to FDA approval, because they do not undergo the scientific testing required of conventional therapies. They cannot be promoted specifically for treatment, prevention, or cure of a disease. However, the Dietary Supplement Health and Education Act of 1994 has allowed these products to be sold and labeled with statements describing their professed effects. With increasing use and availability of herbal medications, poison-control centers and health care providers are commonly encountering patients with adverse effects from impure products, drug interactions, and intentional ingestions. *Ginkgo biloba* has been suggested to have antiplatelet effects, and cases of spontaneous hyphema and bilateral subdural hematomas have been reported.[141] The additional risk of warfarin must be considered in patients taking *Ginkgo biloba*. Ephedra (Ma Huang) is a common ingredient in herbal weight-loss products (herbal fen-phen), stimulants (herbal ecstasy), decongestants, and bronchodilators. The active moiety in Ephedra is ephedrine and related alkaloids. Serious adverse reactions, including hypertension, seizures, arrhythmias, heart attack, stroke, and death, have been reported.[142] St. John's wort (*Hypericum perforatum*), touted as a natural antidepressant, has been shown to inhibit serotonin, dopamine, and norepinephrine reuptake and thus presents the possibility of interaction with MAO inhibitors and other serotoninergic drugs.[142]

Adverse events associated with most herbal products are largely undescribed, and there are few specific antidotes. Emergency and supportive measures should therefore be instituted as necessary [see Management of Common Complications, above]. To enhance research and knowledge in this area, all such events should be reported to poison-control centers and to the FDA's MedWatch Program (800-FDA-1088; http://www.fda.gov/medwatch).

Smoke Inhalation

Smoke inhalation injury is the most common cause of mortality among fire victims, accounting for up to 75% of deaths.[81] Fires produce heat and smoke, although the latter is the chief culprit in inhalation injuries.[143] Smoke comprises a varying mixture of particles and gaseous chemicals that are pyrolysis products of substances that become toxic only when burned.[144] Smoke components can be broken down into simple asphyxiants, chemical asphyxiants, and irritants. Simple asphyxiants (e.g., methane and carbon dioxide) displace oxygen, thus decreasing F_1O_2 (fraction of inspired oxygen) and resulting in hypoxemia. Chemical asphyxiants (e.g., carbon monoxide, cyanide, and hydrogen sulfide) cause systemic toxicity and cellular hypoxia by interrupting transport or utilization of oxygen [see Specific Drugs and Poisons, above].

Irritant gases have a direct cytotoxic effect on the oropharynx and the respiratory tract. Toxicity depends on the physical and chemical properties of the gas, which are often divided into two major groups on the basis of their water solubility. Highly water-soluble gases (e.g., ammonia, acrolein, hydrogen chloride, and sulfur dioxide) are readily absorbed in the mucous membranes along the upper respiratory tract, causing local irritation of the eyes, nose, and throat. Compounds with intermediate solubility (e.g., chlorine and isocyanates) cause upper and lower respiratory tract injury. Substances that are less water soluble (e.g., phosgene and nitrogen dioxide) do not dissolve readily in the mucous membranes of the upper respiratory tract and can reach the distal airway, producing delayed-onset pulmonary toxicity.[81,144]

DIAGNOSIS

Clinical symptoms vary with the location of tissue injury, which in turn depends on the solubility and the concentration of exposure. Manifestations of toxicity may include conjunctival irritation, rhinitis, oropharyngeal erythema and burns, coryza, hoarseness, stridor, wheezing, coughing, and noncardiogenic pulmonary edema. Onset of pulmonary edema may be delayed up to 12 to 24 hours or longer when the patient has been exposed to low-solubility gases such as phosgene and nitrogen dioxide.[81]

TREATMENT

Management at the scene of the exposure should include evacuation of all persons from further exposure to the smoke. Rescuers should take precautions to avoid personal exposure and should use a self-contained breathing apparatus. Although the clinician rarely has access to information regarding the constituents of the smoke, initial treatment of all victims should focus on the airway [see Initial Stabilization, above]. All patients should receive supplemental oxygen in the highest concentration while arterial blood gas and carboxyhemoglobin levels are pending [see Carbon Monoxide, above]. For patients who do not require immediate airway protection (e.g., those who are without respiratory distress, coma, or stridor), a careful plan should be sought for identifying those at high risk for potential deterioration. Many authors recommend fiberoptic bronchoscopy to help identify supraglottic and subglottic airway injury.[81] An important caveat is that lack of upper airway injury (e.g., oropharyngeal burns or singed nasal hairs) neither precludes nor predicts future airway demise. Patients should be risk-stratified on the basis of history (e.g., closed-space fire, particular materials in the fire, loss of consciousness, or history of reactive airway disease) before final disposition. Patients with any sign of airway injury or clinically significant smoke inhalation should be observed overnight. A normal initial chest radiograph is not a reliable indicator of pulmonary injury.[145] If exposure to a low-solubility toxin is likely (e.g., phosgene or nitrogen dioxide), manifestation of pulmonary injury may be delayed for 12 to 24 hours. Bronchodilators should be used for bronchospasm, but unlike in asthma and chronic obstructive pulmonary disease, use of

steroids has not been shown to be beneficial in smoke inhalation patients.[81] Patients with suspected cyanide poisoning should receive sodium thiosulfate [see Cyanide, above].

References

1. Annual Emergency Room Data 1992: Data from the Drug Abuse Warning Network (DAWN). US Department of Health and Human Services, Public Health Service, Alcohol, Drug Abuse, and Mental Health Administration (DHS Publication No [SMA] 94-2080), Rockville, Maryland, 1997
2. Annual Medical Examiner Data 1992: Data from the Drug Abuse Warning Network (DAWN). US Department of Health and Human Services, Public Health Service, Substance Abuse and Mental Health Services Administration (DHS Publication No [SMA] 94-2081), Rockville, Maryland, 1994
3. Kharasch M, Graff J: Emergency management of the airway. Crit Care Clin 11:53, 1995
4. Powner DJ: Drug-associated isoelectric EEGs: a hazard in brain-death certification. JAMA 236:1123, 1976
5. Hoffman RS, Goldfrank LR: The poisoned patient with altered consciousness: controversies in the use of a 'coma cocktail.' JAMA 274:562, 1995
6. Sporer KA: Acute heroin overdose. Ann Intern Med 130:584, 1999
7. Bowden CA, Krenzelok EP: Clinical applications of commonly used contemporary antidotes: a US perspective. Drug Saf 16:9, 1997
8. Vernon DD, Gleich MC: Poisoning and drug overdose. Crit Care Clin 13:647, 1997
9. Krenzelok EP, Leikin JB: Approach to the poisoned patient. Dis Mon 42:509, 1996
10. Kolecki PF, Curry SC: Poisoning by sodium channel blocking agents. Crit Care Clin 13:829, 1997
11. Sing K, Erickson T, Amitai Y, et al: Chloral hydrate toxicity from oral and intravenous administration. J Toxicol Clin Toxicol 34:101, 1996
12. Leo PJ, Hollander JE, Shih RD, et al: Phenylpropanolamine and associated myocardial injury. Ann Emerg Med 28:359, 1996
13. Volz HP, Gleiter CH: Monoamine oxidase inhibitors: a perspective on their use in the elderly. Drugs Aging 13:341, 1998
14. Perron AD, Gibbs M: Thoracic aortic dissection secondary to crack cocaine ingestion. Am J Emerg Med 15:507, 1997
15. Brust JC: Acute neurologic complications of drug and alcohol abuse. Neurol Clin 16:503, 1998
16. Hoffman RS, Hollander JE: Evaluation of patients with chest pain after cocaine use. Crit Care Clin 13:809, 1997
17. Olson KR, Kearney TE, Dyer JE, et al: Seizures associated with poisoning and drug overdose. Am J Emerg Med 12:392, 1994
18. Bleck TP: Management approaches to prolonged seizures and status epilepticus. Epilepsia 40(suppl 1):S59, 1999
19. Chan TC, Evans SD, Clark RF: Drug-induced hyperthermia. Crit Care Clin 13:785, 1997
20. Hanania NA, Zimmerman JL: Accidental hypothermia. Crit Care Clin 15:235, 1999
21. Antretter H, Dapunt OE, Bonatti J: Management of profound hypothermia. Br J Hosp Med 54:215, 1995
22. Visweswaran P, Guntupalli J: Rhabdomyolysis. Crit Care Clin 15:415, 1999
23. Salgia AD, Kosnik SD: When acetaminophen use becomes toxic: treating acute accidental and intentional overdose. Postgrad Med 105:81, 1999
24. Kirk M, Pace S: Pearls, pitfalls, and updates in toxicology. Emerg Med Clin North Am 15:427, 1997
25. Belson MG, Simon HK: Utility of comprehensive toxicologic screens in children. Am J Emerg Med 17:221, 1999
26. Manoguerra AS: Gastrointestinal decontamination after poisoning. Where is the science? Crit Care Clin 13:709, 1997
27. Henry JA, Hoffman JR: Continuing controversy on gut decontamination. Lancet 352:420, 1998
28. Bond GR: The poisoned child: evolving concepts in care. Emerg Med Clin North Am 13:343, 1995
29. Krenzelok E, Vale A: Position statements: gut contamination. American Academy of Clinical Toxicology: European Association of Poisons Centres and Clinical Toxicologists. J Toxicol Clin Toxicol 35:695, 1997
30. Pond SM, Lewis-Driver DJ, Williams GM, et al: Gastric emptying in acute overdose: a prospective randomised controlled trial. Med J Aust 163:345, 1995
31. Mowad E, Haddad I, Gemmel DJ: Management of lead poisoning from ingested fishing sinkers. Arch Pediatr Adolesc Med 152:485, 1998
32. Bradberry SM, Vale JA: Multiple-dose activated charcoal: a review of relevant clinical studies. J Toxicol Clin Toxicol 33:407, 1995
33. Makin AJ, Wendon J, Williams R: A 7-year experience of severe acetaminophen-induced hepatotoxicity (1987-1993). Gastroenterology 109:1907, 1995
34. Whitcomb DC, Block GD: Association of acetaminophen hepatotoxicity with fasting and ethanol use. JAMA 272:1845, 1994
35. Bray GP, Harrison PM, O'Grady JG, et al: Long-term anticonvulsant therapy worsens outcome in paracetamol-induced fulminant hepatic failure. Hum Exp Toxicol 11:265, 1992

36. Jones AL: Mechanism of action and value of N-acetylcysteine in the treatment of early and late acetaminophen poisoning: a critical review. J Toxicol Clin Toxicol 36:277, 1998

37. Brok J, Buckley N, Gluud C: Interventions for paracetamol (acetaminophen) overdoses (Cochrane Review). Cochrane Database Syst Rev (3):CD003328, 2002

38. Woo OF, Mueller PD, Olson KR, et al: Shorter duration of oral N-acetylcysteine therapy for acute acetaminophen overdose. Ann Emerg Med 35:363, 2000

39. Perry HE, Shannon MW: Efficacy of oral versus intravenous N-acetylcysteine in acetaminophen overdose: results of an open-label, clinical trial. J Pediatr 132:149, 1998

40. Bailey B, McGuigan MA: Management of anaphylactoid reactions to intravenous N-acetylcysteine. Ann Emerg Med 31:710, 1998

41. Greene GS, Patterson SG, Warner E: Ingestion of angel's trumpet: an increasingly common source of toxicity. South Med J 89:365, 1996

42. Doig JC: Drug-induced cardiac arrhythmias: incidence, prevention and management. Drug Saf 17:265, 1997

43. de Abajo FJ, Rodriguez LA: Risk of ventricular arrhythmias associated with nonsedating antihistamine drugs. Br J Clin Pharmacol 47:307, 1999

44. Gottlieb S: Antihistamine drug withdrawn by manufacturer. BMJ 319:7, 1999

45. Burns MJ, Linden CH, Graudins A, et al: A comparison of physostigmine and benzodiazepines for the treatment of anticholinergic poisoning. Ann Emerg Med 35:374, 2000

46. Chua JD, Friedenberg W: Superwarfarin poisoning. Arch Intern Med 158:1929, 1998

47. Sheen SR, Spiller HA, Grossman D: Symptomatic brodifacoum ingestion requiring high-dose phytonadione therapy. Vet Hum Toxicol 36:216, 1994

48. Bruno GR, Howland MA, McMeeking A, et al: Long-acting anticoagulant overdose: brodifacoum kinetics and optimal vitamin K dosing. Ann Emerg Med 36:262, 2000

49. Love JN, Litovitz TL, Howell JM, et al: Characterization of fatal beta blocker ingestion: a review of the American Association of Poison Control Centers data from 1985 to 1995. J Toxicol Clin Toxicol 35:353, 1997

50. Kerns W II, Kline J, Ford MD: Beta-blocker and calcium channel blocker toxicity. Emerg Med Clin North Am 12:365, 1994

51. Love JN, Handler JA: Toxic psychosis: an unusual presentation of propranolol intoxication. Am J Emerg Med 13:536, 1995

52. Miller MB: Arrhythmias associated with drug toxicity. Emerg Med Clin North Am 16:405, 1998

53. Ashraf M, Chaudhary K, Nelson J, et al: Massive overdose of sustained-release verapamil: a case report and review of literature. Am J Med Sci 310:258, 1995

54. Albertson TE, Dawson A, de Latorre F, et al: TOX-ACLS: toxicologic-oriented advanced cardiac life support. Ann Emerg Med 37:S78, 2001

55. Buckley N, Dawson AH, Howarth D, et al: Slow-release verapamil poisoning: use of polyethylene glycol whole-bowel lavage and high-dose calcium. Med J Aust 158:202, 1993

56. Yuan TH, Kerns WP, Tomaszewski CA, et al: Insulin-glucose as adjunctive therapy for severe calcium channel antagonist poisoning. J Toxicol Clin Toxicol 37:463, 1999

57. Carbon monoxide poisoning deaths associated with camping—Georgia, March 1999. MMWR Morb Mortal Wkly Rep 48:705, 1999

58. Carbon monoxide poisonings associated with snow-obstructed vehicle exhaust systems in Philadelphia and New York City, January 1996. MMWR Morb Mortal Wkly Rep 45:1, 1996

59. Hardy KR, Thom SR: Pathophysiology and treatment of carbon monoxide poisoning. J Toxicol Clin Toxicol 32:613, 1994

60. Weaver LK: Carbon monoxide poisoning. Crit Care Clin 15:297, 1999

61. Hampson NB: Pulse oximetry in severe carbon monoxide poisoning. Chest 114:1036, 1998

62. Weaver LK, Hopkins RO, Chan KJ, et al: Hyperbaric oxygen for acute carbon monoxide poisoning. N Engl J Med 347:1057, 2002

63. Van Meter KW, Weiss L, Harch PG, et al: Should the pressure be off or on in the use of oxygen in the treatment of carbon monoxide-poisoned patients? (editorial). Ann Emerg Med 24:283, 1994

64. Olson KR, Seger D: Hyperbaric oxygen for carbon monoxide poisoning: does it really work? Ann Emerg Med 25:535, 1995

65. Tibbles PM, Perrotta PL: Treatment of carbon monoxide poisoning: a critical review of human outcome studies comparing normobaric oxygen with hyperbaric oxygen. Ann Emerg Med 24:269, 1994

66. Scheinkestel CD, Bailey M, Myles PS, et al: Hyperbaric or normobaric oxygen for acute carbon monoxide poisoning: a randomised controlled clinical trial. Med J Aust 170:203, 1999

67. Elkharrat D, Raphael JC, Korach JM, et al: Acute carbon monoxide intoxication and hyperbaric oxygen in pregnancy. Intensive Care Med 17:289, 1991

68. Boghdadi MS, Henning RJ: Cocaine: pathophysiology and clinical toxicology. Heart Lung 26:466, 1997

69. Benowitz NL: Clinical pharmacology and toxicology of cocaine. Pharmacol Toxicol 72:3, 1993

70. Henning RJ, Wilson LD, Glauser JM: Cocaine plus ethanol is more cardiotoxic than cocaine or ethanol alone. Crit Care Med 22:1896, 1994

71. Strote J, Lee JE, Wechsler H: Increasing MDMA use among college students: results of a national survey. J Adolesc Health 30:64, 2002

72. Club Drugs. Drug Abuse Warning Network [DAWN]. DAWN Briefings 2001

73. Kalant H: The pharmacology and toxicology of "ecstasy" (MDMA) and related drugs. CMAJ 165:917, 2001

74. Safer DJ, Zito JM, Fine EM: Increased methylphenidate usage for attention deficit disorder in the 1990s. Pediatrics 98:1084, 1996

75. White SR, Yadao CM: Characterization of methylphenidate exposures reported to a regional poison control center. Arch Pediatr Adolesc Med 154:1199, 2000

76. Klein-Schwart W: Abuse and toxicity of methylphenidate. Curr Opin Pediatr 14:219, 2002

77. Kao WF, Dart RC, Kuffner E, et al: Ingestion of low-concentration hydrofluoric acid: an insidious and potentially fatal poisoning. Ann Emerg Med 34:35, 1999

78. Matsuno K: The treatment of hydrofluoric acid burns. Occup Med (Lond) 46:313, 1996

79. Beasley DM, Glass WI: Cyanide poisoning: pathophysiology and treatment recommendations. Occup Med (Lond) 48:427, 1998

80. Shusterman D, Alexeeff G, Hargis C, et al: Predictors of carbon monoxide and hydrogen cyanide exposure in smoke inhalation patients. J Toxicol Clin Toxicol 34:61, 1996

81. Bizovi KE, Leikin JD: Smoke inhalation among firefighters. Occup Med 10:721, 1995

82. Dasgupta A, Emerson L: Neutralization of cardiac toxins oleandrin, oleandrigenin, bufalin, and cinobufotalin by digibind: monitoring the effect by measuring free digitoxin concentrations. Life Sci 63:781, 1998

83. Marik PE, Fromm L: A case series of hospitalized patients with elevated digoxin levels. Am J Med 105:110, 1998

84. Derlet RW, Horowitz BZ: Cardiotoxic drugs. Emerg Med Clin North Am 13:771, 1995

85. Williamson KM, Thrasher KA, Fulton KB, et al: Digoxin toxicity: an evaluation in current clinical practice. Arch Intern Med 158:2444, 1999

86. Freedland ES, McMicken DB, D'Onofrio G: Alcohol and trauma. Emerg Med Clin North Am 11:225, 1993

87. Glaser DS: Utility of the serum osmol gap in the diagnosis of methanol or ethylene glycol ingestion. Ann Emerg Med 27:343, 1996

88. Jacobsen D, McMartin KE: Antidotes for methanol and ethylene glycol poisoning. J Toxicol Clin Toxicol 35:127, 1997

89. Galloway GP, Frederick SL, Staggers FE Jr, et al: Gamma-hydroxybutyrate: an emerging drug of abuse that causes physical dependence. Addiction 92:89, 1997

90. Adverse events associated with ingestion of gamma-butyrolactone—Minnesota, New Mexico, and Texas, 1998–1999. MMWR Morb Mortal Wkly Rep 48:137, 1999

91. Chin RL, Sporer KA, Cullison B, et al: Clinical course of gamma-hydroxybutyrate overdose. Ann Emerg Med 31:716, 1998

92. Dyer JE, Roth B, Hyma BA: Gamma-hydroxybutyrate withdrawal syndrome. Ann Emerg Med 37:147, 2001

93. Addolorato G, Caputo F, Capristo E, et al: A case of gamma-hydroxybutyric acid withdrawal syndrome during alcohol addiction treatment: utility of diazepam administration. Clin Neuropharmacol 22:60, 1999

94. McGuigan MA: Acute iron poisoning. Pediatr Ann 25:33, 1996

95. Siff JE, Meldon SW, Tomassoni AJ: Usefulness of the total iron binding capacity in the evaluation and treatment of acute iron overdose. Ann Emerg Med 33:73, 1999

96. Romero JA, Kuczler FJ Jr: Isoniazid overdose: recognition and management. Am Fam Physician 57:749, 1998

97. Shah BR, Santucci K, Sinert R, et al: Acute isoniazid neurotoxicity in an urban hospital. Pediatrics 95:700, 1995

98. Temmerman W, Dhondt A, Vandewoude K: Acute isoniazid intoxication: seizures, acidosis and coma. Acta Clin Belg 54:211, 1999

99. Graeme KA, Pollack CV Jr: Heavy metal toxicity, part II: lead and metal fume fever. J Emerg Med 16:171, 1998

100. Markowitz SB, Nunez CM, Klitzman S, et al: Lead poisoning due to Hai Ge Fen: the porphyrin content of individual erythrocytes. JAMA 271:932, 1994

101. Berlin CM Jr: Lead poisoning in children. Curr Opin Pediatr 9:173, 1997

102. Gordon RA, Roberts G, Amin Z, et al: Aggressive approach in the treatment of acute lead encephalopathy with an extraordinarily high concentration of lead. Arch Pediatr Adolesc Med 152:1100, 1998

103. Rogan WJ, Dietrich KN, Ware JH, et al: The effect of chelation therapy with succimer on neuropsychological development in children exposed to lead. N Engl J Med 344:1421, 2001

104. Staudinger KC, Roth VS: Occupational lead poisoning. Am Fam Physician 57:719, 1998

105. Timmer RT, Sands JM: Lithium intoxication. J Am Soc Nephrol 10:666, 1999

106. Kores B, Lader MH: Irreversible lithium neurotoxicity: an overview. Clin Neuropharmacol 20:283, 1997

107. Gehrke JC, Watling SM, Gehrke CW, et al: In-vivo binding of lithium using the cation exchange resin sodium polystyrene sulfonate. Am J Emerg Med 14:37, 1996

108. Bailey B, McGuigan M: Comparison of patients hemodialyzed for lithium poisoning and those for whom dialysis was recommended by PCC but not done: what lesson can we learn? Clin Nephrol 54:388, 2000

109. Coleman MD, Coleman NA: Drug-induced methaemoglobinaemia: treatment issues. Drug Saf 14:394, 1996

110. Sinex JE: Pulse oximetry: principles and limitations. Am J Emerg Med 17:59, 1999

111. Mills KC: Serotonin syndrome: a clinical update. Crit Care Clin 13:763, 1997

112. Wanger K, Brough L, Macmillan I, et al: Intravenous vs subcutaneous naloxone for out-of-hospital management of presumed opioid overdose. Acad Emerg Med 5:293, 1998

113. Bardin PG, van Eeden SF, Moolman JA, et al: Organophosphate and carbamate poisoning. Arch Intern Med 154:1433, 1994

114. Holstege CP, Kirk M, Sidell FR: Chemical warfare: nerve agent poisoning. Crit Care Clin 13:923, 1997

115. Lifshitz M, Rotenberg M, Sofer S, et al: Carbamate poisoning and oxime treatment in children: a clinical and laboratory study. Pediatrics 93:652, 1994

116. De Bleecker J, Van den Neucker K, Colardyn F: Intermediate syndrome in organophosphorus poisoning: a prospective study. Crit Care Med 21:1706, 1993

117. Yip L, Dart RC, Gabow PA: Concepts and controversies in salicylate toxicity. Emerg Med Clin North Am 12:351, 1994

118. Chui PT: Anesthesia in a patient with undiagnosed salicylate poisoning presenting as intraabdominal sepsis. J Clin Anesth 11:251, 1999

119. Fraser AD: Use and abuse of the benzodiazepines. Ther Drug Monit 20:481, 1998

120. Coupey SM: Barbiturates. Pediatr Rev 18:260, 1997

121. Hojer J, Baehrendtz S, Gustafsson L: Benzodiazepine poisoning: experience of 702 admissions to an intensive care unit during a 14-year period. J Intern Med 226:117, 1989

122. Zahedi A, Grant MH, Wong DT: Successful treatment of chloral hydrate cardiac toxicity with propranolol. Am J Emerg Med 17:490, 1999

123. Herrington AM, Clifton GD: Toxicology and management of acute drug ingestions in adults. Pharmacotherapy 15:182, 1995

124. Shannon M: Hypokalemia, hyperglycemia and plasma catecholamine activity after severe theophylline intoxication. J Toxicol Clin Toxicol 32:41, 1994

125. Shannon M: Life-threatening events after theophylline overdose: a 10-year prospective analysis. Arch Intern Med 159:989, 1999

126. Kempf J, Rusterholtz T, Ber C, et al: Haemodynamic study as guideline for the use of beta blockers in acute theophylline poisoning. Intensive Care Med 22:585, 1996

127. Shannon MW: Comparative efficacy of hemodialysis and hemoperfusion in severe theophylline intoxication. Acad Emerg Med 4:674, 1997

128. Shanon M, Liebelt E: Targeted management strategies for cardiovascular toxicity from tricyclic antidepressant overdose: the pivotal role for alkalinization and sodium loading. Pediatr Emerg Care 14:293, 1998

129. Harrigan RA, Brady WJ: ECG abnormalities in tricyclic antidepressant ingestion. Am J Emerg Med 17:387, 1999

130. Update: Neurologic illness associated with eating Florida pufferfish, 2002. MMWR Morb Mortal Wkly Rep 51:414, 2002

131. Schnorf H, Taurarii M, Cundy T: Ciguatera fish poisoning: a double-blind randomized trial of mannitol therapy. Neurology 58:873, 2002

132. Ting JY, Brown AF: Ciguatera poisoning: a global issue with common management problems. Eur J Emerg Med 8:295, 2001

133. Davis RT, Villar LA: Symptomatic improvement with amitriptyline in ciguatera fish poisoning. N Engl J Med 315:65, 1986

134. Berlin RM, King SL, Blythe DG: Symptomatic improvement of chronic fatigue with fluoxetine in ciguatera fish poisoning. Med J Aust 157:567, 1992

135. Perez CM, Vasquez PA, Perret CF: Treatment of ciguatera poisoning with gabapentin. N Engl J Med 344:692, 2001

136. Yamada EG, Mohle-Boetani J, Olson KR, et al: Mushroom poisoning due to amatoxin. Northern California, Winter 1996-1997. West J Med 169:380, 1998

137. Walker R: The significance of excursions above the ADI. Case study: monosodium glutamate. Regul Toxicol Pharmacol 30:S119, 1999

138. Yang WH, Drouin MA, Herbert M, et al: The monosodium glutamate symptom complex: assessment in a double-blind, placebo-controlled, randomized study. J Allergy Clin Immunol 99:757, 1997

139. Tarasoff L, Kelly MF: Monosodium L-glutamate: a double blind study and review. Food Chem Toxicol 31:1019, 1993

140. Cupp MJ: Herbal remedies: adverse effects and drug interactions. Am Fam Physician 59:1239, 1999

141. Matthews MK Jr: Association of *Ginkgo biloba* with intracerebral hemorrhage (letter). Neurology 50:1933, 1998

142. Haller CA, Benowitz NL: Adverse cardiovascular and central nervous system events associated with dietary supplements containing ephedra alkaloids. N Engl J Med 343:1833, 2000

143. Hill IR: Reactions to particles in smoke. Toxicology 115:119, 1996

144. Weiss SM, Lakshminarayan S: Acute inhalation injury. Clin Chest Med 15:103, 1994

145. Wittram C, Kenny JB: The admission chest radiograph after acute inhalation injury and burns. Br J Radiol 67:751, 1994

146. Harpe C, Stoudemire A: Aetiology and treatment of neuroleptic malignant syndrome. Medical Toxicology 2:166, 1987

147. Sessler DI: Malignant hyperthermia. J Pediatr 109:9, 1986

148. Goldberg RJ, Huk M: Serotonin syndrome from trazodone and buspirone (letter). Psychosomatics 33:235, 1992

149. Sternbach H: The serotonin syndrome. Am J Psychiatry 148:705, 1991

150. Benowitz NL: Beta-adrenergic blockers. Poisoning & Drug Overdose, 2nd ed., Olson KR, Ed. Norwalk, Connecticut, Appleton & Lange, 1994

151. Stremski ES, Grande GA, Ling LJ: Survival following hydrofluoric acid ingestion. Ann Emerg Med 21:1396, 1992

152. Bertolini JC: Hydrofluoric acid: a review of toxicity. J Emerg Med 10:163, 1992

153. Spiller HA, Quadrani-Kushner DA, Cleveland P: A five year evaluation of acute exposures to phenol disinfectant (26%). J Toxicol Clin Toxicol 31:307, 1993

154. Hunter DM, Timerding BL, Leonard RB, et al: Effects of isopropyl alcohol, ethanol, and polyethylene glycol/industrial methylated spirits in the treatment of acute phenol burns. Ann Emerg Med 21:1303, 1992

155. Suzuki K, Takasu N, Arita S, et al: Evaluation of severity indexes of patients with paraquat poisoning. Hum Exp Toxicol 10:21, 1991

156. Karlson-Stiber C, Persson H: Ethylene glycol poisoning: experiences from an epidemic in Sweden. J Toxicol Clin Toxicol 30:565, 1992

157. Gaudet MP, Fraser GL: Isopropanol ingestion: case report with pharmacokinetic analysis. Am J Emerg Med 7:297, 1989

158. Becker CE: Methanol poisoning. J Emerg Med 1:51, 1983

159. Kim S: Food poisoning: fish and shellfish. Poisoning & Drug Overdose, 3rd ed. Olson KR, Ed. Appleton & Lange, Stamford, Connecticut, 1999, p 175

Acknowledgment

Figure 1   Tom Moore. Adapted from "Acetaminophen poisoning and toxicity," by B.H. Rumack and H. Matthew, in *Pediatrics* 55:871, 1975. Reproduced by permission of *Pediatrics*.

14 Bites and Stings

Lawrence M. Lewis, M.D., *Mark D. Levine*, M.D., *and William H. Dribben*, M.D.

Mammalian Bites

EPIDEMIOLOGY

In the United States each year, an estimated two million people are bitten by mammals.[1] Dog bites alone account for approximately 0.5% of all emergency department (ED) visits and 3.5% of all injury-related ED visits in boys 5 to 9 years of age.[2] However, most bite-wound victims do not seek medical attention.

PATHOPHYSIOLOGY

Infection, the most common complication of bite wounds, arises from microbes either on the victim's skin or in the mouth of the human or animal inflicting the bite wound. The relative risk of infection varies with the species of animal inflicting the wound, the location of the bite, the size and depth of the wound, host factors, and the type of wound care that is given.[3-6] Most infections resulting from mammalian bites are polymicrobial, with mixed aerobic and anaerobic species.[7] Nonetheless, bites from certain species tend to cause infections with particular bacteria. The risk of transmission of the rabies virus depends on the species inflicting the bite and the nature of the inflicted wound.

DOMESTIC ANIMALS

Dogs

Dogs are responsible for the majority of bites for which patients seek medical attention.[8] Most dog bites are inflicted by animals known to the victim, with strays accounting for less than 10% of reported bite-wound injuries.[8] Wounds occur most frequently on the extremities, except in young children, in whom bite wounds to the face, head, and neck are the most common.[9] Bite wounds to the hand account for 20% to 50% of reported cases. Hand bites are at increased risk for infection, particularly tenosynovitis, closed-space compartmental infections, and septic arthritis.[1] Although deaths from dog attacks are rare, this tragic scenario occurs about 10 times a year in the United States. From 1979 through 1998, pit bull–type dogs and Rottweilers were responsible for more than half of deaths.[10]

The oral bacterial flora of dogs includes *Pasteurella multocida*, *Staphylococcus aureus*, *Capnocytophaga canimorsus*, *S. epidermidis*, and *Streptococcus* species. The aerobic organisms most commonly isolated from infected dog bites include species of *Staphylococcus*, *Streptococcus*, and *Corynebacterium*.[11] Anaerobic organisms can be isolated from about 38% to 76% of all bite wounds.[12] The anaerobic organisms most commonly associated with dog bites include *Bacteroides fragilis*, *Prevotella*, *Porphyromonas*, *Peptostreptococcus*, and *Fusobacterium* species.

Dog bites are unlikely to become infected; infection rates range from 2% to 20%. The risk of infection is higher in older patients, however, especially in patients with diabetes, vascular disease, alcoholism, or immunosuppression. It is also higher in puncture wounds, wounds on the hand or foot or over a joint, and in wounds associated with crush injuries.[1]

Dog bites infected with *C. canimorsus* may cause overwhelming sepsis, with high fever, leukocytosis, disseminated intravascular coagulation (DIC), and multiorgan failure. *C. canimorsus* sepsis occurs most commonly in immunocompromised patients (e.g., those with asplenia, alcoholism, or hematologic malignancy) and carries a 25% mortality.[1]

Cats

Cat bites are the second most common mammalian bites in the United States, accounting for 5% to 15% of all reported cases. About two thirds of all cat bites occur on the upper extremity. Cat bites are more often puncture wounds than tearing lacerations and often appear innocuous initially. However, the infection rate for cat bites is reported to be 30% to 50%, more than double that for dogs.[13,14] *P. multocida* is the major pathogen associated with cat bites, being found in 50% to 80% of infected cat-bite wounds. *P. multocida* infection progresses rapidly, with pain, swelling, and erythema usually occurring within 24 hours.[8] Penetration into deep tissues, with resultant osteomyelitis or septic arthritis, is more common with cat bites than dog bites.[15]

Cat-scratch disease (CSD) is an infection arising from a rickettsia-like organism, *Bartonella henselae*. It may occur after minor scratches and is characterized by a nontender papule at the inoculation site, followed 1 to 2 weeks later by lymphadenopathy and fever. The disease is usually self-limited in immunocompetent hosts but may cause a distinctive cutaneous and visceral syndrome in patients with AIDS [*see Chapter 141*].[15] Symptomatic and prolonged CSD may be treated with a course of antibiotics, although the antibiotic of choice is controversial, with macrolides, fluoroquinolones, rifampin, and trimethoprim-sulfamethoxazole all appearing to produce some clinical response.

Cats outnumber dogs by more than 2 to 1 as the most common domestic rabid animal.[16] Overall, however, domestic animals account for less than 10% of rabies transmission to humans in the United States.

Ferrets

Ferrets have become increasingly popular as pets in the United States, with an estimated half-million households containing one or more.[17] Ferret attacks are uncommon but can result in severe damage, especially to infants and small children. In contrast to dog or cat bites, these attacks are usually unprovoked.[17,18]

The bacteriologic flora in ferrets has not been well studied. One study of the gingival flora found predominantly facultative anaerobic gram-positive cocci, followed by facultative anaerobic rods such as *Pasteurella* and *Corynebacterium* species, with few strict anaerobes.[19]

Ferrets are clearly capable of contracting and carrying the rabies virus.[20] However, it is not known how long ferrets can shed the rabies virus before showing clinical signs of disease, which makes quarantine recommendations problematic. Although there is an approved rabies vaccine for use in ferrets, its efficacy in preventing rabies is currently unknown.[21] Current recommendations are to give rabies postexposure prophylaxis immediately for animals suspected to be rabid but, otherwise, to observe the animal for 10 days and withhold prophylaxis unless the animal shows signs of rabies.[22]

HUMAN BITES

Human bites are the third most common mammalian bite in the United States, accounting for 5% to more than 20% of bite wounds seen in urban EDs.[1,23] Most human-bite wounds are on the extremities. A particularly high percentage of them occur when the patient punches another person in the mouth and the clenched fist contacts a tooth, creating a wound over the metacarpal-phalangeal joint.

Human-bite wounds have traditionally had a reputation for frequent and severe complications. However, more recent data suggest an infection rate from human-bite wounds of approximately 10% to 50%, depending on the wound type and location.[1,13,23] Occlusional or simple bite wounds to areas other than the hand probably pose no greater risk of infection than any other type of bite wound and probably just minimally more risk than nonbite lacerations.[14,24] A clenched-fist injury is considered the most serious of all human-bite wounds.[1] Such an injury can appear innocent at first but then progress to a serious infection that may involve the joint, tendons, or compartments of the hand. It requires meticulous wound care, appropriate antibiotic therapy, and consultation with a hand surgeon.

Bacterial pathogens associated with human-bite wounds include many of the same anaerobes recovered from dog and cat bites but with a much higher percentage of β-lactamase producers.[25,26] The predominant aerobes are *Staphylococcus* and *Streptococcus* species. Human-bite wounds may also contain *Eikenella corrodens*, a facultative anaerobe that functions anaerobically in 10% to 30% of cases.[23,25] *E. corrodens* is present in 25% of clenched-fist injuries and often results in serious, chronic infections.[27] Besides causing bacterial infection, human bites can transmit hepatitis B, HIV, herpes simplex, tuberculosis, and even syphilis.[12,28] Prophylaxis against hepatitis B or HIV should be considered for those bitten by persons considered at high risk for these diseases.

NONDOMESTIC ANIMALS

Rats

Rat bites are uncommon, representing less than 2% of the bite wounds seen in one urban ED.[29] Nevertheless, one study found that rat and mouse bites were the third most common bite for which rabies prophylaxis was used in the United States. Although the list of potential pathogens that could be transmitted via rat bites is daunting, infections from rat bites, including rabies, are actually very infrequent.[29]

Rat-bite fever is a disease caused by *Streptobacillus moniliformis*, a gram-negative rod. It is marked by fever, chills,

Table 1 Bite Wounds Requiring Prophylactic Antibiotics

Wound characteristics	Puncture wounds Full-thickness wounds Hand or foot wounds Wounds requiring surgical repair Treatment delay (> 24 hr)
Patient characteristics	Age > 50 yr Immunosuppression (e.g., asplenia, alcoholism, corticosteroid use) Diabetes mellitus Peripheral vascular disease

headache, myalgias, and rash and usually begins abruptly about 3 to 10 days after inoculation [*see Chapter 144*].

Other Species

Bat bites are significant because they have been responsible for almost 75% of all reported rabies cases in the United States since 1990 and were responsible for 90% of all cases acquired in the United States from 1981 through 1998.[30,31] Skunks, raccoons, and foxes are also important animal reservoirs of rabies in the United States.

Bite wounds from nonhuman primates are rare but can transmit not only bacterial infection but also *Herpesvirus simiae*, the causative agent of monkey B virus disease [*see Chapter 153*]. Untreated monkey B virus disease often results in death or permanent neurologic impairment.[32]

DIAGNOSIS

Management of mammalian-bite wounds begins with a directed history and physical examination. The history should include when and where the bite occurred, the events leading to the bite, what type of animal was responsible for the bite, and any available information about the animal. Any treatment rendered before arrival and the patient's tetanus immunization status should be documented.

A careful physical examination to assess for injuries to arteries, major veins, nerves, joints, bone, or tendons should be performed and documented. When appropriate, photographs and diagrams should be used to document wounds.[33] In children who have suffered dog bites, the evaluation should include not only penetrating injury from the bite but also any blunt component, which may represent the most serious aspect in such cases.[34]

Table 2 Common and Important Pathogens and Antibiotic Selection for Various Mammalian Bite Wounds

Animal	Pathogen	Antibiotics
Dog	*Staphylococcus, Streptococcus, Capnocytophaga canimorsus, Pasteurella multocida*, anaerobes	Amoxicillin–clavulanic acid, third-generation fluoroquinolones, clindamycin plus trimethoprim-sulfamethoxazole (TMP-SMX)
Cat	*P. multocida, Staphylococcus, Streptococcus*, anaerobes	Amoxicillin–clavulanic acid, third-generation fluoroquinolones, clindamycin plus TMP-SMX
Human	*Staphylococcus, Streptococcus*, anaerobes, *Eikenella corrodens*	Amoxicillin–clavulanic acid, third-generation fluoroquinolones
Rodents	*Staphylococcus, Streptococcus, S. moniliformis*	Penicillin G (for *S. moniliformis*), amoxicillin–clavulanic acid, doxycycline
Nonhuman primates	*Staphylococcus, Streptococcus*, monkey B virus	Amoxicillin–clavulanic acid, third-generation fluoroquinolones, acyclovir or ganciclovir (for monkey B virus)

Table 3 Recommendations for Tetanus Prophylaxis after Animal Bites

Primary Tetanus Immunization Series Received?	Wound	Time since Last Tetanus Toxoid Dose	Recommended Prophylaxis
Yes	Clean, minor	> 10 yr	Td*
	All other	> 5 yr	Td*
Uncertain	Clean, minor	—	Td*
	All other	—	Td*, TIG†

*Adult (> 7 yr) Td dose is 0.5 ml I.M.; DTaP (diphtheria, tetanus, acellular pertussis) vaccine may be used in patients younger than 7 yr.
†Dose of TIG is 250 units I.M.; give in opposite arm from Td.
Td—diphtheria and tetanus toxoids adsorbed   TIG—tetanus immune globulin

TREATMENT

After adequate anesthesia has been given, the wound should be explored for foreign bodies, including teeth or fragments of teeth, and then meticulously cleaned and irrigated. Copious irrigation has been shown to decrease bacterial contamination by as much as 75%.[35] The irrigation fluid can be normal saline or normal saline with dilute povidone-iodine.[36] Careful debridement of nonviable or grossly contaminated tissue may be necessary. The use of soap and a virucidal agent such as povidone-iodine is an important measure for preventing rabies.[37]

Whether to use primary closure for bite lacerations is an area of debate. A number of studies suggest that one can safely suture bite lacerations that are longer than one half to three quarters of an inch—especially those that are on the face or head, where there is greater concern for a good cosmetic result.[38,39] Bite wounds to the hand, foot, or face often result in complications and may necessitate early surgical consultation.

Antibiotic Prophylaxis

The use of prophylactic antibiotics for any bite wound is debatable,[40] but there is general consensus that certain wounds in all patients and most wounds in certain patients deserve prophylactic antibiotics [see Table 1]. The antibiotic of choice for prophylaxis in most mammalian bite wounds is amoxicillin–clavulanic acid. For the penicillin-allergic patient, third-generation fluoroquinolones (e.g., trovafloxacin) serve as a good alternative

[see Table 2]. It is important to start prophylactic antibiotics as soon as possible after the bite injury. Tetanus prophylaxis should be given when appropriate [see Table 3].

Rabies Prophylaxis

With domestic-animal bites, postexposure rabies prophylaxis is warranted if (1) the animal is observed to be abnormal; (2) the animal is not available for observation and the rate of rabies in domestic animals in the region is high; or (3) the animal exhibited abnormal behavior, such as an unprovoked attack. With bites from wild animals, recommendations for rabies prophylaxis depend on the species[30] [see Table 4]. Bats, skunks, raccoons, and foxes should be regarded as rabid unless immediate brain testing can be performed on the animal. Rabies prophylaxis is warranted in those cases, particularly if rabies is prevalent in the area or the animal's behavior is deemed abnormal.[41] In patients who have not been previously vaccinated against rabies, postexposure prophylaxis includes both rabies immune globulin and rabies vaccine.[22] Information on rabies prophylaxis is available through state and local health departments and from the Centers for Disease Control and Prevention, at http://www.cdc.gov/ncidod/dvrd/rabies/prevention&control/ACIP/ACIP99.htm.

Snakebites

EPIDEMIOLOGY

Over 3,000 species of snakes exist worldwide. Snakes are found everywhere on Earth except for the Arctic and Antarctic, New Zealand, Malagasy, and a few small islands. Snakes live in almost all land environments and in both saltwater and freshwater.

Approximately 10% of snakes are venomous. Of the 14 families of snakes, only five include venomous species: the Colubridae, Hydrophidae (sea snakes), Elapidae (cobras, kraits, mambas, and coral snakes), Viperidae (Russell viper, puff adder, Gaboon viper, saw-scaled viper, and European viper), and Crotalidae (rattlesnake, water moccasin, copperhead, bushmaster, and fer-de-lance). Snakes are carnivores, and venomous snakes use their venom to immobilize prey for digestive purposes.

The number of snakebites in the United States is estimated at approximately 8,000 a year. Most of those bites do not result in envenomation, but nine to 15 deaths occur annually from bites that do result in envenomation.[42] In the United States, rattlesnake bites most frequently result in significant envenomation and death.

Table 4 Recommendations for Rabies Postexposure Prophylaxis[35]

Animal Type	Evaluation and Disposition of Animal	Postexposure Prophylaxis Recommendations
Dogs, cats, ferrets	Healthy and available for 10 days of observation Rabid or suspected rabid Unknown (e.g., escaped)	Do not begin prophylaxis unless animal develops clinical signs of rabies* Immediately vaccinate Consult public health officials
Skunks, raccoons, foxes, most other carnivores; bats	Regarded as rabid unless animal proved negative by laboratory tests†	Consider immediate vaccination
Livestock, small rodents, lagomorphs (rabbits and hares), large rodents (woodchucks and beavers), other mammals	Consider individually	Consult public health officials; bites of squirrels, hamsters, guinea pigs, gerbils, chipmunks, rats, mice, other small rodents, rabbits, and hares almost never require antirabies postexposure prophylaxis

*During the 10-day observation period, begin postexposure prophylaxis at first sign of rabies in a dog, cat, or ferret that has bitten someone. If the animal exhibits clinical signs of rabies, it should be euthanized immediately and tested.
†The animal should be euthanized and tested as soon as possible. Holding for observation is not recommended. Discontinue vaccine if immunofluorescence test results of the animal are negative.

Snakes are most active in the spring, when they begin to mate and are no longer hibernating[43]; however, the incidence of snakebite is highest in the summer months. Snakes remain active throughout the day and night, but because they are poikilothermic, they must contain their activity within a narrow temperature range of approximately 25° to 35° C.

CORAL SNAKES

The range of the eastern coral snake extends from North Carolina south and west to Texas. The western coral snake is found mainly in Arizona and New Mexico. Coral snakes are nocturnal and shy away from human contact.

Coral snakes are identified by their color, pattern, and permanently erect fangs. The nose of the coral snake is black, and the body has black, red, and yellow bands. The black bands do not separate the red and yellow bands, as they do on the nonvenomous but similarly banded kingsnake. This pattern is commonly remembered through the rhyme "red on black, venom lack; red on yellow, kills a fellow" [see Figure 1]. Coral snakes release their venom slowly, so they attach themselves to their prey and envenomate through a chewing motion. Instead of the puncture wounds typical of most snakebites, the chewing leaves what appear to be scratches on the skin.[43,44]

The bite of the eastern coral snake can be fatal. There are no confirmed fatalities from western coral snake envenomations.

PIT VIPERS

In the United States, pit vipers (Crotalidae) are found in all states except Maine, Alaska, and Hawaii. South America has nine subspecies of rattlesnakes, and Mexico and Central America have four subspecies of rattlesnakes. These snakes can be found in a variety of habitats and at elevations up to 14,000 ft. The eastern and western diamondback rattlesnakes (Crotalus adamanteus and C. strox) [see Figure 2] are the largest and most dangerous in the United States and are found in the southwestern states and in Nevada, California, and Oklahoma.[45,46] The timber rattlesnake (C. horridus) is the second most dangerous rattlesnake common to the eastern United States, but it is rarely found in Delaware, Maine, Michigan, and Washington, D.C. Pigmy rattlesnakes (Sistrurus catenatus and S. miliarius) are found in areas ranging from New York to Michigan and from Texas to Arizona and have the least toxic venom of all of the rattlesnakes.[42] The cottonmouths (Agkistrodon piscivorus), also known as water moccasins, live in the southern and southeastern states along streams and in low-lying trees. Copperheads (A. contortix) [see Figure 3] are found in mountains, rock piles, and sawdust piles. Their range extends from Massachusetts southwest to Texas. Cottonmouths and copperheads have only moderately toxic venom; their bite is painful but rarely fatal.

Pit vipers are identified by a small depression (pit) between the eyes and the nostrils bilaterally. They have a triangular-shaped head, an elliptical pupil, and fangs that fold back when the mouth is closed and unfold via a hingelike mechanism when the mouth is opened. The pit is a heat-sensitive organ that enables the snake to locate live, warm-blooded prey. Snakes can detect movement at about 40 ft. They can strike at a distance of approximately half their body length. The rattle is used when the snake is threatened or endangered, not necessarily just when it is about to attack. The pit viper is aggressive and will stand its ground when provoked or cornered.[45,46] The venom is stored in glands that are located on each side of the head above the maxillae and behind the eyes. The glands are similar in function to the human submaxillary glands. The snake may discharge anywhere from 25% to 75% of its venom when attacking a human. The fangs are either hollow or grooved. Even young snakes are venomous, and the venom of young snakes may be 12 times as strong as the venom of adult snakes.

ENVENOMATION

Toxicology

Snake venom has both neurotoxic and hematotoxic properties. The venom is a complex mixture of hydrolases, polypeptides, glycoproteins, and low-molecular-weight compounds. Snake venom, especially that of the Elapidae and Hydrophidae families, contains polypeptides that produce neuromuscular blockade at the presynaptic or postsynaptic terminals, or both, causing a flaccid paralysis. Composition of the venom varies greatly between the two species and between individual snakes.

Snake venom has profound effects on coagulation pathways, causing a hypercoagulable state. Over the first few hours after being bitten, thrombocytopenia occurs, with a platelet count of less than $10,000/mm^3$, a decrease in fibrinogen, and an increase in fibrin degradation products. Prothrombin time and partial thromboplastin time increase with severe envenomation. Drops in hematocrit may also occur, along with so-called burring of erythrocytes.[45] Approximately 53% of patients experience coagulopathy 2 to 14 days after envenomation. In one study, 76% of patients with pit viper envenomations developed coagulopathy during their hospital course.[47]

Clinical Features

From 30% to 50% of snakebites do not result in envenomation. The snake can control the amount of venom injected and may inject up to 90% of its venom to immobilize its prey. Other factors involved in the injection of venom include the health of the snake; its satiety; the condition of the fangs; the toxicity of the venom; whether the snake is injured; and the size, age, and health of the victim.

Minor pit-viper envenomation causes local pain and swelling (edema with a diameter of approximately 1 to 5 in.), without systemic symptoms or signs. Moderate envenomation is characterized by greater edema (diameter of 6 to 12 in.), weakness, sweating, nausea, fainting, dizziness, ecchymoses, and tender adenopathy.[42] As the envenomation becomes more severe, the symptoms increase to include tachycardia, tachypnea, hypothermia, hypotension, ecchymoses, paresthesias, fasciculations, gingival bleeding, hematemesis, hematuria, melena, oliguria, or coma. Fasciculations are a characteristic manifestation of bites from the eastern diamondback rattlesnake.[48] The skin around and over the snakebite will develop a tense, discolored bulla with serous or hemorrhagic fluid. Death usually results from hemorrhage, increased vascular permeability, and thromboembolic events secondary to disruption of the coagulation pathways.

Coral snake envenomation is painful and has the appearance of scratch marks with no surrounding edema. Systemic symptoms are delayed by about 1 to 6 hours. They begin with paresthesias around the wound margins, followed by weakness, apprehension, giddiness, nausea, vomiting, and a sense of euphoria. Excess salivation is nearly always present.[48] Bulbar and cranial nerve paralysis and ptosis may develop. Ptosis is very common and is often the first sign of coral snake envenomation. Diplopia, papillary dilatation, salivation, dysphagia, and respiratory failure may occur. The paralysis may last up to 14 hours,

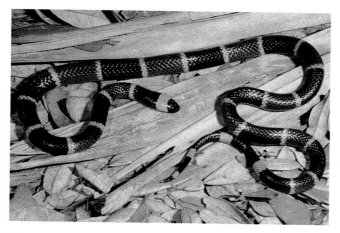

Figure 1 **The nose of the coral snake is black, and the body has black, red, and yellow bands. The black bands do not separate the red and yellow bands, as they do on the nonvenomous but similarly banded kingsnake. Shown is an eastern coral snake, *Micrurus fulvius*.**

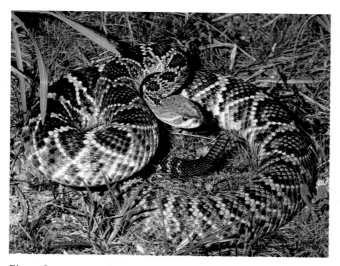

Figure 2 **Diamondback rattlesnakes are the largest and most dangerous rattlesnakes in the United States. Shown is an eastern diamondback rattlesnake, *Crotalus adamanteus*.**

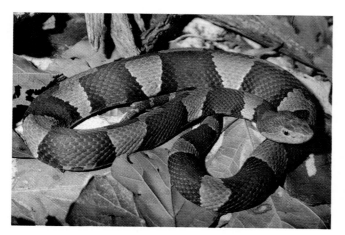

Figure 3 **The copperhead (*Agkistrodon contortix*) has a geographic range that extends from Massachusetts southwest to Texas. Bites from these snakes are painful but rarely fatal.**

and full strength may not return for 6 to 8 weeks. In fatal cases, the usual cause of death is respiratory failure.

TREATMENT

First Aid

Treatment in the field should focus on preventing systemic absorption of the toxin. This may be done with compressive dressings and immobilization of the bitten extremity. Stabilization may be accomplished via an inflatable splint. Nothing should be given by mouth.

If signs of envenomation begin to occur, a constriction band to impede lymphatic flow should be placed on the extremity, proximal to the bite.[49] The Commonwealth Serum Laboratory technique (Australia) uses an elastic band or air splint for wrapping the extremity. The Monash method uses a thick pad and tight bandage over the wound site to impede flow of the venom. Both of these methods have proven efficacy only with Elapidae bites. Transport to a hospital should take place immediately, because the absorption of neurotoxic venoms may result in respiratory compromise or arrest. In patients with a facial envenomation, edema may cause airway obstruction, so prehospital personnal may have to establish immediate airway control.[50]

The site should be wiped off and cleaned. However, the old practice of incising the bite site and applying suction to remove the snake venom should not be used. This practice, which dates from the 1920s, was tested in animal models and found not to increase survival. In fact, incision and suction at the wound site poses more hazard than benefit. The incision may aggravate bleeding, damage nerves and tendons, introduce infection, and delay healing. Cryotherapy (e.g., placing ice on the bite site), which was once thought to lower venom enzyme activity and absorption into the systemic circulation, has also been shown to provide no significant benefit; rather, it causes tissue loss, cold injury, and possible permanent disability.

Extraction therapy has also fallen out of favor. In this procedure, a suction device is placed over the fang wounds, and suction is applied to remove the venom from the bite site and the surrounding tissue without an incision. Prehospital personnel who find a suction device already in place when they arrive at the scene should remove the device, provided there is no fluid accumulating in the cup.[50]

Although popular belief has it that snakebites kill within minutes, in fact the toxicity from snake venom usually does not even begin to affect the body for several hours. In one review, 64% of deaths from snakebite occurred between 6 and 48 hours after the patient was bitten.[51]

Emergency Department Management

History When a snakebite victim arrives at the hospital, the history of the bite should be obtained. This should include (1) a description of the snake, (2) the time elapsed since the bite, (3) the circumstances surrounding the bite, (4) the number of bites, (5) the location of the bite, (6) the type of first aid administered, and (7) any symptoms that have occurred since the bite. The patient's past medical history and allergy history should be reviewed briefly. In particular, the clinician should ask whether the patient has ever experienced allergic symptoms around horses or on exposure to horse serum and whether the patient has asthma, hay fever, or urticaria.

Physical examination Special attention should be paid to the area around the snakebite. The wound should be examined for fang marks, edema, petechiae, ecchymoses, and bullae. Thorough neurologic and cardiovascular examinations are indicated. If the patient was bitten on an extremity, circumferential measurements of the extremity should be taken at the site of injury and 5 in. proximal to the site. Distal pulses and neurologic status should be assessed and recorded.[50] The patient should be monitored in an intensive care setting.

Laboratory tests   All patients should have baseline laboratory studies, including a complete blood count, urinalysis, electrocardiogram, prothrombin time, partial thromboplastin time, fibrinogen levels, fibrin split products, serum electrolytes, blood urea nitrogen, and serum creatinine. Blood should be typed and screened. In severe envenomations, arterial blood gas determinations also are indicated. In patients with extremity edema, arterial Doppler evaluation and, in some cases, compartmental pressure determinations may be necessary.

Antivenin Therapy

Antivenins are available for bites of North American pit vipers and eastern coral snakes. Water moccasin and copperhead bites are typically managed without the use of antivenin. The choice whether to use antivenin is based on many factors, including clinical signs and symptoms of envenomation and the physiologic status of the victim. Antivenin is indicated only for severe envenomations.[52]

Antivenin can be obtained through hospital pharmacies, veterinarians, local zoos, and poison control centers. Antivenin is most therapeutic when given within 4 hours of the bite. It is of limited value when given after 12 hours.[43]

Classification of envenomation   Envenomations are classified according to a five-level system. The amount of antivenin given correlates with the grade of envenomation.

In grade 0 envenomations, the patient may have fang marks or superficial abrasions of the skin at the bite site but has minimal local edema or pain and no associated systemic manifestations.

Grade 1 envenomations involve some pain or throbbing at the bite site, with 1 to 5 in. of edema and erythema surrounding it. There are no systemic manifestations.

Grade 2 envenomations produce more severe pain over a larger area. The edema spreads toward the trunk, and petechiae and ecchymosis are present in the edematous area. There may be systemic involvement consisting of nausea, vomiting, and temperature elevation.

Grade 3 envenomation is considered severe. Edema spreads up the extremity and may move to the trunk. There may be generalized ecchymosis and petechiae. The patient may have a rapid pulse, hypotension, and hypothermia and may go into shock.

Grade 4 envenomation is very severe and usually results from the bite of a large snake or from a very large venom load. Edema, petechiae, ecchymosis, and necrosis rapidly overtake the extremity and a large portion of the trunk. Muscle fasciculations, sweating, nausea, vomiting, cramping, pallor, weak pulse, incontinence, convulsions, and coma may all occur.

Antivenins   There are now multiple types of antivenin on the market. The first marketed antivenin (Antivenin [Crotalidae] polyvalent [ACP]) was a horse-serum–based, whole antibody preparation. The dosage for that preparation was three to five ampules of antivenin diluted in 500 ml of intravenous fluid. Up to 54% of patients treated in studies were allergic to the ACP an-

tivenin. Rash, hypotension, wheezing, and phlebitis occurred in 20% of patients.[53] Nevertheless, clinicians would frequently forgo skin testing for allergy to ACP because it delayed administration of the antivenin.

Although the ACP antivenin is still produced and is used in some areas, a polyvalent crotalid (ovine) Fab antivenin (CroFab) has been introduced. This antivenin minimizes the risk of immediate hypersensitivity and prevents delayed serum sickness. It is based on sheep serum and is four to five times more potent than ACP.[47] CroFab is made by immunizing sheep with crotaline snake venom and digesting the immune serum with papain to produce antibody fragments (Fab and Fc); the antigenic Fc segment is removed during purification.[52] In a study of 1,000 treated patients, none showed evidence of true anaphylaxis.[54] Each vial of CroFab contains 750 mg of Fab and is reconstituted in 10 ml of normal saline; four vials are diluted in 250 ml of normal saline. Studies have shown improvement at the 4-hour mark in all patients given this regimen, although some patients subsequently worsened.[54] The half-life of Fab antivenin is less than 12 hours, compared with 61 to 194 hours for ACP,[55,56] so repeat dosing of Fab may be needed to maintain therapeutic serum levels.[57] In these studies, only 16% of patients experienced serum sickness after administration of Fab antivenin, and the severity of the serum sickness was classified as only mild to moderate. The Fab antivenin is given in interval doses, with the first dose given to achieve initial control (defined as cessation of all symptoms—local, systemic, and coagulopathy) and subsequent doses given 6, 12, and 18 hours after the first dose. It is presumed that in some cases, coagulopathy may recur after initial neutralization of the venom. Recurrence may result from a depot of unneutralized venom at the bite site that is released into the circulation after the venom-antivenin complexes are cleared. A combination of edema, circulatory injury, and a lesser amount of subcutaneous tissue at the site of the bite may inhibit the antivenin from reaching the venom depot.[47,58] Alternatively, uncleared complexes may dissociate, leaving free venom to recirculate.[47,54]

Adjunctive Therapy

A number of adjunctive therapies have been proposed for snakebite envenomations. Excision of tissue around the snakebite to remove the depot of venom was proposed at one time, but this approach is no longer used. The strategy of excising only necrotic-appearing tissue has likewise proved inadvisable, because histologic examination of the excised tissue revealed live muscle fibers interwoven with the macroscopically necrotic tissue.

Extremity edema from a snakebite may mimic compartment syndrome, but true compartment syndrome is rare in such cases. Most often, the subcutaneous tissue rather than the deep compartmental space is involved. When a deep envenomation occurs and a true compartment syndrome does develop, first-line treatment is antivenin administration, which diminishes the compartmental pressure and swelling. Compartmental pressures greater than 30 mm Hg may indicate a need for fasciotomy, but fasciotomy and debridement should be avoided if possible because this procedure is associated with worse functional results. Fasciotomy is recommended only if a patient's fingertip was bitten and has swelled, with loss of neurovascular or functional activity. In such cases, patients are candidates for so-called digit dermotomy. The incision should be made on the lateral or medial aspect of the finger, through the skin only, and should extend from the web to the middle of the distal phalanx.[59]

General Management

A regional poison control center or the local zoo should be used as a resource when dealing with a venomous snakebite. This is especially true if the snake is not believed to be native to the area, as might occur with hobbyists who keep exotic snakes as pets. For cases in which an expert is not available, the Department of Surgery at the University of California, San Diego, has established a Web site that lists protocols (including antivenin availability) for management of snakebites from venomous species around the world. This information is available at: http://www.surgery.ucsd.edu/ENT/DAVIDSON/snake/index.htm.

Other therapeutic measures are keyed to specific symptoms. Isotonic fluid replacement should be given if the patient is hypotensive. Abnormalities of the clotting mechanism should be corrected with blood product replacement as necessary, but this should be done only after antivenin therapy has been started. Corticosteroids are contraindicated during the acute stages of envenomation, but they may be used if the patient experiences serum sickness from antivenin use. Patients should be placed on oxygen and should be given mechanical support if necessary for signs of trismus, laryngeal spasm, or excessive salivation. Tetanus therapy should be given if indicated [see Table 3]. Antibiotics are recommended only if signs of infection are present. In one study, there were no wound infections in patients with nonenvenomated snakebite.[60]

The wounds should be examined daily. Superficial necrosis and hemorrhagic blebs should be debrided at days 3 through 10. Debridement may need to be done in stages.

SPECIAL CONSIDERATIONS

Snakebite in Pregnancy

In pregnant women who have been bitten by snakes, what is best for the mother will usually be best for the fetus. Fetal outcome may depend on the gestational age of the fetus, with younger age associated with a negative outcome. The miscarriage rate after snake envenomation may be as high as 43%.[61] Miscarriage may result from shock, uterine contractions, pyrexia, or placental or uterine bleeding. Venom may cross the placental barrier and cause some systemic poisoning of the fetus, even if the mother remains symptom free.[61]

In pregnant snakebite victims, airway compromise and shock states should be corrected to ensure perfusion of the placenta and uterus and thereby prevent fetal hypoxia. Circulatory support with vasopressors should be avoided because they reduce uterine blood flow and are detrimental to the fetus. Pregnant women are already in a hypercoagulable state and therefore are even more susceptible to DIC.[61] Abruptio placentae from hypercoagulability has occurred after snakebites.

Antivenin is the therapy of choice in pregnant patients, but there is no accurate information regarding the risks of administration of antivenin during pregnancy. Serum sickness and anaphylactic reactions remain the highest risk associated with antivenin administration.[62]

Snakebite in Children

Snakebites in children are often on the lower extremities or—if the child was handling the snake—on the hands. Signs and symptoms are typically similar to those in adults.[63] Because of their smaller blood volume, however, children may experience a more severe envenomation syndrome.[64] In a study of 67 children

with severe envenomation, 72% had systemic involvement and 50% developed coagulopathy; 61% received antivenin, and 36% of those treated experienced adverse reactions.

DISPOSITION

All victims of suspected snakebites should be observed for a minimum of 4 to 6 hours. If there is no sign of envenomation after 6 hours and it is believed that the snake was either nonvenomous or a pit viper, the patient can be discharged. The patient should be given instructions to return to the ED immediately if any symptoms of envenomation occur. A patient who has minimal edema and pain should be observed for at least 12 hours. If the swelling has begun to diminish and the pain has resolved, the patient may be discharged with the same discharge instructions.

Pit viper envenomation may result in significant hypofibrinogenemia and thrombocytopenia lasting up to 2 weeks, which may lead to complications from surgery or trauma.[65] If coagulation abnormalities have resolved, however, no further workup of the coagulation system is needed. The best predictor of late hypofibrinogenemia is early hypofibrinogenemia.[47]

Any patient who has been bitten by a Mojave rattlesnake, coral snake, or other exotic snake should be admitted to the intensive care unit, with cardiorespiratory and dialysis equipment readily available. Antivenin should be administered to such patients.[66]

SNAKEBITE PREVENTION

Snakes should not be handled except by a professional herpetologist. Even a dead snake can envenomate its handler. Persons spending time outdoors in areas known to be heavily populated with snakes should wear long pants and closed shoes. Because of the varying size of snake fangs, loose pants are preferred to tight-fitting trousers. Heavy leather boots are recommended rather than sandals, open-toed shoes, or sneakers. Persons who are going to handle snakes, even dead ones, should also wear protective gloves.

Spider Bites

The class Arachnida contains the largest number of known venomous species, including 20,000 venomous spiders. In the United States, only 50 species can envenomate humans, partly because most spiders' fangs are not long enough to penetrate human skin. All spiders are carnivorous; they capture their prey either by hunting or trapping it. Trappers spin webs and wait for prey to become ensnared. They have limited vision and sense prey on their web with their jaw, which can detect movement. Hunters have better eyesight than trappers, and most hunters eat their prey on the spot.

BLACK WIDOW SPIDERS

The black widow spider, Latrodectus mactans [see Figure 4], is found throughout the United States and southern Canada, with other closely related species found mainly in the western United States. There have been no recorded findings of the spider in Alaska. The female is twice the size of the male and is the only sex that is able to envenomate. The male does have venom, but because of its smaller size and less powerful fangs, it is unable to bite and envenomate a human. The female is glossy black, with a bright-red marking on the abdomen that may appear to be two spots or have an hourglass shape. Occasionally, it has red stripes. Immature females are red, brown, and cream colored. The spi-

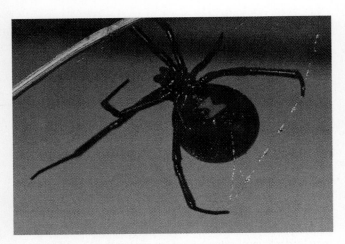

Figure 4 **The mature female black widow spider is glossy black, with a bright-red marking on the abdomen that may appear to be two spots or have an hourglass shape.**

der's body is about 1/2 in. long; with the legs, it measures approximately 1 1/2 in. in length. It is usually found under rocks and in woodpiles, outhouses, and stables, and it is not aggressive unless guarding its eggs. The black widow is a trapper. The webs are close to the ground to have access to crawling insects and are usually in secluded, dim areas.

Envenomation

Toxicology Black widow venom contains various proteinaceous compounds. The venom paralyzes the prey and begins the digestive process by liquefying the victim's tissues. The toxin depletes acetylcholine from the presynaptic nerve terminals, thereby destabilizing nerve cell membranes and opening ionic channels. The toxin of the black widow is thought to cause a massive release of acetylcholine and then block its reuptake, which leads to both sympathetic and parasympathetic stimulation.[67] There is a patchy paralysis of skeletal muscles with various changes in the autonomic nervous system. This paralytic syndrome has been likened to polio.[68]

Clinical features On being bitten by a black widow, a person may feel a pinprick sensation, with minimal local swelling and erythema. Two small fang marks may be visible. The middle of the bite site may be white, with surrounding erythema and a reddish-blue border. Within an hour, the patient may feel a dull ache or crampy pain in the area of envenomation. This feeling may spread throughout the body shortly thereafter. The pain spreads to the chest from upper extremity bites and to the abdomen from lower extremity bites. This pain may mimic pancreatitis, appendicitis, or a peptic ulcer. The abdomen may have boardlike rigidity but will not necessarily be painful to palpation. In addition, there may be other myopathic signs such as facial trismus, muscle fibrillation, tonic contractions, or so-called facies latrodectismica, a constellation of symptoms that includes blepharoconjunctivitis, flushing, and contortions.[69] Other systemic symptoms may include dizziness, nausea, vomiting, headache, itching, conjunctivitis, diaphoresis, piloerection, priapism, anxiety, and dyspnea. The symptoms may last for 2 to 3 days, abating slightly after a few hours. Patients with preexisting hypertension, cerebrovascular disease, or cardiovascular disease are at risk for a worsening of those conditions.

Treatment

First aid Patients bitten by a black widow spider should have cool compresses applied to the bite and be transported to a hospital. Laboratory experiments have shown that a Sawyer extraction device may be helpful in removing venom if applied to the skin within 3 minutes after the bite.[69] Basic or advanced life support should be given on the way to the hospital. If possible, the spider should be brought along with the patient, because many nonvenomous species may resemble the black widow.

Emergency department management A complete history and physical examination should be done, with attention paid to the circumstances surrounding the bite, a description of the spider, and allergies to other bites or to horse serum. The site should be inspected and cleansed. Tetanus immunization should be updated, if necessary. Laboratory studies should be obtained, including a complete blood count, serum electrolytes, clotting studies, urinalysis, electrocardiogram, blood urea nitrogen, and serum creatinine.

Patients with envenomations should be treated symptomatically. Nitroprusside may be used for hypertensive episodes related to the envenomation. Abdominal cramps may be alleviated with calcium gluconate (10 ml of a 10% solution given intravenously over 20 minutes). Serum calcium levels should be followed. Diazepam may be given to alleviate muscle spasms.[70] Dantrolene has also been shown to provide muscle relaxation in these patients.[71]

Antivenin therapy *Latrodectus* antivenin exists and is indicated for patients who have hypertensive heart disease, underlying respiratory disease, or severe envenomation. Patients between the ages of 16 and 65 may receive the antivenin. The antivenin is derived from horse serum and may cause allergic reactions. The intravenous route is preferred. The contents of the vial are diluted in 50 ml of normal saline and given over 15 minutes. The typical dosage is one to two vials.

Special Considerations

Spider bites in children Children who are bitten by a black widow spider may have severe symptoms that may lead to death. Possibly because of the smaller volume in which the venom is circulated, a dose that would be tolerable in an adult may cause fatal cardiovascular or respiratory decompensation in a child.

Spider bites in pregnancy A pregnant woman who is bitten by a black widow spider will have signs and symptoms that are otherwise typical, but she may not have a rigid abdomen because of the stretching and laxity of the gravid abdominal wall. However, the cramping may be severe enough to induce miscarriage. The toxin does not seem to have a direct effect on the fetus, possibly because it is not able to cross the placental barrier, nor is it able to cross the blood-brain barrier. Antivenin is indicated for the symptomatic pregnant patient.[61]

Disposition

Patients with signs or symptoms of black widow spider envenomation should be admitted to the hospital. The patient should be observed for a minimum of 2 hours and, if totally asymptomatic, may be discharged with instructions to return if any symptoms develop.

BROWN RECLUSE SPIDER BITES

The brown recluse spider, *Loxosceles reclusa* [*see Figure 5*], lives under rocks and in woodpiles in the south central United States, especially in Missouri, Kansas, Arkansas, Louisiana, east Texas, and Oklahoma. The brown recluse is approximately 1 in. long and ranges in color from tan to dark brown. It has a violin-shaped dark-brown spot on its abdomen. In addition, the brown recluse has three sets of eyes.

The brown recluse hunts for its food but can live for 6 months without food or water.[72] It forages at night but is not aggressive unless threatened.[73]

Envenomation

Toxicology Brown recluse venom is protein based, and it has antigenic and locally destructive properties. Esterases, hyaluronidases, and proteases have been isolated from recluse spider venom.[73] The components of the venom are cytotoxic to endothelial cells and red blood cells. Sphingomyelinase-D acts directly on red blood cells to cause lysis.[74] Unlike black widow venom, brown recluse venom has no known neurotoxic effects.

Clinical features Brown recluse spider venom produces both localized and systemic symptoms. There may be initial pain in the area of the bite, or pain may be absent at first and then develop over the next 3 to 4 hours. Soon thereafter, a ring of pallor from vasoconstriction appears around the bite, with a surrounding area of erythema. A bleb develops in the center and, after a few days, becomes necrotic. The bleb may spread with gravity-dependent flow. This necrotic area spreads over the next few days, involving both superficial and deep tissues. An eschar usually forms days later, and the wound may not heal for months after the eschar separates.[75,76] Associated systemic effects include fever, chills, rash, nausea, vomiting, shock, renal failure, hemorrhage, DIC, or pulmonary edema. There have been case reports of transverse myelitis and paralysis from the brown recluse spider bite that are believed to result from microthrombosis at the anterior vertebral artery.[77] Also, loss of cutaneous sensation may be caused by damage to or destruction of a nerve or its branch by the venom itself or ischemia from the edema.[74] Children are more likely to progress to intravascular hemolysis and death. Local cutaneous necrosis is thought to be caused by enzymes that cause vasoconstriction of the tissue.

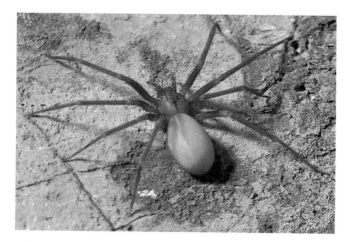

Figure 5 **The brown recluse spider (7 to 12 mm body length) is a timid arachnid that may be encountered in basements, closets, and woodpiles.**

The differential diagnosis of the skin changes caused by a brown recluse spider envenomation includes Stevens-Johnson syndrome, toxic epidermal necrolysis, erythema nodosum, purpura fulminans, diabetic ulcer, allergic dermatitis, Lyme disease, and pyoderma gangrenosum.[69] Patients who have had numerous brown recluse spider bites have demonstrated an antibody response and may have a decreased response to subsequent bites.[73]

Treatment

Prehospital care should include basic or advanced life support, cool compresses, and immobilization of the extremity. On arrival at the ED, a complete history and physical examination should be done, with attention paid to the circumstances surrounding the bite, the description of the spider, and allergies to other bites or to horse serum. Early diagnosis is most easily accomplished if the patient presents to the ED with the spider. The site should be inspected and cleansed. Tetanus toxoid should be administered, if appropriate.

There is some evidence that systemic steroids should be used with brown recluse bites if the patient is seen within 24 hours.[78] Other studies have shown that intralesional injection of steroids may help control inflammation.[79] Dapsone has also been shown to be helpful in treating the local effects of the venom. However, it should be used only in adults who have been screened for glucose-6-phosphate dehydrogenase (G6PD) deficiency. In addition, dapsone complications include hemolysis, agranulocytosis, aplastic anemia, methemoglobinemia, rashes, toxic epidermal necrolysis, and fatal reactions.[78] Phentolamine has not been shown to have any appreciable effect on the necrotic activity.[73] In animal models, hyperbaric oxygen therapy has not been conclusively proven to be effective.[80] Excision has not been shown to improve outcome and, in fact, may be detrimental. Antibiotics may be prescribed if signs of infection are present. Analgesia should also be offered to the patient.[74] Patients who have signs or symptoms of envenomation should be admitted to the hospital. If acute renal failure develops, dialysis may be necessary. Tissue necrosis at the wound site may necessitate surgical intervention.

Disposition

A patient who has been bitten by a brown recluse spider should be observed in the ED for a minimum of 6 hours. If no local or systemic symptoms develop, the patient may be discharged with instructions to return if any symptoms appear.

TARANTULAS

At least 30 species of tarantula (*Theraphosidae*) live in the deserts of the western United States. Tarantulas are hunters that eat nocturnal insects. Because of the location of its fangs, a tarantula must raise itself on its hind legs in to inflict a bite. In addition, when it is handled, a tarantula releases the hairs of its abdomen, which cause a local urticarial reaction in humans.

Bites from the tarantula are relatively innocuous and result in a low-grade histamine reaction. However, they should be cleansed, and tetanus immunization should be updated if necessary.

Bites from tarantulas from the Panama Canal zone may cause paresthesias and local discomfort. The South American tarantula has a more toxic bite, for which antivenin is available.

Treatment of all tarantula bites should be supportive, with the administration of antihistamines and oral analgesics. The tarantula hairs, which may be barbed, can be removed with adhesive tape.

Scorpion Stings

EPIDEMIOLOGY

Scorpion stings are common in tropical and subtropical regions of the world. For example, Tunisia reports almost 40,000 stings a year, which result in approximately 1,000 hospitalizations and 100 deaths.[81] Deaths from severe envenomation are the result of cardiogenic shock and pulmonary edema.[82]

Scorpion envenomation is not rare in the United States, with 13,918 consultations for scorpion stings reported by the American Association of Poison Control Centers for 1997.[83] Most scorpion stings occur in the southwestern states. The scorpion responsible for severe envenomations in the United States is *Centruroides exilicauda.*[84]

ENVENOMATION

Toxicology

The toxin of *C. exilicauda* is a heat-stable neurotoxin that increases permeability of neuronal sodium channels, causing depolarization of the nerve and myocyte.[84] Severe envenomation results in stimulation of both cholinergic and adrenergic neurons by its action on presynaptic cell membranes.[85] Increased permeability of neuronal sodium channels in the autonomic nervous system results in tachycardia, agitation, hypertension, hypersalivation, dysphagia, and gastrointestinal symptoms.[86,87]

Clinical Features

Scorpion envenomation can produce effects ranging from local to life threatening. Envenomations are categorized by severity from grade I (pain or paresthesia at the sting site) to grade IV (combined cranial nerve and somatic-skeletal neuromuscular dysfunction) [see Table 5].[85]

TREATMENT

Most adults stung by *C. exilicauda* experience only local pain and paresthesia and can be managed as outpatients.[88] Young children, however, often present with severe involuntary motor activity, agitation, and respiratory symptoms requiring intensive supportive care.[88,89]

Initial hypertension and tachycardia may occur in close to half the patients with milder envenomation.[90] These patients normally respond well to treatment with an antihypertensive agent such as prazosin[90] or captopril.[91]

Patients with severe envenomation may have hypotension, left ventricular failure, and pulmonary edema.[91] Supportive care and afterload reduction with vasodilators appear to reduce mortality.[90,91]

The use of specific antivenin in scorpion stings is controversial.[92-96] Antivenin specific to *C. exilicauda* is not available except in Arizona,[84] where it is commonly used for severe grade III and almost all grade IV envenomations.[97] It is rarely associated with anaphylaxis but commonly results in mild serum sickness.[84,97]

The use of sedative-hypnotics has been advocated for the severe agitation and motor restlessness associated with *C. exilicauda* envenomation. Careful assessment (to ensure adequate airway, breathing, and circulation) and monitoring of patients treated with sedative-hypnotics is essential because respiratory depression and even respiratory arrest have been reported with this therapy.[84,89]

Insect Bites and Stings

Insect bites are medically important primarily because insects can act as vectors for pathogenic microorganisms by di-

Table 5 Grading System for Severity of *Centruroides exilicauda* Envenomation[80]

Grade	Features
I	Pain or paresthesia at the site of envenomation
II	Local findings plus pain or paresthesia remote from the sting site
III	Cranial nerve dysfunction* or somatic-skeletal neuromuscular dysfunction†
IV	Cranial nerve dysfunction* and somatic-skeletal neuromuscular dysfunction†

*Blurred vision, wandering eye movements, hypersalivation, trouble swallowing, tongue fasciculation, problems with upper airway, slurred speech.
†Restlessness, severe involuntary shaking, and jerking of extremities (may be mistaken for seizures).

rectly inoculating their human hosts while feeding on blood or tissue fluids. In addition, stinging insects have venom, and the exoskeleton, hair, and secretions of some insects may act as irritants or allergens.

Although insect bites and stings are an essentially universal human experience, the exact incidence of serious morbidity and mortality is difficult to determine because of different reporting practices, regional differences of endemic species, and the wide spectrum of clinical effects, especially severity. In 2000, the American Association of Poison Control Centers reported 90,784 human exposures to bites or envenomations (4.2% of total exposures), with three deaths (0.003% fatal exposure cases).[98] These statistics include stings from bees, wasps, and other Hymenoptera, which are discussed elsewhere [see Chapter 110].

FIRE ANTS

Two species of fire ant were imported into Alabama in the early 1900s. Since that time, they have spread throughout the southeastern United States and Texas.[99] Fire ants both bite and sting, anchoring themselves with their mandibles to leverage the thrust of their stinger. Their venom is primarily composed of an insoluble alkaloid, which has local hemolytic and necrotic effects.[100] Fire ants have a propensity to swarm, resulting in multiple stings. Initially, stings cause an erythematous papule or wheal that develops into a pruritic, sterile pustule over the course of 6 to 24 hours and may persist for weeks. Because of the alkaloid nature of the venom, reactions typically remain local; systemic or anaphylactic reactions are rare. Occasionally, secondary infection occurs.[101]

Treatment consists of local wound care, cold packs, antihistamines, and topical steroids. Extensive involvement may necessitate oral steroids. Anaphylactic reactions are managed in the same manner as they are from other causes. Secondary infection requires treatment with antibiotics. Desensitization therapy should be considered for patients who have life-threatening reactions.[102]

KISSING BUGS AND BED BUGS

The kissing bug (*Triatoma* species), also known as the assassin, cone-nosed, or reduviid bug, is found mostly in the southern and western regions of the United States. It feeds on the blood of vertebrates, including humans, mostly at night. These insects possess a long proboscis, through which they suck blood from their victims without causing pain. Bites commonly occur on the face, because that area is usually exposed during the night.[100] In Central and South America, kissing bugs are the vector for *Trypanosoma cruzi*, the causative agent of Chagas disease.[103]

Bedbugs (*Cimex* species) are also nocturnal bloodsucking insects that have adapted to human environments. They are found throughout the United States and live in baseboards, furniture, clothing, and bedding. Bedbugs are not known vectors for human disease, but allergic reactions to their bites can present as multiple, clustered, erythematous, pruritic papules that can last over a week.[104] Systemic effects are rarely encountered. Treatment consists of symptomatic care with antihistamines and topical steroids.

CATERPILLARS AND MOTHS

The order Lepidoptera includes venomous caterpillars and moths. Some of these caterpillars have hollow spines among their body hairs; injection of venom through these spines can cause symptoms ranging from local dermatitis to generalized systemic reactions. The puss caterpillar, or woolly slug, is found in the southeastern United States and Texas and accounts for most of the envenomations from this insect family for which patients seek medical care. Stings produce small, erythematous, painful papules at the site of contact. Fever and muscle cramps may occur, but serious systemic effects are rare.[105]

Gypsy moths infest much of the eastern United States but also are present elsewhere in the country. Skin contact with gypsy moth caterpillars can cause dermatitis from delayed hypersensitivity. Treatment is symptomatic, with topical steroids and oral antihistamines. Analgesics occasionally are needed for pain control.[103]

BLISTER BEETLES

The blister beetle is found throughout the United States. Blister beetles do not have a toxic bite or sting, but they secrete cantharidin, which acts as a vesicating agent, causing skin irritation and blisters several hours after contact.[100] The blisters can range from a few millimeters to several centimeters in diameter. Pulverized blister beetles were used as an aphrodisiac known as Spanish fly, which causes urethral irritation when ingested orally. Local blisters from blister beetle contact are treated as a chemical burn, with diligent wound care and prevention of secondary infection.[103]

TICKS

Ticks are found throughout the world and are members of the class Arachnida. They painlessly attach to their host (mostly mammals) to feed on blood. The primary medical importance of ticks is as vectors for infection. Infectious diseases carried by ticks include Lyme disease, Rocky Mountain spotted fever, babesiosis, ehrlichiosis, tularemia, Colorado tick fever, and relapsing fever.[106]

Some *Ixodid* species of ticks produce a neurotoxin in their salivary gland that can induce a syndrome known as tick paralysis.[107] The toxin is usually transmitted by an engorged, gravid female and causes an ascending flaccid paralysis approximately 2 to 7 days after the tick begins feeding. Children are most often affected. Respiratory failure may occur, and ventilatory support is required in some cases. The diagnosis is confirmed by finding an embedded tick on the victim. Removal of the tick is essential to recovery. Symptoms improve several hours to days after the tick is removed.[108]

Ticks generally attach themselves to their hosts after approximately 1 to 2 hours, so persons in tick-infested areas should perform frequent checks of their clothing and body. If a tick does attach, it should be removed promptly to minimize risk of disease transmission. The tick should be grasped as close to the skin as possible, using blunt forceps, tweezers, or protected fingers. Steady pressure should be applied while pulling out the tick. Special care should be taken not to squeeze or crush the body of the tick. After removal, standard wound care should be employed. If the mouthparts are only partially removed, foreign-body reactions, secondary infections, and granuloma formation can occur.[109]

Marine Envenomations

Almost 75% of the earth's surface is covered with water, and approximately 80% of our planet's living organisms live in this environment. Only a few of these marine creatures pose a threat to humans, but the dangers have been recognized since ancient times. Significant human morbidity and mortality, ranging from minor dermatitis to life-threatening infections, envenomations, and trauma, may occur in an aquatic environment.

Over recent decades, man's exposure to water has greatly increased, thanks to scientific and technological advancement and exploration, increased sport diving and recreational activities, increased harvesting of marine resources for food, private and commercial saltwater aquariums, and more travel to and greater accessibility of exotic locations. These factors have increased the risk of exposure to marine organisms. Consequently, it is imperative for clinicians, not only in coastal areas but inland as well, to be familiar with the hazards.

Marine organisms that are harmful to humans range from one-celled diatoms and dinoflagellates that cause poisoning after being bioamplified up the food chain (e.g., ciguatera and amnestic shellfish poisoning) to invertebrates with lethal toxins (e.g., jellyfish poisoning) to large vertebrates, such as sharks, that can inflict massive trauma. This discussion will review some of the more common and clinically relevant envenomations (and their associated injuries and infections) that humans may incur in freshwater and saltwater around the United States.

TOXIC INVERTEBRATES

Coelenterates

Coelenterates comprise almost 10,000 species, over 100 of which are dangerous to humans. The phylum Cnidaria (which includes the former phylum Coelenterata) is divided into three classes: (1) Hydrozoa (Portuguese man-of-war, feather hydroids, fire coral); (2) Scyphozoa (true jellyfish, sea nettles, box jellyfish); and (3) Anthozoa (sea anemones, stony corals, soft corals).[110]

Coelenterates are characterized by venomous stinging organoids called nematocysts. The nematocyst is a fluid-filled capsular structure that encloses a tightly coiled, hollow, sharply pointed tubule that bursts forth into the victim when it is discharged after contact. The venom is a complex mixture of proteins, carbohydrates, and other nonproteinaceous substances.[111]

Envenomation Clinical features of coelenterate envenomation are fairly constant but have a range of severity from mild dermatitis to rapid cardiovascular collapse resulting in death. Factors that determine severity include the following: species (the Australian box jellyfish is the most deadly of all stinging marine life); season; number of nematocysts triggered; size and age of the victim; location and surface area of the sting; and the sensitivity of the victim to the venom.[110,112] Knowledge of the species of coelenterates indigenous to the geographic location is important in predicting the potential severity of the envenomation. Most hydroids and hydroid corals (which inhabit both temperate and tropical waters off the Atlantic and Pacific coasts of the United States) initially produce a stinging sensation, paresthesias, and pruritus with local edema, blistering, and wheal formation. Occasionally, the injury can progress over several days to local necrosis, ulceration, and secondary infection.

Physalia physalis (Portuguese man-of-war) consists of a violet-blue floating sail with several nematocyst-bearing tentacles that can be up to 30 m in length.[113] They are widely distributed, but prevalent in the tropical and semitropical waters off the southeastern coast of the United States and in the Gulf of Mexico.

The man-of-war's sting produces an intense pain radiating up the involved extremity, with the development of linear, edematous, erythematous eruptions on the skin. Systemic involvement can occur, involving multiple organ systems, with nausea, vomiting, headache, myalgias, respiratory distress, hypotension, anaphylaxis, and cardiovascular collapse.[113,114]

Jellyfish from the class Scyphozoa display a wide variety of colors, shapes, and sizes and vary in toxic potential. They are the most common coelenterates that produce clinical injuries and cause people to seek medical attention. They have a worldwide distribution and can range in size from a few millimeters to more than 2 m at the bell with tentacles up to 36 m in length.[115] Because the tentacles are so long in some species, it is possible to suffer a significant envenomation without ever seeing the bell. Organisms that have washed ashore also pose a risk, because undischarged nematocysts can fire if an unwary person steps on or picks up a tentacle or part of it. Envenomations from most jellyfish are of mild to moderate severity, with clinical symptoms similar to the hydroids and *Physalia* species.[116]

Treatment Treatment of coelenterate stings includes advanced life support measures, symptomatic care, pain control, and prevention of further envenomation by inactivation of nematocysts. The area of the sting should immediately be rinsed with seawater (not freshwater) or 5% acetic acid (vinegar) for nematocyst inhibition. In the case of a Portuguese man-of-war sting, vinegar should be avoided and only seawater used. Tentacles should then be removed with a gloved hand, hemostats, or a towel to prevent envenomation of the caregiver.[111] Alternatively, isopropyl alcohol (40% to 70%) may be effective. For *Chrysaora* (sea nettle) or *Cyanea* (lion's mane) stings, a baking-powder slurry applied to the affected area is an effective treatment.[112] In patients with seabather's eruption, a vesicular or morbilliform, pruritic dermatitis caused by larval forms of certain coelenterates, a papain (meat tenderizer) solution is effective.[117] Topical anesthetics, antihistamines, and corticosteroids may be of benefit. Prophylactic antibiotics are generally not indicated, but appropriate tetanus prophylaxis and proper wound care should be maintained.

Echinodermata

The phylum Echinodermata consists of poisonous species of starfish, sea urchins, and sea cucumbers. Toxic sea urchins (mostly found in the Pacific and Indian Oceans and the Red Sea) have sharp, brittle, venom-filled spines and may also possess pincerlike seizing organs termed pedicellariae.[115] Spines can easily penetrate wet suits and skin to lodge in the victim.[118] The immediate reaction consists of intense local pain, erythema, edema, and bleeding. Subcutaneous staining from pigments in the spine

can also occur. If multiple spines have penetrated the skin, the patient may develop systemic envenomation symptoms, such as nausea, vomiting, paresthesias, muscular paralysis, hypotension, and respiratory distress.

Sea cucumbers are free-living bottom dwellers that produce a mild toxin that is concentrated in the tentacular organs. Direct contact can cause dermatitis. The venom is usually diluted in the seawater, and the greatest risk is exposure of the corneas and conjunctiva, resulting in an intense inflammation.[116] Treatment consists of immersion in hot water (110° to 115° F) for 30 to 90 minutes or until the patient has significant relief of pain. Spines should be localized under direct visualization or with appropriate radiographic techniques and carefully removed; retained spines may produce a granulomatous reaction that necessitates surgical excision. Routine antibiotics are not necessary, but diligent wound care and tetanus prophylaxis should be employed.[115]

Porifera

The phylum Porifera consists of over 5,000 species of sponges. Sponges are stationary acellular animals that attach to the ocean floor or coral beds and may be colonized by other animals.[115] Sponges inhabit waters off both the Atlantic and Pacific coasts of the United States, as well as Hawaii. Sponge diver's disease is usually caused by colonization of the sponges by coelenterates and presents as a dermatitis or a local necrotic skin reaction.[119] Two primary syndromes can also occur from contact with sponges.[113] The first is a contact dermatitis similar to that caused by plants. The second is an irritant dermatitis caused by the penetration of small spicules of silica or calcium carbonate into the skin. Because it is difficult to distinguish between the two different reactions, treatment of both should be initiated. The skin should be dried and the spicules removed with adhesive tape or a facial peel. Acetic acid 5% soaks should be applied for 10 to 30 minutes three or four times a day (isopropyl alcohol 40% to 70% may be substituted). Topical steroids may help with secondary inflammation but should not be used initially.[113]

Annelida

The phylum Annelida includes bristleworms, or fireworms, which are covered by cactuslike bristles and spines. On contact, these bristles easily enter the skin and break off, causing an intense inflammation with a burning sensation and erythema.

Table 6 Pathogens Associated with Aquatic Sources of Infections

Freshwater Organisms	Saltwater Organisms
Aeromonas hydrophila	Aeromonas hydrophila
Agrobacterium sanguineum	Bacteroides fragilis
Chromobacterium violaceum	Clostridium perfringens
Escherichia coli	Erysipelothrix rhusiopathiae
Pseudomonas aeruginosa	Mycobacterium marinum
Staphylococcus aureus	Salmonella enteritidis
Streptococcus species	Staphylococcus aureus
Vibrio parahaemolyticus	Streptococcus species
	Vibrio species

Bristles should be removed with adhesive tape or a facial peel, and this envenomation should be treated in a manner similar to that for sponge envenomations. [113,116]

TOXIC VERTEBRATES

Stingrays

Stingrays are found in temperate to tropical waters worldwide and represent the most common source of human envenomations from vertebrates.[113] The stingray is armed with one to four venomous spines on a whiplike tail. Envenomations usually occur when an unwary swimmer steps on a buried stingray. The fish reflexively whips its tail upward, thrusting its spine into the victim. The venomous spine has a sharp tip with serrated edges that often cause a jagged laceration in addition to a puncture wound. Occasionally, a spine breaks off and remains in the wound.[120] Most envenomations occur on the ankle or foot. Initial symptoms include an intense, localized pain that may radiate centrally. Local edema and variable bleeding occur. The pain intensifies, peaking after approximately 30 to 60 minutes.[121] The wound often appears dusky or cyanotic and progresses to an erythematous, hemorrhagic stage, occasionally with deep tissue involvement and frank necrosis.[120] Systemic effects can occur and include muscle cramps, nausea, vomiting, weakness, headache, diaphoresis, dizziness, and, in rare cases, seizures, paralysis, cardiovascular collapse, and death.[112] Initial treatment consists of hot-water immersion for 60 minutes to deactivate the venom, which is heat labile, and provide pain relief. The wound should then be thoroughly irrigated and debrided, if needed. Hot-water immersion often provides adequate pain relief, but if pain continues, analgesics may be given. Tetanus prophylaxis is indicated. These wounds are at risk for infection, and antibiotics are often necessary, along with diligent wound care and close follow-up.[121]

Scorpionfish and Lionfish

The Scorpaenidae family consists of over 80 species and includes stonefish, lionfish, and zebrafish. Most Scorpaenidae species are reef-dwelling fish of tropical waters of the Pacific and Indian oceans and the Red Sea.[115] They are exquisitely camouflaged, and envenomations occur when a victim inadvertently grasps or steps on one of these fish. Lionfish are often kept in home saltwater aquariums because of their beauty and, therefore, may be involved in accidental envenomations. These fish possess venomous spines covered by an integumentary sheath. The venom consists of a complex mixture of inflammatory mediators and heat-labile proteins and is injected after the spine punctures the skin.[120] The spine may also fracture and remain in the puncture site, causing a foreign-body reaction or acting as a nidus for secondary infection. Clinical manifestations of envenomation vary from mild toxicity with the lionfish to severe life-threatening toxicity with the stonefish.[122] Initial symptoms include an intense pain at the sting site with central radiation that can continue to intensify for several hours. The wound appears ecchymotic and cyanotic initially, and subsequently, it often becomes erythematous and swollen. Localized tissue necrosis and skin sloughing can occur after several days.[121] Systemic symptoms can include nausea, vomiting, abdominal pain, headache, myalgias, weakness, tremor, syncope, hypotension, paralysis, seizures, cardiac arrhythmias, hypotension, cardiopulmonary arrest, and death.[120] Initial treatment is immediate immersion of the affected area in hot water (110° to 115° F) for 60 to 90 minutes in an attempt to denature the venom proteins and provide pain relief.[121] Supportive care for systemic symptoms, diligent local wound care (including evaluation for retained spines), tetanus prophylaxis, and analgesics are also the mainstay of treatment. An antivenin is available but is usually reserved for the more serious stonefish envenomations.[122]

Catfish

There are over 1,000 species of catfish worldwide that inhabit both freshwater and saltwater environments.[115] Freshwater catfish are typically sedentary bottom dwellers of slow-moving and often dirty waters. Saltwater catfish, on the other hand, travel in schools and typically stay on the move. Catfish have a smooth, scaleless skin and derive their name from their perioral barbells (which, contrary to popular belief, are incapable of inflicting any stings or envenomation). However, catfish do possess serrated dorsal and pectoral spines that have venom glands enclosed in an integumentary sheath. The spines can produce a deep puncture wound, and the glands release their venom after being traumatized.[123] Most stings occur when the fish is handled after capture, although occasionally a wader will be stung on the foot. The initial symptom is intense pain, which radiates up the affected limb and is out of proportion to the mechanical trauma. The pain is followed by an intense inflammatory reaction that can include erythema, swelling, local hemorrhage, and tissue necrosis.[124] Systemic reactions are rare but can include nausea, vomiting, weakness, hypotension, syncope, and respiratory distress.[121] The main concern with catfish stings, as with all aquatic trauma, is the risk of secondary infection. Catfish spines can be retained in the puncture site. Because spines are often radiopaque, x-rays should be taken to locate them.[123] If there is evidence of a retained spine, the wound should be surgically explored and foreign matter removed. Initial treatment includes immersion of the affected site in hot water (100° to 115° F) for 60 to 90 minutes, meticulous wound care and debridement, tetanus prophylaxis, and analgesics.[121]

WATERBORNE INFECTIONS

Freshwater and saltwater environments provide a medium for a host of microbes not typically encountered in traumatic wounds of nonaquatic origin. The concentration and diversity of these organisms vary, depending on temperature, sunlight, depth, salinity, nutrients, coexisting life forms, and pollutants. However, most aquatic microbes are heterotrophic, motile, gram-negative rods that are facultative anaerobes [see Table 6].[125,126] Antibiotic coverage should include gram-negative organisms, as well as *Staphylococcus aureus* and *Streptococcus* species, which are the pathogens in most secondary aquatic wound infections.

References

1. Griego RD, Rosen T, Orengo IF, et al: Dog, cat, and human bites: a review. J Am Acad Dermatol 33:1019, 1995
2. Weiss HB, Friedman DI, Coben JH: Incidence of dog bite injuries treated in emergency departments. JAMA 279:51, 1998
3. Goldstein EJ: Bite wounds and infection. Clin Infect Dis 14:633, 1992
4. Abrahamian FM: Dog bites: bacteriology, management, and prevention. Curr Infect Dis Rep 2:446, 2000
5. Rest JG, Goldstein EJ: Management of human and animal bite wounds. Emerg Med Clin North Am 1:117, 1985
6. Galloway RE: Mammalian bites. J Emerg Med 6:325, 1988
7. Bacteriologic analysis of infected dog and cat bites. Emergency Medicine Animal Bite Infection Study Group. N Engl J Med 340:85, 1999
8. Garcia VF: Animal bites and *Pasteurella* infections. Pediatr Rev 18:127, 1997
9. Dire DJ: Emergency management of dog and cat bite wounds. Emerg Med Clin North Am 10:719, 1992

10. Sacks JJ, Sinclair L, Gilchrist J, et al: Breeds of dogs involved in fatal human attacks in the United States between 1979 and 1998. J Am Vet Med Assoc 217:836, 2000

11. Goldstein EJ, Citron DM, Finegold SM: Dog bite wounds and infection: a prospective clinical study. Ann Emerg Med 9:508, 1980

12. Goldstein EJ, Richwald GA: Human and animal bite wounds. Am Fam Physician 36:101, 1987

13. Aghababian RV, Conte JE Jr: Mammalian bite wounds. Ann Emerg Med 9:79, 1980

14. Callaham ML: Human and animal bites. Top Emerg Med 4:1, 1982

15. Goldstein EJ: Current concepts on animal bites: bacteriology and therapy. Curr Clin Top Infect Dis 19:99, 1999

16. Compendium of animal rabies prevention and control, 2000. National Association of State Public Health Veterinarians, Inc. MMWR Morb Mortal Wkly Rep 49(RR-8):21, 2000

17. Paisley JW, Lauer BA: Severe facial injuries to infants due to unprovoked attacks by pet ferrets. JAMA 259:2005, 1988

18. Applegate JA, Walhout MF: Childhood risks from the ferret. J Emerg Med 16:425, 1998

19. Fischer RG, Edwardsson S, Klinge B, et al: The effect of cyclosporin-A on the oral microflora at gingival sulcus of the ferret. J Clin Periodontol 23:853, 1996

20. Krebs JW, Strine TW, Smith JS, et al: Rabies surveillance in the United States during 1994. J Am Vet Med Assoc 207:1562, 1995

21. Compendium of animal rabies control, 1996: National Association of State Public Health Veterinarians, Inc. J Am Vet Med Assoc 208:214, 1996

22. Human rabies prevention—United States, 1999. MMWR Recomm Rep 48(RR-1):1, 1999

23. Callaham M: Controversies in antibiotic choices for bite wounds. Ann Emerg Med 17:1321, 1988

24. Lindsey D, Christopher M, Hollenbach J, et al: Natural course of the human bite wound: incidence of infection and complications in 434 bites and 803 lacerations in the same group of patients. J Trauma 27:45, 1987

25. Brook I: Microbiology of human and animal bite wounds in children. Pediatr Infect Dis J 6:29, 1987

26. Goldstein EJ, Citron DM, Hunt Gerardo S: Activities of HMR 3004 (RU 64004) and HMR 3647 (RU 66647) compared to those of erythromycin, azithromycin, clarithromycin, roxithromycin, and eight other antimicrobial agents against unusual aerobic and anaerobic human and animal bite pathogens isolated from skin and soft tissue infections in humans. Antimicrob Agents Chemother 42:1127, 1998

27. Glass KD: Factors related to the resolution of treated hand infections. J Hand Surg [Am] 7:388, 1982

28. Wiley JF 2nd: Mammalian bites: review of evaluation and management. Clin Pediatr (Phila) 29:283, 1990

29. Ordog GJ, Balasubramanium S, Wasserberger J: Rat bites: fifty cases. Ann Emerg Med 14:126, 1985

30. Krebs JW, Smith JS, Rupprecht CE, et al: Mammalian reservoirs and epidemiology of rabies diagnosed in human beings in the United States, 1981–1998. Ann NY Acad Sci 916:345, 2000

31. Glaser C, Lewis P, Wong S: Pet-, animal-, and vector-borne infections. Pediatr Rev 21:219, 2000

32. Ostrowski SR, Leslie MJ, Parrott T, et al: B-virus from pet macaque monkeys: an emerging threat in the United States? Emerg Infect Dis 4:117, 1998

33. Presutti RJ: Prevention and treatment of dog bites. Am Fam Physician 63:1567, 2001

34. Calkins CM, Bensard DD, Partrick DA, et al: Life-threatening dog attacks: a devastating combination of penetrating and blunt injuries. J Pediatr Surg 36:1115, 200

35. Gross A, Cutright DE, Bhaskar SN: Effectiveness of pulsating water jet lavage in treatment of contaminated crushed wounds. Am J Surg 124:373, 1972

36. Dire DJ, Welsh AP: A comparison of wound irrigation solutions used in the emergency department. Ann Emerg Med 19:704, 1990

37. Smith JS, Fishbein DB, Rupprecht CE, et al: Unexplained rabies in three immigrants in the United States: a virologic investigation. N Engl J Med 324:205, 1991

38. Maimaris C, Quinton DN: Dog-bite lacerations: a controlled trial of primary wound closure. Arch Emerg Med 5:156, 1988

39. Chen E, Hornig S, Shepherd SM, et al: Primary closure of mammalian bites. Acad Emerg Med 7:157, 2000

40. Medeiros I, Saconato H: Antibiotic prophylaxis for mammalian bites. Cochrane Database Syst Rev (2):CD001738, 2001

41. Appropriateness of rabies postexposure prophylaxis treatment for animal exposures. Emergency ID Net Study Group. JAMA 284:1001, 2000

42. Gold BS, Barish RA: Venomous snakebites: current concepts in diagnosis, treatment and management. Emerg Med Clin North Am 10:249, 1992

43. Smith TA II, Figge HL: Treatment of snakebite poisoning. Am J Hospital Pharm 48:2190, 1991

44. Norris R: Snake envenomations: coral. eMedicine J 2(5), 2001

45. Sanford JP: Snakebites. Cecil Textbook of Medicine. Wyngaarden JB, Smith LH, Bennett JC, Eds. WB Saunders Co, Philadelphia, 1992, p 439

46. Bush SP: Snake envenomations: rattle. eMedicine J 2(5), 2001

47. Boyer LV, Seifert SA, Clark RF, et al: Recurrent and persistent coagulopathy following pit viper envenomation. Arch Intern Med 159:706, 1999

48. Watt CH Jr: Treatment of poisonous snakebite with emphasis on digit dermotomy. South Med J 78:694, 1985

49. McKinney PE: Out-of-hospital and interhospital management of Crotaline snakebite. Ann Emerg Med 72:168, 2001

50. Lewis JV, Portera CA Jr: Rattlesnake bite of the face: case report and review of the literature. Am Surgeon 60:681, 1994

51. Parrish HM: Analysis of 460 fatalities from venomous animals in the United States. Am J Med Sci 245:129, 1963

52. Dart RC, McNally J: Efficacy, safety, and use of snake antivenoms in the United States. Ann Emerg Med 37:181, 2001

53. Jurkovich GJ, Luterman A, McCullar K, et al: Complications of Crotalidae antivenin treatment. J Trauma 28:1032, 1988

54. Dart RC, Seifert SA, Carroll L, et al: Affinity-purified, mixed monospecific crotalid antivenom ovine Fab for the treatment of crotalid venom poisoning. Ann Emerg Med 30:33, 1997

55. Gillissen A, Theakston RD, Barth J, et al: Neurotoxicity, haemostatic disturbances and haemolytic anaemia after a bite by a Tunisian saw-scaled or carpet viper (Echis' pyramidium'-complex): failure of antivenom treatment. Toxicon 32:937, 1994

56. Hardy DL, Jeter M, Corrigan JJ: Envenomation by the Northern blacktail rattlesnake (Crotalus molossus molossus): report of two cases and the in vitro effects of the venom on fibrinolysis and platelet aggregation. Toxicon 20:487, 1982

57. Seifert SA, Boyer LV, Dart RC, et al: Relationship of venom effects to venom antigen and antivenom serum concentrations in a patient with Crotalus atrox envenomation treated with a Fab antivenom. Ann Emerg Med 30:49, 1997

58. Berlinger FG, Flowers HH: Some observations of the treatment of snakebites in Vietnam. Military Med 138:139, 1973

59. Hall EL: Role of surgical intervention in the management of Crotaline snake envenomation. Ann Emerg Med 37:175, 2001

60. Weed HG: Nonvenomous snakebite in Massachusetts: prophylactic antibiotics are unnecessary. Ann Emerg Med 22:220, 1993

61. Pantanowitz L, Guidozzi F: Management of snake and spider bite in pregnancy. Obstet Gynecol Survey 51:615, 1996

62. Parrish HM, Kahn MS: Snakebite during pregnancy. Obstet Gynecol 27:468, 1966

63. Cruz NS, Alvarez RG: Rattlesnake bite complications in 19 children. Pediatr Emerg Care 10:30, 1994

64. Weber RA, White RR 4th: Crotalidae envenomation in children. Ann Plast Surg 31:141, 1993

65. Mammen EF: Fibrinogen abnormalities. Semin Thromb Hemost 9:1, 1983

66. Ownby CL, Reisbeck SL, Allen R: Levels of therapeutic antivenin and venom in a human snakebite victim. South Med J 89:803, 1996

67. Zukowski CW: Black widow spider bite. J Am Board Fam Pract 6:279, 1993

68. Sternlicht H, Fosson A: Partial paralysis following a black widow spider bite. J Kentucky Med Assoc 9:531, 1987

69. Allen C: Arachnid envenomations. Emerg Med Clin North Am 19:269, 1992

70. Otten EJ: Venomous animal injuries. Emergency Medicine – Concepts and Clinical Practice. Rosen P, Barkin RM, Braen GR, et al, Eds. Mosby Year Book, St. Louis, 1992, p 885

71. Ryan PG: Preliminary report: experience with the use of dantrolene sodium in the treatment of bites by the black widow spider Latrodectus hesperus. J Toxicol Clin Toxicol 21:487, 1984

72. Cacy J, Mold JW: The clinical characteristics of brown recluse spider bites treated by family physicians: an OKPRN study. J Fam Prac 48:536, 1999

73. Young VL, Pin P: The brown recluse spider bite. Ann Plast Surg 20:447, 1988

74. Gross AS, Wilson DC, King LE Jr: Persistent segmental cutaneous anesthesia after a brown recluse spider bite. South Med J 83:1321, 1990

75. Wasserman G: Wound care of spider and snake envenomations. Ann Emerg Med 17:1331, 1988

76. Wong R, Hughes S, Voorhees J: Spider bites. Arch Dermatol 123:99, 1987

77. Sauer GC: Transverse myelitis and paralysis from a brown recluse spider bite. Missouri Med 72:603, 1975

78. King LE, Rees RS: Dapsone treatment of brown recluse bite. JAMA 250:648, 1983

79. Gutowicz M, Fritz RA, Sonoga AL: Brown recluse spider bite: a literature review and case report. J Am Podiatric Med Assoc 79:142, 1979

80. Wright SW, Wrenn KD, Murray L, et al: Clinical presentation and outcome of brown recluse spider bites. Ann Emerg Med 30:28, 1997

81. Abroug F, Nouira S, Haguiga H, et al: High-dose hydrocortisone hemisuccinate in scorpion envenomation. Ann Emerg Med 30:23, 1997

82. Abroug F, Boujdaria R, Belghith M, et al: Cardiac dysfunction and pulmonary edema following scorpion envenomation. Chest 100:1057, 1991

83. Litovitz TL, Klein-Schwartz W, Dyer KS, et al: 1997 annual report of the American Association of Poison Control Centers Toxic Exposure Surveillance System. Am J Emerg Med 16:443, 1998

84. Gibly R, Williams M, Walter FG, et al: Continuous intravenous midazolam infusion for Centruroides exilicauda scorpion envenomation. Ann Emerg Med 34:620, 1999

85. Sofer S: Scorpion envenomation. Intensive Care Med 21:626, 1995

86. Curry SC, Vance MV, Ryan PJ, et al: Envenomation by the scorpion Centruroides sculpturatus. J Toxicol Clin Toxicol 21:417, 1983

87. Likes K, Banner W Jr, Chavez M: Centruroides exilicauda envenomation in Arizona. West J Med 141:634, 1984

88. Rachesky IJ, Banner W Jr, Dansky J, et al: Treatments for Centruroides exilicauda envenomation. Am J Dis Child 138:1136, 1984

89. Berg RA, Tarantino MD: Envenomation by the scorpion Centruroides exilicauda (C.

sculpturatus): severe and unusual manifestations. Pediatrics 87:930, 1991

90. Bawaskar HS, Bawaskar PH: Prazosin for vasodilator treatment of acute pulmonary oedema due to scorpion sting. Ann Tropic Med Parasitol 81:719, 1987

91. Karnad DR: Haemodynamic patterns in patients with scorpion envenomation. Heart 79:485, 1998

92. Abroug F, ElAtrous S, Nouira S, et al: Serotherapy in scorpion envenomation: a randomised controlled trial. Lancet 354:906, 1999

93. Belghith M, Boussarsar M, Haguiga H, et al: Efficacy of serotherapy in scorpion sting: a matched-pair study. J Toxicol Clin Toxicol 37:51, 1999

94. Amaral CF, Rezende NA: Treatment of scorpion envenoming should include both a potent specific antivenom and support of vital functions. Toxicon 38:1005, 2000

95. Bond GR: Antivenin administration for *Centruroides* scorpion sting: risks and benefits. Ann Emerg Med 21:788, 1992

96. de Rezende NA, Chavez-Olortegui C, Amaral CF: Is the severity of *Tityus serrulatus* scorpion envenoming related to plasma venom concentrations? Toxicon 34:820, 1996

97. LoVecchio F, Welch S, Klemens J, et al: Incidence of immediate and delayed hypersensitivity to *Centruroides* antivenom. Ann Emerg Med 34:615, 1999

98. Litovitz TL, Klein-Schwartz W, White S, et al: 2000 Annual report of the American Association of Poison Control Centers Toxic Exposure Surveillance System. Am J Emerg Med 19:337, 2001

99. Kemp SF, DeShazo RD, Moffitt JE, et al: Expanding habitat of the imported fire ant (*Solenopis invicta*): a public health concern. J Allergy Clin Immunol 105:683, 2000

100. Handbook of Clinical Toxicology and Animal Venoms and Poisons. Meier J, White J, Eds. CRC Press, New York, 1995, p 331

101. deShazo RD, Williams DF, Moak ES: Fire ant attacks on residents in health care facilities: a report of two cases. Ann Intern Med 131:424, 1999

102. Elgart GW: Ant, bee, and wasp stings. Dermatol Clin 8:229, 1990

103. Sherman AM, Bechtel HB, Erickson TB: North American arthropod envenomation and parasitism. Wilderness Medicine, 4th ed. Auerbach PS, Ed. Mosby, St. Louis, 2001, p 863

104. Elston DM, Stockwell S: What's eating you? Bedbugs. Cutis 65:262, 2000

105. Rosen T: Caterpillar dermatitis. Dermatol Clin 8:245, 1990

106. Spach DH, Liles WC, Campbell GL, et al: Tick-borne diseases in the United States. N Engl J Med 329:936, 1993

107. Grattan-Smith PJ, Morris JG, Johnston HM, et al: Clinical and neurophysiological features of tick paralysis. Brain 120:1975, 1997

108. Dworkin MS, Shoemaker PC, Anderson DE: Tick paralysis: 33 human cases in Washington State. Clin Infect Dis 29:1435, 1999

109. Gentile DA, Lang JE: Tick-borne diseases. Wilderness Medicine, 4th ed. Mosby, St. Louis, 2001, p 769

110. Fenner PJ: Dangers in the ocean: the traveler and marine envenomation: I. Jellyfish. J Travel Med 5:135, 1998

111. Burnett JW, Calton GJ: Venomous pelagic coelenterates: chemistry, toxicology, immunology and treatment of their stings. Toxicon 25:581, 1987

112. Burnett JW: Human injuries following jellyfish stings. Maryland Med J 41:509, 1992

113. Auerbach PS: Envenomation by aquatic invertebrates, envenomation by aquatic vertebrates. Wilderness Medicine, 4th ed. Auerbach PS, Ed. Mosby, St. Louis, 2001, p 1450

114. Kaufman MB: Portuguese man-of-war envenomation. Pediatr Emerg Care 8:27, 1992

115. Handbook of Clinical Toxicology and Animal Venoms and Poisons. Meier J, White J, Eds. CRC Press, New York, 1995, p 27

116. Brown CK, Shepherd SM: Marine trauma, envenomations, and intoxications. Emerg Med Clinics North Am 10:385, 1992

117. Kumar S, Hlady WG, Malecki JM: Risk factors for seabather's eruption: a prospective cohort study. Public Health Rep 112:59, 1997

118. Baden HP, Burnell JW: Injuries from sea urchins. South Med J 70:459, 1997

119. Auerbach PS: Marine envenomations. N Engl J Med 325:486, 1991

120. Cooper NK: Stone fish and stingrays: some notes on the injuries that they cause to man. J R Army Med Corps 137:136, 1991

121. McGoldrick J, Marx JA: Marine envenomations. J Emerg Med 9:497, 1991

122. Gwee MC, Gopalakrishnakone P, Yuen R, et al: A review of stonefish venoms and toxins. Pharmacol Ther 64:509, 1994

123. Shepherd S, Thomas SH, Stone K: Catfish envenomation. J Wilderness Med 5:67, 1994

124. Blomkalns AL, Otten EJ: Catfish spine envenomation: a case report and literature review. Wilderness Environ Med 10:242, 1999

125. Auerbach PS, Yajko DM, Nassos PS, et al: Bacteriology of the freshwater environment: implications for clinical therapy. Ann Emerg Med 16:1016, 1987

126. Auerbach PS, Yajko DM, Nassos PS, et al: Bacteriology of the marine environment: implications for clinical therapy. Ann Emerg Med 16:643, 1987

Acknowledgments

Figures 1, 2, and 3   Photography by Bill Love/Blue Chameleon Ventures.

Figure 4   Photography from Animals Animals/Jim Bockowski. Used by permission.

Figure 5   Photography by B. J. Kaston (Trans. no K13623). Courtesy of the Department of Library Services, the American Museum of Natural History, New York.

CARDIOVASCULAR MEDICINE

15 Approach to the Cardiovascular Patient

Catherine M. Otto, M.D., and David M. Shavelle, M.D.

The complete evaluation of the cardiovascular patient begins with a thorough history and a detailed physical examination. These two initial steps will often lead to the correct diagnosis and assist in excluding life-threatening conditions. Cardiovascular conditions that frequently require evaluation include chest pain, dyspnea, palpitations, syncope, and cardiac murmurs. Each of these conditions will be discussed separately with an emphasis on a diagnostic algorithm and the appropriate use of invasive and noninvasive cardiac testing.

Chest Pain

BACKGROUND

Chest pain is perhaps the most common cardiovascular symptom encountered in clinical practice. Establishing a cardiac origin of chest pain in a patient with multiple cardiovascular risk factors is essential because it allows initiation of appropriate therapy, thereby reducing the risk of myocardial infarction and death. Similarly, excluding a cardiac origin of chest pain in a low-risk patient is no less essential to avoid costly and potentially risky diagnostic testing that will neither add to the care of the patient nor relieve the discomfort.[1] Cardiac disorders that result in chest pain include myocardial ischemia, myocardial infarction, acute pericarditis, aortic stenosis, hypertrophic cardiomyopathy, and aortic dissection. Noncardiac disorders that may result in chest pain include pulmonary embolism, pneumonia, pleural effusion, reactive airway disease, gastrointestinal and biliary disease, anxiety, and musculoskeletal disorders.

Angina most frequently is caused by atherosclerosis of the coronary arteries. Less common causes of angina include coronary artery spasm (e.g., Prinzmetal angina or secondary to drug use, as with cocaine), coronary artery embolism (from aortic valve endocarditis), congenital coronary anomalies, spontaneous coronary artery dissection, coronary arteritis, and aortic dissection when the right coronary artery is involved. Angina may also occur in the presence of angiographically normal coronary arteries and is referred to as syndrome X. The underlying pathophysiology is thought to be related to microvascular dysfunction; the prognosis is generally good despite frequent episodes of chest pain.[2]

HISTORY AND PHYSICAL EXAMINATION

Essential features of the history include an accurate description of the chest pain, including the severity, frequency, location, radiation, quality, alleviating and aggravating factors and duration of symptoms [*see Table 1*]. Anginal chest pain is often described as pressure or a heavy sensation. Symptoms may be difficult for the patient to describe and may be better characterized as discomfort, not pain. Angina typically is described as substernal with radiation to the left neck, jaw, or arm; is mild to moderate in severity; and lasts for 5 to 15 minutes. Classically, angina occurs with exercise, stress, or exposure to cold weather and is relieved with rest or use of nitroglycerin. Some of the most useful features of the patient history that help establish that chest pain is angina are (1) reproducibility of the pain with a given degree of activity, (2) brief duration, and (3) alleviation of the pain with rest or use of nitroglycerin. In patients with a history of coronary artery disease (CAD), an accurate characterization of the quality and frequency of the pain is essential to determine whether a change in the anginal pattern has occurred (i.e., a patient with chronic stable angina now has unstable angina) or if a noncardiac origin of pain is now present (e.g., a patient with chronic stable angina now has musculoskeletal pain). Elderly patients, diabetic patients, and women experiencing angina often present with atypical symptoms that may appear to be noncardiac in nature.

Anginal chest pain may also be seen in patients with aortic stenosis or hypertrophic cardiomyopathy secondary to the supply-demand imbalance caused by excessive myocardial hypertrophy. Pericarditis commonly results in a sharp type of chest pain that occurs in the substernal region and worsens on inspiration (pleuritic) when the patient is in a supine position and im-

---

Table 1   Differentiating Features in the Patient's History of Chest Pain

Condition	Location	Radiation	Quality	Alleviating Factors	Aggravating Factors	Duration
Angina pectoris	Substernal	Jaw, arm	Pressure	Rest, nitroglycerin	Exercise, cold weather	5–15 minutes
Pericarditis	Left-sided, substernal	Neck, trapezius ridge	Sharp	Sitting up and leaning forward	Inspiration, supine position	Hours
Musculoskeletal	Variable over entire chest wall	None	Sharp	Rest, anti-inflammatory or analgesic medications	Movement, palpation	Variable, but usually constant
Aortic stenosis	Substernal	Occasionally to jaw, arm	Pressure	Rest, nitroglycerin	Exercise, cold weather	Minutes
Hypertrophic cardiomyopathy	Substernal	Occasionally to jaw, arm	Pressure	Rest, nitroglycerin	Exercise, cold weather	Minutes
Aortic dissection	Substernal	Back	Tearing	None	None	Minutes to hours

proves when the patient is in an upright position. The pain of aortic dissection is also substernal, but typically, it is described as a tearing or ripping sensation, radiates to the back or interscapular area, begins abruptly, and fails to improve with rest or use of nitroglycerin. Musculoskeletal pain may be located anywhere on the chest wall, is often reproducible with palpation, and frequently worsens with rotation of the thorax. Recent episodes of excessive lifting or activity may be elicited in the history. Esophageal spasm and gastroesophageal reflux disease are frequent causes of noncardiac chest pain.[3]

Cardiovascular risk factors should be reviewed in all patients presenting with chest pain. These risk factors include a history of hypertension, hyperlipidemia, diabetes mellitus, or cigarette smoking; age greater than 45 years in males and 55 years in females; and a family history of CAD (i.e., first-degree male relative with myocardial infarction or sudden death occurring before 55 years of age; first-degree female relative with these events occurring before 65 years of age). Relatively uncommon factors that may also result in angina include prior radiation therapy, drug use (e.g., cocaine and amphetamines), and the presence of a systemic disease, such as lupus erythematosus, polyarteritis nodosum, or rheumatoid arthritis, that is associated with coronary arteritis.

The physical examination is usually unremarkable in patients presenting with anginal chest pain. However, certain physical findings can be very helpful in supporting the diagnosis of CAD. Elevated blood pressure by cuff sphygmomanometry and retinal abnormalities on fundoscopic examination (arteriovenous nicking, copper wiring, and hemorrhages) may indicate previously undiagnosed hypertension. Asymmetric peripheral pulses, an early diastolic murmur, and the appropriate clinical history (tearing chest pain with radiation to the back) indicate an aortic dissection. Xanthomas (cholesterol-filled nodules that occur subcutaneously or over tendons) indicate severe elevations in serum cholesterol levels. Femoral, carotid, or renal artery bruits and diminished peripheral pulses signify peripheral vascular disease and markedly increase the probability of CAD.[4] Tenderness to palpation of the chest wall, especially at the costochondral and chondrosternal articulations, suggests a musculoskeletal etiology of chest pain. Occasionally, patients with anginal chest pain may also have a component of reproducible pain with palpation. A third heart sound and a holosystolic murmur of mitral regurgitation (secondary to ischemia of a papillary muscle) may be present if a patient with CAD is examined during an episode of anginal pain.

Physical examination also is directed toward findings that suggest an alternative cause of chest pain. A systolic murmur that radiates to the base of the neck (aortic stenosis) or a systolic murmur that increases in intensity with the strain phase of the Valsalva maneuver (hypertrophic cardiomyopathy) are uncommon but useful findings. A so-called leatherlike or scratchy series of sounds indicates a pericardial rub and supports a diagnosis of pericarditis. The intensity of the rub may increase with inspiration, indicating associated inflammation of the pleura, or pleuritis. Examination of the lung fields may disclose diminished breath sounds associated with dullness to percussion (pleural effusion), rhonchi, and egophony (pneumonia) or expiratory wheezes (asthma).

DIAGNOSTIC TESTS

On the basis of the history, chest pain is characterized as anginal, atypical (some features of angina combined with some noncharacteristic features), or nonanginal. In combination with as-

sessment of cardiovascular risk factors and pertinent findings from physical examination, patients can be characterized as having a low, moderate, or high likelihood of CAD. Whereas an estimate of a patient's pretest likelihood of CAD may be adequate in some cases, quantitative methods for defining the risk of CAD are also available.[5,6] The most widely used method is from the Duke University Database and considers the patient's age, sex, cardiovascular risk factor profile, description of chest pain, and information from the resting electrocardiogram to determine the pretest likelihood of CAD.[6]

Although the diagnostic yield from the baseline ECG is low, it provides useful information in pursuing additional diagnostic testing [see Figure 1]. Notable findings include Q waves consistent with a prior myocardial infarction and left ventricular hypertrophy that may be secondary to aortic stenosis, hypertrophic cardiomyopathy, or long-standing hypertension. ST segment depression, T wave abnormalities, and arrhythmias may be present if the ECG is obtained during an episode of anginal chest pain.

As with the ECG, a routine chest roentgenogram is usually normal. However, the presence of cardiomegaly, a left ventricular aneurysm, significant coronary or aortic calcification, or pulmonary venous congestion would be useful findings and may warrant additional diagnostic testing.

Patients with a low risk of CAD should not undergo an exercise ECG stress test on a treadmill (stress-ECG), because an abnormal test result is likely to be a false positive. Conversely, a negative test result simply confirms the low probability of CAD. However, if patient reassurance is a consideration, a normal test result and determination of exercise duration may be very useful. In addition, exercise stress testing provides information regarding symptom status and the hemodynamic response to exercise when the history is problematic. Absolute and relative contraindications to exercise testing should be reviewed in all patients before testing is begun [see Table 2].[7]

Similarly, patients with a high risk of CAD in general should not undergo noninvasive cardiac stress testing for the purpose of diagnosing CAD, because a negative test is likely to be a false negative, and a positive test simply confirms the high probability of CAD. In this group of patients, coronary angiography should be used to establish a diagnosis of CAD. However, noninvasive cardiac stress testing in certain patients at high risk for CAD may be useful. Indications for noninvasive stress testing in these patients include (1) assessment of the effectiveness of current medical therapy, (2) objective measurement of exercise capacity, (3) evaluation of the extent and location of ischemia or infarction with nuclear or echocardiographic imaging, (4) preoperative risk assessment in patients with known CAD who are undergoing noncardiac surgery, and (5) assessment of prognosis in patients with symptoms consistent with CAD or in patients with known CAD.

To establish the diagnosis of CAD in intermediate-risk patients, a number of noninvasive testing methods are available.[8] The decision to perform a specific test is based on various patient characteristics (e.g., body size, associated medical conditions, and ability to exercise), findings on the baseline ECG, and institutional experience with specific testing methods [see Table 3].[9-14] The most appropriate noninvasive stress test is chosen on the basis of each of these factors, as indicated in the chest pain algorithm [see Figure 1]. For patients who are able to exercise with a normal baseline ECG, treadmill-ECG stress testing can be performed. Women have a higher incidence of false positive results; therefore, many physicians recommend that, for all women, exercise be combined with an imaging method (e.g., echocardiography or

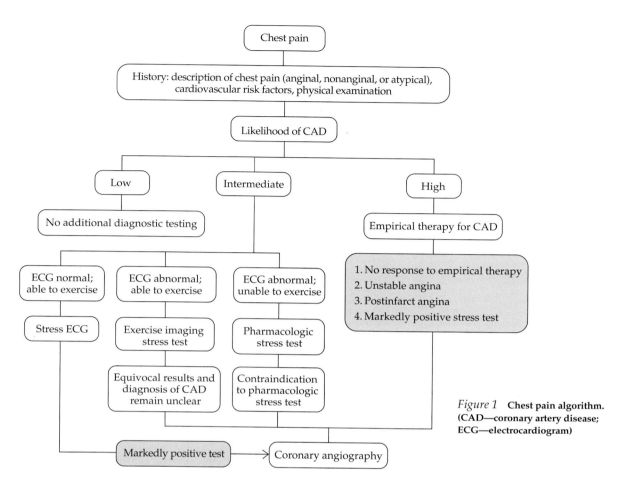

Figure 1 **Chest pain algorithm.
(CAD—coronary artery disease;
ECG—electrocardiogram)**

nuclear imaging).[10] In general, to establish the diagnosis of CAD, exercise is preferred over pharmacologic stress agents. For patients who are unable to exercise because of physical limitations (e.g., arthritis or orthopedic problems), severe coexisting pulmonary disease, or general disability, pharmacologic stress agents such as dobutamine, adenosine, or dipyridamole can be employed. Each of these agents has specific contraindications [*see Table 4*].

Coronary angiography is considered the gold standard for the diagnosis of CAD. Although the incidence of major complications is low (< 2%), coronary angiography is costly and has some risk; thus, it is reserved for (1) patients with markedly positive noninvasive tests (i.e., hypotension and significant ST segment depression on ECG stress testing on a treadmill), (2) patients at high risk for CAD who have failed a course of empirical antianginal therapy, (3) patients with unstable or postinfarction angina, (4) patients with a contraindication to exercise or pharmacologic stress testing, and (5) patients with equivocal results on noninvasive stress testing when the diagnosis of CAD remains unclear. Coronary angiography has certain limitations, including the inability to determine (1) the functional significance of a coronary artery stenosis and (2) which coronary plaque is likely to rupture (i.e., the so-called vulnerable plaque) and result in an acute coronary syndrome. Intravascular ultrasound studies have also shown that coronary angiography may occasionally underestimate the severity of an area of narrowing, because it represents a so-called luminogram (shadow image) and not the size of the atherosclerotic plaque.[15] Despite these shortcomings, the extent and severity of CAD and measurement of left ventricular function by left heart catheterization are powerful predictors of clinical outcome.[13]

Dyspnea

BACKGROUND

Dyspnea refers to difficulty with breathing and can occur with a wide variety of cardiac, pulmonary, and systemic conditions [*see Table 5*]. Dyspnea can be classified as occurring (1) at rest, (2)

Table 2 **Absolute and Relative Contraindications to Exercise Testing[7]**

Absolute	Relative
Recent myocardial infarction (within 48 hr)	Left main coronary stenosis
Unstable angina not previously stabilized with medical therapy	Moderate stenotic valvular heart disease
Uncontrolled cardiac arrhythmias causing symptoms or hemodynamic compromise	Electrolyte abnormalities
Symptomatic severe aortic stenosis	Severe arterial hypertension
Uncontrolled symptomatic heart failure	Tachycardia or bradyarrhythmias
Acute pulmonary embolism or pulmonary infarction	Hypertrophic cardiomyopathy and other forms of outflow tract obstruction
Acute myocarditis or pericarditis	Mental or physical impairment leading to inability to exercise adequately
Acute aortic dissection	High degree of atrioventricular block

with exertion, (3) during the night, awakening a patient from sleep (paroxysmal nocturnal dyspnea), or (4) during episodes of recumbency (orthopnea). Paroxysmal nocturnal dyspnea and or- thopnea result from a similar mechanism. Specifically, the recum- bent position augments venous return to the right heart. This in- crease in cardiac filling further increases the pulmonary capillary

Table 3 Diagnostic Testing Methods Available for Evaluating Chest Pain[9-14]

Diagnostic Test	Indications	Information Obtained	Limitations	Sensitivity	Specificity
Exercise electrocardiographic stress test (stress ECG)	Initial test for most males with chest pain to establish diagnosis of CAD; females have higher rate of false positive test results Assess prognosis and functional capacity in patients with prior MI or known CAD Assess efficacy of current medical therapy in patients with known CAD	Exercise duration and functional aerobic capacity Amount of ST segment depression as indication of extent of ischemia Hemodynamic response to exercise	Normal baseline ECG Ability to exercise (patients who cannot attain adequate cardiopulmonary stress because of respiratory or musculoskeletal problems should receive a pharmacologic stress agent) Contraindications [see Table 2] False positives occur with left ventricular hypertrophy, bundle branch block, preexcitation syndromes, electrolyte abnormalities, and digoxin use	68%[1] (females, 61%[2])	77%[1] (females, 70%[2])
Thallium-201 perfusion scintigraphy	Often used when increased diagnostic accuracy for CAD required Can be combined with pharmacologic stress agents such as dobutamine, adenosine, or dipyridamole	Diagnosis of CAD with higher sensitivity and specificity than stress ECG Extent of ischemia Extent of infarction Left ventricular cavity size	Higher cost and longer testing time than stress ECG Imaging artifacts (attenuation) from diaphragm, breast, and intestine Contraindications [see Table 2 if exercise; see Table 4 if pharmacologic stress agent]	Ex thall 89%[5] Ph thall 90%[5] Dob thall 88%[4]	Ex thall 76%[5] Ph thall 70%[5] Dob thall 74%[4]
Technetium-99m perfusion scintigraphy	Often used when increased diagnostic accuracy for CAD required Can be combined with pharmacologic stress agents such as dobutamine, adenosine, or dipyridamole	Higher sensitivity and specificity for diagnosis of CAD than stress-ECG Extent of ischemia Extent of infarction Left ventricular cavity size ECG-gated SPECT allows calculation of left ventricular ejection fraction and evaluation of wall motion; evaluation of wall motion reduces false positive scans caused by imaging artifacts (attenuation) Used when excessive body weight precludes thallium imaging	Higher cost and longer testing time than stress ECG Imaging artifacts (attenuation) from diaphragm, breast, and intestine Contraindications [see Table 2 if exercise; see Table 4 if pharmacologic stress agent]	Ex tech 89%[5] Ph tech 90%[5] Dob tech 88%[4]	Ex tech 76%[5] Ph tech 70%[5] Dob tech 74%[4]
Exercise or dobutamine echocardiography	Exercise echocardiography often used when patient can exercise and has good-quality echocardiographic images Dobutamine used when exercise not possible	Higher sensitivity and specificity for diagnosis of CAD than stress ECG Left and right ventricular chamber size and function, presence of valve disease and pulmonary arterial pressures	Inadequate image quality may occur in patients with obesity, chronic obstructive pulmonary disease, and chest wall deformities Contraindications [see Table 2 if exercise; see Table 4 if pharmacologic stress agent]	Ex echo 85%[6] Dob echo 82%[6]	Ex echo 86%[6] Dob echo 82%[6]
Holter monitoring	Prinzmetal angina	Transient ST segment elevation during chest pain	Difficult to interpret because of baseline abnormalities		
Coronary angiography	Chest pain of unclear etiology despite noninvasive testing Angina not responsive to medical therapy Unstable and postinfarction angina Unclear diagnosis of CAD despite noninvasive stress testing	Anatomic severity of CAD Completely exclude cardiac origin of chest pain—gold standard of diagnostic tests Left ventricular function if left ventricular angiography also performed	Invasive procedure with low (< 2%) but inherent risk of MI, stroke, and death Represents a luminogram; does not evaluate functional significance of arterial narrowing	100%	100%

CAD—coronary artery disease Dob tech—dobutamine technetium Dob thall—dobutamine thallium ECG—electrocardiogram Ex echo—exercise echocardiography
Ex tech—exercise technetium Ex thall—exercise thallium MI—myocardial infarction Ph stress—pharmacologic stress Ph tech—pharmacologic (adenosine or dipyridamole) stress combined with technetium Ph thall—pharmacologic (adenosine or dipyridamole) stress combined with thallium SPECT—single-photon emission computed tomography

Table 4 Mechanism of Action, Side Effects, and Contraindications of Pharmacologic Stress Agents

Pharmacologic Stress Agent	Mechanism of Action	Side Effects	Contraindications
Dobutamine	Increase myocardial oxygen demand by increasing heart rate, blood pressure, and myocardial contractility	78% of patients experience side effects: chest pain, palpitations, headache, flushing, malaise, and dyspnea; ventricular and atrial arrhythmias may occur	Severe hypertension at baseline, recent history of ventricular and/or atrial arrhythmias, and current beta-blocker use
Dipyridamole	Coronary artery vasodilatation—indirect response by blocking adenosine uptake and degradation	Increase in heart rate (average, 5–10 beats a minute), decrease in systolic blood pressure (average, 10–15 mm Hg); approximately 50% of patients experience side effects: chest pain, flushing, dizziness, headaches, or nausea; may provoke bronchospasm	Severe reactive airway disease (not contraindicated with chronic obstructive pulmonary disease unless a significant component of reactive airway disease is present), current theophylline use; avoid caffeine use 1 day before testing
Adenosine	Coronary artery vasodilatation—direct response	79% of patients experience side effects (more than with dipyridamole); side effects are chest, throat or jaw pain, headache, flushing, malaise, nausea, and bradyarrhythmias	Similar to dipyridamole; avoid caffeine use 1 day before testing; may cause bradyarrhythmias and is therefore contraindicated with baseline second- or third-degree heart block

pressure and results in interstitial (and possibly intra-alveolar) pulmonary edema. Patients find relief by sitting upright, which reduces venous filling and transiently decreases the pulmonary interstitial pressure.

Dyspnea may be acute or chronic. An acute presentation suggests a pulmonary embolism, acute asthma exacerbation, pneumothorax, or rapidly developing pulmonary edema, as occurs with ischemic mitral regurgitation.

HISTORY AND PHYSICAL EXAMINATION

The history will often exclude less likely conditions and establish the etiology of dyspnea. A history of reactive airway disease, bronchodilator use, or corticosteroid use suggests asthma. Reactive airway disease tends to occur in children and young adults; therefore, in older patients given this diagnosis, a cardiac cause for dyspnea (e.g., new onset of congestive heart failure) should be considered. A significant history of tobacco use, wheezing, chronic cough, and sputum production suggests obstructive airway disease.[16] A recent history of fever, chills, and productive cough may indicate bronchitis or pneumonia. The acute onset of dyspnea associated with pleuritic chest pain after a period of immobilization suggests pulmonary embolism. Paroxysmal nocturnal dyspnea, orthopnea, nocturia, recent weight gain, and lower extremity edema suggest a cardiac cause for dyspnea. Patients with chronic obstructive pulmonary disease may also awaken at night with dyspnea, but they usually have a history of sputum production and expectoration that improves with the patient in the upright position. Occasionally, on the basis of the history alone, it may not be possible to determine whether a cardiac or pulmonary cause of dyspnea is present.[17] In up to one third of patients being evaluated, dyspnea may have more than one cause.[18] In elderly patients, dyspnea may be the only symptom of a myocardial infarction. Hemoptysis may indicate the presence of severe underlying pulmonary disease (e.g., pulmonary embolism or lung cancer) but must be differentiated from hematemesis and nasopharyngeal bleeding.

Several findings on physical examination can assist in excluding a cardiac cause for dyspnea. These findings include a normal level of the jugular venous pulsations, a normal point of maximal cardiac impulse, the lack of a third heart sound or cardiac murmurs, the absence of rales on lung examination, and the absence of peripheral edema. Alternatively, elevated jugular venous pulsations, a displaced point of maximal cardiac impulse, a

third heart sound, a holosystolic murmur of mitral regurgitation, basilar rales, and peripheral edema suggest congestive heart failure. A positive abdominojugular reflux maneuver may also identify dyspnea of cardiac origin.[19]

Obese patients and those with chest wall deformities may experience dyspnea secondary to the increased workload of breathing from the mechanical limitation imposed on the chest wall.

Table 5 Causes of Dyspnea

Cardiac
  Valve disease
    Aortic stenosis
    Aortic regurgitaion
    Mitral stenosis
    Mitral regurgitation
  Myocardial disease
    Dilated cardiomyopathy
    Restrictive cardiomyopathy
    Hypertrophic cardiomyopathy
  Pericardial disease
    Constrictive pericarditis
    Pericardial tamponade
    Pericardial effusion
  Coronary disease
    Myocardial infarction and ischemia
  Arrhythmia
    Ventricular and supraventricular arrhythmias
  Congenital heart disease
Pulmonary
  Reactive airway disease
  Chronic obstructive lung disease (chronic bronchitis and emphysema)
  Interstitial lung disease
  Infection (acute bronchitis and pneumonia)
  Pulmonary embolism
  Chest wall disease
  Pleural effusion
Deconditioning
Obesity
Malingering
Psychogenic
  Anxiety and panic disorders
Anemia

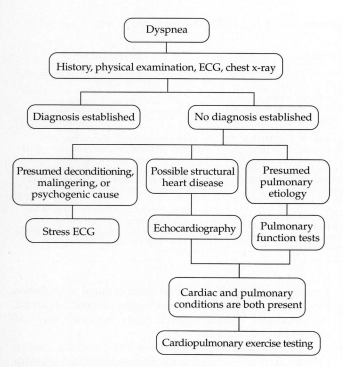

Figure 2 **Evaluation of patients with dyspnea.**
(ECG—electrocardiogram)

Patients with emphysema frequently have an increased antero-posterior chest diameter, prolonged expiratory phase, expiratory wheezes, and diminished breath sounds. Central cyanosis, a normal anteroposterior chest diameter, and expiratory wheezes or rhonchi on lung examination suggest chronic bronchitis. Expiratory wheezing can occur in both cardiac and pulmonary conditions and is therefore not helpful in establishing an etiology. Stridor may result from an upper airway obstruction or vocal cord paralysis and at times may resemble wheezing. Tachypnea, a loud pulmonic component of the second heart sound, and calf tenderness indicate a pulmonary embolism.

DIAGNOSTIC TESTS

An ECG and a chest roentgenogram should be the initial tests in the evaluation of dyspnea. Pertinent ECG findings include Q waves (prior myocardial infarction), a bundle branch block (structural heart disease), left ventricular hypertrophy (aortic stenosis, hypertension), and evidence of atrial chamber enlargement (valvular heart disease). Notable chest roentgenogram findings include an enlarged cardiac silhouette; interstitial or alveolar edema (congestive heart failure); aortic valve calcification (valvular heart disease); lung mass (lung cancer); focal infiltrate (pneumonia); pleural effusion (congestive heart failure, infectious process); and hyperinflation, bullae, and flattened hemidiaphragms (emphysema). Screening laboratory tests may be useful to exclude anemia as a potential cause of dyspnea.

If the diagnosis of dyspnea remains unclear, additional testing can be pursued [*see Figure 2*]. For those patients with cardiovascular risk factors, with findings on physical examination that suggest structural heart disease, or with abnormal ECGs, echocardiography is indicated to exclude valvular heart disease and assess systolic and diastolic ventricular function. Patients with a presumed pulmonary etiology for dyspnea that remains undiagnosed should undergo pulmonary function testing to ex-

clude reactive airway and restrictive and chronic obstructive pulmonary disease. Stress-ECG may be useful to objectively evaluate the degree of limitation and may be particularly helpful for patients with presumed deconditioning, malingering, or a psychogenic cause for dyspnea. For patients who may have a component of dyspnea from both a cardiac and a pulmonary source, cardiopulmonary exercise testing can be considered.

Palpitations

BACKGROUND

Palpitations are a nonspecific symptom associated with severity ranging from an increased awareness of the normal heartbeat to life-threatening ventricular arrhythmias [*see Table 6*]. Although palpitations represent one of the most common complaints requiring evaluation in the outpatient setting,[20] consensus guidelines describing the appropriate evaluation have not yet been established.

Psychiatric illnesses (anxiety, panic, and somatization disorders) account for a significant proportion of patients who seek medical attention for palpitations.[21] Although an underlying psychiatric illness should be considered in appropriate patients, it does not obviate the need for a complete evaluation to exclude a cardiac origin.[22]

For patients with an underlying cardiac disease associated with palpitations, long-term outcome is poor. In contrast, clinical outcome is excellent for those with a noncardiac origin for palpitations, despite a high rate of recurrent episodes.[21] The key, then, in the evaluation of palpitations is to establish or exclude the presence of underlying structural heart disease. This determination can often be made by use of information from the history, physical examination, and ECG, but it may require additional evaluation with ambulatory ECG monitoring and possibly electrophysiologic testing. Psychiatric illnesses can initially be screened by use of simple and rapid patient-administered questionnaires. A diagnostic algorithm is presented that utilizes a rational approach to diagnostic testing [*see Figure 3*].

HISTORY AND PHYSICAL EXAMINATION

Palpitations are often described as a fluttering, a pounding, or an uncomfortable sensation in the chest. Occasionally, patients may complain only of a sensation of awareness of the heart

Table 6 **Causes of Palpitations**

General Category	Prognosis
Hyperdynamic state	Anemia, thyrotoxicosis, and exercise—all leading to sinus tachycardia
Increase in cardiac stroke volume	Aortic regurgitation, patent ductus arteriosus
Arrhythmia Ventricular	Frequent ventricular premature beats, ventricular tachycardia
Supraventricular	Frequent atrial premature beats, atrial fibrillation, atrial flutter, multifocal atrial tachycardia, atrial tachycardia, atrioventricular nodal reentry tachycardia, atrioventricular reentry tachycardia
Psychiatric	Anxiety, panic, or somatization disorder

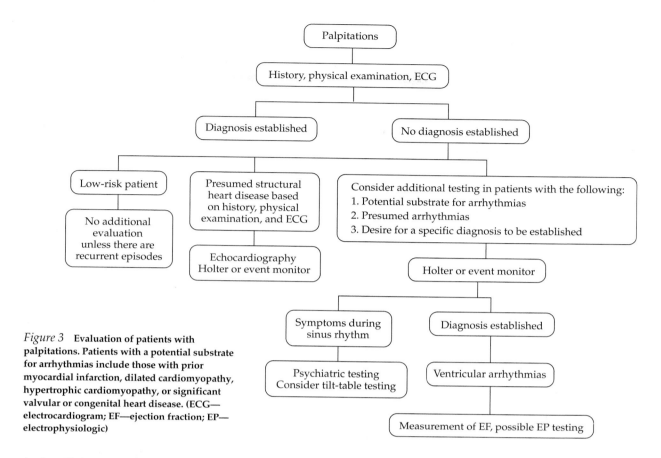

Figure 3 **Evaluation of patients with palpitations. Patients with a potential substrate for arrhythmias include those with prior myocardial infarction, dilated cardiomyopathy, hypertrophic cardiomyopathy, or significant valvular or congenital heart disease. (ECG—electrocardiogram; EF—ejection fraction; EP—electrophysiologic)**

rhythm. Patients may be able to discern whether the episodes are rapid and regular or rapid and irregular. Tapping a finger on the patient's chest in either a regular or an irregular manner may occasionally lead to an accurate description of the events.

A history of palpitations since childhood suggests a supraventricular arrhythmia and possibly an atrioventricular bypass tract, such as in the Wolff-Parkinson-White syndrome. Patients with congenital long QT syndrome typically manifest symptoms beginning in adolescence. A family history of sudden cardiac death, congestive heart failure, or syncope may suggest an inherited dilated or hypertrophic cardiomyopathy.

Knowing the circumstances in which palpitations occur may be useful in determining their origin. Palpitations associated only with strenuous physical activity are normal, whereas episodes occurring at rest or with minimal activity suggest underlying pathology. Episodes associated with a lack of food intake suggest hypoglycemia, and episodes after excessive alcohol intake suggest the toxic effects of alcohol. The resolution of symptoms with vagal maneuvers (breath-holding or the Valsalva maneuver) suggests paroxysmal supraventricular tachycardia. The onset of an episode of palpitations on assuming an upright position after bending over suggests atrioventricular nodal tachycardia.[23] Emotional stress and strenuous exercise may precipitate episodes in patients with long QT syndrome. Palpitations associated with anxiety or a sense of doom or panic suggest, but do not confirm, an underlying psychiatric disorder.

Symptoms associated with an episode of palpitations should also be explored. Syncope or presyncope after an episode suggests ventricular arrhythmias. However, patients with structural heart disease (e.g., severe left ventricular systolic dysfunction) may also experience these symptoms after supraventricular ar-

rhythmias because of dependence on atrial filling. Additional mechanisms of syncope in patients with supraventricular arrhythmias have also been reported.[24] Regardless of the mechanism, syncope and presyncope are worrisome symptoms and merit a complete cardiovascular evaluation. Occasionally, patients may experience an episode of polyuria that follows the palpitations. This condition may suggest supraventricular arrhythmias as the cause of palpitations, although studies have found this to be uncommon.[25]

The physical examination should focus on establishing whether underlying structural heart disease is present. A displaced point of maximal cardiac impulse, third heart sound, and holosystolic murmur of mitral regurgitation suggest an underlying dilated cardiomyopathy. A midsystolic click, often followed by a systolic murmur, indicates mitral valve prolapse, which is associated with both ventricular and supraventricular arrhythmias. A midsystolic murmur along the left sternal border that varies in intensity with alterations in left ventricular filling (e.g., Valsalva maneuver or changes in body position) indicates hypertrophic cardiomyopathy. Although atrial fibrillation is common in hypertrophic cardiomyopathy, ventricular arrhythmias may also occur.

DIAGNOSTIC TESTS

The ECG is the first step in the diagnostic evaluation of a patient with palpitations [*see Figure 3*]. A short PR interval and delta wave (Wolff-Parkinson-White syndrome), prolonged QT interval (long QT syndrome), and left bundle branch block (structural heart disease) are notable findings. Certain medications [*see Table 7*] may result in prolongation of the QT interval (i.e., acquired prolonged QT) and increase the risk of arrhyth-

Table 7 Medications Associated with Prolongation of the QT Interval

Antibiotics
  Tetracycline
  Erythromycin
  Trimethoprim and
    sulfamethoxazole
  Pentamidine
Antihistamines
  Terfenadine
  Astemizole
  Diphenhydramine
Antiarrhythmic agents
  Quinidine
  Procainamide
  Disopyramide
  Sotalol
  Amiodarone
  Dofetilide

Other cardiac drugs
  Bepridil
  Gastrointestinal
    Cisapride
  Antifungal drugs
    Ketoconazole
    Fluconazole
    Itraconazole
  Psychotropic drugs
    Tricyclic antidepressants
    Phenothiazines
    Haloperidol
    Resperidone
  Diuretics
    Indapamide

mias. Extreme voltage amplitudes and Q waves in leads I, aVL, and V4 through V6 are seen with hypertrophic cardiomyopathy. Pathologic Q waves indicate prior myocardial infarction and therefore a substrate for ventricular arrhythmias. Left ventricular hypertrophy or atrial abnormalities are nonspecific findings but suggest underlying structural heart disease. A summary of pertinent findings from the history, physical examination, and ECG for various causes of palpitations is provided [see Table 8].

If the cause of palpitations is not apparent after the initial evaluation (history, physical examination, and ECG), additional diagnostic testing is indicated for certain patients [see Figure 3].[23] These patients include those with presumed arrhythmias that re-

main undiagnosed and those with prior myocardial infarction, dilated cardiomyopathy, hypertrophic cardiomyopathy, or significant valvular or congenital heart disease. In addition, patients who desire a specific diagnosis to be established should be considered for additional testing.

Ambulatory ECG devices include Holter monitoring and continuous-loop event recorders. Holter monitors continuously record the heart rhythm for 24 or 48 hours. Patients are asked to maintain a diary documenting the time and describing their symptoms during the monitoring period. The key is to correlate patient symptoms with documented rhythm abnormalities. Patients with significant complaints of palpitations that correlate with periods of normal sinus rhythm should be further evaluated for underlying psychiatric disorders. Event monitors also continuously record the heart rhythm but require the patient to trigger the device to save the information. These devices can be kept by patients for several weeks and are especially useful for those with infrequent symptoms. Event monitors are more cost-effective than Holter monitors for evaluating palpitations.[26,27] For patients with underlying structural heart disease and documented ventricular arrhythmias on ambulatory ECG monitoring, additional evaluation is warranted, including determination of left ventricular function and, occasionally, electrophysiologic testing.

Syncope

BACKGROUND

Syncope refers to a transient loss of consciousness accompanied by loss of postural tone. Roughly one third of individuals have an episode of syncope during their lifetime. It is a particularly common problem encountered in emergency departments and accounts for approximately 6% of all hospital admissions.[28] Determining which patients require hospital admission is diffi-

Table 8 Diagnosis of the Underlying Etiology of Palpitations

Condition	History	Physical Examination	ECG	Underlying Etiology of Palpitations
Congenital long QT syndrome	Symptom onset in adolescence; episodes may be triggered by emotional stress and strenuous exercise	Normal	Prolonged QT interval	Ventricular arrhythmias
Atrioventricular bypass tract (e.g., Wolf-Parkinson-White syndrome)	Childhood episodes of palpitations	Normal	Short PR interval, delta wave	Supraventricular arrhythmias
Inherited dilated cardiomyopathy	Family history of cardiomyopathy, syncope, or sudden cardiac death	Abnormal cardiac impulse, systolic murmur (MR), third heart sound	Atrial enlargement, IVCD, LBBB, ventricular ectopic beats, or Q waves	Supraventricular or ventricular arrhythmias
Hypertrophic cardiomyopathy	Family history of cardiomyopathy, syncope, or sudden cardiac death	Systolic murmur	Increased voltage amplitude (LVH), Q waves in V4-V6, I, aVL	Supraventricular or ventricular arrhythmias
Anxiety, panic, or somatization disorder	Sense of doom, panic, or anxiety associated with episodes; coexisting psychiatric illness	Normal	Normal	Psychiatric
Mitral valve prolapse	Associated fatigue, dyspnea	Midsystolic click, systolic murmur (MR)	Normal or left atrial enlargement	Supraventricular arrhythmias

IVCD–interventricular conduction defect   LBBB–left bundle branch block   LVH–left ventricular hypertrophy   MR–mitral regurgitation

Table 9   Classification of Syncope Based on Etiology

Cardiac
    Blood flow obstruction
        Aortic stenosis
        Pulmonic stenosis
        Left atrial myxoma
        Hypertrophic cardiomyopathy
        Massive pulmonary embolism
    Reduction in forward cardiac output
        Pericardial tamponade
        Severe pump failure
    Arrhythmia
        Tachyarrhythmias
          Ventricular tachycardia
          Supraventricular tachycardia
        Bradyarrhythmias
          Sinus bradycardia
          Sick sinus syndrome
          Atrioventricular block
          Carotid sinus hypersensitivity (can also be considered neurologic cause)
Neurologic
    Vasovagal
    Situational (micturition)
    Seizures
    Cerebrovascular accident
    Cerebrovascular insufficiency
    Orthostatic hypotension—autonomic dysfunction
Other
    Volume depletion
    Drugs
    Hypoglycemia
    Anxiety attack
    Psychogenic

cult, given the large number of potential causes of syncope. Whereas many conditions that result in syncope are life-threatening, other common etiologies, such as medication side effects, orthostatic hypotension, and psychiatric disorders, are benign.

Syncope is classified on the basis of the underlying etiology [see Table 9]. In elderly patients, the etiology may be multifactorial and related to medication side effects (particularly antihypertensives and antidepressants),[29] orthostatic hypotension, and bradyarrhythmias. Various medications are associated with prolongation of the QT interval and the development of ventricular arrhythmias and resulting syncope [see Table 7]. Vasovagal syncope is particularly common in otherwise healthy patients and has a benign prognosis. Episodes often occur in response to fear or injury and are characterized by a sudden decline in blood pressure with or without associated bradycardia.

Establishing the presence of structural heart disease in the evaluation of syncope is essential because these patients may have a 1-year mortality as high as 30%.[30] Structural heart disease is usually apparent on the basis of history, physical examination, and information from the baseline ECG. Occasionally, additional diagnostic testing with echocardiography, tilt-table testing, or electrophysiologic testing may be required.

HISTORY AND PHYSICAL EXAMINATION

The first step in establishing the presence of structural heart disease is to obtain an accurate description of the syncope episode. Key elements of the history include the presence of postural or exertional symptoms; associated chest pain, shortness of breath, or palpitations; and the situation in which the episode occurred (e.g., during micturition). Neurologic symptoms such as focal motor weakness, arm or leg movement, tongue biting, or a postictal state suggest a neurologic rather than cardiac event. However, seizures can occur from cardiac causes if a patient is kept upright during an episode (usually the result of a well-meaning bystander) because of cerebral hypoperfusion. A witness to the episode of syncope may provide a clear description of the event and should be questioned if possible. Medications associated with QT prolongation [see Table 7], blood pressure lowering (antihypertensives), and volume depletion (diuretics) should be reviewed. A family history of sudden cardiac death, syncope, or heart failure suggests hypertrophic cardiomyopathy, an inherited dilated cardiomyopathy, or long QT syndrome. A history of myocardial infarction or congestive heart failure raises the possibility of ventricular arrhythmias.

The physical examination focuses on determining whether structural heart disease is present and excluding common causes of syncope. Orthostatic vital signs should be obtained in all patients. Focal neurologic findings such as a motor deficit or a visual-field defect may indicate a neurologic cause for syncope. Pertinent findings on cardiovascular examination include a delayed carotid upstroke (aortic stenosis), an abnormal point of maximal cardiac impulse (cardiomyopathy), an irregular or bradycardiac rhythm (arrhythmias), a third heart sound (cardiomyopathy), a midsystolic murmur (aortic stenosis, hypertrophic cardiomyopathy), and a holosystolic murmur (mitral regurgitation secondary to left ventricular dilatation). Less common findings include an early diastolic sound (so-called tumor plop, indicating a left atrial myxoma), asymmetrical peripheral pulses (aortic dissection), and a loud second heart sound (pulmonary hypertension secondary to pulmonary embolism). Information from the history and physical examination yields a cause for syncope in approximately 45% of patients.[31]

DIAGNOSTIC TESTS

An ECG is the initial diagnostic test for all patients with syncope. Although the yield of the baseline ECG is low (approximately 5%), a number of potential findings are useful.[31] These findings include bundle branch block, Q waves indicating prior myocardial infarction, left ventricular hypertrophy, prolonged QT interval, or evidence of atrioventricular block. The presence of sinus bradycardia, first-degree atrioventricular block, and bundle branch block suggests bradyarrhythmias as the cause of syncope. Extreme voltage amplitudes and Q waves in leads I, aVL, and V4 through V6 suggest hypertrophic cardiomyopathy and therefore the possibility of ventricular arrhythmias. An uncommon but unique ECG abnormality is the combination of a right bundle branch block, T wave inversions in leads V1 through V3, and an epsilon wave (a positive wave on the terminal portion of the QRS complex)—findings that indicate right ventricular dysplasia, which is associated with ventricular arrhythmias. Ventricular arrhythmias are also seen in the Brugada syndrome, which can be identified on the ECG by an incomplete right bundle branch block and ST segment elevation in leads V1 through V3. A short PR interval and slurring of the initial portion of the QRS complex (the delta wave) suggests preexcitation (i.e., Wolff-Parkinson-White syndrome), with the possibility of rapid antegrade conduction via the accessory pathway.

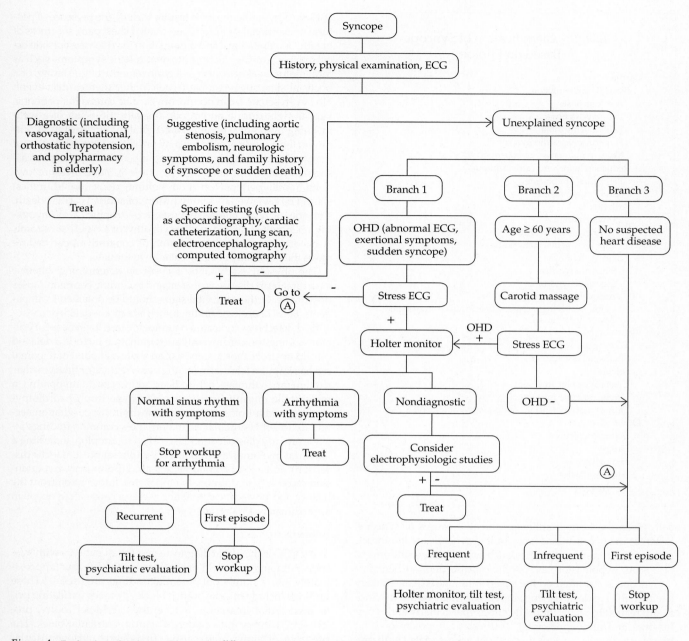

Figure 4 Evaluation of patients with syncope.[31,32] (ECG—electrocardiogram; OHD—organic heart disease)

If the etiology of syncope remains unclear after reviewing the history, physical examination, and ECG, additional diagnostic testing should be pursued. For patients with findings suggestive of an underlying cardiac cause, echocardiography and coronary angiography can be obtained; for those with a possible neurologic cause, brain imaging (computed tomography or magnetic resonance imaging), neurovascular studies (carotid and transcranial Doppler ultrasound studies), and electroencephalography can be performed; and for those with a presumed pulmonary cause, lung scanning can be considered [*see Figure 4*]. If the diagnosis remains uncertain despite these tests, one of three pathways can be followed.[32]

The first pathway is for patients with structural heart disease or an abnormal ECG, who therefore have an increased likelihood for underlying arrhythmias or valve disease as a cause for

syncope. Echocardiography, noninvasive stress testing, and Holter monitoring should be considered for these patients. If Holter monitoring documents normal sinus rhythm in the setting of reported syncope, psychiatric evaluation and possibly tilt-table testing are warranted.

The second pathway is for patients older than 60 years, who are more likely to have valve disease (aortic stenosis), ischemic heart disease, carotid sinus syncope, cerebrovascular disease (transient ischemic attacks), and situational events (micturition, defecation, postural) as a basis for syncope. Carotid sinus massage (in the absence of carotid bruits, recent myocardial infarction, or stroke) should be the initial diagnostic test for these patients.[33,34] A positive test is defined as asystolic arrest lasting 3 seconds or longer and may identify those with cardioinhibitory hypersensitivity of the carotid sinus who will benefit from pace-

Table 10 Differential Diagnosis of a Cardiac Murmur Based on Timing of Cardiac Cycle

Systolic
    Midsystolic
        Innocent flow murmur
        Aortic stenosis
        Pulmonic stenosis
        Atrial septal defect
    Holosystolic
        Ventricular septal defect
        Tricuspid regurgitation
        Hypertrophic cardiomyopathy
        Mitral regurgitation
Diastolic
    Early diastolic
        Aortic regurgitation
        Pulmonic regurgitation
    Middiastolic
        Mitral stenosis
        Tricuspid stenosis
        Austin Flint murmur associated with chronic aortic regurgitation
        Severe mitral regurgitation (augmented antegrade mitral valve flow)
Continuous
    Patent ductus arteriosus

maker placement. For those with a negative test result, echocardiography, noninvasive stress testing, and Holter monitoring can be performed.

The third pathway is for patients with unexplained syncope and no suspected structural heart disease. For those who have had a single episode, additional evaluation can be deferred until a second episode occurs. For patients with frequent episodes, ambulatory ECG monitoring or tilt-table testing should be considered. Finally, for those with infrequent episodes, tilt-table testing and psychiatric evaluation can be performed.

Tilt-table testing was initially developed in the 1980s to evaluate patients with presumed vasovagal syncope. The passive portion of the test involves quickly raising a patient from the supine position to an angle of 60° (the tilt angle) for approximately 45 minutes, which causes pooling of venous blood in the lower extremities, a decrease in venous return, compensatory tachycardia, and enhanced ventricular contraction. For individuals with vasovagal syncope, augmented ventricular contraction causes activation of vasodepressor reflexes that result in hypotension, bradycardia, or both. Approximately 49% of patients referred for evaluation of vasovagal syncope have positive responses, compared with 9% of control patients.[35] The active portion of tilt-table testing uses an isoproterenol infusion to enhance the vasodepressor reflex.

Cardiac Murmurs

BACKGROUND

The increased access to health care and the widespread use and availability of echocardiography have resulted in a large number of patients being diagnosed and evaluated for various cardiac murmurs. A cardiac murmur may indicate underlying valvular, congenital, or myocardial disease, but it may also be caused by systemic illnesses and occur in the setting of a structurally normal heart.

Cardiac murmurs result from disturbed or turbulent blood flow, often through diseased cardiac valves or intracardiac structures. The presence of a cardiac murmur, however, does not always indicate underlying cardiac pathology. Hyperthyroidism, anemia, and a febrile illness may all result in increased blood flow though the aortic valve and produce a soft, crescendo-decrescendo, systolic murmur over the aortic area. In this setting, the aortic valve is structurally normal, and the murmur is the result of augmented blood flow (i.e., a flow murmur) caused by the systemic illness. Another common cause of a systolic murmur is calcification of the aortic valve, which is referred to as aortic sclerosis when there is no obstruction to left ventricular outflow. Aortic sclerosis is a common finding in elderly patients; 25% of those older than 65 years are affected.[36] This condition is often diagnosed when a systolic murmur is detected in an otherwise asymptomatic patient during a routine physical examination. In addition to diseases of the cardiac valves, murmurs may also result from intracardiac communications (atrial and ventricular septal defects), congenital abnormalities (patent ductus arteriosus), and disease of the myocardium (hypertrophic cardiomyopathy).

A thorough history and physical examination can often provide the etiology of a murmur. Additional diagnostic tests, such as the ECG, chest roentgenogram, and echocardiogram, are used to confirm the diagnosis and establish the severity of the abnormality.

HISTORY AND PHYSICAL EXAMINATION

A history of a childhood murmur may indicate a congenital abnormality of a cardiac valve, such as a bicuspid or unicuspid aortic valve. A febrile illness occurring in childhood should raise the suspicion of rheumatic fever, possibly resulting in rheumatic mitral stenosis. Although rheumatic fever is uncommon in the United States, it may still be seen in immigrants from Asia, Latin America, and the Caribbean.

Establishing the presence or absence of cardiovascular symptoms is essential in the evaluation of a cardiac murmur. Otherwise healthy young adults without cardiac symptoms, with a systolic flow murmur and no other cardiac findings on examination, often require no additional evaluation.[37] In contrast, the finding of a cardiac murmur in patients with cardiovascular symptoms must be further explored and a diagnosis established.

Aortic stenosis may result in the triad of angina, syncope, and impaired exercise tolerance or dyspnea on exertion. Patients

Table 11   Physical Findings Useful for Evaluating a Cardiac Murmur

Condition	Timing	Location	Radiation	Characteristics	Effects of Maneuvers	Associated Findings
Innocent flow murmur	Midsystolic	Base	Variable or none	Soft, ejection	No change	None
Aortic stenosis	Systolic	Base (right second ICS)	Carotid arteries	Crescendo-decrescendo	Decrease with hand-grip or standing	Single S_2, delayed and decreased carotid upstroke, ES if mobile valve leaflets
Mitral regurgitation	Systolic	Apex	Axilla (sometimes back)	Holosystolic	Increase with hand-grip	Hyperdynamic apical impulse
Ventricular septal defect	Systolic	Left sternal border	None	Holosystolic	No change	Palpable thrill
Atrial septal defect	Systolic	Left second ICS	None	Crescendo-decrescendo	Possible increase with inspiration	Fixed split S_2
Hypertrophic cardiomyopathy	Systolic	Base	Carotid arteries	Late-peaking crescendo	Increase with standing and strain phase of Valsalva maneuver	Brisk carotid upstroke
Tricuspid regurgitation	Systolic	Left lower sternal border	Right lower sternal border	Holosystolic	Increase with inspiration	Prominent v waves in JVP, pulsatile liver
Pulmonic stenosis	Systolic	Left second ICS	None	Crescendo-decrescendo	No change	ES if mobile valve leaflets
Aortic regurgitation	Diastolic	Left sternal border	None	Decrescendo, high-pitched	Increase with handgrip	Wide pulse pressure, displaced and enlarged apical impulse
Mitral stenosis	Diastolic	Apex	None	Low-pitched rumble, presystolic accentuation	Best heard in left lateral decubitus position	Loud S_1, opening snap
Pulmonic regurgitation	Diastolic	Left second ICS	Left sternal border	Decrescendo	May increase with inspiration	—
Tricuspid stenosis	Diastolic	Right lower sternal border	Right upper abdomen	Low-pitched rumble	Increase with inspiration	Right ventricular heave
Patent ductus arteriosus	Continuous	Left second ICS	Back	Machinery-like	None	Wide pulse pressure, bounding pulses

ES—ejection sound   ICS—intercostal space   JVP—jugular venous pulse S_1, S_2—first, second heart sounds

with hypertrophic cardiomyopathy experience similar symptoms but may also complain of palpitations from associated atrial or ventricular arrhythmias. Hypertrophic cardiomyopathy is most commonly familial, with an autosomal dominant inheritance pattern. A family history of sudden cardiac death, heart failure, and syncope should therefore be explored. Symptoms of mitral stenosis include shortness of breath, impaired exercise tolerance, palpitations (from associated atrial fibrillation), and hemoptysis. These symptoms may occur during episodes of tachycardia, volume overload, or both as mitral valve flow is increased and the stenotic mitral valve impairs filling of the left ventricle. This condition is the reason that previously asymptomatic females develop symptoms during pregnancy. Mitral and aortic regurgitation cause a volume overload to the left atrium and left ventricle, respectively, and may result in shortness of breath, orthopnea, paroxysmal nocturnal dyspnea, lower extremity edema, and impaired exercise capacity. A ventricular septal defect is either congenital or traumatic (e.g., occurring after a myocardial infarction). The congenital form often becomes apparent during adolescence; the traumatic form presents sever-

al days after a myocardial infarction as a new holosystolic murmur associated with significant respiratory distress.

The physical examination begins with determining the timing of the murmur in the cardiac cycle—systolic, diastolic, or continuous [see Table 10]. The grade, quality, location, area of radiation, and change in intensity with maneuvers should then be described. Murmurs are graded on a scale of 1 to 6. Grade 1 is a soft intermittent murmur, grade 4 is a palpable murmur, and grade 6 is a murmur that can be appreciated without a stethoscope. Thus, most murmurs are classified as grade 2 or 3. Midsystolic murmurs are derived from the aortic or pulmonic valves or occur in association with hypertrophic cardiomyopathy. In contrast, holosystolic murmurs are the result of regurgitant blood flow through either the mitral or the tricuspid valves or originate from a ventricular septal defect. The murmur of a ventricular septal defect is usually well localized to the fourth left intercostal space, does not radiate significantly, and is often associated with a thrill (i.e., grade 4 or higher). Late systolic murmurs occur from mitral regurgitation that is secondary to (1) ischemia or infarction to the papillary muscles (ischemic mitral regurgitation), (2) left ventric-

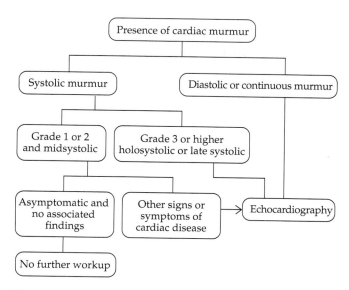

Figure 5 **Approach to patients with cardiac murmurs.**[37]

ular dilatation with functional mitral regurgitation, or (3) mitral valve prolapse. Additional findings on cardiac auscultation, such as a fixed, split second heart sound or an ejection sound, may be helpful in determining the etiology of a systolic murmur [*see Table 11*].

Diastolic murmurs always indicate underlying cardiac pathology and commonly occur in either early diastole or middiastole. Early diastolic murmurs begin at the onset of diastole (i.e., with the second heart sound) and originate from regurgitant flow across the pulmonic and aortic valves. Aortic regurgitation occurs because of failure of the aortic valve leaflets to adequately coadapt during diastole and may be the result of disease processes affecting the aortic valve (e.g., endocarditis) or the aortic root (e.g., aortic dissection). Pulmonary regurgitation is most commonly seen in patients with pulmonary hypertension and is therefore associated with a loud second heart sound. Middiastolic murmurs occur from either mitral or tricuspid stenosis; the Austin Flint murmur associated with chronic aortic regurgitation or occurring in the setting of severe mitral regurgitation results in augmented antegrade flow across the mitral valve in diastole.

In adults, continuous murmurs are usually from a previously undiagnosed patent ductus arteriosus. Occasionally, a patient with chronic aortic regurgitation may have a prominent systolic murmur in addition to the early diastolic murmur, thus simulating a continuous murmur. The systolic murmur in this case is the result of enhanced stroke volume from increased diastolic filling of the left ventricle. Whereas both conditions are associated with a widened pulse pressure and murmurs that occur during both systole and diastole, the murmur of a patent ductus arteriosus is continuous and peaks on the second heart sound; with chronic aortic regurgitation, there is a so-called silent period at the end of systole as the systolic murmur fades, before the beginning of the diastolic murmur.

Additional findings on physical examination can assist in determining the severity of the valve lesion and in excluding other conditions that result in similar murmurs. For patients with a midsystolic murmur presumed to be aortic stenosis, the carotid upstroke and splitting of the second heart sound should be carefully evaluated. A delayed carotid upstroke and single splitting of the second heart sound indicate hemodynamically severe aortic stenosis. In contrast, hypertrophic cardiomyopathy results in

a brisk carotid upstroke (the so-called spike-and-dome configuration) and normal splitting of the second heart sound. Severe mitral regurgitation can be identified by a holosystolic murmur associated with a third heart sound and a middiastolic murmur that results from the increased blood flow crossing antegrade across the mitral valve in diastole.

Several bedside maneuvers may also be useful in the evaluation of cardiac murmurs.[38] Right-sided murmurs (e.g., tricuspid regurgitation) increase in intensity during inspiration because of augmented right heart filling. The murmur of hypertrophic cardiomyopathy is extremely dependent on left ventricular filling, such that both the strain phase of the Valsalva maneuver and moving from squatting to the standing position augment the intensity of the murmur.

DIAGNOSTIC EVALUATION

An ECG should be obtained to evaluate for the presence of cardiac chamber enlargement and hypertrophy. Aortic stenosis imposes a pressure overload to the left ventricle, resulting in left ventricular hypertrophy by ECG in approximately 50% of patients. Hypertrophic cardiomyopathy is characterized by increased ventricular muscle mass, which is usually apparent on the ECG with extreme voltage amplitudes and small Q waves in leads I, aVl, and V4 through V6, referred to as septal Q waves. Mitral stenosis results in left atrial enlargement and occasionally right axis deviation and right ventricular hypertrophy.

A chest roentgenogram should be reviewed for chamber enlargement and the presence of calcification. Chronic aortic and mitral insufficiency cause a volume overload to the left ventricle and left atrium, respectively. Left atrial enlargement, without enlargement of the left ventricle, and mitral valve calcification suggest mitral stenosis. Calcification of the aortic valve frequently occurs with valvular aortic stenosis but is rarely apparent on the chest roentgenogram.

In the absence of cardiovascular symptoms and other physical findings, a grade 1 or grade 2 midsystolic murmur does not require additional evaluation [*see Figure 5*].[37] Midsystolic murmurs of grade 3 and higher, holosystolic murmurs, or late systolic murmurs should be further evaluated by echocardiography. All patients with a diastolic or continuous murmur should be referred for echocardiography because these murmurs always indicate underlying cardiac pathology. In addition to confirming the etiology of a cardiac murmur, echocardiography provides evaluation of left ventricular systolic and diastolic function, wall motion abnormalities (that may indicate associated CAD), and estimation of pulmonary arterial pressures. For patients with valvular, congenital, or myocardial diseases, echocardiography provides a baseline from which additional studies can be obtained and used to follow disease progression over time.

Cardiovascular Information on the Internet

There are numerous sources of cardiovascular information on the World Wide Web. The most useful general information sites are listed [*see Sidebar* Pertinent Web Sites].

References

1. Lee TH, Goldman L: Evaluation of the patient with acute chest pain. N Engl J Med 341:1187, 2000
2. Ammann P, Sabine M, Kraus M, et al: Characteristics and prognosis of myocardial infarction in patients with normal coronary arteries. Chest 117:333, 2000

3. Goyal RK: Changing focus on unexplained esophageal chest pain. Ann Intern Med 124:1008, 1996

4. Hertzer NR, Beven EG, Young JR, et al: Coronary artery disease in peripheral vascular patients: a classification of 1,000 coronary angiograms and results of surgical management. Ann Surg 199:223, 1984

5. Diamond GA, Forrester JS: Analysis of probability as an aid in the clinical diagnosis of coronary artery disease. N Engl J Med 300:1350, 1979

6. Pryor DB, Harrell FE, Lee KL, et al: Estimating the likelihood of significant coronary artery disease. Am J Med 75:771, 1983

7. Gibbons RJ, Balady GJ, Beasley JW, et al: ACC/AHA guidelines for exercise testing: a report of the American College of Cardiology/American Heart Association Task Force on Practice Guidelines (Committee on Exercise Testing). J Am Coll Cardiol 30:260, 1997

8. Chou TM, Amidon TM: Evaluating coronary artery disease noninvasively: which test for whom? West J Med 161:173, 1994

9. Gianrossi R, Detrano R, Mulvihil D, et al: Exercise-induced ST depression in the diagnosis of coronary artery disease: a meta-analysis. Circulation 80:87, 1989

10. Kwok Y, Kim C, Grady D, et al: Meta-analysis of exercise testing to detect coronary artery disease in women. Am J Cardiol 83:660 1999

11. Garber AM, Solomon NA: Cost effectiveness of alternative test strategies for the diagnosis of coronary artery disease. Ann Intern Med 130:719, 1999

12. Geleijnse ML, Elhendy A, Fioretti PM, et al: Dobutamine stress myocardial perfusion imaging. J Am Coll Cardiol 36:2017, 2000

13. Gibbons RJ, Chatterjee K, Daley J, et al: ACC/AHA/ACP-ASIM guidelines for the management of patients with chronic stable angina: a report of the American College of Cardiology/American Heart Association Task Force on Practice Guidelines (Committee on the Management of Patients with Chronic Stable Angina). J Am Coll Cardiol 33:2092, 1999

14. Cheitlin MD, Alpert JS, Armstrong WF, et al: ACC/AHA Guidelines for the clinical application of echocardiography. A report of the American College of Cardiology/American Heart Association Task Force on Practice Guidelines (Committee on Clinical Application of Echocardiography). Developed in collaboration with the American Society of Echocardiography. Circulation 95:1686, 1997

15. Nissen SE, Grines CL, Gurley JC, et al: Application of a new phased-array ultrasound catheter in the assessment of vascular dimensions: in-vivo comparison to cineangiography. Circulation 82:660, 1990

16. Holleman DR Jr, Simel DL, Goldberg JS: Diagnosis of obstructive airways disease from the clinical examination. J Gen Intern Med 8:63, 1993

17. Manning HL, Schwartzstein RM: Mechanism of disease: pathophysiology of dyspnea. N Engl J Med 333:1547, 1995

18. Schmitt BP, Kushner MS, Wiener SL: The diagnostic usefulness of the history of the patient with dyspnea. J Gen Intern Med 1:386, 1986

19. Mulrow CD, Lucey CR, Farnett LE: Discriminating causes of dyspnea through clinical examination. J Gen Intern Med 8:383, 1993

20. Kroenke K, Arrington ME, Mangelsdorff AD: The prevalence of symptoms in medical outpatients and the adequacy of therapy. Arch Intern Med 150:1685, 1990

21. Weber BE, Kapoor WN: Evaluation and outcomes of patients with palpitations. Am J Med 100:138, 1996

22. Lessmeier TJ, Gamperling D, Johnson-Liddon V, et al: Unrecognized paroxysmal supraventricular tachycardia: potential for misdiagnosis as panic disorder. Arch Intern Med 157:537, 1997

23. Zimetbaum P, Josephson ME: Current concepts: evaluation of patients with palpitations. N Engl J Med 338:1369, 1998

24. Leitch JW, Klein GJ, Yee R, et al: Syncope associated with supraventricular tachycardia: an expression of tachycardia rate or vasomotor response? Circulation 85:1064, 1992

25. Brugada P, Gursoy S, Brugada J, et al: Investigation of palpitations. Lancet 341:1254, 1993

26. Kinlay S, Leitch JW, Neil A, et al: Cardiac event recorders yield more diagnoses and are more cost-effective than 48-hour Holter monitoring in patients with palpitations: a controlled clinical trial. Ann Intern Med 124:16, 1996

27. Fogel RI, Evans JJ, Prystowsky EN: Utility and cost of event recorders in the diagnosis of palpitations, presyncope and syncope. Am J Cardiol 79:207, 1997

28. Hayes OW: Evaluation of syncope in the emergency department. Emerg Med Clin North Am 16:601, 1998

29. Hanlon JT, Linzer M, MacMillan JP, et al: Syncope and presyncope associated with probable adverse drug reactions. Arch Intern Med 150:230, 1990

30. Kapoor WN: Evaluation and outcome of patients with syncope. Medicine (Baltimore) 69:160, 1990

31. Linzer M, Yang EH, Estes M III, et al: Diagnosing syncope: value of history, physical examination and electrocardiography (pt 1). Ann Intern Med 126:989, 1997

32. Linzer M, Yang EH, Estes M III, et al: Diagnosing syncope: unexplained syncope (pt 2). Ann Intern Med 127:76, 1997

33. Brignole M, Menozzi C, Gianfranchi L, et al: Neurally mediated syncope detected by carotid sinus massage and head-up tilt table test in sick sinus syndrome. Am J Cardiol 68:1032, 1991

34. McIntosh SJ, Lawson J, Kenny RA: Clinical characteristics of vasodepressor, cardioinhibitory, and mixed carotid sinus syndrome in the elderly. Am J Med 95:203, 1993

35. Kapoor WN, Smith MA, Miller NL: Upright tilt testing in evaluating syncope: a comprehensive literature review. Am J Med 97:78, 1994

36. Stewart BF, Siscovick D, Lind BK, et al: Clinical factors associated with calcific aortic valve disease. J Am Coll Cardiol. 29:630, 1997

37. Bonow RO, Carabello B, de Leon AC Jr, et al: ACC/AHA guidelines for the management of patients with valvular heart disease: a report of the American College of Cardiology/American Heart Association Task Force on Practice Guidelines (Committee on Management of Patients with Valvular Heart Disease). J Am Coll Cardiol 32:1486, 1998

38. Lembo NJ, Dell'Italia LJ, Crawford MH, et al: Bedside diagnosis of systolic murmurs. N Engl J Med 318:1572, 1988

16 High Blood Pressure

Suzanne Oparil, M.D., and David A. Calhoun, M.D.

High blood pressure (BP) is a major health problem throughout the industrialized world because of its high prevalence and its association with increased risk of cardiovascular disease.[1] Numerous interventions, including both lifestyle modification and pharmacologic treatment, have been shown in clinical trials to produce major reductions in BP.

Long-term benefits of antihypertensive therapy have been demonstrated for the general population as well.[2] In the Framingham Heart Study, increases in the rate of use of antihypertensive medications from 2.3% to 24.6% in men and from 5.7% to 27.7% in women were associated with reductions in the prevalence of hypertension (defined as BP > 160/100 mm Hg) from 18.5% to 9.2% in men and from 28.0% to 7.7% in women. The increased use of antihypertensives was associated with reductions in the prevalence of electrocardiographic evidence of left ventricular hypertrophy (an index of target-organ damage) from 4.5% to 2.5% in men and from 3.6% to 1.1% in women.

These findings suggest that the increasing use of antihypertensive medication may in part explain the major decline in mortality from cardiovascular disease observed in the United States since the late 1960s. Yet, despite all of these effective treatments, high BP remains untreated and uncontrolled in a large percentage of people. For example, in the United States, the third National Health and Nutrition Examination Survey (NHANES III) estimated that only 53% of persons with hypertension are being treated and only 24% have their hypertension under control (BP < 140/90 mm Hg),[3] despite a high level of awareness (69% of the sample population) of the condition. Because 24% of all adults in the United States have hypertension, the findings of NHANES III suggest that over 30 million Americans are at increased risk for cardiovascular disease resulting from uncontrolled hypertension. The risk is even greater in the non-Hispanic black population, in whom the prevalence of hypertension is estimated to be 32%.

The goal of antihypertensive treatment is prevention of the cardiovascular complications of high BP, including coronary artery disease, stroke, congestive heart failure, arterial aneurysm, and end-stage renal disease. Whereas lowering BP has proved dramatically successful in preventing stroke, randomized clinical trials of antihypertensive treatment have produced disappointing results in preventing coronary artery disease.[4] Randomized, controlled trials may underestimate the benefits of antihypertensive treatment for a number of reasons: (1) BP reductions achieved in clinical trials are generally modest (5 to 6 mm Hg), compared with those accomplished in the office with aggressive individualized therapy; (2) the period of intervention in most clinical trials is relatively brief (5 years), and the maximum benefit of antihypertensive treatment may take decades to achieve; (3) high-risk patients, who derive the greatest benefit from antihypertensive treatment, are frequently excluded from clinical trials; (4) most clinical trials do not include a true placebo group, and treatments given to the control group may reduce the apparent benefit of the intervention; and (5) adverse metabolic effects of some classes of antihypertensive drugs may increase coronary risk and offset the benefit of BP reduction. Furthermore, the prevalence of end-stage renal disease[5] and congestive heart failure,[6] which are major complications of hypertension, has continued to rise despite the development of effective antihypertensive therapy.

Survey results indicate that physicians frequently do not follow consensus guidelines for antihypertensive treatment, particularly for black patients, older patients, and those with comorbid conditions, such as renal insufficiency.[7,8] The contribution of physician-prescribing practices to the failure of antihypertensive treatment to achieve its full potential is an important issue that remains to be fully examined. Whatever the causes, the disappointing results of antihypertensive treatment in preventing coronary artery disease, end-stage renal disease, and congestive heart failure have raised questions that challenge traditional approaches to managing the hypertensive patient. Antihypertensive treatment should be undertaken in the context of overall management of cardiovascular disease risk factors, and its ultimate goal should be to reduce overall cardiovascular risk. Accordingly, concomitant disease states and cardiovascular risk factors should be taken into account when antihypertensive treatment programs are designed and therapeutic goals are set.

Definition

Because BP in the human population is distributed normally (gaussian distribution), the cutoff point for high BP is arbitrary. Hypertension in persons 18 years of age or older is defined and classified by the Joint National Committee on Detection, Evaluation, and Treatment of High BP (JNC VI) [*see Table 1*].[9] An adult is diagnosed as hypertensive when he or she has a diastolic BP at or above 90 mm Hg, a systolic BP at or above 140 mm Hg, or both on repeated determinations.

Etiology and Pathogenesis

Essential hypertension, which accounts for more than 95% of all cases of hypertension, tends to cluster in families and represents a collection of genetically based diseases or syndromes with

Table 1 Classification of Blood Pressure for Adults 18 Years of Age and Older*

Category	Systolic (mm Hg)	Diastolic (mm Hg)
Optimal	< 120	< 80
Normal[†]	< 130	< 85
High normal	130–139	85–89
Hypertension[‡]		
Stage 1 (mild)	140–159	90–99
Stage 2 (moderate)	160–179	100–109
Stage 3 (severe)	≥ 180	≥ 110

*Not taking antihypertensive drugs and not acutely ill. When systolic and diastolic pressures fall into different categories, the higher category should be selected to classify the person's blood pressure status. For instance, 160/92 mm Hg should be classified as stage 2, and 180/120 mm Hg should be classified as stage 3. Isolated systolic hypertension (ISH) is defined as systolic BP ≥ 140 mm Hg and diastolic BP < 90 mm Hg and staged appropriately (e.g., 170/85 mm Hg is defined as stage 2 ISH).
†Based on the average of two or more readings taken at each of two or more visits after an initial screening.
‡In addition to classifying stages of hypertension on the basis of average BP levels, the clinician should specify presence or absence of target-organ disease and additional risk factors. For example, a patient with diabetes and a blood pressure of 142/94 mm Hg plus left ventricular hypertrophy should be classified as "stage 1 hypertension with target-organ disease (left ventricular hypertrophy) and with another major risk factor (diabetes)." This specificity is important for risk classification and management.

a number of resultant inherited biochemical abnormalities.[10] Many pathophysiologic factors have been implicated in the genesis of essential hypertension, including increased sympathetic nervous system activity, perhaps related to heightened exposure or response to psychosocial stress, overproduction of sodium-retaining hormones and vasoconstrictors (e.g., endothelin and thromboxane), long-term high sodium intake, inadequate dietary intake of potassium and calcium, increased or inappropriate renin secretion, deficiencies of vasodilators such as prostaglandins and nitric oxide, congenital abnormalities of the resistance vessels, diabetes mellitus, insulin resistance, obesity, increased activity of vascular growth factors, and altered cellular ion transport.

GENETICS OF PRIMARY HYPERTENSION

Identifiable single-gene mutations account for only a very small percentage of cases of essential hypertension.[11] In most cases, hypertension results from a complex interaction of genetic, environmental, and demographic factors.[12] Improved techniques of genetic analysis have allowed a search for genes that contribute to the development of primary hypertension. Early results of this search indicate that primary hypertension is polygenic in origin; however, with one exception, the particular genes, or even the number of genes, involved have not been identified.

Of the small number of candidate genes evaluated, only the gene encoding angiotensinogen has been linked to the pathogenesis of primary hypertension. Three independent lines of evidence, reproduced in unrelated cohorts in Salt Lake City and Paris, support a role for angiotensinogen variants in primary hypertension: (1) linkage of the angiotensinogen locus with hypertension in hypertensive sibling pairs, (2) association of specific angiotensinogen variants with hypertension in case-control studies, and (3) association of these variants with elevated plasma angiotensinogen levels.[11] Although some studies have suggested that other genes, such as those encoding for endothelin or atrial natriuretic factor peptides, might be linked to hypertension, compelling evidence demonstrating their clear association with this disease is lacking. Interestingly, genes for other components of the renin-angiotensin system, such as renin and angiotensin-converting enzyme (ACE), have not been linked to hypertension.

WATER AND SODIUM RETENTION

Although so-called major hypertensive genes have not been identified for essential hypertension, it is interesting that, to date, the final common pathway of identifiable genetically related hypertension is salt and water retention. Hypertension has been attributed to defects in the angiotensinogen gene and to single-gene defects in glucocorticoid-remediable aldosteronism (GRA), apparent mineralocorticoid excess (AME), Liddle syndrome, and 11β- and 17α-hydroxylase deficiency.[13-19] In all of these conditions, BP is increased secondary to volume expansion attributable to excessive salt and water retention.[11] It is certainly possible that other genes will be identified that increase BP through other mechanisms, but the genetic observations to date reinforce the longtime argument of Guyton[20] that the development of hypertension is dependent on genetically determined renal dysfunction with resultant salt and water retention.

INHERITED CARDIOVASCULAR RISK FACTORS

Cardiovascular risk factors, including hypertension, tend to cosegregate more commonly than would be expected by chance. Approximately 40% of persons with essential hypertension also have hypercholesterolemia (serum cholesterol levels > 240 mg/ dl).[21] Formal genetic studies have established a clear association between hypertension and dyslipidemia.[22] Hypertension and diabetes mellitus also tend to coexist. In the general population, hypertension is approximately twice as common in persons with diabetes as in persons without it, and the association is even stronger in African Americans and Mexican Americans.[23] Overall, an estimated 35% to 75% of the cardiovascular complications of diabetes are attributable to hypertension.

Hypertension, insulin resistance, dyslipidemia, and obesity often occur concomitantly. Associated abnormalities include microalbuminuria, high uric acid levels, hypercoagulability, and accelerated atherosclerosis. This cosegregation of abnormalities, referred to as syndrome X, insulin-resistance syndrome, or the deadly quartet, has a multiplying effect on cardiovascular risk.[24] The underlying cause of these abnormalities has been hypothesized to be heightened sympathetic activation secondary to hyperinsulinemia or endothelial cell dysfunction. Until a common cause is identified, physicians must assess and treat these risk factors individually, recognizing that many hypertensive patients have insulin resistance, dyslipidemia, or both.

SYMPATHETIC NERVOUS SYSTEM ACTIVATION

Increased sympathetic nervous system activity raises BP through stimulation of the heart, the peripheral vasculature, and the kidneys, causing increased cardiac output, increased vascular resistance, and fluid retention. Increased sympathetic activation contributes to the development of hypertension but plays a lesser role in maintaining BP elevation once hypertension is established.[25] Circulating norepinephrine levels are generally higher in hypertensive than in normotensive persons, suggesting greater sympathetic activation in the latter. This relation is particularly true in persons younger than 40 years and tends to diminish with age. Vascular changes induced by heightened sympathetic activity, such as smooth muscle hypertrophy, may maintain elevations in BP despite decreases in sympathetic activity.

Norepinephrine spillover is a more sensitive index of sympathetic activity than circulating norepinephrine levels. Whole body norepinephrine spillover is elevated in young hypertensive persons, compared with normotensive control subjects.[26] This increase is primarily attributable to greater sympathetic outflow to the musculature, kidneys, and heart. Studies of norepinephrine spillover in normotensive offspring of hypertensive parents suggest that increases in sympathetic activity that predispose to the development of hypertension are, in large part, genetic in origin. Microneurography, a technique using microelectrodes to directly measure peripheral or muscle sympathetic nerve activity, which is also a more sensitive and specific index of sympathetic activity than plasma norepinephrine levels, has also shown that sympathetic activity is increased in hypertensive persons.[25]

VASCULAR REACTIVITY

Exposure to stress increases sympathetic outflow, and repeated stress-induced vasoconstriction may result in vascular hypertrophy, leading to progressive increases in peripheral resistance and BP. This could explain in part the greater incidence of hypertension in lower socioeconomic groups, in that this population may experience greater levels of stress associated with daily living. Laboratory stress testing suggests that persons with a family history of hypertension manifest augmented vasoconstrictor responses to laboratory stressors, such as cold pressor testing and mental stress, that may predispose them to the development of hypertension. This is particularly true of young African Americans, and exaggerated stress responses may contribute to the greater incidence of hypertension in African Americans than in white Americans.[27]

RENIN-ANGIOTENSIN-ALDOSTERONE SYSTEM REACTIVITY

The renin-angiotensin-aldosterone system is an important mediator of BP control in both normotensive and hypertensive persons. Angiotensin II (ANG II) has a number of actions, including vasoconstriction of resistance vessels; stimulation of aldosterone synthesis and release and of renal tubular sodium reabsorption (directly and indirectly via aldosterone); inhibition of renin release; and production of neural effects, including stimulation of thirst, release of antidiuretic hormone, and increases in sympathetic output. In addition, ANG II induces cell hyperplasia and hypertrophy. These effects are mediated by the ANG II type 1 receptor, and all tend to elevate BP. Local production of ANG II in a variety of tissues, including the blood vessels, heart, adrenals, and brain, is under the control of ACE and a number of other enzymes, including the serine proteinase chymase.[28] The activity of local renin-angiotensin systems and alternative pathways of ANG II formation may make an important contribution to the development of target-organ damage (including left ventricular hypertrophy, congestive heart failure, and atherosclerosis) in hypertensive persons. Other manifestations of target-organ damage are stroke, renal failure, myocardial infarction, and arterial aneurysm.

INHIBITION OF NITRIC OXIDE PRODUCTION

Nitric oxide (NO) is a short-lived but highly permeable gas that is a potent vasodilator, inhibitor of platelet adhesion and aggregation, and suppressor of migration and proliferation of vascular smooth muscle cells. NO is released by endothelial cells in response to a variety of stimuli—including changes in BP, shear stress, and pulsatile stretch—and plays an important role in BP regulation, thrombosis, and atherosclerosis formation. Pharmacologically induced increases in BP promote NO release, whereas decreases in BP suppress NO release. Furthermore, inhibitors of NO production induce sustained hypertension when they are administered continuously to animals, which suggests that the cardiovascular system is exposed to a continuous NO-dependent vasodilator tone. NO-related vascular relaxation is diminished in hypertensive persons, but it is unclear whether this impairment of endothelial function is a cause or consequence of hypertension.[29] If the latter interpretation is correct, NO may play an important role in the pathogenesis of the vascular complications of hypertension but not in the development of hypertension per se.

ENDOTHELIN PRODUCTION

Endothelin is a potent vasoactive peptide that is released from endothelial cells and has both vasoconstrictor and vasodilator properties. The role of endothelin in regulating BP and in the pathogenesis of hypertension is under investigation. Evidence suggesting that endothelin causes hypertension includes the observations that a form of hypertension caused by a rare endothelin-secreting tumor can be cured with excision of the tumor and that endothelin antagonists reduce BP and peripheral vascular resistance in normotensive persons. Endothelin antagonists have successfully lowered BP in clinical trials in patients with mild to moderate essential hypertension.[30]

Diagnosis

Hypertension should be diagnosed and treated in the context of reducing overall cardiovascular risk and preventing morbidity and mortality from cardiovascular disease. In most hypertensive patients, multiple risk factors for atherosclerotic disease coexist.[21] Therefore, comprehensive assessment and treatment of all risk factors are essential for effective intervention. Accordingly, all modifiable cardiovascular risk factors (i.e., hypertension, hyperlipidemia, alcohol and tobacco use, obesity, sedentary lifestyle, glucose intolerance, and insulin resistance) should be included in the initial assessment and addressed by the treatment plan. In addition, the initial evaluation should include an accurate measurement of BP, assessment of target-organ damage, and screening for secondary causes of hypertension [see Table 2].

Table 2 Causes of Secondary Hypertension

Systolic and Diastolic Hypertension
Renal
  Renal parenchymal disease
    Chronic nephritis
    Polycystic disease
    Collagen vascular disease
    Diabetic nephropathy
    Hydronephrosis
    Acute glomerulonephritis
  Renal vascular disease
  Renal transplantation
  Renin-secreting tumors
Endocrine
  Adrenal
    Primary aldosteronism
    Overproduction of 11-deoxycorticosterone (DOC), 18-hydroxy-DOC, and other mineralocorticoids
    Congenital adrenal hyperplasia
    Cushing syndrome
    Pheochromocytoma

Extra-adrenal chromaffin tumors
Hyperparathyroidism
Acromegaly
Pregnancy-induced hypertension
Sleep apnea
Coarctation of the aorta
Neurologic disorders
  Dysautonomia
  Increased intracranial pressure
  Obstructive sleep apnea
  Quadriplegia
  Lead poisoning
  Guillain-Barré syndrome
Postoperative hypertension
Drugs and chemicals
  Cyclosporine
  Ethanol
  Oral contraceptives
  Glucocorticoids
  Mineralocorticoids, including licorice and carbenoxolone

Sympathomimetics
Tyramine and monoamine oxidase inhibitors
Erythropoietin
Antidepressants
Appetite suppressants
Nonsteroidal anti-inflammatory agents
Nasal decongestants
Phenothiazines

Isolated Systolic Hypertension
Aging, with associated aortic rigidity
Increased cardiac output
  Thyrotoxicosis
  Anemia
  Aortic valvular insufficiency
Decreased peripheral vascular resistance
  Arteriovenous shunts
  Paget disease of bone
  Beriberi

BLOOD PRESSURE MEASUREMENT

Except in cases of extreme BP elevation (systolic BP > 210 mm Hg, diastolic BP > 120 mm Hg, or both) or elevated BP with evidence of ongoing target-organ damage, hypertension should not be diagnosed on the basis of measurements made on a single occasion. Hypertension is diagnosed when at least two separate readings obtained at least 1 to 2 weeks apart average 140/90 mm Hg. Accurate determination of BP is essential to avoid misdiagnosis. Patients should abstain from tobacco use and caffeine ingestion for at least 30 minutes before the BP measurement is taken. The arm should be exposed and free of constricting clothing. Patients should be asked to sit quietly for 5 minutes before their BP measurement is taken. Use of an appropriately sized cuff, in which the bladder encircles at least 80% of the arm, is essential because a cuff that is too large or too small will result in falsely low or falsely high readings, respectively. During BP measurement, the arm should be supported with the cuff at approximately heart level.

In addition to the BP level, the presence or absence of other cardiovascular risk factors and target-organ damage plays a role in determining when treatment should be initiated or the patient reevaluated. Levels consistent with hypertensive crisis (systolic BP > 210 mm Hg, diastolic BP > 120 mm Hg, or both) warrant prompt initiation of therapy. Lesser elevations in BP should be confirmed by remeasurement. Abnormally high BP levels during the first office visit are not uncommon and should be excluded by subsequent reassessment. However, the presence of target-organ damage indicates long-standing, poorly controlled hypertension, and initiation of therapy should not be delayed.

Measurement of BP by patients or family members or automated ambulatory BP monitoring often helps verify the diagnosis and assess the severity of hypertension. BP values obtained outside the clinic setting have consistently been shown to be lower than those obtained by health care personnel and to correlate better with target-organ damage. The superiority of home or workplace BP measurements depends on use of accurate and calibrated BP monitors and careful repeated instruction in how to measure BP. So-called white-coat hypertension, in which a patient's BP is elevated when measured by health care personnel but is otherwise normal, occurs in approximately 20% of hypertensive patients. It is likely to be an anxiety response to having one's health assessed or is perhaps a conditioned response—that is, an initial anxiety response that has been reinforced and perhaps amplified through patient-physician interactions. White-coat hypertension is also associated with other coronary risk factors, such as obesity, insulin resistance, and elevated low-density lipoprotein cholesterol levels. However, evidence of increased target-organ damage has not been found consistently in patients with white-coat hypertension.

Determining BP accurately can be difficult in elderly patients because of stiffening of arterial walls. The loss of arterial wall compliance can result in falsely elevated BP measurements when a standard sphygmomanometer is used. Pseudohypertension, a falsely elevated BP obtained by indirect cuff measurement secondary to loss of arterial compliance, should be suspected in elderly patients diagnosed as having hypertension but without evidence of target-organ damage. The Osler maneuver, in which the BP cuff is inflated above the level of systolic BP, can sometimes be used to identify this phenomenon. If the pulseless radial or brachial artery remains palpable, stiffening of the artery may be sufficient to falsely elevate the BP measurement. Intra-arterial BP determinations may be necessary to accurately diagnose hypertension in this setting.

MEDICAL HISTORY

The purpose of the medical history and physical examination is (1) to determine the need for and guide a possible workup of secondary causes of hypertension and (2) to assess overall cardiovascular risk and deal with all modifiable cardiovascular risk factors. Accordingly, the medical history should include a history of hypertension, a history and symptoms of end-organ damage, prior diagnoses and treatment of other cardiovascular risk factors, and diagnoses of concomitant disease.

History of hypertension should include duration and severity of hypertension, prior workup of possible secondary causes of hypertension, and efficacy and adverse effects of previously prescribed therapies. Risk factors for primary hypertension, such as a positive family history or pregnancy-related hypertension, should be discussed. The medical history should also include reference to relevant lifestyle characteristics, such as weight gain, sedentary lifestyle, high dietary salt ingestion, and excessive alcohol consumption.

When obtaining the history, the physician should elicit evidence of secondary causes of hypertension [see Table 2], including the onset of severe hypertension at an early age, particularly in the absence of a positive family history of hypertension, and an abrupt worsening in severity or refractoriness of hypertension in an older patient. Patients with resistant hypertension, which remains uncontrolled in the presence of an adequate multidrug regimen, are also prime candidates for secondary hypertension. In particular, renal artery stenosis (RAS) secondary to fibromuscular dysplasia most often occurs in young women. RAS in older patients usually, but not exclusively, occurs in the context of diffuse atherosclerotic disease. Pheochromocytoma is suggested by episodic increases in hypertension often accompanied by headache, diaphoresis, and palpitations. Primary aldosteronism is suggested by a history of hypokalemia.

The degree of target-organ damage must be documented by history and physical examination. A history of coronary artery disease, left ventricular hypertrophy, cerebrovascular disease, peripheral vascular disease, or renal insufficiency suggests long-standing, poorly controlled hypertension. In addition, prior diagnoses and successful treatment of other cardiovascular risk factors (e.g., hyperlipidemia, diabetes, smoking, obesity, or sedentary lifestyle) must be established to guide treatment recommendations. Last, comorbid conditions and their treatment should be delineated so as to anticipate potential drug interactions and optimize choices of antihypertensive drugs.

PHYSICAL EXAMINATION

The physical examination should accurately determine the BP, identify signs of secondary causes of hypertension, and document the presence and degree of target-organ damage. The BP determination should be the average of a minimum of two BP readings obtained 2 to 3 minutes apart. Initially, the BP should be measured in both arms. Though there are often small variations between arms, large differences suggest subclavian artery obstruction. In general, the BP measurement should be obtained from the arm that yields the higher readings. Standing BP levels should be checked during the initial evaluation and after drug titrations to exclude significant orthostasis.

Arteriolar narrowing, arteriovenous nicking, hemorrhages, exudates, or papilledema on funduscopic examination suggests poor BP control and target-organ damage. Carotid or femoral bruits or diminished peripheral pulses indicate atherosclerotic obstructive disease. An S_4 gallop is often heard in patients with long-standing hypertension. Ventricular hypertrophy is suggested by a displaced or prominent precordial impulse. Congestive heart failure is indicated by pulmonary rales, jugular vein distention, and an S_3 gallop.

Signs of secondary causes of hypertension include abdominal bruits in renal artery stenosis, truncal obesity, excessive hair growth, abdominal striae, and a so-called buffalo hump in Cushing syndrome.

LABORATORY EVALUATION

Laboratory evaluation should further the documentation of target-organ damage. Blood urea nitrogen and serum creatinine levels should be obtained to quantify renal function. Urine should be analyzed for microalbuminuria, one of the earliest signs of hypertensive renal disease. Serum potassium should be checked to rule out hypokalemia suggestive of aldosteronism. Fasting serum glucose should be assessed to exclude glucose intolerance, which occurs in as many as 50% of hypertensive patients. Likewise, a fasting lipid profile should be obtained to rule out hyperlipidemia, which is also common in hypertensive patients. An electrocardiogram should be obtained to look for evidence of coronary artery disease, left ventricular hypertrophy, or both.

Treatment

RISKS OF HYPERTENSION

In young and middle-aged people, the risk of cardiovascular disease mortality is positively related to both systolic and diastolic BP over the entire range.[1] Twelve-year follow-up data from more than 350,000 middle-aged men screened for the Multiple Risk Factor Intervention Trial (MRFIT) show that the relative risk of cardiovascular mortality doubled when systolic BP was in the high-normal range (130 to 139 mm Hg) and diastolic BP was in the stage 1 hypertension range (95 to 99 mm Hg).[31] Risk of stroke in this cohort of men doubled and even tripled when systolic BP levels were as low as 120 mm Hg.[32] Subsequent analyses found a doubling in the risk for end-stage renal disease in MRFIT participants with high-normal BP (130/85 to 139/89 mm Hg).[33] Furthermore, data from the Framingham Heart Study show a twofold and threefold increase in risk of development of congestive heart failure in hypertensive (stages 1 and 2) men and women, respectively, compared with normotensive persons in the population.[6]

In contrast, in people in late middle-age and in the elderly, systolic BP, but not diastolic BP, is a strong predictor of both total and cardiovascular mortality.[34] It is important to note that systolic BP in the population as a whole increases with advancing age, whereas diastolic BP tends to plateau or fall after age 60[35]; consequently, in older persons, the diagnosis of hypertension is more often made on the basis of systolic rather than diastolic BP.[36] Furthermore, in the elderly population, increased pulse pressure (which is generally a result of decreased diastolic BP in the presence of elevated systolic BP) is an even better predictor of cardiovascular disease risk than systolic BP alone.[35,37] Thus, if equal elevations of systolic BP are assumed, persons with isolated systolic hypertension are at greater risk for cardiovascular disease than those with combined systolic-diastolic hypertension. This finding has important therapeutic implications: although lowering systolic BP in elderly patients with isolated systolic hypertension is clearly beneficial,[38,39] lowering diastolic BP to below 70 mm Hg with active treatment has been associated with increased stroke, coronary artery disease, and cardiovascular disease.[40] This inverse relation between diastolic BP and cardiovascular disease is even more marked at diastolic BPs below 60 mm Hg, in which cases it is thought to reflect unmasking of underlying subclinical vascular disease. Therefore, systolic BP should be stressed more than diastolic BP in the diagnosis and treatment of hypertension in the elderly, because systolic BP plays a major role in determining the risk of cardiovascular events and benefits of therapy.[36]

BENEFITS OF ANTIHYPERTENSIVE TREATMENT

Reducing BP by pharmacologic means clearly reduces cardiovascular morbidity and mortality.[41] A meta-analysis of 17 randomized, controlled trials of antihypertensive therapy showed a 21% reduction in mortality from cardiovascular disease, a 38% reduction in stroke, and a 16% reduction in coronary artery disease in persons assigned to diuretic or beta-blocker therapy.[4] Furthermore, drug treatment of hypertension has beneficial effects regarding progression to more severe hypertension, development of left ventricular hypertrophy, progression of renal disease and heart failure, and, most important, all-cause mortality.[2,42]

The benefits of antihypertensive treatment in elderly patients appear to be even greater than in younger patients. Trials in older patients have shown a 17% reduction in fatal and nonfatal myocardial infarction and a 47% reduction in heart failure.[43,44] A meta-analysis of 13 randomized clinical trials that evaluated cardiovascular outcomes in 16,000 persons 60 years of age and older showed that 43 persons had to be treated for 5 years to prevent one cerebrovascular event and that 61 persons had to be treated for 5 years to prevent one coronary artery disease event.[43] Only 18 persons had to be treated 5 years to prevent one cardiovascular (cerebrovascular or cardiac) event. Furthermore, only 15 persons with isolated systolic hypertension (systolic BP > 140 mm Hg and diastolic BP < 90 mm Hg) had to be treated for 5 years to prevent a cardiovascular event. Comparison with 12 trials involving 33,000 middle-aged and younger hypertensive persons revealed that for all outcomes except cardiac mortality, two to four times as many younger persons as older persons needed to be treated for 5 years to prevent events of morbidity and mortality. No significant effect on cardiac mortality was seen in younger persons, whereas 78 older persons had to be treated to prevent a fatal cardiac event.[43]

The reasons for the greater short-term (5 years) benefits of antihypertensive therapy in older persons include the following: (1) older persons are at higher immediate and absolute risk of developing a cardiovascular event than younger persons because the prevalence of preexisting cardiovascular disease and cardiovascular risk factors is greater in older persons; (2) systolic hypertension is associated with greater cardiovascular risk than diastolic hypertension and is more prevalent in the elderly[34,35]; (3) smoking is less common in older persons than younger persons, and smokers have been shown to respond less well to antihypertensive treatment; and (4) most large trials involving the elderly are more recent than those involving younger patients and have used treatment regimens that have fewer adverse effects, such as lower doses of thiazides or combinations of thiazides and potassium-sparing agents.[43,45] Because the benefits of antihypertensive treatment increase over time, the long-term benefits of antihypertensive treatment in younger persons could exceed those in older persons, despite the greater short-term benefits in the latter group.

PATIENT SELECTION

In any given hypertensive patient, the risk of cardiovascular disease is dependent on the BP level, the presence or absence of concomitant risk factors, and the presence or absence of target-organ damage. Concomitant risk factors that lower the threshold for antihypertensive treatment include dyslipidemia, diabetes mellitus, age greater than 60 years, smoking, and family history of cardiovascular disease. Target-organ damage that should be considered in antihypertensive treatment decisions includes damage that results from heart disease, such as left ventricular hypertrophy, as well as angina, prior myocardial infarction, or both; prior coronary revascularization and heart failure; stroke or transient ischemic attack; nephropathy; peripheral arterial disease; and retinopathy.[9]

A reasonable approach to antihypertensive treatment is to be most aggressive with persons who have both concomitant risk factors and target-organ damage [see Table 3]. Immediate initiation of pharmacologic treatment is indicated for these patients, even if their BP levels are in the high-normal range. Patients who are free of target-organ damage and clinical cardiovascular disease and who have stage 1 hypertension or high-normal BP may benefit from 6 to 12 months of lifestyle modification and reevaluation before initiation of pharmacologic therapy. Many of these patients may be spared the expense and hazard of drug therapy if they are given a serious trial of lifestyle modification. For patients with white-coat hypertension who have no evidence of target-organ damage, pharmacologic therapy is likely to be unnecessary. If, however, target-organ damage is present—particularly if it is progressive—pharmacologic therapy may be beneficial but should be administered cautiously to avoid overtreatment, and subsequent ambulatory BP measurements should be obtained. Immediate initiation of pharmacologic treatment is indicated for all patients with stage 2 or greater hypertension, independent of concomitant risk factors and target-organ damage. Furthermore, lifestyle modification should be included as adjunctive therapy for all patients receiving pharmacologic treatment.

TREATMENT GOALS

The goal of antihypertensive therapy is to reduce overall cardiovascular risk and thus cardiovascular morbidity and mortality. To accomplish this goal, BP should be reduced to the lowest levels tolerated, and other modifiable cardiovascular risk factors should be eliminated. The standard goal of less than 140/90 mm Hg is arbitrary, and recent studies have shown that treatment to achieve lower levels may have added value in preventing the cardiovascular complications of hypertension.[9,46,47] In particular, reducing BP to levels lower than 140/90 mm Hg is believed to be useful in slowing the progression of renal failure and congestive heart failure. Accordingly, JNC VI has recommended a BP goal of less than 130/85 mm Hg—or lower (125/75 mm Hg) in patients with proteinuria in excess of 1 g/24 hours—and a goal of less than 130/85 mm Hg in diabetic patients.[9] Similarly, the World Health Organization–International Society of Hypertension (WHO-ISH) guidelines include

BP goals of less than 130/85 mm Hg for young, middle-aged, and diabetic patients and less than 140/90 mm Hg for elderly patients.[48]

LIFESTYLE MODIFICATION

Lifestyle modifications of proven benefit in antihypertensive treatment include weight reduction or prevention of weight gain, moderation of alcohol intake, increased physical activity, maintenance of recommended levels of dietary calcium and potassium, and moderation of dietary sodium. Cessation or avoidance of smoking is also critical because smoking is an important independent risk factor for cardiovascular disease and may interfere with the related benefits of antihypertensive therapy. Although permanent modifications in diet and lifestyle are difficult to achieve, in motivated patients they may obviate drug treatment or reduce the doses needed to adequately control BP. In well-motivated patients with stage 1 or 2 hypertension, modifying lifestyle effectively lowers BP and may be more important than the initial choice of antihypertensive drug. Two recent clinical trials—one with a comprehensive food plan that supplied the recommended dietary allowances (RDAs) of all of the major nutrients[49] and the other with a diet rich in fruits, vegetables, and low-fat dairy products and reduced amounts of saturated and total fat[50]—produced reductions in BP comparable to or greater than those usually seen with monotherapy for stage 1 hypertension. The Dietary Approaches to Stop Hypertension (DASH) trial[50] showed reductions in BP of 11.4/5.5 mm Hg in persons on the low-fat diet (called the combination diet), compared with control subjects on a so-called usual American diet, although dietary sodium intake and weight were held constant. Importantly, the DASH combination diet, unlike most other lifestyle-modification strategies, lowered BP effectively in all subgroups of participants, including whites and blacks, men and women, younger people and older people, obese people and nonobese people, and people of higher and lower socioeconomic status.[51] The DASH combination diet and other lifestyle-modification strategies that are effective in treating hypertensive patients may be useful in preventing the development of hypertension in persons with high-normal BP.

Weight Reduction

There is a clear, direct relation between body weight and BP. Overweight people (body mass index greater than 27.8 for men and greater than 27.3 for women) have an increased incidence of hypertension and increased cardiovascular risk. Weight loss is closely correlated with reduction in BP and is potentially the most efficacious of all nonpharmacologic measures to treat hypertension.[10,52,53] This effect is independent of dietary sodium restriction and is seen in both obese and nonobese hypertensive persons.

Table 3 Risk Stratification and Treatment[9]

Blood Pressure Stage (mm Hg)	Risk Group A (no risk factors, no TOD/CCD)	Risk Group B (≥ 1 risk factor, not including diabetes; no TOD/CCD)	Risk Group C* (TOD/CCD and/or diabetes ± other risk factors)
High-normal (130–139/85–89)	Lifestyle modification	Lifestyle modification	Drug therapy†
Stage 1 (140–159/90–99)	Lifestyle modification (up to 12 mo)	Lifestyle modification‡ (up to 6 mo)	Drug therapy
Stages 2 and 3 (≥ 160/≥ 100)	Drug therapy	Drug therapy	Drug therapy

Example: A patient with diabetes and a blood pressure of 142/94 mm Hg plus left ventricular hypertrophy should be classified as having stage 1 hypertension with target-organ disease (left ventricular hypertrophy) and with another major risk factor (diabetes). This patient would be categorized as stage 1, risk group C, and recommended for immediate initiation of pharmacologic treatment.

*Lifestyle modification should be adjunctive therapy for all patients recommended for pharmacologic therapy.

†For those with heart failure, renal insufficiency, or diabetes.

‡For patients with multiple risk factors, clinicians should consider drugs as initial therapy plus lifestyle modifications.

TOD/CCD—target-organ disease/clinical cardiovascular disease

Weight loss also enhances the efficacy of antihypertensive drugs. In addition to reducing BP, weight loss independently reduces cardiovascular risk, in part through favorable effects on concomitant risk factors such as diabetes and hyperlipidemia, and tends to improve the patient's self-image and sense of well-being. Patients should avoid appetite suppressants, which contain sympathomimetics (e.g., phenylpropanolamine) that can elevate BP. Weight reduction through a combination of dietary caloric restriction and increased physical activity is recommended for all overweight hypertensive people. Because sustained weight reduction is so difficult to achieve, even more emphasis should be placed on prevention of weight gain, particularly in younger people with high-normal BP and in families with a high prevalence of hypertension.

Increased Physical Activity

At least 30 minutes of moderate-intensity physical activity, such as brisk walking, bicycling, or yard work, three times a week (preferably once a day) can lower BP in both normotensive and hypertensive persons.[54] Although more-intense physical activity may confer even greater cardiovascular benefit, for the general population the greatest benefit and the least risk are seen when sedentary people become moderately active. Additional benefits of regular physical activity include weight loss, enhanced sense of well-being, improved functional health status, and reduced risk of cardiovascular disease and all-cause mortality.[55] Accordingly, regular aerobic physical activity is recommended for all hypertensive people, including those with target-organ damage. Patients with advanced or unstable cardiovascular disease may require a medical evaluation before initiation of exercise or a medically supervised exercise program.[55]

Moderation of Alcohol Intake

Alcohol consumption elevates BP, both acutely and chronically, and there is a clear association between elevated BP and increased alcohol consumption. Excessive alcohol intake also appears to cause resistance to antihypertensive therapy.[56] However, moderate alcohol consumption has been shown to reduce overall cardiovascular risk in the general population.[57] Whether this risk reduction also occurs in the hypertensive population needs further study. For unrelated health reasons, alcohol consumption is not recommended for nondrinkers; for drinkers, alcohol intake should be limited to 1 oz (2 oz of 100-proof whiskey, 8 oz of wine, or 24 oz of beer) a day.[9]

Restricting Dietary Sodium

Physicians commonly recommend dietary sodium restriction for hypertensive patients. However, studies evaluating the antihypertensive efficacy of dietary salt restriction in unselected patients with essential hypertension have not demonstrated a large benefit. Meta-analyses of published studies have shown small but consistent reductions in BP in hypertensive persons who participated in clinical trials of salt restriction.[58,59] An observational study of a large cohort of hypertensive persons, all of whom were advised to restrict their sodium intake, showed that men in the lowest quartile of sodium excretion had a fourfold greater risk of heart attack than those in the highest quartile.[60] This observation, although not yet confirmed in prospective, controlled trials, raises the possibility that sodium restriction may be harmful for some hypertensive persons. Furthermore, increased BP levels have been observed in some hypertensive patients when dietary sodium intake is reduced. The observed heterogeneity in BP response to restricted dietary sodium has given rise to attempts to classify hypertensive patients as salt sensitive or salt resistant and to develop

biochemical indices of salt sensitivity. Concomitant potassium intake is a major determinant of salt sensitivity, and the pressor effects of dietary salt supplementation have been shown to be greatly reduced or abolished by increases in potassium intake within the normal range.[61] Salt sensitivity is most common in persons whose diets are low in potassium (see below).[62] Patients with low renin activity, such as elderly and black patients, are more likely to respond to sodium restriction with a decrease in BP.[63] Sodium restriction can minimize diuretic-induced hypokalemia and may enhance the ease of BP control with diuretic therapy and, therefore, should be encouraged in patients taking diuretics. Additional benefits of salt restriction include protection from osteoporosis and fractures by reducing urinary calcium excretion and favorable effects on left ventricular hypertrophy. Physicians can recommend moderate sodium restriction (4 to 6 g of salt daily) for hypertensive patients, realizing that only a subset will benefit. This can be effected by the simple and tolerable measures of not adding salt to food during preparation or at the table and avoiding processed foods containing salt as a preservative. Salt substitutes in which sodium is replaced with potassium are useful for hypertensive patients who do not have renal dysfunction. Patients should be instructed to avoid concomitant decreases in calcium and potassium intake, because ensuring adequate calcium and potassium intake will lower BP independently and obviate the need for aggressive salt restriction.

Maintenance of Dietary Potassium Intake

Dietary potassium intake is inversely related to BP in the general population, and dietary potassium supplementation causes small but significant reductions in BP in both normotensive and hypertensive persons.[64] This effect appears to be related to concomitant sodium intake in that potassium supplementation reduces BP more effectively in persons with higher sodium intake. Importantly, increasing potassium intake to high-normal levels reduces renal salt retention and BP in salt-sensitive persons.[61] Hypertensive patients should maintain adequate potassium intake (> 100 mEq/day), preferably by eating enough fresh fruits and vegetables, as in the DASH combination diet.[50,51] Potassium supplements should be avoided or used only with extreme caution in patients with renal insufficiency; diabetics; and patients taking potassium-sparing diuretics, ACE inhibitors, or ANG II receptor blockers. Hypokalemia, whether caused by diuretic use or poor dietary intake, should be treated. Hypokalemia should be prevented, particularly in patients taking digoxin and those with known coronary artery disease, because it predisposes patients to arrhythmia.

Maintenance of Dietary Calcium Intake

There is an inverse relation between dietary calcium intake and BP in the general population.[65] Furthermore, 75% to 90% of adults in the United States fail to consume the RDA of calcium (1,000 mg for adults younger than 65 years; 1,500 mg for adults older than 65 years), and hypertensive persons generally ingest less calcium than normotensive persons. Whereas clinical studies of the BP-lowering effects of calcium supplements have produced mixed results, the recent DASH trial showed that a diet rich in low-fat dairy foods is associated with major reductions in BP in both normotensive and hypertensive persons.[50] The BP effects of the DASH diet were significantly greater in both normotensive and hypertensive blacks (−6.8 mm Hg systolic BP) than in whites (−3.4 mm Hg).[51] The DASH trial was not designed to identify the specific components of the diet that are effective in reducing BP. Nevertheless, it is likely that calcium and vitamin D derived from food sources contributed to the effects of the diet on BP, perhaps accounting for the greater effect of the diet in blacks, who have a generally lower calcium intake than whites. Maintaining oral calcium intake of at least 1 g/day, preferably from food sources, is also beneficial for other health reasons, such as preventing osteoporosis and gastrointestinal malignancy.

Other Interventions

Other lifestyle modifications, including relaxation and stress reduction, caffeine restriction, magnesium supplementation, changing the fat content of the diet, and garlic and onion consumption, have not been shown to produce sustained benefits in BP control.

Overall Recommendations

Lifestyle modifications should be used in all hypertensive patients, either as definitive treatment or as adjunctive therapy. Therapy should be tailored to the characteristics of each patient. A reasonable generalized approach includes (1) weight loss for the overweight patient, (2) regular physical activity, (3) moderation of alcohol consumption, (4) smoking cessation, and (5) adherence to national guidelines for dietary sodium, calcium, and potassium, preferably from food sources. Such an approach has been shown to produce significant sustained reductions in BP while reducing overall cardiovascular risk.

PHARMACOLOGIC TREATMENT

Initial Choice of Therapy

The initial choice of antihypertensive drug treatment has received increasing attention in recent years for a variety of reasons, including the development of new drugs with real or perceived advantages over existing agents, cost issues, and the lack of morbidity and mortality data for the newer agents. Although this is a major issue, it is even more important to note that the initial choice of monotherapy for hypertension is frequently not sustained over time. Most antihypertensive agents effectively control BP in fewer than 50% of patients. Further, changing or discontinuing treatment is frequent: in one large study of hypertensive patients seen by general practitioners, 50% to 60% of new treatments were changed or discontinued within the first 6 months.[66] This was true for all four of the most commonly prescribed classes of antihypertensive agents. Whether these discontinuance rates are high because of drug-related adverse effects, poor efficacy, or other factors is uncertain, but this inconsistency in treatment likely contributes to poor BP control rates and the progression of target-organ damage.

Adherence and Compliance Issues

Nonadherence to prescribed therapy is a major problem in the management of hypertensive patients, and maximizing adherence may be more important than choosing a specific drug regimen. Nonadherence to therapy is attributable to a variety of factors, including cost of medication and related care, inadequate patient education, complexity of the regimen, the patient's level of literacy and of education, and the adverse effects of medication. Clues to noncompliance include frequently missed appointments; failure to manifest the expected biologic effects of prescribed drugs, such as reduction of heart rate with beta-adrenergic blockers; and alcohol or other substance abuse.[67]

Compliance with antihypertensive treatment can be enhanced by a variety of strategies.[68] The cornerstone of these is the establishment of a good relationship with the patient and free and open communication about hypertension, its complications, and

the goals and pitfalls of treatment. Educational messages can be delivered by office personnel verbally, by written material, or by video presentations. A positive and supportive approach to treatment—with the message that a drug regimen that is effective, affordable, convenient, and relatively free of side effects can be found for almost every patient—yields the best results. The large number of antihypertensive medications now available, including sustained-release preparations and fixed-dose combinations, have made once-a-day dosing and smooth 24-hour control of BP a reality, thus improving the tolerability of multidrug antihypertensive regimens.

Comparison of Drug Classes

Two randomized trials have compared the effects of representatives of all the major classes of antihypertensive drugs in large numbers of patients with essential hypertension,[69,70] or hypertension of unknown origin, which includes 95% of all cases of hypertension. Both of these studies included only patients with uncomplicated stage 1 and stage 2 disease. The Treatment of Mild Hypertension Study—a randomized, double-blind, placebo-controlled clinical trial—compared the effects of five antihypertensive agents from different therapeutic classes (diuretics, alpha blockers, beta blockers, calcium channel blockers, and ACE inhibitors), combined with lifestyle modifications in persons with stage 1 essential hypertension for an average of 4.4 years. BP control and other outcome measures in the five drug-treatment groups did not differ significantly; all were significantly better than lifestyle modification alone. Adverse experiences did not differ significantly in the drug-treatment groups, except that diuretics were associated with a significantly higher incidence of sexual dysfunction in men.[71] The Department of Veterans Affairs Cooperative Study Group on Antihypertensive Agents compared the effects of six antihypertensive drugs from different classes, each of which was administered as monotherapy to a group of male veterans.[70] This study found that a sustained-release preparation of the calcium channel blocker diltiazem had a small but statistically significant advantage in controlling BP. Neither study had the power to compare the effects of the treatments on cardiovascular outcomes.

A meta-analysis of 23 randomized clinical trials representing 50,583 patients has addressed the comparative effectiveness of first-line antihypertensive drugs in lowering BP and preventing adverse outcomes.[45] Six possible first-line antihypertensive drugs were compared either with another drug or with placebo. The trials evaluated four drug classes: thiazides (21 trials), beta-adrenergic blockers (five trials), calcium channel blockers (four trials), and ACE inhibitors (one trial). In five trials comparing thiazides with beta blockers, thiazides were associated with a significantly lower rate of withdrawal caused by adverse effects. In the trials that included an untreated control group, low-dose thiazide therapy was associated with a significant reduction in the risk of death, stroke, coronary artery disease, and cardiovascular events. High-dose thiazide therapy, beta-blocker therapy, and calcium channel blocker therapy did not significantly reduce the risk of death or coronary artery disease. In both the drug-drug and the drug–no treatment comparison trials, thiazides were significantly better at reducing systolic BP than the other drug classes. These data indicate that low-dose thiazide therapy can be prescribed as first-line treatment of hypertension with the confidence that risk of death, coronary artery disease, and stroke will be reduced. Because of limitations in the availability of data from controlled trials, the same cannot be said for high-dose thiazide therapy, beta blockers, calcium channel blockers, ACE inhibitors, or ANG II receptor blockers. Preference for diuretics as first-line therapy for patients with uncomplicated essential hypertension is reflected in some,[9,72] but not all,[48] current consensus guidelines.

The Captopril Prevention Project (CAPPP),[73] a prospective, randomized, open trial with blinded end-point evaluation, compared the effects of the ACE inhibitor captopril with those of conventional therapy with diuretics, beta blockers, or both on cardiovascular disease morbidity. There was no difference between treatment groups in primary end-point events (a composite of fatal and nonfatal myocardial infarction, stroke, and other cardiovascular deaths). Cardiovascular mortality was lower with captopril than with conventional treatment. The two groups had similar rates of fatal and nonfatal myocardial infarction, but fatal and nonfatal stroke was more common in the captopril group. The difference in stroke risk was attributed to a disparity in BP that was observed throughout the trial (BP in the captopril group was 2 mm Hg higher than BP in the conventional-treatment group). Interestingly, significantly fewer patients developed diabetes in the captopril group than in the conventional-treatment group—a finding attributed by the investigators to the positive effect of captopril on insulin sensitivity. The subgroup of patients with diabetes had significantly fewer end points on captopril treatment than on conventional therapy. These results suggest that captopril and conventional antihypertensive treatment are equally effective in preventing cardiovascular morbidity and mortality in the hypertensive population as a whole. Whether these results can be generalized to other ACE inhibitors and whether the apparent benefits of captopril in diabetes will be seen in larger populations remain to be determined.

Because of their proven benefit in preventing cardiovascular morbidity and mortality in patients with left ventricular dysfunction and heart failure, some researchers have suggested that the ACE inhibitors may have protective effects in patients at high risk for cardiovascular events, independent of their BP status. The Heart Outcomes Prevention Evaluation (HOPE) study tested this hypothesis in 9,297 patients 55 years of age or older who had evidence of vascular disease or diabetes plus one other cardiovascular risk factor and who were not known to have a low ejection fraction or heart failure.[74] Half of the patients had a history of hypertension. Participants received ramipril (10 mg/day orally) or matching placebo for a mean of 5 years. Treatment with ramipril reduced the rates of death from cardiovascular causes, myocardial infarction, stroke, death from any cause, revascularization procedures, cardiac arrest, heart failure, and complications related to diabetes. Only a fraction of the benefit was attributable to reduction in BP (which averaged only 3/2 mm Hg in the course of the study) because the majority of participants were not hypertensive at baseline and the beneficial effects of ACE-inhibitor treatment were seen in both hypertensive and normotensive participants. Whether these results can be generalized to treatment with other ACE inhibitors or ANG II receptor antagonists, to hypertensive populations, to populations of different racial or ethnic composition, and to populations with different cardiovascular risk profiles remains to be investigated.

In contrast, the Swedish Trial in Old Patients with Hypertension-2 (STOP-2) study—a prospective, randomized trial in elderly hypertensive patients—confirmed the similarity between older and newer classes of antihypertensive drugs in prevention of cardiovascular morbidity and mortality.[75] Participants were randomly assigned to receive conventional antihypertensive drugs (atenolol, 50 mg/day; metoprolol, 100 mg/day; pindolol, 5 mg/day; or hydrochlorothiazide, 25 mg/day, plus amiloride, 2.5 mg/day) or newer drugs (enalapril, 10 mg/day; lisinopril, 10 mg/day; felodipine, 2.5 mg/day; or isradipine, 2.5 mg/day); additional medications were added as needed to control BP. Control of BP and overall reductions in cardiovascular end points were similar in patients treated with conventional drugs, ACE inhibitors, and calcium channel blockers, suggesting that BP reduction, rather than the specific treatment modality, was the prime determinant of outcome. There was, however, a significant reduction in fatal and nonfatal myocardial infarction and heart failure in the ACE-inhibitor group compared with the calcium channel blocker group.

Additional long-term controlled clinical trials are needed to clarify the benefits and risks of cardiovascular outcomes associated with BP reduction induced by the newer classes of antihypertensive agents, particularly in patients with multiple cardiovascular risk factors. Major clinical trials in progress around the world, with a projected patient enrollment of over 200,000, are addressing this issue.[43,76] Three to 5 years of follow-up will be required to determine significant differences in cardiovascular disease outcomes between the treatment arms of these costly and complex clinical trials. Thus, the data needed to help determine the optimal antihypertensive therapy will not be available before the year 2002.

General Treatment Strategies

In the interim, it seems most appropriate to use BP reduction as the primary surrogate end point for antihypertensive treatment and to individualize treatment on the basis of each patient's comorbid conditions and personal needs with respect to convenience, cost, and quality of life. Treatment should always include lifestyle modifications. When drug therapy is indicated, it is reasonable to initiate treatment with the agent that is expected to be best tolerated and is most likely to be effective in lowering BP in a given patient. Long-acting agents are preferable because adherence to therapy and consistency of BP control are superior with once-a-day dosing. When monotherapy is unsuccessful, a second agent, usually of a different class, should be added.

A novel strategy for optimizing initial antihypertensive drug therapy in younger patients was evaluated in a prospective rotation study of the four main classes of antihypertensive drugs: ACE inhibitors (A), beta blockers (B), calcium channel blockers (C), and diuretics (D).[77] This open-label crossover study was carried out in 56 young, untreated hypertensive patients. Significant variability in response to the four drug classes was found: 20 of 41 patients who ultimately reached target BP (≤ 140/90 mm Hg) failed to achieve the target on their first drug. Rotation increased the success of monotherapy from 22/56 (39%) to 41/56 (73%) ($P = 0.0001$). There were significant correlations between the BP responses to A and B ($r = 0.5$; $P < 0.01$) and C and D ($r = 0.6$, $P < 0.001$) but not between the other four pairings of treatments. The responses to the AB pair were, on average, at least 50% higher than those to the CD pair. The researchers concluded that because of individual differences among patients in the pathophysiology of their hypertension and their responsiveness to antihypertensive drugs, optimal treatment requires systematic rotation through several therapies. To facilitate the practical application of that concept, the researchers proposed an AB/CD rule in which one of each pair of treatments is selected initially to abbreviate the rotation procedure.

An interesting alternative approach is the use of low-dose, fixed-dose combination drugs. The rationale for this approach is that low doses of drugs with different mechanisms of action may have additive or synergistic effects on BP but cause minimal dose-dependent adverse effects and provide the convenience of

Table 4   Antihypertensive Drugs in Ambulatory Treatment of Hypertension

Drug	Adult Maintenance Dose (mg)	Drug	Adult Maintenance Dose (mg)
Diuretics		Terazosin (Hytrin)	1–20 s.i.d.
Thiazides		Doxazosin (Cardura)	1–16 s.i.d.
Chlorothiazide (Diuril)	250–500 b.i.d.	Combined alpha- and beta-adren-ergic blocking agents	
Hydrochlorothiazide (Esidrix, HydroDIURIL, Oretic)	12.5–50 s.i.d.	Labetalol (Normodyne)	200–1,200 b.i.d.
Bendroflumethiazide (Naturetin)	5–20 s.i.d.	(Trandate)	12.5–50 b.i.d.
Hydroflumethiazide (Saluron)	25–50 s.i.d.	Carvedilol (Coreg)	6.25–12.5 b.i.d.
(Diucardin)	25–100 s.i.d.	Ganglion blocking agent	
Methyclothiazide (Aquatensen, En-duron)	2.5–10.0 s.i.d.	Mecamylamine (Inversine)	2.5 b.i.d.
Polythiazide (Renese)	2–4 s.i.d.	*Angiotensin-Converting Enzyme Inhibitors*	
Trichlormethiazide (Naqua)	2–4 s.i.d.	Captopril (Capoten)	25–150 t.i.d.
Indapamide (Lozol)	1.25–2.5 s.i.d.	Enalapril (Vasotec)	5–40 b.i.d.
Phthalimidines		Lisinopril (Prinivil, Zestril)	5–40 s.i.d.
Chlorthalidone (Thalitone)	12.5–50 s.i.d.	Quinapril (Accupril)	5–80 s.i.d. or t.i.d.
(Hygroton)	12.5–100 s.i.d.	Ramipril (Altace)	1.25–20 s.i.d. or t.i.d.
Metolazone (Mykrox)	0.5–1 s.i.d.	Benazepril (Lotensin)	5–40 s.i.d. or t.i.d.
(Zaroxolyn)	2.5–10 s.i.d.	Fosinopril (Monopril)	10–80 s.i.d. or t.i.d.
Loop diuretics		Spiropril	12.5–50 s.i.d. or t.i.d.
Furosemide (Lasix)	20–1,000 b.i.d. or t.i.d.	Moexipril (Univasc)	7.5–30 s.i.d. or t.i.d.
Ethacrynic acid (Edecrin)	25–100 b.i.d. or t.i.d.	Perindopril (Aceon)	4–8 s.i.d.
Bumetanide (Bumex)	0.5–4.0 b.i.d. or t.i.d.	Trandolapril (Mavik)	1–4 s.i.d.
Torsemide (Demadex)	5–40 s.i.d. or t.i.d.	*Angiotensin II Receptor Antagonists*	
Potassium-sparing diuretics		Losartan (Cozaar)	50–100 s.i.d.
Spironolactone (Aldactone)	25–100 s.i.d.	Valsartan (Diovan)	80–160 s.i.d.
Triamterene (Dyrenium)	25–100 s.i.d.	Candesartan cilexitil (Atacand)	8–32 s.i.d.
Amiloride (Midamor)	5–10 s.i.d.	Eprosartan (Teveten)	400–1,200 s.i.d.
		Irbesartan (Avapro)	75–300 s.i.d.
Sympatholytics		Telmisartan (Micardis)	40–80 s.i.d.
Centrally acting agents		*Calcium Channel Blocking Agents*	
Methyldopa (Aldomet)	250–2,000 b.i.d.	Phenylalkylamines	
Clonidine tablets (Catapres)	0.2–1.2 b.i.d. or t.i.d.	Verapamil (Tiazac, Isoptin, Calan, Verelan)	90–480 b.i.d.
Clonidine patch (Catapres-TTS)	1 patch weekly (0.1, 0.2, or 0.3 mg)	Verapamil sustained release (Isoptin SR, Calan SR)	120–480 s.i.d. or b.i.d.
Guanfacine (Tenex)	1–3 s.i.d.	(Covera-HS)	180–480 s.i.d. or b.i.d.
Guanabenz (Wytensin)	8–32 b.i.d.	Benzothiazepines	
Peripherally acting agents		Diltiazem (Cardizem)	90–360 b.i.d. or t.i.d.
Reserpine	0.05–0.25 s.i.d.	Diltiazem sustained release (Cardizem SR)	120–360 s.i.d.
Guanethidine (Ismelin)	10–150 s.i.d.	(Cardizem CD)	120–360 s.i.d.
Guanadrel (Hylorel)	10–75 b.i.d.	(Dilacor XR)	120–480 s.i.d.
Beta-adrenergic blocking agents		Dihydropyridines	
Propranolol (Inderal)	40–640 b.i.d.	Nifedipine* (Procardia)	30–120 t.i.d. or q.i.d.
Propranolol sustained release (In-deral LA)	80–640 s.i.d.	(Adalat)	30–180 t.i.d. or q.i.d.
Carteolol (Cartrol)	2.5–10 s.i.d.	Nifedipine sustained release (Procardia XL)	30–120 s.i.d.
Betaxolol (Kerlone)	5–20 s.i.d.	(Adalat CC)	30–120 s.i.d.
Metoprolol (Lopressor)	50–300 b.i.d.	Nicardipine (Cardene)	30–90 t.i.d.
Metoprolol sustained release (Toprol XL)	50–300 s.i.d.	Nicardipine sustained release (Cardene SR)	60–90 b.i.d.
Bisoprolol (Zebeta)	2.5–10 s.i.d.	Isradipine (DynaCirc)	2.5–20 b.i.d.
Atenolol (Tenormin)	25–100 b.i.d.	Amlodipine (Norvasc)	2.5–10 s.i.d.
Nadolol (Corgard)	40–320 s.i.d.	Felodipine sustained release (Plendil)	2.5–20 s.i.d.
Timolol (Blocadren)	20–60 b.i.d.	Tetralol derivative	
Pindolol (Visken)	10–60 b.i.d.	Mibefradil (Posicor)	50–100 s.i.d.
Acebutolol (Sectral)	400–1,200 b.i.d. or t.i.d.		
Penbutolol (Levatol)	10–20 s.i.d.	*Direct Vasodilators*	
Alpha-adrenergic blocking agents		Hydralazine (Apresoline)	20–300 b.i.d. or t.i.d.
Prazosin (Minipress)	2.5–20 b.i.d. or t.i.d.	Minoxidil (Loniten)	5–100 s.i.d. or b.i.d.20

*The Food and Drug Administration has issued a warning discouraging use of short-acting nifedipine, particularly at high doses, for hypertension.

Table 5 Combination Agents for Treatment of Hypertension

Drug	Daily Dose (pills/day)	Pill Content (mg/mg)
Combination Diuretics		
HCTZ/amiloride (Moduretic)	1 or 2	50/5
HCTZ/spironolactone (Aldactazide)	1 or 2	25/25
HCTZ/triamterene (Maxzide)	1 or 2	25/37.5; 50/75
HCTZ/triamterene (Dyazide)	1 or 2	25/37.5
ACE Inhibitors and Diuretics		
Benazepril/HCTZ (Lotensin HCT)	1 or 2	5/6.25; 10/12.5; 20/12.5; 20/25
Captopril/HCTZ (Capozide)	2 or 4	25/15; 25/25; 50/15; 50/25
Enalapril/HCTZ (Vaseretic)	1 or 2	5/12.5; 10/25
Lisinopril/HCTZ (Zestoretic, Prinzide)	1 or 2	10/12.5; 20/12.5; 20/25
Moexipril/HCTZ (Uniretic)	1 or 2	7.5/12.5; 15/25
Angiotensin II Receptor Antagonists and Diuretics		
Irbesartan/HCTZ (Avalide)	1	150/12.5; 300/12.5
Losartan/HCTZ (Hyzaar)	1 or 2	50/12.5; 100/12.5
Valsartan/HCTZ (Diovan HCT)	1	80/12.5; 160/12.5
Beta-blocking Agents and Diuretics		
Atenolol/chlorthalidone (Tenoretic)	1	50/25; 100/25
Bisoprolol/HCTZ (Ziac)	1 or 2	2.5/6.25; 5/6.25; 10/6.25
Nadolol/bendroflumethiazide (Corzide)	1	40/5; 80/5
Propranolol/HCTZ (Inderide)	2 to 4	40/25; 80/25
Propranolol LA/HCTZ (Inderide LA)	1	80/50; 120/50; 160/50
Timolol/HCTZ (Timolide)	1 or 2	10/25
Calcium Channel Blockers and ACE Inhibitors		
Amlodipine/benazepril (Lotrel)	1	2.5/5; 5/10; 10/20
Diltiazem/enalapril (Teczem)	1 or 2	180/5
Felodipine/enalapril (Lexxel)	1 or 2	5/5
Verapamil/Trandolapril (Mavik)	1	180/2; 240/1; 240/2; 240/4
Vasodilators and Diuretics		
Hydralazine/HCTZ (Apresazide)	2 to 4	25/25; 50/50; 100/50
Prazosin/polythiazide (Minizide)	2 to 4	1/0.5; 2/0.5; 3/0.5
Centrally Acting Agents and Diuretics		
Clonidine/chlorthalidone (Combipres)	2 or 3	0.1/0.2; 0.3/15
Deserpidine/methyclothiazide (Enduronyl)	0.5 to 2	0.25/50
(Enduronyl-Forte)	0.5 to 5	0.5/50
Deserpidine/HCTZ (Oreticyl)	2 to 4	0.125/25; 0.125/50
(Oreticyl-Forte)	2 to 4	0.250/25
Guanethidine/HCTZ I (Esimil)	1 to 4	10/25
Methyldopa/chlorothiazide (Aldoclor)	2 to 8	250/150; 250/250
Methyldopa/HCTZ (Aldoril)	2 to 4	250/15; 250/25; 500/30; 500/50
Reserpine/chlorothiazide (Diupres)	1 or 2	0.125/250; 0.125/500
Reserpine/methyclothiazide (Diutensen-R)	1 to 4	0.1/2.5
Reserpine/HCTZ (Hydropres)	1 or 2	0.125/25; 0.125/50
Reserpine/polythiazide (Renese-R)	0.5 to 2	0.25/2
Reserpine/hydroflumethiazide (Salutensin-Demi)	1	0.125/25
(Salutensin)	1	0.125/50
Reserpine/chlorthalidone (Demi-Regroton)	1	0.125/25
(Regroton)	1	0.25/50
Rauwolfia/bendroflumethiazide (Rauzide)	1 to 4	50/4
Other Combinations		
Reserpine/hydralazine/HCTZ (Ser-Ap-Es)	3 to 6	0.1/25/15

HCTZ—hydrochlorothiazide   ACE—angiotensin-converting enzyme

single-tablet dosing.[78] Low-dose combination therapy with biso-prolol plus hydrochlorothiazide[79] and reserpine plus the thiazide clopamide[80] has been shown to be more effective and better tolerated than monotherapy with representatives of the newer classes of antihypertensive agents. In contrast, traditional fixed-dose combinations, which contain full conventional doses of each component, have usually been reserved for patients who do not respond adequately to monotherapy.

After therapy has been initiated, patients should be seen every 1 to 4 weeks (depending on the severity of hypertension) to titrate antihypertensive drug dosage and every 3 to 4 months once BP control is achieved. Patients should be encouraged to measure and

Table 6   Common Adverse Effects of Antihypertensive Drugs

Drugs	*Side Effects*	*Precautions and Special Considerations*
Diuretics		
Thiazides and related sulfonamides	Hypokalemia, hyperuricemia, glucose intolerance, hypercholesterolemia, hypertriglyceridemia, sexual dysfunction	May be ineffective in renal failure; hypokalemia increases digitalis toxicity; hyperuricemia may precipitate acute gout
Loop diuretics	Same as for thiazides	Effective in chronic renal failure; cautions regarding hypokalemia and hyperuricemia same as above; hyponatremia may occur, especially in elderly patients
Potassium-sparing agents	Hyperkalemia	Danger of hyperkalemia in patients with renal failure or diabetes or those receiving angiotensin-converting enzyme inhibitors
Amiloride	Sexual dysfunction	
Spironolactone	Gynecomastia, mastodynia, sexual dysfunction	
Adrenergic Antagonists		
Beta-adrenergic blockers	Bradycardia, fatigue, insomnia, bizarre dreams, sexual dysfunction, hypertriglyceridemia, decreased high-density lipoprotein cholesterol	Should not be used in patients with asthma, chronic obstructive pulmonary disease, congestive heart failure, heart block (> first degree), and sick sinus syndrome Use with caution in patients with diabetes and peripheral vascular disease; sudden withdrawal of these drugs may be hazardous
Centrally acting agents		Rebound hypertension may occur with abrupt discontinuance
Methyldopa	Drowsiness, dry mouth, fatigue	May cause liver damage and positive direct Coombs' test (rare hemolytic anemia)
Reserpine	Sexual dysfunction, nasal congestion, lethargy	Contraindicated in patients with a history of depression; use with caution in patients with a history of peptic ulcer
Alpha$_1$-adrenergic blockers	First-dose syncope, orthostatic hypotension, weakness, palpitations, dizziness, headache, fluid retention	Use cautiously in elderly patients
Combined alpha- and beta-adrenergic blockers	Nausea, fatigue, dizziness, headache, orthostatic hypotension	Use with caution in patients with cardiac failure, chronic obstructive pulmonary disease, sick sinus syndrome, heart block (> first degree), diabetes
Vasodilators	Headache, tachycardia, fluid retention	May precipitate angina in patients with coronary artery disease
Hydralazine	Positive antinuclear antibody (without other changes)	Lupus syndrome may occur (rarely with recommended doses)
Minoxidil	Hypertrichosis, ascites (rare)	May cause or aggravate pleural and pericardial effusions
Angiotensin-Converting Enzyme Inhibitors	Cough	Can cause reversible acute renal failure in patients with renal artery stenosis; neutropenia may occur in patients with autoimmune collagen disorders; may cause fetal injury
Angiotensin II Receptor Antagonists	Dizziness	Can cause reversible acute renal failure in patients with renal artery stenosis; may cause fetal injury
Calcium Channel Blocking Agents	Headache, hypotension, dizziness	
Verapamil	Constipation, bradycardia	Use with caution in patients with congestive heart failure or heart block

record their own BP levels at home or in the workplace as an aid to adherence and improved BP control. Recommended dose ranges are listed for individual drugs [*see Table 4*] and combination agents [*see Table 5*]; common adverse effects are summarized [*see Table 6*].

Step-down therapy, or withdrawing antihypertensive medication under close monitoring, should be attempted in patients with stage 1 or stage 2 hypertension whose BP has been adequately controlled for 1 year or more. This strategy is most likely to be successful in patients with well-controlled hypertension who have been recently (within 5 years) diagnosed or treated, or both, and who adhere to lifestyle interventions such as weight loss and dietary modifications.[81] More than 80% of these patients succeed in medication withdrawal for longer than 1 year. Dosages should be titrated slowly downward and medications discontinued one at a time, if possible. Step-down therapy is generally most effective for patients who are also making lifestyle modifications.

SPECIAL PATIENT GROUPS

Comorbid conditions that influence the choice of antihyperten-

sive therapy have been demonstrated in an estimated 50% to 70% of patients with essential hypertension, particularly in the elderly.[82] The most common of these are related to target-organ damage and major cardiovascular risk factors, including dyslipidemia, congestive heart failure, ischemic heart disease, and diabetes mellitus. For the minority of hypertensive patients without comorbid conditions, diuretics or beta blockers should be considered for initial monotherapy because in randomized clinical trials, they have been shown to prevent cardiovascular morbidity and mortality related to hypertension and because they are less costly than the newer classes of agents. For patients with coexistent diabetes mellitus or cardiovascular disease, there are compelling indications, based on randomized controlled trials, for initial drug choices from specific drug classes [*see Figure 1*]. Other common conditions in middle-aged and elderly hypertensive patients that may influence drug selection include benign prostatic hyperplasia and osteoporosis. Agents that have added benefit for patients with these conditions should be included as part of the treatment program [*see Table 7*], although additional drugs may be needed to bring BP under con-

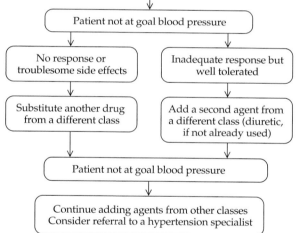

Begin or continue lifestyle modifications

↓

Patient not at goal blood pressure (< 140/90 mm Hg)
Lower goals for patients with diabetes or renal disease

↓

Initial Drug Choices*

Uncomplicated Hypertension
Diuretics
Beta blockers

*Specific Indications for the
Following Drugs*

ACE inhibitors†
Angiotensin II
  receptor blockers
Alpha blockers
Alpha-beta blockers
Beta blockers
Calcium antagonists
Diuretics

Compelling Indications
Insulin-dependent diabetes
  mellitus with proteinuria
  • ACE inhibitors†
Heart failure
  • ACE inhibitors†
  • Diuretics
Isolated systolic hypertension
  (older persons)
  • Diuretics preferred
  • Long-acting dihydropyridine
    calcium antagonists
Myocardial infarction
  • Beta blockers (non-ISA)
  • ACE inhibitors (with
    systolic dysfunction)†

  • Start with a low dose of a long-acting once-daily drug,
    and titrate dose
  • Low-dose combinations may be appropriate

↓

Patient not at goal blood pressure

↓   ↓

No response or   Inadequate response but
troublesome side effects   well tolerated

↓   ↓

Substitute another drug   Add a second agent from
from a different class   a different class (diuretic,
                                     if not already used)

↓

Patient not at goal blood pressure

↓

Continue adding agents from other classes
Consider referral to a hypertension specialist

* Unless contraindicated.

† In cases in which ACE inhibitors are the preferred therapy, angiotensin II receptor antagonists may be substituted in patients intolerant to ACE inhibitors. The efficacy of angiotensin II receptor antagonists and of ACE inhibitors in these patients are currently being compared in clinical trials (see text).

Figure 1 **Treatment algorithm for patients with primary hypertension. If goal blood pressure is not achieved in response to a given intervention, the additional interventions indicated in the lower boxes are added.[9] (ACE—angiotensin-converting enzyme; ISA—intrinsic sympathomimetic activity)**

trol. Agents that have adverse effects on these comorbid conditions should not be selected as first- or second-line therapy but may occasionally be needed to control BP in patients with resistant hypertension who also have one of these comorbid conditions.

HYPERTENSIVE CRISIS

Hypertensive crisis is a severe elevation in BP, arbitrarily defined as a diastolic BP of 120 to 130 mm Hg.[83] However, the rate of rise in BP is more important than the absolute BP recorded in de-

termining whether the patient with very high BP needs emergency treatment. Patients with chronic hypertension can tolerate much higher elevations in BP than previously normotensive persons. Encephalopathy, for example, rarely develops in patients with long-standing hypertension until the diastolic BP exceeds 150 mm Hg. Conversely, a young woman with preeclampsia may become encephalopathic with a diastolic BP of 100 mm Hg or less.

Hypertensive crisis occurs most commonly in patients with a history of hypertension who have failed to comply with their prescribed antihypertensive medications or have been undermedicated. In this setting, rising BP is thought to cause endothelial damage, releasing vasoconstrictor substances such as endothelin, ANG II, and norepinephrine. A vicious circle of release of additional vasoconstrictor substances and further increases in peripheral resistance is initiated, and in a hypertensive emergency, life-threatening target-organ damage ensues.[83]

The history and the physical and laboratory evaluation of a patient with severely elevated BP should be directed toward identifying target-organ damage and possible secondary causes of the BP elevation [*see Table 8*]. Patients with evidence of acute or ongoing target-organ damage require immediate BP reduction, generally by means of intravenous therapy in the intensive care setting. The goal in treating most hypertensive emergencies is to reduce BP promptly but gradually. Precipitous reductions in BP and reductions to normotensive levels should be avoided because they may provoke target-organ ischemia or infarction. In general, reductions in mean arterial pressure should not exceed 20% in the first 1 to 2 hours.[84] Further reductions should be achieved gradually over the ensuing 24 to 48 hours. In most cases, sodium nitroprusside is the drug of choice for treatment in hypertensive emergencies. Its immediate onset of action and short half-life allow for effective minute-by-minute titration. Risk of toxicity from thiocyanate and cyanide, which are metabolites of nitroprusside, is increased in patients with renal or hepatic insufficiency. Patients experiencing a hypertensive crisis are at increased risk for a secondary cause of hypertension. If the initial evaluation is not revealing, a more extensive workup should be performed once the BP is stabilized.

Patients with severely elevated BP without evidence of acute or ongoing target-organ damage (urgent hypertensive crisis) are more likely to be harmed than helped by acute, aggressive BP reduction. Such patients do well without acute BP reduction,[84] and abrupt BP reduction in previously asymptomatic patients with severe hypertension is fraught with serious complications.[85] Accordingly, in patients with severe but asymptomatic BP elevation, immediate BP reduction is not indicated. In particular, sublingual or oral administration of short-acting nifedipine, which can induce dramatic BP lowering, is strongly discouraged.[86] Often, allowing a patient with severely elevated BP to sit for 20 to 30 minutes in a quiet area will facilitate a significant BP reduction. Afterward, oral antihypertensive therapy should be initiated in the previously untreated patient, resumed in the noncompliant patient, or adjusted in the undermedicated patient. Follow-up should be within 24 hours to ensure patient compliance and BP control.

Secondary Hypertension

Secondary hypertension is hypertension of known etiology. It accounts for fewer than 5% of all cases of hypertension.

RENOVASCULAR HYPERTENSION

The prevalence of RAS increases with increasing severity of hypertension, ranging from 1% in patients with a diastolic BP of

Table 7 Effects of Antihypertensive Drugs on Comorbid Conditions

Comorbid Condition	Beneficial Effects	Adverse Effects
Angina pectoris	Beta-adrenergic blockers are given as first-line therapy; calcium channel blockers are given as second-line therapy	—
Benign prostatic hyperplasia	Alpha-adrenergic blockers reduce prostate size	—
Diabetes mellitus	ACE inhibitors and probably angiotensin II type 1 receptor blockers delay the progression of renal failure and proteinuria in insulin-dependent and ?non–insulin-dependent diabetes mellitus with proteinuria	Thiazide diuretics may worsen biochemical abnormalities; beta-adrenergic blockers mask symptoms of hypoglycemia
Dyslipidemia	Alpha blockers increase HDL cholesterol levels and reduce LDL cholesterol and triglyceride levels	Thiazide diuretics in high doses increase LDL cholesterol levels; beta-adrenergic blockers that lack intrinsic sympathomimetic activity reduce HDL cholesterol levels and increase LDL cholesterol levels
Congestive heart failure	Loop diuretics, ACE inhibitors, angiotensin II type 1 receptor blockers, and carvedilol (?low-dose beta-adrenergic blockers) relieve symptoms and may prolong life	Beta-adrenergic blockers and calcium channel blockers in high doses may worsen failure
Ischemic heart disease	ACE inhibitors and beta-adrenergic blockers are indicated for secondary prevention of MI	Short-acting dihydropyridine calcium channel blockers may increase mortality and incidence of MI
Osteoporosis	Thiazide diuretics retard bone loss and prevent fractures	—

ACE—angiotensin-converting enzyme   HDL—high-density lipoprotein   LDL—low-density lipoprotein   MI—myocardial infarction

less than 90 mm Hg to more than 30% in patients with a diastolic BP greater than 125 mm Hg. RAS occurs in about 75% of cases of atherosclerotic disease, compared with 25% of cases of fibromuscular dysplasia. RAS is less common in African Americans than in white Americans. Patients most likely to have renovascular hypertension include those who have hypertension of abrupt onset, especially those who are young, in late middle age, or elderly; those who experience malignant hypertension (diastolic BP > 140 mm Hg and the presence of papilledema) or sudden acceleration of benign hypertension (elevated BP and grade 3 Kimmelstiel-Wilson retinopathy); and those who fail to respond to medical therapy. The presence of an upper abdominal bruit, particularly one that is systolic-diastolic or continuous in timing, is high pitched, and radiates laterally from the midepigastrium, strongly suggests functionally significant RAS. Such bruits have been described in one half to two thirds of patients with surgically proven renovascular hypertension. A precipitous drop in BP, acute deterioration in renal function in response to ACE inhibitor therapy, or both suggest possible RAS and warrant further workup.

Screening tests for RAS, including the captopril renogram, duplex ultrasonography, and magnetic resonance imaging angiography, have a sensitivity that approaches 95% to 100% under optimal conditions. Because the predictive value of such tests is extremely operator dependent, patients should be referred to experienced, high-volume centers for testing. Renal arteriography is required for definitive diagnosis and presurgical evaluation. Renal vein renin sampling may be necessary to identify the culprit kidney in the setting of bilateral RAS.

Table 8 Types of Hypertensive Crises and Treatment Considerations

Crisis	Recommended Treatment	Comments
Encephalopathy	Nitroprusside	Avoid hydralazine; it may raise intracranial pressure
Myocardial infarction, unstable angina	Nitroglycerin	Reduce BP until pain is relieved or to diastolic BP of 100 mm Hg; use in conjunction with conventional treatment (thrombolytics, aspirin, oxygen, morphine, or beta blockers); avoid diazoxide and hydralazine, which may increase oxygen demand; dihydropyridines may worsen angina; reserve nitroprusside for refractory cases because it may induce coronary steal
Congestive heart failure	Nitroprusside	Use in conjunction with loop diuretics, morphine, and oxygen
Subarachnoid hemorrhage, intra-cerebral hemorrhage, stroke	Nitroprusside	Blood pressure reduction is controversial because it may provoke tissue hypoperfusion; generally recommended for severe hypertension (systolic BP > 220 mm Hg or diastolic BP > 120 mm Hg)
Dissecting aneurysm	Nitroprusside with a beta blocker	Immediate blood pressure reduction is essential; trimethaphan is a good alternative; avoid hydralazine and diazoxide because they may increase shear force
Pheochromocytoma, cocaine overdose	Phentolamine	Labetalol is effective, but there are anecdotal reports of paradoxical increases in blood pressure; use nitroprusside for refractory cases; with cocaine, sedation alone may be effective; unopposed beta blockade may precipitate or worsen crisis
Renal insufficiency	Nitroprusside	Calcium antagonists and labetalol are good alternatives; monitor cyanide and thiocyanate levels
Postoperative hypertension	Nitroprusside	Nicardipine and labetalol are good alternatives

The natural history of RAS is progressive arterial occlusion with loss of renal function. The treatment of choice is revascularization via angioplasty or surgery. For patients with obstruction of inflow to the renal artery caused by aortic plaque (ostial lesions) and those who have undergone unsuccessful balloon angioplasty, renal artery stents are useful in maintaining renal artery patency.[87] Renal revascularization is seldom successful in curing hypertension in middle-aged or elderly patients with atherosclerotic RAS but is useful in improving the ease of BP control with medical therapy and in preserving renal function.

For patients in whom revascularization is not possible, strict BP control should be attempted. Use of an ACE inhibitor, alone or in combination with a diuretic, is preferred, except in bilateral RAS, RAS in a solitary kidney, or unilateral RAS with severe parenchymal disease in the contralateral kidney. Renal function and serum potassium levels must be monitored closely, particularly when ACE inhibitor therapy is initiated.

PRIMARY ALDOSTERONISM

Increased aldosterone production by an adrenal adenoma or hyperplastic adrenal glands produces hypertension associated with a tendency to lose potassium. Hypokalemia or difficulty maintaining normal serum potassium levels despite replacement therapy in a patient with resistant hypertension is a clue to the diagnosis. Screening tests include measurement of plasma aldosterone and renin activity (aldosterone-renin ratios greater than 25:1 suggest inappropriate aldosterone release) in patients who have not received ACE inhibitor therapy in the month before study. Confirmatory tests include measurement of 24-hour urinary aldosterone excretion in patients on a high-salt diet (values greater than 14 µg in 24 hours are abnormal).[88] Definitive diagnosis is by abdominal computed tomography or MRI. Adrenal adenomas constitute 65% of the cases of primary aldosteronism. If multiple nodules are seen or risk of an undetected adenoma remains, adrenal vein sampling for aldosterone assay can be attempted. In the absence of adenoma (or, in rare cases, carcinoma), idiopathic aldosteronism and bilateral hyperplasia are diagnoses of exclusion.

The treatment for unilateral adenomas is adrenalectomy. Idiopathic aldosteronism, bilateral hyperplasia, and bilateral adenomas are generally treated medically. The aldosterone antagonist spironolactone is generally used for women, whereas amiloride is used for men because spironolactone causes gynecomastia in some patients.

SLEEP APNEA

Approximately 50% of patients with obstructive sleep apnea are also hypertensive. Conversely, as many as 30% of hypertensive patients are estimated to have sleep apnea.[89] If there is a causal relation between the two disorders, it is most commonly thought that recurrent hypoxia induced by sleep apnea triggers sustained increases in peripheral resistance and cardiac output, in part secondary to chronic sympathetic activation. Alternatively, hypertension and sleep apnea may simply share risk factors, such as age and obesity, and occur independently. Furthermore, sleep deprivation in untreated or inadequately treated hypertensive patients may increase sympathetic nerve activity during the night and the following morning, leading to increased BP and heart rate and increased risk for both target-organ damage and cardiovascular events.[90] Effective treatment of sleep apnea has been shown to benefit BP control.[66] Therefore, all patients being evaluated for hypertension should be screened for sleep apnea. There is no evidence that one class of antihypertensive agents is any more advantageous than any other class in patients with sleep apnea.

References

1. Van den Hoogen PCW, Feskens EJM, Nagelkerke NJD, et al: The relation between blood pressure and mortality due to coronary heart disease among men in different parts of the world. N Engl J Med 342:1, 2000

2. Mosterd A, D'Agostino RB, Silbershatz H, et al: Trends in the prevalence of hypertension, antihypertensive therapy, and left ventricular hypertrophy from 1950 to 1989. N Engl J Med 340:1221, 1999

3. Burt VL, Whelton P, Roccella EJ, et al: Prevalence of hypertension in the US adult population: results from the third National Health and Nutrition Examination Survey. Hypertension 25:305, 1995

4. Collins R, MacMahon S: Blood pressure, antihypertensive drug treatment and the risks of stroke and of coronary heart disease. Br Med Bull 50:272, 1994

5. US Renal Data System: USRDS 1999 Annual Data Report. US Department of Health and Human Services, National Institute of Diabetes and Digestive and Kidney Disease, Bethesda, Maryland, April 1999 [http://www.usrds.org]

6. Levy D, Larson MG, Vasan RS, et al: The progression from hypertension to congestive heart failure. JAMA 275:1557, 1996

7. Siegel D, Lopez J: Trends in antihypertensive drug use in the United States: do the JNC V recommendations affect prescribing? Fifth Joint National Commission on the Detection, Evaluation, and Treatment of High Blood Pressure. JAMA 278:1745, 1997

8. Mehta SS, Wilcox CS, Schulman KA: Treatment of hypertension in patients with comorbidities: results from the study of hypertensive prescribing practices. Am J Hypertens 12:333, 1999

9. The sixth report of the Joint National Committee on Prevention, Detection, Evaluation, and Treatment of High Blood Pressure (JNC VI). Arch Intern Med 157:2413, 1997

10. Oparil S: Arterial hypertension. Cecil Textbook of Medicine, 21st ed. Goldman L, Bennett JC, Eds. WB Saunders Co, Philadelphia, 2000, p 258

11. Lifton RP: Molecular genetics of human blood pressure variation. Science 272:676, 1996

12. Lander ES, Schork NJ: Genetic dissection of complex traits. Science 265:2037, 1994

13. Lifton RP, Dluhy RG, Powers M, et al: A chimaeric 11β-hydroxylase/aldosterone synthase gene causes glucocorticoid-remediable aldosteronism and human hypertension. Nature 355:262, 1992

14. Mune T, Rogerson FM, Nikkila H, et al: Human hypertension caused by mutations in the kidney isozyme of 11β-hydroxysteroid dehydrogenase. Nat Genet 10:394, 1995

15. Ulick S, Chan CK, Gill JR Jr, et al: Defective fasciculata zone function as the mechanism of glucocorticoid-remediable aldosteronism. J Clin Endocrinol Metab 71:1151, 1990

16. Stewart PM, Wallace AM, Valentino R, et al: Mineralocorticoid activity of liquorice: 11-beta-hydroxysteroid dehydrogenase deficiency comes of age. Lancet 2:821, 1987

17. Bubien JK, Ismailov II, Berdiev BK, et al: Liddle's disease: abnormal regulation of amiloride-sensitive Na+ channels by β-subunit mutation. Am J Physiol 270:C208, 1996

18. Shimkets RA, Warnock DG, Bositis CM, et al: Liddle's syndrome: heritable human hypertension caused by mutations in the β subunit of the epithelial sodium channel. Cell 79:407, 1994

19. Schild L, Canessa CM, Shimkets RA, et al: A mutation in the epithelial sodium channel causing Liddle disease increases channel activity in the Xenopus laevis oocyte expression system. Proc Natl Acad Sci USA 92:5699, 1995

20. Guyton AC: Blood pressure control: special role of the kidneys and body fluids. Science 252:1813, 1991

21. Fuster V, Pearson TA: 27th Bethesda Conference: matching the intensity of risk factor management with the hazard for coronary disease events. J Am Coll Cardiol 27:957, 1996

22. Selby JV, Newman B, Quiroga J, et al: Concordance for dyslipidemic hypertension in male twins. JAMA 265:2079, 1991

23. National High Blood Pressure Education Program Working Group report on hypertension in diabetes. The National High Blood Pressure Education Program Working Group. Hypertension 23:145, 1994

24. Reaven GM, Lithell H, Landsberg L: Hypertension and associated metabolic abnormalities—the role of insulin resistance and the sympathoadrenal system. N Engl J Med 334:374, 1996

25. Mark AL: The sympathetic nervous system in hypertension: a potential long-term regulator of arterial pressure. J Hypertens 14(suppl 5):S159, 1996

26. Esler MD: Catecholamines and essential hypertension. Baillieres Clin Endocrinol Metab 7:415, 1993

27. Calhoun DA, Mutinga ML: Race, family history of hypertension, and sympathetic response to cold pressor testing. Blood Pressure 6:209, 1997

28. Balcells E, Meng QC, Johnson WH, et al: Angiotensin II formation from ACE and chymase in human and animal hearts: methods and species considerations. Am J Physiol 273:H1769, 1997

29. Lüscher TF: The endothelium in hypertension: bystander, target or mediator? J Hypertens 12(suppl):S105, 1994

30. Krum H, Viskoper RJ, Lacourciere Y, et al: The effect of an endothelin receptor antagonist, bosentan, on blood pressure in patients with essential hypertension. N Engl J Med 338:784, 1998

31. National High Blood Pressure Education Program Working Group report on primary prevention of hypertension. The National High Blood Pressure Education Program Working Group. Arch Intern Med 153:186, 1993

32. Stamler J, Stamler R, Neaton JD: Blood pressure, systolic and diastolic and cardiovascular risks. Arch Intern Med 153:598, 1993

33. Klag MJ, Whelton PK, Randall BL, et al: Blood pressure and end-stage renal disease in men. N Engl J Med 334:13, 1996

34. Alli C, Avanzini F, Bettelli G, et al: The long-term prognostic significance of repeated blood pressure measurements in the elderly. Arch Intern Med 159:1205, 1999

35. Franklin SS, Khan SA, Wong ND, et al: Is pulse pressure useful in predicting risk for coronary heart disease? The Framingham Heart Study. Circulation 100:354, 1999

36. Lloyd-Jones DM, Evans JC, Larson MG, et al: Differential impact of systolic and diastolic blood pressure level on JNC-VI staging. Hypertension 34:381, 1999

37. Chae CU, Pfeffer MA, Glynn RJ, et al: Increased pulse pressure and risk of heart failure in the elderly. JAMA 281:634, 1999

38. Morbidity and mortality in the placebo-controlled European Trial on Isolated Systolic Hypertension in the Elderly. Systolic Hypertension-Europe (SYST-EUR) Trial Investigators. Lancet 360:757, 1997

39. SHEP Cooperative Research Group: Prevention of stroke by antihypertensive drug treatment in older persons with isolated systolic hypertension: final results of the Systolic Hypertension in the Elderly Program. JAMA 265:3255, 1991

40. Somes G, Pahor M, Shorr R, et al: The role of diastolic blood pressure when treating isolated systolic hypertension. Arch Intern Med 159:2004, 1999

41. Oparil S: Antihypertensive therapy and atherosclerosis in coronary heart disease. Cardiovasc Risk Factors 6:222, 1996

42. Psaty BM, Smith NL, Siscovick DS, et al: Health outcomes associated with antihypertensive therapies used as first-line agents. JAMA 277:739, 1997

43. Mulrow CD, Cornell JA, Herrera CR, et al: Hypertension in the elderly: implications and generalizability of randomized trials. JAMA 272:1932, 1994

44. Psaty BM, Furberg CK: Antihypertensive treatment trials: morbidity and mortality. Hypertension Primer: The Essentials of High Blood Pressure. Izzo JL, Black HR, Eds. American Heart Association, Dallas, 1993, p 197

45. Wright JM, Lee CH, Chambers GK: Systematic review of antihypertensive therapies: does the evidence assist in choosing a first-line drug? CMAJ 161:25, 1999

46. Du X, Cruickshank K, McNamee R, et al: Case-control study of stroke and the quality of hypertension control in northwest England. BMJ 314:272, 1997

47. Lazarus JM, Bourgoignie JJ, Buckalew VM: Achievement and safety of a low blood pressure goal in chronic renal disease. Hypertension 29:641, 1997

48. 1999 World Health Organization-International Society of Hypertension guidelines for the management of hypertension. Guidelines Subcommittee. J Hypertens 17:151, 1999

49. McCarron DA, Oparil S, Chait A, et al: Nutritional management of cardiovascular risk factors: a randomized clinical trial. Arch Intern Med 157:169, 1997

50. Appel LJ, Moore TJ, Obarzanek E, et al: The effect of dietary patterns on blood pressure: results from the Dietary Approaches to Stop Hypertension (DASH) Clinical Trial. N Engl J Med 336:1117, 1997

51. Svetkey LP, Simons-Morton D, Vollmer WM, et al: Effects of dietary patterns on blood pressure subgroup analysis of the Dietary Approaches to Stop Hypertension (DASH) randomized clinical trial. Arch Intern Med 159:285, 1999

52. Effects of weight loss and sodium reduction intervention on blood pressure and hypertension incidence in overweight people with high-normal blood pressure: the Trials of Hypertension Prevention, Phase II. The Trials of Hypertension Prevention Collaborative Research Group. Arch Intern Med 157:657, 1997

53. Pickering TG: Lessons from the Trials of Hypertension Prevention, Phase II: energy intake is more important than dietary sodium in the prevention of hypertension. Arch Intern Med 157:396, 1997

54. US Department of Health and Human Services: Physical activity and health: a report to the Surgeon General. US Department of Health and Human Services, Public Health Service, Publication No. DHHS 017-023-00196-5, Hyattsville, Maryland, 1996

55. Physical activity and cardiovascular health. NIH Consensus Development Panel on Physical Activity and Cardiovascular Health. JAMA 276:241, 1996

56. Puddey IB, Parker M, Beilen LJ, et al: Effects of alcohol and caloric restrictions on blood pressure and serum lipids in overweight men. Hypertension 20:533, 1992

57. Rimm ED, Giovannucci EL, Willett WC, et al: Prospective study of alcohol consumption and risk of coronary disease in men. Lancet 338:464, 1991

58. Midgley JP, Matthew AG, Greenwood CMT, et al: Effect of reduced dietary sodium on blood pressure: a meta-analysis of randomized controlled trials. JAMA 275:1590, 1996

59. Cutler JA, Follmann D, Allender PS: Randomized trials of sodium reduction: an overview. Am J Clin Nutr 65(suppl):643S, 1997

60. Alderman MH, Madhavan S, Cohen H, et al: Low urinary sodium is associated with greater risk of myocardial infarction among treated hypertensive men. Hypertension 25:1144, 1995

61. Morris RC Jr, Sebastian A, Forman A, et al: Normotensive salt sensitivity: effects of race and dietary potassium. Hypertension 33:18, 1999

62. Sorof JM, Forman A, Cole N, et al: Potassium intake and cardiovascular reactivity in children with risk factors for essential hypertension. J Pediatr 131:87, 1997

63. Weinberger MH: Salt sensitivity of blood pressure in humans (pt 2). Hypertension 27:481, 1996

64. Whelton PK, Jiang H, Cutler JA, et al: Effects of oral potassium on blood pressure. JAMA 277:1624, 1997

65. Reusser ME, McCarron DA: Micronutrient effects on blood pressure regulation. Nutr Rev 52:367, 1994

66. Jones JK, Gorkin L, Lian JF, et al: Discontinuation of and changes in treatment after start of new courses of antihypertensive drugs: a study of a United Kingdom population. BMJ 311:293, 1995

67. Setaro JF, Black HR: Refractory hypertension. N Engl J Med 327:543, 1992

68. Miller NH, Hill M, Kottke T, et al: The multilevel compliance challenge: recommendations for a call to action: a statement for healthcare professionals. Circulation 95:1085, 1997

69. Neaton JD, Grimm RH Jr, Prineas RJ, et al: Treatment of Mild Hypertension Study: final results. JAMA 270:713, 1993

70. Materson BJ, Reda DJ, Cushman WC: Department of Veterans Affairs Single-Drug Therapy of Hypertension Study: revised figures and new data. Am J Hypertens 8:189, 1995

71. Grimm RH Jr, Grandits GA, Prineas RJ, et al: Long-term effects on sexual function of five antihypertensive drugs and nutritional hygienic treatment in hypertensive men and women: Treatment of Mild Hypertension Study (TOMHS). Hypertension 29:8, 1997

72. Ramsay L, Williams B, Johnston G, et al: Guidelines for management of hypertension: report of the third working party of the British Hypertension Society. J Hum Hypertens 13:569, 1999

73. Hansson L, Lindholm L, Niskanen L, et al: Effect of angiotensin-converting-enzyme inhibition compared with conventional therapy on cardiovascular morbidity and mortality in hypertension: The Captopril Prevention Project (CAPPP) randomised trial. Lancet 353:611, 1999

74. Effects of an angiotensin-converting-enzyme inhibitor, ramipril, on death from cardiovascular causes, myocardial infarction, and stroke in high-risk patients. The Heart Outcomes Prevention Evaluation Study Investigators. N Engl J Med 342:145, 2000

75. Hansson L, Lindholm LH, Ekbom T, et al: Randomised trial of old and new antihypertensive drugs in elderly patients: cardiovascular mortality and morbidity. The Swedish Trial in Old Patients with Hypertension-2 Study. Lancet 354:1751, 1999

76. Staessen JA, Wang JG: Characteristics of published, ongoing, and planned outcome trials in hypertension. Hypertension: A Companion to Brenner and Rector's the Kidney. Oparil S, Weber M, Eds. WB Saunders Co, Philadelphia, 1999, p 341

77. Dickerson JEC, Hingorani AD, Ashby MJ, et al: Optimisation of antihypertensive treatment by crossover rotation of four major classes. Lancet 353:2008, 1999

78. Fagan TC: Remembering the lessons of basic pharmacology. Arch Intern Med 154:1430, 1994

79. Prisant LM, Weir MR, Papademetriou V, et al: Low-dose drug combination therapy: an alternative first-line approach to hypertension treatment. Am Heart J 130:359, 1995

80. Krönig B, Pittrow DB, Kirch W, et al: Different concepts in first-line treatment of essential hypertension: comparison of a low-dose reserpine-thiazide combination with nitrendipine monotherapy. Hypertension 29:651, 1997

81. Espeland M, Whelton P, Kostis JB, et al: Predictors and mediators of successful long-term withdrawal from antihypertensive medications. Arch Fam Med 8:228, 1999

82. Black H: Blood pressure control. Am J Med 101(suppl 4A):50S, 1996

83. Calhoun DA, Oparil S: Treatment of hypertensive crisis. N Engl J Med 323:1177, 1990

84. Murphy C: Hypertensive emergencies. Emerg Med Clin North Am 13:973, 1995

85. Zeller KR, von Kuhnert L, Matthews C: Rapid reduction of severe asymptomatic hypertension: a prospective, controlled trial. Arch Intern Med 149:2186, 1989

86. Marwick C: FDA gives calcium channel blockers clean bill of health but warns of short-acting nifedipine hazards. JAMA 275:423, 1996

87. Blum U, Krumme B, Flügel P, et al: Treatment of ostial renal-artery stenoses with vascular endoprostheses after unsuccessful balloon angioplasty. N Engl J Med 336:459, 1997

88. Akpunonu BE, Mulrow PJ, Hoffman EA: Secondary hypertension: evaluation and treatment. Dis Mon 42:609, 1996

89. Fletcher EC: The relationship between systemic hypertension and obstructive sleep apnea: facts and theory. Am J Med 98:118, 1995

90. Lusardi P, Zoppi A, Preti P, et al: Effects of insufficient sleep on blood pressure in hypertensive patients: a 24-h study. Am J Hypertens 12:63, 1999

17 Atrial Fibrillation

Mina Chung, M.D., and Allan Klein, M.D.

Definition and Classification

Atrial fibrillation is defined as electrical activation of the atria by rapid, irregular waves of depolarization with continuously changing, wandering pathways. The frequency of these waves often exceeds 400 beats/min [see Figure 1].[1] This rapid, disordered atrial activation results in loss of coordinated atrial contraction, with irregular electrical inputs to the atrioventricular (AV) node and His-Purkinje system leading to sporadic ventricular contractions. On the surface electrocardiogram, atrial fibrillation is characterized by the absence of visible discrete P waves or the presence of irregular fibrillatory waves, or both, and an irregularly irregular ventricular response.

Atrial fibrillation is often categorized according to its dominant rhythm: paroxysmal, generally characterized by predominant sinus rhythm with intermittent episodes of fibrillation; chronic, often defined as persistent or permanent atrial fibrillation (some authors include chronic paroxysmal atrial fibrillation[2]); acute, an episode of atrial fibrillation with onset within 24 to 48 hours; and lone, variably defined but generally considered to occur in the absence of cardiac disease. A Mayo Clinic study defined lone atrial fibrillation as atrial fibrillation occurring in persons younger than 60 years without hypertension or cardiovascular or pulmonary disease.[3] The Framingham Study included patients of all ages without cardiovascular disease and also included those with hypertension in the absence of heart disease.[4]

The most common underlying cardiovascular diseases associated with atrial fibrillation are hypertension and ischemic heart disease [see Table 1].[5] In the Framingham Study, age, valvular disease, congestive heart failure, hypertension, and diabetes were shown to be independent risk factors for atrial fibrillation.[6,7]

Prevalence and Incidence

Atrial fibrillation is the most common sustained arrhythmia seen in clinical practice, occurring with an overall prevalence of 0.4% in the general population.[8] The incidence in the United States population is estimated to be more than two million cases. Prevalence and incidence of atrial fibrillation increase with advancing age [see Figure 2]. The Framingham Study reported an annual incidence of 0.1%.[9,10]

Morbidity and Mortality

Although not usually considered a life-threatening arrhythmia, atrial fibrillation has been associated with a twofold increase in total and cardiovascular mortality.[11] Factors that may increase mortality in atrial fibrillation include age, mitral stenosis, aortic valve disease, coronary artery disease, hypertension, and congestive heart failure.

The most clinically important consequences of atrial fibrillation are thromboembolic events and stroke. A fourfold to sixfold increased risk of stroke (15-fold in patients with a history of rheumatic heart disease[9,11-14]) makes this arrhythmia one of the most

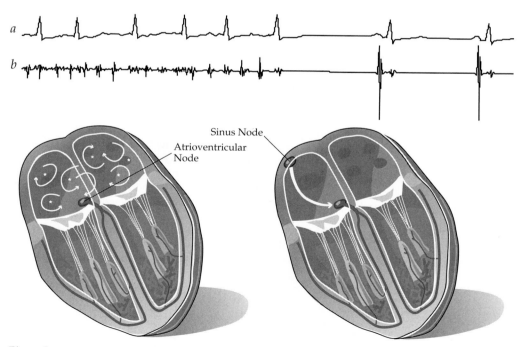

Figure 1 (*a*) Electrocardiographic tracing and (*b*) intracardiac atrial electrographic tracing were taken during atrial fibrillation (left) and normal sinus rhythm (right). During atrial fibrillation, atrial depolarization occurs with multiple wavelets of electrical activation. Conduction to the atrioventricular node is irregular and rapid, resulting in irregular conduction to the ventricles and loss of synchronous atrial contraction. In normal sinus rhythm, the sinus node initiates a regular electrical impulse, which is conducted with a uniform depolarization wavefront through the atria to the atrioventricular node, then via the His-Purkinje system to the ventricles.

Table 1 Factors Predisposing to Atrial Fibrillation

Most Common Associated Heart Disease
Hypertensive heart disease
Ischemic heart disease

Other Associated Conditions
Rheumatic valvular disease
Cardiomyopathy
Nonrheumatic valvular disease
Congestive heart failure
Congenital heart disease
Pulmonary embolism
Thyrotoxicosis
Chronic lung disease
Wolff-Parkinson-White syndrome
Pericarditis
Neoplastic disease
Postoperative state
Normal heart affected by alcohol, stress, drugs, excessive caffeine, hypoxia, hypokalemia, hypoglycemia, systemic infection

potent risk factors for stroke in the elderly and the most common cause of cardiogenic stroke. The risk of stroke in nonvalvular atrial fibrillation varies with age and with the presence of concomitant cardiovascular disease and other risk factors for stroke.

Meta-analysis of five major primary prevention trials for stroke in patients with atrial fibrillation estimated the risk of stroke in those younger than 65 years without hypertension, diabetes, or a history of stroke or transient ischemic attack (TIA) to be approximately 1% a year.[15] In older patients with risk factors for stroke or concomitant cardiovascular disease, the stroke rate is approximately 3% to 5% a year, rising to 8% a year in those older than 75 years. Most strokes associated with atrial fibrillation appear to be caused by cardiac emboli, presumably formed in fibrillating atria.

Persistent rapid ventricular rates associated with atrial fibrillation may lead to impairment of ventricular function by a mechanism similar to that of tachycardia-mediated cardiomyopathy.[16] This condition may be reversible, however; improved ventricular function has been reported after complete AV node ablation, medical control of ventricular rate, or achievement of sinus rhythm.[16-21] Evidence for development of atrial myopathy has also been reported in patients with atrial fibrillation in the absence of valvular disease.[22-24] Mechanical and electrical remodeling could also promote further propensities toward atrial fibrillation and thromboembolism.[25,26]

Morbidity attributable to atrial fibrillation also includes limitation in functional capacity from symptoms of palpitations, fatigue, dyspnea, angina, or congestive heart failure.[27,28]

Pathophysiology

According to the multiple wavelet hypothesis, pioneered by Moe and colleagues,[1] atrial fibrillation occurs as a result of intra-atrial reentry and is sustained by the propagation of multiple reentrant circuits with continuously changing, wandering pathways determined by local atrial refractoriness and excitability. Mapping of atrial fibrillation in animal models and humans has confirmed the presence of multiple, wandering reentrant circuits.[29,30]

In 1915, atrial electrical activity was classified by Hewlett and Wilson as coarse or fine on the basis of surface electrocardiogram recordings[31]; in 1978, Wells and associates distinguished four types of atrial electrical activity on the basis of recordings from single bipolar atrial electrograms.[32] More recently, mapping studies of human right atria during induced atrial fibrillation, by use of high-density recording electrode arrays, identified three different patterns—types I, II, and III [*see Figure 3*].[30]

Mapping studies suggest that the likelihood of termination of atrial fibrillation depends on the average number of wavelets present.[29,30] The smaller the number of wavelets, the more likely they are to be extinguished or to be fused into a broad, single wavefront, which may then resolve into atrial flutter or normal sinus rhythm.[1,29] It has been estimated that a three- to six-wavelet pattern is required for perpetuation of atrial fibrillation.[29,33]

The number of wavelets present during atrial fibrillation depends on reentrant circuit wavelengths and atrial size and excitability. To initiate or sustain a reentrant circuit, the path length available to the electrical impulse must equal or exceed the circuit wavelength, which is defined as the distance traveled by the depolarization wavefront during the refractory period (recovery time) of the tissue involved in the reentrant circuit. With shorter wavelengths, more wavelets may be present. With longer wavelengths, fewer circuits could be present, and atrial fibrillation may be short-lived.

Studies suggest that electrical remodeling occurs during atrial fibrillation, shortening the effective refractory periods and enhancing the propensity to sustain atrial fibrillation.[25] Therefore, therapies that target the components of wavelength, such as antiarrhythmic drugs that prolong refractory periods, could be useful for the termination of atrial fibrillation and maintenance of sinus rhythm. These concepts also illustrate why larger atrial size, by providing longer path lengths, would promote atrial fibrillation by allowing for the propagation of more wavelets.

Other, less common etiologies of atrial fibrillation demonstrated in animal models include rapid firing of one or multiple atrial foci (from enhanced automaticity or triggered activity) and the presence of a very small, rapidly conducting stable reentrant circuit.[34] Single or multiple foci of repetitive impulses occurring during atrial fibrillation have also been demonstrated in humans.[35]

Typical atrial flutter, a more organized atrial arrhythmia, is also caused by reentrant mechanisms. Seen on the ECG as sawtoothed flutter waves, which are negatively oriented in the inferior leads, the reentrant circuit occurs in a counterclockwise direction in the right atrium. An area of slowed conduction in the low right atrium has been a vulnerable target for ablation of the atrial flutter circuit.

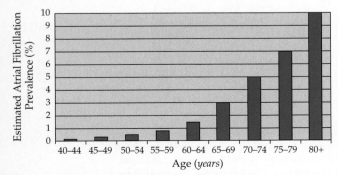

Figure 2 **Estimated prevalence of atrial fibrillation in the United States.**[8]

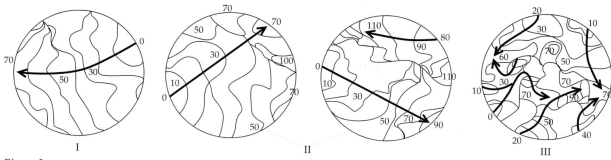

Figure 3 **Mapping criteria for classification of atrial fibrillation show that type I is characterized by uniformly propagating waves, type II is characterized by one or two conducting waves with areas of conduction block, and type III is characterized by the three or more wavelets associated with multiple areas of slowed conduction and conduction block.**[30]

Diagnosis

CLINICAL MANIFESTATIONS

Although atrial fibrillation may in some cases present as an asymptomatic finding on physical examination or electrocardiogram, more commonly the loss of AV synchrony and the rapid rates associated with atrial fibrillation result in significant symptoms and even significant hemodynamic impairment. Symptoms may range from palpitations to angina or other signs of acute or subacute myocardial ischemia, congestive heart failure, pulmonary edema, and hypotension. Atrial fibrillation may also cause marked fatigue or generalized weakness. Occasionally, thromboembolism, including stroke or systemic emboli, may be the first presentation of atrial fibrillation.

Symptoms may be the result of increased heart rates, leading to decreased diastolic ventricular and coronary filling times and increased oxygen demand. Symptoms may also result from the loss of atrial contribution to ventricular filling, leading to decreased cardiac output, particularly in patients with stiff, noncompliant ventricles.

HISTORY AND PHYSICAL EXAMINATION

A careful history and physical examination can identify the presence of conditions and precipitating factors (including alcohol, caffeine, and sympathomimetic or other drug use) that can predispose to atrial fibrillation. Duration and frequency of episodes, degree of associated symptoms, and manner of initiation should be assessed. Review of ECGs and rhythm strips that document atrial fibrillation is essential given the arrhythmia's association with thromboembolism, which is an indication for anticoagulation. Laboratory studies to exclude electrolyte imbalance, thyroid dysfunction, and substance abuse may be indicated. All patients with atrial fibrillation should have a transthoracic echocardiogram to assess atrial size, ventricular function, and valvular function. Ambulatory monitoring may be useful to assess ventricular response during atrial fibrillation or to assess the frequency of episodes. In patients with suggestive histories, a memory-loop transtelephonic event monitor may identify a primary arrhythmia as initiator of the atrial fibrillation. Paroxysmal supraventricular tachycardia or atrial flutter that degenerates to atrial fibrillation might be amenable to cure by radiofrequency catheter ablation methods. Demonstration of bradycardia-induced or vagally mediated atrial fibrillation can also alter therapeutic approaches. In addition, evaluation for underlying coronary artery disease with a functional stress test or cardiac catheterization may be indicated in some patients.

Management of Atrial Fibrillation

The consequences of atrial fibrillation include palpitations; impaired hemodynamics; thromboembolism and stroke; atrial cardiomyopathy, ventricular cardiomyopathy, or both; and a potential for associated increase in mortality. These conditions should represent the targets of therapy, which can include treatment to control ventricular rates, achieve and maintain sinus rhythm, reduce the risk of thromboembolism, ameliorate associated cardiomyopathy, and improve survival.

PHARMACOLOGIC MANAGEMENT

Control of Ventricular Rate

Ventricular rate is usually controlled with pharmaceutical agents that slow AV nodal conduction (e.g., digoxin, beta blockers, calcium channel blockers). Digoxin is inexpensive, is available intravenously, can be safely used in patients with heart failure, and has both direct and indirect effects on the AV node, with a primary vagotonic effect. However, it has a delayed (1 to 4 hours) peak onset, has a narrow therapeutic window, and is less effective in rate control of paroxysmal atrial fibrillation or rapid rates during hyperadrenergic states when vagal tone is low, such as during exercise or in acute and ICU settings, because of increased sympathetic tone. Finally, digoxin must be used with caution in elderly patients and patients with decreased renal function. Beta-adrenergic blockers are very effective in heart rate control, even during exercise; are available intravenously; and have rapid onset of action. Potential side effects include bronchospasm and exacerbation of congestive heart failure as a result of negative inotropy.

Calcium channel blockers, such as verapamil and diltiazem, can also slow ventricular rates during atrial fibrillation. Verapamil and diltiazem are available intravenously (diltiazem is available for continuous infusion), have a rapid onset, and can be used safely in chronic obstructive pulmonary disease and diabetes mellitus. However, calcium channel blockers can have negative inotropic effects and can cause hypotension.

The class III antiarrhythmic agents sotalol and amiodarone are also effective in slowing ventricular rates during atrial fibrillation, as are the class IC drugs propafenone and flecainide [*see* Maintenance of Sinus Rhythm, *below*].

Restoration of Sinus Rhythm

Although the most effective method of restoring sinus rhythm is electrical cardioversion, pharmacologic cardioversion can be attempted by loading with an antiarrhythmic agent. A commonly used agent is procainamide, which can be loaded at 50 mg/min (1 g over 20 minutes or 15 mg/kg) to achieve high peak levels. Blood pressure must be monitored closely during loading, as hypotension may necessitate a decrease in infusion rate. Dosing should be modified and caution exercised in patients with renal insufficiency, because an active metabolite, N-acetylprocainamide (NAPA), may accumulate to toxic levels in the presence of renal failure. Ibutilide is a recently approved class III antiarrhythmic agent that can also be effective in achieving pharmacologic conversion of recent-onset atrial fibrillation or flutter. The usual dosage is 1 mg given intravenously over 10 minutes. If the arrhythmia does not terminate within 10 minutes after the end of infusion, a second 10-minute intravenous infusion of 1 mg may be administered. Both procainamide and ibutilide should be administered with continuous ECG monitoring, as prolongation of the QT interval and torsade de pointes may occur.

Maintenance of Sinus Rhythm

Maintenance of sinus rhythm often requires use of an antiarrhythmic agent, particularly in patients with frequent or resistant atrial fibrillation, underlying cardiovascular disease, or enlarged atria. The available antiarrhythmic agents that have proved effective in maintaining sinus rhythm are classified according to the patterns of their electrophysiologic effects, their presumed mechanism of action, or both.

Class IA sodium channel blocking agents   Class IA sodium channel blocking agents, including quinidine, procainamide, and disopyramide, can enhance AV nodal conduction and potentially increase the ventricular response during atrial fibrillation. These drugs usually require the concomitant use of AV nodal blocking agents. Their effects on repolarization with QT interval prolongation are associated with an incidence of torsade de pointes, which is a ventricular tachycardia characterized by polymorphic QRS complexes that change in amplitude and cycle length, giving the appearance of oscillations around the baseline.

Quinidine is one of the best-studied drugs used for atrial fibrillation. A meta-analysis showed that 50% of patients taking quinidine after cardioversion remained in sinus rhythm at 1 year.[36] Because of the potential for proarrhythmia with quinidine, including torsade de pointes, we recommend initiation of quinidine therapy in the hospital, with continuous electrocardiographic monitoring and assessment of the QT interval. Moreover, quinidine increases serum digoxin levels, so concomitant digoxin dosage usually should be decreased. Other adverse effects include gastrointestinal symptoms, particularly diarrhea.

Procainamide, which is available for intravenous use, is often a first-line antiarrhythmic agent for atrial fibrillation after cardiac surgery. However, its long-term use is often limited by a high incidence of drug-induced lupus. Disopyramide has also been shown to be effective. Its use is limited in older men because of its anticholinergic side effects and because of urinary retention. The drug can also manifest negative inotropic effects.

Class IC sodium channel blocking agents   Class IC sodium channel blocking agents flecainide and propafenone have also been shown to be effective in the treatment of atrial fibrillation.[37] (Another class I/IC drug, moricizine, like propafenone, is indicated for the treatment of ventricular arrhythmias, such as sustained ventricular tachycardia, but has been used effectively for atrial fibrillation.) Patients with underlying heart disease may be at higher risk for proarrhythmia with class IC agents. The Cardiac Arrhythmia Suppression Trial showed in-

creased mortality in patients treated with flecainide, encainide, and moricizine for ventricular arrhythmias after myocardial infarction. The use of these agents in patients with coronary artery disease has raised concern,[38,39] and their use for atrial fibrillation in patients with coronary artery disease or impaired ventricular function should be balanced against the potential for excess risk.

Class III potassium channel blocking drugs   Class III potassium channel blocking drugs prolong repolarization. Amiodarone is effective against atrial fibrillation, but long-term use is associated with a potential for toxicities, the most important of which is pulmonary toxicity (hypersensitivity or interstitial/alveolar pneumonitis or pulmonary fibrosis). However, the risk of pulmonary toxicity appears to be dose related, and the usual maintenance dosages for control of atrial arrhythmias are generally less than 400 mg/day, often 200 mg/day or less.

Another class III drug, sotalol, also seems to be effective, but monitoring for QT interval prolongation, torsade de pointes, and bradycardia is recommended. Sotalol has significant beta-blocking activity, with potential for bradycardia and negative inotropic effects. Several other antiarrhythmic drugs for the maintenance of sinus rhythm are under investigation.

NONPHARMACOLOGIC MANAGEMENT

Restoration of Sinus Rhythm

Electrical cardioversion   Electrical cardioversion is the most effective method of conversion to sinus rhythm and is the method of choice for hemodynamically compromising atrial fibrillation.[40] Evaluation of the need for anticoagulation before cardioversion should be performed (see Cardioversion and the Risk of Thromboembolism, below). Before undergoing elective direct-current cardioversion, the patient should be fasting for 6 to 8 hours; electrolyte imbalances should be corrected and toxic drug levels excluded. Digoxin may be withheld the morning of the procedure. Electrode positioning should ensure an appropriate vector for atrial defibrillation (anteroposterior or right parasternal/subclavicular–left posterior patch positions). Patients should be anesthetized with short-acting agents (e.g., etomidate, methohexital, or propofol) and monitored closely for vital signs and respiratory status. Electrocardiography and pulse oximetry are also used to monitor the patient.

The shock must be synchronized to the QRS to minimize risk of inducing ventricular fibrillation. Atrial flutter can require less energy (50 to 100 joules) for successful cardioversion than atrial fibrillation, for which shock attempts usually begin at 200 joules. If atrial pacing electrodes are present, atrial overdrive pacing may be attempted for termination of atrial flutter. For atrial fibrillation that is refractory to external cardioversion, internal cardioversion has been successful with high-energy (200 to 360 joules) transcatheter direct-current shocks. Recently, much lower energies (2 to 10 joules) with catheters placed in the right atrium and coronary sinus have been successful.[41,42]

Control of Ventricular Rate

Nonpharmacologic management options include complete AV nodal (or His bundle) ablation and implantation of a permanent rate-responsive pacemaker. Originally performed using direct current, AV junction ablation is now achieved with radiofrequency electrode catheters. The procedure is successful in as many as 100% of patients; most patients experience significant symptomatic improvement. It is clinically most successful and appropriate for patients whose symptoms are secondary to difficult-to-control rapid ventricular rates. Disadvantages include dependence on a permanent pacemaker, a small risk of late sudden death (primarily reported after direct-current ablation), lack of effect on AV asynchrony, and risk of thromboembolism. AV nodal modification without complete ablation has also been successful in controlling ventricular rates and, in some patients, may prevent the need for permanent pacing.

Maintenance of Sinus Rhythm

Radiofrequency catheter ablation has been used not only for AV nodal ablation and modification but also for the ablation of supraventricular tachycardias, such as AV nodal reentrant tachycardia and accessory pathway–mediated atrioventricular reentry, which may degenerate to atrial fibrillation and typical atrial flutter circuits. Surgical approaches to atrial fibrillation and flutter include the left atrial isolation, corridor, and maze procedures. The maze procedure was designed to cure atrial fibrillation by dividing the atria into mazelike corridors and blind alleys that limit the development of reentry by limiting available path length.[43]

Pacemaker therapies Permanent pacing may become necessary for sick sinus syndrome, tachyarrhythmia-bradyarrhythmia syndromes, bradyarrhythmias occurring as a result of drug therapy, or after AV junction ablation.[44] Newer pacemakers have sophisticated programming options that can restrict upper tracking limits during atrial arrhythmias yet allow higher rate-responsive limits. Pacemakers with mode-switching algorithms can change from dual-chamber pacing to single-chamber pacing at the onset of atrial arrhythmias.[44-47]

Several studies have suggested that dual-chamber or atrial pacing that maintains atrioventricular synchrony may reduce the incidence of atrial fibrillation when compared with single-chamber ventricular pacing. These studies have largely consisted of patients with sick sinus syndrome, who require permanent pacing. Although most have been nonrandomized, comparisons of patients who have physiologic dual-chamber, atrial synchronous pacemakers with patients who have ventricular-paced devices have suggested a decreased incidence in the development of atrial fibrillation in physiologically paced groups. A review reported an incidence of atrial fibrillation between 0% and 23% in patients with atrial and dual-chamber pacemakers and between 14% and 57% in those with single-chamber ventricular devices.[48] A prospective, randomized trial of atrial pacing versus ventricular pacing in 225 patients with sick sinus syndrome reported that the frequency of atrial fibrillation and the thromboembolic event rate were higher in the ventricular-paced group.[49] Atrial fibrillation that occurs via vagally mediated mechanisms has also been controlled by atrial overdrive pacing.[50] Novel pacing approaches include atrial overdrive pacing and dual atrial site pacing modalities.

Investigational approaches Newer, investigational approaches to atrial fibrillation include the development of an implantable atrial defibrillator[51,52] and a catheter-based maze procedure.

RATE CONTROL VERSUS RHYTHM CONTROL

The decision whether to pursue achievement and maintenance of sinus rhythm or to treat with ventricular rate control measures alone often involves complex analyses of the risks and benefits of maintaining sinus rhythm in a given patient. The benefits of maintaining sinus rhythm may include potential for more complete relief of symptoms and for hemodynamic improvement. However, even with antiarrhythmic therapy, approximately 50% of patients develop recurrent atrial fibrillation after cardioversion to sinus rhythm, and studies have raised concern over the proarrhythmic potential and the risk of increased mortality associated with antiarrhythmic agents.[36,53,54] A multicenter trial, the Atrial Fibrillation Follow-up Investigation of Rhythm Management (AFFIRM), aims to test the hypothesis that total mortality rates in patients with atrial fibrillation are the same whether primary therapy is designed to maintain sinus rhythm or to control heart rate.[55]

Risk of Stroke in Atrial Fibrillation

STRATIFICATION OF RISK IN NONVALVULAR ATRIAL FIBRILLATION

Patients with nonvalvular atrial fibrillation show an approximately sixfold increased risk of stroke, which varies with age and the presence of coexisting cardiac disease.[14,56] The Framingham Study, with more than 30 years of follow-up, showed an annual stroke rate of 4.2% and demonstrated that the relative risk of stroke was associated with hypertension (relative risk, 3.4), coronary artery disease (2.4), congestive heart failure (4.3), and atrial fibrillation (4.8). Risk of stroke related to atrial fibrillation increases with aging (1.5% in the sixth decade to 24% in the ninth decade). Strokes are clustered at the onset of the arrhythmia (25% of patients), with another 14% occurring within the first year.[56] The Framingham Study stroke rate (4.2% a year) is strikingly similar to the 4.5% reported in the control arm of randomized clinical trials of atrial fibrillation.[15,57-61]

Pooled data from five large clinical trials have confirmed that four clinical variables are predictive of stroke risk, including TIAs and previous stroke (relative risk, 2.5), diabetes mellitus (1.7), hypertension (1.6), and age (1.4 for each decade of life) [see Table 2]. In patients with none of these conditions who received no anticoagulation or aspirin, risk of stroke was 1% a year.[15] Patients with congestive heart failure, angina, or myocardial infarction—conditions not found to be statistically significant in the pooled analysis—had stroke rates of about 4% a year.

Patients younger than 65 years with no risk factors have a low event rate of 1%, whereas those older than 75 years who have one or more risk factors have a high risk of 8.1%. Those with atrial fibrillation and a recent stroke or TIA have a very high risk of recurrent stroke (12%), as shown in the European Atrial Fibrillation Trial (EAFT).[60]

Echocardiographic variables, including left ventricular dysfunction, increased left atrial size, and increased wall thickness, have also been associated with an increased incidence of stroke.[26,58,62] The Boston Area Anticoagulation Trial in Atrial Fibrillation (BAATAF) has implicated mitral annular calcification as a predictor of stroke.[57]

Transesophageal echocardiographic assessment of spontaneous echo contrast, left atrial thrombus, and left atrial appendage velocities has also been used to stratify the risk of stroke in atrial fibrillation, but further trials are necessary to confirm these findings.[63,64] Preliminary observations from the Stroke Prevention in Atrial Fibrillation (SPAF) Trial III suggest that patients with a composite of decreased left atrial appendage velocities, thrombi in the left atrial appendage, and

Table 2 Annual Event Rates per
Age Groups and Risk Factors*

Risk	Event Rate
Categories	(95% CI)
Age < 65 years	
No risk factors	1% (0.3–3.1)
One or more risk factors	4.9% (3.0–8.1)
Age 65–75 years	
No risk factors	4.3% (2.7–7.1)
One or more risk factors	5.7% (3.9–8.3)
Age > 75 years	
No risk factors	3.5% (1.6–7.7)
One or more risk factors	8.1% (4.7–13.9)

*Risk factors are history of hypertension, history of diabetes, or history of prior stroke or transient ischemic attacks.

the presence of complex atheroma have a very high risk for stroke (21% a year).[65]

LONE ATRIAL FIBRILLATION

The risk of stroke associated with lone atrial fibrillation is much lower than that with chronic atrial fibrillation in patients older than 60 years. A Mayo Clinic study described 97 such patients with lone atrial fibrillation (without hypertension, pulmonary disease, or cardiac disease) who had a stroke rate of 1.3% after mean follow-up of 15 years, with an overall survival of 94% and a cumulative survival free of risk of stroke of 98.7% at 15 years.[3] These findings contrast with those of the Framingham Study, which found that 43 (8.3%) of 5,209 patients of all ages developed lone atrial fibrillation over 30-year follow-up. The age-adjusted incidence of stroke for lone atrial fibrillation was 28%, compared with 7% in the group that did not have atrial fibrillation.

The major reason for the discrepancies between the two studies was the age of the patients; the Framingham Study included patients older than 65 years as well as patients with hypertension but without hypertensive heart disease. Other investigators have generally confirmed the lower risk of stroke in patients with lone atrial fibrillation.[57,66,67] An analysis of pooled data found that untreated patients younger than 60 years with atrial fibrillation, but without hypertension, diabetes, or prior history of TIA or stroke, had a stroke rate of 1%.[15]

PAROXYSMAL ATRIAL FIBRILLATION

Patients with paroxysmal atrial fibrillation (PAT) also have an increased risk of stroke, of 3.7% a year.[66] There is a clustering of events at the onset of the arrhythmia, with an incidence of embolism of 6.8% in the first month, which decreases to 2% a year over the next 5 years.[68]

VALVULAR HEART DISEASE

The risk of stroke in patients with atrial fibrillation and mitral stenosis is 15 times higher than that in an age-matched and hypertension-matched control group. Because these patients are usually younger than those with nonvalvular atrial fibrillation, the absolute risk of stroke is similar, at 4.5% a year.[12,13]

CARDIOMYOPATHY

Atrial fibrillation occurs in 20% of patients with dilated cardiomyopathy and in 10% of patients with hypertrophic cardiomyopathy.[69,70] These patients may have a high incidence of thromboembolism. There have been no large, randomized trials to evaluate the risk factors for stroke in these patients, however, as there have been for nonvalvular atrial fibrillation.[12]

THYROTOXICOSIS

Atrial fibrillation occurs in 10% to 30% of patients with thyrotoxicosis,[71] and there may be a high incidence of thromboembolism in these patients. The risk is not well defined, however. One study found no differences in stroke rate between thyrotoxicosis patients and age-matched and sex-matched control subjects.[72] The stroke risk is generally believed to be as high as if not higher than that in euthyroid patients.[12,73]

CONGENITAL HEART DISEASE

Patients with Ebstein's anomaly, atrial and ventricular septal defects, and corrected transposition of the great vessels may often have atrial fibrillation; however, the incidence of stroke is unknown, except from anecdotal cases.[74]

Management of the Risk of Stroke

MECHANISMS OF STROKE IN ATRIAL FIBRILLATION

Approximately 15% to 20% of ischemic strokes are related to emboli that arise from the cardiac chambers or valves.[75] Atrial fibrillation accounts for 45% of embolic strokes, with the major mechanism being embolization of a thrombus from the left atrial appendage.[76,77] Transesophageal echocardiography (TEE) has shown the formation of thrombus in the left atrial appendage to be associated with stasis of blood in the left atrium (spontaneous echo contrast), low shear rates, and decreased left atrial appendage flow velocities.[78] Atrial fibrillation is associated with the elevation of biochemical markers of coagulation activation.[79]

Other potential mechanisms of stroke include embolization of left ventricular thrombi in the presence of left ventricular systolic dysfunction and mitral valve disease, including prolapse and annular calcification.[80-82] TEE has also been used to show that diseases of the atrial septum, including patent foramen ovale, atrial septal defect, and atrial septal aneurysm, as well as complex aortic atheromatous plaques, are sources of emboli.[83,84] Cerebrovascular disease may also be a cause of stroke.[80]

CHRONIC ANTICOAGULATION AND THROMBOTIC THERAPY

Recommendations for Anticoagulation in Atrial Fibrillation

According to guidelines of the American College of Chest Physicians (ACCP) for anticoagulation, long-term oral warfarin therapy (international normalized ratio [INR], 2.0 to 3.0) should be strongly considered for all patients with atrial fibrillation who are 65 years of age or older. Oral warfarin therapy should also be considered for patients younger than 65 years who have any of the following risk factors: previous TIA or stroke, hypertension, heart failure, diabetes, clinical coronary artery disease, mitral stenosis, prosthetic heart valves, or thyrotoxicosis.[12]

Oral anticoagulation rather than aspirin therapy is recommended for these patients because of the greater reduction in stroke provided by anticoagulation. Patients who are poor candidates for anticoagulant therapy or who refuse it should be treated with aspirin, 325 mg/day.

For patients between 65 and 75 years of age with no risk factors, the patient and physician should balance the low risk of stroke with the possible side effects of antithrombotic therapy in selecting either aspirin therapy or oral anticoagulation.

Patients older than 75 years should receive oral anticoagulant therapy (INR at the lower end of therapeutic range), but the recommendation must be balanced against the age-related risk of intracranial bleeding. Low-risk patients—those younger than 65 years with no risk factors—do not need anticoagulation.

Contraindications to Anticoagulation

Among the several contraindications to anticoagulation are hemorrhagic tendencies, recent intracranial hemorrhage or neurosurgery, recent major hemorrhagic trauma, recurrent or active bleeding, and diastolic blood pressure greater than 105 mm Hg. Other critical considerations include patients at risk for falling, alcohol abuse, drug interactions, poor compliance with follow-up, and the concomitant use of nonsteroidal anti-inflammatory drugs. It should be noted that many such patients were excluded from the multicenter trials on atrial fibrillation.

Major Trials of Chronic Anticoagulation

Five multicenter trials have evaluated the role of anticoagulation in the primary prevention of thromboembolism and nonvalvular atrial fibrillation: the Copenhagen Atrial Fibrillation, Aspirin and Anticoagulation (AFASAK) study[85]; the SPAF I and II trials[61,66]; the BAATAF[57,59]; the Canadian Atrial Fibrillation Anticoagulation (CAFA) trial[86]; and the Stroke Prevention in Nonrheumatic Atrial Fibrillation (SPINAF) study.[87] A sixth study, the EAFT, was chiefly concerned with secondary prevention.[34]

Primary prevention trials Pooled data from five of the primary prevention trials, all of which were controlled, randomized studies of warfarin, established the efficacy of this drug and, to a lesser extent, of aspirin in preventing ischemic strokes.[15] The overall 68% reduction in risk of stroke corresponds to an absolute reduction from an annual 4.5% in the control group to 1.4% in the warfarin group. Mortality decreased by 33%, from 5.4% to 3.6% annually. The effect of warfarin was statistically significant in women, with a decreased risk of 84%, compared with 60% in men. The stroke reduction with warfarin was probably underestimated because many patients included in the warfarin arms were either undercoagulated or were not actually taking warfarin at the time of their stroke. The anticoagulation regimen was accomplished using low-intensity warfarin to achieve a prothrombin time/international normalized ratio (PT/INR) of 2.0 to 3.0.

Major bleeding (defined as bleeding requiring transfusion or hospitalization or occurring in a critical anatomic location) can be an important complication of warfarin therapy, with rates varying from 0.3% a year in AFASAK to 4.2% a year in SPAF II (in patients older than 75 years). The rate of intracranial bleeding varied from 0.3% a year in the five-trial pooled data to 1.8% a year in SPAF II. Thus, the apparent risk of bleeding may counteract the benefits of warfarin in patients older than 75 years. It is recommended that the PT/INR be kept under 3.0 in these patients.

Role of aspirin in prevention of stroke in atrial fibrillation Three studies (SPAF, AFASAK, and EAFT) also evaluated the efficacy of aspirin in stroke reduction. Although pooled data showed aspirin (doses of 75 mg, 300 mg, and 325 mg) to be associated with an overall decrease in stroke risk of 36% (range, 17% to 44%), only SPAF showed a significant decrease (44%) of events compared with placebo. Thus, anticoagulation with warfarin is twice as effective as aspirin in preventing strokes. In the SPAF II trial, warfarin was compared with aspirin. Patients older than 75 years showed more bleeding with warfarin than with aspirin ($P = 0.04$).[61]

Secondary prevention trials In the EAFT study, patients who had had a TIA or stroke during the preceding 3 months were randomized to receive warfarin, aspirin, or neither. The primary end point was the composite event of death from cardiovascular causes, nonfatal stroke (including intracranial hemorrhage), nonfatal myocardial infarction, or systemic embolism. Warfarin and aspirin reduced the risk of the primary event (composite event of death) by 47% and 17%, respectively; the risk of stroke was reduced 66% and 10%, respectively. Thus, anticoagulation is more effective than aspirin in reducing the risk of recurrent stroke in patients with nonvalvular atrial fibrillation.

Multicenter anticoagulation trials in progress The SPAF III trial compared warfarin with a combination of low-dose warfarin and aspirin in patients at high risk for atrial fibrillation who had at least one thromboembolic risk factor. Also, a subset of the patients had TEE to assess the presence of spontaneous echo contrast in the left atrium. The combination of low-dose warfarin and aspirin was not effective in preventing stroke in high-risk patients, as compared with adjusted-dose warfarin.[88] The rate of ischemic stroke and systemic embolism was significantly higher in patients given the combination therapy than in patients given adjusted-dose warfarin (7.9% versus 1.9% a year, $P < 0.0001$). Another trial, the Assessment of Cardioversion Using Transesophageal Echocardiography (ACUTE) multicenter trial, is under way to assess the role of a TEE-guided strategy with brief anticoagulation compared with a conventional approach in patients undergoing electrical cardioversion.

MONITORING ATRIAL FIBRILLATION WITH ECHOCARDIOGRAPHY

Transthoracic echocardiography (TTE) and TEE are playing increasingly important roles in the management of patients with atrial fibrillation.[77,84,89]

Transthoracic Echocardiography

TTE has been used to determine left atrial size and the presence of left ventricular dysfunction, left ventricular hypertrophy, and valvular abnormalities.[84] These factors have been included in the risk-factor assessment of stroke in the SPAF II and Framingham studies.[26,62] Although TTE's detection of left atrial appendage thrombi is poor, with a sensitivity of less than 20%, it detects left atrial cavity thrombi with a sensitivity of 63% to 83% and a specificity of 94% to 99%.[90-92]

Transesophageal Echocardiography

In contrast to TTE, TEE, which provides excellent visualization of posterior cardiac structures, including the left atrial appendage and left atrial cavity, has made a major contribution to stroke risk assessment in patients with atrial fibrillation. It detects thrombi and prethrombotic conditions in the left atrium, as well as aortic atheroma [see Figure 4].

Detection of left atrial thrombi TEE has recently elucidated the role of left atrial appendage function in thromboembolism.[78,93] The physiology of the left atrial appendage can be assessed by placing a pulsed-wave Doppler sample volume in its mouth.

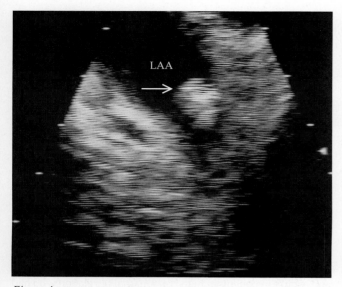

Figure 4 In this transesophageal echocardiogram, a thrombus (arrow) can be seen in the left atrial appendage (LAA).

Pulsed-wave Doppler patterns of filling and emptying of the appendage have been described in normal persons and patients with atrial fibrillation. The presence of thrombi and the resultant thromboembolism have been associated with increased appendage size and decreased flow velocities as well as with the presence of spontaneous echo contrast. [94,95] Patients with detected thrombi are at high risk for thromboembolism and death. [96] The current use of multiplane TEE imaging with its ability to obtain off-axis views of the left atrial appendage and the awareness of multilobed left atrial appendages have further facilitated detection of thrombi. [97]

Safe to perform, with minimal complications, TEE has 95% to 99% sensitivity and specificity for the detection of left atrial appendage or left atrial cavity thrombi [see Figure 4]. It has recently been advocated as a guide to electrical cardioversion with brief anticoagulation [see The Role of TEE in Electrical Cardioversion, *below*].

Detection of spontaneous echo contrast Spontaneous echo contrast, defined as swirling, smokelike echoes distinct from artifact, is associated with the presence of stasis in the left atrium, agglutination of red blood cells, and increased fibrinogen levels [see Figure 5]. [63,98] Spontaneous echo contrast is usually graded qualitatively as absent, mild, or severe, but attempts have been made to quantify its severity objectively, using integrated backscatter. [99] Several investigators have shown that spontaneous echo contrast is an independent risk factor for thrombus formation and thromboembolism in nonvalvular atrial fibrillation and mitral valve disease. [63,64] The presence of left atrial spontaneous echo contrast can independently prognosticate embolic risk and mortality in patients with atrial fibrillation. Interestingly, the presence of significant mitral regurgitation in the left atrium may wash the spontaneous echo contrast, indicating an absence of significant stasis and, in turn, decreased embolic risk. This is controversial, however.

Aortic atheroma Complex aortic atheroma (protruding or mobile plaques or those > 4 mm) are independent risk factors for stroke [see Figure 6]. [100] Furthermore, the presence of aortic atheroma has been shown to be a marker for concomitant coronary artery disease. [101] The detection of aortic atheroma in the ascending aorta during cardiac surgery may result in unplanned interventions, such as change in cannula site and debridement of the aortic atheroma. [102]

TEE and risk stratification By detecting thrombi, spontaneous echo contrast, or aortic atheroma, TEE can identify high-risk patients who may potentially benefit from anticoagulation as well as those at low risk who can be managed on aspirin alone. [65] Moreover, when guided by TEE, cardioversion may be safer and more cost-effective. [103,104] Finally, TEE can identify patients with thrombi who need prolonged anticoagulation after cardioversion. [104]

CARDIOVERSION AND THE RISK OF THROMBOEMBOLISM

Atrial fibrillation can be converted to normal sinus rhythm with electrical cardioversion. The goals of cardioversion are to relieve symptoms of congestive heart failure, improve cardiac function by restoring atrial contractility, and reduce the risk of thromboembolism, which varies from 0% to 5.6%. The risk can be decreased with anticoagulation, however.

Among 437 patients undergoing cardioversion for atrial fibrillation, for example, the incidence of embolic events was 0.8% among those who received anticoagulants, compared with 5.3% among those who did not receive anticoagulants. [105] Similarly, in a retrospective analysis of 454 patients who underwent elective cardioversion of atrial arrhythmias, six (1.3%) new embolic events occurred among those not taking anticoagulants. [106] On the other hand, earlier studies have reported embolic events among patients taking anticoagulants, and other studies have found that the incidence of embolization after cardioversion was similar whether or not patients received anticoagulant therapy. [107] These discrepancies in the effect of anticoagulation are related to different study populations, lack of controls, and poor understanding of the mechanisms of thromboembolism as they relate to electrical cardioversion. [104]

Mechanism of Thromboembolism after Cardioversion

Thromboembolism after cardioversion of atrial arrhythmias to sinus rhythm has traditionally been related to dislodgment of

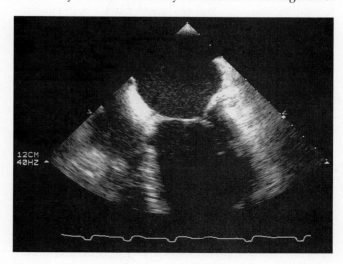

Figure 5 The smokelike echoes, or spontaneous echo contrast, in this transesophageal echocardiogram of a fibrillating left atrium are associated with prethrombotic conditions.

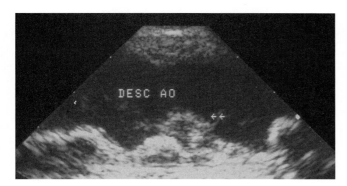

Figure 6 **Protruding atheroma (arrows) in the descending aorta (DESC AO) is evident in this transesophageal echocardiogram.**

preexisting thrombi upon the return of atrial electrical and mechanical function. The prevalence of thrombi in the left atrial appendage detected by TEE in patients with acute atrial fibrillation is estimated to vary from 10% to 15%, compared with 14% in those with chronic arrhythmia.[108,109] Assuming an embolic stroke rate after cardioversion of only 2%, it is estimated that 80% of thrombi do not embolize.[104]

Most conversion-related embolic events do not occur at the time of successful cardioversion and resumption of sinus rhythm but are delayed a few hours to a few weeks. The reason for this phenomenon is believed to lie in the lag between the return of electrical sinus rhythm and the resumption of mechanical atrial activity, resulting in delayed expulsion of preexisting thrombi. Moreover, cardioversion and return of sinus rhythm create a thrombogenic milieu, leading to the formation of new thrombi. Apparently related to the duration of the atrial fibrillation, the delay in return of left atrial mechanical function can be as long as 4 weeks, as shown by the return of the Doppler mitral inflow A wave.[110,111]

Investigations have advanced another potential mechanism of thromboembolism: the left atrial appendage may be stunned immediately after electrical cardioversion, resulting in the potential for de novo thrombosis and thromboembolism.[112] The left atrial appendage velocities were shown to be lower after cardioversion than before, and spontaneous echo contrast developed or increased immediately after cardioversion in 35% of the patients.[78] Another investigator reported similar findings in 40% of study patients after electrical cardioversion.[98] On the basis of these and other studies, anticoagulation at the time of and after cardioversion is strongly recommended, even in patients without TEE evidence of thrombi. Atrial stunning has also been shown to occur after pharmacologic and spontaneous conversion.[113,114]

Anticoagulation in Patients Undergoing Cardioversion

The recommendations of the ACCP for anticoagulation in patients with atrial fibrillation undergoing electrical cardioversion are that those with atrial fibrillation of longer than 2 days' duration or of unknown duration should receive warfarin for 3 weeks before cardioversion (to allow endothelialization of the thrombus) and for 4 weeks after cardioversion (to allow for resumption of left atrial mechanical transport).[12] Long-term anticoagulation beyond the 4 weeks after cardioversion should be considered in patients with cardiomyopathy, a history of previous embolism, or mitral valve disease.

There have been no randomized clinical trials to examine the incidence of thromboembolism after pharmacologic cardiover-

sion. It is believed, however, that the incidence may be similar to that after electrical cardioversion. There are insufficient data to recommend anticoagulation for short-term (< 48 hours) atrial fibrillation. A study showed that the likelihood of thromboembolism is low in patients with short-term atrial fibrillation.[115] Heparin followed by oral anticoagulation may be indicated for patients requiring emergency cardioversion for hemodynamic instability in the presence of mitral valve disease or for those whose postcardioversion TEE reveals spontaneous echo contrast in the left atrium or left atrial appendage. Because of reports of embolization after conversion of atrial flutter, consideration should be given to treating atrial flutter–like atrial fibrillation.[116] Anticoagulation is not necessary for conversion of supraventricular tachycardia.

The Role of TEE in Electrical Cardioversion

The fact that ACCP recommendations regarding anticoagulation before cardioversion are not based on well-controlled trials and that clinicians need to assess the risk of embolism in patients undergoing cardioversion has resulted in the advocacy of TEE-guided cardioversion.[77,104,108,117] Some investigators have suggested that TEE may be useful in screening for thrombi in patients who are not adequately anticoagulated,[118] whereas other investigators have suggested that a negative transesophageal echocardiogram might obviate anticoagulation.[119] More recent studies have demonstrated that TEE is useful in ruling out atrial thrombi and therefore in facilitating early cardioversion from atrial fibrillation by using short-term anticoagulation.[117] Of 196 patients without thrombi on TEE, 186 (95%) were cardioverted to sinus rhythm without prolonged anticoagulation or subsequent embolic events.

The TEE-guided approach has several advantages over conventional therapy. It may decrease embolic risk by detecting thrombi, allow for earlier cardioversion with brief anticoagulation, and prove to be more cost-effective than conventional therapy. The ACUTE study is an ongoing international multicenter clinical trial that compares a TEE-directed approach with brief anticoagulation and the conventional approach recommended by the ACCP.[104,108]

All patients in the ACUTE trial's TEE-guided group who have had atrial fibrillation for longer than 2 days are anticoagulated (with heparin if they are hospitalized or with a 5-day course of warfarin if they are outpatients) before being cardioverted. If no left atrial thrombus is detected on the TEE, electrical cardioversion proceeds, followed by a 4-week course of warfarin. If a thrombus is detected, cardioversion is postponed, the patient receives 4 weeks of warfarin therapy, and TEE is repeated. If the thrombus persists, the likelihood of successful conversion must be weighed against the risk of embolization. Patients receiving conventional management receive 3 weeks of warfarin therapy before undergoing cardioversion, followed by a 4-week course after cardioversion. The primary end points of the study are ischemic stroke, TIA, or peripheral embolism during the 8 weeks after randomization. The ACUTE pilot study randomized 126 patients from 10 clinical sites; 64 patients constituted the conventional treatment group and 62 constituted the TEE-guided group [*see Figure 7*].[108] No embolic events occurred in the TEE-guided group, compared with one event (1.6%) among the conventionally treated patients. Thrombi were detected by TEE in 13% of patients, allowing for short-term anticoagulation with electrical cardioversion in 5 days, compared with the 5 weeks required for patients in the conventional arm. Furthermore, patients in the TEE group demonstrated less clinical instability (hypotension and congestive heart failure or bleeding) than those treated con-

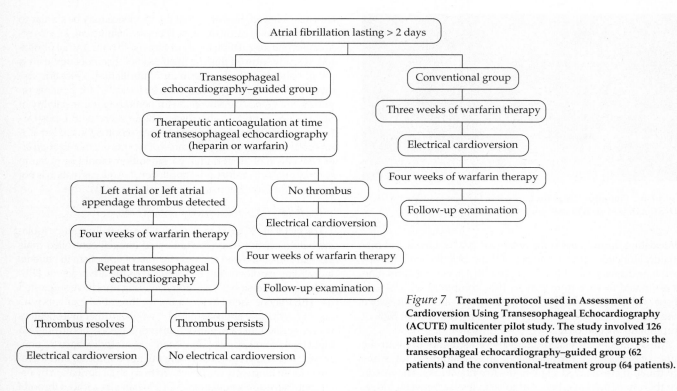

Figure 7 **Treatment protocol used in Assessment of Cardioversion Using Transesophageal Echocardiography (ACUTE) multicenter pilot study. The study involved 126 patients randomized into one of two treatment groups: the transesophageal echocardiography–guided group (62 patients) and the conventional-treatment group (64 patients).**

ventionally. Finally, TEE made it possible for the investigators to follow resolution of the thrombi. The study concluded that the TEE-guided approach is both feasible and safe.

Special Conditions Associated with Atrial Fibrillation

POSTOPERATIVE ATRIAL FIBRILLATION

The incidence of atrial fibrillation after cardiac surgery generally is 20% to 40%; it is the most common complication after open heart surgery, with a peak incidence during postoperative days 2 to 4.[120] Postoperative atrial fibrillation is associated with a twofold to threefold increase in risk of stroke.[121] Predisposing factors may include advanced age; hyperadrenergic effects, such as beta-blocker withdrawal; atrial ischemia from inadequate myocardial protection or prolonged cross-clamp times; and inflammation from atrial edema or pericarditis.

Beta-adrenergic blockers have a protective, prophylactic effect against the development of postoperative atrial fibrillation.[122] Mixed success has been reported with other agents, such as digoxin, magnesium, verapamil, diltiazem, and procainamide. Management includes control of ventricular response and consideration of pharmacologic or electrical cardioversion and anticoagulation.

ATRIAL FIBRILLATION AND WOLFF-PARKINSON-WHITE SYNDROME

Atrial fibrillation associated with an anterograde conducting accessory pathway requires special consideration, because very rapid conduction to the ventricles may precipitate ventricular fibrillation. Procainamide has been a drug of choice in the acute control of this situation. Drugs that block conduction through the AV node will be ineffective and may accelerate conduction through the accessory pathway. Digoxin and verapamil should be avoided. Cardioversion should be used in hemodynamically unstable patients. Long-term management should include ra-

diofrequency catheter ablation of the accessory pathway. Long-term medical management could include the use of class IC, IA, or III antiarrhythmic agents.

References

1. Moe G, Rheinboldt W, Abildskov J: A computer model of atrial fibrillation. Am Heart J 67:200, 1964

2. Sopher SM, Camm AJ: Atrial fibrillation: maintenance of sinus rhythm versus rate control. Am J Cardiol 77:24A, 1996

3. Kopecky SL, Gersh BJ, McGoon MD, et al: The natural history of lone atrial fibrillation: a population-based study over three decades. N Engl J Med 317:669, 1987

4. Brand FN, Abbott RD, Kannel WB, et al: Characteristics and prognosis of lone atrial fibrillation: thirty-year follow-up in the Framingham Study. JAMA 254:3449, 1985

5. Davidson E, Weinberger I, Rotenberg Z, et al: Atrial fibrillation: cause and time of onset. Arch Intern Med 149:457, 1989

6. Kannel WB, Abbott RD, Savage DD, et al: Epidemiologic features of chronic atrial fibrillation: the Framingham Study. N Engl J Med 306:1018, 1982

7. Podrid PJ: Atrial fibrillation in the elderly. Cardiol Clin 17:173, 1999

8. Feinberg WM, Blackshear JL, Laupacis A, et al: Prevalence, age distribution, and gender of patients with atrial fibrillation: analysis and implications. Arch Intern Med 155:469, 1995

9. Wolf PA, Abbott RD, Kannel WB: Atrial fibrillation: a major contributor to stroke in the elderly: the Framingham Study. Arch Intern Med 147:1561, 1987

10. Prystowsky EN, Benson DW, Fuster V, et al: Management of patients with atrial fibrillation: a statement for healthcare professionals from the subcommittee on electrocardiography and electrophysiology, American Heart Association. Circulation 93:1262, 1996

11. Kannel WB, Abbott RD, Savage DD, et al: Coronary heart disease and atrial fibrillation: the Framingham Study. Am Heart J 106:389, 1983

12. Laupacis A, Albers G, Dalen J, et al: Antithrombotic therapy in atrial fibrillation. Chest 108:352S, 1995

13. Wolf PA, Dawber TR, Thomas HJ, et al: Epidemiologic assessment of chronic atrial fibrillation and risk of stroke: the Framingham Study. Neurology 28:973, 1978

14. Wolf PA, Abbott RD, Kannel WB: Atrial fibrillation as an independent risk factor for stroke: the Framingham Study. Stroke 22:983, 1991

15. Risk factors for stroke and efficacy of antithrombotic therapy in atrial fibrillation: analysis of pooled data from five randomized controlled trials. Arch Intern Med 154:1449, 1994

16. Grogan M, Smith HC, Gersh BJ, et al: Left ventricular dysfunction due to atrial fibrillation in patients initially believed to have idiopathic dilated cardiomyopathy. Am J Cardiol 69:1570, 1992

17. Kieny JR, Sacrez A, Facello A, et al: Increase in radionuclide left ventricular ejection fraction after cardioversion of chronic atrial fibrillation in idiopathic dilated cardiomyopathy. Eur Heart J 13:1290, 1992

18. Van GI, Crijns HJ, Blanksma PK, et al: Time course of hemodynamic changes and improvement of exercise tolerance after cardioversion of chronic atrial fibrillation unassociated with cardiac valve disease. Am J Cardiol 72:560, 1993

19. Rosenqvist M, Lee M, Moulinier L, et al: Long-term follow-up of patients after transcatheter direct current ablation of the atrioventricular junction. J Am Coll Cardiol 16:1467, 1990

20. Rodriguez LM, Smeets JL, Xie B, et al: Improvement in left ventricular function by ablation of atrioventricular nodal conduction in selected patients with lone atrial fibrillation. Am J Cardiol 72:1137, 1993

21. Twidale N, Sutton K, Bartlett L, et al: Effects on cardiac performance of atrioventricular node catheter ablation using radiofrequency current for drug-refractory atrial arrhythmias. Pacing Clin Electrophysiol 16:1275, 1993

22. Suarez GS, Lampert S, Ravid S, et al: Changes in left atrial size in patients with lone atrial fibrillation. Clin Cardiol 14:652, 1991

23. Sanfilippo AJ, Abascal VM, Sheehan M, et al: Atrial enlargement as a consequence of atrial fibrillation: a prospective echocardiographic study. Circulation 83:792, 1990

24. Welikovitch L, Lafreniere G, Burggraf GW, et al: Change in atrial volume following restoration of sinus rhythm in patients with atrial fibrillation: a prospective echocardiographic study. Can J Cardiol 10:993, 1994

25. Wijffels MC, Kirchhof CJ, Dorland R, et al: Atrial fibrillation begets atrial fibrillation: a study in awake chronically instrumented goats. Circulation 92:1954, 1995

26. Predictors of thromboembolism in atrial fibrillation: II. Echocardiographic features of patients at risk. The Stroke Prevention in Atrial Fibrillation Investigators. Ann Intern Med 116:6, 1992

27. Gosselink AT, Crijns HJ, van den Berg MP, et al: Functional capacity before and after cardioversion of atrial fibrillation: a controlled study. Br Heart J 72:161, 1994

28. Gosselink AT, Bijlsma EB, Landsman ML, et al: Long-term effect of cardioversion on peak oxygen consumption in chronic atrial fibrillation: a 2-year follow-up. Eur Heart J 15:1368, 1994

29. Allessie MA, Konings K, Kirchhof CJHJ, et al: Electrophysiologic mechanisms of perpetuation of atrial fibrillation. Am J Cardiol 77:10A, 1996

30. Konings KT, Kirchhof CJ, Smeets JR, et al: High-density mapping of electrically induced atrial fibrillation in humans. Circulation 89:1665, 1994

31. Hewlett AW, Wilson FN: Coarse auricular fibrillation in man. Arch Intern Med 15:786, 1915

32. Wells JL, Karp RB, Kouchoukos NT, et al: Characterization of atrial fibrillation in man: studies following open heart surgery. Pacing Clin Electrophysiol 1:426, 1978

33. Brugada J: Electrophysiologic mechanisms of atrial fibrillation. Rev Esp Cardiol 49(suppl 2):8, 1996

34. Schuessler RB, Grayson TM, Bromberg BI, et al: Cholinergically mediated tachyarrhythmias induced by a single extra stimulus in the isolated canine right atrium. Circ Res 71:1254, 1992

35. Holm M, Blomstrom P, Brandt J, et al: Determination of preferable directions of impulse propagation during atrial fibrillation by time averaging of multiple electrogram vectors. Atrial Fibrillation: Mechanisms and Therapeutic Strategies. Olsson SB, Allessie MA, Campbell RWF, Eds. Futura Publishing, Armonk, New York, 1994, p 67

36. Coplen SE, Antman EM, Berlin JA, et al: Efficacy and safety of quinidine therapy for maintenance of sinus rhythm after cardioversion: a meta-analysis of randomized control trials. Circulation 82:2248, 1990

37. Kochiadakis GE, Igoumenidis NE, Parthenakis FI, et al: Amiodarone versus propafenone for conversion of chronic atrial fibrillation: results of a randomized, controlled study. J Am Coll Cardiol 33:966, 1999

38. Echt DS, Liebson PR, Mitchell LB, et al: Mortality and morbidity in patients receiving encainide, flecainide, or placebo: the Cardiac Arrhythmia Suppression Trial. N Engl J Med 324:781, 1991

39. Effect of the antiarrhythmic agent moricizine on survival after myocardial infarction. The Cardiac Arrhythmia Suppression Trial II Investigators. N Engl J Med 327:227, 1992

40. Ewy GA: The optimal technique for electrical cardioversion of atrial fibrillation. Clin Cardiol 17:79, 1994

41. Alt E, Schmitt C, Ammer R, et al: Initial experience with intracardiac atrial defibrillation in patients with chronic atrial fibrillation (pt 2). Pacing Clin Electrophysiol 17:1067, 1994

42. Luderitz B, Pfeiffer D, Tebbenjohanns J, et al: Nonpharmacologic strategies for treating atrial fibrillation. Am J Cardiol 77:45A, 1996

43. Cox JL, Boineau JP, Schuessler RB, et al: Five-year experience with the maze procedure for atrial fibrillation. Ann Thorac Surg 56:814, 1993

44. Pollak A, Falk RH: Pacemaker therapy in patients with atrial fibrillation. Am Heart J 125:824, 1993

45. Ovsyshcher IE, Katz A, Bondy C: Initial experience with a new algorithm for automatic mode switching from DDDR to DDIR mode. Pacing Clin Electrophysiol 17:1908, 1994

46. Provenier F, Jordaens L, Verstraeten T, et al: The "automatic mode switch" function in successive generations of minute ventilation sensing dual chamber rate responsive pacemakers. Pacing Clin Electrophysiol 17:1913, 1994

47. Brignole M, Gianfranchi L, Menozzi C, et al: A new pacemaker for paroxysmal atrial fibrillation treated with radiofrequency ablation of the AV junction. Pacing Clin Electrophysiol 17:1889, 1994

48. Hesselson AB, Parsonnet V, Bernstein AD, et al: Deleterious effects of long-term single-chamber ventricular pacing in patients with sick sinus syndrome: the hidden benefits of dual-chamber pacing. J Am Coll Cardiol 19:1542, 1992

49. Andersen HR, Thuesen L, Bagger JP, et al: Prospective randomized trial of atrial versus ventricular pacing in sick-sinus syndrome. Lancet 344:1523, 1994

50. Coumel P, Friocourt P, Mugica J, et al: Long-term prevention of vagal atrial arrhythmias by atrial pacing at 90/minute: experience with 6 cases. Pacing Clin Electrophysiol 6:552, 1983

51. Griffin JC, Ayers GM, Adams J, et al: Prospects for an implantable atrial defibrillator. J Electrocardiol 26:204, 1993

52. Levy S, Richard P: Is there any indication for an intracardiac defibrillator for the treatment of atrial fibrillation? J Cardiovasc Electrophysiol 5:982, 1994

53. Flaker GC, Blackshear JL, McBride R, et al: Antiarrhythmic drug therapy and cardiac mortality in atrial fibrillation. The Stroke Prevention in Atrial Fibrillation Investigators. J Am Coll Cardiol 20:527, 1992

54. Falk RH: Flecainide-induced ventricular tachycardia and fibrillation in patients treated for atrial fibrillation. Ann Intern Med 111:107, 1989

55. Atrial fibrillation follow-up investigation of rhythm management: the AFFIRM study design. The Planning and Steering Committee of the AFFIRM Study for the NHLBI AFFIRM Investigators. Am J Cardiol 79:1198, 1997

56. Wolf PA, Kannel WB, McGee DL, et al: Duration of atrial fibrillation and imminence of stroke: the Framingham Study. Stroke 14:664, 1983

57. The effect of low-dose warfarin on the risk of stroke in patients with nonrheumatic atrial fibrillation.The Boston Area Anticoagulation Trial for Atrial Fibrillation Investigators. N Engl J Med 323:1505, 1990

58. Predictors of thromboembolism in atrial fibrillation: I. Clinical features of patients at risk. The Stroke Prevention in Atrial Fibrillation Investigators. Ann Intern Med 116:1, 1992

59. Singer DE, Hughes RA, Gress DR, et al: The effect of aspirin on the risk of stroke in patients with nonrheumatic atrial fibrillation: the BAATAF Study. Am Heart J 124:1567, 1992

60. Secondary prevention in non-rheumatic atrial fibrillation after transient ischemic attack or minor stroke. EAFT (European Atrial Fibrillation Trial) Study Group. Lancet 342:1255, 1993

61. Warfarin versus aspirin for prevention of thromboembolism in atrial fibrillation: Stroke Prevention in Atrial Fibrillation II Study. Lancet 343:687, 1994

62. Vaziri SM, Larson MG, Benjamin EJ, et al: Echocardiographic predictors of nonrheumatic atrial fibrillation: the Framingham Heart Study. Circulation 89:724, 1994

63. Black IW, Hopkins AP, Lee LC, et al: Left atrial spontaneous echo contrast: a clinical and echocardiographic analysis. J Am Coll Cardiol 18:398, 1991

64. Black IW, Stewart WJ: The role of echocardiography in the evaluation of cardiac source of emboli: left atrial spontaneous echo contrast. Echocardiography 10:429, 1993

65. A prospective study to assess transesophageal echocardiographic (TEE) findings in the prediction of stroke in high risk patients with atrial fibrillation (abstr). Circulation 94:I-216, 1996

66. Stroke Prevention in Atrial Fibrillation Study: final results. Circulation 84:527, 1991

67. Lui CY: Should patients with lone atrial fibrillation be treated with anticoagulant therapy (editorial)? J Am Coll Cardiol 18:301, 1991

68. Takahashi N, Seki A, Imataka K, et al: Clinical feature of paroxysmal atrial fibrillation: an observation of 94 patients. Jpn Heart J 22:143, 1981

69. Hinton RC, Kistler JP, Fallon JT, et al: Influence of etiology of atrial fibrillation on incidence of systemic embolism. Am J Cardiol 40:509, 1977

70. Robinson K, Frenneaux MP, Stockins B, et al: Atrial fibrillation in hypertrophic cardiomyopathy: a longitudinal study. J Am Coll Cardiol 15:1279, 1990

71. Yuen RW, Gutteridge DH, Thompson PL, et al: Embolism in thyrotoxic atrial fibrillation. Med J Aust 1:630, 1979

72. Petersen P, Kastrup J, Helweg-Larsen S, et al: Risk factors for thromboembolic complications in chronic atrial fibrillation: the Copenhagen AFASAK study. Arch Intern Med 150:819, 1990

73. Presti CF, Hart RG: Thyrotoxicosis, atrial fibrillation, and embolism, revisited. Am Heart J 117:976, 1989

74. Laupacis A: Anticoagulants for atrial fibrillation. Lancet 342:1251, 1993

75. Hart RG: Cardiogenic embolism to the brain. Lancet 339:589, 1992

76. Rittoo D, Sutherland GR, Currie P, et al: A prospective study of left atrial spontaneous echo contrast and thrombus in 100 consecutive patients referred for balloon dilation of the mitral valve. J Am Soc Echocardiogr 7:516, 1994

77. Black IW, Hopkins AP, Lee LC, et al: Evaluation of transesophageal echocardiography before cardioversion of atrial fibrillation and flutter in nonanticoagulated patients. Am Heart J 126:375, 1993

78. Grimm RA, Stewart WJ, Maloney JD, et al: Impact of electrical cardioversion for atrial fibrillation on left atrial appendage function and spontaneous echo contrast: characterization by simultaneous transesophageal echocardiography. J Am Coll Cardiol 22:1359, 1993

79. Ikeda U, Yamamoto K, Shimada K, et al: Biochemical markers of coagulation activation in mitral stenosis, atrial fibrillation, and cardiomyopathy. Clin Cardiol 20:7, 1997

80. Aronow WS: Etiology and pathogenesis of thromboembolism. Herz 16:395, 1991

81. Boysen G: Anticoagulation for atrial fibrillation and stroke prevention. Neuroepidemiology 12:280, 1993

82. Benjamin EJ: Mitral annular calcification and the risk of stroke in an elderly cohort. N Engl J Med 327:374, 1992

83. Archer SL, James KE, Kvernen LR, et al: Role of transesophageal echocardiography in the detection of left atrial thrombus in patients with chronic nonrheumatic atrial fibrillation. Am Heart J 130:287, 1995

84. Asinger RW, Herzog CA: Echocardiography in the evaluation of cardiac sources of emboli: the role of transthoracic echocardiography. Echocardiography 10:373, 1993

85. Petersen P, Boysen G, Godtfredsen J, et al: Placebo-controlled, randomized trial of warfarin and aspirin for prevention of thromboembolic complications in chronic atrial fibrillation: the Copenhagen AFASAK study. Lancet 1:175, 1989

86. Connolly SJ, Laupacis A, Gent M, et al: Canadian atrial fibrillation anticoagulation (CAFA) study. J Am Coll Cardiol 18:349, 1991

87. Ezekowitz MD, Bridgers SL, James KE, et al: Warfarin in the prevention of stroke associated with nonrheumatic atrial fibrillation. Veterans Affairs Stroke Prevention in Nonrheumatic Atrial Fibrillation Investigators. N Engl J Med 327:1406, 1992

88. Adjusted-dose warfarin versus low-intensity, fixed-dose warfarin plus aspirin for high-risk patients with atrial fibrillation: Stroke Prevention in Atrial Fibrillation III randomized clinical trial. Stroke Prevention in Atrial Fibrillation Investigators. Lancet 348:633, 1996

89. Cheitlin MD, Alpert JS, Armstrong WF, et al: ACC/AHA guidelines for the clinical application of echocardiography: executive summary: a report of the American College of Cardiology/American Heart Association Task Force on Practice Guidelines (committee on clinical application of electrocardiography). J Am Coll Cardiol 29:862, 1997

90. Bansal RC, Heywood T, Appelgate PM: Detection of left atrial thrombi by two-dimensional echocardiography and surgical correlation in 148 patients with mitral valve disease. Am J Cardiol 64:243, 1989

91. Pearson AC, Labovitz AJ, Tatineni S: Superiority of transesophageal echocardiography in detecting cardiac source of emboli in patients with cerebral ischemia of uncertain etiology. J Am Coll Cardiol 17:66, 1991

92. Mugge A, Kuhn H, Daniel WG: The role of transesophageal echocardiography in the detection of left atrial thrombi. Echocardiography 10:405, 1993

93. Pollick C, Taylor D: Assessment of left atrial appendage function by transesophageal echocardiography. Circulation 84:223, 1991

94. Fatkin D, Kelly RP, Feneley MP: Relations between left atrial appendage blood flow velocity, spontaneous echocardiographic contrast and thromboembolic risk in vivo. J Am Coll Cardiol 23:961, 1994

95. Pozzoli M, Febo O, Torbicki A: Left atrial appendage dysfunction: a cause of thrombosis? Evidence by transesophageal echocardiography-Doppler studies. J Am Soc Echocardiogr 4:435, 1991

96. Leung DY, Davidson PM, Cranney GB, et al: Thromboembolic risks of left atrial thrombus detected by transesophageal echocardiogram. Am J Cardiol 79:626, 1997

97. Leung DY, Black IW, Grimm RA, et al: Multi-lobed appendage: visualization by multiplane transesophageal echocardiography (abstr). Circulation 90:I-224, 1994

98. Fatkin D, Herbert E, Feneley MP: Hematologic correlates of spontaneous echo contrast in patients with atrial fibrillation and implications for thromboembolic risk. Am J Cardiol 73:672, 1994

99. Klein AL, Murray RD, Black IW, et al: Integrated back scatter for quantification of left atrial spontaneous echo contrast. J Am Coll Cardiol 28:222, 1996

100. Kronzon I, Tunick PA: Transesophageal echocardiography as a tool in the evaluation of patients with embolic disorders. Prog Cardiovasc Dis 36:39, 1993

101. Fazio GP, Redberg RF, Winslow T, et al: Transesophageal echocardiographically detected atherosclerotic aortic plaque is a marker for coronary artery disease. J Am Coll Cardiol 21:144, 1993

102. Waering TH, Davila-Roman VG, Barzilai B, et al: Management of the severely atherosclerotic ascending aorta during cardiac operations: a strategy for detection and treatment. J Thorac Cardiovasc Surg 103:453, 1992

103. Seto TB, Taira DA, Tsevat J, et al: Cost-effectiveness of transesophageal echocardiographic-guided cardioversion: a decision analytic model for patients admitted to the hospital with atrial fibrillation. J Am Coll Cardiol 29:1222, 1997

104. Grimm RA, Stewart WJ, Black IW, et al: Should all patients undergo transesophageal echocardiography before electrical cardioversion of atrial fibrillation? J Am Coll Cardiol 23:533, 1994

105. Bjerkelund CJ, Orning OM: The efficacy of anticoagulant therapy in preventing embolism related to D.C. electrical conversion of atrial fibrillation. Am J Cardiol 23:208, 1969

106. Arnold AZ, Mick MJ, Mazurek RP, et al: Role of prophylactic anticoagulation for direct current cardioversion in patients with atrial fibrillation or atrial flutter. J Am Coll Cardiol 19:851, 1992

107. Aberg H, Cullhed I: Direct current conversion of atrial fibrillation—long-term results. Acta Med Scand 184:433, 1968

108. Klein AL, Grimm RA, Black IW, et al: Cardioversion guided by transesophageal echocardiography: the ACUTE pilot study: a randomized controlled trial. Ann Intern Med 126:200, 1997

109. Stoddard MF, Dawkins PR, Prince CR, et al: Left atrial appendage thrombus is not uncommon in patients with acute atrial fibrillation and a recent embolic event: a transesophageal echocardiographic study. J Am Coll Cardiol 25:452, 1995

110. Manning WJ, Leeman DE, Gotch PJ, et al: Pulsed Doppler evaluation of atrial mechanical function after electrical cardioversion of atrial fibrillation. J Am Coll Cardiol 13:617, 1989

111. Manning WJ, Silverman DI, Katz SE, et al: Temporal dependence of the return of atrial mechanical function on the mode of cardioversion of atrial fibrillation to sinus rhythm. Am J Cardiol 75:624, 1995

112. Fatkin D, Kuchar DL, Thorburn CW, et al: Transesophageal echocardiography before and after direct current cardioversion of atrial fibrillation: evidence for "atrial stunning" as a mechanism of thromboembolic complications. J Am Coll Cardiol 23:307, 1994

113. Falcone RA, Morady F, Armstrong WF: Transesophageal echocardiographic evaluation of left atrial appendage function and spontaneous contrast formation after chemical or electrical cardioversion of atrial fibrillation. Am J Cardiol 78:435, 1996

114. Grimm RA, Leung DY, Black IW, et al: Left atrial appendage "stunning" after spontaneous conversion of atrial fibrillation demonstrated by transesophageal Doppler echocardiography. Am Heart J 130:174, 1995

115. Weigner MJ, Caulfield TA, Danias PG, et al: Risk for clinical thromboembolism associated with conversion to sinus rhythm in patients with atrial fibrillation lasting less than 48 hours. Ann Intern Med 126:615, 1997

116. Santiago D, Warshofsky M, Li MG, et al: Left atrial appendage function and thrombus formation in atrial fibrillation-flutter: a transesophageal echocardiographic study. J Am Coll Cardiol 24:159, 1994

117. Manning WJ, Silverman DI, Keighley CS, et al: Transesophageal echocardiographically facilitated early cardioversion from atrial fibrillation using short-term anticoagulation: final results of a prospective 4.5-year study. J Am Coll Cardiol 25:1354, 1995

118. Orsinelli DA, Pearson AC: Usefulness of transesophageal echocardiography to screen for left atrial thrombus before elective cardioversion for atrial fibrillation. Am J Cardiol 72:1337, 1993

119. Stoddard ME, Longaker RA: Role of transesophageal echocardiography prior to cardioversion in patients with atrial fibrillation. J Am Coll Cardiol 21:28A, 1993

120. Fuller JA, Adams GG, Buxton B: Atrial fibrillation after coronary artery bypass grafting: Is it a disorder of the elderly? J Thorac Cardiovasc Surg 97:821, 1989

121. Creswell LL, Schuessler RB, Rosenbloom M, et al: Hazards of postoperative atrial arrhythmias. Ann Thorac Surg 56:539, 1993

122. Kowey PR, Taylor JE, Rials SJ, et al: Meta-analysis of the effectiveness of prophylactic drug therapy in preventing supraventricular arrhythmia early after coronary artery bypass grafting. Am J Cardiol 69:863, 1992

Acknowledgments

Figure 1   Joseph Bloch, CMI.

Figures 2 and 7   Marcia Kammerer.

18 Supraventricular Tachycardia

Patrick J. Tchou, M.D., and Richard G. Trohman, M.D.

This chapter focuses primarily on atrioventricular nodal reentrant tachycardia, tachycardias associated with accessory pathways, intra-atrial reentrant and automatic atrial tachycardias, and tachycardias originating from or near the sinus node. The two most common forms of supraventricular tachycardia, atrial fibrillation and flutter, are discussed elsewhere in this section [*see Chapter 17*].

Atrioventricular Nodal Reentrant Tachycardia

Atrioventricular nodal reentrant tachycardia (AVNRT) is the most common type of paroxysmal supraventricular tachycardia (PSVT). It accounts for approximately 50% to 60% of PSVT evaluated at referral centers.[1,2] AVNRT presents later than tachycardias related to accessory pathways, frequently after 20 years of age.[3] It is an uncommon mechanism of tachycardia in childhood and is more common in women than in men.

ANATOMY AND PHYSIOLOGY OF THE AV NODE

Knowledge of the posterior inputs into the atrioventricular (AV) node has existed since the early 1900s.[1] During the 1960s, the work of James[4] and of Truex and Smythe[5] suggested that the AV junctional area is divided into three regions: the compact AV node itself (located in the anterosuperior atrial septum) and two nodal approaches (the anterosuperior pathway, in the anterior interatrial septum, and the posteroinferior pathway, originating near the ostium of the coronary sinus).[2,3]

Atrioventricular nodal reentrant tachycardia was initially and for many years thought to be confined to the compact AV node.

Analysis of this older model is still useful in conceptualizing the arrhythmias seen in this disorder [*see Figure 1a*].

In 1981, the retrograde exit of the slow pathway was localized to the region of the coronary sinus ostium.[6] Curative radiofrequency ablation has demonstrated that the slow pathway is easily ablated near the coronary sinus os and has provided evidence that the anterior approaches to the compact node generally represent the fast pathway.[7-11]

Knowledge gained during experimental studies,[12] surgical ice mapping,[13] and catheter ablative cures[14] of AVNRT has provided insight into the arrhythmia substrate. The anatomic basis for fast and slow fibers appears to exist in the normal AV node complex. The physiologic conditions required to initiate the first reentrant beat or to sustain the reentrant process prevent tachycardia in most persons. An increase in ectopy and physiologic changes may allow development of the tachycardia with increasing age. Although the tachycardia's circuit remains incompletely identified, it seems likely that the compact node and its anterior and posterior approaches, as well as perinodal atrial tissue, are involved [*see Figure 1b*].

DIAGNOSIS

Clinical Presentation

The typical heart rate in AVNRT ranges from 150 to 250 beats/min. Palpitations, light-headedness, and near-syncope may accompany the paroxysms. True syncope is unusual. Neck pounding, attributed to cannon a waves, is thought to be virtually pathognomonic of AVNRT.[15] Its absence does not exclude the diagnosis.

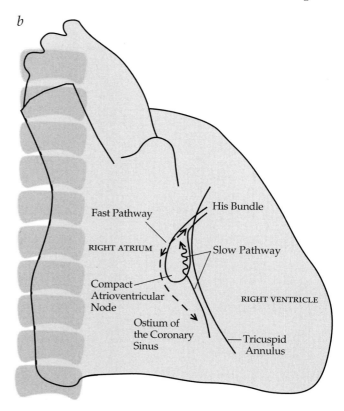

a Fast Pathway / Compact Atrioventricular Node / Slow Pathway / His Bundle / Fast Pathway / Slow Pathway / His Bundle

b Fast Pathway / His Bundle / RIGHT ATRIUM / Slow Pathway / Compact Atrioventricular Node / RIGHT VENTRICLE / Ostium of the Coronary Sinus / Tricuspid Annulus

Figure 1 During sinus rhythm, antegrade conduction occurs through both the fast pathway and the slow pathway. However, the fast-pathway conduction predominates and the atrioventricular conduction time is short. If a premature atrial beat blocks in the antegrade fast pathway, atrioventricular (AV) conduction proceeds via the slow pathway. Then, if the fast pathway recovers quickly enough to permit retrograde conduction, atrial echoes or typical slow-fast atrioventricular nodal reentrant tachycardia (AVNRT) occurs. (*a*) This simplified diagram demonstrates only one method of tachycardia induction and implies the requisite tachycardia circuit is confined to the compact AV node. (*b*) A modernized version of the tachycardia circuit reveals the involvement of the compact AV node, its anterior (fast pathway) and posterior (slow pathway) approaches, and the perinodal atrial tissue.[18]

Electrocardiographic Findings

In the electrophysiology laboratory, typical AVNRT is initiated with a long atrium-to–His bundle conduction interval, indicating antegrade conduction via the slow pathway. Because retrograde atrial activation occurs via the fast pathway, atrial and ventricular activation are virtually simultaneous [see Figure 2]. The resulting contraction of the atrium on a closed atrioventricular valve accounts for the characteristic neck pounding as well as the typical absence of P waves, which are buried within the QRS complex.

MANAGEMENT

Acute Management

Since AVNRT is usually hemodynamically stable, urgent intervention is not required. Vagal maneuvers, such as carotid sinus massage, the Valsalva maneuver, or both, may terminate tachycardia. The patient should be asked to lie on his or her back and relax as much as possible. After a minute or two, the legs can be elevated to further increase blood pressure; this should be followed by the vagal maneuver.

Adenosine is the drug of choice. An initial dose of 6 mg is administered through a freely running intravenous catheter as a rapid bolus and flushed in as quickly as possible with intravenous fluids. Administration of adenosine via a peripheral vein results in a delay of 5 to 10 seconds before any ECG effects can be detected. Complete atrioventricular block lasting for several seconds is common after termination of the tachycardia; however, conduction should normalize within 5 to 10 seconds.

If the initial 6 mg dose of adenosine is not effective, two subsequent doses of 12 mg each may be given approximately 2 minutes apart. A dose of 12 mg or less will result in at least transient termination of the tachycardia in more than 90% of patients.[16] If both the 6 mg and the 12 mg doses prove inadequate, 18 mg can be used. Adenosine has a brief half-life (10 seconds). Patients should be warned that adenosine can result in short-lived unpleasant sensations, such as chest pressure, dyspnea, flushing, headache, and light-headedness, which generally terminate without sequelae.

If adenosine is not effective or tachycardia quickly recurs, verapamil (5 to 10 mg I.V.) is almost always effective. Beta blockers and digitalis preparations have little or no role in the acute management of AVNRT. Pharmacotherapy and vagal maneuvers generally interrupt the tachycardia by causing block in the slow pathway. If hypotension, angina pectoris, or congestive heart failure is precipitated by AVNRT, direct current (DC) cardioversion (25 to 50 joules) may be applied to restore sinus rhythm.

Chronic Pharmacologic Management

Long-term pharmacotherapy is still a reasonable approach when it achieves excellent arrhythmia control and is well tolerated. Digoxin is sometimes effective.[2,17] Beta blockers may be useful when arrhythmia initiation appears to be catecholamine dependent. Although verapamil is effective and may be administered as a single daily dose of 240 mg, its use may be limited by constipation, fatigue, flushing, and edema. Diltiazem may also be effective and is generally better tolerated. Class I agents (e.g., quinidine or flecainide) act primarily on the retrograde fast pathway and perhaps by reducing ectopic beats that precipitate tachycardia. Amiodarone is effective but has too many side effects to warrant its use for this curable arrhythmia.

Nonpharmacologic Management

Both direct and cryoablative surgical approaches have been

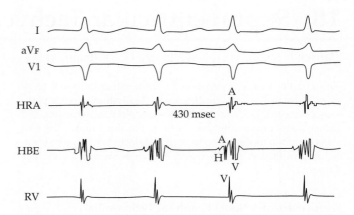

Figure 2 During AVNRT, atrial activity, seen first in the His bundle recording, occurs simultaneously with ventricular activity and is buried within the QRS complex on surface tracings.[14] (I, aVF, V1—surface ECG leads; HRA—high right atrium; HBE—His bundle electrograms; RV—right ventricle; A, H, V—atrial, His bundle, and right ventricular intracardiac recordings, respectively)

employed with high success rates and relatively low morbidity. These techniques are primarily of anatomic and historical interest, in view of the remarkable success achieved by catheter ablation in curing AVNRT.

The safety and efficacy of selective slow-pathway ablation, using both anatomic and slow-pathway potential-guided approaches, have been clearly demonstrated. Potential-guided approaches seem to require fewer radiofrequency lesions and do not require progressive movement toward the midseptum and anteroseptum (where the risk of AV block increases).[18] Reported success rates range from 94% to 100%, with complete AV block noted in 0% to 3.4% of patients.[7-10,19-25] As experience grows, it seems likely that success rates will reach nearly 100% and complete AV block will occur in fewer than 1% of cases. When performed by an experienced electrophysiologist, this technique is reasonable first-line therapy for patients with frequent episodes of AVNRT.

In one study, attempts to selectively destroy the retrograde fast pathway using DC ablation resulted in relatively low success rates and a 10% incidence of AV block.[26] Although ablation using radiofrequency energy made elimination of the fast pathway more reliable, early investigators reported complete AV block in approximately 10% of patients. Fast-pathway ablation has become safer with the use of energy titration, and some investigators advocate this technique as a backup in the rare instances when slow-pathway ablation is unsuccessful.[27,28] It should be noted that fast-pathway ablation is ineffective for unusual AVNRT variants and may instead result in incessant tachycardia.

Wolff-Parkinson-White Syndrome and Concealed Accessory Pathways

The normal conduction system of the heart limits antegrade propagation of electrical impulses, from atrium to ventricle, to a single pathway through the atrioventricular node and the His-Purkinje system. This single connection between atria and ventricles results in a delay in activation between the upper and lower myocardial chambers long enough to optimize mechanical function without creating the opportunity for reentrant tachycardia. The presence of an alternative pathway of atrioventricular conduction creates the potential for reentrant tachycardia.

ANATOMY AND PHYSIOLOGY OF ACCESSORY PATHWAYS

The most prominent manifestation of accessory atrioventricular pathways is the so-called Wolff-Parkinson-White (WPW) syndrome. In this syndrome, the accessory pathway can be located at various regions around the tricuspid and the mitral atrioventricular rings, most commonly at the left free wall of the mitral annulus. The next most common pathways are located in the posteroseptal and right free wall areas. Pathways found in the anteroseptal and the midseptal regions are relatively rare.[29] Occasionally, these pathways can be associated with a penetrating vein from the coronary sinus.[30]

The accessory pathways of the WPW syndrome usually have conduction properties similar to those of the myocardium and unlike the AV node. They are characterized by relatively fast propagation of action potentials and demonstrate very little decremental conduction. Thus, after propagating through the atria, a sinus nodal impulse can travel down both the atrioventricular node and the accessory pathway to activate the ventricles, with ventricular activation occurring earlier at sites near the accessory pathway than at sites activated normally via the His-Purkinje system.

This ventricular preexcitation causes an earlier than normal deflection on the surface QRS complex—the delta wave—which can cause a positive or negative deflection in any ECG lead, depending on the location of the accessory pathway. Delta waves can mimic the Q waves of myocardial infarction [see Figure 3]. The most common example is associated with posteroseptal accessory pathways producing Q waves in the inferior ECG leads, thus mimicking an inferior wall myocardial infarction. The prevalence of delta waves in the general population has been estimated to be about 1.5 cases per 1,000 population.[29]

Accessory pathways do not always conduct impulses in both directions. Those that conduct only in the retrograde direction, from ventricles to atria, can participate in a reentrant circuit. Because antegrade conduction occurs only via the normal pathway, ventricular preexcitation is not detectable on a 12-lead ECG during sinus rhythm. Such pathways are referred to as concealed.

Occasionally, an accessory pathway conducts well in an antegrade direction but is incapable of retrograde conduction. This condition should be suspected in a patient who has no clinical history of tachycardia but whose ECG shows a clear delta wave.

DIAGNOSIS

Clinical Presentation

Symptomatic tachyarrhythmias associated with the WPW syndrome generally begin in the teenage years or during early adulthood. Pregnancy may produce an initial attack in some women. Pregnancy can also be associated with an increasing frequency of attacks and more symptomatic episodes. Symptoms are generally paroxysmal palpitations with or without dizziness, syncope, shortness of breath, weakness, or chest pain. Another frequently described symptom, diuresis, which occurs 30 minutes to an hour after onset of tachycardia, may be related to production of atrial natriuretic factor during the arrhythmia.

Electrocardiographic Findings

Tachyarrhythmias associated with the WPW syndrome can be of several types. The most common is orthodromic reentrant tachycardia, during which the electrical impulse is conducted through the AV node and the His-Purkinje system in the normal antegrade direction to activate the ventricular myocardium and returns to the atria via the accessory connection. The QRS com-

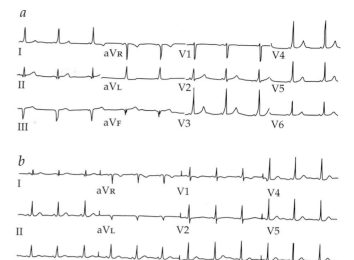

Figure 3　(*a*) **Activation of the ventricular myocardium via an accessory pathway frequently precedes earliest ventricular activation through the His-Purkinje system and results in a slurring of the QRS onset called a delta wave, easily seen in leads I, III, aV$_R$, aV$_L$, aV$_F$, and V2 through V6. (*b*) A more subtle delta wave is produced when there is minimal preexcitation, as shown in this example of a left free wall accessory pathway. These small delta waves can be overlooked on cursory examination of the 12-lead ECG. Delta waves can be mistaken for infarction Q waves. For example, a posteroseptal accessory pathway produces a delta wave that mimics an inferior myocardial infarction (*a*). Large pseudo–Q waves present in leads III and aV$_F$ are actually part of the delta wave. The posteroseptal area of the ventricles is the most caudal aspect of the ventricular myocardium, so depolarization of that area generates a superior vector, which is recorded on inferior leads of the ECG as a Q wave. (*b*) ECG changes related to early activation at the base of the left ventricular free wall include the negative delta wave in lead aV$_L$ and the large R wave in V1, which can be mistaken for a posterolateral wall myocardial infarction.**

plex usually has a normal (narrow) morphology [see Figure 4]. This arrhythmia is generally initiated by an atrial or ventricular premature beat, which is blocked in one of the atrioventricular conduction pathways but can be conducted via the other.

At times, bundle branch block may give the QRS complex a typical bundle branch block morphology, which can be helpful in identifying the location of the accessory pathway. The shortest path for an impulse to propagate from the His bundle to a free wall accessory pathway is via the ipsilateral bundle branch; when block in this bundle occurs, the impulse is forced to conduct to the ventricle via the contralateral bundle, and propagation to the accessory pathway is delayed because of later activation of the ipsilateral ventricle. This prolongation of the reentrant pathway can lengthen the tachycardia cycle.

A less common type of arrhythmia seen with the WPW syndrome is antidromic tachycardia, in which atrial impulses are conducted in an antegrade direction over the accessory pathway to activate the ventricles eccentrically from the annular site where the pathway connects to the ventricle. The impulse then travels in a retrograde direction to the atrium via the AV node or, occasionally, via another accessory pathway. Because the ventricles are strictly activated from the periphery via an accessory pathway, the QRS complex has a widened and bizarre appearance, not typical for bundle branch block morphology. On the basis of ECG criteria, these arrhythmias may be difficult to distinguish from ventricular tachycardia.

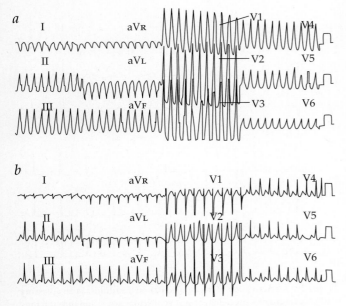

Figure 4 Electrocardiograms taken during episodes of reentrant tachycardia in a patient with the Wolff-Parkinson-White syndrome reveal both antidromic and orthodromic tachyarrhythmias. (*a*) During an antidromic episode, the QRS complex is wide, resembling the morphology seen in ventricular tachycardia. Activation of the ventricle is occurring over a left free wall accessory pathway. The impulse then travels retrogradely up the atrioventricular node to the atria before reentering the ventricle via the accessory pathway. (*b*) In the orthodromic reentrant tachycardia, the QRS complex is narrow in all leads. The ventricle is activated strictly via the atrioventricular node and His-Purkinje system, followed by retrograde propagation of the impulse via the accessory pathway to the atria.

Atrial fibrillation and flutter are of particular concern in the WPW syndrome [*see Chapter 17*], at times producing very rapid, wide QRS tachycardia that may result in syncope or sudden cardiac death. Other types of supraventricular tachycardia can occasionally use an accessory pathway to activate the ventricle. These include atrial tachycardias and atrioventricular nodal tachycardias. In such cases, the pathway does not participate directly in sustaining the tachycardia but provides impulse propagation to the ventricle in a bystander fashion.

MANAGEMENT

Whether asymptomatic patients with ventricular preexcitation on the surface ECG should be evaluated and treated remains unclear. Opinions differ regarding the risk of sudden death as the presenting symptom in these patients.[31,32] Clearly, sudden death has occurred in the absence of other signs or symptoms. Whether this risk is high enough to recommend evaluation of accessory pathway conduction characteristics in all asymptomatic patients with the WPW syndrome is unclear. Competitive athletes and pilots may be at increased risk because of the extent of sympathetic tone activation associated with their activities. In addition, pilots have a responsibility for public safety. In these patients, electrophysiologic assessment of accessory pathway conduction may be needed and ablation may need to be performed if rapid ventricular response is possible during atrial fibrillation.

Acute Management

Acute treatment of an episode of tachycardia depends on the characteristics of its presentation. The most common form of

tachycardia, orthodromic reentrant tachycardia, usually presents as a narrow QRS tachycardia, although functional or pathologic bundle branch block can widen the QRS complex. A 12-lead ECG should be obtained whenever possible. Occasionally, the QRS complex may look narrow on a single ECG lead but be obviously wide on others.

Treatment of orthodromic tachycardia should begin with vagal maneuvers, which often terminate the arrhythmia. When these are not sufficient, intravenous medications should be administered. Adenosine is the drug of choice.[16] Its main therapeutic effect is atrioventricular nodal conduction block, but it can also depress sinus node function. Adenosine usually terminates the tachycardia. On the rare occasion when it does not, verapamil can be administered.

Treatment of a wide QRS tachycardia should be aimed at blocking conduction across the accessory pathway. Identification of the arrhythmia's mechanism is frequently difficult. Although adenosine can terminate an antidromic tachycardia, it will have no effect on atrial fibrillation, atrial flutter, or an ectopic atrial tachycardia conducting rapidly across the accessory pathway. Adenosine is short acting, however, so there is very little chance of its causing difficulty if it is unsuccessful at terminating the tachycardia.

Verapamil should not be administered to patients with a wide QRS tachycardia. Verapamil's hypotensive effect together with its inability to block conduction across an accessory pathway may worsen the situation and even contribute to the onset of ventricular fibrillation.[33]

Patients whose systolic blood pressure is above 90 mm Hg in the supine position can be given intravenous procainamide, administered in a loading dose of 10 mg/kg infused at a rate not to exceed 50 mg/min. The patient's blood pressure should be monitored every minute, with the infusion rate decreased if the systolic pressure drops below 90 mm Hg. As with all class IA and IC antiarrhythmic drugs, procainamide will depress conduction across the accessory pathway. This effect can slow the ventricular response and stabilize the patient. Procainamide may also terminate the wide QRS tachycardia.

Equipment for DC cardioversion should be readily available, preferably at the patient's bedside, whenever treatment is administered for a wide QRS tachycardia. Should the patient become hemodynamically unstable during intravenous drug therapy, DC cardioversion should be performed immediately. If drug therapy is unsuccessful, DC cardioversion should be the next elective therapy.

Long-term Management

Successful treatment of an acute episode of tachycardia in a patient with WPW syndrome should be followed by long-term antiarrhythmic therapy. All patients with orthodromic atrioventricular reentrant tachycardias should be taught to perform vagotonic maneuvers. For those patients with frequent symptomatic episodes that interfere with activities of daily living, medication or a curative intervention should be considered. Although beta blockers or calcium channel blockers may adequately control the clinical episodes, their use is limited by unpleasant side effects. Of the other antiarrhythmic medications, flecainide may be the best choice for patients without coronary artery disease or cardiomyopathy. It is usually well tolerated, can be taken on a twice-a-day schedule, and is highly successful in suppressing the atrioventricular reentrant tachycardias of the WPW syndrome.[34]

Nonpharmacologic Management

Patients who do not tolerate medications or in whom medications are ineffective should be considered for catheter ablation. Use of radiofrequency catheter ablation as first-line therapy may be appropriate and should be considered on an individual basis.

Atrial Tachycardias

In addition to atrial fibrillation and atrial flutter [*see Chapter 17*], two other types of tachycardia arise in the atria: intra-atrial reentry tachycardia and automatic atrial tachycardia.

ANATOMY AND PHYSIOLOGY

Intra-atrial Reentry Tachycardia

The development of atrial reentry depends on the presence of a circuit with unidirectional block and a zone of slow conduction.

Structural heart disease can be detected in about 50% of patients with intra-atrial reentry.[35] This tachycardia is particularly common in patients who have undergone surgery for congenital heart disease. Reentry occurs around obvious structural barriers, such as suture lines. In patients without obvious cardiac disease, more subtle changes, such as scarring and fibrosis, provide substrates for reentry.

Automatic Atrial Tachycardia

Automatic atrial tachycardia arises from focal sources having abnormal automaticity and does not require the presence of a reentrant circuit. Young patients with automatic atrial tachycardia may have structurally normal hearts. If the tachycardia becomes incessant (rates greater than 120 beats/min present more than 75% of the time), cardiomyopathy may occur.[36] In older patients, structural and metabolic derangements may contribute to the development of automatic atrial tachycardias.

Multifocal Atrial Tachycardia

Multifocal atrial tachycardia, generally regarded as automatic in origin, is characterized by atrial rates of 100 to 130 beats/min, three or more morphologically distinct (nonsinus) P waves, and variable AV conduction. It is commonly associated with respiratory disease and congestive heart failure. Hypoxemia is a frequent finding. The arrhythmia may be exacerbated by digitalis excess, theophylline toxicity, or hypokalemia.

Treatment of multifocal atrial tachycardia is usually directed at the underlying precipitants. Metoprolol (used cautiously in patients with bronchospasm) or verapamil may slow atrial and ventricular rates and, occasionally, may restore sinus rhythm.[37-39] Potassium and magnesium supplements may help suppress the arrhythmia.[40] Amiodarone has also been useful in restoring sinus rhythm.[39-41]

Sinus Tachycardia

Sinus tachycardia is usually a normal reflex response to changes in physiologic, pharmacologic, or pathophysiologic stimuli, such as exercise, emotion (e.g., anxiety, anger), fever, hemodynamic or respiratory compromise, anemia, thyrotoxicosis, poor physical condition, sympathomimetic or vagolytic agents, and abnormal hemoglobins.[42] Heart rate during sinus tachycardia generally does not exceed 180 beats/min, except perhaps in young patients, who may achieve sinus rates greater than 200 beats/min during vigorous exercise.[39]

When sinus tachycardia is a reflex response to altered physiology, the resulting increase in cardiac output is usually beneficial. Tachycardia resolves when conditions return to normal.

ANATOMY AND PHYSIOLOGY OF THE SINUS NODE

The sinus node is located in the high lateral right atrium at the junction of the superior vena cava and the crista terminalis. It runs a superoinferior course toward the inferior vena cava in the majority of patients. In about 10% of patients, however, the node remains more superior, with its head extending across the crest of the atrial appendage into the interatrial groove to create a horseshoe-shaped structure around the superior vena cava.

The sinus node is spindle shaped, 1 to 2 cm long, 2 to 3 mm wide, and thick, tending to narrow toward the inferior vena cava. It contains three types of cells: P cells (thought to be the source of normal impulse formation), transitional cells, and atrial cells extending as peninsulas into the nodal boundaries. It is unlikely that a single cell type serves as the pacemaker. The nodal cells function as electrically coupled oscillators, discharging synchronously because of mutual entrainment. In other words, faster discharging cells are slowed by cells firing more slowly, and slower cells are accelerated, so that a synchronous discharge rate occurs.[43,44] The more rapid pacemaker cells tend to arise superiorly, whereas more slowly discharging cells arise more inferiorly within the node's pacemaker complex.[45]

The sinus node is richly innervated with sympathetic and parasympathetic inputs. Autonomic control of sinus rate is characterized by accentuated antagonism with parasympathetic predominance.[43,46]

Sinus Node Reentrant Tachycardia

Sinus tachycardia may also result from reentry within the sinus node, the perinodal atrial tissue, or both. Sinus node reentry has been purported to account for 3% of cases of paroxysmal supraventricular tachycardia.[47]

DIAGNOSIS

Clinical Presentation

Sinus node reentrant tachycardia has a sudden onset and termination (a physiologic sinus tachycardia begins and ends gradually). It is our bias that sinus node reentrant tachycardia is rarely the sole presenting supraventricular tachycardia, a concept supported by the work of Sanders and colleagues.[48] In their series of 343 consecutive patients referred for electrophysiologic evaluation, the incidence of sinus node reentry was 3.2%. However, the arrhythmia accompanied another supraventricular tachycardia in nine of 11 patients. Most patients with this tachycardia do not have structural heart disease.

Electrocardiographic Findings

During sinus node reentrant tachycardia, the heart rate varies between 80 and 200 beats/min (average, 130 to 140 beats/min). Sinus node reentry is difficult to prove clinically. Most investigators agree that the P wave may be nearly identical to that seen during sinus rhythm, which suggests that the exit point of a reentrant beat may differ slightly from spontaneous sinus pacemaker beats. The exact reentrant pathway has not been well defined. (A comprehensive discussion of the electrophysiologic criteria used to identify sinus node reentry is beyond the scope of this presentation.)

MANAGEMENT

Pharmacologic Management

Sinus node reentry may be an incidental finding in the electrophysiology laboratory. These rhythms usually are nonsustained, are nonclinical, and require no treatment. Sinus node reentry may respond to vagal maneuvers. Adenosine, propranolol, verapamil, and digitalis may also terminate symptomatic episodes. Beta blockers, calcium channel blockers (particularly verapamil), and digoxin are also useful in preventing tachycardia recurrences.

Nonpharmacologic management is discussed elsewhere.

Inappropriate Sinus Tachycardia

An infrequent but troublesome problem, inappropriate sinus tachycardia (IST) appears to be a true syndrome with cardiac, neurologic, and psychiatric components. It affects women more often than men. Structural heart disease is generally absent. In one series of 475 patients, IST was the indication for ablation in 2.3%.[49]

DIAGNOSIS

Clinical Presentation

This tachycardia may be persistent or episodic. It is often precipitated by arising from a reclining or sitting position (postural orthostatic tachycardia).[50] Very rapid rates (> 170 beats/min) may be triggered by minimal exertion.

The tachycardia is frequently accompanied by symptoms of dizziness, near-syncope, or syncope. Fatigue and atypical chest pain may also accompany IST. Peculiar but inconsistent autonomic and hemodynamic findings may be seen in these patients.[51] This suggests that the syndrome is not uniform in etiology.

Electrocardiographic Findings

Because tachycardia rates may arise from higher foci, the P waves seen during IST may differ slightly from those seen at rest.

MANAGEMENT

Pharmacologic Management

Beta blockers and calcium channel blockers (i.e., verapamil or diltiazem) may be used to alleviate tachycardia in IST. Unfortunately, these drugs are often not effective and tend to exacerbate the nonspecific symptoms that accompany this syndrome. Agents that alter sinus node automaticity, autonomic tone, or both, such as flecainide, propafenone, and amiodarone, may be tried in selected patients.[52]

Nonpharmacologic Management

Radiofrequency ablation has also been employed to ablate or modify the sinus node in IST. Large-tipped (8 to 10 mm) catheters are often required to create more sizable lesions. Both intracardiac electrograms and intracardiac ultrasonography have been used to target lesion delivery, with achievement of successful modification or ablation in 73% to 100% of patients. Sinus nodal modification is associated with a 10% to 27% risk of sinus node damage necessitating permanent pacing.[49,53,54]

The use of intracardiac ultrasonography targets the fastest portions of the sinus node by ablating the uppermost portion of the crista terminalis. This approach seems to require fewer radiofrequency applications than electrogram-guided approaches. It may also reduce the need for permanent pacing.

Long-term follow-up after radiofrequency modification has been less encouraging. Recurrence rates are high. Ablation to the extent that permanent pacing is required may be necessary for sustained success.[55] Thus, patients require careful follow-up for recurrent tachycardia or progressive sinus node dysfunction. Surgical isolation of the sinus node for IST has also been followed by recurrent tachycardia at new foci.[56]

All radiofrequency applications to the sinus node region should be preceded by pacing at 10 to 20 milliamperes. If diaphragmatic stimulation is seen, damage to the ipsilateral phrenic nerve may ensue.

Intracoronary ethanol has also been used to eliminate IST.[57] Because reflux of ethanol may cause a significant degree of infarction, this technique must be viewed with a great deal of caution.

References

1. Trohman RG, Pinski SL, Sterba R, et al: Evolving concepts in radiofrequency catheter ablation of atrioventricular nodal reentry tachycardia. Am Heart J 128:586, 1994
2. Prystowsky EN, Klein GJ: Cardiac Arrhythmias: An Integrated Approach for the Clinician. McGraw-Hill, New York, 1994, p 359
3. Rodriguez LM, deChillou C, Schlapfer J, et al: Age at onset and gender of patients with different types of supraventricular tachycardias. Am J Cardiol 70:1213, 1992
4. James T: Morphology of the human atrioventricular node, with remarks pertinent to its electrophysiology. Am Heart J 62:756, 1961
5. Truex R, Smythe M: Reconstruction of the human atrioventricular node. Anat Rec 158:11, 1967
6. Sung RJ, Waxman HL, Saksena S, et al: Sequence of retrograde atrial activation in patients with dual atrioventricular nodal pathways. Circulation 64:1059, 1981
7. Jackman WM, Beckman KJ, McClelland JH, et al: Treatment of supraventricular tachycardia due to atrioventricular nodal reentry by radiofrequency catheter ablation of slow-pathway conduction. N Engl J Med 327:313, 1992
8. Jazayeri MR, Hempe SL, Sra JS, et al: Selective transcatheter ablation of the fast and slow pathways using radiofrequency energy in patients with atrioventricular nodal reentrant tachycardia. Circulation 85:1318, 1992
9. Haissaguerre M, Gaita F, Fischer B, et al: Elimination of atrioventricular nodal reentrant tachycardia using discrete slow potentials to guide application of radiofrequency energy. Circulation 85:2162, 1992
10. Wathen M, Natale A, Wolfe K, et al: An anatomically guided approach to atrioventricular node slow pathway ablation. Am J Cardiol 70:886, 1992
11. Lee MA, Morady F, Kadish A, et al: Catheter modification of the atrioventricular junction with radio frequency energy for control of atrioventricular nodal reentry tachycardia. Circulation 83:827, 1991
12. Tchou PJ, Cheng YN, Mowrey K, et al: Relation of the atrial input sites to the dual atrioventricular nodal pathways: crossing of conduction curves generated with posterior and anterior pacing. J Cardiovasc Electrophysiol 8:1133, 1997
13. Keim S, Werner P, Jazayeri M, et al: Localization of the fast and slow pathways in atrioventricular nodal reentrant tachycardia by ice mapping. Circulation 86:919, 1992
14. Trohman RG: Interventions for supraventricular tachycardia unrelated to accessory pathways. Textbook of Interventional Cardiology (update 15). Topol EJ, Ed. WB Saunders Co, Philadelphia, 1994, p 223
15. Gursoy S, Steurer G, Brugada J, et al: Brief report: the hemodynamic mechanism of pounding in the neck in atrioventricular nodal reentrant tachycardia. N Engl J Med 327:772, 1992
16. DiMarco JP, Miles W, Akhtar M, et al: Adenosine for paroxysmal supraventricular tachycardia: dose ranging and comparison with verapamil in placebo-controlled, multicenter trials. Ann Intern Med 113:104, 1990
17. Wellens HJ, Duren DR, Liem DL, et al: The effect of digitalis in patients with paroxysmal atrioventricular nodal tachycardia. Circulation 52:779, 1975
18. Jackman WM, Nakagawa H, Heidbuchel H, et al: Three forms of atrioventricular nodal (junctional) reentrant tachycardia: differential diagnosis, electrophysiological characteristics and implications for anatomy of the reentrant circuit. Cardiac Electrophysiology: From Cell to Bedside. Zipes DP, Jalife J, Eds. WB Saunders Co, Philadelphia, 1994, p 620
19. Kay GN, Epstein AE, Dailey SM, et al: Selective radiofrequency ablation of the slow pathway for the treatment of atrioventricular nodal reentrant tachycardia. Circulation 85:1675, 1992
20. Jazayeri MR, Sra S, Akhtar M: Transcatheter modification of the atrioventricular node using radiofrequency energy. Herz 17:143, 1992
21. Mitrani RD, Klein LS, Hackett FK, et al: Radiofrequency ablation for atrioventricular node reentrant tachycardia: comparison between fast (anterior) and slow (posterior) pathway ablation. J Am Coll Cardiol 21:432, 1993
22. Moulton K, Miller B, Scott J, et al: Radiofrequency catheter ablation for AV nodal reentry: a technique for rapid transection of the slow AV nodal pathway. Pacing Clin Electrophysiol 16:760, 1993

23. Epstein LM, Coggins DL, Cohen TJ, et al: Improved efficacy of slow pathway AV nodal modification using a direct mid septal approach (abstr). Circulation 86:I, 1992

24. Wu D, Yeh SJ, Wang LC, et al: A simple technique for selective ablation of the slow pathway in atrioventricular node reentrant tachycardia. J Am Coll Cardiol 21:1612, 1993

25. Chen SA, Chiang CE, Tsung WP, et al: Selective radiofrequency catheter ablation of fast and slow pathways in 100 patients with atrioventricular nodal reentrant tachycardia. Am Heart J 125:1, 1993

26. Haissaguerre M, Warin JF, Lemetayer P, et al: Closed-chest ablation of retrograde conduction in patients with atrioventricular nodal reentrant tachycardia. N Engl J Med 320:426, 1989

27. Lungberg JJ, Harvey M, Calkins H, et al: Titration of power during radiofrequency catheter ablation of atrioventricular nodal reentrant tachycardia. Pacing Clin Electrophysiol 16:465, 1993

28. Morady F: Fast pathway ablation for atrioventricular nodal reentrant tachycardia. J Am Coll Cardiol 25:982, 1995

29. Sorbo MD, Buja GF, Miorelli M, et al: The prevalence of the Wolff-Parkinson-White syndrome in a population of 116,542 young males. G Ital Cardiol 25:681, 1995

30. Guiraudon GM, Guiraudon CM, Klein GJ, et al: The coronary sinus diverticulum: a pathologic entity associated with the Wolff-Parkinson-White syndrome. Am J Cardiol 62:733, 1988

31. Topaz O, Perin E, Cox M, et al: Young adult survivors of sudden cardiac arrest: analysis of invasive evaluation of 22 subjects. Am Heart J 118:281, 1989

32. Klein GJ, Prystowsky EN, Yee R, et al: Asymptomatic Wolff-Parkinson-White: should we intervene? Circulation 80:1902, 1989

33. McGovern B, Garan H, Ruskin JN: Precipitation of cardiac arrest by verapamil in patients with Wolff-Parkinson-White syndrome. Ann Intern Med 104:791, 1986

34. Anderson JL, Jolivette DM, Fredell PA: Summary of efficacy and safety of flecainide for supraventricular arrhythmias. Am J Cardiol 62:62D, 1988

35. Swerdlow CD, Liem LB: Atrial and junctional tachycardias. Cardiac Electrophysiology: From Cell to Bedside. Zipes DP, Jalife J, Eds. WB Saunders Co, Philadelphia, 1990, p 742

36. Gillette PC, Crawford FC, Zeigler VL: Mechanisms of atrial tachycardia. Cardiac Electrophysiology: From Cell to Bedside. Zipes DP, Jalife J, Eds. WB Saunders Co, Philadelphia, 1990, p 559

37. Hanau SP, Solar M, Arsura EL: Metoprolol in the treatment of multifocal atrial tachycardia. Cardiovasc Rev Rep 5:1182, 1984

38. Levine JH, Michael JR, Guarnieri T: Treatment of multifocal atrial tachycardia with verapamil. N Engl J Med 312:21, 1985

39. Zipes DP: Specific arrhythmias, diagnosis and treatment. Heart Disease. Braunwald E, Ed. WB Saunders Co, Philadelphia, 1992, p 667

40. Kouraras G, Cokkinos DV, Halal G, et al: The effective treatment of multifocal atrial tachycardia with verapamil. Jpn Heart J 30:301, 1989

41. Villain E, Vetter VL, Garcia JN, et al: Evolving concepts in the management of congenital junctional ectopic tachycardia: a multicenter study. Circulation 81:1544, 1990

42. Dougherty AH, Schroth G, Ilkiw RL: Episodic tachycardia in a 12-year-old girl. Circulation 92:268, 1995

43. Zipes DP: Genesis of cardiac arrhythmias: electrophysiological considerations. Heart Disease. Braunwald E, Ed. WB Saunders Co, Philadelphia, 1992, p 588

44. Michaels DC, Matyas EP, Jalife J: Mechanisms of sinoatrial pacemaker synchronization: a new hypothesis. Circ Res 61:704, 1987

45. Boineau JP, Schuessler RB, Cain ME, et al: Activation mapping during normal atrial rhythms and atrial flutter. Cardiac Electrophysiology: From Cell to Bedside. Zipes DP, Jalife J, Eds. WB Saunders Co, Philadelphia, 1990, p 537

46. Randall WC, Ardell JL: Nervous control of the heart: anatomy and pathophysiology. Cardiac Electrophysiology: From Cell to Bedside. Zipes DP, Jalife J, Eds. WB Saunders Co, Philadelphia, 1990, p 291

47. Josephson ME: Clinical Cardiac Electrophysiology. Lea & Febiger, Philadelphia, 1993, p 181

48. Sanders WE Jr, Sorrentino RA, Greenfield RA, et al: Catheter ablation of sinoatrial node reentrant tachycardia. J Am Coll Cardiol 23:926, 1994

49. McKenzie JP, Frazier DW, Smith JM, et al: Successful radio frequency ablation of inappropriate sinus tachycardia (abstr). Circulation 92:I, 1995

50. Low PA, Opfer-Gehrking TL, Textor TC, et al: Postural tachycardia syndrome (POTS). Neurology 45(suppl 5):519, 1995

51. Trohman RG, Pinski SL, Fouad F, et al: Inappropriate sinus tachycardia and head-up tilt: Is heart rate just the tip of the iceberg (abstr)? Pacing Clin Electrophysiol 19:710, 1996

52. Krahn AD, Yee R, Klein GJ, et al: Inappropriate sinus tachycardia: evaluation and therapy. J Cardiovasc Electrophysiol 12:1124, 1995

53. Ching Man K, Hummel J, Knight B, et al: Radiofrequency catheter ablation of inappropriate sinus tachycardia (abstr). Circulation 92:I, 1995

54. Lee RJ, Kalman JM, Fitzpatrick AP, et al: Radiofrequency catheter modification of the sinus node for "inappropriate" sinus tachycardia. Circulation 92:2919, 1995

55. Shinbane JS, Lesh MD, Scheinman MM, et al: Long-term follow-up after radiofrequency sinus node modification for inappropriate sinus tachycardia (abstr). J Am Coll Cardiol 29:199A, 1997

56. Lowe JE: Surgery for automatic atrial tachycardias. Cardiac Arrhythmia Surgery. Cox JL, Ed. Hanley & Belfus, Philadelphia, 1990, p 197

57. De Paola AAV, Horowitz LN, Vattimo AC, et al: Sinus node artery occlusion for treatment of chronic nonparoxysmal sinus tachycardia. Am J Cardiol 70:128, 1992

19 Ventricular Arrhythmias

Jonathan J. Langberg, M.D., and David B. DeLurgio, M.D.

Assessment and treatment of ventricular tachyarrhythmias present extraordinary challenges to the clinician. Moreover, the prognosis for patients is quite variable with these characteristically sudden-onset, unpredictable, and transitory arrhythmias. In some patients, ventricular ectopic activity may be benign and without sequelae, but in other patients, comparable ectopy is a harbinger of ventricular fibrillation and sudden cardiac death.[1]

This chapter summarizes the practical aspects of evaluation and treatment of patients with ventricular arrhythmias.

Pathophysiology

Ventricular tachyarrhythmias are mediated by one of three basic mechanisms: reentry, abnormal automaticity, and triggering. Although causation cannot be directly determined in individual patients, experimental and clinical observations allow us to infer the mechanism underlying many ventricular arrhythmia syndromes encountered in practice.

VENTRICULAR TACHYCARDIA DUE TO REENTRY

Reentrant arrhythmias (also called circus movement tachycardias) are produced by a continuous circular or looping pattern of myocardial activation. Two features must be present for reentry to occur. The first is a barrier around which the wavefront circulates, either a fixed region of inexcitability caused by scarring or a dysfunctional region resulting from local refractoriness. The sec-

ond feature required for reentry is unidirectional block at the entrance of the circuit. If activation spreads down both sides of the barrier, the impulses will collide distally and reentry will not occur. But if propagation is blocked in one limb and proceeds in an antegrade direction over the other, the activation wavefront may be capable of retrograde invasion of the initially blocked pathway, thereby initiating sustained reentry.

In patients with structural heart disease, most symptomatic ventricular arrhythmias are mediated by reentry.[2,3] Sustained monomorphic ventricular tachycardia often occurs after transmural myocardial infarction. The arrhythmia usually arises in the border zone of the scar [*see Figure 1*]. The larger the extent of this heterogeneous border zone, the greater the probability of a circuit capable of mediating reentrant ventricular tachycardia. This is consistent with the observation that the risk of malignant ventricular arrhythmias is proportional to the volume of the scar and the severity of left ventricular dysfunction after myocardial infarction.[4]

Although they are controversial, experimental and clinical observations suggest that ventricular fibrillation is also a reentrant phenomenon.[5] Unlike ventricular tachycardia, during which a single activation wavefront circulates around a fixed barrier, ventricular fibrillation is caused by multiple simultaneous rotors that travel around functional barriers of refractory tissue, moving continuously throughout the myocardium to create very rapid, irregular, and ineffective activation.

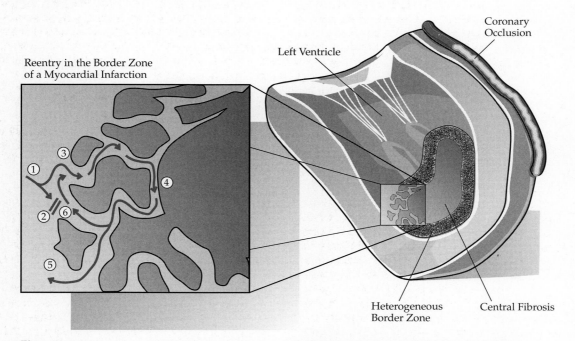

Reentry in the Border Zone of a Myocardial Infarction

Coronary Occlusion

Left Ventricle

Heterogeneous Border Zone

Central Fibrosis

Figure 1 **Reentrant ventricular tachycardia usually arises as the result of reentry within the border zone of a myocardial infarction. This region consists of strands of viable myocytes interspersed with inexcitable fibrous tissue. Reentry begins when a wavefront of activation (1) encounters a bifurcation and blocks in one of the two pathways around an obstacle (2). The activation wavefront then conducts exclusively through the orthodromic pathway (3) and encounters a region of relatively slow conduction within the tachycardia circuit (4). The activation wavefront may exit from the tachycardia circuit at a site quite different from the entrance point (5). Although the antegrade limb of the circuit is initially refractory, it recovers excitability by the time it is depolarized by the reentrant wavefront (6). The activation wavefront reenters the orthodromic limb of the circuit, and the circus movement is established.**

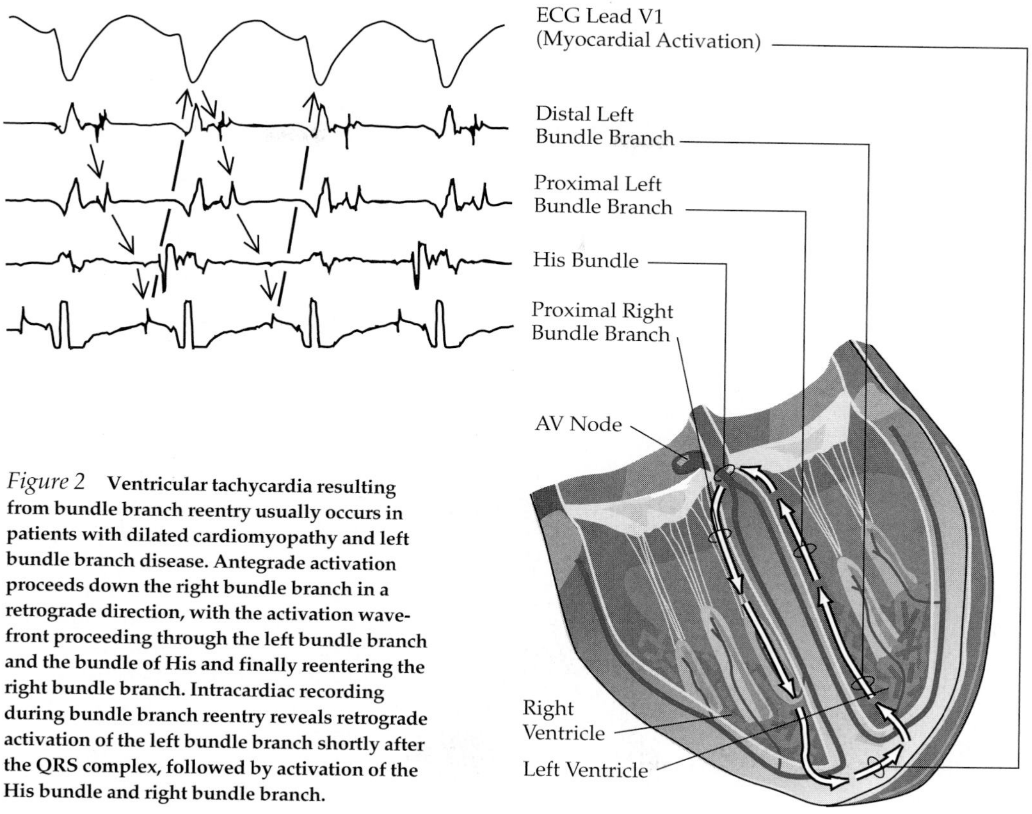

Figure 2 **Ventricular tachycardia resulting from bundle branch reentry usually occurs in patients with dilated cardiomyopathy and left bundle branch disease. Antegrade activation proceeds down the right bundle branch in a retrograde direction, with the activation wavefront proceeding through the left bundle branch and the bundle of His and finally reentering the right bundle branch. Intracardiac recording during bundle branch reentry reveals retrograde activation of the left bundle branch shortly after the QRS complex, followed by activation of the His bundle and right bundle branch.**

Like postinfarction arrhythmias, the ventricular tachycardia in patients with nonischemic cardiomyopathy is often the result of reentry in a zone of patchy fibrosis. However, in patients with left ventricular dilatation and slowed conduction in the specialized conduction system, the tachycardia may be mediated by bundle branch reentry: antegrade conduction over the right bundle branch, activation of the septum, and retrograde conduction over the left bundle branch [*see Figure 2*].[6] Although an infrequent cause of ventricular tachycardia, bundle branch reentry is of interest to cardiac electrophysiologists because it can be cured by selective destruction of either the right or the left bundle branch by use of radiofrequency catheter ablation.

VENTRICULAR TACHYCARDIA MEDIATED BY ABNORMAL AUTOMATICITY

Normal ventricular myocytes maintain a steady transmembrane resting potential of −80 to −90 mV, depolarizing only when stimulated by an activation wavefront. Extrinsic factors, such as electrolyte imbalance and ischemia, or intrinsic disease may reduce the resting potential and produce simultaneous diastolic (phase 4) depolarization [*see Figure 3*].

Unlike reentry, which can usually be induced and terminated by premature beats, automatic rhythms tend not to be influenced by pacing. Changes in heart rate at the onset of ventricular tachycardia may also provide insight into the arrhythmia mechanism. Reentrant tachycardias are usually stable because of a fixed conduction time around the circuit. In contrast, automaticity often shows warm-up, with progressive acceleration during the first few seconds of the tachycardia.

Abnormal automaticity may play a role in a number of clinical arrhythmia syndromes. An accelerated idioventricular rhythm (60 to 100 beats/min) or episodes of slow ventricular tachycardia (100 to 140 beats/min) occur in approximately 20% of patients who are monitored after transmural myocardial infarction.[7] These slow-fast rhythms are probably the result of abnormal automaticity in ischemic Purkinje fibers.

More rapid ventricular tachycardia is also a frequent complication of acute ischemia, reperfusion, or both. These arrhythmias are often polymorphic, characterized by QRS complexes that change in amplitude and cycle length, with heart rates that may approach 300 beats/min. It is likely that abnormal automaticity in ischemic myocardium is responsible for many of these episodes.

Ventricular tachycardia occasionally occurs in patients without apparent structural heart disease.[8] This idiopathic arrhythmia generally originates in the right ventricular outflow tract, just beneath the pulmonary valve. A number of observations suggest that it, too, is sometimes mediated by abnormal automaticity. It can develop spontaneously in response to increased adrenergic tone and, as a rule, cannot be induced or terminated by pacing. It may occur as a pattern of recurrent short bursts of tachycardia interspersed with equally short interludes of sinus rhythm, a pattern more consistent with automaticity than reentry.[9]

VENTRICULAR TACHYCARDIA DUE TO TRIGGERING

Early Afterdepolarization

Triggered activity, defined as premature activation caused by one or more preceding impulses, is the result of afterdepolarizations that occur either during (early afterdepolarization) or just after (delayed afterdepolarization) completion of the repolarization process [*see Figure 4*]. Factors that slow the heart rate tend to prolong the duration of depolarization, which is identified by a lengthened QT interval on the ECG, often sufficiently to bring early afterdepolarizations to threshold. Thus, triggered ventricu-

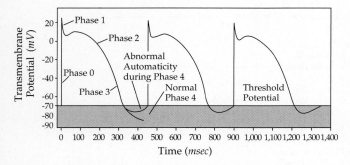

Figure 3 **The resting transmembrane potential of the myocardial cell is created by active maintenance of sodium and potassium gradients. The cell is depolarized (phase 0) by an electrical stimulus that allows a sudden influx of sodium (Na^+). Repolarization, phases 1 through 3, requires an early rapid chloride influx, a plateau phase mediated by calcium currents, and reestablishment of the resting transmembrane potential via potassium (K^+) efflux. Between action potentials, the resting potential is designated as phase 4. In cells with automaticity, depolarization mediated by calcium (Ca^{2+}) and Na^+ currents may occur during phase 4, resulting in spontaneous generation of the next action potential. In normal ventricular myocytes, the resting potential during electrical diastole (phase 4) remains in the region of −80 to −90 mV. The rate of automatic firing is determined by the resting potential, the slope of phase 4, and the threshold potential.**

lar tachycardia that results from early afterdepolarizations is characteristically bradycardia dependent or pause dependent.

Early afterdepolarizations have been produced experimentally under a variety of conditions, including ischemia, hypokalemia, and antiarrhythmic drug toxicity. The arrhythmias seen in these studies are bradycardia dependent and, typically, are both rapid and polymorphic. Slowing of the tachycardia rate just before spontaneous termination is another characteristic feature of early afterdepolarization-mediated ventricular tachycardia.

Although it is difficult to prove, it seems likely that early afterdepolarizations mediate a variety of clinical arrhythmias. Patients with the congenital long QT syndrome and patients with acquired QT prolongation produced by drugs (typically, class IA antiarrhythmic agents) or electrolyte depletion are at risk for a polymorphic ventricular tachycardia. As in the experimental situation, patients with QT prolongation tend to develop polymorphic ventricular tachycardia as a result of slowing of the heart rate, heart rate pauses, or sudden surges in adrenergic tone. Unlike rhythms mediated by automaticity or reentry, ventricular tachycardia in the setting of QT prolongation is almost always polymorphic, sometimes with the twisting pattern that characterizes torsade de pointes.

Delayed Afterdepolarization

Arrhythmias mediated by delayed afterdepolarization are distinctly different from those associated with early afterdepolarization and appear to be caused by abnormal accumulation and oscillation of cytosolic calcium concentration. The amplitude of these arrhythmias is augmented by acceleration rather than slowing of the heart rate. Delayed afterdepolarizations have been implicated in the genesis of ventricular tachycardia caused by digitalis toxicity and in some patients with ventricular tachycardia and no apparent structural heart disease. Verapamil may be therapeutic in this subset of patients.[10] Although these arrhythmias have been recorded from surviving Purkinje fibers and infarcted canine myocardium, their role in clinical arrhythmias during and after myocardial infarction is less well established.

Delayed afterdepolarizations are induced at a critical heart rate range (which is patient specific) either spontaneously or during atrial or ventricular pacing. As with reentrant arrhythmias, tachycardia resulting from delayed afterdepolarizations is often terminated by overdrive pacing, although it will frequently persist for several cycles after cessation of pacing.

Asymptomatic Ventricular Ectopy

Ventricular ectopy is recorded in more than half of normal persons undergoing ambulatory electrocardiographic monitoring. Complex ectopy (multifocal premature ventricular complexes and nonsustained ventricular tachycardia) is less frequent but is still observed in 5% to 10% of healthy persons with no apparent heart disease.[11]

The prognostic significance of ventricular ectopy depends on the severity of left ventricular dysfunction. In the absence of structural heart disease, asymptomatic ventricular ectopic activity is benign, with no demonstrable risk of sudden death, even in the presence of ventricular tachycardia. In patients with structural heart disease, however, ventricular ectopic activity is associated with an increased risk of sudden cardiac death. This risk is markedly increased with progressive left ventricular dysfunction.[12] For example, postmyocardial infarction patients with a left ventricular ejection fraction greater than 40% who experience fewer than 10 ventricular premature complexes (VPCs) an hour after myocardial infarction have a mortality of 5% to 7% a year. Those patients who experience more than 10 VPCs an hour, however, have a mortality of 12% to 18%. The combination of a left ventricular ejection fraction of less than 40% and more than 10 VPCs an hour raises the annual mortality to between 27% and 40%.

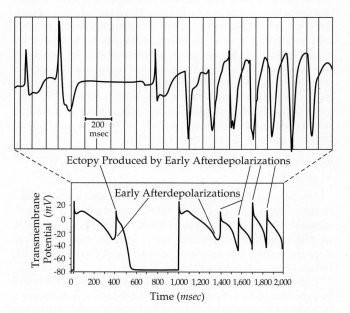

Figure 4 **In ventricular tachycardia caused by triggering, prolongation of the action potential (and the QT interval) results in depolarization during phase 3. Such early afterdepolarizations are manifested as positive deflections at the end of the phase 2 plateau or during the phase 3 rapid repolarization of the action potential. If this deflection exceeds the threshold potential, one or more triggered beats will occur. Bradycardia-dependent torsade de pointes is an example of an arrhythmia caused by early afterdepolarizations. The electrocardiogram of a patient with quinidine intoxication reveals an extrasystole and polymorphic ventricular tachycardia.**

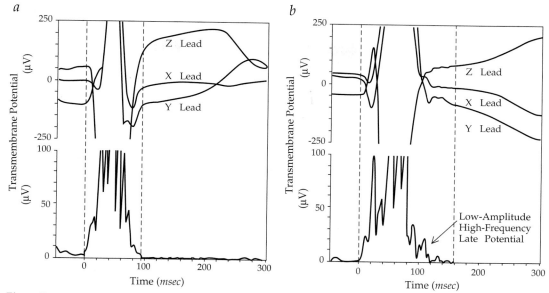

Figure 5 **Signal-averaged electrocardiography is useful for estimating the risk of sustained ventricular tachycardia in patients with a history of previous myocardial infarction. In a normal patient, the signal-averaged QRS duration is less than 100 msec and the offset of the QRS is fairly abrupt. In a patient with a history of myocardial infarction and ventricular tachycardia, the signal-averaged QRS duration is 155 msec. The low-amplitude, high-frequency tail represents late activation in a region of the scarred myocardium capable of mediating reentrant ventricular tachycardia [*see Figure 1*].**

The presence of frequent ventricular premature beats 7 to 10 days after myocardial infarction is associated with a fivefold increase in the risk of symptomatic or fatal arrhythmias during follow-up.[4] Because many patients with frequent ectopy do not develop malignant ventricular arrhythmias, the positive predictive accuracy of this finding is only 16%. Conversely, because the majority of patients without frequent ectopy remain free of fatal arrhythmias, its absence is associated with a negative predictive accuracy of 82%. The occurrence of nonsustained ventricular tachycardia (fewer than three consecutive beats over a period of less than 30 seconds) during monitoring appears to confer an even greater risk than does the presence of frequent isolated ventricular premature beats.[4,11,12]

The association between ambient ventricular ectopy and the risk of arrhythmic death is less well established in patients with nonischemic (i.e., valvular, hypertensive, or idiopathic) cardiomyopathy. However, most reports in the literature do suggest that the presence of high-grade ventricular arrhythmias, defined as multifocal VPCs or nonsustained ventricular tachycardia, confers an increased risk of sudden death that is independent of the severity of left ventricular dysfunction.[13,14]

Because the significance of ventricular ectopy depends on the degree of ventricular function impairment, cardiac imaging should be part of the initial evaluation. Echocardiography is the most versatile test; it provides information regarding regional wall motion abnormalities and valvular lesions as well as the left ventricular ejection fraction. Radionuclide ventriculography also gives precise information regarding ejection fraction and may be of value in patients whose heart disease is already well characterized.

Another study that may be useful for estimating risk in patients with heart disease and ventricular ectopy is signal-averaged electrocardiography. This noninvasive test detects signals from areas of slow conduction in the arrhythmogenic regions on the periphery of a myocardial infarction. The surface electrocardiogram is recorded for approximately 250 beats, and the signal is averaged by a computer and filtered, resulting in dramatic reduction of the signal-to-noise ratio. This allows detection of low-amplitude, high-frequency late potentials that result from the activation of zones of slow conduction just after the offset of the QRS complex [*see Figure 5*].

Low-amplitude, high-frequency late potentials are recorded in about one third of patients after myocardial infarction. These patients have a 20% incidence of life-threatening ventricular arrhythmias during the first year after infarction, compared with a 3% incidence in patients without late potentials.[15] Signal-averaged ECG findings are independently predictive of adverse events after myocardial infarction and provide additional information regarding risks in patients with frequent ventricular premature contractions and impaired left ventricular function.

Electrophysiologic study can be used to assess the inducibility of sustained ventricular arrhythmias in patients with structural heart disease.[4] Electrode catheters are introduced percutaneously into the venous system, usually via the femoral vein, and advanced under fluoroscopic guidance into the right ventricle. Programmed electrical stimulation is performed in an attempt to elicit ventricular tachycardia or fibrillation. This usually consists of a drive train at a constant paced cycle length followed by one, two, or three extra stimuli. The stimuli are introduced at progressively more premature coupling intervals until tachycardia is induced or the stimuli fail to capture as the result of local refractoriness.

The role of invasive electrophysiologic study for risk stratification in asymptomatic patients after myocardial infarction remains controversial.[16] In about 20% of such patients, sustained monomorphic ventricular postinfarction tachycardia can be induced using programmed stimulation, and in an additional 10% to 15%, ventricular fibrillation can be produced. During follow-up, arrhythmic events occur in 5% of the noninducible patients, in 10% of patients with inducible ventricular fibrillation, and in 50% of patients with inducible ventricular tachycardia.

Although electrophysiologic study has reasonable sensitivity for prediction of subsequent arrhythmic events, the positive predictive value of the test is probably no better than that of the signal-averaged ECG, especially when the latter is combined with measurements of left ventricular systolic function and quantification of ambient ectopy. Electrophysiologic study is invasive and relatively expensive. Moreover, there is no evidence to suggest that treatment of this group of patients with antiarrhythmic drugs improves survival. Thus, it is difficult to justify routine electrophysiologic testing in asymptomatic patients after myocardial infarction.

Electrophysiologic testing is of uncertain value for stratification of risk in patients with nonischemic cardiomyopathy and asymptomatic ventricular ectopy. In this population, induction of sustained monomorphic ventricular tachycardia is infrequent and does not appear to be predictive of subsequent sudden cardiac death.

Syncope and Ventricular Arrhythmias

Syncope, defined as transient loss of consciousness, is a common phenomenon, accounting for about 3% of all emergency room visits.[17] Because the spells usually resolve by the time the patient is initially evaluated, determination of the cause of loss of consciousness is difficult but extremely important, because prognosis depends on the nature of the episode. If ventricular arrhythmias are detected during subsequent monitoring, additional evaluation should be undertaken to determine whether the syncope was produced by a paroxysm of ventricular tachycardia.

HISTORY AND PHYSICAL EXAMINATION

A thorough history may provide important clues to the diagnosis of ventricular tachycardia. The onset of syncope mediated by ventricular tachycardia is usually abrupt, with only a brief prodrome of light-headedness or no premonitory symptoms at all. The absence of rapid heartbeat does not exclude the diagnosis, because only 60% of patients with documented sustained ventricular tachycardia experience this symptom. The duration of unconsciousness is brief, rarely lasting longer than several minutes. Because of the abrupt onset, traumatic injury is common.

Spontaneous movements during syncope often cause confusion and misdiagnosis. Cerebral hypoperfusion from any cause, including ventricular tachycardia, may produce one or more clonic jerks of the extremities. However, syncopal episodes differ from seizure activity in several respects: the movements in syncopal episodes are not reciprocating (tonic-clonic) and are much briefer in duration, and bladder or bowel incontinence rarely occurs.

Historical information regarding the patient's condition after awakening is frequently overlooked but may be very helpful. Patients typically recover quickly from ventricular tachycardia–mediated syncope. Postictal confusion lasting longer than 5 minutes suggests a grand mal event rather than an arrhythmic one. Similarly, persistent residual malaise, nausea, and weakness are characteristic of a faint produced by the vasodepressor syndrome rather than arrhythmic syncope.

Ventricular tachycardia of sufficient rate or duration to produce loss of consciousness is rare in patients with normal ventricular function. Thus, patients in whom ventricular arrhythmias are identified after a syncopal episode must be thoroughly evaluated for structural heart disease. The presence of severe left ventricular dysfunction in these patients is associated with an ominous prognosis.

Patients with coronary artery disease, syncope, or ventricular arrhythmias require evaluation of myocardial ischemia with a functional study (e.g., thallium scintigraphy), coronary angiography, or both, in addition to quantification of ventricular function. Acute ischemia may precipitate rapid ventricular tachycardia that is sufficient to cause loss of consciousness. In such cases, exercise treadmill testing may induce ventricular ectopy, thereby suggesting the diagnosis, especially if premonitory symptoms are reproduced.

ELECTROCARDIOGRAPHY

Signal-averaged electrocardiography plays a limited but important role in the evaluation of patients with syncope and ventricular arrhythmias. The positive predictive accuracy of this test is inadequate to confirm the diagnosis of an arrhythmic event. However, a negative result makes the possibility of sustained ventricular tachycardia unlikely enough that additional, more invasive studies are probably not justified.

Ambulatory electrocardiography is useful in selected patients with a history of syncope and ventricular arrhythmias. The yield of 24-hour or 48-hour Holter monitoring is low among patients with infrequent arrhythmic episodes, however. In such patients, a transtelephonic event recorder is more likely to provide diagnostic information. This device is worn by the patient for 4 to 6 weeks, continuously recording and storing approximately 90 seconds of the ECG in an endless loop. Immediately after presyncope or a syncopal spell, the patient presses the event button on the device to stop the recording and store the preceding ECG in memory. The output of the device is then transmitted over the telephone to a receiving station. This system has been shown to be more cost-effective than Holter monitoring and is preferable unless symptoms are present on a daily basis.

ELECTROPHYSIOLOGIC TESTS

Electrophysiologic testing can be useful in determining whether an episode of loss of consciousness was produced by ventricular tachycardia.[18] Assessment of sinus node function and atrioventricular conduction should be performed during electrophysiologic testing even when ventricular tachycardia is suspected, because episodic bradyarrhythmias may produce spells with very similar symptoms.

The induction of sustained monomorphic ventricular tachycardia during programmed stimulation increases the probability that the patient's spontaneous episode was mediated also by ventricular tachycardia. Several studies have shown a 2% to 27% rate of recurrent syncope in patients whose therapy is based on results of electrophysiologic testing, compared with 18% to 80% in those in whom the study was unrevealing or for whom no effective treatment could be found.[18,19]

Evaluation of the Patient Rescued from Cardiac Arrest

Between 80% and 90% of patients who develop out-of-hospital cardiac arrest have as the precipitating event either primary ventricular fibrillation or a rapid ventricular tachycardia that degenerates into ventricular fibrillation. Bradyarrhythmic events occur occasionally, but when asystole is recorded as the initial rhythm, it is usually indicative of a prolonged downtime interval and is associated with a very poor prognosis.

The majority of patients who sustain cardiac arrest have structural heart disease. In industrialized societies, this is most often the result of coronary atherosclerosis. Studies of both victims and survivors of cardiac arrest show significant coronary obstruction in 75% to 80% of patients. Unfortunately, sudden cardiac death is the initial manifestation of coronary artery disease in 10% to 20%

of patients, making it the most common cause of mortality in adults younger than 65 years.[20]

Despite the close association between coronary artery disease and sudden cardiac death, acute myocardial infarction is an infrequent cause of cardiac arrest. Only about 20% of patients rescued from an episode of ventricular fibrillation have evidence of an evolving myocardial infarction during their subsequent hospitalization.[21] The prognosis is favorable for cardiac arrest survivors in whom the event can be clearly linked to acute myocardial ischemia, with a recurrence rate of only 2% during the subsequent year. In contrast, patients with ventricular fibrillation not related to an ischemic event have an annual recurrence rate of greater than 20%, presumably because they have a chronic substrate capable of mediating malignant ventricular arrhythmias.[20,21]

All patients rescued from cardiac arrest require serial ECGs and enzyme measurements to determine whether the event was a consequence of acute myocardial infarction. Coronary angiography should be performed in all patients as well, except those in whom the precipitating factor has already been unequivocally identified.

ELECTROCARDIOGRAPHY

Laboratory evaluation of patients rescued from cardiac arrest should be directed at the identification of specific reversible causative factors. The postresuscitation ECG may provide important information. A prolonged QT interval suggests the possibility of drug-induced torsade de pointes or the congenital long QT syndrome. A short PR interval and slurring of the QRS onset (a delta wave) are manifestations of the Wolff-Parkinson-White (WPW) syndrome [see Chapter 18]. Patients with WPW syndrome have an accessory connection linking the atrium and ventricle across either the mitral or the tricuspid annulus. A subset of patients with the WPW syndrome are capable of very rapid antegrade conduction over the accessory connection. If these patients develop atrial fibrillation, the ventricular response may be in excess of 300 beats/min and can degenerate into ventricular fibrillation.

LABORATORY TESTS

The initial evaluation of serum electrolytes is sometimes revealing, because severe depletion of serum potassium, serum magnesium, or both may precipitate ventricular arrhythmias. Such depletions are characteristic of patients with congestive heart failure who are maintained on chronic diuretic therapy with inadequate electrolyte supplementation.

ELECTROPHYSIOLOGIC TESTS

Electrophysiologic study is an important part of the evaluation of the majority of cardiac arrest survivors in whom a reversible cause cannot be identified, including those with coronary artery disease, unless there is clear evidence for ischemia immediately preceding the event. The most specific end point of electrophysiologic study is the induction of sustained monomorphic ventricular tachycardia, which is more common in patients with a history of coronary artery disease and remote myocardial infarction than in those with other forms of structural heart disease. In a large series of cardiac arrest survivors undergoing electrophysiologic evaluation, slightly more than 42% of the survivors had inducible sustained monomorphic ventricular tachycardia, and either polymorphic ventricular tachycardia or ventricular fibrillation was induced in an additional 16%.[22] These latter arrhythmias are less likely to be specific and reproducible than is stable monomorphic ventricular tachycardia.

Pharmacologic Therapy

As a result of changes in the medical care climate, more primary care practitioners bear direct responsibility for treatment decisions in patients with cardiac arrhythmias. The use of antiarrhythmic drugs in patients with ventricular arrhythmias presents a growing challenge, especially given that the medical literature contains reports of real and potential harm associated with the use of antiarrhythmic drugs. However, there have been advances in the understanding of electrophysiologic mechanisms of arrhythmias, there is an ever-growing and more powerful pharmacopoeia, and effective nonpharmacologic tools to prevent and treat ventricular arrhythmias are also emerging.

CLASSIFICATION AND MECHANISMS OF ANTIARRHYTHMIC DRUGS

Antiarrhythmic drugs directly alter the electrophysiologic properties of myocardiocytes. Therefore, an understanding of basic cellular electrophysiology is critical for an informed use of these compounds [see Figure 6].[23]

The most widely accepted classification of antiarrhythmic drugs, originally proposed by Vaughan Williams in 1970, involves four main classes of drugs, with the first further divided into three subgroups [see Table 1].[24] This classification is based primarily on the ability of the drug to control arrhythmias by blocking ionic channels and currents. Few drugs demonstrate pure class effects, however, and other characteristics, such as influence of the drug on autonomic tone, contractility, and adverse effects, may be more important clinically and will be discussed as they pertain to individual drugs.

Class I agents inhibit the fast Na^+ channel during depolarization (phase 0) of the action potential, with resultant decreases in depolarization rate and conduction velocity [see Figure 6]. Agents in class IA (quinidine, procainamide, disopyramide, and moricizine) significantly lengthen both the action potential duration and the effective refractory period, achieved by the class I effect of Na^+ channel inhibition and the lengthening of repolarization by K^+ channel blockade, a class III effect.

Class IB drugs (lidocaine, mexiletine, tocainide, and phenytoin) are less powerful Na^+ channel blockers and, unlike class IA agents, shorten the action potential duration and refractory period in normal ventricular tissue, probably by inhibition of a background Na^+ current during phase 3 of the action potential.[25,26] Recent evidence suggests that in ischemic tissue, lidocaine may also block an adenosine triphosphate (ATP)–dependent K^+ channel, thus preventing ischemically mediated shortening of depolarization.[27]

Class IC drugs (flecainide and propafenone), the most potent Na^+ channel blockers, markedly decrease phase 0 depolarization rate and conduction velocity. Unlike other class I agents, they have little effect on the action potential duration and the effective refractory period in ventricular myocardial cells, but they do shorten the action potential of the Purkinje fibers.[28,29] This inhomogeneity of depolarization combined with marked slowing of conduction may contribute to the proarrhythmic effects of this class of drugs.

Class II agents are the beta-adrenergic antagonists. The efficacy of these drugs in the reduction of arrhythmia-related morbidity and mortality has become more evident in recent years, but the precise ionic bases for their salutary effects have not been fully elucidated. Beta-adrenergic antagonism has been shown to decrease spontaneous phase 4 depolarization and, therefore, to decrease adrenergically mediated automaticity, an effect that may be of particular importance in the prevention of ventricular arrhythmias during ischemia and reperfusion. Beta blockade also

Table 1 Classification of Antiarrhythmic Drugs[47]

Class (Agents)	Action	I.V. Dosage	Oral Dosage	Route of Elimination	Side Effects
I	Inhibit membrane sodium channels; affect Purkinje fiber action potential during depolarization (phase 0)				
IA					
Quinidine		6–10 mg/kg (I.M. or I.V.) over 20 min	200–400 mg every 4–6 hr or every 8 hr (long-acting)	Hepatic	GI, ↓LVF, ↑Dig, torsade de pointes
Procainamide	Slow the rate of rise of the action potential and prolong its duration; slow conduction; increase refractoriness	100 mg every 1–3 min to 500–1,000 mg; maintain at 2–6 mg/min	50 mg/kg/day in divided doses every 3–4 hr or every 6 hr (long-acting)	Renal	SLE, hypersensitivity, ↓LVF, torsade de pointes
Disopyramide			100–200 mg every 6–8 hr	Renal	Urinary retention, dry mouth, markedly ↓LVF
Moricizine			200–300 mg every 8 hr	Hepatic	Dizziness, nausea, headache, ↓theophylline level, ↓LVF
IB					
Lidocaine		1–2 mg/kg at 50 mg/min; maintain at 1–4 mg/min		Hepatic	CNS, GI
Tocainide	Shorten action potential duration; do not affect conduction or refractoriness		200–400 mg every 6–8 hr	Hepatic	CNS, GI, leukopenia
Mexiletine			100–300 mg every 6–12 hr; maximum, 1,200 mg/day	Hepatic	CNS, GI, leukopenia
IC	Slow the rate of rise of the action potential and slow repolarization (phase 4); slow conduction; increase refractoriness				
Flecainide			100–200 mg twice daily	Hepatic	CNS, GI, ↓↓LVF, incessant VT, sudden death
Propafenone			150–300 mg every 8–12 hr	Hepatic	CNS, GI, ↓↓LVF, ↑Dig
II					
Beta blockers					
Esmolol		500 µg/kg over 1–2 min; maintain at 25–200 µg/kg/min	Other beta blockers may be used	Hepatic	↓LVF, bronchospasm
Propranolol	Inhibit sympathetic activity; decrease automaticity; prolong atrioventricular conduction and refractoriness	1–5 mg at 1 mg/min	40–320 mg in 1–4 doses (depending on preparation)	Hepatic	↓LVF, bradycardia, AV block, bronchospasm
Acebutolol			200–600 mg twice daily	Hepatic	↓LVF, bradycardia, positive ANA, lupuslike syndrome
III					
Amiodarone		150 mg I.V. over 10 min, then 1 mg/min for 6 hr; maintain at 0.5 mg/min; overlap with initiation of oral treatment	800–1,600 mg/day for 7–21 days; maintain at 100–400 mg/day (higher doses may be needed)	Hepatic	Pulmonary fibrosis, hypothyroidism, hyperthyroidism, corneal and skin deposits, hepatitis, ↑Dig, neurotoxicity, GI
Sotalol	Block potassium channels; predominantly prolong action potential duration, prolong repolarization, widen QRS complex, prolong QT interval, decrease automaticity and conduction, and prolong refractoriness		80–160 mg every 12 hr (higher doses may be used for life-threatening arrhythmias)	Renal (dosing interval should be extended if creatinine clearance < 60 ml/min)	↓LVF, bradycardia, fatigue and other side effects associated with beta blockers
Bretylium		5–10 mg/kg over 5–10 min; maintain at 0.5–2.0 mg/min; maximum, 30 mg/kg		Renal	Hypotension, nausea
IV					
Verapamil		10–20 mg over 2–20 min; maintain at 5 µg/kg/min	80–120 mg every 6–8 hr; 240–360 mg once daily with sustained-release preparation (not approved for arrhythmia)	Hepatic	↓LVF, constipation, ↑Dig
Diltiazem	Slow calcium channel blockers; block the slow inward current; decrease automaticity and atrioventricular conduction	0.25 mg/kg over 2 min; second 0.35 mg/kg bolus after 15 min if response is inadequate; infusion rate, 5–15 mg/hr	180–360 mg daily in 1–3 doses, depending on preparation (oral forms not approved for arrhythmias)	Hepatic metabolism, renal excretion	Hypotension, ↓LVF

ANA—antinuclear antibodies AV—atrioventricular CNS—central nervous system ↑Dig—elevation of serum digoxin level GI—gastrointestinal (nausea, vomiting, diarrhea) ↓LVF—reduced left ventricular function SLE—systemic lupus erythematosus VT—ventricular tachycardia

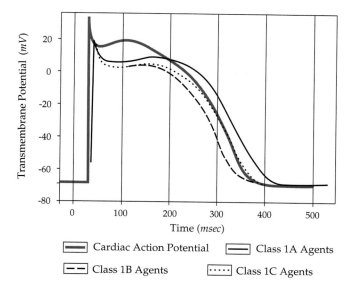

Figure 6 **The electrophysiologic hallmark of class I antiarrhythmic drugs is inhibition of the fast Na$^+$ channel, which results in a decrease in the slope and amplitude of phase 0 of the cardiac action potential. Class IA agents (quinidine, procainamide, and disopyramide) also prolong the action potential duration, whereas class IB agents (lidocaine and mexiletine) may shorten the action potential duration, particularly in ischemic tissue. Class IC agents (flecainide and propafenone) have little effect on action potential duration.**

results in the slowing of heart rate and decreased oxygen consumption, effects long recognized as desirable in myocardial infarction patients.[30] Effects on the cardiac action potential differ in atrial, ventricular, and specialized conduction tissues. For example, conduction velocity is slowed most profoundly in specialized conduction tissue, resulting in prolongation of the PR interval, whereas action potential duration in ventricular myocardium is generally not affected.

The primary actions of class III agents (amiodarone, sotalol, and bretylium) are prolongation of depolarization, the action potential duration, and the effective refractory period by K$^+$ channel blockade. These effects may prevent arrhythmias by decreasing the relative proportion of the cardiac cycle during which the myocardial cell is excitable and therefore susceptible to a triggering event. Reentrant tachycardias may be suppressed if the action potential duration becomes longer than the cycle length of the tachycardia circuit and if the leading edge of the wavefront suddenly impinges on inexcitable tissue. Use of class III agents is increasing because of proven efficacy and an incidence of proarrhythmia lower than that seen with class IA agents.

Class IV agents act by inhibiting the inward slow Ca^{2+} current, which may contribute to late afterdepolarizations and therefore to ventricular tachycardia. These Ca^{2+} channel blockers reduce afterdepolarizations and are useful in the treatment of idiopathic ventricular tachycardia.[10,31,32] They have no appreciable effect on conduction velocity or repolarization and tend to evoke sympathetic activation. Thus, their role in the treatment of ventricular tachycardia in the setting of structural heart disease is limited.

Antiarrhythmic drugs in clinical use today have activity in multiple classes. For example, in addition to its class III effects, amiodarone also exhibits prominent Na$^+$ channel blockade (class I), beta blockade (class II), and Ca^{2+} channel blockade (class IV). Sotalol is a racemic mixture of D and L isomers, both of which have a similar class III effect, whereas the L-isomer is essentially a

beta blocker. D-Sotalol has been shown to increase mortality in patients with left ventricular dysfunction and recent myocardial infarction.[33] The lower incidence of proarrhythmia seen with amiodarone or racemic sotalol therapy may be related to beneficial class II effects.

PROARRHYTHMIA

Proarrhythmia refers to the worsening of an existing arrhythmia or the induction of a new one by an antiarrhythmic drug. Three types of proarrhythmia have been described: torsade de pointes (the most common), incessant ventricular tachycardia, and extremely wide complex ventricular rhythm.

Torsade de Pointes

Torsade de pointes is triggered by early afterdepolarizations in a setting of delayed repolarization and increased dispersion of refractoriness. Class IA and class III drugs, which prolong refractoriness (and thus the QT interval) by K$^+$ channel blockade, provide the milieu for torsade de pointes. Drug-induced torsade de pointes is often pause dependent or bradycardia dependent, because the QT interval is longer at slower heart rates and after pauses. Exacerbating factors, such as hypokalemia, hypomagnesemia, and the concomitant use of other QT-prolonging drugs, are particularly important in this type of proarrhythmia.

Incessant Ventricular Tachycardia

Incessant ventricular tachycardia may be induced by drugs that markedly slow conduction (class IA and class IC) sufficiently to make the patient's own ventricular tachycardia continuous.[34,35] The arrhythmia is generally slower because of the drug effect, but it may become resistant to drugs or cardioversion, with potentially disastrous consequences in the presence of hemodynamic instability. This proarrhythmia is rarely associated with class IB drugs, which affect weaker Na$^+$ channel blockades.

Extremely Wide Complex Ventricular Rhythm

Extremely wide complex ventricular rhythm is usually associated with class IC agents, also in the setting of structural heart disease, and has been linked to excessive plasma drug levels or a sudden change in dose. The arrhythmia is not thought to represent a preexisting reentrant tachycardia and easily degenerates to ventricular fibrillation.

EFFICACY AND OUTCOMES OF ANTIARRHYTHMIC DRUG USE

Suppression of ambient ventricular ectopy by an antiarrhythmic agent does not prevent future life-threatening arrhythmias. In fact, patients effectively treated with class IC agents in the Cardiac Arrhythmia Suppression Trial (CAST) had a greater risk of sudden cardiac death than those who received placebo, a finding that underlines the proarrhythmic potential of these agents.[36] Conversely, beta blockers, agents that typically do not suppress ambient ectopy, appear to reduce the risk of malignant ventricular arrhythmias. A retrospective analysis of the CAST data showed that mortality related to arrhythmias, as well as from all causes, was reduced in patients who received beta blockers. The Electrophysiologic Study versus Electrocardiographic Monitoring (ESVEM) trial compared seven antiarrhythmic drugs and found that the risk of arrhythmia recurrence and cardiac mortality was greater with the class I agents than with sotalol.

As discussed above, patients with a history of myocardial infarction and ventricular arrhythmias have an increased risk of fatal arrhythmias during follow-up. Meta-analysis of 138 trials involving 98,000 patients showed increased mortality with class I drugs, no benefit with class IV agents, and reduced mortality with amiodarone and beta blockers.[37] Beta blockers have been conclusively associated with short-term and long-term survival in this population.[38] Therefore, all such patients should receive a beta blocker unless it is specifically contraindicated. In contrast, evidence that class IA and class IC agents increase mortality suggests that these drugs should be avoided in myocardial infarction patients. Amiodarone has resulted in decreased arrhythmia events and mortality when used for treatment of ventricular arrhythmias after myocardial infarction. Class IV agents have shown neither benefit nor harm.

Survivors of cardiac arrest have the greatest risk of subsequent arrhythmic death. In a study entitled Cardiac Arrest in Seattle: Conventional versus Amiodarone Drug Evaluation (the CASCADE study), amiodarone and class I antiarrhythmic therapy were compared for efficacy in cardiac arrest survivors at high risk for recurrent ventricular fibrillation.[39] Patients treated with amiodarone had fewer subsequent cardiac arrests, fewer implanted defibrillator discharges, and longer survival.

The Cardiac Arrest Study Hamburg (CASH) randomized survivors of cardiac arrest to receive amiodarone, metoprolol, propafenone, or an implanted cardioverter-defibrillator (ICD) device.[40] After preliminary analysis revealed increased mortality in the propafenone group, that arm of the study was discontinued. At this time, amiodarone appears to be the most effective drug for preventing recurrence of cardiac arrest.

Treatment of ventricular arrhythmias in patients with congestive heart failure is particularly challenging. The presence of a reduced ejection fraction and ventricular ectopy significantly increases the risk of sudden death. The proarrhythmic and negative inotropic effects of class IA and class IC drugs preclude their use in these patients. Two major trials have assessed the effects of amiodarone on mortality in this population. The first, a multicenter, randomized trial from Argentina, found that in patients receiving amiodarone, a significant reduction occurred in sudden death and death resulting from progressive heart failure.[13] The Survival Trial of Antiarrhythmic Therapy in Congestive Heart Failure did not show significantly greater improvement in survival among patients treated with amiodarone than among those who received placebo, despite an antiarrhythmic effect.[14] Therefore, at the very least, amiodarone appears to be safe in patients with significant ventricular dysfunction and can be used to suppress ectopy without excess mortality as a result of proarrhythmia.

Nonpharmacologic Therapy

SURGICAL TREATMENT OF VENTRICULAR TACHYCARDIA

Surgical techniques for the treatment of ventricular tachycardia after myocardial infarction were introduced in the late 1970s. Currently, the most widely accepted procedure involves opening a ventriculotomy through the middle of the infarcted region. Programmed stimulation is used to induce ventricular tachycardia, detailed mapping of the border zone is performed to identify all arrhythmogenic regions, and an extensive map-guided endocardial resection is often performed. Electrophysiologic guidance is mandatory because 15% to 20% of arrhythmia circuits may be in myocardial tissue outside the region of visible scarring. The procedure is generally performed in combination with coronary artery bypass grafting.

Large series have reported a perioperative mortality of 13% to 17% and long-term (5 years) freedom from recurrence of 95%.[41]

Patients with a history of sustained monomorphic ventricular tachycardia who require coronary artery bypass grafting and who have a large discrete aneurysm may be considered for endocardial resection. Ideal candidates have well-preserved left ventricular function outside of the aneurysmal segment, which reduces the risk of postoperative congestive heart failure.

Although the transvenous ICD has replaced arrhythmia surgery as the definitive nonpharmacologic intervention for life-threatening ventricular arrhythmias, endocardial resection continues to play a small role for highly selected patients being considered for coronary artery bypass. Because the outcome depends critically on technique, this procedure should be performed only at experienced centers.

CATHETER ABLATION OF VENTRICULAR TACHYCARDIA

The therapy of choice for reentrant supraventricular arrhythmias, radiofrequency catheter ablation also has an important role in selected patients with idiopathic ventricular tachycardia and bundle branch reentry, as well as in a subset of patients with ventricular tachycardia resulting from coronary artery disease.

THE TRANSVENOUS IMPLANTABLE CARDIOVERTER-DEFIBRILLATOR

The ICD automatically detects ventricular tachycardia or fibrillation and terminates the arrhythmia by overdrive pacing, high-energy shocks, or both. Since the first use of an ICD in a human, in 1980, the device has been used in over 100,000 patients worldwide.

All ICD systems contain three elements: the generator, rate-sensing leads, and electrodes to deliver high-energy shocks. In the early ICDs, conventional epicardial screw-in leads were used for rate sensing. Defibrillating shocks were delivered via wire-mesh patch electrodes applied directly to the epicardial surface. The generator was implanted subcutaneously in the abdomen. The implantation procedure required a thoracotomy and was associated with considerable morbidity and a perioperative mortality of 3% to 5%.[42]

Advances in hardware design have made the implantation procedure dramatically simpler and safer [see Figure 7]. In our institution, the median duration of ICD implantation has been reduced to 50 minutes, and the median postoperative stay is 24 hours. There have been no perioperative deaths in patients undergoing implantation of transvenous ICDs, and the incidence of major complications is less than 2%.[43] Comparable results have recently been reported in studies of pectoral ICD implantation.

As with modern pacemakers, the current generation of ICDs are multiprogrammable, microprocessor-based devices capable of automatically detecting ventricular tachycardia or fibrillation on the basis of timing information. The heart rate and duration of a tachycardia episode that will trigger overdrive pacing or shock therapy can be programmed. Additional detection enhancements can be used to reduce the probability that inappropriate pacing or shock will be delivered during episodes of sinus tachycardia or atrial fibrillation that exceed the programmed rate cutoff. The device can also be programmed to initiate therapy only if the heart rate increases abruptly during one cycle and only if the rate variability during the episode is less than a specified amount.

The ICD's output can also be tailored to suit patients' individual needs. For patients with a history of primary ventricular fibrillation, the ICD is programmed to deliver high-energy shocks when it detects tachycardia. Patients with a history of stable monomorphic ventricular tachycardia may benefit from overdrive pace ter-

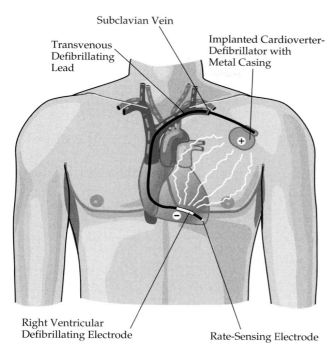

Subclavian Vein

Transvenous Defibrillating Lead

Implanted Cardioverter-Defibrillator with Metal Casing

Right Ventricular Defibrillating Electrode

Rate-Sensing Electrode

Figure 7 **The transvenous implantable cardioverter-defibrillator is usually installed in the pectoral region. A transvenous defibrillating lead is inserted into the subclavian vein and advanced into the apex of the right ventricle. When a persistent ventricular tachyarrhythmia with a rate faster than the programmed rate cutoff is detected by the rate-sensing electrode in the lead's tip, the device charges and delivers a high-voltage shock between the right ventricular defibrillating electrode and the metal casing of the defibrillator, which serves as the return electrode (anode) for defibrillating shocks.**

mination. Cardioverting shocks will be delivered only if the specified number of pacing trains fails to terminate or if it accelerates the arrhythmia. Because overdrive pacing is associated with little or no discomfort, the device may be considered in patients with recurrent episodes of tolerated ventricular tachycardia.

The ICD also functions as a ventricular demand pacemaker, obviating a second device in patients with symptomatic brady-arrhythmias. This feature is also useful for prevention of the transitory bradycardia that sometimes occurs after delivery of a defibrillating shock.

The ICD has the capability of recording individual arrhythmia episodes. When tachycardia is detected, the device stores the electrograms in memory that can then be played back through the programmer at the time of a follow-up visit. This Holter function provides valuable diagnostic information regarding arrhythmia frequency, duration, rate, and response to therapy.

As with many other therapeutic innovations, the ICD is already in widespread clinical use even though prospective trials intended to quantify its utility have not been completed. Moreover, hardware improvements continue at a rapid pace, making it difficult to assess efficacy, morbidity, and cost. As a result, indications for the ICD are controversial; however, there is consensus regarding its use in four situations: nonreproducible ventricular fibrillation or sustained tachycardia, drug-refractory ventricular fibrillation or sustained tachycardia, late failure of drug therapy, and intolerable drug side effects.

Patients who have been rescued from an episode of ventricular fibrillation or sustained hypotensive ventricular tachycardia require electrophysiologic testing. The inability to reproduce the

spontaneous arrhythmia with programmed stimulation was initially thought to be associated with a favorable prognosis. However, more recent studies show that these patients continue to be at high risk for recurrence, especially in the setting of advanced left ventricular dysfunction. A false negative electrophysiologic study precludes the possibility of assessing antiarrhythmic drug efficacy with programmed stimulation. For this reason, the ICD is indicated in patients with one or more spontaneous episodes of sustained ventricular tachycardia or fibrillation in whom sustained ventricular arrhythmias are not reproducible at electrophysiology testing.

Drug-refractory ventricular fibrillation or sustained ventricular tachycardia can usually be induced with programmed stimulation and continue to be inducible despite the best available antiarrhythmic drug therapy. The incidence of recurrent ventricular tachycardia or fibrillation in this cohort may be as high as 90% within 3 years, suggesting that device therapy is likely to be beneficial.

Late drug failure is said to have occurred if sustained ventricular tachycardia or fibrillation recurs spontaneously despite antiarrhythmic drug therapy predicted to be effective by prior testing. This is a fairly frequent indication for ICD implantation, as evidenced by a recurrence rate of 20% to 40% a year in the recently reported ESVEM trial.

Many patients who must discontinue effective antiarrhythmic medication do so because of pulmonary, hepatic, thyroid, or neurologic toxicity from long-term amiodarone therapy. In one large, retrospective study, 37% of patients treated with amiodarone for life-threatening ventricular arrhythmias had to discontinue the drug because of organ toxicity during a 60-month follow-up.

Although the ICD is effective in the prevention of antiarrhythmic death, it must be remembered that the device treats the tachyarrhythmia after it has occurred and does not alter the disorder's natural history. It is contraindicated in patients with incessantly recurrent ventricular tachycardia because the episodes will cause excessive device activation. These patients must be treated initially with antiarrhythmic medications or ablation of the dominant arrhythmia focus before an ICD can be considered.

The ICD is costly and invasive and is unlikely to provide significant benefits to patients with severe concomitant illness, with expected survival of less than a year.

The Congenital Long QT Syndrome

A familial disorder with distinct clinical features, the congenital long QT syndrome usually presents as syncope (or, in rare instances, as cardiac arrest) during childhood or teenage years, mediated by recurrent bouts of rapid, polymorphic ventricular tachycardia. Many patients are incorrectly diagnosed with a grand mal seizure disorder. Loss of consciousness characteristically occurs with a sudden surge in adrenergic tone caused by abrupt physical, emotional, or auditory stimulation. There is often a family history of unexplained syncope or premature sudden cardiac death.

The hallmark of this disorder is abnormal prolongation of the QT interval on the ECG. Prolongation is present if the heart rate–corrected QT interval (QT/RR interval) exceeds 0.47 in children, 0.46 in men, or 0.48 in women. Other depolarization abnormalities are often present in the long QT syndrome. The T wave is flattened and may have a bifid, or double-hump, appearance. In addition, a prominent U wave may be seen. About one third of patients will have a resting heart rate of less than 60 beats/min.

The originally described Jervell and Lange-Nielsen syndrome, an autosomal recessive disorder with associated deafness, has proved to be quite rare.[44] The more common Romano-Ward syndrome is an autosomal dominant disorder and is not associated with hearing loss. The relation between sympathetic activation and arrhythmias led to the hypothesis that an abnormality in cardiac sympathetic innervation was responsible for the syndrome. An alternative theory, for which there is now definitive evidence, postulates a primary defect in the ion channels mediating myocardial depolarization.[45]

Studies of affected families have now defined the disorder's molecular genetics. Linkage analyses have identified four distinct chromosomal loci associated with the disease. Remarkably, specific mutations have now been characterized at two of these loci. One mutation produces an abnormal sodium channel that has a small, persistent inward current. This inability of the depolarizing channel to completely turn off would be expected to prolong the plateau phase of the action potential and the QT interval. A second mutation produces a defective subunit in a repolarizing potassium channel (I_{KR}). Dysfunctional or nonfunctional potassium channels would attenuate the outward current that returns the cell to resting potential after depolarization, thereby increasing action potential duration and the QT interval. Of note is that this same potassium channel is blocked by many of the antiarrhythmic drugs that are associated with torsade de pointes.

Evaluation of a patient with the long QT syndrome should include screening of all first-degree relatives. A careful history regarding unexplained syncope and a 12-lead ECG should be obtained. Although genetic testing of affected families is currently available only for research, it seems likely to become a clinical reality in the near future.

Holter monitoring, which should be performed in these patients, may reveal episodes of nonsustained ventricular tachycardia. Transient severe bradyarrhythmias and T wave alternans are also indicative of electrical instability. Exercise treadmill testing may sometimes be of value; absence of appropriate shortening of the QT interval during effort may help to confirm the diagnosis in questionable cases.

The prognosis for untreated long QT syndrome is poor. More than 50% of affected individuals have experienced loss of consciousness or cardiac arrest by 12 years of age. After the diagnosis has been established, the incidence of recurrent syncope is approximately 5% a year and incidence of sudden death is 1% a year. Prospective studies have identified risk factors for sudden death, which include congenital deafness, a history of syncope, female gender, and ventricular tachycardia during monitoring.[46]

Antiadrenergic intervention with either beta-blocking drugs or surgical sympathectomy is the therapy of choice in the long QT syndrome. Although it has no direct effect on the primary disorder directly, reduction in cardiac sympathetic tone may reduce the amplitude of afterdepolarizations and, in turn, the likelihood that they will reach threshold and produce ventricular ectopy. Any patient or family member with QT prolongation and one or more risk factors should be treated with beta blockade sufficient to blunt the chronotropic response to exercise.

For patients with recurrent symptoms or persistent nonsustained ventricular tachycardia despite pharmacologic beta blockade, left thoracic sympathectomy may be useful. The caudal half of the left stellate ganglion and the first four thoracic ganglia are generally removed via a supraclavicular approach. An alternative procedure for patients who fail to respond to beta blockers is permanent cardiac pacing, which may be especially helpful in patients whose ECG shows torsade de pointes in association with profound bradycardia. Finally, patients with a history of cardiac arrest who have had recurrences despite appropriate therapy or who have multiple risk factors should be considered for an ICD. Again, the device will not alter the natural history of the disorder, so it should be considered an adjunct to antiadrenergic interventions.

References

1. Zipes DP: An overview of arrhythmias and antiarrhythmic approaches. J Cardiovasc Electrophysiol 10:267, 1999

2. de Bakker JM, van Capelle FLJ, Janse MJ, et al: Reentry as a cause of ventricular tachycardia in patients with chronic ischemic heart disease: electrophysiological and anatomic correlation. Circulation 77:589, 1988

3. de Bakker JM, Coronel R, Tasseron S, et al: Ventricular tachycardia in the infarcted, Langendorff-perfused human heart: role of the arrangement of surviving cardiac fibers. J Am Coll Cardiol 15:1594, 1990

4. Callans DJ, Josephson ME: Ventricular tachycardias in the setting of coronary artery disease. Cardiac Electrophysiology: From Cell to Bedside. Zipes DP, Jalife J, Eds. WB Saunders Co, Philadelphia, 1995, p 732

5. Kenknight BH, Bayly PV, Gerstle RJ, et al: Regional capture of fibrillating ventricular myocardium: evidence of an excitable gap. Circ Res 77:849, 1995

6. Caceres J, Jazayeri M, McKinnie J, et al: Sustained bundle branch reentry as a mechanism of clinical tachycardia. Circulation 79:256, 1989

7. Kaplinsky E, Ogawa S, Michelson EL, et al: Instantaneous and delayed ventricular arrhythmias after reperfusion of acutely ischemic myocardium: evidence for multiple mechanisms. Circulation 63:333, 1981

8. Wellens HJJ, Rodriguez LM, Smeets JL: Ventricular tachycardia in structurally normal hearts. Cardiac Electrophysiology: From Cell to Bedside. Zipes DP, Jalife J, Eds. WB Saunders Co, Philadelphia, 1995, p 780

9. Nibley C, Wharton JM: Ventricular tachycardias with left bundle branch block morphology. Pacing Clin Electrophysiol 18:334, 1995

10. Ohe T, Shimomura K, Aihara N, et al: Idiopathic left ventricular tachycardia: clinical and electrophysiological characteristics. Circulation 77:560, 1988

11. Gordon T, Kannel WB: Premature mortality from coronary heart disease: the Framingham study. JAMA 215:1617, 1971

12. Myerburg RJ, Kessler KM, Castellanos A: Sudden cardiac death: epidemiology, transient risk and intervention assessment. Ann Intern Med 119:1187, 1993

13. Doval HC, Nul DR, Grancelli HO, et al: Randomized trial of low-dose amiodarone in severe congestive heart failure. Lancet 344:493, 1994

14. Singh SN, Fletcher RD, Fisher SG, et al: Amiodarone in patients with congestive heart failure and asymptomatic ventricular arrhythmia. Survival Trial of Antiarrhythmic Therapy in Congestive Heart Failure. N Engl J Med 333:77, 1995

15. Breithardt G, Schwarzmaier M, Borggrefe M, et al: Prognostic significance of late ventricular potentials after acute myocardial infarction. Eur Heart J 4:487, 1983

16. Mason JW: A comparison of seven antiarrhythmic drugs in patients with ventricular tachyarrhythmias: electrophysiological study versus electrocardiographic monitoring investigators. N Engl J Med 329:452, 1993

17. Kapoor W: Evaluation and management of syncope. JAMA 268:2553, 1992

18. Krol RB, Morady FF, Flaker GC, et al: Electrophysiological testing in patients with unexplained syncope: clinical and noninvasive predictors of outcome. J Am Coll Cardiol 10:358, 1987

19. Denes P, Ezri MD: The role of electrophysiological studies in the management of patients with unexplained syncope. Pacing Clin Electrophysiol 8:424, 1985

20. Gillum RF: Sudden coronary death in the United States: 1980-1985. Circulation 78:756, 1989

21. Bardy GH, Olsen WH: Clinical characteristics of spontaneous-onset sustained VT and VF in survivors of cardiac arrest. Cardiac Electrophysiology: From Cell to Bedside. Zipes DP, Jalife J, Eds. WB Saunders Co, Philadelphia, 1995, p 778

22. Milner PG, Platia EV, Reid PR, et al: Ambulatory electrocardiographic recordings at the time of fatal cardiac arrest. Am J Cardiol 56:588, 1985

23. Singh BN: Current antiarrhythmic drugs: an overview of mechanisms of action and potential utility. J Cardiovasc Electrophysiol 10:283, 1999

24. Vaughan Williams EM: Cardiac Arrhythmias. Sandoe E, Fiensted-Jensen E, Olson KH, Eds. Astra, Sodertalje, Sweden, 1970, p 449

25. Singh BN, Opie LH, Marcus FI: Antiarrhythmic agents. Drugs for the Heart, Third Edition. Opie LH, Ed. WB Saunders Co, Philadelphia, 1991, p 180

26. Opie LH: The Heart: Physiology, Metabolism, Pharmacology and Therapy. Grune & Stratton, Orlando, 1984

27. Olschewski A, Brau ME, Olschewski H, et al: ATP-dependent potassium channel in rat cardiomyocytes is blocked by lidocaine. Circulation 93:656, 1996

28. Cowan JC, Vaughan Williams EM: Characterization of a new oral antiarrhythmic drug, flecainide (R818). Eur J Pharmacol 73:333, 1981

29. Ikeda N, Singh BN, Davis LD, et al: Effects of flecainide on the electrophysiological properties of isolated canine and rabbit myocardial fibers. J Am Coll Cardiol 5:303, 1985

30. Jewitt DE, Singh BN: The role of beta-adrenergic blockade during and after myocardial infarction. Prog Cardiovasc Dis 16:421, 1974

31. Takanaka C, Singh BN: Barium induced nondriver action potential as a model of triggered potentials from early afterdepolarizations: significance of slow channel activity and differing effects of quinidine and amiodarone. J Am Coll Cardiol 15:213, 1990

32. Belhassen B, Horowitz LN: Use of intravenous verapamil for ventricular tachycardia. Am J Cardiol 54:1131, 1984

33. Waldo AL, Camm AJ, deRuyter H, et al: Survival with oral D-sotalol in patients with left ventricular dysfunction after myocardial infarction: rationale, design, and methods (the SWORD trial). Am J Cardiol 75:1023, 1995

34. Levine JH, Morganroth J, Kadish AH: Mechanisms and risk factors for proarrhythmia with type Ia compared with Ic antiarrhythmic drug therapy. Circulation 80:1063, 1989

35. Josephson ME: Antiarrhythmic agents and the danger of proarrhythmic events. Ann Intern Med 111:101, 1989

36. Preliminary report: effect of encainide and flecainide on mortality in a randomized trial of arrhythmia suppression after myocardial infarction. The Cardiac Arrhythmia Suppression Trial (CAST) investigators. N Engl J Med 321:406, 1989

37. Teo KK, Yusuf S, Furburg CD: Effects of prophylactic antiarrhythmic drug therapy in acute myocardial infarction. JAMA 270:1589, 1993

38. Kennedy HL, Brooks MM, Barker AH, et al: Beta blocker therapy in the Cardiac Arrhythmia Suppression Trial. CAST Investigators. Am J Cardiol 74:674, 1994

39. Greene HL: The CASCADE Study: randomized and antiarrhythmic drug therapy in survivors of cardiac arrest in Seattle. CASCADE Investigators. Am J Cardiol 72:70F, 1993

40. Siebels J, Cappato R, Ruppel R, et al: Preliminary results of the Cardiac Arrest Study Hamburg (CASH). Am J Cardiol 72:109F, 1993

41. Krafchek J, Lawrie GM, Roberts R, et al: Surgical ablation of ventricular tachycardia: improved results with a map directed regional approach. Circulation 73:1239, 1986

42. Bardy GH, Hofer B, Johnson G, et al: Implantable transvenous cardioverter-defibrillators. Circulation 87:1152, 1993

43. Lehmann MH, Saksena S: Implantable cardioverter defibrillators in cardiovascular practice: report of the Policy Conference of the North American Society of Pacing and Electrophysiology. NASPE Policy Conference Committee. Pacing Clin Electrophysiol 14:969, 1991

44. Schwartz PJ, Loceti EH, Napolitano C, et al: The Long QT syndrome. Cardiac Electrophysiology: From Cell to Bedside. Zipes DP, Jalife J, Eds. WB Saunders Co, Philadelphia, 1995, p 788

45. Moss AJ: Prolonged QT-interval syndrome. JAMA 256:2985, 1986

46. Keating M: Linkage analysis and long QT syndrome: using genetics to study cardiovascular disease. Circulation 85:1973, 1992

47. Massie BM: Heart disease. Current Medical Diagnosis & Treatment, 35th ed. Tierney LM Jr, McPhee SJ, Papadakis MA, Eds. Appleton & Lange, Stamford, Connecticut, 1996, p 345

Acknowledgments

Figures 1, 2, and 7   Joseph Bloch, CMI.

Figures 3 through 6   Marcia Kammerer.

20 Ischemic Heart Disease: Angina Pectoris

Paul E. Fenster, M.D., Harold C. Sox, Jr., M.D., and Joseph Alpert, M.D.

Definition

The coronary artery circulation normally supplies sufficient blood flow to meet the demands of the myocardium as it labors under a widely varying work load. An imbalance between coronary blood flow (supply) and myocardial oxygen consumption (demand) can precipitate ischemia, which frequently manifests as angina pectoris. When the imbalance becomes extreme, myocardial infarction, congestive heart failure, and electrical instability (arrhythmia) may result. Arrhythmia is probably the major cause of sudden death in ischemic heart disease.

Pathophysiology

The coronary artery circulation is governed by the various factors that affect blood flow [see Figure 1]. For example, narrowing of the cross-sectional area of a segment of a major coronary artery by more than 50% (or narrowing of the diameter of a segment of an artery by more than 70%) impairs nutrient blood flow under conditions of increased myocardial demand.

The major determinants of myocardial oxygen consumption are wall tension, which is defined by left ventricular systolic pressure, left ventricular size, and left ventricular wall thickness; heart rate; and the state of contractility, or inotropic state. Increases in oxygen consumption cause ischemia if coronary artery blood flow cannot rise to meet the higher demand. Excessive myocardial oxygen demand, as may be seen in severe aortic stenosis, may cause angina despite normal coronary arteries.

Angina pectoris is a consequence of cardiac ischemia. The pain is caused, in part, by the intracardiac release of adenosine during ischemia. Stimulation of adenosine receptors slows atrioventricular nodal conduction and decreases contractility, effects that help compensate for the myocardial oxygen supply–demand imbalance. Adenosine receptor stimulation also provokes the painful sensation in the chest. The intracoronary or intravenous administration of adenosine may cause chest pain even in the absence of ischemia.[1]

A variety of mechanisms can interfere with blood flow through the coronary arteries and give rise to angina. The most common underlying pathologic process is atherosclerosis, but other factors, such as vasoactive agents released from platelets, endothelial damage, and coronary artery spasm, also play an important role.

ATHEROSCLEROSIS

In most patients, atherosclerosis is diffuse and involves both the proximal and distal vessels, although the extent of involvement may not be apparent on coronary angiography. In some patients, plaques may be present in only discrete locations [see Chapter 54].

The pathogenesis of atherosclerosis probably involves vascular injury and subsequent responses to the injury. The three types of vascular injury are functional alterations of endothelial cells (type I), endothelial denudation and intimal damage (type II), and endothelial denudation and damage to both the intima and the media (type III).[2] Type I injury can be caused by mechanical stress resulting from patterns of blood flow and can be potentiat-ed by such disorders as hypercholesterolemia or hypertension. Type I injury leads to the accumulation of lipids and macrophages. Type II injury follows the type I injury and is characterized by the adhesion of platelets to injured endothelium, which releases various growth factors and vasoactivators in a process that leads to the development of a fibrointimal lesion or a lipid lesion surrounded by a thin capsule. The lipid lesion can be easily disrupted, leading to a type III injury, thrombus formation, and continued growth of the atherosclerotic plaque. Large thrombi can cause unstable angina or myocardial infarction.

PLATELETS AND VASOCONSTRICTION

Studies in animals indicate that microscopic thrombi composed of platelets, erythrocytes, and leukocytes can transiently impair blood flow to a coronary artery that is already partially narrowed by extrinsic compression. The thrombi cause endothelial damage at the site of coronary artery narrowing, mechanically obstruct an artery, or synthesize and release vasoactive agents, which can cause vasoconstriction.[3,4] These cyclic variations in blood flow can be prevented by inhibitors of thromboxane synthetase, such as aspirin, or by antagonists of serotonin receptors, alpha$_2$ receptors, or thromboxane receptors.[3,5,6] Leukotriene C4 released from leukocytes in intracoronary thrombi also reduces coronary blood flow.[4]

ENDOTHELIAL INJURY

Endothelial injury leads to vasoconstrictor responses to vasoactive substances that cause vasodilatation in normal endothelium. A normal, intact endothelium prevents platelet aggregation by producing the platelet inhibitor and vasodilator prostaglandin I$_2$. Other vasoactive agents stimulate normal endothelium to produce a relaxing factor, nitric oxide, which inhibits vascular smooth muscle contraction. If the endothelium is damaged and does not produce sufficient nitric oxide, these vasoactive substances directly activate smooth muscle contraction.[7] In humans, endothelium-dependent stimuli, such as acetylcholine, and sympathetic stimulation, such as the stimulation that occurs in the cold pressor test, dilate normal coronary artery segments but cause vasoconstriction in diseased and stenotic coronary artery segments.[8] This endothelial dysfunction precedes angiographic evidence of coronary artery stenosis. Abnormal coronary vasomotor responses occur in patients with hypercholesterolemia[8] or hypertension,[9] in smokers,[10] and in patients with other risk factors for atherosclerosis.[11] Lowering the serum cholesterol level[12] or regular exercise[13] can reduce the vasoconstrictor response of damaged endothelium. These abnormal vasomotor responses may cause inadequate coronary artery blood flow, resulting in ischemia, even in the absence of hemodynamically significant stenosis.

CORONARY ARTERY SPASM

Spontaneous contraction of the coronary arteries (coronary artery spasm) can cause angina or contribute to it. Because platelet aggregation releases potent vasoconstrictive agents, the role of platelets and the role of coronary artery spasm in causing va-

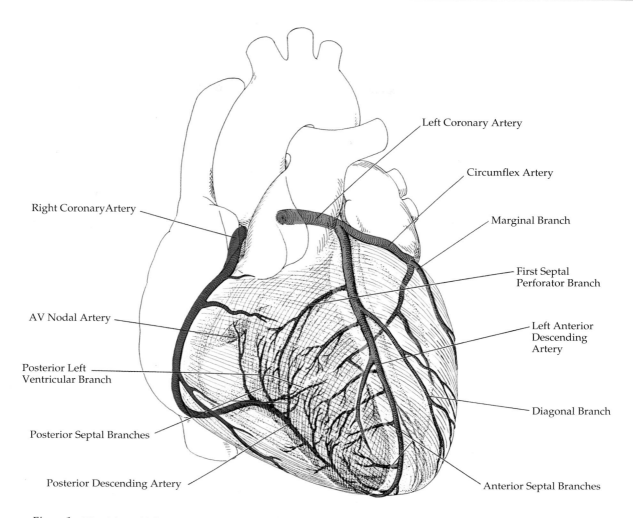

Right Coronary Artery

Left Coronary Artery

Circumflex Artery

Marginal Branch

First Septal
Perforator Branch

AV Nodal Artery

Left Anterior
Descending
Artery

Posterior Left
Ventricular Branch

Diagonal Branch

Posterior Septal Branches

Posterior Descending Artery

Anterior Septal Branches

Figure 1   **The right and left coronary arteries arise from the aorta immediately above the aortic valve. The right coronary artery runs in the atrioventricular (AV) groove toward the posterior surface of the heart. In its course, the right coronary artery yields branches that supply the right atrium and ventricle. At the posterior border of the interventricular septum, the AV nodal artery, which supplies the AV node, branches off from the right coronary artery and then divides into a posterior descending artery and a posterior left ventricular branch. Septal branches arising from the posterior descending artery supply blood to the posterior third of the interventricular septum. Soon after its emergence from the aortic sinus, the main left coronary artery divides into the left anterior descending artery, which runs downward to the cardiac apex, and the circumflex artery, which winds around the left side of the heart in the AV groove. The left anterior descending artery, in turn , gives rise to a first septal perforator branch, which is a major supplier of nutrient blood to the right bundle branch and the anterior fascicle of the left bundle branch; a diagonal branch, which courses laterally to nourish the anterolateral aspects of the ventricle; and anterior septal branches, which supply the anterior two thirds of the interventricular septum. The circumflex artery gives off a marginal branch, which nourishes the lateral aspect of the left ventricle.**

sospastic angina may be intertwined. Spasm plays an important role in variant angina and is probably the sole cause of this form of angina in patients who have no fixed obstructive lesions (about 10% to 15% of patients with variant angina). About 85% of patients with variant angina in the United States and Europe have arterial spasm at the site of a fixed atherosclerotic narrowing. Changes in normal arterial tone in the area around a fixed obstructive plaque may also contribute to more classic forms of angina, especially angina that is induced by cold.

In summary, hemodynamically significant coronary artery narrowing is often a dynamic process, as a result of release of vasoconstrictor substances from platelets or paradoxical vasoconstrictor responses of damaged endothelium. Some patients can predict the amount of exercise required to cause their angina; these patients probably have a fixed narrowing. In other patients, angina

is unpredictable, occurring at rest or after variable amounts of exercise. Angina in these patients undoubtedly reflects transient platelet clumps that cause obstruction directly or by releasing substances that cause vasoconstriction in a region of damaged endothelium.

SMALL VESSEL DISEASE

In some patients, coronary blood flow is impaired by disease that affects only the small distal vessels.[14] Small vessel disease has been seen in patients with inflammatory diseases such as systemic lupus erythematosus, polyarteritis nodosa, rheumatoid arthritis, rheumatic myocarditis, scleroderma, or radiation injury to the heart; in patients with hypertrophic cardiomyopathy or hypertension[15]; and in patients with angina whose coronary arteries appear normal by angiography.[16] Amyloidosis, hereditary medio-

Table 1   Likelihood of Significant Angiographic Coronary Atherosclerosis[18]

Age (years)	Nonanginal Chest Pain (%)*		Atypical Angina (%)*		Typical Angina (%)*	
	Men	Women	Men	Women	Men	Women
35	3–35	1–19	8–59	2–39	30–88	10–78
45	9–47	2–22	21–70	5–43	51–92	20–79
55	23–59	23–59	45–79	10–47	80–95	38–82
65	49–69	49–69	71–86	20–51	93–97	56–84

*Each value represents the percentage of patients with coronary artery disease. The first number given in each range (e.g., 3–35) is the percentage for a low-risk, mid-decade patient who does not have diabetes, does not smoke, and does not have hyperlipidemia. The second number in each range is the percentage for a same-age patient who does have diabetes, does smoke, or does have hyperlipidemia.

necrosis, thrombotic thrombocytopenia, and embolic phenomena can also cause obstructive lesions of the small coronary arteries. Some patients who have normal major coronary arteries and angina (syndrome X) display reduced coronary arteriolar vasodilator reserve[17]; they show an inadequate increase in coronary blood flow in response to a rise in myocardial oxygen consumption.

Diagnosis

CLINICAL MANIFESTATIONS

Angina pectoris is typically a retrosternal chest discomfort, usually perceived as pain but often described as pressure or heaviness. The patient may clench a fist when describing the sensation (Levine sign). Discomfort often radiates to the neck, the left shoulder, the left arm, or the lower jaw and occasionally to the back, down the right arm, or down both arms. Although angina may be perceived as an epigastric discomfort resembling indigestion, the pain usually does not radiate far below the level of the diaphragm. Some patients describe their angina as shortness of breath, mistaking a sense of constriction for being out of wind. The patient's need to take a deep breath, rather than to breathe quickly, often identifies shortness of breath as an anginal equivalent. An anginal episode usually lasts several minutes. A sharp pain that lasts only a few seconds or a dull ache that lasts for hours is rarely caused by cardiac ischemia.

Physical exertion typically induces angina, and rest usually relieves it promptly. Other precipitating factors include emotional tension, cold weather, and a large meal. Several factors occurring at the same time may precipitate angina without any of the factors being at the level usually required to cause angina if it were the only one present.

Chest discomfort is classified as typical angina if it (1) has the qualities described above and lasts at least several minutes, (2) is provoked by exertion or emotion, and (3) is relieved by rest or nitroglycerin. Chest discomfort that has any two of these characteristics is called atypical angina. Chest discomfort meeting only one or none of these characteristics is classified as noncardiac chest pain.[18] The classification correlates with the probability of the presence of significant coronary obstruction (≥ 70% diameter stenosis of at least one major epicardial artery segment or ≥ 50% diameter stenosis of the left main coronary artery) [*see Table 1*]. The probability of coronary artery disease is highest with typical angina, intermediate with atypical angina, and low with atypical chest pain. In each of the three syndromes, the probability of CAD is higher in men than in women. In primary care office practice, the probabilities corresponding to atypical angina and noncardiac chest pain are lower than the probabilities characteristic of patients referred for coronary arteriography [*see Table 1*].[19]

DIFFERENTIAL DIAGNOSIS FOR CHEST PAIN

In primary care office practice, most patients with chest pain do not have myocardial ischemia.[19] Although atypical chest pain may be ischemic, many alternative diagnoses should be considered before tests for CAD are performed [*see Table 2*]. Pain that originates in the chest wall is usually fleeting, exacerbated by chest wall movement, and associated with tenderness over the involved area, which is frequently a costochondral joint. Exertion that increases chest wall movement can bring on such pain, which may radiate to the left arm. Unfortunately, chest wall pain in the center of the chest is often incorrectly interpreted as angina because of a failure to examine each costochondral junction for tenderness in an effort to reproduce the patient's complaints. Retrosternal sharp pain exacerbated by deep breathing, by coughing, or by variation in position also suggests pericarditis, a far less common diagnosis

Table 2   Differential Diagnosis of Chest Pain[18]

Type	Cause
Nonischemic cardiovascular	Aortic dissection Pericarditis
Pulmonary	Embolus Pneumothorax Pneumonia Pleuritis

Gastrointestinal	Esophageal
	    Esophagitis
	    Spasm
	    Reflux
	Biliary
	    Colic
	    Choledocholithiasis
	    Cholangitis
	Peptic ulcer
	Pancreatitis

Chest wall	Costochondritis Fibrositis Rib fracture Sternoclavicular arthritis Herpes zoster (before the rash)

Psychiatric	Anxiety disorders
	    Hyperventilation
	    Panic disorder
	    Primary disorder
	Affective disorders (e.g., depression)
	Somatiform disorders
	Thought disorders (e.g., fixed delusions)

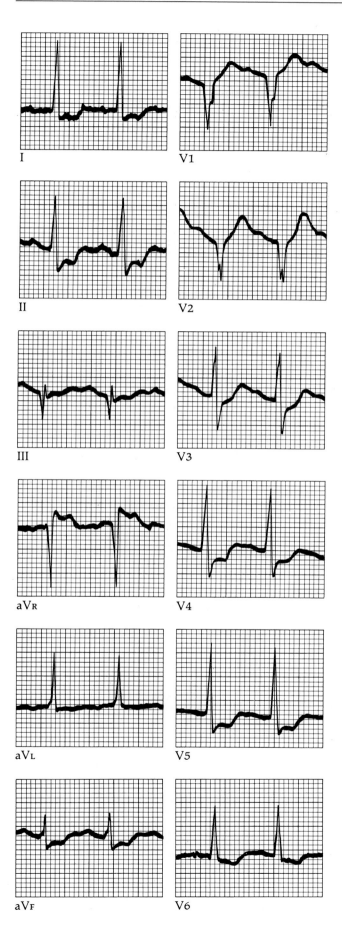

I V1
II V2
III V3
aVR V4
aVL V5
aVF V6

than musculoskeletal pain. The same type of pain in the lateral chest suggests viral pleuritis, pneumonitis, or pulmonary embolus when accompanied by new or worsening dyspnea.

Esophageal spasm can produce severe substernal pressure sensation that can be confused with ischemic pain. This pain is more likely to occur when the patient is in a recumbent position, especially after a large meal; however, it can also occur during exertion. The pain often radiates to the back. Radiation to the left arm is unusual. Because the esophagus is a smooth muscle structure, nitroglycerin or calcium channel blockers often relieve the pain of esophageal spasm.

PHYSICAL EXAMINATION

Physical examination during chest discomfort can provide a high degree of diagnostic certainty when abnormal findings wax and wane with the appearance and disappearance of chest pain. A transient S_3 or S_4 gallop, mitral regurgitation murmur, or paradoxical splitting of the second heart sound indicates that left ventricular function is altered during pain and strongly argues for an ischemic cause of pain.

IMAGING AND PHYSIOLOGIC TESTING

Electrocardiography

The standard electrocardiogram is a critical tool in the diagnosis of angina pectoris. The baseline ECG may show firm evidence of an old myocardial infarction, thus indicating that the patient has coronary artery disease (CAD) but not proving that it is the cause of the patient's pain. Furthermore, many patients with angina have a normal ECG in the absence of pain. Thus, an ECG taken when a patient is free of pain may misdirect the effort to diagnose the cause of the patient's chest pain.

An ECG taken in the presence of pain, however, can be very useful in establishing that chest pain is caused by myocardial ischemia. When transient ST segment depression, a characteristic sign of subendocardial ischemia [see Figure 2], coincides in time with an episode of anginal chest pain, the discomfort is caused by myocardial ischemia. The same is true in patients with variant angina, except that they have ST segment elevation with ischemic discomfort, a finding that indicates more extensive transmural ischemia. Indeed, ST segment elevation with chest discomfort is a necessary criterion for diagnosing variant angina.

T wave changes may also be highly specific for ischemic discomfort. During angina, some patients with a normal baseline ECG may manifest transient deep, symmetrical T wave inversion without ST segment shift. Other patients will have stable inverted T waves in association with pathologic Q waves from a previous myocardial infarction. During angina, the inverted T waves may become upright and appear normal, a phenomenon termed pseudonormalization of the ECG during angina. Pseudonormalization not only confirms that the pain is angina but also suggests that the area of previous infarction is the site of the angina and therefore contains viable myocardium.

SELECTION AND INTERPRETATION OF DIAGNOSTIC TESTS

The diagnostic evaluation of patients with possible CAD should

Figure 2 **The finding of ST segment depression in an electrocardiogram taken during an episode of angina pectoris documents subendocardial ischemia. The changes are seen in leads I, II, aVF, V3, V4, and V6. Note the ST segment elevation in aVR, an indication that the ischemia is subendothelial.**

Table 3 Performance of Diagnostic Tests for Coronary Artery Disease (CAD)[61]

Test	Sensitivity (range)	Specificity (range)	LR+	LR−	Cost ($)*	Studies	Patients	Patients with CAD (%)
Planar thallium stress imaging	0.79 (0.70–0.94)	0.73 (0.43–0.97)	2.9	0.29	221	6	510	66
Single-photon emission CT	0.88 (0.73–0.98)	0.77 (0.53–0.96)	3.8	0.16	475	8	628	70
Stress echocardiography	0.76 (0.40–1.00)	0.88 (0.80–0.95)	6.3	0.27	265	10	1,174	64
Positron emission tomography	0.91 (0.69–1.00)	0.82 (0.73–0.88)	5.1	0.11	1,500	3	206	68
Exercise ECG	0.68	0.77	3.0	0.42	110	132	24,074	66

*The cost is Medicare reimbursement except for positron emission tomography scans, in which case the cost is the insurer's reimbursement.
LR—likelihood ratio

follow the recommendations for management of chronic stable angina made by a joint panel of the American College of Cardiology, the American Heart Association, and the American College of Physicians-American Society of Internal Medicine (ACC/AHA/ACP-ASIM).[18] This expert panel adopted an approach that uses the pretest probability of CAD to decide whether a test can alter the CAD probability enough to change treatment. Choosing between tests, therefore, requires knowledge such as the sensitivity and specificity of each test, as well as the likelihood ratio for positive and negative results of each test [*see Table 3*]. The likelihood ratio shows how much the odds of CAD change as a result of the test result (from the Bayes theorem). These tests have been shown not to change the odds very much (at best, a sixfold increase after a positive test and a fall to 10% of the pretest odds after a negative test).

A number of diagnostic strategies have been recommended by the ACC/AHA/ACP-ASIM [*see Table 4*].

Typical Angina

The pretest probability of CAD is high when a patient has typical angina, although it is lower in women (0.73 for a 50-year-old woman) than in men (0.93 for a 50-year-old man). In men, a positive result with any of the noninvasive diagnostic tests will raise the probability of CAD to approximately 1.0, which is a small increase in probability and thus of doubtful diagnostic significance. In women, the probability after a positive test result exceeds 0.90. A negative test result does not lower the probability of disease enough to alter management. Because the exercise test result will not change the probability of CAD enough to alter treatment, the ACC/AHA/ACP-ASIM guidelines recommend administering empirical treatment for CAD and secondary prevention measures.

Although the exercise ECG is not very useful for diagnosis in patients with typical angina, it can be useful for establishing the prognosis. Some patients with typical angina have a bad enough prognosis to warrant consideration for revascularization despite stable, tolerable symptoms. Exercise performance is an excellent measure of left ventricular function, a key determinant of prognosis. Patients with CAD who can complete stage IV of the Bruce protocol have an excellent prognosis. Therefore, it is reasonable to perform exercise ECG as a staging procedure in a person who almost certainly has CAD on the basis of the history of typical angina. The ACC/AHA/ACP-ASIM guidelines recommend exercise ECG in patients with comorbid conditions or those who want to know their prognosis. As with other indications, a person with resting ST segment depression, a paced ventricular rhythm, Wolff-

Parkinson-White syndrome, or complete left bundle branch block should undergo stress imaging rather than stress ECG. Finally, a person who has come close to sudden cardiac death has a very high risk of death and should undergo coronary arteriography because the prognosis would be poor even after a negative noninvasive test.

Atypical Angina

The pretest probability of CAD is intermediate in patients who have atypical angina and lower in women (0.31 for a 50-year-old woman) than in men (0.65 for a 50-year-old man). An intermediate probability means that there is considerable uncertainty about

Table 4 Recommended Diagnostic Strategies in Patients with Chronic Stable Angina[1,2]

Pretest Probability of Coronary Artery Disease*	Strategy
High (typical angina) 0.93 in men 0.73 in women	For most patients, administer empirical therapy for coronary artery disease and secondary prevention measures For patients with comorbid conditions that worsen coronary artery disease and those who wish to know their prognosis, perform exercise ECG (perform stress imaging test in patients with Wolff-Parkinson-White syndrome, a paced ventricular rhythm, > 1 mm ST segment depression at rest, or complete left bundle branch block) For patients surviving near sudden coronary death and those with contraindications to noninvasive testing, refer patients directly for coronary angiography without noninvasive testing
Intermediate (atypical angina) 0.65 in men 0.31 in women	For most patients, perform exercise ECG (perform stress imaging test in patients with ECG abnormalities) For patients with contraindications to noninvasive testing, refer patients directly for coronary angiography without noninvasive testing
Low (nonanginal chest pain) 0.20 in men 0.07 in women	For most patients, reconsider the diagnosis before testing for coronary artery disease and pursue noncardiac causes of chest pain Initiate primary prevention

*Probabilities are based on history and apply to men and women 50 to 59 years of age. The probabilities will be lower for intermediate-risk patients in primary care.

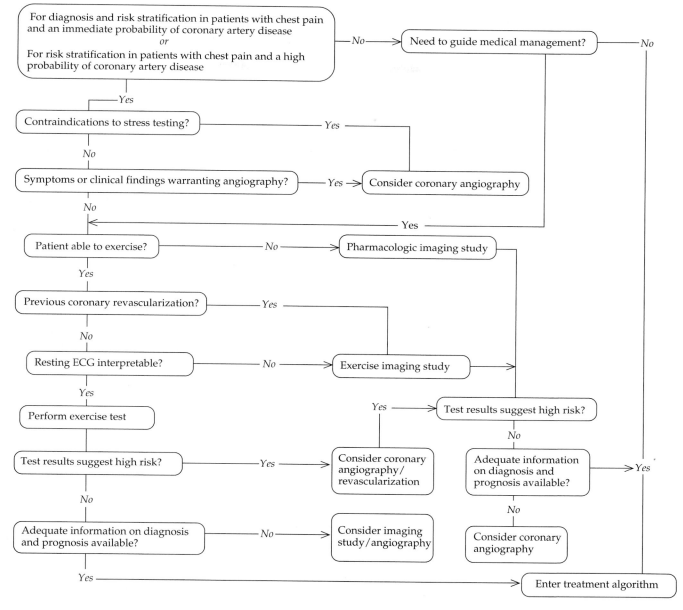

Figure 3 **Algorithm for selection of exercise ECG, pharmacologic imaging test, exercise imaging test, or coronary angiography for diagnosis or for risk stratification.**

whether the patient has significant coronary artery stenosis. In these patients, noninvasive testing can reduce diagnostic uncertainty. The ACC/AHA/ACP-ASIM guidelines recommend exercise ECG in these patients unless they have one of the conditions that interfere with interpreting ST segment depression. The probability of CAD for a 50-year-old man would increase from 0.65 to 0.83 after a positive exercise ECG. The probability for a 50-year-old woman would increase from 0.31 to 0.60 after a positive exercise ECG. The posttest probability of CAD in women would be 0.75 after a positive stress echocardiogram, perhaps warranting use of this test over exercise ECG. Note that the probability of CAD after a normal exercise ECG is 0.44 for men and 0.17 for women. However, normal results do not rule out CAD in patients who have atypical angina.

The choice of tests in women with typical or atypical angina il-

lustrates an important principle. Because the pretest probability of CAD is lower in women than in men, achieving a high posttest probability in women requires use of a test with a higher likelihood ratio than that of exercise ECG. Imaging tests may be worth the higher cost [*see Table 3*] in women with angina.

Atypical Chest Pain

The pretest probability of CAD is low in patients with atypical angina and, again, is lower in women (0.07 for a 50-year-old woman) than in men (0.20 for a 50-year-old man). The ACC/AHA/ACP-ASIM guidelines recommend pursuing other noncardiac causes of chest pain before testing for CAD. The reason for this recommendation is that positive tests for CAD do not raise the probability of CAD very far from its pretest value, which is quite low in these patients. If the diagnostic workup excludes common noncardiac causes of chest pain, the probability of CAD will be increased, and at that point, testing might become worthwhile.

DIAGNOSTIC TESTS

Exercise Electrocardiography

An exercise ECG is helpful in detecting the presence of CAD and in assessing prognosis. The test is generally safe, with myocardial infarction and death occuring at a rate of less than 1 in 2,500 tests.[20] Unless cardiac catheterization is indicated or unless an exercise ECG is not feasible or not interpretable, patients with atypical angina should undergo an exercise ECG to establish the diagnosis. In patients with typical angina, the principal role of the exercise ECG is to assess the risk of future cardiac events [*see Figure 3*].

Contraindications to exercise testing include acute myocardial infarction within the previous 2 days, serious arrhythmias, severe aortic stenosis, symptomatic heart failure, acute pulmonary embolism, acute myocarditis, acute pericarditis, and acute aortic dissection.[21]

Exercise may be done on either a treadmill or a bicycle. Treadmill testing is preferred, unless the patient regularly uses a bicycle. During exercise, a patient's symptoms, heart rate, blood pressure, and multiple-lead ECG are monitored. The usual goal is to reach at least 85% of age-predicted maximum heart rate. The test should be stopped before reaching the target heart rate if any of the following occur: severe angina or presyncope; drop in systolic blood pressure of more than 10 mm Hg from baseline; cyanosis; sustained ventricular tachycardia; or ST segment elevation of at least 1 mm in any lead without a pathologic Q wave.

The exercise ECG occupies a central role in the diagnosis of CAD because it has an excellent track record. Over 100 studies involving tens of thousands of patients have consistently shown that the test provides information about the presence of CAD, its severity, and the patient's prognosis. Exercise ECG is less accurate in detection of CAD than imaging tests, but it is less costly and far better studied. Interpretation of the test includes evaluation of symptoms, exercise capacity, blood pressure response, maximal heart rate, and ST segment changes. The minimum criterion for an abnormal ST segment response is at least 1 mm of horizontal or downsloping ST segment depression or ST segment elevation occurring during or within 4 minutes after exercise. The greater the amount of ST segment depression, the higher the probability of CAD. There is a greater probability of more severe CAD, with a worse prognosis, if the ST segment abnormality is associated with angina, poor exercise capacity, or a fall in systolic blood pressure during exercise. Severe CAD and a poor prognosis are also more likely if there is an unexpectedly low heart rate at the onset of ST segment change, a large number of ECG leads with ST segment changes, and persistence of ST segment deviation long after exercise is discontinued. To estimate the risk of annual mortality, the physician can use a nomogram that takes into account the presence or absence of angina, the maximum exercise capacity, and the degree of ST segment deviation [*see Figure 4*].[21]

The posttest probability of CAD after an exercise ECG depends on the patient's pretest probability [*see Table 1*]. In a 70-year-old man with typical angina pectoris, the test is not useful for determining the presence or absence of CAD, but it can yield useful information about prognosis and about severity of ischemia. In a 35-year-old woman with atypical chest pain and no atherosclerotic risk factors, a positive exercise ECG is more likely to be a false positive than a true positive. Overall, the test is most useful for diagnosis when the clinical features suggest an inter-

ST Segment Deviation during Exercise	Ischemia Reading Line	Angina during Exercise	Prognosis		Duration of Exercise	
			5-Year Survival	Avg. Annual Mortality	MET	Minutes
0 mm		None	0.99	0.2%	20	18
			0.98	0.4%		
					17	15
1 mm		Nonlimiting	0.95	1%	13	12
			0.93	1.5%		
			0.90	2%	10	9
			0.85	3%		
2 mm			0.80	4%	7	6
		Exercise-limiting	0.75	5%		
			0.70	6%		
					5	3
3 mm			0.55	9%	0	0
4 mm						

Figure 4   **Nomogram showing risk of mortality. Prognosis is determined in five steps: (1) Exercise-induced ST segment deviation is marked on the ST segment deviation column during exercise. (2) Degree of angina is marked on the angina column. (3) The marks for ST segment deviation and degree of angina are connected by a straight line across the ischemia-reading column; the point of intersection is the ischemia mark. (4) The amount of time on a treadmill is marked on the exercise-during column. (5) The ischemia mark is connected to the exercise-duration mark. The point at which this line crosses the prognosis column indicates the 5-year cardiovascular survival rate and the average annual mortality.**

mediate probability of significant coronary atherosclerosis, corresponding to a history of atypical angina.[21]

ECHOCARDIOGRAPHIC AND NUCLEAR STRESS IMAGING

Although physicians often turn first to an imaging test, the ACC/AHA/ACP-ASIM guidelines specify a relatively limited role for these tests. Exercise testing is not always possible because peripheral vascular disease, arthritis, severe lung disease, or other noncardiac conditions markedly limit the ability of the patient to exercise. Also, the ECG response to exercise can be difficult to interpret because of the presence of left bundle branch block, electronically paced ventricular rhythm, preexcitation (Wolff-Parkinson-White) syndrome, or a greater than 1 mm ST segment depression at rest, as may occur in left ventricular hypertrophy or with digitalis. These situations are the principal indications for noninvasive imaging tests, according to the ACC/AHA/ACP-ASIM guidelines [see Figure 3 and Table 4].[18]

When the patient can exercise but the ST segment response would not be interpretable, there are several alternative tests. Echocardiography may reveal new or worsened left ventricular segmental wall abnormalities, indicative of ischemia. An intravenous echocardiographic contrast agent can enhance the accuracy of stress echocardiography.[22] Another alternative to the exercise ECG is the assessment of coronary perfusion by radionuclide imaging, using tracers such as thallium-201, technetium-99m sestamibi, or technetium-99m tetrofosmin. Activity of these agents may be detected over the myocardium and corresponds to coronary blood flow. A significant coronary obstructive lesion causes relatively less flow and, hence, less tracer activity. Exercise increases the difference in tracer activity between normal and underperfused regions because coronary blood flow increases markedly with exercise except in regions distal to coronary artery obstruction.

For a patient who is unable to exercise, dobutamine or pacing to progressively faster rates will provide adequate cardiac stress. Another alternative is to administer a coronary vasodilator, such as dipyridamole or adenosine, which dilates normal coronary arteries but causes little change in the diameter of an atherosclerotic segment. After inducing stress by these techniques, the physician can use echocardiography to assess myocardial function or radionuclide tracer scanning to assess myocardial perfusion.

Echocardiographic wall motion analysis is performed after stressing the heart by exercise, by dobutamine infusion, or by pacing. Wall motion analysis provides information beyond that obtained from the ECG, even if the ST segments are normal at baseline. The wall motion abnormalities induced by stress correspond to the site of ischemia, thereby localizing the obstructive coronary lesion. In contrast, stress-induced ST segment depression indicates the presence of ischemia but does not reliably predict the location of the coronary lesion.

Stress echocardiography is more accurate than exercise ECG in the diagnosis of ischemic heart disease [see Table 3]. In 36 studies that included a total of 3,270 patients, the average sensitivity of exercise echocardiography was 85% and that of dobutamine echocardiography was 82%. The specificity averaged 86% for exercise echocardiography and 85% for dobutamine echocardiography.[22] Thus, a positive result on these tests increases the odds of CAD by fivefold to sixfold. A negative result reduces the odds of CAD to 20% of the pretest odds.

Dobutamine echocardiography indicates a relatively poor prognosis (mortality > 3% a year) when a new wall motion abnormality in two or more segments develops after administration

of dobutamine at a dosage of 10 μg/kg/min or less or develops at a heart rate of less than 120 beats/min.[22]

Radionuclide assessment of coronary perfusion is usually performed after either exercise or after administration of dipyridamole or adenosine. Myocardial perfusion may be assessed by either planar or single-photon emission computed tomography (SPECT) techniques, with visual or quantitative analysis. In diagnosing cardiac ischemia, these methods have a sensitivity and specificity similar to those of dobutamine echocardiography [see Table 3], although at considerably greater cost. The radionuclide techniques can also identify the area of hypoperfusion and thereby identify the abnormal coronary artery.[23]

The number, size, and location of radionuclide perfusion abnormalities, the amount of lung uptake of thallium, and the occurrence of left ventricular dilatation correlate with the severity of coronary atherosclerosis and with prognosis. The magnitude of the perfusion abnormality is the most important prognostic indicator. Increased lung uptake of thallium is associated with pulmonary venous hypertension, caused by exercise-induced global left ventricular dysfunction, and thus indicates increased ischemia and increased risk.[23,24]

The choice of echocardiographic or radionuclide test depends on local expertise, available facilities, and cost. There is a trade-off between test performance and cost [see Table 3].

Coronary Angiography

Indications for angiography   The clearest indication for angiography is the presence of incapacitating angina in a patient on a maximal medical program. Angiography is indicated for patients who have failed to achieve the goals of medical therapy and are at increased risk for death or myocardial infarction. In such patients, revascularization therapy provides the best hope for pain relief and improved prognosis. Whether revascularization will help depends on the findings at angiography.

According to the ACC/AHA/ACP-ASIM guidelines, angiography should be performed if noninvasive tests suggest the presence of a large area of ischemia and therefore a poor prognosis.[18] Similarly, patients with known or suspected coronary atherosclerosis who have survived an episode of cardiac arrest are at high risk for death and should undergo coronary angiography.

Angiography is appropriate for patients who have chest pain that is possibly attributable to myocardial ischemia but should not undergo noninvasive testing because it is contraindicated or is unlikely to yield useful information. This group of patients includes those who cannot exercise because of chronic obstructive pulmonary disease, who cannot receive dipyridamole or adenosine because of the risk of bronchospasm, or in whom echocardiographic images are likely to be poor. Angiography is appropriate for angina patients whose posttest probability after noninvasive tests leaves either the patient or the physician too uncertain about the correct diagnosis to proceed to the next step in therapy. Angiography is also appropriate for angina patients whose occupations could put them or others at risk. This group includes pilots, police officers, firefighters, and professional athletes.

Coronary angiography is useful in establishing a diagnosis of nonatherosclerotic CAD when the condition is clinically suspected, such as in cases of coronary artery spasm, congenital coronary artery anomalies, Kawasaki disease, coronary artery dissection, and radiation-induced vasculopathy.

Risks of angiography   Although coronary angiography is the procedure that provides the most information about the condition of the coronary arteries, it is relatively expensive and carries some risk. The major complications of angiography include myocardial infarction, stroke, and death. Procedure-related mortality is low, averaging about 0.1% in centers that perform a minimum of six procedures a week. The risk of infarction or stroke is comparable (about 0.1%).

Interpretation of the angiogram The physiologic consequences of narrowing caused by a coronary artery stenosis are often uncertain. There is good evidence that 70% narrowing of the lumen diameter (as interpreted visually) impairs flow. Quantitative coronary angiography and measurements of coronary flow reserve indicate that stenosis greater than 60% of the diameter of the lumen or a cross-sectional area of less than 2.5 mm^2 reduces coronary flow reserve. Physiologic data can be very helpful in interpreting coronary artery narrowing of less than 60% of the luminal diameter. For example, a patient whose ECG reveals marked ST segment depression when pain is present probably has significant impairment of flow through a coronary artery even though the angiogram shows only a 50% decrease in the diameter of the lumen. Direct intracoronary measurement of flow provides a more accurate assessment of the physiologic significance of a lesion.

A vessel of reasonable size, with a high-grade proximal stenosis, and free of significant distal plaques is suitable for bypass surgery. The most suitable lesion for coronary angioplasty is discrete, concentric, proximal, noncalcified, and less than 5 mm in length; the lesion should not be longer than 10 mm.

Assessment of left ventricular function is an important factor in deciding whether to use medical or revascularization therapy, because randomized trials of bypass surgery have consistently shown improved survival in patients with multivessel disease and poor ventricular function (ejection fraction < 40%) who receive bypass surgery.[25] Echocardiography or left ventricular angiography are the two principal methods for measuring ejection fraction and end-diastolic volume and for assessing ventricular contractility. A failing myocardium with large areas that contract poorly (hypokinetic) or not at all (akinetic) or that bulge paradoxically during systole (dyskinetic) connotes a worse prognosis for any given anatomic extent of CAD.[26] Knowing the cause of a wall motion abnormality is important when trying to determine whether revascularization will be successful. If there is extensive myocardial fibrosis caused by prior myocardial infarctions, the risk of revascularization is especially high, and there is little likelihood of improving ventricular function.[27] In contrast, some patients with chronic ischemia have chronically impaired myocardial function, a phenomenon called hibernating myocardium. If tests such as dobutamine echocardiography or positron emission tomography indicate that a significant amount of myocardium is hibernating (i.e., contractility returns after treatment with low-dose dobutamine), the long-term prognosis is better with revascularization than with medical therapy.[22]

Prognostic implications of angiography The two most important prognostic determinants in patients with CAD are the anatomic extent of disease as revealed by coronary angiography and the state of left ventricular function.[24,25] In a 12-year follow-up study of medically treated patients by the Coronary Artery Surgery Study (CASS) registry, survival for patients with zero-, one-, two-, and three-vessel disease was 91%, 74%, 59%, and 40%, respectively [see Table 5].[26] Twelve-year survival for patients with CAD was 73% if the ejection fraction was over 50%, 54% if the

Table 5 Prognosis Related to Specific Coronary Artery Atherosclerotic Lesions[24]

Type of Disease	Extent of Disease (%)	5-Year Survival Rate (%)*
1 vessel	75	93
> 1 vessel	50–75	93
1 vessel	≥ 95	91
2 vessel	—	88
2 vessel	Both ≥ 95	86
1 vessel	≥ 95 in proximal left anterior descending coronary artery	83
2 vessel	≥ 95 in left anterior descending coronary artery	83
2 vessel	≥ 95 in proximal left anterior descending coronary artery	79
3 vessel	—	79
3 vessel	≥ 95 in at least one vessel	73
3 vessel	75 in proximal left anterior descending coronary artery	67
3 vessel	≥ 95 in proximal left anterior descending coronary artery	59

*Assume medical treatment only.

ejection fraction was 35% to 49%, and 21% if it was less than 35%.[26] Main left coronary artery disease is the most dangerous anatomic lesion, and active ischemia, as shown by severe angina or markedly positive exercise ECG, indicates an unfavorable prognosis with medical therapy.

Although the extent and severity of angiographic disease correlate with prognosis, there are significant limitations in the use of angiography for prognostication. The coronary angiogram cannot predict which plaques are most likely to rupture and cause unstable angina, myocardial infarction, or death. The plaques most vulnerable to rupture have a thin fibrous cap and a large lipid core, and they contain an increased number of macrophages. These features predict an increased risk of coronary events, independent from the degree of stenosis. Studies have demonstrated that unstable angina and myocardial infarction most often are a consequence of rupture of a plaque that produced less than 50% stenosis before the acute event.[28,29]

Treatment

The primary aims of therapy are to alleviate the symptoms of ischemia without undue restriction of activity and to reduce the risks of death and myocardial infarction. Achieving these goals usually requires anti-ischemic therapy and treatment of CAD risk factors to slow the progression of atherosclerosis. General treatment modalities include lifestyle modification, pharmacologic therapy, and revascularization. Treatment that prolongs life has the highest priority. Such treatment includes revascularization for significant left main or three-vessel coronary artery obstruction. In many patients with stable angina and one- or two-vessel disease, antianginal medical therapy, percutaneous transluminal coronary angioplasty (PTCA), or coronary artery bypass graft surgery (CABG) are all reasonable options. Factors affecting the

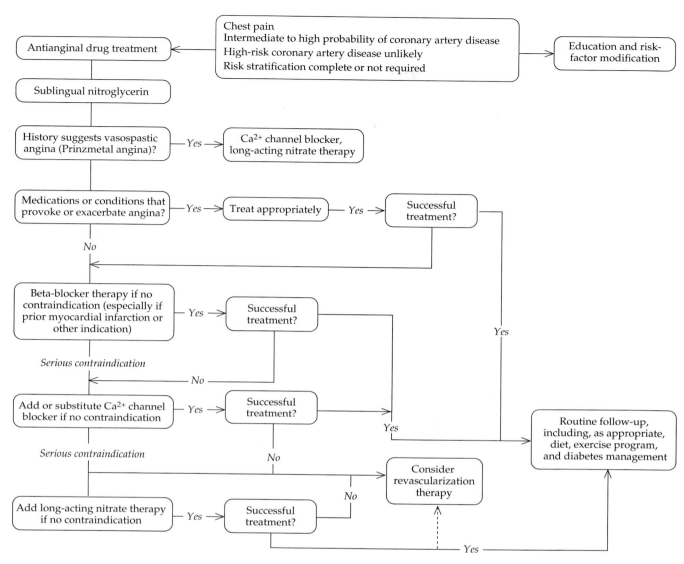

Figure 5 Treatment algorithm for the management of patients with ischemia. Factors that exacerbate or provoke angina are vasodilators, excessive thyroid replacement, vasoconstrictors, profound anemia, uncontrolled hypertension, hyperthyroidism, hypoxemia, tachyarrhythmias, bradyarrhythmias, valvular heart disease (especially aortic stenosis), and hypertrophic cardiomyopathy. On the basis of coronary anatomy, severity of anginal symptoms, and patient preferences, it is reasonable to consider evaluation for coronary revascularization. Unless a patient has documented left main, three-vessel, or two-vessel CAD with significant stenosis of the proximal left anterior descending coronary artery, there is no demonstrated survival advantage associated with revascularization in low-risk patients with chronic stable angina. Thus, medical therapy should be attempted in most patients before percutaneous transluminal coronary angioplasty or coronary artery bypass graft is considered.

choice of therapy include response to medical therapy, presence of noncardiac conditions, and patient preference. The ACC/AHA/ACP-ASIM practice guidelines[18] present an overview of treatment recommendations [see Figure 5].

LIFESTYLE MODIFICATION AND TREATMENT OF ATHEROSCLEROSIS RISK FACTORS

The process of atherosclerosis may be slowed by treatment of some risk factors. All patients should be instructed to maintain a low-fat, low-cholesterol diet and to achieve and maintain ideal body weight through diet and regular aerobic exercise. Patients who smoke cigarettes should be strongly advised to stop smoking and should be offered behavioral and pharmacologic treatment for smoking cessation.

The fasting level of low-density lipoprotein (LDL) cholesterol should be measured. Clinical trials demonstrate substantial reduction in rates of death and major coronary events when the LDL cholesterol level is lowered by either diet or drugs.[30] The 3-hydroxy-3-methylglutaryl coenzyme A (HMG-CoA) reductase inhibitors are the class of drug most effective in lowering the level of LDL cholesterol. Drug treatment is appropriate when the LDL cholesterol level exceeds 130 mg/dl. The goal is to lower the LDL cholesterol level to below 100 mg/dl.[30]

The value of aggressive lowering of the LDL cholesterol level was demonstrated in a clinical trial comparing PTCA with medical therapy that included 80 mg of atorvastatin daily in patients with clinically mild, stable, chronic ischemic heart disease.[31] The atorvastatin-treated group reached a mean serum LDL cholesterol level of 77 mg/dl, compared with 119 mg/dl in the PTCA group. After 18 months of follow-up, there was a very low rate of death and myocardial infarction in both groups. However, the incidence of worsening angina with objective evidence of ischemia was 6.7% in the atorvastatin group and 14.1% in the PTCA group.

Hypertension increases the risk of coronary events as a result of direct vascular injury, increased left ventricular mass, and myocardial oxygen demand. Lowering blood pressure reduces the risk of death, stroke, heart failure, myocardial infarction, and other vascular events, especially in older patients with systolic hypertension.[32] In patients with atherosclerosis, as in all patients, blood pressure should be less than 140/90 mm Hg; if diabetes, heart failure, or renal failure is present, lowering the blood pressure still further to less than 130/85 mm Hg achieves further reduction in CAD events.[32] Beta blockers or long-acting calcium channel blockers are especially useful in patients with hypertension and angina. Short-acting calcium channel blockers may be associated with increased mortality and should be avoided.[33] If left ventricular systolic dysfunction is present[34] or if the patient is otherwise at high risk,[35] an angiotensin-converting enzyme inhibitor or an angiotensin receptor blocker will reduce mortality.

MEDICAL TREATMENT FOR ISCHEMIA

Antiplatelet Agents

Aspirin reduces the risk of cardiovascular events in patients with stable angina pectoris. In an overview of randomized clinical trials involving over 3,000 patients with stable angina, aspirin reduced the risk of adverse cardiac and vascular events by 33%.[36] Low doses of aspirin achieve this benefit. In the Swedish Angina Pectoris Trial, treatment of patients with stable angina with 75 mg of aspirin daily reduced the risk of sudden death and myocardial infarction by 34%.[37] Aspirin (75 to 325 mg daily) should be used in all patients with ischemic heart disease, unless it is contraindicated or not tolerated.

Clopidogrel prevents adenosine diphosphate–mediated activation of platelets. Clopidogrel is comparable to aspirin in reducing the risk of vascular death, stroke, or myocardial infarction in patients with chronic atherosclerotic disease.[38]

Ticlopidine also inhibits adenosine diphosphate–induced platelet aggregation but has less antithrombotic effect than clopidogrel. Ticlopidine has not been shown to decrease cardiovascular events in patients with stable angina.

Dipyridamole has antiplatelet effects and is a coronary vasodilator. Dipyridamole can enhance exercise-induced myocardial ischemia[39] and therefore should not be used as an antiplatelet agent.

Antianginal and Anti-ischemia Therapy

Beta blockers, long-acting calcium channel blockers, and nitrates all reduce the symptoms of cardiac ischemia, but beta blockers are the first choice as initial therapy. Beta blockers reduce the risk of death, myocardial infarction, and other cardiac events when used to treat patients who have already had a myocardial infarction[40] and in older patients with systolic hypertension.[33] Calcium channel blockers may be as effective as beta blockers in reducing morbidity and mortality in angina patients[41] but are not as effective in the postinfarction population.[42] Nitrates relieve angina but do not reduce the risk of death or cardiac events. Therefore, beta blockers should be strongly considered as the initial therapy for chronic stable angina. Calcium channel

blockers, nitrates, or both may be added as needed for angina relief, or they may replace the beta blocker if it is poorly tolerated or contraindicated.

Beta blockers Blockade of the beta$_1$-adrenergic receptor is associated with a slowing of the sinus rate, a slowing of atrioventricular nodal conduction, and a decrease in inotropy. These effects are relatively greater during activity than during rest. The result is a decrease in myocardial oxygen demand, with a consequent reduction in the occurrence of ischemia during exertion. The reduction in heart rate also increases diastolic perfusion time, which may enhance myocardial perfusion.

Beta blockers may selectively block the beta$_1$ receptor or may block both beta$_1$ and beta$_2$ receptors. Beta$_2$-receptor blockade will increase the risk of bronchospasm in patients with reactive airways. Beta$_2$-receptor blockade may also worsen the clinical manifestations of peripheral vascular disease. Another differentiating feature is that some beta blockers have partial agonist activity. This property is associated with less slowing of the heart rate at rest. Despite these differences, all beta blockers are comparably effective in the treatment of angina pectoris [see Table 6].

In the treatment of angina, the beta-blocker dose should be individually titrated. The effective dose usually decreases the resting heart rate to less than 60 beats a minute. However, a more important measure is the heart rate during exercise, which ideally should not exceed 75% of the heart rate at which ischemia occurs.

Beta blockers increase the survival of patients who have had a recent myocardial infarction or who have hypertension. In the Atenolol Silent Ischemia Trial (ASIST),[43] patients with documented CAD and mild angina were randomized to receive either 100 mg of atenolol daily or placebo. Atenolol reduced the risk of death, myocardial infarction, hospitalization, revascularization, and worsening angina.

Beta blockers are contraindicated in the presence of severe bradycardia, high-grade atrioventricular block, or severe, unstable heart failure. Relative contraindications include asthma or reactive airway disease, severe mental depression, and peripheral vascular disease. Diabetes is not a contraindication, but beta

Table 6 Properties of Beta Blockers in Clinical Use[18]

Drugs	Selectivity	Partial Agonist Activity	Usual Dose for Angina
Propranolol	None	No	20–80 mg b.i.d.
Metoprolol	β_1	No	50–200 mg b.i.d.
Atenolol	β_1	No	50–200 mg/day
Nadolol	None	No	40–80 mg/day
Timolol	None	No	10 mg b.i.d.
Acebutolol	β_1	Yes	200–600 mg b.i.d.
Betaxolol	β_1	No	10–20 mg/day
Bisoprolol	β_1	No	10 mg/day
Esmolol (intravenous)	β_1	No	50–300 µg/kg/min
Labetalol*	None	Yes	200–600 mg b.i.d.
Pindolol	None	Yes	2.7–7.5 mg t.i.d.

*Labetalol is a combined alpha and beta blocker.

Table 7   Properties of Calcium Antagonists in Clinical Use[18]

Drugs	Usual Dose	Duration of Action	Side Effects
Dihydropyridines			
Nifedipines	30–90 mg/day orally (immediate release)	Short	Hypotension, dizziness, flushing, nausea, constipation, edema
	30–180 mg/day orally (slow release)		
Amlodipine	5–10 mg q.d.	Long	Headache, edema
Filodipine	5–10 mg q.d.	Long	Headache, edema
Isradipine	2.5–10 mg b.i.d.	Medium	Headache, fatigue
Nicardipine	20–40 mg t.i.d.	Short	Headache, dizziness, flushing, edema
Nisoldipine	20–40 mg t.i.d.	Short	Similar to nifedipine
Nitrendipine	20 mg q.d. or b.i.d.	Medium	Similar to nifedipine
Miscellaneous			
Bepridil	200–400 mg q.d.	Long	Arrhythmias, dizziness, nausea
Diltiazem	30–80 mg q.i.d. (immediate release)	Short	Hypotension, dizziness, flushing, bradycardia, edema
	120–320 mg q.d. (slow release)	Long	—
Verapamil	80–160 mg t.i.d. (immediate release)	Short	Hypotension, myocardial depression, heart failure, edema, bradycardia
	120–480 mg q.d. (slow release)	Long	—

blockers reduce the warning signs of hypoglycemia and should be used carefully in patients who use insulin.

The most common side effects of beta blockers are fatigue, reduced maximal exercise capacity, lethargy, insomnia, and erectile dysfunction.

Calcium channel blockers   Calcium channel blockers reduce vascular smooth muscle contractility, thereby increasing coronary blood flow and causing peripheral vasodilatation with reduction in systemic vascular resistance and in blood pressure. All of the actions contribute to the anti-ischemic effect of these drugs. All calcium channel blockers in clinical use exert a negative inotropic effect that reaches clinical significance primarily with diltiazem and verapamil.

Calcium channel blockers are comparable to beta blockers in relieving angina. In several relatively small clinical trials, calcium channel blockers were comparable to beta blockers in the reduction of the risk of death or myocardial infarction.[44-47] Retrospective case-control studies have suggested that short-acting calcium channel blockers, such as immediate-release formulations of nifedipine, diltiazem, and verapamil, may increase the risk of vascular events, possibly by stimulating adrenergic activity.[48,49] The safe approach is to use only calcium channel blockers with long half-lives or those in a slow-release formulation.

All calcium channel blockers are highly effective in reducing the frequency and severity of episodes of vasospastic angina.

Calcium channel blockers are contraindicated in patients with severe heart failure. Verapamil and diltiazem are contraindicated in patients with severe bradycardia, sinus node dysfunction, or atrioventricular nodal block.

Table 8   Nitroglycerin and Nitrates in Angina[18]

Compound	Route	Dose	Duration of Effect
Nitroglycerin	Sublingual tablets	0.3–0.6 mg to 1.5 mg	1.5–7 min
	Spray	0.4 mg as needed	Similar to tablets
	Ointment	2% 6 × 6 in., 15 × 15 cm, 7.5–40 mg	Up to 7 hr
	Transdermal	0.2–0.8 mg/hr q. 12hr	8–12 hr (intermittent therapy)
	Oral sustained release	2.5–13 mg	4–8 hr
	Buccal	1–3 mg t.i.d.	3–5 hr
	Intravenous	5–200 mg/min	Tolerance in 7–8 hr
Isosorbide dinitrate	Sublingual	2.5–15 mg	Up to 1 hr
	Oral	5–80 mg b.i.d. to t.i.d.	Up to 8 hr
	Spray	1.25 mg/day	2–3 min
	Chewable	5 mg	2–2.5 hr
	Oral slow release	40 mg s.i.d. to b.i.d.	Up to 8 hr
	Intravenous	1.25–5.0 mg/hr	Tolerance in 7–8 hr
	Ointment	100 mg/24 hr	Not effective
Isosorbide mononitrate	Oral	20 mg b.i.d.	12–24 hr
		60–240 mg s.i.d.	
Pentaerythritol tetranitrate	Sublingual	10 mg as needed	Not known
Erythritol tetranitrate	Sublingual	5–10 mg as needed	Not known
	Oral	10–30 mg t.i.d.	Not known

Common side effects of calcium channel blockers include hypotension, peripheral edema, flushing, headache, and constipation. The various calcium channel blockers in clinical use differ in terms of the usual doses, duration of action, and side effects [see Table 7].

Nitrates Nitrates are endothelium-independent vasodilators. They dilate coronary arteries and collateral vessels, improving coronary artery blood flow. The peripheral arteriolar dilation reduces peripheral vascular resistance, thereby decreasing left ventricular outflow impedance and myocardial oxygen consumption. The venodilating effect of nitrates reduces the return of blood to the heart, thereby reducing left ventricular filling pressure and left ventricular volume. These actions also reduce myocardial oxygen consumption.

Nitrates reduce the frequency of occurrence, duration, and severity of anginal episodes. Clinical studies using treadmill testing have documented that nitrates improve exercise capacity and increase the amount of exercise before onset of angina and of ST segment depression.

Sublingual nitroglycerin tablets or nitroglycerin spray provides immediate relief of angina. These rapidly acting preparations may also be taken shortly before planned exertion to prevent angina. For long-term therapy, long-acting nitrate preparations, such as isosorbide dinitrate, isosorbide mononitrate, nitroglycerin ointment, or nitroglycerin transdermal patches, are available. All long-acting formulations are comparably effective [see Table 8].[50,51]

Nitrates are relatively contraindicated in hypertrophic obstructive cardiomyopathy and in severe aortic stenosis. In these conditions, nitrates may precipitate syncope. Nitrates should not be used within 24 hours of taking sildenafil (Viagra), because this combination may induce severe hypotension.[52] It is important to warn patients of this potentially serious drug interaction.

For long-term use, nitrates in any form should be administered with one daily nitrate-free interval of at least 8 hours, which is the most practical method for prevention of nitrate tolerance. Without this nitrate-free interval, tolerance to the antianginal and hemodynamic effects of nitrates develops within days.

The most common side effect of nitrate treatment is headache, which sometimes resolves with continued use of the nitrate. Hypotension may occur, especially in the volume-depleted patient. The choice of antianginal drug is often influenced by the presence of concomitant medical conditions [see Table 9].

In the absence of specific indications or contraindications for a particular class of antianginal drug, beta blockers are favored as initial therapy. These drugs are documented to reduce morbidity and mortality in postinfarction patients and in hypertensive patients and are relatively inexpensive. The dose may be up-titrated, and if necessary, calcium channel blockers and nitrates may be added to eliminate angina during normal activity.

In the majority of patients, risk-factor evaluation and treatment, along with antianginal drug therapy, achieves satisfactory symptom relief and optimal reduction in morbidity and mortality. In some patients, this medical approach does not adequately

Table 9 Recommended Drug Therapy for Patients with Angina and Associated Conditions[18]

Condition	Recommended Treatment (Alternative)
Systemic hypertension	Beta blockers (calcium antagonists)
Migraine or vascular headaches	Beta blockers (verapamil or diltiazem)
Asthma or COPD with bronchospasm	Verapamil or diltiazem; avoid beta blockers
Hyperthyroidism	Beta blockers
Raynaud syndrome	Long-acting slow-release calcium antagonists; avoid beta blockers
Type 1 diabetes mellitus	Beta blockers if prior MI or long-acting slow-release calcium antagonists
Type 2 diabetes mellitus	Beta blockers or long-acting slow-release calcium antagonists
Depression	Long-acting slow-release calcium antagonists; avoid beta blockers
Mild peripheral vascular disease	Beta blockers or calcium antagonists
Severe peripheral vascular disease with rest ischemia	Calcium antagonists; avoid beta blockers
Cardiac arrhythmias and conduction abnormalities	
Sinus bradycardia	Long-acting slow-release calcium antagonists that do not decrease heart rate; avoid beta blockers, diltiazem, verapamil
Sinus tachycardia (not due to heart failure)	Beta blockers
Supraventricular tachycardia	Verapamil, diltiazem, or beta blockers
Atrioventricular block	Long-acting slow-release calcium antagonists that do not slow AV conduction; avoid beta blockers, diltiazem, verapamil
Rapid atrial fibrillation (with digitalis)	Verapamil, diltiazem, or beta blockers
Ventricular arrhythmias	Beta blockers
Left ventricular dysfunction	
Congestive heart failure	
Mild (LVEF ≥ 40%)	Beta blockers
Moderate to severe (LVEF < 40%)	Amlodipine or felodipine (nitrates); avoid verapamil, diltiazem
Left-sided valvular heart disease	
Mild aortic stenosis	Beta blockers
Aortic insufficiency	Long-acting slow-release dihydropyridines
Mitral regurgitation	Long-acting slow-release dihydropyridines
Mitral stenosis	Beta blockers
Hypertrophic cardiomyopathy	Beta blockers, nondihydropyridine calcium antagonist; avoid nitrates, dihydropyridine calcium antagonists

AV—atrioventricular   COPD—chronic obstructive pulmonary disease   LVEF—left ventricular ejection fraction   MI—myocardial infarction

Table 10   Recommendations for Revascularization in Chronic Stable Angina

Class	Condition	Recommendations
I	There is evidence or general agreement that revascularization is useful and effective	1. CABG for patients with significant left main coronary artery disease 2. CABG for patients with three-vessel disease; the survival benefit is greater in patients with abnormal LV function (ejection fraction < 50%) 3. CABG for patients with two-vessel disease with significant proximal left anterior descending CAD and either abnormal LV function (ejection fraction < 50%) or demonstrable ischemia on noninvasive testing 4. PTCA for patients with two- or three-vessel disease with significant proximal left anterior descending CAD who have anatomy suitable for catheter-based therapy and normal LV function and who do not have treated diabetes 5. PTCA or CABG for patients with one- or two-vessel CAD without significant proximal left anterior descending CAD but with a large area of viable myocardium and high-risk criteria on noninvasive testing 6. CABG for patients with one- or two-vessel CAD without significant proximal left anterior descending CAD who have survived near sudden cardiac death or sustained ventricular tachycardia 7. Revascularization in patients with prior PTCA, CABG, or PTCA for recurrent stenosis associated with a large area of viable myocardium or high-risk criteria on noninvasive testing 8. PTCA or CABG for patients who have not been successfully treated by medical therapy and can undergo revascularization with acceptable risk
IIa	There is conflicting evidence or a divergence of opinion, but the weight of evidence/opinion favors the usefulness/efficacy of revascularization	1. Repeat CABG for patients with multiple saphenous vein graft stenoses, especially when there is significant stenosis of a graft supplying the LAD; it may be appropriate to use PTCA for focal saphenous vein graft lesions or multiple stenoses in poor candidates for reoperative surgery 2. PTCA or CABG for patients with one- or two-vessel CAD without significant proximal LAD disease but with a moderate area of viable myocardium and demonstrable ischemia on noninvasive testing 3. PTCA or CABG for patients with one-vessel disease with significant proximal LAD disease
IIb	There is conflicting evidence or a divergence of opinion, and usefulness/efficacy is less well established by evidence/opinion	1. PTCA for patients with two- or three-vessel disease with significant proximal left anterior descending CAD who have anatomy suitable for catheter-based therapy and who have treated diabetes or abnormal LV function 2. PTCA for patients with significant left main coronary disease who are not candidates for CABG 3. PTCA for patients with one- or two-vessel CAD without significant proximal left anterior descending CAD who have survived near sudden cardiac death or sustained ventricular tachycardia

III	There is evidence and/or general agreement that revascularization is not useful/effective and may be harmful	1. PTCA or CABG for patients with one- or two-vessel CAD without significant proximal left anterior descending CAD who have mild symptoms that are not likely caused by myocardial ischemia or who have not received an adequate trial of medical therapy and
		    (a) have only a small area of viable myocardium, or
		    (b) have no demonstrable ischemia on noninvasive testing
		2. PTCA or CABG for patients with borderline coronary stenoses (50%–60% diameter in locations other than the left main coronary artery) and no demonstrable ischemia on noninvasive testing
		3. PTCA or CABG for patients with insignificant coronary stenosis (< 50% diameter)
		4. PTCA in patients with significant left main coronary artery disease who are candidates for CABG

CABG—coronary artery bypass grafting   CAD—coronary artery disease   LAD—left anterior descending artery   LV—left ventricular   PTCA—percutaneous transluminal coronary angioplasty

relieve symptoms, or diagnostic studies suggest the presence of severe coronary atherosclerosis. In such cases, coronary revascularization should be considered.

REVASCULARIZATION

Revascularization by either PTCA (or other catheter-based methods, including stents, atherectomy, and laser therapy) or bypass surgery is indicated when optimal medical treatment inadequately controls symptoms because of cardiac ischemia. Revascularization is also indicated for specific coronary lesions or specific combinations of coronary lesions, for left ventricular function, and when there is evidence of ischemia, because revascularization prolongs survival in these subgroups. The results of published randomized trials comparing medical therapy with PTCA or with bypass surgery or of trials comparing PTCA with bypass surgery cannot be rigidly applied, because advances since completion of those trials have substantially improved the outcome of all three forms of therapy. However, the older and the most recent clinical trials are consistent with the general principle that medical therapy is preferred for patients at low risk for

death and that revascularization is of greatest benefit for patients at moderate or high risk. The ACC/AHA/ACP-ASIM Committee on Management of Patients with Chronic Stable Angina has made recommendations for revascularization [*see Table 10 and Figure 5*].[18]

The randomized trials comparing medical treatment with bypass surgery showed improved survival rate with surgery in patients with a left main artery stenosis of 70% or more or in patients with two- or three-vessel disease that included a proximal left anterior descending artery stenosis of 70% or more or who had abnormal left ventricular function.[25,53-55] Revascularization is likely to improve survival in patients with one-, two-, or three-vessel disease who have evidence of extensive ischemia on noninvasive testing or who have other high-risk features, such as impaired ventricular contractility, especially if there is also evidence of hibernating myocardium.[18]

In contrast, among patients who do not have left main artery stenosis or three-vessel disease and who are at low risk on the basis of clinical characteristics such as mild angina, normal ejection fraction, absence of hypertension, and absence of resting ST segment depression, the long-term survival is slightly better with medical therapy than with bypass surgery.[25]

PTCA has been compared with bypass surgery in randomized trials of patients who are good candidates for either procedure.[56,57] In these trials, most patients had two-vessel disease and most had normal left ventricular function. After about 5 years of follow-up, the survival rates were equivalent for the two procedures. Some of these studies have shown a better survival rate with bypass surgery in patients with diabetes. In these trials, bypass surgery resulted in a higher percentage of patients free of angina, and bypass patients needed to take fewer antianginal medications. The need for repeat revascularization was much higher in the PTCA groups. However, these studies were done before the widespread use of stents with PTCA, which reduces the rate of restenosis and the need for repeat revascularization. These studies also included very few high-risk patients, a group that greatly benefits from bypass surgery and in whom the benefit of PTCA has not been established.

PTCA has been compared with medical therapy in randomized studies of patients who have one- or two-vessel disease and stable angina.[58,59] PTCA is better for relief of anginal symptoms but does reduce the risk of death or myocardial infarction to a greater extent than medical therapy.

ENHANCED EXTERNAL COUNTERPULSATION

Enhanced external counterpulsation (EECP) involves sequential inflation and deflation of cuffs wrapped around the patient's thighs and calves. During diastole, the cuffs inflate sequentially from the calves up to the thighs and rapidly deflate at the onset of systole. This external pulsatile action increases venous return, which should increase cardiac output, and raises aortic diastolic pressure, which should increase coronary artery perfusion pressure. The rapid deflation in systole should decrease left ventricular afterload.

EECP has been evaluated in a randomized, controlled trial of 139 selected patients with chronic stable angina and a positive exercise ECG.[60] EECP treatments were given for 1 hour, once or twice a day. After 35 treatments, the time to at least 1 mm ST segment depression was prolonged in the EECP group, compared with the control group, but there was no significant difference between the groups in exercise duration. The EECP group had a slight reduction in the frequency of angina episodes. Skin abrasion and pain in the legs or back were common adverse effects of EECP. This treatment may be helpful in decreasing angina in some patients who have had an inadequate response to medical treatment and who are not candidates for revascularization.

References

1. Crea P, Pupita G, Galassi AR, et al: Role of adenosine in pathogenesis of anginal pain. Circulation 81:164, 1990

2. Fuster V, Badimon L, Badimon JJ, et al: The pathogenesis of coronary artery disease and the acute coronary syndromes. N Engl J Med 326:242, 1992

3. Yao S-K, Rosolowsky M, Anderson HV, et al: Combined thromboxane A_2 synthetase inhibition and receptor blockade are effective in preventing spontaneous and epinephrine-induced canine coronary cyclic flow variations. J Am Coll Cardiol 16:705, 1990

4. Dinerman JL, Mehta JL: Endothelial, platelet and leukocyte interactions in ischemic heart disease: insights into potential mechanisms and their clinical relevance. J Am Coll Cardiol 16:207, 1990

5. Golino P, Piscione F, Willerson JT, et al: Divergent effects of serotonin on coronary-artery dimensions and blood flows in patients with coronary atherosclerosis and control patients. N Engl J Med 324:641, 1991

6. McFadden IP, Clarke JG, Davies GJ, et al: Effect of intracoronary serotonin on coronary vessels in patients with stable angina and patients with variant angina. N Engl J Med 324:648, 1991

7. Vanhoutte PM, Shimokawa H: Endothelium-derived relaxing factor and coronary vasospasm. Circulation 80:1, 1989

8. Zeiher AM, Drexler H, Wollschläger H, et al: Modulation of coronary vasomotor tone in humans: progressive endothelial dysfunction with different early stages of coronary atherosclerosis. Circulation 83:391, 1991

9. Brush JE, Faxon DP, Salmon S, et al: Abnormal endothelium-dependent coronary vasomotion in hypertensive patients. J Am Coll Cardiol 19:809, 1992

10. Celermajer DS, Sorensen KE, Georgakopoulos D, et al: Cigarette smoking is associated with dose-related and potentially reversible impairment of endothelium-dependent dilation in healthy young adults. Circulation 88:2149, 1993

11. Reddy KG, Nair RN, Sheehan HM, et al: Evidence that selective endothelial dysfunction may occur in the absence of angiographic or ultrasound atherosclerosis in patients with risk factors for atherosclerosis. J Am Coll Cardiol 23:833, 1994

12. Treasure CB, Klein JL, Weintraub WS, et al: Beneficial effects of cholesterol-lowering therapy on the coronary endothelium in patients with coronary artery disease. N Engl J Med 332:481, 1995

13. Hambrecht R, Wolf A, Gielen S, et al: Effect of exercise on coronary endothelial function in patients with coronary artery disease. N Engl J Med 342:454, 2000

14. James TN: The spectrum of diseases of small coronary arteries and their physiologic consequences. Seminar on small coronary artery disease: structure and function of small coronary arteries in health and disease-II. J Am Coll Cardiol 15:763, 1990

15. Tanaka M, Fujiwara H, Onodera T, et al: Quantitative analysis of narrowings of intramyocardial small arteries in normal hearts, hypertensive hearts, and hearts with hypertrophic cardiomyopathy. Circulation 75:1130, 1987

16. Mosseri M, Yarom R, Gotsman MS, et al: Histologic evidence for small-vessel coronary artery disease in patients with angina pectoris and patent large coronary arteries. Circulation 74:964, 1986

17. Cannon RO, Camici PG, Epstein SE: Pathophysiological dilemma of syndrome X. Circulation 53:883, 1992

18. Gibbons RJ, Chatterjee K, Daley J, et al: ACC/AHA/ACP-ASIM guidelines for the management of patients with chronic stable angina: a report of the American College of Cardiology/American Heart Association Task Force on Practice Guidelines (Committee on the Management of Patients with Chronic Stable Angina). J Am Coll Cardiol 33:2092, 1999

19. Sox HC, Hickam DH, Marton KI, et al: Using the patient's history to estimate the probability of coronary artery disease: a comparison of referral and primary care practice. Am J Med 89:7, 1990

20. Stuart RJ, Ellestad MH: National survey of exercise stress testing facilities. Chest 77:94, 1980

21. Gibbons RJ, Balady GJ, Beasley JW, et al: ACC/AHA guidelines for exercise testing: a report of the American College of Cardiology/American Heart Association Task Force on Practice Guidelines (Committee on Exercise Testing). J Am Coll Cardiol 30:260, 1997

22. Cheitlin MD, Alpert JS, Armstrong WF, et al: ACC/AHA guidelines for the clinical application of echocardiography: a report of the American College of Cardiology/American Heart Association Task Force on Practice Guidelines (Committee on Clinical Application of Echocardiography). Circulation 95:1686, 1997

23. Ritchie JL, Bateman TM, Bonow RO, et al: Guidelines for clinical use of cardiac radionuclide imaging: report of the American College of Cardiology/American Heart Association Task Force on Assessment of Diagnostic and Therapeutic Cardiovascular Procedures (Committee on Radionuclide Imaging). J Am Coll Cardiol 25:521, 1995

24. Califf RM, Armstrong PW, Carver JR, et al: Stratification of patients into high, medium and low risk subgroups for purposes of risk factor management. J Am Coll Cardiol 27:1007, 1996

25. Yusuf S, Zucker D, Peduzzi P, et al: Effect of coronary artery bypass graft surgery on survival: overview of 10-year results from randomised trials by the Coronary Artery Bypass Graft Surgery Trialists Collaboration. Lancet 344:563, 1994

26. Emond M, Mock MB, Davis KB, et al: Long-term survival of medically treated patients in the Coronary Artery Surgery Study (CASS) Registry. Circulation 90:2645, 1994

27. Afridi I, Grayburn PA, Panza JA, et al: Myocardial viability during dobutamine echocardiography predicts survival in patients with coronary artery disease and severe left ventricle dysfunction. J Am Coll Cardiol 32:921, 1998

28. Ambrose JA, Tannenbaum MA, Alexopoulos D, et al: Angiographic progression of coronary artery disease and the development of myocardial infarction. J Am Coll Cardiol 12:56, 1988

29. Little WC, Constantinescu M, Applegate RJ, et al: Can coronary angiography predict the site of a subsequent myocardial infarction in patients with mild-to-moderate coronary artery disease? Circulation 78:1157, 1988

30. National Cholesterol Education Program: Second Report of the Expert Panel on Detection, Evaluation, and Treatment of High Blood Cholesterol in Adults (Adult Treatment Panel II). Circulation 89:1333, 1994

31. Pitt B, Waters D, Brown WV, et al: Aggressive lipid-lowering therapy compared with angioplasty in stable coronary artery disease. N Engl J Med 341:70, 1999

32. The Sixth Report of the Joint National Committee on Prevention, Detection, Evaluation, and Treatment of High Blood Pressure. Arch Intern Med 157:2413, 1997

33. Prevention of stroke by antihypertensive drug treatment in older persons with isolated systolic hypertension: final results of the Systolic Hypertension in the Elderly Program (SHEP). SHEP Cooperative Research Group. JAMA 265:3255, 1991

34. Pfeffer MA, Braunwald E, Moyé LA, et al: Effect of captopril on mortality and morbidity in patients with left ventricular dysfunction after myocardial infarction: results of the Survival and Ventricular Enlargement trial. N Engl J Med 327:669, 1992

35. Effects of an angiotensin-converting enzyme inhibitor, ramipril, on cardiovascular events in high-risk patients. The Heart Outcomes Prevention Evaluation Study Investigators. N Engl J Med 342:145, 2000

36. Antiplatelet Trialists Collaboration: Collaborative overview of randomised trials of

antiplatelet therapy: I. Prevention of death, myocardial infarction and stroke by prolonged antiplatelet therapy in various categories of patients. Br Med J 308:81, 1995

37. Juul-Møller S, Edvardsson N, Jahnmatz B, et al: Double-blind trial of aspirin in primary prevention of myocardial infarction in patients with stable chronic angina pectoris. The Swedish Angina Pectoris Aspirin Trial (SAPAT) Group. Lancet 340:1421, 1992

38. CAPRIE Steering Committee: A randomised, blinded, trial of clopidogrel versus aspirin in patients at risk of ischemic events (CAPRIE). Lancet 348:1329, 1996

39. Tsuya T, Okada M, Horie H, et al: Effect of dipyridamole at the usual oral dose on exercise-induced myocardial ischemia in stable angina pectoris. Am J Cardiol 66:275, 1990

40. The β-blocker heart attack trial. β-Blocker Heart Attack Study Group. JAMA 246:2073, 1981

41. Heidenreich PA, McDonald KM, Hastie T, et al: Meta-analysis of trials comparing beta-blockers, calcium antagonists, and nitrates for stable angina. JAMA 281:1927, 1999

42. Held PH, Yusuf S: Effects of β-blockers and calcium channel blockers in acute myocardial infarction. Eur Heart J 14(suppl F):18, 1993

43. Pepine CJ, Cohn PF, Deedwania PC, et al: Effects of treatment on outcome in mildly symptomatic patients with ischemia during daily life. The Atenolol Silent Ischemia Study (ASIST). Circulation 90:762, 1994

44. Dargie HJ, Ford I, Fox KM: Total Ischaemic Burden European Trial (TIBET). Effects of ischaemia and treatment with atenolol, nifedipine SR and their combination on outcome in patients with chronic stable angina. The TIBET Study Group. Eur Heart J 17:104, 1996

45. Rehnquist N, Hjemdahl P, Billing E, et al: Treatment of stable angina pectoris with calcium antagonists and beta blockers. The APSIS study. Angina Prognosis Study in Stockholm. Cardiologia 40(suppl 1):301, 1995

46. von Arnim T: Medical treatment to reduce total ischemic burden: total ischemic burden bisoprolol study (TIBBS), a multicenter trial comparing bisoprolol and nifedipine. The TIBBS Investigators. J Am Coll Cardiol 25:231, 1995

47. Savonitto S, Ardissiono D, Egstrup K, et al: Combination therapy with metoprolol and nifedipine versus monotherapy in patients with stable angina pectoris: results of the International Multicenter Angina Exercise (IMAGE) study. J Am Coll Cardiol 27:311, 1996

48. Psaty BM, Heckbert SR, Koepsell TD, et al: The risk of myocardial infarction associated with antihypertensive drug therapies. JAMA 274:620, 1995

49. Furberg CD, Psaty BM, Meyer JV: Nifedipine: dose-related increase in mortality in patients with coronary heart disease. Circulation 92:1326, 1995

50. Abrams J: Glyceryl trinitrate (nitroglycerin) and the organic nitrates: choosing the method of administration. Drugs 34:391, 1987

51. Silber S: Nitrates: why and how should they be used today? Current status of the clinical usefulness of nitroglycerin, isosorbide dinitrate and isosorbide-5-mononitrate. Eur J Clin Pharmacol 38(suppl 1):535, 1990

52. Cheitlin MD, Hutter AM Jr, Brindis RG, et al: ACC/AHA expert consensus document: use of sildenafil (Viagra) in patients with cardiovascular disease. J Am Coll Cardiol 33:273, 1999

53. The VA Coronary Artery Bypass Surgery Cooperative Study Group: Eighteen-year follow-up in the Veterans Affairs Cooperative Study of Coronary Artery Bypass Surgery for stable angina. Circulation 86:121, 1992

54. Varnauskas E: Twelve-year follow-up of survival in the randomized European Coronary Surgery Study. N Engl J Med 319:332, 1988

55. Passamani E, Davis KB, Gillespie MJ, et al: A randomized trial of coronary artery bypass surgery: survival in patients with a low ejection fraction. N Engl J Med 312:1665, 1985

56. Comparison of coronary bypass surgery with angioplasty in patients with multivessel disease. The Bypass Angioplasty Revascularization Investigation (BARI) Investigators. N Engl J Med 335:217, 1996

57. King SB, Lembo NJ, Weintraub WS, et al: A randomized trial comparing coronary angioplasty with coronary bypass surgery. Emory Angioplasty versus Surgery Trial (EAST). N Engl J Med 331:1044, 1994

58. Parisi AF, Folland ED, Hartigan P: A comparison of angioplasty with medical therapy in the treatment of single-vessel coronary artery disease. Veterans Affairs ACME Investigators. N Engl J Med 326:10, 1992

59. RITA-2 Trial Participants: Coronary angioplasty versus medical therapy for angina: the second Randomized Intervention Treatment of Angina (RITA-2) trial. Lancet 350:461, 1997

60. Arora RR, Chou TM, Jain D, et al: The Multicenter Study of Enhanced External Counterpulsation (MUST-EECP): effect of EECP on exercise-induced myocardial ischemia and anginal episodes. J Am Coll Cardiol 33:1833, 1999

61. Garber AM, Solomon NA: Cost effectiveness of alternative test strategies for the diagnosis of coronary artery disease. Ann Intern Med 130:719, 1999

21 Acute Myocardial Infarction

Peter B. Berger, M.D.

In the 1970s, coronary angiography demonstrated that almost all cases of acute myocardial infarction were caused by thrombotic occlusion of a coronary artery. This discovery has led to the development of therapies to restore coronary blood flow in the occluded artery, which has dramatically reduced the morbidity and mortality associated with acute myocardial infarction.

Epidemiology

In the past decade, the number of people who die each year of myocardial infarction has decreased significantly. Both in-hospital mortality and out-of-hospital mortality have declined as a result of substantial increases in the use of thrombolytic therapy, coronary angioplasty, aspirin, and heparin and a reduction in the risk factors for coronary artery disease.[1]

Despite these advances, approximately 1.5 million people in the United States suffer acute myocardial infarction each year, and nearly 500,000 of these patients die of coronary disease.[2] Nearly half of these deaths occur before the patients receive medical care either from emergency medical technicians or in a hospital.[2,3]

Pathogenesis

The factors responsible for the sudden thrombotic occlusion of a coronary artery have only recently been elucidated. Atherosclerotic plaques rich in foam cells (lipid-laden macrophages) are susceptible to sudden plaque rupture and hemorrhage into the vessel wall, which may result in the sudden partial or total occlusion of the coronary artery.[4] Although severe stenosis of a coronary artery (i.e., stenosis $\geq$ 70% of the diameter of the artery) is generally required to produce anginal symptoms, such stenoses tend to have dense fibrotic caps and are less prone to rupture than mild to moderate stenoses, which are generally more lipid laden. Studies of patients in whom angiography was performed before and after a myocardial infarction revealed that in most cases, acute coronary occlusion occurred at sites in the coronary circulation with stenoses of less than 70%, as demonstrated on the preinfarction angiogram.[5] Although patients who have unstable anginal syndromes with increasingly frequent and severe angina are clearly at increased risk for myocardial infarction, the ability of physicians to predict which patients with stable anginal syndromes are likely to experience infarction and which coronary stenoses are likely to result in acute thrombotic occlusion is poor.

Diagnosis

According to the World Health Organization, the diagnosis of myocardial infarction requires at least two of the following three criteria: (1) a clinical history of ischemic-type chest discomfort, (2) serial electrocardiographic tracings indicative of myocardial infarction, and (3) a rise and fall in serum cardiac markers.[6] The serum cardiac marker creatine kinase (CK) and the more specific creatine kinase–myocardial band (CK-MB) have been the primary markers in use around the world. How-ever, there has been a recent proposal by the European Society of Cardiology and the American College of Cardiology that the criteria for making a diagnosis of myocardial infarction be changed to include the use of more sensitive biomarkers (troponins). According to the proposed criteria, a diagnosis of myocardial infarction would require a typical rise and fall in CK-MB levels or a rise in troponin levels, together with findings of ischemic symptoms or new ischemic ECG changes, or both, that are indicative of ischemia.[7] The use of troponin, rather than CK-MB, was recommended. If adopted, these criteria will dramatically increase the frequency with which myocardial infarction is diagnosed by including a large number of patients who would otherwise have been diagnosed as having an acute coronary syndrome without infarction. Therefore, if the new diagnostic criteria are widely adopted, it will be essential that some clinical centers measure the levels not only of the newly specified biomarkers but also of the enzymes that were traditionally used in diagnosis. In addition, it is essential that older diagnostic criteria of myocardial infarction continue to be applied to understand the magnitude of change engendered by the use of the newly employed biomarkers and to enable comparisons of the frequency of myocardial infarction and the outcomes of patients before and after the change in diagnostic criteria. Individual physicians should, however, use the new diagnostic criteria for acute myocardial infarction, owing to the improved sensitivity and specificity of those criteria and their prognostic impact.

CLINICAL MANIFESTATIONS

Patients with acute myocardial infarction often describe a heaviness, pressure, squeezing, or tightness in the chest that has persisted for more than 30 minutes. The discomfort may radiate or be located primarily in the arms, neck, or jaw. Chest pain, particularly severe or stabbing chest pain, and pain that causes writhing are unusual for coronary ischemia and should lead the clinician to consider causes other than myocardial infarction. Many patients with acute myocardial infarction, particularly those with inferior infarction, are diaphoretic; nausea and emesis are common as well. Dyspnea is also a common associated symptom. Syncope may occur and is more frequent with inferior than anterior infarction, in part because of the more frequent occurrence of bradyarrhythmias, heart block, and tachyarrhythmias with inferior infarction. Elderly patients with infarction often present with symptoms that differ from the symptoms of infarction in younger patients; more than half of elderly patients present with shortness of breath as their main complaint, and many others present with dizziness or symptoms of arrhythmia rather than the classic symptoms of acute myocardial infarction.[8]

Approximately two thirds of patients describe the new onset of angina or a change in their anginal pattern in the month preceding infarction.[9] However, in approximately one fourth of patients, myocardial infarction is associated with only mild symptoms or no symptoms at all.[10]

PHYSICAL EXAMINATION

The patient with acute myocardial infarction often appears anxious and in distress. Vital signs are often normal, but sinus

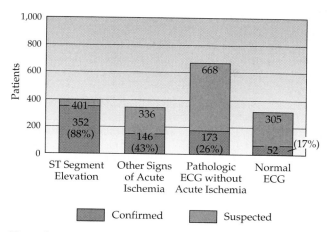

Figure 1   Relation between the initial electrocardiographic changes and the development of infarction in 1,715 patients strongly suspected of having an acute myocardial infarction. Each column shows the total number of patients and the number of patients later found to have had an infarction. Although infarction is less frequently confirmed in patients without ST segment elevation than in those with ST segment elevation, even patients with normal ECG findings may suffer acute myocardial infarction.[11]

tachycardia is not uncommon. The pulse may be rapid or slow if arrhythmias are present. Either hypotension caused by left or right ventricular dysfunction or arrhythmia or hypertension caused by adrenergic discharge may be present. The respiratory rate may be elevated because of anxiety or pain or because of hypoxia in patients with significant congestive heart failure. The jugular venous pressure may be elevated, reflecting right ventricular dysfunction caused by right ventricular involvement (more common with inferior infarction); arrhythmia in which atrioventricular dissociation is present may produce so-called cannon A waves, which are abnormally high jugular venous waves caused by atrial systole occurring when the atrioventricular valves are closed. The lung examination is typically normal, but moist rales indicative of congestive heart failure resulting from left ventricular dysfunction may be present. The cardiac examination may reveal a dyskinetic apical pulsation on palpation; a fourth and, less commonly, a third heart sound may be audible. The murmur of ischemic mitral regurgitation may be present. If a left bundle branch block is present, abnormal splitting of the second heart sound may be heard.

It must be emphasized that the physical examination in acute myocardial infarction is generally most useful in excluding other potentially serious causes of the patient's chest discomfort, including pulmonary embolism, aortic dissection, spontaneous pneumothorax, pericarditis, and cholecystitis, rather than in confirming a diagnosis of acute myocardial infarction.

ELECTROCARDIOGRAPHY

ECG is a valuable tool both in confirming the diagnosis and in selecting the most appropriate therapy for the patient with acute myocardial infarction. Although rhythm and conduction disturbances may be present, the presence and type of repolarization abnormalities are most useful in identifying myocardial infarction. If ST segment elevation is present in a patient with chest pain typical of acute myocardial infarction, the likelihood that the patient has acute myocardial infarction is greater than 90%.[11] Other findings, such as ST segment depression, T wave

inversion, and bundle branch block, are less specific but may also support a diagnosis of acute myocardial infarction, particularly when typical symptoms are present [*see Figure 1*].[11] Fully 50% of patients with myocardial infarction do not have ST segment elevation on their ECGs; among such patients, the ECG can help predict complications and short-term mortality.[12] Patients with ST segment depression are at high risk; 30-day mortality in such patients is nearly as high as in patients with anterior ST segment elevation.[13] Those with other nonspecific ECG abnormalities are at lesser risk; those with normal ECGs who suffer infarction generally have the best prognosis [*see Figure 2*]. Regardless of the findings on the initial ECG, the most important element in the evaluation of a patient with suspected acute myocardial infarction is the patient's description of symptoms. All patients suspected of having acute myocardial infarction should be admitted to the hospital and receive rapid and appropriate therapy.

LABORATORY FINDINGS

Injury to myocardial cells results in the release of intracellular enzymes into circulating blood, permitting their detection by blood tests. Traditionally, CK and an isoenzyme, CK-MB, found in high concentration in myocardial cells, have been used to diagnose myocardial infarction in its earliest stages.[14] Rapid assays of these enzymes have been developed, permitting the determination of the blood levels of these enzymes within 30 to 60 minutes. Drawbacks to the use of CK-MB include its lack of specificity for cardiac muscle and the time required for CK-MB levels to rise during myocardial infarction. CK and CK-MB usually require at least 3 hours of profound ischemia to rise above normal levels; patients who present early in their infarction would not be expected to have elevation of CK. Furthermore, patients may have partial destruction in the infarct-related artery, or there may be extensive collateralization of the infarct-related artery, which further delays the release of these enzymes. In patients suspected of having acute myocardial infarction, it is not appropriate to delay treatment until an elevation of CK or CK-MB is present, because the goal of treatment is to prevent injury to the myocardium. The challenge facing physicians is to identify patients suffering myocardial infarction even before CK becomes elevated, because these patients require emergency therapy and stand to benefit the most from reperfusion therapy.

To overcome these limitations and more accurately and rapidly identify patients in need of emergency reperfusion therapy, other blood tests have been developed to help identify patients with ischemia.

Myoglobin is a low-molecular-weight heme protein found in cardiac muscle. Its advantage for diagnosis is that it is released more rapidly from infarcted myocardium than is CK-MB. However, myoglobin is also found in skeletal muscle, and the lack of specificity is a drawback.[15]

Troponin is a cardiac-specific marker for acute myocardial infarction; an increase in serum levels of troponin occurs early after myocardial cell injury. An elevated cardiac troponin level on admission is a predictor of subsequent cardiac events.[16,17] The role of troponin assays in the evaluation of patients in the emergency department and elsewhere is likely to increase as a result of the proposed revision to the diagnostic criteria of myocardial infarction, as described above.[7]

A simple automated analysis of the white cell count has been shown to increase the ability to accurately diagnose myocardial infarction in patients with chest pain but no ST segment elevation on ECG. A relative lymphocytopenia (a lymphocyte decrease to < 20.3% of leukocytes) is an independent predictor of acute myocardial infarction in such patients.[18,19] The presence of both a relative lymphocytopenia and a rapid elevation in CK-MB level in these patients may be particularly helpful in identifying myocardial infarction.

IMAGING STUDIES

Echocardiography

Echocardiography may be useful in identifying patients with myocardial infarction in the emergency department.[20-23] Most patients with acute myocardial infarction have regional wall motion abnormalities readily seen on echocardiography; however, echocardiographic evidence of myocardial infarction is not required in patients with symptoms and ECG evidence typical of acute myocardial infarction, and echocardiography should not be performed in such patients. Echocardiography is probably most useful in patients with left bundle branch block or abnormal ECGs without ST segment elevation whose symptoms are atypical and in whom the diagnosis is uncertain.[24]

Radionuclide Imaging

Perfusion imaging with both thallium and sestamibi in the emergency department has been reported to be both sensitive and specific in the evaluation of patients in whom the diagnosis is uncertain.[24,25] However, the time required to perform these tests limits their usefulness, and their ultimate value in this setting remains unclear.[26]

Emergent Therapy

Treatments have been developed that reduce the morbidity and mortality of acute myocardial infarction, particularly when initiated early; it is therefore important to avoid delay in administering therapy.[3,27] Although the greatest delay in treatment of acute myocardial infarction is usually the time that it takes a patient to seek medical care, much of the emphasis on reducing delay has focused on the time between a patient's presentation to the emergency department and the administration of reperfusion therapy. A patient with symptoms suggestive of myocardial infarction should be evaluated within 10 minutes after arrival in the emergency department.[28] Early steps should include the assessment of hemodynamic stability by measurement of the patient's heart rate and blood pressure; the performance of a 12-lead ECG; and the administration of oxygen by nasal prongs, of I.V. analgesia (most commonly morphine sulfate), of oral aspirin, and of sublingual nitroglycerin if the blood pressure is greater than 90 mm Hg. The challenge facing physicians who work in emergency departments is that more than 90% of patients who present to the emergency department complaining of chest pain are not suffering myocardial infarction; many do not have a cardiac etiology for their chest pain.[29]

All patients with definite or suspected myocardial infarction should be admitted to the hospital, undergo preparation for I.V. access, and be placed on continuous ECG monitoring. High-risk patients should be admitted to a coronary care unit. In many hospitals, patients at low risk for major complications are admitted to a telemetry unit, where emergency medical care can be quickly administered, rather than to a coronary care unit. Tachyarrhythmias and bradyarrhythmias may occur even in low-risk patients, particularly in the first 24 hours. Lido-

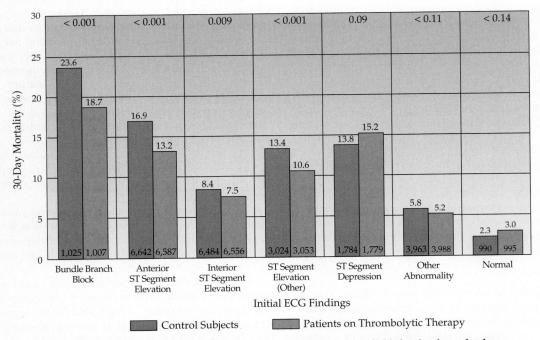

Figure 2   **Thirty-day mortality in patients with suspected acute myocardial infarction from placebo-controlled trials of thrombolytic therapy on the basis of their initial ECGs. Patients with ST segment depression are at high risk, nearly as high as patients with anterior ST segment elevation. The mortality among such patients is not reduced (and may be increased) by thrombolytic therapy. Patients with other nonspecific electrocardiographic abnormalities are at lesser risk, and those with normal ECG findings have the best prognosis.**

caine, atropine, an external or internal pacemaker, and a defibrillator should be readily available.

OXYGEN

Oxygen is generally recommended for all patients with acute myocardial infarction for the first several hours after admission and is mandatory for patients with pulmonary congestion or evidence of oxygen desaturation.

ASPIRIN

Aspirin should be given to all patients as soon as a diagnosis of myocardial infarction is made.[13] In the second International Study of Infarct Survival (ISIS-2), aspirin was found to be nearly as effective as streptokinase, reducing 30-day mortality 23% in 17,000 patients with acute myocardial infarction; the benefit was additive in patients receiving both aspirin and streptokinase [see Figure 3].[13] Other studies have revealed similar benefit from immediate aspirin therapy.[30] The beneficial effect of aspirin is the result of its antiplatelet effect, which is achieved through the rapid inhibition of thromboxane A_2 production.

Patients should be maintained on aspirin indefinitely. Prolonged administration of aspirin in patients with a history of myocardial infarction is associated with a 25% reduction in death, nonfatal reinfarction, and stroke.[30]

ANALGESIA

Pain relief should be among the initial therapies offered to patients with acute myocardial infarction. Persistent chest discomfort is generally caused by ongoing myocardial ischemia; although the ultimate goal of therapy is to eliminate ischemia, analgesia should be administered without delay. In addition to making patients more comfortable, pain relief may reduce the outpouring of catecholamines characteristic of the early stages of acute myocardial infarction and thereby reduce myocardial oxygen demand. Intravenous morphine sulfate is commonly used for pain relief in this setting.

Reperfusion Therapy

REPERFUSION STRATEGIES AND OUTCOMES

Importance of Time to Reperfusion

Many important predictors of early clinical outcome in myocardial infarction are independent of treatment. Such factors include the age of the patient; whether the patient has suffered a previous myocardial infarction; whether the patient has undergone coronary artery bypass surgery; and whether the patient has impaired ventricular function. However, the time to administration of reperfusion therapy is a critical determinant of outcome and one of the few determinants of early clinical outcome under the control of the physician. Many studies have revealed a lower mortality and, among survivors, reduced infarct size in patients with myocardial infarction treated most rapidly [see Figure 4].[31] This observation has led to recommendations that the time between a patient's presentation to the emergency department and the administration of thrombolytic therapy not exceed 60 minutes; ideally, this period should not exceed 30 minutes.[32] The most critical interval is the time between symptom onset and the achievement of reperfusion and not the time to the initiation of therapy. Thus, therapy that takes longer to initiate (such as direct coronary angioplasty)

may actually be superior if it achieves reperfusion more rapidly than another therapy that can be initiated more rapidly (such as thrombolytic therapy).

The importance of avoiding hospital delay in performing direct coronary angioplasty was evident in the Global Use of Strategies to Open Occluded Arteries (GUSTO-IIb) substudy, which compared direct coronary angioplasty with tissue plasminogen activator (t-PA) therapy.[33] There was a clear relation between the length of time until angioplasty was performed after enrollment in the study and 30-day mortality [see Figure 5]. Analysis of 27,080 patients in the second National Registry of Myocardial Infarction also revealed a relation between time to treatment with direct percutaneous transluminal coronary angioplasty (PTCA) and survival, even after adjusting for other mortality risk factors.[34] In that study, the volume of patients treated with angioplasty at the hospital was also a predictor of outcome; a lower mortality was seen at hospitals in which a high number of patients with acute myocardial infarction were treated with coronary angioplasty. There have been studies in which unacceptably high mortality was seen at hospitals when direct angioplasty was not performed rapidly; reducing delay led to a reduction in mortality.[35] Therefore, as is the case with thrombolytic therapy, the speed with which reperfusion is achieved appears to be an important determinant of clinical

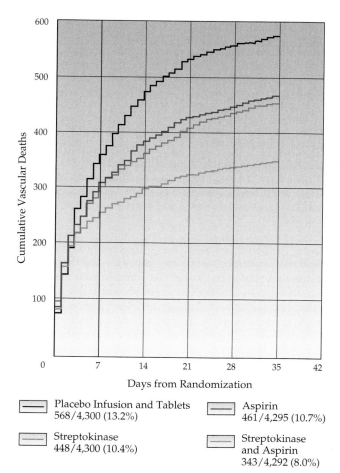

Figure 3 **Mortality at 35 days in 17,187 cases of suspected acute myocardial infarction in the second International Study of Infarct Survival (ISIS-2). In this study, aspirin reduced 30-day mortality by 23% and was nearly as effective as streptokinase; the benefit was additive in patients receiving both aspirin and streptokinase.[13]**

a

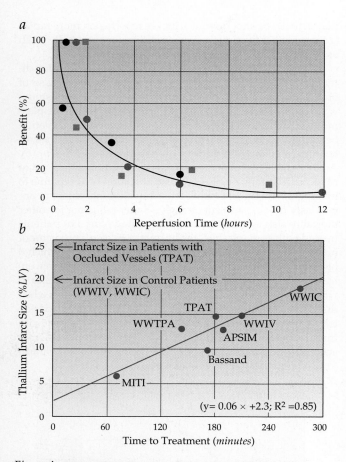

b

Coronary Angiography after Uncomplicated Myocardial Infarction

In patients who have not undergone direct coronary angioplasty, the role of coronary angiography after uncomplicated myocardial infarction remains controversial. Coronary angiography in patients initially treated with thrombolytic agents has been studied in the second Thrombolysis in Myocardial Infarction (TIMI II) study, the Should We Intervene Following Thrombolysis? (SWIFT) study, the Treatment of Post-thrombolytic Stenoses (TOPS) study, and, most recently, a German study.[39-42] It is clear from these studies that patients treated with thrombolytic therapy in whom complications do not occur are at low risk for reinfarction and death after discharge and that the routine performance of coronary angiography and coronary angioplasty does not reduce the occurrence of these adverse events. Despite the publication of these well-designed studies, there has been considerable reluctance among physicians to accept their results, and there remains considerable variability throughout the United States and the world in the frequency with which coronary angiography is performed in such patients.

Many cardiologists feel more comfortable caring for patients who have suffered a myocardial infarction if the patient's coronary anatomy is known. Patients at low risk may be discharged from the hospital more rapidly. Patients who have left main or multivessel disease, particularly those who have reduced ventricular function, may be referred for coronary bypass surgery or percutaneous revascularization. Patients with persistent occlusion of the infarct-related artery may benefit from revascularization because of favorable effects on remodeling, a reduction in ventricular arrhythmia, and the improved ability of the infarct-related artery to provide collateral blood flow to other coronary arteries in the future. Nonetheless, until the benefits of cardiac catheterization are demonstrated in asymptomatic patients after an uncomplicated myocardial infarction, a conservative strategy is recommended in patients who have been given thrombolytic therapy, and coronary angiography is recommended only for patients with hemodynamic instability or for patients in whom spontaneous or exercise-induced isch-

Figure 4 **Many studies have revealed lower mortality (*a*) and reduced infarct size among survivors (*b*) of myocardial infarction treated most rapidly. The equation shows the linear relation between infarct size and time to treatment.[31,124] (APSIM—APSAC dans l'Infarctus du Myocarde; Bassand—Bassand study; MITI—Myocardial Infarction Triage and Intervention; TPAT—Tissue Plasminogen Activator, Toronto trial; WWIC—Western Washington Intracoronary streptokinase trial; WWIV—Western Washington Intravenous streptokinase trial; WWTPA—Western Washington Tissue Plasminogen Activator trial)**

outcome. The best reperfusion therapy (coronary angioplasty or thrombolytic therapy) is not necessarily the one that can be most rapidly initiated but, rather, the one that achieves coronary patency most rapidly. Clinicians should know, at their own institution, whether coronary angioplasty is more rapid or less rapid than thrombolytic therapy at restoring flow to the infarct-related artery; in general, the therapy that restores flow most rapidly should be preferred. At institutions where a skilled catheterization team is on call 24 hours a day and can be rapidly assembled, coronary angioplasty would most likely be able to restore coronary blood flow in more patients more rapidly than thrombolytic therapy. Elsewhere, thrombolytic therapy may be preferable.[36-38]

The most recent American College of Cardiology/American Heart Association (ACC/AHA) guidelines indicate that for patients with symptoms suggestive of myocardial infarction, the time from arrival in the emergency department to obtaining an ECG should be no more than 10 minutes.[27] If thrombolytic therapy is used, it should be administered within 30 minutes; and if angioplasty is performed, it should be initiated within 1 to 2 hours of admission.[28]

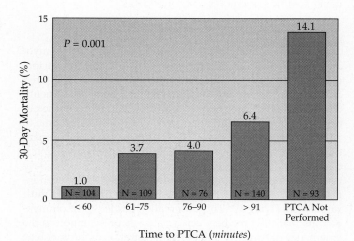

Figure 5 **Relation between the time from study enrollment to the first balloon inflation and 30-day mortality in the GUSTO-IIb substudy. Patients assigned to angioplasty in whom angioplasty was not performed are also shown. (PTCA—percutaneous transluminal coronary angioplasty)**

emia occurs; such a strategy is safe and is associated with a good clinical outcome.

Patients who are not given thrombolytic therapy are at higher risk for reinfarction and death than those receiving thrombolytic therapy. The role of coronary angiography in patients with acute myocardial infarction not receiving thrombolytic therapy has not been studied. In such patients whose infarctions are complicated by hemodynamic compromise or postinfarction chest pain or in patients in whom multivessel disease or reduced ventricular function is believed to be present, coronary angiography is probably helpful. It remains unclear whether coronary angiography should be performed in patients not treated with thrombolytic therapy who do not have these high-risk characteristics. It is impossible to be definitive about recommendations in the absence of appropriate studies, and not surprisingly, practice patterns vary widely throughout the United States and the world in such patients.

Reperfusion Therapy in Patients without ST Segment Elevation

Direct PTCA has not been appropriately studied in patients without ST segment elevation, and it is not possible to be definitive about its use in this setting. However, regardless of the findings on ECG, PTCA is widely believed to be beneficial in patients with ischemic-type chest discomfort that persists despite medical therapy. Many patients with prolonged chest pain without ST segment elevation are not suffering from myocardial infarction; the likelihood that infarction is present is increased if repolarization abnormalities are present on the ECG and the patient has risk factors for coronary artery disease. In patients with critical coronary stenoses, immediate PTCA or bypass surgery may be appropriate. In patients without significant coronary disease, immediate angiography can also be extremely useful and can lead to the withdrawal of cardiac medications, discharge from the coronary care unit, and appropriate diagnostic evaluation, in many cases as an outpatient. Immediate angiography is recommended in all patients with hypotension, severe congestive heart failure, or cardiogenic shock regardless of the initial ECG results, because immediate revascularization appears to reduce mortality in this setting.[43] Immediate angiography is strongly recommended in the most recent ACC/AHA guidelines for patients without ST segment elevation who have persistent or recurrent symptomatic ischemia, congestive heart failure, hypotension, or shock.[28]

In the TIMI IIIb study, an early intervention strategy was compared with a conservative strategy in 3,000 patients with either unstable angina, recent non–Q wave myocardial infarction, or prolonged chest pain without ST segment elevation on ECG.[44] Patients were randomized to receive either early angiography or medical therapy; only those patients who subsequently experienced recurrent chest pain or had a exercise test underwent angiography. Although death and myocardial infarction occurred with similar frequency in the two groups, the study showed that the initial hospitalization was longer and the need for rehospitalization more frequent in the group receiving conservative therapy. More recently, in the second Fragmin and Fast Revascularization during Instability in Coronary Artery Disease (FRISC II) trial, an early invasive strategy was shown to reduce both mortality and myocardial infarction at 1 year.[45] In the Treat Angina with Aggrastat [tirofiban] and Determine Cost of Therapy with Invasive or Conservative Strategy—Thrombolysis in Myocardial Infarction–18 (TAC-TICS-TIMI 18) study, an early invasive strategy was found to reduce the combined end point of death or myocardial infarction.[46] In both the FRISC II and TACTICS-TIMI 18 studies, patients at greatest risk, such as those with positive troponin values and with ST segment depression at study entry, had the highest event rates and derived the greatest benefit from an invasive strategy. Other than the avoidance of thrombolytic therapy, patients with ST segment elevation on the initial ECG should generally receive the same pharmacologic therapy as those without such a finding.

THROMBOLYTIC THERAPY

Thrombolytic therapy has been widely studied in prospective, randomized, controlled trials involving more than 50,000 patients and has been proved to reduce mortality 29% in patients with ST segment elevation treated within 6 hours of the onset of chest pain [see Figure 6].[47] The survival benefit of thrombolytic therapy is maintained for years.[48] The benefit of thrombolytic therapy is achieved through rapid restoration of coronary blood flow in an occluded coronary artery.[49-51]

Thrombolytic therapy is strongly recommended for patients with ST segment elevation in two or more contiguous leads who have had less than 6 hours of chest pain; for patients with classic symptoms of infarction in whom a bundle branch block precludes detection of ST segment elevation[47]; and for patients presenting with 6 to 12 hours of chest pain, although the expected benefits for this last group of patients are less, and the potential benefits should be weighed against the potential risks in patients with relative contraindications to thrombolytic therapy.[13,52] It is important to calculate the duration of infarction as the time from the last pain-free interval. The infarct-related artery often opens and closes spontaneously during the early stages of infarction, which the patient may experience as alternating pain-free and painful intervals; the window of benefit from thrombolytic therapy may be greater than 12 hours if antegrade flow was even briefly restored.

Contraindications to Thrombolytic Therapy

Contraindications to thrombolytic therapy include all conditions that predispose a patient to significant bleeding. The most feared bleeding complication is intracerebral hemorrhage, which is fatal in over half of cases. Risk factors for intracerebral bleeding include advanced age, low body weight, hypertension, warfarin use, and previous stroke.[47,53] Patients with gastrointestinal bleeding and those who have recently undergone surgery are also at increased risk for bleeding. Even when risk factors for bleeding are present, however, the potential benefits of thrombolytic therapy may still outweigh the risks. For example, although the elderly have a higher risk of intracerebral bleeding than younger patients, elderly patients should certainly be considered candidates for thrombolytic therapy, because their increasing absolute mortality results in a greater reduction in absolute mortality with thrombolytic therapy than is seen in younger patients.[47]

Thrombolytic therapy has been studied in patients with ECG findings other than ST segment elevation or bundle branch block and has been found to be either of no use or deleterious; its use is not recommended in such patients.[13,47]

Choice of Thrombolytic Agent

Many different thrombolytic regimens have been proved effective for the treatment of acute myocardial infarction, and

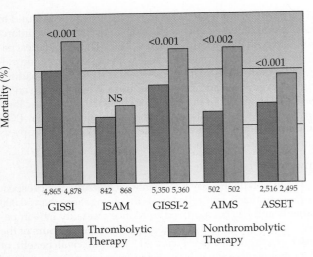

Figure 6 **Data from five controlled megatrials of thrombolytic therapy large enough to detect a mortality difference between the thrombolytic and nonthrombolytic control arms of the trials. Pooled data from these five trials (not shown) reveal a 29% mortality reduction in patients treated within 6 hours of symptom onset. (AIMS—APSAC International Mortality Study; ASSET—Anglo-Scandinavian Study of Early Thrombosis; GISSI—Gruppo Italiano per lo Studio della Streptochinasi nell'Infarto Miocardico; GISSI-2—Gruppo Italiano per lo Studio della Sopravvivenza nell'Infarto Myocardico; ISAM—Intravenous Streptokinase in Acute Miocardial Infarction; NS—not significant)**

many more are being studied. In principle, the preferred thrombolytic regimen would restore normal antegrade blood flow to an occluded coronary artery most rapidly and in the greatest number of patients, would have the lowest reocclusion rate, and would be associated with the lowest risk of severe hemorrhagic complications. The first Global Utilization of Streptokinase and Tissue Plasminogen Activator for Occluded Arteries (GUSTO-I) trial evaluated four thrombolytic regimens to determine which was associated with the greatest overall survival and stroke-free survival at 30 days: (1) a regimen of front-loaded, weight-adjusted t-PA and I.V. heparin, (2) a regimen of streptokinase and I.V. heparin, (3) a regimen of streptokinase and subcutaneous heparin, and (4) a combination of I.V. t-PA and streptokinase given concurrently with I.V. heparin. Front-loaded t-PA was found to be superior to the other thrombolytic regimens [*see Figure 7*].[50] However, because of the approximately 10 times greater cost of t-PA than I.V. streptokinase and the low margin of superiority (one life saved per thousand patients treated), some physicians prefer the less expensive streptokinase therapy, particularly for patients at low risk of dying (such as those with uncomplicated inferior infarctions) and the elderly, who are more likely to have hemorrhagic complications with t-PA than with streptokinase; t-PA is associated with a greater frequency of intracerebral hemorrhage than streptokinase.[50] The recommendation of streptokinase in these patient groups is largely driven by its lower cost; if the costs of t-PA and streptokinase were similar, t-PA would most likely be the preferred therapy in all patient subgroups, with the possible exception of those at increased risk for intracerebral hemorrhage, in whom streptokinase might be preferred.

Streptokinase therapy is contraindicated in patients who have recently received a dose of streptokinase because of antibodies that form against the drug; these antibodies limit the efficacy of repeat doses and increase the risk of allergic reactions. It has been suggested that the drug not be readministered for at least 2 years.

New thrombolytic agents are continuously being developed in the hope of finding safer and more effective therapies. One such agent, reteplase, is a recombinant tissue plasminogen activator that is a mutant of alteplase. Reteplase is easier to administer than alteplase; because of its longer half-life, it can be administered as two 10 mU boluses given 30 minutes apart, with concomitant aspirin and I.V. heparin administration. Several pilot studies suggest that reteplase has an early patency rate that is superior to the patency rates of streptokinase and alteplase. In the International Joint Efficacy Comparison of Thrombolytics (INJECT) trial, 6,010 patients with acute myocardial infarction received either reteplase or streptokinase within 12 hours of the onset of symptoms.[54] Mortality at 35 days, the primary end point of the study, was 9.02% for patients given reteplase, compared with 9.53% for patients given streptokinase, a nonsignificant difference (95% confidence interval, 1.98 to 0.96). This lack of significant difference indicates that reteplase was at least as effective as streptokinase.

In the Global Use of Strategies to Open Occluded Coronary Arteries (GUSTO-III) trial,[55] reteplase was compared with t-PA in 15,059 patients with acute myocardial infarction who presented within 6 hours of symptom onset. Patients received either reteplase or an accelerated infusion of t-PA. For patients receiving reteplase, the mortality at 30 days was 7.47%, compared with 7.24% for patients receiving t-PA ($P = 0.54$; odds ratio, 1.03; 95% confidence interval, 0.91 to 1.18). The mortality rates with the two agents were therefore similar, and the two agents are probably, although not definitely, equivalent in efficacy.

Pilot studies have suggested that the combination of half the normal dose of a fibrin-specific thrombolytic agent—either t-PA or reteplase—with a standard dose of the platelet glycoprotein IIb/IIIa inhibitor abciximab restores patency of an infarct-related artery more rapidly and more frequently than full-dose thrombolytic therapy alone, without a significant increase in bleeding complications.[56,57] The safety and efficacy of the combination of these thrombolytic agents with abciximab is being studied in large randomized trials. Half-dose streptokinase and abciximab resulted in unacceptable bleeding complications in pilot studies, with the complications being worse than those seen with the fibrin-specific agents and abciximab.

DIRECT CORONARY ANGIOPLASTY

Coronary angioplasty without antecedent thrombolytic therapy, termed direct or primary coronary angioplasty, has been studied in the treatment of acute myocardial infarction [*see Figure 8*]. In prospective, randomized trials comparing direct coronary angioplasty with different thrombolytic agents, direct coronary angioplasty was associated with a lower morbidity and mortality than thrombolytic therapy.[58-62] Although most of the individual trials were too small to detect statistically significant differences in mortality, pooled data from these trials suggest that direct coronary angioplasty is the preferred therapy for acute myocardial infarction at institutions where it can be performed without delay [*see Figure 9*].[63] The GUSTO-IIb trial was designed to be large enough to confirm the reduction in mortality found in the smaller randomized trials. The preliminary results of the study indicate that direct coronary angioplasty is associated with a lower mortality, reinfarction rate,

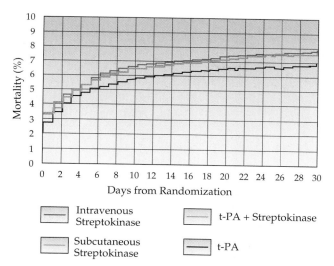

Figure 7 **The frequency of death or disabling stroke in the 30 days after enrollment in 41,021 patients in the Global Utilization of Streptokinase and Tissue Plasminogen Activator for Occluded Arteries (GUSTO-I) trial. Front-loaded t-PA was found to be superior to the other thrombolytic regimens.**[50]

Legend: Intravenous Streptokinase; Subcutaneous Streptokinase; t-PA + Streptokinase; t-PA

and frequency of stroke in the 30 days after enrollment than thrombolytic therapy [*see Figure 10*]. However, the degree of benefit associated with direct coronary angioplasty was much smaller than that seen in the earlier randomized studies; this finding was in part related to the lower frequency with which patients assigned to undergo angioplasty in GUSTO-IIb actually underwent the procedure and in part related to the lower frequency with which normal antegrade coronary blood flow was achieved in patients who did undergo coronary angioplasty.

The consistency of the results favoring direct coronary angioplasty and the greater speed and frequency with which coronary angioplasty can restore flow to an occluded coronary artery support the conclusion that PTCA is preferable to thrombolytic therapy at institutions where it can be performed quickly with a high success rate.[64] Studies have shown that excessive delay in performing direct coronary angioplasty and operator inexperience lead to a higher mortality than that seen when direct coronary angioplasty is performed rapidly by experienced operators.[34] The need for surgical backup is controversial, as excellent results have been obtained at centers without surgical backup.[65] However, surgical backup is recommended because approximately 5% of patients with acute myocardial infarction who undergo immediate coronary angiography require emergency surgery either for failed angioplasty or, more commonly, because lethal coronary anatomy precludes PTCA. In addition, most centers without surgical backup do not have experienced interventional cardiologists, and the volume of angioplasties is not sufficient to allow that procedure to be safely performed in these high-risk patients.

Because of concerns that the routine use of direct PTCA might actually delay reperfusion in certain medical centers, direct PTCA is currently recommended only in medical centers in which the procedure can be initiated (arterial access achieved) within 2 hours, where a high success rate and low complication rate can be demonstrated, and where PTCA is performed in at least 80% to 90% of patients in whom acute myocardial infarction is confirmed.[28,63,66] Although reocclusion and renarrowing of the infarct-related artery are both associat-

ed with adverse outcome and are less frequent with direct PTCA than with thrombolytic therapy, the most important aspect of the initial treatment should be the speed with which normal flow can be restored in the infarct-related artery. Ideally, physicians would use the therapy (thrombolytic therapy or direct PTCA) that is able to restore normal antegrade blood flow in the most infarct-related arteries most rapidly at their hospital.

Combined Thrombolytic and Glycoprotein IIb/IIIa Inhibitor Therapy

The role of the platelet glycoprotein inhibitor abciximab in conjunction with direct coronary angioplasty has been examined in the Randomized, Placebo-Controlled Trial of Abciximab with Primary Angioplasty for Acute Myocardial Infarction (RAPPORT), the Intracoronary Stenting and Antithrombotic Regimen–2 (ISAR-2) study, the Abciximab before Direct Angioplasty and Stenting in Myocardial Infarction Regarding Acute and Long-term Follow-up (ADMIRAL) study, and, most recently, the CADILLAC study.[67-72] The results of the four studies differ, in part because the trials used different end points, in part because of the high frequency of noncompliance with the protocol in some trials, and in part because of differences in the treatments utilized (e.g., balloon angioplasty alone versus balloon angioplasty followed by stent placement). The largest of the four studies, the CADILLAC study, found that abciximab is beneficial at reducing major adverse events, but the benefit appeared to be limited to patients undergoing balloon angioplasty rather than stent placement.

The apparent lack of other benefits of abciximab in patients treated with stents is contrary to the results of the ISAR-2 and ADMIRAL trials, in which abciximab was found to be beneficial in patients receiving stents. There are data to suggest that stent placement in the setting of acute myocardial infarction slightly reduces the frequency with which normal antegrade blood flow in the infarct-related artery is achieved.[71,73] This would suggest that glycoprotein IIb/IIIa inhibitors are particularly beneficial in this setting. Taken together, the results of these studies that are currently available suggest that abciximab is beneficial in patients with acute myocadial infarction but that the benefit in patients undergoing balloon angioplasty alone may differ from that in patients who undergo balloon angioplasty and also receive stents. Clearly, however, stents markedly reduce the frequency with which a repeat revascularization procedure is needed in the months after the angioplasty procedure.[73] The combined use of stents and platelet glycoprotein inhibitors may maximize the frequency with which normal antegrade blood flow is achieved while reducing the need for repeat procedures in the following year.[71] One study compared the outcome of lytic therapy using t-PA with that of direct angioplasty utilizing both stents and abciximab. The reduction in infarct size was far greater in the group undergoing direct angioplasty; the clinical outcome was also better in the patients who underwent angioplasty.[74]

CORONARY ARTERY BYPASS SURGERY

Coronary artery bypass surgery can restore blood flow in an occluded infarct-related artery. Emergency bypass surgery has been reported in many small retrospective analyses to be an effective treatment in acute myocardial infarction and was found to be beneficial in a prospective, randomized trial in which it was compared with medical therapy that did not include

a *b*

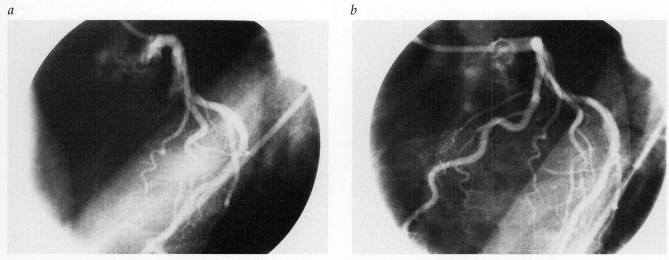

Figure 8 (*a*) Left anterior oblique view of an occluded left anterior descending artery in a patient suffering an acute anterior myocardial infarction. (*b*) Patency was restored with direct coronary angioplasty 17 minutes after the patient had arrived in the catheterization laboratory, and the patient had immediate resolution of his symptoms.

reperfusion therapy.[75,76] However, because of the time required to perform coronary angiography and to transport patients to the operating room, reperfusion is achieved more slowly with bypass surgery than with thrombolytic therapy and direct coronary angioplasty.[77] Emergency coronary artery bypass surgery should generally be reserved for patients in whom immediate angiography reveals coronary anatomy that precludes direct coronary angioplasty; for patients in whom angioplasty has failed; and for patients with a ventricular septal defect, severe mitral regurgitation, or myocardial rupture.

RESCUE CORONARY ANGIOPLASTY

Depending on the regimen used, only 33% to 60% of patients treated with thrombolytic therapy have restoration of normal antegrade flow in the infarct-related artery 90 minutes after the initiation of therapy.[49] Accordingly, immediate coronary angiography has been studied to determine whether patients with persistent occlusion of the infarct-related artery benefit from coronary angioplasty; this procedure has been termed rescue angioplasty. A single small randomized trial has examined the clinical outcome of patients with anterior infarction

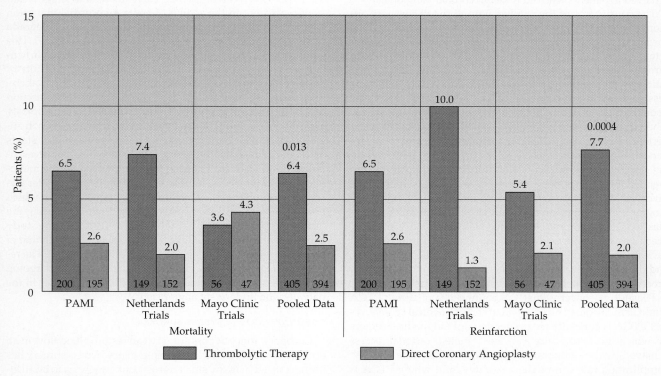

Figure 9 Pooled data from the first Primary Angioplasty in Myocardial Infarction (PAMI-1), Netherlands, and Mayo Clinic trials suggest that direct coronary angioplasty is superior to thrombolytic therapy in the treatment of acute myocardial infarction in terms of mortality and reinfarction at institutions where it can be performed without delay.

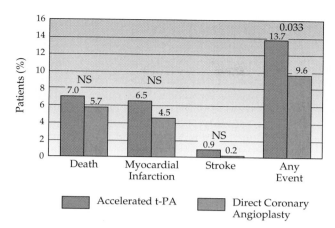

Figure 10 **Results from the GUSTO-IIb substudy trial comparing direct coronary angioplasty and accelerated t-PA indicate that direct coronary angioplasty was associated with a lower mortality, reinfarction rate, and frequency of stroke in the 30 days after enrollment than accelerated t-PA. (NS—not significant)**

and persistent coronary occlusion that persist despite thrombolytic therapy. Patients were randomized to either undergo rescue coronary angioplasty or receive continued medical therapy alone. The results of the trial suggested improved outcome with rescue angioplasty, although the benefits were not compelling.[78] Three additional randomized trials evaluated the role of rescue angioplasty.[79-81] Analyzed together, the four trials suggest that rescue angioplasty offers benefit, although the data are not compelling. Although use of coronary stents and platelet glycoprotein inhibitors improves the results of percutaneous revascularization procedures and would be expected to further increase the benefit of angioplasty after failed lytic therapy, this has not yet been proved. There are insufficient data to recommend immediate angiography and angioplasty in all patients early after thrombolytic therapy. Immediate angiography is most likely to be beneficial in patients with large myocardial infarctions in whom persistent pain, ST segment elevation, or hemodynamic compromise is present more than 90 minutes after the administration of a thrombolytic agent.

The routine performance of angioplasty immediately after the administration of thrombolytic therapy in all patients with a significant residual stenosis (not just those patients with occluded coronary arteries) has been well studied in three prospective, randomized trials and has been found to be either of no benefit or deleterious.[39,82] Angioplasty should not be routinely performed in such patients.

Stents appear to improve the ability to achieve arterial patency early after lytic therapy, as compared with balloon angioplasty alone[83]; therapy with a glycoprotein IIb/IIIa inhibitor may also do so, although an increase in bleeding has been seen when glycoprotein IIb/IIIa inhibitors are used early after full-dose lytic therapy.[84] Data from several pilot studies suggest that the combination of a fibrin-specific thrombolytic agent, either t-PA or reteplase, combined with the glycoprotein IIb/IIIa inhibitor abciximab, may actually facilitate the performance of angioplasty rather than reduce its safety and efficacy, as was seen when balloon angioplasty was performed after thrombolytic therapy.[56,57] Hence, the term facilitated angioplasty has been coined for the routine performance of angioplasty after the combination of half-dose lytic therapy with a glycoprotein IIb/IIIa inhibitor. This approach is currently being further evaluated in clinical trials.

Adjunctive Medical Therapy

INTRAVENOUS HEPARIN

The need for I.V. heparin after thrombolytic therapy varies with the thrombolytic agents used. A retrospective analysis of the GUSTO-I trial suggested that I.V. heparin with a partial thromboplastin time of 50 to 70 seconds was associated with the best clinical outcome in patients treated with t-PA.[85] Data from GUSTO-I also suggest that I.V. heparin is not required when I.V. streptokinase is used, although heparin is recommended in patients with large anterior infarctions to prevent the development of apical mural thrombus and embolization.[50] In patients in whom I.V. heparin is not administered, subcutaneous heparin should be administered during the period of bed rest to reduce the risk of deep vein thrombosis.[86]

The optimal duration of I.V. heparin therapy is unclear. Standard practice was to administer I.V. heparin for 3 to 5 days, although patients are now often discharged after only 3 days. It is recommended that heparin not be discontinued less than 24 hours after patient discharge from the hospital because of the possibility of a rebound effect and recurrent thrombosis within 24 hours after cessation of heparin therapy.[87]

Randomized studies from the prethrombolytic era suggested that administration of I.V. heparin reduces mortality and reinfarction in patients not treated with thrombolytic agents.[86] Aspirin and beta blockers were not routinely administered in those early trials, so the true benefits of heparin when these drugs are administered are unknown. However, on the basis of these early data, I.V. heparin is generally recommended for patients with suspected myocardial infarction who are not treated with thrombolytic therapy.[66]

BETA BLOCKERS

Numerous studies of beta-blocker therapy in patients with acute myocardial infarction have documented significant reductions in in-hospital and long-term mortality. Early administration of beta blockers has been promoted because it may reduce infarct size by reducing heart rate, blood pressure, and myocardial contractility, all of which diminish myocardial oxygen demand. Meta-analysis of the effects of early administration of I.V. beta blockers in 27,486 patients with acute myocardial infarction enrolled in 28 randomized trials revealed a 14% reduction in mortality during the first week of therapy; reinfarction was reduced 18%.[88]

The TIMI II study compared immediate beta-blocker therapy with deferred beta-blocker therapy in acute myocardial infarction; all patients also received I.V. t-PA.[89] Results indicated that immediate beta-blocker therapy reduced the incidence of nonfatal reinfarction and recurrent ischemia, compared with oral metoprolol therapy begun on the sixth hospital day; as in earlier studies, only about 40% of patients with acute myocardial infarction were eligible for acute beta-blocker therapy.[39] There are also data suggesting that immediate beta-blocker therapy reduces the risk of intracranial hemorrhage after lytic therapy.[90] It is recommended that all patients with acute myocardial infarction without contraindications receive I.V. beta blockers as early as possible, whether or not they receive reperfusion therapy.

In patients in whom contraindications preclude early beta-blocker therapy, reevaluation should take place before discharge. Many patients will no longer have contraindications at the time of discharge. Patients without contraindications should be routinely started on beta-blocker therapy before discharge from the hospital. The optimal duration of benefit remains unclear, but it appears that the benefit of beta-blocker therapy is maintained for years. Patients with the largest infarctions benefit the most from the use of beta blockers. Current recommendations are that beta-blocker therapy be continued indefinitely in the absence of contraindications or side effects.

ANGIOTENSIN-CONVERTING ENZYME INHIBITORS

Several large randomized, controlled clinical trials evaluating the use of angiotensin-converting enzyme (ACE) inhibitors early after acute myocardial infarction have been performed; all but one trial revealed a significant reduction in mortality. Meta-analysis of these large trials and many smaller trials, which together included over 100,000 patients, suggested a 6.5% reduction in deaths, with an absolute reduction in mortality of 4.6 deaths per 1,000 patients among those treated with an ACE inhibitor.[91] All patients with significant ventricular dysfunction (an ejection fraction < 40%) without contraindications should be treated with an ACE inhibitor; treatment should begin within the first 48 hours of infarction and be increased cautiously to avoid hypotension. If hypotension results from the early administration of ACE inhibitors, short-term mortality may be increased.[92]

The benefit of ACE inhibitors is clear in patients with large anterior infarctions and an ejection fraction less than 40%; whether patients with an ejection fraction greater than 40% benefit from ACE inhibitor therapy is less clear. However, the results of one large trial suggest that patients with a normal ejection fraction after myocardial infarction, and even patients with coronary disease without a previous myocardial infarction, have a reduction in mortality when treated with an ACE inhibitor. In the Heart Outcomes Prevention Evaluation (HOPE) study, 9,297 patients 55 years of age or older with vascular disease (or with diabetes and another cardiovascular risk factor) without a low ejection fraction or congestive heart failure were randomly assigned to receive either the ACE inhibitor ramipril or placebo for a mean of 5 years.[93] The reduction in the combined end point of death from cardiovascular causes, myocardial infarction, or stroke with ramipril was remarkable; it occurred in 17.7% of placebo-treated patients versus 14.1% of patients receiving ramipril (relative risk, 0.78; 95% confidence interval, 0.70 to 0.86; P < 0.001). A statistically significant reduction in each of the individual end points of cardiovascular death, myocardial infarction, and stroke was present as well. The study was stopped prematurely by the Data Safety Monitoring Board when clear evidence of a beneficial effect of ramipril was found. Another large randomized trial examining the role of ACE inhibitor therapy in patients with a normal ejection fraction is ongoing; if it also suggests benefit, ACE inhibitor therapy will be routinely recommended for the majority of patients who survive a myocardial infarction regardless of ejection fraction or the presence of congestive heart failure.

INTRAVENOUS NITROGLYCERIN

Randomized studies examining the role of I.V. nitroglycerin in acute myocardial infarction revealed beneficial effects on left ventricular function and a reduction in infarct size and mortality.[94] However, these studies were small and were performed before the reperfusion era. To determine whether nitroglycerin therapy is beneficial in patients treated with reperfusion, 58,050 patients with acute myocardial infarction in the fourth International Study of Infarct Survival (ISIS-4) were randomized to receive either oral controlled-release mononitrate therapy or placebo; thrombolytic therapy was administered to patients in both groups.[91] The results of this study revealed no benefit to the routine administration of oral nitrate therapy in this setting. Similar results were seen among 19,000 patients in the third Gruppo Italiano per lo Studio della Sopravvivenza nell'Infarto Miocardico (GISSI-3) study, in whom I.V. nitroglycerin was administered for the first 24 hours, followed by transdermal nitrates.[95] Whether these disappointing results in the ISIS-4 and GISSI-3 trials were caused by the routes of administration of the nitroglycerin preparation or the administration of thrombolytic therapy is unknown. However, on the basis of existing data, it does not appear that the routine administration of nitroglycerin to patients receiving early thrombolytic therapy is beneficial. I.V. nitroglycerin is probably most likely to be beneficial in patients with persistent or recurrent chest pain after reperfusion therapy and in patients in whom reperfusion therapy is not administered.

PROPHYLACTIC ANTIARRHYTHMIC THERAPY

Previously, routine prophylactic antiarrhythmic therapy with I.V. lidocaine was recommended for all patients in the early stages of acute myocardial infarction. However, studies have revealed that prophylactic therapy with lidocaine does not reduce and may actually increase mortality because of an increase in the occurrence of fatal bradyarrhythmia and asystole.[96] Neither I.V. lidocaine nor other antiarrhythmic agents are recommended as prophylactic therapy for patients without malignant ventricular ectopy.[96,97]

CALCIUM CHANNEL ANTAGONISTS

Calcium channel antagonists should not be routinely administered for acute myocardial infarction. Calcium channel antagonists have been studied in prospective, double-blind, placebo-controlled trials; and neither verapamil,[98,99] nifedipine,[100,101] nor diltiazem[102] appears to reduce postinfarction mortality. Verapamil and diltiazem may be useful in patients with preserved left ventricular function and no heart failure in whom contraindications to beta blockers exist.[103,104] However, the data are insufficient to recommend the routine administration of these agents. On the basis of existing data, treatment with calcium channel blockers should be reserved for patients with ischemia that persists despite use of aspirin, beta blockers, nitrate therapy, and I.V. heparin and for patients with other indications for their administration.

MAGNESIUM

Magnesium has been studied in many prospective, randomized trials of acute myocardial infarction, and the results have been conflicting. Magnesium is involved in hundreds of enzymatic steps and produces systemic and coronary vasodilatation, inhibits platelet function, and reduces reperfusion injury. Meta-analysis of seven prospective, randomized trials revealed a significant reduction in mortality with the use of magnesium (odds ratio, 0.44; confidence interval, 0.27 to 0.71).[105] Subsequently, the second Leicester Intravenous Magnesium Intervention Trial (LIMIT-2) revealed a 25% reduction in mortality with use of magnesium in over 2,000 patients who had acute myocardial infarction.[106] However, in ISIS-4, in which 58,050 patients were randomized to receive either I.V. magnesium or no magnesium, there was no reduction in 30-day mortality.[91] It is possible that the later administration of magnesium in this study, compared with the previous studies, and the concomitant use of thrombolytic therapy in 70% of patients contributed to the lack of efficacy of magnesium in ISIS-4; only one third of patients in the LIMIT-2 study received thrombolytic therapy. A subsequent small randomized trial reexamined the role of magnesium in patients in whom reperfusion therapy was not administered and did find a mortality reduction associated with its use.[107] On the basis of the existing evidence, current recommendations are that magnesium not be routinely given to patients in whom reperfusion therapy is administered. It is possible that magnesium is of benefit, particularly in patients not receiving reperfusion therapy. Further studies are under way to evaluate the use of magnesium in patients with acute myocardial infarction.

Magnesium is clearly indicated in patients with myocardial infarction who have torsade de pointes–type ventricular tachycardia and in patients with magnesium deficiency.[28]

Complications of Acute Myocardial Infarction

VENTRICULAR ARRHYTHMIAS

Ventricular arrhythmias are a frequent cause of death in the earliest stages of acute myocardial infarction. The development of coronary care units, continuous ECG surveillance, and defibrillators in the 1960s led to a reduction in mortality from acute myocardial infarction through the prompt identification and treatment of ventricular arrhythmia; and emergency medical technicians have reduced outpatient mortality in the earliest minutes of myocardial infarction. In cities with well-developed emergency response systems, such as Seattle, where the average response time is less than 5 minutes, survival of patients with myocardial infarction complicated by cardiac arrest has increased.[3]

Ventricular Fibrillation

In the setting of acute myocardial infarction, ventricular fibrillation is often described as either primary, when it occurs in the absence of hypotension or heart failure, or secondary, when hypotension or heart failure is present. Primary ventricular fibrillation occurs in approximately 3% to 5% of patients with acute myocardial infarction; the peak incidence is in the first 4 hours of infarction. Primary ventricular fibrillation is infrequent more than 24 hours after symptom onset. Mortality is increased in patients who suffer this complication.[108,109] In those who are successfully resuscitated and survive to hospital discharge, however, the long-term prognosis does not appear to be affected.[108] Although lidocaine has been shown to reduce the occurrence of primary ventricular fibrillation, mortality in patients receiving lidocaine was increased because of an increase in fatal bradycardia and asystole, and prophylactic lidocaine is no longer recommended if defibrillation can rapidly be performed.[96] Beta blockers may reduce the early occurrence of ventricular fibrillation and should be administered to patients who have no contraindications. Hypokalemia is a risk factor for primary ventricular fibrillation and should be rapidly corrected if present. When ventricular fibrillation occurs, rapid defibrillation with 200 to 300 joules should be attempted, and repeated shocks of 360 joules should be administered. The Advanced Cardiac Life Support (ACLS) guidelines recommend medical therapy, including epinephrine, lidocaine, and bretylium; in addition, I.V. amiodarone should be considered in patients in whom defibrillation is initially unsuccessful.

Secondary ventricular fibrillation is associated with a high mortality, in part because of the underlying hypotension and heart failure. Treatment must be aimed not only at terminating the arrhythmia but also at the hemodynamic abnormalities and their causes.

Ventricular Tachycardia

Ventricular tachycardia (three or more consecutive ventricular ectopic beats) is common in patients with acute myocardial infarction; however, short runs of nonsustained ventricular tachycardia are no longer believed to predispose a patient to sustained ventricular tachycardia or ventricular fibrillation. In patients in whom sustained or hemodynamically significant ventricular tachycardia occurs, prompt electrical cardioversion should be performed. If the ventricular tachycardia is monomorphic, synchronic cardioversion with 100 joules should first be attempted. As with ventricular fibrillation, polymorphic ventricular tachycardia should be treated with unsynchronized discharge. Prolonged runs of asymptomatic ventricular tachycardia can be initially treated with I.V. lidocaine, procainamide, or amiodarone. These medications may also be helpful in reducing recurrent ventricular tachycardia.

ATRIAL ARRHYTHMIA

Atrial Fibrillation

Atrial fibrillation is the most common atrial arrhythmia in acute myocardial infarction, occurring in 10% to 16% of patients. Atrial fibrillation may result either from an acute increase in left atrial pressure caused by left ventricular dysfunction or from atrial ischemia as a result of occlusion of a coronary artery (usually the right coronary artery) proximal to the origin of atrial branches. The incidence of atrial fibrillation is decreased in patients given thrombolytic therapy.[50]

The treatment of atrial fibrillation in acute myocardial infarction should be similar to the treatment of atrial fibrillation in other settings. When there is hemodynamic compromise caused by loss of atrial systole or a rapid ventricular response with a reduction in cardiac output, cardioversion should be performed immediately. In patients with preserved left ventricular function in whom the atrial fibrillation is well tolerated, beta-blocker therapy is indicated. Verapamil and diltiazem may also be effective in such patients. In patients with reduced ventricular function and, in particular, those with congestive heart failure, digoxin can slow the ventricular response. Although less effective than beta blockers or calcium channel blockers in that regard, digoxin is preferred because of its positive inotropic effect, in contrast to the negative inotropic effect of the other agents. If atrial fibrillation recurs, antiarrhythmic agents may be used, although their impact on clinical outcome has not been studied.

BRADYARRHYTHMIAS AND HEART BLOCK

Sinus bradycardia is common in acute myocardial infarction, particularly in patients with inferior myocardial infarction. However, treatment with atropine and a temporary pacemaker is required infrequently and, generally, only in patients with significant hemodynamic compromise manifested by increased angina, hypotension, or congestive heart failure.

High-degree (second- or third-degree) heart block occurs in

approximately 20% of patients with inferior infarction; it is uncommon with infarction at other sites.[110] About half of the cases of heart block seen with inferior infarction are Wenckebach-type second-degree heart block; the remainder are cases of third-degree heart block. The heart block is often easily treated with atropine, but a temporary pacemaker is required in as many as 50% of cases. The heart block generally lasts for hours to days; placement of a permanent pacemaker is needed in fewer than 1% of cases. However, the development of heart block with inferior infarction is associated with a threefold to fourfold increase in in-hospital mortality over inferior infarction without heart block.[110,111] The increased mortality appears to result from the association between heart block and more severe left and right ventricular infarction rather than from the heart block itself or treatment of the heart block.

Heart block during anterior infarction is uncommon, occurring in fewer than 1% of cases. It is generally associated with extensive left ventricular myocardial infarction involving the conduction system below the atrioventricular node and carries a very poor prognosis.

MITRAL REGURGITATION

Mitral regurgitation may result from injury to any of the components of the mitral valve apparatus, including the papillary muscles and ventricular walls to which they attach. Mild mitral regurgitation is common in acute myocardial infarction and is present in nearly 50% of patients. Severe mitral regurgitation caused by acute myocardial infarction is rare and generally results from partial or complete rupture of a papillary muscle. The characteristic murmur of severe chronic mitral regurgitation may not be present with acute rupture of a papillary muscle. Instead, a decrescendo systolic murmur is often present, extending less throughout systole as systemic arterial pressure falls and left arterial pressure rises. In many cases, the significance of the murmur is not recognized. The blood supply of the anterior papillary muscle arises from branches of both the left anterior descending and the circumflex arteries; therefore, rupture of the anterior papillary muscle is rare. However, the posterior papillary muscle receives blood only from the dominant coronary artery (the right coronary artery in nearly 90% of patients); thrombotic occlusion of this artery may cause rupture of the posterior papillary muscle, resulting in severe mitral regurgitation. Severe mitral regurgitation is 10 times more likely to occur with inferior infarction than with anterior infarction. Acute severe mitral regurgitation is poorly tolerated and generally results in pulmonary edema, often with cardiogenic shock. Prompt surgical repair is recommended. Although the mortality associated with mitral valve surgery is high in this setting, approaching 50%, survival appears to be greater than with medical therapy alone. Therapy aimed at reducing left ventricular afterload, such as use of I.V. nitroprusside and an intra-aortic balloon pump, reduces the regurgitant volume and increases forward blood flow and cardiac output and may be helpful as a temporizing measure.

VENTRICULAR SEPTAL DEFECTS

Ventricular septal defects are slightly more frequent in patients with anterior infarction than in patients with inferior infarction. The characteristic holosystolic murmur of ventricular septal defects may be difficult to distinguish from that of severe mitral regurgitation; however, ventricular septal defects are generally better tolerated and less frequently result in severe congestive heart failure. Surgical repair is recommended and results in the best outcome when repaired emergently in the hemodynamically compromised patient. As with acute severe mitral regurgitation, therapy aimed at reducing afterload, including I.V. nitroprusside and an intra-aortic balloon pump, may be beneficial. Repair of the septum is generally more difficult when associated with inferior infarction, because there may not be a viable rim of myocardial tissue beneath the defect to facilitate repair. The surgical mortality associated with repair of a postinfarction ventricular septal defect is approximately 20% but is largely related to the age of the patient, whether cardiogenic shock is present, the infarction site, and the severity of the underlying coronary disease.

MYOCARDIAL RUPTURE

As more and more patients survive the acute phase of myocardial infarction because reperfusion therapy reduces myocardial infarct size, myocardial rupture has increased in frequency as a cause of early death. Myocardial rupture has been reported to account for more than 20% of in-hospital deaths in some series in the thrombolytic era. Physicians must have a heightened awareness of the diagnosis if a patient is to survive this catastrophic occurrence, because emergency surgery is required. Symptoms suggestive of rupture include repetitive vomiting, pleuritic chest pain, restlessness, and agitation. ECG evidence of rupture includes a deviation from the normal pattern of ST segment and T wave evolution. Resolution of ST segment elevation and T wave inversion, with maximal T wave negativity in the leads with maximal ST segment elevation, should normally occur; however, in patients with rupture, there is progressive or recurrent ST segment elevation and persistently positive T wave deflections or reversal of initially inverted T waves.[112] Echocardiography can quickly confirm the diagnosis. Even when emergency surgery is performed, fewer than 50% of patients survive to discharge.

RIGHT VENTRICULAR INFARCTION

Right ventricular infarction occurs in approximately one third of patients with acute inferior left ventricular infarction and is hemodynamically significant in approximately 50% of affected patients.[113] Hemodynamically significant right ventricular infarction associated with anterior infarction or isolated right ventricular infarction is rare. The classic findings associated with hemodynamically significant right ventricular infarction are hypotension with clear lung fields and an elevated jugular venous pressure, often with the Kussmaul sign. Although nearly all patients with right ventricular infarction suffer both right and left ventricular infarction, the characteristic hemodynamic findings of right ventricular infarction generally dominate the clinical course and must be the main focus of therapy. Right ventricular involvement during inferior myocardial infarction is associated with a significant increase in mortality, and aggressive attempts at early reperfusion should be pursued.[110,113] Prompt recognition of right ventricular involvement is clinically important because therapy that reduces right ventricular filling, such as use of nitrates or diuretics, should be avoided. Volume therapy should be administered to maintain cardiac output; in patients whose hypotension is refractory to volume therapy, dopamine may be beneficial. Heart block, which occurs in as many as 50% of patients with right ventricular infarction, should be treated rapidly, and maintenance of atrioventricular synchrony with dual atrial and ventricular pacing is often required to maintain filling of the ischemic noncompliant right ventricle and an adequate cardiac output.

Cardiogenic shock resulting from right ventricular infarction is generally reversible with these measures. Improvement in right ventricular function generally occurs over time, particularly in patients in whom reperfusion therapy was successful in achieving vessel patency.[108] In patients who survive the initial hospitalization, left ventricular function is the most potent predictor of long-term outcome.

STROKE

Extensive infarction of the anterior wall and apex of the left ventricle leads to thrombus formation in the apex of the left ventricle in approximately 30% of patients; systemic embolization occurs in about 15% of these patients. Left ventricular thrombus formation is much less common after inferior infarction. The thrombus generally appears within the first several days after infarction; if the thrombus is pedunculated or protrudes into the left ventricular cavity or is mobile, it is more likely to embolize and cause stroke. Left ventricular thrombus is an indication for anticoagulation with I.V. heparin followed by warfarin therapy for 3 to 6 months.

Therapy that reduces infarct size, such as thrombolytic therapy, reduces the frequency of thrombus formation and therefore the risk of systemic embolization and stroke. However, in 0.3% to 1.0% of patients, thrombolytic therapy causes hemorrhagic stroke, most commonly in the 24 hours after its administration, which is fatal in more than 50% of cases. Hemorrhagic stroke is rare in acute myocardial infarction except as a consequence of thrombolytic therapy, although an ischemic stroke may become hemorrhagic because of thrombolytic, antiplatelet, and anticoagulation therapy. Hemorrhagic stroke, the most feared complication of thrombolytic therapy, is more likely in elderly patients; in patients with low body weight, with hypertension, or who have previously had a stroke; and in those on warfarin.[47,53] Although thrombolytic therapy decreases the risk of ischemic stroke, there is a slight net increase in the overall risk of stroke because of the risk of hemorrhagic stroke. Direct coronary angioplasty is believed to reduce the incidence of ischemic stroke without increasing the risk of hemorrhagic stroke.

Predischarge Exercise Testing

In patients with spontaneous postinfarction angina, congestive heart failure, hypotension, or malignant ventricular arrhythmia, exercise testing should generally be deferred, and coronary angiography should be performed. However, in patients without these high-risk characteristics, exercise testing is generally recommended before discharge from the hospital to assess a patient's functional capacity and ability to return to activities of daily living and work.[114] Most data indicating that predischarge exercise testing can identify patients at increased risk for cardiac events after discharge are from the prethrombolytic era, when the risk of adverse cardiac events was much higher. In the modern era, in which thrombolytic therapy or direct coronary angioplasty is frequently performed and in which aspirin, beta blockers, ACE inhibitors, and lipid-lowering agents are routinely administered—all of which reduce the frequency of adverse events in the years after discharge—it is difficult to identify patients at risk, because the adverse event rate is so low. Nonetheless, exercise testing is generally recommended to provide a measure of comfort to both the patient

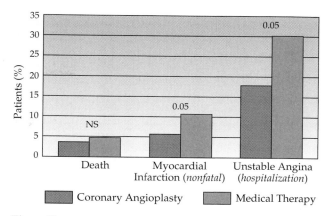

Figure 11   In the Danish Acute Myocardial Infarction (DANAMI) study, 1,008 patients treated with thrombolytic therapy in whom exercise-induced ischemia was present on a predischarge exercise test were randomized to receive either coronary angioplasty or medical therapy alone. Clinical outcome was improved in patients in the invasive arm of the study. (NS—not significant)

and the physician, to help determine the appropriateness of medical therapy, and to facilitate entry of the patient into a cardiac rehabilitation program.

Although predischarge exercise testing has been the standard of care in the United States for some time, only recently has a study examined whether therapy based on the results of a predischarge exercise test improves clinical outcome. The Danish Trial in Acute Myocardial Infarction (DANAMI) was the first study to examine the usefulness of exercise testing in patients treated with thrombolytic agents (a low-risk group) and to provide support for what has been the standard of care in the United States [*see Figure 11*].[115] The results of this study revealed that clinical outcome was improved in patients who received angiography and coronary angioplasty, compared with those who received medical therapy alone. Use of the results of exercise testing to decide whether or not to employ revascularization in patients without spontaneous angina is less common outside of the United States.

Patients with acute myocardial infarction who do not receive thrombolytic therapy or undergo direct angioplasty are at greater risk for adverse events after discharge from the hospital, and predischarge exercise testing is of even greater utility in such patients.

Prognostic variables indicating increased risk during exercise testing are exercise-induced angina or ST segment depression, particularly when it occurs during exercise at a low work load; an abnormal drop in systolic blood pressure; and an inability to complete the exercise test. However, the patients at greatest risk are those unable to exercise; such patients have the highest mortality after discharge.[116]

The type of exercise test that should be performed has been the subject of controversy. It is generally recommended that only simple treadmill testing be performed before discharge; in patients with abnormalities in the baseline ECG, stress testing with perfusion imaging or stress echocardiography may be helpful. In patients without widespread abnormalities on the ECG, perfusion imaging or stress echocardiography is generally deferred until at least 4 weeks after discharge, when a more vigorous exercise test can be performed. Whether the predischarge treadmill test should be a low-level test or a more vigorous symptom-limited test is unclear. It has been shown that a symptom-limited Bruce protocol exercise test detects ischemia more frequently than a submaximal test; however, it is not known which test has the greater positive and negative predictive value for identifying patients at risk. Currently, a lower-level exercise test is preferred, although a more vigorous test might be appropriate in patients likely to resume a more active and vigorous lifestyle shortly after discharge and in whom a low-level test might not cause the patient to expend the amount of energy he or she will be using during activities of daily living.

There has been concern that the use of beta blockers before the predischarge exercise test may mask the presence of significant coronary disease and prevent the identification of high-risk patients. This concern does not appear to be significant enough to outweigh the benefits of early beta-blocker therapy.

Secondary Prevention

PHARMACOTHERAPY

Lipid-Lowering Therapy

Recent studies have demonstrated that in patients with coronary artery disease, lipid-lowering therapy with HMG-CoA (3-hydroxy-3-methylglutaryl coenzyme A) reductase inhibitors reduces not only fatal and nonfatal infarction but also mortality from all causes. The Scandinavian Simvastatin Survival Study revealed a 42% reduction in cardiac mortality and a 30% reduction in all-cause mortality in 4,444 men and women with coronary artery disease over the 5.4 years of the study.[117] The reduction in mortality was similar among patients in the lowest and highest quartiles of serum low-density lipoprotein (LDL) cholesterol. It has been demonstrated that postinfarction patients with an LDL cholesterol level at or above 130 mg/dl benefit from lipid-lowering therapy within as little as 2 years of the initiation of such therapy.[118] Initial measurement of cholesterol should be made within 24 hours after myocardial infarction; measurement of lipids 24 hours or more after myocardial infarction can be misleading in that cholesterol levels may be reduced below baseline levels during this period and remain low for up to 1 month. Early initiation of statins may be more beneficial than later initiation.[119] Exercise, weight reduction in overweight patients, avoidance of dietary saturated fat and cholesterol, and smoking cessation have all been reported to favorably influence blood lipid levels and should be recommended whether or not lipid-lowering medications are prescribed.

Anticoagulation Therapy

Several prospective, randomized trials revealed that warfarin therapy reduces mortality after discharge from the hospital in patients with acute myocardial infarction. However, in these studies in which warfarin therapy was compared with placebo, aspirin was not administered in either arm of the study.[120,121] The Coumadin Aspirin Reinfarction Study (CARS) revealed that the risk of reinfarction in patients treated with aspirin alone was similar to that in patients treated with aspirin and either low-dose or higher-dose warfarin. Warfarin is also ineffective at preventing coronary reocclusion in patients in whom thrombolytic therapy was successful.[122] The routine administration of warfarin is not currently recommended to prevent reinfarction in patients who have survived myocardial infarction.

Antiarrhythmic Therapy

Although Holter monitoring before discharge can help identify patients at increased risk for sudden cardiac death, antiarrhythmic therapy has not been shown to decrease the risk of death in such patients, and in fact, it increased mortality in the Cardiac Arrhythmia Suppression Trial (CAST).[123] Since CAST, several prospective, randomized studies have been performed that have examined the role of amiodarone in patients at increased risk for sudden death. Taken together, the results of those studies do not indicate that amiodarone reduces mortality. Further studies are needed before the routine use of amiodarone can be recommended in high-risk patients such as those included in these trials.

RISK-FACTOR MODIFICATION

An important and often neglected aspect of medical care after a myocardial infarction is the identification and modification of risk factors for atherosclerosis. Hypertension and hypercholesterolemia should be treated. Cessation of smoking [see Chapter 3] has been shown to prolong life in patients who have survived a myocardial infarction; behavior modification and group therapy can increase the likelihood of kicking the habit. Cardiac rehabilitation and the establishment of a healthier lifestyle with an exercise program [see Chapter 4] can further reduce the likelihood of a return to smoking. Hypercholesterolemia should be aggressively treated as described above.

Although there are few data that conclusively indicate that patients who participate in a cardiac rehabilitation program after discharge have increased survival, an exercise rehabilitation program appears to improve a patient's sense of well-being and hasten return to work and leisure activities. A cardiac rehabilitation program can also help improve diet and aid weight reduction in overweight patients, help smokers refrain from smoking, and help establish an exercise program that the patient can maintain long after the formal rehabilitation program has ended. In summary, participation in a cardiac rehabilitation program often leads to the establishment of a healthier lifestyle.

Long-term Prognosis

Long-term prognosis after myocardial infarction is determined primarily by the severity of left ventricular dysfunction, the presence and degree of residual ischemia, and the potential for malignant ventricular arrhythmia. These adverse prognostic factors are related to each other but are also independently associated with death after discharge. Age is also an important determinant of outcome. Most deaths that occur in the first year after discharge occur in the first 3 months, a fact that stresses the importance of assessing risk and optimizing therapy before discharge from the hospital. However, there can be substantial improvement in ventricular function in the weeks and months after acute myocardial infarction, particularly in patients in whom early reperfusion was achieved. Therefore, measurement of ventricular function 2 to 3 months after myocardial infarction is a more accurate predictor of long-term prognosis than measurement of left ventricular function in the acute stages.

References

1. McGovern PG, Pankow JS, Shahar E, et al: Recent trends in acute coronary heart disease. N Engl J Med 334:884, 1996

2. Mortality from coronary heart disease and acute myocardial infarction—United States, 1998. MMWR Morb Mortal Wkly Rep 50:90, 2001

3. Patient/bystander recognition and action: rapid identification and treatment of acute myocardial infarction. National Heart Attack Alert Program (NHAAP). National Heart, Lung, and Blood Institute. National Institutes of Health (NIH Publication No 93-3303), Bethesda, Maryland, 1993

4. Fuster V, Badimon L, Badimon JJ, et al: The pathogenesis of coronary artery disease and the acute coronary syndromes. N Engl J Med 326:242, 1992

5. Ambrose JA, Tannenbaum MA, Alexopoulos D, et al: Angiographic progression of coronary artery disease and the development of myocardial infarction. J Am Coll Cardiol 12:56, 1988

6. Tunstall-Pedoe H, Kuulasmaa K, Amouyel P, et al: Myocardial infarction and coronary deaths in the World Health Organization MONICA Project. Circulation 90:583, 1994

7. Myocardial infarction redefined: a consensus document of The Joint European Society of Cardiology/American College of Cardiology Committee for the Redefinition of Myocardial Infarction. J Am Coll Cardiol 36:959, 2000

8. Aronow WS: Prevalence of presenting symptoms of recognized acute myocardial infarction and of unrecognized healed myocardial infarction in elderly patients. Am J Cardiol 60:1182, 1987

9. Kouvaras G, Bacoulas G: Unstable angina as a warning symptom before acute myocardial infarction. Q J Med 64:679, 1987

10. Kannel WB, Abbott RD: Incidence and prognosis of unrecognized myocardial infarction: an update on the Framingham study. N Engl J Med 311:1144, 1984

11. Karlson BW, Herlitz J, Edvardsson N, et al: Eligibility for I.V. thrombolysis in suspected acute myocardial infarction. Circulation 82:1140, 1990

12. Cragg DR, Friedman HZ, Bonema JD, et al: Outcome of patients with acute myocardial infarction who are ineligible for thrombolytic therapy. Ann Intern Med 115:173, 1991

13. Randomised trial of intravenous streptokinase, oral aspirin, both, or neither among 17,187 cases of suspected acute myocardial infarction: ISIS-2. Second International Study of Infarct Survival Collaborative Group. Lancet 2:349, 1988

14. Roberts R, Kleinman N: Earlier diagnosis and treatment of acute myocardial infarction necessitates the need for a "new diagnostic mind-set." Circulation 89:872, 1994

15. Zabel M, Hohnloser SH, Koster W, et al: Analysis of creatine kinase, CK-MB, myoglobin, and troponin T time-activity curves for early assessment of coronary artery reperfusion after intravenous thrombolysis. Circulation 87:1542, 1993

16. Ohman EM, Armstrong P, Califf RM, et al: Risk stratification in acute ischemic syndromes using serum troponin T. The GUSTO Investigators. J Am Coll Cardiol 25(suppl):148A, 1995

17. Ravkilde J, Nissen H, Horder M, et al: Independent prognostic value of serum creatine kinase isoenzyme MB mass, cardiac troponin T and myosin light chain levels in suspected acute myocardial infarction: analysis of 28 months of follow-up in 196 patients. J Am Coll Cardiol 25:574, 1995

18. Thompson SP, Gibbons RJ, Smars PA, et al: Incremental value of the leukocyte differential and the rapid creatine kinase-MB isoenzyme for the early diagnosis of myocardial infarction. Ann Intern Med 122:335, 1995

19. Cannon CP, McCabe CH, Wilcox RG, et al: Association of white blood cell count with increased mortality in acute myocardial infarction and unstable angina pectoris. OPUS-TIMI 16 Investigators. Am J Cardiol 87:636, 2001

20. Sabia P, Abbott RD, Afrookteh A, et al: Importance of two-dimensional echocardiographic assessment of left ventricular systolic function in patients presenting to the emergency room with cardiac-related symptoms. Circulation 84:1615, 1991

21. Fleischmann KE, Lee TH, Come PC, et al: Echocardiographic prediction of complications in patients with chest pain. Am J Cardiol 79:292, 1997

22. Talreja D, Gruver C, Sklenar J, et al: Efficient utilization of echocardiography for the assessment of left ventricular systolic function. Am Heart J 139:394, 2000

23. St John Sutton M, Pfeffer MA, Plappert T, et al: Quantitative two-dimensional echocardiographic measurements are major predictors of adverse cardiovascular events after acute myocardial infarction: the protective effects of captopril. Circulation 89:68, 1994

24. Villanueva FS, Sabia PJ, Afrookteh A, et al: Value and limitations of current methods of evaluating patients presenting to the emergency room with cardiac-related symptoms for determining long-term prognosis. Am J Cardiol 69:746, 1992

25. Hilton TC, Thompson RC, Williams HJ, et al: Technetium-99m sestamibi myocardial perfusion imaging in the emergency room evaluation of chest pain. J Am Coll Cardiol 23:1016, 1994

26. Radensky PW, Hilton TC, Fulmer H, et al: Potential cost effectiveness of initial myocardial perfusion imaging for assessment of emergency department patients with chest pain. Am J Cardiol 79:595, 1997

27. Rapid identification and treatment of acute myocardial infarction. National Heart, Lung, and Blood Institute. National Institutes of Health (NIH Publication No 94-3302), Bethesda, Maryland, 1994

28. Ryan TJ, Antman EM, Brooks NH, et al: 1999 Update: ACC/AHA guidelines for the management of patients with acute myocardial infarction. J Am Coll Cardiol 34:890, 1999

29. Hedges JR, Young GP, Henkel GF, et al: Serial ECGs are less accurate than serial CK-MB results for emergency department diagnosis of myocardial infarction. Ann Emerg Med 21:1445, 1992

30. Secondary prevention of vascular disease by prolonged antiplatelet treatment. Antiplatelet Trialists Collaboration. Br Med J 296:320, 1988

31. Weaver WD: Time to thrombolytic treatment: factors affecting delay and their influence on outcome. J Am Coll Cardiol 25(suppl 7):3S, 1995

32. Emergency department rapid identification and treatment of patients with acute myocardial infarction. National Heart Attack Alert Program Coordinating Committee 60 minutes to Treatment Working Group. Ann Emerg Med 23:311, 1994

33. Berger PB, Ellis SG, Holmes DR Jr, et al: The relationship between delay in performing direct coronary angioplasty and early clinical outcome in patients with acute myocardial infarction: results from the global use of strategies to open occluded arteries in acute coronary syndromes (GUSTO-IIb) trial. Circulation 100:14, 1999

34. Cannon CP, Gibson CM, Lambrew CT, et al: Relationship of symptom-onset-to-balloon time and door-to-balloon time with mortality in patients undergoing angioplasty for acute myocardial infarction. JAMA 283:2941, 2000

35. Caputo RP, Ho KKL, Stoler RC, et al: Effect of continuous quality improvement on the delivery of primary percutaneous transluminal coronary angioplasty for acute myocardial infarction. Am J Cardiol 79:1159, 1997

36. Jhangiana AH, Jorgenson MB, Kotlewski A, et al: Community practice of primary angioplasty for myocardial infarction. Am J Cardiol 80:209, 1997

37. Patel S, Reese C, O'Connor RE, et al: Adverse outcomes accompanying primary angioplasty (PTCA) for acute myocardial infarction (AMI)—dangers of delay. J Am Coll Cardiol 27(suppl A):62A, 1996

38. Rosman HS, Ciolino D, Nerenz D, et al: Primary PTCA and thrombolysis for acute myocardial infarction: observations from the community. J Am Coll Cardiol 27(suppl A):26A, 1996

39. Immediate versus delayed catheterization and angioplasty following thrombolytic therapy for acute myocardial infarction. The TIMI Study Group. JAMA 260:2849, 1988

40. Ellis SG, Mooney MR, George BS, et al: Randomized trial of late elective angioplasty versus conservative management for patients with residual stenoses after thrombolytic treatment of myocardial infarction. Circulation 86:1400, 1992

41. SWIFT trial of delayed elective intervention v conservative treatment after thrombolysis with anistreplase in acute myocardial infarction. SWIFT Study Group. BMJ 302:555, 1991

42. Zeymer U: The ALKK Trial. Oral presentation at the Late Breaking Clinical Trials Session of the 49th Annual Scientific Sessions of the American College of Cardiology, March 2000

43. Berger PB, Holmes DR Jr, Stebbins AL, et al: Impact of an aggressive invasive catheterization and revascularization strategy on mortality in patients with cardiogenic shock in the Global Utilization of Streptokinase and Tissue Plasminogen Activator for Occluded Coronary Arteries (GUSTO-I) trial: an observational study. Circulation 96:122, 1997

44. Effects of tissue plasminogen activator and a comparison of early invasive and conservative strategies in unstable angina and non-Q-wave myocardial infarction: results of the TIMI IIIB Trial. The TIMI IIIB Investigators. Circulation 89:1545, 1995

45. Wallentin L, Lagerqvist B, Husted S, et al: Outcome at 1 year after an invasive compared with a non-invasive strategy in unstable coronary-artery disease: the FRISC II invasive randomised trial. Lancet 356:9, 2000

46. Cannon C: TACTICS-TIMI 18 (Treat Angina with Aggrastat and Determine Cost of Therapy with an Invasive or Conservative Strategy). Presented at American Heart Association Scientific Sessions 2000, New Orleans, November 15, 2000

47. Indications for fibrinolytic therapy in suspected acute myocardial infarction: collaborative overview of early mortality and major morbidity results from all randomised trials of more than 1000 patients. Fibrinolytic Therapy Trialists' (FTT) Collaborative Group. Lancet 343:311, 1994

48. French JK, Hyde TA, Patel H, et al: Survival 12 years after randomization to streptokinase: the influence of thrombolysis in myocardial infarction flow at three to four weeks. J Am Coll Cardiol 34:62, 1999

49. The effects of tissue plasminogen activator, streptokinase, or both on coronary-artery patency, ventricular function, and survival after acute myocardial infarction. The GUSTO Angiographic Investigators. N Engl J Med 329:1615, 1993

50. An international randomized trial comparing four thrombolytic strategies for acute myocardial infarction. The GUSTO Investigators. N Engl J Med 329:673, 1993

51. Simes RJ, Topol EJ, Holmes DR Jr, et al: Link between the angiographic substudy and mortality outcomes in a large randomized trial of myocardial reperfusion: importance of early and complete infarct artery reperfusion. Circulation 91:1923, 1995

52. Late Assessment of Thrombolytic Efficacy (LATE) study with alteplase 6 to 24 hours after onset of acute myocardial infarction. Lancet 342:759, 1993

53. de Jaegere PP, Arnold AA, Balk AH, et al: Intracranial hemorrhage in association with thrombolytic therapy: incidence and clinical predictive factors. J Am Coll Cardiol 19:289, 1992

54. Randomised double-blind comparison of reteplase double-bolus administration with streptokinase in acute myocardial infarction (INJECT): trial to investigate the equivalent. International Joint Efficacy Comparison of Thrombolytics. Lancet 346:329, 1995

55. A comparison of reteplase with alteplase for acute myocardial infarction. The Global Use of Strategies to Open Occluded Coronary Arteries (GUSTO III) Investigators. N Engl J Med 337:1118, 1997

56. Antman EM, Giugliano RD, Gibson CM, et al: Abciximab facilitates the rate and extent of thrombolysis: results of the Thrombolysis in Myocardial Infarction (TIMI 14) Trial. Circulation 99:2720, 1999

57. Ohman EM, Lincoff AM, Bode C, et al: Enhanced early reperfusion at 60 minutes with low-dose reteplase combined with full-dose abciximab in acute myocardial infarction: preliminary results from the GUSTO-IV Pilot (SPEED) Dose-ranging Trial (abstr). Circulation 98(suppl I):I-504, 1998

58. O'Neill W, Timmis G, Bourdillon P, et al: A prospective randomized clinical trial of intracoronary streptokinase versus coronary angioplasty for acute myocardial infarction. N Engl J Med 314:812, 1986

59. de Boer MJ, Hoorntje JCA, Ottervanger JP, et al: Immediate coronary angioplasty versus intravenous streptokinase in acute myocardial infarction: left ventricular ejection fraction, hospital mortality, and reinfarction. J Am Coll Cardiol 23:1004, 1994

60. de Boer MJ, Suryapranata H, Hoorntje JC, et al: Limitation of infarct size and preservation of left ventricular function after primary coronary angioplasty compared with intravenous streptokinase in acute myocardial infarction. Circulation 90:753, 1994

61. Zijlstra F, de Boer MJ, Hoorntje JCA, et al: A comparison of immediate coronary angioplasty with intravenous streptokinase in acute myocardial infarction. N Engl J Med 328:680, 1993

62. Grines CL, Browne KF, Marco J, et al: A comparison of immediate angioplasty with thrombolytic therapy for acute myocardial infarction. N Engl J Med 328:673, 1993

63. Michels KB, Yusuf S: Does PTCA in acute myocardial infarction affect mortality and reinfarction rates? A quantitative overview (meta-analysis) of the randomized clinical trials. Circulation 91:476, 1995

64. Berger PB, Bell MR, Holmes DR Jr, et al: Time to reperfusion with direct coronary angioplasty and thrombolytic therapy in acute myocardial infarction. Am J Cardiol 73:231, 1994

65. Wharton TP, McNamara SN, Fedele FA, et al: Primary angioplasty for the treatment of acute myocardial infarction: experience at two community hospitals without cardiac surgery. J Am Coll Cardiol 33:1257, 1999

66. Ryan TJ, Anderson JL, Antman EM, et al: ACC/AHA guidelines for the management of patients with acute myocardial infarction: a report of the American College of Cardiology/American Heart Association task force on practice guidelines (Committee of Management of Acute Myocardial Infarction). J Am Coll Cardiol 28:1328, 1996

67. Brener SJ, Barr LA, Burchenal J, et al: Randomized, placebo-controlled trial of abciximab with primary angioplasty for acute myocardial infarction (abstr). Circulation 96(suppl I):I-473, 1997

68. Montalescot G, Barragan P, Wittenberg O, et al: Abciximab associated with primary angioplasty and stenting in acute myocardial infarction: the ADMIRAL study, 30-day final results. Circulation 100(suppl I):1, 1999

69. Barragan P, Montalescot G, Wittenberg O, et al: Abciximab associated with primary angioplasty and stenting in acute myocardial infarction: the ADMIRAL study, 6-month results. Circulation 102(suppl II):18, 2000

70. Neumann FJ, Blasini R, Schmitt C, et al: Effect of glycoprotein IIb/IIIa receptor blockade on recovery of coronary flow and left ventricular function after placement of coronary-artery stents in acute myocardial infarction. Circulation 98:2695, 1998

71. Stone GW: Results of CADILLAC trial. Presented at the Transcatheter Cardiovascular Therapeutics XI: Frontiers in Interventional Cardiology. Washington, DC, October 22, 2000

72. Tcheng JE, Effron MB, Grines CL, et al: Final results of the CADILLAC trial. J Am Coll Cardiol 37(suppl A):343A, 2001

73. Grines CL, Cox DA, Stone GW, et al: Coronary angioplasty with or without stent implantation for acute myocardial infarction. Stent Primary Angioplasty in Myocardial Infarction Study Group. N Engl J Med 341:1949, 1999

74. Schomig A, Kastrati A, Dirschinger J, et al: Coronary stenting plus platelet glycoprotein IIb/IIIa blockade compared with tissue plasminogen activator in acute myocardial infarction. Stent versus Thrombolysis for Occluded Coronary Arteries in Patients with Acute Myocardial Infarction Study Investigators. N Engl J Med 343:385, 2000

75. Dittrich HC, Gilpin E, Nicod P, et al: Outcome after acute myocardial infarction in patients with prior coronary artery bypass surgery. Am J Cardiol 72:507, 1993

76. Loop FD, Lytle BW, Cosgrove DM, et al: Reoperation for coronary atherosclerosis: changing practice in 2509 consecutive patients. Ann Surg 212:378, 1990

77. Berger PB, Stensrud PE, Daly RC, et al: Emergency coronary artery bypass surgery following failed coronary angioplasty: time to reperfusion and other procedural characteristics. AmJ Cardiol 76:565, 1995

78. Ellis SG, Ribeiro da Silva E, Heyndrickx G, et al: Randomized comparison of rescue angioplasty with conservative management of patients with early failure of thrombolysis for acute anterior myocardial infarction. Circulation 90:2280, 1994

79. Belenkie I, Traboulsi M, Hall CA, et al: Rescue angioplasty during myocardial infarction has a beneficial effect on mortality: a tenable hypothesis. Can J Cardiol 8:357, 1992

80. Widimsky P, Groh L, Ascherman M, et al: The "PRAGUE" study: a national multicenter randomized study comparing primary angioplasty vs thrombolysis vs both in patients with acute myocardial infarction admitted to the community hospitals: results of the pilot phase (abstr). Eur Heart J 19(suppl):56, 1998

81. Vermeer F, Brunninkhuis L, van de Berg E, et al: Prospective randomized comparison between thrombolysis, rescue PTCA, and primary PTCA in patients with extensive myocardial infarction admitted to a hospital without PTCA facilities: a safety and feasibility study. Heart 82:426, 1999

82. Simoons ML, Arnold AE, Betriu A, et al: Thrombolysis with tissue plasminogen activator in acute myocardial infarction: no additional benefit from immediate percutaneous coronary angioplasty. Lancet 1:197, 1988

83. Dirschinger J, Kastrati A, Neumann FJ, et al: Influence of balloon pressure during stent placement in native coronary arteries on early and late angiographic and clinical outcome: a randomized evaluation of high-pressure inflation. Circulation 100:918, 1999

84. Miller JM, Smalling R, Ohman EM, et al: Effectiveness of early coronary angioplasty and abciximab for failed thrombolysis (reteplase or alteplase) during acute myocardial infarction: results from the GUSTO-III trial. Am J Cardiol 84:779,1989

85. Granger CB, Hirsh J, Califf RM, et al: Activated partial thromboplastin time and outcome after thrombolytic therapy for acute myocardial infarction: results from the GUSTO-I trial. Circulation 93:870, 1996

86. Chesebro JH, Fuster V: Antithrombotic therapy for acute myocardial infarction: mechanisms and prevention of deep venous, left ventricular, and coronary artery thromboembolism. Circulation 74:1, 1986

87. Granger CB, Miller JM, Bovill EG, et al: Rebound increase in thrombin generation and activity after cessation of intravenous heparin in patients with acute coronary syndromes. Circulation 91:1929, 1995

88. Gersh BJ, Rahimtoola SHE: Acute myocardial infarction. Pharmacological Management of Acute Myocardial Infarction. Warnica JW, Ed. Elsevier, New York, 1991, p 205

89. Comparison of invasive and conservative strategies after treatment with intravenous tissue plasminogen activator in acute myocardial infarction: results of the Thrombolysis in Myocardial Infarction (TIMI) phase II trial. The TIMI Study Group. N Engl J Med 320:618, 1989

90. Barron HV, Rundle AC, Gore JM, et al: Intracranial hemorrhage rates and effect of immediate beta-blocker use in patients with acute myocardial infarction treated with tissue plasminogen activator. Participants in the National Registry of Myocardial Infarction–2. Am J Cardiol 85:294, 2000

91. ISIS-4: a randomised factorial trial assessing early oral captopril, oral mononitrate, and intravenous magnesium sulphate in 58,050 patients with suspected acute myocardial infarction. Fourth International Study of Infarct Survival Collaborative Group. Lancet 345:669, 1995

92. Sigurdsson A, Swedberg K: Left ventricular remodelling, neurohormonal activation and early treatment with enalapril (CONSENSUS II) following myocardial infarction. Eur Heart J 15(suppl B):14, 1994

93. Yusuf S, Sleight P, Pogue J, et al: Effects of an angiotensin-converting-enzyme inhibitor, ramipril, on cardiovascular events in high-risk patients. The Heart Outcomes Prevention Evaluation Study Investigators. N Engl J Med 342:145, 2000

94. Judgutt BI, Warnica JW: Intravenous nitroglycerin therapy to limit myocardial infarct size, expansion, and complications: effect of timing, dosage, and infarct location. Circulation 78:906, 1988

95. GISSI-3: effects of lisinopril and transdermal glyceryl trinitrate singly and together on 6-week mortality and ventricular function after acute myocardial infarction. Gruppo Italiano per lo Studio della Sopravvivenza nell'Infarto Miocardico. Lancet 343:1115, 1994

96. MacMahon S, Collins R, Peto R, et al: Effects of prophylactic lidocaine in suspected acute myocardial infarction: an overview of results from the randomized, controlled trials. JAMA 260:1910, 1988

97. Teo KK, Yusuf S, Furberg CD: Effects of prophylactic antiarrhythmic drug therapy in acute myocardial infarction: an overview of results from randomized controlled trials. JAMA 270:1589, 1993

98. Gheorghiade M: Calcium channel blockers in the management of myocardial infarction patients. Henry Ford Hosp Med J 39:210, 1991

99. Held PH, Yusuf S: Effects of beta-blockers and calcium channel blockers in acute myocardial infarction. Eur Heart J 14(suppl F):18, 1993

100. Secondary Prevention Reinfarction Israeli Nifedipine Trial (SPRINT): A randomized intervention trial of nifedipine in patients with acute myocardial infarction. The Israeli SPRINT Study Group. Eur Heart J 9:354, 1988

101. Goldbourt U, Behar S, Reicher-Reiss H, et al: Early administration of nifedipine in suspected acute myocardial infarction. The Secondary Prevention Reinfarction Israel Nifedipine Trial 2 Study. Arch Intern Med 153:345, 1993

102. The effect of diltiazem on mortality and reinfarction after myocardial infarction. The Multicenter Diltiazem Postinfarction Trial Research Group. N Engl J Med 319:385, 1988

103. Gibson RS, Hansen JF, Messerli F, et al: Long-term effects of diltiazem and verapamil on mortality and cardiac events in non-Q-wave acute myocardial infarction without pulmonary congestion: post hoc subset analysis of the multicenter diltiazem postinfarction trial and the second Danish verapamil infarction trial studies. Am J Cardiol 86:275, 2000

104. Boden WE, van Gilst WH, Scheldewaert RG, et al: Diltiazem in acute myocardial infarction treated with thrombolytic agents: a randomised placebo-controlled trial. Incomplete Infarction Trial of European Research Collaborators Evaluating Prognosis post-Thrombolysis (INTERCEPT). Lancet 355:1751, 2000

105. Teo KK, Yusuf S, Collins R, et al: Effects of intravenous magnesium in suspected acute myocardial infarction: overview of randomised trials. BMJ 303:1499, 1991

106. Woods KL, Fletcher S, Roffe C, et al: Intravenous magnesium sulphate in suspected acute myocardial infarction: results of the second Leicester Intravenous Magnesium Intervention Trial (LIMIT-2). Lancet 339:1553, 1992

107. Schechter M, Hod H, Chouraqui P, et al: Magnesium therapy in acute myocardial infarction when patients are not candidates for thrombolytic therapy. Am J Cardiol 75:321, 1995

108. Berger PB, Ruocco NA, Ryan TJ, et al: Incidence and prognostic significance of ventricular tachycardia and ventricular fibrillation in the absence of hypotension or heart failure in acute myocardial infarction treated with recombinant tissue-type plasminogen activator: results from the TIMI II trial. J Am Coll Cardiol 22:1773, 1993

109. Behar S, Goldbourt U, Reicher-Reiss H, et al: Prognosis of acute myocardial infarction complicated by primary ventricular fibrillation. Am J Cardiol 66:1208, 1990

110. Berger PB, Ryan TJ: Inferior infarction: high risk subgroups. Circulation 81:401, 1990

111. Berger PB, Ruocco NA, Frederick MM, et al: The incidence and significance of heart block during inferior infarction: results from the TIMI II trial. J Am Coll Cardiol 20:533, 1992

112. Oliva PB, Hammill SC, Edwards WD: Cardiac rupture, a clinically predictable complication of acute myocardial infarction: report of 70 cases with clinicopathologic correlations. J Am Coll Cardiol 22:720, 1993

113. Zehender M, Kasper W, Kauder E, et al: Right ventricular infarction as an independent predictor of prognosis after acute inferior myocardial infarction. N Engl J Med

328:981, 1993

114. Flapan AD: Management of patients after their first myocardial infarction. BMJ 309:1129, 1994

115. Madsen JK, Grande P, Saunamaki K, et al: Danish Multicenter Randomized Study of Invasive Versus Conservative Treatment in Patients with Inducible Ischemia after Thrombolysis in Acute Myocardial Infarction (DANAMI). Danish Trial in Acute Myocardial Infarction. Circulation 96:748, 1997

116. Chaitman BR, McMahon RP, Terin M, et al: Impact of treatment strategy on predischarge exercise test in the Thrombolysis in Myocardial Infarction (TIMI) II trial. Am J Cardiol 71:131, 1993

117. Randomised trial of cholesterol lowering in 4444 patients with coronary heart disease: the Scandinavian Simvastatin Survival Study (4S). Scandinavian Simvastatin Survival Study Group. Lancet 344:1383, 1994

118. Sacks FM, Pfeffer MA, Moye LA, et al: The effect of pravastatin on coronary events after myocardial infarction in patients with average cholesterol levels. N Engl J Med 335:1001, 1996

119. Stenestrand U, Wallentin L: Early statin treatment following acute myocardial infarction and 1-year survival. JAMA 285:430, 2001

120. Effect of long-term oral anticoagulant treatment on mortality and cardiovascular morbidity after myocardial infarction. Anticoagulants in the Secondary Prevention of Events in Coronary Thrombosis (ASPECT) Research Group. Lancet 343:499, 1994

121. Smith P, Arnesen H, Holme I: The effect of warfarin on mortality and reinfarction after myocardial infarction. N Engl J Med 323:147, 1990

122. Meijer A, Verheugt FWA, Wester CPJP, et al: Aspirin versus coumadin in the prevention of reocclusion and recurrent ischemia after successful thrombolysis: a prospective placebo-controlled angiographic study: results of the APRICOT study. Circulation 87:1524, 1993

123. Epstein AE, Hallstrom AP, Rogers WL, et al: Mortality following ventricular arrhythmia suppression by encainide, flecainide, and moricizine after myocardial infarction: the original design concept of the Cardiac Arrhythmia Suppression Trial (CAST). JAMA 270:2451, 1993

124. Tiefenbrunn AJ, Sobel BE: Timing of coronary recanalization: paradigms, paradoxes, and pertinence. Circulation 85:231, 1992

Acknowledgment

Figures 1 through 5, 7 through 9, and 11   Marcia Kammerer.

22 Heart Failure

G. William Dec, M.D., and Adolph M. Hutter, Jr., M.D.

Definition

Heart failure is often defined as the inability of the heart to deliver a supply of oxygenated blood sufficient to meet the metabolic needs of peripheral tissues at normal filling pressures, both at rest and during exercise. It is a clinical syndrome characterized by specific symptoms (e.g., dyspnea, fatigue, and exercise intolerance) and signs (e.g., fluid retention). A decline in contractility resulting from inadequate blood flow (i.e., ischemia), intrinsic factors (as in cardiomyopathy, myocarditis, or scarring from previous myocardial infarction), or circulating extrinsic factors (e.g., endotoxin or inflammatory cytokines) can lead to congestive heart failure in the absence of abnormal volume or pressure overload. In addition, inadequate diastolic relaxation may prevent normal filling of the chamber and lead to heart failure in the presence of normal systolic function. Congestive heart failure is thereby distinguished from other causes of inadequate oxygen delivery, such as (1) circulatory collapse resulting from hemorrhage or other causes of severe volume loss, (2) congestion caused by fluid overload, and (3) high-output failure caused by increased peripheral demands, which occurs in such conditions as thyrotoxicosis, arteriovenous fistula, Paget disease, and anemia.

Clinicians find it useful to describe congestive heart failure as left-sided heart failure, right-sided heart failure, or biventricular failure, depending on whether the left atrial pressure, the right atrial pressure, or both are elevated. Elevation of the left atrial pressure results in symptoms and signs of pulmonary congestion, whereas elevation of the right atrial pressure leads to symptoms and signs of systemic venous hypertension and congestion. Many different disorders can raise atrial pressure and precipitate either type of congestive heart failure [*see Figures 1 and 2*]. Under clinical conditions, the most common cause of right-sided failure is chronic left-sided failure. Heart failure caused by an abnormality in systolic function leading to inadequate ejection of blood is known as systolic failure. Diastolic failure is associated with an impaired ability of the ventricle or ventricles to accept blood at normal filling pressures.

Epidemiology

Heart failure is a major public health problem in the United States, affecting about 4.7 million persons. Approximately 470,000 new cases are diagnosed each year; it is the only major cardiovascular disease that is still increasing in frequency.[1] Despite improvements in treatment, heart failure accounts for nearly 300,000 deaths a year. Heart failure should be considered a disease of the elderly. Approximately 6% to 10% of patients older than 65 years have heart failure; further, 85% of patients hospitalized for heart failure are in this age group. Data from the Framingham Heart Study indicate that hypertension and coronary artery disease are the two most common preexisting conditions.[2] Diabetes mellitus and left ventricular hypertrophy (LVH) are also associated with increased risk of heart failure. The first National Health and Nutrition Examination Survey Epidemiologic Study (NHANES I) also identified the following as independent risk factors for the development of heart failure: male sex (risk ratio [RR], 1.24), physical inactivity (RR, 1.59), overweight (RR, 1.30), valvular heart disease (RR, 1.46), and known coronary artery disease (RR, 8.11).[3] Heart failure may occur as a result of either systolic or diastolic dysfunction (see below). Approximately 40% of all patients hospitalized for symptomatic heart failure have normal or near-normal systolic function. In multivariate models, age greater than 75 years, female sex, and valvular heart disease have been associated with a left ventricular ejection fraction of greater than 50%.[4]

Pathophysiology

A heart with properly functioning valves can adequately accept a returning volume of blood (preload) and eject it forcefully against a peripheral arteriolar resistance (one of the determinants of afterload). The heart can be overloaded either by an increase in the volume of blood it has to eject forward (as in a left-to-right shunt, mitral regurgitation, or aortic regurgitation) or by an increase in the resistance against which it must eject (as in systemic hypertension or aortic stenosis). The proper functioning of the ventricle, a cone-shaped muscular chamber, is critically related to its internal dimensions, wall thickness, state of contractility, and ability to relax in diastole. The coronary arteries must also supply adequate nutrition to meet the demands of the heart muscle both at rest and during exercise.

ADAPTIVE MECHANISMS

The heart must be capable of handling normal variable loads as well as the extraordinary loads that may be imposed by such conditions as diseased valves or impaired myocardial function. Several physiologic mechanisms determine cardiac performance. The most important of these mechanisms are the Frank-Starling relation (related to preload), the state of inotropy (contractility), the tension or stress developed by the ventricle during contraction (afterload), and the heart rate. Heart failure is most frequently the result of a substantial decline in myocardial contractility, resulting from either the permanent loss of functional myocytes with myocardial infarction or impairment in force generation with dilated cardiomyopathy. Severe uncontrolled hypertension or progressive aortic stenosis may cause heart failure through excessive afterload. Acute mitral or aortic regurgitation may produce heart failure as a result of excessive preload, even with normal myocardial contractility.

The heart can compensate for some of the pathophysiologic abnormalities of heart failure by other adaptive mechanisms, including cardiac muscle changes (e.g., myocyte hypertrophy and chamber dilatation) and peripheral mechanisms (e.g., arteriolar and venous constriction, reduced renal blood flow, and expanded intravascular fluid volume). Many of the cardiac and peripheral adaptations are mediated through neural reflexes and neurohormonal activation (see below).

Myocardial Mechanisms

Hypertrophy and dilatation develop in response to chronic overloading of the heart. Chronic pressure overload, as occurs in systemic hypertension or aortic stenosis, induces expression of proto-oncogenes (i.e., *c-fos, c-myc, c-jun*), which results in myocardial hypertrophy. Hypertrophy entails an increase both in the size of individual muscle cells and in the overall muscle mass. This

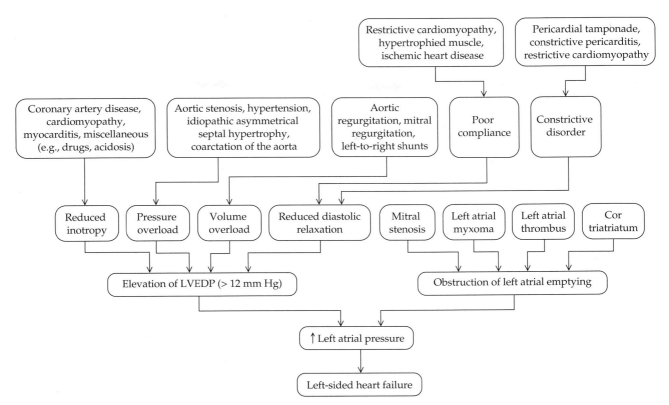

Figure 1 Various pathologic conditions may ultimately cause an increase in the left atrial pressure and thereby precipitate left-sided congestive heart failure. In general, the increased left atrial pressure can be attributed either to mechanical obstructions that interfere with diastolic emptying of the left atrium or to abnormalities that produce an increased left ventricular end-diastolic pressure (LVEDP). Atrial myxomas, thrombi, and valvular stenosis may obstruct blood flow in both the left side and the right side of the heart. Cor triatriatum, which affects only the left side of the heart, is a congenital defect in which an abnormal diaphragm divides the left atrium into two chambers, impeding inflow from the pulmonary veins.

response helps the heart overcome pressure overload, but it has its limitations because a hypertrophied muscle operates at a lower inotropic state than does a normal muscle.[5] Furthermore, hypertrophy is associated with structural and biochemical changes, such as apoptosis, which may have deleterious effects in the long term.

Volume overload (e.g., aortic regurgitation or mitral regurgitation) causes the left ventricle to dilate. Within limits, this response effects a compensatory increase in cardiac output by the Frank-Starling mechanism [*see Figure 3*]. Dilatation in the absence of a volume overload is an indication of ventricular failure.

Peripheral Mechanisms

Arteriolar and venous constriction occur in heart failure. Arteriolar constriction serves to maintain blood pressure despite a reduced cardiac output. An increase in sympathetic nervous system activity is a major factor responsible for arteriolar constriction. Blood flow is redistributed, so that the blood supply to the kidneys, skin, splanchnic organs, and skeletal muscle is reduced. However, blood flow is maintained to the brain and heart, which have few alpha-adrenergic receptors and high metabolic rates and produce a greater amount of vasodilating metabolites. An increase in the activity of the renin-angiotensin-aldosterone system also increases systemic vascular resistance. Plasma concentrations of endothelins, a family of potent vasoconstrictor peptides originating in the vascular endothelium, are elevated, and acetylcholine-mediated, endothelium-dependent vasodilatation appears to be impaired in the peripheral vasculature of patients with heart failure. Increased venous tone tends to cause blood to

shift from the peripheral pool to the central circulation, enhancing ventricular filling and helping maintain cardiac output by the Frank-Starling mechanism.

A combination of decreased cardiac output and renal vasoconstriction lowers renal blood flow. Consequently, proximal tubular reabsorption of sodium and water is enhanced, increasing the intravascular volume and elevating cardiac output by the Frank-Starling mechanism. Other factors also enhance the renal retention of sodium and water. Increased activation of the renin-angiotensin-aldosterone system causes the aldosterone level to increase, which plays an important role in sodium and water retention.

All of these peripheral mechanisms are effective in compensating for hypovolemic states, such as that produced by acute blood loss, but these responses can contribute to a vicious circle in chronic heart failure. Fluid retention, increased return of volume to the heart by the enhanced venous tone, and increased afterload all impose additional work on the failing myocardium and can further decrease cardiac output. Interruption of this vicious circle is the rationale for the use of vasodilators, agents such as angiotensin-converting enzyme (ACE) inhibitors, and even digitalis and beta blockers, all of which decrease the activity of the sympathetic nervous system and the renin-angiotensin system [*see* Treatment Goals for Left-Sided and Right-Sided Congestive Heart Failure, *below*].

Neurohumoral Activation

Heart failure is often a progressive process, even in the ab-

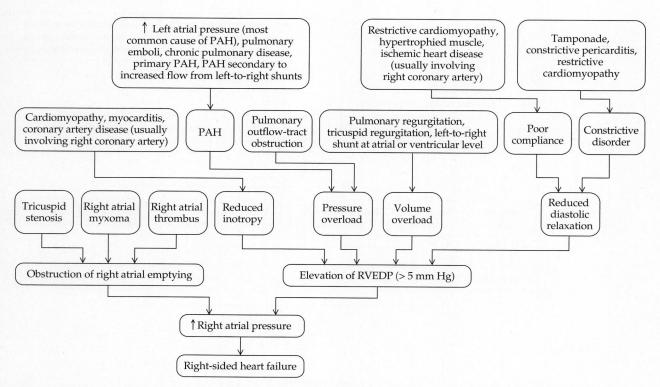

Figure 2   **Various pathways may lead to an increase in the right atrial pressure and consequently provoke right-sided congestive heart failure. The increased right atrial pressure can be induced either by mechanisms that cause an increase in the right ventricular end-diastolic pressure (RVEDP) or by lesions that obstruct blood flow from the right atrium. The most common cause of right ventricular failure and the resultant rise in right atrial pressure is left ventricular failure, which produces an increase in left atrial pressure. This increased left atrial pressure in turn leads to pulmonary artery hypertension (PAH), which imposes a pressure overload on the right ventricle and may trigger right ventricular failure.**

sence of any new identifiable insults to the myocardium. The principal manifestation of this progression is a geometric change in the left ventricle as the chamber dilates, hypertrophies, and becomes more spherical. Cardiac imaging studies have demonstrated that at least 40% of patients will develop a degree of left ventricular dilatation during the first 12 months after myocardial infarction.[6] Likewise, patients with chronic systolic dysfunction typically experience a slow increase in left ventricular end-diastolic dimensions and a decline in ejection fraction.[7] The more spherically shaped left ventricle has higher myocardial wall stress and increased atrioventricular (AV) regurgitation, which lead to further impairment in forward stroke volume. This process is referred to as cardiac remodeling. Although many mechanisms play a part, there is substantial evidence that activation of endogenous neurohormonal systems plays a pivotal role in cardiac remodeling and, as a consequence, heart failure progression [*see Table 1*]. Sympathetic nervous system activation, as reflected by elevated plasma norepinephrine concentrations, occurs early, before activation of the renin-angiotensin-aldosterone axis. Early in congestive heart failure, levels of the potent vasoconstrictors vasopressin and endothelin increase. Levels of counterregulatory vasodilator prostaglandins and both atrial natriuretic peptide (ANP) and brain natriuretic peptide (BNP) also increase; this results in the partial inhibition of the effects of epinephrine, angiotensin II, and endothelin. Often, the first of the circulating neurohormones to be elevated is ANP; elevation of ANP often occurs in patients after myocardial infarction or in patients with asymptomatic left ventricular dysfunction.[8] ANP di-

rectly affects the kidneys by increasing the glomerular filtration rate (GFR); this leads to pronounced natriuresis and diuresis. ANP also suppresses aldosterone secretion and vasopressin release and lowers elevated plasma renin levels. Tumor necrosis factor (TNF) is also synthesized by the heart in response to hemodynamic stress.[9] TNF has been shown to exert cardiodepressant and cardiotoxic effects in experimental heart failure models. Although hemodynamic abnormalities typically correlate with symptoms, disease progression is most closely associated with the extent of neurohormonal activation.

ASSESSMENT OF PRESSURE-VOLUME RELATIONSHIPS

Ejection Fraction

Clinically, decreased inotropy (as seen in ischemia or cardiomyopathy), increased afterload (as seen in aortic stenosis or hypertension), or asynergy of left ventricular contraction (as seen in left ventricular aneurysm) can reduce the ejection fraction. The ejection fraction can be measured by angiographic techniques, radioisotope imaging, or echocardiography. Although helpful in predicting long-term prognosis, ejection fraction correlates poorly with heart failure symptoms, functional capacity, or response to medical treatment.

End-Diastolic Volume and Pressure

End-diastolic volume (EDV), normally 70 ml/m² body surface area, is increased in a failing heart. This increase reflects not only the inability of the heart to empty adequately in sys-

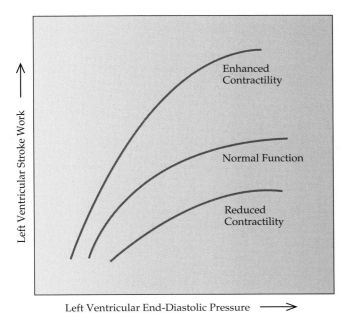

Figure 3 The Frank-Starling relation holds that an increase in the length of resting ventricular muscle fibers (reflected in an increased left ventricular end-diastolic pressure) is associated with an increase in the left ventricular stroke work. The three curves depict the Frank-Starling relation for three different states of myocardial inotropy: normal, enhanced, and reduced. In states of enhanced inotropy, such as may be produced by sympathetic stimulation, a relatively higher stroke output can be achieved for any given left ventricular filling pressure. Conversely, when inotropy is reduced, as in the failing heart, a lower stroke output is achieved relative to any given left ventricular filling pressure.

tole but also the operation of the Frank-Starling mechanism. Because an increase in EDV is often associated with an increase in end-diastolic pressure (EDP), the latter value can be used as an indicator of ventricular function. EDP is influenced not only by left ventricular volume but also by ventricular compliance. The relation between left ventricular pressure and volume at various stages of contraction and relaxation in a normal heart can be expressed by a pressure-volume loop [*see Figure 4*]. An increase in blood pressure in the absence of volume changes increases systolic stress [*see Figure 4b, loop B*]. Similarly, an increase in ventricular volume that is not accompanied by an elevation in blood pressure also increases systolic stress [*see Figure 4b, loop C*]; this phenomenon represents the inability of a poorly contracting left ventricle to eject its volume and characterizes systolic dysfunction. An increase in the EDP that is not associated with an increase in the EDV indicates the presence of a poorly compliant left ventricle with impaired diastolic relaxation; this condition is termed diastolic dysfunction or failure [*see Figure 4c, loop D*]. Pressure-volume loop analysis is currently used as a research tool in assessing the inotropic or vasodilatory properties of new therapies for heart failure.

Cardiac Output

Cardiac output is the product of stroke volume and heart rate. A patient with moderate left ventricular dysfunction may have a normal resting cardiac output but be unable to increase cardiac output appropriately in response to exercise (fixed cardiac output). More severe heart failure is associated with reduced cardiac output at rest. In patients with low cardiac output, enhanced ex-

traction of oxygen by peripheral tissues lowers the oxygen content of venous blood. This condition produces an increase in the difference between the oxygen content of arterial and venous blood. Thus, the arteriovenous oxygen difference provides a semiquantitative method to assess the extent of impairment of cardiac output.

Causes of Congestive Heart Failure

Various pathologic conditions elevate the atrial pressure by more than one mechanism [*see Figures 1 and 2*]. For example, aortic stenosis imposes a pressure overload on the left ventricle that initially causes reduced ventricular compliance as the myocardium hypertrophies. Later, as the myocardium fails, inotropy is depressed. Coronary artery disease is the most common cause of congestive heart failure. Acute myocardial infarction impairs ventricular contractility and reduces compliance. Ischemic papillary muscle dysfunction with resultant mitral regurgitation may also produce volume overload. Abnormal ventricular remodeling caused by thinning of the infarct zone and impaired contractility in surrounding, noninfarcted zones of myocardium leads to progressive left ventricular dilatation. This remodeling process may occur within the first 2 weeks after an acute myocardial infarction or after many months or even years. Early ventricular remodeling or infarct expansion results from the degradation of the intermyocyte collagen struts by serine protease and from the activation of matrix metalloproteinases by neutrophils.[10] Several factors account for late remodeling, including eccentric left ventricular hypertrophy, subsequent ischemic events, increased wall stress, apoptosis, and elevations in the levels of circulating vasoconstrictors, such as angiotensin II, endothelin 1, and norepinephrine. Left ventricular remodeling is particularly common after extensive transmural anterior infarctions, especially when associated with an occluded infarct-related artery.[11]

Predictors of Survival

Annual mortality for patients with congestive heart failure caused by impaired systolic function is less than 5% for asymptomatic left ventricular dysfunction (left ventricular ejection fraction [LVEF] < 45%), 10% to 20% for mild to moderate symptoms (New York Heart Association [NYHA] class II or III [*see Table 2*]), and often exceeds 40% for patients with advanced NYHA class IV symptoms. Clinical, hemodynamic, and ventriculographic features are useful in predicting mortality in patients with congestive heart failure. Prognosis most closely relates to the extent of impairment in ejection fraction, the degree of ventricular dilatation, and the decrease in left ventricular sphericity.[12] Clinical features that are associated with more favorable prognosis include NYHA class I to class III symptoms, younger age, and female sex. Syncope, a persistent third heart sound (RR, 1.35; 95% confidence interval [CI], 1.17 to 1.55), signs of chronic right-sided heart failure (RR, 1.52; 95% CI, 1.27 to 1.82), extensive conduction system disease, and ventricular tachyarrhythmias portend a poor prognosis.[13] Progressive heart failure accounts for the majority of deaths. Sudden cardiac death caused by ventricular tachycardia, fibrillation, bradycardia, or electromechanical dissociation occurs in 20% to 40% of patients with congestive heart failure. Multivariable proportional-hazards survival models have been validated to predict prognosis in advanced (NYHA class III and IV) heart failure. A heart failure survival score has been developed that considers seven variables: disease etiology, resting heart rate,

Table 1 Factors That Increase Neurohormonal/Cytokine
Activation and the Consequences of Activation

Neurohormone	Activation Factor	Consequence
Renin/angiotensin II	Renal hypoperfusion Sodium depletion SNS activity	Arterial vasoconstriction Aldosterone secretion Renal efferent vasoconstriction Increased plasma norepinephrine secretion Enhanced SNS activation Vascular hypertrophy Myocardial hypertrophy
Plasma norepinephrine	Decline in blood pressure Decreased circulating volume Baroreceptor control	Arterial vasoconstriction Myocardial apoptosis
Endothelin 1	Angiotensin II Hypoxemia Thrombin Endotoxin Vasopressin	Arterial vasoconstriction Bronchoconstriction Mitogenic effects on vascular smooth muscle and myocardium Increased renal artery resistance
Atrial natriuretic peptide	Increased right atrial stretch Increased preload	Positive inotropic effect Natriuresis Vasodilatation
Brain natriuretic peptide	Ventricular stretch	Natriuresis Vasodilatation
Tumor necrosis factor	Increased preload Increased wall stretch	Impaired contractility Cachexia

SNS—sympathetic nervous system

LVEF, QRS duration greater than 0.12 msec, mean resting blood pressure, peak oxygen uptake on exercise testing, and serum sodium level.[14] In one study, for the one third of the patients with congestive heart failure at lowest risk, odds of an adverse outcome at 1 year were five times and 21 times less than for patients at medium risk and high risk, respectively.[15] Predictive models have not been developed for patients with mild or moderate heart failure.

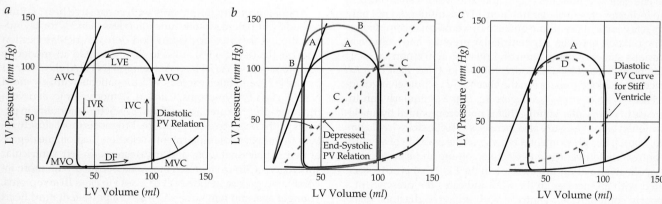

Figure 4 **Pressure-volume (PV) loops depict the relative changes in left ventricular (LV) pressure and volume that develop during the cardiac cycle for a normal heart (*a*), for a heart subjected to systolic stress or dysfunction (*b*), and for a heart exhibiting diastolic failure (*c*). During the normal cardiac cycle, as the mitral valve closes (MVC), isovolemic contraction (IVC) occurs, and the pressure rises until the aortic valve opens (AVO). Left ventricular ejection (LVE) then ensues, accompanied by a further increase in ventricular pressure as the left ventricular volume falls. After ejection, the ventricular pressure starts to fall; when the aortic valve closes (AVC), isovolemic relaxation (IVR) takes place, with a marked drop in left ventricular pressure. When the mitral valve opens (MVO), diastolic filling (DF) occurs, and volume increases with little change in pressure. The end-diastolic volume and end-diastolic pressure occur just before systole and the closing of the mitral valve. The point at the end of diastole represents the end-diastolic pressure-volume relation, and the point of aortic valve closure represents the end-systolic pressure-volume relation. Disturbances in the pressure-volume relation can be compared with the normal pressure-volume loop (loop A) in panels *b* and *c*. In panel *b*, systolic stress is indicated by a rise in ventricular pressure that is not accompanied by a parallel change in volume (loop B). When ventricular volume increases in the absence of an increase in pressure (loop C in panel *b*), systolic dysfunction or failure is present. This condition is indicated by a depression of the end-systolic pressure-volume relation. In panel *c*, diastolic failure caused by a stiff left ventricle is indicated by an elevation of the end-diastolic pressure without a concomitant increase in the end-diastolic volume (loop D).**

Table 2 New York Heart Association Functional Classification of Cardiovascular Disability

Class	Characteristics
I	Patients with cardiac disease without resulting limitations of physical activity
II	Patients with cardiac disease resulting in slight limitation of physical activity; they are comfortable at rest; ordinary physical activity causes fatigue, palpitations, dyspnea, or anginal pain
III	Patients with cardiac disease resulting in marked limitation of physical activity; they are comfortable at rest; less than ordinary physical activity causes fatigue, palpitations, dyspnea, or anginal pain
IV	Patients with cardiac disease resulting in inability to carry on any physical activity without discomfort; symptoms may be present even at rest; if any physical activity is undertaken, discomfort is increased

Diagnostic Evaluation

LEFT-SIDED CONGESTIVE HEART FAILURE

Clinical Manifestations

Dyspnea Dyspnea is one of the earliest subjective symptoms of left-sided heart failure that are intimately related to increased interstitial lung edema; such edema decreases lung compliance and thereby increases the work necessary to breathe. Dyspnea is also related to abnormalities of respiratory muscle function. Dyspnea initially occurs on exertion, and the physician can quantitate its severity by asking the patient how many flights of stairs he or she can climb or how far he or she can walk on level ground at a normal pace before the onset of dyspnea. Dyspnea can result from pulmonary and peripheral mechanisms related to low cardiac output and may be associated with weakness, easy fatigability, and weight loss, which are clinical manifestations of the low cardiac output syndrome [*see* Low Cardiac Output Syndrome, *below*]. Dyspnea can also result from excessive obesity and poor physical fitness, both of which can usually be easily identified. It is sometimes more difficult to rule out chronic lung disease as a cause of dyspnea, especially because chronic lung disease and congestive heart failure frequently coexist. Dyspnea that is associated with light-headedness, tingling of the fingers or lips, and manifestations of anxiety suggests the diagnosis of hyperventilation syndrome. The sensitivity and specificity of dyspnea in diagnosing heart failure have been reported at 66% and 52%, respectively.[16]

Orthopnea Orthopnea refers to recumbent dyspnea. A patient with this disorder finds it necessary to sleep with the head and thorax elevated. Its physiologic basis is increased venous return to the heart in the recumbent position, which is poorly handled by a failing left ventricle.

Orthopnea is not specific to congestive heart failure. Patients with chronic obstructive pulmonary disease also find it easier to breathe with the head and thorax elevated; the abdominal organs are thereby lowered relative to the thoracic cavity, reducing their interference with diaphragmatic movement. For the same reason, obese persons and patients receiving peritoneal dialysis often breathe better when sleeping in a bed that is tilted so that the head is higher than the feet. Some patients may complain of a dry, nonproductive cough that develops when they are in the supine position and that is relieved by sitting up. This orthopneic cough, which often occurs a few hours after the patient lies down, is a clue to the presence of pulmonary alveolar edema. The reported sensitivity and specificity of orthopnea for diagnosing heart failure are 21% and 81%, respectively.[16]

Nocturnal angina Nocturnal angina in a patient with ischemic heart disease can be a clue to early left-sided heart failure. The failing left ventricle responds to increased venous return in the supine position with an increase in left ventricular end-diastolic pressure (LVEDP), causing enhanced oxygen consumption and angina pectoris.

Paroxysmal nocturnal dyspnea Paroxysmal nocturnal dyspnea is characterized by sudden attacks of shortness of breath that occur after a few hours of sleep. Patients often obtain relief by sitting up, opening a window to get some air, or walking around. Paroxysmal nocturnal dyspnea caused by pulmonary congestion must be differentiated from hyperventilation in an anxious person or paroxysmal nocturnal wheezing that develops in a supine patient with chronic bronchitis in response to increased accumulation of bronchial secretions. Its sensitivity and specificity have been reported at 33% and 76%, respectively.[16]

In some patients, bronchospasm may develop because of pulmonary congestion and may manifest as cardiac asthma with wheezing. Bronchial hyperresponsiveness to cholinergic stimuli has been documented in patients with congestive heart failure and may result from vasodilatation of blood vessels in the small airways caused by high left ventricular filling pressure. Cardiac asthma may occur only on exertion, paroxysmally at night, or as the earliest manifestation of pulmonary edema. In general, a chest x-ray is most helpful in the differential diagnosis of wheezing that occurs at rest; if the cause of the wheezing is pulmonary congestion, that will usually be evident on the chest film.

Physical Signs

It should be noted that the sensitivity of clinical assessment in identifying systolic dysfunction is approximately 81%, and the specificity is 47%.[17] The most prominent physical finding in acute left-sided heart failure is moist rales in the lungs, which is indicative of interstitial edema. The rales may be confined to the lung bases in mild forms, or they may be heard throughout the lung fields in acute pulmonary edema. Wheezing may occur with or without rales. Rales are typically absent in chronic congestive heart failure despite elevated pulmonary arterial wedge pressures because of enhanced lymphatic drainage of the lung interstitium. Although pulmonary rales usually cannot of themselves lead to a correct diagnosis, the diagnosis can be made through a combination of symptoms, physical findings, chest x-ray findings, and the electrocardiographic findings.[17] Tachypnea and an accentuation of the pulmonary component of the second heart sound are early and subtle indications of interstitial edema and pulmonary venous congestion.

Cardiac examination may indicate the presence of aortic or mitral valve abnormalities. Mitral regurgitation resulting from annular dilatation is commonly audible. This regurgitant murmur is generally no louder than grade II to grade III in intensity and waxes and wanes, depending on the extent of left ventricular dilatation. Murmurs of greater intensity should suggest intrinsic rather than functional valvular disease.

In the absence of valvular heart disease, the major indicators of left ventricular systolic dysfunction are an S_3 gallop and paradoxical splitting of the second heart sound, caused by either left bundle branch block or reversal of A_2 and P_2 as a result of prolonged ejection of blood by the impaired left ventricle. A presystolic, or S_4, gallop indicates reduced compliance of the left ventricle but not a failing left ventricle per se. Enlargement of the left ventricle can be detected by palpation and percussion. Percussion dullness in the fifth left intercostal space is useful for detecting increased left ventricular end-diastolic volume (LVEDV); a distance greater than 10.5 cm can identify increased LVEDV, with a sensitivity of 91% and a specificity of 30%.[18] In the 50% of patients in whom an impulse can be palpated, an apical impulse of more than 3 cm in the left lateral decubitus position can detect increased left ventricular volume or mass with a sensitivity of 100% and a specificity of 40%.[18] Pulsus alternans, characterized by alternating weaker and stronger pulsations in the peripheral arteries, indicates a diseased left ventricle with poor systolic function.

Electrocardiographic Findings

The electrocardiogram is usually abnormal but most often shows nonspecific repolarization abnormalities. Left atrial enlargement is frequently evident and correlates well with increased left atrial pressure, even in the acute phase. Conduction defects, particularly left bundle branch block, atrial arrhythmias, and ventricular ectopic activity, are common in patients with left ventricular dilatation. Atrial fibrillation occurs in 10% to 15% of patients with heart failure and is associated with an increased risk of all-cause mortality.[19] The presence of QS waves is useful in differentiating ischemic heart disease from primary cardiomyopathy.

Radiographic Signs

The earliest radiographic sign of pulmonary congestion is pulmonary venous hypertension, manifested as distention of the pulmonary veins of the upper lobe in an upright chest film. This finding, which is most easily observed on the right side of the upper hilum, helps distinguish pulmonary edema of cardiac etiology from that of noncardiac etiology.

Interstitial pulmonary edema appears on an x-ray as septal edema, perivascular edema, or subpleural edema.

Alveolar edema usually produces large homogeneous densities in the lung field but may instead produce smaller patchy densities, a pattern that simulates the radiographic picture of bronchopneumonia. The edema frequently exhibits a central distribution pattern, and the radiograph displays a butterfly or bat-wing appearance. The distribution pattern may be symmetrical or asymmetrical and may be bilateral or unilateral.

The chest x-ray pattern of pulmonary venous, interstitial, or alveolar congestion does not always correlate closely with the pulmonary arterial wedge pressure. In chronic heart failure, lymphatic drainage is enhanced, and the chest x-ray often appears clear despite high filling pressures. Further, the radiographic pattern of pulmonary congestion can persist for 1 to 4 days after the wedge pressure has been restored to normal by vigorous diuresis. Patients with chronic lung disease and interstitial fibrosis may show little evidence of pulmonary congestion on chest x-ray, even when the wedge pressure increase has been prolonged.

RIGHT-SIDED HEART FAILURE

Clinical Manifestations

Systemic venous congestion The hallmark of right ventricular failure is systemic venous congestion, which is best appreciated by examination of the neck veins. The upper limit of the fluid column is often more easily seen in the superficial neck veins, but the extent of elevation is more accurately represented in the internal jugular veins, especially the right internal jugular vein. Jugular venous pressure is most accurately described by the number of centimeters that the venous column is elevated above the right atrium. A normal jugular venous pressure is between 5 and 8 cm.

With inspiration, the intrathoracic negative pressure increases, venous return to the chest is increased, and the jugular venous pressure falls if the right ventricle is capable of propelling the increased venous return into the lungs. However, in right ventricular failure, constrictive pericarditis, or tricuspid stenosis, increased venous return cannot be accommodated by the compromised right ventricle; thus, a rise, rather than the normal fall, in jugular venous pressure occurs with inspiration (a positive Kussmaul sign). This sign is a subtle indicator of right ventricular dysfunction and may be seen even in the presence of normal jugular venous pressure.

Pressing on the liver while the patient is breathing normally (and not straining) may distend the neck veins (hepatojugular reflux) as a result of the increased venous return to the chest, indicating right ventricular dysfunction.

Organ involvement The liver is usually the first organ to become engorged with blood during right-sided heart failure. If the engorgement is relatively rapid, right upper quadrant pain and tenderness may be noted as the liver distends against its capsule. Hepatic congestion is more often symptomatic in younger patients. When chronic congestion is present, the results of liver function tests may be abnormal, and the alkaline phosphatase and bilirubin levels may be mildly elevated. In acute liver congestion associated with hypoxia, hepatocellular damage may result in an increase in the aspartate aminotransferase level. In patients with more severe and chronic systemic venous congestion, the prothrombin time may be prolonged. In rare instances, acute hepatic decompensation can occur, with frank hepatic coma. This unusual manifestation ordinarily requires a concurrent combination of passive congestion, arterial hypoxia, and decreased hepatic arterial perfusion, such as can occur in severe pulmonary edema with hypoxia and hypotension.

The spleen also may be enlarged and palpable, but this manifestation is uncommon and is almost always associated with hepatomegaly. Splanchnic congestion in right-sided heart failure can lead to nausea, diarrhea, and malabsorption. On rare occasions, a protein-losing enteropathy can occur. This disorder is more common in patients with severe constant systemic venous congestion caused by tricuspid stenosis or constrictive pericarditis than in those with severe congestion caused by other lesions, such as tricuspid regurgitation. Splanchnic congestion and bowel edema can lead to inadequate absorption of oral medications, particularly diuretics, and further exacerbate volume overload. Ascites is a late manifestation of congestive heart failure; again, it appears more frequently in patients in whom congestion is caused by tricuspid stenosis, constrictive pericarditis, or a restrictive cardiomyopathy.

Table 3 Useful Clinical Findings for the Detection of Increased Filling Pressures in Heart Failure[15]

Usefulness	Key Findings
Very helpful	Jugular venous distention Pulmonary venous redistribution on chest film
Somewhat helpful	Dyspnea, orthopnea Tachycardia, low blood pressure S₃ gallop, pulmonary rales Hepatojugular reflux Cardiomegaly on chest film
Helpful	Edema

Edema Dependent edema is very common and is one of the early manifestations of right-sided congestive heart failure. Pitting edema appears in the dependent portions of the body. Edema results from a combination of passive venous congestion and salt and water retention. The latter condition is related to increased aldosterone levels and decreased excretion of sodium by the kidneys. Ankle edema caused by right-sided heart congestion must be differentiated from ankle edema caused by local venous or lymphatic obstruction, cirrhosis, or hypoalbuminemia. Detection of jugular venous distention, which is not a feature of the last three causes of edema listed, permits easy determination of right-sided heart failure.

ACCURACY OF CLINICAL ASSESSMENT IN DIAGNOSING HEART FAILURE

Although clinicians routinely assess left- and right-sided filling pressures, isolated clinical findings have limited reliability in diagnosing heart failure. Clinical examination alone has a reported sensitivity of 54% and a specificity of 60% for detecting elevated filling pressures.[15] A variety of symptoms, physical findings, and x-ray abnormalities may suggest the diagnosis [*see Table 3*].

Pulmonary venous redistribution, as seen on chest film, and the presence of jugular venous distention are most accurate. Somewhat useful findings include dyspnea, orthopnea, tachycardia, an S₃ gallop, pulmonary rales, and cardiomegaly.[15] The number of findings may predict low, intermediate, and high probability of elevated filling pressures [*see Figure 5*]. In patients without known systolic dysfunction, those with no more than one abnormal finding are likely to have normal filling pressures; those with at least three abnormal findings are highly likely (> 90%) to have elevated filling pressures. When systolic dysfunction is known to exist, patients with even one abnormal clinical finding are likely to have elevated filling pressures.[15]

LOW CARDIAC OUTPUT SYNDROME

Exercise intolerance, usually manifested as dyspnea and fatigue, is caused by a combination of cardiac, pulmonary, peripheral vascular, and skeletal muscle abnormalities. The clinical syndrome of low cardiac output is often seen in conjunction with either left-sided or right-sided congestive heart failure. The hallmarks of low cardiac output are fatigue and loss of lean muscle weight, often resulting in cardiac cachexia. High circulating levels of TNF are typical in patients with this syndrome and predict a poor prognosis.[20] Decreased cerebral blood flow may produce lethargy, light-headedness, and confusion. Reduced kidney perfusion may lead to prerenal azotemia, which is characterized by a disproportionate rise in blood urea nitrogen (BUN) relative to serum creatinine, and oliguria.

NEW-ONSET HEART FAILURE

All patients presenting with heart failure should undergo diagnostic evaluation that (1) determines the type of cardiac dysfunction (systolic versus diastolic), (2) uncovers correctable etiologic factors, (3) defines prognosis, and (4) guides therapy.

Differentiating Systolic from Diastolic Heart Failure

Transthoracic two-dimensional echocardiography is the ini-

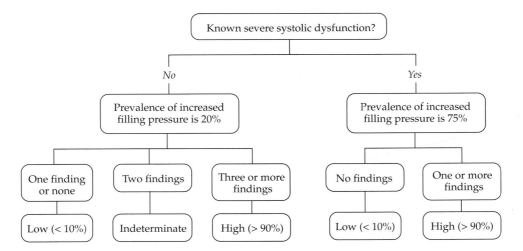

Figure 5 Shown is an algorithm for determining the likelihood of increased left ventricular filling pressure using the known prevalence of elevated filling pressures in two populations. Findings include symptoms (dyspnea, orthopnea), physical findings (tachycardia, low systolic pressure, S₃ gallop, jugular venous distention, pulmonary rales, and hepatojugular reflux), and x-ray abnormalities (cardiomegaly and pulmonary venous redistribution). In patients without known systolic dysfunction, a single finding is seldom sufficient to make a diagnosis of left-sided heart failure. Conversely, when there is a high probability of heart failure, a single abnormal clinical finding can provide a high degree of certainty with regard to an elevation in left ventricular filling pressure.[15]

Table 4　Reversible Causes of Acute Left Ventricular Dysfunction

Active myocardial ischemia
Myocardial hibernation after an acute infarction
Aortic stenosis
Mitral regurgitation
Acute dilated cardiomyopathies
　Peripartum cardiomyopathy
　Idiopathic
　Toxic
　　Alcohol
　　Cobalt
　　Carbon monoxide
　　Cocaine
　Drug-induced
　　Antiretroviral agents
　　Doxorubicin (acute response)
　　Interferon
　Myocarditis
　　Lymphocytic
　　Giant cell
　　Eosinophilic (drug-induced or idiopathic)
Uncontrolled supraventricular tachycardia
Sepsis-associated myocardial depression
Myocardial depression after cardiopulmonary bypass
　(postcardiotomy syndrome)

---

tial diagnostic procedure of choice; it remains the only reliable method of differentiating systolic from diastolic dysfunction in a patient with signs and symptoms of heart failure. Echocardiography provides useful information on left ventricular mass, chamber dimension, and valvular disease (e.g., unsuspected aortic stenosis or severe mitral regurgitation). Segmental wall motion abnormalities or visible myocardial scar, if identified, should suggest underlying ischemic heart disease.[21]

Identifying Reversible Causes of Heart Failure

Every effort should be made to identify and correct reversible causes of heart failure [see Table 4]. Patients should be queried about a history of hypertension, diabetes, hypercholesterolemia, valvular or peripheral heart disease, rheumatic heart disease, chest irradiation, or exposure to cardiotoxic drugs such as anthracyclines. A quantitative alcohol history should be obtained, and the patient should be questioned regarding the use of cocaine. A detailed family history should be obtained to exclude the possibility of a familial cardiomyopathy. Recent guidelines have suggested that initial testing include a chest x-ray; electrocardiography; complete blood count; assessment of serum electrolyte levels, creatinine level, and calcium level; liver function studies; and urinalysis.[21] Thyroid function should be measured (especially thyroid-stimulating hormone levels) in all patients older than 65 years who lack a heart failure etiology and in those patients with atrial fibrillation or other signs or symptoms of possible hypothyroidism or hyperthyroidism. Measurement of serum creatine kinase is often useful in evaluating the possibility of myocarditis, ischemic insult, or the concomitant presence of skeletal myopathy. Serum ferritin and transferrin saturation may be useful in selected cases or when hemochromatosis is suspected (e.g., abnormal skin color or the presence of diabetes). Titers for coxsackievirus and other viruses are frequently measured in patients with heart failure of recent onset, but the yield of such testing is low, and the therapeutic implications of a positive re-

sult are uncertain; hence, such testing cannot be recommended. Tests for connective tissue diseases (i.e., assays for antinuclear antibody and rheumatoid factor and measurement of the erythrocyte sedimentation rate) and pheochromocytoma should be performed only if such a diagnosis is clinically suspected.

CORONARY ARTERY DISEASE

Coronary artery disease results in approximately two thirds of cases of heart failure caused by systolic dysfunction. It is frequently useful to determine whether coronary artery disease is present in patients presenting with this syndrome; if it is present, the anatomic severity and functional significance of the coronary artery disease should be determined. Assessment of coronary artery disease should be considered in three types of patients: (1) those with known coronary artery disease and symptomatic angina pectoris; (2) those with known coronary artery disease without angina pectoris; and (3) those in whom the possibility of coronary artery disease has not yet been evaluated.

Patients with Heart Failure and Angina Pectoris

Observational studies support the role of coronary revascularization in patients with heart failure and angina pectoris. Coronary artery bypass surgery was shown to improve symptoms and survival in such patients, although patients with symptoms of severe heart failure or marked reduction in LVEF (< 30%) were not included in these series.[21] Because revascularization is recommended in the vast majority of these patients, most clinicians would proceed directly to coronary angiography rather than perform noninvasive cardiac imaging. Localization of regional ischemia by stress perfusion studies can be a helpful adjunct to angiography to ensure that operable vessels supply viable but ischemic myocardium.

Patients with Heart Failure and Known Coronary Disease but without Angina

No controlled trials have been performed to investigate whether coronary revascularization can improve clinical outcomes in patients with heart failure who do not have angina. However, many observational studies have shown that complete revascularization can favorably affect left ventricular function in many patients with impaired, yet viable, myocardium.[21] Noninvasive testing to determine the presence and quantify the degree of myocardial ischemia and viability in these patients should be undertaken. Stress or dobutamine echocardiography appears to have the highest degree of sensitivity and specificity in detecting viable myocardium (> 80%). Exercise testing with technetium-99m sestamibi imaging or positron emission tomography may also be performed to assess viability. Coronary angiography should be reserved for patients who have large areas of noninfarcted but hypoperfused and hypocontractile myocardium.

Patients without Chest Pain or Known Coronary Artery Disease

No clear guidelines exist for the evaluation of heart failure patients who do not have chest pain and do not have a history of coronary artery disease. Although many physicians perform noninvasive testing before coronary angiography, perfusion deficits and segmental wall motion abnormalities suggestive of coronary artery disease are commonly present in patients with nonischemic cardiomyopathy. We recommend proceeding directly to coronary angiography for any patient who has chest pain, has electrocardiographic abnormalities that suggest ischemia or previous infarction, or is older than 40 years and has one or more known coronary risk factors. If multivessel coronary artery disease is demonstrated, a noninvasive study to assess myocardial viability should then be undertaken before making a recommendation regarding the role of coronary revascularization.

Prognosis

For most patients, measurement of functional capacity has provided the most useful prognostic information. In patients with absent or mild (NYHA class II or II) symptoms of heart failure, survival estimates can be refined by measurement of LVEF. The utility of this variable diminishes greatly when its value declines below 25%.[21] Left ventricular size, as assessed by the cardiothoracic ratio on chest film or end-diastolic dimension on echocardiography, provides additional prognostic information. For patients with more advanced disease (NYHA class III or IV), serum sodium concentration and renal function provide additional prognostic information. Although elevated circulating levels of neurohormonal factors and cytokines have been associated with heart failure severity and mortality, the routine assessment of serum norepinephrine, endothelin 1, and natriuretic peptides is not currently recommended, because the amount of incremental information provided by these tests is too small to justify their expense.[21] Similarly, routine use of Holter monitoring or signal-averaged ECG has not been shown to provide incremental value in assessing prognosis or guiding treatment.[21]

Treatment

TREATMENT GOALS FOR LEFT-SIDED AND RIGHT-SIDED CONGESTIVE HEART FAILURE

Treatment goals include improvement in symptoms, increased functional capacity, prevention or partial amelioration of left ventricular dilatation, and improved survival.[22] Although never prospectively validated, several general measures are advisable for most patients with heart failure, because these measures are not harmful and may improve functional capacity. Obese patients should lose weight, and smokers should discontinue tobacco use; low-level aerobic physical activity should be encouraged. Every effort should be made to identify and correct reversible causes of heart failure. A cardiac pacemaker may benefit patients who demonstrate inappropriate sinus bradycardia or AV block. Atrial or AV pacing is usually preferred in heart failure patients because preservation of atrial contraction contributes to cardiac output. A reasonable initial rate is 70 beats/min. If a rapid supraventricular tachycardia such as atrial fibrillation is present, cardioversion to normal sinus rhythm or at least slowing of the ventricular response at rest and during exercise with an appropriate drug (e.g., a beta blocker or digitalis) can alleviate heart failure symptoms.

Specific therapy should be given for anemia, thyrotoxicosis, and other causes of high cardiac output failure. Systemic hypertension should be treated, and surgical correction of significant valvular or congenital cardiac lesions should be weighed. Withdrawal of any cardiac depressants, such as alcohol or disopyramide, should also be considered.

Heart failure that persists after correction of reversible causes is treated with salt restriction, diuretics, digitalis, vasodilators (particularly ACE inhibitors), beta-adrenergic blockers, spironolac-

tone, or combinations of these measures. The overall aim of therapy is to improve the patient's quality of life, using a program that can reasonably be followed at home and at work. Salt restriction is important, but since the advent of potent diuretics, marked salt restriction is necessary only in the most severe cases of congestive heart failure. Most patients have difficulty restricting salt intake to less than 4 or 5 g/day (a no-added-salt diet) at home.

When heart failure is complicated by poor renal perfusion, one must strike a proper balance between the process of adequate diuresis and providing sufficient intravascular volume to maintain adequate renal perfusion. The addition of a vasodilator to the regimen is often more beneficial to a patient with poor renal perfusion than the administration of more diuretics.

Bed rest mobilizes fluid from the periphery and increases venous return to the heart. The resultant increase in cardiac output (attributable to the Frank-Starling mechanism) enhances renal perfusion and often induces an effective diuresis. Although it is important to restrict activity during periods of acute decompensation, long-term restriction of activity causes progressive deconditioning; most patients should be encouraged to exercise regularly. This approach improves exercise capacity and quality of life and can be safely undertaken through a structured aerobic rehabilitation program.[23]

TREATMENT OF HEART FAILURE AND ANGINA

Randomized studies have not assessed optimal therapy for angina pectoris in patients who also have symptomatic heart failure. Patients who have congestive heart failure and active angina pectoris and who are not candidates for coronary revascularization should initially be treated with long-acting nitrates and aspirin. Although ACE inhibitors are ineffective antianginal drugs, they do reduce the risk of recurrent myocardial infarction (RR, 25%; 95% CI, 5% to 40%) in post–myocardial infarction populations[24,25] [see Pharmacologic Therapy for Systolic Heart Failure, below]. Beta blockers remain the mainstay of treatment for patients with angina and congestive heart failure; most patients can tolerate beta blockers despite significantly impaired systolic function [see Pharmacologic Therapy for Systolic Heart Failure, below]. Agents such as bucindolol, bisoprolol, and carvedilol, which possess vasodilatory properties that partially offset their negative inotropic effects, may further minimize the risk of detrimental effects of beta blockade in these patients. Diuretics often improve anginal symptoms in fluid-overloaded patients by reducing ventricular volumes and by reducing elevated filling pressures. Verapamil and diltiazem should be avoided in patients with overt heart failure because of their negative inotropic and chronotropic effects. The Multicenter Diltiazem Postinfarction trial found that the use of diltiazem was associated with more frequent development of heart failure and increased mortality among post–myocardial infarction patients with left ventricular ejection fractions of less than 40%.[26] Amlodipine has been shown to improve symptoms of both angina and congestive heart failure in patients with underlying ischemic heart disease.[27] Amlodipine does not increase mortality in these patients and should be considered a third-line treatment for angina refractory to nitrates and beta blockers.

SURGICAL TREATMENT OF LEFT VENTRICULAR DYSFUNCTION

Given the high prevalence of ischemic heart disease and its role as the principal cause of heart failure, the possibility that ventricular function may improve through revascularization should always be considered. Systolic dysfunction may reflect not only

> **Table 5** Factors Predictive of Improvement in Left Ventricular Function after Coronary Revascularization
>
> Multivessel coronary artery disease
> Suitable distal coronary vessels
> Complete coronary arterial revascularization
> Left ventricular ejection fraction > 20%
> Mitral regurgitation < 3+ in severity, as assessed with
>   ventriculography
> Preserved right ventricular function
> Left ventricular end-diastolic dimension < 70 mm
> Evidence of active myocardial ischemia or hibernating
>   myocardium
>   Symptomatic angina pectoris
>   Viable myocardium in two or more myocardial regions, as
>   determined by imaging techniques

fixed scar but also partially reversible areas of intermittent or prolonged myocardial ischemia. For patients who do not have angina, the potential benefit of revascularization (i.e., coronary artery bypass grafting or percutaneous transluminal coronary angioplasty) is directly proportional to the extent of ischemic but noninfarcted myocardium that can be adequately revascularized [see Table 5].[28] Even patients with severe left ventricular dysfunction (ejection fractions < 20%) may show marked improvement in functional capacity and contractile function after revascularization, provided that substantial areas of ischemic myocardium can be demonstrated by pharmacologic or physiologic stress testing.[21] Left ventricular ejection fraction typically increases by 5 to 10 units, and NYHA class improves by 1 to 2 functional classes in successful cases.[28] Mitral valve repair for severe (4+) mitral regurgitation is also being successfully employed for treatment of symptoms of refractory heart failure in patients with marked depression of left ventricular function.[29] Although left ventricular aneurysm resection may be useful in selected patients, left ventricular reduction therapy (i.e., Batista procedure) is seldom performed because of its high perioperative mortality and the frequency of sudden deaths in early survivors. Permanent use of an implantable ventricular assist device has recently been shown to improve 1- and 2-year survival rates and quality of life.[30] As these devices become even more reliable, they may serve as an alternative therapy for selected patients with advanced heart failure who are not candidates for cardiac transplantation.

PHARMACOLOGIC THERAPY FOR SYSTOLIC HEART FAILURE

Diuretics

Diuretics remain the mainstay of treatment for the so-called congestive symptoms of left-sided or right-sided heart failure (i.e., edema and exertional dyspnea) but have not been shown to improve survival [see Table 6]. Most agents also further activate the renin-angiotensin axis. Diuretics interfere with sodium retention by inhibiting the resorption of sodium or chloride in the renal tubules. Unfortunately, most agents produce further activation of the renin-angiotensin system in patients with heart failure by lowering afferent glomerular renal blood flow. Two pharmacologic classes of agents are available: loop diuretics and agents that act in the distal tubule.[31]

Loop diuretics The loop diuretics ethacrynic acid, furosemide, torsemide, and bumetanide are the most potent diuretics available and are generally preferred because of their efficacy. They inhibit tubular reabsorption of sodium chloride in the ascending limb of the loop of Henle (diluting segment). As much as 20% to 30% of the filtered load of sodium chloride is excreted in the urine after intravenous administration of furosemide. Recent data suggest that torsemide and bumetanide may be more effective than furosemide. Although the oral bioavailability of furosemide varies widely (10% to 100%), absorption of torsemide and bumetanide is nearly complete, ranging from 80% to 100%.[31] A once-daily dose of loop diuretic is usually effective, but patients with persistent fluid retention may require twice-daily dosing.

Long-term oral administration of loop diuretics can lead to hypokalemia, hypomagnesemia, contraction of extracellular volume, orthostatic hypotension, azotemia, and hypochloremic hypokalemic alkalosis. However, loop diuretics are effective even in the presence of metabolic alkalosis or impaired renal function.

Thiazides Thiazide diuretics act mainly by inhibiting reabsorption of sodium and chloride in the distal convoluted tubules. They also increase potassium secretion in the distal convoluted tubule and collecting ducts, resulting in potassium depletion. The diuresis caused by maximal doses of a thiazide is relatively modest and is ineffective when the glomerular filtration rate falls below 40 ml/min.[31] Chlorothiazide and hydrochlorothiazide are the most commonly prescribed thiazides. The most common undesirable side effects are hypokalemia and hypomagnesemia. Drug fever and allergic dermatitis have been associated with thiazide use, but the incidence of serious allergic reactions, such as thrombocytopenia, leukopenia, and vasculitis, is low. Thiazides may precipitate or exacerbate hyperglycemia, worsen hyperuricemia, and decrease sexual function. Thiazides can adversely affect lipid metabolism, producing a 5% to 8% elevation of low-density lipoprotein (LDL) cholesterol and a 15% to 20% increase in triglyceride levels, but these effects may be short term, with serum cholesterol levels falling back to or below baseline levels after 1 to 2 years of therapy.

Metolazone is a member of the quinazoline-sulfonamide series; it exerts its effect primarily by inhibiting sodium reabsorption at the cortical diluting site and in the proximal convoluted tubule. The drug's prolonged duration of action is attributed to protein binding and enterohepatic recycling.

Potassium-sparing agents Spironolactone, triamterene, and amiloride are relatively weak diuretics but enhance the action and counteract the kaliuretic effects of thiazide and loop diuretics. The spironolactones are steroid analogues of the mineralocorticoids and work by inhibiting the effect of aldosterone in the distal tubule. Further, in the Randomized Aldactone Survival Evaluation Study (RALES), low-dose spironolactone (12.5 to 25 mg daily) decreased mortality and risk of hospitalization in patients with heart failure symptoms of NYHA functional class III or IV.[32] However, the drug did not improve symptoms or functional capacity. Ongoing studies will address the role of aldosterone inhibition in cases of milder heart failure or asymptomatic left ventricular dysfunction. At present, therapy should be considered only for patients with advanced heart failure whose creatinine level is below 2.5 mg/dl and potassium level is less than 5.0 mmol/L.

Ongoing trials will address whether aldosterone inhibition benefits patients with milder symptoms of heart failure or symptomatic left ventricular dysfunction.

Table 6   Characteristics and Dosages of Commonly Used Diuretic Agents

	Diuretic	Brand Name	Principal Site and Mechanism of Action	Effect on Electrolytes In Urine	Effect on Electrolytes In Blood	Usual Dosage	Action Onset (hr)	Action Peak (hr)	Action Duration (hr)
Thiazides	Chlorothiazide	Diuril	Distal tubule: inhibition of NaCl reabsorption	↑Na, ↑Cl, ↑K	↓Cl, ↓K, ↑HCO₃	500–1,000 mg/day p.o.	1	4	6–12
						500 mg q. 12 hr I.V.	¼	½	2
	Hydrochlorothiazide	HydroDIURIL				50–100 mg/day	2	4	6–12
	Trichlormethiazide	Metahydrin, Naqua				4–8 mg/day	2	6	24
	Chlorthalidone*	Hygroton	Distal tubule (cortical diluting segment) and proximal tubule			100 mg/day	2	6	24
	Metolazone	Zaroxolyn, Diulo				2.5–20 mg/day p.o.	1	2	12–24
Loop Diuretics	Furosemide	Lasix	Ascending limb of loop of Henle: inhibition of Cl reabsorption	↑Na, ↑Cl, ↑HCO₃, ↑K, ↑H	↓Cl, ↑HCO₃, ↓K, ↓Na	40–160 mg/day p.o.	1	1–2	6–8
						10–80 mg I.V.	5 min	½	4–6
	Torsemide	Demadex				5–200 mg/day p.o.	1	1–2	6–8
						5–20 mg I.V.	10 min	1	4–6
	Ethacrynic acid	Edecrin				50–150 mg/day p.o.	½	2	6–8
						20–100 mg I.V.	5 min	¾	3
	Bumetanide	Bumex				0.5–2.0 mg b.i.d., p.o.	½–1	1–2	4–6
						0.25–2.0 mg I.V.	¼	½	½–1
Potassium-Sparing Diuretics	Spironolactone	Aldactone	Distal tubule: aldosterone antagonism	↓K; ↓H; slight ↑Na, ↑Cl, and ↑HCO₃	↑K	25 mg q.i.d.	Gradual	2–3 days after starting therapy	2–3 days after starting therapy
	Triamterene	Dyrenium	Distal tubule: membrane effect			100–300 mg/day	2–4	3	12–16
	Amiloride	Midamor	Proximal and distal tubules: inhibition of Na⁺, K⁺-ATPase			5–10 mg/day p.o.	2	6–10	24

*Chlorthalidone is chemically different from, but pharmacologically similar to, the thiazides.

Triamterene has a site of action similar to that of spironolactone, and triamterene causes urinary changes similar to those caused by spironolactone. Amiloride acts at the proximal and the distal tubules, probably by inhibiting Na⁺,K⁺-ATPase. The potassium-sparing agents should be used cautiously in patients with renal failure because they may precipitate dangerous hyperkalemia. Spironolactone has been associated with gynecomastia, amiloride with impotence, and triamterene with kidney stones. All three agents can cause gastrointestinal upset, skin rashes, and drug fever.

Combination therapy   Lack of response to diuretic therapy may be caused by excessive sodium intake, use of agents that antagonize their effects (e.g., nonsteroidal anti-inflammatory drugs, including cyclooxygenase-2 [COX-2] inhibitors), chronic renal dysfunction, or compromised renal blood flow. The combination of two or more diuretics is particularly useful in such difficult situations. The potassium-retaining diuretics lessen the chance of hypokalemia from the thiazide and loop diuretics and enhance the diuretic action of the latter drugs. Metolazone exerts a marked additive effect when given with furosemide, and this combination may offer an alternative for patients with significant edema. Thiazide diuretics may occasionally be employed to improve hyperkalemia that is related to use of ACE inhibitors. In cases of advanced congestive heart failure, patients can be instructed to follow a flexible diuretic program whereby they adjust their daily diuretic dose to maintain a desired body weight, ascertained to minimize symptoms of venous congestion. The ideal body weight should be periodically reevaluated during office visits.

Vasodilators

Vasodilator therapy is the cornerstone in the treatment of heart failure [*see Tables 7 and 8*]. The mechanisms of action of dif-

Table 7 Effects and Dosages of Major Vasodilators Used in Heart Failure Management

Agent	Mechanism of Action	Venous Dilating Effect	Arteriolar Dilating Effect	Usual Dosage
Nitroglycerin	Direct	+++	+	25–500 µg/min I.V.
Isosorbide dinitrate	Direct	+++	+	5–20 mg q. 2 hr s.l. or 10–60 mg q. 4 hr p.o.
Hydralazine	Direct	—	+++	10–100 mg q. 6 hr p.o.
Sodium nitroprusside	Direct	+++	+++	5–150 µg/min I.V.
Epoprostenol (prostacyclin)	Direct	+++	+++	5–15 ng/kg/min I.V.
Captopril	Inhibition of angiotensin-converting enzyme	+++	++	6.25–50.0 mg q. 6–8 hr p.o.
Enalapril	Inhibition of angiotensin-converting enzyme	+++	+++	5–20 mg b.i.d., p.o.
Lisinopril	Inhibition of angiotensin-converting enzyme	+++	++	10–40 mg/day p.o.
Quinapril	Inhibition of angiotensin-converting enzyme	+++	++	10–40 mg/day p.o.
Ramipril	Inhibition of angiotensin-converting enzyme	+++	++	1.25–5 mg/day p.o.
Losartan	Angiotensin II receptor blockade	+++	++	25–100 mg/day p.o.
Valsartan	Angiotensin II receptor blockade	+++	++	80–320 mg/day p.o.
Candesartan	Angiotensin II receptor blockade	+++	++	16–32 mg/day p.o.
Irbesartan	Angiotensin II receptor blockade	+++	++	75–300 mg/day p.o.

ferent vasodilators vary and include a direct effect primarily on veins (nitrates) or on arterioles (hydralazine), a direct balanced effect on veins and arterioles (sodium nitroprusside), alpha-adrenergic blockade with balanced venous and arteriolar effect (e.g., prazosin), inhibition of ACE (e.g., captopril, enalapril, and lisinopril), and blockade of the angiotensin II receptor (e.g., losartan, candesartan, valsartan, and irbesartan).

Agents that are primarily venodilators reduce cardiac filling pressure. Thus, nitrates can be effective in reducing pulmonary congestion while having little effect on systemic blood pressure. Agents that primarily dilate the arterioles (afterload-reducing agents) reduce systemic vascular resistance and increase cardiac output [*see Figure 6*] but produce little change in ventricular filling pressures. If the rise in cardiac output leads to an increase in renal perfusion, however, diuresis may ensue, with a consequent decrease in cardiac filling pressure. Drugs that produce balanced venous and arteriolar dilatation should generally be chosen as first-line therapy because most heart failure patients have elevated preload and afterload that require pharmacologic modulation.

ACE inhibitors play a crucial initial role in the treatment of heart failure by breaking the vicious circle of hemodynamic abnormalities and neurohormonal activation. The renin-angiotensin-aldosterone system is known to exert a major role in producing heart failure symptoms and disease progression. Impaired forward cardiac output results in a decline in renal afferent blood flow that leads to increased renin and angiotensin II excretion. In addition, enhanced activation of carotid baroreceptors produces a reflex increase in sympathetic neural activity, which leads to further renal production of renin through vasoconstriction of efferent renal arterioles. These elevated levels of angiotensin II and sympathetic neural activity produce clinical vasoconstriction and increased renal production of aldosterone that lead to sodium and water retention.

Although randomized trials in patients with NYHA class II or III heart failure have shown that survival is improved either by the combination of hydralazine and isosorbide dinitrate or by enalapril, a review of 30 randomized, placebo-controlled trials found that only the ACE inhibitors have been associated with both enhanced survival and improved functional status.[33] Subsequent trials in patients with NYHA class III or IV heart failure have shown that captopril increases survival to a greater extent than hydralazine when doses are titrated to achieve the same hemodynamic goals and when nitrates are included in both regimens; this presumably is the result of captopril's effects on neurohormonal activation and its favorable hemodynamic effects.[34]

Table 8 Effect of Pharmacologic Therapy on Outcome in Chronic Heart Failure

Agent	NYHA Class	Risk Ratio (95% Confidence Interval)
Digoxin	II–IV	0.99 (0.91–1.07)[47]
Diuretics	II–IV	Not studied
Hydralazine/nitrates	II–III	0.64 (0.46–0.89)[77]
ACE inhibitors	II–III IV	0.84 (0.74–0.95)[78] 0.60 (not provided)[79]
Beta blockers	II–III IV	0.35 (0.20–0.61)[53] 0.65 (0.52–0.81)[27]
Amlodipine	III–IV	0.91 (0.76–1.10)[80]
Spironolactone	III–IV	0.70 (0.60–0.82)[32]

NYHA—New York Heart Association

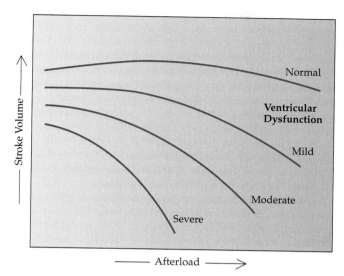

Figure 6 **Depicted is the relationship between ventricular afterload and systolic function for normal and failing ventricles. Afterload has little effect on systolic function when ventricular function is normal. However, small alterations in afterload can have profound effects on forward stoke volume when marked ventricular systolic dysfunction is present. Vasodilators produce a decrease in afterload in the failing ventricle and enhance forward stoke volume.**

There is clear and compelling evidence that ACE inhibitor therapy should be used whenever feasible in all symptomatic patients. A variety of well-designed, prospective, placebo-controlled studies (CONSENSUS I [Cooperative New Scandinavian Enalapril Survival Study I], V-HeFT II [Vasodilator–Heart Failure Trial II], SOLVD [Studies of Left Ventricular Dysfunction] trials, and MHFT [Munich Mild Heart Failure Trial]) have shown that ACE inhibition improves symptoms and prolongs survival in patients with heart failure symptoms of NYHA class II to IV.[33] Important racial differences exist in pharmacologic responsiveness to different vasodilator therapies. Retrospective analyses of both V-HeFT and SOLVD have confirmed that although enalapril was effective in decreasing mortality and hospitalizations in white patients, it was ineffective in black patients with heart failure of comparable severity.[35,36] In contrast, combination therapy with hydralazine and isosorbide dinitrate appears effective in lowering all-cause mortality in blacks.[35]

Despite the acknowledged benefits of ACE inhibitors, only 50% to 65% of all symptomatic patients take them. Initiating treatment in the elderly often causes the greatest concern; yet, this is the population in whom heart failure is most prevalent and that includes the largest number of patients who may benefit from therapy. The dose of ACE inhibitor should be slowly up-titrated in the elderly to avoid orthostatic hypotension. Physicians often question the dosage levels of ACE inhibitors that should be achieved in heart failure patients. Controlled trials have targeted high dosages regardless of the patient's therapeutic response. The recently completed Assessment of Treatment with Lisinopril and Survival (ATLAS) trial demonstrated that high dosages of lisinopril (32.5 to 35 mg daily) were better than low dosages (2.5 to 5 mg daily) in reducing the risk of hospitalization, but the two dosages had similar effects on symptoms and mortality.[37]

Aspirin is frequently prescribed when heart failure results from ischemic heart disease. Retrospective analyses of several large-scale clinical trials have suggested that aspirin lessens the beneficial effects of ACE inhibitors on survival and cardiovascular morbidity.[38] More recent data from the Bezafibrate Infarction Prevention trial demonstrated that aspirin use was associated with lower mortality (RR, 0.7; 95% CI, 0.49 to 0.99) in patients with heart failure resulting from ischemic heart disease.[39] The current recommendation is that aspirin be prescribed for such patients.

ACE Inhibitors in Post–Myocardial Infarction Management

ACE inhibitor therapy is being used in patients with asymptomatic or minimally symptomatic left ventricular dysfunction to slow disease progression; it is also being used to reduce mortality after acute myocardial infarction. In the SOLVD prevention trial, enalapril reduced the incidence of hospitalizations for new-onset congestive heart failure during a 36-month follow-up period.[25] Long-term treatment has also been shown to slow progression of left ventricular dilatation in patients with asymptomatic left ventricular dysfunction.[25] Postinfarction trials that have randomized over 100,000 patients (including the Survival and Ventricular Enlargement [SAVE] trial, the Acute Infarction Ramipril Efficacy [AIRE] trial, the Survival of Myocardial Infarction Long-term Evaluation [SMILE] trial, the Gruppo Italiano per lo Studio della Sopravvivenza nell'Infarto Miocardico–3 [GISSI-3] trial, and the Fourth International Study of Infarct Survival [ISIS-4]) have demonstrated that ACE inhibitor therapy results in a 10% to 27% reduction in all-cause mortality and a 20% to 50% reduction in the risk of development of symptomatic heart failure.[25] Oral ACE inhibitors, begun within 24 hours of acute infarction, are safe and are most beneficial for patients whose LVEF is reduced to below 40%.

Five ACE inhibitors have been approved for therapy for chronic heart failure—captopril, enalapril, lisinopril, quinapril, and fosinopril. Ramapril is approved for heart failure therapy after acute myocardial infarction and has recently been shown to reduce the risk of death, myocardial infarction, and stroke in high-risk patients with diabetes or vascular disease but in whom overt heart failure has not occurred.[40]

Angiotensin Receptor Blockers

Angiotensin II receptor blockers block the angiotensin I receptor rather than inhibit the production of angiotensin II, as is the case for ACE inhibitors. Recent studies have documented that prolonged use of ACE inhibitors does not result in full inhibition of ACE activity and results in a slow rise in angiotensin II levels.[41] Although several controlled studies have shown that long-term therapy improves hemodynamic and neurohormonal profiles, angiotensin II receptor blockers have not shown consistent effects on symptoms or exercise tolerance.[42] Although an early pilot study (the first Evaluation of Losartan in the Elderly Trial [ELITE I]) raised the possibility that an angiotensin II receptor blocker might have mortality benefits superior to that of captopril, the second losartan study (ELITE II) showed no comparative benefit from losartan and demonstrated a trend for better outcome and freedom from sudden death with captopril.[43] At present, angiotensin II receptor blockers should be considered instead of ACE inhibitors only in patients who are truly intolerant of ACE inhibitors as a result of angioedema or intractable cough. Angiotensin II receptor blockers are as likely as ACE inhibitors to produce hypotension, renal dysfunction, and hyperkalemia. The addition of an angiotensin II receptor blocker to an ACE inhibitor may improve exercise capacity; that combination is the subject of several ongoing clinical trials (e.g., V-HeFT and the Candesartan in Heart Failure—Assessment of Reduction in Mortality and Morbidity [CHARM] trial).[44]

Positive Inotropic Agents

Digitalis At the cellular level, digitalis acts by inhibiting sarcolemmal Na^+,K^+-ATPase activity, thereby restricting the transport of sodium and potassium across the plasma membrane. This enzyme inhibitory effect leads to an increase in intracellular sodium and an efflux of potassium from the cell. Coupled with the influx of sodium is an increase in the influx of calcium, which is then made available to the contractile element of the myofibril.

Digitalis enhances inotropy of cardiac muscle and at the same time reduces activation of the sympathetic nervous system and the renin-angiotensin system.[45] The latter effects are related to the ability of digitalis to restore the inhibitory effect of cardiac baroreceptors on sympathetic outflow from the central nervous system.[45] These neurohormonal effects are sustained during prolonged treatment with digoxin.[45] Controlled trials have shown that long-term therapy with digoxin modestly reduces symptoms, prolongs exercise tolerance, improves ejection fraction and hemodynamics, and decreases the risk of clinical progression of congestive heart failure.[46] The Digoxin Investigation Group (DIG) trial enrolled 3,800 patients and was designed to detect a 5% difference in mortality. It demonstrated that digoxin had no effect on all-cause mortality but did reduce the hospitalization rate for decompensated heart failure (RR, 0.72; 95% CI, 0.66 to 0.79).[47] Digoxin has not been evaluated in patients with asymptomatic left ventricular dysfunction.

Digoxin absorption may be impaired in patients who have had extensive jejunal and ileal resection or jejunoileal bypass procedures.[45] Splanchnic congestion probably also alters digoxin absorption. Decreased intestinal absorption has been associated with the administration of antacids, kaolin-pectin, and the anion-exchange resin cholestyramine. In about 10% of patients, gastrointestinal bacteria inactivate digoxin, reducing its bioavailability. A 5-day course of erythromycin or tetracycline can raise serum digoxin concentrations in these patients.

Digoxin is excreted mainly by the kidney, and its clearance is closely related to the creatinine clearance. A patient with normal renal function excretes daily about 37% of the digoxin that has been administered; maintenance therapy should replace this amount each day. The blood level of digoxin plateaus 7 days (four to five half-lives) after initiation of regular maintenance doses without loading, making this approach a satisfactory one for gradual digitalization of outpatients. Poor renal perfusion, as indicated by a high BUN level, suggests that digoxin levels may be high if a patient is on a standard maintenance dose. A number of drugs, including quinidine, verapamil, flecainide, propafenone, spironolactone, and amiodarone, increase serum digoxin levels. Quinidine produces increased serum digoxin levels in 90% of patients. Serum digoxin levels are not significantly affected by either diltiazem or nifedipine. In the majority of patients, the dosage of digoxin should be 0.125 to 0.25 mg daily.

Intravenous Inotropic Agents

Intermittent or continuous outpatient infusion of a positive inotropic agent (e.g., a beta agonist such as dobutamine or a phosphodiesterase inhibitor such as milrinone) is occasionally employed in patients with advanced heart failure to decrease the frequency of hospitalizations and improve quality of life. Although dobutamine often produces dramatic short-term clinical and he-

modynamic benefits, long-term outpatient use of dobutamine has unquestionably been associated with an increased risk of ventricular arrhythmias and sudden death. Dobutamine is often useful in treating acute heart failure decompensation in hospitalized patients and may very occasionally be used as palliative therapy on an outpatient basis for carefully selected patients who require repeated hospitalizations for low-output symptoms. Long-term use of oral beta-adrenergic receptor antagonists may lead to downregulation of these receptors, which renders such agents less effective. Orally active sympathomimetic agents such as prenalterol, pirbuterol, and levodopa have failed in clinical trials because of unfavorable side effects, exacerbation of ventricular arrhythmias, and rapid tachyphylaxis of their hemodynamic benefits.

Phosphodiesterase inhibitors enhance myocardial cyclic adenosine monophosphate by inhibiting its breakdown. Milrinone, amrinone, enoximone, ibopamine, xamoterol, and vesnarinone have all failed to improve symptoms and have increased mortality in patients with moderate to severe heart failure in controlled clinical trials.[48,49] Oral enoximone has been utilized as a bridge to the introduction of beta-blocker therapy in patients with severe medically refractory heart failure.[50] The safety and efficacy of this approach are being evaluated in an ongoing, randomized clinical trial.

Beta-Adrenergic Blockers

Beta blockers act principally to inhibit the detrimental effects of excessive sympathetic nervous system activation in heart failure patients. Sympathetic activation results in peripheral vasoconstriction and impaired renal sodium excretion. In addition, it induces cardiac hypertrophy, may provoke arrhythmias, and can trigger apoptosis by stimulating growth and oxidative stress.[51] Beta blockers that have been shown to be effective in the management of heart failure include those that selectively block the $beta_1$ receptor (bisoprolol and metoprolol) and those that block $alpha_1$-, $beta_1$-, and $beta_2$-adrenergic receptors (i.e., carvedilol) [see Table 9]. A short-term (1- to 2-week) decrease in myocardial contractility and deterioration in hemodynamics is usually followed by a slow, steady rise in ejection fraction over the next 3 to 6 months of treatment. Results from over 20 published placebo-controlled clinical trials in heart failure patients representing a wide spectrum of disease severity indicate that long-term treatment with beta blockers can lessen heart failure symptoms, improve clinical status, and decrease hospitalizations.[52,53] Bisoprolol, carvedilol, and metoprolol have also been shown to reduce mortality.[53-55] The benefits of beta blockers have been observed in patients with NYHA class II to IV symptoms as well as in those with diabetes and in patients with and without coronary artery disease. Carvedilol has been shown to produce similar benefits in functional capacity, heart failure readmissions, and all-cause mortality in both black and nonblack patients.[56] Thus, beta-blocker therapy should be routinely administered to clinically stable patients with left ventricular systolic dysfunction (LVEF < 40%) and mild to moderate symptoms of heart failure who are receiving standard therapy, including an ACE inhibitor, digoxin, and diuretics as needed to control fluid retention.[22] A recently completed trial with carvedilol confirms that stable NYHA class IV patients also experience a substantial reduction in all-cause mortality (RR, 35%; 95% CI, 19% to 48%).

The choice of a particular agent remains controversial. Carvedilol has been shown to improve hemodynamics and ejection fraction at rest and during exercise to a greater degree than metoprolol; however, metoprolol resulted in a greater improvement in maximal exercise capacity, and the two drugs improved

Table 9 Beta-Adrenergic Blockers That Are
Commonly Prescribed in Heart Failure

Drug	*Action*	*Initial Dose*	*Maximal Dose*
Bisoprolol	Beta$_1$-specific antagonist	1.25 mg p.o. daily	10 mg p.o. daily
Carvedilol	Beta$_1$, beta$_2$, and alpha$_1$ antagonist	3.125 mg p.o., b.i.d.	25 mg p.o., b.i.d.
Metoprolol tartrate	Beta$_1$-specific antagonist	6.25 mg p.o., b.i.d	75 mg p.o., b.i.d.
Metoprolol succinate (extended release)	Beta$_1$-specific antagonist	12.5 mg p.o. daily	200 mg p.o. daily

quality of life to a similar degree.[57] Whichever drug is chosen, it must be introduced at a very low dose; if the lower doses are well tolerated, gradual up-titration should be employed over weeks to months. Diuretics should be optimized before and during up-titration of the beta blocker. With a cautious approach, over 85% of patients enrolled in clinical trials have been able to tolerate long-term treatment with these agents.[51]

Endothelin and Cytokine Antagonists and Vasopeptidase Inhibitors

Endothelin 1 is considered the most potent known vasoconstrictor, exhibiting an in vitro potency 10-fold that of angiotensin II. Plasma endothelin 1 levels are elevated in heart failure patients, and agents that antagonize endothelin produce favorable hemodynamic effects. Two types of endothelin 1 antagonists are under evaluation: those that block the endothelin 1 receptor and those that inhibit endothelin-converting enzyme. Bosentan and tezosentan have been demonstrated to improve cardiac hemodynamics and functional status in pilot studies; however, high doses of bosentan were associated with reversible liver function abnormalities.[58] Two multicenter trials are nearing completion and will better define the safety and efficacy of these new agents.

TNF, a circulating cytokine, has exerted cardiodepressant effects in experimental heart failure models. The failing heart is a major source of TNF production, which it synthesizes in response to hemodynamic stresses, particularly elevated ventricular filling pressures and increased wall stress. A soluble TNF receptor antagonist (etanercept) and several chimeric natriuretic factors are undergoing evaluation for heart failure therapy.

Vasopeptidase inhibitors are a new class of agents that not only block ACE (leading to decreased angiotensin II levels) but also competitively block neutral endopeptidase (leading to enhanced endogenous vasodilator activity). Omapatrilat has recently been shown to improve neurohormonal activation, hemodynamics, and functional status in a short-term study.[59] The possibility that omapatrilat is superior to ACE inhibitor therapy alone is now being evaluated in a large-scale clinical trial (the Omapatrilat Versus Enalapril Randomized Trial of Utility in Reducing Events [OVERTURE]). None of these new pharmacologic agents have yet been approved by the Food and Drug Administration for clinical use in heart failure patients.

PACEMAKER THERAPY

Many heart failure patients with NYHA class III or IV symptoms have abnormal ventricular electrical activation (as demonstrated by prolonged QRS duration on the surface electrocardiogram) that may contribute to abnormal hemodynamic performance. A marked intraventricular conduction delay (QRS duration > 0.120 msec) results in dyssynchronous ventricular contraction between the septum and left ventricular posterior free wall. This poor contractile coordination impairs ventricular systolic pressure devel-

opment and results in increased left atrial filling pressure and decreased cardiac index. Biventricular pacing that is atrially sensed may enhance ventricular contractile function and reduce the secondary mitral regurgitation that results from this delayed septal activation.[60] Small, uncontrolled studies have shown that synchronized biventricular pacing (combined with patient-specific atrioventricular interval adjustment) is associated with improved heart failure symptoms and short-term improvement in exercise tolerance.[61,62] Controlled trials are now under way to evaluate the long-term effects of cardiac pacing therapy; until the results are available, this approach cannot be recommended for the routine treatment of heart failure.

PREVENTION OF SUDDEN CARDIAC DEATH

Sudden cardiac death accounts for 20% to 40% of mortality in heart failure patients. Routine ambulatory ECG monitoring is not useful in identifying asymptomatic patients at risk for sudden death because 50% to 70% of this population will have asymptomatic episodes of nonsustained ventricular tachycardia (NSVT). Empirical use of class IA antiarrhythmic drugs (e.g., quinidine and procainamide), class IC drugs (e.g., flecainide) and certain class III drugs (e.g., sotolol and dofetilide) should be avoided because their efficacy declines and proarrhythmic effects increase dramatically when the ejection fraction falls below 35%. Optimum management of patients with asymptomatic NSVT remains to be defined. Two large-scale controlled trials, the Grupo de Estudio de la Sobrevida en la Insuficiencia Cardiaca en Argentina (GESICA) and the Congestive Heart Failure–Survival Trial of Antiarrhythmic Therapy (CHF-STAT), have produced conflicting findings.[63,64] All-cause mortality was reduced by 26% at 2 years with low-dose amiodarone in the GESICA trial.[63] In contrast, the CHF-STAT trial found no benefit of low-dose amiodarone in lowering the risk of sudden cardiac death or improving long-term survival, except possibly in patients with nonischemic cardiomyopathy.[64] This difference may be attributable to the fact that there was a higher percentage of patients with nonischemic cardiomyopathy in the GESICA trial. A meta-analysis of 13 amiodarone trials (eight trials involved post–myocardial infarction patients; five involved patients with congestive heart failure) reported a decrease in total mortality with amiodarone treatment, but the finding was of marginal statistical significance.[65] Although the Multicenter Automatic Defibrillator Implantation Trial (MADIT) documented improved survival in patients with left ventricular ejection fractions of less than 35% and asymptomatic NSVT treated with implantable defibrillators (RR, 0.46; 95% CI, 0.26 to 0.82), this approach should be reserved for carefully selected survivors of myocardial infarction who are at high risk for sudden cardiac death, as demonstrated by inducible and nonsuppressible ventricular tachycardia during electrophysiologic studies.[66] The incremental cost-effectiveness of defibrillator therapy has been estimated at $27,000 per life-year saved; this compares favorably to other cardiac interventions. Recently, the second Multicenter Automatic Defibrillator Implantation Trial (MADIT II) demonstrated a 30% reduction in all-cause mortality in post–myocardial infarction patients whose ejection fractions were below 30%.[67] This benefit was observed in patients with and without symptomatic heart failure and was independent of degree of asymptomatic ventricular arrhythmias. If confirmed, these finding would suggest an expanded role for prophylactic use of implantable cardioverter defibrillators in patients with ischemic heart disease and severe impairment of left ventricular function.

DIASTOLIC HEART FAILURE

A sizable portion of patients with symptomatic heart failure have normal or near-normal left ventricular systolic function. Thus, a diagnosis of heart failure should not be rejected on the basis of findings of a normal ejection fraction if the clinical presentation (orthopnea, paroxysmal nocturnal dyspnea, and edema) is convincing. Recently, several groups have proposed criteria for diagnosing diastolic heart failure.[68] The simultaneous presence of three criteria should be considered obligatory for establishing an unequivocal diagnosis: (1) clinical evidence of heart failure on physical examination; (2) normal or mildly abnormal left ventricular systolic function (LVEF > 45%); and (3) objective evidence of abnormal left ventricular relaxation, filling, diastolic distensibility, or diastolic stiffness, as assessed by echocardiography or cardiac catheterization. Prevalence of diastolic heart failure is age dependent, increasing from less than 15% for patients younger than 45 years to 35% for patients older than 65 years. It is primarily a disease of elderly, hypertensive women.[69] In diastolic heart failure, the left ventricle has diminished compliance and cannot adequately fill at normal diastolic pressures. Factors that predispose to decreased diastolic distensibility include myocardial edema, fibrosis, hypertrophy, aging, and pressure overload. Ischemic heart disease, long-standing hypertension, and progressive aortic stenosis are the most common etiologies [see Table 10] . Clinical signs and symptoms do not reliably differentiate systolic from diastolic dysfunction [see Figure 7]. The absence of cardiomegaly on chest film is a useful clue to diastolic heart failure, but demonstration of a normal ejection fraction is necessary to establish the correct diagnosis. The absence of left ventricular hypertrophy does not exclude the diagnosis, because the correlation between magnitude of hypertrophy on ECG or echocardiogram and extent of ventricular filling abnormalities, as measured by echocardiography or left heart catheterization, is inconsistent. Abnormally short diastolic filling times and reversal of the normal mitral E to A wave pattern on Doppler echocardiography aid in establishing the diagnosis of diastolic heart failure, but these parameters are easily altered by changes in loading conditions of the heart.[70,71]

Table 10   Conditions Associated with
Diastolic Heart Failure

Aging	Chronic renal failure
Systemic hypertension	Infiltrative cardiomyopathies
Left ventricular hypertrophy	(e.g., amyloidosis)
Coronary artery disease	Restrictive cardiomyopathies
Aortic stenosis	Obesity
Diabetes mellitus	

The goal of treatment of diastolic heart failure is to reduce symptoms of dyspnea and edema by lowering filling pressures without significantly compromising forward cardiac output. Therapeutic strategies should include control of hypertension and tachycardia, maintenance of normal sinus rhythm, alleviation of myocardial ischemia, and modest reduction in central blood volume. No pharmacologic agents have yet been shown to effectively improve diastolic distensibility. Long-acting nitrates and judicious use of diuretics improve congestive symptoms by lowering preload but do not alter the natural history of the disease.[72] Annual mortality of 3% to 9% has been reported.[72] Unlike with systolic dysfunction, no randomized, controlled trials have yet assessed the influence of pharmacologic agents on outcome in patients with diastolic heart failure.

Emergency Presentations of Congestive Heart Failure

ACUTE PULMONARY EDEMA

Acute pulmonary edema results from the movement of fluid into the interstitial and alveolar spaces as a result of very high left atrial pressure. Pulmonary edema may develop suddenly (a phenomenon sometimes referred to as "flash" pulmonary edema) in patients with chronic hypertension or after a major cardiac insult, such as acute myocardial infarction or global myocardial ischemia.[73] In patients with previous borderline pulmonary congestion, it may follow seemingly modest stress, such as the stress associated with a fever or eating a salty meal. In typical cases, the patient is pallid and has cold, clammy, sometimes cyanotic skin. Tachypnea, coughing, wheezing, or combinations of these symptoms are present, and the patient generally sits bolt upright to obtain relief. The sputum may be frothy and blood tinged. Blood pressure is often elevated, although in more serious cases, hypotension may occur with cardiogenic shock. Bubbling rales may be heard throughout the chest, with or without wheezes; sometimes, only wheezing is heard.

Pulmonary edema can also develop in the absence of an increased wedge pressure as a result of direct damage to the alveolar epithelium, to the pulmonary capillary walls, or to both structures [see Table 11]. It is often difficult to differentiate clinically between cardiac and noncardiac causes of pulmonary edema. Knowledge of the pulmonary capillary wedge pressure is often crucial in making this important differential diagnosis.

Treatment

Acute pulmonary edema is a dire emergency requiring immediate treatment. The patient should be seated upright and given humidified oxygen via a face mask. Nasal prongs are generally inadequate in this setting. Arterial blood gas levels should be determined promptly to assess oxygenation, acidosis, and carbon dioxide retention. Morphine, 5 to 10 mg, should be given intravenously; such treatment will reduce venous return to the heart, systemic vascular resistance, and anxiety. Intramuscular or subcutaneous routes should be avoided because absorption is unpredictable in patients with peripheral vasoconstriction.

A rapid-acting intravenous diuretic such as furosemide, 10 to 40 mg, should be given. The addition of chlorothiazide, 250 to 500 mg I.V., may greatly enhance diuresis in a patient who does not respond adequately to furosemide alone. Diuretics initially cause venodilatation and reduce preload, even before diuresis occurs.

Digitalis plays only a secondary role in the treatment of acute pulmonary edema. Indeed, rapid intravenous administration of digitalis probably should be used only to alleviate rapid atrial tachyarrhythmias. Digitalis may be added later for long-term therapy.

In addition to furosemide and morphine, several other measures are available to reduce venous return to the heart. Adequate doses of nitroglycerin can cause significant venodilatation; it may be administered sublingually, transdermally, or intravenously. For patients who have prominent bronchoconstriction, intravenous aminophylline can be infused if the heart rhythm is monitored to ensure that ectopy or excessive sinus tachycardia does not occur.

It is important to search for and correct reversible causes of pulmonary edema, especially myocardial ischemia or arrhythmias. Monitoring the pulmonary arterial wedge pressure and systemic arterial pressure aids in managing protracted forms of pulmonary edema.

CARDIOGENIC SHOCK

Cardiogenic shock is the most dramatic and life-threatening manifestation of congestive heart failure resulting from left ventricular systolic dysfunction. It is characterized by severe and prolonged tissue hypoperfusion as a result of marked impairment in cardiac index. The diagnosis is hemodynamically established by the combination of the following findings: low systemic blood pressure (generally < 90 mm Hg); depressed cardiac index (< 2.2 L/min/m²); elevated filling pressures (pulmonary arterial wedge pressure > 18 mm Hg); and elevated arteriovenous oxygen difference (> 5.5 ml/dl). Acute myocardial infarction is the most common cause of cardiogenic shock, which is especially likely when infarction leads to loss of more than 40% of the left ventricular mass. When shock develops after hospital admission, the patient tends to be older and have diabetes, a history of myocardial infarction, and a high creatine kinase level.[74] The absence of hyperkinesis in the ventricular wall opposite the region of acute infarction is an important risk factor for the development of shock.[74] At autopsy, approximately 70% of patients who had cardiogenic shock have three-vessel disease, usually including the left anterior descending artery. Other causes of left ventricular dysfunction, such as acute myocarditis, progressive dilated cardiomyopathy, or myocardial depression that occurs during cardiac surgery, may occasionally result in shock. Cardiogenic shock must be differentiated from acute right ventricular infarction and mechanical defects after myocardial infarction, including acute mitral regurgitation resulting from papillary muscle dysfunction or rupture, myocardial rupture, or development of a postinfarction ventricular septal defect.

The clinical features that are evident at the bedside include peripheral vasoconstriction, with cool, clammy skin and peripheral cyanosis; oliguria, with urine output below 30 ml/hr; mental obtundation; hypotension; and a narrow pulse pressure. Echocardiography typically reveals severe contractile dysfunction; the left ventricular ejection fraction is almost always lower than 30%.

The prognosis of patients with cardiogenic shock is generally poor, with reported 60% to 75% in-hospital mortality.[74] Surprisingly, during the past 2 decades, survival has not increased despite more aggressive care.[74] Prognosis is more favorable for patients younger than 50 years, patients with single-vessel coronary dis-

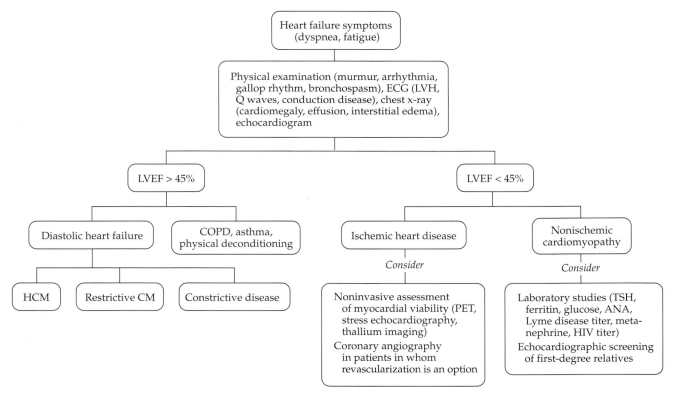

Figure 7 Shown is an algorithm for the diagnostic evaluation of new-onset heart failure. Physical findings, electrocardiography (ECG), and echocardiography are used to differentiate heart failure caused by systolic dysfunction from heart failure caused by diastolic dysfunction. Further noninvasive and invasive procedures help clarify disease etiology and should guide subsequent therapy. (ANA—antinuclear antibody; CM—cardiomyopathy; COPD—chronic obstructive pulmonary disease; HCM—hypertrophic cardiomyopathy; HIV—human immunodeficiency virus; LVEF—left ventricular ejection fraction; LVH—left ventricular hypertrophy; PET—positron emission tomography; TSH—thyroid-stimulating hormone)

Table 11   Major Causes of Pulmonary Edema of Noncardiac Etiology

Allergic reactions to blood products

Idiosyncratic reactions to pharmacologic agents, such as nitro-furantoin, sulfonamides, hydralazine, hexamethonium, methotrexate, busulfan, and ethchlorvynol

Pulmonary edema of infectious etiology, such as that which occurs in bacterial or viral pneumonia

Inhalation of toxic agents, such as phosgene or oxides of nitrogen (silo-filler's disease)

Circulating toxins, such as snake venom, or vasoactive substances, such as histamine, kinins, and prostaglandins

Disseminated intravascular coagulation

Radiation pneumonitis

Uremia

Drowning and near-drowning

Smoke inhalation

Shock lung

Profound hypoalbuminemia

High-altitude pulmonary edema (high oxygen tension)

Neurogenic pulmonary edema

Heroin overdose

Salicylate intoxication

Cardiopulmonary bypass (pump lung)

---

ease, and patients in whom subsequent coronary revascularization salvages a substantial amount of viable myocardium.

Treatment

The goals of treatment are to improve ventricular contractile performance, maintain adequate systemic blood pressure and perfusion to vital organs, reduce pulmonary congestion, preserve viable but ischemic areas of myocardium, and limit infarction size. Management should begin with general supportive measures designed to relieve ongoing ischemic pain and anxiety, correct electrolyte imbalances, and provide adequate oxygenation. Insertion of indwelling intra-arterial and pulmonary artery catheters is essential to define hemodynamics and monitor cardiac function during pharmacologic interventions. Specific therapeutic interventions may include pharmacologic agents (loop diuretics, vasopressors, and intravenous vasodilators), mechanical circulatory support (intra-aortic balloon counterpulsation or, in rare instances, a left ventricular assist device), and coronary artery reperfusion (thrombolysis, angioplasty, or coronary revascularization). Cardiac performance is generally optimal after acute myocardial infarction when the pulmonary arterial wedge pressure is between 15 and 18 mm Hg. When the cardiac index remains lower than 1.8 $L/min/m^2$, despite adequate volume repletion, dobutamine is the inotropic agent of choice because it improves cardiac contractility, lowers filling pressures, and augments coronary artery blood flow to the ischemic area.[74] Dopamine is useful for treatment of moderate hypotension; norepinephrine is often required for persistent severe hypotension (systolic blood pressure < 80 mm Hg). Intravenous vasodilators, particularly nitroprusside, are potentially useful when shock is further complicated by mitral regurgitation. Extreme caution is needed to avoid precipitating a further decline in blood pressure, however.

Coronary angiography should be considered in most patients with shock and ECG evidence of an acute evolving myocardial infarction. Thrombolysis has been shown to reduce mortality from 85% to less than 60% if reperfusion of the infarct-related artery is successful. Unfortunately, angiographic studies have shown that this initial approach establishes antegrade coronary perfusion in only 40% to 50% of cases. Direct angioplasty, coronary stenting, or both should be considered the most effective forms of reperfusion therapy. Recent studies have shown that in-hospital mortality can be reduced from 75% in patients with a persistently occluded infarct-related artery to less than 40% for patients with a patent infarct-related artery.[75] In hospitals that cannot provide primary angioplasty, patients in shock should receive a thrombolytic agent and be transferred urgently for coronary angiography and intervention. Surgical revascularization has also been advocated in the treatment of cardiogenic shock because it improves perfusion not only to the infarct zone but also to ischemic areas remote from the infarction. In carefully selected patients, surgical mortality is often less than 40%.[76] Enthusiasm for coronary artery bypass surgery during myocardial infarction remains limited, however, and most centers recommend primary angioplasty as a more cost-effective approach.

References

1. Massie BM, Shah NB: Evolving trends in the epidemiologic factors of heart failure: rationale for preventive strategies and comprehensive disease management. Am Heart J 133:703, 1997

2. Ho KK, Pinsky JL, Kannel WB, et al: The epidemiology of heart failure: the Framingham Study. J Am Coll Cardiol 22(suppl A):6A, 1993

3. He J, Ogden LG, Bazzano LA, et al: Risk factors for congestive heart failure in US men and women: NHANES I epidemiologic follow-up. Arch Intern Med 161:996, 2001

4. Philbin EF, Rocco TA Jr, Lindenmuth NW, et al: Systolic versus diastolic heart failure in community practice: clinical features, outcomes, and use of angiotensin-converting enzyme inhibitors. Am J Med 109:683, 2000

5. Holubarsch C, Ruf T, Goldstein DJ, et al: Evidence of the Frank-Starling mechanism in the failing human heart: investigations on the organ, tissue, and sarcomere levels. Circulation 94:683, 1996

6. Warren SE, Royal HD, Markis JE, et al: Time course of left ventricular dilation after myocardial infarction: influence of infarct-related artery and success of coronary thrombolysis. J Am Coll Cardiol 11:12, 1988

7. Konstam MA, Rousseau MF, Kronenberg MW, et al: Effect of the angiotensin converting enzyme inhibitor enalapril on the long-term progression of left ventricular dysfunction in patients with heart failure. Circulation 86:431, 1992

8. Schrier RW, Abraham WT: Hormones and hemodynamics in heart failure. N Engl J Med 341:577, 1999

9. Feldman AM, Combes A, Wagner D, et al: The role of tumor necrosis factor in the pathophysiology of heart failure. J Am Coll Cardiol 35:537, 2000

10. St John Sutton MG, Sharpe N: Left ventricular remodeling after myocardial infarction: pathophysiology and therapy. Circulation 101:2981, 2000

11. Brodie BR, Stuckey TD, Kissling G, et al: Importance of infarct-related patency for recovery of left ventricular function and late survival after primary angioplasty for acute myocardial infarction. J Am Coll Cardiol 28:319, 1996

12. Vasan RS, Larson MG, Benjamin EJ, et al: Left ventricular dilatation and the risk of congestive heart failure in people without myocardial infarction. N Engl J Med 336:1350, 1997

13. Drazner MH, Rame JE, Stevenson LW, et al: Prognostic importance of elevated jugular venous pressure and a third heart sound in patients with heart failure. N Engl J Med 345:574, 2001

14. Aaronson KD, Schwartz JS, Chen TM, et al: Development and prospective validation of a clinical index to predict survival in ambulatory patients referred for cardiac transplant evaluation. Circulation 95:2660, 1997

15. Badgett RG, Lucey CR, Mulrow CD: Can the clinical examination diagnose left-sided heart failure in adults? JAMA 277:1712, 1997

16. Harlan WR, Oberman A, Grimm R, et al: Chronic congestive heart failure in coronary artery disease: clinical criteria. Ann Intern Med 86:133, 1977

17. Gillespie ND, McNeill G, Pringle T, et al: Cross sectional study of contribution of clinical assessment and simple cardiac investigations to diagnosis of left ventricular systolic dysfunction in patients admitted with acute dyspnoea. BMJ 314:936, 1997

18. Heckerling PS, Wiener SL, Wolfkiel CJ, et al: Accuracy and reproducibility of precordial percussion and palpation for detecting increased left ventricular end-diastolic volume and mass: a comparison of physical findings and ultrafast computed tomography of the heart. JAMA 270:1943, 1993

19. Dries DL, Exner DV, Gersh BJ, et al: Atrial fibrillation is associated with an increased risk for mortality and heart failure progression in patients with asymptomatic and symptomatic left ventricular systolic dysfunction: a retrospective analysis of the SOLVD trials. J Am Coll Cardiol 32:695, 1998

20. Torre-Amione G, Kapadia S, Lee J, et al: Tumor necrosis factor–alpha and tumor necrosis receptors in the failing human heart. Circulation 93:704, 1996

21. Williams JF, Bristow MR, Fowler MB, et al: Guidelines for the evaluation and man-

agement of heart failure: report of the American College of Cardiology/American Heart Association Task Force on Practice Guidelines (Committee on Evaluation and Management of Heart Failure). J Am Coll Cardiol 26:1376, 1995

22. Heart Failure Society of America (HFSA) practice guidelines. HFSA guidelines for management of patients with heart failure caused by left ventricular systolic dysfunction: pharmacological approaches. J Card Fail 5:357, 1999

23. Belardinelli R, Georgiou D, Cianci G, et al: Randomized, controlled trial of long-term moderate exercise training in chronic heart failure: effects on functional capacity, quality of life, and clinical outcome. Circulation 99:1173, 1999

24. Rutherford JD, Pfeffer MA, Moye LA, et al: Effects of captopril on ischemic events after myocardial infarction: results of the survival and ventricular enlargement trial. Circulation 90:1731, 1994

25. Indications for ACE inhibitors in the early treatment of acute myocardial infarction: systematic overview of individual data from 100,000 patients in randomized trials. ACE Inhibitor Myocardial Infarction Collaborative Group. Circulation 97:2202, 1998

26. Goldstein RE, Boccuzzi SJ, Cruess D, et al: Diltiazem increases late-onset congestive heart failure in postinfarction patients with early reduction in ejection fraction. Circulation 83:52, 1991

27. Packer M, O'Connor CM, Ghali JK, et al: Effect of amlodipine on morbidity and mortality in severe chronic heart failure. Prospective Randomized Amlodipine Survival Evaluation Study Group. N Engl J Med 335:1107, 1996

28. Mickleborough LL, Carson S, Tamariz M, et al: Results of revascularization in patients with severe left ventricular dysfunction. J Thorac Cardiovasc Surg 119:550, 2000

29. Bolling SF, Pagani FD, Deeb GM, et al: Intermediate-term outcome of mitral reconstruction in cardiomyopathy. J Thorac Cardiovasc Surg 115:381, 1998

30. Rose EA, Gelijns AC, Moskowitz AJ, et al: Long-term use of a left ventricular assist device for end-stage heart failure. N Engl J Med 345:1435, 2001

31. Brater DC: Diuretic therapy. N Engl J Med 339:387, 1998

32. Pitt B, Zannad F, Remme WJ, et al: The effect of spironolactone on morbidity and mortality in patients with severe heart failure. N Engl J Med 341:709, 1999

33. Garg R, Yusuf S: Overview of randomized trials of angiotensin-converting enzyme inhibitors on mortality and morbidity in patients with heart failure. JAMA 273:1450, 1995

34. Fonarow GC, Chelimsky-Fallick C, Stevenson LW, et al: Effect of direct vasodilation with hydralazine versus angiotensin-converting enzyme inhibition with captopril on mortality in advanced heart failure: the Hy-C trial. J Am Coll Cardiol 19:842, 1992

35. Carson P, Ziesche S, Johnson G, et al: Racial differences in response to therapy for heart failure: analysis of the vasodilator-heart failure trials. Vasodilator-Heart Failure Trial Study Group. J Card Fail 5:178, 1999

36. Exner DV, Dries DL, Domanski MJ, et al: Lesser response to angiotensin-converting-enzyme inhibitor therapy in black as compared with white patients with left ventricular dysfunction. N Engl J Med 344:1351, 2001

37. Packer M, Poole-Wilson PA, Armstrong PW, et al: Comparative effects of low and high doses of the angiotensin-converting enzyme inhibitor, lisinopril, on morbidity and mortality in chronic heart failure. ATLAS Study Group. Circulation 100:2312, 1999

38. Al-Khadra AS, Salem DN, Rand WM, et al: Antiplatelet agents and survival: a cohort analysis of the Studies of Left Ventricular Dysfunction (SOLVD) trial. J Am Coll Cardiol 31:419, 1998

39. Leor J, Reicher-Reiss H, Goldbourt U, et al: Aspirin and mortality in patients treated with angiotensin-converting enzyme inhibitors: a cohort study of 11,575 patients with coronary artery disease. J Am Coll Cardiol 33:1920, 1999

40. Effects of an angiotensin-converting enzyme inhibitor, ramipril, on cardiovascular events in high-risk patients. The Heart Outcomes Prevention Evaluation Study Investigators. N Engl J Med 342:145, 2000

41. Jorde UP, Ennezat PV, Lisker J, et al: Maximally recommended doses of angiotensin-converting enzyme (ACE) inhibitors do not completely prevent ACE-mediated formation of angiotensin II in chronic heart failure. Circulation 101:844, 2000

42. Goodfriend TL, Elliott ME, Catt KJ: Angiotensin receptors and their antagonists. N Engl J Med 334:1649, 1996

43. Pitt B, Poole-Wilson P, Segal R, et al: Effect of losartan compared with captopril on mortality in patients with symptomatic heart failure: randomised trial—the Losartan Heart Failure Survival study ELITE II. Lancet 355:1582, 2000

44. Hamroff G, Katz SD, Mancini D, et al: Addition of angiotensin II receptor blockade to maximal angiotensin-converting enzyme inhibition improves exercise capacity in patients with severe congestive heart failure. Circulation 99:990, 1999

45. Hauptman PJ, Kelly RA: Digitalis. Circulation 99:1265, 1999

46. Young JB, Gheorghiade M, Uretsky BF, et al: Superiority of "triple" drug therapy in heart failure: insights from the PROVED and RADIANCE trials. J Am Coll Cardiol 32:686, 1998

47. The effect of digoxin on mortality and morbidity in patients with heart failure. The Digitalis Investigation Group. N Engl J Med 336:525, 1997

48. Ewy GA: Inotropic infusions for chronic congestive heart failure: medical miracles or misguided medicinals? J Am Coll Cardiol 33:572, 1999

49. Cohn JN, Goldstein SO, Greenberg BH, et al: A dose-dependent increase in mortality with vesnarinone among patients with severe heart failure. N Engl J Med 339:1810, 1998

50. Shaker SF, Abraham WT, Gilbert EM, et al: Combined oral positive inotropic and beta-blocker therapy for treatment of refractory class IV heart failure. J Am Coll Cardiol 31:1336, 1998

51. Bristow MR: Beta-adrenergic receptor blockade in chronic heart failure. Circulation 101:558, 2000

52. Lechat P, Packer M, Charlton S, et al: Clinical effects of beta-adrenergic blockade in chronic heart failure: a meta-analysis of double-blind, placebo-controlled, randomized trials. Circulation 98:1184, 1998

53. Packer M, Bristow MR, Cohn JN, et al: The effect of carvedilol on morbidity and mortality in patients with chronic heart failure. N Engl J Med 334:1349, 1996

54. The cardiac insufficiency bisoprolol study II (CIBIS-II): a randomised trial. CIBIS II Investigators and Committees. Lancet 353:9, 1999

55. Effect of metoprolol CR/XL in chronic heart failure: metoprolol CR/XL randomised intervention trial in congestive heart failure (MERIT-HF). MERIT-HF Study Group. Lancet 353:2001, 1999

56. Yancy CW, Fowler MB, Colucci WS, et al: Race and the response to adrenergic blockade with carvedilol in patients with chronic heart failure. N Engl J Med 344:1358, 2001

57. Metra M, Giubbini R, Nodari S, et al: Differential effects of beta-blockers in patients with heart failure: a prospective, randomized, double-blind comparison of long-term effects of metoprolol versus carvedilol. Circulation 102:546, 2000

58. Sutsch G, Kiowski W, Yan XW, et al: Short-term oral endothelin-receptor antagonist therapy in conventionally treated patients with symptomatic severe chronic heart failure. Circulation 98:2262, 1998

59. McClean DR, Ikram H, Garlick AH, et al: The clinical, cardiac, renal, arterial and neurohormonal effects of omapatrilat, a vasopeptidase inhibitor, in patients with chronic heart failure. J Am Coll Cardiol 36:479, 2000

60. Kass DA, Chen CH, Curry C, et al: Improved left ventricular mechanics from acute VDD pacing in patients with dilated cardiomyopathy and ventricular conduction delay. Circulation 99:1567, 1999

61. Cazeau S, Leclercq C, Lavergne T, et al: Effects of multisite biventricular pacing in patients with heart failure and intraventricular conduction delay. N Engl J Med 344:873, 2001

62. Gras D, Mabo P, Tang T, et al: Multisite pacing as a supplemental treatment of congestive heart failure: preliminary results of the Medtronic Inc. InSync Study. Pacing Clin Electrophysiol 21(part II):2249, 1998

63. Doval HC, Nul DR, Grancelli HO, et al: Randomised trial of low dose amiodarone in severe congestive heart failure. Lancet 344:493, 1999

64. Singh Fletcher RD, Fisher SG, et al: Amiodarone in patients with congestive heart failure and asymptomatic ventricular arrhythmia. N Engl J Med 333:77, 1995

65. Effect of prophylactic amiodarone on mortality after acute myocardial infarction and in congestive heart failure: meta-analysis of individual data from 6500 patients in randomised trials. Amiodarone Trials Meta-Analysis Investigators. Lancet 350:1417, 1997

66. Moss AJ, Hall WJ, Cannom DS, et al: Improved survival with an implanted defibrillator in patients with coronary disease at high risk for ventricular arrhythmia. N Engl J Med 335:1933, 1996

67. Mushlin AI, Hall WJ, Zwanziger J, et al: The cost-effectiveness of automatic implantable cardiac defibrillators: results from MADIT. Multicenter Automatic Defibrillator Implantation Trial. Circulation 97:2129, 1998

68. Vasan RS, Levy D: Defining diastolic heart failure: a call for standardized diagnostic criteria. Circulation 101:2118, 2000

69. Vasan RS, Benjamin EJ, Levy D: Congestive heart failure with normal left ventricular systolic function. Arch Intern Med 156:146, 1996

70. Nishimura RA, Tajik J: Evaluation of diastolic filling of left ventricle in health and disease: Doppler echocardiography is the clinician's Rosetta Stone. J Am Coll Cardiol 30:8, 1997

71. Zile MR, Gaasch WH, Carroll JD, et al: Heart failure with normal ejection fraction: is measurement of diastolic function necessary to make the diagnosis of diastolic heart failure? Circulation 104:779, 2001

72. Vasan RS, Larson MG, Benjamin EJ, et al: Congestive heart failure in subjects with normal versus reduced left ventricular ejection fraction: prevalence and mortality in a population-based cohort. J Am Coll Cardiol 33:1948, 1999

73. Gandhi SK, Powers JC, Nomeir AM, et al: The pathogenesis of acute pulmonary edema associated with hypertension. N Engl J Med 344:17, 2001

74. Goldberg RJ, Samad NA, Yarzbski J, et al: Temporal trends in cardiogenic shock complicating acute myocardial infarction. N Engl J Med 340:1162, 1999

75. Antoniucci D, Valenti R, Santoro GM, et al: Systematic direct angioplasty and stent-supported direct angioplasty therapy for cardiogenic shock complicating acute myocardial infarction: in-hospital and long-term survival. J Am Coll Cardiol 31:292, 1998

76. Hochman JS, Sleeper LA, Webb JG, et al: Early revascularization in acute myocardial infarction complicated by cardiogenic shock. N Engl J Med 341:625, 1999

77. Cohn JN, Archibald DG, Ziesche S, et al: Effect of vasodilator therapy on mortality in chronic congestive heart failure: results of a Veterans Administration Cooperative Study. N Engl J Med 314:1547, 1986

78. Effect of enalapril on survival in patients with reduced left ventricular ejection fractions and congestive heart failure. The SOLVD Investigators. N Engl J Med 325:293, 1991

79. Effects of enalapril on mortality in severe congestive heart failure. Results of the Cooperative North Scandinavian Enalapril Survival Study (CONSENSUS). The CONSENSUS Trial Study Group. N Engl J Med 316:1429, 1987

80. Packer M, Coats AJ, Fowler MB, et al: Effect of carvedilol on survival in severe chronic heart failure. N Engl J Med 344:1651, 2001

Acknowledgments

Figures 1 and 3   Al Miller.
Figure 2   Andrew Christie.

23 Valvular Heart Disease

Brian P. Griffin, M.D.

Valvular heart disease is an important cause of cardiac morbidity in developed countries despite a decline in the prevalence of rheumatic disease in those countries. Valvular heart disease can give rise to stenosis, regurgitation, or a combination of lesions at one or more valves. The more common significant anomalies currently encountered are mitral regurgitation, caused by mitral valve prolapse; aortic stenosis, caused by a congenital bicuspid valve or by senile valvular calcification; and aortic regurgitation, caused by a bicuspid aortic valve or dilatation of the aorta. Valvular lesions can occur as a result of pathologic changes in the valve leaflets or supporting structures (i.e., the chordae or papillary muscles). Ventricular or aortic enlargement can also produce valvular regurgitation as a result of annular dilatation and inadequate leaflet coaptation in the absence of any specific valve pathology. Valvular heart disease tends to progress over time as degenerative changes are superimposed on the primary pathology. Iatrogenic causes of valvular disease are increasingly recognized. Common causes of major valvular lesions are listed [*see Table 1*].[1]

Etiology

CONGENITAL DISORDERS

Anomalies in the development of valve cusps are common at the aortic or pulmonary positions. The normal configuration of these valves is tricuspid. Stenosis is the rule when only one cusp develops, whereas bicuspid valves may be stenotic or regurgitant [*see Figure 1*]. Congenital anomalies of the atrioventricular valves are uncommon; the most common abnormality is congenital cleft mitral valve. Valvular abnormalities can be seen in specific developmental syndromes, such as pulmonary stenosis in rubella syndrome and supravalvular aortic stenosis in Williams syndrome.

MYXOMATOUS DEGENERATION

Myxomatous degeneration most often involves the mitral or tricuspid valve. In this condition, leaflet tissue, particularly chordal tissue, is abnormally extensible and weak. The affected valves are therefore more likely to prolapse, leading to significant regurgitation. Chordal rupture is common and may precipitate a rapid clinical deterioration from sudden severe regurgitation. The precise abnormality in valvular tissue is unknown but is thought to involve the structural proteins, such as collagen.[2] A familial tendency is often noted in this disease.[3] Inherited connective tissue diseases such as Marfan syndrome produce valvular abnormalities similar to those found in myxomatous degeneration.

RHEUMATIC HEART DISEASE

Rheumatic heart disease remains the most common cause of mitral stenosis and a frequent cause of aortic regurgitation. It is the most common cause of multivalvular heart disease. Isolated outbreaks of rheumatic fever continue to be reported in the United States, even in affluent communities.[4] Rheumatic heart disease remains a significant problem in immigrants, especially those from Latin America and Southeast Asia. Rheumatic fever appears to cause valvular heart disease by an autoimmune phenomenon whereby antibodies against streptococcal antigens cross-react with valvular tissue. Valvular involvement can present acutely as a result of edema of valvular tissue. Progressive fibrosis, superimposed calcification, and scarring with retraction of leaflet tissue lead to valvular stenosis, incompetence, or both. The interval between the occurrence of rheumatic fever and clinical manifestations varies, as does the degree of involvement. Both mitral and aortic valves are usually involved.

DEGENERATIVE DISEASE

Degenerative calcification is a cause of aortic stenosis in the elderly and in patients with renal dysfunction; it results from calcium deposition on the body of the valvular leaflets rather than on the commissures [*see Figure 1*]. Factors found to promote degenerative valvular changes are increasing age, a low body mass index, hypertension, and hyperlipidemia. Histologic changes that simulate atheroma and involve lipid deposition and inflammatory cell infiltration of the leaflets have been described in patients with early degenerative changes in the aortic leaflets. Even mild degenerative changes in the aortic valve have been reported to be adverse prognostic factors.[5] Calcification of the mitral annulus is common in the elderly; it is more common in women than in men and can produce mitral regurgitation. Occasionally, mitral annular calcification extends onto the valvular leaflets, causing stenosis.

ENDOCARDITIS

Endocarditis usually occurs on previously abnormal valves, although overwhelming sepsis can infect normal valves. The predominant hemodynamic manifestation of endocarditis is valvular regurgitation. Contributory causes of endocarditis include leaflet prolapse (resulting from a large vegetation), leaflet perforation, and chronic scarring of infected tissue. In rare cases, large vegetations lead to valvular stenosis.

CORONARY ARTERY DISEASE

Mitral regurgitation is common in coronary artery disease; it has a number of causal mechanisms. Acute ischemia or infarction

Table 1 Causes of Specific Valvular Lesions

	Mitral	*Aortic*	*Tricuspid*	*Pulmonary*
Stenosis	Rheumatic disease, calcification, SLE	Calcification, congenital disease, rheumatic disease	Rheumatic disease, carcinoid tumor	Congenital disease, carcinoid tumor
Regurgitation	Myxomatous degeneration, ischemia, secondary causes, rheumatic disease, annular calcification, endocarditis, SLE	Congenital disease, secondary causes, rheumatic disease, endocarditis, SLE	Secondary causes, rheumatic disease, endocarditis	Secondary causes

SLE—systemic lupus erythematosus

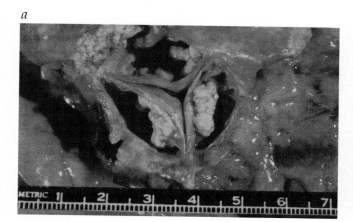 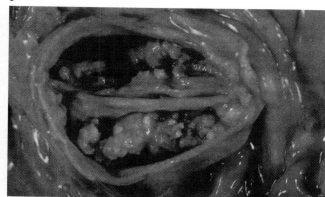

Figure 1 Pathologic specimens showing degenerative calcification of (*a*) a tricuspid aortic valve and (*b*) a congenital bicuspid valve.[62]

of a papillary muscle or of the wall to which the papillary muscle is attached leads to impaired leaflet coaptation and mitral regurgitation. Regurgitation can be severe and can vary with the severity of the ischemia. Papillary head rupture or, more rarely, muscle rupture, leads to catastrophic regurgitation that is often fatal.

CONNECTIVE TISSUE DISEASE

Libman-Sacks endocarditis consists of noninfected warty vegetations involving predominantly the mitral valve; it is characteristic of systemic lupus erythematosus (SLE).[6] Significant regurgitation and stenosis rarely occur acutely but are seen with scarring from chronic disease. Valvular involvement in rheumatoid arthritis is common and leads to valvular thickening but is usually not of hemodynamic significance. Aortitis in ankylosing spondylitis may produce significant aortic regurgitation.

IATROGENIC CAUSES OF VALVULAR HEART DISEASE

Iatrogenic causes include radiation therapy, the use of serotonin agonists such as methysergide, and the use of anorexiants such as fenfluramine and phentermine in combination.[7,8] Radiation leads to scarring and calcification of valvular leaflets many years after the initiating radiation. The effects of both methysergide and anorexiant agents on valvular tissue often simulate rheumatic disease, but regurgitation rather than stenosis predominates as the hemodynamically severe lesion. Serotonin is also thought to play a role in the valvulopathy produced by anorexiants; the precise mechanism by which this occurs remains to be established.

OTHER CAUSES OF VALVULAR HEART DISEASE

Amyloid disease causes valvular thickening but rarely causes significant stenosis. The carcinoid syndrome most often involves the valves on the right side of the heart and leads to stenosis or incompetence of the tricuspid or pulmonary valve.

SECONDARY INVOLVEMENT

Left ventricular dilatation can cause dilatation of the mitral annulus and, thereby, mitral regurgitation. Common secondary causes of mitral regurgitation include coronary artery disease, aortic valvular disease, and dilated cardiomyopathy. Similarly, tricuspid regurgitation results from right ventricular enlargement secondary to pulmonary hypertension or an atrial septal defect. Dilatation of the ascending aorta, especially involving the annulus of the aortic valve, can lead to aortic regurgitation. This condition is seen in hypertension and in aneurysms of the ascending aorta.

Assessment and Management

Valvular heart disease often remains asymptomatic for many years, but once symptoms develop, survival is reduced if the lesion is not corrected. The assessment of patients with valvular heart disease can be summarized [*see Table 2*]. The evaluation of symptoms can require a stress test or stress echocardiogram in addition to a careful history. Characterization of the lesions and assessment of hemodynamic severity are often possible on physical examination but are aided by additional testing, such as Doppler echocardiography and cardiac catheterization. The auscultatory findings of common valvular lesions also can be summarized [*see Table 3*]. Doppler echocardiography measures the flow velocity across a narrowed valve. By use of the modified Bernoulli equation, the pressure gradient (P), measured in mm Hg, may be estimated from the flow velocity (v), which is measured in m/sec: $P = 4v^2$. Therefore, if the peak velocity recorded across the aortic valve by Doppler echocardiography is 4 m/sec, then the peak pressure gradient will be estimated as $4(4^2)$ or 64 mm Hg. The effects of valvular heart disease on chamber size and function are best assessed serially by echocardiography or, at the time of cardiac catheterization, by ventriculography. In cases of stenotic lesions, intervention is rarely required until symptoms occur. Indications for intervention in regurgitant lesions are more

Table 2 Assessment of Patients
with Valvular Heart Disease

Parameters	*Tools*
Symptom severity	History, stress testing
Nature of valve lesion	Auscultation, Doppler echocardiography
Hemodynamic severity of lesion	Physical examination, Doppler echocardiography, cardiac catheterization
Effects of lesion on cardiac chamber size and function	Echocardiography, cardiac catheterization, stress echocardiography
Determination of the optimal time for intervention	Echocardiography, stress echocardiography
Selection of appropriate procedure/prosthesis	Echocardiography

Table 3　Auscultatory Findings Associated with Common Valve Problems

Lesion	Cardiac Cycle	Quality	Location	Other Sounds
Aortic stenosis	Systolic, mid-peaking to late peaking	Harsh	Aortic area, left sternal border, apex	Soft S_2, S_4
Aortic regurgitation	Diastolic, early decrescendo	Blowing	Left sternal border, aortic area	—
Mitral stenosis	Diastolic, mid-peaking to late peaking, increases with atrial contraction if rhythm is normal	Rumble	Apex	Opening snap, loud S_1
Mitral regurgitation	Systolic, holosystolic, late systolic with MVP, papillary muscle dysfunction	Blowing	Apex, axilla	Click, soft S_1, S_3
Tricuspid regurgitation	Systolic, increase with inspiration	Blowing	Lower left sternal border, xiphisternum	—
Pulmonary stenosis	Systolic, mid-peaking	Harsh	Pulmonary area, left sternal border	—

MVP—mitral valve prolapse

complex; such indications include significant symptoms or, in the absence of symptoms, increasing ventricular size, overt ventricular contractile dysfunction, or both.

All patients with even mild valvular heart disease require prophylaxis against endocarditis at the time of dental procedures or other procedures that can produce significant bacteremia. The prophylactic regimens recommended by the American Heart Association have been revised [see Table 4].[9]

Despite the increase in intravascular volume, pregnancy is usually well tolerated in previously asymptomatic patients with valvular heart disease.[10] During pregnancy, regurgitant lesions are better tolerated than stenosis. Prophylactic intervention to increase the valve area is recommended in patients with hemodynamically severe stenosis before pregnancy.

Patients with hemodynamically significant valvular heart disease should generally avoid participation in competitive sports. Reference should be made to the recommendations of the American College of Cardiology for more information about specific lesions.[11] Valvular heart disease is a chronic disease requiring periodic examination and follow-up, even in asymptomatic patients and in those who have had corrective surgical or other procedures. Patients with prosthetic valves should be seen at least yearly.

Specific Valvular Lesions

MITRAL STENOSIS

Normally, the cross-sectional area of the mitral valve is at least 4 cm². Mitral stenosis leads to a reduction in valve area and is considered severe when the valve area is less than 1 cm². To maintain flow through the valve, left atrial pressure rises, leading to an increase in the pressure gradient across the valve and to increased pulmonary venous and capillary pressures, with resultant dyspnea. Flow through the stenotic valve is dependent on the duration of diastole. Tachycardia shortens diastole disproportionately and causes a further elevation in left atrial pressure and can precipitate symptoms even in patients with relatively mild stenosis. Elevated left atrial pressure contributes to left atrial enlargement, which in turn predisposes the patient to atrial fibrillation, atrial thrombus formation, and thromboembolism, all of which are common complications of mitral stenosis. Severe mitral stenosis is often associated with an increase in pulmonary arterial pressure, leading to right-sided heart failure and secondary tricuspid and pulmonary incompetence. In patients with severe pulmonary hypertension, cardiac output at rest is reduced; this output reduction can cause a relatively low pressure gradient across the mitral valve even in patients with severe stenosis.

Diagnosis

Clinical manifestations　Mitral stenosis is often asymptomatic at presentation and for many years thereafter. Symptomatic patients often present with dyspnea, but they can also present with angina, right-sided heart failure, atrial arrhythmia, or embolism. The physical findings in mitral stenosis depend on the severity of the stenosis, the mobility of the valve, and the rhythm. The principal sign is a rumbling diastolic murmur that is best heard at the apex with the stethoscope bell. Such a murmur is accentuated by having the patient lie on the left side and by using provocative maneuvers, such as exercise to increase the heart rate. In sinus rhythm, the murmur increases in intensity with atrial contraction (presystolic accentuation). Increased severity of stenosis is associated with a longer murmur and a thrill. With a pliable valve, an opening sound (the opening snap) is heard, and the sudden closure of the stenotic valve at end diastole gives rise to a loud first heart sound that lends a tapping quality to the apex beat. When the valve calcifies and becomes less mobile, the opening snap and loud first heart sound disappear. A loud pulmonary component of the second heart sound is heard with pulmonary hypertension. The signs and symptoms of mitral stenosis are simulated by left atrial myxoma. In this condition, functional mitral stenosis results from prolapse of a mobile tumor arising from the interatrial septum into the mitral valve opening.

Imaging studies　Electrocardiography can reveal left atrial enlargement if the patient is in sinus rhythm. Left atrial enlargement, mitral valve calcification, and signs of pulmonary congestion can all be present on chest x-ray. Doppler echocardiography is the test of choice in confirming the diagnosis, establishing the severity of stenosis, detecting complications, and determining the most appropriate treatment. Echocardiography also allows accurate differentiation of mitral stenosis from a left atrial myxoma.

Typically, the stenotic mitral valve leaflets are thicker and less mobile than normal. The severity of stenosis is determined by measuring the pressure gradient across the valve with Doppler echocardiography and by calculating the valve area. Mitral stenosis should be suspected if the mean gradient exceeds 5 mm Hg; the pressure can exceed 20 mm Hg in severe stenosis. Valve area is measured by tracing the smallest opening of the valve in cross section [see Figure 2]. This method is the most accurate way of defining the severity of stenosis, although it is technically demanding and sometimes impossible to perform.[12] The valve area can also be calculated by Doppler echocardiography. Such evaluation is made on the basis of an empirical formula that calculates the time it takes for the pressure gradient to fall to half its initial

Table 4 Summary of American Heart Association Recommendations for Endocarditis Prophylaxis[9]

Procedure	Patient Condition	Drug	Regimen*
Dental, oral, respiratory tract, or esophageal[†]	At risk	Amoxicillin	Adults, 2.0 g; children, 50 mg/kg; orally 1 hr before procedure
	At risk and unable to take oral medications	Ampicillin	Adults, 2.0 g; children, 50 mg/kg. I.M. or I.V. within 30 min before procedure
	At risk and allergic to amoxicillin, ampicillin, and penicillin	Clindamycin *or* Cephalexin[‡] or cefadroxil[‡] *or* Azithromycin or clarithromycin	Adults, 600 mg; children, 20 mg/kg; orally 1 hr before procedure Adults, 2.0 g; children, 50 mg/kg; orally 1 hr before procedure Adults, 500 mg; children, 15 mg/kg; orally 1 hr before procedure
	At risk and allergic to amoxicillin, ampicillin, and penicillin and unable to take oral medications	Clindamycin *or* Cefazolin	Adults, 600 mg; children, 20 mg/kg. I.V. within 30 min before procedure Adults, 1.0 g; children, 25 mg/kg. I.M. or I.V. within 30 min before procedure
Genitourinary/ gastrointestinal	High risk	Ampicillin plus gentamicin	Ampicillin: adults, 2.0 g; children, 50 mg/kg *plus* Gentamicin: 1.5 mg/kg (for both adults and children, not to exceed 120 mg) I.M. or I.V. within 30 min before starting procedure *Then, 6 hr later,* Ampicillin: adults, 1 g; children, 25 mg/kg. I.M. or I.V. *or* Amoxicillin, orally: adults, 1.0 g; children, 25 mg/kg
	High risk and allergic to ampicillin and amoxicillin	Vancomycin plus gentamicin	Vancomycin: adults, 1.0 g; children, 20 mg/kg I.V.; over 1–2 hr *plus* Gentamicin: 1.5 mg/kg (for both adults and children, not to exceed 120 mg) I.M. or I.V. Complete injection/infusion within 30 min before starting procedure
	Moderate risk	Amoxicillin *or* Ampicillin	Adults, 2.0 g; children, 50 mg/kg; orally 1 hr before procedure Adults, 2.0 g; children, 50 mg/kg. I.M. or I.V. within 30 min before starting procedure
	Moderate risk and allergic to ampicillin and amoxicillin	Vancomycin	Adults, 1.0 g; children, 20 mg/kg; over 1–2 hr; complete infusion within 30 min of starting the procedure

*Total children's dose should not exceed adult dose.
[†]Follow-up dose no longer recommended.
[‡]Cephalosporins should not be used in patients with immediate-type hypersensitivity reaction to penicillins.
Note: For patients already taking an antibiotic or for other special situations, see reference 9.

value (the pressure half-time). Valve area is estimated as 220 divided by the pressure half-time. Pulmonary arterial (systolic) pressure (PAP) can be determined from the tricuspid regurgitant velocity (TRv) and the estimated right atrial pressure (RAP) (usually estimated as 5 mm Hg) by the following equation: $PAP = 4(TRv)^2 + RAP$. If the tricuspid regurgitant velocity is 3 m/sec, and RAP is estimated to be 5 mm Hg, then the estimated PAP is $4(3^2) + 5 = 41$ mm Hg. The likelihood that the valve may be successfully dilated, either with a balloon or surgically, is estimated by use of a scoring system based on the echocardiographic appearance of the valvular leaflets and supporting structures.

Transesophageal echocardiography is more useful than transthoracic echocardiography in excluding atrial thrombus and determining the severity of mitral regurgitation and is usually performed if balloon valvuloplasty is contemplated. Cardiac catheterization is rarely needed to establish the diagnosis but is used

to confirm the severity of stenosis. The valve gradient is the difference between the left atrial pressure or the pulmonary arterial wedge pressure and the left ventricular diastolic pressure. Valve area can be calculated from the pressure gradient and the cardiac output.

Treatment

Once symptoms develop in mitral stenosis, the chance of survival decreases without surgical or balloon dilatation or valve replacement. In the absence of symptoms, management is directed at preventing recurrence of rheumatic fever.[13]

Medical therapy Patients in atrial fibrillation require heart-rate control with a beta blocker (e.g., atenolol, 50 mg q.d.), digoxin (0.125 to 0.25 mg q.d.), or both. Systemic anticoagulation with warfarin is definitely indicated to prevent thromboembolism when (1) atrial fibrillation is present, (2) there is a history of embolism, or (3) a thrombus is detected in the atrium. Anticoagulation should be considered for patients with paroxysmal atrial fibrillation, a dilated left atrium (> 50 mm in diameter on echocardiography), or severe atrial stasis (as evidenced by swirling echoes or smoke in the left atrium on echocardiography).[14] Regarding symptomatic patients for whom surgical intervention poses a relatively high risk, the judicious use of diuretics and drugs to control heart rate (i.e., digoxin, calcium channel blockers, or beta blockers) may allow symptomatic relief without the need for surgical intervention.

Surgical intervention   Intervention to increase valve area is indicated before the onset of symptoms of dyspnea in the following patients: women with severe stenosis who wish to become pregnant but are unlikely to tolerate the volume load of pregnancy, patients who experience recurrent thromboembolic events, and patients who have severe pulmonary hypertension. A number of interventions are currently available to increase the valve area in mitral stenosis. These interventions include percutaneous balloon valvuloplasty, performed in the cardiac catheterization laboratory; surgical commissurotomy; and replacement of the mitral valve with a prosthesis.[15]

Balloon valvuloplasty is performed by inflating a specially designed balloon catheter in the mitral orifice to split the fused commissures. Excellent symptomatic relief is obtained in suitable patients.[16] This intervention is currently the initial choice in mitral stenosis. Typically, the mitral valve area doubles in size from 1.0 to 2.0 cm², with a concomitant reduction in the pressure gradient [see Figure 3]. Complications of balloon mitral valvuloplasty include severe mitral regurgitation (3%), thromboembolism (3%), and residual atrial septal defect with significant shunting (10% to 20%). Mortality associated with the procedure is less than 1%.[17,18] Contraindications to balloon mitral valvuloplasty include significant mitral regurgitation, which will likely increase after balloon inflation; left atrial thrombus, which can be dislodged at the time of the procedure; and significant subvalvular involvement or leaflet calcification, each of which increases the risk of complications and limits the degree of dilatation produced.[19] In pregnant patients with symptomatically severe mitral stenosis that has not responded to conservative measures such as bed rest and heart-rate control, balloon valvuloplasty is the technique of choice to increase the valve area.[20]

Surgical commissurotomy is now usually performed under di-

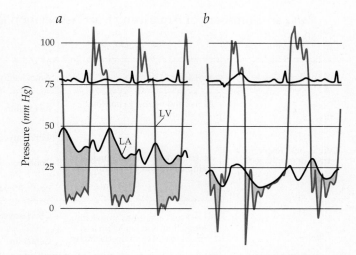

Figure 3   **Simultaneous left atrial pressure (LA, black line) and left ventricular pressure (LV, blue line) are shown (a) before and (b) after percutaneous mitral valvuloplasty. The shaded area shows the pressure gradient across the mitral valve; the pressure falls after valvuloplasty.**

rect vision after cardiopulmonary bypass. Surgical commissurotomy may be feasible when balloon valvuloplasty is impossible, such as in patients with significant mitral regurgitation, subvalvular stenosis, or atrial thrombus. A number of studies comparing surgical commissurotomy with balloon commissurotomy have shown equivalent immediate and medium-term (3- to 4-year) results regarding increase in valve area, improvement in symptoms, and freedom from repeat intervention in appropriately selected patients.[19] However, commissurotomy, whether effected by a balloon or surgically, is a palliative procedure, and in most cases further intervention is eventually required. Repeat commissurotomy is sometimes feasible; but most often, mitral valve replacement is also necessary.[21]

A prosthetic replacement is indicated if the valve is heavily scarred or calcified or if severe mitral regurgitation is present. Morbidity and mortality are higher with prosthetic replacement than with either surgical or balloon commissurotomy.

MITRAL REGURGITATION

Mitral regurgitation leads to volume overload of the left ventricle, which must increase in size to achieve a normal stroke output to accommodate the leakage of blood back into the left atrium. Progressive left ventricular dilatation eventually leads to an increase in afterload, contractile impairment, reduction of cardiac output, and heart failure. In acute mitral regurgitation (such as can occur with chordal rupture, ischemia, or endocarditis), left atrial and pulmonary venous and arterial pressures increase quickly, giving rise to dyspnea and, often, acute pulmonary edema. In more chronic forms of mitral regurgitation, an increase in left atrial pressure is often offset by a concomitant increase in atrial compliance; and hence, symptoms appear late in the course of the disease. Left atrial enlargement predisposes the patient to atrial fibrillation and atrial thromboembolism. In long-standing mitral regurgitation, pulmonary hypertension can develop, which in turn leads to tricuspid regurgitation and right-sided heart failure.

Diagnosis

Clinical manifestations   In most patients, mitral regurgitation remains asymptomatic for many years. Dyspnea, fatigue

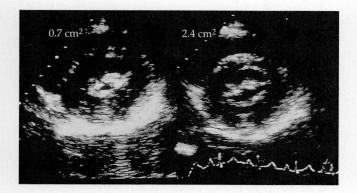

Figure 2   **Two-dimensional echocardiographic parasternal short-axis image of a mitral valve before (left) and after (right) percutaneous balloon mitral valvuloplasty. The valve area is estimated by planimetry and increases from 0.7 cm² before valvuloplasty to 2.4 cm² after valvuloplasty.**

from low cardiac output, and edema occur late in the course of the disease. Mitral regurgitation is recognized clinically by a systolic murmur at the apex, radiating to the axilla and increasing on expiration. In patients with a posteriorly directed jet of mitral regurgitation, the murmur is heard well at the back. In more severe cases, the murmur lasts throughout systole, the first and second heart sounds are soft or difficult to hear, and a third heart sound is present. A midsystolic click can be present in myxomatous disease; in less severe cases, this click can precede the murmur. The murmur can also be confined to late systole, with papillary muscle dysfunction. Mitral regurgitant murmurs caused by ischemia can be variable in duration and intensity, depending on the degree of ischemia and the loading conditions.

Imaging studies Doppler echocardiography is the noninvasive method of choice in confirming the presence of mitral regurgitation. Echocardiography is used to diagnose the mechanism of the regurgitation (e.g., prolapse or annular dilatation); color-flow mapping is used to provide a semiquantitative assessment of severity based on the size and penetration of the left atrium by the regurgitant jet. Additionally, echocardiography can be used to assess the effects of the regurgitation on left ventricular size and function. Quantitative measurements of regurgitation, such as the regurgitant volume, regurgitant fraction ([regurgitant volume plus stroke volume] divided by regurgitant volume), and regurgitant orifice area (the area through which the valve leaks), are now possible with newer Doppler techniques. These techniques are useful in determining the true severity of the lesion and following it over time.[22] Left ventricular size and volume, as well as contractile function assessed by the ejection fraction, are used to determine the need for surgical intervention.

However, asymptomatic mitral regurgitation is more difficult to assess and manage than other valvular lesions because in this condition, the true contractile function of the left ventricle is difficult to determine with conventional measures such as the ejection fraction. These measurements of contractility are confounded by the increase in ventricular preload caused by the extra volume of blood in the left atrium and the variable effect on afterload. Afterload is increased by left ventricular dilatation, but this effect is offset as the ventricle ejects much of its blood into a relatively low pressure system (the left atrium). The left ventricular ejection fraction can appear falsely elevated in mitral regurgitation and usually falls after surgical correction. An ejection fraction of less than 60% should be considered abnormally low in patients with mitral regurgitation.

Transesophageal echocardiography is very sensitive in the detection of mitral regurgitation and is used mainly in those patients who are difficult to evaluate by the transthoracic approach.[23] Contrast ventriculography is used to determine the severity of mitral regurgitation in patients undergoing cardiac catheterization. This procedure involves injecting radiopaque contrast medium into the left ventricle and assessing the extent and duration of opacification of the left atrium. In patients undergoing hemodynamic monitoring, large systolic V waves on the pulmonary arterial wedge tracing raise the suspicion of acute severe mitral regurgitation, as can occur in acute ischemia, but such V waves can occur in the absence of severe regurgitation.

Treatment

Indications for surgery In the management of asymptomatic mitral regurgitation, it should be borne in mind that left ventricular dysfunction is often latent and that, once present, the dysfunc-

tion cannot be corrected by operative intervention.[24] Therefore, it is important to refer patients for surgery before the onset of true left ventricular dysfunction even in the absence of symptoms.

Unfortunately, no load-independent measure of contractile function is readily available. Stress echocardiography is useful in detecting latent left ventricular dysfunction not evident on a resting study. Failure of the left ventricular ejection fraction to increase on exercise or of the left ventricular end-systolic volume to decrease on exercise is predictive of incipient left ventricular dysfunction and should be considered an indication for early surgery.[23]

Other echocardiographic indices that have been associated with a less favorable surgical outcome include an absolute end-systolic dimension that is greater than 4.5 cm or that is greater than 2.6 cm/m^2 when indexed for body surface area; an end-systolic volume of greater than 50 ml/m^2; and a resting ejection fraction of less than 60%.[23] Surgical referral should be considered if ventricular size and function approach these indices.[25] Serial echocardiographic evaluation should be performed at least yearly and should be performed more frequently as ventricular dilatation progresses in patients with severe asymptomatic mitral regurgitation. Studies indicate a better long-term survival rate in patients with severe mitral regurgitation when surgery is performed early.[26,27]

Symptomatic severe mitral regurgitation is considered an indication for surgical intervention if the valve is primarily involved. Symptomatic patients with ischemic mitral regurgitation often require mitral valve surgery in addition to revascularization. Mitral regurgitation secondary to left ventricular dilatation often improves with afterload reduction, and surgical intervention is not usually indicated.

Patients with moderately severe or severe left ventricular dysfunction (ejection fraction < 35%) and significant mitral regurgitation were thought in the past to be poor surgical candidates because of high operative risk. However, recent research has shown that there is acceptable risk associated with operations in these patients. Symptoms usually improve, but a survival benefit associated with surgery in this group has not yet been shown.[28,29] Patients who are not considered suitable for surgery because of left ventricular dysfunction often benefit from afterload reduction and diuretics.[30] However, in patients who have primary asymptomatic mitral regurgitation with preserved left ventricular function, afterload reduction has not been shown to delay surgery or improve left ventricular function in the few small studies that have addressed this issue; afterload reduction is not currently recommended to treat such patients.[31] Afterload reduction is beneficial for stabilizing patients with hemodynamically significant acute mitral regurgitation in preparation for surgery.

Surgical intervention Mitral valve repair is currently the technique of choice in the surgical management of mitral regurgitation because the operative mortality is lower, ventricular function is better preserved, and long-term complications such as thromboembolism and infection are lower with repair than with replacement [*see Figure 4*].[32-34] Valve repair is most likely to be feasible in patients with myxomatous disease, especially if such disease involves the posterior leaflet, and is least likely to be successful in patients with rheumatic disease and endocarditis.[34,35] Valve repair is accomplished by use of a variety of techniques, depending on the mechanism and etiology of the regurgitation. Such techniques include partial leaflet resection, chordal shortening or transfer, and insertion of an annuloplasty ring to reduce the size of the annulus. Long-term failure of repair occurs at a rate of 1% to 2% a year but is higher in patients with rheumatic disease. If mitral

a

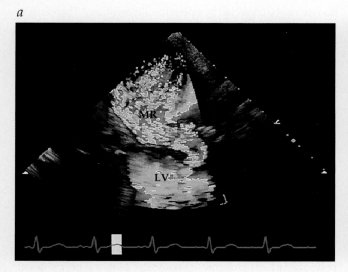

b

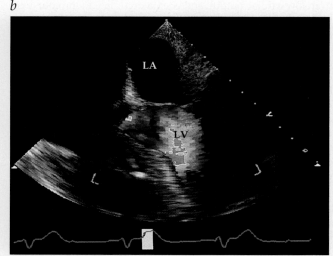

Figure 4 **Transesophageal echocardiogram of a patient with severe myxomatous mitral regurgitation (MR) (*a*) before and (*b*) after mitral valve repair.**

valve repair is not possible, a mitral prosthesis is implanted.[35] Chordal and papillary muscle preservation is increasingly being employed when a mitral prosthesis is inserted, because preserving the muscles has been shown to help conserve left ventricular function after surgery.[36]

MITRAL VALVE PROLAPSE

Mitral valve prolapse is a common condition in which the mitral valve leaflets are displaced in systole into the left atrium.[3] It is usually caused by myxomatous degeneration of the valve and can occur in some form in up to 3% of the general population; it is more common in women than in men. In the majority of cases, mitral valve prolapse represents a benign abnormality; in a minority, mainly older men, significant mitral regurgitation results from rupture of a chord or from endocarditis and requires surgical intervention. Mitral valve prolapse is associated with low body weight, low blood pressure, and thoracic skeletal abnormalities such as pectus excavatum. Patients with mitral valve prolapse have a slightly increased risk of stroke, myocardial ischemia, and sudden death. Ventricular extrasystoles are common and can be symptomatically troublesome. Other arrhythmias, such as ventricular or supraventricular tachycardia, are reported but are uncommon.

Diagnosis

Mitral valve prolapse has been associated with multiple nonspecific symptoms, such as atypical chest pain, presyncope, anxiety, and panic attacks. These symptoms are more commonly reported by women than men. A causal relation between these symptoms and mitral valve prolapse has not been established.[3]

A midsystolic click at the mitral area during cardiac auscultation is often the finding that first brings mitral valve prolapse to the attention of the examiner. The click has been attributed to tensing of the redundant valvular tissue with cardiac contraction. A late systolic murmur can follow the click. Maneuvers that reduce intracardiac volume, such as having the patient stand or perform the Valsalva maneuver, cause the click to occur earlier in systole and cause an increase in the duration of the murmur. The typical auscultatory findings and their response to these maneuvers are sufficient to make a diagnosis of mitral valve prolapse.

Two-dimensional echocardiography is the method of choice to confirm the diagnosis. Apparent systolic displacement beyond the annular plane is possible with both M-mode and two-dimensional approaches because the annulus is nonplanar and saddle-shaped. The possibility of a false positive diagnosis can be minimized by seeking systolic displacement of the leaflets in a parasternal long-axis view. Myxomatous mitral valve leaflets frequently are thicker, are more redundant, and have longer chordae than normal as seen on echocardiography. Doppler echocardiography is used to detect and quantify associated regurgitation.

Treatment

Asymptomatic mitral valve prolapse requires no specific treatment. Periodic examination is indicated to detect any progression in the severity of mitral regurgitation. Prophylaxis for endocarditis is indicated if both a click and a murmur are present but is not indicated in the absence of mitral regurgitation.[37] Symptomatic ventricular ectopy often responds to beta blockade. Many patients with atypical chest pain and other nonspecific symptoms improve when they are reassured of the relatively benign nature of the condition. Empirical treatment with small doses of beta blockers can also provide symptomatic relief. Mitral regurgitation should be treated as described earlier.

AORTIC STENOSIS

The normal aortic valve is 3 to 4 cm² in area when fully open. Aortic stenosis is considered severe when the valve area is 1 cm² or less and is considered critical when the area is less than 0.75 cm². Aortic stenosis causes concentric left ventricular hypertrophy as a compensatory mechanism that maintains cardiac output at rest despite the increased pressure gradient across the valve. Eventually, this compensatory mechanism is overcome, causing the left ventricle to fail and dilate and the resting cardiac output to decline.

Diagnosis

Clinical manifestations There is a variable relation between the severity of stenosis and symptoms. Many patients with critical aortic stenosis are asymptomatic, whereas patients in states of volume overload, such as pregnancy, may have symptoms with stenosis of lesser severity. Dyspnea is often the presenting feature; it reflects increased left atrial pressure and pulmonary venous hypertension from the increased left ventricular pressure in systole and the diastolic ventricular dysfunction imposed by left ventricular hypertrophy. Angina is common even in the absence of significant obstruction in the epicardial coronary blood vessels because of impaired supply of blood to the subendocardium in the hypertrophied left ventricle. Exertional syncope also occurs with stenosis and can result from the inability to increase cardiac output sufficiently to supply both skeletal muscle and the cerebral vasculature, resulting in impaired cerebral blood supply, or from abnormal baroreceptor reflexes. Serious arrhythmia can also cause syncope and, in severe aortic stenosis, even sudden death. Fatigue is common because of low cardiac output.

In severe aortic stenosis, the carotid pulse typically is reduced in intensity and has a slow delayed upstroke. Aortic stenosis gives rise to a systolic murmur that is heard over the aortic area and that can radiate to the carotid arteries and to the apex. In severe stenosis, the murmur peaks later in systole and can be associated with a thrill. A fourth heart sound is usually present. In mobile congenitally abnormal valves, an ejection click can precede the murmur. Severe calcific aortic stenosis is often associated with a diminished intensity of the aortic component of the second heart sound. Although the physical findings are important in alerting the clinician to the presence of aortic valve disease, the degree of hemodynamic severity is more reliably determined with Doppler echocardiography.

Imaging studies   The presence of left ventricular hypertrophy on electrocardiography provides useful supporting evidence for significant aortic stenosis. Doppler echocardiography is used to determine the mechanism and the hemodynamic severity of the stenosis as well as the effects on left ventricular size and function. In aortic stenosis, the opening of the aortic valve is reduced, as seen on the echocardiogram. Continuous wave Doppler echocardiography is used to measure the peak velocity across the valve and thus the aortic pressure gradient; the mean pressure gradient across the valve is often 50 mm Hg or more in patients with severe aortic stenosis. However, the pressure gradient is determined not only by the degree of stenosis but also by flow through the valve and can be relatively low despite severe aortic stenosis if cardiac output is reduced. In most instances, therefore, the valve area as well as the pressure gradient should be calculated. The valve area is estimated readily from the flow through the valve and the pressure gradient across the valve. With cardiac catheterization, the pressure difference across the aortic valve between the left ventricle and the aorta is measured directly. Valve area can be calculated from the cardiac output and the pressure gradient. Because Doppler echocardiography and invasive measurements of aortic valve severity have been shown to agree when both are performed expertly, cardiac catheterization is now used less often as the primary diagnostic tool in assessing aortic stenosis [*see Figure 5*]. Cardiac catheterization is used to confirm the echocardiographic findings in patients being considered for surgery or when there is significant discrepancy between the clinical findings and echocardiographic findings.

Treatment

Indications for surgery   Aortic stenosis is a progressive disease, and patients with the disease can remain asymptomatic for many years. The rate of progression varies greatly but increases with age, associated coronary artery disease, and the severity of the stenosis.[38] Progression to symptoms or intervention is likely within 2 years in older patients with severe asymptomatic aortic stenosis.[37] Once symptoms become manifest, the survival rate without surgical treatment is reduced; mean survival is 5 years in patients with angina, 3 years in patients with syncope, and 2 years or less in patients with heart failure.[38] Operative mortality increases with severe symptoms, advanced age, and the presence of left ventricular dysfunction. The onset of symptoms, therefore, is the major indication for surgical intervention. Left ventricular dysfunction attributable to aortic stenosis is another indication for intervention because it demonstrates failure of compensatory mechanisms and incipient symptoms. Sudden death can occur with aortic stenosis, but this is rare in the absence of symptoms. Patients should be instructed to report the onset of any symptoms and should undergo regular follow-up evaluations with physical examination and Doppler echocardiography. Doppler examination should be performed at least yearly and should be performed more frequently in patients with severe stenosis and in older patients. Surgical relief of aortic stenosis usually leads to relief of symptoms and improvement in left ventricular function when such function was abnormal preoperatively.

Aortic valve surgery in the very elderly is associated with an increased mortality but provides excellent palliation of symptoms; surgery should be considered for such patients provided they are otherwise viable candidates.[39] Patients with severe left ventricular dysfunction resulting from aortic stenosis should also be considered for surgery, because significant improvement in ventricular function and symptoms often results, and without surgery the survival rate in these patients is poor.

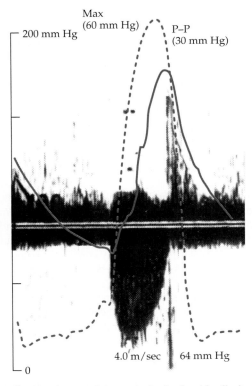

Figure 5   Simultaneous left ventricular (broken blue line) and aortic (solid blue line) pressure tracings and continuous wave Doppler tracing in a patient with severe aortic stenosis. The pressure gradient (P–P, or 30 mm Hg) is the area between the aortic and LV tracings. Maximal pressure gradient (Max) by cardiac catheterization (60 mm Hg) is similar to that measured by Doppler echocardiography (64 mm Hg).[63]

Surgical intervention   Surgical intervention for patients with aortic stenosis usually involves insertion of a prosthesis or a human valve. In congenital aortic stenosis, valve repair or commissurotomy can be feasible, although significant aortic regurgitation can result. Balloon valvuloplasty has proved disappointing in the long-term treatment of adult calcific aortic stenosis. Valve area typically increases from 0.5 cm^2 to 0.8 cm^2 and is associated with improvement of symptoms in the majority of cases.[18] However, stenosis recurs in as many as 50% of patients within 6 months, and fewer than 25% survive more than 3 years.[40] Balloon valvuloplasty is now indicated in the palliative treatment of adult patients with aortic stenosis who are not surgical candidates because of significant comorbidity; it is also used to stabilize critically ill patients for whom surgery is planned at a later stage. Balloon dilatation is effective in young patients with congenital aortic stenosis and is an alternative to surgery in symptomatic aortic stenosis during pregnancy.

AORTIC REGURGITATION

Aortic regurgitation causes a volume overload of the left ventricle. In chronic aortic regurgitation, the volume overload is well tolerated for years. The left ventricle dilates to accommodate the increased volume load and thereby maintains a normal resting cardiac output. Unlike mitral regurgitation, the left ventricle in aortic regurgitation must expel all of the increased volume of blood into the systemic circulation; severe enlargement of the left ventricle is common. Because of a compensatory increase in ventricular compliance, left ventricular diastolic pressure often remains in the normal range despite the increase in ventricular size. The ventricle hypertrophies to maintain normal wall stress. Eventually, compensatory mechanisms fail, and contractile impairment and increased diastolic pressure result in elevated left atrial and pulmonary venous pressures and symptoms. Acute aortic regurgitation can develop as a result of sudden disruption of the valve apparatus with endocarditis or aortic dissection. This condition is poorly tolerated because the left ventricle is unable to dilate fast enough to compensate for the volume load. Left ventricular diastolic pressure rises rapidly and leads to pulmonary congestion and edema. Cardiac output falls, and shock and even death can follow.

Diagnosis

Clinical manifestations   In chronic aortic regurgitation, symptomatic presentation occurs late in the course of disease; dyspnea and fatigue are the usual findings. Angina can occur in the absence of coronary artery disease because of the increased demand for oxygen caused by severe left ventricular enlargement and hypertrophy together with the reduced supply of oxygen resulting from the underperfusion of the coronary arteries. Such underperfusion is caused by the low diastolic pressure characteristic of this condition.

The cardinal physical sign of aortic regurgitation is a diastolic murmur that is high pitched and best heard with the diaphragm of the stethoscope with respiration suspended in expiration. The murmur is loudest immediately after aortic valve closure; it progressively diminishes in intensity throughout diastole, paralleling the decline in the pressure gradient between the aorta and the left ventricle. The murmur is best heard on the left of the sternal border in disease of the aortic cusps and on the right of the sternal border in disease of the aortic root. Even in the absence of significant stenosis, an aortic systolic murmur is audible, reflecting the increased flow through the valve. Severe chronic aortic regurgitation is characterized by a wide pulse pressure and an elevated systolic pressure caused by the increased stroke output; also characteristic is a reduction in the diastolic pressure, which occurs as blood leaks back into the left ventricle throughout diastole. If the aortic regurgitant jet hits the mitral valvular leaflet, it can cause partial closure of the valve, creating an apical diastolic murmur that simulates mitral stenosis (Austin Flint murmur). The ejection of a large volume of blood into the systemic circulation and its rapid leak backward into the heart cause many peripheral circulatory manifestations that confirm rather than establish the diagnosis. Acute aortic regurgitation can be more difficult to recognize because the murmur is often short, and the reduced cardiac output leads to reduced intensity of the murmur.

Imaging studies   Marked cardiomegaly and prominence of the ascending aorta are often present on chest x-ray in patients with chronic severe aortic regurgitation. Doppler echocardiography confirms the mechanism and severity of aortic regurgitation and its effect on left ventricular size and function. Regurgitant volume and fraction can be quantified by echocardiographic Doppler techniques. More often, the severity of regurgitation is graded on the basis of several qualitative and semiquantitative measures, including the dimensions of the regurgitant jet in the left ventricular outflow tract and of the ventricular cavity, as determined by color flow Doppler mapping, and the presence of diastolic flow reversal in the descending thoracic aorta, as determined with pulsed wave Doppler echocardiography [see Figure 6].[41] In severe aortic regurgitation, early closure of the mitral valve and diastolic mitral regurgitation can occur as a result of the increased pressure in the left ventricle in diastole [see Figure 6]. Confirmation of the severity of aortic regurgitation is obtained by aortography, a process in which contrast medium is injected into the aortic root and the retrograde filling and clearing of contrast dye from the left ventricle is examined. Aortography is the current gold standard for assessing the severity of aortic regurgitation; it should be performed if there is any discrepancy between the clinical findings and the findings on Doppler echocardiography. Stress ventriculography and echocardiography have both been used to determine the response of the left ventricle to the effects of exercise: a significant fall in left ventricular ejection fraction or an increase in end-systolic volume suggests incipient contractile dysfunction and can be an indication for early surgical intervention.

Treatment

Chronic aortic regurgitation is well tolerated for many years.[42] Operative mortality is increased and long-term survival reduced if the left ventricle is greatly enlarged or if left ventricular dysfunction has been present for more than 1 year. Left ventricular dysfunction that is present for a shorter period is likely to improve and even resolve after surgery. Several studies have shown that asymptomatic patients with normal left ventricular function can be safely followed for a long period (up to 11 years in one study) when serial physical examination and Doppler echocardiographic examination are performed at least yearly and then performed more frequently as left ventricular dilatation progresses.[42]

Surgery is indicated when symptoms develop. In asymptomatic patients, surgery is indicated when resting left ventricular function declines or if severe left ventricular dilatation (end-systolic dimension > 5 cm; end-diastolic dimension = 7 cm) occurs.[43] Evidence suggests that these dimensions should be normalized for body size and that surgery should be considered at an earlier stage, especially in women. Afterload reduction with vasodilators such as hydralazine, captopril, and nifedipine has been shown to

a

b

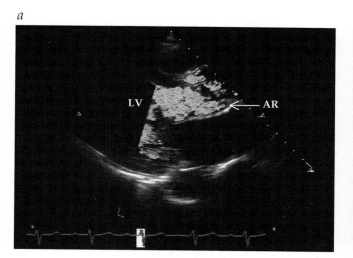

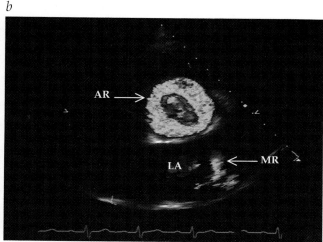

Figure 6   Parasternal long-axis view (*a*) and short-axis view (*b*) of a severely regurgitant aortic allograft. Aortic regurgitation (AR) is seen circumferentially around the insertion site. Diastolic mitral regurgitation (MR) is also seen.

reduce regurgitant volume and ventricular size in aortic regurgitation.[31] Treatment with nifedipine, 20 mg twice a day, has been shown to delay the need for surgical intervention in chronic asymptomatic aortic regurgitation but has not been widely used for this indication.[44] Acute severe aortic regurgitation necessitates urgent surgery. Intravenous vasodilatation with sodium nitroprusside or another vasodilator can reduce the regurgitant volume and help stabilize the patient awaiting surgery.

Surgical intervention in aortic regurgitation usually leads to improvement in symptoms and left ventricular size. Although the operative risk is increased when severe left ventricular dilatation or dysfunction is present, significant improvement in symptoms and ventricular function often occurs after surgery; the prognosis without surgery is very poor.[43] Aortic regurgitation usually requires insertion of a prosthesis or a human valve. Occasionally, repair is feasible, especially in prolapsing bicuspid valves or when the aortic ring is dilated.

Tricuspid and Pulmonary Disease

Tricuspid regurgitation is most often secondary to right ventricular dilatation and is the most common valvular problem of the right heart. Tricuspid regurgitation is recognized on physical examination by the characteristic large V waves in the jugular venous pulse and by a systolic murmur heard at the base of the xiphisternum that increases on inspiration. In severe cases, pulsatile hepatomegaly is present. Doppler echocardiography allows rapid detection and assessment of the severity of the regurgitation. Presentation often includes fatigue from reduced forward output and peripheral edema. Severe tricuspid regurgitation is usually treated with surgical repair. If a repair is not possible, a bioprosthesis is usually implanted because of the increased risk of thrombosis of a mechanical prosthesis at this position. Secondary tricuspid regurgitation can improve if the primary condition leading to pulmonary hypertension is treated and leads to a decrease in right heart size.

Tricuspid stenosis occurs in approximately 5% to 10% of patients with severe mitral stenosis. The characteristic physical findings are a large A wave in the jugular venous pressures and a diastolic murmur over the tricuspid area. Doppler echocardiography and right heart catheterization are both used to assess severity. The mean gradient across the tricuspid valve is typically greater than 5 mm Hg. In patients with significant stenosis, either balloon dilatation or surgical repair or replacement is indicated.

a

b

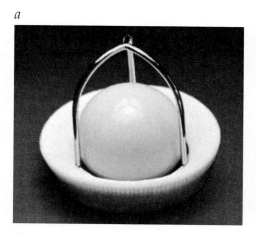

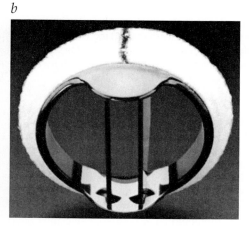

Figure 7   Two aortic mechanical prostheses. (*a*) Starr-Edwards ball-in-cage prosthesis and (*b*) St. Jude bileaflet tilting-disk prosthesis.

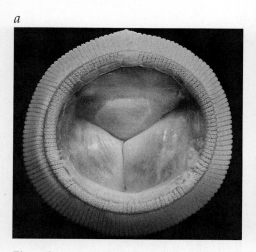
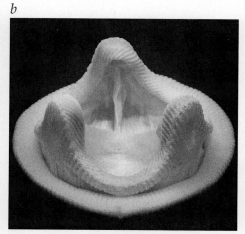

Figure 8   (*a*) **Top view of an aortic porcine xenograft that has been preserved in glutaraldehyde and mounted on a flexible plastic stent. (*b*) Bottom view of the same valve.**

Congenital pulmonary stenosis occurs in isolation or as part of various syndromes and is usually detected before adulthood. Significant pulmonary stenosis is treated with balloon dilatation or surgery. Significant pulmonary insufficiency is rare but can occur with a carcinoid tumor or endocarditis or secondary to pulmonary hypertension. Pulmonary allograft implantation is indicated for severe cases.

PROSTHETIC VALVES

Prostheses can be classified into two groups—mechanical and biologic—each having different properties, problems, and indications.[45]

Mechanical Prostheses

Mechanical prostheses are of two main types: ball-in-cage and tilting-disk [*see Figure 7*]. The Starr-Edwards valve is the prototypical ball-in-cage valve that has been implanted with various modifications since the 1960s. Tilting-disk valves can consist of one or two leaflets. Single-leaflet models include the Björk-Shiley and Medtronic-Hall valves. The most commonly implanted bileaflet models are the St. Jude valve and the CarboMedics valve. The major advantage of mechanical prostheses is durability. Mechanical prostheses can remain functional for decades and are used especially in young or middle-aged patients to reduce the need for reoperation.[46] Their chief disadvantage is the associated risk of thromboembolism, which necessitates long-term anticoagulation and carries a risk of hemorrhage. An increased incidence of subsequent infection, hemolysis, thrombosis of the valve, and mechanical failure is another problem associated with mechanical prostheses.

Bioprostheses

Three classes of biologic valves are currently available. A xenograft is a prosthesis fashioned from animal tissue [*see Figure 8*]. Most xenografts consist of modified porcine valves that are preserved in glutaraldehyde and mounted on a stent.[47] Prostheses have also been constructed of pericardium and other biologic materials.[48] Stentless bioprostheses are under investigation and are postulated to improve the effective size of the prosthetic valve opening.[49] Allografts (homografts) are human valves that have been harvested postmortem and either cryopreserved or treated with antibiotics.[50] An autograft is a valve from the patient's own

body that is moved to a different anatomic site.[51] The most common autograft is the pulmonary valve inserted at the aortic position. A pulmonary allograft is inserted in its place. Patients with biologic valves have a lower risk of thromboembolism than those with mechanical prostheses and do not usually require long-term anticoagulation. Biologic valves are indicated for patients in whom anticoagulation is inappropriate. Xenografts are less durable than mechanical prostheses. Xenograft durability is greatest in patients older than 60 years and improves with age.[52] Xenografts are not usually inserted in patients younger than 60 years because of the poor survival record in this group. Allografts and autografts are alternatives to mechanical prosthetic implantation at the aortic or pulmonary positions in younger patients. Insertion of these valves is technically more demanding and is not widely done. No long-term survival benefit of allografts over xenografts has been demonstrated. Autografts have proved to be durable and have the potential to grow in situ.[51] They are used in the management of pediatric and adolescent patients with aortic valve disease.[53] Both allografts and autografts result in a low reinfection rate when used in the treatment of prosthetic aortic endocarditis and are considered the valve replacement of choice for this condition.[50]

PROBLEMS AND COMPLICATIONS OF VALVE PROSTHESES

Thromboembolism

Systemic anticoagulation with warfarin or dicumarol decreases the incidence of, but does not eliminate the occurrence of, thromboembolism with mechanical valves.[54] The incidence of thromboembolic events is lowest in patients younger than 50 years, lower with aortic prostheses than with mitral or multiple prostheses, and lower with bileaflet disk valves than with single-leaflet valves.[54] Hemorrhagic events are more common in older patients. Anticoagulation is generally monitored using the international normalized ratio (INR). Studies have indicated that the level of anticoagulation required to prevent thromboembolism is less than was previously thought. A large study of anticoagulation in patients with mechanical prostheses has suggested that an INR of between 2.5 and 4.0 is desirable in most instances and minimizes hemorrhagic and thromboembolic complications.[54] The appropriate INR for an individual patient will vary depending on the history of embolic or bleeding events; age; and type, position, and number of prostheses. Antiplatelet agents such as aspirin (81 mg q.d.) or clopidogrel may be added to the anticoagulation regimen in patients who have sustained recurrent thromboembolic events despite adequate anticoagulation. Thromboembolic risk with xenografts is greatest in the first 3 months after surgery.[55] During this period, oral anticoagulation medications are recommended for high-risk patients (e.g., those with mitral prostheses or paroxysmal atrial fibrillation); for patients who are not at high risk, aspirin, 325 mg/day, is recommended.

Valvular Thrombosis

Acute thrombosis of a mechanical valve is more common with a single tilting-disk valve. The incidence is highest at the tricuspid position, followed by the mitral position, and is least common at the aortic position. Thrombosis of left-sided valves can lead to acute pulmonary edema and systemic thromboembolism. Reduced motion of the disk or ball is characteristic of valvular thrombosis and can be demonstrated with transesophageal echocardiography or fluoroscopy.[56,57] There is usually an increased pressure gradient across the valve. Acute thrombosis of a mechanical valve is an indication for emergency surgery to remove the thrombus and to implant another prosthesis. In patients who are not surgical candidates or who are considered at high operative risk, thrombolysis has been used successfully to increase valve opening and motion and reduce the valve gradient. Success rates greater than 70% have been reported in a number of series.[56] Thromboembolism is the most common complication of thrombolysis in this setting and occurs in 12% to 22% of patients. Further episodes of valvular thrombosis after initial successful thrombolysis have been reported.[56]

Valve Failure

In mechanical prostheses, failure of one of the mechanical parts is rare but can have catastrophic consequences. Failure is most common with tilting-disk valves, particularly with the Björk-Shiley single-leaflet tilting-disk valve, which is no longer available commercially in the United States.[58] Failure of the outlet strut in several of these models led to embolization of the disk and acute valve failure, with high morbidity and mortality. Prophylactic repeat surgery has been recommended for certain groups of patients in whom the failure rate is highest.[58] Advanced imaging techniques designed to detect sites of potential strut fractures are currently in development.[59]

Valve failure is expected with bioprostheses and allografts. Fortunately, degeneration is a slow process in biologic prostheses and is usually present for years before significant hemodynamic consequences are seen. Leaflet calcification can give rise to stenosis, whereas cusp degeneration can lead to perforation, with resultant regurgitation. Bioprosthetic degeneration is managed in the same way as stenosis or regurgitation of a native valve. Repeat surgery is indicated for significant symptoms or progressive ventricular enlargement or dysfunction.

Failure of either a mechanical or a biologic prosthesis can occur because of failure of the sutures holding the valve in place. Sutures can fail because of associated infection, but they can also fail spontaneously. A St. Jude valve in which the sewing ring was impregnated with silver nitrate to reduce the likelihood of infection was recalled because of a high incidence of paravalvular leak. The paravalvular leak resulting from suture failure can begin as a relatively mild lesion, but progression is common. In severe instances, partial or complete dehiscence can result in a characteristic rocking motion of the valve, as revealed by echocardiography. Paravalvular leaks are often accompanied by significant hemoly-

sis as red blood cells are destroyed at the site of increased shear stress.[60] Hemodynamically significant paravalvular leaks are considered an indication for reoperation.

Infection

There is an increased risk of endocarditis with mechanical prostheses and xenografts, compared with native valves or allografts. Prosthetic valve endocarditis is often associated with abscess formation. Prosthetic vegetation and abscess formation are best evaluated by using transesophageal echocardiography, which should be performed if a diagnosis of prosthetic valve endocarditis is being considered. Prosthetic valve endocarditis is extremely difficult to eradicate with medical treatment alone; operative intervention is usually required.

Inherent or Acquired Prosthetic Stenosis

All prosthetic valves are inherently stenotic, but in an appropriately selected prosthesis, the degree of stenosis is mild and not of clinical significance. Occasionally, a smaller than desirable prosthesis is implanted because the native valve annulus is small. In such cases, patients can manifest symptoms and signs of valvular stenosis and have severely increased pressure gradients across the valve, especially during exercise. In severe cases, explanation of the prosthesis and annular reconstruction may be necessary to accommodate a prosthesis of sufficient size. In some patients with mechanical prostheses, ingrowth of a fibrous pannus can impede blood flow and lead to hemodynamic stenosis, requiring reoperation.

Problems Associated with Pregnancy

Pregnancy is contraindicated in women with mechanical prostheses because of considerable risk to mother and fetus. The risk to the mother is associated with difficulty in maintaining effective anticoagulation; the risk to the fetus is associated with potential teratogenic effects of warfarin.[61] If possible, valve repair or insertion of an allograft or autograft should be attempted in a woman of childbearing age who wishes to become pregnant. Xenografts are less durable in young patients, especially during pregnancy, and are best avoided.[62] The management of patients with mechanical prostheses who become pregnant or desire pregnancy is controversial. Warfarin is associated with embryopathy and increases the risk of fetal wastage. Optimal anticoagulation is also difficult with heparin, especially when given subcutaneously, and is associated with increased maternal risk for thromboembolism and hemorrhage.[62] Different approaches have been advocated for the management of pregnant patients with mechanical prostheses; self-administration of heparin subcutaneously throughout pregnancy (ideally, from the time of conception) is the preferred approach in the United States.[63] This approach involves administering heparin every 12 hours and keeping the activated partial thromboplastin time at 1.5 to 2.0 times the control value 6 hours after administration, unless low-molecular-weight heparin is used, thereby eliminating the need to monitor the partial thromboplastin time.

ANOREXIANT-INDUCED VALVULAR DISORDER

Drugs that suppress appetite (anorexiants) have been reported to cause a valvular disorder similar to that caused by ergot derivatives and carcinoid syndrome. This finding was first reported in 1997, and a number of large studies since then have confirmed an increased prevalence of valvular disorders in populations treated with fenfluramine, dexfenfluramine, phentermine, or a combination of these drugs.[7,8] Over 18 million prescriptions were filled for these drugs in 1996 alone. The precise pathophysiology of the valvular disorder is still unclear. All of these anorexiants affect central serotininergic receptors. A causal relation of serotonin in this disorder is also suggested by the disorder's similarity to carcinoid disease, in which serotonin is also implicated as a causative factor. Initial reports suggested a high prevalence of valvular disease in patients treated with these anorexiants, and they were withdrawn from the market in September 1997. The prevalence of clinically symptomatic valve-related disease in patients receiving these drugs has been reported to be 1 in 1000.[64]

Anorexiant-drug valvulopathy affects mainly the aortic and mitral valve. Leaflet thickening, restricted leaflet motion, chordal thickening, and valve regurgitation without stenosis are the most common abnormalities seen.[65] Although valvular disease severe enough to warrant surgery has been reported, in many instances the valvular lesion appears to be mild or moderate in severity. Factors thought to increase the likelihood of more severe disease are longer duration of treatment with anorexiant therapy, use of drug combinations, and higher dosages of drugs. Patients who received less than 3 months of treatment appear to have a relatively low likelihood of significant valvular disease.[66] Studies also suggest that the valvular lesions may not progress and may even regress after discontinuance of the drug.[67] Patients exposed to anorexiants should undergo a thorough cardiovascular examination for signs of mitral or aortic regurgitation. Echocardiography is indicated if the physical findings suggest valvular disease or if the duration of treatment has been more than 3 months. Patients with evidence of valvular disease on echocardiography should be followed serially and receive prophylactic antibiotics for dental and other procedures associated with significant bacteremia.

References

1. Rose AG: Etiology of valvular heart disease. Curr Opin Cardiol 11:98, 1996

2. Tamura K, Fukuda Y, Ishizaki M, et al: Abnormalities in elastic fibers and other connective-tissue components of floppy mitral valve. Am Heart J 129:1149, 1995

3. Devereux RB: Recent developments in the diagnosis and management of mitral valve prolapse. Curr Opin Cardiol 10:107, 1995

4. Feldman T: Rheumatic heart disease. Curr Opin Cardiol 11:126, 1996

5. Otto CM, Lind BK, Kitzman DN, et al: Association of aortic valve sclerosis with cardiovascular mortality and morbidity in the elderly. N Engl J Med 341:142, 1999

6. Roldan CA, Shively BK, Crawford MH: An echocardiographic study of valvular heart disease associated with systemic lupus erythematosus. N Engl J Med 335:1424, 1996

7. Connolly HM, Crary JL, McGoon MD, et al: Valvular heart disease associated with fenfluramine-phentermine. N Engl J Med 337:581, 1997

8. Gardin JM, Schumacher D, Constantine G, et al: Valvular abnormalities and cardiovascular status following exposure to dexfenfluramine or phentermine/fenfluramine. JAMA 283:1703, 2000

9. Dajani AS, Taubert KA, Wilson W, et al: Prevention of bacterial endocarditis: recommendations by the American Heart Association. JAMA 277:1794, 1997

10. Oakley CM: Valvular disease in pregnancy. Curr Opin Cardiol 11:155, 1996

11. Bonow RO, Carabello BA, de Leon AC, et al: ACC/AHA guidelines for the management of patients with valvular heart disease. Circulation 98:1949, 1998

12. Faletra F, Pezzano A Jr, Fusco R, et al: Measurement of mitral valve area in mitral stenosis: four echocardiographic methods compared with direct measurement of anatomic orifices. J Am Coll Cardiol 28:1190,1996

13. Dajani AS, Taubert K, Ferrieri P, et al: Treatment of streptococcal pharyngitis and prevention of rheumatic fever. Pediatrics 96:758,1995

14. Gohlke-Burwolf C, Acar J, Oakley C, et al: Guidelines for prevention of thromboembolic events in valvular heart disease: study group of the working group on valvular heart disease of the European Society of Cardiology. Eur Heart J 16:1320, 1995

15. Elliott JM, Tuzcu EM: Recent developments in balloon valvuloplasty techniques. Curr Opin Cardiol 10:128, 1995

16. Palacios IF, Tuzai ME, Weyman AE, et al: Clinical follow-up of patients undergoing percutaneous mitral balloon valvotomy. Circulation 91:671, 1995

17. Dean LS, Mickel M, Bonan R, et al: Four-year follow up of patients undergoing percutaneous balloon mitral commissurotomy: a report from the National Heart, Lung and Blood Institute Balloon Valvuloplasty Registry. J Am Coll Cardiol 28:1452, 1996

18. Orrange SE, Kawanishi DT, Lopez BM, et al: Actuarial outcome after catheter balloon commissurotomy in patients with mitral stenosis. Circulation 95:382, 1997

19. Reyes VP, Raju BS, Wynne K, et al: Percutaneous balloon valvuloplasty compared with open surgical commissurotomy for mitral stenosis. N Engl J Med 331:961, 1994

20. Gupta A, Lokhandwada YY, Satoskar PR, et al: Balloon mitral valvotomy in pregnancy: maternal and fetal outcome. J Am Coll Surg 187:409, 1998

21. Pathan AZ, Mahdi NA, Leon MN, et al: Is redo percutaneous mitral balloon valvuloplasty (PMV) indicated in patients with post-PMV mitral stenosis? J Am Coll Cardiol 34:49,1999

22. Pu M, Vandervoort PM, Greenberg NL, et al: Impact of wall constraint on velocity distribution in proximal flow convergence zone. J Am Coll Cardiol 27:706, 1996

23. Leung DY, Griffin BP, Stewart WJ, et al: Left ventricular function after valve repair for chronic mitral regurgitation: predictive value of preoperative assessment of contractile reserve by exercise echocardiography. J Am Coll Cardiol 28:1198, 1996

24. Enriquez-Sarano M, Schaff HV, Orszulak TA, et al: Congestive heart failure after surgical correction of mitral regurgitation: a long-term study. Circulation 92:2496, 1995

25. Gaasch WH, John RM, Aurigemma GP: Managing asymptomatic patients with chronic mitral regurgitation. Chest 108:842, 1995

26. Ling LH, Enriquez-Sarano M, Seward JB, et al: Early surgery in patients with mitral regurgitation due to flail leaflets: a long-term outcome study. Circulation 96:1819, 1997

27. Ling LH, Enriquez-Sarano M, Seward JB, et al: Clinical outcome of mitral regurgitation due to flail leaflet. N Engl J Med 335:1417, 1996

28. Bach DS, Bolling SF: Improvement following correction of secondary mitral regurgitation in end stage cardiomyopathy with mitral annuloplasty. Am J Cardiol 78:966, 1996

29. Bolling SF, Pagani FD, Deeb GM, et al: Intermediate term outcome of mitral reconstruction in cardiomyopathy. J Thorac Cardiovasc Surg 115:381, 1998

30. Rosario LB, Stevenson LW, Solomon SD, et al: The mechanism of decrease in dynamic mitral regurgitation during heart failure treatment: importance of reduction of regurgitant orifice size. J Am Coll Cardiol 32:1819, 1998

31. Levine HJ, Gaasch WH: Vasoactive drugs in chronic regurgitant lesions of the mitral and aortic valves. J Am Coll Cardiol 28:1083, 1996

32. Enriquez-Sarano M, Schaff HV, Orszulak TA, et al: Valve repair improves the outcome of surgery for mitral regurgitation: a multivariate analysis. Circulation 91:1022, 1995

33. Grossi EA, Galloway AC, Miller JS, et al: Valve repair versus replacement for mitral insufficiency: when is a mechanical valve still indicated? J Thorac Cardiovasc Surg 115:389, 1998

34. Stewart WJ: Choosing the "golden moment" for operation in the era of valve repair for mitral regurgitation. American College of Cardiology Heart House Learning Center Highlights 10:2, 1995

35. Gillinov AM, Cosgrove DM, Lytle BW, et al: Reoperation for failure of mitral valve repair. J Thorac Cardiovasc Surg 113:467, 1997

36. Corin WJ, Sutsch G, Murakami T, et al: Left ventricular function in chronic mitral regurgitation: preoperative and postoperative comparison. J Am Coll Cardiol 25:113, 1995

37. Oakley CM: Management of valvular stenosis. Curr Opin Cardiol 10:117, 1995

38. Otto CM, Burwash IG, Legget ME, et al: Prospective study of asymptomatic valvular aortic stenosis: clinical, echocardiographic, and exercise predictors of outcome. Circulation 95:2262, 1997

39. Tseng EE, Lee CA, Cameron DE: Aortic valve replacement in the elderly: risk factors and long-term results. Ann Surg 225:793, 1997

40. Wang A, Harrison JK, Bashore TM: Balloon aortic valvuloplasty. Prog Cardiovasc Dis 40:27, 1997

41. Dolan MS, Castello R, St. Vrain JA, et al: Quantitation of aortic regurgitation by Doppler echocardiography: a practical approach. Am Heart J 129:1014, 1995

42. Bonow RO: Chronic aortic regurgitation: role of medical management and optimal timing of surgery. Cardiol Clin 16:449, 1998

43. Klodas E, Enriquez-Sarano M, Tajik AT, et al: Aortic regurgitation complicated by extreme left ventricular dilation: long-term outcome after surgical correction. J Am Coll Cardiol 27:670, 1996

44. Scognamiglio R, Rahimtoola SH, Fasoli G, et al: Nifedipine in asymptomatic patients with severe aortic regurgitation and normal left ventricular function. N Engl J Med 33:689, 1994

45. Vongpatanasin W, Hillis LD, Lange RA: Prosthetic heart valves. N Engl J Med 335:407, 1996

46. Zellner JL, Kratz JM, Crumbly AS, et al: Long-term experience with the St Jude Medical valve prosthesis. Ann Thorac Surg 68:1210, 1999

47. Cohn LH, Collins JJ Jr, Rizzo RJ, et al: Twenty-year follow up of the Hancock modified orifice porcine aortic valve. Ann Thorac Surg 66(6 suppl):S30, 1998

48. Banbury MK, Cosgrove DM 3rd, Lytle BW, et al: Long-term results of the Carpentier-Edwards pericardial aortic valve: a 12-year follow up. Ann Thorac Surg 66(6 suppl):S73, 1998

49. Walther T, Falk V, Langebartels G, et al: Prospectively randomized evaluation of stentless versus conventional biological aortic valves: impact on early regression of left ventricular hypertrophy. Circulation 100(19 suppl):II6, 1999

50. Ross DN: Evolution of the homograft valve. Ann Thorac Surg 59:565, 1995

51. Chambers JC, Somerville J, Stone S, et al: Pulmonary autograft procedure for aortic valve disease: long-term results of the pioneer series. Circulation 96:2206, 1997

52. Milano A, Guglielmi C, DeCarlo M, et al: Valve-related complications in elderly patients with biological and mechanical aortic valves. Ann Thorac Surg 66(6 suppl):S82, 1998

53. Lupinetti FM, Warner J, Jones TK, et al: Comparison of human tissues and mechanical prostheses for aortic valve replacement in children. Circulation 96:321, 1997

54. Cannegieter SC, Rosendaal FR, Wintzen AR, et al: Optimal oral anticoagulant therapy in patients with mechanical heart valves. N Engl J Med 333:11, 1995

55. Heras M, Chesebro JH, Fuster V, et al: High risk of thromboemboli early after bio-prosthetic cardiac valve replacement. J Am Coll Cardiol 25:1111, 1995

56. Binder T, Baumgartner H, Maurer G: Diagnosis and management of prosthetic valve dysfunction. Curr Opin Cardiol 11:131, 1996

57. Barbetseas J, Nagueh SF, Pitsavos C, et al: Differentiating thrombus from pannus formation in obstructed mechanical prosthetic valves: an evaluation of clinical, trans-thoracic and transesophageal echocardiographic parameters. J Am Coll Cardiol 32: 1410, 1998

58. Kallewaard M, Algra A, Defauw J, et al: Prophylactic replacement of Bjork-Shiley convexo-concave valves at risk of strut fracture: Bjork-Shiley Study Group. J Thorac Cardiovasc Surg 115:577, 1998

59. O'Neill WW, Chandler JG, Gordon RE, et al: Radiographic detection of strut separations in Björk-Shiley convexo-concave mitral valves. N Engl J Med 333:414, 1995

60. Garcia MJ, Vandervoort PM, Stewart WJ, et al: Mechanism of hemolysis with mitral prosthetic regurgitation: a study using transesophageal echo and fluid dynamic simulation. J Am Coll Cardiol 27:399, 1996

61. Chan WS, Anand S, Ginsberg JS: Anticoagulation of pregnant women with mechanical heart valves: a systemic review of the literature. Arch Intern Med 160:191, 2000

62. Weyman AE: The left ventricular outflow tract. Principles and Practice of Echocardiography, 2nd ed., rev. Weyman AE, Ed. Lea & Febiger, Philadelphia, 1994, p 513

63. Currie PJ, Seward JB, Reeder GS, et al: Continuous wave Doppler echocardiographic assessment of severity of calcific aortic stenosis: a simultaneous Doppler-catheter correlative study in 100 adult patients. Circulation 71:1162, 1985

64. Jick H, Vasilakis C, Weinnarich LA, et al: A population based study of appetite suppressant drugs and the risk of cardiac valve regurgitation. N Engl J Med 339:719, 1998

65. Weissman NJ, Tighe JF Jr, Gottdiener JS, et al: An assessment of heart-valve abnormalities in obese patients taking dexfenfluramine, sustained-release dexfenfluramine, or placebo. N Engl J Med 339:725, 1998

66. Jick H: Heart valve disorders and appetite-suppressant drugs. JAMA 283:1738, 2000

67. Weissman NJ, Tighe JF Jr, Gottdiener JS, et al: Prevalence of valvular-regurgitation associated with dexfenfluramine three to five months after discontinuation of treatment. J Am Coll Cardiol 34:2088, 1999

24 Diseases of the Aorta

Kim A. Eagle, M.D., and William F. Armstrong, M.D.

The Normal Aorta

The normal aorta is composed of three distinct layers: the inner intima, a thick elastic middle layer called the media, and a thin outer layer called the adventitia. In the media, layers of elastic elements intertwine with collagen and smooth muscle cells, providing the elastic strength that enables the aorta to withstand the pulsatile stress produced by the ejection of blood during ventricular systole. During systole, the aorta is distended by the force of blood ejected into the lumen. The kinetic energy of the ejected blood is transmitted to the wall of the aorta. In diastole, the potential energy stored in the aortic wall is transformed to kinetic energy as it propels the blood forward in the aorta and to its branches. With age, the normal elastic elements of the aorta degenerate, reducing its elasticity and distensibility. Because of this degenerative process, hypertension is more common and more difficult to control in the aging population.

Anatomically, the aorta is considered to consist of three important segments: the ascending aorta, the aortic arch, and the descending aorta. The ascending aorta consists of the aortic annulus, the aortic valve, the sinus of Valsalva, the sinotubular ridge, and the tubular portion of the ascending aorta. The ascending aorta connects the cardiovascular outflow tract at the aortic valve to the aortic arch, which begins at the brachiocephalic artery. The arch provides branches to the head and neck vessels, coursing just in front of the trachea and then proceeding to the left of the esophagus and the trachea. The descending aorta begins in the posterior mediastinum and courses in front of the vertebral column as it descends from the level of the ligament arteriosum to the bifurcation of the leg vessels.

Aortic Aneurysms

SCREENING FOR AORTIC ANEURYSMS

Current recommendations are for noninvasive screening of patients of appropriate age, which is typically defined as older than 65 years but younger if there is a significant family history of or risk factors for aneurysms. Screening may be particularly effective for obese patients, in whom abdominal palpation is of limited value. The cost-effectiveness of various screening strategies has yet to be demonstrated, however.[1] Careful abdominal palpation is probably cost-effective, particularly in men older than 55 years who are at risk for developing vascular disease. A related issue concerns which patients should undergo noninvasive imaging when the abdominal examination is difficult to perform.

ABDOMINAL AORTIC ANEURYSMS

An aorta is considered aneurysmal when its diameter exceeds 1.5 times the expected normal diameter at any location along its length. Aneurysms are divided into those that affect the abdominal cavity or the thoracic cavity. More extensive aneurysms (termed thoracoabdominal) involve both aortic areas. In addition, aneurysms are defined as either fusiform or saccular.

Aneurysms of the abdominal aorta are more common than thoracic aortic aneurysms. Among the risk factors for aneurysms, perhaps the most important is age. The incidence of aneurysms increases in men older than 55 years and in women older than 70 years. Overall, men are four to five times more likely to experience aortic aneurysms. Additional risk factors are smoking and a family history suggesting a genetic predisposition to aneurysms. Several reports show that aneurysms develop in as many as 25% of first-degree relatives of patients with abdominal aortic aneurysms.[2] The infrarenal aorta is the most commonly affected region.

Clinical Presentation

Most abdominal aortic aneurysms produce no symptoms and are discovered during a routine physical examination or as a result of noninvasive screening. The most common symptom is pain, often described as a steady, gnawing discomfort in the lower back or hypogastrium. Generally, the pain is not affected by movement.

In some patients, the abdominal aortic aneurysm is first discovered during a period of rapid expansion or an impending rupture, which is often marked by severe discomfort in the lower abdomen or back, radiating to the buttocks, groin, or legs. Rupture is accompanied by the abrupt onset of back and abdominal pain, abdominal tenderness, the presence of a palpable pulsatile mass, hypotension, and shock. However, only one third of aneurysms present in this fashion. Of note, a ruptured aneurysm may mimic other conditions, including abdominal colic, renal colic, diverticulitis, and gastrointestinal hemorrhage. Not surprisingly, more than 25% of patients presenting with rupture or expansion of an aortic aneurysm are initially misdiagnosed.

Patients with impending or actual rupture must be treated in the same way as a high-level trauma victim. Such patients rapidly experience hemorrhagic shock, manifested by peripheral vasoconstriction, hypotension, mottled skin, diaphoresis, oliguria, disorientation, and cardiac arrest. Patients with retroperitoneal rupture may show evidence of hematomas on the flank and in the groin. Although rare, rupture into the duodenum may present as massive upper or lower gastrointestinal hemorrhage.

Diagnostic Evaluation

Physical examination The abdominal aorta is usually detectable on deep palpation, particularly in thin persons. In obese patients, the normal aortic impulse may not be palpable. Obese patients may harbor a large aneurysm without any symptoms or findings on physical examination, unless the aneurysm is exerting pressure on an adjacent structure. Thin patients, in contrast, often feel a pulsatile mass in the abdomen when an abdominal aneurysm has developed.

When palpable, an aneurysm will be identified as a pulsatile mass extending from as high as the xiphoid process to the suprapubic area. Because of the layers of tissue between the examiner's fingers and the aneurysm, measurements of the transverse diameter of the aneurysm are typically overestimated. Also, it is difficult to differentiate ectatic aorta from aneurysm. Some aneurysms are sensitive to palpation and may be tender if they have recently expanded or are in impending rupture. Thus, palpation should be done with consideration of patient discomfort. Patients with aneurysms often have evidence of other peripheral vascular disease, such as femoral bruits and poor peripheral pulses.

Imaging studies Several diagnostic tools can help identify and measure the size of abdominal aortic aneurysms. Abdominal ultrasonography is the most frequently used method and the most practical.[3] Ultrasonography has a sensitivity of nearly 100% for diagnosing aneurysms of significant size and can discriminate size to within ±3 mm. Ultrasonography is inexpensive and noninvasive but may be inadequate for evaluating the most superior or inferior extent of an aneurysm and is generally considered inadequate as a sole diagnostic technique for planning surgical resection.

Computed tomography can discriminate aneurysm size to within ±2 mm. Because CT scanning can determine the inferior and superior extent of the aneurysm and its shape, this method is more useful for planning surgical repair. However, the need for radiographic contrast is a relative disadvantage. When a CT image is compared with an image derived from abdominal ultrasonography, the size of the aneurysm determined by CT is larger by approximately 2.7 mm.[4] New diagnostic techniques such as fast spiral CT have improved the resolution of CT scanning.

For years, aortography was considered the gold standard of diagnostic techniques for evaluating aortic aneurysms. One advantage of aortography is that it can be used to evaluate associated iliofemoral disease and involvement of the renal and mesenteric branches of the aorta. However, aortography is invasive and requires intravascular contrast, which carries a risk of nephrotoxicity. Its use has declined with the development of magnetic resonance angiography. Anatomic landmarks are more easily distinguished in the three-dimensional images created with MR angiography, which correctly defines the distal and proximal extent of an aneurysm in more than 75% of the cases examined.[5]

Management to Reduce Risk of Aneurysm Rupture

Current management of abdominal aortic aneurysm is directed at reducing the risk of rupture by intervening with timely surgical resection. Natural history studies show that the likelihood of rupture is greatest in patients with symptomatic, large, or rapidly expanding aneurysms. Aneurysms smaller than 4 cm in diameter have a low (< 2%) risk of rupture. Aneurysms exceeding 10 cm in diameter have a 25% risk of rupture over 2 years. Because aneurysms tend to expand with time, current strategies call for identifying and observing aneurysms that are asymptomatic and small enough not to have a high risk of rupture. The median rate of expansion is slightly less than 0.5 cm a year.[6] However, the tendency for expansion is variable and may not be linear. The more rapidly expanding aneurysms are more likely to rupture than a stable aneurysm. Aneurysms larger than 6 cm in diameter are generally referred for surgery, whereas aneurysms less than 4 cm in diameter are generally watched.[7] Evidence of expansion, particularly if the diameter of the aneurysm has exceeded 5.0 to 5.5 cm, is often taken as an indication to operate.[8] Current data support careful observation and serial noninvasive testing of patients with aneurysms between 4.0 and 5.5 cm in diameter.[9]

Surgical Treatment

Surgical treatment consists of resection of the aneurysm with insertion of a synthetic (Dacron) graft. Additional distal surgery is often necessary, with resection and interposition of grafts into one or both iliac arteries. For most large aneurysms, the aneurysm wall is left intact, and the Dacron graft is placed inside the aneurysm. The surgical treatment of abdominal aneurysms carries an average operative mortality of 4% to 6%. Surgical mortality is 2% in low-risk patients but may be as high as 20% to 50% in patients with impending or actual rupture.

A more recent therapeutic option is percutaneous placement of implantable endovascular stents, similar to those used in patients with coronary artery, renal artery, and peripheral artery stenoses. Some centers are using endovascular stents in nearly 50% of patients referred for treatment of abdominal aortic aneurysms.[10] Larger stents have been used successfully to isolate abdominal aortic aneurysms in patients for whom the risk of surgical resection is unacceptable. However, widespread application of stenting awaits further evaluation of long-term outcomes.[11]

Preoperative evaluation and management Appropriate preoperative evaluation and management of a patient before elective aortic aneurysm resection is critical. Reports suggest that one third to two thirds of perioperative deaths are attributed to coronary artery disease. A guideline published by the American College of Cardiology and the American Heart Association reviews the literature regarding preoperative assessment and presents a simple algorithm to help determine which patients should be considered for preoperative noninvasive testing for coronary disease [see Figure 1].[12]

The first consideration is whether the vascular surgery is urgent or emergent. By definition, emergent surgery cannot be delayed, and risk will be higher. In either case, the usual medical approach is to assume the patient may have preexisting coronary disease. Unless contraindicated, beta blockers should be used to treat such patients. Ideally, beta blockers should be started days to several weeks before surgery, titrating the dose to achieve a target heart rate of 50 to 60 beats a minute.[13] The clinical status, electrocardiogram, and hemodynamics of these patients should be monitored carefully after surgery.

For determination of perioperative risk, the first issue to address is whether the patient has had a recent coronary revascularization. If the patient has had coronary bypass surgery within 6 years and no subsequent coronary symptoms, the risk of perioperative events is low. A second issue is whether the patient has had a recent coronary evaluation. Further preoperative testing is not usually required for patients whose recent stress test or coronary angiogram indicates minimal or no coronary disease, particularly if the evaluation was performed within the previous 2 years and the patient has undergone no change in status.

Other patients with known prior coronary disease (prior myocardial infarction [MI] or angina), diabetes, or prior congestive heart failure should be more thoroughly evaluated. If such patients have poor functional capacity and have not undergone recent coronary evaluation, they should undergo a preoperative stress test to evaluate the severity of coronary artery disease and to determine the status of left ventricular function. When possible, exercise is generally the preferred method of stress testing[14] and appears to be safe in most patients. For patients who are unable to exercise, pharmacologic stress testing with either dobutamine echocardiography or adenosine thallium imaging is appropriate. Risk of cardiac events is directly related to the presence and extent of left ventricular (LV) dysfunction and ischemia.

The relative risk of perioperative cardiac morbidity or mortality is low (1% to 5%) in patients with no inducible ischemia and without evidence of fixed perfusion defects or wall-motion abnormalities. In patients with extensive areas of ischemia or prior infarction detected during preoperative testing, perioperative event rates (death and MI) may be as high as 20% to 40%. Such patients should probably undergo coronary angiography and possibly coronary revascularization before major operative procedures.

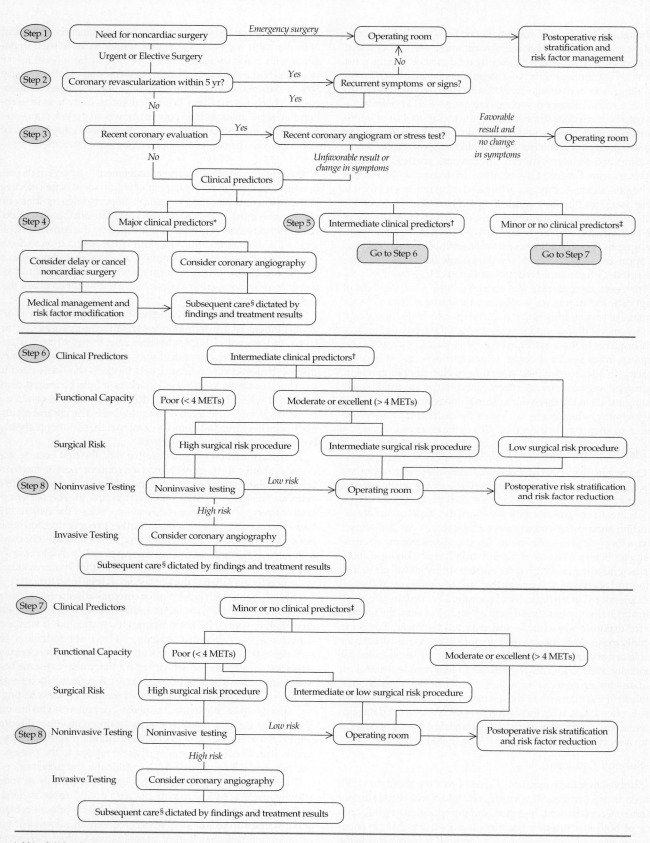

* Major clinical predictors: unstable coronary syndrome, decompensated CHF, significant arrhythmias, severe valvular disease.
† Intermediate clinical predictors: mild angina pectoris, prior MI, compensated or prior CHF, diabetes mellitus.
‡ Minor clinical predictors: advanced age, abnormal ECG, rhythm other than sinus, low functional capacity, history of stroke, uncontrolled systemic hypertension.
§ Subsequent care of patient may include cancellation or delay of surgery, coronary revascularization followed by surgery, or intensified care.

Figure 1   **Stepwise approach to cardiac assessment. (CHF—congestive heart failure; METs—metabolic equivalents; MI—myocardial infarction)**

Although the indications for coronary bypass surgery or percutaneous coronary interventions are generally the same in the preoperative patient as for the general population, evaluation for potential heart disease before aneurysm resection may be the patient's first such evaluation. Coronary artery disease must be treated to the fullest extent before undertaking a potentially stressful noncardiac operation on the aorta.

Postoperative modification of risk factors   A frequently forgotten issue in the management of patients undergoing abdominal aortic aneurysm resection is long-term modification of cardiovascular risk factors. The preoperative period represents an excellent opportunity to identify and treat hypertension, diabetes, hypercholesterolemia, smoking, obesity, and poor functional status. All patients identified as having vascular disease should take aspirin daily to prevent long-term cardiovascular events. Often, beta blockers are prescribed for patients with coronary artery disease, and the cholesterol profiles of such patients should be routinely assessed. Studies suggest that secondary prevention of vascular disease is enhanced by aggressive treatment of hypercholesterolemia, particularly in persons with a low-density-lipoprotein cholesterol exceeding 100 mg/dl. Currently, the best evidence suggests that the broad class of statin drugs (3-hydroxy-3-methylglutaryl coenzyme A [HMG-CoA] reductase inhibitors) are effective. Beta blockers have been championed as therapy both to reduce risk of MI and to potentially reduce the risk of expansion of aneurysms that may develop or be present elsewhere in patients who previously had significant aneurysms.

THORACIC AORTIC ANEURYSMS

Thoracic aortic aneurysms, which are less common than abdominal aneurysms, are classified according to the involvement of the ascending aorta, the descending aorta, or a combination. Aneurysms of the descending aorta are the most common. The etiology of thoracic aneurysms correlates with their location. Descending thoracic aortic aneurysms, which are seen in patients with extensive atherosclerosis, usually originate beyond the left subclavian artery and may be either fusiform or saccular. Aneurysms of the arch are often contiguous with aneurysms of the ascending or descending thoracic aorta.

The etiology generally reflects the process that has led to the ascending or descending aneurysm. Aneurysms of the ascending aorta are usually associated with cystic medial necrosis. This association is particularly common in patients with Marfan syndrome, Ehlers-Danlos syndrome, and annuloaortic ectasia, which represents the loss of elastic tensile strength in the aorta.

Clinical Presentation

More than half of thoracic aortic aneurysms are symptomatic; the rest are discovered only incidentally, often after a routine chest x-ray. Symptoms usually reflect pressure on a contiguous structure, leading to pain or such vascular consequences as concomitant aortic insufficiency, causing congestive heart failure; pressure on a coronary artery, causing angina; and arterial thromboembolism, causing cerebral, lower-extremity, mesenteric, or renal ischemia or infarction. Local mass effects may include a superior vena cava syndrome, caused by obstruction of the superior vena cava; pressure on a trachea, leading to cough or wheezing; and, occasionally, dramatic hemoptysis, resulting from fistula formation between the aneurysm and a major airway. Pressure on the esophagus may produce dysphagia. Pressure on the recurrent laryngeal nerve may result in hoarseness. Chest pain is usually caused by direct pressure of the aneurysm on an intrathoracic structure or by erosion of a bony structure. Normally, this pain is steady and often severe.

A leaking or ruptured aneurysm usually presents with dramatic symptoms. Most such aneurysms leak or rupture into the left pleural space or intrapericardial space, resulting in hypotension and sudden onset of severe pain. Aortoesophageal fistulas may produce life-threatening gastrointestinal bleeding.

Diagnostic Evaluation

Physical examination   The thoracic aorta is generally not palpable unless there is a significant pathologic process. Most often, this pathologic process consists of an ascending aortic arch aneurysm, and the aortic impulse can be palpated just above the sternum or at the right upper sternal border.

Imaging studies   The diagnosis of thoracic aortic aneurysms is rarely suspected on physical examination. It is more often initially suspected on chest x-ray and then confirmed with noninvasive or invasive imaging.

On chest x-ray, most aneurysms are visible and appear as a widening of the mediastinal silhouette. Small aneurysms may be invisible. MRI and fast or spiral CT scanning are the most commonly used methods for delineating the size and extent of thoracic aneurysms. Transthoracic echocardiography and transesophageal echocardiography (TEE) are also used to diagnose, measure, and monitor ascending aortic aneurysms. TEE can evaluate only the proximal 3 to 5 cm of the ascending aorta and is not useful for evaluating aneurysms below the diaphragm.

Management to Reduce Risk of Aneurysm Rupture

The natural history of a thoracic aneurysm can shed light on the disease process that has led to the aneurysm, on the risk factors that may affect the rate of aneurysm expansion, and on the concomitant presence of other vascular disease, including peripheral and coronary disease, that might affect long-term survival. Because size is a critical issue in terms of the risk of rupture, the initial size and potential growth of an aneurysm are important factors in the decision whether to operate on asymptomatic aneurysms. Aneurysms that are invading local structures or creating a marked vascular effect should usually be resected. Careful control of blood pressure is crucial for all patients and may require medical therapy, particularly with beta blockers, which may also slow the rate of aneurysm growth.[15]

The initial size of a thoracic aneurysm is an important predictor of subsequent growth. In general, small aneurysms tend to grow slowly, whereas large aneurysms have a higher probability of growth and rupture. On average, thoracic aneurysms grow at 0.43 cm/yr, but the growth rate varies greatly.[16] Small aneurysms (i.e., < 5 cm in diameter) grow at about 0.1 cm/yr. Large aneurysms (i.e., > 5 cm) grow at about 0.5 to 1.0 cm/yr. Although these average growth rates are reassuring, it should be emphasized that rapid expansion can occur and can dramatically affect the natural history and management. In general, thoracic aneurysms smaller than 5 cm in diameter are unlikely to rupture, whereas those larger than 7 cm are at high risk for rupture. Currently, most thoracic centers recommend surgery for aneurysms that exceed 5.5 to 6 cm in an otherwise reasonable surgical candidate.[17,18] Because of their relatively young age, absence of associated disease, and low surgical risk of elective repair, patients with Marfan syndrome should undergo surgery when aneurysms reach 5 cm, particularly if the aneurysm is growing. Some centers wait until aneurysms reach 6.5 or 7 cm before operating on high-risk surgical candidates. As in the case of treatment of abdominal aneurysm, the use of percutaneously placed aortic stent grafts may emerge as an attractive option in some patients with thoracic aneurysms.[19]

Surgical Treatment

The surgical approach to thoracic aortic aneurysms depends on the site. For ascending aortic aneurysms, the major issue is whether the aortic valve is competent and whether reimplantation of the coronary arteries will be necessary. With the availability of aortic homografts and stentless valves, surgical approaches to thoracic aortic aneurysm are undergoing rapid evolution. Individual patient characteristics and surgical preferences have a great deal to do with a given surgical approach.

Postoperative Complications

Neurologic sequelae are the most serious of potential postoperative complications. Currently, the risk of stroke after thoracic aneurysm resection ranges from 3% to 7%.[20] Efforts to reduce diffuse brain injury caused by prolonged periods of aortic cross clamping include hypothermic arrest and the use of retrograde cerebral perfusion by way of a superior vena cava cannula.[21] Efforts to reduce CNS embolic events focus on meticulous surgical techniques to avoid dislodging atheroemboli present in the aortic margins and to avoid air embolism during surgery. The above issues are especially pertinent in aneurysms of the ascending aorta and the arch. Surgery on the posterior thoracic aorta carries a different neurologic risk—namely, postoperative paraplegia as a result of interrupting the supply of arterial blood to the spinal cord—and occurs in more than 5% of patients. Several methods have been devised to deal with this risk, but no definitive solution has yet emerged. Some centers have suggested that reattaching critical intercostal arteries leads to improved outcome,[22] whether or not the spinal cord is treated under epidural cooling during surgery.[23]

Aortic Dissection

The incidence of recognized aortic dissection is estimated at 10 to 20 per million population, or about 5,000 cases a year in the United States. We stress, however, that the incidence of MI is greater than 500,000 cases annually; that is, MI is at least 100 times more common than aortic dissection. For most patients, dissection entails a tear in the intima, with the subsequent development of a propagating hematoma between the intima and the adventitia. Approximately two thirds of aortic dissections are initiated by a tear in the intima just above the aortic valve.[24] Most of the remaining cases develop in the descending aorta at the attachment of the ligamentum arteriosum. Often, multiple reentry sites are present between the true lumen and the false lumen, and the dissection spirals as it courses retrograde or antegrade along the aorta. Approximately 10% to 15% of aortic dissections are caused by intramural hematoma, which is spontaneous rupture of the vaso vasorum within the media, creating a hematoma that may propagate.

CLASSIFICATION

Aortic dissections are classified as acute or chronic and according to their location. Dissections are termed acute when they are diagnosed within 2 weeks of the onset of symptoms; dissections diagnosed after 2 weeks of symptom onset are termed chronic.[25]

A key feature for classification is involvement of the ascending aorta, regardless of where the dissection began. Ascending aortic dissections are also called type A dissections. Dissections not involving the ascending aorta are typically classified as distal, or type B, dissections. Ascending aortic involvement identifies a patient population with high mortality if not treated surgically. Normally, the life-threatening condition is caused by communication of the ascending aorta with the pericardial space, creating cardiac tamponade, or by spontaneous rupture or hemorrhage, leading to shock.

The predisposing factors for type A and type B dissections differ somewhat. Disorders of the media that result in cystic medial necrosis are a common forerunner of type A aortic dissection. Typically, affected patients include those with Marfan syndrome or other heritable disorders, such as Ehlers-Danlos syndrome, Noonan syndrome, and Turner syndrome. Another risk factor for ascending aortic dissection is aortic valve disease, such as bicuspid valve disease or prosthetic aortic valve disease. Although these conditions are classically associated with aortic dissection, the majority of patients (> 90%) with acute aortic dissection do not have any recognized substrate for dissection. Distal or type B aortic dissection is seen in patients with hypertension. Patients with type B dissection are older on average than patients with type A dissection. An unexplained relation between aortic dissection and pregnancy also exists, perhaps because of changes in cardiac output, blood pressure, or blood volume or the effects of pregnancy on the aortic wall itself.[26] Aortic dissection after inhalation of crack cocaine has also been reported.[27]

ETIOLOGY

Aortic dissection may occur after manipulation of the aorta—for example, during coronary artery angiography or interventions or during cardiac surgery, when the aorta is cross-clamped or when buttons of tissue are removed to allow placement of saphenous vein grafts for aortocoronary bypass.[28]

CLINICAL PRESENTATION

The most common distinguishing clinical feature of aortic dissection is the abrupt onset of pain.[28] The abruptness of onset is one of the clinical features reliably distinguishing the pain of aortic dissection from that accompanying other cardiovascular pathologies. This instantaneous pain may begin in the chest or back and may migrate to involve the neck, head, back, and legs as the dissecting hematoma propagates. The classic combination of abrupt tearing pain, with pulse deficits and apparent aortic insufficiency, is seldom observed in practice.[28,29] Other presentations of type A dissection are sudden syncope or hypotension, resulting from dissection into the pericardial space; stroke, resulting from interruption of the blood supply to one or both internal carotid arteries; and, in rare instances, isolated congestive heart failure, when the dissection involves the ascending aorta and interrupts aortic valve function.

The most typical presentation of type B dissection is onset of severe interscapular pain, which may radiate down the back toward the legs. Type B dissection is frequently accompanied by hypertension, whereas type A dissection more often occurs in the presence of normal or low blood pressure.[28] Spinal cord ischemia, ischemic extremities, and mesenteric ischemia are most frequently encountered in type A dissection that has extended to involve the descending aorta. Whereas aortic insufficiency is seen in 35% to 50% of the cases of ascending aortic dissection, it is rather unusual in cases of type B dissection. Pulse deficits are seen in about

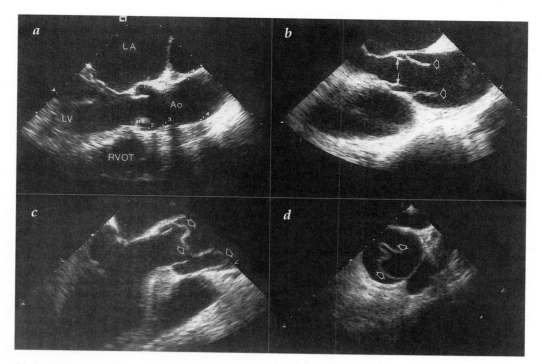

Figure 2 Transesophageal echocardiograms from a patient with a normal ascending aorta (panel A) and three different ascending aortic dissections (panels B through D). In the normal ascending aorta, the cardiac chambers are noted. The ascending aorta is well visualized, including its annulus (point 1), the coronary sinuses (point 2), the sinotubular junction (point 3), and the true ascending aorta (point 4). Note that the aorta dilates at the level of the sinuses, narrows at the sinotubular junction to a dimension equivalent to that of the annulus, and then slightly dilates further in the ascending aorta. Shown is a normal aortic valve in its open position. Panel B was recorded in a patient with a proximal aortic dissection. The orientation is identical to that in panel A. The solid arrows denote the position of an open aortic valve leaflet. The open arrows represent the margins of a dissection that originated at the sinotubular junction and extended distally. Panel C was recorded in a patient with an ascending aortic dissection (orientation identical to that in panels A and B), and the aortic valve is open. In this instance, a convoluted intimal flap (open arrows) is clearly visualized in the proximal ascending aorta. Panel D was recorded in the short axis of the aorta in a patient with an aortic dissection. In the circular ascending aorta, multiple convolutions of an intimal flap are clearly visualized (open arrows). Note that a communication point (between the downward pointing arrow and the wall of the aorta) allows free communication of flow between the two lumens. (LA—left atrium; Ao—ascending aorta; RVOT—right ventricular outflow tract; LV—left ventricle)

25% of patients with type A dissection and in perhaps 5% to 10% of patients with type B dissection.[28,30]

DIAGNOSTIC EVALUATION

Because acute aortic dissection is a life-threatening emergency, rapid and accurate diagnosis is crucial to patient survival. Therefore, sophisticated imaging modalities may be required. Routine ECG in patients with suspected aortic dissection usually reveals only nonspecific abnormalities on the electrocardiogram. Although type A dissection will affect one of the coronary arteries and lead to a transmural MI in 1% to 2% of patients, most patients have nonspecific ST-T wave changes or a finding of left ventricular hypertrophy related to long-standing hypertension.

The typical chest x-ray reveals widening of the mediastinal silhouette and may also demonstrate evidence of a pleural effusion, cardiomegaly, or congestive failure if severe aortic regurgitation is present. A normal-appearing chest x-ray is seen in more than 10% of such cases.[28] Other laboratory abnormalities are generally nonspecific. An increase of smooth muscle myosin is present in more than 85% of patients presenting within 3 hours of onset of acute aortic dissection.[31] This serum assay, if further developed, may become a useful adjunctive tool to early assessment of suspected aortic dissection.[31]

After a careful history and physical examination, the key to diagnosis is rapid identification of the aortic dissection, ascertainment of whether the ascending aorta is involved, and urgent cardiac surgery if proximal aortic dissection is diagnosed. The importance of rapid diagnosis and institution of definitive therapy for aortic dissection cannot be overemphasized. Given the 1% to 2% mortality per hour in the first 24 hours after presentation, even brief delays to achieve diagnostic imaging are unacceptable.[28,32]

Currently, four diagnostic tools are used to evaluate patients with suspected dissection[33]: CT scanning, echocardiography, MRI, and aortography. In general, the choice of which imaging modality to initially employ will depend on local expertise and availability. In most hospitals, the choice is either CT or MRI.

CT scanning is widely available in most community and tertiary care hospitals. Spiral or ultrafast CT scanning gives even greater resolution than the older scanners and has a reported sensitivity and specificity for aortic dissection exceeding 95%.[34,35] TEE offers significant advantages in diagnosis [*see Figures 2 and 3*].[36] The primary attractiveness of TEE is its portability, making it suitable to be performed in the emergency department, intensive care unit, or operating room. Thus, imaging can be achieved substantially faster with TEE than with other modalities.[37] Second, TEE is highly sensitive for the identification of type A dissection. TEE is also potentially useful when the degree of involvement of the aortic valve and the status of the left ventricle, pericardial space, and right and left coronary artery ostia are unknown.[38]

TEE can be very useful in detecting the mechanism of aortic insufficiency and detecting the feasibility of repair.[39,40] Valves in which aortic insufficiency is the result of sinotubular dilatation or extension of the dissection into the sinus are often candidates for repair. Patients with intrinsic disease of the aortic valve leaflets are less optimal candidates for repair.

MRI is less commonly used where the MRI scanner is part of the emergency department.[41] For most hospitals, however, the delay required in getting a patient into the suite and completing the MRI makes this technology less efficient than TEE.

Finally, although aortography is still used in some hospitals, it is seldom the initial test for aortic dissection. The reported false negative rate for aortography is in the range of 5% to 15%.[42] Aortography frequently misses lesions such as an intramural hematoma. In addition, the time required to get a patient to an angiography suite and complete the study is generally considerably longer than TEE. Our medical center and many others follow an algorithmic approach to evaluation and treatment of a suspected aortic dissection [see Figure 4].

TREATMENT

The treatment of aortic dissection includes aggressive medical therapy for all patients and definitive surgical therapy in selected patients. The decision to perform surgery depends first and foremost on the site of the aortic dissection [see Figure 4].

Surgical Repair

Type A aortic dissection Any involvement of the ascending aorta carries with it a much greater risk for rupture into the pericardial space; development of coronary or cerebral ischemia, aortic regurgitation, and congestive heart failure; or free rupture of the aorta into the thorax. Thus, in an appropriate candidate, definitive surgical repair is carried out as quickly as possible for patients with proximal or type A aortic dissection.

For patients with type A dissection complicated by malperfusion, medical therapy plus percutaneous reperfusion utilizing aortic stenting or fenestration, or both, and selective branch stenting may allow stabilization and reduce risk of the operation. Af-

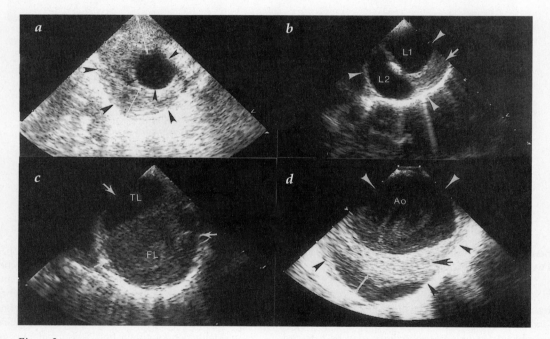

Figure 3 **Panels A through D represent four transesophageal echocardiograms recorded in a short-axis view of the descending thoracic aorta in patients with aortic pathology. Panel A was recorded in a patient with an ascending aortic aneurysm and a large periaortic (adventitial) hematoma extending distally along the thoracic aorta. The smaller black arrows denote the boundaries of the normal-diameter descending thoracic aorta. The larger black arrows pointing inward mark the full dimension of the periaortic hematoma; the full dimension is also noted by the double-headed white arrows. In this instance, the intima of the descending thoracic aorta was not involved in the dissection process. However, a large periadventitial hematoma ruptured along the course of the descending thoracic aorta. Panel B was recorded in a patient with an aortic dissection localized to the descending thoracic aorta. The maximum external dimensions of the aorta are noted by the large white arrowheads. The white arrow notes an area of atherosclerosis and thrombus within the aorta. Two distinct lumens (L1 and L2) can be seen at this level. Panel C was recorded in a patient with an aortic dissection extending from the aortic valve to the bifurcation of the aorta. The large white arrows denote the outer dimension of the aorta. There is an echo-free lumen, or true lumen (TL), and a false lumen (FL) with early thrombus formation. Note the vague echo densities within the false lumen. Panel D was recorded in a patient with a large descending thoracic aortic aneurysm and intramural hematoma. The large arrowheads (black and white) denote the outer dimensions of the aorta. The dilated aortic lumen (Ao) is also noted. The black arrow denotes an area of marked atherosclerosis within the aorta, and the double-headed white arrow denotes an area of intramural hemorrhage, characterized by a lower echo density than the atherosclerotic components. Note also the low-density echoes, which represent stagnant blood flow within the aorta.**

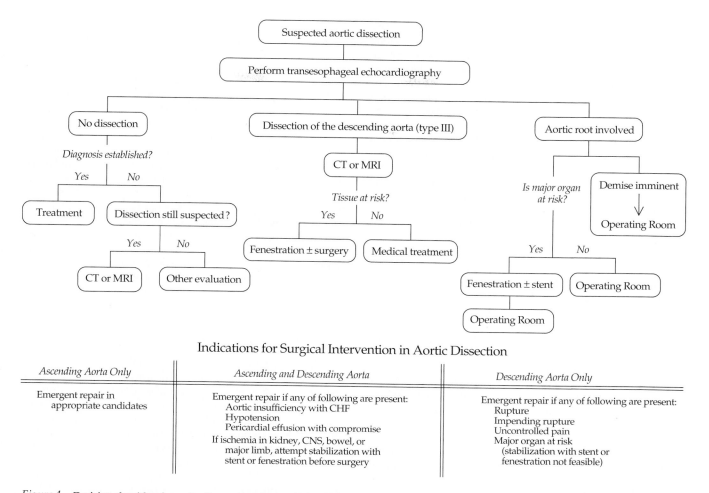

Indications for Surgical Intervention in Aortic Dissection

Ascending Aorta Only	*Ascending and Descending Aorta*	*Descending Aorta Only*
Emergent repair in appropriate candidates	Emergent repair if any of following are present: Aortic insufficiency with CHF Hypotension Pericardial effusion with compromise If ischemia in kidney, CNS, bowel, or major limb, attempt stabilization with stent or fenestration before surgery	Emergent repair if any of following are present: Rupture Impending rupture Uncontrolled pain Major organ at risk (stabilization with stent or fenestration not feasible)

Figure 4 **Decision algorithm for evaluation and treatment of a suspected aortic dissection. Type III dissection originates in the descending aorta and extends distally down the aorta or, in rare instances, retrograde into the aortic arch and ascending aorta. (CHF—congestive heart failure)**

ter a period of recovery, repair of the patient's ascending aorta may be undertaken.[43]

Definitive aortic repair includes resection of the dissected aorta and insertion of a conduit. The procedure often includes implanting a prosthetic aortic valve. More recently, repair and resuspension of the aortic valve have proved feasible in many patients. For most patients, repair includes reimplantation of the coronary arteries. In some patients, this repair includes resection and placement of a graft to the aortic arch.

Type B aortic dissection Surgery for type B dissection is predominantly indicated for patients with life-threatening complications that require a surgical approach. Examples include patients who experience ischemia of both kidneys, leading to reversible renal failure; development of ischemic bowel; ischemia involving one of the legs or arms; development of a progressive aneurysm; impending rupture; and recurrent extension of the dissection. In some centers, percutaneous insertion of aortic stents has been used to stabilize dissections of the descending aorta. This strategy may be preferable to surgery in some candidates.[44-46] In particular, stenting may promote thrombosis of the false channel and thereby reduce the long-term risk of aneurysm formation and aortic rupture. Surgical placement of an endoprosthesis, or so-called elephant trunk, has also been advocated as a preferred strategy for operative type B dissection.[47,48]

Postoperative Complications

In the management of aortic dissection, surgical complications can be divided into the sequelae of operations involving the ascending aorta and those of operations involving the arch or descending aorta. Because some period of circulatory arrest is often required to approach the ascending aorta or arch, the most severe complication of surgery in this region is cerebral anoxia, with postoperative neurologic dysfunction. Currently, most aortic centers of excellence perform this operation under conditions of deep hypothermia and circulatory arrest, along with retrograde cerebral perfusion by way of the jugular veins. This technique has dramatically diminished the incidence of severe neurologic injury after aortic surgery.

For surgery on the descending aorta, the most serious complication is interruption of the blood supply to the spinal cord, with resultant paraplegia. Procedures to reduce this complication include the use of shunts and the careful isolation of ostia of the spinal arteries with reimplantation. This complication remains the one most feared in descending-aorta surgery. Additional risks are acute renal failure, mesenteric ischemia, distal atheroembolic events, and pulmonary complications.

Medical Therapy

All patients with aortic dissection receive aggressive medical therapy. This treatment is first directed at controlling the blood pressure. For patients who are hypertensive, administration of intravenous beta blockers followed by oral beta blockers, along with the concomitant administration of intravenous or oral vasodilators, is imperative. Patients who are normotensive should maintain a low-normal blood pressure and a low heart rate. The likelihood for propagation of dissection is believed to be in part related to acceleration of flow in the aorta, that is, the force of the aortic jet per unit time (i.e., dp/dt). Accordingly, beta blockers have been the most important therapy for the medical treatment of aortic dissection. Such therapy should maintain heart rates at or below 60 beats/min and keep blood pressure as low as possible while allowing perfusion of the brain, kidneys, and other vital organs. Also important are careful measurements of urine output and filling pressures of the heart.

Long-term management of aortic dissection requires aggressive medical therapy and careful surveillance. Patients who retain patency in the false channel of the aorta after either medical treatment or surgical repair have a significant risk of aneurysm formation and rupture of the false channel, especially in the first 6 months after initial therapy.[49] Expansion, rupture, or both are more common among patients who are older and have poorly controlled hypertension and chronic obstructive pulmonary disease.[50] Aggressive treatment of blood pressure and heart rate and careful monitoring of the patient's status with physical examination and noninvasive imaging are essential. At many centers, either CT scanning or MRI is performed on a regular basis after initial treatment of the dissection. For instance, the patient might be seen at 2 to 4 weeks after admission for adjustment of dosages of antihypertensive medications and beta blockers. At our center, spiral CT scanning is done 3 months or, sometimes, 6 months after surgery to screen for the development of aneurysm in the false channel or at the margins of a surgical repair. After this, patients undergo aortic imaging at least once a year and aggressive antihypertensive therapy.

Atypical Aortic Dissection

AORTIC DISSECTION WITHOUT INTIMAL TEAR

About 10% to 15% of patients presenting with symptoms suggestive of aortic dissection actually have aortic dissection without an intimal tear (intramural hematoma).[29,51] This hemorrhage into the medial layer of the aorta may produce a localized or discrete hematoma or may extend for various distances by dissecting along the outer media adjacent to the adventitia. Clinically, this hemorrhage mirrors aortic dissection in terms of both its risk factors and its presentation. Intramural hematoma is generally not identified on aortography. It is most easily diagnosed with ultrafast CT scanning. With noncontrast imaging, the hematoma appears as a crescent-shaped high-attenuation area along the aortic wall; moreover, this region cannot be enhanced with contrast imaging. MRI reveals the same crescent-shaped high-intensity area [see Figure 3], whereas on TEE, intramural hematoma may appear as a circular or crescentic thickening.[52]

Studies of the natural history of the intramural hematoma suggest that the outcome may be similar to that of classic aortic dissection. By 30 days, the rate of aortic expansion or death in patients with medically treated ascending aortic intramural hematoma approaches 50%. Patients with aneurysmal aortas—that is, those with aortas measuring more than 5 cm in diameter—are at particular risk.[53] By contrast, the mortality for intramural hematoma in the descending aorta appears to be between 10% and 15%, similar to that for distal type B aortic dissection.[29]

A second unusual type of aortic disease is a penetrating atherosclerotic ulcer. Penetrating ulcers of the aorta result from erosion of the intima of the aorta, usually because of extensive atherosclerosis. Ulcer formation may produce a hematoma in the media that extends several centimeters from its origin up or down the aorta. Occasionally, pseudoaneurysms are created that may extend into the adventitia and, in rare instances, may rupture. This aortic process develops gradually in elderly patients with extensive atherosclerosis and often is heralded by chest pain or back pain and hypertension. By usually presenting as a localized process, it is seldom associated with other symptoms of aortic dissection, such as pulse deficits, aortic valve regurgitation, and neurologic defects. Symptomatic penetrating atherosclerotic ulcer may require surgery. Asymptomatic patients who experience progressive enlargemenia or recurrent atheroemboli may also require surgical therapy. For most patients, however, medical therapy primarily entails aggressive treatment of atherosclerotic risk factors, including cessation of smoking, control of hypertension, lipid-lowering therapy, and careful surveillance. The role of antiplatelet or anticoagulant therapy for this condition is not clear.

Aortic Atheromatous Emboli

Atherosclerosis of the aorta may be so extensive that it leads to overlying thrombosis and subsequent dislodging of thrombi, cholesterol particles, or fibrinous material into the CNS or peripheral circulation. Risk factors are hypertension, diabetes, hyperlipidemia, advanced age, and other vascular diseases. Atheromatous disease is most common in the distal aorta but may also occur in the ascending aorta and arch. Evidence of ulceration of atherosclerotic plaques is an independent risk factor for stroke, as is the identification of a mobile, large, protruding aortic atheroma detected with TEE.[54] Plaques more than 4 mm in diameter in the ascending aorta are particularly associated with an increased risk of ischemic stroke.[55] Atheroemboli or cholesterol-particle emboli may also involve the peripheral extremities, leading to ischemic lesions on the feet or toes (so-called blue-toe syndrome). These emboli may present as abdominal pain as a result of ischemic bowel. Acute nonoliguric renal failure is another occasional manifestation, as is gastrointestinal bleeding or pancreatitis. Cutaneous involvement may produce a characteristic skin lesion called livedo reticularis.

Cholesterol embolism syndrome is particularly common after manipulation of the aorta. It is most common in patients undergoing cardiac catheterization or other angiographic procedures in which catheters or wires are manipulated within the aorta. Because the occurrence of atheroemboli may be delayed some months after aortic manipulation, the relation between the two may not be apparent when the patient is first examined. If cutaneous manifestations are present, a biopsy of the lesions will often identify needle-shaped clefts in the arteriolar lumen characteristic of cholesterol particles that have embolized to the small vessels.

Treatment of cholesterol embolism syndrome begins with avoidance of further aortic manipulation (e.g., cardiac catheterization), if this has been a precipitant. Aggressive treatment of hypercholesterolemia is warranted. A search for an aortic aneurysm or protruding mobile atheromas is appropriate in patients for whom the syndrome develops without a concomitant iatrogenic source. Occasionally, recurrent emboli warrant the resection of an aneurysm or of a severely diseased segment of atheromatous aorta.[56] The role of anticoagulant and antiplatelet drugs in this syndrome is uncertain.

Takayasu Arteritis and Giant Cell Arteritis

TAKAYASU ARTERITIS

Takayasu arteritis is a rare inflammatory condition that affects the aorta and its major branches. Other names include aortic arch syndrome, pulseless disease, and young female arteritis.[57]

Epidemiology

Although Takayasu arteritis is seen throughout the world, most cases occur in Asia and Africa. A specific etiologic agent has yet to be identified, but current evidence favors an autoimmune mechanism. Some studies suggest it may be linked to rheumatic fever, streptococcal infections, certain HLA subtypes, rheumatoid arthritis, and other collagen vascular diseases. Takayasu arteritis is more prevalent in women than in men. By definition, most patients are young, with an average age of 29 years.

Pathophysiology

Takayasu arteritis generally involves a granulomatous arteritis of the aorta and its branches, with subsequent involvement of the media and adventitia. Later, the disease may progress to a sclerotic stage in which the intima is hyperplastic, the media degenerates, and the adventitia develops fibrosis. This late fibrotic process may encroach on the lumen of the aorta or its branches. Common areas of involvement are the main aorta and branch points of its major branch vessels. The pulmonary artery may also be involved. The coronary arteries are affected in fewer than 10% of patients. In some patients, involvement of the ascending aorta may lead to aortic valve regurgitation.

Classification

Takayasu arteritis has been divided into three types.[58] Type I involves the aortic arch and its branches, type II involves the distal aorta and spares the arch, and type III may affect both the ascending aorta and the descending aorta. A suggested fourth category involves the pulmonary arteries.

Clinical Presentation

The initial symptoms are often typical of an acute or systemic inflammatory process, including fever, loss of appetite, weight loss, night sweats, and arthralgias.[59] Involved vessels may have accompanying localized tenderness over them. By the time the diagnosis is established, most patients have reached a sclerotic phase, in which vascular insufficiency is causing the predominant symptoms. It may involve the upper or lower extremities. Hypertension occurs in more than half of patients. Congestive heart failure occurs in 25% of them because of hypertension, aortic valve insufficiency, or involvement of the coronary arteries.

Diagnostic Evaluation

Laboratory findings in patients with Takayasu arteritis generally include an elevated erythrocyte sedimentation rate, mild anemia, and a slightly increased white blood cell count. The chest x-ray may demonstrate a rim of calcification around the involved vessels. Aortography often shows an irregular intimal surface with stenoses of the aorta or its branch arteries. Poststenotic dilatation or frank arterial aneurysms may be visible. Similar diagnostic features can also be detected by TEE and MRI.[60,61] Among the established criteria for the clinical diagnosis of Takayasu arteritis is that patients must be no more than 40 years of age to have this diagnosis.

Treatment

The management of Takayasu arteritis begins with high-dose glucocorticoid therapy, which usually leads to abatement of constitutional symptoms and the laboratory signs of inflammation. Serial sedimentation rates are useful for monitoring the benefits of treatment. For patients who fail to respond to steroid therapy, cyclophosphamide at a daily dosage of 2 mg/kg has been used. Alternatively, low-dose methotrexate may enhance the efficacy of steroids or allow steroid tapering. Surgery may be necessary to treat unremitting ischemia, symptomatic coronary disease, or aortic valve disease or to treat renal artery stenosis that causes severe hypertension. Percutaneously placed arterial stents have successfully treated segmental disease in a variety of vessels in patients with this syndrome.

GIANT CELL ARTERITIS

Giant cell arteritis is another form of aortoarteritis. In contrast to Takayasu disease, this illness is more commonly seen in Europe and the United States and in patients older than 50 years (the mean age at onset of disease is 67 years).

Pathophysiology

This form of arteritis often affects the branches of the proximal aorta, particularly the branches supplying the head and neck, the extracranial structures (including the temporal arteries), and the upper extremities. Aortic involvement often coexists with temporal arteritis and polymyalgia rheumatica. Unlike Takayasu arteritis, giant cell arteritis seldom has a sclerotic phase progressing to occlusion of vessels. However, giant cell arteritis may lead to aneurysm formation, aortic regurgitation, or aortic dissection.[62,63]

Clinical Presentation

The classic presentation of giant cell arteritis consists of headaches, tenderness over involved arteries in the scalp or the temporal region, jaw claudication, difficulty combing one's hair, and constitutional symptoms. Fever is common, and the blood vessels involved are thick and tender. Pulses may be diminished, and bruits may be present. Occasionally, signs of aortic valve regurgitation are present.

A serious complication of this syndrome is blindness, which results when arteritis affects the ophthalmic artery. The progression to total blindness may be rapid. Visual symptoms of some type occur in as many as 50% of patients. In rare instances, giant cell arteritis may lead to reduced upper extremity pulses and blood pressure along with arm or leg claudication. It also may cause coronary ischemia or abdominal angina in rare cases. Unlike Takayasu arteritis, giant cell arteritis virtually never affects the kidneys. Aortic aneurysms occur in 15% of patients with giant cell arteritis, most commonly involving the ascending aorta. Such aneurysms may develop late in the disease, leading to rupture, aortic dissection, or severe aortic valve regurgitation.

Diagnostic Evaluation

An above-normal erythrocyte sedimentation rate is characteristic of this disease, and the diagnosis is confirmed by biopsy of an involved artery, usually the temporal artery. Clinicians need to be aware, however, that temporal artery biopsy may be negative in as many as 15% of patients with confirmed disease; therefore, a second biopsy may be necessary in patients with a high likelihood of temporal arteritis.

Treatment

Standard therapy for giant cell arteritis is high-dose glucocorticoid therapy (e.g., prednisone, 40 to 60 mg/day). Methotrexate may be used to reduce the need for steroids or to treat patients who respond inadequately to steroids. Cyclophosphamide may also be useful for reducing the need for glucocorticoids. Surgery is typically reserved for patients who experience progressive ischemic symptoms or aortic aneurysms.

Traumatic Disease of the Aorta

Finally, a relatively common form of aortic pathology is partial or complete transsection as a result of major blunt thoracic trauma, most commonly as a result of high-speed motor vehicle accidents. Most patients with complete aortic transsection do not survive long enough for hospital evaluation. Patients with partial transsection often survive long enough to undergo surgical correction. Evidence of aortic trauma is often obscured by other major organ trauma. Patients with aortic transsection are typically in shock and may have diminished lower extremity pulses. The transsection is usually located at the distal arch, immediately after the origin of the left subclavian artery.

Rapid diagnosis is the key to the survival of patients with aortic transsection. The routine chest x-ray typically reveals a widened mediastinum, often with pleural effusions. The gold standard for diagnosis of this disorder remains aortography, but TEE,[54,64-67] CT, and MRI have also been used successfully. Successful treatment requires vigorous fluid and blood resuscitation and surgical repair of the aortic transsection.

References

1. Frame PS, Fryback DG, Patterson C: Screening for abdominal aortic aneurysm in men ages 60 to 80 years: a cost-effectiveness analysis. Ann Intern Med 119:411, 1993

2. Crawford ES, Cohen ES: Aortic aneurysm: a multifocal disease. Arch Surg 117:1393, 1982

3. Ernst CB: Abdominal aortic aneurysm. N Engl J Med 328:1167, 1993

4. Lederle FA, Wilson SE, Johnson GR, et al: Variability in measurements of abdominal aortic aneurysms. J Vasc Surg 21:945, 1995

5. Petersen MJ, Cambria RP, Kaufman JA, et al: Magnetic resonance angiography in the preoperative evaluation of abdominal aortic aneurysms. J Vasc Surg 21:891, 1995

6. Gadowski GR, Pilcher DB, Ricci MA: Abdominal aortic aneurysm expansion rate: effect of size and beta-adrenergic blockade. J Vasc Surg 19:727, 1994

7. Hollier LD, Taylor LM, Ochsner J: Recommended indications for operative treatment of abdominal aortic aneurysms: report of a subcommittee of the Joint Council of the Society for Vascular Surgery and of the North American Chapter of the International Society for Cardiovascular Surgery. J Vasc Surg 15:1046, 1992

8. Mortality results for randomised controlled trial of early elective surgery or ultrasonographic surveillance for small abdominal aortic aneurysms. The UK Small Aneurysm Trial Participants. Lancet 352:1649, 1998

9. Ballard DJ, Fowkes FG, Powell JT: Surgery for small asymptomatic abdominal aortic aneurysms. Cochrane Database Syst Rev 2:CD001835, 2000

10. Wolf YG, Fogarty TJ, Olcott C, et al: Endovascular repair of abdominal aortic aneur-rysms: eligibility rate and impact on the rate of open repair. J Vasc Surg 32:519, 2000

11. Wolf YG, Hill BB, Rubin GD, et al: Rate of change in abdominal aortic aneurysm diameter after endovascular repair. J Vasc Surg 32:108, 2000

12. Eagle KA, Brundage BH, Chaitman BR, et al: Guidelines for perioperative cardiovascular evaluation for noncardiac surgery. Report of the American College of Cardiology/American Heart Association Task Force on Practice Guidelines. Committee on Perioperative Cardiovascular Evaluation for Noncardiac Surgery. Circulation 93:1278, 1996

13. Poldermans D, Boersma E, Bax JJ, et al: The effect of bisoprolol on perioperative mortality and myocardial infarction in high-risk patients undergoing vascular surgery. Dutch Echocardiographic Cardiac Risk Evaluation Applying Stress Echocardiography Study Group. N Engl J Med 341:1789, 1999

14. Best PJ, Tajik AJ, Gibbons RJ, et al: The safety of treadmill exercise stress testing in patients with abdominal aortic aneursyms. Ann Intern Med 129:628, 1998

15. Shores J, Berger KR, Murphy EA, et al: Progression of aortic dilatation and the benefit of long-term beta-adrenergic blockade in Marfan's syndrome. N Engl J Med 330:1335, 1994

16. Dapunt OE, Galla JD, Sadeghi AM, et al: The natural history of thoracic aortic aneurysms. J Thorac Cardiovasc Surg 107:1323, 1994

17. Livesay JJ, Cooley DA, Ventemiglia RA, et al: Surgical experience in descending thoracic aneurysmectomy with and without adjuncts to avoid ischemia. Ann Thorac Surg 39:37, 1985

18. Coady MA, Rizzo JA, Hammond GL, et al: What is the appropriate size criterion for resection of thoracic aortic aneurysm? J Thorac Cardiovasc Surg 113:476, 1997

19. Dake MD, Miller DC, Semba CP, et al: Transluminal placement of endovascular stent-grafts for the treatment of descending thoracic aneurysms. N Engl J Med 331:1729, 1994

20. Okita Y, Takamoto S, Ando M, et al: Mortality and cerebral outcome in patients who underwent aortic arch operations using deep hypothermic circulatory arrest with retrograde cerebral perfusion: no relation of early death, stroke, and delirium to the duration of circulatory arrest. J Thorac Cardiovasc Surg 115:129, 1998

21. Coselli JS, Buket S, Djukanovic B: Aortic arch operation: current treatment and results. Ann Thorac Surg 59:19, 1995

22. Coselli JA, LeMaire SA, deFigueiredo LP, et al: Paraplegia after thoracoabdominal aortic aneurysm repair: is dissection a risk factor? Ann Thorac Surg 63:28, 1997

23. Cambria RP, Davison JK, Zannetti S, et al: Clinical experience with epidural cooling for spinal cord protection during thoracic and thoracoabdominal aneurysm repair. J Vasc Surg 25:234, 1997

24. Spittell PC, Spittell JA Jr, Joyce JW, et al: Clinical features and differential diagnosis of aortic dissection: experience with 236 cases (1980 through 1990). Mayo Clin Proc 68:642, 1993

25. Hirst AE Jr, Johns VJ Jr, Lime SW Jr: Dissecting aneurysm of the aorta: a review of 505 cases. Medicine (Baltimore) 37:217, 1958

26. Elkayam U, Ostzega E, Shotan A, et al: Cardiovascular problems in pregnant women with the Marfan syndrome. Ann Intern Med 123:177, 1995

27. Perron AD, Gibbs M: Thoracic aortic dissection secondary to crack cocaine ingestion. Am J Emerg Med 15:507, 1997

28. Hagan PG, Nienaber CA, Isselbacher EM, et al: The international registry of aortic dissection (IRAD): new insights into an old disease. JAMA 283:897, 2000

29. Armstrong WF, Bach DS, Carey LM, et al: Clinical and echocardiographic findings in patients with suspected acute aortic dissection. Am Heart J 136:1051, 1998

30. Slater EE, DeSanctis RW: The clinical recognition of dissecting aortic aneurysm. Am J Med 60:625, 1976

31. Suzuki T, Katoh H, Tsuchio Y, et al: Diagnostic implications of elevated levels of smooth-muscle myosin heavy-chain protein in acute aortic dissection. The smooth muscle myosin heavy chain study. Ann Intern Med 133:537, 2000

32. Suzuki T, Katoh H, Kurabayashi M, et al: Biochemical diagnosis of aortic dissection by raised concentrations of creatine kinase BB-isozyme. Lancet 350:784, 1997

33. Cigarroa JE, Isselbacher EM, DeSanctis RW, et al: Diagnostic imaging in the evaluation of suspected aortic dissection: old standards and new directions. N Engl J Med 328:35, 1993

34. Zeman RK, Berman PM, Silverman PM, et al: Diagnosis of aortic dissection: value of helical CT with multiplanar reformation and three-dimensional rendering. AJR Am J Roentgenol 164:1375, 1995

35. Small JH, Dixon AK, Coulden RA, et al: Fast CT for aortic dissection. Br J Radiol 69:900, 1996

36. Evangelista A, Garcia-del-Castillo H, Gonzales-Alujas T, et al: Diagnosis of ascending aortic dissection by transesophageal echocardiography: utility of M-mode in recognizing artifacts. J Am Coll Cardiol 27:102, 1996

37. Banning AP, Ruttley MST, Musumeci F, et al: Acute dissection of the thoracic aorta: transesophageal echocardiography is the investigation of choice. BMJ 310:72, 1995

38. Armstrong WF, Bach DS, Carey L, et al: Spectrum of acute dissection of the ascending aorta: a transesophageal echocardiographic study. J Am Soc Echocardiogr 9:646, 1996

39. Movsowitz H, Levine RA, Hilgenberg AD, et al: Transesophageal echocardiographic description of the mechanisms of aortic regurgitation in acute type A aortic dissection: implications for aortic valve repair. J Am Coll Cardiol 36:884, 2000

40. Keane MG, Wiegers SE, Yang E, et al: Structural determinants of aortic regurgitation in type A dissection and the role of ventricular resuspension as determined by intraoperative transesophageal echocardiography. Am J Cardiol 85:604, 2000

41. Nienaber CA, von Kodolitsch Y, Nicolas V, et al: Definitive diagnosis of thoracic aortic dissection: the emerging role of noninvasive imaging modalities. N Engl J Med 328:1, 1993

42. Bansal RC, Chandrasekaran K, Ayala J, et al: Frequency and explanation of false negative diagnosis of aortic dissection by tomography and transesophageal echocardiography. J Am Coll Cardiol 25:1393, 1995

43. Deeb GM, William DM, Bolling SF, et al: Surgical delay for acute type A dissection with malperfusion. Ann Thorac Surg 64:1669, 1997

44. Nienaber CA, Fattori R, Lund G, et al: Nonsurgical reconstruction of thoracic aortic dissection by stent-graft placement. N Engl J Med 340:1539, 1999

45. Dake MD, Kato N, Mitchell RS, et al: Endovascular stent-graft placement for the treatment of acute aortic dissection. N Engl J Med 340:1546, 1999

46. Kato M, Matsuda T, Kaneko M, et al: Outcomes of stent-graft treatment of false lumen in aortic dissection. Circulation 98:II305, 1998

47. Moon MR, Dake MD, Pelc LR, et al: Intravascular stenting of acute experimental type B dissections. J Surg Res 54:381, 1993

48. Palma JH, Almeida DR, Carvalho AC, et al: Surgical treatment of acute type B aortic dissection using an endoprosthesis (elephant trunk). Ann Thorac Surg 63:1081, 1997

49. Yamashita C, Okada M, Ataka K, et al: Cerebral complications and distal false lumen in the repair of aortic dissection with retrograde cerebral perfusion. J Cardiovasc Surg 38:581, 1997

50. Juvonen T, Ergin MA, Galla JD, et al: Risk factors for rupture of chronic type B dissections. J Thorac Cardiovasc Surg 117:776, 1999

51. Nienaber CA, von Kodolitsch Y, Petersen B, et al: Intramural hemorrhage of the thoracic aorta: diagnostic and therapeutic implications. Circulation 92:1465, 1995

52. Vilacosta I, San Roman JA, Ferreiros J, et al: Natural history and serial morphology of aortic intramural hematoma: a novel variant of aortic dissection. Am Heart J 134:495, 1997

53. Kaji S, Nishigama K, Akasada T, et al: Prediction of progression or regression of type A aortic intramural hematoma by computed tomography. Circulation 100:II281, 1999

54. Willens HJ, Kessler KM: Transesophageal echocardiography in the diagnosis of diseases of the thoracic aorta: part II—atherosclerotic and traumatic diseases of the aorta. Chest 117:233, 2000

55. Amarenco P, Cohen A, Tzourio C, et al: Atherosclerotic disease of the aortic arch and the risk of ischemic stroke. N Engl J Med 331:1474, 1994

56. Bojar RM, Payne DD, Murphy RE, et al: Surgical treatment of systemic atheroembolism from the thoracic aorta. Ann Thorac Surg 61:1389, 1996

57. Numano F, Kobayashi Y: Takayasu arteritis—beyond pulselessness. Intern Med 38:226, 1999

58. Ishikawa K: Diagnostic approach and proposed criteria for the clinical diagnosis of Takayasu's arteriopathy. J Am Coll Cardiol 12:964, 1988

59. Ishikawa K, Maetani S: Long-term outcome for 120 Japanese patients with Takayasu's disease: clinical and statistical analyses of related prognostic factors. Circulation 90:1855, 1994

60. Matsunaga N, Hayaski K, Sakamoto I, et al: Takayasu arteritis: MR manifestations and diagnosis of acute and chronic phase. J Magn Reson Imaging 8:406, 1998

61. Choe YH, Lee WR: Magnetic resonance imaging diagnosis of Takayasu arteritis. Int J Cardiol 66(suppl 1):S175, 1998

62. Evans JM, O'Fallon WM, Hunder GG: Increased incidence of aortic aneurysm and dissection in giant cell (temporal) arteritis: a population-based study. Ann Intern Med 122:502, 1995

63. Gravanis MB: Giant cell arteritis and Takayasu aortitis: morphologic, pathogenetic and etiologic factors. Int J Cardiol 75:S21, 2000

64. Smith MD, Cassidy JM, Souther S, et al: Transesophageal echocardiography in the diagnosis of traumatic rupture of the aorta. N Engl J Med 332:356, 1995

65. Demetriades D, Gomez H, Velmahos CG, et al: Routine helical computed tomographic evaluation of the mediastinum in high-risk blunt trauma patients. Arch Surg 133:1084, 1998

66. Mirvis S, Shanmuganathan K, Buell J, et al: Use of spiral computed tomography for the assessment of blunt trauma patients with potential aortic injury. J Trauma 45:922, 1998

67. Patel NH, Stephens KE Jr., Mirvis SE, et al: Imaging of acute thoracic aortic injury due to blunt trauma: a review. Radiology 209:335, 1998

25 Diseases of the Pericardium, Cardiac Tumors, and Cardiac Trauma

E. William Hancock, M.D.

Diseases of the Pericardium

The pericardium provides a protective sac around the heart. The sac contains a thin layer of fluid that permits the heart to move with minimal friction during the cardiac cycle. Neither the sac nor the fluid appears to be necessary for normal function. When one or more of the cardiac chambers dilate acutely, the pericardium restrains the heart. In chronic dilatation of the heart, however, the pericardium stretches and therefore does not exert a restraining effect, except during exercise or other acute stresses.

Pericardial disease results from diverse causes, many of which lead to responses to injury that are pathologically and clinically similar. There are three clinicopathologic responses to injury: acute pericarditis, pericardial effusion, and constrictive pericarditis.

ACUTE PERICARDITIS

Viral infection is usually assumed to be the cause of acute pericarditis that occurs as an apparently primary illness. Because most cases follow a brief and uncomplicated natural course, the syndrome is often termed acute benign pericarditis. Cases resulting from other conditions or treatments, such as rheumatic disease or radiotherapy, often exhibit clinical features similar to those of acute benign pericarditis.

Diagnosis

The clinical diagnosis of acute pericarditis rests primarily on the findings of chest pain, pericardial friction rub, and electrocardiographic changes. The chest pain of acute pericarditis typically develops suddenly and is severe and constant over the anterior chest. In acute pericarditis, the pain worsens with inspiration—a response that helps distinguish acute pericarditis from myocardial infarction. Low-grade fever and sinus tachycardia also are usually present.

A pericardial friction rub can be detected in most patients when symptoms are acute. Pericardial friction rubs are typically triphasic: systolic and early diastolic components are followed in later diastole by a third component associated with atrial contraction.

Electrocardiographic changes are common in most forms of acute pericarditis, particularly those of an infectious etiology in which the associated inflammation in the superficial layer of myocardium is prominent. The characteristic change is an elevation in the ST segment in diffuse leads. The diffuse distribution and the absence of reciprocal ST segment depression distinguish the characteristic pattern of acute pericarditis from acute myocardial infarction. However, the normal variant pattern of ST segment elevation often complicates the differential diagnosis [see Figure 1]. Depression of the PR segment, which reflects superficial injury of the atrial myocardium, is as frequent and specific as ST elevation and is often the earliest electrocardiographic manifestation.[1]

Treatment

Analgesic agents, such as codeine (15 to 30 mg taken orally every 4 to 6 hours) or hydrocodone (5 to 10 mg taken orally every 4 to 6 hours), are usually effective in providing symptomatic relief. Salicylates given at an initial dosage of 4 to 6 g a day or a nonsteroidal anti-inflammatory drug (NSAID) such as indomethacin given at an initial dosage of 25 mg four times daily is often effective in reducing pericardial inflammation. Corticosteroids such as prednisone given at an initial dose of 40 to 60 mg/day often greatly relieve symptoms; however, steroid therapy should be reserved for severe cases that are unresponsive to other therapy, because symptoms may recur after steroid withdrawal. The corticosteroid dose should be reduced as soon as a clinical response is observed and should be tapered to zero over a period of 2 to 4 weeks.

Other Forms of Acute Pericarditis

Relapsing pericarditis   Acute pericarditis of any etiology may follow a recurrent or chronic relapsing course in some patients. In many instances, the manifestations of this syndrome are subjective (e.g., weakness, fatigue, or headache) and often present in addition to the chest discomfort. Treatment with 1 mg of colchicine daily, methylprednisolone in 1 g pulses daily for 3 days, or an immunosuppressant such as prednisone (60 to 100 mg daily) or azathioprine (50 to 100 mg daily) has proved successful in patients with relapsing pericarditis, particularly in patients whose symptoms are mainly related to withdrawal of prednisone.[2,3]

Progression to constriction   In a few instances, acute pericarditis progresses to subacute or chronic constrictive pericarditis. In such cases, the pericarditis may be idiopathic or have a bacterial, viral, rheumatoid, radiation-induced, or dialysis-related origin. These patients usually have subacute rather than acute pericarditis initially; pericardial effusion is present at onset, usually with some degree of cardiac tamponade. Acute benign pericarditis unaccompanied by tamponade or substantial pericardial effusion in the acute phase rarely progresses to constrictive pericarditis.

PERICARDIAL EFFUSION AND CARDIAC TAMPONADE

Fluid may accumulate in the pericardial cavity in virtually any form of pericardial disease. The fluid may be a transudate or an exudate and is often serosanguineous in neoplastic, idiopathic, dialysis-related, radiation-induced, and tuberculous cases. The fluid is serosanguineous or frankly bloody in cases of coagulopathy, trauma, rupture of acute myocardial infarction, and aortic dissection. Chylopericardium and pneumopericardium also can occur, although rarely.[4] Cardiac tamponade or compression of the heart by effusion is the most important complication of pericardial effusion.

Pathophysiology

The physiologic effect of the accumulation of pericardial fluid depends on whether the fluid is under increased pressure.[5] If effusion develops gradually, the pericardium stretches enough to accommodate volumes that may exceed 2,000 ml. However, if the effusion develops acutely, as little as 200 ml of accumulated fluid may raise the intrapericardial pressure and cause cardiac tamponade.

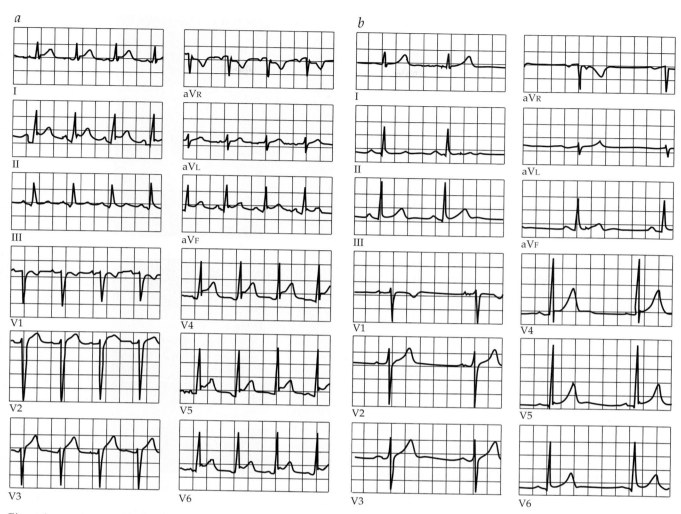

Figure 1   Electrocardiograms contrast the pattern of ST segment elevation characteristic of acute pericarditis (*a*) with the normal variant (early repolarization) pattern of ST segment elevation (*b*). The normal variant pattern is associated with a normal or slow heart rate and has relatively tall R waves and T waves in V4, V5, and V6. The ST segment elevation is less than 25% of the T wave amplitude. In contrast, the acute pericarditis has PR depression and lower T wave amplitude.

As the pericardial fluid pressure rises, the right atrial and central venous pressures increase correspondingly. Thus, reading the central venous pressure gives an accurate reflection of the intrapericardial pressure.

Cardiac tamponade should be viewed as a spectrum of hemodynamic abnormalities of various severities rather than an all-or-none phenomenon. Depending on the severity of the tamponade, the blood pressure may be lowered or maintained near the normal range; in patients with preexisting hypertension, it may even be increased. The central venous pressure is almost always increased, except in the rare instances of low-pressure cardiac tamponade, which may occur when intravascular volume is depleted.

As a rule, paradoxical pulse—a marked decrease in arterial pressure during inspiration—is present in patients with cardiac tamponade, although it may not be easy to detect on clinical examination [*see Figure 2*]. The arbitrary value of 10 mm Hg is commonly used to indicate the upper limit of the normal decrease in arterial pressure with inspiration.

The inspiratory drop in arterial pressure reflects a selective impairment of diastolic filling of the left ventricle, probably the combined effects of two factors. First, when the filling of the right ventricle is augmented in inspiration, the simultaneous filling of the left ventricle is limited because the entire heart is enclosed in a fixed volume. Second, during inspiration, blood is sequestered in the lungs and pulmonary veins as a result of impaired transmission of changes in intrapleural pressure to the left atrium and to the intrapericardial portions of the pulmonary veins.

Diagnosis

Pericardial effusion without tamponade   Echocardiography is the most accurate and easily applied method for the clinical detection of pericardial effusion [*see Figure 3*]. Echocardiograms detect effusions as small as 20 ml and show characteristic findings with effusions larger than 100 ml. Computed tomography is also a reliable method for detecting both pericardial effusion and pericardial thickening. Magnetic resonance imaging provides information similar to that provided by CT [*see Figure 4*].

Electrocardiograms usually show low voltage in patients with large pericardial effusions, but this finding is nonspecific. Electrical alternans occurs occasionally when the pericardial effusion is large and permits a beat-to-beat oscillation of the heart from one position to another within the pericardial sac [see Figure 5]. Alternans is most common with effusion caused by neoplasm. This type of alternans must be differentiated from other types of electrical alternans, such as that occurring in supraventricular tachycardias or alternating intraventricular conduction defects.

Cardiac tamponade   The diagnosis of cardiac tamponade is often difficult.[6] The diagnosis is one of the most common important diagnoses made at autopsy but is often overlooked while the patient is alive in a medical intensive care unit.[7] This diagnosis should be based on a synthesis of various clinical findings, because no single finding is pathognomonic or necessarily present. Echocardiography, although essentially definitive for the demonstration of pericardial effusion, is not as certain a method of assessing tamponade. Several echocardiographic features are helpful, however, particularly the observation of an early diastolic inward motion (so-called collapse) of the right atrial wall or right ventricular wall, indicating similarity of intracavitary and intrapericardial pressures.[8] Another useful sign is an exaggerated respiratory variation in the velocity of flow through the mitral and tricuspid valves or in the left ventricular ejection, as detected in pulsed Doppler recordings [see Figure 6]. This phenomenon has the same significance as paradoxical pulse.

Loculated pericardial effusions may selectively compress one or more chambers of the heart, producing regional cardiac tamponade. This condition is seen most frequently after cardiac surgery, when bloody fluid accumulates behind the sternum and selectively compresses the right atrium and right ventricle[9]; less often, the left ventricle and left atrium are compressed locally. Similar conditions may occur after closed chest trauma. Fluid accumulations in the mediastinum can compress the heart even when they are not truly within the pericardial space. Transesophageal echocardiography is superior to transtho-

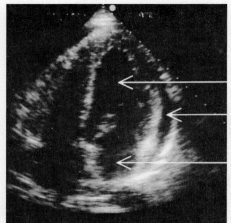

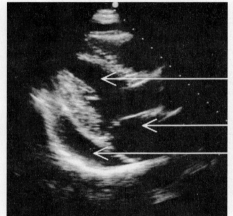

Figure 3   Pericardial effusion is seen in the two-dimensional echocardiogram as an echo-free space outside the cardiac chambers. Two characteristic sites are lateral to the left ventricle in the apical four-chamber view (top) and posterior to the left ventricle in the parasternal long-axis view (bottom).

racic echocardiography in demonstrating such local fluid accumulations, particularly those along the right heart border.

Treatment

Pericardial effusion without tamponade   Occasionally, a syndrome of idiopathic chronic large pericardial effusion is seen, usually without tamponade. Colchicine may be effective in such cases.[10]

In patients with pericardial effusion but no tamponade, pericardiocentesis is rarely performed for the sole purpose of providing diagnostic studies of the fluid, because such specific diagnoses are rarely made in those patients, at least in regions of the world where tuberculous pericarditis has become rare.[11] Pericardial biopsy can be obtained by any of the usual surgical methods. However, pericardiocentesis can be useful in diagnosing infection or neoplastic disease. In addition, pericardioscopy can be performed in association with subxiphoid pericardiostomy; biopsy under direct vision may permit the diagnosis of tuberculosis or neoplasm in some instances in which studies of the fluid alone might be inconclusive.[12]

Cardiac tamponade   Mild cardiac tamponade may be managed conservatively in some cases, but removal of the fluid

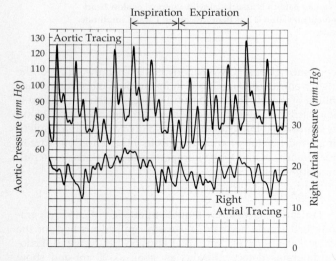

Figure 2   The aortic pressure and right atrial pressure are recorded during quiet breathing in a patient with cardiac tamponade. The marked fall in arterial pressure that occurs during inspiration is a paradoxical pulse. The decrease in pulse pressure, defined as the difference between systolic and diastolic pressures, that accompanies the fall in systolic pressure indicates that left ventricular stroke volume decreases during inspiration. Central venous pressure, as indicated by the right atrial pressure, also falls during inspiration.

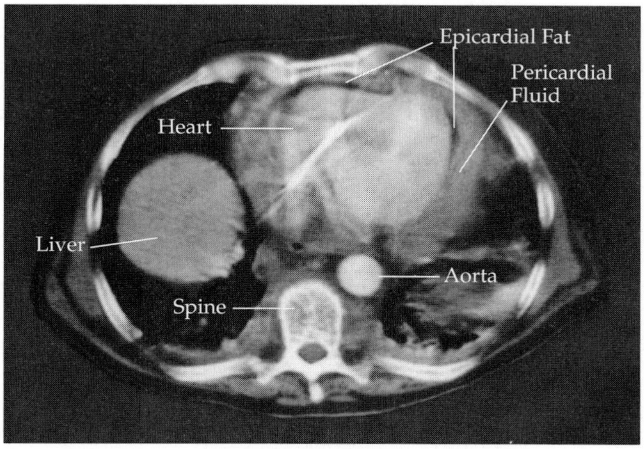

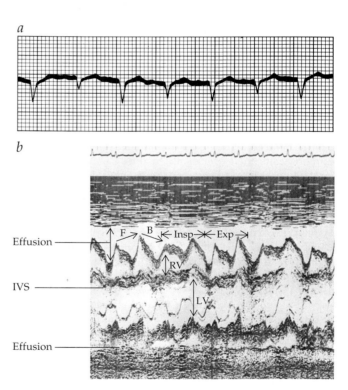

Figure 4 **In a CT scan of the chest of a patient with pericardial effusion, pericardial fluid appears less dense than the heart and is separated from the myocardium by epicardial fat in some areas.**

is required for definitive treatment and should be carried out in most instances when the central venous pressure is increased. Pericardial fluid may be removed by needle pericardiocentesis or by a surgical technique (subxiphoid pericardiostomy, thoracoscopic pericardiostomy, or thoracotomy).[13,14]

The most acute forms of cardiac tamponade, such as hemopericardium secondary to aortic dissection, penetrating cardiac trauma, or rupture of acute myocardial infarction, require immediate surgery. Pericardiocentesis is effective in most subacute forms of tamponade, such as those associated with idiopathic or viral acute pericarditis, rheumatic diseases, dialysis, and neoplasm.

Thoracoscopy and thoracotomy are usually reserved for patients with recurrent tamponade after an initial pericardiocentesis or subxiphoid pericardiostomy, usually for neoplastic disease. Pericardiostomy by means of a balloon catheter as part of a pericardiocentesis is another alternative for such cases.[15]

SPECIAL ETIOLOGIC FORMS OF ACUTE PERICARDITIS AND PERICARDIAL EFFUSION

Pericarditis Related to Renal Failure and Dialysis

Acute pericarditis with pericardial effusion occurs in patients with end-stage renal disease and in patients who are on chronic dialysis [*see Chapter 164*]. In the dialysis patients, conservative management with more-intensive dialysis and NSAIDs is usually successful. An unexpected decrease in blood pressure during a dialysis session may be the clue to the presence of tamponade. Pericardiocentesis is occasionally necessary for the relief of tamponade, although fluid overload and left ventricular failure are often important factors associated with causing increased central venous pressure. Cardiac catheterization in combination with pericardiocentesis is often useful in assessing the hemodynamic significance of those factors that contribute to an increase of pulmonary and systemic venous pressure in dialysis patients.

Radiation-Induced Pericardial Effusion

Pericardial effusion develops relatively frequently in patients with Hodgkin disease, other lymphomas, or breast carcinoma who survive for long periods after receiving large doses of radiation to the mediastinum. Radiation-induced effusion may evolve into chronic constrictive pericarditis after many years.[16]

Neoplastic Pericardial Effusion

Neoplastic pericardial effusion accounts for about one half of the patients with cardiac tamponade who are seen in an internal medicine setting [*see Chapter 192*]. Lung cancer and breast cancer account for the majority of the cases; lymphoma and leukemia account for most of the remainder.[17] In most cases, the primary neoplasm has been previously diagnosed; patients in whom pericardial effusion is the first manifestation of the disease usually have primary cancer of the lung. Cytologic examination of the pericardial fluid is highly accurate in diagnosing common carcinomas but less accurate in diagnosing other neoplasms, especially the lymphomas and leukemias.[18]

Neoplastic pericardial effusion often can be managed conservatively when no symptoms directly related to the pericardial effusion are present. Symptomatic tamponade can be managed palliatively with pericardiocentesis, although recurrent effusion is more likely to form in such cases than in many other types of pericardial effusion. Subxiphoid pericardiostomy is often the preferred procedure, leading to a pericardial reaction that produces adhesion of the parietal and visceral layers of pericardium and thus prevents recurrent effusion. Balloon pericardiostomy is an alternative. Chemotherapy or radiotherapy may be of value, depending on the nature of the primary

Figure 5 **The electrocardiogram (V2 lead) from a patient with pericardial effusion caused by malignant melanoma reveals a low voltage and electrical alternans (*a*). The echocardiogram (*b*) demonstrates that the heart moves forward (F) and backward (B) within the effusion on alternate beats, thus producing the alternation of the QRS axis characteristic of electrical alternans. The heart also moves with inspiration (Insp) and expiration (Exp), which accounts for a change in anterior wall motion with every two cardiac cycles.**

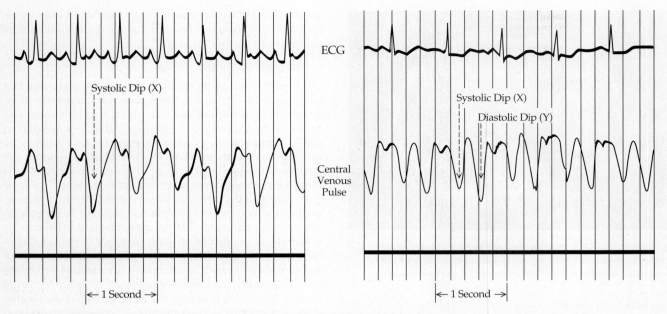

ECG

Systolic Dip (X)

Central Venous Pulse

Systolic Dip (X)

Diastolic Dip (Y)

|← 1 Second →|

|← 1 Second →|

Figure 6 **Differences between the central venous pulse contours characteristic of cardiac tamponade (left) and chronic constrictive pericarditis (right) provide the basis for differential diagnosis. The pressure contour in a patient with pericardial effusion and tamponade has a prominent systolic dip (X) but little or no diastolic deflection. The central venous pulse pattern in a patient with chronic constrictive pericarditis displays an M or W contour consisting of both systolic dip (X) and diastolic dip (Y), with the Y descent being more prominent.**

neoplasm. Intrapericardial instillation of chemotherapeutic agents has often been used with apparent success, but no results from controlled trials are available. Few patients survive longer than a year, and whether pericardiocentesis has a major effect on their longevity is difficult to determine, even when tamponade is relieved.[19]

Purulent Pericarditis

Tamponade is usually present in purulent bacterial pericarditis; after pericardiocentesis, the pericarditis is highly likely to recur rapidly and progress to constrictive pericarditis. Purulent pericarditis therefore usually requires a surgical drainage procedure; a partial pericardiectomy by a limited left lateral thoracotomy is often the best choice. Surgery may not be required for patients in whom tamponade or constriction does not develop, because antibiotics apparently have entered the pericardial cavity in effective concentrations. Active tuberculous pericarditis with effusion is particularly likely to progress to constriction and to require pericardiectomy in addition to antituberculous chemotherapy. AIDS is a common cause of large pericardial effusions, the majority of which are not caused by identifiable opportunistic infective agents.[20] However, the incidence of tuberculous and other forms of bacterial pericarditis has increased in the United States as a result of AIDS.

Drug-Induced Pericarditis

Several drugs have been implicated in the etiology of pericardial disease, including procainamide, which leads to a lupuslike syndrome; minoxidil, which has been linked to pericardial effusion; and methysergide, which may lead to constrictive pericarditis.

Pericarditis after Cardiac Surgery

The postcardiotomy syndrome presents primarily as acute pericarditis. Whether it has an infective or autoimmune cause

is unclear. A similar condition occurs after blunt or penetrating trauma, hemopericardium from other causes, or epicardial pacemaker implantation. Cardiac tamponade and constrictive pericarditis occur occasionally.

Pericardial Complications of Invasive Procedures

Cardiac tamponade occurs as a complication of various invasive procedures in the cardiac catheterization laboratory and in the intensive care unit. Particularly important, and usually preventable, is the perforation of the heart by central venous catheters that have been allowed to lie in the right atrium rather than in the superior vena cava.[21] The use of newer devices, such as stents, and procedures, such as rotational atherectomy, has increased the incidence of percutaneous coronary interventions having cardiac tamponade complications.[22] Most of these cases are managed successfully by pericardiocentesis.[23]

CONSTRICTIVE PERICARDITIS

Constrictive pericarditis was formerly considered to be primarily a tuberculous lesion and is still so regarded in many areas of the world.[24] Most cases now seen in the United States are idiopathic or are related to previous cardiac surgery or radiotherapy.[25,26] Fewer cases result from purulent pericarditis, rheumatic diseases, dialysis, and various rarer conditions.

In the classic form of chronic constrictive pericarditis, fibrous scarring and adhesion of both pericardial layers obliterate the pericardial cavity. The resulting fibrotic lesion has been likened to a rigid shell around the heart, particularly when there is considerable calcification of the pericardium, a feature seen in long-standing cases. The subacute form of constrictive pericarditis is now more common than the chronic calcific type. In the subacute variant, the constriction is rather fibroelastic and may be produced by fibrous contracture of the visceral pericardial layer (epicardium) alone. The fibroelastic constriction may also exist in combination with persisting loculated or totally free

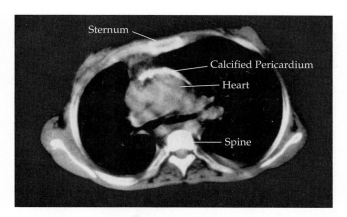

Figure 7 **In this CT scan of the chest of a patient with chronic constrictive pericarditis, the dense layer on the anterior surface of the heart represents thickened and partially calcified pericardium.**

pericardial effusion; this form is termed effusive-constrictive pericarditis, and it can be documented by measuring pericardial and central venous pressures before and after removal of the fluid.[27]

Pathophysiology

The pathophysiology of constrictive pericarditis is similar to that of tamponade in that both conditions impede diastolic filling of the heart and lead to increased venous pressure and ultimately to reduced cardiac output. Differences exist in the diagnostic signs, however. Paradoxical pulse is a regular feature of cardiac tamponade but may be inconspicuous or absent in constrictive pericarditis. The Kussmaul sign (an increase in venous pressure with inspiration) is seen in some patients with constrictive pericarditis but not in patients with pure cardiac tamponade. When tamponade is present, the venous pulse shows a predominant systolic dip, whereas in constrictive pericarditis, the early diastolic dip is the more prominent deflection [*see Figure 6*].

An early diastolic sound (pericardial knock) is often heard in constrictive pericarditis but not in tamponade; this sound is directly related to the extent to which ventricular filling is re-

stricted to early diastole, being abruptly checked at the peak of early filling when the heart reaches the fixed volume imposed by the constricting shell surrounding it.

Diagnosis

Constrictive pericarditis is difficult to diagnose, frequently being misdiagnosed for prolonged periods as liver disease or idiopathic pleural effusion. Clinical diagnosis of constrictive pericarditis depends on the recognition of increased venous pressure in a patient who may not have other obvious signs or symptoms of heart disease. The heart size and lung fields often appear normal in the chest radiograph, and the ECG shows only minor nonspecific abnormalities. Echocardiography is also nondiagnostic in many instances, although the appearance of abnormal septal motion and pericardial thickening often provide clues. Transesophageal echocardiography and chest CT are superior to echocardiography for the demonstration of pericardial thickening [*see Figure 7*]; however, the pericardium is not measurably thicker than normal in noninvasive imaging studies in some patients with constriction.[28]

As in cardiac tamponade, pulsed wave Doppler studies show exaggerated respiratory variation in the mitral and tricuspid diastolic flow velocity in most cases of constrictive pericarditis. Doing the study in the upright position improves the sensitivity of this test.[29] False positive results occur in patients with chronic obstructive pulmonary disease, but that can be recognized by performing Doppler studies of flow velocity in the superior vena cava; the changes in velocity with respiration are much greater in pulmonary disease than in constrictive pericarditis.[30]

Cardiac catheterization shows characteristic abnormalities, with increased central venous pressure, nondilated and normally contracting right and left ventricles, and near equilibration of the cardiac filling pressures of the right and left sides. These features may also be present in idiopathic restrictive cardiomyopathy or in specific myocardial diseases, especially cardiac amyloidosis; in such cases, the demonstration of pericardial thickness by CT or MRI and the use of endomyocardial biopsy are helpful.[31] Many other clues can assist in this differential diagnosis [*see Table 1*]. The increased interdependence of the two ventricles in constrictive pericarditis causes the right

Table 1 Clinical Features That Differentiate Constrictive Pericarditis from Amyloidosis and Idiopathic Restrictive Cardiomyopathy

Clinical Feature	Constrictive Pericarditis	Cardiac Amyloidosis	Idiopathic Restrictive Cardiomyopathy
Early diastolic sound (S_3 or pericardial knock)	Frequent	Occasional	Occasional
Late diastolic sound (S_4)	Rare	Frequent	Frequent
Atrial enlargement	Mild or absent	Marked	Marked
Atrioventricular or intraventricular conduction defect	Rare	Frequent	Frequent
QRS voltage	Normal or low	Low	Normal or high
Mitral or tricuspid regurgitation	Rare	Frequent	Frequent
Paradoxical pulse	Frequent but usually mild	Rare	Rare
Exaggerated variation in mitral and tricuspid flow velocity with respiration, out of phase	Usual	Rare	Rare

a

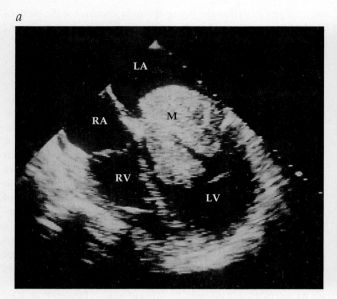

b

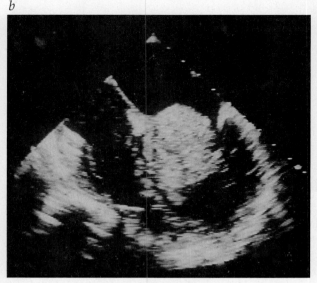

Figure 8   This transesophageal echocardiogram demonstrates a large myxoma (M) in the left atrium (LA) of a 23-year-old man. The picture on the left (*a*) was taken during early systole, and the picture on the right (*b*) was taken during early diastole. The marked mobility of the tumor is evident as it moves from the left atrium to the left ventricle (LV). The right atrium (RA) and right ventricle (RV) are also visible.

and left ventricular systolic pressures to vary out of phase with each other in respiration; in conditions other than constrictive pericarditis, the two systolic pressures increase and decrease together with respiration.[32]

Treatment

Constrictive pericarditis occasionally resolves spontaneously when it develops as a complication of acute pericarditis.[33] In nearly all instances, however, relief of constrictive pericarditis requires surgical stripping and removal of both layers of the adherent, constricting pericardium. This operation is far more difficult to perform than the operation for relief of pericardial effusion. The operation must be thorough, which carries the risk of hemorrhage from perforations in the wall of the heart. Inadequate long-term relief after surgical removal of the pericardium may reflect the presence of associated myocardial disease, particularly in instances of radiation-induced pericardial disease.[34] In most other forms of constrictive pericarditis, however, myocardial function is normal.

Cardiac Tumors

Cardiac tumors may be either primary or secondary and either benign or malignant. Metastatic cardiac involvement occurs 20 to 40 times more frequently than primary tumors. However, primary tumors are often benign and curable by surgery.

METASTATIC TUMORS

About 10% of patients who die of malignant disease have metastatic cardiac involvement, but the metastases produce symptoms in only 5% to 10% of the affected patients. Neoplasms particularly likely to metastasize to the heart are cancers of the lung or breast, melanoma, leukemia, and lymphoma.[35]

The most frequent clinical manifestation is pericardial effusion with cardiac tamponade. In such cases, the mass of the tu-

mor is often relatively small. Extensive solid tumor in and around the heart is less common but may resemble constrictive pericarditis or effusive-constrictive pericarditis. Invasion of the myocardium most often manifests clinically as arrhythmias; atrial flutter and atrial fibrillation are particularly common.

Usually the only effective treatment in metastatic involvement of the heart is relief of cardiac tamponade. Otherwise, treatment depends on the nature of the primary tumor.

PRIMARY BENIGN TUMORS

Eighty percent of all primary cardiac tumors are benign; myxomas account for more than half of these in adults, whereas rhabdomyomas and fibromas are the most common benign cardiac tumors in children.[36-38] Cardiac rhabdomyomas in infancy and childhood have a high incidence of spontaneous regression; although they are sometimes responsible for a remarkable syndrome of paroxysmal ventricular tachycardia in infancy, this syndrome can be cured by surgical removal of the tumor. Echocardiography and MRI are both excellent methods for demonstrating intracardiac tumors [*see Figures 8 and 9*].

Myxomas consist of scattered stellate cells embedded in a mucinous matrix. They are found in the cavities of the heart, attached to the endocardial wall (or, in rare cases, attached to one of the heart valves) by either a narrow stalk or a broader pedicle. The tumor often shows considerable movement within the cardiac chamber during the cardiac cycle [*see Figure 8*]. About 70% of myxomas are in the left atrium; the rest are mostly in the right atrium.

Myxomas are most often manifested clinically by mechanical hemodynamic effects, which often simulate mitral or tricuspid stenoses when they obstruct the valve orifice. They may simulate mitral or tricuspid regurgitation when they interfere with valve closure or cause a so-called wrecking-ball type of trauma to the mitral or tricuspid valve. Intermittent obstruction of the valve orifice can lead to such dramatic symptoms as syncope or to remarkable changes in physical signs that are some-

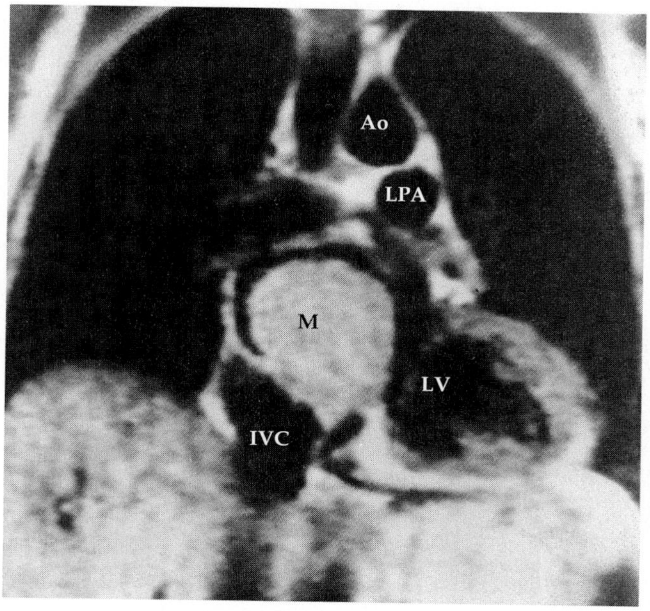

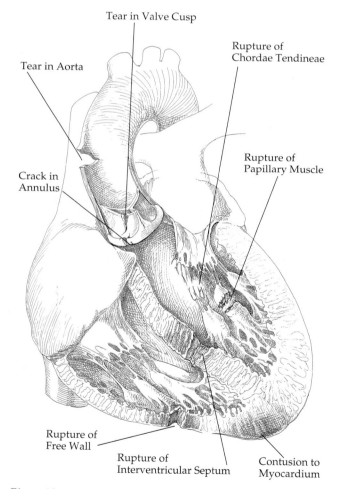

Figure 9   **This magnetic resonance image, coronal view, shows a large left atrial myxoma (M). The left ventricle (LV), aorta (Ao), left pulmonary artery (LPA), and inferior vena cava (IVC) are also visible.**

times related to changes in body position.

Myxomas also cause thromboembolic complications when portions of the tumor or thrombi from the surface of the tumor are detached. Another manifestation is a constitutional disturbance consisting of fatigue, fever, erythematous rash, myalgias, and weight loss, accompanied by anemia and an increased erythrocyte sedimentation rate. The constitutional symptoms may be caused by production of interleukin-6 by the myxoma.[39]

About 5% of cardiac myxoma cases are familial, multicentric, or associated with a genetic syndrome that includes cutaneous lentiginosis, cutaneous myxomas, myxoid fibroadenomas of the breast, pituitary adenomas, adrenocortical micronodular hyperplasia with Cushing syndrome, and Sertoli cell tumors of the testis. These cases are referred to as complex myxoma, myxoma syndrome, or the Carney complex. A genetic mutation underlying this syndrome has been identified.[40]

Surgical treatment of cardiac myxomas is usually curative, particularly if the resection includes the portion of the atrial septum or atrial free wall from which the tumor has arisen. Recurrence and distant metastases are rare except in myxoma syndrome.[41]

PRIMARY MALIGNANT TUMORS

Most malignant tumors of the heart are sarcomas, of either the spindle cell or the round cell type. Spindle cell tumors include fibrosarcomas, hemangiosarcomas, leiomyosarcomas, rhabdomyosarcomas, and fibromyxosarcomas. Round cell tumors include lymphosarcomas or reticulum cell sarcomas. Primary lymphoma of the heart, which is usually seen only in immune-compromised patients, is increasing in incidence.[42]

Malignant tumors are more apt to occur in the right side of the heart than in the left, being about equally frequent in the right atrium and the right ventricle. Signs and symptoms usually stem from intracavitary growth of the tumor, causing obstructive phenomena that simulate congestive heart failure. Pericardial effusion and tamponade are also common.

Malignant pericardial mesothelioma usually presents as pericardial effusion with tamponade or as subacute constrictive pericarditis.

Although surgical excision of malignant cardiac tumors is often attempted, cure is only rarely achieved. The tumors are usually unresponsive to radiation or chemotherapy, and most are fatal within a few months.

Cardiovascular Trauma

Cardiovascular injury may be either blunt (i.e., nonpenetrating) or penetrating.[43] Automobile accidents are the most common cause of blunt cardiovascular trauma; gunshots and stabbings are the most common causes of penetrating trauma. Both types of injury can damage the myocardium, the valves, the coronary arteries, the pericardium, and the great vessels, especially the aorta [*see Figure 10*]. Diagnosis is often difficult because the associated injuries in such instances can mask the cardiovascular trauma; cardiac trauma should therefore be suspected in all patients with chest injuries or severe generalized trauma.

Figure 10   **Blunt trauma, such as that caused by the impact of the chest against the steering wheel in an automobile accident, may injure various cardiac structures. Myocardial contusion is the most frequent injury, but rupture may occur at several sites, including the interventricular septum, the walls of the cardiac chambers, the papillary muscles, and the chordae tendineae. The shearing forces that accompany abrupt deceleration may also cause tearing of the aorta and the valve cusps and cracking of the annulus.**

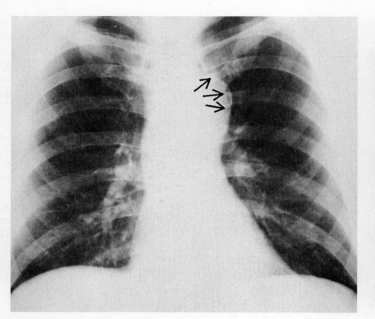 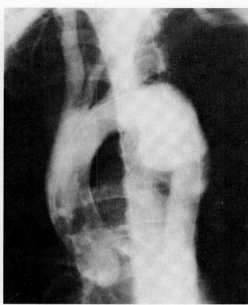

Figure 11 A posteroanterior chest x-ray (left) reveals a posttraumatic aortic aneurysm at the aortic isthmus. Calcification (arrows) is evident in the wall of the aneurysm, which arose in a 45-year-old policeman who had sustained chest injuries in a motorcycle accident 24 years earlier. The lesion had gradually enlarged during a 10-year period of observation after its discovery. The aneurysm, outlined by angiography (right), was successfully excised.

BLUNT CARDIAC TRAUMA

Myocardial Contusion

Myocardial contusion is the most common blunt injury.[44] The right ventricle, because of its immediately substernal location, is the chamber most often involved. The pathologic changes in myocardial contusion consist of myocardial necrosis with hemorrhage, which may range in severity from scattered petechiae to intramural extravasations with associated transmural necrosis. In some instances, coronary arterial occlusion with secondary myocardial infarction is present. Seemingly innocuous blows to the chest by missiles such as baseballs or hockey pucks may cause sudden arrhythmic death, probably when they strike directly over the heart during the vulnerable portion of the T wave and induce ventricular fibrillation.[45]

The most important complication of myocardial contusion is cardiac arrhythmia. Hypotension, intracardiac thrombus, congestive heart failure, and cardiac tamponade occur occasionally.

Myocardial contusion is best recognized clinically by echocardiography, which shows localized areas of impaired wall motion. Transesophageal echocardiography is often superior to the transthoracic evaluation.[46] The abnormalities of wall motion usually resolve within a few days. Increases in the concentrations of creatine kinase (CK) and its MB fraction (CK-MB) in the blood are difficult to interpret because of the release of CK from injured skeletal muscle. Cardiac troponin-I is a more specific marker.[47] Diffuse nonspecific ST-T abnormalities in the electrocardiogram are common in injured patients, even in the absence of echocardiographically detected abnormalities in wall motion. However, localized changes, especially ST segment elevation, are more specific for contusion. Patients with Q-wave infarct patterns and irreversible wall motion defects are likely to have a coronary arterial occlusion secondary to trauma with myocardial infarction. Severe contusions may also lead to the formation of traumatic left ventricular aneurysms or pseudoaneurysms that are sometimes detected months or years after the initial trauma.

Valvular Injury

Blunt trauma may injure any of the cardiac valves and lead to valvular regurgitation. Traumatic valvular regurgitation is more likely to be recognized after the patient has recovered from the acute injuries; it is less likely to play a major role in the early postinjury course.

Aortic Injury

Injuries of the aorta result from abrupt deceleration in violent thoracic trauma and are relatively common. The most common injury results from a tear in the wall of the aorta at a point just distal to the left subclavian artery, where the aorta is fixed to the dorsal thoracic cage. Usually, complete transection of the aorta is quickly fatal. Less extensive tears can result in a localized hematoma or a localized false aneurysm. Such aneurysms may be recognized months or years after the initial injury, when they cause symptoms by gradually enlarging, or may be discovered incidentally by chest radiography [*see Figure 11*].

A widened mediastinal shadow in the chest radiograph is often the first clue to the presence of a traumatic aortic rupture. The chest CT and the transesophageal echocardiogram are useful aids in making the diagnosis.

At least 50% of patients with aortic rupture die before they reach a hospital, often of injuries unrelated to the aortic trauma. Surgical therapy should be undertaken as soon as possible, even if the bleeding from the ruptured aorta has stabilized; such therapy results in survival of about 80% of those patients who are still alive when they reach a medical facility. Resection of the injured segment and replacement with a prosthetic graft are usually required.

Usually, false aneurysms that are diagnosed long after the initial injury should be resected electively. Their natural history in most instances is to enlarge gradually and eventually rupture.

PENETRATING TRAUMA

Penetrating injuries of the heart and great vessels are caused either by stab wounds or by gunshot wounds. Any of the cardiac chambers or great vessels may be punctured, and injury of multiple structures is common. The most common sites of involvement, in order of decreasing frequency, are the right ventricle, the left ventricle, the right atrium, and the left atrium.

Stab wounds and especially bullet wounds of the heart often are immediately fatal. However, if the penetrating wound is relatively small, cardiac tamponade can occur, and the buildup of pressure in the pericardial sac may help reduce the severity of bleeding and thus improve survival.

Other sequelae of penetrating trauma include laceration of the aorta or the pulmonary artery; defects in the ventricular or atrial septum; fistulas between the great vessels and between the coronary arteries and the cardiac chambers; coronary arterial fistulas; puncture of any of the heart valves; and atrioventricular block as a result of disruption of the conduction system. Occasionally, a missile that lodges in a cardiac chamber or in one of the great arteries will embolize to a distal site, whereas missiles that initially lodge in distal sites may work their way through the veins to lodge in the chambers of the heart or the pulmonary artery.[48]

The existence of intracardiac shunts, fistulas between the heart and great vessels, coronary arterial fistulas, or valve disruption is usually suggested by the presence of new murmurs. Echocardiography and Doppler studies generally allow precise definition, localization, and quantitation of the lesions.

Penetrating cardiac trauma usually requires prompt surgical intervention, even performance of a thoracotomy in the emergency department. The immediate availability of echocardiography in the emergency department or trauma unit is extremely valuable in management of penetrating wounds of the heart. The survival rate of patients who reach the hospital alive is about 50% for those with knife wounds of the heart and 30% for those with gunshot wounds.[49]

ELECTRICAL INJURY

Electrical injury, a special type of cardiac trauma, is produced by a direct electrical effect on the tissues, the generation of heat from the passage of current from a high-voltage source through tissue with high electrical resistance, extreme release of catecholamines, or extreme autonomic stimulation.[50] Sudden cardiac arrest occurs with exposure to both household AC current and lightning strikes. Lightning strikes also cause myocardial injury, which may be extensive; in such cases, ECG patterns change, concentrations of cardiac enzymes increase, and wall motion exhibits abnormalities. Pericarditis and pericardial effusion also occur. The abnormalities usually resolve within several weeks.

References

1. Baljepally R, Spodick DH: PR-segment deviation as the initial electrocardiographic response in acute pericarditis. Am J Cardiol 81:1505, 1998

2. Adler Y, Finkelstein J, Guindo A, et al: Colchicine treatment for recurrent pericarditis: a decade of experience. Circulation 97:2183, 1998

3. Marcolongo R, Russo R, Laveder F, et al: Immunosuppressive therapy prevents recurrent pericarditis. J Am Coll Cardiol 26:1276, 1995

4. Akashi H, Tayama K, Ishihara K: Isolated primary chylopericardium. Jpn Circ J 63:59, 1999

5. Spodick DH: Pathophysiology of cardiac tamponade. Chest 113:1372, 1998

6. Larose E, Ducharme A, Mercier LA, et al: Prolonged distress and clinical deterioration before pericardial drainage in patients with cardiac tamponade. Can J Cardiol 16:331, 2000

7. Roosen J, Frans E, Wilmer A, et al: Comparison of premortem clinical diagnoses in critically ill patients and subsequent autopsy findings. Mayo Clin Proc 75:562, 2000

8. Mercé J, Sagrista-Sauleda J, Permanyer-Miralda G, et al: Correlation between clinical and Doppler echocardiographic findings in patients with moderate and large pericardial effusion: implications for the diagnosis of cardiac tamponade. Am Heart J 138:759, 1999

9. Beppu S, Tanaka N, Nakatani S, et al: Pericardial clot after open heart surgery: its specific localization and haemodynamics. Eur Heart J 14:230, 1993

10. Sagristà-Sauleda J, Angel J, Permanyer-Miralda G, et al: Long-term follow-up of idiopathic chronic pericardial effusion. N Engl J Med 341:2054, 1999

11. Merce J, Sagrista-Sauleda J, Permanyer-Miralda G, et al: Should pericardial drainage be performed routinely in patients who have a large pericardial effusion without tamponade? Am J Med 105:106, 1998

12. Nugue O, Millaire A, Porte H, et al: Pericardioscopy in the etiologic diagnosis of pericardial effusion in 141 consecutive patients. Circulation 94:1635, 1996

13. Allen KB, Faber LP, Warren WH, et al: Pericardial effusion: subxiphoid pericardiostomy versus percutaneous catheter drainage: Ann Thorac Surg 67:437, 1999

14. Flores RM, Jaklitsch MT, DeCamp MM Jr, et al: Video-assisted thoracic surgery pericardial resection for effusive disease. Chest Surg Clin N Am 8:835, 1998

15. Ziskind AA, Pearce AC, Lemmon CC, et al: Percutaneous balloon pericardiotomy for the treatment of cardiac tamponade and large pericardial effusions: description of technique and report of the first 50 cases. J Am Coll Cardiol 21:1, 1993

16. Piovaccari G, Ferretti RM, Prati F, et al: Cardiac disease after chest irradiation for Hodgkin's disease: incidence in 108 patients with long followup. Int J Cardiol 49:39, 1995

17. Wilkes JD, Fidias P, Vaickus L, et al: Malignancy-related pericardial effusion. 127 cases from the Roswell Park Cancer Institute. Cancer 76:1377, 1995

18. Bardales RH, Stanley MW, Schaefer RF, et al: Secondary pericardial malignancies: a critical appraisal of the role of cytology, pericardial biopsy, and DNA ploidy analysis. Am J Clin Pathol 106:29, 1996

19. Laham RJ, Cohen DJ, Kuntz RE, et al: Pericardial effusion in patients with cancer: outcome with contemporary management strategies. Heart 75:67, 1996

20. Rerkpattanapipat P, Wongpraparut N, Jacobs LE: Cardiac manifestations of acquired immunodeficiency syndrome. Arch Intern Med 160:602, 2000

21. Fletcher SL, Bodenham AR: Safe placement of central venous catheters: where should the tip of the catheter lie? (editorial). Br J Anaesth 85:188, 2000

22. Von Sohsten R, Kopistansky C, Cohen M, et al: Cardiac tamponade in the "new device" era: evaluation of 6999 consecutive percutaneous coronary interventions. Am Heart J 140:279, 2000

23. Tsang TS, Freeman WK, Barnes ME, et al: Rescue echocardiographically guided pericardiocentesis for cardiac perforation complicating catheter-based procedures: the Mayo Clinic experience. J Am Coll Cardiol 32:1345, 1998

24. Dardas P, Tsikaderis D, Ioannides E, et al: Constrictive pericarditis after coronary artery bypass surgery as a cause of unexplained dyspnea: a report of five cases. Clin Cardiol 21:691, 1998

25. Veeragandham RS, Goldin MD: Surgical management of radiation-induced heart disease. Ann Thorac Surg 65:1014, 1998

26. Fowler NO: Constrictive pericarditis: its history and current status. Clin Cardiol 18:341, 1995

27. Mehta A, Mehta M, Jain AC: Constrictive pericarditis. Clin Cardiol 22:334, 1999

28. Ling L, Oh J, Tei C, et al: Pericardial thickness measured with transesophageal echocardiography: feasibility and potential clinical usefulness. J Am Coll Cardiol 29:1317, 1997

29. Oh JK, Tajik AJ, Appleton CP, et al: Preload reduction to unmask the characteristic Doppler features of constrictive pericarditis: a new observation. Circulation 95:796, 1997

30. Boonyaratavej S, Oh JK, Tajik AJ, et al: Comparison of mitral inflow and superior vena cava Doppler velocities in chronic obstructive pulmonary disease and constrictive pericarditis. J Am Coll Cardiol 32:2043, 1998

31. Vaitkus PT, Kussmaul WG: Constrictive pericarditis versus restrictive cardiomyopathy: a reappraisal and update of diagnostic criteria. Am Heart J 122:1431, 1991

32. Hurrell DG, Nishimura RA, Higano ST, et al: Value of dynamic respiratory changes in left and right ventricular pressures for the diagnosis of constrictive pericarditis. Circulation 93:2007, 1996

33. Oh JK, Hatle LK, Mulvagh SL, et al: Transient constrictive pericarditis: diagnosis by two-dimensional Doppler echocardiography. Mayo Clin Proc 68:1158, 1993

34. Ling LH, Oh JK, Schaff HV, et al: Constrictive pericarditis in the modern era: evolving clinical spectrum and impact on outcome after pericardiectomy. Circulation 100:1380, 1999

35. Silvestri F, Bussani R, Pavletic N, et al: Metastases of the heart and pericardium. G Ital Cardiol 27:1252, 1997

36. Perchinsky MJ, Lichtenstein SV, Tyers GF: Primary cardiac tumors: forty years' experience with 71 patients. Cancer 79:1809, 1997

37. Reynen K: Cardiac myxomas. N Engl J Med 333:1610, 1995

38. Freedom RM, Lee KJ, MacDonald C, et al: Selected aspects of cardiac tumors in infancy and childhood. Pediatr Cardiol 21:299, 2000

39. Hövels-Gürich HH, Seghaye MC, Amo-Takyi BK, et al: Cardiac myxoma in a 6-year-old child—constitutional symptoms mimicking rheumatic disease and the role of interleukin-6. Acta Paediatr 88:786, 1999

40. Casey MC, Vaughn CJ, He J, et al: Mutations in the protein kinase A R1alpha regulatory subunit cause familial cardiac myxomas and Carney complex. J Clin Invest 106:R31, 2000

41. Bhan A, Mehrotra R, Choudhary SK, et al: Surgical experience with intracardiac myxomas: long-term follow-up. Ann Thorac Surg 66:810, 1998

42. Ceresoli GL, Ferreri AJ, Bucci E, et al: Primary cardiac lymphoma in immunocompetent patients: diagnostic and therapeutic management. Cancer 80:1497, 1997

43. Baum VC: The patient with cardiac trauma. J Cardiothorac Vasc Anesth 14:71, 2000

44. Pretre R, Chilcott M: Blunt trauma to the heart and great vessels. N Engl J Med 336:626, 1997

45. Curfman GD: Fatal impact—concussion of the heart (editorial). N Engl J Med 338:1841, 1998

46. Garcia-Fernandez MA, Lopez-Perez JM, Perez-Castellano N, et al: Role of transesophageal echocardiography in the assessment of patients with blunt chest trauma: correlation of echocardiographic findings with the electrocardiogram and creatine kinase monoclonal antibody measurements. Am Heart J 135:476, 1998

47. Swaanenburg JC, Klaase JM, DeJongste MJ, et al: Troponin I, troponin T, CKMB-activity and CKMB-mass as markers for the detection of myocardial contusion in patients who experienced blunt trauma. Clin Chim Acta 272:171, 1998

48. Gandhi SK, Marts BC, Mistry BM, et al: Selective management of embolized intracardiac missles. Ann Thorac Surg 62:290, 1996

49. Tyburski JG, Astra L, Wilson RF, et al: Factors affecting prognosis with penetrating wounds of the heart. J Trauma 48:587, 2000

50. Fish RM: Electric injury: III. Cardiac monitoring indications, the pregnant patient, and lightning. J Emerg Med 18:181, 2000

26 Cardiomyopathies

G. William Dec, M.D., and Roman W. DeSanctis, M.D.

Classification of Cardiomyopathies

The cardiomyopathies are a diverse group of diseases characterized by myocardial dysfunction that is not related to the usual causes of heart disease, notably coronary atherosclerosis, valvular dysfunction, and hypertension. Cardiomyopathies are classified according to hemodynamic characteristics and etiology.

HEMODYNAMIC CLASSIFICATION

The four major hemodynamic categories of cardiomyopathies are dilated, hypertrophic, restrictive, and obliterative [see Table 1]. The major features of dilated cardiomyopathy are ventricular dilatation and systolic dysfunction, which usually involve both ventricles, although some degree of ventricular hypertrophy is often present. Right ventricular dysplasia is a subtype of dilated cardiomyopathy that primarily involves the right ventricle but that may ultimately progress to the left ventricle as well. The hallmark of hypertrophic cardiomyopathy is ventricular hypertrophy, which is usually massive. Often, the thickening of the interventricular septum is disproportionately greater than that of the free wall of the left ventricle. However, concentric hypertrophy, as well as many other patterns of localized hypertrophy, can occur with this disease.[1] Restrictive cardiomyopathy is characterized by a rigid, poorly distensible myocardium that causes greatly diminished compliance; restrictive cardiomyopathy may mimic constrictive pericarditis clinically and hemodynamically. Obliterative cardiomyopathy is rarely seen in the Western world. It is endemic in other parts of the world, particularly eastern Africa and India, where it presents as endomyocardial fibrosis. The massive fibrosis of the endocardium encroaches on and diminishes the size of the ventricular cavities and causes a restrictive and obliterative hemodynamic pattern. Space-occupying thrombi associated with eosinophilic endomyocardial disease (also called Löffler endocarditis and fibroplastic endocarditis) may behave similarly.

Although a single category called restrictive-obliterative has been proposed,[2] we believe separate categories for restrictive and obliterative cardiomyopathies are still warranted, because restrictive cardiomyopathies involve only the myocardium, whereas the obliterative cardiomyopathies are characterized by both myocardial and major endocardial abnormalities. In any given case, features of more than one type of cardiomyopathy may be present. For example, the thick, stiff left ventricle of hypertrophic cardiomyopathy causes impaired diastolic relaxation and ventricu-

Table 1 Morphologic and Hemodynamic Characteristics of the Cardiomyopathies

		Dilated	Hypertrophic	Restrictive	Obliterative (Restrictive-Obliterative)
Morphologic					
		Biventricular dilatation	Marked hypertrophy of left ventricle and occasionally of right ventricle; usually, but not always, disproportionate hypertrophy of septum	Reduced ventricular compliance; usually caused by infiltration of myocardium (e.g., by amyloid, hemosiderin, or glycogen deposits)	Thickened endocardium or mural thrombi, or both, act as space-occupying lesions
Hemodynamic	Cardiac output	↓ ↓	Normal	Normal to ↓	Normal or ↓
	Stroke volume	↓ ↓	Normal or ↑	Normal or ↓	Normal or ↓
	Ventricular filling pressure	↑ ↑	Normal or ↑	↑ ↑	Usually ↑
	Chamber size	↑ ↑	Normal or ↓	Normal or ↑	Typically ↓
	Ejection fraction	↓ ↓	↑ ↑	Normal to ↓	Normal to ↓
	Diastolic compliance	Normal or ↓	↓ ↓	↓ ↓	↓ ↓
	Other findings	May have associated functional mitral or tricuspid regurgitation	Obstruction may develop between interventricular septum and septal leaflet of mitral valve Mitral regurgitation may be present	Characteristic ventricular pressure tracings that resemble those recorded in constrictive pericarditis, with early diastolic dip-and-plateau configuration	May be seen as a feature of the hypereosinophilic syndromes Some investigators consider it a form of restrictive cardiomyopathy

lar filling, which are also features of restrictive cardiomyopathy. Furthermore, the massive hypertrophy that characterizes hypertrophic cardiomyopathy may reduce left ventricular chamber size, which is also a feature of obliterative cardiomyopathy.

ETIOLOGIC CLASSIFICATION

The causes of cardiomyopathies are poorly understood; in many cases, the cause is unknown and the disorder is considered idiopathic. Recognized causes and associations include certain drugs and toxins and several infectious, systemic, infiltrative, nutritional, and ischemic disorders [see Table 2].

Dilated cardiomyopathy can either be idiopathic or have a known etiology. It can be associated with pregnancy, excessive alcohol consumption, or several disease processes or can occur as a toxic effect of drugs. Although the cause of obliterative cardiomyopathies remains unknown, the vast majority of cases of hypertrophic cardiomyopathy result from specific defects in the genes regulating the formation of cardiac muscle. Restrictive cardiomyopathies usually result from diseases that infiltrate the myocardium, such as amyloidosis, hemochromatosis, and glycogen storage diseases; however, many cases of restrictive cardiomyopathy are idiopathic.

When cardiomyopathy has a definite etiology—for example, when it is secondary to another disease (e.g., sarcoidosis or scleroderma)—signs of that process are usually evident. On rare occasions, however, cardiac involvement may precede other systemic manifestations.

Dilated Cardiomyopathy

ETIOLOGY

Pregnancy

Peripartum cardiomyopathy is an idiopathic dilated cardiomyopathy that usually develops in the last month of pregnancy or 3 to 4 months after parturition. It is unlikely that the stress of pregnancy exacerbates an underlying subclinical cardiomyopathy, because the disease typically develops well after the period of maximum physiologic stress has passed. A small minority of cases of peripartum cardiomyopathy have been shown by endomyocardial biopsy to result from acute inflammatory myocarditis.[3]

Drugs and Toxins

Dilated cardiomyopathy is associated with excessive alcohol intake. There is ample evidence that alcohol depresses cardiac function, and it appears that alcohol can damage the heart in some heavy drinkers.[4] The typical patient with alcoholic cardiomyopathy is a middle-aged man who has consumed at least 80 g of alcohol daily for 10 or more years. Another drug that has been implicated in the development of dilated cardiomyopathy is cocaine.

Serious myocardial damage can result from certain drugs used in anticancer chemotherapy, especially the anthracycline drugs doxorubicin and daunorubicin. The incidence and, to some extent, the severity of these reactions are directly related to the cumulative dose. The incidence is 3.5% in patients who receive a cumulative dose of doxorubicin of 400 mg/m^2, 7% in patients who receive 550 mg/m^2, and 15% in patients who receive 700 mg/m^2.[5,6] There is evidence that cardiotoxicity is reduced if doxorubicin is administered in smaller doses (20 mg/m^2) on a weekly basis rather than in larger doses (60 mg/m^2) every 3 weeks. Patients with preexisting cardiac disease, those 70 years of age or older, and those treated with concomitant mediastinal irradiation are

more vulnerable.[7] Combinations of doxorubicin with other antineoplastic drugs, such as dactinomycin, dacarbazine, cyclophosphamide, and mitomycin, also appear to increase the risk. There is evidence that the bispiperazinedione dexrazoxane can protect against cardiac toxicity when given simultaneously with doxorubicin to women with breast cancer, but this may also partially reduce the beneficial chemotherapeutic effects of doxorubicin.[8]

Table 2   Etiologic Classification of Cardiomyopathies

Cardiomyopathies of Unknown Etiology
  Idiopathic dilated cardiomyopathy
  Peripartum cardiomyopathy*
  Hypertrophic cardiomyopathy
  Endomyocardial fibrosis
  Subendocardial fibroelastosis
  Eosinophilic endomyocardial disease (also called Löffler endocarditis or fibroplastic endocarditis)
  Right ventricular dysplasia
  Idiopathic restrictive cardiomyopathy

Cardiomyopathies of Known Etiology
  Infectious
    Viral and rickettsial myocarditis (e.g., human immunodeficiency virus, coxsackievirus B,* cytomegalovirus*)
    Septic (bacterial endocarditis*)
    Syphilis
    Parasitic disease (e.g., Chagas disease, trichinosis, toxoplasmosis)*
    Bacterial toxins (e.g., diphtheria toxin) or hypersensitivity (rheumatic fever)
  Toxic
    Alcohol*
    Cobalt*
    Carbon tetrachloride
    Carbon monoxide*
    Thioridazine drugs
    Anticancer agents (e.g., daunorubicin, doxorubicin, cyclophosphamide)
    Antimonials
    Cocaine*
    Antiretroviral agents (e.g., zidovudine,* dideoxyinosine*)
    Interferon alfa
  Systemic
    Neuromuscular and muscular degenerative syndromes: muscular dystrophies (e.g., progressive muscular dystrophy, myotonic dystrophy), Friedreich ataxia
    Collagen vascular disease
    Sarcoidosis*
    Endocrine diseases* (e.g., thyrotoxicosis, myxedema, pheochromocytoma, acromegaly)
  Infiltrative†
    Amyloidosis
    Hemochromatosis
    Glycogen storage disease
    Fabry disease
    Hurler syndrome
    Primary or metastatic tumors (e.g., lymphoma, melanoma)
  Nutritional
    Beriberi*
    Selenium deficiency*
    Kwashiorkor
  Ischemic

*Is potentially reversible.
†Usually causes a restrictive hemodynamic picture.

Congestive heart failure associated with anthracycline administration may develop within 2 months after the last dose of the drug, although latent periods of several months or years have been reported.[9] Among 201 pediatric cancer patients who had received anthracycline therapy and were followed for 4 to 20 years, 23% showed evidence of late cardiac abnormalities.[9] Mortality can be as high as 60%.

Infectious and Autoimmune Processes

Some cases of cardiomyopathy that are classified as idiopathic may be sequelae of viral infections, such as infection with coxsackievirus B,[10] or autoimmune processes.[11] Although enteroviral RNA sequences have been detected in explanted myocardium or in endomyocardial biopsy samples of 25% to 30% of patients with idiopathic dilated cardiomyopathy, the significance of those sequences is uncertain.[12,13] Some investigators have reported that patients with dilated cardiomyopathy demonstrate a significantly higher incidence of the histocompatibility antigens HLA-B27 and HLA-DR4 and reduced suppressor cell activity, but other researchers have found no evidence of an abnormal cellular immune response. In addition, beta$_1$ receptor antibodies have been reported to occur in up to 45% of cases of dilated cardiomyopathy.[14] Transvenous endomyocardial biopsy has revealed that a significant number of these patients also have active myocarditis. The precise implications of these findings remain unclear.

There is a high incidence of cardiac dysfunction in patients with AIDS. Evidence of clinically reduced myocardial function, usually determined by cardiac echocardiography, has been noted in 10% to 20% of patients with AIDS,[15] and autopsy evidence of myocarditis has been found in approximately 50% of patients who have died of AIDS.[16] It is unclear how much of the myocardial dysfunction results from HIV infection itself, but substantial evidence suggests that HIV plays an important role. Additionally, opportunistic infections—viral, protozoal, fungal, and bacterial—have all been implicated. Furthermore, reversible cardiac toxicity has been ascribed to certain drugs, such as zidovudine (AZT) and interferon alfa-2b, that are used to treat AIDS and its complications.[17] As the lives of HIV-infected patients are prolonged, it is likely that more of these patients will have cardiac complications.

Genetic Mutations

A familial form of dilated cardiomyopathy may be present in 10% to 30% of cases of previously disguised idiopathic cardiomyopathy.[18] Specific genetic mutations in dystrophin (X-linked inheritance), actin (autosomal dominant inheritance), and nuclear envelope proteins such as lamin A/C (autosomal dominant) have been characterized.[19] Nearly one third of asymptomatic relatives will have echocardiographic abnormalities, and over 25% of these individuals will develop overt dilated cardiomyopathy.[20]

Coronary Artery Disease

It is not known whether ischemia related to coronary artery disease can cause dilated cardiomyopathy. If coronary ischemia does cause cardiomyopathy, then by inference, coronary revascularization may reverse the process. There is no doubt that recurrent and extensive myocardial infarction can lead to cardiomyopathy (typically, left ventricular failure). Moreover, there have been reports of patients with severe coronary artery disease and dilated cardiomyopathy who had no history of angina or of known myocardial infarction.[21]

Despite these findings, there is little direct evidence that significant disease of the major coronary arteries results in cardiomyopathy. In fact, left ventricular function usually remains normal despite severe obstructive coronary artery disease, as long as myocardial infarction has not occurred. It has been shown that the cardiomyopathic syndrome in coronary artery disease is directly related to the extent and severity of proximal coronary artery disease and hence to the previous occurrence of multiple myocardial infarctions.[21] However, recurring severe ischemia can contribute to congestive heart failure in some individuals who already have significant impairment of resting left ventricular function. It is important to detect these patients because surgical revascularization may lead to improved left ventricular function.

In a group of patients with intimal obliterative disease of the small coronary arteries (100 to 200 mm in diameter), the presenting symptoms suggested cardiomyopathy. Such abnormalities have been described in Marfan syndrome, primary pulmonary hypertension, and neuromuscular degenerative syndromes.[22] Small vessel disease is also seen in some cases of hypertrophic cardiomyopathy.

PATHOPHYSIOLOGY

Dilated cardiomyopathy is characterized by diminished myocardial contractility. Frequently, the cardiomyopathic process involves both ventricles. Apoptosis, or programmed cell death, has been reported in clinical and experimental dilated cardiomyopathy.[23,24] Cardiocyte dropout may contribute to impaired contractility. Impaired contractility is reflected in diminished systolic performance of the heart—that is, reduced ejection fraction, increased end-diastolic and residual volumes, biventricular failure, and reduced ventricular stroke work. The myocardium is frequently hypertrophied, but ventricular dilatation and failure, not hypertrophy, are the fundamental problems.

Cardiac output is usually reduced in patients with dilated cardiomyopathy; it is almost invariably decreased when congestive heart failure is advanced. During exercise, filling pressures rise abnormally, but cardiac output remains fixed or may even fall. In rare instances, as in beriberi or thyrotoxicosis, dilated cardiomyopathy is associated with a high cardiac output.

Occasionally, the cardiomyopathic process can involve predominantly the right ventricle. This condition, termed right ventricular dysplasia, is characterized by clinical evidence of right ventricular dysfunction and often by coexistent ventricular tachycardia of right ventricular origin.[25] Noninvasive studies of cardiac function in a series of patients with right ventricular dysplasia revealed subtle abnormalities of left ventricular function that were especially evident during exercise. Hence, the cardiomyopathic process is not always confined to the right ventricle; in particular, as the disease progresses, the left ventricle may ultimately become involved. Familial right ventricular dysplasia has also been reported.[26]

DIAGNOSIS

Clinical Features

The most common symptoms of dilated cardiomyopathy are dyspnea and fatigue. Although pulmonary congestion is frequent, acute pulmonary edema is less common. This has been ascribed to the fact that the coincidence of right ventricular failure with left ventricular failure protects the pulmonary vascular bed from pulmonary edema. However, acute pulmonary edema can occur, especially in response to a respiratory infection, heart rhythm change, or worsening of mitral regurgitation.

Palpitations are common and reflect the occurrence of ectopic beats and arrhythmias; occasionally, arrhythmias cause syncope.

a

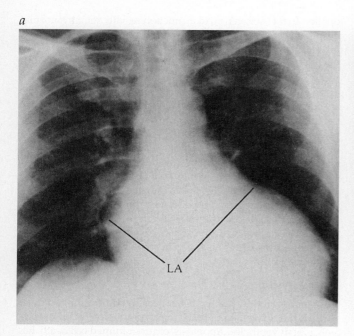

LA

b

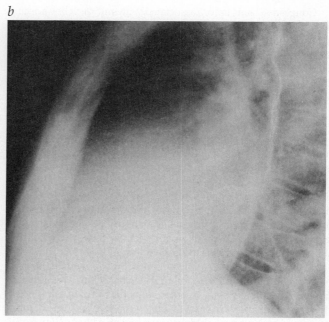

Figure 1   Posteroanterior (*a*) and lateral (*b*) chest roentgenograms of a 52-year-old man with idiopathic dilated cardiomyopathy exhibit diffuse cardiomegaly. The left atrium (LA) can be seen as a faint double density on the posteroanterior film, but the enlargement of this chamber is not disproportionate to that of the left ventricle.

Although systemic and pulmonary emboli are an infrequent initial presentation, they occur in approximately 1% to 4% of patients each year and are more common in those with advanced heart failure and cardiomegaly. Chest pain is present in over one third of patients, but it usually does not have the typical qualities of angina unless coronary artery disease is present. Ischemiclike chest pain in some patients with dilated cardiomyopathy has been ascribed to inadequate coronary vasodilator reserve.[27] Pleuritic chest pain may indicate the occurrence of pulmonary infarction. Asymptomatic cardiomegaly is detected in fewer than 10% of patients.

Physical Findings

Physical findings in patients with dilated cardiomyopathy reflect the severity of left ventricular dysfunction and range from asymptomatic cardiomegaly to overt heart failure. In congestive heart failure, the blood pressure is often slightly elevated: the systolic pressure may be raised to 150 to 170 mm Hg and the diastolic pressure to 100 to 110 mm Hg. As congestive heart failure clears, blood pressure returns to normal. Systemic venous pressure is frequently increased, and the liver may be enlarged and tender; both of these abnormalities are signs of right ventricular failure. Prominent venous A waves, reflecting reduced right ventricular compliance, may be seen. Prominent V waves, if present, result from tricuspid incompetence. Cardiac enlargement is the rule, and an abnormally displaced, heaving cardiac impulse—particularly of the left ventricle but often of the right ventricle as well—may be palpable. Presystolic impulses may be generated by vigorous atrial contraction.

The most prevalent auscultatory findings in dilated cardiomyopathy are gallops. A fourth heart sound (S_4, or atrial gallop) is almost universal, and a third heart sound (S_3 gallop) is heard in about 75% of decompensated cases. It is sometimes possible to differentiate right from left ventricular S_3 gallops that are simultaneously present. Right ventricular S_3 gallops, best heard at the lower left sternal border, may be accentuated on inspiration and diminish or disappear on expiration.

Although the loudness of S_3 gallops fluctuates with the severity of congestive heart failure, the third heart sounds may persist even when compensation is restored. Furthermore, if they do disappear, they can often be elicited with gentle exercise. When the heart rate is rapid, summation gallops, which represent fusion of S_3 and S_4 gallops, are sometimes heard.

Murmurs in dilated cardiomyopathy are generally functional and are usually associated with relative mitral insufficiency. The murmurs arise from misalignment of the papillary muscles as they are displaced by the enlarging ventricles, a misalignment that causes mitral incompetence. Cardiomyopathic involvement of the papillary muscles may contribute to mitral regurgitation. Tricuspid regurgitation is less common and results from right ventricular failure.

Murmurs are pansystolic and are of grades I to II/VI in intensity. They are related to ventricular geometry and wax and wane, respectively, with increasing or decreasing ventricular dimensions.

There is nothing unique about the second heart sound in patients with dilated cardiomyopathy. The loudness of the pulmonic component is frequently increased, and the second sound may split abnormally if bundle branch block is present.

Noninvasive Studies

All patients with newly diagnosed dilated cardiomyopathy should have a chest roentgenogram and undergo electrocardiography and transthoracic echocardiography.

Chest roentgenography   Chest roentgenograms show evidence of pulmonary venous hypertension, sometimes with associated interstitial pulmonary edema. The heart is often markedly enlarged, with involvement of all four chambers [*see Figure 1*]. The left atrium is usually abnormally large, but the enlargement is in proportion to the large size of the left ventricle.

Electrocardiography The electrocardiogram is invariably abnormal. In at least 50% of patients, it shows a pattern of left ventricular hypertrophy. ST segment and T wave abnormalities are prevalent. Right or left bundle branch block is present in up to 20% of cases. P wave changes indicative of left or right atrial abnormalities, or both, are very common, as is first-degree atrioventricular (AV) block. Arrhythmias, particularly atrial and ventricular premature beats, are frequent. High-grade ventricular ectopy and especially asymptomatic, nonsustained ventricular tachycardia occur to a more severe degree in patients who have greater impairment of left ventricular function.[28] Paroxysmal or established atrial fibrillation, which is often poorly tolerated, develops in up to 20% of patients and has been associated with a poor prognosis in those with advanced heart failure. Although the findings on ECG may occasionally mimic those associated with myocardial infarction, the presence of pathologic Q waves more commonly indicates an ischemic cardiomyopathy than an idiopathic cardiomyopathy.[29]

Echocardiography and magnetic resonance imaging Echocardiography shows cardiac chamber enlargement with diminished ventricular contractility [see Figure 2]. Radioisotope imaging of the cardiac chambers is seldom needed, but when performed, it also shows dilatation of one or both ventricles and diffuse, global reduction in ventricular contractility. Right ventricular dysfunction is associated with poor long-term survival.[30] During exercise, the ejection fraction, which in healthy persons normally rises, often falls in patients with dilated cardiomyopathy. Although impaired ventricular contractility is the hallmark of this disorder, the extent of ventricular dilatation varies: mild dilatation that is associated with little myofibrillar loss has been described.[31] Segmental rather than global wall motion abnormalities may occur in more than 50% of cases and appear to be associated with a more favorable prognosis. Thus, noninvasive techniques cannot reliably differentiate ischemic from nonischemic dilated cardiomyopathic processes.

Echocardiography and MRI are very helpful for detecting the hallmarks of right ventricular dysplasia: right ventricular dilatation and diminished contractility with well-preserved left ventricular function. MRI often shows infiltration and replacement of the right ventricular myocardium with fat.[26,32] However, these noninvasive studies also often reveal some degree of left ventricular dysfunction.

Myocardial imaging using gallium-67 may occasionally identify patients with dilated cardiomyopathy and active myocardial inflammation, particularly inflammation due to sarcoidosis or myocarditis.

Cardiac catheterization and angiography After noninvasive testing, most adult patients with acute dilated cardiomyopathy should undergo cardiac catheterization and coronary and left ventricular angiography to exclude occult atherosclerosis. Cardiac catheterization may yield nonspecific findings. Elevation of the left and right ventricular end-diastolic pressures at rest or during exercise is the rule; cardiac output is normal or reduced and rises little if at all during exercise. Left ventricular angiography shows chamber enlargement, diffusely diminished left ventricular contractions, and a reduced ejection fraction. Mitral regurgitation may be observed; it is typically mild but may vary in severity. Angiography usually reveals normal coronary arteries. Right ventriculography may occasionally aid in the diagnosis of right ventricular dysplasia.

Endomyocardial Biopsy

The role of endomyocardial biopsy of the right ventricle is now quite limited. Although the biopsy-verified detection rate of active myocarditis ranges from 1% to 67%, the usual yield is 10% to 15% [see Figure 3]. This low diagnostic yield, as well as uncertainty regarding the role of immunosuppressive therapy in the treatment of biopsy-proven myocarditis, has led most investigators to abandon routine use of this technique. Biopsy is occasionally helpful in establishing a definitive diagnosis (e.g., amyloidosis) and in searching for potentially treatable causes of the dilated cardiomyopathy in patients with systemic diseases known to affect the myocardium (e.g., sarcoidosis, scleroderma).

Special Diagnostic Considerations for Patients Receiving Chemotherapy

Anthracycline chemotherapy Various noninvasive techniques have been used to evaluate patients receiving anthracycline chemotherapy. The procedures employed have included measurement of systolic time intervals, derived simply from correlating the phonocardiogram and the ECG, and echocardiographic and radionuclide assessment of left ventricular function.[8] All studies have found that left ventricular function diminishes as increasingly large doses of anthracycline drugs are administered. No study, however, has identified criteria that are particularly helpful in selecting patients en route to congestive heart failure far enough in advance to permit adjustment of anthracycline dosage or cessation of treatment. Of all of the noninvasive methods of monitoring cardiac function serially, radionuclide angiography seems to be the most useful.[6,8]

Doxorubicin chemotherapy Radionuclide imaging of the ventricles during exercise may be especially useful in revealing left ventricular dysfunction caused by doxorubicin. Abnormalities may persist long after cessation of chemotherapy. Although endomyocardial biopsy of the right ventricle can detect myocyte injury before discernible changes in ventricular function occur, this technique is seldom used to monitor doxorubicin therapy.

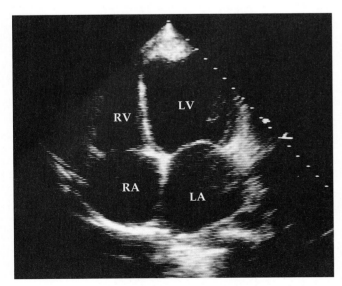

Figure 2 Apical four-chamber echocardiographic view of a patient with severe dilated cardiomyopathy. All four cardiac chambers are markedly enlarged. The left ventricular ejection fraction was 22%, and the left ventricular end-diastolic diameter was 74 mm.

a

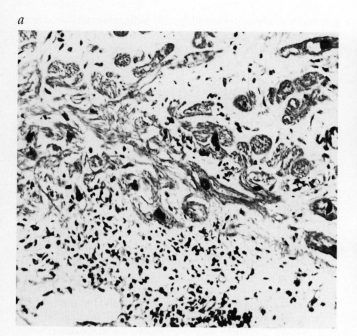

b

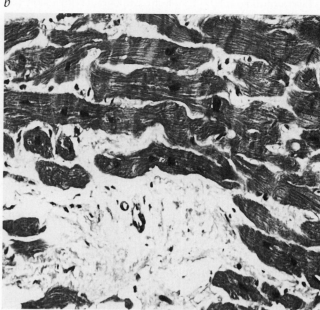

Figure 3   The endomyocardial biopsy specimen (*a*) is from a 19-year-old man who presented with dilated cardiomyopathy and ventricular arrhythmias. The findings of focal lymphocytic infiltrates, interstitial edema, and myocyte degeneration are typical of myocarditis. The patient responded to prednisone. The endomyocardial biopsy specimen (*b*) is from an 80-year-old woman with end-stage dilated cardiomyopathy. There is marked hypertrophy of myocytes, interstitial and focal replacement fibrosis, and no evidence of interstitial inflammation. Immunosuppressive therapy was not indicated.

The following program for monitoring patients receiving doxorubicin has been suggested. In patients who have a baseline radionuclide left ventricular ejection fraction (LVEF) of 50% or more, radionuclide ventriculography is repeated after 250 to 300 mg/m² of doxorubicin has been administered. Another ventriculogram is obtained after a cumulative dose of 400 mg/m² in patients with other risk factors for cardiotoxicity (e.g., known previous cardiac disease, radiation exposure, ECG abnormalities, or cyclophosphamide therapy) and after a dose of 450 mg/m² in patients who do not have such risk factors. Sequential studies are then recommended before each additional dose is given. Doxorubicin is discontinued if there is an absolute decline in the LVEF of 10% or more to a level of 50% or lower. For patients whose baseline LVEF is already 50% or lower, several recommendations are made: (1) no doxorubicin should be given if the LVEF is 30% or lower, (2) in patients with an LVEF of 30% to 50%, radionuclide angiography should be performed before each additional dose is given, and (3) doxorubicin should be stopped if the LVEF declines by 10% or more or if the final LVEF is 30% or lower.

DIFFERENTIAL DIAGNOSIS

Dilated cardiomyopathy must be distinguished from acute myocarditis of many different etiologies (the various myocarditides, in fact, can represent forms of acute dilated cardiomyopathy), as well as from valvular heart disease, coronary artery disease, and hypertensive heart disease. Acute myocarditis is usually caused by viruses, especially coxsackievirus B; fever and signs of systemic illness frequently accompany congestive heart failure. Pericarditis and elevation of the creatine kinase level occur in fewer than 30% of biopsy-verified cases of acute myocarditis. However, unexplained heart failure is commonly the only manifestation of myocarditis in patients with dilated cardiomyopathy.

Points that can assist in distinguishing dilated cardiomyopathy with functional mitral incompetence from rheumatic mitral regurgitation include the absence of a history of rheumatic fever, the absence of mitral valve calcification, the relative infrequency of atrial fibrillation, the presence of impaired left ventricular contractility, variation in the intensity of the murmur in response to the clinical state of the patient, and the presence of left atrial enlargement that is proportional to the degree of left ventricular dilatation.

The clinical manifestations of end-stage aortic valve disease—either stenosis or regurgitation—may resemble a dilated cardiomyopathy. This is particularly true in aortic regurgitation, in which severe left ventricular failure can mask signs of aortic runoff and cause the diastolic murmur to disappear. The murmur in end-stage aortic stenosis may be faint, but it is rarely absent. Suspicion that aortic stenosis may be present in patients with severe left ventricular failure should be confirmed by echocardiography and cardiac catheterization.

The relation between ischemic disease and cardiomyopathy is uncertain. Usually, patients who show simultaneous signs of ischemic disease and cardiomyopathy also have a history of angina, myocardial infarction, or both, although some have painless, coincident coronary artery obstruction and dilated cardiomyopathy.

Hypertensive heart disease is usually the result of severe, longstanding hypertension. It primarily affects the left ventricle.

COURSE AND PROGNOSIS

By far the most common complication of dilated cardiomyopathy is progressive congestive heart failure, which is the cause of death in 75% of patients with this disease. Sudden death caused by arrhythmias is also frequent, especially in patients with complex ventricular ectopy and severe left ventricular dysfunction.[28] Evidence of systemic embolism, pulmonary embolism, or both is found at autopsy in more than 50% of patients with dilated cardiomyopathy. Emboli can cause catastrophic complications but are an infrequent cause of death.[33]

The prognosis for patients with dilated cardiomyopathy varies considerably [*see Figure 4*]. The disease may pursue a fulminating course and result in death within a few weeks or months after the onset of symptoms. Conversely, some patients do remarkably well for years. Most deaths occur within 5 years after the onset of symptoms.

Spontaneous improvement in ventricular function occurs in 20% to 40% of cases, most frequently within 6 months of initial presentation but occasionally up to 4 years after the onset of symptoms.[33] Active myocardial inflammation and lesser degrees of myofibrillar loss on endomyocardial biopsy correlate with spontaneous improvement in function.[34] Improvement in baseline left ventricular ejection fraction and sphericity during dobutamine echocardiography in patients with dilated cardiomyopathy has been associated with spontaneous improvement in contractile function over time.[35]

The most reliable indicator of prognosis is the degree of ventricular dysfunction. Although the relation is not linear, the lower the ejection fraction or the greater the left ventricular enlargement, the poorer the long-term prognosis.[33] Other morphologic features that are associated with a poor prognosis include left ventricular hypertrophy, a more spherically shaped left ventricular cavity, right ventricular dilatation, and a persistent restrictive left ventricular diastolic filling pattern despite optimized medical therapy.[36] Clinical features that are associated with a more favorable outcome include female sex, an age younger than 50 years, and less advanced heart failure symptoms.[33,34] Cardiopulmonary exercise testing can provide useful prognostic information and quantify the patient's functional capacity. A peak level of oxygen uptake that is lower than 14 ml/kg/min predicts a 1-year survival rate of 70% and is frequently used to identify patients in need of cardiac transplantation.[37] Differences in etiology undoubtedly contribute to differences in prognosis.

TREATMENT

Medical Therapy

Treatment of congestive heart failure includes salt restriction and the administration of digitalis glycosides, diuretics, and vasodilators [*see Chapter 22*]. Controlled trials of digoxin have now demonstrated that digoxin has beneficial long-term effects on ejection fraction, exercise capacity, and chronic symptoms of heart failure.[38] Efficacy has been demonstrated in patients with mild to advanced symptoms, including those who are receiving concomitant vasodilator therapy. The Digitalis Investigation Group trial demonstrated that digoxin decreases heart failure hospitalizations but has no effect on long-term survival.[38] To help prevent the development of ventricular arrhythmias in patients who are receiving diuretics, the serum potassium level should be kept in the upper-normal range (4.5 to 5.0 mmol/L), and the therapeutic trough digoxin level should be kept at approximately 1.0 ng/dl. Magnesium deficiency often accompanies hypokalemia and also contributes to the development of ventricular arrhythmias.

Vasodilators Vasodilator therapy should be considered the standard initial treatment in symptomatic patients with left ventricular dysfunction.[39] Vasodilators can be classified in two broad categories: agents that reduce preload by causing venous dilatation and peripheral venous pooling, and agents that reduce afterload and aortic impedance by causing arterial and arteriolar di-

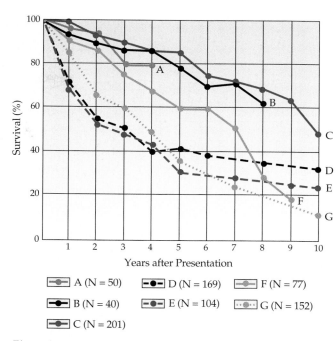

Figure 4 **Survival among patients with symptomatic idiopathic dilated cardiomyopathy in seven reported series. Study A, 1986–89 (basis for selection unspecified); study B, 1975–84 (population based); study C, 1973–87 (referral based); study D, 1962–82 (referral based); study E, 1960–73 (referral based); study F, 1972–82 (referral based); study G, 1965–86 (autopsy series). (N—the number of patients studied)**

latation. Preload-reducing agents help alleviate pulmonary and systemic congestive symptoms, whereas the arteriolar vasodilators help reverse deleterious effects of peripheral vasoconstriction. Consequently, arterial perfusion increases in several important areas, such as the kidneys and splanchnic beds. Patients often feel better, prerenal azotemia may improve, and diuretic requirements may fall.

Occasionally, specific vasodilators that act primarily on the venous or arteriolar circulation are useful (e.g., nitrates for relief of angina); however, agents that produce balanced reductions in preload and afterload, particularly the angiotensin-converting enzyme (ACE) inhibitors, are the most effective and widely prescribed drugs for the treatment of chronic congestive heart failure[39] [*see Table 3*]. Prospective, randomized, placebo-controlled clinical trials have shown that ACE inhibitors produce sustained improvement in functional class and a decline in hospitalizations for decompensated heart failure.[40,41] Captopril, which is short acting, and enalapril and lisinopril, which are both long acting, have all proved to be effective. Additional long-acting ACE inhibitors, including ramipril, quinapril, benazepril, and fosinopril, have been introduced. Although these agents are used primarily for the treatment of hypertension, they are also efficacious in the treatment of heart failure. Because ACE inhibitors interfere with the renin-angiotensin-aldosterone system, they may also correct dilutional hyponatremia in patients with severe congestive heart failure. Compared with other variables, hyponatremia is correlated strongly with a poor long-term prognosis; correction of the hyponatremia by administration of an ACE inhibitor improves the prognosis.

Although there has been some concern that long-acting ACE inhibitors might cause more renal insufficiency and postural hypotension than captopril, it appears that their actions are essentially the same as those of captopril when used in equivalent dos-

Table 3 Vasodilator Drugs Used in Therapy for Chronic Congestive Heart Failure

	Effect on Venous System	Effect on Arterial System	Usual Dosage	Peak Action	Duration of Effect
Nitroglycerin	+ + +	+	0.3–0.6 mg q. hr	10–20 min	30–60 min
Isosorbide dinitrate	+ + +	+	5–20 mg q. 6–8 hr	15–45 min	2–4 hr
Hydralazine	0	+ + +	25–100 mg q. 6 hr	1–2 hr	4–6 hr
Captopril	+ +	+ + +	25–75 mg q. 6–8 hr	1–2 hr	4–8 hr
Enalapril	+ +	+ + +	5–20 mg q. 12 hr	4–8 hr	18–30 hr
Lisinopril	+ +	+ + +	5–40 mg q. 24 hr	4–6 hr	18–30 hr

0 = no effect   + = slight effect   + + = moderate effect   + + + = marked effect

es.[42] ACE inhibitors are powerful hypotensive agents; they should be initiated cautiously and in low starting doses. Uncommon but significant side effects include a troublesome cough, neutropenia, angioedema, and precipitation of renal failure in patients with renal artery stenosis.

Four well-designed trials—the first and second Veterans Affairs Vasodilator–Heart Failure Trials (V-HeFT I and II), the first Cooperative North Scandinavian Enalapril Survival Study (CONSENSUS I), and the Studies of Left Ventricular Dysfunction (SOLVD)—have unequivocally demonstrated that certain vasodilators (ACE inhibitors and the combination of hydralazine and isosorbide dinitrate) relieve symptoms and improve prognosis in patients with mild to advanced heart failure.[39] Therapy with enalapril appears to be superior to that with hydralazine and isosorbide dinitrate in prolonging survival.[41] Now that vasodilator therapy has been shown to reduce mortality in symptomatic patients, investigators have shifted their focus to designing strategies to arrest abnormal ventricular remodeling before the onset of symptoms. The randomized SOLVD Prevention Trial, which enrolled more than 4,000 patients with asymptomatic left ventricular dysfunction (defined as an ejection fraction of 35% or less), demonstrated that enalapril reduced the number of initial hospitalizations for heart failure by 36% and produced a nonsignificant 12% risk reduction in cardiac mortality.[43] Thus, the use of ACE inhibitors in asymptomatic patients with cardiomyopathy is strongly recommended.

Whenever possible, an ACE inhibitor should be chosen as first-line therapy. Although dose-response curves for these agents have not been established, the recently completed Assessment of Treatment with Lisinopril and Survival (ATLAS) trial demonstrated that high-dose ACE inhibition was superior to low-dose therapy in decreasing hospitalizations but not in lowering long-term mortality.[44] For patients who cannot tolerate ACE inhibitors, the combination of hydralazine and isosorbide dinitrate or an angiotensin receptor antagonist (e.g., losartan, valsartan, candesartan) may be a useful second choice. In the Evaluation of Losartan in the Elderly (ELITE) trial, losartan was actually found to be superior to enalapril in elderly patients with heart failure.[45] However, the recently completed ELITE II trial found losartan and enalapril to have similar effects on survival.[46] Amlodipine, a calcium channel blocking drug, may be useful for patients with ischemic heart disease and symptoms of both heart failure and angina.[47]

Antiarrhythmic agents Frequent or complex asymptomatic ventricular ectopy—defined as more than 10 premature beats a minute, multiform premature beats, or nonsustained ventricular tachycardia—is commonly observed in patients with cardiomyopathy who undergo ambulatory ECG monitoring. As is true in ischemic heart disease, an inverse relation exists between the severity of the ventricular arrhythmias and the LVEF. Empirical pharmacologic suppression of asymptomatic ventricular arrhythmias has not been demonstrated to reduce the risk of sudden death or improve long-term survival in these patients. Class IA antiarrhythmic agents such as quinidine and procainamide are generally ineffective when the ejection fraction falls below 35%, and these drugs can cause significant proarrhythmic effects. Disopyramide and flecainide should not be used, because they can precipitate severe heart failure in patients with preexisting left ventricular dysfunction. The newer class IB agents, such as mexiletine and tocainide, have minimal negative inotropic properties but have not been carefully studied in this population. Amiodarone is the most widely used agent because it has minimal negative inotropic effects, is a modest vasodilator, is highly effective in suppressing ventricular arrhythmias despite the presence of impaired left ventricular function, and is not likely to cause proarrhythmic effects. Two prospective, placebo-controlled trials of low-dose amiodarone for suppression of asymptomatic nonsustained ventricular tachycardia (NSVT) have yielded conflicting results. The Grupo de Estudio de la Sobrevida en la Insuficiencia Cardiaca en Argentina (GESICA) trial demonstrated a 26% reduction in all-cause mortality and a trend toward decreased risk of sudden death in patients with moderate heart failure.[48] In contrast, the Survival Trial of Antiarrhythmic Therapy in Congestive Heart Failure (STAT-CHF) reported no improvement in survival or reduction in sudden deaths in a similar population.[49] There was a nonsignificant trend toward improved survival in patients with nonischemic cardiomyopathy. Thus, the empirical use of amiodarone in heart failure patients with asymptomatic ventricular arrhythmias is not recommended.

Anticoagulant therapy Because of the high frequency of pulmonary and systemic embolism, anticoagulant therapy, generally warfarin, is often prescribed when not contraindicated for patients with dilated cardiomyopathy and marked depression of left ventricular function (LVEF < 35%). Such therapy remains controversial because no controlled trials have examined its efficacy.[50] Similarly, the efficacy of platelet inhibitors in preventing embolism has not been proved.

Corticosteroids Corticosteroids may be of modest value in cases of dilated cardiomyopathy that are associated with collagen vascular disease, which occur rarely, and in cases of cardiac sarcoidosis, which occur even more rarely. The response of lymphocytic myocarditis to immunosuppressive therapy (prednisone alone or in combination with either cyclosporine or azathioprine) is unpredictable. Some patients exhibit a dramatic reduction in inflammation with concomitant clinical improvement, whereas others show either no response[51] or an intermediate response. It is not clear why these differences exist. Although uncontrolled studies have shown that short-term immunosuppression improves left ventricular function and is sometimes associated with regression of ventricular dilatation, the randomized Multicenter Myocarditis Treatment Trial failed to identify which patients were most likely to experience improvement in ventricular function during 6 months of immunosuppressive therapy.[52] Likewise, a single, uncontrolled short-term study using immunoglobulin G, a nonspecific immunomodulator, was shown to improve ventricular function in patients with acute dilated cardiomyopathy, but a recently completed randomized trial failed to confirm a benefit.[53] Focus has now shifted to immunomodulatory agents and cytokine antagonists for treatment of inflammatory heart disease. Short-term benefits in ventricular mass and contractile function have also been reported during human recombinant growth hormone therapy for idiopathic dilated cardiomyopathy.[54] An uncontrolled study using immunoadsorption of circulating autoantibodies resulted in improvement in ventricular function.[55] Controlled trials are needed to evaluate this new treatment approach.

Inotropic agents   Several new positive inotropic drugs have been developed for the treatment of heart failure. Most of these agents also possess vasodilator properties. Intravenous amrinone and milrinone are approved for use in the United States for the short-term treatment of patients with very advanced heart failure. Although these drugs may increase cardiac output, reduce elevated cardiac filling pressures, and alleviate symptoms, there is clear evidence that they do not prolong life and are often highly arrhythmogenic. Studies of oral milrinone and vesnarinone in patients with severe chronic heart failure demonstrated excessive mortality in the active treatment groups.[56]

Patients with advanced decompensated heart failure should be hospitalized to receive intravenous inotropic therapy. Administration of dobutamine, a beta-adrenergic stimulating drug, usually provides acute hemodynamic improvement and may also result in a modest sustained clinical improvement in patients with New York Heart Association functional class IV symptoms. Dosages should be initiated at 2.5 to 5.0 µg/kg/min; they should then be titrated upward in accordance with heart rate, blood pressure, cardiac output, and systemic vascular resistance and maintained for 72 hours. Acute hemodynamic improvement has also been reported with amrinone and milrinone therapies.[57] Controlled trials have not compared the safety or efficacy of these inotropic agents during continuous or intermittent treatment.

Beta blockers   Emphasis has shifted away from the use of agents that stimulate cardiac contractility and has focused on beta-adrenergic blockers, which partially protect the myocardium from excessive sympathetic stimulation. Controlled studies have demonstrated that a variety of agents, including metoprolol, bisoprolol, carvedilol, and bucindolol, relieve symptoms and improve ejection fraction in chronic heart failure. The effect of beta blockers on mortality has been variable and may reflect intrinsic differences in the agents themselves or in the populations studied. In the Metoprolol Dilated Cardiomyopathy Trial, metoprolol was found to reduce clinical deterioration, but it did not improve overall survival.[58] In contrast, in a larger trial—the Metoprolol CR/XL Randomized Intervention Trial in Congestive Heart Failure (MERIT-HF)—sustained-release metoprolol was found to provide a substantial survival benefit.[59] Similarly, the second Cardiac Insufficiency Bisoprolol Study (CIBIS 2) demonstrated a mortality benefit of this agent.[60] Carvedilol, a nonselective beta blocker with vasodilator and antioxidant properties, has been shown to slow disease progression and reduce mortality.[61,62] Symptomatic and survival benefits were observed in patients with mild to advanced heart failure as well as in those with ischemic and nonischemic disease. In contrast, the Beta-Blocker Evaluation of Survival Trial (BEST) recently failed to show a decrease in all-cause mortality for patients receiving bucindolol.[63] Given these conflicting results on outcome, agents that have demonstrated a significant survival benefit (sustained-release metoprolol, carvedilol, bisoprolol) should be selected for therapy. When used in congestive heart failure, the initial doses of beta blockers should be very low, and the daily dose should be gradually increased over weeks or months [see Table 4].

Spironolactone   The recently completed Randomized Aldatone Evaluation Study (RALES) found a 30% reduction in mortality and 35% reduction in hospitalizations for worsening heart failure in a large series of patients in New York Heart Association classes III and IV given rather small doses (25 to 50 mg daily) of the aldosterone antagonist spironoloactone.[64]

Defibrillation

The presence of late potentials on signal-averaged ECGs has not been an accurate predictor of sudden cardiac death in patients with advanced heart failure.[65] Likewise, intracardiac electrophysiologic testing has also not been proved to be reliable in assessing prognosis or in guiding antiarrhythmic therapy in patients with dilated cardiomyopathy. In patients who have experienced symptomatic, sustained ventricular tachyarrhythmia or ventricular fibrillation that is refractory to drug therapy, an automatic, implantable cardioverter-defibrillator (ICD) may greatly improve prognosis.[39,66]

Although the Multicenter Automatic Defibrillator Implantation Trial (MADIT) demonstrated lower all-cause mortality for patients with asymptomatic NSVT and LVEF below 35% who received a prophylactic ICD, few patients in this study had nonischemic car-

Table 4   Use of Beta-Adrenergic Blockers in Heart Failure*

Drug	Initial Dosage	Desired Dosage Range	Comments
Carvedilol	3.125 mg b.i.d.	25–50 mg b.i.d.	Initiation may require transient decrease in vasodilator therapy and increase in diuretic
Metoprolol XL/CR	6.25 mg b.i.d.	50–150 mg daily	Initiate therapy with non–extended-release preparation
Bisoprolol	1.25 mg daily	5 mg daily	—

*The agents listed have been shown to improve survival in heart failure in controlled clinical trials.
CR—controlled release   XL—extended release

diomyopathy, and all patients had inducible ventricular tachycardia on electrophysiologic testing before randomization.[66] Hence, these results are not directly applicable to the broad population of patients with dilated cardiomyopathy. Several multicenter defibrillator trials are now evaluating this approach in asymptomatic cardiomyopathy patients who have not undergone electrophysiologic risk stratification.

Surgery

Not infrequently, patients with severe dilated cardiomyopathy (LVEF < 25%) and coronary atherosclerosis may demonstrate a significant improvement in left ventricular function after coronary bypass surgery. Surgery may be undertaken in such patients if an extensive and complete revascularization of the myocardium can be achieved and if there is reversible ischemia of viable myocardium. The presence of reversible ischemia might be surmised from a history of severe angina or from ECG changes. A favorable surgical outcome may be more likely to occur if reversible defects in two or more myocardial regions are shown by thallium scintigraphy or positron emission tomography (PET) during ischemia provoked by exercise or pharmacologic stress testing.[21] The risk of bypass surgery remains high and is directly related to the extent of left ventricular dysfunction. However, there is growing evidence that surgical revascularization, even in the absence of angina, can relieve heart failure symptoms and improve exercise capacity and long-term prognosis in selected patients with extensive multivessel coronary artery disease and poor left ventricular function.[67,68]

When congestive heart failure is very advanced and the prognosis is exceedingly poor, heart transplantation is an excellent option if the patient does not have pulmonary hypertension or other significant, irreversible comorbidities.[69] In the United States, there are now over 150 hospitals that perform heart transplantations; roughly 2,400 heart transplantations are performed annually, a comparatively low figure given that an estimated 14,000 to 15,000 patients could benefit from transplantation. With cyclosporine-based immunosuppressive therapy, 1-year survival is 85% to 90% and 5-year survival is approaching 70%.[70] The longest survival exceeds 20 years. Although the cost of transplantation is high, the results clearly warrant its continued application in selected patients. Approximately 20% of patients awaiting heart transplantation die each year because of the scarcity of suitable donor hearts.

The mechanical heart has received much attention but currently has a limited role in the treatment of end-stage heart failure. Its greatest use at present is to sustain life in patients with end-stage heart failure until a transplantable heart is available.[71] As an alternative to replacing the entire heart, left ventricular assist devices (LVADs), particularly the Novacor and HeartMate models, are now being used for prolonged (> 4 months) pretransplant hemodynamic support. Permanently implantable battery-powered prototypes are just beginning to undergo clinical trials.

Dynamic cardiomyoplasty has been applied to a small number of patients with advanced heart failure.[72] The left or right latissimus dorsi muscle is mobilized and wrapped around the ventricles, and over several weeks, the latissimus dorsi is conditioned by electrical stimulation to function like myocardium. Although initial results were encouraging, 1-year mortality is 30% to 40%, and sudden death is a common late complication. Furthermore, this procedure cannot be used in patients with severe angina, recurrent ventricular tachyarrhythmias, marked left ventricular dilatation, or advanced right heart failure. Dynamic cardiomyoplasty is considered to be experimental and is performed in only a few

medical centers. Likewise, left ventricular reduction surgery (the Batista procedure) for patients with nonischemic cardiomyopathy, marked left ventricular dilatation, and refractory heart failure symptoms is now rarely performed because of its high (30% to 40%) 2-year mortality.[73] Mitral valve repair appears to significantly improve heart failure symptoms and lower intermediate-term (3-year) mortality in carefully selected patients with severe mitral regurgitation and markedly impaired left ventricular function.[74] This encouraging single-center experience needs to be confirmed by others before this approach can be recommended.

Hypertrophic Cardiomyopathy

ETIOLOGY AND GENETICS

Although hypertrophic cardiomyopathy can develop sporadically, it is hereditary in more than 50% of cases and is transmitted as an autosomal dominant trait. Major advances have been made in defining the genetics of the disease. The first abnormality that was found was a defect in the gene that encodes the cardiac β-myosin heavy chain located on chromosome 14.[75] Since then, approximately 140 additional defects have been discovered, all involving the cardiac contractile proteins, including troponin T, α-tropomyosin, myosin-binding protein C, essential and regulatory myosin light chains, and troponin I.[76,77] The same genetic defect is found in all members of a given kindred who have the disease, although the phenotypic expression may vary in any given family. About 70% of the mutations are missense mutations (i.e., they result in the substitution of a single amino acid). The others result in deletions of amino acids from the affected genes. There is good evidence that the specific defect caused by the mutation may relate to prognosis. In a study of 25 unrelated families with hypertrophic cardiomyopathy, seven different missense mutations were discovered in 12 families.[78] These missense mutations were located on the head or the head-rod junction region of the β-myosin heavy-chain gene. Six of the mutations altered the charge of the amino acid and were associated with a shortened average life expectancy of 33 years [see Figure 5]. The one mutation that did not change the charge of the amino acid was associated with virtually normal survival. Similar results were reported in a study of two families.[79] Defects in the genes for troponin T and α-tropomyosin seem to be characterized by mild or minimal hypertrophy and are associated with a high incidence of sudden death.[76,77] Defects in cardiac myosin-binding protein C are associated with late-life onset and a generally good prognosis.[80] Genetic defects have also been identified in cases of sporadic disease, which suggests that spontaneous mutations of the gene responsible for hypertrophic cardiomyopathy can occur and that these defects may then be transmitted to offspring.[81] Because transcripts of the β-myosin heavy-chain gene and other contractile proteins can be detected in blood lymphocytes, it is possible to screen family members of patients with identified genetic defects for preclinical or prenatal evidence of these defects.[82]

Currently, the search for genetic defects in hypertrophic cardiomyopathy is an expensive and cumbersome process that is confined to a few major academic medical centers. However, within the near future, it is anticipated that screening tests using gene-chip technology will be widely available. These tests will allow the identification of affected family members before the phenotypic manifestations of the disease appear and will also enable physicians to search for the defects that are associated with a poor prognosis, perhaps permitting more aggressive treatment of such patients in the hope of preventing sudden cardiac death.

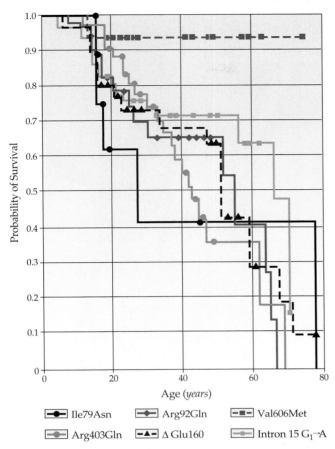

Legend:
- Ile79Asn
- Arg92Gln
- Val606Met
- Arg403Gln
- Δ Glu160
- Intron 15 G₁→A

Figure 5 **Kaplan-Meier survival curves for patients with hypertrophic cardiomyopathy caused by different mutations. The survival of patients with hypertrophic cardiomyopathy caused by cardiac troponin T mutations (introns 15 G₁ → A, Ile79Asn, ΔGlu160, and Arg92Gln) is similar to that in persons with a malignant β-myosin heavy-chain mutation (Arg403Gln) but significantly shorter than that observed in persons with a benign myosin mutation (Val606Met).**

PATHOLOGY

The hallmark of the disease is unexplained myocardial hypertrophy, usually with thickening of the interventricular septum that is disproportionately greater than that of the free wall of the left ventricle just beneath the posterior mitral leaflet [*see Figure 6*]. Thus, the disease has been termed asymmetrical septal hypertrophy (ASH). However, the hypertrophy is concentric in 20% of cases. Furthermore, two-dimensional echocardiographic studies indicate that there is an enormous variation in the location and extent of the hypertrophy.

In its severest forms, the hypertrophy of the left ventricle reaches massive dimensions and encroaches on the left ventricular chamber, which becomes small, elongated, and slitlike. In rare cases, the hypertrophy involves the right ventricle as well.

The left ventricular papillary muscles are also greatly hypertrophied, and the anterior papillary muscle is often displaced medially and anteriorly. Movement of the septal leaflet of the mitral valve may be restricted by the hypertrophied septum; this defect, together with the papillary muscle abnormality, leads to mitral insufficiency.

In many cases, the septal mitral leaflet strikes against the upper part of the underlying septum. This juxtaposition causes thickening and even occasional calcification of the undersurface of the septal leaflet and of the immediately subjacent endocardium of the interventricular septum [*see Figure 6*].

As a consequence of the massive septal hypertrophy, the interventricular septum may oppose the mitral leaflets in systole, causing obstruction to left ventricular outflow. The thickened anterior papillary muscle may also contribute to the genesis of this obstruction. Thus, hypertrophic cardiomyopathy may exist without left ventricular outflow obstruction, with a labile and inducible obstruction, or with a fixed obstruction; mitral insufficiency may or may not be present.

The histologic features are distinctive. The myofibrils in the hypertrophied muscle are bizarre and are arranged chaotically [*see Figure 7*]. They are typically enlarged, vary in size and shape, and show strikingly heterogeneous morphology.[1] In contrast, microscopic examination of tissue from patients in whom left ventricular hypertrophy has developed secondary to hypertension or aortic valve disease reveals myofibrils that are aligned in an orderly, parallel fashion and that are the same size and shape [*see Figure 7*]. Once considered specific for hypertrophic cardiomyopathy, the myofibrillar disarray has been noted in many other conditions—usually those associated with marked isometric left ventricular work—as well as in a small number of normal neonates; however, the disorganization in these other conditions is not nearly as marked or extensive.

Hypertrophic cardiomyopathy may be associated with a variety of patterns of regional involvement of the left ventricle. For example, midventricular obstruction has been described,[1] and nonobstructive hypertrophic cardiomyopathy predominantly localized to the cardiac apex has been reported[1]; the latter variant, which is prevalent in Japan, is associated with giant negative T waves on ECG.

PATHOPHYSIOLOGY

As a result of the hypertrophy, left ventricular compliance is much reduced. Systolic performance, however, is not depressed, at least not initially. The heart is hypercontractile, and systole occurs with striking rapidity. Ejection fractions are often 80% to 90%, and the left ventricle may be virtually obliterated in systole. Systolic ejection is usually excellent, even in cases of congestive heart failure; thus, failure in patients with hypertrophic cardiomyopathy usually reflects diminished diastolic compliance rather than reduced systolic performance.

The ability to provoke obstruction or to increase or decrease already existing obstruction is influenced by many factors, which may be grouped into three broad categories: (1) factors that change myocardial contractility (agents that increase contractility intensify obstruction, whereas those that depress contractility reduce obstruction); (2) factors that influence left ventricular chamber size, that is, preload (the larger the chamber, the lesser the obstruction); and (3) factors that affect afterload (the arterial pressure against which the heart must empty in systole). Increasing afterload reduces obstruction.

Many factors influence these variables [*see Table 5*]. Some agents may affect obstruction in more than one way. For example, nitroglycerin aggravates obstruction in three ways: it increases heart rate, reduces chamber size, and reduces blood pressure (afterload).

DIAGNOSIS

Clinical Features

The major symptoms of hypertrophic cardiomyopathy are angina, syncope, palpitations, and those symptoms related to con-

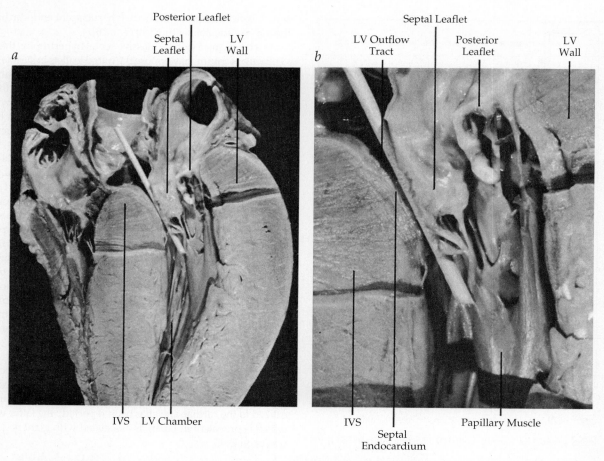

Figure 6 **The thickening of the interventricular septum (IVS) is disproportionately greater than that of the left ventricular (LV) wall behind the posterior mitral leaflet, as shown in this coronal section of the heart of a 48-year-old woman with hypertrophic cardiomyopathy (*a*). The LV chamber is small and elongated. A wooden stick lies in the LV outflow tract, and the close-up (*b*) emphasizes the proximity of the mitral valve to the IVS. Both the septal leaflet of the mitral valve and the immediately subjacent septal endocardium are markedly thickened.**

gestive heart failure. Angina is usually of the classic type, but because the severity of obstruction is influenced by several factors, angina sometimes develops without any obvious provocation. Angina that is relieved by the patient's assuming the recumbent position is virtually pathognomonic for hypertrophic cardiomyopathy, but this telltale sign is rarely encountered. Presumably, the increase in left ventricular size in recumbency acts to decrease the obstruction and thus alleviate the angina.

Although the coronary arteries of patients with hypertrophic cardiomyopathy tend to be enlarged, hypertrophic cardiomyopathy and coronary artery disease often coexist, especially in older people.[1] Myocardial infarction in the absence of significant disease of the large coronary arteries has been reported[1] and presumably occurred because coronary arteries could not supply adequate amounts of blood to the massively hypertrophied myocardium. Obstructive changes in small intramural coronary arteries have also been reported. Their significance is not known, but the severity of these obliterative changes is greatest adjacent to areas of myocardial fibrosis, suggesting a causal relation.[22]

It has been shown that patients with hypertrophic cardiomyopathy have a limited ability to dilate the coronary arteries in response to increased myocardial oxygen demand, a phenomenon that contributes to ischemia and angina. The presence of left ven-

tricular outflow obstruction makes this limitation of coronary vasodilator reserve even more significant.

Syncope typically occurs with or shortly after completion of physical activity, but it may also develop at rest. Sometimes, arrhythmias lead to loss of consciousness. Congestive heart failure is manifested by the constellation of dyspnea, fatigue, and fluid retention.

Hypertrophic cardiomyopathy predisposes to arrhythmias, of which paroxysmal or sustained atrial fibrillation and ventricular premature beats are the most common. Because the left ventricle is so massively hypertrophied, the presystolic atrial contraction is extremely important for the preservation of cardiac output. Consequently, the onset of atrial fibrillation is often not well tolerated; a poorly controlled rapid heart rate, which impairs diastolic filling, also adds to the deleterious effect of atrial fibrillation. Atrial fibrillation may lead to hypotension, syncope, or congestive heart failure. Although symptoms of hypertrophic cardiomyopathy typically worsen during atrial fibrillation, one large study showed that the onset of atrial fibrillation did not have a negative effect on long-term prognosis.[83]

Systemic embolism is a common complication of atrial fibrillation in this disease. Sudden cardiac death can occur, even in asymptomatic patients. In some families, the incidence of prema-

a

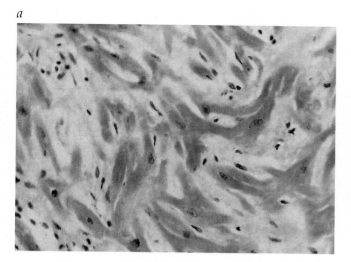

b

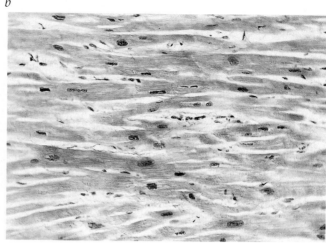

Figure 7   Different myofibrillar patterns are evident in tissue taken from the septum of a patient with hypertrophic cardiomyopathy (*a*) and from the hypertrophied left ventricle of a patient with hypertension (*b*). Note the chaotic arrangement of the cells in the higher-powered photomicrograph (magnified 250 times) of septal myocardium taken from the heart shown in Figure 6. In contrast, note the orderly parallel arrangement of myofibrils in ventricular myocardium in the hypertensive patient.

ture sudden cardiac death is very high, a phenomenon that is related to the underlying genetic defect.[1] Lethal arrhythmias are especially likely to occur in young patients.

Physical Findings

Physical findings in hypertrophic cardiomyopathy depend on the presence or absence of left ventricular outflow obstruction, the severity of obstruction, and the presence or absence of mitral regurgitation.

With or without obstruction, the initial carotid upstroke (percussion wave) is very rapid and forceful. If obstruction is present, a second, slower impulse in systole (tidal wave) may be felt after the initial rapid upstroke because left ventricular emptying is retarded [*see Figure 8*].

Because the degree of obstruction may fluctuate, the quality of the carotid arterial pulse may vary greatly. The carotid arterial pulse should be palpated not only with the patient at rest but also after various maneuvers designed to provoke obstruction, particularly the Valsalva maneuver. A single brisk impulse may be converted to a double impulse if obstruction develops.

The jugular venous pressure is usually normal in the absence of congestive heart failure, although somewhat prominent A waves, reflecting diminished ventricular compliance, may be present.

Findings on palpation of the heart vary greatly. Results can be normal in patients who have massive hypertrophy but neither outflow obstruction nor mitral regurgitation. More typically, an abnormal cardiac impulse is felt. A presystolic impulse is generated by vigorous atrial contraction. A hyperdynamic systolic im-

Table 5   Factors That Influence the Degree of Obstruction in Hypertrophic Cardiomyopathy*

Factors That Increase Obstruction		*Factors That Decrease Obstruction*	
Mechanism	*Physiologic or Pharmacologic Factor*	*Mechanism*	*Physiologic or Pharmacologic Factor*
Increase in contractility	Digitalis glycosides Beta-adrenergic stimulation (e.g., isoproterenol, epinephrine) Tachycardia Premature beats	Decrease in contractility	Beta-adrenergic blockade (e.g., propranolol) Heavy sedation and general anesthesia Calcium channel blockers, disopyramide, and other drugs that depress myocardial function
Reduction in preload	Valsalva maneuver[†] Decrease in intravascular volume (e.g., from hemorrhage, diuresis, GI losses) Standing[†] Nitroglycerin and related drugs[†] Vasodilator drugs Tachycardia	Increase in preload	Intravascular volume expansion Squatting[†] Bradycardia Beta-adrenergic blockade
Reduction in afterload	Hypovolemia Nitroglycerin and related drugs[†] Vasodilator drugs	Increase in afterload	Intravascular volume expansion Squatting[†] Alpha-adrenergic stimulation (e.g., phenylephrine, mephentermine) Handgrip exercise[†]

*In general, anything that increases obstruction will increase the intensity of the associated murmurs, whereas factors that reduce obstruction will diminish murmur intensity.
[†]May assist in diagnosis at the bedside.

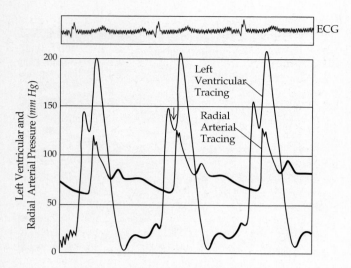

Figure 8 **Classic left ventricular and radial arterial pressure tracings are recorded simultaneously in a patient with obstructive hypertrophic cardiomyopathy. An initial rapid upstroke is observed in both recordings. As obstruction develops, a notch (arrow) appears in the left ventricular tracing, accompanied by a fall in the arterial pressure. Slower ejection follows, producing a second rise in the arterial tracing. The events are observed slightly later in the radial artery than in the left ventricle because some delay occurs in the transmission of the impulse to the radial artery.**

pulse may be felt, usually displaced somewhat to the left and inferiorly. In rare cases, two distinct impulses in systole can be felt in patients who have hypertrophic cardiomyopathy with outflow obstruction.

Auscultation almost invariably reveals an S_4 gallop. The S_2 may be paradoxically split, particularly if left ventricular obstruction is present. Because the obstruction may be dynamic and may fluctuate in severity, however, there can be much variation in the movement of the S_2.

The murmurs of hypertrophic cardiomyopathy are caused by either left ventricular outflow obstruction or mitral regurgitation. The systolic murmur of outflow obstruction has a crescendo-decrescendo quality and is best heard at the third and fourth left intercostal spaces adjacent to the sternum. The murmur of mitral regurgitation typically has a more blowing quality, is holosystolic, and is best heard at the apex, with transmission to the axilla.

Characteristic of these murmurs is their marked variability with different maneuvers, of which the Valsalva maneuver is especially useful at the bedside [*see Table 5*]. This maneuver reduces left ventricular chamber size, thereby increasing the degree of left ventricular outflow obstruction; thus, the murmur associated with obstruction becomes louder [*see Figure 9*]. In addition, because left ventricular systolic pressure increases, the murmur of mitral regurgitation also intensifies. The increase in intensity of murmurs with the Valsalva maneuver is not an invariable finding in hypertrophic cardiomyopathy; when present, however, it is highly suggestive of the disease. In fact, except for some cases of mitral valve prolapse, there is virtually no other murmur that behaves similarly.

Nitroglycerin may also make the murmur or murmurs louder. Standing increases the intensity of the murmurs, whereas squatting or recumbency may diminish it. A few patients have a faint murmur of aortic insufficiency.

Imaging and Tracing Studies

Roentgenographic findings in patients with hypertrophic cardiomyopathy are not specific. Variable degrees of cardiac enlargement, particularly of the left ventricle and the left atrium, are seen. Occasionally, both right and left atrial enlargement may be truly massive, resembling that seen in rheumatic heart disease. Pulmonary venous congestion may be present secondary to elevated left ventricular diastolic pressure.

The ECG usually shows an extreme degree of left ventricular hypertrophy. In asymptomatic patients without gallops or murmurs, marked and unexplained left ventricular hypertrophy may be the only sign of the disease. Because of the massive septal hypertrophy, abnormal Q waves resembling those that occur in myocardial infarction may be seen, particularly in the anterolateral and inferior leads [*see Figure 10*]. Giant negative T waves have been seen in hypertrophic cardiomyopathy involving primarily the ventricular apex.[1]

The diagnosis of hypertrophic cardiomyopathy should be considered in any young patient whose ECG suggests myocardial infarction but who does not have a history of infarction. ECG abnormalities often precede clinical or echocardiographic evidence of the disease.

Echocardiography is extremely useful in recognizing and assessing the severity of this condition. The thickness of the interventricular septum can be measured and compared with that of the free wall of the left ventricle at a point just beneath and behind the posterior mitral valve leaflet. Normally, the ratio of septal thickness to left ventricular free wall thickness is less than 1.3 : 1. In hypertrophic cardiomyopathy, the septum may be quite large, approaching four to five times the normal thickness of 1 cm. Asymmetrical hypertrophy of the interventricular septum has

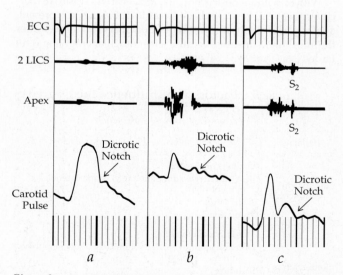

Figure 9 **Variations in the quality of the murmur associated with obstructive hypertrophic cardiomyopathy are observed before (*a*), during (*b*), and after (*c*) the Valsalva maneuver. From top to bottom are shown the electrocardiogram, the phonocardiogram at the second left intercostal space (2 LICS), the phonocardiogram at the apex, and the external recording of the carotid pulse. Before the Valsalva maneuver, a soft systolic murmur is recorded at the apex. The arterial pulse contour is normal. During the Valsalva maneuver, there is a dramatic increase in the intensity of the murmur. After Valsalva release, the murmur becomes softer, but the carotid pulse exhibits the classic spike-and-dome configuration characteristic of obstructive hypertrophic cardiomyopathy.**

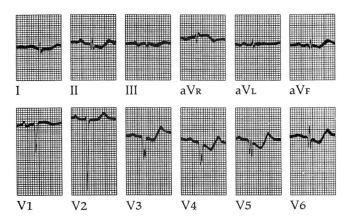

Figure 10 **Abnormal Q waves suggestive of an old anterior myocardial infarct are observed in leads V3 through V6 in an ECG recorded in a 45-year-old woman with obstructive hypertrophic cardiomyopathy.**

been reported in several other disorders, especially those associated with long-standing right ventricular hypertension, such as pulmonic stenosis and pulmonary hypertension. It is also found in neonates and in patients with posterior myocardial infarction. Nevertheless, in the context of other clinical and ECG features, asymmetrical septal hypertrophy is a highly specific, although not pathognomonic, marker of hypertrophic cardiomyopathy.

Several patterns of distribution, severity, and extent of ventricular hypertrophy have been detected in hypertrophic cardiomyopathy by two-dimensional echocardiography [*see Figure 11*]. Ultrasonography may reveal the presence and severity of an obstruction and whether it is fixed or labile. Normally, the anterior leaflet of the mitral valve moves in a posterior direction in systole, a phenomenon easily shown by echocardiography. In hypertrophic cardiomyopathy, when left ventricular outflow obstruction exists, systolic anterior movement of the anterior (septal) mitral valve leaflet occurs, and the mitral valve approaches the interventricular septum in systole [*see Figure 11*]. This finding may be constant or variable, depending on whether the obstruction is fixed or labile.

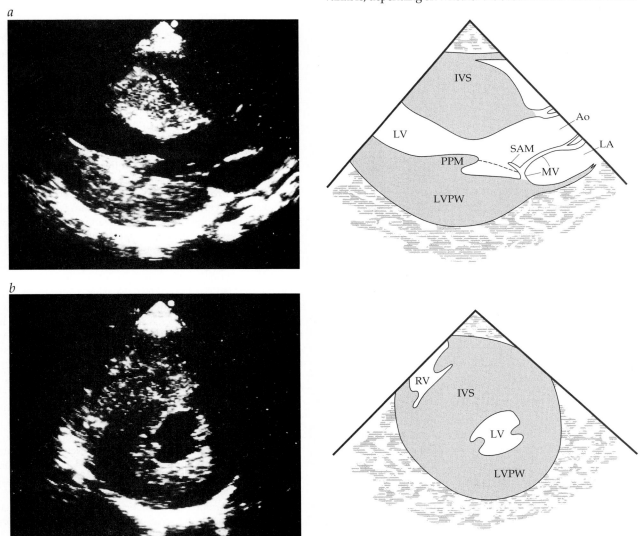

Figure 11 **These two-dimensional echocardiograms (left) show the classic features of hypertrophic cardiomyopathy (explanatory diagrams are on the right). In the parasternal long-axis view in systole (*a*), note the tremendous hypertrophy of the interventricular septum (IVS) and left ventricular posterior wall (LVPW) with disproportionate thickening of the septum. Slight systolic anterior movement (SAM) of the mitral valve (MV) can be seen. In the parasternal short-axis view in diastole (*b*), the marked and symmetrical thickening of the IVS can again be seen. (LV—left ventricle; Ao—aorta; PPM—posterior papillary muscle; LA—left atrium; RV—right ventricle)**

The pressure gradient across the left ventricular outflow tract can be calculated from the echocardiogram. Although systolic anterior motion of the mitral valve has been described in other cardiac conditions, it is highly specific (97%) for obstructive hypertrophic cardiomyopathy. However, because many patients lack obstruction, this finding is not a particularly sensitive marker of the disease. Doppler echocardiography has also proved to be very accurate in determining the pressure gradient across the left ventricular outflow tract.[1] Ultrasonography is very useful for following disease progression, particularly in children and young adults with familial disease.

MRI may also be used to define the pattern of hypertrophy. On exercise-induced thallium-201 imaging, transient perfusion defects typical of ischemia have been noted in many patients with hypertrophic cardiomyopathy who have angiographically normal large coronary arteries.[84] These abnormalities may be related to obliterative changes in small coronary arteries.

Cardiac Catheterization

Catheterization in patients with hypertrophic cardiomyopathy usually reveals elevated left ventricular end-diastolic pressure as a consequence of diminished left ventricular compliance. Reduced compliance produces an increase in the height of the left atrial A wave, which may reach 25 to 30 mm Hg. If obstruction is present, a pressure gradient exists between the left ventricle and the aorta [see Figures 8 and 12]. The obstruction may be fixed or labile. Such procedures as the Valsalva maneuver, the administration of nitroglycerin, and the infusion of inotropic agents, such as isoproterenol, may be used to provoke or aggravate obstruction.

One particularly useful maneuver is to induce ventricular premature beats with a catheter and observe the hemodynamic response. Left ventricular contractility is markedly augmented after a ventricular premature beat, producing not only an increase in left ventricular systolic pressure but also an increase in the severity of obstruction in the beat after the compensatory pause. Consequently, in the recording of the arterial pressure of the beat after the compensatory pause, the systolic pressure usually falls and the pulse pressure narrows (the Brockenbrough phenomenon) [see Figure 12]. Although not invariably present in hypertrophic cardiomyopathy, the Brockenbrough phenomenon is virtually pathognomonic for the disease.

Left ventricular angiography characteristically shows a small, hyperdynamic chamber. The apex of the ventricle is often obliterated in systole. Papillary muscles are thickened, and mitral regurgitation (usually mild) may be seen.

DIFFERENTIAL DIAGNOSIS

Hypertrophic cardiomyopathy is often overlooked and confused with valvular and subvalvular membranous aortic stenosis, mitral regurgitation, infundibular pulmonic stenosis, and ventricular septal defect. The brisk carotid pulses (especially if bifid), the ECG abnormalities, and the increase in the intensity of the murmurs with the Valsalva maneuver are useful differential points. The diagnosis usually can be confirmed by echocardiography.

COURSE AND PROGNOSIS

The course and prognosis are exceedingly variable. Most patients do very well for years,[85] although some experience progression of symptoms. Unfortunately, sudden death is all too common, especially in children and in men younger than 25 years with the familial form of the disease.[86] Furthermore, sudden death may

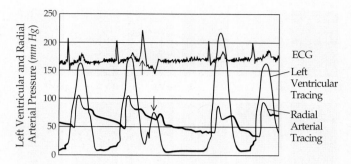

Figure 12 **Simultaneous left ventricular and radial arterial pressure tracings in a patient with obstructive hypertrophic cardiomyopathy show the Brockenbrough phenomenon in response to a ventricular premature beat (VPB). The gradient across the left ventricular outflow tract is about 80 mm Hg. After the VPG (indicated by arrows on the ECG and the left ventricular tracing), there is a compensatory pause. In the beat that follows the compensatory pause, the radial pulse pressure narrows, and the arterial pressure falls despite an increase in the left ventricular systolic pressure.**

result from arrhythmias even in patients without significant left ventricular hypertrophy or outflow tract obstruction. Although it is believed that most cases of sudden death are caused by arrhythmias, some may be the result of serious hemodynamic abnormalities, such as the development of sudden outflow obstruction with exercise. Genetic studies have identified specific abnormalities that seem to be harbingers of a poor prognosis.[78,79]

Progressive left ventricular hypertrophy develops in many patients; those with more severe degrees of hypertrophy appear to have a poorer prognosis.[1] In some patients who initially have no obstruction or only an inducible one, a fixed obstruction eventually develops. Progressive left ventricular hypertrophy is especially likely to develop in adolescents and young adults[87]; in older patients, hypertrophy often remains stable or progresses very slowly. However, progressive hypertrophy appearing for the first time in the sixth or seventh decade has recently been described for myosin-binding protein C defects.[80] In rare cases, hypertrophic cardiomyopathy may progress to a state of ventricular dilatation and failure indistinguishable from dilated cardiomyopathy. Long-term survival is common, especially in adults. The mortality in most large series is 2% to 3% a year, but the rate may be lower in the general population of patients with hypertrophic cardiomyopathies, which includes many elderly patients with the disease.

SCREENING

A 24-hour Holter monitor should be used to test for potentially lethal arrhythmias in patients with hypertrophic cardiomyopathy, especially if there is a strong family history of sudden cardiac death. The presence of nonsustained ventricular tachycardia, which is often asymptomatic, on prolonged ECG monitoring seems to correlate with an increased incidence of sudden cardiac death in adults,[86] but not necessarily in children.

Because hypertrophic cardiomyopathy has a familial incidence, close relatives should be screened for the disease. Appropriate measures are a routine history, physical examination, ECG, and echocardiography. In the near future, screening may also include searching for an abnormal gene. One frequently asked question is what degree of hypertrophy can be considered normal in people who exercise vigorously. In a study of 947 elite, highly trained athletes, only 16 had an echocardiographically measured left ventricular wall thickness greater than 13 mm; the thickest left ventricular wall measured 16 mm.[88] All 16 individuals participated in extremely strenuous endurance sports. However, in comparably athletic women, none had a left ventricular wall thickness greater than 12 mm.[89] Some investigators suggest that the following findings support a diagnosis of hypertrophic disease rather than physiologic hypertrophy: (1) documentation of hypertrophic cardiomyopathy in a relative of the athlete, (2) transmitral Doppler evidence of impaired left ventricular filling, usually demonstrated as a diminished peak early diastolic filling rate, (3) left ventricular wall thickness greater than 15 mm, and (4) left ventricular cavity size less than 45 mm.[90]

TREATMENT

Medical Therapy for Symptomatic Patients

Medical therapy is the preferred initial approach for symptomatic patients who have hypertrophic cardiomyopathy with or without obstruction.

Beta blockers and calcium channel blockers Beta-adrenergic blocking drugs are the most widely used medications and have been used to treat this disease for many years.[86] They provide effective relief of angina, dyspnea, and syncope and improve exercise capacity in many symptomatic patients. In addition, they may help prevent arrhythmias. Propranolol has been the most widely used beta blocker, with usual dosages ranging from 160 to 320 mg/day orally. Much higher dosages may be necessary in some patients for the initial relief of symptoms or to relieve the recurrence of symptoms in patients taking usual dosages. Other beta blockers may be as effective as propranolol if given in equivalent amounts, although those that possess intrinsic sympathomimetic activity, such as pindolol and acebutolol, should probably be avoided.

Verapamil, a calcium channel blocker, has also proved to be very effective in the treatment of symptomatic hypertrophic cardiomyopathy with or without obstruction.[86] Verapamil has also been shown to be effective in preventing silent myocardial ischemia detected by exercise-induced thallium-201 imaging in patients with hypertrophic cardiomyopathy.[91] In addition to reducing myocardial oxygen consumption and relieving obstruction, there is evidence that verapamil, when used for a long period, may lead to better diastolic compliance.[92] Warnings against the hypotensive and negative inotropic actions of verapamil should be heeded. These effects may be particularly deleterious in patients with severe outflow obstruction and left ventricular failure. In high doses, the drug may also cause potentially serious bradycardia by depressing the sinus node or by inducing AV block.

The role of other calcium channel blockers is less clear. Intravenous diltiazem and sublingual nifedipine have led to improved diastolic compliance of the hypertrophied left ventricle in some studies but not in others.

Occasionally, combinations of beta blockers and calcium channel blockers may be effective in patients who are unresponsive to either type of drug alone. However, caution is required when the two are used in combination. In patients with angina, nitroglycerin and its companion drugs are contraindicated.

Disopyramide Disopyramide, an antiarrhythmic agent with negative inotropic properties, may reduce obstruction and relieve symptoms in some patients. Dosages of 150 to 200 mg orally four times a day are recommended.

Diuretics Diuretics may be used in patients with congestive heart failure, but they must be used cautiously because patients with hypertrophic cardiomyopathy are very sensitive to intravascular volume depletion.

Digitalis glycosides Digitalis glycosides, which increase contractility, may worsen obstruction. They are generally contraindicated, although they may help control the ventricular rate in patients with atrial flutter or atrial fibrillation. Beta blockers or verapamil are preferable to digitalis glycosides for rate control in atrial fibrillation. Every attempt, including repeated cardioversion, should be made to maintain sinus rhythm. However, in some patients, maintenance of sinus rhythm may ultimately prove to be impossible. Patients with sustained atrial fibrillation are at high risk for systemic embolization and should be given warfarin to produce an international normalized ratio of 2 to 3, unless there is a strong contraindication to its use.

Prophylactic measures Bacterial endocarditis, usually involving the aortic valve but occasionally the mitral valve, can occur. Therefore, appropriate endocarditis prophylaxis is mandatory.

The prevention of sudden cardiac death remains a major challenge in the management of patients with hypertrophic cardiomyopathy. Markers of an increased risk of sudden cardiac death include young age, massive hypertrophy, sustained or nonsustained ventricular tachycardia on Holter monitoring, a history of ventricular fibrillation, a strong family history of sudden cardiac death, and a history of syncope.[93] As previously noted, certain genetic defects, such as troponin T gene mutations, seem to convey a high risk of sudden death.[77] A recent study also found a marked increase in the left ventricular collagen matrix in young people with this disease who died suddenly.[87]

There is no clear evidence that either beta blockers or calcium channel blockers prevent sudden death, although one uncontrolled study suggested that very high doses of propranolol (5 to 23 mg/kg/day) were helpful in preventing sudden death in young people with this disease.[94] In England, amiodarone has been widely used in the treatment of hypertrophic cardiomyopathy. One study using historical controls found evidence that amiodarone, given in a median dosage of 300 mg/day orally, prevented sudden cardiac death in patients with episodes of ventricular tachycardia demonstrated by ambulatory ECG monitoring. Not all researchers have experienced good results with amiodarone. In one group of 50 patients treated with this drug, seven patients died (six suddenly) during an average follow-up of 2.2 years.[95] Amiodarone has many potentially serious side effects [*see Chapter 19*]. Therefore, the drug must be used cautiously and in the lowest possible dose.

Invasive electrophysiologic studies have been of limited value in assessing patients, especially low-risk patients, with hypertrophic cardiomyopathy for the risk of sudden cardiac death. Such studies have been more useful in assessing patients who have experienced cardiac arrest or who have major risk factors for sudden death. Electrophysiologic abnormalities were found in 81% of a group of 155 patients with major risk factors for sudden death.[96] In a group of 30 survivors of sudden cardiac arrest, 21 had sustained ventricular arrhythmias. Seventeen of these patients were treated with ICDs and four with antiarrhythmic drugs.[97] These high-risk patients are most likely to benefit from implantation of automatic ICDs.[98] The presence of abnormal late potentials on signal-averaged ECGs may be useful in screening young patients who may be at risk for sudden cardiac death, but this has not yet been confirmed.

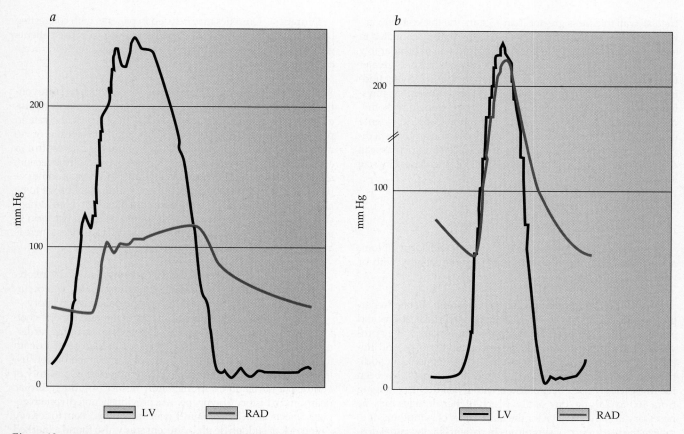

Figure 13   **Results of chemical septal ablation in a 77-year old woman with obstructive hypertrophic cardiomyopathy are shown. Simultaneous left ventricular and radial artery pressure recordings (*a*) show a gradient of approximately 140 mm Hg across the left ventricular outflow tract. Moments after injection of alcohol into the interventricular septum (*b*), the gradient is abolished. (LV—left ventricle; RAD—radial artery)**

MEDICAL THERAPY FOR ASYMPTOMATIC PATIENTS

The proper management of asymptomatic patients who have hypertrophic cardiomyopathy is not certain. We usually maintain asymptomatic patients on beta blockers. Unfortunately, there is no evidence that any form of therapy prevents progression of the disease.[92] In asymptomatic individuals in families with a high incidence of sudden cardiac death, more aggressive workup and treatment are indicated. If ventricular tachycardia is detected on ambulatory ECG monitoring in such individuals, antiarrhythmic treatment with amiodarone or use of an ICD for primary prevention of sudden death should be considered.[98] It is likely that as genetic studies become more available, aggressive therapy for preventing sudden cardiac death will be directed at those patients who are found to have the more lethal genetic abnormalities.

There is general agreement that patients with hypertrophic cardiomyopathy should be prohibited from engaging in competitive sports because of the risk of sudden cardiac death. A task force has made specific recommendations in this regard.[99]

Cardiac Pacing

Accumulating experience with sequential AV pacing continues to confirm the effectiveness of this technique in the treatment of some patients who continue to be symptomatic on drug therapy.[100,101] Depolarization of the ventricles, initiated by an electrode in the tip of the right ventricle, diminishes left ventricular outflow tract obstruction. In a large series of patients so treated, symptoms improved in many patients in the course of several months. One study has suggested that patients older than 65 years are most likely to benefit from pacer therapy.[102] In a study comparing myectomy with AV pacing in similar patients, there was a much greater improvement in symptoms in the surgical patients (90%) than in the patients receiving AV pacing (47%).[103] Although further long-term follow-up is necessary in these patients, it is probable that dual-chamber pacing can eliminate the need for cardiac surgery in some patients and postpone it in others. The effect on prognosis is unknown. Cardiac pacing is not recommended in symptomatic patients who do not have obstruction.[104]

Surgery

Surgery is recommended in symptomatic patients with fixed obstruction who do not respond to medical therapy or to synchronized pacing, but it may also be justifiable in patients with inducible gradients whose symptoms are quite severe and are not effectively controlled by medical measures. Only about 10% to 15% of patients with hypertrophic cardiomyopathy, however, ultimately undergo surgery. Many different operative procedures have been devised, but the one most often used involves myotomy or myectomy, or both, of the left ventricular outflow tract, usually around the septum.[86] This operation relieves the obstruction and usually is done via a transaortic approach using cardiopulmonary bypass. In some cases, mitral valve replacement may be necessary to correct associated mitral regurgitation or may be required because the ventricular septum is unusually thin, making septal myotomy or myectomy unsafe. Mitral valve replacement, without myotomy or myectomy, also may relieve the gradient. Generally, the results of surgical therapy have been satisfactory. In the longest reported follow-up, in which patients were followed for a mean period of 11.5 years (some were followed for as long as 25 years), 40% of patients survived. Approximately 25% of the patients died of complications of the hypertrophic cardiomyopathy, with a steady annual attrition rate from the disease of approximately 2%. More recent surgical results are even better; survival rates of 85% at 5 years and 72% at 10 years are not uncommon.[105] The great majority of the survivors experience symptomatic relief, and very few need a second operation or progress to dilated cardiomyopathy. Marked asymmetrical septal hypertrophy, severe anterior motion of the mitral leaflet or leaflets, and prolonged isovolumetric relaxation time are important preoperative variables that identify patients most likely to benefit from septal myectomy.[106] Although surgery relieves symptoms and improves the quality of life for survivors, it unfortunately does not prevent sudden cardiac death.

Controlled Septal Ablation

The most recent treatment for hypertrophic cardiomyopathy involves the production of a small infarct within the hypertrophied septum.[107-109] In this procedure, a catheter is introduced into one or more septal perforating arteries. After the artery has been occluded, a small amount of absolute ethanol is injected via the catheter into the septum. This creates a small infarct localized to the septum. If successful, there is an almost immediate reduction in the outflow tract gradient [see Figure 13]. In expert hands, the procedure is successful 90% of the time. Mortality is approximately 2%; 10% of patients may require permanent pacing.

At this time, we favor the procedure in older patients (i.e., patients older than 65 years) or in younger patients with comorbid conditions that increase the risks of surgery. To be eligible for the procedure, patients should have (1) medically refractory symptoms, (2) well-preserved left ventricular systolic function, (3) thickening of the interventricular septum of at least 18 mm, (4) a resting or inducible intraventricular pressure gradient of 50 mm Hg or greater, and (5) suitable coronary artery anatomy.

Restrictive Cardiomyopathy

ETIOLOGY

Restrictive cardiomyopathies are usually the product of an infiltrative disease of the myocardium, such as amyloidosis, hemochromatosis, or a glycogen storage disease.[2,110,111] Evidence also suggests that in certain diabetic patients, a form of restrictive cardiomyopathy may develop. However, cases of idiopathic restrictive cardiomyopathy are not uncommon.[110] A familial form of restrictive cardiomyopathy associated with AV block and skeletal myopathy has been reported.[112]

PATHOPHYSIOLOGY

The myocardium is rigid and noncompliant, impeding ventricular filling and raising cardiac filling pressures. Systolic performance is often reduced, but the overriding problem is impaired diastolic filling, which produces a clinical and hemodynamic picture that mimics constrictive pericarditis.

DIAGNOSIS

The most common clinical manifestation is congestive heart failure. Evidence of right-sided heart failure—edema, hepatomegaly, and ascites—often predominates. The systemic venous pressure is elevated and exhibits the characteristic early diastolic dip-and-plateau pattern associated with restricted ventricular filling. At cardiac catheterization, this pattern is recorded in both ventricles and atria [see Figure 14]. With inspiration, venous pressure rises rather than falls (Kussmaul sign). An early diastolic third sound is often heard. The heart is usually enlarged, and the ECG frequently shows low voltage. Arrhythmias are common.

Two-dimensional echocardiography may be helpful in the diagnosis of cardiac amyloidosis. The cardiac walls are often thickened and have a characteristic granular, speckled appearance.[113] Echocardiographic data can also provide prognostic information. In a large group of patients with amyloid heart disease, survival was negatively influenced by greater wall thickness and reduced systolic function, which were seen on two-dimensional echocardiography.[113] Enhanced diffuse myocardial uptake of technetium-99m pyrophosphate in radionuclide scintigraphy may also be found in patients with cardiac amyloidosis. Because restrictive cardiomyopathies are often caused by a specific process, they constitute one of the few cardiac diseases in which a definitive diagnosis can be made by percutaneous myocardial biopsy.

DIFFERENTIAL DIAGNOSIS

Restrictive cardiomyopathy must be differentiated from constrictive pericarditis, a distinction that is not always easy to make. Clues to the nature of a restrictive cardiomyopathy may be provided by the presence of other signs of the underlying disease process. The presence of a small heart favors a diagnosis of constrictive pericarditis.

The conditions may also be distinguished hemodynamically because constrictive pericarditis may involve the two ventricles equally and produce a so-called plateau of filling pressures. Thus, the left ventricular diastolic, left atrial, pulmonary wedge, right ventricular, right atrial, and systemic venous pressures are similar in magnitude and configuration. Ventricular interdependence, evidenced by an inspiratory increase in right ventricular systolic pressure and a decline in left ventricular systolic pressure, has recently been suggested as the most sensitive and specific hemodynamic criterion for diagnosing pericardial constriction.[114]

In contrast, restrictive cardiomyopathies tend to cause greater impairment to left than to right ventricular filling. Thus, the left-sided filling pressures are almost always higher than those recorded in the right side of the heart and may result in pulmonary arterial systolic pressures greater than 50 mm Hg—a pressure level that is a distinct rarity in constrictive pericarditis. Patterns of dia-

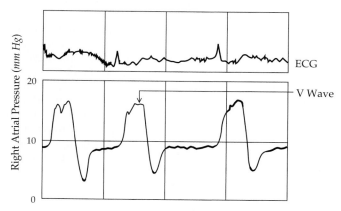

Figure 14 Shown is a right atrial pressure tracing in a patient with restrictive cardiomyopathy secondary to amyloidosis; some functional tricuspid regurgitation is present. The cardiac rhythm is atrial fibrillation. Large systolic (V) waves appear, followed by a typical early diastolic dip-and-plateau configuration.

stolic filling, as determined by Doppler echocardiography and radionuclide ventriculography, may also distinguish restrictive cardiomyopathy from constrictive pericarditis.[115] MRI can be of particular value in assessing the extent of pericardial thickening in patients with suspected constrictive pericarditis.

In some cases, restrictive cardiomyopathy cannot be distinguished from constrictive pericarditis, and surgical exploration may be warranted.

TREATMENT

In most cases, there is no therapy for restrictive cardiomyopathies, which ultimately result in death from congestive heart failure or arrhythmias. However, in some patients with idiopathic restrictive cardiomyopathy, the prognosis may be quite good.[110] Removal of excessive iron by frequent phlebotomies may improve myocardial function in those patients whose cardiomyopathies are caused by hemochromatosis. To ensure that phlebotomy is depleting myocardial iron stores in patients with hemochromatosis, some researchers have recommended periodic endomyocardial biopsies.[116] AL (amyloid light chain–related) amyloidosis may show some response to intermittent oral melphalan and prednisone.[111]

Obliterative (Restrictive-Obliterative) Cardiomyopathy

The hypereosinophilic syndrome accounts for the rare cases of obliterative cardiomyopathy encountered in the United States. The syndrome is characterized by profound eosinophilia and multiple organ involvement. Degranulation of many of the eosinophils is a characteristic feature, which suggests that the release of substances from the eosinophils is causally related to the damage to the heart and other organs that occurs in this highly fatal disease. Deposits of eosinophil granule proteins have been identified within the intracardiac thrombi and endocardium, a finding that also suggests a direct link between the eosinophils and the cardiac damage. Clinically, obliterative cardiomyopathy is characterized by inexorably progressive congestive heart failure, systemic embolism, and cardiac arrhythmias and conduction disturbances. Although there may be a transient response to adrenal glucocorticoids or antitumor therapy, there is no effective treatment of this disorder.

Worldwide, the most common cause of obliterative cardiomyopathy is endomyocardial fibrosis, which is particularly common in eastern Africa. Some researchers believe that many cases of endomyocardial fibrosis represent the end stage of a hypereosinophilic syndrome.[2] Characteristically, there is massive endocardial thickening of both ventricles, although one ventricle may be more severely affected than the other. Fibrous bands extend into the myocardium, and mitral and tricuspid insufficiency are common. Patients usually die of congestive heart failure. In a large series of patients, the survival rates were 76% at 1 year, 68% at 2 years, and 36% at 5 years.[117] Biventricular fibrotic involvement and the presence of mitral or tricuspid regurgitation are associated with poor long-term survival. There is no effective medical treatment. However, surgery consisting of endocardial stripping and relief of mitral or tricuspid insufficiency has been undertaken.[118] The results have been reasonable, although the surgical mortality has been high.

References

1. Wigle EG, Rakowski H, Kimball BP, et al: Hypertrophic cardiomyopathy: clinical spectrum and treatment. Circulation 92:1680, 1995

2. Richardson P, McKenna W, Bristow M, et al: Report of the 1995 World Health Organization/International Society and Federation of Cardiology Task Force on the definition and classification of cardiomyopathies. Circulation 93:841, 1996

3. Rizeq MN, Richenbacher PR, Fowler MB, et al: Incidence of myocarditis in peripartum cardiomyopathy. Am J Cardiol 74:474, 1994

4. Urbano-Márquez A, Estruch R, Fernández-Solá J, et al: The greater risk of alcoholic cardiomyopathy and myopathy in women compared with men. JAMA 274:149, 1995

5. Shan K, Lincoff AM, Young JB: Anthracycline-induced cardiotoxicity. Ann Intern Med 125:47, 1996

6. Singal PK, Iliskovic N: Doxorubicin-induced cardiomyopathy. N Engl J Med 339:900, 1998

7. Lipshultz SE, Lipsitz SR, Mone SM, et al: Female sex and higher drug dose as risk factors for late cardiotoxic effects of doxorubicin therapy for childhood cancer. N Engl J Med 332:1738, 1995

8. Hochster H, Wasserheit C, Speyer J: Cardiotoxicity and cardioprotection during chemotherapy. Curr Opin Oncol 7:304, 1995

9. Leandro J, Dyck J, Poppe D, et al: Cardiac dysfunction late after cardiotoxic therapy for childhood cancer. Am J Cardiol 74:1152, 1994

10. Keeling PJ, Lukaszyk A, Poloniecki J, et al: A prospective case-control study of antibodies to coxsackie B virus in idiopathic dilated cardiomyopathy. J Am Coll Cardiol 23:593, 1994

11. Bandorff C, Noutsias M, Kuhl U, et al: Cell-mediated cytotoxicity in hearts with dilated cardiomyopathy: correlation with interstitial fibrosis and foci of activated T lymphocytes. J Am Coll Cardiol 29:429, 1997

12. Why HJF, Meany BT, Richardson PJ, et al: Clinical and prognostic significance of detection of enteroviral RNA in the myocardium of patients with myocarditis or dilated cardiomyopathy. Circulation 89:2582, 1994

13. Figulla HR, Stille-Siegener M, Mall G, et al: Myocardial enterovirus infection with left ventricular dysfunction: a benign disease compared with idiopathic dilated cardiomyopathy. J Am Coll Cardiol 25:1170, 1995

14. Magnusson Y, Wallukat G, Waagstein F, et al: Autoimmunity in idiopathic dilated cardiomyopathy: characterization of antibodies against the beta1-adrenoceptor with positive chronotropic effect. Circulation 89:2760, 1994

15. Barbaro G, Di Lorenzo G, Grisorio B, et al: Incidence of dilated cardiomyopathy and detection of HIV in myocardial cells of HIV-positive patients. N Engl J Med 339:1093, 1998

16. DeCastro S, D'Amati G, Gallo P, et al: Frequency of development of acute global left ventricular dysfunction in human immunodeficiency virus infection. J Am Coll Cardiol 24:1018, 1994

17. Herskowitz A, Willoughby SB, Baughman KL, et al: Cardiomyopathy associated with antiretroviral therapy in patients with HIV infection: a report of six cases. Ann Intern Med 116:311, 1992

18. Michels VV, Moll PP, Miller FA, et al: The frequency of familial dilated cardiomyopathy in a series of patients with idiopathic dilated cardiomyopathy. N Engl J Med 326:77, 1992

19. Fatkin D, MacRae C, Sasaki T, et al: Missense mutations in the rod domain of the lamin A/C gene as causes of dilated cardiomyopathy and conduction-system disease. N Engl J Med 341:1715, 1999

20. Baig MK, Goldman JH, Caforio AP, et al: Familial dilated cardiomyopathy: cardiac abnormalities are common in asymptomatic relatives and may represent early disease. J Am Coll Cardiol 31;195, 1998

21. Bax JJ, Wijns W, Cornel JH, et al: Accuracy of currently available techniques for prediction of functional recovery after revascularization in patients with left ventricular dysfunction due to chronic coronary artery disease: comparison of pooled data. J Am Coll Cardiol 30:1451, 1997

22. Maron BJ, Wolfson JK, Epstein SE, et al: Intramural ("small vessel") coronary artery disease in hypertrophic cardiomyopathy. J Am Coll Cardiol 8:545, 1986

23. Narula J, Haider N, Virmani R, et al: Apoptosis in myocytes in end-stage heart failure. N Engl J Med 335:1182, 1996

24. Olivetti G, Abbi R, Quaini F, et al: Apoptosis in the failing human heart. N Engl J Med 336:1131, 1997

25. Basso C, Thiene G, Corrado D, et al: Arrhythmogenic right ventricular cardiomyopathy: dysplasia, dystrophy, or myocarditis? Circulation 94:983, 1996

26. Pinamonti B, Singra G, Camerini F: Clinical relevance of right ventricular dysplasia/cardiomyopathy [editorial]. Heart 83:9, 2000

27. Mathier MA, Rose GA, Fifer MA, et al: Coronary endothelial dysfunction in patients with acute-onset idiopathic dilated cardiomyopathy. J Am Coll Cardiol 32:216, 1998

28. Doval HC, Nul DR, Grancelli HO, et al: Nonsustained ventricular tachycardia in severe heart failure: independent marker of increased mortality due to sudden death. Circulation 94:3198, 1996

29. Feld H, Priest S, Denson M: Importance of pathologic Q waves in patients with dilated cardiomyopathies. Am J Med 94:546, 1993

30. De Groote P, Millaire A, Foucher-Hossein C, et al: Right ventricular ejection fraction is an independent predictor of survival in patients with moderate heart failure. J Am Coll Cardiol 32:948, 1998

31. Keren A, Gottlieb S, Tzivoni D, et al: Mildly dilated congestive cardiomyopathy: use of prospective diagnostic criteria and description of the clinical course without heart transplantation. Circulation 81:506, 1990

32. Menghetti L, Basso C, Nava A, et al: Spin-echo nuclear resonance for tissue characterisation in arrhythmogenic right ventricular cardiomyopathy. Heart 76:467, 1996

33. Dec GW, Fuster V: Idiopathic dilated cardiomyopathy. N Engl J Med 331:1564, 1994

34. Steimle AE, Stevenson LW, Fonarow GG, et al: Prediction of improvement in recent onset cardiomyopathy after referral for heart transplantation. J Am Coll Cardiol 23:553, 1994

35. Naqvi TZ, Goel RK, Forrester JS, et al: Myocardial contractile reserve on dobutamine echocardiography predicts late spontaneous improvement in cardiac function in patients with recent onset dilated cardiomyopathy. J Am Coll Cardiol 34:1537, 1999

36. Pinamonti B, Zecchin M, Di Lenarda A, et al: Persistence of restrictive left ventricular filling pattern in dilated cardiomyopathy: an ominous prognostic sign. J Am Coll Cardiol 29:604, 1997

37. Mancini DM, Eisen H, Kussmaul W, et al: Value of peak exercise oxygen consumption for optimal timing of cardiac transplantation in ambulatory patients with heart failure. Circulation 83:778, 1991

38. The effect of digoxin on mortality and morbidity in patients with heart failure. The Digitalis Investigation Group. N Engl J Med 336:525, 1997

39. Heart Failure Society of America guidelines for management of patients with heart failure caused by left ventricular systolic dysfunction: pharmacologic approaches. Heart Failure Society of America. J Card Fail 5:357, 1999

40. Effects of enalapril on mortality in severe congestive heart failure: results of the Cooperative North Scandinavian Enalapril Survival Study (CONSENSUS). The CONSENSUS Trial Study Group. N Engl J Med 316:1429, 1987

41. Cohn JN, Johnson G, Ziesche S, et al: A comparison of enalapril with hydralazine-isosorbide dinitrate in the treatment of chronic congestive heart failure. N Engl J Med 325:303, 1991

42. Lonn EM, Jha P, Montague TJ, et al: Emerging role of angiotensin-converting-enzyme inhibitors in cardiac and vascular protection. Circulation 90:2056, 1994

43. Effect of enalapril on mortality and the development of heart failure in asymptomatic patients with reduced left ventricular ejection fractions. The SOLVD Investigators. N Engl J Med 327:685, 1992

44. Packer M, Poole-Wilson PA, Armstrong PW, et al: Comparative effects of low and high doses of the angiotensin-converting-inhibitor lisinopril on morbidity and mortality in chronic heart failure. Circulation 100:2312, 1999

45. Pitt B, Martinez FA, Meurers G, et al: Randomised trial of losartan versus enalapril in patients over 65 with heart failure. Lancet 349:747, 1997

46. Pitt B, Poole-Wilson PA, Segal R, et al: Effect of losartan compared with captopril on mortality in patients with symptomatic heart failure: randomised trial—the Losartan Heart Failure Survival Study ELITE II. Lancet 355:1582, 2000

47. Packer M, O'Connor CM, Ghali JK, et al: Effect of amlodipine on morbidity and mortality in severe chronic heart failure. N Engl J Med 335:1107, 1996

48. Doval HC, Nul DR, Grancelli HO, et al: Randomised trial of low-dose amiodarone in severe congestive heart failure. Lancet 344:493, 1994

49. Amiodarone in patients with congestive heart failure and asymptomatic ventricular arrhythmia. Survival Trial of Antiarrhythmic Therapy in Congestive Heart Failure. N Engl J Med 333:77, 1995

50. Koniaris LS, Goldhaber SZ: Anticoagulation in dilated cardiomyopathy. J Am Coll Cardiol 31:745, 1998

51. Latham RD, Mulrow JP, Virmani R, et al: Recently diagnosed idiopathic dilated cardiomyopathy: incidence of myocarditis and efficacy of prednisone therapy. Am Heart J 117:876, 1989

52. Mason JW, O'Connell JB, Herskowitz A, et al: A clinical trial of immunosuppressive therapy for myocarditis. The Myocarditis Treatment Trial Investigators. N Engl J Med 333:269, 1995

53. McNamara DM, Rosenblum WD, Janosko KM, et al: Intravenous immune globulin in the therapy of myocarditis and acute cardiomyopathy. Circulation 95:2476, 1997

54. Osterziel KJ, Strohm O, Schuler J, et al: Randomised, double-blind, placebo-controlled trial of human recombinant growth hormone in patients with chronic heart failure due to dilated cardiomyopathy. Lancet 351:1233, 1998

55. Müller J, Wallukat G, Dandel M, et al: Immunoglobulin adsorption in patients with idiopathic dilated cardiomyopathy. Circulation 101:385, 2000

56. Cohn JN, Goldstein SO, Greenberg BH, et al: A dose-dependent increase in mortality with vesnarinone among patients with severe heart failure. N Engl J Med 339:1810, 1998

57. Mehra MR, Ventura HO, Kapoor C, et al: Safety and clinical utility of long-term intravenous milrinone in advanced heart failure. Am J Cardiol 80:61, 1997

58. Waagstein F, Bristow MR, Swedberg K, et al: Beneficial effects of metoprolol in idiopathic dilated cardiomyopathy. Lancet 342:1441, 1993

59. Hjalmarson A, Goldstein S, Fagerberg B, et al: Effects of controlled-release metoprolol on total mortality, hospitalizations, and well-being in patients with heart failure: the Metoprolol CR/XL Randomized Intervention Trial in Congestive Heart Failure (MERIT-HF). MERIT-HF Study Group. JAMA 283:1295, 2000

60. The Cardiac Insufficiency Bisoprolol Study II (CIBIS-II): a randomised trial. Lancet 353:9, 1999

61. Effect of carvedilol on morbidity and mortality in chronic heart failure. US Carvedilol Heart Failure Study Group. N Engl J Med 347:1199, 1996

62. Colucci WS, Packer M, Bristow MR, et al: Carvedilol inhibits clinical progression in patients with mild symptoms of heart failure. Circulation 94:2800, 1996

63. Eichhorn E: Preliminary results from the Bucindolol Evaluation Survival Trial (BEST). Paper presented at the 72nd scientific session of the American Heart Association, November 10, 1999, Atlanta, Georgia

64. Pitt B, Zannad F, Remme WJ, et al: The effect of spironolactone on morbidity and mortality in patients with severe heart failure. N Engl J Med 341:709, 1999

65. Wu AH, Das SK: Sudden death in dilated cardiomyopathy. Clin Cardiol 27:267, 1999

66. Moss AJ, Hall J, Cannon DS, et al: Improved survival with an implantable defibrillator in patients with coronary disease at high risk for ventricular arrhythmia. N Engl J Med 335:1933, 1996

67. Beller G: Selecting patients with ischemic cardiomyopathy for medical treatment, revascularization, or heart transplantation. J Nucl Cardiol 4:S152, 1997

68. Mickleborough LL, Maruyama J, Takagi Y, et al: Results of revascularization in patients with severe left ventricular dysfunction. Circulation 92(suppl II):II-73, 1995

69. Costanzo MR, Augustine S, Bourge R, et al: Selection and treatment of candidates for heart transplantation: a statement for health professionals from the Committee on Heart Failure and Cardiac Transplantation of the Council on Clinical Cardiology, American Heart Association. Circulation 92:3593, 1995

70. Hosenpud JD, Bennett LE, Keck BM, et al: The Registry of the International Society for Heart and Lung Transplantation: sixteenth official report—1999. J Heart Lung Transplant 18:611, 1999

71. Oz MC, Argenziano M, Catanese KA, et al: Bridge experience with long-term implantable left ventricular assist devices: are they an alternative to transplantation? Circulation 95:1844, 1997

72. Rector TS, Benditt D, Chachques JC, et al: Retrospective risk analysis for early heart-related death after cardiomyoplasty. J Heart Lung Transplant 16:1018, 1997

73. McCarthy PM, Starling RC, Wong J, et al: Early results with partial left ventriculectomy. J Thorac Cardiovasc Surg 114:755, 1997

74. Bolling SF, Pagani FD, Deeb GM, et al: Intermediate-term outcome of mitral reconstruction in cardiomyopathy. J Thorac Cardiovasc Surg 115:381, 1998

75. Marian AJ, Robert R: Recent advances in the molecular genetics of hypertrophic cardiomyopathy. Circulation 92:1336, 1995

76. Watkins H, McKenna WJ, Thierfelder L, et al: Mutations in the genes for cardiac troponin T and alpha-tropomyosin in hypertrophic cardiomyopathy. N Engl J Med 2:1058, 1995

77. Moolman JC, Corfield VA, Posen B, et al: Sudden death due to troponin T mutations. J Am Coll Cardiol 29:549, 1997

78. Watkins H, Rosenzweig A, Hwang DS, et al: Characteristics and prognostic implications of myosin missense mutations in familial hypertrophic cardiomyopathy. N Engl J Med 326:1108, 1992

79. Epstein ND, Cohn GM, Cyran F, et al: Differences in clinical expression of hypertrophic cardiomyopathy associated with two distinct mutations in the beta-myosin heavy chain gene: a 908$^{Leu \rightarrow Val}$ mutation and a 403$^{Arg \rightarrow Gln}$ mutation. Circulation 86:345, 1992

80. Niimura H, Bachinski LL, Sangwatanaroj S, et al: Mutations in the gene for cardiac myosin-binding protein C and late-onset familial hypertrophic cardiomyopathy. N Engl J Med 338:1248, 1998

81. Watkins H, Thierfelder L, Hwang DS, et al: Sporadic hypertrophic cardiomyopathy due to de novo myosin mutations. J Clin Invest 90:1666, 1992

82. Rosenzweig A, Watkins H, Hwang D-S, et al: Preclinical diagnosis of familial hypertrophic cardiomyopathy by genetic analysis of blood lymphocytes. N Engl J Med 325:1753, 1991

83. Robinson K, Frenneaux MP, Stockins B, et al: Atrial fibrillation in hypertrophic cardiomyopathy: a longitudinal study. J Am Coll Cardiol 15:1279, 1990

84. O'Gara PT, Bonow RO, Maron BJ, et al: Myocardial perfusion abnormalities in patients with hypertrophic cardiomyopathy: assessment with thallium-201 emission computed tomography. Circulation 76:1214, 1987

85. Cecchi F, Olivotto I, Montereggi A, et al: Hypertrophic cardiomyopathy in Tuscany: clinical course and outcome in an unselected regional population. J Am Coll Cardiol 26:1529, 1995

86. Spirito P, Seidman CE, McKenna WJ, et al: The management of hypertrophic cardiomyopathy. N Engl J Med 336:775, 1997

87. Shirani J, Pick R, Roberts WC, et al: Morphology and significance of the left ventricular collagen network in young patients with hypertrophic cardiomyopathy and sudden cardiac death. J Am Coll Cardiol 35:36, 2000

88. Pelliccia A, Maron BJ, Spataro A, et al: The upper limit of physiologic cardiac hypertrophy in highly trained elite athletes. N Engl J Med 324:295, 1991

89. Pelliccia A, Maron BJ, Culasso F, et al: Athlete's heart in women: echocardiographic characterization of highly trained elite female athletes. JAMA 276:211, 1996

90. Maron BJ, Isner JM, McKenna WJ: 26th Bethesda Conference: recommendations for determining eligibility for competition in athletes with cardiovascular abnormalities. Task Force 3: hypertrophic cardiomyopathy, myocarditis and other myopericardial diseases and mitral valve prolapse. J Am Coll Cardiol 24:880, 1994

91. Udelson JE, Bonow RO, O'Gara PT, et al: Verapamil prevents silent myocardial perfusion abnormalities during exercise in asymptomatic patients with hypertrophic cardiomyopathy. Circulation 79:1052, 1989

92. Bonow RO, Dilsizian V, Rosing DR, et al: Verapamil-induced improvement in left ventricular diastolic filling and increased exercise tolerance in patients with hypertrophic cardiomyopathy. Circulation 72:853, 1985

93. Maron BJ, Fananapazir L: Sudden cardiac death in hypertrophic cardiomyopathy. Circulation 85(suppl I):I-57, 1992

94. Östman-Smith I, Wettrell G, Riesenfeld T: A cohort study of childhood hypertrophic cardiomyopathy: improved survival following high-dose beta-adrenoceptor antagonist treatment. J Am Coll Cardiol 34:1813, 1999

95. Fananapazir L, Leon MB, Bonow RO, et al: Sudden death during empiric amiodarone therapy in symptomatic hypertrophic cardiomyopathy. Am J Cardiol 67:169, 1991

96. Fananapazir L, Tracy CM, Leon MB, et al: Electrophysiologic abnormalities in patients with hypertrophic cardiomyopathy: a consecutive analysis in 155 patients. Circulation 80:1259, 1989

97. Fananapazir L, Epstein SE: Hemodynamic and electrophysiologic evaluation of patients with hypertrophic cardiomyopathy surviving cardiac arrest. Am J Cardiol 67:280, 1991

98. Maron BJ, Shen WK, Link MS, et al: Efficacy of implantable cardioverter-defibrillators for the prevention of sudden death in patients with hypertrophic cardiomyopathy. N Engl J Med 342:365, 2000

99. Maron BJ, Isner JM, McKenna WJ: 26th Bethesda Conference: recommendations for determining eligibility for competition in athletes with cardiovascular abnormalities. Task Force 3: hypertrophic cardiomyopathy, myocarditis, and other myopericardial diseases and mitral valve prolapse. Med Sci Sports Exerc 26(10 suppl):S261, 1994

100. Slade AKB, Sadoul N, Shapiro L, et al: DDD pacing in hypertrophic cardiomyopathy: a multicenter clinical experience. Heart 75:44, 1996

101. Nishimura RA, Trusty JM, Hayes DL, et al: Dual-chamber pacing for hypertrophic cardiomyopathy: a randomized double-blind, cross-over trial. J Am Coll Cardiol 29: 435, 1997

102. Maron BJ, Nishimura RA, McKenna WJ, et al: Assessment of permanent dual-chamber pacing as a treatment for drug-refractory symptomatic patients with obstructive hypertrophic cardiomyopathy: a randomized, double-blind, cross-over study (M-PATHY). Circulation 99:2927, 1999

103. Ommen SR, Nishimura RA, Squires RW, et al: Comparison of dual-chamber pacing versus septal myectomy for the treatment of patients with hypertrophic obstructive cardiomyopathy. J Am Coll Cardiol 34:191, 1999

104. Cannon RO 3rd, Tripodi D, Dilsizian V, et al: Results of permanent dual-chamber pacing in symptomatic nonobstructive hypertrophic cardiomyopathy. Am J Cardiol 73: 571, 1994

105. Robbins RC, Stinson EB: Long-term results of left ventricular myotomy and myectomy for obstructive hypertrophic cardiomyopathy. J Thorac Cardiovasc Surg 111:586, 1996

106. McCully RB, Nishimura RA, Bailey KR, et al: Hypertrophic obstructive cardiomyopathy: preoperative echocardiographic predictors of outcomes after septal myectomy. J Am Coll Cardiol 27:1491, 1996

107. Knight C, Kurbaan AS, Seggewiss H, et al: Nonsurgical septal reduction for hypertrophic obstructive cardiomyopathy: outcome in the first series of patients. Circulation 95: 2075, 1997

108. Seggewiss H, Geichmann U, Faber L, et al: Percutaneous transluminal septal myocardial ablation in hypertrophic cardiomyopathy: results and 3-month follow-up in 25 patients. J Am Coll Cardiol 31:252, 1998

109. Lakkis NM, Nagueh SF, Kleiman NS, et al: Echocardiography-guided ethanol septal reduction for hypertrophic obstructive cardiomyopathy. Circulation 98:1750, 1998

110. Kushwaha SS, Fallon JT, Fuster V: Restrictive cardiomyopathy. N Engl J Med 336: 267, 1997

111. Falk RH, Comenzo RL, Skinner M: The systemic amyloidoses. N Engl J Med 337:898, 1997

112. Fitzpatrick AP, Shapiro LM, Rickards AF, et al: Familial restrictive cardiomyopathy with atrioventricular block and skeletal myopathy. Br Heart J 63:114, 1990

113. Katritsis D, Wilmshurst PT, Wendon JA, et al: Primary restrictive cardiomyopathy: clinical and pathologic characteristics. J Am Coll Cardiol 18:1230, 1991

114. Hurrell DG, Nishimura RA, Higano ST, et al: Value of dynamic respiratory changes in left and right ventricular pressures for the diagnosis of constrictive pericarditis. Circulation 93:2007, 1996

115. Aroney CN, Ruddy TD, Dighero H, et al: Differentiation of restrictive cardiomyopathy from pericardial constriction: assessment of diastolic function by radionuclide angiography. J Am Coll Cardiol 13:1007, 1989

116. Olson LJ, Edwards WD, Holmes DR Jr, et al: Endomyocardial biopsy in hemochromatosis: clinicopathologic correlates in six cases. J Am Coll Cardiol 13:116, 1989

117. Gupta PN, Valiathan MS, Balakrishnan KG, et al: Clinical course of endomyocardial fibrosis. Br Heart J 62:450, 1989

118. Martinez EE, Venturi M, Buffolo E, et al: Operative results in endomyocardial fibrosis. Am J Cardiol 63:627, 1989

Acknowledgments

Figure 2   Echocardiogram courtesy of the Cardiac Ultrasound Laboratory, Massachusetts General Hospital, Boston.

Figures 3 and 6   Photographs courtesy of Dr. John Fallon, Department of Pathology, Massachusetts General Hospital, Boston.

Figure 11   Tom Moore. Echocardiograms and diagrams courtesy of Dr. Robert A. Levine, Cardiac Ultrasound Laboratory, Massachusetts General Hospital, Boston.

Figure 13   Tracings courtesy of Dr. Michael A Fifer, Knight Cardiac Catheterization Laboratory, Massachusetts General Hospital, Boston.

Table 2   Adapted from chart supplied by Dr. Walter Abelmann, Beth Israel Hospital, Boston.

27 Adult Congenital Heart Disease

Mary P. Mullen, M.D., Ph.D.

Therapeutic advances in pediatric medicine over the past 25 years have resulted in increased survival. These advances, however, have brought with them new challenges to internists and practitioners who treat adults, especially in the area of cardiovascular disease, where the combined efforts of pediatric cardiologists and surgeons have resulted in a rapidly growing population of adults with congenital heart disease. Such patients require specialized and comprehensive care that incorporates both understanding of the underlying congenital lesions and attention to adult medical issues.

The increased survival of adults with congenital heart disease is the result of earlier and expanded recognition of cardiac disorders and improved care. Transthoracic and transesophageal echocardiography has facilitated accurate diagnosis. Fetal cardiac ultrasonography has prompted earlier diagnosis of congenital heart defects, allowing subsequent perinatal management in specialized tertiary care centers.[1] Imaging modalities, such as cardiac MRI and three-dimensional echocardiography, have increased the understanding of complex cardiac malformations and allowed visualization of blood flow and vascular structures.[2]

Advanced surgical and transcatheter therapies and improved postoperative care have reduced morbidity and mortality associated with cardiovascular procedures. Early and definitive surgical repair, instead of palliation, has decreased morbidity from primary lesions and allowed correction before occurrence of secondary complications involving other organ systems.[3] Improved myocardial protection strategies have decreased the incidence of impaired ventricular function after cardiopulmonary bypass. Bioengineering has refined the prosthetic materials utilized in cardiac surgery. Catheter-based intervention has allowed complete repair without the need for surgery in some settings and has prolonged the interval between surgical procedures in other settings.[4] The growing population of adults with congenital heart disease continues to benefit from advances in medical and pediatric care overall.

Epidemiology

Adult congenital heart disease comprises varied groups of patients, each with unique concerns. The overall incidence of cardiac malformations is estimated to be eight per 1,000 live births. With increased survival, the number of adults with congenital heart disease in the United States will have reached more than 900,000 by the year 2000.[5] The largest and fastest-growing group consists of adults who have undergone complete repair of their underlying defect. Such patients need careful follow-up, with scrutiny for postoperative complications and attention to the need for possible repeat operation. A second group is composed of patients who have undergone palliative surgeries, such as systemic-pulmonary shunts or systemic-cavopulmonary shunts. In these patients, the defect either cannot be completely repaired because of long-standing pulmonary hypertension or other reasons or has not been definitively repaired. A third group consists of adult patients with congenital heart disease who have not undergone surgery. These patients may be newly diagnosed, may have been lost to follow-up for many years, or may have been evaluated and deemed to have an inoperable defect. Included in this category are cyanotic patients with systemic-to-pulmonary circulation connections that have developed reversed shunting in the setting of pulmonary vascular disease, a condition known as the Eisenmenger syndrome.[6]

Etiology

Advances in molecular biology have provided new insights into the genetic basis of congenital heart disease. Chromosomal abnormalities are associated with 10% of congenital cardiovascular lesions. Two thirds of these lesions occur in patients with trisomy 21; one third are found in patients with karyotypic abnormalities, such as trisomy 13 and trisomy 18, and in patients with Turner syndrome.[5] The remaining 90% of congenital cardiovascular lesions have been postulated to be multifactorial in origin, as a result of interactions of several genes with or without additional environmental factors.[7] Examples of the effects of external influences include cardiovascular anomalies associated with maternal diabetes mellitus and congenital rubella syndrome and cardiac defects diagnosed after prenatal exposure to ethanol, diphenylhydantoin, thalidomide, and lithium. However, prospective investigations that have demonstrated an increased incidence of congenital heart disease in the offspring of affected adult patients[8,9] have generated renewed interest in the familial occurrence of inherited cardiac lesions. These studies suggest a greater potential role of single-gene defects in isolated congenital heart disease.

New light has been shed on a number of major congenital syndromes by use of molecular tools such as linkage analysis to identify markers close to genes responsible for certain inherited defects and fluorescent in situ hybridization (FISH) analysis to detect particular DNA sequences in metaphase chromosomes. Two findings are of particular import for physicians involved in counseling patients with congenital cardiac disease and their families.[10] The first finding is the recognition of a yet undefined role for the elastin gene product in congenital supravalvular arteriopathy. This finding stems from the discovery of elastin gene mutations in DNA from patients with familial supravalvular aortic stenosis and elastin gene hemizygosity in individuals with Williams syndrome (supravalvular aortic stenosis, characteristic facies, distinctive personality, and mental retardation).[11-13] Rapid genetic screening for Williams syndrome utilizing FISH analysis of the elastin gene deletion is currently available[12,14] [*see Figure 1*]. The second important finding is the identification of a microdeletion in the long arm of chromosome 22 (22q11) in patients with the overlapping DiGeorge syndrome, velocardiofacial syndrome, and conotruncal anomaly face syndrome. A widely used acronym, CATCH-22 (cardiac defects, *a*bnormal facies, *t*hymic hypoplasia, *c*left palate, *h*ypocalcemia), summarizes the common phenotype of these syndromes and their association with chromosome 22.[15] The cardiac defects associated with the syndromes include primarily conotruncal and brachial arch defects. A prospective study found chromosome 22q11 deletions in 50% of patients with interrupted aortic arch, in 34.5% of patients with truncus arteriosus, and in 15.9% of patients with tetralogy of Fallot.[16] Precise localization of the gene or genes within the deletion responsible for cardiac abnormalities is an area of ongoing research.

Figure 1   **Fluorescence in situ hybridization of metaphase chromosomes from a patient with Williams syndrome demonstrating absence of elastin gene on one copy of chromosome 7.**

Guidelines for screening patients with FISH analysis for elastin gene mutations or microdeletion of chromosome 22 are currently in evolution.[17]

Frequently Encountered Lesions

ATRIAL SEPTAL DEFECTS

Exclusive of bicuspid aortic valves, atrial septal defects are the most frequently encountered unrepaired congenital cardiac lesion in adults.

Classification

Atrial septal defects may be classified as secundum atrial septal defects, ostium primum defects, or sinoseptal defects [*see Figure 2*]. Secundum atrial septal defects constitute approximately 10% of all isolated congenital heart malformations.[18] Embryologically, the defect appears to stem from abnormal development of the septum primum that results in a failure to cover the fossa ovalis. Familial secundum atrial septal defect has been reported with autosomal dominant inheritance but with low penetrance and variable expressivity.[19]

Ostium primum defects are a form of endocardial cushion defect almost always associated with cleft anterior leaflet of the mitral valve and often seen in patients with Down syndrome.

Sinoseptal defects constitute 10% of all atrial septal defects. The most common, sinus venosus defects, are located at the entrance of the superior vena cava to the right atrium and are frequently associated with anomalous pulmonary venous return. Inferior vena caval type sinus venosus defects are similarly located at the entrance of the inferior vena cava to the right atrium. The least common type of atrial septal defect is an unroofed coronary sinus, resulting in a connection between the coronary sinus and the left atrium.

Diagnosis

Atrial septal defects are often incidentally diagnosed late in childhood or in adulthood. Physical examination may reveal a widely split and fixed second heart sound lacking usual respiratory variability. There frequently is a soft systolic murmur heard at the left upper sternal border caused by increased pulmonary flow. An early diastolic rumble may be present because of augmented flow through the tricuspid valve. The chest x-ray may show a cardiac silhouette that is normal or enlarged. The electrocardiogram demonstrates characteristic findings. These findings may include right ventricular volume overload and right ventricular conduction delay in secundum atrial septal defect and superior axis deviation in ostium primum atrial septal defect. Definitive diagnosis of atrial septal defect is achieved by transthoracic echocardiography. This modality may demonstrate the opening by direct imaging, right ventricular volume overload, or Doppler color flow across the atrial septum. Transesophageal echocardiographic studies may be required in some patients for adequate views of the atrial septum or to evaluate pulmonary venous drainage in patients with sinus venosus defects. Diagnostic cardiac catheterization is reserved for patients in whom elevated pulmonary vascular resistance or concomitant coronary artery disease is suspected.

Children and young adults with isolated atrial septal defects are usually initially asymptomatic but may experience symptoms of dyspnea or palpitations later in life. The basic physiology consists of left-to-right shunting of blood across the atrial septum, producing a right ventricular volume overload. Increased shunting may occur in the setting of decreased left ventricular compliance in patients with systemic hypertension , diabetes mellitus, or ischemic heart disease.

Treatment

Closure at the time of diagnosis is generally advocated for adult patients with a hemodynamically significant atrial septal defect (median pulmonary-to-systemic shunt ratio [Qp/Qs] greater than 1.5 and right ventricular volume overload revealed by echocardiographic imaging) for relief of symptoms, for improvement in functional capacity, and to decrease the potential for right ventricular failure and atrial arrhythmias.[20-22] The management of patients presenting with atrial septal defects at older ages has been controversial because of insufficient follow-up data. A retrospective study examined the clinical course of 179 consecutive patients with atrial septal defect diagnosed after age 40; 84 patients treated surgically were compared with 95 patients managed medically.[23] Preoperative characteristics of the two groups were similar. The surgical repair of atrial septal defect in these patients resulted in a significant decrease in mortality at 5 and 10 years, as well as prevention of functional decline as measured by the New York Heart Association classification.

Current options for atrial septal defect closure include both surgical repair and transcatheter approaches. Atrial septal defect surgery in adults has been shown to be safe and effective.[24] Data evaluating transcatheter device closure of atrial septal defects are accumulating.[25] Several device options are available. The choice of either surgery or transcatheter closure may in the future depend on the type of defect, its size, its location in the atrial septum and on patient preference and presence of comorbid illness [*see Figure 3*].

Complications and Long-term Management

Atrial arrhythmias and thrombotic events may occur late in both unoperated patients and patients with repaired defects.[21,23] The risk of atrial flutter or atrial fibrillation in adults with atrial septal defects is associated with increased age at time of surgery and elevated pulmonary arterial pressure.[12] After closure of atrial septal defects, patients should be periodically screened for atrial arrhythmias. If arrhythmias do occur, patients should receive anticoagulation therapy for the prevention of thromboem-

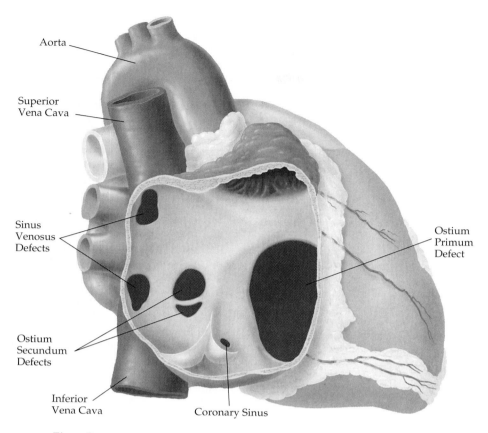

Figure 2   **Anatomic classification of atrial septal defects.**

bolism. Endocarditis prophylaxis is not recommended for isolated atrial septal defects.[26] Pregnancy in patients with atrial septal defects without pulmonary hypertension is generally well
tolerated. However, closure of a significant atrial septal defect is
recommended before childbearing, if possible, because of the
potentially increased risk of paradoxical thromboembolism in
the hypercoagulable peripartum period.

BICUSPID AORTIC VALVE

Bicuspid aortic valves are found in 1% to 2% of the general
adult population[27] and may be associated with other left-sided
obstructive lesions, such as aortic coarctation. Familial patterns
of inheritance have been reported.[28]

Diagnosis

The diagnosis of a bicuspid aortic valve is frequently suggested by characteristic auscultatory findings and later confirmed with echocardiography. On physical examination, there
may be a systolic murmur at the right upper sternal border and
a systolic ejection sound at the cardiac apex. Patients may present without additional symptoms, or the bicuspid valve may
be associated with more significant pathology.

Treatment

Guidelines for intervention in patients with significant hemodynamic abnormalities of the bicuspid aortic valve may differ
from those in adults with acquired aortic valvular disease, as
studies of treated and untreated conditions continue to emerge.

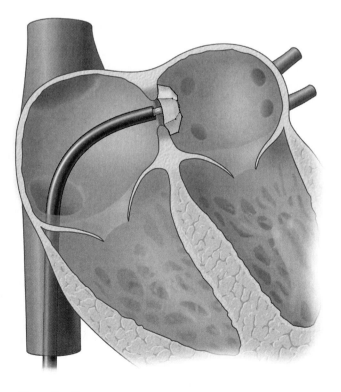

Figure 3   **Self-centering transcatheter atrial septal defect closure
device (partially open) positioned across atrial septum.**

Complications and Long-term Management

Complications include aortic stenosis or insufficiency, infective endocarditis, and aortic dissection.[27] Stenosis of the bicuspid valve is associated with increasing age and the presence of fibrocalcific disease.[29] Aortic insufficiency occurs in younger patients and may be isolated, the result of endocarditis, or associated with cystic medial necrosis and aortic root dilatation.[30,31] Patients should be evaluated periodically by physical examination and echocardiography for the development of complications throughout adult life. Adults with congenitally bicuspid aortic valves should receive subacute bacterial endocarditis prophylaxis for appropriate indications.[26]

PATENT DUCTUS ARTERIOSUS

Excluding cases in premature infants, persistent patent ductus arteriosus constitutes 5% to 10% of all cases of congenital heart disease. The physiology is that of a left-to-right shunt lesion with resulting left ventricular volume overload.[32] A large, unrestrictive duct presenting in infancy results in pulmonary hypertension and congestive heart failure and is most often repaired in the first year of life.[32] In rare cases, adults will present with differential cyanosis (affecting lower but not upper extremities) because of right-to-left shunting across a patent ductus with pulmonary vascular obstructive disease.

Diagnosis

Clinicians are usually faced with management of the small to moderate ductus arteriosus in adults. Diagnosis should be suspected in the setting of a machinery-type continuous murmur at the left upper sternal border. The chest x-ray may show a cardiac silhouette that is normal or enlarged. Diagnosis is confirmed with echocardiography. Transesophaeal echocardiography or MRI is generally thought to be superior to transthoracic echocardiography for ductal imaging.[33,34] The patient should undergo cardiac catheterization if concerns about significant pulmonary hypertension arise.

Treatment

Closure of the small persistent patent ductus arteriosus in the adult is generally performed to prevent infectious complications. In patients with patent ductus arteriosus, endocarditis has been reported at an incidence of 0.45% a year[35] in past decades; however, this number is likely considerably lower at present. A retrospective review found no cases of patent ductus arteriosus complicated by infective endarteritis in Sweden over an aggregate of 1,196 patient-years of risk.[36]

Surgical options for closure of patent ductus arteriosus include open surgical ligation and division as well as video-assisted transthoracoscopic patent ductus ligation.[37] Nonsurgical transcatheter methods for duct occlusion, such as Gianturco coils and devices are widely used. Transcatheter coil occlusion appears to have clinical efficacy and cost-effectiveness similar to those of surgical closure.[38] The choice of surgical or transcatheter methods for patent ductus arteriosus closure may depend on duct size and configuration and on patient characteristics.

Management of the so-called silent patent ductus arteriosus remains controversial. Color flow Doppler echocardiography has greatly increased limits of sensitivity for diagnosis of the clinically inapparent ductus.[39] Although infection of the silent ductus has been noted, closure of a small or trivial ductus is generally not indicated if the patient has neither a murmur nor evidence of left ventricular volume overload.

PULMONARY STENOSIS

Pulmonary stenosis occurs in up to 10% of patients with congenital heart disease.[18] Obstruction may occur at the valvular, the branch pulmonary arterial, or on rare occasions, the subvalvular level. Supravalvular or branch pulmonary arterial stenosis may be associated with congenital rubella or with the Noonan, Williams, or Alagille syndrome. Valvular pulmonary stenosis occurs most frequently.

Diagnosis

Adult presentation of pulmonary stenosis may range from no symptoms to profound fatigue and dyspnea on exertion, depending on degree of stenosis. The diagnosis is suggested by a characteristic ejectionlike murmur at the second left intercostal space and the presence of an early systolic ejection sound that decreases with inspiration. The shape and duration of the murmur and the extent of S_2 splitting may be correlated with the pulmonary stenosis gradient because of the timing of right ventricular ejection.[40] With severe stenosis, a systolic thrill and right ventricular heave may also be present. Peripheral pulmonary stenosis is associated with bilateral systolic murmurs radiating to the axilla and back.

In valvular pulmonary stenosis, the chest x-ray may show characteristic poststenotic dilatation of the main and left pulmonary arteries.[40] The ECG demonstrates right ventricular conduction delay and right ventricular hypertrophy in patients with moderate to severe obstruction. Physical examination findings are confirmed by echocardiography. Generally, degrees of stenosis are expressed as mild (right ventricular systolic pressure less than 50 mm Hg), moderate (right ventricular systolic pressure between 50 and 100 mm Hg), or severe (right ventricular systolic pressure greater than 100 mm Hg).

Treatment

Although open surgical valvotomy was historically the initial therapeutic approach, transcatheter balloon dilatation is the current treatment of choice for valvular pulmonary stenosis with gradients greater that 50 mm Hg shown by echocardiography.[41] The procedure is associated with low morbidity and mortality and with successful short-term and long-term results.[42] Complications of balloon pulmonary valvotomy include pulmonary regurgitation and restenosis requiring repeat balloon dilatation.

Peripheral pulmonary stenosis in the adult may also be approached through transcatheter balloon dilatation, with a resulting decrease in right ventricular systolic pressure, improvement in pulmonary blood flow, and relief of symptoms[43] [see Figure 4].

VENTRICULAR SEPTAL DEFECTS

Isolated ventricular septal defects are the most common congenital defects seen in childhood and young adult life.[44] Anatomic classification is based on septal location. Lesions may be perimembranous, subpulmonary, atrioventricular canal–type, or muscular.

Diagnosis

In adults, large ventricular septal defects without a pressure gradient between left and right ventricles are often associated with elevated pulmonary vascular resistance and Eisenmenger physiology. Such patients may present with cyanosis, arrhythmia, syncope, or hemoptysis. Cardiac examination reveals a single S_1 and a loud single S_2. A systolic murmur may be soft or absent, and there is often a high-pitched early diastolic murmur of pulmonary regurgitation. The chest x-ray may show cardio-

a

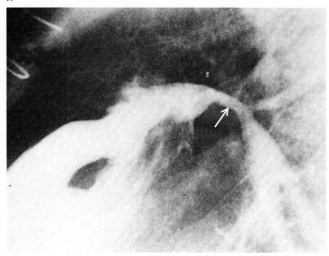

b

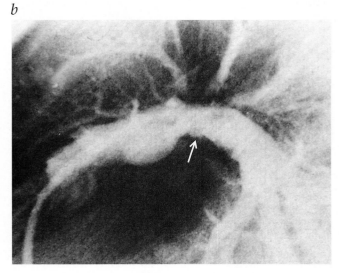

Figure 4 **Angiograms demonstrating pulmonary artery stenosis (*a*) before and (*b*) after transcatheter balloon dilatation.**

megaly. The ECG may reveal biventricular hypertrophy. Hemodynamic assessment and determination of pulmonary vascular responsivity to vasodilators should be performed in the catheterization laboratory before determination of operability.[45]

Alternatively, the adult patient may present with a small, restrictive ventricular septal defect. The gradient across the defect from systemic left ventricle to right ventricle is high, and pulmonary arterial pressures remain low. On examination, patients may have a notable systolic thrill and a harsh holosystolic murmur at the left sternal border. The chest x-ray and ECG are unremarkable. Definitive diagnosis is made by echocardiography. There is no evidence of left ventricular enlargement.

Treatment

Up to 50% of membranous or muscular ventricular septal defects present at birth will eventually undergo spontaneous closure. Subpulmonary defects, associated with aortic insufficiency, and atrioventricular canal–type defects, unlikely to close spontaneously, are generally repaired surgically. Man-

agement of a ventricular septal defect generally is defined by patient age, defect size, and pulmonary vascular resistance.

Repair of large ventricular septal defects is generally contraindicated when pulmonary vascular resistance is greater than 7 to 8 Wood units without reactivity to pulmonary vasodilators.[46]

Small defects may eventually undergo spontaneous closure. Ongoing medical follow-up is indicated to screen for associated complications of endocarditis, arrhythmia, or aortic regurgitation.[47] In rare cases, surgical closure is indicated for the prevention of endocarditis.

Complications and Long-term Management

Complications of postoperative ventricular septal defect repair include residual ventricular septal defect, postoperative pulmonary hypertension, surgically acquired complete heart block, and sudden death.[48,49] Patients should be periodically evaluated after surgery for arrhythmia, left ventricular dysfunction, or the rare progression of postoperative complete right bundle branch block to higher grade atrioventricular block.

TETRALOGY OF FALLOT

Tetralogy of Fallot is the most common cyanotic congenital lesion, occurring in 9% of children with critical congenital heart disease in the first year of life. Each year in the United States, approximately 2,000 persons who previously underwent surgery for tetralogy of Fallot reach adulthood.

Diagnosis

Tetralogy of Fallot, which consists of ventricular septal defect, infundibular pulmonary stenosis, overriding aorta, and right ventricular hypertrophy, is usually diagnosed by echocardiography in infancy during workup of a systolic murmur. In rare cases, adults who have not undergone surgery present for evaluation. These patients should undergo cardiac catheterization for assessment of shunt flow, pulmonary vascular resistance, and distal pulmonary anatomy before consideration of repair.

Treatment

In the past, patients were managed with systemic-pulmonary shunts that were obliterated at the time of full repair. In recent years, there has been a move toward complete repair performed in infancy. Goals of definitive surgery consist of ventricular septal defect closure and elimination of right ventricular outflow tract obstruction. Residual postoperative lesions may include shunt complications such as pulmonary arterial distortion or pulmonary vascular disease, peripheral pulmonary stenosis, residual ventricular septal defect, right ventricular outflow tract obstruction, or pulmonary regurgitation.

Prognosis

Data on long-term follow-up of repaired tetralogy of Fallot continues to accumulate. Long-term survival after the initial postoperative period is excellent, with reported 32-year actuarial survival of 86%, as compared with 96% in a control population.[50] At late follow-up, the majority of patients (77%) were in New York Heart Association functional class I. Some patients may experience postoperative sequelae, including exercise limitation, right ventricular failure, right ventricular outflow tract aneurysms, arrhythmia, and, on rare occasions, sudden death.[51] Right ventricular outflow tract complications are the major indication for reoperation.[52] In a study of 490 patients, mortality increased during the 25 years after surgery from 0.24% a year to 0.94% a year.[53] The most frequent cause of late mortality is sudden death, occurring at a frequency of 1% to 3% in most long-term studies.[54]

Complications and Long-term Management

Postoperative rhythm disturbances occur frequently in patients with tetralogy of Fallot. Complete right bundle branch block is found in 80% to 90% of patients who have undergone right ventriculotomy, and bifascicular block (right bundle branch block with left axis deviation) is seen in 15% to 20%.[54] The incidence of late-onset complete heart block is 4% after a mean follow-up of 20 years.[55] Atrial arrhythmias, including sinus node dysfunction, atrial flutter, and atrial fibrillation, have been noted in up to one third of patients who have undergone repair; in many cases, intervention has been necessary.[56]

Ongoing research is aimed at predicting the risk of malignant ventricular arrhythmias and sudden death after repair of tetralogy of Fallot. Ventricular ectopy is noted on routine 24-hour Holter monitoring in 40% to 50% of patients.[57] Predisposing factors in some studies include older age at repair, increased right ventricular systolic pressure, significant pulmonary regurgitation, increased cardiopulmonary bypass time, and ventricular dysfunction.[58] Nonsustained ventricular ectopy on ambulatory monitoring, however, does not appear to identify patients at risk for sudden death.[59] Documented sustained ventricular tachycardia is relatively infrequent; in a retrospective review, it has been associated with structural lesions, including right ventricular outflow tract aneurysm and pulmonary regurgitation.[58] Prolonged QRS duration (> 180 msec) on resting ECG has been shown to be a sensitive predictor of life-threatening ventricular arrhythmias after repair of tetralogy of Fallot.[60] Increased dispersion of the QT interval (QTd) has also been found to identify patients at risk for postoperative sustained ventricular tachycardia.[61] The etiology of ventricular arrhythmia and sudden death after repair of tetralogy of Fallot repair likely includes both anatomic and electrical variables.[50]

Long-term care for patients after repair of tetralogy of Fallot should incorporate both careful hemodynamic assessment, with attention to need for reoperation, and ECG screening with antiarrhythmic therapy as indicated.

CORONARY ANOMALIES

On rare occasions, congenital coronary anomalies present in adult life, with the potential to result in myocardial ischemia, congestive heart failure, or sudden death. Coronary arteriovenous fistulas are the most common congenital coronary lesions. These lesions may arise between right or left coronary arteries and cardiac chambers or great vessels and may produce high-output cardiac failure or ischemia. Patients may be asymptomatic or may present with dyspnea, congestive heart failure, or angina. Diagnosis is suggested by the presence of a continuous murmur and is confirmed by echocardiography. Symptomatic coronary arterial fistulas may be treated with transcatheter coil embolization[62] or surgery.

Abnormal origin of coronary arteries from the pulmonary artery or opposite aortic sinus may result in congenital anomalies that may be diagnosed in adults. An anomalous left coronary artery from the pulmonary artery (Bland-White-Garland syndrome) usually presents in infancy with myocardial ischemia or infarction. Over time, however, some patients develop extensive right coronary artery to left coronary artery collaterals and present later in life with sequelae of myocardial steal–producing infarction, congestive heart failure, mitral re-

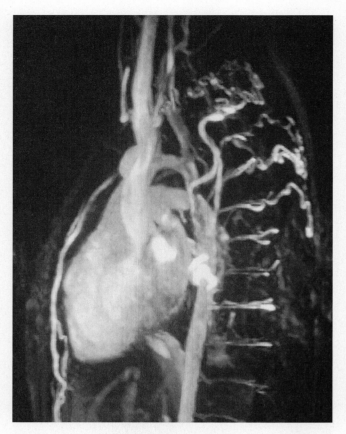

Figure 5   **Angio-MRI imaging of patient with aortic coarctation demonstrating collateral vessels.**

gurgitation, or ventricular arrhythmia. On evaluation, the ECG may show diffuse ST segment and T wave changes, as well as deep Q waves. The chest x-ray may show cardiomegaly. Cardiac echocardiography or catheterization should confirm the diagnosis of anomalous left coronary artery from the pulmonary artery. Surgical therapy includes reimplantation of the anomalous coronary artery or baffling of the left coronary artery from the pulmonary artery to the aorta. Abnormal origin of the right or left coronary artery from the opposite aortic sinus of Valsalva and coursing between the aorta and the pulmonary artery may also be associated with myocardial infarction or sudden death. Symptoms may be caused by accompanying coronary ostial narrowing or by distention of the aorta with exercise, resulting in proximal coronary artery compression. Surgical therapy usually involves bypass grafting. The importance of defining coronary origins and course in all young adults presenting with unexplained angina or ventricular arrhythmia should be underscored.

AORTIC COARCTATION

Aortic coarctation is a narrowing of the descending aorta at the site of insertion of the ductus arteriosus, distal to the left subclavian artery. This occurs in 5% to 10% of patients with congenital heart disease and is often associated with additional cardiac abnormalities. A bicuspid aortic valve is present in 40% to 80% of patients with aortic coarctation. Most cases are sporadic, however, and familial aortic coarctation has been reported. The association of coarctation with Turner syndrome suggests a genetic etiology.[63]

Diagnosis

Critical aortic coarctation presents in infancy with symptoms of shock and hypoperfusion; however, varying degrees of stenosis provide a spectrum of severity. Up to 50% of patients with aortic coarctation are diagnosed in late childhood or adulthood. The diagnosis may be suspected in the evaluation of a young patient with systemic hypertension. Physical examination reveals a systolic murmur extending into early diastole and is best heard in the infrascapular region. Four-extremity blood pressures may reveal the presence of a gradient between upper and lower blood pressures. There may be decreased lower extremity pulses and a brachial-femoral pulse delay. The ECG may show signs of left ventricular hypertrophy. Classic chest x-ray findings include the presence of a reversed 3 sign caused by prestenotic and poststenotic dilatation and rib notching caused by the development of large collateral vessels. Diagnosis is confirmed by echocardiography. Descending aortic Doppler ultrasonography may show antegrade flow in diastole, suggesting the presence of coarctation.[64] MRI, angiography, or both may be required for the delineation of precise anatomic details and collateral vessels [see Figure 5].

Treatment

Repair is indicated in the setting of moderate aortic coarctation (maximal instantaneous gradient greater than 25 to 30 mm Hg), especially when it is accompanied by systemic hypertension, left ventricular hypertrophy, or elevated left ventricular end diastolic pressure. Surgical repair has been the standard approach. Perioperative concerns include risk of spinal cord ischemia or bleeding from collateral vessels. Experience is accumulating in the treatment of native coarctation with transcatheter balloon dilatation and balloon-expandable intravascular stents.[65] Use of balloon angioplasty for native coarctation was limited because of concern about aneurysm formation.

Complications and Long-term Management

Late postoperative complications include the development of aneurysms and recurrent coarctation, which has been reported in up to 20% of patients.[66] Transcatheter balloon angioplasty with or without stent placement has become the standard therapy for restenosis. A high incidence of postoperative systemic hypertension at rest and with exercise has been noted after surgery for aortic coarctation.[63,67] Elevation in blood pressure appears to be inversely correlated with age at complete repair.[68] Potential etiologies include residual coarctation, altered arterial reactivity, transverse arch gradients, increased arterial stiffness, and hyperdynamic left ventricular function.[67]

Long-term follow-up of patients with repaired aortic coarctation should include monitoring for associated vascular lesions, including aneurysms of the circle of Willis (occurring in 3% to 5% of patients), hemangiomas, aortic dissection, and premature coronary artery disease.[63]

EISENMENGER SYNDROME

Pulmonary vascular disease and cyanosis resulting from unrepaired systemic-pulmonary shunts may occur in patients who have not undergone surgery for ventricular septal defects, atrial septal defects, aortopulmonary window, patent ductus arteriosus, truncus arteriosus, D-transposition of the great arteries, and other complex forms of congenital heart disease. Generally, these patients undergo a period of increased pulmonary blood flow from left-to-right shunting in childhood. With increased pulmonary vascular resistance, the shunt becomes bidirectional and, eventually, reversal of shunt flow and cyanosis occur.[2,69] Characteristic changes, including medial hypertrophy, intimal proliferation, plexiform lesions, and eventual arterial dilatation, are seen in the pulmonary artery microvasculature as the disease progresses.[70]

Diagnosis

Adult patients with the Eisenmenger syndrome may initially present for evaluation of unexplained pulmonary hypertension. Assessment of all such patients should include imaging to exclude structural heart disease, including shunt lesions, peripheral pulmonary stenosis, pulmonary vein obstruction, cor triatriatum, and mitral valve disease. Confirmation of elevated pulmonary arterial pressure, investigation of hemodynamics, and pulmonary vasoreactivity to pulmonary vasodilators, including oxygen and inhaled nitric oxide, should be performed at cardiac catheterization before determination of inoperability.[45]

Symptomatic Treatment

Cardiac symptoms An elevated hematocrit in the cyanotic patient is the result of an increase in erythrocyte mass and blood volume triggered by erythropoietin produced in response to tissue hypoxia.[71] Symptoms of hyperviscosity, including headache, visual changes, and mild paresthesias, may accompany significant erythrocytosis in the cyanotic patient. In general, phlebotomy with volume replacement is recommended for hyperviscosity symptoms in patients with a hematocrit greater than 65% after adequate hydration and correction of possible precipitating factors. Phlebotomy is not advised for isolated elevation of the hematocrit in asymptomatic patients or for hyperviscosity symptoms in patients with a hematocrit less than 65%.[2,72] It is important to note that iron deficiency results in decreased deformability of microcytic red blood cells and may also cause increased blood viscosity.[73] Iron supplementation should be cautiously provided to patients with documented deficiency followed by careful monitoring for rebound erythrocytosis.

Noncardiac symptoms Systemic effects of cyanosis may involve multiple organ systems. Clubbing, the loss of the 160° angle between nail and nail bed, and hypertrophic osteoarthropathy are components of ongoing bone hypertrophy and resorption found in many cyanotic patients.[74] Gout, caused by increased production and decreased fractional urate excretion, may manifest itself as hyperuricemia or as joint discomfort.[75] Renal dysfunction, including an elevated serum creatinine level, a decreased glomerular filtration rate, proteinuria, and abnormal findings on urinalysis, often complicates clinical management.[76] Calcium bilirubinate gallstones, caused by increased breakdown of heme, may present as symptomatic cholecystitis.[77] Abnormalities of hemostasis, including a prolonged prothrombin time, thrombocytopenia, impaired platelet aggregation, and shortened platelet survival, may accompany an increased tendency for perioperative bleeding.[78] Cerebrovascular events in adult patients with cyanotic congenital heart disease have been associated with hypertension, atrial fibrillation, iron deficiency anemia, and microcytosis.[79] Patients are at risk for systemic embolization, including brain abscesses caused by right-to-left shunting and bypass of the pulmonary circulation.

Prognosis

The prognosis for patients with Eisenmenger syndrome is generally felt to be better than that for adult patients with primary pulmonary hypertension.[80] A series from a tertiary adult referral center estimated a median survival of 53 years.[81] Factors suggesting increased mortality include younger age at presentation, supraventricular arrhythmia, poor New York Heart Association functional class, and an ECG index for right ventricular hypertrophy. History of syncope, hemoptysis, systemic oxygen saturation of less than 85%, and elevated right-sided filling pressures has also been associated with a worse prognosis.[82,83] Causes of mortality include congestive heart failure and sudden death.[81]

Long-term Management

Principles of long-term management of patients with Eisenmenger syndrome include ongoing assessment and improvement of cardiopulmonary status, with meticulous attention to associated cyanotic complications. A comprehensive team of cardiologists, anesthesiologists, and medical specialists should care for patients' noncardiac surgical procedures by planning for potential complications.[84] Evaluation of the patient with increased cyanosis should prompt an extensive search for a potentially correctable underlying cause [*see Figure 6*]. Optimizing the hematocrit level and administering supplemental oxygen can maximize oxygen-carrying capacity of the blood. Decreasing pulmonary vascular resistance through the use of pulmonary vasodilators, such as inhaled nitric oxide and intravenous prostacyclin, may increase pulmonary blood flow.[85] Improving ventricular function through management of volume status, maintenance of sinus rhythm, administration of inotropes, or judicious use of angiotensin-converting enzyme (ACE) inhibitors may augment cardiac output.

Pregnancy and Congenital Heart Disease

Increasing numbers of patients with congenital heart disease face concerns regarding childbearing. The management of pregnancy in female survivors of congenital heart disease has become an issue of vital concern for caregivers and patients and their families. Outcome of pregnancy in women with heart disease depends on the nature of structural lesions, history of repair, presence of pulmonary hypertension, ventricular function, and performance status. A number of published reviews detail the results of pregnancy in selected congenital heart defects.[86-90] Successful strategies rely on prepregnancy planning and subsequent treatment by a team of high-risk obstetric, genetic, cardiovascular, and anesthesia specialists. The maternal outcome of pregnancy in Eisenmenger syndrome remains discouraging despite advances and use of vasodilator therapy. A review of 73 published cases from 1978 to 1996 cited a maternal mortality of 36%.[91]

Management includes assessing cardiac adaptation to the hemodynamic changes of pregnancy, screening for arrhythmias, and counseling about recurrence rates. A general evaluation of the pregnant patient with congenital heart disease should assess ventricular function as well as evaluate risk factors predictive of maternal complications, including pulmonary hypertension; left-sided obstructive lesions such as mitral stenosis, aortic stenosis or coarctation; right-to-left shunting; and arrhythmia.[92,93] Prepregnancy cardiovascular drugs should be adjusted to approved medications. In particular, ACE inhibitors should be avoided because of adverse fetal events. Although endocarditis prophylaxis is not recommended for uncomplicated vaginal deliveries, many centers routinely administer antibiotics for patients with complex cardiac disease.

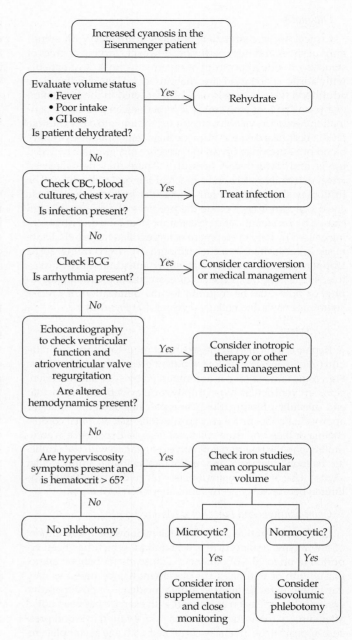

Figure 6 **Algorithm for evaluation of increased cyanosis in a patient with Eisenmenger syndrome.[6]**

Prophylaxis for Endocarditis

Adults with congenital heart disease are at significant risk for morbidity and mortality from infective endocarditis. A continuing incidence of endocarditis is noted after operative repair of cardiac defects, particularly in patients with left heart obstructive lesions such as aortic stenosis. A population-based registry noted a cumulative incidence of endocarditis of 20.6% at 30 years in these patients.[94] All patients with adult congenital heart disease should be instructed in the appropriate use of antibiotics for the prevention of bacterial endocarditis, according to recommendations by the American Heart Association.[26] Given the potential variability in clinical presentation, establishing the diagnosis of endocarditis may be complex. In addition to microbiologic data, the use of transthoracic echocardiography supplemented by transesophageal imaging is essential for prompt recognition and appropriate therapeutic strategies. [95]

Candidates for Heart or Heart-Lung Transplantation

Heart transplantation for adults with congenital heart disease is generally considered for (1) patients with inoperable lesions or (2) patients in whom operative procedures have failed, such as those with refractory ventricular dysfunction after repair.[96] Technical considerations unique to this group include challenges posed by complex cardiac and vascular structures and the increased potential for bleeding in patients who have previously undergone repeated cardiac surgical procedures. Significant pulmonary hypertension has been noted to be a risk factor for mortality in patients with congenital heart disease undergoing heart transplantation; candidates must demonstrate low pulmonary vascular resistance or sufficient reactivity to vasodilator testing at catheterization before transplantation.[97,98]

Patients with congenital heart disease and pulmonary hypertension may be candidates for lung or heart-lung transplantation, although there is still considerable risk. Patients with significant left ventricular dysfunction or complex inoperable cardiac anatomy merit consideration of heart-lung transplantation. Single and double lung transplantation with simultaneous repair of simple congenital defects has been successfully performed in patients with pulmonary vascular disease caused by Eisenmenger syndrome.[99,100] Impaired right ventricular function in the setting of severe pulmonary hypertension has shown sustained improvement after lung transplantation alone.[101]

Major drawbacks to transplantation include the limited availability of organs and long-term complications of immunosuppression, including infection, malignancy, and graft vascular disease. Most patients with congenital heart disease referred for evaluation of heart or heart-lung transplantation can have improved survival and quality of life with alternative medical and surgical planning. Therefore, the care of such patients is best coordinated between adult congenital and transplant services. For selected patients, transplantation may prove to be an acceptable therapy with reasonable short- and medium-term results.[96] It is hoped that improved outcomes will occur as a result of advances in transplantation biology and immunosuppressive regimens.

Challenges to the Care of Adults with Congenital Heart Disease

Adults with congenital heart disease pose numerous challenges for long-term follow-up care. Issues of insurability remain to be clarified for many individuals with lifelong heart defects. Outpatient clinics for this group face large increases in numbers of patients and an evolving patient profile with growing numbers of reparative surgeries and reoperations.[102] Despite definitive repair, patients with adult congenital heart disease require ongoing assessment and treatment of residual cardiac problems, including arrhythmias, decreased ventricular function, and pulmonary hypertension. Many also need continuing management of accompanying neurologic complications or syndrome-associated diseases. Other patients seek guidance about athletic participation and employment considerations.[103] Paramount for many young adults are concerns about reproduction and the inheritance of congenital heart disease. The future ramifications of acquired medical and coronary artery disease for this group remain unknown. It is clear

that the emerging populations of patients reaching adulthood after repair of complex congenital lesions are rewriting the natural history for previously characterized cardiac defects.

References

1. Bonnet D, Coltri A, Butera G, et al: Detection of transposition of the great arteries in fetuses reduces neonatal morbidity and mortality. Circulation 99:916, 1999

2. Wimpfheimer O, Boxt LM: MR imaging of adult patients with congenital heart disease. Radiol Clin North Am 37:421, 1999

3. Castenada AR, Mayer JE, Jonas RA, et al: Neonates with critical congenital heart disease:repair—a surgical challenge. J Thorac Cardiovasc Surg 98:869, 1989

4. Landzberg MJ, Lock JE: Interventional catheter procedures used in congenital heart disease. Cardiol Clin 11:569, 1993

5. Moller JH, Taubert KA, Allen HD, et al: Cardiovascular health and disease in children: current status. Circulation 89:923, 1994

6. Vongpatanasin W, Brickner ME, Hillis LD, et al: The Eisenmenger syndrome in adults. Ann Intern Med 128:745, 1998

7. Nora JJ: From generational studies to a multilevel genetic-environmental interaction. J Am Coll Cardiol 23:1468, 1994

8. Whittemore R, Wells JA, Castellsague X: A second generation study of 427 probands with congenital heart defects and their 837 children. J Am Coll Cardiol 23:1459, 1994

9. Burn J, Brennan P, Little J, et al: Recurrence risks in offspring of adults with major heart defects: results from first cohort of British collaborative study. Lancet 351:311, 1998

10. Feit LR: Genetics of congenital heart disease: strategies. Adv Pediatr 45:267, 1998

11. Curran ME, Atkinson DL, Ewart AK, et al: The elastin gene is disrupted by a translocation associated with supravalvular aortic stenosis. Cell 73:159, 1993

12. Keating MT: Genetic approaches to cardiovascular disease: supravalvular aortic stenosis, Williams syndrome and long-QT syndrome. Circulation 92:142, 1995

13. Chowdhury T, Reardon W: Elastin mutation and cardiac disease. Pediatr Cardiol 20:103, 1999

14. Smoot LB: Elastin gene deletions in Williams syndrome. Curr Opin Pediatr 7:698, 1995

15. Payne RM, Johnson MC, Grant JW, et al: Toward a molecular understanding of congenital heart disease. Circulation 91:494, 1995

16. Goldmuntz E, Clark BJ, Mitchell LE, et al: Frequency of 22q11 deletions in patients with conotruncal defects. J Am Coll Cardiol 32:492, 1998

17. Bristow JD, Bernstein HS: Counseling families with chromosome 22q11 deletions: the catch in CATCH-22. J Am Coll Cardiol 32:499, 1998

18. Hoffman JIE: Congenital heart disease: incidence and inheritance. Pediatr Clin North Am 37:25, 1990

19. Benson DW, Sharkey A, Fatkins D, et al: Reduced penetrance, variable expressivity and genetic heterogeneity of familial atrial septal defects. Circulation 97:2043, 1998

20. Helber U, Baumann R, Seboldt H, et al: Atrial septal defect in adults: cardiopulmonary exercise capacity before and 4 months and 10 years after defect closure. J Am Coll Cardiol 29:1345, 1997

21. Murphy JG, Gersh BJ, McGoon MD, et al: Long-term outcome after surgical repair of isolated atrial septal defect. N Engl J Med 323:1645, 1990

22. Gatzoulis MA, Freeman MA, Siu SC, et al: Atrial arrhythmia after surgical closure of atrial septal defects in adults. N Engl J Med 340:839, 1999

23. Konstantinides S, Geibel A, Olschewski M, et al: A comparison of surgical and medical therapy for atrial septal defect in adults. N Engl J Med 333:469, 1995

24. Horvath KA, Burke RP, Collins JJ, et al: Surgical treatment of adult atrial septal defect: early and long-term results. J Am Coll Cardiol 20:1156, 1992

25. Rigby ML: The era of transcatheter closure of atrial septal defects. Heart 81:227, 1999

26. Dajani AS, Taubert KA, Wilson W, et al: Prevention of bacterial endocarditis. Recommendations by the American Heart Association. JAMA 277:1794, 1997

27. Roberts WC: The congenitally bicuspid aortic valve. a study of 85 autopsy cases. Am J Cardiol 26:72, 1970

28. Huntington K, Hunter AGW, Chan K-L: A prospective study to assess the frequency of familial clustering of congenital bicuspid aortic valve: J Am Coll Cardiol 30:1809, 1997

29. Mensah GA, Friesinger GC: Calcific aortic valve stenosis and the congenitally bicuspid aortic valve: did Osler miss the link? J Am Coll Cardiol 77:417, 1996

30. Sabet HY, Edwards WD, Tazelaar HD, et al: Congenitally bicuspid aortic valves: a surgical pathology study of 542 cases (1991 through 1996) and a literature review of 2,715 additional cases. Mayo Clin Proc 74:14, 1999

31. Hahn RT, Roman MJ, Mogtader AH, et al: Association of aortic dilation with regurgitant, stenotic and functionally normal bicuspid aortic valves. J Am Coll Cardiol 19:283, 1992

32. Radtke WAK: Current therapy of the patent ductus arteriosus. Curr Opin Cardiol 13:59, 1998

33. Shyu KG, Lai LP, Lin SC, et al: Diagnostic accuracy of transesophageal echocardiography for detecting patent ductus arteriosus in adolescents and adults. Chest 108:1201, 1995

34. Chien CT, Lin CS, Hsu YH, et al: Potential diagnosis of hemodynamic abnormalities in patent ductus arteriosus by cine magnetic resonance imaging. Am Heart J 122:1065, 1991

35. Campbell M: Natural history of persistent ductus arteriosus. Br Heart J 30:4, 1968

36. Thilen U, Astrom-Olsson K: Does the risk of infective endarteritis justify routine patent ductus arteriosus closure? Eur Heart J 18:503, 1997

37. Burke RP, Wernovsky G, Van der Velde M, et al: Video-assisted thoracoscopic surgery for congenital heart disease. J Thorac Cardiovasc Surg 109:499, 1995

38. Prieto LR, DeCamillo DM, Konrad DJ, et al: Comparison of cost and clinical outcome between transcatheter coil occlusion and surgical closure of isolated patent ductus arteriosus. Pediatrics 101:1020, 1998

39. Sullivan ID: Patent arterial duct: when should it be closed? Arch Dis Child 78:285, 1998

40. Liberthson RR: Congenital pulmonary stenosis. Congenital Heart Disease Diagnosis and Management in Children and Adults. Little Brown & Co, Boston, 1989, p 31

41. Rome JJ: Balloon pulmonary valvuloplasty. Pediatr Cardiol 19:18, 1998

42. Chen CR, Chieng TO, Huang T, et al: Percutaneous balloon valvuloplasty for pulmonic stenosis in adolescents and adults. N Engl J Med 335:21, 1996

43. Kreutzer J, Landzberg MJ, Preminger TJ, et al: Isolated peripheral pulmonary artery stenoses in the adult. Circulation 93:1417, 1996

44. Fyler DC: Trends. Nadas' Pediatric Cardiology. Fyler DC, Ed. Hanley & Belfus, Philadelphia, 1992, p 273

45. Atz AM, Adatia I, Lock JE, et al: Combined effects of nitric oxide and oxygen during acute pulmonary vasodilator testing. J Am Coll Cardiol 33:813, 1999

46. Neutze JM, Ishikawa T, Clarkson PM, et al: Assessment and follow-up of patients with ventricular septal defect and elevated pulmonary vascular resistance. Am J Cardiol 63:327, 1989

47. Neumayer U, Stone S, Somerville J: Small ventricular septal defects in adults. Eur Heart J 19:1573, 1998

48. Moller JH, Patton C, Varco RL, et al: Late results (30 to 35 years) after operative closure of isolated ventricular septal defect from 1954 to 1960. Am J Cardiol 68:1491, 1991

49. Kidd L, Driscoll DJ, Gerson WM, et al: Second natural history study of congenital heart defects: results of treatment of patients with ventricular septal defects. Circulation 87 (suppl I):I38, 1993

50. Murphy JG, Gersh BJ, Mair DD, et al: Long-term outcome in patients undergoing surgical repair of tetralogy of Fallot. N Engl J Med 329:593, 1993

51. Rowe SA, Zahka KG, Manolio TA, et al: Lung function and pulmonary regurgitation limit exercise capacity in postoperative tetralogy of Fallot. J Am Coll Cardiol 17:461, 1991

52. Oechslin EN, Harrison DA, Harris L, et al: Reoperation in adults with repair of tetralogy of Fallot: indications and outcomes. J Thorac Cardiovasc Surg 118:245, 1999

53. Nollert G, Fischlein T, Bouterwek S, et al: Long-term survival in patients with repair of tetralogy of Fallot: 36-year follow-up of 490 survivors of the first year after surgical repair. J Am Coll Cardiol 30:1374, 1997

54. Friedli B: Electrophysiological follow-up of tetralogy of Fallot. Pediatr Cardiol 20:326, 1999

55. Rosenthal A: Adults with tetralogy of Fallot—repaired, yes; cured, no. N Engl J Med 329:655, 1993

56. Roos-Hesselink J, Perlroth MG, McGhie J, et al: Atrial arrhythmias in adults after repair of tetralogy of Fallot: correlations with clinical, exercise, and echocardiographic findings. Circulation 91:2214, 1995

57. Vaksmann G, Fournier A, Davignon A, et al: Frequency and prognosis of arrhythmias after operative "correction" of tetralogy of Fallot. Am J Cardiol 66:346, 1990

58. Harrison DA, Harris L, Siu SC, et al: Sustained ventricular tachycardia in adult patients late after repair of tetralogy of Fallot. J Am Coll Cardiol 30:1368, 1997

59. Cullen S, Celermajer DS, Franklin RC, et al: Prognostic significance of ventricular arrhythmia after repair of tetralogy of Fallot: a 12-year prospective study. J Am Coll Cardiol 23:1151, 1994

60. Gatzoulis MA, Till JA, Somerville J, et al: Mechanoelectrical interaction in tetralogy of Fallot. Circulation 92:231, 1995

61. Gatzoulis MA, Till JA, Redington AN: Depolarization-repolarization inhomogeneity after repair of tetralogy of Fallot. Circulation 95:401, 1997

62. Perry SB, Rome J, Keane JF, et al: Transcatheter closure of coronary artery fistulas. J Am Coll Cardiol 20:205, 1992

63. Rothman A: Coarctation of the aorta: an update. Curr Probl Pediatr 28:37, 1998

64. Sanders SP, MacPherson D, Yeager SB: Temporal flow velocity profile in the descending aorta in coarctation. J Am Coll Cardiol 7:603, 1986

65. Tyagi S, Arora R, Kaul UA, et al: Balloon dilation of native coarctation of the aorta in adolescents and young adults. Am Heart J 123:674, 1992

66. Hijazi ZM, Geggel R: Balloon angioplasty for postoperative recurrent coarctation of the aorta. J Interv Cardiol 8:509, 1995

67. Ruttenberg HD: Pre- and postoperative exercise testing of the child with coarctation of the aorta. Pediatr Cardiol 20:33, 1999

68. Seirafi PA, Warner KG, Geggel RL, et al: Repair of coarctation of the aorta during infancy minimizes the risk of late hypertension. Ann Thorac Surg 66:1378, 1998

69. Somerville J: How to manage the Eisenmenger syndrome (review). Int J Cardiol 63:1, 1998

70. Heath D, Edwards JE: The pathology of hypertensive pulmonary vascular disease: a description of six grades of structural changes in the pulmonary arteries with special reference to congenital cardiac septal defects. Circulation 18:544, 1958

71. Territo MC, Rosove MH: Cyanotic congenital heart disease: hematologic management. J Am Coll Cardiol 18:311, 1991

72. Perloff JK, Rosove MH, Child JS, et al: Adults with cyanotic congenital heart disease: hematologic management. Ann Intern Med 109:406, 1988

73. Linderkamp O, Klose HJ, Betke K, et al: Increased blood viscosity in patients with cyanotic congenital heart disease and iron deficiency. J Pediatr 95:567, 1979

74. Pineda CJ, Guerra J, Weisman MH, et al: The skeletal manifestations of clubbing: a study in patients with cyanotic congenital heart disease and hypertrophic osteoarthropathy. Semin Arthritis Rheum 14:263, 1985

75. Ross EA, Perloff JK, Danovitch GM, et al: Renal function and urate metabolism in late survivors with cyanotic congenital heart disease. Circulation 73: 396, 1986

76. Flanagan MF, Hourihan M, Keane JF: Incidence of renal dysfunction in adults with cyanotic congenital heart disease. Am J Cardiol 68:403, 1991

77. Perloff JK: Systemic complications of cyanosis in adults with congenital heart disease. Cardiol Clin 11:689, 1993

78. Colon-Otero G, Gilchest GS, Holcomb GR, et al: Preoperative evaluation of hemostasis in patients with congenital heart disease. Mayo Clin Proc 62:379, 1987

79. Ammash N, Warnes CA: Cerebrovascular events in adult patients with cyanotic congenital heart disease. J Am Coll Cardiol 28:768, 1996

80. Hopkins WE, Ochoa LL, Richardson GW, et al: Comparison of the hemodynamics and survival of adults with severe primary pulmonary hypertension or Eisenmenger syndrome. J Heart Lung Transplant 15:100, 1996

81. Cantor WJ, Harrison DA, Moussadji JS, et al: Determinants of survival and length of survival in adults with Eisenmenger syndrome. Am J Cardiol 84:677, 1999

82. Saha A, Balakrishnan KG, Jaiswal PK, et al: Prognosis for patients with Eisenmenger syndrome of various etiology. Int J Cardiol 45:199, 1999

83. Clarkson PM, Frye RL, Dushane JW, et al: Prognosis of patients with ventricular septal defect and severe pulmonary vascular obstructive disease. Circulation 38:129, 1968

84. Ammash NM, Connolly HM, Abel MD, et al: Noncardiac surgery in Eisenmenger syndrome. J Am Coll Cardiol 33:222, 1999

85. Rosenzweig EB, Kerstein D, Barst RJ: Long-term prostacyclin for pulmonary hypertension with associated congenital heart defects. Circulation 99:1858, 1999

86. Zuber M, Gautschi N, Oechslin E, et al: Outcome of pregnancy in women with congenital shunt lesions. Heart 81:271, 1999

87. Genoni M, Jenni R, Hoerstrup SP, et al: Pregnancy after atrial repair for transposition of the great arteries. Heart 81:276, 1999

88. Canobbio MM, Mair DD, Van Der Velde M, et al: Pregnancy outcomes after the Fontan Repair. J Am Coll Cardiol 28:763, 1996

89. Saidi AS, Bezold LI, Altman CA, et al: Outcome of pregnancy following intervention for coarctation of the aorta. Am J Cardiol 82:786, 1998

90. Connolly HM, Warnes CA: Ebstein's anomaly: outcome of pregnancy. J Am Coll Cardiol 23:1194, 1994

91. Weiss BM, Zemp L, Seifert B, et al: Outcome of pulmonary vascular disease in pregnancy: a systematic overview from 1978 through 1996. J Am Coll Cardiol 31:1650, 1998

92. Siu SC, Sermer M, Harrison DA, et al: Risk and predictors for pregnancy-related complications in women with heart disease. Circulation 96:2789, 1997

93. Siu S, Chitayat D, Webb G: Pregnancy in women with congenital heart defects: what are the risks? Heart 81:225, 1999

94. Morris CD, Reller MD, Menashe VD: Thirty-year incidence of infective endocarditis after surgery for congenital heart defect. JAMA 279:599, 1998

95. Bayer AS, Bolger AF, Taubert KA, et al: Diagnosis and management of infective endocarditis and its complications. Circulation 98:2936, 1998

96. Speziali G, Driscoll DJ, Danielson GK, et al: Cardiac transplantation for end-stage congenital heart defects: the Mayo Clinic experience. Mayo Clin Proc 73:923, 1998

97. Adatia I, Perry S, Landzberg M, et al: Inhaled nitric oxide and hemodynamic evaluation of patients with pulmonary hypertension before transplantation. J Am Coll Cardiol 25:1656, 1995

98. Costard-Jackle A, Fowler MB: Influence of preoperative pulmonary artery pressure on mortality after heart transplantation: testing of potential reversibility of pulmonary hypertension with nitroprusside is useful in defining a high risk group. J Am Coll Cardiol 19:48, 1998

99. Aeba R, Griffith BP, Hardesty RL, et al: Isolated lung transplantation for patients with Eisenmenger's syndrome. Circulation 88:II452, 1993

100. Bridges ND, Mallory GB, Huddleston CB, et al: Lung transplantation in children and young adults with cardiovascular disease. Ann Thorac Surg 59:813, 1995

101. Ritchie M, Waggoner AD, Davila-Roman VG, et al: Echocardiographic characterization of the improvement in right ventricular function in patients with severe pulmonary hypertension after single lung transplantation. J Am Coll Cardiol 22:1170, 1993

102. Gatzoulis MA, Hechter S, Siu SC, et al: Outpatient clinics for adults with congenital heart disease: increasing workload and evolving patterns of referral. Heart 81:57, 1999

103. Graham TP, Bricker JT, James FW, et al: Task Force 1: Congenital heart disease. J Am Coll Cardiol 24:845, 1994

Acknowledgments

Figure 1 courtesy of Leslie B. Smoot, M.D.

Figure 2 Tom Moore.

Figure 3 courtesy of James E. Lock, M.D., and Emily Flynn-McIntosh. Redrawn by Tom Moore.

Figure 4 courtesy of James E. Lock, M.D.

Figure 5 courtesy of Tal Geva, M.D.

Figure 6 Marcia Kammerer.

Table 3 Leg Segmental Pressure Measurements in Patient with Right Calf Claudication and Right Foot Pain*

	Right	*Left*
Brachial	158	158
Upper thigh	160	162
Lower thigh	94	154
Calf	62	116
Ankle	42	116
Ankle:brachial ratio	0.27	0.68

*Findings are consistent with femoropopliteal and tibioperoneal artery stenoses in the right leg. The right ankle:brachial ratio indicates ischemia. Systolic pressure gradients between the lower thigh and calf and between the calf and ankle in the left leg are consistent with distal femoropopliteal artery and tibioperoneal artery stenoses. The left ankle:brachial ratio is consistent with symptoms of claudication.

Angiography

Magnetic resonance angiography and contrast angiography can be used to evaluate the location and severity of peripheral atherosclerosis.[9] Angiography is not required for most diagnoses of peripheral arterial disease; results from the noninvasive tests currently available and from clinical evaluation are usually sufficient. Contrast angiography is performed when a diagnosis is in doubt or as a prelude to endovascular interventions or surgical reconstruction [*see Figure 3*]. Digital subtraction angiography is a computer-enhancing technique that is used to improve resolution, particularly when used in conjunction with the intra-arterial administration of radiographic contrast agent.

TREATMENT

Risk Factor Modification and Antiplatelet Therapy

Risk factors for atherosclerosis should be identified and treated, to reduce the likelihood of progression of atherosclerosis and also to prevent adverse cardiovascular events in patients with peripheral arterial disease. Patients who stop smoking cigarettes have a more favorable prognosis than those who continue to smoke. Aggressive lipid-lowering therapy reduces progression of peripheral atherosclerosis, but it has not been established that it prevents progression of symptoms from claudication to critical limb ischemia. Cholesterol-lowering therapy with 3-hydroxy-3-methylglutaryl coenzyme A (HMG-CoA) reductase inhibitors reduces adverse cardiovascular events in patients with atherosclerosis.

Antihypertensive agents should be tailored to bring blood pressure into a normotensive range. Aggressive reduction of blood pressure, however, may reduce perfusion pressure to an ischemic extremity and potentially aggravate symptoms. Some antihypertensive medications, specifically beta-adrenergic receptor antagonists, may cause reflex peripheral cutaneous vasoconstriction and exacerbate critical limb ischemia. Beta-adrenergic receptor antagonists do not adversely affect claudication.[10] Beta-adrenergic receptor antagonists are indicated to reduce the risk of myocardial infarction and death in patients with coronary artery disease—a condition that frequently coexists with peripheral arterial disease.

Aggressive treatment of diabetes mellitus reduces microangiopathic complications such as retinopathy and nephropathy.[11] It is not known whether aggressive treatment of diabetes reduces progression of atherosclerosis or prevents critical limb ischemia or foot ulceration. B-complex vitamins, such as folic acid, cobalamin, and pyridoxine, may lower homocystine levels, but it is not

yet known whether such therapy reduces cardiovascular events or prevents progression of peripheral atherosclerosis. Angiotensin-converting enzyme inhibitors, such as ramipril, may also reduce the risk of adverse cardiovascular events in patients with atherosclerosis, including those with peripheral arterial disease.[12]

There is little information regarding the efficacy of platelet inhibition in treating symptoms of peripheral arterial disease. In one study, primary prevention with aspirin was shown to reduce the need for surgical revascularization for peripheral arterial disease.[13] Small angiography trials have suggested that platelet inhibitors reduce the risk of acute peripheral arterial occlusion.[14] These agents may prevent thrombosis after plaque rupture in the peripheral arteries, as they do in coronary arteries. Antiplatelet therapy has been shown to reduce adverse cardiac events such as nonfatal myocardial infarction and stroke and have been shown to reduce cardiovascular mortality in patients with atherosclerosis.[15] In one study, clopidogrel was more effective than aspirin in reducing adverse cardiovascular events, particularly in patients with peripheral arterial disease.[16]

Hygiene and Physical Therapy

Local measures are used to prevent skin ulceration and foot infection, particularly in patients with critical limb ischemia. The

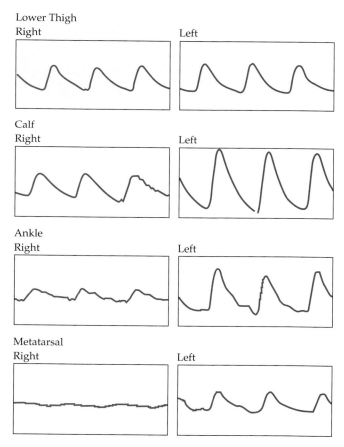

Figure 2 **Pulse volume recordings provide a qualitative assessment of blood flow to the extremity. In this example from a patient with right calf claudication and right foot pain, the pulse volume recordings are abnormal in the right calf, right ankle, and right metatarsal segments. In the right calf and ankle, the amplitude of the pulse is diminished and the rate of rise is delayed. No pulse volume can be recorded in the right metatarsal segment. The pulse volume recordings in the left leg are normal.**

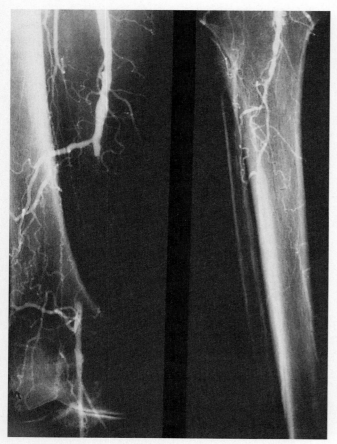

Figure 3 **Arteriogram of a patient with critical ischemia of the right foot. The left panel shows a long, total occlusion of the right superficial femoral artery. The popliteal artery reconstitutes via collaterals. The right panel reveals evidence of anterior tibial, posterior tibial, and peroneal artery occlusions with poor runoff.**

feet should be kept clean, and moisturizing cream should be applied to prevent drying and fissuring. The skin of the feet should be inspected frequently and minor abrasions treated promptly. Stockings should be made of natural, absorbent fibers. Elastic hose are contraindicated because they restrict skin blood flow. Shoes should be carefully fitted to reduce the possibility of pressure-induced skin breakdown. In patients with critical limb ischemia, the limbs should be maintained in a dependent position to increase perfusion pressure. This can be achieved by angling the mattress so that the affected limb is below heart level. Cotton wicks placed between the toes absorb moisture and reduce friction. Sheepskin placed beneath the heels of the feet reduces pressure and necrosis. A warm environment is recommended to reduce vasoconstriction. Ulcerations and necrotic areas should be kept dry and covered with dry, nonadhesive material. Infections should be drained. Local antibiotics should be avoided. Pain should be treated with analgesics.

Supervised exercise training programs improve walking capacity in patients with peripheral arterial disease.[17] Among the most likely factors that account for the improvement are more efficient skeletal muscle metabolic function and changes in ergonomics. Most studies have not found that exercise training improves blood flow to the exercising extremity. Training programs should be individualized for each patient. Because supervised settings provide structure and guidance, patients have achieved the most success with supervised training. Programs typically involve treadmill exercise for approximately 1 hour three times a week for at least 3 months. Patients are encouraged to walk independently outside the supervised program.

Pharmacotherapy of Claudication and Critical Limb Ischemia

Drug therapy has generally not been successful in improving symptoms of claudication or reducing the complications of critical limb ischemia. Although arterioles dilate in response to the metabolic demands of exercise, blood-flow augmentation is limited by critical stenoses. Thus, perfusion pressure distal to a stenosis falls further during exercise. Pharmacologic vasodilators may not reduce resistance to blood flow any more than endogenous vasodilators released during exercise. However, vasodilator drugs may increase blood flow to unaffected regions and thereby steal blood away from the ischemic limb.

Two drugs have been approved by the Food and Drug Administration for the treatment of intermittent claudication: pentoxifylline and cilostazol. Pentoxifylline is a xanthine derivative with hemorrheologic properties. It has been reported to improve red cell flexibility and decrease blood viscosity. Pentoxifylline improved patients' exercise capacity in several but not all clinical trials.[10,18]

Cilostazol is a quinolinone derivative that inhibits phosphodiesterase III and thereby prevents the degradation of cyclic adenosine monophosphate. It has vasodilatory and platelet inhibitory properties, but its precise mechanism of action in patients with peripheral arterial disease is not known. Several trials have found that cilostazol leads to an increase in the distance walked before onset of claudication and also in the maximal walking distance in patients with peripheral arterial disease.[19,20]

Metal-chelating compounds, such as ethylenediaminetetraacetic acid (EDTA), are not useful in the treatment of patients with peripheral arterial disease.[21]

Several classes of drugs are currently undergoing investigation for use in treatment of claudication, critical limb ischemia, or both. Some drug treatments are designed to increase the efficiency of substrate utilization, which enhances cellular energetics. L-Carnitine and its analogue, propionyl-L-carnitine, may decrease the ratio of acetyl CoA to CoA via the action of CoA:carnitine acetyltransferase and thereby stimulate glucose oxidation and energy production. Small placebo-controlled trials have found that treatment with L-carnitine or propionyl-L-carnitine improves exercise capacity in patients with intermittent claudication.[22] In one study, L-arginine, the precursor of nitric oxide, improved endothelium-dependent vasodilatation and increased claudication distance after 3 weeks of intensive therapy.[23] Vasodilator and antithrombotic prostaglandins have shown promise in the treatment of patients with peripheral arterial disease. Prostaglandin E_1 (PGE_1) and prostacyclin (PGI_2) or their synthetic analogues have been found to increase the distance walked before onset of claudication in some trials but not in others.[24] Administration of PGE_1 for several hours each day for up to 28 days is reported to reduce pain and facilitate healing of ulcers but not to affect the probability of amputation.[25] The angiogenic growth factors vascular endothelial growth factor (VEGF) and basic fibroblast growth factor (bFGF) are undergoing intensive investigation for their potential efficacy in patients with peripheral arterial disease. These angiogenic factors may be delivered parenterally as recombinant proteins or through gene transfer using intra-arterial catheter techniques or intramuscular injection. Both VEGF and bFGF increase collateral blood vessel development and improve blood flow in experimental models of hindlimb ischemia. Small preliminary trials in humans have been encouraging,[26,27] and larger placebo-controlled trials in patients with claudication or critical limb ischemia are in progress.

Revascularization

Revascularization procedures are indicated for patients with disabling claudication, ischemic rest pain, or impending limb loss. Revascularization can be achieved by catheter-based endovascular interventions [see Figure 4] or surgical reconstruction.

Percutaneous transluminal angioplasty (PTA) of iliac arteries has an initial success rate of 90%. Patency rates after 4 to 5 years are approximately 60% to 80% and are even higher with implantation of a stent.[28-30] Femoral and popliteal artery PTA has a lower success rate than PTA of iliac arteries. Patency rates at 1, 3, and 5 years are approximately 60%, 50%, and 45%, respectively.[28] The patency rate is better when PTA is performed for relief of claudication rather than for limb salvage and is also better in patients with good runoff (i.e., in patients with open distal vessels). Stents have not been shown to improve the patency rates of femoral and popliteal arteries over PTA alone. PTA of tibial and peroneal arteries is associated with poorer outcome than PTA of more proximal lesions and is usually performed in patients with critical limb ischemia who are considered at high risk for vascular surgery. Limb salvage rates of 1 to 2 years range from 50% to 75%. Thrombolytic therapy is not used routinely for treatment of peripheral atherosclerosis but may be effective in restoring patency of native arteries and bypass grafts after acute arterial occlusion [see Acute Arterial Occlusion, below].

The operative procedures used in vascular reconstruction depend on the location and severity of the arterial stenoses. Aortobifemoral bypass with a bifurcated Dacron or polytetrafluoroethylene prosthetic graft is the standard treatment for aortoiliac disease. Operative mortality ranges from 1% to 3% at centers with expertise in this technique. Long-term patency and relief of symptoms exceed 80% over 10 years.[31] Intra-abdominal aortoiliac reconstructive surgery is not feasible in patients whose comorbid conditions pose excessive surgical risk. Axillobifemoral bypass can circumvent the abdominal aorta and achieve revascularization of both legs. Femorofemoral bypass can be performed with the patient under regional anesthesia and is appropriate in cases of unilateral iliac artery obstruction.

Infrainguinal bypass procedures include femoral-popliteal and femoral-tibioperoneal reconstruction. Two techniques are generally used: the in situ saphenous vein bypass graft and the reversed autologous saphenous vein bypass graft. Femoropopliteal reconstruction is most successful when the distal anastomosis is constructed proximal to the knee. The 5-year patency rate for all saphenous vein infrainguinal bypass grafts, including grafts that have undergone revision, is approximately 75% to 80%.[28,32] Patency rates are higher in claudicants than in patients with critical limb ischemia. Synthetic grafts made of polytetrafluoroethylene are used when veins are not available.[33] The patency of prosthetic grafts is inferior to those composed of veins, particularly because of early thrombotic occlusion. Synthetic grafts inserted below the knee have a very low patency rate and are typically not used for tibioperoneal reconstruction. Operative mortality for infrainguinal vascular reconstruction is 1% to 2%.[32]

Lumbar sympathectomy is used rarely to treat patients with critical limb ischemia. The pathophysiology of limb ischemia suggests that ischemic vessels are maximally vasodilated; thus, lumbar sympathectomy may not increase blood flow.

Amputation is a surgical alternative for patients with advanced limb ischemia in whom revascularization procedures are not possible or have failed. It is a final alternative for patients with unremitting rest pain or gangrene. Selection of the amputation level requires assessment of perfusion. Transphalangeal amputation causes minimal disability. Transmetatarsal amputation of the forefoot may affect balance, but patients are usually able to ambulate after rehabilitation. Patients who undergo below-the-knee amputation and subsequently use a prosthesis expend 10% to 40% more energy to walk on a horizontal surface than a person who has use of both legs. Patients who undergo amputations above the knee and use a prosthetic device expend 65%

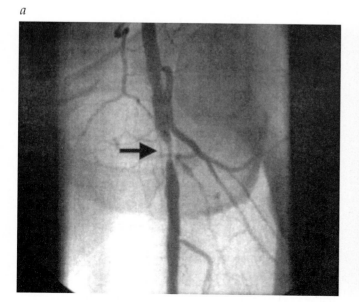
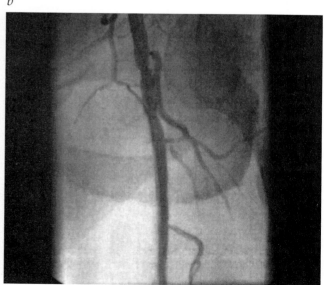

a *b*

Figure 4 Arteriograms of a patient with disabling claudication of the left leg. A focal stenosis (arrow) of the superficial femoral artery is apparent (*a*). After percutaneous transluminal angioplasty, patency is restored (*b*).

more energy to walk than a person who has use of both legs. Overall prognosis after major leg amputation is poor, usually because of coexisting coronary and cerebrovascular disease.

Acute Arterial Occlusion

Acute arterial occlusion is to be distinguished from the gradual development of limb artery obstruction caused by peripheral atherosclerosis. The causes of acute arterial occlusion include embolism, thrombosis, dissection, and trauma. The most common cause is arterial embolism. The majority of systemic emboli arise from cardiac sources, including atrial fibrillation, valvular heart disease, congestive heart failure, left ventricular aneurysm, acute myocardial infarction, and cardiac tumors (e.g., left atrial myxomas). Noncardiac sources of embolism include aneurysms of the aorta and the iliac, femoral, and popliteal arteries. A deep vein thrombus may enter the systemic circulation via an intracardiac shunt, resulting in what is termed paradoxical embolism. Thrombosis in situ may develop in peripheral atherosclerotic arteries at a site of plaque rupture and in bypass grafts. Thrombus may also develop in otherwise normal vessels of patients with procoagulant disorders such as hyperhomocystinemia (including homocystinuria), antiphospholipid antibody syndrome, and heparin-induced thrombocytopenia. Arterial thrombus formation is uncommon in patients with resistance to activated protein C and in patients deficient in protein C, protein S, or antithrombin III. Aortic dissection and trauma may acutely occlude arteries by disrupting the integrity of the vessel lumen.

Acute arterial occlusion may cause severe limb ischemia, resulting in pain, paresthesia, and motor weakness distal to the site of occlusion. There is loss of peripheral pulses, cool skin, and pallor or cyanosis distal to the obstruction site. Noninvasive tests can provide additional evidence of peripheral arterial occlusion and may reveal the severity of ischemia, but definitive treatment should not be delayed. Arteriography is used to define the site of acute arterial occlusion and may distinguish thrombus in an atherosclerotic vessel from an arterial embolism. Once the diagnosis is made, anticoagulation with heparin should be initiated to prevent propagation of the thrombus.

Acute severe limb ischemia requires urgent revascularization. Catheter-directed intra-arterial thrombolysis with agents such as recombinant human tissue plasminogen activator may restore patency in acutely occluded arteries and bypass grafts. An embolectomy catheter can be used to remove arterial emboli. Surgical reconstruction to bypass the occlusion is considered if embolectomy is unsuccessful or not possible. The decision to utilize thrombolysis or surgery for acute arterial occlusion depends in part on the severity of ischemia and urgency of revascularization.[34,35]

Atheroembolism

Atherothrombotic debris from friable plaques in the aorta or other large arteries may dislodge and embolize to small distal limb arteries. Atheroembolism occurs spontaneously, although it occasionally occurs as a complication of arterial catheterization. Violaceous discoloration, petechiae, and livedo reticularis appear when emboli occlude small vessels. Occlusion of digital vessels causes painful cyanotic toes (the blue toe syndrome), despite the presence of palpable pedal arteries [see Figure 5]. Embolic occlusion of intramuscular vessels causes pain and tenderness. Abnormal laboratory findings include an elevated eosinophil count and an increased erythrocyte sedimentation rate. Anemia,

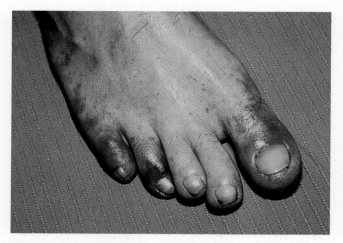

Figure 5 Ischemia of the toes of the right foot caused by atheroemboli. There is fixed violaceous discoloration of several toes and the lateral aspect of the right foot.

thrombocytopenia, and hypocomplementemia may also occur. Azotemia may occur if there is concurrent atheroembolism to the kidneys. Sites of shaggy atheroma may be identified by imaging the aorta with transesophageal echocardiography or magnetic resonance angiography.[36] Confirmation of the diagnosis is made by skin or muscle biopsy. Tissue examination will reveal elongated needle-shaped clefts in small arteries that are associated with intimal thickening, perivascular fibrosis, inflammatory cells, and lipid-laden giant cells.

The risk of recurrence of atheroembolism is high. Platelet inhibitors have been used in this disorder, although it has not been established that these agents prevent recurrent atheroemboli. The role of warfarin is even less clear. Some investigators have found that warfarin reduces the likelihood of atheroembolism in patients with mobile atheromas, whereas others have suggested that warfarin may contribute to the development of atheroemboli in persons with a predisposition to the disease.[37,38] Surgical bypass of occluded vessels usually is not possible, because the emboli typically lodge in small distal arteries. If a proximal source, such as an aneurysm, is identified, bypass surgery and removal of the source from the circulation may reduce the risk of recurrence. Risk-factor modification—in particular, lipid-lowering therapy—can serve to stabilize atheromatous plaques and may reduce cardiovascular events; it is not known whether atheroembolism is prevented by lipid-lowering therapy.

Popliteal Artery Entrapment

Popliteal artery entrapment is caused by a congenital anomaly in which the medial head of the gastrocnemius muscle compresses or displaces the popliteal artery. In young patients who present with symptoms of intermittent claudication or rest pain, popliteal artery entrapment should be considered a possible diagnosis. It occurs more frequently in men than in women and is unilateral in two thirds of cases.[39]

The diagnosis is made by measuring ankle pressures before and after exercising the calf muscle, because contraction of the gastrocnemius muscle compresses the popliteal artery. Duplex ultrasonography can demonstrate popliteal artery compression and cessation of blood flow during gastrocnemius contraction. Angiography is used to confirm the diagnosis by delineating the altered course of the popliteal artery and may reveal a popliteal artery thrombus and poststenotic dilatation.

Popliteal artery entrapment should be treated surgically, preferably by relieving compression of the popliteal artery. Occasionally, thrombectomy or bypass grafting is required.

Thromboangiitis Obliterans

Thromboangiitis obliterans is a vasculitis that is also known as Buerger disease.[40] In the United States, the prevalence is approximately 1 per 10,000 population. It occurs throughout the world but is most prevalent in Asia, portions of Eastern Europe, and Israel. Thromboangiitis obliterans affects men primarily but may also occur in women. Onset of the disease usually occurs before 45 years of age. The most important predisposing factor is tobacco use.

Thromboangiitis obliterans affects small and middle-sized arteries and veins in the extremities. Inflammatory cells, particularly polymorphonuclear leukocytes, infiltrate the intima, media, and adventitia; thrombi typically occlude the lumen. Leukocytes and multinucleated giant cells may be found within or surrounding the thrombus. The internal elastic lamina and media remain intact.

Involvement of limb arteries causes forearm, calf, or foot claudication. Severe ischemia of the hand and foot causes rest pain, ulcerations, and skin necrosis. Raynaud phenomenon, which is indicative of digital artery obstruction, occurs in approximately 45% of patients. Migratory superficial vein thrombosis develops in approximately 40% of patients.

There are no specific serologic laboratory tests to diagnose thromboangiitis obliterans; however, serologic tests are used to exclude other causes of vasculitis. Serum immunologic markers such as antinuclear antibodies, rheumatoid factor, and antiphospholipid antibodies should not be present, and acute-phase reactants are usually normal. The diagnosis can be supported by arteriography, which reveals interspersed affected and normal segments of blood vessels. Collateral vessels circumventing sites of occlusion are often present. Biopsy of affected vessels should reveal the typical pathologic findings described above but is rarely indicated.

The most effective treatment for patients with thromboangiitis obliterans is smoking cessation. The risk of progression to critical limb ischemia and amputation is greater in patients who continue to smoke. Surgical revascularization is not usually an option because of involvement of small distal vessels. There is no established pharmacologic intervention. The use of vasodilator prostaglandins may be beneficial in some patients. Intramuscular administration of naked plasmid DNA encoding the 165 amino acid isoform of human vascular endothelial growth factor [phVEGF (165)] was reported to heal ulcers and relieve pain in some patients with thromboangiitis obliterans.[41] The efficacy of platelet inhibitors, anticoagulants, and thrombolytic therapy has not been established.

Raynaud Phenomenon

Raynaud phenomenon is episodic vasospastic ischemia of the digits. It is characterized by digital blanching, cyanosis, and rubor after exposure to cold and rewarming and can also be induced by emotional stress. Although many patients describe a triphasic color response, most experience only one or two color changes. The digital discoloration is confined primarily to the fingers or toes. Occasionally, the tongue, tip of the nose, or ear-

Table 4 Secondary Causes of Raynaud Phenomenon

Connective tissue diseases	Cold agglutinin disease
Scleroderma	Cryoglobulinemia
Systemic lupus erythematosus	
Rheumatoid arthritis	Trauma
Dermatomyositis	Thermal injury
Mixed connective tissue disease	Frostbite
	Percussive injury
Sjögren syndrome	Exposure to vibrating tools
Peripheral arterial occlusive diseases	Hypothenar hammer syndrome
Atherosclerosis	Drugs
Thromboangiitis obliterans	Antimetabolites
Thromboembolism	Vinblastine
Thoracic outlet syndrome	Bleomycin
	Cisplatin
Neurologic disorders	Beta-adrenergic blockers
Carpal tunnel syndrome	Ergot alkaloids
Reflex sympathetic dystrophy	Ergotamine
Stroke	Bromocriptine
Intervertebral disk disease	Tricyclic antidepressants
Spinal cord tumors	Imipramine
Syringomyelia	Amphetamines
Blood dyscrasias	Miscellaneous conditions
Hyperviscosity syndromes	Primary pulmonary hypertension
Myeloproliferative disorders	Hypothyroidism

lobes are affected. Blanching represents the ischemic phase of the phenomenon, caused by digital vasospasm. Cyanosis results from deoxygenated blood in capillaries and venules. With rewarming and resolution of the digital vasospasm, a hyperemic phase ensues, causing the digits to appear red.

Raynaud phenomenon is categorized as primary or secondary [*see Table 4*]. The primary form of Raynaud phenomenon is also called Raynaud disease. Criteria for Raynaud disease include episodic digital ischemia, absence of arterial occlusion, bilateral distribution, absence of symptoms or signs of other diseases that also cause Raynaud phenomenon, and duration of symptoms for 2 years or longer. Most people with Raynaud disease develop symptoms before they reach 40 years of age. It can occur in young children. Raynaud disease affects women three to five times more frequently than men. The prevalence is lower in warm climates than in cold climates.

ETIOLOGY

The mechanisms postulated to cause Raynaud phenomenon include increased sympathetic nervous system activity, heightened digital vascular reactivity to vasoconstrictive stimuli, circulating vasoactive hormones, and decreased intravascular pressure. The sympathetic nervous system mediates the digital vasoconstrictive response to cold exposure and emotional stress but has been discounted as a primary mechanism. Some investigators have suggested that increased sensitivity, increased numbers of postsynaptic alpha$_2$-adrenergic receptors, or both enhance the vasoconstrictive reactivity to sympathetic stimulation.[42] In some cases of Raynaud phenomenon, endogenous vasoactive substances (e.g., angiotensin II, serotonin, and thromboxane A$_2$) and exogenous vasoconstrictors (e.g., ergot alkaloids and sympathomimetic drugs) may cause digital vasospasm.

Many patients with Raynaud phenomenon have low blood pressure. Decreased digital vascular pressure caused by proximal arterial occlusive disease or by digital vascular obstruction may increase the likelihood of digital vasospasm when vasoconstrictive stimuli occur.

DIAGNOSIS

Noninvasive vascular tests that are occasionally used to evaluate patients with Raynaud phenomenon include digital pulse volume recordings and measurement of digital systolic blood pressure and digital blood flow. Nailfold capillary microscopy is normal in patients with Raynaud disease, whereas deformed capillary loops and avascular areas are present in patients with connective tissue disorders or other conditions that cause digital vascular occlusion. Determinations of the erythrocyte sedimentation rate and titers of antinuclear antibody, rheumatoid factor, cryoglobulins, and cold agglutinins are useful to exclude specific secondary causes of Raynaud phenomenon. Angiography is not necessary to diagnose Raynaud phenomenon but may be indicated in patients with persistent digital ischemia secondary to atherosclerosis, thromboembolism, or thromboangiitis obliterans to identify a cause that may be treated effectively with a revascularization procedure.

TREATMENT

Patients with Raynaud phenomenon should avoid unnecessary exposure to cold and should wear warm clothing. The hands, feet, trunk, and head should be kept warm to avoid reflex vasoconstriction. Pharmacologic intervention is indicated in patients who do not respond satisfactorily to conservative measures. Calcium channel blockers, such as nifedipine, and sympathetic nervous system inhibitors, such as prazosin and its longer-acting analogues, can be used to treat Raynaud phenomenon. Intravenous infusion of vasodilator prostaglandins, including PGE_1, PGI_2, and their analogues, has been reported to facilitate healing of digital ulcers in patients with scleroderma.[43] In patients with persistent severe digital ischemia, selective digital sympathectomy and microarteriolysis may facilitate ulcer healing and improve symptoms. Cervical and limb sympathectomy may also be considered in persons with severe Raynaud phenomenon, but long-term efficacy is not ensured.

Acrocyanosis

Raynaud phenomenon should be distinguished from acrocyanosis, a condition in which there is persistent bluish discoloration of the hands or feet. Like Raynaud phenomenon, cyanotic discoloration intensifies during cold exposure, and rubor may appear with rewarming. Acrocyanosis affects both men and women, and the age at onset is usually between 20 and 45 years. The prognosis of patients with idiopathic acrocyanosis is good, and loss of digital tissue is uncommon. Patients should avoid cold exposure and dress warmly. Pharmacologic intervention usually is not necessary. Alpha-adrenergic blocking agents and calcium channel blockers may be effective in some patients with acrocyanosis.

References

1. Dormandy JA, Rutherford RB: Management of peripheral arterial disease (PAD). TASC Working Group. J Vasc Surg 31:S1, 2000

2. Leng GC, Lee AJ, Fowkes FG, et al: Incidence, natural history and cardiovascular events in symptomatic and asymptomatic peripheral arterial disease in the general population. Int J Epidemiol 25:1172, 1996

3. Criqui M, Langer RD, Fronek A, et al: Mortality over a period of 10 years in patients with peripheral arterial disease. N Engl J Med 326:381, 1992

4. Fowkes FG, Housley E, Riemersma RA, et al: Smoking, lipids, glucose intolerance, and blood pressure as risk factors for peripheral atherosclerosis compared with ischemic heart disease in the Edinburgh Artery Study. Am J Epidemiol 135:331, 1992

5. Murabito JM, D'Agostino RB, Silbershatz H, et al: Intermittent claudication: a risk profile from The Framingham Heart Study. Circulation 96:44, 1997

6. Hiatt WR, Hoag S, Hamman RF: Effect of diagnostic criteria on the prevalence of peripheral arterial disease. The San Luis Valley Diabetes Study. Circulation 91:1472, 1995

7. Graham IM, Daly LE, Refsum HM, et al: Plasma homocysteine as a risk factor for vascular disease. The European Concerted Action Project. JAMA 277:1775, 1997

8. Rutherford RB, Baker JD, Ernst C, et al: Recommended standards for reports dealing with lower extremity ischemia: revised version. J Vasc Surg 26:517, 1997

9. Koelemay MJ, Lijmer JG, Stoker J, et al: Magnetic resonance angiography for the evaluation of lower extremity arterial disease: a meta-analysis. JAMA 285:1338, 2001

10. Radack K, Deck C: Beta-adrenergic blocker therapy does not worsen intermittent claudication in subjects with peripheral arterial disease: a meta-analysis of randomized controlled trials. Arch Intern Med 151:1769, 1991

11. Intensive blood-glucose control with sulphonylureas or insulin compared with conventional treatment and risk of complications in patients with type 2 diabetes (UKPDS 33). UK Prospective Diabetes Study (UKPDS) Group. Lancet 352:837, 1998

12. Yusuf S, Sleight P, Pogue J, et al: Effects of an angiotensin-converting-enzyme inhibitor, ramipril, on cardiovascular events in high-risk patients. The Heart Outcomes Prevention Evaluation Study Investigators. N Engl J Med 342:145, 2000

13. Goldhaber SZ, Manson JE, Stampfer MJ, et al: Low-dose aspirin and subsequent peripheral arterial surgery in the Physicians' Health Study. Lancet 340:143, 1992

14. Collaborative overview of randomised trials of antiplatelet therapy. II: Maintenance of vascular graft or arterial patency by antiplatelet therapy. Antiplatelet Trialists' Collaboration. BMJ 308:159, 1994

15. Collaborative overview of randomised trials of antiplatelet therapy. I: Prevention of death, myocardial infarction, and stroke by prolonged antiplatelet therapy in various categories of patients. Antiplatelet Trialists' Collaboration. BMJ 308:81, 1994

16. A randomised, blinded, trial of clopidogrel versus aspirin in patients at risk of ischaemic events (CAPRIE). CAPRIE Steering Committee. Lancet 348:1329, 1996

17. Gardner AW, Poehlman ET: Exercise rehabilitation programs for the treatment of claudication pain: a meta-analysis. JAMA 274:975, 1995

18. Lindgarde F, Labs KH, Rossner M: The pentoxifylline experience: exercise testing reconsidered. Vasc Med 1:145, 1996

19. Beebe HG, Dawson DL, Cutler BS, et al: A new pharmacological treatment for intermittent claudication: results of a randomized, multicenter trial. Arch Intern Med 159:2041, 1999

20. Dawson DL, Cutler BS, Hiatt WR, et al: A comparison of cilostazol and pentoxifylline for treating intermittent claudication. Am J Med 109:523, 2000

21. van Rij AM, Solomon C, Packer SG, et al: Chelation therapy for intermittent claudication: a double-blind, randomized, controlled trial. Circulation 90:1194, 1994

22. Brevetti G, Diehm C, Lambert D: European multicenter study on propionyl-L-carnitine in intermittent claudication. J Am Coll Cardiol 34:1618, 1999

23. Boger RH, Bode-Boger SM, Thiele W, et al: Restoring vascular nitric oxide formation by L-arginine improves the symptoms of intermittent claudication in patients with peripheral arterial occlusive disease. J Am Coll Cardiol 32:1336, 1998

24. Lievre M, Morand S, Besse B, et al: Oral beraprost sodium, a prostaglandin I(2) analogue, for intermittent claudication: a double-blind, randomized, multicenter controlled trial. Beraprost et Claudication Intermittente (BERCI) Research Group. Circulation 102:426, 2000

25. Prostanoids for chronic critical leg ischemia: a randomized, controlled, open-label trial with prostaglandin E1. The ICAI Study Group. Ischemia Cronica degli Arti Inferiori. Ann Intern Med 130:412, 1999

26. Baumgartner I, Pieczek A, Manor O, et al: Constitutive expression of phVEGF165 after intramuscular gene transfer promotes collateral vessel development in patients with critical limb ischemia. Circulation 97:1114, 1998

27. Lazarous DF, Unger EF, Epstein SE, et al: Basic fibroblast growth factor in patients with intermittent claudication: results of a phase I trial. J Am Coll Cardiol 36:1239, 2000

28. Hunink MG, Wong JB, Donaldson MC, et al: Revascularization for femoropopliteal disease: a decision and cost-effectiveness analysis. JAMA 274:165, 1995

29. Bosch JL, Hunink MG: Meta-analysis of the results of percutaneous transluminal angioplasty and stent placement for aortoiliac occlusive disease. Radiology 204:87, 1997

30. Tetteroo E, van der Graaf Y, Bosch JL, et al: Randomised comparison of primary stent placement versus primary angioplasty followed by selective stent placement in patients with iliac-artery occlusive disease. Dutch Iliac Stent Trial Study Group. Lancet 351:1153, 1998

31. de Vries SO, Hunink MG: Results of aortic bifurcation grafts for aortoiliac occlusive disease: a meta-analysis. J Vasc Surg 26:558, 1997

32. Belkin M, Knox J, Donaldson MC, et al: Infrainguinal arterial reconstruction with nonreversed greater saphenous vein. J Vasc Surg 24:957, 1996

33. Abbott WM, Green RM, Matsumoto T, et al: Prosthetic above-knee femoropopliteal bypass grafting: results of a multicenter randomized prospective trial. Above-Knee Femoropopliteal Study Group. J Vasc Surg 25:19, 1997

34. Ouriel K, Veith FJ, Sasahara AA: A comparison of recombinant urokinase with vascular surgery as initial treatment for acute arterial occlusion of the legs. Thrombolysis or

Peripheral Arterial Surgery (TOPAS) Investigators. N Engl J Med 338:1105, 1998

35. Results of a prospective randomized trial evaluating surgery versus thrombolysis for ischemia of the lower extremity. The STILE trial. Ann Surg 220:251, 1994

36. Atherosclerotic disease of the aortic arch as a risk factor for recurrent ischemic stroke. The French Study of Aortic Plaques in Stroke Group. N Engl J Med 334:1216, 1996

37. Transesophageal echocardiographic correlates of thromboembolism in high-risk patients with nonvalvular atrial fibrillation. The Stroke Prevention in Atrial Fibrillation Investigators Committee on Echocardiography. Ann Intern Med 128:639, 1998

38. Ferrari E, Vidal R, Chevallier T, et al: Atherosclerosis of the thoracic aorta and aortic debris as a marker of poor prognosis: benefit of oral anticoagulants. J Am Coll Cardiol 33:1317, 1999

39. Persky JM, Kempczinski RF, Fowl RJ: Entrapment of the popliteal artery. Surg Gynecol Obstet 173:84, 1991

40. Olin JW: Thromboangiitis obliterans (Buerger's disease). N Engl J Med 343:864, 2000

41. Isner JM, Baumgartner I, Rauh G, et al: Treatment of thromboangiitis obliterans (Buerger's disease) by intramuscular gene transfer of vascular endothelial growth factor: preliminary clinical results. J Vasc Surg 28:964, 1998

42. Freedman RR, Baer RP, Mayes MD: Blockade of vasospastic attacks by alpha 2-adrenergic but not alpha 1-adrenergic antagonists in idiopathic Raynaud's disease. Circulation 92:1448, 1995

43. Wigley FM, Wise RA, Seibold JR, et al: Intravenous iloprost infusion in patients with Raynaud phenomenon secondary to systemic sclerosis: a multicenter, placebo-controlled, double-blind study. Ann Intern Med 120:199, 1994

44. Rutherford RR: Standards for evaluating results of interventional therapy for peripheral vascular disease. Circulation 83(suppl I):1-6, 1991

29 Venous Thromboembolism

Jack Hirsh, M.D., and Clive Kearon, M.B., Ph.D.

Venous thromboembolism, which involves venous thrombosis and pulmonary embolism, is a leading cause of morbidity and mortality in hospitalized patients and is being seen with increasing frequency in outpatients.[1] This increased incidence of venous thromboembolism in outpatients may be attributable to clinicians' heightened awareness of the importance of this condition and the comparatively recent development of reliable noninvasive tests for its diagnosis.

Risk Factors and Etiology

Most patients with venous thromboembolism have one or more well-recognized clinical risk factors. The most common risk factors are recent surgery, trauma, and immobility, as well as serious illness, including congestive heart failure, stroke, malignancy, and inflammatory bowel disease.[2] The common risk factors in outpatients include hospital admission within the past 6 months,[3] malignancy, presence of antiphospholipid antibody, and familial thrombophilia. Less common risk factors are paroxysmal nocturnal hemoglobinuria, nephrotic syndrome, and polycythemia vera.

Classification

Although venous thrombosis can occur in any vein in the body, it usually involves superficial or deep veins of the legs. Generally benign and self-limiting, thrombosis in a superficial vein of the leg can be serious if it extends from the long saphenous vein into the common femoral vein or if it is associated with deep vein thrombosis that is clinically silent. Superficial thrombophlebitis is easily recognized by the presence of a tender vein surrounded by an area of erythema, heat, and edema. A thrombus can often be palpated in the affected vein. Superficial thrombophlebitis may be associated with deep vein thrombosis. In most cases, superficial disease can be treated conservatively with anti-inflammatory drugs.

Thrombosis involving the deep veins of the leg may be confined to calf veins or may extend into the popliteal or more proximal veins. Thrombi confined to calf veins are usually small and are rarely associated with pulmonary embolism.[2,4] About 20% of calf vein thrombi, however, extend into the popliteal vein and beyond, where they can cause serious complications.[2,4] About 50% of patients with symptomatic proximal vein thrombosis also have silent pulmonary embolism, with high-probability ventilation perfusion lung scans,[4] and about 70% of patients with symptomatic pulmonary embolism have deep vein thrombosis, which is usually clinically silent.[2,5]

Pulmonary embolism is the most serious and most feared complication of venous thrombosis, but the postthrombotic syndrome, which occurs as a long-term complication in 30% to 50% of patients with symptomatic proximal vein thrombosis after 8 years of follow-up,[6,7] is responsible for greater morbidity. Most cases of the postthrombotic syndrome occur within 2 years of the acute thrombotic event.[6,7] Clinically, the postthrombotic syndrome may mimic acute venous thrombosis but typically presents as chronic leg pain that is associated with edema and worsens at the end of the day. Some patients also have stasis pigmentation, induration, and skin ulceration; a smaller number of patients have venous claudication on walking caused by persistent obstruction of the iliac veins. A study has reported that the routine use of compression stockings reduces the incidence of the postthrombotic syndrome by about 50%.[7]

Pathophysiology

Venous thrombi are composed predominantly of fibrin and red blood cells. They usually arise at sites of vessel damage or in the large venous sinuses of the calves or the valve cusp pockets in the deep veins of the calves. Thrombosis occurs when blood coagulation overwhelms the natural anticoagulant mechanisms and the fibrinolytic system. Coagulation is usually triggered when blood is exposed to tissue factor on the surface of activated monocytes that are attracted to sites of tissue damage or vascular trauma. Clinical risk factors that activate blood coagulation include extensive surgery, trauma, burns, malignant disease, myocardial infarction, cancer chemotherapy, and local hypoxia produced by venous stasis. Malignant cells contain a cysteine proteinase that activates factor X, which is a key clotting enzyme. Venous stasis and damage to the vessel wall increase the thrombogenic effect of blood coagulation. Venous stasis is produced by immobility, by obstruction or dilatation of veins, by increased venous pressure, and by increased blood viscosity. The critical role of stasis in the pathogenesis of venous thrombosis is exemplified by the observation that thrombosis occurs with equal frequency in the two legs in paraplegic patients but occurs with greater frequency in the paralyzed limb than in the nonparalyzed limb in stroke patients.[2]

Tissue damage, by stimulating the release of inflammatory cytokines, also results in impaired fibrinolysis. The cytokines induce endothelial cell synthesis of plasminogen activator inhibitor–1 (PAI-1)[8] and, by downregulating the endothelial-bound anticoagulant thrombomodulin,[2] reduce the protective effect of the vascular endothelium.

Increased central venous pressure, which produces venous stasis in the extremities, may explain the high incidence of venous thrombosis in patients with heart failure. Stasis resulting from venous dilatation occurs in elderly patients, in patients with varicose veins, and in women who are pregnant or using supplemental estrogen, perhaps contributing to the increased incidence of thrombosis in these persons. Venous obstruction contributes to the risk of venous thrombosis in patients with pelvic tumors. Increased blood viscosity, which also causes stasis, may explain the risk of thrombosis in patients with polycythemia vera, hypergammaglobulinemia, or chronic inflammatory disorders. Direct venous damage may lead to venous thrombosis in patients undergoing hip surgery, knee surgery, or varicose vein stripping and in patients with severe burns or trauma to the lower extremities.[2]

Table 1   Model for Determining Clinical Suspicion of Deep Vein Thrombosis[32]

Variables	Points*
Active cancer (treatment ongoing or within previous 6 months or palliative)	1
Paralysis, paresis, or recent plaster immobilization of the lower extremities	1
Recently bedridden for more than 3 days, or major surgery within the past 4 weeks	1
Localized tenderness along the distribution of the deep venous system	1
Entire leg swollen	1
Affected calf 3 cm greater than asymptomatic calf (measured 10 cm below tibial tuberosity)	1
Pitting edema confined to the symptomatic leg	1
Dilated superficial veins (nonvaricose)	1
Alternative diagnosis is at least as likely as that of deep vein thrombosis	-2
Total points	

*Pretest probability is calculated as follows: total points ≤ 0, low probability; 1 to 2, moderate probability; ≥ 3, high probability.

Blood coagulation is modulated by circulating inhibitors or by endothelial cell–bound inhibitors. The most important circulating inhibitors of coagulation are antithrombin (AT), protein C, and protein S.[9,10] An inherited deficiency of one of these three proteins is found in about 20% of patients who have a family history of venous thrombosis and whose first episode of venous thrombosis occurs before 41 years of age.[11] Some types of congenital dysfibrinogenemias can also predispose patients to thrombosis, as can a congenital deficiency of plasminogen.[12] An inherited thrombophilic defect, known as activated protein C (APC) resistance or factor V Leiden, is now established as the most common cause of inherited thrombophilia, occurring in about 5% of whites who do not have a family history of venous thrombosis and in about 20% of patients with a first episode of venous thrombosis.[13,14] The second most common thrombophilic defect is a mutation (G20210A) in the 3' untranslated region of the prothrombin gene that results in about a 25% increase in prothrombin levels.[13,15] This mutation occurs in about 2% of whites without a family history of venous thrombosis and in about 5% of patients with a first episode of venous thrombosis.[13] Elevated levels of clotting factors VIII[16] and XI[17] and of homocysteine[18] also predispose patients to thrombosis. The risk of thrombosis in patients with activated protein C resistance or the prothrombin gene mutation is increased by estrogen-containing oral contraceptives.[13,19] A randomized trial also found that the administration of estrogens in the doses used for postmenopausal replacement more than doubled the risk of thromboembolism.[20]

Natural History and Prognosis

Most venous thrombi produce no symptoms and are confined to the intramuscular veins of the calf. Many calf vein thrombi undergo spontaneous lysis, but some extend into the popliteal and more proximal veins. Complete lysis of proximal vein thrombosis is less common.[2,21] Most symptomatic pulmonary emboli and virtually all fatal emboli arise from thrombi in the proximal veins of the legs. Extensive venous thrombosis causes valvular damage, which is thought to lead to the postthrombotic syndrome. Patients with a history of venous thrombosis are more likely to experience additional episodes, particularly if they are exposed to high-risk situations.[1]

Untreated or inadequately treated venous thrombosis is associated with a high rate of complications, which can be decreased considerably by adequate anticoagulant therapy. About 20% to 30% of untreated calf vein thrombi extend into the popliteal vein, and about 40% to 50% of untreated proximal vein thrombi also undergo extension.[2,4,22] Patients with proximal vein thrombosis who are inadequately treated have a recurrence rate of about 40%,[22] and patients with symptomatic calf vein thrombosis who are treated with a 5-day course of intermittent intravenous heparin without continuation of oral anticoagulant therapy have a recurrence rate greater than 20% over the following 3 months.[23]

In contrast, fewer than 3% of patients who have proximal vein thrombosis experience a clinically detectable recurrence during the initial period of treatment with high-dose heparin or low-molecular-weight heparin (LMWH), and fewer than 3% of patients experience recurrence during the subsequent 3 months of moderate-intensity oral anticoagulant therapy or moderate-dose subcutaneous heparin therapy.[24] After 3 months of anticoagulant therapy, patients have an annual recurrence rate of about 3% if their thrombosis developed after a reversible provocation, such as surgery, or as high as 15% if their thrombosis is idiopathic or associated with ongoing conditions, such as prolonged immobilization or cancer.[15,25-28] The recurrence rate is significantly higher after a 4- or 6-week course of warfarin treatment, compared with a 3- or 6-month course.[25,27,28] In patients with more than one documented episode of deep vein thrombosis or pulmonary embolism, the recurrence rate in the first year after a 6-month course of anticoagulant therapy is approximately 6%.[27] Additional risk factors for recurrent venous thrombosis include older age, proximal versus isolated distal thrombosis, hyperhomocysteinemia, malignancy, and elevated levels of factor VIII.[29,30]

Diagnosis

VENOUS THROMBOSIS

Clinical Features

The clinical features of venous thrombosis, such as localized swelling, redness, tenderness, and distal edema, are nonspecific and should always be confirmed by objective tests.[4,31]

About 70% of ambulatory patients with clinically suspected venous thrombosis have another cause for their symptoms. The conditions that are most likely to simulate venous thrombosis are ruptured Baker cyst, cellulitis, muscle tear, muscle cramp, muscle hematoma, external venous compression, superficial thrombophlebitis, and the postthrombotic syndrome. Of the 30% of patients who have venous thrombosis, about 85% have proximal vein thrombosis, and the rest have thrombosis confined to the calf.[4]

Although clinical features cannot unequivocally confirm or exclude a diagnosis of venous thrombosis, careful documentation of the patient's history and of the signs and symptoms at presentation are useful in diagnosis [see Table 1].[32] Evidence suggests that patients can be classified as having a high, intermediate, or low probability of venous thrombosis on the basis of (1) the presence or absence of risk factors (such as recent immobilization, hospitalization within the past 6 months, or malignancy), (2) whether the clinical manifestations at presentation are typical or atypical, and (3) whether the patient has an alternative explanation for the symptoms that is at least as likely as deep vein thrombosis.[31-33]

Diagnostic Tests

Three objective tests (venography, impedance plethysmography [IPG], and venous ultrasonography) have been validated for the diagnosis of venous thrombosis.[4] Of these, venography and venous ultrasonography are most widely used.

Venography Venography, which involves the injection of a radiocontrast agent into a distal vein, is the reference standard for the diagnosis of venous thrombosis [see Figure 1]. Venography detects both proximal vein thrombosis and calf vein thrombosis. However, it is technically difficult and expensive, can be painful, may produce superficial phlebitis, and is complicated by deep vein thrombosis in 1% to 2% of patients. For these reasons, venography has been replaced by IPG and venous ultrasonography for the diagnosis of most cases of suspected venous thrombosis.[4]

Venous ultrasonography Venous ultrasonography is the noninvasive method of choice for diagnosing venous

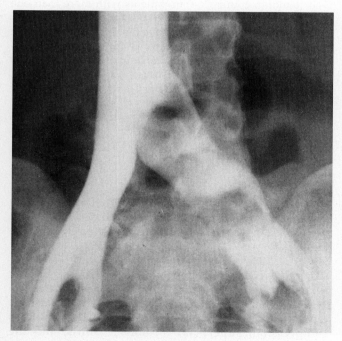

Figure 1 Filling defects in the left iliac vein, apparent in this venogram, reveal the presence of thrombi.

thrombosis.[4] It is not painful and is easier to perform than venography. The common femoral vein, superficial femoral vein, popliteal vein, and proximal deep calf veins are imaged in real time and compressed with the transducer probe. Inability to fully compress or obliterate the vein is diagnostic of venous thrombosis.[4] Duplex ultrasonography, which combines real-time imaging with pulsed Doppler and color-coded Doppler technology, facilitates the identification of veins.

Venous ultrasonography is highly accurate for the detection of proximal vein thrombosis in symptomatic patients, with the reported sensitivities and specificities approaching 95%.[4] The sensitivity for symptomatic calf vein thrombosis is approximately 70%.[4] Although venous ultrasonography fails to detect a substantial number of calf vein thrombi and small thrombi of the popliteal vein, this limitation is not critical. If the initial test result excludes proximal deep vein thrombosis, the test can be repeated in 7 days to detect the small number of calf vein thrombi that have extended since initial presentation.[4] If the test remains negative after 7 days, the risk of thrombus extension to the proximal veins is negligible, and it is safe to withhold treatment.[4,34]

In asymptomatic patients who have had elective hip or knee replacement, the sensitivity of real-time ultrasonography or of color Doppler ultrasonography for proximal deep vein thrombosis is about 60%.[4]

Ultrasonography is accurate, provided its results are concordant with clinical assessment; however, its accuracy drops if the results of these two assessments do not agree.[33] Therefore, venography should be considered if the clinical suspicion for deep vein thrombosis is low and the ultrasound is abnormal or if clinical suspicion is high and the ultrasound is normal; in about one quarter of such cases, the results of venography differ from those of the ultrasound.[33] Because the prevalence of deep vein thrombosis (mostly distal) is only about 2% in patients who have a low clinical suspicion of thrombosis and an initial normal proximal venous ultrasound, a follow-up test is not necessary in such patients [see Table 2].[4]

D-dimer blood testing D-dimer is formed when cross-linked fibrin in thrombi is broken down by plasmin, so elevated levels of D-dimer can be used to detect deep vein thrombosis and pulmonary embolism. A variety of D-dimer assays are available, and they vary markedly in their accuracy as diagnostic tests for venous thromboembolism.[35]

All D-dimer assays have low positive predictive value for deep vein thrombosis; an abnormal test is nonspecific and cannot be used to diagnose venous thrombosis. However, some D-dimer tests are sensitive for venous thrombosis, and a normal result can be used to exclude venous thromboembolism. In one study, a normal highly sensitive (~ 99%) D-dimer assay that occurred in 27% of consecutive patients was shown to exclude deep vein thrombosis (negative predictive value = 98.4%) [see Table 2].[36] Management studies have shown that it is safe to withhold anticoagulant therapy and serial testing in patients who have a normal D-dimer test in combination with a normal impedance plethysmograph (negative predictive value = 98.5%)[37] or a normal venous ultrasound of the proximal veins (negative predictive value = 99.8%)[38] [see Table 2].

Table 2 Test Results That Effectively Confirm or Exclude Deep Vein Thrombosis (DVT)

Purpose	Test	Indication for Use
Diagnostic for first DVT	Venography	Intraluminal filling defect
	Venous ultrasonography	Noncompressible proximal veins at two or more of the common femoral, popliteal, and calf trifurcation sites
Excludes first DVT	Venography	All deep veins seen, and no intraluminal filling defects
	D-dimer	Normal test, which has a very high sensitivity (i.e., ≥ 98%) and at least a moderate specificity (i.e., ≥ 40%)
	Venous ultrasonography or impedance plethysmography	Normal and (1) low clinical suspicion for DVT at presentation, (2) normal D-dimer test, which has a moderately high sensitivity (i.e., ≥ 85%) and specificity (i.e., ≥ 70%) at presentation, or (3) normal serial testing (venous ultrasonography at 7 days; impedance plethysmography at 2 and 7 days)
Diagnostic for recurrent DVT	Venography	Intraluminal filling defect
	Venous ultrasonography	(1) A new noncompressible common femoral or popliteal vein segment or (2) a ≥ 4.0 mm increase in diameter of the common femoral or popliteal vein since a previous test*
	Impedance plethysmography	(1) Conversion of a normal test to abnormal* (2) An abnormal test 1 year after diagnosis*
Excludes recurrent DVT	Venogram	All deep veins seen and no intraluminal filling defects
	Venous ultrasonography or impedance plethysmography	Normal or ≤ 1 mm increase in diameter of the common femoral or popliteal veins on venous ultrasound since a previous test and remains normal (no progression of venous ultrasound) at 2 and 7 days.

*If other evidence is not consistent with recurrent DVT (e.g., venous ultrasonography or impedance plethysmography, clinical assessment, or D-dimer), venography should be considered.

RECURRENT VENOUS THROMBOSIS

The diagnosis of acute recurrent deep vein thrombosis can be difficult.[4] A common approach is to perform venous ultrasonography. If the result is positive and the result of the previous test was negative, a recurrence is diagnosed. This diagnosis can also be made if venous ultrasonography shows more extensive thrombosis than was seen at the initial examination upon which the original diagnosis of deep vein thrombosis was made. If venous ultrasonography continues to show abnormal findings after the initial examination, venography should be performed. If the venogram shows a new intraluminal filling defect or evidence of thrombus extension since the previous venogram, recurrent venous thrombosis is diagnosed. If no new defect is found, however, the diagnosis must be based on clinical features. If venous ultrasonography shows normal findings at presentation, the test should be repeated twice over the next 7 to 10 days [*see Table 2*].

PULMONARY EMBOLISM

Clinical Features

The clinical features of pulmonary embolism, like those of venous thrombosis, are nonspecific, and fewer than one third of symptomatic patients have the diagnosis confirmed by objective tests.[39,40] Although pulmonary emboli may have a subtle presentation and are easily missed, especially in the elderly, it is important to evaluate clinical features carefully in patients with suspected pulmonary embolism. When combined with lung scan findings, the clinical presentation can be extremely useful in diagnosis.

Dyspnea is the most common symptom in patients with pulmonary embolism.[39] Chest pain is also common; it is usually pleuritic but can be substernal and compressing. Hemoptysis is a less frequent feature of pulmonary embolism. Fewer than 25% of patients with symptomatic pulmonary embolism have clinical features of venous thrombosis.[39,41]

Diagnostic Tests

Chest radiography and electrocardiography In patients with pulmonary embolism, chest radiography shows either normal or nonspecific findings. Chest radiography, however, is useful for exclusion of pneumothorax and other conditions that can simulate pulmonary embolism. The electrocardiogram also frequently shows normal or nonspecific findings, but it may be diagnostic of acute myocardial infarction. In the appropriate clinical setting, ECG evidence of right ventricular strain suggests pulmonary embolism.

Ventilation-perfusion lung scanning One of the main diagnostic tests for pulmonary embolism is ventilation-perfusion lung scanning.[5,39] There are two components to lung scanning. In ventilation-perfusion lung scanning, perfusion scanning is performed after intravenous injection of isotopically labeled microaggregates of human albumin [*see Figure 2*]. These particles become trapped in the pulmonary capillary bed, and their distribution reflects lung blood flow, which is recorded with an external photoscanner. Perfusion lung scanning is the pivotal test in the diagnostic process because a normal perfusion scan excludes a diagnosis of pulmonary embolism; an abnormal perfusion scan is nonspecific.[5,39]

During ventilation lung scanning, the patient inhales and exhales either radioactive gases or aerosols while a gamma camera records the distribution of radioactivity within the alveolar gas–exchange units. Ventilation imaging improves

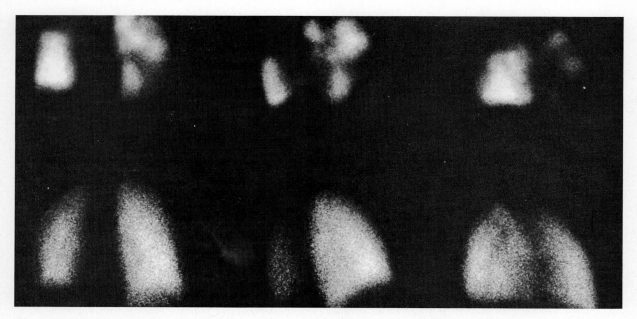

Figure 2   Posterior, right posterior oblique, and left posterior oblique perfusion scans (top), which were developed by using radiopharmaceutical technetium-99m (^{99m}Tc) microspheres of albumin, show multiple perfusion defects, some relatively large, in both lungs. Three ventilation scans (bottom) made with the patient breathing krypton-81m (^{81m}Kr) were recorded simultaneously with the perfusion scans. The scans were interpreted as showing a marked ventilation-perfusion mismatch, highly suggestive of pulmonary emboli. This diagnosis was confirmed by pulmonary arteriography.

the specificity of perfusion scanning for the diagnosis of pulmonary embolism, particularly a larger or segmental defect that is not matched by a ventilation scan.[5,39]

Unfortunately, only 40% of patients with pulmonary embolism have a high-probability lung scan.[5,39] The remaining 60% have abnormal perfusion scans that are classified as non–high probability. Patients with non–high-probability findings on lung scanning require pulmonary angiography or objective tests for venous thrombosis. The latter are useful because approximately 70% of patients with proven pulmonary embolism have deep vein thrombosis of the legs.[39]

Pulmonary angiography   Pulmonary angiography is the reference standard for establishing the presence or absence of pulmonary embolism [*see Figure 3*].[5,39] Unfortunately, it is invasive, technically difficult, and unavailable in most hospitals. Selective angiography and magnification views improve resolution and reduce the risks associated with the procedure. If the test is performed adequately, a normal pulmonary angiogram excludes the diagnosis of pulmonary embolism; in a patient with a small perfusion defect, however, the diagnosis of a small pulmonary embolism cannot be excluded by pulmonary angiography unless the tertiary pulmonary arteries are visualized.

Arrhythmias, cardiac perforation, cardiac arrest, and hypersensitivity to the contrast medium occur in 3% to 4% of patients undergoing pulmonary angiography.

Computed tomography and magnetic resonance imaging
Traditional computed tomography is not suitable for evaluating suspected pulmonary embolism because it is not feasible to opacify the pulmonary arteries with radiographic contrast for the time required to complete imaging (i.e., 3 minutes). Even if the pulmonary arteries could be opacified, motion artifact would interfere with image quality. These problems are over-

come by helical CT (also known as spiral or continuous volume CT) because image acquisition can be completed within a single holding of the breath (e.g., 20 seconds). Although it is widely used in clinical practice, the safety of managing patients with suspected pulmonary embolism according to the results of helical CT is not well established. In particular, the safety of withholding further testing and anticoagulation on the basis of a negative study is uncertain. A systematic review of studies that have evaluated the accuracy of helical CT for the diagnosis of pulmonary embolism concluded that the technique has been inadequately evaluated for this purpose.[42]

Current evidence suggests that helical CT has a sensitivity of about 90% or higher for emboli in segmental or larger pulmonary arteries. Sensitivity of isolated subsegmental emboli, which account for about 20% of symptomatic emboli,

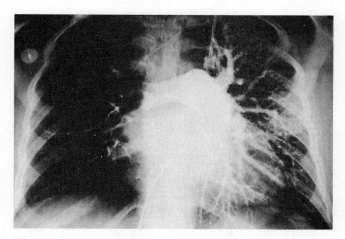

Figure 3   Pulmonary arteriogram demonstrates nonfilling of pulmonary arterial branches in the right lung, an indication of massive occlusion.

appears to be much lower. These observations suggest the following:

1. An intraluminal filling defect in a segmental or larger pulmonary artery is likely to be associated with at least a 90% probability of embolism and, therefore, may be interpreted in the same way as a high-probability lung scan.

2. A normal helical CT markedly reduces the probability of pulmonary embolism but does not exclude this diagnosis. It may be reasonable to interpret a normal spiral CT in the same way as a low-probability lung scan.

3. Intraluminal defects that are confined to subsegmental pulmonary arteries are likely to be nondiagnostic and require further investigation (e.g., pulmonary angiography or lung scanning).

Magnetic resonance imaging is less well evaluated than helical CT for the diagnosis of pulmonary embolism but appears to have a similar accuracy. Both helical CT and MRI have the advantage of possibly suggesting an alternative pulmonary diagnosis. MRI does not expose the patient to radiation or radiographic contrast media, and the examination may be extended to look for concomitant deep vein thrombosis.

Compression ultrasonography and D-dimer assay Two noninvasive, relatively inexpensive, complementary approaches can be used to simplify the diagnosis of pulmonary embolism in patients with nondiagnostic lung scan findings. These approaches involve the use of compression ultrasonography and the D-dimer test. Because pulmonary emboli usually arise from mostly asymptomatic thrombi in the deep proximal leg veins, a positive compression ultrasound test result can serve as indirect evidence in making a diagnosis of pulmonary embolism. However, a positive compression ultrasound test result is found in only 5% to 10%[43,44] of patients with nondiagnostic scans. Furthermore, a negative compression ultrasound test result does not exclude a diagnosis of pulmonary embolism in these patients, possibly because either the original thrombus has embolized or the residual thrombus is too small to be detected by compression ultrasonography. A negative ultrasound test result can, however, eliminate the possibility of an associated large proximal vein thrombosis; in most patients with a negative ultrasound test result, treatment can be withheld while further investigations are performed.

Two prospective studies—one utilizing plethysmography[45] and the other utilizing compression ultrasonography[44]—in patients with good cardiopulmonary reserve have reported that patients with non–high-probability lung scan results and a negative noninvasive test result for deep vein thrombosis can be safely managed with serial noninvasive testing for proximal vein thrombosis for 14 days. Both studies reported a very low rate (2%) of confirmed venous thromboembolism over a 6-month follow-up period, provided that the noninvasive test result remained negative.

About 90% of patients with a non–high-probability lung scan have a normal compression ultrasound test; of these, about 80% do not have pulmonary embolism. Therefore, the use of serial ultrasonography in all patients with a non–high-probability lung scan result and a normal compression ultrasound test result would lead to the testing of a large number of patients to identify very few at risk for recurrent

Table 3 Model for Determining a Clinical Suspicion of Pulmonary Embolism[36]

Variables	Points*
Clinical signs and symptoms of deep vein thrombosis (minimum leg swelling and pain with palpation of the deep veins)	3.0
An alternative diagnosis is less likely than pulmonary embolism	3.0
Heart rate > 100 beats/min	1.5
Immobilization or surgery in the previous 4 weeks	1.5
Previous deep vein thrombosis/pulmonary embolism	1.5
Hemoptysis	1.0
Malignancy (treatment ongoing or within previous 6 months or palliative)	1.0
Total points	

*Pretest probability is calculated as follows: total points < 2, low probability; 2 to 6, moderate probability; > 6, high probability.

pulmonary embolism. The noninvasive diagnostic process has been simplified by introducing two additional components: pretest probability and D-dimer testing.

In a prospective study of 1,177 patients with suspected pulmonary embolism, the D-dimer test (using the SimpliRED whole blood assay) showed a sensitivity of 84% and a specificity of 68%. Of 698 patients with a nondiagnostic lung scan, 668 (96%) had a low or moderate pretest probability and a negative bilateral compression ultrasound test result on presentation. In this group, the D-dimer assay had a negative predictive value of 99.7%. Of all patients, 44% with a nondiagnostic scan had a low pretest probability and a negative D-dimer test result; in this group, the negative predictive value of the D-dimer test was 99%, independent of compression ultrasound findings.[43]

The diagnosis of pulmonary embolism can be safely excluded in patients with nondiagnostic lung scans and either low or moderate pretest probabilities if the presenting bilateral compression ultrasound test result is normal and the D-dimer test result is negative. It is likely that a diagnosis of pulmonary embolism can also be excluded in patients with low pretest probability and nondiagnostic lung scans simply if the D-dimer assay is negative, although this approach requires confirmation before it can be recommended.

Used alone, a rapid enzyme-linked immunosorbent assay (ELISA) for D-dimer has a high sensitivity (99%) and a low-to-moderate specificity (45%) and was found to rule out pulmonary embolism in 36% of consecutive patients with suspected embolism.[36]

Diagnostic Strategy

Until recently, clinical assessment of the probability of pulmonary embolism was not standardized; physicians made the assessment informally on the basis of their experience and the results of initial routine tests (e.g., chest x-ray and electrocardiogram). Two groups have recently published explicit criteria for determining the clinical probability of pulmonary embolism. Clinical probability was used to manage patients in conjunction with perfusion scanning alone in one study,[46] whereas in the other study, clinical probability was used in conjunction with ventilation-perfusion lung scanning.[44] The latter clinical model, by Wells and colleagues,[44,47] incorporates an assessment of symptoms and signs, the presence of an alternative diagnosis to account for the patient's presentation, and the presence of risk factors for venous thromboembolism. The resulting model enables a patient's clinical probability of pulmonary embolism to be categorized as low (prevalence of 2%), moderate (prevalence of 19%), or high (prevalence of 60%) [see Table 3].[40]

The diagnostic approach to pulmonary embolism should take into account pretest clinical probabilities and lung scan findings [see Figure 4]. Pulmonary embolism can be excluded in patients with a normal perfusion scan. In patients with high or intermediate pretest clinical probabilities of pulmonary embolism, a diagnosis can be made if there are large perfusion defects (involving one or more segments) and a ventilation mismatch; these patients have a 90% probability of pulmonary embolism. The probability of pulmonary embolism is less than 5% in patients with a low pretest clinical probability of the disease who have a small perfusion defect with a matched ventilation abnormality; in these patients, a diagnosis of pulmonary embolism can be ruled out if noninvasive tests for venous thrombosis show normal findings.

For patients with other combinations of clinical and lung scan findings, including patients with a large ventilation-perfusion mismatch and a low pretest probability and those with perfusion defects—matched or unmatched with ventilatory abnormalities—that are not classified as high-probability defects, the frequency of pulmonary embolism is not sufficiently low to exclude pulmonary embolism or high enough to confirm this diagnosis.[5,39] These patients require further investigation with either pulmonary angiography or objective tests for venous thrombosis. A positive venogram or compression ultrasonogram can be used to make the diagnosis of venous thromboembolism in these patients,[5,39] and treatment with anticoagulants can be started without performing pulmonary angiography. If tests for venous thrombosis are negative, however, pulmonary angiography is required if the clinical probability of pulmonary embolism is high or the perfusion defect is large. In patients with a low pretest likelihood of pulmonary embolism and small defects, anticoagulants can be withheld, and serial ultrasonography or IPG can be used to detect propagating venous thrombosis. As previously described, the negative predictive value of a normal D-dimer test result can supplement this approach.

Prophylaxis and Treatment

PHARMACOLOGY OF ANTITHROMBOTIC AGENTS

Anticoagulants

A less intense anticoagulant effect is required for the prevention of venous thrombosis than is required for its treatment. The anticoagulants in clinical use are heparin and LMWH, which are administered subcutaneously or intravenously, and coumarin compounds, which are given orally. Thrombolytic agents are streptokinase, urokinase, and recombinant tissue plasminogen activator (rt-PA).

Heparin Heparin is a highly sulfated glycosaminoglycan that produces its anticoagulant effect by binding to AT, markedly accelerating the ability of the naturally occurring anticoagulant to inactivate thrombin, activated factor X (factor Xa), and activated factor IX (factor IXa).[48] At therapeutic concentrations, heparin has a half-life of about 60 minutes. Its clearance is dose dependent. Heparin has decreased bioavailability when administered subcutaneously in low doses but has approximately 90% bioavailability when administered in high therapeutic doses.

Heparin binds to a number of plasma proteins, a phenomenon that reduces the anticoagulant effect of heparin by limiting its accessibility to AT. The concentration of heparin-binding proteins increases during illness, contributing to the variability in anticoagulant response in patients

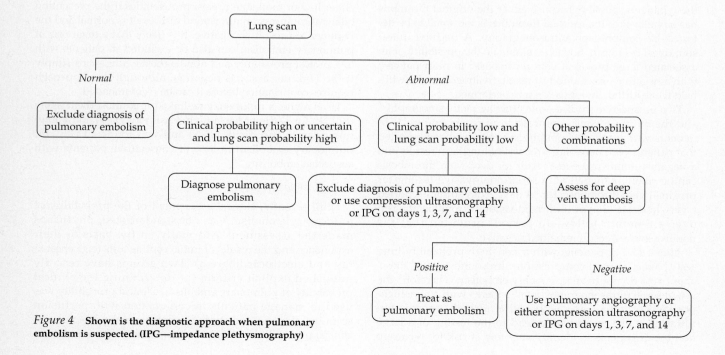

Figure 4 Shown is the diagnostic approach when pulmonary embolism is suspected. (IPG—impedance plethysmography)

Table 4   Drug and Food Interactions with Warfarin
by Level of Supporting Evidence* and Direction of Interaction[81]

	Antibiotics	Cardiac	Anti-inflammatory	Central Nervous System	Gastrointestinal	Miscellaneous
Potentiation Level 1	Trimethoprim-sulfamethoxazole, erythromycin, isoniazid, fluconazole, metronidazole, miconazole	Amiodarone, clofibrate, propafenone, propranolol, sulfinpyrazone[†]	Phenylbutazone,[†] piroxicam High-dose intravenous methylprednisolone Acetaminophen	Alcohol (with liver disease)	Cimetidine,[‡] omeprazole	—
Level 2	Ciprofloxacin, itraconazole, tetracycline	Aspirin, quinidine, simvastatin	Aspirin, dextro-propoxyphene	Chloral hydrate, disulfiram, phenytoin	—	Anabolic steroids, influenza vaccine, tamoxifen
Level 3	Nalidixic acid, norfloxacin, ofloxacin	Disopyramide, lovastatin, metolazone	Topical salicylates, sulindac, tolmetin	—	—	Fluorouracil, ifosfamide
Level 4	Cefamandole, cefazolin, sulfisoxazole	Gemfibrozil, heparin	Indomethacin	—	—	—
Inhibition Level 1	Griseofulvin,* nafcillin, rifampin	Cholestyramine	—	Barbiturates, carbamazepine, chlordiazepoxide	Sucralfate	Foods with a high vitamin K content, enteral nutritional support, large amounts of avocado Ticlopidine
Level 2	Dicloxacillin	—	—	—	—	—
Level 3	—	—	Azathioprine	Trazodone	—	Azathioprine, cyclo-sporine, etretinate, large amounts of broccoli
No effect Level 1	Enoxacin	Atenolol, bumetanide, felodipine, metoprolol, moricizine	Diflunisal, ketorolac, naproxen	Alcohol, fluoxetine, nitrazepam	Antacids, famotidine, nizatidine, psyllium, ranitidine[‡]	—
Level 2	Ketoconazole	—	Ibuprofen, ketoprofen	—	—	—
Level 4	Vancomycin	Diltiazem	—	—	—	Tobacco

*Level 1 evidence indicates that the likelihood of an association is very strong; level 2 evidence suggests that a true association is likely; level 3 evidence suggests that a true association is probable; and level 4 evidence suggests that a true association is possible.
†Supporting level 1 evidence was obtained from both patients and volunteers.
‡In a small number of volunteers, an inhibitory drug interaction occurred.

with thromboembolism.[48] Because the clinical effectiveness of heparin is related to its anticoagulant effect, the dose of heparin administered to patients should be monitored by the activated partial thromboplastin time (aPTT) and adjusted to achieve a therapeutic range, which for many aPTT reagents corresponds to an aPTT ratio of 1.5 to 2.5.[48]

LMWHs are effective in the prevention and treatment of venous thrombosis. They are derived from standard commercial-grade heparin by chemical depolymerization to yield fragments approximately one third the size of heparin.[49] Depolymerization of heparin results in a change in its anticoagulant profile, bioavailability, and pharmacokinetics and in a lower incidence of heparin-induced thrombo-cytopenia and of osteopenia.[50,51]

The plasma recoveries and pharmacokinetics of LMWHs differ from those of heparin because LMWHs bind much less avidly to heparin-binding proteins than does heparin. This property of LMWHs contributes to their superior bioavailability at low doses and their more predictable anticoagulant response. LMWHs also exhibit less binding to macrophages and endothelial cells than does heparin, a property that accounts for their longer plasma half-life, which is approximately 3 hours, and their dose-independent clearance. These potential advantages over heparin permit once-daily administration of LMWHs without laboratory monitoring. These advantages of LMWHs have been exploited to successfully treat patients with deep vein thrombosis out of hospital[52,53] and to treat patients with acute pulmonary embolism in hospital with once- or twice-daily subcutaneous dosing regimens of three different LMWH preparations.[41,54] Collectively, these four studies, which include over 3,000 patients treated with either once-daily or twice-daily subcutaneous doses of LMWH, establish this class of anticoagulants as a safe, effective, and convenient method of treating venous thrombosis and pulmonary embolism.[24]

Oral anticoagulants Oral anticoagulants are coumarin compounds, the most common being warfarin, that produce their anticoagulant effect through the production of hemostatically defective vitamin K–dependent coagulant proteins (prothrombin, factor VII, factor IX, and factor X).[55]

The dose of warfarin must be monitored closely because the anticoagulant response varies widely among individuals. Laboratory monitoring is performed by measuring the prothrombin time (PT), a test responsive to depression of three of the four vitamin K–dependent clotting factors (prothrombin and factors VII and X). Commercial PT reagents vary markedly in their responsiveness to warfarin-induced reduction in clotting factors. This problem of variability in the responsiveness of PT reagents has been overcome by the introduction of the international normalized ratio (INR).

The starting dose has been 10 mg, with an average maintenance dose of about 5 mg. However, the dose varies widely among individuals. Elderly patients, for example, have been shown, on average, to require lower doses. Evidence indicates that it might be safer to use a starting dose of 5 mg of warfarin because, compared with 10 mg, the 5 mg starting dose does not delay achieving a therapeutic INR and is associated with a lower incidence of supratherapeutic INR values during the first 5 days of treatment.[56] Some patients receiving warfarin are difficult to manage because of unexpected fluctuations in dose response, which may reflect changes in diet, inaccuracy in PT testing, undisclosed drug use, poor compliance, surreptitious self-medication, or intermittent alcohol consumption. Concomitant medication with over-the-counter and prescription drugs can augment or inhibit the anticoagulant effect of coumarin compounds on hemostasis or interfere with platelet function [see Table 4].

Patients receiving coumarin compounds are also sensitive to fluctuating levels of dietary vitamin K, obtained predominantly from leafy green vegetables. The effect of coumarins can be potentiated in sick patients with poor vitamin K intake, particularly if they are treated with antibiotics and intravenous fluids without vitamin K supplementation and in states of fat malabsorption.

Thrombolytic Agents

Pharmacologic thrombolysis is produced by plasminogen activators—including streptokinase, tissue plasminogen activator (t-PA), and urokinase—which convert the proenzyme plasminogen to the fibrinolytic enzyme plasmin.[57]

Streptokinase Streptokinase is a protein produced by β-hemolytic streptococci. In contrast to other plasminogen activators, streptokinase is not an enzyme and does not convert plasminogen directly to plasmin by proteolytic cleavage. Instead, streptokinase binds noncovalently to plasminogen, converting it to a plasminogen-activator complex that acts on other plasminogen molecules to generate plasmin. Streptokinase has a plasma half-life of 30 minutes.

Because streptokinase is a bacterial product, it stimulates antibody production and can prompt allergic reactions. Antistreptococcal antibodies, present in variable titers in most patients before streptokinase treatment, induce an amnestic response that makes repeated treatment with streptokinase difficult or impossible for a period of months or years after an initial course of treatment. Laboratory monitoring of streptokinase can be limited to a thrombin time, which is used as a marker for an effective lytic state. If

the thrombin time is not prolonged within the first few hours of commencing treatment, resistance to streptokinase resulting from a high titer of antistreptococcal antibodies should be suspected, and the dose of streptokinase should be increased.

Urokinase Synthesized by endothelial and mononuclear cells, urokinase is a direct activator of plasminogen. Like streptokinase, urokinase is non–fibrin specific. It has a plasma half-life of 10 minutes.

rt-PA, which is fibrin specific, is synthesized by endothelial cells as a single-chain polypeptide. Proteolytic cleavage converts the single-chain form into a two-chain species. Both forms are enzymatically active. rt-PA has a plasma half-life of approximately 5 minutes. However, it is no longer commercially available.

Complications of Antithrombotic Agents

Bleeding is the main complication of antithrombotic therapy.[58] With all antithrombotic agents, the risk of bleeding is influenced by the dose and by patient-related factors, the most important being recent surgery or trauma. Other patient characteristics that increase the risk of bleeding are age, recent stroke, generalized hemostatic defect, a history of gastrointestinal hemorrhage, and serious comorbid conditions. Bleeding is more common and more serious with thrombolytic drugs than with anticoagulants. The risk of bleeding with thrombolytic therapy is just as great with rt-PA as with streptokinase and urokinase, which, unlike rt-PA, lack fibrin specificity. The risk of bleeding increases with the duration of treatment.

With heparin, the incidence of bleeding is influenced by dosage and by means of administration, being higher with intermittent intravenous therapy than with continuous intravenous therapy.[58] Recent trials show that the rates of bleeding are similar for heparin and LMWH.[24] Bleeding that is associated with coumarin anticoagulants is influenced by the intensity of anticoagulant therapy. Such bleeding is reduced to about one third if the targeted range is lowered from between 3.0 and 4.5 to between 2.0 and 3.0. Both heparin-induced bleeding and warfarin-induced bleeding are increased by concomitant use of aspirin, which impairs platelet function and produces gastric erosions. When the INR is less than 3.0, coumarin-associated bleeding frequently has an obvious underlying cause or is caused by an occult gastrointestinal or renal lesion.

Nonhemorrhagic side effects of thrombolytic therapy are limited mainly to allergic reactions to streptokinase. Nonhemorrhagic side effects of heparin include the following: (1) urticaria at sites of subcutaneous injection; (2) thrombocytopenia, which occurs in 2% to 4% of patients treated with high-dose heparin and is complicated by arterial or venous thrombosis in about 0.2% of treated patients; (3) osteoporosis, which occurs with prolonged high-dose heparin use; and, rarely, (4) alopecia, adrenal insufficiency, and skin necrosis.[48] The incidence of thrombocytopenia is lower with LMWHs than with heparin.[49] Similarly, there is evidence that the risk of osteopenia is lower with LMWH than with heparin.[48,51]

The most important nonhemorrhagic side effect of coumarin anticoagulants is skin necrosis, an uncommon complication usually observed on the third to eighth day of therapy. Skin necrosis is caused by extensive thrombosis of the venules and capillaries within the subcutaneous fat. An association has been reported between coumarin-induced skin necrosis and protein C deficiency—and, less commonly, protein S deficiency—but this complication can occur in individuals without these protein deficiencies.

PROPHYLAXIS

The most effective way of reducing the mortality associated with pulmonary embolism and the morbidity associated with the postthrombotic syndrome is to institute primary prophylaxis in patients at risk for venous thromboembolism. On the basis of well-defined clinical criteria, patients can be classified as being at low, moderate, or high risk for venous thromboembolism, and the choice of prophylaxis should be tailored to the patient's risk [see Table 5].[59] In the absence of prophylaxis, the frequency of fatal postoperative pulmonary embolism ranges from 0.1% to 0.4% in patients undergoing elective general surgery and from 1% to 5% in patients undergoing elective hip or knee surgery, emergency hip surgery, major trauma, or spinal cord injury.[59] Prophylaxis is cost-effective for most high-risk groups.[59]

Prophylaxis is achieved either by modulating activation of blood coagulation or by preventing venous stasis by using the following proven approaches: low-dose subcutaneous heparin, intermittent pneumatic compression of the legs, oral anticoagulants, adjusted doses of subcutaneous heparin, graduated compression stockings, or LMWHs.[59] Administration of antiplatelet agents, such as aspirin, also prevents venous thromboembolism[60] but probably less effectively than the previously stated methods.[59]

Low-dose heparin is given subcutaneously, at a dose of 5,000 U 2 hours before surgery and 5,000 U every 8 or 12 hours after surgery. In patients undergoing major orthopedic surgical procedures, low-dose heparin is less effective than warfarin, adjusted-dose heparin, and LMWHs. Intermittent pneumatic compression of the legs enhances blood flow in the deep veins and increases blood fibrinolytic activity. This method of prophylaxis is free of clinically important side effects and is particularly useful in patients who have a high risk of serious bleeding. It is the method of choice for preventing venous thrombosis in patients undergoing neurosurgery, it is effective in patients undergoing major knee surgery, and it is as effective as low-dose heparin in patients undergoing abdominal surgery.

Graduated compression stockings reduce venous stasis and prevent postoperative venous thrombosis in general surgical patients and in medical or surgical patients with neurologic disorders, including paralysis of the lower limbs.[59] In surgical patients, the combined use of graduated compression stockings and low-dose heparin is significantly more effective than use of low-dose heparin alone. Graduated compression stockings are relatively inexpensive and should be considered in all high-risk surgical patients, even if other forms of prophylaxis are used.

Moderate-dose warfarin (INR = 2.0 to 3.0) is effective for preventing postoperative venous thromboembolism in patients in all risk categories.[59] Warfarin therapy can be started preoperatively, at the time of surgery, or in the early postoperative period. Although the anticoagulant effect is not achieved until the third or fourth postoperative day, warfarin treatment started at the time of surgery or in the early postoperative period is effective in very high risk patient groups, including patients with hip fractures and those who undergo joint replacement. Prophylaxis with warfarin is less convenient than low-dose heparin or LMWHs, however, because careful laboratory monitoring is necessary.

LMWH is a safe and effective form of prophylaxis in high-risk patients undergoing elective hip surgery, major general surgery, or major knee surgery or experiencing hip fracture, spinal injury, or stroke. LMWH was more effective than standard low-dose heparin in general surgical patients, patients undergoing elective hip surgery, and patients with stroke or spinal injury.

In patients who are undergoing hip or major knee surgery, LMWH is more effective than warfarin but is associated with more frequent bleeding; both of these differences may be caused by a more rapid onset of anticoagulation with postoperatively initiated LMWH than with warfarin.[59,61] It is uncertain whether the superior efficacy of LMWH over warfarin in the prevention of venographically detectable venous thrombosis is mirrored by fewer symptomatic episodes of venous thromboembolism with LMWH.[59,61]

Indications for Prophylaxis

General surgery and medicine Low-dose-heparin prophylaxis is the method of choice for moderate-risk general surgical and medical patients.[59] It reduces the risk of venous thromboembolism by 50% to 70%[41] and is simple, inexpensive, convenient, and safe. If anticoagulants are contraindicated because of an unusually high risk of bleeding, intermittent pneumatic compression of the legs should be used.

Hip surgery LMWH or oral anticoagulants are effective prophylaxis for venous thrombosis in patients who have undergone hip surgery. Aspirin has also been shown to reduce the frequency of symptomatic venous thromboembolism and fatal pulmonary embolism after hip fracture.[60] The relative efficacy and safety of aspirin versus LMWH or oral anticoagulants in patients who have a hip fracture or have undergone hip or knee arthroplasty is not known. However, because studies have shown that aspirin is much less effective than LMWH or oral anticoagulants at preventing venographically detectable venous thrombosis,

Table 5 Risk Categories for Venous Thromboembolism and Recommendations for Prophylaxis

	High Risk	*Moderate Risk*
Calf vein thrombosis	30%–50%	10%–30%
Proximal vein thrombosis	10%–20%	2%–8%
Fatal pulmonary embolism	1%–5%	0.2%–0.7%
Recommended prophylaxis	Low-molecular-weight heparin, oral anticoagulants, or adjusted-dose heparin	Low-dose heparin or external pneumatic compression

aspirin is not recommended as the sole agent for post-operative prophylaxis.[59]

Major knee surgery Both LMWH and intermittent pneumatic compression are effective in preventing venous thrombosis in patients undergoing major knee surgery. LMWH is more convenient and will probably become the treatment of choice.

Genitourinary surgery, neurosurgery, and ocular surgery Intermittent pneumatic compression, with or without static graduated compression stockings, is effective prophylaxis for venous thrombosis and does not increase the risk of bleeding.

TREATMENT

Overview

The objectives of treating patients with venous thromboembolism are to prevent fatal pulmonary embolism, the postthrombotic syndrome, thromboembolic pulmonary hypertension, and recurrent venous thromboembolism and to alleviate the discomfort of the acute event.

Anticoagulants can effectively reduce morbidity and mortality caused by pulmonary embolism.[5] Vena caval interruption, which is usually achieved with an inferior vena caval filter, is also effective but is more complicated, expensive, and invasive and is associated with a doubling of the frequency of recurrent deep vein thrombosis during long-term follow-up.[62] For these reasons, it is used generally only if anticoagulant therapy has failed or is contraindicated because of the risk of serious hemorrhage.[5]

Thrombolytic therapy with streptokinase, urokinase, or rt-PA is more effective than heparin in achieving early lysis of venous thromboembolism and is better than heparin for preventing death in patients with massive pulmonary embolism associated with shock.[63] Thrombolytic therapy is therefore the treatment of choice for patients with life-threatening pulmonary embolism.

Thromboendarterectomy is effective treatment in selected cases of chronic thromboembolic pulmonary hypertension involving proximal pulmonary arterial obstruction.[64] Urgent pulmonary embolectomy is rarely indicated, being reserved for patients with a saddle embolism lodged in the main pulmonary artery or for those with massive embolism whose blood pressure cannot be maintained despite administration of thrombolytic therapy and vasopressor agents or in whom there is an absolute contraindication to thrombolytic therapy.[5]

Administration and Dosage Guidelines

Anticoagulant therapy Anticoagulants are the mainstay of treatment for most patients with venous thrombo-embolism. In the past, the treatment of choice was heparin administered by continuous intravenous infusion or subcutaneous injection, in doses sufficient to produce an adequate anticoagulant response. Results of recent studies indicate that LMWH administered by subcutaneous injection without laboratory monitoring is as effective and safe as heparin.[24]

The anticoagulant effect of intravenous heparin or LMWH is immediate. With subcutaneous injection, the anticoagulant effect of both anticoagulants is delayed for about an hour; peak levels occur at 2 to 3 hours. The anticoagulant effect of subcutaneous heparin is maintained for about 12 hours with therapeutic doses. LMWH is effective when administered subcutaneously once daily.[24]

Heparin therapy is usually monitored by the aPTT and less frequently by heparin assays, which measure the ability of heparin to accelerate the inactivation of factor Xa or thrombin by AT. The anticoagulant effect should be monitored carefully, and the dosage should be adjusted to achieve an adequate anticoagulant effect because there is a greater risk of recurrent venous thromboembolism if the anticoagulant effect is suboptimal.[5] The therapeutic range of aPTT should be maintained above a ratio equivalent to a heparin level between 0.35 and 7.0 U/ml as measured by an anti–factor Xa assay.[65] For many aPTT reagents, this range is equivalent to an aPTT ratio of 1.8 to 2.5 times the mean of the normal laboratory control value.[48,65]

LMWH is administered subcutaneously on a weight-adjusted basis at a dosage of either 100 anti-Xa U/kg every 12 hours or 150 to 200 anti-Xa U once daily.[49] It does not require monitoring.

Treatment with heparin or LMWH is usually continued for 5 to 6 days; warfarin therapy is started on the first or second day, overlapping the heparin therapy (or LMWH) for 4 or 5 days, and is continued until an INR of 2.0 is maintained for at least 24 hours.[48] For patients with major pulmonary embolism or extensive deep vein thrombosis, heparin should be given for at least 7 days. A 4- to 5-day period of overlap is necessary because the antithrombotic effects of oral anticoagulants are delayed. The initial course of heparin should be followed by warfarin for about 3 to 6 months to prevent recurrence.[29] Less intense warfarin therapy (INR = 2.0 to 3.0) is just as effective as the high-intensity regimen (INR = 3.0 to 4.5) but produces significantly less bleeding.[55] Adjusted-dose subcutaneous heparin or intermediate-dose LMWH can also be used in the outpatient setting,[29] but they are more expensive and less convenient than warfarin.

Thrombolytic therapy Thrombolytic therapy produces complete lysis of acute venous thrombi in 30% to 40% of cases and causes partial lysis in an additional 30%.[5,18] In contrast, complete lysis of venous thrombi occurs in fewer than 10% of patients treated with heparin.[5,18] The risk of major bleeding, however, is about three times greater with thrombolytic therapy than with heparin. The risk of hemorrhage increases with the duration of thrombolytic infusion and usually occurs at a site of previous surgery or trauma. Intracranial hemorrhage occurs in 1% to 2% of patients with pulmonary embolism who are treated with thrombolytic agents, which is about five to 10 times higher than that seen in patients with pulmonary embolism who are treated with heparin.[66] Some evidence suggests that the incidence of postthrombotic syndrome is reduced by thrombolytic therapy with streptokinase,[4] but properly designed trials are lacking. The incidence of postthrombotic syndrome appears to be reduced by the early use of graduated compression stockings.[5,7] Accordingly, patients with previous proximal vein thrombosis should be encouraged to wear these stockings at the first sign of leg swelling.

The potential role of thrombolytic therapy in preventing late sequelae of pulmonary embolism is unknown. Selected patients with thromboembolic pulmonary hypertension, estimated to occur in fewer than 1% of patients with pulmonary embolism, benefit from surgical pulmonary endarterectomy.[64]

Indications for Treatment

Anticoagulant therapy Most patients with proximal vein thrombosis, calf vein thrombosis, or symptomatic pulmonary embolism should be treated first with high-dose heparin or LMWH and then with moderate-intensity oral anticoagulant therapy (INR = 2.0 to 3.0) for 3 to 6 months, as previously described.

Long-term anticoagulant therapy should be considered for patients with recurrent unprovoked episodes of venous thromboembolism and for those with continuing risk factors; deficiency of protein C, protein S, or AT; malignancy; or the antiphospholipid antibody syndrome.[29]

Thrombolytic therapy As previously discussed, thrombolytic therapy is indicated in patients who have major pulmonary embolism with hemodynamic compromise. A regimen of 100 mg of rt-PA administered over 2 hours is probably the method of choice because this regimen produces greater lysis at 2 hours than a 24-hour course of conventional urokinase[67] and, compared with heparin, produces more rapid improvement in pulmonary vascular resistance and right ventricular function.[68] For patients with major pulmonary embolism who are at high risk for bleeding, a short course of rt-PA (0.6 mg/kg over 10 minutes), which accelerates lysis of pulmonary embolism, can also be considered.[69]

The use of thrombolytic therapy in patients who have venous thrombosis is even more controversial. Although there is no rigorous supporting evidence for it and it is not part of our clinical practice, regional or systemic thrombolysis may be considered in patients who have large proximal venous thrombi—particularly if the thrombi are confined to the iliac and femoral veins—if there are no contraindications.

Absolute contraindications to thrombolytic therapy include major surgery within the past 10 days, active internal bleeding, a stroke within the past 3 months, and intracranial disease. Relative contraindications include recent organ biopsy, recent puncture of a noncompressible vessel, recent gastrointestinal bleeding, liver or renal disease, severe arterial hypertension, and severe diabetic retinopathy.

Venous Thromboembolism in Pregnancy

The management of venous thromboembolism during pregnancy is complicated because clinical diagnosis is unreliable, some of the objective diagnostic tests are potentially risky to the fetus, and treatment is more difficult than in the nonpregnant patient because of potential teratogenicity or bleeding in the fetus.[70] Clinical diagnosis of venous thrombosis is unreliable in pregnancy because leg swelling can be caused by compression of the left common iliac vein by the gravid uterus. Unless special precautions are taken, venography exposes the fetus to radiation, and impedance plethysmography can yield false positive results in the latter part of the third trimester of pregnancy.

DIAGNOSIS

In pregnant patients suspected of having venous thrombosis, venous ultrasonography should be used as the initial test.[4] If the result is not normal, a diagnosis of proximal deep vein thrombosis is made, and the patient is treated with anticoagulants. If venous ultrasound results are normal, we perform IPG to exclude an isolated iliac vein thrombosis. If both tests are normal, either a limited venogram can be performed, to exclude isolated calf vein thrombosis, or serial compression ultrasonography can be performed on four or five occasions over the next 14 days.[4]

The diagnostic approach to pulmonary embolism in pregnancy is similar to that used in nonpregnant patients. Lung scanning and pulmonary angiography can be performed, but the techniques should be modified to reduce exposure of the fetus to radiation. Although there is little radiation exposure from perfusion scanning and ventilation scanning, it can be reduced further without a serious loss of resolution by administering 50% of the standard dose of radioactive particles for perfusion lung scanning and by limiting ventilation scanning to patients with an abnormal perfusion scan. The radiation exposure from pulmonary angiography can be reduced by using the brachial route and by shielding the abdomen with a lead-lined apron.

TREATMENT

The treatment of venous thromboembolism is much more complicated in pregnant patients than in nonpregnant patients because oral anticoagulants cross the placenta and, if administered during the first trimester, can cause warfarin embryopathy, which is characterized by nasal hypoplasia and skeletal abnormalities.[70] If warfarin is administered during the second and third trimesters, possible congenital defects include dorsal midline dysplasia, abnormalities of the ventricular system, and optic atrophy.

Heparin, which does not cross the placenta, is much safer than oral anticoagulants during pregnancy. Although there have been reports associating heparin therapy during pregnancy with a high incidence of stillbirth or prematurity, most of the fetal complications occurred in mothers receiving heparin for disorders that are known to be associated with a high rate of fetal loss. Other studies have shown that heparin is safe for the fetus but, when used on a long-term basis during pregnancy, can produce osteoporosis in the mother.[55] The incidence of heparin-induced osteopenia diagnosed by dual-photon absorption x-ray or by conventional x-rays may be as high as 15%, but overt fractures are uncommon, occurring in fewer than 5% of patients. Heparin-induced bleeding is not a common problem during pregnancy, provided that heparin therapy is monitored carefully. The anticoagulant response to heparin can be prolonged if it is administered in high doses just before parturition, so there is the potential for local bleeding during and immediately after delivery.

In pregnant patients with acute venous thromboembolism, continuous intravenous heparin or twice-daily LMWH should be administered for 4 to 7 days, followed by subcutaneous heparin or LMWH, given in adjusted therapeutic doses for the remainder of the pregnancy.[71] The injection site should be rotated over the fatty tissue of the lower abdomen and thighs; the site should be compressed for 5 minutes after injection to prevent local bruising. An unwanted anticoagulant effect during delivery can be avoided by discontinuing subcutaneous heparin therapy 24 hours before elective induction of labor.

If there is no evidence of excessive postpartum bleeding, heparin therapy can be resumed about 2 hours after delivery and continued until oral anticoagulation is established. The intensity of heparin therapy will depend on the amount of time that has passed since the diagnosis of venous thromboembolism was made: if the diagnosis was made less than 1 month ago, therapeutic doses may be used; if the diagnosis was made more than 1 month ago, prophylactic or intermediate doses of heparin may be used. Warfarin therapy is started at the same time as heparin and is continued for a minimum of 6 weeks and until patients have received a minimum of 3 months of anticoagulation. Warfarin does not enter breast milk and therefore can be administered to nursing mothers.

Miscellaneous Thromboembolic Disorders

THROMBOSIS IN UNUSUAL SITES

Subclavian or Axillary Veins

Thrombosis of the subclavian or axillary veins may be idiopathic or may occur as a complication of local vascular damage.[72] It is now most frequently seen as a complication of chronic indwelling catheter use, but it also occurs as a complication after mastectomy and local radiotherapy for breast cancer. Idiopathic subclavian or axillary vein thrombosis often occurs in muscular young individuals and may be preceded by repetitive, strenuous activity involving the affected arm. Some of these persons have a fixed stenosis of the subclavian vein that is thought to be caused by external compression of the vein as it courses behind the clavicle. Occasionally, subclavian or axillary vein thrombosis can occur in patients with congenital deficiency of AT, protein C, or protein S or in patients with antiphospholipid antibodies. Thrombosis of the axillary or subclavian vein or the superior vena cava is a rare complication of an implantable perivenous endocardial pacing system.

Subclavian or axillary thrombosis causes pain, edema, and cyanosis of the arm. In rare cases, the thrombosis extends into the superior vena cava and causes edema and cyanosis of the face and neck. Definitive diagnosis is made by venography or venous ultrasonography. Subclavian or axillary vein thrombosis is usually treated with anticoagulants. Regional or systemic thrombolytic therapy may be considered in young patients without contraindications, because a substantial number of these patients experience aching and swelling when they exert the affected arm.

Mesenteric Vein

An uncommon disorder, mesenteric vein thrombosis usually occurs in the sixth or seventh decade of life. It generally affects segments of the small bowel, leading to hemorrhagic infarction. Affected patients often have associated disorders, such as inflammatory bowel disease, malignant disease, portal hypertension, or familial thrombophilia or polycythemia vera, or they may have a history of recent abdominal surgery. In about 20% of cases, no underlying cause is found.

The clinical manifestations of mesenteric vein thrombosis include intermittent abdominal pain, abdominal distention, vomiting, diarrhea, and melena. Diagnosis of mesenteric vein thrombosis is often difficult, but the finding of blood-stained ascitic fluid on abdominal paracentesis or peritoneoscopic evidence of hemorrhagic bowel infarction is characteristic of the disorder. Management includes supportive care and surgical resection, followed by anticoagulant therapy. Mortality is about 20%, and recurrence is likely in up to 20% of patients.

Renal Vein

Renal vein thrombosis can be idiopathic or a complication of the nephrotic syndrome. Patients may be asymptomatic or may present with abdominal, back, or flank pain and tenderness. Pulmonary embolism is a relatively common complication of renal vein thrombosis. Anticoagulant therapy results in a gradual improvement in renal function, but patients may have long-standing proteinuria. Thrombolytic agents have been used, but the data are inadequate for critical appraisal of this form of treatment.

THROMBOPHILIA

The term thrombophilia denotes any increased tendency to thrombosis, whether inherited or acquired. Thrombophilia is usually diagnosed on the basis of the clinical findings, because a patient presents with one or more of the following features[13,9,10]: a family history of thrombosis, thrombosis at a young age, idiopathic thrombosis, or recurrent thrombosis; thrombosis that occurs in an unusual site or despite adequate anticoagulant therapy; a combination of venous thrombosis and arterial thrombosis; and thrombophlebitis migrans.

Many patients with clinical features of thrombophilia do not have a recognizable inherited or acquired disorder.[11] The causes of inherited thrombophilia are APC resistance caused by factor V Leiden, the G20210A prothrombin gene mutation, and abnormalities or deficiencies of AT, protein C, protein S, and, much less commonly, plasminogen and fibrinogen.[13,9,10] There is an association between elevated levels of coagulation factors XI and VIII and venous thrombosis.[16,17] It is probable that there is a hereditary component to these elevations in some patients. Current evidence does not support the view that inherited deficiencies of fibrinolysis cause venous thrombosis or recurrent venous thrombosis, nor is there evidence that deficiencies or elevations of coagulation factors, including factor XII, factor V, and factor VII, predispose to venous thrombosis.

The main causes of acquired thrombophilia are antiphospholipid antibody syndrome, collagen vascular disorders, hyperhomocysteinemia, malignancy, and cancer chemotherapy.[2] Less common causes are paroxysmal nocturnal hemoglobinuria, myeloproliferative disorders, nephrotic syndrome, and Buerger disease (thromboangiitis obliterans).

Inherited Thrombophilia

The reported prevalence of inherited thrombophilias is highest in patients referred to specialized laboratories for screening studies and lowest in unselected populations of patients with thrombosis. In a study of unselected outpatients referred with symptoms of venous thrombosis whose diagnosis was confirmed by venography, 23 of 277

(8.3%) had inherited deficiencies of AT, protein C, protein S, or plasminogen.[11] The prevalence of the deficiencies was 22% (6 of 27) in patients younger than 41 years who had a family history of thrombosis and 30% (3 of 10) in young patients with a family history of thrombosis who had had a previous episode of venous thromboembolism. The relative odds of having a deficiency were 3.2 when patients who had thrombosis and a family history of thrombosis were compared with patients who had thrombosis but no family history of the condition. The study was performed before the discovery of APC resistance and the G20210A prothrombin gene mutation. Since their discovery, about 50% of young patients with idiopathic venous thrombosis (including idiopathic thrombosis in pregnancy) have been found to have an inherited thrombophilic defect.

Antithrombin, protein S, protein C deficiency, factor V Leiden, and the G20210A prothombin gene mutation are autosomal dominant traits. Venous thrombosis and pulmonary embolism are the most common manifestations of the inherited thrombophilias. Approximately 50% of episodes occur without a clinically obvious provocation.[13] Superficial thrombophlebitis also occurs, particularly in protein C or protein S deficiencies. Arterial thrombosis has been described in all three deficiencies,[73] but it is uncertain whether the association is causal or coincidental. Cerebral arterial thrombosis has been described in case series of factor V Leiden, the G20210A prothrombin gene mutation, and protein S deficiency. Venous thrombosis during pregnancy appears to be particularly common in AT deficiency, but postpartum venous thrombosis is common in all three deficiencies.[13] Patients with AT deficiency may show heparin resistance, those with protein C or protein S deficiency are prone to warfarin-induced skin necrosis, and those with homozygous recessive protein C and protein S deficiency are prone to neonatal purpura fulminans.

The incidence of a first spontaneous thrombosis in AT, protein C, and protein S deficiencies has been estimated to be about 3% a year.[13] The risk of thrombosis in asymptomatic carriers is very low in the first 2 decades of life. Deep vein thrombosis or pulmonary embolism develops in about 50% to 70% of carriers during their lifetime. Because more than 50% of the thromboembolic episodes in deficient individuals occur during or after a reversible provocation such as surgery, these episodes may be prevented by appropriate prophylaxis.

The combined prevalence of factor V Leiden and the G20210A prothrombin gene mutation in the normal population is about 10-fold higher than the combined prevalence of AT, protein C, and protein S deficiencies. However, the risk of thrombosis with factor V Leiden or the G20210A prothrombin gene mutation is about fivefold lower than for that with the other three deficiencies.[9,10,13] The risk of thrombosis with inherited thrombophilia is increased by the use of estrogen-containing oral contraceptives.[9,10,13]

Because 90% to 95% of episodes of venous thrombo-embolism are not fatal, antithrombotic therapy is not warranted in most asymptomatic carriers of the inherited thrombophilias. Prophylaxis with either adjusted-dose heparin or oral anticoagulants should be used after surgery or during a major medical illness in asymptomatic carriers.

Long-term anticoagulant treatment should be considered for patients with inherited or acquired thrombophilic disorders who have one or more unprovoked episodes of venous thromboembolism.[13] Because AT is a cofactor for heparin, patients with AT deficiency may have heparin resistance, which can usually be overcome by increasing the heparin dose. Infusions of AT concentrate usually are not necessary. Patients with protein C deficiency are theoretically at risk for hypercoagulability during initial warfarin therapy because protein C has a much shorter half-life than three of the four vitamin K–dependent procoagulants. The thrombogenic risk can be reduced by avoiding a loading dose of warfarin and ensuring that heparin therapy begins before warfarin treatment.

Women with inherited thrombophilia should avoid estrogen-containing oral contraceptives and hormone replacement therapy. Pregnancy is a risk factor for thrombosis in inherited thrombophilic patients and in patients with antiphospholipid antibodies.

We recommend prophylactic doses of heparin or LMWH throughout pregnancy in patients with AT deficiency, regardless of whether they have had a previous episode of thrombosis.[13] Women with deficiencies of protein C or S need prophylactic therapy only if they have had a previous episode of thrombosis. It is generally reasonable to withhold prophylaxis in women with factor V Leiden or the G20210A prothrombin gene mutation. Prophylaxis (e.g., warfarin) should be used for about 6 weeks after delivery.[13]

Acquired Thrombophilia

Malignancy An association between cancer and thrombosis has been recognized for over a century. Patients with cancer (especially pancreatic, ovarian, lung, and gastrointestinal carcinoma) may experience unusual forms of thrombosis, including migratory superficial thrombo-phlebitis, nonbacterial thrombotic endocarditis, and thrombosis in unusual sites, such as renal veins, the inferior vena cava, and the portal and hepatic veins. Venous thrombosis may progress in cancer patients despite apparently adequate oral anticoagulant therapy or, less often, heparin therapy. Migratory thrombophlebitis, characterized by recurrent thrombosis in superficial and deep veins, is a feature of mucin-secreting tumors. The symptoms may be resistant to treatment with oral anticoagulants but generally respond to heparin. Hepatic vein thrombosis may be associated with myeloproliferative disorders, with hepatoma, and with renal cell and adrenal carcinomas.

Evidence suggests that patients who have idiopathic venous thrombosis are at risk for an associated occult malignancy, which is usually expressed clinically during the following 12 months.[26,74] In one study,[26] approximately 70% of such malignancies were in the gastrointestinal tract, the male or female urogenital tract, and the lung.

It is uncertain whether intensive investigation will detect occult malignancy in patients with idiopathic venous thrombosis and, if it does, whether early identification and treatment of occult malignancies improves prognosis. Expensive or invasive investigations for malignant disease probably are not indicated in patients with the first episode of deep vein thrombosis.[74] Initial investigations should include a complete blood count, hepatic biochemistry, a chest radiograph, and testing for fecal occult blood. If malignancy is strongly suspected on clinical grounds because of associated laboratory abnormalities or because of recurrent idiopathic venous thrombosis or thrombosis refractory to warfarin therapy, further investigations can be performed.

The risk of thrombosis is also increased by cancer chemotherapy. In a study of patients with stage II breast cancer who were treated with chemotherapy, the incidence of thrombosis was 6.8% during the first 3 months of chemotherapy and 4.9% during the next 6 months (in patients randomized to an additional 6 months of chemotherapy); during the 6-month period, the incidence was 0% among those who did not receive additional chemotherapy.[75]

Antiphospholipid antibody syndrome The antiphospholipid antibody syndrome (APLS) is a disorder in persons with antiphospholipid antibodies plus one or more of the following clinical manifestations: venous and arterial thrombosis, fetal wastage, and thrombocytopenia.[76] The antibodies are of the IgG or IgM class and are directed at various phospholipid moieties, including cardiolipin. Some of the antibodies have anticoagulant properties because they bind epitopes on the phospholipid portion of prothrombinase and, as a result, prolong coagulation assays such as the aPTT and kaolin clotting time. These anticoagulants were initially described in patients with systemic lupus erythematosus (SLE) and were termed lupus anticoagulants. Paradoxically, these circulating anticoagulants do not produce abnormal bleeding but are associated with thrombosis. It subsequently became clear that antiphospholipid antibodies occur in persons with disorders other than SLE, including other autoimmune disorders and drug-induced lupus, as well as in otherwise healthy persons.

Antiphospholipid antibodies with or without anticoagulant properties occur in patients with idiopathic venous and arterial thrombosis and are an important marker for acquired thrombophilia. Cross-sectional studies suggest about a twofold increase in the risk of venous thrombosis with an anticardiolipin antibody and a fivefold to 10-fold increase with a lupus anticoagulant in patients with or without SLE.[77,78] The mechanism by which thrombosis occurred in the patients with antiphospholipid antibodies is uncertain. The titer of antibody and the pattern of test positivity can change over time within an individual, and the test may be only transiently positive. No single test has been demonstrated to be the best predictor of thrombosis, and it is not clear whether the level of the antibody titer influences the risk of thrombosis.

The most common thrombotic manifestation of APLS is idiopathic venous thrombosis involving the deep veins of the legs. Other associations with APLS are thrombosis in childhood, a combination of arterial and venous thrombosis, and thrombosis in an unusual site (including the inferior vena cava or hepatic, portal, splenic, axillary, mesenteric, or renal vein). APLS is also associated with arterial thrombotic disease, especially stroke.[76] Antiphospholipid antibodies are associated with an increased risk of infertility, preeclampsia, fetal growth retardation, and fetal wastage[70] in women with APLS. Evidence suggests that low-dose heparin and aspirin are effective at preventing fetal loss, possibly by limiting the extent of placental infarction.[70]

The management of APLS in nonpregnant women is uncertain, but the following guidelines seem reasonable in the light of current evidence. If an antibody is found in the absence of symptoms or a history of thrombosis, long-term anticoagulant treatment is not indicated. Aggressive prophylaxis should be used in high-risk situations, including long airplane flights, confinement to bed because of medical illness, surgery, and after trauma. Patients with antiphospholipid antibodies and unprovoked venous thromboembolism should be treated with long-term warfarin unless they have a high risk of bleeding.

THROMBOANGIITIS OBLITERANS

A rare form of vasculitis called thromboangiitis obliterans (Buerger disease) involves both arteries and veins, especially those of the lower extremities.[79] The incidence of this disorder, which usually occurs in young men who are heavy smokers, is much higher in Israel, Eastern Europe, and the Far East than in the United States. An immune mechanism appears to be responsible for some of the pathologic features. Occasionally, there is migratory thrombophlebitis, associated with tender areas of erythema. Arterial insufficiency often causes claudication of the foot, Raynaud phenomenon, and tropic changes. Cerebral, coronary, and visceral vessels can be affected. Patients should be told to stop smoking; if they do so, the progress of the disease process will be slowed or arrested.

References

1. Anderson FA, Wheeler B, Goldberg RJ, et al: A population-based perspective of the hospital incidence and case-fatality rates of deep vein thrombosis and pulmonary embolism. Arch Intern Med 151:933, 1991

2. Kearon C, Salzman EW, Hirsh J: Epidemiology, pathogenesis, and natural history of venous thrombosis. Hemostasis and Thrombosis: Basic Principles and Clinical Practice, 4th ed. Colman RW, Hirsh J, Marder VJ, et al, Eds. JB Lippincott Co, Philadelphia, p 1153

3. Anderson FA Jr, Wheeler HB, Goldberg RJ, et al: The prevalence of risk factors for venous thromboembolism among hospital patients. Arch Intern Med 152:1660, 1992

4. Kearon C, Julian JA, Math M, et al: Noninvasive diagnosis of deep venous thrombosis. Ann Intern Med 128:663, 1998

5. Ginsberg JS: Management of venous thromboembolism. N Engl J Med 335: 1816, 1996

6. Prandoni P, Lensing AWA, Cogo A, et al: The long-term clinical course of acute deep venous thrombosis. Ann Intern Med 125:1, 1996

7. Brandjes DPM, Buller HR, Heijboer H, et al: Randomised trial of effect of compression stockings in patients with symptomatic proximal-vein thrombosis. Lancet 349:759, 1997

8. Prins MH, Hirsh J: A critical review of the evidence supporting a relationship between impaired fibrinolytic activity and venous thromboembolism. Arch Intern Med 151:1721, 1991

9. Lane DA, Mannucci PM, Bauer KA, et al: Inherited thrombophilia (pt 1). Thromb Haemost 76:651, 1996

10. Lane DA, Mannucci PM, Bauer KA, et al: Inherited thrombophilia (pt 2). Thromb Haemost 76:824, 1996

11. Heijboer H, Brandjes DPM, Buller HR, et al: Deficiencies of coagulation-inhibiting and fibrinolytic proteins in outpatients with deep-vein thrombosis. N Engl J Med 323:1512, 1990

12. van den Belt AGM, Prins MH, Huisman MV, et al: Familial thrombophilia: a review analysis. Clin Appl Thromb Hemost 2:227, 1996

13. Kearon C, Crowther M, Hirsh J, et al: Management of patients with hereditary hypercoagulable disorders. Annu Rev Med 51:169, 2000

14. Kearon C, Gent M, Hirsh J, et al: A comparison of three months of anticoagulation with extended anticoagulation for a first episode of idiopathic venous thromboembolism. N Engl J Med 340:901, 1999

15. Poort SR, Rosendaal FR, Reitsma PH, et al: A common genetic variation in the 3' untranslated region of the prothrombin gene is associated with elevated plasma prothrombin levels and an increase in venous thrombosis. Blood 88:3698, 1996

16. Rosendaal FR: High levels of factor VIII and venous thrombosis. Thromb Haemost 83:1, 2000

17. Meijers JCM, Tekelenburg WLH, Bouma BN, et al: High levels of coagulation factor XI as a risk factor for venous thrombosis. N Engl J Med. 342:696, 2000

18. Cattaneo M: Hyperhomocysteinemia, atherosclerosis and thrombosis. Thromb Haemost 81:165, 1999

19. Vandenbrouke JP, Koster E, Briet E, et al: Increased risk of venous thrombosis in oral contraceptive users who are carriers of factor V Leiden mutation. Lancet 344:1453, 1994

20. Grady D, Wenger NK, Herrington D, et al: Postmenopausal hormone therapy increases risk for venous thromboembolic disease. Ann Intern Med 132:689, 2000

21. Hirsh J, Lensing A: Thrombolytic therapy for deep vein thrombosis. Int J Angiol 5:S22, 1996

22. Hull R, Delmore T, Genton E, et al: Warfarin sodium versus low-dose heparin in the long-term treatment of venous thrombosis. N Engl J Med 301:855, 1979

23. Hirsh J: The optimal duration of anticoagulant therapy for venous thrombosis. N Engl J Med 332:1710, 1995

24. Dolovich LR, Ginsberg JS, Douketis JD, et al: A meta-analysis comparing low-molecular-weight heparins with unfractionated heparin in the treatment of venous thromboembolism. Arch Intern Med 160:181, 2000

25. Optimum duration of anticoagulation for deep-vein thrombosis and pulmonary embolism. Research Committee of the British Thoracic Society. Lancet 340:873, 1992

26. Prandoni P, Lensing AWA, Büller HR, et al: Deep-vein thrombosis and the incidence of subsequent symptomatic cancer. N Engl J Med 327:1128, 1992

27. Schulman S, Rhedin A-S, Lindmarker P, et al: A comparison of six weeks with six months of oral anticoagulant therapy after a first episode of venous thromboembolism. Duration of Anticoagulation Trial Study Group. N Engl J Med 332:1661, 1995

28. Levine MN, Hirsh J, Gent M, et al: Optimal duration of oral anticoagulant therapy: a randomized trial comparing four weeks with three months of wafarin in patients with proximal deep vein thrombosis. Thromb Haemost 74:606, 1995

29. Couturaud F, Kearon C: Long-term treatment for venous thromboembolism. Curr Opin Hematol 7:302, 2000

30. Kyrle P, Minar E, Hirschl M, et al: High plasma levels of factor VIII and the risk of recurrent venous thromboembolism. N Engl J Med 343:62, 2000

31. Anand SS, Wells PS, Hunt D, et al: Does this patient have deep vein thrombosis? JAMA 279:1094, 1998

32. Wells PS, Hirsh J, Anderson DR, et al: A simple clinical model for the diagnosis of deep-vein thrombosis combined with impedance plethysmography: potential for an improvement in the diagnostic process. J Intern Med 243:15, 1998

33. Wells PS, Hirsh J, Anderson DR, et al: Accuracy of clinical assessment of deep vein thrombosis. Lancet 345:1326, 1995

34. Heijboer H, Buller HR, Lensing AWA, et al: A comparison of real-time-compression ultrasonography with impedance plethysmography for the diagnosis of deep-vein thrombosis in symptomatic outpatients. N Engl J Med 329:1365, 1993

35. Lee AY, Ginsberg JS: Laboratory diagnosis of venous thromboembolism. Baillieres Clin Haematol 11:2461, 1998

36. Perrier A, Desmarais S, Miron MJ, et al Non-invasive diagnosis of venous thromboembolism in outpatients. Lancet 353:190, 1999

37. Ginsberg JS, Kearon C, Douketis J, et al: The use of D-dimer testing and impedance plethysmographic examination in patients with clinical indications of deep vein thrombosis. Arch Intern Med 157:1077, 1997

38. Bernardi E, Prandoni P, Lensing AWA, et al: D-dimer testing as an adjunct to ultrasonography in patients with clinically suspected deep vein thrombosis: prospective cohort study. BMJ 317:1037, 1998

39. Kearon C, Hirsh J: The diagnosis of pulmonary embolism. Haemostasis 25:72, 1995

40. Wells PS, Anderson DR, Rodger M, et al: Derivation of a simple clinical model to categorize patients probably of pulmonary embolism: inreasing the models utility with the SimpliRED D-dimer. Thromb Haemost 83:416, 2000

41. Simonneau G, Sors H, Charbonnier B, et al: A comparison of low-molecular-weight heparin with unfractionated heparin for acute pulmonary embolism. N Engl J Med 337:663, 1997

42. Rathbun SW, Raskob GE, Whitsett TL: Sensitivity and specificity of helical computed tomography in the diagnosis of pulmonary embolism: a systematic review. Ann Intern Med 132:227, 2000

43. Ginsberg JS, Wells PS, Kearon C, et al: Sensitivity and specificity of a rapid whole-blood assay for D-dimer in the diagnosis of pulmonary embolism. Ann Intern Med 129:997, 1998

44. Wells PS, Ginsberg JS, Anderson DR, et al: Use of a clinical model for safe management of patients with suspected pulmonary embolism. Ann Intern Med 129:997, 1998

45. Hull RD, Raskob GE, Ginsberg JS, et al: A noninvasive strategy for the treatment of patients with suspected pulmonary embolism. Arch Intern Med 154:289, 1994

46. Miniati M, Prediletto R, Formichi B, et al: Accuracy of clinical assessment in the diagnosis of pulmonary embolism. Am J Respir Crit Care Med 159:864, 1999

47. Wells PS, Anderson DR, Ginsberg J: Assessment of deep vein thrombosis or pulmonary embolism by the combined use of clinical model and noninvasive diagnostic tests. Semin Thromb Hemost 26:643, 2000

48. Hirsh J: Heparin. N Engl J Med 324:1565, 1991

49. Weitz JI: Low-molecular-weight heparins. N Engl J Med 337:688, 1997

50. Warkentin TE, Levine MN, Hirsh J, et al: Heparin-induced thrombocytopenia in patients treated with low-molecular-weight heparin or unfractionated heparin. N Engl J Med 332:330, 1995

51. Muir JM, Hirsh J, Weitz JI, et al: A histomorphometric comparison of the effects of heparin and low-molecular-weight heparin on cancellous bone in rats. Blood 89:3236, 1997

52. Levine M, Gent M, Hirsh J, et al: A comparison of low-molecular-weight heparin administered primarily at home with unfractionated heparin administered in the hospital for proximal deep-vein thrombosis. N Engl J Med 334:677, 1996

53. Koopman MMW, Prandoni P, Piovella F, et al: Treatment of venous thrombosis with intravenous unfractionated heparin administered in the hospital as compared with subcutaneous low-molecular-weight heparin administered at home. N Engl J Med 334:682, 1996

54. Low-molecular-weight heparin in the treatment of patients with venous thromboembolism. The Columbus Investigators. N Engl J Med 337:657, 1997

55. Hirsh J: Oral anticoagulant drugs. N Engl J Med 324:1865, 1991

56. Harrison L, Johnston M, Massicotte MP, et al: Comparison of 5-mg and 10-mg loading doses in initiation of warfarin therapy. Ann Intern Med 126:133, 1997

57. Weitz JI, Stewart RJ, Fredenburgh JC: Mechanism of action of plasminogen activators. Thromb Haemost 82:974, 1999

58. Levine M, Raskob G, Landerfeld S, et al: Hemorrhagic complications of antithrombotic therapy. Chest 119(suppl) :1085, 2001

59. Geerts WH, Heit JA, Clagett P, et al: Prevention of venous thromboembolism. Chest 119(suppl):1325, 2001

60. Prevention of pulmonary embolism and deep vein thrombosis with low dose aspirin. Pulmonary Embolism Prevention (PEP) Trial Collaborative Group. Lancet 355:1295, 2000

61. Colwell CW, Collis DK, Paulson R, et al: Comparison of enoxaparin and warfarin for the prevention of venous thromboembolic disease after total hip arthroplasty. J Bone Joint Surg Am 81:932, 1999

62. Decousus H, Leizorovicz A, Parent F, et al: A clinical trial of vena caval filters in the prevention of pulmonary embolism in patients with proximal deep-vein thrombosis. N Engl J Med 338:409, 1998

63. Jerjes-Sanchez C, Ramírez-Rivera A, de Lourdes García M, et al: Streptokinase and heparin versus heparin alone in massive pulmonary embolism: a randomized controlled trial. J Thromb Thrombolysis 2:227, 1995

64. Moser KM, Daily PO, Peterson K, et al: Thromboendarterectomy for chronic, major-vessel thromboembolic pulmonary hypertension: immediate and long-term results in 42 patients. Ann Intern Med 107:560, 1987

65. Brill-Edwards P, Ginsberg JS, Johnston M, et al: Establishing a therapeutic range for heparin therapy. Ann Intern Med 119:104, 1993

66. Dalen JE, Alpert JS, Hirsh J: Thrombolytic therapy for pulmonary embolism. Is it effective? Is it safe? When is it indicated? Arch Intern Med 157:2550, 1997

67. Goldhaber SZ, Kessler CM, Heit J, et al: Randomised controlled trial of recombinant tissue plasminogen activator versus urokinase in the treatment of acute pulmonary embolism. Lancet 2:293, 1988

68. Goldhaber SZ, Haire WD, Feldstein ML, et al: Alteplase versus heparin in acute pulmonary embolism: randomised trial assessing right-ventricular function and pulmonary perfusion. Lancet 341:507, 1993

69. Levine MN, Hirsh J, Weitz JI, et al: A randomized trial of a single bolus dosage regimen of recombinant tissue plasminogen activator in patients with acute pulmonary embolism. Chest 98:1473, 1990

70. Ginsberg JS, Greer I, Hirsh J: Use of antithrombotic agents during pregnancy (review). Chest 119(suppl):122S, 2001

71. Sanson BJ, Lensing AWA, Prins MH, et al: Safety of low-molecular-weight heparin in pregnancy: a systematic review. Thromb Haemost 81:668, 1999

72. Pradoni P, Polistena P, Bernardi E, et al: Upper-extremity deep vein thrombosis: risk factors, diagnosis, and complications. Arch Intern Med 157:57, 1997

73. Coller BS, Owen J, Jesty J, et al: Deficiency of plasma protein S, protein C, or antithrombin III and arterial thrombosis. Arteriosclerosis 7:456, 1987

74. Prins MH, Hettiarachchi RJK, Lensing AWA, et al: Newly diagnosed malignancy in patients with venous thromboembolism. Search or wait and see? Thromb Haemost 78:121, 1997

75. Levine MN, Gent M, Hirsh J, et al: The thrombogenic effect of anticancer drug therapy in women with stage II breast cancer. N Engl J Med 318:404, 1988

76. Greaves M: Antiphospholipid antibodies and thrombosis. Lancet 353:1348, 1999

77. Wahl DG, Guillemin F, de Maistre E, et al: Risk for venous thrombosis related to antiphospholipid antibodies in systemic lupus erythematosus—a meta-analysis. Lupus 6:467, 1997

78. Wahl DG, Guillemin F, de Maistre E, et al: Meta-analysis of the risk of venous thrombosis in individuals with antiphospholipid antibodies without underlying autoimmune disease or previous thrombosis. Lupus 7:15, 1998

79. Olin JW: Thromboangiitis obliterans (Buerger's disease). N Engl J Med 343:864, 2000

DERMATOLOGY

30 Cutaneous Manifestations of Systemic Diseases

Mark Lebwohl, M.D.

The cutaneous manifestations of systemic diseases are so numerous and varied that a single chapter could not cover them all, even in a cursory way. Instead, this chapter reviews key cutaneous manifestations of systemic diseases that should be recognized by most physicians and highlights recent developments in the diagnosis and management of those disorders. For fuller discussions of specific diseases, including their cutaneous manifestations, readers are referred to the chapters devoted to those conditions.

In many of the disorders presented in this chapter, workup and therapy of the underlying systemic condition are essential to a favorable outcome. A finding of cutaneous sarcoidosis, for example, should prompt a search for systemic sarcoidosis. In other conditions—for example, recessive dystrophic epidermolysis bullosa—treatment of the skin disorder is key to the management of the systemic disease.

Cardiopulmonary and Vascular Diseases

SARCOIDOSIS

The cutaneous manifestations of sarcoidosis are as varied as its systemic manifestations [*see Chapter 215*]. Papules around the eyes or nose are most characteristic. The term lupus pernio refers to noncaseating granulomas that result in translucent, violaceous plaques of the ears, cheeks, and nose [*see Figure 1*]. Involvement of underlying bone can occur, and diagnosis is made by skin biopsy. Treatment with intralesional corticosteroids is traditional, and oral antimalarials and methotrexate have been used with success. In some patients with sarcoidosis, erythema nodosum, characterized by deep, tender erythematous nodules, occurs on the lower extremities. Lupus pernio is associated with a more chronic course, whereas erythema nodosum indicates a more acute and benign disease.[1]

GRANULOMATOUS VASCULITIS

Wegener Granulomatosis

Wegener granulomatosis is associated with both distinctive and nonspecific mucocutaneous signs. Palpable purpura is one of the most common skin findings, but ulcers, papules, nodules, and bullae have also been described. In addition to upper and lower pulmonary symptoms [*see Chapter 214*], saddle-nose deformity, nasal ulcerations, and septal perforation should suggest the diagnosis of Wegener granulomatosis. Definitive diagnosis is made by demonstrating a necrotizing granulomatous vasculitis in a patient with upper and lower respiratory tract disease and glomerulonephritis. Anticytoplasmic autoantibodies are often present.

Lymphomatoid Granulomatosis

Lymphomatoid granulomatosis can be associated with nonspecific skin lesions, including erythematous macules, papules, plaques, nodules, and ulcers. This disorder is clinically distinguishable from Wegener granulomatosis by the absence of upper respiratory tract involvement. Diagnosis is established by demonstrating a granulomatous necrotizing infiltrate with atyp-

ical lymphoid cells around blood vessels. This disorder has been attributed to a clonal proliferation of B cells that induces a T cell response.[2]

Churg-Strauss Syndrome

Churg-Strauss syndrome, or allergic granulomatous angiitis, most commonly presents as asthma and eosinophilia; however, related skin lesions develop in up to 40% of patients. Symmetrical, palpable purpura and petechiae of the lower extremities are the most common findings and show a leukocytoclastic vasculitis on skin biopsy. Cutaneous nodules caused by extravascular necrotizing granulomas and papules of the elbows also occur.[3]

HYPERLIPOPROTEINEMIA

Xanthomas are cutaneous manifestations of hyperlipoproteinemias. Several types of xanthomas occur with different lipid abnormalities. Xanthelasma of the eyelids is the most common manifestation of familial hypercholesterolemia [*see Figure 2*]; however, at least half the people who have eyelid lesions have normal plasma lipids. Planar xanthomas are flat yellow plaques that can in-

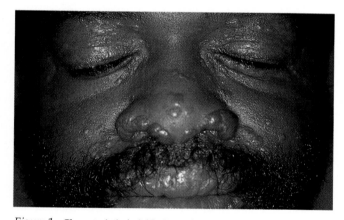

Figure 1 **Characteristic facial lesions of sarcoidosis, called lupus pernio, are shown.**

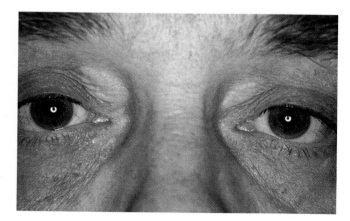

Figure 2 **Xanthelasma, a xanthoma of the eyelid, is the most common manifestation of familial hypercholesterolemia.**

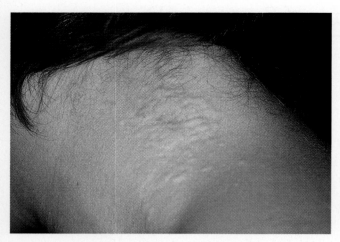

Figure 3   Xanthomalike papules are characteristic of pseudoxanthoma elasticum. The neck and axillae are the most common sites of involvement.

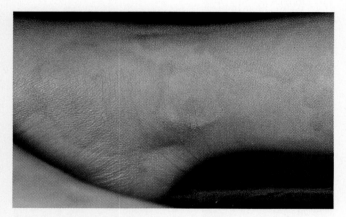

Figure 4   Transient annular erythematous rashes (erythema marginatum) typically occur in patients with rheumatic fever.

volve the palms, soles, neck, and chest. They can occur in patients with primary biliary cirrhosis or multiple myeloma. Tuberous xanthomas are large yellow or red nodules that appear on the extensor surfaces of joints, such as on the elbows and hands, but are not attached to underlying tendons. They can occur in patients with elevated triglyceride or cholesterol levels. In contrast, tendinous xanthomas, which can appear in patients with familial hypercholesterolemia, are fixed to underlying tendons of the elbows, ankles, knees, and hands. Eruptive xanthomas occur when plasma triglyceride levels suddenly become elevated. Skin lesions consist of small yellow papules that often resolve with lowering of triglyceride levels.

KAWASAKI DISEASE

Kawasaki disease, also called mucocutaneous lymph node syndrome [*see Chapter 117*], is a disorder in children that can be complicated by coronary artery occlusion and myocardial infarction, coronary artery aneurysms, electrocardiographic abnormalities, cardiac arrhythmias, or myocarditis. It has been suggested that a toxin secreted by *Staphylococcus aureus* is responsible for this disease.[4] Diagnosis is based on clinical criteria that include fever, conjunctivitis, lymphadenopathy, and rash. In addition to generalized erythematous eruption, abnormalities of the oral mucosa as well as swelling and erythema of the hands and feet may

develop. Striking desquamation of the palms and soles ultimately occurs. Perianal and scrotal erythema and scaling are common as well. Thrombocytosis is a late finding, with platelet counts increasing to more than one million over 2 weeks after the onset of the disease.

PSEUDOXANTHOMA ELASTICUM

Pseudoxanthoma elasticum (PXE) is an inherited disorder of elastic tissue that is associated with a wide array of systemic manifestations. Angioid streaks, the ocular hallmark of PXE, are breaks in the Bruch membrane. Retinal bleeding and vision loss commonly occur. Calcification of the internal elastic laminae of arteries can result in bleeding or occlusion of those vessels. As a result, patients develop intermittent claudication on walking and occlusive coronary artery disease at an early age. Cardiac valvular abnormalities have also been described.[5] Skin lesions consist of yellow xanthomalike macules, papules, or redundant folds of skin in flexural areas, particularly the neck and axillae [*see Figure 3*]. Some patients may have systemic manifestations of PXE without clinically apparent skin lesions.[6] Diagnosis is established by biopsy of scar or normal-appearing flexural skin.[7] The genetic defect responsible for PXE has been mapped to chromosome 16.[8]

RHEUMATIC FEVER

The two cutaneous manifestations of rheumatic fever are erythema marginatum and subcutaneous nodules. Erythema marginatum is a transient faint annular erythematous rash that often develops over joints [*see Figure 4*]. The subcutaneous nodules that appear with rheumatic fever are nontender, freely movable, and approximately 1 cm in diameter and occur on the extensor surfaces of elbows, hands, or feet.

YELLOW NAIL SYNDROME

Yellow nail syndrome is caused by an abnormality of lymphatics [*see Figure 5*]. Affected patients develop lymphedema, usually of the legs, and pleural effusions. Pulmonary symptoms such as recurrent bronchitis are also common. Diagnosis is made by finding evidence of abnormal lymphatic function associated with yellow nails without other causes of nail pathology.[9]

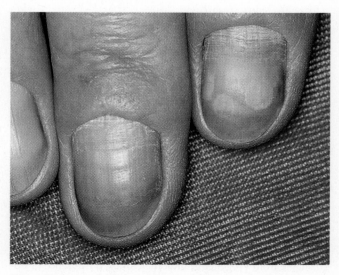

Figure 5   Yellow nails are a sign of underlying disease of the lymphatics in patients with yellow nail syndrome.

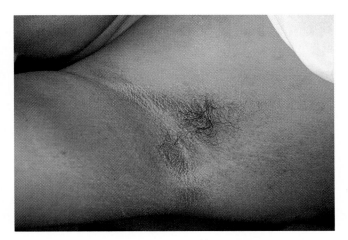

Figure 6 **Acanthosis nigricans, a dark velvety acanthosis that can occur in patients with diabetes mellitus and other endocrine disorders, often appears in axillae.**

Endocrinologic Diseases

DIABETES MELLITUS

There are numerous cutaneous manifestations of diabetes mellitus [*see Chapter 48*]. Acanthosis nigricans can occur in patients with diabetes and other endocrinopathies, such as Cushing syndrome, acromegaly, polycystic ovary syndrome, and thyroid disease. Skin lesions consist of brown velvety patches in intertriginous areas, especially the neck and axillae [*see Figure 6*]. Acanthosis nigricans has also been associated with internal malignancies, particularly gastric adenocarcinoma or other gastrointestinal adenocarcinomas.

Necrobiosis lipoidica is a specific cutaneous manifestation of diabetes. Lesions consist of chronic atrophic patches with enlarging erythematous borders. The legs are most commonly affected. The center of lesions appears yellow because of subcutaneous fat that is visible through the atrophic dermis and epidermis. Occasionally, the lesions ulcerate. Necrobiosis lipoidica is often associated with diabetic nephropathy or retinopathy.[10]

Scleredema, another manifestation of diabetes, consists of induration of the skin of the back and posterior neck in obese patients with type 2 (non–insulin-dependent) diabetes. Scleredema may improve if diabetes is controlled.[11] Less commonly, scleredema occurs in nondiabetic patients after streptococcal pharyngitis; in such patients, the disease is self-limited, resolving within 2 years of onset.

Diabetic bullae, neuropathic ulcers, and so-called waxy skin and stiff joints occur in patients with diabetes. In the last condition mentioned, scleroderma-like induration of the skin over the dorsal aspect of the hands prevents full flexion or extension of the proximal interphalangeal joints.

Diabetic patients are prone to a number of infections, including erythrasma, a corynebacterial infection resulting in asymptomatic reddish-brown patches in intertriginous sites, especially the groin and axillae. Patients are also prone to staphylococcal infections and frequently develop furuncles and carbuncles. Candidal infections are another risk, particularly when blood glucose levels are poorly controlled.

GRAVES DISEASE

Graves disease consists of a triad of exophthalmos, hyperthyroidism, and pretibial myxedema [*see Chapter 46*]. Pretibial myxedema presents as skin-colored nodules and plaques that extend from the pretibial area down to the dorsa of the feet. Onycholysis, the separation of the nail plate from the nail bed, occurs in many patients with hyperthyroidism. Other autoimmune skin diseases, such as vitiligo and alopecia areata, are increased in patients with Graves disease. Lesions often develop after treatment of hyperthyroidism, although they can occur at any stage in the evolution of Graves disease. Other manifestations of thyroid disease include the stigmata of hypothyroidism. Patients can develop alopecia and specifically lose the lateral third of the eyebrows. Edematous thickening of the lips, tongue, and nose occur as well.

Gastrointestinal Diseases

Patients with any of a number of gastrointestinal diseases may present with cutaneous manifestations; similarly, patients with certain cutaneous diseases can develop gastrointestinal complications.

CARCINOID SYNDROME

The carcinoid syndrome is characterized by episodic flushing that can be associated with abdominal pain, diarrhea, and wheezing. Ninety percent of carcinoid tumors originate in the gastroin-

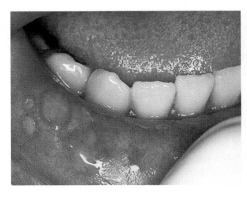

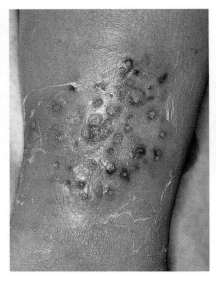

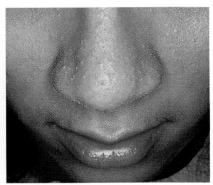

Figure 7 **Aphthous stomatitis is a common finding in patients with ulcerative colitis.**

Figure 8 (center) **Pyoderma gangrenosum is characterized by ulcers that begin with craterlike holes draining pus.**

Figure 9 **The patient's nose and cheeks are covered with small papules called trichilemmomas, which are the cutaneous hallmark of Cowden disease.**

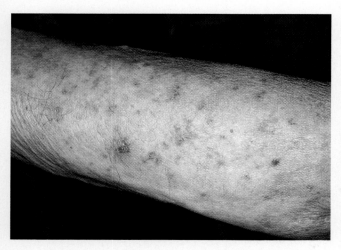

Figure 10   **The primary lesions of dermatitis herpetiformis are vesicles, but these are quickly broken to form crusts and excoriations.**

testinal tract; however, bronchial carcinoids occur occasionally. Less common cutaneous manifestations of carcinoid tumors include sclerodermatous changes, cutaneous metastases presenting as deep nodules, and hyperkeratosis and pigmentation similar to that seen in pellagra.

INFLAMMATORY BOWEL DISEASE

There are several specific and nonspecific cutaneous manifestations of inflammatory bowel disease [*see Chapter 58*]. In both Crohn disease and ulcerative colitis, patients can progress to a hypercoagulable stage, causing venous and arterial thromboses that can lead to loss of digits and limbs. Aphthous stomatitis is another nonspecific manifestation of inflammatory bowel disease [*see Figure 7*]. In patients with Crohn disease, the lesions may appear as noncaseating granulomas, whereas in patients with ulcerative colitis, they may be indistinguishable from canker sores.

Pyoderma gangrenosum occurs in patients with Crohn disease and ulcerative colitis and has also been reported in patients with chronic active hepatitis, rheumatoid arthritis, and a number of myeloproliferative disorders. The lesions are distinguishable from other ulcers by the presence of craterlike holes, pustules, and purulent drainage [*see Figure 8*]. The lesions may occur at sites of trauma. Treatment with intralesionally injected or systemic corticosteroids may be required. Immunosuppressive agents such as cyclosporine have proved to be dramatically effective; in refractory cases, thalidomide has been shown to be beneficial.[12]

Erythema nodosum is a septal panniculitis that is associated with a number of conditions, including Crohn disease, ulcerative colitis, Behçet syndrome, sarcoidosis, infection, and the ingestion of estrogens and other drugs. Other manifestations of Crohn disease include inguinal abscesses and sinuses and anal fistulae.

METASTATIC CROHN DISEASE

The term metastatic Crohn disease refers to histologically proven noncaseating granulomas that are remote from the gastrointestinal tract in patients with Crohn disease. The clinical presentation can be quite variable, and the diagnosis of this disorder is frequently missed. In some cases, patients present with marked swelling of the scrotum or vulva.

CUTANEOUS CONDITIONS WITH GASTROINTESTINAL COMPLICATIONS

Cowden Disease

Cowden disease is an autosomal dominant disorder in which gastrointestinal polyps develop along with numerous skin lesions. Wartlike papules known as trichilemmomas occur, particularly around the nose, mouth, and ears but also on the hands and feet [*see Figure 9*]. Small papules can also develop on the gingival mucosa, creating a cobblestone appearance. Hemangiomas and lipomas are common.[13] A distinctive nodule of the scalp known as Cowden fibroma has been described. Up to 50% of women with Cowden disease develop breast cancer. Thyroid carcinomas, thyroid adenomas, and thyroid goiters can occur as well.

Dermatitis Herpetiformis

Dermatitis herpetiformis is an autoimmune vesicular disease that is associated with a gluten-sensitive enteropathy [*see Chapter 39*]. Skin lesions begin as vesicles that are so pruritic that they are quickly broken by scratching, leaving only excoriations and crusts [*see Figure 10*]. Like patients with celiac disease not on a gluten-free diet, patients with dermatitis herpetiformis have an increased risk of non-Hodgkin lymphoma.[14]

Peutz-Jeghers Syndrome

In Peutz-Jeghers syndrome, patients develop hamartomatous polyps of the small intestine associated with pigmented macules of the lips and oral mucosa [*see Chapter 41*]. Also, pigmented macules can develop on the palms, fingers, soles, and toes and in areas around the mouth, nose, and rectum. The disease is inherited as an autosomal dominant trait, and the genetic defect has been localized to chromosome 19.[15]

Recessive Dystrophic Epidermolysis Bullosa

Recessive dystrophic epidermolysis bullosa is a congenital bullous disease with recurrent blistering and scarring, particularly on the hands and feet [*see Chapter 39*]. The scarring results in pseudosyndactyly, giving rise to mittenlike hands. Ingestion of coarse food can result in mucosal bullae of the esophagus, which heal with scarring and stricture formation. Dysphagia is a frequent complaint. Scarring of the esophagus can lead to squamous cell carcinoma, which is a leading cause of death in this disorder. Gastroenterologists and dermatologists must play key roles in the management of these patients. Liquid and pureed diets and appropriate skin care are essential to the survival of patients with this debilitating disorder. Prenatal diagnosis can be made by sampling DNA from the chorionic villus.[16]

Hematologic Diseases

AMYLOIDOSIS

There are several forms of local and systemic amyloidosis. In a form that is associated with multiple myeloma, amyloid fibrils consisting of immunoglobulin light chains are deposited in the skin. Shiny translucent papules develop, particularly on the eyelids. Because of amyloid deposits in blood vessels, spontaneous bleeding occurs. Minimal trauma results in petechiae and purpura. Macroglossia also occurs in some patients with myeloma-associated amyloidosis and in some with primary systemic amyloidosis. The systemic manifestations of myeloma-associated and primary systemic amyloidosis are quite varied. Hepatomegaly

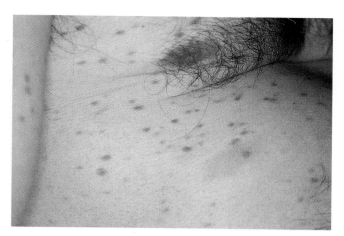

Figure 11 **Multiple reddish-brown macules resembling nevi occur in patients with urticaria pigmentosa.**

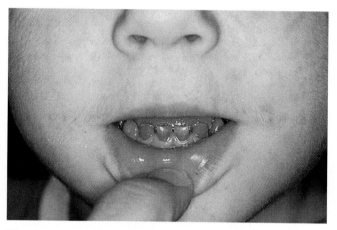

Figure 12 **A reddish pigmentation (erythrodontia) occurs when porphyrins are deposited in the teeth in congenital erythropoietic porphyria.**

develops in 50% of patients. Amyloid can affect the heart, resulting in congestive heart failure or myocardial infarction. Amyloidosis of the gastrointestinal tract can result in malabsorption and protein-losing enteropathy.

MASTOCYTOSIS

Mastocytosis is caused by the infiltration of mast cells into the skin and other organs [*see Chapter 60*]. Urticaria pigmentosa refers to the skin lesions that occur in most patients with mastocytosis. Reddish-brown macules and papules resembling nevi are characteristic [*see Figure 11*]. On stroking individual lesions, urticarial wheals occur—a phenomenon known as the Darier sign. Pruritus, flushing, abdominal pain, nausea, vomiting, and diarrhea are common complaints.

Most patients with mastocytosis have an indolent form of the disease, even when mast cells have infiltrated the bone marrow.[17] Malignant or aggressive systemic mast cell disease can involve the spleen, liver, and lymph nodes in addition to the skin and bone marrow. Histologically, infiltrates contain atypical nonmetachromatic mast cells that are monoclonal in some patients.[18]

The diagnosis of mastocytosis is made by the demonstration of mast cells on skin biopsy. Because mast cells easily degranulate, making them difficult to identify, biopsies should be performed with a minimum of tissue manipulation.

PORPHYRIAS

The porphyrias result from defective hemoglobin synthesis, leading to excess porphyrins in the blood and in body tissues [*see Chapter 55*].

Congenital Erythropoietic Porphyria

Congenital erythropoietic porphyria is a rare, autosomal recessive disorder that is characterized by severe photosensitivity. Vesicles and bullae develop after sun exposure; these lesions heal with scar formation. Erythrodontia (red-stained teeth) is a characteristic feature [*see Figure 12*]. Digit, ear, and nose loss is common in patients who manage to survive to adulthood [*see Figure 13*]. Hypertrichosis is another frequent complication. Formation of gallstones, splenomegaly, and hemolytic anemia are also associated with this condition.

Porphyria Cutanea Tarda

Porphyria cutanea tarda is characterized by photosensitivity, vesicle formation (especially on the dorsa of the hands) [*see Figure 14*], and hypertrichosis. The condition may be associated with ingestion of alcohol or medications such as estrogens. Diagnosis of the porphyrias can be established by elevated urinary porphyrin levels. Examination of the urine with a Wood lamp will often reveal pink-red fluorescence attributable to the high level of urinary porphyrins.

Immunodeficiency Diseases

AIDS

The rise of AIDS has resulted in cutaneous infections and neoplasms that are often dramatic in their extent and severity. This section focuses on selected cutaneous manifestations of infections and other diseases associated with AIDS. (For a more comprehensive discussion of disorders associated with HIV infection, see

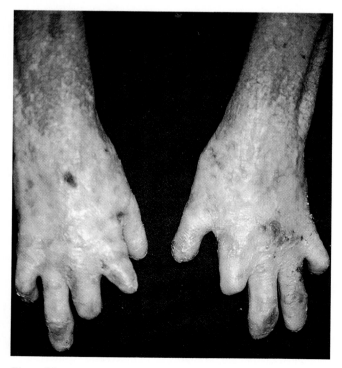

Figure 13 **Skin changes in congenital erythropoietic porphyria can be severe; scarring and loss of digits are common in older patients.**

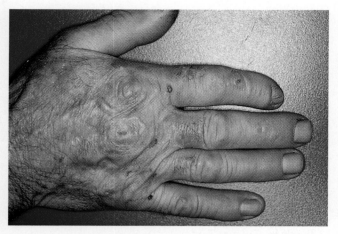

Figure 14 **Crusting and scarring follow the appearance of vesicles and bullae in porphyria cutanea tarda.**

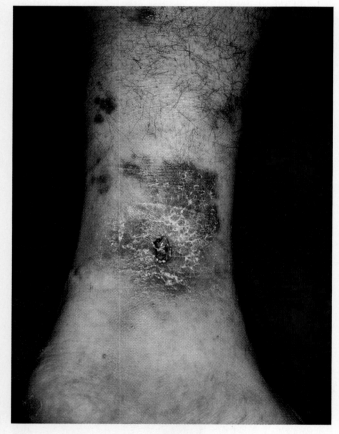

Figure 15 **Kaposi sarcoma is the most common malignancy in AIDS patients. If often presents as a plaque or a purplish lesion that can grow larger and bleed.**

Chapters *140 and 141* and other chapters devoted to specific conditions.)

Opportunistic Infections

Viral infections Banal viral infections, such as molluscum contagiosum, that are ordinarily self-limited and easily curable have become widespread, chronic, and enormous in patients with AIDS. These umbilicated white papules, ordinarily only a few millimeters in diameter, can reach diameters of 1 to 2 cm in patients with AIDS. Similarly, condyloma acuminatum, caused by human papillomavirus (HPV) infection, is often difficult to treat in patients with AIDS.

Herpes simplex virus infections become chronic and erosive, forming large, nonhealing ulcers [*see Chapter 148*]. Acyclovir-resistant strains of herpes simplex virus have been reported in some patients with AIDS.[19] Such patients require other antiviral agents, such as foscarnet. Topical cidofovir gel has been reported to be beneficial for herpes infections in patients infected with HIV.[20]

Herpes zoster infections are a common sign of HIV infection. In the non–HIV-infected host, herpes zoster is characterized by grouped vesicles in a dermatomal distribution. The eruption is self-limited, resolving within 1 to 2 weeks. In contrast, herpes zoster infection can develop into a disseminated vesicular eruption in patients with AIDS; and in some AIDS patients, chronic herpetic lesions can develop that last for months.

Fungal infections Fungal infections are common in patients with HIV infection. Monilial infections include oral thrush and candidiasis of the groin. Several fungal infections that rarely cause widespread infection in patients with normal immune systems (e.g., cryptococcosis, histoplasmosis, aspergillosis, and sporotrichosis) have emerged as serious pathogens in patients with AIDS.

Bacterial infections Bacterial infections are more frequent and severe in patients with AIDS than in patients with normal immune systems. Bacillary angiomatosis, caused by *Rochalimaea henselae,* presents as purple papules and nodules that can be mistaken for Kaposi sarcoma (see below).[21] Chronic fever and chills can occur, as can bone lesions. The condition resolves upon treatment with oral antibiotics.

Scabies and other pruritic eruptions Scabies, a severely pruritic eruption, has a predilection for the buttocks, the genitals, the periumbilical area, and the webs between the fingers. Norwegian scabies, a thickly crusted psoriasislike form of the parasitic disease, has been described in patients with Down syndrome and in other immunosuppressed persons. In recent years, Norwegian scabies has been reported most commonly in patients with AIDS. The scales of Norwegian scabies contain thousands of mites that are easily seen with the microscope. Burrows form linear lesions up to 1 cm long. The causative mite, *Sarcoptes scabiei,* can be identified by microscopic examination of scrapings from the burrows.

Eosinophilic pustular folliculitis and papular eruption of AIDS are pruritic rashes that affect patients with HIV infection. Both conditions are characterized by severe itching, and skin-colored papules and excoriations are common in both. Patients with eosinophilic pustular folliculitis can develop pustules and erythematous papules. Both conditions respond to treatment with ultraviolet B.

Kaposi Sarcoma

Kaposi sarcoma, a slowly progressive vascular neoplasm, was originally described in elderly Italian and Jewish men [*see Chapter 31*]. Subsequently, a more rapidly progressive form of the disorder was described in immunosuppressed patients with lymphomas and in kidney transplant patients on immunosuppressive drugs. An aggressive form has been described in patients with AIDS [*see Figure 15*]. Classic Kaposi sarcoma typically affects the lower extremities and only gradually progresses to other sites. In contrast, AIDS-related Kaposi sarcoma can occur on any surface of the body, including mucous membranes. Human herpesvirus type 8 has been implicated in both classic and AIDS-related Kaposi sarcoma.[22] Treatments include radiation therapy, cryotherapy, and intralesional injection with vinblastine.

Oral Hairy Leukoplakia

Oral hairy leukoplakia, another condition that has been described in HIV-infected patients, consists of linear white papules on the lateral surfaces of the tongue that result in the so-called hairy appearance. Oral hairy leukoplakia can be distinguished from oral thrush in that the lesions cannot be rubbed off, as they can be in thrush.

OTHER IMMUNODEFICIENT STATES

Other inherited or acquired immunodeficiency states share a number of clinical features. Susceptibility to monilial infections or bacterial infections is increased in disorders such as chronic granulomatous disease and chemotherapy-induced neutropenia. Oral ulcers similarly occur in cyclic neutropenia and in chemotherapy-induced immunosuppression.

Some immunosuppressive drugs have characteristic cutaneous effects. Corticosteroids, when used long-term, cause vascular fragility, resulting in steroid purpura. They can also cause cutaneous atrophy, formation of striae, and acneiform eruptions. Cyclosporine is associated with hypertrichosis. Aphthous stomatitis is a characteristic effect of numerous immunosuppressive drugs, particularly agents that suppress bone marrow function.

Infectious Diseases

Cutaneous manifestations can be major features of a number of systemic infections: for example, patients with overwhelming septicemia can develop disseminated intravascular coagulation (DIC), which results in hemorrhage into the skin and cutaneous infarcts. Key cutaneous features of selected systemic infections follow.

INFECTIVE ENDOCARDITIS

The cutaneous manifestations of infective endocarditis include petechiae, splinter hemorrhages (linear red streaks under the nail), Osler nodes (tender purpuric nodules on the finger pads and toes), and Janeway lesions (nontender purpuric macules of the palms and soles). Skin lesions are caused by either septic emboli or vasculitis. Treatment of the underlying infection results in resolution of the cutaneous manifestations [see Chapter 126].

STAPHYLOCOCCAL TOXIC-SHOCK SYNDROME

Staphylococcal toxic-shock syndrome is a recently described syndrome that was first recognized in menstruating women who used super-absorbent tampons [see Chapter 134]. It is caused by an exotoxin produced by certain strains of S. aureus.[23] Staphylococcal infections in bone, soft tissue, and other sites have been implicated. Patients develop diffuse sunburnlike erythema, with swelling of the hands and feet, followed by desquamation of the palms and soles. Erythema of mucous membranes, fever, and hypotension also occur. Gastrointestinal symptoms, impaired renal function, elevated liver function values, thrombocytopenia, and myositis can develop.

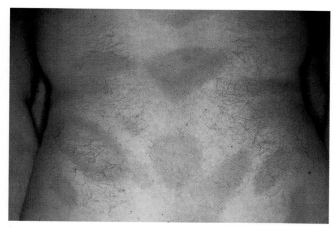

Figure 16 **Several weeks after primary infection, hematogenous dissemination of spirochetes results in multiple patches of erythema chronicum migrans.**

STAPHYLOCOCCAL SCALDED SKIN SYNDROME

Staphylococcal scalded skin syndrome (SSSS) is caused by a circulating exfoliative toxin produced by S. aureus phage group 11. Generalized bulla formation with large areas of desquamation is characteristic of the disorder. Along with tenderness, erythema, and exfoliation of skin, patients have fever. The source of the staphylococcal infection is not always apparent; occasionally the infection arises in a wound or in an occult abscess. Because the staphylococcal infection is usually remote from the affected skin, culture of the skin does not grow S. aureus.

SSSS must be differentiated from toxic epidermal necrolysis. Toxic epidermal necrolysis commonly affects adults and involves mucous membranes; SSSS usually affects children and spares mucous membranes. In addition, toxic epidermal necrolysis can last for several weeks and has a high rate of mortality, whereas SSSS lasts a few days and usually has a good outcome. Histologically, SSSS shows bulla formation in the upper epidermis, and the bulla cavity contains free-floating, normal-appearing, acantholytic cells. In toxic epidermal necrolysis, bulla formation occurs at the basal layer of the epidermis, and the epidermal cells are necrotic.

NECROTIZING FASCIITIS

Necrotizing fasciitis is caused by a mixed anaerobic infection of an ulcer or a surgical or traumatic wound. The affected skin is erythematous, warm, and tender and develops hemorrhagic bullae that rupture to form rapidly enlarging areas of gangrene that extend down to the fascia. Surgical debridement is essential for this life-threatening infection.[24]

MENINGOCOCCEMIA

Acute meningococcemia can occur either in epidemics or in isolated cases [see Chapter 137]. Fever, headache, and a hemorrhagic rash develop. If untreated, patients develop DIC, with extensive hemorrhage, hypotension, and ultimately death. The causative organism, Neisseria meningitidis, is usually identified in cerebrospinal fluid but can also be identified by smear or cultures of skin lesions or by blood cultures.

SCARLET FEVER

Scarlet fever begins with pharyngitis caused by group A streptococcal infection [see Chapter 134]. A generalized rash develops 1 to 2 days after onset of the pharyngitis. The rash is characterized by pinpoint erythematous papules that may be easier to palpate than to see. Other characteristic lesions include a white strawberry tongue and linear petechial macules occurring in body folds (Pastia lines). As the rash fades, desquamation of the palms and soles appears. Treatment with penicillin results in rapid resolution of all symptoms.

VIBRIO INFECTION

Vibrio vulnificus infection arises from minor trauma sustained while swimming in lakes or the ocean or while cleaning seafood. Cellulitis occurs, with lymphangitis and bacteremia. In patients with hepatic cirrhosis, infection can occur after eating raw oysters. These patients develop hemorrhagic bullae, with leukopenia and DIC.[25]

LYME DISEASE

Lyme disease is caused by the spirochete *Borrelia burgdorferi* and is transmitted primarily by the tick *Ixodes dammini* [*see Chapter 144*]. The characteristic skin lesion, erythema chronicum migrans, begins as an erythematous macule or papule at the site of the tick bite. Over days and weeks, the erythematous lesion expands to form a red ring, often with central clearing. If left untreated, lesions last weeks or months. Hematogenous dissemination of spirochetes occurs after several weeks, resulting in multiple annular patches of erythema chronicum migrans [*see Figure 16*]. Systemic complications include an acute arthritis involving one or a few large joints a few weeks after the onset of symptoms. A chronic erosive arthritis develops in approximately 10% of patients. Neurologic symptoms, including Bell palsy, can occur, as can cardiac complications, including heart failure and cardiac conduction abnormalities.

Lyme disease can be prevented by the removal of ticks within 18 hours of attachment. Once symptoms have developed, oral antibiotics are effective at destroying *B. burgdorferi*. A vaccine containing a genetically engineered protein from the surface of the bacteria prevents infection in most vaccinated people.[26]

ROCKY MOUNTAIN SPOTTED FEVER

Rocky Mountain spotted fever (RMSF) is a tick-borne illness caused by *Rickettsia rickettsii* [*see Chapter 145*]. It is characterized by the sudden onset of fevers, chills, and head-ache. Approximately 4 days later, a characteristic erythematous rash develops that becomes purpuric on the wrists and ankles. The rash then spreads centrally to involve the extremities, trunk, and face.

Because the mortality of RMSF is high, the disease should be treated immediately with intravenous chloramphenicol or tetracycline if suspected. Diagnosis can then be established by skin biopsy: immunofluorescence with antibodies against *R. rickettsii* shows the organism in the walls of cutaneous blood vessels. Serologic tests, such as the Weil-Felix reaction, can confirm the diagnosis after the acute phase of the illness.

Neurologic Diseases

BASAL CELL NEVUS SYNDROME

The basal cell nevus syndrome is an autosomal dominant disorder in which patients develop basal cell carcinomas at an early age [*see Chapter 31*]. Multiple skeletal abnormalities are associated with the syndrome, and affected individuals may also develop jaw cysts. Lamellar calcification of the falx cerebri occurs, as well as other neurologic abnormalities, including medulloblastomas.

EPIDERMAL NEVUS SYNDROME

The epidermal nevus syndrome is characterized by systemic manifestations, such as seizures, mental retardation, blindness, and skeletal abnormalities in association with large epidermal nevi. The nevi consist of long pigmented streaks that are linear or whirled and involve large areas of the body [*see Figure 17*].

INCONTINENTIA PIGMENTI

Incontinentia pigmenti is an inherited syndrome that affects the skin and nervous system. The inheritance pattern is X-linked dominant and is lethal in male fetuses. The first skin manifestations begin within weeks of birth, occasionally occurring in utero, and consist of linear patterns of vesiculobullous lesions. Within weeks, these lesions evolve into verrucous papules and, eventually, into pigmented whirls. Apart from neurologic symptoms, ocular abnormalities, scarring alopecia, and skeletal malformations can occur.

Hypomelanosis of Ito

Hypomelanosis of Ito, also called incontinentia pigmenti achromians, consists of whirls of hypopigmentation that are associated with neurologic symptoms in 50% of patients. Skin lesions are present at birth or develop in early childhood. In addition to seizures and mental retardation, skeletal and ocular abnormalities occur.

NEUROFIBROMATOSIS

Neurofibromatosis is a common autosomal dominant disorder involving the skin and nervous system [*see Chapter 40*]. Skin lesions include cutaneous neurofibromas, which are soft, skin-colored nodules that are often pedunculated [*see Figure 18*]. Café au lait macules are flat, evenly pigmented patches up to several centimeters in diameter. Six or more café au lait macules greater than 1.5 cm in diameter are found in most patients with neurofibromatosis type 1 (also called von Recklinghausen disease). Plexiform neuromas are larger, deeper tumors that are associated with hypertrophy of bony and soft tissues. In a small proportion of tumors, neurofibrosarcomas will arise. On skin biopsy, café au lait macules are found to contain macromelanosomes—giant granules of pigment in melanocytes and keratinocytes. Axillary and inguinal freckling also appear as pigmented macules that resemble small café au lait spots in intertriginous sites. Lisch nodules—pigmented iris hamartomas—are also found in most patients with neurofibromatosis.

Several variants of neurofibromatosis exist, including segmental neurofibromatosis, in which patients develop a segmental distribution of café au lait spots and cutaneous neurofibromas, and neurofibromatosis type 2, which consists of bilateral acoustic neuromas without Lisch nodules and with fewer café au lait macules than appear in type 1. Patients with neurofibromatosis type 2 may have some cutaneous neurofibromas as well. Neurofibromatosis types 1 and 2 are caused by different genetic defects, found on chromosomes 17 and 22, respectively.[27,28]

SNEDDON SYNDROME

Sneddon syndrome is a disease of the skin and nervous system caused by occlusion of small to medium-sized arteries in persons younger than 45 years. The skin lesions resemble livedo reticularis and have been called livedo racemosa. Transient ischemic attacks or strokes are common. Definitive diagnosis is made by demonstrating characteristic vascular changes on skin biopsy of patients with associated neurologic findings.

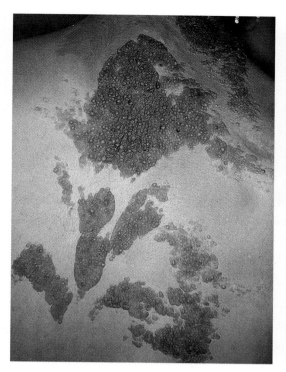

Figure 17 **The epidermal nevus syndrome is characterized by linear or whirled streaks of pigmentation that involve large areas of the body.**

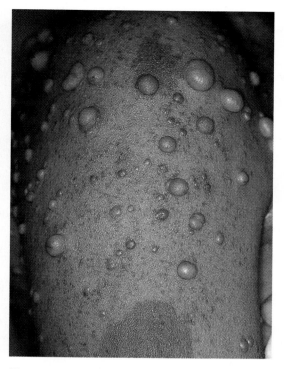

Figure 18 **Large café au lait spot and numerous cutaneous neurofibromas are evident on the arm of a patient with neurofibromatosis type 1.**

TUBEROUS SCLEROSIS

Tuberous sclerosis is an autosomal dominant disease that affects the skin and nervous system. Affected patients can develop seizures, mental retardation, and brain lesions, called tubers, which can be seen on CT scans. Adenoma sebaceum, the most characteristic cutaneous manifestation of tuberous sclerosis, consists of skin-colored papules of the face [*see Figure 19a*]. Other skin lesions are hypopigmented macules referred to as ash-leaf macules [*see Figure 19b*], smaller hypopigmented lesions called confetti macules, periungual and subungual fibromas (skin-colored nodules that arise around the finger and toenails) [*see Figure 19c*], and the shagreen patch (a skin-colored plaque made of thick dermal connective tissue). Two separate disease-determining genes have been identified on chromosomes 9 and 16.[29]

Renal Diseases

FABRY DISEASE

Fabry disease is caused by an abnormality of α-galactosidase A, resulting in deposition of glycosphingolipids in body tissues. The disorder is inherited as an X-linked recessive trait. Affected males often complain of severe pain in the extremities, with burning of the palms and soles. Episodes of pain are transient, but patients complain of persistent paresthesias in the hands and feet.

Skin lesions consist of angiokeratomas, which are pinpoint red or purple papules that resemble cherry hemangiomas [*see Figure 20*]. Angiokeratomas are most commonly found in the periumbilical area but can also occur on the palms, soles, trunk, extremities, and mucous membranes. In adults, glycosphingolipids deposit in blood vessels and organs, affecting the heart, heart valves, coronary arteries, and kidneys.

POLYARTERITIS NODOSA

Polyarteritis nodosa is an inflammatory condition that affects muscular arteries [*see Chapter 117*]. Aneurysms form in many arteries, including those leading to the kidneys and subcutaneous tissue. Diagnosis of the systemic form of polyarteritis can be made by demonstrating aneurysms of the renal arteries on renal arteriograms.

A localized cutaneous form of polyarteritis nodosa most commonly presents as painful nodules of the lower extremities.[30] In mild cases, patients may only have livedo reticularis; but in severe cases, skin lesions can ulcerate. A polyneuropathy may be associated with the disorder. Patients with classic polyarteritis and microaneurysms have an increased incidence of hepatitis B antigenemia; in contrast to patients with other vasculitides, they usually do not have antineutrophil cytoplasmic antibodies.[31]

PERFORATING DISORDERS

The term perforating disorders refers to several conditions characterized by extrusion of dermal material through the epidermis. These lesions often develop in association with renal failure and diabetes mellitus.[32] Skin lesions are characterized by hyperkeratotic papules with central white craters that histologically can be shown to contain dermal material. Reactive perforating collagenosis, perforating folliculitis, and Kyrle disease are all examples of perforating disorders associated with renal failure.

CALCIPHYLAXIS

Calciphylaxis is a condition of patients with renal failure in which localized areas of skin become necrotic as a result of vascular calcification. Calciphylaxis begins with painful purpuric patches that may be reticulated, resembling livedo reticularis. These

a   *b*   *c*

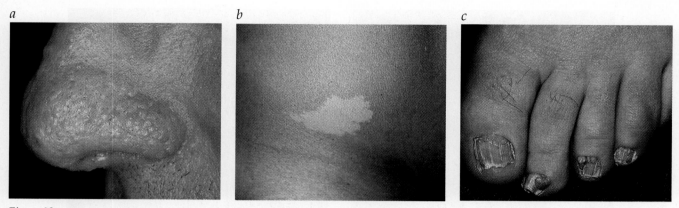

Figure 19   **Several of the characteristic cutaneous findings of tuberous sclerosis are shown: adenoma sebaceum (*a*); ash-leaf macule (*b*); and periungual fibromas (*c*).**

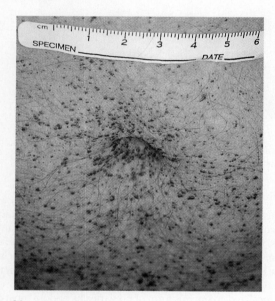

Figure 20   **Angiokeratomas are particularly common in the periumbilical area of patients with Fabry disease.**

patches progress to indurated plaques that may ulcerate, becoming necrotic [*see Figure 21*]. Calciphylaxis often eventuates in amputation or death. Parathyroidectomy may result in healing of affected skin without amputation.[33]

Rheumatologic Diseases

DERMATOMYOSITIS

The best-known cutaneous manifestations of dermatomyositis, an inflammatory disorder of muscle and skin, are Gottron papules and heliotrope erythema. Gottron papules are erythematous scaling macules and papules that occur on the dorsa of the knuckles [*see Figure 22*]. Heliotrope erythema consists of periorbital erythema and edema. Most recently, scalp lesions, which can be associated with alopecia, have been described.[34] The lesions are often misdiagnosed as seborrheic dermatitis or psoriasis.

The association between dermatomyositis and malignancy remains controversial. Malignancies are reported in 15% to 50% of patients but are usually detected on history and physical examination or in routine tests, such as mammography, chest x-ray, uri-

nalysis, and stool examination for occult blood. More-extensive workups are seldom justified unless evidence of malignancy is found on initial evaluation.[35]

Classifications of dermatomyositis include a juvenile variant that is characterized by calcification of skin or muscle. A vasculitic form of dermatomyositis in children is complicated by cutaneous infarcts and ulceration and by gastrointestinal vasculitis with abdominal pain, bleeding, or perforation. The vasculitic form of dermatoyositis carries a poor prognosis, with many of the patients dying of this disease.

SCLERODERMA AND SCLERODERMA-LIKE DISEASES

The sclerodermas include a number of distinct syndromes sharing a common feature, induration of the skin [*see Chapter 115*].

Progressive Systemic Sclerosis

Progressive systemic sclerosis, also known as systemic scleroderma, is a frequently fatal disease in which patients present with Raynaud phenomenon and sclerodactyly (induration of skin of the digits) [*see Figure 23*]. Cutaneous induration can become widespread. Involvement of the face can lead to a characteristic appearance with pursed lips and bound-down skin of the nose that creates a beaklike appearance. Patients with antibodies to Scl-70 have a poor prognosis, often succumbing to renal disease and malignant hypertension. Patients with anticentromere antibodies have a more slowly progressive variant of scleroderma known as

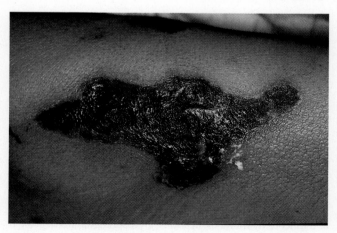

Figure 21   **Calcification of arteries in patients with renal failure results in calciphylaxis. Affected skin forms a black, necrotic eschar.**

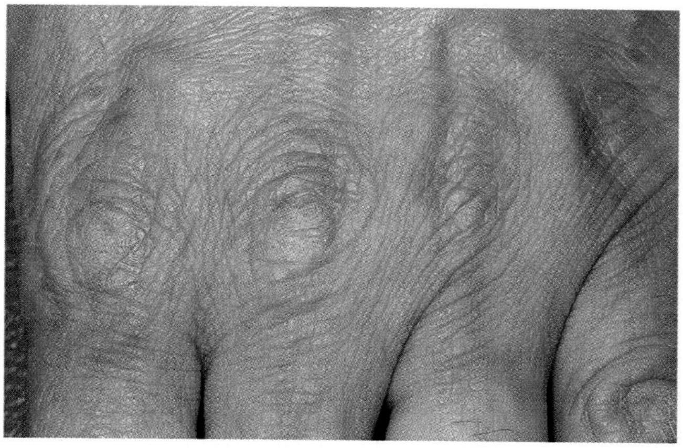

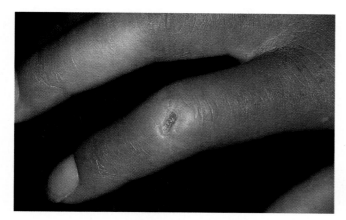

Figure 22   **Erythematous scaling papules on the dorsal aspects of the knuckles (Gottron papules) are a sign of dermatomyositis.**

Figure 23   **Sclerodactyly with a nonhealing digital ulcer commonly occurs in progressive systemic sclerosis.**

the CREST syndrome, which is characterized by cutaneous calcinosis, Raynaud phenomenon, esophageal dysmotility, sclerodactyly, and telangiectasia. With time, pulmonary fibrosis, pulmonary hypertension, and right-sided heart failure develop.

Morphea

Morphea, also called localized scleroderma, is characterized by sharply demarcated patches of indurated skin that can become generalized. It is distinguished from progressive systemic sclerosis by the absence of Raynaud phenomenon, sclerodactyly, or the systemic complications of scleroderma.

There have been innovations in the treatment of both progressive systemic sclerosis and morphea. Exposure to psoralen and longwave ultraviolet light (PUVA) has been reported to improve progressive systemic sclerosis and morphea dramatically,[36] and exposure to UVA1 (the longer UVA spectrum, from 340 to 400 nm) has been reported to benefit localized scleroderma.[37] Further studies must be done to confirm the efficacy of these treatments. Anecdotal reports have indicated that minocycline may benefit progressive systemic sclerosis, but controlled trials are needed.[38]

Graft versus Host Disease

As organ transplantation becomes more common, another scleroderma-like illness, graft versus host disease, increases in frequency, particularly after bone marrow transplantation [*see Chapter*

95]. There are two stages of graft versus host disease. The first—acute graft versus host disease—develops 10 to 40 days after transplantation and consists of an erythematous macular and papular rash that is often associated with fever, hepatomegaly, lymphadenopathy, or gastrointestinal symptoms. Chronic graft versus host disease develops 3 months after transplantation and consists of purple papules resembling lichen planus [*see Figure 24*]. Sclerodermatous skin changes with telangiectasia, reticulated hyperpigmentation, and alopecia are most characteristic. Both cyclosporine and PUVA have proved to be useful in the prevention and treatment of graft versus host disease.[39,40]

Eosinophilic Fasciitis

Scleroderma-like hardening of the skin also occurs in eosinophilic fasciitis. Puckering of the skin on the extremities typically develops and is associated with pain. In contrast to progressive systemic sclerosis, Raynaud phenomenon does not occur. Definitive diagnosis requires biopsy of skin and fascia overlying the affected muscle. In some cases of eosinophilic fasciitis, hematologic abnormalities develop, including aplastic anemia, thrombocytopenia, Hodgkin disease, and leukemias.[41]

Eosinophilia-Myalgia Syndrome

Some patients who were misdiagnosed with eosinophilic fasciitis were discovered to have ingested L-tryptophan, which has been associated with eosinophilia-myalgia syndrome [*see Chapter 115*]. As a result, severe muscle pain and weakness occur, along with fever, eosinophilia, and a wide array of systemic symp-

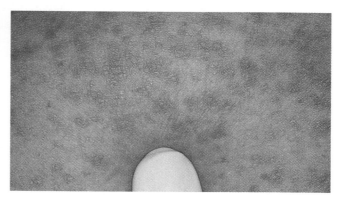

Figure 24   **Flat-topped papules are seen in this chronic lichenoid graft versus host reaction.**

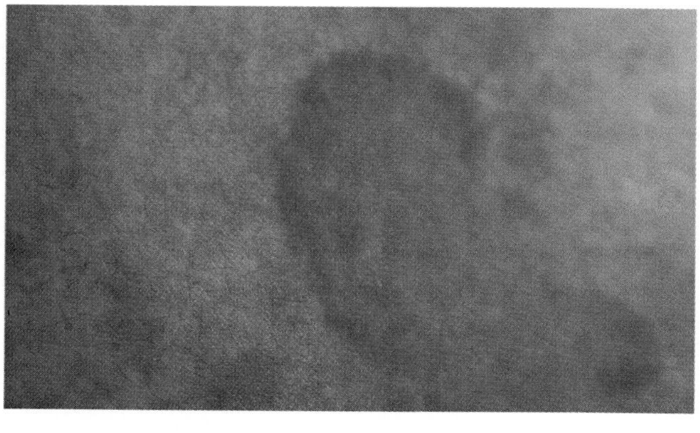

Figure 25   **Annular scaling erythematous patches are characteristic of subacute cutaneous lupus erythematosus.**

toms. The common cutaneous manifestations are erythema and swelling.[42]

SYSTEMIC LUPUS ERYTHEMATOSUS

There are many cutaneous manifestations of lupus, including Raynaud phenomenon, so-called discoid lupus (characterized by round scarred skin lesions with central hypopigmentation and a rim of hyperpigmentation), malar erythema, photosensitivity, alopecia, and mucosal ulcers [see Chapter 114]. As we learn more about lupus, the spectrum of skin diseases associated with this disorder continues to expand. Subacute cutaneous lupus, a variant characterized serologically by anti-Ro and anti-La antibodies, is associated with annular psoriasiform skin lesions [see Figure 25].

Anticardiolipin Antibody Syndrome

The anticardiolipin antibody syndrome, which can occur in patients with lupus, has been described in patients who suffer repeated episodes of phlebitis, arterial thromboses, and repeated miscarriages. Cutaneous infarcts are common manifestations. Patients have false positive serologies for syphilis and have a circulating lupus anticoagulant. Circulating antiphospholipid antibodies are the serologic hallmark of this newly described syndrome.[43]

Livedo Vasculitis

Livedo vasculitis, another disorder that has been associated with lupus, is characterized by painful recurrent ulcers over the lower legs and ankles. The ulcers heal, leaving white sclerotic scars. Affected patients often have livedo reticularis. This condition, also known as atrophie blanche, has been attributed to thrombotic processes rather than immune complex deposition or leukocytoclastic vasculitis.[44]

Neonatal Lupus

Neonatal lupus is a distinct syndrome of annular, erythematous macules and papules occurring on the face of newborn infants. The disorder has been attributed to transplacental passage of anti-Ro and occasionally anti-La antibodies. Mothers are often asymptomatic, but some may have lupus or Sjögren syndrome. Congenital heart block is the most serious complication of this disorder.[45]

References

1. Mana J, Marcoval J, Graells J, et al: Cutaneous involvement in sarcoidosis: relationship to systemic disease. Arch Dermatol 133:882, 1997

2. McNiff JM, Cooper D, Howe G, et al: Lymphomatoid granulomatosis of the skin and lung: an angiocentric T-cell-rich B-cell lymphoproliferative disorder. Arch Dermatol 132:1464, 1996

3. Davis MD, Daoud MS, McEvoy MT, et al: Cutaneous manifestations of Churg-Strauss syndrome: a clinicopathologic correlation. J Am Acad Dermatol 37:199, 1997

4. Leung DY, Sullivan KE, Brown-Whitehorn TF, et al: Association of toxic shock syndrome toxin-secreting and exfoliative toxin-secreting Staphylococcus aureus with Kawasaki syndrome complicated by coronary artery disease. Pediatr Res 42:268, 1997

5. Lebwohl MG, Distefano D, Prioleau PG, et al: Pseudoxanthoma elasticum and mitral valve prolapse. N Engl J Med 307:228, 1982

6. Lebwohl M, Halperin J, Phelps RG: Brief report: occult pseudoxanthoma elasticum in patients with premature cardiovascular disease. N Engl J Med 329:1237, 1993

7. Lebwohl M, Phelps RG, Yannuzzi L, et al: Diagnosis of pseudoxanthoma elasticum by scar biopsy in patients without characteristic skin lesions. N Engl J Med 317:347, 1987

8. Struk B, Neldner KH, Rao VS, et al: Mapping of both autosomal recessive and dominant variants of pseudoxanthoma elasticum to chromosome 16p13.1. Hum Mol Genet 6:1823, 1997

9. Bull RH, Fenton DA, Mortimer PS: Lymphatic function in the yellow nail syndrome. Br J Dermatol 134:307, 1996

10. Verrotti A, Chiarelli F, Amerio P, et al: Necrobiosis lipoidica diabeticorum in children

11. Rho YW, Suhr KB, Lee JH, et al: A clinical observation of scleredema adultorum and its relationship to diabetes. J Dermatol 25:103, 1998

12. Hecker MS, Lebwohl MG: Recalcitrant pyoderma gangrenosum: treatment with thalidomide. J Am Acad Dermatol 38:490, 1998

13. Barax C, Lebwohl M, Phelps RG: Multiple hamartoma syndrome. J Am Acad Dermatol 17:342, 1987

14. Collin P, Pukkala E, Reunala T: Malignancy and survival in dermatitis herpetiformis: a comparison with coeliac disease. Gut 38:528, 1996

15. Nakagawa H, Koyama K, Tanaka T, et al: Localization of the gene responsible for Peutz-Jeghers syndrome within a 6-cM region of chromosome 19p13.3. Hum Genet 102:203, 1998

16. Christiano AM, LaForgia S, Paller AS, et al: Prenatal diagnosis for recessive dystrophic epidermolysis bullosa in 10 families by mutation and haplotype analysis in the type VII collagen gene (COL7A1). Mol Med 2:59, 1996

17. Topar G, Staudacher C, Geisen F, et al: Urticaria pigmentosa: a clinical, hematopathologic, and serologic study of 30 adults. Am J Clin Pathol 109:279, 1998

18. Horny HP, Ruck P, Krober S, et al: Systemic mast cell disease (mastocytosis): general aspects and histopathological diagnosis. Histol Histopathol 12:1081, 1997

19. Pottage JC Jr, Kessler HA: Herpes simplex virus resistance to acyclovir: clinical relevance. Infect Agents Dis 4:115, 1995

20. Lalezari J, Schacker T, Feinberg J, et al: A randomized, double-blind, placebo-controlled trial of cidofovir gel for the treatment of acyclovir-unresponsive mucocutaneous herpes simplex virus infection in patients with AIDS. J Infect Dis 176:892, 1997

21. Koehler JE, Quinn FD, Berger TG, et al: Isolation of Rochalimaea species from cutaneous and osseous lesions of bacillary angiomatosis. N Engl J Med 327:1625, 1992

22. Kennedy MM, Cooper K, Howells DD, et al: Identification of HHV8 in early Kaposi's sarcoma: implications for Kaposi's sarcoma pathogenesis. Mol Pathol 51:14, 1998

23. Parsonnet J: Nonmenstrual toxic shock syndrome: new insights into diagnosis, pathogenesis, and treatment. Curr Clin Top Infect Dis 16:1, 1996

24. Green RJ, Dafoe DC, Raffin TA: Necrotizing fasciitis. Chest 110:219, 1996

25. Hally RJ, Rubin RA, Fraimow HS, et al: Fatal Vibrio parahemolyticus septicemia in a patient with cirrhosis: a case report and review of the literature. Dig Dis Sci 40:1257, 1995

26. Steere AC, Sikand VK, Meurice F, et al: Vaccination against Lyme disease with recombinant Borrelia burgdorferi outer-surface lipoprotein A with adjuvant: Lyme Disease Vaccine Study Group. N Engl J Med 339:209, 1998

27. Upadhyaya M, Osborn MJ, Maynard J, et al: Mutational and functional analysis of the neurofibromatosis type 1 (NF1) gene. Hum Genet 99:88, 1997

28. De Klein A, Riegman PH, Bijlsma EK, et al: A G-A transition creates a branch point sequence and activation of a cryptic exon, resulting in the hereditary disorder neurofibromatosis 2. Hum Mol Genet 7:393, 1998

29. Soucek T, Holzl G, Bernaschek G, et al: A role of the tuberous sclerosis gene-2 product during neuronal differentiation. Oncogene 16:2197, 1998

30. Daoud MS, Hutton KP, Gibson LE: Cutaneous periarteritis nodosa: a clinicopathological study of 79 cases. Br J Dermatol 136:706, 1997

31. Guillevin L, Lhote F, Amouroux J, et al: Antineutrophil cytoplasmic antibodies, abnormal angiograms and pathological findings in polyarteritis nodosa and Churg-Strauss syndrome: indications for the classification of vasculitides of the polyarteritis nodosa group. Br J Rheumatol 35:958, 1996

32. Poliak S, Lebwohl MG, Parris A, et al: Reactive perforating collagenosis associated with diabetes mellitus. N Engl J Med 306:81, 1982

33. Angelis M, Wong LL, Myers SA, et al: Calciphylaxis in patients on hemodialysis: a prevalence study. Surgery 122:1083 (discussion: 1089), 1997

34. Kasteler JS, Callen JP: Scalp involvement in dermatomyositis: often overlooked or misdiagnosed. JAMA 272:1939, 1994

35. Drake LA, Dinehart SM, Farmer ER, et al: Guidelines of care for dermatomyositis. American Academy of Dermatology. J Am Acad Dermatol 34:824, 1996

36. Kanekura T, Fukumaru S, Matsushita S, et al: Successful treatment of scleroderma with PUVA therapy. J Dermatol 23:455, 1996

37. Kerscher M, Volkenandt M, Gruss C, et al: Low-dose UVA phototherapy for treatment of localized scleroderma. J Am Acad Dermatol 38:21, 1998

38. Le CH, Morales A, Trentham DE: Minocycline in early diffuse scleroderma. Lancet 352:1755, 1998

39. Zikos P, van Lint MT, Frasoni F, et al: Low transplant mortality in allogeneic bone marrow transplantation for acute myeloid leukemia: a randomized study of low-dose cyclosporin versus low-dose cyclosporin and low-dose methotrexate. Blood 91:3503, 1998

40. Vogelsang GB, Wolff D, Altomonte V, et al: Treatment of chronic graft-versus-host disease with ultraviolet irradiation and psoralen (PUVA). Bone Marrow Transplant 17:1061, 1996

41. Kim SW, Rice L, Champlin R, et al: Aplastic anemia in eosinophilic fasciitis: responses to immunosuppression and marrow transplantation. Haematologia (Budap) 28:131, 1997

42. Gordon M, Lebwohl M, Phelps RG, et al: Eosinophilic fasciitis associated with tryptophan ingestion: a manifestation of eosinophilia-myalgia syndrome. Arch Dermatol 127:217, 1991

43. Derksen RH: Clinical manifestations and management of the antiphospholipid syndrome. Lupus 5:167, 1996

44. McCalmont CS, McCalmont TH, Jorizzo JL, et al: Livedo vasculitis: vasculitis or thrombotic vasculopathy? Clin Exp Dermatol 17:4, 1992

45. Brucato A, Franceschini F, Buyon JP: Neonatal lupus: long-term outcomes of mothers and children and recurrence rate. Clin Exp Rheumatol 15:467, 1997

and adolescents: a clue for underlying renal and retinal disease. Pediatr Dermatol 12:220, 1995

31 Acne Vulgaris and Related Disorders

Mark Lebwohl, M.D.

Acne and its clinical variants are among the most common causes of patient visits to the physician for cutaneous disorders. Severe forms of these disorders can be disfiguring and debilitating; and because the face is the primary site of involvement, patients will often seek therapy for even mild forms. Therapeutic approaches will therefore be stressed in this chapter.

Epidemiology and Etiology

Acne vulgaris is the most common dermatologic problem of adolescent years; it usually begins in puberty. Age of onset and severity of disease are affected by sex, genetics, and external factors such as cosmetics and medications. Acne is usually more severe in males than in females and often begins earlier (in early adolescence) in males. Acne often subsides after the teenage years, but the disease can remain a problem for adults in the third and fourth decades and beyond. A significant portion of women experience premenstrual flares of acne; this phenomenon may be more common in older women.[1]

Genetic factors clearly play a role in severe acne. A family history of severe acne can often be elicited during the workup of affected patients. Various external factors, such as occlusive cosmetics, can contribute to acne, and certain medications (e.g., corticosteroids, adrenocorticotropic hormone [ACTH], phenytoin sodium, isoniazid, lithium, progestins, potassium iodide, bromides, actinomycin D) can cause acnelike lesions [*see Chapter 36*].

Pathogenesis

Multiple factors contribute to the development of acne in susceptible persons. Among the most significant are alterations in keratinization, accumulation of sebum, and inflammation. Androgenic influences may contribute to some of these factors.

Modified keratinization of the follicular infundibulum leads to proliferation and increased cohesiveness of keratinocytes, which causes plugs to form. These plugs block follicular outlets, allowing cellular debris in sebum to form comedones (the noninflammatory lesions of acne).

The composition of sebum does not appear to be altered in patients with acne; however, sebaceous glands are often larger and sebum production is often greater in persons affected with acne than in unaffected persons.[2] Sebum is comedogenic and inflammatory, which may account for its role in acne.[3] Inflammation in acne has also been attributed to the anaerobic diphtheroid *Propionibacterium acnes*. The presence of *P. acnes* correlates with the occurrence of acne in adolescents.[4] The microbe's role in inflammation has been attributed to lipases, proteases, and hyaluronidases, as well as chemotactic factors.

Androgens play a role in the development of acne, as evidenced by increased levels of dehydroepiandrosterone sulfate (DHEAS) in girls with acne[5] and an association of acne with endocrinopathies characterized by increased levels of circulating androgens. For example, the occurrence of acne is increased in patients with congenital adrenal hyperplasia, polycystic ovaries, and some ovarian and adrenal tumors. Androgens act to increase sebum production and enlarge sebaceous glands; they may also contribute to the follicular hyperkeratinization that leads to acne. However, serum androgens are usually within the normal range in patients with acne. Some researchers have postulated that local production of androgens in the skin can lead to acne. Skin biopsies from patients with acne show increases in 5α-reductase activity.[6] This increased androgenic activity may result in the conversion of testosterone to dihydrotestosterone in the skin, leading to the development of acne.

Diagnosis

CLINICAL FEATURES

The characteristic skin lesions of acne include open and closed comedones, erythematous papules, pustules, nodules, cysts, and scars. The most commonly affected site is the face, but in more severely affected individuals, the back and chest can be involved as well.

Comedonal Acne

Comedones consist of keratinized cells and sebum. Comedonal acne consists of a predominance of open and closed comedones. Open comedones (blackheads) are black papules measuring 0.1 to 2 mm that are easily extruded with gentle pressure. The material that is removed is greasy and has a gray-white color. Contrary to popular belief, the dark color of open comedones is caused by melanin, not by dirt or oxidized fatty acids. Closed comedones (whiteheads) consist of white papules measuring 0.1 to 2 mm. Unless extracted, they persist somewhat longer than open comedones, often for weeks to months.

Inflammatory Acne

Erythematous papules, pustules, nodules, and cysts are the predominant lesions in inflammatory acne [*see Figure 1*]. Erythematous papules range in size from 3 to 10 mm and can develop

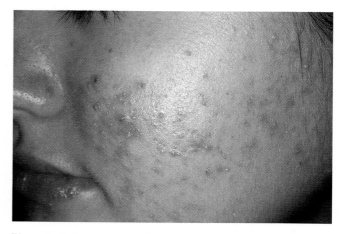

Figure 1 **Inflammatory acne is characterized by erythematous papules and pustules.**

into pustules or resolve into an erythematous macule that fades. Postinflammatory hyperpigmentation can occur. Pustules are superficial and usually dry in a few days. Nodules, which are 1 cm or larger, are erythematous and tender. They can be firm at onset but often become fluctuant. In severely affected individuals, these lesions form fluctuant sinuses that open to the surface through multiple tracts. Postinflammatory pigmentary changes and scarring commonly occur.

Clinical Variants of Acne

Acne conglobata Acne conglobata is a severe, scarring form of acne in which large cysts and abscesses become confluent to form draining sinus tracts. Scarring is often severe. Topical acne therapy and oral antibiotics are frequently ineffective; patients may require treatment with oral isotretinoin [*see* Treatment, *below*]. Intralesional injection of corticosteroids and drainage of abscesses are temporarily helpful.

Acne cosmetica A persistent, low-grade form of acne can result from the use of greasy, occlusive cosmetics, moisturizers, and sunscreens. Women are most commonly affected.

Acne excoriée Picking of minor acne lesions can cause large ulcers and erosions that heal with scarring. Young women are most typically affected.

Acne mechanica An acneiform eruption can result from repeated trauma associated with the wearing of sports helmets, shoulder pads, and bras and from the chin rests of violins and violas (so-called fiddler's neck).

Pomade acne A form of acne results from the use of thick oils in the hair. Comedones, papules, and pustules are usually found close to the hairline. Black men and women are most commonly affected.

Acne in neonates and children Neonatal acne has been attributed to maternal androgens, as well as androgens secreted by the neonatal adrenal gland. Erythematous papules and pustules may last for 2 to 3 months after birth but usually resolve spontaneously.

Infantile acne develops between 3 and 6 months after birth. This condition is characterized by inflamed papules and pustules and signals early secretion of androgens by the gonads, particularly in boys. This condition may last until age 5. It has

Table 1 Laboratory Evaluation for Women with Acne and Signs of Hyperandrogenism

Finding	Suspected Condition
DHEAS 4,000–8,000 ng/ml > 8,000 ng/ml	Congenital adrenal hyperplasia Adrenal tumor
LH:FSH ratio > 2.0	Polycystic ovary disease
Testosterone (unbound) 20–40 yr, > 107.5 pmol/L 41–60 yr, > 86.7 pmol/L 61–80 yr, > 69.3 pmol/L	Polycystic ovary disease; ovarian tumor Polycystic ovary disease; ovarian tumor Polycystic ovary disease; ovarian tumor

DHEAS—dehydroepiandrosterone sulfate   FSH—follicle-stimulating hormone
LH—luteinizing hormone

been suggested that affected infants may be predisposed to severe acne later in life.

LABORATORY TESTS

The clinical features of acne are so commonly recognized that laboratory investigation is usually not necessary. Laboratory tests should be considered, however, for female patients who have other signs of hyperandrogenism, such as hirsutism or irregular menses. Serum for determining DHEAS and free testosterone levels and for the ratio of luteinizing hormone to follicle stimulating hormone (LH:FSH) should be obtained 2 weeks before the onset of menses [*see Table 1*]. Tests should also be undertaken in patients whose conditions do not respond to adequate doses of isotretinoin, the most potent treatment available for acne [*see* Treatment, *below*].

Differential Diagnosis

Clinical features of acne are sufficiently distinctive that diagnosis is usually obvious. Nevertheless, a number of disorders can be mistaken for acne.

Folliculitis The perifollicular pustules of folliculitis can be distinguished from the lesions of acne by their distribution. Folliculitis can affect the trunk and extremities and is not limited to the usual sites of acne on the face, back, and chest. Malassezia folliculitis is characterized by erythematous acneiform papules that do not respond to typical acne therapies. Gram stain of pus from the lesions reveals gram-positive budding yeast [*see Chapter 37*].

Gram-negative folliculitis In patients on long-term antibiotics, superficial pustules or nodules can develop at the anterior nares and spread outward on the face. This condition responds promptly to oral ampicillin.

Milia Milia are white pinpoint cysts that resemble closed comedones. They frequently occur around the eyes but can develop anywhere on the face. If untreated, they last for months or years. Milia can be opened with a small surgical blade and their contents easily drained.

Perioral dermatitis Long-term use of topical corticosteroids on the face can result in acneiform, erythematous, inflamed papules on the chin and cheeks. Despite the name, the area immediately around the mouth is typically spared in perioral dermatitis.

Chloracne Cysts and closed comedones that resemble acne lesions can be caused by exposure to halogenated hydrocarbons.

Hidradenitis suppurativa Hidradenitis suppurativa is a chronic condition in which inflamed cysts in the axillae and groin form fluctuant sinuses with draining tracts.

Favre-Racouchot disease Numerous open and closed comedones can appear around the eyes of elderly patients, especially men who have worked out of doors for much of their lives. This condition has been attributed to a lifetime of sun exposure.

Rosacea Rosacea is a common condition that usually begins after 30 years of age. It is so similar to acne in some individuals

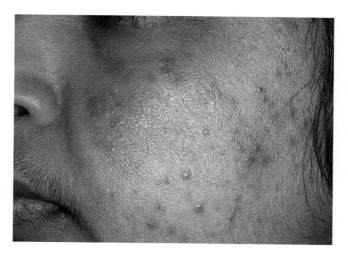

Figure 2 **Erythematous papules, pustules, telangiectasia, and flushing are features of rosacea.**

that it has been called acne rosacea. Skin lesions consist of erythematous papules, pustules, and telangiectasia [*see Figure 2*]. Facial flushing is a common feature. In patients with a predominance of inflamed papules and pustules, differentiation from acne can be difficult. Presence of telangiectasia and the occurrence of flushing help distinguish this common condition from acne.

Recently, it has been suggested that *Helicobacter pylori* plays a role in the pathogenesis of rosacea.[7] Further work must be done, however, to confirm the contribution of *H. pylori* to this antibiotic-responsive condition.

Treatment

Treatment of acne depends on the type and severity of lesions and on the patient's response to treatment. Comedonal acne is usually best managed with topical retinoids and acne surgery; inflammatory acne is treated with a range of topical therapies and may require oral therapy in moderate to severe cases. Because nodules and cysts are more likely than comedones to scar, they are treated more quickly with oral antibiotics and, if necessary, isotretinoin (see below). Intralesional corticosteroids administered by dermatologists can prevent scarring from cysts. Incision and drainage of infected cysts may be necessary but can contribute to scarring. Unroofing of sinus

Table 2 **Surgical Treatments for Acne Lesions and Acne Scars**

Lesions	Extraction of comedones Drainage of pustules and cysts Intralesional injection of corticosteroids in cysts Excision and unroofing of sinus tracts and cysts
Scars	Dermabrasion Laser abrasion Acid peels Injection of filling materials (e.g., collagen) Excision Punch autographs Intralesional injection of 5-fluorouracil

tracts and other surgical procedures are best performed by physicians with expertise in dermatologic surgery [*see Table 2*]. Scars can be treated with dermabrasion, laser abrasion, or intralesional injection of fluorouracil.[8] The appearance of depressed scars can be improved by chemical peels and other resurfacing procedures, as well as the injection of filler substances such as injectable collagen.[9]

Numerous over-the-counter cleansing agents are available to help patients remove seborrhea and oily debris from the skin, resulting in subjective improvements. Overmanipulation of lesions by picking, squeezing, or excessive washing can lead to exacerbation of lesions and even scarring.

Topical preparations, including sunscreens, soaps, and cosmetics, should be oil-free and noncomedogenic. Numerous over-the-counter oil-free, noncomedogenic moisturizers are available for persons who have dry skin and acne.

There is no role for dietary change in the management of acne. Previous beliefs that chocolate or oily foods cause acne have been disproved.

TOPICAL THERAPY

Comedonal Acne

Topical retinoids are among the most effective therapies for comedonal acne; these preparations unplug follicles and allow penetration of topical antibiotics and benzoyl peroxide. Retinoids can be used in combination with antibacterial agents and are also effective in the management of inflammatory acne. They are often irritating when first applied; patients can reduce the irritation by reducing the frequency of application. Significant improvement is evident within 6 weeks and can continue for 3 to 4 months, at which time the frequency of application can be reduced, depending on the patient's response.

Newer formulations of retinoids that are purportedly less irritating are a tretinoin microsponge vehicle and adapalene, but few comparative studies examining irritation have been performed.[10,11] Tazarotene, a topical retinoid used for acne and psoriasis, can be used effectively in a short-contact method, in which it is applied for seconds to minutes.[12]

Inflammatory Acne

Topical antibiotics are not as effective as retinoids or benzoyl peroxide for inflammatory acne, but they are less irritating and better tolerated. The resistance of *P. acnes* to antibiotics has been well documented; such resistance threatens the usefulness of this form of acne therapy in the future.[13,14] It is therefore useful to use antibiotics in combination with benzoyl peroxide. A new combined formulation of clindamycin 1% and benzoyl peroxide 5% produced faster and greater reductions in *P. acnes* than formulations containing clindamycin alone.[15] Moreover, the combination of benzoyl peroxide and clindamycin resulted in greater improvement in acne than either of its individual components alone.[16]

A commonly used regimen includes the combined antibiotic–benzoyl peroxide gel in the morning and topical retinoid in the evening. Azelaic acid, a recently introduced anticomedonal and antibacterial agent, offers yet another choice for the topical treatment of acne. It, too, can be used in combination with topical retinoids, benzoyl peroxide, or topical antibiotics.[17] Salicylic acid, an over-the-counter comedolytic agent, plays a minor role in the treatment of acne. Skin-colored sul-

Table 3 Topical Therapies for Acne

Medication	Formulation	Frequency of Application	Primary Mechanism of Action	Adverse Effects
Azelaic acid	20% cream	b.i.d.	Anticomedonal, antibacterial	Stinging, irritation
Benzoyl peroxide	2.5%, 5%, 10% creams, gels, lotions, washes	b.i.d.	Antibacterial	Dryness, irritation, allergic contact dermatitis
Antibiotics				
Clindamycin	1% solutions, lotions, gels	b.i.d.	Antibacterial	Antibiotic resistance
Erythromycin	2% solutions, creams, gels, pledgets, wipes	b.i.d.	Antibacterial	Antibiotic resistance
Erythromycin–benzoyl peroxide	3% erythromycin–5% benzoyl peroxide gel	b.i.d.	Antibacterial	Dryness, irritation, allergic contact dermatitis; deteriorates if not refrigerated
Sodium sulfacetamide–sulfur	10% sodium sulfacetamide, 5% sulfur lotions	b.i.d.	Antibacterial	Dryness, irritation, allergic contact dermatitis
Retinoids				
Adapalene	0.1% gels	q.d.	Comedolytic	Dryness, irritation, photosensitivity
Tazarotene	0.05%, 0.1% gels	q.d.	Comedolytic	Dryness, irritation, photosensitivity
Tretinoin	0.025%, 0.05%, 0.1% creams; 0.01%, 0.025% gels; 0.05% solutions	q.d.	Comedolytic	Dryness, irritation, photosensitivity
Sulfur and resorcinol	2% resorcinol, 8% sulfur lotions, creams	q.d., b.i.d.	Comedolytic	Dryness, peeling, allergic contact dermatitis
Salicylic acid	0.5%–2% gels, pads, soaps	q.d., b.i.d.	Comedolytic	Dryness, irritation

fur-resorcinol lotions are available; these very effective drying and peeling agents can be useful for treating individual lesions [*see Table 3*].

SYSTEMIC THERAPY

Systemic agents are warranted for patients with nodulocystic acne or inflammatory acne that is not responsive to topical therapy. Oral antibiotics are usually the first line of systemic treatment. Isotretinoin has generally been reserved for patients whose acne is refractory to antibiotics. To prevent scarring, patients with particularly severe acne are occasionally started on isotretinoin, as are patients with a history of antibiotic intolerance.

Antibiotics

Antibiotics have both antibacterial and anti-inflammatory effects that are beneficial in treating acne. The antibiotics most commonly used for acne are doxycycline, erythromycin, minocycline, tetracycline, and trimethoprim-sulfamethoxazole [*see Table 4*]. Because antibiotic resistance is a major problem with many of the older antibiotics, minocycline has been prescribed for many acne patients even though it is considerably more expensive. Most recently, strains of *P. acnes* that are resistant to minocycline have begun to emerge, and this may limit the usefulness of this drug in the future.[18] The duration of treatment with oral antibiotics depends on patient response. For example, azithromycin given at a dosage of 500 mg/day for 4 days, repeated at 10-day intervals for four cycles, is as effective as minocycline given at a dosage of 100 mg/day for 6 weeks.[19] Further refinements of regimens with these newer antibiotics will undoubtedly be performed before they achieve more widespread usage.

In recent years, a lupuslike syndrome has been reported in patients taking oral minocycline. Synovitis, the presence of antinuclear antibodies, and elevations in hepatic transaminase levels were reported, but renal disease and central nervous system disease do not occur.[20] Upon discontinuance of mino-

cycline, symptoms resolve, but upon retreatment, the syndrome recurs.

Isotretinoin

Oral isotretinoin is the most effective agent available for the treatment of acne. It results in long-lasting remissions or cures in the majority of patients treated. Because of its serious potential adverse effects, however, isotretinoin is not generally used as first-line therapy except for unusual cases.

Most of the side effects of isotretinoin are dose related and affect a majority of patients treated. For example, cheilitis uniformly occurs in patients treated with significant doses. Myalgias, dryness of mucous membranes, dry eczematous skin changes, and hyperlipidemia frequently occur. Total serum cholesterol levels can rise in patients taking isotretinoin, and triglyceride levels can rise sufficiently to cause pancreatitis.

Teratogenicity occurs with even a single dose of isotretinoin administered to pregnant women. Birth control counseling is an essential part of the management of women for whom isotretinoin is prescribed. The use of two forms of contraception is advised. Despite major educational efforts, pregnancies in women receiving isotretinoin continue to occur, resulting in severe birth defects.[21] Consequently, the manufacturers of isotretinoin have started a program in which physicians and pharmacists prescribing and administering isotretinoin must be registered and agree to require pregnancy tests on a regular basis.

There have been several instances of suicide and depression occurring in patients receiving oral isotretinoin.[22] However, teenagers with severe acne may be at increased risk of suicide, regardless of the treatment they are using. A study compared the risk of depression, psychotic symptoms, suicide, and attempted suicide in acne patients receiving isotretinoin and in similar patients being treated with oral antibiotics. The relative risk of depression or psychosis for isotretinoin-treated patients was 1.0, and the relative risk for suicide and attempt-

Table 4 Commonly Prescribed Systemic Therapies for Acne

Medication	Dosage	Advantages	Adverse Effects
Antibiotics			
Doxycycline	50–100 mg p.o., b.i.d.	Inexpensive	Photosensitivity, GI symptoms, candidiasis
Erythromycin	250–500 mg p.o., b.i.d.	Alternative to tetracyclines	GI symptoms, candidiasis
Minocycline	50 mg p.o., q.d.–100 mg p.o., b.i.d.	Highly effective; antibiotic resistance rare at 200 mg/day	GI symptoms, candidiasis, vertigo, lupuslike syndrome (rare), autoimmune hepatitis (rare)
Tetracycline	250 mg p.o., q.d.–500 mg p.o., q.i.d. (b.i.d. dosing preferred)	Inexpensive	Photosensitivity, GI symptoms, candidiasis
Trimethoprim-sulfamethoxazole	160 mg trimethoprim–800 mg sulfamethoxazole b.i.d.	Alternative to tetracyclines and erythromycin	Bone marrow suppression, drug eruption
Other Agents			
Isotretinoin	0.5–2.0 mg/kg/day, in two divided doses	Most effective treatment; long-lasting remissions	Teratogenicity, hyperlipidemia, cheilitis, alopecia, pyogenic granulomas, dry eyes, epistaxis, rare pseudotumor cerebri (especially with concomitant antibiotics)
Norgestimate–ethinyl estradiol	0.18 mg norgestimate, 0.035 mg ethinyl estradiol p.o., q.d., for 21 days, repeat every 4 wk	Alternative to antibiotics and isotretinoin; less androgenic activity than progestins in other contraceptives	Thromboembolic disorders, ?antibiotic interaction, ?increased breast carcinoma, gallbladder disease, reduced glucose tolerance, headache, fluid retention, hypertension, breakthrough bleeding, breast swelling and tenderness

ed suicide was 0.9, suggesting that isotretinoin does not cause depression.[23]

Pseudotumor cerebri, a rare side effect of isotretinoin, occurs more commonly in patients who are concomitantly given oral antibiotics. Extensive counseling and monitoring—including complete blood counts, chemistry screens, and pregnancy tests when appropriate—should be done before treatment with isotretinoin, at 2-week intervals during the first month of treatment, and monthly thereafter. Depending on patient response, treatment with 1 to 2 mg/kg/day in two divided doses should be continued for 4 to 6 months. Some clinicians have continued low-dose isotretinoin therapy for more than 6 months. Rarely, a second course of therapy is indicated when acne recurs. A new micronized formulation of isotretinoin is more bioavailable than other acne treatments and requires taking the medicine only once daily.[24]

Other Therapies

Estrogens in the form of oral contraceptives can be beneficial for patients with acne; progestins, however, can exacerbate the condition. The newer progestins—desogestrel, norgestimate, and gestodene—have less androgenic activity and therefore are less likely to exacerbate acne. A combination of ethinyl estradiol and norgestimate has been shown to be beneficial in the treatment of acne.[25] These agents are ideal in women who are seeking birth control methods and in women who are not candidates for or who have not responded to oral antibiotics or isotretinoin. Oral contraceptives can be particularly helpful to women with the polycystic ovarian syndrome. It is noteworthy that the beneficial effects of combined oral contraceptives are diminished in patients who are obese.[26]

Some concerns have been raised about the concomitant use of antibiotics and oral contraceptives because of the possibility that some antibiotics interfere with contraceptive activity. Reviews of large numbers of patients treated concomitantly with oral contraceptives and antibiotics have not revealed significant increases in pregnancies.[27] Nevertheless, caution is advisable when a patient uses an antibiotic and an oral contraceptive together, especially one of the new low-dose estrogen contraceptives.

Additional Information

Additional information about acne and its related disorders is available from the American Academy of Dermatology (http://www.aad.org) and the National Rosacea Society (http://www.rosacea.org).

References

1. Stoll S, Shalita AR, Webster GF, et al: The effect of the menstrual cycle on acne. J Am Acad Dermatol 45:957, 2001

2. Harris HH, Downing DT, Stewart ME, et al: Sustainable rates of sebum secretion in acne patients and matched normal control subjects. J Am Acad Dermatol 8:200, 1983

3. Tucker SB, Rogers RS III, Winkelmann RK, et al: Inflammation in acne vulgaris: leukocyte attraction and cytotoxicity by comedonal material. J Invest Dermatol 74:21, 1980

4. Leyden JJ, McGinley KJ, Mills OH, et al: Propionibacterium levels in patients with and without acne vulgaris. J Invest Dermatol 65:382, 1975

5. Lucky AW, Biro FM, Huster GA, et al: Acne vulgaris in premenarchal girls: an early sign of puberty associated with rising levels of dehydroepiandrosterone. Arch Dermatol 130:308, 1994

6. Sansone G, Reisner RM: Differential rates of conversion of testosterone to dihydrotestosterone in acne and in normal human skin: a possible pathogenic factor in acne. J Invest Dermatol 56:366, 1971

7. Utas S, Ozbakir O, Turasan A, et al: Helicobacter pylori eradication treatment reduces the severity of rosacea. J Am Acad Dermatol 40:433, 1999

8. Fitzpatrick RE: Treatment of inflamed hypertrophic scars using intralesional 5-FU. Dermatol Surg 25:224, 1999

9. Hirsch RJ, Lewis AB: Treatment of acne scarring. Semin Cutan Med Surg 20:190, 2001

10. Leyden J, Grove GL: Randomized facial tolerability studies comparing gel formulations of retinoids used to treat acne vulgaris. Cutis 67(6 suppl):17, 2001

11. Dunlap FE, Baker MD, Plott RT, et al: Adapalene 0.1% gel has low skin irritation potential even when applied immediately after washing. Br J Dermatol 139(suppl):52, 1998

12. Bershad S, Kranjac Singer G, Parente JE, et al: Successful treatment of acne vulgaris using a new method: results of a randomized vehicle-controlled trial of short-contact therapy with 0.1% tazarotene gel. Arch Dermatol 138:481, 2002

13. Leyden JJ: The evolving role of *Propionibacterium acnes* in acne. Semin Cutan Med Surg 20:139, 2001

14. Dreno B, Reynaud A, Moyse D, et al: Erythromycin-resistance of cutaneous bacterial flora in acne. Eur J Dermatol 11:549, 2001

15. Leyden J, Kaidbey K, Levy SF: The combination formulation of clindamycin 1% plus benzoyl peroxide 5% versus 3 different formulations of topical clindamycin alone in the reduction of *Propionibacterium acnes*: an in vivo comparative study. Am J Clin Dermatol 2:263, 2001

16. Leyden JJ, Berger RS, Dunlap FE, et al: Comparison of the efficacy and safety of a combination topical gel formulation of benzoyl peroxide and clindamycin with benzoyl peroxide, clindamycin and vehicle gel in the treatments of acne vulgaris. Am J Clin Dermatol 2:33, 2001

17. Webster G: Combination azelaic acid therapy for acne vulgaris. J Am Acad Dermatol 43(2 pt 3):S47, 2000

18. Ross JI, Snelling AM, Eady EA, et al: Phenotypic and genotypic characterization of antibiotic-resistant *Propionibacterium acnes* isolated from acne patients attending dermatology clinics in Europe, the U.S.A., Japan and Australia. Br J Dermatol 144:339, 2001

19. Gruber F, Grubisic-Greblo H, Kastelan M, et al: Azithromycin compared with minocycline in the treatment of acne comedonica and papulo-pustulosa. J Chemother 10:469, 1998

20. Lawson TM, Amos N, Bulgen D, et al: Minocycline-induced lupus: clinical features and response to rechallenge. Rheumatology (Oxford) 40:329, 2001

21. Honein MA, Paulozzi LJ, Erickson JD: Continued occurrence of Accutane-exposed pregnancies. Teratology 64:142, 2001

22. Wysowski DK, Pitts M, Beitz J: An analysis of reports of depression and suicide in patients treated with isotretinoin. J Am Acad Dermatol 45:515, 2001

23. Jick SS, Kremers HM, Vasilakis-Scaramozza C: Isotretinoin use and risk of depression, pyschotic symptoms, suicide, and attempted suicide. Arch Dermatol 136:1231, 2000

24. Strauss JS, Leyden JJ, Lucky AW, et al: A randomized trial of the efficacy of a new micronized formulation versus a standard formulation of isotretinoin in patients with severe recalcitrant nodular acne. J Am Acad Dermatol 45:187, 2001

25. Lucky AW, Henderson TA, Olson WH, et al: Effectiveness of norgestimate and ethinyl estradiol in treating moderate acne vulgaris. J Am Acad Dermatol 37:746, 1997

26. Cibula D, Hill M, Fanta M, et al: Does obesity diminish the positive effect of oral contraceptive treatment on hyperandrogenism in women with polycystic ovarian syndrome? Hum Reprod 16:940, 2001

27. London BM, Lookingbill DP: Frequency of pregnancy in acne patients taking oral antibiotics and oral contraceptives. Arch Dermatol 130:392, 1994

Reviews

Brown SK, Shalita AR: Acne vulgaris. Lancet 351:1871, 1998

Munro CS: Acne. J R Coll Physicians Lond 31:360, 1997

32 Papulosquamous Disorders

Elizabeth A. Abel, M.D.

Papulosquamous disorders comprise a group of dermatoses that have distinct morphologic features.[1] The characteristic primary lesion of these disorders is a papule, usually erythematous, that has a variable amount of scale on the surface. Plaques or patches form through coalescence of the primary lesions. Some common papulosquamous dermatoses are pityriasis rosea, lichen planus, seborrheic dermatitis, tinea corporis, pityriasis rubra pilaris, psoriasis [see Chapter 33], and parapsoriasis. Drug eruptions, tinea corporis, and secondary syphilis may also have a papulosquamous morphology. Some papulosquamous disorders may be a cutaneous manifestation of AIDS as well.[2]

Pityriasis Rosea

Pityriasis rosea is a relatively common, self-limited, exanthematous disease characterized by oval papulosquamous lesions on the trunk and proximal areas of the extremities. Pityriasis rosea typically appears during the spring and fall; its incidence is highest in persons between 10 and 35 years of age.[3,4]

A population-based, 10-year epidemiologic survey identified 939 patients with pityriasis rosea, about one third of whom had antecedent acute infection or atopy.[5] It also showed that peak incidence occurred at 20 to 24 years of age, that the incidence was higher in colder months, and that recurrences were rare. Occurrences among household contacts are uncommon. This study also noted that the incidence of disease had appeared to decline.

ETIOLOGY

A viral etiology has been suggested for pityriasis rosea on the basis of immunologic and histologic data. The superficial dermis contains aggregates of CD4$^+$ helper T cells in perivascular locations and increased numbers of Langerhans cells. It has been postulated that IgM antibodies to keratinocytes cause the secondary form of the eruption. An association between human herpesvirus type 7 (HHV-7) and pityriasis rosea was initially reported in 1997.[6] More recent studies, however, suggested that pityriasis rosea was not associated with HHV-7; these studies used polymerase chain reaction and immunohistochemical analyses of tissue samples to detect HHV-7 DNA sequences and antigens. In a retrospective study of 13 patients and 14 control subjects, the prevalence of HHV-7 was lower in lesional skin of patients with pityriasis rosea than in control subjects.[7] A subsequent seroepidemiologic study of HHV-6 and HHV-7 was conducted in 44 patients with pityriasis rosea and in 25 patients with other skin eruptions. Although in this study several patients with pityriasis rosea had antibody titers consistent with active infection, the overall prevalence of HHV-6 and HHV-7 was no greater in patients with pityriasis rosea than in control subjects.[8] A viral etiology of pityriasis rosea thus remains elusive.

Certain drugs that cause a pityriasis rosea–like eruption have been implicated in the etiology of this disorder. These drugs include the antihypertensive agent captopril, metronidazole, isotretinoin (13-*cis*-retinoic acid), penicillamine, arsenic, gold, bismuth, barbiturates, and clonidine.[4]

DIAGNOSIS

The primary lesion, called a herald patch, appears first as a slightly raised, salmon-colored oval patch with a fine, wrinkled scale resembling cigarette paper. Typically, 7 to 10 days after the appearance of the herald patch, there occurs a bilaterally symmetrical eruption; this eruption occurs mainly on the trunk and upper extremities [see Figure 1]. Lesions tend to fall in cleavage planes in a so-called fir tree distribution and are occasionally pruritic. Atypical manifestations occur in 20% of those affected. Such manifestations include a purpuric form of pityriasis rosea that resembles vasculitis, as well as papular, vesicular, pustular, and urticarial forms. An inverse variant of pityriasis rosea, more common in children than in adults, is characterized by lesions on the face and extremities, with relatively few lesions appearing on the trunk.[4]

DIFFERENTIAL DIAGNOSIS

Because lesions of pityriasis rosea may closely resemble those of secondary syphilis, a serologic test for syphilis may be indicated. Lesions may also resemble tinea corporis or tinea versicolor and should be examined by fungal scrapings and potassium hydroxide (KOH) wet mounts. A careful drug history must be obtained to exclude the possibility of a drug eruption.

TREATMENT

Pityriasis rosea lesions resolve spontaneously after 6 to 8 weeks. The patient should be reassured that the disorder is benign and self-limited; such reassurance, together with educating the patient about the disease, is the most important aspect of treatment. Lesions are variably pruritic. Symptoms should be treated with bland emollients or systemic antipruritics. Sun exposure may accelerate clearing. Irradiation with ultraviolet B (UVB) sunlamps is beneficial in decreasing the severity of disease, especially when treatment is initiated within the first week of the eruption. One study found that 10 erythemogenic exposures of UVB substantially decreased the extent of pityriasis rosea, although it neither altered the duration of the disorder nor improved the itching.[9]

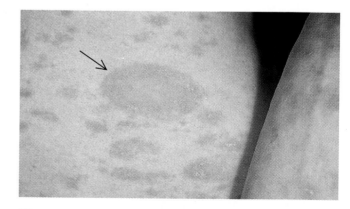

Figure 1 **Pityriasis rosea commonly presents with a single large salmon-colored plaque called a herald patch (arrow). Appearance of the isolated lesion is followed in a week to 10 days by a bilaterally symmetrical papulosquamous eruption, mainly on the trunk and upper extremities.**

411

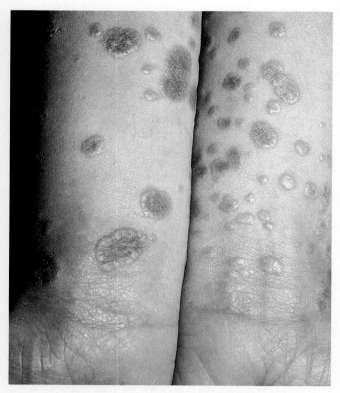

Figure 2 **Violaceous, flat-topped, polygonal papules are typical of lichen planus. A common location is the flexor aspect of the wrists and forearms.**

In a double-blind, placebo-controlled study in India, oral erythromycin administered in divided doses for 14 days was effective in treating patients with pityriasis rosea.[10] In this cohort, upper respiratory tract infections preceded the skin eruption in 68.8% of the 90 patients. A complete response, with complete resolution of skin lesions occurring within 2 weeks, was reported in 33% of the treatment group, as compared with 0% in the placebo group. The duration of disease was comparable for both groups of patients. Although not all patients with pityriasis rosea are benefited by erythromycin therapy, a trial of erythromycin is a safe treatment approach.

Lichen Planus

Lichen planus is a localized or generalized eruption with violaceous, flat-topped, polygonal papules and little or no observable scale [*see Figure 2*]. It is often localized to the oral mucosa; 25% of patients with oral lichen planus have skin involvement as well.[11] The incidence is highest in young to middle-aged persons. Lichen planus usually appears in the fifth or sixth decade and affects women more than men.

ETIOLOGY

The etiology of lichen planus is unknown. An alteration in basal keratinocytes that induces humoral and cell-mediated immune responses has been postulated as a mechanism. Skin and mucous membrane lesions resembling lichen planus have been observed in patients with graft versus host disease (GVHD) [*see Chapter 36*]. Lichen planus has also been associated with other immune-mediated diseases, including ulcerative colitis, bullous pemphigoid, myasthenia gravis with thymoma, primary biliary cirrhosis, and chronic active hepatitis.[12] There is an increased prevalence of viral hepatitis, especially hepatitis C,[13] in patients with lichen planus. In an epidemiologic study of 30 sequential patients with lichen planus in Miami (a geographic area of high reactivity), the prevalence of hepatitis C virus was 23%, compared with 4.8% in control subjects. Two patients with lichen planus and hepatitis C recovered after treatment with interferon alfa. There are a number of reports of lichen planus occurring after administration of different types of hepatitis B vaccine.[14] This is a rare occurrence, considering the widespread use of this vaccine; several cases have been reported from France and Italy, and one case has been reported from the Middle East. As with GVHD, an immunologic mechanism has been postulated as the cause. The latency period ranges from several days to 3 months after any one of the three usual injections of vaccine.

A variety of drugs have been reported to cause lichenoid reactions in the skin, usually sparing the mucous membranes. Such drugs include beta blockers, methyldopa, penicillamine, quinidine, and quinine. Other drugs that have been implicated but for which causal evidence is insufficient include angiotensin-converting enzyme inhibitors, sulfonylurea agents, carbamazepine, gold, and lithium.[15] In one study, the administration of penicillamine for primary biliary cirrhosis was followed by the development of lichen planus in 17 of 24 patients[16];

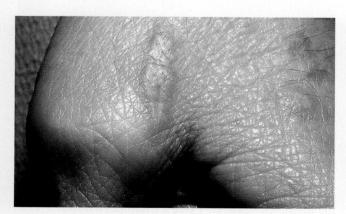

Figure 3 **The Koebner phenomenon, the appearance of lesions along a scratch line, may be seen in patients with lichen planus.**

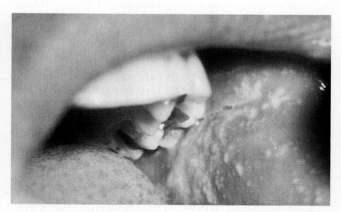

Figure 4 **Lichen planus of the mucous membrane assumes a white, reticulated mosaic pattern, as seen above on the buccal mucosa.**

in addition, after treatment with penicillamine, the skin eruption became worse in three of seven patients with biliary cirrhosis and preexisting lichen planus. Nonsteroidal anti-inflammatory agents have been documented to cause a lichenoid drug eruption; these drugs include naproxen, indomethacin, diflunisal, ibuprofen, acetylsalicylic acid, and salsalate.[17] Although the latency period is highly variable, symptoms usually develop within a few months after drug initiation and resolve within weeks to months after discontinuance of the offending agent.

DIAGNOSIS

Lichen planus appears as flat-topped, shiny, violaceous papules, often with a fine, reticulated scale on the surface. Common sites of involvement include the skin, nails, mucous membranes, vulva, and penis. Wickham striae—white lacy patterns on the papule surface—are apparent on magnification with a hand lens.[18] The occurrence of papules along a scratch line, as in linear lichen planus, is referred to as the Koebner phenomenon [see Figure 3]. In the hypertrophic form of the disease, papules coalesce to form thick plaques or nodules that are often found on the lower extremities. Pruritus may be severe, particularly in the generalized or hypertrophic forms of the disease. Common sites of involvement are the flexor surfaces of the wrists, the sacrum, the mucous membranes of the mouth, the medial thighs, and the genitalia. Mucous membrane lesions show a white, reticulated mosaic pattern [see Figure 4]. A severe erosive form of lichen planus can involve the oral mucous membranes. In rare cases, lesions occur in the esophagus, causing esophageal stricture and dysphagia.[19]

A follicular form known as lichen planopilaris may result in scarring alopecia. Variants of lichen planus with distinct morphologic features include actinic, annular, bullous, hypertrophic, linear, ulcerative, and zosteriform forms. The nails may also be involved [see Chapter 43]. The clinical features of some forms of lichen planus may resemble those of lupus erythematosus.[18]

Skin biopsy confirms the clinical diagnosis of lichen planus. Typically, the epidermis shows hyperkeratosis, a prominent granular layer, liquefaction degeneration of the basal cell layer, and an intense upper dermal inflammatory infiltrate. Immunoperoxidase studies using monoclonal antibodies to cell surface antigens have shown that most cells in the infiltrate are of the helper-inducer T cell subset. Colloid bodies (Civatte bodies) coated with immunoglobulin are frequently seen in the dermal papillae. On ultrastructural examination, numerous Langerhans cells can be observed at the dermoepidermal junction.

TREATMENT

Patients who experience an acute outbreak of lichen planus have a good prognosis; in most cases, the papules clear within several months to a year. The chronic form, however, may last for 10 years or longer. The long-term course of lichen planus was followed in 214 patients for 8 to 12 years. In two thirds of the patients, lichen planus had cleared within 1 year. The recurrence rate was 49%, which was higher than recurrence rates reported in previous studies; the authors attributed the high rate of recurrence to treatment with potent topical corticosteroids.[20]

Emollients, topical glucocorticoids, a short course of systemic corticosteroids, and systemic antipruritics have been used to treat the symptoms of lichen planus. Oral metronidazole is an alternative therapy that may have immunomodulatory and antimicrobial action.[21] In a trial of oral psoralen photochemotherapy for widespread recalcitrant lichen planus, clinical remission occurred in six of seven patients and correlated with the disappearance of the upper dermal infiltrate.[22] Systemic retinoids, such as acitretin, are beneficial in some patients with oral and cutaneous forms of lichen planus. Azathioprine has been used for its steroid-sparing effect in erosive and generalized lichen planus.[23] Recombinant interferon alfa-2b, administered subcutaneously every other day, was successful in the treatment of generalized lichen planus in three patients with no evidence of hepatitis, further supporting the cell-mediated immunologic etiology of this disease.[24] Oral cyclosporine has also been effective, but potential renal toxicity and hypertension limit its long-term use.[18]

For lichen planus that is localized to the oral mucosa, a high-potency corticosteroid such as clobetasol in a vehicle that is adherent to the mucosal surface (Orabase) is helpful.[25] Intralesional injections of corticosteroids may be used to treat localized, recalcitrant lesions. Use of miconazole gel in combination with chlorhexidine mouth rinses is effective for prophylaxis against oral candidiasis.[25] Topical isotretinoin gel is an effective alternative to corticosteroids, although relapses often occur after discontinuance of this medication.[26] In a double-blind, placebo-controlled study of 22 patients with biopsy-proven oral lichen planus, an 8-week course of 0.1% isotretinoin gel is found to be effective.[26] Cyclosporine mouth rinses have been helpful for some patients. Topical tacrolimus, a macrolide that suppresses T cell activation, was used to treat erosive mucosal lichen planus in six patients whose conditions were resistant to conventional treatment. In three of the patients, disease resolved completely; the other three patients experienced significant improvement of the symptoms of pain and burning.[27] A 6-month course of hydroxychloroquine, 200 to 400 mg daily, was successful as monotherapy in nine of 10 patients with oral lichen planus; ulcers healed and pain decreased after 1 to 2 months.[28]

Seborrheic Dermatitis

Seborrheic dermatitis is a papulosquamous condition that is often associated with excessive oiliness or seborrhea, dandruff, and well-defined red, scaly patches on the face, trunk, and intertriginous areas.[29] Some cases may progress to a severe exfoliative erythroderma. Seborrheic dermatitis is a common skin disorder that occurs in otherwise healthy adults. It is increasingly prevalent in middle-aged and elderly persons. Seborrheic dermatitis does not occur before puberty except during infancy (usually between 2 and 12 weeks of age), at which time transplacentally derived maternal hormones are present. The prognosis in adults is one of lifelong recurrence, with each episode lasting weeks to months.

ETIOLOGY

The cause of seborrheic dermatitis is unknown. An occasional association with neurologic abnormalities, especially parkinsonism, has been observed. Genetic predisposition, emotional stress, diet, hormones, and climatic factors may also influence this disorder. Infection with the yeastlike organism Pityrosporum has also been implicated.

Patients with classic seborrheic dermatitis may have normal or reduced rates of sebum excretion; therefore, seborrhea is not essential for the development of this disorder.[30] However, seborrhea may play a role in the seborrheic dermatitis present in certain patients, such as those with parkinsonism. Reduction of

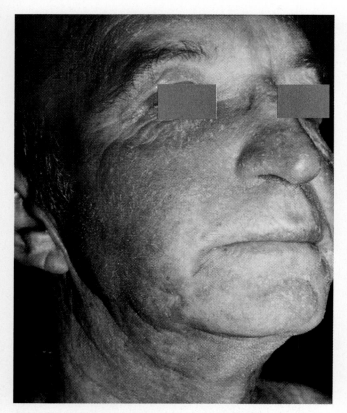

Figure 5 **Seborrheic dermatitis seen on the face of this patient involves sites of sebaceous gland activity.**

seborrhea with improvement of the dermatitis has been observed after a favorable neurologic response to levodopa treatment for parkinsonism.

DIAGNOSIS

The scale associated with seborrheic dermatitis may be yellowish and either dry or greasy. Sites of predilection are in areas of sebaceous gland activity [*see Figure 5*], such as the scalp, eyebrows, eyelids, forehead, nasolabial folds, and presternal or interscapular regions. Blepharitis involves granular inflammation of the lid margin with scaling and shedding of debris into the eye, which may cause conjunctivitis. Seborrheic dermatitis is the most common cause of otitis externa. When the scalp is involved, lesions often extend along the frontal hairline, forming a band of erythema. The postauricular area is a common site of involvement. Lesions of the trunk may consist of erythematous follicular papules covered by greasy scales, which may coalesce to form large plaques or circinate patches. Seborrheic dermatitis can be seen in areas of male pattern baldness, but it is not a cause of hair loss unless there has been a severe intervening secondary infection resulting in a scarring alopecia.

DIFFERENTIAL DIAGNOSIS

Seborrheic dermatitis should be considered in the differential diagnosis of chronic eczematous dermatitis and in that of papulosquamous disorders, particularly psoriasis. The clinical features of seborrheic dermatitis limited to the scalp and face may resemble those associated with psoriasis, giving rise to the term sebopsoriasis. Histologic features range from psoriasiform changes of acanthosis and parakeratosis to the spongiosis

of eczema. Seborrheic dermatitis of the face may resemble the facial lesions found in lupus erythematosus or other photosensitivity dermatoses. Lesions on the trunk may be confused with tinea versicolor, but the latter is easily excluded by skin scraping and KOH preparation or Wood light examination. Atopic dermatitis and psoriasis, especially when partially treated, are also included in the differential diagnosis.

SEBORRHEIC DERMATITIS ASSOCIATED WITH AIDS

Severe seborrheic dermatitis can be one of the most common and earliest manifestations of AIDS. From 30% to 80% of patients with AIDS have seborrheic dermatitis, compared with 3% to 5% of HIV-negative young adults.[31] Lesions may be explosive in onset and are often resistant to therapy. Clinical features include a predominantly inflammatory papular eruption on the face, with a tendency to spare the scalp, in contrast to the mild erythema and scaling of the scalp typical of seborrheic dermatitis in persons without AIDS. Truncal involvement in seborrheic areas is common in AIDS patients, and the lesions may resemble psoriasis. Although the cause of the association of seborrheic dermatitis with AIDS is unknown, immunologic dysfunction may lead to an overgrowth of the yeast *P. orbiculare* in seborrheic areas.

Skin biopsy specimens from AIDS patients with seborrheic dermatitis have distinct histologic features, including keratinocyte necrosis, leukoexocytosis, a superficial perivascular infiltrate of plasma cells, and, frequently, neutrophils.[32]

TREATMENT

The condition on the scalp usually responds well to frequent—as often as daily—shampooing with a preparation containing 3% to 5% sulfur and 2% to 3% salicylic acid. For the face and nonhairy areas, a mild cream containing precipitated 3% sulfur and 3% salicylic acid is effective. Involved areas also respond well to low-potency topical glucocorticoids, such as 1% hydrocortisone cream or desonide cream. Caution, however, must be exercised in the use of high-potency fluorinated steroid preparations, especially on the face and in skin folds; prolonged application may lead to chronic skin changes, such as atrophy and telangiectasia. Wet dressings followed by a topical antibiotic preparation are helpful in treating intertriginous areas, in which maceration and superficial secondary infection may occur.

Ketoconazole has a potent antifungal effect on the lipophilic yeast *Pityrosporum*, which is an etiologic factor in seborrheic dermatitis. In one study, 575 patients with seborrheic dermatitis underwent twice-weekly treatments with 2% ketoconazole shampoo; an excellent response was seen in 88% of the patients.[33] Continued prophylactic treatment once weekly over 6 months was helpful in preventing relapse of the disorder in a significant number of patients.

In a study of the effect of ketoconazole on living and killed *Staphylococcus aureus* in an animal model, ketoconazole was found to have antibacterial and anti-inflammatory effects when compared with hydrocortisone acetate. The anti-inflammatory effect was caused by ketoconazole's inhibition of the lipoxygenase pathway, which resulted in a decrease in the production of leukotrienes. Ketoconazole inhibits keratinocytes by interfering with cholesterol biosynthesis.[34]

In a trial of 38 patients with seborrheic dermatitis, 1% metronidazole gel was found to be effective. Improvement was noted after 2 weeks, and marked improvement or complete clearing was noted at 8 weeks.[35]

Seborrheic blepharitis may be treated by applying baby shampoo with a cotton-tipped applicator to debride scales. If topical corticosteroids are required, the patient should be referred to an ophthalmologist to monitor potential side effects to the eye, such as increased intraocular pressure, glaucoma, cataracts, and activation of latent herpes infection.[1]

Treatment of HIV-associated seborrheic dermatitis is similar to that of seborrheic dermatitis in general, although HIV-associated seborrheic dermatitis is apt to be recalcitrant, requiring intensive, prolonged therapy. Treatment of the underlying HIV infection may lead to improvement of the associated seborrheic dermatitis.

Pityriasis Rubra Pilaris

Pityriasis rubra pilaris is a relatively uncommon chronic inflammatory dermatosis that is considered to be a disorder of keratinization. The age distribution is bimodal, occurring either in childhood or in the fifth decade; the clinical course is variable. An autosomal dominant inheritance has been postulated for the juvenile form of the disease.[36] Patients with the classic adult form of the disease have the best prognosis; resolution usually occurs over a 3-year period.

DIAGNOSIS

Typically, pityriasis rubra pilaris initially manifests as a seborrheic dermatitis–like eruption that occurs in sun-exposed areas of the body; there then occurs the development of follicular papules that coalesce into psoriasiform patches on the trunk and extremities, with progression to erythroderma. Generalized involvement is characterized by yellow-orange erythema with desquamation. Diffuse areas of involvement

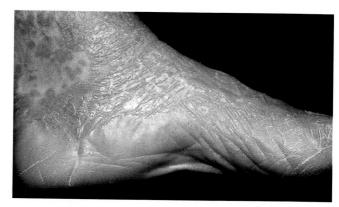

Figure 7 Plantar hyperkeratosis and confluent erythematous follicular papules typical of pityriasis rubra pilaris are seen on the ankle and foot of this patient.

generally show islands of spared skin [*see Figure 6*]. Additional features are palmoplantar hyperkeratosis [*see Figure 7*] and prominent follicular plugging over the dorsal aspects of the fingers. Pruritus is usually mild or absent. A pityriasis rubra pilaris–like eruption with follicular hyperkeratosis is a little-known but distinctive cutaneous manifestation of dermatomyositis.[37]

TREATMENT

The response of patients with pityriasis rubra pilaris to conventional antipsoriatic therapies, such as topical corticosteroids, tars, and oral methotrexate, is often unsatisfactory; some patients, however, have shown a favorable response to topical calcipotriene (known outside the United States as calcipotriol).[38] Ultraviolet B phototherapy may exacerbate the disease.[39] High-dose vitamin A in excess of 200,000 IU daily has been used but can cause liver or central nervous system toxicity. An oral retinoid such as etretinate or, more recently, acitretin is indicated for the treatment of pityriasis rubra pilaris in men and postmenopausal women. In an early study involving 45 patients with pityriasis rubra pilaris, isotretinoin produced definite improvement in 50% of the patients after 4 weeks of therapy.[40] Remission of up to 6 months was sustained in some patients after the drug was withdrawn. Long-term use of this drug in patients with keratinizing disorders has been associated with irreversible skeletal toxicity. Because teratogenicity is a concern, women of childbearing age must use effective birth control with either agent. Although acitretin has a shorter half-life and is, therefore, less teratogenic than etretinate, ingestion of alcohol can convert acitretin to the prodrug etretinate; thus, the risk of birth defects associated with acitretin would be the same as that incurred with etretinate.

In one study, retinoid therapy consisting mainly of etretinate, 25 to 75 mg/day, or isotretinoin resulted in 25% to 75% improvement in 17 of 24 patients after 16 weeks of therapy.[41] Concomitant or subsequent methotrexate therapy was used in 11 of these patients who had recalcitrant disabling disease. There is concern, however, about potential hepatotoxicity in patients receiving this combination. Cyclosporine, 5 mg/kg/day, was effective in the treatment of three adult patients with pityriasis rubra pilaris. A favorable response was noted within 2 to 4 weeks of initiation of therapy, but relapse occurred when the dose was decreased to 1.2 mg/kg/day.[42]

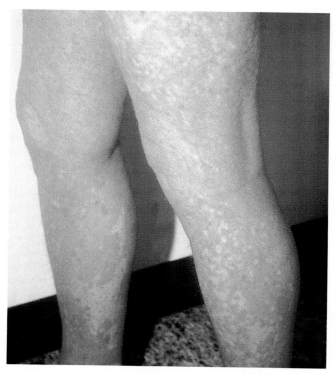

Figure 6 Islands of spared skin within a background of diffuse erythema are present on the legs of this patient with pityriasis rubra pilaris.

Parapsoriasis

Parapsoriasis encompasses a variety of relatively uncommon chronic inflammatory dermatoses of unknown etiology that are resistant to conventional treatment. Despite the designation parapsoriasis, the clinical appearance of the noninfiltrated scaly patches or plaques is distinct from that of psoriatic lesions. Classification of these disorders is controversial and further complicated by the use of several terms to denote a single entity and by the use of various systems of nomenclature. A proposed standard nomenclature divides parapsoriasis into two distinct subgroups: pityriasis lichenoides, which may be acute or chronic, and small- and large-plaque parapsoriasis.[43]

PITYRIASIS LICHENOIDES

Diagnosis

The acute form of pityriasis lichenoides, also known as pityriasis lichenoides et varioliformis acuta (PLEVA) or Mucha-Habermann disease, is characterized by the abrupt onset of a generalized eruption of reddish-brown maculopapules that evolve during a period of weeks to months. Lesions are typically present at all stages of evolution and may be vesicular, hemorrhagic, crusted, or necrotic [see Figure 8]. Healing with varioliform scarring is common. Nonspecific histologic features include intraepidermal lymphocytes and erythrocytes, dermal hemorrhage, and a lymphocytic vasculitis.[44] Skin lesions of PLEVA may resemble those of lymphomatoid papulosa, which has immunohistologic features of a CD30+ cutaneous T cell lymphoma. Lymphomatoid papulosa occurs as a chronic, recurrent, self-healing papulonodular eruption; an association with mycosis fungoides has been observed in some patients. T cell clonality has been documented by PCR in 20 patients with PLEVA; similar findings have been made in patients with lymphomatoid papulosis.[45] Investigators have suggested that PLEVA is a lymphoproliferative process rather

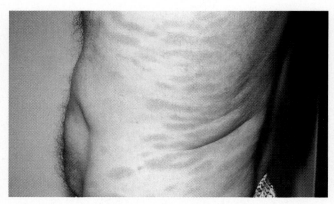

Figure 9   The digitate variant of small-plaque parapsoriasis is seen in this patient.

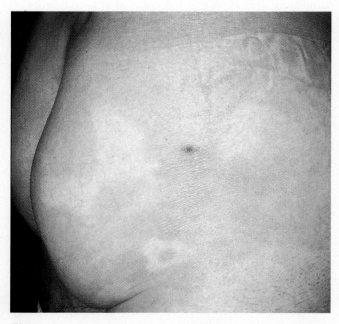

Figure 10   Large-plaque parapsoriasis as seen on the buttocks of this patient may eventuate in cutaneous T cell lymphoma.

than an inflammatory reaction to various trigger factors, such as infectious agents.

A chronic form of pityriasis lichenoides, pityriasis lichenoides chronica, shows milder skin changes without necrosis. Lesions evolve during a period of weeks and may recur over many years.

Treatment

Treatment of both acute and chronic forms of pityriasis lichenoides is generally unsatisfactory. Topical corticosteroids, tars, and systemically administered methotrexate have all been tried, with variable success. Ultraviolet radiation from sunlamps[46] and oral psoralen photochemotherapy[47] may have a beneficial effect on the course of disease. Treatment with high-dose tetracycline, 2 g/day for 1 month or more, has also been effective in clearing the condition.[48] Minocycline, 100 mg once or twice daily, is also beneficial. A rare type of PLEVA known as Degos disease (also called malignant atrophic papulosis), characterized by fever and hemorrhagic and papulonecrotic lesions, responds rapidly to the administration of methotrexate [see Chapter 117].[49]

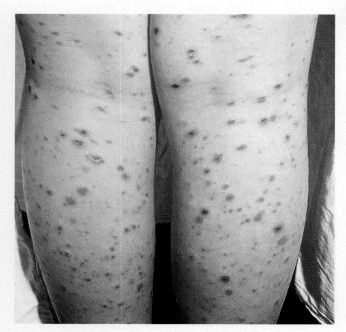

Figure 8   Hemorrhagic brown-crusted varioliform papules are present on the lower legs of this patient with the acute form of pityriasis lichenoides.

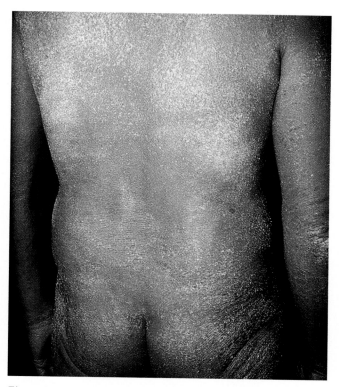

Figure 11 Erythroderma, which appears as total skin erythema and scaling, can occur as a result of papulosquamous and eczematous disorders caused by a variety of diseases. Cutaneous T cell lymphoma, as seen in this patient with Sézary syndrome, can result in erythroderma.

SMALL- AND LARGE-PLAQUE PARAPSORIASIS

Diagnosis

Small-plaque parapsoriasis consists of slightly scaly, thin, oval erythematous plaques of less than 5 cm in diameter, commonly located on the trunk and proximal extremities. The variant—digitate dermatosis—shows elongated lesions falling along lines of skin cleavage. The two diseases follow similar chronic, benign courses [*see Figure 9*].

Clinically, large-plaque parapsoriasis consists of slightly thickened, red-brown, scaly plaques that are more than 10 cm in diameter and have ill-defined borders; such lesions are present mainly on the proximal extremities and the buttocks and on the breasts of women [*see Figure 10*]. Frequently, there is a component of poikiloderma, which includes mottled hyperpigmentation and hypopigmentation, atrophy, and telangiectasia. Early lesions may show a nonspecific histology; late lesions show atypical lymphocytes within the epidermis.

It is important to differentiate large-plaque parapsoriasis from the small-plaque form because about 10% of cases of large-plaque parapsoriasis result in a cutaneous T cell lymphoma (mycosis fungoides).[43] Large-plaque lesions may be present for many years before malignant transformation is recognized histologically. The malignant change is suggested clinically by increased pruritus and progressive induration of lesions. The retiform variant may show prominent poikiloderma with atrophy and has a greater potential for malignant transformation.[50] Studies of T cell subsets using monoclonal antibodies to membrane markers have shown a variable predominance of helper T cells in the cutaneous infiltrates in atrophic

parapsoriasis; such findings suggest a similarity to lesions of mycosis fungoides, although epidermotropism is absent.[51] Patients with this form of the disease should be evaluated with repeated biopsies of untreated lesions. Once a definitive diagnosis of mycosis fungoides has been established, specific treatment of this disease may be instituted.

Treatment

Treatment of large- and small-plaque parapsoriasis is similar to that of pityriasis lichenoides chronica [*see Pityriasis Lichenoides, above*].

Erythroderma

Papulosquamous and psoriasiform eczematous dermatitis may progress to generalized skin involvement with erythema and scaling, known as exfoliative erythroderma. Other causes of erythroderma include drug eruption, contact dermatitis, and pityriasis rubra pilaris. Eyrthroderma is a rare skin disorder that occurs more often as an exacerbation of a preexisting skin disorder; less commonly, it is idiopathic. There are no accurate studies on the incidence of erythroderma. However, on the basis of a survey of all dermatologists in The Netherlands, the annual incidence was estimated to be 1 to 2 patients per 100,000 inhabitants.[52]

DIAGNOSIS

Most cases of exfoliative erythroderma are associated with exacerbation of an underlying dermatosis, such as psoriasis, pityriasis rubra pilaris, seborrheic dermatitis, drug eruptions, atopic dermatitis, or contact dermatitis. Some patients have idiopathic erythroderma, also called red man syndrome.[51] Common associated skin findings include palmoplantar keratoderma, alopecia, and nail dystrophy. Skin biopsy usually shows nonspecific inflammation. Lymph node biopsy may reveal dermatopathic lymphadenopathy. In some patients, idiopathic erythroderma may progress to cutaneous T cell lymphoma (e.g., erythrodermic mycosis fungoides and Sézary syndrome) [*see Figure 11*] [*see Chapter 41*].

Systemic symptoms associated with erythroderma include fever and chills, dehydration from transepidermal water loss, and high-output cardiac failure.

TREATMENT

Nonspecific treatment includes restoration of fluid and electrolyte balance and supportive measures such as administration of antipruritics, application of cool compresses and mild topical corticosteroids, and bed rest. Antibiotics may be required for treatment of secondary bacterial infection. Generally, more aggressive topical and systemic therapies are avoided until the inflammation subsides. More specific treatment depends on the underlying diagnosis and cause of the erythroderma. For example, in patients with erythroderma that is secondary to Sézary syndrome, treatment would be directed toward the underlying cutaneous T cell lymphoma [*see Chapter 41*]. For erythroderma caused by a drug eruption, the offending drug must be discontinued. Systemic agents such as acitretin and methotrexate may be used to treat psoriatic erythroderma [*see Chapter 33*].

References

1. Fox BJ, Odom RB: Papulosquamous diseases: a review. J Am Acad Dermatol 12:597, 1985

2. Sadick NS, McNutt NS, Kaplan MH: Papulosquamous dermatoses of AIDS. J Am Acad Dermatol 22:1270, 1990

3. Allen RA, Janniger CK, Schwartz RA: Pityriasis rosea. Cutis 56:198, 1995

4. Chuang T-Y, Ilstrup DM, Perry HO, et al: Pityriasis rosea in Rochester, Minnesota, 1969 to 1978: a 10-year epidemiologic study. J Am Acad Dermatol 7:80, 1982

5. Parsons JM: Pityriasis rosea update: 1986. J Am Acad Dermatol 15:159, 1986

6. Drago F, Ranieri E, Malaguti F, et al: Human herpesvirus 7 in 7 patients with pityriasis rosea. Dermatology 195:374, 1997

7. Kempf W, Adams V, Kleinhans M, et al: Pityriasis rosea is not associated with human herpesvirus 7. Arch Dermatol 135:1070, 1999

8. Kosuge H, Tanaka-Taya K, Miyoshi H, et al: Epidemiological study of human herpesvirus–6 and human herpesvirus–7 in pityriasis rosea. Br J Dermatol 143:795, 2000

9. Leenutaphong V, Jiamton S: UVB phototherapy for pityriasis rosea: a bilateral comparison study. J Am Acad Dermatol 33:996, 1995

10. Sharma PK, Yadav TP, Gautam RK, et al: Erythromycin in pityriasis rosea: a double-blind placebo-controlled clinical trial. J Am Acad Dermatol 42:241, 2000

11. Bricker SL: Oral lichen planus: a review. Semin Dermatol 13:87, 1994

12. Shai A, Halevy S: Lichen planus and lichen planus-like eruptions: pathogenesis and associated diseases. Int J Dermatol 31:379, 1992

13. Bellman B, Reddy R, Falanga V: Generalized lichen planus associated with hepatitis C virus immunoreactivity. J Am Acad Dermatol 35:770, 1996

14. Al-Khenaizan S: Lichen planus occurring after hepatitis B vaccination: a new case. J Am Acad Dermatol 45:614, 2001

15. Thompson DF, Skaehill PA: Drug-induced lichen planus. Pharmacotherapy 14:561, 1994

16. Powell FC, Rogers RS III, Dickson ER: Primary biliary cirrhosis and lichen planus. J Am Acad Dermatol 9:540, 1983

17. Powell ML, Ehrlich A, Belsito DV: Lichenoid drug eruption to salsalate. J Am Acad Dermatol 45:616, 2001

18. Boyd AS, Neldner KH: Lichen planus. J Am Acad Dermatol 25:593, 1991

19. Abraham SC, Ravich WJ, Anhalt GJ, et al: Esophageal lichen planus: case report and review of the literature. Am J Surg Pathol 24:1678, 2000

20. Irvine C, Irvine F, Champion RH: Long-term follow-up of lichen planus. Acta Derm Venereol 71:242, 1991

21. Büyük AY, Kavala M: Oral metronidazole treatment of lichen planus. J Am Acad Dermatol 43:260, 2000

22. Ortonne JP, Thivolet J, Sannwald C: Oral photochemotherapy in the treatment of lichen planus (LP): clinical results, histological and ultrastructural observations. Br J Dermatol 99:77, 1978

23. Lear JT, English JS: Erosive and generalized lichen planus responsive to azathioprine. Clin Exp Dermatol 21:56, 1996

24. Hildebrand A, Kolde G, Luger TA, et al: Successful treatment of generalized lichen planus with recombinant interferon alfa-2b. J Am Acad Dermatol 33:880, 1995

25. Carbone M, Conrotto D, Carrozzo M, et al: Topical corticosteroids in association with miconazole and chlorhexidine in the long-term management of atrophic-erosive oral lichen planus: a placebo-controlled and comparative study between clobetasol and fluocinonide. Oral Dis 5:44, 1999

26. Giustina TA, Stewart JB, Ellis CN, et al: Topical application of oral isotretinoin gel improves oral lichen planus: a double-blind study. Arch Dermatol 122:534, 1986

27. Vente C, Reich K, Rupprecht R, et al: Erosive mucosal lichen planus: response to topical treatment with tacrolimus. Br J Dermatol 140:338, 1999

28. Eisen D: Hydroxychloroquine sulfate (Plaquenil) improves oral lichen planus: an open trial. J Am Acad Dermatol 28:609, 1993

29. Plewig G: Seborrheic dermatitis. Dermatology in General Medicine, 4th ed, Vol 1. Fitzpatrick TB, Eisen AZ, Wolff K, et al, Eds. McGraw-Hill Book Co, New York, 1993, p 1569

30. Burton JL, Pye RJ: Seborrhoea is not a feature of seborrhoeic dermatitis. Br Med J 26:1169, 1983

31. Odom RB: Common superficial fungal infections in immunosuppressed patients. J Am Acad Dermatol 31:S56, 1994

32. Soeprono FF, Schinella RA, Cockerell CJ, et al: Seborrheic-like dermatitis of acquired immunodeficiency syndrome: a clinicopathologic study. J Am Acad Dermatol 14:242, 1986

33. Peter RU, Richarz-Barthauer U: Successful treatment and prophylaxis of scalp seborrhoeic dermatitis and dandruff with 2% ketoconazole shampoo: results of a multicentre, double-blind, placebo-controlled trial. Br J Dermatol 132:441, 1995

34. Van Cutsem J, Van Gerven F, Cauwenbergh G, et al: The anti-inflammatory effects of ketoconazole. J Am Acad Dermatol 25:257, 1991

35. Parsad D, Pandhi R, Negi KS, et al: Topical metronidazole in seborrheic dermatitis—a double-blind study. Dermatology 202:35, 2001

36. Dicken CH: Treatment of classic pityriasis rubra pilaris. J Am Acad Dermatol 31:997, 1994

37. Requena L, Grilli R, Soriano L, et al: Dermatomyositis with a pityriasis rubra pilaris-like eruption: a little-known distinctive cutaneous manifestation of dermatomyositis. Br J Dermatol 136:768, 1997

38. Van de Kerkfho PC, Steijlen PM: Topical treatment of pityriasis rubra pilaris with calcipotriol. Br J Dermatol 130:675, 1994

39. Yaniv R, Barzilai A, Trau H: Pityriasis rubra pilaris exacerbated by ultraviolet B phototherapy (letter). Dermatology 189:313, 1994

40. Goldsmith LA, Weinrich AE, Shupack J: Pityriasis rubra pilaris response to 13-*cis*-retinoic acid (isotretinoin). J Am Acad Dermatol 6:710, 1982

41. Clayton BD, Jorizzo JL, Hitchcock MG, et al: Adult pityriasis rubra pilaris: a 10-year case series. J Am Acad Dermatol 36:959, 1997

42. Usuki K, Sekiyama M, Shimada S, et al: Three cases of pityriasis rubra pilaris successfully treated with cyclosporin A. Dermatology 200:324, 2000

43. Lambert WC, Everett MA: The nosology of parapsoriasis. J Am Acad Dermatol 5:373, 1981

44. Hood AF, Mark EJ: Histopathologic diagnosis of pityriasis lichenoides et varioliformis acuta and its clinical correlation. Arch Dermatol 118:478, 1982

45. Dereure O, Levi E, Kadin ME: T-cell clonality in pityriasis lichenoides et varioliformis acuta: a heteroduplex analysis of 20 cases. Arch Dermatol 136:1483, 2000

46. LeVine MJ: Phototherapy of pityriasis lichenoides. Arch Dermatol 119:378, 1983

47. Satra KH, DeLeo VA: PUVA for photosensitivity and other skin diseases. Photochemotherapy in Dermatology. Abel EA, Ed. Igaku-Shoin Medical Publishers, New York, 1991, p 159

48. Humbert P, Treffel P, Chapuis J-F, et al: The tetracyclines in dermatology. J Am Acad Dermatol 25:691, 1991

49. Fink-Puches R, Soyer HP, Kerl H: Febrile ulceronecrotic pityriasis lichenoides et varioliformis acuta. J Am Acad Dermatol 30:261, 1994

50. Kikuchi A, Naka W, Harada T, et al: Parapsoriasis en plaques: its potential for progression to malignant lymphoma. J Am Acad Dermatol 29:419, 1993

51. Thestrup-Pedersen K, Halkier-Sorensen L, Sogaard H, et al: The red man syndrome: exfoliative dermatitis of unknown etiology: a description and follow-up of 38 patients. J Am Acad Dermatol 18:1307, 1988

52. Sigurdsson V, Steegmans PH, van Vloten WA: The incidence of erythroderma: a survey among all dermatologists in The Netherlands. J Am Acad Dermatol 45:675, 2001

33 Psoriasis

Elizabeth A. Abel, M.D., and Mark Lebwohl, M.D.

Psoriasis is an immune-mediated inflammatory skin disorder characterized by chronic, scaling, erythematous patches and plaques of skin. It can begin at any age and can vary in severity. Psoriasis can manifest itself in several different forms, including pustular and erythrodermic forms. In addition to involving the skin, psoriasis frequently involves the nails, and some patients may experience inflammation of the joints (psoriatic arthritis).

Recent breakthroughs in the treatment of psoriasis have led to a better understanding of its pathogenesis. New developments in the genetics, pathogenesis, and treatment of psoriasis are reviewed.

Epidemiology

The estimated prevalence of psoriasis ranges from 0.5% to 4.6% worldwide. The reasons for the geographic variation in prevalence are unknown, but climatic factors and genetics may play a role. Psoriasis is uncommon in blacks in tropical zones, but it is more often seen in blacks in temperate zones. It occurs commonly in Japanese persons but rarely in persons native to North and South America. On the basis of a survey mailed to 50,000 households, the prevalence in the United States is estimated to be 2.6%.[1] Psoriasis can occur in patients of any age, with some cases being reported at birth and others being reported in patients older than 100 years. In Farber and Nall's pioneer study of 5,600 patients, the average age of onset of psoriasis was 27.8 years; in 35% of patients, onset occurred before 20 years of age, and in 10%, onset occurred before 10 years of age.[2] Psoriasis occurs with equal frequency in men and women, but in Farber and Nall's study, onset occurred later in men. In populations in which there is a high prevalence of psoriasis, onset tends to occur at an earlier age. In the Faroe Islands, for example, the prevalence is 3%, and the average age of onset is 12.5 years. The average age of onset is 23 years in the United States. In persons with earlier age of onset, psoriasis is more likely to be severe, with involvement of a large area of skin surface.

Pathogenesis

Psoriasis was once thought to be caused by an abnormality in epidermal cell kinetics; it is now thought that the immune system acts as a trigger to initiate epidermal proliferation. The role of activated lymphocytes in the development of psoriasis was first proved through investigations of DAB389 interleukin-2 (IL-2), a fusion protein consisting of molecules of IL-2 fused to diphtheria toxin. This fusion protein binds to high-affinity IL-2 receptors on activated T cells, destroying those cells. In a study in which DAB389 IL-2 was administered to 10 patients, four patients showed dramatic clinical improvement and four others showed moderate improvement.[3] Unfortunately, because of side effects, DAB389 IL-2 has not been approved for the treatment of psoriasis.[4]

In the skin of patients with lesional psoriasis, there is an increase in the number of antigen-presenting cells that can activate T cells. For T cell activation to occur, antigen-presenting cells must deliver at least two signals to resting T cells. The first signal occurs when major histocompatibility complex class II molecules (MHC class II molecules) of the antigen-presenting cells

present antigens to the T cells. A second costimulatory signal must be delivered in the form of costimulatory ligands on the surface of the antigen-presenting cells interacting with T cell surface receptors. Examples of these interactions include the interaction of B7 molecules with CD28 on the surface of resting T cells and the interaction of lymphocyte function–associated antigen–3 (LFA-3) with CD2 or intercellular adhesion molecule–1 (ICAM-1) with LFA-1 on the surface of T cells.[5,6] Blockade of any of these steps results in clearing of psoriasis.[7-9] Upon activation, T cells release Th1 (T helper type 1) cytokines, IL-2, and interferon gamma, which together induce proliferation of keratinocytes and further stimulation of T cells.

Etiology

GENETIC FACTORS

Several lines of evidence suggest that psoriasis has a genetic etiology. One third of persons affected have a positive family history. Studies have found a higher concordance rate in monozygotic twins than in dizygotic twins or siblings (70% versus 23%).[10]

Current evidence suggests genetic heterogeneity. Both autosomal dominant inheritance with incomplete penetrance and polygenic or multifactorial inheritance have been described. A psoriasis susceptibility gene located on the distal long arm of human chromosome 17 has been identified in 65 cases of psoriasis in eight families. The gene was not present in all families, a finding that supports the genetic heterogeneity of this disease.[11] Three candidate genes—HLA-C, corneodesmosin, and HCR—have been identified on the short arm of chromosome 6.[12,13] Whether a single gene or multiple genes are identified, it is clear that complex interactions between the immune system and the epidermis result in the clinical outcome we identify as psoriasis.

CONTRIBUTING FACTORS

The course and severity of psoriasis can be affected by a number of endogenous and exogenous factors, including stress, climate, the presence of concurrent infections, and medications that the patient may be receiving.

Psychological Stress

Many patients believe that anxiety or psychological stress has an adverse effect on the course of their psoriasis. The etiologic significance of stress in psoriasis is difficult to evaluate, however, because of the subjective nature of the evidence used in many of the investigations into the role played by stress.[14] In a prospective study, a multivariate statistical method revealed a positive correlation between severity of psoriasis symptoms and psychological stress related to adverse life events.[15] The effects of psoriasis on physical and mental function have been compared with the effects of cancer, heart disease, diabetes, and depression.[16]

Climate

It has long been known that psoriasis improves when patients are exposed to sunny climates and to regions of lower latitude. In northern latitudes, exacerbation of psoriasis commonly occurs during the fall and winter.

Infection

Viral or bacterial infections, especially streptococcal pharyngitis, may precipitate the onset or exacerbation of psoriasis.[17] Guttate psoriasis, in particular, is often attributed to a previous streptococcal infection. Attempts to reverse psoriasis by treatment with oral antibiotics have not proved effective in double-blind trials.[18] Nevertheless, some investigators advocate antibiotic therapy for psoriasis.[19]

Infection with HIV has also been associated with psoriasis. In some patients with HIV infection, preexisting psoriasis becomes exacerbated, whereas other patients develop psoriasis within a few years of infection. Often, patients present with symptoms similar to Reiter syndrome.[20]

Drugs

Numerous drugs can worsen psoriasis.[21] Antimalarial agents such as chloroquine can cause exfoliative erythroderma or pustular psoriasis. Up to 31% of patients experience new onset or worsening of psoriasis as a result of antimalarial therapy. Lithium and beta blockers such as propranolol may precipitate the onset of psoriasis or cause exacerbations of psoriasis.[22] Some nonsteroidal anti-inflammatory drugs (NSAIDs) also exacerbate psoriasis, although this effect is sufficiently minor to allow NSAIDs to be used to treat psoriatic arthritis.[23] Flares of pustular psoriasis may be precipitated by withdrawal from systemic corticosteroids or withdrawal from high-potency topical corticosteroids.

Other Factors

Trauma to the clinically uninvolved skin of patients with psoriasis can cause a lesion to appear at the exact site of injury; this phenomenon is known as the Köbner response. Cuts, abrasions, injections, burns resulting from phototherapy, and other forms of trauma can elicit this reaction.

Recent evidence suggests that smoking may be an exacerbating factor in psoriasis.[24] Alcohol has also been implicated in the exacerbation of psoriasis.[25]

Attempts have been made to affect the clinical course of psoriasis through modification of diet, and a number of surveys have suggested that diet plays a role in the development of psoriasis.[26] Double-blind studies, however, have failed to show that diet has either a beneficial or a detrimental effect on the severity of psoriasis.

Diagnosis

HISTOPATHOLOGY

The classic microscopic features of a psoriatic plaque include the following:

1. A markedly thickened stratum corneum, with layered zones of parakeratosis (retention of nuclei)
2. A moderately to markedly hyperplastic epidermis, with broadening of rete projections and elongation to a uniform depth in the dermis
3. Increased mitotic activity in the lower epidermis
4. Epidermal thinning over the dermal papillae
5. A scant amount of inflammatory infiltrate from mononuclear cells in the superficial dermis
6. Intracorneal or subcorneal collections of polymorphonuclear leukocytes (Munro microabscesses)

Differential diagnosis includes other scaling dermatoses, such as seborrheic dermatitis that involves the scalp, nasolabial folds,

and retroauricular folds; pityriasis rosea, which begins with a herald patch and is self-limited; lichen simplex chronicus, which is caused by repeated rubbing or scratching; parapsoriasis, which is characterized by atrophy, telangiectasia, and pigmentary abnormalities; and other conditions that can be differentiated by clinical and pathologic criteria.

CLINICAL VARIANTS

Nearly 90% of patients have plaque-type psoriasis, a form that is characterized by sharply demarcated, erythematous scaling plaques. The elbows [see Figure 1], knees, and scalp [see Figure 2] are the most commonly affected sites. The intergluteal cleft [see Figure 3], palms [see Figure 4], soles [see Figure 5], and genitals are also commonly affected, but psoriasis can involve any part of the body. Lesions frequently occur in a symmetrical pattern of distribution.

Many patients have only one or a few lesions that persist for years and that occasionally resolve after exposure to sunlight. Other patients can be covered with plaques that become confluent, affecting nearly 100% of the body surface area. Nail involvement is common, particularly in patients with severe disease.

The second most common form of psoriasis, guttate psoriasis, affects fewer than 10% of patients and is characterized by the de-

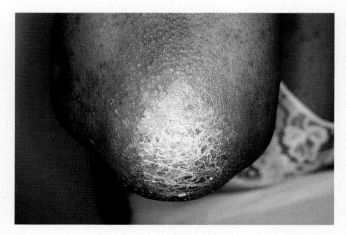

Figure 1 **Involvement of the elbows is characteristic of plaque psoriasis.**

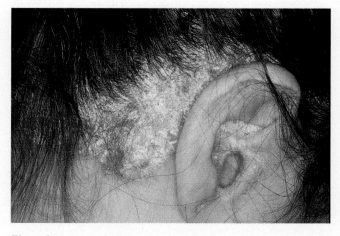

Figure 2 **The scalp is affected in the majority of patients with plaque psoriasis.**

Erythrodermic psoriasis is a severe form of psoriasis that often affects the entire cutaneous surface. Patients present with an exfoliative erythroderma in which the skin is very red and inflamed and is constantly scaling [see Figure 7]. Patients are acutely ill, their skin having lost all protective function. Loss of temperature control, loss of fluids and nutrients through the impaired skin, and susceptibility to infection make this a life-threatening condition.

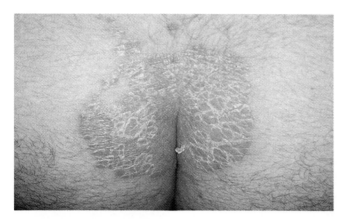

Figure 3 The intergluteal cleft is a common site of involvement in patients with plaque psoriasis.

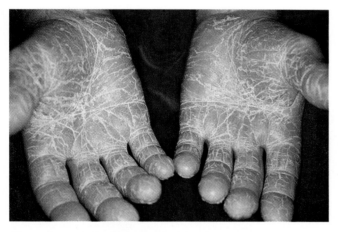

Figure 4 Psoriasis of the palms is shown in this patient.

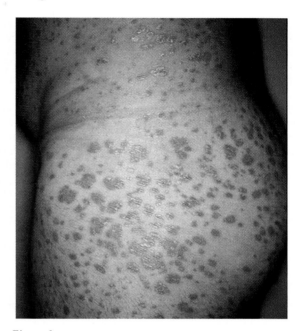

Figure 6 Guttate psoriasis is characterized by small scaly papules and plaques.

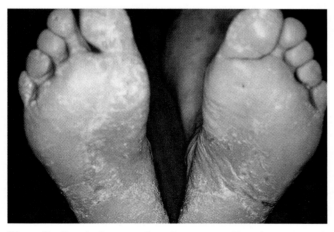

Figure 5 Sharply demarcated, erythematous, scaling plaques on the feet are apparent in this patient with psoriasis of the soles.

velopment of small, scaling erythematous papules on the trunk and extremities [see Figure 6]. This form of psoriasis often occurs after streptococcal infection. Patients with plaque-type psoriasis can develop guttate psoriasis. Conversely, patients with guttate psoriasis frequently develop plaque-type psoriasis. Occasionally, guttate lesions enlarge and become confluent, resulting in the formation of plaques.

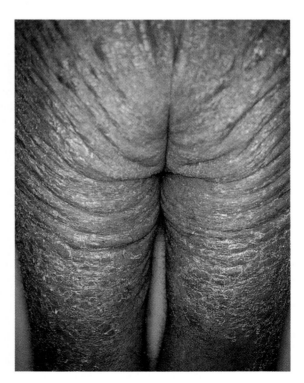

Figure 7 Erythrodermic psoriasis is characterized by generalized erythema and desquamation.

Some patients present with erythrodermic psoriasis de novo; others develop erythrodermic psoriasis after having typical plaque-type or guttate psoriasis. Erythrodermic psoriasis can occur after withdrawal of systemic corticosteroids, after phototherapy burns, as a result of antimalarial treatment, as a result of a drug-induced hypersensitivity reaction, or for no apparent reason. Erythrodermic psoriasis has been associated with cutaneous T cell lymphoma.

Pustular psoriasis, another severe form of the disease, can occur in patients with preexisting psoriasis, or it can arise de novo. Pustular psoriasis can be generalized (von Zumbusch–type) or localized to the palms and soles [see Figure 8]. In either case, the condition is severe and debilitating. In generalized pustular psoriasis, the body is covered with sterile pustules. As with erythrodermic psoriasis, the protective functions of the skin are lost, and patients may succumb to infection or hypovolemia and electrolyte imbalance caused by loss of fluid through the skin. Although fever and leukocytosis are commonly found in patients with pustular psoriasis, the possibility of infection should not be overlooked; patients with pustular psoriasis have died of staphylococcal sepsis.[27]

As with erythrodermic psoriasis, pustular psoriasis is most commonly precipitated by withdrawal of systemic corticosteroids, but it can also result from therapy with antimalarial drugs or lithium, and it can develop spontaneously.

SPECIAL PRESENTATIONS

Nail Psoriasis

Nail changes can be of immeasurable value when the diagnosis is in doubt [see Figure 9]. In one study, 55% of patients with psoriasis experienced such changes.[28] The most common change consists of the appearance of tiny pits, as might be made with an ice pick, which often occur in groups. This characteristic pitting of the nails is highly specific for psoriasis, although a few isolated pits may be seen in healthy nails or as a result of past trauma. Yellowish discoloration is common in psoriatic toenails and may appear in fingernails as well. Onycholysis, or distal separation of the nail plate from its bed, frequently occurs.

Other changes include subungual hyperkeratosis—an accumulation of keratinous debris under the nail—as well as transverse and longitudinal ridging. These findings, however, are much less specific because they also occur secondary to dermatitis, fungal infection, vascular insufficiency, and other conditions. Occasionally, a patient shows typical psoriatic nail changes without any other cutaneous signs at initial examination; all such patients are probably psoriatic and may eventually manifest psoriatic lesions.

Psoriatic Arthritis

Psoriatic arthritis has been estimated to occur in 5% to 10% of patients with psoriasis. Joint inflammation in psoriatic arthritis is chronic, with occasional remissions.[29] The most common presentation is an oligoarthritis in which one or a few joints are affected. This form accounts for approximately 70% of cases of psoriatic arthritis. Skin lesions of psoriasis usually precede articular disease, but occasionally patients develop inflamed joints before skin lesions occur. If a diagnosis of psoriatic arthritis is suspected, careful examination of the scalp, nails, intergluteal cleft, and genital region should be performed to confirm the presence of psoriasis.

The second most common type of psoriatic arthritis is virtually identical to rheumatoid arthritis. This form is character-

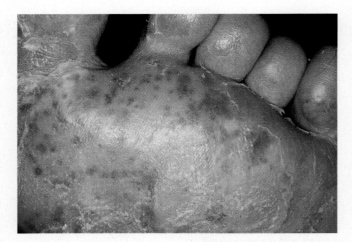

Figure 8 **Pustular psoriasis can be localized to the palms and soles or generalized.**

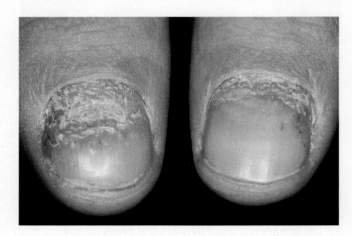

Figure 9 **Involvement of the nails is common in psoriasis.**

ized by symmetrical involvement of the joints with ulnar deviation and typical deformities, such as swan-neck deformity and boutonnière deformity. The only distinguishing features are the presence of psoriasis and the absence of circulating rheumatoid factor.

Arthritis mutilans is a rare, severely destructive form of psoriatic arthritis in which the interphalangeal joints of the hands and feet are destroyed, resulting in deformed digits. Ankylosing spondylitis accounts for 5% of cases of psoriatic arthritis. As in other forms of ankylosing spondylitis, the genetic marker HLA-B27 is present.

Distal interphalangeal joint involvement is the most characteristic form of psoriatic arthritis. It is usually associated with nail involvement.

Treatment

More treatments have been introduced for psoriasis than perhaps for any other dermatologic disease. New topical therapies, new systemic therapies, and new forms of phototherapy have been introduced, and additional treatments are in development. Biologic therapies that target specific molecules are likely to change the way we treat psoriasis in the future. Topical therapy will continue to be used by most patients, however.

Table 1   Ranking of Topical Steroids for Psoriasis in Order of High to Low Potency

Group	Generic Name	Trade Name	Strength (%)
I	Betamethasone dipropionate in optimized vehicle Clobetasol propionate Diflorasone diacetate	Diprolene ointment Temovate cream, ointment Psorcon ointment	0.05 0.05 0.05
II	Amcinonide Betamethasone dipropionate, augmented Betamethasone dipropionate Mometasone furoate Diflorasone diacetate Halcinonide Fluocinonide Desoximetasone	Cyclocort ointment Diprolene AF cream Diprosone ointment Elocon ointment Florone ointment, Maxiflor ointment Halog cream Lidex cream, ointment; Topsyn gel Topicort cream, ointment	0.1 0.05 0.05 0.1 0.05 0.1 0.05 0.25
III	Triamcinolone acetonide Betamethasone dipropionate Diflorasone diacetate Betamethasone valerate	Aristocort cream (HP) Diprosone cream Florone cream, Maxiflor cream Valisone ointment	0.5 0.05 0.05 0.1
IV	Triamcinolone acetonide Betamethasone benzoate Flurandrenolide Mometasone furoate Fluocinolone acetonide	Aristocort ointment, Kenalog ointment Benisone ointment Cordran ointment Elocon cream { Synalar-HP cream { Synalar ointment	0.1 0.025 0.05 0.1 0.2 0.025
V	Betamethasone benzoate Flurandrenolide Fluticasone propionate Betamethasone dipropionate Triamcinolone acetonide Hydrocortisone butyrate Fluocinolone acetonide Betamethasone valerate Hydrocortisone valerate	Benisone cream Cordran cream Cutivate cream Diprosone lotion Kenalog cream, lotion Locoid cream Synalar cream Valisone cream, lotion Westcort cream	0.025 0.05 0.05 0.02 0.1 0.1 0.025 0.1 0.2
VI	Alclometasone dipropionate Desonide Flumethasone pivalate Fluocinolone acetonide	Aclovate cream Tridesilon cream, ointment; DesOwen cream, ointment Locorten cream Synalar solution	0.05 0.05 0.03 0.01
VII	Hydrocortisone	{ Hytone cream, lotion, ointment { Hytone, Penecort, Synacort, Cort-Dome, Nutracort	2.5 1.0

TOPICAL THERAPY

The 1990s saw the development of many new therapies for psoriasis.[30] Topical therapy is the mainstay of treatment for most patients, particularly those with mild disease. Topical corticosteroids are the most commonly prescribed class of medication, but they are now frequently administered in a regimen that also involves application of calcipotriene, a vitamin D_3 analogue that has been approved for treatment of psoriasis.[31] Tar and salicylic acid are available by prescription and as over-the-counter products. Use of anthralin has declined as effective nonsteroidal agents have become available. Tazarotene, a retinoid that has been approved for psoriasis, is a new addition to the therapeutic armamentarium.

Emollients are an important part of any topical regimen for psoriasis. Application of petrolatum alone may be sufficient therapy for some patients. More elegant, cosmetically acceptable creams and lotions are helpful but are somewhat less effective than greasy ointments. Tar and salicylic acid shampoos are also valuable in the treatment of patients with scalp involvement. These preparations are available without prescription.

Corticosteroids

Topical corticosteroids are the most commonly prescribed medication for treatment of psoriasis because of their ease of use and their wide availability. They have anti-inflammatory, antiproliferative, and antipruritic effects. Corticosteroids are more potent when they are applied under occlusion, which increases their percutaneous penetration. Unfortunately, occlusion increases side effects.

Topical steroids have been ranked in seven categories in decreasing order of potency, with potency determined by a vasoconstriction assay [*see Table 1*]. Superpotent corticosteroids are in group I, and weak over-the-counter topical corticosteroids are in group VII.[32]

Indications   Topical corticosteroids are very effective for limited plaques of psoriasis.

Side effects   The most commonly encountered side effects of topical corticosteroids are local cutaneous reactions. Development of cutaneous atrophy, telangiectasia, and irreversible striae are the most common side effects. Perioral dermatitis, which is characterized by erythematous papules and pustules on the face, is caused by chronic use of topical corticosteroids. Tachyphylaxis, a phenomenon in which patients become habituated to the use of topical corticosteroids and stop responding to them, is noted by most patients. Flare or rebound of psoriasis upon sudden withdrawal of topical corticosteroids can occur. Finally, suppression of the hypothalamic-pituitary-adrenal axis can occur, especially with use of superpotent topical corticosteroids, the widespread application of corticosteroids, occlusion, or chronic use. Because of concern over side effects, the package insert for some superpotent corticosteroids suggests that use be limited to 2 weeks' duration. A number of regimens have been developed in which, after the initial weeks of continuous treatment with superpotent topical corticosteroids, psoriasis plaques are subsequently treated only on weekends.[33]

Vitamin D Analogues

Calcipotriene, the first topical vitamin D analogue to be approved for use in the United States, has rapidly gained acceptance, despite the fact that it is not as effective as superpotent topical corticosteroids. Calcipotriene is available in ointment and cream form and as a solution. The primary reason for its success is that it is not associated with any corticosteroid side effects—namely, cutaneous atrophy, telangiectasia, striae, or suppression of the hypothalamic-pituitary-adrenal axis. Calcipotriene is comparable in efficacy to a group II corticosteroid. It is applied twice daily.

Calcipotriene Calcipotriene has been used very successfully in combination with several therapies. It is most effective topically when used in combination with a superpotent topical corticosteroid. It has been shown that a regimen of calcipotriene ointment and halobetasol propionate ointment, each applied once daily, is more effective than monotherapy using either calcipotriene twice daily or halobetasol propionate twice daily.[34] Up to 90% of patients achieve marked improvement within 2 weeks of combination therapy with once-daily calcipotriene and once-daily halobetasol propionate ointment. For long-term maintenance of remission, a regimen has been developed in which halobetasol propionate is applied only on weekends and calcipotriene is applied on weekdays.[35] Using this regimen, 76% of patients achieved marked improvement for at least 6 months; this level of improvement was achieved in only 40% of patients receiving halobetasol propionate ointment on weekends only. Calcipotriene has also been shown to improve the response to phototherapy with ultraviolet B light (UVB)[36] and with psoralen plus ultraviolet A light (PUVA).[37]

Caution must be used when combining calcipotriene ointment with other medications, however, because it is easily inactivated. Salicylic acid, for example, completely inactivates calcipotriene on contact. Several other topical medications, including topical corticosteroids, can inactivate calcipotriene. In contrast, halobetasol propionate ointment is compatible with calcipotriene even when one medication is applied on top of the other.[38] UVA has been shown to inactivate calcipotriene.[39] Consequently, this medication should be applied after PUVA therapy, not before. Use of calcipotriene should be limited to a maximum of 120 g a week because of isolated reports of hypercalcemia.[40]

Other vitamin D analogues Several new vitamin D analogues are under investigation in the United States or are in use elsewhere. Tacalcitol and maxacalcitol are promising medications for the treatment of psoriasis. The only common side effect is irritation, which occurs in up to 20% of patients, most commonly on the face and on intertriginous areas. Topical calcitriol has been approved for the treatment of psoriasis in several countries around the world; it appears to be comparable in efficacy to calcipotriene,[13] and it may be less irritating in intertriginous sites.

Tazarotene

Tazarotene is a new retinoid that has been developed for the treatment of psoriasis. It is available in 0.05% and 0.1% gels and in cream formulations. Tazarotene is comparable in efficacy to a group II corticosteroid cream. Patients receiving tazarotene 0.1% gel experience longer periods of remission after discontinuance of therapy than patients receiving corticosteroids.

Indications Tazarotene has several advantages over the corticosteroids. First, it is not associated with cutaneous atrophy, telangiectasia, or the development of striae. Furthermore, tazarotene, like other retinoids, may actually prevent corticosteroid atrophy. Tazarotene has been shown to enhance the efficacy of UVB phototherapy.[41] It does, however, increase the erythemogenicity of ultraviolet light.[42] Doses of UVB and UVA should therefore be reduced in patients receiving phototherapy who are being treated with tazarotene.

Side effects The main side effect of tazarotene is local irritation, which has caused many patients to discontinue its use. As a consequence, tazarotene has been studied for use in combination regimens with topical corticosteroids. With these regimens, irritation is reduced and the efficacy of both agents is enhanced.

Tars

Tar has been used since the 19th century to treat psoriasis. Crude coal tar, a complex mixture of thousands of hydrocarbon compounds, affects psoriatic epidermal cells through enzyme inhibition and antimitotic action.[43] Crude coal tar is messy to apply, is odoriferous, and stains skin and clothing. It is applied in conjunction with UVB phototherapy in the Goeckerman regimen [see Phototherapy, below]. More refined tar preparations, which are cosmetically acceptable, are available by prescription and over the counter in the form of gels, creams, bath oils, shampoos, and solutions (liquor carbonis detergens). Tar is often used in combination therapies and as maintenance therapy after psoriasis plaques have resolved.

Anthralin

Anthralin (dithranol) has been used to treat psoriasis since 1916.[44] It is an extremely effective topical agent for psoriasis, probably because it inhibits enzyme metabolism and reduces epidermal mitotic turnover.[44]

Indications Because of the staining and irritation associated with use of anthralin, the agent is usually prescribed for patients who do not respond to other topical therapies.

A modified Ingram regimen combines the daily application of anthralin in a stiff paste with tar baths and with exposure to ultraviolet light. This therapy was introduced in the United States for hospitalized psoriatic patients[44] and for ambulatory patients in a psoriasis day care center.[45] Anthralin is carefully applied to involved skin areas; to avoid irritation of surrounding normal skin, affected areas are powdered with talcum and wrapped with protective stockinette dressing. The medication is initially applied in a concentration of 0.1%; depending on the patient's response, the concentration is gradually increased to 0.8%.

For guttate lesions or for thin plaques with poorly marginated borders, a less occlusive soft paste, which minimizes inflammation of surrounding normal skin, is applied. After 6 to 8 hours, mineral oil is used to remove the anthralin.

Modified anthralin formulations have been used to minimize the staining from anthralin, to decrease irritation, and to promote home use of the medication. Short-contact therapy consists of the application of ointment containing 1% anthralin to involved areas for 1 hour, after which the medication is removed.[46] When short-contact therapy is used for localized plaques, the cream must be thoroughly removed after 30 minutes to 2 hours to minimize irritation of the surrounding skin. Anthralin in a cream base, which can be removed by washing with water, is suitable for home use; it is commercially available as Drithocreme in concentrations of 0.1%, 0.25%, 0.5%, and 1.0% and as Dritho-Scalp in concentrations of 0.25% and 0.5%.

For scalp care, a pomade containing 0.4% anthralin is applied after the scales have been loosened by the application of warm mineral oil under a turban-type occlusion. The pomade is removed with a tar shampoo.

A formulation of 1% anthralin cream, composed of microencapsulated lipid crystals that release anthralin for absorption at skin temperature, is available. When used as short-contact therapy, this preparation carries a low risk of staining and irritation.[47]

Anthralin is most effective therapeutically when it is in the form of a hard paste containing paraffin. Anthralin ointment is less effective than anthralin paste, and anthralin cream is even less effective. With regard to patient compliance, this order is reversed. The end point of treatment is resolution of plaques to a macular state; this is usually associated with residual postinflammatory hyperpigmentation and temporary staining from anthralin. Resolution of symptoms usually occurs within 2 to 3 weeks after a modified Ingram regimen; remissions last for weeks to months.

Side effects   Staining of skin, clothing, and the home is common with anthralin, as is irritation at the site of application.

PHOTOTHERAPY

Phototherapy is an effective treatment of psoriasis. Sunbathing for 2 to 4 weeks lessens the morbidity associated with the disorder.

Indications

Climatotherapy at the Dead Sea is an effective alternative therapy for psoriasis for those who can travel to that part of the world. Because of its unique geographic location 300 m below sea level, patients are exposed to naturally filtered ultraviolet light, which results in significant improvement or complete resolution of symptoms in 83% of patients over several weeks.[48] It is clear that the sunlight at the Dead Sea accounts for most of the response, with little additional improvement resulting from bathing in the Dead Sea. Not surprisingly, there is an increase in nonmelanoma skin cancer in patients treated at the Dead Sea.[49]

Efficacy

Daily in-hospital application of crude coal tar and exposure to ultraviolet light (the Goeckerman regimen) can lead to a resolu-

tion of symptoms in widespread psoriasis within 3 or 4 weeks and can effect remissions that last for weeks to months.

In a reevaluation of the Goeckerman regimen, application of a 1% tar preparation was found to be as effective as a 6% preparation of the same substance. Furthermore, application of the tar preparation for 2 hours before irradiation was equivalent to longer periods of application.[50] Contraindications to the use of the Goeckerman regimen include the presence of severely excoriated or inflamed psoriasis, erythrodermic and pustular forms of the disease, folliculitis, and a history of photosensitivity.

According to one report, the effects of exposure to erythemogenic UVB with emollients are equivalent to those of UVB irradiation with tar. The emollient or vehicle decreases reflectance of the psoriatic scale, thereby increasing light transmissions. However, tar may have an additive effect when combined with a less aggressive regimen of suberythemogenic UVB.[51]

In a comparison study,[52] outpatient UVB phototherapy was administered three times weekly along with the application of either a tar oil or an emollient twice every day. This approach led to clearing of psoriatic lesions in 78% of the patients [*see Figure 10*]. No difference was observed between the side of the body treated with tar oil and the side treated with the vehicle. Although the previous study had shown an additive effect for tar combined with UVB irradiation when patients were evaluated after 3 to 4 weeks (before their lesions had cleared),[53] the subsequent study showed no such advantage among patients who were evaluated at the time of lesion clearing.

Remission lasted longer in patients who received maintenance UVB phototherapy twice weekly for 1 to 2 months and then once weekly for up to 4 months than in patients who discontinued UVB phototherapy after the initial clearing.

Narrow-band UVB, which comprises wavelengths of approximately 311 nm, has recently been developed and is more effective than broad-band UVB.[54] As with other forms of phototherapy, narrow-band UVB works through local effects; therefore, covered areas, such as the scalp, do not respond.[55]

PHOTOCHEMOTHERAPY

Indications

PUVA is indicated for patients who have not responded adequately to conventional or narrow-band UVB phototherapy.

PUVA therapy entails the administration of the photosensitizing drug methoxsalen (8-methoxypsoralen) in an oral dose or by soaking in a tub containing methoxypsoralen or by applying topical methoxypsoralen before the patient is exposed to high-intensity longwave ultraviolet light in a walk-in irradiation chamber. The initial UVA dose (in joules/cm^2) is based on the patient's skin type in accordance with established protocols.[56] Although its therapeutic effect is local, PUVA is a systemic treatment in which photoactivated methoxsalen binds to epidermal DNA, forming monofunctional and bifunctional adducts. It has been postulated that the resulting interference with epidermal mitosis is one of the mechanisms of action of PUVA therapy for psoriasis, although effects on immune function in the skin play an important role.

Efficacy

The efficacy of oral PUVA therapy has been established by several multicenter clinical trials.[57] A course of PUVA therapy administered two or three times weekly resulted in significant clearing of psoriasis lesions in approximately 90% of patients within a mean of 25 total treatments. After the initial course, a ta-

a 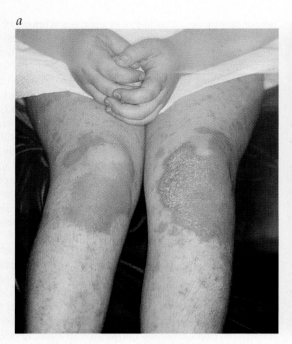 *b*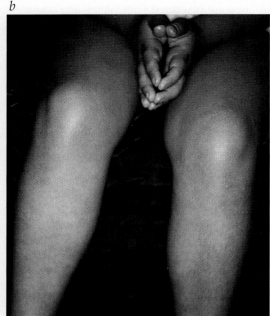

Figure 10 **Psoriasis in a child before (*a*) and after (*b*) phototherapy.**

pering maintenance regimen is instituted, and PUVA therapy is eventually discontinued. In most patients, psoriasis recurs months to years after PUVA is discontinued, indicating that this therapy is palliative rather than curative.

Side Effects

Acute side effects caused by phototoxicity, such as erythema and blistering, are dose related and can therefore be controlled. Pruritus, usually associated with dryness of the skin, is fairly common and can be alleviated by the use of emollients and oral antihistamines. Nausea may follow ingestion of methoxsalen. Of greater concern are the potential long-term side effects, particularly carcinogenicity.

A multicenter study of more than 1,300 PUVA-treated patients in the United States who were evaluated after 1 to 3 years of follow-up revealed a significant increase in the number of squamous cell carcinomas (SCCs) in those patients with a history of exposure to ionizing radiation or a history of skin cancer.[58] A higher-than-expected ratio of SCCs to basal cell epitheliomas and an excess of SCCs in areas of the body that were not exposed to the sun were significant findings of the study. A 5.7-year follow-up study of the original cohort group revealed a dose-dependent increase in the risk of SCC.[59] There was only a slight increase in the risk of basal cell carcinoma in these patients. The patients who received high cumulative doses of PUVA experienced almost a 13-fold increase in the risk of SCC compared with those who received low-dose therapy.

Continued study of 1,049 of the 1,153 surviving patients 13 or more years after initiation of PUVA therapy revealed that SCC developed in more than 25% of patients exposed to high-dose PUVA for 300 or more treatments. Most patients had multiple tumors. Data regarding previous exposure to ionizing radiation, use of high-dose topical tar (more than 45 months of therapy), and use of high-dose methotrexate (defined as a cumulative dose of 3 g) were collected. The only additional significant association was between high-level exposure to methotrexate and risk of

SCC. No interaction between PUVA and methotrexate was demonstrated, however. Other types of tumors that developed in these patients, including 104 cases of SCC in situ and 181 keratoacanthomas, were not included in the analysis.[57] A 15-year or longer follow-up study of the surviving members of that cohort assessed the risk of skin cancers. Of great concern was a small but statistically significant increase in the incidence of malignant melanoma. Because that increase did not become apparent until after a period of at least 15 years, there is great concern that in patients who began PUVA therapy years ago, an epidemic of melanomas will occur. Fortunately, this has not occurred thus far.

Studies in animals suggest that PUVA may have ocular side effects. Methoxsalen has been detected in the lenses of rats after they have ingested the drug; subsequent exposure to UVA enhances such ultraviolet-induced changes as cataracts.[60] The risk of ocular toxicity and possible retinal damage is of particular concern in young persons, whose lenses transmit more UVA than the more opaque lenses of older persons, and in aphakic persons, in whom lenses are absent.[61] The use of UVA-opaque goggles during PUVA treatment sessions is extremely important. Glasses that block UVA must be worn from the time that methoxsalen is administered throughout the rest of the day. Some investigators advise protection of the eyes the day after therapy. Thus far, studies of patients treated with PUVA have not revealed an increase in the incidence of cataracts.

Although the Food and Drug Administration has approved the use of PUVA in the treatment of psoriasis, patients must be closely monitored for long-term side effects. Use of PUVA is limited to patients with extensive, disabling psoriasis whose condition has failed to respond to conventional forms of therapy.

SYSTEMIC THERAPY

Methotrexate

The antimetabolite methotrexate was considered effective for the treatment of psoriasis because of its antimitotic effect on proliferating keratinocytes. However, tissue culture studies have suggested that activated lymphoid cells in the lymph nodes, blood, and skin are a likely target of methotrexate; proliferating macrophages and T cells are 100 times more sensitive to methotrexate than proliferating epithelial cells.[62] These findings may be relevant to the mechanism of action of methotrexate in other immunologically based disorders, including psoriatic arthritis, rheumatoid arthritis, and Crohn disease.

Indications Methotrexate is indicated for patients who do not respond adequately to phototherapy and for patients with psoriatic arthritis.

Methotrexate is best given in a single weekly oral dose of up to 30 mg or in three divided doses at 12-hour intervals during a 24-hour period (e.g., at 8:00 A.M., at 8:00 P.M., and again at 8:00 A.M.).

Advisability of liver biopsy The use of liver biopsy to monitor patients on methotrexate has been a source of great controversy. Liver biopsies are not routinely performed in patients with rheumatoid arthritis who are undergoing treatment with methotrexate, but liver biopsy has been advocated in patients with psoriasis.[63] From a review of the literature, it is clear that patients with psoriasis who are treated with methotrexate are more prone to hepatic fibrosis, possibly because of their underlying disease or because of the concomitant treatments they are given. Current guidelines call for the use of liver biopsy in patients with psoriasis who have received a cumulative dose of 1 to 1.5 g of methotrexate and who do not have a history of liver disease or alcoholism. Biopsy should be performed early in the course of treatment in patients with a history of hepatitis C, alcoholism, or other liver disease. Risk factors for hepatotoxicity include heavy alcohol intake, obesity, a history of diabetes or hepatitis, and abnormal results on liver function testing.

Pathologic liver changes caused by methotrexate therapy have been graded as follows: grade I, normal liver histology or mild fatty infiltration; grade II, moderate to severe fatty infiltration with portal tract inflammation and necrosis; grade IIIA, mild fibrosis; grade IIIB, moderate to severe fibrosis; and grade IV, cirrhosis. Methotrexate should be discontinued in the presence of pathologic liver changes of grade IIIB or IV. The importance of strict adherence to current guidelines for the administration of methotrexate is emphasized by the occurrence of methotrexate-induced cirrhosis, which necessitated liver transplantation in three patients with long-term psoriasis who did not undergo serial liver biopsies.[64]

Side effects Side effects of methotrexate therapy include bone marrow suppression, nausea, diarrhea, stomatitis, and hepatotoxicity. Methotrexate is teratogenic and can cause reversible oligospermia. Pneumonitis can occur early in the course of treatment if methotrexate is administered in oncologic doses. Evaluation by tests of liver function, renal function, and blood elements must be made before and throughout the course of methotrexate therapy.

Certain drugs increase the toxicity of methotrexate by reducing renal tubular secretion; these drugs include salicylates, sulfonamides, probenecid, and penicillins. Other drugs increase toxicity by displacing methotrexate from the sites at which it binds to plasma proteins; these drugs include salicylates, probenecid, barbiturates, and phenytoin. Many of the NSAIDs and trimethoprim-sulfamethoxazole enhance methotrexate toxicity.[63]

Cases of pancytopenia after low-dose methotrexate therapy underscore the hazards of use of the drug in patients with renal insufficiency or in patients who are concomitantly receiving drugs that increase methotrexate toxicity.[65]

Contraindications to treatment with methotrexate and indications for stopping treatment should be heeded. Constant medical supervision is necessary, and therapy must be stopped at once if toxicity develops.

Acitretin

Indications Acitretin, an oral retinoid, is approved for the treatment of plaque psoriasis. It is highly effective in the treatment of pustular psoriasis and can be very effective as monotherapy for erythrodermic psoriasis. For plaque-type and guttate psoriasis, however, acitretin is most useful in combination with other treatments, particularly UVB and PUVA phototherapy.[66,67] Acitretin is initiated 1 to 2 weeks before UVB or PUVA therapy is started. With combination treatment, symptoms resolve much more quickly. Doses of only 10 to 25 mg daily are effective, thus minimizing retinoid side effects.[66,67] When used as monotherapy, acitretin is prescribed in doses of 25 mg daily, which can be increased to 50 mg a day or higher.

Side effects Side effects are dose related and are common with doses above 25 mg daily. Hair loss, cheilitis, desquamation of the palms and soles, sun sensitivity, and periungual pyogenic granulomas are among the mucocutaneous side effects. Hyperlipidemia is common but is easily controlled with lipid-lowering agents. Elevations in liver enzyme levels can occur, and enzyme levels must be monitored. Serial liver biopsies have not demonstrated hepatic fibrosis in patients treated with oral retinoids.[68] More serious than acitretin's side effects is the risk of teratogenicity. Characteristic retinoid birth defects occur in a high proportion of fetuses exposed to even small amounts of the drug in utero. Acitretin is eliminated from the body much more quickly than its prodrug etretinate. In the presence of alcohol, however, acitretin is converted back to etretinate,[69] raising concerns that women of childbearing age who take acitretin and who later become pregnant would then be at risk for exposing their fetus to acitretin's teratogenic effects. The FDA therefore requires that acitretin not be administered to women planning a pregnancy within 3 years.

Long-term side effects of oral retinoids include calcification of ligaments and tendons and osteoporosis.[70,71] The long-term safety of etretinate, acitretin's prodrug, was examined in a 5-year prospective study of 956 patients with psoriasis. The investigators concluded that with appropriate patient selection and monitoring, there was no substantially increased risk of side effects related to cardiovascular disease, cancer, diabetes, cataracts, and inflammatory bowel disease. Although joint symptoms improved in some patients, more patients had joint problems associated with etretinate. Etretinate also caused short-term changes in liver enzyme levels in some patients and, in rare cases, caused acute hepatitis. The long-term risk of liver disease and cirrhosis with etretinate, however, was less than that associated with comparable periods of methotrexate.[72]

Cyclosporine

Cyclosporine in a microemulsion formulation was approved by the FDA for the treatment of psoriasis after extensive worldwide experience. In dosages of 2.5 to 5 mg/kg/day, cyclosporine is highly effective for psoriasis. Even at those doses, however, it is associated with significant side effects, which have limited its use to severely affected or refractory patients.

Indications Cyclosporine is indicated for patients in whom phototherapy or methotrexate therapy has failed.

The microemulsion formulation is better absorbed than earlier formulations of cyclosporine. It is available in gel capsules of 25 and 100 mg. It is most commonly prescribed in divided doses, to be taken twice daily.

At dosages of 5 mg/kg/day, a response is usually seen within 4 weeks, and some patients respond in as little time as 1 week. It should be noted that in the United States, the package insert for cyclosporine recommends an upper dosage limit of 4 mg/kg/day, although worldwide experience regarding the efficacy and safety of this drug has established an upper limit of 5 mg/kg/day.[73]

Side effects Cyclosporine is associated with a number of side effects that are easily managed; other side effects are of greater concern. Hypertrichosis, tremors, paresthesias, headache, gingival hyperplasia, joint pain, and fatigue can occur. Elevations in serum lipid levels and minor elevations in liver enzyme levels are also common. Hypomagnesemia may require magnesium supplementation. The most serious common side effects are hypertension and nephrotoxicity. Hypertension can be managed by lowering the dose or by instituting treatment with calcium channel blockers such as amlodipine besylate. There is some evidence that in normotensive patients receiving cyclosporine, amlodipine therapy may prevent some of the nephrotoxicity that has been associated with this potent psoriasis treatment.[74]

Renal interstitial fibrosis and renal tubular atrophy are common in patients on long-term therapy with cyclosporine.[75,76] Consequently, serum creatinine levels must be monitored on a regular basis. If the serum creatinine level rises more than 30% above baseline (or more than 25%, according to the U.S. package insert), the dosage may have to be reduced.[73]

In organ transplant patients on cyclosporine and other immunosuppressive drugs for the prevention of organ transplant rejection, there has been an increase in lymphoproliferative diseases and skin cancers.[77,78] It is hoped that the lower doses and intermittent usage of cyclosporine in psoriasis patients will not be associated with an increase in malignancies, but caution must be exercised. In one study, rheumatoid arthritis patients who were treated for a short period (median, 1.6 years) with cyclosporine were compared with a parallel group of rheumatoid patients who were not treated with cyclosporine; there was no increase in lymphoproliferative disorders.[79] Nevertheless, caution must be used with this powerful new psoriasis treatment.

Tacrolimus (FK506)

Indications Tacrolimus may be substituted for cyclosporine in patients who cannot tolerate hypertrichosis associated with the latter agent. It is not approved for psoriasis.

Another potent immunosuppressive agent, tacrolimus (FK506), has proved effective in the treatment of psoriasis. In a double-blind trial, 50 patients with severe recalcitrant psoriasis were treated with either oral tacrolimus or placebo.[80] In the tacrolimus group, starting dosages were 0.5 mg/kg/day; dosages could be increased to 0.10 mg/kg at weeks 3 or 6 if response was judged to be insufficient. After 9 weeks of treatment, patients receiving tacrolimus experienced an 84% reduction in psoriasis area severity index scores.

As with cyclosporine, there are concerns about hypertension, nephrotoxicity, and immunosuppressive effects with tacrolimus. This drug is not associated with hypertrichosis or gingival hyperplasia. Tacrolimus is not studied as extensively as cyclosporine for the treatment of psoriasis, and further investigations are warranted for this very effective antipsoriatic agent.

Hydroxyurea

For hepatic disease, chemotherapy with hydroxyurea, which uncommonly induces hepatotoxicity,[81] may be considered. Response is slower and less complete than with methotrexate, and resistance to hydroxyurea may develop more frequently. Hydroxyurea is administered orally at a dosage of 1 to 2 g/day. Careful monitoring of blood counts is necessary during therapy.

Sulfasalazine

Sulfasalazine in dosages of 3 to 4 g daily was reported to be beneficial for most patients. Over 25% of patients stopped the treatment because of side effects. In clinical practice, results have been less promising.[82] Sulfasalazine is not approved for psoriasis but is highly effective in selected patients.

COMBINATION THERAPY

Combinations of various psoriasis treatments have proved to be superior in efficacy to monotherapy. Acitretin is routinely used with UVB and PUVA, a combination that allows the use of smaller doses and minimizes toxicities of both retinoid and phototherapy.[66,67] Methotrexate and acitretin have been used successfully despite some concern that both drugs are hepatotoxic.[83] Careful monitoring of liver enzyme levels is essential. Methotrexate and cyclosporine can be used together. Concurrent administration of these two agents in small doses can result in greater efficacy and less toxicity than that which can be achieved with higher doses of either methotrexate or cyclosporine used alone.[84] Methotrexate has also been used very successfully in combination with UVB[85] and PUVA,[86] although there is some concern that methotrexate may potentiate the carcinogenic effect of PUVA.[87] Because cyclosporine has been associated with skin cancers, it is not routinely used in combination with PUVA. It can be used in combination with retinoids and mycophenolate mofetil.

BIOLOGIC THERAPIES

Advances in biotechnology have allowed the creation of molecules that target specific steps in the pathogenesis of psoriasis. Several steps in the pathogenesis of psoriasis have proved to be optimal targets. First, activation of T cells places a key role in the development of psoriasis. For T cells to be activated, it is clear that at least two signals must be delivered by the antigen-presenting cell to the resting T cell. By blocking any of those costimulatory signals, T cell activation and development of psoriasis can be blocked. Thus, alefacept, a fusion protein that consists of the Fc portion of human IgG1 and LFA-3, blocks the interaction between LFA-3 on antigen-presenting cells and CD2 on T cells.[88] Efalizumab, a humanized monoclonal antibody to CD11A, which is a component of LFA-1 on the surface of T cells, blocks the interaction between LFA-1 on T cells and ICAM1 on antigen-presenting cells. Efalizumab works by a second mechanism, because the interaction between LFA-1 and ICAM-1 is also involved in tethering of circulating T cells to endothelium. By blocking that interaction, efalizumab prevents trafficking of activated T cells into inflamed skin.[89]

Once activated, T cells release cytokines, including tumor necrosis factor–α (TNF-α). Two agents approved for the treatment of rheumatoid arthritis and Crohn disease—etanercept and infliximab—have also proved to be effective for psoriasis.[90,91] Both agents block TNF-α, resulting in improvement in psoriasis and psoriatic arthritis.

All of the aforementioned biologic agents appear to be free of the nephrotoxicity of cyclosporine and the hepatotoxicity of methotrexate. Undoubtedly, patients at risk for the side effects of methotrexate and cyclosporine will consider switching to these new medications, but many factors, including expense and severity of psoriasis, will have to be considered when selecting new therapies. Certainly, wholesale abandonment of current psoriasis therapies is not likely to occur despite the advent of these exciting new drugs. However, these new agents may help reduce the cumulative major organ toxicity of drugs such as cyclosporine and methotrexate.

FUTURE THERAPIES

Mycophenolate mofetil, a drug that was approved for the prevention of organ transplant rejection, is highly effective for some patients with psoriasis.[92] Mycophenolate mofetil is the prodrug of mycophenolic acid, a medication that was tested for psoriasis in the 1970s.[93] Although mycophenolic acid was found to be highly effective in the treatment of psoriasis, the manufacturers did not pursue FDA approval for that indication because of its side effects, which included gastrointestinal toxicity and an immunosuppressive effect that resulted in the occurrence of herpes zoster infections in more than 10% of treated patients.

6-Thioguanine is another agent that is available for the treatment of malignancy and that is highly effective for psoriasis. Unfortunately, it was associated with bone marrow suppression in approximately 50% of patients.[94] Administration of 6-thioguanine two to three times a week can reduce bone marrow toxicity.[95]

In addition to the biologic agents discussed above, several fusion proteins that block key steps in T cell activation have been developed. In clinical trials, at least one of these has been effective for psoriasis.[7]

Prognosis

Severe exacerbation of psoriasis taxes the ingenuity of even the most skilled clinician. Fortunately, the wide range of psoriasis therapies now available enables clinicians to successfully treat almost all patients with psoriasis. The goal of therapy must be to minimize toxicity while achieving satisfactory improvement.

References

1. Koo J: Population-based epidemiologic study of psoriasis with emphasis on quality of life assessment. Dermatol Clin 14:485, 1996

2. Farber EM, Nall ML: The natural history of psoriasis in 5,600 patients. Dermatologica 148:1, 1974

3. Gottlieb SL, Gilleaudeau P, Johnson R, et al: Response of psoriasis to a lymphocyte-selective toxin (DAB389IL-2) suggests a primary immune, but not keratinocyte, pathogenic basis. Nat Med 1:442, 1995

4. Bagel J, Garland WT, Breneman D, et al: Administration of DAB389IL-2 to patients with recalcitrant psoriasis: a double-blind, phase II multicenter trial. J Am Acad Dermatol 38:938, 1998

5. Krueger JG: The immunologic basis for the treatment of psoriasis with new biologic agents (review). J Am Acad Dermatol 46:1, 2002

6. Singri P, West DP, Gordon KB: Biologic therapy for psoriasis: the new therapeutic frontier. Arch Dermatol 138:657, 2002

7. Abrams JR, Lebwohl MG, Guzzo CA, et al: CTLA4Ig-mediated blockage of T-cell costimulation in patients with psoriasis vulgaris. J Clin Invest 103:1243, 1999

8. Ellis CN, Krueger GG: Treatment of chronic plaque psoriasis by selective targeting of memory effector T lymphocytes. N Engl J Med 345:248, 2001

9. Gottlieb A, Krueger JG, Bright R, et al: Effects of administration of a single dose of a humanized monoclonal antibody to CD11a on the immunobiology and clinical activity of psoriasis. J Am Acad Dermatol 42:428, 2000

10. Farber EM, Nall ML, Watson W: Natural history of psoriasis in 61 twin pairs. Arch Dermatol 109:207, 1974

11. Tomfohrde J, Silverman A, Barnes R, et al: Gene for familial psoriasis susceptibility mapped to the distal end of human chromosome 17q. Science 264:1141, 1994

12. Barker JN: Genetic aspects of psoriasis. Clin Exp Dermatol 26:321, 2001

13. Queille-Roussel C, Duteil L, Parneix-Spake A, et al: The safety of calcitriol 3 µg/g ointment: evaluation of cutaneous contact sensitization, cumulative irritancy, photoallergic contact sensitization and phototoxicity. Eur J Dermatol 11:219, 2001

14. Lebwohl M, Tan MH: Psoriasis and stress. Lancet 351:82, 1998

15. Gaston L, Lassonde M, Bernier-Buzzanga J, et al: Psoriasis and stress: a prospective study. J Am Acad Dermatol 17:82, 1987

16. Rapp SR, Feldman SR, Exum ML, et al: Psoriasis causes as much disability as other major medical diseases. J Am Acad Dermatol 41:401, 1999

17. Telfer NR, Chalmers RG, Whale K, et al: The role of streptococcal infection in the initiation of guttate psoriasis. Arch Dermatol 128:39, 1992

18. Vincent F, Ross JB, Dalton M, et al: A therapeutic trial of the use of penicillin V or erythromycin with or without rifampin in the treatment of psoriasis. J Am Acad Dermatol 26:458, 1992

19. Rosenberg EW, Noah PW, Zanolli MD, et al: Use of rifampin with penicillin and erythromycin in the treatment of psoriasis: preliminary report. J Am Acad Dermatol 14:761, 1986

20. Obuch ML, Maurer TA, Becker B, et al: Psoriasis and human immunodeficiency virus infection. J Am Acad Dermatol 27:667, 1992

21. Abel EA: Diagnosis of drug-induced psoriasis. Semin Dermatol 11:269, 1992

22. Krueger GG: Psoriasis: current concepts of its etiology and pathogenesis. Yearbook of Dermatology. Dobson RL, Thiers BH, Eds. Year Book Medical Publishers, Chicago, 1982, p 13

23. Katayama H, Kawada A: Exacerbation of psoriasis induced by indomethacin. J Dermatol (Tokyo) 8:323, 1981

24. Gupta MA, Gupta AK, Watteel GN: Cigarette smoking in men may be a risk factor for increased severity of psoriasis of the extremities. Br J Dermatol 135:859, 1996

25. Naldi L, Peli L, Parazzini F: Association of early-stage psoriasis with smoking and male alcohol consumption: evidence from an Italian case-control study. Arch Dermatol 135:1479, 1999

26. Naldi L, Parazzini F, Peli L, et al: Dietary factors and the risk of psoriasis: results of an Italian case-control study. Br J Dermatol 134:101, 1996

27. Green MS, Prystowsky JH, Cohen SR, et al: Infectious complications of erythrodermic psoriasis. J Am Acad Dermatol 34:911, 1996

28. Calvert HT, Smith MA, Wells RS: Psoriasis and the nails. Br J Dermatol 75:415, 1963

29. Gladman DD, Hing EN, Schentag CT, et al: Remission in psoriatic arthritis. J Rheumatol 28:1045, 2001

30. Lebwohl M: Advances in psoriasis therapy. Dermatol Clin 18:13, 2000

31. Feldman SR, Fleischer AB, Cooper JZ: New topical treatments change the pattern of treatment of psoriasis: dermatologists remain the primary providers of this care. Int J Dermatol 39:41, 2000

32. Cornell RC, Stoughton RB: Correlation of the vasoconstriction assay and clinical activity in psoriasis. Arch Dermatol 121:63, 1985

33. Katz HI, Prawer SE, Medansky RS, et al: Intermittent corticosteroid maintenance treatment of psoriasis: a double-blind multicenter trial of augmented betamethasone dipropionate ointment in a pulse dose treatment regimen. Dermatologica 183:269, 1991

34. Lebwohl M, Siskin SB, Epinette W, et al: A multicenter trial of calcipotriene ointment and halobetasol ointment to either agent alone for the treatment of psoriasis. J Am Acad Dermatol 35:268, 1996

35. Lebwohl M, Yoles A, Lombardi K, et al: Calcipotriene ointment and halobetasol ointment in the long-term treatment of psoriasis: effects on the duration of improvement. J Am Acad Dermatol 39:447, 1998

36. Ramsay CA, Schwartz BE, Lowson D, et al: Calcipotriol cream combined with twice weekly broad-band UVB phototherapy: a safe, effective and UVB-sparing antipsoriatic combination treatment. The Canadian Calcipotriol and UVB Study Group. Dermatology 200:17, 2000

37. Speight EL, Farr PM: Calcipotriol improves the response of psoriasis to PUVA. Br J Dermatol 130:79, 1994

38. Patel B, Siskin S, Krazmien BA, et al: Compatibility of calcipotriene with other topical medications. J Am Acad Dermatol 38:1010, 1998

39. Lebwohl M, Hecker D, Martinez J, et al: Interactions between calcipotriene and ultraviolet light. J Am Acad Dermatol 37:93, 1997

40. Georgiou S, Tsambaos D: Hypercalcaemia and hypercalciuria after topical treatment of psoriasis with excessive amounts of calcipotriol. Acta Derm Venereol 79:86, 1999

41. Koo JY: Tazarotene in combination with phototherapy. J Am Acad Dermatol 39:S144, 1998

42. Hecker D, Worsley J, Yueh G, et al: Interactions between tazarotene and ultraviolet light. J Am Acad Dermatol 41:927, 1999

43. Lowe NJ, Breeding J, Wortzman MS: The pharmacological variability of crude coal

tar. Br J Dermatol 126:608, 1992

44. Fiore M: Practical aspects of anthralin therapy. Cutis 46:351, 1990

45. Abel EA, O'Connell BM, Farber EM: Psoriasis Day Care Center treatment at Stanford: part-time and full-time programs. Int J Dermatol 26:500, 1987

46. Schaefer H, Farber EM, Goldberg L, et al: Limited application period for dithranol in psoriasis: preliminary report on penetration and clinical efficacy. Br J Dermatol 102:571, 1980

47. Volden G, Bjornberg A, Tegner E, et al: Short-contact treatment at home with micanol. Acta Derm Venereol Suppl (Stockh) 172:20, 1992

48. Even-Paz Z, Gumon R, Kipnis V, et al: Dead Sea sun vs. Dead Sea water in the treatment of psoriasis. Dermatol Treat 7:83, 1996

49. Frentz G, Olsen JH, Avrach WW: Malignant tumours and psoriasis: climatotherapy at the Dead Sea. Br J Dermatol 141:1088, 1999

50. Petrozzi JW, Barton JO, Kaidbey KH, et al: Updating the Goeckerman regimen for psoriasis. Br J Dermatol 98:437, 1978

51. Lowe NJ, Wortzman MS, Breeding J, et al: Coal tar phototherapy for psoriasis reevaluated: erythemogenic versus suberythemogenic ultraviolet with a tar extract in oil and crude coal tar. J Am Acad Dermatol 8:781, 1983

52. Stern RS, Gange RW, Parrish JA, et al: Contribution of topical tar oil to ultra-violet B phototherapy for psoriasis. J Am Acad Dermatol 14:742, 1986

53. Lowe NJ, Stern RS: Contribution of topical tar oil to ultraviolet B phototherapy for psoriasis. J Am Acad Dermatol 15:1053, 1986

54. Barbagallo J, Spann CT, Tutrone WD, et al: Narrowband UVB phototherapy for the treatment of psoriasis: a review and update. Cutis 68:345, 2001

55. Dawe RS, Cameron H, Yule S, et al: UV-B phototherapy clears psoriasis through local effects. Arch Dermatol 138:1071, 2002

56. Abel EA: Administration of PUVA therapy: protocols, indications, and cautions. Photochemotherapy in Dermatology. Abel EA, Ed. Igaku-Shoin Medical Publishers, New York, 1992, p 75

57. Stern RS, Laird N: The carcinogenic risk of treatments for severe psoriasis. Cancer 73:2759, 1994

58. Stern RS, Thibodeau LA, Kleinerman RA, et al: Risk of cutaneous carcinoma in patients treated with oral methoxsalen photochemotherapy for psoriasis. N Engl J Med 300:809, 1979

59. Stern RS, Laird N, Melski J, et al: Cutaneous squamous-cell carcinoma in patients treated with PUVA. N Engl J Med 310:1156, 1984

60. Lerman S, Borkman RF: A method for detecting 8-methoxypsoralen in the ocular lens. Science 197:1287, 1977

61. Lerman S: Ocular phototoxicity and psoralen plus ultraviolet radiation (320–400 nm) therapy: an experimental and clinical evaluation. J Natl Cancer Inst 69:287, 1982

62. Jeffes EB III, McCullough JL, Pittelkow MR, et al: Methotrexate therapy of psoriasis: differential sensitivity of proliferating lymphoid and epithelial cells to the cytotoxic and growth-inhibitory effects of methotrexate. J Invest Dermatol 104:183, 1995

63. Roenigk HH Jr, Auerbach R, Maibach H, et al: Methotrexate in psoriasis: consensus conference. J Am Acad Dermatol 38:478, 1998

64. Gilbert SC, Lintmalm G, Menter A, et al: Methotrexate-induced cirrhosis requiring liver transplantation in three patients with psoriasis: a word of caution in light of the expanding use of this "steroid-sparing" agent. Arch Intern Med 150:889, 1990

65. Al-Awadhi A, Dale P, McKendry RJ: Pancytopenia associated with low dose methotrexate therapy: a regional survey. J Rheumatol 20:1121, 1993

66. Lebwohl M: Acitretin in combination with UVB or PUVA. J Am Acad Dermatol 4:S22, 1999

67. Lebwohl M, Drake L, Menter A, et al: Consensus conference: acitretin in combination with UVB or PUVA in the treatment of psoriasis. J Am Acad Dermatol. 45:544, 2001

68. Roenigk HH Jr, Callen JP, Guzzo CA, et al: Effects of acitretin on the liver. J Am Acad Dermatol 41:585, 1999

69. Larsen FG, Jakobsen P, Knudsen J, et al: Conversion of acitretin to etretinate in psoriatic patients is influenced by ethanol. J Invest Dermatol 100:623, 1993

70. DiGiovanna JJ, Sollitto RB, Abangan DL, et al: Osteoporosis is a toxic effect of long-term etretinate therapy. Arch Dermatol 131:1263, 1995

71. Wilson DJ, Kay V, Charig M, et al: Skeletal hyperostosis and extraosseous calcification in patients receiving long-term etretinate (Tigason). Br J Dermatol 119:597, 1988

72. Stern RS, Fitzgerald E, Ellis CN, et al: The safety of etretinate as long-term therapy for psoriasis: results of the Etretinate Follow-Up Study. J Am Acad Dermatol 33:44, 1995

73. Lebwohl M, Ellis C, Gottlieb A, et al: Cyclosporine consensus conference: with emphasis on the treatment of psoriasis. J Am Acad Dermatol 39:464, 1998

74. Raman GV, Campbell SK, Farrer A, et al: Modifying effects of amlodipine on cyclosporin A–induced changes in renal function in patients with psoriasis. J Hypertens Suppl 16:S39, 1998

75. Zachariae H, Kragballe K, Hansen HE, et al: Renal biopsy findings in long-term cyclosporin treatment of psoriasis. Br J Dermatol 136:531, 1997

76. Lowe NJ, Wieder JM, Rosenbach A, et al: Long-term low-dose cyclosporine therapy for severe psoriasis: effects on renal function and structure. J Am Acad Dermatol 35:710, 1996

77. Jensen P, Hansen S, Moller B, et al: Skin cancer in kidney and heart transplant recipients and different long-term immunosuppressive therapy regimens. J Am Acad Dermatol 40:177, 1999

78. Srivastava T, Zwick DL, Rothberg PG, et al: Posttransplant lymphoproliferative disorder in pediatric renal transplantation. Pediatr Nephrol 13:748, 1999

79. van den Borne BE, Landewe RB, Houkes I, et al: No increased risk of malignancies and mortality in cyclosporin A–treated patients with rheumatoid arthritis. Arthritis Rheum 41:1930, 1998

80. Systemic tacrolimus (FK 506) is effective for the treatment of psoriasis in a double-blind, placebo-controlled study. The European FK 506 Multicenter Psoriasis Study Group. Arch Dermatol 132:419, 1996

81. Smith CH: Use of hydroxyurea in psoriasis. Clin Exp Dermatol 24:2, 1999

82. Gupta AK, Ellis CN, Siegel MT, et al: Sulfasalazine improves psoriasis: a double-blind analysis. Arch Dermatol 126:487, 1990

83. Roenigk HH Jr: Acitretin combination therapy. J Am Acad Dermatol 41:S18, 1999

84. Wong KC, Georgouras K: Low dose cyclosporin A and methotrexate in the treatment of psoriasis. Acta Derm Venereol 79:87, 1999

85. Paul BS, Momtaz K, Stern RS, et al: Combined methotrexate–ultraviolet B therapy in the treatment of psoriasis. J Am Acad Dermatol 7:758, 1982

86. Morison WL, Momtaz K, Parrish JA, et al: Combined methotrexate–PUVA therapy in the treatment of psoriasis. J Am Acad Dermatol 6:46, 1982

87. Stern RS, Laird N: The carcinogenic risk of treatments for severe psoriasis. Photochemotherapy Follow-up Study. Cancer 73:2759, 1994

88. Krueger GG: Selective targeting of T cell subsets: focus on alefacept: a remittive therapy for psoriasis. Expert Opin Biol Ther 2:431, 2002

89. Krueger J, Gottlieb A, Miller B, et al: Anti-CD11a treatment for psoriasis concurrently increases circulating T-cells and decreases plaque T-cells, consistent with inhibition of cutaneous T-cell trafficking. J Invest Dermatol 115:333, 2000

90. Mease PJ, Goffe BS, Metz J, et al: Etanercept in the treatment of psoriatic arthritis and psoriasis: a randomised trial. Lancet 356:385, 2000

91. Chaudhari U, Romano P, Mulcahy LD, et al: Efficacy and safety of infliximab monotherapy for plaque-type psoriasis: a randomised trial. Lancet 357:1842, 2001

92. Kirby B, Yates VM: Mycophenolate mofetil for psoriasis. Br J Dermatol 139:357, 1998

93. Epinette WW, Parker CM, Jones EL, et al: Mycophenolic acid for psoriasis: a review of pharmacology, long-term efficacy, and safety. J Am Acad Dermatol 17:962, 1987

94. Zackheim HS, Glogau RG, Fisher DA, et al: 6-Thioguanine treatment of psoriasis: experience in 81 patients. J Am Acad Dermatol 30:452, 1994

95. Silvis NG, Levine N: Pulse dosing of thioguanine in recalcitrant psoriasis. Arch Dermatol 135:433, 1999

34 Eczematous Disorders, Atopic Dermatitis, and Ichthyoses

Seth R. Stevens, M.D., *Kevin D. Cooper*, M.D., *and Kefei Kang*, M.D.

Eczematous Disorders

Eczematous dermatitis, or eczema, is a skin disease that is characterized by erythematous vesicular, weeping, and crusting patches. Although the term eczema is often used as a diagnosis, it can in fact be used appropriately to describe lesions seen in several diseases. Itching is a characteristic symptom, and epidermal intercellular edema (spongiosis) is a characteristic histopathologic finding of eczematous conditions. The term eczema is also commonly used to describe atopic dermatitis [*see* Atopic Dermatitis, *below*].

CONTACT DERMATITIS

Contact dermatitis, a paradigmatic example of an eczematous disorder, is common and well studied [*see Chapter 35*]. Contact dermatitis can be either allergic or irritant in etiology. Allergic contact dermatitis differs from other eczematous disorders in that determination of the offending contactant is an important part of the evaluation. If the patient's history does not provide the answer, the body site of the lesion may (e.g., head involvement in allergy to paraphenylenediamine in hair dye). Patch testing may be required to confirm the diagnosis.[1]

The manifestations of irritant contact dermatitis are similar to those of allergic contact dermatitis[2]; in the irritant form, however, the mechanism is not immunologic. Given sufficient concentration and duration of contact, offending agents will induce irritation in anyone's skin. Detergents, acids, alkalis, solvents, formaldehyde, and fiberglass are common causes.

SEBORRHEIC DERMATITIS

Seborrheic dermatitis is another common eczematous condition [*see Chapter 32*]. Clinically, seborrheic dermatitis may exist without vesicle formation. Lesional morphology is usually a greasy scale on erythematous patches; however, the scale may be dry and the patches may have an orange hue. Scalp, eyebrows, mustache area, nasolabial folds, and chest are typical areas of involvement. Psoriasis may be in the differential diagnosis. Treatment is with shampoos containing selenium sulfide, zinc pyrithione, tar, or ketoconazole; emollients; and mild (nonfluorinated) topical steroids. Antimicrobial therapy directed at the commensal yeast *Pityrosporum ovale* can be effective, although a causative role of the organism remains unproved.

OTHER ECZEMATOUS DERMATITIDES

Two other eczematous dermatitides are nummular eczema and dyshidrotic eczema (pompholyx). Nummular eczema describes well-demarcated, coin-shaped eczematous patches that are usually 2 to 4 cm (rarely more than 10 cm) in diameter. The lesions are quite pruritic and require potent topical steroids, antihistamines, and, occasionally, intralesional or systemic corticosteroids for treatment. Dyshidrotic eczema presents as a vesicular eruption of the hands and feet, accompanied on rare occasions by hyperhidrosis. Typically, 1 to 2 mm vesicles appear on the sides of fingers, although more extensive involvement can occur. Treatment is with compresses and soaks, antipruritics, topical steroids, and, in severe recalcitrant cases, systemic corticosteroids. Photochemotherapy with topical psoralen and ultraviolet A irradiation (PUVA) may also be effective.

Atopic Dermatitis

Atopic dermatitis (AD) is a common chronic inflammatory dermatosis. The term atopy was coined in the early 1920s to describe the associated triad of asthma, allergic rhinitis, and dermatitis.[3] The role of reaginic antibodies and allergies in the etiology of AD is controversial; in 80% of patients with AD, however, serum immunoglobulin IgE is elevated, sometimes markedly.

ETIOLOGY AND PATHOGENESIS

The expression of AD is a complex integration of environmental and genetic factors. The lifetime prevalence is estimated to be 30% of the population,[4-6] possibly because of increasing contact with causative agents in the environment. Epidemiologic data suggest a genetic influence—25% of dizygotic twins and 75% of monozygotic twins are concordant for AD.[7] The condition develops in 60% of children who have one affected parent and in 80% of children with two affected parents.[8] The defect is likely carried in the immune system, because both antigen-specific IgE reactivity and AD have been transplanted from an AD-affected bone marrow donor to a previously unaffected recipient.[9] Candidate genes continue to be investigated.

AD can be quickly exacerbated by environmental trigger factors.[10] Wool, lanolin, and harsh detergents are particularly irritating. Emotional stress can also lead to flares. The role of airborne and foodborne allergens is difficult to assess. Although patients with AD frequently have circulating dust mite antigen-specific IgE and T_{H2} $CD4^+$ T cells,[11] hyposensitization infrequently results in improvement. Contact urticaria to food occurs in AD,[12] but generalized exacerbation after eating is rare. In the absence of a strong supporting history, elimination diets are rarely effective in treating AD. A role has been frequently suggested for cow's milk in inducing AD; however, such an association was not supported in a study of AD in infants fed breast milk rather than cow's milk–based formula.[13] Mechanisms have been proposed to explain a link between *Staphylococcus aureus* and exacerbations of AD,[14] including effects of cell wall constituents to increase expression of IgE, IgE receptor, and enterotoxin B, a superantigen that activates T cells in an antigen-independent fashion.[15]

The apparent paradox of reduced cell-mediated immunity[16,17] and hyperimmunoglobulinemia E seen in AD is addressed by the so-called T_{H1}/T_{H2} model of helper T cells. In this model of the murine immune system, $CD4^+$ cells are divided into two mutually exclusive classes on the basis of cytokine secretion: T_{H1} cells, which secrete cytokines that promote cell-mediated immunity (e.g., interleukin-2 [IL-2], interferon gamma), and T_{H2} cells, which secrete cytokines that promote humoral immunity and eosinophil function (e.g., IL-4 and IL-5). Atopy, including AD, has been seen as the paradigmatic condition of a so-called T_{H1}-deficient state. Refinements have shown a heterogeneity of re-

Table 1   Diagnostic Criteria for Atopic Dermatitis[11]

Major criteria

    Personal or family history of atopy (atopic dermatitis, allergic rhinitis, allergic conjunctivitis, allergic blepharitis, or asthma)

    Characteristic morphology and distribution of lesions

    Pruritus

    Chronic or chronically recurring dermatosis

Minor features

    Hyperimmunoglobulinemia E

    Food intolerance

    Intolerance to wool and lipid solvents

    Recurrent skin infections

    Xerosis

    Sweat-induced pruritus

    White (not red) dermatographism

    Ichthyosis

    Chronically scaling scalp

    Accentuation of hair follicles

    Recurrent conjunctivitis

    Anterior subcapsular cataracts and keratoconus

    Morgan line, or Dennie sign (single or double creases in the lower eyelids)

    Periorbital darkening (allergic shiner)

    Pityriasis alba (hypopigmented, scaling patches, typically on the cheeks)

    Cheilitis

    Anterior neck folds

    Keratosis pilaris (perifollicular papules with keratotic plugs, typically on the arms and thighs)

    Nipple eczema

    Hyperlinear palms (increased folds, typically on the thenar or hypothenar eminence)

    Recurrent hand and foot dermatitis

    Exacerbation of symptoms by environmental or emotional factors

sponses within different AD lesions, however. The current model is that blood and acute lesions of AD patients are more often dominated by T_{H2} cells, whereas chronic lesions are more often dominated by T_{H1} cells.[18]

Hyperstimulatory dendritic antigen-presenting cells (Langerhans cells) are present in patients with AD.[19] One proposed mechanism for the augmented function of Langerhans cells in AD is the binding of antigen-specific IgE and antigen to the IgE receptors on Langerhans cells as a means of antigen focusing.[20] Another antigen-presenting cell, the monocyte, also manifests altered function in AD. Cyclic adenosine monophosphate (cAMP) phosphodiesterase has increased activity in monocytes of patients with AD—leading to hyperproduction of prostaglandin E_2, among other effects. Increased cAMP phosphodiesterase in AD may explain aberrant adrenergic responses, and the increased prostaglandin E_2 leads to diminished interferon-gamma production. Additionally, monocytes secrete IL-10 in AD, which further augments the so-called T_{H2} responses.[21] Altered cyclic nucleotide metabolism leads to excessive release of histamine by basophils and, potentially, to mast cell degranulation. High levels of cAMP phosphodiesterase are found in the umbilical cord blood of infants of AD-affected parents.[22] This finding may indicate an early, if not primary, defect in the disease that may become the basis of a diagnostic laboratory test.

Because IL-5 is a critical eosinophil growth factor and activating cytokine, blood eosinophilia may be expected to occur in a

T_{H2} disease such as AD[23]; tissue eosinophilia, however, is variable. Cutaneous endothelial cells are also activated in AD, leading to increased expression of adhesion molecules and recruitment of leukocytes into the skin (i.e., dermatitis).

DIAGNOSIS

AD remains a clinical diagnosis. Major diagnostic criteria are (1) personal or family history of atopy (AD, allergic rhinitis, allergic conjunctivitis, allergic blepharitis, or asthma); (2) characteristic morphology and distribution of lesions; (3) pruritus; and (4) chronic or chronically recurring dermatosis. Several minor features can be added [see Table 1].[12] Pruritus is a consistent feature of AD. The lack of itching or of another major diagnostic criterion should prompt consideration of alternative diagnoses [see Differential Diagnosis, below]. Cutaneous signs can vary, depending on the age of the lesions.

Acute lesions of AD are eczematous—erythematous, scaling, and papulovesicular. Weeping and crusted lesions may develop [see Figure 1]. Scratching results acutely in linear excoriations, presenting as erosions or a hemorrhagic crust. In extremely severe cases, exfoliative dermatitis (erythroderma) may occur, with generalized redness, scaling, weeping, and crusting. There may be accompanying systemic toxicity, sepsis, lymphadenopathy, altered thermoregulation (either hyperthermia or hypothermia), and high-output cardiac failure. Erythroderma is a potentially life-threatening condition.

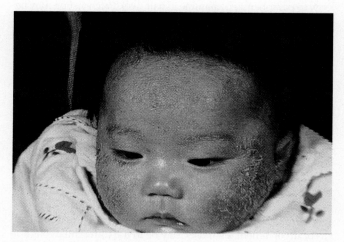

Figure 1   Extensive, severe, weeping, crusted acute eczematous patches on the face of this infant are characteristic of patients in this age group.

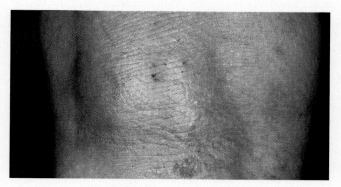

Figure 2   Lichenified patches appear after chronic rubbing of eczematous patches. These lesions are characteristic of chronic allergic contact dermatitis and atopic dermatitis.

Chronic lesions tend not to be eczematous (thus, atopic eczema is not an ideal synonym for AD). Instead, lichenified plaques [see Figure 2] or nodules predominate. Lichenification denotes areas of thickened skin divided by deep linear furrows. Lichenified plaques result from repeated rubbing or scratching and thus often occur in areas of predilection, such as the popliteal and cubital fossae. As is typical of lesions in AD, lichenification is poorly demarcated. There may be accompanying acute signs. Lichenified lesions are very difficult to treat; once established, they may persist for months even with adequate therapy and avoidance of rubbing or scratching.

Clinical expression of AD also varies with the age of the patient. The infantile stage of AD occurs up to approximately 2 years of age. Of all cases of AD, approximately 90% arise before the fifth year and 60% in the first year of life; onset before 2 months of age is unusual, however.[7] During infancy, ill-defined, erythematous scaling patches and confluent, edematous papules and vesicles are typical. These lesions may become crusted and exudative. Intense pruritus leads to scratching, which induces linear excoriations and, with time, lichenification. Before the infant begins to crawl, the scalp and face are most often involved [see Figure 1], although lesions may be seen anywhere. After the child begins crawling, the extensor surfaces—particularly the knees—become involved. Involvement of fingers can be severe if the child sucks them frequently. Intense pruritus can lead to sleep disturbances of child and parents. Other features may arise [see Table 1]. Perifollicular accentuation and papules are commonly seen at any point in the life of an atopic patient, particularly in persons of Asian or African ancestry.

During childhood, the clinical features evolve into those seen in adults. Lesions tend to become less eczematous and drier, with increasing flexural and neck involvement. Scaling, fissured, and crusted hands may become especially troublesome. Infraorbital folds (sometimes called Morgan lines or the Dennie sign) and pityriasis alba can appear. Chronic or chronically relapsing pruritic, erythematous, papulovesicular eruptions that progress to scaling, lichenified dermatitis in a flexural distribution typify adult AD. Extensive areas of skin may be involved, including the face, chest, neck, flanks, and hands. Areas of dyspigmentation may result from repeated skin trauma. Approximately 10% to 15% of childhood AD persists after puberty.[7]

AD that begins after 20 years of age has been termed adult-onset atopic dermatitis.[24] This condition should be considered in patients with characteristic features of AD.

There are many associated features of AD. Asthma and allergic rhinitis, the major and minor criteria, respectively, have already been mentioned. Another important association, cutaneous infection, is related to diminished cutaneous cell-mediated immunity and defective chemotaxis. S. aureus is usually found on AD skin, and its density correlates with lesion severity. Although such observations have implicated S. aureus as a cause of AD,[14,25] it is also clear that reduction in AD lesions reduces bacterial colonization.[26] Regardless, the high bacterial counts in lesional skin and the relative ease of their reduction suggest the desirability of extra efforts (e.g., use of topical steroids) to reduce the presence of S. aureus before elective procedures are performed through involved skin. Frank infection also occurs more commonly in AD, which results in pustules and oozing, crusted lesions.

Cutaneous fungal and viral infections also occur frequently and with increased severity in patients with AD. Eczema herpeticum, an extensive eruption of 2 to 3 mm vesicles, pustules, and punched-out erosions caused by herpes simplex virus,

may coalesce into extensive areas of eroded skin. Frequently, the condition is most severe on the face (where it often arises from a herpetic lesion) and diminishes as it progresses to the trunk and extremities. Secondary bacterial infection is common. Lymphadenopathy, fever, and malaise may develop. Antiviral and antibiotic therapy can be lifesaving and should be started empirically upon presentation. Tzanck test, viral culture, and direct fluorescent antibody detection of viral antigens can confirm the diagnosis.

Molluscum contagiosum and common warts are also problematic in patients with AD, as are dermatophyte infections. Because of similar appearance, foot eczema must be distinguished from tinea pedis by potassium hydroxide preparation or fungal culture.

Numerous ocular complications of AD exist.[27] These include anterior subcapsular cataracts, retinal detachment, keratoconus, blepharitis, conjunctivitis, and iritis.

DIFFERENTIAL DIAGNOSIS

The differential diagnosis of AD includes the eczematous conditions and ichthyoses described in this chapter and other immunologic, metabolic, neoplastic, and rheumatologic disorders [see Table 2]. Because 80% to 85% of patients with occupational hand dermatitis have AD, the possibility of coexisting AD and contact dermatitis needs to be considered. Another important element of the differential diagnosis is cutaneous T cell lymphoma. Cutaneous T cell lymphoma can arise clinically as scaling, erythematous patches or exfoliative erythroderma. The classic distribution—near axillae, buttocks, and groin—is distinct from that of AD, and patches are frequently well demarcated. There is often sufficient clinical overlap between the two conditions, however, to necessitate further investigation, including histology, immunophenotyping, and gene rearrangement analysis of T cell receptors. Cutaneous T cell lymphoma can arise in patients with AD, and the lack of conclusive clinical or laboratory tests for either disease can make distinction difficult. Reassessment from time to time in such cases is recommended.

Table 2 Differential Diagnosis of Atopic Dermatitis

Type	Disorders
Dermatitides	Allergic contact dermatitis Dermatitis herpetiformis Irritant contact dermatitis (may be concomitant with atopic dermatitis) Nummular eczema Seborrheic dermatitis
Ichthyoses	Ichthyosis vulgaris
Immunologic disorders	Graft versus host disease HIV-associated dermatosis Hyperimmunoglobulinemia E syndrome Wiskott-Aldrich syndrome
Infectious diseases	Scabies Dermatophytosis
Metabolic disorders	Zinc deficiency Various inborn errors of metabolism
Neoplastic disorders	Cutaneous T cell lymphoma
Rheumatologic disorders	Dermatomyositis

TREATMENT

Reduction of Trigger Factors

Reduction of trigger factors (e.g., harsh chemicals, detergents, and wool) and avoidance of occupations that require contact with trigger factors (e.g., hairdressing, nursing, and construction) can be helpful. Appropriate behaviors should be taught to patients and parents early during life, when habits are more easily formed.[28,29]

The use of mild, nonalkali soaps and frequent use of emollients are important elements in the long-term management of AD. Because moisture evaporating off the skin can trigger flares, bathing is sometimes discouraged. A better approach is the prompt application of an emollient such as petrolatum (finishing within 3 minutes of the end of the bath), which can serve to seal the moisture from the bath. Lotions and creams containing high amounts of water are usually inadequate, however, and can actually worsen AD. Products containing hydroxy acids, phenol, or urea can reduce dryness and scaling, but these can sting inflamed skin and should therefore be used with caution. Because of a specific reduction of ceramides in AD, a lotion that provides excess ceramides relative to other lipids has been tried in AD and appears to have a therapeutic advantage.[30] Bubble baths and scented salts and oils can be irritating. Scalp care should include a bland shampoo. Topical tar products, such as shampoos and bath solutions, and topical creams and lotions containing 5% to 10% liquor carbonis detergens can help. Baths, soaks, and compresses with Burow solution can ameliorate crusted, infected, eczematous patches. Cotton clothing, washed to remove finishing (which often releases formaldehyde), is preferable to wool or synthetics.

Corticosteroids

Topical corticosteroids are another mainstay of therapy. Application immediately after bathing improves cutaneous penetration. Lowering the risk of side effects with less potent preparations must be balanced against gaining control of a flare quickly with more potent preparations. Long-term use of inadequately potent topical corticosteroids may pose a greater risk of adverse effects than brief use of more potent agents followed by a rapid taper to bland emollients. Because steroid-induced cutaneous atrophy is a greater risk on the face, in intertriginous areas (e.g., groin, axillae, and inframammary folds), and under diapers, less potent steroids (e.g., hydrocortisone and desonide) should be used in these areas, and they should be used with particular caution. For the remainder of the body, midpotency preparations, such as 0.1% triamcinolone acetonide, are helpful. More potent ointments, such as fluocinonide and desoximetasone, are useful for lichenified plaques. Flurandrenolide tape is useful for nodular prurigo (so-called picker's nodules) because it also physically protects the area from manipulation. For the scalp, solutions are preferred.

Systemic corticosteroids (e.g., prednisone, 20 to 80 mg/day orally) may be useful to treat severe, acute flares. Because of the risks of gastrointestinal, endocrine, skeletal, central nervous system, and cardiovascular complications, however, they should not be used more than twice yearly.

Other Therapies

Antihistamines can sometimes be helpful in breaking the itch-scratch cycle in AD. Sedating antihistamines, such as hydroxyzine and diphenhydramine, are particularly useful—especially when itching prevents sleep. Nonsedating antihistamines are less useful. Doxepin, a tricyclic antidepressant known to have antihistaminic effects, can be beneficial when applied topically in a 5% cream.

Virtually every phototherapy regimen has been reported to ameliorate AD. Some patients cannot tolerate the heat generated by the equipment, however—particularly that used in UVB irradiation. In addition to UVB, the following can be beneficial: UVA, longwave UVA1, narrow-band UVB, UVA-UVB, and PUVA. Extracorporeal photochemotherapy (photopheresis) is also emerging as an effective therapy for recalcitrant disease.[31] Although some patients may benefit from natural sunlight, the risk of sunburn and induction of malignancy by ultraviolet light must be considered.

The macrolide antibiotic tacrolimus has been approved for use in both pediatric (0.03% ointment) and adult (0.1% ointment) atopic dermatitis.[32] Current labeling is for use in steroid-unresponsive disease. However, because this medication appears to have a much-improved therapeutic index, its position in the armamentarium is still being determined. The ascomycin macrolactam derivative, SDZ ASM 981, also shows promise in AD[33] and may be widely available shortly.

Antimicrobials are obviously important for patients with infection. Less clear is whether antimicrobial agents can directly treat AD by reducing bacterial products thought to exacerbate the condition. Antistaphylococcal therapy has been advocated for use in patients with AD; however, a double-blind, placebo-controlled study of flucloxacillin did not show improvement in AD despite reduced bacterial counts.[34] Ketoconazole, likewise, has been used; its success, however, may be the result of anti-inflammatory, rather than antifungal, effects.

More advanced therapeutic options exist for severe, recalcitrant AD. The altered expression of cytokines in AD [see Etiology and Pathogenesis, above] has led investigators to explore the use of interferon gamma. Clinical trials have demonstrated that for some patients, daily subcutaneous administration of interferon gamma is effective in reducing both signs and symptoms of AD[35,36] and that long-term treatment can maintain the benefit.[37]

Oral cyclosporine (2.5 to 5 mg/kg/day orally),[38,39] methotrexate (15 to 25 mg/wk orally), and azathioprine (100 to 200 mg/day orally) can be used in severe, recalcitrant disease provided that patients are monitored for adverse effects specific to those agents.

Traditional Chinese herbal medicine has been found to be effective in the treatment of AD, both in children[40] and in adults,[41] although the efficacy of this treatment remains controversial.[42] The mechanisms of action of these preparations are unclear. Patients should be cautioned that herbal remedies are not risk free and may carry a potential for hepatotoxicity, cardiomyopathy, and other adverse effects; such remedies should be monitored, as should any other treatment.

Although evening primrose oil has for many years been proposed to be effective in AD, a well-controlled study failed to show any benefit to patients taking either evening primrose oil or a combination of evening primrose oil and fish oil compared with those receiving placebo.[43] The importance of well-controlled studies to assess efficacy of treatments must be stressed because AD patients on the placebo arms of most controlled studies tend to show benefit from the placebo. The cAMP phosphodiesterase inhibitor CP80633 shows promise as an emerging therapy.[44] These new agents, which are based on the emerging pathogenic concepts of altered cytokine production and cyclic nucleotide regulation, may prove to reduce pruritus and dermatitis effectively without producing unacceptable side effects.

Ichthyoses

The ichthyoses are a group of diseases of cornification that are characterized by excessive scaling.[45] Etiologies of the ichthyoses are diverse, including genetic defects of structural proteins and enzymes as well as acquired forms. Only the major clinical variants will be discussed here.

MAJOR VARIANTS

Ichthyosis Vulgaris

Ichthyosis vulgaris, the most common form of ichthyosis, is found in approximately one in 300 births. This autosomal dominant condition presents as dry skin with fine scaling. The extensor surfaces of extremities are the most commonly affected areas. Ichthyosis vulgaris can occur concomitantly with keratosis pilaris and can also be associated with AD. Age at onset is typically between 3 months and 12 months. Implicated etiologic factors include reduced filaggrin (filament-aggregating protein) and its precursor profilaggrin, whose normal functions are to allow for aggregation of keratin filaments and to serve as sources of compounds that hydrate the skin. The clinical severity of ichthyosis vulgaris correlates with the degree of reduction in filaggrin and profilaggrin. Another possible etiologic factor is the reduced activity of proteases that normally lead to dissociation of keratinocytes.[46]

X-Linked Ichthyosis

Recessive X-linked ichthyosis occurs in approximately one in 2,000 to one in 6,000 male infants. Although collodion membrane may be present at birth, the skin is usually normal, with fine scaling beginning at 1 to 3 weeks of life. Typically, the scales are thick and dark, giving the skin a dirty appearance. Extensor distribution—combined with involvement of the sides of the neck and preauricular skin and sparing the flexural areas—is typical. Steroid sulfatase deficiency is an etiologic factor, causing an increase in cholesterol sulfate and a decrease in cholesterol in the stratum corneum.[47] The accumulated cholesterol sulfate may inhibit proteolysis—a process similar to the inhibition seen in ichthyosis vulgaris. Prenatal diagnosis is available, and gene therapy may be on the horizon.

Lamellar Ichthyosis

Lamellar ichthyosis occurs in one in 300,000 births. It is inherited in an autosomal recessive pattern. Collodion membrane

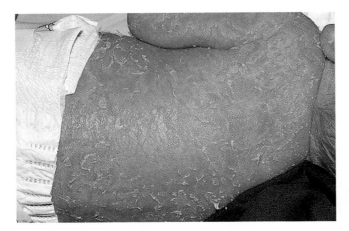

Figure 3 Erythroderma (total body erythema) and extensive scaling are seen in this infant with congenital ichthyosiform erythroderma.

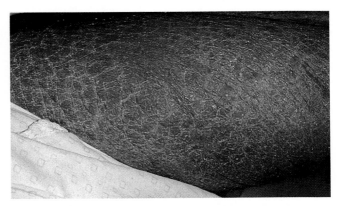

Figure 4 This patient developed marked scaling (acquired ichthyosis) over a 6-month period. Investigation revealed non-Hodgkin lymphoma.

may be present at birth but is then shed, revealing characteristic large, platelike scales. Erythroderma may be present, albeit difficult to discern because of the thickness of the scales. Ectropion is present in most patients and can give rise to ophthalmic complications. The leading candidate for the etiologic genetic disorder is defective transglutaminase, which normally cross-links the structural proteins that give rise to the cornified envelope of stratum corneum cells that is critical to cutaneous barrier function.[48]

Congenital Ichthyosiform Erythroderma

Formerly, congenital ichthyosiform erythroderma [*see Figure 3*] was considered a variant of lamellar ichthyosis. Both are inherited as autosomal recessive traits, and collodion membrane may be present at birth in both conditions. Ectropion, eclabion (eversion of the lip), and erythroderma can also occur. Although patients with congenital ichthyosiform erythroderma, like patients with lamellar ichthyosis, may have platelike scales on the lower extremities, elsewhere the scales are fine and white. Also in contrast to lamellar ichthyosis, X-linked ichthyosis, and ichthyosis vulgaris, whose lesions are scaly because of an abnormal ability to desquamate (so-called retention hyperkeratoses), the lesions of congenital ichthyosiform erythroderma are scaly because of increased production of keratinocytes (so-called hyperproliferative ichthyosis).

Epidermolytic Hyperkeratosis

Epidermolytic hyperkeratosis (formerly called bullous congenital ichthyosiform erythroderma) is autosomal dominant in inheritance. The combinations of large blisters and erythema with denuded skin that appear at birth may be confused with epidermolysis bullosa, staphylococcal scalded skin syndrome, or toxic epidermal necrolysis. Several months to 1 year after birth, the blisters become less prominent, and thick, verrucous plaques comprising rows of hyperkeratotic ridges develop. Flexural skin is usually involved, but the disease can be more extensive. Bacterial colonization leads to a clinically significant foul odor. Abnormal keratin gene expression is the etiologic basis of this condition.[49]

Acquired Ichthyosis

Acquired ichthyoses have been associated with numerous systemic diseases and medications. Although the onset of scaling is commonly a manifestation of dryness or ichthyosis vulgaris, patients with unusual manifestations or with severe or recalcitrant disease warrant further investigation. Endocrinopathies (e.g., thyroid disease), autoimmune diseases, infectious diseases (e.g.,

HIV), and malignancies such as lymphomas [*see Figure 4*] and other carcinomas have been associated with the onset of ichthyosiform dermatosis.

TREATMENT

The standard therapy for the ichthyoses is emollients (e.g., petrolatum) and keratolytics (e.g., lactic acid with or without propylene glycol). Lactic acid should be used cautiously in neonates to avoid causing excess absorption. Oral retinoids (which require lipid monitoring) can be helpful, particularly in the management of X-linked ichthyosis, congenital ichthyosiform erythroderma, and lamellar ichthyosis. Epidermolytic hyperkeratosis is the most difficult of these conditions to treat because of the risk of blistering induced by therapeutic agents. Antimicrobial agents can be useful to reduce the odor caused by bacterial colonization.

References

1. Andersen KL, Frankild S: Predictive testing in contact dermatitis: allergic contact dermatitis. Clin Dermatol 15:645, 1997

2. Denig NI, Hoke AW, Maibach HI: Irritant contact dermatitis: clues to causes, clinical characteristics, and control. Postgrad Med 103:199, 1998

3. Coca AF, Cooke RA: On the classification of the phenomena of hypersensitiveness. J Immunol 8:163, 1922

4. Worldwide variation in prevalence of symptoms of asthma, allergic rhinoconjunctivitis, and atopic eczema: The International Study of Asthma and Allergies in Childhood (ISAAC) Steering Committee. Lancet 351:1225, 1998

5. Laughter D, Istvan JA, Tofte SJ, et al: The prevalence of atopic dermatitis in Oregon schoolchildren. J Am Acad Dermatol 43:649, 2000

6. Foley P, Zuo Y, Plunkett A, et al: The frequency of common skin conditions in preschool-age children in Australia: atopic dermatitis. Arch Dermatol 137:293, 2001

7. Larsen FS: The epidemiology of atopic dermatitis. Monogr Allergy 31:9, 1993

8. Uehara M, Kimura C: Descendant family history of atopic dermatitis. Acta Derm Venereol 73:62, 1993

9. Agosti JM, Sprenger JD, Lum LG, et al: Transfer of allergen-specific IgE-mediated hypersensitivity with allogeneic bone marrow transplantation. N Engl J Med 319:1623, 1998

10. Wollenberg A, Kraft S, Oppel T, et al: Atopic dermatitis: pathogenetic mechanisms. Clin Exp Dermatol 25:530, 2000

11. Bos JD, Wierenga EA, Sillevis Smitt JH, et al: Immune dysregulation in atopic eczema. Arch Dermatol 128:1509, 1992

12. Hanifin JM, Rajka G: Diagnostic features of atopic dermatitis. Acta Derm Venereol Suppl (Stockh) 92:44, 1980

13. Gustafsson D, Lowhagen T, Andersson K: Risk of developing atopic disease after early feeding with cows' milk based formula. Arch Dis Child 67:1008, 1992

14. Zoller TM, Wichelhaus TA, Hartung A, et al: Colonization with superantigens producing *Staphylococcus aureus* is associated with increased severity of atopic dermatitis. Clin Exp Allergy 30:994, 2000

15. Herz U, Bunikowski R, Renz H: Role of T cells in atopic dermatitis: new aspects on the dynamics of cytokine production and the contribution of bacterial superantigens. Int Arch Allergy Immunol 115:170, 1998

16. Rees J, Friedmann PS, Matthews JN: Contact sensitivity to dinitrochlorobenzene is impaired in atopic subjects. Arch Dermatol 126:1173, 1990

17. Akdis CA, Akdis M, Trautmann A, et al: Immune regulation in atopic dermatitis. Curr Opin Immunol 12:641, 2000

18. Grewe M, Bruijnzeel-Koomen CAFM, Schöpf E, et al: A role for Th1 and Th2 cells in the immunopathogenesis of atopic dermatitis. Immunol Today 19:359, 1998

19. Taylor RS, Baadsgaard O, Hammerberg C, et al: Hyperstimulatory CD1a+CD1b+CD36+ Langerhans cells are responsible for increased autologous T lymphocyte reactivity to lesional epidermal cells of patients with atopic dermatitis. J Immunol 147:3794, 1991

20. Stingl G, Maurer D: IgE-mediated allergen presentation via Fc epsilon RI on antigen-presenting cells. Int Arch Allergy Immunol 113:24, 1997

21. Hanifin JM, Chan SC: Monocyte phosphodiesterase abnormalities and dysregulation of lymphocyte function in atopic dermatitis. J Invest Dermatol 105 (1 suppl):84S, 1995

22. Heskel NS, Chan SC, Thiel ML, et al: Elevated umbilical cord blood leukocyte cyclic adenosine monophosphate-phosphodiesterase activity in children with atopic parents. J Am Acad Dermatol 11:422, 1984

23. Uehara M, Izukura R, Sawai T: Blood eosinophilia in atopic dermatitis. Clin Exp Dermatol 15:264, 1990

24. Bannister MJ, Freeman S: Adult-onset atopic dermatitis. Australas J Dermatol 41:225, 2000

25. Hofer MF, Lester MR, Schlievert PM, et al: Upregulation of IgE synthesis by staphylococcal toxic shock syndrome toxin-1 in peripheral blood mononuclear cells from patients with atopic dermatitis. Clin Exp Allergy 25:1218, 1995

26. Nilsson EJ, Henning CG, Magnusson J: Topical corticosteroids and *Staphylococcus aureus* in atopic dermatitis. J Am Acad Dermatol 27:29, 1992

27. Rich LF, Hanifin JM: Ocular complications of atopic dermatitis and other eczemas. Int Ophthalmol Clin 25:61, 1985

28. McHenry PM, Williams HC, Bingham EA: Management of atopic eczema. Joint Workshop of the British Association of Dermatologists and the Research Unit of the Royal College of Physicians of London. BMJ 310:843, 1995

29. Guidelines of care for atopic dermatitis. American Academy of Dermatology. J Am Acad Dermatol 26:485, 1992

30. Chamlin SL, Frieden IJ, Fowler A, et al: Ceramide-dominant, barrier-repair lipids improve childhood atopic dermatitis. Arch Dermatol 137:1110, 2001

31. Richter HI, Billmann-Eberwein C, Grewe M, et al: Successful monotherapy of severe and intractable atopic dermatitis by photopheresis. J Am Acad Dermatol 38:585, 1998

32. Alaiti S, Kang S, Fiedler VC, et al: Tacrolimus (FK506) ointment for atopic dermatitis: a phase I study in adults and children. J Am Acad Dermatol 38:69, 1998

33. Van Leent EJ, Graber M, Thurston M, et al: Effectiveness of the ascomycin macrolactam SDZ ASM 981 in the topical treatment of atopic dermatitis. Arch Dermatol 134:805, 1998

34. Ewing CI, Ashcroft C, Gibbs AC, et al: Flucloxacillin in the treatment of atopic dermatitis. Br J Dermatol 138:1022, 1998

35. Hanifin JM, Schneider LC, Leung DY, et al: Recombinant interferon gamma therapy for atopic dermatitis. J Am Acad Dermatol 28:189, 1993

36. Ellis CN, Stevens SR, Blok BK, et al: Interferon-gamma therapy reduces blood leukocyte levels in patients with atopic dermatitis: correction with clinical improvement. Clin Immunol 92:49, 1999

37. Stevens SR, Hanifin JM, Hamilton T, et al: Long-term effectiveness and safety of recombinant human interferon gamma therapy for atopic dermatitis despite unchanged serum IgE levels. Arch Dermatol 134:799, 1998

38. Berth-Jones J, Graham-Brown RA, Marks R, et al: Long-term efficacy and safety of cyclosporin in severe adult atopic dermatitis. Br J Dermatol 136:76, 1997

39. Berth-Jones J, Finlay AY, Zaki I, et al: Cyclosporine in severe childhood atopic dermatitis: a multicenter study. J Am Acad Dermatol 34:1016, 1996

40. Sheehan MP, Atherton DJ: A controlled trial of traditional Chinese medicinal plants in widespread non-exudative atopic eczema. Br J Dermatol 126:179, 1992

41. Sheehan MP, Atherton DJ: One-year follow up of children treated with Chinese medicinal herbs for atopic dermatitis. Br J Dermatol 130:488, 1994

42. Fung AY, Look PC, Chong LY, et al: A controlled trial of traditional Chinese herbal medicine in Chinese patients with recalcitrant atopic dermatitis. Int J Dermatol 38:387, 1999

43. Berth-Jones J, Graham-Brown RA: Placebo-controlled trial of essential fatty acid supplementation in atopic dermatitis. Lancet 341:1557, 1993

44. Hanifin JM, Chan SC, Cheng JB, et al: Type 4 phosphodiesterase inhibitors have clinical and in vitro anti-inflammatory effects in atopic dermatitis. J Invest Dermatol 107:51, 1996

45. Williams ML, Elias PM: Genetically transmitted, generalized disorders of cornification: the ichthyoses. Dermatol Clin 5:155, 1987

46. Rabinowitz LG, Esterly NB: Atopic dermatitis and ichthyosis vulgaris. Pediatr Rev 15:220, 1994

47. Paller AS: Laboratory tests for ichthyosis. Dermatol Clin 12:99, 1994

48. Epstein EH Jr: The genetics of human skin diseases. Curr Opin Genet Dev 6:295, 1996

49. Fuchs E, Coulombe P, Cheng J, et al: Genetic bases of epidermolysis bullosa simplex and epidermolytic hyperkeratosis. J Invest Dermatol 103(5 suppl):25S, 1994

35 Contact Dermatitis and Related Disorders

James S. Taylor, M.D.

Contact dermatitis is an acute or chronic skin inflammation resulting from interaction with a chemical, biological, or physical agent.[1] It is one of the most common conditions seen by physicians, accounting for an estimated 6.5 million physician visits in 1994 and 95% of all reported occupational skin diseases.[2] Substances that produce contact dermatitis after single or multiple exposures may be irritant or allergic. Direct tissue damage results from contact with irritants. Tissue damage by allergic substances is mediated through immunologic mechanisms. Eczema or dermatitis is the most common clinical expression of this induced inflammation. Of the more than 85,000 chemicals in our environment, most can be irritants, depending on the circumstances of exposure.[1] More than 3,700 substances have been identified as contact allergens.[3] The potential for these substances to cause contact dermatitis varies greatly, and the severity of the dermatitis ranges from a mild, short-lived condition to a severe, persistent, job-threatening, and possibly life-threatening disease.

Major Types of Contact Dermatitis

IRRITANT CONTACT DERMATITIS

Irritants cause as much as 80% of contact dermatitis, act by direct nonimmunologic chemical or physical action on the skin, and are divided into marginal and acute types. Marginal irritants are the most common. Repeated insults by low-grade irritants such as soap, detergents, surfactants, organic solvents, and oils may not cause clinical changes for days or months. Dryness of the skin with a glazed, parched appearance are often the initial signs; erythema, hyperkeratosis, and fissuring may supervene.

In contrast, acute irritants cause a more immediate reaction. Some irritants, such as strong acids and alkalis, aromatic amines, phosphorus, and metallic salts, produce a marked observable effect within minutes.[4-6] Others, such as hydrofluoric acid, ethylene oxide, podophyllin, and anthralin, produce a reaction within 8 to 24 hours after exposure.[4] Acute irritant contact dermatitis (ICD) is usually easily diagnosed by the patient history and often results from occupational accidents. The clinical appearance varies depending on the irritant and ranges from burns and deep-red ulcerations with sharp circumspection of the dermatitis, sometimes with a gravitational, dripping effect, to a vesicular dermatitis that is indistinguishable from acute allergic contact dermatitis.

Almost any substance can be an irritant, depending on the conditions of exposure [see Figure 1]. The nature of the irritant (i.e., its pH, solubility, physical state, and concentration), the duration of contact, and the nature of the vehicle affect disease severity. Host factors that predispose to ICD include preexisting dermatitis, skin dryness, sweating, and decreased thickness or breaks in the stratum corneum; environmental factors include high temperature, low humidity, friction, and pressure.

The causative factors are complex and usually involve exposure to a combination of irritants. The sentinel event for irritant hand eczema in hairdressers is dermatitis developing in moist areas that are difficult to rinse and dry, such as under rings and in the web spaces of the fingers.[7] Dermatitis may spread to the dorsum of the hand, where the skin is thinner and less resistant than on the palms.

ICD may become chronic if it is not treated early. Even when the skin appears to be healed, its protective capacity remains impaired for weeks or months. Additionally, ICD impairs the barrier function of the skin, allowing penetration of potential contact allergens. Individuals who had childhood atopic eczema are more likely than others to develop ICD of the hands when their jobs involve wet work.

No universally accepted test exists for diagnosing ICD, which is often diagnosed by excluding allergic contact dermatitis (ACD). Because of the clinical similarity of allergic and irritant contact dermatitis, it is important that patients thought to have either disorder undergo patch testing, which is positive with ICD and negative with ACD.[6]

ALLERGIC CONTACT DERMATITIS

Allergic contact dermatitis is a type 4, T cell–mediated, delayed hypersensitivity reaction in the skin. The disorder affects only certain sensitized individuals, typically after two or more exposures, and accounts for about 20% of contact dermatitis cases.

Predisposing Factors

Immunologic status Predisposing factors to ACD include the patient's immunologic status, which in turn is influenced by genetics, age, gender, and the presence of systemic disease. Patients with AIDS, severe combined immunodeficiency, advanced lymphoma or other malignancy, sarcoidosis, lepromatous leprosy, cachexia, and atopic dermatitis may have impaired cell-medi-

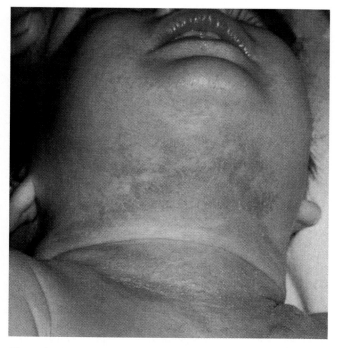

Figure 1 **Wearing a plastic bib resulted in irritant dermatitis in an 18-month-old child.**

Table 1   Body Sites Often Affected by 10 Common Contact Allergens

Allergen	Common Uses	Localization Site
Nickel	Costume jewelry	Earlobes, neck, fingers, wrists, abdomen
Neomycin	Topical antibiotics (dermatologic; ophthalmologic; ear, nose, throat)	Face, neck, trunk, extremities
Balsam of Peru	Fragrances, cosmetics, medications, flavorings	Face, trunk, extremities, perianal area
Fragrance mix	Toothpaste, fragrances, toiletries, cosmetics	Same as for balsam of Peru
Thimerosal	Topical antiseptic, contact lens solutions, eye cosmetics, nasal sprays	Eyelids, face, neck (relevance hard to prove)
Gold	Jewelry	Eyelids, earlobes, wrists, fingers
Formaldehyde	Cosmetics (preservative), shampoos, nail enamel	Eyelids, face, neck, trunk (especially intertriginous areas)
Quaternium-15	Cosmetics (preservative), shampoos, soaps, lotions	Face, trunk, extremities, hands
Cobalt	Metal-plated objects, jewelry	Earlobes, neck, fingers, wrists
Bacitracin	Topical antibiotics (dermatologic; ophthalmologic; ear, nose, throat)	Face, neck, trunk, extremities

ated immunity or anergy.[8] However, contact allergy should not be excluded in these individuals, especially those with atopic eczema. In experimental models, agents that affect the immune system, such as ultraviolet light (ultraviolet B or psoralen and ultraviolet A [PUVA]), glucocorticoids, cyclosporine, and various other drugs, may downregulate ACD.[8] Administration of systemic corticosteroids below certain dosages (e.g., prednisone, 20 mg or less daily), however, does not inhibit strong patch-test reactions.[9]

In patients with occupational dermatitis, a form of natural hyporeactivity termed hardening may occur with diminished but continued exposure to chemical irritants. The process is inducible and is not localized.[10] This acquired state of unresponsiveness is called tolerance. Tolerance may be achieved in guinea pigs through intravenous administration of a dilute allergen or through repeated topical administration of a dilute allergen before a sensitizing exposure.[8]

Environment   The chemical environment in which we live defines opportunities for exposure to various allergens. A patient's age, gender, occupation, avocation, habits, and nationality determine the environment and thus the chemicals to which an individual is exposed. The most common source of contact allergen in the United States is *Toxicodendron*, a plant genus that includes poison ivy, poison oak, and poison sumac. In addition to *Toxicodendron*, there are 10 sources of contact allergens that are commonly encountered in North America [*see Table 1*].[11]

Other cutaneous disorders   Skin that is infected, inflamed, burned, or eczematous predisposes a patient to ACD. Patients with stasis, hand and foot eczema, or chronic actinic dermatitis are at high risk for ACD. ACD occasionally occurs with other skin disorders, including seborrheic dermatitis, psoriasis, prurigo nodularis, and benign familial pemphigus (Hailey-Hailey disease).[12] Noneczematous contact reactions have also been reported: purpuric reactions caused by black rubber; lichen planus–like eruptions caused by color-film developers, gold, and other dental metals (oral mucosa); and granulomas caused by beryllium and zirconium.[13]

Pathogenesis

Despite their different pathogenesis, ACD and ICD, especially of the chronic type of ICD, show remarkable similarities with respect to clinical appearance, histology, and immunohistology. Some inflammatory immune reactions are the same for ICD and ACD, with similar cytokine (tumor necrosis factor–α and interferon gamma) and accessory molecule (HLA-DR and intercellular adhesion molecule-1) activity that produces the cascade of inflammation. However, there is no memory T cell function in ICD,[14] and the extent of reaction is directly related to the amount of irritant and duration of exposure.[15]

In contrast, even small amounts of an allergen can trigger the T cell reaction in ACD. Minor variations in an allergen's physical and chemical properties may affect its ability to induce sensitization.[8] Most environmental allergens are haptens, small (<500 daltons) molecules that penetrate the skin and undergo in vivo conjugation with tissue, or carrier, protein. Once the complex forms, the carrier protein is no longer recognized by the immune system as self. ACD represents a delayed-type hypersensitivity reaction to this complex.

During the sensitization phase, which usually takes a minimum of 5 to 21 days, an individual acquires a specific hypersensitivity to a particular contact allergen. Sensitization not only can evoke a type 4 delayed hypersensitivity response (mediated by lymphocytes) but also can produce a type 1 immediate hypersensitivity reaction (mediated by circulating antibodies).

During the elicitation phase, on re-exposure to an allergen, a hapten-carrier complex capable of eliciting a specific reaction reforms. The reaction time—the time required for a previously sensitized individual to manifest a clinical dermatitis after reexposure to the antigen—is usually 12 to 48 hours but may range from 8 to 120 hours.

A spontaneous flare may occur within 10 to 21 days without reexposure, possibly because enough allergen remains at the site to cause a reaction once the sensitization phase has occurred.

Cross-sensitization occurs when a patient allergic to one chemical also reacts when exposed to structurally related chemicals. Examples include *Toxicodendron* antigens (poison ivy, oak and

Table 2 Common Misconceptions about ACD[12]

Fallacy	Truth
Rash quickly follows contact	Rash is often delayed 1 to 2 days and may not appear for 1 wk after contact
Allergy develops only to new substances	Allergy can develop years after contact; an induction period may last virtually a lifetime
Allergy is dose-dependent	Allergy is not, within a wide range, dose-dependent
If changes in medications or cosmetics do not lead to clearing of the rash, those products are not the cause	Many products contain the same or cross-reacting allergens; also, the composition of the product may be altered without a change in the trade name of the product
Contact allergy occurs only at the site of exposure to the offending agent	Contact allergy can spread by direct or indirect contact, airborne exposure, connubial contact, or autoeczematization
Expensive products are not allergenic	Allergy is not related to cost
Negative prick or scratch test or RAST exclude ACD	Only patch testing is diagnostic of ACD
ACD is always bilateral if allergen exposure is bilateral	Shoe and glove allergy are often bilateral but may be unilateral
ACD is of the same intensity at all areas of exposure	Body sites may differ in responsiveness to allergens; ACD may be patchy (e.g., hand dermatitis from gloves)
ACD does not affect the palms and soles	ACD may occur on the palms and soles (e.g., from gloves, topical medicaments, shoes)

ACD—allergic contact dermatitis   RAST—radioallergosorbent test

sumac Japanese lacquer, mango, cashew nutshell oil), aromatic amines (p-phenylenediamine, procaine, benzocaine, and p-aminobenzoic acid), and perfumes or flavors (balsam of Peru, benzoin, cinnamates, and vanilla). This phenomenon may explain persistence or reactivation of dermatitis when such exposures are unknown.[8,13]

Diagnosis

Diagnosis of ACD is based on the patient history; on the appearance, periodicity, and localization of the eruption; and on the clinical course. The history is especially important in cases of chronic dermatitis and putative occupational contact dermatitis. The history alone may be accurate only 50% of the time, on average, ranging from 80% correct for nickel to 50% correct for moderately common allergens to about 10% correct for less common allergens. Even with causes considered obvious, the specific allergen may not be known, and ACD caused by other chemicals may also be present. Skillful history taking is required to differentiate ACD from contact urticaria and ICD, with differentiation being especially difficult in chronic cases [see Table 2]. Published history forms may be utilized.[16] Detailed questioning of the patient about all topical medications (over-the-counter and prescription), systemic medication, cosmetics, other lotions and creams, occupation, hobbies, travel and clothing is also important. A history of ACD caused by one or more of the major contact allergens, such as nickel, rubber, topical medicaments, and cosmetics (fragrances, preservatives, and dyes), or obvious occupational or avocational exposures to substances or chemicals, such as chrome, epoxy, acrylics, gloves, clothing, first-aid creams, preservatives, and plants, may point to inadvertent ACD in an otherwise unexplained eruption.[17]

Clinical features In the acute stage, papules, oozing vesicles, and crusting lesions that are surrounded by inflammation pre-

dominate. These clinical features may occur anywhere, but they are best visualized on the palms, sides of the fingers, periungual areas, and soles of the feet. Frequently occurring or persistent episodes of ACD often become chronic, with thickening associated with lichenification, scaling, and fissuring [see Figures 2 and 3]. Postinflammatory hyperpigmentation or hypopigmentation may occur. Features of both the acute and the chronic stages characterize the subacute form. All forms of contact dermatitis frequently cause pruritus. Acute dermatitis is more likely to be caused by recent exposure, and accordingly, the cause is more obvious. On the other hand, the onset of ACD is often more subtle. A low-grade, subacute to chronic eczema may appear as primarily a scaly or chapped eruption, especially on the face or on the dorsa of the hands.[6,13,17]

The distribution of dermatitis is often the single most important clue to the diagnosis of ACD. The area of most intense dermatitis usually corresponds to the site of most intense contact with the allergen. Exceptions occur, such as nail-polish allergy, which typically appears on ectopic sites, especially the eyelids, face, and neck. In addition to the transfer of allergens to distant sites, volatile airborne chemicals may cause dermatitis on exposed body areas. Regional differences in susceptibility to contact allergens exist. Thinner eyelid and genital skin is more susceptible to both allergic and irritant contact dermatitis. Scalp hair is often protective, with allergic reactions to hair cosmetics involving the upper face, eyelids, postauricular area, and neck. Other areas of the body have higher or lower exposures to allergens; these exposures are not always clear and are reflected in unusual distributions of dermatitis. Allergens in lotions and creams applied all over the body sometimes produce reactions in skin folds and intertriginous areas, where the chemicals tend to concentrate. Recognition of ACD on the basis of the physical examination alone may be only partially accurate. Linear vesicular streaks are commonly seen in poison ivy, poison oak, and poison sumac der-

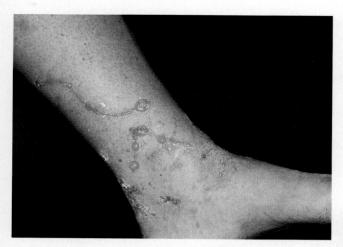

Figure 2 **Exposure to poison oak produced this acute** *Toxicodendron* **dermatitis with erythema, edema, and linear vesicles and bullae.**

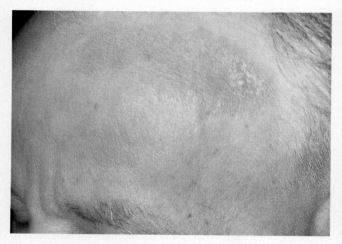

Figure 3 **Chronic eczematous dermatitis, with scaling, lichenification, and hyperpigmentation, was caused by an allergy to leather components in a hatband.**

matitis, but contact with other plants can give a similar picture. Contact with liquids may also produce linear vesicles. Failure to examine the entire skin surface may result in misdiagnosis. Eczema on the trunk and arms may in fact represent autoeczematization from contact or stasis dermatitis of the legs. Significant regional variations are associated with contact dermatitis, and knowledge of substances that cause dermatitis of specific body sites facilitates the diagnosis. Three such areas are the hands, face and neck, and feet [*see Figures 4 through 7*]. It is helpful to know the occupations when determining which patients with ACD should be given patch tests [*see Table 3*]. Also helpful is a list of blind spots in the diagnosis of ACD, with specific examples [*see Table 4*].

Histopathology Biopsies are of limited help in diagnosing contact dermatitis. Microscopic findings vary according to the stage of the process: acute, subacute, or chronic. The hallmark of eczema is spongiosis, or intercellular edema, associated with spongiotic vesicles. Intracellular edema may cause reticular degeneration of the epidermis with multilocular bullae formation. Most types of eczema show similar pathologic changes and cannot be distinguished with certainty.[18]

Patch test The patch test is the only useful and reliable method—the gold standard—for the diagnosis of ACD. The proper performance and interpretation of this bioassay require considerable experience. Because the procedure is subject to patient variability and observer error, the technique has been standardized by the North American Contact Dermatitis Group. First, the allergen is diluted in petrolatum or water to a concentration that does not produce active sensitization or irritation. A widely used patch-test system consists of strips of paper tape, onto which are fixed aluminum disks 8 mm in diameter (Finn Chambers on Scanpor tape). A small amount of allergen is placed within these disks, covering slightly more than one half of its diameter [*see Figure 8*].

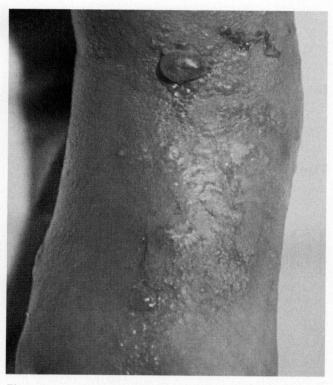

Figure 4 **Acute contact dermatitis caused by wearing sandals typically involves the dorsal surface of the feet.**

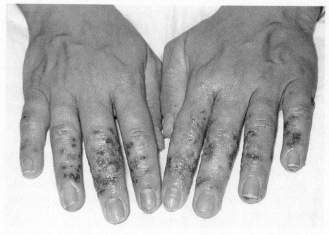

Figure 5 **Hairdresser with acute allergic contact dermatitis of the hands, caused by glyceryl thioglycolate.**

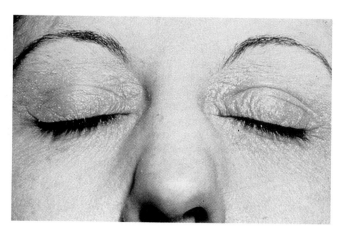

Figure 6 Ectopic allergic contact dermatitis of the eyelids from tosylamide formaldehyde resin in nail polish.

Currently, the only commercially available patch-test system in the United States is the thin-layer rapid-use epicutaneous (T.R.U.E.) test. The T.R.U.E. test contains 23 preloaded allergens that are crystallized, micronized, or emulsified into gels that are affixed to paper tape.

With both systems the tests are applied to the upper back or midback, which must be free of dermatitis. The patches are left in place and kept dry. When removed at 48 hours, the first reading is performed after 20 to 30 minutes, which allows time for pressure erythema to resolve. It is important to perform a second reading between 4 and 7 days after the patches are initially applied. Otherwise, almost 20% of positive reactions will be missed. Neomycin, formaldehyde and formaldehyde-releasing preservatives, and tixocortol pivolate are often late reactors. Results at both readings are graded according to intensity of the reaction covering at least 50% of the patch-test site on a scale of 0 to 3+, as follows:

0 = no reaction
? (doubtful) = weak erythema only
1+ = erythema and edema
2+ = erythema, edema, and papules
3+ = vesicles or bullae

Both false positive and false negative reactions can result. Thus, patch testing is best done by physicians who are familiar with the intricacies of the procedure and who have been trained to advise patients about allergen substitution, relevance of the test, and prognosis. Reading test results and interpreting relevance are as important as performing the test. Any reaction must be evaluated with regard to the individual patient. Thus, when an allergen is found to be positive, it cannot always be assumed to be the cause of ACD.[8,13,16] The relevance of positive reactions to present or past episodes of ACD ranges from a low of 16.7% for thimerosal to 93.4% for DMDM hydantoin [*see Table 5*]. Thus, relevance is determined by correlating the patch-test results with chemicals, products, and processes encountered in the environment. Occasionally, when patients are allergic to chemicals in products they use, the allergen may be present in only minimal amounts and may not be responsible for the dermatitis.[8] In these cases, repeat

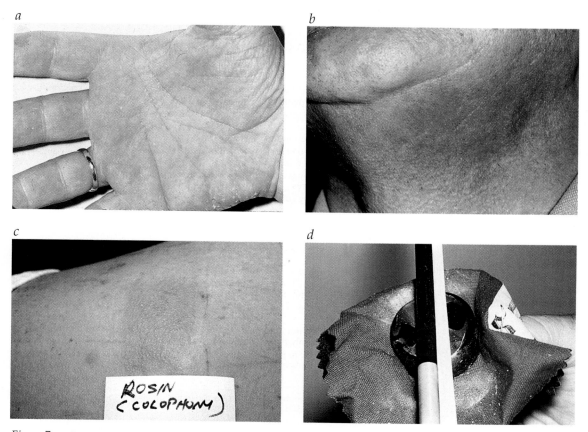

Figure 7 Allergic contact dermatitis of the hands (*a*) and neck (*b*), with a positive patch test to rosin (colophony) (*c*), which is used by violinists on their bows (*d*).

Table 3 Criteria* for Determining Which ACD Patients Should Be Given a Patch Test[12]

Presence of a specific type of eczema that places patient at higher risk for ACD (stasis, hand, foot, or chronic)

Patient is in a high-risk occupation
- Health care worker
- Cosmetologist (hairdresser)
- Rubber compounder
- Plastics processor
- Chemical worker
- Printer
- Machinist
- Woodworker

Specific allergen or substance is suspected

Patient has a highly suggestive history or distribution of dermatitis

Dermatitis flares or does not respond to treatment

Patient has previously undiagnosed dermatoses and erythroderma

Patient has putative occupational dermatitis

Special situation applies, such as photosensitivity or systemic contact dermatitis

*Test is ordered if any one of the risk factors is present.

open application testing (ROAT), in which the patient applies the commercial product to normal skin twice daily for several days, can be helpful. ROAT is typically used with products that are left on rather than washed off after application.

In the United States, patch testing is often initially performed with 23 T.R.U.E. test allergens, the standard screening diagnostic series approved by the Food and Drug Administration. However, since there are over 3,700 environmental contact allergens, and this series identifies only 20% to 50% of patients with ACD, testing with additional chemicals is imperative for a thorough diagnosis of ACD. These additional substances can be obtained from chemical suppliers and prepared by a compounding pharmacist in appropriate concentrations, as detailed in a standard text, for testing with the Finn Chamber system. As an alternative, many centers in the United States use individual patch-test chemicals or series (e.g., corticosteroid, plastics and glues, acrylic, dental, machinist, hairdresser) that are available in Europe but have not been approved in the United States.[11,19]

Reproducibility and validity of patch testing   In a study in which 383 patients received simultaneous duplicate patch tests on opposite sides of the upper back, 8% of patients had completely discordant results: positive on one side of the back and negative on the other. The intensity of the reactions was not disclosed, and clinical relevance of this problem was considered small. The most reproducible positive patch tests were for fragrance mix, nickel, and balsam of Peru. Formaldehyde and lanolin were the least reproducible positive reactors, both of which may be weak irritants.[20] The sensitivity, specificity, and validity of a standard screening series has been estimated at about 70%,[21] indicating that about 30% of these patch-test results were not valid. However, patch tests are diagnostically very useful, and the patients whose screening results were negative later had positive results to other allergens. It was assumed that the earlier screening results had been false negative. The positive predictive value of a diagnosis of ACD is a function of the prevalence of ACD in the population and a function of the sensitivity and specificity of the patch test.[22]

Table 4 Blind Spots in the Diagnosis of ACD

Fallacy	Truth
ACD may be identical to another disease	Seborrheic dermatitis–like ACD caused by hair tonic Tinea pedis misdiagnosed as ACD; a positive potassium hydroxide preparation made the diagnosis Psoriasis of the soles mimicking ACD caused by shoes; patch tests were negative Factitial eczema of the dorsal hand, from an unknown cause, mimicking ACD; cured with an Unna occlusive dressing ACD caused by fragrances and preservatives; misdiagnosed for 5 years as lupus erythematosus ACD caused by sunscreen; misdiagnosed as sunburn
Failure to make a second diagnosis	ACD caused by neomycin; misdiagnosed as worsening atopic eczema Chronic actinic dermatitis of face, with ACD caused by fragrance Morphea of the leg, with ACD caused by a topical corticosteroid cream
Occult exposure to an allergen	Keys in pants pocket caused ACD of the lateral thigh in a man allergic to nickel ACD caused by the preservative imidazolidinyl urea, present in a sunscreen with a label that listed only the active ingredients Chronic hand eczema from ACD caused by red dye in window curtains
Inadequate or deceptive history (patient does not recall exposure to specific allergens)	Patient with chronic eczema worsened by use of a prescription topical cream (doxepin) identified only from a pharmacy prescription list Patient allergic to neomycin had periorbital contact eczema caused by an ophthalmic ointment that contained tobramycin, which was not recognized as a cross-reacting allergen
Failure of patch testing	Occupational contact dermatitis of the hands attributed to a false positive irritant-patch-test reaction to a cleanser. Occupational contact dermatitis of the hands with a false negative patch-test reaction to latex surgical gloves; further patch-testing indicated an allergy to thiurams, which were present as accelerators in the gloves

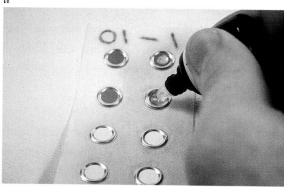

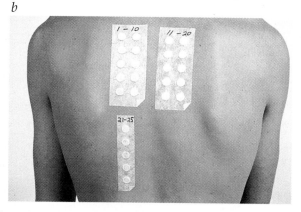

Figure 8 Patch-test allergens to be tested, usually in petrolatum and occasionally aqueous, are placed on Finn Chambers on Scanpor tape (*a*) for application to the patient's back (*b*) for 48 hours. See patch testing in text and Figure 7c for a positive patch test.

A large dose-response study that tested the impact of seasonal variation on the irritant susceptibility of skin identified a stronger reaction to irritants in winter.[23]

PREVENTION AND TREATMENT OF IRRITANT AND ALLERGIC CONTACT DERMATITIS

Prevention

Most cases of contact dermatitis can be effectively treated and controlled once the offending irritant or allergen is identified and eliminated. Identifying hidden sources of allergens is important, and patients who have positive patch-test results are given exposure lists identifying various names of allergens, cross-reacting substances, lists of potential products and processes containing the allergen, and nonsensitizing substitutes. Standard texts should be consulted for detailed information.[13,16] Examples of allergen alternatives include topical erythromycin or mupirocin ointments as substitutes for neomycin.[24] Neomycin may cross-react with gentamicin and tobramycin. Bacitracin should generally be avoided for neomycin-sensitive patients because of coreactivity.

Reasons for persistence of ACD include unidentified sources of allergens or irritants at home or at work, exposure to cross-reacting allergens, presence of underlying endogenous (e.g., atopic) eczema, and adverse reactions to therapy [*see* Topical Medication Allergy, *below*].

In the case of hand dermatitis, practical management must include protective measures as well as the use of topical corticosteroids and lubrication. The use of vinyl gloves with cotton liners to avoid the accumulation of moisture that often occurs during activities involving exposure to household or other irritants and foods (e.g., peeling or chopping fruits or vegetables) may be helpful. However, it is important to verify that gloves are safe to use in the workplace around machinery before recommending them. Protective devices themselves may introduce new allergic or irritant hazards in the form of rubber in gloves and solvents in waterless cleansers. Automation of industrial processes may reduce exposure but is the most expensive preventive measure. Barrier creams are generally the last resort and are probably best for workers with no dermatitis.[25] A barrier agent containing quaternium-18 bentonite has been shown to be effective with exposure to a specific allergen, such as poison ivy.[26] Principles of treatment of atopic dermatitis [*see Chapter 34*] may also be applied to treatment of contact dermatitis.

Topical Therapy

In the acute vesicular stage, apply cool, wet compresses for 15 minutes two to three times daily. Isotonic saline or Domeboro powder dissolved in tap water to make a 1:40 dilution (aluminum acetate) may be used. A soft cloth, such as Kerlex gauze or a towel, is immersed in the solution. The cloth is wrung slightly and applied to the affected area of the skin. The solution should not be poured directly on the dressing. Lukewarm to cool water baths or sitz baths are antipruritic and anti-inflammatory; they also aid in cleansing and removing crusts and medications. Oatmeal in the form of Aveeno Oilated (colloidal powdered oatmeal with oils) may be added to the bath for its antipruritic and drying effects.

In acute dermatitis such as that caused by poison ivy, a lotion of camphor, menthol, and hydrocortisone (Sarnol-HC) is soothing, drying, and antipruritic. Pramoxine, a topical anesthetic in a lotion base (Prax), may also relieve pruritus. In the subacute and chronic stages of contact dermatitis, an emollient lotion (Eucerin) or ointment (Aquaphor) may be applied to moist skin after bathing for lubrication. Oil in water emulsions that contain perfluoropolyethers have been shown to significantly inhibit irritation caused by a wide variety of hydrophilic and lipophilic irritants.[27]

Corticosteroid creams and ointments are effective anti-inflammatory agents for treating subacute and chronic contact dermatitis. Hydrocortisone is effective topically in a 1% concentration. The high-potency fluorinated corticosteroids act more rapidly but should be used with discretion. Frequent and prolonged use in skin-fold areas may cause atrophy, telangiectasia, or striae, and their use on the face may cause steroid rosacea. For patients with chronic dermatitis, crude coal tar preparations may be used to control eczema. Bath PUVA may be effective for contact dermatitis of the palms and soles.[28]

Systemic Therapy

Intense itching may be relieved with sedating antihistamines such as diphenhydramine hydrochloride (Benadryl), hydroxyzine hydrochloride (Atarax), and doxepin hydrochloride (Sinequan), administered at night. Most cases of ICD and ACD are effectively managed without the use of systemic corticosteroids. However, short courses of systemic corticosteroids are indicated for patients with severe vesiculobullous eruptions of the hands and feet or the face [*see Figure 9*] or severe disseminated ACD, such as poison ivy. Attempts at desensitization have generally been unsuccessful.[8] Secondary infection sometimes arises as a complication of ICD and ACD, and systemic antibiotics may be indicated.[27]

Table 5   Patch Test Results in North America from 1996 through 1998[11]

Test Substance*	TT†	Use	Allergic (%)	Test Substance‡
Nickel sulfate 2.5%	TT	Metal	14.2	49.1
Neomycin sulfate 20%	TT	Antibiotic	13.1	46.2
Balsam of Peru (*Myroxylon pereirae*) 25%	TT	Fragrance	11.8	82.9
Fragrance mix 8%	TT	Fragrance	11.7	86.9
Thimerosal 0.1%	TT	Preservative	10.9	16.8
Gold sodium thiosulfate 0.5%		Metal	9.5	40.6
Formaldehyde 1% aq	TT	Preservative	9.2	63.2
Quaternium-15 2%	TT	Preservative	9.0	88.7
Cobalt chloride 1%	TT	Metal	9.0	55.1
Bacitracin 20%		Antibiotic	8.7	50.4
Methyldibromaglutaronitrile/phenoxyethanol 2.5%		Preservative	7.6	59.1
Carba mix 30%	TT	Rubber accelerators	7.3	71.7
Ethyleneurea melamine-formaldehyde resin 5%		Fabric finish resin	7.2	65.9
Thiuram mix 1%	TT	Rubber accelerators	6.9	79.8
p-Phenylenediamine 1%	TT	Hair dye	6.0	53.1
Propylene glycol 30% aq		Medicine/cosmetic solvent	3.8	82.8
Diazolidinyl urea 1%		Preservative	3.7	91.5
Lanolin 30%	TT	Cosmetic emollient	3.3	78.9
Imidazoldinyl urea 2%		Preservative	3.2	91.7
2-Bromo-2-nitropropane-1,3-diol 0.5%		Preservative	3.2	68.5
Methylchloroisothiazolinone/methylisothiazolinone 100 ppm aq	TT	Preservative	2.9	87.2
Diazolidinyl urea 1% aq		Preservative	2.9	85.0
Cinnamic aldehyde 1%		Fragrance	2.8	83.2
Potassium dichromate 0.25%	TT	Metal	2.8	54.3
Methyldibromoglutaronitrile/phenoxyethanol 1%		Preservative	2.7	73.8
Ethylenediamine dihydrochloride 1%	TT	Medicine/cosmetic stabilizer	2.6	23.9
DMDM hydantoin 1%		Preservative	2.6	93.4
Glutaraldehyde 1%		Antibacterial	2.6	48.1
Imidazolidinyl urea 2% aq		Preservative	2.5	86.1
Tixocortol-21-pivalate 1%		Corticosteroid	2.3	91.7
Benzocaine 5%	TT (as caine mix)	Anesthetic	2.0	34.3
Colophony (rosin) 20%	TT	Adhesive, etc.	2.0	36.2
Epoxy resin 1%	TT	Industrial coating/adhesive	1.9	55.2
DMDM hydantoin 1% aq		Preservative	1.9	82.0
Glyceryl thioglycolate 1%		Permanent wave chemical	1.9	39
Mercaptobenzothiazole 1%	TT	Rubber accelerator	1.8	75.8

Table 5 (continued)

Test Substance*	TT†	Use	Allergic (%)	Test Substance‡
p-Tert-butylphenol formaldehyde resin 1%	TT	Adhesives	1.8	46
Mercapto mix 1%	TT	Rubber accelerators	1.8	77.1
Paraben mix 15%	TT	Preservative	1.7	86.8
Glutaraldehyde 0.2%		Antibacterial	1.7	59.4
Methyl methacrylate 2%		Resin/adhesive	1.6	67.2
N-Isopropyl-*N*-phenyl paraphenylene-diamine 0.1%	TT (as black rubber mix)	Rubber antioxidant	1.5	58.5
Tosylamide formaldehyde resin 10%		Nail polish resin	1.5	67.7
Mixed dialkyl thiourea 1%		Rubber adhesive/accelerator	1.3	69.1
Ethyl acrylate 0.1%		Acrylic nails/resin	1.3	72.8
Budesonide 0.1%		Corticosteroid	1.2	78
Chloroxylenol 1%		Preservative	1.0	63.4
Sesquiterpene lactone mix 0.1%		Plant oleoresins	0.7	44.8
Oxybenzone 3%		Sunscreen	0.5	73.7
Butylated hydroxyanisole 2%		Antioxidant	0.2	85.7

*Allergens in petrolatum unless noted aqueous (aq).
†Allergens present on the thin-layer rapid-use epicutaneous (T.R.U.E) test series.
‡Definite, probable, or possible relevance to patient's dermatitis at time of testing.
TT— T.R.U.E. test.

Specific Etiologic Forms of Contact Dermatitis

TOPICAL MEDICATION ALLERGY

Reactions to topically applied medications include allergic and irritant contact dermatitis, photosensitivity, airborne contact dermatitis, and contact urticaria and anaphylaxis. ACD is the most common skin reaction to topically applied drugs. The three most important contact allergens are topical antibiotics, anesthetics, and antihistamines. Neomycin and bacitracin are among the most frequently prescribed medications and are common causes of ACD. Mupirocin ointment infrequently causes ACD.[24] Benzocaine, the most common topical anesthetic allergen, is still widely used in topical agents, and there have been a number of reports of contact allergy to topical doxepin, which was initially marketed in 1994.[29]

ACD from topical corticosteroids is most often caused by the steroid itself rather than the vehicle. In a series of 2,073 patients screened for contact dermatitis, the prevalence of allergy to one or more corticosteroids ranged from 2.9% to 4.8%. Patch testing for allergy to tixocortol pivolate and budesonide detects a great majority of cases of ACD caused by topical corticosteroids. Further patch or ROAT with commercial preparations from the major cross-reacting classes may identify additional allergenic steroids or, alternatively, nonreacting steroids. Delayed readings are important at 5 to 7 days. Allergy to inhaled corticosteroids may present as perinasal or perioral itching or dermatitis, mimicking impetigo and herpes simplex or worsening asthma or allergic rhinitis. In these cases, prior sensitization by the cutaneous route is usual, although allergy from mucosal exposure is possible.[30,31]

Topical drug allergy is particularly common in patients with other dermatitis, especially stasis dermatitis [see Figure 10]. Often, this allergy appears as a nonhealing dermatitis, masking its presentation. A detailed history is important and should include the patient's use of nonprescription preparations, topical agents meant for animal use, medicated bandages, borrowed medications, transdermal devices, and herbal medicines. Patch testing with the standard screening tray and the patient's topical medications is invaluable in diagnosing ACD caused by topical medications.

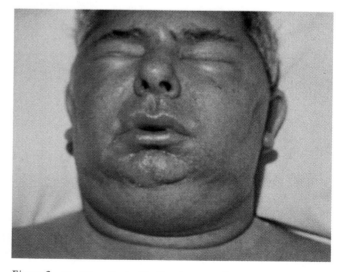

Figure 9 **For this patient with allergic contact dermatitis with marked facial edema, a short course of therapy with systemic corticosteroids is indicated.**

SYSTEMIC CONTACT DERMATITIS

Systemic contact dermatitis occurs in individuals with contact allergy to a hapten when they are exposed systemically to the hapten via the oral, subcutaneous, transcutaneous, intravenous, inhalation, intra-articular, or intravesicular route. The disorder has been caused by a number of medications, metals, and other allergens, including food components, but occurs infrequently compared with allergic and irritant contact dermatitis. Systemic contact dermatitis presents with the following clinically characteristic features[32,33]:

1. Flare-up of previous dermatitis or of prior positive-patch-test sites.
2. Skin disorders in previously unaffected skin, such as vesicular hand eczema, dermatitis in the elbow and knee flexures, nonspecific maculopapular eruption, vasculitis with palpable purpura, and the so-called baboon syndrome. This syndrome includes a pink-to–dark-violet eruption that is well demarcated on the buttocks and genital area and is V-shaped on the inner thighs. It may occupy the whole area or only part of it.
3. General symptoms of headache, malaise, arthralgia, diarrhea, and vomiting.

Systemic contact dermatitis may start a few hours or 1 to 2 days after experimental provocation, suggesting that more than one type of immunologic reaction is involved. Documentation rests on patch testing and investigational oral-challenge studies. Well-controlled oral-challenge studies in sensitized individuals have been performed with medications but are more difficult to

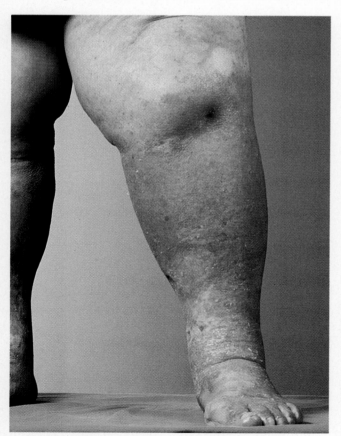

Figure 10 **Patients with stasis dermatitis are at high risk for allergic contact dermatitis, especially from topical medications. Bacitracin was the cause in this case.**

perform with ubiquitous contact allergens, such as metals and natural flavors. A relatively high dose of hapten is usually needed. Other variables include route of administration, bioavailability, individual sensitivity to the allergen, and interaction with amino acids and other allergens.[32] When 12 leg ulcer patients with neomycin allergy were challenged with an oral dose of the hapten,[33] 10 reacted.[33] However, of 29 patients with confirmed localized ACD caused by transdermal clonidine, only one had a skin reaction to oral clonidine.[34]

CLOTHING AND TEXTILE DERMATITIS

ACD from clothing is usually not caused by the fibers but rather by the dyes used to color the garments or by formalin finish resins added to make them wrinkle-resistant, shrinkproof, or wash-and-wear. Disperse blue dyes (especially blue 106 and blue 124) were designated "allergen of the year" for 2000.[35] These dyes are highly valuable screening agents for diagnosing an important cause of textile dermatitis. The distribution of dermatitis corresponds to areas where garments fit snugly, such as the upper and inner anterior thighs, popliteal fossae, buttocks, and waistband areas. Other areas include, in men, the parts of the neck that come in contact with stiff collars and, in women, the anterior or posterior axillary folds, vulva, and suprapubic area. Diagnosis is confirmed by patch testing with disperse dyes (especially blue 106 and blue 124) and formaldehyde-releasing fabric-finish resins (e.g., dimethyloldihydroxyethyleneurea and ethyleneurea melamine formaldehyde). Patch testing with the clothing (particularly acetate and polyester liners) of patients with dye allergy may yield positive results.

Textile dye dermatitis can be managed in the following ways:

1. Avoiding clothes with the offending dye (especially 100% acetate or 100% polyester liners).
2. Avoiding nylon hose (especially beige tones) and tight synthetic spandex/Lycra exercise clothing.
3. Wearing 100% natural fabrics (i.e., cotton, linen, silk, wool) or 100% silk long-sleeved undershirts and slip pants.
4. Wearing loose-fitting clothing that has been washed (three times) before wearing.[36]

Many of these principles also apply to managing fabric-finish allergy, especially avoiding wrinkle-resistant, shrinkproof, and wash-and-wear clothing.

OCCUPATIONAL CONTACT DERMATITIS

Contact dermatitis, particularly of the hands, is one of the most common types of occupational skin disorders. Special issues associated with these disorders include the following:

1. Inadequate workplace data, especially job descriptions and material-safety data sheets that include information on workplace chemicals and other substances.
2. Objective information on exposure history (a factory visit is ideal) is important. Direct exposure to chemicals can occur because of spills or routine work levels; indirect exposure can come from contaminated tools, rags, and gloves; and airborne exposures can result from mists, droplets, and sprays.
3. The skin is an important portal of entry for a number of toxic chemicals that may or may not have a direct effect on skin. These chemicals include aniline, carbon disulfide, ethylene glycol ethers, certain pesticides, tetrachloroethylene, and toluene.
4. Patch testing with industrial chemicals should be performed very carefully. Irritants should not be tested, and many require

Table 6 Topical and Systemic Photosensitizers[18,38,39]

Agent	PT/PA	Common Sources/Forms
Topical photosensitizers		
Psoralens	PT	Plants and drugs
Pitch, creosote, and coal tar derivatives	PT	Medications/industrial products
Halogenated salicylanilides (e.g., bithionol, dibromosalicylanilide)	PA	Antibacterials in soaps and detergents
Musk ambrette	PA	Fragrance
Oxybenzone/padimate O	PA	Sunscreens
Phenothiazines	PA	Topical drugs
Ketoprofen	PA	Nonsteroidal anti-inflammatory drugs
Systemic photosensitizers		
Thiazides	PT	Diuretics
Phenothiazines	PT	Tranquilizers
Dimethylchlorotetracycline	PT	Antibiotic
Griseofulvin	PT	Antifungal
Nalidixic acid	PT	Antibiotic
Sulfonamides	PT	Antibiotic
Psoralens	PT	Photosensitizing drug
Piroxicam	PT?	Nonsteroidal anti-inflammatory drugs, especially in thimerosal-sensitive patients

PA—photoallergenic reaction   PT—phototoxic reaction

dilution to nonirritating concentrations. Testing with individual chemical components of mixtures is preferable in many cases.

5. Establishing occupational causation for ACD is often a challenge, and recommendations have been published.

Prevention and treatment of occupational contact dermatitis is the same as for ACD.[17]

Subtypes of Contact Dermatitis

PHOTOSENSITIVITY

Photosensitivity refers to a condition in which ultraviolet light in combination with endogenous or exogenous substances, usually drugs or chemicals, evokes an eruption on sun-exposed skin. Most cases are evoked by ultraviolet A, but on occasion, eruptions are caused by ultraviolet B (sunburn irradiation) or by visible light. The most common causes are systemic exposure to photosensitizing drugs [see Table 6] or cutaneous exposure, usually accidental, to psoralen in plants.

Photosensitivity reactions are of two types: phototoxicity and photoallergy. Many substances that are photoallergic at low concentrations may be phototoxic at high concentrations.[37,38]

Phototoxicity

Phototoxicity is analogous to irritation and occurs in any individual after one exposure to sufficient amounts of chemical and light. Phototoxicity has been likened to an exaggerated sunburn response, consisting of delayed erythema and edema followed by pigmentation and desquamation. Asphalt workers and roofers working with pitch develop the so-called smarts when exposed to sufficient sunlight. Phytophotodermatitis, or meadow dermatitis, is a particularly striking phototoxicity characterized by streaky bullae after contact, sometimes while sunbathing, with psoralen containing umbelliferones. Berloque dermatitis is a phototoxic dermatitis characterized by the appearance of hyperpigmented, droplike patches on the neck, face, and breast. This reaction is caused by exposure to 5-methoxypsoralen present in perfumes or colognes containing oil of bergamot, and the hyperpigmentation may persist for many months. Photo-onycholysis has been reported with tetracyclines, psoralen, and other phototoxic drugs. Not all cases exhibit obvious skin phototoxicity.[18] Most cases of phototoxicity are caused by administration of phototoxic systemic drugs [see Table 6].

Photoallergy

Photoallergy is analogous to ACD and is an immunologic reaction in which exposure of the photosensitizing compound to UV light plays a role in formation of a complete antigen. A delayed eruption, usually eczematous, appears in sun-exposed body areas, usually the face and dorsal hands, typically sparing the submental and retroauricular areas [see Figure 11]; shaded areas and covered areas remain relatively clear but occasionally are involved. Most cases are caused by topical photoallergens [see Table 6], and the most common photocontact allergens are sunscreen chemicals, which act by absorbing ultraviolet light, especially oxybenzone. Other sunscreen chemicals, such as padimate O and the dibenzoylmethanes, have also been reported to cause photoallergic contact dermatitis.[37] Photoallergic contact dermatitis is reproduced and diagnosed by photopatch testing in which ultraviolet light (usually ultraviolet A) is combined with patch testing. This procedure is particularly helpful in separating patients with eruptions caused by polymorphous light from patients with photoallergic contact dermatitis. Photopatch testing is not indicated in phototoxic drug eruptions. Photoallergic reactions can persist in some individuals as chronic actinic dermatitis (CAD), which can be a difficult management problem. Patients with photoallergic contact dermatitis often have contact allergy and should also be patch tested.

Treatment of Phototoxicity and Photoallergy

Elimination of exposure to the photoallergen or phototoxic agent is effective for most patients, except for a few with CAD. Broad-spectrum sunscreens or sunblocks, especially those con-

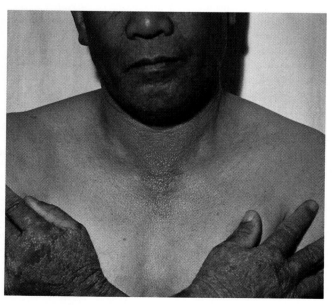

Figure 11 **Photocontact dermatitis characteristically involves areas exposed to the sun.**

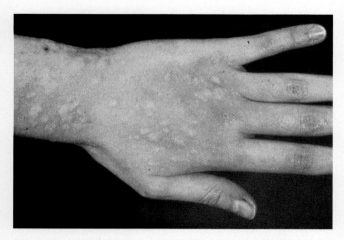

Figure 12 **Contact urticaria of the hands in a nurse allergic to her powdered natural rubber latex gloves (latex allergy). She also experienced allergic rhinitis and asthma while at work. Urticaria is often short-lived after gloves are used and may be absent at the time of examination.**

taining micronized titanium, along with sun-protective clothing, may be helpful. Topical steroids are helpful for mildly affected patients, but severely affected patients with CAD may require azathioprine, with or without systemic steroids; psoralen ultraviolet A therapy and cyclosporine have also been used in some severe cases.[18]

LATEX ALLERGY

Latex allergy is an IgE-mediated hypersensitivity to one or more of a number of proteins present in raw or uncured natural rubber latex (NRL). The paradigm for immunologic contact urticaria is latex allergy, which, over the past decade, has become a significant medical and occupational health problem.

Populations at Risk

Individuals at highest risk are patients with spina bifida (30% to 65% prevalence), health care workers, and other workers with significant NRL exposure. Most reported series of occupational cases involve health care workers, affecting 5% to 11% of those studied. Studies of populations of non–health care workers are infrequent and include kitchen workers; cleaners; rubber-band, surgical-glove, and latex-doll manufacturing workers; and miscellaneous other occupations in which NRL is utilized.

Predisposing Risk Factors

Predisposing risk factors are hand eczema, allergic rhinitis, allergic conjunctivitis, or asthma in individuals who frequently wear NRL gloves; mucosal exposure to NRL; and multiple surgical procedures.[39,40]

Clinical Features

Clinical signs of NRL allergy include contact urticaria [*see Figure 12*], generalized urticaria, allergic rhinitis, allergic conjunctivitis, angioedema, asthma, and anaphylaxis.[39] More than 600 serious reactions to NRL, including 16 fatal anaphylactic reactions, were reported to the FDA by the early 1990s.

The majority of cases involve reactions from wearing NRL gloves or being examined by individuals wearing NRL gloves. Reactions from other medical and nonmedical NRL devices have occurred; these include balloons, rubber bands, condoms, vibrators, dental dams, anesthesia equipment, and toys for animals or children. The route of exposure to NRL proteins includes direct contact with intact or inflamed skin and mucosal exposure, such as inhalation of powder from NRL gloves, especially in medical facilities and in operating rooms.[40] Most immediate-type NRL reactions result from exposure to dipped NRL products (gloves, condoms, balloons, and tourniquets). Dry-molded rubber products (syringes, plungers, vial stoppers, and baby-bottle nipples) contain lower residual protein levels or have less easily extracted proteins than do dipped NRL products.

NRL allergy is sometimes associated with allergic reactions to fruit, especially bananas, kiwi, and avocados, and to chestnuts. This allergic reaction results from cross-reactivity between proteins in NRL and those found in some fruits and nuts. Symptoms range from oral itching and angioedema to asthma, gastrointestinal upset, and anaphylaxis.

Diagnosis

Diagnosis of NRL allergy is strongly suggested by a history of angioedema of the lips when inflating balloons and by a history of itching, burning, urticaria, or anaphylaxis when donning gloves; when undergoing surgical, medical, and dental procedures; or after exposure to condoms or other NRL devices. Diagnosis is confirmed by a positive wear or use test with NRL gloves, a valid positive intracutaneous prick test with NRL, or a positive serum radioallergosorbent test with NRL.[39] Severe allergic reactions have occurred from prick and wear tests; epinephrine latex-safe resuscitation equipment free of NRL should be available during these procedures.[39]

Table 7   Dermatitis and Latex Allergy Information Sources

Condition	Organization	Web Address
Contact Dermatitis	American Contact Dermatitis Society	www.contactderm.org
	American Academy of Dermatology	www.aad.org
	National Institute for Occupational Safety and Health	www.cdc.gov/NIOSH
Latex Allergy	A.L.E.R.T. Inc	www.latexallergyresources.org
	Elastic Inc	www.latexallergyhelp.com
	Spina Bifida Association of America	www.sbaa.org

Treatment and Prevention

Hyposensitization to NRL is not yet feasible, and NRL avoidance and substitution is imperative. Because many patients with NRL allergy have hand eczema or have immediate allergic symptoms or both, the most important issues for physicians are accurate diagnosis, appropriate treatment, and counseling.

Prevention and control of NRL allergy includes latex avoidance in health care settings for affected workers and patients. Synthetic non-NRL gloves should be available to replace latex gloves. Also, in many cases, low-allergen NRL gloves should be worn by coworkers so as to minimize symptoms and decrease induction of NRL allergy in those with NRL allergy. Allergen content of gloves should be requested from manufacturers and suppliers; lists of glove allergen levels have also been published. Patients with NRL allergy should also obtain Medic-Alert bracelets and inform health care providers of their sensitivity. These patients should be given lists of substitute gloves, other non-NRL devices, potentially allergenic fruits, latex-safe anesthesia protocols, occult sources of NRL exposure such as toys (for animals and children), and dental prophylaxis cups. Some of this information is available in published sources, government agencies, and latex allergy support groups that publish newsletters and other relevant information. Some sources have Web sites [see Table 7].

References

1. Rietschel RR, Adams RM, Daily AD, et al: Guidelines of care for contact dermatitis. J Am Acad Dermatol 32:109, 1995

2. Schappert SM: National Ambulatory Medical Care Survey: 1994 Summary. Adv Data 273:1, 1996

3. De Groot AC: Patch Testing: Test Concentrations and Vehicles for 3700 Chemicals, 2nd ed. Elsevier, Amsterdam, 1994

4. Wigger-Alberti W, Elsner P: Contact dermatitis due to irritation. Handbook of Occupational Dermatology. Kanerva L, Elsner P, Wahlberg JE, et al, Eds. Springer Verlag, Berlin, 2000, p 99

5. Iliev D, Elsner P: Clinical irritant contact dermatitis syndromes. Immunol Allergy Clin North Am 17:365, 1997

6. Andersen KE, Maibach HI: Contact dermatitis. Dermatology. Orkin M, Maibach HI, Dahl MV, Eds. Appleton & Lange, Norwalk, 1991, p 405

7. Schwanitz HJ, Uter W: Interdigital dermatitis: sentinel skin damage in hairdressers. Br J Dermatol 142:1011, 2000

8. Belsito DV: Allergic contact dermatitis. Fitzpatrick's Dermatology in General Medicine, 5th ed. Freedberg IM, Eisen AZ, Wolff, K, et al, Eds. McGraw-Hill, New York, 1999, p 1447

9. Condie MW, Adams RM: Influence of oral prednisone on patch test reaction to Rhus antigen. Arch Dermatol 107:540, 1973

10. Wulfhorst B: Skin hardening in occupational dermatology. Handbook of Contact Dermatology. Kanerva L, Elsner P, Wahlberg J, et al, Eds. Springer Verlag, Berlin, 2000, p 115

11. Marks JG Jr, Belsito DV, DeLeo VA, et al: North American contact dermatitis group test results 1996–1998. Arch Dermatol 136:272, 2000

12. Marks JG, DeLeo V: Contact and Occupational Dermatology, 2nd ed. Mosby, St. Louis, 1997

13. Rietschel RL, Fowler JF: Fisher's Contact Dermatitis, 4th ed. Williams & Wilkins, Baltimore, 1995

14. Gaspari AA: The role of keratinocytes in the pathophysiology of contact dermatitis. Immunol Allergy Clin North Am 17:377, 1997

15. Corsini E, Galli CL: Cytokines and irritant contact dermatitis. Toxicol Lett 102:277, 1998

16. Adams RM: Occupational Skin Disease, 3rd ed. WB Saunders, Philadelphia, 1999

17. Taylor JS: Recognizing allergic contact dermatitis. Practical Contact Dermatitis. Guin JD, Ed. McGraw Hill, New York, 1995, p 31

18. Wilkinson JD, Shaw S: Contact dermatitis: allergic. Rook/Wilkinson/Ebling Textbook of Dermatology. Champion RH, Burton JL, Burns DA, et al, Eds. Blackwell Science, London, 1998, p 733

19. Rietschel RL: Experience with supplemental allergens in the diagnosis of contact dermatitis. Cutis 65:27, 2000

20. Bourke JF, Batta K, Prais L, et al: The reproducibility of patch tests. Br J Dermatol 140: 102, 1999

21. Nethercott JR, Holness DL: Validity of patch test screening trays in the evaluation of patients with allergic contact dermatitis. J Am Acad Dermatol 21:568, 1989

22. Diepgen TL, Coenraads PJ: Sensitivity, specificity and positive predictive value of patch testing: the more you test, the more you get? Contact Dermatitis 42:315, 2000

23. Basketter DA, Griffiths HA, Wang XM, et al: Individual, ethnic, and seasonal variation in irritant susceptibility of skin: the implications for a predictive human patch test. Contact Dermatitis 35:208, 1996

24. Zappi E, Brancaccio RR: Allergic contact dermatitis from mupirocin ointment. J Acad Derm 36:266, 1977

25. Wigger-Alberti W, Elsner P: Preventive measures in contact dermatitis. Clin Dermatol 15:661, 1997

26. Marks JG Jr, Fowler JF Jr, Sherertz EF, et al: Prevention of poison ivy and poison oak allergic contact dermatitis by quaternium-18 bentonite. J Am Acad Dermatol 33:212, 1995

27. Elsner P, Wiggerti-Alberti W, Pantini G: Perfluoropolyethers in the prevention of irritant contact dermatitis. Dermatology 197:141, 1998

28. Taylor JS: Occupational dermatoses. Conn's Current Therapy. Rakel RE, Ed. WB Saunders, Philadelphia, 1996, p 823

29. Taylor JS, Praditsuwan P, Handel D, et al: Allergic contact dermatitis from doxepin cream: a one-year patch test clinic experience. Arch Dermatol 132:515, 1996

30. Isaksson M, Dooms-Goosens A: Corticosteroids. Clin Dermatol 15:527, 1997

31. Rietschel RL: Patch testing for corticosteroid allergy in the United States. Arch Dermatol 131:91, 1995

32. Veien NK: Ingested food in systemic contact dermatitis. Clin Dermatol 15:547, 1997

33. Menne T, Veien N, Sjolin K-E, et al: Systemic contact dermatitis. Am J Contact Dermatitis 5:1, 1994

34. Maibach HI: Oral substitution in patients sensitized by transdermal clonidine treatment. Contact Dermatitis 16:1, 1987

35. Storrs FJ: Contact allergen of the year: disperse blue dyes. Am J Contact Dermatitis 11:1, 2000

36. Pratt M, Taraska V: Disperse blue dyes 106 and 124 are common causes of textile dermatitis and should serve as screening allergens for this condition. Am J Contact Dermatitis 11:30, 2000

37. Isaksson M, Bruze M: Photocontact dermatitis: photopatch testing. Clin Dermatol 15:615, 1997

38. Harber LC, Bickers DR: Photosensitivity Diseases. BC Decker, Toronto, 1989

39. Taylor JS, Wattanakrai P, Charous L, et al: Latex allergy. 1999 Yearbook of Dermatology and Dermatologic Surgery. Thiers BH, Lang PG, Eds. Mosby, St. Louis, 1999, p 1

40. Fink JN, Ed: Latex allergy. Immunol Allergy Clin North Am 15:1, 1995

41. Taylor JS: Occupational dermatoses. Conn's Current Therapy. Rakel RE, Ed. WB Saunders, Philadelphia, 1996, p 823

42. Shelley WB, Shelly ED: Contact dermatitis. Advanced Dermatologic Diagnosis. WB Saunders Co, Philadelphia, 1992, p 437

Acknowledgments

Figure 7   Courtesy of James R. Nethercott, M.D. (deceased), Department of Dermatology, University of Maryland, Baltimore.

Figure 11   Courtesy of Kristina Turjanmaa, M.D., and Arto Lahti, M.D., Tampere and Oulu, Finland.

36 Cutaneous Adverse Drug Reactions

Neil H. Shear, M.D., *Sandra Knowles*, B.Sc.Pharm., *and Lori Shapiro*, M.D.

An adverse drug reaction (ADR) is defined as any noxious, unintended, and undesired effect of a drug that occurs at doses used in humans for prophylaxis, diagnosis, or therapy.[1] A cutaneous eruption is one of the most common manifestations of an ADR. Over the past 15 years, a dramatic shift has occurred in our understanding of drug-induced cutaneous eruptions. This understanding has not been widely appreciated in clinical practice. The best approach to drug-induced eruptions is first to make the diagnosis. It is clear that drugs cause special syndromes, and a complete examination of the patient is required. This chapter reviews the pathophysiology and clinical manifestations that are important for correct diagnosis and treatment of cutaneous ADRs.

Epidemiology

Epidemiologic studies have shown that ADRs occur in 6.7% of all hospitalized patients,[2] and 3% to 6% of all hospital admissions are the result of ADRs.[3] In the Boston Collaborative Drug Surveillance Program,[4] the prevalence of cutaneous ADRs in hospitalized patients was 2.2%. Antibiotics were responsible for 75% of detected reactions. The cost of drug-related morbidity and mortality has been estimated at $30 billion a year,[5] and ADRs are thought to be between the fourth and sixth leading cause of death in the United States.[2,5]

Etiology

Cutaneous reactions to drugs often occur in complicated clinical scenarios that may include exposure to multiple agents. New drugs started within the preceding 6 weeks are potential causative agents, as are drugs that have been used intermittently, including over-the-counter preparations and herbal and naturopathic remedies.

Diagnosis

CLINICAL MANIFESTATIONS

The morphology of cutaneous eruptions may be exanthematous, urticarial, blistering, or pustular. The extent of the reaction is variable. For example, once the morphology of the reaction has been documented, a specific diagnosis (e.g., fixed drug eruption or acute generalized exanthematous pustulosis) can be made. The reaction may also present as a syndrome (e.g., serum sickness–like reaction or hypersensitivity syndrome reaction). Fever is associated with the more serious cutaneous ADRs.

DIFFERENTIAL DIAGNOSIS

Differential diagnoses can include viral exanthems (e.g., infectious mononucleosis and parvovirus B19 infection), bacterial infections, Kawasaki syndrome, collagen vascular disease, and neoplasia.[6]

LABORATORY TESTS

Penicillin skin testing with major and minor determinants is useful for confirmation of an IgE-mediated immediate hyper-sensitivity reaction to penicillin.[7] Oral rechallenges may be useful in the diagnosis of ADRs; however, they should not be used if a serious reaction, such as Stevens-Johnson syndrome (SJS) or toxic epidermal necrolysis (TEN), previously occurred. Patch testing may be helpful in the diagnosis of fixed drug eruptions or contact dermatitis.[8]

Exanthematous Eruptions

SIMPLE ERUPTIONS

Exanthematous eruptions, also known as morbilliform, maculopapular, or scarlatiniform eruptions, are the most common cutaneous ADRs.[4] Simple exanthems are erythematous changes in the skin without blistering or pustulation.

Many drugs can cause exanthematous eruptions, including the penicillins, sulfonamides, barbiturates, antiepileptic medications, and antimalarials.[4,9] Exanthematous eruptions occur in 3% to 7% of patients receiving such aminopenicillins as ampicillin and amoxicillin. However, these eruptions may occur in 60% to 100% of patients taking ampicillin or amoxicillin who are receiving concurrent allopurinol therapy or who have concomitant lymphocytic leukemia, infectious mononucleosis, cytomegalovirus infection, or hyperuricemia.

Studies suggest that some exanthematous eruptions represent cell-mediated hypersensitivity.[10,11] The etiology of the ampicillin rash concurrent with a viral infection is unknown, but the rash does not appear to be IgE mediated, and patients can tolerate all β-lactam antibiotics, including ampicillin, once the infectious process has resolved. A similar reaction was seen in 50% of HIV-infected patients exposed to sulfonamide antibiotics.[12]

Simple exanthems are symmetrical and often become generalized. Pruritus is the most frequently associated symptom. Fever is not associated with simple exanthematous eruptions. These eruptions usually occur within 1 week after the beginning of therapy and generally resolve within 7 to 14 days.[13] The exanthem's turning from bright red to brownish red marks resolution. Resolution may be followed by scaling or desquamation.[14] Some patients with ampicillin- or amoxicillin-induced exanthematous eruptions may have a positive result on a patch test or on a delayed intradermal test.[11,12] In general, however, skin testing is not considered helpful in the diagnosis of an exanthematous eruption.

The differential diagnosis of drug-induced exanthematous eruption includes viral exanthem (patients should be tested for mononucleosis), collagen vascular disease, bacterial infection, and rickettsial infection. Hypersensitivity syndrome should be considered in the differential diagnosis.

The treatment of simple exanthematous eruptions is generally supportive. For example, oral antihistamines used in conjunction with soothing baths may help relieve pruritus. Topical corticosteroids are indicated when antihistamines do not provide relief. Systemic corticosteroids are used only in severe cases. Discontinuance of the offending agent is recommended.

Table 1   Clinical Features of Hypersensitivity Syndrome Reaction and Serum Sickness–like Reaction

	Rash	*Fever*	*Internal Organ Involvement*	*Arthralgia*	*Lymphadenopathy*
Hypersensitivity syndrome reaction	Exanthem Exfoliative dermatitis Pustular eruptions Erythema multiforme Stevens-Johnson syndrome Toxic epidermal necrolysis	Present	Present	Absent	Present
Serum sickness–like reaction	Urticaria Exanthem	Present	Absent	Present	Present

COMPLEX ERUPTIONS

Hypersensitivity Syndrome Reaction

Hypersensitivity syndrome reaction is a complex drug reaction that affects various organ systems. A triad of fever, skin eruption, and internal organ involvement signals this potentially life-threatening syndrome. It occurs in approximately one in 3,000 exposures to such agents as aromatic anticonvulsants (e.g., phenytoin, phenobarbital, and carbamazepine[15]), sulfonamide antibiotics, dapsone, minocycline, and allopurinol.[16,17]

It has been suggested that the metabolism of aromatic anticonvulsants by cytochrome P-450 plays a pivotal role in the development of the hypersensitivity syndrome reaction.[18] In most people, the chemically reactive metabolites that are produced are detoxified by epoxide hydroxylases. If detoxification is defective, however, one of the metabolites may act as a hapten and initiate an immune response, stimulate apoptosis, or cause cell necrosis directly.

In one study,[18] 75% of patients with hypersensitivity syndrome reactions to one aromatic anticonvulsant showed in vitro cross-reactivity to the other two aromatic anticonvulsants. In addition, in vitro testing has shown that there is a familial occurrence of hypersensitivity to anticonvulsants.[18] Although lamotrigine is not an aromatic anticonvulsant, it can also cause a hypersensitivity syndrome reaction.[19,20]

Sulfonamide antibiotics can cause hypersensitivity syndrome reactions in susceptible persons. The primary metabolic pathway for sulfonamides involves acetylation of the drug to a nontoxic metabolite and renal excretion. An alternative metabolic pathway, quantitatively more important in patients who are slow acetylators, engages the cytochrome P-450 mixed-function oxidase system. These enzymes transform the parent compound to reactive metabolites, namely hydroxylamines and nitroso compounds, which produce cytotoxicity independently of preformed drug-specific antibody. In most people, detoxification of the metabolite occurs. However, hypersensitivity syndrome reactions may occur in patients who are unable to detoxify this metabolite (e.g., those who are glutathione deficient).[21] Although the detoxification defect is present in 2% of the population, only one in 10,000 people will manifest a hypersensitivity syndrome reaction in response to sulfonamide antibiotics. Siblings and other first-degree relatives of patients with the detoxification defect are at an increased risk (perhaps one in four) of having a similar defect.

Other aromatic amines, such as procainamide, dapsone, and acebutolol, are also metabolized to chemically reactive compounds. We recommend that patients who develop symptoms compatible with a sulfonamide hypersensitivity syndrome reaction avoid these aromatic amines, because the potential exists for cross-reac-

tivity. However, cross-reactivity should not occur between sulfonamides and drugs that are not aromatic amines (e.g., sulfonylureas, thiazide diuretics, furosemide, and acetazolamide).

Hypersensitivity syndrome reaction occurs most frequently on first exposure to the drug, with initial symptoms starting 1 to 6 weeks after exposure [*see Table 1*]. Fever and malaise, which can be accompanied by pharyngitis and cervical lymphadenopathy, are the presenting symptoms in most patients. Atypical lymphocytosis, with subsequent eosinophilia, may occur during the initial phases of the reaction in some patients. A cutaneous eruption, which occurs in approximately 85% of patients, can range from an exanthematous eruption [*see Figure 1*] to the more serious Stevens-Johnson syndrome or toxic epidermal necrolysis. The liver is often involved, resulting in hepatitis, although other internal organs may be affected, such as the kidney (e.g., interstitial nephritis and vasculitis), the central nervous system (e.g., encephalitis and aseptic meningitis), and the lungs (e.g., interstitial pneumonitis, respiratory distress syndrome, and vasculitis). A subgroup of patients may become hypothyroid as part of an autoimmune thyroiditis within 2 months after the initiation of symptoms.[22]

After hypersensitivity syndrome reaction has been recognized from the symptom complex of fever, rash, and lymphadenopathy, some laboratory tests can be used to evaluate internal organ involvement, which may be asymptomatic. A complete blood count, urinalysis, and measurements of liver transaminases and serum creatinine levels should be performed. In addition, the clinician should be guided by symptoms that may suggest

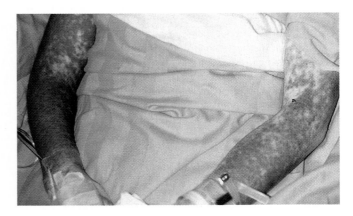

Figure 1   **This 35-year-old woman developed hypersensitivity syndrome reaction, characterized by fever, rash, and hepatitis, 14 days after starting trimethoprim-sulfamethoxazole therapy. The rash is an extensive, symmetrical, red edematous eruption.**

specific internal organ involvement (e.g., respiratory symptoms). Thyroid function should be evaluated on presentation of hypersensitivity syndrome reaction symptoms and 2 to 3 months later. A skin biopsy may be helpful when the patient has a blistering or a pustular eruption. Unfortunately, diagnostic or confirmatory tests are not readily available. An in vitro test employing a mouse hepatic microsomal system is used for research purposes to characterize patients who develop hypersensitivity syndrome reactions.[18,23] Because of the severity of the reactions, oral rechallenges are not recommended.

Although the role of corticosteroids is controversial, most clinicians choose to start prednisone at a dose of 1 to 2 mg/kg/day when symptoms are severe. Antihistamines, topical corticosteroids, or both can be used to alleviate symptoms. Because the risk of hypersensitivity syndrome reactions in first-degree relatives of patients who have had reactions is substantially higher than in the general population, counseling of family members regarding their risk of hypersensitivity syndrome reaction is advised.

Urticarial Eruptions

SIMPLE ERUPTIONS

Urticaria and Angioedema

Urticaria is characterized by pruritic red wheals of varying sizes that can occur with any medication. When deep dermal and subcutaneous tissues are also swollen, the reaction is known as angioedema.

Urticaria and angioedema usually result from a type I immediate hypersensitivity reaction. This mechanism is typified by immediate reactions to penicillin and other antibiotics. Binding of the drug or its metabolite to IgE bound to the surfaces of cutaneous mast cells leads to activation, degranulation, and release of such vasoactive mediators as histamine, leukotrienes, and prostaglandins.[24]

Urticarial reactions may also result from nonimmunologic activation of inflammatory mediators. Drugs such as acetylsalicylic acid and nonsteroidal anti-inflammatory drugs (NSAIDs),[25] radiocontrast media, and narcotic analgesics[26] may directly cause release of histamine from mast cells, independently of IgE. Angiotensin-converting enzyme (ACE) inhibitors are frequent causes of angioedema.[27] The mechanism of this reaction is unclear but may relate to accumulation of bradykinin or activation of the complement system.

Although medications tend to cause urticaria, angioedema, or both, other causal agents are food, physical factors (e.g., dermatographism and cholinergic urticaria), and idiopathic factors. Certain foods containing proteins that can cross-react with latex proteins, such as bananas, kiwifruit, avocados, and chestnuts, can cause oral itching and swelling, hives, or wheezing after ingestion. People at greatest risk for latex allergy include children with spina bifida and health care workers.[28,29] Latex allergy can manifest as contact urticaria at sites of latex exposure, such as lip swelling in a person who has blown up a balloon or sucked on a pacifier. Contact with aerosolized powder from latex gloves to which the latex protein has adhered may cause mucosal symptoms, such as itchy, swollen eyes; runny nose; sneezing; or wheezing. Anaphylaxis may also occur.[30]

Signs and symptoms of IgE-mediated allergic reactions are typically pruritus, urticaria, cutaneous flushing, angioedema, nausea, vomiting, diarrhea, abdominal pain, nasal congestion, rhinorrhea, laryngeal edema, and bronchospasm or hypotension or both. Fever is not associated with urticaria or angioedema reactions. In general, individual lesions of urticaria last for less than 24 hours, although new lesions can continually develop. With ACE-inhibitor therapy, the onset of the adverse reaction is usually within hours but can occur as late as 1 week to several months into therapy.[31] With treatment, the resulting angioedema usually resolves within 48 hours.

Skin testing may be helpful in cases of IgE-mediated urticaria. For example, penicillin skin testing with the major and minor determinants identifies approximately 99% of patients who have had an IgE-mediated reaction to penicillin.[8] A latex skin test is a sensitive indicator of IgE sensitization.[32] For large-molecular-weight agents, such as insulin,[33] protamine,[34] and egg-containing vaccines, positive immediate skin-test reactions identify patients at risk for IgE-mediated reactions.

Withdrawal of the causative agent is recommended. When angioedema or anaphylaxis occurs, immediate therapy with epinephrine and systemic steroids may be needed. Symptomatic relief can generally be achieved with antihistamines (H_1 receptor blockers).

Differential Diagnosis

Allergic urticaria must be differentiated from urticaria caused by physical factors. Cold urticaria, for example, is precipitated by exposure to cold, occurring within minutes after immersion of hands or body in cold water or after exposure to cold air. In severe cases, systemic symptoms, including wheezing and syncopy, can occur. A rare familial form of cold urticaria that is autosomal dominant has been linked to chromosome 1q44.[35]

Cold urticaria can be differentiated from other forms of urticaria by eliciting an urticarial reaction with an ice cube applied to the skin for 5 to 10 minutes. Other physical urticarias also have distinguishing causes or features. Solar urticaria occurs within minutes of exposure to sunlight and can be produced by exposing limited areas of skin to sunlight or to appropriate wavelengths of ultraviolet light in a phototherapy response to physical pressure. Cholinergic urticaria, which is characterized by small urticarial papules, can be induced by exposure to heat or by exercise. Papular urticaria is caused by insect bites.

Histologically, all the urticarias are characterized by an increase in mast cells in the dermis. Edema, vascular changes, and mononuclear infiltrates are more striking in the dermis of patients with cold urticaria. Mononuclear infiltrates are also more prominent in the deep dermis of patients with delayed pressure urticaria.[36]

As with drug-induced urticaria, first-line therapy of most urticarias consists of oral antihistamines and avoidance of precipitating factors. Psoralen plus ultraviolet A (PUVA) has been used successfully to treat patients with solar urticaria. More recently, montelukast has been used successfully to treat delayed pressure urticaria,[37] and cyclosporine is promising for cases of severe refractory chronic urticaria.[38]

COMPLEX ERUPTIONS

Serum Sickness–like Reactions

Serum sickness–like reactions are defined by fever, rash (usually urticarial), and arthralgias occurring 1 to 3 weeks after drug initiation. Other symptoms, such as lymphadenopathy and eosinophilia, may also be present. In contrast to true serum sickness, serum sickness–like reactions are without immune complexes, hypocomplementemia, vasculitis, and renal lesions [*see Table 1*].

Epidemiologic studies in children suggest that the risk of serum sickness–like reactions is greater with cefaclor than with other antibiotics, including other cephalosporins.[39,40] The overall incidence of cefaclor serum sickness–like reactions has been estimated to be 0.024% to 0.2% per course of cefaclor prescribed.

Although the pathogenesis is unknown, it has been postulated that in genetically susceptible hosts, metabolism of cefaclor produces a reactive metabolite that may bind to tissue proteins and elicit an inflammatory response that manifests as a serum sickness–like reaction.[41]

Other drugs that have been implicated in serum sickness–like reactions are cefprozil,[42] bupropion,[43] and minocycline.[17,44] The incidence of serum sickness–like reactions caused by these drugs is unknown.

Discontinuance of the culprit drug and symptomatic treatment with antihistamines and topical corticosteroids are recommended for patients with serum sickness–like reactions. A short course of oral corticosteroids may be required for patients with more severe symptoms. The drug that caused the serum sickness–like reaction should be avoided. For cefaclor and cefprozil, the risk of cross-reaction with β-lactam antibiotics is small, and the administration of another cephalosporin is usually well tolerated.[45] However, some clinicians recommend that patients who experience serum sickness–like reactions from cefaclor avoid all β-lactam drugs.[46]

Blistering Eruptions

SIMPLE ERUPTIONS

Fixed Drug Eruptions

Fixed drug eruptions usually appear as solitary pruritic, erythematous, bright-red or dusky-red macules that may evolve into an edematous plaque [*see Figure 2*]. In some patients, multiple lesions may be present. Blistering and erosion may occur on mucosal surfaces.

Fixed drug eruptions recur in the same skin area after readministration of the causative medication. Many drugs have been implicated in fixed drug eruptions, including phenolphthalein, ibuprofen, sulfonamides, tetracyclines, and barbiturates. The pathogenesis of fixed drug eruptions has not been fully elucidated.

Fixed drug eruptions are most common on the genitalia and in the perianal area, although they can occur anywhere on the skin surface. The onset of a fixed drug eruption can be sudden, developing within 30 minutes to 8 to 16 hours after ingestion of the medication. In patients who continue to take the offending drug, the number of eruption sites may gradually increase.[47]

After the initial acute phase, which lasts days to weeks, residual hyperpigmentation develops. Some patients may complain of burning or stinging on the affected skin sites. Systemic manifestations, which are present in approximately 25% of cases, can include fever, malaise, and abdominal symptoms.[48]

No conclusive diagnostic tests are available, but a challenge or provocation test with the suspected drug may be useful in confirming the diagnosis. Patch testing at the site of a previous lesion yields a positive response in up to 43% of patients. Prick and intradermal skin tests are reported to yield positive reactions in 24% and 67% of patients, respectively, but results vary with different drugs and reaction patterns. Patients with macu-

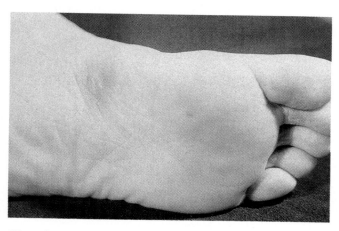

Figure 2 **This 28-year-old man taking tetracycline for acne vulgaris developed a fixed drug eruption.**

lopapular rashes are more likely to have positive patch tests than patients with urticarial rashes.[49]

Treatment includes discontinuance of the causative agent and symptomatic therapy (e.g., topical corticosteroids).

Pseudoporphyria

Pseudoporphyria is a cutaneous phototoxic disorder that can resemble either porphyria cutanea tarda (PCT) or erythropoietic protoporphyria (EPP). Tetracycline, furosemide, and naproxen have been implicated in PCT- and EPP-pseudoporphyria.[14] The eruption may begin within 1 day after initiation of therapy or be delayed for as long as 1 year. PCT-pseudoporphyria is characterized by skin fragility, blister formation, and scarring in areas exposed to sunlight; it occurs with normal porphyrin metabolism. The second clinical pattern mimics EPP and manifests as cutaneous burning, erythema, vesiculation, angular scars, and waxy thickening of the skin.

Because of the risk of permanent facial scarring, the implicated drug should be discontinued when skin fragility, blistering, or scarring occurs.[50] In addition, broad-spectrum sunscreen and protective clothing should be recommended to the patient.

COMPLEX ERUPTIONS

Drug-Induced Linear IgA Disease

Linear IgA disease is an autoimmune bullous dermatosis that is identified on the basis of the linear deposition of IgA at the basement membrane zone.[51] This disease can be induced by such drugs as vancomycin, lithium, diclofenac, and amiodarone. The drug-induced disease probably represents an immunologic response to the offending drug.

Drug-induced linear IgA disease is heterogeneous in clinical presentation. Cases have shown morphologies resembling erythema multiforme, bullous pemphigoid, and dermatitis herpetiformis. Mucosal or conjunctival lesions are less common in the drug-induced disease than in the idiopathic disease. Spontaneous remission occurs once the offending agent is withdrawn, and immune deposits disappear from the skin once the lesions resolve.[52]

Biopsy specimens are necessary for diagnosis. Histologically, the two disease entities are similar. One study suggests that, as for the idiopathic variety, the target antigen is not unique in the drug-induced disease. Although 13% to 30% of patients with sporadic linear IgA disease have circulating basement

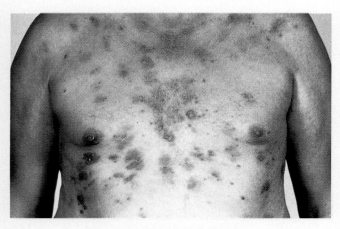

Figure 3 **Pemphigus foliaceus developed in this 64-year-old man taking enalapril.**

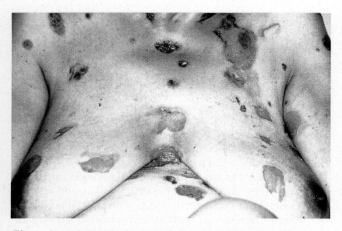

Figure 4 **Pemphigus vulgaris developed in this 59-year-old woman who took penicillamine as treatment for rheumatoid arthritis.**

membrane zone antibodies, these have not been reported in drug-induced cases.[53]

Drug-Induced Pemphigus

Pemphigus may be drug induced or drug triggered (i.e., the latent disease is unmasked by the drug exposure).

Drugs that cause pemphigus are penicillin, rifampin, phenylbutazone, propranolol, progesterone, piroxicam, interferon beta, interleukin-2, and levodopa.[54,55] An active amide group found in masked thiol drugs such as penicillin and cephalosporins and in nonthiol drugs such as enalapril may contribute to the pathogenesis of pemphigus.[55,56,57] Pemphigus foliaceus [*see Figure 3*][56,58] caused by penicillamine and other thiol drugs tends to resolve spontaneously in 35% to 50% of cases. The average interval to onset is 1 year. Antinuclear antibodies are detected in 25% of affected patients.

Most patients with nonthiol drug–induced pemphigus manifest clinical, histologic, immunologic, and evolutionary aspects similar to those of idiopathic pemphigus vulgaris [*see Figure 4*]. Drug-induced pemphigus is associated with mucosal involvement. Spontaneous recovery after drug withdrawal occurs in 15% of affected patients.

Treatment of drug-induced pemphigus begins with drug withdrawal. Systemic corticosteroids are often required until all symptoms of active disease disappear. Vigilant follow-up is re-

quired after remission for an early relapse to be detected. The patient's serum should be monitored regularly for autoantibodies.[59]

Erythema Multiforme, Stevens-Johnson Syndrome, and Toxic Epidermal Necrolysis

These eruptions, which may represent variants of the same disease process, encompass a spectrum ranging from erythema multiforme (EM) to more serious reactions, such as SJS and TEN [*see Figure 5*].

A large percentage of EM and SJS cases are not drug related and may develop after a variety of predisposing factors, including infections, neoplasia, and autoimmune diseases. The drugs most frequently cited as causes for EM, SJS, and TEN are anticonvulsants, antibiotics (e.g., sulfonamides), allopurinol, and NSAIDs (e.g., piroxicam).[60] With anticonvulsants, risk appears to be greatest during the first 8 weeks of therapy.[61]

The pathogenesis of severe cutaneous ADRs is unknown, although a metabolic basis has been hypothesized. Sulfonamides and anticonvulsants, the two groups of drugs most frequently associated with SJS and TEN, are metabolized to toxic metabolites that are subsequently detoxified in most persons. However, in predisposed patients with a genetic defect, the metabolite may bind covalently to proteins. In some of these patients, the metabolite-protein adducts may trigger an immune response that leads to a cutaneous ADR.[62]

Clinically, the reaction patterns of EM, SJS, and TEN are characterized by the triad of mucous membrane erosions, target lesions, and epidermal necrosis with skin detachment.[63] The more severe the reaction, the more likely it is that it was drug-induced. Cases of severe cutaneous ADRs to lamotrigine, such as SJS and TEN, have been reported.[20,64] The prevalence of severe cutaneous ADRs associated with lamotrigine has been reported to be as high as one in 1,000 in adults and is higher in children. The risk is increased in the presence of valproic acid.

Complete blood counts, liver enzyme measurements, and chest x-rays should be performed to rule out concurrent internal organ involvement.

Treatment of EM, SJS, and TEN includes discontinuance of a suspected drug and such supportive measures as careful wound care, hydration, and nutritional support.[65-67] The use of corticosteroids in SJS and TEN is controversial. Some clinicians believe corticosteroids may be beneficial when administered early in the disease and at relatively high dosage.[68] However, others suggest

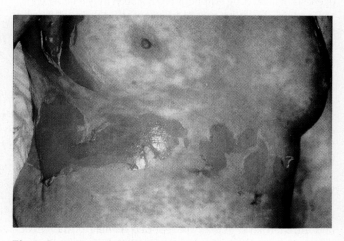

Figure 5 **This 50-year-old woman developed toxic epidermal necrolysis 17 days after starting phenytoin therapy.**

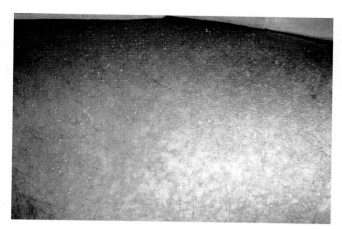

Figure 6 **Acute generalized exanthematous pustulosis (small nonfollicular pustules on a red base) in a 70-year-old man who took doxacillin as treatment for cellulites.**

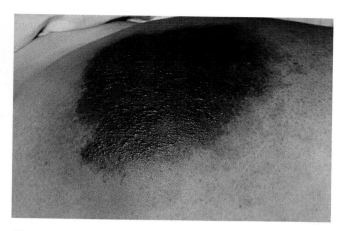

Figure 7 **Coumarin-induced skin necrosis in a 57-year-old woman who was given coumarin as treatment for atrial fibrillation.**

that corticosteroids do not shorten the recovery time and may increase the risk of complications, including secondary infections and gastrointestinal bleeding.[65,69] Uncontrolled studies have shown that plasmapheresis may be efficacious in the treatment of TEN.[70] Patients who have developed a severe cutaneous ADR (EM, SJS, or TEN) should not be rechallenged with the drug or undergo desensitization with the medication.

Pustular Eruptions

SIMPLE ERUPTIONS

Acneiform Eruptions

Eruptions morphologically mimicking acne vulgaris may be associated with drug ingestion. Iodides, bromides, adrenocorticotropic hormone, corticosteroids, isoniazid, androgens, lithium, dactinomycin, and phenytoin are reported to induce acnelike lesions.[71] Acne fulminans was induced by testosterone in 1% to 2% of adolescent boys who were treated for excessively tall stature.[72]

Drug-induced acne may appear in atypical areas, such as arms and legs, and is usually monomorphous.[73] Comedones are usually absent. Fever is absent. Acneiform eruptions do not affect prepubertal children, indicating that previous hormonal priming is a prerequisite. Topical tretinoin may be useful when the drug cannot be stopped.

COMPLEX ERUPTIONS

Acute Generalized Exanthematous Pustulosis

Acute generalized exanthematous pustulosis is characterized by acute onset, with fever and a cutaneous eruption with nonfollicular sterile pustules on an edematous erythema[74] [*see Figure 6*]; leukocytosis is another common finding. Generalized desquamation occurs 2 weeks later. Differential diagnosis includes pustular psoriasis, hypersensitivity syndrome reaction with pustulation, and pustular eruptions of infancy.

Acute generalized exanthematous pustulosis is most commonly associated with β-lactam and macrolide antibiotic usage.[75] Many other drugs have been implicated, however, including calcium channel blockers and analgesics. Discontinuance of therapy is usually the extent of treatment necessary in most patients.

Other Eruptions

ANTICOAGULANT-INDUCED SKIN NECROSIS

Anticoagulant drugs may induce hypercoagulable states with subsequent vascular infarction and cutaneous necrosis [*see Figure 7*]. Both coumarin and heparin can induce skin necrosis. Clinical pearls that can help differentiate these reactions are the location, timing, platelet count, and primary diagnosis [*see Table 2*].

The pathogenesis of coumarin-induced skin necrosis is the paradoxical development of occlusive thrombi in cutaneous and subcutaneous venules caused by a transient hypercoagulable state. This condition results from the suppression of the natural anticoagulant protein C at a greater rate than natural procoagulant factors. Coumarin-induced skin necrosis is associated with protein C and protein S deficiency, but pretreatment screening is not warranted.

It is estimated that one in 10,000 persons who take coumarin are at risk for this adverse event.[76] The prevalence is four times higher in women than in men. In both sexes, the peak inci-

Table 2 Clinical Pearls to Identify Anticoagulant-Induced Skin Necrosis

	Interval to Onset	*Location*	*Other*
Coumarin-induced skin necrosis	3–5 days	Adipose-rich sites	
Heparin-induced thrombocytopenia and thrombosis	4–14 days	Extremities	Thrombocytopenia occurs concurrently
Purple-toe syndrome	3–8 wk	Acral location	Often occurs after angiography

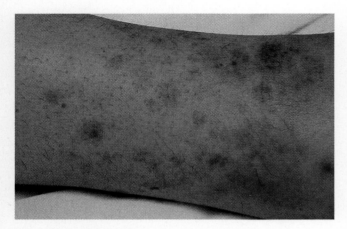

Figure 8 Leukocytoclastic vasculitis developed in this 47-year-old woman taking hydrochlorothiazide.

dence occurs in the sixth and seventh decades of life. Afflicted patients tend to be obese.

Coumarin-induced skin necrosis begins 3 to 5 days after initiation of treatment. Painful red plaques develop in adipose-rich sites such as breasts, buttocks, and hips. These plaques may blister, ulcerate, or develop into necrotic areas. An accompanying infection, such as pneumonia, viral infection, or erysipelas, may occur in as many as 25% of patients. Purple-toe syndrome occurs 3 to 8 weeks after initiation of coumarin therapy.

Treatment entails the discontinuance of coumarin, administration of vitamin K, and infusion of heparin at therapeutic doses. Fresh frozen plasma and purified protein C concentrates have been used.[77] Supportive measures for the skin are recommended. Plastic surgery for remediation is necessary in 60% of affected patients.

A complication of heparin therapy is heparin-induced thrombocytopenia and thrombosis.[78] Heparin-induced thrombocytopenia type 1 is a mild, transient drop in the platelet count during the first 4 days of heparin therapy and relates to the platelet proaggregant effect of heparin. Heparin-induced thrombocytopenia type 2 is a severe thrombocytopenia that occurs 4 to 14 days after initiation of heparin, sooner when there has been prior exposure. The major complication of heparin-induced thrombocytopenia type 2 is thrombosis, either arterial or venous. Events include deep vein thrombosis, pulmonary embolus, myocardial infarction, cerebral thrombosis, and extremity infarction requiring amputation in 20% of patients. Treatment requires heparin discontinuance and alternative forms of anticoagulant therapy, such as danaparoid or ancrod.

DRUG-INDUCED LICHENOID ERUPTIONS

Drug-induced lichen planus produces lesions that are clinically and histologically indistinguishable from those of idiopathic lichen planus. Many drugs, including beta blockers, penicillamine, NSAIDs, gold, and ACE inhibitors, especially captopril, have been reported to produce this reaction.

The latent period between the start of administration of the drug and appearance of the eruption is variable. The mean latent period is between 2 months and 3 years for penicillamine, approximately 1 year for beta-adrenergic blocking agents, and 3 to 6 months for ACE inhibitors. The latent period may be shorter if the patient was previously exposed to the drug.[79,80] In general, resolution usually occurs within 2 to 4 months.

Rechallenge with the culprit drug has been attempted in a few patients, with reactivation of symptoms within 4 to 15 days.[80] Patch testing has not proved helpful in most cases of drug-induced lichen planus. However, results of patch tests performed with contact inducers of lichen drug eruptions (e.g., color-film developers and dental restorative materials) are usually positive.[79]

DRUG-INDUCED VASCULITIS

Drug-induced vasculitis represents approximately 10% of the acute cutaneous vasculitides and usually affects small vessels [*see Figure 8*].[81] Drug-induced vasculitis should be considered in any patient with small vessel vasculitis that is usually confined to the skin.[82] Drugs that are associated with vasculitis include allopurinol, penicillin and aminopenicillins, sulfonamides, thiazides, hydantoins, propylthiouracil, retinoids, quinolones, and interferons.[83] The average interval to onset of drug-induced vasculitis is 7 to 21 days.[84]

The clinical hallmark of cutaneous vasculitis is palpable purpura, classically found on the lower extremities, although any cutaneous site may be affected. Urticaria can be a manifestation of small vessel vasculitis. Unlike nonvasculitic allergic urticaria, vasculitic urticaria lasts longer than 1 day, may evolve into purpuric lesions, and may be accompanied by hypocomplementemia.[85] Other features are hemorrhagic bullae, urticaria, ulcers, nodules, Raynaud disease, and digital necrosis.[16] The same vasculitic process may also affect internal organs, such as the liver, kidney, gut, and CNS, and is potentially life threatening.

Histologically, the small blood vessels of the dermis display fibrinoid necrosis, polymorphonuclear infiltration into the blood vessel wall, extravasation of red blood cells, and nuclear dust. Direct immunofluorescence may show deposits of IgM and C3 in the blood vessel walls. Therefore, these reactions are immune complex-dependent drug reactions. The immune complexes may be composed of antibodies directed against drug-related haptens, but this has not been proved.

Drug-induced vasculitis can be difficult to diagnose, and diagnosis is often one of exclusion.[86] Alternative causes of cutaneous vasculitis, such as infection or autoimmune disease, must be eliminated.

Treatment consists of drug withdrawal. Systemic steroids may be beneficial.

Conclusion

Drug reactions are a challenging management problem that often requires specialized expertise and a multidisciplinary approach. We must be able to recognize new drug-induced diseases, such as acute generalized exanthematous pustulosis, and better define syndromes, such as severe cutaneous adverse drug reactions, drug hypersensitivity syndrome, serum sickness–like reaction, and drug-induced lupus. It is now believed that the last four are caused by the formation of reactive oxidative metabolites and perhaps the formation of antibodies to drug-protein complexes and skin proteins, cytochrome P-450 enzymes, or both. The role of cross-reaction with viral antigens is still unclear. The predisposition to drug-induced eruptions may be genetic, and family counseling is part of the care plan. In vitro testing is being used in certain centers to manage patients and their families. The treatment of severe reactions, systemic and cutaneous, is still under investigation and the subject of debate. Options range from the obligatory cessation of the offending drug to the use of immunosuppressive drugs or plasmapheresis.

References

1. Karch F, Lasagna L: Adverse drug reactions: a critical review. JAMA 234:1236, 1975

2. Lazarou J, Pomeranz B, Corey P: Incidence of adverse drug reactions in hospitalized patients: a meta-analysis of prospective studies. JAMA 279:1200, 1998

3. Lakshmanan M, Hershey C, Breslau D: Hospital admissions caused by iatrogenic disease. Arch Intern Med 146:1391, 1986

4. Bigby M, Jick S, Jick H, et al: Drug-induced cutaneous reactions: a report from the Boston Collaborative Drug Surveillance Program on 15,438 consecutive inpatients, 1975 to 1982. JAMA 256:3358, 1986

5. Classen D, Pestotnik S, Evans R, et al: Adverse drug events in hospitalized patients: excess length of stay, extra costs and attributable mortality. JAMA 277:301, 1997

6. Shear N: Diagnosing cutaneous adverse reactions to drugs. Arch Dermatol 126:94, 1990

7. Sogn D, Evans R, Shepherd G: Results of the National Institute of Allergy and Infectious Diseases Collaborative Clinical Trial to test the predictive value of skin testing with major and minor penicillin derivatives in hospitalized adults. Arch Intern Med 152:1025, 1992

8. Alanko K, Stubb S, Reitamo S: Topical provocation of fixed drug eruption. Br J Dermatol 116:561, 1987

9. Smith HR, Croft AM, Black MM: Dermatological adverse effects with the antimalarial drug mefloquine: a review of 74 published case reports. Clin Exp Dermatol 24:249, 1999

10. Vega J, Blanca M, Carmona M, et al: Delayed allergic reactions to beta-lactams. Allergy 46:154, 1991

11. Romano A, Quaratino D, Papa G, et al: Aminopenicillin allergy. Arch Dis Child 76:513, 1997

12. Coopman S, Johnson R, Platt R, et al: Cutaneous disease and drug reactions in HIV infection. N Engl J Med 328:1670, 1993

13. Kerns D, Shira J, Go S: Ampicillin rash in children. Am J Dis Child 125:187, 1973

14. Prussick R, Knowles S, Shear N: Cutaneous drug reactions. Curr Probl Dermatol 6:81, 1994

15. Vittorio C, Muglia J: Anticonvulsant hypersensitivity syndrome. Arch Intern Med 155:2285, 1995

16. Roujeau JC, Stern R: Severe adverse cutaneous reactions to drugs. N Engl J Med 331:1272, 1994

17. Knowles S, Shapiro L, Shear N: Serious adverse reactions induced by minocycline: a report of 13 patients and review of the literature. Arch Dermatol 132:934, 1996

18. Shear N, Spielberg S: Anticonvulsant hypersensitivity syndrome: in vitro assessment of risk. J Clin Invest 82:1826, 1988

19. Chaffin J, Davis S: Suspected lamotrigine-induced toxic epidermal necrolysis. Ann Pharmacother 31:720, 1997

20. Wadelius M, Karlsson T, Wadelius C, et al: Lamotrigine and toxic epidermal necrolysis. Lancet 348:1041, 1996

21. Shear N, Spielberg S, Grant D, et al: Differences in metabolism of sulfonamides predisposing to idiosyncratic toxicity. Ann Intern Med 105:179, 1986

22. Gupta A, Eggo M, Uetrecht J, et al: Drug-induced hypothyroidism: the thyroid as a target organ in hypersensitivity reactions to anticonvulsants and sulfonamides. Clin Pharmacol Ther 51:56, 1992

23. Rieder M: In vivo and in vitro testing for adverse drug reactions. Pediatr Clin North Am 44:93, 1997

24. Anderson J: Allergic reactions to drugs and biologic agents. JAMA 268:2845, 1992

25. Manning M, Stevenson D, Mathison D: Reactions to aspirin and other nonsteroidal anti-inflammatory drugs. Immunol Allergy Clin North Am 12:611, 1992

26. Fisher M, Harle D, Baldo B: Anaphylactoid reactions to narcotic analgesics. Clin Rev Allergy 9:309, 1991

27. Pracy J, McGlashan J, Walsh R, et al: Angioedema secondary to angiotensin-converting enzyme inhibitors. J Laryngol Otol 108:696, 1994

28. Porri F, Pradal M, Lemiere C, et al: Association between latex sensitization and repeated latex exposure in children. Anesthesiology 86:599, 1997

29. Taylor J, Praditsuwan P: Latex allergy: review of 44 cases including outcome and frequent association with allergic hand eczema. Arch Dermatol 132:265, 1996

30. Sullivan T, Magera B: Recurrent allergic reactions to latex in a hospitalized pediatric patient. J Allergy Clin Immunol 96:423, 1995

31. Dyer P: Late-onset angioedema after interruption of angiotensin converting enzyme inhibitor therapy. J Allergy Clin Immunol 93:947, 1994

32. Sussman G, Beezhold D: Allergy to latex rubber. Ann Intern Med 122:43, 1995

33. deShazo R, Mather P, Grant W, et al: Evaluation of patients with local reactions to insulin with skin tests and in vitro techniques. Diabetes Care 10:330, 1987

34. Dykewicz M, Kim H, Orfan N, et al: Immunologic analysis of anaphylaxis to protamine component in neutral protamine Hagedorn human insulin. J Allergy Clin Immunol 93:117, 1994

35. Hoffman HM, Wright FA, Broide DH, et al: Identification of a locus on chromosome 1q44 for familial cold urticaria. Am J Hum Genet 66:1693, 2000

36. Haas N, Toppe E, Henz BE: Microscopic morphology of different types of urticaria. Arch Dermatol 134:41, 1998

37. Berkun Y, Shalit M: Successful treatment of delayed pressure urticaria with motelukast. Allergy 55:203, 2000

38. Ilter N, Gurer MA, Akkoca MA: Short-term oral cyclosporine for chronic idiopathic urticaria. J Eur Acad Dermatol Venereol 12:67, 1999

39. Heckbert S, Stryker W, Coltin K, et al: Serum sickness in children after antibiotic exposure: estimates of occurrence and morbidity in a health maintenance organization population. Am J Epidemiol 132:336, 1990

40. Joubert GI, Hada K, Matsui D, et al: Selection of treatment of cefaclor-associated urticarial, serum sickness-like reactions and erythema multiforme by emergency pediatricians: lack of a uniform standard of care. Can J Clin Pharmacol 6:197, 1999

41. Kearns G, Wheeler J, Childress S, et al: Serum sickness-like reactions to cefaclor: role of hepatic metabolism and individual susceptibility. J Pediatr 125:805, 1994

42. Lowery N, Kearns G, Young R, et al: Serum sickness-like reactions associated with cefprozil therapy. J Pediatr 125:325, 1994

43. McCollom RA, Elbe DH, Ritchie AH: Bupropion-induced serum sickness–like reaction. Ann Pharmacother 34:471, 2000

44. Shapiro L, Knowles S, Shear N: Comparative safety and risk management of tetracycline, doxycline and minocycline. Arch Dermatol 133:1224, 1997

45. Vial T, Pont J, Pham E, et al: Cefaclor-associated serum sickness-like disease: eight cases and review of the literature. Ann Pharmacother 26:910, 1992

46. Grammer L: Cefaclor serum sickness. JAMA 275:1152, 1996

47. Commens C: Fixed drug eruption. Aust J Dermatol 24:1, 1983

48. Sehgal V, Gangwani O: Fixed drug eruption: current concepts. Int J Dermatol 26:67, 1987

49. Barbaud A, Reichert-Penetrat S, Trechot P, et al: The use of skin testing in the investigation of cutaneous adverse drug reactions. Br J Dermatol 139:49, 1998

50. Lang B, Finlayson L: Naproxen-induced pseudoporphyria in patients with juvenile rheumatoid arthritis. J Pediatr 124:639, 1994

51. Kuechle M, Stegemeir E, Maynard B, et al: Drug-induced linear IgA bullous dermatosis: report of six cases and review of the literature. J Am Acad Dermatol 30:187, 1994

52. Baden L, Apovian C, Imber M, et al: Vancomycin-induced linear IgA bullous dermatosis. Arch Dermatol 124:1186, 1988

53. Primka E, Liranzo E, Bergfeld W, et al: Amiodarone-induced linear IgA disease. J Am Acad Dermatol 31:809, 1994

54. Mutasim D, Pelc N, Anhalt G: Drug-induced pemphigus. Dermatol Clin 11:463, 1993

55. Brenner S, Bialy-Gohan A, Ruocco V: Drug-induced pemphigus. Clin Dermatol 16:393, 1998

56. Bialy-Golan A, Brenner S: Penicillamine-induced bullous dermatoses. J Am Acad Dermatol 35:732, 1996

57. Worf R, Brenner S: An active amide group in the molecule of drugs that induce pemphigus: a casual or causal relationship? Dermatology 189:1, 1994

58. Anhalt G: Drug-induced pemphigus. Semin Dermatol 8:166, 1989

59. Ruocco V, Sacerdoti G: Pemphigus and bullous pemphigoid due to drugs. Int J Dermatol 30:307, 1991

60. Roujeau J, Kelly J, Naldi L, et al: Medication use and the risk of Stevens-Johnson syndrome or toxic epidermal necrolysis. N Engl J Med 333:1600, 1995

61. Rzany B, Correia O, Kelly JP, et al: Risk of Stevens-Johnson syndrome and toxic epidermal necrolysis during first weeks of antiepileptic therapy: a case-control study. Study Group of the International Case Control Study on Severe Cutaneous Adverse Reactions. Lancet 353:2190, 1999

62. Wolkenstein P, Charue D, Bagot M, et al: Metabolic predisposition to cutaneous adverse drug reactions. Arch Dermatol 131:544, 1995

63. Bastuji-Garin S, Rzany B, Stern R, et al: Clinical classification of cases of toxic epidermal necrolysis, Stevens-Johnson syndrome, and erythema multiforme. Arch Dermatol 129:92, 1993

64. Mitchell P: Paediatric lamotrigine use hit by rash reports. Lancet 349:1080, 1997

65. Barone C, Bianchi M, Lee B, et al: Treatment of toxic epidermal necrolysis and Stevens-Johnson syndrome in children. J Oral Maxillofac Surg 51:264, 1993

66. Fine J: Management of acquired bullous skin diseases. N Engl J Med 333:1475, 1995

67. Garcia-Doval I, LeCleach L, Bocquet H, et al: Toxic epidermal necrolysis and Stevens-Johnson syndrome: does early withdrawal of causative drugs decrease the risk of death? Arch Dermatol 136:323, 2000

68. Patterson R, Miller M, Kaplan M, et al: Effectiveness of early therapy with corticosteroids in Stevens-Johnson syndrome: experience with 41 cases and a hypothesis regarding pathogenesis. Ann Allergy 73:27, 1994

69. Prendville J, Hebert A, Greenwald M, et al: Management of Stevens-Johnson syndrome and toxic epidermal necrolysis in children. J Pediatr 115:881, 1989

70. Chaidemenos G, Chrysomallis FK, Mourellou O: Plasmapheresis in toxic epidermal necrolysis. Int J Dermatol 36:218, 1997

71. Remmer H, Falk W: Successful treatment of lithium-induced acne. J Clin Psychiatry 47:48, 1986

72. Traupe H, von Muhlendahl K, Bramswig J, et al: Acne of the fulminans type following testosterone therapy in three excessively tall boys. Arch Dermatol 124:414, 1988

73. Heng C: Cutaneous manifestation of lithium toxicity. Br J Dermatol 106:107, 1982

74. Beylot C, Doutre M, Beylot-Barry M: Acute generalized exanthematous pustulosis. Semin Cutaneous Med Surg 15:244, 1996

75. Roujeau J, Bioulac-Sage P, Bourseau C, et al: Acute generalized exanthematous pustulosis: analysis of 63 cases. Arch Dermatol 127:1333, 1991

76. Bauer K: Coumarin-induced skin necrosis. Arch Dermatol 129:766, 1993

77. Schramm W, Spannagel M, Bauer K, et al: Treatment of coumarin-induced skin necrosis with a monoclonal antibody purified protein C concentrate. Arch Dermatol 19:753, 1993

78. Chong B: Heparin-induced thrombocytopenia. Br J Haematol 89:431, 1995

79. Halevy S, Shai A: Lichenoid drug eruptions. J Am Acad Dermatol 29:249, 1993

80. Thompson D, Skaehill P: Drug-induced lichen planus. Pharmacotherapy 14:561, 1994

81. Sanchez N, Van Hale H, Su W: Clinical and histopathologic spectrum of necrotizing vasculitis: reports of findings in 101 cases. Arch Dermatol 121:220, 1985

82. Jennette J, Falk K: Small-vessel vasculitis. N Engl J Med 337:1512, 1997

83. Zurcher K, Krebs A: Cutaneous Drug Reactions, 2nd ed. Karger, Basel, 1992, p 349

84. Dubost J, Souteyrand P, Sauvezie B: Drug-induced vasculitides. Baillieres Clin Rheumatol 5:119, 1991

85. Mehregan D, Hall M, Gibson E: Urticarial vasculitis: a histopathologic and clinical review of 72 cases. J Am Acad Dermatol 26:441, 1992

86. Wolkenstein P, Revuz J: Drug-induced severe skin reactions: incidence, management and prevention. Drug Safety 13:56, 1995.

37 Fungal, Bacterial, and Viral Infections of the Skin

Jan V. Hirschmann, M.D.

Despite its large surface area and its constant exposure to the environment, the skin is relatively resistant to infection. The most important protective factor is an intact stratum corneum, the tough barrier of protein and lipid formed on the cutaneous surface by the underlying epidermis.[1] This barricade impedes invasion by environmental pathogens, and its dryness discourages colonization and growth of the many organisms that require moisture to survive, such as gram-negative bacilli. Furthermore, the constant shedding of cells of the epidermis impedes most microbes from establishing permanent residence.

Some organisms, however, can attach to skin cells and reproduce there; the normal cutaneous flora comprises primarily aerobic, gram-positive cocci and bacilli in densities ranging from about 10^2 organisms/cm^2 on dry skin to 10^7 organisms/cm^2 in moist areas, such as the axilla.[2] This resident population inhibits harmful organisms from colonizing the skin by occupying binding sites on the epidermal cells, by competing for nutrients, by producing antimicrobial substances, and by maintaining the skin surface at a low pH (about 5.5). Anaerobes are sparse except in areas that have abundant sebaceous glands, such as the face and chest; in the deeper portions of such areas, as well as in hair follicles, anaerobes occur in concentrations of 10^4 to 10^6 organisms/cm^2.

Cutaneous infections occur when the skin's protective mechanisms fail, especially when trauma, inflammation, maceration from excessive moisture, or other factors disrupt the stratum corneum. The organisms causing infection may originate from the victim's own resident flora, either on the skin or on adjacent mucous membranes, but many come from other people, animals, or the environment.

Dermatophyte Infections

Dermatophytes are fungi (molds) that can infect the skin, hair, and nails. These fungi, which include *Trichophyton, Microsporum,* and *Epidermophyton* species, are classified as anthropophilic, zoophilic, or geophilic, depending on whether their primary source is humans, animals, or the soil, respectively.[3] Geophilic dermatophyte infections occur sporadically, primarily among gardeners and farm workers. Zoophilic dermatophytes (*Trichophyton* and *Microsporum* species) may have a restricted range of hosts (e.g., *M. persicolor* infects only voles), or they may afflict many different animals (e.g., *T. mentagrophytes* can infect mice and other rodents, dogs, cats, and horses). Human infections with zoophilic species have occurred after exposure to dogs, cats, horses, cattle, pigs, rodents, poultry, hedgehogs, and voles.

Anthropophilic dermatophytes are the most common cause of fungal skin infections in humans. Transmission of these infections may occur from direct contact between people or from exposure to desquamated skin cells present in the environment—the arthrospores of fungi can survive for months. Direct inoculation of the spores through breaks in the skin can lead to germination and subsequent invasion of the superficial cutaneous layers.

Dermatophyte infections occur more frequently in certain ethnic groups and in people with impaired cell-mediated immunity. Many of the anthropophilic dermatophyte infections are more likely to occur in persons of certain age groups and are more common in males or in females.[4] Infection of the scalp, for example, is primarily a disease of children. Involvement of the feet and groin is most common in adolescents and young adults, especially men, but is unusual in children. Nail infection is more frequent in both sexes with advancing age. The reasons for these differences are unknown.

The anthropophilic dermatophytes also have unique geographic distribution patterns. The most common cause of scalp infection in the United States, for example, is *T. tonsurans,* but in Southeast Asia and the Middle East, *T. violaceum* is the most common cause. These differences may relate to climatic or racial factors.

The various forms of dermatophytosis, also called ringworm, are named according to the site involved. These infections include tinea capitis (scalp), tinea corporis (body), tinea barbae (beard area of men), tinea faciei (face), tinea cruris (groin), tinea pedis (feet), tinea unguium (nails), and tinea manuum (hands). The characteristic skin lesion is an annular scaly patch [*see Figure 1*], though the clinical appearance varies not only with the site involved but also with the host's immune status and the identity of the infecting organism. In general, anthropophilic species elicit little inflammation and cause chronic infections. Zoophilic and geophilic species, however, often provoke intense inflammation, which sometimes leads to eradication of the organisms and healing without treatment.

CLINICAL PRESENTATIONS

Tinea Capitis

Tinea capitis occurs primarily in children but also may develop in adults, especially the elderly, those with poor personal hygiene, and the impoverished. Transmission may occur between humans by the sharing of combs, brushes, or headgear. Tinea capitis is caused only by *Microsporum* and *Trichophyton* species. Infection begins with invasion of the stratum corneum of the skin of the scalp. The hairs then become affected, with infection of the hairs occurring in one of three microscopic patterns: endothrix, ectothrix, or favus. In ectothrix, the spores are outside the hair shaft and destroy the cuticle; in endothrix, they are in-

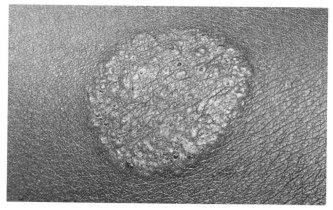

Figure 1 **Classic annular lesion of tinea corporis shows a raised or vesicular margin with central clearing.**

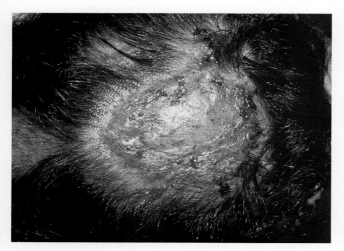

Figure 2 **A typical kerion presenting as a zoophilic *Microsporum canis* infection of the scalp (tinea capitis).**

side the hair and do not affect the cuticle; and in favus, broad hyphae and air spaces form within the hair, but spores are absent. In all three types of infection, scaling, hair loss, and inflammation of varying degrees are present.

T. tonsurans, the major cause of tinea capitis in adults, characteristically produces a noninflammatory infection with either well-demarcated or irregular and diffuse areas of scaling and alopecia. Because the swollen hairs may fracture a few millimeters from the epidermis in this endothrix infection, the scalp sometimes appears to be marked by small black dots. Like all infections with *Trichophyton* species, these scalp lesions do not fluoresce under a Wood's light.

T. schoenleinii causes favus, characterized by an inflammatory crust (scutulum) in which hair appears to be matted in the dried, yellow exudate. Hair shedding late in the infection is common because the hair shaft is not damaged until the infection is well advanced.

M. audouinii, which causes an ectothrix infection, produces well-delineated, noninflammatory patches of alopecia in which the hair breaks at the epidermal surface and is often dull gray because of the presence of numerous spores on the surface of the hair shaft. As in all *Microsporum* infections, these lesions fluoresce under a Wood's light. The most severe inflammation, usually from a zoophilic species, results in a kerion, which is a painful, boggy mass in which follicles may discharge pus and in which sinus tracts form [*see Figure 2*]. Crusting and matting of adjacent hairs are common, and cervical lymph nodes may enlarge.

Tinea Corporis

Tinea corporis typically appears as a single lesion or multiple circular lesions with scaling, well-delineated margins, and a raised, erythematous edge. Often, lesions are characterized by an area of central clearing. The amount of inflammation is variable; when it is intense, pustules, vesicles, and even bullae may occur. Sometimes, involvement of the hair follicles in the middle of a patch of scaling erythema leads to perifollicular nodules, a condition called Majocchi's granuloma. This condition usually occurs on the legs of patients infected with *T. rubrum*. In immunocompromised hosts, subcutaneous abscesses may develop.

Tinea Barbae

Tinea barbae occurs in adult men and involves the skin and coarse hairs of the beard and mustache area. The usual cause is a zoophilic species, primarily *T. verrucosum* and *T. mentagrophytes,*

a

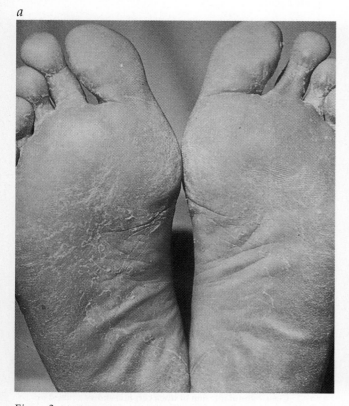

b

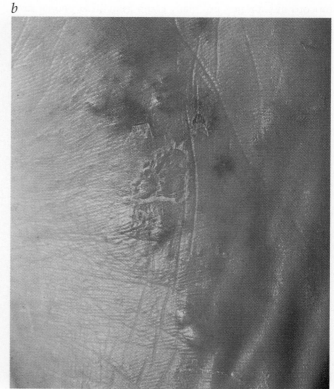

Figure 3 (*a*) **The scaling of tinea pedis appears between and under the toes and on the plantar surface.** (*b*) **Tinea pedis may also present as vesicles.**

which are organisms that commonly infect cattle and horses. The victims are generally farm workers, and the infection usually causes erythema, scaling, and follicular pustules. Many hairs become loose and are easily removed with a forceps.

Tinea Faciei

Tinea faciei occurs as an infection of the face in women and children and infection of the area outside the mustache and beard in men. The usual causes are *T. rubrum* and *T. mentagrophytes*; these organisms may reach the face through direct inoculation or by spreading from another site of infection on the body. Patients often complain of itching and burning, and symptoms may worsen after exposure to sunlight. The lesions may be scaly, annular erythematous patches, but often they are indistinct red areas with little or no scaling.

Tinea Cruris

Tinea cruris, infection of the groin, is much more common in men than in women and is often associated with infection of the feet. *T. rubrum* and *E. floccosum* are the most common causes. The lesions are usually red, scaling, sharply demarcated areas with raised, erythematous borders. The infection, which affects the medial portion of the upper thighs but consistently spares the scrotum, may extend to the buttocks, abdomen, and lower back. Vesicles, nodules, pustules, and maceration may be present.

Tinea Pedis

Tinea pedis is most commonly caused by *T. rubrum, E. floccosum,* and *T. mentagrophytes.* The most common form of this disorder is characterized by fissuring, scaling, and maceration in the interdigital spaces of the toes, especially between the fourth and fifth toes. A second form is characterized by scaling, hyperkeratosis, and erythema of the soles, heels, and sides of the feet. In this form of tinea pedis, the lesions occur in a so-called moccasin distribution pattern [*see Figure 3a*]. The plantar skin may become very thick and scaly. A third type of tinea pedis demonstrates an inflammatory pattern characterized by vesicles, pustules, or even bullae, usually on the soles [*see Figure 3b*].

An important complication of tinea pedis is streptococcal cellulitis of the lower leg. Streptococci do not ordinarily survive on normal skin, but the presence of fungal disease apparently permits streptococci of various groups, including A, B, C, and G, to colonize the toe webs.[5] From this location, these bacteria may invade the skin damaged by the tinea pedis, or they may migrate to locations higher up the leg and enter the skin through any defects.

Tinea Unguium

Involvement of the nails usually occurs from adjacent fungal infection of the hands or feet. The organisms typically invade the nail from the distal or lateral borders, and infection spreads proximally. The nails are thickened, opaque, and yellowish to brownish. They may crack or crumble, and often, subungual hyperkeratosis lifts the nail plate from the underlying bed (a condition known as onycholysis) [*see Figure 4*]. Splinter hemorrhages are common.

Tinea Manuum

Tinea manuum is infection of the hands. Most cases of tinea manuum have accompanying involvement of the feet; inexplicably, often only one hand is affected (so-called two-feet, one-hand disease). The most common finding is scaling or hyperkeratosis

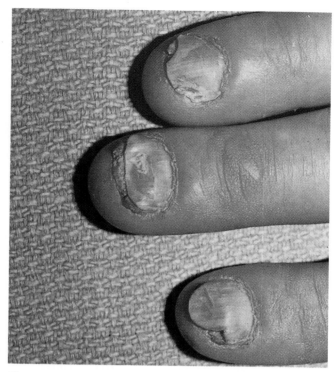

Figure 4 **Nails are usually thickened, cracked, and crumbly in tinea unguium; subungual debris may be present, as shown.**

of the palms and fingers. Occasionally, vesicles, papules, or follicular nodules are present on the dorsal surface of the hands.

DIAGNOSIS

Clinicians should suspect dermatophyte infection in patients with any scaling, erythematous eruption and in patients whose nails exhibit the characteristics of tinea unguium (see above). Patients with skin lesions that are suspected of having been caused by dermatophytes should be asked about contact with animals. The diagnosis can be confirmed by microscopy or culture of properly obtained specimens.

Microscopy is performed by placing the specimen on a glass slide and treating it with potassium hydroxide (KOH), which digests the keratin of the skin, nails, and hair. The basic culture medium for isolating dermatophytes is an agar containing Sabouraud's medium, often combined with antibiotics to eliminate bacteria and with cycloheximide to inhibit saprophytic fungi. Growth is usually apparent in 3 to 14 days. When both KOH preparations and cultures are negative, a biopsy may be useful in identifying the infecting organism, usually by special tissue stains such as periodic acid–Schiff or Gomori's methenamine-silver stains.

TREATMENT

Most cutaneous dermatophyte infections respond to topical agents applied once or twice daily to the affected area, usually for 2 to 4 weeks. The cost of the preparation can dictate which agent to prescribe. Tinea pedis often recurs after effective therapy, especially in cases of the moccasin form of the disease. When infection reappears, the previous therapy can be resumed without loss of effectiveness.

Oral therapy is necessary for extensive lesions, for infection involving the hair or hair follicles, for tinea unguium, and, often, for tinea manuum and various forms of dermatophytoses in immunocompromised hosts. Five oral agents are currently available: griseofulvin, ketoconazole, itraconazole, fluconazole, and terbinafine. Griseofulvin, a fungistatic agent, is the oldest oral treatment available and is still useful, primarily in infections not involving the nails. Griseofulvin reduces the serum levels of barbiturates and warfarin, and some patients receiving griseofulvin note a diminished tolerance to alcohol.

The azoles include ketoconazole, itraconazole, and fluconazole, and like griseofulvin, they are fungistatic. Ketoconazole is usually well tolerated, but hepatotoxicity occurs in about 1 in 10,000 patients, typically after several weeks of use. Fluconazole and itraconazole are very expensive, but they provide protracted levels of antibiotic in the nails, allowing short or intermittent courses of therapy for tinea unguium. Both fluconazole and itraconazole can cause gastrointestinal disorders, rashes, and, occasionally, hepatotoxicity and have serious interactions with several medications, including cyclosporine, digoxin, quinidine, and cisapride. Clinicians using ketoconazole, itraconazole, or fluconazole in patients receiving other medications should consult pharmacologic sources for potential interactions.

Terbinafine, also an expensive medication, is an allylamine. Unlike both griseofulvin and the azoles, which are fungistatic, terbinafine is fungicidal. It achieves high levels of drug in the nails, and the drug persists for many weeks after discontinuance. Its few side effects include gastrointestinal reactions and, occasionally, skin rashes. Hepatotoxicity and hematologic abnormalities are rare, and drug interactions are uncommon.

These oral antifungals, usually given for 4 weeks for tinea capitis, are quite successful. The adult dosage for griseofulvin is 500 mg twice daily; for itraconazole, 200 mg daily; for fluconazole, 200 mg daily; and for terbinafine, 250 mg daily. Of these, griseofulvin is the least expensive, but some *T. tonsurans* isolates are resistant to this agent. All of these medications are effective in tinea barbae, Majocchi's granuloma, extensive tinea corporis, and tinea manuum that is unresponsive to topical agents.

Tinea unguium is difficult to eradicate, particularly in the toenails. Griseofulvin requires protracted use and is attended by high failure or relapse rates. Itraconazole, fluconazole, and terbinafine are all more effective. Itraconazole is most commonly prescribed as a pulse regimen, 200 mg twice daily, 7 days per month for up to 6 months. Fluconazole may be effective even when administered once a week. Terbinafine is administered at a dosage of 250 mg daily for 6 weeks for fingernail infections and for 12 weeks for toenail involvement.[6] An alternative dosage is 250 mg twice a day for 1 week a month for 3 consecutive months. Because terbinafine persists in the nails for several weeks, it continues to exert antifungal effects long after it is discontinued. The terbinafine regimens produce short-term eradication of infection in about 70% to 90% of patients with fingernail infection and in about 50% to 80% of patients with toenail infection. The frequency of relapse is unclear. This therapy is very expensive, and clinicians must decide in each case whether treatment is warranted.

Yeast Infections

Yeasts are unicellular fungi that reproduce by budding. They may form filamentous projections, which, unlike the hyphae of molds, do not contain separate cells. Accordingly, they are called pseudohyphae. *Candida* species are not part of the normal skin flora, but they commonly reside in the oropharynx, vagina, and colon. From these locations, they may cause infections in adjacent traumatized skin. Alternatively, with reduction in the other

flora or with impaired host defense mechanisms, these yeasts may proliferate in large numbers to produce lesions on the mucosal surfaces of the mouth and vagina.

Malassezia furfur (also called *Pityrosporum orbiculare* or *P. ovale*) is a yeast that requires lipids for growth. It normally colonizes the skin of adults, especially of the scalp and upper trunk, where the presence of sebum is highest. For unknown reasons, these organisms, which are ordinarily commensals, can become pathogenic and cause tinea versicolor (also known as pityriasis versicolor) or folliculitis. Cogent evidence suggests these organisms cause seborrheic dermatitis and dandruff.

CANDIDIASIS

Clinical Presentations

Oral candidiasis One form of oral candidiasis, thrush, appears as white to gray patches (pseudomembranes) on the tongue, soft palate, gingiva, oropharynx, and buccal mucosa. Removing the material from the mucosal surface reveals an underlying erythematous base. Predisposing factors in adults include diabetes mellitus, use of systemic or local corticosteroids, use of broad-spectrum antibiotics, use of radiotherapy or chemotherapy, and impaired cell-mediated immunity, especially from HIV infection. Acute atrophic candidiasis especially follows antibiotic therapy and causes painful, red, denuded lesions of the mucous membranes; the tongue may have erythematous areas with atrophic filiform papillae. In chronic atrophic candidiasis, contamination of dentures with *Candida* causes painful, red, and sometimes edematous lesions with a shiny, atrophic epithelium and well-demarcated borders where the dentures contact the mucous membranes. Poor dental hygiene and prolonged use of dentures are common predisposing factors. Some patients

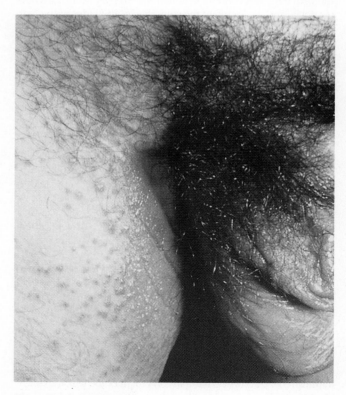

Figure 5 **Prominent satellite lesions of discrete vesicles are seen in a patient with candidiasis.**

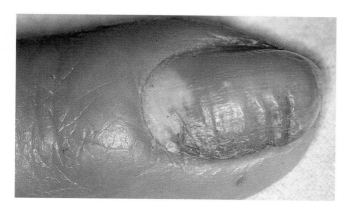

Figure 6 In a *Candida* paronychia, seen on this patient's thumb, the nail fold becomes red, swollen, and painful. Nail dystrophy is also seen.

with these predisposing factors have angular cheilitis (perleche), characterized by erythema and fissuring of the corners of the mouth. Other contributing conditions are maceration from excessive salivation or licking, poorly fitting dentures, and a larger fold from diminished alveolar ridge height. *Candida* is present in most, but not all, patients with this disorder.

Chronic hyperplastic candidiasis (candidal leukoplakia) consists of irregular, white, persistent plaques on the tongue or mucous membranes that are difficult to remove; this form of candidiasis occurs especially in male smokers. Soreness, burning, and roughness of the affected areas are the usual symptoms. Candidiasis of the tongue can also take the form of median rhomboid glossitis, a diamond-shaped area of atrophic papillae in the central portion of the lingual surface.

Candidal intertrigo *Candida* infection may occur in any skin fold, causing soreness and itching. Obese patients are especially vulnerable. Commonly affected areas include the groin, inframammary regions, and folds of the abdominal pannus. The lesions are patches of bright erythema accompanied by maceration and an irregular, scalloped border, beyond which papules and pustules (satellite lesions) commonly form [*see Figure 5*].

Candidal vulvovaginitis and balanitis Most women with candidal vulvovaginitis have no underlying disease, but candidal vulvovaginitis may accompany diabetes mellitus and HIV infection. Candidal vulvovaginitis causes white plaques on a swollen, red vaginal mucosa; a creamy vaginal discharge; and erythema, sometimes with pustules, on the vulvar skin. Soreness and burning are common symptoms. Male sexual partners of women with candidal vulvovaginitis—especially male sexual partners who are uncircumcised—may develop balanitis, characterized by erythema, pustules, and erosions on the glans of the penis. Balanitis may occur spontaneously as well.

Candidal paronychia and nail infection Maceration of the tissue surrounding the nail, typically caused by excessive moisture, may predispose to colonization by *Candida*, resulting in paronychia. Folds of the nail become reddened, swollen, and painful [*see Figure 6*]. Pus may be present. With chronic infection, nail involvement may occur, causing yellowish discoloration and separation of the nail plate from the nail bed (onycholysis).

Diagnosis

Scrapings from cutaneous or mucous membrane lesions may

be mixed with KOH solution and examined under the microscope for budding yeasts with pseudohyphae. Gram's stains of the same specimen are easier to evaluate because they disclose very large, oval, gram-positive cocci that may demonstrate budding or pseudohyphal formation. These organisms are much larger than bacteria and are much easier to see on Gram's stain than on KOH preparation. Culture of specimens may be useful if the microscopy is normal or ambiguous. These organisms grow rapidly on both fungal and conventional bacterial media.

Treatment

For oral candidiasis, topical nystatin suspension, 200,000 to 400,000 units three to five times a day, is usually effective; an alternative treatment is clotrimazole troches. For patients in whom topical treatment is ineffective or poorly tolerated, systemic therapies include ketoconazole, 200 mg/day; fluconazole, 100 mg/day; and itraconazole, 100 mg twice a day. Angular cheilitis usually responds to an azole cream, such as miconazole or clotrimazole. Dentures should be cleaned carefully with an effective disinfectant, such as chlorhexidine.

Candidal intertrigo and balanitis respond to a topical azole cream, such as miconazole or clotrimazole. Treatment of vulvovaginitis includes a topical azole in the form of a cream, suppository, or ointment, administered intravaginally, typically once daily for 7 days. A cream may be used for vulvar involvement. An alternative to suppositories is treatment with a single oral dose (150 mg) of fluconazole, which is at least as effective as topical therapy and is often preferred by patients.

Patients with candidal paronychia should keep their fingers dry; when wet work is unavoidable, patients should use cotton liners under rubber gloves. Prolonged topical therapy with creams or solutions of various azole preparations, such as clotrimazole, is often necessary to eradicate the infection.

MALASSEZIA INFECTIONS

Clinical Presentations

Tinea versicolor (pityriasis versicolor) Because the term tinea traditionally refers to diseases caused by dermatophytes, some clinicians prefer the term pityriasis, which means scaling, for this yeast infection. Usually asymptomatic, tinea versicolor may cause itching or skin irritation. The lesions are small, discrete macules that tend to be darker than the surrounding skin in light-skinned patients and hypopigmented in patients with dark skin. They often coalesce to form large patches of various colors (versicolor) ranging from white to tan [*see Figure 7*]. When the lesions are scratched, a fine scale is apparent. This infection most commonly involves the upper trunk, but the arms, axillae, abdomen, and groin may also be affected. Most lesions fluoresce a yellowish color under a Wood's light.

Malassezia folliculitis (pityrosporum folliculitis) In folliculitis, inflammation of the hair follicle causes red papules and pustules that surround individual hairs. One cause of folliculitis, especially in young adults, is *M. furfur*. Lesions appear predominantly on the trunk but occasionally on the arms as well. The lack of comedones distinguishes the lesion from acne. Pruritus and stinging may be present.

Diagnosis

In patients with tinea versicolor, KOH preparations of scrapings from the lesions demonstrate pseudohyphae and yeasts,

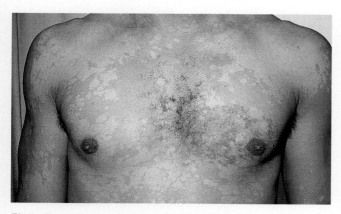

Figure 7 Tinea versicolor appears on the chest of this patient as oval, hypopigmented, finely scaling macules.

which resemble spaghetti and meatballs. This technique is sufficient to establish the diagnosis. The yeast form prevails in folliculitis and is easily seen on Gram's stain of purulent material from a pustule, appearing as a large, oval, gram-positive coccus that is much larger than bacteria. Biopsies of these lesions show organisms around and within the hair follicle, with accompanying neutrophilic inflammation. The yeasts are best seen with periodic acid–Schiff or Gomori's methenamine-silver stain. Because these yeasts are part of the normal cutaneous flora, growth of the organism on cultures from scrapings of the skin surface is not very helpful diagnostically. Culture of the yeast from the pus of folliculitis, however, is definitive, but it requires special media, such as Sabouraud's agar with olive oil, to provide the necessary lipids for growth. Growth typically occurs in 3 to 5 days.

Treatment

Simple treatment of tinea versicolor and *Malassezia* folliculitis involves applying selenium sulfide shampoo from the chin to the waist and from the shoulders to the wrist, allowing the shampoo to dry, and then washing it off after 10 to 15 minutes. Repeating this regimen after 1 week is usually effective, and reapplication once every few weeks as necessary should prevent relapses, which are otherwise common. With tinea versicolor, scaling resolves promptly, but the pigmentary changes may take weeks to months to disappear. Topical azoles, such as ketoconazole, mi-

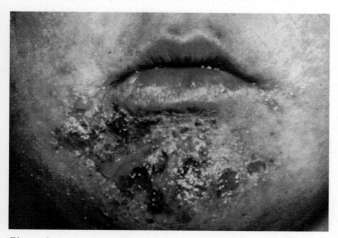

Figure 8 Vesicopustules or bullae of impetigo rupture quickly and leave an erythematous base covered with a thin, seropurulent exudate. The exudate dries, forming layers of honey-colored crusts.

conazole, and clotrimazole, are also effective, but the expense of these drugs makes their use impractical except for small or isolated lesions. For patients who have difficulty applying a topical agent because of physical disabilities or other factors, oral ketoconazole or fluconazole in a single 400 mg dose is an effective alternative. This oral program can be repeated for recurrences.

Bacterial Infections

SKIN INFECTIONS CAUSED BY STREPTOCOCCI, STAPHYLOCOCCI, OR BOTH

Impetigo

Initially a vesicular infection of the skin, impetigo rapidly evolves into pustules that rupture, with the dried discharge forming honey-colored crusts on an erythematous base [*see Figure 8*]. The lesions are often itchy. Impetigo characteristically occurs on skin damaged by previous trauma, such as abrasions or cuts. Exposed areas are most commonly involved, typically the extremities or the areas around the mouth and nose. Impetigo is most often a disease of young children and is more frequent in hot, humid climates than in temperate ones. The usual cause is *Staphylococcus aureus*, but sometimes, *Streptococcus pyogenes* (group A streptococci) is also present; occasionally, *S. pyogenes* is the sole organism cultured.[7] Some strains of *S. aureus* elaborate a toxin that causes a split in the epidermis and the development of thin-roofed bullae. In this disorder, known as bullous impetigo, superficial, fragile, and flaccid vesiculopustules form and then rupture, with the exudate drying into a thin, brown, varnishlike crust. Sometimes, the vesiculopustules are not apparent, and erythematous erosions are the only evident disturbance.

Growth of *S. aureus*, *S. pyogenes*, or both from the skin lesions confirms the diagnosis, but cultures are unnecessary in characteristic cases. For treatment of sparse, nonbullous lesions, topical mupirocin ointment applied three times daily for 7 days is as effective as oral antimicrobials. Systemic antibiotics active against both *S. aureus* and *S. pyogenes*, such as cephalexin or dicloxacillin, represent an alternative to topical treatment. For extensive lesions, these antibiotics are preferred to topical therapy, and they are the treatment of choice for bullous impetigo. Because of the superficial nature of these infections, the lesions heal without scarring.

Ecthyma

Ecthyma (from the Greek word *ekthyma*, meaning pustule) is a deeper infection than impetigo. As with impetigo, *S. aureus*, *S. pyogenes*, or both may be the cause. Ecthyma commonly occurs in patients with poor hygiene or malnutrition or patients who have had skin trauma. The lesions, which are most common on the lower extremities and are often multiple, begin as vesicles that rupture, creating circular, erythematous lesions with adherent crusts. Beneath the scabs, which may spontaneously slough, are ulcers that leave a scar when healing occurs. Culture of the ulcer base yields the causative organisms. Treatment should be with an oral antistaphylococcal agent, such as dicloxacillin or cephalexin.

SKIN INFECTIONS CAUSED BY STREPTOCOCCI

Cellulitis and Erysipelas

Cellulitis and erysipelas are acute, spreading infections of the skin caused by streptococci of groups A, B, C, and G. Erysipelas involves the superficial dermis, especially the dermal lymphatics, and cellulitis affects the deeper dermis and subcuta-

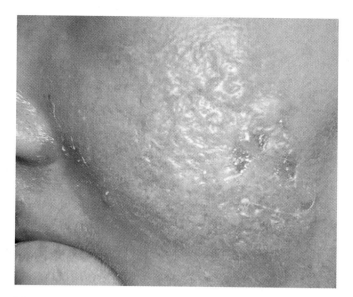

Figure 9 Erythema, edema, and sharp demarcation of the lesion from the normal surrounding skin characterize facial erysipelas.

neous fat. Erysipelas has an elevated, sharply demarcated border, but differences in the clinical appearances of erysipelas and cellulitis are unimportant and often unclear. The most common sites of infection are the face and lower extremities. The causative organisms may enter the skin at obvious areas of recent trauma or in regions of cutaneous inflammation, such as eczema; often, however, no point of entry is apparent. Edema from any cause, including venous insufficiency, hypoalbuminemia, and lymphatic damage, is a predisposing factor. Infection commonly occurs on skin that has been permanently damaged by burns, trauma, radiotherapy, or surgery. For example, cellulitis may occur at the site of a saphenous vein removal for cardiac or vascular surgery months to years after the procedure.[8] An important predisposing factor in patients with cellulitis or erysipelas is tinea pedis; streptococci can invade at sites of tinea pedis through adjacent skin surface disrupted by the fungal infection, or streptococci can migrate to more proximal locations on the leg and enter through abnormal skin there.

Cutaneous findings include rapidly expanding erythema and swelling of the cutaneous surface [*see Figure 9*], sometimes accompanied by proximal streaks of redness, representing lymphangitis, and tender, enlarged regional lymph nodes. Vesicles, bullae, petechiae, and ecchymoses may occur. The cutaneous surface may resemble the skin of an orange (peau d'orange) because the hair follicles remain tethered to the deeper structures, keeping their openings below the surrounding superficial edema and creating the characteristic dimpling of the skin. On the face, the typical location is on one or both cheeks, with involvement of the nasal bridge, producing a butterfly pattern of erythema and swelling. Extension to the eyelids, ears, or neck is common. Systemic symptoms, such as fever, headache, and confusion, can accompany these infections; sometimes, such symptoms precede by hours any cutaneous findings on examination. Some patients, however, have no systemic features despite severe cutaneous findings.

The diagnosis is largely clinical; in a typical case, cultures are unnecessary and usually unrewarding. Needle aspiration of the lesion yields an isolate in about 5% of specimens, as do blood cultures in febrile patients. Punch biopsies of the skin are culture positive in about 20% of cases.[9] These results, together with re-

sults of serum antibody tests for streptococci[10] and immunofluorescent studies of skin biopsies,[11] indicate that streptococci cause the vast majority of cases of cellulitis and erysipelas. *S. aureus* is often suspected but rarely implicated in cellulitis in the absence of an abscess or penetrating injury. Additional circumstances in which organisms other than streptococci are likely to be responsible for cases of cellulitis include immunodeficiency, penetrating trauma, immersion injuries in freshwater or saltwater, granulocytopenia, and animal bites or scratches. Cultures are appropriate in these situations.

Treatment consists of elevation of the affected area to help reduce edema and administration of systemic antibiotic therapy. For patients who do not have serious systemic illness, oral treatment is satisfactory. Penicillin is the drug of choice; for outpatients who may not take an oral medication as prescribed, I.M. benzathine penicillin G in an adult dose of 1.2 million units provides a complete course. Instead of penicillin, many clinicians prescribe an antistaphylococcal agent—either a first-generation cephalosporin or a penicillinase-resistant penicillin—because of concerns about *S. aureus*. Patients often get worse shortly after therapy, with further extension of the cellulitis, higher fever, greater toxicity, and increased white blood cell counts, presumably because rapid killing of the organisms releases potent enzymes, such as streptokinase and hyaluronidase, that cause many of the clinical features. Oral prednisolone, taken for 8 days in doses of 30 mg, 15 mg, 10 mg, and 5 mg each for 2 days, decreases the duration of cellulitis and shortens hospital stay; it is a reasonable regimen in those with no contraindications to systemic corticosteroids.[12]

In patients with leg cellulitis, treatment of tinea pedis is useful in preventing further episodes, which are likely to cause permanent lymphatic damage and can lead to lymphedema and further risk of infection. Other measures to diminish the frequency of future attacks include control of edema by diuretics or mechanical means, such as elastic stockings, and, for those with frequent episodes, prophylactic antibiotics. The easiest approach is the administration of oral penicillin or erythromycin, 250 mg twice daily.[13]

INFECTIONS DUE TO *STAPHYLOCOCCUS AUREUS*

Furunculosis

A furuncle is a deep-seated inflammatory nodule with a pustular center that develops around a hair follicle [*see Figure 10*]. With involvement of several adjacent follicles, a mass called a

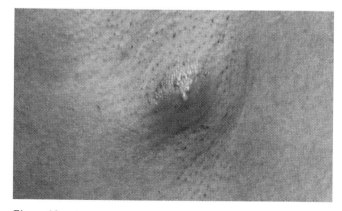

Figure 10 A furuncle, or boil, occurs as an acute, painful, localized staphylococcal abscess surrounding a hair follicle.

carbuncle may occur, with pus discharging from multiple follicular orifices. This infection typically develops on the back of the neck and appears more commonly in patients with diabetes than in the general population. Moist heat is usually adequate for small furuncles, which ordinarily drain spontaneously. Incision and drainage are appropriate for large or multiple furuncles and for all carbuncles. Systemic antibiotics are unnecessary unless there is fever or substantial surrounding cellulitis.

Some patients have recurrent episodes of furunculosis. Although a few patients have definable abnormalities in host defenses, such as neutrophil disorders, most are otherwise healthy people who, like 20% to 40% of the population, carry *S. aureus* in the anterior nares. From this site or occasionally from the perineum or axilla, organisms can spread and enter the skin, presumably through minor, usually inapparent, trauma. Successful prevention of recurrent infection requires eradication of these bacteria from their site of residence, but most systemic antibiotics do not achieve adequate levels of drug in the anterior nares. An exception is clindamycin, which, when given as a single daily dose of 150 mg for 3 months, is very effective in preventing subsequent episodes.[14] A less effective alternative is mupirocin ointment, applied in the anterior nares twice daily for 5 days each month.[15]

SKIN INFECTIONS CAUSED BY THE RESIDENT CUTANEOUS FLORA

The normal cutaneous flora helps prevent infection by other organisms through the mechanisms mentioned above: occupying available sites of residence, competition for nutrients, establishment of a low pH, and the elaboration of antibacterial substances. Occasionally, however, the resident skin flora causes cutaneous infections, especially with trauma or alterations in the stratum corneum. Examples are erythrasma, pitted keratolysis, trichomycosis axillaris, and most cases of cutaneous abscesses.

Cutaneous Abscesses

S. aureus, usually in pure culture, causes about 25% of cutaneous abscesses, especially in the axillae, on the hand, and on the breasts of women after childbirth.[16] In other sites, however, the predominant organisms are anaerobes, either alone or in the mixture of anaerobes and aerobes that constitutes the normal regional flora, including that from adjacent mucous membranes. In anogenital infections, such as scrotal, inguinal, vaginal, buttock, and perirectal abscesses, the organisms are commonly fecal bacteria, including streptococci, anaerobic gram-positive cocci, and anaerobic gram-negative bacilli, such as *Bacteroides fragilis.* On the extremities, trunk, neck, and head, the usual microbes include coagulase-negative staphylococci, anaerobic gram-positive cocci, and *Propionibacterium acnes,* an anaerobic gram-positive bacillus. These organisms ordinarily possess little virulence, but when introduced into the dermis or subcutaneous tissue by trauma or through a disrupted cutaneous surface, they may become pathogenic.

Cutaneous abscesses usually cause a painful, fluctuant, red, tender swelling, on which may rest a pustule. Treatment is incision and drainage of the area. Gram's stain and culture of the pus are ordinarily unnecessary, as are topical antimicrobials. Systemic antibiotics are reserved for patients with extensive surrounding cellulitis, neutropenia, cutaneous gangrene, or systemic manifestations of infection, such as high fever.

Erythrasma

Porphyrin-producing coryneform bacteria, which are gram-positive bacilli that constitute part of the normal cutaneous flora, cause a superficial, usually asymptomatic, skin disorder called erythrasma. One particular species, *Corynebacterium minutissimum,* has often been cited as the sole cause of this infection, but its precise role, if any, remains unclear. The most common site of erythrasma is between the toes, especially in the fourth interdigital space, where it causes fissuring, maceration, and scaling, resembling tinea pedis. Other locations are intertriginous areas, such as the axillae, groin, submammary area, and intergluteal cleft. In these regions, the lesions are usually scaly, brownish-red, sharply circumscribed patches. In hot, humid climates, more extensive disease may occur. The definitive diagnostic technique is examination of the skin with a Wood's light, which, because the organisms produce porphyrins, reveals a coral-red fluorescence. Culture of the lesions, which requires special media, is unnecessary. Because they possess some activity against gram-positive bacteria, topical azoles, such as miconazole and clotrimazole, are effective in the treatment of this infection. Topical erythromycin or clindamycin is also effective.

Pitted Keratolysis

C. minutissimum and a gram-positive coccus, *Micrococcus sedentarius,* either alone or together, cause a disorder that may affect the soles or, occasionally, the palms.[17] Pitted keratolysis consists of small pitted erosions about 1 to 7 mm in diameter that may be present on reddened plaques and are often more apparent after soaking in water for a few minutes. This infection occurs with increased moisture, such as caused by excessive sweating, occlusive footwear, or frequent contact with water. It appears more commonly in hot, humid climates than in more temperate ones. An impressive malodor of the feet is often apparent, and although the disorder may cause no symptoms, some patients complain of itching and tenderness. As in erythrasma, topical azoles, such as clotrimazole and miconazole, are effective, as are topical erythromycin and clindamycin.

Trichomycosis axillaris

Trichomycosis axillaris is characterized by colored concretions of axillary hair that result from infection of the hair shafts by large colonies of various species of *Corynebacterium.* The nodules may be yellow, black, or red; and because the organisms may invade the cuticle, the hair can become brittle. The same process occasionally affects the facial or pubic hair.[18] Excessive sweating, poor hygiene, and failure to use an axillary deodorant are predisposing factors. Shaving the hair is effective treatment; other options include topical erythromycin or clindamycin.

INFECTIONS DUE TO OTHER BACTERIA

Necrotizing Fasciitis

Necrotizing fasciitis, a necrotizing infection of the subcutaneous tissue, can be caused by streptococci; more often, however, the responsible organisms are a combination of aerobic bacteria—such as gram-negative enteric organisms (e.g., *Escherichia coli*) and gram-positive cocci—and anaerobes, including *B. fragilis.*[19] Necrotizing fasciitis usually occurs after a penetrating wound to the extremities. The injury is typically deep, but sometimes, infection occurs after apparently trivial trauma, such as abrasions or lacerations. The necrotizing process may develop from extension of an adjacent infection, especially in the second most common location, the anogenital area. There, infection typically arises from a perianal abscess; as an extension of a periurethral gland infection, especially in men with urethral strictures;

through retroperitoneal suppuration from perforated abdominal viscera; or as a complication of a preceding surgery. Necrotizing infection involving the genitalia is called Fournier's gangrene.

These infections typically begin with fever, systemic toxicity, severe pain in the affected site, and the development of a painful, red swelling that rapidly progresses to necrosis of the subcutaneous tissue and overlying skin. Early on, the pain may appear disproportionate to the clinical findings; in some cases involving *S. pyogenes* infection, the characteristics of the streptococcal toxic-shock syndrome may appear [*see Chapter 134*]. When anaerobes or certain aerobic gram-negative bacilli cause the infection, gas may form in tissues, evident as crepitus on physical examination or visible on radiographic studies. Although the disease may resemble uncomplicated cellulitis, the following signs and symptoms should suggest the presence of a necrotizing subcutaneous infection: edema beyond the apparent limits of the infection; rapid development of bullae and ecchymoses; cutaneous gangrene; fluctuance; crepitus; and radiographically visible gas. Computed tomography or magnetic resonance imaging may be helpful in some cases in detecting the infection and defining its extent. Aspiration of the affected tissue may yield purulent fluid, which on Gram's stain demonstrates only gram-positive cocci in chains when *S. pyogenes* is responsible or demonstrates a variety of many different organisms when a mixed infection is present. The find-

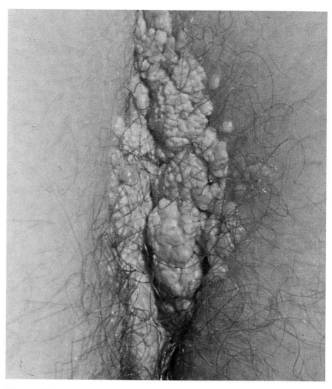

Figure 12 **Condyloma acuminatum may appear as a large cauliflower-like mass that resembles a malignant tumor.**

ings on Gram's stain and culture of pus should dictate antibiotic choice, but a good initial program is gentamicin in combination with clindamycin. Most important is incision and drainage of the affected area, which should include removal of any necrotic tissue. Often, the amount of disease revealed at surgery is much greater than was apparent on the preoperative clinical examination, because the infection typically extends far beyond the borders of cutaneous inflammation. Repeat operation after 24 hours is typically prudent to detect new areas of infection and necrotic tissue.

Folliculitis

Folliculitis is an inflammation at the opening of the hair follicle that causes erythematous papules and pustules surrounding individual hairs [*see Figure 11*]. The most common location is the trunk. The initiating factor seems to be occlusion of the opening of the follicle, which may occur from contact with chemicals, such as oils or cosmetics, overhydration of the skin from excessive moisture, or repetitive trauma, such as friction from tight-fitting clothing, which elicits hyperkeratosis and follicular plugging. Subsequently, inflammation develops, which may be provoked by bacteria, yeast, or other nonmicrobial substances trapped beneath the occluded ostium.

Among bacteria, *S. aureus* is often suspected but rarely found. When bacteria are present in the pustules, the culture usually yields normal skin flora. In these patients, oral erythromycin or doxycycline may be effective in eradicating the lesions. Another cause is *M. furfur,* a yeast that is a normal resident on the skin. In other patients, the avoidance of oily substances on the skin or tight clothing leads to resolution of the problem.

Occasionally, *Pseudomonas aeruginosa* is responsible, as a consequence of inadequate disinfection of hot tubs, swimming pools, or whirlpools.[20] This gram-negative bacillus grows well in

a

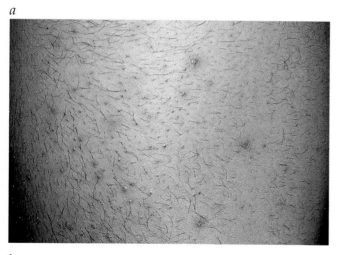

b

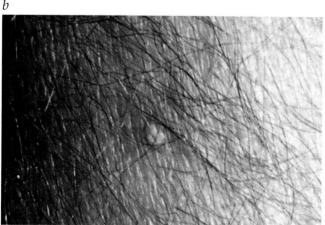

Figure 11 **Folliculitis is a superficial or deep inflammation of the hair follicles, appearing at follicular openings as small pustules surrounded by erythema (*a*). Folliculitis may also occur as an isolated lesion (*b*).**

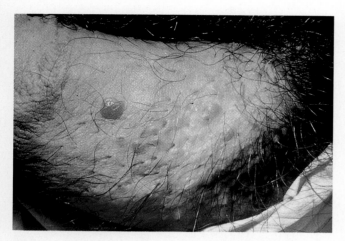

Figure 13 **Benign lesions of bowenoid papulosis, as seen on the shaft of the penis, may histologically resemble carcinoma in situ.**

hot water; outbreaks occur an average of 48 hours after exposure, with a range of several hours to several days. Erythematous, pruritic papules, often with a pinpoint central pustule, appear in areas exposed to the contaminated water; lesions are particularly numerous in regions occluded by tight-fitting swimming suits. The lesions disappear spontaneously over several days, leaving no scars; ordinarily, no topical or systemic therapy is necessary. Some patients have sore throat, rhinitis, earache, and headache, but fever or bacteremia is very rare. Cultures of the skin lesions and the contaminated water usually yield the organism.

Viral Infections

WARTS

Warts, or verrucae, are caused by human papillomaviruses (HPVs), a subgroup of DNA-containing papovaviruses, of which there are more than 70 types. Humans are the only known reservoir; transmission probably occurs from close contact with infected people or possibly from exposure to sloughed, infected epidermal cells. The virus presumably enters through small breaks in the skin. The incubation period is difficult to discern but is probably several months. Autoinoculation from one portion of the body to another also occurs. Cell-mediated immunity appears important in controlling these infections, which can be very extensive and refractory to treatment in immunocompromised patients.

Verrucae vary according to location. They include the common, elevated wart (verruca vulgaris), typically appearing on the hands; the flat wart (verruca plana), on the face and legs; the moist wart (condyloma acuminatum), in the anogenital area; and the callus-covered plantar wart (verruca plantaris), on the sole of the foot. A histologic feature that distinguishes a wart from other papillomas is the presence in the upper epidermis of large, vacuolated cells that contain numerous viral particles.

Condyloma Acuminatum

Anogenital warts consist of skin-colored or gray, discrete or confluent cauliflower-like excrescences that may cause no symptoms or produce itching, burning, pain, or tenderness [*see Figure 12*]. The incidence is highest in young adults; most often, it is a sexually transmitted disease, though some anogenital warts may develop from autoinoculation or may be acquired in other ways.[21]

Infection with some types of HPV predispose to malignancy. Most cases of squamous carcinoma of the cervix are caused by HPV, especially HPV-16 and HPV-18, but fortunately, these types represent only a small percentage of the isolates from anogenital warts. Genital verrucous carcinoma, also called giant condyloma acuminatum of Buschke-Löwenstein, is a low-grade genital malignancy caused by HPV-6 and HPV-11. Squamous carcinoma of the anus is associated primarily with HPV-16.

Anogenital warts may be difficult to eradicate, and several treatments are often necessary.[22] One option is liquid nitrogen; another is podophyllotoxin, which the patient applies twice daily for 3 days. This regimen can be repeated for a maximum of four courses, each separated by a 4-day hiatus. Although burning or soreness develops as a side effect in some patients, most tolerate the program without significant difficulties, and there is no need to wash off the medication between applications. A third approach involves fluorouracil (5-FU) cream administered twice daily for 1 to 3 weeks. This medication is particularly suitable for large wart plaques and warts of the urethral meatus, but side effects, including discomfort and painful erosions, are common.

Bowenoid Papulosis

Bowenoid papulosis consists of benign-appearing erythematous or pigmented papules in the anogenital area that histologically resemble Bowen's disease (squamous cell carcinoma in situ) [*see Figure 13*]. Its course, however, is not aggressive, and the papules should be treated as anogenital warts (see above). HPV-16 is a common cause, however, and malignancy does occasionally develop, especially in women.

References

1. Roth RR, James WD: Microbiology of the skin: resident flora, ecology, infection. J Am Acad Dermatol 20:367, 1989
2. Leyden JJ, McGinley KJ, Nordstrom KM, et al: Skin microflora. J Invest Dermatol 88(suppl):65s, 1987
3. Macura AB: Dermatophyte infections. Int J Dermatol 32:313, 1993
4. DeVroey C: Epidemiology of ringworm. Semin Dermatol 4:185, 1985
5. Semel JD, Goldin H: Association of athlete's foot with cellulitis of the lower extremities: diagnostic value of bacterial cultures of ipsilateral interdigital space samples. Clin Infect Dis 23:1162, 1996
6. Brautigam M, Nolting S, Schopf RE, et al: Randomised double blind comparison of terbinafine and itraconazole for treatment of toenail tinea infection. BMJ 311:919, 1995
7. Demidovich CW, Wittler RR, Ruff ME, et al: Impetigo: current etiology and comparison of penicillin, erythromycin, and cephalexin therapies. Am J Dis Child 144:1313, 1990
8. Dan M, Heller K, Shapira I, et al: Incidence of erysipelas following venectomy for coronary artery bypass surgery. Infection 15:107, 1987
9. Hook EW, Hooton TM, Horton CA, et al: Microbiologic evaluation of cutaneous cellulitis in adults. Arch Intern Med 146:295, 1986
10. Eriksson B, Jorup-Rönstrom C, Karkkonen K, et al: Erysipelas: clinical and bacteriologic spectrum and serological aspects. Clin Infect Dis 23:1091, 1996
11. Bernard P, Bedane C, Mounier M, et al: Streptococcal cause of erysipelas and cellulitis in adults: a microscopic study using a direct immunofluorescence technique. Arch Dermatol 125:779, 1989
12. Bergkvist PI, Sjöbeck K: Antibiotic and prednisolone therapy of erysipelas: a randomized, double blind placebo-controlled study. Scand J Infect Dis 29:377, 1997
13. Kremer M, Zuckerman R, Avraham Z, et al: Long-term antimicrobial therapy in the prevention of recurrent soft-tissue infections. J Infect 22:37, 1991
14. Klempner MS, Styrt B: Prevention of recurrent staphylococcal skin infections with low-dose oral clindamycin therapy. JAMA 260:2682, 1988
15. Raz R, Miron D, Colodner R, et al: A 1-year trial of nasal mupirocin in the prevention of recurrent staphylococcal nasal colonization and skin infection. Arch Intern Med 156:1109, 1996
16. Meislin HW, Lerner SA, Graves MH, et al: Cutaneous abscesses: anaerobic and aerobic bacteriology and outpatient management. Ann Intern Med 87:145, 1977
17. Nordstrom KM, McGinley KJ, Cappiello L, et al: Pitted keratolysis: the role of *Micrococcus sedentarius*. Arch Dermatol 123:1320, 1987
18. White SW, Smith J: Trichomycosis pubis. Arch Dermatol 115:444, 1979
19. Stone DR, Gorbach SL: Necrotizing fasciitis: the changing spectrum. Dermatol Clin 15:213, 1997
20. Agger WA, Mardan A: *Pseudomonas aeruginosa* infections of intact skin. Clin Infect Dis 20:302, 1995
21. Von Krogh G, Gross G: Anogenital warts. Clin Dermatol 15:355, 1997
22. Gross G, Von Krogh G: Therapy of anogenital HPV-induced lesions. Clin Dermatol 15:457, 1997

38 Parasitic Infestations

Elizabeth A. Abel, M.D.

Ectoparasites may cause severely pruritic infectious diseases of the skin. With early detection and treatment, parasitic infestations can be cured and their spread to other persons can be prevented. The most common parasitic diseases of the skin that occur in nontropical environments are scabies, which is caused by itch mites, and pediculosis capitis, pediculosis corporis, and pediculosis pubis, which are caused by bloodsucking lice.

An increase in international travel, including vacation travel to tropical destinations and immigration from such areas, has led to the occurrence of parasitic disorders endemic to tropical regions in persons living in temperate climates. The differential diagnosis of skin disorders in patients treated at a tropical disease clinic in Paris over a 2-year period included cutaneous larva migrans, pyodermas, arthropod-reactive dermatitis, myiasis, tungiasis, urticaria, and cutaneous leishmaniasis.[1]

Scabies

Scabies is caused by infestation with *Sarcoptes scabiei*, an ectoparasite that bores into the corneal layer of human skin, forming burrows in which it deposits its eggs. The incubation period is 2 to 6 weeks in a person who has not been previously exposed. During this time, the host develops delayed hypersensitivity to mite antigens. Upon reinfestation, symptoms occur in sensitized persons within 24 to 48 hours after exposure.[2] The incidence of scabies follows a 30-year cycle: 15 years of high incidence alternates with 15 years of low incidence. The current pandemic, however, has exceeded 15 years.

The scabies mite does not survive for more than 48 hours away from the host. Therefore, most infestations are transmitted through direct personal skin-to-skin and sexual contact.[2] However, transfer of organisms can occur by exposure to fomites in contaminated bedding, clothing, or furniture and is a common cause of epidemics of scabies in nursing homes and other institutions.[2,3]

DIAGNOSIS

Clinical Features

Scabies causes severe itching, which is usually worse at night. Characteristic sites of infestation are the webs of the fingers, the flexor aspects of the wrists, the axillae, the buttocks, the umbilicus, the penis and scrotum of males, and the breasts and nipples of females. The disease is more generalized in infants and children than in adults.

The burrow of the female *Sarcoptes* may be seen as an irregular zigzag line in the stratum corneum, with a black dot at one end that indicates the presence of the mite [*see Figure 1*]. Secondary lesions represent immunologic reactions to the mites and usually appear as small erythematous papules and vesicles with surrounding edema and scratch marks [*see Figure 2*]. The type and number of lesions depend predominantly on the immune status of the host. Occasionally, nodular lesions, which may resemble lesions of histiocytosis X (Langerhans cell granulomatosis) or lymphoma, occur as a hypersensitivity reaction to retained mite parts. Fewer lesions occur in people who practice good hygiene, and the condition may be masked in those who are using topical steroids. Secondary bacterial infection with impetiginization is common, especially in children and in elderly patients who actively excoriate their lesions.

Atypical presentations of scabies have been described in immunosuppressed persons, including organ transplant recipients, patients with lymphoma or leukemia, and patients with AIDS. Itching and scratching, with elimination of mites and burrows, may be minimal in patients who lack an immunologic host response, allowing for thousands of mites to reproduce and thrive.[2] Crusted scabies, which was originally described in Norway, is associated with widespread hyperkeratotic lesions and deep fissures in the skin. Crusted scabies can develop in patients with malnutrition or severe mental deficiency and in institutionalized patients. The condition is highly contagious because of the large number of mites present in the exfoliating skin.

A severe form of scabies with unusual clinical features consisting of crusted lesions and a widespread pruritic papular dermatitis has been described in HIV-infected patients.[2,4] In these patients, multiple treatment applications may be needed because of the large mite population as well as the patients' impaired immunologic response.

Skin Scrapings

A skin scraping that demonstrates the presence of mite eggs or mite products can confirm a diagnosis of scabies. A No. 15 surgical blade is used to scrape across one or more burrows. Saline solution or mineral oil is used to remove scrapings from the blade. The scrapings are then placed on a glass slide with a coverslip and examined under a microscope at low-power magnification. The scraping is positive if the gravid female, eggs, or scybala (fecal pellets) are seen [*see Figure 3*]. The yield is greatest in burrows that are not yet excoriated, which may be difficult to find. For this reason, if the scraping is negative but the clinical suspicion of scabies is high, the patient should be treated empirically. Histopathologic examination of a skin biopsy sample is also diagnostic if it reveals the mite or the superficial skin burrow and its contents.[5]

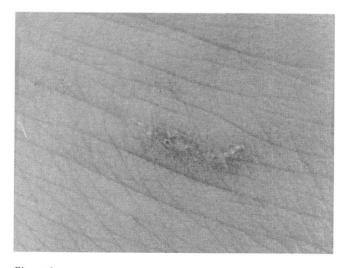

Figure 1 **Typical scabies lesions are small erythematous papules and vesicles with surrounding edema.**

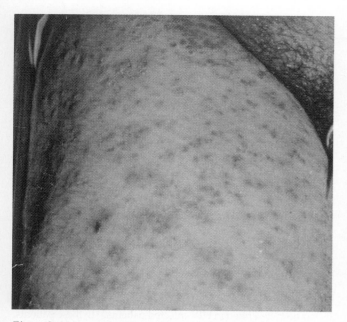

Figure 2 **The burrow of the female *Sarcoptes* frequently appears as an irregular line several millimeters to a few centimeters long in the stratum corneum.**

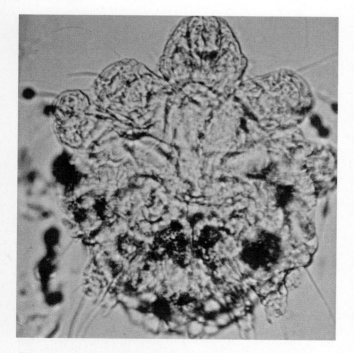

Figure 3 **Observation of the *Sarcoptes scabiei* or its eggs and feces confirms the diagnosis of scabies. Magnification is 400 times.**

DIFFERENTIAL DIAGNOSIS

Clinical differential diagnosis includes drug eruption, papular urticaria, follicullitis, atopic dermatitis, dermatitis herpetiformis, and contact dermatitis, particularly from fiberglass. Papular urticaria is an intensely itchy eruption caused by a hypersensitivity reaction to bites from such insects as fleas, bedbugs, and animal scabies. Lesions occur as small papules that may have a central punctum, often occurring in groups on exposed skin.

TREATMENT

Initial Treatment

After a cleansing bath or shower, the patient should allow the skin to dry and cool and then apply a scabicide over the entire body, excluding the face and scalp. Care must be taken to include skin folds such as toe webs and the skin under the nails. The medication is left in place for 8 to 12 hours, usually overnight. In the morning, the patient showers and changes clothes. All clothing worn within 2 days after treatment, in addition to towels and bed linens, is laundered in hot water or dry-cleaned. Chairs and mattresses should be vacuumed.

Available scabicides include 5% permethrin cream (Elimite, Acticin); lindane, or gamma benzene hexachloride, lotion or cream (Kwell, Gamene); 10% to 20% benzyl benzoate lotion; crotamiton cream (Eurax); and 6% precipitated sulfur ointment.

Permethrin, a synthetic pyrethroid with low toxicity, is considered the first line of therapy.[6] Natural pyrethrins, which are derived from chrysanthemum flowers, have greater toxicity and less insecticidal activity than the synthetic pyrethroids. The low toxicity of the drug is a result of its rapid breakdown into inactive metabolites. Permethrin cream can be safely used in children and infants older than 2 months and in the elderly. Acticin is a form of permethrin in a base that has a lower viscosity to promote ease of application. Alternative scabicides that can be used for young children and pregnant or lactating women include crotamiton cream and sulfur ointment. Six percent precipitated sulfur ointment is applied three times: at diagnosis, after 24 hours, and at 1 week. Crotamiton cream is applied for 2 or more consecutive days but is less effective than permethrin.

Lindane is lipophilic and can accumulate in fat and bind to brain tissue. Toxic reactions may occur in patients who have increased absorption; infants and young children, who have a higher ratio of skin surface to body volume than do adults, are especially susceptible. Excessive treatment with lindane has been reported to cause central nervous system toxicity resulting in convulsions.[7,8] Nevertheless, low cost, ease of application, and experience with the drug have made lindane one of the most commonly prescribed scabicides.

Oral ivermectin is another option that may increase compliance to treatment because oral administration is easier than whole body therapy. A single oral dose of 200 μg/kg of ivermectin was used to treat uncomplicated scabies in 11 otherwise healthy patients and in 11 patients with HIV infection.[9] Clearing was documented by negative skin scrapings at 2 weeks and 4 weeks after treatment, and cure was achieved in all of the otherwise healthy patients and in eight of the HIV-infected patients.

In a comparative study of oral ivermectin and topical permethrin, a single application of permethrin was found to be superior to a single dose of ivermectin. Two doses of ivermectin were required for eradication of scabies. The lack of ovicidal activity of ivermectin may explain the difference in effectiveness between the two drugs.[10] Ivermectin is toxic to invertebrate nerve and muscle cells but may not be effective against younger stages of the parasite that do not have a developed nervous system. Permethrin acts at all stages of the life cycle of the parasite, and topical application ensures adequate drug concentration in the skin.[10]

Topical ivermectin has also been investigated for treatment of scabies. A total of 75 patients were found to be cured, on the basis of clinical and parasitologic examinations, within 48 hours after a single application of ivermectin. Postscabies itching, which persisted in 50% of the patients, was effectively treated by a second application of ivermectin within 5 days.[11]

Postscabies Itch

Postscabies itch is thought to represent a hypersensitivity reaction to the mite or mite products and is not caused by active infestation. The pruritus may persist for weeks to months and can be treated with an antipruritic or anti-inflammatory agent, such as a low-potency to midpotency corticosteroid cream, in addition to oral antihistamines. Overtreatment with the scabicide may result in a primary irritant dermatitis that may be confused with persistent infestation. The use of bland emollients and a corticosteroid cream and avoidance of skin irritants may reduce the dermatitis. Patients should be evaluated at 4 weeks, the time required for viable eggs to mature to the adult stage, to determine the efficacy of treatment. If lesions are healed and no new outbreaks have occurred, the patient is considered cured.[2]

Resistant Scabies

Pyrethroids are effective in cases of resistant scabies that may be associated with overuse of lindane.[12] Treatment failures can also occur in cases involving impetiginized or crusted scabies. In these cases, treatment with the appropriate oral antibiotic is initiated along with application of the scabicide and is followed within a week by a second application of the scabicide. Keratolytics are useful as an aid in removal of the crusts.

Oral ivermectin has been used to treat resistant scabies. Although it has not been approved by the FDA for this purpose, oral ivermectin is rapidly gaining acceptance as first-line therapy for scabies. Combination treatment with one or two doses of ivermectin 8 days apart, in addition to permethrin and mechanical removal of subungual debris, has been advocated for outbreaks of crusted scabies in the geriatric population.[13]

Combination therapy with oral ivermectin, 200 mg/kg, and benzylbenzoate, 15% solution applied twice daily for 3 days, is more effective than either agent alone for the treatment of crusted scabies in patients with HIV.[14]

Cases of apparent resistant scabies may be the result of reinfestation. Therefore, family members and sexual partners of persons with scabies should be treated because they may be asymptomatic carriers. Scabies occurring in patients and personnel in long-term health care facilities may be difficult to diagnose and manage. In this setting, it is extremely important to treat all nursing contacts, as well as family members and other visitors of affected patients. In addition to the patients with scabies, other patients in the facility need to be assessed, and care must be coordinated to treat all affected persons simultaneously. In cases of crusted scabies, the head and neck must be treated, as well as subungual areas, which may also harbor the mites.[3]

ANIMAL SCABIES

Animal scabies is a common disorder in farm animals and domestic animals—especially dogs, in which the external ear is frequently infested with a species-specific mite. In persons who handle affected animals, an extremely pruritic papular eruption can develop that differs from ordinary scabies in several ways: distribution of lesions is proximal, with involvement of the thighs, abdomen, and forearms. Burrows are usually absent. The course is self-limited provided there is no reexposure. Other persons in the household do not have to be treated, because human-to-human transmission of animal scabies does not occur.

The *Cheyletiella* mite is an ectoparasite that resides in the fur of dogs, cats, and rabbits. Persons who hold infested house pets, especially cats, are susceptible to a dermatitis from the mite bites. However, the mites do not live on humans, so diagnosis requires a high index of suspicion. Lesions may appear as urticarial papules, vesicles, or bullae on the arms, trunk, and legs. Cases most commonly occur in the fall or winter. An important part of the overall treatment of *Cheyletiella* infestation is treatment of the household pets by a veterinarian.[15]

Pediculosis

The three types of bloodsucking lice that cause pediculosis are *Pediculus humanus* var. *capitis* (head louse), *Pediculus humanus* var. *corporis* (body louse), and *Phthirus pubis* (pubic, or crab, louse). The first two types are closely related. The third is a separate genus and is distinctive not only in appearance and in location on the body but also in its characteristic attachment to the skin for long periods. Any form of pediculosis causes intense pruritus, aggravated by scratching and often complicated by secondary bacterial infection.[16]

The most common infestation is pediculosis capitis, except under conditions of overcrowding and poor sanitation or in wartime, when pediculosis corporis is widespread. The lice may be transmitted directly from person to person or indirectly through contact with contaminated personal objects such as combs and brushes, clothing, and bedding. Pediculosis pubis (also called crabs) is usually transmitted sexually; only occasionally are the lice transmitted through contact with fomites such as contaminated bedding or toilet seats.

The natural history of lice is important because it suggests specific preventive measures. The life expectancy of the organism is about 1 month. Eggs live up to 10 days but need the body heat of the host to hatch. Eggs ordinarily hatch in 7 to 8 days, and organisms reach adulthood and attain sexual reproductive capacity in 3 to 4 weeks. Lice can survive 48 hours without a blood meal.

DIAGNOSIS

Pediculosis capitis is confined to the scalp and is most prevalent in women and children. Examination of the itchy scalp may reveal the lice, which look like tiny black dots that are barely visible to the naked eye, and lice eggs (nits), which are white and are attached to the hair shafts [see Figure 4]. Viable nits are attached close to the scalp. Those that occur several millimeters away from the surface on hairs that have grown out are empty egg cases. The hair may become matted because of exudation and secondary infection of lesions, and the cervical glands may become enlarged and painful.

Pediculosis corporis, also called vagabond disease, affects areas of the body covered by clothing. Body lice live in the seams of clothing, and they attach to the body only to feed [see Figure 5]. They may serve as vectors of infectious disease under conditions of overcrowding or poor hygiene, as in wartime or during natural disasters. Characteristic lesions include erythematous macules and wheals. Lesions are most common on the shoulders, buttocks, and abdomen; furunculosis is an occasional complication. Excoriations and secondary infection may result from intense scratching. After the eggs hatch, the organisms reach adulthood in 10 days and complete their life cycle in approximately 1 month. Adult lice lay about 10 eggs a day.

Pediculosis pubis, which is caused by infestation with *Phthirus pubis* [see Figure 6], tends to be limited to the pubic area but occasionally affects the axillae, eyelashes, or other hairy parts of the

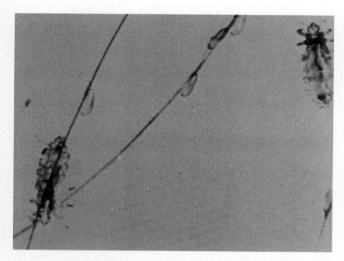

Figure 4 **Pediculosis capitis is caused by infestation of the scalp with** *Pediculus humanus* var. *capitis*. **Magnification is 10 times.**

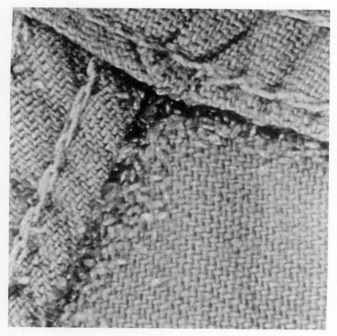

Figure 5 **Pediculosis corporis is caused by infestation with** *Pediculus humanus* var. *corporis* **organisms, which live in the seams of clothing.**

body. Examination will reveal lice attached to the skin and lice eggs attached to the hair shafts [*see Figure 7*]. Blue macules, which are caused by the lice's sucking blood from the dermis, may be seen on the thighs or pubic area.

TREATMENT

Pediculosis Capitis

One of the most widely used remedies for pediculosis in the United States is 1% lindane (Kwell, Gamene). For the treatment of *Pediculus capitis*, 2 tbsp (30 ml) of the shampoo is applied to affected and adjacent areas of the scalp for at least 4 minutes, followed by thorough rinsing and drying. Adherent nits may be removed with a fine-tooth comb. Distilled white vinegar can be used to soften the nit cementing material to aid in removal of the nits.

Over-the-counter preparations available for the treatment of pediculosis capitis include synergized pyrethrin products such as RID, R&C Spray, A-200, and a 1% permethrin cream rinse (Nix). These products are cosmetically acceptable and require only 10 minutes to apply but may not always be effective. Repeat treatment in 7 to 10 days is advisable because the initial treatment does not kill all the eggs.

Resistance to lindane has emerged over the past 2 decades. More recently, treatment of lice infestation has been complicated by the development of resistance to permethrin.[17] Mechanical methods of removing head lice and nits[18] and application of occlusive oils or ointments[19] have been advocated for treatment of resistant head lice. Oral ivermectin has been administered as a single dose of 12 mg (2 to 6 mg tablets) followed by a second dose 7 to 10 days later.[16]

Pediculosis Pubis and Pediculosis Corpis

To treat hairy areas of the body infested with *P. pubis*, a cleansing bath or shower should first be taken and the skin dried with a towel. One ounce of lindane cream or lotion is applied to the affected and surrounding areas and left on for 12 to 24 hours. After another bath or shower, freshly laundered clothing should be donned; bedsheets and towels should also be changed. Lindane may be applied a second time after 1 week if infestation continues. Lindane should not be applied to the face and eyelids, because it causes irritation; eyelash infestation may be treated by local application of 0.25% physostigmine ophthalmic ointment. An alternative treatment for eyelash infestation that is effective and nonirritating is the application of a thick layer of petrolatum twice a day, followed by mechanical removal of the nits.

Neurologic complications can ensue from absorption of lindane after extensive or prolonged topical application [*see Scabies, above*]. Alternative treatments are therefore indicated in infants (who are especially susceptible), in young children, in pregnant women, and in the elderly. No serious side effects have been reported from the use of lindane for head lice.

A combination of pyrethrins with piperonyl butoxide (RID or A-200) has been shown to be considerably less toxic than lindane in animal experiments and in clinical experience. However, this combination irritates the eyes and mucous membranes and may also cause allergic contact dermatitis in susceptible people.

General Treatment Measures

All family members should be carefully examined for pediculosis and treated, if necessary, to avoid spread or reinfection of previously treated persons. In the case of pediculosis pubis, sexual contacts should be examined and treated. Because sexually transmitted diseases are frequently present in persons infested with *P. pubis*, a serologic test for syphilis and screening for HIV are usually done. To prevent spread of pediculosis, contaminated clothing and other articles, such as towels and bedding, should be boiled, machine washed in hot water, and placed in a dryer using a 20-minute hot cycle or should be dry-cleaned. Items such as combs and brushes may be cleaned with medicated shampoo or soaked in 5% Lysol. To eradicate *P. corporis*, the patient's clothing must be put through the same decontamination process as that used for *P. pubis*. A hot iron with pressure applied, especially to the seams of clothing, may also be used to kill *P. corporis*. Systemic antibiotics should be prescribed for concomitant secondary bacterial infections such as furunculosis and impetigo, both of which are commonly associated with pediculosis capitis.

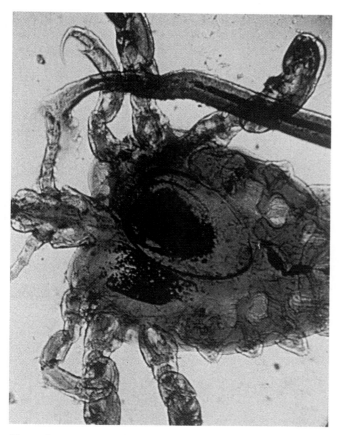

Figure 6 **Pediculosis pubis, also called crabs, is caused by infestation with *Phthirus pubis*. Magnification is 100 times.**

Miscellaneous Infestations

FLEA INFESTATIONS

Fleas are small (approximately 3 mm), bloodsucking, wingless ectoparasites of the insect order Siphonaptera. Fleas are medically significant because they are vectors of infectious disease [*see Chapter 142*]. They can also cause considerable cutaneous symptoms, particularly if the symptoms are associated with an allergic hypersensitivity reaction, as seen in papular urticaria. There are approximately 250 species of flea, 20 of which can infest humans. Two common species that infest cats and dogs are *Ctenocephalides felis* and *C. canis*. They are not host specific and can therefore infest humans as well. *Pulex irritans*, the house flea, infests humans and is not a problem for pets. Flea bites appear as erythematous edematous papules with hemorrhagic puncta in clusters or groups on the lower extremities, especially on the ankles. Occasionally, vesicles and bullae can appear, as well as larger urticarial lesions. Secondary impetiginization may occur because of scratching.[20]

Fleas are difficult to eradicate because of their unpredictable life cycle, which consists of egg, larva, pupa, and adult stages. The eggs are laid on the host but can drop to the ground; onto carpets, pet bedding , and furniture; and into floor cracks. Eggs hatch in 2 to 21 days into larvae. A larva molts twice and, in the third larval stage, spins a cocoon, in which it becomes a pupa. Within 7 days to 1 year or more, the adult emerges, depending on various trigger factors (e.g., a vibration caused by a nearby pet or human). The life cycle from egg to adult can range from 14 to 21

days and under ideal conditions to as long as 20 months.[20]

Eradication of the fleas may require consultation with a veterinarian. Pets must be treated more than once to kill the eggs, larvae, and pupae, as well as the residual fleas. A household flea spray should be combined with a fogger to fumigate the house. Proper extermination procedure includes vacuuming the furniture and vacuuming or steam cleaning carpets or rugs. The yard should be sprayed and cleared of organic debris.

Treatment of flea bites consists of cool-water compresses, application of a corticosteroid cream and an antipruritic lotion, and oral antihistamines in the case of allergic hypersensitivity reaction. Systemic antibiotics are prescribed for secondary bacterial infection.

Tungiasis

Cutaneous infestation by the sandflea *Tunga penetrans* is endemic in Central and South America, parts of Mexico, tropical Africa, Pakistan, and the west coast of India. Isolated cases have been reported in the United States, Australia, and New Zealand. Tungiasis is more prevalent in poverty-stricken areas and is associated with domestic animals such as pigs, dogs, and cattle, which serve as intermediaries in the biologic life cycle.[21] The female adult sandflea exists in sandy soils and requires a warm-blooded host to complete its life cycle. The organism penetrates the stratum corneum, resulting in erythematous nodules with a central dark spot. Common sites of skin involvement are the soles of the feet, the web spaces between fingers and toes, the ankles, the perineal area, and the buttocks.

Infestation can be prevented by wearing shoes and proper clothing and by the use of insecticides.

MYIASIS

Myiasis is caused by the larvae (maggots) of feeding flies of the order Diptera. The larvae may invade the skin primarily or become secondarily implanted in a preexisting skin wound.[22] Many species of the genus *Cuterebra* can cause myiasis, but in

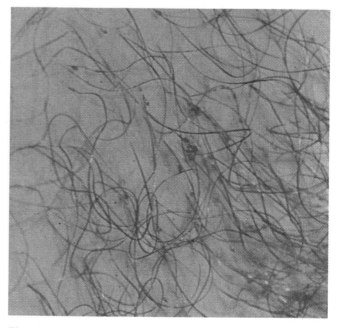

Figure 7 **Lice attached to the skin and lice eggs attached to the hair shafts can be seen on a patient with pediculosis pubis.**

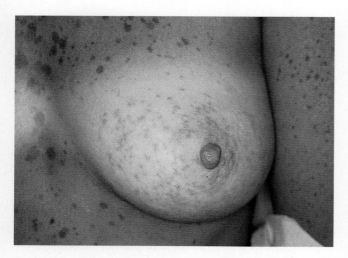

Figure 8   Seabather's eruption is characterized by the development of pruritic papules on areas covered by the patient's bathing suit.

North America, *C. cuterebra* and *C. dermatobia* cause furuncular cutaneous infestations.

The skin lesions appear as nonhealing single or multiple nodules on the upper trunk, usually at the site of a painful bite wound. Skin lesions may be misdiagnosed as cellulitis, boils, or sebaceous cysts. Myiasis is commonly reported in travelers to endemic areas such as Central and South America and tropical and subtropical Africa. Preventive measures include the use of insect repellents, the wearing of protective clothing to prevent mosquito bites, and the avoidance of direct skin contact with sand that may be infested with eggs.

The condition is effectively treated by removal of the larvae by incision and drainage with debridement. Antibiotics are prescribed for secondary bacterial infection. Occlusion with such agents as liquid paraffin, lubricating jelly, and even the fatty portion of raw bacon has been suggested to cause suffocation of the larvae or migration of the larvae from the wound.[23]

CUTANEOUS LARVA MIGRANS

Cutaneous larva migrans is caused by penetration and migration of larval hookworms (usually *Ancylostoma braziliense*) within the skin. Patients are usually travelers returning from seawater beaches in tropical areas and commonly present to the dermatologist with pruritic skin lesions. The abdomen or feet are most often involved, with a characteristic eruption consisting of one or several erythematous linear to serpiginous thin lines in the skin.

Treatment includes oral thiabendazole, 25 to 60 mg/kg for 2 to 4 days only. This drug may cause side effects such as headaches, nausea, and vomiting. Oral albendazole has a high cure rate in a dosage of 400 mg for 5 consecutive days. Oral ivermectin is reportedly effective in a single dose of 150 to 200 µg/kg.[24]

SEABATHER'S ERUPTION

Seabather's eruption, also known as sea lice by laypersons, is an acute pruritic dermatitis that occurs within 24 hours of seawater exposure and resolves spontaneously after 3 to 5 days.[25] Lesions affect areas of the skin covered by swimwear, particularly those that are subjected to pressure or friction, such as the waistline, axillae, neck, and inner thighs [*see Figure 8*]. The larvae of the thimble jellyfish *Linuche unguiculata*, which are

washed ashore by ocean currents, have been identified as the cause of seabather eruption in southern Florida and the Caribbean. Similar outbreaks on Long Island, New York, are thought to be caused by larvae of *Edwardsiella lineata*.[26]

Treatment is symptomatic and includes antihistamines, topical antipruritic agents, and steroids.

SWIMMER'S ITCH

Cercarial dermatitis, known as swimmer's itch, is caused by an avian schistosome, *Microbilharzia variglandis*. The skin eruption appears approximately 12 hours after contact with seawater as a pruritic papulovesicular dermatitis on exposed skin sites.[27] The inflammatory response is attributed to dermatologic penetration by cercariae, which are the free-swimming larvae of *M. variglandis* and other bird schistosomes.

Treatment is symptomatic and includes antihistamines, topical antipruritic agents, topical corticosteroids, and antibiotic treatment of superimposed bacterial infection.

CUTANEOUS AND MUCOCUTANEOUS LEISHMANIASIS

There are distinctive skin lesions associated with the cutaneous and mucocutaneous forms of leishmaniasis [*see Figure 9*]. Leishmaniasis is caused by an obligate intracellular parasite introduced by the *Phlebotomus* sandfly that feeds on infected animals. *Leishmania braziliensis* and *L. mexicana* are the most common causes of American, or New World, leishmaniasis. *L. donovani* causes Old World leishmaniasis, which is endemic in Asia and West Africa [*see Chapter 157*].

Cutaneous leishmaniasis—the initial, or primary, form of the disease—appears as a localized, usually single, lesion involving the mouth and nose. A red-brown papule develops at the site of inoculation into a nodule that becomes verrucous or ulcerates, and satellite nodules may form. Spontaneous healing with an atrophic scar occurs in most cases. Old World leishmaniasis is usually limited to the skin, whereas New World leishmaniasis can cause mutilating mucocutaneous involvement.[28] After a period of months to years, the mucocutaneous, or secondary, form of the disease may develop, depending on host immunologic factors. Lesions in this stage range from edema of the lips and nose to perforation of the nasal cartilage. A rare form, disseminated cutaneous leishmaniasis, which has widespread nodules resembling lepromatous leprosy, may occur in immunosuppressed patients.

The differential diagnosis includes various inflammatory and

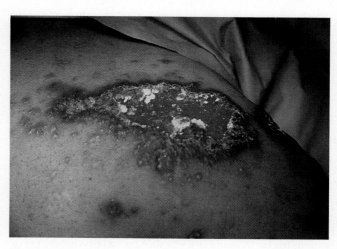

Figure 9   Leishmaniasis can present as chronic cutaneous ulcerations.

neoplastic disorders, including squamous cell carcinoma. Diagnosis is made by skin biopsy with histopathologic examination. Appropriate therapy depends on species identification. A pentavalent antimony compound, such as sodium stibogluconate, is the drug of choice for New World leishmaniasis, which tends to be more aggressive. Lesions acquired in the Middle East and North Africa may spontaneously involute or may respond to local therapy, including cryosurgery, heat therapy, or intralesional injection of antimonials.

Delusions of Parasitosis

Patients with delusions of parasitosis express the conviction that there are scabies, insects, lice, fleas, worms, or other vermin infesting their skin and producing a crawling, itching, or prickling sensation.[29] They may have excoriations or skin inflammation and erosions consistent with factitial dermatitis. Frequently, patients will bring small containers filled with lint, hairs, pieces of skin, fibers, or other debris for examination. Despite the lack of objective evidence for infestation—including negative results from clinical examination, microscopic examination of skin scrapings, and skin biopsy—the delusions persist. Associated underlying psychiatric disturbances may range from a phobic-obsessive state or anxiety reaction to a frank psychosis with either depression or paranoia. Not infrequently, the delusion is shared by the spouse or other family members, as in the classic folie à deux or folie à famille. The patient usually functions in a highly organized manner in other aspects of his or her life. Such patients typically resist seeking psychiatric evaluation.

Treatment with pimozide, a high-potency antipsychotic neuroleptic of the diphenylbutylpiperidine group, has been used successfully.[29] The effectiveness of the drug may be mediated by its ability to specifically block central dopamine receptors. As is characteristic of high-potency antipsychotic drugs, pimozide has fewer cardiovascular and anticholinergic effects but greater neurologic toxicity, especially with long-term use, than does low-potency antipsychotic drugs. Tardive dyskinesia, an extrapyramidal syndrome characterized by involuntary movements of facial muscles and extremities, may occur in 10% to 20% of patients on antipsychotic drugs. Other side effects may include skin discoloration, dermatitis, and blurred vision. Thorough medical and psychiatric evaluation should be obtained before antipsychotic medication is instituted.

References

1. Lucchina LC, Wilson ME, Drake LA: Dermatology and the recently returned traveler: infectious diseases with dermatologic manifestations. Int J Dermatol 36:167, 1997
2. Hoke AW, Maibach HI: Scabies management: a current perspective. Cutis 64:2, 1999
3. Holness DL, DeKoven JG, Nethercott JR: Scabies in chronic health care institutions. Arch Dermatol 128:1257, 1992
4. Orkin M: Scabies in AIDS. Semin Dermatol 12:9, 1993
5. Head ES, Macdonald EM, Ewert A, et al: *Sarcoptes scabiei* in histopathologic sections of skin in human scabies. Arch Dermatol 126:1475, 1990
6. Taplin D, Meinking TL: Pyrethrins and pyrethroids in dermatology. Arch Dermatol 126:213, 1990
7. Schultz MW, Gomez M, Hansen RC, et al: Comparative study of 5% permethrin cream and 1% lindane lotion for the treatment of scabies. Arch Dermatol 126:167, 1990
8. Tenenbein M: Seizures after lindane therapy. J Am Geriatr Soc 39:394, 1991
9. Meinking TL, Taplin D, Hermida JL, et al: The treatment of scabies with ivermectin. N Engl J Med 333:26, 1995
10. Usha V, Gopalakrishnan Nair TV: A comparative study of oral ivermectin and topical permethrin cream in the treatment of scabies. J Am Acad Dermatol 42:236, 2000
11. Youssef MYM, Sadaka HAH, Eissa MM, et al: Topical application of ivermectin for human ectoparasites. Am J Trop Hyg 53:652, 1995
12. Purvis RS, Tyring SK: An outbreak of lindane-resistant scabies treated successfully with permethrin 5% cream. J Am Acad Dermatol 26(pt 1):1015, 1991
13. Paasch U, Haustein U-F: Management of endemic outbreaks of scabies with allethrin, permethrin, and ivermectin. Int J Dermatol 39:463, 2000
14. Alberici F, Pagani L, Ratti G, et al: Ivermectin alone or in combination with benzyl benzoate in the treatment of human immunodeficiency virus-associated scabies. Br J Dermatol 142:969, 2000
15. Lee BW: *Cheyletiella* dermatitis: a report of fourteen cases. Cutis 47:111, 1991
16. Elston DM: What's eating you? *Pediculus humanus* (head louse and body louse). Cutis 63:259, 1999
17. Downs AM, Stafford KA, Harvey I, et al: Evidence for double resistance to permethrin and malathion in head lice. Br J Dermatol 141:508, 1999
18. Roberts RJ, Casey D, Morgan DA, et al: Comparison of wet combing with malathion for treatment of head lice in the UK: a pragmatic randomised controlled trial. Lancet 356:540, 2000
19. Mumcuoglu KY: Prevention and treatment of head lice in children. Paediatr Drugs 1:211, 1999
20. Hutchins ME, Burnett JW: Fleas. Cutis 51:241, 1993
21. Campos Macias P, Mendez Sashida P: Cutaneous infestation by *Tunga penetrans*. Int J Dermatol 39:296, 2000
22. Burnett JW: Myiasis. Cutis 46:51, 1990
23. Brewer TF, Wilson ME, Gonzalez MD, et al: Bacon therapy and furuncular myiasis. JAMA 270:2087, 1993
24. Caumes E, Carriere J, Datry A, et al: A randomized trial of ivermectin versus albendazole for the treatment of cutaneous larva migrans. Am J Trop Med Hyg 49:641, 1993
25. Tomchik RS, Russell MT, Szmant AM, et al: Clinical perspectives on seabather's eruption, also known as "sea lice." JAMA 269:1669, 1993
26. Freudenthal AR, Joseph PR: Seabather's eruption. N Engl J Med 329:542, 1993
27. Cercarial dermatitis outbreak at a State Park—Delaware, 1991. JAMA 267:2581, 1992
28. Koff AB, Rosen T: Treatment of cutaneous leishmaniasis. J Am Acad Dermatol 31:693, 1994
29. Driscoll MS, Rothe MJ, Grant-Kels JM, et al: Delusional parasitosis: a dermatologic, psychiatric, and pharmacologic approach. J Am Acad Dermatol 29:1023, 1993

39 Vesiculobullous Diseases

Elizabeth A. Abel, M.D., and Jean-Claude Bystryn, M.D.

Vesiculobullous diseases, which number more than 50, are characterized by fluid-filled blisters in the skin. Blisters smaller than 0.5 cm are called vesicles, and larger ones are called bullae. Vesicles and bullae are reaction patterns of skin to injury and thus can be caused by a wide variety of conditions.

Most primary vesiculobullous diseases are either immunologic or genetic. They are caused by autoimmune reactions to components of skin, by allergic reactions to external agents in which the skin is the major organ system affected, and by genetic conditions in which some components of the skin are missing or abnormal. The final common pathway is disadhesion: one or more of the structures that hold the skin together separate, and a fluid-filled cavity appears. The different diseases are classified by the structure or structures affected and the mechanism or mechanisms by which disadhesion occurs [*see Table 1*]. In this chapter, several paradigmatic vesiculobullous diseases are discussed in the context of a general diagnostic approach to the patient with blistering lesions.

General Clinical Assessment

Diagnosis is based on clinical features, histologic findings, and immunologic findings. Clinical features of diagnostic importance include the following:

1. The history. Is the condition acute or chronic? Is it aggravated by sun or physical trauma?
2. The appearance of individual lesions [*see Table 2*]. Is the lesion a vesicle or bulla? Is it tense, flaccid, or umbilicated? Does the skin at the base of the blister appear normal, urticarial, or scarred? Is the blister in the middle of urticarial plaques or on the periphery? Does more than one bulla arise from the same plaque?
3. The grouping of individual lesions. Are the lesions in closely spaced groups (as occurs in herpes simplex), or are they randomly distributed?
4. Sites of involvement. Are lesions on the skin as well as on mucosal surfaces? Are they predominantly on flexural or extensor surfaces; on the palms and soles or on the dorsa of the hands and feet; on the scalp, face, and upper torso; or on areas exposed to trauma?

The most important histologic finding is the layer of skin where the blister forms. If the blister forms in the epidermis, does it form immediately above the basal cell layer or higher up (beneath the stratum corneum)? If it forms in the basement membrane zone, is it within the lamina lucida or below the lamina densa? The precise location may be determined by immunofluorescence procedures.

The most important immunologic finding is the presence or absence of abnormal circulating or tissue-fixed antibodies to skin. These are detected by immunofluorescence techniques: (1) indirect immunofluorescence to detect circulating antibodies and (2) direct immunofluorescence on skin biopsies to detect tissue-fixed antibodies.

Pemphigus

DEFINITION AND PATHOGENESIS

Pemphigus is characterized by blisters that arise within the epidermis and by a loss of cohesion of the epidermal cells (acantholysis) that results in the formation of clefts above the basal cell layer. Autoantibodies directed against adhesion molecules cause epidermal keratinocytes to separate, resulting in intraepidermal bullae. There are two types of pemphigus: deep (e.g., pemphigus vulgaris) and superficial (e.g., pemphigus foliaceus). They differ in the epidermal layers that are injured, in the clinical manifestations of the diseases, and in the associated immunologic abnormalities.[1] In the deep forms, the blisters form immediately above the basal cell layer and are associated with autoantibodies to desmoglein 3, a keratinocyte adhesion molecule. In the superficial forms, the bullae form immediately below the stratum corneum. The superficial forms of pemphigus are associated with antibodies to desmoglein 1.

CLINICAL FEATURES

Pemphigus Vulgaris

Pemphigus vulgaris is the most common form of pemphigus. It can develop at any age but usually occurs in persons between 30 and 60 years old. The disorder tends to affect persons of Mediterranean ancestry but can occur in persons of any ethnicity. Pemphigus is more common in persons with certain HLA allotypes. The occurrence of the disease in first-degree relatives, although rare, suggests an inherited susceptibility transferred as a dominant trait. However, other unknown factors are required for expression of the disorder in predisposed persons.[2] Studies of HLA class II alleles in Japanese patients as well as in other ethnic groups show an association with HLA-DRB1*04 and HLA-DRB1*14 in patients with pemphigus vulgaris across racial lines.[3]

Pemphigus vulgaris usually, but not invariably, begins with chronic, painful, nonhealing ulcerations in the oral cavity [*see Figure 1*]. Bullae are rarely seen because they rupture easily, leaving ulcerated bases. The ulcerations are usually multiple, superficial, and irregular in shape. Any oral mucosal surface can be involved, but the most common sites are the buccal and labial mucosae, the palate, and the tongue. The occurrence of multiple ulcerations differentiates these lesions from ulcerated malignant tumors of the oral cavity, which are usually single. A diagnosis of pemphigus is usually considered only after lesions have been present for weeks to months.

Skin lesions can also be the initial manifestation, beginning as small fluid-filled bullae on otherwise normal-looking skin. The blisters are usually flaccid because the thin overlying epidermis cannot sustain much pressure. Bullae therefore rupture rapidly, usually in several days, and may be absent when a patient is examined. Sharply outlined, coin-sized, superficial erosions with a collarette of loose epidermis around the periphery of the erosions may appear instead. The upper chest, back, scalp, and face are common sites of involvement, but lesions can occur on any part of the body. The condition progresses over weeks to months [*see Figure 2*]. Sites often overlooked include the periungual areas (manifested as painful, erythematous, paronychial swelling), the pharynx and larynx (pain on swallowing and hoarseness), and the nasal cavity (nasal congestion and a bloody mucous discharge, particularly noticeable upon blowing the nose in the morning).

A characteristic feature of all severe active forms of pemphigus is Nikolsky's sign, in which sliding firm pressure on normal-appearing skin causes the epidermis to separate from the dermis. Nikolsky's sign is elicited most easily on normal skin adjacent to an active lesion.

If left untreated, the erosions and bullae of pemphigus vulgaris gradually spread, involving an increasing surface area, and

Table 1 Differentiating Features and Standard Therapy for Selected Blistering Diseases

	Disease	Features	Therapy
Epidermal	Pemphigus vulgaris	Chronic, painful ulcerations in the oral cavity; small, flaccid bullae *or* coin-sized superficial erosions arising from normal skin; positive Nikolsky's sign; IgG and C3 at intercellular spaces; serum antidesmoglein 1 or 3 antibodies	[*See* Pemphigus, Treatment, *in text*]
	Pemphigus vegetans	Hypertrophic proliferation of epidermis in intertriginous areas; IgG and C3 at intercellular spaces; serum antidesmoglein 3 antibodies	[*See* Pemphigus, Treatment, *in text*]
	Pemphigus foliaceus	Small, pruritic, crusted lesions on upper torso, face, or scalp; chronic superficial erosions; rare oral involvement; immunopathology higher in epidermis	[*See* Pemphigus, Treatment, *in text*]
	Pemphigus erythematosus	Erythematous scaly to crusted eruption on face and upper chest; lupuslike immunologic abnormalities (granular deposits of IgG and C3 at epidermal-dermal junction)	[*See* Pemphigus, Treatment, *in text*]
	Fogo selvagem	Features similar to pemphigus foliaceus (primarily affects persons < 30 yr old in rural areas of Brazil, Colombia, Tunisia)	[*See* Pemphigus, Treatment, *in text*]
	Paraneoplastic mixed bullous disease	Large, tense bullae; target lesions on skin; oral erosions; keratinocyte necrosis; subepidermal separation; IC and BMZ antibodies on direct IF	Difficult (standard treatments for autoimmune blistering diseases fail in most patients)
	Hailey-Hailey disease	Multiple vesicles on inflammatory bases in intertriginous areas and other areas subject to friction or pressure; loss of bridges between epidermal cells; no circulating or tissue-fixed autoantibodies	Involved areas kept dry and free of friction; administration of topical and systemic antibiotics; topical, intralesional corticosteroids; ablation of involved areas
Subepidermal	Bullous pemphigoid	Crops of large, tense blisters recurring from urticarial plaques on torso and flexures; negative Nikolsky's sign; oral lesions (10%–25% of patients); circulating BMZ antibodies; IgG and C3 at BMZ in a linear pattern on direct IF	Administration of systemic corticosteroids at doses lower than those used for pemphigus (≤ 80 mg/day prednisone) [*see also* Bullous Pemphigoid, Treatment, *in text*]
	Cicatricial pemphigoid	Blisters on mucosal surfaces (oral cavity, esophagus, eyes) that heal with scarring, often occurring repeatedly at same site; diffuse, painful erythema and atrophy of the gingival mucosa; IgG and C3 at BMZ in a linear pattern on direct IF	Combination therapy with systemic corticosteroids and dapsone or azathioprine; long-term therapy with systemic corticosteroids, sometimes combined with immunosuppressive agents; intralesional corticosteroids
	Herpes gestationis	Pruritic urticarial plaques occurring in pregnancy (beginning around the umbilicus, spreading to abdomen and thighs); laminal blisters with linear deposits of C3 or IgG at the epidermal-dermal junction; circulating complement-fixing BMZ antibodies on indirect IF	Normally clears after delivery
	Dermatitis herpetiformis	Clusters of intensely pruritic, small, polymorphic vesicles on elbows, knees, buttocks, scapular area, and scalp; accumulations of neutrophils and eosinophils in dermal papillae; granular deposits of IgA in BMZ; no circulating antibodies to normal skin components	Administration of sulfones (dapsone, 100–200 mg/day; sulfapyridine, 1–3 g/day in divided doses; or sulfamethoxypyridazine); reduction of gluten intake
	Linear IgA dermatosis	Blisters resembling those of dermatitis herpetiformis or erythema multiforme; linear deposition of IgA in BMZ on direct IF	Administration of sulfones
	Erythema multiforme	Sudden eruption of crops of lesions on elbows, knees, hands, and feet; target papule or vesicle with halo of erythema; subepidermal edema, deep perivascular inflammatory infiltrate	Elimination of underlying causes (e.g., infectious agents, drugs); *in mild cases,* topical glucocorticoids, anti-inflammatories, antipruritics, antibiotics; *in severe cases,* prednisone 40–120 mg/day in divided doses
	Toxic epidermal necrolysis	Rapidly progressive painful denudation of epithelium (usually a drug reaction); full-thickness epidermal necrosis; absence of immune reactants within skin blood vessels; little dermal inflammation	Meticulous wound care with debridement of necrotic tissue, fluid and electrolyte replacement, and prevention of sepsis; I.V. Ig [42]
	Staphylococcal scalded skin syndrome	Scarlatiniform eruption accompanied by skin tenderness, fever, and irritability; lack of mucous membrane involvement or target lesions	Intravenous penicillinase-resistant penicillins
	Epidermolysis bullosa	[*See* Epidermolysis Bullosa, *in text*]	Supportive therapy; counseling; promotion of wound healing; prevention of complications

BMZ—basal membrane zone IC—intercellular IF—immunofluorescence I.V. Ig—intravenous immunoglobulin

Table 2 Pathologic Typology of Blisters[43]

Blister Type	Mode of Formation	Site of Formation	Disease
Subcorneal blister	Detachment of horny layer	Epidermis (subcorneal layer)	Miliaria crystallina Impetigo
Blister due to intracellular degeneration	Separation of cells from one another	Upper epidermis	Friction blisters
Spongiotic blister	Intercellular edema	Epidermis	Dermatitis (eczema) Miliaria rubra
Acantholytic blister	Dissolution of intercellular bridges	Epidermis (suprabasal layer)	Keratosis follicularis (Darier's disease) Pemphigus vulgaris
		Epidermis (subcorneal layer)	Pemphigus foliaceus
Viral blister	Ballooning degeneration leading to acantholysis	Epidermis	Herpes simplex Herpes zoster Varicella
Blister due to degeneration of basal cells	Cytolysis of basal cells	Basal cell layer	Epidermolysis bullosa simplex Erythema multiforme (epidermal type)
	Loss of dermal contact by damaged basal cells	Basal cell layer	Lichen planus Lupus erythematosus
Blister due to degeneration of basement membrane zone	Damage in the structures that cause coherence of basal cells	Basement membrane zone	Bullous pemphigoid Dermatitis herpetiformis Erythema multiforme (dermal type)
Dermolytic blister	Anchoring fibrils are decreased and rudimentary	Dermis	Dystrophic epidermolysis bullosa Acquired epidermolysis bullosa

can become complicated by severe infections and metabolic disturbances. Before the advent of corticosteroids, pemphigus was almost invariably fatal—approximately 75% of patients died within a year.[4] However, as improved techniques have permitted the diagnosis of earlier, milder forms of the disease, the prognosis has become variable. Mild forms may regress spontaneously, and the progression of even the most severe forms can be reversed in most cases. With treatment (see below), lesions normally heal without scarring. Most patients treated for pemphigus will enter a partial remission within 2 to 3 years. They can then be maintained lesion-free with minimal doses of corticosteroids (< 15 mg of prednisone daily). In a longitudinal study of outcome in 40 patients with pemphigus vulgaris, 45% entered a complete and long-term remission after 5 years and 71% after 10

years. Patients in remission remained lesion-free without any therapy.[5] The hyperpigmentation that is commonly associated with pemphigus usually resolves after several months.

In pregnancy, pemphigus appears to be associated with an increased incidence of premature delivery and fetal death.[6] The lesions of pemphigus can appear on the skin of the neonate; however, they normally resolve spontaneously in several weeks.

Pemphigus Foliaceus

Pemphigus foliaceus is the second most common form of pemphigus. It usually begins with small (≤ 1 cm), pruritic, crusted lesions resembling corn flakes on the upper torso and face. The crusts are easily removed, leaving chronic, superficial erosions.

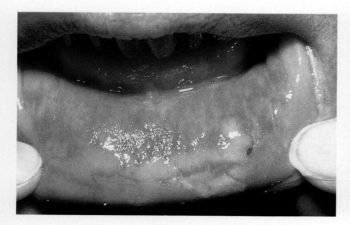

Figure 1 **Painful ulcerations or erosions in the mouth may be present many months before the onset of generalized pemphigus vulgaris.**

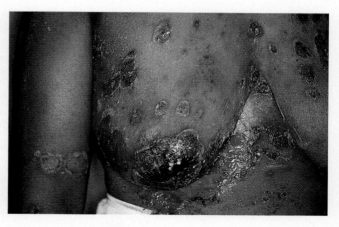

Figure 2 **Flaccid bullae of pemphigus vulgaris have broken down to form erosions and crusts, particularly under the breasts.**

Over weeks to months the condition progresses, with an increasing number of lesions appearing on the upper torso, face, and scalp. In extensive cases, lesions develop over the entire body, become confluent, and can progress to an exfoliative erythroderma. In contrast to the deep forms of pemphigus, oral involvement in pemphigus foliaceus is very rare.

The prognosis of untreated pemphigus foliaceus is more favorable than that of pemphigus vulgaris. The lesions of pemphigus foliaceus are not as deep, and there is less chance for infection, fluid loss, and metabolic disturbance. Although pemphigus foliaceus is less severe, the doses of medications required for control are similar to those used for pemphigus vulgaris. There are two clinical variants, pemphigus erythematosus (also known as Senear-Usher syndrome) and fogo selvagem (Portuguese for "wild fire"; also known as endemic pemphigus and Brazilian pemphigus) [see Table 1].

Drug-Related Pemphigus

Both pemphigus vulgaris and pemphigus foliaceus can be either induced or triggered (i.e., latent disease unmasked) by certain drugs. Pemphigus that continues after a patient stops using a drug is referred to as triggered, whereas lesions that clear soon after withdrawal are referred to as induced. Although drug-related pemphigus is uncommon, its possibility must be excluded in all patients with newly diagnosed disease. The clinical, histologic,[7] and immunofluorescence abnormalities[8] of drug-induced pemphigus are similar to those of the idiopathic variety. However, pemphigus caused by drugs containing a sulfhydryl radical (thiol drugs) is clinically distinct from pemphigus caused by nonthiol drugs. The presence or absence of sulfhydryl radical appears to influence both the type of pemphigus that is expressed and the prognosis of the drug-induced condition. Thiol drugs are more likely to induce pemphigus foliaceus, which is more likely to regress spontaneously when the drug is discontinued [see Chapter 36]. Nonthiol drugs are more likely to trigger pemphigus vulgaris, which can persist even after the drug is stopped. The most commonly implicated agents are thiol drugs such as penicillamine and captopril. Other responsible drugs include sulfur-containing drugs such as penicillins and cephalosporins. These undergo metabolic changes to form thiol groups and are termed masked thiol drugs. Nonthiol drugs that contain an amide group (e.g., dipyrone and enalapril) can provoke a disease that is indistinguishable from spontaneously occurring pemphigus vulgaris.[8]

HISTOLOGIC AND IMMUNOLOGIC FINDINGS

The diagnosis should always be confirmed by histopathologic examination and immunofluorescence studies. Biopsies for pemphigus and all other bullous diseases should be performed at the edge of a lesion, so as to include uninvolved adjacent normal skin. Acantholysis (the separation of keratinocytes from each other) is the fundamental abnormality in all forms of pemphigus.

All forms of pemphigus are associated with circulating and tissue-fixed intercellular (IC) autoantibodies that react against cell-surface keratinocyte antigens. The detection of these antibodies is very helpful in establishing the diagnosis, because they rarely appear in other conditions. Circulating IC autoantibodies are detected by indirect immunofluorescence assays on serum, and tissue-fixed IC autoantibodies are detected by direct immunofluorescence on skin biopsies. In both cases, they cause a lacelike pattern of fluorescence within the epidermis. Low titers of IC autoantibodies may also be present in burns,

fungal infections, and allergic drug reactions. Antigens against ABO, which are present in approximately 5% of the normal population, are the most common cause of false positive tests for IC autoantibodies. Tissue-fixed IC autoantibodies are present in lesions and adjacent normal skin in approximately 90% of patients with pemphigus and are more sensitive and specific for the diagnosis of pemphigus than are circulating IC autoantibodies. The most common autoantibodies are IgG, but IgM and IgA (with or without C3) may also be deposited.

TREATMENT

Initial Therapy

Initial therapy is determined by the extent and rate of progression of lesions. Localized, slowly progressive disease can be treated with intralesional injections of corticosteroids (triamcinolone acetonide, 10 to 20 mg/ml) or topical application of high-potency corticosteroids. New lesions that continue to appear in increasing numbers can be controlled in some cases with low-dose systemic corticosteroids (prednisone, 20 mg/day). Patients with extensive or rapidly progressive disease are treated with moderately high doses of corticosteroids (prednisone, 70 to 90 mg/day). This dose is rapidly escalated every 4 to 14 days in 50% increments until disease activity is controlled, as evidenced by an absence of new lesions and the disappearance of skin pain or itching. If disease activity persists despite high doses of corticosteroids (> 120 to 160 mg/day of prednisone), one of the following approaches should be considered for rapid control:

1. Plasmapheresis, normally performed three times a week for removal of 1 to 2 L of plasma per procedure.[9]
2. Intravenous immunoglobulin (I.V. Ig), is usually given at a dosage of 400 mg/kg/day for 5 days or in higher doses for 3 days.[10] The use of I.V. Ig for the treatment of skin diseases has recently been reviewed.[11] With both I.V. Ig and plasmapheresis it is important to concurrently administer an immunosuppressive agent such as cyclophosphamide or azathioprine to minimize rebound in the level of pemphigus antibodies,[12] and it is also important to monitor the level of these antibodies to ensure that the patient is responding to treatment.
3. Pulse therapy with megadoses of methylprednisolone, given at a dosage of 1 g/day I.V. for 5 days.[13]

No comparative studies have yet evaluated the relative effectiveness of these procedures. On the basis of such limited experience, I.V. Ig may be preferred in some cases because it has fewer side effects than the other procedures and is associated with an unusually high response rate. Once disease activity is controlled, the patient is maintained on the type and dose of medications required to establish control until approximately 80% of lesions are healed. Therapy should not be tapered while new lesions are appearing.

Adjuvant Therapy

The role of adjuvants in the treatment of pemphigus remains controversial. Because of a lack of controlled studies, it is not known whether the potential benefits of adjuvants outweigh the additional toxicities.[2] Indications for adjuvant therapy include the presence of relative contraindications to systemic corticosteroids, development of serious corticosteroid side effects, and repeated flares of disease activity that make it undesirable to reduce corticosteroid doses.[5] Because they require 4 to 6 weeks to become effective, adjuvants are not used to control active, rapidly progressive disease.

Adjuvant treatments for pemphigus include a variety of cytotoxic and immunosuppressive agents (e.g., cyclophosphamide, azathioprine, cyclosporine, methotrexate, and mycophenolate mofetil[14]); dapsone; anti-inflammatory agents (e.g., gold); antimalarials; and certain antibiotics (e.g., tetracycline and minocycline).

Bullous Pemphigoid

PATHOGENESIS

The immediate cause of bullous pemphigoid (BP) appears to be an autoantibody response to the 180 kd (BP180) and 230 kd (BP230) basement membrane zone antigens.[15] Passive transfer of these antibodies into animals can cause lesions of the disease,[16] and anti-BP180 autoantibodies have been found to be a poor prognostic factor in one human study.[17]

CLINICAL FEATURES

BP is a nonscarring, subepidermal blistering disease that is characterized by recurrent crops of large, tense blisters arising from urticarial bases. Lesions normally appear on the torso and flexures, particularly on the inner thighs and axillae. Blisters can range in size from a few millimeters to several centimeters [*see Figure 3*]. They are usually filled with a clear fluid, but they can be hemorrhagic. Erosions are much less common than in pemphigus, and Nikolsky's sign is negative. A characteristic feature is that multiple bullae usually arise from large (palm-sized or larger), irregular, urticarial plaques. This is in contrast to the bullae of erythema multiforme (see below); in erythema multiforme, a single bulla arises from the center of a smaller (coin-sized) urticarial base.

In acute flares of BP, bullae may arise from normal-appearing skin. Oral lesions can occur in 10% to 25% of patients; ocular involvement, however, is rare. Without treatment, the disease may become very extensive.

BP is a sporadic disease that occurs mainly in the elderly but can occur at any age and in any race. It has been reported in a 2-month old infant.[18] Precipitating factors include trauma, burns, ionizing radiation, ultraviolet light, and certain drugs. In a case-control study of 116 incident cases, neuroleptics and diuretics—particularly aldosterone antagonists—were more commonly used in patients with BP than in control subjects.[19] There is still controversy as to whether BP is associated with an increased incidence of cancer[20]; however, correlations between flare in disease activity and recurrence of underlying cancer suggest such an association in individual patients.

BP is characterized by spontaneous remissions followed by flares in disease activity that can persist for years. Even without therapy, BP is often self-limited. Approximately 30% of patients have a complete remission after a mean of 27 months.[21] The disease is nonetheless serious, particularly in older persons.[22] Mortality is low in younger persons but is significant in the elderly. In one study of patients older than 68 years, nearly a third died of the disease or complications (mainly sepsis and cardiovascular disease) within 1 year.[17]

HISTOLOGIC AND IMMUNOLOGIC FINDINGS

The earliest lesion of BP is a blister arising in the lamina lucida, between the basal membrane of keratinocytes and the lamina densa. This is followed by loss of anchoring filaments and hemidesmosomes. Histologically, there is a superficial inflam-

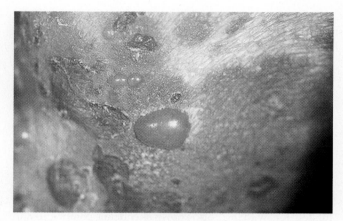

Figure 3   **Tense bullae characteristically occur in bullous pemphigoid.**

matory cell infiltrate and a subepidermal blister without necrotic keratinocytes. The infiltrate consists of lymphocytes and histiocytes and is particularly rich in eosinophils. There is no scarring.

Approximately 70% to 80% of patients with active BP have circulating antibodies to one or more basement membrane zone antigens. On direct immunofluorescence, the antibodies are deposited in a thin linear pattern; and on immunoelectronmicroscopy, they are present in the lamina lucida. By contrast, the antibodies to basement membrane zone antigens that are present in the skin of patients with systemic lupus erythematosus are deposited in a granular pattern.

Two less common subepidermal blistering diseases that are closely related to BP are cicatricial pemphigoid and herpes gestationis [*see Table 1*]. The differential diagnosis also includes dermatitis herpetiformis and acquired epidermolysis bullosa (see below).

TREATMENT

Treatment of BP is generally similar to that of pemphigus.[3] The differences are as follows: (1) BP normally, but not invariably, responds to lower doses of systemic corticosteroids, with most patients improving on prednisone at a dosage of 80 mg/day or less; and (2) BP is more likely to respond to dapsone[23] or to the combination of tetracycline and niacinamide.[24,25] Considering that the prognosis of untreated BP is better than that of pemphigus, side effects of treatment are of greater concern.

Dermatitis Herpetiformis

Dermatitis herpetiformis (DH) is a rare vesiculobullous disease characterized by intensely pruritic, small vesicles that are grouped in small clusters and typically appear on the extensor aspects of extremities and on the buttocks, scalp, and back. The condition is believed to be an immune-mediated disorder and is associated with abnormal granular deposits of IgA at the basement membrane zone and with asymptomatic, gluten-sensitive, spruelike enteropathy. The disease is chronic, with periods of exacerbation and remission. Lesions may clear if patients follow a strict gluten-free diet. Linear IgA dermatosis [*see Table 1*] is an uncommon subepidermal blistering disease that may clinically resemble DH or erythema multiforme (see below).

PATHOGENESIS

The cause of DH is unknown. It may be related to gluten-sensitive celiac disease; there is a strong association between the

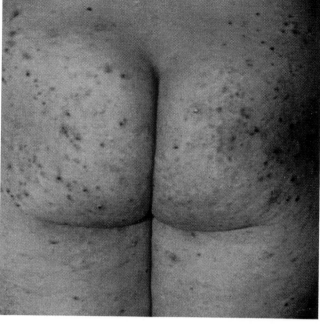

Figure 4 **Dermatitis herpetiformis, an extremely pruritic eruption, commonly presents as excoriated, grouped papulovesicles, often in a symmetrical distribution.**

two conditions, and they share a similar genetic basis (both are associated with HLA-B8 and HLA-DR3). DH is thought to result from an abnormal IgA immune response to an unidentified antigen (possibly found in gluten) that contacts the gut. Skin lesions may result from deposition of immune complexes against this antigen in skin.

CLINICAL FEATURES

Skin lesions of DH are polymorphic. They usually begin as small, very pruritic urticarial papules or vesicles that are grouped in a herpetiform pattern [*see Figure 4*]. Actual vesicles or other primary lesions are rarely seen because they are excoriated by patients' scratching. The distribution of lesions is characteristic: they occur most commonly on the elbows, knees, buttocks, scapular area, and scalp. Sometimes, lesions are scattered over the entire body. The lesions tend to appear suddenly and symmetrically, sometimes after ingestion of large amounts of gluten. Lesions heal, leaving hyperpigmentation; scarring may result from scratching or secondary infection. Involvement of mucous membranes is rare.

The disease is twice as common in men as in women. It predominantly affects persons between the ages of 20 and 50. There may be an associated patchy duodenal and jejunal atrophy that resembles the gluten-sensitive enteropathy of adult celiac disease.[26,27] The enteropathy is usually asymptomatic and, like celiac disease, responds to gluten restriction. Because celiac disease is associated with gastrointestinal lymphoma, there is concern that the same may be true for DH. However, although lymphomas of the small intestine have been reported in DH,[28] the association appears to be rare.

HISTOLOGIC AND IMMUNOLOGIC FINDINGS

Two characteristic laboratory features of DH are used for diagnosis. First, the disease is characterized histologically by accu-mulations of neutrophils and eosinophils in microabscesses at the tips of dermal papillae. In more severe cases, edema appears and can progress to subepidermal blisters appearing just below the lamina densa. Secondly, granular deposits of IgA are found at the basement membrane zone in almost all patients. These are often associated with granular deposits of C3 and, occasionally, of IgG and IgM. When found alone, IgA is one of the most sensitive and specific diagnostic markers for DH. When IgA is found with deposits of IgG, IgM, or C3, immune complex vasculitis and systemic lupus erythematosus are added to the differential diagnosis. Although basement membrane zone deposits of IgA alone also occur in linear IgA disease,[29] the deposits in that condition are linear rather than granular. There are no circulating antibodies to normal skin components in DH.

TREATMENT

DH responds rapidly and dramatically to sulfones. Dapsone at a dosage of 100 to 200 mg/day is most commonly used for treatment. Sulfapyridine at a dosage of 1 to 3 g/day in divided doses (or sulfamethoxypyridazine) can be used in patients who cannot tolerate dapsone. Doses of these drugs are gradually reduced to the lowest amount that will suppress pruritus and development of new lesions. As indicated, patients also respond to a gluten-free diet; however, such diets are difficult to follow. Nevertheless, even a partial decrease in gluten intake will result in a decreased requirement for sulfones and should therefore be encouraged.

Erythema Multiforme

Erythema multiforme is an acute, recurrent, self-limiting disease that affects all age groups and races. It is characterized by the sudden eruption of crops of lesions, which represent a cell-mediated hypersensitivity reaction of the skin and mucous membranes to a variety of precipitating factors, including infectious agents and drugs [*see Table 3*].[30]

CLINICAL FEATURES

Lesions may be localized or widespread and may affect both the skin and the mucous membranes. The eruption often occurs bilaterally and symmetrically on the extensor surfaces of the extremities and on both the dorsal and the volar areas of the hands and feet. Lesions vary from well-defined, red to purple, edematous macules and papules to vesicular or bullous lesions that may ulcerate, encrust, erode, and become infected. A target lesion consisting of a papule or vesicle surrounded by a region of normal skin and a halo of erythema at the periphery [*see Figure 5*] is characteristic.

Stevens-Johnson syndrome is a severe form of erythema multiforme that is usually disseminated, fulminant, and multisystemic [*see Figure 6*]. The syndrome may be accompanied by high fever, malaise, chills, headache, tachycardia, tachypnea, and prostration. The mucous membranes in the mouth, the anus, and the vagina contain round or oval erythematous macules that form vesicles, bullae, and ulcers. Ocular lesions are bilateral yellowish-gray papules that often ulcerate and become secondarily infected, resulting in conjunctivitis. Ocular involvement has produced blindness.

Toxic epidermal necrolysis (TEN), considered by some to be a form of erythema multiforme, is often a reaction to medication (e.g., certain long-acting sulfonamides [particularly trimethoprim-sulfamethoxazole], anticonvulsants, barbiturates, and nonsteroidal anti-inflammatory drugs). The absence of im-

Table 3 Precipitating Factors in
Erythema Multiforme

Viral diseases	Herpes simplex Hepatitis Influenza A Vaccinia Mumps
Fungal diseases	Dermatophytoses Histoplasmosis Coccidioidomycosis
Bacterial diseases	Hemolytic streptococcal infections Tuberculosis Leprosy Typhoid
Collagen vascular disorders	Rheumatoid arthritis Systemic lupus erythematosus Dermatomyositis Allergic vasculitis Polyarteritis nodosa
Malignant tumors	Carcinoma Lymphoma after radiation therapy
Hormonal changes	Pregnancy Menstruation
Drugs	Penicillins Sulfonamides Barbiturates Salicylates Halogens Phenolphthalein
Miscellaneous	*Rhus* dermatitis Dental extractions *Mycoplasma pneumoniae* infection

mune reactants within the blood vessels in the skin and the paucity of dermal inflammation have led other researchers to consider TEN a separate disease . Staphylococcal scalded skin syndrome, which results from toxins produced by *Staphylococcus aureus*,[31] is sometimes confused with TEN [*see Table 1*].

HISTOLOGIC AND IMMUNOLOGIC FINDINGS

Characteristic cutaneous histologic findings of erythema multiforme include subepidermal edema, bulla formation, epidermal cell necrosis, and a deep perivascular inflammatory infiltrate. There are no specific immunofluorescent findings, although direct immunofluorescence may show granular deposits of C3 and fibrin at the dermoepidermal junction and deposits of IgM, C3, and fibrin in the dermal blood vessels. Recurrent erythema multiforme is frequently associated with herpes simplex viral infections, as reported in 71% of a series of 65 patients with erythema multiforme. Circulating immune complexes to the herpes simplex virus may be present in such patients.[32]

TREATMENT

Erythema multiforme eruptions may recur without warning, despite preventive measures. It is therefore important to identify and eliminate underlying causes. Mild cases are treated symptomatically with topical glucocorticoids and topical anti-inflammatory, antipruritic, or antibiotic preparations. Oral

acyclovir may be effective in the prophylaxis of recurrent postherpetic erythema multiforme. In more severe cases, treatment with prednisone, 40 to 120 mg/day in divided doses, is indicated. If the eyes are involved, prompt ophthalmologic consultation should be obtained.

Epidermolysis Bullosa

Epidermolysis bullosa (EB) comprises a group of genetically based disorders with a prevalence of approximately one in 500,000 persons. There are more than 20 different phenotypes of EB, which may be inherited as an autosomal recessive trait. These disorders are characterized by blistering and erosions that heal with or without scarring after minor skin trauma or friction. Extent of involvement ranges from localized blisters (e.g., on the palms and soles) to severe widespread sloughing of the skin, with a risk of severe morbidity and mortality due to infection, fluid and electrolyte imbalance, anemia, or other complications.

EB is classified primarily on the basis of an ultrastructural level of skin cleavage in the basement membrane zone [*see Figure 7*]. Three major subtypes include EB simplex or epidermolytic (intraepidermal), junctional EB (intra–lamina lucida), and dystrophic or dermolytic EB (sub–lamina densa). Electron microscopy examination localizes the lesions to a specific lay-

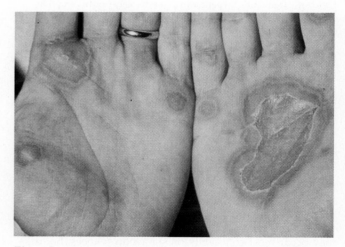

Figure 5 **Target lesions are characteristic of erythema multiforme.**

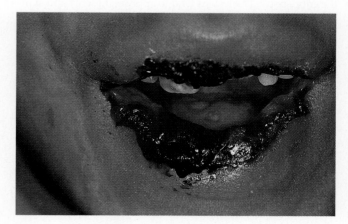

Figure 6 **Stevens-Johnson syndrome is a fulminating form of erythema multiforme associated with marked mucocutaneous involvement, eye involvement, and severe constitutional symptoms.**

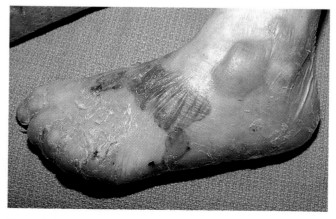

EPIDERMIS

BASEMENT MEMBRANE

DERMIS

Basal Cell Layer

Lamina Lucida

Lamina Densa

Anchoring Fibrils

Figure 7 Three major forms of epidermolysis bullosa (EB) have been recognized: EB simplex, in which a split occurs within the basal cell layer; junctional EB, which is characterized by separation within the lamina lucida; and dystrophic EB, in which separation occurs below the basement membrane zone.

er.[33] Because this technology may not be widely available, immunofluorescence mapping with monoclonal antibodies can be used to target components of the basement membrane layers such as BP antigen (basal cell layer), laminin (lamina lucida), and type IV collagen (lamina densa).[34] The prenatal diagnosis may be made by immunocytochemical probes for antigenic components of the basement membrane in fetal skin biopsy, such as in the junctional EB pyloric atresia syndrome.[35]

EPIDERMOLYSIS BULLOSA SIMPLEX

There are at least five forms of EB simplex. The most common type is a mild autosomal dominant form that appears at birth or shortly thereafter as either localized or generalized blisters that do not usually result in scarring. A second type is Weber-Cockayne disease, which can be either localized or generalized. In the localized form, blisters appear acrally on the palms and soles during childhood or adolescence. In the generalized form, disease activity is usually greater in a warm climate.

The Dowling-Meara variant (EB herpetiformis) is a less common form of EB simplex that presents as severe generalized blistering in infancy; it resembles recessive junctional and dystrophic EB. EB herpetiformis becomes less severe with age.

JUNCTIONAL EPIDERMOLYSIS BULLOSA

Junctional EB is a recessively inherited group of disorders that exhibit a decreased number and hypoplasia of hemidesmosomes, as revealed by electron microscopy, and separation at the level of the lamina lucida. Mucosal involvement and dystrophic nails are common. The most severe form, EB letalis, occurs within the first few days or months of life and has a high mortality. Patients with EB letalis have a high incidence of respiratory arrest at an early age because of laryngeal and tracheal involvement. Less severe forms of junctional EB exhibit severe generalized blistering at birth that gradually improves. Esophageal strictures may develop.

DYSTROPHIC EPIDERMOLYSIS BULLOSA

There are two forms of dystrophic EB that are inherited in an autosomal dominant fashion. Hyperplastic EB dystrophica

(Cockayne-Touraine syndrome) appears in early infancy or childhood as serosanguineous blisters, predominantly on extensor aspects of the lower extremities, in association with nail dystrophy. The albopapuloid type of EB dystrophica is characterized by white papules that develop during adolescence on the trunk or extremities; however, blistering is present in the perinatal period. In both forms, ultrastructural examination reveals sublaminal dermal separation, with abnormalities in anchoring fibrils or a decrease in their number.

Recessive forms of EB dystrophica appear during the neonatal period as severe serosanguineous blistering that is either localized to sites of skin trauma or generalized. Milium formation is uncommon, but lesional scarring may result. Other complications include dental abnormalities, nail dystrophy or loss, digital fusion, flexion contractures, and esophageal strictures [*see Figure 8*]. Growth retardation, malnutrition, and chronic anemia also occur. Patients with recessive EB dystrophica are at increased risk for squamous cell carcinoma, with a high incidence of fatal metastases.

Prenatal diagnosis of recessive dystrophic EB may be made by fetoscopy and skin biopsy; ultrastructural analysis of the tissue reveals dermolytic blister formation. An alternative method for diagnosing suspected recessive dystrophic EB involves a biochemical test for enhanced expression of collagenase by fetal fibroblasts.[36]

Supportive treatment of EB is directed toward promotion of wound healing and prevention of complications. Daily skin care may include wet dressings or whirlpool baths, antibiotic ointment, and nonadhesive dressings, such as fine-mesh gauze (N-terface). A multidisciplinary approach that includes genetic counseling, psychological or psychiatric counseling, and support systems for the patient and family is essential, particularly for managing the severe forms of the disease.

A national registry has been established by the Dystrophic Epidermolysis Bullosa Research Association of America (http://www.debra.org) to collect epidemiologic data, to assess economic and social aspects of EB, and to register patients willing to participate in various research protocols.

ACQUIRED EPIDERMOLYSIS BULLOSA

Onset of blistering in adults in whom there is no genetic basis for disease is called acquired epidermolysis bullosa, or epidermolysis bullosa acquisita (EBA). Both circulating and tissue-bound IgG anti–basement membrane zone antibodies may be

Figure 8 Recessive dystrophic epidermolysis bullosa may cause severe scarring and syndactyly.

demonstrated by immunohistology. The blisters develop below the epidermis and heal with atrophic scars and malformation. They are usually confined to the extremities at sites of mechanical trauma. Oral lesions and nail dystrophy may be associated with EBA. Underlying malignant, autoimmune, and inflammatory diseases may be associated with this condition. The presence of ulcerative colitis or Crohn's disease in approximately 30% of cases suggests that EBA should be included among the extraintestinal manifestations of inflammatory bowel disease.[37]

The diagnosis is made by excluding other bullous disorders, particularly BP (see above). Immunoelectron microscopy may be used as an additional diagnostic aid, although this technique may not be widely available. Direct immunofluorescence with the use of salt-split skin to separate the lamina lucida aids in the differential diagnosis. With this method, the IgG antibodies appear on the dermal side of the split specimens in EBA and on the epidermal side in pemphigoid.[38] The antigen of EBA has been identified as the globular carboxyl terminus of type VII procollagen.[39]

Differential Diagnosis of Vesiculobullous Disorders

The major forms of bullous diseases occurring on an autoimmune or inherited basis have been discussed. The differential diagnosis includes a number of additional conditions in which vesicles or bullae are less common or appear secondary to other disease processes. A fixed drug eruption may produce localized bullae that appear after ingestion of a particular drug [see Chapter 36]. Eczematous dermatitis results in spongiotic vesicles caused by intercellular edema [see Chapter 34]. This is manifested clinically by large bullae in acute allergic contact dermatitis due to poison ivy or poison oak dermatitis. Systemic lupus erythematosus [see Chapter 114] occasionally produces bullae by causing degeneration of basal cells.

A bullous eruption on the dorsa of the hands and other sun-exposed sites in patients receiving long-term hemodialysis may resemble porphyria cutanea tarda [see Chapter 55].[40] Porphyrin levels are usually within normal limits. Intraepidermal or subepidermal bullae, primarily on the extremities, may be a cutaneous sign of diabetes mellitus.[41] Bacterial infections of the skin, such as impetigo, may be associated with subcorneal bulla formation.

Various viral infections, including varicella (chickenpox), herpes simplex, and herpes zoster, also must be considered in the differential diagnosis [see Chapters 37, 133, and 148].

References

1. Korman NJ, Eyre RW, Klaus-Kovtun V, et al: Demonstration of an adhering-junction molecule (plakoglobin) in the autoantigens of pemphigus foliaceus and pemphigus vulgaris. N Engl J Med 321:631, 1989

2. Starzycki Z, Chorzelski TP, Jablonska S: Familial pemphigus vulgaris in mother and daughter. Int J Dermatol 37:211, 1998

3. Miyagawa S, Higashimine I, Iida T, et al: HLA-DRB1*04 and DRB1*14 alleles are associated with susceptibility to pemphigus among Japanese. J Invest Dermatol 109:615, 1997

4. Bystryn JC, Steinmen NM: The adjuvant therapy of pemphigus: an update. Arch Dermatol 132:203, 1996

5. Herbst A, Bystryn JC: Remissions in pemphigus. J Invest Dermatol 106:850, 1996

6. Ruach M, Ohel G, Rahav D, et al: Pemphigus vulgaris and pregnancy. Obstet Gynecol Surv 50:755, 1995

7. Landau M, Brenner S: Histopathologic findings in drug-induced pemphigus. Am J Dermatopathol 19:411, 1997

8. Brenner S, Bialy-Golan A, Anhalt GJ: Recognition of pemphigus antigens in drug-induced pemphigus vulgaris and pemphigus foliaceus. J Am Acad Dermatol 36:919, 1997

9. Tan-Lim R, Bystryn JC: Effect of plasmapheresis therapy on circulating levels of pemphigus antibodies. J Am Acad Dermatol 22:35, 1990

10. Beckers RC, Brand A, Vermeer BJ, et al: Adjuvant high-dose intravenous gammaglobulin in the treatment of pemphigus and bullous pemphigoid: experience in six patients. Br J Dermatol 133:289, 1995

11. Jolles S, Hughes J, Whittaker S: Dermatological uses of high-dose intravenous immunoglobulin. Arch Dermatol 134:80, 1998

12. Auerbach R, Bystryn JC: Plasmapheresis and immunosuppressive therapy: effect on levels of intercellular antibodies in pemphigus vulgaris. Arch Dermatol 115:728, 1979

13. Werth VP: Treatment of pemphigus vulgaris with brief, high-dose intravenous glucocorticoids. Arch Dermatol 132:1435, 1996

14. Enk AH, Knop J: Treatment of pemphigus vulgaris with mycophenolate mofetil. Lancet 350:494, 1997

15. Moll R, Moll I: Epidermal adhesion molecules and basement membrane components as target structures of autoimmunity. Virchows Arch 432:487, 1998

16. Lin MS, Mascaro JM Jr, Liu Z, et al: The desmosome and hemidesmosome in cutaneous autoimmunity. Clin Exp Immunol 107(suppl 1):9, 1997

17. Bernard P, Bedane C, Bonnetblanc JM: Anti-BP180 autoantibodies as a marker of poor prognosis in bullous pemphigoid: a cohort analysis of 94 elderly patients. Br J Dermatol 136:694, 1997

18. Cunha PR, Thomazeski PV, Hipolito E, et al: Bullous pemphigoid in a 2-month-old infant. Int J Dermatol 37:935, 1998

19. Bastuji-Garin S, Joly P, Picard-Dahan C, et al: Drugs associated with bullous pemphigoid: a case-control study. Arch Dermatol 132:272, 1996

20. Ogawa H, Sakuma M, Morioka S, et al: The incidence of internal malignancies in pemphigus and bullous pemphigoid in Japan. J Dermatol Sci 9:136, 1995

21. Chang YT, Liu HN, Wong CK: Bullous pemphigoid: a report of 86 cases from Taiwan. Clin Exp Derm 21:20, 1996

22. Roujeau JC, Lok C, Bastuji-Garin S, et al: High risk of death in elderly patients with extensive bullous pemphigoid. Arch Dermatol 134:465, 1998

23. Bouscarat F, Chosidow O, Picard-Dahan C, et al: Treatment of bullous pemphigoid with dapsone: retrospective study of thirty-six cases. J Am Acad Dermatol 34:683, 1996

24. Hornschuh B, Hamm H, Wever S, et al: Treatment of 16 patients with bullous pemphigoid with oral tetracycline and niacinamide and topical clobetasol. J Am Acad Dermatol 36:101, 1997

25. Thornfeldt CR, Menkes AW: Bullous pemphigoid controlled by tetracycline. J Am Acad Dermatol 16:305, 1987

26. Brow JR, Parker F, Weinstein WM, et al: The small intestinal mucosa in dermatitis herpetiformis: I. Severity and distribution of the small intestinal lesion and associated malabsorption. Gastroenterology 60:355, 1971

27. Katz SI, Hall RP III, Lawley TJ, et al: Dermatitis herpetiformis: the skin and the gut. Ann Intern Med 93:857, 1980

28. Jenkins D, Lynde CW, Stewart WD: Histiocytic lymphoma occurring in a patient with dermatitis herpetiformis. J Am Acad Dermatol 9:252, 1983

29. Prost C, De Leca AC, Combemale P, et al: Diagnosis of adult linear IgA dermatosis by immunoelectronmicroscopy in 16 patients with linear IgA deposits. J Invest Dermatol 92:39, 1989

30. Fine JD: Management of acquired bullous skin diseases. N Engl J Med 333:1475, 1995

31. Manders SM: Toxin-mediated streptococcal and staphylococcal disease. J Am Acad Dermatol 39:383, 1998

32. Schofield JK, Tatnall FM, Leigh IM: Recurrent erythema multiforme: clinical features and treatment in a large series of patients. Br J Dermatol 128:542, 1993

33. Fine JD: Epidermolysis bullosa: clinical aspects, pathology, and recent advances in research. Int J Dermatol 25:143, 1986

34. Hintner H, Stingl G, Schuler G, et al: Immunofluorescence mapping of antigenic determinants within the dermal-epidermal junction in the mechanobullous diseases. J Invest Dermatol 76:113, 1981

35. Shimizu H, Fine JD, Suzumori K, et al: Prenatal exclusion of pyloric atresia-junctional epidermolysis bullosa syndrome. J Am Acad Dermatol 31:429, 1994

36. Bauer EA, Ludman MD, Goldberg JD, et al: Antenatal diagnosis of recessive dystrophic epidermolysis bullosa: collagenase expression in cultured fibroblasts as a biochemical marker. J Invest Dermatol 87:597, 1986

37. Raab B, Fretzin DF, Bronson DM, et al: Epidermolysis bullosa acquisita and inflammatory bowel disease. JAMA 250:1746, 1983

38. Gammon WR, Kowalewski C, Chorzelski TP, et al: Direct immunofluorescence studies of sodium chloride–separated skin in the differential diagnosis of bullous pemphigoid and epidermolysis bullosa acquisita. J Am Acad Dermatol 22:664, 1990

39. Woodley DT, Burgeson RE, Lunstrum G, et al: The epidermolysis bullosa acquisita antigen is the globular carboxyl terminus of type VII procollagen. J Clin Invest 81:683, 1988

40. Goldsman CI, Taylor JS: Porphyria cutanea tarda and bullous dermatoses associated with chronic renal failure: a review. Cleve Clin Q 50:151, 1983

41. Perez MI, Kohn SR: Cutaneous manifestations of diabetes mellitus. J Am Acad Dermatol 30:519, 1994

42. Viard I, Wehrli P, Bullani R, et al: Inhibition of toxic epidermal necrolysis by blockade of CD95 with human intravenous immunoglobulin. Science 282:490, 1998

43. Elder D, Elenitsas R, Jaworsky C, et al: Lever's Histopathology of the Skin, 8th ed. Lippincott-Raven, Philadelphia, 1997

40 Benign Cutaneous Tumors

Elizabeth A. Abel, M.D.

General Considerations

CLASSIFICATION

Tumors of the cutaneous surface may arise from the epidermis, dermis, or subcutaneous tissue or from any of the specialized cell types in the skin or its appendages. Broad categories include tumors derived from epithelial, melanocytic, or connective tissue structures. Within each location or cell type, lesions are classified as benign, malignant, or, in certain cases, premalignant.[1,2]

Benign epithelial tumors include tumors of the surface epidermis that form keratin; tumors of the epidermal appendages; and cysts of the skin.

Melanocytic, or pigment-forming, lesions are very common. One of the most frequently encountered forms is the nevus cell nevus. The term nevus has two meanings: a malformation commonly involving the entire skin layer (tissue nevus) and a benign growth of melanocytic cells (nevus cells).

Nevus cells are closely related to melanocytes and may be defined as modified neuroectodermal melanin-producing elements. The word mole, often used as a synonym for nevus, is an imprecise term because it refers to birthmarks that may or may not contain nevus cells. Neural tumors, such as neurofibromas, are related to melanocytic tumors because both are of neuroectodermal origin.

Tumors that are derived from connective tissue include fibromas, histiocytomas, lipomas, leiomyomas, and hemangiomas.

HISTOLOGIC EVALUATION

For cases in which it is not possible to distinguish clinically between benign and malignant cutaneous tumors, histopathologic examination is extremely important. The type of biopsy performed depends on the location, size, and nature of the lesion and on cosmetic considerations. In all cases, the clinical features must be correlated with the distinctive microscopic appearance of the tumor to confirm or exclude the diagnosis on the basis of physical examination.

Epithelial Tumors

SEBORRHEIC KERATOSIS

Diagnosis and Classification

Seborrheic keratosis (seborrheic wart) consists of a sharply circumscribed, rough or smooth papule or plaque that is 1 mm to several centimeters in size and dirty yellow or light to dark brown in color. The lesions often have the appearance of being stuck on and are characterized by prominent follicular plugging. They are most common in light-skinned races, first appearing in adults on the face and upper trunk and occurring more frequently with increasing age [*see Figure 1*].

Transient eruptive seborrheic keratoses have been associated with inflammatory skin conditions, including erythroderma associated with psoriasis and drug eruptions. These keratoses tend to resolve when the skin inflammation clears.[3] These transient keratoses should be distinguished from eruptive seborrheic keratoses—the sign of Leser-Trelat—which are associated with internal malignancy, particularly adenocarcinoma. The true value of the sign of Leser-Trelat as a marker of underlying malignancy is a subject of debate.

Dermatosis papulosa nigra is similar to seborrheic keratosis, but it is seen in dark-skinned races; it usually appears on the face and presents at an earlier age than seborrheic keratosis [*see Figure 2*].

Differential Diagnosis

The differential diagnosis of seborrheic keratosis and dermatosis papulosa nigra includes lentigo, wart, and nevus cell nevus. A biopsy may be required to rule out a pigmented basal cell carcinoma or, in the case of an inflamed seborrheic keratosis, malignant melanoma or squamous cell carcinoma. A shave biopsy that includes the base of the lesion may be performed before treatment with curettage.

Treatment

Curettage is a satisfactory treatment. When multiple lesions are present, anesthesia may be achieved by freezing the affected area with an ethyl chloride spray before performing curettage. For larger lesions, electrodesiccation is unnecessary and may cause scarring. Smaller lesions may be successfully treated with electrodesiccation, cryotherapy, or topical application of 50% trichloroacetic acid.

EPIDERMAL NEVUS

Diagnosis

Epidermal nevus consists of closely set, skin-colored or hyperpigmented papules that either may be localized to one side of the body and arranged in linear fashion or may be widespread. When localized, the condition is termed nevus unius lateris [*see Figure 3*]. When widespread, it is called systematized nevus. Lesions affect about one in 1,000 people; they are present at birth or appear in early childhood. The lesions have no malignant potential but may constitute a serious cosmetic problem.

Histologically, epidermal nevi exhibit hyperplasia of the epidermis; the structure or maturation of these lesions is not significantly different from that of normal epidermis. One variant, the inflammatory linear verrucous epidermal nevus, shows psori-

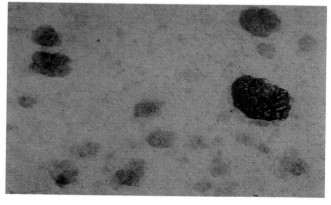

Figure 1 **Verrucous, hyperpigmented lesions of seborrheic keratosis with a stuck-on appearance are present on the trunk of this patient.**

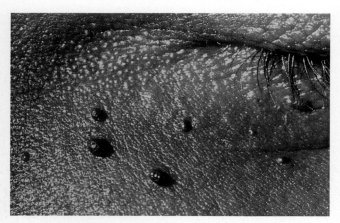

Figure 2 Dermatosis papulosa nigra, as seen on the face, appears in dark-skinned races at a younger age than seborrheic keratosis.

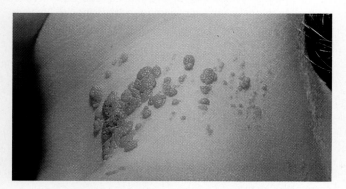

Figure 3 Epidermal nevus with discrete and confluent brown papillomas is present in a somewhat linear arrangement.

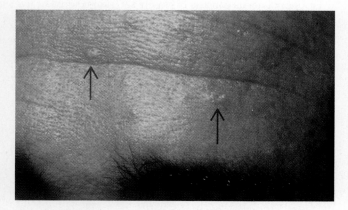

Figure 4 Skin-colored or yellowish, often umbilicated papules of sebaceous hyperplasia, as seen on the forehead, may clinically resemble basal cell carcinomas.

asiform hyperplasia. Another variant, which is common in systematized nevi, shows granular degeneration of epidermolytic hyperkeratosis histologically. This type of epidermal nevus is a mosaic genetic disorder of suprabasal keratin. Mutations in the *K10* gene are associated with lesions of the skin, whereas the normal gene is found in unaffected skin.[4]

Variants

The epidermal nevus syndrome involves a spectrum of different types of epidermal nevi associated with disturbances in the skeletal, urogenital, cardiovascular, and nervous systems.[5] This rare syndrome is apparent at birth; the presence of widespread epidermal nevi should trigger a search for associated anomalies.

Nevus comedonicus is a variant of an epidermal nevus affecting the pilosebaceous structures; it occurs as clusters of comedonelike papules, usually in a linear pattern on the face, neck, upper arms, and trunk.[5]

Nevus sebaceous is a benign tumor that shows sebaceous differentiation. The lesion has a yellow hue and a granular surface and occurs in a linear pattern on the face or scalp. At puberty, nevus sebaceous may become more elevated; in adulthood, there is an associated risk of basal cell carcinoma.

Treatment

Treatment of epidermal nevi with electrodesiccation and curettage is often unsuccessful and may cause scarring. Surgical or laser removal may be indicated for localized lesions. Disturbances involving other organ systems must be evaluated and managed appropriately through a multidisciplinary approach.

Tumors of the Epidermal Appendages

There are a large number of benign tumors of the hair follicles, the sebaceous glands, and the apocrine and eccrine glands. Solitary skin tumors of these epidermal appendages are typically nonhereditary, whereas multiple neoplasms may show an autosomal dominant inheritance pattern.[6]

SEBACEOUS HYPERPLASIA

Sebaceous hyperplasia is a common clinical condition that appears as multiple skin-colored or yellowish, often umbilicated papules or plaques, usually on the forehead, nose, or cheeks of persons after the fifth decade of life. These lesions consist of enlarged sebaceous gland lobules with a central dilated duct. Sebaceous hyperplasia may respond to cryotherapy with liquid nitrogen or the application of a dilute solution of trichloroacetic or bichloroacetic acid. Lesions may sometimes be confused clinically with basal cell carcinoma [*see Figure 4*]. In the familial form of this disorder, onset occurs in puberty; with the passage of time, the lesions increase in extent over the face, neck, and upper thorax. This condition must be distinguished from acne vulgaris, rosacea, and the angiofibromas of tuberous sclerosis. Three patients with this condition responded favorably to oral isotretinoin at a dosage of 1 mg/kg/day. To maintain the response, this dosage was tapered after 6 weeks.[7] Isotretinoin is a known teratogen that cannot be given to women who are of childbearing age unless strict precautions are observed [*see Chapter 31*].

TRICHOEPITHELIOMAS

Trichoepitheliomas usually present as multiple yellowish-pink, translucent papules distributed symmetrically on the cheeks, eyelids, and nasolabial areas [*see Figure 5*]. Often inherited as an autosomal dominant trait, the papules first appear at puberty and grow slowly for years. The gene for multiple familial trichoepitheliomas has been mapped to chromosome 9p21.[8] Lesions may be confused both clinically and histologically with basal cell carcinoma, though trichoepithelioma usually shows differentiation toward the formation of hair. A single or localized trichoepithelioma may be removed by electrodesiccation and curettage. Multiple lesions are difficult to treat and may be a cosmetic problem.

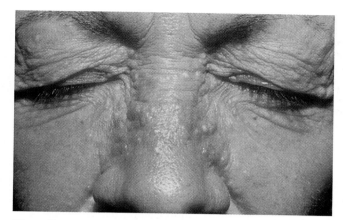

Figure 5 **Symmetrical papules of trichoepithelioma appear on the eyelids and nasolabial areas and may be inherited as an autosomal dominant trait.**

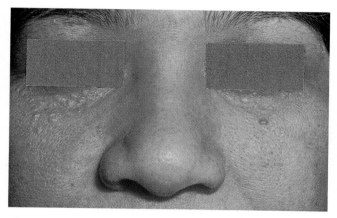

Figure 6 **Syringomas—benign tumors of eccrine ducts—are commonly seen on the face, especially on the lower eyelids.**

SYRINGOMAS

Syringomas usually present in groups of multiple small papules that are distributed symmetrically over the face, especially on the lower eyelids [*see Figure 6*]. Eruptive syringoma, a rare condition, is characterized by widespread lesions.

Histologically, there is a benign proliferation of the eccrine ducts.

EPIDERMOID CYST

Diagnosis

Commonly called wens, epidermoid cysts have a lining that resembles the epidermis. Several types of cyst exist, but they are usually clinically indistinguishable from one another. On histologic examination, most of these cysts appear to be derived from hair follicles.

The epidermoid cyst is commonly located on the back and consists of one or more slow-growing, elevated, firm nodules, often with a central pore [*see Figure 7*]. The diameters of the lesions vary from 0.2 to 5.0 cm.

Treatment

The epidermoid cyst may be incised with a pointed scalpel to express its wall and contents, which consist of a thick keratinous material. If the cyst wall is not completely removed, there

may be a recurrence of the lesion. Occasionally, the entire cyst has to be excised. Preliminary treatment with a systemic antibiotic, such as erythromycin, and warm-water compresses applied three or four times daily may be instituted if the cyst is inflamed and infected. When the inflammation and infection resolve, the lesion can be removed. Repeated episodes of infection may cause fibrosis, after which the cyst may have to be surgically excised.

Other Cysts

The pilar cyst, which is less common, has a wall that contains keratin similar to that found in hair. The contents of these cysts are semifluid and often have a rancid odor.

A milium is similar to an epidermoid cyst but differs mainly in size. Milia are white, hard subepidermal keratin cysts, 1 to 2 mm in diameter, that commonly arise spontaneously on the face [*see Figure 8*]. They may also arise secondarily in scars or in association with certain bullous diseases. Incision and expression of contents with a comedo extractor may be performed.

Familial Tumor Syndromes

Multiple cutaneous neoplasms may be a feature of familial tumor syndromes that are thought to be mediated by inactiva-

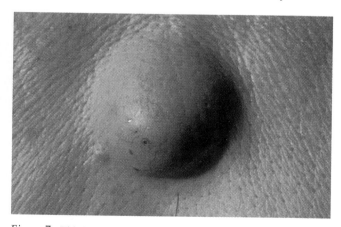

Figure 7 **This large epidermoid cyst has a central pore, contains thick keratinous material, and has a lining that resembles the epidermis.**

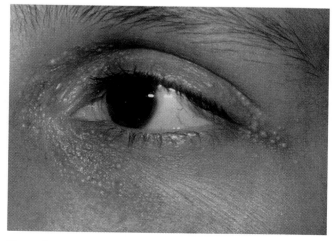

Figure 8 **Milia, which are multiple small subepidermal inclusion cysts, can be observed in the periorbital area of this patient.**

tion of tumor suppressor genes. It is important to recognize these syndromes because they may be associated with underlying malignancies.

MUIR-TORRE SYNDROME

Muir-Torre syndrome (MTS), previously known as Torre syndrome, consists of sebaceous gland neoplasms that are associated with visceral carcinoma and that arise from colonic epithelium. Sebaceous gland tumors may include, in decreasing order of frequency, adenomas, epitheliomas, and carcinomas.[9] Keratoacanthomas and sebaceous hyperplasia are also seen in patients with MTS. Colorectal cancer develops in 51% of patients with MTS a decade earlier than it develops in the general population. Genitourinary cancer develops in 24% of MTS patients. A germline mutation in the DNA mismatch repair gene *hMSH2* has been identified in patients with MTS. Predictive diagnosis in family members should be preceded by careful genetic counseling.[9]

GARDNER SYNDROME

Gardner syndrome consists of the triad of intestinal polyposis, bony tumors, and soft tissue lesions; it has an autosomal dominant inheritance. The colonic polyps eventually become malignant if left untreated. Soft tissue lesions include epidermoid cysts, sebaceous cysts, desmoid tumors, and scattered lentigines on the head and extremities.[10]

COWDEN SYNDROME

Cowden syndrome is characterized by facial trichilemmomas and acral fibromas, and it is associated with an increased risk of cancer of the breast, thyroid, and gastrointestinal tract. This rare genodermatosis, which is also known as multiple hamartoma syndrome, is inherited as an autosomal dominant trait. It is important to make a prompt diagnosis of this syndrome because of the high risk of malignancy, particularly cancer of the breast in women.

BIRT-HOGG-DUBÉ SYNDROME

Birt-Hogg-Dubé syndrome (BHDS) is an autosomal dominant multisystem disorder characterized by the cutaneous triad of fibrofolliculomas, trichodiscomas, and acrochordons. Fibrofolliculomas are benign tumors of the hair follicle. Fibrofolliculomas are firm, pink or skin-colored papules measuring 1 to 3 mm that appear on the face, particularly the nose, earlobes, and forehead. In the original kindred described by Birt (a dermatologist), Hogg (a pathologist), and Dubé (a pathologist), family members were afflicted with medullary carcinoma of the thyroid. Subsequently, there appeared reports of patients with BHDS who had intestinal polyps, adenocarcinoma of the colon, parathyroid adenomas, and renal cell carcinoma. The skin tumors begin in early adulthood; systemic tumors appear years later. In families with recognized renal cell carcinoma, BHDS may account for 6% of the cases.[11,12]

Melanocytic (Pigment-Forming) Tumors

Benign tumors of pigment-forming cells, including those containing nevus cells (melanocytic nevi) and those of epidermal or dermal melanocytes, are of neuroectodermal origin.

MELANOCYTIC NEVUS

Melanocytic nevus, also called nevus cell nevus, has a characteristic life history of evolution and involution. Melanocytic nevi are the most common of all skin tumors; each young adult has an average of 20 to 40 of them. Their incidence increases with age up to the second or third decade of life, after which they occur less commonly.

Risk Factors for Melanoma

An increase in the total number of melanocytic nevi is a risk factor for melanoma.[13] In a study of 716 patients with newly diagnosed melanoma, an increased number of small nevi (25 to 49) was associated with a twofold increase in risk of melanoma; greater numbers of nevi were associated with further increased risk.[14] The presence of one clinically dysplastic nevus was associated with a twofold increase in risk of melanoma; and 10 or more, with a 12-fold increase in risk. Criteria for dysplastic nevi included large size (over 5 mm), flatness (entirely macular or having a macular component), and at least two of the following: irregular pigmentation, asymmetry, and indistinct borders [*see Chapter 41*]. The presence of freckling conferred additional risk of melanoma for all types of nevi.

The relation between sun exposure and melanocytic nevi has been investigated to determine what environmental factors influence melanoma and to facilitate preventive measures. Studies suggest that melanocytic nevi are more common on sun-exposed skin sites and reach a peak incidence earlier in age on these sites than on covered areas of the body.[15] A study of Australian schoolchildren showed an increasing prevalence of nevi with decreasing latitude, particularly in children 6 and 9 years of age.[16] Sun exposure during childhood was considered to be a factor in the development of melanocytic nevi and an associated risk factor for melanoma.[16] In Australia, however, sun exposure may be sufficient to maximally induce nevi regardless of latitude. Further studies need to be performed on persons living at higher latitudes to see whether the relation between sun exposure and nevi continues into adulthood.

Diagnosis

A melanocytic nevus that is present at birth or appears during the first year of life is considered to be congenital. Certain syndromes are associated with congenital nevi, including epidermal (linear sebaceous) nevus syndrome, neurocutaneous melanosis, premature-aging syndrome, and occult spinal dysraphism or tethered cord syndrome.[17] Various neuroectodermal defects and multisystem abnormalities may also be present. Giant congenital melanocytic nevi are associated with an increased risk of melanoma (see below).

Acquired melanocytic nevi vary considerably in form, ranging from flat to pedunculate. They may be hairy or hairless and may be skin colored, dark brown, or even black. Nevi that are flat and darkly pigmented are called junctional nevi. Slightly raised nevi are often compound; that is, they contain both epidermal and dermal components. Nevi that are predominantly intradermal are usually more elevated and contain less pigment than compound or junctional nevi. Nevi that are papillomatous, dome shaped, or pedunculate are usually intradermal [*see Figures 9 through 11*].

Differential Diagnosis

The differential diagnosis of melanocytic nevi includes ephelis (freckle), lentigo, café au lait spot (see below), wart, seborrheic keratosis, and skin tag (a small pedunculate protrusion of skin that does not contain nevus cells). Ephelis is a tan macule, commonly seen in children after sun exposure; it often dis-

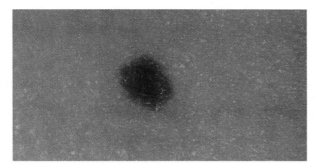

Figure 9 **A flat junctional nevus with dark pigmentation is seen in this patient.**

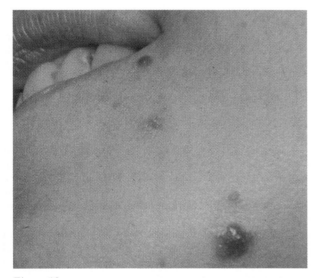

Figure 10 **This slightly raised compound nevus typically has less pigmentation than a junctional nevus.**

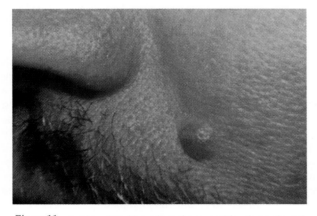

Figure 11 **A skin-colored intradermal nevus with a dome-shaped configuration is seen on the face.**

appears in the winter. Lentigo, also called senile lentigo or liver spot, is a tan or brown macule commonly seen on exposed skin areas, such as the face, the backs of the hands, and the neck. The labial melanotic macule is a distinct entity that appears in adults as a well-defined brown or black pigmented macule on the lip. In a study of 79 patients, the majority of melanocytic lesions (94%) were on the central third of the lower lip, suggesting that exposure to ultraviolet light has a causative role.[18] Patients fol-

lowed for up to 13 years had no adverse developments, a finding indicative of the benign nature of this lesion.

Treatment

No treatment is required for melanocytic nevi. However, shave biopsy or excisional biopsy may be performed for cosmetic reasons or when a nevus is subject to irritation because of pressure from clothing or because it is located in an intertriginous area. Patients should be followed with serial photographs. Biopsy should be performed for nevi that appear prone to malignant transformation; nevi that show severe dysplasia should be removed. Removal of mildly or moderately dysplastic nevi is advocated by some but not all experts [*see Chapter 41*].

CAFÉ AU LAIT SPOTS

Café au lait spots are common benign congenital or acquired birthmarks. They are tan, round to oval macules ranging in size from several millimeters to 10 to 20 cm. They can occur on any area of the body but are more common on the trunk, buttocks, and lower extremities. The presence in a prepubertal child of five or more café au lait spots larger than 0.5 cm may be a marker for neurofibromatosis-1 (NF-1) (see below).[19] Histologically, café au lait spots show an increased number of dihydroxyphenylalanine (DOPA)-positive melanocytes that produce an increased concentration of melanosomes. The café au lait spots seen in Albright hereditary osteodystrophy are usually unilateral and show jagged rather than smooth margins. An association of juvenile xanthogranulomas with café au lait macules carries an increased risk of underlying systemic disorders, including leukemia.[20]

HALO NEVUS

A halo nevus consists of an acquired zone of hypopigmentation surrounding a pigmented tumor, most commonly a compound nevus [*see Figure 12*]; other tumors, even malignant melanoma, may also be surrounded by a depigmented halo. The halo lesion typically involutes during a period of months in the absence of clinical signs of inflammation. Histologically, a chronic lymphocytic infiltrate surrounds the nevus cells, which may represent an autoimmune phenomenon.

SPINDLE CELL NEVUS

Formerly called benign juvenile melanoma, spindle cell nevus usually arises in childhood as a pink or reddish-brown, smooth or slightly scaly, firm papule with a predilection for the face, especially the cheeks [*see Figure 13*].[21] Although benign, spindle cell nevus may closely resemble a malignant melanoma. Excisional biopsy is therefore advisable in many cases.

MONGOLIAN SPOT

The mongolian spot is a bluish macule that is seen in newborns of dark-skinned races. The discoloration is caused by persistence of dermal melanocytes, often in the lumbosacral region [*see Figure 14*]. The lesion usually disappears by 3 or 4 years of age.

BLUE NEVUS

The common blue nevus occurs as a solitary, sharply circumscribed, blue-black papule [*see Figure 15*]. This malformation consists of a group of melanocytes with long, thin surface projections in the middle and lower thirds of the dermis and

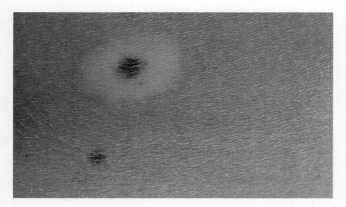

Figure 12   The halo nevus may represent an autoimmune phenomenon; a zone of hypopigmentation may appear around a nevus, with subsequent involution of the pigmented tumor.

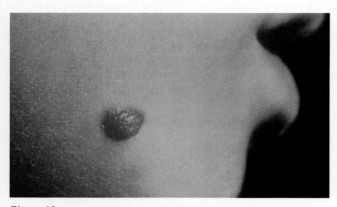

Figure 13   The spindle cell nevus is an active compound nevus that may be difficult to distinguish histologically from a melanoma.

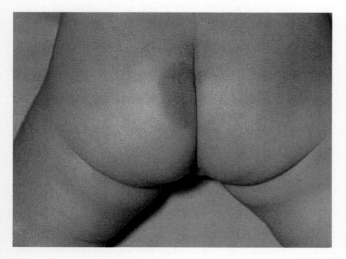

Figure 14   The bluish pigmentation of a mongolian spot is seen in the lumbosacral area and is caused by the persistence of dermal melanocytes.

in subcutaneous fat. The common blue nevus does not show a tendency toward malignant transformation. The cellular blue nevus, which appears as a blue-black nodule or an indurated plaque, contains two types of cells: spindle shaped and rounded. The cellular blue nevus may in rare instances become malignant.

NEVUS OF OTA

The nevus of Ota occurs in infancy or appears in adolescence as a blue-gray macule in the distribution of the trigeminal nerve. The lesion is unilateral in 90% of cases. Asian females are most commonly affected. Histologically, a benign dendritic melanocytosis is present in the papillary and upper reticular dermis. High-energy fluences of the Q-switched ruby laser results in lightening of the lesion, without scarring, after a few treatments.[22]

BECKER NEVUS

A malformation of epidermal melanocytes, Becker nevus occurs as a large area of hyperpigmentation and increased hair growth and is usually located on one shoulder. It appears most commonly in males during adolescence [*see Figure 16*]. Underlying bony and soft tissue abnormalities may be associated with this disorder.[23]

Light microscopy reveals hyperpigmentation of the basal layer of the epidermis, with melanin-containing phagocytes in the dermis but no nevus cells.

CONGENITAL GIANT PIGMENTED NEVUS

Giant pigmented nevus is an uncommon birthmark appearing sporadically in one in 20,000 live births. Its features are different from those of an ordinary acquired nevus. Lesions are often darkly pigmented, hairy, and slightly infiltrated, eventually becoming verrucous or nodular. They tend to occur in the distribution of a dermatome and may be quite extensive, as in bathing trunk nevus [*see Figure 17*]. Satellite lesions may be present. The condition not only is of cosmetic concern but also has a high association with malignant melanoma, with a reported 10% to 15% of nevus patients developing melanoma. Histologic features of an ordinary compound nevus, an intradermal nevus, a neural nevus, or a blue nevus may be present.[1] Treatment consists of multiple operations to excise as much of the lesion as possible.

NEUROCUTANEOUS MELANOSIS

Lesions on the scalp and neck may be associated with neurocutaneous melanosis of the leptomeninges that can be complicated by epilepsy, mental retardation, or central nervous system melanoma. Large congenital melanocytic nevi (LCMN) carry a poor prognosis in the presence of CNS signs or symptoms such as abnormal reflexes, hydrocephalus, and papilledema. Posterior axial LCMN, especially in association with satellite nevi, is a risk factor for CNS melanosis. Magnetic resonance imaging should be considered in the evaluation of newborns with these findings. In one study, CNS involvement occurred in 33 of 289 patients with LCMN. All the patients with CNS involvement had nevi in the posterior axial location. Satellite nevi were present in 31 of the 33 patients.[24] These findings suggest that melanocytic malformation occurs during the migration of neural crest cells that give rise to cutaneous leptomeningeal melanocytes. Malformation resulting in LCMN on the extremities occurs after migration from the neural crest and is not associated with CNS melanosis.

Neural Tumors

Neural tumors, such as neurofibromas, are of neuroectodermal origin, as are melanocytic tumors. Neurilemmomas (also called schwannomas) are benign nerve sheath tumors that extend subcutaneously adjacent to a peripheral nerve. They usually occur in solitary form but may occur as multiple lesions in the

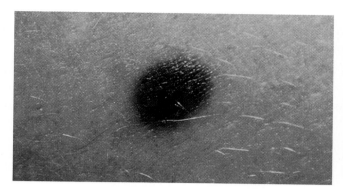

Figure 15 The presence of melanocytes in the middle and lower dermis is responsible for the color of the blue nevus.

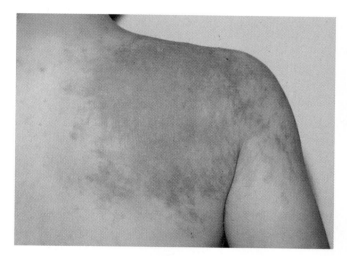

Figure 16 Becker nevus, an acquired localized malformation of epidermal melanocytes that may be associated with hypertrichosis, is seen on the shoulder.

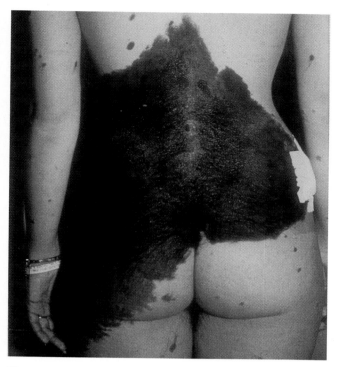

Figure 17 This form of congenital giant pigmented hairy nevus is associated with an increased risk of malignant melanoma, which develops within the lesion.

syndrome of neurilemmomatosis.[25] These tumors are usually painful and may be associated with nerve compression. Other benign tumors that must be considered in the differential diagnosis of painful skin nodules are neuromas, angiolipomas and angiomyolipomas, leiomyomas, eccrine spiradenomas, glomus tumors, and the blue rubber bleb nevus.

NEUROFIBROMATOSIS

Neurofibromatosis represents a spectrum of disorders involving the skin, central and peripheral nervous systems, bones, and blood vessels. This neurocutaneous syndrome is transmitted via an autosomal dominant gene at an estimated frequency of one in 3,000 persons with almost complete penetrance.[26]

Diagnosis and Classification

Two distinct forms of neurofibromatosis are recognized, but variant forms also exist.

Neurofibromatosis-1 The most common form (occurring in 85% to 90% of all cases) is NF-1, or von Recklinghausen disease [*see Figure 18*]. This is a common autosomal disorder, with an incidence of one in 3,500 persons. It is characterized by the presence of café au lait spots, intertriginous freckling, multiple spinal and peripheral neurofibromas, plexiform neuromas, bilateral iris hamartomas (also known as Lisch nodules), neurologic impair-

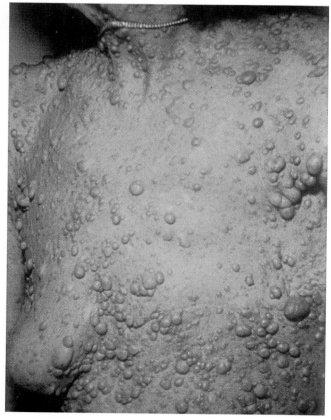

Figure 18 Multiple neurofibromas, as seen in von Recklinghausen disease, usually appear in late childhood and increase in size and number with age.

ment, and bone abnormalities. The disease is progressive and is associated with a predisposition to a malignant state.

Sarcomatous degeneration of skin lesions is rare but may occur in extracutaneous tumors. Café au lait spots of NF-1 may be present at birth and may be best visualized under a Wood light. Neurofibromas begin to appear at puberty as soft, globoid, and pedunculated tumors that are skin colored or violaceous. Lesions may be large and numerous, causing complications resulting from impingement on surrounding structures.

Neurofibromatosis-2 A second form of the disease, neurofibromatosis-2 (NF-2), is characterized by bilateral acoustic neuromas, which are Schwann cell tumors that arise from vestibular nerves.[27] Associated features may include meningiomas, gliomas, paraspinal neurofibromas, and subcapsular cataracts. Skin tumors and café au lait spots are less commonly seen in NF-2 than in NF-1.

Variants Other forms of neurofibromatosis include segmental cases in which café au lait spots or neurofibromas are localized to a single dermatome. The gene for NF-2 is located on chromosome 22. In this autosomal dominant disorder, the *merlin* tumor suppressor gene encoded in chromosome band 22q12 is inactivated. This results in an alteration in DNA with substitution of tyrosine for asparagine at position 220 of the merlin cytoskeletal associated protein.[28]

Genetic Counseling

Patients with either NF-1 or NF-2 should seek genetic counseling because there is a 50% risk that their offspring will also be affected with neurofibromatosis. In NF-1, optic glioma can appear in early childhood; patients with NF-1 may also have scoliosis. In NF-2, bilateral acoustic neuromas can cause deafness. The genes for the two distinct forms of neurofibromatosis have been located on two separate chromosomes. This finding may lead to improved diagnosis, which would facilitate genetic counseling and enable prenatal testing.[27]

Treatment

For treatment of selected neurofibromas, surgical excision is more successful than scalpel removal or electrodesiccation and curettage. In a preliminary study, the use of ketotifen, a benzocycloheptathiophene compound that acts as a mast cell stabilizer, was evaluated in the treatment of patients with neurofibromatosis.[29] All treated patients showed a decrease in symptoms of pruritus, pain, or skin tenderness and experienced a decreased rate of neurofibroma growth. Long-term double-blind studies are required, however, to confirm and extend these preliminary findings.

The bilateral acoustic neuromas of NF-2 may be visualized by computed tomography or MRI. Hearing loss is an early symptom that may begin in the second or third decade of life; it can be detected by an audiologic study with brain stem auditory-evoked response. Unilateral acoustic neuromas that are not associated with neurofibromatosis and that are not inherited are more common in older persons and pose fewer management problems.[27] Surgical removal of small acoustic neuromas may improve neurologic or audiologic status.

Connective Tissue Tumors

Fibroma of the skin comprises multiple conditions that may represent reactions to hemorrhage, infection, or chronic irritation.

SKIN TAG

Skin tag, also called acrochordon, commonly occurs as multiple skin-colored or tan, filiform or smooth-surfaced papules that are 2 to 3 mm in diameter. Lesions are often located on the neck or axillae but may also appear in the groin or on the extremities, often as isolated larger polypoid growths [*see Figure 19*]. The fibrous stalk consists of loose connective tissue with dilated capillaries. Lesions may become inflamed if they are irritated or are traumatized from twisting of the stalk. Biopsy is performed if the clinical diagnosis is uncertain. Skin tags may be removed for cosmetic reasons by using scissors to clip the pedunculate lesions at the base.

DERMATOFIBROMA

Dermatofibroma, also called histiocytoma, is a firm, skin-colored or reddish-brown sessile papule or nodule that arises spontaneously or after minor trauma, usually in adults [*see Figure 20*]. A dermatofibromatous lesion may occur, for example, after an insect bite on an extremity. A solitary lesion is most common, though multiple or eruptive histiocytomas have been reported. It may be necessary to perform a biopsy when the diagnosis is uncertain. Treatment is necessary only for cosmetic reasons.

KELOID AND HYPERTROPHIC SCAR

Normal wound healing in response to tissue injury involves several integrated processes: inflammation, production of granulation tissue, formation of the extracellular matrix, wound con-

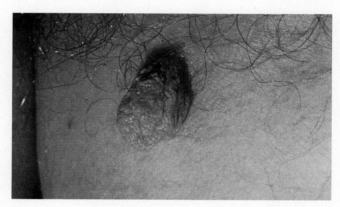

Figure 19 **Skin tags, also called acrochordons or soft fibromas, are skin-colored or tan papules. They are commonly seen in such intertriginous areas as the groin or axillae.**

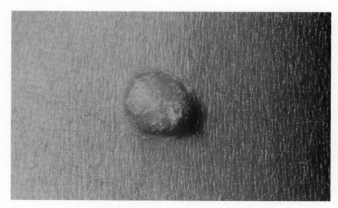

Figure 20 **Dermatofibroma appears as a firm skin-colored or reddish-brown papule and may arise spontaneously or follow minor trauma to the skin.**

traction, and, finally, scar formation. In the final phases of wound healing, fibroblasts degrade and produce bundles of collagen fibers. These bundles become thicker and are aligned along the lines of tension to which the tissues are exposed. As a result of these changes, wound tensile strength gradually increases. The resulting scar is relatively acellular and has fewer macrophages, blood vessels, and fibroblasts than the unwounded tissue.

Diagnosis and Classification

Scars may be normotrophic, atrophic, hypertrophic, or keloidal. Both hypertrophic and keloidal scars are abnormal responses to tissue injury. Hypertrophic scars mature and flatten over time, usually after 6 months. The keloid appears as a shiny, smooth, raised proliferation of scar tissue with typical crablike extensions beyond the site of the original injury [see Figure 21]. Keloids differ from hypertrophic scars in that their development is delayed, sometimes occurring months after tissue injury. Keloids do not regress, and they frequently cause pain, itching, and burning. Keloids are more common in African Americans, Hispanics, and persons with a personal or family history of keloids. Other factors associated with the development of keloids include wound tension, especially in skin sites such as the chest, shoulders, and back; ear piercing; healing by second intention; pregnancy; young age; and deep laceration.[30]

In atrophic scars, there is thinning of the skin and loss of normal architecture. Striae distensae, a so-called stretch mark, is a common dermal atrophic scar that tends to appear during periods of rapid weight gain and in the presence of excess glucocorticoid, as well as late in gestation.

Treatment

Treatment with intralesional steroids, 10 to 40 mg/ml once a month for up to 6 months, can effectively flatten keloid and hypertrophic scars. Cryotherapy (a 30-second application once a month for 3 months) has been found to be safe and effective.[31] Topical silicone gel sheeting, which was first used for burn scars, has been used in the treatment of keloids and hypertrophic scars.[32] There is no release of silicone into the skin, and there are no adverse side effects from this treatment. The mechanism of action is unknown. Potential side effects of intralesional corticosteroid treatment include atrophy, depigmentation, telangiectasia, and ulceration and dose-related systemic effects.

Vascular Birthmarks

Vascular proliferations are broadly classified as hyperplasias that show a tendency to regress or as benign vascular tumors that persist.[33,34] Vascular hyperplasias include pyogenic granuloma and pseudo-Kaposi sarcoma. Vascular hemangiomas can be further subdivided according to their histologic cell of origin (endothelial cell, pericyte, glomus cell), depth of tissue involvement (superficial or deep), and size of involved vessels (capillaries, venules, arterioles, veins, or arteries). Vascular birthmarks such as nevus flammeus and salmon patch may resemble angiomas but are nonproliferative malformations that usually do not involute.

EPIDEMIOLOGY

Hemangiomas (see below) occur in a female-to-male ratio of 5:1, whereas vascular malformations occur with equal frequency in males and females. A rare familial occurrence of heman-

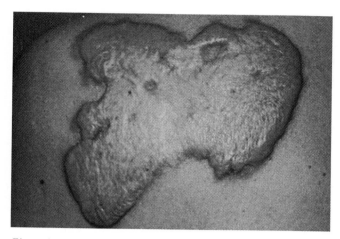

Figure 21 The proliferation of scar tissue in a keloid may extend beyond the original site of injury.

giomas, vascular malformations, or both has been reported in six kindreds, suggesting autosomal dominant inheritance in these cases.[35]

Vascular malformations are congenital developmental defects that are generally of unknown etiology. Port-wine stains may result from progressive ectasia of the superficial vascular plexus in the skin as a result of abnormal neural regulation of blood flow.[36] In the Klippel-Trénaunay-Weber syndrome, a mesodermal abnormality affecting differentiation of the limb bud may occur during the third to sixth week of gestation.[37]

PATHOGENESIS

The etiopathogenesis of hemangiomas and vascular malformations is not well understood. Hemangiomas arise in response to an angiogenic stimulus that may begin in utero. Through use of immunohistochemical techniques, infantile hemangiomas and placental microvessels were found to coexpress the vascular antigens GLUT-1 and Lewis Y antigen (LeY).[38] These antigens are not present in other vascular tumors, such as pyogenic granulomas, or in vascular malformations. A pathogenic link involving aberrant differentiation of vascular precursor cells or embolization of placental cells to fetal tissue has been hypothesized.[38] These antigens are also absent in congenital nonprogressive hemangioma, a distinctive hemangioma consisting of lesions that are fully formed at birth and that either remain static or rapidly involute.[39]

OVERVIEW OF MANAGEMENT

Evaluation and management of hemangiomas and malformations require a multidisciplinary approach. Specific diagnosis may be aided by imaging techniques such as CT and MRI to assess depth of involvement and extension to adjacent structures and to evaluate associated abnormalities. Laboratory evaluation for associated systemic disease may be required in addition to ophthalmologic, neurologic, and cardiologic assessment for complications of vascular tumors and dysmorphic syndromes.

HEMANGIOMAS

Hemangiomas are proliferating vascular tumors that are not necessarily present at birth. The vascular lesion may appear in neonates as a faint pink patch that subsequently undergoes rapid proliferation over a period of months to years before the lesion stabilizes and regresses.

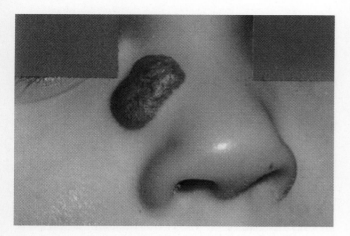

Figure 22 **The strawberry, or capillary, hemangioma appears between the second and fifth weeks of life and undergoes spontaneous involution over a period of several years.**

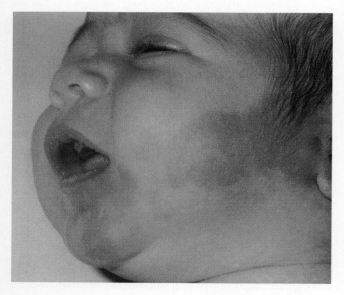

Figure 23 **A nevus flammeus is present at birth as a reddish or violaceous macular discoloration, often in a unilateral and segmental distribution; it shows little tendency to involute later in life.**

The biologic classification of hemangiomas is very different from that of vascular malformations. Vascular tumors can be classified according to their cell or origin, the size of the involved vessels, and the depth of involvement. Such classifications have led to refinement in terminology.[40] The terms strawberry hemangioma and cavernous hemangioma are descriptive clinical terms that do not specify the type of vessels that are involved.

Diagnosis and Classification

Capillary hemangioma, also known as strawberry hemangioma, appears as a single vascular lesion or multiple lesions during the second to the fifth week of life. Infantile hemangiomas are bright-red, soft, lobulated tumors that increase in size for a period of months [*see Figure 22*]. Lesions spontaneously involute, sometimes with fibrosis, over a period of several years.[33] Histologically, the capillary hemangioma shows a proliferation of endothelial cells that form many new small vessels.

Treatment

It is important to realize that most hemangiomas are uncomplicated and regress without treatment early in life with minimal residual scarring. Follow-up studies have shown that in 90% of patients, hemangiomas regress by 9 years of age.[41] Parents may require considerable reassurance that the best course is to refrain from treatment. Care must be taken to prevent trauma and infection, which may lead to scarring.

There is considerable controversy as to when to intervene in the treatment of complicated hemangiomas because of potential side effects, such as scarring. The ideal time to treat would be at the beginning of the period of rapid growth, but this is difficult to predict. Indications for treatment include involvement of a vital orifice, infection, ulceration, ocular involvement, and severe cosmetic deformity. Medical options include intralesional or systemic steroids, the latter at a dose of 1 to 3 mg/kg/day. Antimetabolites have been used for their antiproliferative effect. Interferon alfa has been used for severe hemangiomatosis, but its use is associated with systemic side effects and the potential risk of spastic diplegia. Laser surgery with 585 nm pulsed dye laser may be used to treat the superficial proliferative component.[41] Radiation therapy may lead to scarring and is discouraged in children because of long-term radiation effects, including risk of malignancy. Interventional techniques involving embolization of vessels may be required in cases involving airway obstruction or other life-threatening complications. A multidisciplinary team approach involving the dermatologist, pediatrician, radiologist, surgeon, and other specialists is needed for optimal management of complicated cases.[42]

VASCULAR MALFORMATIONS

Vascular malformations are usually present at birth. They are permanent or progress in the form of ectasias but do not proliferate. Vascular malformations may be subdivided into the following groups: venous, lymphatic, combined arteriovenous, and capillary (such as port-wine stain).[43] Dysmorphic syndromes such as Sturge-Weber and Klippel-Trénaunay-Weber syndromes are more commonly associated with vascular malformations than with hemangiomas.

Diagnosis and Classification

Salmon patch The salmon patch, one of the most common vascular birthmarks, is a dull-pink macule that appears on the nape of the neck, central forehead, or eyelids. Although the salmon patch is sometimes classified as a nevus flammeus, it is distinguished from the latter by its tendency to fade in early life. The salmon patch is caused by the persistence of fetal capillary ectasia in the dermis.[33]

Port-wine stain Port-wine stain, also called nevus flammeus, appears at birth as a reddish or violaceous macular discoloration, usually in a unilateral, segmental distribution [*see Figure 23*]. Mature dilated capillaries are present in the dermis. After puberty, nevus flammeus lesions may become thickened and nodular or papular. There is little tendency toward involution. Nevus flammeus lesions may be associated with abnormalities of the larger vessels and with neurologic manifestations.

Sturge-Weber syndrome A facial port-wine stain that involves the skin innervated by the first branch of the trigeminal nerve is a feature of the Sturge-Weber syndrome (also known as encephalotrigeminal angiomatosis). Other features of the Sturge-

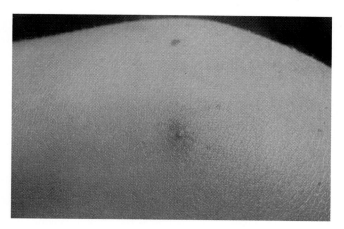

Figure 24 A spider angioma, which has a central arteriole from which fine vessels radiate, blanches with pressure.

Weber syndrome include ipsilateral congenital glaucoma and contralateral seizures caused by leptomeningeal angiomatosis. Ophthalmologic and neurologic evaluation may be warranted in patients with the Sturge-Weber syndrome.

Klippel-Trénaunay-Weber syndrome The triad of findings seen in Klippel-Trénaunay-Weber syndrome includes a port-wine stain, usually in a patchy distribution on the involved extremity; varicose veins; and soft tissue or bony hypertrophy. The most common site of involvement is the lower leg; the next most common sites of involvement are the arms and trunk.[37]

Venous malformation Formerly referred to as cavernous hemangiomas, vascular malformation consists of a collection of abnormal veins and venous pouches that commonly occur around the head and neck but can occur anywhere on the body. They are frequently multiple or have satellite lesions. Superficially, they appear as a subcutaneous swelling with a bluish hue on the skin surface or mucous membrane. Deeper components may be invisible on clinical examination. Lesions enlarge for several months, become stationary for an indefinite period, and spontaneously resolve.

Treatment

Because vascular malformations do not proliferate, treatment may be cosmetic and can be postponed to later in life. However, a multidisciplinary approach is needed to treat potential complications of vascular malformations associated with dysmorphic syndromes. Salmon patch tends to fade in early life and usually requires no treatment.

Treatment of port-wine stains by excision, tattooing, ionizing radiation, cryosurgery, or dermabrasion is largely unsatisfactory. Use of the argon laser has resulted in lightening of vascular lesions; however, there is wide variability in response. The effectiveness of this treatment results from the selective absorption of the monochromatic 585 nm laser light by red hemoglobin pigment, which produces thermal energy with resultant photocoagulation of tissue.[44] Thinner lesions are more responsive than thicker lesions that have undergone progressive vascular ectasia. In a study of 100 patients of different age groups who had port-wine stains of the head and neck and who were treated with a flashlamp pulsed dye laser, treatment was no more effective when given in early childhood than when given at a later date.[45]

Acquired Vascular Disorders

DIAGNOSIS AND CLASSIFICATION

Spider Angioma

Spider angioma, also called spider nevus or arterial spider, appears as a central red punctum from which fine vessels radiate; the appearance of the lesion is suggestive of a red spider [*see Figure 24*]. The central arteriole may be pulsatile. These telangiectasias (dilated capillaries) are commonly seen on the face, neck, trunk, and upper extremities and occur most commonly in middle-aged or elderly persons. They may arise spontaneously or in association with pregnancy or hepatic dysfunction. Spider angiomas may be treated with laser therapy for cosmetic reasons.

Unilateral Telangiectasia

Acquired unilateral telangiectatic nevi are uncommon, but those that have been reported resulted from mechanical or physical trauma, including sun damage.[46]

Cherry Angioma

Cherry angioma, also called senile angioma, appears as multiple bright-red, soft, dome-shaped papules on the trunk of middle-aged or older persons. Trauma produces slight bleeding. Electrodesiccation may be performed for cosmetic purposes.

Pyogenic Granuloma and Other Vascular Tumors

The pyogenic granuloma is a soft red lesion that is solitary, raised, and nonpulsatile; it often appears after minor skin trauma, such as a puncture wound. Other predisposing factors include hormonal effects, infection, viral oncogenes, microscopic arteriovenous anastomoses, and growth factors.[47] Epulis gravidarum is a variant of a pyogenic granuloma. The lesion was formerly believed to be caused by a pyogenic infection of a small wound; histologically, however, an early lesion resembles a capillary hemangioma. The thin, sometimes verrucous epidermis is friable and apt to become eroded or ulcerated. Lesions rapidly reach a size of 1 to 2 cm and then remain static. Common sites of involvement are the fingers, feet, and face [*see Figure 25*]. Biopsy is performed to rule out malignant tumors, such as Kaposi sarcoma and amelanotic melanoma.

Other benign tumors with a vascular component include angiofibroma, angioleiomyoma, and angiolipoma. Some of these can be painful. Differential diagnosis of painful skin tumors includes glomus tumor, angiolipoma, angioleiomyoma, neuromas, and eccrine spiradenoma.[34] Lesions are usually easily removed by electrodesiccation and curettage. If they recur or if satellite lesions appear after such treatment, excisional biopsy is recommended.

Kimura Disease

Kimura disease and angiolymphoid hyperplasia with eosinophilia are rare tumors of unknown cause that occur mainly on the head and neck in young adults and may resemble pyogenic granuloma.[48] Kimura disease, which was first reported in Korea, is most common in Asians. It appears as a granulomatous proliferation of lymphoid tissue that may be accompanied by peripheral eosinophilia and contiguous lymphadenopathy. Lesions may occasionally be seen on the trunk, extremities, and genitalia in addition to the head and neck. Angiolymphoid hy-

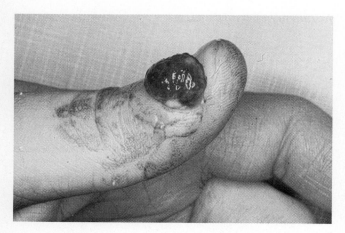

Figure 25 **The pyogenic granuloma, which may show a smooth, verrucous, eroded, or friable surface, may be confused with a malignant tumor.**

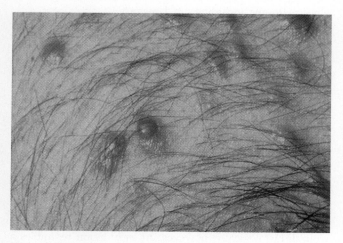

Figure 26 **Leiomyomas are sometimes painful papules that arise from smooth muscle of blood vessels or the arrector pili.**

perplasia with eosinophilia, which may or may not represent a different disease, appears as localized single or multiple nodules. Infectious, allergic, hormonal, and traumatic mechanisms have been postulated. Immunodermatopathologic studies suggest an unusual distribution of adhesion molecules, IgE, and CD23 in these angioproliferating tumors.[49]

Lipoma

The lipoma, which is a soft, rounded to lobulated subcutaneous tumor of mature fat cells, is commonly seen on the trunk, neck, or forearms. Lesions are rubbery in consistency and freely movable under the overlying skin, which appears normal. There may be a single lesion or multiple lesions, and they are usually asymptomatic unless they impinge on a nerve. Lipomas are of variable size and grow slowly. Histologically, the tumors are usually encapsulated and show fat cells that are indistinguishable from normal adipose tissue. Admixture of other tissue components may result in fibrolipomas (fibrous tissue), angiolipomas (blood vessels), and myolipomas (smooth muscle). Excision may be performed for cosmetic reasons. If a lesion grows rapidly, biopsy should be performed, though lipomas rarely become malignant.

Leiomyoma

The leiomyoma is an uncommon tumor of smooth muscle that appears as a single brownish-red papule or as multiple papules or small nodules, which are sometimes painful [*see Figure 26*]. Leiomyomas may arise from the arrector pili (the smooth muscle attached to the hair follicle sheath) or from the smooth muscle surrounding cutaneous blood vessels (angioleiomyoma). Painful lesions can be excised.

Lymphangioma Circumscriptum

Lymphangioma circumscriptum is characterized by groups of persistent localized or diffuse translucent vesicles. Indications for treatment include severe cosmetic problems, persistent leakage of lymphatic fluid or blood, and recurrent infection. The vesicles frequently recur after surgery, radiotherapy, electrocautery, or cryosurgery because of the persistence of deep lymphatic cisterns. Carbon dioxide laser in a vaporization mode has been used to ablate superficial cutaneous lesions in patients with lymphangioma circumscriptum.[50] The major advantage of this technique is that it may reduce the frequency of recurrences because it seals the communicating channels to the deeper cisterns by vaporizing the superficial lymphatics.

References

1. Lever's Histopathology of the Skin. Elder D, Elenitsas R, Jaworsky C, et al, Eds. Lippincott-Raven Publishers, Philadelphia, 1997

2. Dermatology in General Medicine. Fitzpatrick TB, Eisen AZ, Wolff K, et al, Eds. McGraw-Hill Book Co, New York, 1993

3. Flugman SL, McClain SA, Clark RF: Transient eruptive seborrheic keratoses associated with erythrodermic psoriasis and erythrodermic drug eruption: report of two cases. J Am Acad Dermatol 45:S212, 2001

4. Paller AS, Syder AJ, Chan YM, et al: Genetic and clinical mosaicism in a type of epidermal nevus. N Engl J Med 331:1408, 1994

5. Seo YJ, Piao, YJ, Suhr KB, et al: A case of nevus comedonicus syndrome associated with neurologic and skeletal abnormalities. Int J Dermatol 40:648, 2001

6. Brownstein MH: Basaloid follicular hamartoma: solitary and multiple types. J Am Acad Dermatol 27:237, 1992

7. Grimalt R, Ferrando J, Mascaro JM: Premature familial sebaceous hyperplasia: successful response to oral isotretinoin in three patients. J Am Acad Dermatol 37:996, 1997

8. Sidhu SK, Wakelin SH, Wilkinson JD: Multiple familial trichoepitheliomas. Cutis 63:191, 1999

9. Esche C, Kruse R, Lamberti C, et al: Muir-Torre syndrome: clinical features and molecular genetic analysis. Br J Dermatol 136:913, 1997

10. Parks ET, Caldemeyer KS, Mirowski GW: Radiologic images in dermatology: Gardner syndrome. J Am Acad Dermatol 45:940, 2001

11. Liu V, Kwan T, Page EH: Parotid oncocytoma in the Birt-Hogg-Dubé syndrome. J Am Acad Dermatol 43:1120, 2000

12. Lindor NM, Hand J, Burch PA, et al: Birt-Hogg-Dube syndrome: an autosomal dominant disorder with predisposition to cancers of the kidney, fibrofolliculomas, and focal cutaneous mucinosis. Int J Dermatol 40:653, 2001

13. Grob JJ, Gouvernet J, Aymar D, et al: Count of benign melanocytic nevi as a major indicator of risk for nonfamilial nodular and superficial spreading melanoma. Cancer 66:387, 1990

14. Tucker MA, Halpern A, Holly EA, et al: Clinically recognized dysplastic nevi: a central risk factor for cutaneous melanoma. JAMA 277:1439, 1997

15. Augustsson A, Stierner U, Rosdahl I, et al: Melanocytic naevi in sun-exposed and protected skin in melanoma patients and controls. Acta Derm Venereol (Stockh) 71:512, 1991

16. Kelly JW, Rivers JK, MacLennan R, et al: Sunlight: a major factor associated with the development of melanocytic nevi in Australian schoolchildren. J Am Acad Dermatol 30:40, 1994

17. Marghoob AA, Orlow SJ, Kopf AW: Syndromes associated with melanocyti nevi. J Am Acad Dermatol 29:373, 1993

18. Gupta G, Williams REA, Mackie RM: The labial melanotic macule: a review of 79 cases. Br J Dermatol 136:772, 1997

19. Cohen JB, Janniger CK, Schwartz RA: Café-au-lait spots. Cutis 66:22, 2000

20. Thami GP, Kaur S, Kanwar A: Association of juvenile xanthogranuloma with *café-au-lait* macules. Int J Dermatol 40:281, 2001

21. Mooney MA, Barr RJ, Buxton MG: Halo nevus or halo phenomenon: a study of 142 cases. J Cutan Pathol 22:342, 1995

22. Lowe NJ, Wieder JM, Sawcer D, et al: Nevus of Ota: treatment with high energy fluences of the Q-switched ruby laser. J Am Acad Dermatol 29:997, 1993

23. Glinick SE, Alper JC, Bogaars H, et al: Becker's melanosis: associated abnormalities. J Am Acad Dermatol 9:509, 1983

24. DeDavid M, Orlow SJ, Provost N, et al: Neurocutaneous melanosis: clinical features of large congenital melanocytic nevi in patients with manifest central nervous system melanosis. J Am Acad Dermatol 35:529, 1996

25. Buenger KM, Porter NC, Dozier SE, et al: Localized multiple neurilemmomas of the lower extremity. Cutis 51:36, 1993

26. Riccardi VM: Von Recklinghausen neurofibromatosis. N Engl J Med 305:1617, 1981

27. Martuza RL, Eldridge R: Neurofibromatosis 2 (bilateral acoustic neurofibromatosis). N Engl J Med 318:684, 1988

28. MacCollin M, Mohney T, Trofatter J, et al: DNA diagnosis of neurofibromatosis 2: altered coding sequence of the merlin tumor suppressor in an extended pedigree. JAMA 270:2316, 1993

29. Riccardi VM: Mast-cell stabilization to decrease neurofibroma growth: preliminary experiences with ketotifen. Arch Dermatol 123:1011, 1987

30. Sahl WJ, Clever H: Cutaneous scars: part I. Int J Dermatol 33:681, 1994

31. Zouboulis CC, Blume U, Buttner P, et al: Outcomes of cryosurgery in keloids and hypertrophic scars: a prospective consecutive trial of case series. Arch Dermatol 129:1146, 1993

32. Gold MH: Topical silicone gel sheeting in the treatment of hypertrophic scars and keloids. J Dermatol Surg Oncol 19:912, 1993

33. Requena L, Sangueza OP: Cutaneous vascular proliferations. Part II: hyperplasias and benign neoplasms. J Am Acad Dermatol 37:887, 1997

34. Requena L, Sanqueza MD: Cutaneous vascular proliferations. Part III: malignant neoplasms, other cutaneous neoplasms with significant vascular component, and disorders erroneously considered as vascular neoplasms. J Am Acad Dermatol 38:143, 1998

35. Blei F, Walter J, Orlow SJ, et al: Familial segregation of hemangiomas and vascular malformations as an autosomal dominant trait. Arch Dermatol 134:718, 1998

36. Smoller BR, Rosen R: Port-wine stains: a disease of altered neural modulation of blood vessels. Arch Dermatol 122:177, 1986

37. Meine JG, Schwartz RA, Janniger CK: Klippel-Trénaunay-Weber syndrome. Cutis 60:127, 1997

38. North PE, Waner M, Mizeracki A, et al: A unique microvascular phenotype shared by juvenile hemangiomas and human placenta. Arch Dermatol 137:559, 2001

39. North PE, Waner M, James CA, et al: Congenital nonprogressive hemangioma: a distinct clinicopathologic entity unlike infantile hemangioma. Arch Dermatol 137:1607, 2001

40. Mulliken JB, Young AE: Vascular Birthmarks: Hemangiomas and Malformations. WB Saunders Co, Philadelphia, 1988, p 77

41. Barlow RJ, Walker NJ, Markey AC: Treatment of proliferative haemangiomas with the 585 nm pulsed dye laser. Br J Dermatol 134:700, 1996

42. Donnelly LF, Adams DM, Bisset GS 3rd: Vascular malformations and hemangiomas: a practical approach in a multidisciplinary clinic. AJR Am J Roentgenol 174:597, 2000

43. Requena L, Sangueza OP: Cutaneous vascular anomalies. Part I. Hamartomas, malformations, and dilatation of preexisting vessels. J Am Acad Dermatol 37:523, 1997

44. Fitzpatrick RE, Lowe NJ, Goldman MP, et al: Flashlamp-pumped pulsed dye laser treatment of port-wine stains. J Dermatol Surg Oncol 20:743, 1994

45. van der Horst CM, Koster PL, de Borgie CM, et al: Effect of the timing of treatment of port-wine stains with the flash-lamp-pumped pulsed-dye laser. N Engl J Med 338:1028, 1998

46. Pasyk KA: Acquired lateral telangiectatic nevus: port-wine stain or nevus flammeus. Cutis 51:281, 1993

47. Mooney MA, Janniger CK: Pyogenic granuloma. Pediatr Dermatol 55:133, 1995

48. Chun SI, Ji HG: Kimura's disease and angiolymphoid hyperplasia with eosinophilia: clinical and histopathologic differences. J Am Acad Dermatol 27:954, 1992

49. von den Driesch P, Gruschwitz M, Schell H, et al: Distribution of adhesion molecules, IgE, and CD23 in a case of angiolymphoid hyperplasia with eosinophilia. J Am Acad Dermatol 26:799, 1992

50. Bailin PL, Kantor GR, Wheeland RG: Carbon dioxide laser vaporization of lymphangioma circumscriptum. J Am Acad Dermatol 14:257, 1986

Allan C. Halpern, M.D., and Patricia L. Myskowski, M.D.

Malignant tumors can arise from cells of any layer of the skin—keratinocytes, melanocytes, fibroblasts, endothelial cells, adipocytes—as well as from cells such as lymphocytes, which normally transit through the skin. Cutaneous metastases may also arise from other primary sites. In this chapter, we review the most common malignant cutaneous tumors in their order of frequency.

Malignant Tumors of the Epidermis

Epidermal skin cancers are the most common cancers in humans. They arise in the keratinocytes and the melanocytes of the epidermis. Epidermal skin cancers present a unique opportunity for effective intervention with both early detection and primary prevention. They are amenable to clinical diagnosis by simple visual inspection and to pathologic diagnosis by minimally invasive biopsy.

Basal cell carcinoma and squamous cell carcinoma originate from the keratinocytes of the epidermis. Because these two cancers share many features, they are often lumped together under the term nonmelanoma skin cancer.

Malignant melanoma is a malignancy arising from a melanocyte. Although malignant melanomas can arise in any melanocyte of the body, including the eye, the vast majority occur in the skin. Cutaneous malignant melanoma has been categorized into four major histogenetic types: lentigo maligna melanoma, superficial spreading melanoma, nodular melanoma, and acral lentiginous melanoma.

SUN EXPOSURE AND SKIN CANCER

Several lines of evidence implicate ultraviolet (UV) radiation in the pathogenesis of all three of the major epidermal skin cancers.[1] Epidemiologic data implicate chronic cumulative sun exposure in the development of squamous cell carcinoma and intense intermittent sun exposure in basal cell carcinoma and melanoma. Laboratory studies indicate that both UVA (320 nm to 400 nm) and UVB (290 nm to 320 nm) radiation from sunlight can damage DNA both directly and through oxidative damage. In addition, UV radiation can suppress the cutaneous immune system.[2] The association of some squamous cell carcinomas with chemical carcinogens and the occurrence of acral lentiginous and mucosal melanomas in unexposed areas of the body underscore the need for studies to identify additional etiologic agents.

Recognition of the important role of sunlight in the etiology of skin cancer affords an opportunity for primary prevention through the use of sun protection. Unfortunately, the timing and doses of UV exposure involved in the development of skin cancer in humans are not yet known. Accordingly, patients should be educated about the deleterious effects of sun exposure and tanning. Sun-protection efforts should be geared to an overall reduction of sun exposure through the avoidance of sun-seeking behavior and the use of sun-protective clothing. Broad-spectrum sunscreens with a sun protection factor (SPF) of 15 or greater are a useful adjunct to sun protection, but they should not be used to increase the amount of time spent in direct sunlight.[3]

NONMELANOMA SKIN CANCER

Nonmelanoma skin cancer (NMSC) typically occurs as pink lesions on the sun-exposed skin surface. Any pink skin lesion that persists or recurs in the same location, especially if easily irritated by minor trauma, should raise the suspicion of NMSC. Some forms of NMSC will fade with changes in season (i.e., with reduced sun exposure) or with the application of topical steroids, and the clinician should advise patients that any lesion that recurs warrants further attention.

Basal Cell Carcinoma

Basal cell carcinoma (BCC) is a malignant cutaneous tumor arising from the basal keratinocytes of the epidermis.

Epidemiology　BCC is the most common skin cancer. Reported incidence ranges from 3.4 per 100,000 per year in African Americans to over 1,100 per 100,000 per year in Townsville, Queensland, Australia.[4,5] Although rare, metastases and death from BCC do occur.

Etiology　UV radiation—specifically, intense intermittent sun exposure—appears to play an important role in the development of BCC. Recent studies of basal cell nevus syndrome (Gorlin syndrome) are yielding dramatic new insights into the genetics of BCC. A gene named patched, which was first recognized as a developmental gene in the fruit fly *Drosophila*, has been identified as playing a critical role in the development of BCC. Almost all patients with basal cell nevus syndrome appear to inherit a mutated copy of the patched gene, and studies of sporadic BCC suggest that mutations in the patched gene pathway are a necessary, if not sufficient, step in the development of most BCCs.[6]

Diagnosis　Approximately 90% of BCCs occur on the head and neck. They occur in nodular and superficial forms.

Nodular BCC appears as a raised, pearly, translucent, pink bump on the skin surface. It is often easily irritated, fragile, and associated with episodes of superficial ulceration or hemorrhage. When ulceration is prominent, it can lead to the appearance of a so-called rodent ulcer, in which the pearly translucent border is barely appreciable. Such lesions can also appear more white than pink and, on close observation, often demonstrate small telangiectasias. They tend to have a smoother, shinier surface and firmer texture than common dermal nevi [*see Figure 1*].

Superficial BCC appears as a pink patch of skin. On close inspection, most superficial BCCs demonstrate a thready translucent border, with areas of seemingly normal or slightly fibrotic skin within the lesion. Superficial BCC is usually found on the upper trunk, arms, and legs.

Less common clinical variants of BCC include morpheaform, pigmented, and cystic lesions. Morpheaform BCCs have an infiltrative pattern that histologically and clinically resembles a scar. Pigmented BCCs typically contain specks of blue-black pigment, but they may be deeply pigmented throughout. Pigment is most commonly a variant of nodular BCC. Cystic BCCs tend to be softer than typical nodular BCCs and may have a clear to blue-gray appearance.

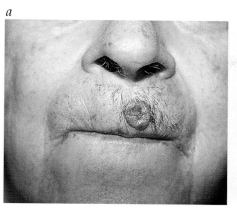 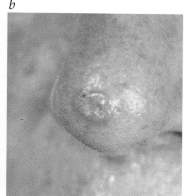 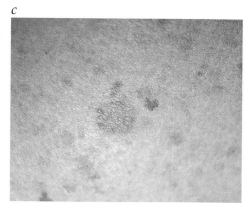

Figure 1   Nodular basal cell carcinoma—shown here above a patient's lip, with a so-called rodent's ulcer (*a*)—commonly presents as a raised, pearly, translucent pink bump on the skin surface (*b*). A superficial form appears as a pink patch of skin (*c*).

Patient history plays a critical role in the diagnosis of BCC. When questioned about lesions that become easily irritated or bleed from minor trauma, patients can often alert the clinician to early lesions that would otherwise elude detection. With the patient under local anesthesia, a biopsy should be obtained of any suspicious lesion.

Differential diagnosis   Nodular BCC can be confused with angiofibromas, dermal nevi, amelanotic melanoma, cutaneous metastases, and a host of benign adnexal tumors (e.g., trichoepithelioma). Superficial BCCs mimic several inflammatory dermatoses (e.g., eczema and tinea) and share several clinical features with actinic keratoses. Pigmented BCC can easily be confused with a primary melanocytic neoplasm. Cystic BCCs can be confused with cystic adnexal tumors and inflammatory lesions.

Treatment   The goal of therapy is to adequately eradicate the lesion and ensure the best cosmetic and functional outcome. Multiple factors—such as the size, location, and histologic subtype of the lesions and attributes of the patient, including age, general health, skin color, and skin laxity—should be taken into consideration in choosing an optimal therapy.

The vast majority of BCCs are amenable to surgical treatment. The primary options include curettage and electrodesiccation, excision, cryotherapy, radiotherapy, and Mohs micrographic surgery.

A small but significant subset of BCCs benefit from Mohs micrographic surgery, which entails microscopic examination of frozen sections of the entire undersurface of the excised specimen at the time of surgery. The technique may be indicated for recurrent lesions and lesions with a high likelihood of recurrence. These include ill-defined lesions, large lesions (> 2 cm), lesions with a high-risk histology (i.e., aggressive growth pattern, sclerosing pattern, or perineural involvement), and lesions overlying embryonal fusion planes (e.g., ocular canthi or nasofacial sulcus). The Mohs micrographic technique has significantly higher cure rates than other treatments for these high-risk lesions.[7]

Radiation therapy can be an effective, painless, and well-tolerated alternative that is typically reserved for older patients who are poor surgical candidates. Radiation therapy should be avoided, however, in patients with basal cell nevus syndrome.

Experimental therapies under investigation include intralesional chemotherapy, topical immune modulators, and photodynamic therapy.

All patients treated for BCC are at risk for local recurrence as well as at significant risk for the development of additional skin cancers. Patients should be instructed in the self-examination of their skin as well as in methods of sun protection, and they should receive routine professional follow-up.

Prognosis   As noted (see above), the risk of local recurrence relates to the lesion's size, location, and histology. Metastases are very rare: a prevalence of 0.0028% was reported in a series of 50,000 Australians.[8] Metastases occur through both the lymphatic and the hematogenous routes; risk factors include basal cell nevus syndrome, immunosuppression, and previous exposure to ionizing radiation. Metastases that are not amenable to surgical management are associated with a poor outcome.

Squamous Cell Carcinoma

Like BCC, cutaneous squamous cell carcinoma (SCC) arises from the keratinocytes of the epidermis. Histologically, the cells of well-differentiated SCC resemble the cells of the superior portion of the epidermis.

Epidemiology   An estimated 150,000 to 250,000 new cases of cutaneous SCC were diagnosed in the United States in 1994.[9] The estimated mortality from SCC in the United States in 1988 was approximately 0.5 per 100,000. Several lines of data suggest significant recent increases in SCC incidence. In Australia, for example, SCC incidence increased by 51% between the years 1985 and 1990.[10]

Etiology   In addition to sunlight, other known etiologic agents that contribute to the development of cutaneous SCC are ionizing radiation, chemical carcinogens, thermal burns, and chronic nonhealing wounds. Sun-related SCCs demonstrate a lower risk of metastases and death than SCCs related to other exposures. Factors involved in predisposition to SCC from sun exposure include light skin color, tendency to burn, and inability to tan.

Pathophysiology and pathogenesis   Sun-related SCC is often associated with a precursor lesion called an actinic keratosis. Such lesions occur on the scalp, face, extensor surfaces of the forearms, and backs of the hands. They tend to be rough-surfaced, irregularly shaped, and pink. They are often more readily felt than seen. The majority of patients with actinic keratoses have multiple lesions. The risk of SCC in these individuals has

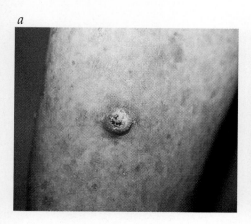
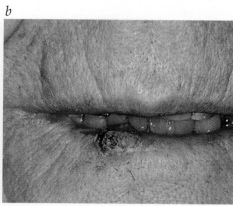

Figure 2 **A squamous cell carcinoma is shown on an arm (*a*) and lower lip (*b*).**

been estimated to be as high as 20%.[11] SCC may also appear on normal-looking skin.

SCC of the oral or genital mucosa may arise in precursor lesions termed leukoplakia or erythroplakia. Mucosal SCCs are associated with a significant risk of metastases.

Immune surveillance affects the progression of SCC. Immunosuppression as occurs in transplant recipients and patients with lymphoma is associated with a high incidence of SCC. In these patients, infection with human papillomavirus appears to play an etiologic role in conjunction with sun exposure. SCCs tend to be more aggressive in immunosuppressed persons.

Diagnosis Most lesions occur in areas of the body that are usually exposed to the sun. The lesions are pinkish, firm plaques that often have a rough, scaly surface [*see Figure 2*]. Biopsy is required for definitive diagnosis.

Differential diagnosis The differential diagnosis of SCC includes keratoacanthoma, Bowen disease, verrucous carcinoma, BCC, hypertrophic actinic keratosis, and common warts.

Keratoacanthomas share many features with SCC both clinically and histologically. They arise de novo on normal-looking skin and grow very rapidly. They are typically pink, dome-shaped, shiny bumps on the surface of the skin with a central crateriform keratotic plug. They may become very large. Although keratoacanthomas are not associated with a risk of metastasis, they can be locally destructive. Spontaneous regression of keratoacanthoma over the course of months has been well documented.

Bowen disease is SCC that is confined to the epidermis. It appears as red, scaly, minimally elevated plaques with well-defined, irregular borders. The previously reported association of Bowen disease with internal malignancy has not held up to closer scrutiny.

SCCs that lack a scaly keratotic surface can be confused with a host of other adnexal and dermal skin tumors.

Treatment Small SCCs evolving from an actinic keratosis can be adequately treated with simple curettage and electrodesiccation. Larger actinic lesions, as well as lesions arising in non–sun-exposed areas of skin, are best treated with definitive surgical excision with confirmation of negative margins. High-risk, ill-defined lesions, especially those occurring in the surgically sensitive areas of the face, genitalia, hands, and feet, are often best treated by Mohs micrographic surgery.

Fractionated radiation therapy is an alternative treatment for primary SCC in older patients who are poor surgical candidates. The benefits of adjuvant radiation therapy are less clear, as are the benefits of elective lymph node dissection for patients with high-risk SCC of the head and neck.

Cytotoxic chemotherapy and biologic response modifiers have been used in patients who have advanced SCC, with complete response rates of 25% to 46% but with few long-term survivors.

Actinic keratoses are treated with cryotherapy, curettage, topical chemotherapy with fluorouracil, chemical peels, and laser resurfacing to prevent progression to SCC.

Treatment guidelines from the National Comprehensive Cancer Network have recently been published.[12]

Prognosis Regardless of the therapy employed, high-risk lesions have a significant rate of local recurrence at 5 years. High-risk SCCs include those in specific anatomic sites (e.g., ears, lips, genitalia and other non–sun-exposed areas), those greater than 2 cm in diameter, those with aggressive histologic features (depth > 4 mm, Clark level IV and above, and poorly differentiated histology), and those in immunosuppressed patients.[13] The primary route of SCC metastasis is via lymphatic spread to regional lymph nodes. Reported rates of metastasis vary from as low as 0.3% in small, sun-derived lesions to 33% in larger, poorly differentiated lesions.[13] Reported overall 5-year survival for patients with regionally metastatic SCC has ranged from 25% to 47%.[13]

MALIGNANT MELANOMA

Epidemiology

In the United States, a person's lifetime risk for developing melanoma is about 1 in 75 (1.3%).[14] Between 1973 and 1994, the incidence of melanoma rose by 121%, and the mortality rose by 39%.[14] Encouraging trends include a shift toward the detection of earlier disease as well as a stabilization of incidence rates in some segments of the population. In terms of both morbidity and mortality, however, the burden of melanoma-related disease continues to increase. Although melanoma can occur in anyone, it is primarily a disease of whites. Melanomas occurring in blacks are typically of the acral lentiginous variety.

Etiology

Although strong epidemiologic and basic-science evidence supports an association between melanoma and sun exposure, the relationship appears to be complex. Lentigo maligna melanoma is associated with chronic cumulative sun exposure.

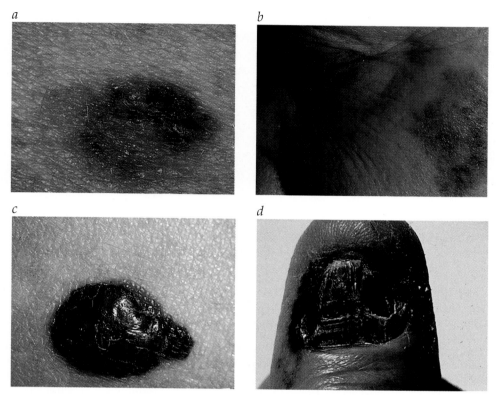

Figure 3 **Superficial spreading malignant melanoma begins as a small, irregular brown lesion (*a*). Variation in color and contour is characteristic of lentigo maligna melanoma (*b*). Nodular melanoma often grows more in thickness than in diameter (*c*). Acral lentiginous melanoma can resemble a hematoma under the nail (*d*).**

Superficial spreading melanoma and nodular melanoma appear to be associated with intense intermittent sun exposure, especially in youth. Acral lentiginous melanoma has no apparent association with sun exposure. Basic-science studies and animal models have implicated different wavelengths of UV in melanoma carcinogenesis; UV wavelength may vary among types of melanoma.

Approximately 5% of patients with melanomas have a family history of melanoma. Mutations in the cell-cycle regulatory gene *p16* (cyclin-dependent kinase inhibitor–2a) are associated with melanoma in approximately 40% of familial-melanoma families, with linkage of the gene to chromosome 9p.[15] Abnormalities of DNA repair found in patients with dysplastic nevi suggest this as another mechanism of genetic predisposition to melanoma.

Diagnosis

As a pigmented lesion occurring on the surface of the skin, melanoma is amenable to early detection by simple visual inspection at an easily curable stage. Left untreated, melanoma is among the deadliest and most therapeutically unresponsive forms of cancer.

Early recognition of melanoma requires attention to pigmented lesions on all body surfaces. Despite the strong association of melanoma with sun exposure, melanomas can occur anywhere on the cutaneous surface. Patients' self-examination, as well as physician examination, must therefore include all skin surfaces, including the scalp, genitalia, and soles of the feet. Any pigmented skin lesion with recent change or with features described by the ABCD mnemonic (asymmetry, border irregularity, color variation, diameter > 6 mm) warrants consideration of the possibility of melanoma. Although any mole may change gradually over time, any that change color, shape, or size relative to a patient's other moles deserve special attention [*see Figure 3*].

Among whites, several additional risk factors have been identified, such as fair complexion, tendency to burn, inability to tan, freckling, and family history of melanoma. The strongest phenotypic markers of melanoma risk are moles (nevi)—more specifically, increased numbers of moles and the presence of atypical moles (dysplastic nevi). Melanoma can arise in a preexisting mole or may arise de novo on normal-appearing skin.

Screening of the family members of patients with melanoma (particularly multiple melanoma) may be a useful preventive and diagnostic measure.[16]

Dysplastic nevi   Several epidemiologic studies have correlated dysplastic nevi with melanoma risk. Clinically, dysplastic nevi are large (> 5 mm) moles with variegate pigmentation and ill-defined borders [*see Figure 4*]. Histologically, dysplastic nevi are characterized by the presence of architectural atypia and random cytologic atypia.[17] The degree of melanoma risk associated with dysplastic nevi depends on the genetic context. In families with familial melanoma–dysplastic nevus syndrome, the abnormal mole phenotype appears to be inherited in an autosomal dominant fashion. Members of these families with dysplastic nevi have a lifetime melanoma risk that approaches 100%.[18] Outside the context of familial melanoma, dysplastic nevi occur in approximately 5% to 10% of whites. In this general population, dysplastic nevi are markers of increased melanoma risk [*see Table 1*].[19]

Dysplastic nevi present both opportunity and challenge in melanoma detection. On one hand, their recognition allows effi-

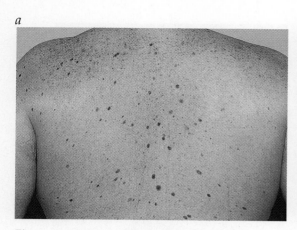
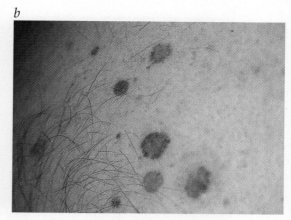

Figure 4   **Dysplastic nevi typically are larger than common moles (*a*) and have variegate pigmentation and ill-defined borders (*b*).**

cient targeting of a high-risk group. On the other, they can complicate attempts at melanoma detection by clinically mimicking early melanomas. Although some dysplastic nevi may progress to melanoma, the overwhelming majority remain benign. Furthermore, not all melanomas arising in patients with dysplastic nevi develop in a preexisting mole. Wholesale removal of dysplastic nevi is an impractical approach to melanoma prevention. In patients with dysplastic nevi, melanoma detection is predicated on specialized visual examination aided by self-examination and professional follow-up to identify changing lesions.

Several specialized aids to diagnosis of melanoma in patients with dysplastic nevi are under development. Epiluminescent microscopy (ELM), which is also known as dermatoscopy, entails the use of a handheld otoscopelike device to magnify a pigmented lesion while applying pressure and oil to the surface. The technique allows the visualization of pigment patterns and features not apparent with simple visual inspection. With experience and training, ELM can be a useful aid in distinguishing

melanoma from benign pigmented lesions; however, when used inexpertly, ELM may actually decrease diagnostic accuracy.[20,21] Another aid to melanoma detection in high-risk individuals is photographically assisted follow-up.[22] A baseline set of whole body photographs of the skin are used during self-examination and follow-up professional examination to assess change in the lesions. This procedure helps to prevent unnecessary excision of stable lesions and improves the sensitivity of examinations in detecting change. New imaging technologies such as in vivo confocal scanning laser microscopy hold promise for future improvements in the noninvasive diagnosis of melanoma.[23]

Any lesion that raises a clinical suspicion of melanoma requires definitive diagnosis. Full-thickness excision is the preferred technique for biopsy of a suspicious pigmented lesion. Partial biopsy can lead to misdiagnosis through sampling error or by depriving the pathologist of a view of the overall architecture and cytology of the lesion. Incisional biopsies with good clinical-pathologic correlation may be appropriate, however, in the assessment of large lesions and of lesions occurring in surgically sensitive areas. There is no evidence to suggest that incisional biopsy increases the risk of metastasis.

Differential Diagnosis

Dysplastic nevi share many features with early superficial spreading melanoma. Other common lesions that may mimic melanoma include lentigines, sunburn freckles, traumatized nevi, thrombosed angiomas, pigmented BCCs, pigmented Bowen disease, dermatofibromas, and atypical seborrheic keratoses. Two other challenges in the differential diagnosis of melanoma deserve special mention. Amelanotic melanomas (melanomas without pigment) present as pink lesions that may be misdiagnosed as BCCs or Spitz nevi. Spitz nevi can be difficult to differentiate from melanoma both clinically and histologically. Spitz nevi occur most commonly in children, but they also occur in adults. Like nodular melanomas, Spitz nevi tend to appear suddenly and range in color from red to reddish brown.

Treatment

Primary site   Primary cutaneous melanoma is managed surgically with definitive reexcision. The wide excisions of the past have given way to more modest resection margins. Data from two prospective, randomized trials of surgical margins for primary cutaneous melanoma have demonstrated the safety of 1

Table 1   Adjusted Estimated Relative Risks of Melanoma by Nevus Type and Number[17]

Type	Number	Adjusted Relative Risk*
Nevi > 2 mm and < 5 mm	0–24	1.0
	25–49	1.8 (1.3–2.5)
	50–99	3.0 (2.1–4.4)
	≥ 100	3.4 (2.0–5.7)
Nondysplastic nevi > 5 mm	0	1.0
	1	0.9 (0.7–1.3)
	2–4	1.3 (1.0–1.8)
	5–9	1.7 (1.0–2.7)
	≥ 10	2.3 (1.2–4.3)
Dysplastic nevi	None	1.0
	Indeterminate	1.0 (0.7–1.6)
	1	2.3 (1.4–3.6)
	2–4	7.3 (4.6–12.0)
	5–9	4.9 (2.5–9.8)
	≥ 10	12.0 (4.4–31.0)

*Mutually adjusted and adjusted for age, sex, center, referral pattern, morphologic dysplastic nevi < 5 mm, sunburns, freckles, solar damage, scars, nevus excisions, and family history of melanoma (confidence interval = 95%).

cm margins for melanomas less than 1 mm in thickness and of 2 cm margins for melanomas between 1 and 4 mm in thickness.[24,25] Randomized trials of resection margins for melanomas more than 4 mm thick have not been conducted. Most authors recommend a 2 to 4 cm margin for these thicker primary melanomas. Primary closure and reconstructive flaps are preferable, cosmetically and functionally, to skin grafts and should be used instead of grafts whenever possible.

Lymph nodes   Patients with clinically evident regional lymph node disease are treated with therapeutic lymph node dissection. The performance of elective lymph node dissection (ELND) has long been controversial in patients with intermediate-thickness primary cutaneous melanoma but no clinical evidence of regional nodal disease. Overall, the data on survival benefit suggest that ELND is not warranted, given the morbidity associated with this procedure.

Sentinel lymph node biopsy is being increasingly used as an alternative to ELND in patients with primary cutaneous melanoma. This technique utilizes lymphoscintigraphy to identify the draining regional lymph node basins for the skin at the site of the primary melanoma. At the time of definitive reexcision of the melanoma, a blue dye and radioisotope are injected into the dermis around the melanoma site. A small incision is made over the spot that has been identified on lymphoscintigraphy as the proximal area of drainage of the regional lymph node basin. The first lymph node identified as taking up the blue dye and radioisotope (the sentinel node) is then excised.

The sentinel node is then histologically evaluated, often with the use of immunohistochemical techniques and occasionally with the use of polymerase chain reaction, which is more sensitive. The absence of melanoma in the sentinel node is highly sensitive for ruling out the presence of metastases in the remainder of the lymph node basin when the procedure is performed by an experienced team. When the sentinel node is found to be positive for melanoma, a full ELND is typically performed. Prospective studies have demonstrated sentinel node status to be strongly correlated with 5-year survival.[26] Patients with positive sentinel nodes are appropriate candidates for consideration of adjuvant therapy (see below). Several multicenter trials are currently under way to assess the clinical utility of this procedure.[27,28]

In-transit metastases   In-transit metastases can remain confined to a single limb for prolonged periods. Amputation does not appear to provide a long-term survival benefit in this setting. Slow-growing individual in-transit metastases can be managed surgically. More extensive disease can be treated with sensitization therapy with dinitrochlorobenzene (DNCB). For extensive in-transit metastases confined to an extremity, limb perfusion therapy can result in dramatic palliation and limb salvage. The procedure entails isolation of the vasculature of the involved extremity from the systemic vasculature and perfusion of the isolated limb with chemotherapeutic agents, biologic agents, or both at doses that could not be tolerated if given systemically.[29]

Distant metastases   Despite the development of several novel approaches to the treatment of patients with metastatic melanoma, including multidrug chemotherapy, biologic therapy, immunotherapy, and combinations of these treatments, monotherapy with dacarbazine (DTIC) remains the only regimen approved by the Food and Drug Administration for the treatment of metastatic melanoma.[30] Objective responses to DTIC are seen in approximately 5% to 20% of patients; durable complete responses are rare. Radiation therapy can play an important palliative role. In the absence of more effective clinically proven therapy, patients with distant metastases should be offered the opportunity to participate in clinical trials of experimental therapy when appropriate.

Adjuvant therapy   Patients with cutaneous or regional disease who have been surgically rendered free of disease but are at high risk for recurrence or metastasis are potential candidates for adjuvant therapy.[31] Various adjuvant therapies have been used in melanoma, including immunostimulants such as bacillus Calmette-Guérin, *Corynebacterium parvum,* and levamisole. Several chemotherapeutic agents have been tried as well. More recently, immunotherapy with cytokines, such as interferons, and active immunization with vaccines have been studied. A high-dose regimen of interferon alfa (20 million units/m^2 I.V. daily for 1 month followed by 10 million units/m^2 S.C. three times a week for 48 weeks) has been approved by the FDA for use as adjuvant therapy for melanoma. Two studies have demonstrated a small but statistically significant improvement in overall survival with this regimen. Multiple studies have failed to demonstrate improved long-term overall survival with the use of adjuvant interferon in intermediate-dose or low-dose regimens.[32,33]

A host of novel strategies, including active immunization, passive immunization, and myriad biologic therapies, are currently being studied and may provide opportunities for patients who are appropriate candidates for trials.[34]

Prognosis

Stage   The single strongest prognostic factor for melanoma is stage of disease. Various staging classifications have been used over the years. All staging systems for melanoma take into account the classic TNM classification of tumor size (T), lymph node involvement (N), and distant metastases (M). The differences across staging systems relate largely to the staging of the primary site. New staging systems attempt to use the attributes of the primary tumor that strongly correlate with outcome. These attributes include thickness, ulceration, and, in the case of thin melanomas less than 1 mm, the Clark level of invasion. The advent of sentinel node biopsy has led to the inclusion of microstaging of lymph nodes in the new staging system [*see Tables 2 and 3*].[35,36]

Attributes of the primary tumor   Several attributes of the primary tumor have been identified as predictors of outcome from primary cutaneous melanoma. The single strongest, most consistent predictor of outcome is the Breslow tumor thickness. Other important histologic parameters are the Clark level of tumor invasion, extent of ulceration, rate of mitosis, presence of tumor-infiltrating lymphocytes, and vascular invasion. For thin primary melanomas, one of the strongest predictors of outcome is growth phase.[37] Radial-growth-phase melanoma does not appear to metastasize, whereas vertical-growth-phase melanoma (characterized by the formation of a tumor nodule in the dermis) is associated with significant risk of metastasis even in lesions less than 1 mm thick.[38] Patient characteristics associated with improved survival from melanoma include young age (< 60 years), female sex, and location of the melanoma on an extremity. Multivariable models for predicting outcome from melanoma have been developed [*see Table 4*].[39]

Malignant Tumors of the Dermis

METASTATIC TUMORS

Cutaneous metastases occur in approximately 5% of patients with solid tumors and are usually associated with widespread disease. The relative frequency of skin metastases is gender specific, reflecting the rates of the primary cancers.[40] In women, two thirds of metastases are from breast cancer, but lung, colorectal, melanoma, and ovarian cancers are also frequent. In men, lung cancer is most common, followed by cancer of the large intestine, melanoma, SCC of the head and neck, and cancer of the kidneys.[40] The anatomic distribution of skin metastases is not random. Cutaneous metastases from breast cancer often involve the chest wall and may appear as nodules, lymphedema, or cellulitis. The scalp is a common site for metastasis, especially of cancer from the lung and kidney (in men) and breast (in women). Head and neck cancers may invade the skin by local extension, giving rise to a firm, dusky-red edema of the skin that resembles cellulitis. Abdominal wall metastases, often called Sister Joseph's nodules, may occur with GI or ovarian malignancies.[40] Clinically, cutaneous metastases are often minimally symptomatic dermal papules or nodules and are flesh-colored or pink; dissemination occurs via lymphatic or vascular pathways. Cutaneous metastases may clinically reflect the histology of the primary tumor (e.g., black, brown, or gray nodules with metastatic melanoma, and vascular nodules with renal cell or thyroid carcinoma).

PRIMARY TUMORS

Primary malignancies of the dermis may develop from any of the myriad structures of the skin, including sebaceous glands (sebaceous carcinoma), connective tissue (dermatofibrosarcoma protuberans), smooth muscle (leiomyosarcoma), and other adnexal tissue (eccrine carcinoma).[41] Most of these primary dermal neoplasms are rare; they may exhibit aggressive biologic behavior. Although these neoplasms are quite varied histologically, many share a common clinical presentation of a rapidly growing flesh-colored to pink or red subcutaneous nodule that occasionally resembles a sebaceous cyst.

Merkel cell carcinoma This neoplasm is a dermal malignancy of neuroendocrine origin. It usually appears as a red to violaceous dermal papule or nodule on the head and neck of elderly patients, although all age groups are affected.[41] The treatment of choice is wide local excision with or without ELND. Local recurrences are frequent, and distant metastases occur in

Table 2   AJCC 2002 TNM Classification[35]

TNM Classification	Node Size, Number, or Site	Characteristics
T classification T1	≤ 1.0 mm	a: Without ulceration and Clark level II or III b: With ulceration or Clark level IV or V
T2	1.01–2.0 mm	a: Without ulceration b: With ulceration
T3	2.01–4.0 mm	a: Without ulceration b: With ulceration
T4	> 4.0 mm	a: Without ulceration b: With ulceration
N classification N1	One lymph node	a: Micrometastasis* b. Macrometastasis†
N2	2–3 lymph nodes	a: Micrometastasis* b. Macrometastasis† c: In-transit met(s)/satellites(s) without metastatic lymph nodes
N3	4 or more metastatic lymph nodes, matted lymph nodes, or combination of in-transit met(s)/satellite(s) with metastatic lymph nodes	—
M classification M1a	Distant skin, subcutaneous, or lymph node mets	Normal LDH
M1b	Lung mets	Normal LDH
M1c	All other visceral mets Any distant mets	Normal LDH Elevated LDH with any M

*Micrometastases are diagnosed after sentinel or elective lymphadenectomy.
†Macrometastases are defined as clinically detectable nodal metastases confirmed by therapeutic lymphadenectomy; the term also applies to nodal metastases that exhibit gross extracapsular extension.
AJCC—American Joint Committee on Cancer   LD—lactic dehydrogenase   mets—metastases

Table 3 AJCC 2002 Staging System[35]

Pathologic Stage	TNM	Thickness (mm)	Ulceration	No. + Nodes	Node Size	Distant Metastasis	5-Year Survival	10-Year Survival
IA	T1a	< 1	No	0	—	—	95.3 ± 0.4	87.9 ± 1.0
IB	T1b	< 1	Yes or level IV, V	0	—	—	90.9 ± 1.0	83.1 ± 1.5
	T2a	1.01–2.0	No	0	—	—	89.0 ± 0.7	79.2 ± 1.1
IIA	T2b	1.01–2.0	Yes	0	—	—	77.4 ± 1.7	64.4 ± 2.2
	T3a	2.01–4.0	No	0	—	—	78.7 ± 1.2	63.8 ± 1.7
IIB	T3b	2.01–4.0	Yes	0	—	—	63.0 ± 1.5	50.8 ± 1.7
	T4a	> 4.0	No	0	—	—	67.4 ± 2.4	53.9 ± 3.3
IIC	T4b	> 4.0	Yes	0	—	—	45.1 ± 1.9	32.3 ± 2.1
IIIA	N1a	Any	No	1	Micro	—	69.5 ± 3.7	63.0 ± 4.4
	N2a	Any	No	2–3	Micro	—	63.3 ± 5.6	56.9 ± 6.8
IIIB	N1a	Any	Yes	1	Micro	—	52.8 ± 4.1	37.8 ± 4.8
	N2a	Any	Yes	2–3	Micro	—	49.6 ± 5.7	35.9 ± 7.2
	N1b	Any	No	1	Macro	—	59.0 ± 4.8	47.7 ± 5.8
	N2b	Any	No	2–3	Macro	—	46.3 ± 5.5	39.2 ± 5.8
IIIC	N1b	Any	Yes	1	Macro	—	29.0 ± 5.1	24.4 ± 5.3
	N2b	Any	Yes	2–3	Macro	—	24.0 ± 4.4	15.0 ± 3.9
	N3	Any	Any	4	Micro/macro	—	26.7 ± 2.5	18.4 ± 2.5
IV	M1a	Any	Any	Any	Any	Skin, S.C.	18.8 ± 3.0	15.7 ± 2.9
	M1b	Any	Any	Any	Any	Lung	6.7 ± 2.0	2.5 ± 1.5
	M1c	Any	Any	Any	Any	Other visceral	9.5 ± 1.1	6.0 ± 0.9

AJCC—American Joint Committee on Cancer   S.C.—subcutaneous

more than one third of patients. Chemotherapy of metastases is generally disappointing.[41]

Paget disease A rare malignancy of the skin associated with an underlying adenocarcinoma,[40,41] Paget disease usually presents as an erythematous, often weeping unilateral dermatitis of the breast that involves the nipple and areola. The differential diagnosis includes eczema, psoriasis, contact dermatitis, and impetigo. For this reason, biopsy of an inflammatory, nonresolving dermatitis of the nipple or areola is imperative. In Paget disease, the biopsy will reveal typical pale-staining Paget cells in the epidermis. Appropriate surgical resection of the cutaneous and underlying neoplasm is the treatment of choice; lymph node metastases often occur.[41]

Extramammary Paget disease Extramammary Paget disease is even more uncommon than Paget disease. It typically presents as red, often ulcerated, plaques in the perineal areas of elderly persons.[40,41] Lesions may be pruritic or asymptomatic, are often long-standing, and may have been misdiagnosed as psoriasis, contact dermatitis, or chronic fungal infections. Underlying associated tumors include rectal and genitourinary carcinomas. Even without an associated internal malignancy, extramammary Paget disease is difficult to treat, and it is associated with a high local recurrence rate.[41]

Angiosarcoma A rare, often highly aggressive vascular malignancy,[41] angiosarcoma may appear as multicentric reddish-purple patches or nodules in a lymphedematous limb, such as on a lymphedematous arm after a mastectomy (Stewart-Treves syndrome). Another presentation is violaceous patches or plaques on the head or neck (especially scalp) of elderly persons. Patients with angiosarcoma have a poor prognosis, with pulmonary metastases frequently developing despite surgery or radiation.[41]

Dermatofibrosarcoma protuberans Dermatofibrosarcoma protuberans is a slow-growing, locally aggressive malignancy that rarely metastasizes but often recurs. Lesions typically present as firm reddish-brown or purple nodules, usually on the trunk or non–sun-exposed extremities. The differential diagnosis includes keloids and benign dermatofibroma. Young adults are most often affected, although the tumor may occur at any age. Wide local excision with or without Mohs micrographic surgery offers the best chance of cure.[41]

KAPOSI SARCOMA

Kaposi sarcoma (KS) is a multicentric cutaneous neoplasm that has several distinct clinical variants.[42,43] In spite of its name, KS is not a true sarcoma. Although the cell of origin has not been clearly established, lymphatic endothelium is a likely candidate.[42,43]

Epidemiology

In its classic form, KS is an indolent disease of elderly men of Mediterranean or eastern European background, in which violaceous nodules and plaques develop on the lower extremities.[42,43] Before the advent of AIDS, the disorder was rare in the United States, with an age-adjusted annual incidence of 0.29 per 100,000 population in men and 0.07 per 100,000 population in women.[43] In the mid-1960s, a second, endemic form of KS was recognized in central Africa. African KS, which typically affects young adults and children, pursues a more aggressive course than classic KS, with frequent bone, lymph node, and visceral involvement.[42,43]

In 1981, KS became the first tumor to be recognized as part of AIDS. Primarily affecting homosexual men, KS was an AIDS-defining illness for 30% to 40% of patients in the earliest years of the HIV epidemic.[42] HIV-infected homosexual men have a 73,000-fold increased incidence of KS, and HIV-infected women and nonhomosexual men have a 10,000-fold increase, compared with the general United States population.[42,43] A fourth variant of KS has been recognized in iatrogenically immunosuppressed patients, especially organ transplant recipients. Men are affected slightly more often than women.[42,43]

Etiology

The epidemiology of KS has long suggested a transmissible infectious agent or cofactor.[42,43] Kaposi sarcoma–associated herpesvirus (KSHV), also known as human herpesvirus type 8 (HHV-8), has been detected[44] and propagated[45] in all variants of KS. HHV-8 has also been found in patients with body cavity–based lymphoma, Castleman disease, and angioblastic lymphadenopathy, as well as in certain skin lesions of organ transplant recipients.[42] There is a high risk of KS in HIV-infected individuals who are coinfected with HHV-8; up to half of such patients will develop KS during long-term (i.e., 10-year) follow-up.[46] The mechanism by which HHV-8 infection leads to KS tumorigenesis is unclear but probably involves a complex combination of inflammation, angiogenesis, and neoplastic proliferation.[42,43] The prevalence of KS largely parallels the rate of HHV-8 infection in various populations.[43] Although the incidence of HHV-8 infection may be as high as 2% to 10% in the general population, the incidence of KS is very low, suggesting that the majority of infections are subclinical.[42,43]

Host factors, particularly immunosuppression, are crucial in some populations with KS.[42,43] HIV may play an indirect role in the development of KS through CD4+ T cell depletion and stimulated production of cytokines such as interleukin-1 (IL-1) and IL-6.[42,43] Immunosuppressive drugs, especially cyclosporine, azathioprine, and prednisone, increase the risk of developing KS, especially in kidney and liver transplant recipients.[43] Spontaneous KS regression has been observed after withdrawal of cyclosporine and corticosteroids.[43]

Despite the prevalence of KS in some ethnic groups, the role of any possible genetic factors is unclear. An increased incidence of HLA-DR5 in classic KS patients has been debated.[43] Familial KS is extremely rare, suggesting that genetic factors alone are not responsible.

Finally, gender appears to be a significant risk factor, especially in classic KS, in which the male-to-female ratio may range from 3:1 to 10:1.[42,43] The reasons for this male predominance remain unclear.[42,43]

Diagnosis

The clinical manifestations of KS differ among the variants of the disorder.[42,43] In classic KS, faint reddish-purple macules or patches or purple nodules first appear on the feet, especially the soles. Lymphadenopathy (especially inguinal) is present on rare occasions. Lesions may also occasionally develop on the arms and genital areas. As the disease progresses, the lesions coalesce into violaceous plaques.

HIV-associated KS usually presents as cutaneous lesions, but the first lesions may appear in the oral mucosa or lymph nodes. In contrast to classic KS lesions, HIV-associated KS lesions often begin on the upper body (face, trunk, or arms). Most typically, HIV-associated KS lesions are purple-red, often oval, papules that follow the skin lines in a pityriasis rosea–like distribution.[42,43] Lesions vary from pink macules to deep-purple plaques [see Figure 5] or may resemble ecchymoses, especially in patients with low CD4+ T cell counts. Oral lesions are typically red-purple plaques or nodules on the palate, gingiva, or buccal mucosa. Patients with darker skin may have dark-purple to black lesions or hyperpigmented plaques.[43]

As HIV-associated KS progresses, lymphedema may develop in the feet, scrotum, genitalia, and periorbital regions, and lymphadenopathy (especially inguinal) may occur. Gastrointestinal lesions are usually submucosal and asymptomatic but may result in gastrointestinal hemorrhage. Pulmonary KS carries a poor prognosis.[43]

Laboratory workup of patients with KS should include HIV antibody testing, complete blood count, fecal occult blood test-

Table 4 Estimated Probability of 10-Year Survival in Patients with Primary Cutaneous Melanoma[37]

| Tumor Thickness/Age of Patient | Probability of 10-Year Survival* | | | |
| | Tumor with Extremity Location | | Tumor with Axis Location† | |
	Female Patients	Male Patients	Female Patients	Male Patients
< 0.76 mm				
≤ 60 yr	0.99 (0.98–1.0)	0.98 (0.95–0.99)	0.97 (0.93–0.99)	0.94 (0.88–0.97)
> 60 yr	0.98 (0.95–0.99)	0.96 (0.89–0.98)	0.92 (0.82–0.96)	0.84 (0.70–0.93)
0.76–1.69 mm				
≤ 60 yr	0.96 (0.92–0.98)	0.93 (0.85–0.97)	0.86 (0.76–0.92)	0.75 (0.62–0.84)
> 60 yr	0.90 (0.80–0.95)	0.81 (0.64–0.91)	0.67 (0.50–0.81)	0.50 (0.33–0.67)
1.70–3.60 mm				
≤ 60 yr	0.89 (0.80–0.94)	0.80 (0.65–0.89)	0.65 (0.50–0.77)	0.48 (0.35–0.61)
> 60 yr	0.73 (0.57–0.85)	0.57 (0.38–0.75)	0.38 (0.24–0.55)	0.24 (0.14–0.37)
> 3.60 mm				
≤ 60 yr	0.74 (0.53–0.87)	0.58 (0.36–0.77)	0.39 (0.21–0.60)	0.24 (0.13–0.40)
> 60 yr	0.48 (0.28–0.69)	0.32 (0.16–0.53)	0.18 (0.08–0.35)	0.10 (0.04–0.20)

*Confidence interval = 95%.
†Axis location includes the trunk, head, neck, and volar and subungual sites.

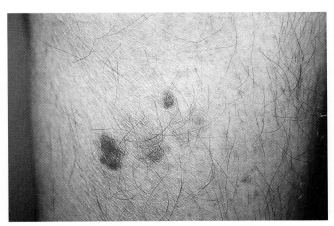

Figure 5 **HIV-associated Kaposi sarcoma lesions vary from pink patches (shown) to deep-purple plaques.**

ing, and chest radiograph. CD4[+] T cell counts are indicated in HIV-positive patients. A complete medical history and physical examination should be performed, with special attention paid to the presence of opportunistic infections in HIV-infected or otherwise immunosuppressed patients.

Skin biopsy should be obtained in patients with suspected KS. The histopathologies of all KS variants are similar: spindle-shaped cells in the dermis, with extravasated red blood cells present in slits between irregular vascular spaces.[47]

Differential Diagnosis

The clinical differential diagnosis of KS includes dermatofibroma, purpura, pyogenic granuloma, bacillary angiomatosis, metastatic melanoma, and BCC. Other histopathologic entities that may resemble KS include angiosarcoma and stasis dermatitis.[42,43]

Treatment

Classic Kaposi sarcoma   The therapy for KS is palliative. In classic KS, where the disease is indolent and the patients are elderly, aggressive systemic therapy is rarely warranted.[42,43] Instead, radiation therapy is the treatment of choice.[43,48] KS is very radiosensitive: single doses of 800 cGy have been used for rapid palliation in patients with poor prognoses.[49] Total doses of 800 to 3,500 cGy have yielded 50% complete responses and 46% partial responses, with more than half of patients needing no follow-up treatment for as long as 13 years.[48] A treatment regimen equivalent to 3,000 cGy in 10 fractions over 2 weeks has been advocated.[48]

For patients with classic KS who have only one or two papules, excisional biopsy may be sufficient for both diagnosis and treatment. Cryotherapy with liquid nitrogen may be useful for isolated papules. Systemic therapy for classic KS may be indicated in cases of extensive cutaneous disease or visceral involvement. Single-agent chemotherapy with vinca alkaloids (vincristine or vinblastine) is most commonly used. Low-dose recombinant interferon alfa may also be effective in classic KS; however, side effects (fever, chills, myalgias, and fatigue) may not be well tolerated by elderly patients.[42,43]

HIV-associated Kaposi sarcoma Although KS is more aggressive in HIV-infected patients, the extent of immune suppression and the presence of opportunistic infections or other systemic illnesses may be of equal importance in staging, determining prognosis, and choosing appropriate therapy.[42,43] Clinical features that were traditionally associated with a more favorable outcome included a CD4[+] T cell count higher than 200

cells/mm³, a lack of systemic illness, KS limited to the skin or lymph nodes, and minimal (i.e., not nodular) oral KS; poor risk factors included a CD4[+] T cell count below 200 cells/mm³, KS-associated lymphedema, visceral KS, ulcerated KS, nodular oral KS, and opportunistic infection.[50] With the advent of highly active antiretroviral therapy (HAART), however, physicians treating patients with HIV-associated KS now have the opportunity to influence and even reverse immune suppression by affecting both HIV viral load and CD4[+] T cell count. Regression of KS has been observed after initiation of HAART, often during the first few months of therapy[51]; consequently, this is often first-line therapy in HIV-associated KS.[43]

Local therapy is a reasonable approach in KS patients with limited disease, those with infectious complications, and those who cannot tolerate systemic therapy.[49] Specific antitumor therapy has not been shown to improve overall survival.[42,43] Radiation therapy is effective in HIV-associated KS in doses similar to those for classic KS (see above). Responses in HIV-associated KS are generally short-lived, however.[43] Topical alitretinoin (9-*cis*-retinoic acid) gel may be effective in HIV-associated KS and has been approved by the FDA for this use.[52] Intralesional injections of vinblastine or interferon have also been useful in selected lesions.[42,43] Cryotherapy with liquid nitrogen is effective for small lesions[49]; however, cryotherapy is contraindicated in dark-skinned patients in whom posttreatment hypopigmentation may appear much worse cosmetically than the original KS lesion.

Systemic therapy has included conventional chemotherapy and biologic response modifiers. Single-agent chemotherapeutic regimens have response rates of 30% to 70%.[42,43] In the past, combination chemotherapy (e.g., doxorubicin, bleomycin, and vincristine) was complicated by profound bone marrow suppression and frequent opportunistic infections. The advent of hematopoietic colony-stimulating factors (e.g., granulocyte colony-stimulating factor) and *Pneumocystis carinii* prophylaxis reduced these complications.

The development of liposomally encapsulated anthracyclines (e.g., doxorubicin and daunorubicin) represents an important new option in KS treatment. In a randomized study of 258 patients with advanced AIDS-associated KS, those who received pegylated liposomal doxorubicin had significantly higher response rates than those who received standard combination chemotherapy with doxorubicin, bleomycin, and vincristine.[53] Paclitaxel has also had good responses in patients with advanced KS.[54]

Promising investigative approaches for HIV-associated KS include combination therapy with antiretroviral agents and specific antitumor therapy and, potentially, therapy targeting HHV-8.[42,43]

Complications

Bacterial infections and sepsis are common with ulcerated tumors of the legs and feet. Opportunistic infections may intervene, especially in patients with very low CD4[+] T cell counts.

Prognosis

The total CD4[+] T cell count is the most important predictor of survival in HIV-associated KS.[50] Large tumor burdens,[50] lymphedema, and pulmonary KS are also predictive of poorer outcomes.[50,54]

Cutaneous Lymphoma

Lymphomas may be of B cell or T cell lineage and may involve the skin primarily or secondarily [*see Chapter 191*]. B cell lymphomas, particularly non-Hodgkin lymphomas, may in-

a 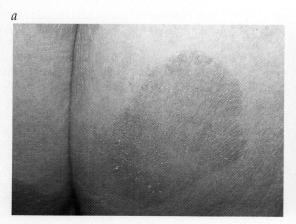 *b*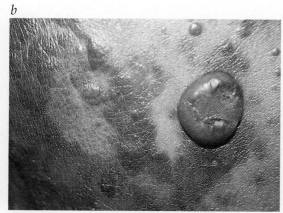

Figure 6 Cutaneous T cell lymphoma is shown in the large-patch stage (*a*) and as tumor-stage mycosis fungoides (*b*).

volve the skin secondarily in advanced disease. They typically appear as reddish-purple subcutaneous plaques or nodules. Primary B cell lymphomas of the skin are even rarer. They appear as reddish nodules that often remain localized to the skin but may progress to systemic disease. The vast majority of primary cutaneous lymphomas fall into the spectrum of cutaneous T cell lymphoma (CTCL).

CTCL is a rare skin disorder that is often still referred to as mycosis fungoides (MF).[55,56] MF is actually the largest subset of CTCL; the two terms, however, are often used interchangeably. The leukemic variant of MF is termed Sézary syndrome.[55] Another variant of CTCL is associated with human T cell lymphotropic virus type I (HTLV-I) and is part of the spectra of adult T cell lymphoma/leukemia and peripheral T cell lymphoma.[55]

EPIDEMIOLOGY

Approximately 1,000 new cases of CTCL are diagnosed in the United States each year.[55,56] From 1973 to 1984, the incidence of CTCL rose from 0.19 per 100,000 population to 0.42 per 100,000 population. CTCL primarily affects middle-aged adults; the median age at presentation is 50 years.[57] The male-to-female ratio is approximately 2:1; blacks are twice as likely as whites to develop CTCL.[55,57]

ETIOLOGY

Host susceptibility and an environmental antigen, perhaps viral, are hypothesized as playing important roles in the pathogenesis of CTCL.[55] Genetic factors may be related to major histocompatibility antigens, such as an increase in HLA-DR5 in CTCL patients.[58] Chronic antigenic stimulation (e.g., infection) may play an etiologic role.[55] For example, HTLV-I infection may be associated with a peripheral T cell lymphoma with cutaneous involvement; it has unique clinical features, including hypercalcemia and bone lesions.[55]

DIAGNOSIS

Clinical Manifestations

The clinical manifestations of MF typically evolve over many months to years. In one study, the mean duration of symptoms before diagnosis was 7.5 years.[59] Flat erythematous patches, often scaling and occasionally atrophic, begin most commonly on the trunk and thighs, especially in a so-called bathing-trunk distribution [*see Figure 6*]. Lesions are asymptomatic or mildly pruritic and may spontaneously remit or re-

spond to topical corticosteroid therapy. Patients may also report improvement after sun exposure.

As MF progresses, patches tend to enlarge and thicken into plaques. The color may become darker red; in dark-skinned persons, lesions may initially be hyperpigmented or hypopigmented and may acquire an erythematous or violaceous hue. In advanced MF, tumors may develop or transform to a large-cell lymphoma.[55,60,61] In approximately 10% of cases, tumors are the initial presentation of CTCL (tumor d'emblé). Generalized erythroderma with circulating atypical T cells (in Sézary syndrome) is the presentation in 5% of CTCL patients.[55]

Physical examination of patients with suspected CTCL includes complete skin examination, including classification of lesions (patch, plaque, or tumor) and extent of body surface area involved. Lymph nodes, liver, and spleen should be palpated.

Skin Biopsy

Skin biopsy is necessary for the definitive diagnosis of MF. The presence of atypical lymphoid cells with hyperconvoluted cerebriform nuclei in clusters in the epidermis (Pautrier microabscesses) and a bandlike lymphocytic infiltrate in the upper dermis are diagnostic of CTCL.[55,56,61] The malignant cell is a T cell, with most of the cells expressing the pan–T cell markers CD2, CD3, and CD5.[55] The use of T cell receptor gene rearrangement studies to confirm clonality in early disease may be an aid to diagnosis.[55] Neither immunophenotypic studies nor electron microscopy may be considered as definitively diagnostic of MF; clinicopathologic correlation is necessary.

Laboratory Studies

The laboratory evaluation for CTCL includes complete blood count, eosinophil count, Sézary cell count, assessment of lactic dehydrogenase level, and liver function tests. Bone marrow biopsy is unnecessary in the absence of circulating leukemic cells. HTLV-I testing should be considered for patients with risk factors or atypical presentations. Lymph node biopsy should be considered for palpable nodes, especially those larger than 2 cm. Abdominal computed tomography or chest radiography may be important in patients with tumors or suspected visceral involvement.

DIFFERENTIAL DIAGNOSIS

In its early stages, MF may resemble any of a number of benign inflammatory disorders (e.g., drug reaction, eczema, psoriasis, or contact dermatitis). These disorders should be ruled out before contemplating therapy.

TREATMENT

Topical Therapy

Topical therapy is the mainstay of the treatment of early (stage IA, IB, and IIA), patch, or plaque disease. Early aggressive therapy with radiation and chemotherapy has not proved to be superior to local approaches in controlling disease or improving survival in patients with limited disease.[55,56] A rational approach for early limited (or histologically equivocal) disease is topical corticosteroids.[62] Topical nitrogen mustard (mechlorethamine), in either aqueous or ointment form, is the most frequently used topical chemotherapy and leads to complete remission in patch and plaque disease in up to 60% to 80% of patients.[55,63] Therapy must continue for prolonged periods (up to 3 years after clearing of lesions). Contact dermatitis develops in about one third of patients.[55]

Carmustine (BCNU) solution, applied daily to lesions, is another useful regimen. Treatment generally lasts 8 to 16 weeks but has been continued for up to 6 months. Because systemic absorption can result in bone marrow suppression, complete blood counts must be monitored.[55,63] Recently, a topical retinoid, bexarotene, was shown to be effective in CTCL; it is approved by the FDA for use in CTCL.[64]

Ultraviolet Radiation

Radiation therapy for CTCL takes several forms, from ultraviolet light to ionizing radiation. UVB is useful in stage I disease. In one study, it resulted in a 71% complete clinical remission rate. Median time to remission was 5 months, and median duration was 22 months.[65]

Another effective approach in MF is the combination of psoralen and UVA (PUVA). In one study, 95% of patients with stage I CTCL had complete clinical clearing, with a median response duration of 43 months.[66]

Radiation Therapy

Total skin electron beam (TSEB) radiation delivers radiotherapy to the skin surface without a significant internal dose. It is especially useful with plaque diseases. Typical doses are 2,400 to 3,600 cGy, fractionated over several weeks with 4 to 9 MeV electron beam radiation.[67] Complete skin remissions are related to stage as follows: IA, 84% to 96%; IB, 56% to 81%; IIA, 63% to 74%; IIB, 24% to 53%; III, 26% to 50%; and IVA, 8% to 33%. A 50% relapse-free survival at 5 years was achieved with IA disease, but most patients with more advanced disease experienced relapse by 5 years.[67]

Systemic Therapy

Systemic therapy for CTCL has been undertaken as primary therapy in advanced disease (stages III through IVB) and as sequential therapy to promote more durable responses in earlier disease.[55,56] Oral bexarotene has yielded response rates of up to 45%, and it is approved by the FDA for use in this disease.[68] Another recently approved systemic therapy for CTCL is denileukin diftitox [DAB(389) IL-2].[69] This receptor-targeted cytotoxic fusion protein binds to the IL-2 receptor on T cells; it achieved a 30% response rate in heavily-pretreated patients with CTCL.[70]

Extracorporeal photopheresis appears most useful in erythrodermic CTCL and Sézary syndrome.[49,62] In this treatment, the patient undergoes extracorporeal photopheresis with UVA irradiation to leukocytes after oral ingestion of 8-methoxypsoralen.

Advanced tumor and visceral CTCL have also been treated with single-agent and combination chemotherapy, including methotrexate, adenosine analogues, interferon alfa, and retinoids.

Combination Therapy

Early aggressive treatment of CTCL (TSEB followed by combination chemotherapy with cyclophosphamide, doxorubicin, etoposide, and vincristine) provides no survival advantage over sequential topical therapy.[55] Similarly, the addition of systemic chemotherapy (doxorubicin and cyclophosphamide) or extracorporeal photopheresis after a complete response to TSEB appears to have no impact on survival on early MF and no impact on relapse-free survival for all stages.[69] Other regimens include interferon alfa and retinoids (isotretinoin) with TSEB, followed by topical nitrogen mustard. The heterogeneity of reported combination therapy regimens in CTCL makes it virtually impossible to compare results.

COMPLICATIONS

The most serious complications of CTCL are infections. Sepsis from ulcerated cutaneous tumors is a common cause of death. Visceral CTCL may occur, as may transformation to large cell lymphoma in some CTCL patients (39% probability after 12 years).[60] In long-term survivors with early disease, local therapies (e.g., TSEB or PUVA) may contribute to the development of other skin cancers (e.g., BCC or SCC) and cataracts.

PROGNOSIS

Staging of CTCL is based on an evaluation of type and extent of skin lesions and extent of lymph node, peripheral blood, and visceral involvement.[55,56,59,61] Many different attempts have been made to classify CTCL into useful prognostic groups. An early and still valid study that used the TNM system identified three major groups: good-risk patients (stages IA, IB, and IIA, with plaque-only skin disease and no lymph node, blood, or visceral involvement [median survival, > 12 years]); intermediate-risk patients (stages IIB, III, and IVA, with cutaneous tumors, erythroderma, or plaque disease and node or blood involvement but no visceral disease or node effacement [median survival, 5 years]); and poor-risk patients (stage IVB, with visceral involvement or node effacement [median survival, 2.5 years]).[59]

Eosinophilia is also associated with shortened survival.[59] Other long-term studies have revealed that stage IA patients do not have a reduced life expectancy and that fewer than 10% of these patients experience disease progression to more advanced stages.[71] Survival of patients with generalized patch/plaque MF (stages IB or IIA), at a median of 11.7 years, is significantly worse than that of a race-, age-, and sex-matched control population.[72] Gender and race appear to have no effect on survival, but older patients (> 58 years) have shorter disease-specific survivals.[55,57]

References

1. Marks R: An overview of skin cancers: incidence and causation. Cancer 75:607, 1995
2. Grossman D, Leffell DJ: The molecular basis of nonmelanoma skin cancer: new understanding. Arch Dermatol 133:1263, 1997
3. Naylor MF, Farmer KC: The case for sunscreens: a review of their use in preventing actinic damage and neoplasia. Arch Dermatol 133:1146, 1997
4. Buettner PG, Raasch BA: Incidence rates of skin cancer in Townsville, Australia. Int J Cancer 78:302, 1998
5. Scotto J, Fears TR, Fraumeni JF: Incidence of non-melanoma skin cancer in the United States (NIH Publication No. 83-2433). U.S. Public Health Service, Bethesda, Maryland, 1983
6. Gailani MR, Bale AE: Developmental genes and cancer: role of patched in basal cell carcinoma of the skin. J Natl Cancer Inst 89:1103, 1997
7. Shriner DL, McCoy DK, Goldberg DJ, et al: Mohs micrographic surgery. J Am Acad Dermatol 39:79, 1998
8. Paver K, Royser K, Burry N, et al: The incidence of basal cell carcinoma and their

metastases in Australia and New Zealand. Australas J Dermatol 14:53, 1973

9. Miller DL, Weinstock MA: Nonmelanoma skin cancer in the United States: incidence. J Am Acad Dermatol 30:774, 1994

10. Staples M, Marks R, Giles G: Trends in the incidence of non-melanocytic skin cancer (NMSC) treated in Australia 1985–1995: are primary prevention programs starting to have an effect? Int J Cancer 78:144, 1998

11. Elder D, Elenitsas R, Jaworsky C, et al: Tumors and cysts of the epidermis. Lever's Histopathology of the Skin, 8th ed. Lippincott-Raven, Philadelphia, 1997, p 685

12. Miller SJ: The National Comprehensive Cancer Network (NCCN) guidelines of care for nonmelanoma skin cancers. Dermatol Surg 26:289, 2000

13. Rowe DE, Carroll RJ, Day CL Jr: Prognostic factors for local recurrence, metastasis, and survival rates in squamous cell carcinoma of the skin, ear, and lip: implications for treatment modality selection. J Am Acad Dermatol 26:976, 1992

14. Hall HI, Miller DR, Rogers JD, et al: Update on the incidence and mortality from melanoma in the United States. J Am Acad Dermatol 40:35, 1999

15. Haluska FG, Hodi FS: Molecular genetics of familial cutaneous melanoma. J Clin Oncol 16:670, 1998

16. Blackwood MA, Holmes R, Synnestvedt M, et al: Multiple primary melanoma revisited. Cancer 94:2248, 2002

17. Elder DE, Clark WH Jr, Elenitsas R, et al: The early and intermediate precursor lesions of tumor progression in the melanocytic system: common acquired nevi and atypical (dysplastic) nevi. Semin Diagn Pathol 10:18, 1993

18. Carey WP Jr, Thompson CJ, Synnestvedt M, et al: Dysplastic nevi as a melanoma risk factor in patients with familial melanoma. Cancer 74:3118, 1994

19. Tucker MA, Halpern A, Holly EA, et al: Clinically recognized dysplastic nevi: a central risk factor for cutaneous melanoma. JAMA 277:1439, 1997

20. Binder M, Puespoeck-Schwarz M, Steiner A, et al: Epiluminescence microscopy of small pigmented skin lesions: short-term formal training improves the diagnostic performance of dermatologists. J Am Acad Dermatol 36:197, 1997

21. Binder M, Schwarz M, Winkler A, et al: Epiluminescence microscopy: a useful tool for the diagnosis of pigmented skin lesions for formally trained dermatologists. Arch Dermatol 131:286, 1995

22. Halpern AC: The use of whole body photography in a pigmented lesion clinic. Dermatol Surg 26:1175, 2000

23. Busam KJ, Charles C, Lee G, et al: Morphologic features of melanocytes, pigmented keratinocytes, and melanophages by in vivo confocal scanning laser microscopy. Mod Pathol 14:862, 2001

24. Balch CM, Soong SJ, Smith T, et al: Long-term results of a prospective surgical trial comparing 2 cm vs. 4 cm excision margins for 740 patients with 1–4 mm melanomas. Ann Surg Oncol 8:101, 2001

25. Veronesi U, Cascinelli N, Adamus J, et al: Thin stage I primary cutaneous malignant melanoma: comparison of excision with margins of 1 or 3 cm. N Engl J Med 318:1159, 1988

26. Gershenwald JE, Thompson W, Mansfield PF, et al: Multi-institutional melanoma lymphatic mapping experience: the prognostic value of sentinel lymph node status in 612 stage I or II melanoma patients. J Clin Oncol 17:976, 1999

27. Kelley MC, Ollila DW, Morton DL: Lymphatic mapping and sentinel lymphadenectomy for melanoma. Semin Surg Oncol 14:283, 1998

28. Chan AD, Morton DL: Sentinel node detection in malignant melanoma. Recent Results Cancer Res 157:161, 2000

29. Thompson JF, Hunt JA, Shannon KF, et al: Frequency and duration of remission after isolated limb perfusion for melanoma. Arch Surg 132:903, 1997

30. Houghton A, Coit D, Bloomer W, et al: NCCN melanoma practice guidelines. Oncology 12:153, 1998

31. Agarwala SS, Kirkwood JM: Adjuvant interferon treatment for melanoma. Hematol Oncol Clin North Am 12:823, 1998

32. Kirkwood JM, Strawderman MH, Ernstoff MS, et al: Interferon alfa-2b adjuvant therapy of high-risk resected cutaneous melanoma: the Eastern Cooperative Oncology Group Trial EST 1684. J Clin Oncol 14:7, 1996

33. Kirkwood JM, Ibrahim JG, Sosman JA, et al: High-dose interferon alfa-2b significantly prolongs relapse-free and overall survival compared with the GM2-KLH/QS-21 vaccine in patients with resected stage IIB-III melanoma: results of intergroup trial E1694/S9512/C509801. J Clin Oncol 19:2370, 2001

34. Brinckerhoff LH, Thompson LW, Slingluff CL Jr: Melanoma vaccines. Curr Opin Oncol 12:163, 2000

35. Balch CM, Buzaid AC, Soon SJ, et al: Final version of the American Joint Committee on Cancer staging system for cutaneous melanoma. J Clin Oncol 19:3635, 2001

36. Balch CM, Soong SJ, Gershenwald JE, et al: Prognostic factors analysis of 17,600 melanoma patients: validation of the American Joint Committee on Cancer melanoma staging system. J Clin Oncol 19:3622, 2001

37. Guerry D 4th, Synnestvedt M, Elder DE, et al: Lessons from tumor progression: the invasive radial growth phase of melanoma is common, incapable of metastasis, and indolent. J Invest Dermatol 100:342S, 1993

38. Elder DE, Van Belle P, Elenitsas R, et al: Neoplastic progression and prognosis in melanoma. Semin Cutan Med Surg 15:336, 1996

39. Schuchter L, Schultz DJ, Synnestvedt M, et al: A prognostic model for predicting 10-year survival in patients with primary melanoma. Ann Intern Med 125:369, 1996

40. Schwartz RA: Cutaneous metastatic disease. J Am Acad Dermatol 33:161, 1995

41. Demetrius RW, Randle HW: High-risk nonmelanoma skin cancers. Dermatol Surg 24:1272, 1998

42. Antman K, Chang Y: Kaposi's sarcoma. N Engl J Med 342:1027, 2000

43. Myskowski PL, Krown SE: Kaposi's sarcoma. Sober AJ, Haluska FG, Ed. Skin Cancer. American Cancer Society Atlas of Clinical Oncology. BC Decker, Ontario, 2001

44. Moore PS, Change Y: Detection of herpesvirus-like DNA sequences in Kaposi's sarcoma in patients with and without HIV infection. N Engl J Med 332:1181, 1995

45. Foreman KE, Friborg J Jr, Kong WP, et al: Propagation of a human herpesvirus from AIDS-associated Kaposi's sarcoma. N Engl J Med 336:163, 1997

46. Gao SJ, Kingsley L, Hoover DR, et al: Seroconversion to antibodies against Kaposi's sarcoma–associated herpesvirus-related latent nuclear antigen before the development of Kaposi's sarcoma. N Engl J Med 335:233, 1996

47. Niedt GW, Myskowski PL, Urmacher C, et al: Histologic predictors of survival in acquired immunodeficiency syndrome–associated Kaposi's sarcoma. Hum Pathol 23:1419, 1992

48. Cooper JS, Sacco J, Newall J: The duration of local control of classic (non–AIDS-associated) Kaposi's sarcoma by radiotherapy. J Am Acad Dermatol 19:59, 1988

49. Dezube BJ: AIDS-related Kaposi sarcoma: the role of local therapy for a systemic disease. Arch Dermatol 136:1554, 2000

50. Krown SE, Testa MA, Huang J: AIDS-related Kaposi's sarcoma: prospective validation of the AIDS Clinical Trials Group staging classification. J Clin Oncol 15:3085, 1997

51. Krischer J, Rutschmann O, Hirschel B, et al: Regression of Kaposi's sarcoma during therapy with HIV-1 protease inhibitors: a prospective pilot study. J Am Acad Dermatol 38:594, 1998

52. Duvic M, Friedman-Kien AE, Looney DJ, et al: Topical treatment of cutaneous lesions of acquired immunodeficiency syndrome–related Kaposi sarcoma using alitretinoin gel: results of phase 1 and 2 trials. Arch Dermatol 136:1461, 2000

53. Northfelt DW, Dezube BJ, Thommes JA, et al: Pegylated-liposomal doxorubicin versus doxorubicin, bleomycin, and vincristine in the treatment of AIDS-related Kaposi's sarcoma: results of a randomized phase III clinical trial. J Clin Oncol 16:2445, 1998

54. Welles L, Saville MW, Lietzau J, et al: Phase II trial with dose titration of paclitaxel for the therapy of human immunodeficiency virus–associated Kaposi's sarcoma. J Clin Oncol 16:1112, 1998

55. Seigel RS, Pandolfino T, Guitart J, et al: Primary cutaneous T-cell lymphoma: review and current concepts. J Clin Oncol 18:2908, 2000

56. Duvic M, Cather JC: Emerging new therapies for cutaneous T-cell lymphoma. Dermatol Clin 18:147, 2000

57. Weinstock MA, Reynes JF: The changing survival of patients with mycosis fungoides: a population-based assessment of trends in the United States. Cancer 85:208, 1999

58. Jackow CM, McHam JB, Friss A, et al: HLA-DR5 and DQB1*03 class II alleles are associated with cutaneous T-cell lymphoma. J Invest Dermatol 107:373, 1996

59. Sausville EA, Eddy JL, Makuch RW, et al: Histopathologic staging at initial diagnosis of mycosis fungoides and the Sézary syndrome: definition of three distinctive prognostic groups. Ann Intern Med 109:372, 1988

60. Diamandidou E, Colome-Grimmer M, Fayad L, et al: Transformation of mycosis fungoides/Sézary syndrome: clinical characteristics and prognosis. Blood 92:1150, 1998

61. Fung MA, Murphy MJ, Hoss DM, et al: Practical evaluation and management of cutaneous lymphoma. J Am Acad Dermatol 46:325, 2002

62. Zackheim HS, Kashani-Sabet M, Amin S: Topical corticosteroids for mycosis fungoides: experience in 79 patients. Arch Dermatol 134:949, 1998

63. Ramsay DL, Meller JA, Zackheim HS: Topical treatment of early cutaneous T-cell lymphoma. Hematol Oncol Clin North Am 9:1031, 1995

64. Breneman D, Duvic M, Kuzel T, et al: Phase 1 and 2 trial of bexarotene gel for skin-directed treatment of patients with cutaneous T-cell lymphoma. Arch Dermatol 138:398, 2002

65. Ramsay DL, Lish KM, Yalowitz CB, et al: Ultraviolet-B phototherapy for early-stage cutaneous T-cell lymphoma. Arch Dermatol 128:931, 1992

66. Herrmann JJ, Roenigk HH Jr, Hurria A, et al: Treatment of mycosis fungoides with photochemotherapy (PUVA): long-term follow-up. J Am Acad Dermatol 33:234, 1995

67. Jones GW, Hoppe RT, Glatstein E: Electron beam treatment for cutaneous T-cell lymphoma. Hematol Oncol Clin North Am 9:1057, 1995

68. Duvic M, Hymes K, Heald P, et al: Bexarotene is effective and safe for treatment of refractory advanced-stage cutaneous T-cell lymphoma: multinational phase II–III trial results. J Clin Oncol 19:2456, 2001

69. Wilson LD, Licata Al, Braverman IM, et al: Systemic chemotherapy and extracorporeal photochemotherapy for T3 and T4 cutaneous T-cell lymphoma patients who have achieved a complete response to total skin electron beam therapy. Int J Radiat Oncol Biol Phys 32:987, 1995

70. Olsen E, Duvic M, Frankel A, et al: Pivotal phase III trial of two dose levels of denileukin diftitox for the treatment of cutaneous T-cell lymphoma. J Clin Oncol 19:376, 2001

71. Kim YH, Jensen RA, Watanabe GL, et al: Clinical stage IA (limited patch and plaque) mycosis fungoides: a long-term outcome analysis. Arch Dermatol 132:1309, 1996

72. Kim YH, Chow S, Varghese A, et al: Clinical characteristics and long-term outcome of patients with generalized patch and/or plaque (T2) mycosis fungoides. Arch Dermatol 135:26, 1999

42 Disorders of Hair

David A. Whiting, M.D.

Physiology and Evaluation of Hair Growth

A basic knowledge of the hair growth cycle is needed to evaluate disorders of hair growth.[1,2] Scalp hair follicles cycle independently of one another. On average, of 100,000 scalp hairs, approximately 90% are in the anagen (growing) phase and 10% in the telogen (resting) phase at any given time. Anagen lasts an average of 3 years, with a range of 1 to 7 years. Telogen usually lasts 3 months, after which the resting hairs are shed and new hairs grow in. The average rate of scalp hair growth is approximately 0.35 mm/day, or 1 cm/month (1 in. every 2 to 3 months).

An average loss of 100 hairs a day is normal, with larger numbers of hairs being lost on shampoo days. When obtaining a history, it is important to determine whether shedding is abnormal and whether the shed hairs break off or come out by the roots.[3] Hair normally comes out by the roots; however, trauma or excessive fragility may cause hair to break.

Examination of the patient should include a routine check for broken-off hairs and the performance of hair-pull tests on the top, sides, and back of the scalp. The hair-pull test is performed by grasping groups of 10 to 20 hairs between the index finger and thumb and pulling steadily.[4,5] Extraction of more than 20% of the grasped hairs indicates a potential for abnormal shedding, usually involving telogen hairs. Telogen hairs (club hairs) are easily recognized by their whitish club-shaped bulbs and lack of root sheaths. Anagen hairs are normally difficult to detach and have blackish, indented roots with intact root sheaths.

Androgenetic Alopecia

Androgenetic alopecia is the common type of nonscarring hair loss affecting the crown. It results from a genetically determined end-organ sensitivity to androgens. It is often referred to as common baldness, male-pattern alopecia, and female-pattern alopecia.

EPIDEMIOLOGY AND PATHOGENESIS

Androgenetic alopecia affects at least 50% of men by 50 years of age and 50% of women by 60 years of age.[6,7] Males have more androgen than females and therefore are usually affected earlier and more severely. Male-pattern alopecia often starts between 15 and 25 years of age. Male-pattern alopecia has two characteristic components, bitemporal recession and vertex balding [*see Figure 1*], which in pronounced cases can progress to complete balding of the crown.[6,7] Female-pattern alopecia is more likely to start between 25 and 30 years of age (or sometimes later, after menopause). It is characterized by an intact frontal hairline and an oval area of diffuse thinning over the crown [*see Figure 2*]. Bitemporal recession in women is much less obvious than it typically is in men, or it can be nonexistent. In general, androgenetic alopecia in women progresses to mild, moderate, or severe thinning but not to complete baldness. The best predictor of outcome is the degree of progression in affected relatives.

Androgenetic alopecia is an autosomal dominant disorder with variable penetrance. Susceptible hairs on the crown are predisposed to miniaturize under the influence of androgens, notably dihydrotestosterone. In both sexes, miniaturization results from a shortening of the anagen cycle, from years to months or weeks. Miniaturized hairs are characterized by re-

duced length and diameter; this accounts for the appearance of hair loss.[8] Androgenetic alopecia largely spares the back and sides of the scalp.

DIAGNOSIS

The diagnosis of androgenetic alopecia is usually obvious from the clinical pattern of hair loss from the top of the head.[9] In some men, a female pattern of alopecia (see above) causes diagnostic confusion but has no other significance. In women, a male pattern of alopecia (i.e., bitemporal recession and vertex balding) occurring with menstrual irregularities, acne, hirsutism, and a deep voice is significant. The virilism indicates significant hyperandrogenism, the cause of which must be identified and treated [*see Chapters 49 and 51*].

Scalp biopsies are rarely necessary to diagnose androgenetic alopecia. Biopsies cut horizontally are sometimes useful, however, in differentiating female-pattern alopecia from chronic telogen effluvium (see below).

TREATMENT

Depending on the severity of the condition, management of androgenetic alopecia ranges from watchful inactivity to medical and surgical treatment, or a hairpiece or wig may be used in the most refractory cases.

Topical Therapy

The Food and Drug Administration approved topical 2% minoxidil for use in men in 1987 and in women in 1989. Minoxidil is applied twice daily with a dropper, spread over the top of the scalp, and gently rubbed in. The drug should be tried for at least a year. Minoxidil acts by initiating and prolonging anagen. It produces visible hair growth in approximately one third of male and female patients, fine-hair growth in approximately one third, and no growth in approximately one third. It is more effective as a preventive agent, retarding hair loss in approximately 80% of patients.[6]

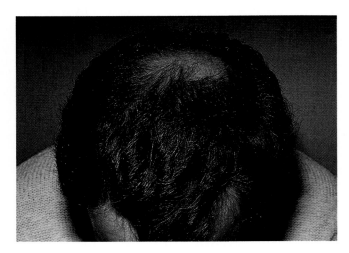

Figure 1 **Bitemporal recession and vertex balding are present in this patient with male pattern androgenetic alopecia.**

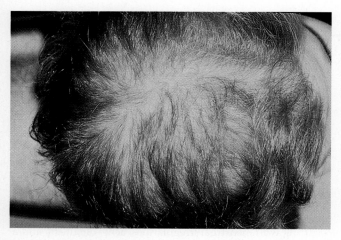

Figure 2   Intact frontal hairline and diffuse thinning over the crown are characteristic of female pattern androgenetic alopecia.

Topical 5% minoxidil, which was approved for use in men in 1997, produces visible hair growth in 45% of patients in less time than the 2% solution. Both concentrations are available over the counter. Side effects are not significant and include scalp irritation and increased facial hair.[10] The medication has to be continued indefinitely.[11]

Systemic Therapy

Oral finasteride, at a dosage of 1 mg/day, was approved by the FDA for the treatment of male-pattern alopecia in 1997. Finasteride is a powerful type II 5α-reductase inhibitor that prevents formation of dihydrotestosterone in the prostate gland and in the hair follicle. It reduces circulating dihydrotestosterone by 65% to 70%. When administered at a dosage of 1 mg/day for 2 years to male patients with androgenetic alopecia who are between 18 and 41 years of age, finasteride grew visible hair in 66% and prevented further hair loss in 83%.[12] The efficacy of finasteride was maintained in a 5-year study.[13] Hair-weight studies have shown that finasteride increases hair length and diameter, producing better coverage from existing hairs.[14]

Side effects in men are minimal and include lack of libido, lack of potency, and mild reduction in semen in approximately 0.5% of patients. These effects are reversed when the drug is stopped and often disappear as the drug is continued. A 1-year trial of finasteride at a dosage of 1 mg/day in postmenopausal women failed to show any positive effects.

Because of the likelihood of finasteride to cause severe side effects in the male fetus, the drug is contraindicated in premenopausal women.

Therapy for Hair Loss in Women

Topical minoxidil is currently the best available treatment for androgenetic alopecia in women.[10,15] However, various antiandrogenic drugs have been used. Oral contraceptives (e.g., ethinyl estradiol–ethynodiol diacetate [Demulen], desogestrel–ethinyl estradiol [Desogen], and ethinyl estradiol–norgestimate [Ortho Tri-Cyclen]) can reduce hair loss and occasionally lead to slight hair growth.[6] Oral spironolactone (Aldactone) in dosages of 75 mg/day to 200 mg/day can produce androgen blockade. Dexamethasone in dosages of 0.125 mg/day to 0.5 mg/day can suppress adrenal overactivity. Cyproterone acetate, which is not available in the United States, is not as effective as minoxidil in female pattern hair loss unless other signs of hyperandrogenism are present.[16]

Therapy for Refractory Cases

In patients who do not respond to the treatments listed above, the next step may be hair transplantation. Micrografts and minigrafts can produce a good cosmetic appearance in patients who have a sufficient reserve of hair on the back and sides of the scalp.[17] If all therapies fail, a hairpiece may be an option.

Diffuse Alopecia

Diffuse alopecia is generalized hair loss over the entire scalp. Because the loss is so diffuse, it is often unnoticeable until 30% to 50% of scalp hair is shed. Causes of diffuse alopecia include telogen effluvium, anagen arrest, drug reactions, and a number of systemic and nonsystemic conditions [see Table 1].[18,19]

TELOGEN EFFLUVIUM

Telogen effluvium is the most common form of diffuse alopecia.[20] It presents as a generalized shedding of telogen hairs from normal resting follicles. The basic cause of telogen effluvium is a premature interruption of anagen, leading to an increase in the number of hairs cycling into telogen. When the 3-month telogen period ends, new anagen hairs grow in and numerous telogen hairs fall out. Patients may need reassurance that this apparent loss of hair is actually a sign of regrowth.

Acute telogen effluvium can be caused by childbirth, febrile illnesses, surgery, chronic systemic diseases, crash diets, traction, severe emotional stress, and drug reactions [see Table 2]. It can also be a physiologic reaction in neonates.[21]

During acute telogen effluvium, pull tests are positive all over the scalp, yielding two to 10 club hairs. Telogen effluvium is often accompanied by bitemporal recession; this is a useful diagnostic sign in women [see Figure 3]. The acute form usually ends within 3 to 6 months. The diagnosis is usually made on the basis of the history of an initiating event 3 months before the onset of shedding. No treatment is needed for acute telogen effluvium, because the hair invariably regrows within a short time.

Chronic telogen effluvium has a long, fluctuating course of 6 months to 7 years or more. Very often, no identifiable cause can be found.

Diagnosis

The diagnosis of telogen effluvium is usually clinical; biopsies may be necessary to distinguish telogen effluvium from an acute onset of widespread androgenetic alopecia.[22] Other causes of

---

Table 1   Causes of Diffuse Alopecia[45]

Telogen effluvium (acute and chronic)
Anagen arrest
Reactions to drugs and other chemicals
Thyroid disorder
Iron deficiency and other nutritional deficiencies
Malabsorption
Renal failure
Hepatic failure
Systemic disease
Miscellaneous causes (e.g., diffuse alopecia areata, congenital hypotrichosis) and idiopathic causes

Table 2 Categories of Drugs That Can Cause Alopecia[5]

Category	Selected Agents
Alpha blockers	Doxazosin, prazosin, terazosin
Angiotensin converting enzyme inhibitors	Captopril, enalapril
Anticancer drugs	Bleomycin, cyclophosphamide, cytarabine, dactinomycin, daunorubicin, doxorubicin, etoposide, floxuridine, fluorouracil, methotrexate, mitomycin, mitoxantrone, procarbazine, thioguanine, vinblastine, vincristine
Anticoagulant drugs	Dicumarol, heparin, warfarin
Anticonvulsant drugs	Ethotoin, mephenytoin, paramethadione, phenytoin, trimethadione, valproate sodium
Antithyroid drugs	Carbimazole, methylthiouracil, methimazole, propylthiouracil
Beta blockers	Acebutolol, atenolol, labetalol, metoprolol, nadolol, pindolol, propranolol, timolol
Calcium channel blockers	Diltiazem, verapamil
Cholesterol reducers	Clofibrate, lovastatin
H_2 receptor blockers	Cimetidine, famotidine, ranitidine
Nonsteroidal anti-inflammatory drugs	Fenoprofen, ibuprofen, indomethacin, ketoprofen, meclomen, naproxen, piroxicam, sulindac
Retinoids and retinol	Acitretin, etretinate, isotretinoin, vitamin A overdose
Tricyclic antidepressants	Amitriptyline, amoxapine, desipramine, doxepin, imipramine, nortriptyline, protriptyline, trimipramine

vere protein calorie malnutrition. Because 90% of scalp hairs are in anagen at any given time, this condition causes obvious and severe baldness [*see Figure 4*].

Diagnosis

The diagnosis of anagen arrest is easily made by the history, evidence of extensive hair loss, and hair-pull tests that yield easily broken hairs with proximal tapering.

Treatment

Treatment of anagen arrest lies in elimination of the underlying cause. Once the antimitotic influence is removed, the anagen

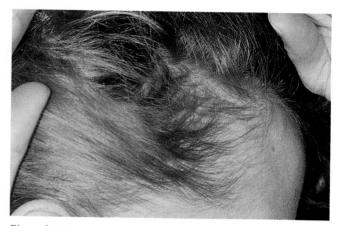

Figure 3 **In women, marked bitemporal recession is often a sign of telogen effluvium.**

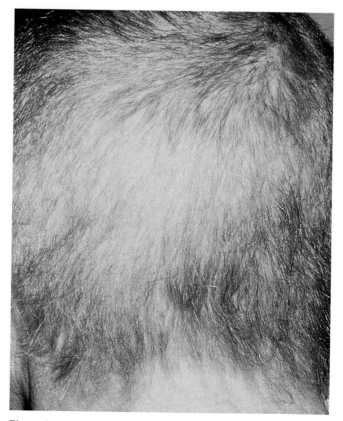

Figure 4 **Anagen arrest causes severe, diffuse hair loss.**

hair loss should be excluded by a careful drug history and tests for iron deficiency, syphilis, and disorders of the thyroid, kidney, and liver.

Treatment

As mentioned above, no treatment is needed for acute telogen effluvium because the hair invariably regrows within a short time. In chronic telogen effluvium, topical minoxidil in a 2% or 5% solution may be indicated. The patient should be reassured that telogen effluvium rarely causes permanent baldness.

ANAGEN ARREST (ANAGEN EFFLUVIUM)

So-called anagen effluvium represents a diffuse loss of anagen hairs from growing follicles.[23] The term anagen effluvium is a misnomer. Normally, hairs pass through a brief transition phase (catagen) between the anagen and telogen phases before falling out by the roots. In anagen arrest, inhibition of cell division in the hair bulb matrix leads to a progressive narrowing of the hair shaft and sometimes failure of hair formation. As the growing hair narrows near the skin surface, it may break off. The resultant shedding can occur within a few weeks, unlike in telogen effluvium, in which shedding takes 3 months to occur.

Causes of anagen arrest include reactions to cytostatic drugs and other toxic agents, radiation therapy, endocrine diseases, alopecia areata, cicatricial alopecia, trauma and pressure, and se-

Table 3 Miscellaneous Chemicals
That Can Cause Alopecia[45]

Chemical	Common Source
Abrin	Plant source (*Abrus precatorius* [rosary pea, jequirity bean, or precatory bean])
Arsenic	Pesticides
Bismuth	Old treatment for syphilis
Boric acid	Mouthwashes, occupational exposure
Chloroprene dimers	Occupational exposure (synthetic-rubber manufacturing)
Lead	Paints
Mercury	Cosmetics, teething powders, antiseptics
Mimosine	Plant source (*Leucaena glauca*)
Selenocystothione	Plant source (*Lecythis* species)
Thallium salts	Rodenticides

hair will regrow promptly with a normally tapering shaft. Unbroken hairs that regrow often show the Pohl-Pinkus deformity (i.e., a constriction that results in a dumbbell shape).

ALOPECIA CAUSED BY DRUGS AND CHEMICALS

Substance-induced alopecia is relatively common but is often hard to diagnose because of the large number of drugs and chemicals that can cause hair loss [*see Tables 2 and 3*]. It often takes time to identify the underlying cause by trial and error: many patients are exposed to several alopecia-inducing substances, and removal of the causative agent may not result in immediate regrowth of hair.

OTHER CAUSES OF DIFFUSE ALOPECIA

Hypothyroidism and iron deficiency should be excluded in patients with diffuse hair loss [*see Table 1*]. Appropriate treatment may lead to hair regrowth.

Alopecia Areata

Alopecia areata is typically characterized by patchy hair loss; however, involvement can vary from a single patch on the scalp or elsewhere to total body baldness (alopecia universalis).[24]

EPIDEMIOLOGY AND PATHOGENESIS

In the United States, alopecia areata affects 1.7% of the population younger than 50 years.[25] Some 70% to 75% of cases are not associated with any other disease. In these patients, alopecia areata often starts in the 20s and 30s, although it can occur at any age. In only about 6% of these patients with alopecia areata does the disease progress to total loss of scalp hair. Even total alopecia can reverse itself.

Alopecia areata is currently regarded as an autoimmune disease. A positive family history in 20% of alopecia areata patients indicates a genetic predisposition to this disease. Certain HLA groups have been associated with mild or severe cases of alopecia areata.[26] Although the exact cause is unknown, many researchers presume that an infectious agent such as a virus is the offending agent. Stress, seasonal factors, and infection are among the trigger factors for active episodes of hair loss.

Some 5% of alopecia areata cases—usually those occurring in middle-aged patients—are associated with autoimmune disease, either in the patient or in the patient's family. Some 10% of these patients will experience loss of all scalp hair in the course of the disorder. Approximately 20% to 25% of cases—often those occurring in childhood—may be associated with atopic disease (e.g., hay fever, asthma, or eczema). The incidence of complete scalp hair loss is much higher in these patients.

Despite its long course, often recurring over many years, the prognosis of alopecia areata is often favorable. Most patients will regrow hair at one time or another. In cases of extensive alopecia areata, alopecia totalis, and alopecia universalis, however, hair loss may be permanent.

DIAGNOSIS

Active alopecia areata is characterized by a spreading, annular area of hair loss; a smooth, depressed area of scalp that is slick to the touch is surrounded by hairs that often include so-called exclamation-point hairs (i.e., broken hairs 3 to 4 mm long, usually with an expanded tip and a telogen bulb). These hairs are not always seen but are diagnostic when present. They delineate the active spreading margin of alopecia areata. The bald patches generally affect the scalp but can also involve eyebrows, eyelashes, beard hair, and body hair. Spontaneous regrowth is common.

This condition is extremely unpredictable, often fluctuating without any obvious reason. However, seasonal outbreaks are noted in many patients. The initial patch may enlarge, or additional patches may develop and become confluent [*see Figure 5*]. The condition can progress to large irregular areas of baldness. In severe cases, patients lose all scalp hair or all body hair.

Ophiasis is a chronic and difficult to treat form of alopecia areata in which a band of baldness circles the scalp, very often around the inferior margin. This slowly extending lesion is often present for several years before any regrowth occurs. Permanent hair loss may result in some areas.

TREATMENT

The treatment of alopecia areata depends on the severity of the disease.[27] Small patches of alopecia areata often regrow hair without treatment. If not, they usually respond to medium- or high-potency topical corticosteroids or to intralesional injections of triamcinolone acetonide at a concentration of 5 mg/ml.

In more severe cases, intralesional corticosteroids may be tried; however, these may not be feasible in extensive hair loss. Daily, short-contact topical therapy with 0.25% to 1% anthralin cream for up to an hour at a time may help and is suitable for children and adults. Psoralen and ultraviolet A (PUVA) therapy has also been used with some success.

Topical 5% minoxidil can be tried to speed hair regrowth and lengthen existing hairs. Minoxidil has no effect on the course of the disease but may improve hair coverage. It has few side effects and is often used in older children; however, the FDA has approved minoxidil for use only in persons 18 years of age and older. Systemic steroids are effective; however, they have shown a potential for side effects and do not prevent future recurrences.[28] Prednisone (20 to 40 mg daily in the morning for 1 or 2 months followed by slow tapering) has controlled the disease in adults; a change to alternate-day therapy is advisable whenever possible.

Topical immunotherapy with the sensitizing chemical diphencyprone has been used in some centers; it has a response rate comparable to that of systemic corticosteroids.[29] Success with this treatment usually requires supervision in a specialized clinic.[27]

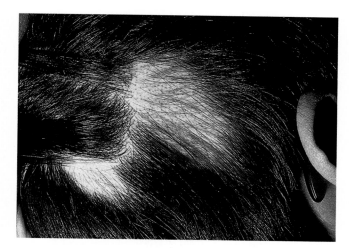

Figure 5 Circumscribed patches of hair loss are present in alopecia areata.

Sulfasalazine has been reported to have a 23% success rate in the treatment of severe alopecia areata.[30] Other immunosuppressive drugs, such as oral cyclosporine, have been used experimentally. Such therapies are risky and expensive, however, and have not been approved in the United States for alopecia areata.

TRAUMATIC ALOPECIA

Traumatic alopecia may be caused by a variety of physical or chemical injuries to the hair and scalp. These injuries may be deliberate or accidental, inflicted by self or others, and acute or repetitive. The cause may be obvious or unclear.[31] Potential causes include trichotillomania, habit tics, pruritic dermatoses, traction, pressure and friction, heat, radiation, and chemicals. In most cases of traumatic alopecia, management is removal of the underlying cause. In areas with permanent damage, hair transplantation may be necessary.

TRICHOTILLOMANIA

Trichotillomania is a compulsion to pull out one's hair. It is characterized by an increasing sense of tension before, and a sense of relief after, the hair is pulled. Trichotillomania is now classified as a specific disorder of impulse control.[31,32] It is more common in children, in whom it is often caused by insecurity re-

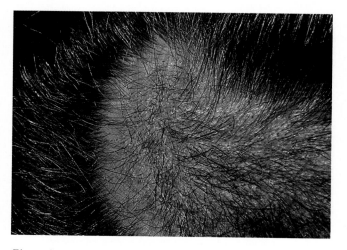

Figure 6 Irregular, broken-off hairs are seen in trichotillomania.

sulting from sibling rivalry, lack of attention, divorce of parents, learning disabilities, or unhappiness or teasing at school. In adolescents and adults, trichotillomania may be accompanied by mood disorders, anxiety disorders, or mental retardation and is often harder to treat than in children.

The diagnosis is based on the presence of irregular, broken-off hairs in patches on the scalp [*see Figure 6*]. The hairs are irregular in length because they are broken off at different times. The scalp itself is normal. Occasionally, biopsies are necessary to confirm the diagnosis. The best treatment is to explain cause and remedy to the patient in a nonconfrontational manner; usually, reassurance and understanding go a long way in the treatment of this condition. In more difficult cases, psychiatric consultation may be indicated.[33] If habit tics or head rolling and banging are found to be causing traumatic hair loss, those behaviors should be treated.

OTHER CAUSES OF TRAUMATIC ALOPECIA

Pruritic Dermatoses

Pruritic dermatoses such as acne necrotica, folliculitis, lichen simplex chronicus, pediculosis capitis, prurigo nodularis, psoriasis, seborrheic dermatitis, and neurotic excoriations can lead to hair loss from excoriation. They need to be identified and treated.

Traction Alopecia and Loose Anagen Syndrome

Traction alopecia may be acute (caused by accidental or deliberate avulsion of the scalp) or may arise from a familial condition, the loose anagen syndrome. Common causes of traction alopecia are excessive brushing and combing; backcombing and pulling the hair into braids, cornrows, and ponytails; weaving; and application of rollers.[31]

Loose anagen syndrome is usually seen in fair-haired children 2 to 5 years of age.[34] It often presents as patchy hair loss following an incident of hair tugging. Prompt hair regrowth is the rule. The condition becomes asymptomatic with gentle hair care. Diagnosis is made on the basis of positive hair pull tests showing many anagen hairs.

Alopecia Caused by Pressure and Friction

Prolonged pressure on a localized area of the scalp in immobilized neonates or patients under anesthesia, in coma, or with debilitating illness may result in ischemia leading to pressure alopecia. The hair usually regrows with time, but if the damage is severe, permanent hair loss and scarring may result.[31] Alopecia caused by friction from vigorous massage has been described but is easily remedied.

Alopecia Caused by Heat, Radiation, and Chemicals

Excessive heat from hot oils and pomades, hot combs, and hot rollers is a common cause of chronic hair loss. Overheated hair dryers frequently cause the fluid droplets in wet hair shafts to expand, leading to the formation of bubble hairs.[35] These brittle hairs are a frequent cause of follicle damage. The source of the overheating needs to be identified and removed.

Radiation dermatitis can cause hair loss. Permanent scarring alopecia is still seen in patients who were overtreated with x-rays for tinea capitis before oral antifungal agents became available.

Many chemicals, such as hair dyes, moisturizers, oils and pomades, permanent waves, relaxers and straighteners, setting lotions, certain cationic and detergent shampoos, and saltwater, are possible causes of hair loss.[36] A careful history of hair care and grooming is needed to uncover these causes.

Cicatricial Alopecia

Cicatricial alopecia results from permanent scarring of the hair follicles. It may be widespread or localized and is sometimes difficult to identify. The causes of cicatricial alopecia may be primary or secondary.[37] It can result from hereditary or congenital conditions, infections, injuries, neoplasms, and dermatoses [*see Table 4*].

DIAGNOSIS

On clinical examination, scarring is detected by the absence of follicular orifices and a pearly or scarred appearance of the skin. The scar may be depressed or hypertrophic. Associated lesions such as folliculitis, follicular plugs, scales, and telangiectasias may be found, along with broken, twisted, or easily extractable hairs. Other lesions may be present on skin or mucous membranes. If the disease is active, a specific diagnosis may be possible; but in an inactive case, the initial cause is often inapparent.

Clinical Variants

The common variants of primary cicatricial alopecia of the scalp include discoid lupus erythematosus, lichen planopilaris, folliculitis decalvans, and pseudopelade.[38,39] The end phases of these conditions are similar; they are characterized by a lack of pores and by inflammation in white, scarred areas. For an accurate diagnosis, an early biopsy from an area of activity might show the identifying pathology. In the final scarring stage, it is usually not possible to identify the original cause.

Discoid lupus erythematosus Lesions are often itchy at onset and lead to erythema, scaling, telangiectasia, follicular spines, and atrophy [*see Figure 7*]. They often occur centrally in bare patches of scarring with an inactive border [*see Chapter 114*].

Lichen planopilaris Central scarring characterizes these lesions. The condition generally starts with bare, white patches that bud out from one another like pseudopods. Prominent follicular hyperkeratosis is present around the residual terminal hairs at the edges of the lesion, and varying degrees of erythema, scaling, and telangiectasia may occur. Itching may be present.

Folliculitis decalvans Crops of follicular pustules surrounding multiple, slowly expanding, and round or oval areas of alopecia characterize this condition. It may involve large areas of the skin. Secondary infection may be severe, with crusting and oozing. Eventually this condition gradually loses activity and looks like other forms of chronic cicatricial alopecia.

Pseudopelade (nonspecific cicatricial alopecia) The majority of cases classified as pseudopelade are in fact cases of nonspecific cicatricial alopecia in which the initial cause has not been established. In general, there is an insidious spread of a scarring process, which is apparently noninflammatory. It often involves the crown and occurs mainly in middle-aged women. It may represent the final common pathway of various causes, such as lichen planopilaris in particular or discoid lupus erythematosus. It is characterized by patchy areas of alopecia with irregular extensions. The affected skin is smooth, white, and devoid of erythema, scaling, or pores, causing the so-called footprints in the snow. The course is variable and may last for a few years or several decades.

The original cases were described as a specific entity in the late 19th century and were reported as pseudopelade of Brocq.

Table 4 Causes of Cicatricial Alopecia[46]

Dermatoses	Cicatricial pemphigoid, dermatomyositis, folliculitis decalvans, lichen planopilaris, lupus erythematosus, neurotic excoriations, pseudopelade, scleroderma
Hereditary and congenital disorders	Aplasia cutis, epidermal nevi, epidermolysis bullosa
Infections Bacterial	Acne keloidalis, dissecting cellulitis, folliculitis, syphilis
Fungal	Favus (tinea capitis), kerion, mycetoma
Protozoan	Leishmaniasis
Viral	Herpes zoster, varicella
Injuries	Burns, mechanical trauma, radiodermatitis
Neoplasms	Angiosarcoma, basal cell epithelioma, lymphoma, melanoma, metastatic tumors, squamous cell carcinoma

This eponym is rarely used nowadays except perhaps for a small cohort of cases with no inflammatory phase at all, particularly occurring in children. Most cases of so-called pseudopelade of Brocq are explainable as an end stage of lichen planopilaris or other causes.[37]

TREATMENT

Treatment depends on the level of activity of the underlying disease. Discoid lupus erythematosus and lichen planopilaris may respond to topical, intralesional, or systemic steroids or oral chloroquine therapy. Topical minoxidil is sometimes helpful in regrowing any surviving hairs, which may be normal, dystrophic, or in a resting stage. The application of a 2% or 5% solution twice daily should be tried for at least a year on scarred areas that show

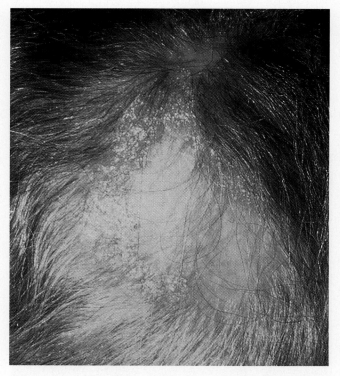

Figure 7 **Atrophic scarring with erythema, scaling, telangiectasia, and follicular spines are characteristic of discoid lupus erythematosus.**

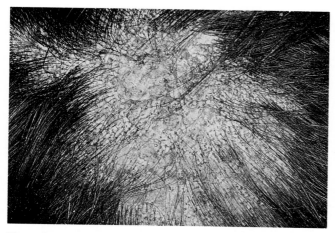

Figure 8　In endothrix tinea capitis, black dots represent brittle, infected hairs snapped off flush with the scalp.

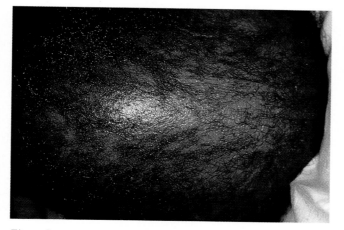

Figure 9　The characteristic irregular, so-called moth-eaten diffuse alopecia caused by syphilis is seen here.

some hair. Folliculitis decalvans may respond to treatment with long-term antibiotics such as tetracycline (500 mg), minocycline (100 mg), erythromycin (250 mg), trimethoprim-sulfamethoxazole (regular strength), or rifampin (300 mg, with regular-strength trimethoprim-sulfamethoxazole, given twice daily for at least 3 months). When the conditions have burned themselves out, either scalp reduction or hair transplants may be helpful.

Miscellaneous Causes of Hair Loss

As mentioned earlier, less common causes of hair loss include infections (e.g., tinea capitis),[40] infestations, hair shaft abnormalities, hereditary and congenital conditions, and various dermatoses involving the scalp.

In the United States, tinea capitis is now largely caused by *Trichophyton tonsurans,* an endothrix that infects the inside of the hair shaft. This makes the shaft brittle, which causes it to snap off flush with the skin, leaving a characteristic black dot of hair [*see Figure 8*]. The clinical diagnosis depends on this finding of black dots in patchy areas of hair loss. Removing the black dot with a small scalpel blade and dissolving it in potassium hydroxide (KOH) should reveal many spores that were packed inside the affected hair shaft. Ectothrix ringworm caused by *Microsporum canis* and *M. audouinii* is much less common; it can usually be di-

agnosed by Wood's light or by a finding of fungal spores around the hair shaft with KOH. Suitable oral antifungal treatments include griseofulvin, itraconazole, terbinafine, and fluconazole.

Secondary syphilis can cause a somewhat nondescript, moth-eaten type of diffuse alopecia [*see Figure 9*]. In such cases, a routine serologic test for syphilis is indicated.

Scalp lice should always be sought in cases of hair loss accompanied by pruritus. Lice are most likely to be found around and behind the ears and on the nape of the neck. Lymphadenopathy may also be present. Suitable treatment with permethrin shampoo or 0.5% malathion can be given.

Hair shaft abnormalities frequently present as broken-off hairs. Structural abnormalities of the hair shaft include fractures, irregularities, coiling and twisting, and extraneous matter.[41,42]

There are many different types of congenital and inherited hair loss.[43] These include congenital hypotrichosis with or without associated defects, congenital triangular alopecia, and many ectodermal dysplasias that affect the hair, teeth, nails, and sweat glands. One major form of congenital hypotrichosis is the Marie-Unna syndrome, which affects large families that have a dominant gene.[44] Minor forms of hypotrichosis can occur in patients with other hereditary syndromes and chromosomal abnormalities. In most of these conditions, a reduction of hair follicles accounts for the hair loss. Some patients have surviving hairs that are often in telogen and may benefit from topical minoxidil.

References

1.　Abell E: Embryology and anatomy of the hair follicle. Disorders of Hair Growth: Diagnosis and Treatment. Olsen EA, Ed. McGraw-Hill, New York, 1994, p 1

2.　Stenn KS, Paus R: Controls of hair follicle cycling. Physiol Rev 81:449, 2001

3.　Olsen EA: Clinical tools for assessing hair loss. Disorders of Hair Growth: Diagnosis and Treatment. Olsen EA, Ed. McGraw-Hill, New York, 1994, p 59

4.　Rietschel RL: A simplified approach to the diagnosis of alopecia. Dermatol Clin 14:691, 1996

5.　Whiting DA, Howsden FL: Assessment of patient with hair loss. Color Atlas of Differential Diagnosis of Hair Loss, rev. Whiting DA, Howsden FL, Eds. Canfield Publishing, Fairfield, New Jersey, 1998, p 8

6.　Olsen EA: Androgenetic alopecia. Disorders of Hair Growth: Diagnosis and Treatment. Olsen EA, Ed. McGraw-Hill, New York, 1994, p 257

7.　Sawaya ME: Clinical updates in hair. Dermatol Clin 15:37, 1997

8.　Birch MP, Messenger JF, Messenger AG: Hair density, hair diameter and the prevalence of female pattern hair loss. Br J Dermatol 144:297, 2001

9.　Whiting DA, Howsden FL: Androgenetic alopecia. Color Atlas of Differential Diagnosis of Hair Loss, rev. Whiting DA, Howsden FL, Eds. Canfield Publishing, Fairfield, New Jersey, 1998, p 18

10.　Shapiro J, Price VH: Hair regrowth: therapeutic agents. Dermatol Clin 16:341, 1998

11.　Olsen EA, DeLong ER, Weiner MS: Long-term follow-up of men with male pattern baldness treated with topical minoxidil. J Am Acad Dermatol 16:688, 1987

12.　Kaufman KD, Olsen EA, Whiting DA, et al: Finasteride in the treatment of men with androgenetic alopecia. Finasteride Male Pattern Hair Loss Study Group. J Am Acad Dermatol 39:578, 1998

13.　Kaufman KD: Long-term (5-year) multinational experience with finasteride 1 mg in the treatment of men with androgenetic alopecia. Eur J Dermatol 12:38, 2002

14.　Price VH, Menefee E, Sanchez M, et al: Changes in hair weight and hair count in men with androgenetic alopecia after treatment with finasteride, 1 mg, daily. J Am Acad Dermatol 46:517, 2002

15.　Tosti A, Piraccini BM: Androgenetic alopecia. Int J Dermatol 38(suppl 1):1, 1999

16.　Vexiau P, Chaspoux C, Boudou P, et al: Effects of minoxidil 2% vs. cyproterone acetate treatment on female androgenetic alopecia: a controlled, 12-month randomized trial. Br J Dermatol 146:992, 2002

17.　Unger WP: What's new in hair replacement surgery. Dermatol Clin 14:783, 1996

18.　Fiedler VC, Hafeer A: Diffuse alopecia: Telogen hair loss. Disorders of Hair Growth: Diagnosis and Treatment. Olsen EA, Ed. McGraw-Hill, New York, 1994, p 241

19.　Sinclair R: Diffuse hair loss. Int J Dermatol 38(suppl 1):8, 1999

20.　Headington JE: Telogen effluvium: new concepts and review. Arch Dermatol 129:356, 1993

21.　Kligman AM: Pathologic dynamics of human hair loss 1: telogen effluvium. Arch Dermatol 83:175, 1961

22.　Whiting DA: Chronic telogen effluvium. Dermatol Clin 14:723, 1996

23.　Grossman KL, Kvedar JC: Anagen hair loss. Disorders of Hair Growth: Diagnosis and Treatment. Olsen EA, Ed. McGraw-Hill, New York, 1994, p 223

24. Hordinsky MK: Alopecia areata. Disorders of Hair Growth: Diagnosis and Treatment. Olsen EA, Ed. McGraw-Hill, New York, 1994, p 195

25. Safavi KH, Muller SA, Suman VJ, et al: Incidence of alopecia areata in Olmsted County, Minnesota, 1975 through 1989. Mayo Clin Proc 70:628, 1995

26. Price VH, Colombe BW: Heritable factors distinguish two types of alopecia areata. Dermatol Clin 14:679, 1996

27. Shapiro J, Madani S: Alopecia areata: diagnosis and management. Int J Dermatol 38(suppl 1):19, 1999

28. Shapiro J, Price VH: Hair regrowth: therapeutic agents. Dermatol Clin 16:341, 1998

29. Madani S, Shapiro J: Alopecia areata update. J Am Acad Dermatol 42:549, 2000

30. Ellis CN, Brown MF, Voorhees JJ: Sulfasalazine for alopecia areata. J Am Acad Dermatol 46:541, 2002

31. Whiting DA: Traumatic alopecia. Int J Dermatol 38(suppl 1):34, 1999

32. Walsh KH, McDougle CJ: Trichotillomania: presentation, etiology, diagnosis and therapy. Am J Clin Dermatol 2:327, 2001

33. Hautmann G, Hercogova J, Lotti T: Trichotillomania. J Am Acad Dermatol 46:807, 2002

34. Price VH, Gummer CL: Loose anagen syndrome. J Am Acad Dermatol 20:249, 1989

35. Detwiler SP, Carson JL, Woosley JT, et al: Bubble hair: case caused by overheating hair dryer and reproducibility in normal hair with heat. J Am Acad Dermatol 30:54, 1994

36. Wilborn WS: Disorders of hair growth in African Americans. Disorders of Hair Growth: Diagnosis and Treatment. Olsen EA, Ed. McGraw-Hill, New York, 1994, p 389

37. Amato L, Mei S, Massi D, et al: Cicatricial alopecia: a dermatopathologic and immunopathologic study of 33 patients (pseudopelade of Brocq is not a specific clinicopathologic entity). Int J Dermatol 41:8, 2002

38. Headington JT: Cicatricial alopecia. Dermatol Clin 14:773, 1996

39. Whiting DA: Cicatricial alopecia: clinico-pathological findings and treatment. Clin Dermatol 19:211, 2001

40. DeVillez RL: Infectious, physical and inflammatory causes of hair and scalp abnormalities. Disorders of Hair Growth: Diagnosis and Treatment. Olsen EA, Ed. McGraw-Hill, New York, 1994, p 71

41. Whiting DA: Hair shaft defects. Disorders of Hair Growth: Diagnosis and Treatment. Olsen EA, Ed. McGraw-Hill, New York, 1994, p 134

42. DeBerker D, Sinclair R: Defects of the hair shaft. Diseases of the Hair and Scalp, 3rd ed. Dawber R, Ed. Blackwell Science, Oxford, 1997, p 239

43. Sinclair R, DeBerker D: Hereditary and congenital alopecia and hypotrichosis. Diseases of the Hair and Scalp, 3rd ed. Dawber R, Ed. Blackwell Science, Oxford, 1997, p 151

44. Roberts JL, Whiting DA, Henry D, et al: Marie Unna congenital hypotrichosis: clinical description, histopathology, scanning electron microscopy of a previously unreported large pedigree. J Invest Dermatol Symp Proc 4:261, 1999

45. Dawber RR, Simpson NB, Barth JH: Diffuse alopecia: endocrine, metabolic and chemical influences on the follicular cycle. Diseases of the Hair and Scalp, 3rd ed. Dawber R, Ed. Blackwell Science, Oxford, 1997, p 123

46. Dawber RR, Fenton DA: Cicatricial alopecia. Diseases of the Hair and Scalp, 3rd ed. Dawber R, Ed. Blackwell Science, Oxford, 1997, p 370

Acknowledgments

Figures 2, 4, 7, and 8 D. A. Whiting and F. L. Howsden: *Color Atlas of Differential Diagnosis of Hair Loss, rev.* Canfield Publishing, Fairfield, New Jersey, 1998. Used with permission.

43 Disorders of the Nail

James Q. Del Rosso, D.O., and C. Ralph Daniel III, M.D.

The human nail is a complex unit composed of five major modified cutaneous structures: the nail matrix, nail bed, nail plate, nail folds, and cuticle (eponychium).[1] These components are structurally supported by specialized mesenchyme, which provides a ligamentlike function, anchoring the soft tissue structures of the nail to the underlying phalangeal bone. The primary function of the human nail is to provide protection for the distal digits. Nails also assist in performance of fine touch and digital dexterity. For many individuals, nails serve as an important aesthetic symbol of optimal appearance, enhanced self-image, or individuality; several cosmetic techniques are available to modify the appearance of the nail plate. The basic anatomic components of the nail unit are diagrammed [*see Figure 1*].

Nail Structure, Function, and Pathophysiology

NAIL MATRIX

The nail matrix is the dynamic, germinative portion of the nail unit that produces the nail plate.[2-4] The lunula is the visible portion of the nail matrix, appearing under the proximal nail plate as a gray-white half moon projecting just distal to the proximal nail-fold cuticle. That lunula decreases with age in approximately 20% of persons.[5]

Nails are usually devoid of pigmentation because of the relatively sparse number of melanocytes present in matrix epithelium.[1,2] Because nail-matrix or nail-bed melanocytes tend to be more numerous in blacks, Asians, and Hispanics, persons of these racial backgrounds may present more commonly with diffuse or banded nail-plate or nail-bed hyperpigmentation.

Pathophysiology Affecting the Nail Matrix

Because of the diagonal orientation of the ventral nail matrix, the proximal portion of the nail matrix produces the superior portion of the nail plate.[6] As a result, disorders of the proximal matrix produce surface abnormalities of the nail plate. A characteristic example is nail-plate pitting secondary to psoriasis. Diseases of the distal nail matrix result in abnormalities of the undersurface of the nail plate, changes that are visible at the free edge of the nail, or both. Permanent damage to the matrix as the result of trauma, surgical intervention, or disease may result in permanent nail-plate dystrophy.

NAIL BED

The nail bed is a layer of epithelium lying between the lunula and the hyponychium (the distal epithelium at the free edge of the nail). The surface epithelium of the nail bed is longitudinally ridged, with small superficially oriented vessels coursing along the same axis, interdigitating with a complementary array of ridges on the undersurface of the nail plate.[3] This anatomic feature explains the longitudinal linearity of splinter hemorrhages, which are foci of extravasation wedged between the bed and the plate. As outgrowth of the nail plate occurs, splinter hemorrhages progress distally.

Pathophysiology Affecting the Nail Bed

The epidermis of the nail bed is thin and minimally keratinized, without a granular layer. If there is prolonged loss of nail plate as a result of disease or surgical intervention, in-

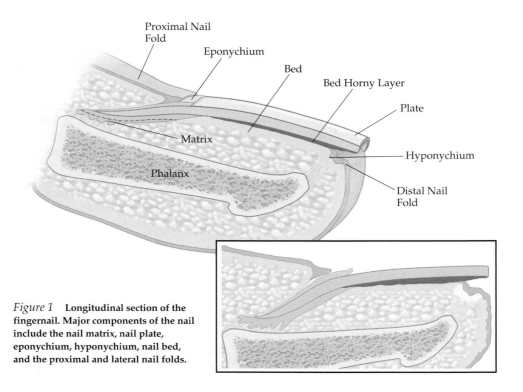

Figure 1 **Longitudinal section of the fingernail. Major components of the nail include the nail matrix, nail plate, eponychium, hyponychium, nail bed, and the proximal and lateral nail folds.**

Proximal Nail Fold
Eponychium
Bed
Bed Horny Layer
Plate
Matrix
Hyponychium
Phalanx
Distal Nail Fold

creased nail-bed keratinization with development of a granular layer prevents the firm attachment of the ingrowing nail plate to the underlying nail bed. Melanocytes are more sparsely distributed in nail-bed epithelium than in the nail matrix [see Nail Matrix, above]. The dermal layer of the nail bed is very thin and is supported by very sparse subcutaneous tissue; it is firmly attached to the underlying bony phalanx.

NAIL PLATE

The nail plate, which is composed of densely compacted keratinized epithelial cells, is produced by the matrix and progesses distally toward the free edge of the nail as newly formed plate slowly pushes forward in a distal direction. Formation and outgrowth of the nail plate is a continual process. A fully formed nail plate extends from below the proximal nail-fold cuticle to beyond the hyponychium and extends laterally below the cuticle of the lateral nail folds. Nail-plate abnormalities frequently occur secondary to changes or disorders affecting function of the nail matrix; infections such as onychomycosis; or trauma.

Age-Related Nail-Plate Findings

The growth rate of an adult fingernail plate is approximately 3 mm/mo, with marked variability among individuals.[2] Toenail plate growth occurs at one third to one half the rate of fingernail growth. A general rule is that adult fingernails take approximately 6 months to grow out fully; adult toenails, 12 to 18 months. Nail-plate growth is faster in children, peaking between 10 and 14 years of age; there is a slowly progressive decline after the second decade of life.[2] Linear nail-plate growth decreases by 50 % over a lifetime, with periods of slow decline alternating with periods of rapid decline in approximate 7-year increments.[7] Nail-plate growth increases during pregnancy and decreases during lactation, after use of chemotherapeutic agents, and in conditions characterized by limb paralysis, persistently diminished circulation, or malnutrition.[2,3,8] Yellow nail syndrome is characterized by very slow or absent growth of nail plate; it usually affects both fingernails and toenails and is seen in association with several underlying conditions, such as lymphedema, respiratory disorders (e.g., bronchiectasis and pleural effusions), and nephrotic syndrome.[9]

Constitutional age-related findings in the nail plate include changes in nail color and luster, longitudinal ridging, changes in convexity, and brittle nails.[8,10] Nail plates, especially of toenails, often develop a yellow or gray color with a dull, opaque appearance. Longitudinal ridging may affect some or all nails and may present as slightly indented grooves or projection ridges or as beading. Over time, the surface of the nail plate may become flattened (platyonychia) or spooned (koilonychia). Temporary koilonychia, especially of the toenails, is also seen in infants.[6]

Pathophysiology Affecting the Nail Plate

Brittle nails is a common complaint; its incidence is 20% in the overall population (27% in female patients) and increases with advancing age.[10] When nail water content falls below 16%, nail plates become brittle; when the water content rises above 25%, nail plates become soft. The most common cause of brittle nails is dehydration, which can be caused or exacerbated by external factors such as use of nail-polish remover or exposure to dry climate. Onychoschizia, which presents as a layered, superficial splitting of the nail plate, may increase in incidence with

age. This condition is seen much more frequently in female patients. It is likely related to recurrent exposures to water or irritants, such as during nail-care procedures.

Fingernails demonstrate a tendency to become thinner and more fragile over time. Toenails usually become thicker and harder. Onychogryphosis is a marked thickening, usually of the large toenail, resulting in a compacted mass of heaped-up dystrophic nail plate.[8] Contributing factors appear to be advanced age, poor nail care, chronic trauma, decreased peripheral circulation, and neuropathy. Poor-fitting shoewear causes long-term exposure to lateral pressure and friction, resulting in gryphotic changes (marked thickening or heaping of nail plate), usually of the first and fifth toenails.

NAIL FOLDS

The nail folds are the cutaneous soft tissue that houses the nail unit, invaginating proximally and laterally to encompass the emerging nail plate. The proximal nail fold, with the exception of the lunula, covers the underlying matrix and is devoid of sebaceous glands and dermatoglyphic skin markings.[11] The term paronychia describes inflammation of the nail folds. Paronychia may be acute or chronic and may occur secondary to a variety of conditions, including contact dermatitis, psoriasis, bacterial infection, and fungal infection.[12,13] The cuticle (eponychium) is a thin, keratinized membrane of modified stratum corneum that extends from the distal portion of the nail fold, reflecting onto the nail-plate surface. Intact cuticle serves as a seal that protects the space between the nail folds and the nail plate from exposure to external irritants, allergens, and pathogens. Loss of cuticle allows for exposure and trapping of these deleterious external agents, providing an environment in which either inflammatory or infectious paronychia can develop.

Nail Findings Associated with Disease States

Several nail findings have been associated with both underlying systemic and dermatologic conditions. The following is a review of selected, recognized associations. Diagnosis is based on proper evaluation of clinical findings; treatment is based on a confirmed etiology or the recognition of an underlying systemic association.

Special care must be taken when performing biopsy of the nail bed or matrix to avoid trauma to the tissue specimen and surrounding structures upon specimen removal. The most appropriate plane of dissection during nail-bed or nail-matrix biopsy is subdermal. The sampled tissue should be manipulated very gently throughout the biopsy procedure to avoid crush artifact, which may interfere significantly with histopathologic evaluation. It is also important to carefully dissect along the undersurface of the specimen, ensuring nontraumatic separation of the biopsy tissue from its underlying firm attachment to bone.

SPLINTER HEMORRHAGES

Splinter hemorrhages may be secondary to trauma, high altitude, primary dermatoses (i.e., psoriasis), or several underlying conditions (e.g., arterial emboli, collagen vascular disease, or thromboangiitis obliterans). The simultaneous appearance of splinter hemorrhages in several nails should raise suspicion of a possible underlying systemic disorder, especially in female patients.[14]

KOILONYCHIA

Koilonychia may be found in association with other conditions, including congenital conditions, iron deficiency anemia, cardiac disease, endocrinopathy, occupational exposures, and trauma.[3,15]

TRANSVERSE NAIL-PLATE DEPRESSIONS (BEAU LINES)

Beau lines present as well-delineated, transverse depressions in the nail plate. They are believed to occur secondary to temporary growth arrest of the nail matrix. The grooves become evident weeks after the occurrence of an abrupt, stressful event, such as an acute febrile illness. The width of the groove reflects the duration of interrupted nail-matrix function. When limited to one or a few digits, Beau lines may be associated with trauma, carpal tunnel syndrome, or Raynaud disease, or they may occur subsequent to tourniquet application during hand surgery.[15] Approximately 1 to 2 months after birth, infants may demonstrate physiologic Beau lines, which mark the transition from intrauterine to extrauterine life.[16] Multiple transverse grooves (stepladder appearance) may be seen in association with repeated cycles of chemotherapy, or they may be related to zinc deficiency. Multiple Beau lines should not be confused with the multiple transverse depressions that are stacked longitudinally along the central nail plate (washboard nails), resulting from the obsessive habit of repeatedly pushing back the cuticle or picking at the proximal nailfold margin (habit-tic deformity) [see Figure 2].[15,17] There is no specific treatment for Beau lines. They grow out over time after resolution of the growth-arrest period.

ONYCHOLYSIS

Onycholyis is defined as the separation of the nail plate from the nail bed. In most cases, onycholysis begins distally; it is often related to acute or chronic trauma that produces a lever effect, lifting the nail plate upward and away from its bed. Other causes of onycholysis are chemical exposure (allergic or irritant dermatitis), onychomycosis, and primary dermatoses (e.g., psoriasis or lichen planus).[13] Associations with underlying systemic disease (e.g., thyroid disease) have been sporadically reported but are less commonly encountered in clinical practice. When moisture accumulates under onycholytic nail plate, bacterial proliferation may occur. This can cause a green discoloration of the nail plate as a result of a pigment produced by certain organisms (e.g., *Pseudomonas aeruginosa*) [see Figure 3].

Treatment requires avoidance of precipating factors for onycholysis, debridement of separated nail plate, and the twice-daily topical application of diluted acetic acid solution (consisting of equal parts white vinegar and water), gentamicin, or the combination of polymyxin B and bacitracin.[18]

LEUKONYCHIA

Leukonychia, a white discoloration of the nail plate or subungual tissue, has multiple presentations. Small 1 to 3 mm white spots (punctate leukonychia) or irregular transverse streaks (leukonychia variegata) of the nail plate are the most common varieties.[15] These two presentations are generally secondary to repeated microtrauma to the matrix, growing out distally with outgrowth of the nail plate. Mee lines specifically refer to transverse 1 to 2 mm white bands, which usually are demonstrated at the same site in multiple nails and reported in association with arsenic intoxication, Hodgkin disease, sickle cell anemia, renal failure, and cardiac insufficiency. Leukonychia is also associated with systemic infection and chemotherapy.[19-21]

Half-and-half nails (Lindsay nails) present as a diffuse, dull whitening of the proximal nail bed that obscures the lunula and as a distal region of pink or reddish-brown discoloration that occupies from 20% to 60% of the nail length.[15,22] The most commonly reported association with half-and-half nails is chronic renal failure. When the distal brown band of discoloration constitutes less than 20% of the total nail length, the anomaly is known as Terry nails, which occurs in association with chronic congestive heart failure, hepatic cirrhosis, type 2 (non–insulin-dependent) diabetes mellitus, and advanced age. In both half-and-half nails and Terry nails, the proximal portion of the nail bed may be light pink, exhibiting a more normal appearance, rather than white.

Muehrcke nails present as paired, white, narrow transverse bands of the nail bed, separated by normal-appearing thin pink bands.[15,22] Muehrcke nails have been associated with chronic hypoalbuminemia. Resolution of this nail finding correlates with normalization of serum albumin levels.[15]

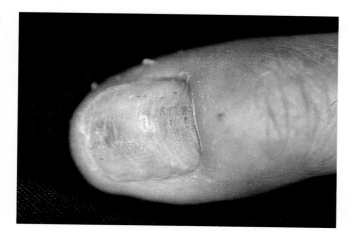

Figure 2 Stacking of transverse linear grooves traversing the entire length of the central nail plate, resulting from the repeated picking of the proximal nail fold margin (habit-tic deformity). Note the marked hypertrophy of the lunula, which is typical of this disorder.

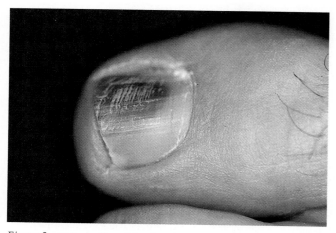

Figure 3 Colonization of the closed space between the nail bed and nail plate with *Pseudomonas aeruginosa*, causing a green nail. Moisture trapped in the onycholytic space provides an optimal environment for proliferation of this bacterium.

CLUBBING

When the normal angle between the proximal nail fold and the nail plate exceeds 180°, digital clubbing is present. The morphologic changes of clubbing typically include hypertrophy of the surrounding soft tissue of the nail folds as a result of hyperplasia of dermal fibrovasculature and edematous infiltration of the pulp tip.[21] Radiologic changes are identified in fewer than 20% of cases.[15]

Clubbing may be hereditary, or it may be seen in association with several underlying disease states, such as hypertrophic pulmonary osteoarthropathy, chronic congestive heart failure, congenital heart disease associated with cyanosis, polycythemias associated with hypoxia, Graves disease, chronic hepatic cirrhosis, lung cancer, Crohn disease, and irritable bowel disease.[15,22,23] When clubbing is unilateral, consideration should be given to underlying causes of obstructed circulation, such as aneurysm, arteriovenous fistula, and a pulmonary sulcus tumor (Pancoast tumor); disorders producing soft tissue edema; and diseases causing localized changes in underlying digital bone (e.g., sarcoidosis). Unilateral clubbing can also be found in cases of hemiplegia,[24] and a case of subungual perineurioma caused by unilateral clubbing has been reported.[25] Paronychia and distal phalangeal resorption may cause changes that simulate true clubbing (pseudoclubbing).

NAIL-PLATE PITTING

Nail-plate pitting (onychia punctata) develops as a result of focal defects in nail-plate formation from the proximal nail matrix. The number, size, and shape of the superficial depressions may vary.[15] The extent and duration of involvement with nail pitting correlates with the duration of nail-matrix abnormality. Psoriasis, the most common association with nail pitting, may produce a random array of shallow or deep pitted indentations, usually affecting one or more fingernails.[26,27]

Psoriasis of the nails often responds poorly to treatment, and it tends to recur. Topical corticosteroids, topical tazarotene, and intralesional corticosteroid injection may help in some cases.[28,29] It is a common misconception that nail pitting is pathognomonic for psoriasis.[27] Nail pitting may also be seen in association with alopecia areata, punctate keratoderma, idiopathic trachyonychia, occasionally in normal nails, and rarely in association with collagen vascular disease or syphilis. Fingernail pitting occurs in one third of children with alopecia areata; mild disease involving only a few nails is observed in approximately 20% of cases.[27] Compared to psoriasis, nail pitting seen in alopecia areata is typically more uniform and patterned, often presenting as orderly rows of shallow pitted depressions. Currently, there is no available treatment for this type of nail pitting.

LONGITUDINAL PIGMENTED BANDS

Longitudinal pigmented bands (melanonychia striata), also referred to as longitudinal melanonychia, is the presence of single or multiple longitudinally oriented brown or black bands [see Figure 4]. Homogeneous longitudinal bands occur in approximately 75% of African Americans older than 20 years. It usually affects the thumb and index finger.[30,31] Melanonychia striata is also commonly seen in Hispanics, may be found in up to 20% of Japanese, and is rare in whites.[30]

The deposition of melanin in the nail plate may result from increased melanin synthesis by matrix melanocytes that are usually nonfunctional; it may also occur as a result of a prolif-

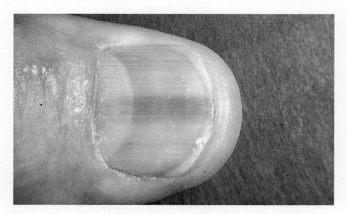

Figure 4 Melanonychia striata (longitudinal pigmented band) produced by a melanocytic nevus of the nail matrix. A high index of suspicion for subungual melanoma is very important when a longitudinal pigmented band of the nail is identified.

eration of matrix melanocytes.[30] Melanonychia striata affecting a single nail may result from a benign melanocytic nevus or a subungual melanoma. Thus, it is important to distinguish between a benign cause and a malignant cause of a longitudinal pigmented band. Factors suggesting the presence of melanoma or an atypical melanocytic proliferation are (1) single digit involvement; (2) periungual spread of pigment onto the nail-fold region (Hutchinson sign); (3) border irregularity or variegated color within the linear streak; and (4) changes in appearance (e.g., color or borders) involving an established longitudinal band.[32] Because of the severity of subungual melanoma and the importance of making a prompt diagnosis, the index of suspicion must be high. A simple biopsy of the nail plate is not satisfactory in establishing the diagnosis, because it will only demonstrate the presence of melanin. An appropriate biopsy inclusive of the nail matrix, as well as the nail bed if clinically indicated, should be performed by a surgeon who is familiar with the intricacies of performing a nail biopsy.[33] Because of limited experience and the difficulties that are commonly con-

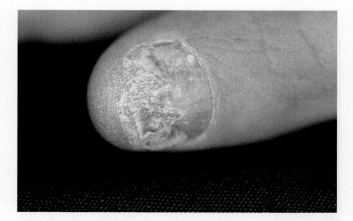

Figure 5 Psoriasis of the nail, characterized by subungual hyperkeratosis and loss of distal onycholytic nail plate. This patient was unsuccessfully treated with oral antifungal therapy after an erroneous diagnosis of onychomycosis was made on the basis of clinical diagnosis alone. Careful examination of the proximal intact nail plate reveals pitting, a feature characteristic for psoriasis and not onychomycosis.

a   *b*

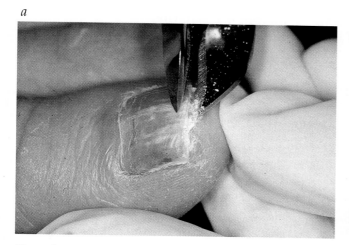
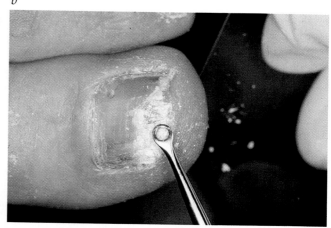

Figure 6 (*a*) **When obtaining a nail specimen for potassium hydroxide (KOH) preparation, it is important to expose the affected nail bed by first trimming away and discarding the distal, separated (onycholytic) nail plate. (*b*) Small specimen fragments of subungual hyperkeratosis of the nail bed and exposed undersurface of the nail plate are effectively obtained using a small curette. The smaller fragments are more easily dissolved by KOH, allowing for more accurate microscopic visualization, and can be easily plated on fungal culture medium.**

fronted in the histologic interpretation of nail specimens, biopsies of melanonychia striata are best interpreted by a dermatopathologist.[34]

When nail-bed pigmentation is noted, other causes such as systemic drugs (e.g., antimalarials, zidovudine, bleomycin, doxorubicin, minocycline, and hydroxyuria) or systemic disease (e.g., Addison disease and HIV infection) must be considered; however, these causes usually result in a broader, more diffuse pigmentation, often involving multiple nails.[35] Another reported association with melanonychia striata is systemic lupus erythematosus.[36] Frictional melanonychia resulting from trauma from athletic activities or poorly fitting shoewear may cause nail pigmentation, including pigmentation of the nail fold, especially in dark-skinned persons (pseudo-Hutchinson sign).[32]

Bacterial and Fungal Nail Infections

BACTERIAL PARONYCHIA

Bacterial infection of the nail folds (bacterial paronychia) is usually acute in nature. It is is characterized by swelling, erythema, discomfort, and sometimes purulence. The most common etiologic pathogen is *Staphylococcus aureus*. Treatment requires drainage of a focal abscess, if present, and oral antibiotic therapy.[37]

CHRONIC PARONYCHIA

Chronic paronychia results from persistent or frequently recurrent nail-fold inflammation, which is usually the result of chronic irritant dermatitis and loss of cuticle from trauma or nail-care practices. Secondary candidal infection may occur.[29,38]

Table 1   Oral Antifungal for Toenail Onychomycosis*[46]

Drug	Dosage	Comments
Griseofulvin tablets or liquid	500 mg – 1 g daily × 12 – 18 mo	Generally not recommended because of limited efficacy and because more effective agents are available; only active against dermatophyte organisms
Itraconazole capsules	Pulse therapy[†]: 200 mg twice daily × 1 wk/mo for 3 consecutive mo Continuous therapy: 200 mg daily × 3 mo	Contraindications include specific drug interactions and congestive heart failure; potential hepatotoxicity (rare); effective for dermatophytes, *Candida* species, and some nondermatophytic molds; should be administered with food; absorption may be decreased by increased gastric pH (as might result from use of H$_2$ blockers, antacids, proton pump inhibitors); blood clearance in 1 – 2 wk; therapeutic nail levels 9 mo posttherapy
Terbinafine tablets	250 mg daily × 3 mo	Most active for dermatophytes; some efficacy for certain nondermatophytic molds; limited activity against most *Candida* species; potential hepatotoxicity (rare); sporadic reports of blood dyscrasias (rare); reversible change or loss of taste (< 2%); blood clearance in 1 – 2 mo; therapeutic nail levels 9 mo posttherapy
Fluconazole tablets[‡]	150 – 300 mg × 9 – 12 mo	Effective against dermatophytes and *Candida* species; potential hepatotoxicity (rare); some significant drug interactions; limited therapeutic drug reservoir in nail posttherapy

*Topical ciclopirox 8% nail lacquer is FDA approved for onychomycosis caused by *Trichophyton rubrum*. Treatment involves application once daily for 12 mo (or until outgrowth of clear nail occurs), combined with debridement/trimming of onycholytic nail plate. Efficacy is lower than that seen with newer oral agents (e.g., itraconazole, terbinafine). No oral or topical agent is currently FDA approved for nondermatophytic onychomycosis (e.g., *Candida* species, molds).
†Pulse itraconazole is FDA approved for fingernail tinea unguium; established efficacy has been demonstrated for toenail disease.
‡Fluconazole is not FDA approved for onychomycosis; established efficacy has been demonstrated for tinea unguium.

Table 2 Selected Dermatologic Disorders Affecting the Nail Unit

Disease State	Disease Features	Nail Findings
Inflammatory diseases		
Psoriasis	Nail findings in 10% – 50% of patients; 39% of children with psoriasis with nail changes (usually pitting); nail disease present in 50% – 85% of patients with psoriatic arthritis	Proximal matrix involvement: pitting, transverse grooving, deeply ridged plate surface (onychorrhexis) Distal matrix involvement: plate thinning, lunula erythema Nail bed: subungual hyperkeratosis, oil drop sign, splinter hemorrhages Nail folds: cutaneous lesions of psoriasis Phalangeal/joint involvement: psoriatic arthritis
Lichen planus	Nail changes occur in up to 10% of patients with lichen planus; may occur in childhood or adulthood; nail involvement may be present with or without skin or mucosal disease; potentially reversible in early inflammatory stage; irreversible in cicatricial (later stage) of disease; may present as ridged, rough-surfaced, lusterless plates (trachyonychia) or 20-nail dystrophy in children	Matrix involvement: combination of nail-plate ridging, splitting, and progressive uniform thinning; distal-edge splitting, fragility, crumbling, brittleness, nail-plate shedding (onychomadesis) Focal matrix scarring: pterygium formation (scarring bridge between proximal nail fold and subungual epidermis with focal loss of nail plate) Nail-bed involvement: subungual hyperkeratosis, onycholysis Diffuse matrix/nail-bed disease: total nail-plate loss, atrophy, scarring
Alopecia areata	Nail changes in 10% of patints with alopecia areata; nail changes in over 40% of children with alopecia areata; fingernail involvement most common; may present in children as 20-nail dystrophy	Matrix involvement: orderly nail pitting arranged in a crosshatched pattern (glen-plaid sign); roughened nail-plate surface (trachyonychia); fragility; splitting; longitudinal ridging; spotted or red lunula (erythema); nail-plate shedding (onychomadesis)
Nail tumors		
Glomus tumor	75% occur on the hand, usually subungual (nail bed); a benign vascular hamartoma	Visible through plate as a light-red, reddish-blue spot; rarely exceeds 1 cm in size; characteristic symptom of intense or pulsatile pain; pain is spontaneous or provoked by slight trauma or pressure
Digital myxoid (mucus) cyst	A form of focal mucinosis; not a true cyst (no epithelial lining); contains clear, viscous, jellylike fluid; usually seen in adults	Soft, domed, translucent, pink or skin-colored, shiny, soft neoplasm of proximal nail fold or overlying distal interphalangeal joint; those over fold may compress matrix, producing flattening of plate; those over joint may connect to underlying joint space
Subungual exostoses	Outgrowths of calcified cartilage or normal bone; most seen on great toe; most frequent in adolescents and young adults; benign lesions	Emerge from the dorsal digit at distal phalanx; may erode through plate or project from under distal or lateral edge of plate; often painful; may become eroded
Periungual angiofibromas	Arise out of nail fold; often multiple; seen in 50% of cases of tuberous sclerosis (Borneville-Pringle disease); usually arise in early teenage years; benign neoplasm	Small, round, flesh-colored or pink, firm papules with shiny, smooth surface arising from nail-fold region; may partially cover nail plate; usually asymptomatic

ONYCHOMYCOSIS

Onychomycosis, the most common infection of the nail, is a fungal infection characterized by nail-bed and plate involvement. Dermatophyte onychomycosis (tinea unguium) is the most common type of fungal nail infection.[39] It is seen far more commonly in adults than in children and most frequently affects one or more toenails. The mode of fungal invasion usually presents as distal-lateral subungual onychomycosis, occurring as dermatophyte organisms migrate from pedal skin to below the nail plate and invade nail-bed tissue.[40] Tinea pedis and onychomycosis frequently coexist in a patient.[41,42]

The dermatophytes that most commonly cause onychomycosis are *Trichophyton rubrum* and *T. mentagrophytes*.[43] The tendency to harbor dermatophytes (especially *T. rubrum*), predominantly on pedal skin, has been noted in some kindreds. As a result, patients with such a tendency are prone to tinea pedis, tinea unguium, tinea cruris, and diffuse tinea corporis. They may present with dermatophyte infections earlier in life than usually seen and often experience recurrence of dermatophyte infection after completion of initially effective therapy.

The most characteristic clinical features of dermatophyte onychomycosis are distal onycholysis, subungual hyperkeratosis, and a dystrophic, discolored nail plate.[42] Because this combination of features is also seen in persons with nail psoriasis, accurate diagnosis may require performance of a potassium hydroxide (KOH) preparation and fungal culture [*see Figure 5*]. It is important that specimens be obtained from the nail bed [*see Figure 6*] and that culture specimens be transported and plated appropriately, because different culture media are required for identification of dermatophyte and nondermatophyte fungal nail pathogens.[42] Dermatophyte test medium (DTM) may be used as an in-office culture technique that has no special incubation requirements. DTM is inexpensive and accurate in the diagnosis of dermatophyte onychomycosis.[44] The clinical presentation of proximal white subungual onychomycosis, another presentation of dermatophyte onychomycosis, has been reported in association with systemic immunosuppression, including HIV disease.[45]

Candida onychomycosis is far less common than dermatophyte onychomycosis. *Candida* onychomycosis is often associated with immunosuppression (e.g., HIV disease and chronic mucocutaneous candidiasis). The *Candida* organisms may invade the nail as a secondary pathogen, and they more frequently affect the fingernails.[42] Nondermatophyte molds, including *Aspergillus* species, *Scopulariopsis brevicaulis*, *Fusarium* species, *Scytalidium hyalinum*, and *Scytalidium dimidiatum*, have been reported to cause fingernail or toenail infection; however, such infections are relatively uncommon.[42,46] Associated paronychia may be seen when nondermatophytic fungi cause onychomycosis. Effective therapy for onychomycosis includes the use of an oral antifungal agent [*see Table 1*].[47] Because nails grow slowly, clinical response is delayed.[46] Infections with *Scytalidium* species are rare in the United States, and such infections respond poorly to currently available antifungal agents.

DERMATOLOGIC DISORDERS AFFECTING THE NAIL

Complete reviews of dermatologic, systemic, neoplastic, and exogenous disorders affecting the nail are beyond the scope of this chapter. An overview of selected dermatologic disorders affecting the nail unit and their associated clinical findings is provided [*see Table 2*].

References

1. Gonzalez-Serva A: Structure and function. Nails: Therapy, Diagnosis, Surgery. Scher RK, Daniel CR, Eds. WB Saunders Co, Philadelphia, 1997, p 12

2. Fleckman P: Basic science of the nail unit. Nails: Therapy, Diagnosis, Surgery. Scher RK, Daniel CR, Eds. WB Saunders Co, Philadelphia, 1997, p 44

3. Dawber RPR, De Berker DAR, Baran R: Science of the nail apparatus. Diseases of the Nails and Their Management. Baran R, Dawber RPR, Eds. Blackwell Science, Oxford, England, 1994, p 5

4. Fleckman P, Allan C: Surgical anatomy of the nail unit. Dermatol Surg 27:257, 2001

5. Cohen PR: The lunula. J Am Acad Dermatol 34:943, 1996

6. Tosti A, Peluso AP, Piraccini BM: Nail diseases in children. Adv Dermatol 13:353, 1998

7. Orentreich N, Markofsky J, Vogelman JH: The effect of aging on the rate of linear nail growth. J Invest Dermatol 73:126, 1979

8. Cohen PR, Scher RK: Geriatric nail disorders: diagnosis and treatment. J Am Acad Dermatol 26:521, 1992

9. Tosti A, Baran R, Dawber RPR: The nails in systemic disease and drug-induced changes: yellow nail syndrome. Diseases of the Nails and Their Management. Baran R, Dawber RPR, Eds. Blackwell Science, Oxford, England, 1994, p 185

10. Lubach D, Cohrs W, Wurzinger R: Incidence of brittle nails. Dermatologica 172:144, 1986

11. Baran R, Dawber RPR, Tosti A: Science of the nail apparatus and relationship to foot function. A Text Atlas of Nail Disorders. Baran R, Dawber RPR, Tosti A, Eds. Martin Dunitz, London, 1996, p 3

12. Daniel CR III, Daniel MO, Gupta AK: Nonfungal infections and paronychia. Nails: Therapy, Diagnosis, Surgery. Scher RK, Daniel CR, Eds. WB Saunders Co, Philadelphia, 1997, p 165

13. Kern D: Occupational disease. Nails: Therapy, Diagnosis, Surgery. Scher RK, Daniel CR, Eds. WB Saunders Co, Philadelphia, 1997, p 285

14. Tosti A, Baran R, Dawber RPR: The nails in systemic disease and drug-induced changes: splinter hemorrhages. Diseases of the Nails and Their Management. Baran R, Dawber RPR, Eds. Blackwell Science, Oxford, England, 1994, p 183

15. Baran R, Dawber RPR: Physical signs. Diseases of the Nails and Their Management. Baran R, Dawber RPR, Eds. Blackwell Science, Oxford, England, 1994, p 35

16. Baran R, Dawber RPR: Physical signs: Beau's lines and transverse grooves. Diseases of the Nails and Their Management. Baran R, Dawber RPR, Eds. Blackwell Science, Oxford, 1994, p 50

17. Habif TP: Nail diseases: habit-tic deformity. Clinical Dermatology. Habif TP, Ed. Mosby, St Louis, 1996, p 774

18. Daniel CR III, Daniel MO, Gupta AK: Appendix 2. Nails: Therapy, Diagnosis, Surgery. Scher RK, Daniel CR, Eds. WB Saunders Co, Philadelphia, 1997, p 368

19. Naumann R, Wozel G: Transverse leukonychia following chemotherapy in a patient with Hodgkin's disease. Eur J Dermatol 19:392, 2000

20. Cribier B, Mena ML, Rey D, et al: Nail changes in patients infected with human immunodeficiency virus: a prospective controlled study. Arch Dermatol 134:1216, 1998

21. Mautner GH, Lu I, Ort RJ, et al: Transverse leukonychia with systemic infection. Cutis 65:318, 2000

22. Daniel CR III, Sams WM, Scher RK: Nails in systemic disease. Nails: Therapy, Diagnosis, Surgery. Scher RK, Daniel CR, Eds. WB Saunders Co, Philadelphia, 1997, p 219

23. Myers KA, Farquhar DR: The rational clinical examination: does this patient have clubbing? JAMA 286:341, 2001

24. Siragusa M, Schepis C, Cosentino FI, et al: Nail pathology in patients with hemiplegia. Br J Dermatol 144:557, 2001

25. Baran R, Perrin C: Subungual perineurioma: a peculiar location. Br J Dermatol 146:125, 2002

26. Farber EM, Nall ML: Nail psoriasis. Cutis 50:174, 1992

27. Del Rosso JQ, Basuk P, Scher RK, et al: Dermatologic diseases of the nail unit. Nails: Therapy, Diagnosis, Surgery. Scher RK, Daniel CR, Eds. WB Saunders Co, Philadelphia, 1997, p 172

28. Scher RK, Stiller M, Zhu YI: Tazarotene 0.1% gel in the treatment of fingernail psoriasis: a double-blind, randomized, vehicle-controlled study. Cutis 68:355, 2001

29. Tosti A, Piraccini BM: Treatment of common nail disorders. Dermatol Clin 18:339, 2000

30. Baran R, Haneke E: Tumors of the nail apparatus and adjacent tissues: longitudinal melanonychia. Diseases of the Nails and Their Management. Baran R, Dawber RPR, Eds. Blackwell Science, Oxford, England, 1994, p 485

31. Haneke E, Baran R: Longitudinal melanonychia. Dermatol Surg 27:580, 2001

32. Baran R, Dawber RPR, Tosti A: Nail colour changes (chromonychia). A Text Atlas of Nail Disorders. Baran R, Dawber RPR, Tosti A, Eds. Martin Dunitz, London, 1996, p 147

33. Salasche SJ: Surgery. Dermatologic diseases of the nail unit. Nails: Therapy, Diagnosis, Surgery. Scher RK, Daniel CR, Eds. WB Saunders Co, Philadelphia, 1997, p 335

34. Fleckman P, Omura EF: Histopathology of the nail. Adv Dermatol 17:385, 2001

35. Aste N, Fumo G, Contu F, et al: Nail pigmentation caused by hydroxyurea: report of 9 cases. J Am Acad Dermatol 47:146, 2002

36. Skowron F, Combemale P, Faisant M, et al: Functional melanonychia due to involvement of the nail matrix in systemic lupus erythematosus. J Am Acad Dermatol 47(suppl):S187, 2002

37. Habif T: Nail diseases: acute paronychia. Clinical Dermatology. Habif TP, Ed. Mosby, St. Louis, 1996, p 763

38. Van Laborde S, Scher RK: Developments in the treatment of nail psoriasis, melanonychia striata, and onychomycosis: a review of the literature. Dermatol Clin 18:37, 2000

39. Gupta AK, Taborda P, Taborda V, et al: Epidemiology and prevalence of onychomycosis in HIV-positive individuals. Int J Dermatol 39:746, 2000

40. Elewski BE: Onychomycosis: treatment, quality of life, and economic issues. Am J Clin Dermatol 1:19, 2000

41. Lauritz B: Dermatoses of the feet. Am J Clin Dermatol 1:181, 2000

42. Elewski BE, Charif MA, Daniel CR III: Onychomycosis. Nails: Therapy, Diagnosis, Surgery. Scher RK, Daniel CR, Eds. WB Saunders Co, Philadelphia, 1997, p 152

43. Jennings MB, Weinberg JM, Koestenblatt EK, et al: Study of clinically suspected onychomycosis in a podiatric population. J Am Podiatr Med Assoc 92:327, 2002

44. Pariser D, Opper C: An in-office diagnostic procedure to detect dermatophytes in a nationwide study of onychomycosis patients. Manag Care 11:43, 2002

45. Baran R, Dawber RPR, Tosti A: Onychomycosis and its treatment. A Text Atlas of Nail Disorders. Baran R, Dawber RPR, Tosti A, Eds. Martin Dunitz, London, 1996, p 157

46. Del Rosso JQ: Current management of onychomycosis and dermatomycoses. Curr Infect Dis Rep 2:438, 2000

47. Crawford F, Young P, Godfrey C, et al: Oral treatments for toenail onychomycosis: a systematic review. Arch Dermatol 138:811, 2002

Acknowledgment

Figure 1   Tom Moore.

44 Disorders of Pigmentation

Pearl E. Grimes, M.D.

Disorders of Hyperpigmentation

MELASMA

Definition

Melasma is a common acquired symmetrical hypermelanosis characterized by irregular light-brown to gray-brown macules involving the face. There is a predilection for the cheeks, forehead, upper lips, nose, and chin [see Figure 1]. Lesions may occasionally occur in other sun-exposed areas, including the forearms and back.[1-3]

Epidemiology

The condition is most commonly observed in females. Men constitute only 10% of the cases and usually demonstrate the same clinicopathologic features as noted in women. Melasma affects all racial and ethnic groups but is most prevalent in individuals with darker complexions (skin types IV through VI). It is also more common in geographical areas exposed to intense ultraviolet radiation (sunlight), such as tropical and subtropical regions.

Etiology and Pathogenesis

Although the precise cause of melasma is unknown, multiple factors have been implicated in the etiopathogenesis of this condition. These factors include genetic influences, intense ultraviolet radiation exposure, pregnancy, oral contraceptive use, hormone replacement therapy, cosmetics, and phototoxic and antiseizure medications.[1]

Endocrinologic studies of patients with melasma report varying results. A detailed study of nine women with melasma showed significantly increased levels of luteinizing hormone (LH) and low levels of estradiol, suggesting an increase in subclinical mild ovarian dysfunction. In contrast, a study of 26 women assessed LH, follicle-stimulating hormone (FSH), and α-melanocyte–stimulating hormone (α-MSH) levels and reported no differences between patients and control subjects.[3] Thyroid dysfunction and increased levels of 17β-estradiol have also been reported in patients with melasma.

Diagnosis

Clinically, the light-brown patches are commonly evident on the malar, forehead, chin, nose, and upper lip areas of the face. Patients may exhibit a malar, centrofacial, or mandibular distribution. Histologically, an epidermal, epidermal-dermal, or dermal pattern of increased pigmentation occurs. A Wood light examination enhances the epidermal pattern of pigment deposition. Such epidermal lesions are most amenable to treatment.

Melasma must be distinguished from other conditions that cause facial hyperpigmentation, such as postinflammatory hyperpigmentation, drug-induced hyperpigmentation, lichen planus, actinicus, and photosensitivity disorders.

Treatment

Current treatments for melasma include broad-spectrum sunscreens, 2% (over-the-counter) and 4% (prescription) hydroquinone formulations, azelaic acid, kojic acid formulations, α-hydroxy acid products, retinoic acid, and superficial chemical peels.[1,4,5] Laser therapy offers minimal long-term success and in-

stead may worsen the condition. The aforementioned therapies improve melasma. However, none are curative. Hence, it is essential for patients to rigidly adhere to a regimen of daily sunscreen or other protection against the sun to control the progression of melasma.

POSTINFLAMMATORY HYPERPIGMENTATION

Definition

Postinflammatory hyperpigmentation is characterized by an acquired increase in cutaneous pigmentation secondary to an inflammatory process [see Figure 2]. Excess pigment deposition may occur in the epidermis or in both epidermis and dermis.

Epidemiology

The condition occurs in all racial and ethnic groups; however, it has a higher incidence in people with darker complexions. In a diagnostic survey of 2,000 African-American patients seeking dermatologic care, the third most common diagnosis was pigmentary disorders, of which postinflammatory hyperpigmentation was the most prevalent.[1]

Etiology and Pathogenesis

Pigmentary changes may be a result of production of inflammatory mediators and altered cytokine production.[6,7] The afore-

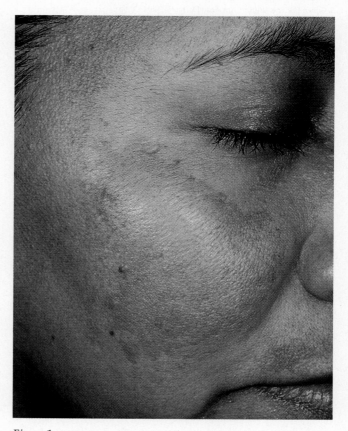

Figure 1 **Melasma is characterized by hyperpigmentation of the cheek, forehead, and upper lip.**

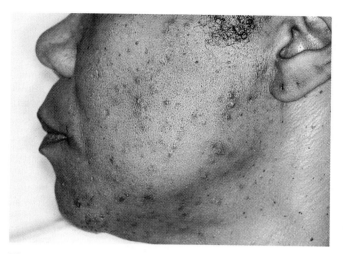

Figure 2 **Postinflammatory hyperpigmentation of the face may be secondary to acne vulgaris.**

mentioned changes may lead to an increase in the number and size of epidermal melanocytes. In addition, hyperpigmentation may be a consequence of pigmentary incontinence, with deposition of pigment in the upper dermis. Causes of postinflammatory hyperpigmentation include acne, allergic reactions, drug eruptions, papulosquamous disorders, eczematoid disorders, and vesiculobullous conditions.[8]

Diagnosis

Clinically, postinflammatory pigmentary changes may be localized, circumscribed, or generalized. Lesions range in color from brown to black to ashen gray and usually follow the distribution of the primary dermatosis.

Treatment

Therapies for postinflammatory hyperpigmentation include over-the-counter and prescription hydroquinone preparations. Higher concentrations are indicated for moderate to severe involvement. Other treatments are azelaic acid, kojic acid, and retinoic acid [*see* Melasma, *above*].

DRUG-INDUCED HYPERPIGMENTATION

Medications are a common cause of cutaneous hyperpigmentation. Lesions may be localized or generalized. Medications can also cause hyperpigmentation of the oral mucosa and nails. There may be some improvement upon withdrawal of the offending agent; however, drug-induced hyperpigmentation can persist for many years.

Medications causing drug-induced hyperpigmentation include minocycline, oral contraceptives, estrogens, zidovudine, bleomycin, hydrochlorothiazide, hydantoin, amiodarone, tetracycline, busulfan, chlorpromazine, quinicrine, and imipramine.[9-11]

Heavy metals can also cause hyperpigmentation. Such preparations include arsenic, gold, silver, mercury, and bismuth.[9]

ERYTHEMA DYSCHROMICUM PERSTANS

Definition

Erythema dyschromicum perstans (EDP, or ashy dermatosis), first described in 1957, is an acquired benign condition characterized by slate-gray to violaceous macules.

Epidemiology

EDP is reported most commonly in dark-skinned persons. However, cases have been reported globally and in all skin types. The disease appears to have a relative equal frequency in males and females. Children have also been reported with this condition.

Etiology and Pathogenesis

The precise cause of EDP is unknown. Studies suggest that pollutants, hair dyes, chemicals, and drug exposure may play a role in the pathogenesis.[12-14] Findings in light microscopic, ultrastructural, and immunofluorescent studies of EDP have been similar to those in studies of lichen planus, leading some investigators to postulate that EDP may be a variant of lichen planus. Other studies suggest that EDP is a distinct entity. Expression of intercellular adhesion molecule–I (ICAM-I) and major histocompatibility complex (MHC) class II molecules (HLA-DR) has been reported.[15] These findings suggest that aberrant cell-mediated immunity may be involved in the pathogenesis of EDP.

Diagnosis

Clinically, the macules of EDP are ashen and may have an erythematous, slightly raised border during the early stages of the disease. Erythematous macules have also been described during the early stages. Areas of erythema eventually resolve, leaving slate-gray areas of pigmentation. The lesions are usually symmetrically distributed and vary in size from small macules to very large patches. Common sites of involvement include the face, neck, trunk, and upper extremities. Mucous membrane, palms, soles, and nails are usually spared. Light microscopic changes show slight epidermal atrophic changes, spongiosis, lymphocytic exocytosis, and basal vacuolopathy in the epidermis and lymphohistocytic, lichenoid dermal infiltrates. Later stages lack the epidermal changes and show increased deposition of dermal pigment.

Postinflammatory hyperpigmentation, pityriasis rosea, lichen planus, fixed drug eruption, Addison disease, pinta, syphilis, macular amyloidosis, hemochromatosis, and argyria must be distinguished from EDP.

Treatment

Therapies for EDP have been minimally effective. They include sunscreens, hydroquinone, bleaching creams, topical corticosteroids, griseofulvin, clofazamine, antibiotics, and antimalarials.

LENTIGINES

Definition

A lentigo is a well-circumscribed, brown to brown-black macule, usually less than 1 cm in size, that appears at birth or in early childhood. Lentigines occur in all skin types and may be found in any cutaneous surface, including the palms, soles, and mucous membranes. They do not darken with sun exposure. Lentigines can be localized and must be distinguished from freckles (ephelides). Clinical differentiating features include the later appearance of freckles (at 4 to 6 years of age) and their predominance on sun-exposed skin and increased frequency in redheads and fair-skinned persons. Freckles also tend to fade in winter and with advancing age.

Epidemiology

Multiple lentigines have been reported in 18.5% of black newborns and 0.04% of white newborns. Solar lentigines have been reported in 90% of whites older than 60 years.

Diagnosis

Several types of lentigines are recognized, including lentigo simplex, solar lentigines, nevus spilus, lentigines induced by psoralens plus ultraviolet A (PUVA), generalized lentiginosis, and syndrome-related lentiginosis.

Lentigo simplex lesions may occur as solitary localized macules or may be numerous and widespread. They often occur during the first decade of life and can be found on any cutaneous surface.

Solar (senile) lentigines, or so-called liver spots, are brown macules that appear late in adult life on chronically sun-exposed skin. These lesions are present in 90% of whites older than 70 years and occur in response to solar exposure. Solar lentigines correlate with the tendency to freckle and two or more sunburns after 20 years of age.

Nevus spilus, or speckled lentiginosis nevus, is a congenital brown patch that develops dotted brown macules during childhood. Histologically, the brown patch has features of a lentigo, whereas the dotted brown macules most often reveal features of junctional nevi. Zosteriform patterns have also been described. Generalized lentiginosis is characterized by innumerable lentigines unassociated with other abnormalities.

The histopathology of lentiginosis shows elongated rete ridges, increased numbers of basal melanocytes, and increased basal melanization. In contrast, freckles result from hypermelanization of basal melanocytes without a concomitant increase in number.

Lentigo must be distinguished from other flat, pigmented lesions, including freckles, junctional nevi, postinflammatory hyperpigmentation, and pigmented actinic keratoses.

Treatment

The treatment of lentigines includes hydroquinone-containing bleaching agents, cryotherapy, and laser therapy.

CONFLUENT AND RETICULATED PAPILLOMATOSIS OF GOUGEROT AND CARTEAUD

The eruption of confluent and reticulated papillomatosis was initially described by Gougerot and Carteaud in 1927 and 1932. The condition consists of 2 to 5 mm hyperpigmented papules having a predilection for the sternal area and midline of the back and neck.

Epidemiology

Confluent and reticulated papillomatosis has an equal frequency in males and females and shows no racial or ethnic predilections. The disease usually begins during the third decade of life.

Etiology and Pathogenesis

The precise cause of confluent and reticulated papillomatosis is unknown. Endocrine disturbances, abnormal host response to *Pityrosporum orbiculare,* and genetically determined defects of keratinization have been suggested.[16]

Diagnosis

Patients present with 2 to 5 mm hyperpigmented, slightly verrucoid papules having a predilection for the back, scapula, and inframammary areas. The papules become confluent near the midline and possess a reticulated pattern near the periphery. The lesions do not form a true scale but, rather, a mealy deposit that can easily be removed with the fingertips.

Histologically, studies show hyperkeratosis, decreased granular cell layers, papillomatosis, absence of sweat glands, and fragmentation of elastic fibers.

Other conditions that simulate confluent and reticulated papillomatosis are tinea versicolor and acanthosis nigricans.

Treatment

Recent studies have reported the beneficial effects of minocycline therapy.[17,18] Other treatments that have shown some efficacy include selenium sulfide shampoo, salicylic acid, vitamin A, retinoids, and PUVA.

DOWLING-DEGOS DISEASE

Dowling-Degos disease, or reticulated pigmented anomaly of the flexures, is an autosomal dominant disorder with variable penetrance characterized by brownish-black macules of the flexures that develop in a reticulated pattern. It may be caused by an underlying defect in follicular epithelial proliferation.

Diagnosis

Dowling-Degos disease manifests symmetrical reticulated hyperpigmentation of the groin, axilla, antecubital area, inframammary areas, and neck.[19] The lesions begin as 1 to 3 mm macules that gradually become confluent, assuming a reticulated lacelike pattern. In addition, perinasal and facial involvement is common. Pigmented pinhead-sized comedones are frequently observed in the affected areas, and perinasal, pitted acneiform scars can occur around the mouth.

Lesions begin in early adult life and are slowly progressive. The condition has been reported in association with reticulated acropigmentation of Kitamura and hidradenitis suppurativa,[20] suggesting an underlying defect in follicular epithelial proliferation. Histologically, thin-pigmented epithelial strands of downgrowth extend from the epidermis and follicular wall in a filiform pattern resembling adenoid seborrheic keratoses.

Treatment

In general, there is no effective treatment for Dowling-Degos disease. Adapalene has been reported to offer some benefit.

Disorders of Hypopigmentation

VITILIGO

Definition

Vitiligo is a common acquired, idiopathic skin disorder characterized by one or more patches of depigmented skin caused by loss of cutaneous melanocytes. These lesions are cosmetically disfiguring and usually cause severe emotional trauma in children as well as adults [*see Figure 3*].

Epidemiology

Vitiligo affects 1% to 2% of the population. Onset may begin at any age, but peak incidences occur in the second or third decade of life. The disease shows no racial or ethnic predilection, but because of the stark contrast between depigmented and darker skin tones, it is more cosmetically disfiguring in darker racial and ethnic groups. Females are affected more often than males. The disease has a familial incidence of 25% to 30%. Genetic studies suggest a polygenic inheritance pattern.

Human leukocyte antigen (HLA) studies have reported increases in a variety of haplotypes of class I and class II antigens. However, results vary significantly by race and ethnicity of the population studied. The reported HLA associations include increased frequencies of HLA A30, CW6, CW7, DR1, DR3, DR4, and DQW3.[21]

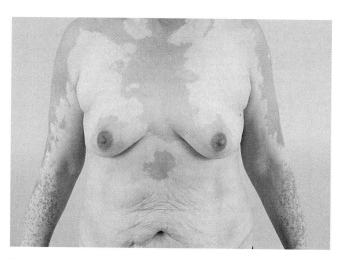

Figure 3 **Vitiligo is indicated by generalized patches of depigmentation of the trunk.**

Etiology and Pathogenesis

The precise cause of vitiligo is unknown. However, multiple theories have been proposed, including genetic autoimmune, neural, biochemical, and viral mechanisms. Reviews addressing the etiology of vitiligo viewed in totality suggest that vitiligo is probably a heterogeneous disease encompassing multiple etiologies.[21,22] In light of the acute prodromal symptoms, a viral etiology has been postulated but not confirmed.

An immune-mediated pathogenesis is indeed the most popular theory. This theory is predicated on the plethora of immunologic diseases and immune phenomena reported in patients with vitiligo. Patients demonstrate an increased frequency of a variety of diseases, including hypothyroidism (Hashimoto thyroiditis, Graves disease, pernicious anemia, diabetes mellitus, and alopecia areata). Thyroid disease is the most common associated condition in patients with vitiligo. Other diseases reported in association with vitiligo include Addison disease, atopic dermatitis, asthma, lichen planus, morphea, lichen sclerosus et atrophicus, mucocutaneous candidiasis, biliary cirrhosis, myasthenia gravis, Down syndrome, AIDS, and cutaneous T cell lymphoma.

Humoral and cell-mediated immunologic defects are a common phenomenon in vitiligo.[21,22] Numerous studies have documented an increased frequency of organ-specific autoantibodies. Antithyroid, gastric antiparietal cell, and antinuclear antibodies are most commonly demonstrated. Patients with positive organ-specific autoantibodies unassociated with autoimmune disease have an increased risk of subsequent subclinical or overt autoimmune disease.

Antimelanocyte antibodies, often demonstrated in the sera of patients with vitiligo, induce the destruction of melanocytes grown in culture by complement-mediated lysis and antibody-dependent cellular cytotoxicity. The presence and titer of antimelanocyte antibodies correlate with the severity and activity of vitiligo. These antibodies are directed to melanocyte cell surface antigens with molecular weights of 25, 35 to 40, 75, 90, and 150 kd. Studies suggest that the antimelanocyte antibody may mediate the destruction of melanocytes in vitiligo. Tyrosinase antibodies have also been reported in patients with localized and generalized disease.[23]

Cellular immune-mediated defects include diminished contact sensitization and quantitative and qualitative alterations in T cells and natural-killer cells. Quantitative studies of Langerhans cells from involved and uninvolved skin are inconsistent. Immunohistochemical studies have demonstrated abnormal expression of MHC class II and ICAM-I by melanocytes in vitiligo, which may contribute to the aberrant cellular immune response. In addition, there is increased expression of the antiadhesive matrix component tenasin in perilesional and lesional vitiliginous skin. Increased tenasin expression may be a consequence of elevated cytokine production and cellular infiltrates in vitiligo.[22]

Cytomegalovirus DNA has been demonstrated in the involved and uninvolved skin of patients with vitiligo. No viral DNA was detected in matched control subjects.[24] These findings suggest that in some cases, vitiligo may be triggered by a viral infection.

The neural theory is supported by several clinical, biochemical, and ultrastructural observations. These observations include the occurrence of segmental vitiligo; the demonstration of lesional autonomic dysfunction, such as increased sweating; and the demonstration of nerve ending–melanocyte contact. The last observation is rare in normal skin. In addition, studies have demonstrated aberrant tetrahydrobiopterin and catecholamine biosynthesis and release in patients with vitiligo.[22] It is therefore suggested that abnormal release of catecholamines from autonomic nerve endings may damage melanocytes by altering the free radical defense of the epidermis.

The self-destruction hypothesis proposes that melanocytes may be destroyed by phenolic compounds formed during the synthesis of melanin. In vivo and in vitro studies have demonstrated the destruction of melanocytes by phenols and catechols. In addition, industrial workers who are exposed to catechols and phenols may experience depigmentation of areas of skin or leukoderma.

A variety of environmentally ubiquitous compounds containing catechols, phenols, and sulfhydryls can induce hypopigmentation, depigmentation, or both. These compounds are most often encountered in industrial chemicals and cleaning agents. Possible mechanisms for altered pigment production by the aforementioned chemicals include melanocyte destruction via free radical formation, inhibition of tyrosinase activity, and interference with the production or transfer of melanosomes.

Diagnosis

Clinical manifestations Vitiliginous lesions are typically asymptomatic depigmented macules without clinical signs of inflammation. However, inflammatory vitiligo with erythematous borders has been reported. Hypopigmented lesions may coexist with depigmented lesions. The patches are occasionally pruritic. Macules frequently begin on sun-exposed or perioral facial skin and either remain localized or disseminate to other cutaneous sites. Areas of depigmentation vary in size from a few millimeters to many centimeters, and their borders are usually distinct. Trichrome lesions are most often observed in darker-complexioned persons. These lesions are characterized by zones of white, light brown, and normal skin color. This finding suggests that melanocyte loss begins in the hair follicle. Depigmented hairs are often present in lesional skin and do not preclude repigmentation of a lesion. In addition, there is a high incidence of premature graying of scalp hair in patients with vitiligo and their families. Vitiliginous lesions can remain stable or slowly progress for years. In some instances, however, patients undergo almost complete spontaneous depigmentation over a few years.

Vitiligo is subclassified into different types on the basis of the distribution of skin lesions. These subclassifications include the generalized or vulgaris, acral or acrofacial, localized, and segmented types. The generalized pattern is characterized by symmetrical macules occurring in a random distribution. Acral or acrofacial vitiligo consists of depigmented macules confined to the extremities or to the face and extremities, respectively. A subcategory of the acrofacial type is the lip-tip variety, in which lesions are confined to the lips and the tips of the digits. The generalized and acrofacial varieties are the most common. Localized vitiligo occurs in a dermatomal or quasidermatomal distribution; lesions rarely spread beyond the affected dermatome. This variety is the less common variety of vitiligo and most often occurs along the distribution of the trigeminal nerve.

Melanocytes of the eye, ear, and leptomeninges may also be involved in vitiligo. Depigmented areas of the retinal pigment epithelium and choroid have been reported in 39% of patients studied. These lesions usually do not interfere with vision. Vitiligo is also a manifestation of the Vogt-Koyanagi-Harada syndrome, which is characterized by poliosis, chronic uveitis, alopecia, dysacusis, vitiligo, and signs of meningeal irritation. It usually begins in the third decade of life, and although no race is spared, the disease tends to be more severe in darker-complexioned races, especially Asians. The syndrome has been divided into three stages. The first, or meningeal, stage is associated with headache, nausea, vomiting, fever, confusion, cranial nerve palsies, hemiparesis, and cerebrospinal fluid pleocytosis. Usually, there are few neurologic sequelae. In the second stage, ophthalmic and auditory changes predominate, including photophobia, ocular pain, visual loss, anterior or posterior uveitis, and sometimes retinal detachment, tinnitus, and dysacusis. Cutaneous lesions are dominant in the third, or convalescent, stage, occurring as the uveitis begins to subside. Common features are vitiligo, which frequently involves the eyelids and periorbital region [see Figure 4]; poliosis of the scalp, hair, eyelashes, and eyebrows; and diffuse or patchy alopecia.

Patients with malignant melanoma frequently experience a vitiligolike depigmentation surrounding melanoma lesions and at distant sites. The presence of depigmentation in melanoma patients portends a longer survival.

Laboratory findings Histologically, the predominant finding of vitiligo lesions is an absence of melanocytes in lesional skin. Light microscopy and ultrastructural studies have also revealed vacuolar degeneration of basal and parabasal keratinocytes and revealed epidermal and dermal lymphohistiocytic cell infiltrates. Immunohistochemical staining has confirmed the presence of a predominantly T cell infiltrate in vitiliginous and adjacent skin.

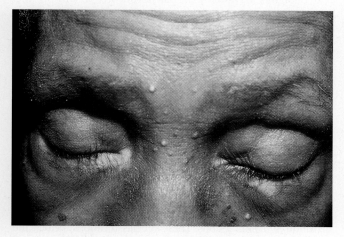

Figure 4 **A patient with Vogt-Koyanagi-Harada syndrome shows periorbital depigmentation.**

In view of the association of vitiligo with myriad other autoimmune diseases, the routine baseline evaluation of a patient should include a thorough history and physical examination. Recommended laboratory tests include a complete blood count; sedimentation rate; comprehensive metabolic panel, including liver function tests; thyroid function tests; and autoantibody tests (antinuclear antibody, thyroid peroxidase, and parietal cell antibodies).

Differential diagnosis Other disorders characterized by depigmentation may occasionally mimic vitiligo clinically. These include piebaldism, nevus depigmentosus, nevus anemicus, postinflammatory depigmentation or hypopigmentation, pityriasis alba, tinea versicolor, discoid lupus erythematosus, scleroderma, hypopigmentated mycosis fungoides, and sarcoidosis. Therefore, in some instances, a skin biopsy may be necessary to substantiate a diagnosis of vitiligo.

Treatment

Therapies for vitiligo include medical and surgical approaches for repigmentation of vitiliginous lesions. Medical therapies include topical and systemic steroids, topical and systemic PUVA, narrow-band and broad-band UVB, nutritional vitamin supplementation, oral and topical phenylalanine, and immunomodulations.[25-27] Surgical therapies are only indicated in patients with localized stable lesions and include autologous blister grafts, punch grafts, sheet grafts, and micropigmentation.[28]

Therapeutic measures should include efforts to stabilize or limit the progression of vitiligo as well as limitation of therapies to induce repigmentation of vitiliginous lesions.

Repigmentation therapies should be predicated on the age of the patient, extent of cutaneous surface involvement (severity), and activity or progression of the disease. The disease can be divided into four stages: limited (< 10% involvement), moderate (10% to 25% involvement), moderately severe (26% to 50% involvement), and severe (greater than 50% involvement) [see Table 1].

Medical treatment Mid- to high-potency steroids are indicated in patients with limited involvement. Low-potency topical steroids are usually ineffective. Topical mid- to high-potency steroids can be safely used for 2 to 3 months, then interrupted for 1 month or tapered to a low-potency preparation. Patients must be closely monitored for topical steroid side effects, which include skin atrophy, telangiectasias hypertrichosis, and acneiform eruptions.

Short courses of oral prednisone for 1 to 2 weeks or intramuscular triamcinolone acetonide injections, 40 mg/month for 2 to 3 months, are often extremely helpful in stabilizing patients with rapidly progressive vitiligo. However, prolonged use of systemic steroids is not indicated.

When compared with other medical therapies for vitiligo, topical and systemic PUVA therapy remains the mainstay for repigmenting vitiliginous lesions.[25,26] Topical photochemotherapy can be administered in office or in combination with sunlight. The choice of topical PUVA is predicated on the severity of vitiligo and lifestyle and convenience of the patient. Topical in-office PUVA is appropriate for patients with less than 20% to 25% cutaneous surface involvement. A thin coat of 0.01% to 0.1% methoxalen ointment is applied to affected areas 30 minutes before UVA exposure. For patients with less than 10% involvement, an alternative approach involves the use of 0.001% methoxalen ointment applied 30 minutes before sunlight exposure. Patients are allowed to

Table 1   Therapeutic Approaches for Vitiligo

Stages I and II disease*	Topical steroids

	Topical photochemotherapy
	   PUVA-sol
	   In-office PUVA

	Bath photochemotherapy
	Pseudocatalase/UVB

	UVB phototherapy
	   Narrow band
	   Broad band

	L-phenylalanine/UV
	Topical khellin/UVA
	Melagenina
	Calcipotriol/PUVA
	Tar emulsions
	Vitamin supplementation
	Autologous melanocyte grafting (stable lesions)
Stages III and IV disease*	Oral photochemotherapy
	Systemic steroids (oral, I.M.) (for stabilization)
	Bath photochemotherapy

	UVB phototherapy
	   Narrow band
	   Broad band

	Oral khellin/UVA
	L-phenylalanine/UV

	Immunomodulators
	   Isoprinosine
	   Levamasole

	Immunosuppressives
	   Cyclosporine
	   Cyclophosphamide
	   Nitrogen mustard

	Depigmentation (severe, recalcitrant lesions)

*Stage I, < 10% involvement; stage II, 10%–25% involvement; stage III, 26%–50% involvement; stage IV, > 50% involvement.
PUVA—psoralens plus ultraviolet A   UV—ultraviolet   UVA—ultraviolet A
UVB—ultraviolet B

expose the affected areas for 15 to 30 minutes. Oral photochemotherapy is indicated in patients with greater than 20% to 25% cutaneous surface involvement. The standard dose of 8-methoxypsoralen (8-MOP) is usually 0.3 to 0.4 mg/kg ingested 1.5 hours before UVA exposure. The treatments are administered twice weekly. Broad-spectrum sunscreen protection is essential after PUVA treatments. In addition, in light of the ocular pharmacokinetics of 8-MOP, protective UVA sunglasses should be worn indoors and outdoors for 18 to 24 hours after ingestion of 8-MOP.

Contraindications to oral PUVA treatment include cataracts, liver disease, and general photosensitivity disorders. Side effects include headaches, nausea, vomiting, xerosis, pruritus, photoaging, diffuse hyperpigmentation, and hypertrichosis. The major advantage of oral PUVA includes its effectiveness in controlling the progression of active disease and its lower frequency of blistering reactions. Oral PUVA therapy has been associated with an increase in nonmelanoma and melanoma skin cancer in patients with psoriasis. However, similar documentation has not been reported in patients with vitiligo.

Factors that portend enhanced PUVA-induced repigmentation include young age (children), patient motivation, maintenance of adequate lesional phytotoxicity, and location of lesions. Maximal repigmentation occurs on the face and neck, and minimal responses occur in the hands and feet. Overall, mean repigmentation of 60% to 65% of the affected areas can be achieved.[26]

Recent studies have reported the benefits of narrow-band and broad-band UVB phototherapy.[29] Narrow-band UVB treatment was shown to be as effective as topical PUVA with fewer side effects. The beneficial effects of pseudocatalase and calcium applied twice daily and twice-weekly UVB exposure have also been reported. The rationale for this therapy is derived from previous studies that demonstrated aberrant catalase and calcium homeostasis in patients.[30]

Preliminary open-label studies have documented stabilization and repigmentation in vitiligo patients treated with high-dose vitamin supplementation, including daily doses of ascorbic acid (1,000 mg), vitamin B_{12} (1,000 mg), and folic acid (1 to 5 mg).[25]

Abnormalities of both humoral and cell-mediated immunity have been documented in patients with vitiligo. Hence, a rational therapeutic approach involves the use of immunomodulatory drugs. The efficacy of isoprinosine therapy, cyclosporine, levamasole, and anapsos has been reported in patients with vitiligo.[25]

Monobenzylether of hydroquinone (MBEH, or monobenzone) has been used as a depigmenting agent for patients with extensive vitiligo since the 1950s. In general, MBEH causes permanent destruction of melanocytes and induces depigmentation locally and remote from the sites of application. Hence, the use of MBEH for other disorders of pigmentation is contraindicated.

Depigmentation is a viable therapeutic alternative in patients with greater than 50% cutaneous depigmentation who have demonstrated recalcitrance to repigmentation or in patients with extensive vitiligo who have no desire to undergo repigmentation therapies. The major side effects of MBEH therapy are dermatitis and pruritus, which usually respond to topical and systemic steroids. Other side effects include severe xerosis, alopecia, premature graying, and suppression of lymphoproliferative responses.

Surgical treatment   Surgical treatment is appropriate for patients with localized, stable areas of vitiligo that have been recalcitrant to medical treatment. Such approaches are contraindicated in patients with keloids or hypertrophic scars. Techniques for surgical grafting include suction blister grafts, punch grafts, sheet grafts, pure melanocyte cultures, and cocultures of melanocytes and keratinocytes. These techniques are indeed beneficial for localized lesions.

Micropigmentation is often associated with the induction of koebnerization; hence, it should be used only for treatment of mucous membrane lesions.

Complications

Patients should be screened yearly in light of the potential development of associated autoimmune diseases.

ALBINISM

Definition

Albinism is an uncommon complex congenital disorder characterized by hypopigmentation of the hair, eyes, and skin. Albinism is generally subclassified as oculocutaneous albinism (OCA) and ocular albinism (OA), in which reduction of melanin is limited to the eye.[31] Sometimes, different mutations in the same gene can cause OCA or OA.

Epidemiology

Oculocutaneous albinism has been reported by investigators in all mammalian orders and in all human ethnic groups. It is one of the most widely distributed genetic abnormalities in the animal kingdom. Human albinism has been noted throughout history. Oculocutaneous albinism is the most common inherited disorder of generalized hypopigmentation.

Etiology and Pathogenesis

Albinism may result from primary defects that are specific for the melanin synthetic pathway or from defects that are not specific for melanin synthesis. Mutations in six genes have been reported to cause OCA or OA.[32,33] They include the tyrosinase gene (OCA1), the oculocutaneous albinism gene (OCA2), the tyrosinase-related protein 1 gene (OCA3), the HPS gene (Hermansky-Pudlak syndrome), the CHS gene (Chédiak-Higashi syndrome), and the OA1 gene (X-linked ocular albinism).

Diagnosis

Clinically, the most severe disease is observed in OCA1A, oculocutaneous albinism resulting from mutations in the tyrosinase gene. It is characterized by absent tyrosinase activity, which results in complete absence of melanin in the eyes, skin, and hair. There is no improvement with age. Affected individuals have marked photophobia, nystagmus, and profound sun sensitivity because of inability to tan.

OCA1B, or yellow albinism, is less severe. Tyrosinase activity is low or absent, and pigmentation of the hair and skin improves with age. In contrast to OCA1A, pigmented freckles and lentigines develop with age.

OCA1-MP, or minimal pigment oculocutaneous albinism, is characterized by white skin and hair at birth. Iris pigment is present at birth, or it appears during the first decade of life. All reported cases have been in white persons. The tyrosinase gene mutation produces a less active enzyme.

Temperature-sensitive oculocutaneous albinism (OCA1-TS) is characterized by white skin and hair and blue eyes at birth and development of patterned pigmentation by puberty. Darker hair develops in cooler areas (extremities), and white hair is retained in warmer areas (axilla and scalp). The pattern results from a tyrosinase mutation that causes a temperature-sensitive enzyme.

OCA2, tyrosinase-positive oculocutaneous albinism, with normal tyrosinase activity, is the most common variety. The hair darkens with age, but the skin remains white. Pigmented nevi, lentigines, and freckles develop and are especially pronounced in sun-exposed areas. This type has recently been ascribed to mutation of the P gene, which encodes the tyrosinase-transporting membrane protein. The P gene is on chromosome 15q.

The secondary varieties of albinism in which the primary defect is not specific for the melanin synthetic pathway include Hermansky-Pudlak syndrome,[34] Chédiak-Higashi syndrome, Cross-McKusick-Breen syndrome, Prader-Willi syndrome, and Angelman syndrome. The autosomal recessive Hermansky-Pudlak syndrome is characterized by low to absent tyrosinase activity. The HPS gene has been mapped to chromosome 10q.[35,36] Skin and hair color varies from white to light brown. Freckles and lentigines develop with age. Iris pigment correlates with hair and skin pigmentation. Affected individuals experience a hemorrhagic diathesis secondary to a platelet storage pool deficiency. They lack storage granules, that is, sites of storage of serotonin, calcium, and adenine nucleotides. Ceroidlike deposits are present in macrophages of the bone marrow, lungs, liver, spleen, and gastrointestinal tract. Patients bruise easily and are subject to epistaxis and gingival bleeding. Pulmonary fibrosis

and granulomatous colitis develop as a consequence of the ceroid deposits.

Chédiak-Higashi syndrome consists of hypopigmentation, recurrent sinopulmonary bacterial infections, peripheral neuropathy, and giant lysosomal granules and leads to death at an early age as a result of lymphoreticular malignancies. The CHS gene locus is on chromosome 1q.[29]

Cross-McKusick-Breen syndrome includes hypopigmentation, microphthalmia, nystagmus, and severe mental and physical retardation.

Prader-Willi syndrome is a developmental syndrome characterized by mental retardation, neonatal hypotonia, and poor feeding followed by hyperphagia and obesity later in life. Short stature, hypogonadism, and inappropriate emotional behavior constitute the syndrome. Fifty percent of patients have a deletion on the long arm of chromosome 15. Patients have ocular abnormalities and skin and hair hypopigmentation consistent with oculocutaneous albinism.

Mutation of the P gene has been reported in Angelman syndrome and is also characterized by mental retardation, abnormal behavior, and hypopigmentation. The pattern of hypopigmentation is similar to that in Prader-Willi syndrome. In addition, Angelman syndrome is associated with a deletion on chromosome 15. However, in contrast to Prader-Willi syndrome, the deletion occurs on the maternal chromosome.

Treatment

The management of patients with albinism should include genetic counseling and patient education regarding the use of sunscreens and clothing for protection against ultraviolet-radiation–induced damage. Magnifiers are beneficial for ocular symptoms.

Complications

The long-term consequences of albinism are solar keratoses and basal and squamous cell carcinomas. Malignant melanoma is uncommon.

PIEBALDISM

Definition

Piebaldism is a rare autosomal dominant congenital disorder of pigmentation. It is a stable leukoderma and is characterized by patches of white skin and white hair. The affected areas are principally the frontal scalp, forehead, ventral chest, abdomen, and extremities. A white forelock occurs in 80% to 90% of patients.

Epidemiology

Although rare, piebaldism occurs in all ethnic groups worldwide. Its estimated occurrence is one in 100,000 persons. It is found with equal frequency in males and females.

Etiology and Pathogenesis

Molecular genetics studies have shown that piebaldism results from frameshift and splice junction mutations of the KIT gene, located on chromosome segment 4q12. Mutations occur in the highly conserved tyrosinase kinase domain of c-Kit. Reduced KIT function arrests the migration of melanocytes into affected hair follicles and epidermis during embryonal development.[37,38]

In general, patients with piebaldism are healthy and do not have associated systemic abnormalities. However, the disorder occasionally has been associated with heterochromia irides, men-

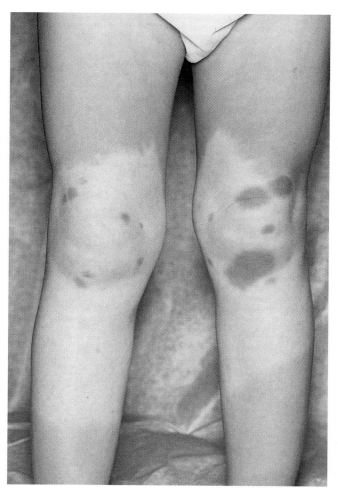

Figure 5 **A patient with piebaldism has the classic midextremity areas of depigmentation with islands of hyperpigmentation.**

tal retardation, osteopathia striata, Woolf syndrome, and Hirschsprung disease.

Diagnosis

Cutaneous depigmentation is the only manifestation of piebaldism in 10% to 20% of cases. Amelanotic macules are usually present on the ventral surface of the thorax and abdomen and extend to the back but spare the midline. Characteristic extremity lesions extend from midarm to wrist and occur on the midleg [*see Figure 5*]. White patches of the mucous membranes have also been reported. Hyperpigmented macules may appear within the areas of depigmentation.

Light and electron microscopic studies of the white macules have typically revealed an absence of melanocytes. However, melanocytes have been demonstrated in the white forelock and amelanotic skin of three patients studied.

Differential Diagnosis

Piebaldism is sometimes confused with vitiligo, but in piebaldism the leukodermic patches are both congenital and relatively static in shape and size.

Treatment

The lesions are usually stable throughout life, although some patients have reported spontaneous repigmentation. In general,

therapeutic approaches, including psoralen photochemotherapy and grafting, are unsatisfactory. Autologous melanocyte grafting procedures may offer some benefit for localized or limited areas of involvement.

IDIOPATHIC GUTTATE HYPOMELANOSIS

Definition

Idiopathic guttate hypomelanosis (IGH) is a common asymptomatic disorder characterized by hypopigmenation and depigmented polygonal macules ranging from approximately 2 mm to 8 mm in diameter.

Epidemiology

IGH appears to be a very common, benign dermatosis. It occurs in all races with a frequency ranging from 46% to 70%. It is, however, more prevalent in darker-skinned racial and ethnic groups. Macules may begin to appear during the third or fourth decade of life and gradually increase in number thereafter.

Etiology and Pathogenesis

The precise pathogenesis has not been established for IGH. Long-term sun exposure, trauma, genetic influences, and aging, with a gradual loss of melanocytes, have been implicated in the pathogenesis of this disorder.[39]

Diagnosis

The lesions are macules that are punctate to polygonal in shape, 2 to 8 mm in size, and hypopigmented to depigmented and are most commonly observed on the lower extremities. There is no atrophy or change in the overlying skin. Histologic evaluation of lesions reveals hyperkeratosis, epidermal atrophy, and diseased epidermal melanin. Melanocytes may be normal or decreased.

Differential Diagnosis

IGH must be differentiated from other hypopigmentary disorders, such as vitiligo, scleroderma, leukodermic guttate parapsoriasis, tinea versicolor, hypopigmentated sarcoidosis, pityriasis alba, chemical depigmentation, and postinflammatory hypopigmentation.

Treatment

No definitive treatment is currently available. Patients often need reassurance regarding the banality of lesions. For patients concerned about the cosmetic appearance of lesions, camouflage, intralesional steroids, and topical photochemotherapy have been used.

References

1. Grimes PE: Melasma: etiologic and therapeutic considerations. Arch Dermatol 131:1453, 1996

2. O'Brien TJ, Dyall-Smith D, Hall AP: Melasma of the forearms. Australas J Dermatol 38:35, 1997

3. Boissy RE, Nordlund JJ: Molecular basis of congenital hyperpigmentary disorders in humans: a review. Pigment Cell Res 10:12, 1997

4. Pramphongsant T: Treatment of melasma: a review with personal experience. Int J Dermatol 37:897, 1998

5. Grimes PE: The safety and efficacy of salicylic acid peels in darker-racial ethnic groups. Dermatol Surg 25:19, 1999

6. McKenzie R, Sauder DN: The role of keratinocyte cytokines in inflammation and immunity. J Invest Dermatol 95:1055, 1990

7. Kinbauer R, Kock A, Neuner P, et al: Regulation of epidermal cell interleukin production by UV light and corticosteroids. J Invest Dermatol 96:484, 1991

8. Ruiz-Maldonado R, Orozco-Covarrubias ML: Postinflammatory hypopigmentation and hyperpigmentation. Semin Cutan Med Surg 16:36, 1997

9. Granskin R, Sober AJ: Drug and heavy metal–induced hyperpigmentation. J Am Acad Dermatol 5:1, 1981

10. Lerner EA, Sober AJ: Chemical and pharmacologic agents that cause hyperpigmentation or hypopigmentation of the skin. Dermatol Clin 6:327, 1988

11. Miseg ME, Ghawan J, Stefanato CM: Imipramine-induced hyperpigmentation: four cases and a review of the literature. J Am Acad Dermatol 40:159, 1999

12. Combemale P, Faisant M, Guennoc B, et al: Erythema dyschromicum perstans: report of a new case and review of the literature. J Dermatol 25:747, 1992

13. Dominguez-Soto L, Hojya-Tomoka T, Vega-Memye E, et al: Pigmentary problems in the tropics. Dermatol Clin 12:777, 1994

14. Penagos H, Jimenez V, Fallas V, et al: Chlorethalanil: a possible cause of erythema dyschromicum perstans (ashy dermatitis). Contact Dermatitis 35:214, 1996

15. Baranda L, Torres-Alvarez B, Cortes-Franco R, et al: Involvement of cell adhesion and activation molecules in the pathogenesis of erythema dyschromicum perstans (ashy dermatitis). Arch Dermatol 133:32, 1997

16. Lee MP, Stiller SA, McClain JL, et al: Confluent and reticulated papillomatosis: response to high-dose oral isotretinoin therapy and reassessment of epidemiologic data. J Am Acad Dermatol 31:327, 1994

17. Purg L, de Moragas JM: Confluent and reticulated papillomatosis of Gougerot and Carteaud: minocycline deserves trial before etritinate. Arch Dermatol 131:109, 1995

18. Angeli-Besson C, Koeppel MC, Jacquart SP, et al: Confluent and reticulated papillomatosis (Gougerot-Carteaud) treated with tetracycline. Int J Dermatol 34:567, 1995

19. Kim YC, Davis MD, Schanbacher CF, et al: Dowling-Degos disease (reticulate pigmented anomaly of the flexures): a clinical and histopathologic study of six cases. J Am Acad Dermatol 40:462, 1999

20. Lestringant GG, Masouye I, Frossard PM, et al: Co-existence of leukoderma with features of Dowling-Degos disease reticulate acropigmentation kitamura spectrum in five unrelated patients 105:337, 1997

21. Kovacs SO: Vitiligo. J Am Acad Dermatol 38:647, 1998

22. Boissy R, Le Poole C: Vitiligo. Semin Cutan Med Surg 16:3, 1997

23. Baharav E, Merimski O, Shoenfeld Y, et al: Tyrosinase as an autoantigen in patients with vitiligo. Clin Exp Immunol 105:84, 1996

24. Grimes PE, Sevall S, Vojdani A: Cytomegalovirus DNA identified in skin biopsy specimens of patients with vitiligo. J Am Acad Dermatol 35:21, 1996

25. Grimes PE: Therapies for vitiligo. Drug Therapy in Dermatology. Millikan L, Ed. New York: Marcel Dekker (in press)

26. Grimes PE: Psoralen photochemotherapy for vitiligo. Clin Dermatol 15:921, 1997

27. Jimbow K: Vitiligo: therapeutic advances. Dermatol Clin 16:399, 1998

28. Falabella R: Surgical therapies for vitiligo. Clin Dermatol 15:927, 1997

29. Westerhof W, Nievweboer-Krobotova L: Treatment of vitiligo with UV-B radiations topical psoralen plus UV-A. Arch Dermatol 133:1525, 1997

30. Schallreuter KU, Wood JM, Lemke KR, et al: Treatment of vitiligo with a topical application of pseudocatalase and calcium in combination with short-term UV-B exposure: a case study of 33 patients. Dermatology 196:223, 1995

31. Lyle WM, Sangsker JOS, Williams TD: Albinism: an update and review of the literature. J Am Opt Assoc 68:623, 1997

32. Oetting WS, King RA: Molecular basis of albinism: mutations and polymorphism or pigmentation genes associated with albinism. Hum Mutat 13:99, 1999

33. Orlow SJ: Albinism: an update. Sem Cut Med Surg 16:24, 1997

34. Shotelersak V, Gahl WA: Hermansky-Pudlak syndrome: models for intracellular vesicle formulation. Molec Gen Metab 65:85, 1998

35. Taylor SI, Arioglu E: Syndromes associated with insulin resistance and acanthosis nigricans. J Basic Clin Physiol Pharmacol 9:419, 1998

36. Schwartz RA: Acanthosis nigricans. J Am Acad Dermatol 31:18, 1994

37. Spritz RA: Piebaldism, Waardenburg syndrome and related disorders of melanocyte development. Sem Cut Med Surg 16:15, 1997

38. Spritz RA, Hearing VJ: Genetic disorders or pigmentation. Adv Hum Genet 22:1, 1994

39. Falabella R: Idiopathic guttate hypomelanosis (review). Dermatol Clin 6:241, 1988

ENDOCRINOLOGY AND METABOLISM

45 Pituitary

Daniel D. Federman, M.D.

Neuroendocrinology

The principal organs of communication for response to stressful exogenous and endogenous stimuli, disease processes, and surgery are the nervous and endocrine systems. Neural responses to stress involve intercellular communication over minuscule distances and use chemical transmitters; the response time and the period before another response can occur (latency) are each measured in fractions of a second. In contrast, endocrine responses involve hormones that circulate in the blood from one site to another. The latency is measured in minutes or hours. In addition, hormonal adaptations can continue for as long as a day or a month.

The hypothalamic-pituitary axis provides a convergence of neural and hormonal adaptive capacities. The neurons of the hypothalamus have rich synaptic connections with the central nervous system, allowing for aminergic, peptidergic, and opioid influences. In addition, the hypothalamus is outside the blood-brain barrier and therefore can sense and respond to circulating levels of glucose, cortisol, sodium, and other substances. The hypothalamus is also the site of major homeostatic controls, including those for hunger, thirst, osmolarity, blood pressure, temperature, and respiration. Finally, the hypothalamus is the source of stimulatory and inhibitory humoral communication with the anterior pituitary [*see Figure 1*]. Small peptides produced in hypothalamic neurons enter fenestrated capillaries, descend through the hypophyseal portal veins, and then diffuse through additional fenestrated capillaries to reach individual cells of the anterior pituitary.[1]

The principal hypophysiotropic hormones of the hypothalamus have been identified [*see Table 1*]; the clinical significance, diagnostic use, and therapeutic applications of each are discussed in this chapter. Certain general statements about the control of the hypothalamic-pituitary axis are pertinent to this discussion. First, hypothalamic and pituitary secretion is pulsatile rather than tonic [*see Figure 2*]; in certain cases, sampling every 2 to 3 minutes may be required to demonstrate the pulses.[2] These pulses are superimposed on broader biologic rhythms, such as the circadian release of adrenocorticotropic hormone (ACTH), the sleep-entrained release of growth hormone (GH) and prolactin (PRL), and the monthly cycle of gonadotropins in females. Second, the hypothalamus is a rich source of the biogenic amines dopamine, epinephrine, norepinephrine, and serotonin, each of which modulates pituitary rhythms. Endogenous opioids are also important in regulating pituitary function: endorphins promote the release of GH, thyrotropin (thyroid-stimulating hormone, or TSH), and PRL and suppress the release of follicle-stimulating hormone (FSH), luteinizing hormone (LH), and ACTH. Hypothalamic connections with other brain centers can also provide a conduit for pituitary regulation (e.g., the hippocampus-amygdala appears to inhibit hypothalamic control of ACTH and adrenal function).

The physiology and specific pathophysiology of pituitary tropic hormones (i.e., FSH, LH, ACTH, and TSH) are discussed in chapters on the thyroid, testis, ovary, and adrenal [*see Chapters 46 through 51*]. This chapter addresses broader disorders of the anterior pituitary, specific disorders of the nontropic hormones GH and PRL, and syndromes that affect posterior pituitary and general endocrine function.

The use of synthetic gonadotropin-releasing hormone (GnRH) agonists and antagonists has revolutionized the practice of re-productive endocrinology and related disorders. These applications are referenced here for convenience but discussed in the relevant chapters [*see Chapter 50*].[3]

The Anterior Pituitary

OVERPRODUCTION OF PITUITARY TROPIC HORMONES

Overproduction of pituitary tropic hormones is usually perceived as disease of the target gland.[4] For example, hypersecretion of ACTH by a pituitary adenoma is the most frequent cause of Cushing's syndrome.[5,6] The tumor is generally a microadenoma (< 10 mm in diameter) and does not produce local symptoms; transsphenoidal surgery, enhanced by laser, endoscopic, and radiofrequency techniques, is the treatment of choice [*see Chapter 49*].[7] Hypersecretion of the other pituitary tropic hormones seldom occurs. Tumors secreting excess gonadotropins or gonadotropin fragments occur most often in middle-aged men who have undergone normal sexual development.[8] Some of these patients exhibit secondary hypogonadism, and most have large tumors that cause visual-field defects. Immediate transsphenoidal surgery can restore or improve vision and provide time for definitive treatment. TSH-producing pituitary adenomas cause a hyperthyroid syndrome without the autoimmune features of Graves' disease. Mechanical features of a pituitary tumor may be seen [*see Chapter 46*].

UNDERPRODUCTION OF PITUITARY TROPIC HORMONES

Monotropic Pituitary Hormone Deficiency

Monotropic pituitary hormone deficiency is an uncommon but well-defined cause of hypofunction of a target gland. The resulting syndromes are described in chapters on the gonads, thyroid, and adrenal, but a few additional comments may be appropriate here.

Isolated gonadotropin deficiency usually implies inadequate secretion of both FSH and LH by the anterior pituitary secondary to congenital deficiency of the hypothalamic-releasing hormone. Affected persons do not undergo puberty; all aspects of gonadal function are deficient, and plasma gonadotropin levels are low or low normal, thus distinguishing the condition from primary gonadal failure.[9,10]

Isolated lack of TSH can be an acquired condition; it presents as typical hypothyroidism except for the absence of a goiter and of antithyroid antibodies. Patients also have low-normal serum TSH concentration, which may increase somewhat but does not rise excessively after administration of thyrotropin-releasing hormone (TRH).

The diagnosis of monotropic ACTH deficiency is remarkably elusive. Aldosterone function is affected late in the course, if at all; thus, the syndrome is one of selective glucocorticoid deficiency unaccompanied by hyperpigmentation or volume deficiency. Patients typically show a failure to thrive characterized by diminished appetite, lack of pep or ambition, proneness to water intoxication and hyponatremia, and generalized asthenia. Symptomatic differentiation of the syndrome from depression or a chronic organic illness such as cancer or anemia is almost impossible. Most patients with selective ACTH deficiency are diagnosed only after they are found to be hyponatremic or unable to

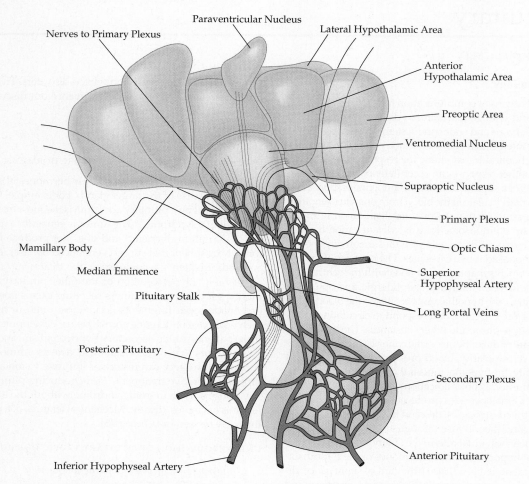

Figure 1 **The anterior pituitary and the hypothalamus are connected by the hypophyseal portal vasculature. Releasing or inhibiting hormones secreted by hypothalamic neurons enter the primary plexus of the hypophyseal portal vasculature. They flow down the long portal veins in the pituitary stalk to the secondary plexus, a capillary network that enmeshes the cells of the anterior pituitary. The anterior pituitary cells secrete their hormones in response to the releasing hormones. Because neither the hypothalamus nor the anterior pituitary is isolated by the blood-brain barrier, feedback signals have direct access to both sites of regulation. The posterior pituitary is made up of the terminal portions of neurons whose origin is the hypothalamus.**

respond normally to stress. The plasma cortisol level is low (i.e., < 4.5 μg/dl); it does not rise after insulin-induced hypoglycemia but increases after ACTH is infused over several days.

Panhypopituitarism

Panhypopituitarism is more common than any of the monotropic deficiencies.[11] Generalized pituitary hypofunction usually results from destruction of the pituitary by one of several causes. The pituitary is the only endocrine gland for which destruction by tumor is a significant cause of hypofunction; compression of the gland against the bony confines of the sella turcica (pituitary fossa) is the proximate mechanism. The primary pituitary tumor most often responsible is the chromophobe adenoma. Craniopharyngioma, a tumor of neighboring structures, is another cause of pituitary hypofunction. It often manifests in childhood but can first appear in adulthood, with pituitary hypofunction or visual loss as the presenting defect. Metastatic tumor, often from the breast or lung, also occasionally produces hypofunction.

The term Sheehan's syndrome classically referred to hypopituitarism secondary to peripartum uterine hemorrhagic shock.[12] The pituitary necrosis was attributed to infarction induced by collapse of the superior hypophyseal artery. As obstetric care im-

proves, fewer such florid cases are seen. Occasionally, however, a subtle variant of Sheehan's syndrome is encountered in patients who develop anemia late in pregnancy and who do not receive transfusions. Inability to nurse, failure of menses to resume, fatigue, and weakness are the usual presenting features. Computed tomographic scanning can be diagnostic in showing an empty sella of normal size; magnetic resonance imaging is probably more sensitive.

The empty sella syndrome remains an enigmatic variant of pituitary disease.[13] An enlarged pituitary fossa found on x-ray is usually interpreted as a pituitary neoplasm; in some patients, however, the apparent enlargement is principally an extension of the subarachnoid cistern into the sella turcica. The pathogenesis of the lesion is unclear. Patients in whom the initial event is the projection of the subarachnoid space into the sella are said to have primary empty sella syndrome. In these patients, pituitary function is usually normal, although PRL or ACTH hypersecretion may be present if there is a coexisting microadenoma. Secondary empty sella syndrome is a disorder in which the pituitary has become smaller as a result of infarction, surgery, irradiation, or other mechanism. Partial or complete anterior pituitary deficiency is common in patients with secondary empty sella. Pneu-

Table 1 Hypothalamic and Related Pituitary Hormones

Hypothalamic Hormones	Pituitary Hormones
Growth hormone–releasing hormone (GHRH)	Growth hormone (GH)
Growth hormone release–inhibiting hormone (somatostatin)	GH
Prolactin release inhibitory factor (dopamine)	Prolactin (PRL)
Gonadotropin-releasing hormone (GnRH)	Follicle-stimulating hormone (FSH) Luteinizing hormone (LH)
Corticotropin-releasing hormone (CRH) Vasopressin (arginine vasopressin, or AVP; antidiuretic hormone, or ADH)	Adrenocorticotropic hormone (ACTH; corticotropin)
Thyrotropin-releasing hormone (TRH)	Thyrotropin (thyroid-stimulating hormone, or TSH)

moencephalography used to be required for diagnosis, but CT scanning with metrizamide provides definitive answers with less morbidity, and MRI is probably superior to CT.

Destruction of pituitary tissue by granuloma or infection is an infrequent problem but one worth remembering in a patient who has either unexplained hypopituitarism or known disseminated granulomatous disease. Indeed, the combination of partial hypopituitarism and visual defects caused by sarcoidosis involving the optic nerves can suggest a pituitary tumor. In such cases, however, the sella is usually not enlarged, field defects are spotty (unlike those produced by chiasmatic compression), and functional testing suggests that hypopituitarism is caused by hypothalamic deficiency.

Pituitary insufficiency secondary to radiotherapy of neighboring structures is being seen more frequently.[14,15] The larger doses of x-rays now in use, the longer survival of irradiated patients, and the use of subtle tests of pituitary reserve all serve to increase the number of such patients detected. Current understanding indicates that the defect is more often hypothalamic than pituitary.[16] Pituitary necrosis secondary to bleeding within a tumor can produce hormone insufficiency. Hypopituitarism was once considered to be a permanent condition, but hormone secretion may resume after shrinkage of macroprolactinomas by drugs[17] and after transsphenoidal decompression of tumors or hemorrhagic infarction of the pituitary.

Clinical features The clinical features of panhypopituitarism are highly variable; they may include both mechanical and hormonal changes. Mechanical changes are secondary to enlargement of a tumor beyond the sella; symptoms are headache and disturbances in vision, such as blurring, decreased acuity, and field defects. The earliest defect is typically a bitemporal upper quadrant loss, which is best detected by examination with a flashing red light. Because the macula is often spared, patients can have far-advanced loss of visual field without realizing it.

The endocrine features of panhypopituitarism depend on the extent of the hormone deficiency, the rate at which the deficiency develops, the age of the person, and the presence or absence of associated disease. GH and the gonadotropins are about equally sensitive to partial pituitary impairment; when the syndrome de-

velops gradually, production of these hormones is affected first. The features of growth hormone deficiency (GHD) are impaired well-being, reduced lean body mass and bone density, increased abdominal fat, thin dry skin, and diminished muscle strength.[18,19] In menstruating women, amenorrhea is the earliest sign of gonadotropin deficiency; in men, the earliest symptom is erectile dysfunction. In postmenopausal women, gonadotropin deficiency produces no symptoms, and detection is usually delayed. Apathy and lack of concern over diminishing well-being, typical of hypopituitary patients, delay definitive diagnosis even further.

In contrast to the early appearance of gonadotropin deficiency, the development of TSH and ACTH deficiencies may be long delayed. When these deficiencies supervene, features of thyroid and

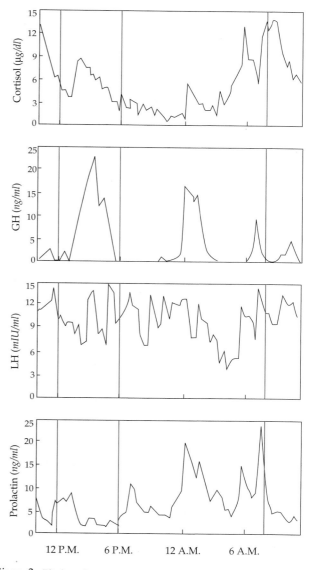

Figure 2 Pituitary hormone secretion is pulsatile rather than sustained and is closely dependent on biologic rhythms. This feature is demonstrated by the secretion of anterior pituitary hormones over 24 hours in a 21-year-old woman early in the menstrual cycle. Cortisol levels reflect the pulsatile secretion of adrenocorticotropic hormone (ACTH), which reaches a peak at 6:00 A.M., when the normal diurnal rhythm is approaching its apex. Cortisol-ACTH, growth hormone (GH), and prolactin all have sleep-related secretion patterns. This correlation with sleep is true of luteinizing hormone (LH) secretion during puberty but not in adulthood.[80]

glucocorticoid deficiencies appear in various patterns. Mistaken attribution of such symptoms to depression or old age is common.

The diagnosis of hypopituitarism in the elderly is particularly challenging because nonspecific symptoms, such as fatigue, lack of ambition, weakness, and pallor, may be the only symptoms noted until frank hypothyroidism or hyponatremia develops.[20]

Laboratory findings Laboratory confirmation of suspected panhypopituitarism has been greatly simplified by the introduction of sensitive assays for peptide hormones. The general diagnostic approach is first to demonstrate target gland deficiency and then to measure the relevant pituitary hormone. To prove gonadotropin deficiency in men, plasma testosterone is measured. When the testosterone level is low, pituitary LH and FSH levels are determined. Low values for LH and FSH confirm a central origin of the defect. In women of reproductive age, amenorrhea, an immature vaginal cytology, and the failure to bleed after administration of synthetic progestin [*see Chapter 51*] reflect estrogen deficiency; a normal or low FSH level then points to pituitary deficiency. TSH deficiency is demonstrated by a low thyroxine value and then a low TSH level. One would think that TRH administration could then differentiate hypothalamic from pituitary TSH deficiency, but this approach has yielded disappointing results.

ACTH deficiency is often more subtle than the deficiencies discussed above, and therefore, diagnosis of this disorder usually requires provocative testing. A fasting morning cortisol level less than 5 μg/dl is strong evidence of ACTH deficiency, especially when the ACTH level is low or normal. However, when suspicion is high and the cortisol level is not low, provocative testing is needed. Metyrapone, an inhibitor of adrenal 11β-hydroxylase, can be used for this purpose [*see Figure 3*]. A single oral dose of 3 g is given at midnight, and the plasma cortisol and 11-deoxycortisol levels are measured the next morning. If both hormone levels are low, the patient has ACTH deficiency; if cortisol is low and 11-deoxycortisol is greater than 10 μg/dl, the patient has normal pituitary reserve. Another approach to testing ACTH response is the administration of insulin to induce hypoglycemia. After a standard intravenous dose of 0.1 U/kg, the blood glucose falls to less than half the control value; if the hypothalamic-pituitary-adrenal system is intact, the plasma cortisol level will double in response to the hypoglycemia. If the cortisol level does not rise in response to hypoglycemia but does rise after prolonged ACTH infusion (40 units I.V. over an 8-hour period on each of 2 consecutive days), the diagnosis of ACTH deficiency is confirmed. A simpler test uses the synthetic ACTH, cosyntropin. A 0.25 mg dose is given intravenously; the normal response is a rise in the level of plasma cortisol to more than 18 mg/dl. This test works because an adrenal gland that has been chronically deprived of ACTH will not respond promptly to a single burst of ACTH.

Insulin-induced hypoglycemia is also the gold standard for detecting GHD, but it is not used in patients with known heart disease or in patients older than 60 years.[21] Arginine-stimulated GH measurements can be used, but a sophisticated endocrine laboratory is needed to distinguish hypopituitary GHD from the sluggish GH response of the elderly. One acceptable approach is to estimate the likelihood of GHD on the basis of deficiency of other pituitary hormones. If one hormone, usually gonadotropin, is missing, the likelihood of GHD is 55%. If all three other hormones are deficient, this rises to over 90%. The availability of purified or synthetic hypothalamic-releasing hormones provides a sensitive and simplified diagnostic test of pituitary reserve. An intravenous bolus of one or more of the releasing hormones is given, and the

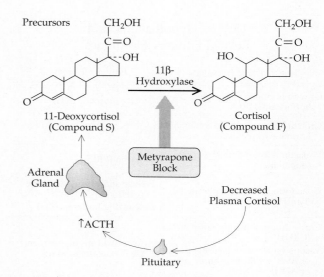

Figure 3 **Because it blocks cortisol synthesis, metyrapone can be used to test ACTH reserve. Normally, a drop in plasma cortisol stimulates ACTH release from the pituitary. ACTH activates adrenal production of cortisol precursors such as 11-deoxycortisol (compound S), which, through the action of the enzyme 11β-hydroxylase, is converted into cortisol (compound F). Rising levels of cortisol serve to shut down ACTH production. Metyrapone, however, blocks the action of 11β-hydroxylase, so that the cortisol levels remain low. Thus, if pituitary ACTH reserve is intact, the plasma compound S level should rise to a value greater than 10 μg/dl.**

corresponding pituitary hormone or hormones are measured at appropriate intervals [*see Table 2*]. The releasing hormones are well tolerated, except for occasional slight nausea and flushing.

Therapy Hypopituitary patients need permanent, carefully individualized replacement therapy. Treatment should follow physiologic principles as closely as possible, using doses and timing that mimic the natural patterns of secretion. The target-gland hormones are preferable to the pituitary hormones because parenterally administered pituitary hormones are inconvenient, expensive, and antigenic. In patients with partial panhypopituitarism, smaller doses of thyroid and hydrocortisone than those used for primary hypothyroidism or hypoadrenalism are often adequate.

Adrenal replacement can be achieved with oral hydrocortisone. Patients who have shown evidence of hypopituitarism for more than 1 year should be started at low dosages, perhaps 5 mg/day, unless there is some urgency. Higher initial dosages occasionally induce hypomanic behavior. In patients who are only mildly deficient, 10 mg of hydrocortisone twice daily is a reasonable initial regimen. The morning dose can be increased to 15

Table 2 Typical Protocol for Testing Pituitary Response

Amount of Releasing Hormone	Normal Response
100 μg GHRH	GH level increases by 10–20 ng/ml
50 μg CRH	Cortisol level at least doubles
500 μg TRH	TSH level increases by 7–12 μU/ml
200 μg GnRH	FSH level increases by onefold to twofold LH level increases by more than twofold

mg when needed to achieve full well-being. The dose should be abruptly increased at times of acute stress, as in the patient with primary adrenal insufficiency. Patients with secondary adrenal insufficiency generally do not need mineralocorticoid replacement, but such therapy should be given when hyponatremia or postural hypotension persists despite hydrocortisone replacement.

Thyroxine is the appropriate remedy for thyroid deficiency. I usually begin with 0.05 mg/day, unless the patient is older than 60 years or has underlying heart disease, in which case 0.025 mg/day is safer. I raise the dosage by 0.025 mg/day every month until a level of 0.075 to 0.150 mg/day is attained.

For men, testosterone enanthate in a dosage of 300 mg every 3 weeks provides full replacement. Again, for patients who have been hypogonadal for more than 2 years, it is wise to begin with one third the full replacement dose. This approach should avoid the abrupt increase in aggressiveness and libido and the frightening sexual fantasies that sometimes occur when full replacement is started abruptly.[22]

For women younger than 50 years, I use conjugated estrogen, 1.25 mg/day for the first 25 days of each calendar month, and a progestin such as medroxyprogesterone acetate on days 16 to 25. For those older than 50 years, 0.625 mg/day of conjugated estrogen and the progestin should be adequate. As with other postmenopausal women, continuous low-dose estrogen and progestin can be used to avoid menses. For patients of reproductive age who desire fertility, pulsatile GnRH therapy can be tried to induce spermatogenesis or ovulation when the patient's basic problem is hypothalamic. If the hypopituitarism is caused by pituitary destruction, sequential treatment with FSH and LH is available.

The unlimited availability of recombinant GH has introduced a new era for GH-deficient hypopituitary patients. Regular replacement leads to increased lean body mass, decreased adiposity, restoration of fluid volume, improved muscle mass and strength, and, after 1 to 2 years, increased bone mineral density. Many patients experience an impressive psychological benefit as well. Whether GH treatment reverses the higher mortality of hypopituitary patients is not known, nor is it clear how late in life treatment should be continued.[23,24]

Growth hormone supplementation in older persons with an age-related borderline hormone deficiency, in an attempt to retard involutional changes, is even more debatable. A few studies have suggested improved strength and well-being, but much more information is needed about benefits and risks. On the basis of current knowledge, there is little justification for prescribing the hormone for persons who are not clearly GH deficient. Another factor to be considered is the high cost of growth hormone therapy, which averages $10,000 to $20,000 a year for each patient.[25]

PITUITARY TUMORS AND THE ENLARGED SELLA

Enlargement of the sella turcica is often discovered incidentally on a skull radiograph taken for another purpose—for example, after head trauma or during evaluation of the sinuses. Occasionally, the enlargement is caused by an empty sella, but the most common cause of an enlarged sella is a benign neoplasm.

Pituitary tumors vary in size from microadenomas of 1 or 2 mm to massive lesions. Limited evidence indicates that these tumors are clonal in origin—that is, they arise from a single cell.[26] The smallest tumors produce no so-called neighborhood symptoms but rather announce themselves through hormonal syndromes, such as hyperprolactinemic amenorrhea and Cushing's syndrome. In contrast, tumors that produce no functional hormones and are therefore discovered when they produce local

symptoms are usually macroadenomas (> 10 mm in diameter) that in many cases have extended well beyond the sella; such tumors regularly compromise visual fields and acuity and can affect other brain sites. Some of these large tumors produce hormone fragments, especially the α or β chain of the glycoprotein hormones FSH, LH, or TSH [see Figure 4]. These fragments are demonstrated by immunostaining of tumor tissue, and they may also be found in the circulation. A sensitive monoclonal antibody–based assay has detected α-subunit hypersecretion in about one quarter of clinically nonfunctioning tumors. About 30% of macroadenomas secrete neither hormones nor hormone fragments and are known as null tumors.

The endocrine impact of a macroadenoma should be evaluated by the methods described above for assessment of hypopituitarism; a serum prolactin level is crucial.

It is less clear how one should approach a microadenoma discovered incidentally by MRI done for another reason. About 10% to 15% of pituitaries show a microadenoma at autopsy; immunostaining suggests that many of these microadenomas contain prolactin. If the person has no symptoms and if menstrual or erectile function is normal, the most cost-effective workup may be a single assay for serum prolactin level.[27] Identifying a presymptomatic acromegaly or Cushing's syndrome is both extraordinarily unlikely and of no proven benefit.

MRI is the most sensitive method for evaluation of the sella, pituitary, and hypothalamus, but CT scanning with contrast medium is also satisfactory.

The appropriate therapy for pituitary tumors depends on the results of the endocrine, radiologic, and neuro-ophthalmologic evaluation. Secreting tumors require treatment, but nonsecreting microadenomas can be left alone. Macroadenomas require a judicious combination of transsphenoidal (occasionally, transfrontal) surgery and radiotherapy.[28,29] Hypopituitarism, discovered before or after treatment, should be managed with hormone replacement therapy. In some patients, hypopituitarism detected preoperatively is improved or corrected by transsphenoidal resection.[30]

The most urgent complication of pituitary tumors is pituitary apoplexy. In some patients with large tumors, hemorrhage and necrosis occur suddenly and create a neurosurgical emergency. The clinical findings are headache, obtundation, ophthalmoplegia and loss of vision, and a bloody cerebrospinal fluid. CT scanning or MRI has greatly simplified the diagnosis, and emergency hydrocortisone therapy provides time for neurosurgical intervention.[31] A subacute apoplexy, in which symptoms are milder

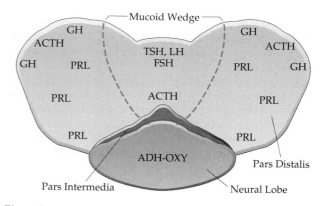

Figure 4 The distribution of hormone-secreting cells within the pituitary gland indicates where tumors of the cells will occur. (ADH-OXY—antidiuretic hormone and oxytocin)

or absent, can be confirmed by MRI. Hypopituitarism can occur as a consequence of bleeding and necrosis in tumors. Only the adrenal deficiency requires prompt therapy; the other hormonal states can be evaluated after emergency care is rendered.[32,33]

GROWTH HORMONE

Growth hormone, a protein composed of 191 amino acids, is secreted by the somatotropes of the anterior pituitary. Despite its name, GH does not directly promote growth; rather, it acts by stimulating hepatic generation of somatomedin C (also known as insulinlike growth factor–1, or IGF-1), one of many growth factors. IGF-1 enters the circulation and binds to one of two receptors; the membrane-bound IGF-1 receptor is very similar to the insulin receptor. In some tissues, GH binds directly to a membrane-associated receptor.[34] It is not yet clear exactly which GH effects are caused by which receptor.

The plasma level of GH is regulated principally by the opposing effects of two neuropeptides that are produced in the hypothalamus and reach the pituitary by the portal circulation.[35] The neuropeptide growth hormone–releasing hormone (GHRH) stimulates the pulsatile release of GH by the pituitary, whereas somatostatin inhibits GH secretion. The combination of pulsatile secretion, a half-life of 20 minutes, and the opposing secretory controls results in highly variable plasma levels of GH. Furthermore, in both children and adults, GH is secreted in response to a falling blood glucose level, amino acid ingestion, exercise, sleep, stress, and many other factors, including alpha-adrenergic stimuli such as levodopa. GH secretion is suppressed by an elevated blood glucose level and by beta-adrenergic stimuli.

Several times each day, the normal person's plasma GH varies from undetectable to a value typical of acromegaly. Because of this variability, random GH determinations are not clinically definitive. Provocative and suppressive tests are needed.

Acromegaly

Growth hormone excess produces acromegaly in adults and gigantism in children.[36] The most frequent cause of GH excess is a pituitary adenoma. By the time acromegaly is clinically recognized, most patients have an enlarged sella and a macroadenoma; as a result, suprasellar extension is common. One mechanism of adenoma formation, found in 30% to 40% of patients with acromegaly, is a somatic mutation of the α_S gene, which encodes the α chain of a membrane-bound regulatory G protein (G_S). This protein couples cell surface receptors to stimulation of second messengers within the cell. The trimeric G protein moves between guanosine diphosphate (GDP), which is inactive, and guanosine triphosphate (GTP), which is active. Several mutations in the α_S gene result in inhibition of the hydrolysis of GTP to GDP; thus, the G_S protein becomes constitutively active, and the cell secretes GH continuously.

A second source of GH excess is pathologic stimulation by GHRH derived either from the hypothalamus (eutopic) or from tumors elsewhere in the body (ectopic). GHRH was first isolated from a bronchial carcinoid and then from a pancreatic tumor, and it has since been found in many other tumors. These tumors are usually benign foregut lesions and are especially frequent in the lungs and pancreas.

Diagnosis The signs and symptoms of acromegaly are secondary to parasellar manifestations and GH excess [*see Table 3*]. Perhaps the most common combination of symptoms is sweating, headache, and weakness or fatigue. Unexplained swelling of the feet and hands, gradual acral enlargement, thickening of the lips and tongue, and unpleasant body odor are additional troublesome features. The diagnosis is often delayed because the patient, family, and regular physician are unlikely to notice gradual alterations in appearance. Thus, it is usually a distant relative or new doctor who is struck by a change in the patient's facial appearance. Once the diagnosis has been considered, the following may help in recognizing acromegaly: coarsened features, a profusion of skin tags (fibroma molluscum), thickness and oiliness of the skin, prominent frontal bossing, spreading of the teeth and bite, a history of new snoring or sleep apnea,[37] and a peculiar huskiness of the voice. Comparison of old and recent photographs can be invaluable, as it is in myxedema and Cushing's syndrome.

The essential hormonal feature of acromegaly is absence of the normal suppressibility of GH by glucose. Throughout the day, the normal person[38,39] intermittently has extremely low GH levels after glucose ingestion. The patient with acromegaly loses this responsiveness to glucose and releases GH at a level that is always higher than the minimum reached by a healthy person. This distinction is important. The patient with acromegaly need not produce vast amounts of GH; indeed, the plasma GH level may be no higher than that reached by a normal person after exercise or during a preprandial drop in the blood glucose level, but the GH level does not fall after glucose ingestion. One need only measure the GH level 1 or 2 hours after the patient has ingested 75 to 100 g of glucose. When the value is greater than 3 ng/ml, acromegaly should be strongly suspected, and confirmatory and then definitive testing should be undertaken. The postglucose value may be above 2 ng/ml in adolescents and in patients with chronic liver disease, uremia, or anorexia nervosa, but these conditions are easy to diagnose.

Assay of the level of IGF-1, which correlates better than GH levels with the clinical activity of acromegaly, is a supplementary or

Table 3 Frequency of
Manifestations of Acromegaly[82]

Manifestation	Frequency (%)
Parasellar	
Enlarged sella	93
Headache	85
Visual impairment	62
Rhinorrhea	15
Uncinate epileptic seizures	7
Papilledema	3
Pituitary apoplexy	Rare
Secondary to growth hormone excess	
Acral growth	100
Soft tissue growth	100
Hypermetabolism	70
Hyperhidrosis	60
Hypertrichosis	53
Prognathism	Common
Arthritic complaints	Common
Osteoporosis	Common
Visceromegaly	Common
Hyperpigmentation	40
Weight gain	39
Fibroma molluscum	27
Goiter	25
Impaired glucose tolerance	25
Clinical diabetes mellitus	12

alternative method for confirming the diagnosis. Indeed, in many centers, this test is the preferred initial screening approach. Normal values vary with age and with different laboratory methods. Thus, it is mandatory to interpret the IGF-1 level accordingly.[40]

Serum prolactin should be measured in all patients with acromegaly. The level is elevated in about one third of patients, most often because of secretion from the adenoma. In the case of some large macroadenomas with major suprasellar extension, however, the prolactin level can be elevated because of compression of the pituitary stalk, which leads to interference with prolactin inhibition by dopamine.

Therapy I believe that all patients with screening tests suggestive of acromegaly should be referred for specialized endocrine consultation. Initial therapy for most patients is transsphenoidal surgery of the pituitary, a highly specialized but often not curative procedure. Subsequent treatment may include pituitary irradiation, bromocriptine, or the somatostatin analogue octreotide. Most clinicians strive for complete return of GH levels to under 2 ng/ml to minimize the morbidity and mortality of GH excess. However, the proper therapy, monitoring of side effects, and even the laboratory confirmation of complete control are highly debatable topics.[41-43]

Growth Hormone and Aging

The availability of recombinant human GH has opened an entirely new area of endocrinology—the possible treatment of non–GH-deficient adults. IGF-1 levels are lower in older persons than in younger persons, and insulin-induced GH release is lower as well,[44] which raises several questions. When should the gradually declining levels of GH in older adults be considered GH deficiency?[45] Whether or not there is pathologic deficiency, could the lower levels be contributing to the decrease in lean body mass, muscle, and bone in the elderly? Could GH therapy offset these changes without inducing deleterious side effects?[46,47] Several short-term studies have shown a significant anabolic effect of GH therapy, but there are few data on long-range effects on the cardiovascular system or on the predisposition to cancer, which are of grave concern in the elderly.

PROLACTIN

Prolactin is the second anterior pituitary hormone that acts directly on target tissues rather than as a tropic hormone. Although prolactin plays many physiologic roles in other animals, its only known function in humans is postpartum stimulation of milk production. It is, however, present in males and nonpregnant females. In addition, bursts of prolactin release occur in response to sleep, stress, and sundry stimuli. Unlike other pituitary hormones, prolactin is mainly regulated by tonic inhibition rather than by intermittent stimulation. Its principal inhibitor is dopamine. Prolactin enhances dopamine secretion and thus inhibits its own secretion. Other known physiologic inhibitors are somatostatin and triiodothyronine (T_3). Prolactin release is stimulated by serotonin, acetylcholine, opiates, estrogens, TRH, and angiotensin II, among other agents, but exactly which of these, if any, is physiologically important is not known.

Prolactin secretion rises during pregnancy, reaching levels as high as 20 to 30 times normal at term. When estrogen levels, which also rise dramatically during pregnancy, begin to fall, lactation becomes possible; as nursing continues, basal levels of prolactin fall toward nonpregnant levels. Although suckling stimulates prolactin release, lactation can continue at normal resting levels of prolactin. Similarly, basal prolactin levels are normal in certain patients with galactorrhea; whether levels were formerly elevated in such cases is not known.

Disorders of Prolactin Secretion

Hypoprolactinemia occurs in Sheehan's syndrome and in other types of panhypopituitarism. Baseline prolactin measurements may not reliably differentiate low from low-normal values, but serum prolactin does not rise after TRH stimulation in affected patients.

Hyperprolactinemia is a much more common problem than prolactin deficiency.[48] The principal direct symptom of prolactin excess is galactorrhea, or nonpuerperal lactation. Lactation may be spontaneous, or it may be detected by gentle compression of the nipple. The correlation between elevated prolactin levels and lactation is poor: many patients have elevated prolactin levels without lactation, and significant lactation can persist without hyperprolactinemia.

Indirect consequences of hyperprolactinemia are much more common presenting abnormalities than galactorrhea. Impotence in the male or menstrual abnormality in the female is the most frequent complaint. The menstrual defect can be a short luteal phase, anovulatory periods, oligomenorrhea, menorrhagia, or amenorrhea. The prolactin level should therefore be determined in all patients with reproductive disturbances.

Hyperprolactinemia often occurs during the use of phenothiazines, monoamine oxidase inhibitors, or other drugs that influence hypothalamic or adrenergic function. Oral contraceptives have also been implicated in lactation syndromes; hyperprolactinemia can occur either during or shortly after withdrawal of oral contraceptives.

Hypothyroidism causes hyperprolactinemia, but prolactin values seldom exceed 50 ng/ml; a serum TSH assay should be obtained to distinguish primary hypothyroidism (which causes secondary prolactin elevation) from pituitary disease causing both hypothyroidism and hyperprolactinemia [*see Figure 5*]. Renal failure may also cause prolactin elevation.

Diagnosis In the evaluation of patients with hyperprolactinemia, a careful history and physical examination, along with evaluation of thyroid and renal function, usually suffice to detect nonpituitary causes.[49] A variety of suppression and stimulation tests have been used to differentiate hypothalamic from pituitary origin of hyperprolactinemia, but none is consistently reliable. High-resolution CT scanning of the head with contrast medium or MRI is therefore indispensable.

The degree of prolactin elevation and the radiologic findings must be carefully correlated. Serum prolactin levels above 300 ng/ml regularly reflect a pituitary tumor, occasionally a microadenoma (< 10 mm in diameter), and often a macroadenoma (> 10 mm). Very high levels (> 600 ng/ml) may be found with large tumors. A level of only 50 to 300 ng/ml found with a large tumor may signify compression of the pituitary stalk by the tumor and consequent blockage of dopamine inhibition of prolactin release, rather than the presence of a prolactinoma. At the low end of the scale, microadenomas can occur with prolactin values as low as 30 ng/ml. In such a case, the radiologist must carefully distinguish minor normal variations from true tumor, and clinical correlation is necessary for discovery or exclusion of nontumorous causes of the elevated prolactin level. When no explanation is found, a provisional diagnosis of idiopathic hyperprolactinemia is made.

Therapy Most cases of hyperprolactinemia, whether from a tumor or of functional origin, can be controlled by the dopamine

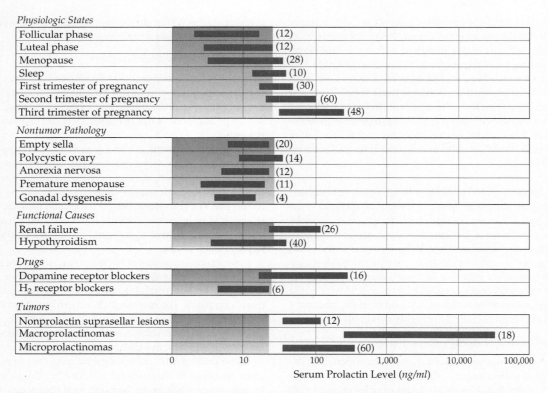

Figure 5 **Large-scale study of 439 subjects showed pregnancy to be the only normal physiologic state in which pro-lactin levels are consistently elevated above the normal range, which is less than 25 ng/ml (blue area). The length of the gray bar denotes the range of prolactin levels observed in a particular category of patients, and the numerals in parentheses indicate the number of subjects in each group. A prolactin level above 30 ng/ml in the absence of renal failure or the use of certain drugs is strongly suggestive of prolactinomas; hyperprolactinemia plus an apparently empty sella may signify the presence of a microprolactinoma.[81]**

agonist bromocriptine.[50] The drug is given at an initial dosage of 1.25 mg/day; it is taken with food at bedtime to minimize the side effects of nausea and postural hypotension. After 1 week, the dosage can be increased to 1.25 mg twice a day, which is usually well tolerated. The serum prolactin level should be measured after 2 weeks at this dosage level before an increase in the dose is considered. The dose of bromocriptine can be increased by 2.5 mg every 2 weeks until the prolactin level falls, symptoms appear, or a maximum of 7.5 mg/day is reached. Prolactin levels fall within days after initiation of treatment, and menses can resume or potency can return after several weeks. An alternative dopamine agonist, pergolide mesylate, appears to be as effective as bromocriptine and is occasionally better tolerated. Indeed, the once-daily schedule for pergolide is preferable for patients who have difficulty tolerating bromocriptine. Another dopamine agonist, cabergoline, also has some advantages over bromocriptine.[51] Treatment with any of these drugs is usually discontinued during pregnancy. However, pregnant patients with macroadenomas need close monitoring because in about 1% to 2% of cases, high estrogen levels induce clinically significant enlargement of prolactinomas. Patients with tumors are occasionally resistant to bromocriptine; this resistance appears to be related to low levels of D_2 dopamine receptors in prolactinoma cell membranes.[52] For such patients and others who may prefer to avoid medication, transsphenoidal adenomectomy offers a highly successful alternative approach.

The cure rate of surgery reaches 88% in patients who have microadenomas and prolactin levels lower than 100 ng/ml. However, with time, a significant frequency of recurrence is observed.

Thus, patients who appear to have had successful surgery should have occasional serum prolactin determinations, particularly if symptoms recur. Follow-up should continue for at least 5 years. Macroadenomas provide a greater surgical challenge because of both the greater surgical hazard and the lower rate of success. For this reason, bromocriptine is widely used as the initial treatment for macroadenomas,[15] even when surgical treatment is ultimately necessary. Preoperative bromocriptine therapy can improve the surgical outlook in such cases; indeed, shrinkage of prolactinomas can be so rapid as to provide one option for emergency treatment of patients with severe headaches and visual field defects. Postoperative irradiation and bromocriptine therapy are often indicated. Radiotherapy alone is used in selected cases, but it seems to be less effective than either bromocriptine or transsphenoidal surgery [*see Chapter 51*].

Must all patients with hyperprolactinemia be treated? The results of studies of the natural history of hyperprolactinemia have varied, but several series have reported the following findings: (1) microadenomas progress very little, if at all; (2) in some patients, prolactin levels revert spontaneously to normal; and (3) regular pituitary imaging is a safe way to follow patients who do not desire treatment. I think it is reasonable to follow normally menstruating women whose prolactin levels are less than 100 ng/ml. Progestin therapy should be used to induce regular menses in patients with oligomenorrhea. In patients who do not respond to progestin therapy, the plasma estradiol level should be measured and bone densitometry studies performed. It is probably best to urge such unresponsive patients to begin bromocriptine therapy [*see Chapter 51*].

The Posterior Pituitary

The posterior pituitary is composed of the terminal portions of neurons that originate in the supraoptic and paraventricular nuclei of the hypothalamus. Vasopressin (AVP), antidiuretic hormone (ADH), and oxytocin are synthesized in the hypothalamus as part of a large precursor molecular complex that includes associated proteins called neurophysins. The precursor molecule is processed as it moves along the axon of the nerve cell. AVP and oxytocin are then stored in the posterior pituitary and released in response to appropriate stimuli. Physiologic study using the AVP assay has shown the following [see Figure 6][53]:

1. The normal adult with a serum osmolality of 287 ± 5 mOsm/kg has a serum AVP level between 1 and 2 pg/ml.

2. A 1% increase in osmolality elicits a change of 1 pg/ml in the serum AVP level. The sensitivity and, to a lesser extent, the threshold of AVP response to a change in tonicity show considerable variability from one person to another; at least part of this variation is hereditary.[54]

3. The change of 1 pg/ml in AVP increases the urinary concentration about 200 mOsm/kg; thus, a change of 3% to 4% in serum osmolality will increase the urine concentration 600 to 800 mOsm/kg, or from very dilute to maximally concentrated.

4. In the normal person, the tonicity is balanced at a midpoint, with changes in either direction directly altering AVP release and urinary concentration.

5. Congestive heart failure lowers the osmotic threshold for AVP release, whereas aging and other factors reduce sensitivity of AVP release (i.e., the rate of AVP release per unit change in osmolality).

6. Mild shifts in blood volume and pressure (i.e., < 10%) do not affect AVP release significantly, but greater shifts do. Hypotension and hypovolemia stimulate AVP release by lowering the osmotic threshold; hypertension and hypervolemia inhibit release by raising the threshold. These influences are mediated by baroreceptor pathways that have afferents in the left atrium.

7. Nausea, but not vomiting, is a powerful stimulus to AVP release; it raises the serum AVP up to 1,000 times the level required for maximal antidiuresis. Pain, however, is not an important stimulant of AVP release.

8. Many neural pathways influence AVP release in response to nonosmotic stimuli. In general, alpha-adrenergic pathways stimulate and beta-adrenergic pathways inhibit AVP release.

The principal disorders of AVP secretion consist of partial or complete deficiency (diabetes insipidus) and the syndrome of inappropriate antidiuretic hormone (SIADH) excess [see Chapter 159]. The syndromes of AVP deficiency are considered here.

DIABETES INSIPIDUS

Polyuria is a common clinical problem.[55] A patient passing large quantities of urine generally has one of three abnormalities: an osmotic diuresis, resistance to AVP, or deficient AVP secretion.[56] The most common osmotic diuresis is that caused by glycosuria, a presenting symptom of diabetes mellitus. Resistance to AVP (i.e., nephrogenic diabetes insipidus) occurs in certain forms of chronic renal disease, after relief of urinary obstruction, and as a hereditary disorder. Genetic defects in the renal receptor for AVP have been identified.[57,58] Deficiency of AVP (i.e., neurogenic diabetes insipidus) reflects either functional or structural disease of the supraoptic hypothalamic neurons that secrete the hormone. Again, genetic defects in the secretion of AVP are now known.[59,60] Two clues—sudden onset of polyuria and a preference for iced beverages—suggest AVP deficiency. However, neurogenic diabetes insipidus must be distinguished from primary polydipsia because overdrinking also results in polyuria and suppressed AVP secretion.

Diagnosis

Neurogenic and nephrogenic diabetes insipidus can usually be differentiated by means of clinical testing [see Figure 7]. The patient is deprived of water until 3% to 5% of body weight is lost and the serum tonicity is higher than 295 mOsm/kg. If polyuria disappears and the urine concentration rises above 500 mOsm/kg,

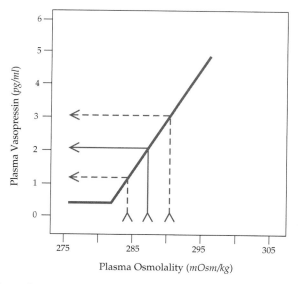
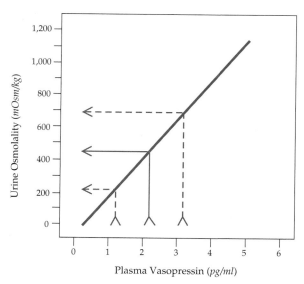

Figure 6 The relation of serum tonicity to vasopressin levels and urine concentration is depicted. In the graph at left, normal resting serum tonicity hovers around 287 mOsm/kg (solid arrow). Small increases or decreases (broken arrows) elicit proportional changes in serum vasopressin. In the graph at right, it can be seen that small increases or decreases in serum vasopressin produce striking changes in urine concentration.

AVP secretion is adequate. If polyuria and dilute urine (< 300 mOsm/kg) persist, then 20 μg of desmopressin acetate (DDAVP) is given by inhalation; alternatively, 300 μU of AVP can be administered intravenously. If urine flow decreases and urine concentration rises, AVP deficiency can be inferred. If, however, the serum becomes concentrated and the urine remains dilute despite administration of DDAVP, nephrogenic diabetes insipidus is present.

Some cautions should be kept in mind when conducting dehydration tests. First, the term partial diabetes insipidus describes a patient who, when deprived of water, achieves a urine concentration greater than the serum osmolality but less than that obtained after administration of antidiuretic hormone. Functional testing can be misleading in patients with neurogenic or nephrogenic partial diabetes insipidus. In such patients, who have a urine concentration between 300 and 500 mOsm/kg, measurement of the serum AVP level can be extremely helpful. A high AVP level in the presence of a concentrated serum and a relatively dilute urine points to nephrogenic diabetes insipidus; a low value points to hormone deficiency. Conversely, partial resistance to AVP can result from chronic overdrinking, with secondary dilution of the medullary concentration in the kidney. If such patients control their excess water intake, they recover a normal renal medullary concentration and, at the same rate, a normal response to AVP. Finally, water deprivation appears to produce less thirst in older men than in younger men.[61] Men older than 80 years must be watched carefully after testing to ensure that they resume appropriate water intake.

Granulomas, trauma, infection, and other infiltrations can all produce diabetes insipidus. Metastatic tumor seldom produces insufficiency in other endocrine glands, but secondary tumors arising from lung, breast, and other organs can all produce insufficiency in the posterior pituitary. The sensitivity of MRI has considerably refined the approach to the diagnosis of diabetes insipidus.[62]

Diabetes insipidus can develop suddenly after neurosurgery or external trauma. In this setting, a dilute polyuria with a serum sodium level greater than 145 mEq/L allows a presumptive diagnosis, and parenteral DDAVP should be given immediately.[63] Conversely, hyponatremia from increased AVP secretion after transsphenoidal surgery should also be anticipated by following serum sodium levels.[64] Explosive and fatal central diabetes melli-

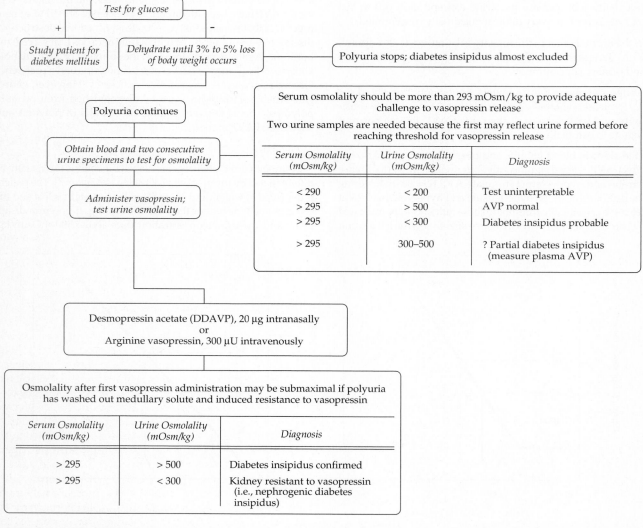

Figure 7 **Differential diagnosis of polyuria and polydipsia is presented in flowchart. Note: This test is done for patients with a serum osmolality of less than 290 mOsm/kg. Dehydration is inadvisable when the serum osmolality is greater than 290 mOsm/kg (serum sodium ≥ 142). A simultaneous urine osmolality should be measured; if it is dilute, the response to administered vasopressin should be directly determined.**

tus and diabetes insipidus have been reported in young women with postoperative hyponatremia that was not aggressively treated. The pathogenesis of the disorder is not understood, but the pathologic sequence included cerebral edema and herniation, compression of the third cranial nerve, hypoxic infarction of the pituitary and hypothalamus, respiratory arrest, and coma. The rapidity of deterioration in these patients indicates that the hyponatremia in such cases should be promptly corrected, even though fixed pupillary dilatation, secondary to compression of the oculomotor nerve, may suggest brain death.[65]

Therapy

There are several approaches to the treatment of diabetes insipidus.[66] If the polyuria is mild and does not interfere with sleep, no treatment may be needed. Chlorpropamide potentiates the effect of AVP on renal concentrating ability and can be used to treat partial diabetes insipidus. It is given in a dosage of 250 to 375 mg once a day and usually does not produce hypoglycemia in normal persons. However, if patients do not eat regularly or if they have unsuspected anterior pituitary insufficiency, chlorpropamide can be hazardous.

For patients with severe diabetes insipidus, vasopressin tannate in oil, 5 units every 2 to 4 days intramuscularly, provides excellent control of polyuria and polydipsia. It is wise to allow the antidiuretic effect to wear off and the polyuria to reappear before giving the succeeding dose; otherwise, hyponatremia is common. This caution is particularly important after neurosurgery, where a triphasic sequence of AVP deficiency, AVP excess, and AVP deficiency can occur. This formerly standard approach to the treatment of diabetes insipidus is being replaced by intranasal or oral DDAVP. Intranasal administration of DDAVP is effective, nontoxic, and nonirritating. Tablets of DDAVP, in a dose of 0.1 or 0.2 mg, taken one to three times daily is the most recently developed treatment for diabetes insipidus. All patients with diabetes insipidus should be warned that in circumstances of extreme water loss or at times of unconsciousness, they are exposed to added risk unless they are under the care of a physician who is aware of the diagnosis.

Multiple Endocrine Neoplasia Syndromes

Several hereditary syndromes affect multiple endocrine glands in distinct patterns.[67] Multiple endocrine neoplasia type I (MEN I) involves diverse abnormalities of the anterior pituitary, the parathyroid, and the pancreatic islets. Affected families show a high incidence of peptic ulcer disease and a low, irregular frequency of other somatic and endocrine lesions. The following lesions are the primary endocrine abnormalities:

1. Pituitary gland—adenomas or hyperplasia of acidophil or chromophobe cells, with acromegaly, hyperprolactinemia, or hypopituitarism. Endocrine function may be normal.

2. Parathyroid—adenoma, multiple adenoma, hyperplasia, and carcinoma of the parathyroid have all been reported; hyperparathyroidism is the most common endocrine disturbance in patients with MEN I. The parathyroid involvement often frustrates the efforts of the pathologist and surgeon to distinguish adenomas from hyperplasia because the two conditions may occur in the same family.

3. Pancreas—adenomas, hyperplasia, and carcinoma may occur in any of the cells of the pancreatic islets. The resultant endocrine syndromes are hyperinsulinism, hypergastrinism (a Zollinger-Ellison syndrome is produced), pancreatic cholera, and other less well defined defects.

MEN I is inherited as an autosomal dominant trait but is seldom manifest before puberty. Hyperparathyroidism is the most frequent spontaneous endocrine manifestation, but some series indicate that prospective screening of first-order relatives may detect either pancreatic or pituitary lesions before the onset of hyperparathyroidism.[68,69] Whether these series are typical, however, is not known.

The genetics and molecular biology of MEN I are particularly interesting. Expression of the trait varies widely between persons and between families. According to the Knudson two-stage theory of carcinogenesis,[70] hereditary cancers are caused by a germ cell mutation that creates the predisposition and a somatic cell mutation that leads to clinical manifestation. The comparison of DNA sequences of parathyroid and pancreatic tumors with those of peripheral blood leukocytes and other tissues from patients with MEN I reveals loss of a segment of the q13 band of chromosome 11 in the tumors themselves.[71-73] It is presumed, but not proved by current techniques, that the inherited lesion is a mutation at the q13 locus in one member of the chromosome 11 pair and that this defect is present in all the body tissues [see Figure 8]. The gene at the q13 locus of chromosome 11 is thought to encode a tumor suppressor product. When the q13 locus is lost from the second member of the chromosome 11 pair, the change produces a loss of heterozygosity, and the homozygous deficiency of the tumor suppressor protein allows tumors to develop. Unlike tumors in multiple endocrine neoplasia type II (MEN II) [see Chapter 46], however, the tumors in patients with MEN I do not require a background of hyperplasia for their appearance. Nevertheless, the finding of parathyroid hyperplasia and of a parathyroid mitogen in some MEN I patients provides at least suggestive evidence that, as in MEN II, hyperplasia precedes neoplasia. It is also of interest that some isolated parathyroid adenomas show the same clonal defect in chromosome 11 segment q13.[74]

The delayed appearance and protean manifestations of MEN I raise an important clinical question: in a patient showing any of the clinical features of MEN I, should a search for other signs be considered? Such investigation should be minimal when the index of suspicion is not high. For example, in a patient with a parathyroid adenoma cured by surgery, there is little reason to search for additional involvement. However, if parathyroid hyperplasia is found, a second endocrine gland is involved, or the family history includes a second affected person, a formal search for involvement of other glands and other family members is appropriate. First-order relatives are at a 50% risk for the disease. A detailed pedigree should be plotted, and even out-of-town relatives should be informed of their risk. Screening approaches vary, but I favor determination of at least the blood calcium, prolactin, and glucose levels. Tests should be repeated at 1- or 2-year intervals beginning at 15 years of age. Early discovery leads to more effective treatment and should reduce the morbidity experienced by the family.

Although the gene for MEN I has not been cloned, genetic linkage to flanking sequences on chromosome 11 allows predictive studies in affected persons.[75-77] This approach is both more important and more pressing in MEN II, but in informative families with MEN I, affected family members can be targeted for appropriate follow-up.

A negative family history does not obviate a search for MEN I. New mutations account for almost 50% of cases. When sponta-

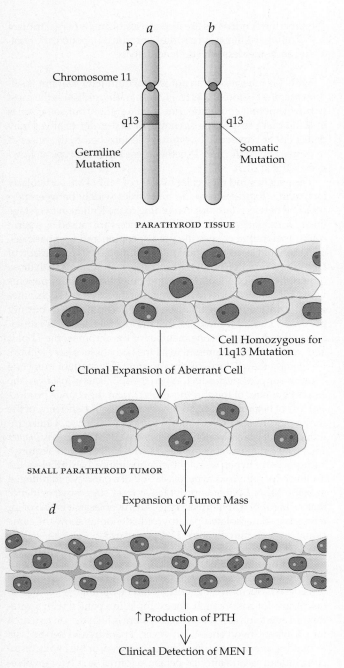

Figure 8 **The genetic defect that predisposes to the development of multiple endocrine neoplasia type I (MEN I) is thought to be a germline mutation at the q13 locus of chromosome 11. This germline mutation is present in all the body cells, including leukocytes, parathyroid epithelial cells, and hepatocytes (*a*). However, before this defect can give rise to clinical disease, a second, somatic mutation must occur at the same locus in the homologous chromosome (*b*). This mutation may arise as a result of mitotic nondisjunction, mitotic recombination, or a point mutation. The gene at the q13 locus is thought to encode a tumor suppressor protein, and the loss of heterozygosity at this site allows the affected cell to escape from normal restraints. Clonal expansion of the aberrant cell ensues, leading to the formation of an adenoma (*c*). In MEN I, the cell affected by the somatic mutation may be in the parathyroid (shown here), pancreas, or anterior pituitary. As the mass of tumor tissue increases (*d*), constitutive overproduction of the natural hormone (in this case, parathyroid hormone [PTH]) occurs, producing symptoms.**

neous cases occur, only the children of such patients—not parents or siblings—are at increased risk for disease.

Finally, MEN I can occur in association with the Zollinger-Ellison syndrome, either in an individual or in an affected family. When the family history suggests the Zollinger-Ellison syndrome, serum gastrin measurement should be included in the screening. The hypercalcemia of hyperparathyroidism can exaggerate the symptoms and the secretory abnormalities of the Zollinger-Ellison syndrome.

MEN II (including pheochromocytomas, medullary thyroid carcinoma, parathyroid hyperplasia, and adenomas) is discussed elsewhere [*see Chapter 46*].

Interactions between the Endocrine and Immune Systems

There are rich interactions between the immune and the endocrine systems. Cortisol is a major anti-inflammatory substance, and its production is one of the body's principal responses to stress. Both corticotropin-releasing hormone and AVP have proinflammatory effects, but both lead to increased cortisol production. At least four cytokines influence acute inflammation: interleukin-1 (IL-1), IL-6, tumor necrosis factor–α, and IL-1 receptor antagonist (IL-1ra). The first three are proinflammatory, but IL-1ra is a brake on the inflammatory response. The net effect of the cytokines and related responses is to induce a so-called sick-everything state—a sick euthyroid, hypogonadal, diabetogenic condition that appears predominantly as laboratory abnormalities more than a clinically significant therapeutic challenge. The importance of these changes, and indeed of the immune-endocrine interactions, is being carefully studied.[78,79]

References

1. Molitch ME: Neuroendocrinology. Endocrinology and Metabolism, 3rd ed. Felig P, Baxter JD, Frohman LA, Eds. McGraw-Hill, New York, 1995, p 221

2. Veldhuis JD: Pulsatile hormone release as a window into the brain's control of the anterior pituitary gland in health and disease: implications and consequences of pulsatile luteinizing hormone secretion. Endocrinologist 4:454, 1994

3. Conn PM, Crowley WF Jr: Gonadotropin-releasing hormone and its analogs. Annu Rev Med 45:391, 1994

4. Frohman LA: Diseases of the anterior pituitary. Endocrinology and Metabolism, 3rd ed. Felig P, Baxter JD, Frohman LA, Eds. McGraw-Hill, New York, 1995, p 289

5. Corticotropin-releasing hormone (CRH) in the differential diagnosis of Cushing's syndrome. Endocrinologist 7(suppl):1S, 1997

6. Orth DN: Cushing's syndrome. N Engl J Med 332:791, 1995

7. Blevins LS Jr, Christy JH, Khajavi M, et al: Outcomes of therapy for Cushing's disease due to adrenocorticotropin-secreting pituitary macroadenomas. J Clin Endocrinol Metab 83:63, 1998

8. Young WF Jr, Scheithauer BW, Kovacs KT, et al: Gonadotroph adenoma of the pituitary gland: a clinicopathologic analysis of 100 cases. Mayo Clin Proc 71:649, 1996

9. Yen SSC: Female hypogonadotropic hypogonadism: hypothalamic amenorrhea syndrome. Endocrinol Metab Clin North Am 22:29, 1993

10. Waldstreicher J, Seminara SB, Jameson JL, et al: The genetic and clinical heterogeneity of gonadotropin-releasing hormone deficiency in the human. J Clin Endocrinol Metab 81:4388, 1996

11. Vance ML: Hypopituitarism. N Engl J Med 330:1651, 1994

12. Dash RJ, Gupta V, Suri S: Sheehan's syndrome: clinical profile, pituitary hormone responses and computed sellar tomography. Aust NZ J Med 23:26, 1993

13. Vance ML: The empty sella. Curr Ther Endocrinol Metab 6:38, 1997

14. Constine LS, Woolf PD, Cann D, et al: Hypothalamic-pituitary dysfunction after radiation for brain tumors. N Engl J Med 328:87, 1993

15. Shalet SM: Radiation and pituitary dysfunction (editorial). N Engl J Med 328:131, 1993

16. Sklar CA, Constine LS: Chronic neuroendocrinological sequelae of radiation therapy. Int J Radiat Oncol Biol Phys 31:1113, 1995

17. Reversible hypopituitarism (editorial). Lancet 337:276, 1991

18. Consensus guidelines for the diagnosis and treatment of adults with growth hormone deficiency: summary statement of the Growth Hormone Research Society workshop on adult growth hormone deficiency. J Clin Endocrinol Metab 83:379, 1998

19. Carroll PV, Christ ER, Bengtsson BÅ, et al: Growth hormone deficiency in adulthood and the effects of growth hormone replacement: a review. J Clin Endocrinol Metab 83:382, 1998

20. Mannakkara JV, Datta-Chaudhuri M: Recognizing pituitary insufficiency in the elderly. J Am Geriatr Soc 39:273, 1991

21. Shalet SM, Toogood A, Rahim A, et al: The diagnosis of growth hormone deficiency in children and adults. Endocr Rev 19:203, 1998

22. Bardin CW, Swerdloff RS, Santen RJ: Androgens: risks and benefits. J Clin Endocrinol Metab 73:4, 1991

23. Riedel M, Brabant G, Rieger K, et al: Growth hormone therapy in adults: rationales, results, and perspectives. Exp Clin Endocrinol 102:273, 1994

24. Bates AS, Van't Hoff W, Jones PJ, et al: The effect of hypopituitarism on life expectancy. J Clin Endocrinol Metab 81:1169, 1996

25. Bouillanne O, Rainfray M, Tissandier O, et al: Growth hormone therapy in elderly people: an age delaying drug? Fund Clin Pharm 10:416, 1996

26. Levy A, Lightman SL: The pathogenesis of pituitary adenomas. Clin Endocrinol (Oxf) 38:559, 1993

27. King JT Jr, Justice AC, Aron DC: Management of incidental pituitary microadenomas: a cost-effective analysis. J Clin Endocrinol Metab 82:3625, 1997

28. Wilson CB: Surgical management of pituitary tumors. J Clin Endocrinol Metab 82:2381, 1997

29. Tran LM, Blount L, Horton D, et al: Radiation therapy of pituitary tumors: results in 95 cases. Am J Clin Oncol 14:25, 1991

30. Arafah BM, Kailani SH, Nekl KE, et al: Immediate recovery of pituitary function after transsphenoidal resection of pituitary macroadenomas. J Clin Endocrinol Metab 79:348, 1994

31. Bills DC, Meyer FB, Laws ER Jr, et al: A retrospective analysis of pituitary apoplexy. Neurosurgery 33:602, 1993

32. Fraioli B, Esposito V, Palma L, et al: Hemorrhagic pituitary adenomas: clinicopathological features and surgical treatment. Neurosurgery 27:741, 1990

33. Glick RP, Tiesi JA: Subacute pituitary apoplexy: clinical and magnetic resonance imaging characteristics. Neurosurgery 27:214, 1990

34. Matthews LS: Molecular biology of growth hormone receptors. Trends in Endocrinology and Metabolism 2:176, 1991

35. Scanlon MF, Issa BG, Dieguez C: Regulation of growth hormone secretion. Horm Res 46:149, 1996

36. Jaffe CA, Friberg RD, Barkan AL: Suppression of growth hormone (GH) secretion by a selective GH-releasing hormone (GHRH) antagonist: direct evidence for involvement of endogenous GHRH in the generation of GH pulses. J Clin Invest 92:695, 1993

37. Grunstein RR, Ho KY, Sullivan CE: Sleep apnea in acromegaly. Ann Intern Med 115:527, 1991

38. Hartman ML, Pincus SM, Johnson ML, et al: Enhanced basal and disorderly growth hormone secretion distinguish acromegalic from normal pulsatile growth hormone release. J Clin Invest 94:1277, 1994

39. Ho KKY, Weissberger AJ: Characterization of 24-hour growth hormone secretion in acromegaly: implications for diagnosis and therapy. Clin Endocrinol (Oxf) 41:75, 1994

40. Barkan A: Controversies in the diagnosis and therapy of acromegaly. Endocrinologist 7:300, 1997

41. Colao A, Merola B, Ferone D, et al: Acromegaly. J Clin Endocrinol Metab 82:2777, 1997

42. Frohman LA: Acromegaly: what constitutes optimal therapy? (editorial). J Clin Endocrinol Metab 81:443, 1996

43. Clayton RN, Wass JAH: Pituitary tumours: recommendations for service provision and guidelines for management of patients. J R Coll Physicians Lond 31:628, 1997

44. Rudman D, Mattson DE: Serum insulin-like growth factor I in healthy older men in relation to physical activity. J Am Geriatr Soc 42:71, 1994

45. Hodes RJ: Frailty and disability: can growth hormone or other trophic agents make a difference? J Am Geriatr Soc 42:1208, 1994

46. Corpas E, Harman SM, Blackman MR: Human growth hormone and human aging. Endocr Rev 14:20, 1993

47. Toogood AA, O'Neill PA, Shalet SM: Beyond the somatopause: growth hormone deficiency in adults over the age of 60 years. J Clin Endocrinol Metab 81:460, 1996

48. Yazigi RA, Quintero CH, Salameh WA: Prolactin disorders. Fertil Steril 67:215, 1997

49. Sarapura V, Sclaff WD: Recent advances in the understanding of the pathophysiology and treatment of hyperprolactinemia. Curr Opin Obstet Gynecol 5:360, 1993

50. Molitch ME, Thorner MO, Wilson C: Management of prolactinomas. J Clin Endocrinol Metab 82:996, 1997

51. Webster J, Piscitelli G, Polli A, et al: A comparison of cabergoline and bromocriptine in the treatment of hyperprolactinemic amenorrhea. N Engl J Med 331:904, 1994

52. Brue T, Pellegrini I, Priou A, et al: Prolactinomas and resistance to dopamine agonists. Horm Res 38:84, 1992

53. Robertson GL: Physiology of ADH secretion. Kidney Int Suppl 21:S20, 1987

54. Zerbe RL, Miller JZ, Robertson GL: The reproducibility and heritability of individual differences in osmoregulatory function in normal human subjects. J Lab Clin Med 117:51, 1991

55. Singer I, Oster JR, Fishman LM: The management of diabetes insipidus in adults. Arch Intern Med 157:1293, 1997

56. Robertson GL: Posterior pituitary. Endocrinology and Metabolism, 3rd ed. Felig P, Baxter JD, Frohman LA, Eds. McGraw-Hill, New York, 1995, p 385

57. Holtzman EJ, Harris HW Jr, Kolakowski LF Jr, et al: Brief report: a molecular defect in the vasopressin V2-receptor gene causing nephrogenic diabetes insipidus. N Engl J Med 328:1534, 1993

58. Merendino JJ Jr, Spiegel AM, Crawford JD, et al: Brief report: a mutation in the vasopressin V2-receptor gene in a kindred with X-linked nephrogenic diabetes insipidus. N Engl J Med 328:1538, 1993

59. McLeod JF, Kovács L, Gaskill MB, et al: Familial neurohypophyseal diabetes insipidus associated with a signal peptide mutation. J Clin Endocrinol Metab 77:599A, 1993

60. Miller WL: Molecular genetics of familial central diabetes insipidus (editorial). J Clin Endocrinol Metab 77:592, 1993

61. Phillips PA, Rolls BJ, Ledingham JG, et al: Reduced thirst after water deprivation in healthy elderly men. N Engl J Med 311:753, 1984

62. Tien R, Kucharczyk J, Kucharczyk W: MR imaging of the brain in patients with diabetes insipidus. AJNR Am J Neuroradiol 12:533, 1991

63. Buonocore CM, Robinson AG: The diagnosis and management of diabetes insipidus during medical emergencies. Endocrinol Metab Clin North Am 22:411, 1993

64. Sane T, Rantakari K, Poranen A, et al: Hyponatremia after transsphenoidal surgery for pituitary tumors. J Clin Endocrinol Metab 79:1395, 1994

65. Fraser CL, Arieff AI: Fatal central diabetes mellitus and insipidus resulting from untreated hyponatremia: a new syndrome. Ann Intern Med 112:113, 1990

66. Robinson AG, Verbalis JG: Diabetes insipidus. Curr Ther Endocrinol Metab 6:1, 1997

67. Schimke RN: Multiple endocrine neoplasia: how many syndromes? Am J Med Genet 37:375, 1990

68. Skogseid B, Eriksson B, Lundqvist G, et al: Multiple endocrine neoplasia type 1: a 10-year prospective screening study in four kindreds. J Clin Endocrinol Metab 73:281, 1991

69. Shepherd JJ: The natural history of multiple endocrine neoplasia type 1: highly uncommon or highly unrecognized? Arch Surg 126:935, 1991

70. Knudson AG Jr, Strong LC, Anderson DE: Heredity and cancer in man. Progress in Medical Genetics 9:113, 1973

71. Friedman E, Sakaguchi K, Bale AE, et al: Clonality of parathyroid tumors in familial multiple endocrine neoplasia type 1. N Engl J Med 321:213, 1989

72. Brandi ML: Multiple endocrine neoplasia type 1: general features and new insights into etiology. J Endocrinol Invest 14:61, 1991

73. Beckers A, Abs R, Reyniers E, et al: Variable regions of chromosome 11 loss in different pathological tissues of a patient with multiple endocrine neoplasia type I syndrome. J Clin Endocrinol Metab 79:1498, 1994

74. Bale AE, Norton JA, Wong EL, et al: Allelic loss on chromosome 11 in hereditary and sporadic tumors related to familial multiple endocrine neoplasia type 1. Cancer Res 51:1154, 1991

75. Thakker RV: The role of molecular genetics in screening for multiple endocrine neoplasia type I. Endocrinol Metab Clin North Am 23:117, 1994

76. Larsson C, Nordenskjöld M: Family screening in multiple endocrine neoplasia type 1 (MEN 1). Ann Med 26:191, 1994

77. Skogseid B, Rastad J, Öberg K: Multiple endocrine neoplasia type 1: clinical features and screening. Endocrinol Metab Clin North Am 23:1, 1994

78. Chrousos GP: The hypothalamic–pituitary–adrenal axis and immune-mediated inflammation. N Engl J Med 332:1351, 1995

79. Reichlin S: Neuroendocrine–immune interactions. N Engl J Med 329:1246, 1993

80. Weitzman ED: Circadian rhythms and episodic hormone secretion in man. Annu Rev Med 27:225, 1976

81. Robertson GL, Shelton RL, Athar S: The osmoregulation of vasopressin. Kidney Int 10:27, 1976

82. Daughaday WH: The adenohypophysis. Textbook of Endocrinology, 5th ed. Williams RH, Ed. WB Saunders Co, Philadelphia, 1974

Acknowledgments

Figure 1   Carol Donner.

Figures 2 and 3   Alan Iselin.

Figures 4 and 8   Tom Moore.

Figure 5   Al Miller.

Figure 6   Hank Iken.

46 Thyroid

Daniel D. Federman, M.D.

Physiology of the Thyroid

THYROID HORMONE BIOSYNTHESIS AND STORAGE

Inorganic iodide is actively concentrated in the thyroid epithelial cells to a level approximately 30 times its concentration in plasma. This step is competitively opposed by inorganic ions such as thiocyanate and perchlorate, which accounts for the antithyroid action of these compounds.[1]

Within minutes after entering the thyroid, inorganic iodide is oxidized, in a peroxidase-dependent reaction, to an organic form. This oxidation is hardly distinguishable from the next reaction, in which organic iodine is incorporated into tyrosine residues within thyroglobulin, a large glycoprotein molecule. The resultant monoiodotyrosine (MIT) and diiodotyrosine (DIT) are brought into proximity and are coupled through an ether linkage to form thyroxine (also called tetraiodothyronine, or T_4) and triiodothyronine (T_3), the principal thyroid hormones. Apparently, only iodinated tyrosines are coupled because noniodinated thyronine is not found within the thyroid gland. Both coupling and incorporation-iodination require oxidative conditions, both may involve the same peroxidase, and both are inhibited by thiourea derivatives.

The thyroid is unique among endocrine glands in its large storage capacity and relatively slow release of hormone: the gland normally contains about 8,000 µg of iodine, a reserve sufficient for at least 100 days. T_4 and T_3 are principally stored in the colloid of the thyroid gland lumen as part of thyroglobulin. The thyroid also contains a much smaller amount of another iodoprotein, thyralbumin, which is very similar to albumin. This substance is increased in many hyperfunctioning thyroids and in some neoplasms.

PROTEOLYSIS AND RELEASE OF HORMONE

Release of hormone from the thyroid involves reentry of thyroglobulin by endocytosis from the colloid into the apical portions of the thyroid follicular cell. The engulfed droplets fuse with lysosomes and are hydrolyzed, releasing T_4 and T_3 into the circulation. Hydrolysis of thyroglobulin also produces some iodotyrosines within the follicular cells; these compounds are deiodinated in a reaction catalyzed by iodotyrosine deiodinase, restoring iodide to an intracellular pool from which

reincorporation into hormone can occur. The intracellular pool is an important source of iodine; hypothyroidism and goiter develop in patients deficient in iodotyrosine deiodinase. The proteolytic step is stimulated by thyroid-stimulating hormone (also called thyrotropin, or TSH) and inhibited by iodine; this action of iodine is probably its principal antithyroid effect. The proteolytic step is also inhibited by lithium but perhaps at a site different from that of inhibition by iodine; the antithyroid effects of iodine and lithium are sometimes additive.

The active circulating thyroid hormones are T_4 and T_3. Circulating T_3 is produced within the thyroid from the coupling of MIT and DIT and from the monodeiodination of T_4. The latter process also operates within the tissues to yield additional T_3. Approximately 15 to 20 percent of circulating T_3 arises from thyroid secretion, and the rest arises peripherally. In both hyperthyroidism and hypothyroidism, however, a significantly larger fraction of the circulating T_3 than usual is derived from the thyroid.

Approximately 30 µg of T_3 is produced daily by peripheral deiodination of T_4. This process is important in overall regulation of thyroid hormone production [*see Figure 1*]. There are two deiodinases. Type I deiodinase, found in the liver and the kidney, acts on circulating T_4 to produce T_3 for peripheral tissues. Hypothyroidism can occur as a result of underactivity of type I deiodinase induced by insufficiency of selenium, one of its components. Type II deiodinase is found principally in the pituitary, the brain, and the placenta. It is responsible for the monodeiodination of T_4 in the pituitary; the resulting T_3 has direct regulatory effects on TSH synthesis.[2] Monodeiodination can remove either the iodine at the 5' position, yielding T_3, or the iodine at the 5 position, yielding the compound called reverse triiodothyronine (rT_3). T_3 is a principal active biologic hormone, whereas rT_3 is inactive. The rT_3 level is not measured in the serum T_3 assay. In a variety of circumstances—gestation, cirrhosis, uremia, malnutrition, acute and chronic illness, stress, and steroid therapy—T_3 levels fall and rT_3 levels rise. These changes result at least in part from decreased production of T_3 and decreased clearance of rT_3. The biologic significance of these changes is unclear, but they are clinically relevant. In the conditions listed, and undoubtedly in others not yet identified, a low serum T_3 level cannot be taken as evidence of hy-

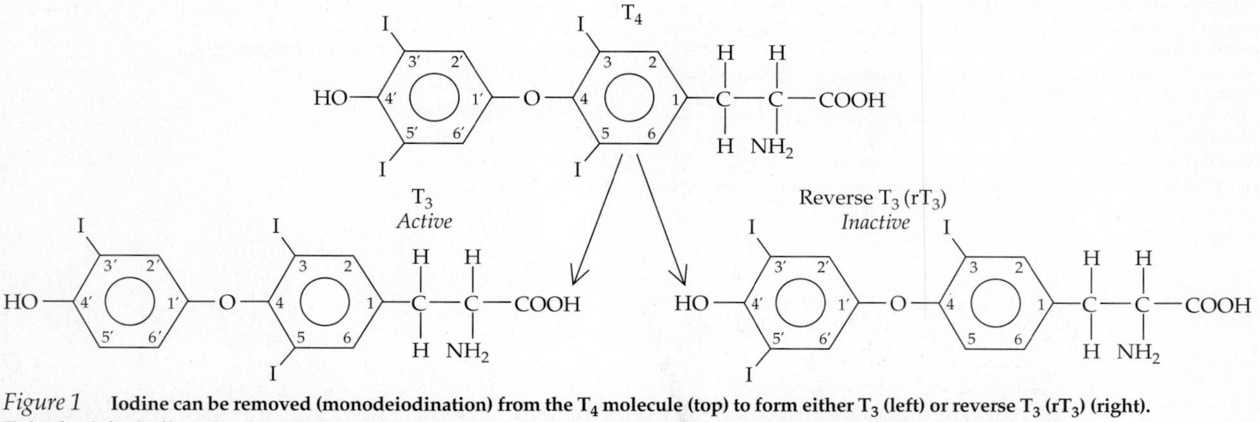

Figure 1   Iodine can be removed (monodeiodination) from the T_4 molecule (top) to form either T_3 (left) or reverse T_3 (rT_3) (right). T_3 is physiologically active, but rT_3 is inactive. Serum T_3 assays measure only T_3; a special assay is needed to measure rT_3.

pothyroidism if the serum T_4 and TSH levels are normal [*see* Thyroid Function Tests, *below*].

THYROID HORMONE TRANSPORT AND METABOLISM

Circulating thyroid hormones bind to three plasma proteins. About 75 percent of T_4 and 70 percent of T_3 are bound to thyroxine-binding globulin (TBG), a 54 kd glycoprotein normally present at a concentration of 2 mg/dl. Smaller amounts of both hormones are bound to thyroxine-binding prealbumin (transthyretin) and albumin. The equilibrium between bound and free T_4 is strongly shifted toward the bound state; only about 0.03 percent of T_4 is free. At an average T_4 value of 6 μg/dl, the absolute free T_4 value is about 2 ng/dl. T_3 is also bound to TBG, but the affinity is lower; the percentage of free T_3 is 0.30.[1]

REGULATION OF THYROID FUNCTION

Two major influences control the thyroid gland: TSH from the anterior pituitary[3] and the intrathyroidal iodine level. TSH is a glycoprotein that attaches to a membrane-bound receptor typical of G protein–coupled units.[4] Like other receptors, the TSH receptor has an extracellular region, a seven-segment transmembrane domain, and an intracellular region that functions as an adenylate cyclase; that is, it stimulates the formation of intracellular cyclic adenosine monophosphate (cAMP). This second messenger stimulates all the steps in iodine metabolism and hormonogenesis [*see Figure 2*].

The secretion of TSH is principally regulated by two influences. The dominant one is the circulating level of thyroid hormone; higher thyroid hormone levels reduce pituitary TSH release, whereas lower levels stimulate it. The inhibition of TSH release is mediated by reduced transcription of TSH messenger RNA (mRNA). The intracellular level of T_3 in the pituitary appears to be the specific regulator of TSH synthesis. The intracellular T_3 level is determined by the serum T_3 level and the amount of T_3 that is produced in the cell as a result of the deiodination of T_4.

The second influence that controls production of TSH is a hypothalamic neurohumor: thyrotropin-releasing hormone (TRH). This tripeptide modulates TSH synthesis and release primarily by altering the set point for feedback regulation by T_3 and by stimulating transcription of TSH mRNA. TRH works by stimulation of a membrane-bound receptor of the G protein family, catalyzing the hydrolysis of phosphatidylinositol 4,5-bisphosphate and increasing intracellular calcium.[5] The effect of TRH on TSH in turn may be offset by inhibitory factors, including dopamine, somatostatin, and glucocorticoids. The secretion of TRH is stimulated by norepinephrine and serotonin; it is inhibited by dopamine and by T_3. T_3 inhibits TRH production by suppressing the transcription of TRH mRNA in thyroid-specific cells of the paraventricular nucleus of the hypothalamus. Expression of the gene is found elsewhere in the body, including the heart, testis, and brain, but nowhere else does T_3 suppress it.[6]

Thyroid secretion is also influenced by the level of intrathyroidal iodine stores, which probably modulates the stimulatory effect of TSH.[1]

MECHANISM OF THYROID HORMONE ACTION

Multiple tissues of the body, including the liver, heart, kidney, and brain, contain nonhistone nucleoproteins that bind T_3 at least 10 times more avidly than T_4. Molecular analysis of

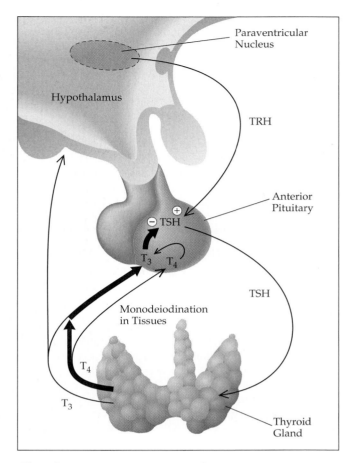

Figure 2 Impulses from the periventricular nucleus control the output of thyroid-releasing hormone (TRH) from the hypothalamus. TRH promotes the release of thyroid-stimulating hormone (TSH) by the pituitary. TSH, in turn, stimulates the thyroid to produce the hormones triiodothyronine (T_3) and tetraiodothyronine (T_4). Some T_4 is converted to T_3 before and after uptake of the hormones by the pituitary. The large amount of T_3 has a negative feedback (inhibitory) effect on TSH and TRH production.

these thyroid hormone receptors reveals that they are part of a so-called superfamily of receptor proteins that, in various forms, bind sex steroids, vitamin D, and retinoic acid as well as T_3. Members of this superfamily show marked structural homology with one another and with the *c-erb*-A proto-oncogenes, which also bind T_3 with high specificity and affinity.

Thyroid hormone receptors exist in at least four isoforms: TRα-1, TRα-2, TRβ-1, and TRβ-2.[7] Each receptor protein has a site for binding to DNA and a distinct site for binding the ligand hormone. The DNA-binding domain includes two projecting zinc fingers (characteristic loop structures that contain zinc ion), whose amino acid sequence is rigorously conserved. Other sequences in the receptor are responsible for translocation of the receptor protein to the nucleus, for its dimerization to the active form, and for a transactivating effect. When it is bound to hormone, the receptor stimulates gene transcription and subsequent protein synthesis, thereby producing a physiologic effect. The T_3 receptor is unique among the superfamily members in that it remains attached to chromatin even in the absence of the ligand hormone. In that situation (i.e., when the receptor is not bound to T_3), gene transcription is inhibited. Thus, it is possible that thyroid hormone and its receptor act by positive and negative regulation of one or more genes. The increase in specific mRNA elicited by thyroid hormone may combine with an augmented stimulation of mRNA synthesis by other factors. The connections between these events and such thyroid hormone effects as calorigenesis, growth, and differentiation require further elucidation.[8]

Thyroid Function Tests

The two major goals of thyroid function tests are to assess the amount of circulating thyroid hormone and to explain the findings obtained by physical examination of the gland.

TESTS DEFINING FUNCTIONAL STATE

Thyroid-Stimulating Hormone

The measurement of the serum TSH level is the preferred approach to assessing the functional state of the thyroid gland, for three reasons: (1) TSH is central to a negative feedback system [see Figure 2]; (2) TSH responds logarithmically to arithmetic changes in serum thyroid hormone level [see Figure 3]; thus, small changes in thyroid function are amplified by resulting changes in TSH secretion; and (3) TSH assays can now detect both elevation of TSH levels and pathophysiologically significant lowering of TSH levels.

Standard radioimmunoassays use one antibody, but supersensitive assays use two. When the second antibody of the supersensitive assay is labeled with radioiodine, the assay is termed an immunoradiometric assay (IRMA). This assay is classified as a second-generation TSH assay and can distinguish low-normal values from low values with a detection threshold of about 0.05 mU/L. When the second antibody bears a fluorophor, an enzyme, or a chemiluminescent molecule, the test is designated as a third-generation TSH assay. The sensitivity of the third-generation assays reaches 0.005 mU/L. This advance in sensitivity is clinically important because nonspecific lowering of TSH in the range of 0.05 to 0.50 mU/L is common, but truly thyrotoxic values are less than 0.05 mU/L and thus can be detected by the most advanced (third-generation) TSH assays.

Total Serum T_4

The total serum T_4 level, which is measured by competitive protein binding or radioimmunoassay (RIA), comes closest to reflecting the functional state of the thyroid gland in most patients. The T_4 level is high in approximately 90 percent of hyperthyroid patients and low in approximately 85 percent of hypothyroid patients. This sensitivity should make the measurement of the T_4 level an excellent test for hyperthyroidism. Unfortunately, however, the specificity of the total serum T_4 level for hyperthyroidism is much lower. Many factors elevate the level of thyroxine-binding proteins—especially the level of thyroxine-binding globulin, which is the principal thyroxine-binding protein—and therefore raise the serum T_4 level. These factors include pregnancy, oral contraceptives, estrogens, acute infectious hepatitis, and genetic alteration.[9] Conversely, androgens, nephrotic syndrome, hypoproteinemia, and acromegaly each lower thyroxine-binding globulin. In addition, many circumstances other than hyperthyroidism raise the serum T_4 level

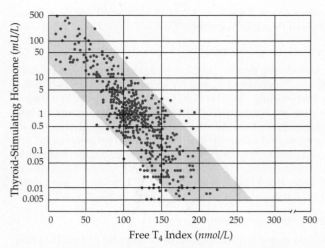

Figure 3 Relation between serum thyroid-stimulating hormone and free T_4 index values in 505 stable ambulatory patients.

without altering the level of thyroxine-binding globulin; these circumstances include increased binding of T_4 to serum albumin, acute nonthyroidal illness, and some drug effects. Additional function tests may be required to clarify resultant changes in the serum T_4 level. Because most of the alterations of total T_4 do not affect the level of free, or unbound, T_4 (FT$_4$), it is often useful to measure this value. There are two approaches to measuring FT$_4$: resin T_3 uptake (RT$_3$U) and direct measurement. RT$_3$U, or one of its modifications, is more widely available than the direct measurement technique.

Resin T_3 Uptake and Free T_4 Index

The measurement of RT$_3$U depends on the relative binding of labeled T_3 to TBG and an artificial resin mixed with the patient's serum. The extent of binding of T_3 to the resin is inversely proportional to the number of unoccupied T_4 binding sites in the patient's blood. The RT$_3$U is best used to illuminate changes in the blood level of T_4 that are not caused by pathological thyroid function. The free T_4 index (FTI), obtained by multiplying the serum T_4 concentration by the RT$_3$U value, provides a guide for interpreting abnormal T_4 values that are caused by elevation or depression of the TBG level. If the T_4 level is high because of an elevated TBG level, the resin T_3 uptake will be low. In such a case, the FTI will be within the normal range (1.3 to 5.1 units), reflecting a normal FT$_4$ level. Conversely, a low level of TBG, causing a low T_4 level, will lead to increased resin uptake. Again, the product of T_4 and resin uptake values will be a normal FTI.

This phenomenon underlies all the indirect efforts to assay the FT$_4$ level. In each instance, an alteration of the T_4 level produced by a change in binding results in a reciprocal alteration of the resin uptake. The product of the two is a normal FTI, indicating that the FT$_4$ is also normal. An elevation of thyroid hormone production, however, will lead to an increase in the number of occupied T_4 binding sites and will produce a parallel increase in RT$_3$U; the product will then indicate an elevated FT$_4$. Because TBG abnormalities, which require an RT$_3$U for clarification, occur fairly frequently, many laboratories routinely do both a total T_4 and an RT$_3$U and report the result as the FTI.[10]

Free T_4

In direct measurement of FT_4, the percentage of FT_4 (%FT_4) is measured by equilibrium dialysis and is then multiplied by the T_4 value, which has already been determined:

$$\%FT_4 \times T_4 = FT_4$$

Direct measurement is especially useful in providing the correct diagnosis in a hyperthyroid patient whose TBG level is low because of malnutrition, for example. In such a patient, the T_4 level appears normal, but the FT_4 level is high. Direct measurement of the FT_4 fraction is notoriously difficult, particularly in such conditions as the euthyroid sick syndrome, in which it would be most valuable.[11] Fortunately, sensitive TSH assays obviate direct measurement of FT_4.

Serum T_3 and Reverse T_3

Less than 25 percent of the circulating T_3 is secreted by the thyroid; the remainder is produced by peripheral monodeiodination of T_4. Sensitive and specific assays for T_3 are useful in the detection or exclusion of hyperthyroidism, in which the T_3 level can rise before the T_4 level does. In some patients, T_3 is the only hormone produced in excess. Caution is needed in evaluating acutely ill thyrotoxic patients, who may have high T_4 and FT_4 levels but a normal T_3 level [see Hyperthyroidism, Laboratory Tests in the Diagnosis of Hyperthyroidism, *below*].

The T_3 level is misleading in at least two circumstances. First, it can be low in euthyroid patients with cirrhosis, uremia, malnutrition, or other disorders in which the conversion of T_4 to T_3 is diminished. Second, the serum T_3 level is low in only about 50 percent of hypothyroid patients. This variability results from the tendency of hypothyroid patients to produce relatively more T_3 than T_4 as the thyroid fails.

The measurement of reverse T_3, although not yet widely available, can illuminate an occasional clinical problem. When rT_3, T_3, and T_4 levels are all elevated, overproduction of thyroid hormone can be assumed. An individual with a normal T_4 level, a low T_3 level, and an elevated rT_3 level is referred to as being euthyroid sick [see Euthyroid Sick Syndrome, *below*].[1]

In ordering thyroid function tests, it is critical to distinguish the assay for T_3 from the measurement of RT_3U. Both tests are often referred to as T_3, but they are different.

Radioactive Iodine Uptake

The radioactive iodine uptake (RAIU) measures the percentage of a tracer dose that enters the thyroid in a given period. An overactive gland generally shows an increased avidity for iodine, whereas an underactive gland shows decreased avidity. However, many shortcomings have reduced the value of the test, so that now it is used less often. The widespread use of iodine in food preservation, for example, has raised the usual stable iodine intake in the United States, thus lowering the percentage uptake of labeled iodine. The normal RAIU value, which must be recalibrated for any population, is now between five and 25 percent at 24 hours. The decrease in normal uptake is significant because it has made separating pathologically low values from low-normal values much more difficult. Moreover, hyperthyroidism can exist with normal or only minimally elevated radioactive iodine uptake levels.

Serum Thyroglobulin

The serum thyroglobulin level, measured by radioimmuno-assay, is detectable in three quarters of normal persons. The normal level ranges from 0 to 30 ng/ml, with a mean of about 10 ng/ml; men have slightly lower values than women. The thyroglobulin level is elevated in patients with hyperthyroidism or thyroiditis and in many patients with thyroid cancer. In hyperthyroidism, this elevation is associated with increased T_4 and T_3 levels. In thyroiditis, however, there is a dissociation, such that T_4 and T_3 are usually normal. The principal use of the thyroglobulin assay is to track the effectiveness of treatment of metastatic thyroid cancer [see Nodules, Nodular Goiters, and Thyroid Cancer, *below*].

Thyrotropin-Releasing Hormone Testing

TRH testing has been almost completely replaced by the immunoradiometric and other supersensitive TSH assays.

Effects of Drugs on Thyroid Function Tests

Medication often alters the results of thyroid function tests, as it does measurements in other areas of medicine. This possibility should be considered when clinical and laboratory findings are at odds.

TESTS TO DETERMINE THE CAUSE OF GOITER

Several types of tests are available for defining the probable pathological basis of thyroid enlargement.

Thyroid Scan

Scintiscanning with technetium-99m (^{99m}Tc) demonstrates iodide-concentrating capacity in the thyroid; scanning with isotopes of iodine reflects both concentration and binding. Hyperfunctioning thyroid tissue is very rarely malignant; nonfunctioning tissue may or may not be malignant. Either ^{99m}Tc or iodine-123 (^{123}I) is preferable to iodine-131 (^{131}I), which exposes the patient to excessive radiation.

Ultrasonography

Scanning by ultrasonography may provide a valuable approach to evaluation of nodular lesions of the thyroid. A combination of A and B mode ultrasonographic studies has provided 90 percent reliability in discriminating between cystic and solid thyroid nodules. Cystic lesions of the thyroid are rarely malignant and can be treated by percutaneous needle aspiration. On the other hand, single solid cold nodules are malignant often enough (10 to 30 percent of the time) to warrant consideration of surgery.

Antibodies to Thyroid Tissue Components

Antibodies that react with components of thyroid tissue are usually present in the serum of patients with hyperthyroidism and are almost always present in the serum of patients with Hashimoto's thyroiditis. A high antibody titer, which is particularly suggestive of Hashimoto's thyroiditis, is very useful in differentiating this condition from thyroid cancer in patients who have goiters that are unusually nodular and hard enough to suggest neoplasm.

Aging and Thyroid Function

A clear delineation of thyroid function in the elderly has been frustrated by the difficulty of identifying truly normative populations and of excluding the influence of nonthyroid illness.

There appears to be a slight decrease in thyroxine release and an offsetting slowing of thyroxine metabolism. As a result, serum T_3 values are slightly lower in the elderly, but for practical purposes, no accommodation for age needs to be made in interpreting function tests. Quite the contrary, thyroid testing (especially TSH) assumes enhanced importance because clinical diagnosis of thyroid dysfunction is notoriously difficult in the elderly.[12]

Hyperthyroidism

Hyperthyroidism is a generic term for any condition in which the body tissues are exposed to a supraphysiologic amount of thyroid hormone.

GRAVES' DISEASE

The most common hyperthyroid condition is Graves' disease, which is also called diffuse toxic goiter. The typical clinical picture of hyperthyroidism in a young adult is very familiar. The patient, more often female than male, reports sweating, palpitations, nervousness, irritability, insomnia, tremor, frequent stools, and weight loss despite a good appetite. Physical examination shows mild proptosis, stare, and lid lag; a smooth, diffuse, nontender goiter; tachycardia, especially after exercise, with loud heart sounds and often a systolic murmur or left sternal border scratch; and tremor, onycholysis, and palmar erythema. A bruit is often heard over the thyroid, and a cervical venous hum is almost always present. When this picture is observed, the disorder can be recognized readily, confirmed with a serum T_4 test, and treated.

Occasionally, patients with Graves' disease have other, more troublesome manifestations. The most disturbing is severe exophthalmos accompanied by ophthalmoplegia, follicular conjunctivitis, chemosis, and even loss of vision.[13] Additional features include dermopathy, pretibial myxedema, clubbing, and, in the most severe instances, acropachy. These signs and symptoms are known as the autoimmune features of Graves' disease, reflecting the belief that this form of hyperthyroidism has an autoimmune pathogenesis.

This concept of Graves' disease emerged when Adams and Purves showed that the serum of many patients with Graves' disease contained a factor that stimulated the mouse thyroid and had a longer duration of action than TSH; this factor was termed long-acting thyroid stimulator (LATS). Various test systems eventually revealed two types of antibodies to the TSH receptor (TRAb) in the sera of patients with Graves' disease.[14] One type is thyroid-stimulating antibody (TSAb); it is identified by its capacity to activate adenylate cyclase and thereby stimulate thyroid function. Another type of antibody to the TSH receptor can inhibit binding of TSH to its receptor but does not activate thyroid cell function; this antibody is termed TSH-binding inhibitor (TBI). Thus, the generic term TRAb embraces immunoglobulins of diverse potential and clinical expression. More than one antibody may be present in the blood of a patient.

The defect that predisposes to autoimmune thyroid disease is not known.[15] Possible mechanisms, which are not mutually exclusive, include (1) a tissue-specific defect in suppressor T cell activity, (2) genetically programmed presentation of a thyroid-specific antigen, and (3) an idiotype–anti-idiotype reaction.[16] The common outcome of these proposed mechanisms is the production of one or more types of TRAb, which results in autonomous overproduction of thyroid hormone.[17] This autonomy explains why hyperthyroid patients do not respond to measures that usually influence TSH. Thus, T_3 does not suppress thyroid function, and TRH does not stimulate it. Many questions remain, however: What triggers TRAb production? How does the production of TRAb relate to (or explain) the variable accompanying features, such as ophthalmopathy and dermopathy? Why is antithyroid therapy or ablative therapy successful? What is the relation of hyperthyroidism to emotional and other presumed precipitating factors?

Whatever the answers to these questions, the Graves' thyroid is driven to hypersecretion of both T_4 and T_3. T_3 elevations in hyperthyroid patients can be explained almost entirely by increased thyroid secretion and release without implicating a significant change of peripheral T_4 metabolism.

DIFFICULTIES IN RECOGNIZING HYPERTHYROIDISM

Florid hyperthyroidism is easy to recognize, confirm, and treat. But the spectrum of hyperthyroidism is much broader, and therefore, it seems appropriate to consider variant manifestations to facilitate recognition of subtler cases.

Hyperthyroidism in the Elderly Patient

In elderly persons, the picture of hyperthyroidism may be altered by several factors, the most important of which is underlying cardiac disease.[18] An increased level of thyroid hormone, by itself too slight to produce typical symptoms of hyperthyroidism, produces symptoms by aggravating the cardiac status. The most common manifestations are the appearance or worsening of angina pectoris, unexplained congestive heart failure, and supraventricular arrhythmias, most often atrial fibrillation. The diagnostic problem arises from the fact that the natural focus is on the cardiac finding. Because the patient is often known to have or has just been found to have organic heart disease, the changes are attributed to progression of the heart condition rather than to the aggravating effect of thyroid hormone excess. The proper diagnosis may also be overlooked because of the absence of a goiter; thyroid enlargement occurs in only 20 to 40 percent of hyperthyroid patients older than 70 years.[19]

A similar sequence occurs in younger persons with cardiac disease. Typically, hyperthyroidism develops gradually over a period of months or years [see Figure 4]. In the absence of underlying heart disease, the thyroid excess itself eventually produces symptoms in most patients. At that time, in more than 90 percent of cases, the T_4 level is elevated, confirming the clinical suspicion. In patients with heart disease, a less marked elevation of thyroid hormone may produce cardiac, not thyroid, symptoms. Furthermore, in such cases the serum T_4 level may be within the normal range; only an elevated T_3 level or a subnormal TSH level will reveal the diagnosis. Diagnosis in such patients rests on compulsive alertness to the possibility of noncardiac factors exacerbating known cardiac disease. Along with fever, anemia, occult infection, paroxysmal rhythm disturbance, anoxia, and pulmonary emboli, hyperthyroidism should be considered as a potential exacerbating factor. Because clinical findings may be minimal, it is prudent to do a sensitive TSH assay in every patient with unexplained congestive heart failure, new atrial fibrillation, or inexplicably worsening angina pectoris [see Chapters 19, 20, and 22, respectively]. Most determinations will be normal, but a small number of patients with curable thyrotoxicosis will be discovered.

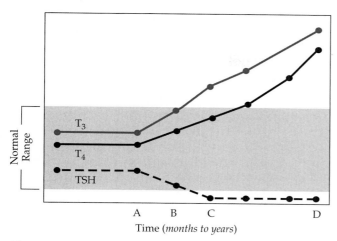

Figure 4 Levels of T_4 (solid black curve), T_3 (solid blue curve), and TSH (broken black curve) are normal early in the progression of hyperthyroidism (stage A). A stage B, where thyroid secretion has already increased, is presumed, but even an ultrasensitive TSH assay does not definitively demonstrate suppression. At stage C, a further excess of the thyroid hormones develops, which is sufficient to exacerbate cardiac symptoms. T_4 may be within the upper-normal range and T_3 minimally elevated, making diagnosis difficult. However, the TSH level is typically depressed at this point, and its measurement by the sensitive TSH assay can yield the diagnosis. In the absence of cardiac symptoms, hyperthyroidism is generally not detected until both T_4 and T_3 are substantially above normal (stage D) and thyrotoxic symptoms are evident.

The arrhythmias associated with hyperthyroidism may not be as benign as has often been thought. In one series of 262 patients with hyperthyroidism and atrial fibrillation, 21 patients had 26 episodes of major arterial embolization. In addition, severe hyperthyroidism itself (i.e., without underlying heart disease) can produce congestive heart failure.

Monosymptomatic Hyperthyroidism

Excess thyroid hormone usually produces multiple symptoms and signs. In some patients, however, the disease so emphasizes one symptom that it is confused with other disorders that can cause the same symptom. Some outstanding examples are myopathy, inanition, gonadal dysfunction, and personality changes.

Myopathy Muscular weakness is typical of hyperthyroidism. In some patients, particularly older men, this feature is exaggerated, and symmetric weakness and wasting of large muscles are the dominant features. Breathing may be affected. For unknown reasons, these patients usually have a small goiter and no eye signs.

Inanition Hypermetabolism and weight loss are common features of hyperthyroidism. In a few elderly patients, weight loss predominates and hypermetabolism is difficult to recognize. Factors contributing to weight loss include anorexia (progressively more common as the age of the patient increases), vitamin deficiency, diarrhea, and hepatic congestion. Testing may be misleading in malnourished patients. TBG and T_4 levels may be normal or even low as a consequence of liver disease and protein depletion. The clues to the diagnosis are then

found in a suppressed TSH level and an elevated FT_4 or T_3 level. An elevated T_3 level is particularly significant because in chronic disease and malnutrition without hyperthyroidism, the serum T_3 level is often low. In fact, a T_3 level in the normal range in an ill person suggests hyperthyroidism; this result is produced by an increase in the T_4 level combined with a blockage of 5' deiodination.[20]

Gonadal dysfunction A change in reproductive function may be a presenting complaint. In women, the gonadal disorder is usually oligomenorrhea. In men, it can be impotence or gynecomastia, and serum estrogen, testosterone, and sex hormone–binding globulin levels may be significantly elevated. The amount of testosterone that is not bound to sex hormone–binding globulins is decreased, however, and the level of free testosterone is usually normal.[21]

Neuropsychiatric features Nervousness and irritability are routine in hyperthyroidism, but in some patients, major mental changes dominate the picture. Frank psychosis is rare, but severe personality disturbances can occur. Thyrotoxic periodic paralysis associated with hypokalemia is rare in the United States but is more frequent in Asian populations.[22]

VARIANTS OF HYPERTHYROIDISM

The instances of thyroid hyperfunction that are not caused by an autoimmune mechanism are distinct syndromes with unique clinicopathologic correlates. In this section, they are reviewed and contrasted with Graves' disease to highlight diagnostic features.

Toxic Nodular Goiter

Although understanding of Graves' disease has grown, there has been no comparable advance in the interpretation of toxic nodular goiter.[23] The clinical picture is rather different. In many cases of toxic nodular goiter, a goiter will have been present for years. The results of prior thyroid testing may have been normal, although subtle tests of suppressibility give abnormal results in a quarter of patients. Very gradually, autonomous overproduction of thyroid hormone develops.[24] In an older patient with underlying disease in other organs, the confusing findings that were outlined previously may appear. The thyroid gland shows pathological findings that are a variable mixture of hyperplasia, involution, fibrosis, and calcification. In a significant number of patients (more than in Graves' disease), the T_4 level is not strikingly high; the clue to the disease is an elevated FT_4 level, an elevated T_3 level, or a suppressed TSH level. RAIU measurements are often within the normal range; uptake values as low as 10 to 20 percent are consistent with the diagnosis of toxic nodular goiter.

Plummer's Nodule, or Toxic Adenoma

Plummer's nodule may be a variant of toxic nodular goiter in which hyperthyroidism is caused by overproduction of thyroid hormone by a single adenoma of the thyroid known as a toxic adenoma. Consequently, thyroid gland activity and production of TSH are suppressed. The pathogenesis of this lesion is a somatic mutation in the TSH receptor in the cells of the nodule itself [see Figure 5]. As a consequence, the receptor is constitutively activated (i.e., the receptor does not need a stimulating ligand) and the nodule is overactive.[25,26] On physical ex-

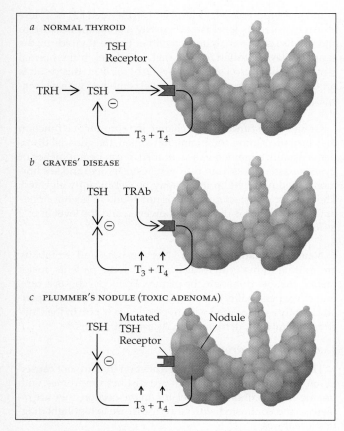

a NORMAL THYROID

b GRAVES' DISEASE

c PLUMMER'S NODULE (TOXIC ADENOMA)

Figure 5 (*a*) Normally, the production of T_3 and T_4 by the thyroid is kept in balance by TSH, and in turn, T_3 prevents the overproduction of TSH. (*b*) In Graves' disease, a TSH receptor antibody (TRAb) attaches itself to the TSH receptor, causing the thyroid to produce excessive amounts of T_3 and T_4 and thereby increasing the inhibitory effect of T_3 on TSH production. (*c*) A toxic nodule, such as Plummer's nodule, causes a mutation of the TSH receptor. The resulting increase in T_4 and in T_3 diminishes the inhibitory effect on TSH production.

amination, the distinctive feature in Plummer's nodule is an isolated lump in an atrophic thyroid. Scanning confirms that the rest of the thyroid is inactive, and uptake of radioiodine is confined to the palpable mass. A repeat scan after administration of TSH (e.g., Thytropar, 10 units intramuscularly) will frequently demonstrate uptake in the rest of the gland. Plummer's nodule is the form of hyperthyroidism that carries the most favorable prognosis: ablation of the adenoma by either radioactive iodine or surgery is followed by resumption of normal function in the remainder of the gland, and there is almost no risk of either recurrence or hypothyroidism after therapy.

Spontaneously Resolving Hyperthyroidism

A syndrome of spontaneously resolving hyperthyroidism accompanying thyroiditis has been described [*see* Thyroiditis, *below*].

Pharmacologically Masked Hyperthyroidism

The term masked hyperthyroidism has been used to describe patients whose symptoms are caused by an overactive thyroid but do not call attention to their thyroid origin. Similarly, the use of beta blockers can mask many of the symptoms of hyperthyroidism. Patients taking beta blockers who happen to develop hyperthyroidism experience minimal palpitations, tachycardia, sweating, or tremor; the presenting features usually are unexplained weight loss and personality changes. The physical examination in such cases may be almost normal unless goiter or eye signs are present. Fortunately, laboratory tests for hyperthyroidism are not affected by beta blockers and thus can be used to confirm the diagnosis.

Rarer Forms of Hyperthyroidism

Several rarer forms of hyperthyroidism are seen often enough to warrant consideration. In the Jod-Basedow phenomenon, hyperthyroidism is precipitated by sudden exposure to large amounts of iodine. First recognized in Europe in the 1800s, this phenomenon is usually seen in countries in which the diet is iodine deficient; occasionally, goitrous persons in the United States manifest this disorder. The common factor appears to be the prior existence of thyroid hyperplasia or thyroid adenoma, presumably associated with an increased blood supply to the thyroid gland.[27] When, in this setting, the patient begins to ingest large amounts of iodine, massive overproduction of thyroid hormone occasionally occurs; the result is an abrupt onset of clinical features of hypermetabolism. In addition to medicinal iodine or iodide, radiographic contrast media and iodine-containing drugs, such as amiodarone, have been implicated. Indeed, both hyperthyroidism and hypothyroidism have been important complications of amiodarone use. A history of iodine ingestion and preexistent goiter suggests the diagnosis of the Jod-Basedow phenomenon. Although the T_4 level is elevated, the serum T_3 level is often normal. The RAIU is often low.

The antiarrhythmic drug amiodarone has several effects on thyroid function. In euthyroid individuals, there is often an increase in the free T_4 level, a decrease in the free T_3 level, and a decrease in binding of T_3 to nuclear receptors.[28] However, in areas of low iodine intake, hyperthyroidism gradually develops in approximately 10 percent of amiodarone-treated subjects, who exhibit an elevated T_4 level and a normal or increased level of T_3. Hyperthyroidism is occasionally very severe in these patients, particularly when their underlying heart disease cannot be corrected.[29] The radioactive iodine uptake is low in patients without a goiter, but the uptake is often normal and sometimes high in those with either diffuse or nodular goiters.[30]

All forms of hyperthyroidism can occur or recur during pregnancy, but a self-limited variant accompanies hyperemesis gravidarum.[31,32] In patients with hyperemesis gravidarum, there is a direct correlation between the hyperthyroidism and the severity of the vomiting and accompanying metabolic disorders. High levels of human chorionic gonadotropin (HCG) appear to account for the thyroid stimulation, and the disorder abates by the 18th week of gestation.

Patients with hydatidiform mole occasionally show a syndrome of hyperthyroidism without accompanying autoimmune phenomena. The mole apparently secretes a thyrotropic substance that induces diffuse thyroid hyperplasia and hyperfunction. The thyrotropic substance may be HCG, which, because of its molecular similarity to thyrotropin, binds to the TSH receptor and stimulates cAMP production. Alternatively, a different compound or a modified form of HCG may be involved.

Factitious hyperthyroidism is an uncommon but important

condition. It tends to occur in medical personnel or in the families of patients with thyroid disease. The abuse of either thyroxine or triiodothyronine can produce the syndrome; there are no consistent differences between the two clinical pictures, although one clinical impression is that tachycardia and headache may be more frequent with triiodothyronine abuse. Clinical clues include absence of eye signs other than lid lag and widened palpebral fissure, absence of goiter, absence of associated autoimmune phenomena, and the presence of neurotic symptoms. The RAIU is low. If the patient has taken thyroxine, both T_4 and T_3 levels are high; if only triiodothyronine has been ingested, T_3 will be high and T_4 low. In either case, the TSH will be suppressed.

Finally, in one series, thyroid disease associated with TRAb developed in 2.5 percent of patients treated with recombinant interferon alfa for chronic viral hepatitis. Hyperthyroidism developed in three of six patients, two of whom had detectable thyroid-stimulating immunoglobulin (TSIg); hypothyroidism developed in the other three patients, who had high levels of antithyroid antibodies. This early finding needs to be watched, particularly because the thyroid disorders did not remit after interferon therapy was stopped, and therefore, active therapy was required.[33]

Inappropriate Secretion of TSH

Increases in the serum level of thyroid hormone normally inhibit TSH secretion; thus, TSH is generally undetectable in hyperthyroidism. There are increasing reports, however, of thyrotoxic patients who have measurable or elevated TSH levels.[34] The most straightforward examples are patients who have pituitary tumors secreting TSH and thereby driving the thyroid to overproduce hormone. These patients lack the autoimmune features of Graves' disease and may have signs of pituitary tumor such as headache or visual field defect. Their TSH levels are variably elevated and usually do not increase after TRH administration. Neuroradiological studies, especially computed tomography scans, should be done on hyperthyroid patients whose TSH level is not suppressed.[35]

In patients without tumors, inappropriate secretion of TSH is a consequence of resistance to the effects of thyroid hormone. When this resistance is confined to the pituitary, the persistent secretion of TSH and thyroid hormones leads to clinical hyperthyroidism. When the resistance is general, the patient is euthyroid, even though TSH, T_4, and T_3 levels are elevated. The syndromes of generalized resistance to thyroid hormone are discussed elsewhere [see Hypothyroidism and Myxedema, below].

LABORATORY TESTS IN THE DIAGNOSIS OF HYPERTHYROIDISM

The serum T_4 level is raised in more than 90 percent of hyperthyroid patients, and thus, the sensitivity of this assay is extremely high. But many hyperthyroxinemic patients are not hyperthyroid; that is, the specificity of the total T_4 assay is far lower than its sensitivity. For this reason, the combined use of a free thyroxine index and a sensitive TSH assay is now the preferred approach to the diagnosis of hyperthyroidism.[36] The occasional hyperthyroid patient who has an elevated T_3 level but a normal T_4 level will be detected by the suppressed TSH level.

The laboratory tests useful in the diagnosis of hyperthyroidism are summarized as follows:

1. To confirm clinically obvious hyperthyroidism, measurement of the FT_4 level is the simplest and most widely available test. A suppressed TSH level is as sensitive as FT_4 and more specific than FT_4. The serum T_3 level is sometimes elevated when the T_4 is not [see Figure 4].

2. An FT_4 level is often useful when the patient is taking a medication that alters TBG levels.

3. When the goal is to exclude hyperthyroidism as the diagnosis, the sensitive TSH assay is best: a normal value, combined with a normal FTI, is adequate to rule out this diagnosis.

4. Familial dysalbuminemic hyperthyroxinemia (FDH) can also cause misleading elevation of the serum T_4 level. Patients with FDH are euthyroid and have no goiter or eye signs. Their elevated T_4 level reflects the presence of a serum albumin variant that has a greatly enhanced affinity for T_4. To the unwary, the increased T_4 level and FTI suggest hyperthyroidism, but the true FT_4, the serum T_3, and the TSH levels are all normal, permitting differentiation of this disorder.

5. RAIU is not usually needed to confirm the diagnosis of hyperthyroidism and therefore is often omitted from the workup. The growing frequency of thyroiditis associated with hyperthyroidism, however, now indicates that an uptake measurement should be done routinely to determine not the presence but the type of hyperthyroidism.

TREATMENT OF HYPERTHYROIDISM

Three principal therapies are available for hyperthyroidism: antithyroid drugs, subtotal thyroidectomy, and radioactive iodine. Several factors influence the selection of therapy.[37,38]

Antithyroid Drugs

Antithyroid drugs are reversible, effective in most patients, and generally safe. They principally block oxidation of iodine and its incorporation into tyrosine residues.[39] Propylthiouracil, in an initial dosage of 100 mg every eight hours, or methimazole, in an initial dosage of 10 mg every eight to 12 hours, will render almost all patients euthyroid in one to six months. In an effort to simplify treatment and encourage compliance, a single daily dose of methimazole, 20 to 40 mg, can be tried in any but the most florid cases.[40] Methimazole is probably preferable to propylthiouracil for most patients because it can be administered once a day, produces fewer adverse reactions, and is less expensive. Propylthiouracil is preferable during pregnancy and perhaps for treating thyroid storm. In addition to blocking thyroid hormone synthesis, methimazole increases the number and activity of suppressor T cells and diminishes the activity of helper T cells. As a result, the drug inhibits production of antimicrosomal and anti–TSH receptor antibodies.

The complications of antithyroid drugs are allergic ones: minor or major skin reactions, arthralgias, hepatitis, and agranulocytosis, a potentially serious but rare occurrence. Agranulocytosis occurs most often in patients older than 40 years who are given more than 30 mg of methimazole a day. Standard dosages of propylthiouracil in patients older than 40 years may also cause agranulocytosis. All of the complications tend to resolve spontaneously if drugs are withdrawn promptly.

There are several subtleties to the use of antithyroid drugs. If, after being rendered euthyroid, the patient is kept on the initial dosage, hypothyroidism often results. Any of the symptoms of hypothyroidism may develop, but certain ones—arthralgias, paresthesias, muscle cramps, and enlarging goiter—are particularly common in recently hyperthyroid patients who have been rapidly rendered hypothyroid. To avoid hypothyroidism when the patient has entered the euthyroid range or when the level of TSH, previously suppressed by the toxic state, begins to rise, either 0.1 mg of thyroxine daily can be added or the dosage of antithyroid drug can be reduced; the correct combination of antithyroid drug and thyroxine replacement can be maintained if the TSH level is kept between 1 and 5 mU/L.[41] This regimen is continued for a year. A high frequency of recurrences has been a problem in choosing drug therapy.[42,43] Favorable prognostic signs for permanent remission include a short history, mild disease, and a small goiter, the last being the most useful.[44] Although one report suggested that simultaneous thyroxine therapy greatly reduced the recurrence of hyperthyroidism after antithyroid drugs were stopped,[41] further experience has not confirmed that observation.[45-48]

Attempts to predict recurrence of hyperthyroidism are of limited value if only a single course of antithyroid drug is planned. I tend to recommend antithyroid drugs to persons younger than 30 years, especially women, who have had a recent onset of the disease and who have a small goiter. I give the drugs for a year, using supplementary thyroxine as described, and then stop them and see what happens. If there is a recurrence, ablative therapy is indicated.

Beta blockers are a valuable adjunct in the treatment of hyperthyroidism.[49] Without altering basic thyroid function or test results, these drugs alleviate many of the symptoms, such as palpitation, excess sweating, tachycardia, nervousness, and tremors. Thus, patients can feel better while waiting for the effects of antithyroid drugs or ablative therapy to emerge. In transient hyperthyroid states, such as spontaneously resolving hyperthyroidism or some postpartum episodes, beta blockade alone may be used. The usual contraindications, such as asthma and congestive heart failure, should be observed. The daily dose of atenolol is about 200 mg; nadolol, 80 mg; and propranolol, 160 mg. Much larger doses of propranolol are sometimes needed.

Subtotal Thyroidectomy

Although much less often used now, subtotal thyroidectomy is a venerable approach to hyperthyroidism. For reasons that remain obscure, extensive but incomplete removal induces remission in most patients with Graves' disease. The operation is difficult, and recent graduates of even very good surgical training programs are likely to have had relatively little experience performing it. Even in excellent hands, there is a trade-off between the possibility of myxedema and that of incomplete control or recurrence of hyperthyroidism. Additional complications include hemorrhage, hypoparathyroidism, and damage to the recurrent laryngeal nerve; however, they seldom occur if the surgeon is experienced.

Until about 1980, most hyperthyroid patients were rendered euthyroid before surgery by a combination of antithyroid drugs and, for seven to 10 days before surgery, potassium iodide. Patients who were euthyroid had a lower risk of surgically induced thyroid storm; iodide also reduced the vascularity of the thyroid gland. The introduction of propranolol led to its use as the sole preparation for subtotal thyroidectomy.[50,51] The purported advantages include rapid preparation for surgery, less blood loss than after preparation with antithyroid drugs and

iodine, and no increase in postoperative exacerbation of hyperthyroidism. However, this approach requires expert anesthetic administration and surgery, tight teamwork, unfailing administration of propranolol just before and soon after surgery, and alert use of atropine to counteract propranolol-induced bradycardia. A long-acting beta blocker, such as nadolol, is easier to use than propranolol because the blood level of nadolol is more predictable and nadolol can be administered the morning after surgery rather than immediately after surgery. Rapid preparation for surgery with beta blockers alone seems to work well in patients who have mild to moderate hyperthyroidism. In more severe cases, the addition of iodide for 10 days preoperatively reduces the elevated thyroxine level to the normal range and thereby reduces the risk of hyperthyroid-related complications.

Hypothyroidism develops after surgery at a frequency (two to three percent a year) that is quite comparable to the frequency at which hypothyroidism develops after low doses of radioiodine. In a Mayo Clinic series, more than 75 percent of patients who had had a thyroidectomy had at least chemical, or subclinical, hypothyroidism five years later. The trend to hypothyroidism may be related to the inherent tendency of Graves' disease to abate with time. Two follow-up studies of patients who had been rendered euthyroid with drugs and had had no subsequent therapy showed that a significant percentage had become hypothyroid several years later. Thus, regardless of therapy, a patient with hyperthyroidism must be followed indefinitely to see whether hyperthyroidism recurs or hypothyroidism develops.

Radioactive Iodine Therapy

The preferential entry of iodine into the thyroid gland and the availability of an isotope (^{131}I) with primarily short-distance penetration provide a singular method of delivering high-dose radiation to the diseased tissue while largely sparing the rest of the body.[52] Several million patients have been treated with radioactive iodine, which has been in use since the mid-1940s. The experience can be summarized as follows[53,54]:

1. Almost all patients with hyperthyroidism caused by Graves' disease and an only slightly smaller percentage of patients with toxic nodular goiter can be rendered euthyroid with radioactive iodine, provided enough is given.

2. The surgical complications of bleeding, hypoparathyroidism, and hoarseness are avoided.

3. All effective treatment programs carry a risk of hypothyroidism, which may develop at any time after treatment.

4. There has been no increased incidence of thyroid malignancy, leukemia, or other cancer in patients treated with radioactive iodine.

5. No genetic damage has been documented; however, undetected detriment cannot be excluded.

From the patient's viewpoint, therefore, radioactive iodine is associated with only two risks: the unknown and unmeasurable risk of genetic damage to gametes, probably of particular significance in women, and the possible development of hypothyroidism. The frequency of immediate hypothyroidism and its annual rate of appearance are proportional to the dose of radioiodine: smaller doses (3 to 6 mCi) lead to lower initial cure rates and lower rates of early hypothyroidism than do larger doses. Some physicians regard the higher rate of hypothyroidism associated with higher doses of radioiodine (> 10 mCi) as an inevitable accompaniment of effective treatment.

The main significance of radioiodine-induced hypothyroidism is its delayed and subtle onset. The insidious symptoms of hypothyroidism are not disabling but can include a degree of apathy that delays recognition and leaves patients handicapped for significant periods. If prolonged and conscientious follow-up is maintained, including regular measurements of TSH, the risk of undetected hypothyroidism is minimized. Such follow-up is a responsibility that must be assumed when ablative therapy is offered for hyperthyroidism.

Choice of Treatment in Hyperthyroidism

Given the uncertainties and conflicting opinions in the literature, are there any generalizations to guide individual choices of therapy?[38] Certainly, no one uses radioactive iodine during pregnancy, and almost everyone uses it for patients who have had a recurrence after surgery. There is also almost universal agreement that radioactive iodine is the treatment of choice for hyperthyroid patients older than 40 years; in such patients, antithyroid drugs may be used initially for the rapid alleviation of cardiac or respiratory symptoms. For all other patients, it is necessary to assess the individual circumstances, explain the options, and provide regular follow-up to keep the patient euthyroid and protected from risk. Two polls of experienced thyroidologists have revealed the prevailing therapeutic choices.[55] In both polls, the clinicians were asked to recommend therapy for hypothetical patients. Radioactive iodine was strongly favored for all patients older than 40 years, with antithyroid drugs a weak second and surgery a distant third. For women younger than 30 years, antithyroid drug therapy was chosen by almost two thirds of the respondents.

Subtotal thyroidectomy is effective for patients who are apprehensive about radioactive iodine and who are not suitable candidates for drug therapy. I have found it an excellent option for young women who are eager to be free of the disease and who want to conceive without worry about possible delayed effects of radioiodine.

Hyperthyroidism that is present during pregnancy often requires no treatment, either because the disease is mild or because it sometimes resolves spontaneously.[56] When therapy is needed during pregnancy, the preferred treatment is propylthiouracil, 200 to 400 mg daily in divided doses. It is advisable to minimize or omit drug therapy in the final trimester to avoid transplacental passage of the drug and the risk of hypothyroidism or goiter in the fetus. Thyroxine (0.1 mg/day) has been reported to greatly reduce the postpartum recurrence of hyperthyroidism. If the patient's goiter is large—an indication that the withdrawal of drugs in the final trimester will lead to a flareup—it is best to render her euthyroid with an antithyroid drug and to do a subtotal thyroidectomy in the second trimester.

The TRAb level should be measured in the last trimester of pregnancy in women who have or have had Graves' disease. A high level of thyroid stimulator suggests that the fetus or newborn may have transient hyperthyroidism from transplacental transfer of TRAb and is an indication for pediatric endocrine consultation.

In choosing a therapy for hyperthyroidism, individual considerations are important. In this disease, perhaps as much as in any other, it is practical to inform the patient fully and let him or her join in the decision. A word of caution, however, is useful: thyrotoxic patients are nervous and irritable and often have difficulty concentrating. Presenting such patients with the therapeutic possibilities and their implications and requesting that a choice be made may constitute an intolerable burden. A simple solution is to institute antithyroid drug therapy and then discuss the problems electively as the patient becomes euthyroid. Therapy allows patients to achieve a calmness and perspective that enables them to play a responsible and involved role. Because improvement begins as soon as antithyroid drugs are started, no time is lost for any of the therapies ultimately elected.

Most patients can be treated in an ambulatory setting, often with little alteration in their ordinary activities. Some patients, however, are nutritionally depleted, and others have acute cardiac difficulties; for both of these groups, a judicious selection among the following supplementary modalities can markedly affect the speed of recovery and the interim morbidity:

1. Bed rest—a measure that has great value in blunting the severity of complicating angina pectoris or congestive heart failure.
2. Nutritional supplementation—especially protein and vitamin B.
3. Sedation—using phenobarbital, chlordiazepoxide, or a similar agent.
4. Propranolol—given as outlined earlier (reserpine should not be used with propranolol).

Once the diagnosis of hyperthyroidism is made, the physician and patient should be committed to lifelong follow-up. A schedule of regular visits should be set up and followed strictly. A sensitive method for the detection of hypothyroidism, such as measurement of the serum TSH level, should be used. However, there is persistent difference of opinion about the significance of a mildly elevated TSH level. Although a mildly elevated TSH level can herald hypothyroidism and although some authorities feel it is intrinsic evidence of hypothyroidism, at least of the pituitary, a slightly elevated TSH level can persist a long time without clinical or other laboratory evidence of hypothyroidism. Therefore, it is not critical to begin replacement therapy on the first observation of an elevated TSH level unless there is clinical evidence of hypothyroidism.

Treatment of Thyroid Storm

In some patients, a severe exacerbation of hyperthyroidism known as thyroid storm develops.[57] The disorder is difficult to define precisely; as a result, incidence figures vary widely. The term should probably be restricted to a severe and prostrating illness characterized by fever, severe tachycardia, extreme sweating, and pronounced restlessness, leading ultimately, if unchecked, to dehydration and shock. Thyroid storm is rarely the initial manifestation of hyperthyroidism, although it may be the event that brings the patient to seek medical attention. Usually, it supervenes in the course of smoldering hyperthyroidism, particularly in one of the following settings: superimposed infection; surgery, either of the thyroid or elsewhere; withdrawal of partially effective antithyroid therapy; after trauma to the thyroid; or after high-dose radioiodine therapy for hyperthyroidism.

If the prior thyroid disease is recognized, the diagnosis of thyroid storm need not present difficulty. If the underlying diagnosis is missed, the identification of thyroid storm may be delayed.[58,59] Recognition is facilitated by thinking of the patient as burning up: fever is disproportionate to the infection; tachycardia is disproportionate to the fever; and restlessness and tremor are present without explanation. Once considered, the diagnosis is usually straightforward; measurement of the serum TSH, T_3, and T_4 levels should be initiated, and emergency antithyroid therapy should be started before there is laboratory confirmation. The following program usually results in prompt improvement of the condition:

1. Propylthiouracil, 100 mg administered orally or by Levin tube every six hours.
2. Sodium iodide, 0.5 g I.V. twice a day, the first dose to be given at least one-half hour after the antithyroid drug. The two drugs are used together because they complement each other. Iodide works immediately to block the release of thyroid hormone, but it is also the precursor for new hormone synthesis. For the former effect, iodide will work; for the latter, oxidation to iodine is necessary. Giving the antithyroid drug first prevents oxidation, thus preserving the effect of iodide on hormone release while preventing its oxidation to iodine and incorporation into new hormone. Some physicians favor the use of radiographic dyes such as sodium ipodate or iopanoate instead of potassium iodide.[60]
3. Propranolol, 40 mg every six hours; in the absence of contraindications, a higher dosage may be used.
4. Dexamethasone, 0.5 mg every six hours, is useful as a corticosteroid; moreover, it decreases the conversion of T_4 to T_3.
5. Aggressive replacement of volume deficit.
6. Treatment of infection, if suspected.

Treatment of Rare Forms of Hyperthyroidism

There is a specific approach to treatment of each of the rare forms of hyperthyroidism [see Variants of Hyperthyroidism, above]. Hyperthyroidism caused by pituitary TSH production by a tumor can be treated with antithyroid drugs temporarily, but ultimately, an attack on the primary lesion is preferable to ablative thyroid therapy. Patients with increased TSH levels and thyroid hormone resistance may be cautiously given some thyroxine or triiodothyronine, but as yet, there is no satisfactory therapy for this group of hyperthyroid patients. The Jod-Basedow phenomenon should be treated by withdrawal of iodine and administration of antithyroid drugs and propranolol; the patient should then be observed to see whether these measures suffice without ablative therapy. Amiodarone-induced hyperthyroidism can be treated with methimazole plus potassium perchlorate in patients with underlying nodular goiter or Graves' disease; prednisone can be helpful in patients who have no goiter.[61] On rare occasions, emergency thyroidectomy is needed.[62]

Factitious or iatrogenic disease should be treated with rest and propranolol as well as psychotherapy. Patients with molar pregnancy should be treated with propranolol, antithyroid drugs if needed to make surgery safe, and molectomy. Finally, there is a transient form of hyperthyroidism that occurs in association with thyroiditis two to 20 weeks post partum.[63] Affected patients have a low RAIU, which predicts that the disorder will resolve spontaneously. The administration of a beta blocker, along with temporary simple sedation if needed, should suffice.

MALIGNANT EXOPHTHALMOS

Most patients with hyperthyroidism have minimal eye signs, including proptosis, lid lag, and widening of the palpebral fissures. Occasionally, patients with Graves' disease have a more troublesome syndrome, malignant exophthalmos, which consists variably of severe proptosis, inflammatory changes in the conjunctivae, ophthalmoplegia, and visual loss.[64] These phenomena do not necessarily parallel the course of hyperthyroidism, and although they are part of Graves' disease, they show distinctive clinical features that have never been explained.[65] Unlike hyperthyroidism, malignant exophthalmos virtually never occurs before puberty, and it affects males and females equally. Graves' ophthalmopathy is best regarded as part of a spectrum of pathological features that includes ophthalmopathy, nonsuppressible thyroid function (usually with hyperthyroidism), dermopathy, and Hashimoto's thyroiditis.

There is a wide variation of opinion about the proper therapy for malignant exophthalmos.[66] All authorities agree that the patient should be rendered and kept euthyroid; the choice of therapy for the hyperthyroidism can be made on the usual grounds because the type of therapy has little effect on the course of the ophthalmopathy. Some studies showed that radioiodine was associated with a higher incidence of ophthalmopathy, but in these studies, patients were allowed to become hypothyroid.[67,68] It is, however, desirable to avoid hypothyroidism.[69] In addition to treating the thyroid, it is desirable to institute local hygienic measures to keep the cornea moist and the sclera covered at night. For severe inflammatory changes, which may produce the disturbing side effect of chemosis, elevation of the head of the bed and intermittent diuretic therapy can be helpful; most clinics also advise corticosteroid therapy. Surgical decompression of the orbit may occasionally be necessary, but plasmapheresis can sometimes obviate that procedure.[70] In any event, severe ophthalmopathy requires endocrine consultation as well as ophthalmologic advice. The physician's primary responsibilities include early referral, careful follow-up, supervision of local and diuretic therapy, maintenance of the euthyroid state, and provision of advice and support.[71]

SUBCLINICAL HYPERTHYROIDISM

The sensitivity of third-generation TSH assays has disclosed several groups of patients with suppressed TSH but normal levels of T_4 and T_3. These patients include those overtreated with thyroxine replacement (the largest group) and others with Graves' disease or autonomously functioning single or multiple nodules. In such patients, the management decisions are clear, but there are numerous patients with no symptoms of any kind. It is very difficult to determine how best to manage these symptomless patients. In one important study, one third of such patients followed for 10 years experienced atrial fibrillation. This observation has led some clinicians to suggest radioactive iodine treatment of all patients with subclinical hyperthyroidism, but most authorities favor careful follow-up, with repeat TSH measurements, and careful scrutiny for any clinical evidence of hyperthyroidism.[72,73]

Hypothyroidism and Myxedema

Hypothyroidism is the generic term for exposure of the body tissues to a subnormal amount of thyroid hormone. Myxedema refers to the full-blown syndrome of cold intolerance, thick dry skin, hoarse voice, constipation, apathy, and retarded speech and reactions. Mild symptoms, often discovered incidentally by an alert physician, are much more common than the severe picture of myxedema. Subclinical hypothyroidism has also been detected.

PATHOGENESIS AND CLINICAL PICTURE

Inadequate production of thyroid hormone can result from a wide variety of causes [see Table 1]. The most frequent causes are chronic Hashimoto's thyroiditis and ablative therapy for hyperthyroidism. A less common cause is neck irradiation for cancers such as lymphoma. Amiodarone can cause hypothyroidism as well as hyperthyroidism; neither effect requires preexisting thyroid disease. Other iodine-containing medications can also induce hypothyroidism, especially in patients with subclinical or compensated autoimmune thyroiditis. The presence of immunoglobulins that bind to the TSH receptor but do not stimulate thyroid function can also lead to thyroid deficiency. Lastly, hypothalamic or pituitary deficiency can cause secondary hypothyroidism; this mechanism accounts for less than five percent of cases.

The clinical picture of hypothyroidism depends on the age and sex of the patient, the site of the defect (pituitary or thyroid), and the rate of development of the deficiency. As with hyperthyroidism, the complete syndrome of myxedema is obvious. Diagnosis is still very much delayed for reasons that include slow progression of the disease, an intrinsic apathy that minimizes patients' complaints, and overlap with other conditions. A further parallel with hyperthyroidism is that any of the component symptoms of myxedema may dominate the picture. These symptoms include constipation, skin changes, edema, anovulation, headache, arthralgias, hoarseness, and fatigue. In patients who become hypothyroid quickly (e.g., from overtreatment of hyperthyroidism), myalgias, arthralgias, and paresthesias often dominate the picture.

Making the diagnosis of hypothyroidism on physical examination depends a great deal on the circumstances under which the patient is seen. The best chance is on first meeting a new patient and on hearing the patient speak; once a patient's looks and voice have become familiar, it is easy to miss the subtle progression of the disease while seeing the person for some other problem. In considering hypothyroidism, an invaluable trick is to look at an old photo of the patient; the cumulative effect of minor changes may then become apparent. The presence of a goiter may be a diagnostic help. Even in the seeming absence of hypothyroid symptoms, the evaluation of a goiter

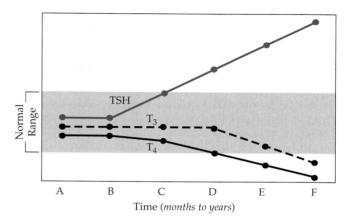

Figure 6   **The development of autoimmune thyroiditis progressively alters the level of thyroid-stimulating hormone (TSH), T_4, and T_3. At A, thyroid function is normal. At B, thyroid function is normal, but antithyroid antibodies and lymphocytic infiltration are present; at this stage, the thyroid may be palpably enlarged. At C, the T_4 level is slightly low and the TSH level is borderline elevated, but no clinical disturbance is apparent; however, administration of TRH will induce an exaggerated TSH response. At D, the T_4 level is borderline or low, the TSH level is increased, and hypothyroid symptoms are likely to be present. At E, the T_4 level is severely depressed, and the patient is usually markedly symptomatic; nevertheless, the serum T_3 is still within the normal range. At F, all tests are abnormal, and profound myxedema would be apparent. The TSH response to TRH injection changes as thyroid impairment progresses.**

should include a serum TSH assay. An elevated value can point to the diagnosis of hypothyroidism before the patient is aware of the disease [see Figure 6].

Pituitary hypothyroidism occurs secondary to hypothalamic or pituitary deficiency. Hypogonadism, which presents as either amenorrhea or impotence, almost invariably develops before pituitary hypothyroidism. Although secondary hypothyroidism is often milder than the primary condition, it can be equally severe. Hyperprolactinemia can occur either with a pituitary tumor or as a consequence of primary thyroid deficiency. Because the pituitary can enlarge when thyroid failure occurs, it is mandatory to measure the TSH level to distinguish between primary and secondary hypothyroidism; the TSH level is elevated when thyroid gland failure is the basic problem.

The frequency of Sheehan's syndrome, or hypopituitarism secondary to peripartum obstetric catastrophe, has diminished as obstetric care has improved; however, a history of shock during delivery and a failure to nurse or resume menstruation is still worth seeking in patients with hypothyroidism. Indeed, as concern about acquired immunodeficiency syndrome (AIDS) has made patients reluctant to receive transfusions, Sheehan's syndrome has been identified in patients who have peripartum anemia but who are not given transfusions.

Hypothyroidism is generally irreversible and progressive. One exception to this rule is drug-induced hypothyroidism, which remits on withdrawal of the drug. Two additional causes of reversible hypothyroidism have now been described. In one study, 20 percent of hyperthyroid patients who were prepared for subtotal thyroidectomy with propranolol became hypothyroid (with a low TSH level) one month postoperatively and returned to a euthyroid state without therapy.[51]

Subclinical hypothyroidism refers to patients who are clini-

Table 1   Causes of Hypothyroidism

Mechanism	Cause
Deficiency of TRH	Hypothalamic disease
Deficiency of TSH	Pituitary tumor or destruction
Thyroid destruction	Chronic inflammation Surgical ablation Radioiodine ablation Irradiation of the neck (usually for malignant disease)
Thyroid deficiency	Iodine deficiency (i.e., substrate lack) Iodine excess (i.e., interference with hormone synthesis or release) Antithyroid drugs, including lithium Biosynthetic defects

cally euthyroid but who have an elevated TSH level and a normal T_4 level. This condition principally occurs in patients with compensated autoimmune thyroiditis or in those who have had ablative therapy for hyperthyroidism. Because there is no independent test for hypothyroidism, it is difficult to determine whether such patients are in fact minimally hypothyroid. The possibility that the T_4 level is low for a particular patient even though it is within normal limits is bolstered by the fact that several studies have shown minimal cardiovascular impairment in patients with subclinical hypothyroidism.

LABORATORY DIAGNOSIS OF HYPOTHYROIDISM

The earliest sign of primary hypothyroidism, antedating clinical symptoms, is a rise in the level of serum TSH. This increase occurs before the T_4 level or T_3 level becomes abnormally low. Thus, when primary hypothyroidism is suspected or when the consistency of a goiter suggests Hashimoto's thyroiditis, a serum TSH determination is more sensitive than an assay of the T_4 level. The latter, however, gives valuable information and should be obtained simultaneously with the TSH assay or after an elevated TSH level has been found.

Secondary hypothyroidism associated with hypothalamic or pituitary insufficiency is presumed to be caused by a lack of TSH, but the available assays for TSH, including the sensitive immunoradiometric assay, do not distinguish between pathologically low levels and low-normal levels. If the T_4 level is low, however, the serum TSH will differentiate pituitary from thyroid deficiency.

The choice of laboratory tests for hypothyroidism depends on the stage of the disease [see Figure 6]. When Hashimoto's disease is present without hypothyroidism, a goiter and antithyroid antibodies may be present, but the T_4, T_3, and TSH levels are within the normal range. When the T_4 level is slightly decreased and the TSH level is minimally increased—a condition some would classify as subclinical hypothyroidism—an injection of TRH elicits an exaggerated TSH response. Once the patient is symptomatic, either minimally or with severe disease, the basal TSH level is a reliable guide to the presence of hypothyroidism. Although the TSH response to TRH becomes progressively more abnormal, TRH testing is seldom necessary.

Two points about laboratory testing are important. The serum T_3 level and the RT_3U, each so useful in diagnosing hyperthyroidism, are of little value in hypothyroidism; both are normal in as many as 50 percent of hypothyroid patients. In patients with hypothalamic or pituitary hypothyroidism, the serum TSH value is not elevated as the T_4 level falls. Interestingly, sensitive TSH assays are not definitive in the evaluation of hypothalamic or pituitary hypothyroidism. The pituitary thyrotropes apparently synthesize TSH variants that are recognized immunologically but are not active biologically.[74] Thus, in a patient with a low T_4 level and a normal or low TSH level, study of other pituitary functions is required. In particular, gonadotropin, prolactin, and plasma cortisol should be measured [see Chapter 45]. Prolactin levels must be interpreted with caution. They may be elevated either because of a pituitary tumor or as a feature of hypothyroidism. In the latter circumstance, elevations are slight; in one series, values ranged from 4.7 to 42 ng/ml, with a mean value of 14 ng/ml, compared with a normal mean value of 8 ng/ml. The TSH level is also elevated in patients with primary hypothyroidism but is low or normal in those with secondary hypothyroidism.

Diagnosing Hypothyroidism in Patients on Thyroid Therapy

It is not unusual to encounter patients who have been put on thyroid hormone replacement therapy without firm laboratory confirmation of hypothyroidism.[75] How is the diagnosis of hypothyroidism to be confirmed or excluded in these patients? If the serum TSH level is elevated despite inadequate thyroid therapy, the patient is hypothyroid; if the TSH level is high despite adequate therapy, the existence of thyroid hormone resistance is likely. If the TSH level is normal, I favor discontinuing thyroid medication in patients in whom the diagnosis of hypothyroidism has not been established. Pituitary-thyroid recovery occurs within five weeks after therapy is stopped.[76,77] At that time, measurement of the TSH level reliably separates euthyroid individuals from hypothyroid individuals; thus, one can clarify the issue by discontinuing thyroid therapy and measuring the T_4 and TSH levels at five weeks. If symptoms have recurred, the evidence is all the more compelling. Of course, responsibility must be assumed for completing the test, interpreting the results to the patient, and resuming therapy if indicated.

TREATMENT OF HYPOTHYROIDISM

The aim of all endocrine replacement therapy is to restore the patient as near to normal as possible. In no other endocrine disorder—indeed, in few diseases of any kind—can this goal be fulfilled as completely as in hypothyroidism. Thyroid hormone replacement is reliable, nontoxic, nonallergenic, inexpensive, and indistinguishable from endogenous secretion in its effects.[78] Therapy is simple.[79,80] I usually give 0.05 mg of thyroxine daily for one month and build up to 0.10 to 0.15 mg daily over three to five months. Once these dosages have been reached, the patient should feel well and, after several months, be returned to a normal state. All symptoms caused by hypothyroidism should remain absent as long as daily therapy is maintained. The average daily maintenance dose is 1.68 µg/kg, but the range of doses is wide. An increased dose may be needed for patients with the short-bowel syndrome or cirrhosis and for patients on certain drugs, including aluminum hydroxide, sucralfate, cholestyramine, phenytoin, iron, rifampin, and phenobarbital. Smoking interferes with thyroid function and the effect of thyroid hormone and thus increases the thyroxine requirement, especially in patients with partial thyroid failure.[81,82]

Optimal therapy must be monitored by measurement of the serum TSH level.[83,84] Until the TSH level is normal, full replacement has not been reached. Once the patient has started on replacement therapy, however, there is no urgency in finding the exact right dose. Clinical improvement from partial replacement is gratifying, and a long-elevated TSH level may not return to normal for six to nine months. Indeed, as the daily dose comes close to the probable maintenance level of 0.075 to 0.125 mg, a given dose level should be maintained for eight weeks before the serum TSH level is measured again.[74] To avoid overtreatment, a sensitive TSH assay should be used; if the TSH level with this test is below the normal range, the patient is overtreated and the dose should be lowered. Measurement of serum T_4 and T_3 levels is not a reliable guide to adequacy of therapy. Indeed, one of the few complications of thyroxine therapy—accelerated bone loss and the potential aggravation of osteoporosis—correlates with a suppressed sensitive TSH level, as measured with a sensitive assay.[85] The decreases in bone density are minor and have not proved to be clinically important. Nevertheless, avoiding excessive thyroxine replacement seems advisable, inasmuch as osteoporosis and hypothyroidism occur simultaneously in postmenopausal women.[86,87]

Several precautions should be remembered in the treatment of hypothyroidism. First, treatment of patients with significant cardiac disease and elderly persons should begin with smaller doses, such as 0.025 mg of thyroxine daily for two to four weeks, and the amount should be gradually increased until a maintenance dose is reached. Such patients are often kept on 0.075 to 0.100 mg daily rather than on the larger doses used in otherwise healthy young people. Second, patients with angina pectoris and hypothyroidism may not be able to tolerate even carefully administered thyroid replacement therapy. For such patients, one can begin with 0.0125 mg of thyroxine daily and increase the dose by that amount every four weeks. If angina appears or worsens during thyroxine therapy, coronary angiography and bypass surgery may be necessary before adequate thyroxine replacement can be reached. Fortunately, several studies have shown that this seemingly aggressive approach can be safely pursued when suitable precautions are taken.[88] Indeed, some clinics favor performing coronary surgery before replacement therapy.

Regular monitoring of TSH levels in patients on thyroxine therapy occasionally reveals a surprising abnormality. In one study, elevated TSH levels developed in several patients with known hypothyroidism who were being treated with thyroxine and who were also receiving amiodarone. This elevation was attributed to an amiodarone-induced decrease in the conversion of T_4 to T_3, and it responded to an increase in the dose of thyroxine.[89] Following the TSH level has further utility in caring for hypothyroid patients with depression or another disorder with symptoms that overlap those of hypothyroidism. If the TSH value is normal, one can be confident that any remaining symptoms are not caused by hypothyroidism and that larger doses of thyroid will not help. Finally, whether starting patients on thyroid replacement or caring for patients with hyperthyroidism, the clinician is establishing a continuing relationship and assuming a prolonged responsibility. Patients must be carefully instructed in the need for indefinite therapy. Lapses may result in the reappearance of apathy and may thus prevent patients from returning for examination. To guard against this possibility, an effective follow-up system is needed.

How rigidly should the TSH level be held within the normal range? Third-generation assays are so sensitive that a value below the lower-normal limit but well above the 0.05 mU/L of hyperthyroidism is sometimes found. If the patient has no symptoms or signs of hyperthyroidism, a value between 0.25 and 5.0 mU/L should be acceptable, and yearly follow-up should be adequate.[90]

Pregnancy

In most pregnant hypothyroid patients receiving thyroxine, there is a fall in the serum FTI level and a rise in the TSH level that appear during the first trimester and last throughout the pregnancy.[91] The association of hypothyroidism with increased maternal and fetal morbidity suggests that achieving a euthyroid state in the mother is an important goal.[92] Serum TSH should be monitored in each trimester, and the daily dose of thyroxine should be increased by 25 to 50 µg as required to keep the serum TSH within the normal range. The prepregnant dose can be resumed one month after delivery.[93,94]

Myxedema Coma

Myxedema coma is a rare complication of hypothyroidism in which profound lethargy or coma is accompanied by hypothermia, defined as temperature below 35°C (95°F). This condition primarily affects patients who are older than 75 years, often in a setting of sepsis, exposure to severe cold, or ingestion of alcohol or narcotics. The pathogenesis of the disorder is unclear, but decreased thermogenesis, alveolar hypoventilation, and a resulting sensitivity to sedative and narcotic drugs are all important. Cardiovascular impairments such as decreased heart rate, decreased stroke volume, and pericardial effusion can be present singly or in combination. Treatment has been relatively ineffective, but recent series suggest a much better outlook.[95] The favored approach is immediate restitution of body T_4 stores by administration of 250 to 500 µg of thyroxine intravenously.[96,97] Fluid volumes should be restored, but patients in myxedema coma are prone to water intoxication and resultant hyponatremia. Hypopituitarism can seldom be discounted in the short time before therapy must be started. It is therefore reasonable to obtain blood for plasma cortisol measurement and to administer 100 mg of hydrocortisone hemisuccinate every 12 hours intravenously until improvement is evident or until the initial plasma cortisol level is known to be normal.

Thyroid Dysfunction in the Elderly

As already noted, both hyperthyroidism and hypothyroidism often have atypical presentations in the elderly. Several efforts to define the prevalence of thyroid dysfunction have been reported. The frequency of hypothyroidism has varied from three to 10 percent in ambulatory patients older than 65 years, with a female-to-male ratio of at least 3:1. It is not clear whether this frequency justifies the screening of healthy elderly populations; however, it is worth doing a TSH test at only slight provocation in symptomatic elderly persons.[98-100]

Generalized Resistance to Thyroid Hormone

More than 400 patients have been described who demonstrate resistance to the biochemical and physiologic effects of T_4 and T_3.[101-103] The clinical picture of generalized resistance to thyroid hormone is highly varied. Some patients have impaired growth, mental retardation, and features of cretinism. The least severe manifestations are elevated serum levels of TSH and T_4 in patients who are clinically normal. Virtually all patients have a goiter, which occasionally reaches considerable size. Inheritance is mostly autosomal dominant, but families with recessive patterns of inheritance are known. Molecular genetic studies of patients with generalized resistance to thyroid hormone have produced extraordinary insights into the nature of thyroid hormone action. The thyroid hormone receptor is a dimeric transcription factor with separate domains for binding to thyroid hormone (principally T_3) and DNA. The defects underlying generalized resistance to thyroid hormone are mutations in the hormone-binding region of the *TRb* gene in an area that influences dimerization. Binding of the mutant *TR* gene to DNA is unimpaired; as a result, abnormal *TR* genes occupy binding sites but, lacking T_3, cannot initiate transcription. The disorder thus provides an example of dominant negative inheritance.[104]

The clinical implications of the syndromes resulting from generalized resistance to thyroid hormone vary. Patients whose resistance is limited to the pituitary have mild to moderate hyperthyroidism [*see* Hyperthyroidism, *above*]. Other patients are frankly hypothyroid but have different manifestations in different body tissues. Thyroxine supplementation may be used in the latter group of patients, but tissue and organ response rather than TSH levels must be followed. Finally, the genetics of the disorders allow for sound family counseling and support.

Interpretation of Surprise Changes in T_4

Assay of the T_4 level remains a widely used thyroid function test. As emphasized, this level varies with changes in thyroxine-binding proteins; surprise elevations and depressions of T_4 are common. In addition, many drugs and illnesses alter thyroxine binding. To clarify such problems, an FTI and a sensitive, third-generation TSH assay are very useful.

Interpretation of an Asymmetric Goiter

Thyroid scanning plays a major role in interpretation of an asymmetric goiter. The scan can determine the functional state of the nodular portions of the thyroid and provide a guide to treatment. Determining serum antibodies is highly useful, especially in patients with lobular, firm goiters that suggest thyroiditis but raise the question of malignant disease. A high antibody level points strongly to chronic thyroiditis.

Thyroiditis

Inflammatory disease of the thyroid is an important cause of clinical abnormality. Three classes can be defined: acute, subacute, and chronic. Acute thyroiditis is usually secondary to penetrating injury of the neck; the disease is very rare, and its pathogenesis and manifestations are obvious. Occasionally, acute thyroiditis results from hematogenous spread of infection in immunosuppressed patients.

SUBACUTE THYROIDITIS

Subacute thyroiditis is characterized by pain, fever, and viral-type symptoms suggestive of upper respiratory tract infection or grippe. Pain may be in the anterior neck, in the throat on swallowing, or in one or both ears. Although formerly thought to be a constant feature of the disease, pain is sometimes absent. Tenderness on careful palpation is almost universal, but occasional instances of nontender thyroiditis have been described. Usually, the thyroid is diffusely enlarged. Although at the outset only one side may be palpable and tender, in most patients the entire gland ultimately becomes abnormal. Local adenopathy is not impressive. Fever, leukocytosis, and a striking elevation of the sedimentation rate (often to more than 50 mm/hr) are frequent. Thyroid function tests may be invaluable in diagnosis because subacute thyroiditis produces the unusual combination of an elevated T_4 level and a low RAIU. The elevation of the T_4 level is presumably caused by follicular rupture with discharge of stored hormone; the suppression of RAIU is caused by the acute inflammation of the thyroid plus the T_4-induced suppression of TSH. Scanning may show a cold area when the inflammation is localized; patients manifesting a cold area must be followed, and resumption of RAIU must be shown before their condition can be distinguished from thyroid neoplasm.

Subacute thyroiditis is self-limited, but the course is extraordinarily variable. As a result, it has been difficult to demonstrate either the need for treatment or the best approach. For most patients, salicylates and time are adequate. If these do not work or if the disease is more severe than usual, triiodothyronine, 25 µg three times daily for a month, appears to abort symptoms. In elderly patients or those with underlying cardiac disease, adjunctive use of propranolol may offset the putative risk of triiodothyronine. An alternative treatment is prednisone in full anti-inflammatory doses. When treatment is withdrawn, recrudescence of symptoms is common; reinstitution of the same therapy for an additional month is then appropriate.

Subacute thyroiditis does not induce permanent hypothyroidism. Patients should be followed until euthyroidism is restored and symptoms have disappeared. When suppression of uptake has been unilateral, a repeat scan to demonstrate recovery and to exclude neoplasm is desirable.

CHRONIC THYROIDITIS (HASHIMOTO'S THYROIDITIS)

Chronic thyroiditis is a major thyroid disorder whose pathogenesis has been under intensive study for decades.[105] Since the demonstration of elevated antithyroid antibodies in Hashimoto's thyroiditis, the disorder has been accepted as a classic example of human autoimmunity. The pathological findings in the thyroid include extensive infiltration with chronic inflammatory cells, follicular rupture, eosinophilia, varying degrees of hyperplasia, and fibrosis. The serum of patients with chronic thyroiditis shows a panoply of antibodies—to cell fractions rich in microsomes, to the thyroid peroxidase, to thyroid follicular cells, and to TSH receptors. Although not all patients demonstrate all four types of antibody, almost all have at least one type; many patients have multiple positive results, and titers may be very high, reaching 1:1,000,000 in some individuals.

The clinical manifestations of chronic thyroiditis are extraordinarily variable, but the major syndromes are painless goiter, hypothyroidism, and a combination of both. Goiter without hypothyroidism may be the most common early stage of the disease. The goiter is usually discovered incidentally during a routine physical examination. The goiter is typically diffuse and firm to hard in consistency and often involves the pyramidal lobe—a major diagnostic feature that should be sought. Occasionally, a local lymph node is felt, but significant adenopathy suggests malignant disease, even in a gland that is a site of chronic inflammation.

Hashimoto's thyroiditis is the most common cause of goitrous hypothyroidism in the adult. As the inflammatory process progressively destroys thyroid tissue, compensatory hyperplasia may be unable to produce adequate thyroid hormone, and partial or severe hypothyroidism results. Almost 100 percent of cases of primary hypothyroidism in adults are secondary to Hashimoto's thyroiditis. This association should be sought regardless of which manifestation is first recognized. Adults with diffuse goiter should have antibody measurements to confirm the diagnosis; once thyroiditis is suspected, thyroid function status should be determined and followed at regular intervals because hypothyroidism can develop insidiously [*see Figure 6*]. Conversely, patients found to be hypothyroid should be carefully examined for goiter, and antibody titers should be measured to confirm the underlying pathological condition.

Hypothyroidism without goiter in the adult is most often caused by a late stage of chronic thyroiditis, particularly the variant in which fibrosis, rather than inflammation or hyperplasia, has dominated the pathological process. Patients usually have very high antibody titers, which establish the diagnosis.

Variants and special features of Hashimoto's thyroiditis provide interesting challenges. Some patients have high RAIU values and frank hyperthyroidism. Because patients with Graves' disease can have lymphocytic infiltration in the thyroid and high antibody titers, this syndrome is a bridge between the two disorders and is sometimes referred to as hashitoxicosis. Some patients with subclinical Hashimoto's thyroiditis are unusually susceptible to iodides; in patients in whom hypothyroidism has been induced by iodide or another antithyroid drug, evaluation for Hashimoto's thyroiditis is indicated. The disease overlaps in occurrence with other autoimmune diseases, including pernicious anemia, myasthenia gravis, Addison's disease, and premature ovarian failure, as well as with diabetes mellitus. The existence of any of these conditions except diabetes should enhance suspicion of thyroid disease.

The course of Hashimoto's thyroiditis is extremely variable. The disease can be clinically undetectable despite high antibody levels; it can present as euthyroidism with goiter and remain stable for years; it can progress to hypothyroidism; or it can manifest itself initially as hypothyroidism. Diagnostic approaches include careful palpation of the neck and measurement of antibody, TSH, and T_4 levels. Thyroid needle biopsy is occasionally useful when the gland appears irregular and hard enough to suggest malignant disease.

Treatment is straightforward. Thyroxine is used to suppress the goiter or to correct hypothyroidism. In some patients, thyrotropin receptor–blocking antibodies, presumably implicated in the hypothyroidism, disappear. When thyroxine replacement is discontinued in these patients, they remain euthyroid.[106] Although interesting, this finding does not change the general approach: thyroxine therapy, once begun, is appropriate indefinitely.

THYROIDITIS WITH SPONTANEOUSLY RESOLVING HYPERTHYROIDISM

A variant form of thyroiditis should be distinguished from subacute and Hashimoto's thyroiditis. The syndrome presents as hyperthyroidism with typical peripheral features but without the autoimmune type of ophthalmopathy. The thyroid is either normal in size or minimally enlarged and is painless and often nontender. The sedimentation rate is not strikingly elevated. T_3 and T_4 levels are elevated, but the 24-hour RAIU is low, in the range of one to three percent. Antithyroid antibodies are elevated in some patients but rarely to the very high levels seen in Hashimoto's thyroiditis. More important, the hyperthyroidism resolves spontaneously as the thyroid inflammation heals. Biopsy findings vary; some reports suggest subacute thyroiditis. More often, the pathological examination reveals lymphocytic thyroiditis but without the eosinophilia, hyperplasia, and fibrosis of full-blown Hashimoto's thyroiditis. The disease can occur at any age but is perhaps most common during the postpartum period, when it often reveals autoimmune features and a lymphocytic histopathology.

The main significance of the disorder is revealed by one of its names: spontaneously resolving hyperthyroidism. This disorder has been reported frequently enough so that the RAIU, the only test that can detect it, should be reinstated in the routine workup of hyperthyroid patients. The most reasonable

therapy would appear to be propranolol; ablative therapy is contraindicated, and antithyroid drugs are unlikely to work. It is essential to bear in mind the other causes of increased T_4 and T_3 levels with a low RAIU: the Jod-Basedow phenomenon, struma ovarii, and thyrotoxicosis factitia.

POSTPARTUM THYROIDITIS

Transient thyroiditis, usually painless, occurs in about one in 20 postpartum women.[107] It can produce hyperthyroidism, hypothyroidism, or first one disorder and then the other.[108] A positive test for antimicrosomal antibody is strongly associated with this phenomenon, and repeat occurrences of thyroiditis after subsequent pregnancies are common. The disease is usually self-limited, requiring only symptomatic therapy; sometimes, a beta blocker is administered for hyperthyroid symptoms. Permanent hypothyroidism develops in some patients; its occurrence is best predicted by a very high antimicrosomal antibody titer and by severe symptoms during the acute phase of postpartum hypothyroidism.[109]

Nodules, Nodular Goiters, and Thyroid Cancer

Enlargement of the thyroid is a common physical finding as well as a common nonfinding because it is often missed. When the gland is diffusely enlarged, a general process such as inflammation or hyperplasia is likely. Irregular, localized, or nodular enlargement of the gland raises the specter of neoplasm. However, cancer of the thyroid is rare and death from it even more so. An alert and informed approach will avoid many unnecessary operations and much anxiety and still identify the patients for whom surgical therapy is indicated.

A localized nodular enlargement of the thyroid gland represents a benign thyroid adenoma, a nodular goiter, or cancer of the thyroid.[97] Thyroid adenomas may occur singly or as portions of benign nodular goiters. Their cause is unknown. Some are differentiated enough to function like normal thyroid glands; indeed, some are more active than normal tissue, suppressing TSH and leading to hypofunction of the rest of the gland. This capacity is, with rare exception, seen only in benign lesions. As noted [see Plummer's Nodule, or Toxic Adenoma, above], thyroid adenoma is often caused by a somatic mutation in the TSH receptor.[110] Thus, a so-called hot nodule, an area of thyroid tissue that is the sole active focus in the gland, can be safely watched without surgery. Radionuclide scanning establishes the diagnosis by showing a concentration of the isotope in an area that corresponds to the palpable nodule. Serum T_4, T_3, and TSH levels should be determined to test whether the patient is hyperthyroid. Hot nodules less than 2.5 cm in diameter are unlikely to cause hyperthyroidism; those greater than 3 cm in diameter have a 20 percent chance of producing hyperthyroidism within six years.

Nodular goiter remains one of the great enigmas of thyroid disease. A common disorder, beginning usually in persons in their 30s, nodular goiter affects women much more often than men. The pathogenesis is obscure, and the variegated pathological findings may show patches of atrophy, fibrosis, hyperplasia, calcification, and involution. The disease may reflect a defect in intrathyroidal regulation of thyroid function by iodine, but just how this defect would lead to the particular pathological findings is not clear.[111] The clinical attributes of the disease are important. Patients with nodular goiters are usually euthyroid, but as many as 25 percent have nonsuppressible thyroid function; that is, when they are given exogenous thyroid hormone, their RAIU values do not fall more than 50 percent. It is probably among these patients that the hyperthyroidism that occurs in association with some nodular goiters develops. Thus, patients with nodular glands should have their thyroid function assessed and should be watched for the insidious development of thyrotoxicosis. The use of fine-needle aspiration has revealed foci of cancer in multinodular goiters more often than was previously thought. Suspicion should be raised when one nodule is markedly larger than the others or when one nodule is increasing preferentially. In such a case, fine-needle aspiration is advisable. Surgery may be needed if the goiter causes mechanical compression of neck tissues. Plain films and barium swallow should be done to determine how far the goiter impinges on the larynx or trachea. Surgery should not be unduly delayed, because hemorrhage into a nodular goiter can lead to tracheal compromise and choking.[112,113]

CLINICAL FORMS OF THYROID CANCER

Papillary and Follicular Cancers

Papillary cancers of the thyroid occur most frequently in patients between 10 and 50 years of age.[114] Papillary cancers are often remarkably indolent lesions, tending to metastasize to local lymph nodes and to grow slowly in both the gland and the secondary sites. Histopathologic differentiation of benign and malignant thyroid lesions can defy the most expert pathologist; definitive features of malignancy include invasion of the capsule or blood vessels and metastasis. Patients younger than 40 years with papillary cancer survive longer than older patients.

Pure follicular carcinomas are much less common and can provide the same difficulty in discrimination between benign and malignant lesions. These tumors tend to metastasize hematogenously to bone, where they produce lytic lesions and pathological fractures. It is not uncommon for the bony lesion, particularly in the spine, skull, or pelvis, to cause the symptom that leads the patient to seek medical attention. The small primary lesion in the thyroid may be overlooked, partly because the patient is in too much pain from a fracture to sit up for examination of the neck. Persons younger than 40 years with follicular carcinoma have a higher survival rate than older individuals; in one series, patients younger than 40 years had an 86 percent cure rate, whereas those older than 60 years had a cure rate of 26 percent. In another series, patients younger than 45 years with an intrathyroidal cancer less than 2.5 cm in diameter had an excellent prognosis, but the overall mortality and morbidity of follicular carcinoma were twice those of papillary cancer.[115]

More common than the pure papillary lesion or the pure follicular lesion is a mixed papillary and follicular lesion. This type shows extreme variability of appearance within the primary lesion, between the primary lesion and metastases, and among metastases. Its behavior is closer to that of a papillary lesion; slow growth, local recurrence, and occasional pulmonary spread are typical. Metastasis to bone, so common in the follicular cancer, is less frequent with the follicular component of the mixed lesions.

The Hürthle cell tumor is the least frequent type of tumor and the least well documented in its behavior. It develops principally in persons older than 50 years and can be benign or malignant. It is best evaluated and treated as other thyroid tumors are.[116]

Medullary Cancer of the Thyroid

Medullary carcinoma is a differentiated tumor of the thyroid, accounting for about three percent of thyroid cancers. It derives not from follicular cells but from the embryologically separate parafollicular cells, which are the source of thyrocalcitonin.[117,118]

Medullary carcinoma has two clinical patterns: a unifocal lesion occurring sporadically in elderly people (75 percent of cases) and a bilateral form apparently arising in hyperplastic foci in the midportion of the thyroid lobes. The bilateral variant is often associated with pheochromocytomas that tend to be bilateral and malignant. The combination of medullary thyroid carcinomas and pheochromocytoma is an autosomal dominant disorder known as multiple endocrine neoplasia type II (MEN II). Two variants of this syndrome, running true to form within affected families, are known. In one syndrome, type IIA, which is caused by a defect on chromosome 10, the two endocrine tumors are associated with parathyroid hyperplasia; in the other, type IIB or III, the endocrine abnormalities are accompanied by neuroectodermal defects and characteristic facies [see Chapter 45].

The clinical syndromes associated with medullary carcinoma include asymptomatic elevation of serum calcitonin levels, intractable diarrhea, Cushing's syndrome caused by excessive production of adrenocorticotropic hormone (ACTH), and the carcinoid syndrome.

In both familial variants of MEN II, the medullary cancer typically produces large amounts of thyrocalcitonin. This overproduction can often be demonstrated in the basal state but sometimes requires provocative testing with calcium infusion, glucagon, or pentagastrin. Assay of calcitonin thus has several clinical uses: confirmation that a nodule in the thyroid is a medullary carcinoma, confirmation of cure after surgery, and sensitive detection of residual or recurrent disease after surgery. Perhaps the most exciting use of the measurement has been in the study of first-order relatives of affected individuals; through this test, nongoitrous individuals have been diagnosed as having the disease and have been surgically cured before any tumor was palpable.[119,120] This is an exciting example of the diagnosis and treatment of significant but silent disease by a combination of genetic study and provocative endocrine testing. As a result of this approach, survival is better with the familial form, in which tumors are typically less than 3 cm in diameter when diagnosed, than with the sporadic form.[121]

Undifferentiated Thyroid Cancer

Although Hodgkin's disease, other lymphoproliferative tumors, and other cancers can all metastasize to the thyroid, anaplastic cancers occasionally arise in the thyroid.[122] They grow extremely rapidly, and local invasion leads to strangulation or esophageal obstruction, causing death within six to 12 months. Patients usually have a discernibly growing mass and often exhibit stridor, hoarseness, or both. Physical examination discloses a goiter and irregular extension into surrounding tissues. The outlook in such cases is grave, despite a combination of surgery, radiation therapy, and adjuvant chemotherapy.

PATHOGENESIS OF THYROID CANCER

The application of molecular biology techniques has revealed some suggestive correlations between certain oncogenes and the pathogenesis of thyroid cancer.[123,124] However, by far the most important clinical lesson relates to exposure to irradiation in childhood. The tragic explosion of a nuclear reactor at Chernobyl provided a reminder of this risk.[125] It has been known for some time that patients who had irradiation to the neck in childhood, usually for benign inflammatory or infectious diseases, have a significantly increased incidence of thyroid cancer.[126] There is a direct correlation between the dose of radiation and the occurrence of a thyroid neoplasm. Additional predisposing factors are female sex and younger age at the time of irradiation.[127] It is critical to elicit from all patients a history of head and neck irradiation in infancy or childhood. Although many patients are unaware of the details or even the occurrence of such treatment, its effect on cancer incidence is evident as long as 40 years later. A positive history warrants particularly careful examination of the neck, including repeated inspection and palpation while the patient is swallowing a cupful of water. On the basis of a positive history plus the findings on palpation, patients will fall into three categories.

Category 1 Patients in category 1 have a positive history but no palpable nodule in the neck. Radionuclide scanning with ^{99m}Tc-pertechnetate or ^{123}I is advisable. If a cold area is identified, a repeat physical examination may detect a nodule; the patient would then be reclassified in category 2. Some physicians favor surgery for nodules detected only on a scan; others prefer thyroid suppression and regular follow-up.

Category 2 A history of irradiation and the presence of one or more palpable nodules place a patient in category 2. These patients should undergo a scan; if it discloses a hot nodule, testing for hyperthyroidism is appropriate, but surgery is not needed. If a single cold nodule is discovered, fine-needle aspiration cytology can be used as a guide to therapy.[128] If cancer can be excluded, the patient should be given suppressive doses of thyroxine and followed at yearly intervals. If cancer cannot be excluded or if there are multiple nodules, surgical exploration and intraoperative pathological evaluation are advisable.

Category 3 Patients who have a diffuse goiter but no palpable nodules are placed in category 3. The thyroid function of these patients should be defined, their antibody levels should be measured (to screen for Hashimoto's thyroiditis), and a scan with ^{99m}Tc-pertechnetate or ^{123}I should be performed. If the radionuclide scan shows no nodules, thyroid suppression is indicated, and the patient should undergo a reexamination for nodules in six months. If a nodule is found, surgery is indicated. If the initial scan shows a cold nodule but nothing is felt, thyroid hormone suppression is indicated and examination advised after six months. If a nodule appears, surgery is indicated.

APPROACH TO THE PATIENT WITH A THYROID NODULE

The main clinical problem posed by the discovery of a single thyroid nodule is the possibility that the nodule may harbor cancer. Although goiters are common, thyroid cancer is rare; the challenge is to identify those patients who should undergo surgery, thereby avoiding unnecessary operations.[129-131] The most direct, expeditious, and ultimately cost-effective approach to the isolated nodule is fine-needle aspiration for cytologic examination.[132]

With or without ultrasound guidance, a small-gauge needle and syringe suction are used to obtain several samples for cytologic study. In a review of data pooled from seven large series employing fine-needle aspiration, experienced cytologists reported 69 percent of the results as benign, 10 percent as suspect, 4 percent as malignant, and 17 percent as nondiagnostic. In another study, of over 9,000 patients, the interpretation was benign in 74 percent, malignant in four percent, and suspicious or inadequate in 22 percent. There is general agreement that patients with suspicious and malignant results should have surgery. If surgery is also deemed appropriate for nondiagnostic findings, the overall sensitivity of fine-needle aspiration is 83 percent (ranging from 65 to 98 percent) and the overall specificity is 92 percent (ranging from 72 to 100 percent), providing a diagnostic accuracy of 95 percent. When fine-needle aspiration is used as a guide, 25 to 50 percent fewer patients undergo operation for single nodules and at least twice as many (i.e., 30 percent rather than 15 percent) are found to have cancer. If neither a skilled operator nor a skilled cytologist is available, the following approach leads to more surgery but also detects almost all cancers.

Once a nodule is felt, a thyroid scan is appropriate. ^{99m}Tc-pertechnetate is usually used because of its low radiation dose (0.1 cGy to the thyroid versus 100 to 200 cGy for a scan with ^{131}I). Percutaneous ethanol injection has been tried but is neither widely available nor clearly preferable at present.[133] If the nodule is hot, no further workup is needed unless the patient is hyperthyroid, in which case surgical or radioiodine ablation of the nodule is indicated. If the nodule is cold, ultrasonography may help distinguish cystic lesions from solid and mixed cystic-solid lesions. Purely cystic lesions less than 4 cm in diameter are rare and are seldom malignant; simple needle drainage is adequate therapy. Mixed and solid lesions may contain carcinoma, and ultrasonography is not able to make that differentiation. X-rays of soft tissue provide definitive evidence of carcinoma in the rare circumstance in which they show the microscopic calcification of psammoma bodies. Hormonal markers of tumor, other than the elevated calcitonin level of medullary carcinoma, are not reliable. The serum thyroglobulin level is almost always elevated in patients with cancer of the thyroid, but it is often high in patients with thyroiditis and Graves' disease and is therefore not of differentiating value [see Figure 7].

The sequence of noninvasive testing described thus far is both cumbersome and inexact. It results in more thyroidectomies than are needed because in surgery planned by such a protocol, only about five to 10 percent of nodules are positive for cancer. As a result, the use of fine-needle aspiration with cytology is preferable.[134,135] Fine-needle aspiration can also be used to evaluate a nodule that is disproportionate in size or growing in a nodular goiter. Should the patient with one or more nodules that do not require surgery be treated with thyroxine or iodide? Interestingly, after all these years, there is no definitive or consensual answer to this question. Some such nodules regress under therapy and some do not enlarge,[136,137] but whether this matters in the long run is still debated.[138]

The details of treatment of thyroid cancer are beyond the scope of this chapter.[139-143] The basic principles do not differ from the principles of management of other malignant diseases, but certain special aspects are important. Thyroid cancer in young people is often a slow-moving disease with an indolent course and favorable prognosis. As a result, although surgery is the initial treatment for all papillary thyroid cancers, radical neck dissection has given way to a more conservative and less disfiguring approach, most often a near total thyroidectomy.[144] After removal of the primary lesion, most patients

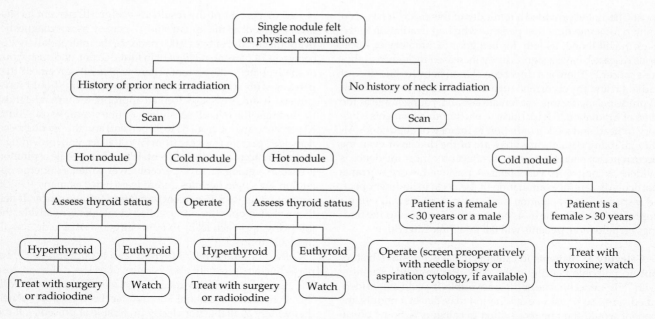

Figure 7   **This approach to the management of a thyroid nodule will disclose almost all clinically significant thyroid cancers; however, fewer patients would undergo surgical procedures if aspiration cytology were used as the initial step.**

receive a thyroid ablative dose of radioactive iodine and are then treated with suppressive doses of thyroxine, with regular follow-up to identify any palpable recurrence in the neck or any radiologically demonstrable disease in the lungs. Functional thyroid carcinomas may take up radioactive iodine and, in favorable cases, respond to high doses of irradiation delivered by this modality. However, the generalist's responsibility rests heavily on the interpretation of nodular thyroid glands and on the elicitation of a history of neck irradiation.

Euthyroid Sick Syndrome

Many different abnormal thyroid function test results are encountered in severe nonthyroidal illness, and patients who manifest such abnormalities are referred to as being euthyroid sick. Both elevated T_4, caused by increased TBG, and depressed T_4, caused by lowered TBG or impaired binding of T_4, are found. The most common thyroid test abnormality is a low T_3 level, often depressed to values much lower than those seen in most cases of myxedema.[145] This is caused by the decreased activity of type I deiodinase and is reflected in an increased rT_3 value. The serum TSH does not rise, however, and may indeed be lower than normal. Patients appear clinically euthyroid, perhaps because of an increase in T_3 receptors and in tissue responsiveness. This state is called the low T_3 syndrome and tends to remit as the acute illness disappears.

More severe test derangements occur in more severe acute illnesses. In the so-called low T_3–low T_4 syndrome, T_4 deiodination is impaired and T_4 binding is apparently, although not yet verifiably, inhibited, resulting in a normal level of directly measured free T_4.[146] Again, the TSH level is usually normal or slightly below normal; the failure of TSH to rise despite depressed T_4 and T_3 levels is attributed to dopamine or corticosteroid therapy. However, there is no definitive way to prove transient hypothalamic or pituitary failure because it is difficult to be sure of the true free thyroxine.[147] Progressive lowering of the T_4 level

is accompanied by a corresponding increase in mortality. Patients who survive their acute illness often experience a two- to four-week period during which the TSH level is above normal before returning to the normal range.

Because abnormalities of the euthyroid sick syndrome are prevalent, establishing a diagnosis of primary thyroid disease is extremely difficult in the acutely ill and malnourished patient. If the TSH level is lower than 0.01 mU/L and the serum T_3 level is not depressed, occult hyperthyroidism can be suspected; if the TSH level is higher than 20 mU/L, primary hypothyroidism can be suspected. Unless pressed by clinical deterioration or impressed with historical and physical evidence of thyroid disease antedating the acute illness, the clinician would be well advised to wait for the acute illness to clear before instituting thyroid-directed treatment.[148]

References

1. DeGroot LJ, Larsen PR, Henneman G, et al: The Thyroid and Its Diseases, 6th ed. Churchill Livingstone, New York, 1996

2. Berry MJ, Larsen PR: The role of selenium in thyroid hormone action. Endocr Rev 13:207, 1992

3. Magner JA: Thyroid-stimulating hormone: biosynthesis, cell biology, and bioactivity. Endocr Rev 11:354, 1990

4. Nagayama Y, Rapoport B: The thyrotropin receptor 25 years after its discovery: new insight after its molecular cloning. Mol Endocrinol 6:145, 1992

5. Stevenin B, Lee SL: Hormonal regulation of the thyrotropin releasing hormone (TRH) gene. Endocrinologist 5:286, 1995

6. Wilbur JF, Feng P, Li Q-L, et al: The thyrotropin-releasing hormone gene: differential regulation, expression, and function in hypothalamus and two unexpected extrahypothalamic loci, the heart and testis. Trends Endocrinol Metab 7:93, 1996

7. Lazar MA: Thyroid hormone receptors: multiple forms, multiple possibilities. Endocr Rev 14:184, 1993

8. Samuels HH, Forman BM, Horowitz ZD, et al: Regulation of gene expression by thyroid hormone. J Clin Invest 81:957, 1988

9. Stockigt JR: Hyperthyroxinemia secondary to drugs and acute illness. Endocrinologist 3:67, 1993

10. DeGroot LJ, Mayor G: Admission screening by thyroid function tests in an acute general care teaching hospital. Am J Med 93:558, 1992

11. Ekins R: The free hormone hypothesis and measurement of free hormones. Clin Chem 38:1289, 1992

12. Mariotti S, Franceschi C, Cossarizza A, et al: The aging thyroid. Endocr Rev 16:686, 1995

13. Carter JA, Utiger RD: The ophthalmopathy of Graves' disease. Annu Rev Med 43:487, 1992

14. Furmaniak J, Rees Smith B: Immunity to the thyroid-stimulating hormone receptor. Springer Semin Immunopathol 14:309, 1993

15. DeGroot LJ, Quintans J: The causes of autoimmune thyroid disease. Endocr Rev 10:537, 1989

16. O'Connor G, Davies TF: Human autoimmune thyroid disease. Trends in Endocrinology and Metabolism 1:266, 1990

17. Volpe R: The pathophysiology of autoimmune thyroid disease. Endocr Regul 25:187, 1991

18. Woeber KA: Thyrotoxicosis and the heart. N Engl J Med 327:94, 1992

19. Greenwood RM, Daly JG, Himsworth RL: Hyperthyroidism and the impalpable thyroid gland. Clin Endocrinol (Oxf) 22:583, 1985

20. Griffin MA, Solomon DH: Hyperthyroidism in the elderly. J Am Geriatr Soc 34:887, 1986

21. Ford HK, Cooke RR, Keightley EA, et al: Serum levels of free and bound testosterone in hyperthyroidism. Clin Endocrinol (Oxf) 36:187, 1992

22. Ober KP: Thyrotoxic periodic paralysis in the United States: report of 7 cases and review of the literature. Medicine (Baltimore) 71:109, 1992

23. Dumont JE, Maenhaut C, Lamy F: Control of thyroid cell proliferation and goitrogenesis. Trends Endocrinol Metab 3:12, 1992

24. Elte JWF, Bussemaker JK, Haak A: The natural history of euthyroid multinodular goitre. Postgrad Med J 66:186, 1990

25. Van Sande J, Parma J, Tonacchera M, et al: Somatic and germline mutations of the TSH receptor gene in thyroid diseases. J Clin Endocrinol Metab 80:2577, 1995

26. Parma J, Van Sande J, Swillens S, et al: Somatic mutations causing constitutive activity of the thyrotropin receptor are the major cause of hyperfunctioning thyroid adenomas: identification of additional mutations activating both the cyclic adenosine 3',5'-monophosphate and inositol phosphate-Ca^{2+} cascades. Mol Endocrinol 9:725, 1995

27. Fradkin JE, Wolff J: Iodide-induced thyrotoxicosis. Medicine (Baltimore) 62:1, 1983

28. Franklyn JA, Davis JR, Gammage MD, et al: Amiodarone and thyroid hormone action. Clin Endocrinol (Oxf) 22:257, 1985

29. Georges J-L, Normand J-P, Lenormand M-E, et al: Life-threatening thyrotoxicosis induced by amiodarone in patients with benign heart disease. Eur Heart J 13:129, 1992

30. Martino E, Aghini-Lombardi F, Lippi F, et al: Twenty-four hour radioactive iodine uptake in 35 patients with amiodarone associated thyrotoxicosis. J Nucl Med 26:1402, 1985

31. Goodwin TM, Montoro M, Mestman JH: Transient hyperthyroidism and hyperemesis gravidarum: clinical aspects. Am J Obstet Gynecol 167:648, 1992

32. Goodwin TM, Montoro M, Mestman JH, et al: The role of chorionic gonadotropin in transient hyperthyroidism of hyperemesis gravidarum. J Clin Endocrinol Metab 75:1333, 1992

33. Lisker-Melman M, Di Bisceglie AM, Usala SJ, et al: Development of thyroid disease during therapy of chronic viral hepatitis with interferon alfa. Gastroenterology 102:2155, 1992

34. Wynne AG, Gharib H, Scheithauer BW, et al: Hyperthyroidism due to inappropriate secretion of thyrotropin in 10 patients. Am J Med 92:15, 1992

35. Beck-Peccoz P, Brucker-Davis F, Persani L: Thyrotropin-secreting pituitary tumors. Endocr Rev 17:610, 1996

36. Feldkamp CS, Carey JL: An algorithmic approach to thyroid function testing in a managed care setting: 3-year experience. Am J Clin Pathol 105:11, 1996

37. Singer PA, Cooper DS, Levy EG, et al: Treatment guidelines for patients with hyperthyroidism and hypothyroidism. JAMA 273:808, 1995

38. Törring O, Tallstedt L, Wallin G, et al: Graves' hyperthyroidism: treatment with antithyroid drugs, surgery, or radioiodine—a prospective, randomized study. J Clin Endocrinol Metab 81:2986, 1996

39. Laurberg P, Hansen PEB, Iversen E, et al: Goitre size and outcome of medical treatment of Graves' disease. Acta Endocrinol (Copenh) 111:39, 1986

40. Roti E, Gardini E, Minelli R, et al: Methimazole and serum thyroid hormone concentrations in hyperthyroid patients: effects of single and multiple daily doses. Ann Intern Med 111:181, 1989

41. Hashizume K, Ichikawa K, Sakurai A, et al: Administration of thyroxine in treated Graves' disease: effects on the level of antibodies to thyroid-stimulating hormone receptors and on the risk of recurrence of hyperthyroidism. N Engl J Med 324:947, 1991

42. Hirota Y, Tamai H, Hayashi Y, et al: Thyroid function and histology in forty-five patients with hyperthyroid Graves' disease in clinical remission more than ten years after thionamide drug treatment. J Clin Endocrinol Metab 62:165, 1986

43. Rittmaster RS, Zwicker H, Abbott EC: Effect of methimazole with or without exogenous L-thyroxine on serum concentrations of thyrotropin (TSH) receptor antibodies in patients with Graves' disease. J Clin Endocrinol Metab 81:3283, 1996

44. Winsa B, Dahlberg PA, Jansson R, et al: Factors influencing the outcome of thyrostatic drug therapy in Graves' disease. Acta Endocrinol (Copenh) 122:622, 1990

45. Tamai H, Hayaki I, Kawai K, et al: Lack of effect of thyroxine administration on elevated thyroid stimulating hormone receptor antibody levels in treated Graves' disease patients. J Clin Endocrinol Metab 80:1481, 1995

46. Hershman JM: Does thyroxine therapy prevent recurrence of Graves' hyperthyroidism (editorial)? J Clin Endocrinol Metab 80:1479, 1995

47. McIver B, Rae P, Beckett G, et al: Lack of effect of thyroxine in patients with Graves' hyperthyroidism who are treated with an antithyroid drug. N Engl J Med 334:220, 1996

48. Wiersinga WM: Immunosuppression of Graves' hyperthyroidism—still an elusive goal (editorial). N Engl J Med 334:265, 1996

49. Geffner DL, Hershman JM: β-Adrenergic blockade for the treatment of hyperthyroidism. Am J Med 93:61, 1992

50. Toft AD, Irvine WJ, Sinclair I, et al: Thyroid function after surgical treatment of thyrotoxicosis: a report of 100 cases treated with propranolol before operation. N Engl J Med 298:643, 1978

51. Zonszein J, Santangelo RP, Mackin JP, et al: Propranolol therapy in thyrotoxicosis: a review of 84 patients undergoing surgery. Am J Med 66:411, 1979

52. O'Doherty MJ, Kettle AG, Eustance CNP, et al: Radiation dose rates from adult patients receiving ^{131}I therapy for thyrotoxicosis. Nucl Med Commun 14:160, 1993

53. Graham GD, Burman KD: Radioiodine treatment of Graves' disease. Ann Intern Med 105:900, 1986

54. Franklyn J, Sheppard M: Radioiodine for hyperthyroidism: perhaps the best option. BMJ 305:727, 1992

55. Solomon B, Glinoer D, LaGasse R, et al: Current trends in the management of Graves' disease. J Clin Endocrinol Metab 70:1518, 1990

56. Burrow GN: Thyroid function and hyperfunction during gestation. Endocr Rev 14:194, 1993

57. Tietgens ST, Leinung MC: Thyroid storm. Med Clin North Am 79:169, 1995

58. Burger AG, Philippe J: Thyroid emergencies. Baillieres Clin Endocrinol Metab 6:77, 1992

59. Smallridge RC: Metabolic and anatomic thyroid emergencies: a review. Crit Care Med 20:276, 1992

60. Roti E, Robuschi G, Gardini E, et al: Comparison of methimazole, methimazole and sodium ipodate, and methimazole and saturated solution of potassium iodide in the early treatment of hyperthyroid Graves' disease. Clin Endocrinol (Oxf) 28:305, 1988

61. Bartalena L, Brogioni S, Grasso L, et al: Treatment of amiodarone-induced thyrotoxicosis, a difficult challenge: results of a prospective study. J Clin Endocrinol Metab 81:2930, 1996

62. Farwell AP, Abend SL, Huang SK, et al: Thyroidectomy for amiodarone-induced thyrotoxicosis. JAMA 263:1526, 1990

63. Amino N, Mori H, Iwatani Y, et al: High prevalence of transient post-partum thyrotoxicosis and hypothyroidism. N Engl J Med 306:849, 1982

64. Perros P, Kendall-Taylor P: Pathogenesis of thyroid-associated ophthalmopathy. Trends Endocrinol Metab 4:270, 1993

65. Perros P, Crombie AL, Kendall-Taylor P: Natural history of thyroid associated ophthalmopathy. Clin Endocrinol 42:45, 1995

66. DeGroot LJ, Gorman CA, Pinchera A, et al: Radiation and Graves' ophthalmopathy. J Clin Endocrinol Metab 80:339, 1995

67. Tallstedt L, Lundell G, Torring O, et al: Occurrence of ophthalmopathy after treatment for Graves' hyperthyroidism. N Engl J Med 326:1733, 1992

68. Utiger RD: Pathogenesis of Graves' ophthalmopathy. N Engl J Med 326:1772, 1992

69. Sridama V, DeGroot LJ: Treatment of Graves' disease and the course of ophthalmopathy. Am J Med 87:70, 1989

70. Glinoer D, Etienne-Decerf J, Schrooven M, et al: Beneficial effects of intensive plasma exchange followed by immunosuppressive therapy in severe Graves' ophthalmopathy. Acta Endocrinol (Copenh) 111:30, 1986

71. Bahn RS, Garrity JA, Gorman CA: Diagnosis and management of Graves' ophthalmopathy. J Clin Endocrinol Metab 71:559, 1990

72. Sawin CT, Geller A, Wolf PA, et al: Low serum thyrotropin concentration as a risk factor for atrial fibrillation in older persons. N Engl J Med 331:1249, 1994

73. Haden ST, Marqusee E, Utiger RD: Subclinical hyperthyroidism. Endocrinologist 6:322, 1996

74. Nicoloff JT, Spencer CA: The use and misuse of the sensitive thyrotropin assays. J Clin Endocrinol Metab 71:553, 1990

75. Sawin CT, Geller A, Hershman JM, et al: The aging thyroid: the use of thyroid hormone in older persons. JAMA 261:2653, 1989

76. Krugman LG, Hershman JM, Chopra IJ, et al: Patterns of recovery of the hypothalamic-pituitary-thyroid axis in patients taken off chronic thyroid therapy. J Clin Endocrinol Metab 41:70, 1975

77. Vagenakis AG, Braverman LE, Azizi F, et al: Recovery of pituitary thyrotropic function after withdrawal of prolonged thyroid-suppression therapy. N Engl J Med 293:581, 1975

78. Roti E, Minelli R, Gardini E, et al: The use and misuse of thyroid hormone. Endocr Rev 14:401, 1993

79. Choe W, Hays MT: Absorption of oral thyroxine. Endocrinologist 5:222, 1995

80. Toft AD: Thyroxine therapy. N Engl J Med 331:174, 1994

81. Müller B, Zulewski H, Huber P, et al: Impaired action of thyroid hormone associated with smoking in women with hypothyroidism. N Engl J Med 333:964, 1995

82. Utiger RD: Cigarette smoking and the thyroid (editorial). N Engl J Med 333:1001, 1995

83. Kabadi UM: Optimal daily levothyroxine dose in primary hypothyroidism: its relation to pretreatment thyroid hormone indexes. Arch Intern Med 149:2209, 1989

84. Helfand M, Crapo LM: Monitoring therapy in patients taking levothyroxine. Ann Intern Med 113:450, 1990

85. Stall GM, Harris S, Sokoll LJ, et al: Accelerated bone loss in hypothyroid patients overtreated with L-thyroxine. Ann Intern Med 113:265, 1990

86. Franklyn JA, Sheppard MC: The thyroid and osteoporosis. Trends Endocrinol Metab 3:113, 1992

87. Greenspan SL, Greenspan FS, Resnick NM, et al: Skeletal integrity in premeno-pausal and postmenopausal women receiving long-term L-thyroxine therapy. Am J Med 91:5, 1992

88. Becker C: Hypothyroidism and atherosclerotic heart disease: pathogenesis, medical management, and the role of coronary artery bypass surgery. Endocr Rev 6:432, 1985

89. Figge J, Dluhy RG: Amiodarone-induced elevation of thyroid stimulating hormone in patients receiving levothyroxine for primary hypothyroidism. Ann Intern Med 113:553, 1990

90. Oppenheimer JH, Braverman LE, Toft A, et al: Thyroid hormone treatment: when and what? J Clin Endocrinol Metab 80:2873, 1995

91. Mandel SJ, Larsen PR, Seely EW, et al: Increased need for thyroxine during preg-nancy in women with primary hypothyroidism. N Engl J Med 323:91, 1990

92. Leung AS, Millar LK, Koonings PP, et al: Perinatal outcome in hypothyroid preg-nancies. Obstet Gynecol 81:349, 1993

93. Utiger RD: Therapy of hypothyroidism: when are changes needed (editorial)? N Engl J Med 323:126, 1990

94. Roti E, Minelli R, Salvi M: Management of hyperthyroidism and hypothyroidism in the pregnant woman. J Clin Endocrinol Metab 81:1679, 1996

95. Jordan RM: Myxedema coma: the prognosis is improving. Endocrinologist 3:149, 1993

96. Hylander B, Rosenqvist U: Treatment of myxoedema coma—factors associated with fatal outcome. Acta Endocrinol (Copenh) 108:65, 1985

97. Holvey DN, Goodner CJ, Nicoloff JT, et al: Treatment of myxedema coma with in-travenous thyroxine. Arch Intern Med 113:139, 1964

98. Bagchi N, Brown TR, Parish RF: Thyroid dysfunction in adults over age 55 years: a study in an urban US community. Arch Intern Med 150:785, 1990

99. Sawin CT, Castelli WP, Hershman JM, et al: The aging thyroid: thyroid deficiency in the Framingham Study. Arch Intern Med 145:1386, 1985

100. Danese MD, Powe NR, Sawin CT, et al: Screening for mild thyroid failure at the periodic health examination: a decision and cost-effectiveness analysis. JAMA 276:285, 1996

101. Refetoff S: Clinical and genetic aspects of resistance to thyroid hormone. Endocri-nologist 2:261, 1992

102. Refetoff S, Weiss RE, Usala SJ: The syndromes of resistance to thyroid hormone. Endocr Rev 14:348, 1993

103. Brucker-Davis F, Skarulis MC, Grace MB, et al: Genetic and clinical features of 42 kindreds with resistance to thyroid hormone. The National Institutes of Health pro-spective study. Ann Intern Med 123:572, 1995

104. Jameson JL: Thyroid hormone resistance: pathophysiology at the molecular level (editorial). J Clin Endocrinol Metab 74:708, 1992

105. Dayan CM, Daniels GH: Chronic autoimmune thyroiditis. N Engl J Med 335:99, 1996

106. Takasu N, Yamada T, Takasu M, et al: Disappearance of thyrotropin-blocking an-tibodies and spontaneous recovery from hypothyroidism in autoimmune thyroiditis. N Engl J Med 326:513, 1992

107. Walfish PG, Meyerson J, Provias JP, et al: Prevalence and characteristics of post-partum thyroid dysfunction: results of a survey from Toronto, Canada. J Endocrinol In-vest 15:265, 1992

108. Smallridge RC: Postpartum thyroid dysfunction: a frequently undiagnosed en-docrine disorder. Endocrinologist 6:44, 1996

109. Othman S, Phillips DIW, Parkes AB, et al: A long-term follow-up of postpartum thyroiditis. Clin Endocrinol (Oxf) 32:559, 1990

110. Parma J, Duprez L, Van Sande J, et al: Somatic mutations in the thyrotropin recep-tor gene cause hyperfunctioning thyroid adenomas. Nature 365:649, 1993

111. Studer H, Derwahl M: Mechanisms of nonneoplastic endocrine hyperplasia—a changing concept: a review focused on the thyroid gland. Endocr Rev 16:411, 1995

112. Humphrey ML, Burman KD: Retrosternal and intrathoracic goiter. Endocrinolo-gist 2:195, 1992

113. Mack E: Management of patients with substernal goiters. Surg Clin North Am 75:377, 1995

114. Hay ID: Papillary thyroid carcinoma. Endocrinol Metab Clin North Am 19:545, 1990

115. DeGroot LJ, Kaplan EL, Shukla MS, et al: Morbidity and mortality in follicular thy-roid cancer. J Clin Endocrinol Metab 80:2946, 1995

116. Chetty R: Hurthle cell neoplasms of the thyroid gland revisited. Aust NZJ Surg 62:802, 1992

117. Pommier RF, Brennan MF: Medullary thyroid carcinoma. Endocrinologist 2:393, 1992

118. Gagel RF, Robinson MF, Donovan DT, et al: Medullary thyroid carcinoma: recent progress. J Clin Endocrinol Metab 76:809, 1993

119. Kaplan MM, Stall GM, Cummings T, et al: High-sensitivity serum calcitonin as-says applied to screening for thyroid C-cell disease in multiple endocrine neoplasia type 2A. Henry Ford Hosp Med J 40:227, 1992

120. Emerson CH, Veronikis IE: Medullary thyroid carcinoma—an uncommon cause of thyroid nodules but an important cause of thyroid neoplasms. Mayo Clin Proc 67:1006, 1992

121. Bergholm U, Adami H-O, Bergström R, et al: Long-term survival in sporadic and familial medullary thyroid carcinoma with special reference to clinical characteristics as prognostic factors. Acta Chir Scand 156:37, 1990

122. Swamy Venkatesh YS, Ordonez NG, Schultz PN, et al: Anaplastic carcinoma of the thyroid: a clinicopathologic study of 121 cases. Cancer 66:321, 1990

123. Frauman AG, Moses AC: Oncogenes and growth factors in thyroid carcinogene-sis. Endocrinol Metab Clin North Am 19:479, 1990

124. Fagin JA: Molecular defects in thyroid gland neoplasia. J Clin Endocrinol Metab 75:1398, 1992

125. Williams D: Thyroid cancer and the Chernobyl accident (editorial). J Clin En-docrinol Metab 81:6, 1996

126. Schneider AB, Shore-Freedman E, Weinstein RA: Radiation-induced thyroid and other head and neck tumors: occurrence of multiple tumors and analysis of risk factors. J Clin Endocrinol Metab 63:107, 1986

127. Schneider AB: Thyroid nodules following childhood irradiation: a 1989 update. Thyroid Today 12:1, 1989

128. DeGroot LJ: Diagnostic approach and management of patients exposed to irradia-tion to the thyroid. J Clin Endocrinol Metab 69:925, 1989

129. Ridgway EC: Clinician's evaluation of a solitary thyroid nodule. J Clin Endocrinol Metab 74:231, 1992

130. Sheppard MC, Franklyn JA: Management of the single thyroid nodule. Clin En-docrinol (Oxf) 37:398, 1992

131. Gharib H, Mazzaferri EL: A strategy for the solitary thyroid nodule. Hosp Pract 27(9A):53, 1992

132. Mazzaferri EL: Management of the solitary thyroid nodule. N Engl J Med 328:553, 1993

133. Monzani F, Goletti O, Caraccio N, et al: Percutaneous ethanol injection treatment of autonomous thyroid adenoma: hormonal and clinical evaluation. Clin Endocrinol (Oxf) 36:491, 1992

134. Altavilla G, Pascale M, Nenci I: Fine needle aspiration cytology of thyroid gland diseases. Acta Cytol 34:251, 1990

135. Gelderblom AJ, Hoek WVD, Lips PTAM, et al: A study of the importance of fine needle aspiration cytology in the diagnosis of the solitary thyroid nodule. Neth J Med 36:13, 1990

136. La Rosa GL, Lupo L, Giuffrida D, et al: Levothyroxine and potassium iodide are both effective in treating benign solitary solid cold nodules of the thyroid. Ann Intern Med 122:1, 1995

137. Blum M: Why do clinicians continue to debate the use of levothyroxine in the di-agnosis and management of thyroid nodules (editorial)? Ann Intern Med 122:63, 1995

138. Cooper DS: Thyroxine suppression therapy for benign nodular disease. J Clin En-docrinol Metab 80:331, 1995

139. Mazzaferri EL: Treating differentiated thyroid carcinoma: where do we draw the line? Mayo Clin Proc 66:105, 1991

140. Brennan MD, Bergstralh EJ, van Heerden JA: Follicular thyroid cancer treated at the Mayo Clinic, 1946 through 1970: initial manifestations, pathologic findings, therapy, and outcome. Mayo Clin Proc 66:11, 1991

141. McConahey WM, Hay ID, Woolner LB, et al: Papillary thyroid cancer treated at the Mayo Clinic, 1946 through 1970: initial manifestations, pathologic findings, therapy, and outcome. Mayo Clin Proc 61:978, 1986

142. Beldet L, Manderscheid J-C, Glinoer D, et al: The management of differentiated thyroid cancer in Europe in 1988: results of an international survey. Acta Endocrinol (Copenh) 120:547, 1989

143. Samaan NA, Schultz PN, Hickey RC, et al: The results of various modalities of treatment of well differentiated thyroid carcinoma: a retrospective review of 1599 pa-tients. J Clin Endocrinol Metab 75:714, 1992

144. Solomon BL, Wartofsky L, Burman KD: Current trends in the management of well differentiated papillary thyroid carcinoma. J Clin Endocrinol Metab 81:333, 1996

145. Wong TK, Hershman JM: Changes in thyroid function in nonthyroid illness. Trends Endocrinol Metab 3:8, 1992

146. Boelen A, Schiphorst P-T, Wiersinga WM: Soluble cytokine receptors and the low 3,5,3'-triiodothyronine syndrome in patients with nonthyroidal illness. J Clin En-docrinol Metab 80:971, 1995

147. Stockigt JR: Guidelines for diagnosis and monitoring of thyroid disease: nonthy-roidal illness. Clin Chem 42:188, 1996

148. Utiger RD: Altered thyroid function in nonthyroidal illness and surgery: to treat or not to treat (editorial). N Engl J Med 333:1562, 1995

Acknowledgments

Figures 1, 4, and 6   Albert Miller.

Figures 2 and 5   Seward Hung.

Figure 3   Marcia Kammerer.

47 Hypoglycemia

F. John Service, M.D., Ph.D.

Definition

Hypoglycemia is a clinical syndrome of diverse etiologies characterized by episodes of low blood glucose. These episodes are typically marked by autonomic manifestations such as trembling, sweating, nausea, and, in more severe episodes, central nervous system manifestations (neuroglycopenia) such as dizziness, confusion, and headache.

Classification

Hypoglycemic disorders have long been categorized as fasting or postprandial (reactive). This classification lacks practical value. Insulinoma, which is the archetypal cause of fasting hypoglycemia, may produce symptoms postprandially and, indeed, in some cases solely postprandially. Patients with factitious hypoglycemia evince symptoms irrespective of meals.

A more useful approach for the practitioner is a classification based on the patient's clinical characteristics. Persons who appear otherwise healthy have hypoglycemic disorders different from those of persons who are ill.

HYPOGLYCEMIA IN APPARENTLY HEALTHY PATIENTS

In apparently healthy persons, single episodes of hypoglycemia may result from accidental drug ingestion (e.g., ethanol in children). In addition to ethanol, salicylates and quinine can lower blood glucose levels; the combined effects of ethanol and quinine are responsible for so-called gin-and-tonic hypoglycemia. The healthy-appearing adult patient with a history of repeated episodes of neuroglycopenia usually has a disorder involving excessive insulin production, such as insulinoma; rarely, the hypoglycemia is factitious, caused by surreptitious or inadvertent use of a hypoglycemic agent (e.g., insulin or a sulfonylurea) [see Conditions That Cause Hypoglycemia, *below*].

Hypoglycemia may occur in patients who have coexistent disease but whose disease is being controlled with medical treatment. Typically, the hypoglycemia in these cases is a side effect of the medication being used to treat the coexistent disease, or it results from the mistaken dispensing of a sulfonylurea instead of the prescribed drug.

HYPOGLYCEMIA IN ILL PATIENTS

Illness can lead to hypoglycemia through a variety of mechanisms, only some of which involve insulin and not all of which are known. Many illnesses (e.g., renal failure and sepsis) are known to pose the risk of low blood glucose levels [see Table 1]; hypoglycemia in a patient with one of these illnesses requires little if any investigation of its cause. However, not all patients with a disease that has a proclivity to generate hypoglycemia actually experience low blood glucose levels. Why only some ill patients experience hypoglycemia is unknown.

Hospitalized patients are at increased risk for hypoglycemia, often from iatrogenic factors. In any inpatient with hypoglycemia, medication should be considered a potential cause.

Low blood glucose levels may be found on laboratory testing of ill patients who have no symptoms of hypoglycemia. In patients with leukemia or severe hemolysis, the hypoglycemia may be an artifact resulting from consumption of glucose in the blood collection tube by large numbers of leukocytes or by nucleated red blood cells, respectively.[1,2] Patients with glycogen storage disease may be asymptomatic because they have adapted to lifelong hypoglycemia from their disease.[3]

Diagnosis

Although the diagnosis of hypoglycemia requires the measurement of blood glucose, such measurement often is not feasible when symptoms arise during activities of ordinary life. Under these circumstances, the physician must take a detailed history to determine whether to proceed with further evaluation. The history should include a full description of the patient's symptoms and the circumstances under which they occur.

A medication history is also an important aspect of the evaluation in a patient with clinical manifestations of hypoglycemia, especially if the onset coincides with the filling of a new prescription. Because of the potential for drug error, all medications taken by the patient should be identified by a medical professional, such as a physician or pharmacist.

CLINICAL MANIFESTATIONS

The symptoms of hypoglycemia have been classified into two major groups: autonomic and neuroglycopenic. In a study of experimentally induced hypoglycemia in diabetic and nondiabetic persons, a principal-components analysis assigned sweating, trembling, feelings of warmth, anxiety, and nausea to the autonomic group and dizziness, confusion, tiredness, difficulty in speaking, headache, and inability to concentrate to the neuroglycopenic group. Hunger, blurred vision, drowsiness, and weakness could not be confidently assigned to either group.[4] In a retrospective analysis of 60 patients with insulinomas, 85% had various combinations of diplopia, blurred vision, sweating, palpitations, and weakness; 80% had confusion or abnormal behavior; 53% had amnesia or went into coma during the episode; and 12% had generalized seizures.[5]

The symptoms of hypoglycemia differ between persons but are nevertheless consistent from episode to episode in any one person.[6,7] There is no consistent chronologic order to the evolution of symptoms; autonomic symptoms do not always precede neuroglycopenic ones. In many patients, neuroglycopenic symptoms are the only ones observed.[7] Patients who have autonomic symptoms only are unlikely to have a hypoglycemic disorder. An additional factor that influences the generation of symptoms in hypoglycemia is their blunting by earlier hypoglycemic episodes.

PHYSICAL EXAMINATION

In patients who appear healthy, with or without coexistent compensated disease, the physical examination is normal or reveals only minor abnormalities that are unlikely to be germane to the underlying hypoglycemic disorder. In patients suspected of having factitious hypoglycemia from injection of insulin, a search for needle-puncture sites is fruitless. In ill patients with a primary disorder that can cause hypoglycemia, the results of physical examination will reflect that disease. For the patient observed while hypoglycemic, findings may include diaphoresis,

Table 1   Causes of Hypoglycemia

Drugs	Disopyramide Ethanol Haloperidol Quinine Salicylates
Drugs in specific illnesses	Pentamidine in *Pneumocystis* pneumonia Propoxyphene in renal failure Quinine in malaria Trimethoprim-sulfamethoxazole in renal failure Topical salicylates in renal failure

Endogenous hyperinsulinism	Insulinoma
	Islet hyperplasia/nesidioblastosis
	   Persistent hyperinsulinemic hypoglycemia
	     of infancy
	   Noninsulinoma pancreatogenous
	     hypoglycemia syndrome
	Insulin autoimmune hypoglycemia

Conditions that predispose to hypoglycemia	Neonatal
	   Infant small for gestational age
	   Erythroblastosis fetalis
	   Infant of diabetic mother
	   Cyanotic congenital heart disease
	   Beckwith-Wiedemann syndrome
	Inherited
	   Defects in amino acid and fatty acid
	     metabolism
	   Glycogen storage disease
	   Hereditary fructose intolerance
	   Isolated adrenocorticotropic hormone (ACTH)
	     deficiency
	   Isolated growth hormone deficiency
	Acquired
	   Addison disease
	   Carnitine deficiency
	   Intense exercise
	   Hypopituitarism
	   Heart failure
	   Lactic acidosis
	   Severe liver disease
	   Postoperative status
	   Renal failure
	   Reye syndrome
	   Sepsis
	   Shock
	   Spinal muscular atrophy
	   Starvation
	     Anorexia nervosa
	   Large mesenchymal tumors (fibroma, sarcoma,
	     small cell carcinoma, mesothelioma)

widened pulse pressure, and neurologic abnormalities ranging from slowed mentation or withdrawal from spontaneous communication to more overt confusion, erratic behavior, coma, seizure, and hypothermia.

LABORATORY TESTS

Serum Glucose

Studies of acute insulin-induced hypoglycemia in healthy persons have shown that the threshold for the development of symptoms is a serum glucose concentration of approximately 60 mg/dl; the threshold for impairment of brain function is approx-

imately 50 mg/dl.[8,9] These measurements were taken from arterialized venous blood (i.e., blood drawn from a vein in a heated hand [the application of heat shunts arterial blood into the venous system]); comparable levels in venous blood would probably be about 3 mg/dl lower. The rate of decrease in the serum glucose level does not influence the occurrence of the symptoms and signs of hypoglycemia.

Because symptoms of hypoglycemia are nonspecific, it is necessary to verify their origin. This is accomplished by applying a set of criteria first proposed by Whipple in 1938. The Whipple triad comprises spontaneous symptoms consistent with hypoglycemia, a low serum glucose concentration at the time the symptoms occur, and relief of the symptoms through normalization of the glucose level.[10]

A normal serum glucose concentration, reliably obtained during the occurrence of spontaneous symptoms, eliminates the possibility of a hypoglycemic disorder. Capillary glucose measurements that patients take themselves with a blood glucose meter during the occurrence of spontaneous symptoms are often unreliable, because nondiabetic patients usually are not experienced in this technique and because the measurements are obtained under adverse circumstances. Patients with a confirmed low serum glucose level (< 50 mg/dl) or a history of neuroglycopenic symptoms should undergo further testing. This is best accomplished with a prolonged fast.

The Prolonged (72-Hour) Fast

The prolonged (72-hour) fast is the classic diagnostic test for hypoglycemia. It should be conducted in a standardized manner [*see Table 2*]. The fast may be undertaken to demonstrate the Whipple triad and thereby establish that hypoglycemia is the basis for the patient's symptoms. If the Whipple triad has already been documented, the fast may be conducted for the purpose of determining the mechanism of the hypoglycemia, through measurement of beta cell polypeptide and plasma sulfonylurea levels. In the latter case, the fast can be terminated when the serum glucose level drops to 55 mg/dl or less (or, better yet, ≤ 50 mg/dl), which is the concentration at which beta cell polypeptides should be suppressed. Not all patients will need the full 72 hours to accomplish the purpose for the fast. In a study of 170 patients with surgically proven insulinomas, termination of the fast occurred within 12 hours in 33% of patients, within 24 hours in 65%, within 36 hours in 84%, within 48 hours in 93%, and within 72 hours in 99%.[11] Truncation of the fast at 48 hours, if hypoglycemia has not occurred by then, risks misdiagnosis.

Starting the fast overnight has allowed 40% of patients (including those with insulinoma and other causes of hypoglycemia) to conclude their fast in the outpatient endocrine-testing unit. Patients whose fast is not completed by the end of the business day are admitted to the hospital to complete the fast.

The decision whether to end the fast may not be easy to make when the Whipple triad is the goal. Because of delays in the availability of glucose measurements, the bedside glucose meter may have to serve as a guide. Some patients have slightly depressed glycemic levels without symptoms or signs of hypoglycemia. In other patients, fasting evokes the symptoms they experience in ordinary life but their serum glucose levels are not in the hypoglycemic range. In such instances, symptoms cannot be attributed to hypoglycemia. To complicate matters, young, lean, healthy women—and, to a lesser degree, some men—may have serum glucose concentrations in the range of 40 mg/dl or even lower during prolonged fasting.[12] Careful examination and testing for subtle signs or symptoms of hypoglycemia should therefore be conducted repeatedly when the patient's serum glucose level is near or in the hypoglycemic range. To end the fast solely on the basis of a low serum glucose level, in the absence of symptoms or signs of hypoglycemia, may jeopardize accurate diagnosis. On the other hand, failing to appreciate the manifestations of neuroglycopenia and, hence, concluding that the results of the fast are negative is an equally egregious error. It is essential to monitor patients closely during the fast and to be vigilant for subtle signs of neuroglycopenia.

Beta Cell Polypeptides and Their Surrogates

Concentrations of beta cell polypeptides (insulin, C-peptide, and proinsulin) are interpreted in the context of the concomitant serum glucose concentration. The normal overnight fasting ranges for these polypeptides do not apply when the serum glucose level is low. When immunochemiluminometric assays (ICMA) are used, the criteria for endogenous hyperinsulinemia are as follows: serum insulin, 3 μU/ml or greater; C-peptide, 200 pmol/L or greater; and proinsulin, 5 pmol/L or greater [see Figure 1].[13]

Insulin concentrations rarely exceed 100 μU/ml in patients with insulinomas. Values above this level suggest recent insulin administration or the presence of insulin antibodies.

Ratios of glucose to insulin, and vice versa, have no diagnostic utility [see Figure 1]. The molar ratio of insulin to C-peptide is the same for patients with insulinomas and healthy persons (approximately 0.2). The molar ratio of proinsulin to insulin appears to be higher in persons with insulinoma, but it provides poor diagnostic utility.

Because insulin has an antiketogenic effect, serum levels of the ketone body β-hydroxybutyrate can be used as a surrogate for measurement of insulin. The serum β-hydroxybutyrate level is low—2.7 mmol/L or less—in patients with insulin-mediated hypoglycemia; normal persons and those with non–insulin-mediated hypoglycemia have higher levels [see Figure 1].[13]

At the end of the fast, the patient is given an intravenous dose of 1 mg of glucagon, and the subsequent glucose response is measured. Because insulin is glycogenic and antiglycogenolytic, the glucagon injection results in an increase in the serum glucose level of 25 mg/dl or greater in patients with insulin-mediated hypoglycemia, whereas normal persons or those with non–in-

sulin-mediated hypoglycemia have lesser increases [see Figure 1].[13] An exuberant serum insulin response to intravenous glucagon has been considered an indication of insulinomas, but unfortunately, no normative data have been generated for this test. Measurement of beta cell polypeptides and insulin surrogates (β-hydroxybutyrate and glucose response to intravenous glucagon) has diagnostic utility only when the serum glucose level is 60 mg/dl or lower at the end of the fast.

Sulfonylureas and Meglitinides

Persons with hypoglycemia from inappropriate use of sulfonylureas or meglitinides (e.g., repaglinide) have concentrations of beta cell polypeptides that are identical to those observed in persons with insulinoma. Consequently, plasma assays for these drugs is an essential aspect of the evaluation. I use a highly sensitive and accurate liquid chromatographic tandem mass spectroscopy method to identify these drugs. A positive assay suggests either covert or inadvertent usage.

Insulin Antibodies

An assay for insulin antibodies should be done in every patient with clear evidence of hypoglycemia. The detection of insulin antibodies in a nondiabetic patient was once considered to be firm evidence of insulin factitious hypoglycemia, especially when animal insulin was the only commercially available type. Currently, most patients with factitious hypoglycemia have no detectable insulin antibodies, possibly because of the use of human insulin, which is less antigenic than beef or pork insulin. Rather, the presence of insulin antibodies, especially in high titers, is diagnostic of insulin autoimmune hypoglycemia (IAH) (see below).[13] Very low titers of insulin antibodies may sometimes be detected in persons without hypoglycemia[14] and, in rare instances, in patients with insulinomas.

Glycated Hemoglobin

Measurement of glycated hemoglobin is not a standard aspect of the clinical evaluation of hypoglycemia. Concentrations of glycated hemoglobin are statistically significantly lower in patients with insulinomas than in normal persons, but there is too much overlap between the two groups for this test to provide a diagnostic criterion.[6]

Oral Glucose Tolerance Test

The oral glucose tolerance test should not be used for the evaluation of hypoglycemia, because it is fraught with risk of misdiagnosis. At least 10% of healthy persons have serum glucose nadirs below 50 mg/dl, and the results of the test do not correlate with serum glucose responses to a mixed meal (i.e., a meal containing a balance of proteins, carbohydrates, and fat).

Mixed-Meal Test

For persons with a history of neuroglycopenic symptoms within 5 hours after food ingestion, a mixed-meal test may be conducted. The test is considered to be positive if the patient experiences neuroglycopenic symptoms when a concomitant serum glucose level measures 50 mg/dl or less. A positive mixed-meal test does not provide a diagnosis, only biochemical confirmation of the history.

C-Peptide Suppression Test

C-peptide is formed during the conversion of proinsulin to insulin by the pancreatic beta cells. In the C-peptide suppression

---

Table 2   **Protocol for Prolonged Supervised Fast**

1. Date the onset of the fast as of the last ingestion of calories. Discontinue all nonessential medications.
2. Allow the patient to drink calorie-free and caffeine-free beverages.
3. Ensure that the patient is active during waking hours.
4. Measure plasma glucose, insulin, C-peptide, and, if an assay is available, proinsulin in the same specimen. Repeat measurements every 6 hr until the plasma glucose drops below 60 mg/dl; then repeat the measurements every 1–2 hr.
5. When the plasma glucose is less than 45 mg/dl and the patient has symptoms or signs of hypoglycemia, measure plasma glucose, insulin, C-peptide, proinsulin, β-hydroxybutyrate, and sulfonylurea in the same specimen; then inject 1 mg of glucagon I.V. and measure plasma glucose after 10, 20, and 30 min.
6. Feed the patient.

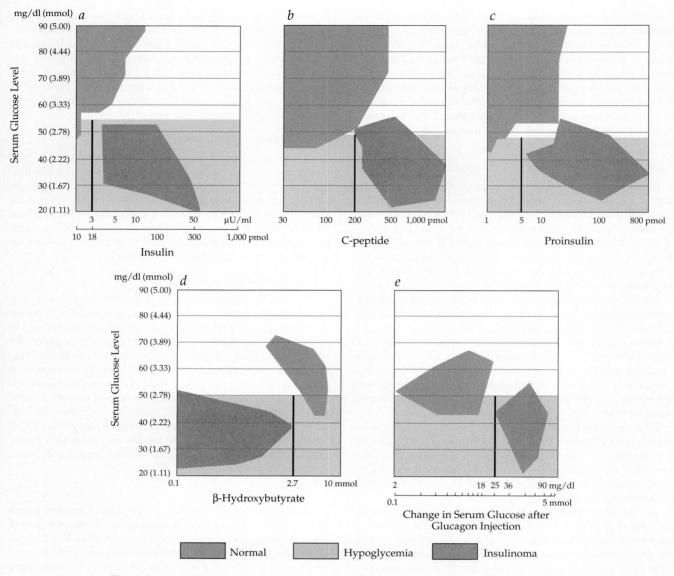

Figure 1 **During the 72-hour fast, levels of serum glucose are compared with serum levels of insulin (*a*), C-peptide (*b*), proinsulin (*c*), and β-hydroxybutyrate (*d*). At the end of the fast, 1 mg of glucagon is injected intravenously, and its effect on glucose levels is measured (*e*). Normal patients may have glucose levels that drop into the hypoglycemic range, so careful documentation of hypoglycemic symptoms is necessary.**

test, the patient fasts overnight and then receives an hour-long intravenous infusion of insulin, during which levels of serum glucose and C-peptide are measured. In normal patients, hypoglycemia from the exogenous insulin results in suppression of C-peptide production; patients with insulinomas have higher levels of C-peptide. When the likelihood of a hypoglycemic disorder is not high, a normal result on the C-peptide suppression test may preclude the need for a 72-hour fast. Interpretation of the C-peptide suppression test requires normative data appropriately adjusted for the patient's body mass index and age.[7]

Intravenous Tolbutamide Test

In the past, serum glucose response to an intravenous injection of tolbutamide was used in the diagnosis of insulinoma. This test is potentially dangerous and is less accurate than other tests for insulinoma and, therefore, has been rarely used in recent years.

Conditions That Cause Hypoglycemia

The causes of hypoglycemia in healthy-appearing adults encompass the following conditions: insulinoma, factitious hypoglycemia from insulin or sulfonylurea, noninsulinoma pancreatogenous hypoglycemia syndrome (NIPHS), and insulin autoimmune hypoglycemia.

INSULINOMA

Epidemiology

Between 1927 and 1986, 224 hypoglycemic patients underwent their first pancreatic exploration at the Mayo Clinic and were found to have insulinoma. Because of the relatively large number of cases of insulinoma treated at the Mayo Clinic, in comparison with other medical centers, and the comprehensive epidemiologic database that the Mayo Clinic maintains for Olmsted County, Minnesota, it was possible to determine the population-based incidence of insulinoma, the risk of recurrence, and the survival in patients with insulinoma.[15]

The median age of the Mayo Clinic insulinoma patients was 47 years, with a range of 8 to 82 years; 59% were female. The incidence in Olmsted County was 4 cases per 1 million person-years. Of the 224 patients, 7.6% had multiple endocrine neoplasia type I (MEN I) and 5.8% had malignant insulinoma. The risk of recurrence was greater in patients with MEN I (21%) than in those without this condition (7%). Over a 45-year period, overall survival of the total cohort was similar to the expected survival (78% versus 81%).

Insulinomas have been found in pregnant patients and in patients with type 2 (non–insulin-dependent) diabetes mellitus. One case of insulinoma in type 1 (insulin-dependent) diabetes mellitus has been reported.[16]

Diagnosis

Laboratory tests Insulinoma is characterized by hypoglycemia caused by elevated levels of endogenous insulin. Confirmation of the diagnosis requires exclusion of hypoglycemia from exogenous sources.

Localization Once a biochemical diagnosis of insulinoma has been made, the next step is localization. Success with the various modalities reflects local skill and experience. Great success has been seen with transabdominal ultrasonography and triple-phase spiral computed tomography. Magnetic resonance imaging and scintigraphy with indium-111 (In-111)–pentetreotide (OctreoScan) can also be used. I reserve endoscopic ultrasonography for complex cases. Percutaneous transhepatic portal venous sampling has been abandoned even by its former proponents.

In patients whose tumor is not found by ultrasonography or CT, the selective arterial calcium stimulation test provides a means to both regionalize and confirm endogenous hyperinsulinemia. This test involves serial injections of calcium into the splenic, gastroduodenal, and superior mesenteric arteries. Subsequent doubling of serum insulin concentrations in the right hepatic vein indicates hyperfunctioning beta cells in the part of the pancreas served by that artery.

There is general agreement that the best localization of insulinomas is achieved with intraoperative ultrasonography and careful mobilization and palpation of the pancreas by a surgeon experienced with insulinoma surgery. This approach has seen a 98% success rate in the identification of insulinoma. After this test, these patients go straight to surgery.

Management

The treatment of choice for insulinomas is surgical removal. Depending on the lesion, the surgery required may range from enucleation of the insulinoma to subtotal pancreatectomy. It is advisable for the surgery to be performed at an institution with expertise in the management of insulinoma.

Medical therapy is less effective than tumor resection, but the former can be used in patients who are not candidates for surgery, who refuse surgery, or whose surgery is unsuccessful. The most effective medication for controlling symptomatic hypoglycemia in these patients is diazoxide, which lowers insulin secretion. Diazoxide is given in divided doses of up to 1,200 mg daily. Side effects include edema, which may require high doses of loop diuretics, and hirsutism. Oth-

er medications for insulinomas include verapamil, phenytoin, and octreotide.

FACTITIOUS HYPOGLYCEMIA

The term factitious (or factitial) has been used in medical parlance to imply covert patient activity. The consideration of such a possibility often changes the patient-physician relationship, leading the physician to feel deceived and the patient to feel mistrusted. However, the pejorative connotation with which factitious illness has been encumbered requires softening because some patients with factitious disease suffer through no fault of their own.

Epidemiology

Factitious hypoglycemia is more common in women and occurs most often in the third or fourth decade of life. Many of these patients work in health-related occupations.

Factitious hypoglycemia in patients with diabetes is probably more common than the incidence noted in published series.[17] Confirmation of the diagnosis in these cases can be very difficult. When deprived of access to hypoglycemic agents, diabetic patients with factitious hypoglycemia become hyperglycemic.

Etiology

Factitious hypoglycemia results from the use of insulin or the use of sulfonylureas or meglitinides that stimulate insulin secretion. The most common form of factitious hypoglycemia is the covert self-administration of a hypoglycemic drug or insulin by a patient without diabetes or the inappropriate manipulation of hypoglycemic drugs or insulin by a patient with diabetes. Less often, a parent may administer a hypoglycemic agent to a child; this is a form of child abuse.[18] In all reported cases, the alleged perpetrator was the patient's mother, who had ready access to insulin. Insulin has also been used to attempt suicide or homicide.[19]

There are increasing numbers of patients who, by taking a prescribed medication in good faith, incur hypoglycemia because a sulfonylurea was mistakenly dispensed.[20] In most instances, confusion in dispensing the drug arose because of similarity in spelling between the intended medication and the sulfonylurea. In some cases, however, the dispensing error was a result of negligence. On occasion, cases have arisen in which a nondiabetic person mistakenly takes hypoglycemic medication belonging to another member of the household.

Diagnosis

The possibility of factitious hypoglycemia should be considered in every patient undergoing evaluation for a hypoglycemic disorder, especially when the hypoglycemia has a chaotic occurrence—that is, when it has no relation at all to meals or fasting. All medications should be identified; the assistance of a pharmacist is desirable. The practice of searching personal effects and labeling insulin with a traceable substance that can be detected in blood or urine is probably unacceptable in the current climate of patients' rights.

The diagnosis of factitious hypoglycemia can usually be established by measuring serum insulin, sulfonylurea, and C-peptide when the patient is hypoglycemic. If a spontaneous episode of hypoglycemia is not observed, the patient should undergo a 72-hour fast. The results of the fast may be negative, however, should the patient not take the offending agent.

In a patient whose hypoglycemia results from covert use of a hypoglycemic agent, the agent will be present in the blood. A sensitive method such as liquid chromatography linked to mass spectroscopy should be used for the detection of sulfonylureas and meglitinides.

In insulin-related factitious hypoglycemia, the serum insulin level is high and the C-peptide level is suppressed, usually being close to the lower limit of detection. This observation applies both to nondiabetic patients and to those with type 2 diabetes. Patients with type 1 diabetes are characteristically severely insulin deficient and have low or undetectable serum concentrations of C-peptide. Although the C-peptide values in these patients cannot be further suppressed, confirmation that the values are low during a hypoglycemic episode eliminates any consideration of endogenous hyperinsulinism.

Management

Treatment of factitious hypoglycemia is simple: the patient stops taking the offending medication. The difficulty involved when medication is taken in error is identification of the drug. In the case of deliberate covert use, psychiatric referral is indicated.

NONINSULINOMA PANCREATOGENOUS HYPOGLYCEMIA SYNDROME

There have been cases of adults who do not have insulinomas but have hypoglycemia resulting from postprandial hypersecretion of insulin by pancreatic beta cells. Because of the unique clinical, diagnostic, radiologic, surgical, and histologic features of this disorder, it warrants designation as a new syndrome. We have termed it noninsulinoma pancreatogenous hypoglycemia syndrome, or NIPHS.[21]

Epidemiology

Like insulinoma, NIPHS affects patients across a broad age range—16 to 78 years, in one series—and causes severe neuroglycopenia, with loss of consciousness and, in some cases, generalized seizures. Unlike insulinoma, NIPHS occurs predominantly in males (70%).

Pathophysiology and Pathogenesis

Histologic analysis of pancreatic tissue from patients with NIPHS shows cells budding off ducts, which is best seen by chromogranin A and insulin immunohistochemical staining. Islet cell hypertrophy is also evident. No gross or microscopic tumor has been identified on hematoxylin-eosin–stained sections in any NIPHS patients.

Whether islet hypertrophy, nesidioblastosis, or both are pathogenic in these patients is open to question, as is the case with persistent hyperinsulinemic hypoglycemia of infancy (PHHI). However, a role for some form of diffuse islet cell dysfunction appears well established in these cases. Whatever the pathologic process may be, it is nonfocal, yet it does not necessarily involve the entire pancreas uniformly.

The histologic findings in NIPHS are similar to those in PHHI. Although familial forms of PHHI may be associated with mutations in the *Kir6.2* and *SUR1* genes, analysis of these genes in NIPHS patients has not shown such mutations.[22] However, these patients may have common mutations at another, as yet unspecified, locus.

Diagnosis

Clinical manifestations Symptoms of NIPHS occur primarily in the postprandial state 2 to 4 hours after eating. Although insulinoma patients may experience symptoms postprandially, they also have symptoms during food deprivation. It is extreme-ly rare for insulinoma patients to have symptoms solely in the postprandial state.

Laboratory tests Patients with NIPHS have low serum glucose levels and elevated serum insulin levels in the postprandial period. Because of the short half-life of insulin, the criteria for hyperinsulinemia used in the fasting state appear to apply in the postprandial state, as long as the low glucose level occurs more than 30 minutes from the peak postprandial insulin level. Supervised 72-hour fasts have shown normal results in patients with NIPHS, whereas a negative 72-hour fast in a patient with insulinoma is a rare occurrence.

The selective arterial calcium stimulation test has shown positive results for patients with NIPHS.[23,24] All radiologic localizing studies in patients with NIPHS (transabdominal ultrasonography, triple-phase CT, celiac axis angiography, and intraoperative ultrasonography) have been negative for insulinoma.

Management

Gradient-guided partial pancreatectomy has been effective in relieving symptoms in patients with NIPHS. The pancreas is resected to the left of the superior mesenteric vein when results of the selective arterial calcium stimulation test are positive only for the splenic artery, and the pancreas is resected to the right of the superior mesenteric vein when the test is positive for an additional artery. Fortunately, gradient-guided debulking of the pancreas can ameliorate the symptoms of NIPHS even in patients whose disease would appear to have involved the whole pancreas. In rats, the mechanism for this effect may be related to decreased insulin secretion, attributed to reduced glucose transporter GLUT2, in remnant pancreas after partial pancreatectomy.[25] Unfortunately, recurrence of hypoglycemia after a few symptom-free years has developed in a few of the NIPHS patients.

INSULIN AUTOIMMUNE HYPOGLYCEMIA

Epidemiology

IAH is an extraordinarily rare disorder that is observed primarily, although not exclusively, in persons of Japanese and Korean ethnicity. The disorder may occur at any age. IAH tends to be be self-limited in Asians, but it may be persistent in whites. There is no gender predilection. Many patients have an ongoing autoimmune disorder or a history of treatment with a sulfhydryl-containing drug such as antithyroid medication. No patients have had a history of exposure to insulin.[14]

Pathogenesis

IAH is characterized by the presence of autoantibodies to insulin or the insulin receptor. There is speculation that meal ingestion in these patients may result in the unbinding of insulin from these antibodies. However, measurements of total insulin and free insulin have shown no postprandial alteration in their relative concentrations. The mechanism for the generation of insulin antibodies is unknown but may involve enhanced immunogenicity resulting from an effect of the disulfide bond in drugs with a sulfhydryl component.

Diagnosis

Clinical manifestations Patients with IAH typically experience postprandial hypoglycemia resulting in neuroglycopenia. The symptomatic severity of IAS appears to vary greatly. Whites may become more seriously debilitated than Asians.

Laboratory tests Serum insulin levels are markedly elevated in IAH, because the insulin antibodies interfere with this assay. Values can be as high as 1,000 µU/ml. Oddly, C-peptide levels are usually not suppressed. Insulin antibody titers are very high, higher than those seen in insulin-treated diabetic patients. The antibodies may bind only to human insulin or to both human insulin and beef and pork insulin. The antibodies may be polyclonal or monoclonal, and they usually have characteristics similar to those that occur in patients with type 1 diabetes mellitus. It should be noted that very low titers of insulin antibodies may also be observed in healthy persons without hypoglycemia and occasionally in persons with insulinoma.

Management

Supportive treatment, such as frequent small meals, may be effective in IAH, especially for mild cases. For more severely affected patients, a variety of approaches have been tried, including glucocorticoids, immunosuppressants, plasmapheresis, octreotide, and diazoxide. Unfortunately, all these treatments usually fail. Use of partial pancreatectomy and splenectomy has led to amelioration but not complete resolution of symptoms.

References

1. Goodenow TJ, Malarkey WB: Leukocytosis and artifactual hypoglycemia. JAMA 237:1961, 1977

2. Macaron CI, Kadri A, Macaron Z: Nucleated red blood cells and artifactual hypoglycemia. Diabetes Care 4:113, 1981

3. Service FJ, Veneziale CM, Nelson RA, et al: Combined deficiency of glucose-6-phosphate and fructose-1,6-diphosphate: studies of glucagon secretion and fuel utilization. Am J Med 64:698, 1978

4. Hepburn DA, Deary IJ, Frier BM, et al: Symptoms of acute insulin-induced hypoglycemia in humans with and without IDDM: factor-analysis approach. Diabetes Care 14:949, 1991

5. Service FJ, Dale AJD, Elveback LR, et al: Insulinoma: clinical and diagnostic features of 60 consecutive cases. Mayo Clin Proc 51:417, 1976

6. Hassoun AAK, Service FJ, O'Brien PC: Glycated hemoglobin in insulinoma. Endocr Pract 4:181, 1998

7. Service FJ, O'Brien PC, Kao PC, et al: C-peptide suppression test: effects of gender, age and body mass index: implications for the diagnosis of insulinoma. J Clin Endocrinol Metab 74:204, 1992

8. Schwartz NS, Clutter WE, Shah SD, et al: Glycemic thresholds for activation of glucose counterregulatory systems are higher than the threshold for symptoms. J Clin Invest 79:777, 1987

9. Mitrakou A, Ryan C, Veneman T, et al: Hierarchy of glycemic thresholds for counterregulatory hormone secretion, symptoms and cerebral dysfunction. Am J Physiol 260:E57, 1991

10. Whipple AE: The surgical therapy of hyperinsulinism. J Int Chir 3:237, 1938

11. Service FJ, Natt N: Clinical perspective: the prolonged fast. J Clin Endocrinol Metab 85:3973, 2000

12. Merimee TJ, Fineberg SE: Homeostasis during fasting: II. Hormone substrate differences between men and women. J Clin Endocrinol Metab 37:698, 1973

13. Service FJ: Diagnostic approach to adults with hypoglycemic disorders. Endocrinol Metab Clin North Am 28:519, 1999

14. Redmon JB, Nuttall FQ: Autoimmune hypoglycemia. Hypoglycemic Disorders 28:603, 1999

15. Service FJ, McMahon MM, O'Brien PC, et al: Functioning insulinoma—incidence, recurrence, and long-term survival of patients: a 60-year study. Mayo Clin Proc 66:711, 1991

16. Svartberg J, Stridsberg M, Wilander E, et al: Tumour-induced hypoglycaemia in a patient with insulin-dependent diabetes mellitus. J Intern Med 239:181, 1996

17. Tattersall RB, Gregory R, Selby C, et al: Course of brittle diabetes: 12 year follow up. BMJ 302:1240, 1991

18. Mayefsky JH, Sarnaik AP, Postellon DC: Factitious hypoglycemia. Pediatrics 69:804, 1982

19. Marks V, Teale JD: Hypoglycemia: factitious and felonious. Endocrinol Metab Clin North Am 28:579, 1999.

20. Hooper PL, Tello RJ, Burstein PH, et al: Pseudoinsulinoma: the Diamox-Diabinese switch. N Engl J Med 323:448, 1990

21. Service FJ, Natt N, Thompson GB, et al: Noninsulinoma pancreatogenous hypoglycemia: a novel syndrome of hyperinsulinemic hypoglycemia in adults independent of mutations in *Kir6.2* and *SUR1* genes. J Clin Endocrinol Metab 84:1582, 1999

22. Thomas PM, Cote GJ, Wohlik N, et al: Mutations in the sulfonylurea receptor gene in familial hyperinsulinemic hypoglycemia of infancy. Science 268:426, 1995

23. Doppman JL, Chang R, Fraker DL, et al: Localization of insulinomas to regions of the pancreas by intraarterial stimulation with calcium. Ann Intern Med 123:269, 1995

24. O'Shea D, Rohrer-Theus A, Lynn JA, et al: Localization of insulinomas by selective intraarterial calcium injection. J Clin Endocrinol Metab 81:1623, 1996

25. Zangen DH, Bonner-Weir S, Lee CH, et al: Reduced insulin, GLUT2, and IDX-1 in beta-cells after partial pancreatectomy. Diabetes 46:258, 1997

48 Diabetes Mellitus

Saul Genuth, M.D.

Definition and Overview

Diabetes mellitus is a metabolic disease characterized by hyperglycemia that results from defects in insulin secretion, insulin action, or both. Important abnormalities in fat and protein metabolism are also present. Nonetheless, the diagnosis still rests upon demonstrating elevated plasma glucose levels. The chronic hyperglycemia of diabetes mellitus is specifically associated with long-term damage, dysfunction, and failure of various organs, especially the retina and lens of the eye, the kidneys, and both somatic and autonomic nervous systems. The heart, arterial system, and microcirculation are also adversely affected.

A variety of pathogenic processes are involved in the development of different forms of diabetes. These processes range from autoimmune destruction of the beta cells of the pancreatic islets with consequent insulin deficiency to mutations in the insulin receptor gene with consequent resistance to insulin action. The basis for the metabolic abnormalities of diabetes mellitus is deficient action of insulin on its major target tissues, including skeletal muscle, cardiac muscle, adipose tissue, and liver. Loss of proper insulin regulation of metabolism results from inadequate secretion of insulin, from diminished tissue responses to insulin at one or more points in the complex pathways of insulin action, or from both processes. Impairment of insulin secretion and defects in insulin action coexist in many patients, and in these patients, it is often unclear which abnormality is the primary cause of the hyperglycemia.

Acute life-threatening consequences of diabetes mellitus are ketoacidosis and nonketotic hyperglycemic hyperosmolar coma. Overtreatment of hyperglycemia can lead to hypoglycemia, which may be severe enough to cause seizures and loss of consciousness. Symptoms of poorly controlled hyperglycemia include polyuria, polydipsia, blurred vision, weight loss, polyphagia, stunting of growth, and vulnerability to infections or susceptibility to a more virulent or chronic course when infected.

Specific long-term complications of diabetes include (1) retinopathy with potential loss of vision, (2) nephropathy leading to end stage renal disease (ESRD), and (3) neuropathy with risk of foot ulcers, amputation, Charcot joints, sexual dysfunction, and potentially disabling dysfunction of the stomach, bowel, and bladder. Numerous mechanisms have been discovered that may mediate the specific tissue damage caused by hyperglycemia. Diabetic patients are also at increased risk for atherosclerotic cardiovascular, peripheral vascular, and cerebrovascular disease. These conditions may be related to hyperglycemia as well as to hypertension and abnormal lipoprotein profiles that are often found in diabetic patients.

Sufficient hyperglycemia to cause pathologic and functional changes in target tissues may be present for some time before clinical symptoms lead to a diagnosis of diabetes in many patients. At an even earlier stage, an incipient abnormality in glucose metabolism can be identified on plasma glucose testing, which indicates that the patient is at considerably increased risk for the full clinical disorder.

Classification

The classification of diabetes mellitus has recently been revised by a task force of the American Diabetes Association that included representation from Europe.[1] Major etiologic classes of the disease, along with more esoteric examples, have been categorized [see Table 1]. The vast majority of cases of diabetes mellitus are either type 1 (insulin-dependent) or type 2 (non–insulin-dependent) in an approximate ratio of 1:9.

TYPE 1 AND TYPE 2 DIABETES MELLITUS

Type 1 and type 2 diabetes were formerly known as insulin-dependent diabetes mellitus (IDDM) and non–insulin-dependent diabetes mellitus (NIDDM), respectively. This classification was abandoned largely because it was difficult to distinguish patients with IDDM from those patients with NIDDM who eventually required insulin treatment to mitigate hyperglycemia. Physicians, nurses, hospital-record-room personnel, health insurers, and even sometimes researchers were hard put to distinguish between these two forms of diabetes using the old terminology. The new classification, dependent on etiology rather than mode of treatment, puts a greater emphasis on the history and characteristics of the patients to determine the probable etiology and type. Two categories of blood glucose elevation, impaired glucose tolerance (IGT) and impaired fasting glucose (IFG), that lie between normal glucose levels and overt diabetes have also been established [see Impaired Glucose Tolerance, below].[2]

GESTATIONAL DIABETES MELLITUS

Gestational diabetes mellitus (GDM) constitutes a separate category for cases of diabetes first detected during pregnancy.[3] When diabetes is detected early in pregnancy, it is likely to be type 1 or type 2 diabetes mellitus that is presenting symptomatically and was probably precipitated or worsened by the pregnant state. Diabetes is commonly detected in the second and third trimester (i.e., in 4% of pregnant women) and is likely to be specific for the pregnant state, to be transient, and to reverse to normal glucose tolerance or to IGT on follow-up oral glucose tolerance testing 6 weeks after delivery. However, GDM is associated with a high risk of future diabetes, especially in women who have IGT post partum or who remain obese.[3] Permanent diabetes will develop in approximately 50% of patients within 10 years of GDM. The greatest importance of any single episode of GDM lies in the risks it poses to the fetus. These risks include intrauterine mortality, neonatal mortality, respiratory distress syndrome, hypoglycemia, hypocalcemia, jaundice, and macrosomia, which can cause trauma such as shoulder dystocia during passage through the birth canal.

SECONDARY FORMS OF DIABETES MELLITUS

Of the categories of secondary diabetes [see Table 1], endocrinopathies and drug- or chemical-induced diabetes are noteworthy because they represent instances of diabetes that are potentially reversible if they are recognized and the physician can cure the endocrinopathy or discontinue the offending drug. The category of genetic defects in beta cell function illustrates how the classification will grow ever more detailed as knowledge increases. For example, the single diabetes mellitus phenotype formerly called maturity-onset diabetes of the young (MODY) can now be more precisely classified into at least four genetic varieties, each of which arises from mutation of a different gene.

Diabetes caused by chronic pancreatitis, pancreatectomy, or occasionally carcinoma of the pancreas is usually type 1 in character. Because patients with this disease have glucagon as well as insulin deficiency, they are somewhat less likely to go into ketoacidosis[4] but are quite vulnerable to hypoglycemia. Because they are deficient in pancreatic enzymes, their digestion and subsequent absorption of nutrients is somewhat erratic, even though replacement enzymes are ingested with meals. If alcoholism, often the cause of chronic pancreatitis, is irremediable, it also contributes to blood glucose instability, as does the often accompanying irregular lifestyle. Small frequent doses of lispro insulin should be helpful, but safety may require less stringent blood glucose goals in such patients.

Although many individual drugs have been incriminated as a cause of hyperglycemia, the continued use of pharmacologic anti-inflammatory or immunosuppressive doses of synthetic gluco-corticoids is an especially important continuing problem. Up to 25% of renal transplant patients develop so-called steroid diabetes.[5] In a case-control study, use of glucocorticoids for up to 45 days was a risk factor for diabetes that required pharmacologic treatment.[6] The odds ratio rose from 1.77 at a prednisone equivalent of 10 mg/day to an odds ratio of 10.3 at 30 mg/day. Obesity and family history of diabetes increased the risk of steroid diabetes. Although insulin resistance in the liver and muscle is a well-recognized effect of glucocorticoids, an action on the beta cells to limit the compensatory response to hyperglycemia[7] adds to the diabetogenic effect at higher steroid doses. Patients treated with glucocorticoids for more than a few days need to be warned to watch for and report clinical symptoms of hyperglycemia promptly. Ketoacidosis is rare, but hyperglycemic hyperosmolar nonketotic coma can occur. Insulin treatment is usually necessary for symptomatic patients and for those with a fasting plasma glucose (FPG) level greater than 200 mg/dl, but sulfonylurea drugs are sometimes effective. There is little systematic information on the efficacy of the other oral agents. In most instances, steroid diabetes is transient, but in a minority of cases, diabetes persists even after withdrawal of the glucocorticoids.

Screening for Diabetes

Screening for type 1 diabetes mellitus by office glucose testing is not currently indicated. Depending on the results of a prevention trial in progress, future screening may become indicated and cost-effective. Current American Diabetes Association criteria for office screening of asymptomatic individuals for type 2 diabetes mellitus employ FPG levels.[1] Mass indiscriminate public screening is not justified, because there is as yet no proof of population benefit. Screening is recommended in all individuals 45 years of age and older at 3-year intervals. Younger individuals should be screened if they are obese (> 120% desirable body weight or a body mass index ≥ 27), have a first-degree relative with diabetes, are members of a high-risk ethnic population (African American, Hispanic American, Native American, Asian American), have delivered a baby weighing more than 9 lb, have previously had GDM, are hypertensive (blood pressure ≥ 140/90 mm Hg), have atherogenic dyslipidemia (high-density lipoprotein [HDL] cholesterol levels ≤ 35 mg/dl or triglyceride levels ≥ 250 mg/dl) or had IFG or IGT on previous testing.[1]

Epidemiology

TYPE 1 DIABETES MELLITUS

Available, but not up-to-date, studies suggest the prevalence of type 1 diabetes mellitus in the United States is 1.7 per 1,000 in individuals younger than 19 years and 2.1 per 1,000 in adults.[8] A total prevalence of approximately 500,000 is estimated. Current estimates of annual incidence are 18 per 100,000 population in the 0- to 19-year age range and 9 per 100,000 population in those older than 20 years.[8] Approximately 30,000 cases of type 1 diabetes mellitus are estimated to occur yearly in the United States, and it is more common in whites than in African Americans. Worldwide, the highest annual incidence of type 1 diabetes mellitus is found in Finland (35 cases per 100,000) and the lowest is found in Korea (< 1 per 100,000).

TYPE 2 DIABETES MELLITUS

Analysis of data from the third National Health and Nutrition

---

Table 1 **Etiologic Classification of Diabetes**

Type 1 diabetes mellitus* (β cell destruction, usually leading to absolute insulin deficiency)
  Immune mediated
  Idiopathic
Type 2 diabetes mellitus* (may range from predominantly insulin resistance with relative insulin deficiency to a predominantly insulin secretory defect with insulin resistance)
Other specific types of diabetes
  Genetic defects of β cell function
    Chromosome 12, HNF-1α (formerly MODY3)
    Chromosome 7, glucokinase (formerly MODY2)
    Chromosome 20, HNF-4α (formerly MODY2)
  Genetic defects in insulin action
    Type A insulin resistance
  Disease of the exocrine pancreas
    Pancreatitis
    Trauma/pancreatectomy
    Neoplasia
  Endocrinopathies
    Acromegaly
    Cushing syndrome
    Glucagonoma
  Drug- or chemical-induced
    Nicotinic acid
    Glucocorticoids
    Thiazides
  Infections
    Congenital rubella
    Cytomegalovirus
  Uncommon forms of immune-mediated diabetes
    Stiff-man syndrome
    Anti-insulin receptor antibodies
  Other genetic syndromes associated with diabetes
    Down syndrome
    Turner syndrome
    Friedreich ataxia
    Myotonic dystrophy
Gestational diabetes mellitus (GDM)

Note: The list of other specific types of diabetes is not comprehensive. There are many other such syndromes.
*Patients with any form of diabetes may require insulin treatment at some stage of their disease. Such use of insulin does not, of itself, classify the patient.

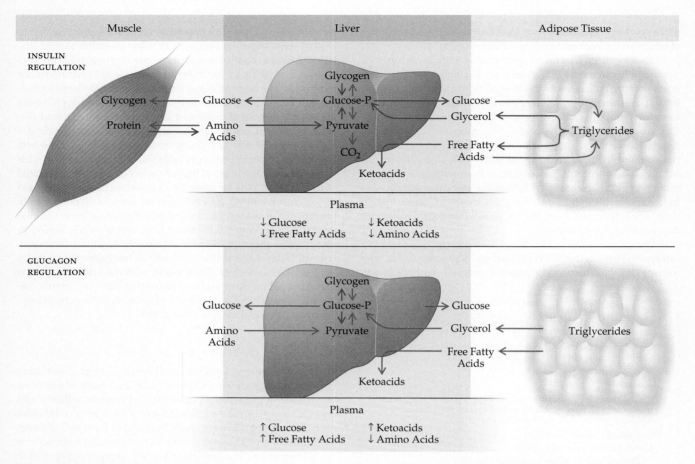

Muscle	Liver	Adipose Tissue

Figure 1 **The opposing actions of insulin and glucagon, particularly within the liver, on substrate flow and plasma levels are seen here. The two hormones have directly opposite effects on key enzymes, such as glycogen synthase and phosphorylase. Thus, stimulatory effects of glucagons on glucose and ketoacid production are magnified when insulin is deficient, as in type 1 diabetes mellitus. Red arrows indicate stimulation. Blue arrows indicate inhibition.**

Examination Survey (NHANES III), conducted from 1988 to 1994,[9] indicates a prevalence of 5.1% for adults at least 20 years of age in the United States and a prevalence of 2.7% of undiagnosed diabetes (FPG ≥ 126 mg/dl). A prevalence of 12.3% (diagnosed plus undiagnosed) was estimated for individuals 40 to 74 years of age. There are an estimated 10.2 million diagnosed and 5.4 million undiagnosed cases of diabetes in the United States. The estimated number of persons with IGT equals the number with diabetes. Non-Hispanic African-American and Mexican-American women have nearly twice the prevalence of diabetes as non-Hispanic white women. Non-Hispanic African-American men have a slightly higher risk than non-Hispanic white men, but Mexican-American men have about a 50% greater risk than non-Hispanic white men.[9]

Annual incidence of type 2 diabetes mellitus per 100,000 population ranges from 180 in 25 to 44 year olds to a peak of 860 in 65 to 74 year olds. Approximately 625,000 cases of type 2 diabetes mellitus develop yearly in the United States.[10] A recent temporal increase in incidence and prevalence[11,12] reflects aging of the population, strikingly increased obesity,[13] and a sedentary lifestyle. This rise in the number of cases is especially troubling in regard to high-risk ethnic minorities whose access to medical care may be limited.[14,15]

Obesity is a major risk factor for type 2 diabetes mellitus.[16] The current definition of obesity employs the body mass index (BMI) (body weight in kilograms divided by height in meters squared).

A person with a BMI of at least 25 but less than 30 is defined as overweight.[17] A BMI of 30 or more is defined as obesity,[16] and a BMI of 40 and above is associated with a 15-fold increased risk of type 2 diabetes mellitus.[15] Abdominal obesity, defined as a waist circumference greater than 100 cm in men and greater than 88 cm in women or a waist-to-hip ratio greater than 0.9, is an especially strong risk factor for type 2 diabetes mellitus. A large preponderance of patients with type 2 diabetes mellitus are obese; even those with normal BMI may have an increased percentage of their body weight accounted for by fat.[18] Longer duration of obesity further increases the risk of diabetes, emphasizing the importance of early efforts to control weight. Many patients with type 2 diabetes mellitus have a strong family history of that disease in first-degree relatives. An extraordinary example is found among the Arizona Pima Indians on the Gila River reservation, where 50% of the adult population has type 2 diabetes mellitus. Other risk factors for the disease include physical inactivity, hypertension, dyslipidemia, gestational diabetes, low birth weight, low income, low level of education, and low socioeconomic status.[1,19]

Hormonal Regulation of Metabolism

Diabetes involves the most fundamental aspects of human metabolism. The following are all affected by the hormonal abnormalities of diabetes: energy production and expenditure; the proportioning of carbohydrate, fat, and protein as energy sourc-

fatty acids in triglycerides, and amino acids in protein, and it inhibits glycogenolysis, lipolysis, ketogenesis, proteolysis, and gluconeogenesis [*see Figure 1*]. Glucagon stimulates mobilization of glucose, free fatty acids, and glycerol and stimulates hepatic uptake of amino acids and the conversion of their carbon skeletons to glucose. Glucagon also stimulates ketogenesis from free fatty acids. The normal steady-state levels of insulin and glucagon help maintain the overnight FPG level at 60 to 110 mg/dl, free fatty acid levels at less than 0.7 mmol/L, ketoacids at less than 0.2 mmol/L, and each amino acid at its unique level. After a mixed meal, plasma insulin rises sharply [*see Figure 2*] and, with it, the insulin-glucagon ratio. This condition reverses all the previously described processes. Dietary carbohydrate is stored in muscle and liver glycogen, free fatty acids are reesterified and stored as triglycerides in adipose tissue, and protein metabolism shifts back toward anabolism. When all the nutrients have been assimilated and plasma glucose returns to its basal preprandial level, plasma insulin [*see Figure 2*] and the insulin-glucagon ratio promptly return to basal levels, preventing an overshoot of insulin action that would otherwise cause hypoglycemia. Thus, an immediate rise, an early peak, and a prompt fall in insulin secretion are requisite to normal postprandial metabolism [*see Figure 2*].

Insulin is synthesized in pancreatic islet beta cells from a larger molecule called proinsulin, which is then split to yield insulin and an intramolecular connecting peptide called C-peptide [*see Figure 3*]. The two molecules are stored in the same granules and secreted in an equimolar ratio when the beta cell is stimulated. Thus, plasma C-peptide levels are a faithful marker of beta cell function [*see Figure 3*].

Insulin acts via a plasma insulin receptor that leads to the generation of multiple mediators of insulin's numerous intracellular cytoplasmic and nuclear effects [*see Figure 4*]. Insulin regulates both the activities and syntheses of target enzymes. Sensitivity of target tissues to insulin is the other major determinant of insulin action. Insulin sensitivity is best measured in humans by infusing insulin to establish steady-state plasma insulin levels [*see Figure 5*]. Simultaneously, the baseline plasma glucose is maintained at a constant level by a variable glucose infusion. The amount of glucose required to prevent plasma glucose from decreasing under the effect of insulin is equal to the increased amount of glucose being used per unit time under insulin stimulation (assuming that insulin has completely suppressed hepatic glucose output by the liver). The quantity of glucose used per unit time divided by the plasma insulin level provides an index of whole body sensitivity to insulin in the sphere of glucose metabolism.

A feedback loop exists between insulin responsiveness in target tissues and insulin secretion by beta cells. This relation operates to increase insulin secretion in individuals relatively resistant to insulin action and to decrease insulin release in individuals very sensitive to insulin action. The result is one critical mechanism for maintaining fasting and postprandial plasma glucose levels within narrow normal ranges.

Pathogenesis of Microvascular Complications in Diabetes

A distinctive feature of diabetes—the microvascular complications—were only revealed or commonly appreciated after the introduction of insulin therapy in 1922 allowed patients with type 1 diabetes mellitus to live long enough to experience these complications. It should be borne in mind that the descriptions and pathogenetic sequences presented below reflect a former

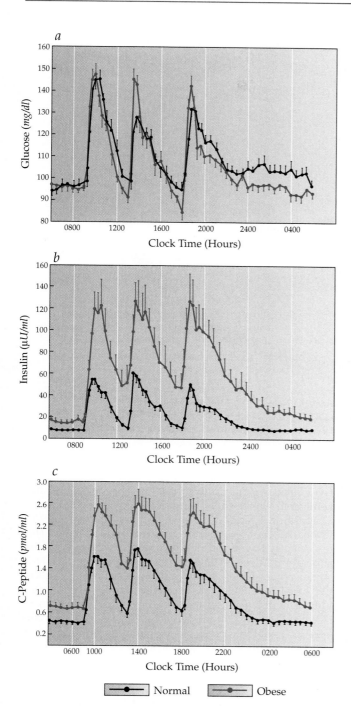

Figure 2 Plasma glucose (*a*) is normally kept within a narrow range throughout the day, largely because of beta cell function. Plasma insulin (*b*) and plasma C-peptide (*c*) rise sharply from their basal levels with each meal and, after reaching peaks, return promptly to basal levels, which are maintained throughout the night. Note also that plasma insulin and C-peptide levels are elevated in obese individuals who are insulin resistant.

es; the storage of energy as carbohydrate and fat; and the balance between protein synthesis (anabolism) and degradation (catabolism). To understand the pathogenesis of diabetes, it is useful to start with a brief review of normal metabolism.[20]

A proper balance between insulin and glucagon is one crucial hormonal regulator of basal metabolic homeostasis.[20] Insulin primarily facilitates storage of glucose as glycogen, free

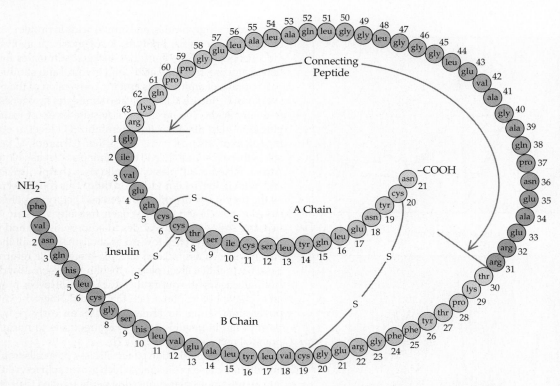

Figure 3   The structure of human proinsulin, the precursor molecule to insulin. The peptide that connects the amino terminus (NH_2^-) of the A chain to the carboxyl terminus (–COOH) of the B chain is called connecting peptide (C-peptide). Proinsulin is converted to insulin and C-peptide, and these two molecules are packaged together in the secretory granule. On stimulation of the beta cell, C-peptide and insulin are secreted in equimolar proportions. Thus, C-peptide levels reflect beta cell functional capacity.

commonly practiced degree of metabolic control no longer considered acceptable. Prevention of these complications is a major goal of current therapeutic policy and recommendations for all but transient forms of diabetes [*see* Prevention and Treatment of Microvascular Complications, *below*].

RETINOPATHY

Given a long enough duration, retinopathy occurs in almost all patients with type 1 diabetes mellitus and in most patients with type 2 diabetes mellitus who are on conventional treatment that does not come close to normalizing glycemic levels [*see* Table 2].[21] The most common form of retinopathy is nonproliferative retinopathy (also termed background retinopathy). It begins with loss of capillary pericytes, the supporting cells of the retinal vasculature, a loss leading to capillary dilatations that are seen on direct fundoscopy as microaneurysms [*see* Figure 6a]. Microaneurysms measure 50 to100 μm in diameter and can occur anywhere in the retina. However, they tend to cluster near the macula, the area responsible for central vision and visual acuity. Small dot hemorrhages form when microaneurysms leak blood. Hard lipid exudates form on leakage of serum [*see* Figure 6a]. These lesions are usually benign unless they occur quite close to the macula and in sufficient number to cause clinically significant macular edema. The latter is a feared complication that can decrease central vision and acuity. Capillary closure, which actually begins in the phase of background retinopathy, increases; and in the phase of preproliferative retinopathy, enough capillaries become obstructed to cause ischemia of the retina. Infarctions of the retinal nerve layer appear as soft (cotton wool) exudates. The retina responds to further ischemia with proliferation

of new blood vessels from its surface [*see* Figure 6b]. In this phase of proliferative retinopathy, ischemic retina releases vascular endothelial growth factor (VEGF), which stimulates new vessel formation. These new vessels grow forward into the vitreous. They are extremely fragile and can bleed into the vitreous, causing temporary loss of vision until the blood is reabsorbed. If no reabsorption occurs, blindness can result unless successful vitrectomy is carried out. Proliferative vessels that cover more than one fourth of the disk diameter and that occur within 1 disk diameter of the disk [*see* Figure 6b] are especially likely to bleed. Even after reabsorption of the vitreous blood, fibrous scars form that can cause traction on the retina and can lead to retinal detachment, another cause of profound and often permanent loss of vision.

NEPHROPATHY

Diabetic nephropathy [*see* Figure 7] is the complication associated with the highest mortality. Between 35% and 45% of patients with type 1 diabetes mellitus and a somewhat smaller percentage of patients with type 2 diabetes mellitus experience significant nephropathy.[22-24] Histologically, the earliest change is thickening of the capillary basement membrane. Subsequently, accumulation of mesangial material diffusely throughout the glomerulus occurs [*see* Figure 8]. Excretion of low but abnormal levels of albumin in the urine is a marker of the incipient phase of nephropathy.[25] As glomeruli become increasingly filled with mesangial matrix products, albuminuria increases and eventually gross proteinuria appears. Microalbuminuria is defined as excretion of 30 to 300 mg of albumin a day or an albumin-creatinine ratio between 30 and 300 in a random urine specimen. Clinical proteinuria is defined as excretion of more than 0.5 g of total

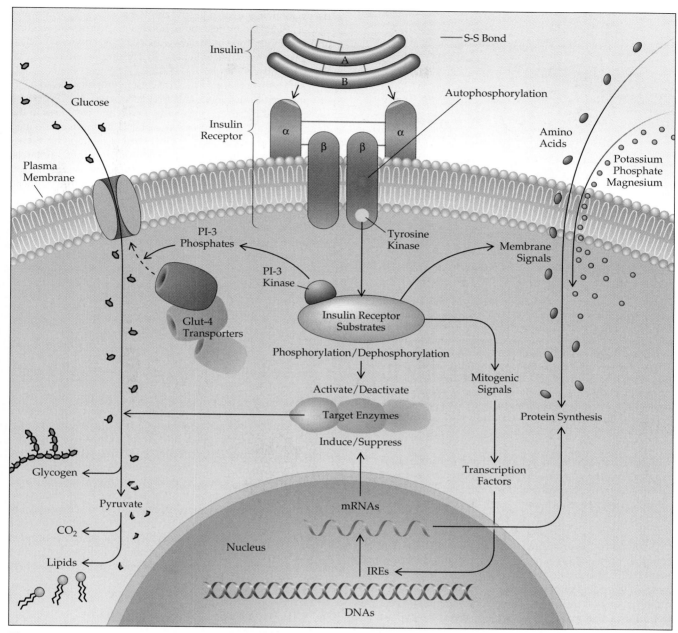

Figure 4   The cellular actions of insulin begin with binding to its plasma membrane receptor. As a result, certain tyrosine molecules in the intracellular portion of the transmembrane receptor are autophosphorylated, creating tyrosine kinase activity in the receptor. Several intracellular insulin receptor substrates (IRS) are then tyrosine phosphorylated by the receptor. Phosphorylated IRS docks and either activates or inactivates numerous enzymes (e.g., phosphatidylinositol-3-kinase [PI-3 kinase]) and other mediating molecules. Among the chief effects of these insulin-stimulated cascades are translocation of glucose (Glut-4) transporters to the plasma membrane, where they facilitate glucose diffusion into the cell; shifting of intracellular glucose metabolism toward storage as glycogen by activating glycogen synthase; stimulation of cellular uptake of amino acids, phosphate, potassium, and magnesium; stimulation of protein synthesis and inhibition of proteolysis; and regulation of gene expression via insulin regulatory elements (IRE) in target DNA molecules. Numerous intermediates in these various pathways, along with the molecules mentioned above, are products of candidate genes whose mutation could produce the state of insulin resistance characteristic of type 2 diabetes mellitus. Red connectors between insulin chains A and B and among insulin receptor subunits α and β indicate S-S bonds. The A chain also has an intramolecular S-S bond.

protein a day. This level of excretion can be detected by a positive dipstick urine test for protein. The nephrotic syndrome may also eventually occur.

Early in type 1 diabetes mellitus, kidney size and glomerular filtration rate (GFR) may actually be greater than normal. However, in both types of diabetes, GFR begins to decline, and after clinical proteinuria develops, GFR almost inexorably falls to the level of ESRD [*see Figure 7*]. Unlike the risk of retinopathy, the risk of nephropathy does not continue to rise with increasing duration. The incidence of nephropathy peaks at approximately 15 to 17 years and declines somewhat thereafter.[26] The prevalence of nephropathy remains approximately constant after that time. If the dipstick test has not revealed proteinuria by 25 to 30 years of diabetes duration, the risk of ESRD decreases. Coincident

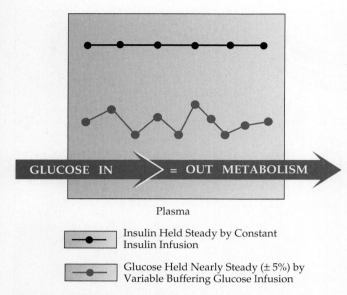

Plasma

—●— Insulin Held Steady by Constant
     Insulin Infusion

—●— Glucose Held Nearly Steady (± 5%) by
     Variable Buffering Glucose Infusion

Figure 5   **The diagram represents the gold standard for measuring the sensitivity of glucose metabolism to insulin, utilizing a glucose insulin clamp. When steady state is reached, glucose metabolized/unit time = glucose infused/unit time. Assuming endogenous glucose production is suppressed to zero, insulin sensitivity = (glucose metabolized/unit time) ÷ plasma insulin. For each dose of insulin, the more exogenous glucose required to sustain plasma glucose at its basal levels, the greater the insulin sensitivity. Conversely, individuals who require lesser amounts of glucose than usual to maintain the basal plasma glucose level are insulin resistant. The latter is usually the case in type 2 diabetes mellitus.**

with or shortly after the development of microalbuminuria, hypertension often appears. Hypertension in turn further aggravates diabetic nephropathy and is an important component in the progression to renal failure.

NEUROPATHY

Neuropathy has protean manifestations in diabetes. The most common presentation is peripheral symmetrical sensorimotor neuropathy, which causes numbness or tingling in the toes and feet.[27] At this point, symptoms are only mildly disturbing and require no specific treatment. These symptoms may even abate over time as neuropathy becomes more severe and hypoesthesia or anesthesia takes the place of paresthesias and dysesthesias. Ultimately, insensate feet become very vulnerable to trauma, and neuropathic foot ulcers are frequent causes of hospitalization and even amputation. Testing sensation with a nylon monofilament providing a calibrated 10 g point pressure is an effective way to screen for high risk of foot ulcers. Patients who cannot detect the pressure of the nylon filament have a 30- to 40-fold increased risk of foot ulcer.[28] In some instances, neuropathy is manifested by severe pain that can interfere with sleep and normal daily activities. The distribution of pain can suggest mononeuropathy and radiculopathy. Abrupt onset of cranial neuropathies that most commonly give rise to extraocular muscle weakness and diplopia has been attributed to microinfarcts caused by thrombosis of nutrient blood vessels. Carpal tunnel syndrome and other entrapment syndromes are more frequent in diabetic patients than in nondiabetic patients.

Involvement of the autonomic nervous system is also common and can become debilitating. Manifestations include male impotence and female anorgasmia, difficulty voiding and uri-

nary retention, impaired gastric emptying with early satiety and emesis, diarrhea, orthostatic hypotension, decreased sweating and vasomotor tone in the lower extremities, and loss of vagal control of the heart rate with persistent resting sinus tachycardia. Sudden death can result.

A somewhat unique form of diabetic neuropathy called amyotrophy occurs most commonly in elderly males with diabetes. It is manifested by severe, unremitting pain and weakness in the thigh muscles. Severe depression, cachexia, and weight loss may mark the 1- to 2-year course of this form of neuropathy. Sometimes confused with painful neuropathy are rare muscle infarcts, usually occurring in the thigh muscles. These infarcts are marked by abrupt onset of severe pain lasting several months. Magnetic resonance imaging of the affected area can demonstrate the presence of necrosis.

Diabetic neuropathy may be another microvascular complication, but the pathogenesis is still not completely understood.[29] Demyelinization of nerves is manifested by decreases in motor and sensory nerve conduction velocities. Axonal degeneration is reflected in decreased amplitudes of action potentials. Histologically, swelling is seen at the axonal nodes. An inflammatory component to diabetic neuropathy has also been suggested.[30]

RELATION OF MICROVASCULAR COMPLICATIONS TO GLYCEMIA

The appearance of microvascular complications in the 1930s generated a 50-year debate about whether diabetic retinopathy, nephropathy, and neuropathy were the direct result of the metabolic abnormalities, most notably hyperglycemia, or whether they were a parallel independent consequence of diabetes that had formerly been usually preempted by death from extreme metabolic disequilibrium (i.e., diabetic coma). This debate ultimately came to encompass type 2 diabetes mellitus as well. The debate was not merely academic, because it was reflected in quite different approaches to treatment. A belief in the metabolic hyperglycemic cause of retinopathy, nephropathy, and neuropathy impelled the physician to work with inadequate means to help the patient achieve as close to normal blood glucose levels as possible. Conversely, a belief in the metabolically independent nature of these complications encouraged a somewhat more laissez-faire

Table 2   Diabetic Retinopathy

Stage*	Pathologic Process	Manifestations
Background	Loss of capillary integrity Leakage, exudation, diapedesis Early capillary closure	Microaneurysms Dot hemorrhages Hard exudates Macular edema
Preproliferative	Capillary closure Microinfarcts Ischemia	Blot hemorrhages Soft exudates Intraretinal microvascular abnormalities Venous beading Macular edema
Proliferative	Forward growth of new large vessels Fibrosis Traction on retina or vitreous	Preretinal hemorrhage Vitreous hemorrhage Retinal detachment Macular edema

*Loss of visual acuity may occur from macular edema at any stage. Blindness may occur from severe macular edema, vitreous hemorrhage, or retinal detachment.

a

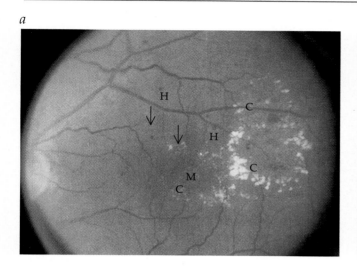

b

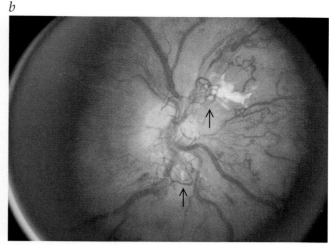

Figure 6   (*a*) This fundus photograph reveals nonproliferative (or background) retinopathy in a diabetic patient. Microaneurysms (arrows) occur at end capillaries. Punctate (or dot-and-blot) hemorrhages (H) and hard exudates (C) can also be seen. The hard exudates form three distinct circles (termed circinate retinopathy), which indicate leakage of plasma proteins from abnormal vessels located in the centers of the three circles. Lesions in the area of the macula (M) are potentially more dangerous, as they may lead to macular edema requiring laser therapy. (*b*) In proliferative retinopathy, new vessels grow from the retina into the vitreous. This fundus photograph reveals fine, tangled, new vessels originating from several areas of the disk (arrows). The vessels often form arcades and characteristically have thin walls and are fragile. They tend to bleed into the vitreous; the scars that form can cause retinal detachment and loss of vision. Proliferation within one disk diameter of the disk (termed neovascularization of the disk) is particularly dangerous, as these vessels are especially prone to bleed and form traction scars.

approach, which attempted primarily to eliminate the immediate symptoms, such as polyuria, that were produced by plasma glucose levels exceeding the renal threshold (> 180 mg/dl). Furthermore, the risks associated with the more aggressive approach to hyperglycemia reinforced the arguments of the conservative practitioners. A large body of evidence was eventually built up that supported but did not prove the so-called glucose hypothesis.[31] The Diabetes Control and Complications Trial (DCCT) and United Kingdom Prospective Diabetes Study (UKPDS) ended this debate for type 1 and type 2 diabetes mellitus, respectively.

The DCCT[32] was a randomized clinical trial that enrolled 1,441 nonobese patients, aged 13 to 39 years, with type 1 diabetes mellitus. Half of the patients with diabetes of 1 to 5 years' duration participated in a primary prevention trial that excluded all patients with retinopathy or microalbuminuria, and half of the patients with diabetes of 1 to 15 years' duration participated in a secondary intervention trial that included only patients who already had mild to moderate nonproliferative diabetic retinopathy but less than 200 mg/day of urinary albumin excretion. In both of these DCCT trials, patients were randomly assigned either to receive conventional treatment (no more than two insulin injections a day) or to receive intensive treatment (three to four insulin injections a day or use of a continuous subcutaneous insulin infusion [CSII] pump; self-monitoring of blood glucose at least four times a day; premeal target blood glucose levels of 70 to 120 mg/dl; glycated hemoglobin [HbA$_{1c}$] goal of less than 6.05%; and very frequent contacts between patient and treatment team). An HbA$_{1c}$ difference of 1.8% (8.9% versus 7.1%) was maintained between the two treatment groups for up to 9 years.[33]

Over a mean follow-up of 6.5 years, intensive treatment produced substantial benefits. The risks of de novo development (primary prevention trial) or of progression (secondary intervention trial) of retinopathy were reduced by 27% to 76%; the development of microalbuminuria was reduced by 35%; macroalbuminuria (i.e., proteinuria) was reduced by 56%; and development

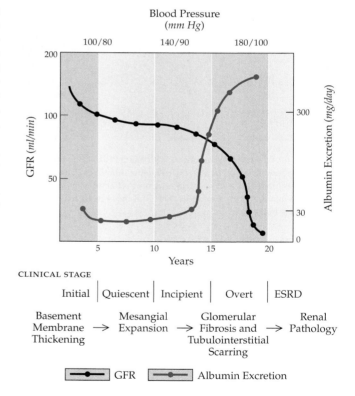

Figure 7   Relation of the developing histopathologic changes in the kidney to the development of renal functional abnormalities. Note that GFR is actually elevated early, corresponding to early renal hypertrophy. The appearance of microalbuminuria (albumin excretion > 30 mg/day) indicates that the patient is at considerable risk for overt nephropathy and end-stage renal disease (ESRD), but not all such individuals suffer this fate. Blood pressure begins to rise at about the time that microalbuminuria appears, and hypertension further damages the kidney.

a

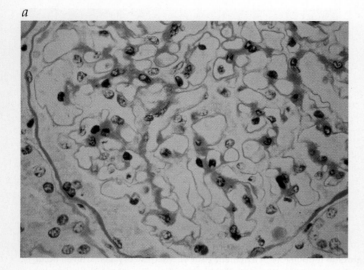

b

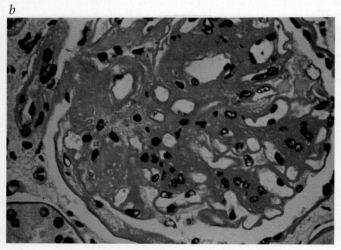

Figure 8   (*a*) The normal glomerulus with a large filtration surface has a lacy appearance. (*b*) There is diffuse deposition of extramesangial material throughout, as well as thickening of capillary basement membranes in a diabetic glomerulus. The GFR through such a glomerulus is reduced.

of clinical neuropathy, confirmed by abnormal nerve conduction velocities or autonomic nervous system function tests, was reduced by 60%.[32]

The main adverse effect of intensive treatment was a threefold increase in the risk of severe hypoglycemic episodes characterized by coma, convulsions, or the required assistance of others to treat and reverse the episode.[32,34] At least one such event per year was experienced by 25% of intensively treated patients, and 50% had experienced more than one such episode by the end of the study[34];14% experienced 10 or more episodes. The overall rate of severe hypoglycemia was 62 events per 100 patient-years for intensive treatment, compared with 19 events per 100 patient-years for conventional treatment. In addition, intensive treatment caused greater weight gain; one third of the patients exceeded 120% of ideal body weight (approximate BMI, 27) by the end of the study.[32] Intensive treatment was also more expensive than conventional treatment.[35] However, the cost was partly offset by projected decreased costs of a lower rate of complications,[36] and the estimated cost per year of quality life gained was $28,661, a figure thought to represent a good value.

The UKPDS[37,38] enrolled 5,102 patients with newly diagnosed type 2 diabetes mellitus, a mean age of 53 years, and a mean BMI of 28. After a 3-month dietary run-in, 1,138 patients were randomly assigned to a continuation of diet treatment only as long as their FPG remained below 270 mg/dl and they had no hyperglycemic symptoms. In the study, 2,729 patients were randomly assigned to intensive treatment, 1,573 to receive one of three sulfonylurea (SU) drugs, and 1,156 to receive insulin. In two thirds of the clinical sites, 342 patients were also randomized to intensive treatment with metformin. The goal of intensive treatment was an FPG of less than 108 mg/dl. Of the conventional-treatment patients, 80% ultimately required drugs to maintain their treatment goals of an FPG of less than 270 mg/dl and freedom from symptoms, although nearly 60% of their total treatment time was spent on diet therapy alone. Likewise, in the intensive-treatment groups, metformin therapy had to be added to the SU therapy, and insulin had to be substituted for or added to oral-drug therapy to maintain the stringent treatment goal.

Despite these drug crossovers, after 10 years of follow-up, patients who received intensive treatment showed a 25% decrease in the risk of serious microvascular complications (vitreous hemorrhage, need for laser treatment, and renal failure), compared with patients given conventional treatment.[37] This important benefit was associated with an HbA_{1c} difference of 0.9% (7.9% for conventional therapy; 7.0% for intensive therapy). Serious hypoglycemia occurred in 3% of insulin-treated patients each year and in 1% to 2% of SU-treated patients. These rates were much lower than that experienced with intensive treatment in patients with type 1 diabetes mellitus in the DCCT.

These two trials provided experimental proof that microvascular and neuropathic complications could be prevented or at least substantially delayed by maintaining blood glucose levels as near to normal as treatment techniques would safely allow. Although these two experimental trials did not prove that hyperglycemia caused microvascular complications, both trials provided additional strong evidence supporting that hypothesis. In the DCCT, the risk of retinopathy was directly related to the preceding mean HbA_{1c} difference in a similar exponential fashion in each of the two treatment groups.[39] The risk of retinopathy was decreased by about 44% for each proportional 10% decrease in HbA_{1c} (e.g., a decrease in HbA_{1c} from 10% to 9.0%). Microalbuminuria and neuropathy showed similar risk relations with glycemia. In the UKPDS, the risk of microvascular complications was also directly related to the mean HbA_{1c} in an exponential fashion.[40] The risk of these complications was decreased by about 37% for every absolute decrease of 1% in HbA_{1c}. These similarities suggest that similar biologic processes are at work. Neither the UKPDS nor the DCCT analyses indicated any glycemic threshold in the diabetic range of HbA_{1c}, below which there was no further risk of microvascular complications.[40,41] This observation sets normoglycemia as the ultimate goal of treating type 1 and type 2 diabetes mellitus. It has also been shown that the benefits of preceding intensive treatment (or the adverse effects of preceding conventional treatment) were still demonstrable 4 years after the DCCT was completed, during which time interval the mean HbA_{1c} concentrations in both groups were nearly identical (approximately 8.0%).[42] Thus, the effects of a sustained period of any glycemic exposure are associated with prolonged consequences..

Multiple mechanisms by which increased glucose concentrations may cause damage to the retina, kidney, and nerves have been discovered [*see Figure 9*]. (1) Glucose itself can react nonenzymatically with free amino groups in N-terminal amino acids and lysine residues of proteins. HbA_{1c} is one such molecule. This reaction sets into motion cross-linking of proteins that ultimately generate harmful advanced glycation end products (AGEs).[43,44] Such products include carboxymethyllysine and pentosidine. Concentrations of long-lived AGEs were higher in tissues of conventionally treated patients in the DCCT than in tissues of intensively treated patients in the DCCT.[45] AGEs correlated with HbA_{1c} and, independent of HbA_{1c}, with the presence of retinopathy, nephropathy, and neuropathy.[45] (2) Three-carbon dicarbonyl products of glucose and lipid metabolism, glyoxal and methylglyoxal, also react readily with amino groups in proteins and produce other AGEs, one of which is argpyrimidine. AGEs react with specific cellular receptors and can stimulate numerous potentially dangerous processes.[43,44] (3) Hyperglycemia can also secondarily produce oxidative stress in tissues, with depletion of glutathione and formation of reactive oxygen species and damaging free radicals.[46] (4) When glucose is insufficiently metabolized by insulin-stimulated routes [see Figure 1], it can overflow into the sorbitol (polyol) pathway via the enzymes aldose reductase and sorbitol dehydrogenase.[47] Accumulation of sorbitol and fructose in vulnerable tissues such as nerves produces osmotic damage, loss of myoinositol essential to nerve membrane integrity, and reduction of Na^+, K^+–ATPase activity.[47] (5) Elevated glucose levels increase protein kinase C, an enzyme whose activity influences numerous cellular processes with damaging potential,[48] such as stimulating neovascularization and epithelial cell proliferation, increasing collagen synthesis, increasing vascular permeability, increasing apoptosis (programmed cell death), increasing oxidative stress, and mediating the actions of VEGF and transforming growth factor–β. (6) Elevated glucose levels also increase the production of VEGF, a molecule that stimulates angiogenesis. VEGF is present in high concentrations in human diabetic ocular tissues and in kidneys of animals with experimentally produced diabetes. It is a logical candidate to mediate development of proliferative retinopathy. (7) Hyperglycemia stimulates nitric oxide synthase to produce nitric oxide, a molecule that itself generates damaging free radicals.[46] (8) A single primary mitochondrial defect that leads to overproduction of reactive oxygen species can result in at least three of the above pathways.[49] A number of these pathways are also mutually reinforcing, setting up vicious circles that can accelerate tissue damage.

The therapeutic importance of elucidating the mechanistic links between hyperglycemia and microvascular/neuropathic complications lies in our current inability to normalize blood glucose consistently. Therefore, drug therapies that intercept pathogenetic processes downstream from glucose hold promise for preventing these complications, even in the presence of hyperglycemia. An inhibitor of AGE formation, aminoguanidine, has been successful in animal experiments, but human trials have revealed unacceptable toxicity. Several inhibitors of aldose reductase, catalyzing the first step in the polyol pathway, have been studied in clinical trials, but none have shown sufficient clinical benefit or an acceptable adverse-effect profile to warrant approval in the United States. Nonetheless, such drugs have been effective in animal models. Current clinical trials are testing the effects of antioxidants such as vitamin E and a relatively nontoxic oral inhibitor of protein kinase C. Antagonists to VEGF and other growth factors to be administered by systemic or local injection are also in development.

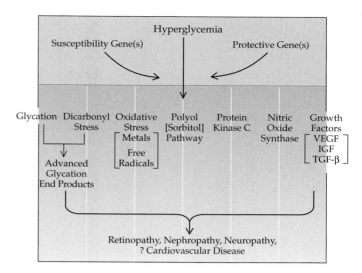

Figure 9 Multiple pathways have been described that may link high blood glucose levels to the microvascular and neuropathic complications of diabetes (see text). There are good reasons to believe that genetic factors, possibly operating through such pathways, may explain the observation that some individuals with consistently high blood glucose levels do not experience complications, whereas other individuals with near-normal blood glucose levels do experience complications.

GENETICS OF MICROVASCULAR COMPLICATIONS

There is considerable evidence from several studies that diabetic nephropathy clusters in families.[50] Thus, either genetic susceptibility or genetic protection is likely to explain the fact that nephropathy develops in only 35% to 40% of patients with diabetes. One likely influence on the development of nephropathy is the family of genes that code for the components of the renin-angiotensin system. Both positive and negative findings have been reported concerning involvement of the gene for angiotensin-converting enzyme (ACE) and the gene for angiotensinogen in the risks for nephropathy and retinopathy. A family study conducted in the DCCT showed no evidence for familial clustering of diabetic retinopathy per se. In view of the nearly 100% prevalence of retinopathy in patients with type 1 diabetes mellitus of many years' duration, it is not likely that a genetic factor is involved in the initiation of retinopathy. The DCCT analyses did, however, show evidence of familial clustering of severe diabetic retinopathy and confirmed familial clustering of nephropathy.[51]

Type 1 Diabetes Mellitus

PATHOGENESIS OF TYPE 1 DIABETES MELLITUS

Type 1 diabetes mellitus is characterized by absolute insulin deficiency, making patients dependent on exogenous insulin replacement for survival.[52] Insulin deficiency results from destruction or disappearance of the insulin-producing beta cells[53] that constitute 80% of the pancreatic islets of Langerhans. When 90% of the beta cells have been eliminated, clinical diabetes occurs [see Figure 10].

Autoimmune Factors

There is strong evidence for a cell-mediated autoimmune process being involved in the destruction of beta cells in the majority of cases of type 1 diabetes mellitus.[54-56] In a number of cases in which death occurred from an accident or from an illness oth-

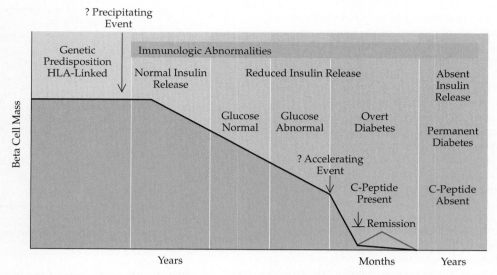

Figure 10   Current view of the pathogenesis of type 1 autoimmune diabetes mellitus. In some individuals, HLA-linked genes set in motion an autoimmune attack on islet cells, predominantly beta cells. In other individuals, HLA-linked genes protect against the autoimmune destructive response. An initiating event, such as exposure to a virus with an antigenic epitope that resembles a beta cell antigen or to a toxin, may start the process of self-destruction. Disappearance of the beta cells may occur because the viral antigen accelerates the normal rate of apoptosis (programmed cell death). As time passes, insulin production and secretion diminish, despite increasing hyperglycemia. When insulin release falls to trivial amounts or none, diabetic ketoacidosis results. Another external event may trigger this final beta cell catastrophe. A few beta cells may survive, because after this, a brief period of remission marked by reappearance of C-peptide in plasma may ensue if plasma glucose levels are controlled very tightly with exogenous insulin. Eventually, all beta cell function ceases, leading to metabolic instability.

er than diabetes shortly after diagnosis of type 1 diabetes mellitus, a mononuclear lymphocytic infiltrate was found in the islets. In this form of insulinitis, T cell distribution shows an increase in CD8 suppressor-inducer T cells and a decrease in CD4 helper-inducer T cells.[54] A similar immunocellular response has been found in animal models of spontaneous insulin-deficient diabetes.[56] In some instances, experimental manipulations that prevent T cell lymphocytic responses also prevent the development of diabetes. Furthermore, transfer of diabetes from affected animals to nonaffected animals by lymphocytes has also been described. Interleukins and other cytokines have been shown to exhibit toxic effects on the beta cells and to inhibit insulin secretion.

Autoantibodies to a variety of beta cell and islet autoantigens are present in the sera of patients with type 1 diabetes mellitus at the time of diagnosis.[57,58] The autoantigens include the enzymes glutamic acid decarboxylase (GAD), carboxypeptidase H, a protein tyrosine phosphatase labeled ICA512 or IA-2, and insulin itself.[58-60] Some, but not all, studies have shown that islet autoantibodies are capable of inhibiting insulin secretion in vitro or even causing lysis of beta cells. Other evidence supports the importance of autoimmune phenomena in the pathogenesis of type 1 diabetes mellitus. In cases of transplantation of pancreases from nondiabetic identical twins to patients with type 1 diabetes mellitus who were not given immunosuppressive therapy, the pancreas was rejected by the diabetic host's immune system, which apparently recognized as self, identical antigens in the normal twin's pancreatic islets. If treatment of type 1 diabetes mellitus with the immunosuppressive agent cyclosporine is initiated within 2 to 6 weeks after clinical onset of diabetes, dependency upon insulin can be eliminated or insulin doses markedly reduced, but only as long as immunosuppression is maintained.[61,62] The toxicity associated with cyclosporine and other immunosuppressive agents has precluded use of this form of therapy in clinical practice.

It is now clear that the autoimmune phenomena begin long before clinical onset of the disease. Islet or beta cell autoantibodies can be found in 2% to 4% of first-degree relatives of patients with type 1 diabetes mellitus, which is 10 to 20 times the prevalence of control subjects. Longitudinal studies have shown that type 1 diabetes mellitus is much more likely to develop in clinically unaffected relatives with high autoantibody titers than in relatives without such antibodies, and that the disease will develop in such patients within a few years.[63-65] Longitudinal serial testing of plasma insulin responses to intravenous glucose injection demonstrates progressively declining beta cell function in autoantibody-positive relatives before the clinical onset of diabetes.[66]

Environmental Factors

Because only 30% to 50% of unaffected monozygotic identical twins of patients with type 1 diabetes melllitus will eventually develop the disease, it is likely that an environmental factor may be required to trigger the autoimmune destructive process.[67] A number of viral candidates have been proposed.[67] The only certain association is that offspring of women who are infected with rubella during pregnancy are at increased risk for type 1 diabetes mellitus. A small amount of indirect evidence also associates coxsackievirus B with type 1 diabetes mellitus.[68] Toxins in the environment or diet might also initiate the destruction of genetically vulnerable beta cells.

Temporal Sequence of Beta Cell Destruction

At the time of clinical onset of type 1 diabetes mellitus, at least a small number of beta cells are still potentially capable of func-

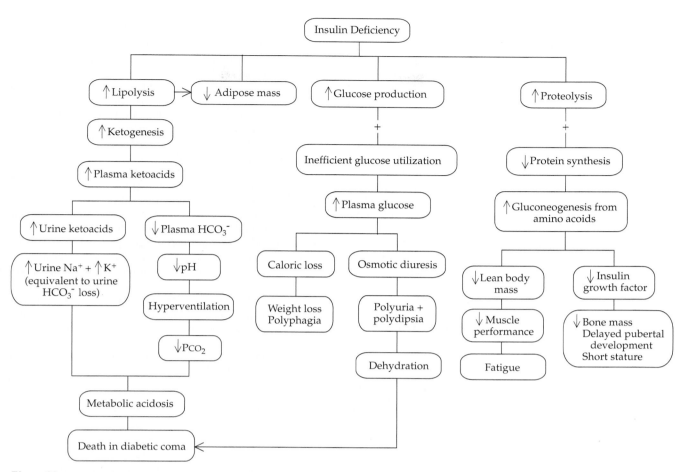

Figure 11 **Shown are the pathways that lead from insulin deficiency to the major clinical manifestations of type 1 diabetes mellitus. Note that a decrease in insulin growth factor also results from insulin deficiency and decreases growth rate.**

tion.[69,70] After several weeks of exogenous insulin treatment, particularly if exemplary metabolic control has been established,[71] dependency on exogenous insulin decreases or ceases entirely for weeks to months in some patients. This temporary so-called honeymoon remission phase is marked by an increase in serum C-peptide levels, which indicates an increase in endogenous insulin secretion [*see Figure 10*].[70] However, within 5 years after diagnosis of childhood type 1 diabetes mellitus, C-peptide virtually disappears from the serum.[72]

Type 1 diabetes mellitus does not develop in all autoantibody-positive individuals. Moreover, the latency period between initiation of beta cell destruction and appearance of the clinical disorder may be many years,[73] as the disease does not appear in some patients until considerably later in life.[57] The gradual, indolent nature of the disease in these autoantibody-positive individuals is also suggested by the fact that some can be treated with beta cell–stimulating drugs before absolutely requiring insulin.[74] A current diabetes prevention trial sponsored by the National Institute of Diabetes and Digestive and Kidney Diseases is seeking to determine whether type 1 diabetes mellitus can be prevented by inducing immune tolerance to exogenous human insulin given subcutaneously or orally to relatives of patients with high islet autoantibody titers.

Genetic Factors

Although a family history of type 1 diabetes mellitus is more likely to be absent than present in index cases, it is nonetheless true that offspring and siblings of patients with type 1 diabetes mellitus are at increased risk for the disease. There is a genetic basis for susceptibility to type 1 diabetes mellitus but not for inevitable development of the disease.[75] The disease will develop in 5% to 10% of first-degree relatives of patients with type 1 diabetes mellitus and in 20% of persons who have two first-degree relatives (e.g., both parents) with the disease. Association and linkage studies have incriminated a number of genes involved in the risk of type 1 diabetes mellitus. Polymorphism of HLA genes in the MHC locus on chromosome 6 account for 50% of the genetic risk.[75] DR3 and DR4 are susceptibility alleles that appear to operate synergistically. Individuals heterozygous for DR3 and DR4 are at greater risk than either homozygous DR3 or homozygous DR4 individuals. The DR2 allele decreases the risk and dominates the susceptibility effect of DR3 or DR4 when either is accompanied by DR2. The HLA-DQ locus also is associated with increased risk of diabetes.[76] Substitution of alanine, valine, or serine for the more usual aspartic acid at position 57 of DQ β chain or the presence of arginine at position 52 of DQ α chain increases the risk of type 1 diabetes mellitus. A number of mechanisms have been suggested to explain how HLA class II molecules might predispose to or protect against the disease.[77] Despite the accumulation of considerable knowledge, type 1 diabetes mellitus still cannot be predicted with complete certainty.[78]

Type 1 diabetes mellitus is associated with at least 15 additional loci on nine other chromosomes.[78] Of particular interest is that a variable number of tandem repeats in the promoter region of the insulin gene has been associated with the disease. However, the insulin molecule itself is apparently normal in structure in patients with type 1 diabetes mellitus. With the human genome soon to be fully known and advanced genetic technology becoming cost-effective, it is likely that the genetic components of type 1 diabetes mellitus will be sorted out in a way that will make it possible to identify susceptible individuals who might benefit from preventive therapies.

The clinical and biochemical manifestations of type 1 diabetes mellitus can all be accounted for as consequences of insulin deficiency [see Figures 1 and 11].[79] Loss of the stimulating effect of insulin on glucose uptake by muscle and adipose tissue coupled with loss of the suppressive effect of insulin on hepatic glucose output lead to severe hyperglycemia. FPG rises typically to 300 to 400 mg/dl, and postprandial glucose levels rise to 500 to 600 mg/dl in patients before treatment.[79] This increase presents a high filtered load of glucose to the renal tubules, causing a severe osmotic diuresis, manifested by polyuria and compensatory polydipsia. Loss of the lipogenic and antilipolytic effects of insulin on adipose tissue leads to high plasma levels and increased hepatic uptake of free fatty acids. This condition enhances ketogenesis, and ultimately, high plasma ketoacid levels cause metabolic acidosis. Protein breakdown is favored in the absence of the anticatabolic and anabolic actions of insulin. The proteolysis of muscle protein provides amino acids that sustain high rates of gluconeogenesis. Bodyweight loss thus includes fat and lean body mass, and it is further aggravated by an increase in basal energy expenditure.[80] The negative nitrogen balance, accompanied by losses of potassium, magnesium, and phosphate in the urine, impairs growth and development in children.

DIAGNOSIS OF TYPE 1 DIABETES MELLITUS

The diagnosis of type 1 diabetes mellitus is still almost always made on the basis of symptom history confirmed by a blood or plasma glucose level greater than 200 mg/dl, with the presence of glucosuria and often ketonuria. The classic symptoms are polyuria, polydipsia, weight loss with normal or even increased food intake, fatigue, and blurred vision, commonly present 4 to 12 weeks before the symptoms are noticed. In the future, however, before clinical onset of type 1 diabetes mellitus, diagnosis may be possible with serologic methods, complemented by beta cell function tests.

MANAGEMENT OF TYPE 1 DIABETES MELLITUS

Of all chronic diseases, diabetes is unique because its therapy involves daily self-management by the patient and a host of lifestyle adaptations. For optimal metabolic control, patients must prick their fingers to test blood glucose at least four times daily, inject insulin at least three times daily, pay regular attention to the timing and content of their meals, and try to follow a scheduled exercise program. The patient is truly at the center of his or her care. Patient self-management requires intensive education with regard to the skills of injection and blood glucose monitoring, urine ketone testing on sick days, meal planning, detection and treatment of hypoglycemia, and management of intercurrent illness. Family members and close associates of the patient need to be included as is appropriate, particularly with regard to recognition and treatment of hypoglycemia. Ideally, the patient should understand the pathophysiology of diabetes and its long-term complications almost as well as health care professionals. Some aspects of care require periodic educational reinforcement, which is often stimulated by some therapeutic mishap, such as a preventable episode of severe hypoglycemia.

The clinical goals of treatment include (1) decreasing plasma glucose levels and urine glucose excretion to eliminate polyuria, polydipsia, polyphagia, caloric loss, and adverse effects such as blurred vision from lens swelling and susceptibility to infection, particularly vaginitis in women, (2) abolishing ketosis, (3) inducing positive nitrogen balance to restore lean body mass and physical capability and to maintain normal growth, development, and life functioning, (4) preventing or greatly minimizing the late complications of diabetes previously discussed. After publication of the DCCT results, The American Diabetes Association revised their standards of care accordingly [see Table 3] to include firm biochemical goals[81]: (1) maintaining preprandial capillary whole blood glucose levels at 80 to 120 mg/dl, bedtime blood glucose levels at 100 to 140 mg/dl, and postprandial peak blood glucose levels at less than 180 mg/dl, and (2) maintaining an HbA_{1c} of less than 7.0% (relative to a nondiabetic DCCT range of approximately 4.0% to 6.0%). Realistically, current therapeutic tools make it difficult to achieve these stringent goals in many patients with type 1 diabetes mellitus, particularly those with absolutely no endogenous insulin secretion. The exponential relation between the risk of microvascular complications and HbA_{1c} predicts that only normal HbA_{1c} levels would completely prevent the complications. However, maintaining an HbA_{1c} of at

Table 3 American Diabetes Association Standards*
for Glycemic Control in Diabetes Mellitus[288]

Biochemical Index	Normal	Goal	Additional Action Suggested
Capillary whole blood values† (mg/dl)			
Average preprandial glucose level	< 110	80–120	< 80
			> 140
Average bedtime glucose level	< 120	100–140	< 100
			< 160
HbA_{1c} (%)	< 6	< 7	> 8

*The values shown in this table are by necessity generalized to the entire population of individuals with diabetes. Patients with comorbid diseases, the very young, older adults, and patients with unusual conditions or circumstances may warrant different treatment goals. These values are for nonpregnant adults. Additional action suggested depends on individual patient circumstances. Such actions may include enhanced diabetes self-management education, comanagement with a diabetes team, referral to an endocrinologist, change in pharmacologic therapy, initiation of or increase in self-monitored blood glucose testing, or more frequent contact with the patient. HbA_{1c} is referenced to a nondiabetic range of 4.0% to 6.0% (mean, 5.0%; SD, 0.5%).
†To convert to plasma glucose values, add 10 mg/dl to whole blood values, except for 160 mg/dl, which becomes 180 mg/dl.

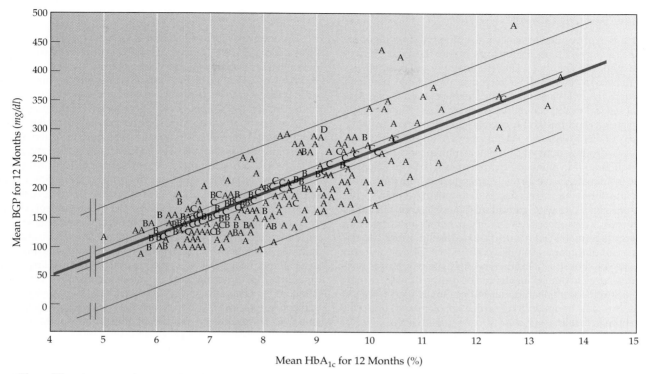

Figure 12 **The 12-month mean value of all seven-sample-a-day blood glucose profile values measured quarterly in the Diabetes Control and Complications Trial central biochemistry laboratory is plotted against the 12-month mean of quarterly HbA$_{1c}$ values in the same patients. (A = 1 point, B = 2 points, C = 3 or more points; r = 0.80, P < 0.001)**

least below 8% will remove much of the absolute risk from very poorly controlled patients. This intermediate target should be obtainable in most patients. Nonetheless, efforts to achieve an HbA$_{1c}$ of less than 7.0% should continue as long as hypoglycemia can be minimized.

Monitoring of Glycemic Control

In the past 5 to 10 years, blood glucose meters have undergone continuous development and improvement. They are now smaller, use less blood and more sites for puncture, are less vulnerable to inaccuracy because of patient errors, and have memory programs that allow the patient or caregiver to assess the pattern of blood glucose control over the previous 2 months, largely eliminating the problem of incorrect or fabricated written transcription of results. Devices that can accurately estimate blood glucose without a blood sample have been in development for a number of years but have not reached a state of reliability suitable for clinical practice. An indwelling subcutaneous catheter for blood glucose monitoring that can be used for 3 days and provide frequent readings is now available. Although the recorded profile can provide only a brief window into a lifetime of blood glucose fluctuation, such a profile can guide periodic adjustments of the regimen.

Currently, even with its imperfections, blood glucose testing before each meal or large snack is essential if the patient is to adjust each dose of rapid-acting insulin to the level of blood glucose before the meal and to the amount of carbohydrate about to be ingested. Blood glucose levels also need to be periodically checked after meals to ensure that undue postprandial hyperglycemia is not occurring. Patients should also check blood glucose levels before or after intensive exercise to prevent or abort hypoglycemia. It is very important to check blood glucose levels before driving to prevent motor vehicle accidents brought on by

severe hypoglycemia, which can have adverse effects on drivers' judgment and reaction times. Occasional 3:00 A.M. blood glucose readings are useful in monitoring for otherwise unrecognized frequent nocturnal hypoglycemia. Most important, during intercurrent illnesses, especially those accompanied by nausea, vomiting, and limitation of fluid and caloric intake, patients must test blood frequently to guide insulin treatment. In addition, under these circumstances, the risk of ketoacidosis mandates testing of urine or blood for ketoacids. The presence of significant levels of ketoacids is a signal to call the caregiver immediately and establish frequent contact for instructions regarding insulin doses and carbohydrate intake.

A critical supplement to home blood glucose testing is monitoring of HbA$_{1c}$ in the physician's office. It is now well established that this product of nonenzymatic glycation provides an excellent index of average blood glucose levels [*see Figure 12*] for approximately the preceding 2 months.[82,83] In at least one study, patients whose HbA$_{1c}$ was measured periodically had a better health status, lower glycemic levels, and fewer hospitalizations than a randomly selected group of patients whose HbA$_{1c}$ level remained unknown to both the patient and the physician.[84] Quarterly HbA$_{1c}$ measurements are satisfactory except during pregnancy, when monthly levels should be obtained. Because methods and results vary among laboratories, a national glycohemoglobin standardization program is under way, and HbA$_{1c}$ should be measured in laboratories certified to provide DCCT-equivalent results.[85] Future widespread use of rapid-turnaround, point-of-service HbA$_{1c}$ assays should improve the efficiency with which diabetes caregivers modify patients' regimens on office visits and improve treatment results.[86] Assays of other products of nonenzymatic glycation, such as fructosamine and glycated albumin, that reflect shorter periods of chronic glycemia are less useful in routine diabetes management.[85]

Insulin Types and Delivery

Correction of insulin deficiency is the most critical component in managing type 1 diabetes mellitus. Before the availability of insulin, patients with type 1 diabetes mellitus and complete insulin deficiency inevitably followed a predictable downhill course [see Figure 11] and died either in diabetic coma or essentially of starvation and inanition. Insulin extracted from beef and pork pancreas and purified to increasingly high levels was the mainstay of therapy until recombinant DNA technology made it possible to produce authentic human insulin in large quantities. Although animal insulins are therapeutically bioequivalent to human insulin, they have virtually disappeared from the market as manufacturers have switched over to making virtually only human insulin. Allergy or immunoresistance to animal insulins has practically disappeared as a problem. In rare instances of local allergy to human insulin, pure porcine insulin, which has alanine instead of threonine in position B30 [see Figure 3], or lispro insulin can be substituted. In emergency situations, patients with systemic allergy to human insulin can be desensitized by administering extremely small amounts and gradually increasing the dose over 6 to 24 hours until the patient is tolerant and responsive to human insulin.

The basic principle of insulin replacement[87,88] is to provide a slow, long acting, continuous supply that mimics the nighttime and interprandial basal secretion by normal beta cells. In addition, a rapid and relatively short-acting form of insulin delivered before meals mimics the normal meal-stimulated burst of insulin secretion [see Figure 2]. A number of insulin preparations for subcutaneous administration are currently available [see Table 4]. It is important to recognize that there is considerable variability in the pharmacokinetic characteristics of these insulins both from individual to individual and within the same individual from day to day. Rates of insulin absorption from the skin vary with the injection site, the depth and angle of injection, ambient temperature, and exercise of an injected limb. Injection into the subcutaneous tissue of the abdomen produces the least variable results. The expected therapeutic action can also be affected by fluctuations in sensitivity to insulin from time to time in patients. Despite the variability of results, certain average patterns can be expected from the multiple daily injection regimens in common use [see Figure 13]. CSII by use of an external pump provides smooth basal delivery and somewhat more predictable acute increases in plasma insulin for meals. Only crystalline zinc insulin (regular insulin) and lispro insulin are used in such pumps, which is one reason for their greater consistency of effect.

Synthetic Insulin Analogues

Lispro was the first of what undoubtedly will be many new insulin analogues with structures designed to provide pharmacokinetics that more closely mimic physiologic insulin secretion and needs.[89] One of the features of natural (or synthetic) human insulin is that six molecules associate with a zinc molecule to form hexamers. Insulin hexamers must disassociate to monomers before they can be absorbed from subcutaneous injection sites. This requirement is the main reason that crystalline zinc insulin (regular insulin) has a peak action 2 to 4 hours after injection and must be taken 30 to 60 minutes before eating to have any chance of limiting postprandial hyperglycemia. By simply exchanging lysine and proline at positions 28 and 29 of the B chain of insulin [see Figure 3], hexamer formation is prevented and the monomer is rapidly absorbed from an injection site. Lispro insulin action begins within 15 minutes, the peak effect is reached at 1 to 2 hours, and the duration of action is only 4 to 6 hours. Thus, lispro insulin injected just before a meal provides a postprandial plasma insulin profile similar to that of normal human insulin secretion [see Figure 2]. The chief benefits of using lispro insulin are to reduce postprandial blood glucose peaks and to somewhat decrease the hypoglycemia that can result from the late tail of regular insulin action.[90,91] However, loss of that late action can lead to recurrent hyperglycemia before the next meal. Hence patients switched from regular insulin to lispro insulin may have no reduction in HbA_{1c} unless their doses of basal insulin (neutral protamine Hagedorn [NPH], Lente, or Ultralente or the basal rate in CSII) are increased.[92] It may even prove useful to combine lispro insulin with regular insulin in a single injection to optimize postprandial control.

A newly released synthetic rapid-acting analogue, insulin aspart, replaces proline with aspartic acid at position B28 [see Figure 3]. This substitution leads to a profile of action and therapeutic benefits that are very similar to those of lispro insulin.[93] A long-acting analogue, glargine, has also been synthesized as a basal insulin with no discernible peak and a longer duration of action than Ultralente insulin.[94,95] Glargine has two additional arginines at the carboxyl terminus of the B chain, B31 and 32, and has a glycine for arginine substitution at position A21 [see Figure 3]. Glargine has just been approved for use as a single bedtime injection to provide basal insulin for 24 hours with less nocturnal hypoglycemia.[96] For reasons that should now be clear, intensive treatment regimens are the preferred form of therapy and should be implemented in as many patients as is safely possible. Different combinations of insulin preparations can be used to approximate (but never reliably reproduce) normal plasma insulin pro-

Table 4 Insulin Preparations

Insulin Type	Onset (hr)	Duration (hr)	Peak (hr)
Rapid acting (regular, crystalline zinc insulin [CZI])	0.5–1.0	6–8	2–3
Very rapid acting			
Lispro	0.25–0.5	4–6	1–2
Insulin aspart	0.25–0.5	4–6	1–2
Intermediate acting			
Lente, neutral protamine Hagedorn (NPH)	1	10–14	4–8
Long acting			
Ultralente	1	18–24	Minimal at 10–14
Glargine	1.5	30	None

files [*see Figure 13*]. Type 1 diabetes mellitus can almost never be satisfactorily controlled on less than two injections a day of intermediate- or long-acting insulin combined with rapid-acting insulin. Only in patients experiencing a honeymoon remission or in patients with late-onset autoimmune type 1 diabetes mellitus in adults can satisfactory metabolic control be established with a single injection of insulin daily. Such success is made possible only by the presence of some normally regulated endogenous insulin secretion.

Insulin Regimens

As a rule of thumb, basal insulin and mealtime insulin pulses each constitute approximately 50% of the average total daily dose (0.6 to 0.7 U/kg) in intensive-therapy regimens. The dose of regular or lispro insulin (or insulin aspart) before each meal is chosen by the patient on the basis of the blood glucose level, the estimated amount of carbohydrate to be eaten, or both. A typical regimen would call for 1 to 2 extra units of insulin for each 50 mg/dl increment in blood glucose above the dose called for by the preprandial target of 80 to 120 mg/dl, or 1 U/10 to 15 g of extra carbohydrate to be ingested above the usual amount of carbohydrate prescribed by the nutrition plan. Very sophisticated patients can combine both guidelines.

Fixed-dose mixtures of insulin are not physiologically very suitable for patients with type 1 diabetes mellitus. However, for patients who can or will implement only such conventional treatment, a typical regimen might be a total daily dose of 0.6 to 0.7 U/kg. Two thirds to three fourths of the dose would be given before breakfast and the remainder before supper; the ratio of intermediate-acting insulin to rapid-acting insulin might be 2:1 to 4:1 before breakfast and 1:1 before supper. Because giving NPH or Lente insulin before supper increases the risk of hypoglycemia between 2:00 and 4:00 A.M., patients on conventional treatment should be urged to switch to a three-injection regimen, taking the evening dose of intermediate-acting insulin at bedtime to avoid nocturnal hypoglycemia and to better control the prebreakfast blood glucose level. Glargine insulin may also be helpful in minimizing nocturnal hypoglycemia.[87,88]

Insulin requirements are increased by greater caloric and especially carbohydrate intake, by weight gain of both lean body mass and fat mass, by the onset of puberty, by infections and other medical or surgical stresses, by pregnancy, by glucocorticoid administration, and sometimes by the physiologic changes that precede the onset of menses. During acute illnesses, patients will require extra doses of rapid-acting insulin when hyperglycemia accelerates and especially if ketosis occurs. Frequent telephone contact with caregivers allows timely professional guidance of the extra insulin doses, nutrient intake to prevent hypoglycemia, and fluid intake to prevent dehydration. Lispro insulin is especially useful in these circumstances because the effect of an overdose is short lived and hypoglycemia is less likely.

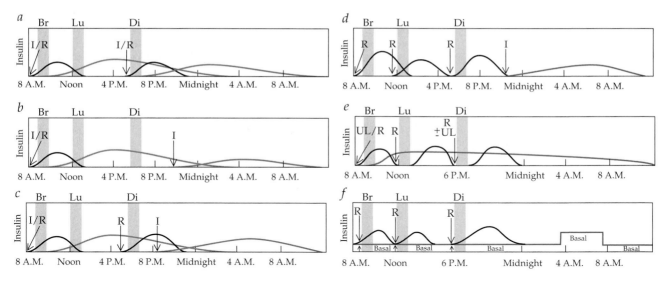

Figure 13 **Different combinations of various insulin preparations can be employed in establishing glycemic control in type 1 diabetes mellitus (and in those patients with type 2 diabetes mellitus who eventually reach an equivalent degree of insulin deficiency). Arrows indicate time of injection. Red curves represent rapid-acting (R) regular or lispro insulin. Blue curves represent intermediate-acting (I) NPH or Lente insulin. Gray curves represent long-acting Ultralente (UL) insulin. (*a*) A mixed injection of I and R insulin is administered before breakfast and dinner in this average regimen. In addition to the risk of hypoglycemia before lunch and in the late afternoon, the predinner administration of I insulin predisposes patients to hypoglycemia from 2:00 A.M. to 4:00 A.M. (*b*) This average regimen combines a mixed injection of I and R insulin given before breakfast with an injection of I insulin given before bed. The I insulin administered at bedtime provides safer, more effective overnight glucose control; without predinner insulin, however, glucose levels may rise to unacceptably high levels after dinner. (*c*) In this intensive regimen, the patient receives three injections: a mixed injection before breakfast, R insulin before dinner, and I insulin before bed. (*d*) This intensive regimen combines three preprandial injections of R insulin with one injection of I insulin before bed. Preprandial doses of R insulin are adjusted according to glucose levels and meal size. (*e*) This intensive regimen uses relatively long acting Ultralente insulin before breakfast and, if needed, before dinner or bed to replace basal insulin secretion. Preprandial doses of R insulin are adjusted according to blood glucose levels and anticipated meal carbohydrate content. (*f*) This intensive regimen provides only R insulin as regular or lispro insulin. A pump-driven continuous subcutaneous infusion of R insulin replaces basal insulin secretion. Basal rates can vary during different times of day or activities. For example, the basal rate can be lowered or even suspended during periods of intensive aerobic exercise. The nocturnal basal rate can be increased 1.5 to 2.0 times from 3:00 A.M. to 4:00 A.M. until breakfast to accommodate the rising early morning insulin requirement known as the dawn phenomenon. Preprandial bolus doses are individually dialed in and rapidly pumped in, adjusted according to blood glucose levels and anticipated meal carbohydrate content. (Br = breakfast, Lu = lunch, Di = dinner)**

CSII has improved considerably since its introduction in the 1970s.[97] Modern insulin infusion pumps permit programming with multiple basal rates, allowing flexibility during the day as well as automatic adjustment of doses while sleeping at night. Frequently, the basal rate needs to be lower in the first half of the night and then increased to accommodate the so-called dawn phenomenon [see Figure 13]. The latter is a slow rise in the plasma glucose level before the patient awakens, demonstrable in normal individuals but exaggerated in individuals with type 1 diabetes mellitus who cannot limit it by increasing endogenous insulin secretion. On the other hand, interruption of insulin delivery from a pump for as little as 8 hours can result in extreme hyperglycemia, diabetic ketoacidosis (DKA), and hyperkalemia. In the DCCT, patients who used an insulin pump had a slightly but significantly higher DKA event rate (1.8 per 100 patient-years) than patients on multiple daily injection regimens (0.8 per 100 patient-years).[98] There was no difference in risk of severe hypoglycemia between patients treated with insulin pumps and patients treated with multiple daily injections, although episodes resulting in coma or seizure were more common in CSII-treated patients.[98] The rate of infection at catheter sites was kept very low by frequent change of catheters and preemptive use of antibiotics at the first visible signs of infection.

Avant-garde Therapy

Implantable pumps delivering insulin into the peritoneal cavity and resulting in a more physiologic first pass of insulin through the liver have provided acceptable HbA_{1c} levels with a lower frequency of severe hypoglycemia.[99] They are not yet approved for commercial use. Closed-loop insulin-delivery devices that would automatically adjust insulin delivery to the patient's blood glucose level measured very frequently still await the development of a practical and long-lived indwelling continuous glucose sensor.

Insulin can be absorbed through the mucosa of the nose and also through the lungs. A nasal preparation of insulin has been effective in short-term clinical trials, but the disadvantages of high cost (10 times the subcutaneous insulin dose is needed to achieve the same blood glucose lowering) and failure to develop a vehicle that does not cause allergic nasal symptoms have prevented this preparation from being used in practice.[100] Inhaled insulin is still undergoing clinical trials,[101] but there are concerns regarding the long-term exposure of the bronchi and lungs to possible mitogenic effects of insulin.[102] Various attempts to package insulin for oral administration so as to prevent its degradation in the gastrointestinal tract have also been investigated.

Pancreas transplantation remains controversial as a routine form of insulin replacement therapy.[103] Over the period of 1994 to 1997, 1-year graft survival rates were 82% when a pancreas was transplanted with a needed kidney transplant and 62% when a pancreas was transplanted alone.[104] Successful pancreas transplants provide nondiabetic HbA_{1c} levels and free the patient from the rigors of diet, blood glucose testing, and insulin injection, and they virtually eliminate episodes of hypoglycemia.[104] Quality of life is usually improved. On the negative side, the patient incurs the risk of operative mortality and morbidity and must remain on immunosuppressive therapy with its attendant risks of infection and malignant disease.[103] Length of stay, readmission rates, morbidity, and the number of acute rejection episodes are higher for pancreas transplants than for kidney transplants. From 1994 to 1996, the 1-year pancreas transplant survival was 81%, compared with a kidney transplant survival of 88%.[103] The large majority of

pancreas transplantations are still performed as an option in conjunction with a necessary kidney transplant.

Transplantation of isolated islets can be accomplished without major surgery. Furthermore, the ability to immunomodulate isolated islets in the laboratory (by masking or removing cell surface antigens) may someday allow transplantation with little or no immunosuppression. Alternatively, islets can be placed in semipermeable hollow tubes that allow glucose to enter and insulin to leave but shield the islets from inflammatory reactions to a foreign body. Islet transplantation with function lasting at least 1 year has been achieved in less than 10% of attempts worldwide. A Canadian group has reported on seven successive cases of islet injection into the liver, with persistent function and independence from insulin injections for up to 15 months, using a new immunosuppressive regimen.[105] This technique is undergoing a multicenter trial.

Nutritional Therapy and Exercise

Intensive and conventional insulin treatment will produce unsatisfactory results unless it is appropriate for the nutrient intake. To facilitate the matching of insulin doses to meals and to prevent hypoglycemia, patients with type 1 diabetes mellitus should eat consistent regular meals comprising about 50% carbohydrate calories, less than 30% total fat calories, and less than 300 mg cholesterol a day.[106] Various methods of teaching patients how to assess amounts of foods and their nutrient and caloric content have been utilized. These methods include exchange lists that place foods into six categories; each category has approximately the same quantity of carbohydrate, protein, and calories per serving. These exchange categories are bread, meat, milk, fruit, fat, and vegetable. Another approach is to focus only on the carbohydrate content of foods because carbohydrates cause most of the postprandial hyperglycemia. Because different carbohydrates are digested and absorbed at different rates and therefore have different effects on plasma glucose levels, glycemic indices have been developed for common foods that help adjust for their different effects.[107] It is noteworthy that numerous studies have disproved the myth that sucrose raises blood glucose more than equivalent amounts of other carbohydrates.[108] For optimal instruction and reinforcement of diet therapy, a dietitian should be part of the diabetes care team.

Exercise is another important component of diabetes care because it helps maintain cardiovascular conditioning, insulin sensitivity, and general well-being.[109] However, patients must be instructed how to adjust their meals, their insulin doses and timing, or both to prevent hypoglycemia during, immediately after, or even 6 to 12 hours after exercise as muscle glycogen stores are replenished from plasma glucose. High-impact sports are contraindicated for patients with advanced retinopathy who are at risk for vitreous hemorrhage or for patients with peripheral neuropathy or vascular disease who are at risk for foot trauma, because such sports can be hazardous.

DIABETIC EMERGENCIES IN TYPE 1 DIABETES MELLITUS

Diabetic Ketoacidosis

DKA is the ultimate result of insulin deficiency[110,111] [see Figure 11], which is aggravated by stress-induced elevations of glucagon, cortisol, growth hormone, epinephrine, and norepinephrine[110] that add a component of insulin resistance.[112] DKA occurs in 2% to 5% of patients with type 1 diabetes mellitus a year. In the closely followed DCCT patients, overall event rates were 2.0 per 100 patient-years in the intensively treated group and 1.8

Table 5 Typical Laboratory Findings and Monitoring in Diabetic Ketoacidosis

Test	Average	Range
Plasma glucose	600 mg/dl (33 mmol/L)	200–2,000 mg/dl (11–110 mmol/L)
Plasma ketones (positive)	1:16	1:2–1:64
Blood betahydroxybutyrate (mmol/L)	—	3–25
Plasma HCO_3 (mEq/L)	10	4–15
Blood pH	7.15	6.80–7.30
Pco_2 (mm Hg)	20	14–30
Plasma anion gap ($Na^+ - [Cl + HCO_3]$) (mEq/L)	23	16–30

Perform complete blood count, serum urea nitrogen measurement, serum creatinine measurement, urinalysis, appropriate cultures, and chest radiography.

1. Weigh on admission and every 12 hr.
2. Record cumulatively intake and output every 1 to 2 hr (Foley catheter if incontinent).
3. Check blood pressure, pulse, respiration, mental status every 1 to 2 hr and temperature every 8 hr.
4. Check blood (fingerstick) or plasma (laboratory) glucose every 1 to 2 hr.
5. Check serum potassium every 2 to 4 hr; check other electrolytes and serum ketones or betahydroxybutyrate every 4 hr.
6. Check arterial blood pH and gases on admission (in children, venous pH may be substituted; add 0.1 to result). If pH < 7.0 on admission, recheck as required until pH exceeds 7.1.
7. Check serum phosphate, magnesium, and calcium levels on admission. If low, repeat every 4 hr; otherwise, every 8 to 12 hr.
8. Spot-check voidings for ketones and glucose.
9. Perform ECG on admission; repeat if follow-up serum potassium level is abnormal or unavailable.

Note: 1–9 should be carried out until the patient is stable, glucose levels have reached and are maintained at 250 mg/dl, and acidosis is largely reversed (plasma HCO_3 > 15–18, plasma anion gap < 16). An intensive care setting is preferred.

per 100 patients-years in the conventionally treated group.[34] Reported mortality varies worldwide from as low as 0% to as high as 10%. Most cases occur in patients already diagnosed with type 1 diabetes mellitus, but DKA still can be the first manifestation of diabetes, especially in children. Self-monitoring of blood glucose and urine ketones and close contact with the diabetes care team should facilitate recognition and abortion of evolving DKA by early and aggressive treatment with extra insulin and fluids at home. Approximately half the cases of DKA are precipitated by infection. Sepsis, myocardial infarction, and other major intercurrent illnesses are more often the cause of death than the metabolic disequilibrium itself. In children, cerebral edema rarely occurs. It usually appears 6 to 12 hours after treatment is initiated when biochemical improvement is manifest; yet it is often fatal.

Presenting features DKA presents with signs and symptoms of dehydration secondary to osmotic diuresis and vomiting and, sometimes, to diarrhea caused by concurrent gastroenteritis; of compensatory hyperventilation to eliminate CO_2; and of various degrees of depressed mentation or decreased consciousness. Seizures are notably not a result of DKA. Complete coma almost certainly indicates a long period of DKA before medical attention. DKA yields a number of characteristic laboratory findings [see Table 5]. The anion gap metabolic acidosis is secondary to elevated levels of acetoacetate and betahydroxybutyrate with small contributions from lactate and free fatty acids. Although serum potassium and phosphate levels are usually normal or even high initially, this finding masks a profound total body depletion of these electrolytes, along with magnesium. Deviations from the customary pattern create pitfalls in diagnosis. Ketones, which current tests detect only as acetoacetate or acetone, may be missing from the serum if the redox potential of the patient is very high and the equilibrium of the ketoacids is shifted toward the reduced partner betahydroxybutyrate (as may occur in alcohol intoxication). Serum bicarbonate levels may be normal if there is coexisting respiratory acidosis. Arterial blood pH may be normal if there is coexistent metabolic alkalosis caused by diuretic ingestion or pernicious vomiting. Occasionally, plasma glucose levels are less than 250 mg/dl because of fasting,[113] high alcohol intake, profound inanition, or pregnancy.

Treatment Treatment of DKA[110,114,115] requires careful monitoring of the patient [see Table 5]. Volume repletion is as important as insulin therapy.[116] Intravenous 0.9% saline should be started even before the diagnosis is established. After an initial liter in 30 to 60 minutes, fluid therapy should continue aggressively until the circulating volume is replenished, as indicated by an increase in blood pressure to normal and a reduction in compensatory tachycardia. Subsequent total volume repletion is carried out more slowly at 150 to 500 ml/hr with 0.45% saline, switching to 5% glucose-containing solutions once plasma glucose has decreased to 250 mg/dl. Typical fluid deficits range from 50 to 100 mEq/kg. Average sodium deficits are 7 mEq/kg, and most important, potassium deficits may be as high as 7 mEq/kg. The effective depletion of total body bicarbonate through loss of the strong organic acids acetoacetate and betahydroxybutyrate in the urine is revealed later, when a hyperchloremic metabolic acidosis often ensues. Potassium repletion (10 to 40 mEq/hr) should begin promptly after insulin administration and as soon as hyperkalemia and oliguria or anuria have been ruled out [see Table 5]. Otherwise, serious hypokalemia will result as insulin stimulates potassium uptake by cells [see Figure 4]. If the serum potassium level is less than 40 mEq/L on admission, a very large deficit exists and repletion should be at a faster rate to maintain a level no lower than 3.5 to 4.0 mEq/L. Insulin should be withheld in such circumstances until serum potassium reaches 4.0 mEq/L. Hypokalemia is the most tragic cause of death resulting from therapeutic misjudgment.

Although DKA can be managed satisfactorily with insulin given intramuscularly or subcutaneously, intravenous administration is far more reliable and results in fewer instances of hypokalemia and hypoglycemia. A bolus of 10 U or 0.1 U/kg is followed by the same dose given hourly by intravenous infusion, preferably with a pump and through its own intravenous line. Routine addition of sodium bicarbonate or potassium phosphate has not been found to hasten recovery in ordinary cases of DKA.[115] Possible indications for administration of sodium bicarbonate (50 to 200 mEq) include arterial pH less than 7.0, ECG changes of hyperkalemia, hypotension that does not respond to rapid infusion of 0.9% saline, and left ventricular failure. If bicarbonate therapy is given, serum potassium and arterial pH should be monitored hourly and extra potassium given to prevent hypokalemia. Rhabdomyolysis, hemolysis, and central nervous system deterioration can be caused by severe hypophosphatemia (< 1.5 mg/dl) and call for intravenous administration of 60 mmol (approximately 2 g) of phosphate as the potassium salt over 6 hours. Once the anion gap has decreased to near normal and bicarbonate has risen to 15 to 18 mEq/L, the insulin infusion rate can be decreased to 2 U/hr. In general, it is best to maintain the insulin infusion at 1 to 2 U/hr with accompanying 5% glucose infusion, aimed at keeping the plasma glucose level at around 150 mg/dl until the following morning, when a subcutaneously mixed insulin regimen can be started or resumed along with a diet.

It is preferable to treat patients with DKA in an intensive care unit to ensure close monitoring. Persistent vomiting calls for gastric intubation, and the airway of an obtunded patient should be protected to prevent aspiration. Any suspicion of sepsis mandates treatment with broad-spectrum antibiotics.

Hypoglycemia

Hypoglycemia is a more common emergency than DKA and potentially as dangerous. Clinical hypoglycemia can range from annoying symptoms accompanying a biochemically low blood glucose level (< 50 to 60 mg/dl) to confusion, seizures, or coma. Any episode that requires intervention by another person to reverse is categorized as severe hypoglycemia. Severe hypoglycemia can have disastrous consequences, particularly if the patient is driving any sort of vehicle, working at heights, or operating potentially dangerous machinery.

The most common causes of hypoglycemia are missed meals and snacks,[117] insulin dosage errors, exercise, alcohol, and drugs such as beta-adrenergic blockers. During the DCCT, 55% of hypoglycemic episodes occurred during sleep.[117] Such episodes often go undetected.[118]

Glucagon and epinephrine are the major counterregulatory hormones that are secreted in response to hypoglycemia.[119] Both restore glucose levels by increasing hepatic glucose output, while epinephrine also decreases the sensitivity of muscles to insulin. Furthermore, catecholamine secretion alerts the patient to treat the episode because it produces the sympathoadrenal symptoms noted below. Cortisol and growth hormone are also secreted in response to hypoglycemia[119] and play a role in maintaining glucose levels but not in rapid recovery from hypoglycemia.

Presenting features　The most common symptoms of early mild hypoglycemia are adrenergic and include tachycardia, tremulousness, anxiety, and sweating.[120] The last symptom requires sympathetic activation of cholinergic nerves innervating the sweat glands.

Factors affecting severity of hypoglycemic episodes　The development of primary or secondary adrenal insufficiency, hypopituitarism, and hypothyroidism may increase the risk of hypoglycemia by increasing sensitivity to insulin, decreasing appetite, or both. Stress, exercise, or use of alcohol or illicit drugs may blunt or prevent recognition of hypoglycemia. Patients who do recognize incipient hypoglycemia but who consciously do not respond expeditiously (for example, they may wait for a meal in a restaurant or continue to drive after symptoms first appear) are also at increased risk for severe hypoglycemia. Moreover, some risk factors for hypoglycemia have multiple effects that can precipitate, prolong, or worsen the severity of hypoglycemia. Alcohol, for instance, impairs judgment and inhibits gluconeogenesis and hepatic glucose output, thereby delaying recovery. When hypoglycemia is inadequately treated, more severe hypoglycemia often ensues.

Finally, because glucagon and epinephrine are the major defense hormones against prolonged hypoglycemia, their absence promotes longer and more severe episodes by two mechanisms: (1) compensatory hepatic glucose output is decreased when not stimulated by glucagon or epinephrine and (2) the familiar adrenergic symptoms may cease in the absence of epinephrine, resulting in failure to recognize the episode.[119] The glucagon response to hypoglycemia often wanes in patients after they have had type 1 diabetes mellitus for a few years. In the absence of glucagon, epinephrine secretion still provides adequate counterregulatory defense; however, epinephrine response can also be lost eventually, sometimes in association with other autonomic neuropathies and sometimes selectively. Many patients lose the ability to counterregulate against hypoglycemia during the first 10 years that they have type 1 diabetes mellitus.

Given the importance of intensive regimens to prevent microvascular complications from hyperglycemia, it is most unfortunate that a lowered glucose threshold for release of glucagon and epinephrine in response to hypoglycemia has been observed, particularly in patients undergoing intensive insulin therapy.[121] The lowered glucose level needed to stimulate counterregulation narrows the safety margin of therapy. For instance, the first symptom of hypoglycemia may occur only at glucose levels as low as 35 mg/dl (as opposed to 55 to 60 mg/dl) and may consist of confusion or loss of judgment, which interferes with self-treatment. Some evidence suggests that unawareness of hypoglycemia is self-generating, because each episode may lower the threshold at which autonomic counterregulation begins in subsequent episodes.[119] The converse of this is that a period free of hypoglycemia, produced by daily therapeutic contact with caregivers, may restore hypoglycemia awareness,[122,123] though it may not restore normal counterregulatory responses.[122] Increased uptake of glucose by the brain in the presence of hypoglycemia[124,125] is a likely explanation for the relative infrequency of clinical hypoglycemic catastrophes.

Treatment　Patients recognize most episodes of hypoglycemia quickly and can effectively treat themselves with a promptly absorbed oral carbohydrate. Approximately 15 g of carbohydrate is sufficient to restore blood glucose levels to normal. This amount is provided by approximately 6 oz of orange juice, 4 oz of a cola drink, 3 to 4 tsp of table sugar, five Life Savers, or three glucose tablets (each containing 5 g of glucose). The use of complex carbohydrates and foods with a high fat content, such as chocolate, may delay digestion and absorption of the glucose and are not first choices for treatment of hypoglycemia. If the patient cannot swallow or cooperate, a gel form of glucose and simple carbohydrates can be administered by mouth, applying it between the gums and cheeks, from where it slowly and generally safely trickles down into the stomach. Glucagon (1 mg administered subcutaneously or intramuscularly) will also usually raise blood glucose levels sufficiently within 15 to 30 minutes, when the patient can then take oral carbohydrates. Glucagon comes in emergency kits, and it should always be on hand for patients with a history of severe hypoglycemic episodes. Glucagon may cause nausea, vomiting, and headache, especially in children. When all else fails, intravenous glucose must be given by emergency medical service personnel or in an emergency room, whichever is quicker. When the timing of an episode suggests it was caused by intermediate- or long-acting insulin or by prior exercise, blood glucose may fall to hypoglycemic levels again and re-treatment may be necessary. Thus, a patient who has required assistance from others in reversing hypoglycemia should be kept under surveillance for some time thereafter.

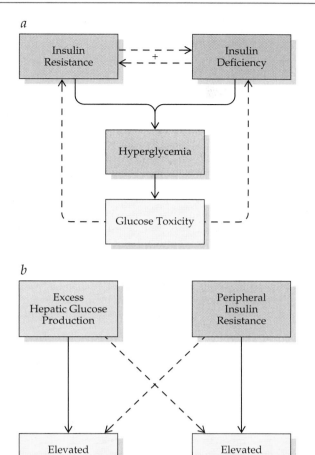

Figure 14 (*a*) **The interrelations of insulin resistance, insulin deficiency, and glucose toxicity that create overall hyperglycemia in type 2 diabetes mellitus are depicted. Insulin resistance and insulin deficiency are mutually reinforcing factors. Glucose toxicity refers to the secondary aggravating effects of hyperglycemia that both increase insulin resistance and reduce beta cell function. The glucose toxicity is diminished or eliminated by any therapy that lowers blood glucose. (*b*) Once fasting glucose levels are abnormal, they are correlated with and largely driven by the excess hepatic glucose production. Abnormal postprandial glucose levels are largely a consequence of peripheral insulin resistance that makes glucose utilization in muscle and adipose tissue inefficient. Insulin deficiency plays an increasingly important role in elevating both fasting and postprandial glucose levels as time goes on.**

Patients with severe hypoglycemia usually respond rapidly to treatment, although patients who are postictal or in a prolonged coma may require days to regain normal mental status and cognitive function. Quite often, there is amnesia for such extended episodes, including a period preceding the onset of hypoglycemia. In rare instances, neurologic deficits can be permanent. In general, however, long-term consequences of hypoglycemia have not been detected in adults.[126,127] In view of the potential consequences of prolonged episodes, hypoglycemia should always be treated immediately.

Prevention Patients should be instructed to treat themselves as though they have hypoglycemia whenever they suspect it,

even if they are unable to do a confirmatory blood glucose test at the time. The threshold for symptoms of hypoglycemia varies from person to person and even varies in the same person on different occasions. Therefore, whenever possible, a confirmatory blood glucose test should be done to help the patient discriminate nonspecific symptoms from true hypoglycemia. Patients at increased risk for severe hypoglycemia should monitor their blood glucose levels more frequently.

Type 2 Diabetes Mellitus

PATHOGENESIS OF TYPE 2 DIABETES MELLITUS

Insulin Resistance and Insulin Deficiency

The pathogenesis of type 2 diabetes mellitus[128] is even more complex than that of type 1 diabetes mellitus. Insulin resistance, reported in 92% of one large group of people with type 2 diabetes mellitus,[129] plays a major role in generating hyperglycemia.[128] In addition, some degree of functional insulin deficiency exists [*see Figure 13*].[128] Certain studies suggest that insulin resistance is primary[128,130] and that impaired insulin secretion is only really evident when fasting hyperglycemia supervenes.[128, 131-133] Other investigators find evidence of early abnormal beta cell function in type 2 diabetes mellitus,[134-136] in IGT,[134,137] and in first-degree glucose-tolerant relatives of patients with type 2 diabetes mellitus.[138] Regardless of which comes first, the loss of compensatory beta cell hyperfunction to overcome insulin resistance is a key factor in the progression from genetic susceptibility to established type 2 diabetes mellitus.[139] Furthermore, insulin resistance may cause secondary insulin deficiency, and insulin deficiency tends to lead to insulin resistance; thus, they are mutually reinforcing defects, partly through an effect commonly referred to as glucose toxicity.[140] Some period of hyperglycemia has a secondary noxious effect that aggravates both insulin resistance and insulin deficiency; thus, hyperglycemia begets hyperglycemia. Therefore, any form of treatment of type 2 diabetes mellitus that lowers plasma glucose levels is self-reinforcing and may gain momentum with time by virtue of the added early benefit of eliminating the effects of glucose toxicity. For this reason, aggressive early treatment (e.g., with insulin) can sometimes be replaced with oral drugs or even diet.[141]

The exact locus of insulin resistance in type 2 diabetes mellitus remains unidentified. Indeed, there may be various sites because the disease is considered likely to be a heterogeneous disorder.[142,143] Numerous candidate genes for defective insulin action, including the insulin receptor, glucose transporter, insulin receptor substrate, and insulin target enzymes, such as glycogen synthase, have been largely excluded as common primary causes of insulin resistance[144,145] in type 2 diabetes mellitus.

As in type 1 diabetes mellitus, the loss of effective insulin action directly leads to unrestrained hepatic glucose production and inefficient peripheral glucose utilization [*see Figure 14*]. Excessive hepatic glucose output largely accounts for elevation of FPG levels.[128] Resistance to the antilipolytic action of insulin in adipose tissue leads to elevated plasma free fatty acid (FFA) levels and increased FFA delivery to the liver. There, the oxidation of FFA generates energy (adenosine triphosphate [ATP]) needed to sustain gluconeogenesis; in addition, the latter process is stimulated by FFA metabolites such as acyl coenzyme A (acyl-CoA). In this indirect manner, insulin resistance also contributes to elevated glucose production in the liver.[146] Moreover, the elevation

---

Table 6 Insulin-Resistance Syndrome

Decreased sensitivity of glucose metabolism to insulin action

Hyperinsulinemia, hyperproinsulinemia

Glucose intolerance (IFG, IGT); increased risk of type 2 diabetes mellitus (or its presence)

Abdominal, visceral obesity

Dyslipidemia: ↑ TG; ↓ HDL; ↑ smaller denser LDL particles; ↑ apo B

Hypertension

↑ Plasminogen activator inhibitor–1; ↓ fibrinolysis

Hyperandrogenism in women; polycystic ovaries

Increased risk of cardiovascular disease and death

HDL—high-density lipoproteins   IFG—impaired fasting glucose
IGT—impaired glucose tolerance   LDL—low-density lipoproteins
TG—triglycerides

---

of FFA levels also contributes to insulin resistance in muscle.[147] The presence of some residual insulin secretion in type 2 diabetes mellitus, however, is ordinarily enough to restrain ketogenesis and prevent DKA. Elevated hepatic glucose output largely sustains an elevated FPG, whereas reduced peripheral glucose utilization especially causes elevation of postprandial glucose levels [see Figure 14].

The ratio of proinsulin to insulin in plasma is high and remains so even after glucose-lowering therapy,[148,149] suggesting an early abnormality in processing of proinsulin to insulin in the beta cell [see Figure 3]. Insulin is normally secreted in cyclic pulses that can be entrained by rapid changes in plasma glucose levels. Disruption of this close concordance between plasma glucose and plasma insulin fluctuations is a subtle lesion that is demonstrable early in patients with type 2 diabetes mellitus and, to a lesser extent, in some patients with only impaired glucose tolerance.[134,136] Finally, the plasma insulin response to abrupt elevation of plasma glucose levels normally shows a first sharp, spikelike phase.[150] Before the plasma insulin level returns to baseline, it slowly rises again to produce a second plateau phase of more prolonged insulin release. The immediate first-phase response to glucose decreases in type 2 diabetes mellitus, as it does in the preclinical phase of type 1 diabetes mellitus, and is completely lost when the FPG level exceeds the normal range.[151]

Other Beta Cell Abnormalities

Another, previously neglected abnormality in type 2 diabetes mellitus is the presence of amyloid in close proximity to the islet beta cells. The amyloid fibrils have been found to contain amylin, a peptide that is cosecreted with insulin.[152] Amylin deficiency parallels insulin deficiency in type 2 diabetes mellitus.[152] Whether the accumulation of amyloid impairs beta cell function or is an epiphenomenon resulting from beta cell hyperfunction with increased amylin secretion in the early phases of the disease remains unclear.

More than 10% of some patient populations presenting with the clinical phenotype of type 2 diabetes mellitus have serum islet cell autoantibodies typical of type 1 diabetes mellitus, such as antibodies to GAD.[153] This combination has been referred to as latent autoimmune diabetes in adults (LADA). These individuals exhibit a rapid decline in beta cell function, as shown by serum C-peptide levels, and they are likely to need insulin replacement therapy, even if their hyperglycemia is initially alleviated by oral beta cell stimulants.[154,155]

Obesity as a Risk Factor

The insulin-resistance syndrome [see Table 6] is closely associated with and is often a forerunner to type 2 diabetes mellitus. One obvious link between them is obesity, which is a cause of insulin resistance[156] and a contributor to the insulin resistance of type 2 diabetes mellitus.[157,158] Weight gain presages diabetes,[159] and weight loss in obese individuals prevents progression of IGT to full-blown diabetes.[160] Most patients with type 2 diabetes mellitus have abdominal obesity and many have dyslipidemia, hypertension, and other features of the insulin-resistance syndrome.[129] Abdominal obesity is itself a risk factor for type 2 diabetes mellitus and cardiovascular disease.[161,162] This relation explains much but not all of the vulnerability of patients with type 2 diabetes mellitus to cardiovascular complications resulting from accelerated atherosclerosis. On the other hand, not all patients with the insulin-resistance syndrome and IGT go on to experience full-blown type 2 diabetes mellitus. A large randomized controlled trial is currently testing the ability of lifestyle changes (weight reduction and regular exercise) and the drug metformin to reduce the risk of progressing from IGT to type 2 diabetes mellitus.[163]

Genetic Factors

Type 2 diabetes mellitus has a strong hereditary component. In virtually all monozygotic twinships, the disease develops in both individuals, often within a few years of each other.[164] Offspring and siblings of diabetic patients are at great risk for the disease. No HLA markers have been identified for type 2 diabetes mellitus, in contrast to type 1 diabetes mellitus. Most current thinking is that the common forms of type 2 diabetes mellitus represent a complex multigenic disorder.[165] Examination of the mechanism of action of insulin [see Figure 4] suggests many logical candidate genes, mutations of which could lead to type 2 diabetes mellitus by causing primary insulin resistance. Thus far, genes for insulin, the insulin receptor, insulin receptor substrate, glucose transporter, muscle hexokinase, glycogen synthase, and other insulin target enzymes have all been excluded as the cause of so-called garden-variety type 2 diabetes mellitus.[165,166] Because of the association with obesity, genes that could cause obesity are also being investigated (e.g., leptin, uncoupling protein, and beta$_3$-adrenergic receptor). The positional cloning approach being used in populations with high diabetes prevalence, such as Pima Indians and Mexican Americans, has yielded hints of loci on certain chromosomes that require confirmation.

There is one form of diabetes, MODY [see Table 1], that does have genetic specificity. In this disorder, mutations of at least four separate genes on different chromosomes lead to a common phenotype resembling type 2 diabetes mellitus, but the disorder begins at an early age.[167] One of the four genes is the gene for glucokinase, an enzyme that plays a key role in stimulation of insulin secretion by glucose.[168] Another mutation occurs in a molecule known as insulin production factor–1, a transcription factor that is responsible for differentiation of precursor cells into beta cells capable of insulin secretion.[167] Two other genes responsible for MODY code for hepatic transcription factor–1 and hepatic transcription factor–4, which, despite their names, operate in beta cells to regulate the glucose responsive pathway of insulin secretion.[167] All of these genetic abnormalities more likely explain type 2 diabetes mellitus caused by beta cell dysfunction than that caused by peripheral insulin resistance. Their functional relation to the diabetic diathesis is still obscure. Even in a phenotypically well defined monogenic form of diabetes such as MODY, the exis-

Table 7 American Diabetes Association Plasma Glucose Diagnostic Criteria for Diabetes Mellitus

Diagnosis	Test Condition	
	Plasma Glucose (mg/dl)	
	Fasting ≥ 8 hr	2 hr after 75 g Oral Glucose
Normal	< 110	< 140
Impaired glucose tolerance (IGT)	< 126	≥ 140–< 200
Impaired fasting glucose (IFG)	≥ 110–< 126	< 200
Diabetes mellitus	≥ 126	—
Diabetes mellitus	< 126	≥ 200
Diabetes mellitus (Classic symptoms + casual plasma glucose, ≥ 200 mg/dl)	—	—

Gestational diabetes mellitus (GDM)	Plasma Glucose (mg/dl)	
	Fasting	After 100 g Oral Glucose
	> 105*	1 hr ≥ 190*
		2 hr ≥ 165*
		3 hr ≥ 145*

Note: The Fourth International Workshop-Conference on Gestational Diabetes Mellitus has proposed lower criteria, which would increase the percentage of cases from 4% to 7% in white women. These criteria are fasting, 95; 1 hour, 180; 2 hours, 155; and 3 hours, 140, after 100 g oral glucose.

*Two of these four criteria must be met for diagnosis of GDM.

tence of many alleles for hepatic transcription factor–1 indicates the genetic complexity of diabetes. Although the mutations responsible for MODY account for only a minute fraction of all cases of type 2 diabetes mellitus, they encourage the view that genes contributing to most or all cases of type 2 diabetes mellitus will eventually be found.

IMPAIRED GLUCOSE TOLERANCE

The state known as impaired glucose tolerance [see Table 7] is associated with a future risk of development of diabetes of 1% to 10% a year, with different levels of risk for different ethnic groups. Equally important is the association of IGT with the insulin-resistance syndrome [see Table 6], which includes hyperinsulinemia, glucose intolerance, dyslipidemia, hypertension, and impaired fibrinolysis. Presence of this syndrome constitutes a high risk for atherosclerosis, cardiovascular disease, thrombotic events, and mortality. The category of impaired fasting glucose was newly established by the American Diabetes Association as an intermediate zone between the upper limit of normal and the lower limit for diabetes.[1] IFG is also associated with increased risk of diabetes, but the magnitude of that risk appears to be less than that for IGT. IFG and IGT are not identical states. About one third of people with IGT have IFG, one third of those with IFG have IGT, and one third of affected individuals have both.[2] The pathophysiologic bases and clinical significance of the differences between IFG and IGT remain to be determined. Both conditions can be thought of as early stages of type 2 diabetes mellitus.

DIAGNOSIS OF TYPE 2 DIABETES MELLITUS

Although patients with type 2 diabetes mellitus may present with symptoms as florid as those of type 1 diabetes mellitus (but usually not exhibiting spontaneous ketonuria), most patients with type 2 disease have relatively mild polyuria and polydipsia, and many cases are diagnosed only by office screening or other health checks.

The preferred test for type 2 diabetes mellitus on the grounds of reproducibility, convenience, and cost is an FPG . Oral glucose tolerance testing is more sensitive than FPG but is not recommended for routine use, because it is less reproducible, more inconvenient, and more costly.[1] Moreover, a combined regimen of nutrition therapy, weight loss, and exercise is the only common treatment for diabetes that can be diagnosed only by inordinate hyperglycemia after oral glucose loading. For almost all overweight or obese patients who would be candidates for such a test, the same therapy is recommended even without knowledge of the oral glucose tolerance test results.

MANAGEMENT OF TYPE 2 DIABETES MELLITUS

The same glycemic goals discussed earlier [see Table 5] are appropriate for type 2 diabetes mellitus. However, these goals may sometimes have to be modified if severe cardiovascular disease, concurrent life-shortening malignancy, hypoglycemia unawareness, or inadequate family or social support make intensive treatment of diabetes dangerous or unlikely to benefit the patient in the long run. Self-monitoring of blood glucose when patients with type 2 diabetes mellitus are treated with diet plus exercise or with oral drugs is of less well established utility in patients with type 2 diabetes mellitus than in patients with type 1 diabetes mellitus. However, fasting and postprandial blood glucose levels both correlate with HbA_{1c} levels, and postprandial values can help reveal inadequate attention to diet and insufficient effectiveness of certain oral agents.

Nutritional Therapy and Exercise

An excellent short-term glycemic response to caloric reduction in patients with type 2 diabetes mellitus who are even modestly overweight can be expected.[169,170] On the basis of the degree of obesity and with the help of a dietitian, the patient should be provided with individualized culturally appropriate instructions to reduce intake by at least 250 to 500 calories a day. Such a decrease generally leads to an overall weight loss of 0.5 to 1.0 lb a week. There should be periodic reinforcement by the dietitian and physician. In the absence of a dietitian, the patient's basal metabolic rate can be estimated at 10 cal/lb (20 cal/kg) of ideal body weight. A caloric prescription less than this amount will perforce decrease energy intake below the total daily energy expenditure. Consensus guidelines recommend that the calories should consist of less than 30% total fat, less than 10% saturated fat, less than 10% polyunsaturated fat, 10% to 15% monounsaturated fat, 10% to 20% protein, and 50% to 55% carbohydrate.[171,172] Table sugar and other concentrated forms of carbohydrates are allowable in small portions at any one time (e.g., 5 g or 1 tsp of table sugar). Adding high-fiber foods can also lower plasma glucose modestly.[173] Teaching patients to count the contemplated grams of carbohydrate before each meal helps them limit elevation of postprandial plasma glucose (PPG).

In massively obese individuals with BMI greater than 40 who are very symptomatic from hyperglycemia, a very low calorie diet (400 to 800 total calories a day using special high-protein supplements) can be very effective for the initial 2 to 3 months, but this strategy requires close medical monitoring.[174,175]

Weight losses of 5% to 10% (10 to 20 lb) produce significant decreases in FPG and HbA_{1c} over 1 to 3 months.[169,170] In the UKPDS, mean HbA_{1c} fell from 9% to 7% during the 3-month dietary run-in period before randomization of the study patients.[176,177] However, many patients are unable to maintain a calorie-restricted diet and even their initial weight loss. Newer pharmacologic aids for weight loss can be considered in such cases, but their efficacy is limited. These drugs include orlistat,[178] a gastrointestinal lipase inhibitor that causes malabsorption of fat calories, and sibutramine, an inhibitor of dopamine, norepinephrine, and serotonin reuptake. Even after the addition of a weight-loss drug to therapy, appropriate diet therapy is essential. The patient should not be blamed for recidivism, because inability to lower body weight to ideal and keep it there may well be a central nervous system manifestation of or contributor to type 2 diabetes mellitus and out of the patient's consistent control.[179] Surgical therapy for obesity by reduction of gastric volume[180,181] can effectively control type 2 diabetes mellitus and is gaining acceptance in very obese individuals who are unresponsive to other therapy.

Additional benefits accrue from gradually increased aerobic exercise[182] aimed at achieving at least 60% of maximal heart rate (220 minus age), such as walking 45 to 60 minutes at a brisk pace three to five times a week. Exercise decreases insulin resistance and glycemia, contributes modestly to weight loss, reduces the risk of future cardiovascular disease, improves prognosis should a myocardial infarction occur, and enhances the patient's sense of well-being and physical fitness. Conversely, physical inactivity predicts mortality in men with type 2 diabetes mellitus.[183] In the presence of known coronary artery disease (CAD), the exercise should be prescribed with input from the patient's cardiologist. If type 2 diabetes mellitus has existed for more than 5 to 10 years or if the patient already has peripheral vascular or cerebral vascular disease, autonomic neuropathy, microalbuminuria, dyslipidemia, or a history of smoking, an electrocardiogram is essential and an electrocardiographic exercise tolerance test is prudent before initiating a formal exercise program.

Pharmacologic Monotherapy

The array of pharmacologic agents available for treatment of type 2 diabetes mellitus is increasing steadily.[184] Drugs can be specifically directed at the known pathophysiologic defects in type 2 diabetes mellitus [*see Figure 15*]. Although patient compliance favors initial use of monotherapy, none of the available agents can alone be expected to adequately control hyperglycemia indefinitely.[185] Therefore, diabetologists are beginning to consider using combinations of drugs from the outset of the need for any pharmacotherapy.[186] Clinical trial data have established the efficacy and safety of various drugs [*see Table 8*] . The degrees to which these drugs lower HbA_{1c} are fairly similar; the higher the initial dose of these agents, the greater the decrease in HbA_{1c}.

Sulfonylurea agents SU agents, the oldest oral hypoglycemic drugs, continue to have an important place in treatment.[187] Their primary mechanism of action is to close ATP-sensitive potassium channels in the beta cell (and other cell) membranes, which leads to an influx of calcium and stimulation of exocytosis of insulin storage granules.[188] They are most effective in normal-weight or modestly obese individuals who have had diabetes for less than 5 years and who can still secrete consider-

able amounts of insulin. The SU drugs in common use stimulate the beta cells more or less continuously and secondarily decrease insulin resistance. These effects [*see Figure 14*][188] result in decreases in FPG of 50 to 70 mg/dl and HbA_{1c} of 1.0% to 2.0%. Peak PPG levels fall approximately as much as FPG. For most patients, treatment is initiated with the lowest recommended dose, and the dose is increased every 1 to 2 weeks until target blood glucose levels are attained or a practical maximal dose is reached [*see Table 9*]. Modern SU drugs can be taken as a single daily dose but occasionally are more effective when split into twice-daily doses. In symptomatic patients with FPG greater than 250, the patient may begin with half the maximal recommended dose. Hypoglycemia, in particular, and weight gain are adverse effects of SU drugs. The highest prevalence of hypoglycemia occurs with glyburide and chlorpropamide,[189] drugs with long biologic half-lives. Elderly patients who live alone and lack concerned family, friends, or neighbors are at a special risk for severe, even fatal, hypoglycemia.[190] The shortest-acting SU drug, tolbutamide, may be the safest to use in such cases.

Patients who present to an emergency room in hypoglycemic coma from any SU drug should be given restorative treatment with intravenous boluses of glucose and then admitted to the hospital because SU drugs can have durations of biologic action for up to 7 days. A blood glucose should be maintained at 150 to 200 mg/dl on intravenous glucose, oral carbohydrate, or both until this level can be sustained by administration of only 5 g/hr of one of the therapeutic agents. In the UKPDS, SU drugs did not increase cardiovascular disease events or mortality.[37] This observation relieves much of the concern previously raised by the University Group Diabetes Program trial in 1970, which found that tolbutamide was associated with an excess of cardiovascular and total deaths.[191] However, interactions of even modern SU drugs with cardiac muscle are reported, particularly inhibition of ischemic preconditioning, a cardioprotective mechanism.[192] SU drugs are contraindicated in hepatic insufficiency and are dangerous when combined with alcohol ingestion. Glimepiride, the newest SU drug,[193] has been given safely to patients with renal insufficiency, although these patients are susceptible to hypoglycemia for other reasons. SU drugs are subject to interactions with other drugs that can either exaggerate or interfere with their effects.

Beta cell stimulants Repaglinide and the phenylalanine derivative nateglinide represent a new class of beta cell stimulants [*see Figure 15*] that differ in structure and timing of action from those of SU drugs.[194,195] Although they may act in part through SU drug mechanisms in the beta cells,[196] they do so rapidly, with a peak effect at about 1 hour, and transiently, with a duration of about 4 hours. Their major action is the decrease of PPG by 50 to 60 mg/dl, although FPG also declines somewhat as glucose toxicity is relieved. As monotherapy, these new beta cell stimulants are most logically used early in type 2 diabetes mellitus, when FPG is not greatly elevated. They lower HbA_{1c} by about 1.0%. Repaglinide and nateglinide must be taken 15 to 30 minutes before a meal and should never be taken without eating. Their short half-lives and the fact that, unlike SU drugs, they are active only in the presence of glucose are expected to reduce the likelihood of severe prolonged hypoglycemic episodes.[195] Weight gain may occur secondary to improved glycemic control.

α-Glucosidase inhibitors α-Glucosidase inhibitors[197-199] are a class of drugs represented by acarbose and miglitol, which are poorly absorbed but act within the gut to inhibit the digestion of

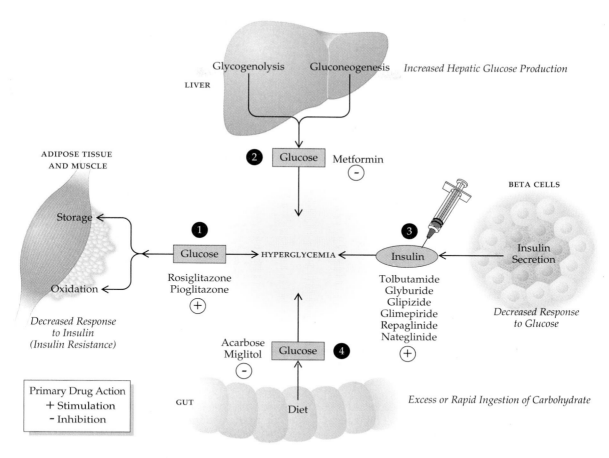

Figure 15 **Multiple drug classes with different predominant therapeutic effects are available for use singly or in numerous combinations. (1) Glitazones (thiazolidinediones) increase the sensitivity to insulin of glucose uptake by muscle and adipose tissue. (2) Metformin, the only approved biguanide drug, inhibits glucose production by the liver. (3) Sulfonylureas, repaglinide, and nateglinide stimulate insulin secretion, and insulin itself can be provided by injection. (4) α-Glucosidase inhibitors slow the digestion and absorption of carbohydrates from the diet. Plus signs indicate stimulation. Minus signs indicate inhibition.**

polysaccharides [*see Figure 15*]. This action results in a slow release of glucose from food and therefore slow absorption from the GI tract. PPG levels decrease by 60 to 70 mg/dl, but FPG decreases by only 15 to 20 mg/dl.[199] HbA$_{1c}$ generally falls 0.5% to 0.8%.[198,199] These drugs are useful only as monotherapy when postprandial hyperglycemia is the main problem. They must be taken at the start of a meal. Flatulence, abdominal cramping, and diarrhea are frequent side effects that result from undigested carbohydrate reaching bacteria in the lower bowel. These side effects often limit patient acceptance of treatment with α-glucosidase inhibitors. Treatment should start with the smallest dose, and doses should be raised very gradually to enhance tolerance. With the exception of rare elevations of alanine aminotransferase (ALT) and aspartate aminotransferase (AST) levels, these agents are nontoxic. Although hypoglycemia does not occur with monotherapy, it can do so when α-glucosidase inhibitors are added to SU drugs or insulin. In those instances, patients must be warned to treat hypoglycemia only with pure glucose (e.g., glucose tablets) because the therapeutic benefits of complex carbohydrates and even sucrose will be delayed by slow digestion.

Biguanide agents Metformin,[184, 200] the only drug approved in the biguanide class, acts primarily by decreasing excessive hepatic glucose production [*see Figure 15*],[201,202] most likely through inhibiting gluconeogenesis. Because insulin also inhibits gluconeo-

genesis [*see Figure 1*][20] and metformin requires the presence of insulin to be effective, metformin may be considered a hepatic insulin sensitizer. During metformin treatment, plasma insulin levels tend to decrease relative to glucose levels as a result of the decrease in insulin resistance. The chief action of this drug is to lower FPG by 50 to 70 mg/dl, with peak PPG levels following suit.[203] Hypoglycemia almost never occurs with metformin monotherapy. Weight is not gained and may even be lost.[200] Metformin also decreases plasma triglyceride and low-density lipoprotein (LDL) cholesterol levels, and it increases HDL cholesterol levels to some degree.[184] In addition, plasma plasminogen activator inhibitor–1 (PAI-1) activity declines.[204] The weight loss, the improvement in the dyslipidemia typical of type 2 diabetes mellitus, and the reduction in antifibrinolytic activity could explain one of the most interesting UKPDS observations. Compared with conventional diet treatment, metformin monotherapy substantially decreased the incidence of myocardial infarction, diabetes-related death, and all-cause mortality in an obese type 2 subcohort of the trial.[38]

The most common side effects of metformin therapy are diarrhea, which may be severe; abdominal cramps; and gastric upset. To reduce the likelihood of these symptoms, the starting dose should not exceed 500 mg twice a day, and the drug should be used with special caution, if at all, in patients who have inflammatory GI disease. The maximum effective dose is 2,000 mg/day.[205]

Table 8 Oral Drugs for Type 2 Diabetes Mellitus

Drugs	Lowest Effective Single Dose (mg)	Practical Maximum Daily Dose (mg)	Hypoglycemia with Monotherapy
Sulfonylureas*			
Glyburide	1.25	10	Yes
Micronized glyburide	1.5	6	Yes
Glipizide	5	20	Yes
Glipizide (gastrointestinal therapeutic system)	5	20	Yes
Glimepiride	0.5	8	Yes
Meglitinides†			
Repaglinide	0.5	4‡	Yes
Biguanides			
Metformin	500	2,000	No
Thiazolidinediones§			
Rosiglitazone	2	8	No
Pioglitazone	15	45	No
α-Glucosidase inhibitors			
Acarbose	25	100‡	No
Miglitol	25	100‡	No

*Tolbutamide, chlorpropamide, and acetohexamide are also still available.
†Nateglinide has a similar action to meglitinides but is technically phenylalanine derivative.
‡This maximal dose must be taken each time with meals.
§Troglitazone was the initial drug approved in this class but was later withdrawn because of serious liver toxicity.

The most feared, although rare, adverse effect is lactic acidosis.[206] This often fatal complication occurs in 30 patients per million patients a year, and it usually occurs when the drug is used inappropriately, such as when the serum creatinine level is elevated or the patient is dehydrated. Hemodialysis along with bicarbonate administration can be effective therapy for metformin-induced lactic acidosis.[207] The following are contraindications to use of metformin: serum creatinine level greater than 1.4 mg/dl in women and greater than 1.5 mg/dl in men; intravenous administration of radiographic iodinated contrast media; acute myocardial infarction; congestive heart failure; and any ischemic condition. Nausea, vomiting, tachypnea, and change in mental status call for measurements of serum electrolytes and lactate to rule out lactic acid metabolic acidosis. Although metformin monotherapy can be effective in both normal-weight and obese patients with type 2 diabetes mellitus, obese patients especially benefit from metformin therapy because of the absence of weight gain as glucose levels gradually fall.

Thiazolidinediones The newest class of oral drugs are thiazolidinediones (TZDs) [*see Table 8*],[208] which were exemplified by the no longer available but best studied drug, troglitazone . These agents work predominantly in muscle and adipose tissue to decrease insulin resistance [*see Figure 15*].[202,209] Because insulin resistance is seen in almost all patients with type 2 diabetes mellitus, the advent of the TZDs raised expectations that they might be singularly effective. Like metformin, TZD drugs need the presence of insulin and are especially effective in obese patients. They also decrease hepatic glucose production to some extent.[202] As monotherapy, they decrease FPG by 50 to 70 mg/dl and PPG by slightly more than that.[209] HbA$_{1c}$ decreases by about 1.0% to 1.5%. Plasma insulin levels also decrease as glucose levels fall.[209] TZD drugs act by binding to a metabolically important receptor, the peroxisome proliferator-activated receptor (PPAR), and they thereby regulate the expression of multiple genes.[210] Their clinical effects take 4 to 12 weeks to become evident. In patients with marked elevation of FPG, a midrange dose is appropriate to start with (e.g., 4 mg rosiglitazone or 30 mg pioglitazone). Otherwise, the lowest dose is appropriate, and dose changes should be made at 4- to 12-week intervals.

TZD drugs can cause weight gain, which is partly fat tissue and partly extracellular fluid.[208] The accumulation of extracellular fluid presents as edema, which can be troublesome when concurrent congestive heart failure exists, and a small dilutional fall in hemoglobin and hematocrit. Some findings suggest that the adipose tissue gain is largely subcutaneous rather than visceral.[211] In clinical research trials, troglitazone therapy was accompanied by elevations of ALT and AST to more than three times the upper limit of normal in 2% of treated patients, compared with 0.6% of patients given placebo. However, after troglitazone was approved by the

Table 9 **Combination Oral Drug Therapy for Type 2 Diabetes Mellitus**

Combinations reported in the literature
  Sulfonylurea + metformin
  Sulfonylurea + thiazolidinedione
  Metformin + thiazolidinedione
  Metformin + repaglinide
  Repaglinide + thiazolidinedione
  Sulfonylurea + metformin + thiazolidinedione
  Acarbose + any other drug except repaglinide
  Miglitol + sulfonylurea
  Insulin + any other drug
Potentially useful combination
  Repaglinide + metformin + thiazolidinedione
  Nateglinide + metformin + thiazolidinedione

FDA, more than 60 cases of hepatic failure that necessitated liver transplantation or resulted in death, or both, were reported out of a user base of about one million persons. The FDA eventually withdrew approval, first for the prescription of troglitazone as monotherapy and later for all indications. In clinical research trials, neither rosiglitazone nor pioglitazone caused AST and ALT elevations in excess of those caused by placebo, but these drugs have not been used enough to provide a guarantee that they will never cause idiosyncratic liver toxicity similar to that caused by troglitazone. Therefore, the FDA has mandated that these drugs be monitored by ALT measurements every 2 months for the first year of use. Neither rosiglitazone nor pioglitazone should be prescribed if the ALT level is greater than 2.5 times the upper limit of normal, and the drugs should be stopped if such levels are reached.

TZD drugs have exhibited effects in addition to glucose lowering that may be beneficial for treating cardiovascular complications.[212-219] Troglitazone and pioglitazone suppress formation of PAI-1, an action that enhances fibrinolysis.[213,214] TZD drugs tend to decrease serum triglyceride levels and increase serum HDL cholesterol levels, but they also increase serum LDL cholesterol levels.[208] In addition, troglitazone has been reported to shift the LDL spectrum from small, dense atherogenic particles to larger, more buoyant, less atherogenic particles.[219] Endothelial function also likely improves.[216,217] A decrease in carotid artery intimal-medial thickness[217]—a marker of atherosclerosis—as well as decreases in vasospastic angina[215] and in recurrence of intimal hyperplasia after coronary angioplasty[218] have been reported in small series of patients treated with troglitazone for only 6 months.[216,217] Whether TZD drugs will decrease rates of cardiovascular events through such actions remains to be seen.

Insulin   About 40% of patients with type 2 diabetes mellitus in the United States are estimated to be taking insulin. A small proportion of these patients may have delayed-onset type 1 diabetes mellitus and may offer serologic evidence of beta cell autoimmunity. However, most of these patients represent the end stage of type 2 diabetes mellitus. A small number of such patients, some of whom are even obese, present initially with clear-cut biologic evidence of insulin deficiency. This evidence includes marked recent loss of weight and muscle mass, debilitating fatigue and weakness, severe polyuria and polydypsia, considerable hypertriglyceridemia, ketonuria, and FPG often exceeding 300 mg/dl. These patients should be started on insulin immediately—as in patients with type 1 diabetes mellitus. After usually rapid clinical and biochemical improvement, insulin-dose requirements may decrease progressively. Patients can sometimes be tapered off insulin and be given a trial of an SU drug. This sequence has been reported in certain groups of African Americans.[220,221]

Much more commonly, the need for insulin treatment has arisen because of eventual failure of oral drug therapy, particularly SU drugs. For normal-weight individuals in this situation, it is best to simply switch them to insulin. Some patients may still be managed on a single dose of intermediate- or long-acting insulin (starting dose of NPH, Lente, or Ultralente of 0.15 to 0.20 U/kg) in the morning[222] or at bedtime if the FPG is being specifically targeted.[223] The latter is a particularly attractive way to lessen glycemia without stimulating weight gain.[224] Other patients may need intermediate- or long-acting insulin twice a day, usually in a ratio of breakfast dose to bedtime dose of from 1:1 to 2:1. As endogenous postprandial insulin secretion declines further, regular or lispro insulin or insulin aspart [see Type 1 Diabetes Mellitus, *above*] must be added before meals. To approach normal glycemia, the doses of rapid, short-acting insulin are best adjusted according to the premeal blood glucose level, the carbohydrate content of the meal, or both. For all practical purposes, some patients with type 2 diabetes mellitus closely resemble patients with type 1 diabetes mellitus in the insulin regimens they require.

For stable patients incapable of accurately mixing different insulins in one syringe because of visual or cognitive impairment, premixed combinations of NPH with regular or lispro insulin are available in varying proportions; these combinations include 70% NPH/30% regular, 50% NPH/50% regular, and 75% NPH/25% lispro. These mixtures all suffer from the inflexibility of neither the dose of NPH nor the dose of the regular or lispro insulin being able to be altered individually. For example, a patient with satisfactory postbreakfast or prelunch blood glucose levels but elevated predinner blood glucose levels would benefit from an increase in the morning NPH insulin dose but not necessarily from an increase in the morning regular or lispro insulin dose. Premixed insulins are not suitable for bedtime use unless an uncommonly large snack is eaten. Despite the above objections, premixed insulins are convenient for patients and for family members who have therapeutic responsibilities.

Whatever insulin regimens are chosen, obese patients with type 2 diabetes mellitus often need large daily doses, which many practitioners are unaccustomed to prescribing. Doses of 1 U/kg body weight are not unusual, and doses of up to 400 U daily have been required to achieve glycemic targets in morbidly obese individuals.[225,226] Concern has been raised in the past that insulin might have atherogenic effects because epidemiologic studies (mostly in nondiabetic individuals) have shown an association between insulin resistance, fasting or postprandial plasma insulin levels, and future risk of cardiovascular disease.[227] In the UKPDS[37] and in the University Group Diabetes Program,[228] exogenous insulin did not increase the rate of myocardial infarction or of cardiovascular death. It can be argued that the insulin doses used in those trials were not very large or that an adverse effect from an atherogenic property of insulin was offset by a beneficial effect resulting from a decrease in glycemia. In any event, there is not enough evidence of cardiovascular danger from exogenous insulin to justify withholding doses necessary to achieve near-normal glycemia. In two randomized clinical trials[37,229] and in a large retrospective study,[190] the incidence of serious hypoglycemic episodes was in the range of two to three events per 100 patient-years. It should be noted, however, that one out of 20 severe hypoglycemic events can be accompanied by such complications as stroke, transient ischemic attack, myocardial infarction, injury, and death.[190] Weight gain—in rare cases, even to degrees that have resulted in sleep apnea—is a major adverse effect of insulin therapy and is one justification for combining insulin with a drug such as metformin, which can restrict weight gain to some extent.[230]

Combination Therapy

Improved understanding of the pathogenesis of hyperglycemia in type 2 diabetes mellitus and longer experience with oral drug monotherapy have greatly increased interest in and popularity of using combinations of oral drugs. In patients with considerable hyperglycemia, none of the current drugs reliably normalize HbA$_{1c}$ when used alone, probably because they act primarily by correcting single abnormalities [see Figure 15]. Thus, to reach aggressive therapeutic targets [see Table 3], combinations are needed [see Table 9]. Moreover, all forms of monotherapy—including insulin used conventionally—fail after a number of years, with the possible exception of TZD drugs, for which long enough experience is still lacking. This need for combination therapy was best shown by the UKPDS experience.[37,185] The availability of combination therapies supports the logic of attacking two or more different causes of hyperglycemia simultaneously—for example, reducing insulin resistance in the liver with metformin while increasing insulin secretion with an SU drug[203] or meglitinide.[231] Moreover, as a practical matter, when monotherapy fails after initial success, substituting another drug from a different drug class has not been effective (except for insulin), as has been shown in trials that unsuccessfully attempted to substitute metformin[203] or a TZD drug[232] for an SU drug. By contrast, addition of either metformin[203] or a TZD[232] to an SU drug did lower HbA$_{1c}$ significantly. The combinations of metformin with repaglinide,[231] metformin with a TZD drug,[202] and repaglinide with a TZD drug[233] have also been more effective than any of these agents given alone.

α-Glucosidase inhibitors complement the different actions of each of the other drugs, including insulin,[198] and their combinations. All other oral drugs are effective when added to SU drugs, except possibly repaglinide or nateglinide, for which data are still lacking. Metformin and troglitazone also work in triple combination with an SU drug. Combinations of oral drugs may at least provide an additional therapeutic period before having to be switched for progressively more intensive insulin therapy as last recourse. Furthermore, the progressive rise in plasma glucose levels seen in patients on monotherapy in the UKPDS was attributable to declining beta cell function.[234] Thus, pathophysiologically rational combinations of oral drugs, if used much earlier in patients with type 2 diabetes mellitus, might even preserve beta cell function longer than was previously achieved with the initial monotherapy approach.

When adding drugs, particularly to insulin, it is usually wise to start with the lowest dose of the drug being added to the regimen and to increase the dose as though it were being used as monotherapy. Self–blood glucose testing at times of the day appropriate for the added drug should be used as a safety check and a guide to efficacy. For metformin, TZD drugs, SU drugs, and bedtime insulin, the FBG is especially helpful. For repaglinide, nateglinide, α-glucosidase inhibitors, premeal regular insulin, lispro insulin, or insulin aspart, postprandial blood glucose levels are important guides to therapy. Patients should be given blood glucose guidelines for when to call the physician (e.g., when FBG is consistently less than 100 mg/dl).

Combination therapy can be quite expensive, even when it results in a lower insulin requirement.[235] The primary aim should always be to decrease the HbA$_{1c}$. Reduction in insulin dose, number of injections, or both should be thought of only as a secondary benefit.

MANAGEMENT OF HYPEROSMOLAR HYPERGLYCEMIC NONKETOTIC COMA

Type 2 diabetes mellitus seldom gives rise to DKA unless the patient experiences a severe medical stress. On the other hand, hyperosmolar hyperglycemic nonketotic coma (HHNC) is a common and feared acute complication characterized by extreme hyperglycemia (> 600 mg/dl) and serum hyperosmolarity (> 320 mOsm/L) but with little or no ketosis.[110,236,237] The CNS effects of extreme hyperosmolarity range from somnolence or confusion to coma but notably can also include focal or generalized seizures as well as focal neurologic deficits that disappear with treatment. The absence of severe ketonemia is usually attributed to enough residual insulin secretion that lipolysis is not as unrestrained as in type 1 diabetes mellitus with DKA. HHNC is marked by extreme dehydration, in which the deficit of free water is prominent and the circulatory volume is often seriously compromised. Thus, hypotension; extemely dry skin and mucous membranes; and gross elevation of hematocrit, urea nitrogen, creatinine, and albumin are frequent. Secondary lactic acidosis[110] is not uncommon, so that the serum bicarbonate level may be low and the anion gap increased. The increased viscosity of the blood predisposes to thrombotic events in the cerebral and coronary artery circulations. However, stroke and myocardial infarction, along with pancreatitis and sepsis, may also precipitate the syndrome. It has also been caused by drugs such as hydrochlorothiazide, phenytoin, and glucocorticoids. Elderly patients living in nursing homes are particularly vulnerable to HHNC because their thirst mechanisms are less sensitive to a rising serum osmolality and because dementia, increasing obtundity, or institutional conditions may combine to reduce water intake to less than urinary and insensible water losses. At presentation, serum sodium level is usually elevated or surprisingly normal in the face of extreme hyperglycemia (i.e., the expected pseudohyponatremia is absent). Whatever the presenting level of serum sodium is, it will rise, sometimes markedly, when glucose levels decline with insulin treatment.

Fluid replacement is the most important component of therapy. Restoration of circulating volume is an urgent first priority. One to two liters of isotonic 0.9% saline is therefore given rapidly initially, followed by 0.45% saline. Later, when plasma glucose levels have declined to 250 to 300 mg/dl, 5% glucose in water or in 0.2% saline is given. Total fluid deficits of as much as 12 L may have to be replaced. Insulin treatment, as for DKA, is started after at least 1 or 2 L of 0.9% saline has been administered. Potassium must be added to intravenous fluids to prevent hypokalemia caused by insulin action. It may take days of fluid replacement, the tonicity of which must be carefully adjusted to achieve a gradual steady decrease in serum osmolality and sodium levels, before central nervous system function returns to normal or at least to baseline. The mortality in HHNC is still high. Infection, especially of the urinary tract, even if only suspected, should be treated with broad-spectrum antibiotics. Papillary necrosis may be seen. Patients with histories of arterial and venous thrombosis can benefit from low-dose prophylactic heparin administration.

Cardiovascular Complications of Diabetes Mellitus

Diabetes as an independent risk factor for cardiovascular disease[238] in women is now well established and is so great that it equalizes the risk of cardiovascular disease in men.[239] The risk of a first myocardial infarction in patients with diabetes is equal to that in nondiabetic individuals who have already suffered such an event.[240] Furthermore, acute and subsequent mortality is greater with diabetic-related myocardial infarctions than with nondiabetic myocardial infarctions.[241] In type 1 diabetes, cardiovascular disease is often a fatal accompaniment of end-stage renal disease (ESRD),[242] although even in patients without ESRD, cardiovascular complications may occur earlier in life than usual. Cardiovascular complications are the most prominent cause of morbidity and the most frequent cause of mortality in type 2 diabetes mellitus.[243,244] Mortality in individuals with diabetes is higher than that in nondiabetic persons of all age and racial groups and both sexes.[244] The decline in heart disease mortality noted in recent years in the United States was less in diabetic persons than in nondiabetic persons, and mortality even increased in women with diabetes.[245] The same common cardiovascular disease risk factors important in nondiabetic individuals are clustered in individuals with type 2 diabetes mellitus[129] as part of the insulin-resistance syndrome. The pathologic picture of atherosclerosis in diabetic persons is similar to that in nondiabetic individuals, and the same processes lead to ischemic events. Thus, in regard to cardiovascular disease, the difference between diabetes and nondiabetes appears largely quantitative, although diabetes remains an independent risk factor even after adjusting for other known risk factors.[238]

Intensive treatment of type 1 or type 2 diabetes mellitus to achieve near-normal glycemia has not been proved to reduce the incidence of cardiovascular complications. The UKPDS reported that intensive treatment with insulin or SU drugs decreased myocardial infarction by 16%, with a P value of less than 0.052.[37] Data from several populations,[246-249] and the UKPDS[250] have shown that HbA$_{1c}$ is a risk factor for cardiovascular events and death. Randomized clinical trials are under way to test the question of whether improved glycemic control or particular blood glucose lowering strategies will decrease cardiovascular outcomes in various stages of type 2 diabetes mellitus. Because we still cannot always eliminate whatever risk is incurred from hyperglycemia or insulin resistance per se, we must work assiduously to minimize or negate the adverse effects of hypertension, dyslipidemia, smoking, obesity, and physical inactivity on the cardiovascular system.

HYPERTENSION

Aggressive treatment of hypertension in diabetes mellitus is mandatory for three important reasons: (1) it decreases the risk of CVD and mortality,[251] (2) it reduces or at least delays progression of diabetic nephropathy to ESRD,[252-254] and (3) it may decrease the risk of hemorrhage from proliferative retinopathy. The most recent American Diabetes Association guidelines[81] recommend a target blood pressure of 130/80 mm Hg, equivalent to a mean blood pressure of 97 mm Hg (mean blood pressure is easily calculated as one third systolic plus two thirds diastolic). However, even lower blood pressure targets may eventually prove to be advisable.

ACE inhibitors have achieved first-choice status in treatment because even in nonhypertensive diabetic patients, these agents decrease albumin excretion and the rate of decline in glomerular filtration rate.[254-257] Whether angiotensin receptor antagonists are likewise efficacious over the long term is not yet known. Low-dose diuretics (25 mg chlorthalidone or hydrochlorothiazide) and beta blockers are also very effective antihypertensive agents in diabetes; they decrease risks of cardiovascular disease events and mortality as well as renal failure. However, the possible adverse effects of these agents on glycemic control and serum lipids must be monitored. Atenolol and captopril were equally effective in lowering blood pressure and reducing cardiovascular events and death in the UKPDS.[258] The role of calcium channel blockers is somewhat uncertain, as a study with nisoldipine has shown an adverse effect in diabetic patients.[259] At present, calcium channel blockers are probably best used after ACE inhibitors, diuretics, and possibly beta blockers fail to achieve the target blood pressure.[256,257] Central alpha$_2$ agonists (e.g., clonidine), alpha$_1$ antagonists (e.g., prazosin, terazosin, and doxazosin), and combined alpha and beta antagonists (e.g., labetalol) also can be used, although orthostatic hypotension may limit their utility, particularly in patients with autonomic neuropathy.

DYSLIPIDEMIA

Severe hypertriglyceridemia may complicate DKA in type 1 diabetes mellitus, but it clears rapidly with insulin treatment. Serum triglyceride levels are usually elevated—sometimes strikingly so—in uncontrolled type 2 diabetes mellitus, and they are almost invariably accompanied by decreased HDL levels, an atherogenic combination.[260,261] LDL levels are normal or slightly elevated; however, the LDL component may include a higher proportion of small, dense, more atherogenic particles. Restriction of saturated fat and calories, elimination of excess weight, exercise, and improved glycemic control reduce triglycerides and increase HDL.[262] When these measures are insufficient, gemfibrozil, fenofibrate, or benzafibrate should be prescribed with the purpose of decreasing triglycerides to less than 200 mg/dl and increasing HDL to greater than 35 mg/dl in men and greater than 45 mg/dl in women. For LDL levels greater than 130 mg/dl, or greater than 100 mg/dl in patients with established coronary artery disease, 3-hydroxy-3-methylglutaryl coenzyme A (HMG-CoA) reductase inhibitors (statins) are the drugs of choice.[262] Simvastatin, pravastatin, and lovastatin have all been shown to decrease cardiovascular events in diabetic patients. Atorvastatin may have the greatest efficacy in lowering LDL and triglyceride levels. If necessary, tolerated doses of bile acid resins may be added. Niacin would be ideal monotherapy because it powerfully lowers triglyceride and LDL levels and increases HDL levels; however, its side effects often discourage compliance, and niacin can also increase blood glucose levels. If niacin is used as monotherapy or in combination with statins, the daily dosage should not exceed 3 g. Both niacin and statins require the monitoring of serum ALT levels.

MEASURES TO REDUCE RISK OF CARDIOVASCULAR DISEASE

Smoking

Referral to successful smoking-cessation programs and use of oral or dermal nicotine preparations during withdrawal from tobacco should be employed as needed to rid patients of this serious risk factor for cardiovascular disease. Success appears to be directly related to the amount of counseling and support provided by physicians or other professionals.[263]

Aspirin

In the Early Treatment of Diabetic Retinopathy Study, administration of 650 mg of aspirin a day resulted in a statistically significant 17% reduction in the risk of fatal plus nonfatal myocardial infarctions.[264] All-cause mortality and cardiovascular disease mortality tended to decrease, whereas strokes tended to increase, but none of these differences were statistically significant. Preventive use of aspirin is now recommended by the American Diabetes Association for patients who already have cardiovascular disease or who have other risk factors for cardiovascular disease.[265,266]

ACE Inhibitors

In the recently completed large, multicentered, randomized 5-year Heart Outcomes Prevention Evaluation (HOPE) trial,[267] ramipril in a single daily dose of 10 mg decreased major cardiovascular events, including myocardial infarction, stroke, heart failure, revascularization procedures, and death by 20% to 32% when compared with placebo. The 9,300 patients were at high risk at entry, and 38% had diabetes. All the diabetic patients benefited from ramipril therapy. Notably, many of the patients were normotensive at baseline, and the beneficial effect of the ACE inhibitor was not thought to be accounted for by the small decrease in average blood pressure. Patients with previous cardiovascular disease also benefited. The data indicated that treatment of 100 patients with ramipril for 4 years would prevent 15 events in seven patients.

Antioxidants

The HOPE study also compared the effect of 400 IU of vitamin E daily with that of placebo. Subjects received no benefit from vitamin E.[268] Although some observational and experimental studies have shown an association between antioxidants and protection from atherosclerosis, there are no firm data on which to base a recommendation for their routine use in diabetes.

MANAGEMENT OF SYMPTOMATIC CORONARY ARTERY DISEASE

Beta blockers, nitrates, and calcium channel blockers can all be used as in nondiabetic individuals, with the proviso that patients treated with insulin or beta cell stimulants should be cautioned about hypoglycemia. When a revascularization procedure has been deemed necessary, coronary artery bypass surgery has been reported to be superior to angioplasty in 5-year survival and recurrent myocardial infarction rates in patients receiving pharmacologic treatment for type 2 diabetes mellitus.[269] In patients without mandatory indications for immediate surgical intervention, such as significant left main coronary artery stenosis, a clinical research trial is currently attempting to determine whether a prompt revascularization procedure is superior to aggressive medical therapy. One study has shown that normalization of blood glucose levels with intravenous insulin during the first 3 days of an acute myocardial infarction, followed by intensive blood glucose control on an outpatient basis for at least 3 months, significantly decreased mortality for up to 3.5 years.[270] If intensive control of glycemia is used in patients with cardiovascular disease, prevention of hypoglycemia should especially be emphasized because, in rare instances, it may precipitate myocardial infarction or stroke.

Prevention and Treatment of Microvascular Complications

As noted above, intensive treatment of both type 1 and type 2 diabetes mellitus, aiming at normoglycemia, reduces the risks of development or progression of diabetic retinopathy, nephropathy, and neuropathy. The earlier such treatment is begun, the greater the benefit.[39] However, once these complications have reached stages of major clinical impact, their response to intensive glycemic control is unknown or at least unproved, with the possible exception of pancreas transplantation.[104] Fortunately, there are forms of therapy for advanced complications that may ameliorate or prevent their worst manifestations.[271,272]

RETINOPATHY

Laser treatment of high-risk proliferative retinopathy and of macular edema has been demonstrated to preserve vision.[273] For proliferative retinopathy, panretinal scatter photocoagulation is performed to ablate ischemic retina in the periphery capable of producing VEGF. For macular edema, finely focused laser treatment is performed to close visibly leaking perimacular vessels that are demonstrated by fluorescein angiography. The role of the internist and ophthalmologist is to detect retinopathy requiring laser therapy before irreversible damage and loss of vision occur. Although fundus photography is the most sensitive means of detecting early retinopathy, ophthalmologists and even well-trained endocrinologists and internists can detect retinopathy by direct ophthalmoscopy.[274] An examination with the pupil dilated is preferable, but examination in a completely blackened room can be reasonably effective. In type 1 diabetes mellitus, significant retinopathy (beyond microaneurysms) seldom occurs before 5 years' duration, so that regular yearly ophthalmologic examina-

tions do not need to commence until then. By contrast, 20% to 40% of patients with type 2 diabetes mellitus already have detectable retinopathy at the time of clinical onset and diagnosis.[275] Therefore, yearly ophthalmologic examinations should begin at the time of diagnosis. Pregnancy is a recognized risk factor for progression of retinopathy in type 1 diabetes mellitus,[276] and ophthalmologic examinations should be performed at the beginning of pregnancy and thereafter with a frequency dependent on the findings of the first examination. For patients with vitreous hemorrhage that does not clear or significant vitreous scarring and debris, vitrectomy can be performed. Fibroproliferative scars can be excised, and a detached retina can be reattached. The vitreous is replaced with a salt solution. In selected cases, these procedures can restore vision.

NEPHROPATHY

The best preventive approach for diabetic nephropathy in both type 1 and type 2 diabetes mellitus is to maintain a normal blood pressure.[257,277] In normotensive patients with type 1[278] and type 2[279] diabetes mellitus who develop microalbuminuria (30 to 300 mg/day), clinical trials have shown that ACE inhibitor treatment decreases the rate of progression from microalbuminuria to clinical proteinuria to early renal insufficiency. Maintaining blood glucose near normal with intensive treatment also significantly reduces the risk of diabetic nephropathy.[32,37] If ESRD does develop, a renal transplant is the preferred replacement therapy; home peritoneal dialysis is superior to chronic hemodialysis because the latter is often complicated by vitreous hemorrhage, amputations, and septic episodes. With all forms of therapy for ESRD, mortality is higher in diabetic patients than nondiabetic patients largely because of cardiovascular complications.[280]

NEUROPATHY

Management of diabetic neuropathy is still largely symptomatic[271,272] and often inadequate. Gabapentin[281] in doses of up to 3 g/day has been added to the list of agents that include bedtime tricyclic antidepressants (e.g., nortriptyline), carbamazepine, and topical capsaicin for relief of pain and dysesthesias. Intensive blood glucose control may benefit patients with diabetic amyotrophy and radiculopathy. Prevention of foot ulcers remains very important; patient self-examination of the feet daily and physician-nurse examination at each office visit unequivocally reduce the risk of foot ulcer and amputation.[282] When a foot ulcer does occur, it should be treated aggressively with broad-spectrum antibiotics effective against staphylococci and anaerobes, vigorous debridement as necessary, radiographic examination for osteomyelitis, and sometimes special weight-bearing casts.[283] The use of locally applied growth factors appears promising to reduce healing time.[283] Aggravating effects of ischemia may be alleviated by revascularization of the leg when it is still possible to abort gangrene. Appropriate specialists should be consulted early for achievement of the best outcomes.

Management of autonomic neuropathy is especially challenging. Gastroparesis can benefit from frequent small feedings and either parenteral or liquid oral preparations of metoclopramide[284] or erythromycin.[285] Intermittent intubation to decompress a dilated full stomach may be required to relieve persistent vomiting or painful bloating. A feeding jejunostomy can be considered for intractable cases. Diarrhea sometimes responds to tetracycline antibiotics; clonidine and occasionally somatostatin are effective. Bladder dysfunction may be improved by oral bethanechol and regular timed voiding, but self-catheterization is necessary in severe cases of atony. Use of indwelling catheters should be minimized because of the danger of bacterial or fungal infection. Orthostatic hypotension is benefited by compression stockings, ample sodium intake, and fluorohydrocortisone. The use of midodrine is limited by the risks of excessive hypotension or urinary retention. Male impotence can be satisfactorily treated by penile injection or urethral insertion of alprostadil; by use of a simple vacuum pump; or, increasingly rarely, by implantation of a penile prosthesis. Sildenafil is effective for diabetic impotence,[286] but it may be dangerous in diabetic men with established or unsuspected coronary disease.

Diabetes Mellitus during Pregnancy

Women in their reproductive years with known diabetes of any type should be instructed to inform their physicians when they have decided to have a child. Conception when diabetes control is inadequate markedly increases the risk of major congenital abnormalities. This risk can be reduced to the nondiabetic background rate when control is excellent.[287,288] Therefore, the patient's HbA_{1c} should be brought as close to normal as possible before conception. One recent recommendation is that the average of preprandial and postprandial home blood glucose test results should be less than 126 mg/dl and HbA_{1c} should be brought to at least less than 7.0%.[288] The patients taking oral hypoglycemic agents should be switched to insulin and excellent control established before conception. Nondiabetic women should be screened for gestational diabetes mellitus (GDM) during weeks 24 to 28 of pregnancy by glucose loading.

Throughout pregnancy, normoglycemia (relative to the normal pregnant state) is required to prevent intrauterine death and perinatal morbidity and mortality. Preprandial blood glucose targets during pregnancy are 60 to 90 mg/dl and postprandial targets are less than 120 to 140 mg/dl.[289,290] Most patients with GDM detected by routine screening can be tried on diet treatment for 1 to 2 weeks. In obese women, either 1,500 kcal or 35 kcal/kg prepregnancy weight has been recommended.[287] In 15% to 20% of cases, persistence of FBG of at least 105 mg/dl or 2-hour postprandial values of at least 120 to 140 mg/dl mandates institution of insulin treatment. The blood glucose control targets can then often be achieved with injections of NPH plus regular insulin before breakfast, regular insulin before supper, and NPH insulin at bedtime. Lispro insulin has not yet been approved for use during pregnancy. Pregnant women with type 1 diabetes mellitus need to continue intensive treatment as described previously. Pregnant women with type 2 diabetes mellitus often respond to insulin regimens as described for GDM. After delivery, insulin requirements disappear almost instantaneously in patients with GDM and may decrease strikingly from those of the third trimester in women with type 1 diabetes mellitus.

References

1. American Diabetes Association: Report of the expert committee on the diagnosis and classification of diabetes mellitus. Diabetes Care 23(suppl 1):S4, 2000

2. DECODE Study Group: Will new diagnostic criteria for diabetes mellitus change phenotype of patients with diabetes? Reanalysis of European epidemiological data. BMJ 317:371, 1998

3. Kjos SL, Buchanan TA: Gestational diabetes mellitus. Current Concepts 341:1749, 1999

4. Barnes AJ, Bloom SR, Goerge K, et al: Ketoacidosis in pancreatectomized man. N Engl J Med 296:1250, 1977

5. Hirsch IB, Paauw DS: Diabetes management in special situations. Curr Therap Diabetes 26:631, 1997

6. Gurwitz JH, Bohn RL, Glynn RJ, et al: Glucocorticoids and the risk for initiation of hypoglycemic therapy. Arch Intern Med 154:97, 1994

7. Matsumoto K, Yamasaki H, Akazawa S, et al: High-dose but not low-dose dexamethasone impairs glucose tolerance by inducing compensatory failure of pancreatic β-cells in normal men. J Clin Endocrinol Metab 81:2621, 1996

8. LaPorte RE, Matsushima M, Chang Y-F: Prevalence and incidence of insulin-dependent diabetes. Diabetes in America, 2nd ed. NIDDK NIH Publication No. 95-1468, 1995

9. Harris MI, Flegal KM, Cowie CC, et al: Prevalence of diabetes, impaired fasting glucose, and impaired glucose tolerance in U.S. adults. Diabetes Care 21:518, 1998

10. Kenny SJ, Aubert RE, Geiss LS: Prevalence and incidence of non-insulin-dependent diabetes. Diabetes in America, 2nd ed. NIDDK NIH Publication No. 95-1468, 1995

11. Mokdad AH, Ford ES, Bowman BA, et al: Diabetes trends in the U.S.: 1990–1998. Diabetes Care 23:1278, 2000

12. Burke JP, Williams K, Gaskill SP, et al: Rapid rise in the incidence of type 2 diabetes from 1987 to 1996: results from the San Antonio Heart Study. Arch Intern Med 159:1450, 1999

13. Mokdad AH, Serdula MK, Dietz WH, et al: The spread of the obesity epidemic in the United States, 1991–1998. JAMA 282:1519, 1999

14. Harris MI: Health care and health status and outcomes for patients with type 2 diabetes. Diabetes Care 23:754, 2000

15. Harris MI, Eastman RC, Cowie CC, et al: Racial and ethnic differences in glycemic control of adults with type 2 diabetes. Diabetes Care 22:403, 1999

16. National Task Force on the Prevention and Treatment of Obesity: Overweight, obesity, and health risk. Arch Intern Med 160:898, 2000

17. Expert Panel on the Identification, Evaluation, and Treatment of Overweight in Adults: Clinical guidelines on the identification, evaluation, and treatment of overweight and obesity in adults: executive summary. Am J Clin Nutr 68:899, 1998

18. Ruderman N, Chisholm D, Pi-Sunyer X, et al: The metabolically obese, normal-weight individual revisited. Diabetes 47:699, 1998

19. Rewers M, Hamman RF: Risk factors for non-insulin-dependent diabetes. Diabetes in America, 2nd ed. NIDDK NIH Publication No. 95-1468, 1995

20. Genuth S: Hormones of the pancreatic islets. Physiology, 4th ed. Berne RM, Levy MN, Eds. Mosby, St. Louis, 1998, p 822

21. Davis MD: Diabetic retinopathy. Diabetes Care 15:1844, 1992

22. Goldfarb S: Diabetic nephropathy. Primer on Kidney Diseases. Greenberg A, Cheung AK, Falk RJ, et al, Eds. Academic Press, San Diego, 1994, p 112

23. Breyer JA: Diabetic nephropathy in insulin-dependent patients. Am J Kidney Dis 20:533, 1992

24. Ritz E, Stefanski A: Diabetic nephropathy in type II diabetes. Am J Kidney Dis 27:167, 1996

25. Mogensen CE, Christensen CK: Predicting diabetic nephropathy in insulin-dependent patients. N Engl J Med 311:89, 1984

26. Andersen AR, Christiansen JS, Andersen JK, et al: Diabetic nephropathy in type 1 (insulin-dependent) diabetes: an epidemiological study. Diabetologia 25:496, 1983

27. Eaton S, Tesfaye S: Clinical manifestations and measurement of somatic neuropathy. Diabetes Reviews 7:312, 1999

28. Rith-Najarian SJ, Stolusky T, Gohdes DM: Identifying diabetic patients at high risk for lower-extremity amputation in a primary health care setting: a prospective evaluation of simple screening criteria. Diabetes Care 15:1386, 1992

29. Malik RA: Pathology and pathogenesis of diabetic neuropathy. Diabetes Reviews 7:253, 1999

30. Krendel DA, Costigan DA, Hopkins LC: Successful treatment of neuropathies in patients with diabetes mellitus. Arch Neurol 52:1053, 1995

31. Genuth SM: The case for blood glucose control. Advances in Internal Medicine, Vol 40. Schrier RW, Abboud FM, Baxter JD, et al, Eds. Mosby, St. Louis, 1995, p 573

32. The Diabetes Control and Complications Trial Research Group: The effect of intensive treatment of diabetes on the development and progression of long-term complications in insulin-dependent diabetes mellitus. N Engl J Med 329:977, 1993

33. The Diabetes Control and Complications Trial Research Group: Implementation of treatment protocols in the Diabetes Control and Complications Trial. Diabetes Care 18:361, 1995

34. The Diabetes Control and Complications Trial Research Group: Adverse events and their association with treatment regimens in the Diabetes Control and Complications Trial. Diabetes Care 18:1415, 1995

35. The Diabetes Control and Complications Trial Research Group: Resource utilization and costs of care in the Diabetes Control and Complications Trial. Diabetes Care 18:1468, 1995

36. The Diabetes Control and Complications Trial Research Group: Lifetime benefits and costs of intensive therapy as practiced in the Diabetes Control and Complications Trial. JAMA 276:1409, 1996

37. UK Prospective Diabetes Study (UKPDS) Group: Intensive blood-glucose control with sulphonylureas or insulin compared with conventional treatment and risk of complications in patients with type 2 diabetes (UKPDS 33). Lancet 352:837, 1998

38. UK Prospective Diabetes Study (UKPDS) Group: Effect of intensive blood-glucose control with metformin on complications in overweight patients with type 2 diabetes (UKPDS 34). Lancet 352:854, 1998

39. The Diabetes Control and Complications Trial Research Group: The relationship of glycemic exposure (HbA_{1c}) to the risk of development and progression of retinopathy in the Diabetes Control and Complications Trial. Diabetes 44:968, 1995

40. Stratton IM, Adler AI, Neil HA, et al: Association of glycaemia with macrovascular and microvascular complications of type 2 diabetes (UKPDS 35): prospective observational study. BMJ 321:405, 2000

41. The Diabetes Control and Complications Trial Research Group: The absence of a glycemic threshold for the development of long-term complications: the perspective of the Diabetes Control and Complications Trial. Diabetes 45:1289, 1996

42. The Diabetes Control and Complications Trial/Epidemiology of Diabetes Interventions and Complications Research Group: Retinopathy and nephropathy in patients with type 1 diabetes four years after a trial of intensive therapy. N Engl J Med 342:381, 2000

43. Vlassara H, Bucala R, Striker L: Pathogenic effects of advanced glycosylation: biochemical, biologic, and clinical implications for diabetes and aging. Lab Invest 70:138, 1994

44. Brownlee M: Negative consequences of glycation. Metabolism 49(suppl 1):9, 2000

45. Monnier VM, Bautista O, Kenny D, et al: Skin collagen glycation, glycoxidation, and crosslinking are lower in subjects with long-term intensive versus conventional therapy of type 1 diabetes: relevance of glycated collagen products versus HbA_{1c} as markers of diabetic complications. Diabetes 48:870, 1999

46. Baynes JW, Thorpe SR: Role of oxidative stress in diabetic complications: a new perspective on an old paradigm. Diabetes 48:1, 1999

47. Carrington AL, Litchfield JE: The aldose reductase pathway and nonenzymatic glycation in the pathogenesis of diabetic neuropathy: a critical review for the end of the 20th century. Diabetes Reviews 7:275, 1999

48. Ishii H, Koya D, King GL: Protein kinase C activation and its role in the development of vascular complications in diabetes mellitus. J Mol Med 76:21, 1998

49. Nishikawa T, Edelstein D, Du XL, et al: Normalizing mitochondrial superoxide production blocks three pathways of hyperglycaemic damage. Nature 404:787, 2000

50. Quinn M, Angelico MC, Warram JH, et al: Familial factors determine the development of diabetic nephropathy in patients with IDDM. Diabetologia 39:940, 1996

51. The Diabetes Control and Complications Trial Research Group: Clustering of long-term complications in families with diabetes in the Diabetes Control and Complications Trial. Diabetes 46:1829, 1997

52. Thai A-C, Eisenbarth GS: Natural history of IDDM. Diabetes Reviews 1:1, 1993

53. Foulis AK, Liddle CN, Farquharson MA, et al: The histopathology of the pancreas in type 1 (insulin-dependent) diabetes mellitus: a 25-year review of deaths in patients under 20 years of age in the United Kingdom. Diabetologia 29:267, 1986

54. Eisenbarth GS: Type 1 diabetes mellitus: a chronic autoimmune disease. N Engl J Med 314:1360, 1986

55. Faustman D, Eisenbarth G, Daley J, et al: Abnormal T-lymphocyte subsets in type 1 diabetes. Diabetes 38:1462, 1989

56. Rossini AA, Greiner DL, Friedman HP, et al: Immunopathogenesis of diabetes mellitus. Diabetes Reviews 1:43, 1993

57. Lernmark A: Selecting culprits in type 1 diabetes β-cell killing. J Clin Invest 104:1487, 1999

58. Littorin B, Sundkvist G, Hagopian W, et al: Islet cell and glutamic acid decarboxylase antibodies present at diagnosis of diabetes predict the need for insulin treatment. Diabetes Care 22:409, 1999

59. Falorni A, Lernmark A: Humoral autoimmunity. Diabetes Mellitus: A Fundamental and Clinical Text, 1st ed. LeRoith D, Taylor SI, Olefsky JM, Eds. Lippincott-Raven Publishers, Philadelphia, 1996, p 298

60. Palmer JP, Asplin CM, Clemons P, et al: Insulin antibodies in insulin-dependent diabetics before insulin treatment. Science 222:1337, 1983

61. Feutren G, Papoz L, Assan R, et al: Cyclosporin increases the rate and length of remissions in insulin-dependent diabetes of recent onset: results of a multicentre double-blind trial. Lancet 2:119, 1986

62. Bougneres PF, Landais P, Boisson C, et al: Limited duration of remission of insulin dependency in children with recent overt type 1 diabetes treated with low-dose cyclosporin. Diabetes 39:1264, 1990

63. Riley WJ, Maclaren NK, Krischer J, et al: A prospective study of the development of diabetes in relatives of patients with insulin-dependent diabetes. N Engl J Med 323:1167, 1990

64. Tarn AC, Thomas JM, Dean BM, et al: Predicting insulin-dependent diabetes. Lancet 1:845, 1988

65. Ziegler AG, Herskowitz RD, Jackson RA, et al: Predicting type 1 diabetes. Diabetes Care 13:762, 1990

66. Srikanta S, Ganda OP, Gleason RE, et al: Pre-type 1 diabetes: linear loss of beta cell response to intravenous glucose. Diabetes 33:717, 1984

67. Rayfield EJ, Ishimura K: Environmental factors and insulin-dependent diabetes mellitus. Diabetes Metab Rev 3:925, 1987

68. Jones DB, Armstrong NW: Coxsackie virus and diabetes revisited. Nat Med 1:284, 1995

69. Agner T, Damm P, Binder C: Remission in IDDM: prospective study of basal C-peptide and insulin dose in 268 consecutive patients. Diabetes Care 10:164, 1987

70. Heinze E, Beischer W, Keller L, et al: C-peptide secretion during the remission phase of juvenile diabetes. Diabetes 27:670, 1978

71. Shah SC, Malone JI, Simpson NE: A randomized trial of intensive insulin therapy in newly diagnosed insulin-dependent diabetes mellitus. N Engl J Med 320:550, 1989

72. The Diabetes Control and Complications Trial Research Group: Effects of age, duration and treatment of insulin-dependent diabetes mellitus on residual beta-cell function: observations during eligibility testing for the Diabetes Control and Complications Trial (DCCT). J Clin Endocrinol Metab 65:30, 1987

73. Gorsuch AN, Spencer KM, Lister J, et al: Evidence for a long prediabetic period in type I (insulin-dependent) diabetes mellitus. Lancet 2:1363, 1981

74. Karjalainen J, Salmela P, Ilonen J, et al: A comparison of childhood and adult type I diabetes mellitus. N Engl J Med 320:881, 1989

75. Pugliese A: Unraveling the genetics of insulin-dependent type 1A diabetes: the search must go on. Diabetes Reviews 7:39, 1999

76. Baisch JM, Weeks T, Giles R, et al: Analysis of HLA-DQ genotypes and susceptibility in insulin-dependent diabetes mellitus. N Engl J Med 322:1836, 1990

77. Nepom GT: Immunogenetics and IDDM. Diabetes Reviews 1:93, 1993

78. Palmer JP: Predicting IDDM: use of humoral immune markers. Diabetes Reviews 1:104, 1993

79. Genuth SM: Plasma insulin and glucose profiles in normal, obese, and diabetic persons. Ann Intern Med 79:812, 1973

80. Nair KS, Halliday D, Garrow JS: Increased energy expenditure in poorly controlled type I (insulin-dependent) diabetic patients. Diabetologia 27:13, 1984

81. American Diabetes Association: Standards of medical care for patients with diabetes mellitus. Diabetes Care 24:533, 2001

82. The DCCT Research Group: Diabetes Control and Complications Trial (DCCT): results of feasibility study. Diabetes Care 10:1, 1987

83. Goldstein DE, Little RR, Lorenz RA, et al: Tests of glycemia in diabetes. Diabetes Care 18:896, 1995

84. Larsen ML, Horder M, Mogensen EF: Effect of long-term monitoring of glycosylated hemoglobin levels in insulin-dependent diabetes mellitus. N Engl J Med 323:1021, 1990

85. American Diabetes Association: Tests of glycemia in diabetes. Diabetes Care 23(suppl 1):S80, 2000

86. Cagliero E, Levina EV, Nathan DM: Immediate feedback of HbA_{1c} levels improves glycemic control in type 1 and insulin-treated type 2 diabetic patients. Diabetes Care 22:1785, 1999

87. Skyler JS: Insulin treatment. Therapy for Diabetes Mellitus and Related Disorders, 3rd ed. Lebovitz HE, Ed. American Diabetes Association, Alexandria, Virginia, 1998, p 186

88. Hirsch IB: Type 1 diabetes mellitus and the use of flexible insulin regimens. Am Fam Physician 60:2343, 1999

89. Lee WL, Zinman B: From insulin to insulin analogs: progress in the treatment of type 1 diabetes. Diabetes Reviews 6:73, 1998

90. Garg SK, Carmain JA, Braddy KC, et al: Pre-meal insulin analogue insulin lispro vs Humulin® R insulin treatment in young subjects with type 1 diabetes. Diabet Med 13:47, 1996

91. Anderson JH Jr, Brunelle RL, Koivisto VA, et al: Reduction of postprandial hyperglycemia and frequency of hypoglycemia in IDDM patients on insulin-analog treatment. Diabetes 46:265, 1997

92. Del Sindaco P, Ciofetta M, Lalli C, et al: Use of the short-acting insulin analogue lispro in intensive treatment of type 1 diabetes mellitus: importance of appropriate replacement of basal insulin and time-interval injection-meal. Diabet Med 15:592, 1998

93. Raskin P, Guthrie RA, Leiter L, et al: Use of insulin aspart, a fast-acting insulin analog, as the mealtime insulin in the management of patients with type 1 diabetes. Diabetes Care 23:583, 2000

94. Heinemann L, Linkeschova R, Rave K, et al: Time-action profile of the long-acting insulin analog insulin glargine (HOE901) in comparison with those of NPH insulin and placebo. Diabetes Care 23:644, 2000

95. Rosenstock J, Park G, Zimmerman J: Basal insulin glargine (HOE 901) versus NPH insulin in patients with type 1 diabetes on multiple daily insulin regimens. Diabetes Care 23:1137, 2000

96. Ratner RE, Hirsch IB, Neifing JL, et al: Less hypoglycemia with insulin glargine in intensive insulin therapy for type 1 diabetes. Diabetes Care 23:639, 2000

97. Mecklenburg RS: Insulin-pump therapy. Therapy for Diabetes Mellitus and Related Disorders, 3rd ed. Lebovitz HE, Ed. American Diabetes Association, Alexandria, Virginia, 1998, p 204

98. Diabetes Control and Complications Trial Research Group: Implementation of treatment protocols in the Diabetes Control and Complications Trial. Diabetes Care 18:361, 1995

99. Dunn FL, Nathan DM, Scavini M, et al: Long-term therapy of IDDM with an implantable insulin pump. Diabetes Care 20:59, 1997

100. Salzman R, Manson JE, Griffing GT, et al: Intranasal aerolized insulin: mixed-meal studies and long-term use in type I diabetes. N Engl J Med 312:1078, 1985

101. Jendle JH, Karlberg BE: Effects of intrapulmonary insulin in patients with non-insulin-dependent diabetes. Scand J Clin Lab Invest 56:555, 1996

102. Kurtzhals P, Schäffer L, Sørensen A, et al: Correlations of receptor binding and metabolic and mitogenic potencies of insulin analogs designed for clinical use. Diabetes 49:999, 2000

103. Robertson RP, Holohan TV, Genuth S: Therapeutic controversy: pancreas transplantation for type I diabetes. J Clin Endocrinol Metab 83:1868, 1998

104. Robertson RP, Davis C, Larsen J, et al: Pancreas and islet transplantation for patients with diabetes. Diabetes Care 23:112, 2000

105. Shapiro J, Lakey JRT, Ryan EA, et al: Islet transplantation in seven patients with type 1 diabetes mellitus using a glucocorticoid-free immunosuppressive regimen. N Engl J Med 343:230, 2000

106. American Diabetes Association: Nutrition recommendations and principles for people with diabetes mellitus. Diabetes Care 23:543, 2000

107. Jenkins DJ, Wolever TM, Taylor RH, et al: Glycemic index of foods: a physiological basis for carbohydrate exchange. Am J Clin Nutr 34:362, 1981

108. Franz MJ, Horton ES, Bantle JP, et al: Nutrition principles for the management of diabetes and related complications. Diabetes Care 17:490, 1994

109. American Diabetes Association: Diabetes mellitus and exercise. Diabetes Care 23(suppl 1):S50, 2000

110. Genuth SM: Diabetic ketoacidosis and hyperglycemic hyperosmolar coma. Current Therapy in Endocrinology and Metabolism, 6th ed. Bardin CW, Ed. Mosby–Year Book, St. Louis, 1997, p 438

111. Foster DW, McGarry JD: The metabolic derangements and treatment of diabetic ketoacidosis. N Engl J Med 309:159, 1983

112. Barrett EJ, DeFronzo RA, Bevilacqua S, et al: Insulin resistance in diabetic ketoacidosis. Diabetes 31:923, 1982

113. Burge MR, Hardy KJ, Schade DS: Short-term fasting is a mechanism for the development of euglycemic ketoacidosis during periods of insulin deficiency. J Clin Endocrinol Metab 76:1192, 1993

114. DeFronzo RA, Matsuda M, Barrett EJ: Diabetic ketoacidosis: a combined metabolic-nephrologic approach to therapy. Diabetes Reviews 2:209, 1994

115. Kitabchi AE, Wall BM: Diabetic ketoacidosis. Med Clin North Am 79:9, 1995

116. Waldhausl W, Kleinberger G, Korn A, et al: Severe hyperglycemia: effects of rehydration on endocrine derangements and blood glucose concentration. Diabetes 28:577, 1979

117. The DCCT Research Group: Epidemiology of severe hypoglycemia in the Diabetes Control and Complications Trial. Am J Med 90:450, 1991

118. Gale EA, Tattersall RB: Unrecognised nocturnal hypoglycaemia in insulin-treated diabetics. Lancet 1:1049, 1979

119. Cryer PE: Hypoglycemia: the limiting factor in the management of IDDM. Diabetes 43:1378, 1994

120. Heller SR, Macdonald IA, Herbert M, et al: Influence of sympathetic nervous system on hypoglycaemic warning symptoms. Lancet 2:359, 1987

121. Mokan M, Mitrakou A, Veneman T, et al: Hypoglycemia unawareness in IDDM. Diabetes Care 17:1397, 1994

122. Dagogo-Jack S, Rattarasarn C, Cryer PE: Reversal of hypoglycemia unawareness, but not defective glucose counterregulation, in IDDM. Diabetes 43:1426, 1994

123. Fanelli C, Pampanelli S, Epifano L, et al: Long-term recovery from unawareness, deficient counterregulation and lack of cognitive dysfunction during hypoglycaemia, following institution of rational, intensive insulin therapy in IDDM. Diabetologia 37:1265, 1994

124. Boyle PJ, Kempers SF, O'Connor AM, et al: Brain glucose uptake and unawareness of hypoglycemia in patients with insulin-dependent diabetes mellitus. N Engl J Med 333:1726, 1995

125. Wahren J, Ekberg K, Fernqvist-Forbes E, et al: Brain substrate utilisation during acute hypoglycaemia. Diabetologia 42:812, 1999

126. The Diabetes Control and Complications Trial Research Group: Effects of intensive diabetes therapy on neuropsychological function in adults in the Diabetes Control and Complications Trial. Ann Intern Med 124:379, 1996

127. Kramer L, Fasching P, Madl C, et al: Previous episodes of hypoglycemic coma are not associated with permanent cognitive brain dysfunction in IDDM patients on intensive insulin treatment. Diabetes 47:1909, 1998

128. DeFronzo RA: The triumvirate beta-cell, muscle, liver: a collusion responsible for NIDDM. Diabetes 37:667, 1988

129. Haffner SM, D'Agostino R, Mykkänen L, et al: Insulin sensitivity in subjects with type 2 diabetes. Diabetes Care 22:562, 1999

130. Haffner SM, Stern MP, Hazuda HP, et al: Increased insulin concentrations in nondiabetic offspring of diabetic parents. N Engl J Med 319:1297, 1988

131. Lillioja S, Mott DM, Howard BV, et al: Impaired glucose tolerance as a disorder of insulin action: longitudinal and cross-sectional studies in Pima Indians. N Engl J Med 318:1217, 1988

132. Saad MF, Knowler WC, Pettitt DJ, et al: Sequential changes in serum insulin concentration during development of non-insulin-dependent diabetes mellitus. Lancet 1:1356, 1989

133. Warram JH, Martin BC, Krolewski AS, et al: Slow glucose removal rate and hyperinsulinemia precede the development of type II diabetes in the offspring of diabetic patients. Ann Intern Med 113:909, 1990

134. O'Meara NM, Sturis J, Van Cauter E, et al: Lack of control by glucose of ultradian insulin secretory oscillations in impaired glucose tolerance and in non-insulin-dependent diabetes mellitus. J Clin Invest 92:262, 1993

135. Porte D Jr: Beta-cells in type II diabetes mellitus. Diabetes 40:166, 1991

136. Hollingdal M, Juhl CB, Pincus SM, et al: Failure of physiological plasma glucose excursions to entrain high-frequency pulsatile insulin secretion in type 2 diabetes. Diabetes 49:1334, 2000

137. Polonsky KS: Evolution of beta-cell dysfunction in impaired glucose tolerance and diabetes. Exp Clin Endocrinol Diabetes 107(suppl 4):S124, 1999

138. Pimenta W, Korytkowski M, Mitrakou A, et al: Pancreatic beta-cell dysfunction as the primary genetic lesion in NIDDM: evidence from studies in normal glucose-tolerant individuals with a first-degree NIDDM relative. JAMA 273:1855, 1995

139. Cavaghan MK, Ehrmann DA, Polonsky KS: Interactions between insulin resistance and insulin secretion in the development of glucose intolerance. J Clin Invest 106:329, 2000

140. Rossetti L, Giaccari A, DeFronzo RA: Glucose toxicity. Diabetes Care 13:610, 1990

141. Cohen M, Crosbie C, Cusworth L, et al: Insulin—not always a life sentence: withdrawal of insulin therapy in non-insulin-dependent diabetes. Diabetes Res 1:31, 1984

142. Saltiel AR: The molecular and physiological basis of insulin resistance: emerging implications for metabolic and cardiovascular diseases. J Clin Invest 106:163, 2000

143. Stern MP: Strategies and prospects for finding insulin resistance genes. J Clin Invest 106:323, 2000

144. Del Prato S, Bonadonna RC, Bonora E, et al: Characterization of cellular defects of insulin action in type 2 (non-insulin-dependent) diabetes mellitus. J Clin Invest 91:484, 1993

145. Pessin JE, Saltiel AR: Signaling pathways in insulin action: molecular targets of insulin resistance. J Clin Invest 106:165, 2000

146. Reaven GM, Chen YD: Role of abnormal free fatty acid metabolism in the development of non-insulin-dependent diabetes mellitus. Am J Med 85:106, 1988

147. Shulman GI: Cellular mechanisms of insulin resistance. J Clin Invest 106:171, 2000

148. Røder ME, Porter D Jr, Schwartz RS, et al: Disproportionately elevated proinsulin levels reflect the degree of impaired B cell secretory capacity in patients with noninsulin-dependent diabetes mellitus. J Clin Endocrinol Metab 83:604, 1998

149. Rachman J, Levy JC, Barrow BA, et al: Relative hyperproinsulinemia of NIDDM persists despite the reduction of hyperglycemia with insulin or sulfonylurea therapy. Diabetes 46:1557, 1997

150. Genuth SM: Hormones of the pancreatic islets. Physiology, 4th ed. Berne RM, Levy MN, Eds. Mosby, St. Louis, 1998, p 822

151. Brunzell JD, Robertson RP, Lerner RL, et al: Relationships between fasting plasma glucose levels and insulin secretion during intravenous glucose tolerance tests. J Clin Endocrinol Metab 42:222, 1976

152. Kahn SE, Andrikopoulos S, Verchere CB: Islet amyloid: a long-recognized but underappreciated pathological feature of type 2 diabetes. Diabetes 48:241, 1999

153. Groop LC, Bottazzo GF, Doniach D: Islet cell antibodies identify latent type 1 diabetes in patients aged 35-75 years at diagnosis. Diabetes 35:237, 1986

154. Turner R, Stratton I, Horton V, et al: UKPDS 25: autoantibodies to islet-cell cytoplasm and glutamic acid decarboxylase for prediction of insulin requirement in type 2 diabetes. Lancet 351:1288, 1997

155. Torn C, Landin-Olsson M, Ostman J, et al: Glutamic acid decarboxylase antibodies (GADA) is the most important factor for prediction of insulin therapy within 3 years in young adult diabetic patients not classified as type 1 diabetes on clinical grounds. Diabetes Metab Res Rev 16:442, 2000

156. Kahn BB, Flier JS: Obesity and insulin resistance. J Clin Invest 106:473, 2000

157. Chung JW, Suh KI, Joyce M, et al: Contribution of obesity to defects of intracellular glucose metabolism in NIDDM. Diabetes Care 18:666, 1995

158. Gastaldelli A, Baldi S, Pettiti M, et al: Influence of obesity and type 2 diabetes on gluconeogenesis and glucose output in humans. Diabetes 49:1367, 2000

159. Colditz GA, Willett WC, Rotnitzky A, et al: Weight gain as a risk factor for clinical diabetes mellitus in women. Ann Intern Med 122:481, 1995

160. Long SD, O'Brien K, MacDonald KG Jr, et al: Weight loss in severely obese subjects prevents the progression of impaired glucose tolerance to type II diabetes: a longitudinal interventional study. Diabetes Care 17:372, 1994

161. Kissebah AH, Krakower GR: Regional adiposity and morbidity. Physiol Rev 74:761, 1994

162. Montague CT, O'Rahilly S: The perils of portliness: causes and consequences of visceral adiposity. Diabetes 49:883, 2000

163. The Diabetes Prevention Program Research Group: The Diabetes Prevention Program: design and methods for a clinical trial in the prevention of type 2 diabetes. Diabetes Care 22:623, 1999

164. Tattersall RB, Pyke DA: Diabetes in identical twins. Lancet 2:1120, 1972

165. Shuldiner AR, Silver KD: Candidate genes for non–insulin-dependent diabetes mellitus. Diabetes Mellitus: A Fundamental and Clinical Text. LeRoith D, Taylor SI, Olefsky JM, Eds. Lippincott-Raven Publishers, Philadelphia, 1996, p 565

166. Stern MP: Strategies and prospects for finding insulin resistance genes. J Clin Invest 106:323, 2000

167. Habener JF, Stoffers DA: A newly discovered role of transcription factors involved in pancreas development and the pathogenesis of diabetes mellitus. Proc Assoc Am Physicians 110:12, 1998

168. Froguel P, Zouali H, Vionnet N, et al: Familial hyperglycemia due to mutations in glucokinase: definition of a subtype of diabetes mellitus. N Engl J Med 328:697, 1993

169. Hadden DR, Blair ALT, Wilson EA, et al: Natural history of diabetes presenting age 40–69 years: a prospective study of the influence of intensive dietary therapy. Quarterly Journal of Medicine 59:579, 1986

170. Wing RR, Koeske R, Epstein LH, et al: Long-term effects of modest weight loss in type II diabetic patients. Arch Intern Med 147:1749, 1987

171. Franz MJ, Horton ES Sr, Bantle JP, et al: Nutrition principles for the management of diabetes and related complications. Diabetes Care 17:490, 1994

172. American Diabetes Association: Nutrition recommendations and principles for people with diabetes mellitus. Diabetes Care 24(suppl 1):S44, 2001

173. Chandalia M, Garg A, Lutjohann D, et al: Beneficial effects of high dietary fiber intake in patients with type 2 diabetes mellitus. N Engl J Med 342:1392, 2000

174. Genuth SM: Supplemented fasting in the treatment of obesity and diabetes. Am J Clin Nutr 32:2579, 1979

175. The National Task Force on the Prevention and Treatment of Obesity: Very low-calorie diets. JAMA 270:967, 1993

176. UK Prospective Diabetes Study Group: UK Prospective Diabetes Study (UKPDS): VIII: study design, progress and performance. Diabetologia 34:877, 1991

177. UKPDS Group: UK Prospective Diabetes Study 7: response of fasting plasma glucose to diet therapy in newly presenting type II diabetic patients. Metabolism 39:905, 1990

178. Hollander PA, Elbein SC, Hirsch IB, et al: Role of orlistat in the treatment of obese patients with type 2 diabetes. Diabetes Care 21:1288, 1998

179. Porte D Jr, Seeley RJ, Woods SC, et al: Obesity, diabetes and the central nervous system. Diabetologia 41:863, 1998

180. MacDonald KG, Long SD, Swanson MS, et al: The gastric bypass operation reduces the progression and mortality of non-insulin-dependent diabetes mellitus. J Gastrointest Surg 1:213, 1997

181. O'Brien PE, Brown WA, Smith A, et al: Prospective study of a laparoscopically placed, adjustable gastric band in the treatment of morbid obesity. Br J Surg 85:113, 1999

182. Schneider SH, Ruderman NB: Exercise and NIDDM. Diabetes Care 13:785, 1990

183. Wei M, Gibbons LW, Kampert JB, et al: Low cardiorespiratory fitness and physical inactivity as predictors of mortality in men with type 2 diabetes. Ann Intern Med 132:605, 2000

184. DeFronzo RA: Pharmacologic therapy for type 2 diabetes mellitus. Ann Intern Med 131:281, 1999

185. Turner RC, Cull CA, Frighi V, et al: Glycemic control with diet, sulfonylurea, metformin, or insulin in patients with type 2 diabetes mellitus. JAMA 281:2005, 1999

186. Riddle M: The 2 defects of type 2 diabetes: combining drugs to treat both insulin deficiency and insulin resistance. Am J Med 108(suppl 6a):S1, 2000

187. Zimmerman BR: Sulfonylureas. Current Therapies for Diabetes 26:511, 1997

188. Ashcroft FM: Mechanisms of the Glycaemic Effects of Sulfonylureas. Horm Metab Res 28:456, 1996

189. Shorr RI, Ray WA, Daugherty JR, et al: Individual sulfonylureas and serious hypoglycemia in older people. J Am Geriatr Soc 44:751, 1996

190. Shorr RI, Ray WA, Daugherty JR, et al: Incidence and risk factors for serious hypoglycemia in older persons using insulin or sulfonylureas. Arch Intern Med 157:1681, 1997

191. University Group Diabetes Program: A study of the effects of hypoglycemic agents on vascular complications in patients with adult-onset diabetes. I: Design, methods and baseline results. II: Mortality results. Diabetes 19:747, 1970

192. Brady PA, Terzic A: The sulfonylurea controversy: more questions from the heart. J Am Coll Cardiol 31:950, 1998

193. Schade DS, Jovanovic L, Schneider J: A placebo-controlled, randomized study of glimepiride in patients with type 2 diabetes mellitus for whom diet therapy is unsuccessful. J Clin Pharmacol 38:636, 1998

194. Wolffenbuttel BHR, Nijst L, Sels JPJE, et al: Effects of a new oral hypoglycaemic agent, repaglinide, on metabolic control in sulphonylurea-treated patients with NIDDM. Eur J Clin Pharmacol 45:113, 1993

195. Lebovitz HE: Insulin secretagogues: old and new. Diabetes Reviews 7:139, 1999

196. Fuhlendorff J, Rorsman P, Kofod H, et al: Stimulation of insulin release by repaglinide and glibenclamide involves both common and distinct processes. Diabetes 47:345, 1998

197. Lebovitz HE: Alpha-glucosidase inhibitors. Current Therapies for Diabetes 26:539, 1997

198. Chiasson JL, Josse RG, Hunt JA, et al: The efficacy of acarbose in the treatment of patients with non-insulin-dependent diabetes mellitus: a multicenter controlled clinical trial. Ann Intern Med 121:928, 1994

199. Coniff RF, Shapiro JA, Robbins D, et al: Reduction of glycosylated hemoglobin and postprandial hyperglycemia by acarbose in patients with NIDDM: a placebo-controlled dose-comparison study. Diabetes Care 18:817, 1995

200. Bailey CJ, Turner RC: Metformin. N Engl J Med 334:574, 1996

201. Stumvoll N, Nurjhan N, Perriello G, et al: Metabolic effects of metformin in non-insulin-dependent diabetes mellitus. N Engl J Med 333:550, 1995

202. Inzucchi SE, Maggs DG, Spollett GR, et al: Efficacy and metabolic effects of metformin and troglitazone in type II diabetes mellitus. N Engl J Med 338:867, 1998

203. Multicenter Metformin Study Group: Efficacy of metformin in patients with non-insulin-dependent diabetes mellitus. N Engl J Med 333:541, 1995

204. Lebovitz HE: Effects of oral antihyperglycemic agents in modifying macrovascular risk factors in type 2 diabetes. Diabetes Care 22(suppl 3):S41, 1999

205. Garber AJ, Duncan TG, Goodman AM, et al: Efficacy of metformin in type II diabetes: results of a double-blind, placebo-controlled, dose-response trial. Am J Med 102:491, 1997

206. Lalau JD, Lacroix C, Compagnon P, et al: Role of metformin accumulation in metformin-associated lactic acidosis. Diabetes Care 18:779, 1995

207. Lalau JD, Westeel PF, Debussche X, et al: Bicarbonate haemodialysis: an adequate treatment for lactic acidosis in diabetics treated by metformin. Intensive Care Med 13:383, 1987

208. Henry RR: Thiazolidinediones. Current Therapies for Diabetes 26:553, 1997

209. Maggs DG, Buchanan TA, Burant CF, et al: Metabolic effects of troglitazone monotherapy in type 2 diabetes mellitus: a randomized, double-blind, placebo-controlled trial. Ann Intern Med 128:176, 1998

210. Olefsky JM: Treatment of insulin resistance with peroxisome proliferator-activated receptor γ agonists. J Clin Invest 106:467, 2000

211. Akazawa S, Sun F, Ito M, et al: Efficacy of troglitazone on body fat distribution in type 2 diabetes. Diabetes Care 23:1067, 2000

212. Minamikawa J, Tanaka S, Yamauchi M, et al: Potent inhibitory effect of troglitazone on carotid arterial wall thickness in type 2 diabetes. J Clin Endocrinol Metab 83:1818, 1998

213. Kato K, Satoh H, Endo Y, et al: Thiazolidinediones down-regulate plasminogen activator inhibitor type 1 expression in human vascular endothelial cells: a possible role for PPARgamma in endothelial function. Biochem Biophys Res Commun 258:431, 1999

214. Yamakawa K, Hosoi M, Fukumoto S, et al: Pioglitazone inhibits plasminogen activator inhibitor–1 expression in human vascular smooth muscle cell (abstr). Diabetes 47:A366, 1998

215. Murakami T, Mizuno S, Ohsato K, et al: Effects of troglitazone on frequency of coronary vasospastic-induced angina pectoris in patients with diabetes mellitus. Am J Cardiol 84:92, 1999

216. Avena R, Mitchell ME, Nylen ES, et al: Insulin action enhancement normalizes brachial artery vasoactivity in patients with peripheral vascular disease and occult diabetes. J Vasc Surg 28:1024, 1998

217. Kotchen TA, Zhang HY, Reddy S, et al: Effect of pioglitazone on vascular reactivity in vivo and in vitro. Am J Physiol 270:R660, 1996

218. Takagi T, Yoshida K, Akasaka T, et al: Troglitazone reduces intimal hyperplasia after coronary stent implantation in patients with type 2 diabetes mellitus: a serial intravascular ultrasound study (abstr). J Am Coll Cardiol 33(suppl A):100A, 1999

219. Tack CJJ, Smits P, Demacker PNM, et al: Troglitazone decreases the proportion of small, dense LDL and increases the resistance of LDL to oxidation in obese subjects. Diabetes Care 21:796, 1998

220. Winter WE, Maclaren NK, Riley WJ, et al: Maturity-onset diabetes of youth in black Americans. N Engl J Med 316:285, 1987

221. Banerji MA, Lebovitz HE: Insulin-sensitive and insulin-resistant variants in NIDDM. Diabetes 38:784, 1989

222. Genuth S: Insulin in non–insulin-dependent patients. Adv Endocrinol Metab 3:89, 1992

223. Riddle MC: Evening insulin strategy. Diabetes Care 13:676, 1990

224. Yki-Jarvinen H, Kauppila M, Kujansuu E, et al: Comparison of insulin regimens in patients with non-insulin-dependent diabetes mellitus. N Engl J Med 327:1426, 1992

225. Genuth SM, Martin P: Control of hyperglycemia in adult diabetics by pulsed insulin delivery. Diabetes 26:571, 1977

226. Henry RR, Gumbiner B, Ditzler T, et al: Intensive conventional insulin therapy for type II diabetes. Diabetes Care 16:21, 1993

227. Elliott TG, Viberti G: Relationship between insulin resistance and coronary heart disease in diabetes mellitus and the general population: a critical appraisal. Baillieres Clin Endocrinol Metab 7:1079, 1993

228. Genuth S: Exogenous insulin administration and cardiovascular risk in non–insulin-dependent and insulin-dependent diabetes mellitus. Ann Intern Med 124:104, 1996

229. Abraira C, Colwell JA, Nuttall FQ, et al: Veterans Affairs Cooperative Study on Glycemic Control and Complications in Type II Diabetes (VA CSDM): results of the feasibility study. Diabetes Care 18:1113, 1995

230. Giugliano D, Quatraro A, Consoli G, et al: Metformin for obese, insulin-treated diabetic patients: improvement in glycaemic control and reduction of metabolic risk factors. Eur J Clin Pharmacol 44:107, 1993

231. Moses R, Slobodniuk R, Boyages S, et al: Effect of repaglinide addition to metformin monotherapy on glycemic control in patients with type 2 diabetes. Diabetes Care 22:119, 1999

232. Horton ES, Whitehouse F, Ghazzi MN, et al: Troglitazone in combination with sulfonylurea restores glycemic control in patients with type 2 diabetes. Diabetes Care 21:1462, 1998

233. Raskin P, Jovanovic L, Berger S, et al: Repaglinide/troglitazone combination therapy: improved glycemic control in type 2 diabetes. Diabetes Care 23:979, 2000

234. U.K. Prospective Diabetes Study Group: U.K. Prospective Diabetes Study 16 – overview of 6 years' therapy of type II diabetes: a progressive disease. Diabetes 44:1249, 1995

235. Casner PR: Insulin-glyburide combination therapy for non-insulin-dependent diabetes mellitus: a long-term double blind, placebo-controlled trial. Clin Pharmacol Ther 44:594, 1988

236. Cruz-Caudillo JC, Sabatini S: Diabetic hyperosmolar syndrome. Nephron 69:201, 1995

237. Lorber D: Nonketotic hypertonicity in diabetes mellitus. Med Clin North Am 79:39, 1995

238. Stamler J, Vaccaro O, Neaton JD, et al: Diabetes, other risk factors, and 12-yr cardiovascular mortality for men screened in the Multiple Risk Factor Intervention Trial. Diabetes Care 16:434, 1993

239. Barrett-Connor EL, Cohn BA, Wingard DL, et al: Why is diabetes mellitus a stronger risk factor for fatal ischemic heart disease in women than in men? The Rancho Bernardo Study. JAMA 265:627, 1991

240. Haffner SM, Lehto S, Rönnemaa T, et al: Mortality from coronary heart disease in subjects with type 2 diabetes and in nondiabetic subjects with and without prior myocardial infarction. N Engl J Med 339:229, 1998

241. Singer DE, Moulton AW, Nathan DM: Diabetic myocardial infarction: Interaction of diabetes with other preinfarction risk factors. Diabetes 38:350, 1989

242. Jensen T, Borch-Johnsen K, Kofoed-Enevoldsen A, et al: Coronary heart disease in young type 1 (insulin-dependent) diabetic patients with and without diabetic nephropathy: incidence and risk factors. Diabetologia 30:144, 1987

243. Grundy SM, Benjamin IJ, Burke GL, et al: Diabetes and cardiovascular disease: a statement for healthcare professionals from the American Heart Association. Circulation 100:1134, 1999

244. Gu K, Cowie CC, Harris MI: Mortality in adults with and without diabetes in a national cohort of the U.S. population, 1971–1993. Diabetes Care 21:1138, 1998

245. Gu K, Cowie CC, Harris MI: Diabetes and decline in heart disease mortality in US adults. JAMA 281:1291, 1999

246. Moss SE, Klein R, Klein BEK, et al: The association of glycemia and cause-specific mortality in a diabetic population. Arch Intern Med 154:2473, 1994

247. Kuusisto J, Mykkänen L, Pyörälä K, et al: NIDDM and its metabolic control predict coronary heart disease in elderly subjects. Diabetes 43:960, 1994

248. Andersson DKG, Svärdsudd K: Long-term glycemic control relates to mortality in type II diabetes. Diabetes Care 18:1534, 1995

249. Wei M, Gaskill SP, Haffner SM, et al: Effects of diabetes and level of glycemia on all-cause and cardiovascular mortality: the San Antonio Heart Study. Diabetes Care 21:1167, 1998

250. Stratton IM, Adler AI, Neil HAW, et al: Association of glycaemia with macrovascular and microvascular complications of type 2 diabetes (UKPDS 35): prospective observational study. BMJ 321:405, 2000

251. UK Prospective Diabetes Study Group: Tight blood pressure control and risk of macrovascular and microvascular complications in type 2 diabetes: UKPDS 38. BMJ 317:703, 1998

252. Nielson FS, Rossing P, Gall MA, et al: Long-term effect of lisinopril and atenolol on kidney function in hypertensive NIDDM subjects with diabetic nephropathy. Diabetes 46:1182, 1997

253. American Diabetes Association: Diabetic nephropathy. Diabetes Care 23:569, 2000

254. American Diabetes Association: Treatment of hypertension in diabetes. Diabetes Care 16:1394, 1993

255. Elliott WJ, Stein PP, Black HR: Drug treatment of hypertension in patients with diabetes. Diabetes Reviews 3:477, 1995

256. Pahor M, Psaty BM, Alderman MH, et al: Therapeutic benefits of ACE inhibitors and other antihypertensive drugs in patients with type 2 diabetes. Diabetes Care 23:888, 2000

257. Barkis GL, Williams M, Dworkin L, et al: Preserving renal function in adults with hypertension with diabetes: a consensus approach. Am J Kidney Dis 36:646, 2000

258. UK Prospective Diabetes Study Group: Efficacy of atenolol and captopril in reducing risk of macrovascular and microvascular complications in type 2 diabetes: UKPDS 39. BMJ 317:713, 1998

259. Estacio RO, Jeffers BW, Hiatt WR, et al: The effect of nisoldipine as compared with enalapril on cardiovascular outcomes in patients with non-insulin-dependent diabetes and hypertension. N Engl J Med 338:645, 1998

260. Howard BV: Pathogenesis of diabetic dyslipidemia. Diabetes Reviews 3:423, 1995

261. Ginsberg HN: Insulin resistance and cardiovascular disease. J Clin Invest 106:453, 2000

262. Haffner SM: Management of dyslipidemia in adults with diabetes. Diabetes Care 21:160, 1998

263. Haire-Joshu D, Glasgow RE, Tibbs TL: Smoking and diabetes. Diabetes Care 22:1887, 1999

264. ETDRS Investigators: Aspirin effects on mortality and morbidity in patients with diabetes mellitus: Early Treatment Diabetic Retinopathy Study report 14. JAMA 268:1292, 1992

265. American Diabetes Association: Aspirin therapy in diabetes. Diabetes Care 24(suppl 1):S62, 2001

266. Colwell JA: Aspirin therapy in diabetes. Diabetes Care 20:1767, 1997

267. The Heart Outcomes Prevention Evaluation Study Investigators: Effects of an angiotensin-converting–enzyme inhibitor, ramipril, on cardiovascular events in high-risk patients. N Engl J Med 342:145, 2000

268. The Heart Outcomes Prevention Evaluation Study Investigators: Vitamin E supplementation and cardiovascular events in high-risk patients. N Engl J Med 342:154, 2000

269. The Bypass Angioplasty Revascularization Investigation (BARI) Investigators: Comparison of coronary bypass surgery with angioplasty in patients with multivessel disease. N Engl J Med 335:217, 1996

270. Malmberg K, for the DIGAMI (Diabetes Mellitus, Insulin Glucose Infusion in Acute Myocardial Infarction) Study Group: Prospective randomised study of intensive insulin treatment on long term survival after acute myocardial infarction in patients with diabetes mellitus. BMJ 314:1512, 1997

271. Nathan DM: Long-term complications of diabetes mellitus. N Engl J Med 328:1676, 1993

272. Clark CM Jr, Lee DA: Prevention and treatment of the complications of diabetes mellitus. N Engl J Med 332:1210, 1995

273. Ferris FL III, Davis MD, Aiello LM: Treatment of diabetic retinopathy. Drug Therapy 341:667, 1999

274. Nathan DM, Fogel HA, Godine JE, et al: Role of diabetologist in evaluating diabetic retinopathy. Diabetes Care 14:26, 1991

275. Harris MI, Klein R, Welborn TA, et al: Onset of NIDDM occurs at least 4–7 yr before clinical diagnosis. Diabetes Care 15:815, 1992

276. Effect of pregnancy on microvascular complications in the diabetes control and complications trial. The Diabetes Control and Complications Trial Research Group. Diabetes Care 23:1084, 2000

277. Cooper ME: Pathogenesis, prevention, and treatment of diabetic nephropathy. Lancet 352:213, 1998

278. Lewis EJ, Hunsicker LG, Bain RP, et al: The effect of angiotensin-converting-enzyme inhibition on diabetic nephropathy. N Engl J Med 329:1456, 1993

279. Ravid M, Savin H, Jutrin I, et al: Long-term stabilizing effect of angiotensin-converting enzyme inhibition on plasma creatinine and on proteinuria in normotensive type II diabetic patients. Ann Intern Med 118:577, 1993

280. Foley RN, Culleton BF, Parfrey PS, et al: Cardiac disease in diabetic end-stage renal disease. Diabetologia 40:1307, 1997

281. Backonja M, Beydoun A, Edwards KR, et al: Gabapentin for the symptomatic treatment of painful neuropathy in patients with diabetes mellitus. JAMA 280:1831, 1998

282. Litzelman DK, Slemenda CW, Langefeld CD, et al: Reduction of lower extremity clinical abnormalities in patients with non–insulin-dependent diabetes mellitus. Ann Intern Med 119:36, 1993

283. Mason J, O'Keeffe C, Hutchinson A, et al: A systematic review of foot ulcer in patients with type 2 diabetes mellitus. II: Treatment. Diabetic Medicine 16:889, 1999

284. McCallum RW, Ricci DA, Rakatansky H, et al: A multicenter placebo-controlled clinical trial of oral metoclopramide in diabetic gastroparesis. Diabetes Care 6:463, 1983

285. Janssens J, Peeters TL, Vantrappen G, et al: Improvement of gastric emptying in diabetic gastroparesis by erythromycin: preliminary studies. N Engl J Med 322:1028, 1990

286. Sildenafil Diabetes Study Group: Sildenafil for treatment of erectile dysfunction in men with diabetes: a randomized controlled trial. JAMA 281:421, 1999

287. Kühl C: New approaches for the treatment of pregnant diabetic women. Diabetes Reviews 3:621, 1995

288. Langer O: Is normoglycemia the correct threshold to prevent complications in the pregnant diabetic patient? Diabetes Reviews 4:2, 1996

289. de Veciana M, Major CA, Morgan MA, et al: Postprandial versus preprandial blood glucose monitoring in women with gestational diabetes mellitus requiring insulin therapy. N Engl J Med 333:1237, 1995

290. Kjos SL, Buchanan TA: Gestational diabetes mellitus. N Engl J Med 341:1749, 1999

Acknowledgments

I am grateful to the previous author of this chapter, Dr. David Nathan, for providing such an excellent template and for generously permitting me to retain certain sections that required only minor updating. I also wish to thank Eileen Campbell and Molly Genuth for skilled assistance in preparing the manuscript.

Figures 1, 4, 14, 15   Seward Hung.

49 Adrenal

Daniel D. Federman, M.D.

Physiology of the Adrenal Cortex

The adrenal gland controls the body's adjustment to an upright posture and permits accommodation to intermittent rather than constant intake of food. Sudden and sometimes sustained increases in adrenal function are also required to negotiate acute stresses such as volume loss, infection, anesthesia, and surgery. Loss of these functions is the most troublesome consequence of adrenal insufficiency. The secretions of the adrenal gland also influence immune reactivity, blood cell formation, cerebral function, protein synthesis, and many other body processes[1]; an excess of these effects is known as Cushing's syndrome.

BIOSYNTHESIS AND METABOLISM OF ADRENAL STEROIDS

Synthesis of the adrenal hormones begins with either acetate or cholesterol [*see Figure 1*]. Cholesterol derived from low-density lipoprotein (LDL) is the substrate for 80 percent of corticoid biosynthesis. The reaction in which cholesterol is converted to Δ^5-pregnenolone is the major point of regulation by the tropic hormones that control adrenal function; both corticotropin and angiotensin stimulate this conversion. Beyond Δ^5-pregnenolone, the pathways diverge toward the formation of definitive, biologically active adrenal products.

Cortisol In humans, cortisol is the principal glucocorticoid. It influences appetite and well-being, maintains blood sugar concentration by promoting hepatic gluconeogenesis, and indirectly affects heart rate and pumping force by controlling synthesis of epinephrine in the adrenal medulla. Increased cortisol secretion is critical in the physiologic response to stress and illness.

Between 13 and 20 mg of cortisol is secreted daily in the zona fasciculata and the zona reticularis; immediately after discharge from the gland, cortisol is bound to the α-globulin transcortin, or cortisol-binding globulin. As is the case with thyroxine, most circulating cortisol is bound and inactive; a small percentage is free and biologically active.

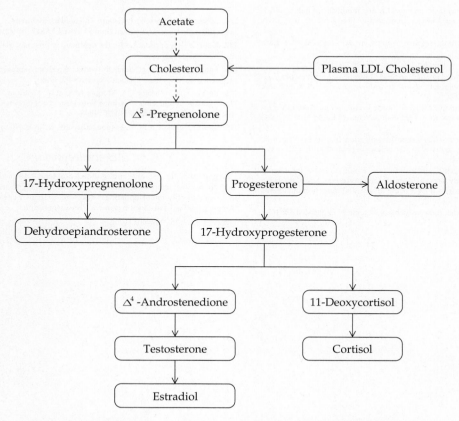

Figure 1   **Biosynthesis of all adrenal hormones begins with acetate or cholesterol, from which a common hormone precursor, Δ^5-pregnenolone, is formed. The pathway to aldosterone, derived from progesterone, exists only in the zona glomerulosa. The synthesis of cortisol and sex steroids is carried out in the zona reticularis and the zona fasciculata. Testosterone and estradiol are manufactured in only trace amounts by the adrenal, but they can be produced elsewhere in the body from weak androgens made in the adrenal.**

Hepatic reduction of a double bond in ring A of the molecule inactivates cortisol. After a number of other biotransformations and subsequent conjugation with glucuronide or sulfate, the metabolites of cortisol are excreted as urinary 17-hydroxysteroid (17-OHS).

Androgens Androgens are produced in the zona fasciculata and in the zona reticularis; their production varies greatly at different stages of life. The fetus makes large amounts of adrenal androgens, especially sulfated dehydroepiandrosterone (DHEAS), whereas the child produces very little.[2] Adrenal androgen production increases in individuals during puberty and reaches a peak in young adults; it then declines to rather low levels in persons older than 50 years. However, secretion of adrenocorticotropic hormone (ACTH), the only known regulator of adrenal androgen biosynthesis, shows no such age-related fluctuations. The regulation of adrenal androgen production is not yet clear: both pituitary-derived and adrenal-derived factors have been postulated but have not been confirmed. Adrenal androgens are relatively weak, but some serve as precursors for hepatic conversion to testosterone [*see Figure 2*]. Hyperfunction of this pathway in the female causes hirsutism and, occasionally, masculinization.

The adrenal androgen androstenedione is converted by hepatic and adipose tissue to the potent estrogen estrone. This pathway is the major source of estrogen in children and in postmenopausal women. The other principal androgen, dehydroepiandrosterone (DHEA), along with its conjugate, DHEAS, is an enigma. DHEA has minimal androgenic potency, and although several nonandrogenic actions have been published, none is of proven physiologic importance. Similarly, DHEAS can be metabolized to either testosterone or estrogen, but its importance in that role is unclear.

Adrenal androgens are metabolized to 17-keto compounds, which are excreted in the urine as 17-ketosteroids (17-KS).

Aldosterone The principal mineralocorticoid of the human adrenal is aldosterone, an 18-oxycorticoid produced in the zona glomerulosa from acetate and cholesterol precursors.[3] Angiotensin is the dominant stimulus to aldosterone biosynthesis [*see Figure 3*]; both angiotensin and ACTH increase aldosterone production by accelerating the conversion of cholesterol to Δ^5-pregnenolone. Other stimuli to aldosterone secretion include an increase in serum potassium, a fall in blood volume or serum sodium, and a rise in estrogen levels. There is evidence that aldosterone release is inhibited by a dopaminergic mechanism. Aldosterone circulates unbound and is degraded by enzymes during hepatic clearance and by renal conjugation and excretion. The metabolic clearance rate of aldosterone depends exquisitely on hepatic blood flow. A decrease in that flow occurs in a variety of liver disorders and may lead to transient aldosteronism. Interactions among the other controls of aldosterone secretion determine whether the condition endures.

REGULATION OF ADRENAL SECRETION

ACTH is the principal regulator of adrenal cortisol and androgen production [*see Figure 3*].[3] Pituitary synthesis and release of ACTH are in turn controlled principally by corticotropin-releasing hormone (CRH), a 41 amino acid peptide produced in the hypothalamus.[4] Vasopressin, also termed arginine vasopressin (AVP) and antidiuretic hormone (ADH), is also active in the basal regulation of ACTH.[5,6] Although vasopressin, oxytocin, and the catecholamines influence the diurnal rhythm of ACTH and cortisol, the major determinant of this cycle appears to be the diurnal release of CRH. During stress, there is a two-fold to 10-fold increase in adrenal steroid output. Surges in both CRH and ADH have a potentiative, rather than simply additive, effect on this output during the response.

ACTH is synthesized as a small segment of the complex molecule called pro-opiomelanocortin (POMC). The primary gene product is a complex molecule that also includes the amino acid sequences for β-lipotropin (β-LPH), a joining peptide, α- and β-melanocyte–stimulating hormones (α-MSH and β-MSH), β-endorphin, γ-LPH, met-enkephalin, and at least two additional fragments—corticotropin-like intermediate lobe peptide (CLIP) and a 16 kb sequence of undetermined physiologic significance [*see Figure 4*]. POMC is also produced in nonpituitary tissues, but its posttranslational processing differs in the various sites. In the pituitary, cleavage separates the long fragment beginning at ACTH; both portions are glycosylated, and the smaller fragments are then released. Although the release of β-LPH tends to parallel that of ACTH, the functions of this molecule and of the other fragments of the larger precursor also remain to be fully elucidated.

Like other pituitary hormones, ACTH is secreted in pulses.[7] About one to three pulses occur each hour, cluster-

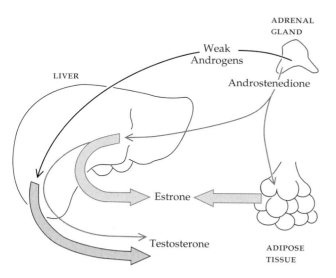

Figure 2 **The weak androgens produced by the adrenal serve as precursors for the formation of the potent androgen testosterone in the liver. In the male, this pathway is a negligible source of testosterone; in the female, it plays a small role in androgen status. The adrenal androgen androstenedione is converted by both hepatic and adipose tissue to the estrogen estrone. This process can be an important source of estrogen after the menstruating years; overactivity of this pathway may be significant in the pathogenesis of cancer in tissues sensitive to estrogen.**

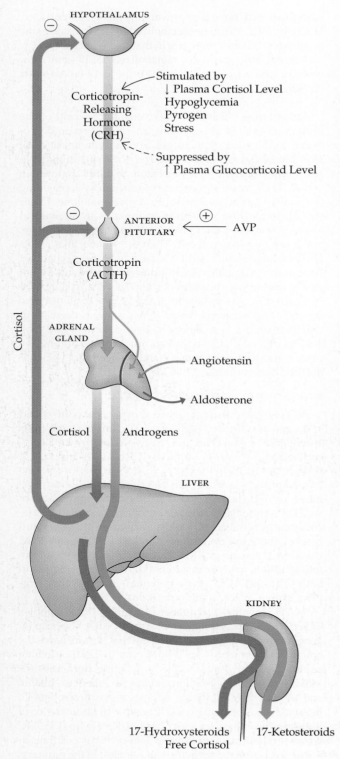

HYPOTHALAMUS

Corticotropin-
Releasing
Hormone
(CRH)

— Stimulated by
↓ Plasma Cortisol Level
Hypoglycemia
Pyrogen
Stress

— Suppressed by
↑ Plasma Glucocorticoid Level

ANTERIOR
PITUITARY ← ⊕ ← AVP

Corticotropin
(ACTH)

Cortisol

ADRENAL
GLAND

— Angiotensin

— Aldosterone

Cortisol   Androgens

LIVER

KIDNEY

17-Hydroxysteroids   17-Ketosteroids
Free Cortisol

Figure 3   **Adrenal function is controlled by two tropic hormones: adrenocorticotropic hormone (ACTH) for the synthesis of cortisol and androgens, and angiotensin for the synthesis of aldosterone. The hypothalamic substance corticotropin-releasing hormone controls ACTH secretion. Arginine vasopressin (AVP) also contributes to the stimulation of ACTH release. Cortisol exerts negative feedback control on ACTH at the anterior pituitary and the hypothalamus. 17-Hydroxysteroids, free cortisol, and 17-ketosteroids are excreted in the urine.**

ing in the morning hours. Because the resulting cortisol disappears more slowly than ACTH, the early morning surges of cortisol summate to a diurnal rhythm that is higher in the morning and lower in the evening. In addition to this endogenous pulse generator, the release of ACTH and cortisol is also triggered by fever, hypoglycemia, stress of many kinds, psychological disturbance, and a falling level of plasma cortisol. The dominant factor suppressing ACTH is the plasma level of cortisol. All synthetic glucocorticoids have the same effect, which is mediated by suppression of transcription of the messenger RNA (mRNA) for POMC synthesis.[8] A similar suppression by glucocorticoid is presumed to inhibit CRH production. Thus, cortisol has a negative feedback effect at both the hypothalamic and the pituitary levels [*see Figure 3*].

Testing Adrenal Function

The principal tests used to evaluate adrenal function include measurements of plasma ACTH and cortisol and of urinary 17-OHS and 24-hour urinary free cortisol.

Measurement of plasma cortisol and ACTH Resting values of plasma cortisol are between 10 and 25 μg/dl in the morning and between 2 and 10 μg/dl at night. The plasma cortisol level is altered by changes in the amount of cortisol-binding globulin, which generally parallel changes in the level of thyroxine-binding globulin. For example, both proteins are raised by increased estrogen levels and lowered by hepatic disease. Resting levels of cortisol are often less significant than the responses of the hormone to physiologic stimuli. Thus, plasma cortisol levels are usually measured after administration of exogenous steroid to determine whether the pituitary-adrenal axis is susceptible to feedback inhibition (i.e., whether it is suppressible) and after ACTH administration to see whether the adrenal responds to stimulation.

The following are some well-standardized tests for the evaluation of adrenal function:

1. To determine pituitary-adrenal suppression, 1 mg of dexamethasone (a cortisol analogue) is given orally at 11:00 P.M., and the plasma cortisol level is measured at 8:00 A.M. the next day. A value of less than 5 μg/dl is normal.
2. To measure adrenal response, 0.25 mg of cosyntropin (synthetic ACTH) is given intravenously. The plasma cortisol is measured at 0 and 60 minutes; a value of 20 μg/dl at any time during the test denotes normal adrenal responsiveness.
3. To assess pituitary-adrenal reserve, 3 g of metyrapone is administered orally at midnight, and plasma cortisol and 11-deoxycortisol (compound S) levels are obtained at 8:00 A.M. the next day. Metyrapone inhibits 11-hydroxylation, which leads to a fall in cortisol and a rise in ACTH. If the pituitary-adrenal reserve is intact, the plasma cortisol level should be less than 5 μg/dl and the 11-deoxycortisol level greater than 10 μg/dl.
4. An alternative method of measuring pituitary-adrenal reserve involves the intravenous administration of insulin, 0.15 U/kg. The ensuing hypoglycemia should elicit both cortisol (normal, 20 μg/dl) and

growth hormone (> 8 ng/ml) responses. This test should be carried out in the presence of a physician prepared to administer 25 ml of 50 percent glucose intravenously in case of a hypoglycemic reaction.

5. To measure pituitary reserve of ACTH, ovine CRH can be administered in a dose of 1 μg/kg body weight. Both ACTH and plasma cortisol levels rise in normal individuals. This test can be performed at any time of day, but the sensitivity is greatest in the afternoon.

Plasma ACTH can be determined by immunoradiometric assay (IRMA), employing antibodies to both the N- and C-terminal domains of the hormone. Unlike radioimmunoassay, IRMA can reliably distinguish low, normal, and elevated ACTH levels.[9]

Urinary 17-OHS level The urinary 17-OHS measurement has the advantage of integrating the secretion of cortisol during a 24-hour period, but its usefulness is limited because the level is elevated by obesity and depressed by hepatic and renal disease. Moreover, the collection of an accurately timed urine specimen is difficult for many patients.

24-Hour urinary free cortisol The 24-hour urinary free cortisol test also requires accurately timed urine collections. Values in obese people rarely overlap with those in Cushing's syndrome patients, and hepatic disease does not distort the result. The urinary free cortisol excretion rate has become a valuable index of adrenal hyperfunction. It is less reliable for the detection of hypoadrenalism.[10]

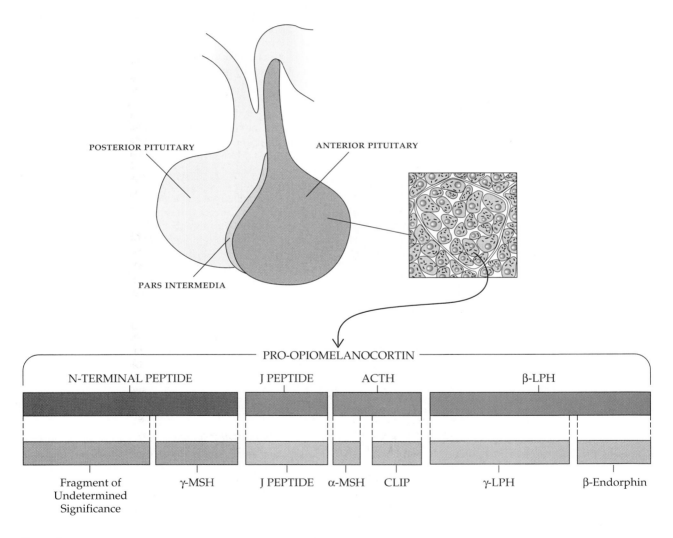

Figure 4　ACTH is synthesized in the anterior pituitary as part of a larger precursor polypeptide, pro-opiomelanocortin (241 residues in humans), which also contains the amino acid sequences of β-LPH (β-lipotropin) and other hormones. DNA complementary to human mRNA for the ACTH–β-LPH precursor molecule has been cloned and its nucleotide sequence determined. The ACTH synthesized from this mRNA contains within itself the amino acid sequences for the peptides α-MSH α-melanocyte–stimulating hormone) and CLIP (corticotropin-like intermediate lobe peptide); similarly, the sequences for γ-LPH and β-endorphin appear within the β-LPH molecule. The various component peptides are thought to be released from ACTH and β-LPH by proteolytic cleavage at the sites of basic amino acid residues.

Hyperfunction of the Adrenal Cortex: Cushing's Syndrome

The condition of hyperadrenocorticism known as Cushing's syndrome is uncommon, but its recognition is important for two reasons. First, it is often curable. Second, glucocorticoid excess is a potential cause of problems the physician sees daily, including obesity, hypertension, diabetes, renal stones, osteoporosis, purpura, mental disorder, menstrual disturbance, impotence, hirsutism, edema, hypokalemia, susceptibility to infection, and poor wound healing. Although none of those problems by itself raises a high suspicion of hyperadrenocorticism, the coexistence of several clinical features can indicate that a workup for Cushing's syndrome is needed. The most valuable clues are plethoric facies, bruising, unexplained hypokalemia, poor wound healing, and change in appearance as judged by comparing present facial appearance with a past photograph.[11]

The causes of Cushing's syndrome are excess ACTH, excess cortisol production originating in the adrenal, and iatrogenic or factitious ingestion of excess corticoid.[12]

ACTH EXCESS

Pituitary Overproduction (Cushing's Disease)

Excess pituitary ACTH with bilateral adrenal hyperplasia accounts for approximately two thirds of cases of Cushing's syndrome. The disease is most frequent in women of reproductive age. Onset is usually gradual. Any of the symptoms caused by cortisol excess may appear first, but menstrual irregularity, impotence in men, bruising, facial rounding, and plethora eventually develop. Adrenal androgen synthesis increases, and hirsutism and slight balding are common in women. The androgen excess may exert some protective effect against the antianabolic influence of cortisol, but the severity of clinical manifestations is roughly proportional to the duration of the disorder and to the amount of ACTH secretion. Pigmentation, reflecting the ACTH excess, can be a valuable clue in the diagnosis, but this finding can be difficult to recognize, especially in individuals who are dark-skinned.

In theory, pituitary ACTH excess could be caused by an excess of corticotropin-releasing hormone or by a primary pituitary neoplasm. Cushing believed that most cases were caused by a pituitary tumor, and the now extensive experience of cure after removal of pituitary microadenomas supports that interpretation. Molecular studies have indicated that most ACTH-producing microadenomas are monoclonal[13]; as with other tumors, this is strong evidence for a neoplastic pituitary origin rather than a hyperplastic response to CRH. However, the recurrence of tumors after apparent cure and the responses of some patients to drugs such as bromocriptine, a dopamine agonist, support but do not prove a hypothalamic origin. Conversely, the success of treatment with pituitary irradiation, especially in children, supports the view that Cushing's disease is most often what Cushing said it was: hyperadrenalism secondary to a pituitary tumor.

The following laboratory findings are characteristic of Cushing's disease:

1. Elevation of urinary free cortisol levels, usually to greater than 150 μg/24 hr.

2. Loss of diurnal rhythm of plasma ACTH and cortisol: evening cortisol levels are greater than 10 μg/dl; excretion of urinary 17-OHS also loses its daily rhythm.
3. Loss of ACTH suppressibility by physiologic doses of glucocorticoid: 1 mg of dexamethasone given at midnight does not prevent the morning rise of cortisol to greater than 10 μg/dl.
4. Suppression of cortisol secretion when a larger dosage of dexamethasone, 2 mg every six hours for two days, is given: urinary 17-OHS and 17-KS levels fall to less than 50 percent of control levels.

Ectopic Production of ACTH

Two variants of ectopic (nonpituitary) ACTH production cause Cushing's syndrome. One form results from the uncontrolled synthesis and release of ACTH by malignant tumors, most commonly of lung, thymus, pancreas, and kidney.[14] The syndrome is that of an acute hyperadrenocorticism, which is usually dominated by mineralocorticoid effects from the secretion of large amounts of cortisol rather than by glucocorticoid-induced changes. Hypokalemic alkalosis, weakness, and weight loss are outstanding elements, and the patient seldom has a cushingoid appearance. Plasma cortisol and urinary steroid levels in the patient with this type of Cushing's syndrome are often much higher than levels in the patient who has a frankly cushingoid appearance. In addition, the urinary or plasma 17-OHS levels are not suppressed by an 8 mg daily dose of dexamethasone. Thus, a major clue to the diagnosis of this type of ectopic ACTH syndrome is the discrepancy between an unimpressive clinical appearance and a striking level of steroid secretion. The pronounced mineralocorticoid effect in this condition results from high cortisol production and its overwhelming of the two pathways of cortisol inactivation (conversion to cortisone, by 11-hydroxysteroid dehydrogenase, and ring A reduction to dihydrocortisol). As a consequence, cortisol accumulates, binds to the mineralocorticoid receptor, and causes sodium retention with kaliuresis.[15,16]

The second form of ectopic Cushing's syndrome is associated with benign or malignant lesions such as bronchial or thymic carcinoids. The clinical picture in such cases is indistinguishable from pituitary Cushing's syndrome, and special approaches are required to make the differentiation [see Diagnosis, below].

Ectopic Production of CRH

Ectopic production of CRH by tumors can stimulate sufficient production of pituitary ACTH to produce adrenal hyperplasia and Cushing's syndrome. The tumor most frequently implicated in ectopic CRH production is the bronchial carcinoid, and most of these tumors co-secrete ACTH.[1] The clinical picture may be typical of Cushing's disease, or it may more closely resemble the manifestations of the ectopic ACTH syndrome, including hypokalemia, alkalosis, and weakness.[17] Low- and high-dose dexamethasone testing show nonsuppressible pituitary-adrenal function, and plasma ACTH levels are quite elevated.

ADRENAL CORTISOL EXCESS

Adrenal neoplasms that hypersecrete cortisol account for fewer than one third of cases of spontaneous Cushing's syndrome. Although symptoms vary, there are certain clues to the diagnosis. Benign adrenal adenomas often secrete only cortisol, and the clinical features reflect cortisol excess without androgen excess. Because the cortisol suppresses endogenous ACTH, other adrenal functions are diminished, and urinary 17-KS levels tend to be low. Adrenal carcinomas that produce excess cortisol almost always produce large amounts of androgens as well. Hirsutism and defeminization occur in women, and urinary 17-KS levels tend to be very high (50 mg/24 hr).[18] Other diagnostic features that indicate the presence of adrenal tumors include wide variability in secretory activity, nonsuppressibility by the large dose of dexamethasone, distortion of the intravenous pyelogram (IVP) on the affected side, and, for about half of adrenal cancers, a palpable mass.

The least frequent and most enigmatic cause of Cushing's syndrome is bilateral nodular hyperplasia that is not ACTH dependent. A number of very rare mechanisms can be postulated, including activating mutations of G protein receptors that stimulate adenylate cyclase.[19] Macronodular hyperplasia is most likely a late outcome of untreated Cushing's disease, in which one or more nodules become autonomous. Depending on the level of autonomous cortisol production, the pituitary-derived ACTH can be elevated or apparently normal; testing with the high dose of dexamethasone should suppress ACTH but not cortisol. In several cases, there was a progression from pituitary dependence to adrenal autonomy.[20]

The most puzzling cause of Cushing's syndrome is bilateral micronodular dysplasia, a sometimes familial disorder in which the cortisol level is high, the ACTH level is low, and the adrenals contain a mixture of small active nodules and atrophic tissue.[21] In some families, the adrenal hyperplasia seems to be caused by an adrenal-stimulating immunoglobulin, an autoantibody to the ACTH receptor reminiscent of the thyroid-stimulating immunoglobulin of Graves' disease.

The least frequent mechanism of nodular adrenal hyperplasia is a food-dependent hypercortisolism in which the inappropriate expression of gastric inhibitory polypeptide (GIP) receptor by adrenal cells leads to exaggerated cortisol secretion in response to meals (but not in the morning). This new understanding of Cushing's syndrome could be extremely important if the same or similar mechanisms can be implicated in other disorders.[22-24]

A discussion of the iatrogenic or factitious ingestion of excess corticoid is presented later [see Pharmacological Use of Glucocorticoids, below].

DIAGNOSIS

Given the protean manifestations of glucocorticoid excess, it is clearly useful to have a simple and sensitive test that will exclude the diagnosis of Cushing's syndrome in a patient in whom it appears unlikely. For this purpose, the most appropriate test is measurement of plasma cortisol the morning after a midnight dose of 1 mg of dexamethasone. If the cortisol level is less than 5 μg/dl, Cushing's syndrome can be excluded. If the value is more than 5 μg/dl and the patient is not taking estrogen, a definitive workup for Cushing's syndrome is indicated. However, the test will not confirm a diagnosis in a patient in whom

Cushing's syndrome seems likely. Because of the very high prevalence of cushingoid obesity (perhaps 3,000 per million adults), nonsuppression by dexamethasone in such patients has very limited significance unless the clinical evidence of Cushing's syndrome is strong.[25]

When Cushing's syndrome is clinically suspected, the 1 mg dexamethasone test or the 24-hour urinary free cortisol test may be used for confirmation. Because the plasma test has more false positives, the urinary cortisol determination is more widely used. When there is doubt about the diagnosis, both tests are advisable.

If the screening test is positive, definitive evaluation should include the following [see Figure 5]:

1. Administration of dexamethasone, 0.5 mg every six hours for two days. A 24-hour urinary 17-OHS level less than 3.5 mg on the second day or a plasma cortisol level less than 5 μg/dl on the third morning rules out Cushing's syndrome; higher levels confirm Cushing's syndrome. The importance of a clear outcome at this point cannot be emphasized too strongly. Tests to locate the pathological cause of Cushing's syndrome are, ironically, not useful in establishing its presence. Hypercortisolism should be unambiguously established before further testing is performed.

2. The first step in establishing the cause is to distinguish ACTH-dependent from non–ACTH-dependent hypercortisolism. Thus, several plasma ACTH assays [see Figure 6] and simultaneous cortisol assays should be performed. The newer immunoradiometric assays for ACTH should clearly separate the low, suppressed values of adrenal tumors (< 5 pg/ml) from the apparently normal or elevated values seen in ACTH-dependent cases.[26] A nomogram developed by the Mayo Clinic can be used to identify the pathological origin of hypercortisolism in about 90 percent of cases by measuring the plasma cortisol, urinary free cortisol, and ACTH levels.[27]

3. Administration of dexamethasone, 2 mg every six hours for two days. The following results are characteristic of pituitary ACTH excess (Cushing's disease): a second-day urinary 17-OHS level less than 35 percent of baseline, a second-day urinary free cortisol level less than 10 percent of baseline, or a third-morning plasma cortisol level less than 10 μg/dl.[28] Failure to achieve these end points indicates a nonpituitary source of ACTH or autonomous adrenal tumor or hyperplasia. The ACTH value determined in step 2, above, should make this distinction.

   The high-dose dexamethasone test has been modified to avoid the inconvenience and inaccuracy of urine collections. A baseline serum cortisol level is drawn at 8 A.M.; an 8 mg dose of dexamethasone is taken orally at 11 P.M. that night; and a second cortisol level is drawn at 8 A.M. the next day. A second-day value less than 50 percent of the control value points to a pituitary origin,[10] but the sensitivity and specificity of this test for ACTH-dependent hypercortisolism are highest if it is combined with the standard high-dose (8 mg/day) suppression test.[29]

4. If ACTH is normal or high, computed tomography or magnetic resonance imaging of the pituitary may indicate the presence of a tumor. If ACTH is suppressed, CT or MRI should be focused on the adrenal area.

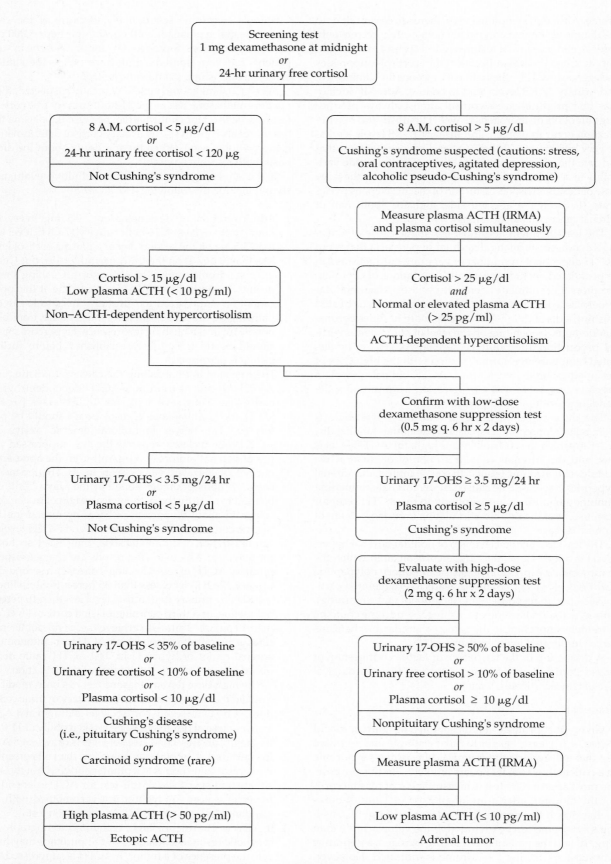

Figure 5 **An approach to the diagnosis of Cushing's syndrome is shown in the flowchart.**

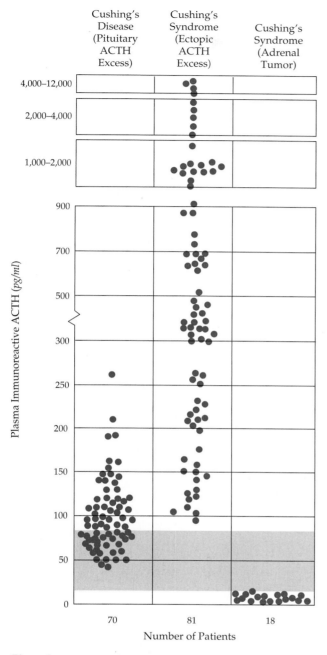

5. The foregoing steps provide a definitive diagnosis in about 90 percent of patients; that is, the endocrine findings and imaging results combine to implicate either a pituitary or ectopic source of ACTH or an adrenal tumor as the cause of the elevated plasma cortisol level. The most difficult remaining problem is the differentiation of pituitary from ectopic ACTH excess of the carcinoid variety [see ACTH Excess, above].[30] If no tumor of the pituitary is visualized, CT scanning of the chest is recommended—90 percent of the benign ectopic ACTH- and CRH-producing tumors occur in that area.

6. For the occasional patient in whom differentiation of the pathology remains a problem, two advances can be exploited. Intravenous injection of ovine corticotropin-releasing hormone (oCRH), 100 μg or 1 μg/kg, elicits a rise in plasma ACTH and cortisol levels in Cushing's disease but not in ACTH-independent hypercortisolism. There is still some overlap, however; in particular, some patients with ectopic ACTH production show a response.[31-34]

7. The most sophisticated and technically demanding test for localizing a pituitary microadenoma too small to be visualized is simultaneous oCRH administration (i.e., pituitary stimulation) and bilateral inferior petrosal sinus sampling.[35] A twofold gradient in ACTH between petrosal and peripheral veins suggests a pituitary adenoma and justifies transsphenoidal exploration. A twofold gradient in ACTH between the petrosal veins, either at baseline or after CRH administration, is considered justification for hemihypophysectomy if no microadenoma is identified surgically.

An elegant new approach for the localization of ectopic ACTH production is provided by the use of radiolabeled octreotide. This long-acting analogue of somatostatin attaches to receptors expressed on neuroendocrine tumors such as bronchial carcinoids but not to ordinary pituitary adenomas. It can thus be exploited for diagnosis, localization, and treatment of ectopic ACTH production.[36,37]

When carefully performed and correlated, the tests described should enable almost every case of Cushing's syndrome to be definitively interpreted [see Figure 6]. However, it is crucial to begin by proving that the patients do have hyperadrenocorticism. Unless the urinary free cortisol measurement is elevated, the differential and localizing testing are likely to be confusing and wasteful.

Some words of caution about pituitary-adrenal testing may be helpful. Several conditions can obliterate the normal diurnal rhythm of ACTH and cortisol secretion and can induce resistance to pituitary suppression by the 1 mg initial screening dose of dexamethasone. The obvious one is acute stress, such as that caused by hospitalization and surgery; the evening cortisol value during the first several days after admission to a hospital may well be greater than 10 μg/dl. A second source of difficulty is agitated depression, which can mimic the dynamic test abnormalities of Cushing's syndrome caused by pituitary ACTH excess. In patients with agitated depression, loss of diurnal rhythm and nonsuppressibility by dexamethasone are observed. This situation is particularly worrisome because hypercortisolism in turn can cause agitated depression. The distinction is made by clinical examination for signs of Cushing's

Figure 6 **Plasma ACTH measurement can help distinguish ectopic from pituitary ACTH excess as the cause of Cushing's syndrome. ACTH values in the upper normal (shaded gray area is normal range) to high range, such as those in the 70 patients in the left panel, are typical of Cushing's disease (Cushing's syndrome caused by a pituitary lesion). A high-normal value (50 to 80 pg/ml) cannot by itself be used to diagnose ACTH excess; however, the combination of a high cortisol value and a high-normal ACTH value implicates ACTH as the cause of the high steroid production. ACTH values greater than 250 pg/ml strongly suggest an ectopic source; 53 of 81 patients with ectopic ACTH had levels greater than 250 (middle panel). ACTH values in 18 patients with adrenal tumor (right panel) are suppressed. Standard ACTH assays do not demonstrate suppressed levels reliably; the double antibody immunoradiometric assay (IRMA), however, is more sensitive.**

syndrome and by measurement of urinary free cortisol; the latter is normal in depressed patients. In the occasional depressed patient with an elevated urinary cortisol level, CRH testing can be helpful.[38]

Obesity and alcoholism are the most difficult conditions to differentiate clinically from Cushing's syndrome because facial fullness, weakness, fatigue, and easy bruising can be present in all three conditions. Occasionally, the results of screening tests in obese patients are anomalous, but the cortisol level in patients with obesity should undergo suppression on the low-dose dexamethasone test. In the pseudo–Cushing's syndrome seen in alcoholics, initial testing may show resistance to suppression of plasma cortisol by 1 mg of dexamethasone and loss of diurnal rhythm; with abstinence, however, plasma cortisol values return to normal, and normal suppressibility emerges.[39]

Cyclic or periodic hypercortisolism is another cause of puzzling or inconsistent laboratory findings in Cushing's syndrome. Cycles may range from days to months and may have persisted for years; great care is needed before ablative therapy is recommended.[40]

THERAPY

The primary therapy in adults with Cushing's syndrome is surgery, and in the most common form of Cushing's syndrome, Cushing's disease (i.e., pituitary ACTH excess), transsphenoidal microadenomectomy is the treatment of choice.[41-45] If pituitary imaging (MRI is the most sensitive technique) or petrosal sinus sampling has identified a microadenoma [see Figure 7], cure rates are as high as 90 percent. Recurrence rates are between five and 20 percent.[46] The best results are obtained when the sella is radiologically normal. When the sella is distorted or the adenoma is more than 10 mm in diameter, the chances of cure are distinctly lower. Transient diabetes insipidus and meningitis are postoperative complications, but they are manageable.

When microadenomectomy is successful, patients display normal or low plasma cortisol levels soon after surgery. Such patients often exhibit adrenal and pituitary suppression and may need adrenal replacement therapy for as long as six months postoperatively.[47] When the surgical findings are indefinite or cortisol levels do not fall, CRH injection can be used to demonstrate persistence of ACTH-producing cells. Other therapies include yttrium implantation, heavy-particle therapy, and external irradiation. All of these treatments are inferior to adenomectomy, but at most centers, external irradiation is the treatment of choice in children.

The current enthusiasm for direct attack on the pituitary should not obscure the value of bilateral adrenalectomy. For patients who have severe disease, life-threatening complications, very large pituitary tumors, or nodular cortical hyperplasia and for those in whom pituitary treatment has failed, adrenalectomy may be preferable to transsphenoidal microadenomectomy.[48] Preoperative treatment with metyrapone can modulate the hypercortisolism, including psychological aberrations, and thus make surgery relatively safe. All cured patients experience adrenal insufficiency after adrenalectomy, and Nelson's syndrome develops in a significant percentage of patients. Autotransplantation of adrenal tissue has been used to avoid adrenal insufficiency, but finding an amount of adrenal tissue that

avoids hypofunction but does not lead to recurrence has been accomplished only rarely.

There are several pharmacological therapies for Cushing's syndrome. Aminoglutethimide inhibits cortisol synthesis by blocking conversion of cholesterol to Δ^5-pregnenolone; mitotane, an adrenolytic agent, inhibits cortisol synthesis; and metyrapone reduces cortisol production by inhibition of 11-hydroxylase. Toxicity, however, is high with aminoglutethimide and mitotane; even when these drugs are given in combination to minimize their separate toxicities, results are rarely satisfactory. Thus, the role of drugs in Cushing's syndrome is limited to special circumstances, such as control of extreme manifestations before surgery, supplementation of a partial remission induced by pituitary irradiation, or amelioration of symptoms caused by inoperable metastatic carcinoma or ectopic ACTH production.

Surgical removal is the treatment of choice for adrenal adenoma or carcinoma. If the tumor is successfully removed, adrenal insufficiency ensues and the patient temporarily requires glucocorticoid therapy. Recovery of normal hypothalamic-pituitary-adrenal function may be delayed for as long as two years.[49]

Nelson's Syndrome

Nelson's syndrome develops in 10 to 40 percent of patients with Cushing's disease (i.e., pituitary ACTH excess) who are treated with bilateral adrenalectomy.[50] This syndrome, characterized by dramatic hyperpigmentation of the skin and chromophobe tumor of the pituitary gland, can develop six months to 15 years after adrenalectomy. In some patients, aggressive local tumor growth causes ophthalmoplegia, visual defect, or, occasionally, pituitary infarction. Because it is not known which features of Cushing's syndrome predict the development of Nelson's

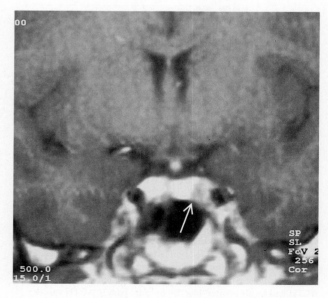

Figure 7 **Magnetic resonance imaging of the pituitary gland after administration of intravenous gadolinium shows an adenoma (arrow) 1 cm in diameter in the left side of the anterior pituitary gland.**

syndrome, patients treated with bilateral adrenalectomy need follow-up at regular intervals. Diagnosis is made by demonstrating hyperpigmentation, enlargement of the sella, and elevated ACTH levels.

Plasma ACTH levels after adrenalectomy for Cushing's syndrome tend to be higher than ACTH levels observed in spontaneous Addison's disease and often increase 20-fold to 300 to 1,000 pg/ml. ACTH levels in Nelson's syndrome almost always exceed 1,000 pg/ml. It is likely, although not certain, that a yearly measurement of plasma ACTH will detect the disease before it becomes clinically apparent. Treatments include surgery, heavy-particle irradiation, cyproheptadine, and bromocriptine. Reports differ on whether prophylactic pituitary irradiation prevents the development of postadrenalectomy Nelson's syndrome.

Pharmacological Use of Glucocorticoids

The glucocorticoids are both boon and bane to the clinician. Although their use in certain diseases is lifesaving, they produce Cushing's syndrome in some patients and hypothalamic-pituitary-adrenal suppression in all patients on long-term therapy.[51] Certain complications seem to be unique to iatrogenic Cushing's syndrome, including those of benign intracranial hypertension, glaucoma, cataracts, and pancreatitis.[51]

Hypothalamic-pituitary-adrenal suppression, although seldom documented as a cause of death, remains a concern in the patient treated with steroids. It is impossible to state the minimal duration of therapy that will suppress endogenous function; if time allows, the short ACTH test can be performed. A 0.25 mg dose of cosyntropin is given intravenously, and if the plasma cortisol at 30 minutes is greater than 18 ng/dl, the hypothalamic-pituitary axis is judged to be normal. Often, however, there is no time to wait for this result; thus, it is wise to give steroid supplementation to any patient previously treated with steroids. A reassessment of the history and experience of secondary adrenal insufficiency has suggested that pharmacological steroid coverage has been needlessly broad and that steroid dose should be guided by two things: the long-term prestress dosage of steroid and the magnitude of the acute illness or surgery. For minor surgery, 25 to 50 mg/day of hydrocortisone equivalent is adequate; for intermediate stress, 50 to 75 mg/day; and for major surgery, 100 to 150 mg/day for one to three days.[52] This treatment can be tapered by 50 percent each day, beginning two days after surgery if all is going well.

Patients who experience severe hypothalamic-pituitary-adrenal suppression may not recover fully for as long as two years after all steroid therapy has been discontinued, and there seems to be no way to hasten the process. During that period, they may have withdrawal symptoms despite normal basal cortisol levels and some pituitary responsiveness to challenge. To judge recovery, the best test appears to be the plasma cortisol response to ACTH or to insulin-induced hypoglycemia.[53] A basal or stimulated level greater than 18 μg/dl indicates normal adrenal responsiveness. No test, however, is 100 percent reliable. The synthetic ACTH stimulation test is occasionally normal in patients who respond subnormally to stress.[54]

Primary Aldosteronism

Primary aldosteronism is a syndrome of hypertension and hypokalemia that occurs in 0.05 to two percent of hypertensive patients[55]. The causes include unilateral adenoma (in about 70 percent of such patients), idiopathic bilateral hyperplasia (in 20 to 30 percent), and, rarely, adrenocortical carcinoma.[56-58] Patients with primary aldosteronism are found among the hypertensive population by noting borderline potassium levels, in the 3.4 to 3.6 mEq/L range, or frank hypokalemia that occurs either spontaneously or in patients on mild diuretics. In patients on diuretics, the drug should be withdrawn for four weeks and potassium repleted. Then, with the patient on a diet that provides at least 100 mEq of salt a day, the plasma aldosterone and renin levels are measured at 8 A.M. after overnight recumbency and again when the patient has been upright for four hours; a 24-hour urine aldosterone level is also determined. In addition to the hypokalemia that is usually caused by sodium loading, in patients with primary aldosteronism, the plasma renin level is less than 1 ng/ml/hr, the plasma aldosterone level is more than 15 ng/dl, and the urinary aldosterone metabolites are elevated. Localization of a tumor or confirmation of hyperplasia is then accomplished by computed tomography and bilateral adrenal vein sampling for both aldosterone and cortisol.[59]

The hypertension and hypokalemia of Conn's syndrome (unilateral adenoma) usually respond to unilateral adrenalectomy. Patients with hyperplasia are treated medically. Obtaining a single plasma aldosterone/plasma renin activity (PA/PRA) ratio has been suggested as a screening approach in primary hyperaldosteronism.[60,61]

The hypertension and hypokalemia induced by licorice ingestion result from the accumulation of glycyrrhizic acid in renal tubular cells and the consequent inhibition of an enzyme (11β-hydroxysteroid dehydrogenase) that inactivates mineralocorticoids.[16] Glucocorticoid-remediable aldosteronism (GRA) typically becomes manifest in childhood, and there is a high frequency of severe hypertension with stroke among young adults of affected families. As in Conn's syndrome, hypokalemia is common but not present often enough to be useful in screening. Inherited as an autosomal dominant disorder, GRA is caused by the mutant formation of a chimeric gene in the zona fasciculata whose protein product combines 11β-hydroxylase and aldosterone synthase activities. This defect results in aldosterone excess that depends on ACTH rather than angiotensin; by suppressing ACTH, glucocorticoids reduce both hypertension and hypokalemia. As with other autosomal dominant disorders, screening has disclosed many more affected individuals than had been previously suspected.[62]

Hypofunction of the Adrenal Cortex

Acute adrenal insufficiency is a rare condition that usually develops during a severe illness. The most common cause is adrenal hemorrhage in patients on anticoagulants; there seems to be an increased association with heparin-induced thrombocytopenia and with the antiphospholipid antibody syndrome.[63,64] Insufficiency can also develop during acute sepsis or after surgery, trauma, myocardial infarction, or pregnancy.[65] The clinical features of acute adrenal failure include nausea, weakness, hypotension, collapse, and abdominal or back pain. This pain may be the only clue to onset of a complicating adrenal insufficiency.[66-68]

The workup is simple. Routine laboratory tests are likely to reveal a low serum sodium level and elevation of blood urea nitrogen (BUN) and potassium levels. Definitive evaluation, however, requires plasma cortisol levels drawn before and 60 minutes after administration of 0.25 mg of synthetic ACTH (Cortrosyn). If the diagnosis is seriously entertained, the patient should be given 100 mg of hydrocortisone intravenously, followed by 10 mg/hr I.V. until the cortisol result is obtained. In desperate circumstances, the ACTH test should be deferred and the treatment begun immediately after a sample has been drawn for the plasma cortisol measurement. A cortisol level below 10 μg/dl when the test sample is examined in retrospect suggests at least partial adrenal insufficiency; a value over 18 μg/dl indicates a normal response to stress. Both CT and MRI can confirm the diagnosis of adrenal hemorrhage.

ADDISON'S DISEASE

Chronic adrenal insufficiency, or Addison's disease, has two main origins. Granulomatous infections, such as tuberculosis and histoplasmosis, now account for a minority of cases in the United States. The more common cause is an autoimmune disorder in which lymphocytic and plasma cell invasion of the adrenal is accompanied by antiadrenal antibodies in the plasma. This condition may occur alone or with hypothyroidism secondary to Hashimoto's thyroiditis [see Polyendocrine Deficiency Syndromes, below]. Adrenal insufficiency can also occur as one feature of a hereditary disorder marked by progressive myelin degeneration in the brain (adrenoleukodystrophy) or the spinal cord (adrenomyelodystrophy).

Adrenal insufficiency can complicate the acquired immunodeficiency syndrome (AIDS).[69] The adrenals are infiltrated by opportunistic pathogens and by Kaposi's sarcoma. Although decreased adrenal reserve has been reported in several series of patients, classic adrenal insufficiency, confirmed by testing and by response to therapy, has been seen less often in AIDS patients. Treatment of AIDS patients with megestrol, a progestin analogue with a putative anabolic effect, occasionally suppresses the pituitary-adrenal axis and causes hypoadrenalism.[70-72]

Computed tomography has shed new light on the etiology of adrenal insufficiency. Enlarged adrenals suggest active tuberculous adrenalitis[73] or metastatic tumor, each with important clinical implications. Patients thought to have active tuberculosis should receive definitive therapy. One interesting implication of this decision has emerged: rifampin therapy can precipitate adrenal insufficiency in untreated or treated addisonian patients.[74] This insufficiency state occurs because the drug induces hepatic steroid-metabolizing enzymes; such enzymes cause accelerated disposal of subnormal endogenous secretion or of ordinary therapeutic amounts of adrenal hormones. The anesthetic etomidate and the antifungal antibiotic ketoconazole can also induce reversible adrenal insufficiency, but their effect is secondary to impairment of corticosteroid biosynthesis.[75,76] Patients with metastases to the adrenals may develop adrenal insufficiency abruptly; therefore, when adrenal enlargement is found in a patient with known metastatic disease, prophylactic glucocorticoid replacement therapy should be considered.[77]

Patients with chronic adrenal insufficiency have weakness, anorexia, weight loss, hypotension, and hypovolemia. A useful clue to the diagnosis is the presence of hyperpigmentation concentrated over palmar and other body creases, over pressure points, and around the areolas of the nipples. Except for a tendency to hyperkalemia, routine laboratory findings are unimpressive until adrenal collapse occurs, at which time hyponatremia, hyperkalemia, hypoglycemia, hemoconcentration, and BUN elevation are seen. The changes in BUN and electrolytes are largely secondary to volume deficiency and prerenal azotemia. The only specific diagnostic test for adrenal insufficiency is measurement of plasma cortisol or urinary 17-OHS before and after administering ACTH. The choice of diagnostic test depends on assessment of the patient's clinical status.

If adrenal insufficiency does not appear to be present and a test is needed to rule it out, intravenous injection of 0.25 mg of synthetic ACTH is sensitive and specific. Plasma cortisol is measured before the injection and 60 minutes later. The normal response is an increase to a level of 18 μg/dl or greater [see Figure 8]. If the resting value is greater than 20 μg/dl, however, the rise may be minimal, and adrenocortical function should be considered normal.

The patient who is thought likely to have adrenal insufficiency (e.g., someone already hyponatremic or hypotensive) should be tested somewhat differently. A morning cortisol measurement and ACTH measurement should be taken, and then, to avoid adrenal collapse, the patient can be given 0.5 mg of dexamethasone twice daily and 0.1 mg of fludrocortisone daily during the testing. Cortisol is measured at 30 and 60 minutes after administration of a 0.25 mg dose of synthetic ACTH. A plasma cortisol level above 18 μg/dl establishes normal adrenal function; however, if the initial measurements showed cortisol to be low and it remains low and the ACTH to be above 100 pg/ml, the diagnosis of primary adrenal insufficiency is established.[78] Patients with hypopituitarism that causes hypoadrenalism can usually be distinguished from patients with primary adrenal insufficiency, or Addison's disease, by the presence of other pituitary hormone deficiencies and by an ACTH value at or below the lower limit of normal. Secondary adrenal insufficiency can also be confirmed by testing with metyrapone (30 mg/kg given orally with food at midnight). A plasma 11-deoxycortisol level above 7 μg/dl confirms normal hypothalamic-pituitary-adrenal (HPA) axis function. This test should be done in the inpatient setting because of the possibility of inducing adrenal insufficiency. On occasion, metyrapone testing will disclose a subnormal response in a patient with a normal acute ACTH test.[79] In such patients, especially those with less than six weeks' onset of pituitary deficiency, the intravenous ACTH test can be normal because adrenal atrophy has not yet occurred.

In patients suspected of having adrenal crisis, no delay for diagnostic purposes should be allowed. The same needle that is used to draw blood for measurement of plasma cortisol and ACTH should be used to administer the first treatment. Replacement therapy for acute adrenal insufficiency is best carried out with intravenous hydrocortisone hemisuccinate, 100 mg as an initial bolus followed by 10 mg/hr during the first two days of the crisis. Intravenous glucose in saline, plasma expanders, and, in some cases, blood should be administered to restore circulating vol-

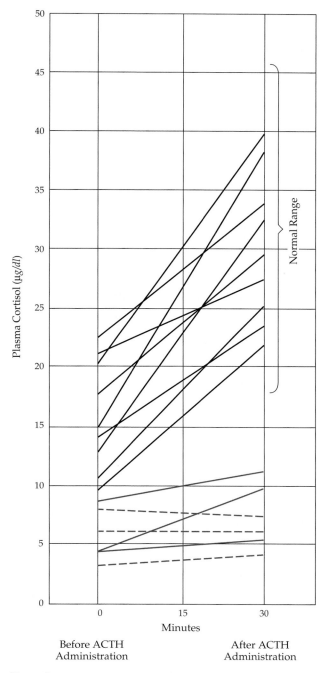

Figure 8 **Administration of synthetic ACTH, 0.25 mg intravenously, is a powerful tool for diagnosing adrenal insufficiency. ACTH is administered at time 0, after measurement of plasma cortisol. After an interval of 30 minutes, plasma cortisol is measured again. In these data, the nine normal individuals (solid black lines) all show elevated plasma cortisol levels of 20 μg/dl or greater. However, patients with adrenal insufficiency (broken blue lines) and patients with pituitary insufficiency (solid blue lines) have plasma cortisol levels that are well below the normal range.**

ume. Because the addisonian patient usually has a borderline volume deficiency before the acute crisis develops, large volumes of fluid may be needed. If the patient's condition is improving, steroid doses can be tapered over three to five days to replacement levels.

Replacement therapy for chronic adrenal insufficiency consists of administration of 20 to 25 mg of cortisone in the morning on arising and 10 to 15 mg of cortisone in the late afternoon. The patient also receives oral fludrocortisone, 0.05 to 0.10 mg daily. The effect of this dosage should be monitored by watching the patient for weight gain or hypokalemia. Steroid dosage should be increased on an elective basis whenever the patient with chronic adrenal insufficiency is exposed to major stress. For an ordinary upper respiratory infection or influenza, it is sufficient to double the daily dose of cortisone. If a patient with Addison's disease experiences vomiting, however, prompt hospitalization for the administration of intravenous fluids and hydrocortisone is advisable.

SECONDARY ADRENAL INSUFFICIENCY

Patients with hypopituitarism that includes ACTH deficiency have a syndrome similar to Addison's disease except for a lesser degree of volume deficiency. Because aldosterone is primarily under angiotensin control, electrolyte regulation and volume regulation are less affected in the patient with panhypopituitarism than in the patient with Addison's disease. Patients with cortisol deficiency of any cause, including panhypopituitarism, are prone to water overload and are likely to become hyponatremic. Plasma ACTH levels are typically elevated in patients with primary adrenal failure and are normal or unmeasurable in patients with primary ACTH deficiency.

CRH, which is now available, may help distinguish between hypothalamic and pituitary etiologies of secondary adrenal insufficiency. If an insulin tolerance test shows no cortisol response to hypoglycemia, secondary hypoadrenalism is present. If in such a patient a CRH test elicits a prompt ACTH release, then, by inference, hypothalamic disease is likely; if CRH does not elicit release of ACTH, then presumably the lesion is in the pituitary.[80]

ALDOSTERONE DEFICIENCY SYNDROMES

Occasionally, aldosterone deficiency is the only, or predominant, sign of adrenal insufficiency. Isolated defects of aldosterone biosynthesis are rare,[81] but partial defects are an aspect of congenital adrenal hyperplasia caused by 21-hydroxylase deficiency. Symptoms attributable to aldosterone deficiency may provide the principal early diagnostic clues to hypoadrenalism; for example, postural hypotension may occur before anorexia, weight loss, asthenia, and hyperpigmentation.

Two syndromes of isolated aldosterone deficiency, idiopathic hypoaldosteronism and hyporeninemic hypoaldosteronism, deserve separate mention.[82] The rare condition idiopathic hypoaldosteronism presents as heart block, secondary to hyperkalemia, or as postural hypotension, secondary to hypovolemia with or without significant hyponatremia. Patients would be expected to demonstrate low plasma and urinary aldosterone levels combined with increased plasma renin activity, although few reports are available. The administration of fludrocortisone, in a dosage of 0.05 to 0.10 mg daily, combined with liberal salt intake, is effective treatment for idiopathic hypoaldosteronism.

Hyporeninemic hypoaldosteronism is much more common than idiopathic hypoaldosteronism. In mild forms, the former condition is perhaps still underdiagnosed. Typical patients are older than 45 years and have chronic renal disease. The kidney disorder affects the tubular and interstitial tissue more than it does the glomeruli. Diabetes mellitus is a common finding. The hallmark of hyporeninemic hypoaldosteronism is mild to marked chronic hyperkalemia, which is sometimes worsened abruptly by hyperglycemia. A hyperchloremic metabolic acidosis, with a normal or low sodium level, is usually present. Restricting sodium intake aggravates the clinical manifestations. The underlying physiologic derangement is a plasma renin level that is low despite hyperkalemia, volume contraction, and hyponatremia. Although the cause of the low renin level is disputed, it is usually attributed to a defect in the juxtaglomerular apparatus. Prostaglandin deficiency induced by nonsteroidal anti-inflammatory drugs (NSAIDs) has been shown to be a reversible cause of the syndrome. In other cases, the disorder has been aggravated by heparin, calcium channel blockers, or beta-adrenergic blockers. The treatment of hyporeninemic hypoaldosteronism includes correction of acidosis, liberalization of sodium intake, and judicious use of fludrocortisone as required for controlling the potassium elevation without inducing congestive heart failure [see Chapter 160]. Heparin is a potent inhibitor of aldosterone production with a consequent natriuresis and occasional hyponatremia. Hyperkalemia occurs in fewer than 10 percent of patients, but it can be rapid and severe in patients with renal failure or diabetes mellitus or patients who are taking medications that raise serum potassium levels.[83]

Polyendocrine Deficiency Syndromes

Just as hyperfunction and neoplasia can affect more than one gland [see Chapter 45], so can endocrine deficiency. The term polyendocrine deficiency syndromes (or polyglandular autoimmune syndromes) refers to two overlapping but distinct clusterings of endocrine deficiency.[84-86] Type I includes hypoparathyroidism, hypoadrenalism, and mucocutaneous moniliasis, with pernicious anemia and chronic hepatitis as occasional features; onset in childhood is characteristic. Type II, also called Schmidt's syndrome, includes adrenal insufficiency, Hashimoto's thyroiditis, and, less often, insulin-dependent diabetes mellitus; onset by 30 years of age is common. Autoimmune causation is suggested by lymphocytic infiltration of the glands, the frequent finding of antiglandular antibodies, and association with known autoimmune disorders such as pernicious anemia and alopecia. Premature primary gonadal failure occurs in some patients with polyendocrine deficiency. Patients with the polyglandular autoimmune syndromes should be monitored closely because a second or third endocrine abnormality can develop. Further, because the polyendocrine deficiency syndromes are familial disorders, with a mostly autosomal recessive pattern,[87] other family members should be screened for endocrine hypofunction.

Adrenal Neoplasms and Incidentalomas

A minority of adrenal neoplasms have endocrine function.[88] Both adenomas and carcinomas can produce Cushing's syndrome and virilizing disorders. Carcinomas are typically inefficient in their biosynthetic patterns; as a result, urinary steroid values may provide a clue to the diagnosis. Adrenal cancer should be suspected in a patient with Cushing's syndrome who has a disproportionately high concentration of urinary 17-ketogenic steroids relative to 17-OHS or in a woman with virilization who is excreting more than 50 mg of 17-KS a day. Although virilization is uncommon with benign adenomas, several cases of adenomas that produced only testosterone have been reported. These cases are of particular note[89-92] because the urinary 17-KS levels were not high, as they usually are with adrenal neoplasms that cause hirsutism, and because two of the tumors responded to chorionic gonadotropin by increasing production of testosterone. In several respects, these adrenal tumors behaved as if they were derived from gonadal tissue. Feminizing tumors are the least frequent of all adrenal neoplasms; they should be considered in the diagnosis of males who show feminization, particularly if urinary 17-KS levels, as well as estrogen levels, are elevated.[93,94]

The widespread use of abdominal CT scanning has introduced a new problem: the incidentally discovered adrenal mass, or so-called incidentaloma. If the lesion is a cyst or a myelolipoma, nothing need be done. If a solitary solid mass is suggested, an economical screening for hormone-producing tumor is recommended. Some clinics screen only for hyperaldosteronism and pheochromocytoma; however, I believe that the screening should include a 1 mg dexamethasone suppression test for Cushing's syndrome, a serum potassium measurement for aldosteronism, a plasma DHEAS or 24-hour urine 17-KS test for androgen excess, and a 24-hour urine catecholamine test for pheochromocytoma. The dexamethasone suppression test sometimes unmasks dysfunction in patients who fail to show a suppressed cortisol level and yet do not have a cushingoid appearance.[95-97] Such patients may experience adrenal insufficiency if the adenoma is removed.[98] If an endocrine abnormality is confirmed, surgery is indicated. For nonfunctioning lesions, the size of the lesion is a useful guide. Lesions less than 6 cm in diameter are almost always benign. Lesions greater than 6 cm in diameter harbor cancer often enough to warrant removal.

Fine-needle aspiration (after the pheochromocytoma has been removed) can be helpful. If a metastatic tumor is identified, the primary tumor can be sought. If an adrenal tumor is recognized, although cytology may be inconclusive, a combination of the appearance plus lesion size will usually lead to a proper decision regarding surgery.[99-101]

Congenital Adrenal Hyperplasia

Congenital adrenal hyperplasia (CAH) denotes a group of hereditary disorders characterized by enzymatic defects in cortisol synthesis. These defects result in increased corticotropin levels with consequent androgen excess. In the genetic female, the hyperandrogenism produces external genital masculinization of the fetus and, if untreated, primary amenorrhea, hypoestrinism, and hirsutism at puberty. In more than 90 percent of CAH cases, there is deficient 21-

hydroxylase activity; 11-hydroxylase, 3-β-ol-dehydrogenase, 17-hydroxylase, and other enzymes involved in cortisol synthesis are less commonly affected. Cortisol therapy suppresses ACTH, decreases the high plasma levels of cortisol precursors, and corrects the clinical disorder.

The gene encoding the 21-hydroxylase enzyme, along with a related pseudogene, is located on chromosome 6 within the HLA segment. Several distinct mutations of these genes have been identified as causes of enzyme deficiency with resulting CAH.[102] The worldwide incidence of the 21-hydroxylase deficiency is estimated to be one in 14,000 births, but there is considerable genetic heterogeneity and not all manifestations are thus far explicable.

Complete 21-hydroxylase deficiency is usually manifest in the newborn as hypertrophy and virilization of the genitalia. Milder expressions of the same pathophysiology are clinically relevant in adolescence and adulthood. Heterozygotes and homozygotes for the defect (identified by genetic studies of HLA phenotype) have been found to have variable degrees of hirsutism and menstrual disturbance. Thus, some patients with so-called idiopathic hirsutism, oligomenorrhea, or even polycystic ovary syndrome have adrenal androgen excess secondary to partial defects in cortisol biosynthesis. In cases in which there is no congenital virilization, the syndrome is called nonclassic congenital adrenal hyperplasia (NC-CAH). The simplest approach is to start with a plasma 17-hydroxyprogesterone (17-OHP) drawn before 9:00 A.M. during the follicular phase of the menstrual cycle. If this cortisol precursor level is 200 ng/dl or lower, the diagnosis is excluded. If the value is 500 ng/dl or higher, the diagnosis is established. Patients with values between those levels should be given 0.25 mg of synthetic ACTH intravenously and have their plasma 17-OHP measured at 60 minutes. Affected individuals have 17-OHP levels above 1,500 ng/dl at that time. Patients with values between 1,000 and 1,500 ng/dl may be manifesting heterozygosity.[103] There is considerable disagreement about the frequency of this abnormality and about the proper test to demonstrate mild expressions of it.[104]

A practical yield of a positive test is that partial pituitary-adrenal suppression, such as that which is induced by giving 5 mg of prednisone at bedtime, can improve menstrual regularity and decrease hirsutism. Partial deficiencies of 11-hydroxylation and of 3β-hydroxysteroid dehydrogenase have also been suggested as possible variants of NC-CAH that produce hirsutism; prednisone suppression as described above is suitable for treating patients with these deficiencies. For those with pure hirsutism, the androgen antagonist spironolactone is appropriate.

Hirsutism

A woman's concern about excessive hair is one of the most frequent reasons for endocrine consultation. Three questions are helpful in deciding what type of evaluation to pursue [see Table 1]: When did the excessive hair growth begin? Is a similar pattern found in family members? Are menses regular or irregular?

Familial hirsutism that begins in puberty and is accompanied by regular periods is the least worrisome condition; most patients need only reassurance. Little endocrine investigation is needed, but cosmetic treatment and spironolactone administration can be tried.

Hirsutism that is disproportionate to the patient's ethnic background and accompanied by normal periods is termed idiopathic. Although it is not necessary to do any endocrine studies, a simple workup may include measurements of total and free testosterone and 17-OHP. If the testosterone and 17-OHP levels are normal, the patient can be reassured that the condition is benign. Occasionally, patients with hirsutism and normal periods have NC-CAH. The pubertal onset of hirsutism and irregular periods essentially defines polycystic ovary syndrome. Ovarian hyperandrogenism is the most common underlying abnormality [see Chapter 51], often but not invariably reflected in an elevated testosterone level. Because NC-CAH can cause polycystic ovary syndrome, however, measurement of 17-OHP should be considered, particularly in a patient who desires fertility.

Patients with idiopathic hirsutism and no menstrual abnormality may nonetheless seek reduction of their hair growth. Cosmetic approaches, such as use of waxes or depilatories or electrolysis, are often all that are needed. The endocrine options include oral contraceptives, which have

Table 1 Clinical Characteristics of Different Types of Hirsutism

Type of Hirsutism	Time of Onset	Familial Incidence	Menstrual Cycle
Familial hirsutism	Puberty	Yes	Regular
Idiopathic hirsutism	Puberty	No	Regular
Hirsutism associated with nonclassic congenital adrenal hyperplasia	Puberty	Yes or No	Oligomenorrhea or normal menses
Hirsutism associated with polycystic ovary syndrome	Puberty	No	Irregular from onset
Hirsutism with virilization	Adulthood	No	Formerly regular, but now irregular or absent

multiple effects, including reduction of circulating free testosterone levels and androgen antagonism at the target tissue. The best type of oral contraceptive to use for reduction of hair growth is one that has a nonandrogenic progestin component, such as Demulen. Administration of the aldosterone antagonist spironolactone is a good approach either alone or with an oral contraceptive. Dosages of 100 to 150 mg daily of spironolactone are often necessary. In patients with diabetes mellitus or renal impairment, this drug can rapidly induce severe hyperkalemia and should be avoided. Finally, the 5α-reductase inhibitor finasteride has been used abroad with some promising results.[105,106] However, it has not yet been approved in the United States.

New-onset hirsutism in an adult female, especially when associated with amenorrhea, requires complete investigation to exclude an adrenal or ovarian tumor. If there are signs of Cushing's syndrome, the workup previously described should follow. In this setting, DHEAS should be measured as a clue to adrenal androgen excess. If, on the other hand, there is pure virilization, the plasma testosterone and DHEAS levels should be measured. If the plasma testosterone level is 1.5 ng/ml or higher, both the ovaries and the adrenals should be imaged. If the DHEAS level is elevated, adrenal suppression with dexamethasone and adrenal CT scanning should be considered.[107,108]

The Adrenal Medulla

PHYSIOLOGY

The adrenal medulla consists of chromaffin tissue of neuroectodermal origin. It is the body's major source of epinephrine, which is synthesized from tyrosine via the intermediate dopamine. Dopamine β-hydroxylase catalyzes hydroxylation of dopamine to norepinephrine (of which the adrenal is a minor source), and norepinephrine is methylated to form epinephrine by catecholamine N-methyltransferase. This enzyme is induced by cortisol that has arrived at the medulla directly from the adrenal cortex. Thus, cortical function ultimately regulates medullary function.

Epinephrine has numerous effects on intermediary metabolism, including promotion of hepatic glycogenolysis, inhibition of hepatic gluconeogenesis, and inhibition of insulin release; epinephrine also promotes free fatty acid release from triglyceride stores in adipose tissue. Epinephrine has a positive inotropic effect on the heart, elicits a pressor response, and produces a mixture of constriction and dilatation in different vascular beds. Ironically, although epinephrine has these manifold metabolic and cardiovascular effects, this hormone does not need to be replaced in the adrenalectomized or addisonian patient.[109,110]

PHEOCHROMOCYTOMA

The only significant pathological condition associated with the adrenal medulla is the highly vascular and exuberantly secreting pheochromocytoma.[111-113] Intermittent hypertension has been considered the hallmark of pheochromocytoma, but about 15 percent of patients have sustained hypertension, 45 percent have paroxysmal hypertension, and 40 percent have sustained hypertension plus paroxysms. Associated symptoms that should call attention to the diagnosis include sweating, headaches, episodic palpita-

tions, hypermetabolism, mental changes (including psychosis), and congestive heart failure caused by myocarditis or focal myocardial necrosis.[114] Postural hypotension is a common finding on physical examination; it is caused partly by a decrease in the plasma volume. Many rare disorders may be associated with pheochromocytomas; medullary thyroid carcinoma, the most common of these, is curable [see Chapter 46].

References

1. Orth DN, Kovaks WJ, DeBold CR: The adrenal cortex. William's Textbook of Endocrinology, 8th ed. Wilson JD, Foster DW, Eds. WB Saunders Co, Philadelphia, 1992, p 489

2. Meikle AW, Daynes RA, Araneo BA: Adrenal androgen secretion and biologic effects. Endocrinol Metab Clin North Am 20:381, 1991

3. Quinn SJ, Williams GH: Regulation of aldosterone secretion. Ann Rev Physiol 50:409, 1988

4. Orth DN: Corticotropin-releasing hormone in humans. Endocr Rev 13:164, 1992

5. Watabe T, Tanaka K, Kumagae M, et al: Role of endogenous arginine vasopressin in potentiating corticotropin-releasing hormone-stimulated corticotropin secretion in man. J Clin Endocrinol Metab 66:1132, 1988

6. Salata RA, Jarrett DB, Verbalis JG, et al: Vasopressin stimulation of adrenocorticotropin hormone (ACTH) in humans. J Clin Invest 81:766, 1988

7. Iranmanesh A, Lizarralde G, Short D, et al: Intensive venous sampling paradigms disclose high frequency adrenocorticotropin release episodes in normal men. J Clin Endocrinol Metab 71:1276, 1990

8. Dallman MF, Akana SF, Levin N, et al: Corticosteroids and the control of function in the hypothalamo-pituitary-adrenal (HPA) axis. Ann NY Acad Sci 746:22, 1994

9. Findling JW, Engeland WC, Raff H: The use of immunoradiometric assay for the measurement of ACTH in human plasma. Trends in Endocrinol Metab 1:283, 1990

10. Kaye TB, Crapo L: The Cushing syndrome: an update on diagnostic tests. Ann Intern Med 112:434, 1990

11. Kannan CR: Diseases of the adrenal cortex. DM 34:613, 1988

12. Sheeler LR: Cushing's syndrome. Cleve Clin J Med 55:329, 1988

13. Biller BMK, Alexander JM, Zervas NT, et al: Clonal origins of adrenocorticotropin-secreting pituitary tissue in Cushing's disease. J Clin Endocrinol Metab 75:1303, 1992

14. Odell WD: Ectopic ACTH secretion: a misnomer. Endocrinol Metab Clin North Am 20:371, 1991

15. Ulick S, Wang JZ, Blumenfeld JD, et al: Cortisol inactivation overload: a mechanism of mineralocorticoid hypertension in the ectopic adrenocorticotropin syndrome. J Clin Endocrinol Metab 74:963, 1992

16. Williams GH: Guardian of the gate: receptors, enzymes, and mineralocorticoid function (editorial). J Clin Endocrinol Metab 74:961, 1992

17. Belsky JL, Cuello B, Swanson LW, et al: Cushing's syndrome due to ectopic production of corticotropin-releasing factor. J Clin Endocrinol Metab 60:496, 1985

18. King DR, Lack EE: Adrenal cortical carcinoma: a clinical and pathologic study of 49 cases. Cancer 44:239, 1979

19. Malchoff CD, MacGillivray D, Malchoff DM: Adrenocorticotropic hormone–independent adrenal hyperplasia. Endocrinologist 6:79, 1996

20. Hermus AR, Pieters GF, Smals AG, et al: Transition from pituitary-dependent to adrenal-dependent Cushing's syndrome. N Engl J Med 318:966, 1988

21. Young WF Jr, Carney JA, Musa BU, et al: Familial Cushing's syndrome due to primary pigmented nodular adrenocortical disease: reinvestigation 50 years later. N Engl J Med 321:1659, 1989

22. Reznik Y, Allali-Zerah V, Chayvialle JA, et al: Food-dependent Cushing's syndrome mediated by aberrant adrenal sensitivity to gastric inhibitory polypeptide. N Engl J Med 327:981, 1992

23. Lacroix A, Bolté E, Tremblay J, et al: Gastric inhibitory polypeptide-dependent cortisol hypersecretion—a new cause of Cushing's syndrome. N Engl J Med 327:974, 1992

24. Bertagna X: New causes of Cushing's syndrome (editorial). N Engl J Med 327:1024, 1992

25. Kreisberg R: Half a loaf. N Engl J Med 330:1295, 1994

26. Findling JW: Clinical application of a new immunoradiometric assay for ACTH. Endocrinologist 2:360, 1992

27. Snow K: Biochemical evaluation of adrenal dysfunction: the laboratory perspective. Mayo Clin Proc 67:1055, 1992

28. Flack MR, Oldfield EH, Cutler GB Jr, et al: Urine free cortisol in the high-dose dexamethasone suppression test for the differential diagnosis of the Cushing syndrome. Ann Intern Med 116:211, 1992

29. Dichek HL, Nieman LK, Oldfield EH, et al: A comparison of the standard high dose dexamethasone suppression test and the overnight 8-mg dexamethasone suppression test for the differential diagnosis of adrenocorticotropin-dependent Cushing's syndrome. J Clin Endocrinol Metab 78:418, 1994

30. Zárate A, Kovaks K, Flores M, et al: ACTH and CRF-producing bronchial carcinoid associated with Cushing's syndrome. Clin Endocrinol 24:523, 1986

31. Grossman AB, Howlett TA, Perry L, et al: CRF in the differential diagnosis of Cushing's syndrome: a comparison with the dexamethasone suppression test. Clin Endocrinol 29:167, 1988

32. Nieman LK, Cutler GB Jr, Oldfield EH, et al: The ovine corticotropin-releasing hormone (CRH) stimulation test is superior to the human CRH stimulation test for the diagnosis of Cushing's disease. J Clin Endocrinol Metab 69:165, 1989

33. Schulte HM, Allolio B, Günther TK, et al: Bilateral and simultaneous sinus petrosus inferior catheterization in patients with Cushing's syndrome: plasma-immunoreactive-ACTH-concentrations before and after administration of CRF. Horm Metab Res (suppl) 16:66, 1987

34. Loriaux DL, Nieman L: Corticotropin-releasing hormone testing in pituitary disease. Endocrinol Metab Clin North Am 20:363, 1991

35. Malchoff CD, Orth DN, Abboud C, et al: Ectopic ACTH syndrome caused by a bronchial carcinoid tumor responsive to dexamethasone, metyrapone, and corticotropin-releasing factor. Am J Med 84:760, 1988

36. Lamberts SWJ, Reubi J-C: A role of (labeled) somatostatin analogs in the differential diagnosis and treatment of Cushing's syndrome (editorial). J Clin Endocrinol Metab 78:17, 1994

37. Krenning EP, Kwekkeboom DJ, Bakker WH, et al: Somatostatin receptor scintigraphy with [^{111}In-DTPA-D-Phe^1]- and [^{123}I-Tyr^3]-octreotide: the Rotterdam experience with more than 1000 patients. Eur J Nucl Med 20:716, 1993

38. Gold PW, Loriaux DL, Roy A, et al: Responses to corticotropin-releasing hormone in the hypercortisolism of depression and Cushing's disease. N Engl J Med 314:1329, 1986

39. Groote Veldman R, Meinders AE: On the mechanism of alcohol-induced pseudo-Cushing's syndrome. Endocr Rev 17:262, 1996

40. Shapiro MS, Shenkman L: Variable hormonogenesis in Cushing's syndrome. Q J Med 288:351, 1991

41. Guilhaume B, Bertagna X, Thomsen M, et al: Transsphenoidal pituitary surgery for the treatment of Cushing's disease: results in 64 patients and long term follow-up studies. J Clin Endocrinol Metab 66:1056, 1988

42. Melby JC: Therapy of Cushing disease: a consensus for pituitary microsurgery. Ann Intern Med 109:445, 1988

43. Mampalam TJ, Tyrrell JB, Wilson CB: Transsphenoidal microsurgery for Cushing disease. Ann Intern Med 109:487, 1988

44. Chandler WF, Schteingart DE, Lloyd RV, et al: Surgical treatment of Cushing's disease. J Neurosurg 66:204, 1987

45. Lamberts SWJ, van der Lely AJ, de Herder WW: Transsphenoidal selective adenomectomy is the treatment of choice in patients with Cushing's disease: considerations concerning preoperative medical treatment and the long-term follow-up (editorial). J Clin Endocrinol Metab 80:3111, 1995

46. Tahir AH, Sheeler LR: Recurrent Cushing's disease after transsphenoidal surgery. Arch Intern Med 152:977, 1992

47. Avgerinos PC, Nieman LK, Oldfield EH, et al: The effect of pulsatile human corticotropin-releasing hormone administration on the adrenal insufficiency that follows cure of Cushing's disease. J Clin Endocrinol Metab 68:912, 1989

48. Sarkar R, Thompson NW, McLeod MK: The role of adrenalectomy in Cushing's syndrome. Surgery 108:1079, 1990

49. Doherty GM, Nieman LK, Cutler GB Jr, et al: Time to recovery of the hypothalamic-pituitary-adrenal axis after curative resection of adrenal tumors in patients with Cushing's syndrome. Surgery 108:1085, 1990

50. Grua JR, Nelson DH: ACTH-producing pituitary tumors. Endocrinol Metab Clin North Am 20:319, 1991

51. Axelrod L: Glucocorticoid therapy. Medicine (Baltimore) 55:39, 1976

52. Salem M, Tainsh RE Jr, Bromberg J, et al: Perioperative glucocorticoid coverage: a reassessment 42 years after emergence of a problem. Ann Surg 219:416, 1994

53. May ME, Carey RM: Rapid adrenocorticotropic hormone test in practice. Am J Med 79:679, 1985

54. Streeten DHP, Anderson GH Jr, Bonaventura MM: The potential for serious consequences from misinterpreting normal responses to the rapid adrenocorticotropin test. J Clin Endocrinol Metab 81:285, 1996

55. Gittler RD, Fajans SS: Primary aldosteronism (Conn's syndrome). J Clin Endocrinol Metab 80:3438, 1995

56. White PC: Disorders of aldosterone biosynthesis and action. N Engl J Med 331:250, 1994

57. Blumenfeld JD, Sealey JE, Schlussel Y, et al: Diagnosis and treatment of primary hyperaldosteronism. Ann Intern Med 121:877, 1994

58. Bravo EL: Primary aldosteronism: issues of diagnosis and management. Endocrinol Metab Clin North Am 23:271, 1994

59. Litchfield WR, Dluhy RG: Primary aldosteronism. Endocrinol Metab Clin North Am 24:593, 1995

60. Melby JC: Diagnosis of hyperaldosteronism. Endocrinol Metab Clin North Am 20:247, 1991

61. McKenna TJ, Sequeira SJ, Heffernan A, et al: Diagnosis under random conditions of all disorders of the renin-angiotensin-aldosterone axis, including primary hyperaldosteronism. J Clin Endocrinol Metab 73:952, 1991

62. Dluhy RG, Lifton RP: Glucocorticoid-remediable aldosteronism. Endocrinol Metab Clin North Am 23:285, 1994

63. McCroskey RD, Phillips A, Mott F, et al: Antiphospholipid antibodies and adrenal hemorrhage. Am J Hematol 36:60, 1991

64. Asherson RA, Hughes GR: Hypoadrenalism, Addison's disease and antiphospholipid antibodies (editorial). J Rheumatol 18:1, 1991

65. Claussen MS, Landercasper J, Cogbill TH: Acute adrenal insufficiency presenting as shock after trauma and surgery: three cases and review of the literature. J Trauma 32:94, 1992

66. Rao RH, Vagnucci AH, Amico JA: Bilateral massive adrenal hemorrhage: early recognition and treatment. Ann Intern Med 110:227, 1989

67. Fitzpatrick PM, Swensen SJ: Report of an unusual case of postoperative adrenal hemorrhage in a young man. Am J Med 86:487, 1989

68. Szalados JE, Vukmir RB: Acute adrenal insufficiency resulting from adrenal hemorrhage as indicated by post-operative hypotension. Intensive Care Med 20:216, 1994

69. Grinspoon SK, Bilezikian JP: HIV disease and the endocrine system. N Engl J Med 327:1360, 1992

70. Leinung MC, Liporace R, Miller CH: Induction of adrenal suppression by megestrol acetate in patients with AIDS. Ann Intern Med 122:843, 1995

71. Loprinzi CL: Effect of megestrol acetate on the human pituitary-adrenal axis. Mayo Clin Proc 67:1160, 1992

72. Oster MH, Enders SR, Samuels SJ, et al: Megestrol acetate in patients with AIDS and cachexia. Ann Intern Med 121:400, 1994

73. Vita JA, Silverberg SJ, Goland RS, et al: Clinical clues to the cause of Addison's disease. Am J Med 78:461, 1985

74. Kyriazopoulou V, Parparousi O, Vagenakis AG: Rifampicin-induced adrenal crisis in addisonian patients receiving corticosteroid replacement therapy. J Clin Endocrinol Metab 59:1204, 1984

75. Wagner RL, White PF, Kan PB, et al: Inhibition of adrenal steroidogenesis by the anesthetic etomidate. N Engl J Med 310:1415, 1984

76. Tucker WS Jr, Snell BB, Island DP, et al: Reversible adrenal insufficiency induced by ketoconazole. JAMA 253:2413, 1985

77. Seidenwurm DJ, Elmer EB, Kaplan LM, et al: Metastases to the adrenal glands and the development of Addison's disease. Cancer 54:552, 1984

78. Grinspoon SK, Biller BMK: Clinical Review 62: laboratory assessment of adrenal insufficiency. J Clin Endocrinol Metab 79:923, 1994

79. Fiad TM, Kirby JM, Cunningham SK, et al: The overnight single-dose metyrapone test is a simple and reliable index of the hypothalamic-pituitary-adrenal axis. Clin Endocrinol 40:603, 1994

80. Hermus ARMM, Pieters GFFM, Pesman GJ, et al: CRH as a diagnostic and heuristic tool in hypothalamic-pituitary diseases. Horm Metab Res (suppl) 16:68, 1987

81. Ulick S, Wang JZ, Morton DH: The biochemical phenotypes of two inborn errors in the biosynthesis of aldosterone. J Clin Endocrinol Metab 72:1415, 1992

82. Jagger PI: Hypoaldosteronism. Endocrinologist 5:23, 1995

83. Oster JR, Singer I, Fishman LM: Heparin-induced aldosterone suppression and hyperkalemia. Am J Med 98:575, 1995

84. Leshin M: Southwestern Internal Medicine Conference: polyglandular autoimmune syndromes. Am J Med Sci 290:77, 1985

85. Trence DL, Morley JE, Handwerger BS: Polyglandular autoimmune syndromes. Am J Med 77:107, 1984

86. Loriaux DL: The polyendocrine deficiency syndromes (editorial). N

Engl J Med 312:1568, 1985

87. Ahonen P, Myllärniemi S, Sipilä I, et al: Clinical variation of autoimmune polyendocrinopathy-candidiasis-ectodermal dystrophy (APECED) in a series of 68 patients. N Engl J Med 322:1829, 1990

88. Nakano M: Adrenal cortical carcinoma. Acta Pathol Jpn 38:163, 1988

89. Werk EE Jr, Sholiton LJ, Kalejs L: Testosterone-secreting adrenal adenoma under gonadotropin control. N Engl J Med 289:767, 1973

90. Givens JR, Andersen RN, Wiser WL, et al: A gonadotropin-responsive adrenocortical adenoma. J Clin Endocrinol Metab 38:126, 1974

91. Larson BA, Vanderlaan WP, Judd HL, et al: A testosterone-producing adrenal cortical adenoma in an elderly woman. J Clin Endocrinol Metab 42:882, 1976

92. Schteingart DE, Woodbury MC, Tsao HS, et al: Virilizing syndrome associated with an adrenal cortical adenoma secreting predominantly testosterone. Am J Med 67:140, 1979

93. Gabrilove JL, Sharma DC, Wotiz HH, et al: Feminizing adrenocortical tumors in the male: a review of 52 cases including a case report. Medicine (Baltimore) 44:37, 1965

94. Desai MB, Kapadia SN: Feminizing adrenocortical tumors in male patients: adenoma versus carcinoma. J Urol 139:101, 1988

95. Reincke M, Nieke J, Krestin GP, et al: Preclinical Cushing's syndrome in adrenal "incidentalomas": comparison with adrenal Cushing's syndrome. J Clin Endocrinol Metab 75:826, 1992

96. Herrera MF, Grant CS, van Heerden JA, et al: Incidentally discovered adrenal tumors: an institutional perspective. Surgery 110:1014, 1991

97. Rosen HN, Swartz SL: Subtle glucocorticoid excess in patients with adrenal incidentaloma. Am J Med 92:213, 1992

98. Bernini G, Sgró M, Molea N, et al: A documented clinical case of pre-Cushing's syndrome. Endocrinologist 5:377, 1995

99. Osella G, Terzolo M, Borretta G, et al: Endocrine evaluation of incidentally discovered adrenal masses (incidentalomas). J Clin Endocrinol Metab 79:1532, 1994

100. Cook DM, Loriaux DL: The incidental adrenal mass. Endocrinologist 6:4, 1996

101. Staren ED, Prinz RA: Selection of patients with adrenal incidentalomas for operation. Surg Clin North Am 75:499, 1995

102. White PC, New MI: Genetic basis of endocrine disease 2: congenital adrenal hyperplasia due to 21-hydroxylase deficiency. J Clin Endocrinol Metab 74:6, 1992

103. Azziz R, Dewailly D, Owerbach D: Clinical review 56: Nonclassic adrenal hyperplasia: current concepts. J Clin Endocrinol Metab 78:810, 1994

104. Rittmaster RS: Hyperandrogenism—what is normal? (editorial). N Engl J Med 327:194, 1992

105. Fruzzetti F, De Lorenzo D, Parrini D, et al: Effects of finasteride, a 5α-reductase inhibitor, on circulating androgens and gonadotropin secretion in hirsute women. J Clin Endocrinol Metab 79:831, 1994

106. Moghetti P, Castello R, Magnani CM, et al: Clinical and hormonal effects of the 5α-reductase inhibitor finasteride in idiopathic hirsutism. J Clin Endocrinol Metab 79:1115, 1994

107. Derksen J, Nagesser SK, Meinders AE, et al: Identification of virilizing adrenal tumors in hirsute women. N Engl J Med 331:968, 1994

108. McKenna TJ: Screening for sinister causes of hirsutism (editorial). N Engl J Med 331:1015, 1994

109. Wortsman J, Frank S, Cryer PE: Adrenomedullary response to maximal stress in humans. Am J Med 77:779, 1984

110. The function of adrenaline (editorial). Lancet 1:561, 1985

111. Daly PA, Landsberg L: Phaeochromocytoma: diagnosis and management. Baillière's Clin Endocrinol Metab 6:143, 1992

112. Golub MS, Tuck ML: Diagnostic and therapeutic strategies in pheochromocytoma. Endocrinologist 2:101, 1992

113. Whalen RK, Althausen AF, Daniels GH: Extra-adrenal pheochromocytoma. J Urol 147:1, 1992

114. Havlik RJ, Cahow CE, Kinder BE: Advances in the diagnosis and treatment of pheochromocytoma. Arch Surg 123:626, 1988

Acknowledgments

Figure 1   Albert Miller.

Figure 2   Alan D. Iselin.

Figure 3   Alan D. Iselin.

Figure 4   Dana Burns-Pizer. Adapted from cover drawing for the article "Nucleotide Sequence of Cloned cDNA for Bovine Corticotropin-β-Lipoprotein Precursor," by S. Nakanishi, A. Inoue, T. Kita, et al, in *Nature* 287:423, 1979. Reprinted by permission from *Nature.* © 1979 Macmillan Journals Limited.

Figure 5   Albert Miller. Reprinted from "ACTH, Lipotrophin and MSH in Health and Disease," by L. H. Rees, in *Clinics in Endocrinology and Metabolism* 6:142, 1977.

Figure 6   Sally Black.

Figure 8   Albert Miller. Reprinted from "Corticotropin Stimulation Tests," by W. R. Greig, M. K. Jasani, J. A. Boyle, et al, in *Memoirs of the Society for Endocrinology* 17:175, 1968.

50 Testis

Daniel D. Federman, M.D.

Physiology and Sexual Development

In the fetus, the testis is responsible for differentiation of the male genitalia. At puberty, the testis promotes the development of secondary sex characteristics and sexual behavior. In the adult male, the central function of the testis is spermatogenesis and maintenance of coital capacity. Older men show some evidence of a physiologic decline in gonadal function.

INTRAUTERINE PHYSIOLOGY

Normal embryos have the anatomic primordia for the internal and external differentiation of both males and females. Female development does not require the positive influence of either the fetal gonad or maternal estrogens. Male differentiation, however, requires a functioning fetal testis, which differentiates from the bipotential gonad of the early embryo in response to a gene known as *SRY*, the sex-determining region of the Y chromosome.[1]

Two hormones secreted by the fetal testis are required for male genital differentiation. Müllerian-inhibiting substance (MIS) is a member of a glycoprotein superfamily of growth factors; it suppresses development of the müllerian ducts (progenitors of the uterus and fallopian tubes) and may inhibit germ cell meiosis and foster testicular descent.[2,3] Testosterone, produced by the fetal testis in response to stimulation by chorionic gonadotropin, determines the remaining steps of masculine development by stimulating the wolffian ducts to develop into the vas deferens, seminal vesicle, and epididymis and by fostering external virilization of the embryo. Dihydrotestosterone, produced by reduction of testosterone in target-tissue cells by the enzyme 5α-reductase, promotes external virilization.

Testosterone and dihydrotestosterone exert their effects by binding to an intracellular receptor, one of a superfamily of receptor proteins that bind steroids, thyroid hormone, and vitamin D. The receptor molecules, which are structurally related to the c-*erb*-A proto-oncogenes, bind their respective hormones

and then attach to DNA sequences controlling the expression of specific genes [*see Figure 1*]. Each receptor has three domains. One domain binds the specific hormone, and a second domain binds to nuclear DNA sequences. The third domain, termed the variable-length domain, has a variable length in different receptors. Although dihydrotestosterone is the active molecule for most androgen effects, testosterone binds to the same receptor, albeit with lesser affinity. The conversion of testosterone to dihydrotestosterone in androgen target tissues can therefore be considered as amplification of the given amount of testosterone that is present.[4]

Defects in androgen effect underlie abnormal sexual differentiation. For example, complete absence of the androgen receptor produces the syndrome of testicular feminization, in which the patient is a 46,XY genetic male with a female external phenotype [*see* Defects in Androgen Synthesis or Effect, *below*]. Less extensive defects in the androgen receptor result in varying degrees of external genital ambiguity and are usually detected at birth.[5] An occasional patient with minimal receptor abnormality presents as an adult with hypospadias and testes smaller than normal. A defect in the steroid 5α-reductase type II, which is found in genital tissues, is another cause of incomplete genital masculinization at birth.

CHILDHOOD AND PUBERTY

The hypothalamus controls pituitary gonadotropin release by secreting gonadotropin-releasing hormone (GnRH) [*see Figure 2*]. This hormone is secreted by hypophysiotropic neurons of the median eminence of the hypothalamus and reaches the pituitary via the hypophyseal portal system. GnRH attaches to receptors on the gonadotropes, the pituitary cells that produce the gonadotropins follicle-stimulating hormone (FSH) and luteinizing hormone (LH). The stimulatory effect of GnRH is mediated through the mobilization of calcium ions and by an increase in the intracellular calcium level, which activates cal-

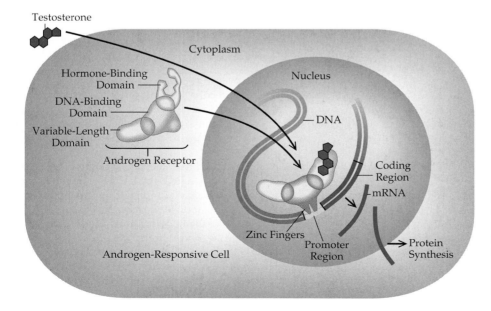

Figure 1 **The intracellular effects of testosterone are mediated by the androgen receptor in androgen-responsive cells. The hormone-receptor complex binds to the promoter region of an androgen-responsive gene, stimulating transcription of messenger RNA (mRNA) and protein synthesis.**

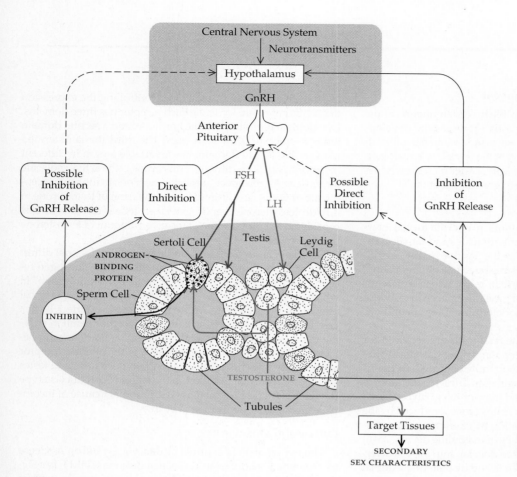

Figure 2 The hormonal regulation of activities in the pituitary-testicular axis involves interactions between the hypothalamus, anterior pituitary, testis, and ducts. The secretion of gonadotropin-releasing hormone (GnRH) by the hypothalamus stimulates the synthesis and release of follicle-stimulating hormone (FSH) and luteinizing hormone (LH) by the pituitary. FSH acts directly on the Sertoli cells within the testicular tubules to enhance the synthesis of an androgen-binding protein; FSH also promotes tubular opening. LH induces the Leydig cells to produce testosterone, which then diffuses into the adjacent tubules and enhances spermatogenesis. Testosterone acts, through a feedback loop, on the hypothalamus and possibly on the anterior pituitary, thereby limiting LH secretion. The protein inhibin, which is secreted by the Sertoli cells, acts on the pituitary to limit FSH secretion; it may also act indirectly via the hypothalamus to limit GnRH secretion and, consequently, FSH secretion.

modulin and, probably, protein kinase C and results in release of FSH, LH, and the free α-subunit of these two glycoprotein hormones (FSH and LH consist of a common α-subunit and distinct β-subunits).[6]

For the first four to six months of life, the male infant has a plasma testosterone level approximating that of a midpubertal boy, with secretion of hypothalamic GnRH maintaining pituitary-testicular secretion. Thereafter, pituitary-testicular function diminishes, and plasma levels of gonadotropins and testosterone remain low throughout childhood. The child's secretion of GnRH is either intrinsically minimal or inhibited by minuscule levels of gonadal steroid that have no known clinical effect.[7] Interestingly, the levels of MIS remain elevated during this time and fall when puberty appears.

Both FSH and LH are required for full testicular function. FSH stimulates the production of an androgen-binding protein in the Sertoli cells of the seminiferous tubules and in certain cells of the epididymis. This intracellular androgen receptor enables the cells to bind and respond to testosterone. FSH also induces the opening of the testicular tubules, which enlarges the testis during early puberty.

LH binds preferentially to the Leydig cells and, like FSH, stimulates adenylate cyclase. This action leads to a marked increase in testosterone formation. A small amount of estradiol, the corresponding estrogen, is also produced. Some testosterone is delivered directly to the testicular tubules, where it plays a major role in spermatogenesis. The remaining testosterone enters the bloodstream.

The complete pubertal maturation of the pituitary-testicular

system takes about three years. The initiating factor is unknown, but the initial increase in pituitary gonadotropin secretion occurs in sleep-related nocturnal bursts, or pulses, of LH and FSH, each triggered by a pulse of GnRH. During each sleep cycle, these pulses are followed by a rise in testosterone levels about an hour after the LH burst. They show a circadian rhythm, with higher values in the morning and lower values later in the day. As puberty advances, pulses of LH occur during the day as well as at night and then increase in both frequency and amplitude during a three- to four-year period. The plasma testosterone level eventually reaches adult levels of 400 to 1,200 ng/dl. Testosterone acts on the hypothalamus, and perhaps to a slight extent on the anterior pituitary itself, to inhibit LH release by lowering pulse frequency.[8] FSH secretion is subject to negative feedback (primarily at the pituitary) by inhibin, a protein produced in the Sertoli cells [*see Figure 2*]. This inhibitory action of inhibin is more easily detected during puberty than later in life; the role of this hormone in the adult male is not clear.

The development and maintenance of the mature male reproductive system thus reflect the balance achieved among three factors: hypothalamic stimulation of the pituitary via GnRH, pituitary stimulation of the testis by FSH and LH, and testicular inhibition of the hypothalamus and pituitary by inhibin and testosterone. The entire axis is under the control of the central nervous system. Testosterone exerts some of its effects directly and others only after it has been converted to dihydrotestosterone or estradiol. The onset of full testicular function is harder to determine than menarche, but sperm appears in the urine of boys at a mean age of 13 years and corresponds to a testicular volume of 10 ml.

Secondary Sex Characteristics

Important information on the development of secondary sex characteristics has been gleaned from the study of 5α-reductase deficiency, a disorder in which the intracellular conversion of testosterone to dihydrotestosterone is severely deficient. In this condition, FSH and LH levels are both slightly elevated and testosterone levels average higher than normal. Patients with 5α-reductase deficiency have internal male ducts, but their external genitalia are not fully masculinized. At puberty, children with 5α-reductase deficiency undergo almost all of the expected changes of male development: a growth spurt, male muscularity, deepening of the voice, male sexual drive, potency, and spermatogenesis—all produced by testosterone. However, the beard and prostate do not develop, suggesting that they require dihydrotestosterone. Because the urethra does not empty into a male phallus, these patients are infertile despite having active spermatogenesis.

NORMAL SEXUAL FUNCTION

Erection is basically a hydraulic event in which vascular channels that are empty in the flaccid penis become filled with arterial blood at pressures approaching systemic levels.[9] Erection occurs when the arteriolar and sinusoidal smooth muscles of the vessels of the corpora relax, thus lowering resistance in these channels [see Figure 3]. Arterial blood surges in, and its exit is impeded by an increase in venous resistance. Further distention of the sinusoids is restrained by the minimally distensible tunica albuginea. This inhibition of expansion restricts venous outflow and raises the pressure further. The corpora cavernosa and corpus spongiosum can be filled and the penis can be erect without placing much demand on cardiac output.

Although many details remain unclear, vasoactive intestinal polypeptide, perhaps aided by alpha-adrenergic blockade and acetylcholine, partially controls the vascular changes that occur during erection. Nitric oxide, a powerful endothelium-derived relaxing factor in many arteriolar systems, serves as a nonadrenergic, noncholinergic relaxant of the corpus cavernosum and may be the major factor in human erection.[10,11]

At least three controls of erection are clinically important. One is the availability of adequate arterial inflow from the aortoiliac system. The second is a neurologic control that involves two pathways: the reflexogenic and the erotogenic. In the reflexogenic pathway, the pudendal nerve serves as an afferent, there is a spinal level synapse, and parasympathetic fibers act as efferents. The erotogenic pathways, which are much more complex, include multiple afferent pathways, unknown central connections, and sympathetic outflow via the 10th dorsal through second lumbar segments. The third control of normal erection is hormonal: testosterone is required for the development of libido and potency and for maintenance of potency. The mechanism by which testosterone produces these effects is not clear, but its induction of nitric acid synthase, and thus nitric acid synthesis, may be involved.

Male Contraception

The search for an effective male contraceptive has not yet provided a clinically acceptable alternative to the condom. Synthetic pharmacological antagonists of GnRH reduce gonadotropin and testosterone secretion dramatically but do not routinely produce azoospermia.[12,13] Moreover, testosterone has to be used simultaneously with GnRH antagonists to prevent the loss of libido and potency caused by lowering testosterone levels. Testosterone itself can lower sperm counts and provide reliable control of fertility. However, the requirement for frequent injections has prevented the use of testosterone, either

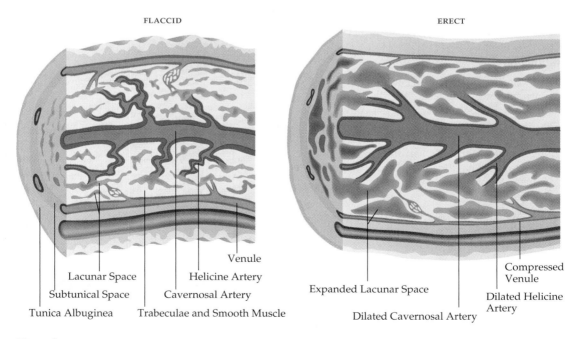

FLACCID   ERECT

Venule
Lacunar Space   Helicine Artery
Subtunical Space   Cavernosal Artery
Tunica Albuginea   Trabeculae and Smooth Muscle

Compressed Venule
Expanded Lacunar Space   Dilated Helicine Artery
Dilated Cavernosal Artery

Figure 3 **One hypothetical mechanism of penile erection is depicted. In the flaccid state, the contracted helicine arteries restrict blood flow to the lacunar spaces, and blood drains through venules in the subtunical space. In the erect state, efferent autonomic nerves dilate the cavernosal and helicine arteries, which increases blood flow to the lacunar spaces. Relaxation of trabecular smooth muscle permits expansion of the trabecular structure against the tunica albuginea, which elongates and compresses the subtunical venules, greatly reducing outflow.[101]**

alone or with GnRH antagonists, from gaining favor.[14] The only male contraceptives, therefore, are the condom (the only contraceptive that prevents sexually transmitted diseases) and vasectomy, which has been proved safe in large-scale studies.

The Male Climacteric

Does the testis undergo a decline in function similar to the ovarian exhaustion that underlies the menopause? Several studies have shown that total and free plasma testosterone levels begin to decline between 50 and 60 years of age.[15,16] In some men, the levels fall to values that would be considered pathological in younger men [see Figure 4]. A few authors, however, have found that plasma testosterone levels remain the same in normal aging men; these results challenge the existence and extent of a male climacteric. Some studies have shown increases in FSH and LH, suggesting partial testicular insufficiency in normal aging men, but other studies have shown that low testosterone levels can occur without any rise in LH.[17] In part, this conflict may reflect disagreement in definitions of healthy aging. In any case, increases in both FSH and LH levels in some older men suggest at least a partial decline in testicular function. In other men, aging is accompanied by a decrease in the LH level and testosterone pulse frequency and by increased sensitivity of the hypothalamic-pituitary axis to inhibition by androgens.[18,19]

Many bodily changes occur in aging males that could be directly or indirectly associated with declining testicular function. Decreases occur in bone density, lean body mass, muscular strength, and hematopoiesis. To what degree these changes are caused by decreasing testosterone levels and to what degree they could (or should) be reversed by testosterone therapy are unknown. Studies in younger, eugonadal males have shown that supraphysiological doses of testosterone, particularly when bolstered by physical training, lead to increased muscle mass and strength.[20,21] Most older patients are not so concerned with diminishing muscle mass and strength; their greater concern is that of diminishing erectile capacity.[22,23]

Erectile Dysfunction

Erectile dysfunction is probably the most common male sexual symptom encountered by physicians. Erectile dysfunction—a term preferable to impotence, which implies complete failure—is defined as the inability to develop and sustain an erection adequate for intercourse on at least 25 percent of attempts. Improved understanding of the problem and new approaches to diagnosis and treatment have greatly increased the chances of helping patients with this symptom.[24-28]

Etiology

Establishing the cause of erectile dysfunction is best approached by considering the normal controls of erection.[29,30]

Vascular insufficiency Inadequate erection caused by major vascular insufficiency occurs with aortoiliac atherosclerosis; it is usually accompanied by claudication and by diminished or absent femoral pulses.

The possibility that erectile dysfunction is caused by disease of smaller arteries can be pursued with modern hemodynamic techniques. Doppler and ultrasound study can delineate arterial, sinusoidal, or venous inadequacy. Because these methods are not widely available, the differential diagnosis is still guided by clinical findings. If injection of papaverine into the corpora cav-

ernosa induces a normal erection within 10 minutes, there is no need for further evaluation of the vascular component.

Peripheral neuropathy Peripheral neurogenic erectile dysfunction occurs as a result of spinal cord trauma. It also occurs in the various syndromes of autonomic insufficiency and in about 50 percent of men with insulin-dependent diabetes mellitus.[31] The medical history of men who have diabetes usually discloses other signs of neuropathy, such as postural hypotension, diarrhea, and incontinence. The erectile defect associated with diabetes may be impaired relaxation of smooth muscle of the corpora cavernosa. In vitro, smooth muscle relaxation is impaired by either direct electrical or neurochemical stimulation.[32] The absence of nocturnal penile tumescence has been used to identify cases of neurologic erectile dysfunction.

Drugs Many drug-related causes of erectile dysfunction involve the complex interconnections of the erotogenic pathways. Antihypertensive drugs, tranquilizers, antidepressants, and many other agents may all cause decreased erectile capacity [see Table 1].[33] Hypertension and antihypertensive medications are frequent causes of erectile dysfunction.[34] In one group of hypertensive patients, 17 percent reported some decrease in potency before they had begun any treatment. Diuretics, centrally active sympatholytics (including clonidine, methyldopa,

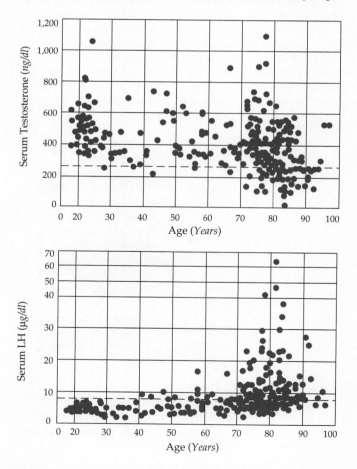

Figure 4 Testosterone and luteinizing hormone levels vary in healthy men between 18 and 97 years of age. In men older than 60 years, a fall in testosterone is accompanied by a rise in LH, indicating a primary decline in gonadal function.[102]

and reserpine), and peripherally active agents may all induce partial or complete erectile dysfunction; some agents (e.g., guanethidine) can cause retrograde ejaculation. Beta blockers may produce erectile dysfunction with or without fatigue and depression. The mechanisms by which these drugs produce erectile dysfunction are not well understood, and it is impossible to predict which agent will affect which patient. Trial and error are therefore necessary to distinguish between the pharmacological causes of erectile dysfunction and the psychological influences of the disease and its treatment. Fortunately, angiotensin-converting enzyme inhibitors and calcium channel blockers do not seem to interfere with erectile function.

Occasionally, drugs cause erectile dysfunction by affecting the hormonal control of erection. For example, spironolactone and cimetidine act as antiandrogens.

Alcohol consumption Alcohol can cause erectile dysfunction by many mechanisms, but it is extremely difficult to untangle its pharmacological effects from its emotional and social impact. Alcohol is a direct central nervous system depressant. It can impair testosterone biosynthesis directly or through liver disease (see below). Alcohol dependence can be associated with spousal abuse or general violence, which may contribute to its negative psychological impact on sexual function.

Epilepsy Erectile dysfunction may accompany temporal lobe epilepsy. Some patients with this disorder have hyperprolactinemia, but in other patients, the erectile difficulty has no obvious cause and may reflect abnormalities in still unknown pathways related to erectile function.

Systemic disorders Several systemic disorders, including alcoholism, cirrhosis, and uremia, can produce hypogonadism associated with a low testosterone level. Although the mechanisms involved remain to be elucidated, the underlying disorder should be corrected whenever possible. Some evidence suggests that uremia adversely affects steroidogenesis, producing a consequent rise in gonadotropin level. Therapy with clomiphene has been beneficial, but confirmation of its effects is still needed. Hyperprolactinemia and a low testosterone level occur in chronic renal failure, and bromocriptine therapy [see Chapter 45] can be helpful in lowering the prolactin level.

Psychogenic factors Psychogenic factors are thought to be the most frequent cause of erectile dysfunction. Anxiety, fatigue, interpersonal stresses, and chronic illness are common underlying factors. Depression requires separate mention because of its frequency; erectile dysfunction may be the presenting complaint that leads to correct diagnosis and treatment.

Endocrine abnormalities The principal endocrine abnormalities that lead to erectile dysfunction include testosterone deficiency from pituitary or testicular disease, estrogen excess (e.g., caused by liver disease), and hyperprolactinemic syndromes. Prolactin excess exerts an antigonadotropic effect manifested mainly by erectile dysfunction, which is usually associated with a low plasma testosterone level. However, even after the plasma testosterone level has been normalized, erectile dysfunction can persist until the hyperprolactinemia is corrected. Hyperthyroidism, Cushing's syndrome, and myxedema can each cause reversible erectile dysfunction.

When should evaluation for an endocrine cause of erectile

Table 1 Drugs That Can Cause Erectile Dysfunction*

Type	Examples
Antihypertensive agents	
Centrally acting drugs	Clonidine, *Rauwolfia* alkaloids
Diuretics	Chlorothiazide, spironolactone
Ganglionic blockers	Hexamethonium, trimethaphan
Adrenergic blockers	Guanethidine, propranolol
False neurotransmitters	Methyldopa
Psychotropics	Monoamine oxidase inhibitors Tricyclic antidepressants Phenothiazines Benzodiazepines
CNS depressants	Sedatives Narcotics Anxiolytics Alcohol
Miscellaneous	Cholinergic blockers (in high doses) Estrogens Cimetidine Anticancer drugs

*This table provides a sampling of the drugs most often associated with erectile dysfunction. Many other drugs have been implicated, but systematic proof is often lacking.[33]

dysfunction be undertaken? Patients with psychogenic erectile dysfunction are often capable of erection in some circumstances—for example, when masturbating or when having sex with a different partner. Endocrine erectile dysfunction, on the other hand, tends to develop gradually and then to be constant. Plasma testosterone and prolactin levels should be measured in any patient who has been impotent in most circumstances for more than three months. Abnormal levels of these hormones may be indicative of treatable organic disease. If a low testosterone level is found, pituitary evaluation, including measurement of serum FSH, LH, and prolactin levels, is warranted.

One study that employed the plasma testosterone assay to screen patients with erectile dysfunction suggests that psychogenic erectile dysfunction may not occur as frequently as has been alleged.[35] Of 105 patients tested, 37 were found to have organic hypogonadism. Of these, 20 patients had hypothalamic-pituitary deficiency, seven had testicular failure, eight suffered from hyperprolactinemia, and two had occult hyperthyroidism. Although these relative frequencies may not be representative, the screening approach using the plasma testosterone assay was nonetheless invaluable.

EVALUATION AND TREATMENT OF ERECTILE DYSFUNCTION

As specific, treatable causes of erectile dysfunction are further defined, it becomes imperative to follow a protocol capable of detecting the principal cause of dysfunction in each patient. The starting point is a careful history and physical examination, combined with a detailed sexual history. The patient should be asked about duration of the symptom, the circumstances in which it is manifested, the potential role of disease or medication, and the possibility of alcoholism or depression. Physical examination should include testing peripheral reflexes and pinprick sensation in the perianal area. If any of the specific conditions already mentioned is suggested, the appropriate therapy is clear. It is extremely important to review all medications being taken and to prescribe a substitute for any that may be contributing to erectile dysfunction. In many patients, no clear etiology is determined; two additonal tests are then indicated.

The gold standard for noninvasive testing is the recording of nocturnal penile tumescence.[36] This test can be done in a sleep laboratory, but several devices are available for use at home. With the RigiScan, measurements of pressure at the base and tip of the penis are recorded during natural sleep; the record is read by a computer, and a profile of pressures is printed out for quantitative interpretation.[37] In this and other direct measurements, one can distinguish between the presence of some erection and the sustained achievement of sufficient pressure for vaginal penetration. Alternatively, a urologist can inject papaverine, papaverine plus phentolamine, or prostaglandin E_1 directly into the penile corpora. A firm erection achieved in this way indicates that the vascular component of erection is adequate and also provides an effective therapeutic alternative. The failure to induce erection should be followed by definitive vascular studies.

There is appropriate therapy for erectile dysfunction of a specific cause (see below). When no specific diagnosis is made, several options exist. Long-term follow-up studies indicate a generally high degree of patient and partner satisfaction with intracavernous injection of vasoactive drugs.[38,39] Injection of papaverine alone or papaverine with phentolamine induces an erection lasting 30 to 120 minutes in about 70 percent of patients. Side effects include pain, ecchymosis, and occasional episodes of priapism that require pharmacological intervention.[40,41] Similar results have been obtained with injections of prostaglandin E_1.[42] Intracavernous injection of the synthetic prostaglandin E_1 alprostadil is approved by the FDA for treatment of erectile dysfunction.[43,44] Intraurethral instillation of alprostadil by a drug-delivery system, MUSE (medicated urethral system for erection), is reportedly effective in inducing satisfactory erection in two thirds of men with erectile dysfunction of diverse causes.[45] It is probably a bit less effective than the direct injection.

An alternative to this invasive approach is the use of a plastic tube and suction pump to create a vacuum around the penis.[46,47] When an erection results, a rubber band is placed at the base of the penis and satisfactory coitus can occur. A third choice is surgical implantation of one of several types of prostheses. These have been used successfully by many couples.[48] Sex therapy is especially helpful for psychogenic erectile dysfunction. Supportive counseling and reassurance are a necessary adjunct for all patients with erectile dysfunction, particularly because anxiety and fear of failure compound any partial erectile difficulty. Two drugs for oral treatment of erectile dysfunction are under consideration by the FDA. A new drug application has been submitted for sildenafil, and an oral form of phentolamine is in phase III trials.

Aging and Erectile Dysfunction

The most frequent clinical presentation of erectile dysfunction is in apparently normal men older than 50 years. The clinical significance of any gradual decline in testicular function in men older than 50 years is receiving renewed study. Although there is much individual variation, aging men generally experience a gradual decline in sexual activity. In some studies, the decrease in erectile function has been associated with decreased plasma levels of free testosterone.[49] Other studies have found that although sexual dysfunction and hypogonadism each increase with age, they are not associated.[17] Detailed correlative and, especially, longitudinal studies of psychosexual behavior are not yet

available; thus, the question whether such changes are inevitable accompaniments of aging or whether they reflect a partial decline in testosterone secretion has not been answered definitively.

Diminished erectile capacity in older men should be evaluated in the total context of other illnesses, interpersonal relationships, physical examination, and drugs being taken. If there is no absolute barrier to sexual function and if the plasma testosterone level is low normal or borderline (i.e., between 150 and 200 ng/dl), testosterone therapy can be considered. If FSH and LH levels are low, particularly if the plasma testosterone level is strikingly depressed (i.e., < 100 ng/dl), serum prolactin and thyroxine levels should be measured to exclude pituitary insufficiency [see Chapter 45]. A rectal examination should be done, and both prostate-specific antigen and prostatic acid phosphatase levels should be measured to exclude early prostate carcinoma. If the resulting data are reassuring, testosterone enanthate, 200 mg intramuscularly monthly, can be tried for three months. If genuine improvement in potency is obtained, long-term therapy can be considered after the patient is informed of the risks and benefits. In patients committed to long-term treatment, periodic rectal examination and prostate-specific antigen determination are indicated because testosterone therapy may stimulate a focus of prostate carcinoma.[50] In view of this concern, other treatments for erectile dysfunction should be given serious consideration in the choice of therapy.

Disorders of the Pituitary-Testicular Axis

Disorders of the pituitary-testicular axis are assessed at four levels: (1) hypothalamus, (2) anterior pituitary, (3) testis, and (4) ducts. Deficiency at any level is usually first detected by finding a low value for one or both gonadal products (i.e., a low testosterone level or a low sperm count).

HYPOTHALAMIC-PITUITARY DISORDERS

Hypothalamic Defects

Puberty occurs later in the male than in the female, and delay in onset of puberty is a much more common clinical problem in boys. There is wide variation in the normal pattern, but 95 percent of normal boys enter puberty by 14.5 years of age; investigation should be undertaken in boys who do not reach puberty by this age, if only for psychological reasons. The embarrassment of sexual immaturity affects almost all boys with delayed puberty, and early diagnosis and therapy can be extremely reassuring.

Delayed puberty Boys with simple pubertal delay are normal on physical examination except for their immature appearance and prepubertal genitalia. Because the onset of puberty is genetically programmed, a family history of pubertal delay is important. If the father or a brother matured late and the patient is growing normally, familial delay is the probable diagnosis. Plotting a growth curve is extremely helpful. Boys with simple delayed puberty have a normal growth pattern except for the absence of a pubertal spurt; in addition, they are normal weight for their height. In contrast, the growth pattern of undernourished boys slackens with time, and they are generally underweight for their height. Undernutrition may be caused by poverty, severe emotional deprivation, malabsorptive bowel disease, or prepubertal anorexia nervosa. In all forms of central delayed puberty, the plasma testosterone level is less than 70 ng/dl and the FSH and LH levels are low or low normal.

Idiopathic hypogonadotropic hypogonadism (congenital)
Patients with idiopathic hypogonadotropic hypogonadism (IHH) fail to initiate or complete puberty because of abnormal GnRH secretion. Affected boys continue to grow but without the normal pubertal growth spurt and without normal sexual maturation. Some patients with IHH have no signs of puberty, very small testes, and no evidence of GnRH secretion; about half of this group are anosmic (i.e., a decreased or absent sense of smell) and meet the criteria for Kallmann's syndrome.[51]

The X-linked form of Kallmann's syndrome is caused by a gene deletion near the end of the short arm of the X chromosome (Xp22.3). The absence of the protein encoded by this gene somehow contributes to the failure of neurons to migrate from the olfactory placode to the arcuate nucleus of the hypothalamus. These neurons ordinarily synthesize GnRH, and the deficiency of the releasing factor leads to hypogonadotropic hypogonadism.[52,53] Autosomal pedigrees of Kallmann's syndrome are also known and may even be more common.[54]

Some patients with IHH show signs of beginning puberty, including testicular maturation, but lack LH pulses. Other patients with partial sexual maturation produce only nocturnal LH pulses or inadequately low pulses throughout the day, suggesting a form of pubertal arrest.

Patients with any form of IHH are identified by their sexual immaturity and low serum testosterone and gonadotropin levels. Proof that FSH and LH deficiency is secondary to a lack of GnRH can be obtained by administering GnRH and observing a rise in FSH and LH. If there is no rise initially, the test is repeated after two weeks of daily GnRH. Higher levels of FSH and LH at that time reflect a prior GnRH deficiency. Gonadorelin, a synthetic GnRH, can be used for this test.

Pubertal delay is far more common than IHH,[55] although patients with simple delayed puberty may show the clinical and laboratory patterns exhibited by those with IHH. Recognition of the features of Kallmann's syndrome, especially diminished or absent sense of smell, makes possible a definitive diagnosis and early institution of therapy. If anosmia is not present, it may be impossible to distinguish between the two disorders.

In evaluating patients with delayed puberty, it is important to be sure that there has been no slowing of growth beyond the absence of increased growth velocity expected with the onset of puberty. If growth is truly slowing down, an evaluation of all pituitary function, including computed tomography or magnetic resonance imaging of the pituitary, is advisable. If the results are negative, most patients will ultimately mature on their own.

Idiopathic hypogonadatropic hypogonadism (acquired)
IHH can be acquired as well as congenital. Acquired IHH affects adult men who have completed puberty, have been sexually active, and are even fertile. They present with erectile dysfunction and have low testosterone, normal prolactin, and low-normal gonadotropin levels and GnRH secretory patterns similar to those of immature or early pubertal boys. They are the male equivalent of women who, having developed normal menstrual function, regress to an immature state because of either malnutrition or hyperprolactinemia.[56]

Pituitary Defects

In contrast to congenital gonadotropin deficiency, which is usually of hypothalamic origin, acquired gonadotropin deficiency is more often of pituitary origin. Both growth hormone release and gonadotropin release are sensitive to partial pituitary impairment. Erectile dysfunction is the first endocrine manifestation in most adult men with pituitary insufficiency, because gonadotropin deficiency results in low testosterone levels; growth hormone deficiency is also a manifestation of pituitary insufficiency, but the symptoms ascribed to it—asthenia and easy fatiguing—are not easy to identify clinically.

Pituitary tumor Pituitary disease that causes hypogonadism is most often caused by a tumor in or above the sella turcica. Chromophobe adenoma of the pituitary and craniopharyngioma are most commonly found. Skeletal growth is almost always slow, and visual defects, especially bitemporal hemianopsia, are common. Adrenocorticotropic hormone secretion and thyroid-stimulating hormone secretion are likely to be normal. If a patient shows growth retardation as well as pubertal delay, MRI of the pituitary is advisable [*see Chapter 45*].

About one third of chromophobe pituitary tumors, once thought to be endocrinologically inert, produce prolactin. Even in patients with microadenomas, the hyperprolactinemia has an antigonadotropic effect, manifested as erectile dysfunction and infertility. Hyperprolactinemia suppresses the hypothalamic GnRH pulse generator, as shown by the finding that LH pulsatility and testosterone levels can be normalized by pulsatile GnRH stimulation.[57] One puzzling observation is that in men, microadenomas are less common than macroadenomas. This finding suggests either that the tumors grow faster in men or that the symptom of erectile dysfunction does not stimulate effective diagnostic workup and the tumors go unrecognized until they produce visual loss or other local symptoms. In any case, because galactorrhea is present only infrequently, the diagnosis of hyperprolactinemia must be made by measuring the serum prolactin level in patients with hypogonadism [*see Chapter 45*]. Surgery of macroadenomas is rarely curative; more often, it is partially effective. When prolactin levels are mildly elevated, bromocriptine in a dosage of 2.5 mg twice daily will often correct the hypogonadism.[58]

Evaluation of Hypothalamic and Pituitary Disorders

Gonadotropin concentrations are determined by radioimmunoassay of plasma levels. The commercially available tests reliably distinguish high levels from normal or low levels, but most laboratories cannot distinguish low from low-normal values. The problem can be handled in two ways. First, if the level of target gland product is low, measurement of the relevant gonadotropin is critical. For example, when testosterone is low because of a gonadal defect, LH is high. If testosterone is low because of a hypothalamic or pituitary defect, immunoassay shows a low or low-normal level of LH.

A second approach uses GnRH to demonstrate central hypofunction. In a normal man, administration of 400 μg of GnRH triggers the release of LH and, usually, FSH. Failure to release LH points to gonadotropin deficiency; repeated negative results provide confirmation. Unfortunately, current tests do not reliably distinguish between hypothalamic defects and pituitary defects in gonadotropin secretion.

A final caution is required in interpreting gonadotropin values. Secretion of gonadotropins is pulsatile, and peak and nadir levels may differ significantly. Because of this variability, puzzling or discordant LH assay results should be checked by repeating the assay on a pooled aliquot of three blood samples drawn at 30-minute intervals. Even then, wide variation is normally found in both amplitude and frequency of LH pulses.

In addition, hypogonadotropic hypogonadism can be caused by a disorder of GnRH pulsatility, which may be revealed only by sampling LH at 10-minute intervals through an indwelling venous catheter.[7] This test is not widely available. Fortunately, major decisions about prognosis and therapy can almost always be based on two concordant gonadotropin assay results.

Treatment of Hypothalamic and Pituitary Disorders

In addition to the psychological disadvantages of hypogonadism, systemic consequences include anemia, osteoporosis,[59] fatigue, and weakness; all of these symptoms can be alleviated to varying degrees by therapy. The goal of therapy for male hypogonadism, as for endocrine deficiencies in general, should be restoration of the normal physiologic state. Both components of testicular function (i.e., testosterone production and spermatogenesis) should be considered.

Testosterone replacement reproduces all the systemic effects of the endogenous hormone.[60-62] Because puberty is a gradual process that requires three to four years, replacement therapy for the adolescent male who has never matured should begin gradually and build to adult levels. Long-acting esters of testosterone given intramuscularly are the most convenient therapy to induce normal pubertal and adult androgenic function.[63] One can begin with 50 mg I.M. of testosterone enanthate or testosterone cypionate every two weeks for three months and then increase the dosage gradually over 18 months to 200 mg every two weeks, a full adult dose. For permanent replacement or substitution in adults, testosterone is given in a dosage of 100 mg I.M. weekly or 200 mg I.M. every two weeks; depending on the patient, the latter regimen may lose its effectiveness in the second week.

Two transdermal preparations are approximately equivalent in effectiveness to injected testosterone. Testoderm, a patch applied daily to shaved scrotal skin, produces a good clinical response—normal testosterone and prostaglandin E_2 levels—but elevated dihydrotestosterone levels. A permeation-enhanced nonscrotal patch, Androderm, produces a good symptomatic response and physiologic levels of all three hormones. The transdermal treatments cost between 10 and 12 times that of self-injected testosterone cypionate. Testosterone maintains normal libido, potency, hair and beard growth, and strength but does not initiate or restore spermatogenesis. It can be used for hypogonadal males with a central or testicular defect.

An alternative approach is available for treating testicular deficiency that is secondary to a lack of gonadotropin. Human chorionic gonadotropin (hCG) produces all the effects of LH. Injections of 3,000 to 5,000 units of hCG twice weekly stimulate the testis to release normal levels of testosterone and often induce some testicular enlargement, which has a highly desirable psychological effect for the adolescent male. Smaller doses of 1,000 to 2,000 units twice weekly are indicated at the start of treatment.

The physiologic treatment for IHH is pulsatile administration of synthetic GnRH [see Figure 5]. The hormone can be given in daily subcutaneous injections of 500 μg, but subcutaneous delivery from a portable infusion pump of 25 to 200 ng/kg every 90 minutes more closely approximates physiologic conditions. With either program, patients who have IHH can undergo normal puberty, including spermatogenesis.[64] A fascinating aspect of pulsatile GnRH therapy is that it restores the circadian rhythm of plasma testosterone without producing a circadian variation of LH.[65,66]

Testosterone replacement in the hypogonadal male is usually a very gratifying clinical experience. Boys go through a pubertal sequence, with a growth spurt, progressive virilization, and the development of sex drive and potency. Adults who have become impotent experience the return of potency and may have increased bone density.[67,68] None of the existing testosterone preparations, however, completely mimics normal testosterone dynamics (pulsatile GnRH administration comes closest), and new testosterone formulations are being developed.[69-71]

TESTICULAR DISORDERS

Tubular Defects

Primary disorders of the testis typically affect the tubules and spermatogenesis more than Leydig cells and testosterone synthesis.[72,73] Except for Klinefelter's syndrome, in which a defect in testosterone synthesis is common, the disorders described below are principally tubular defects. Sensitive assays for testosterone and LH, however, have also shown partial involvement of Leydig cells.

Klinefelter's syndrome Klinefelter's syndrome, the best defined of the gonadal disorders, is caused by a chromosomal defect in which the patient has 47 chromosomes, with two X chromosomes and one Y chromosome (XXY).[74] The testicular tubules remain small and collapsed and, after puberty, show hyalinization and only minimal spermatogenesis. Small testes are the one constant feature of the disorder, but most patients also have gynecomastia (see below). Because testosterone levels are extremely variable, patients differ greatly in symptoms and appearance, ranging from severely eunuchoid individuals to men who are entirely normal except for small testes and infertility. If the karyotype is 47,XXY, the testosterone level is reduced, and the FSH level is high, a definitive diagnosis can be made.

Two disorders closely related to Klinefelter's syndrome can be diagnosed only by testicular biopsy. Germ cells are absent in the Sertoli cell–only syndrome and are severely arrested in development in the germ cell–arrest syndrome. Patients with these disorders are normally virilized but have azoospermia, elevated FSH levels, and high-normal or unusually elevated LH. The karyotype is grossly normal, but subtle defects in the Yq region of the chromosome are seen.[74,75]

Idiopathic hypospermatogenesis The most common defect in testicular function is idiopathic hypospermatogenesis, a quantitative abnormality not confined to a particular stage of spermatogenesis. Unfortunately, there are no reliable endocrine correlates and no particular approaches to the diagnosis.[76] When the sperm count is below 20 million/ml, the FSH level may be elevated. This finding is variable, however; repeat testing is advised. When the sperm count is below 10 million/ml, the testes are often smaller and softer than normal; FSH elevation is more likely in this circumstance, probably because of decreased inhibin levels. There are no consistent abnormalities of testosterone or LH levels, and there is no specific approach to therapy. Prognosis is poor if the FSH level is high; if it is not elevated, some of the empirical approaches employed to treat other tubular defects may be worth trying. In some patients, concentrated samples of sperm can be used for in vitro fertilization.

Cytogenetic studies have revealed that several loci on the long arm of the Y chromosome are involved in the regulation of spermatogenesis. One clinical implication is that assisted re-

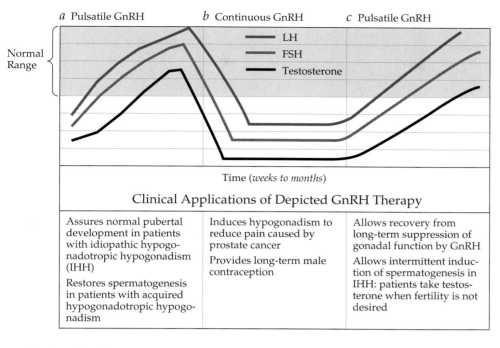

a Pulsatile GnRH   *b* Continuous GnRH   *c* Pulsatile GnRH

Normal Range

— LH
— FSH
— Testosterone

Time (*weeks to months*)

Clinical Applications of Depicted GnRH Therapy

Assures normal pubertal development in patients with idiopathic hypogonadotropic hypogonadism (IHH) Restores spermatogenesis in patients with acquired hypogonadotropic hypogonadism	Induces hypogonadism to reduce pain caused by prostate cancer Provides long-term male contraception	Allows recovery from long-term suppression of gonadal function by GnRH Allows intermittent induction of spermatogenesis in IHH: patients take testosterone when fertility is not desired

Figure 5 (*a*) **Synthetic GnRH, in pulses of appropriate amplitude and frequency, reproduces all features of normal male reproductive function in a GnRH-deficient male. (*b*) Tonic or continuous GnRH administration suppresses gonadotropin and testosterone production (and spermatogenesis, not shown). (*c*) The suppression seen in frame *b* is reversible. When GnRH is again administered in the appropriate pulses, normal adult endocrine status is restored.**

productive technologies using concentrated sperm from an affected man would transmit the defect to male offspring.[77,78]

Immotile cilia syndromes Two immotile cilia syndromes that affect sperm cilia and cause infertility have been identified. In Kartagener's syndrome, infertility accompanies bronchiectasis and situs inversus. In this disorder, both the sperm tail and the respiratory cilia have a defect in the protein dynein. This protein constitutes part of the microtubular assembly that gives each structure mobility. The immotile cilia are ineffective in preventing respiratory infection, and the immotile sperm cannot produce fertilization. In a related disorder, the dynein protein is normal, but the radial spokes in both cilia and sperm are abnormal.

Acquired tubular defects Mumps that occurs after puberty produces bilateral orchitis in about 10 percent of male patients. Infertility ensues in about half of the patients, with concomitant testicular atrophy and elevation of the FSH level. Because Leydig cell function is rarely impaired, testosterone and LH levels remain normal.

The antineoplastic agent cyclophosphamide is an increasingly important cause of testicular insufficiency. The drug selectively damages the germ cells of the testis, leaving Leydig cell function intact. The effect occurs within months of exposure, but if cyclophosphamide is administered for less than 18 months, the damage appears to be gradually reversible. With longer administration, recovery is very slow and incomplete. A number of other antineoplastic drugs can also damage testicular tubules and impair fertility. In some patients taking antineoplastic drugs, gynecomastia associated with a derangement in Leydig cell function has developed.

Prolonged exposure to the pesticide 1,2-dibromo-3-chloropropane (DBCP) can cause selective damage to the testicular tubules. This finding emphasizes the necessity for a careful toxicologic history in patients who have hypospermatogenesis.

Varicocele is found in a small proportion of subfertile men. Physical examination with the patient standing and performing the Valsalva maneuver is important in making this diagnosis.

There is great disagreement about how, or even whether, varicocele impairs spermatogenesis, even when it is unilateral.[79] Nevertheless, correction of the varicocele is reportedly accompanied by an improved sperm count in 60 to 80 percent of cases. Despite the uncertainties, varicocele should be corrected in patients whose sperm count is low but whose testis size and FSH levels are normal.

Defects in Androgen Synthesis or Effect

Defects in testosterone-mediated events can arise from failure of testosterone production, tissue resistance to its action, or failure of the conversion of testosterone to dihydrotestosterone.

The most striking defect in testosterone action is testicular feminization. In this disorder, genetic males develop as females; as newborns, they fail to show any virilization. Although these males have no uterus (müllerian inhibition has occurred normally), they show no evidence of testosterone effect on the ducts or external genitalia. This combination of clinical features allows precise diagnosis. These patients are apparent females with breast development, and their presenting complaint is primary amenorrhea. Body hair is scant, the vagina ends blindly, and rectal examination discloses no uterus. They are chromatin negative, with 46 chromosomes and an XY karyotype. Plasma testosterone levels equal or exceed those of normal males.

Testicular feminization is an example of complete male pseudohermaphroditism because the patient is a genetic male with testes whose anomalous genital development is caused not by a truly hermaphroditic state, with gonads of both sexes, but by the absence of virilizing effects. The resistance to androgen action has been shown by molecular genetic analysis to result from one of several defects in the androgen receptor.[80] The defects include (1) amino acid substitutions that impair androgen binding or binding of the androgen-receptor complex to DNA, (2) premature stop codons or other alterations of the gene that prevent synthesis of the receptor, and (3) synthesis of altered, unstable receptors that are rapidly degraded.

Incomplete pseudohermaphroditism refers to genetically male patients who have partial male development of both the internal ducts and the external genitalia. Production of testosterone and estrogen is normal or increased, and LH levels are elevated despite the large amount of testosterone. The disease is caused by partial resistance to the action of testosterone, decreased amounts of the normal androgen-receptor molecule, or various qualitative abnormalities in the receptor. The several variants of the syndrome are inherited as X-linked disorders. Another incomplete pseudohermaphroditism results from steroid 5α-reductase deficiency (*see* Secondary Sex Characteristics, *above*).

Evaluation for Testicular Disorders

The generalist physician can initiate evaluation of testicular function by obtaining a semen analysis and a serum testosterone level.

The plasma testosterone level is measured by competitive protein binding, immunoassay, or radioreceptor assay. All of these methods are specific and sensitive, and unlike gonadotropin assays, they provide clear differentiation between male and female, child and adult, and normal and abnormal. Although there is some pulsatility and a modest circadian variation, a random plasma testosterone value provides a good representation of the patient's testosterone profile. Thus, assay of plasma testosterone should be the first step in evaluation of any male suspected of hypogonadism.

Like most steroid hormones, testosterone circulates reversibly bound to a protein, sex steroid–binding globulin (SSBG). This protein is synthesized in the liver. Its plasma level is controlled by genetic factors and is raised by estrogen administration and lowered by testosterone administration. Testosterone is also reversibly bound to albumin, and the free fraction of the hormone is sometimes referred to as bioavailable testosterone. Occasionally, the measurement of SSBG and the free testosterone moiety will illuminate a problem. This assay is employed much more frequently to detect androgen excess in the hirsute female than androgen deficiency in the hypogonadal male.

Semen analysis is the indispensable first step in the investigation of male infertility.[81] Normal examination results (volume, count, motility, and morphology) imply the normality of the entire endocrine and duct system. An abnormal result can provide a major clue to the site of the pathological condition.

Testicular biopsy is rarely needed to establish a prognosis but may be invaluable in making a precise diagnosis. As therapeutic techniques improve, testicular biopsy will assume greater significance. It is now used primarily to study infertility in patients with normal endocrine function (i.e., presumed normal spermatogenesis) but no sperm in their semen. In this setting, a biopsy that shows quantitatively normal spermatogenesis suggests a ductal block.[82] This condition is usually congenital and used to be considered an insuperable obstacle to conception. However, microsurgical aspiration of sperm from the epididymis and in vitro fertilization after induction of superovulation can result in conception.[83]

A positive buccal smear for the Barr body (a clump of sex chromatin present in the nucleus of any cell with two X chromosomes) and a karyotype analysis identify patients with Klinefelter's syndrome (XXY), the most common gonadal defect. Both tests are useful in providing a definitive guide to prognosis and management. Standard cytogenetic techniques should be adequate most of the time; specialized banding studies are rarely needed.

Analysis of three semen samples, each taken after two days of sexual abstinence, is usually recommended for definitive evaluation of spermatogenesis. The specimens are examined for volume (normal: 1.5 to 5.0 ml), density (normal: > 20 million sperm/ml), motility (normal: ≥ 30 percent motile), and normal forms (normal: ≥ 60 percent).

It is surprisingly difficult to define the minimum values consistent with fertility. For example, in IHH patients treated with pulsatile GnRH, conceptions have occurred with a sperm count as low as 3 million/ml.

The sperm penetration assay may provide additional guidance in the evaluation of spermatogenesis. This test measures the percentage of sperm that are able to penetrate hamster eggs from which the zona pellucida has been removed. This test may provide functional evaluation of sperm activity, independent of low counts or decreased motility.

Patients who seek fertility should be referred to a specialist for definitive evaluation and therapy.

In men with azoospermia or severe oligospermia who have normal-sized testes and normal serum levels of FSH and testosterone, urologic advances suggest a brighter picture. Ultrasound evaluation of the vasa and seminal vesicles can identify surgically correctable obstruction, and microsurgical techniques offer new hope.[84,85]

Gynecomastia

Gynecomastia, a palpable increase of the glandular tissue of the male breast, is a normal occurrence in puberty, found in 60 to 70 percent of boys at some time. It usually regresses spontaneously but may reappear.[86] Nuttall found symmetric, nontender gynecomastia of 4 cm or less in approximately one third of men between 21 and 40 years of age; the frequency of this finding increased after 40 years of age.[87] Most subjects were unaware of their condition. Thus, gynecomastia is abnormal only when it is recent or painful, when it progresses over a short period, or when it is lumpy or grossly asymmetric.

The pathogenesis of gynecomastia is only partially understood.[88] The most plausible mechanism is an increase in the ratio of effective estrogen to androgen.[89] Estradiol is such a potent hormone that significant changes in its production are not necessarily recognized by measurement of plasma levels. In addition, there is as yet no way of measuring levels or effects within the tissue of interest. Thus, increases in the estradiol to testosterone ratio have been found in patients with hyperthyroidism, cirrhosis,[90] feminizing Leydig cell tumors, and Klinefelter's syndrome. Gynecomastia, however, is also seen in conditions in which an increase in the free estradiol to free testosterone ratio has not yet been demonstrated. Drugs such as digoxin, marijuana, alcohol, spironolactone, cimetidine, metoclopramide, alkylating agents and other antitumor drugs, and psychotropics have all been implicated as causes. Gynecomastia in these circumstances is usually more annoying than significant. If it is accompanied by erectile dysfunction or by lowering of the plasma testosterone level, further study and perhaps discontinuance of the drug are in order.

Occasionally, progressive gynecomastia is the clue to an underlying neoplasm. Tumors of the adrenal gland and testis may induce a disproportionate secretion of estrogen and thereby cause gynecomastia. Patients usually have an increased plasma estradiol level and a low or normal gonadotropin level. An elevated estrogen level indicates the need for testicular ultrasonography and adrenal CT or MRI. Estradiol, however, is so potent that significant gynecomastia can develop without elevation of the plasma estradiol level. Progressive gynecomastia without a known explanation (e.g., puberty, cirrhosis, hyperthyroidism) should therefore be evaluated by imaging of the adrenals and testes.[91]

Ectopic production of hCG by malignant tumors is occasionally accompanied by gynecomastia. In this circumstance, the increased plasma estrogen levels have sometimes been attributed to the tumor; more often, however, a gonadotropin-driven increase in the conversion of testosterone to estradiol in the testis has been implicated. The combination of recent gynecomastia with elevated estrogen and hCG titers should prompt a search for a primary tumor. Although the finding of hCG in the plasma of normal people has thickened the plot, high hCG titers and dynamic studies can be used to identify a tumor as the probable cause.

The treatment of gynecomastia depends on its cause and course. Adolescent gynecomastia almost always regresses spontaneously. If it remains troublesome, plastic surgical reduction is appropriate. Psychological harm may occur if surgical correction is deferred for too long. In adults, drug exposure should be investigated and, when clinically allowable, the medication discontinued. The estrogen antagonist tamoxifen may be helpful in treating painful gynecomastia.

Inducing Androgen Deficiency as Treatment of Prostate Cancer

More than 50 years ago, Huggins demonstrated that orchiectomy slowed the growth and relieved the pain of prostate cancer [see Chapter 197].[92] The progress since then in understanding testicular function has suggested additional ways in which the male endocrine environment can be altered. A summary of the agents that cause androgen deficiency provides an excellent review of the hypothalamic-pituitary-testicular axis.[93]

Long-acting analogues of GnRH induce desensitization of pituitary gonadotropes: after brief stimulation of FSH and LH release, the gonadotropin levels become undetectable and plasma testosterone concentration falls to castrate level. This treatment can reduce benign prostatic hypertrophy. It is now a standard approach for metastatic prostate cancer as well. In some patients, it initially produces an increase in testosterone that can worsen symptoms. For this reason, synthetic GnRH antagonists—which have no stimulatory effect—are preferred for inducing hypogonadism.

The administration of estrogen produces hypoandrogenism by several mechanisms: inhibition of hypothalamic and pituitary gonadotropic secretion, raising of the sex steroid–binding globulin level (which reduces the free testosterone fraction), direct inhibition of the testis, and antagonism of androgen action at target tissues. Comparable antitumor effects have been seen with hypogonadism induced by GnRH analogues and hypogonadism induced by estrogen, but synthetic GnRH is less toxic. The antifungal drug ketoconazole inhibits testicular and adrenal testosterone biosynthesis and lowers circulating testosterone levels, although not so effectively as the GnRH analogues.

The effect of testosterone on target tissue can be antagonized by flutamide, a nonsteroidal anilide that blocks the intracellular access or processing of testosterone; cyproterone acetate, a drug that is not yet available in the United States, works even better than flutamide. Inhibition of the conversion of testosterone to dihydrotestosterone may prove to be an effective pharmacological approach to controlling benign prostatic hypertrophy. Finasteride has a broad spectrum of inhibition; it inhibits the action of 5α-reductase on steroids as diverse as cortisol, androstenedione, and testosterone.[94] Its capacity to block the conversion of testosterone to dihydrotestosterone is promising because dihydrotestosterone and its metabolite androstanediol are important in the pathogenesis of benign prostatic hyperplasia. This method of inducing androgen deficiency is unique because it has the least effect on sexual potency, which depends mainly on testosterone, not dihydrotestosterone. Thus, 5α-reductase inhibition is the only method of inducing hypogonadism that is likely to be acceptable to the patient who has a choice.[95-100]

References

1. Schafer AJ: Sex determination and its pathology in man. Adv Genet 33: 275, 1995

2. Grumbach MM, Conte FA: Disorders of sex differentiation. Williams Textbook of Endocrinology, 8th ed. Wilson JD, Foster DW, Eds. WB Saunders Co, Philadelphia, 1992, p 853

3. Wilson JD, George FW, Renfree MB: The endocrine role in mammalian sexual differentiation. Recent Prog Horm Res 50:349, 1995

4. Grino PB, Griffin JE, Wilson JD: Testosterone at high concentrations interacts with the human androgen receptor similarly to dihydrotestosterone. Endocrinology 126:1165, 1990

5. Hiort O, Sinnecker GHG, Holterhus P-M, et al: The clinical and molecular spectrum of androgen insensitivity syndromes. Am J Med Genet 63:218, 1996

6. Conn PM, Crowley WF Jr: Gonadotropin-releasing hormone and its analogues. N Engl J Med 324:93, 1991

7. Baker ML, Hutson JM: Serum levels of mullerian inhibiting substance in boys throughout puberty and in the first two years of life. J Clin Endocrinol Metab 76:245, 1993

8. Bridges NA, Hindmarsh PC, Pringle PJ, et al: The relationship between endogenous testosterone and gonadotrophin secretion. Clin Endocrinol (Oxf) 38:373, 1993

9. Morales A: Nonsurgical management options in impotence. Hosp Pract (Off Ed) 28(3):15, 1993

10. Rajfer J, Aronson WJ, Bush PA, et al: Nitric oxide as a mediator of relaxation of the corpus cavernosum in response to nonadrenergic, noncholinergic neurotransmission. N Engl J Med 326:90, 1992

11. Nitric oxide and erection (editorial). Lancet 340:882, 1992

12. Tom LKS, Swerdloff RS: GnRH antagonists: possibilities for a male contraceptive. The Endocrinologist 2:133, 1992

13. Tom L, Bhasin S, Salameh W, et al: Induction of azoospermia in normal men with combined Nal-Glu gonadotropin-releasing hormone antagonist and testosterone enanthate. J Clin Endocrinol Metab 75:476, 1992

14. Cummings DE, Bremner WJ: Prospects for new hormonal male contraceptives. Endocrinol Metab Clin North Am 23:893, 1994

15. Morley JE, Kaiser FE: Sexual function with advancing age. Med Clin North Am 73:1483, 1989

16. Vermeulen A: Clinical review 24: androgens in the aging male. J Clin Endocrinol Metab 73:221, 1991

17. Korenman SG, Morley JE, Mooradian AD, et al: Secondary hypogonadism in older men: its relation to impotence. J Clin Endocrinol Metab 71:963, 1990

18. Veldhuis JD, Urban RJ, Lizarralde G, et al: Attenuation of luteinizing hormone secretory burst amplitude as a proximate basis for the hypoandrogenism of healthy aging in men. J Clin Endocrinol Metab 75:707, 1992

19. Vermeulen A, Kaufman JM: Role of the hypothalamo-pituitary function in the hypoandrogenism of healthy aging (editorial). J Clin Endocrinol Metab 75:704, 1992

20. Bardin CW: The anabolic action of testosterone. N Engl J Med 335:52, 1996

21. Bhasin S, Storer TW, Berman N, et al: The effects of supraphysiologic doses of testosterone on muscle size and strength in normal males. N Engl J Med 335:1, 1996

22. Tenover JS: Androgen administration to aging men. Endocrinol Metab Clin North Am 23:877, 1994

23. Vermeulen A: Androgens in the aging male. J Clin Endocrinol Metab 73:221, 1991

24. Carrier S, Zvara P, Lue TF: Erectile dysfunction. Endocrinol Metab Clin North Am 23:773, 1994

25. Whitehead ED, Klyde BJ, Zussman S, et al: Diagnostic evaluation of impotence. Postgrad Med 88:123, 1990

26. Steers WD: Impotence evaluation (editorial). J Urol 149:1284, 1993

27. Rosen MP, Greenfield AJ, Walker TG, et al: Arteriogenic impotence: findings in 195 impotent men examined with selective internal pudendal angiography. Radiology 174:1043, 1990

28. NIH Consensus Development Panel on Impotence: Impotence. JAMA 270:83, 1993

29. Morley JE, Kaiser FE: Impotence: the internist's approach to diagnosis and treatment. Adv Intern Med 38:151, 1993

30. Lerner SE, Melman A, Christ GJ: A review of erectile dysfunction: new insights and more questions. J Urol 149:1246, 1993

31. Price DE: Managing impotence in diabetes. BMJ 307:275, 1993

32. Saenz de Tejada I, Goldstein I, Azadzoi K, et al: Impaired neurogenic and endothelium-mediated relaxation of penile smooth muscle from diabetic men with impotence. N Engl J Med 320:1025, 1989

33. Brock GB, Lue TF: Drug-induced male sexual dysfunction: an update. Drug Safety 8:414, 1993

34. Drugs that cause sexual dysfunction: an update. Med Lett Drugs Ther 34:73, 1992

35. Spark RF, White RA, Connolly PB: Impotence is not always psychogenic: newer insights into hypothalamic-pituitary-gonadal dysfunction. JAMA 243:750, 1980

36. Morales A, Condra M, Reid K: The role of nocturnal penile tumescence monitoring in the diagnosis of impotence: a review. J Urol 143:441, 1990

37. Allen RP, Smolev JK, Engel RM, et al: Comparison of RigiScan and formal nocturnal penile tumescence testing in the evaluation of erectile rigidity. J Urol 149:1265, 1993

38. Virag R, Shoukry K, Floresco J, et al: Intracavernous self-injection of vasoactive drugs in the treatment of impotence: 8-year experience with 615 cases. J Urol 145:287, 1991

39. Althof SE, Turner LA, Levine SB, et al: Through the eyes of women: the sexual and psychological responses of women to their partner's treatment with self-injection or external vacuum therapy. J Urol 147:1024, 1992

40. Kattan S, Collins JP, Mohr D: Double-blind, cross-over study comparing prostaglandin E1 and papaverine in patients with vasculogenic impotence. Urology 37:516, 1991

41. Kerfoot WW, Carson CC: Pharmacologically induced erections among geriatric men. J Urol 146:1022, 1991

42. Broderick GA: Intracavernous Pharmacotherapy. Treatment for the aging erectile response. Urol Clin North Am 23:111, 1996

43. Linet OI, Ogrinc FG: Efficacy and safety of intracavernosal alprostadil in men with erectile dysfunction. N Engl J Med 334:873, 1996

44. Lipshultz LI: Injection therapy for erectile dysfunction (editorial). N Engl J Med 334:913, 1996

45. Padma-Nathan H, Hellstrom WJG, Kaiser FE, et al: Treatment of men with erectile dysfunction with transurethral alprostadil. Medicated Urethral System for Erection (MUSE) Study Group. N Engl J Med 336:1, 1997

46. Korenman SG, Viosca SP, Kaiser FE, et al: Use of a vacuum tumescence device in the management of impotence. J Am Geriatr Soc 38:217, 1990

47. Blackard CE, Borkon WD, Lima JS, et al: Use of vacuum tumescence device for impotence secondary to venous leakage. Urology 41:225, 1993

48. Montague DK: Impotence therapy (editorial). J Urol 149:1313, 1993

49. Tenover JS: Effects of testosterone supplementation in the aging male. J Clin Endocrinol Metab 75:1092, 1992

50. Jackson JA, Waxman J, Spiekerman AM: Prostatic complications of testosterone replacement therapy. Arch Intern Med 149:2365, 1989

51. Christensen RB, Matsumoto AM, Bremner WJ: Idiopathic hypogonadotropic hypogonadism with anosmia (Kallmann's syndrome). The Endocrinologist 2:332, 1992

52. Hardelin J-P, Levilliers J, Young J, et al: Xp22.3 deletions in isolated familial Kallmann's syndrome. J Clin Endocrinol Metab 76:827, 1993

53. Bick D, Franco B, Sherins RJ, et al: Brief report: intragenic deletion of the KALIG-1 gene in Kallmann's syndrome. N Engl J Med 326:1752, 1992

54. Waldstreicher J, Seminara SB, Jameson JL, et al: The genetic and clinical heterogeneity of gonadotropin-releasing hormone deficiency in the human. J Clin Endocrinol Metab 81:4388, 1996

55. Rosenfield RL: Diagnosis and management of delayed puberty. J Clin Endocrinol Metab 70:559, 1991

56. Nachtigall LB, Boepple PA, Pralong FP, et al: Adult-onset idiopathic hypogonadotropic hypogonadism—a treatable form of male infertility. N Engl J Med 336:410, 1997

57. Bouchard P, Lagoguey M, Brailly S, et al: Gonadotropin-releasing hormone pulsatile administration restores luteinizing hormone pulsatility and normal testosterone levels in males with hyperprolactinemia. J Clin Endocrinol Metab 60:258, 1985

58. Molitch ME: Pathologic hyperprolactinemia. Endocrinol Metab Clin North Am 21:877, 1992

59. Finkelstein JS, Klibanski A, Neer RM, et al: Osteoporosis in men with idiopathic hypogonadotropic hypogonadism. Ann Intern Med 106:354, 1987

60. Bhasin S, Bremner WJ: Emerging issues in androgen replacement therapy. J Clin Endocrinol Metab 82:3, 1997

61. Cofrancesco J Jr, Dobs AS: Transdermal testosterone delivery systems. Endocrinologist 6:207, 1996

62. Bagatell CJ, Bremner WJ: Androgens in men—uses and abuses. N Engl J Med 334:707, 1996

63. Bhasin S: Clinical review 34: androgen treatment of hypogonadal men. J Clin Endocrinol Metab 74:1221, 1992

64. Spratt DI, Finkelstein JS, O'Dea LS, et al: Long-term administration of gonadotropin-releasing hormone in men with idiopathic hypogonadotropic hypogonadism: a model for studies of the hormone's physiologic effects. Ann Intern Med 105:848, 1986

65. Delemarre-Van de Waal HA: Induction of testicular growth and spermatogenesis by pulsatile, intravenous administration of gonadotrophin-releasing hormone in patients with hypogonadotrophic hypogonadism. Clin Endocrinol (Oxf) 38:473, 1993

66. Simoni M, Montanini V, Faustini M, et al: Circadian rhythm of plasma testosterone in men with idiopathic hypogonadotrophic hypogonadism before and during pulsatile administration of gonadotrophin-releasing hormone. Clin Endocrinol (Oxf) 36:29, 1992

67. Cunningham GR, Hirshkowitz M, Korenman SG, et al: Testosterone replacement therapy and sleep-related erections in hypogonadal men. J Clin Endocrinol Metab 70:792, 1990

68. Gallagher JC: Effect of gonadotropin-releasing hormone agonists on bone metabolism. Seminars in Reproductive Endocrinology 11:201, 1993

69. Behre HM, Nieschlag E: Testosterone buciclate (20 Aet-1) in hypogonadal men: pharmacokinetics and pharmacodynamics of the new long-acting androgen ester. J Clin Endocrinol Metab 75:1204, 1992

70. Butler GE, Sellar RE, Walker RF, et al: Oral testosterone undecanoate in the management of delayed puberty in boys: pharmacokinetics and effects on sexual maturation and growth. J Clin Endocrinol Metab 75:37, 1992

71. Bhasin S, Swerdloff RS, Steiner B, et al: A biodegradable testosterone microcapsule formulation provides uniform eugonadal levels of testosterone for 10–11 weeks in hypogonadal men. J Clin Endocrinol Metab 74:75, 1992

72. de Kretser DM: Male infertility. Lancet 349:787, 1997

73. Baker HWG: Male infertility. Endocrinol Metab Clin North Am 23:783, 1994

74. Schwartz ID, Root AW: The Klinefelter syndrome of testicular dysgenesis. Endocrinol Metab Clin North Am 20:153, 1991

75. Johnson MD, Tho SPT, Behzadian A, et al: Molecular scanning of Yq11 (interval 6) in men with Sertoli-cell-only syndrome. Am J Obstet Gynecol 161:1732, 1989

76. Jequier AM, Holmes SC: Primary testicular disease presenting as azoospermia or oligozoospermia in an infertility clinic. Br J Urol 71:731, 1993

77. Pryor JL, Kent-First M, Muallem A, et al: Microdeletions in the Y chromosome of infertile men. N Engl J Med 336:534, 1997

78. de Kretser DM, Burger HG: The Y chromosome and spermatogenesis (editorial). N Engl J Med 336:576, 1997.

79. Kaufman DG, Nagler HM: Significance and pathophysiology of the varicocele: current concepts. Seminars in Reproductive Endocrinology 6:349, 1988

80. Imperato-McGinley J, Canovatchel WJ: Complete androgen insensitivity: pathophysiology, diagnosis, and management. Trends in Endocrinology and Metabolism 3:75, 1992

81. Critser JK, Noiles EE: Bioassays of sperm function. Seminars in Reproductive Endocrinology 11:1, 1993

82. Magid MS, Cash KL, Goldstein M: The testicular biopsy in the evaluation of infertility. Semin Urol 8:51, 1990

83. Silber SJ, Ord T, Balmaceda J, et al: Congenital absence of the vas deferens: the fertilizing capacity of human epididymal sperm. N Engl J Med 323:1788, 1990

84. Lipshultz LI: Infertility diagnosis (editorial). J Urol 149:1355, 1993

85. Goldstein M: Surgical therapy of male infertility (editorial). J Urol 149:1374, 1993

86. Biro FM, Lucky AW, Huster GA, et al: Hormonal studies and physical maturation in adolescent gynecomastia. J Pediatr 116:450, 1990

87. Nuttall FQ: Gynecomastia as a physical finding in normal men. J Clin Endocrinol Metab 48:338,1979

88. Braunstein GD: Gynecomastia. N Engl J Med 328:490, 1993

89. Wilson JD: Gynecomastia: a continuing diagnostic dilemma (editorial). N Engl J Med 324:334, 1991

90. Boyden TW, Pamenter RW: Effects of ethanol on the male hypothalamic-pituitary-gonadal axis. Endocr Rev 4:389, 1983

91. Coen P, Kulin H, Ballantine T, et al: An aromatase-producing sex-cord tumor resulting in prepubertal gynecomastia. N Engl J Med 324:317, 1991

92. Huggins C, Hodges CV: Studies on prostatic cancer: I. The effect of castration, of estrogen and of androgen injection on serum phosphatases in metastatic carcinoma of the prostate. Cancer Res 1:293, 1941

93. Santen RJ: Endocrine treatment of prostate cancer. The Endocrinologist 2:384, 1992

94. Rittmaster RS: Finasteride. N Engl J Med 330:120, 1994

95. Gormley GJ, Stoner E, Bruskewitz RC, et al: The effect of finasteride in men with benign prostatic hyperplasia. N Engl J Med 327:1185, 1992

96. Lange PH: Is the prostate pill finally here? N Engl J Med 327:1234, 1992

97. Stone NN: Treatment options in benign prostatic hypertrophy. Hosp Pract (Off Ed) 27(10A):85, 1992

98. Horton R: Benign prostatic hyperplasia: new insights (editorial). J Clin Endocrinol Metab 74:504A, 1992

99. McConnell JD, Wilson JD, George FW, et al: Finasteride, an inhibitor of 5α-reductase, suppresses prostatic dihydrotestosterone in men with benign prostatic hyperplasia. J Clin Endocrinol Metab 74:505, 1992

100. Beisland HO, Binkowitz B, Brekkan E, et al: Scandinavian clinical study of finasteride in the treatment of benign prostatic hyperplasia. Eur Urol 22:271, 1992

101. Krane RJ, Goldstein I, Saenz de Tejada I: Impotence. N Engl J Med 321:1648, 1989

102. Sterns EL, MacDonnell JA, Kaufman BJ, et al: Declining testicular function with age. Am J Med 57:761,1974

Acknowledgments

Figure 1 Alan Iselin.

Figures 2 and 3 Dana Burns-Pizer.

Figure 4 Al Miller.

Figure 5 Tom Moore.

51 Ovary

Daniel D. Federman, M.D.

Physiology

The female reproductive system can be viewed as a four-tiered system, involving (1) the central nervous system, with the hypothalamus; (2) the anterior pituitary; (3) the ovaries; and (4) the duct structures—the uterus and the fallopian tubes [*see Figure 1*].

LEVELS 1 AND 2: HYPOTHALAMUS AND PITUITARY

The driving signal of female gonadal function is a hypothalamic decapeptide called gonadotropin-releasing hormone (GnRH).[1] GnRH is secreted in a pulsatile manner by hypophysiotropic neurons in the arcuate nucleus of the hypothalamus. Its release is modified by the opposing influences of at least two catecholamines: dopamine, an inhibitor, and norepinephrine, a facilitator. GnRH is transported to the gonadotropic cells of the anterior pituitary via the pituitary portal system. After binding to specific membrane receptors, GnRH stimulates the production and pulsatile release of two gonadotropins—follicle-stimulating hormone (FSH) and luteinizing hormone (LH)—that are chemically identical to those in the male [*see Chapter 50*]. In males and females, the secretion of FSH and LH is pulsatile.

Each pulse of LH reflects a prior pulse of GnRH; therefore, frequent LH sampling through an indwelling venous catheter is used to study GnRH behavior. In the adult male, the pulses oscillate around a tonic, sustained level, with a slight diurnal rhythm. In the female, however, there are sequential changes in both the amplitude and the frequency of LH pulses throughout the menstrual cycle [*see Figure 2*]. In the first half, or follicular phase, of the cycle, low-amplitude pulses occur about every 60 to 90 minutes, with a brisk acceleration just before the midcycle ovulation. In the second half, or luteal phase, pulses are of greater amplitude but much lower frequency—sometimes just one pulse a day. Disorders of this pulsatile secretion, some perhaps secondary to an increase in endorphin suppression of GnRH, contribute to menstrual irregularity.

Gonadotropin secretion in childhood is minimal. The pubertal awakening of gonadotropic secretion is thought to be of central origin; it is genetically controlled and linked to the attainment of a critical body weight. Originally sleep-entrained, but later occurring throughout the 24-hour day, gonadotropin secretion increases for 3 to 4 years before a cyclic pattern begins and regular menstrual periods are established [*see Figure 3*]. When a regular cycle is established, FSH secretion begins to rise during the last few days of the prior menstrual period; this secretion stimulates the ripening of a cohort of ovarian follicles, of which one soon dominates. Increasing estradiol secretion by this follicle potentiates the local action of FSH and also exerts positive feedback at the pituitary, contributing to a sudden midcycle rise in FSH and LH. This midcycle surge, crucial to ovulation, appears to require ovarian steroids, an increase in GnRH pulse frequency, and probably other factors. The peak of LH contributes to rupture of the leading follicle (ovulation) and to formation of a corpus luteum. LH levels then decline as abruptly as they arose.

Prolactin is necessary for lactation [*see Chapter 45*]. Whether it plays a physiologic role in the menstrual cycle is unknown, but when prolactin secretion is high, gonadotropin effects are suppressed.

LEVELS 3 AND 4: OVARIES AND DUCT STRUCTURES

The ovary secretes estrogens, inhibins, progesterone, and androgens. The principal estrogen, 17β-estradiol, has dramatic stimulatory effects on the breast, uterus, vagina, and distal urethra. Estrogens stimulate the growth of the breast and the moisture and nutrition of the vagina and maintain the integrity of the distal urethra. In the first half of each menstrual cycle, estrogen stimulates endometrial proliferation and induces production of estrogen and progesterone receptors in endometrial cells.

Progesterone is the primary product of the corpus luteum; its level rises progressively after ovulation, accompanied by a second peak of estradiol. In the first 1 to 2 years after menarche, only about 10% of cycles are ovulatory. In these cycles, the amount of progesterone secreted is lower than in adults, and the length of the luteal phase is shorter. In the course of the 2- to 3-year period after menarche, the proportion of ovulatory cycles increases, the

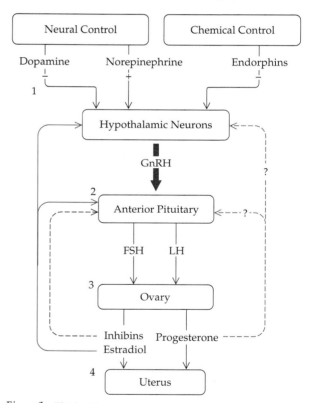

Figure 1　The female reproductive system comprises four levels: (1) the central nervous system, including the hypothalamus, which is the source of gonadotropin-releasing hormone (GnRH); (2) the pituitary, which is the source of the gonadotropins (follicle-stimulating hormone [FSH] and luteinizing hormone [LH]); (3) the ovaries, which are the source of estrogen, inhibins, and progesterone; and (4) the uterus, which is the target organ for the steroid hormones. A positive-feedback loop involving action on the hypothalamic-hypophyseal unit has been verified for estradiol (solid blue arrows) and postulated for progesterone (broken blue arrows). The effect of estradiol is paradoxical: a rising level stimulates the midcycle surge of LH and FSH, but chronically, estradiol suppresses FSH secretion. Inhibins (broken black arrow) are protein hormones that act directly on the anterior pituitary to inhibit the synthesis and release of FSH. Alternative molecular forms, called activins, stimulate gonadotropin output, but the physiologic significance of this effect is not clear.

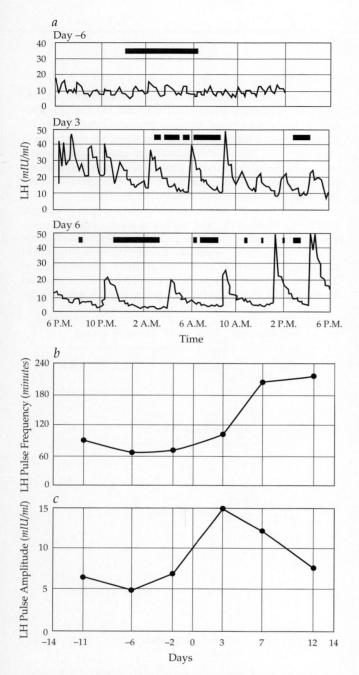

Figure 2 (*a*) LH is secreted in pulses in females in response to pulsatile GnRH secretion. LH pulses vary in frequency and amplitude during different stages of the menstrual cycle. (Bars indicate sleep intervals. Day 0 is the day ovulation occurs.) (*b*) The pulses occur about every 1 to 1.5 hours in the follicular phase and approximately every 2 to 6 hours in the luteal phase. (*c*) The amplitude of the pulses also increases dramatically after ovulation.[116]

peak levels and total secretion of progesterone rise, and the luteal phase reaches its normal duration of 14 days.

The combined effects of estrogen and progesterone, in addition to many other roles, convert the proliferative endometrium of the follicular phase of the cycle to the secretory endometrium of the luteal phase. During the luteal phase, FSH and LH levels are presumably suppressed by the rise in estrogen and progesterone. Toward the end of the 2-week life span of the corpus lute-

um, estrogen and progesterone levels fall, endometrial shedding begins, and a menstrual period results. A new cycle begins immediately, as FSH levels start to rise and several follicles ripen.

Variations in GnRH pulse amplitude and frequency elicit different ratios of FSH and LH. In general, infrequent GnRH pulses favor synthesis of the messenger RNA (mRNA) of the β chain of FSH; more frequent pulses favor production of the mRNA of the β chain of LH. In addition, the ovary makes several protein hormones—inhibins and activins—that affect the FSH level. Inhibins suppress pituitary secretion of FSH. The serum level of inhibin rises late in the follicular phase of each cycle and reaches a peak on the day of ovulation [*see Figure 3*]. Thereafter, inhibin is produced in the corpus luteum, and rising levels of this hormone during the early luteal phase may contribute to the falling levels of FSH that occur during the luteal phase. Activins, on the other hand, increase FSH secretion. Both compounds have other endocrine, paracrine, and probably autocrine influences, but their exact roles in the menstrual cycle have yet to be defined.[2]

A small amount of testosterone is secreted directly by the ovary. Androstenedione is also an important ovarian androgen. The principal role of ovarian androgens may well be within the ovary, but secreted androstenedione serves as a prohormone for peripheral conversion to testosterone or estrone. Ovarian androgens contribute to the anabolic state in females. In excess, they inhibit the normal menstrual cycle.[1]

The fourth level of the female reproductive system is the genital anatomy: uterus, fallopian tubes, vagina, and introitus. These organs secrete no hormones other than prostaglandins; however, they are targets for sex steroids as well as the sites at which symptoms of reproductive endocrine dysfunction are most likely to arise.

The menstrual cycle is dated by patients from the first day of bleeding in one period to the first day of the next period. This interval averages 35 days in teenagers and 28 to 29 days in women from 20 to 40 years of age, but it then increases to 50 days in perimenopausal women.[3]

Among the principal gynecologic endocrine disorders seen by internists are abnormal (deficient or excessive) menstrual bleeding, galactorrhea, and hirsutism. The four-tiered system that has been outlined provides a rational approach to differential diagnosis.

Disorders of Menstruation: Primary Amenorrhea

Primary amenorrhea, or the failure of menses to occur, is a relatively rare problem that usually presents to a pediatrician or gynecologist. Nevertheless, a brief outline of the workup of patients with this disorder is appropriate.[4]

HYPOTHALAMIC DEFECTS

Isolated absence of GnRH occurs in the female much less often than in the male. Patients grow normally until puberty but may reach eunuchoid proportions because of delayed closure of epiphyses. Physical examination shows absence of breast development, immature female external genitalia, minimal pubic hair, an atrophic vagina, and a small uterus. Gonadotropin levels are low, reflecting the central origin of the defect. GnRH stimulation may trigger prompt gonadotropin release, but pretreatment for several days may be needed to stimulate the gonadotrophs to respond to a bolus of GnRH. The presence of anosmia identifies the permanent GnRH deficiency of Kallmann's syndrome.

Menarche is delayed in some girls who exercise vigorously or diet stringently. Ballet dancers, long-distance runners, and girls who jog more than 30 miles a week may all show this effect.

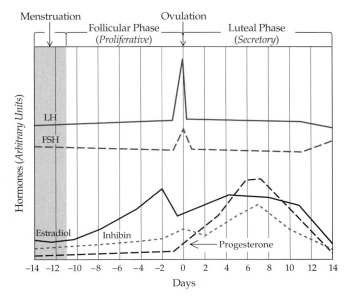

Figure 3 **Levels of two gonadotropins, FSH and LH, and three ovarian hormones—estradiol, progesterone, and inhibin—are shown for an idealized menstrual cycle. Both LH (solid blue curve) and FSH (broken blue curve) show abrupt midcycle surges preceding ovulation. Estradiol (solid black curve) peaks twice; the first peak exerts a positive feedback on gonadotropin secretion. Progesterone (broken black curve) rises slowly, peaking after ovulation in the luteal phase as the uterine wall prepares for implantation. The values for inhibin, a peptide hormone produced by the granulosa cells of the ovary, are shown (broken gray curve), but their clinical significance is unclear.[117]**

PITUITARY DEFECTS

Isolated inability of the pituitary to make gonadotropins is extremely rare. More often, the pituitary is partially destroyed by a tumor, either a chromophobe adenoma, which arises within the gland, or a craniopharyngioma, a congenital defect involving the hypothalamus and pituitary. In such patients, growth hormone is usually involved as well, and primary amenorrhea is accompanied by short stature. Plasma gonadotropin levels are low. Magnetic resonance imaging or computed tomography of the sella and visual-field examination are needed. Prolactin-producing pituitary tumors can also cause primary amenorrhea. Such tumors are often microadenomas, and plasma prolactin assays are more sensitive than radiologic examination in detecting them.

OVARIAN DEFECTS

Defects at the ovarian level account for about 50% of primary amenorrhea cases. Turner's syndrome and its variants are the ones best understood.[5] In the full-blown disorder, primary amenorrhea and genital immaturity are accompanied by short stature and various congenital anomalies. The gonadal lesion is a failure of true development of follicles; elevated plasma gonadotropins reflect this defect. Patients are chromatin negative, have a 45,X karyotype, and have easily recognizable physical features.

Polycystic ovary syndrome and its variants [*see* Polycystic Ovary Syndrome, *below*] account for 8% to 10% of cases of primary amenorrhea. Much more troublesome are mosaic chromosome disorders, in which body cells show a mixture of karyotypes. Recognition is particularly difficult when some cells are normal. A patient with a mosaic of 45,X and 46,XX cells, for example, may be almost normal in height, have few anomalies, and have either primary or secondary amenorrhea. Conception can occur in patients with Turner's syndrome, but many such pregnancies are abnormal.

UTERINE DEFECTS

Uterine defects can also cause primary amenorrhea. Isolated absence of the uterus is found in Rokitansky syndrome. Puberty is otherwise normal, the karyotype is 46,XX, and gonadotropin levels are normal. Developmental anomalies of the urinary tract are common, and pyelography is indicated for patients who have this syndrome. The uterus and upper vagina are also missing in patients who have testicular feminization and other male pseudohermaphroditism syndromes associated with androgen resistance. These patients have breast development because their estrogens are effective. They have 46,XY karyotypes, and their gonadotropin levels are often slightly elevated.[6]

DIAGNOSIS AND THERAPY

In an initial evaluation, any family history of a problem similar to that of the patient should be noted. Important findings on physical examination include the height of the patient, the degree of breast development, and the presence or absence of a uterus, of hirsutism, and of any somatic anomalies [*see Figure 4*]. The fundamental diagnostic aim thereafter is to distinguish between a central and a peripheral cause. If gonadotropin levels are elevated, the defect is in the gonads, and cytogenetic investigation for the cause is indicated. If estrogen effects are absent and the FSH level is low or normal, the defect is in the hypothalamus or pituitary, and CT or MRI of the pituitary and refined tests of pituitary function are needed. If breast development and the gonadotropin level are normal, uterine absence may be the defect.

In general, treatment is obvious once the underlying disease is identified. For otherwise normal girls who have been exercising or dieting strenuously, reassurance and guidance toward ideal body weight should suffice. Hypothalamic hypogonadism can be treated with estrogen and progesterone to produce breast development and to stimulate menstrual periods. Pulsatile administration of GnRH in dynamics that reproduce the normal pattern can induce completely normal pubertal maturation, including ovulation and fertility.[7] Patients who have gonadal failure require replacement therapy; gonadectomy is indicated for those who have Y chromosomes. The psychological difficulties often attendant on sexual immaturity require sensitive counseling and support.

Disorders of Menstruation: Secondary Amenorrhea

The term secondary amenorrhea refers to the cessation of menstrual periods in women who previously had normal periods. The same four-tiered system is useful in the evaluation of these patients, but the causes at each level and the relative importance of the various levels are significantly different. Before the differential diagnosis is described, it should be emphasized that the most common explanation for secondary amenorrhea in nonmenopausal women is pregnancy. It is risky and needless to subject a pregnant woman to a workup for amenorrhea, and therefore, a urine or plasma human chorionic gonadotropin assay should be done. In this discussion, it is assumed that the patient is not pregnant or menopausal.

The broadest way to interpret secondary amenorrhea is to assert that any woman of reproductive age with a healthy uterus who is not having periods is either pregnant or anovulatory. This formulation reflects the finite life span of the corpus luteum (14 days). Two weeks after ovulation, unless pregnancy occurs, the

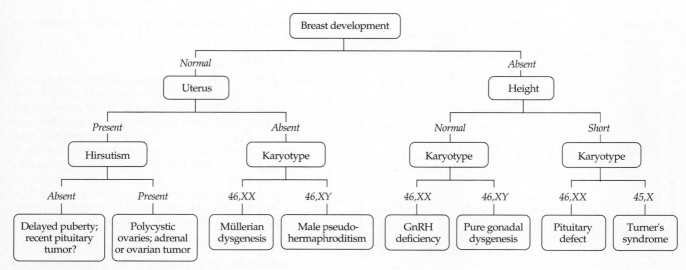

Figure 4 **Algorithm for evaluation of primary amenorrhea.**

plasma levels of estrogen, progesterone, and inhibin fall, and the endometrium is shed. Because uterine unresponsiveness to hormones is very rare, the evaluation of secondary amenorrhea principally depends on showing either that the cyclic production of gonadotropins is deficient or that the ovary is unresponsive.

HYPOTHALAMIC DEFECTS

Although hypothalamic deficiency is the least frequent cause of primary amenorrhea, the most common reason for secondary amenorrhea is a failure of the LH surge that is required for ovulation—so-called hypothalamic amenorrhea. The basal secretion of FSH is low-normal, but a defect in either estrogen secretion or the amplitude or frequency of LH release prevents the normal midcycle surge in LH and FSH from occurring. This hormonal pattern is associated with many kinds of mild psychological distress, such as that encountered in being away from home at camp or school, and with mild weight loss or increase in exercise. Sometimes it occurs for no apparent reason. Because basal estrogen secretion is intact, the endometrium is chronically subjected to a low level of proliferative stimulus, and progesterone-binding protein is presumably present. A brief course of progesterone produces withdrawal bleeding, simulating a normal period. This test is the most valuable initial approach to the diagnosis of secondary amenorrhea. For the price of an injection of progesterone (100 mg) or a few tablets of pure oral progestin, such as medroxyprogesterone, 10 mg daily for 5 days, the clinician gets a safe bioassay of FSH and estrogen levels and confirmation of uterine responsiveness, and the patient gets the reassurance of restored menstrual flow. This test should precede other diagnostic measures [*see Figure 5*].

The term hypothalamic amenorrhea is also applied to a more severely disturbed hypothalamic-pituitary axis. In this variant, basal estrogen secretion is low, and progesterone challenge does not induce withdrawal bleeding. The syndrome is associated with severe weight loss, as in anorexia nervosa; with profound psychological or emotional stress; with strenuous exercise or musical training; or with no apparent cause.[8] As there is a spectrum of clinical severity, so is there a range of pathophysiologic disturbance. In some patients, the frequency of gonadotropin (and, by inference, GnRH) release is decreased, but pulse amplitude is normal. In others, most dramatically in those with severe anorexia, GnRH release reverts from its adult pattern to one characteristic

of the prepubertal child; pulses diminish in both amplitude and frequency. There is thus a wide spectrum of hypothalamic amenorrhea syndromes.

The treatment of hypothalamic amenorrhea depends on the severity and the mechanism. For patients who respond to progestin, it may suffice to provide patience, interpretation, and a supportive relationship because the phenomenon tends to correct itself. Patients who appear underweight should be encouraged to gain a few pounds to give themselves the best chance of spontaneous return of periods. In the light of the growing evidence that unopposed estrogen stimulation of the endometrium is disadvantageous, however, I favor periodic administration of small doses

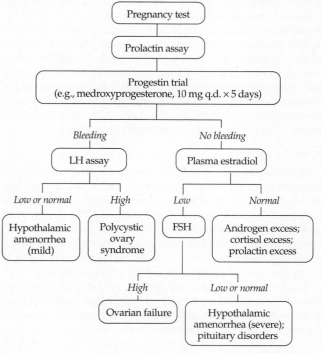

Figure 5 **An algorithm for evaluation of secondary amenorrhea. Because of the frequency of hyperprolactinemia, a prolactin assay should be done at the outset of a workup.**

of progestin to achieve withdrawal bleeding. Medroxyprogesterone, 5 or 10 mg daily for 5 days every 2 months, works well for this purpose. It accomplishes three things: the patient is reassured, excessive buildup of estrogen-stimulated endometrium is prevented, and the diagnostic focus is kept intact for the rare patient who is actually en route to true pituitary deficiency. Patients with pituitary insufficiency bleed in response to progestin as long as FSH secretion remains intact. When FSH (and thus estrogen) deficiency develops, progestin does not induce bleeding, which signals the more troublesome diagnosis (see below).

In patients with hypothalamic amenorrhea who desire fertility, success in inducing bleeding with progesterone correlates with success in inducing ovulation with clomiphene. A low dosage of clomiphene, such as 50 mg daily for 3 days, is given at first. If there is no result, the dosage is gradually increased to 100 mg daily for 5 days. One should wait at least a month after each course of therapy to be sure that neither pregnancy nor menses has supervened. If clomiphene is not successful, gonadotropin therapy is appropriate. However, treatment with synthetic GnRH is more physiologic, less uncomfortable, and less expensive than gonadotropin therapy. The hypothalamic releasing hormone can be given subcutaneously or intravenously through an indwelling needle. Pulses of infusion are timed to mimic the 90- to 120-minute natural intervals.[9,10] Best results are obtained with intravenous administration timed by a battery-driven pump worn like a temporary pacemaker, but self-administration during waking hours also works. Interestingly, GnRH treatment is most successful when GnRH deficiency is absolute. Patients with a partial GnRH deficiency are prone to multiple pregnancies unless minimal GnRH doses are used.

Athlete's Amenorrhea

Menstrual abnormalities among athletes deserve special mention because of their frequency and therapeutic implications. Prospective studies have shown defects in the luteal phase in some asymptomatic women—either subnormal progesterone secretion in women with normal-length cycles or an actual shortening of the luteal phase.[11] An increasing number of young women, seemingly in excellent physical health, are reporting oligomenorrhea and amenorrhea.[12,13] Contributing factors include leanness, extreme physical exertion, psychological stress, fad diets, and eating disorders. The combination of disordered eating, amenorrhea, and osteoporosis has been dubbed the female athlete triad. The amenorrhea is presumed to result from a disturbance of the neuroendocrine rhythm; even though the condition sometimes appears very severe, it seems to be reversible. When the contributing factors are eased or corrected, menses usually resume and fertility is not impaired.

The numerous reports of osteopenia, frank osteoporosis, and sport-related fractures in these patients reflect an underlying problem.[14,15] Estrogen levels and bone density in amenorrheic athletes are lower than those in their eumenorrheic peers, and the decreases in bone mass may not be reversed by later resumption of menses. In other words, by never achieving a normal peak bone mass, these athletes may be risking long-range difficulty with postmenopausal osteoporosis. Thus, it may be wise for amenorrheic athletes who do not wish to lower their exercise level to consider estrogen-progesterone and calcium therapy.[16]

PITUITARY DEFECTS

Acquired gonadotropin deficiency is usually caused by postpartum necrosis of the pituitary (Sheehan's syndrome), a primary or metastatic tumor, or granulomas. Both FSH and LH are usually depressed; thus, the progesterone test produces no withdrawal bleeding [see Figure 5]. Other pituitary hormones may also be deficient, although in early stages only growth hormone is affected, and its absence produces few symptoms in adults. Local symptoms of pituitary tumor (e.g., headache and visual-field defect) should be sought to confirm the diagnosis. CT or MRI of the pituitary and measurement of estrogen, gonadotropin, and prolactin levels should be done in patients who do not respond to progesterone. The longer amenorrhea persists, the more likely a pituitary tumor is the cause. In the occasional patient with a pituitary tumor who at first has enough estrogen effect to respond to progestin, a repeat progestin trial may reveal progressive estrogen deficiency.

Hyperprolactinemia, secondary to either a hypothalamic defect or a pituitary tumor, is the proximate cause of secondary amenorrhea in about 25% of cases. The tumors are often microadenomas that are revealed only by CT or MRI. Measurement of plasma prolactin should therefore be an early part of the workup for secondary amenorrhea. Excellent therapy is available for hyperprolactinemia [see Chapter 45].

OVARIAN DEFECTS

Primary ovarian failure is a rare cause of secondary amenorrhea in young women.[17] It may occur in patients with mosaic gonadal dysgenesis who have some of the features of Turner's syndrome but are so mildly affected that they escape detection. These patients usually have buccal smear defects or karyotype abnormalities as well as a high gonadotropin level. As a measurement of the gonadotropin level, FSH assay gives better separation from the normal range than does LH assay. In patients who do not bleed after a trial of progesterone, FSH assay should be done before other tests. Other causes of acquired ovarian failure include autoimmune oophoritis, usually seen with other evidence of autoimmune disease, such as adrenal or thyroid deficiency (interestingly, adrenal insufficiency almost always precedes ovarian failure), myasthenia gravis, or pernicious anemia; mumps oophoritis, which is less common than orchitis; and idiopathic premature ovarian failure.[18,19] In all circumstances, estrogen levels are either low or early follicular phase, the patient does not respond to progesterone, and the FSH value is high. An elevated FSH value, repeated and confirmed, reflects follicular depletion and ordinarily predicts permanent amenorrhea. However, some patients in this group have so-called resistant ovary syndrome rather than true follicular depletion. In these persons, pelvic ultrasonography or laparoscopy discloses ample numbers of follicles. Mysteriously, even some patients who have premature ovarian failure resume menstruating and conceive. Although patients with premature ovarian failure should receive combined estrogen and progestin therapy for estrogen deficiency, I favor omitting replacement therapy for 1 or 2 months a year to see whether ovarian function has resumed.

Another cause of ovarian failure is the follicular destruction produced by treatment of malignant disease. When this syndrome is caused by drugs such as alkylating agents, it can be reversible; when caused by radiotherapy, the syndrome is permanent. Treatment should include estrogen replacement and periodic progesterone-induced withdrawal bleeding. A patient with premature ovarian failure of any cause can now become pregnant by fertilization and implantation of a donor oocyte and suitable hormonal preparation of the uterus.

Polycystic ovary syndrome can present as either primary or secondary amenorrhea [see Polycystic Ovary Syndrome, below].

UTERINE DEFECTS

Uterine deficiency is the least common cause of secondary amenorrhea. It is found in patients who have had severe endometritis, either postpartum or postabortion (Asherman's syndrome); in some patients who have had energetic curettage that removed the basal epithelial levels; and in occasional patients with tuberculosis, brucellosis, or other chronic granulomatous disease. Diagnostic features include (1) other evidence of the causative disease, (2) a relevant history, (3) normal estrogen and gonadotropin levels, and (4) failure to respond with bleeding after the administration of progesterone and after a trial of estrogen plus progesterone. Gynecologic consultation, with curettage and tissue diagnosis, should be sought. Therapy is available for the granulomatous diseases, and some success has been achieved using curettage and corticosteroids for the bridging synechiae seen in Asherman's syndrome.

SUMMARY OF SECONDARY AMENORRHEA

Secondary amenorrhea can be considered a reversal or abrogation of the pubertal maturation of the hypothalamic-pituitary-ovarian axis. A variety of disorders can reverse the achievement of puberty [see Figure 6]. The mildest abnormality, which does not cause amenorrhea, is an inadequate luteal phase; although ovulation occurs, the corpus luteum produces subnormal levels of estrogen, progesterone, and inhibin, and luteolysis occurs in less than the normal 2 weeks. Endometrial development is retarded, and infertility presumably results because the endometrium is insufficiently prepared.[20]

In a more severe abnormality, anovulation and amenorrhea result, but basal secretion of FSH and LH is intact. In the most severe reversal of puberty, basal gonadotropin and estradiol secretions are low, and even the nocturnal LH release of early puberty disappears. As a patient recovers from one of these disorders—for example, as a previously anorexic patient regains body weight—the normal maturation of puberty is reexperienced, and ultimately, cyclic periods may return. If the abnormality was prolactin excess, recovery after correction of the underlying problem usually occurs at a much faster rate [see Chapter 45].

Disorders of Menstruation: Excessive Uterine Bleeding

Abnormal uterine bleeding often requires gynecologic work-up and therapy, but the primary physician can evaluate most patients and make certain diagnoses before referring the patient. The principal disorders can be found in the previously described four-tiered structure (i.e., hypothalamus, pituitary, ovary, and duct structures), but the problem is more often in the ovaries and uterus than in the hypothalamic-pituitary axis. In the most general terms, pathologic uterine bleeding results from (1) anovulation with high levels of unopposed estrogen, (2) intrauterine structural defects, or (3) bleeding disorders. The primary physician can look for anovulation and bleeding defects; definitive diagnosis of uterine structural disease requires consultation.[21-23]

HYPOTHALAMIC DEFECTS

Like amenorrhea, irregular uterine bleeding may reflect anovulation and may result from a failure of the midcycle surge of LH. If this defect is accompanied by abundant estrogen, bleeding is often excessive; if estrogen levels are low, oligomenorrhea results. Irregular LH cycling is physiologic early in pubescence and in the early months post partum; in both circumstances, oligomenorrhea is the rule, but excessive bleeding occurs occasionally. Hypo-

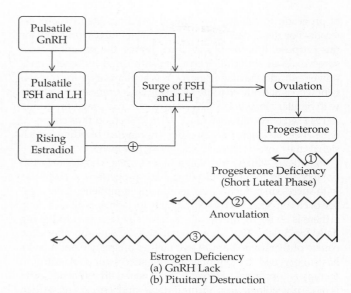

Figure 6 **During the normal menstrual cycle, pulsatile GnRH release stimulates secretion of FSH and LH, which leads to a rising level of estradiol. At a critical level, estradiol triggers surges of GnRH, LH, and FSH, which are followed by ovulation and progesterone secretion. The pathophysiology of secondary amenorrhea involves one of three defects in the normal menstrual cycle, shown here by jagged blue arrows indicating the extent of cycle disruption: (1) deficient progesterone secretion, producing a short, inadequate luteal phase (such patients are infertile rather than amenorrheic); (2) anovulatory cycles, in which tonic gonadotropin and estradiol secretions are intact but no LH or FSH surge takes place, and hence there is no ovulation; and (3) estrogen-deficiency states secondary to diminished GnRH secretion or to pituitary deficiency.**

thyroidism should also be considered as a cause of anovulatory bleeding. A serum thyroid-stimulating hormone assay will confirm or exclude the diagnosis. Psychogenic and nutritionally induced defects in the LH cycle occasionally produce menorrhagia. More often, however, FSH and estrogen levels are on the low side, and periods are scant or absent.

PITUITARY DEFECTS

Pituitary defects rarely cause irregular uterine bleeding. Lack of LH is almost always accompanied by low FSH and estrogen levels, and endometrial stimulation is minimal. Hyperprolactinemia may, however, result in anovulatory cycles accompanied by excess bleeding.

OVARIAN DEFECTS

Ovarian causes of irregular uterine bleeding are of great importance. The most common one is menopause. As menopause approaches, despite adequate LH secretion, follicle depletion may make ovulation irregular and infrequent. If FSH and estrogen levels remain normal, menorrhagia is common [see Menopause, below]. In disorders such as polycystic ovary syndrome, ovulation is also irregular; estrogen levels may be normal or high, and there are usually high opposing androgen levels. If the androgen does not inhibit the estrogen excessively, the latter can produce endometrial hyperplasia and bleeding. Estrogen-secreting ovarian tumors, such as granulosa cell tumor, can produce hyperestrinism, endometrial hyperplasia, and irregular uterine bleeding. This sequence can precede uterine neoplasia as well, and the detection of endometrial carcinoma in the presence of perimenopausal menstrual irregularity is an important challenge.

UTERINE DEFECTS

Uterine lesions are the most frequent cause of abnormal vaginal bleeding. The differential diagnosis of uterine lesions is well beyond the scope of this chapter. It includes pregnancy, fibroids, cervical and endometrial polyps, cervical and fundal cancer, adenomyosis, cystic hyperplasia of the endometrium, and inflammatory lesions. Of the diagnostic modalities available to the general physician, a properly taken vaginal cytology is extremely reliable for detecting cervical cancer but provides poor reassurance about endometrial cancer.

Abnormal uterine bleeding may be caused by defects in hemostasis. Platelet disorders are most common; both thrombocytopenia and qualitative platelet abnormalities often present as menorrhagia. Clotting factor defects seldom produce endometrial bleeding. Whatever the cause, iron deficiency anemia from menorrhagia can inhibit ovulation and lead to estrogen-driven endometrial hyperplasia, adding to poor platelet function.

DIAGNOSTIC AND THERAPEUTIC APPROACH

The approach to abnormal uterine bleeding depends mainly on the age of the woman; in patients younger than 30 years, uterine structural defects are uncommon enough to make it safe to temporize with hormonal approaches. Before initiating a program of hormone therapy, one must carry out certain steps:

1. A careful history to detect symptoms of systemic disease and to identify a pattern of bleeding suggestive of anovulation. Specifically, anovulatory periods tend to be irregular in interval, duration, and amount of flow.

2. A physical examination to exclude systemic illness, pregnancy, and visible or palpable disease of the cervix or fundus uteri.

3. A pregnancy test.

4. A vaginal smear to obtain a negative vaginal cytology.

5. A routine blood cell count to detect anemia, thrombocytopenia, or other hematologic disease, and a blood urea nitrogen (BUN) or creatinine measurement to detect renal impairment, a common cause of a qualitative platelet defect.

A patient with vaginal bleeding who is also anemic and hypotensive needs to be hospitalized for intravenous fluid administration and possibly for blood transfusion. This type of bleeding reflects an inadequate estrogen level, and the administration of 25 mg of conjugated equine estrogen intravenously every 4 hours usually stops the bleeding in less than a day. This dosage of estrogen almost always causes nausea, and thus, the treatment should be discontinued as soon as the bleeding stops. If a single day of therapy is not successful, uterine curettage is usually required.

The administration of high-dose intravenous estrogen therapy is, in fact, seldom needed. If steps 1 through 5 produce reassuring results in a patient who presents in the office, progesterone (100 mg I.M.) or medroxyprogesterone (10 mg p.o. daily for 10 days) should be administered. This approach should change the estrogen-primed endometrium to a secretory pattern and result in a definitive flow. This method, sometimes referred to as a medical dilatation and curettage, is highly reliable for controlling bleeding due to anovulation. If no abnormal bleeding occurs after the progestin-induced period, one can assume that a structural defect is not the major current problem. If bleeding recurs, however, gynecologic consultation is indicated.

In patients older than 30 years, intrauterine disease becomes so much more likely that the above approach is not to be solely trusted. I still carry out steps 1 through 5 and give progestin to control

the problem until consultation can be sought, but there is enough likelihood of a uterine lesion to make me reluctant to monitor such patients without gynecologic consultation.

Finally, some patients have ovulatory cycles and no uterine or hematologic abnormalities but have menorrhagia. For these patients, danazol, 200 mg/day, is excellent therapy.[24]

Polycystic Ovary Syndrome

Ever since Stein and Leventhal defined a syndrome of hirsutism, oligomenorrhea, and enlarged ovaries, the condition has aroused both controversy and intense interest. Modern usage avoids the eponym Stein-Leventhal and refers to polycystic ovary (PCO) syndrome instead. The clinical features of patients with PCO syndrome overlap some of the chief complaints already discussed—amenorrhea and abnormal bleeding. However, additional problems of infertility, hirsutism, and insulin resistance implicate pathogenetic factors different from those so far emphasized.

Clinical findings in PCO syndrome may include primary amenorrhea, irregular periods followed by oligomenorrhea and secondary amenorrhea, dysfunctional bleeding, infertility, hirsutism and occasionally true virilism, and obesity. The typical patient has had difficulty since her teen years: a cardinal diagnostic clue is the statement "Doctor, I've never had regular periods." Physical examination usually shows signs of androgen excess, including increased body hair; true virilism is uncommon. Ovarian enlargement is common but not needed to make the diagnosis. Indeed, even the diagnostic gold standard, transvaginal ultrasonography, is neither completely sensitive nor completely specific: some patients with the syndrome do not have cystic ovaries, and about 20% of normal women have cysts.[25]

Endocrine findings in PCO syndrome are variable and much disputed, partly because of the controversy in making the diagnosis. In general, FSH and estradiol levels are at least as high as normal midfollicular levels but do not cycle normally; amenorrheic or oligomenorrheic patients who have PCO syndrome usually bleed in response to progestin [see Figure 5]. LH is high-normal, typically with an LH-FSH ratio greater than 2, but there is usually no midcycle surge and hence no ovulation or significant progesterone production. Levels of testosterone, androstenedione, and estrone (the estrogen produced directly from androstenedione) tend to be elevated. Often, only the unbound testosterone level is high; this test should be done routinely if PCO syndrome is suspected. The correlation between androgen levels and physical signs is not close; clinical androgen effect may correlate better with the androgen metabolite 5α-androstanediol.

The pathophysiology of PCO syndrome includes anovulation, elevated but not surging LH, increased androgen production, and follicular atresia without maturation. At least four pathophysiologic abnormalities have been identified [see Figure 7]: increased frequency of GnRH pulses,[26,27] dysregulation of androgen secretion in the ovaries and sometimes in the adrenal glands,[28,29] cystic changes in the ovaries, and hyperinsulinism, with insulin or a related peptide contributing to excess androgen production.[30] The precise relation between hyperinsulinism and hyperandrogenism is not clear, but it is likely that high levels of insulin, acting through the insulin receptor, cause or aggravate androgen overproduction in ovaries with the PCO defect.[31,32] Hyperinsulinism and insulin resistance are intrinsic features of PCO syndrome. Diabetes mellitus is uncommon, but obese patients with PCO syndrome usually have markedly elevated insulin levels and often manifest intolerance to glucose challenge. A simple fasting glucose-insulin

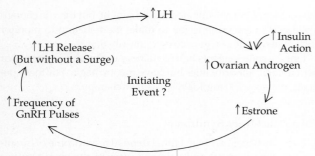

Figure 7 **The pathophysiology of the polycystic ovary syndrome can be viewed as a self-reinforcing cycle. The event initiating the cycle is unknown and may be different in different patients. The elements of the cycle include an acyclic, surgeless increase in the release of LH, increased ovarian androgen production, and increased production of estrone. Hyperinsulinism is a factor in many patients.**

ratio of less than 4.5 can be used in non-Hispanic white women.[33] Clinical decision making, however, does not require resolution of this controversy. Obese patients should be helped to lose weight, and patients with frank diabetes should receive appropriate therapy; hyperandrogenism itself is regularly treated in caring for patients with PCO syndrome.

The differential diagnosis of PCO syndrome is not easy. In the closely related disorder hyperthecosis, clinical androgen excess tends to be greater and frank virilism is more often seen. Adrenal cortical excess is also common in hyperthecosis. Ovarian tumors that make androgen can produce all the features of PCO syndrome, but they tend to have a course with sharper onset and clearer progression; that is, they appear to produce a change in menses and increased hair growth in previously normal women, whereas PCO syndrome is usually manifest beginning at puberty.[34] The usual ovarian tumors are arrhenoblastoma, lipoid tumor, and hilus cell tumor. Arrhenoblastoma, a tumor whose cells resemble Leydig cells, usually develops in young girls. Lipoid tumors are composed of cells similar to adrenal cells and are suggestive of the embryologic and hormonal analogies between gonads and adrenals. Hilus cell tumors, which occur most frequently after menopause, derive from cells similar to testis cells that are carried into the ovary at the time of gonadal differentiation. A unique hormonal feature of the ovary is that a metastatic tumor, particularly of gastrointestinal origin, occasionally triggers overproduction of androgens. A common feature of all ovarian tumors is the finding of a plasma testosterone level of higher than 200 ng/ml. This finding should lead directly to CT or MRI of the ovaries and the adrenal glands. When the plasma testosterone level is lower than 200 ng/ml, functional hyperandrogenism is far more likely.

Ultimately, however, PCO syndrome is a clinical diagnosis that accounts for more than 90% of patients with pubertal onset of irregular periods and hyperandrogenism. Hirsutism is usually apparent but may be very mild. Obesity, especially in young women, is no longer a required feature of the diagnosis, and even cystic changes in the ovary are sometimes absent. The appropriate workup is much debated, but I believe a measurement of total and free testosterone, androstenedione, and dehydroepiandrosterone sulfate (DHEAS) is indicated. An elevated testosterone level with a normal DHEAS level points to an ovarian source; striking elevation of DHEAS suggests an adrenal origin [*see Chapter 49*]. However, because hirsutism without serum androgen elevation can occur, as can increased androgens without hirsutism, the main value of the test is to exclude a tumor as the cause of the syndrome.

The treatment of PCO syndrome has been significantly im-

proved. In the past, wedge resection of one or both ovaries was standard. The antiestrogen clomiphene is now a standard therapy for patients with anovulation caused by PCO syndrome and is used primarily when fertility is desired. Because of the risk of hyperstimulation and multiple ovulation, however, clomiphene should be administered by an experienced practitioner, and the results should be monitored with ultrasonography and measurements of the plasma estrogen level.

The availability of purified GnRH, synthetic GnRH analogues with both agonist and antagonist effects, and gonadotropins has spawned a wide array of therapeutic approaches. Long-acting GnRH analogues can be used to suppress the hypothalamic-pituitary-ovarian axis and accompanying hyperandrogenism. The pulsatile administration of GnRH or sequential FSH and LH has a high likelihood of inducing ovulation. Although it remains easier to induce ovulation in patients with PCO syndrome than to help them achieve pregnancy, the prognosis for these patients has improved greatly.[35]

Alleviation of hirsutism is often the patient's major concern. Depilatory creams, waxes, and electrolysis can all be used to treat limited areas, but many patients seek hormone therapy. There are two principal treatments for hirsutism—antiandrogens and oral contraceptives. The aldosterone antagonist spironolactone competes with androgen for binding to the androgen receptor and decreases the androgen effect beyond that point. Dosages of 50 to 150 mg/day often produce improvement after 4 to 6 months. The drug should not be given to patients with diabetes or to those prone to hyporeninemic hypoaldosteronism. Effective contraception must simultaneously be used by sexually active women to prevent potential harm to a male fetus because of androgen blockade. Oral contraceptives are useful by themselves and in conjunction with spironolactone. To varying degrees in different women, oral contraceptives suppress gonadotropins, reduce circulating androgens, increase androgen binding, and inhibit testosterone metabolism.[36] Prednisone—2.5 to 5.0 mg at bedtime—is useful for patients whose excess androgen appears to arise from the adrenal glands.

One feature of PCO syndrome merits separate mention. Long intervals of anovulation, such as those that occur in PCO syndrome, can be a prelude to endometrial carcinoma. The link may be either continuous exposure of the endometrium to estrogen unopposed by progesterone or the particular carcinogenic role alleged for estrone, the estrogen that appears to be present in high levels in this disorder. Thus, it is important to induce regular shedding of the endometrium by judicious use of a synthetic progestin and to plan follow-up with regular physical examinations, Papanicolaou smears, and careful attention to any unexpected bleeding.

Premenstrual Syndrome

Dysmenorrhea refers to the cramps and other physical discomforts that accompany ovulatory cycles in many women. Cramps reflect the effect of prostaglandins produced and acting in a progesterone-rich environment. Inhibitors of prostaglandin endoperoxide synthase, such as nonsteroidal anti-inflammatory drugs (NSAIDs), are extremely effective in alleviating dysmenorrhea. Indomethacin, 25 mg twice a day for 2 to 3 days from the onset of discomfort, is adequate for most women.

The term premenstrual syndrome (PMS) refers to a variable constellation of symptoms that appear during the 7 to 10 days before menstruation and disappear with the start of the menstrual period. There is great disagreement on the nature, timing, pathogenesis, treatment, and even the existence of the disorder. Physical symptoms include bloating, breast swelling and discomfort, pelvic pain, headache, ankle swelling, and bowel changes. Psychological symptoms include irritability, aggressiveness, depression, anxiety, tension, and changes in libido. There is no physical sign or laboratory marker of PMS, but charting of symptoms by the patient for 2 to 3 months should reveal the menstrual association and serve as a guide to therapy.

The pathogenesis of PMS and whether its several symptoms have differing mechanisms are unknown.[37,38] Candidate explanations include altered absolute levels or ratios of gonadal steroids, steroid-induced variations in neurotransmitters, and hormone-induced changes in salt and water balance or intermediary metabolism. In the absence of better understanding than now exists, empirical therapy seems reasonable.

Relatively few of the drugs used for PMS have demonstrated therapeutic effectiveness in double-blind, placebo-controlled trials.[39] In selecting a remedy, one should begin with a 2-month calendar of daily entries in which the patient's symptoms and weight are recorded in relation to the dates of menstrual flow. Treatment can then be individualized for the type of symptom and for the dates of maximum distress. When breast symptoms predominate, bromocriptine, 2.5 mg at bedtime, or danazol, 200 mg once or twice a day, can be tried, beginning 1 or 2 days before symptoms are expected. For pelvic pain or headache, an NSAID seems best. For bloating accompanied by at least a 2 lb weight gain, spironolactone, 50 to 100 mg a day, is often effective. Pyridoxine, 100 mg daily, has been used extensively for psychological symptoms. Evidence of benefit is inconclusive, and the drug should be used only as a last resort because of numerous reports of sensory neuropathy.

Fluoxetine and alprazolam have each been used with success in patients with PMS.[40,41] It is of some concern whether continuous therapy is appropriate for intermittent symptoms; shorter-term use near the days on which severe symptoms occur is worth trying. Progesterone has probably been the most widely used treatment, but investigation does not support its efficacy.

Despite the fact that PMS symptoms are not consistently associated with a specific hormonal profile, the obliteration of menstrual cycles by use of GnRH antagonism produces a 75% reduction in symptoms. Patients treated with this approach, however, are exposed to the adverse effects of estrogen deficiency. There is now evidence that combining GnRH antagonism with conjugated estrogens and medroxyprogesterone prevents the problem of estrogen deficiency and does not cause PMS symptoms to recur. Thus, this combination therapy offers a new approach for patients with severe and disabling symptoms.[42] For all patients, reassurance, direct answers from the physician, and a generally healthy lifestyle are important predicates of any therapeutic trial. Discontinuance of treatment after 6 months to assess the continuing need is advisable.

Menopause

The ovary is the most precisely and quantitatively doomed organ in the body. More than 99% of the seven million follicles present in the ovaries of a female fetus at a gestational age of 5 months eventually undergo atresia.[43] The consequence of this process is menopause, an almost complete cessation of ovarian estrogen and progesterone production accompanied by amenorrhea, the latter occurring by an average age of 51 years. Four associated endocrine syndromes can be identified; their relative importance varies greatly from one woman to another.

ANOVULATORY CYCLES

The timing of the menopause, like that of the menarche, has a strong genetic influence.[44,45] The years leading up to and 1 year after the final menstrual period are known as perimenopause. During this time, many women actually have elevated levels of estrogen, breast fullness, some hot flashes, and occasionally heavy periods; decreases in serum inhibin levels may explain this change.[46] At some point, most women begin to ovulate irregularly, either because the follicular-phase rise in estrogen is less than what is needed to trigger an LH surge or because the remaining follicles are resistant to the ovulatory stimulus. Although for most women periods become lighter, in some women periods are irregular in interval and duration and heavy in amount. Excessive bleeding raises a question of intrauterine pathology [see Disorders of Menstruation: Excessive Uterine Bleeding, above], but after such pathology has been ruled out, intermittent progestin therapy is extremely effective. Medroxyprogesterone acetate, 10 mg a day from day 16 through day 25, usually corrects endometrial hyperplasia and leads to regular, appropriate menstrual flow. This approach can avert many unnecessary hysterectomies. Any iron deficiency anemia caused by heavy bleeding should also be treated. It is notable that bone mineral density begins to fall at an accelerated rate before the last menstrual period.

HOT FLASHES

The hot flash is a vasomotor phenomenon associated with declining, not deficient, estrogen levels.[47] Five-year-old girls and 85-year-old women do not have hot flashes, but at some point during the decline of estrogen secretion—in many women, for several years preceding the last menstrual period—80% of women in the United States experience hot flashes.[48] A typical flash consists of subjective awareness of heat followed in 45 to 60 seconds by warmth and often sweating in the upper body, a rise of 2° to 4° C in surface temperature, and a fall of 0.2° to 0.3° C in core temperature. Women who are asleep during a flash typically awake. A rise in LH accompanies most flashes. The contrasting changes in surface and core temperatures plus a presumed GnRH release implicate a hypothalamic process involving one or more neurotransmitters.

Estrogen therapy reliably suppresses hot flashes or blunts their severity. If given for less than 2 years, it carries little if any of the increased risk of endometrial carcinoma associated with prolonged use. Similarly, short-term treatment has not shown any correlation with an increased frequency of breast cancer. Thus, the use of oral conjugated estrogens at the lowest effective dosage, usually 0.3 mg daily for the first 25 days of each calendar month, is a safe and inexpensive therapy for hot flashes. Endometrial buildup is minimal at this dosage; nevertheless, to prevent unpredictable vaginal bleeding, most patients should also take a synthetic progestin. The most widely used progestin is medroxyprogesterone, given in dosages of 2.5 to 10 mg a day from day 16 through day 25 of each month. The larger dosage is required to restore the endometrium to a premenopausal luteal biochemical state, but at that dosage, many women notice bloating, mood effects, and even some PMS-like symptoms. Thus, lower progestin dosages are commonly used. When such dosages are taken for 10 days each month, endometrial hyperplasia is prevented in about 98% of patients; occasionally, progestin must be given for 13 days. Aspiration cytology monitoring is not routinely advised but may be reassuring for women who have a higher risk of endometrial cancer, especially those with a history of infertility, dysfunctional uterine bleeding, or anovulatory cycles.

Estrogen can also be administered transdermally. This route provides effective control of symptoms and prevents the buildup of high concentrations of estrogen in the liver that occurs after oral administration and absorption through the portal circulation.[49,50] Low-dose, continuous hormone replacement regimens are an option more frequently used for long-range treatment [*see* Osteoporosis, *below*].

Patients who are troubled by severe hot flashes but who do not wish to take estrogen can be given a pure progestin, such as megestrol acetate, 20 mg twice daily, or clonidine, 0.1 mg once daily.[51]

VAGINAL ATROPHY

In some women, the postmenopausal deficiency of estrogen leads to severe atrophy of the vaginal and urethral mucosae.[52] Symptoms include vaginal dryness and burning, dyspareunia, and a urethral syndrome with or without urinary infection. This condition usually appears several years after menopause rather than within the first year, when hot flashes occur. It is less severe in patients who remain sexually active, and it can be prevented by hormone replacement therapy. Once it has appeared, both oral and vaginal estrogen relieve the symptoms; although many women prefer estrogen vaginal cream, this therapy depends on absorption of estrogen for its effect. Delay in achieving complete correction of genitourinary symptoms reflects the fact that it can take up to 2 years to restore the vaginal mucosa to a premenopausal biochemical state. Correction and symptomatic relief appear to occur more quickly in women who are sexually active. For women who are not taking estrogen, a topical lubricant can afford considerable relief.[53]

OSTEOPOROSIS

One of the most important medical consequences of menopause is osteoporosis and the associated increase in fractures of the wrist, spine, and hips.[54] There are probably at least two types of osteoporosis, with overlapping but distinct pathogeneses.[55] Type I is related to estrogen deficiency; it occurs between 50 and 70 years of age and leads to fractures of the wrist and crush fractures of the spine. Type II occurs at about 70 years of age and beyond and is associated with fractures of the hip and wedge fractures of the spine. In type II, low vitamin D levels, decreased calcium intake, and impaired calcium absorption are more important than estrogen deficiency; slight increases of parathyroid hormone may also play a role.

In young males and females, bone formation exceeds resorption and bone mineral content increases. In early adulthood, the two processes are in balance and bone mass is constant. After about 45 years of age, bone resorption by osteoclasts exceeds formation by osteoblasts, and bone density decreases.[56] In women, however, the perimenopause and menopause are followed by 5 to 10 years of an accelerated decrease in bone density that does not occur in men. This process, superimposed on a lower peak bone mass, accounts in part for the greater frequency of osteoporosis and fracture in women.[57-59] The connection between this process and the predisposition to fracture is not yet clear,[60] but new studies have found an inverse correlation between bone mineral density and serum estradiol levels, including values below the cutoff of prior studies.[61-63] Many factors other than estrogen deficiency, such as smoking, thinness, a sedentary lifestyle, lower calcium intake, and some genetic and constitutional attributes, are associated with osteoporosis.[64,65] African-American women, for example, are less prone to develop osteoporosis because they enter adulthood with a higher average bone mass.[66,67]

Estrogen is the most effective agent for the prevention of postmenopausal osteoporosis.[64,68,69] The primary effect of estrogen on bone is antiresorptive rather than osteoblastic; as a result, it is more effective in preventing bone loss than in promoting recalcification.[70] If, however, estrogen therapy is begun shortly after the onset of menopause and is used regularly, it significantly reduces the rate of bone loss and the incidence of vertebra and hip fractures. The dose required to achieve this effect is 0.625 mg of conjugated estrogen or equivalent. Although this dose is larger than that needed for relief of hot flashes, it is economical, nonallergenic, and virtually free of immediate side effects. There are, however, several disadvantages of long-continued estrogen replacement. If estrogen is taken alone for more than 2 years, it induces endometrial hyperplasia, irregular vaginal bleeding, and a threefold to eightfold increase in endometrial carcinoma. These complications are averted by periodic progestin therapy, such as medroxyprogesterone, 2.5 to 10 mg a day for 10 days each month. This approach, however, reintroduces menstrual periods, and most studies of patient preference have found that concern about this effect weighs heavily in a patient's decision whether to discontinue therapy. A regimen of conjugated estrogens at 0.6 mg/day and medroxyprogesterone acetate at 2.5 mg/day causes most women to become amenorrheic after 6 to 8 months of therapy.[71,72] If the progestin dosage is not effective in controlling bleeding, it may have to be increased. Hysteroscopic curettage of the endometrium is a wise step to take when bleeding is unexplained.

Alternative Treatment of Osteoporosis

Bisphosphonate therapy provides an alternative to the use of estrogen for the prevention of osteoporosis. Bisphosphonates are synthetic derivatives of pyrophosphate that inhibit osteoclast-mediated bone resorption and thus can theoretically restore the balance between bone formation and resorption at a higher bone density. The availability of alendronate represents a significant advance. A 3-year study of women who received 10 mg of alendronate and 500 mg of calcium daily showed an almost 9% increase in lumbar spine density and a 50% decrease in the rate of new spinal fractures.[73,74] Alendronate has also been used to prevent rapid bone loss of the immediate postmenopausal period.[75] Although the long-term safety of alendronate remains to be demonstrated, this drug provides an important alternative for the patient who cannot or will not take estrogen.[76]

Sodium fluoride is another nonhormonal approach to the prevention of and therapy for osteoporosis. When given in a slow-release formulation, with calcium, for more than 4 years, this drug induced a 4% to 5% increase a year in vertebral bone mass and a slightly lesser effect on the hip.[77,78] The treatment was most effective in patients with minimal loss of bone density at initiation of therapy, almost eliminating new fractures in this group of patients.

CARDIOVASCULAR DISEASE

The discussion of the risks and benefits of hormone replacement therapy for osteoporosis has been overshadowed by emerging evidence that long-range estrogen therapy has a beneficial effect on the incidence of coronary artery disease.

Cardiovascular disease is the principal cause of death in postmenopausal women. The relative freedom from atherosclerosis of the premenopausal woman is erased by menopause; after that, mortality from myocardial infarction is more than four times the mortality from breast and endometrial cancer combined.[79-81] The precipitous postmenopausal increase in coronary artery disease may be partly explained by a relative increase in the ratio of low-density lipoprotein (LDL) to high-density lipoprotein (HDL) after menopause. However, estrogen has other, direct, and probably more important effects.[82] It has a vasodilatory action associated with increases in prostacyclin and nitric oxide and an atheroprotective effect probably related to inhibition of vascular proliferation. Thus, the decision whether to undertake estrogen replacement therapy should be made with an awareness of its potential positive impact on cardiovascular disease. Many case-controlled but not randomized studies indicate that postmenopausal women on estrogen replacement have approximately one half the risk of atherosclerotic cardiovascular complications (angina, myocardial infarction, or death) of postmenopausal women not receiving estrogen.[83-85] Several large prospective trials of hormone replacement therapy are under way.[86] One of the first randomized trials did not show a cardiovascular benefit in 4 years—a puzzling finding and one that remains to be confirmed.[87]

The benefits of estrogen on cardiovascular disease have thus far been seen in patients who are taking estrogen alone. Because most patients now take progestin as well as estrogen, it is important to anticipate the influence of combined treatment on lipid levels.[88,89] Although there is some disparity between reports, it appears that the beneficial lowering of LDL cholesterol by estrogen is preserved, and the estrogen-induced increase in HDL cholesterol is unlikely to be offset by cyclic medroxyprogesterone.[90] Estrogen therapy should not be started in patients with hypertriglyceridemia because of the risk of inducing further lipid elevation and pancreatitis.[91]

The principal drawback to long-range hormone replacement therapy is the risk that the estrogen will increase the incidence of breast cancer. Because there has been no large-scale randomized trial, inferences have had to be drawn from a variety of less rigorous sources, including a meta-analysis,[92] and there is no consensus.[93] Most investigators believe that estrogen replacement for longer than 10 years carries a relative risk of about 1.2 to 1.3, that simultaneous progesterone use neither protects against nor aggravates the risk,[94,95] and that this enhanced risk is certainly to be kept in mind by women with a family history of the disease.

Transdermal administration of estrogen prevents the pharmacologic first-pass effect on the liver that occurs when estrogen is given orally; in a sense, oral estrogen overtreats the liver relative to the peripheral tissues. Thus, the transdermal route is preferred for women who need to minimize hepatic consequences such as an excess stimulation of clotting factors. An increase in the risk of deep vein thrombosis has been recently identified as a disadvantage to oral estrogen.[96] Topical estrogen appears to be as safe as oral estrogen and presumably will have the same effect in preventing osteoporosis.[97] Topical estrogen is more expensive than oral conjugated estrogens, and although there is no reason to suspect that the topical form will have less of an impact on cardiovascular disease than the oral form, it has not yet been proved to be as effective in large-scale studies.

ALTERNATIVE APPROACHES TO ESTROGEN THERAPY

A major antagonist to estrogen effect, tamoxifen, has been in use to treat breast cancer for over 15 years. Despite its antiestrogen effect on the breast, tamoxifen is estrogenlike in countering osteoporosis, in modifying coronary artery disease, and in inducing endometrial hyperplasia and neoplasia. This clinical observation, buttressed by extensive research, has dramatically restructured our knowledge of how estrogen works.[98,99] Estrogens use at least two receptors, and the actions of estrogens are modified importantly by a variety of modulators and coactivators. This emerging science has led to the synthesis of compounds tailored to mimic some of the natural hormone's effects. The first of these selective estrogen receptor modulators (SERMs) to be released is raloxifene, which acts as an antagonist in the breast and uterus and an agonist in bone and probably the heart. Although one cannot yet specify the relative role of raloxifene, it is certainly in the vanguard of new agents that will soon be available to the clinician.

Bisphosphonates, such as alendronate, and SERMs, such as raloxifene, are legitimate alternatives to estrogen replacement therapy for osteoporosis (see above). Even more attractive, however, are preventive strategies.[64,100] These include achieving optimal bone mass in childhood, adolescence, and young adulthood and maintaining that bone mass in adulthood through adequate exercise and calcium intake (at least 1,000 mg/day) and the avoidance of tobacco and excessive alcohol intake. After menopause, physical activity and an even higher calcium intake (1,500 mg/day) are important.

SUMMARY OF ESTROGEN THERAPY FOR MENOPAUSE

There are few circumstances in medicine to rival menopausal hormone therapy in allowing informed consent by the patient. The issue is reasonably well understood, the goals of treatment are comprehensible, the risks and benefits can be outlined in accessible terminology, and there is no urgency. However, the bombardment of conflicting assertions and recommendations makes it very difficult for even a well-informed person to find her way. The following section is offered as an approach that I have found useful and that I believe any patient can use.

The increase in human longevity causes many women to live one third or more of their lives without natural estrogen and progesterone.[83] The estrogen-deficiency state produced by menopause has short-range (hot flashes), medium-range (vaginal atrophy), and long-range (osteoporosis) consequences that can be relieved or prevented by estrogen replacement. Treatment for up to 2 years, particularly if it is accompanied by progestin-induced endometrial shedding, has minimal risk and, in the absence of a contraindication such as breast cancer, can be undertaken pretty much as the patient decides.

Long-term estrogen use as prophylaxis against osteoporosis is a different matter. Effective, inexpensive therapy is available that reduces the risk of fracture by 50% and simultaneously reduces the relative risk of coronary artery disease. Simultaneous progestin therapy is required to avoid endometrial hyperplasia and neoplasia, but new programs that employ continuous low-dose progestin can prevent or limit menstrual bleeding.

Patients can be assisted in making a decision about whether to undertake such a prolonged preventive treatment program by having the epidemiology of risks and benefits portrayed in semiquantitative terms. I suggest describing a spectrum of prospective candidates for estrogen replacement therapy, ranging from those who would benefit most to those who would benefit least from such an approach [see Table 1]. For example, a thin, sedentary white smoker whose uterus has been removed would be placed at one end of the spectrum, whereas an obese, physically active African-American woman with a history of deep vein thrombosis and with a sister who has had breast cancer would be placed at the other end. The white woman has a greater likelihood of developing osteoporosis and a lesser concern about estrogen's side effects. In contrast, the African-American woman has much less chance of fracture and more concern about estrogen's putative risks.

Against this rather general background, two large medical issues should be considered for their personal relevance.[82] If the individual has a strong family history of, or personal risk profile for, coronary artery disease, the estrogen-related reduction in relative

Table 1 Factors Influencing Decision to Use Estrogen Therapy to Prevent Osteoporosis

Characteristics of Patients Most Likely to Benefit from Estrogen Therapy	Characteristics of Patients Least Likely to Benefit from Estrogen Therapy
Thin	Obese
White	African American
Sedentary	Physically active
Smoker	History of deep vein thrombosis
Low calcium intake	Sister with history of breast cancer
Uterus previously removed	
Mother with dowager's hump	
Family history of coronary artery disease	

risk provides a strong rationale for long-range hormone replacement. Conversely, a strong family history of breast cancer, especially in first-order relatives, is a negative factor. The availability of alendronate is particularly attractive for such patients. For women who are uncertain, bone densitometry of the spine can be extremely helpful in making a decision. In all cases, avoiding smoking, performing moderate weight-bearing exercise, and taking 1,500 mg of calcium a day are all sound preventive measures.

Contraception

ORAL CONTRACEPTIVES

More than 50 million women worldwide use oral contraceptives. This usage constitutes the largest legal but uncontrolled pharmacologic experiment in history.

Oral contraceptives consist of synthetic estrogens and progestogens; they vary in dosage, ratio of components, and prescribed regimens.[101,102] They prevent pregnancy primarily by suppressing pituitary gonadotropin secretion. Gonadotropin suppression inhibits development of a dominant follicle and the rise in estrogen that normally triggers an LH surge and ovulation. Additional mechanisms include alterations of the cervical mucus and inhibition of implantation of the fertilized egg. If taken without error, the pill would be almost perfectly effective; empirically, it produces the lowest pregnancy rates of all contraceptives in use.[103]

Combined oral contraceptives containing estrogen and progestin reduce the risk of both endometrial and ovarian cancer by as much as 50%. The incidence of pelvic inflammatory disease is similarly reduced. Oral contraceptives also improve much minor menstrual morbidity: users have less iron deficiency anemia (because menses are less heavy), more regular periods and less menometrorrhagia, fewer functional ovarian cysts, and much less dysmenorrhea and premenstrual tension. The incidence of benign breast lesions is decreased. Despite great controversy, there appears to be no increase in breast cancer, even after a 15- to 20-year follow-up, in current or former users, including women with benign breast lesions or a family history of breast cancer.

From most perspectives, oral contraceptives are nearly ideal; toxicity poses the major problem.[104] Most of the evidence associating an increase in coronary disease with oral contraceptives was derived from the era of high estrogen content. In women taking pills with 35 µg or less of ethinyl estradiol, there does not appear to be a significant increase in coronary events, except for one group: women older than 35 years who smoke more than 15 cigarettes a day are at increased risk for myocardial infarction. There is also some concern that the combination of oral contraceptive use and

surgery predisposes to arterial thrombosis. Pill users show increased platelet aggregation and increased levels of many proteins, including several clotting factors, most strikingly factor XII. These findings suggest a hypercoagulable state induced by oral contraceptives, but in vitro clotting tests have not shown a consistent abnormality; an intrinsic vascular defect may be important. This small tendency to induce hypercoagulability interacts with the hereditary deficiency of factor V (Leiden) to produce a significant risk of deep vein thrombosis; oral contraceptives should be avoided in such patients.[105]

The progestin component of oral contraceptives is also important. Hypertension, glucose intolerance, lowering of HDL, and an apparent increase in atherosclerotic events have all been linked to the dose of progestins provided by the low-estrogen combination pills. However, a comparison between women who used oral contraceptives and those who did not found no overall difference in mortality over 12 years of follow-up.[106]

Emergency postcoital contraception has not received much publicity in this country. A tablet containing 100 µg of ethinyl estradiol and 0.5 mg of levonorgestrel, given twice—first within 72 hours of intercourse and again 12 hours later—is approximately 75% effective in preventing pregnancy.[107,108]

Recommendations

The risks and benefits of the pill have been summarized. The following recommendations are consistent with the data that have emerged:

1. Oral contraceptives are the most effective form of contraception known; for this and many other reasons, many young women prefer them. Both hormone components may be associated with a slightly increased risk of cardiovascular disease; potential users should be alerted to this fact. In an asymptomatic woman younger than 35 years, the risk is not a deterrent to use but should be considered additive to other cardiac risk factors, such as hypercholesterolemia, hypertension, diabetes, heavy smoking, or a family history of early coronary disease. Discontinuance of oral contraceptives and use of an effective alternative should be considered in the management of hypertension or major glucose intolerance. In women older than 35 years, use of these agents should be avoided by those who smoke and should be reevaluated for others. Interestingly, oral contraceptive use appears to decrease spontaneously among women in this age group.

2. Absolute contraindications to oral contraceptives include thrombotic disorders, known or suspected cancer of an estrogen-dependent organ (e.g., breast or uterus), impaired liver function, pregnancy, undiagnosed vaginal bleeding, pregnancy-associated jaundice, and hyperlipidemia.

3. In many other disorders, a relative contraindication should be individually evaluated and use of oral contraceptives cautiously explored.

4. Because the frequency of arterial thrombosis appears to be increased after elective surgery, it is recommended that oral contraceptives be discontinued a month before surgery.[109]

5. Which pill should be used? In the past, the concept of individualizing the choice of pill was much discussed, but now the use of the low-dose estrogen pill takes precedence over other considerations. The dose of estrogen should be no higher than 50 µg, and 35 µg is preferable. In general, any of the low-estrogen agents may be tried. For patients with acne or hirsutism, norgestrel may be preferable to norethindrone as the progestin agent.

Postpill Amenorrhea

Despite the former popularity of the term postpill amenorrhea, there does not appear to be such a syndrome.[110] Menstrual function should resume within 2 months after cessation of oral contraceptives, but as much as 6 months can elapse before menses return. The differential diagnosis and evaluation of amenorrhea in a woman who has discontinued oral contraceptives should follow the approach outlined [see Disorders of Menstruation: Secondary Amenorrhea, above]. Transient functional disturbances and pregnancy will probably occur a bit more often than in a random series of patients with secondary amenorrhea.

CONTRACEPTIVE IMPLANTS

The subdermal levonorgestrel implants are the first significant advance in contraception in the United States in more than 20 years.[111] In this system, six pellets are implanted under the skin of the upper arm and slowly release effective progestin into the circulation. Pregnancy rates with the implant are lower than with any other nonoperative form of contraception, and side effects are minor. With the implant approach, the patient does not have to remember to take a pill each day, and the contraceptive effect persists for 5 years. Bleeding patterns vary; two thirds of patients have irregular cycles the first year, but after that time, the bleeding patterns of most women improve.[112,113] Removal of the implants eliminates the contraceptive effect. Difficulties in removal have emerged as a limitation on acceptance of this form of contraception.[114]

CONTRAGESTION

After successful introduction abroad, the progesterone antagonist mifepristone (RU 486) has been found effective in the United States for induction of first-trimester abortion.[115] The drug is given up to 2 months after the onset of amenorrhea. By interfering with the action of progesterone, it prevents or reverses implantation. Uterine contents are evacuated by oral or vaginal use of a prostaglandin analogue.

GONADOTROPIN SUPPRESSION

Gonadotropin Analogues

Synthetic analogues of the decapeptide GnRH have opened new vistas in the management of human reproductive disorders. Short pulses of active analogues are useful in diagnostic studies, and pulsatile administration of short-acting agents can induce ovulation in most hypogonadotropic women. Intramuscular administration of long-acting analogues produces an antigonadotropic effect and can be used to decrease estrogen-dependent lesions such as fibroids, to induce a hypogonadal state for the relief of severe PMS, to provide a basis for contraception, and to eliminate the estrogen environment in which intercurrent disease may have developed. Internists are not likely to use these agents in such specialized ways but should know that they are available.

References

1. Carr BR: Disorders of the ovary and female reproductive tract. Williams Textbook of Endocrinology, 9th ed. Kronenberg H, Larson PR, Eds. WB Saunders Co, Philadelphia, 1998, p 751

2. Hayes FJ, Hall JE, Boepple PA, et al: Differential control of gonadotropin secretion in the human: endocrine role of inhibin. J Clin Endocrinol Metab 83:1835, 1998

3. Parsons AK: The effect of age on the menstrual cycle. Seminars in Reproductive Endocrinology 9:176, 1991

4. Kulin HE, Reiter EO: Managing the patient with a delay in pubertal development. Endocrinologist 2:231, 1992

5. Grumbach MM, Conte FA: Disorders of sex differentiation. Williams Textbook of Endocrinology, 9th ed. Kronenberg H, Larson PR, Eds. WB Saunders Co, Philadelphia, 1998, p 1303

6. Griffin JE: Androgen resistance—the clinical and molecular spectrum. N Engl J Med 326:611, 1992

7. Henzl MR: Gonadotropin-releasing hormone and its analogues: from laboratory to bedside. Clin Obstet Gynecol 36:617, 1993

8. Chrousos GP, Torpy DJ, Gold PW: et al: Interactions between the hypothalamic-pituitary-adrenal axis and the female reproductive system: clinical implications. Ann Intern Med 129:229, 1998

9. Filicori M, Flamigni C, Dellai P, et al: Treatment of anovulation with pulsatile gonadotropin-releasing hormone: prognostic factors and clinical results in 600 cycles. J Clin Endocrinol Metab 79:1215, 1994

10. Conn PM, Crowley WF Jr: Gonadotropin-releasing hormone and its analogs. Annu Rev Med 45:391, 1994

11. Prior JC, Vigna YM: Ovulation disturbances and exercise training. Clin Obstet Gynecol 34:180, 1991

12. Nattiv A, Agostini R, Drinkwater B, et al: The female athlete triad: the inter-relatedness of disordered eating, amenorrhea, and osteoporosis. Clin Sports Med 13:405, 1994

13. Marshall LA: Clinical evaluation of amenorrhea in active and athletic women. Clin Sports Med 13:371, 1994

14. Biller BMK, Klibanski A: Amenorrhea and osteoporosis. Endocrinologist 1:294, 1991

15. De Cree C: Sex steroid metabolism and menstrual irregularities in the exercising female: a review. Sports Med 25:369, 1998

16. Drinkwater BL, Nilson K, Ott S, et al: Bone mineral density after resumption of menses in amenorrhoeic athletes. JAMA 256:380, 1986

17. Rebar RW, Cedars MI: Hypergonadotropic forms of amenorrhea in young women. Endocrinol Metab Clin North Am 21:173, 1992

18. Lieman H, Santoro N: Premature ovarian failure: a modern approach to diagnosis and treatment. Endocrinologist 7:314, 1997

19. Hoek A, Schoemaker J, Drexhage HA: Premature ovarian failure and ovarian autoimmunity. Endocr Rev 18:107, 1997

20. Jordan J, Craig K, Clifton DK, et al: Luteal phase defect: the sensitivity and specificity of diagnostic methods in common clinical use. Fertil Steril 62:54, 1994

21. Cowan BD, Morrison JC: Management of abnormal genital bleeding in girls and women. N Engl J Med 324:1710, 1991

22. Chuong CJ, Brenner PF: Management of abnormal uterine bleeding. Am J Obstet Gynecol 175:787, 1996

23. Wathen PI, Henderson MC, Witz CA: Abnormal uterine bleeding. Med Clin North Am 79:329, 1995

24. Shaw RW: Assessment of medical treatments for menorrhagia. Br J Obstet Gynaecol 101(suppl 11):15, 1994

25. Fox R, Hull M: Ultrasound diagnosis of polycystic ovaries. Ann NY Acad Sci 687:217, 1993

26. Crowley WF Jr, Hall JE, Martin KA, et al: An overview of the diagnostic considerations in polycystic ovarian syndrome. Ann NY Acad Sci 687:235, 1993

27. Hayes FJ, Taylor AE, Martin KA, et al: Use of a gonadotropin-releasing hormone antagonist as a physiologic probe in polycystic ovary syndrome: assessment of neuroendocrine and androgen dynamics. J Clin Endocrinol Metab 83:2343, 1998

28. Ehrmann DA, Barnes RB, Rosenfield RL: Polycystic ovary syndrome as a form of functional ovarian hyperandrogenism due to dysregulation of androgen secretion. Endocr Rev 16:322, 1995

29. Azziz R, Black V, Hines GA, et al: Adrenal androgen excess in the polycystic ovary syndrome: sensitivity and responsivity of the hypothalamic-pituitary-adrenal axis. J Clin Endocrinol Metab 83:2317, 1998

30. Barbieri RL: Hyperandrogenism, insulin resistance and acanthosis nigricans: 10 years of progress. J Reprod Med 39:327, 1994

31. Dunaif A: Insulin resistance and the polycystic ovary syndrome: mechanism and implications for pathogenesis. Endocr Rev 18:774, 1997

32. The polycystic ovary, Kazer RR, Ed. Semin Reprod Endocrinol 15(3):1997

33. Legro RS, Finegood D, Dunaif A: A fasting glucose to insulin ratio is a useful measure of insulin sensitivity in women with polycystic ovary syndrome. J Clin Endocrinol Metab 83:2694, 1998

34. Apter D, Bützow T, Laughlin GA, et al: Accelerated 24-hour luteinizing hormone pulsatile activity in adolescent girls with ovarian hyperandrogenism: relevance to the developmental phase of polycystic ovarian syndrome. J Clin Endocrinol Metab 79:119, 1994

35. Goldzieher JW, Young RL: Selected aspects of polycystic ovarian disease. Endocrinol Metab Clin North Am 21:141, 1992

36. Burkman RT Jr: The role of oral contraceptives in the treatment of hyperandrogenic disorders. Am J Med 98(suppl 1A):130S, 1995

37. Freeman EW: Premenstrual syndrome: current perspectives on treatment and etiology. Curr Opin Obstet Gynecol 9:147, 1997

38. Mortola JF: Premenstrual syndrome. Curr Ther Endocrinol Metab 6:251, 1997

39. Mortola JF: A risk-benefit appraisal of drugs used in the management of premenstrual syndrome. Drug Saf 10:160, 1994

40. Steiner M, Steinberg S, Stewart D, et al: Fluoxetine in the treatment of premenstrual dysphoria. N Engl J Med 332:1529, 1995

41. Rubinow DR, Schmidt PJ: The treatment of premenstrual syndrome—forward into the past (editorial). N Engl J Med 332:1574, 1995

42. Mortola JF, Girton L, Fischer U: Successful treatment of severe premenstrual syndrome by combined use of gonadotropin-releasing hormone agonist and estrogen/progestin. J Clin Endocrinol Metab 71:252A, 1991

43. Schwartzman RA, Cidlowski JA: Apoptosis: the biochemistry and molecular biology of programmed cell death. Endocr Rev 14:133, 1993

44. Snieder H, MacGregor AJ, Spector TD: Genes control the cessation of a woman's reproductive life: a twin study of hysterectomy and age at menopause. J Clin Endocrinol Metab 83:1875, 1998

45. Treloar SA, Do KA, Martin NG: Genetic influences on the age at menopause. Lancet 352:1084, 1998

46. Prior JC: Perimenopause: the complex endocrinology of the menopausal transition. Endocr Rev 19:397, 1998

47. Kronenberg F: Hot flashes: epidemiology and physiology. Ann NY Acad Sci 592:52, 1990

48. Oldenhave A: Pathogenesis of climacteric complaints: ready for the change? Lancet 343:649, 1994

49. Judd HL: Transdermal estradiol: a potentially improved method of hormone replacement. J Reprod Med 39:343, 1994

50. Lufkin EG, Ory SJ: Relative value of transdermal and oral estrogen therapy in various clinical situations. Mayo Clin Proc 69:131, 1994

51. Loprinzi CL, Michalak JC, Quella SK, et al: Megestrol acetate for the prevention of hot flashes. N Engl J Med 331:347, 1994

52. Miodrag A, Castleden CM, Vallance TR: Sex hormones and the female urinary tract. Drugs 34:491, 1988

53. Nachtigall LE: Comparative study: Replens versus local estrogen in menopausal women. Fertil Steril 61:178, 1994

54. Heaney RP: Osteoporosis at the end of the century. West J Med 154:106, 1991

55. Riggs BL: Overview of osteoporosis. West J Med 154:63, 1991

56. Manolagas SC, Jilka RL: Bone marrow, cytokines, and bone remodeling: emerging insights into the pathophysiology of osteoporosis. N Engl J Med 332:305, 1995

57. Marcus R: Skeletal aging: understanding the functional and structural basis of osteoporosis. Trends in Endocrinology and Metabolism 2:53, 1991

58. Marcus R: Understanding osteoporosis. West J Med 155:53, 1991

59. Cooper C, Melton LJ III: Epidemiology of osteoporosis. Trends in Endocrinology and Metabolism 3:224, 1992

60. Heaney RP: Bone mass, bone loss, and osteoporosis (editorial). Ann Intern Med 128:313, 1998

61. Ettinger B, Pressman A, Sklarin P, et al: Associations between low levels of serum estradiol, bone density, and fractures among elderly women: the study of osteoporotic fractures. J Clin Endocrinol Metab 83:2239, 1998

62. Cummings SR, Browner WS, Bauer D, et al: Endogenous hormones and the risk of hip and vertebral fractures among older women. Study of Osteoporotic Fractures Research Group. N Engl J Med 339:733, 1998

63. Marcus R: New perspectives on the skeletal role of estrogen (editorial). J Clin Endocrinol Metab 83:2236, 1998

64. National Osteoporosis Foundation: Physician's Guide to Prevention and Treatment of Osteoporosis. National Osteoporosis Foundation, Washington, DC, 1998

65. Heaney RP: Nutritional factors in osteoporosis. Annu Rev Nutr 13:287, 1993

66. Gilsanz V, Roe TF, Mora S, et al: Changes in vertebral bone density in black girls and white girls during childhood and puberty. N Engl J Med 325:1597, 1991

67. Ott SM: Bone density in adolescents. N Engl J Med 325:1646, 1991

68. Kleerekoper M: Extensive personal experience: the clinical evaluation and management of osteoporosis. J Clin Endocrinol Metab 80:757, 1995

69. Turner RT, Riggs BL, Spelsberg TC: Skeletal effects of estrogen. Endocr Rev 15:275, 1994

70. Girasole G, Jilka RL, Passeri G, et al: 17β-Estradiol inhibits interleukin-6 production by bone marrow-derived stromal cells and osteoblasts in vitro: a potential mechanism for the antiosteoporotic effect of estrogens. J Clin Invest 89:883, 1992

71. Evans MP, Fleming KC, Evans JM: Hormone replacement therapy: management of common problems. Mayo Clin Proc 70:800, 1995

72. Bilezikian JP: Major issues regarding estrogen replacement therapy in postmenopausal women. Journal of Women's Health 3:273, 1994

73. Liberman UA, Weiss SR, Bröll J, et al: Effect of oral alendronate on bone mineral density and the incidence of fractures in postmenopausal osteoporosis. N Engl J Med 333:1437, 1995

74. Sambrook PN: The treatment of postmenopausal osteoporosis (editorial). N Engl J Med 333:1495, 1995

75. McClung M, Clemmesen B, Daifotis A, et al: Alendronate prevents postmenopausal bone loss in women without osteoporosis. Ann Intern Med 128:253, 1998

76. Reginster JY, Meurmans L, Zegels B, et al: The effect of sodium monofluorophosphate plus calcium on vertebral fracture rate in postmenopausal women with moderate osteoporosis: a randomized, controlled trial. Ann Intern Med 129:1, 1998

77. Pak CYC, Sakhaee K, Adams-Huet B, et al: Treatment of postmenopausal osteoporosis with slow-release sodium fluoride. Ann Intern Med 123:401, 1995

78. Kleerekoper M: Osteoporosis and the primary care physician: time to bone up (editorial). Ann Intern Med 123:466, 1995

79. Colditz GA, Willett WC, Stampfer MJ, et al: Menopause and the risk of coronary heart disease in women. N Engl J Med 316:1105, 1987

80. Stampfer MJ, Colditz GA, Willett WC: Menopause and heart disease: a review. Ann NY Acad Sci 592:193, 1990

81. Skafar DF, Xu R, Morales J, et al: Clinical review 91: female sex hormones and cardiovascular disease in women. J Clin Endocrinol Metab 82:3913, 1997

82. Mendelsohn ME, Karas RH: Estrogen and the blood vessel wall. Curr Opin Cardiol 9:619, 1994

83. Grady D, Rubin SM, Petitti DB, et al: Hormone therapy to prevent disease and prolong life in postmenopausal women. Ann Intern Med 117:1016, 1992

84. Stampfer MJ, Colditz GA, Willett WC, et al: Postmenopausal estrogen therapy and cardiovascular disease: ten-year follow-up from the Nurses' Health Study. N Engl J Med 325:756, 1991

85. Stampfer MJ, Colditz GA: Estrogen replacement therapy and coronary heart disease: a quantitative assessment of the epidemiologic evidence. Prev Med 20:47, 1991

86. Wren BG: Megatrials of hormone replacement therapy. Drugs Aging 12:343, 1998

87. Hulley S, Grady D, Bush T, et al: Randomized trial of estrogen plus progestin for secondary prevention of coronary heart disease in postmenopausal women. Heart and Estrogen/progestin Replacement Study (HERS) Research Group. JAMA 280:605, 1998

88. Gambrell RD Jr, Teran A-Z: Changes in lipids and lipoproteins with estrogen deficiency and hormone replacement therapy. Am J Obstet Gynecol 165:307, 1991

89. Crook D, Cust MP, Gangar KF, et al: Comparison of transdermal and oral estrogen-progestin replacement therapy: effects on serum lipids and lipoproteins. Am J Obstet Gynecol 166:950, 1992

90. The Writing Group for the PEPI Trial: Effects of estrogen or estrogen/progestin regimens on heart disease risk factors in postmenopausal women: the Postmenopausal Estrogen/progestin Interventions (PEPI) Trial. JAMA 273:199, 1995

91. Glueck CJ, Lang J, Hamer T, et al: Severe hypertriglyceridemia and pancreatitis when estrogen replacement therapy is given to hypertriglyceridemic women. J Lab Clin Med 123:59, 1994

92. Steinberg KK, Thacker SB, Smith SJ, et al: A meta-analysis of the effect of estrogen replacement therapy on the risk of breast cancer. JAMA 265:1985, 1991

93. Barrett-Connor E: Postmenopausal estrogen and the risk of breast cancer. Ann Epidemiol 4:177, 1994

94. Colditz GA, Hankinson SE, Hunter DJ, et al: The use of estrogens and progestins and the risk of breast cancer in postmenopausal women. N Engl J Med 332:1589, 1995

95. Davidson NE: Hormone-replacement therapy breast versus heart versus bone (editorial). N Engl J Med 332:1638, 1995

96. Lidegaard O, Edstrom B, Kreiner S: Oral contraceptives and venous thromboembolism—a case-control study. Contraception 57:291, 1998

97. Lufkin EG, Wahner HW, O'Fallon WM, et al: Treatment of postmenopausal osteoporosis with transdermal estrogen. Ann Intern Med 117:1, 1992

98. MacGregor JI, Jordan VC: Basic guide to the mechanisms of antiestrogen action. Pharmacological Rev 50:151, 1998

99. Delmas PD, Bjarnason NH, Mitlak BH, et al: Effects of raloxifene on bone mineral density, serum cholesterol concentrations, and uterine endometrium in postmenopausal women. N Engl J Med 337:1641, 1997

100. Kulak CA, Bilezikian JP: Osteoporosis: preventive strategies. Int J Fertil Womens Med 43:56, 1998

101. Goodman AL: The biochemistry of oral contraceptive steroids. Seminars in Reproductive Endocrinology 7:199, 1989

102. Foster DC: Low-dose monophasic and multiphasic oral contraceptives: a review of potency, efficacy, and side effects. Seminars in Reproductive Endocrinology 7:205, 1989

103. Anand Kumar TC: The value and use of different contraceptive methods. Hum Reprod 9(suppl 2):1, 1994

104. Kost K, Forrest JD, Harlap S: Comparing the health risks and benefits of contraceptive choice. Fam Plann Perspect 23:55, 1991

105. Price DT, Ridker PM: Factor V Leiden mutation and the risks for thromboembolic disease: a clinical perspective. Ann Intern Med 127:895, 1997

106. Colditz GA: Oral contraceptive use and mortality during 12 years of follow-up: the Nurses' Health Study. Ann Intern Med 120:821, 1994

107. Glasier A: Emergency postcoital contraception. N Engl J Med 337:1058, 1997

108. Grimes DA: Emergency contraception—expanding opportunities for primary prevention (editorial). N Engl J Med 337:1078, 1997

109. Robinson GE, Burren T, Mackie IJ, et al: Changes in haemostasis after stopping the combined contraceptive pill: implications for major surgery. BMJ 302:269, 1991

110. Archer DF, Thomas RL: The fallacy of the postpill amenorrhea syndrome. Clin Obstet Gynecol 24:943, 1981

111. Sivin I, Alvarez F, Mishell DR Jr, et al: Contraception with two levonorgestrel rod implants: a 5-year study in the United States and Dominican Republic. Contraception 58:275, 1998

112. Shoupe D, Mishell DR Jr, Bopp BL, et al: The significance of bleeding patterns in Norplant implant users. Obstet Gynecol 77:256, 1991

113. Shoupe D, Mishell DR Jr: Norplant: subdermal implant system for long-term contraception. Am J Obstet Gynecol 160:1286, 1990

114. Hatcher RA, Trussell J: Contraceptive implants and teenage pregnancy (editorial). N Engl J Med 331:1229, 1994

115. Spitz IM, Bardin CW, Benton L, et al: Early pregnancy termination with mifepristone and misoprostol in the United States. N Engl J Med 338:1241, 1998

116. Filicori M, Santoro N, Merriam GR, et al: Characterization of the physiological pattern of episodic gonadotropin secretion throughout the human menstrual cycle. J Clin Endocrinol Metab 62:1136, 1986

117. Lenton DM, de Kretser DM, Woodward AJ, et al: Inhibin concentrations throughout the menstrual cycles of normal, infertile, and older women compared with those during spontaneous conception cycles. J Clin Endocrinol Metab 73:1180, 1991

Acknowledgments

Figure 1   Andy Christie.

Figures 2 through 7   Al Miller.

52 Diseases of Calcium Metabolism and Metabolic Bone Disease

Silvio E. Inzucchi, M.D.

Calcium Metabolism

The precise regulation of body calcium stores and its concentration in both extracellular and intracellular compartments is critically important for the following reasons: calcium is the chief mineral component of the skeleton; calcium serves major roles in neurologic transmission, muscle contraction, and blood coagulation; and it is a ubiquitous intracellular signal. Normal serum calcium concentration is between 9 and 10.5 mg/dl; 50% to 60% of the calcium in the blood is bound to plasma proteins or is complexed with citrate and phosphate. The remaining ionized (free) calcium controls physiologic actions. The body regulates not only ionized calcium concentrations but also entry and exit of calcium into its main storage site, bone, through the activity of parathyroid hormone (PTH) and 1,25-dihydroxyvitamin D_3 ($1,25\text{-}(OH)_2D_3$) [*see Figure 1*]. PTH, secreted by the four parathyroid glands, is an 84–amino-acid peptide with a very short plasma half-life (2 to 4 minutes). Cholecalciferol (vitamin D_3) is gen-

erated by skin exposed to ultraviolet light and is also supplied by dietary sources (chiefly liquid milk products). In the liver, vitamin D_3 is hydroxylated to $25\text{-}(OH)D_3$, which is again hydroxylated in the kidney to $1,25\text{-}(OH)_2D_3$ (calcitriol), markedly increasing its potency. In concert, these hormonal systems express their action at the level of the gastrointestinal tract, bone, and the kidney and maintain circulating ionized calcium concentrations under extremely tight control (variation < 0.1 mg/dl), despite significant variations in calcium supply.

Under normal conditions, despite ranges in calcium consumption that can vary from 400 to 2,000 mg daily, net calcium absorption through the GI tract averages about 150 to 200 mg/day. In steady state, this should essentially equal the amount of calcium excreted by the kidneys. Ongoing remodeling of bone utilizes and releases approximately 500 mg of calcium a day. Through humoral regulation, this calcium reservoir can be engaged to maintain extracellular calcium levels despite increased physio-

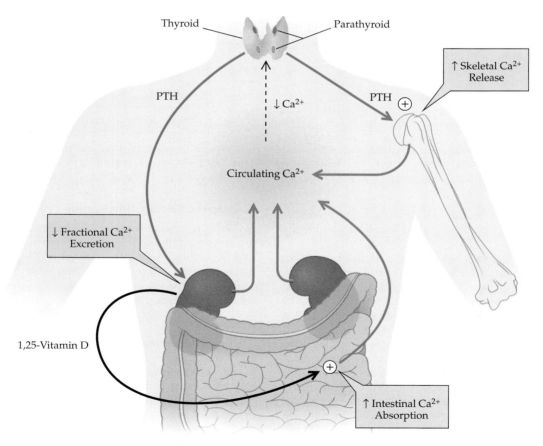

Figure 1 Circulating concentrations of ionized calcium are maintained under extremely tight control by parathyroid hormone (PTH) and the vitamin D axis. Absorption of dietary calcium by the gastrointestinal tract, reduction of calcium excretion by the kidneys, and release of stored calcium from bones serve as sources for circulating calcium. Decreases in circulating calcium trigger the release of PTH, which promotes release of calcium into the extracellular space by increasing bone resorption; the release of PTH also causes an increase in calcium reabsorption in the distal nephron, resulting in a decrease in urinary calcium loss. PTH also augments renal production of 1,25-dihydroxyvitamin D, which secondarily increases calcium absorption in the gut.

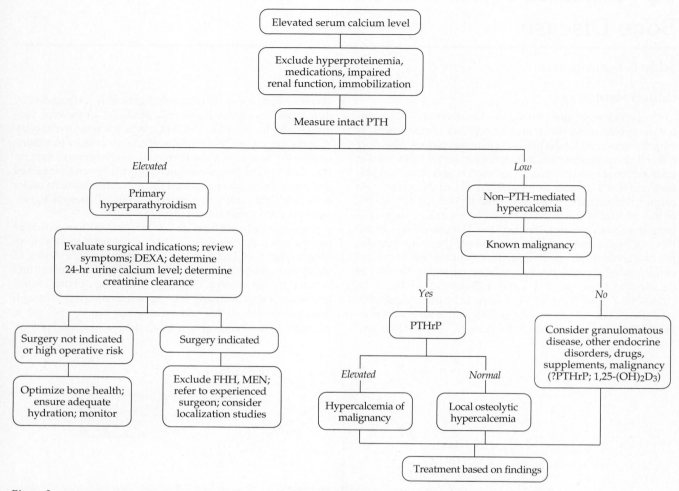

Figure 2 **Evaluation and management of hypercalcemia. (DEXA—dual-energy x-ray absorptiometry; FHH—familial hypocalciuric hypercalcemia; MEN—multiple endocrine neoplasia; PTH—parathyroid hormone; PTHrP—parathyroid hormone–related protein)**

logic need or decreased intake, such as can occur from severe curtailment of the dietary calcium supply or impairment of intestinal calcium absorption.

Changes in the extracellular ionized calcium concentration are registered by parathyroid cells via the calcium-sensing receptor.[1] Interaction of calcium ions at the extracellular domain of the receptor triggers a series of intracellular signaling events, which ultimately govern PTH secretion. As circulating concentrations of calcium fall, PTH secretion rises, and vice versa.

PTH increases bone resorption and distal nephron calcium reabsorption, the former promoting calcium release into the extracellular space and the latter decreasing urinary calcium losses. PTH also augments renal production of calcitriol, which secondarily increases fractional calcium absorption in the gut. If calcium intake increases beyond the body's needs, PTH secretion decreases, leading to decreased calcitriol production and decreased calcium absorption. If calcium is absorbed in excess of requirements, it will be promptly excreted. In this elegant manner, circulating ionized calcium concentration is guarded closely, albeit sometimes at the expense of total body calcium stores. Perturbations in this system are predominately manifested as abnormalities in serum calcium concentration or as alterations in bone mineral density.

Disorders of Calcium Homeostasis

Concentrations of free serum calcium that are outside the normal range typically result from disorders involving the parathyroid. Depending on clinical circumstances, however, the evaluation of hypercalcemia or hypocalcemia must also take into account other etiologies, as well as the possibility that the abnormal reading is factitious.

HYPERCALCEMIA

Hypercalcemia is a common metabolic abnormality. Signs and symptoms of hypercalcemia vary significantly from patient to patient and correlate to some degree with both the degree of calcium elevation and its rate of change. The diagnostic workup of hypercalcemia is straightforward [*see Figure 2*].[2] The etiology of hypercalcemia is usually discovered after a comprehensive history, physical examination, focused laboratory assessment, and occasionally diagnostic imaging studies.[3]

Clinical Manifestations

Most patients with mild hypercalcemia (< 11 mg/dl) are asymptomatic, although some may experience mild fatigue, vague changes in cognitive function, depression, or polyuria and polydipsia (from decreased urine-concentrating ability). Those with moderate hypercalcemia (serum calcium levels of 11 to 14 mg/dl) may be more symptomatic, with anorexia, nausea, vomiting, abdominal pain, constipation, muscle weakness, and further alterations in mental status. Those with severe hypercalcemia (serum calcium levels greater than 14 mg/dl) experience progressive lethargy, disorientation, seizures, and even coma.

History and Physical Examination

The history and physical examination are directed at uncovering signs or symptoms of hypercalcemia itself, as well as those associated with the most common causes of hypercalcemia: hyperparathyroidism, malignancy, granulomatous disease, and certain endocrinopathies. Evidence of any related condition, such as osteoporosis or urinary tract stones, should also be elicited. Because the most common diagnosis, primary hyperparathyroidism, presents as stable or gradually progressive elevation of the serum calcium over a period of years, the medical record, if available, should be scrutinized to determine the duration of the hypercalcemia. All recent medications or nutritional supplements should be thoroughly reviewed, and a careful family history should be elicited. When taking the family history, specific disorders that should be discussed with the patient include disorders of calcium metabolism; renal stones; fragility fractures; and any related endocrinopathies, such as diseases of the pituitary, adrenal, thyroid, or endocrine pancreas.

Aside from mental status deficits, physical examination findings are generally normal in patients with hypercalcemia, especially those patients whose calcium levels are mildly to moderately elevated. Rarely, severe and prolonged hypercalcemia results in visible calcium deposition in the cornea, a condition known as band keratopathy. Other signs and symptoms depend on the etiology of the elevation [see Table 1]. For example, patients with hyperparathyroidism frequently have hypertension, dyspepsia, osteopenia, or nephrolithiasis. Those whose hyperparathyroidism is associated with multiple endocrine neoplasia (MEN) syndromes may have specific manifestations of the other conditions that accompany this diagnosis. Patients with sarcoidosis may present with fever, lymphadenopathy, skin rashes, or evidence of certain pulmonary sequelae. Those with cancer may have features associated with the specific tumor type and extent of disease.

Laboratory Studies

The first step in the laboratory assessment is to exclude factitious hypercalcemia, which may result from an increase in circulating concentrations of plasma proteins. Because 50% to 60% of circulating calcium is bound to these proteins, elevation in their concentrations (such as occurs in myeloma) will produce a proportionate rise in the total calcium concentration. The ionized calcium concentration, however, remains normal. To adjust for elevations in plasma protein, the serum calcium level should be lowered by 0.8 mg/dl for every 1 g/dl of albumin (or protein) above the normal range. Alternatively, ionized calcium can be measured. Because acute renal failure may occasionally lead to hypercalcemia, renal function should also be assessed.

Once hypercalcemia is confirmed, the next step is measurement of the serum PTH concentration. Several PTH assays are commercially available. The most commonly utilized is the two-site immunoradiometric assay (IRMA), or so-called intact PTH, although both C-terminal and midmolecule assays remain in use. Whereas earlier assays measured not only PTH but also other molecular fragments that circulate in increased concentrations in patients with renal insufficiency, IRMA measures only the intact

Table 1 Differential Diagnosis of Hypercalcemia

Parathyroid hormone–mediated hypercalcemia	Primary hyperparathyroidism Parathyroid adenoma Parathyroid hyperplasia Parathyroid carcinoma Tertiary hyperparathyroidism

Non–parathyroid hormone–mediated hypercalcemia	Malignancy-associated hypercalcemia
	Humoral hypercalcemia of malignancy
	Parathyroid hormone–related protein
	  Squamous cell carcinoma of the lung
	  Carcinoma of the oropharynx, nasopharynx, larynx, and esophagus
	  Cervical carcinoma
	  Ovarian carcinoma
	  Renal cell carcinoma
	  Transitional cell carcinoma of the bladder
	  Pheochromocytoma
	  Islet cell neoplasms of the pancreas
	  T–cell lymphoma
	  Others
	1,25-$(OH)_2$-D_3-mediated
	B-cell lymphoma
	Local osteolytic hypercalcemia
	  Multiple myeloma
	  Breast carcinoma
	  Lymphoma
	  Others
	Medications/supplements
	  Vitamin D
	  Vitamin A
	  Lithium
	  Thiazides
	  Calcium antacids (milk-alkali syndrome)
	Granulomatous diseases
	  Sarcoidosis
	  Tuberculosis
	  Histoplasmosis
	  Leprosy
	Other conditions
	  Increased plasma protein levels (factitious hypercalcemia)
	  Acute renal failure
	  Thyrotoxicosis
	  Adrenal insufficiency
	  Immobilization
	  Familial hypocalciuric hypocalcemia (benign familial hypercalcemia)

molecule and is therefore the preferred test in most instances, especially in patients whose serum creatinine level is elevated. Individual PTH assays sometimes exhibit unique features, especially regarding the detection of early or mild hyperparathyroidism (either primary or secondary). It is therefore helpful for clinicians to be aware of any idiosyncrasies of the PTH assays available at their local institutions.

Other helpful tests include blood urea nitrogen (BUN), serum creatinine, alkaline phosphatase, and serum inorganic phosphorus assays; an electrolyte panel; and an assessment of 24-hour urinary calcium output. The BUN and creatinine concentration may be elevated in hypercalcemia, depending on the degree of volume depletion. Prolonged hypercalcemia may lead to nephrocalcinosis, which may further impair renal function. The alkaline phosphatase may be elevated in hypercalcemic states involving increased bone turnover. Patients with hypercalcemia caused by malignancy may demonstrate biochemical or hematologic findings consistent with the site of neoplasia and the degree of its dissemination. Most cases of hypercalcemia are also accompanied by hypercalciuria (24-hour urinary calcium excretion > 4 mg/kg/day), which may lead to renal stone formation.

Electrocardiographic abnormalities of hypercalcemia include shortening of the QT_c interval and, rarely, atrioventricular blocks. In addition, many hypercalcemic conditions cause a decrease in bone mineral density and thus increase the risk of fracture. Specific radiographic findings are few, although in primary hyperparathyroidism, certain specific bony abnormalities may occasionally be seen (see below).

Etiology

The most important test for determining the cause of hypercalcemia is measurement of PTH.[3] When PTH levels are high or, in some cases, inappropriately normal, the hypercalcemia is PTH mediated; this is commonly referred to as hyperparathyroidism. When PTH levels are suppressed, the hypercalcemia is said to be non–PTH mediated.

HYPERPARATHYROIDISM (PTH-MEDIATED HYPERCALCEMIA)

Classification

Primary hyperparathyroidism Primary hyperparathyroidism is the most common form of hypercalcemia in outpatients. Current estimates place the annual incidence at approximately 4 per 100,000, peaking in the fifth to sixth decade of life, with a female-to-male ratio of 3:2.[4] The most common clinical presentation is that of asymptomatic mild hypercalcemia. Pathologically, a solitary parathyroid adenoma is present in 80% to 85% of cases, with hyperplasia involving multiple glands occurring in 15% to 20% and parathyroid carcinoma in less than 1%. Occasionally, a double adenoma is found. Patients with type I MEN (MEN I) or MEN II tend to have hyperplasia.[5]

Secondary hyperparathyroidism Secondary hyperparathyroidism occurs when low circulating calcium concentrations stimulate increased PTH secretion as a normal, homeostatic response. This frequently occurs in patients with chronic renal insufficiency or in those with calcium malabsorption or renal calcium leaks. Normally, of course, PTH secretion would drop once appropriate circulating calcium concentrations are restored. By definition, therefore, if hypercalcemia occurs, PTH secretion must be abnormally elevated.

Tertiary hyperparathyroidism Some patients with secondary hyperparathyroidism may indeed develop dysregulation of parathyroid function, resulting in elevated calcium levels. This condition is known as tertiary hyperparathyroidism.

Diagnosis

Clinical manifestations The clinical manifestations of hyperparathyroidism depend, in part, on the severity of the hypercalcemia. When hyperparathyroidism was first described more than 50 years ago, most patients presented with late-stage complications of prolonged and severe hypercalcemia, such as notable involvement of bone (osteitis fibrosa cystica)[6] or the kidneys (nephrocalcinosis, renal failure). At present, however, the disease is almost always diagnosed before the development of such

sequelae. It may be uncovered during the evaluation of osteoporosis or osteopenia, during workups for renal stone disease, or as an incidental finding during routine blood testing.

When symptomatic, patients with hyperparathyroidism demonstrate clinical manifestations of hypercalcemia (see above). They may also have hypertension and peptic ulcer disease.

Physical examination Hyperparathyroidism does not cause palpable enlargement of the parathyroid glands; a neck mass is essentially never palpated unless the patient has parathyroid carcinoma. However, proximal muscle weakness may be present, and bone tenderness may be demonstrated, classically along the anterior margin of the tibia.

Laboratory tests Patients with hyperparathyroidism typically have a serum calcium concentration of less than 12 mg/dl (unless coexisting volume contraction is present), along with mild to moderate hypophosphatemia and a non–anion gap metabolic acidosis (from renal tubular acidosis). Urinary calcium excretion is usually increased; in these cases, the reduction of fractional calcium excretion by PTH is overcome by the high filtered calcium load. This may result in nephrolithiasis.

Renal stones in hyperparathyroidism are usually composed of calcium oxalate and tend to occur bilaterally, especially in persons who are the most hypercalciuric because of their higher levels of calcitriol. Rarely, nephrocalcinosis and azotemia develop, usually in those with the most severe and protracted hypercalcemia, especially if dehydration or other renal insult is superimposed. Because PTH increases both osteoclast and osteoblast activity, there are increases in serum and urinary concentrations of biochemical markers of bone turnover, such as bone alkaline phosphatase, osteocalcin, pyridinoline and deoxypyridinoline cross-links, and N-terminal telopeptide.

Elevation of both the serum calcium and the PTH concentrations supports a diagnosis of primary hyperparathyroidism. PTH levels are usually increased to less than five times the upper limit of normal. In certain mild cases, the calcium level is only slightly high, and the PTH is minimally elevated or inappropriately normal. Rarely, patients with primary hyperparathyroidism have serum calcium levels in only the high-normal range, although these levels can increase significantly after oral calcium ingestion. The diagnosis in such patients can be extremely challenging; the differential diagnosis includes familial hypocalciuric hypercalcemia (see below).

Once the diagnosis of primary hyperparathyroidism is secured, further evaluation will be necessary to assess the patient for surgical intervention. Typically, this evaluation includes measurement of bone density with a dual-energy x-ray absorptiometry (DEXA) scan. In addition to the standard left hip and lumbar spine measurements, assessment at the distal radius may be particularly helpful, because hyperparathyroidism may affect this predominantly cortical site more than the other locations, which have a greater percentage of trabecular bone.[6]

Other diagnostic studies are usually not necessary. If the patient has specific bone-related complaints, however, plain radiographs are indicated to search for insufficiency fractures, so-called Brown tumors (rounded lucencies within bones, representing areas of intense osteoclastic resorption), or other evidence of osteitis fibrosa cystica. In addition, if not already performed, an assessment of renal function and the 24-hour urinary calcium output should be made. Consideration should also be given to the possibility of one of the MEN syndromes, particularly if the patient is young or has a personal or family history of a related endocrinopathy.[5] This information will be helpful to the surgeon, because the patient with primary hyperparathyroidism in the setting of a MEN syndrome usually has multigland parathyroid hyperplasia, and a surgical procedure beyond a single parathyroidectomy is necessary.

Treatment

Treatment of the patient with primary hyperparathyroidism must take into account the degree of the hypercalcemia, the presence of symptoms, and the severity of any end-organ damage.[7] Because many patients with hyperparathyroidism are either asymptomatic or minimally symptomatic, there is controversy over which patients require definitive therapy. Understandably, it is widely agreed that patients with symptoms clearly attributable to hypercalcemia should undergo surgery. It is also generally agreed that surgery should be offered to patients whose serum calcium levels are substantially elevated, even if the patient is asymptomatic, and especially if the patient is relatively young. In those with milder calcium elevations, a careful search should be undertaken for end-organ damage, such as nephrolithiasis or osteoporosis.

Guidelines for surgical intervention The 2002 NIH Workshop on Asymptomatic Primary Hyperparathyroidism[8] defined the following indications for surgical intervention:

1. Significant bone, renal, gastrointestinal, or neuromuscular symptoms typical of primary hyperparathyroidism.
2. Elevation of serum calcium by 1 mg/dl or more above the normal range (i.e., $\geq$ 11.5 mg/dl in most laboratories)
3. Marked elevation of 24-hour urine calcium excretion (e.g., > 400 mg).
4. Decreased creatinine clearance (e.g., reduced by $\geq$ 30% compared with age-matched normal persons.
5. Significant reduction in bone density (i.e. > 2.5 standard deviations below peak bone mass [T score < –2.5]).
6. Consistent follow-up is not possible or is undesirable because of coexisting medical conditions.
7. Age younger than 50 years.

Those patients with mild hypercalcemia who are truly asymptomatic can be followed clinically for the subsequent development of surgical indications. Most will likely remain asymptomatic and will not require intervention.[8]

Preoperative localization Preoperative localizing imaging studies have become more widely used, particularly as some centers are utilizing intraoperative PTH assays[9] and minimally invasive surgery (see below).[10] In most cases of adenoma in a single gland, precise knowledge of the location of the adenoma may decrease operative time by allowing the surgeon to direct his or her attention to the area of suspicion. It is important to remember, however, that in good hands, parathyroidectomy for primary hyperparathyroidism has a cure rate in the range of 90% to 95%, even without such localization studies. Thus, it is unlikely that preoperative localization will ever be demonstrated to improve overall surgical outcomes. Localization studies are mandatory in the setting of a second neck exploration for persistent or recurrent hyperparathyroidism or before minimally invasive parathyroidectomy. The localization test of choice is technetium-99m sestamibi scintigraphy.[11,12] This is often followed by a neck ultrasound of the region demonstrating scintigraphic activity.

Surgical management The surgical procedure required in patients with hyperparathyroidism resulting from a solitary parathyroid adenoma is resection of that gland. If intraoperative PTH assays show a drop in the PTH level of more than 50% after resection, no further neck exploration is required. If intraoperative PTH is not used, the other three glands require direct inspection to ensure that a second adenoma or generalized hyperplasia is not present.[13] If a second adenoma is found, it too should be excised. If hyperplasia is encountered, the surgeon performs a subtotal parathyroidectomy—removal of approximately three to three and one-half glands. In some centers, this is followed by autotransplantation of remaining parathyroid tissue to the forearm, which may simplify follow-up surgical exploration in the event of recurrent hypercalcemia. Intraoperative measurement of PTH is considered by some experts to be critical in the case of ectopic parathyroid adenoma (which would not be easily found during routine neck exploration) and in reoperations.

At certain centers, so-called minimally invasive parathyroidectomy[10] is being utilized in conjunction with intraoperative PTH measurements. This approach is best suited for a good surgical candidate in whom both history and preoperative imaging studies suggest a single adenoma (which is, in fact, the most common situation in primary hyperparathyroidism). With information from scintigraphy and ultrasound already in hand, the diseased gland can be excised through a smaller, unilateral incision, under local anesthesia, even in an ambulatory setting. Success is gauged by the drop in PTH levels intraoperatively. This approach usually provides a better cosmetic result, quicker recovery time, and a lower incidence of postoperative hypocalcemia. Minimally invasive surgery is inappropriate in suboptimal surgical candidates, patients who may have multigland disease, and reoperative cases. However, it is quite likely that the majority of parathyroidectomies will be performed in this fashion in the future.

Hyperparathyroidism occasionally recurs after operative intervention, usually because of undiagnosed multigland hyperplasia and rarely because of undiagnosed parathyroid carcinoma.[14-16] Scar tissue and the sometimes atypical location of remaining pathologic parathyroid tissue make second surgeries notoriously more challenging. Consequently, preoperative imaging studies are invaluable in patients with recurring hyperparathyroidism. Catheterization studies with venous sampling may also be helpful in certain difficult cases.

Nonsurgical management Although there is as yet no recognized medical therapy for primary hyperparathyroidism, patients who do not meet the criteria for surgical intervention can be followed expectantly. This involves periodic monitoring of blood pressure, serum and urine calcium levels, renal function, and bone mineral density, as well as periodically searching for evidence of nephrolithiasis [see Table 2].[8] Drugs with a tendency to raise serum calcium levels, such as thiazides and lithium, should be avoided. Calcium and vitamin D supplementation should generally be avoided, but dietary calcium should not be restricted, because such restriction may lead to further elevation of PTH and may possibly have detrimental effects on bone mass. Good hydration should be maintained at all times to avoid the development of renal insufficiency and renal stones, especially in patients with hypercalciuria. In postmenopausal women, careful consideration should be given to antiresorptive therapy for the maintenance of bone mass. In the near future, so-called calcimimetic drugs, which activate the calcium-sensing receptor

Table 2 2002 NIH Working Group Recommendations Regarding Follow-up Testing for Patients with Primary Hyperparathyroidism Who Do Not Undergo Surgery[8]

Measurement	Frequency
Serum calcium	Biannually
24-hour urine calcium	At initial evaluation only
Creatinine clearance	At initial evaluation only
Serum creatinine	Annually*
Bone mineral density	Annually (lumbar spine, femur, and forearm)
Abdominal radiograph (or ultrasound)	At initial evaluation only

* If the serum creatinine suggests a change in renal function, measurement of creatinine clearance is recommended.

on parathyroid cells and suppress PTH secretion, may be used for certain patients with hyperparathyroidism.[17]

NON–PTH-MEDIATED HYPERCALCEMIA

Cancer remains the most common cause of non–PTH-mediated hypercalcemia and is most frequently to blame when an acutely elevated calcium level is discovered in the hospitalized patient. Other causes include sarcoidosis, certain endocrine disorders, and various drugs and supplements.

Etiology

Malignancy Malignancy-associated hypercalcemia has two forms: humoral hypercalcemia of malignancy (HHM) and local osteolytic hypercalcemia (LOH).

HHM results from the elaboration by the tumor of a circulating factor that has systemic effects on skeletal calcium release, renal calcium handling, or GI calcium absorption. It can be caused by the unregulated production of calcitriol (usually by B cell lymphomas). However, the best-recognized hormone responsible for HHM is parathyroid hormone–related protein (PTHrP).[18] Normally, PTHrP appears to serve as a paracrine factor in a variety of tissues (e.g., bone, skin, breast, uterus, and blood vessels); it is involved in cellular calcium handling, smooth muscle contraction, and growth and development. The amino terminus of PTHrP is highly homologous with that of PTH, however, and when PTHrP circulates in supraphysiologic concentrations, it mimics most of the metabolic effects of PTH, such as osteoclast activation, decreased renal calcium output, and increased renal phosphate clearance.

Tumors that produce HHM by secreting PTHrP are usually squamous cell carcinomas (e.g., lung, esophageal, laryngeal, oropharyngeal, nasopharyngeal, or cervical).[19] Other tumor types that occasionally produce PTHrP include adenocarcinoma of the breast and ovary, renal cell carcinoma, transitional cell carcinoma of the bladder, islet cell tumors of the pancreas, and T cell lymphomas. All tumors that elaborate PTHrP do so in relatively small amounts, so the syndrome typically develops in patients with a large tumor burden. It is also unusual for HHM to be the presenting feature of the cancer.

LOH occurs when a tumor growing within bone itself causes the local release of calcium through the production of cytokines that activate osteoclasts; there is no production of a systemic fac-tor in these cases. The classic tumor associated with this syndrome is multiple myeloma, although other neoplasms, such as adenocarcinoma of the breast and various lymphomas, may also cause LOH. It has been learned that factors derived from local bone cells may further enhance the growth of such tumors; this results in the skeleton inadvertently working in concert with the tumor to promote progressive bone resorption and calcium release and further advancement of the cancer.

Other causes Non–PTH-mediated hypercalcemia may be caused by sarcoidosis and other granulomatous diseases, such as tuberculosis (granulomas may produce calcitriol). Certain endocrine conditions may occasionally lead to hypercalcemia. These include hyperthyroidism (which stimulates bone turnover), Addison disease (in which volume contraction reduces calcium clearance), and pheochromocytoma (from production of PTHrP by the tumor). Immobilization may increase calcium levels, usually in persons with active bone turnover, such as adolescents or those with previously unrecognized hyperparathyroidism or Paget disease of bone (see below). Drugs and supplements (e.g., thiazides, lithium, vitamin D, and vitamin A) may be associated with hypercalcemia. Although only rarely encountered today, the so-called milk-alkali syndrome resulted from chronic consumption of large quantities of milk and alkali, which was the standard treatment for peptic ulcers in the days before the development of H_2 receptor blockers and proton pump inhibitors. Patients presented with severe hypercalcemia, metabolic alkalosis, and azotemia.

Familial hypocalciuric hypercalcemia (FHH), also referred to as benign familial hypercalcemia, is an inherited condition caused by a loss-of-function mutation in the calcium-sensing receptor. This results in increased PTH secretion and a higher set point for the extracellular ionized calcium concentration. Patients with FHH have chronic asymptomatic, mild hypercalcemia associated with decreased urinary calcium output.

Diagnosis

If the serum calcium concentration is elevated but the PTH level is low, the patient has non–PTH-mediated hypercalcemia. Possible causes include malignancy, granulomatous disease, nonparathyroid endocrinopathy, and vitamin D intoxication. These cases require further laboratory assessment, such as measurement of PTHrP, vitamin D metabolite levels, and 24-hour urinary calcium levels.

In malignancy-associated hypercalcemia, the degree of calcium elevation is usually moderate or severe, and urinary calcium excretion is markedly increased. Evidence of significant volume depletion and generalized debility may dominate the clinical picture, along with other cancer-related symptoms. Typically, the diagnosis of malignancy has already been established. The diagnosis of malignancy-associated hypercalcemia should be suspected in cancer patients with hypercalcemia who have abnormally low PTH concentrations. Radioimmunoassays for PTHrP are commercially available; elevation of PTHrP concentration will essentially confirm the diagnosis of most cases of HHM. In vitamin D–mediated processes, circulating plasma concentrations of calcitriol are increased, whereas in local osteolytic disease, PTHrP and calcitriol are within normal ranges, and there is definitive evidence of bony metastases.

When the PTH is low but PTHrP is elevated and the patient is not known to have a malignancy, further imaging studies are indicated, including, initially, a plain chest radiograph or a computed tomographic scan of the thorax. If the results are negative, consideration should be given to comprehensive otolaryngoscopic examination, esophagoscopy, or CT of the abdomen. If such further assessment is unrevealing, further radiographic or endoscopic assessment of the genitourinary tract should be considered.

When the PTH level is normal or mildly elevated and the PTHrP level is normal, consideration should be given to the possibility of FHH.[20] The decrease in urinary calcium output seen in FHH helps distinguish this condition from mild primary hyperparathyroidism. The only other form of non–PTH-mediated hypercalcemia in which PTH levels are normal or mildly elevated is that caused by lithium therapy (like FHH, such therapy appears to affect the calcium-sensing receptor and decrease the set point for PTH release).

Suspicion for the sometimes challenging diagnosis of FHH is raised when there is a strong family history of mild, stable hypercalcemia, especially when family members have undergone unsuccessful parathyroid surgery or when the patient's urinary calcium output is low. When this diagnosis is suspected, further evaluation will be necessary, such as the screening of other family members or the administering of specific genetic testing, although the latter is not currently widely available from commercial laboratories. FHH must be distinguished from subtle hyperparathyroidism to avoid ineffective parathyroidectomy.

Treatment

Acute hypercalcemia A nonparathyroid etiology, often a malignancy, is responsible for most cases of acute hypercalcemia [*see Table 3*]. When the serum calcium level is substantially elevated, treatment includes attempts to increase renal calcium excretion while simultaneously attenuating either bone resorption or intestinal calcium absorption, depending on which is the primary source of calcium. Because most patients have at least moderate volume contraction, which further exacerbates their ability to excrete calcium, the initial intervention should be to expand intravascular volume with an intravenous infusion of normal saline. This will augment the delivery of sodium to the distal nephron, which will, in turn, increase urinary calci-

um excretion. Once the intravascular volume is repleted, calcium output can be further increased by adding a loop diuretic, such as furosemide. If the serum calcium concentration does not normalize quickly with intravenous fluid alone, pharmacologic therapy is indicated.[21] Because almost all causes of severe hypercalcemia involve some degree of increased osteoclast activation, drugs that decrease bone turnover are favored. The treatment of choice is a bisphosphonate, such as pamidronate or zolendronic acid, both of which are available as intravenous infusions. Pamidronate is given in a dosage of 60 to 90 mg intravenously over several hours; it is generally well tolerated. Typically, serum calcium levels begin to decrease within 24 to 48 hours of the infusion, although the peak effect may not occur for several days. The action of pamidronate may persist for up to several weeks, and treatment can be repeated as needed. Zolendronic acid is given at a dosage of 4 mg intravenously over no less than 15 minutes. It appears to have an even longer duration of action than pamidronate. A repeat dose may be provided after 7 days. When more rapid action is desired, subcutaneous injection of calcitonin can be tried, either alone or in conjunction with a bisphosphonate. Calcitonin is given at a dosage of 100 to 200 IU once or twice daily. Tachyphylaxis to the hypocalcemic effects of calcitonin is a recognized phenomenon and may curtail its long-term effectiveness. Other possible therapies are plicamycin and gallium nitrate, although certain toxicities limit their use as first-line agents. In severe or refractory cases, hemodialysis against a low-calcium bath may also be utilized.

In the more unusual situation of hypercalcemia resulting from an increase in gut calcium absorption, such as in vitamin D intoxication or granulomatous diseases, glucocorticoid therapy may have an integral role. Glucocorticoids directly impede intestinal calcium transport and also decrease renal 1α-hydroxylase activity, decreasing concentrations of calcitriol. In patients with lymphoma, steroids may also have an antineoplastic effect.

Contributing factors to hypercalcemia, such as the use of oral calcium or vitamin D supplements, diuretic therapy, or immobilization, should be corrected, if possible.

In malignancy-associated hypercalcemia, effective surgery, chemotherapy, or radiotherapy targeted at the tumor itself will reduce the hypercalcemia. However, because hypercalcemia is often an end-stage complication, further chemotherapy or radiotherapy may be neither possible nor desired.

HYPOCALCEMIA

Hypocalcemia is defined as a serum calcium level of less than 9 mg/dl.

Etiology

An abnormally low level of serum calcium on laboratory testing is most often factitious, resulting from a decrease in plasma proteins. Because circulating calcium is so highly protein-bound, decreases in serum albumin concentrations—such as that which occurs with malnourishment, liver disease, or nephrotic syndrome—produce proportionate reductions in total serum calcium. In such situations, the corrected serum calcium equals the measured concentration plus 0.8 mg/dl for each 1 g/dl reduction in the serum albumin level below 4 g/dl. Alternatively, ionized calcium can be measured.

Hypocalcemia is most often related to the parathyroid glands. Removal of or vascular injury to the parathyroids during neck

---

Table 3 Therapy for Acute Hypercalcemia

Fluids
  0.9% NaCl I.V.
  Loop diuretic (forced diuresis)
Medications
  Bisphosphonates
    Pamidronate (60–90 mg I.V.)
    Zolendronic acid (4 mg I.V.)
  Calcitonin (4 IU/kg S.C., q. 12 hr)
  Plicamycin (15–25 μg/kg I.V.)
  Gallium nitrate (200 mg/m²/day continuous infusion for 5 days)
  Glucocorticoids (20–100 mg of prednisone a day)
Other
  Primary therapy directed at tumor
    Surgery
    Chemotherapy
    Radiation
  Decrease calcium and vitamin D intake
  Maintain adequate hydration
  Mobilize patient

surgery can result in hypoparathyroidism, which is manifested by hypocalcemia, hyperphosphatemia, and inappropriately low concentrations of PTH. However, unless all four parathyroids are removed or their blood supply is severely impaired, hypocalcemia after parathyroidectomy is usually a transient phenomenon. Normal parathyroid function typically returns after several days to weeks. In patients who have had prolonged, severe primary hyperparathyroidism and significant bone resorption before parathyroidectomy, the surgery may be followed by protracted hypocalcemia and hypophosphatemia, as large quantities of mineral are deposited into the skeleton. This is referred to as the hungry bone syndrome.

Automimmune destruction of the parathyroid glands may be seen in certain autoimmune conditions, as in polyglandular syndrome type 1, which is marked by hypoparathyroidism, premature ovarian failure, Addison disease, and mucocutaneous candidiasis.[22] Certain infiltrative diseases, such as hemochromatosis, may also adversely affect parathyroid function, as may external beam radiation to the neck. Functional hypoparathyroidism may also result from hypomagnesemia, because magnesium is necessary for both PTH release and PTH action. Pseudohypoparathyroidism is a genetic syndrome characterized by several dysmorphic features and PTH resistance, the latter resulting in hypocalcemia.

Because vitamin D ultimately regulates intestinal calcium absorption, disorders of its supply, production, or activity may lead to mild hypocalcemia. In such conditions, serum calcium concentrations are usually not severely affected, thanks to compensatory increases in PTH levels. Indeed, the primary clinical manifestations are in the skeleton (rickets in children and osteomalacia in adults). Dietary vitamin D deficiency in the elderly is common, but it is often overlooked. One recent survey identified a surprising frequency of vitamin D deficiency in older hospitalized patients.[23] At-risk adults include the elderly with poor dietary habits who avoid liquid milk products and get little sun exposure, particularly in industrial cities in the northern United States.

Hypocalcemia may occur in patients with acute pancreatitis, as fatty acids released through the action of pancreatic lipase complex with calcium. Complexing of phosphate with calcium occurs in severely hyperphosphatemic states, such as acute renal failure, rhabdomyolysis, and the tumor lysis syndrome, and may result in decreased serum calcium concentrations. Subtle alterations in parathyroid function may also result in mild hypocalcemia in critically ill patients.

Diagnosis

Mild hypocalcemia is usually well tolerated by patients, especially if it has developed gradually. However, when the serum calcium level falls below 7.5 to 8 mg/dl (assuming that plasma protein levels are normal), the patient may develop symptoms of neuromuscular irritability, such as tremor, muscle spasms, or paresthesias. On examination, Chvostek and Trousseau signs may be positive. If the serum calcium level drops further, tetany or seizures may result. Prolongation of the QT_c interval may also occur, predisposing the patient to cardiac arrhythmias.

As with hypercalcemia, the cause of hypocalcemia can usually be discerned after a careful history (including a review of medications, previous surgeries, and dietary and social habits) and by the measurement of the circulating concentrations of calcium, phosphorus, PTH, and vitamin D metabolites (i.e., 25-

Table 4   Differential Diagnosis of Hypocalcemia

Abnormal supply or action of parathyroid hormone	Hypoparathyroidism
	  Surgical
	  External beam radiation (to neck)
	  Autoimmune
	    Polyendocrine syndromes
	  Congenital
	  Infiltrative
	    Hemochromatosis
	    Thalassemia
	    Wilson disease
	  Magnesium deficiency
	  DiGeorge syndrome
	PTH resistance
	  Pseudohypoparathyroidism

Abnormal supply or action of Vitamin D	Vitamin D–dependent rickets (VDDR)/osteomalacia
	  Nutritional deficiency
	  Malabsorption
	  Altered vitamin D metabolism
	    Cirrhosis
	    Renal failure
	    Anticonvulsant medications
	Vitamin D pseudodeficiency (VDDR I)
	Abnormal vitamin D receptor (VDDR II)
	Vitamin D–resistant hypophosphatemic rickets/osteomalacia
	  Oncogenic osteomalacia

Medications/supplements	Phosphate Calcitonin Bisphosphonates Plicamycin
Other conditions	Hypoalbuminemia (factitious) Acute pancreatitis Rhabdomyolysis Calcium malabsorption Hyperphosphatemia Large transfusions of citrate-containing blood products Osteoblastic metastases (prostatic or breast carcinoma)

$(OH)D_3$ and calcitriol). The differential diagnosis consists principally of conditions that result in abnormal supply or action of PTH or vitamin D, but the use of medications or supplements and the presence of other conditions must be considered [*see Table 4*].

Treatment

In patients with symptoms from their hypocalcemia (e.g., neuromuscular irritability), calcium should be repleted expeditiously with a slow intravenous infusion of calcium salts, such as calcium chloride or calcium gluconate. Concurrently, any deficiency in magnesium stores should be corrected. In less severe cases, calcium can be administered orally as calcium carbonate or calcium citrate, in doses of 1,000 to 2,000 mg daily. In most cases, vitamin D should also be provided. If dietary deficiency is suspected, plain cholecalciferol (vitamin D_3) is adequate. In cases of hypoparathyroidism, however, calcitriol will be required. In hypoparathyroid patients, it is important to not fully normalize the serum calcium level, because this will result in hypercalciuria, increasing the risk of renal stones. Instead, serum calcium should be kept in the range of 8 to 8.5 mg/dl.

Metabolic Bone Disease

OSTEOPOROSIS

Osteoporosis is defined as decreased bone mass (or density), with abnormal skeletal microarchitecture that increases the risk of fracture. The diagnostic criteria of the World Health Organization are based on the results of standardized bone mass measurements: osteoporosis is present when the bone mineral density (BMD) is decreased to more than 2.5 standard deviations (SDs) below that of a normal, young control population (in whom bone mass is at its peak). Osteopenia is present when the BMD falls between −1.0 and −2.5 SDs from peak bone mass.[24,25]

Epidemiology

Peak bone mass occurs in persons who are in their early 20s; after this age, bone density decreases slowly. Consequently, the incidence of osteoporosis increases with age, becoming most common in persons older than 60 years. Because women attain a peak bone mass lower than that of men, they generally have lower bone density at each succeeding stage of life.[25] Therefore, women experience higher rates of fracture. The most common sites of so-called fragility fractures are the hip, distal forearm, and vertebrae.

The lifetime risk for experiencing any fragility fracture for white women is 40%, whereas for white men it is 13%. By site, the respective risks for women and men are as follows: 18% and 6% for hip fracture, 16% and 3% for distal radius fracture, and 18% and 6% for vertebral fracture.[26] The incidence of hip fracture in women and men at 65 years of age is approximately 300 and 150 per 100,000 person-years, respectively. These rates increase to approximately 3,000 and 2,000 per 100,000 by 85 years of age.

Pathogenesis

Bone mass accumulates during the first 2 decades of life, achieves its peak in the late second or early third decade, stabilizes during the next 1 or 2 decades, and then declines slowly. The age-related decline in bone mass occurs at approximately 0.1% to 0.5% a year in both sexes. In women, however, the rate of bone loss accelerates during the relatively abrupt loss of gonadal steroids during menopause, especially just before and during the first 6 or 7 years after the cessation of menses. During this period, bone density may actually fall by up to 4% a year. Thus, by the end of this period, a woman may have lost one quarter to one third of her total skeletal mass.[25] Subsequently, bone loss tends to slow to a rate similar to that seen in aging men.

Bone remodeling occurs continuously in adults; at any given time, as much as 5% to 10% of the skeleton is in a state of turnover. The cells involved in this remodeling process are the osteoclasts, which resorb bone, and osteoblasts, which form new bone. A cycle of bone remodeling begins with the recruitment of osteoclasts into an area. Resorption of bone from the site releases mineral and collagen breakdown products into the circulation. Through local osteoclast-derived cytokine signals, osteoblasts are then recruited to the site and create new bone matrix to fill the resorption pit left behind by the osteoclasts. The matrix is then mineralized through the physiochemical crystallization of hydroxyapatite. Each bone turnover cycle lasts approximately 3 months.

Through the process of bone remodeling, the skeleton is constantly rejuvenated. In an accelerated form, the bone remodeling process allows for the healing of fractures. In addition, the massive mineral stores of the skeleton are continuously made available to the body for systemic needs, especially during times of decreased calcium supply.

With advancing age, slightly less bone is formed than was resorbed during each remodeling cycle, presumably because of a gradual decline in osteoblast activity. As a result, net bone loss occurs with each cycle, resulting in the gradual decline in bone mass with aging. Therefore, bone loss is to some degree linked to the rate of bone turnover. Any process that increases bone resorption, decreases bone formation, or causes a negative imbalance between the two processes will ultimately result in decreased bone mass and, as a result, an increased risk of fracture.

Etiology

The most important risk factors for decreased bone density and osteoporotic fracture are advanced age, female gender, postmenopausal status, white or Asian race, personal or family history of fragility fracture, and low body weight.[27,28] These risk factors assist the health care provider in identifying patients who are at increased risk for bone loss and consequent fracture. Those patients warrant prophylactic measures to help maintain bone mass, and they may benefit from formal bone density measurement to more precisely quantitate risk. Other contributing factors to bone loss include cigarette smoking, ethanol abuse, insufficient dietary calcium, and decreased physical exercise. Diseases or conditions associated with low bone density include Cushing syndrome, glucocorticoid therapy, thyrotoxicosis, excess thyroid hormone replacement, primary hyperparathyroidism, hypogonadism, intestinal malabsorption, chronic obstructive pulmonary disease, chronic renal or hepatic failure, multiple myeloma and other malignancies, hypopituitarism (growth hormone deficiency), rheumatoid arthritis and other connective tissue diseases, and organ transplantation.

Diagnosis

Although risk-factor analysis assists in determining which patients are at greatest risk for osteoporosis and fracture, the measurement of bone density remains the single best tool to assess risk. Several modalities for measuring bone density have been developed over the years, including single-photon absorptiometry (SPA), dual-photon absorptiometry (DPA), quantitative CT (QCT), DEXA, and ultrasound. DEXA has the highest accuracy and precision of any densitometric method and is currently the diagnostic tool preferred by most authorities.[29,30] It is also the method most widely utilized in the larger clinical trials of antiresorptive treatment regimens and is both widely available and safe. DEXA should therefore be used for the initial diagnosis and follow-up of osteoporosis.

In a typical DEXA report, the actual bone density measurements (g/cm^2) are converted to statistical T scores and Z scores. The T score represents a statistical comparison of the patient's bone mass with that of a young, healthy control group (i.e., people in whom bone mass is at a peak), reported in SDs. The Z score represents the deviation of the patient's bone mass from the age-, sex-, and race-matched peer group mean, based on normative data. The most common sites measured by DEXA are the proximal femur and lumbar spine, although the distal nondominant radius can also be assessed. Most reports also include a brief discussion of the general implications of the findings, and they may provide general recommendations for therapy. Each SD below peak bone mass represents a loss of 10% to 12% of bone mineral content and corresponds to an approximate twofold to 2.5-fold increase in fracture risk at that site. It should be noted, however, that factors other than bone density play important roles in the risk of fracture. Such factors include bone strength, the physicogeometric characteristics of certain bones, and the risk of suffering a fall. In elderly persons, in particular, factors that increase the risk of falling can strongly influence the risk of fracture. These include low visual acuity, impaired neuromuscular function, decreased mobility, cognitive decline, sedative drug use, and residence in a nursing home.[31] In a review of the risk of fracture in almost 8,000 women enrolled in a longitudinal study of osteoporosis, the clinical factors found to be most important for risk of fracture included a history of fracture after 50 years of age in either the patient or her mother, weight less than 125 lb, current cigarette smoking, and the inability to raise oneself from the seated position without use of the arms. By combining these factors with the T score at the hip, these researchers were able to calculate an index that predicted the patient's anticipated percent risk over the subsequent 5 years with greater accuracy than the bone density result alone.[32]

In 1998, the National Osteoporosis Foundation recommended that DEXA be used as a screening modality in women with established osteoporotic fractures (to establish a baseline for follow-up measurements) and in women without established osteoporotic fractures who are 65 years of age or older or who are younger than 65 years but have one or more accepted risk factors for fragility fracture. These include low body weight (< 128 lb); current smoking; and personal history of, or a first-degree family relative with, a low-trauma fracture.[28]

Indications for bone density measurement in any patient include fracture from mild or moderate trauma, evidence of decreased bone mass on plain radiography, and ongoing or anticipated chronic corticosteroid therapy. Bone density measurements are also useful in the evaluation of patients with conditions that might adversely affect bone mass (e.g., hyperparathyroidism) and for purposes of monitoring patients currently receiving any antiosteoporosis therapy.

Once the diagnosis of osteoporosis or osteopenia is made, the clinician should undertake a selective evaluation to exclude secondary causes of bone loss (other than estrogen deficiency). In a premenopausal woman or a man with decreased bone density, such investigations are imperative. A comprehensive history and physical examination will reveal many secondary causes of bone loss. The evaluation should explore symptoms of chronic illness, hyperthyroidism, hyperparathyroidism, intestinal disease, and glucocorticoid use.[33] Lifelong calcium and vitamin D intake should be reviewed. In women, the menstrual history should also be discussed, because even relatively short periods of amenorrhea (reflecting estrogen deficiency) in the past may have a detrimental effect on bone mass.[34] Lifestyle factors such as physical activity level, cigarette smoking, and alcohol abuse should also be addressed. In men, osteoporosis is more often associated with a secondary cause, the more common being alcoholism, steroid use, and hypogonadism.[35]

An extensive biochemical assessment of the patient, other than that indicated by the clinical evaluation, is not necessary. It is reasonable, however, to perform routine blood chemistry studies, including measurement of levels of serum calcium and phosphorus, BUN, serum creatinine, and liver enzymes, along with a complete blood count. Serum protein electrophoresis can also be performed to rule out early myeloma if there is suspicion of malignancy. Subclinical hyperthyroidism can be ruled out with a thyroid-stimulating hormone (TSH) determination. Measurement of PTH and vitamin D levels is not necessary unless an aberration of calcium metabolism is suspected. In some centers, PTH levels are measured routinely to detect mild, normocalcemic primary hyperparathyroidism and secondary hyperparathyroidism from calcium deficiency. The latter may also be detected through the routine measurement of 24-hour urinary calcium output; this is recommended for all patients for assessment of dietary calcium supply and gut calcium absorption.

Treatment

Nutritional therapy   The recommended daily dietary intake of calcium is 1,000 to 1,500 mg, depending on age and menopausal status [see Table 5]. Significant and prolonged calcium deficiency may lead to secondary hyperparathyroidism with negative effects on bone mass, as skeletal stores of mineral are utilized for systemic requirements. Any patient being treated for bone loss must consume adequate amounts of both calcium and vitamin D (400 to 800 IU/day). Several investigators have demonstrated that calcium and vitamin D supplementation has a beneficial effect on postmenopausal bone loss, although the effects are not as dramatic as those seen with antiresorptive therapies.[36] In all the major clinical trials of antiresorptive therapies, participants were also provided basal calcium and vitamin D supplements. Thus, the efficacy of virtually any currently available pharmacologic agent for osteoporosis has been demonstrated only in those with adequate calcium and vitamin D intake. Preferably, calcium and vitamin D should be from dietary sources.[37] Unless milk products are a major component of the diet, however, this may be difficult and, therefore, commercially available supplements should be used.

Antiresorptive therapy   Osteoporosis is most often treated with antiresorptive agents; these agents include the bisphosphonates (e.g., alendronate, risedronate); estrogen; selective estogen receptor modulators (SERM), such as raloxifene; and calcitonin.[27,38-41] All these agents reduce fracture rates substantially, but estrogen[42] and bisphosphonates appear to produce the greatest improvement in bone density.[43-45] Antiresorptive therapy should be considered in all women for the treatment or prevention of osteoporosis, particularly women with established fracture and those who are at high risk for fracture.

For the prevention of osteoporosis, the antiresorptives currently approved by the Food and Drug Administration are estrogen, alendronate, risedronate, and raloxifene. These agents increase BMD at both the hip and the spine during the first 2 to 3 years of use, with subsequent stabilization.

FDA-approved agents for the treatment of established osteoporosis are estrogen, alendronate, risedronate, raloxifene, and cal-

Table 5   Dietary Reference Intakes for Calcium[*68]

Population	Age (yr)	DRI (mg)
Children	1–3	500
	4–8	800
Males and Females	9–18	1,300
	19–50	1,000
	> 50	1,200
Pregnant/lactating women	≤ 18	1,300
	≥ 19	1,000

*Recommended Daily Allowances (RDA) are being replaced with dietary reference intakes (DRI).

citonin. These agents are associated with significant reductions in fracture rates (on the order of 30% to 60%) over 2 to 3 years.[27,35-39,43-49] All of these agents tend to be more effective for increasing bone density and lowering fracture risk at the spine than at the hip.

Estrogen Until recently, estrogen replacement therapy (ERT) was widely recommended as first-line therapy for both prevention and treatment of osteoporosis, although it is approved by the FDA for prevention only.[50] Advocates argued that estrogen directly corrected the chief pathophysiologic defect of the menopause—estrogen deficiency. They also cited other benefits, such as relief from vasomotor disturbances, mood swings, sleep disturbance, and urogenital atrophy. ERT was also at one time considered to have potential cardiovascular benefits, possibly related to its positive effects on plasma lipids. However, several large-scale clinical trials have unequivocally demonstrated that ERT offers no clear cardiovascular benefit.[51-53] Indeed, ERT may actually increase the risk of cardiovascular disease, as well as the risk of breast cancer and ovarian cancer. For example, the multicenter Women's Health Initiative (WHI) was created to study the effects of hormone replacement therapy in healthy, postmenopausal women. Women receiving estrogen plus progestin had a lower incidence of fracture, but this arm of the study was stopped prematurely because of a 26% increased risk of breast cancer and a lack of overall benefit in this treatment group. The WHI also found that compared with women taking a placebo, women taking estrogen plus progestin had a 29% increase in myocardial infarction, a 41% increase in stroke, and a doubling of thromboembolic events. For women in the WHI receiving estrogen only (i.e., those who have had hysterectomies), the study is ongoing, and results are still pending. As a result of the WHI findings, estrogen should probably no longer be considered the optimal first-line preventive or therapeutic agent for bone loss in postmenopausal women.[53]

Estrogens are available in both oral and transdermal formulations. Unless the uterus has been surgically removed, estrogen must be administered in conjunction with progestins, either cyclically or continuously, to prevent endometrial hyperplasia and carcinoma. Estrogen slows accelerated bone turnover and leads to a 2% to 7% increase in BMD a year during the first 1 to 2 years of therapy. Subsequently, BMD plateaus to some extent, without further accrual of bone mass. As is true with other antiresorptive agents, the small increase in bone density belies estrogen's more dramatic effect on fracture risk, which drops 40% to 60% at both hip and spine. These data are mostly from observational studies; before the WHI, there was a paucity of well-designed, randomized clinical trials of ERT using fractures as the primary outcome (and none with hip fracture as the end point). ERT is contraindicated in women with a personal history of breast or uterine cancer or any thrombotic disorders. Other potential side effects include weight gain, edema, breast tenderness, and hypertriglyceridemia. It would appear that the use of estrogen for osteoporosis prevention or treatment should be limited to women who require its beneficial effects for menopausal symptoms. For other women, there are equally effective and probably safer alternatives. When used, ERT should be accompanied by a comprehensive screening program consisting of regular lipid profiles, breast examinations, mammography, and gynecologic assessments.[54]

Bisphosphonates Given their demonstrated safety record and unsurpassed efficacy, the bisphosphonates should be considered the optimal choice for the initial therapy for osteoporosis. Bisphosphonates bind to skeletal hydroxyapatite and decrease osteoclast activity and, as a result, lower bone turnover. Over a period of 2 to 3 years, they produce a 6% to 10% increase in bone density and a 30% to 60% reduction in fracture risk at both vertebral and nonvertebral sites, with greater effectiveness at the former.[44-47] Alendronate is available in formulations of 10 mg once daily and 70 mg once weekly, as well as 5 mg once daily for osteoporosis prevention.[55] Risedronate is available at dosages of 5 mg once daily and 35 mg once weekly.[56] Risks of bisphosphonate therapy include esophagitis; these agents are contraindicated in patients with active esophagitis, achalasia, or esophageal stricture, and they should be used with caution in anyone with a history of esophagitis or gastroesophageal reflux disease. Because they are poorly absorbed, bisphosphonates should be taken on an empty stomach immediately upon awakening in the morning. After taking the agent, the patient should remain upright and should not consume food for at least 1 hour. Thus, these agents are somewhat inconvenient to use, although the newer once-weekly formulations have partially addressed this issue.

Calcitonin Generally speaking, calcitonin's effects on bone density appear to be weaker than those of estrogen or the bisphosphonates.[57] This hormone, which is normally produced by the parafollicular cells (C cells) of the thyroid, typically circulates in low concentration in humans. The precise role of calcitonin in the body is not fully understood, but it appears to be a weak regulator of serum calcium concentrations and bone turnover. Commercially available products include calcitonin injections and nasal spray. Both are approved for the treatment of established osteoporosis but not for its prevention. In most of the calcitonin trials, the average increase in bone density was only 1% to 2% over 2 years, although some studies have suggested a greater effect. In some studies, fracture protection was in the same range as seen with other antiresorptive drugs. The best data are at the spine, but these data are somewhat inconsistent; there are no convincing data at the hip.[48]

Calcitonin is generally safe; occasional flushing, headaches, or nasal irritation is observed with the nasal spray. The injectable form is rarely used, except in patients with acute vertebral fracture; it may actually be the preferred agent in these patients because of its ability to alleviate bone-related pain.[58] One concern with calcitonin is decreased effectiveness with time, or tachyphylaxis.

Raloxifene Raloxifene, a SERM, can be used for osteoporosis prevention or treatment.[59] It appears to have a less potent effect on bone density than either ERT or the bisphosphonates. Raloxifene acts as an estrogen agonist in bone, but it acts as an estrogen antagonist in breast and uterus. Thus, its use is not associated with endometrial hyperplasia, and concurrent treatment with progestins is not required. Raloxifene also does not increase the risk of breast cancer. In fact, it is actively being investigated for its potential role in preventing breast cancer in high-risk individuals.[60] Raloxifene increases bone density by only about 1% over 12 to 24 months, but data on vertebral fracture are comparable to those of ERT or the bisphosphonates. However, raloxifene has not been shown to reduce the incidence of hip fracture. It may also exacerbate menopausal hot flashes, and it carries a risk of thromboembolic disease similar to that seen with estrogen. Preliminary reports suggest no detrimental effect on cardiovascular risk.[61]

National Osteoporosis Foundation guidelines The most comprehensive set of guidelines for the management of osteoporosis comes from the National Osteoporosis Foundation (NOF), which recommends that all postmenopausal women with established osteoporotic fractures be considered candidates for antiresorptive therapy regardless of bone mass [see Table 6].[27] In addition, postmenopausal women with one or more of the following risk factors for osteoporotic fracture should also be considered candidates: (1) a family history of osteoporosis in a first-degree relative, (2) a history of any fracture after 40 years of age, (3) low body weight (< 127 lb), and (4) current smoking, if the T score is lower than –1.5. In those without a risk factor for fracture other than female gender, age, and estrogen deficiency, therapy should be initiated if the T score is –2.5 or lower. In the NOF guidelines, the choice of antiresorptive therapy follows current FDA indications. (The FDA indications and NOF guidelines are likely to be revised with the recent data regarding the adverse effects of ERT.)

Combination therapy Because the currently available antiresorptive agents have distinct mechanisms of action, they may have additive effects when used in combination. To date, this has been demonstrated in small trials that have examined bone density or bone turnover markers as the primary end point, but there are few long-term data regarding antifracture efficacy.[62]

Future therapies Extensive investigations are currently under way into the development of new classes of antiosteoporosis therapies, especially anabolic agents that will result in greater accrual of bone mass than the currently available antiresorptive agents. The drug most likely to be available first is recombinant human PTH. Somewhat paradoxically, intermittent subcutaneous injection of PTH leads to significant increases in bone density and reduces the incidence of fracture. It will likely first be used in patients with severe osteoporosis, in those with contraindications to conventional therapies, or in those who fail to respond adequately to antiresorptive therapy. Duration of treatment is likely to be fixed rather than indefinite.

Lifestyle Exercise is an important aspect of osteoporosis management. Weight-bearing physical activity attenuates bone loss; exercise also helps maintain the proximal muscle strength necessary to avoid falls. Patients with established osteoporosis, especially the elderly, should also be instructed on safety issues and fall-avoidance techniques.[63]

Follow-up For purposes of monitoring, a follow-up bone density study is indicated no sooner than 1 to 2 years after the initial determination, depending on the results and whether any therapy is initiated. Subsequent measurements may be made at similar or longer intervals, depending on the patient's progress and any further therapeutic alterations. When possible, follow-up studies should be performed on the same DEXA unit, for more precise comparison.

The significant but necessary delay in the assessment of response to therapy is frustrating for both patients and physicians. Indeed, the effectiveness of a therapeutic program for osteoporosis may take several years to be realized. Biochemical changes as a result of antiresorptive therapy occur sooner, however, and correlate with improvements in bone density. Biochemical bone turnover markers, typically breakdown fragments of collagen, are released during active bone resorption; such markers are rea-

---

Table 6 Internet Resources for Osteoporosis and Bone Metabolism

American Dietetic Association Nutrition Resources
   http://www.eatright.org
American Society for Bone and Mineral Research
   http://www.asbmr.org
BoneKEY-Osteovision Site of the International Bone and Mineral Society (IBMS)
   http://www.bonekey-ibms.org
International Osteoporosis Foundation
   http://www.osteofound.org

---

sonably reliable indicators of recent bone turnover.[64] Their use remains somewhat controversial, because their cost-effectiveness has not been rigorously assessed. Nevertheless, a significant decrease (> 30%) in bone turnover markers after 2 to 3 months of therapy is predictive of an adequate response, and such measurements may actually enhance compliance.

The most widely available bone-turnover markers include urine pyridinoline and deoxypyridinoline and urine and serum N-terminal telopeptide. Some experts stress the importance of measuring these markers in the initial evaluation of osteoporosis to identify patients with the highest turnover states, who may benefit the most from antiresorptive therapy. Elevated levels may also indicate the urgency of the therapeutic intervention; there are data to suggest that elevated bone-turnover markers are independent predictors of fracture risk.

Complications

Osteoporosis produces enormous burdens, both for patients and for society at large. Society pays a high financial price: in the United States, the direct costs of treatment for osteoporotic fractures alone are estimated to be $10 billion to $15 billion annually. Patients experience disruption of their lives: two thirds of patients who sustain osteoporotic fracture never recover their prefracture functional status, and one third require placement in a nursing home. Rates of depression and anxiety also increase after osteoporotic fracture.[10]

Osteomalacia

Osteomalacia is a condition in which the bone matrix is normal in quantity but is weakened by an insufficient supply of mineral, typically calcium. Osteomalacia in the growing skeleton is termed rickets. Causes of osteomalacia include nutritional deficiencies of calcium, phosphate, or vitamin D; intestinal disease affecting the absorption of these substances; abnormalities in vitamin D metabolism, such as that which occurs in liver disease, renal failure, or through the use of antiepileptic drugs; vitamin D resistance; renal phosphate leaks; and oncogenic osteomalacia (a humoral syndrome associated with rare tumors of mesenchymal origin).[65] In adults, osteomalacia presents as fatigue, proximal muscle weakness, and diffuse or focal skeletal pain.[66] Decreased or low-normal concentrations of both calcium and phosphorus are noted on biochemical testing, and the alkaline phosphatase concentration is elevated. Depending on the cause, decreased levels of either $25\text{-}(OH)D_3$ or calcitriol may be seen. Plain films may demonstrate osteopenia and pseudofractures. When necessary, the diagnosis can be confirmed with bone biopsy. Treatment with vitamin D, with or without mineral supplementation, usually results in a prompt improvement of symptoms and a rapid correction of the defective bone mineralization.

PAGET DISEASE OF BONE

Paget disease is a relatively common condition, typically diagnosed in older persons, in which disordered osteoclast function results in highly disorganized bone microarchitecture. This leads to bone deformity, increased bone vascularity, nerve impingement syndromes, and a propensity to fracture. The precise etiology is not yet known, although the disease is suspected to be of viral origin. Many persons with Paget disease are asymptomatic, the disease being confined to one or several adjacent bones. The sole manifestation may be an increased serum alkaline phosphatase level. If the disease is severe or extensive, significant pain syndromes may result. Very often, the discomfort results not from bone itself but from arthritic changes in adjacent joints caused by altered biomechanics. The skull may be enlarged, or there may be significant bowing of the long bones of the legs. Bony overgrowth may lead to local impingement on spinal nerve roots, with pain or neurologic deficits; overgrowth in the inner ear can lead to sensorineural hearing loss. Rare complications include high-output congestive heart failure (from multiple vascular shunts in bone) and transformation to osteosarcoma.

The diagnosis is typically made after finding an isolated elevation of alkaline phosphatase and an unremarkable evaluation for liver disease. The diagnosis is confirmed by the typical appearance of commonly involved bones (e.g., skull, pelvis, long bones) on plain radiographs or on nuclear bone scan. Disease activity and response to therapy are assessed with serial measurement of alkaline phosphatase or other bone turnover markers. In the elderly, treatment is based primarily on symptoms; use of common analgesics is a reasonable initial therapy, particularly if it is unclear whether the pain is the result of active bone disease or nearby osteoarthritis. For those whose pain is refractory to conventional therapy or those with extensive disease burden or established complications, a more aggressive approach is warranted. Antiresorptive agents, such as the bisphosphonates (see above) or injectable calcitonin, can be used.[67] In younger patients, preemptive therapy may be considered, depending on the extent of bone involvement, the risk of impending complications, or the observed tempo of disease progression.

References

1. Brown EM: Physiology and pathophysiology of the extracellular calcium–sensing receptor. Am J Med 106:238, 1999
2. Marx SJ: Hyperparathyroid and hypoparathyroid disorders. N Engl J Med 343:1863, 2000
3. Inzucchi SE: Diagnosis and management of hypercalcemia. Postgrad Med J (in press)
4. Wermers RA, Khosla S, Atkinson EJ, et al: The rise and fall of primary hyperparathyroidism: a population-based study in Rochester, Minnesota, 1965–1992. Ann Intern Med 126:433, 1997
5. Brandi ML, Gagel RF, Angeli A, et al: Guidelines for diagnosis and therapy of MEN type 1 and type 2. J Clin Endocrinol Metab 86:5658, 2001
6. Khan A, Bilezikian J: Primary hyperparathyroidism: pathophysiology and impact on bone. CMAJ 163:184, 2000
7. Silverberg SJ, Shane E, Jacobs TP, et al: A 10-year prospective study of primary hyperparathyroidism with or without parathyroid surgery. N Engl J Med 341:1249, 1999
8. Bilezikian JP, Potts JT Jr, Fuleihan Gel-H, et al: Summary statement from a workshop on asymptomatic primary hyperparathyroidism: a perspective for the 21st century. J Bone Miner Res 17(suppl 2):N2, 2002
9. Westerdahl J, Lindblom P, Bergenfelz A: Measurement of intraoperative parathyroid hormone predicts long-term operative success. Arch Surg 137:186, 2002
10. Monchik JM, Barellini L, Langer P, et al: Minimally invasive parathyroid surgery in 103 patients with local/regional anesthesia, without exclusion criteria. Surgery 131:502, 2002
11. Civelek AC, Ozalp E, Donovan P, et al: Prospective evaluation of delayed technetium-99m sestamibi SPECT scintigraphy for preoperative localization of primary hyperparathyroidism. Surgery 131:149, 2002
12. Dackiw AP, Sussman JJ, Fritsche HA Jr, et al: Relative contributions of technetium Tc 99m sestamibi scintigraphy, intraoperative gamma probe detection, and the rapid parathyroid hormone assay to the surgical management of hyperparathyroidism. Arch Surg 135:550, 2000
13. Irvin GL 3rd, Carneiro DM: Management changes in primary hyperparathyroidism. JAMA 284:934, 2000
14. Udelsman R: Six hundred fifty-six consecutive explorations for primary hyperparathyroidism. Ann Surg 235:665, 2002
15. Kearns AE, Thompson GB: Medical and surgical management of hyperparathyroidism. Mayo Clin Proc 77:87, 2002
16. Shepherd JJ, Burgess JR, Greenaway TM, et al: Preoperative sestamibi scanning and surgical findings at bilateral, unilateral, or minimal reoperation for recurrent hyperparathyroidism after subtotal parathyroidectomy in patients with multiple endocrine neoplasia type 1. Arch Surg 135:844, 2000
17. Ott SM: Calcimimetics: new drugs with the potential to control hyperparathyroidism. J Clin Endocrinol Metab 83:1080, 1998
18. Dunbar ME, Wysolmerski JJ, Broadus AE: Parathyroid hormone–related protein: from hypercalcemia of malignancy to developmental regulatory molecule. Am J Med Sci 312:287, 1996
19. Rankin W, Grill V, Martin TJ: Parathyroid hormone–related protein and hypercalcemia. Cancer 80(8 suppl):1564, 1997
20. Brown EM: Familial hypocalciuric hypercalcemia and other disorders with resistance to extracellular calcium. Endocrinol Clin North Am 29:503, 2000
21. Ziegler R: Hypercalcemic crisis. J Am Soc Nephrol 12(suppl 17):S3, 2001
22. Betterle C, Greggio NA, Volpato M: Clinical review 93: autoimmune polyglandular syndrome type 1. J Clin Endocrinol Metab 83:1049, 1998
23. Thomas MK, Lloyd-Jones DM, Thadhani RI, et al: Hypovitaminosis D in medical inpatients. N Engl J Med 338:777, 1998
24. Cummings SR, Melton LJ: Epidemiology and outcomes of osteoporotic fractures. Lancet 359:1761, 2002
25. Seeman E: Pathogenesis of bone fragility in women and men. Lancet 359:1841, 2002
26. Melton LJ III, Thamer M, Ray NF, et al: Fractures attributable to osteoporosis: report from the National Osteoporosis Foundation. J Bone Miner Res 12:16, 1997
27. Heinemann DF: Osteoporosis: an overview of the National Osteoporosis Foundation clinical practice guide. Geriatrics 55:31, 2000
28. Fitzpatrick LA: Secondary causes of osteoporosis. Mayo Clin Proc 77:453, 2002
29. Kanis JA: Diagnosis of osteoporosis and assessment of fracture risk. Lancet 359:1929, 2002
30. Miller PD, Zapalowski C, Kulak CA, et al: Bone densitometry: the best way to detect osteoporosis and to monitor therapy. J Clin Endocrinol Metab 84:1867, 1999
31. Slemenda C: Prevention of hip fractures: risk factor modification. Am J Med 103(2A):65S, 1997
32. Black DM, Steinbach M, Palermo L, et al: An assessment tool for predicting fracture risk in postmenopausal women. Osteoporos Int 12:519, 2001
33. Canalis E, Giustina A: Glucocorticoid-induced osteoporosis: summary of a workshop. J Endocrinol Metab 86:5681, 2001
34. Miller KK, Klibanski A: Clinical review 106: amenorrheic bone loss. J Endocrinol Metab 84:1775, 1999
35. Bilezikian JP: Osteoporosis in men. J Endocrinol Metab 84:3431, 1999
36. Atkinson SA, Ward WE: Clinical nutrition: 2. The role of nutrition in the prevention and treatment of adult osteoporosis. CMAJ 165:1511, 2001
37. Weaver CM: Calcium requirements of physically active people. Am J Clin Nutr 72(2 suppl):579S, 2000
38. Manson JE, Martin KA: Clinical practice: postmenopausal hormone-replacement therapy. N Engl J Med 345:34, 2001
39. Altkorn D, Vokes T: Treatment of postmenopausal osteoporosis. JAMA 285:1415, 2001
40. Delmas PD: Treatment of postmenopausal osteoporosis. Lancet 359:2018, 2002
41. NIH Consensus Development Panel on Osteoporosis Prevention, Diagnosis, and Therapy. JAMA 285:785, 2001
42. Effects of hormone therapy on bone mineral density: results from the postmenopausal estrogen/progestin interventions (PEPI) trial. PEPI Writing Group. JAMA 276:1389, 1996
43. Liberman UA, Weiss SR, Broll J, et al: Effect of oral alendronate on bone mineral density and the incidence of fractures in postmenopausal osteoporosis. N Engl J Med 333:1437, 1995
44. Hosking D, Chilvers CED, Christiansen C, et al: Prevention of bone loss with alendronate in postmenopausal women under 60 years of age. N Engl J Med 338:485, 1998
45. Fracture risk reduction with alendronate in women with osteoporosis: the Fracture Intervention Trial. FIT Research Group. J Clin Endocrinol Metab 85:4118, 2000
46. Randomized trial of the effects of risedronate on vertebral fractures in women

with established postmenopausal osteoporosis. Vertebral Efficacy with Risedronate Therapy (VERT) Study Group. Osteoporos Int 11:83, 2000

47. Effect of risedronate on the risk of hip fracture in elderly women. Hip Intervention Program Study Group. N Engl J Med 344:333, 2001

48. Rico H, Revilla M, Hernandez ER, et al: Total and regional bone mineral content and fracture rate in postmenopausal osteoporosis treated with salmon calcitonin: a prospective study. Calcif Tissue Int 56:181, 1995

49. Maricic M, Adachi JD, Sarkar S, et al: Early effects of raloxifene on clinical vertebral fractures at 12 months in postmenopausal women with osteoporosis. Arch Intern Med 162:1140, 2002

50. Manson JE, Martin KA: Clinical practice: postmenopausal hormone-replacement therapy. N Engl J Med 345:34, 2001

51. Viscoli CM, Brass LM, Kernan WN, et al: A clinical trial of estrogen-replacement therapy after ischemic stroke. N Engl J Med 345:1243, 2001

52. Grady D, Herrington D, Bittner V, et al: Cardiovascular disease outcomes during 6.8 years of hormone therapy: Heart and Estrogen/Progestin Replacement Study follow-up (HERS II). JAMA 288:49, 2002

53. Risks and benefits of estrogen plus progestin in healthy postmenopausal women. Writing Group for the Women's Health Initiative Investigators. JAMA 288:321, 2002

54. Burkman RT, Collins JA, Greene RA: Current perspectives on benefits and risks of hormone replacement therapy. Am J Obstet Gynecol 185(2 suppl):S13, 2001

55. Vasikaran SD: Bisphosphonates: an overview with special reference to alendronate. Ann Clin Biochem 38(pt 6):608, 2001

56. Crandall C: Risedronate: a clinical review. Arch Intern Med 161:353, 2001

57. Downs RW Jr, Bell NH, Ettinger MP, et al: Comparison of alendronate and intranasal calcitonin for treatment of osteoporosis in postmenopausal women. J Clin Endocrinol Metab 85:1783, 2000

58. Lyritis GP, Paspati I, Karachalios T, et al: Pain relief from nasal salmon calcitonin in osteoporotic vertebral crush fractures: a double blind, placebo-controlled clinical study. Acta Orthop Scand 275(suppl):112, 1997

59. Khovidhunkit W, Shoback DM: Clinical effects of raloxifene hydrochloride in women. Ann Intern Med 130:431, 1999

60. Continued breast cancer risk reduction in postmenopausal women treated with raloxifene: 4-year results from the MORE trial. Multiple Outcomes of Raloxifene Evaluation. Breast Cancer Res Treat 65:125, 2001

61. Barrett-Connor E, Grady D, Sashegyi A, et al: Raloxifene and cardiovascular events in osteoporotic postmenopausal women: four-year results from the MORE (Multiple Outcomes of Raloxifene Evaluation) randomized trial. JAMA 287:847, 2002

62. Compston JE, Watts NB: Combination therapy for postmenopausal osteoporosis. Clin Endocrinol 56:565, 2002

63. Messinger-Rapport BJ, Thacker HL: Prevention for the older woman: a practical guide to prevention and treatment of osteoporosis. Geriatrics 57:16, 2002

64. Looker AC, Bauer DC, Chesnut CH 3rd, et al: Clinical use of biochemical markers of bone remodeling: current status and future directions. Osteoporos Int 11:467, 2000

65. Drezner MK: Tumor-induced osteomalacia. Rev Endocr Metab Disord 2:175, 2001

66. Reginato AJ, Falasca GF, Pappu R, et al: Musculoskeletal manifestations of osteomalacia: report of 26 cases and literature review. Semin Arthr Rheum 28:287, 1999

67. Lyles KW, Siris ES, Singer FR, et al: A clinical approach to diagnosis and management of Paget's disease of bone. J Bone Miner Res 16:1379, 2001

68. Dietary Reference Intakes (DRI) and Recommended Dietary Allowances (RDA). Food and Nutrition Information Center, USDA/ARS/National Agriculture Library, Beltsville, Maryland, December 2002
http://www.nal.usda.gov/fnic/etext/000105.html

53 Obesity

W. Stewart Agras, M.D.

The prevalence of obesity increased by eight percent in the United States during the past decade, affecting 33.4 percent of adults over the age of 20.[1] A similar increase is evident in children.[2] The abundance of food and reduced activity levels found in industrialized societies are important contributors to these alarming increases. A disorder of energy balance, obesity is associated with increased morbidity and mortality and with detrimental effects on health, such as increased risk of cardiovascular disease and the associated conditions of hypertension, diabetes, and hyperlipidemia.[3-7]

Obesity is loosely defined as an excess of fat over that needed to maintain health. A convenient clinical and epidemiological measure of adiposity is the body mass index (BMI), which is calculated as weight divided by the square of the height (kg/m^2) [see Tables 1 and 2]. BMI is highly correlated with more complex measures of body fat, such as that determined by underwater weighing, although the relation is less accurate at the extremes of the height distribution.[8] An accepted measure of obesity is a BMI value above the 85th percentile (a value of 28 for men and 27 for women, which corresponds to a weight that is 20 percent above ideal weight).[9] The prevalence of obesity increases with age and is almost twice as high in black women as in white women, although the difference between the prevalence in black males and white males is less marked. The prevalence of obesity is strongly related to social class; it is more common among poorer persons.[10] The recent National Institutes of Health Consensus Development Conference on Obesity recommended that in view of the deleterious effects of obesity on health, persons 20 percent or more above their desirable weight should be treated.[9]

Pathogenesis

Many factors are involved in the pathogenesis of obesity. These factors include the control of feeding behavior, mechanisms of fat storage, the components of energy intake and expenditure, and genetic and psychological influences.

CONTROL OF FEEDING

The basic role of feeding in both animals and humans is to maintain a stable concentration of nutrients. To achieve this goal, information about internal nutrient levels and available food is used by the brain to control metabolic processes, activity level, and feeding. Feeding behavior is regulated both by peripheral feedback from the gut and by central mechanisms, which are primarily localized to the hypothalamus. The ventromedial hypothalamus (VMH) inhibits feeding, whereas the lateral hypothalamus promotes feeding. Lesions of the VMH therefore give rise to overfeeding, hyperinsulinemia, and, eventually, obesity.

VMH lesions also promote gut motility, which may play a role in overfeeding. Stimulation of the VMH is aversive and interrupts ongoing behavior, whereas stimulation of the lateral hypothalamus is generally rewarding and may strengthen a variety of behaviors. Feeding is therefore intimately related to the basic mechanisms involving responses to reward and punishment.

Feeding is also modulated by learning, although there appear to be central nervous system processes controlling the response to palatability and the reaction to variety. Learning gives rise to the idiosyncratic likes and dislikes that most of us exhibit. The consumption of a restricted range of foods leads to diminished food intake in both ani-

Table 1 Obesity Thresholds for Selected Heights

Height [in (cm)]	Weight	
	Women [lb (kg)]	Men [lb (kg)]
54 (137)	112 (51)	116 (53)
55 (140)	116 (53)	120 (55)
56 (142)	120 (55)	125 (57)
57 (145)	125 (57)	129 (59)
58 (147)	129 (59)	134 (61)
59 (150)	134 (61)	139 (63)
60 (152)	138 (63)	143 (65)
61 (155)	143 (65)	148 (67)
62 (157)	148 (67)	153 (69)
63 (160)	152 (69)	158 (72)
64 (163)	157 (71)	163 (74)
65 (165)	162 (74)	168 (76)
66 (168)	167 (76)	173 (79)
67 (170)	172 (78)	179 (81)
68 (173)	178 (81)	184 (84)
69 (175)	183 (83)	190 (86)
70 (178)	188 (85)	195 (89)
71 (180)	194 (88)	201 (91)
72 (183)	199 (90)	206 (94)
73 (185)	205 (93)	212 (96)
74 (188)	210 (95)	218 (99)
75 (191)	216 (98)	224 (102)
76 (193)	222 (101)	230 (104)
77 (196)	228 (103)	236 (107)
78 (198)	234 (106)	242 (110)

Note: Thresholds are based on a body mass index (BMI) of 27 for women and 28 for men (see Table 2).

Table 2 Obesity and BMI Values

The body mass index, or BMI, is the ratio of weight to the square of the height. That is,

$$BMI = \frac{weight\ (kg)}{height^2\ (m^2)}$$

BMI values are useful for determining the degree of obesity. Specific BMI values have been associated with specific degrees of obesity. For instance, a body weight 20 percent above ideal weight, which is a commonly accepted definition of obesity, corresponds to a BMI of 28 for males and 27 for females. The values in the following table can be used to determine the degree of obesity and select the most appropriate type of therapy.

Percent above Ideal Weight	BMI Values	
	Men	Women
< 35	28–36	27–35
35–100	36–42	35–42
> 100	> 42	> 42

mals and humans, a phenomenon that is known as sensory-specific satiety. The introduction of a new food into a meal may overcome the satiety response.[11] Obese individuals are more sensitive to food palatability than those individuals who are of normal weight. The obese are more likely to avoid foods of low palatability and more likely to prefer highly palatable foods.[12]

DIETARY FACTORS

The composition of the diet consumed by Americans has changed remarkably over the years. In 1910, the proportion of fat in the diet was 27 percent; by 1984, this proportion had risen to 44 percent. An increase in the percentage of fat in the diet increases the amount of energy stored: 23 percent of the calories present in dietary carbohydrate are lost when it is converted to triglyceride, whereas only three percent of the calories present in dietary fat are used when it is stored as triglyceride.[13] Studies suggest that short-term fat balance is directly influenced by fat intake.[14]

FAT STORAGE

Surplus nutrients are converted to triglyceride and stored in adipocytes. This storage is regulated by the enzyme lipoprotein lipase. The activity of this enzyme varies in different parts of the body; it is very active in abdominal fat and less active in hip fat. Fat deposits in highly active sites are associated with higher cholesterol levels and other cardiac risk factors. This association is reflected in the finding that a waist-to-hip ratio greater than 1.0 in women and 0.8 in men increases the risk for ischemic heart disease, stroke, and death, independent of total body fat.[15] Because men tend to accumulate abdominal fat, which is broken down by the more active form of lipoprotein lipase, they generally lose weight more readily

than women, who accumulate hip fat. Experimental work in animals and epidemiological surveys in humans suggest that stress may lead to the deposition of abdominal fat.[16] Cigarette smoking has also been associated with preferential deposition of fat around the abdomen, despite the fact that smokers have a lower level of adiposity than nonsmokers.[17] Cigarette smoking stimulates cortisol secretion, and this may be the mechanism responsible for excess deposition of abdominal fat.

When triglycerides are deposited in fat cells, the cells initially increase in size; when a maximal size is reached, the cells divide. Moderate degrees of obesity (BMI < 40) are thought to result from an increase in cell size, whereas extreme obesity (BMI > 40) is thought to result from adipocyte proliferation.

ENERGY BALANCE

There are two sides to the energy balance equation: energy intake (i.e., feeding) and energy expenditure. Too much intake or too little expenditure can lead to or maintain obesity. Both sides of the equation have been extensively studied.

Energy Intake

It has been difficult to demonstrate that obese adults consume more calories than adults of normal weight. Most studies do not reveal an excess caloric intake for obese persons, particularly when the extra caloric expenditure involved in moving a greater body mass and the heat loss over a larger body surface area are taken into account. Some studies, however, do show increased caloric intake in obese persons, and such a relation has been most strikingly demonstrated in infancy and childhood.[18] Clearly, however, factors other than excessive caloric intake must also be involved in the pathogenesis of obesity.

Energy Expenditure

The other side of the energy balance equation is energy expenditure. There are three components to energy expenditure: the resting metabolic rate (RMR), the thermic effect of activity (facultative thermogenesis), and dietary-induced thermogenesis (i.e., the heat produced by food digestion, absorption, and storage).[19] The largest component of energy expenditure, the RMR, accounts for about 60 percent of energy expenditure. This component includes the energy costs of maintaining the integrated bodily functions. Studies of the RMR in obese persons have produced varying results. The most recent studies suggest that obese people compensate for weight loss by decreasing total energy expenditure to a significantly greater extent than nonobese people.[19] These compensatory changes combined with the hunger and dysphoria associated with dieting may account for the difficulty obese persons have in achieving and maintaining weight loss. The thermic effect of activity accounts for about a fifth of total energy expenditure in the average sedentary individual. This component can be increased by voluntary activity (e.g., by exercise) and also includes the energy cost of small muscle movements (fidgeting), which varies greatly among individuals and may be genetically determined. Exercise can also increase the RMR for at least 18 hours after increased activity. The smallest component of total energy expenditure, dietary-induced thermogenesis, includes the cost of food absorption and metabolism and may be lower in the obese than in persons of normal weight.

Studies have demonstrated that obese adults and children are less active than those of normal weight.[20] Studies have also shown that the thermic response to exercise is blunted in obese persons.[19]

The sites of facultative thermogenesis primarily involve muscle and cell membrane transport. The role of brown fat, which is adipose tissue rich in mitochondria that is used by small animals for generating heat, is uncertain in humans, although it may be an important contributor to thermogenesis. Most of the thermogenic mechanisms are controlled by the sympathetic nervous system. Epinephrine, norepinephrine, glucagon, and glucocorticoids appear to be the primary hormones stimulating thermogenesis. The beta blocker propranolol has been shown to reduce the thermic response to infused glucose and insulin. Studies have shown that the response of the sympathetic nervous system to exercise is blunted in the obese; specifically, norepinephrine turnover is reduced.[13]

To summarize, obese persons may be more metabolically efficient, may demonstrate a greater metabolic compensation in the RMR after dietary reduction, and may exhibit reduced thermic responses to food and exercise as compared with the nonobese. In addition, the obese may demonstrate lower activity levels than the nonobese.

Weight Cycling

Many overweight people repeatedly lose and regain weight in what is termed weight cycling. Whereas animal studies have suggested that weight cycling may have detrimental effects, human studies have produced conflicting findings. One of the problems with research in humans is that such studies do not define weight cycling accurately, often using measures that are strongly correlated with overall weight gain, hence confusing the health risks of weight gain with those of weight cycling. Many studies fail to distinguish between voluntary and involuntary weight losses; others are not prospective studies and include both normal-weight and overweight persons. A recent review of the literature by the National Task Force on the Prevention and Treatment of Obesity[21] concluded that there is no evidence that weight cycling is detrimental to overweight individuals. Hence, the possibility of weight loss followed by regain should not deter overweight individuals from attempting to lose weight, although they should minimize cycling by choosing modest weight losses, which have been demonstrated to be beneficial to health.

Nicotine and Weight

Both animal and human studies have demonstrated that nicotine reduces caloric intake and that its use is associated with a modest weight loss.[22] In addition, most studies have shown that smoking cessation (or withdrawal from nicotine in animals) leads to weight gain. In a large-scale study of smokers, those who had quit smoking and nonsmokers were followed over a 10-year period.[23] The average weight gain after smoking cessation was 2.8 kg in men and 3.8 kg in women, although some 10 percent of men and 13 percent of women had gained more than 13 kg. However, by the end of the follow-up period, the mean body weight of the persons who had quit smoking equaled that of those who had never smoked. Many smokers, particularly women, consider the effects of nicotine on weight to be important and cite this as a reason for not quitting. Both clinical and laboratory evidence suggest that the mechanism for weight gain is increased caloric intake.

Medications Implicated in Obesity

Certain medications may cause or contribute to obesity. About one third of depressed patients treated with tricyclic antidepressants gain weight. Imipramine appears to be associated with weight gain in the greatest number of patients; desipramine and trazodone induce weight gain in fewer patients. For the treatment of depression in overweight patients, fluoxetine, as well as the other serotonin reuptake inhibitors, should be considered, because fluoxetine has been demonstrated to lead to weight loss in obese individuals. The phenothiazines, used in the treatment of schizophrenia, are also associated with weight gain. Chlorpromazine and thioridazine are associated with the highest frequency of weight gain, whereas haloperidol is less frequently associated with such gains. The steroids are also associated with weight gain. Finally, the antiepileptic agents valproic acid and carbamazepine, which are used in the treatment of some psychiatric disorders, are also associated with weight gain.[24]

GENETIC FACTORS

Studies of twins[25] and adopted children[26] have provided evidence that genetic factors are involved in the pathogenesis of obesity. For instance, adopted children more closely resemble their biologic parents in terms of adiposity than their adoptive parents. Because body weight has a continuous distribution in the population, much like height or intelligence, it is likely that more than one gene is involved in obesity. One such gene, the *ob* gene, was recently isolated in a mouse model. Moreover, a human homologue of this gene was found to be 84 percent identical to the mouse gene. Absence of the *ob* gene leads to obesity in the mouse model. More important, a protein apparently secreted by fat cells interacts with the brain ob receptor site, creating a feedback mechanism that may be involved in long-term regulation. In the obese mouse, injection of the ob protein leads to weight loss (i.e., a shortage of the protein leads to obesity). Whether this protein will prove useful in the treatment of obesity is uncertain.[27,28] Indeed, some studies in humans have found that obese persons actually have more of the ob protein than nonobese persons, which suggests that a more important defect may be at the brain receptor site and raises the possibility of designing a drug that mimics the protein secreted by fat cells once the receptor-site gene has been cloned.

A second genetic finding of interest is that a mutation in the beta$_3$-adrenergic receptor gene leads to the replacement of tryptophan with arginine in the receptor protein. Persons with this mutation have an increased capacity to gain weight, are at greater risk for non–insulin-dependent diabetes mellitus, and may also demonstrate a lower resting metabolic rate.[29] The most important aspect of this finding is that the beta$_3$-adrenergic receptor is principally involved in the thermic activity of brown adipose tissue. Selective beta$_3$-adrenergic agonists may be useful in the treatment of obesity because they increase energy expenditure. Although several beta$_3$-adrenergic compounds are available and they increase thermogenesis and decrease insulin resistance, they are not clinically useful because of side effects. However, newer compounds without such side effects may be useful in the treatment of obesity in the future.

Heritable Syndromes Associated with Obesity

Certain rare genetic syndromes are associated with obesity. The Prader-Willi syndrome is the most common of these and is characterized by hypotonia, mental retardation, short stature, a narrow facies with almond-shaped eyes, and, often, strabismus. In infancy, individuals with this syndrome may demonstrate no abnormalities in food intake; in childhood, however, they develop a voracious appetite coupled with temper tantrums when refused food, leading to difficulties in managing their behavior. The Bardet-Biedl syndrome is characterized by retinitis pigmentosa, polydactyly, and obesity. This syndrome has been lumped with the Laurence-Moon syndrome, but the latter is not commonly associated with obesity.

PSYCHOLOGICAL FACTORS

It was previously thought that psychological factors such as depression, anxiety, or a so-called obese personality style predisposed to obesity. It is currently recognized that the psychological problems associated with obesity are a result of the condition rather than a cause. Studies have demonstrated that obese persons suffer from discrimination when applying to college and for employment.[30] Such discrimination can lead to anxiety or depression. In addition, dieting is often associated with transient anxiety and depression, and this response is seen in both normal and overweight populations. Large-scale studies examining psychological traits in obese and nonobese individuals have failed to demonstrate higher levels of psychopathology in the obese.[31]

The question of whether the eating style of obese persons is different from that of nonobese persons has been of much interest, especially because one part of behavior modification therapy is to modify eating style. Several studies have found differences in both children and adults. Obese persons were found to eat more rapidly, take fewer bites for the same number of calories, and chew less than normal-weight or thin individuals. Other studies, however, have found no differences. A vigorous suckling style in infants two weeks of age has been associated with higher levels of adiposity at two years of age.[18] This feeding style may parallel the vigorous suckling of the obese mouse as compared with its lean siblings.[32]

Evaluation

Evaluation of an obese patient should begin with an accurate history. The most common history is an increase in weight in adolescence or early adult life, followed by a slow but steady weight gain punctuated by attempts to diet. Among the precipitants of obesity are an increase in dietary intake and a decrease in exercise, occasioned by a change in the way of life or by the effects of pregnancy. Less commonly, obesity occurs in infancy or early childhood. A history of very rapid weight gain should alert the clinician to consider some primary cause for the change in weight, and medications taken should be noted. Binge eating may complicate obesity [see Chapter 47].[33] Such compulsive overeating is associated with a poorer outcome from treatment and more frequent psychological disturbances than in the obese patient who does not binge. Purging, which, like binging, is associated with bulimia, is also occasionally seen in the obese individual and can indicate a patient's misguided effort at self-treatment.

A careful family history of adiposity should be obtained to evaluate familial predisposition: 80 percent of the children of two obese parents will eventually be obese, compared with only 14 percent of the children of normal-weight parents. Such familial data can be used to introduce preventive measures early in the child's life. In certain patients, the possibility of Prader-Willi or Bardet-Biedl syndrome should be considered. The weight loss methods previously used by the patient, including dietary and pharmacological approaches, should also be reviewed, and the relative success of each treatment should be ascertained. This information may help guide the choice of treatment.

The best clinical measure of adiposity is the BMI. Treatment is recommended for women with a BMI above 27 and men with a BMI above 28 [see Table 1]. The waist-to-hip ratio should also be ascertained; a waist-to-hip ratio greater than 1.0 in women and 0.8 in men is associated with an increased risk of cardiovascular disease and provides another indication for treatment. The patient should be assessed for the presence of conditions associated with obesity, including type II diabetes mellitus (or impaired glucose tolerance), hypertension, hyperlipidemia, coronary artery disease, cardiac failure, gallbladder disease, pulmonary dysfunction (including sleep apnea), and osteoarthritis. In addition, psychological reactions to the social stigma associated with obesity should be sought. These reactions occur frequently and are most often manifested as depression. Associated cardiovascular risk factors such as cigarette smoking should also be documented.

An algorithm has been developed for the evaluation of obese patients [see Figure 1].

Differential Diagnosis

Most endocrine changes found in obese patients are not primary causes of obesity. However, the following conditions should always be considered in the differential diagnosis [see Chapters 45, 46, 49, and 51].

THYROID DISEASE

Although many overweight individuals are given thyroid hormone in an effort to speed up metabolism, this treatment does not reduce weight. In fact, few obese individuals suffer from primary hypothyroidism. Severe hypothyroidism can lead to increased fat deposits, but in most cases, the weight increase is caused by edema, which

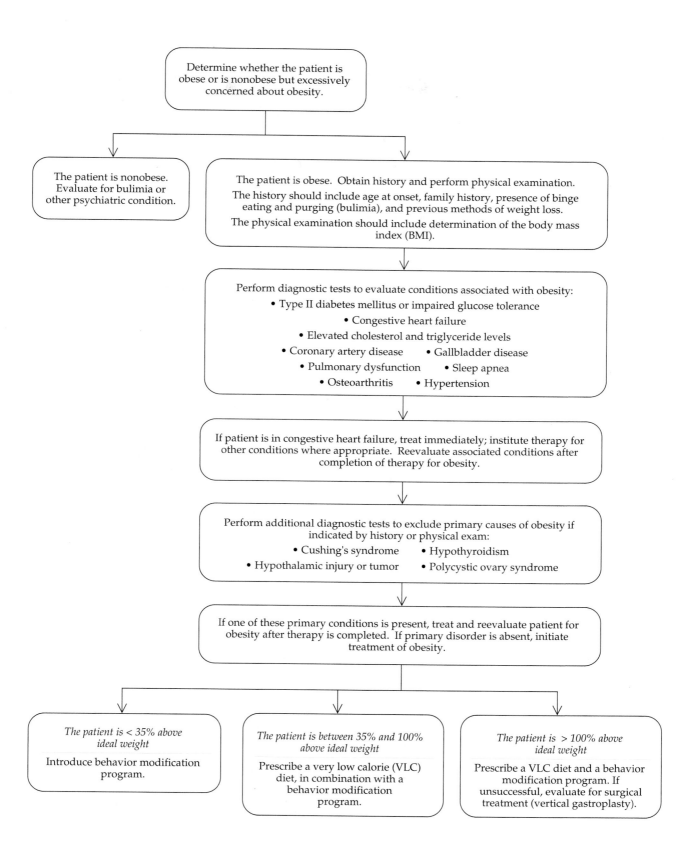

Figure 1   **The flowchart outlines the diagnosis and treatment of obesity.**

resolves when the patient is given thyroid hormone.

PITUITARY AND ADRENAL DISEASE

Cushing's syndrome is characterized by excessive central adiposity, diabetes, and hypertension. This syndrome is caused by overproduction of adrenocorticotropic hormone (ACTH), either by a pituitary tumor or by hyperactive pituitary cells, which leads to excessive synthesis of cortisol by the adrenal cortex.

HYPOTHALAMIC DISEASE

Tumors of the hypothalamus or injury to this region of the brain may give rise to the ventromedial syndrome of hyperphagia, which leads to obesity. The most common tumor associated with this syndrome is the craniopharyngioma. Injury to the hypothalamus may also be caused by intracranial surgery.

POLYCYSTIC OVARY SYNDROME

The polycystic ovary syndrome is characterized by amenorrhea or irregular menses, hirsutism, and, often, obesity.

Treatment

In the past few years, the question of whether to treat obesity has become controversial. There is no doubt that reducing weight is accompanied by health benefits, but it is also clear that the majority of people who lose weight will regain it. This dichotomy fuels the controversy over treatment. However, as noted earlier, weight loss and regain is not associated with particularly deleterious effects for the overweight or obese person; hence, weight loss should be seriously considered for the overweight patient. Moreover, modest weight losses are associated with health benefits. Therefore, the setting of modest goals for the overweight patient should be considered, thus increasing the likelihood of maintenance of weight losses. For patients with a family history of obesity, increases in BMI should be taken seriously before the individual becomes obese, and attempts should be made to stabilize weight by reducing fat intake and increasing activity levels.

Unless a primary cause for obesity is found, the type of treatment will depend on the severity of the problem, associated health problems, and the presence of risk factors for cardiovascular disease. For individuals who are between 20 and 35 percent overweight, a comprehensive behavior modification program is indicated; for those who are between 35 and 100 percent overweight, a very low calorie (VLC) diet program should be considered; and for individuals more than 100 percent overweight who have repeatedly failed at other weight-loss measures, a surgical approach should be considered [see Table 2]. The addition of pharmacotherapy to these approaches may be useful for some patients.

There are few contraindications to weight loss. The presence of marked depression or current major life stresses may be associated with poor outcome, suggesting that treatment should be deferred until the problem has been resolved. In addition, because exercise is an important aspect of all approaches to weight loss, orthopedic or other impediments to exercise should be corrected before beginning treatment. It is important to recognize that although few individuals will reach their ideal weight with treatment, weight losses of only 5 to 10 kg may reduce blood pressure and lipid levels and enhance control of type II diabetes.[34-36] The health benefits of relatively small weight losses should therefore be emphasized to patients for whom weight loss is indicated for specific health reasons.

Factors that predispose to obesity in the United States today include the availability of a highly varied diet for the majority of the population, a high percentage of fat in the diet, lowered activity levels, and, in susceptible individuals, an excessive metabolic response to dieting (i.e., lowering of thermogenesis and the RMR). Treatment must take these pathophysiological factors into account. Caloric intake must be reduced, with special emphasis on lowering fat intake and increasing activity levels. These changes may partially counteract the decrease in the RMR caused by dieting.

Weight loss attempts should be taken seriously and should be viewed as part of a long-term commitment by both patient and physician.

BEHAVIOR MODIFICATION

Most behavior modification programs offer a comprehensive approach to weight loss, including altering eating behaviors and instituting a sensible diet and a suitable exercise regimen. Behavior modification programs initially involve self-monitoring of activity levels and food intake, including the circumstances under which food is consumed. This information is used to help the patient decrease the number of snacks, moderate fat intake, slow down rapid eating, and increase exercise. The nutrition program is usually a so-called heart healthy diet that is aimed at decreasing fat intake, particularly saturated fats, and increasing the proportion of vegetables in the diet. The exercise program usually emphasizes walking; a typical goal would be brisk walking for 30 minutes a day, five to seven times a week. Studies have demonstrated that the addition of moderate exercise to weight loss programs enhances both the initial loss of weight and maintenance of those losses.[37]

Patients following these programs can expect a weight loss of 0.5 kg a week. Most programs are about four months long, with an average weight loss of 7.0 kg. Obviously, patients more than 7.0 kg overweight should expect a longer program; patients at the top end of the recommended range for behavior modification might expect a program approximately one year in length to achieve their weight goal.[38] Excellent results have been reported with comprehensive long-term behavioral therapy programs, with weight losses averaging 16 kg.[39] Dropout rates are relatively low from such programs, averaging a little more than 10 percent. The results from large-scale clinical trials suggest that both black women and black men lose less weight than white men and women when following the same weight-loss program.[40] The cause for such differences is unknown and may involve both sociocultural and biologic factors. Programs such as Weight Watchers are usually based on principles similar to those described above and are available at low cost. Commercial groups differ from professionally led groups primarily in their attrition rate, which approaches 90 percent in some cases.

One year after undergoing behavior modification therapy, the average patient regains one third of the weight lost.[38] Various factors play a role in the failure to maintain weight loss, including a failure to continue the changes in eating behavior and exercise. To rectify this problem, longer maintenance periods are now used, with continued group meetings, monitoring of diet and exercise, and problem-solving sessions. Physicians can play an important role in maintenance by scheduling periodic examinations for weight measurement, ensuring that the patient continues treatment, and encouraging the patient to return to treatment as weight begins to be regained. The health benefits of reduced weight—lowered blood pressure and cholesterol levels and better control of diabetes—should be emphasized to the patient.

VERY LOW CALORIE DIET

The original liquid protein diets, which were often used without medical supervision, were abandoned in the late 1970s, when more than 60 deaths attributed to the diets were reported to the Centers for Disease Control.[41,42] Although the exact cause of these deaths remains unknown, the combination of poor-quality protein and electrolyte depletion appeared to underlie the fatal cardiac arrhythmias. Liquid protein mixtures have since been reformulated for greater safety. Newer products contain high-quality protein and carbohydrate to minimize the negative nitrogen balance associated with starvation, and mineral supplements have been added to avoid electrolyte depletion. The caloric composition varies between 400 and 800 kcal/day. The VLC diet is usually used for 12 weeks because the safety of longer use has not been established. To enhance weight maintenance, the behavior modification techniques described above are usually added to the program.

Careful medical supervision of patients receiving a VLC diet is essential. Patients with a history of myocardial infarction, major cardiac arrhythmia, angina, or stroke should not be treated with the diet. Other contraindications to this approach include a bleeding peptic ulcer or another serious medical disorder that would complicate weight loss, such as thrombophlebitis, liver or kidney disease, or cancer. Patients taking aspirin in therapeutic doses also should not participate in this program. Psychiatric disorders that contraindicate use of a VLC diet include current psychosis, alcoholism, and drug abuse. If the patient is significantly depressed, treatment with a very low calorie diet should be delayed until the depression has been successfully treated.

After the start of the diet, participants should be briefly evaluated medically once a week for the first six weeks and biweekly thereafter. Cardiac rate and blood pressure should be checked, and any new complaints that would indicate a complication of the diet should be followed. Laboratory monitoring, which should be done every two weeks, should include measurement of serum electrolyte and uric acid levels and a complete and differential blood count. An ECG should be performed once a month. Evidence suggests that the incidence of gallstones is increased during dieting, especially with a VLC diet. One controlled study found that administration of ursodeoxycholic acid (1,200 mg/day) significantly reduced the formation of cholesterol crystals and gallstones in dieting patients.[43] Ursodeoxycholic acid should probably be taken routinely by patients following a VLC diet.

An average weight loss of 20 to 25 kg in 12 weeks has been reported for patients using a VLC diet. The addition of behavior modification and exercise to the VLC diet regimen in a comprehensive program enhances the efficacy of the diet.[44] Weight loss can reach 45 kg in a substantial proportion of patients who make appropriate behavioral changes after the dietary phase.[45] The dropout rate varies between 15 and 25 percent during the dietary phase. Patients usually stop because of intolerance to the diet, with feelings of weakness and hunger; some patients, particularly those who are not able to tolerate milk products, experience an allergic reaction to the liquid protein mixture. Unfortunately, only a small percentage maintain their weight loss for one to two years.

Most individuals do not attain their ideal weight. For those who do, maintenance is considerably enhanced: 40 percent of these patients maintain ideal weight 18 months after finishing the diet.

SURGICAL APPROACHES TO OBESITY

For the severely obese patient who has not responded to behavior modification and a VLC diet, surgery should be considered because such individuals are at high risk for the comorbid medical problems associated with obesity. There are three different surgical approaches to obesity: vertical banded gastroplasty,[46] gastric bypass,[47] and biliopancreatic diversion.[48] The last procedure results in fat malabsorption with steatorrhea. The side effects accompanying this procedure may include severe protein deficiency, osteoporosis secondary to calcium and vitamin D malabsorption, and problems secondary to poor absorption of the other fat-soluble vitamins. These complications have led many investigators to consider this procedure unacceptable.[47] Both gastric bypass and vertical banded gastroplasty are frequently used procedures in the United States. Both procedures are associated with marked weight loss, although controlled trials suggest that gastric bypass is associated with better immediate weight loss and better maintenance of those losses. In one study, patients treated with gastric bypass had lost over 60 percent of their excess weight, compared with 40 percent for vertical banded gastroplasty, by three years after surgery.[49] Five-year follow-up appears equally satisfactory. Complications after vertical banded gastroplasty include rupture of the suture line and gastric ulcer. Complaints of nausea and heartburn occur in as many as a quarter of patients. Complications associated with gastric bypass include an occasional anastomotic leak, stomal stenosis, cholecystitis, the dumping syndrome (which may deter patients from eating simple carbohydrates), and iron deficiency anemia. The mortality for such surgical procedures is approximately 0.5 percent.

Given these complications and the permanent effects of surgery on dietary intake, careful selection of patients for surgery is necessary. Psychiatric screening may be useful to eliminate those with severe psychopathology. Nonetheless, despite the complications associated with the surgical approaches to obesity, such surgery may be lifesaving for the high-risk, morbidly obese patient for whom other approaches to weight loss have failed.

PHARMACOLOGICAL AGENTS

Over the past quarter century, the pharmacological agents used to treat obesity have changed. Amphetamines, for example, have been completely abandoned as a treatment for obesity because their addictive potential clearly outweighs the health benefits derived from the drug-induced weight loss. Pharmacological appetite suppressants that have little or no addictive potential have taken the place of amphetamines in the treatment of obesity. Controlled trials have shown that anorectic agents such as fenfluramine, dexfenfluramine, and phentermine are superior to placebo in inducing weight loss, and the average weight loss is comparable to that achieved through behavior modification.[50] Weight loss of about 10 percent of initial body weight can be achieved by patients who both undergo behavior modification and take an appetite suppressant, and controlled studies have shown that long-term maintenance of such loss is possible.[51,52] However, studies have conclusively demonstrated that once the anorectic agent is withdrawn, weight is regained.

The first problem to arise with these medications was demonstrated in epidemiological studies, which showed that anorectic agents increased the prevalence of pulmonary hypertension from a baseline rate of one to two cases per million population to approximately 30 cases per million population.[53]

The second problem was first noted in a study of 24 women who took the combination of fenfluramine and phentermine for an average of one year.[54] Several of these women required cardiac surgery. A sticky plaque covered the valves, stiffening them and causing valvular regurgitation. Histopathology revealed changes in the valvular tissue similar to those found in carcinoid valve disease, which is marked by high levels of circulating serotonin. Data from five sites indicate that the prevalence of abnormal echocardiograms (with aortic regurgitation of mild or greater severity and mitral regurgitation of moderate or greater severity) in patients treated with fenfluramine and dexfenfluramine, either alone or in combination with phentermine, is approximately 30 percent.[55] The U.S. Department of Health and Human Services recommends that all persons exposed to these medications (estimated at 4.7 million persons) undergo cardiovascular examination, including medical history Those individuals who exhibit cardiopulmonary signs should be evaluated by echocardiography. In addition, echocardiography should be performed before an invasive procedure to minimize the risk of bacterial endocarditis. Similar valvular lesions resulting from the use of either fenfluramine or dexfenfluramine alone have been reported. These findings were enough to lead two pharmaceutical companies to voluntarily withdraw both fenfluramine and dexfenfluramine from the market.

No valvular lesions have been reported with the use of phentermine alone; thus, this medication is approved for use. The FDA has recently approved two new antiobesity agents. The first, sibutramine, is an appetite suppressant that inhibits the reuptake of both serotonin and norepinephrine.[56] The second, orlistat, is a lipase inhibitor that acts in the gastrointestinal tract and is not absorbed. Patients taking orlistat must consume a diet made up of no more than 30 percent fat, however, because a higher fat intake has been associated with side effects. Side effects attributed to orlistat include flatus with discharge, fecal urgency, fatty or oily stools, increased defecation, fecal incontinence, abdominal pain, and liquid stools. Both sibutramine and orlistat should become available in 1998.

Prevention

Little is known about the primary prevention of obesity, although it is clear that such efforts should begin at an early age. Prevention programs involving dietary changes must be carefully administered to avoid nutritional deprivation in the developing child. One uncontrolled study suggested that a diet low in fat may help control excessive adiposity. Of a group of infants fed such a diet, only one became overweight at three years of age; in contrast, 25 percent of an untreated group of children in the same pediatric practice became overweight.[57] Such primary prevention should probably be directed toward high-risk children (i.e., those with a strong family history of obesity) and should involve permanent changes in dietary and exercise habits at a family level. Secondary prevention, in the form of early treatment aimed at avoiding the deleterious effects of obesity on health, should also be directed toward those with a family history of obesity and should begin with the recognition that the patient is becoming overweight. The most appropriate treatment at this point would be a behavior modification weight-loss program aimed at making permanent changes in diet and exercise. Studies in childhood suggest that relatively long-term effects on weight result from such treatment, particularly if the family is involved in the behavioral changes.[58] Finally, efforts at education concerning the prevention of obesity at a community level may result in the slowing of weight gain in adults, suggesting that such efforts may be useful in prevention.

References

1. Kuczmarski RJ, Flegal KM, Campbell SM, et al: Increasing prevalence of overweight among US adults: The National Health and Nutrition Examination Surveys, 1960 to 1991. JAMA 272:205, 1994

2. Flegal KM: Defining obesity in children and adolescents: epidemiologic approaches. Crit Rev Food Sci Nutr 33:307, 1993

3. Stamler R, Stamler J, Riedlinger WF, et al: Weight and blood pressure: findings in hypertension screening of 1 million Americans. JAMA 240: 1607, 1978

4. Modan M, Karasik A, Halkin H, et al: Effects of past and concurrent body mass index on prevalence of glucose intolerance and type 2 (non-insulin-dependent) diabetes and on insulin response: the Israel study of glucose intolerance, obesity and hypertension. Diabetologia 29:82, 1986

5. Manson JE, Colditz GA, Stampfer MJ, et al: A prospective study of obesity and risk of coronary heart disease in women. N Engl J Med 322:882, 1990

6. Must A, Jacques PF, Dallal GE, et al: Long-term morbidity and mortality of overweight adolescents: a follow-up of the Harvard Growth Study of 1922 to 1935. N Engl J Med 327:1350, 1992

7. Maclure KM, Hayes KC, Colditz GA, et al: Weight, diet, and the risk of symptomatic gallstones in middle-aged women. N Engl J Med 321:563, 1989

8. Benn RT: Some mathematical properties of weight-for-height indices used as measures of adiposity. British Journal of Preventive and Social Medicine 25:42, 1971

9. U.S. Department of Health and Human Services: National Institutes of Health Consensus Development Conference Statement: Health Implications of Obesity, 1985

10. Stunkard AJ: From explanation to action in psychosomatic medicine: the case of obesity. Psychosom Med 37:195, 1975

11. Rolls BJ, Rowe EA, Rolls ET, et al: Variety in a meal enhances food intake in man. Physiol Behav 26:215, 1981

12. Wooley SC, Wooley OW: Salivation to the sight and thought of food: a new measure of appetite. Psychosom Med 35:136, 1973

13. Sims EA, Danforth E Jr: Expenditure and storage of energy in man. J Clin Invest 79:1019, 1987

14. Schemmel R: Physiological considerations of lipid storage and utilization. Amer Zool 16:661, 1976

15. Björntrop P: Regional patterns of fat distribution. Ann Intern Med 103:994, 1985

16. Rodin J: Determinants of body fat localization and its implications for health. Ann Behav Med 14:275,1992

17. Den Tonkelaar I, Seidell JC, van Noord PA, et al: Fat distribution in relation to age, degree of obesity, smoking habits, parity and estrogen use: a cross-sectional study in 11,825 Dutch women participating in the DOM project. Int J Obes 14:753, 1990

18. Agras WS, Kraemer HC, Berkowitz RI, et al: Does a vigorous feeding style influence the early development of adiposity? J Pediatr 110:799, 1987

19. Leibel RL, Rosenbaum M, Hirsch J: Changes in energy expenditure resulting from altered body weight. N Engl J Med 332:621, 1995

20. Berkowitz RI, Agras WS, Korner AF, et al: Physical activity and adiposity: a longitudinal study from birth to childhood. J Pediatr 106:734, 1985

21. Weight cycling. National Task Force on the Prevention and Treatment of Obesity. JAMA 272:1196, 1994

22. Comstock GW, Stone RW: Changes in body weight and subcutaneous fatness related to smoking habits. Arch Environ Health 24:271, 1972

23. Williamson DF, Madans J, Anda RF, et al: Smoking cessation and severity of weight gain in a national cohort. N Engl J Med 324:739, 1991

24. Mattson RH, Cramer JA, Collins JF, et al: A comparison of valproate with carbamazepine for the treatment of complex partial seizures and secondarily generalized tonic-clonic seizures in adults. N Engl J Med 327:765, 1992

25. Stunkard AJ, Foch TT, Hrubec Z: A twin study of human obesity. JAMA 256:51, 1986

26. Stunkard AJ, Sorensen TIA, Hanis C, et al: An adoption study of human obesity. N Engl J Med 314:193, 1986

27. Zhang Y, Proenca R, Maffei M, et al: Positional cloning of the mouse obese gene and its human homologue. Nature 372:739, 1994

28. Campfield LA, Smith FJ, Guisez Y, et al: Recombinant mouse OB protein: evidence for a peripheral signal linking adiposity and central neural networks. Science 269:546, 1995

29. Walston J, Silver K, Bogardus C, et al: Time of onset of non–insulin-dependent diabetes mellitus and genetic variation in the β_3-adrenergic–receptor gene. N Engl J Med 333:343, 1995

30. Canning H, Mayer J: Obesity: its possible effect on college acceptance. N Engl J Med 275:1172, 1966

31. Kittel F, Rustin RM, Dramaix M, et al: Psycho-socio-biological correlates of moderate overweight in an industrial population. J Psychosom Res 22:145, 1978

32. Wilson LM, Chang SP, Henning SJ, et al: Suckling: developmental indicator of genetic obesity in mice. Dev Psychobiol 14:67, 1979

33. Telch CF, Agras WS, Rossiter EM: Binge eating increases with increasing adiposity. International Journal of Eating Disorders 7:115, 1988

34. Ashley FW Jr, Kannel WB: Relation of weight change to changes in athero-genic traits: The Framingham Study. J Chronic Dis 27:103, 1974

35. Berchtold P, Jörgens V, Kemmer FW, et al: Obesity and hypertension: cardiovascular response of weight reduction. Hypertension 4(suppl 5):50, 1982

36. Kaplan RM, Hartwell SL, Wilson DK, et al: Effects of diet and exercise interventions on control and quality of life in non–insulin-dependent diabetes mellitus. J Gen Intern Med 2:220, 1987

37. Perri MG, McAdoo WG, McAllister DA, et al: Enhancing the efficacy of behavior therapy for obesity: effects of aerobic exercise and multicomponent maintenance program. J Consult Clin Psychol 54:670, 1986

38. Brownell KD, Jeffery RW: Improving long-term weight loss: pushing the limits of treatment. Behavior Therapy 18:353, 1987

39. Perri MG, McAllister DA, Gange JJ, et al: Effects of four maintenance programs on long-term management of obesity. J Consult Clin Psychol 56:529, 1988

40. Kumanyaka SK, Obarzanek E, Stevens VJ, et al: Weight-loss experience of black and white participants in NHLBI-sponsored clinical trials. Am J Clin Nutr 53:1631S, 1991

41. Isner JM, Sours HE, Paris AL, et al: Sudden, unexpected death in avid dieters using the liquid-protein-modified-fast-diet: observations in 17 patients and the role of the prolonged QT interval. Circulation 60:1401, 1979

42. Felig P: Editorial retrospective: very-low-calorie protein diets. N Engl J Med 310:589, 1984

43. Broomfield PH, Chopra R, Sheinbaum RC, et al: Effects of ursodeoxycholic acid and aspirin on the formation of lithogenic bile and gallstones during loss of weight. N Engl J Med 319:1567, 1988

44. Wadden TA, Stunkard AJ: Controlled trial of very low calorie diet, behavior therapy, and their combination in the treatment of obesity. J Consult Clin Psychol 54:482, 1986

45. Kirschner MA, Schneider G, Ertel NH, et al: An eight-year experience with a very-low-calorie formula diet for control of major obesity. Int J Obes 12:69, 1988

46. Mason EE: Morbid obesity: use of vertical banded gastroplasty. Surg Clin North Am 67:521, 1987

47. Sugerman HJ: Surgery for morbid obesity. Gen Surg 3:111, 1992

48. Scopinaro N, Gianetta E, Civalleri D, et al: Partial and total biliopancreatic bypass in the surgical treatment of obesity. Int J Obes 5:421, 1981

49. Sugerman HJ, Starkey JV, Birkenhauer R: A randomized prospective trial of gastric bypass *versus* vertical banded gastroplasty for morbid obesity and their effects on sweets *versus* non-sweets eaters. Ann Surg 205:613, 1987

50. Craighead LW, Stunkard AJ, O'Brien RM: Behavior therapy and pharmacotherapy for obesity. Arch Gen Psychiatry 38:763, 1981

51. Weintraub M: Long-term weight control: the National Heart, Lung, and Blood Institute funded multimodal intervention study. Clin Pharmacol Ther 51:581, 1992

52. Pfohl M, Luft D, Blomberg I, et al: Long-term changes of body weight and cardiovascular risk factors after weight reduction with group therapy and dexfenfluramine. Int J Obes Relat Metab Disord 18:391, 1994

53. Abenhaim L, Moride Y, Brenot F, et al: Appetite suppressant drugs and the risk of primary pulmonary hypertension. N Engl J Med 335:609, 1996

54. Connolly HM, Crary JL, McGoon MD, et al: Valvular heart disease associated with fenfluramine-phentermine. N Engl J Med 337:581, 1997

55. Cardiac valvulopathy associated with exposure to fenfluramine or dexfenfluramine: U.S. Department of Health and Human Services Interim Public Health Recommendations, November 1997. Centers for Disease Control and Prevention. JAMA 278:1729, 1997

56. Bray GA, Ryan DH, Gordon D, et al: A double-blind randomized placebo-controlled trial of sibutramine. Obes Res 4:263, 1996

57. Pisacano JC, Lichter H, Ritter J, et al: An attempt at prevention of obesity in infancy. Pediatrics 61:360, 1978

58. Epstein LH, Valoski A, Wing RR, et al: Ten-year outcomes of behavioral family-based treatment for childhood obesity. Health Psychol 13:373, 1994

54 Diagnosis and Treatment of Lipid Disorders

Stephen P. Fortmann, M.D., and David J. Maron, M.D.

Disorders of lipoprotein metabolism and the susceptibility of human metabolism to adverse effects from diets high in saturated fats, from obesity, and from physical inactivity have resulted in epidemic atherosclerotic disease in the United States and other developed countries. Despite declining mortality from coronary artery disease in the United States since 1970, this disorder remains the most common cause of death among both men and women.

Traditionally, hyperlipoproteinemia has been defined as the elevation of a lipoprotein level to above that of the 95th percentile in the population. A classification system described by Fredrickson and colleagues[1] has been widely used to describe the phenotypes of hyperlipoproteinemia but is frequently misunderstood as a classification scheme for primary, or genetic, disorders of lipoprotein metabolism and is falling out of use as the primary disorders are better understood. The recognition that a low level of high-density lipoprotein (HDL) is clinically important has popularized the term dyslipoproteinemia to describe the range of disorders of abnormally high and low lipoproteins, and this term is now preferred.

Dyslipoproteinemias are clinically important principally because of their contribution to atherogenesis. Risk of atherosclerotic vascular disease begins to increase at a cholesterol concentration of approximately 180 mg/dl,[2] a level far below the 95th percentile traditionally used to define hypercholesterolemia. Roughly half the people in the United States have a cholesterol level that puts them at significant risk. Accordingly, the National Cholesterol Education Program (NCEP) has revised the definition of hypercholesterolemia to any level above 200 mg/dl. In our view, an optimal total cholesterol level is less than 150 mg/dl.

Lipoprotein Composition and Metabolism

Lipoproteins are spherical macromolecular complexes of lipid and protein [*see Figure 1*]. The lipid constituents of lipoproteins are esterified and unesterified (free) cholesterol, triglycerides, and phospholipids. The protein components are termed apolipoproteins. Lipoproteins transport cholesterol and triglycerides (which are not water soluble) from sites of absorption and synthesis to sites of utilization. Cholesteryl ester and triglycerides are nonpolar and constitute the hydrophobic core of lipoproteins in varying proportions. The lipoprotein surface coat contains the polar constituents—free cholesterol, phospholipids, and apolipoproteins—that permit these particles to be miscible in plasma as they transport their hydrophobic cargo. Lipoproteins are classified into six major groups by size, density, electrophoretic mobility, and lipid and protein composition [*see Table 1*]. Apolipoproteins provide structural stability, act as cofactors for specific enzymes, or serve as ligands for specific receptors involved in lipoprotein metabolism [*see Table 2*].

Cholesterol is used for the synthesis of bile acids in the liver, the manufacture and repair of cell membranes, and the synthesis of steroid hormones. There are both exogenous (dietary) and endogenous (primarily hepatic) sources of cholesterol. In the United States, the average consumption of cholesterol is about 300 mg each day; an additional 500 to 1,000 mg is produced daily in the liver and other tissues. Another source is the 500 to 1,000 mg of biliary cholesterol that is secreted into the intestine daily; about 50 percent is reabsorbed (enterohepatic circulation). Triglycerides, which are nonpolar lipids consisting of a glycerol backbone and three fatty acids of varying length and degrees of saturation, are used for storage in adipose tissue and for energy. They are found in liver and adipose cells and also derive from dietary and hepatic sources.

The lipid transport system is divided into the exogenous pathway, for dietary triglyceride and cholesterol absorbed by the intestine, and the endogenous pathway, for triglyceride and cholesterol secreted by the liver [*see Figure 2*]. The reverse cholesterol transport system, mediated by HDL, is involved in both pathways. Three major enzymes—lipoprotein lipase, lecithin-cholesterol acyltransferase (LCAT), and hepatic triglyceride lipase—are involved in lipoprotein metabolism [*see Table 3*].

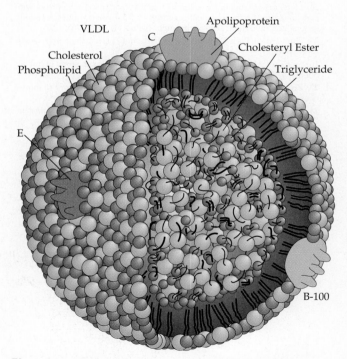

Figure 1 **Lipoproteins transport water-insoluble triglycerides and cholesterol through the bloodstream, and all lipoproteins have a structure similar to that shown for very low density lipoproteins (VLDLs). Triglyceride and cholesteryl ester are isolated within a bipolar layer of phospholipids and apolipoproteins. Most lipoproteins contain several apolipoproteins; VLDL contains apolipoproteins B-100, C-I, C-II, C-III, and E. LDL, which transports most of the cholesterol found in blood, contains only apo B-100.**

Table 1 Lipoprotein Characteristics

Lipoprotein	Diameter (Å)	Density (g/ml)	Electrophoretic Mobility	Major Lipids	Apolipoproteins
Chylomicrons	800–5,000	< 0.94	Remains at origin	Dietary triglycerides	A-I, A-II, A-IV, B-48, C-I, C-II, C-III, E
VLDL	300–800	0.94–1.006	Pre-beta	Endogenous triglycerides	B-100, C-I, C-II, C-III, E
IDL	250–350	1.006–1.019	Slow pre-beta	Cholesteryl ester, triglycerides	B-100, C-III, E
LDL	180–280	1.019–1.063	Beta	Cholesteryl ester	B-100
HDL	50–120	1.063–1.210	Alpha	Cholesteryl ester	A-I, A-II, C-I, C-II, C-III, D, E
Lp(a)	25–30	1.040–1.090	Slow pre-beta	Cholesteryl ester	a, B-100

EXOGENOUS PATHWAY

After a meal, intestinal cells absorb fatty acids and cholesterol, esterify them into triglycerides and cholesteryl ester, and incorporate them into the core of chylomicrons [*see Figure 2*]. Triglycerides greatly predominate over cholesteryl ester in the core. Apolipoprotein C-II (apo C-II) activates endothelial lipoprotein lipase, which hydrolyzes the chylomicron core triglycerides. The resulting free fatty acids are taken up by adipose tissue for storage and by muscle for energy. During lipolysis, the chylomicron shrinks, and surface components become pinched off and are transferred to HDL in exchange for additional apolipoproteins and cholesteryl ester. Normally, chylomicrons are present in the plasma for only a matter of minutes.[3] The residual chylomicron remnants are relatively enriched with cholesteryl ester, both from loss of triglyceride and from addition of cholesteryl ester from HDL. These remnants are removed rapidly from plasma by two receptors in the liver that bind avidly to apo E: the low-density lipoprotein (LDL) receptor and an apparently unique chylomicron remnant receptor termed the LDL receptor–related protein, or LRP. Once inside the hepatocyte, the remnant particles are digested by lysosomal enzymes, and the free cholesterol is reesterified and stored. Intracellular cholesteryl ester is then used for bile acid synthesis, cell membrane synthesis, or the synthesis of lipoproteins in the endogenous pathway. Free cholesterol is also secreted into bile.

ENDOGENOUS PATHWAY

Very low density lipoproteins (VLDLs) are large, triglyceride-rich lipoproteins that are synthesized and secreted by hepatocytes [*see Figure 2*]. VLDL triglyceride is made from glycerol and fatty acids that have been either released by adipose tissue or synthesized in the liver. VLDL cholesterol is derived from circulating lipoproteins or hepatic synthesis. As with chylomicrons, VLDL interacts with lipoprotein lipase in capillary endothelium, and the core triglycerides are hydrolyzed to provide fatty acids to adipose and muscle tissue. About half of the catabolized VLDL particles (sometimes called VLDL remnants) are taken up by hepatic LDL receptors that bind to apo E, and the other half remain in plasma, becoming intermediate-density lipoprotein (IDL). IDL retains apo B-100 and apo E, is enriched in cholesteryl ester relative to triglyceride, and circulates for minutes to hours. It is gradually converted by hepatic lipase to the smaller, denser, cholesteryl ester–rich LDL. As IDL is converted to LDL, apo E becomes detached, and only one apolipoprotein remains, apo B-100.

LDL normally carries about 75 percent of the circulating cholesterol, transporting it to extrahepatic cells for steroid hormone and cell membrane synthesis. LDL particles circulate for approximately two to three days,[3] and about half the LDL particles are taken up by hepatic LDL receptors. LDL uptake is slower than uptake of apo E–containing lipoproteins, because the LDL receptor has a lower affinity for apo B-100 than for apo E. Cellular LDL uptake is mediated by a glycoprotein receptor molecule that binds to apo B-100.[4] Approximately 70 percent of LDL is cleared by receptor uptake, and the remainder is removed by a scavenger cell pathway. After LDL is taken up by receptors, free cholesterol is liberated from LDL and accumulates within cells, with three important metabolic consequences.[4] First, there is a decrease in the synthesis of 3-hydroxy-3-methylglutaryl coenzyme A (HMG-CoA) reductase, the enzyme that controls the rate of de novo cholesterol synthesis by the cell. Second, there is activation of the enzyme acyl cholesterol acyltransferase (ACAT), which esterifies free cholesterol into cholesteryl ester, the cell's storage form of cholesterol. Third, accumulation of cholesterol suppresses the cell's synthesis of new LDL receptors. This feedback mechanism reduces the cell's uptake of LDL from the circulation [*see Figure 3*].

HDL ORIGIN AND METABOLISM

The origin and metabolism of HDL are not as well understood as for the other lipoproteins, but they appear to be more complex and varied.[5] The major HDL apolipoproteins are apo A-I and apo A-II, which are made in the liver and small intestine. These apolipoproteins are secreted with phospholipid in a

Table 2 Functions of Major Apolipoproteins

Apolipoprotein	Function
A-I	Activator of lecithin-cholesterol acyltransferase; structural role in HDL
A-II	Unknown structural role in HDL
A-IV	Unknown
B-48	Structural role in chylomicrons; necessary for assembly and secretion of chylomicrons
B-100	Ligand for LDL receptor; structural role in VLDL, IDL, LDL; necessary for assembly and secretion of VLDL
C-I	Unknown
C-II	Activator of lipoprotein lipase
C-III	May inhibit hepatic uptake of chylomicron and VLDL remnants; may inhibit lipoprotein lipase
D	May be a cofactor for cholesteryl ester transfer protein
E	Ligand for hepatic chylomicron remnant receptor and LDL receptor

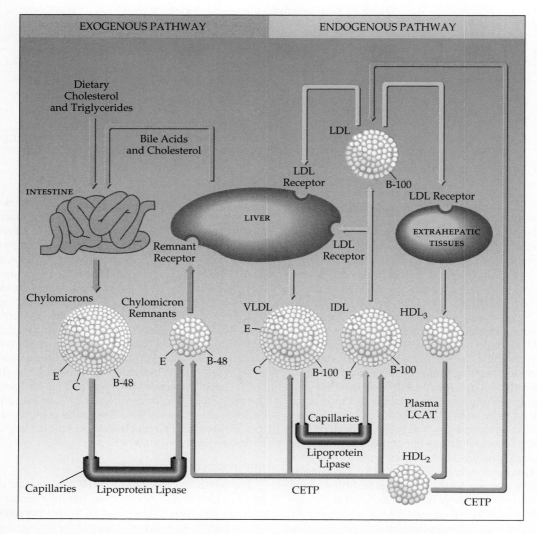

Figure 2 **When dietary cholesterol and triglycerides are absorbed through the intestine, they are packed into chylomicrons, the largest of the lipoproteins. Chylomicrons are rapidly metabolized in the capillaries by lipoprotein lipase, which releases free fatty acids, leaving chylomicron remnants that are taken up by the liver. This exogenous pathway of fat transport is also used to recycle bile acids and cholesterol secreted into the intestine. In the endogenous pathway, triglyceride-rich VLDL particles are secreted by the liver and are metabolized in a fashion similar to that of chylomicrons. The remnant particles are either taken up by the liver or gradually converted to LDL. (IDL—intermediate-density lipoprotein; LCAT—lecithin-cholesterol acyltransferase; CETP—cholesteryl ester transfer protein)**

disklike structure called nascent HDL. Most of the apolipoprotein and phospholipid destined to become nascent HDL is initially secreted on the surface of chylomicrons and VLDL and is transferred to HDL during lipolysis. As lipid-poor HDLs associate with cells, they attract cholesterol from cell membranes, and the cholesterol diffuses into the HDL surface coat. The circulating enzyme LCAT associates with HDL and is activated by apo A-I to esterify free cholesterol on the surface of HDL, causing it to move into the core. These particles become spherical and are called HDL_3. As HDL_3 particles accumulate cholesteryl ester within the core, they become HDL_2 particles, enriched with cholesteryl ester. The majority of cholesteryl ester within HDL_2 particles is then transferred into triglyceride-rich lipoproteins in exchange for triglyceride in a process mediated by cholesteryl ester transfer protein.[6] The triglyceride that the HDL acquires may then be hydrolyzed by the action of hepatic triglyceride lipase, converting HDL_2 back to HDL_3, which is then ready to ac-

cept more free cholesterol from cell membranes. Cholesteryl ester–rich HDL_2 with apo E may also be taken up directly by liver receptors, but the mechanism is not clearly understood. It is also possible that HDL_2 delivers cholesteryl ester directly to

Table 3 Major Enzymes in Lipoprotein Metabolism

Enzyme	Location	Function
Lipoprotein lipase	Muscle and adipose capillary endothelium	Hydrolyzes chylomicron and VLDL triglycerides
Lecithin-cholesterol acyltransferase	Plasma	Esterifies free cholesterol on HDL surface
Hepatic triglyceride lipase	Liver	Hydrolyzes triglyceride within IDL and HDL particles

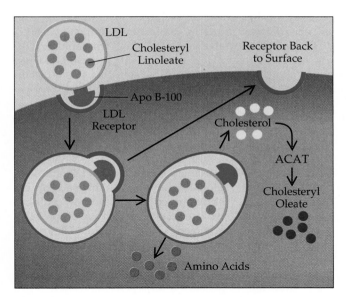

Figure 3 **LDL is absorbed by cells through the LDL receptor. This receptor recognizes apo B-100, the apolipoprotein on the surface of LDL. Once absorbed, the lipoprotein is catabolized, releasing cholesterol and amino acids. The free cholesterol is converted to cholesterol oleate by the enzyme acyl cholesterol acyltransferase (ACAT). The LDL receptor is recycled back to the cell surface.**

the liver without catabolism of the HDL particle. The overall process is termed reverse cholesterol transport.

HDL is thought to be antiatherogenic through reverse cholesterol transport. HDL particles can be divided into two types: those that contain only apo A-I and particles that contain both apo A-I and apo A-II. Cholesterol efflux from extrahepatic tissues appears to be mediated primarily by HDL particles that contain only apo A-I.[7] Overexpression of human apo A-I in transgenic mice inhibits atherosclerosis,[8] and overexpression of apo A-II in transgenic mice promotes atherosclerosis.[9] HDL has also been found to inhibit LDL oxidation, another potential mechanism by which HDL may reduce atherosclerosis.[10]

LIPOPROTEIN(a)

Lipoprotein(a) [Lp(a)] is a specific class of lipoprotein particles synthesized in the liver with lipid composition very similar to that of LDL. Lp(a) differs from LDL by the presence of a highly glycosylated protein of variable mass, termed apo(a), linked by a covalent bond to apo B-100. Research on Lp(a) and atherosclerosis accelerated with the discovery of the structural homology between apo(a) and plasminogen, a key protein of the coagulation cascade. Little is known about Lp(a) catabolism or its physiologic role. Plasma concentrations of Lp(a) vary markedly among individuals, from undetectable to 200 mg/dl. Lp(a) plasma concentration is strongly controlled by genetic factors.[11]

Clinical Manifestations of Lipid Disorders

The major clinical manifestations of common lipid disorders are atherosclerotic cardiovascular disease and pancreatitis. Lipoproteins are fundamentally involved in atherogenesis, and the resulting vascular diseases are the most important cause of death and disability in the United States. Pancreatitis is a much less common but clinically severe manifestation of triglyceride levels.

LOW-DENSITY LIPOPROTEINS AND ATHEROGENESIS

Epidemiological, autopsy, and animal studies have firmly established that a high LDL level is atherogenic. The LDL receptor binds LDL optimally at an interstitial fluid cholesterol concentration of 2.5 mg/dl, which corresponds to a plasma LDL cholesterol level of 25 mg/dl[4] [*see Figure 4*]. Newborns have a plasma LDL cholesterol level of about 30 mg/dl, and mammals that do not develop atherosclerosis and persons on very low fat diets similar to the probable diet of our distant ancestors[12] have plasma LDL cholesterol levels of less than 80 mg/dl. The average adult male in the United States has a plasma LDL cholesterol level of 125 mg/dl, providing an ample supply for atherogenesis. This general human susceptibility to dietary saturated fat leads to mass hypercholesterolemia and epidemic coronary artery disease.[13] The appropriate approach to controlling epidemic atherosclerosis is through public health means, such as health education, agricultural policy, and food labeling.[14] The role of the medical community in this effort is to reinforce the messages regarding general diet and exercise and to identify and treat those persons at sufficient risk to warrant special intervention. The risks of treatment must be balanced against the potential for benefit, and management must be tailored to each patient. The majority of people without known vascular disease can be managed with a more healthful diet.

Primary prevention trials using pharmacological therapy have demonstrated that coronary artery disease events are significantly reduced by lowering LDL levels in asymptomatic hyperlipidemic men.[15-17] The largest and most recent of these trials was the first to use a powerful HMG-CoA reductase inhibitor; 6,595 men 45 to 64 years of age with a mean baseline LDL level of 192 mg/dl were randomized to receive pravastatin, 40 mg/day, or placebo.[16] After a mean of 4.9 years, the active treatment group experienced a 31 percent reduction in the incidence

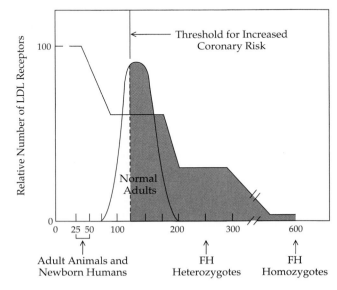

Figure 4 **The range of LDL levels in normal adults in Western developed countries is indicated by the bell-shaped curve. Adult animals and human infants have much lower levels, whereas patients with heterozygous familial hypercholesterolemia have higher levels and a reduced number of LDL receptors. Patients with homozygous FH, who completely lack LDL receptors, have extremely high LDL levels.**

of coronary death or nonfatal myocardial infarction (MI) (absolute risk 5.5 percent versus 7.9 percent), a 32 percent reduction in cardiovascular death, a 38 percent reduction in cardiovascular procedures, and a 22 percent reduction in all-cause mortality. In addition, several randomized repeat angiographic trials have compared the effects of aggressive lipid therapy with the effects of placebo or usual care on the angiographic progression of coronary atherosclerosis in both men and women.[18] Although these trials have differed widely in patient selection and sample size, type of lipid therapy, duration of intervention, and angiographic end points, consistent findings have emerged. A substantial reduction in LDL levels, in the range of 25 to 40 percent, is associated with significantly less progression and more regression of atherosclerosis on follow-up angiography and significantly fewer clinical cardiac events.

The Scandinavian Simvastatin Survival Study (4S)[19] randomized 4,444 patients (81 percent men) with hypercholesterolemia (mean LDL at baseline was 188 mg/dl) and a history of MI or angina to receive simvastatin or placebo. After 5.4 years, the treatment group experienced a 30 percent reduction in total mortality (eight percent in the simvastatin group versus 12 percent in the placebo group), a 42 percent reduction in coronary mortality, a 37 percent reduction in the need for coronary artery bypass surgery or percutaneous transluminal coronary angioplasty, and a 30 percent reduction in the incidence of stroke. The Cholesterol and Recurrent Events (CARE) trial[20] randomized 4,159 patients (86 percent men) with moderate hypercholesterolemia (mean LDL at baseline was 139 mg/dl) and a history of myocardial infarction to receive pravastatin or placebo. After five years, the pravastatin-treated group had a 24 percent reduction in fatal coronary events and nonfatal MI (10.2 percent versus 13.2 percent). The treatment group also had a 27 percent reduction in the need for coronary revascularization procedures and a 31 percent reduction in the incidence of stroke.

The pathogenesis of acute coronary artery syndromes and the possible mechanisms by which LDL reduction may produce clinical benefits have been reviewed.[21,22] Fissuring and rupture of lipid-rich atherosclerotic plaques lead to platelet aggregation, vasospasm, and intraluminal thrombosis. Many angiographic trials have unexpectedly reported significantly fewer clinical cardiac events despite minimal (but measurable) angiographic benefits in patients randomized to intensive lipid-lowering treatment. This finding is consistent, however, with the concept of plaque stabilization, whereby intensive lipid therapy depletes lipid from the plaque core, reduces the concentration of oxidized LDL and inflammatory cells, strengthens the tensile strength of the fibrous cap, and renders vulnerable plaques less likely to rupture.[18] Plaque stabilization, rather than geometric regression of plaque and increasing diameter of the lumen, is probably the most important goal of aggressive lowering of LDL levels.

The vascular endothelium is responsible for the release of nitric oxide (NO) and prostacyclin (PGI_2), both of which inhibit smooth muscle contraction, smooth muscle cell proliferation, platelet aggregation, and platelet and monocyte adhesion to the endothelial surface.[23] Endothelial function is impaired by hypercholesterolemia[24] and improved by cholesterol lowering.[25,26] Because platelet aggregation and coronary vasospasm play important roles in acute coronary syndromes, cholesterol lowering may reduce the incidence of acute cardiac events by restoring endothelial function. Treatment of coronary artery disease patients with statins reduces the frequency and duration of ischemic episodes as measured by ambulatory ECG monitoring[27,28]

This remarkable convergence of findings from epidemiological, basic science, and clinical studies with the results of large-scale clinical trials has led to a clear scientific consensus that the treatment of lipid disorders is a cornerstone of the primary and secondary prevention of vascular diseases.[29]

OXIDIZED LDL AND SMALL, DENSE LDL

In addition to concentration of LDL, two other aspects of LDL have been the focus of considerable research: LDL oxidation and LDL subclasses. It has been found that LDL must undergo modification before it can be ingested by macrophages to form foam cells, which are important components of atherosclerotic plaques.[30] In vivo, oxidative modification is probably the most frequent form of modification. Oxidized LDL not only promotes foam cell formation but also is chemotactic for circulating monocytes, is cytotoxic, and impairs endothelial function. Antioxidant therapy has been shown to improve endothelial cell function in patients with hypercholesterolemia and coronary artery disease.[26] The Cambridge Heart Antioxidant Study (CHAOS) randomized 2,002 patients with angiographically proven coronary disease to vitamin E, 400 to 800 IU, or placebo. After a median follow-up of 1.4 years, antioxidant treatment reduced the primary end point of cardiovascular death and nonfatal MI by 47 percent (41 events versus 64 events).[31] Large clinical trials examining the effect of antioxidants on cardiovascular end points are in progress.

Two distinct LDL subclass patterns, denoted A and B, can be distinguished in the population by ultracentrifugation and gradient gel electrophoresis.[32] Persons with LDL subclass pattern A have predominantly large, buoyant LDL particles enriched with cholesteryl ester, whereas those with pattern B have small, dense LDL particles enriched with triglyceride. Small, dense LDL particles are more susceptible to oxidation. Pattern B is associated with higher triglyceride and apo B levels, lower HDL and apo A-I levels, and a greater risk of coronary artery disease. Pattern B appears to be inherited as a single-gene trait and is strongly associated with familial combined hyperlipidemia.[33] The total cholesterol:HDL ratio and triglyceride concentration have been shown in prospective studies to be stronger predictors of coronary artery disease risk than LDL size; therefore, we do not recommend routine screening of LDL size.[34]

HIGH-DENSITY LIPOPROTEINS AND ATHEROGENESIS

Certain inherited low-HDL syndromes are associated with premature coronary artery disease, yet others are not [see Primary Low-HDL Syndromes, below]. Epidemiological study has shown that within a population group, HDL level is strongly and inversely correlated with the risk of coronary artery disease, independent of the LDL cholesterol level. Both the HDL_2 level and the HDL_3 level are inversely related to the risk of heart disease.[35] The mechanisms proposed for the protective effect of HDL are reverse cholesterol transport and the ability of HDL to inhibit LDL oxidation.[10] The importance of HDL when the LDL level is very low is uncertain; the HDL level may carry less importance in such cases, because when there is a lower concentration of LDL in circulation, the role of HDL is less essential. When HDL levels are compared among populations, those countries with high mean HDL levels generally have higher rates of coronary artery disease than those with low mean HDL levels, probably because HDL and LDL are positively correlated across populations; both are positively related to dietary fat intake.[36] In cholesterol-fed rabbits, homologous HDL administration inhibits formation of aortic fatty streaks and reduces established aortic atherosclerosis.[37,38]

Two primary prevention trials[15,17] found an apparent benefit from increasing the level of HDL independent of lowering the level of LDL, but both trials used drugs that also lower LDL levels and neither trial included subjects selected for having a low HDL. A case-control study in men with angiographically proven coronary artery disease found that more than one third had a total cholesterol level below 200 mg/dl, and of those, nearly three fourths had an HDL level below 35 mg/dl.[39] Surveillance of such men shows that they are at high risk for subsequent cardiovascular events.[40] Angiographic trials have shown that pharmacological intervention that raises HDL prevents progression or induces regression of atherosclerosis.[41,42] American Heart Association guidelines recommend that treatment to increase HDL levels be considered in patients with coronary artery disease who have a low HDL level. Such treatment begins with smoking cessation, weight loss, and increased exercise. If pharmacological therapy is necessary in such patients to achieve an LDL level of less than 100 mg/dl, niacin or statin therapy is recommended.[43] Both the 4S and CARE trials found that subjects with a low HDL level at baseline experienced clinical benefits from statin therapy.[20,44] Drug treatment of asymptomatic patients with a low HDL level but desirable LDL levels remains controversial because clinical trial data addressing this issue are lacking.

HYPERTRIGLYCERIDEMIA AND ATHEROGENESIS

The evidence is insufficient to conclude that hypertriglyceridemia causes coronary artery disease. The most recent NCEP guidelines[29] classify triglycerides as normal (< 200 mg/dl), borderline high (200 to 400 mg/dl), high (400 to 1,000 mg/dl), and very high (> 1,000 mg/dl). In many population studies, hypertriglyceridemia is associated with coronary artery disease in univariate analysis, but this relation weakens or vanishes when triglycerides are considered together with other risk factors, such as LDL level, HDL level, blood pressure, physical activity, and obesity.[45] An observational study showed that a triglyceride level greater than 200 mg/dl significantly increased the risk of coronary artery disease in persons with elevated LDL and low HDL levels.[46] Premature atherosclerosis is associated with some inherited high-triglyceride disorders (e.g., familial combined hyperlipidemia and dysbetalipoproteinemia) but not with others (e.g., familial hypertriglyceridemia). Atherosclerotic plaque does not contain triglyceride, and there have been no clinical trials to study the effect of lowering triglyceride levels on coronary artery disease. Clinical and angiographic trials designed to lower either total or LDL cholesterol have generally found that triglyceride lowering has no significant effect on the clinical or angiographic end point. However, the Helsinki Heart Study, a primary prevention trial, found in subgroup analysis that persons who had an elevated LDL level, a low HDL level, and a triglyceride level greater than 200 mg/dl derived the greatest benefit from treatment with gemfibrozil, an agent that lowers triglyceride level and raises HDL level.[47] In addition, the Stockholm Ischaemic Heart Disease Secondary Prevention Study found that lowering triglyceride levels with clofibrate and nicotinic acid led to reduced total and coronary mortality.[48]

It is likely that triglyceride elevation per se does not cause atherosclerosis but that the metabolic derangements associated with hypertriglyceridemia do. Hypertriglyceridemia is often associated with elevated levels of chylomicron remnants, VLDL remnants, and small, dense LDL particles and with depressed levels of HDL, all of which promote atherogenesis.[32] People with a low HDL level and an elevated triglyceride level may be at particularly high risk for coronary artery disease.[49] Elevated triglyceride levels are also associated with increases in certain coagulation factors and with reduced fibrinolytic activity. Finally, fasting triglyceride levels may reveal the efficiency with which a person clears postprandial triglyceride. When this process is inefficient, extended postprandial lipemia may cause arterial endothelial cell uptake of triglyceride-rich remnants.[50]

LP(a) AND ATHEROGENESIS

Some epidemiological studies suggest that Lp(a) is a risk factor for coronary artery disease and stroke,[51-54] but others show no relation.[55,56] Possible explanations for this apparent discrepancy include differences in measurement methods and the possibility that Lp(a) may increase risk only among people with hypercholesterolemia.[57] If Lp(a) is atherogenic, it may be because of its LDL-like properties: Lp(a) has been shown to undergo endothelial uptake and oxidative modification and to promote foam cell formation. In addition, Lp(a) has a high degree of homology with plasminogen and may have prothrombotic activity by interfering with the binding of plasminogen to fibrin. Preliminary data suggest that reducing elevated LDL cholesterol in patients with high levels of Lp(a) may be an effective strategy to slow progression of atherosclerosis and prevent coronary events. The Lp(a) level itself can be reduced with niacin, estrogen, tamoxifen, or LDL apheresis. However, there are insufficient data regarding the efficacy of lowering the Lp(a) level to inhibit atherosclerosis or to prevent coronary events, and we cannot recommend routine screening for, or treatment of, elevated Lp(a) levels.[57]

PANCREATITIS

After atherogenesis, acute pancreatitis is the major clinical manifestation of dyslipidemia. It is associated with chylomicronemia and elevated VLDL levels. Most patients with acute pancreatitis have triglyceride levels above 2,000 mg/dl, but prophylactic treatment of hypertriglyceridemia should begin when fasting levels exceed 500 mg/dl.[58] The mechanism by which chylomicronemia and elevated VLDL cause pancreatitis is unclear. Pancreatic lipase may act on triglyceride in pancreatic capillaries, resulting in the formation of toxic fatty acids that cause inflammation.

Primary Disorders of Lipoprotein Metabolism

Primary, or familial, disorders of lipoprotein metabolism arise from genetic defects in the metabolic pathways of lipoproteins. The major primary disorders are familial lipoprotein lipase deficiency, familial apolipoprotein C-II deficiency, familial hypertriglyceridemia, familial combined hyperlipidemia, familial hypercholesterolemia, familial defective apolipoprotein B-100, familial hypobetalipoproteinemia and abetalipoproteinemia, dysbetalipoproteinemia, and primary low-HDL syndromes.

FAMILIAL LIPOPROTEIN LIPASE DEFICIENCY

Familial lipoprotein lipase deficiency is a rare, autosomal recessive disorder (one homozygote per million people) caused by a mutation in the *LPL* gene that results in a severe deficiency or absence of lipoprotein lipase. In this disorder, levels of apo C-II are normal. After a fat-containing meal, chylomicrons are produced normally but not catabolized, causing a massive accumulation of chylomicrons in the plasma and severe hypertriglyceridemia, which may persist for several days. VLDL concentrations are usually not elevated, and HDL and LDL levels are low. A variant of this disorder has been reported in a kindred with a circulating inhibitor of lipoprotein lipase.[59]

The disease is typically detected in early childhood because of recurrent bouts of abdominal pain from pancreatitis associated with severe hypertriglyceridemia (1,000 to 5,000 mg/dl) and chylomicronemia. During an episode of acute pancreatitis, the serum and urine amylase levels may be normal because of interference with the assay by hypertriglyceridemia or by circulating inhibitors of amylase activity. Hepatosplenomegaly from accumulation of triglyceride in reticuloendothelial cells is common, and eruptive xanthomas over the buttocks and extensor surfaces of the extremities may be present. Severe chylomicronemia is associated with dyspnea; the mechanism for this is unclear.[60] The chylomicronemia syndrome of pancreatitis, organomegaly, eruptive xanthomas, and lipemia retinalis is reversible with normalization of triglyceride levels. The risk of atherosclerosis may be increased with this disorder,[61] and recurrent pancreatitis may result in pancreatic insufficiency. Heterozygotes for familial lipoprotein lipase deficiency may have elevated VLDL or LDL levels and a clinical syndrome similar or identical to familial combined hyperlipidemia.[60,62]

This disorder should be suspected in a young person with fasting lipemic plasma and severe abdominal pain. Diagnosis is made by demonstrating severely reduced or absent plasma lipoprotein lipase activity after infusion of heparin (which causes the release of lipoprotein lipase bound to the endothelial wall) or by determination of lipoprotein lipase activity in an adipose tissue biopsy. The assay must contain normal plasma or apo C-II. The diagnosis may be confirmed by documentation of a defect in the *LPL* gene.

Treatment is directed at reducing the formation of chylomicrons through restriction of total dietary fat to less than 10 to 20 g/day. Additional calories from fat may be given as a medium-chain triglyceride supplement; these triglycerides are not incorporated into chylomicrons, because they are absorbed directly into the portal vein. Alcohol intake and exogenous estrogens should be restricted. The goal of therapy is to reduce the fasting triglyceride concentration to less than 1,000 mg/dl. In addition to diet therapy, treatment with gemfibrozil or omega-3 fatty acids is sometimes effective. During a bout of acute pancreatitis, oral feedings should be withheld and the patient should be given intravenous nutrition free of lipid. In the setting of severe pancreatitis during pregnancy, acute plasmapheresis has successfully reduced triglyceride levels and symptoms promptly.[63]

FAMILIAL APOLIPOPROTEIN C-II DEFICIENCY

Familial apo C-II deficiency is a rare autosomal recessive disease (one homozygote per one million people) caused by a single gene mutation that results in a severe deficiency or absence of apo C-II. This mutation causes a functional lipoprotein lipase deficiency and results in the chylomicronemia syndrome. Patients with familial apo C-II deficiency tend to present at a later age and have less severe hypertriglyceridemia than patients with familial lipoprotein lipase deficiency. The diagnosis is confirmed by demonstrating that the plasma of the affected person is unable to activate lipoprotein lipase in vitro or by determining the presence of apo C-II deficiency by isoelectric focusing or two-dimensional gel electrophoresis. Postheparin lipoprotein lipase activity is normal when exogenous apo C-II is used. Heterozygotes have 50 percent of the normal concentration of apo C-II and may have mild hypertriglyceridemia but do not develop chylomicronemia and pancreatitis. Treatment consists of dietary fat restriction to less than 20 g/day. Patients with acute pancreatitis may be treated with an infusion of normal plasma (which contains apo C-II) or with purified apo C-II, which results in a rapid fall in triglyceride levels.

FAMILIAL HYPERTRIGLYCERIDEMIA

Familial hypertriglyceridemia is a common inherited disorder, thought to be autosomal dominant, affecting one to two percent of the population. There is increased triglyceride synthesis, and VLDL particles are enriched with triglyceride but are not secreted in excess numbers.[64] Affected people have elevated VLDL concentrations but low levels of LDL and HDL and are generally asymptomatic unless severe chylomicronemia develops. Familial hypertriglyceridemia does not appear to be associated with an increased risk of coronary artery disease.[60] Diagnosis is made by family history and examination of fasting lipoprotein profiles of the patient and relatives. The triglyceride concentration should range from 250 to 1,000 mg/dl in approximately half of first-degree relatives; a strong family history of premature coronary artery disease should be lacking; and severe hypercholesterolemia should not be present. Patients should lose weight if necessary, exercise regularly, and reduce their intake of saturated fatty acids and cholesterol. Alcohol, exogenous estrogens, and other drugs that increase VLDL levels should be restricted. Diabetes should be tightly controlled if present. Hypertriglyceridemia in this disorder often responds to these measures. If triglyceride concentrations exceed 500 mg/dl after six months of nonpharmacological therapy, drug therapy should be instituted with nicotinic acid or gemfibrozil; nicotinic acid should be avoided if the patient has diabetes. Omega-3 fatty acids might also be helpful in this disorder.

FAMILIAL COMBINED HYPERLIPIDEMIA

Familial combined hyperlipidemia (FCH) was originally construed to be a single gene disorder,[62] but it is probably a heterogeneous group of genetic disorders.[33] Approximately one to two percent of the population is affected. In this disorder, the synthesis and secretion of apo B and VLDL are increased. VLDL particles appear to be normal in composition, but LDL particles appear small and dense and have a decreased ratio of cholesterol to apo B. The efficiency of lipolysis in a given affected person may determine whether the increased output of VLDL from the liver results in high concentrations of VLDL, LDL, or both. LDL receptors appear to be normal.[65] Some heterozygotes for lipoprotein lipase deficiency satisfy the criteria for FCH.

People with FCH usually have normal lipoprotein concentrations until early adulthood, at which time they may present with one of three phenotypes: elevated levels of VLDL, elevated levels of LDL, or elevated levels of both. The phenotypic expression of this disorder may change within a person over time. For reasons that are not understood, this disorder is often associated with obesity and diabetes. Patients with FCH almost never develop xanthomas, but FCH is associated with an increased risk of premature coronary artery disease. In fact, persons with FCH account for approximately 10 percent of men younger than 60 years who survive a myocardial infarction.

The diagnosis of FCH is made by taking a careful family history and examining the fasting lipoprotein profiles of the patient and relatives. There should be a strong family history of premature coronary artery disease and multiple lipoprotein disorders affecting approximately half of first-degree relatives. Triglyceride levels, LDL cholesterol levels, or both will be above the 90th percentile in these patients; triglycerides will generally not be greater than 1,000 mg/dl.

Treatment consists of weight loss (if necessary), control of diabetes, regular exercise, reduced intake of saturated fatty acids and cholesterol, and restriction of alcohol, exogenous estrogens, and other drugs that adversely affect VLDL metabolism. If hyperlipidemia persists after an appropriate trial of nonpharmacological therapy, drug therapy should be instituted. Drug selection depends on the hyperlipoproteinemic phenotype exhibited by the individual.

FAMILIAL HYPERCHOLESTEROLEMIA

Etiology and Pathogenesis

Familial hypercholesterolemia (FH) is an autosomal dominant disorder caused by a mutation in the gene encoding the LDL receptor protein. Brown, Goldstein, and associates elucidated this disorder[4] and described five classes of mutant alleles that cause a functional or absolute LDL receptor deficiency.[66]

Homozygotes with FH have two mutant alleles at the LDL receptor locus, leaving them with an absolute or nearly absolute inability to clear VLDL remnants and LDL from the circulation by the LDL receptor. Heterozygotes with FH possess one normal allele, giving them one half of the normal receptor activity. Because VLDL remnants are cleared from the plasma by the LDL receptor, a deficiency of LDL receptors leads to an enhanced conversion of IDL to LDL, which in turn accumulates in the plasma because of the receptor deficiency. The greater the reduction in LDL receptors, the greater the elevation of LDL. High concentrations of LDL result in non–receptor-mediated uptake of LDL in connective tissue and in arterial walls, which causes xanthomas and atherosclerosis.

Clinical Manifestations

Homozygous FH Homozygotes occur in about one in a million people; there is an increased incidence of consanguinity in parents of homozygous individuals. These patients exhibit marked hypercholesterolemia at birth; coronary artery disease develops within the first three decades, and myocardial infarction has been reported as early as 18 months. Affected persons generally do not survive beyond 30 years of age. Yellow-orange cutaneous xanthomas, which are unique to homozygotes, develop within the first few years of life, often in the webbing of the fingers. Tendon xanthomas, typically located within the Achilles tendon and extensor tendons of the hands, and corneal arcus also appear during childhood. Homozygotes may have episodes of polyarthritis and tenosynovitis. Xanthomas may develop on cardiac valves, causing aortic stenosis and, less commonly, mitral regurgitation or stenosis. Supravalvular aortic stenosis may also develop from severe atheromatous involvement of the aortic root. The total cholesterol concentration in homozygotes ranges from 600 to 1,200 mg/dl. The LDL cholesterol concentration is approximately six times that of normal persons, the triglyceride level is normal or mild-

ly elevated, and the HDL cholesterol level is often reduced. Prenatal diagnosis from amniotic fluid is possible.

Heterozygous FH The heterozygous form of this disorder has a prevalence of about one in 500 people, making it one of the most common genetic diseases. Hypercholesterolemia can be detected at birth in umbilical cord blood. Coronary artery disease develops early, with symptoms usually manifesting in men in the third or fourth decade. By 60 years of age, at least 50 percent of men experience myocardial infarction; in women, symptoms tend to develop about 10 years later. Tendon xanthomas begin to appear by 20 years of age and are present in about 70 percent of heterozygotes older than 30 years. Xanthelasma (cutaneous xanthomas on the palpebra) and corneal arcus are common after 30 years of age. Tendon xanthomas are a highly specific sign of FH, but xanthelasma and corneal arcus may occur in normocholesterolemic persons. The total cholesterol levels generally range from 350 to 550 mg/dl. The triglyceride level is elevated in about 10 percent of heterozygote individuals, and the HDL cholesterol level is often reduced. Heterozygotes account for approximately five percent of men who survive a myocardial infarction.

Diagnosis

The diagnosis of homozygous FH is usually made clinically by the presence of cutaneous xanthomas and severe hypercholesterolemia (total cholesterol level > 650 mg/dl) with a normal triglyceride level. LDL receptor function can be measured only in special laboratories. Heterozygous FH should be suspected when severe hypercholesterolemia from elevated LDL is detected. If tendon xanthomas are present, the diagnosis is virtually certain. If tendon xanthomas are absent, secondary causes of hypercholesterolemia should be sought, but the diagnosis of familial hypercholesterolemia is not excluded. A comprehensive family history should reveal a strong history of premature coronary artery disease and hypercholesterolemia without hypertriglyceridemia, affecting approximately one half of first-degree relatives. The presence of hypercholesterolemia and tendon xanthomas in a parent or sibling is virtually diagnostic, as is hypercholesterolemia in a child in the family. It is extremely important to screen first-degree relatives for the disease so that proper treatment and counseling can be provided to them.

Treatment

Homozygous FH The approach to treatment of the homozygote depends on the presence or absence of LDL receptor–binding activity. If the patient has no binding activity, there is no value in applying therapy that stimulates the production of LDL receptors (e.g., dietary therapy, bile acid–binding resins, statins, and ileal bypass surgery). However, LDL reduction of 20 percent is reported with atorvastatin therapy in receptor-negative patients. If the patient has some level of LDL receptor function, significant LDL lowering is possible with a combination of a bile acid–binding resin and a statin. Nicotinic acid, a drug that lowers LDL by reducing the synthesis of its precursor, VLDL, may be effective in lowering LDL cholesterol in homozygotes regardless of the type of receptor defect.

In homozygotes, total parenteral nutrition has been shown to lower LDL levels,[67] as has portacaval shunt surgery. Historically, the most widely used approach in these patients was removal of LDL by plasma exchange. A modern form of this therapy is LDL apheresis, in which plasma is removed from the patient, LDL cholesterol is selectively removed from plasma but HDL cholesterol is not, and the plasma is then returned to the patient. The most dramatic form of therapy is liver transplantation, which provides the patient with hepatic LDL receptors and lowers the LDL concentration promptly to near-normal range.[68] Direct gene therapy to supply the liver with normal LDL receptor genes is an attractive potential treatment for homozygotes.

Heterozygous FH The goal of therapy is to lower the LDL cholesterol level to less than 130 mg/dl or even lower if the patient already exhibits coronary artery disease. It is possible to stimulate the one normal gene in heterozygotes, so effective treatment is possible with bile acid–binding resins and statins. Nicotinic acid is also useful. Combination therapy with two drugs is often required, and three drugs may be necessary. Although diet therapy alone will not be sufficient for FH heterozygotes, reducing saturated fatty acid and cholesterol intake will lower LDL levels and reduce the amount of medication required; animal studies have shown that a high-fat diet suppresses LDL receptor activity.[4] Another way to stimulate LDL receptor synthesis is to prevent bile salts from returning to the liver with ileal bypass surgery, but this therapy is outdated given the availability of LDL-lowering drugs. Tendon xanthomas have been shown to regress when LDL levels are maintained in a desirable range. Aggressive reduction of LDL cholesterol in men and women who have heterozygous familial hypercholesterolemia can induce regression of coronary atherosclerosis.[69]

FAMILIAL DEFECTIVE APOLIPOPROTEIN B-100

A defective apo B-100 ligand is another genetic cause of elevated LDL concentration. The prevalence of this disorder is unknown but is estimated at one in 500 to 700 persons. LDL receptor structure and function are normal in these patients. A full-length apo B-100 is produced and secreted but binds poorly to LDL receptors, leading to LDL accumulation in the plasma. Affected individuals may be clinically indistinguishable from patients with heterozygous familial hypercholesterolemia: they have severe hypercholesterolemia, may have tendon xanthomas, and develop premature atherosclerosis. Treatment with statins appears to lower LDL cholesterol levels in patients with this disorder.[70] Specialized tests available only in selected research laboratories are required to identify affected people.

FAMILIAL HYPOBETALIPOPROTEINEMIA AND ABETALIPOPROTEINEMIA

Familial hypobetalipoproteinemia can be caused by a number of different apo B gene mutations that interfere with the translation of a full-length, functional apo B-100 molecule. A full-length apo B-100 molecule is required for the synthesis and secretion of VLDL from the liver, so in contrast to defective apo B-100, heterozygotes with this disorder are usually asymptomatic, have LDL cholesterol concentrations about one fourth to one third of normal, and are at low risk for coronary artery disease.[3] Homozygotes have a variable range of symptoms; patients who are the most severely affected are indistinguishable from those with abetalipoproteinemia.

Abetalipoproteinemia is a rare autosomal recessive syndrome in which apo B is synthesized normally but synthesis and secretion of apo B–containing lipoproteins are defective. Affected people have very low cholesterol and triglyceride levels, steatorrhea, acanthocytosis, degenerative retinopathy, and progressive neuromuscular disease.

DYSBETALIPOPROTEINEMIA

Dysbetalipoproteinemia, also called type III hyperlipoproteinemia and broad-beta disease, is defined as the presence of VLDL particles that migrate at the beta position on electrophoresis (normal VLDL particles migrate in the pre-beta location). Beta-VLDL particles are chylomicron and VLDL remnants. Dysbetalipoproteinemia is caused in part by a mutant apo E, which impairs the hepatic uptake of apo E–containing lipoproteins and slows the conversion of VLDL to IDL and LDL. Without the presence of an additional genetic, hormonal, or environmental defect, remnants do not accumulate to a degree sufficient to cause hyperlipidemia, because they are cleared by hepatic receptors that also bind, with less avidity, to apo B-48 and apo B-100. Dysbetalipoproteinemia results when an apo E defect is combined with a second genetic or acquired defect that causes either overproduction of VLDL, such as obesity or FCH, or reduced LDL receptor activity, such as heterozygous FH.[60]

There are three common alleles for apo E: E2, E3, and E4. The alleles are found in all six possible combinations. Apo E3 and apo E4 bind more avidly to the LDL receptor than does apo E2, the mutant form of apo E responsible for the disorder. The E2/E2 genotype is found in one percent of the white population and in virtually all persons with dysbetalipoproteinemia. Hyperlipoproteinemia develops in only about one percent of persons with the E2/E2 genotype. Other rare mutants of apo E have been described that appear to produce the same syndrome as E2/E2 homozygosity.[71]

Persons with dysbetalipoproteinemia have elevations in both cholesterol and triglyceride levels and are likely to develop premature coronary artery disease. For reasons that are not understood, these people are also at increased risk for peripheral vascular disease. Hyperlipidemia does not develop before adulthood. Palmar xanthomas (xanthoma striata palmaris), orange-yellow discoloration of the palmar creases, are pathognomonic for dysbetalipoproteinemia, but they are not always present. Tuboeruptive xanthomas are commonly found at pressure sites, particularly the elbows, buttocks, and knees. Tendon xanthomas may be present, but xanthelasmas are uncommon. Obesity is frequently associated with this disorder, and diabetes or hypothyroidism may unmask the disease.

The diagnosis of dysbetalipoproteinemia should be suspected in a person with elevated total cholesterol and triglyceride levels, elevated VLDL cholesterol level, and reduced LDL and HDL cholesterol levels. Cholesterol and triglyceride levels range from 300 to 500 mg/dl and are roughly equal, except during an acute exacerbation, when the hypertriglyceridemia tends to predominate. Beta-migrating VLDL is present on electrophoresis. Ultracentrifugation demonstrates that the ratio of VLDL cholesterol to plasma triglyceride is greater than 0.3. Definitive diagnosis is made by detecting the E2/E2 genotype by isoelectric focusing. The presence of diabetes and hypothyroidism should be excluded.

Treatment of dysbetalipoproteinemia is essentially the same as for other hypertriglyceridemic disorders: weight reduction to ideal body weight, optimum glucose control if diabetes is present, and avoidance of alcohol, estrogens, and other triglyceride-raising drugs. The diet should be low in total fat, saturated fat, cholesterol, and simple carbohydrates. Patients should exercise regularly. If the hyperlipidemia does not resolve with these measures, gemfibrozil, nicotinic acid (niacin), and statins should be tried, since each of these has been found to be effective in this disorder. In general, dysbetalipoproteinemia is very responsive to therapy, and xanthomas have been shown to regress with lipid-lowering treatment.

PRIMARY LOW-HDL SYNDROMES

Low HDL may be caused by reduced synthesis, increased catabolism, or both. It is likely that impaired synthesis promotes atherosclerosis but that rapid catabolism does not. For many of the primary low-HDL disorders, the metabolism of HDL has not been well defined. Lecithin-cholesterol acyltransferase deficiency is an autosomal recessive disease that results from either the absence of lecithin-cholesterol acyltransferase or the presence of an inactive form of the enzyme in the plasma of affected homozygotes. Heterozygotes have mild reductions in HDL, but in the homozygous form, there is no mature HDL_2, because free cholesterol cannot be esterified and cannot move within the core of HDL_3. Only early forms of HDL are present, and the HDL concentration is typically around 5 mg/dl. VLDL and LDL concentrations are normal. Homozygotes develop anemia, corneal opacification, and renal failure. Premature coronary artery disease has been reported.

Fish-eye disease is a rare disorder caused by partial deficiency of lecithin-cholesterol acyltransferase. Patients have low HDL, modest elevation of triglycerides (250 to 350 mg/dl), triglyceride-enriched IDL and LDL, and severe corneal opacification.[72]

Tangier disease is a rare autosomal recessive disease caused by an unknown molecular defect resulting in a severe deficiency or absence of HDL. Triglyceride concentrations are normal or elevated, and cholesteryl ester accumulates in tissues. Clinical features are large orange tonsils, splenomegaly, and peripheral neuropathy. Despite extremely low HDL levels, coronary artery disease is not increased in patients with this disorder.

Molecular defects of apo A-I result in a low HDL level. Paradoxically, at least one defect is not associated with an increased risk of atherosclerosis. Apo A-I$_{Milano}$ is a mutant form of apo A-I that is associated with very low levels of HDL (7 to 14 mg/dl) and high levels of triglyceride but no increased risk of coronary artery disease.[73] The mutation causes a higher affinity of apo A-I for cholesterol, resulting in accelerated catabolism and increased uptake of tissue cholesterol.[74] A different genetic disease with a severe deficiency of apo A-I and an absence of apo C-III causes tendon xanthomas, corneal clouding, and severe premature coronary artery disease.[75]

Primary causes of hypertriglyceridemia frequently result in low HDL levels. As discussed above, normal lipolysis of triglyceride-rich lipoproteins is necessary for the production of mature HDL particles. Whether a specific, monogenic disorder of familial hypoalphalipoproteinemia also exists is controversial. This term has been used to describe members of families who have an HDL level that is in the lowest 10th percentile, with or without hypertriglyceridemia.

POLYGENIC HYPERCHOLESTEROLEMIA

Most people with an LDL cholesterol level higher than the 95th percentile do not have an identifiable monogenic or secondary cause of their lipoprotein disorder and fall into the ill-defined category of polygenic hypercholesterolemia.[62] These patients are distinguished from those with heterozygous FH or FCH because they do not have strong family histories of cardiovascular disease. As more is learned about the molecular biology of hypercholesterolemia, such persons might be found to have one or more specific abnormalities, such as enhanced cholesterol absorption, mild defects in LDL receptor function or

apo B structure, or reduction in the number of LDL receptors from the interaction of multiple genetic and environmental causes. After secondary causes have been ruled out, these patients should be treated for high LDL cholesterol in a standard fashion.

Secondary Disorders of Lipoprotein Metabolism

Secondary dyslipoproteinemias are caused by acquired defects in lipoprotein metabolism that result in hypercholesterolemia, hypertriglyceridemia, or combined hyperlipidemia, with or without a low HDL level [*see Table 4*]. Secondary hypertriglyceridemia may be severe enough to cause chylomicronemia. When dyslipoproteinemia is caused by a medication, the drug should be discontinued whenever possible. Secondary dyslipoproteinemias may cause the same diseases as primary dyslipoproteinemias—that is, atherosclerosis or pancreatitis.

Diabetes mellitus causes an increase in VLDL synthesis and a reduction in VLDL catabolism (caused by a reduction in lipoprotein lipase activity), which results in hypertriglyceridemia and a low HDL level. The LDL level is normal or increased. Fasting chylomicronemia results when there is a coexisting primary or secondary form of hypertriglyceridemia. VLDL and chylomicrons compete for binding to lipoprotein lipase, and both lipoproteins may accumulate. A low HDL level results from impaired lipolysis of triglyceride-rich lipoproteins, which supply components for HDL synthesis. Dyslipoproteinemia occurs in both insulin-dependent and non–insulin-dependent diabetes. Lipid levels should normalize with comprehensive treatment of diabetes; if they fail to do so, additional causes should be sought. In diabetics with persistent hypertriglyceridemia, gemfibrozil is suitable because it enhances the activity of lipoprotein lipase and possibly reduces the secretion of VLDL from the liver. Nicotinic acid should generally be avoided, particularly in non–insulin-dependent diabetics, because it may exacerbate hyperglycemia.[76] Statins are also effective for the dyslipidemia of diabetes.[76]

Hypothyroidism causes severe elevation of LDL because of reduced LDL receptor activity and frequently causes hypertriglyceridemia with an associated reduction in the HDL level as a result of reduced lipoprotein lipase activity.[77] Remnants of chylomicrons and VLDL may also accumulate and unmask type III dysbetalipoproteinemia. The dyslipoproteinemia of hypothyroidism is corrected by thyroid hormone replacement.

Nephrotic syndrome causes enhanced hepatic secretion of apo B-100–containing lipoproteins (i.e., VLDL) in response to the loss of albumin and other proteins in the urine. Hepatic synthesis of cholesterol is also increased, and this may reduce the number of hepatic LDL receptors and clearance of circulating LDL. Severe elevation of the LDL level is seen; the VLDL level may also become elevated late in the course of the disease, associated with a low HDL level, as lipolysis becomes impaired.[78] Patients with nephrotic syndrome are at increased risk for coronary artery disease because of hypercholesterolemia, and the lipid disorder should be treated aggressively if the patient's prognosis is otherwise good. Dietary change, weight loss, and exercise may improve lipoprotein levels, but pharmacological therapy is necessary to achieve desirable levels. Bile acid–binding resins are effective in lowering the LDL level in nephrotic patients, but if they are used as single agents, they are not likely to lower the LDL level sufficiently and may exacerbate hypertriglyceridemia. Nicotinic acid should be an effective drug in this disorder because it inhibits hepatic secretion of apo B-100–containing

Table 4 Secondary Causes of Lipoprotein Disorders

Cause	VLDL	LDL	HDL	Pathophysiology
Metabolic/Endocrine				
Diabetes mellitus*	+++	0/+	– –	Increased VLDL production, reduced lipoprotein lipase activity
Hypothyroidism	+	+++	–	Reduced LDL receptor activity, reduced lipoprotein lipase activity
Obesity	++	+	– –	Increased VLDL production
Anorexia nervosa	0	++	0	Reduced biliary excretion of cholesterol and bile acids
Pregnancy*	++	++	+/–	Increased VLDL production and reduced lipoprotein lipase activity caused by multiple hormonal changes
Acute myocardial infarction	+	–	–	Unknown
Renal				
Nephrotic syndrome	++	+++	–	Increased secretion of apo B-100, reduced lipoprotein lipase activity
Renal failure with dialysis*	+++	0	– –	Reduced lipoprotein lipase activity
Hepatic				
Primary biliary cirrhosis†	0	0	– – –	Regurgitation of biliary cholesterol and phospholipids into plasma forms lipoprotein X; decreased hepatic lipase activity

*May be associated with chylomicronemia if there is a coexisting primary disorder of hypertriglyceridemia.
†Cholesterol levels are severely elevated (300–2,000 mg/dl) in advanced disease; extrahepatic biliary obstruction may cause same pattern.

lipoproteins; however, it has not been studied extensively for this use. The statins may prove to be extremely useful for the nephrotic syndrome, but there is not yet enough collective experience to establish whether this is true. Combination drug therapy is usually necessary for the reduction of LDL levels, and the most effective two-drug combination is a resin plus a statin.

Chronic renal failure produces hypertriglyceridemia as a result of a deficiency in lipoprotein lipase (LPL) and hepatic triglyceride lipase.[78] Triglyceride levels typically range from 200 to 750 mg/dl, and the HDL level is usually low; the risk for coronary artery disease is increased. Nonpharmacological measures should be initiated before drug treatment is considered, unless triglyceride levels exceed 1,000 mg/dl. Drug therapy for hypertriglyceridemia in chronic renal failure is controversial because of the lack of consensus about the role of hypertriglyceridemia in atherogenesis. Gemfibrozil, a drug that enhances lipoprotein lipase activity, has been shown to be effective in this setting. Because this drug is excreted renally, the dose should be reduced to lower the risk of myopathy. Nicotinic acid and statins have not been studied adequately in this condition.

In its early stages, primary biliary cirrhosis causes mild elevation of VLDL and LDL levels and marked increases in the HDL level. With advanced disease, severe elevation of cholesterol results from the regurgitation of bile into plasma, which creates an abnormal lipoprotein particle rich in free cholesterol and phospholipid that is called lipoprotein X. Impaired hepatic triglyceride lipase activity and cholesterol esterification contribute to the dyslipoproteinemia. Lipoprotein X may also be caused by other forms of obstructive jaundice.

Alcohol consumption causes increased hepatic production of triglycerides by increasing the availability of free fatty acids through a variety of mechanisms.[79] Excess fatty acids are incorporated into triglycerides, which are in turn incorporated into VLDL particles and secreted at an increased rate. If LPL activity is impaired by a coexisting disorder, VLDL may accumulate in the plasma and compete with chylomicrons for LPL binding sites, leading to chylomicronemia.[77] Alcohol also raises HDL levels, which may explain the association of low levels of regular alcohol use with reduced risk of coronary artery disease. Studies have shown that HDL_2, HDL_3, or both subfractions increase with alcohol consumption[77]; the apo A-I level consistently rises with alcohol consumption. Alcohol has no significant effect on LDL levels.

Oral contraceptives that contain a combination of estrogen and progestin can have variable effects on lipoproteins, depending on the specific combination used. Estrogen tends to raise VLDL and HDL and lower LDL. Progestins tend to lower VLDL and HDL and raise LDL, but the effect varies considerably. Postmenopausal estrogen replacement lowers LDL and raises HDL; the addition of progesterone to protect the uterus lessens these effects but does not eliminate them.[80] Estrogen also raises triglyceride levels, particularly in overweight women, and should be monitored.

Practical Approach to Common Disorders

Most patients presenting with a lipid disorder have one of three general patterns: predominantly elevated cholesterol level caused by an elevated LDL level; a combined hyperlipidemia, with elevated triglyceride and cholesterol levels; or predominantly elevated triglyceride level with normal or low LDL levels. In this section, we will also discuss a less common disorder, isolated low HDL cholesterol.

PATIENTS WITH ELEVATED CHOLESTEROL

Patients with an elevated cholesterol level have an LDL cholesterol level exceeding 130 mg/dl but a normal triglyceride level (< 200 mg/dl). The HDL cholesterol level is variable, but often it is normal. The lipid disorders in these patients are usually discovered through routine cholesterol screening. Although some observers question the cost-effectiveness of screening younger men and women for elevated cholesterol levels,[81] the high prevalence of elevated LDL and total plasma cholesterol in the United States warrants population screening, as recommended by the NCEP and other authorities. Such screening may also be indicated if a patient is particularly concerned about his or her risk status or if there is a family history of either early cardiovascular disease or lipid abnormalities. The management of patients with a total cholesterol level below 240 mg/dl who are not otherwise at increased risk for cardiovascular disease should stress changes in diet, exercise, and body weight.

Dietary Intervention

Physicians are often frustrated when advising patients to change their diets because this approach produces only small changes in the cholesterol level in many patients. In our experience, patients' LDL cholesterol levels may respond markedly to dietary and lifestyle changes, depending on the baseline diet and the degree of dietary change. Nevertheless, many patients have difficulty controlling weight and achieving and maintaining a low-fat diet and a regular exercise program. Before progressing to drug therapy, the physician must consider several factors, most notably the overall cardiovascular risk status of the individual and the known and unknown risks of drug therapy. Risk can be quantified using risk factor levels from the results of epidemiological studies.[82] One must also realize that laboratory variations tend to obscure small declines in cholesterol level, that a five percent decline in LDL cholesterol reduces the risk of coronary artery disease by 10 percent, and that regular follow-up can help maximize long-term changes in lifestyle. It is often appropriate to stop short of the goal cholesterol level if the risks of the next level of therapy outweigh the probable benefits. Physicians can reinforce dietary and exercise guidelines and help achieve the long-term public health goal of a lower population burden of cardiovascular disease without prescribing medication excessively.

The NCEP guidelines suggest dietary intervention if the LDL cholesterol level exceeds 160 mg/dl (130 mg/dl in the presence of two other risk factors) and drug treatment if the LDL level exceeds 190 mg/dl after dietary intervention (160 mg/dl in the presence of two other risk factors). In the presence of known vascular disease, the goal LDL cholesterol level is 100 mg/dl. These rules are reasonable, but we recommend that these thresholds for therapy be tailored to the individual patient.[82] For example, the potential total benefit of cholesterol lowering is greater for younger people, which should be considered in advising treatment.[83] Drug therapy, however, is inappropriate for many young adult men and premenopausal women who have LDL cholesterol levels below 220 mg/dl and who are otherwise at low risk. The presence of important comorbidity should temper the physician's aggressiveness, as should a markedly elevated HDL cholesterol level (e.g., > 70 mg/dl).[84] An HDL cholesterol level below 35 mg/dl justifies more intense efforts to lower the LDL level, as may an elevated Lp(a).

Most patients with an elevated LDL cholesterol level do not have a primary lipid disorder; rather, such elevations reflect the susceptibility of human lipid metabolism to high saturated fat and cholesterol intake and to obesity and lack of exercise. A primary disorder can be suspected if there is a strong family history of atherosclerotic disease or lipid abnormalities or if tendon xanthomas are present, but this differentiation provides little therapeutic help, at least initially. Secondary causes of hypercholesterolemia need to be considered [see Tables 4 and 5], but most will be apparent; screening for hypothyroidism is advised.

Initial therapy for elevated plasma LDL cholesterol consists of reducing dietary saturated fat and cholesterol; the assistance of a nutritionist is often helpful, as are written materials from various sources. Some patients are highly motivated to make dietary changes (often to avoid medications), and diets with a saturated fat content of less than seven percent of calories lower LDL cholesterol levels in most patients. Other patients are less interested in dietary change, but we generally try dietary change for six months before turning to drug therapy, unless the patient has known coronary disease or an LDL cholesterol level consistently exceeding 200 mg/dl. Reducing dietary fat intake is likely to lower both HDL and LDL cholesterol levels,[85]

Table 5 Effects of Selected Drugs on Lipoprotein Levels

Drug	VLDL	LDL	HDL
Alcohol*	+	0	+
Estrogens*	+	−	+
Androgens	0	+	−
Progestins†	−	+	+
Glucocorticoids*	+	0/+	+
Retinoids*	+	+	−
Cyclosporine	0	+	0
Thiazide diuretics*	+	+	0/−
Beta blockers (without ISA)*	+	0	−
Beta blockers (with ISA)	0	0	0/+
Alpha blockers	0/−	0/−	0/+
Alpha-beta blockers	0	0	0
Calcium channel blockers	0	0	0
Central sympatholytics	0/−	0/−	0
Angiotensin-converting enzyme inhibitors	0	0	0

*May be associated with chylomicronemia if there is a coexisting primary or secondary disorder of hypertriglyceridemia.
†19-Nortestosterone series (i.e., norethindrone, norgestrel) worse than medroxyprogesterone.
ISA = intrinsic sympathomimetic activity.

but the reduction in HDL is caused by increased HDL catabolism, which may enhance reverse cholesterol transport[86]; lowering HDL by diet is not known to be harmful.[87] Weight control and exercise can minimize the decrease in, or even elevate, HDL levels in patients on a low-fat diet.[85]

Drug Therapy

Bile acid–binding resins, statins, and niacin are all first-line drug classes for lowering LDL cholesterol. We prefer resins in younger patients and those with borderline indications for medication use because of their low potential for toxicity; constipation and inconvenience make them difficult to take, however, and physicians need to encourage patients in their use. Constipation is often alleviated by adding soluble fiber to the diet (especially oat bran[88]) or by using a psyllium preparation,[89] both of which also contribute to LDL lowering. The statins are often more cost-effective and allow better adherence than resins, and statins have been shown to lower total mortality[19]; therefore, it is reasonable to use statins first in higher-risk patients and in patients with a history of constipation or other relative contraindications to resin therapy. Statins also lower triglyceride levels and modestly increase HDL levels. Niacin is also quite effective at lowering LDL cholesterol, but because of its side effects, it is realistically reserved for patients with combined hyperlipidemia or low HDL level, or both, or for patients who cannot tolerate the other two classes of drugs. Many patients will require combination drug therapy to achieve a goal LDL cholesterol level below 130 mg/dl (100 mg/dl for patients with known vascular disease); resins and statins are synergistic in their effects on LDL cholesterol, and niacin may be combined with either resins or statins, or both (with some caution for myositis with the statins).

PATIENTS WITH COMBINED HYPERLIPIDEMIA

In combined hyperlipidemia, both the cholesterol level and the triglyceride level are elevated. Typically, the triglyceride level will range from 200 to 800 mg/dl, the LDL level will be greater than 100 mg/dl, and the HDL level will be below 40 mg/dl. Combined hyperlipidemia appears to include several genetic disorders that are poorly characterized. Some patients are simply exhibiting two common disorders simultaneously, namely polygenic LDL cholesterol elevation and overweight-induced hypertriglyceridemia. Other patients may have familial combined hyperlipidemia, which can be diagnosed only through family studies.[33] Another subset of patients exhibits a constellation of cardiovascular risk factors that includes central obesity, hyperinsulinemia, hypertension, and the noted lipid abnormalities of elevated triglyceride and low HDL cholesterol levels.[90] Affected patients tend to exhibit elevated levels of small, dense LDL particles,[32] which are susceptible to oxidation and may be highly atherogenic. Patients with combined hyperlipidemia appear to be at higher risk for cardiovascular disease, but there have been few intervention studies targeted at these patients.

The initial evaluation includes a measurement of other cardiovascular risk factors and a detailed family history. The presence of premature cardiovascular disease in the family history is an important marker for increased risk. Screening these patients for secondary causes of lipoprotein disorders [see Tables 4 and 5] before starting therapy is important.

Behavioral Interventions

Exercise and weight loss are the most important behavioral interventions because most patients with combined hyperlipidemia are overweight and because even small losses of body fat (3 to 6 kg) will markedly lower the triglyceride level and will often produce a small increase in the HDL level.[91] Of course, patients with the constellation of risk factors that includes hyperinsulinemia or hyperglycemia and hypertension will experience a marked improvement in all risk factors through exercise-induced weight loss. Therefore, considerable effort by the physician to convince patients to increase their exercise level and make a diligent effort to lose weight is warranted. Frequent clinic and telephone follow-up can increase adherence to these lifestyle changes.

Dietary saturated fat should be restricted in patients with combined hyperlipidemia, and such restriction can help reduce the LDL cholesterol level. However, some patients will experience an exacerbation of their hypertriglyceridemia if they reduce their total dietary fat intake to below 25 to 30 percent of calories. Such patients may benefit from increasing intake of monounsaturated and polyunsaturated fats to a modest degree, although when a low-fat diet is associated with weight loss, a rise in triglyceride level is uncommon.

Drug Therapy

There are few clinical trials to guide drug therapy of combined hyperlipidemia, as most trials have focused on elevations of LDL cholesterol. The Helsinki Heart Study included men with non-HDL cholesterol levels greater than 200 mg/dl and showed a benefit of gemfibrozil on cardiovascular disease rates but not on total mortality.[17] In this study, patients with combined hyperlipidemia seemed to benefit from therapy in a fashion similar to the other study patients,[47] but the number of patients with combined hyperlipidemia was relatively small,

and such post hoc analyses can be misleading. We consider the use of drug therapy in patients who otherwise qualify for therapy on the basis of their LDL cholesterol level and in patients with known cardiovascular disease, several other cardiovascular risk factors, or a clear family history of premature cardiovascular disease. The treatment of choice for combined hyperlipidemia is niacin, which produces beneficial changes in all of the lipid fractions, particularly the lowering of LDL cholesterol and perhaps the selective lowering of small, dense LDL cholesterol (an important exception is that niacin can worsen glucose metabolism in diabetic patients).[92] Statins can also be useful in this disorder if the triglyceride level is less than 400 mg/dl, producing a modest decrease in the triglyceride level, a modest increase in the HDL level, and a decrease in the LDL level (atorvastatin is the most potent statin for lowering the triglyceride level). Resins may be useful in combined hyperlipidemia as adjunctive therapy for a high LDL cholesterol level after the triglyceride level is controlled. Finally, fibrates will lower the triglyceride level and raise the HDL level, but their effect on LDL cholesterol is variable.

PATIENTS WITH ELEVATED TRIGLYCERIDES

Patients with elevated triglycerides are distinguished from persons with combined hyperlipidemia by higher triglyceride levels (often > 1,500 mg/dl) and a normal LDL cholesterol (< 100 mg/dl and often < 80 mg/dl). HDL cholesterol levels are usually low. This category of lipid disorders also includes familial hypertriglyceridemia and other rare disorders. Patients can be at increased risk for pancreatitis, although in our experience, many patients will present with a long history of elevated triglycerides and no history of pancreatitis. Some patients with hypertriglyceridemia will have diabetes, so screening for this disorder is also appropriate, although diabetes alone usually does not produce marked elevations in triglycerides unless frank ketoacidosis is present. Other secondary causes of elevated triglycerides need to be considered [see Tables 4 and 5]. The family history can be helpful in assessing the individual patient's risk of cardiovascular disease.

Most patients with hypertriglyceridemia are obese and sedentary and will show marked benefit from exercise and weight loss. As with combined hyperlipidemia, the benefits of weight loss are so significant that considerable physician effort is appropriate in attempting to obtain adherence to dietary changes and exercise regimens that will result in weight loss. Alcohol intake should be reduced or eliminated.

Patients who are unable to lose enough weight to maintain their triglyceride level below 500 mg/dl are at risk for severe hypertriglyceridemia, which, at levels above 3,000 mg/dl, may produce pancreatitis and even hyperviscosity. Therefore, most lipid specialists will introduce drug treatment for such patients. In addition, we tend to treat patients who are unable to lose sufficient weight and have a family history of cardiovascular disease or an HDL cholesterol level below 35 mg/dl. Either niacin or gemfibrozil will usually control the triglyceride level and raise the HDL level. Gemfibrozil may raise the LDL level; niacin should be avoided in diabetic patients. If gemfibrozil raises the LDL level above 130 mg/dl, niacin can be substituted or a resin or statin added. There are concerns about the long-term safety of the fibrates.[93] A third pharmacological option for hypertriglyceridemia is omega-3 fatty acid supplementation, but the long-term safety and impact on clinical end points are not known.

PATIENTS WITH LOW HDL CHOLESTEROL

The proper treatment of asymptomatic persons who have low HDL levels accompanied by desirable LDL or total cholesterol levels is unclear.[94] Until the results of primary prevention trials in patients selected for their low HDL levels are reported, the value of drug therapy to raise HDL levels in this category of patients will remain uncertain.

In patients with coronary artery disease, the primary goal should be to reduce the LDL level to below 100 mg/dl regardless of the HDL level. In two secondary prevention trials, patients with low HDL levels at baseline benefited from statin treatment as much as those with higher HDL levels.[20,44] Evidence from angiographic trials suggests that raising the HDL level may inhibit progression or induce regression of coronary atherosclerosis.[41,42] In patients who have coronary artery disease and a low HDL level, nonpharmacological measures to raise the HDL level should always be attempted first. If these measures fail, drug therapy aimed at raising the HDL level should be considered, although drug selection is speculative.[95] Cholestyramine and gemfibrozil raise the plasma HDL level by increasing the synthesis of HDL particles (and apo A-I),[96,97] which presumably facilitates reverse cholesterol transport.[95] Nicotinic acid, which has been used in several angiographic trials, decreases HDL catabolism[98] and lowers LDL levels more than gemfibrozil. The statins also lower LDL levels significantly but raise HDL levels less than nicotinic acid, although, like nicotinic acid, statins may increase HDL synthesis.[99] Unless the LDL level is already below 90 to 100 mg/dl, we favor using nicotinic acid in these patients if they can tolerate it. In patients who cannot tolerate nicotinic acid, we use a statin, with or without cholestyramine. In patients with acceptably low LDL levels, gemfibrozil is a reasonable choice. In all cases, we discuss with the patient the speculative nature of the treatment.

PATIENTS WITH CORONARY ARTERY DISEASE BUT NORMAL LIPOPROTEINS

Occasionally, a patient presents with coronary artery disease but with no identifiable lipoprotein abnormality or other risk factor. Caution must be exercised, however, before concluding that a hospitalized patient with coronary artery disease has a normal LDL level, because the LDL level falls during the course of acute myocardial infarction and falls dramatically when patients undergo cardiopulmonary bypass. We also often observe substantial declines in LDL levels when patients with chest pain (in whom myocardial infarction has been ruled out) are made to fast, are kept supine, and are given intravenous hydration and heparin. In general, it is advisable to obtain previous outpatient lipoprotein values or to measure fasting lipoproteins in the emergency room or four to six weeks after the infarct rather than to rely on inpatient values for diagnosis and treatment.

When such an apparently low-risk patient is identified, we consider screening for elevated concentrations of Lp(a) and homocysteine. Elevated levels of Lp(a) may increase the risk of coronary artery disease, and this may be totally independent of the concentration of other lipoproteins. In patients of European ancestry, a level greater than 20 mg/dl is considered high,[57] and if a high value is found, we consider treatment with niacin or, in postmenopausal women without contraindications, estrogen. The predictive value of Lp(a) in other ethnic groups needs additional study, but levels above the 80th percentile can be considered to be elevated.[57] Hyperhomocysteinemia appears to cause atherosclerosis, probably through a number of direct and indirect effects on vascular endothelium.[100] Rare enzymatic defects can cause severe elevations and early vascular disease, but moderate elevations are common and probably derive from a variety of dietary and genetic causes. Several observational studies have found a positive association between homocysteine level and atherosclerosis,[101,102] but there have been no randomized clinical trials to study the effect of lowering homocysteine levels. A fasting total homocysteine level greater than 15 μmol/L is associated with sufficient increase in risk among patients with vascular disease to be considered for treatment. Folate supplementation of 1 to 5 mg a day appears to be safe and usually sufficient to reduce homocysteine levels to a desirable range. We cannot make a firm recommendation regarding screening or treatment for elevated Lp(a) or homocysteine levels because of the absence of clinical trial data.

Drug Treatment of Lipoprotein Disorders

The choice of drugs for various lipid disorders is guided by triglyceride levels [*see Table 6*]. The physician must also pay attention to such issues as side effects, cost, safety of combination therapy, and convenience [*see Table 7*].

DRUGS FOR AN ELEVATED LDL CHOLESTEROL LEVEL

For the treatment of lipid disorders in which the primary problem is an elevated LDL cholesterol level (triglycerides are normal or near normal), the bile acid–binding resins are first-line drugs because of their low potential for toxicity. These drugs are quite safe, but they are available only as powders that must be hydrated before use or as low-dose tablets and are therefore inconvenient to take. Many patients tolerate these drugs without side effects and are able to cope with the extra effort, providing that the physician is encouraging and discusses some practical tips for making the drugs easier to use. Such tips include adding a psyllium preparation to the resin if constipation occurs and premeasuring a three-day supply of resin and water (or juice) and keeping it in the refrigerator. Resins can be effective in low doses,[103] and colestipol is available in a 1 g tablet, which is preferred by many patients taking 12 g or less a day.

Statins are also first-line drugs for lowering the LDL cholesterol level. We still prefer resins for younger and borderline-

Table 6 **Approach to Drug Therapy**

Lipid/Lipoprotein Abnormality	Single Drug	Drug Combination
Elevated LDL; triglycerides < 200 mg/dl	Statin*† Resin Niacin	Statin + resin Resin + niacin Statin + niacin‡
Elevated LDL; triglycerides 200–400 mg/dl	Statin* Niacin	Statin + niacin‡ Statin + gemfibrozil§ Niacin + resin‖ Niacin + gemfibrozil
Triglycerides > 1,000 mg/dl	Niacin Gemfibrozil Omega-3 fatty acids	Niacin + gemfibrozil

*If HDL is low, niacin is preferred.
†In young patients, resins are preferred.
‡Possible increased risk of myopathy; reduce dose of statin.
§Increased risk of myopathy.
‖Increased risk of hypertriglyceridemia because of resin.

risk patients, but the statins are highly effective and safe[19] and are convenient and relatively free of side effects. The five available statins are similar in use but differ somewhat in potency [see Table 7]. The price of these agents is most frequently determined by contracts between providers and purchasers such as HMOs, a practice that has reduced both costs and flexibility in prescribing drugs. A resin and a statin in combination are highly effective in that they increase hepatic LDL receptor numbers by complementary mechanisms.

Nicotinic acid is also quite effective for lowering the LDL cholesterol level; it also lowers VLDL and raises HDL. We use nicotinic acid as a single agent or in combination with resins in patients with combined hyperlipidemia in whom the use of resins alone may increase the triglyceride level. Nicotinic acid has many side effects, including frequent elevation of hepatic enzymes in the serum, which must be monitored; however, nicotinic acid can be effective in low doses (1.0 to 1.5 g/day) that many patients will tolerate.

Although gemfibrozil raises HDL and lowers VLDL and triglycerides, it is less effective than the other drugs at lowering LDL. It is well tolerated, however, and may be used in patients with combined hyperlipidemia. The patients in the Helsinki Heart Study who were shown to benefit most from gemfibrozil therapy for the primary prevention of coronary events had an LDL to HDL ratio greater than 5 and a triglyceride level greater than 200 mg/dl.[47] There are continued safety concerns about the fibrates, however.[93]

DRUGS USED PRIMARILY FOR ELEVATED TRIGLYCERIDES

Gemfibrozil is the best-tolerated drug for treating elevated triglycerides and VLDL in the absence of significant increases in LDL cholesterol. As the HDL cholesterol level is usually low in these patients, the effect of gemfibrozil on HDL may be beneficial as well. Some patients will experience a rise in LDL cholesterol with gemfibrozil use (usually, when the pretreatment LDL is low); this effect presumably results from improved catabolism of VLDL and hence increased production of LDL. If the LDL exceeds 130 mg/dl, complementary LDL-lowering therapy should be considered. Clofibrate, the original fibric acid, has fallen out of use because it was associated with excess noncardiovascular risk in a clinical trial; it must be used occasionally, however, in patients with serious triglyceride elevation who cannot tolerate gemfibrozil or nicotinic acid.

It is always important to note that exercise and weight loss are critical interventions for the control of elevated triglyceride levels and that efforts to achieve these lifestyle changes must never be abandoned.

ESTROGEN REPLACEMENT IN POSTMENOPAUSAL WOMEN

Epidemiological studies show that the incidence of myocardial infarction in postmenopausal women on estrogen replacement therapy is roughly half that in postmenopausal women not taking estrogen. Estrogen raises HDL, lowers LDL, lowers Lp(a) and fibrinogen, and inhibits LDL oxidation. Estrogen increases triglyceride production but does not reduce clearance of triglycerides, and this property is not thought to be atherogenic. The addition of a progestin reduces the magnitude of increase in the HDL level seen in unopposed estrogen therapy but reduces the risk of adenomatous or atypical endometrial hyperplasia in women with a uterus.[83] Estrogen therapy may increase the risk of breast cancer; the risk is apparently small but may increase with prolonged use.[104] If the vascular benefit

of estrogen therapy approaches that observed in epidemiological studies, the reduction in risk of cardiovascular disease would outweigh the increased risk of cancer. Large primary and secondary prevention studies are under way to test the efficacy of estrogen therapy in reducing coronary disease events. Until the results are available, an individualized approach to therapy is necessary, with consideration of other indications for estrogen replacement therapy, such as osteoporosis and postmenopausal symptoms, the degree of risk for coronary artery disease, and the potential risks of prolonged estrogen replacement therapy. The NCEP guidelines recommend estrogen replacement therapy as an alternative to lipid medications for postmenopausal women who qualify for drug therapy to lower LDL, but the clinical trial evidence favors statin therapy, at least in women with coronary disease.

OMEGA-3 FATTY ACIDS (FISH OIL)

Interest in marine fish oils began with the observation that Greenland Eskimos, who eat a high-fat diet (40 percent of total calories), have a low incidence of heart disease. The type of fat present in fish is highly unsaturated omega-3 fatty acids. The primary lipid effect of omega-3 fatty acids is to lower triglycerides, but the effect on LDL level is variable. It is not clear what dosage is necessary to cause lipid effects; some studies have used dosages of omega-3 fatty acids of 15 to 30 g/day, whereas other studies suggest that dosages of 2 g/day or less may be effective.

Many fish oil supplements are currently on the market. Because they are not regarded as drugs, they are not regulated by the FDA. The long-term safety of taking fish oil capsules is unknown, and there is no evidence that fish oil supplementation prevents heart disease.

Special Issues in Managing Lipid Disorders

TREATING HYPERCHOLESTEROLEMIA IN WOMEN

Women manifest a lower risk of cardiovascular disease than men, leading some to advocate that cholesterol screening is inappropriate in women.[105] In fact, cardiovascular disease is the most common cause of death in both men and women, but women die of cardiovascular disease about 10 years later than men; that is, women in their 60s have about the same cardiovascular mortality as men in their 50s. Furthermore, the value of cholesterol screening is principally educational, allowing those at highest risk to benefit from available information about how to decrease that risk. The medical purpose of screening—case finding—is secondary because most people with a cholesterol level above 200 mg/dl need only dietary change and other alterations in lifestyle, not medical treatment. However, the immediate, absolute risk for women with a given LDL cholesterol elevation is less than that for men with the same LDL level, and the intervention must be tailored to the level of risk.[82] This goal is accommodated by the most recent NCEP guidelines, which combine age and sex as risk factors. We also attempt to use lower-risk drugs (such as the resins) when treating women and set appropriate LDL goals (perhaps 150 mg/dl instead of 130 mg/dl), particularly if the HDL cholesterol level is elevated. Indeed, HDL may be more important in women than in men,[84] and women with HDL cholesterol consistently above 60 mg/dl are unlikely to need intervention to lower LDL unless it is consistently above 220 mg/dl. Secondary prevention trials have found similar benefit

Table 7 Drug Treatment of Lipid Disorders

Cholestyramine and Colestipol

Indications: Elevated LDL with normal triglycerides.

Response: Dose related; 15%–30% decrease in LDL. Maximum response evident in 2–4 wk. HDL increases about 5%. Rise in triglycerides of 5%–20%, which may persist.

Mechanism: These equally effective resins bind to bile acids in the intestine, interrupting enterohepatic circulation and increasing fecal excretion, which increases hepatic bile acid synthesis from cholesterol stores. This increases the production of hepatic LDL receptors, which increases uptake of LDL from blood and lowers plasma LDL. HMG-CoA reductase activity also increases.

Contraindications: Absolute: none. Relative: severe diverticulosis with recent diverticulitis; symptomatic hemorrhoids.

Side effects: Very common: constipation, unpalatability, elevation in triglycerides. Less common: elevation of liver aminotransferases, abdominal pain.

Drug interactions: Decreased absorption of certain drugs, including thiazides, warfarin, digitalis, thyroxine, and beta blockers.

Approach to use: Start with 1 packet or scoop b.i.d. mixed with fluid (usually juice) before ingestion; increase over 1–2 wk to desired dose. If constipation develops, add 1 tsp psyllium to mixture. Take other drugs 1 hr before or 4 hr after resin. For colestipol tablets, start with 2 g b.i.d.

Dosage: Cholestyramine: maximum dosage, 24 g/day, b.i.d. or t.i.d.; colestipol: maximum dosage, 30 g/day, b.i.d. or t.i.d. The t.i.d. dosage is more effective; b.i.d. is more convenient. Maximum dose of colestipol tablets is 16 g/day.

Use with other lipid-lowering drugs: Bile acid–binding resins may be combined with nicotinic acid, lovastatin, gemfibrozil, or probucol. Simultaneous administration with nicotinic acid does not impair its absorption.

Atorvastatin, Fluvastatin, Lovastatin, Pravastatin, and Simvastatin

Indications: Elevated LDL; possibly useful for disorders in which both LDL and triglycerides are elevated.

Response: Dose related; 20%–50% decrease in LDL, 5%–10% increase in HDL, 10%–35% decrease in triglycerides. The maximum decrease in LDL occurs 4 wk after therapy begins.

Mechanism: The statins inhibit HMG-CoA reductase, the rate-limiting enzyme in cholesterol synthesis. Reduced cholesterol production in hepatocytes stimulates LDL receptor synthesis and uptake of LDL and VLDL remnants. Increase in HDL may result from increased synthesis of apolipoprotein A-I.

Contraindications: Absolute: active liver disease, pregnancy or lactation, and unexplained persistent elevations in serum aminotransferases. Relative: avoid use in women of reproductive age unless they are unlikely to conceive. Precaution: treatment of children is not recommended. Use with caution in adults with a history of liver disease, alcohol abuse, or renal impairment; discontinue if myopathy develops.

Side effects: Liver: 1%–2% incidence of marked, persistent increases in transaminase levels (> 3 × the upper limit of normal); resolves upon discontinuance.

Muscle: Uncomplicated myopathy (muscle aching or weakness, or both, plus a rise in creatine kinase to > 10 × normal) has been reported in rare instances (< 1%) for all statin drugs. The rise in CK and symptoms resolve promptly upon discontinuance of drug. Occasionally, myopathy can progress to frank rhabdomyolysis and acute renal failure. Myopathy risk is increased when statins are combined with cyclosporine in transplant patients or with gemfibrozil, niacin, erythromycin, or azole antifungal agents. Myopathy risk is about 30% in transplant patients taking cyclosporine and lovastatin; however, no myopathy occurred with the combination of pravastatin and cyclosporine in about 100 transplant patients reported in the literature. Myopathy appears to be less common for the combination of fluvastatin, pravastatin, or simvastatin with niacin than for lovastatin combined with niacin. Uncomplicated myalgia appears to be least common with fluvastatin (indistinguishable from rates with placebo).

Other: Rash, GI symptoms, headache, insomnia. There is no evidence that these drugs have any adverse effect on the human lens.

Cancer risk: Except for fluvastatin, statins have been associated with hepatocellular tumors in rodents.

Drug interactions: Because the risk of myopathy is increased [*see* Side effects, *above*], the combination of statins and cyclosporine, gemfibrozil, niacin, erythromycin, and azole antifungal agents should be avoided or approached cautiously. The risk of interaction is probably reduced by lowering the dose of statin, especially with niacin. Pravastatin (40 mg) and simvastatin (20 mg) appear to be safe when combined with cyclosporine in transplant patients. Adding statins to warfarin-treated patients may cause a rise in prothrombin time and risk of bleeding.

Approach to use: Use in adults only. The dose-response curves for all statins are not linear — the greatest effect occurs with initiation; subsequent dose increases have less incremental effect. Direct comparison data are limited, but atorvastatin appears to produce the greatest dose response, followed by simvastatin, pravastatin and lovastatin (which are about equivalent), and fluvastatin. The clinical importance of these differences depends on the initial cholesterol value and the goal. The incidence of myopathy is increased at higher doses. The manufacturer of simvastatin is seeking approval for an 80 mg dose. Atorvastatin at high doses generally produces greater triglyceride lowering than the other statins.

Dosage: Atorvastatin: Start with 10 mg, given anytime; maximum daily dose is 80 mg. Fluvastatin: Start with 20 mg b.i.d. or at bedtime; maximum daily dose is 80 mg. Lovastatin: Start with 20 mg with dinner or b.i.d.; maximum daily dose is 80 mg. Pravastatin: Start with 10 mg at bedtime; maximum daily dose is 40 mg. Simvastatin: Start with 10 mg at bedtime; maximum daily dose is 40 mg.

It is generally recommended that liver transaminases be tested at initiation of therapy, at 6 and 12 wk, and periodically (e.g., semiannually) thereafter. If transaminases rise to three times normal, the medication should be discontinued.

Advise patients to report unexplained muscle pain or weakness, and in such cases measure CK to confirm the diagnosis of myopathy. It is not known whether monitoring CK (as with AST and ALT) has any predictive value. Withhold therapy in any acute medical or surgical condition that could predispose to rhabdomyolysis or renal failure.

Use with other lipid-lowering drugs: Statins may be used in combination with bile acid–binding resins, leading to as much as a 50% reduction in LDL cholesterol levels. The combination of lovastatin with a bile acid sequestrant and nicotinic acid (i.e., triple therapy) has been reported with even greater LDL reductions, but caution is needed in combining the statins with nicotinic acid as noted above. The combination of a statin with gemfibrozil should be approached cautiously. Unlike the other three statins, absorption of pravastatin and fluvastatin is reduced when administered concomitantly with resins. While the clinical effect of this interaction may be small, it is recommended that the statin be administered either 1 hr before or 2–4 hr after the resin.

Niacin

Indications: Elevated LDL or triglycerides, or both.

Response: Dose related; 15%–30% decrease in LDL, 20%–50% decrease in triglycerides, 20%–30% increase in HDL. Lipoprotein levels return to baseline within 4 wk of discontinuance.

Mechanism: Inhibits VLDL synthesis in the liver by unknown mechanism; inhibits release of free fatty acids from adipose tissue and increases the activity of lipoprotein lipase.

Contraindications: Absolute: active liver disease, active peptic ulcer disease. Relative: diabetes mellitus, gout, history of peptic ulcer disease.

Side effects: Very common: cutaneous flushing, pruritus. Common: abdominal discomfort, nausea, vomiting, diarrhea, malaise, and elevation of glucose, uric acid, and liver function tests. Rare: peptic ulceration, hyperpigmentation, acanthosis nigricans, postural hypotension, arrhythmias, maculopathy. Severe hepatotoxicity has been reported, more commonly with time-release capsules.

(continued)

Table 7 Drug Treatment of Lipid Disorders *(continued)*

Drug interactions: Increased risk of myopathy with statins.

Approach to use and dosage: Crystalline nicotinic acid is preferred because time-release capsules are associated with more GI complaints and liver toxicity, including hepatic failure. We do not recommend time-release formulations. Confirm that glucose, uric acid, and liver function tests are normal before starting therapy. Start with 100 mg b.i.d. or t.i.d. with meals. Gradually increase dose to at least 1 g/day; the usual dose is 1.5–3.0 g/day in two or three divided doses, and the maximum dose is usually 6 g/day, although higher doses may occasionally be appropriate. Asymptomatic increase in liver amino-transferases up to twice the upper limit of normal does not require discontinuance. If side effects occur at doses higher than 1.5 g/day, consider reducing the dose and adding another lipid-lowering drug rather than discontinuing nicotinic acid.

To minimize flushing: (1) always take with meals, (2) increase the dose gradually, (3) take 80–325 mg aspirin up to 30 min before taking nicotinic acid, and (4) avoid missing doses. Check glucose, uric acid, and liver function tests once a dose of 1.5 g/day is reached and then periodically (three times a year) thereafter once a stable dose is reached.

Use with other lipid-lowering drugs: May be combined with bile acid–binding resins or gemfibrozil. Absorption is not impaired when taken with a bile acid–binding resin. Use caution when combining with statins.

Gemfibrozil

Indications: Elevated triglycerides; disorders with both elevated triglycerides and LDL; occasionally, as adjunctive therapy for elevated LDL.

Response: Dose related; 40%–50% decrease in triglycerides, 20% increase in HDL; effect on LDL is variable. In patients with isolated hypertriglyceridemia, LDL may increase. In patients with elevated LDL with or without elevated triglycerides, LDL may decrease by 10%.

Mechanism: Increases the activity of lipoprotein lipase; may inhibit hepatic secretion of VLDL.

Contraindications: Absolute: hepatic or severe renal dysfunction; gallbladder disease (i.e., documented gallstones). Relative: none.

Side effects: Common: mild GI discomfort (5%). Rare: eosinophilia, skin rash, musculoskeletal pain, blurred vision, mild anemia, leukopenia, mild increase in serum glucose, mild elevation in liver function tests. Gemfibrozil increases the lithogenicity of bile and may increase the formation of gallstones.

Drug interactions: Potentiates the effect of warfarin; 5% incidence of myopathy when taken with lovastatin.

Approach to use: Use in adults only. Monitor cell counts and hepatic enzymes periodically. If elevation of LDL results from treatment of isolated hypertriglyceridemia, consider adding a bile acid–binding resin or nicotinic acid or substituting nicotinic acid.

Dosage: 600 mg b.i.d. before meals.

Use with other lipid-lowering drugs: May be used in combination with bile acid–binding resins and nicotinic acid. Combination with statins should be approached cautiously.

LDL—low-density lipoproteins   HDL—high-density lipoproteins   VLDL—very low density lipoproteins
HMG-CoA reductase—3-hydroxy-3-methylglutaryl coenzyme A reductase   CK—creatine kinase

---

for women as for men, so aggressive risk reduction is appropriate for both sexes.[19,20]

SCREENING FOR AND TREATING HYPERCHOLESTEROLEMIA IN CHILDREN AND YOUNG ADULTS

Physicians caring for adults with early coronary artery disease or a lipid disorder may be confronted with the decision of whether to screen for and treat hypercholesterolemia in children. Numerous autopsy studies demonstrate that coronary atherosclerosis begins in childhood and adolescence and that lipoprotein levels are consistently associated with the extent of such atherosclerosis. Children in families with lipid disorders or early coronary disease have higher cholesterol levels, and childhood cholesterol levels are significant predictors of adult levels. However, a significant proportion of children and adolescents with elevated cholesterol will not have high enough levels as adults to warrant individual intervention, and screening all children for cholesterol level would risk important negative effects from labeling many young people as diseased. All children would benefit from a diet that is low in saturated fat; this goal should be a part of any population strategy for controlling epidemic atherosclerosis. However, the safety and efficacy of long-term drug therapy are not established in this age group, and treatment must be approached cautiously.

Considering these and other aspects, we agree with the recommendations of the NCEP's Expert Panel on Blood Cholesterol Levels in Children and Adolescents.[106] Physicians should advise patients younger than 55 years with known coronary disease or a lipid disorder that their children or grandchildren should undergo regular cholesterol testing from a source of continuing medical care. Of course, patients with a genetically well-defined lipid disorder should obtain appropriate genetic counseling. Physicians who encounter a young patient (i.e., younger than 20 years) with a markedly elevated LDL level should exhaust all lifestyle interventions before considering medications. If such measures are ineffective, resins should be used, and referral to a specialty clinic should be considered.

Treatment of young adults with elevated cholesterol is also controversial.[105] We agree with the strategy of matching the intensity of intervention with the level of risk,[82] but the short-term (e.g., 10-year) risk in young adults may provide an inadequate estimate of the potential benefit of cholesterol lowering. Law, Wald, and Thompson[83] show that several different types of studies indicate that the greatest benefit of cholesterol lowering accrues to younger people—as much as a 50 percent lowering of lifetime risk at age 40 from a 10 percent reduction in cholesterol. Also, sudden death remains an important initial manifestation of coronary disease, and the rate of coronary disease in the active treatment arms of clinical trials remains unacceptably high. Thus, it is incorrect to argue that treatment can be safely deferred to later life. Population-level prevention and lifestyle interventions should still be favored for young adults, but advances in technology to better identify asymptomatic patients (of any age) who should receive aggressive risk reduction are greatly needed. These advances may be in the identification or quantification of vulnerable plaques, markers of inflammation, or noninvasive measurements of endothelial dysfunction.

TREATING HYPERCHOLESTEROLEMIA IN THE ELDERLY

It is now well established that cholesterol level predicts atherosclerosis risk in persons older than 65 years,[107,108] and the majority of cardiovascular disease occurs above this age, especially for women. The Scandinavian Simvastatin Survival Study and the Cholesterol and Recurrent Events Trial both found a significant reduction in total mortality and major coronary events in individuals older than 60 years.[19,20] However, it is not known whether intervention to lower cholesterol for primary prevention is effective in this age group. We suggest careful individualization of management in these situations. Significant comorbidity should discourage preventive therapy, but otherwise healthy, vigorous elders can appropriately be treated for dyslipoproteinemia, using lower-risk interventions as much as possible and setting moderate treatment goals. Dietary advice must be tailored to ensure adequate nutrition in people whose diet may already be marginally deficient in nutrients. Addition of oat bran or psyllium may have benefit, but doses should start low and gradually build up to avoid fecal impaction. The resins are also appropriately employed in selected cases.

LOW CHOLESTEROL AND NONCARDIOVASCULAR MORTALITY

The relation between cholesterol and health has long been controversial.[109] Although the cause-and-effect relation between dietary saturated fat and plasma cholesterol and between plasma cholesterol and atherosclerotic disease is now widely accepted, controversy remains concerning a possible increase in noncardiovascular disease in persons with low levels of plasma cholesterol. This controversy derives from both observational studies[110] and primary prevention trials[111] and has led some physicians to suggest that elevated cholesterol levels should not be treated.[112] A comprehensive discussion of this issue is available.[113]

It is most likely that two phenomena explain the connection between low cholesterol levels and noncardiovascular death in observational studies: reverse causation and confounding. Reverse causation (i.e., an effect appearing to be a cause) refers in this case to the fact that preexisting disease can lower the cholesterol level; although early deaths are eliminated from these cohort studies to compensate for this effect, the decline in cholesterol level can occur more than 10 years before diagnosis.[114] Because many different diseases are associated with low cholesterol levels, low cholesterol is very likely merely a marker for poor health and nutrition, an interpretation that is supported by the longest follow-up data available,[115] studies in China,[116] a study that considered social class,[117] and analyses of the Hawaiian Heart Study.[118]

More data on this issue come from older primary prevention trials of cholesterol lowering, which did not demonstrate lower total mortality in the treated groups because of higher noncardiovascular disease death rates.[109] Early meta-analyses of these trials were flawed because it was inappropriate to combine trials that were not substantially similar: some were diet interventions, whereas others were drug trials in which several different agents were used. Also, some trials showed an excess in cancer mortality, whereas others showed an excess of other causes of death. The only consistent finding across the trials is an increase in death from violence, but the numbers of violent deaths are small (two to 21 deaths in the intervention group and zero to 15 in the control group). A 1995 meta-analysis of cholesterol-lowering trials has helped to clarify this issue.[93] This meta-analysis was different from earlier ones in three important ways: it was the most comprehensive; it examined heterogeneity of effects across the different interventions; and it looked for a dose-response relation between cholesterol lowering and all of the outcomes (a graded effect, either positive or negative, strengthens the causal inference). This meta-analysis found that for every 10 percentage points of cholesterol lowering, coronary artery disease mortality was reduced by 13 percent ($P < 0.002$) and total mortality was reduced by 10 percent ($P < 0.03$). It is important to note

that the analysis also showed that fibrates (clofibrate, seven trials; gemfibrozil, two trials) increased noncoronary disease mortality by about 30 percent ($P < 0.01$) and total mortality by about 17 percent ($P < 0.02$). The issue of noncardiovascular risk from cholesterol lowering has now been laid to rest by the results of both secondary and primary prevention trials with statins, which produce larger falls in cholesterol than in earlier trials and have shown no increase in noncardiovascular deaths and significantly lower total mortality.[16,19,20]

The physician should recognize that primary prevention is practiced on asymptomatic patients, requiring the physician to balance costs and benefits in the absence of any benefit from relieving symptoms. It is not easy, however, to extrapolate from clinical trials the costs and benefits of a particular treatment for a specific patient. Therefore, caution is indicated, particularly when medications are prescribed for lifelong use. Changes in nutrition and exercise for lipid control should be the principal means for the primary prevention of cardiovascular disease in both individuals and populations. Patients with established coronary artery disease are at very high risk for subsequent events; they benefit from lipid lowering, and they deserve aggressive control of LDL, usually with drug therapy.

References

1. Fredrickson DS, Levy RI, Lees RS: Fat transport and lipoproteins—an integrated approach to mechanisms and disorders. N Engl J Med 276:32, 94, 148, 215, 273, 1967

2. Stamler J, Wentworth D, Neaton JD: Is relationship between serum cholesterol and risk of premature death from coronary heart disease continuous and graded? Findings in 356,222 primary screenees of the Multiple Risk Factor Intervention Trial (MRFIT). JAMA 256:2823, 1986

3. Young SG: Recent progress in understanding apolipoprotein B. Circulation 82:1574, 1990

4. Brown MS, Goldstein JL: A receptor-mediated pathway for cholesterol homeostasis. Science 232:34, 1986

5. Eisenberg S: High density lipoprotein metabolism. J Lipid Res 25:1017, 1984

6. Tall AR: Plasma high density lipoproteins: metabolism and relationship to atherogenesis. J Clin Invest 86:379, 1990

7. Rothblat GH, Mahlberg FH, Johnson WJ, et al: Apolipoproteins, membrane cholesterol domains, and the regulation of cholesterol efflux. J Lipid Res 33:1091, 1992

8. Rubin EM, Krauss RM, Spangler EA, et al: Inhibition of early atherogenesis in transgenic mice by human apolipoprotein AI. Nature 353:265, 1991

9. Warden CH, Hedrick CC, Qiao JH, et al: Atherosclerosis in transgenic mice overexpressing apolipoprotein A-II. Science 261:469, 1993

10. Parthasarathy S, Barnett J, Fong L: High-density lipoprotein inhibits the oxidative modification of low-density lipoprotein. Biochim Biophys Acta 1044:275, 1990

11. Scanu AM: Lipoprotein(a): a genetic risk factor for premature coronary heart disease. JAMA 267:3326, 1992

12. Eaton SB, Konner M: Paleolithic nutrition: a consideration of its nature and current implications. N Engl J Med 312:283, 1985

13. Blackburn H: Diet and mass hyperlipidemia: a public health view. Nutrition, lipids, and coronary heart disease. Levy R, Rifkind B, Dennis B, et al, Eds. Raven Press, New York, 1979, p 309

14. Farquhar JW, Fortmann SP, Flora JA, et al: Effects of communitywide education on cardiovascular disease risk factors: the Stanford Five-City Project. JAMA 264:359, 1990

15. The Lipid Research Clinics Coronary Primary Prevention Trial results: I. Reduction in incidence of coronary heart disease. Lipid Research Clinics Program. JAMA 251:351, 1984

16. Shepherd J, Cobbe SM, Ford I, et al: Prevention of coronary heart disease with pravastatin in men with hypercholesterolemia. N Engl J Med 333:1301, 1995

17. Frick MH, Elo O, Haapa K, et al: Helsinki Heart Study: primary-prevention trial with gemfibrozil in middle-aged men with dyslipidemia. N Engl J Med 317:1237, 1987

18. Brown BG, Zhao X-Q, Sacco DE, et al: Lipid lowering and plaque regression: new insights into prevention of plaque disruption and clinical events in coronary disease. Circulation 87:1781, 1993

19. Randomised trial of cholesterol lowering in 4444 patients with coronary heart disease: the Scandinavian Simvastatin Survival Study (4S). Scandinavian Simvastatin Survival Study Group. Lancet 344:1383, 1994

20. Sacks FM, Pfeffer MA, Moye LA, et al: The effect of pravastatin on coronary events after myocardial infarction in patients with average cholesterol levels. N Engl J Med 335:1001, 1996

21. Fuster V, Badimon L, Badimon JJ, et al: The pathogenesis of coronary artery disease and the acute coronary syndromes (pt 2). N Engl J Med 326:310, 1992

22. Levine GN, Keaney JF Jr, Vita JA: Cholesterol reduction in cardiovascular disease: clinical benefits and possible mechanisms. N Engl J Med 332:512, 1995

23. Flavahan NA: Atherosclerosis or lipoprotein-induced endothelial dysfunction: potential mechanisms underlying reduction in EDRF/nitric oxide activity. Circulation 85:1927, 1992

24. Zeiher AM, Drexler H, Wollschläger H, et al: Modulation of coronary vasomotor tone in humans: progressive endothelial dysfunction with different early stages of coronary atherosclerosis. Circulation 83:391, 1991

25. Treasure CB, Klein JL, Weintraub WS, et al: Beneficial effects of cholesterol-lowering therapy on the coronary endothelium in patients with coronary artery disease. N Engl J Med 332:481, 1995

26. Anderson TJ, Meredith IT, Yeung AC, et al: The effect of cholesterol-lowering and antioxidant therapy on endothelium-dependent coronary vasomotion. N Engl J Med 332:488, 1995

27. van Boven AJ, Jukema JW, Zwinderman AH, et al: Reduction of transient myocardial ischemia with pravastatin in addition to the conventional treatment in patients with angina pectoris. Circulation 94:1503, 1996

28. Andrews TC, Raby K, Barry J, et al: Effect of cholesterol reduction on myocardial ischemia in patients with coronary disease. Circulation 95:324, 1997

29. Summary of the second report of the National Cholesterol Education Program (NCEP) Expert Panel on Detection, Evaluation, and Treatment of High Blood Cholesterol in Adults (Adult Treatment Panel II). Expert Panel on Detection, Evaluation, and Treatment of High Blood Cholesterol in Adults. JAMA 269:3015, 1993

30. Steinberg D, Parthasarathy S, Carew TE, et al: Beyond cholesterol: modifications of low-density lipoprotein that increase its atherogenicity. N Engl J Med 320:915, 1989

31. Stephens NG, Parsons A, Schofield PM, et al: Randomised controlled trial of vitamin E in patients with coronary disease: Cambridge Heart Antioxidant Study (CHAOS). Lancet 347:781, 1996

32. Austin MA, Breslow JL, Hennekens CH, et al: Low-density lipoprotein subclass patterns and risk of myocardial infarction. JAMA 260:1917, 1988

33. Austin MA, Brunzell JD, Fitch WL, et al: Inheritance of low density lipoprotein subclass patterns in familial combined hyperlipidemia. Arteriosclerosis 10:520, 1990

34. Gardner CD, Fortmann SP, Krauss RM: Association of small low-density lipoprotein particles with the incidence of coronary artery disease in men and women. JAMA 276:875, 1996

35. Stampfer MJ, Sacks FM, Salvini S, et al: A prospective study of cholesterol, apolipoproteins, and the risk of myocardial infarction. N Engl J Med 325:373, 1991

36. McMurry MP, Cerqueira MT, Connor SL, et al: Changes in lipid and lipoprotein levels and body weight in Tarahumara Indians after consumption of an affluent diet. N Engl J Med 325:1704, 1991

37. Badimon JJ, Badimon L, Galvez A, et al: High density lipoprotein plasma fractions inhibit aortic fatty streaks in cholesterol-fed rabbits. Lab Invest 60:455, 1989

38. Badimon JJ, Badimon L, Fuster V: Regression of atherosclerotic lesions by high density lipoprotein plasma fraction in the cholesterol-fed rabbit. J Clin Invest 85:1234, 1990

39. Genest J Jr, McNamara JR, Ordovas JM, et al: Lipoprotein cholesterol, apolipoprotein A-I and B and lipoprotein (a) abnormalities in men with premature coronary artery disease. J Am Coll Cardiol 19:792, 1992

40. Miller M, Seidler A, Kwiterovich PO, et al: Long-term predictors of subsequent cardiovascular events with coronary artery disease and "desirable" levels of plasma total cholesterol. Circulation 86:1165, 1992

41. Levy RI, Brensike JF, Epstein SE, et al: The influence of changes in lipid values induced by cholestyramine and diet on progression of coronary artery disease: results of the NHLBI Type II Coronary Intervention Study. Circulation 69:325, 1984

42. Brown G, Albers JJ, Fisher LD, et al: Regression of coronary artery disease as a result of intensive lipid-lowering therapy in men with high levels of apolipoprotein B. N Engl J Med 323:1289, 1990

43. Smith SC Jr, Blair SN, Criqui MH, et al: Preventing heart attack and death in patients with coronary disease. American Heart Association Consensus Panel Statement. Circulation 92:2, 1995

44. Baseline serum cholesterol and treatment effect in the Scandinavian Simvastatin Survival Study (4S). Scandinavian Simvastatin Survival Study Group. Lancet 345:1274, 1995

45. Criqui MH, Heiss G, Cohn R, et al: Plasma triglyceride level and mortality from coronary heart disease. N Engl J Med 328:1220, 1993

46. Assmann G, Schulte H: Triglycerides and atherosclerosis: results from the Prospective Cardiovascular Münster Study. Atherosclerosis Reviews 22:51, 1991

47. Manninen V, Tenkanen L, Koskinen P, et al: Joint effects of serum triglyceride and LDL cholesterol and HDL cholesterol concentrations on coronary heart disease risk in the Helsinki Heart Study: implications for treatment. Circulation 85:37, 1992

48. Carlson LA, Rosenhamer G: Reduction of mortality in the Stockholm Ischaemic Heart Disease Secondary Prevention Study by combined treatment with clofibrate and nicotinic acid. Acta Med Scand 223:405, 1988

49. Castelli WP: Epidemiology of triglycerides: a view from Framingham. Am J Cardiol 70:3H, 1992

50. Zilversmit DB: Atherogenesis: a postprandial phenomenon. Circulation 60:473, 1979

51. Wild SH, Fortmann SP, Marcovina SM: A prospective case-control study of lipoprotein(a) levels and apo(a) size and risk of coronary heart disease in Stanford Five-City Project participants. Arterioscler Thromb Vasc Biol 17:239, 1997

52. Seed M, Hoppichler F, Reaveley D, et al: Relation of serum lipoprotein(a) concentration and apolipoprotein(a) phenotype to coronary heart disease in patients with familial hypercholesterolemia. N Engl J Med 322:1494, 1990

53. Bostom AG, Gagnon DR, Cupples LA, et al: A prospective investigation of elevated lipoprotein (a) detected by electrophoresis and cardiovascular disease in women: the Framingham Heart Study. Circulation 90:1688, 1994

54. Schaefer EJ, Lamon-Fava S, Jenner JL, et al: Lipoprotein(a) levels and risk of coronary heart disease in men: the Lipid Research Clinics Coronary Primary Prevention Trial. JAMA 271:999, 1994

55. Ridker PM, Hennekens CH, Stampfer MJ: A prospective study of lipoprotein(a) and the risk of myocardial infarction. JAMA 270:2195, 1993

56. Ridker PM, Stampfer MJ, Hennekens CH: Plasma concentration of lipoprotein(a) and the risk of future stroke. JAMA 273:1269, 1995

57. Fortmann SP, Marcovina SM: Lipoprotein(a), a clinically elusive lipoprotein particle (editorial). Circulation 95: 295, 1997

58. Consensus conference: Treatment of hypertriglyceridemia. JAMA 251:1196, 1984

59. Santamarina-Fojo S, Brewer HB Jr: The familial hyperchylomicronemia syndrome: new insights into the underlying genetic defects. JAMA 265:904, 1991

60. Schonfeld G: Inherited disorders of lipid transport. Endocrinol Metab Clin North Am 19:229, 1990

61. Benlian P, De Gennes JL, Foubert L, et al: Premature atherosclerosis in patients with familial chylomicronemia caused by mutations in the lipoprotein lipase gene. N Engl J Med 335:848, 1996

62. Goldstein JL, Schrott HG, Hazzard WR, et al: Hyperlipidemia in coronary heart disease: II. Genetic analysis of lipid levels in 176 families and delineation of a new inherited disorder, combined hyperlipidemia. J Clin Invest 52:1544, 1973

63. Sanderson S, Iverius PH, Wilson DE: Successful hyperlipemic pregnancy. JAMA 265:1858, 1991

64. Ginsberg HN: Lipoprotein physiology and its relationship to atherogenesis. Endocrinol Metab Clin North Am 19:211, 1990

65. Kane JP, Havel RJ: Disorders of the biogenesis and secretion of lipoproteins containing the B apolipoproteins. The Metabolic Basis of Inherited Disease, 6th ed. Scriver CR, Beaudet AL, Sly WS, et al, Eds. McGraw Hill Book Co, New York, 1989, p 1139

66. Hobbs HH, Russell DW, Brown MS, et al: The LDL receptor locus in familial hypercholesterolemia: mutational analysis of a membrane protein. Annu Rev Genet 24:133, 1990

67. Torsvik H, Fischer JE, Feldman HA, et al: Effects of intravenous hyperalimentation on plasma-lipoproteins in severe familial hypercholesterolaemia. Lancet 1:601, 1975

68. Bilheimer DW, Goldstein JL, Grundy SM, et al: Liver transplantation to provide low-density-lipoprotein receptors and lower plasma cholesterol in a child with homozygous familial hypercholesterolemia. N Engl J Med 311:1658, 1984

69. Kane JP, Malloy MJ, Ports TA, et al: Regression of coronary atherosclerosis during treatment of familial hypercholesterolemia with combined drug regimens. JAMA 264:3007, 1990

70. Illingworth DR, Vakar F, Mahley RW, et al: Hypocholesterolaemic effects of lovastatin in familial defective apolipoprotein B-100. Lancet 339:598, 1992

71. Mahley RW, Weisgraber KH, Innerarity TL, et al: Genetic defects in lipoprotein metabolism: elevation of atherogenic lipoproteins caused by impaired catabolism. JAMA 265:78, 1991

72. Forte TM, Carlson LA: Electron microscopic structure of serum lipoproteins from patients with fish eye disease. Arteriosclerosis 4:130, 1984

73. Franceschini G, Sirtori CR, Capurso A, et al: A-I$_{Milano}$ apoprotein: decreased high density lipoprotein cholesterol levels with significant lipoprotein modifications and without clinical atherosclerosis in an Italian family. J Clin Invest 66:892, 1980

74. Franceschini G, Vecchio G, Gianfranceschi G, et al: Apolipoprotein AI$_{Milano}$: accelerated binding and dissociation from lipids of a human apolipoprotein variant. J Biol Chem 260:16321, 1985

75. Norum RA, Lakier JB, Goldstein S, et al: Familial deficiency of apolipoproteins A-I and C-III and precocious coronary-artery disease. N Engl J Med 306:1513, 1982

76. Garg A, Grundy SM: Nicotinic acid as therapy for dyslipidemia in non–insulin-dependent diabetes mellitus. JAMA 264:723, 1990

77. Chait A, Brunzell JD: Acquired hyperlipidemia (secondary dyslipoproteinemias). Endocrinol Metab Clin North Am 19:259, 1990

78. Joven J, Villabona C, Vilella E, et al: Abnormalities of lipoprotein metabolism in patients with the nephrotic syndrome. N Engl J Med 323:579, 1990

79. Steinberg D, Pearson TA, Kuller LH: Alcohol and atherosclerosis. Ann Intern Med 114:967, 1991

80. Effects of estrogen or estrogen/progestin regimens on heart disease risk factors in postmenopausal women: the Postmenopausal Estrogen/Progestin Interventions (PEPI) Trial. The Writing Group for the PEPI Trial. JAMA 273:199, 1995

81. Hulley SB, Newman TB, Grady D, et al: Should we be measuring blood cholesterol levels in young adults? JAMA 269:1416, 1993

82. Fuster V, Gotto AM, Libby P, et al: Matching the intensity of risk factor management with the hazard for coronary disease events. Task Force 1. Pathogenesis of coronary disease: the biologic role of risk factors. 27th Bethesda Conference. J Am Coll Cardiol 27:957, 1996

83. Law MR, Wald NJ, Thompson SG: By how much and how quickly does reduction in serum cholesterol concentration lower risk of ischaemic heart disease? BMJ 308:367, 1994

84. Abbot RD, Wilson PWF, Kannel WB, et al: High density lipoprotein cholesterol, to-

tal cholesterol screening, and myocardial infarction: the Framingham Study. Arteriosclerosis 8:207, 1988

85. Wood PD, Stefanick ML, Williams PT, et al: The effects on plasma lipoproteins of a prudent weight-reducing diet, with or without exercise, in overweight men and women. N Engl J Med 325:461, 1991

86. Blum CD, Levy RI, Eisenberg S, et al: High density lipoprotein metabolism in man. J Clin Invest 60:795, 1977

87. Sacks FM, Willett WW: More on chewing the fat: the good fat and the good cholesterol. N Engl J Med 325:1740, 1991

88. Ripsin CM, Keenan JM, Jacobs DR, et al: Oat products and lipid lowering: a meta-analysis. JAMA 267:3317, 1992

89. Bell LP, Hectorne K, Reynolds H, et al: Cholesterol-lowering effects of psyllium hydrophilic mucilloid: adjunct therapy to a prudent diet for patients with mild to moderate hypercholesterolemia. JAMA 261:3419, 1989

90. Zavaroni I, Bonora E, Pagliara M, et al: Risk factors for coronary artery disease in healthy persons with hyperinsulinemia and normal glucose tolerance. N Engl J Med 320:702, 1989

91. Wood PD, Stefanick ML, Dreon DM, et al: Changes in plasma lipids and lipoproteins in overweight men during weight loss through dieting as compared with exercise. N Engl J Med 319:1173, 1988

92. Superko HR, Krauss RS: Differential effects of nicotinic acid in subjects with different LDL subclass patterns. Atherosclerosis 95:69, 1992

93. Gould AL, Rossouw JE, Santanello NC, et al: Cholesterol reduction yields clinical benefit: a new look at old data. Circulation 91:2274, 1995

94. Kreisberg RA: Low high-density lipoprotein cholesterol: what does it mean, what can we do about it, and what should we do about it? Am J Med 94:1, 1993

95. Kashyap ML: Effects of drugs on high-density lipoprotein apoprotein metabolism. High-Density Lipoproteins, Reverse Cholesterol Transport, and Coronary Heart Disease. Miller NE, Ed. Excerpta Medica, New York, 1989, p 60

96. Shepherd J, Packard CJ, Morgan HG, et al: The effects of cholestyramine on high density lipoprotein metabolism. Atherosclerosis 33:433, 1979

97. Saku K, Gartside PS, Hynd BA, et al: Mechanism of action of gemfibrozil on lipoprotein metabolism. J Clin Invest 75:1702, 1985

98. Shepherd J, Packard CJ, Patsch JR, et al: Effects of nicotinic acid therapy on plasma high density lipoprotein subfraction distribution and composition and on apolipoprotein A metabolism. J Clin Invest 63:858, 1979

99. Rubenfire M, Maciejko JJ, Blevins RD, et al: The effect of pravastatin on plasma lipoprotein and apolipoprotein levels in primary hypercholesterolemia. Arch Intern Med 151:2234, 1991

100. Mayer EL, Jacobsen DW, Robinson K: Homocysteine and coronary atherosclerosis. J Am Coll Cardiol 27:517, 1996

101. Graham IM, Daly LE, Refsum HM, et al: Plasma homocysteine as a risk factor for vascular disease. The European Concerted Action Project. JAMA 277:1775, 1997

102. Nygard O, Nordrehaug JE, Refsum H, et al: Plasma homocysteine levels and mortality in patients with coronary artery disease. N Engl J Med 337: 230, 1997

103. Denke MA, Grundy SM: Efficacy of low-dose cholesterol-lowering drug therapy in men with moderate hypercholesterolemia. Arch Intern Med 155:393, 1995

104. Grodstein F, Stampfer MJ, Colditz GA, et al: Postmenopausal hormone therapy and mortality. N Engl J Med 336:1769, 1997

105. Guidelines for using serum cholesterol, high-density lipoprotein cholesterol, and triglyceride levels as screening tests for preventing coronary heart disease in adults. Clinical guideline, pt. 1. American College of Physicians. Ann Intern Med 124:515, 1996

106. Report of the Expert Panel on Blood Cholesterol Levels in Children and Adolescents. American Academy of Pediatrics. National Cholesterol Education Program. Pediatrics 89:525, 1992

107. Benfante R, Reed D: Is elevated serum cholesterol level a risk factor for coronary heart disease in the elderly? JAMA 263:393, 1990

108. Shipley MJ, Pocock SJ, Marmot MG: Does plasma cholesterol concentration predict mortality from coronary heart disease in elderly people? 18 year follow up in Whitehall Study. BMJ 303:89, 1991

109. Mann GV: Diet-heart: end of an era. N Engl J Med 297:644, 1977

110. Jacobs D, Blackburn H, Higgins M, et al: Report of the conference on low blood cholesterol: mortality associations. Circulation 86:1046, 1992

111. Muldoon MF, Manuck SB, Matthews KA: Lowering cholesterol concentrations and mortality: a quantitative review of primary prevention trials. BMJ 301:309, 1990

112. Hulley SB, Walsh JMB, Newman TB: Health policy on blood cholesterol: time to change directions. Circulation 86:1026, 1992

113. Epstein FH: Low serum cholesterol, cancer and other noncardiovascular disorders. Atherosclerosis 94:1, 1992

114. Winawer SJ, Flehinger BJ, Buchalter J, et al: Declining serum cholesterol levels prior to diagnosis of colon cancer: a time-trend, case-control study. JAMA 263:2083, 1990

115. Anderson KM, Castelli WP, Levy D: Cholesterol and mortality: 30 years of follow-up from the Framingham Study. JAMA 257:2176, 1987

116. Chen Z, Peto R, Collins R, et al: Serum cholesterol concentration and coronary heart disease in population with low cholesterol concentrations. BMJ 303:276, 1991

117. Smith GD, Shipley MJ, Marmot MG, et al: Plasma cholesterol concentration and mortality: the Whitehall Study. JAMA 267:70, 1992

118. Iribarren C, Dwyer JH, Burchfiel CM, et al: Can the U-shaped relation between mortality and serum cholesterol be explained by confounding? Circulation 87:684, 1993

Acknowledgment

Figures 1 through 4   Andy Christie.

55 The Porphyrias

Mark G. Perlroth, M.D.

Definition and Classification

The porphyrias are a group of diseases characterized by the overproduction of porphyrin compounds and their precursors. In animals, porphyrin synthesis is required for the production of heme, which is a component of hemoglobin, cytochromes (including cytochrome P-450), catalase, peroxidase, and other oxidative enzymes. Just as the iron-containing porphyrin heme catalyzes oxidative phosphorylation in animals through the action of mitochondrial cytochromes, the magnesium-containing porphyrin chlorophyll catalyzes photosynthesis. As more poetically described by the Nobel prize winner Hans Fischer, porphyrins are the substances that make blood red and grass green.[1]

Epidemiology

Although specific genetic and enzymatic defects are present throughout life, most heterozygous persons never experience symptoms of disease.[2] When symptoms develop, they usually do so after puberty. The course of the acute forms of disease is characterized by long latent periods interrupted by acute attacks. During latency, urinary porphyrin and porphyrin precursor excretion ranges from minimal to marked. When symptoms are manifest, biochemical tests for these products are typically positive.

Pathophysiology and Genetic Defects in Porphyria

The porphyrias are best understood by the examination of the basic scheme of heme synthesis [see Figure 1]. The rate of synthesis is controlled by the mitochondrial enzyme δ-aminolevulinic acid synthase (ALAS). Subsequently, in the cytoplasm, the tetrapyrrole rings remain in their reduced state (porphyrinogens), but the number of carboxyl residues progressively decreases from eight to two. The last three enzymatic reactions take place in the mitochondrion, resulting in heme, which represses the production and activity of ALAS, the initial and rate-limiting enzyme in this metabolic pathway. The loss of carboxyl groups makes each successive compound less water soluble.

The conversion of protoporphyrinogen to protoporphyrin by removal of six hydrogen atoms results in a series of alternating double bonds that absorbs light with a wavelength of approximately 400 nm (the Soret band), accounting for the fluorescence characteristic of all porphyrins. Porphyrinogen intermediates oxidize spontaneously, especially in the presence of light. The resulting porphyrins are lost to the heme synthetic pathway and are excreted in the urine, the stool, or both, depending on their relative water solubility.

Each specific abnormality in the pattern of excretion of porphyrins and porphyrin precursors is caused by a reduction in the level of one of the enzymes of the heme synthetic pathway. A deficiency in any of the enzymes from ALA dehydratase (ALAD) to ferrochelatase may occur. The major sites of heme production are bone marrow (erythrocytes) and liver, so the porphyrias are conveniently grouped as erythropoietic, hepatic, or both, depending on the site affected. Because of their striking clinical manifestations, their visible urinary chemical markers, and their familial mode of inheritance, the porphyrias were among the earliest diseases to be defined as inborn errors of metabolism.

With the exception of congenital erythropoietic porphyria (CEP) and ALAD deficiency (plumboporphyria), the porphyrias are usually inherited in an autosomal dominant pattern. Furthermore, two parents who are heterozygous for the same enzymatic deficiency can produce offspring with a much more severe form of the disease, whereas parents who are heterozygous for different enzymatic deficiencies may have offspring with a mixed or so-called dual porphyria.

Among the advances in molecular biology in the past decade are the mapping of the chromosomal locations and sequencing of the genes that code for the enzymes involved in porphyrin biosynthesis,[1] as well as identification of many specific mutations. These may involve point mutations, insertions, or deletions that change the amino acid sequence of an enzyme and thus interfere either with its ability to bind or release intermediates or with its stability.[3]

The presence of nonfunctional enzyme can be verified by cross-reaction with specific antibodies to the normal enzymatic protein (called cross-reacting immunologic material [CRIM]). Because individual mutations define differing protein structures, gradations of enzyme malfunction are encountered; this accounts for some of the differences in clinical severity.

Our greater understanding of the molecular biology of porphyrin synthesis has led not only to advances in clinical evaluation and diagnosis but also to the use of effective therapy for the acute porphyrias with heme. Heme represses the hepatic rate-limiting enzyme ALAS, thereby reducing the overproduction of porphyrin precursors in the liver, with consequent relief of symptoms in the acute porphyrias.

Hepatic Porphyrias

ACUTE PORPHYRIAS

The acute hepatic porphyrias—in order of prevalence in North America—are acute intermittent porphyria (AIP), variegate porphyria (VP), hereditary coproporphyria (HCP), and ALAD deficiency. As a group, the acute porphyrias are characterized by the occurrence of neurovisceral attacks (neurologic manifestations and abdominal pain). Each is characterized by several of five "P's": (1) onset after puberty, (2) psychiatric abnormalities, (3) pain, (4) polyneuropathy, and (5) photosensitivity (found only in HCP and VP). During latency, symptoms are absent. However, acute episodes can be precipitated by four "M's": (1) medicines (including estrogens and alcohol) [see Table 1], (2) menstrual and premenstrual periods, (3) malnutrition (low carbohydrate ingestion or fasting), and (4) medical illnesses (and surgery). Although porphyria cutanea tarda (PCT) also derives from a hepatic enzyme disturbance, it results only in photosensitivity and is discussed separately [see Porphyria Cutanea Tarda, below].

The apparent contradiction between a fixed genetic abnormality and a relapsing clinical pattern is explained by the fact that hepatic ALAS, normally the rate-limiting enzyme for heme synthesis, can be induced by certain endogenous stimuli (e.g., menses) and exogenous stimuli (e.g., starvation or drugs), thereby precipitating acute clinical attacks of the disease. The basic defect in these porphyrias is a partial deficiency of a non–rate-limiting enzyme.

Table 1 Safe and Unsafe Drugs for Patients with Acute Intermittent Porphyria, Variegate Porphyria, Hereditary Coproporphyria, or ALA Dehydratase Deficiency (Plumboporphyria)

Safe Drugs		Unsafe Drugs	
Acetaminophen	Heme arginate	Barbiturates[†]	Nifedipine
Acetazolamide	Heparin		Oral contraceptives[‡]
Acyclovir		Captopril	Orphenadrine[†]
Allopurinol	Insulin	Chloramphenicol[†]	Oxycodone
Amiloride	Iron	Chlordiazepoxide[†]	
Ampicillin		Chlorpropamide[†]	Pentazocine[†]
Aspirin	Lithium salts		Phenobarbital[†]
Atropine		Diazepam[‡]	Phenytoin[†]
	Meperidine	Diltiazem	Piroxicam
Bumetanide	Mequitazine	Diphenhydramine	Pivampicillin[†]
Bupivacaine	Metformin	Doxycycline	Progesterone[†]
Buprenorphine	Metoprolol		Pyrazinamide[†]
	Morphine	Ergot compounds[†]	
Chlorothiazide*		Erythromycin	Sodium valproate[‡]
Codeine phosphate	Nadolol	Estrogen	
Corticosteroids*		Ethanol[†]	Terfenadine
	Oxytocin		Tetracyclines[‡]
Deferoxamine		Furosemide[‡]	Theophylline[†]
Demerol	Penicillin		Trimethoprim
Digoxin	Procaine	Griseofulvin[†]	
	Propofol		Verapamil
Fentanyl	Propylthiouracil	Hydralazine	
Follicle-stimulating hormone		Hydrochlorothiazide[‡]	
(FSH)	Quinine		
		Imipramine[†]	
Gabapentin	Ranitidine*		
Gentamicin		Lidocaine	
Glipizide	Salbutamol		
	Senna	Methyldopa[†]	
Haloperidol		Metoclopramide[‡]	
	Temazepam	Metronidazole	
	Thyroxine		
	Warfarin		

Note: See also the American Porphyria Foundation Web site, at http://www.enterprise.net/apf. The American Porphyria Foundation charges a nominal fee to access their site.
*Has produced conflicting results (occasionally positive but mainly negative) in experiments on porphyrinogenicity. None of the safe drugs listed has been associated with human porphyric attacks.
[†]Has been associated with acute attacks of porphyria.
[‡]Has produced conflicting results (some positive, some negative) in experiments on porphyrinogenicity.

Such a defect may be well tolerated when the level of heme production in the liver is normal; however, when ALAS production is induced, increased precursor production overwhelms the defective step in the pathway. Intermediates proximal to the partial block accumulate and spill into the circulation. Depending on the enzyme involved and the extent to which ALAS has been induced, the precursor surplus may consist of δ-aminolevulinic acid (ALA) and porphobilinogen (PBG) in combination with variable amounts of uroporphyrinogen, coproporphyrinogen, and protoporphyrinogen. Because porphyrinogens readily oxidize to their respective fluorescent porphyrins, the excretion of ALA, PBG, and porphyrin is usually measured. The progressive decarboxylation of porphyrinogen intermediates in the heme synthetic pathway leads to a corresponding loss of aqueous solubility. Therefore, coproporphyrin and protoporphyrin are excreted less by the kidney and more by the liver, necessitating fecal analysis.

Precipitating factors are presumed to act by inducing hepatic ALA synthase either by direct stimulation of the enzyme or by decreased availability of heme, causing derepression of ALAS. Binding of heme by intracellular hepatic proteins may be one avenue that leads to such a reduction. ALAS activity is increased by carbohydrate deprivation, but the mechanism is unknown. The preponderance of several of the hepatic porphyrias among women, the onset of the disease after puberty, and the phenomenon of premenstrual and menstrual exacerbation of disease all suggest a role for estrogens and progesterone in the course of the disease.

Several acquired lesions of porphyrin production exist. Lead inhibits ALAD, which leads to increased ALA excretion (but not excess PBG) in the urine. Abdominal pain, peripheral neuropathy, and other findings typical of acute porphyria may occur. A similar biochemical lesion occurs in hereditary tyrosinemia secondary to accumulation of succinylacetone, a potent ALAD inhibitor. Chronic liver disease, hemolysis, hepatic neoplasms, and some medications are associated with increased coproporphyrin excretion.

Acute Intermittent Porphyria

The autosomal dominant pattern of inheritance of AIP results in approximately 50% of normal activity of the enzyme PBG deaminase (PBGD). More than 100 distinct mutations affecting the stability or catalytic activity of human PBGD as well as 10 neutral genetic polymorphisms have been identified.[4]

The prevalence of the genetic defect in AIP varies from one in 500 in Scandinavia to one in 1,500 in France. Family studies demonstrate that 80% to 90% of cases are latent. On the basis of these figures, the expected incidence of attacks should be one or two per 15,000, much higher than the reported incidence of one to two per 100,000. This discrepancy suggests that many mutations are only mildly expressed or that many cases are misdiagnosed.[4]

In studies of 92 affected families, 89 had diminished erythrocyte PBGD activity caused by either a decrease in the kinetic properties

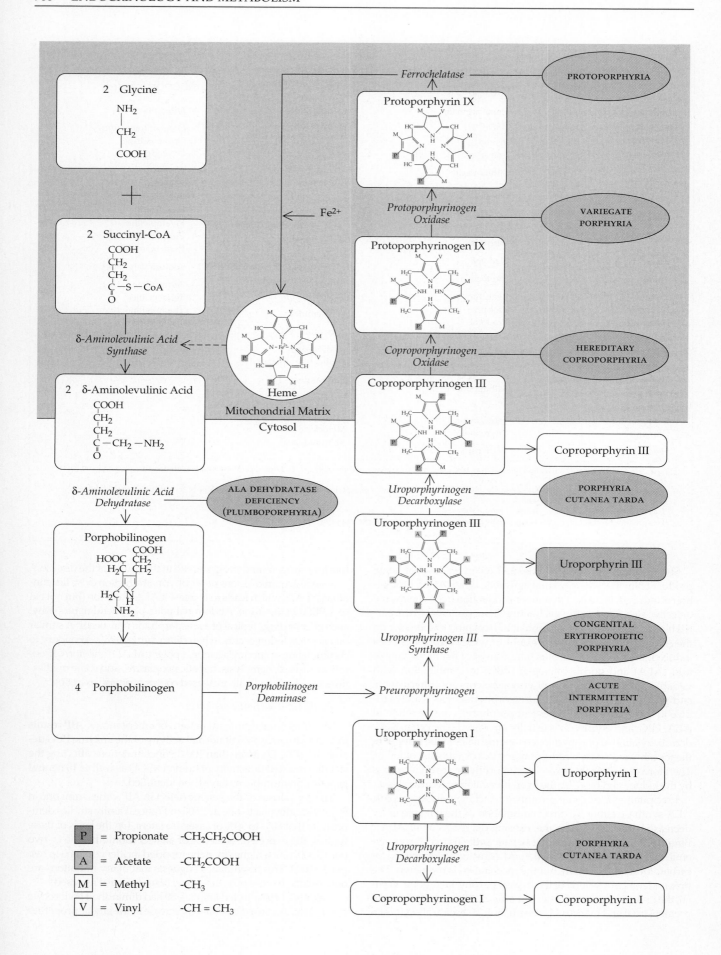

and stability of PBGD, enhanced binding, or defective release of substrate. The remaining three families had normal erythrocyte PBGD levels.[3] An explanation for this discrepancy is that both the hepatocyte and the erythrocyte PBGD are derived from a gene containing 15 exons, but the messenger RNA is spliced differently in the two tissues, allowing heme synthesis to be regulated differently.[5] The hepatic enzyme is translated from exons 1 and 3 through 15; the erythrocytic process splices off exon 1, translating its enzyme from exons 2 through 15. In the hepatocyte, a mutation at the first intron immediately proximal to the splicing site prevents transcription of exon 1, disabling the hepatic enzyme and reducing PBGD activity by 50%. In the erythrocyte, transcription starts at exon 2 and thus has no adverse effect on expression of the enzyme. Conversely, isolated erythrocyte PBGD deficiency may occur in persons with normal hepatic enzyme function, yielding false positive results.[6]

Although the defect in PBGD activity in patients with AIP is unremarkable under normal circumstances, induction of ALAS by one of the four "M's" leads to the accumulation of the precursors ALA and PBG, which are water soluble and are excreted in increased amounts in the urine. ALA is colorless, but PBG forms in a brownish-red polymer (porphobilin) on standing; it is often visible in the urine during acute attacks. Spontaneous condensation of PBG as well as some conversion to uroporphyrin in extrahepatic tissues is thought to explain elevated uroporphyrin levels in urine. In AIP, porphyrinogen production—and hence porphyrin production—is not markedly increased; thus, photosensitivity does not occur in AIP.

AIP varies in its clinical and diagnostic features [see Table 2]. Manifestations of neurotoxicity at the cortical level include mood changes, irritability, and frank psychosis. Hypothalamic lesions may cause the syndrome of inappropriate secretion of antidiuretic hormone (SIADH) with hyponatremia, causing seizures and psychiatric disturbances. Cranial nerve dysfunction, bulbar paresis, and difficulty in swallowing and aspiration lead to pneumonia. Peripheral neuropathy causes pain and paresis. If intercostal and phrenic nerves are involved, ventilatory insufficiency may occur. Involvement of autonomic nerves causes abdominal pain, ileus, tachycardia, hypertension, or, less commonly, diarrhea. Because signs and symptoms are of neuropathic origin, fever, leukocytosis, and other signs of inflammation are usually mild or absent.

AIP should be included in the differential diagnosis of unexplained abdominal pain, acute psychiatric disturbances, and acute polyneuropathies. Of assistance in the diagnosis are a positive family history, the presence of pain in the back and extremities as well as in the abdomen, and the acute development of hypertension during the course of the attack. Suspicion should be greater if

Table 2 Clinical and Diagnostic Features of Acute Intermittent Porphyria

Feature or Finding	Percentage of Patients (Size of Sample)
Abdominal pain	90 (520)
Red or dark urine	72 (237)
Nonabdominal pain*	66 (200)
Nausea/vomiting	61 (520)
Constipation	56 (504)
Diarrhea	9 (508)
Paresis/paralysis	45 (449)
Behavioral change	56 (518)
Irritability/anxiety	40 (73)
Seizure	12 (343)
Tachycardia (> 100 beats/min)	50 (496)
Labile hypertension (> 90 mm Hg diastolic)	44 (496)

*Extremities, joints, back, or head.

symptoms occur during menstruation or pregnancy, after exposure to certain drugs (including alcohol or anesthetics) [see Table 1], during a weight reduction regimen, or after surgery.

A urine sample can be rapidly screened for PBG by the Watson-Schwartz or the Hoesch test, both of which utilize Ehrlich's reagent as a chromogen. Twenty-four-hour urine samples should be collected, placed in opaque containers, refrigerated, and delivered to a qualified laboratory for quantitative analysis of ALA, PBG, and porphyrins.

Because the other inducible hepatic porphyrias (ALAD deficiency, HCP, and VP) may produce identical neuropathic syndromes without photosensitive lesions and may be marked by excess excretion of PBG, ALA, or both, definitive diagnosis should be sought by stool examination and the erythrocyte PBG deaminase assay. The PBGD assay is 80% to 90% sensitive and is accurate during the latent period when urinary biochemical abnormalities may be absent. It is also useful for screening asymptomatic family members. It may be falsely elevated (i.e., normal) when the reticulocyte count is high.[3] If the unique mutation for a kindred has been identified, relatives can be screened using modern techniques of DNA analysis.

Early identification of the etiology of porphyric symptoms will prevent unnecessary tests and permit prompt treatment. Screening of family members should be recommended, even though such screening may cause anxiety and difficulty in obtaining health insurance or employment. It is most important to avoid drugs known to precipitate attacks [see Table 1]. A high-carbohydrate isocaloric diet is also desirable, as is genetic counseling.

Figure 1 The initial rate-limiting step in the synthesis of heme is the synthesis of δ-aminolevulinic acid (ALA) from glycine and succinyl-CoA. This step is catalyzed by the intramitochondrial enzyme ALA synthase. The next step, which takes place in the cytosol, consists of the condensation of two molecules of ALA by the enzyme ALA dehydratase to form the pyrrole ring porphobilinogen (PBG). PBG contains two carboxyl residues, acetate ($- CH_2COOH$) and propionate ($- CH_2CH_2COOH$), and is water soluble. Condensation of four molecules of PBG by the enzyme PBG deaminase and the coenzyme uroporphyrinogen III synthase yields uroporphyrinogen III, an asymmetrical tetrapyrrole that contains four propionate and four acetate groups. Uroporphyrinogen I is formed nonenzymatically and can subsequently form coproporphyrinogen I. In addition, all of the porphyrinogen intermediates can auto-oxidize to their corresponding porphyrins. However, only uroporphyrinogen III is a precursor of heme. Partial decarboxylation of uroporphyrinogen III by the enzyme uroporphyrinogen decarboxylase yields coproporphyrinogen III, which contains four carboxyl groups. Coproporphyrinogen III reenters the mitochondrion and is oxidized by coproporphyrinogen oxidase to form protoporphyrinogen IX, with a loss of two more propionate residues. The enzyme protoporphyrinogen oxidase catalyzes further oxidation of the molecule, with a loss of six hydrogen atoms, to form protoporphyrin IX. Finally, the insertion of Fe^{2+} by the mitochondrial enzyme ferrochelatase completes the synthesis of heme. The proximity in the mitochondrion of heme (the end product) and ALA synthase (the inducible rate-limiting enzyme) facilitates regulation of porphyrin synthesis. Heme inhibits ALA synthase activity directly and also acts to repress synthesis of the enzyme. The porphyrias are caused by inherited defects in specific enzymes in the heme synthetic pathway. The porphyria associated with each defective step is shown in blue. A partial blockage at any step in the pathway, when combined with certain endogenous or exogenous factors, results in an overproduction of precursors or of products normally produced only in small amounts and is associated with overt clinical disease.

Supportive therapy consists of pain relief with meperidine and phenothiazines and intravenous infusion of glucose at a rate of 10 to 20 g/hr (400 to 500 g/day). Small doses of insulin may be administered for excessive hyperglycemia. Beta blockers have been advocated for the treatment of tachycardia and hypertension. Gabapentin has been used safely for the control of seizures.[7] If rapid symptomatic improvement does not occur within 24 hours or if motor neuropathy is present, heme therapy should be started immediately and vital capacity should be measured at frequent intervals. Because of the risk of death caused by rapidly progressing ventilatory insufficiency, skilled facilities for tracheal intubation and respiratory assistance should be available. Proper management of fluid and electrolyte infusions is necessary to treat hyponatremia. Nasogastric intubation or parenteral nutrition will be required if bulbar symptoms prevent swallowing.

The use of hematin, the ferric hydroxylated form of heme, for patients whose acute attacks do not respond rapidly to other measures is the most important component of therapy.[8] Because heme and hematin are powerful repressors of hepatic ALA synthase and because ALA synthase has a relatively short half-life, plasma and urine levels of ALA and PBG can be markedly reduced within 1 to 2 days, resulting in a prompt reduction of symptoms [see Figure 2]. Established peripheral neuropathies are not reversed immediately, but progression is halted. The dosage of hematin is 1 to 4 mg/kg dissolved in normal saline and given intravenously, preferably through a large peripheral vein or central line, over 20 minutes every 12 or 24 hours.[8] Improvement is usually seen within 2 to 7 days. Occasional instances of coagulopathy associated with prolonged partial thromboplastin time, increased prothrombin time, and fibrinolysis have been reported with hematin infusion.[8] Heme arginate is now available in Europe but not in the United States. It is a much more stable preparation of heme that has excellent efficacy and causes few or no thrombotic effects.

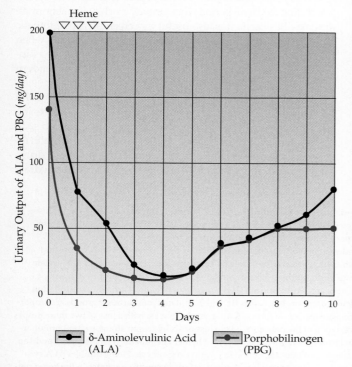

Figure 2 **Response of patients with acute intermittent porphyria to the administration of four doses of heme arginate (3 mg/kg at 12-hour intervals).**[8]

Hematin is also useful when given prophylactically at weekly intervals to women with menstrual exacerbation of AIP. In one study, porphyrin precursor excretion was reduced to near-normal levels and symptoms ceased.[9]

Although oral contraceptives and estrogens increase ALA and PBG excretion and have precipitated attacks, they paradoxically have been useful in some patients by inhibiting menstrual exacerbation of AIP. Injection of a luteinizing hormone–releasing hormone analogue to inhibit acute attacks associated with menses has also been utilized. Although pregnancy may be complicated by AIP, symptomatic attacks are rare. Prophylaxis and treatment are the same as those outlined above.

The prognosis for patients with AIP is probably better than the older medical literature suggests. With the advent of the erythrocyte PBGD assay and DNA analysis, it is clear that there are many more patients with AIP than had been assumed from clinical information. Avoidance of unnecessary surgery and noxious medications [see Table 1] diminishes the likelihood of an acute attack. If attacks do occur, sophisticated methods of intensive care for respiratory failure and pneumonia increase the chance of survival. Finally, prompt use of hematin therapy should abort acute attacks before paralysis occurs. When full support and continuous respiratory assistance are required, hematin therapy is less effective and the prognosis is poor.

Variegate Porphyria

VP (also known as South African porphyria because of its frequency in the South African white population) is rarer than AIP in the United States. It is attributed to a 50% reduction of protoporphyrinogen oxidase (PPOX) and leads to overproduction of protoporphyrinogen, coproporphyrinogen, and uroporphyrinogen (in descending quantitative order) and increased excretion of their corresponding porphyrins. Protoporphyrin, which is the least hydrophilic, is excreted by the liver and partially reabsorbed in the gut. It must be sought in feces, where it is elevated in 95% of cases. Plasma protoporphyrin assays may be even more sensitive.[10] Coproporphyrin is found in both feces and urine. During acute attacks, ALA and PBG are excreted in abnormal quantities in the urine, and the Watson-Schwartz test gives positive results. During remissions, ALA and PBG excretion may be normal. Increased excretion of these early intermediates indicates induction of ALAS. Because the deficient enzyme PPOX is situated in mitochondria, mature red blood cells cannot be used for enzymatic assay. Normoblasts, leukocytes, skeletal muscle, and other tissues have been studied to define the biochemical abnormality. The gene for this human enzyme has now been cloned.[10]

The presence of increased levels of circulating porphyrins predisposes patients to skin lesions. Typically, lesions appear in sun-exposed areas. Blisters as well as superficial ulcers in various stages of healing and scarring are present. Mechanical fragility is common, especially at sites of bony protuberances such as knuckles and ankles. Mild hypertrichosis of the face and temples is seen. Photosensitivity lesions can develop in patients with VP and other cutaneous porphyrias while they are indoors, because the Soret band (wavelength of 400 to 410 nm) can penetrate ordinary window glass and transparent sunscreens. Skin lesions and neuropathic lesions may occur separately or together. Members of the same kindred may have either or both. Because the skin lesions are identical to those seen in hereditary coproporphyria and PCT, VP must be differentiated from these two conditions. The presence of neuropathic lesions without cutaneous manifestations necessitates differentiation from AIP. When both cutaneous and neuropathic lesions occur in a person or a kindred, hereditary coproporphyria or one of the dual porphyrias should be considered in the differential diagnosis.

Biochemical differentiation rests on the fact that VP is caused by a partial enzyme block distal to hepatic protoporphyrinogen synthesis. Therefore, excess protoporphyrin (levels greater than those of coproporphyrin) is present in the stool. In contrast, AIP and hereditary coproporphyria are caused by enzymatic defects proximal to protoporphyrinogen and are therefore associated with normal or near-normal levels of stool protoporphyrin. Patients should avoid eating red meat before and during fecal collections, and stool should be tested for occult blood to exclude confusion with heme-derived protoporphyrin.

The precipitating factors, principles of prophylaxis, and treatment of VP are the same as those for AIP. The absence of a readily accessible assay for the defective enzyme in VP makes it necessary to obtain urine and stool samples from family members and to offer genetic counseling. Negative tests should not be considered definitive unless the family member has reached puberty. The treatment of skin lesions is discussed elsewhere [see Erythropoietic Porphyrias, below].

Hereditary Coproporphyria

Even less common among the hepatic porphyrias is HCP. It is inherited as an autosomal dominant trait caused by diminished activity of coproporphyrinogen oxidase, leading to overproduction of coproporphyrin (predominantly coproporphyrin III) and its precursors. Like AIP and VP, HCP is exacerbated both chemically and clinically by induction of ALAS. The gene has been cloned, and 10 mutations as well as several neutral polymorphisms have been isolated.[11] Two cases were phenotypically homozygous (10% enzyme activity versus 50% in usual cases).[12]

When symptoms occur, increased levels of ALA and PBG are present in the urine, producing a positive Watson-Schwartz test. Coproporphyrin levels in both urine and stool are elevated. There also may be small increases in stool protoporphyrin levels (although coproporphyrin levels are higher), but these are considerably lower than in VP. Modestly increased urine coproporphyrin alone is a nonspecific finding and is seen in hepatic, hematologic, and toxic conditions.

The symptomatic spectrum of HCP is indistinguishable from that of VP; it also overlaps with the pain and neuropathy seen in AIP and the skin lesions of PCT. The decrease in coproporphyrinogen oxidase activity can be detected in lymphocytes by specialized laboratories. Values are usually 50% of normal in patients older than 1 year.

Treatment and prophylaxis for HCP are the same as those for VP and AIP. The response to drugs is also the same [see Table 1].

ALA Dehydratase Deficiency (Plumboporphyria)

The least common form of hepatic porphyria is caused by a partial deficiency of hepatic ALAD, which converts ALA to PBG. Because ALAD is also inhibited by lead (in Latin, plumbum), this disorder is also called plumboporphyria. Only four cases have been reported. The ALAD gene has two promoter exons—one that is erythroid specific and one that is a ubiquitous or housekeeping site—an arrangement analogous to that of PBGD, allowing independent control of hemoglobin synthesis by erythroid cells in response to hematologic needs. In the normal liver, ALAD is present in 80- to 100-fold excess over the rate-limiting enzyme ALAS, and a 50% reduction (heterozygous) would not be clinically apparent. This disorder is inherited as an autosomal recessive disorder, with ALAD activity reduced to 1% to 2% of normal.[13] It is marked by increased urinary excretion of ALA but not PBG. Therefore, despite typical neurovisceral symptoms (neurologic manifestations and abdominal pain), the usual screening tests for PBG (the Watson-Schwartz and Hoesch tests) are negative and a quantitative assay of 24-hour urinary levels of ALA is required. Lead poisoning and familial tyrosinemia should be excluded in the differential diagnosis. Treatment of ALAD deficiency is the same as that of AIP.

Dual Porphyrias

When more than one enzyme in the biosynthetic sequence is affected within a single kindred, a person in the kindred may have a dual porphyria, which is characterized by a mixed profile of porphyrin excretion. In the case of so-called Chester porphyria,[14,15] members of one family were shown to have defects both in PBGD (mapped to chromosome 11) and in PPOX (chromosome 1), manifested as coincidental AIP and VP, respectively. Although no photosensitivity occurred, neurovisceral symptoms were present. The pattern of porphyrin excretion varied among different family members.

There have been reports of other families with dual porphyrias that involved cutaneous and neurovisceral manifestations compatible with coexisting AIP and PCT[16] and coexisting VP and PCT.[17] It is likely that dual porphyrias are more common than has been thought.

PORPHYRIA CUTANEA TARDA

PCT is the most common of the porphyrias. In contrast to the other hepatic porphyrias, PCT is far more commonly sporadic (type I) than familial. It is more common among men than women. Approximately one fifth of cases appear to be familial (type II).

PCT is caused by partial (> 50%) loss of activity of hepatic uroporphyrinogen decarboxylase (UROD). In type I (nongenetic) PCT, UROD dysfunction is limited to the liver. Lesions are caused by overproduction and excretion of uroporphyrin. Sporadic PCT has developed after exposure to estrogens or exogenous chemicals; one large outbreak was traced to consumption of grain contaminated with hexachlorobenzene, a fungicide. PCT is usually associated with alcoholic liver disease, iron overload, or, in rare instances, hepatoma. Recently, an association with hepatitis C has emerged. Antibodies to hepatitis C virus (HCV) have been found in 60% to 80% of nonfamilial cases; however, this association varies with the local prevalence of HCV infection. The prevalence of hepatitis B virus (HBV) antibodies is much lower in the same populations.[18] Clinical and diagnostic features are listed [see Table 3]. Because ALAS is not induced, excretion of ALA and PBG is normal, the Watson-Schwartz test is negative, and there are no acute neuropathic symptoms.

In the familial form of PCT (type II), inherited as an autosomal dominant trait, there is a ubiquitous 50% reduction in the activity of UROD in both erythroid and hepatic tissue. This finding is compatible with the inheritance of a single defective gene. The human UROD gene has been mapped, and 10 mutations have been defined.[19] Clinical expression is variable, and most cases are latent. The offspring of two heterozygotes may be phenotypically homozygous, with severe manifestations beginning in early childhood [see Hepatoerythropoietic Porphyria, below].

The presence of elevated blood and tissue levels of uroporphyrin induces photosensitivity. The skin lesions of PCT are the same as those observed in both VP and HCP. Their onset is usually gradual. PCT can be chemically distinguished from VP and HCP

Table 3 Clinical and Diagnostic Features of Porphyria Cutanea Tarda

Feature or Finding	Percentage of Patients (Size of Sample)	Feature or Finding	Percentage of Patients (Size of Sample)
General Characteristics		*Symptoms*	
Male preponderance	75 (654)	Photoenhanced mechanical dermatosis[††]	100 (689)
Age at onset (yr)		Vesicles/bullae	89 (156)
0–9	0	Hyperpigmentation	79 (152)
10–19	4	Hypertrichosis	75 (156)
20–29	14	Prominent scarring	33 (40)
30–39	20 } (87)	Sclerodermoid changes	21 (58)
40–49	22	Dystrophic calcification with ulceration	8 (40)
50–59	36	*Physical Signs*	
60–69	4	Hepatomegaly	27 (176)
Positive family history*	21 (178)	*Porphyrin Excretion*	
Precipitating Factors of Acute Attack[†]		Urine	
Alcohol abuse	58 (267)	Increased uroporphyrin (> 35 μg/L)[‡‡]	100 (344)
Estrogens[‡]	25 (143)	Increased total porphyrin (> 150 μg/24 hr)	100 (64)
Liver disease[§]	22 (84)	Increased coproporphyrin (> 250 μg/L)	81 (255)
Unknown	13 (168)	Increased δ-aminolevulinic acid (> 3 mg/L)	9 (64)
Hepatoma[‖]	3 (40)	Increased porphobilinogen (> 3 mg/L)	3 (112)
Drugs[¶]	2 (56)	Feces	
Associated Disorders		Increased coproporphyrin (> 20 μg/g dry weight)	65 (81)
Hepatitis C	73	Increased protoporphyrin (> 55 μg/g dry weight)	32 (68)
Cholecystopathy	18 (60)	*Special Laboratory Studies*	
Diabetes mellitus	15 (190)	Decreased hepatic uroporphyrinogen decarboxylase activity (< 20 pmol coproporphyrinogen/min/mg protein)	85 (13)
Tuberculosis	15 (74)	Abnormal glucose tolerance test	42 (71)
Neoplastic disease[#]	8 (138)	Positive for antinuclear antibody[§§]	38 (26)
Collagen vascular disease**	8 (40)	*Abnormal Histology on Liver Biopsy[‖‖]*	100 (155)
Hepatoma	3 (40)	Siderosis	81 (171)
Abnormal Liver Function Tests	94 (133)	Fluorescent porphyrin pigment	65 (48)
Increased saturation of TIBC (> 50%)	70 (27)	Cirrhosis	12 (164)
Increased serum iron (> 200 μg/dl)	54 (136)		
Increased TIBC (> 400 μg/dl)	29 (121)		
Increased serum bilirubin	10 (211)		

TIBC—total iron-binding capacity
*Cutaneous manifestations in at least one family member.
[†]Data do not include 348 cases caused by hexachlorobenzene-contaminated grain reported by Cam and Nigogosyan (JAMA 183:18, 1963).
[‡]Oral estrogens for contraception, postmenopausal hormone replacement therapy, or prostatic carcinoma treatment.
[§]Viral hepatitis or cryptogenic cirrhosis.
[‖]Data do not include eight cases associated with hepatoma found in the literature by Keczkes and Barker (Arch Dermatol 122:78, 1976).
[¶]Polychlorinated hydrocarbons such as dichlorophenyltrichloroethane.

[#]Carcinoma of the breast, colon, lung, prostate, rectum, or thyroid; does not include hepatoma.
**Systemic lupus erythematosus or dermatomyositis.
[††]A seasonal cutaneous vulnerability (a slight mechanical blow is sufficient to cause dermal-epidermal separation) of sun-exposed skin, especially the dorsa of the hands; often considered part of the definition of porphyria cutanea tarda.
[‡‡]Considered part of the definition of porphyria cutanea tarda.
[§§]Usually in a so-called speckled pattern at low titer.
[‖‖]Data may be biased because patients with more severe symptoms are more likely to be biopsied.

by the preponderance of uroporphyrin instead of coproporphyrin in the urine and the absence of marked elevation of protoporphyrin levels in the stool.

Evidence of excess iron stores is found in 60% to 85% of patients and is severe in 20%. Recent studies found hemochromatosis-related mutations in 44% and 73% of patients with sporadic (type I) PCT.[20,21] Nevertheless, overt PCT in hemochromatosis is uncommon. Iron is thought to play a central role in this disease by causing the formation of reactive oxygen radicals, which oxidize uroporphyrinogen to uroporphyrin and generate other products that irreversibly inactivate UROD. Familial (type II) cases with genetically determined UROD deficiency are vulnerable to the same mechanism.

The cornerstone of therapy for all cases of PCT is depletion of iron, even in patients lacking biochemical evidence of iron overload. Repeated phlebotomy of one unit of blood twice monthly for a total of 5 to 10 L, with treatment guided by the patient's hematocrit and ferritin levels, decreases both uroporphyrin excretion and photosensitivity. Improvement occurs within several months to a year. Patients who are on hemodialysis or who are anemic should receive erythropoietin. For patients who cannot tolerate phlebotomy, subcutaneous infusion of deferoxamine by portable syringe pump (1.0 to 1.5 g in 8 to 10 ml of sterile water for 8 to 10 hours 5 nights a week for 2 to 5 months) is effective.[22] Avoidance of sunlight, alcohol, iron, and estrogens is equally important.

Chloroquine, which forms complexes with uroporphyrin, has produced improvement over 3 to 6 months. Hepatotoxicity may occur. Resolution of type I PCT has followed successful interferon therapy for HCV infection.[23] Treatment of photosensitivity with β-carotene may be tried; however, results have been erratic [see Erythropoietic Porphyrias, *below*]. Uroporphyrin excretion should be monitored at 6- to 12-month intervals after remission to determine the need for additional courses of therapy.

Erythropoietic Porphyrias

Two porphyrias are caused by major enzymatic abnormalities in the erythropoietic system: congenital erythropoietic porphyria and erythropoietic protoporphyria, the latter of which also involves a defect in hepatic cells. In contrast to porphyrin synthesis in the liver, porphyrin synthesis in the erythropoietic system is responsive to changes in red blood cell mass and levels of tissue oxygenation. Therefore, anemia, hypoxia, and erythropoietin are important regulators of heme (and hemoglobin) production. Only the reticulocytes and their precursors in the bone marrow are responsive to these stimuli. Mature red blood cells, which lack mitochondria and a nucleus, no longer possess the complete machinery for porphyrin synthesis.

CONGENITAL ERYTHROPOIETIC PORPHYRIA

CEP, also called Günther's disease, is extremely rare. It is inherited as an autosomal recessive trait. The enzymatic basis for this disorder is a severe deficit (< 1% to 36%) of uroporphyrinogen III synthase, the enzyme catalyzing the synthesis of the asymmetrical uroporphyrinogen III molecule from the linear tetrapyrrole hydroxymethylbilane. The human gene has been sequenced, and at least 18 mutations have been identified.[24]

CEP causes accumulation of uroporphyrinogen I and coproporphyrinogen I; these isomers are not intermediates in heme synthesis. Oxidation of these products to their respective porphyrins, uroporphyrin I and coproporphyrin I, begins in the fetus. Excess porphyrin causes staining of bones and teeth (erythrodontia), hemolysis, dark urine, and photosensitivity, all of which are usually identified early in infancy. The most dramatic findings are related to repeated vesiculation, scarring, and mutilation, which follow exposure to sunlight. These late changes may be mistaken for scleroderma. Alopecia, conjunctivitis, corneal inflammation, and keratomalacia are additional findings. Bone deformities, attributed to the toxic effects of porphyrin deposition in bone and perhaps to rickets secondary to avoidance of sunlight, are sometimes present. Hemolytic anemia is common and is often accompanied by splenomegaly. Hypersplenism with leukopenia and thrombocytopenia may occur. Severity is a function of the residual activity and stability of the mutated enzyme. Most cases are compound heterozygotes.[24]

Fluorescence of teeth as well as of red blood cells and their precursors in the blood and bone marrow can be demonstrated by irradiation at Soret band wavelengths. As with other photosensitive porphyrias, window glass and conventional ultraviolet sunscreens are ineffective in blocking the offending wavelengths. Suppression of erythropoiesis and uroporphyrin I production can be achieved by transfusion and, when hemolysis is present, by splenectomy. Avoidance of sunlight and intense artificial light and topical care for skin lesions is required.

Oral sorbents such as cholestyramine and charcoal have been demonstrated to decrease intestinal reabsorption of porphyrins.[25] Even with treatment, progressive mutilation and premature death frequently occur. Bone marrow transplantation has been successful in reversing the metabolic defect in four patients.[24] Transduction of human CEP hematopoietic progenitor cells has been accomplished in vitro, suggesting that ex vivo gene therapy can be developed.[24,26]

HEPATOERYTHROPOIETIC PORPHYRIA

As noted above, patients with genetically determined (type II) PCT are typically heterozygous, and the condition is usually latent. Homozygous (or compound heterozygote) offspring will demonstrate a marked deficiency of UROD, manifested by severe photosensitivity beginning early in childhood. Approximately 30 cases have been reported.[19] Lesions are caused by accumulation and widespread deposition of uroporphyrin III and mimic those caused by CEP (see above). Patients rarely respond to phlebotomy or chloroquine.

ERYTHROPOIETIC PROTOPORPHYRIA

Because erythropoietic protoporphyria (EPP) involves overproduction of protoporphyrin by red blood cells and liver cells, it has also been referred to by two other terms: protoporphyria and erythrohepatic porphyria. Inherited as an autosomal dominant trait, it is attributed to partial absence of the mitochondrial enzyme ferrochelatase (heme synthase), which binds Fe^{2+} to protoporphyrin IX. Complementary DNA encoding human ferrochelatase has been isolated, and only one form of the enzyme is expressed in both erythroid and nonerythroid tissues, in contrast to PBG deaminase. The ratio of ferrochelatase to ALAS activity (the rate-limiting step) is 2.6:1 in erythroid cells, whereas it is 500:1 in liver; therefore, reduction of ferrochelatase function is expressed initially and primarily as an erythroid disorder.[27] Protoporphyria is not associated with increased urinary excretion of porphyrins, ALA, or PBG. Levels of fecal protoporphyrin are often, but not regularly, increased.

The major feature of this disorder is photosensitivity, caused by increased levels of plasma protoporphyrin resulting from overproduction by hepatocytes as well as by erythrocyte precursors. Although erythrocyte protoporphyrin is also increased in iron deficiency anemia and lead intoxication, protoporphyrin is bound to zinc in these two conditions and does not diffuse into plasma and tissues, so that photosensitivity does not occur.

In contrast to the hepatic porphyrias, protoporphyria usually occurs in children younger than 4 years and is more common in males. Symptoms are acutely precipitated by sunlight and may be limited to burning and itching, often accompanied by edema, erythema, or urticaria. Less frequently, blisters and ulcers occur. Excoriations secondary to scratching may be present. Recurrence of these lesions as a result of chronic sun exposure creates scarring, altered pigmentation, lichenification, and premature aging of the skin.

Protoporphyrin is also deposited in the liver. Although mild liver function abnormalities are the rule, cirrhosis, hepatosplenomegaly, and death from liver failure have also been reported. Liver decompensation progressively diminishes biliary protoporphyrin excretion, worsening both cutaneous and hepatic lesions. Gallstones containing protoporphyrin are seen in some patients, and a mild hypochromic, microcytic anemia is found in almost half. Some hemolysis may also be present. A more severe form of protoporphyria occurs if both parents are heterozygous and the offspring inherit two defective genes. Twenty-two mutations have been identified; most carriers are asymptomatic.[28]

Diagnosis is suggested by the combination of history and familial occurrence and is confirmed by increased levels of fecal and erythrocyte protoporphyrin. Erythrocytes or normoblasts fluoresce on exposure to the Soret band.

Avoidance of sunlight to prevent irreversible scarring is desirable but difficult. Ingestion of β-carotene, with the aim of reaching blood levels of 500 μg/dl, diminishes photosensitivity. The effects of treatment may take months. Because hepatic protoporphyrin synthesis may also contribute to the clinical picture, a high-carbohydrate diet may be of value, even though the acute neuropathic attacks characteristic of AIP do not occur in this disorder.

In one patient, oral iron therapy reduced protoporphyrin levels in stool and erythrocytes.[29] Resolution of anemia and improved liver function test results occurred within 4 months. It was postulated that heme production was increased either nonenzymatically or by the action of residual ferrochelatase. Heme formation in turn could have caused the protoporphyrin concentration to be reduced to a less toxic level while repressing ALAS production and reducing porphyrin synthesis.[29]

Liver transplantation for protoporphyrin-induced cirrhosis has been utilized with some good results but with high morbidity, including burns from operating room lights and recurrence of protoporphyric liver disease.[28,30]

Additional Information

Additional information regarding physician and laboratory resources as well as patient-oriented information can be obtained from the American Porphyria Foundation Web site at http://www.enterprise.net/apf. The American Porphyria Foundation charges a nominal fee to access their site.

References

1. Moore MR: Biochemistry of porphyria. Int J Biochem 25:1353, 1993

2. Puy H, Deybach JC, Lamoril J, et al: Molecular epidemiology and diagnosis of PBG deaminase gene defects in acute intermittent porphyria. Am J Hum Genet 60:1373, 1997

3. McDonagh AF, Bissell DM: Porphyria and porphyrinology—the past fifteen years. Semin Liver Dis 18:3, 1998

4. Grandchamp B: Acute intermittent porphyria. Semin Liver Dis 18:17, 1998

5. Chretien S, Dubart A, Beaupain D, et al: Alternative transcription and splicing of the human porphobilinogen deaminase gene result either in tissue-specific or in housekeeping expression. Proc Natl Acad Sci U S A 85:6, 1988

6. Mustajoki P, Kauppinen R, Lannfelt L, et al: Frequency of low erythrocyte porphobilinogen deaminase activity in Finland. J Intern Med 231:389, 1992

7. Tatum WO IV, Zachariah SB: Gabapentin treatment of seizures in acute intermittent porphyria. Neurology 45:1216, 1995

8. Tenhunen R, Mustajoki P: Acute porphyria: treatment with heme. Semin Liver Dis 18:53, 1998

9. Mustajoki P, Nordmann Y: Early administration of heme arginate for acute porphyric attacks. Arch Intern Med 153:2004, 1993

10. Kirsch RE, Meissner PN, Hift RJ: Variegate porphyria. Semin Liver Dis 18:33, 1998

11. Martasek P: Hereditary coproporphyria. Semin Liver Dis 18:25, 1998

12. Grandchamp B, Lamoril J, Puy H: Molecular abnormalities of coproporphyrinogen oxidase in patients with hereditary coproporphyria. J Bioenerg Biomembr 27:215, 1995

13. Sassa S: ALAD porphyria. Semin Liver Dis 18:95, 1998

14. McColl KEL, Thompson GG, Moore MR, et al: Chester porphyria: biochemical studies of a new form of acute porphyria. Lancet 2:796, 1985

15. Norton B, Lanyon WG, Moore MR, et al: Evidence for involvement of a second genetic locus on chromosome 11q in porphyrin metabolism. Hum Genet 91:576, 1993

16. Doss MO: New form of dual porphyria: coexistent acute intermittent porphyria and porphyria cutanea tarda. Eur J Clin Invest 19:20, 1989

17. Sturrock ED, Meissner PN, Maeder DL, et al: Uroporphyrinogen decarboxylase and protoporphyrinogen oxidase in dual porphyria. S Afr Med J 76:405, 1989

18. Conry-Cantilena C, Vilamidou L, Melpolder JC, et al: Porphyria cutanea tarda in hepatitis C virus–infected blood donors. J Am Acad Dermatol 32:512, 1995

19. Elder GH: Hepatic porphyrias in children. J Inher Metab Dis 20:237, 1997

20. Roberts AG, Whatley SD, Morgan RR, et al: Increased frequency of the haemochromatosis Cys282Tyr mutation in sporadic porphyria cutanea tarda. Lancet 349:321, 1997

21. Bonkovsky HL, Poh-Fitzpatrick M, Pimstone N, et al: Porphyria cutanea tarda, hepatitis C, and HFE gene mutations in North America. Hepatology 27:1661, 1998

22. Gibertini P, Rocchi E, Cassanelli A, et al: Advances in the treatment of porphyria cutanea tarda: effectiveness of slow subcutaneous desferrioxamine infusion. Liver 4:280, 1984

23. Sheikh MY, Wright RA, Burruss JB: Dramatic resolution of skin lesions associated with porphyria cutanea tarda after interferon-alpha therapy in a case of chronic hepatitis C. Dig Dis Sci 43:529, 1998

24. Desnick RJ, Glass IA, Xu W, et al: Molecular genetics of congenital erythropoietic porphyria. Semin Liver Dis 18:77, 1998

25. Pimstone NR, Gandhi SN, Mukerji SK: Therapeutic efficacy of oral charcoal in congenital erythropoietic porphyria. N Engl J Med 316:390, 1987

26. Mazurier F, Moreau-Gaudry F, Salesse S, et al: Gene transfer of the uroporphyrinogen III synthase cDNA into haematopoietic progenitor cells in view of a future gene therapy in congenital erythropoietic porphyria. J Inherit Metab Dis 20:247, 1997

27. Taketani S, Fujita H: The ferrochelatase gene structure and molecular defects associated with erythropoietic protoporphyria. J Bioenerg Biomembr 27:231, 1995

28. Cox TM, Alexander GJ, Sarkany RP: Protoporphyria. Semin Liver Dis 18:85, 1998

29. Gordeuk VR, Brittenham GM, Hawkins CW, et al: Iron therapy for hepatic dysfunction in erythropoietic protoporphyria. Ann Intern Med 105:27, 1986

30. Bloomer JR, Rank JM, Payne WD, et al: Follow-up after liver transplantation for protoporphyric liver disease. Liver Transpl Surg 2:269, 1996

Acknowledgments

Figure 1   Dana Burns-Pizer.

Figure 2   Marcia Kammerer.

Tables 2 and 3   Prepared for *Scientific American Medicine* by Mark G. Perlroth, M.D., and Robert Hagberg, M.S.

GASTROENTEROLOGY

56 Esophageal Disorders

Harvey S. Young, M.D.

Relatively few diseases involve the esophagus, and to a remarkable extent, their presence and underlying nature can be inferred from the patient's history alone. Careful interrogation about complaints related to swallowing, therefore, often leads to rapid diagnosis and the opportunity for specific treatment.

Dysphagia

Dysphagia is a common symptom in some stage of all disorders of the esophagus. Dysphagia can be defined simply as difficulty swallowing and passing food from the mouth via the esophagus to the stomach. To obtain the proper history from a patient who may have dysphagia, the physician should ask what the patient experiences when attempting to initiate a swallow. Does the food move to the back of the oral cavity? Can a swallow be initiated? Is the patient aware of the food moving down into the thorax and then to the abdomen? Is there a painful sensation? Does the food seem to lodge, even temporarily, at a particular site? Because of the sensation of something lodging in the throat or thorax, patients may have a concomitant sensation of mild to intense pain, called odynophagia. In contrast to true dysphagia, the nonorganic disorder of globus hystericus is a sensation of a mass or lump in the throat at all times, regardless of whether a swallow is occurring.

Patients with esophageal dysphagia have no difficulty initiating a swallow, but they experience a sensation of food sticking or lodging in the neck or thorax. Early in the course of the dysphagia, the patient may perceive only a transient delay in the passage of food; but as the disease advances, symptoms become more pronounced. The patient can usually locate the point at which the food lodges, and a lesion can usually be identified at that site. However, 20% to 30% of patients with upper esophageal lesions perceive dysphagia in the lower substernal region, and vice versa.

ETIOLOGY

The most commonly encountered disorders of the esophagus are benign peptic stricture, esophageal ring, esophageal spasm, and carcinoma [*see Table 1*]. A presumptive diagnosis can usually be made from the patient's history alone [*see Figure 1*]. For instance, benign stricture typically produces dysphagia during the course of chronic peptic esophagitis. Patients with benign stricture frequently have severe burning pain over the sternum, associated with regurgitation of small amounts of gastric contents into the mouth. Heartburn responds only transiently to antacids and typically occurs for a few years before dysphagia is first noted.

An esophageal ring may be found in 5% to 10% of adults who are examined with an upper intestinal x-ray series, but it is usually not associated with any symptoms. When symptoms do occur, they are typically intermittent, transient, and nonprogressive. They tend to be more severe when the patient is anxious and is eating rapidly.

Spastic disorders of the esophagus appear at any age. Unlike the dysphagia seen with peptic stricture or carcinoma, the dysphagia associated with spastic disorders is intermittent and progresses slowly (over several years); only on a few occasions do patients experience severe sticking, and pain may occur when solid food or even liquids are swallowed.

Esophageal carcinoma usually leads to the insidious onset of the sensation of food sticking under the sternum. There may be an associated lancinating sensation, especially if acidic nutrients such as citrus juices are ingested. Patients with adenocarcinoma of the esophagus often have history of reflux.[1,2] Weight loss occurs early in the course of the disease. A significant number of patients with esophageal squamous cell carcinoma ingest large quantities of alcohol or smoke tobacco heavily.

DIAGNOSTIC AIDS

Despite the essential role of the patient's history in the diagnosis of esophageal diseases, diagnostic procedures must be carried out to establish the diagnosis.

Endoscopy

Endoscopic examination of the esophagus is a standard test used in the diagnosis and management of esophageal disorders. Endoscopy not only produces high-resolution images of the esophageal mucosa but also allows biopsy that provides definitive tissue diagnosis. In addition, endoscopically guided therapies, such as dilation and stent placement, provide immediate symptomatic relief for patients with most esophageal obstructions.

Barium X-ray

Barium sulfate contrast examination of the esophagus is essential in all cases of dysphagia. Distinct abnormalities characteristic of each clinical entity can be found when the examination is done properly.[3] Solid material—such as a half slice of bread or a marshmallow added to the barium solution—or a barium tablet often evokes symptoms of dysphagia and simultaneously localizes the anatomic site of blockage.

The modified barium technique is particularly useful in patients with diffuse spasm who have high-amplitude, nonpropulsive contractions that may produce dysphagia and lodging of food in the absence of a fixed structural narrowing of the esophageal wall. In these cases, a standard barium swallow study may reveal no abnormality.

Table 1   Etiologies of Dysphagia

Esophageal dysphagia	Oropharyngeal dysphagia
Neuromuscular disorders	Neuromuscular disorders
Achalasia	Cerebrovascular accident
Spastic motility disorders (diffuse esophageal spasm, nutcracker esophagus, hypertensive lower esophageal sphincter)	Parkinson disease
	Multiple sclerosis
	Amyotrophic lateral sclerosis
Scleroderma and other collagen vascular diseases	Brain stem lesions
	Myasthenia gravis
	Muscular dystrophies
Chagas disease	Upper esophageal sphincter spasm
Mechanical lesions	Cricopharyngeal achalasia
Peptic stricture	
Mucosal (Schatzki) ring	Mechanical lesions
Tumor	Tumor
Webs and diverticula	Web
Mediastinal lesions	Cricopharyngeal bar
Vascular compression	Zenker diverticulum

709

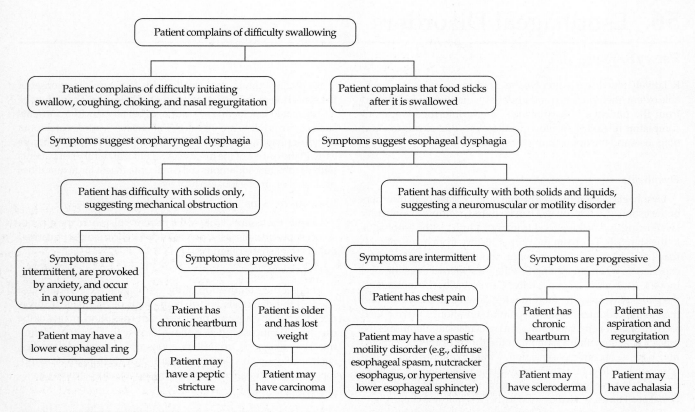

Figure 1   **The evaluation of dysphagia. A presumptive diagnosis can usually be made from the patient's history alone, and diagnostic tests can then be used to establish the definitive diagnosis. The tests used in the evaluation of oropharyngeal dysphagia are cineradiography and upper esophageal sphincter manometry; those used in the evaluation of esophageal dysphagia are endoscopy, barium radiography, 24-hour pH monitoring, and esophageal manometry.[98]**

Cineradiography

Cineradiography, the process of radiographic videotape recording, is a crucial test for evaluation of oropharyngeal dysphagia because it permits frame-by-frame analysis of the complex oropharyngeal swallowing motion. When the patient is given barium-coated foods of different consistencies during the examination, the types of food that produce the least amount of functional impairment can be determined.[4]

Scintigraphy

Esophageal emptying can be measured by scintigraphy with a radioactive liquid or solid bolus. Reflux scintigraphy was once considered to be a sensitive diagnostic tool for gastroesophageal reflux, but its accuracy has not been substantiated in recent studies.[5,6]

Acid Perfusion Test

Perfusion of 0.1N (decinormal) hydrochloric acid solution via a nasoesophageal tube (placed 30 cm from the incisor teeth) has been used to establish the diagnosis of esophagitis. This test has a high specificity but a low sensitivity.[5] With the advent of endoscopy and ambulatory pH monitoring (see below), the use of the acid perfusion test has declined.

Ambulatory Esophageal pH Monitoring

The reflux of acidic gastric contents into the esophageal lumen can be directly monitored by use of a thin pH probe inserted through the nose and placed 5 cm above the lower esophageal sphincter. Computed ambulatory 24-hour pH measurement has been advocated as the definitive diagnostic test for gastroesopha-

geal reflux.[7] In this test, the diagnostic criteria for reflux are a composite symptom score and the percentage of total time when the esophageal pH is less than 4; sensitivity, specificity, and accuracy are all greater than 95%.[8] For most patients with esophagitis, symptoms are typical, and pH monitoring is not necessary. Ambulatory pH monitoring is indicated in patients with atypical reflux symptoms, however (see below), as well as in patients who have typical symptoms but are refractory to standard therapy and have no evidence of esophagitis on endoscopy.

Esophageal Manometry

Esophageal manometry is essential in evaluating patients with motor disorders of the esophagus. It is also useful in the preoperative evaluation of patients undergoing surgery for gastroesophageal reflux.[9] As many as 10% of these patients have poor esophageal peristalsis, which allows only a subtotal fundoplication (a wrap of less than 360°) to be performed.[10] Modern manometric equipment has standardized manometric measurements of the lower esophageal sphincter and of esophageal body function. However, manometric measurement of the upper esophageal sphincter remains a technical challenge and is currently used only in research.[11]

Specific Esophageal Diseases

REFLUX ESOPHAGITIS

Reflux esophagitis is a common clinical problem; indeed, about 25% of healthy persons experience the symptoms of heartburn at least once a month.[12] Gastric infection with *Helicobacter pylori* may be somewhat protective against reflux esophagitis, and successful

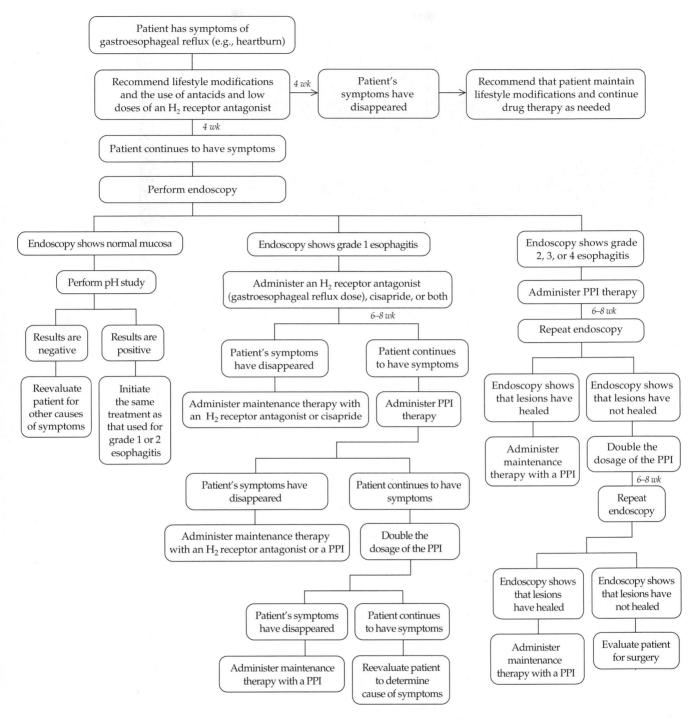

Figure 2 **Algorithm for the management of reflux esophagitis. On endoscopy, grade 1 esophagitis is characterized by erythema and friability, grade 2 by linear erosions, grade 3 by confluent ulcerations, and grade 4 by ulceration and stricture. (PPI—proton pump inhibitor)**

treatment of *H. pylori* infection appears to exacerbate or cause reflux esophagitis.[13-15] The vast majority of those who seek medical treatment respond satisfactorily to intermittent courses of antacid or over-the-counter H_2 receptor antagonist therapy, though a small but significant minority (about 5% to 10%) have severe, persistent symptoms of heartburn. The distress usually begins 1 hour or more after meals and frequently recurs within an hour despite the use of antacids. Often, there is regurgitation of small quantities of gastric contents into the mouth. Regurgitation during

sleep is hazardous because of the danger of aspiration and resultant pneumonia. Atypical presentations may include noncardiac chest pain; dysphagia without esophageal obstruction; and symptoms such as hoarseness, sore throat, frequent clearing of the throat, gingivitis, and asthma that are caused by damage to the larynx, oropharynx, or respiratory tract.[12] Hiatal hernia is another risk factor for reflux esophagitis (see below).[16]

The essential diagnostic feature is the presence of an intermittent substernal burning sensation that can be readily relieved by antacids. In patients with severe or stubborn symptoms, esophagoscopy and biopsy should be performed to confirm the diagnosis. However, the esophageal mucosa may appear normal in about 30% of patients with reflux esophagitis. In such patients, it may also be difficult to detect any subtle histologic changes in endoscopic biopsy specimens that would support a diagnosis of reflux esophagitis[17]; ambulatory 24-hour pH monitoring is helpful in confirming the diagnosis.

The treatment of gastroesophageal reflux includes elimination of foods and agents that decrease lower esophageal sphincter pressure, such as fatty foods, chocolate, alcohol, and cigarettes [see Figure 2]. Weight reduction and nocturnal postural drainage, facilitated by elevation of the head of the bed, are often helpful.[18]

Drug therapy for esophagitis is directed at neutralizing gastric acid and preventing gastroesophageal reflux [see Table 2]. Liquid antacids (15 ml four times daily, 1 hour after meals and at bedtime) are effective for transient symptom relief in many patients [see Chapter 57]. Antacids containing alginic acid, which forms a foam barrier at the gastroesophageal junction, may be particularly helpful.[19]

In patients with stubborn symptoms, acid suppression with an H_2 receptor antagonist is often needed [see Chapter 57]. One 6-week course of an H_2 receptor antagonist in a conventional dose is effective in healing the mucosal ulcerations in 60% to 70% of patients with mild to moderate esophagitis.[20] However, the success rate for severe esophagitis is only 20% to 30%.

Sucralfate, which adheres to ulcerated mucosa and protects the underlying tissues from the effects of acid and pepsin, may be beneficial in reflux esophagitis. Although sucralfate was found not to be superior to placebo in one study,[21] it was shown to be comparable to H_2 receptor antagonists in other studies.[22,23]

Cisapride, a prokinetic agent, until recently was used as a single agent and in combination with H_2 receptor antagonists or proton pump inhibitors in the treatment of mild to moderate reflux esophagitis.[24] However, cisapride in combination with other drugs (e.g., antifungals such as ketoconazole, itraconazole, and fluconazole; antibacterials such as erythromycin, clarithromycin, and troleandomycin; and the HIV protease inhibitors ritonavir and indinavir) can prolong ventricular repolarization, resulting in serious ventricular arrhythmias and sudden death.[25] Cisapride alone may result in serious cardiac arrhythmias in patients with heart disease, hypokalemia, or hypomagnesemia and in those with renal, pulmonary, or liver failure.[25] Because of an excessive number of cardiac deaths, cisapride has not been marketed in the United States after July 14, 2000; it will continue to be available for patients meeting certain eligibility criteria under a limited-access protocol controlled by the manufacturer.[26]

For patients with severe esophagitis, potent acid suppression with an 8- or 12-week course of a proton pump inhibitor (omeprazole or lansoprazole) yields a healing rate of about 90%.[27,28]

Patients with reflux esophagitis often have relapses. Patients who do not have erosive esophagitis can be given maintenance therapy with the lowest dose of acid-suppression therapy that provides adequate symptom control.[17] Sucralfate suspension has also been shown to be effective in these patients.[29] Ninety percent of patients with erosive esophagitis have a relapse within 1 year after cessation of therapy. Maintenance with conventional doses of H_2 receptor antagonists or cisapride has failed to reduce this relapse rate,[30] but long-term maintenance with omeprazole at 20 mg/day or lansoprazole at 15 to 30 mg/day reduces the rate to less than 30%.[31] Daily dosing of omeprazole is better than intermittent dosing in preventing relapse.[32] Patients who experience a

Table 2 Drug Therapy for Reflux Esophagitis[99]

Drug	Dosage	Mechanism of Action
Antacids		
Antacid liquid (e.g., Mylanta, Maalox)*	15 ml q.i.d., 1 hr after meals and at bedtime	Buffers HCl
Antacid with alginic acid (e.g., Gaviscon)	2–4 tablets q.i.d., after meals and at bedtime	Provides a viscous mechanical barrier; buffers HCl in esophagus
H_2 receptor antagonists		
Cimetidine	800 mg b.i.d. or 400 mg q.i.d., after meals and at bedtime	Decreases HCl secretion and gastric volume by inhibiting H_2 receptors
Famotidine	20 mg b.i.d.	Decreases HCl secretion and gastric volume by inhibiting H_2 receptors
Nizatidine	150 mg b.i.d.	Decreases HCl secretion and gastric volume by inhibiting H_2 receptors
Ranitidine	150 mg q.i.d.	Decreases HCl secretion and gastric volume by inhibiting H_2 receptors
Prokinetic agents		
Cisapride†	10 mg q.i.d.	Increases LESP and gastric emptying
Metoclopramide	10 mg q.i.d., 30 min before meals and at bedtime	Increases LESP and gastric emptying
Bethanechol	25 mg q.i.d., 30 min before meals and at bedtime	Increases LESP and esophageal acid clearance
Proton pump inhibitors		
Lansoprazole	30 mg/day	Decreases HCl secretion and gastric volume
Omeprazole	20–40 mg/day	Decreases HCl secretion and gastric volume
Sucralfate	1 g q.i.d., 1 hr after meals and at bedtime	Increases tissue resistance, buffers HCL in esophagus, and binds pepsin and bile salts

*Antacid liquids should have an HCl neutralizing capacity of 25 mEq/5 ml. Patients with reflux are generally not hypersecretors of gastric acid. Therefore, therapeutic doses of antacids are based on the agents' capacity to buffer basal HCl secretion of approximately 1–7 mEq/hr (mean, 2 mEq/hr) and peak meal-stimulated HCl secretion of approximately 10–60 mEq/hr (mean, 30 mEq/hr).
†See text for contraindications; not available by prescription after July 14, 2000 (see text).
LESP—lower esophageal sphincter pressure

relapse of erosive esophagitis on 20 mg/day of omeprazole often respond to a dosage of 40 mg/day.

The major concerns regarding long-term use of proton pump inhibitors are the potential side effects associated with chronic hypochlorhydria. These include gastric bacterial overgrowth and hypergastrinemia with resultant enterochromaffin cell hyperplasia. Carcinoid formation has been reported in rats treated with prolonged courses of very high doses of omeprazole,[33] but European studies have failed to demonstrate any carcinogenic effect in patients treated with omeprazole for as long as 6 years.[34] Although persistent elevation of gastrin levels has been observed, only 11% of patients have a gastrin level higher than 500 ng/L.[35] Other reported complications are gastric micronodular hyperplasia (20% of patients) and subatrophic or atrophic gastritis (25%). Long-term omeprazole therapy in patients infected with *H. pylori* increases the risk of atrophic gastritis.[36] Long-term proton pump inhibitor therapy (> 10 years) is both effective and safe.[37]

Patients with persistent severe esophagitis who respond poorly to medical measures are candidates for surgical procedures that create a valvelike mechanism by wrapping a gastric pouch around the distal esophagus. Belsey fundoplication, Nissen fundoplication, Toupet fundoplication, and Hill posterior gastropexy have been effective in eliminating gastroesophageal reflux and may be responsible for a restoration of lower esophageal sphincter pressures to normal levels.[38,39] Nissen fundoplication can now be performed laparoscopically, with a success rate of about 90%.[40] The total cost, duration of hospitalization, and duration of recovery associated with laparoscopic Nissen fundoplication are significantly lower than those associated with open laparotomy.[41,42] Installation of a C-shaped plastic prosthesis (Angelchik prosthesis) around the distal esophagus is seldom done now because of high complication rates.[43] Simple repair of a hiatal hernia is usually ineffective in preventing esophagitis.

There is no clear choice between medical and surgical maintenance therapy for patients with persistent severe esophagitis. Although a Veterans Affairs cooperative study reported that antireflux surgery was superior to a multiagent medical regimen that did not include proton pump inhibitors,[44] further comparison of surgery (e.g., laparoscopic Nissen fundoplication) with long-term potent acid suppression with a proton pump inhibitor is needed.

STRICTURE

Patients with severe reflux esophagitis run the risk of developing a stricture at the distal esophagus, just above the gastroesophageal junction [*see Figure 3*]. The stricture typically has a tapered or spindle-shaped appearance on barium contrast x-rays. Patients in whom strictures develop typically have slowly progressing dysphagia, which is experienced first with solid foods and later with liquids. Unlike carcinoma, the stricture causes gradual disability, and accompanying weight loss is unusual.

It is possible to open a strictured esophagus with tapered, rigid dilators. A local analgesic is applied to the posterior pharynx, and a dilator is then passed through the stricture. The procedure requires progressively greater dilations until a size 40 or 45 French dilator has been passed through the stricture; this usually cannot be achieved in a single session. In patients with tight strictures, the increase in dilator size is kept under 6 French in each session to decrease the risk of perforation. Repeated dilations several days to a week apart may be required before the symptoms of dysphagia are eliminated. Typically, dilations must be repeated every 3 weeks to 12 months. Hydrostatic balloon dilators that can be passed through the endoscope's biopsy channel and wire-guided polyvinyl dilators have gained wide acceptance. They are particularly useful in dilating long and complicated strictures. Fluoroscopic guidance is often needed to prevent complications.[45] Long-term treatment with omeprazole after successful dilation of a peptic stricture will prevent recurrence of the stricture and decrease the need for repeated dilation.[46] If it is impossible to dilate the stricture sufficiently to enable the patient to tolerate solid food or if dilation has to be performed too frequently, surgical intervention is indicated; however, extensive repair is often required to provide permanent relief. After the stricture has been excised, the usual procedure is to pull the stomach into the thorax, though interposition of a segment of small intestine or colon may be necessary in cases of advanced disease.

BARRETT ESOPHAGUS

The condition known as Barrett esophagus occurs when the squamous epithelium in the esophagus is replaced by a metaplastic specialized columnar epithelium that resembles the large intestine and contains goblet cells. This condition is probably caused by chronic gastroesophageal reflux. It is usually seen in patients of 40 to 50 years of age and occurs predominantly in white men, but it is also seen in infants and children. Barrett esophagus is found in about 10% of patients undergoing endoscopic evaluation for gastroesophageal reflux. However, 10% to

a

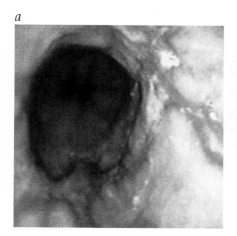

b

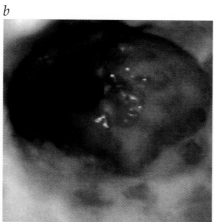

c

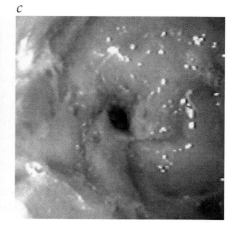

Figure 3 (*a*) In patients with moderately severe esophagitis, circumferential erosions and ulcerations can be seen on endoscopy. In patients with severe esophagitis, confluent ulcerations (*b*) or high-grade stricture at the gastroesophageal junction (*c*) can be seen on endoscopy.

25% of patients with Barrett esophagus are completely asymptomatic. The true prevalence of Barrett esophagus in the general population is still unknown.

On endoscopic examination, Barrett epithelium appears as rosy gastric mucosa extending several centimeters above the gastroesophageal junction into the esophagus [see Figure 4]. However, biopsies that show metaplastic changes are needed to confirm the diagnosis because normal persons and patients with reflux esophagitis may have normal gastric mucosa lining the distal 3 cm of the esophagus.[47] In addition, this metaplastic epithelium may be found in 18% of patients who have gastroesophageal reflux but who have a normal-appearing gastroesophageal junction.[48]

Barrett esophagus is frequently complicated by formation of strictures and ulcers and by bleeding. The condition's established role as a precursor of adenocarcinoma in the esophagus and gastric cardia has evoked particular concern. The median incidence of esophageal adenocarcinoma in patients with Barrett esophagus is about one in 100 patient-years of follow-up.[48] The esophageal cancer risk is about 30 to 40 times greater than that in the general population. However, most patients with Barrett esophagus die of other causes. In a study with a mean duration of 9.3 years of follow-up, only 2.5% of patients with Barrett esophagus died of esophageal carcinoma.[48]

Neoplastic progression in this condition is associated with a process of genomic instability that produces aneuploidy and proliferative abnormalities. The genomic instability produces loss of heterozygosity of several tumor suppressor genes, such as p53 (17q), APC, MCC (5q), DCC (18q), and Rb (13q). Mutation and allelic loss of p53 precede the development of aneuploidy and carcinoma in patients with Barrett esophagus.[49]

Histologically, metaplasia progresses to dysplasia and finally to carcinoma. The time required for this progression is unknown. Endoscopic surveillance for cancer and a vigorous protocol of biopsy are recommended for all patients with Barrett esophagus.[50] If indefinite or low-grade dysplasia is found, follow-up surveillance at 12-month intervals is appropriate. If high-grade dysplasia is detected, endoscopy should be repeated shortly thereafter to define the extent of the dysplasia and to conduct a more intense search for carcinoma. Clearly, esophagectomy should be performed if carcinoma is found. If repeat endoscopy shows only high-grade dysplasia, however, appropriate management is less clearly defined. Therapy must be individualized according to the patient's surgical risk, preferences, and compliance with endoscopic surveillance.[50]

Overall, the efficacy of endoscopic surveillance has not yet been established, and significant interobserver variation in the interpretation of dysplasia exists.[50,51] Long-term prospective studies of the impact of surveillance programs are in progress. In the future, flow cytometry and the techniques of molecular genetics may improve the yield of surveillance programs in patients with Barrett esophagus.

Medical treatment of Barrett esophagus is similar to that of severe esophagitis. Long-term therapy with proton pump inhibitors is generally required. There is no convincing evidence to suggest that any long-term medical therapy or antireflux surgery produces total regression of Barrett esophagus or decreases the risk of carcinoma.[52] Preliminary reports of the regeneration of squamous epithelium after endoscopic ablative therapy with laser, multipolar coagulation, or photodynamic therapy are intriguing and require confirmation.[53,54] Reports of treatment-induced regression of Barrett esophagus, especially in patients who have changes only in short segments, must be viewed with caution be-

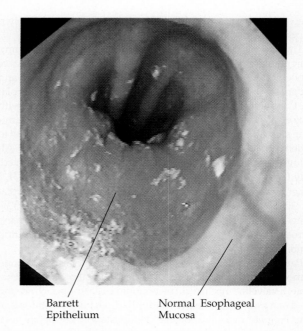

Barrett
Epithelium

Normal Esophageal
Mucosa

Figure 4   **On endoscopy, Barrett esophagus appears as rosy gastric mucosa.**

cause the diagnosis of the changes associated with Barrett esophagus in these patients is frequently inconsistent.[55]

HIATAL HERNIA

Hiatal hernia is a protrusion of a portion of the stomach through the hiatus of the diaphragm and into the thoracic cavity. The sliding type of hiatal hernia, formed by movement of the upper stomach through an enlarged hiatus, can be identified in about 30% of patients who undergo an upper gastrointestinal x-ray series. Because hiatal hernia and peptic esophagitis frequently coexist, they have been erroneously considered to have a cause-and-effect relation. Many patients with hiatal hernia do not have symptoms of reflux esophagitis. Hiatal hernia has been linked to inappropriately frequent lower esophageal sphincter relaxations in response to gastric distention.[16] For patients with asymptomatic hiatal hernia, treatment is not needed.

Paraesophageal hernia occurs when a knuckle of stomach moves through the hiatus alongside the esophagus but the gastroesophageal junction remains below the diaphragm. This unusual variety of hernia is frequently associated with a sensation of fullness or pain after eating. Surgical repair of paraesophageal hernia is recommended because the condition is associated with a risk of ulceration or strangulation and consequent perforation.

ESOPHAGEAL RINGS AND WEBS

Two types of esophageal rings—the mucosal type and the muscular type—have been reported. They are found in approximately 5% to 10% of patients who undergo upper gastrointestinal barium x-ray studies. The mucosal type of ring (Schatzki ring), which consists of redundant mucosa and submucosa covered by normal-appearing squamous mucosa, is located at the squamocolumnar junction. It appears as a symmetrical, circumferential narrowing of less than 3 mm in thickness. The muscular type of ring consists of hypertrophied or hypertonic muscle covered by normal mucosa and is usually located 1 to 2 cm above the squamocolumnar junction. Muscular rings are generally thicker

(4 to 5 mm) than mucosal rings and may be associated with motor disorders of the esophagus. Both types of rings are associated with hiatal hernia and may be related to ringlike strictures induced by reflux esophagitis.

Only a small number of patients with an esophageal ring become symptomatic. Intermittent dysphagia is the most common complaint. Most frequently, symptoms appear in the young adult and occur intermittently throughout life. Dysphagia seems to be more prevalent when patients are under emotional stress or are eating rapidly. For symptomatic patients, treatment with dilation with a large bougie is usually adequate. Episodic dysphagia frequently recurs, but repeated dilation is safe and effective. Long-term treatment with proton pump inhibitors may decrease the recurrence of dysphagia by preventing scar formation that is caused by gastroesophageal reflux. In the rare cases in which dilation fails, endoscopic electrocautery incision of the ring has been successful. Surgery is seldom required.[56,57]

Esophageal webs are membranes of squamous mucosa that are usually found in the anterior wall of the cervical esophagus. Midesophageal webs are rare. An increased incidence of pharyngeal and cervical esophageal carcinoma has been reported in patients with cervical esophageal webs. Most patients with esophageal webs are asymptomatic. Intermittent dysphagia is the usual symptom and is easily treated with dilation with a large bougie.[58]

ACHALASIA

Achalasia is a syndrome marked by the coexistence of aperistalsis and hypertonia of the lower esophageal sphincter. As a result, the esophagus gradually becomes dilated; eventually, it becomes so patulous that in end-stage disease it may occupy up to a quarter of the width of the chest. The cause of this disorder is unknown, but it is usually associated with a reduction in the number or complete absence of neurons in the myenteric plexus of the esophageal muscle layers. Although Chagas disease (American trypanosomiasis) may produce the identical clinical syndrome and identical motor and histologic abnormalities [see Chapter 156], its predominant manifestations are usually those produced by cardiomyopathy and megacolon, neither of which is seen in achalasia.

Achalasia most commonly develops in patients of 25 to 60 years of age. Patients with this disease often experience fullness in the chest during meals that gradually progresses to dysphagia on the ingestion of either liquids or solid food, which subsequently leads to weight loss. Regurgitation of undigested food occurs in 60% to 90% of patients, 10% of whom consequently experience significant bronchopulmonary complications.[59] Early in the course of disease, 30% to 50% of patients with achalasia report substernal chest pain that is usually precipitated by eating, but the pain can also awaken patients from sleep.[59] Heartburn is experienced by 25% to 45% of patients.[59] The heartburn results from lactic acid production caused by bacterial fermentation of retained food in the esophagus, not from gastroesophageal reflux.

Achalasia is usually not difficult to diagnose. Dilatation of the esophageal body and retention of barium above a tapered, so-called bird's-beak, gastroesophageal junction are the typical changes seen on barium studies. Endoscopy confirms the esophageal dilatation and excludes a permanent stricture at the gastroesophageal junction. However, because esophageal dilatation may not be obvious early in the course of disease, the diagnosis of achalasia should always be confirmed by esophageal manometry. Manometric findings in achalasia include the absence of peristalsis in the smooth muscle of the esophagus, incomplete relaxation

of the lower esophageal sphincter, elevated lower esophageal sphincter pressure, and elevated intraesophageal pressures relative to the gastric baseline. Absence of peristalsis is the only absolute criterion needed to make the diagnosis of achalasia. About 10% of patients older than 60 years with suspected achalasia have pseudoachalasia caused by malignancy. Unlike esophageal manometry, endoscopy with biopsy can differentiate between these two conditions. In addition, patients with achalasia have a higher risk of developing squamous cell carcinoma of the esophagus.[60]

The only therapy for achalasia is palliative. The treatment goal is to relax the lower esophageal sphincter with pharmacologic agents or to disrupt the sphincter muscle with balloon dilation or surgical esophagomyotomy. Only dilation and myotomy have been shown to provide long-term benefit, and there is debate regarding which of these two modalities should be used as initial therapy.[59,61] Dilation of the lower esophageal sphincter with balloon dilators that are 3 to 4 cm in diameter produces relief in about 80% of patients who are good candidates for surgery.[62] Younger patients have a lower response rate to dilation. About 40% of patients may require repeat dilation, and about 10% may need myotomy in 5 to 7 years after the initial dilation.[61,62] Esophageal perforation as a result of pneumatic dilation occurs in about 5% of patients.[61,62] Patients who present with relatively little weight loss and minimal esophageal dilatation may be more prone to have perforation during pneumatic dilation.[63,64] Although most of these perforations have to be repaired surgically, perforations that are small and localized may be treated with observation, having the patient take nothing by mouth, and antibiotics.

For patients who are not good candidates for surgery, the use of sublingual nitrates and nifedipine is appropriate. Nifedipine (20 to 40 mg sublingually before meals) decreases or eliminates symptoms of dysphagia in most patients with achalasia.[65] Isosorbide dinitrate (5 mg sublingually before meals) may be even more effective than nifedipine, but side effects of headache and facial flushing are common with this agent.[65] The long-term efficacy of these pharmacologic agents is unclear.[65,66]

Endoscopic injection of botulinum toxin into the lower esophageal sphincter is another less invasive therapy for achalasia.[67] Botulinum toxin induces paralysis in skeletal muscle by binding to presynaptic cholinergic nerve terminals, and it inhibits the release of acetylcholine at the neuromuscular junction. It probably reduces lower esophageal sphincter pressure by decreasing excitatory cholinergic innervation of the sphincter muscle, resulting in chemical denervation. About 80% to 90% of patients treated with botulinum toxin experienced a significant improvement in dysphagia shortly after treatment.[67-69] In a small controlled trial, the efficacy of botulinum toxin injection was similar to that of pneumatic dilation.[69] Patients older than 50 years and those with vigorous achalasia responded better to this treatment.[70] Mild, transient substernal chest pain was the only side effect and was reported by about 18% of these patients.[67,68] Only two thirds of these patients had a sustained response at 6 months, however. Most of these patients would require a second treatment in about 1 year, and about 60% of them responded to a second treatment.[70] The long-term efficacy and safety of the intrasphincteric injection of botulinum toxin for the treatment of achalasia have yet to be defined. At present, pharmacologic therapies for achalasia are best used as initial treatment for patients at high risk for complications from dilation or surgery and for those who are reluctant to accept the risks of these mechanical therapies.

Patients with achalasia that is refractory to dilation or medical therapy may have to undergo surgical myotomy of the lower esophageal sphincter. Myotomy usually provides relief from dysphagia, but 10% of patients may develop reflux esophagitis.[67] The use of thoracoscopic or laparoscopic esophagomyotomy to treat patients with achalasia has been reported.[71] The recovery period after these procedures may be shorter than that after conventional surgical myotomy, but the long-term efficacy and safety of these approaches have yet to be established.

SPASTIC MOTILITY DISORDERS

Spastic motility disorders comprise a group of disorders of the distal esophagus that usually present with dysphagia, chest pain, or both. Manometric studies of the esophagus show a spectrum of contraction abnormalities. The better-defined entities include diffuse esophageal spasm (simultaneous contractions in 10% of swallows of liquid), nutcracker esophagus (elevated distal esophageal peristaltic pressure), and hypertensive lower esophageal sphincter (increased resting lower esophageal sphincter pressure with normal relaxation and peristalsis).[72] However, most patients with spastic motility disorders have multiple contraction abnormalities (nontransmitted, retrograde, and prolonged contractions) that cannot be easily categorized. The pathophysiology of these motility disorders is not well understood. Alteration in pain perception and dysfunction of the autonomic innervation of the esophagus have been implicated, but permanent changes in neural fibers similar to those seen in achalasia have not been demonstrated.[72]

Intermittent dysphagia after ingestion of liquids and solid foods is present in 30% to 60% of patients with spastic motility disorders.[72] It is usually not progressive and seldom causes significant weight loss. About 80% to 90% of patients with spastic motility disorders complain of recurrent substernal chest pain that can be excruciating. Because of its location and severity, the pain produced by esophageal spasm may mimic the pain produced by coronary artery disease. The chest pain associated with esophageal spasm does not always accompany dysphagia.

The essential diagnostic test for these motility disorders is esophageal manometry. However, it is often difficult to establish a correlation between the recorded contraction abnormalities and the patient's symptoms. The chest pain caused by diffuse esophageal spasm is inconsistent and may not be observed during manometric studies. Provocative tests performed during manometric studies to reproduce the chest pain are crucial in establishing esophageal spasm as the cause of these symptoms. The most commonly used test involves the administration of intravenous edrophonium chloride (80 mg/kg).[73] About 30% of patients with noncardiac chest pain will develop chest pain during the challenge, whereas normal persons will be asymptomatic. Administration of a placebo evokes pain in only 6% of patients with noncardiac chest pain. Prolonged ambulatory motility monitoring may be the best test to establish the diagnosis, though it has yet to be standardized.

Treatment consists primarily of reassurance and attempts to reduce symptoms. If concomitant reflux is documented during the process of evaluation, aggressive antireflux therapy should be initiated.[74] Smooth muscle relaxants, such as long-acting nitrates, calcium channel blockers, and anticholinergics, have been evaluated as potential therapies for these patients. Despite the ability of these agents to correct some of the abnormal manometric findings, their efficacy in providing symptomatic relief has been inconsistent.[72,73] For patients with symptomatic spasm associated with stress, anxiolytic or antidepressant drugs such as trazodone may effect overall improvement.[75] A preliminary report suggested that botulinum toxin injection to the lower esophageal sphincter may be useful in these patients, but this observation needs confirmation.[76] In rare instances, the symptoms of diffuse spasm are so incapacitating that pneumatic dilation or surgical intervention must be considered.[72,77]

COLLAGEN VASCULAR DISEASE

Scleroderma is the collagen disease that most commonly affects the esophagus, but polymyositis may produce similar esophageal changes [see Chapter 115]. As many as 80% of scleroderma patients may have esophageal involvement.[78] There are two aspects of the functional defect: first, the peristaltic wave that is initiated by swallowing travels only through the upper third of the esophagus containing skeletal muscle and then ceases, causing a delay in the transport of food to the stomach; second, the resting pressure of the lower esophageal sphincter declines from a normal level of 15 to 20 mm Hg to 0 to 5 mm Hg, causing gastroesophageal reflux of acid to occur readily. Histopathologic examination may reveal a decrease in the number of smooth muscle fibers and replacement by fibrous tissue, as well as atrophy of the local nerve fibers. As might be expected from the pathophysiologic events, patients with scleroderma are prone to develop severe reflux esophagitis, manifested by persistent heartburn. However, 25% of these patients may be asymptomatic. Dysphagia is not common early in collagen vascular disease, probably because the aperistalsis is accompanied by a relaxed lower esophageal sphincter, which permits esophageal emptying by gravity. However, chronic reflux of gastric acid will eventually produce a peptic stricture in an average of 10% of patients.[78]

Although treatment of erosive esophagitis in patients with scleroderma is not entirely satisfactory, aggressive acid suppression therapy is indicated. Long-term therapy with proton pump inhibitors may provide significant symptomatic relief. As many as 50% of these patients may require a high maintenance dose of proton pump inhibitors. Despite an optimal antireflux treatment regimen, strictures develop frequently; there does not appear to be a significantly increased risk of esophageal carcinoma.[78]

ESOPHAGITIS DUE TO DRUGS

Taking drugs in pill form can cause acute caustic injury of the esophagus. Most patients with this injury have had no prior esophageal symptoms.[79] Transient delay in pill transit through the esophagus is common even in persons with normal esophageal motility. Pills should be swallowed along with at least 100 ml of water, and one must remain upright for at least 90 seconds to ensure that the drug passes readily into the stomach. A long list of drugs have been reported to cause acute esophagitis; common ones include aspirin and other nonsteroidal anti-inflammatory drugs, potassium chloride, ferrous sulfate, ascorbic acid, and the tetracycline class of antibiotics. Most of the affected patients experience acute onset of odynophagia and dysphagia, especially when solid foods and acidic liquids such as citrus juices are ingested. Fewer than 20% of these patients may present with progressive painless dysphagia.[79] Erythema, friability, and small ulcerations are seen on endoscopy in the middle and distal thirds of the esophagus. In rare instances, bleeding, deep ulceration, and stricture may develop. Once the diagnosis is made, temporary cessation of the offending drug allows healing in about 1 week. Antacid, H_2 receptor antagonists, sucralfate, and viscous 2% lidocaine are often prescribed, but their therapeutic role in this condition has not been well studied.

ESOPHAGITIS AND STRICTURE DUE TO CAUSTIC CHEMICALS

Accidental or intentional ingestion of caustic alkali or acid agents is an important cause of esophageal and gastric injury. If swallowed, concentrated liquid sodium hydroxide solutions used to clear sink drains can produce extensive esophageal and gastric damage. Solid caustic material (e.g., solid lye) tends to adhere to the mucosae of the mouth and pharynx. Strong alkalis (sodium or potassium hydroxide) produce immediate destruction of buccal and pharyngeal mucosae and are responsible for the most severe acute chemical esophagitis and subsequent stricture. Weak bases (e.g., ammonium hydroxide), weak acids (acetic or phosphoric acid), and bleaches, although not as harmful to the esophagus as strong alkalis, often pass readily into the stomach and may cause appreciable gastric injury.

When a patient presents with a history of ingestion of a caustic agent, the mouth and pharynx should be carefully examined. In most cases of caustic ingestion, acute oral burns are observed, but some patients may have little or no pain; however, nearly 50% of patients with no involvement of the mouth or pharynx will have a chemical esophagitis. Death resulting from extensive deep tissue destruction and perforation occurs in about 6% of cases. Esophageal stricture develops 2 to 8 weeks after the injury in 10% to 30% of patients who ingest a strong base. Gastric antral stricture is an unusual late complication.

Because some esophageal damage occurs in nearly all patients who ingest liquid caustic agents, especially when they contain a strong alkali, diagnostic endoscopy with a small-diameter (< 1 cm) instrument is essential when the patient first seeks medical aid. Despite the obvious concern of possible impending pharyngeal or esophageal perforation, use of the small-diameter flexible endoscope does not appear to be associated with increased morbidity. If major damage is seen in the esophagus, examination of the stomach should be deferred for subsequent endoscopy. Patients who are found to have appreciable acute edema and hemorrhage or ulcerations in the esophagus or stomach should be admitted to the hospital and treated with an intravenous H_2 receptor antagonist [see Chapter 57]. Enteral nutritional support via a soft and flexible nasoenteric feeding tube placed by fluoroscopy is efficacious and safe.[80]

Antibiotics and corticosteroids have been shown to decrease the risk of esophageal stricture formation in animals that were given caustic agents orally, but the role of these drugs in human disease has not been established. A controlled trial did not show any efficacy for corticosteroid therapy.[81] Prophylactic bougienage and stent placement to prevent stricture formation also have not proved to be effective in clinical studies.

If strictures are confirmed, barium studies should be done and dilation therapy started at the first complaint of dysphagia after the acute phase of the clinical course.[80] Although rarely indicated for acute tissue destruction, surgery may be necessary if an esophageal stricture develops, because such strictures are usually resistant to dilation. An elongated stricture may eventually require excision and either jejunal or colonic interposition. Lye stricture is probably associated with a higher risk of squamous cell carcinoma of the esophagus decades after the initial injury [see Chapter 196].

ESOPHAGEAL INFECTIONS

The increased incidence of esophageal infection in recent years can be directly attributed both to the HIV epidemic and to the maximal immunosuppressive therapy required in cancer treatment, solid-organ transplantation, and bone marrow transplanta-

tion. Under conditions of extreme immunosuppression, organisms that are usually incapable of invading the esophageal wall can cause severe local esophagitis that may lead to secondary spread of infection to other organs.[82-84] Candida species, cytomegalovirus (CMV), and herpes simplex virus type 1 (HSV-1) are the most common causes of esophageal infections in these circumstances. Other responsible pathogens are HIV, Mycobacterium tuberculosis, M. avium complex, Pneumocystis carinii, Cryptosporidium species, Aspergillus species, Histoplasma species, Epstein-Barr virus, Nocardia species, and Leishmania donovani.[82] Concurrent infection with multiple organisms is common.

Small esophageal ulcerations may develop during the acute seroconversion phase of HIV infection. Painful, deep esophageal ulcerations without an identifiable causative agent may develop in addition to other opportunistic esophageal infections in AIDS patients. HIV has been implicated as the cause of these ulcers, but the evidence is not conclusive.[84] In patients who have undergone solid-organ or bone marrow transplantation, infectious esophagitis usually presents several weeks later. Candida esophagitis is more common in renal transplant patients than in liver or heart transplant patients, probably because of the concurrent risk of diabetes mellitus in renal transplant recipients. Infectious esophagitis is more severe in bone marrow transplant patients than in solid-organ transplant patients. However, the risk of esophageal infection has been significantly reduced in all transplant patients by the use of prophylactic therapies (see below).

The presenting symptoms of infectious esophagitis may vary according to the pathogen. Dysphagia and odynophagia are reported in 95% of patients with HIV-associated idiopathic ulcers but in only 60% to 80% of patients with other esophageal infections. About one third of patients with esophagitis caused by Candida species, HSV-1, or HIV may also have oral lesions, but these lesions have not been reported to occur in patients with CMV esophagitis. Oral thrush is seen in 75% of patients with Candida esophagitis, but the presence of oral thrush does not eliminate the possibility of other infectious causes of the esophagitis. Nausea, vomiting, abdominal pain, and fever are more commonly seen in patients with CMV esophagitis than in those with esophagitis caused by other organisms, suggesting multiorgan infection by this virus.

Endoscopy is the gold standard in the diagnosis of infectious esophagitis. Raised white or yellow plaques that measure 0.1 to 0.5 cm in diameter and that may exhibit a central ulcerated depression are seen in both fungal and viral infections. The endoscopic appearance of esophageal lesions is often inadequate for a specific pathogen to be identified.[82,85] Biopsy and brush cytology specimens should be obtained for culture and for virologic and histologic examination. Brush cytology is the most sensitive technique for diagnosis of both fungal and viral esophagitis.[84]

Treatment of Candida esophagitis varies according to the severity of the immunosuppression. For patients who do not suffer from immunosuppression or who have minimal immunosuppression, such as those with diabetes, nonabsorbable oral agents such as clotrimazole troches are adequate. For patients with impaired lymphocyte function, such as those with AIDS, oral fluconazole is the treatment of choice.[86] For patients with severe granulocytopenia, intravenous amphotericin B may be needed to prevent systemic dissemination of the Candida organisms.

The efficacy of various antiviral agents for viral esophagitis is less well documented. In uncontrolled studies, ganciclovir and foscarnet were effective in the treatment of CMV esophagitis.[87,88] However, a controlled trial of ganciclovir in bone marrow transplant patients with CMV gastroenteritis and esophagitis failed to demonstrate clinical improvement.[89] The dosage of ganciclovir is 5 mg/kg I.V. every 12 hours for 2 weeks, then once daily for maintenance, if indicated; the dosage of foscarnet is 60 mg/kg I.V. every 8 hours (or 90 mg/kg I.V. every 12 hours) for 2 weeks, then 90 to 120 mg/kg/day for maintenance, if indicated.[82]

Limited studies have suggested that acyclovir is effective for herpetic esophagitis.[90] The dosage of acyclovir is 200 to 400 mg orally five times daily for 2 weeks or 250 mg/m² I.V. every 8 hours for 2 weeks.[82] Patients who are resistant to acyclovir should be given foscarnet, 60 mg/kg I.V. every 8 hours (or 90 mg/kg I.V. every 12 hours) for 2 weeks, then 90 to 120 mg/kg/day for maintenance, if indicated.

Efficacy of steroid therapy for HIV-associated idiopathic esophageal ulcer has been reported in several studies.[84] Responders usually have symptomatic relief within a few days after treatment. A 4-week course of oral prednisone, 40 mg daily and tapered by 10 mg a week, appears to be the best regimen. Opportunistic infection may develop during steroid therapy.

Several prophylactic regimens are available to prevent the development of infectious esophagitis in patients who are undergoing solid-organ or bone marrow transplantation.[82] CMV esophagitis is best prevented by the administration of ganciclovir, 5 mg/kg I.V. every 12 hours for 5 days, then once daily as maintenance therapy. Herpetic esophagitis can be prevented by the administration of acyclovir either orally (200 to 400 mg four or five times daily or 800 mg twice daily during the period of maximal immunosuppressive therapy) or intravenously (250 mg/m² every 12 hours during the period of maximal immunosuppressive therapy).

ESOPHAGEAL DIVERTICULA

There are three types of esophageal diverticulum, classified according to their location and, to some extent, according to their probable cause.

Zenker Diverticulum

Zenker diverticulum occurs in the upper esophagus, usually just above the level of the cricopharyngeal muscle.[91] Most patients with this type of diverticulum have an incoordination of esophageal motility. Normally, the upper esophageal sphincter at the cricopharyngeal muscle relaxes on swallowing and contracts again after the peristaltic wave has propelled the bolus past the sphincter. In patients at risk for Zenker diverticulum, the upper esophageal sphincter relaxes appropriately but contracts prematurely before the peristaltic wave arrives. Peristalsis is capable of overcoming this resistance, but after years of exposure to the high pressures required, the esophageal wall above the sphincter develops a posterior outpouching. This change constitutes Zenker diverticulum, which may produce transient, subtle dysphagia that is usually not disturbing to the patient. More typical complaints are gurgling sounds in the throat after ingestion of a meal, halitosis, the sensation of a lump in the throat, or the actual appearance of a neck mass. Regurgitation of undigested food from the diverticulum occurs frequently and presents a major danger, especially if the patient is sleeping, because pulmonary aspiration may occur. A Zenker diverticulum that has a diameter of more than 3 cm may produce severe dysphagia or obstruction later in the course of the disease [see Therapy, below].

Midesophageal Diverticulum

Midesophageal diverticulum can be classified radiologically as either the pulsion type or the traction type.[92] Traction diverticulum may be caused by retraction of the esophagus as a result of scarring of the adjacent pulmonary structures as may occur in tuberculosis, for example. Pulsion diverticulum is usually associated with nonspecific esophageal motility disorders. Most midesophageal diverticula are small, do not produce significant symptoms, and are usually noted incidentally at the time of a gastrointestinal x-ray series.

Epiphrenic Diverticulum

The epiphrenic diverticulum occurs at the level of the esophagus near the lower esophageal sphincter. It is commonly associated with an incoordination between lower esophageal sphincter function and peristaltic movement of the food bolus. If the diverticulum is large, nocturnal regurgitation may occur, and dysphagia or esophageal obstruction may develop.

Therapy

Esophageal diverticula often do not require therapy unless regurgitation of food contents and pulmonary aspiration occur. Various types of surgery have been devised.[93] If the pouch has not become attached to adjacent tissues, simple excision of the diverticulum can often be done. In some patients, a two-step procedure may be necessary: mobilization of the diverticulum at the initial operation and excision of the diverticular pouch after granulation tissue has formed. A cricopharyngeal myotomy may be successful for Zenker diverticulum. The use of a flexible endoscope to incise the septum between Zenker diverticulum and the esophageal lumen has been reported.[94] This technique appears to be most suitable for patients who are at high surgical risk. However, the long-term efficacy and safety of this method remain to be determined. Midesophageal diverticula usually do not require surgery. A trial of medical treatment of an associated diffuse spasm or achalasia (see above) is indicated before surgical treatment of an epiphrenic diverticulum is considered. Simple excision of epiphrenic diverticula is not advised because of the related motor abnormalities in the lower esophagus.

CARCINOMA OF THE ESOPHAGUS

Squamous cell carcinoma of the esophagus is the most common esophageal carcinoma in the world [see Chapter 196]. Its incidence varies greatly from region to region. In the United States, African Americans have a fourfold to fivefold greater risk of this cancer than whites. The most important predisposing factor is the heavy use of alcohol and cigarettes. Adenocarcinoma of the esophagus, once rare in the United States, has rapidly increased in incidence during the past two decades.[48] Most cases of esophageal adenocarcinoma arise from Barrett esophagus, and the disease predominantly affects white men.

The prognosis for patients with either type of esophageal carcinoma is poor: the 5-year survival is less than 10% because the diagnosis is usually made when the disease is already advanced. In regions of the world that have surveillance programs for early detection, it appears to take 5 years for severe dysplasia to progress to early squamous cell carcinoma and several more years for it to become advanced cancer[95]—a finding that emphasizes the importance of early detection. Although esophagectomy is still the standard treatment for early esophageal carcinoma, preliminary reports of endoscopic photodynamic therapy suggest that this technique has equivalent efficacy.[95,96] It is therefore important that preoperative staging be accurate. Endoscopic ultrasonography, which entails the use of a fiberoptic endoscope with a built-in ultrasound transducer, provides more accurate local staging of esophageal carcinoma and assessment of tumor resectability than do other imaging tools, such as computed tomography and magnetic resonance imaging.[97]

References

1. Blot WJ, Devesa SS, Kneller RW, et al: Rising incidence of adenocarcinoma of the esophagus and gastric cardia. JAMA 265:1287, 1991

2. Blot WJ, Devesa SS, Fraumeni JF Jr: Continuing climb in esophageal carcinoma: an update. JAMA 270:1320, 1993

3. Ekberg O, Olsson R: Dynamic radiology of swallowing disorders. Endoscopy 29:439, 1997

4. Rubesin SE: Oral and pharyngeal dysphagia. Gastroenterol Clin North Am 24:331, 1995

5. Baron TH, Richter JE: The use of esophageal function tests. Adv Intern Med 38:361, 1993

6. Klein HA: Esophageal transit scintigraphy. Semin Nucl Med 25:306, 1995

7. Glade MJ: Continuous ambulatory esophageal pH monitoring in the evaluation of patients with gastroesophageal reflux: diagnostic and therapeutic technology assessment (DATTA). JAMA 274:662, 1995

8. Jamieson JR, Stein HJ, DeMeester TR, et al: Ambulatory 24-h esophageal pH monitoring: normal values, optimal thresholds, specificity, sensitivity, and reproducibility. Am J Gastroenterol 87:1102, 1992

9. Kahrilas PJ, Clouse RE, Hogan WJ: American Gastroenterological Association technical review on the clinical use of esophageal manometry. Gastroenterology 107:1865, 1994

10. Waring JP, Hunter JG, Oddsdottir M, et al: The preoperative evaluation of patients considered for laparoscopic antireflux surgery. Am J Gastroenterol 90:35, 1995

11. Castell JA, Castell DO: Upper esophageal sphincter and pharyngeal function and oropharyngeal (transfer) dysphagia. Gastroenterol Clin North Am 25:35, 1996

12. Richter JE: Typical and atypical presentations of gastroesophageal reflux disease: the role of esophageal testing in diagnosis and management. Gastroenterol Clin North Am 25:75, 1996

13. Weston AP, Badr AS, Topalovski M, et al: Prospective evaluation of the prevalence of gastric *Helicobacter pylori* infection in patients with GERD, Barrett's esophagus, Barrett's dysplasia, and Barrett's adenocarcinoma. Am J Gastroenterol 95:387, 2000

14. Fallone CA, Barkun AN, Friedman G, et al: Is *Helicobacter pylori* eradication associated with gastroesophageal reflux disease? Am J Gastroenterol 95:914, 2000

15. Spechler SJ, Fischbach L, Feldman M: Clinical aspects of genetic variability in *Helicobacter pylori*. JAMA 283:1264, 2000

16. Kahrilas PJ, Shi G, Manka M, et al: Increased frequency of transient lower esophageal sphincter relaxation induced by gastric distention in reflux patients with hiatal hernia. Gastroenterology 118:688, 2000

17. Pope CE II: Acid-reflux disorders. N Engl J Med 331:656, 1994

18. Dent J: Long-term aims of treatment of reflux disease, and the role of non-drug measures. Digestion 51(suppl 1):30, 1992

19. Castell DO, Dalton CB, Becker D, et al: Alginic acid decreases postprandial upright gastroesophageal reflux: comparison with equal-strength antacid. Dig Dis Sci 37:589, 1992

20. Johnson DA: Medical therapy for gastroesophageal reflux disease. Am J Med 92(suppl 5A):88S, 1992

21. Williams RM, Orlando RC, Bozymski EM, et al: Multicenter trial of sucralfate suspension for the treatment of reflux esophagitis. Am J Med 83(suppl 3B):61, 1987

22. Simon B, Dammann H-G, Müller P: Sucralfate in the treatment of reflux esophagitis in adults: an update. Scand J Gastroenterol 24(suppl 156):37, 1989

23. Elsborg L, Jørgensen F: Sucralfate versus cimetidine in reflux oesophagitis: a double-blind clinical study. Scand J Gastroenterol 26:146, 1991

24. Schutze K, Bigard MA, Van Waes L, et al: Comparison of two dosing regimens of cisapride in the treatment of reflux oesophagitis. Aliment Pharmacol Ther 11:497, 1997

25. Nightingale SL: From the Food and Drug Administration: New warnings added to cisapride labeling. JAMA 280:410, 1998

26. U.S. Food and Drug Administration Web site: Medwatch: The FDA Medical Products Reporting Program. New Safety Information Summaries 2000: Propulsid (cisapride). http://www.fda.gov/medwatch/safety/2000/safety00.htm#propul. Accessed April 27, 2000.

27. Feldman M, Harford WV, Fisher RS, et al: Treatment of reflux esophagitis resistant to H_2-receptor antagonists with lansoprazole, a new H^+/K^+-ATPase inhibitor: a controlled, double-blind study. Am J Gastroenterol 88:1212, 1993

28. Koop H, Hotz J, Pommer G, et al: Prospective evaluation of omeprazole treatment in reflux oesophagitis refractory to H_2-receptor antagonists. Aliment Pharmacol Ther 4:593, 1990

29. Tytgat GNJ, Koelz H-R, Vosmaer GDC, et al: Sucralfate maintenance therapy in reflux esophagitis. Am J Gastroenterol 90:1233, 1995

30. Vigneri S, Termini R, Leandro G, et al: A comparison of five maintenance therapies for reflux esophagitis. N Engl J Med 333:1106, 1995

31. Hatlebakk JG, Berstad A: Lansoprazole 15 and 30 mg daily in maintaining healing and symptom relief in patients with reflux oesophagitis. Aliment Pharmacol Ther 11:365, 1997

32. Sontag SJ, Robinson M, Roufail W, et al: Daily omeprazole surpasses intermittent dosing in preventing relapse of oesophagitis: a U.S. multi-centre double-blind study. Aliment Pharmacol Ther 11:373, 1997

33. Maton PN: Omeprazole. N Engl J Med 324:965, 1991

34. Joelson S, Joelson I-B, Lundborg P, et al: Safety experience from long-term treatment with omeprazole. Digestion 51(suppl 1):93, 1992

35. Klinkenberg-Knol EC, Festen HPM, Jansen JBMJ, et al: Long-term treatment with omeprazole for refractory reflux esophagitis: efficacy and safety. Ann Intern Med 121:161, 1994

36. Kuipers EJ, Lundell L, Klinkenberg-Knol EC, et al: Helicobacter pylori plus omeprazole created risk for atrophic gastritis. N Engl J Med 334:1018, 1996

37. Klinkenberg-Knol EC, Nelis F, Dent J, et al: Long-term omeprazole treatment in resistant gastroesophageal reflux disease: efficacy, safety, and influence on gastric mucosa. Gastroenterology 118:661, 2000

38. Laws HL, Clements RH, Swillie CM: A randomized, prospective comparison of the Nissen fundoplication versus the Toupet fundoplication for gastroesophageal reflux disease. Ann Surg 225:647, 1997

39. Civello IM, Brisinda G, Sganga G, et al: Modified Hill operation vs Nissen fundoplication in the surgical treatment of gastro-esophageal reflux disease. Hepatogastroenterology 44:380, 1997

40. Coster DD, Bower WH, Wilson VT, et al: Laparoscopic Nissen fundoplication: a curative, safe, and cost effective procedure for complicated gastroesophageal reflux disease. Surg Laparosc Endosc 5:111, 1995

41. Laine S, Rantala A, Gullichsen R: Laparoscopic vs conventional Nissen fundoplication: a prospective randomized study. Surg Endosc 11:441, 1997

42. Gotley DC, Smithers BM, Rhodes M, et al: Laparoscopic Nissen fundoplication: 200 consecutive cases. Gut 38:487, 1996

43. Kmiot WA, Kirby RM, Akinola D, et al: Prospective randomised trial of Nissen fundoplication and Angelchik prosthesis in the surgical treatment of medically refractory gastro-oesophageal reflux disease. Br J Surg 78:1181, 1991

44. Spechler SJ, Department of Veterans Affairs Gastroesophageal Reflux Disease Study Group: Comparison of medical and surgical therapy for complicated gastroesophageal reflux disease in veterans. N Engl J Med 326:786, 1992

45. ASGE Technology Assessment Status Evaluation: balloon dilation of gastrointestinal tract strictures. Gastrointest Endosc 42:608, 1995

46. Smith PM, Kerr GD, Cockel R, et al: A comparison of omeprazole and ranitidine in the prevention of recurrence of benign esophageal stricture. Gastroenterology 107:1312, 1994

47. Levine DS: Barrett's esophagus. Scientific American Science & Medicine 1(5):16, 1994

48. Cameron AJ: Epidemiology of columnar-lined esophagus and adenocarcinoma. Gastroenterol Clin North Am 26:487, 1997

49. Souza RF, Meltzer SJ: The molecular basis for carcinogenesis in metaplastic columnar-lined esophagus. Gastroenterol Clin North Am 26:583, 1997

50. Levine DS: Management of dysplasia in the columnar-lined esophagus. Gastroenterol Clin North Am 26:613, 1997

51. DeMeester TR: Surgical treatment of dysplasia and adenocarcinoma. Gastroenterol Clin North Am 26:669, 1997

52. Ter RB, Castell DO: Gastroesophageal reflux disease in patients with columnar-lined esophagus. Gastroenterol Clin North Am 26:549, 1997

53. Panjehpour M, Overholt BF, Vo-Dinh T, et al: Endoscopic fluorescence detection of high grade dysplasia in Barrett's esophagus. Gastroenterology 111:93, 1996

54. Sampliner RE: Ablative therapies for the columnar-lined esophagus. Gastroenterol Clin North Am 26:685, 1997

55. Kim SL, Waring JP, Spechler SJ, et al: Diagnostic inconsistencies in Barrett's esophagus. Gastroenterology 107:945, 1994

56. Eckardt VF, Kanzler G, Willems D: Single dilation of symptomatic Schatzki rings: a prospective evaluation of its effectiveness. Dig Dis Sci 37:577, 1992

57. Burdick JS, Venu RP, Hogan WJ: Cutting the defiant lower esophageal ring. Gastrointest Endosc 39:616, 1993

58. Boyce GA, Boyce HW: Esophagus: anatomy and structural anomalies. Textbook of Gastroenterology, 2nd ed., Vol 2. Yamada T, Alpers DH, Owyang C, et al, Eds. JB Lippincott Co, Philadelphia, 1995, p 1156

59. Abid S, Champion G, Richter JE, et al: Treatment of achalasia: the best of both worlds. Am J Gastroenterol 89:979, 1994

60. Streitz JM, Ellis JH, Gibb SP, et al: Achalasia and squamous cell carcinoma of the esophagus: analysis of 241 patients. Ann Thorac Surg 59:1604, 1995

61. Parkman HP, Reynolds JC, Ouyang A, et al: Pneumatic dilatation or esophagomyotomy treatment for idiopathic achalasia: clinical outcomes and cost analysis. Dig Dis Sci 38:75, 1993

62. Eckardt VF, Aignherr C, Bernhard G: Predictors of outcome in patients with achalasia treated by pneumatic dilation. Gastroenterology 103:1732, 1992

63. Borotto E, Gaudric M, Danel B, et al: Risk factors of oesophageal perforation during pneumatic dilatation for achalasia. Gut 39:9, 1996

64. Anselmino M, Perdikis G, Hinder RA, et al: Heller myotomy is superior to dilatation for the treatment of early achalasia. Arch Surg 132:233, 1997

65. Gelfond M, Rozen P, Gilat T: Isosorbide dinitrate and nifedipine treatment of achalasia: a clinical, manometric and radionuclide evaluation. Gastroenterology 83:963, 1982

66. Coccia G, Bortolotti M, Michetti P, et al: Prospective clinical and manometric study comparing pneumatic dilatation and sublingual nifedipine in the treatment of oesophageal achalasia. Gut 32:604, 1991

67. Pasricha PJ, Ravich WJ, Hendrix TR, et al: Intrasphincteric botulinum toxin for the treatment of achalasia. N Engl J Med 322:774, 1995

68. Cuilliere C, Ducrotte P, Zerbib F, et al: Achalasia: outcome of patients treated with intrasphincteric injection of botulinum toxin. Gut 41:87, 1997

69. Annese V, Basciani M, Perri F, et al: Controlled trial of botulinum toxin injection versus placebo and pneumatic dilation in achalasia. Gastroenterology 111:1418, 1996

70. Pasricha PJ, Rai R, Ravich WJ, et al: Botulinum toxin for achalasia: long-term outcome and predictors of response. Gastroenterology 110:1410, 1996

71. Hunter JG, Richardson WS: Surgical management of achalasia. Surg Clin North Am 77:993, 1997

72. Koshy SS, Nostrant TT: Pathophysiology and endoscopic/balloon treatment of esophageal motility disorders. Surg Clin North Am 77:971, 1997

73. Patti MG, Way LW: Evaluation and treatment of primary esophageal motility disorders. West J Med 166:263, 1997

74. Achem SR, Kolts BE, MacMath T, et al: Effects of omeprazole versus placebo in treatment of noncardiac chest pain and gastroesophageal reflux. Dig Dis Sci 42:2138, 1997

75. Clouse RE, Lustman PJ, Eckert TC, et al: Low-dose trazodone for symptomatic patients with esophageal contraction abnormalities: a double-blind, placebo-controlled trial. Gastroenterology 92:1027, 1987

76. Miller LS, Parkman HP, Schiano TD, et al: Treatment of symptomatic nonachalasia esophageal motor disorders with botulinum toxin injection at the lower esophageal sphincter. Dig Dis Sci 41:2025, 1996

77. Patti MG, Pellegrini CA, Arcerito M, et al: Comparison of medical and minimally invasive surgical therapy for primary esophageal motility disorders. Arch Surg 130:609, 1995

78. Lock G, Holstege A, Lang B, et al: Gastrointestinal manifestations of progressive systemic sclerosis. Am J Gastroenterol 92:763, 1997

79. Kikendall JW: Pill-induced esophageal injury. Gastroenterol Clin North Am 20:835, 1991

80. Kikendall JW: Caustic ingestion injuries. Gastroenterol Clin North Am 20:847, 1991

81. Anderson KD, Rouse TM, Randolph JG: A controlled trial of corticosteroids in children with corrosive injury of the esophagus. N Engl J Med 323:637, 1990

82. Baehr PH, McDonald GB: Esophageal infections: risk factors, presentation, diagnosis, and treatment. Gastroenterology 106:509, 1994

83. Dieterich DT, Wilcox CM: Diagnosis and treatment of esophageal diseases associated with HIV infection. Practice Parameters Committee of the American College of Gastroenterology. Am J Gastroenterol 91:2265, 1996

84. Noyer CM, Simon D: Oral and esophageal disorders. Gastroenterol Clin North Am 26:241, 1997

85. Wilcox CM, Schwartz DA, Clark WS: Esophageal ulceration in human immunodeficiency virus infection: causes, response to therapy, and long-term outcome. Ann Intern Med 122:143, 1995

86. Laine L, Dretler RH, Conteas CN, et al: Fluconazole compared with ketoconazole for the treatment of Candida esophagitis in AIDS: a randomized trial. Ann Intern Med 117: 655, 1992

87. Wilcox CM, Straub RF, Schwartz DA: Cytomegalovirus esophagitis in AIDS: a prospective evaluation of clinical response to ganciclovir therapy, relapse rate, and long-term outcome. Am J Med 98:169, 1995

88. Blanshard C, Benhamou Y, Dohin E, et al: Treatment of AIDS-associated gastrointestinal cytomegalovirus infection with foscarnet and ganciclovir: a randomized comparison. J Infect Dis 172:622, 1995

89. Reed EC, Wolford JL, Kopecky KJ, et al: Ganciclovir for the treatment of cytomegalovirus gastroenteritis in bone marrow transplant patients: a randomized, placebo-controlled trial. Ann Intern Med 112:505, 1990

90. Genereau T, Lortholary O, Bouchaud O, et al: Herpes simplex esophagitis in patients with AIDS: report of 34 cases. The Cooperative Study Group on Herpetic Esophagitis in HIV infection. Clin Infect Dis 22:926, 1996

91. Zenker's diverticulum: reappraisal. Am J Gastroenterol 92:1494, 1997

92. Schima W, Schober E, Stacher G, et al: Association of midoesophageal diverticula with oesophageal motor disorders: videofluoroscopy and manometry. Acta Radiol 38:108, 1997

93. Bonafede JP, Lavertu P, Wood BG, et al: Surgical outcome in 87 patients with Zenker's diverticulum. Laryngoscope 107:720, 1997

94. Ishioka S, Sakai P, Maluf Filho F, et al: Endoscopic incision of Zenker's diverticula. Endoscopy 27:433, 1995

95. Lambert R: Endoscopic detection and treatment of early esophageal cancer: a critical analysis. Endoscopy 27:12, 1995

96. Sibille A, Lambert R, Souquet J-C, et al: Long-term survival after photodynamic therapy for esophageal cancer. Gastroenterology 108:337, 1995

97. Van Dam J: Endosonographic evaluation of the patient with esophageal cancer. Chest 112(suppl 4):184S, 1997

98. Castell DO: Approach to the patient with dysphagia. Textbook of Gastroenterology, 2nd ed. Yamada T, Alpers DH, Owyang C, et al, Eds. JB Lippincott Co, Philadelphia, 1995, p 641

99. Orlando RC: Reflux esophagitis. Textbook of Gastroenterology, 2nd ed. Yamada T, Alpers DH, Owyang C, et al, Eds. JB Lippincott Co, Philadelphia, 1995, p 1233

Acknowledgment

Figures 1 and 2   Talar Agasyan.

57 Peptic Ulcer Diseases

Mark Feldman, M.D.

Definition

Peptic ulcers are holes in the inner lining of the gastrointestinal (GI) tract that are attributed to exposure of the mucosa to gastric acid and pepsin. Peptic ulcers extend through the mucosa and the muscularis mucosae, a thin layer of smooth muscle separating the mucosa from the deeper submucosa, muscularis propria, and serosa. Most peptic ulcers are round or oval, but some are linear, triangular, or irregular in shape. Ulcers have depth when viewed through an endoscope. Typically, only a single ulcer is present. An erosion is a focal loss of superficial epithelial cells and glands, without extension through the muscularis mucosae. On endoscopy, erosions appear as breaks in the mucosal lining without depth. At the other extreme, a peptic ulcer may burr itself entirely through the wall of the GI tract, thus connecting the GI lumen with the peritoneal cavity (perforated ulcer), a solid organ such as the pancreas (penetrating ulcer), or another hollow organ such as the intestine or bile duct (fistulizing ulcer).

Epidemiology

In the United States, peptic ulcer disease affects 10% of men and 4% of women at some time in their lives. The incidence is influenced by age (older persons are more susceptible than younger persons) and gender (males are more susceptible than females). Because ulcer disease is often recurrent, its prevalence exceeds its incidence. Eradication of *Helicobacter pylori* from the stomach markedly reduces recurrence of ulcer disease. With the widespread use of treatment regimens for *H. pylori*, the prevalence of peptic ulcer is decreasing in the United States. Reinfection with *H. pylori* remains an uncommon event in the United States (approximately one reinfection per 100 patients a year).

Pathogenesis and Etiologic Factors

The normal stomach and duodenum are able to resist autodigestion by acid-pepsin. However, high rates of acid-pepsin secretion or impaired mucosal resistance factors, such as prostaglandin deficiency, can predispose to duodenal ulcer formation (typically in the most proximal part of the duodenum, the bulb) or to gastric ulcer formation (typically in the most distal part of the stomach, the antrum).

On rare occasions, peptic ulcers occur in the second, third, or fourth portion of the duodenum (postbulbar ulcer) or even in the proximal jejunum. Ordinarily, alkaline secretions from the duodenum, biliary tract, and pancreas neutralize gastric acid in the duodenum, but high rates of gastric acid secretion (e.g., in Zollinger-Ellison syndrome) can overwhelm these endogenous alkaline secretions and lead to postbulbar or jejunal ulcerations.

In patients with pathologic amounts of gastroesophageal reflux of acid-pepsin and in many patients with gastric acid hypersecretion, erosions and ulcers may develop in the lower esophagus [*see Chapter 56*]. Peptic ulcers may also occur where acid and pepsin are secreted heterotopically, such as in a congenital ileal (Meckel) diverticulum.

Regardless of location and etiology, chronic peptic ulcers are similar pathologically. In addition to the focal loss of mucosal epithelial cells, these ulcers have four characteristic layers at their base: fibrinoid necrosis, exudate, granulation tissue, and a fibrous scar, the deepest layer. A layer of granulation tissue and fibrosis may be absent in acute ulcers that occur in settings of serious trauma or severe surgical or medical illnesses [*see Acute Stress Ulcers, below*].

Why a peptic ulcer is such a focal lesion is unclear. Although peptic ulcers require the presence of acid-pepsin, acid-pepsin alone is only rarely sufficient to produce an ulcer, such as in Zollinger-Ellison syndrome. In the majority of patients, there must be another predisposing factor, such as *H. pylori* infection of the stomach,[1,2] use of nonsteroidal anti-inflammatory drugs (NSAIDs), or stress [*see Figure 1*].

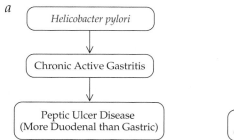
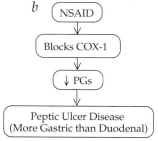
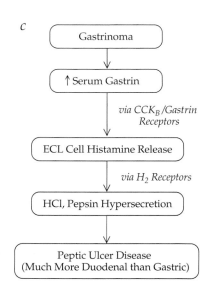

Figure 1 **Etiopathogenesis of peptic ulcers. (a)** *Helicobacter pylori* **induces a diffuse, chronic, active superficial gastritis, usually throughout the stomach. Exactly how this infectious gastritis results in peptic ulcer disease is unknown. (b) Nonsteroidal anti-inflammatory drugs (NSAIDs) block cyclooxygenase-1 (COX-1) to reduce the amount of gastroduodenal prostaglandins (PGs) synthesized from their precursor, arachidonic acid. COX-2 selective inhibitors do not reduce prostaglandins and are associated with much fewer peptic ulcers than nonselective COX-1/COX-2–inhibiting NSAIDs. (c) Gastrinoma in the pancreas or duodenum secretes large amounts of gastrin into the circulation. Elevated serum gastrin levels promote the release of histamine by acting on receptors for cholecystokinin$_B$ (CCK$_B$) and gastrin, which are located on gastric enterochromaffin-like (ECL) cells. Histamine acts on H$_2$ receptors on parietal and chief cells to augment hydrochloric acid (HCl) and pepsin secretion.**

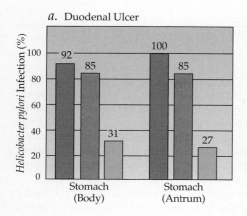

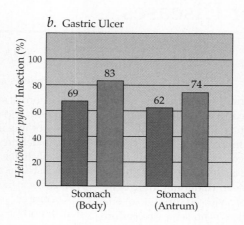

Figure 2 **Point prevalence of *H. pylori* infection assessed by endoscopic biopsy and mucosal histology. The dark-blue bars represent patients with active ulcer (13 duodenal and 13 gastric). The gray bars indicate patients whose ulcers are inactive (20 duodenal and 23 gastric). The light-blue bars represent 26 age- and sex-matched control subjects. None of these ulcer patients were receiving aspirin or NSAIDs.[3]**

H. PYLORI ULCERS

The prevalence of *H. pylori* infection of the stomach is much higher in duodenal ulcer patients and, to a somewhat lesser extent, in gastric ulcer patients than in age-matched control subjects [*see Figure 2*].[3] In addition, cure of *H. pylori* infection with antimicrobial therapy markedly reduces recurrences of duodenal and gastric ulcers.[4,5] The correlation of *H. pylori* infection with peptic ulcers is not consistent, however. Duodenal ulcers develop in some infected persons and gastric ulcers in others, but most infected persons experience no ulcers at all. Patients with duodenal ulcers tend more often to be infected with *cagA*-positive strains than do *H. pylori*–infected patients without ulcer,[6] but how this is mediated is not clear.

The etiologic mechanism linking *H. pylori* infection and ulcerogenesis is not yet absolutely established, for the following reasons: (1) voluntary ingestion of *H. pylori* led to gastric *H. pylori* infection and to gastritis but not to ulcers; (2) duodenal or gastric ulcers develop in only 10% to 20% of individuals with *H. pylori* gastritis, implying that only certain people with additional genetic, anatomic, physiologic, or environmental risk factors are predisposed to ulcers or that only certain *H. pylori* strains are ulcerogenic; (3) *H. pylori* induces diffuse inflammation in the stomach, yet the strongest link between *H. pylori* and peptic ulcer is with focal duodenal bulbar ulcer; and (4) gastric *H. pylori* infection is as common in women as in men, yet duodenal ulcer is two to three times less common in women. Currently, *H. pylori* can be considered the most important risk factor for duodenal and gastric ulcers, but it is clear that the mere presence of *H. pylori* in the stomach is not sufficient to cause peptic ulcers [*see Figure 1a*].

NSAID ULCERS

The ulcerogenicity of NSAIDs has been established experimentally by exposing animals, human volunteers, and patients to these drugs. Experimental studies have been corroborated by numerous case-control studies and autopsy studies. Unlike *H. pylori*–related peptic ulcers, which more often occur in the duodenal bulb, NSAID ulcers typically occur in the stomach. A gastric or duodenal ulcer associated with NSAID use is classified as a peptic ulcer, and it usually heals with potent acid antisecretory therapy, even if NSAID use is continued. NSAIDs can also cause ulcers in the jejunum, ileum, or colon, areas where there is little or no acid-pepsin. These ulcers are not actually peptic ulcers.

Although the pathogenesis of NSAID ulcers is multifactorial, by far the most important mechanism appears to be inhibition of cyclooxygenase-1 (COX-1), the rate-limiting enzyme in GI prostaglandin synthesis [*see Figure 1b*]. Prostaglandins normally protect the GI mucosa from damage by maintaining mucosal blood flow and increasing mucosal secretion of mucus and bicarbonate. Blockade of COX-1 activity by NSAIDs reduces prostaglandin synthesis and thus lowers GI mucosal blood flow and secretion of mucus and bicarbonate. Whether *H. pylori* gastritis increases the risk of gastroduodenal ulcer formation in NSAID users is controversial. In one study of arthritis patients who received the NSAID diclofenac for 6 months, clinically symptomatic peptic ulcers occurred in only 2 of 51 patients (4%) whose *H. pylori* infection was first treated with omeprazole, amoxicillin, and clarithromycin, as compared with occurrence of ulcers in 13 of 49 patients (27%) whose *H. pylori* infection was not first treated with antibiotics.[7] Clinically diagnosed peptic ulcers will develop in approximately 2% to 4% of persons taking NSAIDs per year of exposure. The extent to which the damaging effects of NSAIDs on the stomach are topical rather than systemic is unclear. Many NSAIDs, such as aspirin, are acidic and thus nonionized in the acidic stomach, where they can be absorbed and initiate gastric mucosal damage. However, NSAIDs (such as ketorolac) given by parenteral injection and aspirin given transdermally are ulcerogenic, as are so-called NSAID prodrugs, such as sulindac and nabumetone. (Neither drug inhibits gastric prostaglandins until it is metabolized to its active form after GI absorption.) Evidence suggests that acute mucosal damage by NSAIDs (i.e., hemorrhages and erosions but seldom ulcers) is mainly caused by the topical damaging effects of NSAIDs. Chronic ulcer formation, often with complications such as bleeding and perforation, is mainly the result of the systemic effect of NSAIDs on prostaglandin synthesis by the GI mucosa.

Epidemiologic studies suggest that NSAIDs vary in their ability to cause ulcers,[8] but this issue is complicated by the difficulty of comparing equipotent doses of NSAIDs. All prescription or over-the-counter NSAIDs should be considered ulcerogenic, with the risk of ulcer dependent on dosages and other patient-related factors, particularly advanced age and previous ulcer history. Even low doses of aspirin used for prophylaxis of cardiovascular disease (75 to 325 mg/day) are ulcerogenic in humans.[9] Neither buffering of aspirin nor enteric coating appears to reduce the incidence of clinically detected ulcer formation.[10] Nonacetylated salicylates such as salicylsalicylic acid (salsalate) do not block COX-1 and are not ulcerogenic. Epidemiologic studies indicate that the greatest risk of NSAID ulcers is early in the course of treatment (between day 7 and day 30 after initiation), with the risk decreasing thereafter.

Most NSAIDs, including aspirin, block both COX-1 and COX-2. Unlike COX-1, COX-2 is induced and expressed at inflammatory sites but not in the normal GI tract.[11] Selective COX-2 inhibitors (coxibs) such as celecoxib, rofecoxib, and valdecoxib are analgesic and anti-inflammatory and yet cause much less GI ulcer formation than currently available cyclooxygenase inhibitors when used in recommended doses.[12,13] Whether routine use of coxibs in place of NSAIDs will be cost-effective remains to be determined.

Corticosteroids, which block COX-2 but not COX-1,[11] are no longer considered ulcerogenic when used alone, although they impair healing of preexisting ulcers. When corticosteroids are used in combination with NSAIDs, the risk of ulcer formation is much greater than when NSAIDs are used alone.

ULCERS IN GASTRINOMA OR OTHER HYPERSECRETORY STATES

A gastrinoma is an endocrine tumor of the pancreas or duodenum (usually malignant) consisting of gastrin (G) cells. Gastrinoma causes less than 1% of all peptic ulcers. Peptic ulcers develop in 95% of patients with gastrinoma (Zollinger-Ellison syndrome); ulcers occur most commonly in the duodenal bulb but are also seen in the postbulbar duodenum, jejunum, lower esophagus, and stomach. Multiple ulcers are present in up to 25% of cases of Zollinger-Ellison syndrome.

Patients with a gastrinoma have high circulating levels of gastrin [see Figure 1c], which acts on receptors for cholecystokinin$_B$ (CCK$_B$) and gastrin located on enterochromaffin-like (ECL) cells within the mucosa of the gastric body. ECL cells then release histamine, which acts on H$_2$ receptors present on the membrane of neighboring parietal cells to stimulate (via an adenylate cyclase–cyclic adenosine monophosphate [cAMP]–mediated pathway) the secretion of hydrochloric acid by a unique proton pump, the H$^+$,K$^+$–ATPase pump. Of less physiologic importance, gastrin also acts directly on CCK$_B$/gastrin receptors on parietal cells, increasing cytosol calcium levels in the parietal cells.

Hypergastrinemia in Zollinger-Ellison syndrome results in a continuous high rate of secretion of hydrochloric acid and pepsin, even under basal (fasting) conditions. These secretions overwhelm the buffering and neutralizing capacity of food and upper digestive secretions, as well as mucosal defense factors. Peptic ulceration results, and in many cases, diarrhea (with or without malabsorption) occurs.

Approximately 20% to 30% of patients with gastrinomas have features suggesting a multiple endocrine neoplasia type I (MEN I) syndrome, such as hypercalcemia secondary to hyperparathyroidism, a pituitary adenoma, or both. MEN I is inherited as an autosomal dominant disorder.

Some patients with duodenal ulcer have marked acid hypersecretion but normal serum gastrin levels. A few of these patients have hyperhistaminemia caused by systemic mastocytosis or chronic basophilic leukemia. However, the majority of patients have no known reason for the acid hypersecretion (idiopathic basal acid hypersecretion), although some are infected with H. pylori. Eradication of H. pylori in these latter individuals may reduce basal acid hypersecretion.

IDIOPATHIC ULCERS

Up to 20% of chronic gastric and duodenal ulcers in the United States occur in patients who have no evidence of H. pylori infection, are not taking NSAIDs, and have normal serum gastrin concentrations. These ulcers are referred to as idiopathic peptic ulcers. Some patients with this disorder may be taking NSAIDs surreptitiously. In others, emotional stress, perhaps associated with gastric acid hypersecretion, may be a contributing factor.[14]

Cigarette smoking is also a risk factor for peptic ulcers, but whether smoking is linked to idiopathic ulcers is uncertain.

ACUTE STRESS ULCERS

Acute gastroduodenal erosions and ulcers are very common in patients with serious medical and surgical conditions.[15] Such conditions include severe head injury (Cushing ulcers); burn injury (Curling ulcers); major surgical procedures; and life-threatening illnesses such as septic shock, respiratory failure requiring mechanical ventilation, hepatic failure, renal failure, and multiorgan failure. Unlike peptic ulcers, stress ulcers are typically asymptomatic, rarely causing dyspepsia or epigastric pain. Approximately 10% to 25% of patients with acute stress ulcers experience painless upper GI bleeding of variable severity. Bleeding may manifest itself in the intensive care unit as a dark (so-called coffee-ground) or bloody nasogastric aspirate, as a declining hematocrit, as an increasing transfusion requirement, or as unexplained hypotension.

The pathogenesis of stress ulcers is not well understood. The common denominator seems to be tissue hypoxia and acidosis, precipitated by mucosal vasoconstriction and ischemia. Systemic hypoxia, metabolic acidosis, anemia, and reduced cardiac output often are contributing factors. Once mucosal hypoxia develops, mucosal defense factors are impaired and the cells lining the stomach and duodenum become vulnerable to damage by acid-pepsin. Acute stress ulcers have become less common because of the routine use of prophylaxis with effective medications (see below).

CAMERON ULCERS

Linear gastric erosions that occur in a hiatus hernia are known as Cameron ulcers.[15] The erosions are thought to be related to either traumatic injury of the stomach by the surrounding diaphragm or to mucosal ischemia at the point where the stomach herniates through the diaphragm. Like acute stress ulcers, Cameron ulcers tend to present as bleeding without dyspepsia. Both acute and chronic GI blood loss are possible outcomes of Cameron ulcers.

Diagnosis

CLINICAL MANIFESTATIONS

Peptic ulcers produce a variety of symptoms but none specific for the disease. Also, symptoms of duodenal ulcer are indistinguishable from those of gastric ulcer. Patients with uncomplicated ulcers typically experience mild to moderate abdominal pain, usually in the epigastrium. However, the pain may be localized to the left or right upper quadrant of the abdomen, to the lower chest (subxiphoid or substernal), the midabdomen, or the back. The pain is often gnawing or burning. It may occur in the middle of the night; rarely, it occurs upon first awakening in the morning. Discomfort is typically relieved by food or an antacid.

Severe pain or a rapid increase in pain suggests an ulcer complication (e.g., perforation or penetration) or another diagnosis (e.g., acute pancreatitis). Associated dyspeptic symptoms include nausea, bloating, heartburn, and belching. Although vomiting may occur with uncomplicated peptic ulcers and may temporarily relieve pain, repeated vomiting suggests an ulcer complication (e.g., gastric outlet obstruction) or another diagnosis (e.g., intestinal obstruction).

Peptic ulcers are the most common cause of acute upper GI bleeding. Therefore, hematemesis, melena, or both, even in a pa-

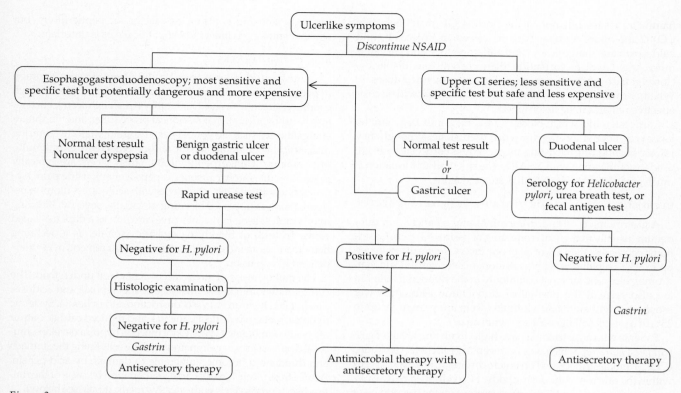

Figure 3 **Approach to a patient with new and undiagnosed ulcerlike symptoms refractory to a therapeutic trial of customary prescription doses of an H$_2$ receptor blocker or with recurrent ulcerlike symptoms when the H$_2$ receptor blocker is stopped.**

tient with no history of ulcer and no dyspeptic symptoms, should suggest the possibility of a bleeding peptic ulcer. Patients who develop ulcers while taking prescription or over-the-counter NSAIDs or low (cardiovascular) doses of aspirin often have no history of ulcerlike pain. Other patients with bleeding ulcers will have experienced dyspeptic symptoms for the preceding days or weeks, only to have these symptoms wane when bleeding ensues.

In addition to a review of the patient's symptoms and ulcer risk factors (particularly NSAID use and smoking), a family history should be obtained. A family history of ulcer can usually be attributed to within-family infection by *H. pylori*, to NSAID use, or to smoking. However, a family history of ulcer, hyperparathyroidism, kidney stones, or endocrine tumor should alert the physician to the possibility of gastrinoma (Zollinger-Ellison syndrome), with or without autosomal dominant MEN I syndrome.

PHYSICAL EXAMINATION FINDINGS

In uncomplicated peptic ulcer disease, the examination is generally normal. The presence of epigastric tenderness does not distinguish dyspepsia caused by peptic ulcer from other types of dyspepsia.

Patients who have complicated ulcers often have tachycardia and hypotension, which are exaggerated when the patient assumes an upright position. These findings may indicate a bleeding ulcer, a perforated ulcer with peritonitis, or an obstructing ulcer with protracted vomiting and volume depletion. Pulse and blood pressure measurements may give misleading information about the extent of volume contraction if the patient has preexisting hypertension, has cardiovascular disease, or is receiving medication that can affect these parameters (e.g., a beta-adrener-

gic blocker or a calcium channel blocker). Fever and tachypnea suggest ulcer perforation with peritonitis.

Special attention should be given to the patient's mental status, skin and mucous membranes, heart and lungs, and, of course, abdomen and rectum. Involuntary guarding, rigidity, rebound tenderness, and a paucity or absence of bowel sounds suggests ulcer perforation with peritonitis. These findings may be less prominent or even absent in the very young, the elderly, and patients on corticosteroids or analgesics. Abdominal distention suggests gastric outlet obstruction or ileus. In a patient who has not eaten in 6 hours, a splashing sound over the stomach when the body is shaken (succussion) suggests gastric outlet obstruction or delayed gastric emptying caused by ileus. Melena or a positive fecal occult blood test suggests ulcer bleeding. Hematochezia or maroon-colored stool may be present if bleeding is voluminous and intestinal transit is rapid. Detection of melena, hematochezia, or maroon-colored stool should prompt placement of a nasogastric tube to obtain an aspirate of gastric contents. If this aspirate is grossly bloody, the diagnosis of upper GI bleeding is confirmed and the likelihood of a bleeding ulcer is increased.

LABORATORY STUDIES

Laboratory results are normal in most patients with uncomplicated ulcer. A complete blood count should be done if blood loss or ulcer perforation is suspected; and serum electrolytes, blood urea nitrogen (BUN), and serum creatinine should be measured if the patient has poor oral intake, nausea, or vomiting. An elevated serum calcium level suggests the possibility of hyperparathyroidism and MEN I with Zollinger-Ellison syndrome, but the pretest probability of this condition is too low in patients presenting with ulcerlike symptoms to recommend routine measurement of serum calcium. If the patient has a strong family history of ulcer disease or of renal stones or has a personal history of renal stones, measurement of serum calcium is warranted, as is measurement of fasting serum gastrin once ulcer disease is confirmed and other etiologies of ulcer are excluded. If the calcium level is elevated, a serum parathyroid hormone measurement should be ordered.

Patients with complicated ulcers often have significant laboratory abnormalities, but these abnormalities are not specific for ulcer disease. Patients with bleeding ulcers have anemia and may have a leukocytosis. The red cell indices (e.g., mean corpuscular volume) are typically normal. In the first several hours after an acute ulcer bleed, the hemoglobin concentration will not completely reflect the severity of the blood loss until compensatory hemodilution occurs or until intravenous fluids such as isotonic saline are administered. Thus, the pulse rate and blood pressure in the supine and upright positions are better initial indicators of extent of blood loss than are red cell counts. Patients with bleeding ulcers typically have azotemia, with ratios of BUN to serum creatinine greater than 20:1, resulting from digestion and intestinal absorption of nitrogenous blood components in concert with reduced renal perfusion.

In patients with perforated ulcers and peritonitis, exudation of plasma into the peritoneal cavity (so-called third space) may result in an increased hemoglobin concentration from hemoconcentration. The presence of leukocytosis, elevated band forms, or leukopenia should raise suspicion of intra-abdominal sepsis. Lactic acidosis with an increased anion gap may ensue as a consequence of a sepsis syndrome or hypovolemia.

Patients with gastric outlet obstruction typically exhibit a hypokalemic, hypochloremic metabolic alkalosis. If volume loss is extreme, a coexistent metabolic lactic acidosis with an increased anion gap may be present, which may cause an elevated serum bicarbonate level to drop toward normal or even to low levels. Likewise, mild to moderate hyponatremia often develops in patients with vomiting from gastric outlet obstruction. Prerenal azotemia and a BUN–serum creatinine ratio greater than 20:1 are typical.

IMAGING STUDIES

Although ulcer disease can be suggested by history, physical examination, and laboratory studies, none of these has sufficient specificity to confirm the diagnosis. Ulcers are diagnosed endoscopically, radiologically, or surgically. Once an ulcer is diagnosed, additional studies can help in determining the cause of the ulcer (e.g., *H. pylori* infection, NSAID use, gastrinoma, or cancer masquerading as benign ulcer).

Endoscopy

Endoscopy is the most accurate way to diagnose a peptic ulcer [*see Figure 3*]. Most patients require local anesthesia of the pharynx and conscious sedation with an intravenous agent such as midazolam. The advantages of endoscopy are its nearly 100% specificity (rare false positives), greater than 90% sensitivity, portability (i.e., it can be performed in the intensive care unit, emergency department, or operating room), and ability to obtain tissue samples to help determine the etiology of the ulcer. The disadvantages of endoscopy are its cost and its potential for serious side effects. The most serious complications of endoscopy are respiratory depression and perforation of the GI tract. When a bleeding or obstructing ulcer is suspected, the stomach should be intubated and emptied with a large-bore tube before endoscopy to decrease the possibility of bronchopulmonary aspiration of gastric contents and to facilitate endoscopic visualization of mucosal lesions. Endoscopy is contraindicated in cases of suspected perforation.

Radiology

Despite having a lower sensitivity and specificity than endoscopy, an upper GI series using barium and air (double contrast) is often favored by primary care physicians over referral for endoscopy for suspected uncomplicated ulcer. An upper GI series offers lower cost, wider availability, and fewer complications [*see Figure 3*]. However, for troublesome and undiagnosed dyspepsia, an upper GI series may be superfluous, because a normal result will often necessitate endoscopy (endoscopy is more sensitive than radiography) and because an upper GI series showing a gastric ulcer will also necessitate endoscopy to obtain biopsy samples to exclude gastric malignancy. In many patients, only a finding of a duodenal bulbar ulcer on an upper GI series will preclude endoscopy [*see Figure 4*].

Plain films of the abdomen, abdominal sonography, and computed tomographic scans may be helpful in patients presenting with suspected complicated ulcers, particularly perforated or obstructing ulcers. Upright chest x-rays of a patient with a perforated ulcer may show free intraperitoneal air [*see Figure 4b*], typically beneath the right hemidiaphragm. When plain films are negative or equivocal, pneumoperitoneum may be diagnosed by abdominal sonography or CT scan. Such studies should be performed

a *b*

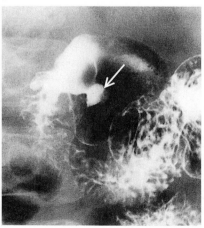 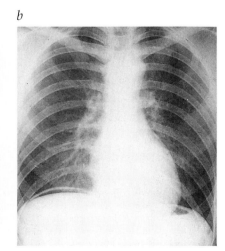

Figure 4   (*a*) Upper GI series in which double contrast (barium and air) is used, showing rounded collection of barium in an ulcer (arrow) in the duodenal bulb of a patient presenting with dyspepsia (uncomplicated duodenal ulcer). (*b*) Upright chest x-ray showing air beneath the right hemidiaphragm (pneumoperitoneum) of a patient presenting with an acute abdomen caused by a perforated duodenal ulcer.

only if the diagnosis of perforation is unclear; if physical signs of peritonitis are obvious, the patient should be referred to a surgeon. Patients with gastric outlet obstruction may have an enlarged stomach with old food debris visible on plain film of the abdomen, upper GI series, abdominal sonography, or CT scan.

SURGICAL DIAGNOSIS

Certain patients will not have ulcers diagnosed until surgery is performed. Such patients include those presenting with an acute abdomen, in whom the diagnosis of perforated ulcer is made at exploratory laparotomy; those presenting with copious upper GI bleeding, in whom it is difficult for the endoscopist to visualize and treat the ulcer; and those with an obstructing ulcer who have a pinpoint pylorus or a duodenal stricture that prevents passage of the endoscope beyond the stenosis.

Tests to Establish the Etiology of the Ulcer

ENDOSCOPIC TESTS

The endoscopist can biopsy the stomach of an ulcer patient to determine whether *H. pylori* organisms are present [*see Figure 5*]. *H. pylori* organisms contain abundant amounts of urease, which splits urea into carbon dioxide and ammonia. If the biopsy sample is placed on a urea-containing medium that also contains a pH-sensitive dye, a change in color indicates that ammonia is being produced. This so-called rapid urease test has a high sensitivity and specificity (> 90%) for *H. pylori*. If the rapid urease test is negative, a separate biopsy specimen should be sent to a pathology laboratory in formalin for histology. *H. pylori* can be detected with routine hematoxylin and eosin stains [*see Figure 5*] or, if necessary, by special stains. Moreover, the presence of active chronic gastritis is virtually diagnostic of *H. pylori* infection, and its absence excludes *H. pylori* infection.

Another useful endoscopic procedure is to obtain multiple biopsies from the edges and the base of the ulcer to exclude malignancy. This is routinely done in cases of gastric ulcer because one in 25 to one in 50 benign-appearing gastric ulcers is in actuality an ulcer within a malignancy, usually in an adenocarcinoma. Duodenal ulcers need not be biopsied unless the ulcer is located in a mass.

Endoscopy may also demonstrate a neuroendocrine tumor, compatible with a gastrinoma on special stains. Such a tumor is usually located in the proximal duodenum.

In an ulcer patient with a negative rapid urease test and no *H. pylori*–related gastritis or gastric malignancy on histology, further history regarding NSAID use should be obtained from the patient or the patient's family. Some patients with NSAID-related ulcers have erosions, subepithelial hemorrhages, or both, which clue the endoscopist to the possibility of occult or surreptitious NSAID use.

SEROLOGIC TESTS

A number of serum antibody tests for *H. pylori* are available that have a greater than 90% sensitivity and specificity if the patient has not yet received therapy for *H. pylori*.[16] In patients in whom active ulcers are diagnosed by radiology or surgery and in whom gastric tissue is not available, *H. pylori* serology can confirm infection with high accuracy [*see Figure 3*].

In ulcer patients with no evidence of *H. pylori* infection or NSAID use, fasting serum gastrin concentration should be measured [*see Figure 3*] to screen for gastrinoma (Zollinger-Ellison syndrome). If the serum gastrin concentration is greater than 1,000 pg/ml in a patient with duodenal ulcer, the diagnosis of gastrinoma is confirmed. A modest elevation in fasting serum gastrin concentration (> 150 pg/ml but < 1,000 pg/ml) is suggestive of gastrinoma, but a provocative test should be performed using intravenous secretin (2 IU/kg as a bolus) or calcium (4 mg Ca^{2+}/kg/hr as a continuous infusion for 3 hours).[17] A rise in serum gastrin concentration of more than 200 pg/ml after secretin administration has a greater than 90% sensitivity and specificity for gastrinoma. Supplies of secretin have been limited recently, making this test impractical. A serum gastrin rise of greater than 395 pg/ml during calcium infusion is quite specific for gastrinoma, but using this cutoff is less sensitive than the secretin test in diagnosing gastrinoma, and the lengthy infusion and the resultant hypercalcemia make this test unpopular. Because achlorhydria can produce marked hypergastrinemia as a result of the loss of negative feedback of gastric acid on gastrin release, basal acid output or pH should be measured to confirm that the stomach secretes acid in ulcer patients with fasting hypergastrinemia. The combination of achlorhydria, hypergastrinemia, and duodenal ulcer is exceedingly rare, whereas the combination of achlorhydria, hypergastrinemia, and gastric ulcer is sometimes encountered and should suggest gastric adenocarcinoma or NSAID use. A fasting gastric pH measurement will almost invariably distinguish gastrinoma (pH 1 to 2) from

a

b

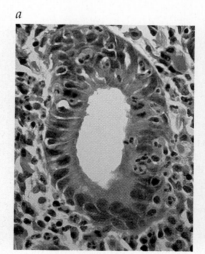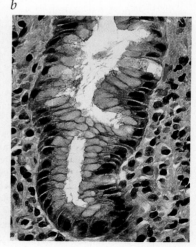

Figure 5   **Gastric biopsy samples stained with hematoxylin and eosin demonstrating (*a*) chronic active gastritis with a few *H. pylori* organisms faintly seen in the lumen of a gland and (*b*) chronic active gastritis with *H. pylori* organisms more abundant.**

achlorhydria (pH 6 to 8), unless the patient has received a potent acid antisecretory agent before pH measurement.

Measurement of serum thromboxane B_2 (platelet COX-1 activity) has been used in research laboratories to demonstrate occult or surreptitious NSAID use.[18] However, this assay is not widely available.

BREATH TESTS

A noninvasive method for detecting *H. pylori* in the stomach, the urea breath test, begins with oral ingestion of urea that has been labeled with carbon-13 (^{13}C) or carbon-14 (^{14}C). If *H. pylori*, with its abundant urease, is present in the stomach, the labeled urea will be rapidly converted to $^{13}CO_2$ or $^{14}CO_2$, which can be detected in breath samples collected during the first 30 to 60 minutes after urea ingestion. Sensitivity and specificity of the breath test are comparable to those of serology.[16] In a patient for whom there is no clinical indication for endoscopy, a urea breath test is an alternative to serology for documenting *H. pylori* infection [*see Figure 3*]. However, because proton pump inhibitors can suppress *H. pylori* without eradicating it, use of these drugs should be avoided for 2 weeks before the urea breath test is administered to minimize false negative results.

Because serology is quicker, it is preferred to breath testing for initial diagnosis. Breath testing is more useful than serology in diagnosing failure of eradication of *H. pylori* or reinfection in patients who were previously treated for *H. pylori* infection, because the serology will usually remain positive for several months even after successful treatment.[19]

FECAL ANTIGEN TEST

Recently, a stool test for *H. pylori* antigen has been developed that compares favorably with urea breath tests.[20] The test can also distinguish current infection (antigen present in stool) from past infection (antigen not present in stool). False positive results have been reported in patients with ulcer bleeding, however.[21]

Differential Diagnosis

The disorder most commonly confused with uncomplicated peptic ulcer is nonulcer dyspepsia; the most serious GI disorder confused with uncomplicated peptic ulcer is gastric cancer [*see Chapter 196*].

Nonulcer, or functional, dyspepsia is a symptom complex similar to that experienced by patients with peptic ulcers. However, no ulcers or other lesions are visible when the patient undergoes endoscopy. Nonulcer dyspepsia is a heterogeneous, poorly understood group of disorders. Some physicians, if they find no ulcer at the time of endoscopy, perform a gastric biopsy to detect *H. pylori*, and if the biopsy is positive for *H. pylori*, they treat the patient for this infection. The utility of this approach is not clear, because studies show little or no symptomatic benefit after successful eradication of *H. pylori* and resolution of active chronic gastritis.[22-24] However, there are probably a few patients in whom *H. pylori* gastritis causes dyspepsia. Because it is not currently possible to predict which patients infected with *H. pylori* will become asymptomatic after *H. pylori* eradication, many physicians treat all dyspeptic patients who are infected with *H. pylori*. The cost-effectiveness of this approach has not been established. Many patients with nonulcer dyspepsia appear to suffer from a dysmotility of the upper GI tract that is akin to irritable bowel syndrome of the lower GI tract. Such individuals may complain of abdominal fullness, postprandial bloating, early

Table 1 Differential Diagnosis
of Peptic Ulcer Disease

Presentation	*Diagnosis*
Suspected uncompli-cated ulcer	Nonulcer dyspepsia, gastroesophageal reflux, biliary colic, pancreatitis, angina pectoris, gastric cancer
Bleeding ulcer	Varices, Mallory-Weiss tear, esophagitis, vascular lesion (arteriovenous malformation, Dieulafoy lesion, angiodysplasia)
Perforated ulcer	Appendicitis, pancreatitis, cholecystitis, spontaneous bacterial peritonitis, bowel ischemia or infarction, diverticulitis
Penetrating ulcer	Pancreatitis, muscle strain, herniated verte-bral disk, ureteral stone
Fistulizing ulcer	Gallstones, GI malignancy, Crohn disease, intra-abdominal abscess

satiety, and nausea, all suggestive of delayed gastric emptying. In some of these patients, gastric prokinetic agents such as domperidone or metoclopramide may help relieve symptoms.

Complicated ulcers may be confused with a variety of disorders. These include both intra-abdominal and musculoskeletal processes [*see Table 1*].

Treatment

The goals of ulcer therapy are to relieve symptoms quickly; to heal the ulcer quickly; to prevent ulcer recurrences; and to reduce ulcer-related complications, morbidity (including the need for surgery), and mortality. The general strategy in a patient with an ulcer should be to treat complications aggressively if present; to determine the etiology of the ulcer; to discontinue NSAID use if possible; to eradicate *H. pylori* infection if present or strongly suspected, even if other risk factors (e.g., NSAID use) are also present; and to use acid antisecretory therapy to heal the ulcer if *H. pylori* infection is not present.

If duodenal ulcer is diagnosed by endoscopy, rapid urease testing of endoscopically obtained gastric biopsy samples, with or without histologic examination, should reliably establish the presence or absence of *H. pylori*. If duodenal ulcer is diagnosed by x-ray, then a serologic, urea breath, or fecal antigen test to diagnose *H. pylori* infection is recommended before treating the patient for *H. pylori*.

TREATMENT OF UNCOMPLICATED DUODENAL ULCERS

H. pylori–*Related Duodenal Ulcer*

Duodenal ulcer associated with *H. pylori* infection should be treated with antimicrobial therapy because successful therapy is associated with markedly reduced ulcer recurrences [*see Figure 6*].[4,5] Antimicrobial therapy is usually empirical rather than based on results of culture and in vitro antimicrobial sensitivity testing. No single antimicrobial agent has an acceptably high success rate against *H. pylori*. Combinations of antimicrobial agents are required, and some regimens that have been approved by the Food and Drug Administration can be recommended [*see Table 2*].

H. pylori has adapted to the acidic stomach, and potent acid antisecretory agents facilitate eradication of *H. pylori* by antimicrobial agents. Bismuth compounds, like proton pump inhibitors, suppress the growth of *H. pylori* but usually do not by themselves eradicate it from the stomach. For this reason, they are frequently employed together with antibiotics.

Antimicrobial agents with activity against *H. pylori* include metronidazole, tetracycline, amoxicillin, and clarithromycin. Most popular are 10- to 14-day regimens, although 7-day courses may be effective and are especially favored in Europe. A 2-week course of a three-drug regimen that includes a proton pump inhibitor, clarithromycin, and amoxicillin has a success rate close to 90%. The major causes of treatment failure are poor compliance with the regimen and clarithromycin resistance; the latter occurs in around 10% of current strains and is increasing with more macrolide use in the population. Metronidazole resistance occurs in 30% to 40% of strains. However, unlike resistance to clarithromycin, which is usually absolute, resistance to metronidazole is relative and can be overcome in some patients.

If a patient who complies with one of the clarithromycin-based regimens fails treatment, clarithromycin resistance is likely. In such cases, the re-treatment regimen should not include clarithromycin. Most physicians choose a regimen consisting of metronidazole, tetracycline, bismuth (e.g., Pepto Bismol), and a proton pump inhibitor or H_2 receptor blocker. Because of the frequency of metronidazole resistance, other antimicrobials with activity against *H. pylori* are being used more often.[25-28] These agents include azithromycin, the quinolones norfloxacin and levofloxacin, and rifabutin [*see Table 3*]. In one study, a 7-day rescue treatment for persistent *H. pylori* infection using the proton pump inhibitor rabeprazole plus rifabutin and levofloxacin had a 95% success rate, as did a four-drug regimen consisting of rabeprazole, bismuth subcitrate, metronidazole, and tetracycline.[29]

It may also be possible to predict resistance to clarithromycin or to metronidazole by taking a careful history to look for prior exposure to these drugs. Such a history might help the physician choose a first-line regimen that will be more likely to be successful, although more studies using this history-directed approach are needed.

Side effects of *H. pylori*–directed therapy are not uncommon but are generally mild. Physicians should be aware of potential drug-drug interactions if the patient is receiving other medications. If the patient has an active, symptomatic ulcer, an antisecretory drug should be continued at a reduced (standard) dosage for 2 to 5 weeks after completion of antimicrobial agents.

Table 2   Clarithromycin-Based FDA-Approved Regimens to Eradicate *Helicobacter pylori**

Esomeprazole, amoxicillin, clarithromycin (EAC)
Esomeprazole, 40 mg b.i.d. for 10 days; then 40 mg q.d. for 18 days if an active ulcer is present
Amoxicillin, 1 g b.i.d. for 10–14 days
Clarithromycin, 500 mg b.i.d. or t.i.d. for 14 days

Lansoprazole, amoxicillin, clarithromycin (LAC)
Lansoprazole, 30 mg b.i.d. for 10–14 days; then 15 mg q.d. for 14–18 days if an active ulcer is present
Amoxicillin, 1 g b.i.d. for 10–14 days
Clarithromycin, 500 mg b.i.d. for 10–14 days

Omeprazole, amoxicillin, clarithromycin (OAC)
Omeprazole, 20 mg b.i.d. for 10 days; then 20 mg q.d. for 18 days if an active ulcer is present
Amoxicillin, 1 g b.i.d. for 10–14 days
Clarithromycin, 500 mg b.i.d. for 10 days

*Another regimen, omeprazole, 40 mg q.d., plus clarithromycin, 500 mg t.i.d., is not listed because of its lower efficacy and association with more clarithromycin resistance.

After a patient has completed a course of ulcer therapy for an *H. pylori*–related uncomplicated duodenal ulcer, it is acceptable to follow the patient clinically without confirming eradication, because most compliant patients will be successfully cured of their *H. pylori* infection [*see Figure 6*]. A patient with an *H. pylori*–related duodenal ulcer that does not recur symptomatically within 2 years after antimicrobial therapy is probably cured. Serology has often reverted to negative by this time.[19]

Those in whom recurrent ulcer symptoms develop during the first 2 years after therapy should be assessed either by endoscopy (for ulcer recurrence and for *H. pylori* persistence or reinfection) or by a urea breath test or fecal antigen test. The most common cause of recurrent ulceration in patients treated for *H. pylori*–related duodenal ulcer is failure to eradicate the organism. Re-treatment of these patients is indicated [*see* Treatment of Intractable Duodenal Ulcers or Gastric Ulcers, *below*]. Rarer causes of duodenal ulcer recurrence include an acid hypersecretory state (e.g., Zollinger-Ellison syndrome), NSAID use, and reinfection with *H. pylori*.

Table 3   Newer Antimicrobial Agents with Reported Activity against *Helicobacter pylori*

Agent*	Dosage	Comments
Azithromycin	500 mg q.d.	Combined with either amoxicillin or a nitroimidazole, plus a proton pump inhibitor, for 3–7 days
Norfloxacin	400 mg b.i.d.	Combined with a proton pump inhibitor for 14 days
Levofloxacin	500 mg q.d.	Combined with either amoxicillin or a nitroimidazole, plus a proton pump inhibitor, for 7 days
Rifabutin	300 mg q.d.	Combined with amoxicillin and a proton pump inhibitor for 7–10 days

*These agents are marketed in the United States, but they are not yet approved for *H. pylori* therapy. Additional studies are needed before they can be strongly endorsed.

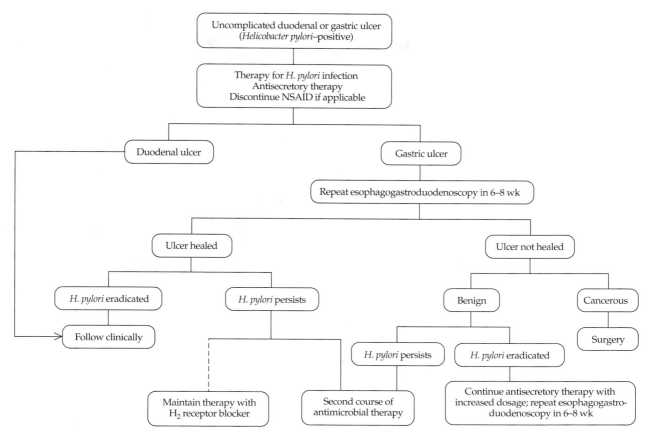

Figure 6 **Approach to treatment and follow-up of a patient with an uncomplicated duodenal or gastric ulcer associated with *H. pylori* infection of the stomach. Maintenance therapy is long-term nightly administration of an H₂ receptor blocker or once-a-day proton pump inhibitor [*see Table 3*].**

H. pylori–*Negative Duodenal Ulcer*

In a duodenal ulcer patient who is *H. pylori* negative, the physician should consider NSAID use and gastrinoma (Zollinger-Ellison syndrome).[30] Patients with duodenal ulcer who are taking NSAIDs should have the NSAID discontinued, if possible. At the same time, an acid antisecretory drug should be administered for 4 to 8 weeks [*see Table 4*]. The anticipated healing rate with this regimen is 85% to 95%.

Patients with duodenal ulcer as part of the Zollinger-Ellison syndrome should be managed initially with a high dose of a proton pump inhibitor, followed by a maintenance dose guided by gastric acid measurements. If there is no evidence of hepatic metastasis on abdominal CT scan, then exploratory laparotomy for gastrinoma resection, with or without parietal cell vagotomy, is warranted.[31] Radionuclide scintigraphy with octreotide, an analog of somatostatin, is a highly sensitive and specific preoperative test for detecting gastrinoma, as is endoscopic ultrasonography.

The vast majority of duodenal ulcers, regardless of cause, heal after 8 weeks of antisecretory therapy with a proton pump inhibitor or an H₂ receptor blocker. Antacids are often prescribed as needed to relieve ulcer symptoms.

In rare cases of idiopathic duodenal ulcer, it is prudent that, after the ulcer has been healed by an acid antisecretory agent, the patient be placed on a maintenance dose of an H₂ receptor blocker given at bedtime to reduce ulcer recurrences. Proton pump inhibitors are also effective in preventing duodenal ulcer recurrences. It is not necessary to confirm duodenal ulcer healing by endoscopy or x-ray before reducing the antisecretory drug dose to a maintenance level.

TREATMENT OF UNCOMPLICATED GASTRIC ULCERS

H. pylori–*Related Gastric Ulcer*

Gastric ulcer associated with *H. pylori* should be treated with antibiotics [*see Table 2*].[9,10] Because they are larger than duodenal ulcers, gastric ulcers take longer to heal. Thus, after antibiotic administration, the patient should be treated with an acid antisecretory agent [*see Tables 3 and 4*] for an additional 4 to 8 weeks. Patients with gastric ulcers should be followed endoscopically until complete healing has been achieved so that an ulcerated gastric cancer is not missed. Gastric biopsies should be obtained during follow-up endoscopy to determine whether eradication of *H. pylori* has occurred [*see Figure 6*]. Patients with a history of an uncomplicated gastric ulcer that is currently quiescent should be screened for *H. pylori* infection, and if the result is positive, they should be treated for *H. pylori* infection to prevent ulcer recurrences.

NSAID-Related Gastric Ulcer

The therapy for an active NSAID-related gastric ulcer is administration of a proton pump inhibitor [*see Tables 4 and 5*], as well as discontinuance of the NSAID. Healing rates with H₂ receptor blockers are nearly as high as with proton pump inhibitors if the NSAID can be stopped.

Table 4   FDA-Approved Antisecretory Drugs
for Active Peptic Ulcer Disease*

Class	Drugs	Dosage	Drug Interactions
H₂ receptor blockers†	Cimetidine‡	800 mg h.s. *or* 400 mg b.i.d.	Slows metabolism of warfarin, theophylline, phenytoin, diazepam, and others‖
	Ranitidine‡	300 mg h.s. *or* 150 mg b.i.d.	Minimal
	Nizatidine‡	300 mg h.s. *or* 150 mg b.i.d.	Minimal
	Famotidine‡	40 mg h.s. *or* 20 mg b.i.d.	Minimal
Proton pump inhibitors§	Omeprazole	20 mg q.d., a.c.	Slows metabolism of diazepam, warfarin, and phenytoin‖
	Lansoprazole	15 mg q.d., a.c.	Minimal
	Esomeprazole	40 mg q.d., a.c.	Slows metabolism of diazepam, warfarin, and phenytoin
	Rabeprazole	20 mg q.d., a.c.	Approved in U.S. for duodenal ulcer healing only (for 4 weeks)
	Pantoprazole	40 mg q.d., a.c.	Not approved for peptic ulcer disease or as part of *Helicobacter pylori* treatment

*Patients with gastrinoma (Zollinger-Ellison syndrome) will usually require much higher dosages of antisecretory drugs than listed here.

†Use for 4–8 wk in the treatment of duodenal ulcer and 6–12 wk in the treatment of gastric ulcer. Duodenal ulcers that do not heal by 8 wk and gastric ulcers that do not heal by 12 wk are considered intractable.

‡Dosage of H₂ receptor blockers should be reduced in patients with renal failure. Half the recommended H₂ receptor blocker dosage, usually given at night, is used to maintain healing.

§Proton pump inhibitors approved for gastric ulcers include omeprazole and lansoprazole; those approved for duodenal ulcers include omeprazole, lansoprazole, and rabeprazole.

‖Most of these drug interactions are minor and not clinically relevant; nevertheless, caution is advised.

TREATMENT OF INTRACTABLE DUODENAL ULCERS OR GASTRIC ULCERS

Ulcers That Fail to Heal

Ulcers refractory to pharmacotherapy are rare, and in most cases, prolonging the course of the gastric antisecretory drug, increasing the dose, or taking both measures will lead to healing. The causes of nonhealing include poor compliance with medications, an acid hypersecretory state requiring higher-than-customary doses of antisecretory drugs, continued NSAID use, and persistent *H. pylori* infection. Often, combinations of these factors and others (e.g., smoking and stress) are present.

Poor compliance with medications necessitates patient education and consideration of elective ulcer surgery. A fasting serum gastrin concentration can be used to screen for an acid hypersecretory state resulting from Zollinger-Ellison syndrome. Physicians should be aware that antisecretory drugs (especially proton pump inhibitors) can also raise serum gastrin levels modestly (to 150 to 600 pg/ml). Definitive documentation of an acid hypersecretory state requires quantitative gastric acid measurement

(gastric analysis). NSAID use should be discontinued if at all possible. Persistent *H. pylori* infection is the result of poor compliance with medications or is caused by drug-resistant strains.[25-29] *H. pylori* has proved to be resistant to metronidazole in 30% to 40% of cases and to clarithromycin in 10% of cases; resistance to tetracycline or amoxicillin occurs in 1% of strains or less.[25] Combined resistance to macrolides (e.g., clarithromycin) and imidazoles (e.g., metronidazole) occurs in approximately 5% of patients, in whom infection may prove difficult to eradicate. Culture of gastric biopsy material for *H. pylori,* followed by antimicrobial drug-susceptibility testing when available, can guide re-treatment. In the absence of this information, the patient should be re-treated for 2 weeks with a proton pump inhibitor, with amoxicillin or tetracycline, and with either clarithromycin or metronidazole (whichever antimicrobial agent the patient did not receive initially). Some physicians use a bismuth preparation (e.g., colloidal bismuth subcitrate, bismuth subsalicylate, or ranitidine bismuth citrate) in place of a proton pump inhibitor [*see Table 2*]. Several other antibiotics have activity against *H. pylori* and may prove to be useful in rescue therapy for patients in whom treatments have failed; many such patients harbor antibiotic-resistant strains.[25-29] Agents that are available in the United States include the macrolide azithromycin, the quinolones norfloxacin and levofloxacin, and rifabutin [*see Table 3*].

Frequent Ulcer Recurrences

Another type of intractability is frequent ulcer recurrences (at least three a year). This type of intractability occurs most often when *H. pylori* has not been successfully eradicated (necessitating re-treatment) or, less often, when NSAID use is resumed or when an acid hypersecretory state is present. Idiopathic ulcers sometimes recur frequently, and patients experiencing such recurrences require lifelong maintenance with H₂ receptor blockers or proton pump inhibitors. Some of these patients may choose ulcer surgery (parietal cell vagotomy for duodenal ulcer or antrectomy for gastric ulcer) over lifelong medication.

TREATMENT OF COMPLICATED PEPTIC ULCERS

Bleeding Ulcers

The first priority in a patient with a suspected bleeding peptic ulcer is to stabilize the vital signs with volume resuscitation, ideally in an intensive care unit. Hemodynamic monitoring will assist in fluid and blood replacement, particularly if the patient has severe cardiac disease.

After the patient becomes clinically stable, diagnostic upper GI endoscopy is performed [*see Figure 7*]. If an actively bleeding ulcer or an ulcer with a visible vessel is found, the lesion is treated endoscopically, by injection of epinephrine, by thermal application with a heater probe or a bipolar electrode, or by a combination of these methods. Endoscopic therapy is successful in controlling bleeding in approximately 90% of patients; the other 10% are referred for surgery if major bleeding continues. Random gastric biopsies are obtained at the time of endoscopy to detect *H. pylori* by rapid urease testing and, if necessary, gastric histology.

Once an ulcer is demonstrated, intravenous therapy with an H₂ receptor blocker (e.g., famotidine) or a proton pump inhibitor (e.g., pantoprazole) can be started. Oral therapy with a proton pump inhibitor is superior to no therapy in reducing early rebleeding if endoscopic therapy is not attempted[32]; proton pump inhibitors also reduce rebleeding after endoscopic therapy.[33] As

Table 5 Treatment and Prevention of Peptic Ulcers

Type of Ulcer	Treatment	Prevention	Comments*
Helicobacter pylori–related ulcers	Antisecretory agents [*see Table 4*]	Antibiotics [*see Tables 2 and 3*]	Highly cost-effective; document healing in gastric ulcer; document *H. pylori* eradication in complicated duodenal or gastric ulcer and in intractable duodenal or gastric ulcer
NSAID-related ulcers	Antisecretory agents (proton pump inhibitor has greater antisecretory effect than H$_2$ receptor blocker) [*see Table 4*] Discontinue NSAID use, if possible	Misoprostol (600–800 µg/day) or proton pump inhibitor (e.g., omeprazole, 20–40 mg q.d., or lansoprazole, 15–30 mg q.d.) along with an NSAID	Diarrhea may limit compliance in patients treated with misoprostol; avoid use during pregnancy (abortifacient); proton pump inhibitors are not yet approved by the FDA for prevention of NSAID-related ulcers
Ulcers associated with Zollinger-Ellison syndrome and other hypersecretory states	High-dose proton pump inhibitor, such as omeprazole, lansoprazole, or rabeprazole	Proton pump inhibitor, adjusted to keep basal acid output < 5–10 mEq/hr	Consider exploratory laparotomy (guided by abdominal imaging studies) to remove easily resectable gastrinomas, if feasible; consider MEN I syndrome (present in 20%–30% of cases)[21]
Idiopathic ulcers	H$_2$ receptor blocker or proton pump inhibitor	Nocturnal H$_2$ receptor blocker or A.M. proton pump inhibitor (e.g., lansoprazole, 15 mg q.d.)	Parietal cell vagotomy for intractable duodenal ulcer and antrectomy for intractable duodenal ulcer
Stress ulcers (ICU)	I.V. H$_2$ receptor blocker or perhaps proton pump inhibitor (e.g., pantoprazole) ?Angiography ?Surgery	I.V. H$_2$ receptor blocker or intragastric sucralfate or intragastric antacid	Maintain pH above 4 with H$_2$ receptor blocker or antacid; continuous I.V. infusion is superior to I.V. boluses of H$_2$ receptor blockers
Cameron ulcers (linear gastric erosions in a hiatal hernia)	Iron salts; packed red cell transfusions; endoscopic hemostasis ?Angiography ?Surgery	Hiatal hernia repair, laparoscopic or open	Roles of H$_2$ receptor blockers and proton pump inhibitors are unproved

*I.V. proton pump inhibitors (e.g., pantoprazole) are under investigation for FDA approval.
MEN I—multiple endocrine neoplasia type I   NSAID—nonsteroidal anti-inflammatory drug

soon as oral intake is resumed, a patient who has been on intravenous therapy should be switched to oral therapy with a proton pump inhibitor, which ideally is administered at a high dosage (e.g., omeprazole, 40 mg/day, or lansoprazole, 30 mg/day). If the rapid urease test or gastric histology is positive for *H. pylori*, the patient should receive at least two effective antibiotics (e.g., clarithromycin and amoxicillin) for 14 days, along with a proton pump inhibitor [*see Figure 7*]. The proton pump inhibitor is continued at the same dosage until week 6 for duodenal ulcer or week 8 for gastric ulcer. If a subsequent endoscopy shows complete ulcer healing and disappearance of *H. pylori* by both rapid urease testing and gastric histology, the risk of rebleeding is very low[33-35] and therapy can be stopped. Future use of NSAIDs or aspirin is almost always prohibited. Although the use of coxibs instead of an NSAID is attractive, freedom from rebleeding is not guaranteed. If an NSAID or low-dose aspirin is absolutely necessary, it should be coprescribed with misoprostol[36] or a proton pump inhibitor.[37] If the ulcer heals but *H. pylori* organisms are still present, the patient should be treated again for *H. pylori* or left on a maintenance H$_2$ receptor blocker or proton pump inhibitor. If the ulcer is not healed, persistent *H. pylori* infection is likely. Under these circumstances, gastric tissue can be cultured for *H. pylori*, if available facilities exist, so that antibiotic sensitivities can be determined before re-treatment. Finally, if the ulcer has not healed even though *H. pylori* has been eradicated, then NSAID use, an acid hypersecretory state, or cancer should be considered.

Figure 7 **Approach to treatment and follow-up of a patient with a complicated duodenal or gastric ulcer associated with *H. pylori* infection of the stomach.**

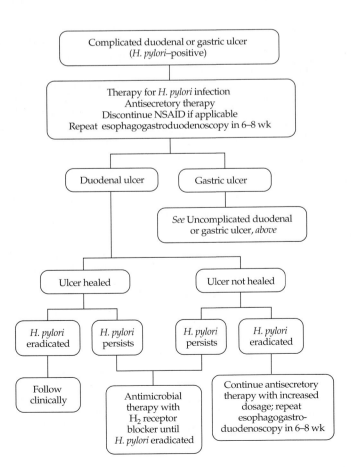

Biopsy samples of the ulcer should be obtained, especially if the ulcer is in the stomach.

A patient with a bleeding peptic ulcer that is negative for *H. pylori* by rapid urease testing and gastric histology usually has an NSAID-related ulcer. The NSAID is stopped if possible, and a high-dose proton pump inhibitor (e.g., 40 mg of omeprazole or 30 mg of lansoprazole) is prescribed for 8 weeks for gastric ulcer or 4 to 6 weeks for duodenal ulcer. Repeat endoscopy is usually indicated to assess healing of a gastric ulcer; if the ulcer has not healed, it is biopsied. Whether to perform a repeat endoscopy to assess healing 4 to 8 weeks after an NSAID-related bleeding duodenal ulcer is controversial. If the ulcer is shown to have healed after the patient is off the NSAID, no further therapy is required unless the patient is placed back on an NSAID or aspirin, even a low dose of aspirin. In such cases, the prostaglandin E_1 analogue misoprostol (200 mg q.i.d.) is modestly protective against subsequent bleeding.[36] There is also evidence that maintenance therapy with a proton pump inhibitor such as lansoprazole or omeprazole is associated with a low rate of NSAID-related ulcer rebleeding. In general, however, NSAIDs should be avoided in patients with ulcers that have bled.

Patients with bleeding ulcers that are idiopathic and that heal on an antisecretory drug should be left on a long-term H_2 receptor blocker or proton pump inhibitor. There is evidence that maintenance therapy with the H_2 receptor blocker ranitidine is effective in preventing rebleeding from duodenal ulcers.[38]

Perforated Ulcers

When a perforated viscus is documented or strongly suspected, the patient is started on broad-spectrum intravenous antibiotics covering gram-negative aerobic bacilli, enterococci, and anaerobes such as *Bacteroides* species and is then taken to surgery for closure of the perforation with a patch of omentum. If the surgeon does not obtain an intraoperative gastric biopsy sample, the patient should undergo postoperative testing for *H. pylori* by serology, urea breath test, or fecal antigen test, and the infection should be treated if present.[39] Many perforated ulcers are associated with NSAID use rather than with *H. pylori* infection.[40] Regardless of the patient's *H. pylori* status, antisecretory drugs should be administered for 6 to 8 weeks postoperatively. Endoscopy is then performed to assess healing. At the time of this endoscopy, success of eradication of *H. pylori* is ascertained by gastric biopsy with rapid urease testing and histology.

Up to 10% of perforated gastric ulcers are in fact perforated gastric cancers. If no biopsy or resection of the ulcer is done at the time of repair of the perforation, postoperative endoscopy with biopsy is imperative before the patient is discharged from the hospital or very soon thereafter.

The mortality in patients with perforated peptic ulcers is 5% to 10%. Factors associated with higher mortality include delayed diagnosis and treatment of perforation; advanced age; comorbid conditions, such as cardiac, pulmonary, or liver disease; immunodeficiency; and advanced malignancy.

A small number of patients with suspected or probable perforated peptic ulcer improve rapidly before surgery is performed. Others refuse surgery or are poor surgical candidates. An alternative to surgery in these situations is nonoperative therapy consisting of nothing by mouth; intravenous fluids and electrolytes; a broad-spectrum antibiotic such as ticarcillin–clavulanic acid; and nasogastric suction. Compared with surgical therapy, nonoperative therapy is associated with more abdominal complications (e.g., abscesses), fewer pulmonary complications (e.g., atelectasis), and similar mortality.[41]

Obstructing Ulcers

The patient with an obstructing ulcer is initially placed on nasogastric suction and intravenous fluids, electrolytes, and an H_2 receptor blocker or proton pump inhibitor. If the obstruction is the result of edema associated with an active ulcer, the gastric outlet may open as edema subsides and the ulcer heals over several days to weeks. If, on the other hand, obstruction is the result of scarring from previous ulcers, it will not resolve with these measures. In some patients, it is difficult to determine whether edema or fibrosis is the primary cause of gastric outlet obstruction. Because obstruction may resolve with time, early consideration should be given to parenteral hyperalimentation. This intervention prevents or minimizes tissue catabolism during the waiting period and also induces a positive nitrogen balance, which will be beneficial if the gastric outlet fails to open up and the patient requires surgery.

A saline load test can be used to guide management. Thirty minutes after 750 ml of isotonic saline is infused into the stomach through the nasogastric tube, gastric contents (saline plus secretions) are aspirated. A return of less than 200 ml indicates normal gastric emptying of liquids and a good prognosis; 200 to 400 ml is indeterminate; and more than 400 ml is suggestive of a high-grade obstruction that will likely require intervention. Repeating the saline load test every day or two may also provide information about whether the obstruction is resolving.

If the obstruction resolves within 5 to 7 days, the nasogastric tube is removed and the patient is fed and observed clinically. An oral proton pump inhibitor or H_2 receptor blocker is started as soon as feasible. Gastric prokinetic agents (e.g., metoclopramide) should not be used. At least 50% of patients whose obstruction resolves with conservative medical therapy will experience another obstruction in about a year. Whether routine treatment of *H. pylori* infection will reduce this high recurrence rate is unknown. Unlike bleeding or perforation, obstruction is usually a late complication of ulcer disease. Thus, *H. pylori* eradication in ulcer patients is more likely to be effective in primary prevention of obstruction than in secondary prevention. NSAIDs may cause gastric outlet obstruction as well and should therefore be avoided. Endoscopic therapy is an option for obstruction that does not resolve with conservative therapy.[42] With inflatable balloons placed over guide wires, a stenotic pylorus or duodenum can be dilated under fluoroscopic guidance, although complications such as perforation may occur. Endoscopic balloon dilatation, when feasible, is a temporizing measure and rarely obviates surgery. Thus, obstruction that recurs after medical therapy or after endoscopic therapy is an indication for surgery. Pyloroplasty, gastroenterostomy, and resection plus gastroenterostomy are the most popular operations for an obstructing ulcer. Pyloroplasty and gastroenterostomy are typically combined with a vagotomy to reduce the likelihood of recurrent ulceration.

Fistulizing Ulcers

Gastric or duodenal ulcers associated with fistulas must be biopsied to exclude malignancy. Initially, benign ulcers are treated as described for an uncomplicated ulcer [see Figure 6]. An antisecretory agent—ideally, a proton pump inhibitor—should be prescribed, along with antibiotics if *H. pylori* organisms are present. Ulcer healing may be associated with closure of the fistula. If the fistula persists, surgical resection of the fistula is warranted only if significant symptoms are present (e.g., troublesome diarrhea in a patient with a gastrocolonic fistula or cholangitis in a patient with a duodenocholedochal fistula).

TREATMENT OF ACUTE STRESS ULCERS

Therapy for bleeding acute stress ulcers and erosions involves blood transfusion if necessary and attempts to treat the underlying disease state. The role of intravenous H_2 receptor blockers or proton pump inhibitors is unproved. Endoscopic therapy is not usually curative, because multiple bleeding lesions are often present. In rare cases, visceral angiography with embolization of the major bleeding site is attempted. Gastrectomy for continuous bleeding or significant rebleeding is used as a last resort and is associated with a very high mortality.

Because of the dire consequences of stress ulcers and the lack of an effective therapy, high-risk patients in intensive care units should be placed on stress ulcer prophylaxis.[43] The patients at highest risk for bleeding are those with multiorgan failure and those who are receiving ventilatory assistance. The incidence of significant bleeding in high-risk patients is reduced from about 10% to 25% to about 1% to 5% with the use of prophylactic intragastric or oral antacids or sucralfate or with the use of intravenous H_2 receptor blockers or proton pump inhibitors given by continuous infusion. I prefer intravenous antisecretory therapy because of ease of administration, the ability to monitor gastric pH to assess effectiveness (the goal is a pH > 4), and proven efficacy in clinical trials.

TREATMENT OF CAMERON ULCERS

Although acid secretory inhibitors are often used in the treatment of linear erosions in hiatal hernias (Cameron ulcers), their value is uncertain.[15] Standard therapy consists of packed red cell transfusions for acute bleeding, oral iron replacement for chronic bleeding, and laparoscopic or open repair of the hiatal hernia when medical therapy fails. Many of these patients are elderly or high-risk, so surgery should be undertaken only when medical therapy fails or becomes cumbersome.

References

1. Blaser MJ: The bacteria behind ulcers. Sci Am 274(2):104, 1996

2. *Helicobacter pylori* in peptic ulcer disease. NIH Consensus Development Panel on Helicobacter pylori in Peptic Ulcer Disease. JAMA 272:65, 1994

3. Cryer B, Faust TW, Goldschmiedt M, et al: Gastric and duodenal mucosal prostaglandin concentrations in gastric or duodenal ulcer disease: relationships with demographics, environmental, and histological factors, including *Helicobacter pylori*. Am J Gastroenterol 87:1747, 1992

4. Forbes GM, Glaser ME, Cullen DJE, et al: Duodenal ulcer treated with *Helicobacter pylori* eradication: seven-year follow-up. Lancet 343:258, 1994

5. Sung JJY, Chung SCS, Ling TKW, et al: Antibacterial treatment of gastric ulcers associated with *Helicobacter pylori*. N Engl J Med 332:139, 1995

6. Spechler SJ, Fischbach L, Feldman M: Clinical aspects of genetic variability in *Helicobacter pylori*. JAMA 283:1264, 2000

7. Chan FLK, To KF, Wu JCY, et al: Eradication of *Helicobacter pylori* and risk of peptic ulcers in patients starting long-term treatment with non-steroidal anti-inflammatory drugs: a randomised trial. Lancet 359:9, 2002

8. Henry D, Lim LL, Rodriguez LAG, et al: Variability in risk of gastrointestinal complications with individual non-steroidal anti-inflammatory drugs: results of a collaborative meta-analysis. BMJ 312:1563, 1996

9. Cryer B, Feldman M: Effects of very low dose daily, long-term aspirin therapy on gastric, duodenal, and rectal prostaglandin levels and on mucosal injury in healthy humans. Gastroenterology 117:17, 1999

10. Kelly JP, Kaufman DW, Jurgelson JM, et al: Risk of aspirin-associated major upper-gastrointestinal bleeding with enteric-coated or buffered product. Lancet 348:1413, 1996

11. Cryer B, Feldman M: Cyclooxygenase-1 and cyclooxygenase-2 selectivity of widely used NSAIDs and other anti-inflammatory or analgesic drugs: studies in whole blood and gastric mucosa of healthy humans. Am J Med 104:413, 1998

12. Silverstein F, Faich G, Goldstein JL, et al: Gastrointestinal toxicity with celecoxib versus nonsteroidal anti-inflammatory drugs for osteoarthritis and rheumatoid arthritis: The CLASS Study: A Randomized Controlled Trial. JAMA 284:1247, 2000

13. Bombardier C, Laine L, Reicin A, et al: Comparison of upper gastrointestinal toxicity of rofecoxib and naproxen in patients with rheumatoid arthritis. N Engl J Med 343:1520, 2000

14. Aoyama N, Kinoshita Y, Fujimoto S, et al: Peptic ulcers after the Hanshin-Awaji earthquake: increased incidence of bleeding gastric ulcer. Am J Gastroenterol 93:311, 1998

15. Spechler SJ: Peptic ulcer disease and its complications. Gastrointestinal and Liver Disease, 7th ed. Feldman M, Friedman LF, Sleisenger MS, Eds. WB Saunders Co, Philadelphia, 2002, p 747

16. Cutler AF, Havstad S, Ma CK, et al: Accuracy of invasive and noninvasive tests to diagnose *Helicobacter pylori* infection. Gastroenterology 109:136, 1995

17. Deveney CW, Deveney KS, Jaffe BM, et al: Use of calcium and secretin in the diagnosis of gastrinoma (Zollinger-Ellison Syndrome). Ann Intern Med 87:680, 1977

18. Lanas A, Sekar MC, Hirschowitz BI: Objective evidence of aspirin use in both ulcer and nonulcer upper and lower gastrointestinal bleeding. Gastroenterology 103:862, 1992

19. Feldman M, Cryer B, Lee E, et al: Role of seroconversion in confirming cure of *Helicobacter pylori* infection. JAMA 280:363, 1998

20. Vaira D, Nimish V, Menegatti M, et al: The stool test for detection of *Helicobacter pylori* after eradication therapy. Ann Intern Med 136:280, 2002

21. Leerdam ME, Ende E, Ten FK et al: Lack of accuracy of the non-invasive *Helicobacter pylori* stool antigen test in patients with gastroduodenal ulcer bleeding. Gastroenterology 122:A46, 2002

22. Blum AL, Talley NJ, O'Morain C, et al: Lack of effect of treating *Helicobacter pylori* infection in patients with nonulcer dyspepsia. N Engl J Med 339:1875, 1998

23. McColl K, Murray L, El-Omar E, et al: Symptomatic benefit from eradicating *Helicobacter pylori* infection in patients with nonulcer dyspepsia. N Engl J Med 339:1869, 1998

24. Friedman LS: *Helicobacter pylori* and nonulcer dyspepsia. N Engl J Med 339:1928, 1998

25. Meyer JM, Silliman NP, Wang W, et al: Risk factors for *Helicobacter pylori* resistance in the United States: the surveillance of *H. pylori* antimicrobial resistance partnership study. Ann Intern Med 136:13, 2002

26. Guslandi M: Alternative antibacterial agents for *Helicobacter pylori* eradication. Aliment Pharmacol Ther 15:1543, 2001

27. Gisbert JP, Pajares JM: *Helicobacter pylori* 'rescue' regimen when proton pump inhibitor-based therapies fail. Aliment Pharmacol Ther 16:1047, 2002

28. Perri F, Festa V, Clemente R, et al: Randomized study of two 'rescue' therapies for *Helicobacter pylori*-infected patients after failure of standard triple therapies. Am J Gastroenterol 96:58, 2001

29. Wong W, Gu Q, Lam SK, et al: Randomized controlled trial of rabeprazole, levofloxacin and rifabutin triple therapy versus rabeprazole-based quadruple therapy as a rescue treatment after failure of *Helicobacter pylori* (*H. pylori*) eradication with standard triple therapies. Gastroenterology 122:A587, 2002

30. McColl KEL, El-Nujumi AM, Chittajallu RS, et al: A study of pathogenesis of *Helicobacter pylori* negative chronic duodenal ulceration. Gut 34:762, 1993

31. McArthur KE, Richardson CT, Barnett CC, et al: Long-term outcome after exploratory laparotomy and proximal gastric vagotomy in Zollinger-Ellison syndrome. Am J Gastroenterol 91:1104, 1996

32. Khuroo M, Yattoo GN, Javid G, et al: A comparison of omeprazole and placebo for bleeding peptic ulcer. N Engl J Med 336:1054, 1997

33. Lau JW, Sung JJY, Lee KKC, et al: Effect of intravenous omeprazole on recurrent bleeding after endoscopic treatment of bleeding peptic ulcers. N Engl J Med 343:310, 2000

34. Rokkas T, Karameris A, Mavrogeorgis A, et al: Eradication of *Helicobacter pylori* reduces the possibility of rebleeding in peptic ulcer disease. Gastrointest Endosc 41:1, 1995

35. Macri G, Milani S, Surrenti E, et al: Eradication of *Helicobacter pylori* reduces the rate of duodenal ulcer rebleeding: a long-term follow-up study. Am J Gastroenterol 93:925, 1998

36. Silverstein FE, Graham DY, Senior JR, et al: Misoprostol reduces serious gastrointestinal complications in patients with rheumatoid arthritis receiving nonsteroidal anti-inflammatory drugs: a randomized, double-blind, placebo-controlled trial. Ann Intern Med 123:241, 1995

37. Lai K, Lam SK, Chu KM, et al: Lansoprazole for the prevention of recurrences of ulcer complications from long-term low-dose aspirin use. N Engl J Med 346:2033, 2002

38. Jensen DM, Cheng S, Kovacs TOG, et al: A controlled study of ranitidine for the prevention of recurrent hemorrhage from duodenal ulcer. N Engl J Med 330:382, 1994

39. Ng EK, Lam YH, Sung JJ, et al: Eradication of *Helicobacter pylori* prevents recurrence of ulcer after simple closure of duodenal ulcer perforation: randomized controlled trial. Ann Surg 231:153, 2000

40. Reinbach DH, Cruickshank G, McColl KEL: Acute perforated duodenal ulcer is not associated with *Helicobacter pylori* infection. Gut 34:1344, 1993

41. Crofts TJ, Park KGM, Steele RJC, et al: A randomized trial of nonoperative treatment for perforated peptic ulcer. N Engl J Med 320:970, 1989

42. DiSario JA, Fennerty MB, Tietze CC, et al: Endoscopic balloon dilation for ulcer-induced gastric outlet obstruction. Am J Gastroenterol 89:868, 1994

43. Cook D, Guyatt G, Marshall J, et al: A comparison of sucralfate and ranitidine for prevention of upper gastrointestinal bleeding in patients requiring mechanical ventilation. N Engl J Med 338:791, 1998

Acknowledgments

Figures 1, 2, 3, 6, 7   Marcia Kammerer.

Figure 5   Courtesy of Edward Lee, M.D.

The author thanks Tracy Cooper for help in preparing this chapter.

58 Inflammatory Bowel Diseases

Stephen B. Hanauer, M.D.

Ulcerative colitis (UC) and Crohn disease (CD) constitute the two major idiopathic inflammatory bowel diseases (IBDs). Clinicians now recognize that there is a spectrum of IBDs, encompassing various types and degrees of intestinal inflammation that must be distinguished from inflammation caused by infections, drugs, ischemia, and radiation. UC and CD are the most common and best understood of these idiopathic diseases; their etiologies, however, remain elusive.[1]

Epidemiology

UC and CD share most epidemiologic characteristics. These diseases are relatively common in developed countries and infrequent in countries with poor sanitation. In North America and Europe, the incidence is approximately five cases per 100,000 population for each disease, with a combined prevalence of approximately 100 per 100,000 population. The diseases can affect persons of any age, but they are most common in the second and third decades. Much smaller, secondary peaks in incidence occur in the sixth and seventh decades. Males and females are affected equally. Risk of disease is higher in some ethnic groups than in others. Ashkenazi Jews have a higher risk of IBD than Africans, African Americans, and Asians; the incidence rates for these lower-risk groups have increased in recent decades, however. No dietary factor has been identified as yet, although case-control studies suggest an association with the ingestion of large amounts of unrefined sugar and possibly with unsaturated fats (essentially, the Western diet).

Etiology

No single etiologic infectious agent has been associated with UC or CD.[1] Potential etiologic agents have been proposed in virtually every decade since the identification of the diseases. In recent years, a chronic measleslike viral infection, infection with *Listeria monocytogenes*, and infection with atypical mycobacteria have been hypothetically linked to CD without sufficient confirmation.[2]

There are two major etiologic clues. The first is the primary familial association of IBD, which suggests a genetic predisposition.[3] Once a proband has been identified, risk of disease occurring in a second family member is approximately 20% (40% if the proband is a child). The estimated risk for individual members of affected families is 3% to 5%, spread among first-, second-, and third-degree relatives. If both parents have IBD, the risk of disease occurring in an offspring is nearly 50%. There is a concordance for disease type (and subtype, in the case of CD) within families, although either UC or CD may be seen. Risk of disease is highest among identical twins, with a concordance for CD reaching 60% (20% for UC). This degree of risk suggests a polygenic causation, with higher penetrance in CD.[3] The search for genetic loci in IBDs has established disease loci on chromosomes 1, 12, and 16. Other potential loci are being investigated.

The second etiologic clue is the relation between cigarette smoking and UC and CD.[4] Cigarette smoking is known to decrease the risk of UC; however, smoking is strongly associated with CD. Cigarette smoking also influences the course of IBD. Ex-smokers with UC are more likely to have refractory disease

and to require surgery than are patients who smoke and those who have never smoked. Conversely, cigarette smokers with CD are more likely to have disease that is refractory to medical therapy. In cigarette smokers, CD often recurs more rapidly after surgical resection than in nonsmokers. It has not been established that nicotine is the primary factor in the opposite associations of cigarette smoking with UC and CD. Nicotine (as delivered by a patch) appears to have a modest ameliorative effect in UC, although not as potent an effect as that provided by cigarette smoking [*see* Treatment Overview, *below*].

Pathogenesis

In captivity, the cotton-top tamarin, a New World monkey, develops a so-called spontaneous colitis that has many features similar to those of human UC. These features include the development of antiepithelial antibodies, a similar response to anti-inflammatory medications, and the development of dysplasia and adenocarcinoma. Other animal models mimic CD, including transgenic rats that overexpress human leukocyte antigen HLA-B27 and β_2-microglobulin molecules and knockout mice with targeted deletions of interleukin-2 (IL-2), IL-10, T cell receptor chains, and transforming growth factor–β. The transfer of enriched functional T helper type 1 (Th1) cells into severe combined immunodeficient mice induces colitis and wasting that can be prevented by transfer of unfractionated CD4+ T cells.[1] Animals raised in germ-free environments do not develop intestinal inflammation.[1,2] In conjunction with the observations that many cases of IBD appear to be triggered by acute infections (e.g., traveler's diarrhea, acute gastroenteritis, or antibiotic exposure), the current concept of etiopathogenesis hypothesizes that IBD may be initiated by environmental factors in genetically susceptible hosts. However, consistent with the so-called hygiene hypothesis and the epidemiology of other autoimmune diseases, early childhood exposure to a variety of microorganisms may protect against future development of IBD.

Once inflammation begins, the primary difference between patients with IBD and unaffected persons is an impaired ability to downregulate mucosal inflammation.[1] Chronic inflammatory cells are normal in the intestinal mucosa: they constitute the gut component of the mucosa-associated lymphoid tract. The number of lymphoid elements in the mucosa is proportional to enteric exposure to bacteria. Persons raised in developed countries have less chronic inflammation than do those raised in countries with poor sanitation. An extreme example is that of tropical sprue, in which mucosal inflammation is extensive and is associated with atrophy and ulceration of the small bowel villi.

In IBD, most of the immune elements (including tissue macrophages and mucosal T cells) respond to an exaggerated degree when they are triggered by an antigen. Activated macrophages and T cells are prominent in the recruitment of nonspecific inflammatory cells—primarily neutrophils, the final mediators of tissue damage. The cytokine responses in UC and CD seem to differ, which may account for some of the differences in disease phenotypes. Many studies have demonstrated increases in mucosal levels of IL-1, IL-6, and tumor necrosis factor–α (TNF-α) in

Table 1   Key Distinguishing Features of Ulcerative Colitis and Crohn Disease

Feature	Ulcerative Colitis	Crohn Disease
History Smoking status	Nonsmoker or ex-smoker	Smoker
Physical examination Symptoms Signs	Rectal bleeding, cramps Normal perianal findings, no abdominal mass	Diarrhea, abdominal pain, weight loss, nausea, vomiting Perianal skin tags, fistulas, abscesses; abdominal mass; clubbing of digits
Laboratory tests Endoscopy Radiology Histology Serology	Rectal involvement; continuous superficial inflammation with granular, friable mucosa; terminal ileum normal or showing backwash ileitis Diffuse, continuous superficial ulceration; ahaustral (lead-pipe) colon; backwash ileitis Diffuse, continuous, superficial inflammation; crypt architectural deformity Elevated p-ANCA (60%–80% of patients)	Rectal sparing; local ulceration with normal intervening mucosa; aphthous, linear, or stellate ulcers; terminal ileum inflamed with aphthous or linear ulcers Focal, asymmetrical, transmural ulceration; strictures, inflammatory masses, fistulas; small bowel disease Focal inflammation, aphthous ulcers, lymphoid aggregates, transmural inflammation, granulomas (15%–30% of patients) Elevated ASCA (~ 30% of patients)

p-ANCA—perinuclear antineutrophil cytoplasmic antibody   ASCA—anti-*Saccharomyces cerevisiae* antibody

the mucosa of patients with UC and CD; it is becoming apparent, however, that the balance of cytokines may differ between the two diseases. CD manifests a higher Th1 cytokine profile (interferon gamma, IL-2, IL-12, and TNF-α); in UC, the balance is more consistent with a Th2 profile, with increased proportions of mucosal B cells, plasma cells, and antibodies.[1] Increased production of antineutrophil cytoplasmic antibodies (ANCAs) and IgG antibodies reacting with a 40 kd tropomyosin protein have been identified in UC; pathogenic consequences have not been defined, however.[5,6] Patients with CD have been found to have an increased likelihood of developing antibodies to common brewer's yeast (*Saccharomyces cerevisiae*).[5]

A final pathway of tissue destruction is through activation of macrophages and neutrophils. Activation of the arachidonic acid cascade leads to increased tissue levels of cyclooxygenase products (prostaglandins and thromboxanes), lipoxygenase products (primarily leukotriene B_4), and platelet activating factor (PAF). These compounds and other nonspecific mediators (e.g., nitric oxide, neutrophil tissue proteases, and reactive oxygen species) contribute to tissue destruction and can be targeted for specific and nonspecific anti-inflammatory therapy.[1]

Diagnosis

Key diagnostic features that help differentiate UC from CD are smoking status, clinical manifestations, and endoscopic findings [*see* Table 1].

ULCERATIVE COLITIS

The diagnosis of UC is made on the basis of clinical, endoscopic, and histologic findings. Patients presenting with rectal bleeding or diarrhea should raise the suspicion of UC. Symptoms are often chronic and persistent but may be intermittent or progressive. The easiest way to exclude UC is by direct examination of the rectosigmoid colon with a proctoscope or flexible sigmoidoscope. Radiography (barium enema) has been virtually replaced by endoscopic examination. Because UC always involves the rectum, inflammatory changes should be visible with a limited examination. In newly diagnosed disease, stool cultures are performed to rule out mimicking or complicating infections such as *Salmonella*, *Shigella*, *Campylobacter*, hemorrhagic *Escherichia coli*, and *Clostridium difficile*.

Clinical Manifestations

UC is manifested by diffuse, superficial inflammation of the colonic mucosa beginning in the rectum and extending proximally to involve any contiguous length of colon. The small intestine is not involved except in the setting of extensive colitis, in which the most distal terminal ileum may exhibit a similar superficial inflammation termed backwash ileitis. Because the extent of colitis usually remains constant from the onset, the classification of UC is defined by the length of involved colon: inflammation limited to the rectum (ulcerative proctitis), inflammation extending up to the splenic flexure (proctosigmoiditis or left-sided colitis), and inflammation extending into the transverse colon (extensive colitis or pancolitis). By itself, extent of inflammation does not necessarily determine severity but does pertain to prognosis (i.e., the risk of cancer) and potential therapeutic approaches.

The symptoms and course of UC relate to both the extent and the severity of inflammation within the involved segment of colon. The most commonly used criteria to define the severity of disease were created to assess improvement in clinical trials. The criteria remain clinically useful to classify severity and have been modified to include fulminant disease [*see* Table 2]. It is important to recognize that patients with some forms of UC can achieve a clinical remission—defined by resolution of inflammatory symptoms and a regeneration of the colonic mucosa—with therapy or even spontaneously.[7]

The onset of UC typically is insidious rather than abrupt, although the disease occasionally presents acutely after infectious colitis or traveler's diarrhea. Rectal bleeding is the most consistent feature. Bleeding may be gross or present with evacuation of mucopus. Associated rectal urgency and tenesmus are related to diminished compliance of the rectum. Diarrhea, distinguished from the passage of mucopus without stool, relates to the extent of colonic involvement. Patients with proctitis often present with constipated bowel movements and interim passage of blood, mucus, or both. Abdominal cramps preceding bowel movements are common, although abdominal pain or tenderness (related to transmural inflammation) signifies progressive, severe disease. In severe or fulminant colitis, systemic symptoms of night sweats, fever, nausea, vomiting, and weight loss accompany diarrhea. Extraintestinal manifestations can include inflammation of the eyes, skin, joints, and liver [*see* Complications, *below*].

Ulcerative proctitis Ulcerative proctitis is the most common and usually the mildest variant of UC, with inflammation limited to the distal 15 to 20 cm of rectum. Proctitis typically presents as hematochezia, a sense of rectal urgency, and constipated bowel movements caused by delayed transit of fecal material in the right colon. Systemic manifestations are uncommon, but skin or joint symptoms can occur. The disease usually remains confined to the rectum but may advance proximally in as many as 30% to 40% of patients.

Proctosigmoiditis (left-sided colitis) Left-sided colitis is an intermediate syndrome of UC that accounts for about one third of cases. It presents as either constipation or diarrhea accompanied by tenesmus, urgency, and rectal bleeding. Abdominal pain in the form of left-lower-quadrant cramping is more common in left-sided colitis than in proctitis, as are extraintestinal symptoms. The proximal disease margin usually remains fixed throughout the course but can spread proximally or even retract distally.

Extensive colitis (pancolitis) Pancolitis presents as inflammation into the transverse or right colon. Patients with pancolitis are more likely to present with diarrhea (caused by diminished absorptive capacity of the colon), accompanied by rectal bleeding and urgency. Abdominal cramps may be diffuse or localized, and patients are more likely to present with weight loss, systemic or extraintestinal symptoms, and anemia.

Toxic megacolon (colonic dilatation) Toxic megacolon is the most severe manifestation of UC. This medical emergency occurs when the superficial mucosal inflammation extends into the submucosa and muscular layers of the colon. Toxic megacolon occurs more commonly with pancolitis but can also occur with severe distal colitis. The colonic wall becomes tissue-paper thin and hypomotile as the colon dilates and is at risk for perforation. The patient often displays symptoms of severe infection, including fever, prostration, severe cramps, abdominal distention, and localized diffuse or rebound abdominal tenderness. Toxic megacolon is not unique to UC and can occur in infectious colitis and CD.[8]

Physical Examination

In most settings the physical examination is normal. There may be mild abdominal tenderness to deep palpation, particularly in the left colon, but significant abdominal findings are limited to patients with moderate to severe disease. Surprisingly, despite the presence of frequent diarrhea, perianal manifestations are absent. Any significant perianal findings (e.g., large hemorrhoids, skin tags, fissures, abscesses, or fistulas) suggest CD rather than UC.

Patients may present with ocular inflammation, erythema nodosum, pyoderma gangrenosum, or arthritis of larger joints. Low back pain with diminished range of motion or sacroiliac tenderness is uncommon. Hepatomegaly, splenomegaly, or evidence of chronic liver disease is rare and limited to patients with end-stage primary sclerosing cholangitis.

Imaging Studies

Endoscopy UC is virtually always diagnosable by endoscopic examination of the rectum and sigmoid colon. The disease presents as diffuse and continuous inflammation that begins in the rectum and involves a proximal extent that varies among individuals. In most cases it is advisable to determine the upper margin of disease, from the standpoints of prognosis and therapeutics.[9] The initial examination should be performed without enema preparation to avoid confusion of idiopathic inflammation with trauma or inflammation caused by enema administration. In the setting of active colitis, there is rarely any fecal material in the involved lumen.

Healthy colonic mucosa is smooth and glistening; it reflects light back from the endoscope and demonstrates a branching mucosal vascular pattern. With inflammation, the mucosa be-

Table 2 Classification of Ulcerative Colitis[7]

Feature	Mild Disease	Moderate Disease	Severe Disease	Fulminant Disease
History				
Stools	< 4/day (usually early in the day); minimal abdominal cramps and urgency	4–8/day; abdominal cramps and urgency	> 8/day; nocturnal bowel movements; severe urgency with or without incontinence	> 10/day; nocturnal bowel movements; severe urgency; tenesmus, severe abdominal pain
Blood in stool	Intermittent	Frequent	Frequent	Continuous
Physical examination				
Abdominal findings	Nontender abdomen; normal bowel sounds	Nontender or minimally tender over sigmoid	Tender abdomen; no rebound tenderness	Distended abdomen; decreased bowel sounds; rebound tenderness
Temperature	Normal	Normal	> 37.5° C (99.5° F)	> 37.5° C
Pulse	Normal	Normal	> 90	> 90
Other physical findings	Normal	Pallor	Weakness, pallor, weight loss	Prostration, hypotension
Laboratory tests				
Hemoglobin	Normal	Mild anemia	< 75% of normal	Transfusion required
Erythrocyte sedimentation rate	< 30 mm/hr	< 30 mm/hr	> 30 mm/hr	> 30 mm/hr
Radiography	Normal gas pattern	Absent stool in involved segment	Edematous colon wall, thumbprinting	Dilated colon, mucosal edema, intramural air, free abdominal air

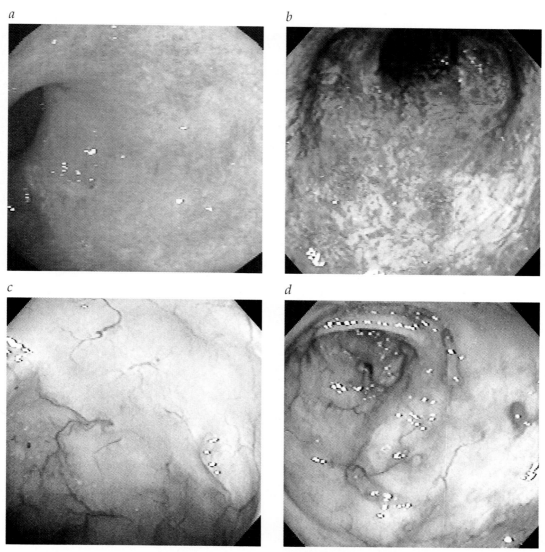

Figure 1 The endoscopic spectrum of ulcerative colitis includes (*a*) mucosal edema, erythema, loss of vasculature; (*b*) granular mucosa with pinpoint ulceration and friability; (*c*) regenerated (i.e., healed) mucosa with distorted mucosal vasculature; and (*d*) regenerated mucosa with typical postinflammatory pseudopolyps.

comes erythematous and granular, breaking apart the light reflection. The vascular pattern becomes obscured by edema [*see Figure 1*]. The granularity of the mucosa may be fine or coarse. Coarse granularity represents microscopic or pinpoint ulcerations and is associated with friability (hemorrhage from the mucosa that may be spontaneous or induced by scope trauma). These findings often are associated with patchy or diffuse exudate of mucopus.

Gross ulcerations represent more severe disease. The lesions are usually shallow, but they can progress to total denudation of the mucosa with exposure of the underlying circular musculature. These changes can be continuous up to a distinct margin where the mucosa appears normal, or they may extend diffusely to the cecum and, occasionally, into the distal ileum (backwash ileitis). In the setting of pancolitis, the ileocecal valve is usually wide open (patulous), allowing easy entry of the endoscope into the terminal ileum. Some patients with distal UC (involving the rectum or sigmoid) also may have limited inflammatory changes around the appendix (cecal red patch).

The mucosal changes may become more focal as UC heals. The colonic mucosa regenerates from ulceration to granularity, with gradual restitution of a distorted mucosal vascular pattern with less distinct branching or irregular, pruned vessels. In areas that were more severely inflamed, granulation tissue may protrude and become reepithelialized as so-called pseudopolyps. These postinflammatory changes can arise in a variety of sizes and shapes and are more likely to become fingerlike projections, or even bridges, in cases of severe undermining ulcerations. Pseudopolyps have no neoplastic potential but can be difficult to differentiate from adenomatous polyps. When extensive, pseudopolyps can carpet the mucosa to such an extent that distinct, potentially neoplastic polyps are impossible to discern.

Radiography Radiographic studies remain valuable adjuncts to endoscopy in specified clinical situations. Plain abdominal radiographs are useful in the setting of severe UC. These examinations outline the air-filled colon and can demonstrate the presence or absence of haustrations or dilatation of the colon (to rule out toxic megacolon). Extraluminal gas under the diaphragm (free air) and evidence of an ileus pattern are additional features of severe colitis.

Contrast barium studies, once the primary diagnostic modality, are less commonly used because endoscopic examinations provide increased diagnostic sensitivity and specificity and add the capability for histologic sampling.[9] Air-contrast barium enemas demonstrate the fine or coarse mucosal granularity caused by microscopic ulcerations and the diffuse, continuous, and symmetrical pattern of ulceration involving the rectum to the proximal extent of disease [see Figure 2]. Additional features demonstrated by barium enemas are loss of haustration in inflamed segments, shortening of the colon, and increase in the space between the sacrum and the rectum. Barium enema examinations are contraindicated in severely ill patients because of the potential for inadvertent perforation or induction of toxic megacolon.

Labeled leukocyte scanning using indium or technetium is occasionally indicated for severely ill patients in whom the extent of colitis is uncertain or to exclude small bowel disease. These studies provide relatively rapid determination of the extent, severity, and continuity of intestinal inflammation. The examinations are noninvasive, and they are sensitive and specific for intestinal inflammation. In the absence of small bowel disease, however, they do not distinguish between UC and CD.

Histology

The histologic features of UC include an inflammatory infiltrate and a disruption of glandular architecture. Architectural distortion is a hallmark distinction between UC and chronic inflammatory bowel diseases from acute self-limited (infectious) colitis [see Figure 3]. In UC, the normal vertical (test tube) alignment of glands is distorted by the separation of glands caused by expand-

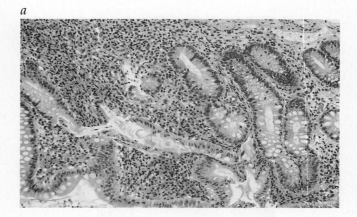

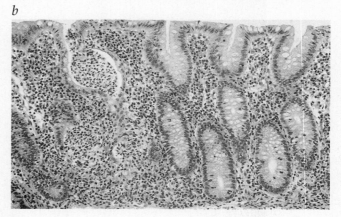

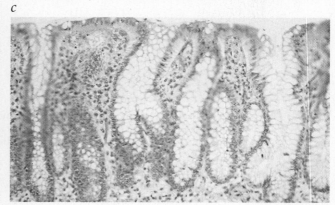

Figure 3 Pathologic changes in ulcerative colitis include (*a*) acute superficial inflammation with distortion of the normal crypt architecture, (*b*) crypt abscesses, and (*c*) quiescent colitis without acute inflammation but with distortions of crypt architecture (abnormal branched crypts).

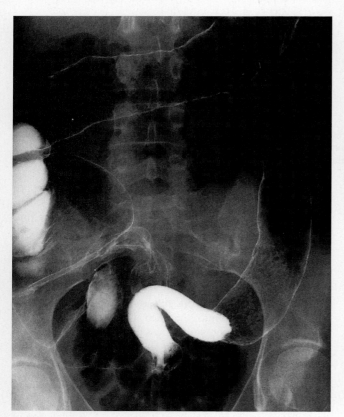

Figure 2 In this air-contrast radiograph of ulcerative colitis, the mucosal pattern is granular with loss of normal haustrations in a diffuse, continuous pattern.

ed lamina propria lymphocytes, plasma cells, eosinophils, and neutrophils. The glands themselves become irregular in shape and, often, branched. The neutrophil infiltrate localizes at the bases of the glandular crypts and extends into the crypts, producing crypt abscesses. In more severe disease, the epithelial lining is destroyed, leaving ulcerations over the lamina propria. The inflammatory changes are usually superficial, limited by the muscularis mucosae. Despite severe superficial changes, deeper inflammation is uncommon except in the setting of fulminant colitis. In fulminant colitis, the muscular layers are breached by expanding inflammatory ulceration that can leave the bowel wall tissue-paper thin and protected only by the serosa.

As the mucosa heals, the glands may become shortened and irregularly shaped with a thinned-out lamina propria. Inflammatory polyps are composed of vascular granulation tissue with a thin colonic epithelium. In quiescent colitis, architectural distortion is present but acute inflammation (neutrophil infiltration) is absent.

Both acute inflammation and regeneration of the colonic epithelium produce cellular atypia that must be distinguished from epithelial dysplasia (neoplastic transformation). In regenerating mucosa, the glandular epithelium can become irregularly shaped and hyperchromatic, with depletion of normal apical mucus. Stratification of nuclei and loss of polarity are manifestations of dysplasia.

CROHN DISEASE

CD is diagnosed on the basis of clinical, endoscopic, radiographic, and histologic criteria. As in UC, there is no pathog-

nomonic marker. The clinical presentation and key history, physical examination, and laboratory features determine the diagnostic workup [*see Table 1*].

Clinical Manifestations

CD encompasses inflammatory diseases of the digestive tract that are manifested by focal, asymmetrical, and transmural inflammation and are at times accompanied by granuloma formation. In contrast to the diffuse, continuous superficial (i.e., mucosal) inflammation of UC, the inflammation of CD is more patchy and can involve any segment of the gastrointestinal tract from mouth to anus. In addition, the transmural inflammation of CD leads to intestinal complications of stenoses (strictures) and fistulas.[10] Although a hallmark of CD is the histologic finding of noncaseating granuloma, this finding is not as common as previously considered (currently identified in only 30% of patients) and is not necessary to make the diagnosis.

Because CD can potentially involve any segment of the gastrointestinal tract, its presentation is more heterogeneous than

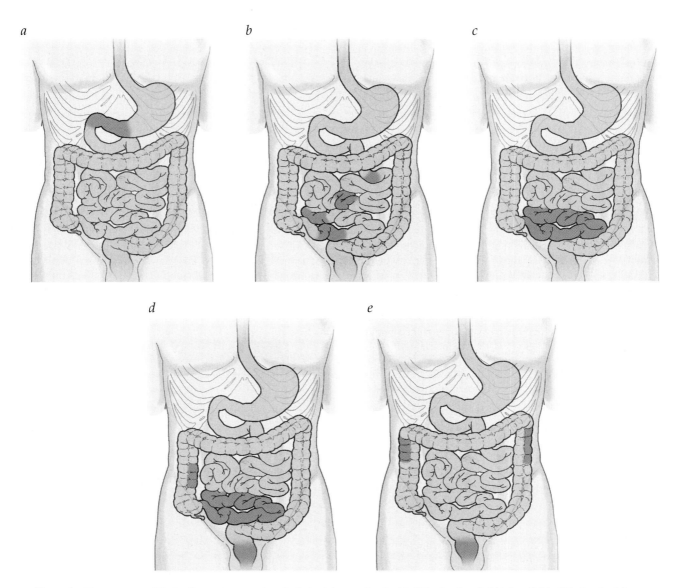

Figure 4 **The spectrum of Crohn disease presentations includes (*a*) gastroduodenitis (7% of patients), (*b*) jejunoileitis (5% of patients), (*c*) ileitis (28% of patients), (*d*) ileocolitis (45% of patients), and (*e*) colitis (15% of patients).**

that of UC and is described by the location, extent, severity, and pattern of inflammation. The location and pattern of inflammation tend to remain constant for each individual.[11] The spectrum of inflammatory patterns in CD ranges from a superficial inflammation similar to that found in UC to the formation of fibrostenosing strictures and the development of a penetrating (i.e., fistulizing) form of disease that is accompanied by mesenteric inflammatory masses or perienteric abscesses.

In contrast to UC, CD is usually not curable by surgery [see Treatment of Crohn Disease, below]. Intestinal resection and anastomosis are inevitably followed by recurrence of the disease involving the anastomotic site and proximal intestine. The segments of the gastrointestinal tract that are most commonly involved in CD are the terminal ileum and cecum.

The pattern of CD can be quite varied [see Figure 4]. The presentation depends on the site, extent, and severity of CD and on any intestinal or extraintestinal complications. The condition is usually chronic, but CD can be acute, with severe abdominal pain, intestinal blockage, or hemorrhage. Because CD is transmural, it often presents as abdominal pain caused by stimulation of pain receptors located on the serosa and peritoneum. Abdominal cramping and postprandial pain are common symptoms and are often accompanied by diarrhea, rectal bleeding, nocturnal bowel movements, fevers, night sweats, and weight loss. Nausea and vomiting occur in the presence of intestinal strictures that produce partial or complete bowel obstructions. Transmural disease commonly is manifested in the perianal region as skin tags, perirectal abscesses, or fistulas but also can present as an inflammatory mass in the right lower quadrant. In children and adolescents, the presentation is often insidious, with weight loss, failure to grow or to develop secondary sex characteristics, arthritis, or fevers of undetermined origin. Skin lesions, primarily erythema nodosum, may precede intestinal symptoms [see Chapter 30]. Finally, toxic megacolon can occur in CD and infectious colitis and is not unique to UC.[8]

In clinical trials, the instrument most commonly used to compare disease activity has been the Crohn's Disease Activity Index (CDAI). The CDAI is derived from measures of individual symptoms (e.g., abdominal pain, liquid bowel movements, overall well-being), clinical findings (e.g., body weight, abdominal mass, extraintestinal symptoms), and use of antidiarrheal agents. Each factor is then weighted to arrive at an overall score of 0 to 500 (higher scores indicate greater disease activity). However, because of its complex derivation and lack of discrimination between symptoms and inflammation, the CDAI is not commonly used in clinical practice. Patients require individualized assessments of the severity of disease according to inflammatory symptoms, obstruction, fistulization, abscess, systemic complications, and effect on the patient's quality of life.[10,12]

Ileitis and ileocecal Crohn disease CD most commonly presents as right lower quadrant abdominal pain and tenderness, diarrhea with or without rectal bleeding, weight loss, fever, chills, and night sweats. An acute presentation may mimic appendicitis.

Crohn disease of the esophagus, stomach, and duodenum Infrequently, primary manifestations and symptoms of CD mimic gastroesophageal reflux or peptic ulcer disease. Heartburn, dysphagia, nausea, dyspepsia, epigastric pain, early satiety, or postprandial vomiting typically accompanies other systemic inflammatory symptoms such as fever, night sweats, or rectal bleeding.

Jejunoileitis Another relatively uncommon presentation of CD often includes diarrhea, cramping abdominal pain, and weight loss. Patients describe borborygmi related to focal, segmental strictures that compromise the passage of enteric contents. Diarrhea is multifactorial and can be secondary to malabsorption as a consequence of enteritis or small bowel bacterial overgrowth proximal to strictures.

Crohn colitis Crohn colitis can be difficult to distinguish from UC [see Table 1]. Approximately 15% of patients with CD present with symptoms limited to the colon. Diarrhea, rectal bleeding, and urgency overlap with symptoms of UC. However, CD of the colon is more likely than UC to be accompanied by perianal manifestations (skin tags, perirectal abscess, or fistulas), and the rectum is often spared (whereas UC always involves the rectum). In approximately 10% to 20% of patients presenting with colitis, the classification may be indeterminate in the setting of diffuse or severe inflammation or questionable focal inflammation.

Perianal Crohn disease A perianal form of CD most often accompanies colonic disease and begins within the anal crypts. Small fistulas from the anorectal junction progress through or around the anal sphincter and present as perirectal abscesses or fistulas [see Figure 5]. Often, perianal tissue becomes hypertrophied and presents as skin tags that are misdiagnosed as hemorrhoids. At times, perianal manifestations are the primary presentation; in extreme situations, the anal sphincter and perineum can become grossly deformed.

Physical Examination

The abdominal examination of patients with CD may be significant for distention and abnormal bowel sounds in the presence of intestinal obstruction. Tenderness in the area of involvement and the presence of an inflammatory mass are common. It is important to examine the perianal region and rectum for evidence of abscess, fistula, skin tags, or an anal stricture [see Table 1].

Patients with CD often are chronically ill and can present with

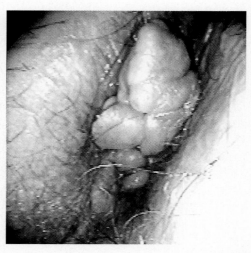

Figure 5 **The typical perianal skin tag of Crohn disease differs from the typical hemorrhoid tag.**

a *b*

c *d*

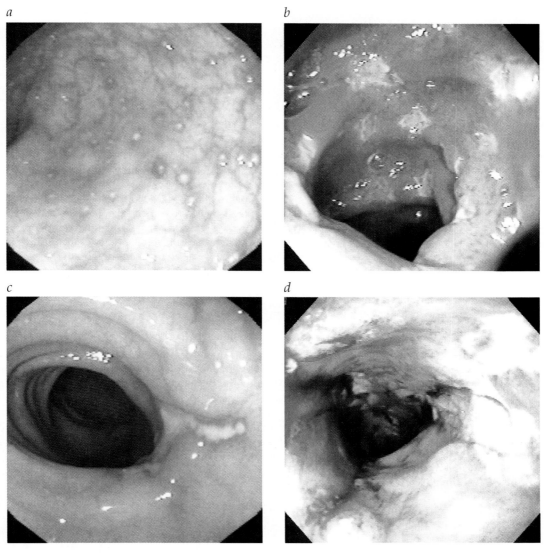

Figure 6 **Endoscopic spectrum of Crohn disease includes (***a***) aphthous ulcerations amid normal colonic mucosal vasculature; (***b***) deeper, punched-out ulcers in ileal mucosa; (***c***) a single colonic linear ulcer; and (***d***) deep colonic ulcerations forming a stricture.**

pallor and evidence of weight loss. The eye examination may demonstrate evidence of episcleritis or uveitis. Aphthous ulcerations in the mouth are common. In extreme cases, there may be evidence of nutritional abnormalities (e.g., cheilosis, atrophic tongue). Examination of the musculoskeletal system may demonstrate swelling or redness of large joints (e.g., knees, ankles, wrists) or clubbing of the fingers. Skin examination can reveal erythema nodosum or, rarely, pyoderma gangrenosum [*see Chapter 30*].

Imaging Studies

Endoscopy Colonoscopy has become a primary means of diagnosing CD. Endoscopic features include focal inflammatory changes in the proximal colon and terminal ileum and sparing of the rectum. Typical features include the presence of aphthous, linear, or irregularly shaped ulcerations with normal intervening mucosa [*see Figure 6*]. Inflammatory strictures may preclude endoscopic examination of proximal segments of bowel. Inflammatory pseudopolyps can be seen, as in UC. Polypoid or masslike inflammatory changes may be difficult to differentiate

from neoplastic masses and may require biopsy and histologic definition. Similar endoscopic features may be present in the esophagus, stomach, or duodenum. An important aspect of endoscopic examination is the capability to obtain samples for pathologic interpretation.

Radiography Barium contrast studies are the most commonly used diagnostic tool to assess and confirm CD of the small intestine and are useful for assessing the upper digestive tract and colon. In colonic disease, barium studies are useful for defining intestinal complications (e.g., stricture formation or fistulas) that are not adequately assessed by endoscopy [*see Figure 7*]. Features of CD that are shown by barium examination include mucosal edema, aphthous and linear ulcerations, asymmetrical narrowing and strictures, and separation of adjacent loops of bowel caused by mesenteric thickening. Abnormalities are focal and asymmetrical in CD, with ulcerations most often involving the antimesenteric border. Typical cobblestoning of the mucosa occurs when networks of linear ulcerations outline islands of residual normal mucosa. Pseudodiverticula formation, or dilated loops of bowel,

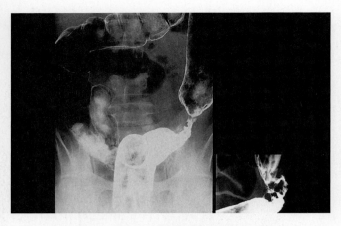

Figure 7 **In this air-contrast radiograph of colonic Crohn disease, note the focal stricture (enlarged on spot film).**

are common proximal to strictures. There may be evidence of fistulizing communications connecting from any involved segment to an adjacent loop of bowel, the mesentery, or the urinary bladder or connecting from the rectum to the vagina or perineum.

Leukocyte scans labeled with indium or technetium can help define locations of intestinal inflammation when barium studies are not possible or are indeterminate.

Other imaging studies Ultrasound examination and computed tomography are useful tools for assessing the presence of an abscess within an inflammatory mass or in the setting of fever, leukocytosis, or abdominal tenderness. Ultrasonography or CT scanning is also warranted to assess the possibility of hydronephrosis in the setting of a right lower quadrant inflammatory mass that may obstruct the right ureter. Transrectal ultrasonography, CT scanning, and magnetic resonance imaging can also be useful to assess the extent of perianal and sphincter involvement in patients presenting with perianal or perirectal pain.

Histology

Pathologic findings in CD reflect the focal and asymmetrical gross pattern of intestinal involvement. The primary histologic lesion is an aphthous ulcer [*see Figure 8*]. These lesions begin as erosions overlying lymphoid aggregates. As the minute ulceration extends in a linear or transmural pattern, the histologic changes include a mixed acute and chronic inflammatory cell infiltrate of the mucosa comprising lymphocytes, plasma cells, and neutrophils. Crypt abscesses are common, and the inflammatory infiltrates often are adjacent to normal epithelium. Noncaseating granulomas are virtually diagnostic in the proper clinical setting and may be identified in mucosal biopsies or in resected specimens; however, they are not necessary to confirm the diagnosis of CD when colonoscopy is available. Granulomas may be identified in specimens from normal-appearing mucosa.

Gross specimens from resected intestine demonstrate transmural inflammatory changes extending from the mucosa into the serosa (which is hyperemic with creeping mesenteric fat). At times there may be paradoxical involvement of the deeper layers of the bowel wall, with lymphoid aggregates overlying normal-appearing epithelium. Submucosal fibrosis, deep fissuring ulcerations, and fistulizing ulcerations communicate between loops of bowel or into the adjacent mesentery.

Serology

Anemia is common in CD patients. The anemia can be multifactorial, caused by deficiencies of iron, vitamin B_{12}, or folic acid, or it can be a complication of chronic disease. The serum ferritin level best reflects iron stores in IBD. Leukocytosis is common, depending on the severity of inflammation and the presence of suppurative complications. Thrombocytosis also is common and is related to inflammation or iron deficiency. Elevated erythrocyte sedimentation rates and C-reactive protein levels reflect nonspecific acute-phase reactions. Electrolyte disturbances depend on the severity of diarrhea and dehydration. The serum albumin level often is reduced because of malnutrition and enteric protein losses. With severe weight loss and malabsorption, there may be evidence of prolonged clotting times caused by vitamin K deficiency. Urinalysis commonly demonstrates calcium oxalate crystals.

In the setting of diarrhea, quantitative stool examinations are useful for assessing fecal leukocytes (confirming inflammatory diarrhea), fecal volume, and fecal fat. The presence of serum anti–*Saccharomyces cerevisiae* antibody (ASCA) is highly specific for the presence of CD[5]; sensitivity is only 30%, however [*see Table 1*].

Differential Diagnosis

IBD should be considered in any patient presenting with rectal bleeding or diarrhea. Identification of fecal leukocytes is the simplest means of discerning an inflammatory process of the intes-

a

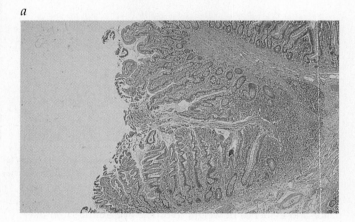

b

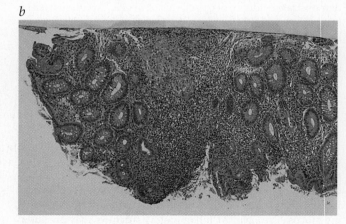

Figure 8 **Pathologic changes in Crohn disease include (*a*) ileal aphthous ulceration overlying a lymphoid aggregate and (*b*) focal colonic ulcer with noncaseating granuloma in lymphoid tissue.**

tine. Other causes of rectal bleeding include hemorrhoids, diverticula, neoplasms, and ischemic colitis. Diarrhea has a large differential diagnosis [see Chapter 61]. The primary chronic diarrheal illness that requires differentiation from UC or CD is irritable bowel syndrome [see Chapter 62]. Irritable bowel syndrome is never associated with rectal bleeding, and nocturnal symptoms are uncommon. The presence of occult blood or fecal leukocytes excludes irritable bowel syndrome.

The presence of gross or occult blood requires an endoscopic evaluation. Colonic neoplasia is a prominent consideration in patients older than 50 years, whereas younger patients are commonly afflicted with hemorrhoids or anal fissures. Nonsteroidal anti-inflammatory drugs (NSAIDs) commonly induce colitis and may contribute to ischemic colitis in older persons. In elderly patients, ischemic colitis presents acutely as precipitating events such as dehydration and heart failure. Endoscopic examination demonstrates focal hemorrhagic or ulcerated mucosa in the watershed segments of the sigmoid colon or splenic flexure. Diverticular hemorrhage is typically profuse and painless; however, some patients—particularly elderly patients on NSAIDs—may present with less vigorous rectal bleeding from a segment of inflamed sigmoid colon associated with diverticulosis.

Inflammatory diarrhea can be infectious or noninfectious. The infectious colitides include invasive bacteria such as *Salmonella*, *Shigella*, *Campylobacter*, and hemorrhagic *E. coli*. Most of these infections are acute and self-limited and need to be considered only in newly presenting patients who have bloody diarrhea and fever. UC and CD usually present insidiously over a period of weeks. *Clostridium difficile* colitis can mimic UC and may be more chronic than other infections, lasting weeks.[13] In immunocompetent hosts, viral or parasitic infections rarely mimic UC. One exception is amebiasis, which may present as acute or subchronic symptoms and can often be distinguished by wet-mount examination of the stool for motile amebae and the more typical focal (collar-button) ulcerations in the colon.

Intercurrent infections and traveler's diarrhea have been recognized to initiate flares of IBD. At presentation or upon acute exacerbation, patients should be evaluated for a complicating enteric infection.[13]

Treatment Overview

The treatment of UC and CD is based on the location, extent, and severity of disease as well as on the prior response to therapy.[7-10] Assessment begins with a comprehensive review of the patient's history, current symptoms, and complications of the disease or therapy or both. Factors contributing to exacerbations of activity or refractoriness to therapy should be sought. These factors include concomitant medications (e.g., NSAIDs, antibiotics), intercurrent infections (e.g., *C. difficile*), changes in menstruation, and changes in diet or lifestyle (including changes in smoking habits). There are more similarities than differences in the treatment of UC and CD; however, those differences are vital. In the following discussion of therapies, common principles of IBD management are presented first; details of treatment of UC and CD are then presented separately.

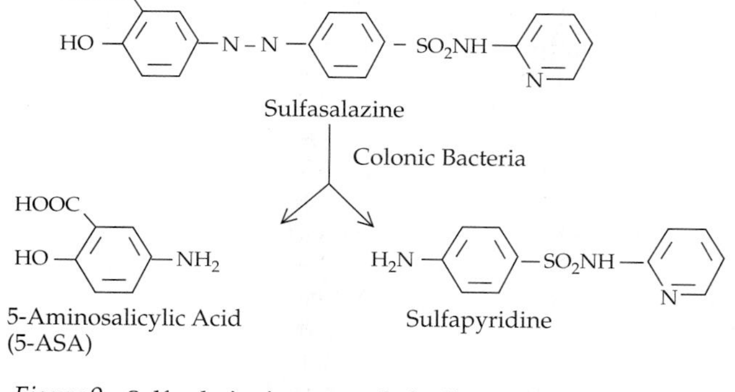

MEDICAL THERAPY

Anti-inflammatory Agents

Aminosalicylates Aminosalicylates are the primary therapy for mild to moderate UC[7,9] and CD.[10] These agents have a long history of clinical use and have been extensively studied in clinical trials for both UC[14,15] and CD.[10,16] Sulfasalazine, the prototype aminosalicylate [see Figure 9], was developed to deliver both an antibacterial agent (sulfapyridine) and an anti-inflammatory agent (5-aminosalicylic acid [5-ASA], mesalamine, or mesalazine) to the connective tissues. It is now recognized that sulfasalazine remains intact through the stomach and small intestine with minimal enteric absorption. Upon reaching the colon, the azo bond between sulfapyridine and 5-ASA is cleaved by colonic bacteria. Released sulfapyridine is almost completely absorbed from the colon and undergoes hepatic metabolism and subsequent renal excretion. In contrast, 5-ASA released into the colon is poorly absorbed and is primarily eliminated in the feces. Therefore, sulfasalazine primarily serves to deliver 5-ASA to the colon.

The 5-ASA moiety, mesalamine, accounts for the primary therapeutic benefits, whereas sulfapyridine causes the majority of side effects attributed to sulfasalazine. These attributes have led to the development of a series of sulfa-free aminosalicylates targeted to specific sites along the gastrointestinal tract,[17] based on the presumption that the effects of 5-ASA are topical (i.e., mucosal), not systemic, and that the active moiety requires delivery to the site of intestinal inflammation [see Table 3].

Sulfasalazine and mesalamine have multiple anti-inflammatory effects, including inhibition of the arachidonic acid cascade along the cyclooxygenase, lipoxygenase, and PAF pathways. In addition, the aminosalicylates are inhibitors of oxygen radical production and scavengers of free radicals. They also inhibit lymphocyte and monocyte function and production of immunoglobulin by plasma cells. Sulfasalazine has also been shown to inhibit IL-1 production and nuclear factor κB. Adverse effects of sulfasalazine are common and primarily related to plasma sulfapyridine concentrations.[18] Intolerance side effects (e.g., nausea, vomiting, malaise, anorexia, dyspepsia, and headaches) are dose related. In contrast, hypersensitivity reactions (e.g., rash, fever, hemolytic anemia, agranulocytosis, hepatitis, hypersensitivity pneumonitis, pancreatitis, and worsening of colitis) are independent of dose. Reversible sperm abnormalities and folate malabsorption are unique complications related to sulfasalazine.

Mesalamine has relatively few side effects or dose-related toxicities.[18] Rare, idiosyncratic reactions (e.g., pancreatitis, nephritis, and worsening of colitis) have been reported. Eighty percent of patients who are unable to tolerate sulfasalazine can tolerate a nonsulfa 5-ASA. Diarrhea is a unique, dose-related complication of olsalazine.

Figure 9 Sulfasalazine is composed of sulfapyridine and 5-aminosalicylic acid (mesalamine), linked by an azo-bond.

Table 3 Aminosalicylate Preparations for Management of Ulcerative Colitis and Crohn Disease

Preparation	Formulation	Delivery	Dosing
Oral Agents			
Azo bond			
Sulfasalazine (Azulfidine, 500 mg)	Sulfapyridine carrier	Colon	3–6 g/day (acute)
			2–4 g/day (maintenance)
Olsalazine (Dipentum, 250 mg)	5-Aminosalicylic acid dimer	Colon	1–3 g/day
Balsalazide (Colazide,* 750 mg)	Aminobenzoyl-alanine carrier	Colon	6 g/day
Delayed Release			
Mesalamine (Asacol, 400 mg, 800 mg*)	Eudragit S (pH, 7)	Distal ileum–colon	2.4–4.8 g/day (acute)
			0.8–4.8 g/day (maintenance)
(Claversal,* Mesasal,* Salofalk,* 250 mg, 500 mg)	Eudragit L (pH, 6)	Ileum-colon	1.5–3.0 g/day (acute)
			0.75–3.0 g/day (maintenance)
Sustained Release			
Mesalamine (Pentasa, 250 mg, 500 mg,* 1,000 mg*)	Ethylcellulose granules	Stomach-colon	2–4 g/day (acute)
			1.5–4.0 g/day (maintenance)
Rectal Agents			
Mesalamine suppository (Rowasa, 400 mg,* 500 mg, 1,000 mg*)	—	Rectum	1.0–1.5 g/day (acute)
			500–1,000 mg/day (maintenance)
Mesalamine enema (Rowasa, 1 g,* 4 g)	60 ml, 100 ml suspension	Rectum–splenic flexure	1–4 g/day (acute)
			1 g q.d.–1 g t.i.w. (maintenance)

*Not available in the United States.

Sulfasalazine and the oral aminosalicylates are equally efficacious for treatment of mild to moderate UC.[9,15] Oral aminosalicylates are effective for both proximal and distal colitis; topical mesalamine effectively treats distal colitis when the formulation reaches the proximal extent of disease.[19] Prevention of relapse of UC and prolongation of remission have been primary indications for all of the aminosalicylates.[7,9]

The efficacy of sulfasalazine in CD is less definitive and more dependent on location of disease. Sulfasalazine is commonly used as a maintenance therapy for patients with quiescent CD.[7,10] The efficacy of mesalamine, at dosages greater than 3 g/day, has been supported by clinical trials in active CD and in the prevention of medical and postoperative relapse.[7,10]

Corticosteroids Corticosteroids are the primary therapy for moderate to severe and fulminant UC and CD. They are ineffective, however, for maintaining remission of these diseases.[7] The mechanisms of action of corticosteroids are multifactorial in IBD and similar to their mechanisms of action in other inflammatory diseases. Corticosteroids can be targeted to specific locations in the digestive tract to enhance effectiveness and minimize systemic exposure.[17] Oral corticosteroids are the primary outpatient treatment for moderately severe UC.[7,9] Prednisone, 20 to 60 mg/day, is administered once a day or four times a day. In most cases, the optimal dosage is 40 mg/day; side effects tend to offset incremental benefits of higher dosages. Rectal (i.e., topical) administration of systemically absorbed glucocorticoids (e.g., hydrocortisone) and rapidly metabolized glucocorticoids (e.g., budesonide) is effective for active distal colitis and has been incorporated into the treatment of severe colitis as an adjunct to parenteral steroids.[7,9] Parenteral corticosteroids are the mainstay of therapy for hospitalized patients with severe or fulminant UC. Corticosteroids are not effective in preventing relapse of quiescent UC.[7,9]

Corticosteroids are also the primary therapy for moderate to severe CD.[10] Delayed-release formulations have become available for delivery of topically active steroids to targeted sites in CD.[17] Controlled-release formulations of budesonide (currently not available in the United States) effectively treat ileocecal CD with nearly the same benefit as systemic prednisone. However, similar to the experience with oral steroids,[20] low-dose budesonide has shown no benefit in preventing relapse of CD.

Immunomodulatory Agents

Immunomodulating therapies have had expanding roles in the induction and maintenance of remission of UC and CD.[21]

Azathioprine and 6-mercaptopurine Azathioprine (AZA) and 6-mercaptopurine (6-MP) have been used to treat IBD for over 25 years. AZA is rapidly absorbed and converted to 6-MP, which is then metabolized to thioinosinic acid, an inhibitor of purine ribonucleotide synthesis and cell proliferation.[21] It is presumed that inhibition of long-lived lymphocytes accounts for the 3- to 6-month delay in onset of action. A genetic polymorphism has been recognized in the enzyme (thiopurine methyltransferase) that metabolizes the purine analogues into 6-thioguanine.[21] One in 300 individuals lacks this enzyme and is susceptible to increased accumulation of thioguanine metabolites and bone marrow suppression.

AZA and 6-MP usually are well tolerated. Pancreatitis is relatively common, occurring in 3% to 15% of patients. It usually occurs within the first few weeks of therapy and resolves upon drug withdrawal without chronic sequelae. Other potential side effects include nausea, fever, rash, and hepatitis. Bone marrow suppression (particularly leukopenia) is dose related and may be delayed, necessitating monitoring of blood counts on a long-term basis. There is a growing consensus regarding the utility and safety of these agents during pregnancy and lactation.[22] Controlled trials with AZA and uncontrolled series with 6-MP support the role of purine analogues for maintenance therapy of UC.[7,9] Similarly, AZA and 6-MP are effective in patients with active CD when it is recognized that a long duration of therapy (i.e., 3 to 6 months) is necessary to assess efficacy. Over 50% of these patients respond after 4 months with either AZA (2.0 to 2.5

mg/kg/day) or 6-MP (1.0 to 1.5 mg/kg/day).[23,24] AZA and 6-MP have also been effective steroid-sparing agents that can be used to treat CD fistulas and perianal disease.[10] Because of their delayed onset of action, they are most often used to maintain remission or as steroid-sparing agents.

Cyclosporine Cyclosporine has had dramatic results for management of acute, severe IBD, but controversy remains regarding its long-term benefits.[21] Cyclosporine is a potent inhibitor of T cells via inhibition of multiple cytokines, including IL-2, interferon gamma, and TNF-α. Cyclosporine has a more rapid onset of action than AZA or 6-MP.

Intravenous cyclosporine is administered as a continuous infusion at 2 to 4 mg/kg/day.[9,25] Correlations between blood levels and response (or toxicity) are poor. The narrow therapeutic margin and significant safety issues remain obstacles to the use of cyclosporine by practitioners outside of facilities with transplantation expertise.[25] Major toxicities include nephrotoxicity and opportunistic infections. Nephrotoxicity can be manifested as hypertension or elevations in blood urea nitrogen and creatinine levels. An increased risk of opportunistic infections, including *Pneumocystis carinii* pneumonia (PCP), has been described. PCP prophylaxis with trimethoprim-sulfamethoxazole is recommended for patients receiving cyclosporine in conjunction with high-dose steroids.[25]

The primary use for cyclosporine in IBD is to treat hospitalized patients with severe UC who have not responded to oral or intravenous steroids. In the short-term management of severe, refractory UC, 50% to 80% of patients respond.[25] The long-term prognosis is more controversial. Approximately 40% to 50% of patients who respond to cyclosporine avoid colectomy, and more than 60% obtain long-term benefits when given therapy with AZA or 6-MP.[25] Cyclosporine has also been used to treat steroid-refractory and fistulizing CD.[21] Benefits are primarily achieved with intravenous cyclosporine. Trials of oral cyclosporine for maintenance therapy of CD have not shown efficacy, possibly because of poor and variable absorption.

Methotrexate Methotrexate inhibits dihydrofolate reductase, impairing synthesis of DNA. Its anti-inflammatory properties are possibly related to inhibition of IL-1.[26] A dose response for methotrexate has not been defined in IBD; however, there is evidence favoring parenteral over oral administration.[26] Bone marrow suppression and hepatic fibrosis are uncommon when blood counts and liver enzymes are monitored. Many common adverse events (e.g., nausea, vomiting, and diarrhea) can be reduced by supplementation with folic acid. Methotrexate is contraindicated during pregnancy.

Approximately 40% of steroid-dependent CD patients are able to taper steroids over 16 weeks, utilizing methotrexate at a weekly dose of 25 mg, administered intramuscularly or subcutaneously.[27] A recent trial has demonstrated that the majority of patients who respond to parenteral methotrexate continue to respond to 15 mg administered intramuscularly for more than 40 weeks.[28] There is minimal evidence to support the use of methotrexate in UC.

Antibiotic Agents

Antibiotic therapy has been used in a variety of clinical scenarios for IBD. Although a specific therapeutic role for antibiotics in UC remains unproven, most centers continue to advocate broad-spectrum antibiotics as a component of the intensive intravenous therapy for fulminant colitis and toxic megacolon.[8]

Antibiotics are also effective to treat pouchitis in UC after ileoanal anastomoses.[29]

In mild to moderate CD, metronidazole is comparable in efficacy to sulfasalazine and superior to placebo at dosages of 20 mg/kg/day.[7,10] Metronidazole is effective for the treatment of perianal CD, and it reduces the likelihood of CD relapse after intestinal resection. In trials, ciprofloxacin has been comparable to mesalamine for mild to moderate CD[30] and, combined with metronidazole, for ileal disease and perianal CD.[31] Combinations of antimycobacterial therapies for CD have had inconsistent results both in active disease and as maintenance therapies.

Biologic Agents

We have entered a new era of therapeutic potential for the treatment of IBD. Cellular messengers, including cytokines, chemokines, and adhesion molecules, offer novel targets for inhibition and stimulation to downregulate the exaggerated immunoinflammatory responses in IBD.[32]

Infliximab, a chimeric monoclonal antibody targeting TNF-α, was the first biologic agent approved by the Food and Drug Administration for the treatment of CD. A double-blind dose-ranging study found that a single 5 mg/kg infusion of infliximab induced clinical improvement in 80% of patients with CD refractory to steroids, aminosalicylates, antibiotics, and AZA and 6-MP. Nearly half of the CD patients achieved remission lasting approximately 8 to 12 weeks.[33] Reinfusion of infliximab at 8-week intervals sustained the response for up to 44 weeks.[34] Infliximab administered in three doses of 5 mg/kg at 0, 2, and 6 weeks induced clinical response in approximately 50% of refractory CD fistulas for approximately 12 weeks.[35] Infliximab has generally been safe, with common side effects similar to those of placebo.[36] Unique adverse events include the development of human antichimeric antibodies and anti-DNA antibodies in approximately 10% of patients with CD. Delayed hypersensitivity (e.g., serum sickness–like reactions) has been observed in patients retreated after a long hiatus between doses but not in patients receiving continuous re-treatment at 8-week intervals. The small risk of lymphoma observed in initial trials with infliximab has not been confirmed in postmarketing experience.

Additional trials are ongoing to assess optimal maintenance strategies for this novel therapy for CD and UC. Other strategies to inhibit TNF are being investigated for IBD.

Other Agents

The protective role of cigarette smoking against the development of UC[4] has led to trials using nicotine as adjunctive therapy. Despite some success, nicotine patches have not been shown to be as effective as aminosalicylates at inducing or maintaining remissions. Nicotine is not a proven therapy for UC but may be a useful adjunctive therapy for the small subgroup of patients who develop UC after cessation of smoking.

A paradoxical improvement in both colitis and extraintestinal manifestations of IBD during heparin therapy for venous thrombosis has led to the investigation of a potential therapeutic role for heparin in IBD.[37] Although heparin has anti-inflammatory activity and appears to be well tolerated in patients with active UC, it remains to be determined whether heparin or low-molecular-weight heparin will provide important therapeutic advances for IBD.

NUTRITIONAL THERAPY

Hypotheses about the importance of dietary intraluminal antigens in the stimulation of the mucosal immune response have led to investigation of nutritional therapies for IBD.[1,38] Dietary manipulations have not been effective in treating UC, but patients with active CD respond to several nutritional approaches.[38] Bowel rest and total parenteral nutrition (TPN) are as effective as corticosteroids at inducing short-term remissions for these patients. Alternatively, enteral nutrition in the form of elemental or peptide-based preparations is equally effective as corticosteroids or TPN. It has been proposed that elemental diets may provide the small intestine with nutrients (e.g., glutamine) vital to cell growth while avoiding complications related to TPN. Despite their efficacy in active CD, neither enteral nutrition nor parenteral nutrition maintains remission. Liquid polymeric diets are more palatable and less expensive than elemental diets, but their effectiveness is more controversial.

Omega-3 fatty acids inhibit synthesis of leukotriene B$_4$ and, at high doses, have had a modest benefit in refractory UC or as maintenance therapy. An enteric-coated fish oil preparation was reported to be effective in CD maintenance therapy[39] and may eventually offer an alternative therapeutic option in IBD.

In itself, IBD is not a risk factor for lactose intolerance. Lactose-free diets should be limited to patients with demonstrated lactase deficiency. Consumption of other poorly absorbed carbohydrates, such as sorbitol, fats, and fat substitutes (e.g., olestra), can lead to excess flatus, bloating, or diarrhea.

SUPPORTIVE THERAPY

Many symptoms of IBD are not related to active inflammation and can be treated without anti-inflammatory agents. The management of symptoms such as pain and diarrhea is as important to the well-being of patients as treatment of mucosal inflammation. These approaches should be individualized according to the patient's symptoms and clinical status.

Irritable bowel syndrome is common in the general population and is equally prevalent in patients with IBD.[13] A dietary history is important in identifying aggravating foods contributing to digestive symptoms. Approximately one half of patients with IBD receive complementary therapies.[40] A careful review of the patient's use of vitamins, health foods, fiber, homeopathic agents, and herbs may help identify factors contributing to changes in bowel habits. Many patients with IBD suffer from concurrent irritable bowel syndrome. Although the usual stress of daily living does not affect the inflammatory activity of IBD, many patients report that stress precedes a worsening of symptoms. Antispasmodics, primarily anticholinergic agents (e.g., dicyclomine, clidinium bromide, hyoscyamine, propantheline, and belladonna alkaloids), treat cramping abdominal discomfort or symptoms of irritable bowel syndrome accompanying UC and CD. Similarly, antidiarrheal preparations (e.g., diphenoxylate, loperamide, and codeine) can be used to reduce the frequency of bowel movements and rectal urgency in patients with mild to moderate UC and CD.[41] Antimotility agents should be avoided in severe or fulminant disease because of the risk of inducing toxic megacolon.

There is no personality profile that predisposes people to IBD, and there is no routine role for sedative, anxiolytic, antidepressant, or antipsychotic therapy. In general, psychopharmacologic therapies are reserved for specific disorders, usually after consultation with a psychiatrist.

Similarly, narcotic analgesia is rarely required to treat IBD. Pain from UC is caused by irritability and muscle spasm or by transmural inflammation. Irritability and muscle spasm are treated with antispasmodics; transmural inflammation is treated with specific anti-inflammatory therapy. Transmural inflammation or stenoses may cause abdominal pain in CD; however, because of the chronic nature of the disease, addictive analgesics should be avoided. Attempts should be made to reduce the inflammation and treat irritability with antispasmodics or nonaddictive analgesics.

NSAIDs are used frequently on a prescription and nonprescription basis. They are an insidious factor in IBD, recognized to exacerbate disease activity[42] and contribute to refractory disease.[13] Arthralgias should be treated without NSAIDs (e.g., with acetaminophen) to avoid the risk of exacerbating the underlying IBD or triggering refractory disease.

Patients with CD often have increased diarrhea after bowel resection, related to the length of bowel removed.[41] Bile-salt malabsorption complicating resections less than 100 cm can be treated with cholestyramine or alternative bile-salt sequestrants. Longer resections resulting in steatorrhea are managed with a low-fat diet.

Treatment of Ulcerative Colitis

The management of UC is determined by the extent of colitis, severity of illness, complications, and response of the individual patient to prior interventions.

TREATMENT OF SPECIFIC CLINICAL MANIFESTATIONS OF ULCERATIVE COLITIS

Ulcerative Proctitis

Induction therapies Topical aminosalicylates are the most effective medical treatments for distal UC.[43] A daily dose of 1 to 4 g is administered nightly as an enema or as a suppository or foam in divided doses. Topical hydrocortisone or budesonide administered as a suppository, an enema, or foam are acceptable alternatives to mesalamine. Foam preparations are easier to retain and are better tolerated.

Oral aminosalicylates can be used to treat mild to moderate symptoms of proctitis but are less effective than topical therapies.[44] Sulfasalazine, 2 to 6 g/day in divided doses, is the most cost-effective aminosalicylate; however, sulfa intolerance, toxic reactions, or allergy can compromise therapy. Mesalamine, olsalazine, or balsalazide formulations are preferable for patients with a history of sulfa allergy or for patients who develop sulfa-related side effects.

Induction therapy is continued until the patient is asymptomatic. A complete response may require 4 to 12 weeks.

Maintenance therapies Maintenance therapy is indicated for most patients with distal colitis; however, mild or infrequent recurrent flares may be treated on an as-needed basis. Continuation of the inductive therapy, excluding steroids, is most effective for maintenance treatment. Mesalamine suppositories or enemas can be continued on a daily basis or can be gradually tapered to every other day, then every third day. An oral aminosalicylate is added when patients continue to experience flares despite attempts to wean them off topical therapy or while tapering topical steroids.

Left-Sided Colitis

Induction therapies For mild to moderate disease, mesalamine enemas are the most effective therapy for left-sided colitis, with hydrocortisone or budesonide enemas used as an alternative.[43] Oral aminosalicylates also are effective, with improvement generally noted within 2 to 4 weeks.[45] The oral aminosalicylates are generally equivalent.[15]

Patients with moderate to severe disease and those in whom topical mesalamine or an oral aminosalicylate has failed are treated as outpatients with oral prednisone, 40 to 60 mg daily, to induce remission—treatment similar to that given to patients with extensive colitis. Severe left-sided colitis requires hospitalization and treatment with systemic steroids as indicated for extensive colitis.

Maintenance therapies Induction therapy is continued until clinical remission is achieved (i.e., normal bowel movements without bleeding, urgency, tenesmus, or inability to evacuate flatus). Neither oral nor topical steroids are effective for maintaining remission. Patients responding to rectal mesalamine can continue with topical therapy or can be transferred to oral treatment. The combination of oral and topical mesalamine therapy has advantages over either therapy alone.[46] If patients experience a relapse while taking an oral aminosalicylate, the dose should be increased to as much as 4.8 g of mesalamine (6 g sulfasalazine). It may be necessary to maintain therapy with topical mesalamine in such cases.

After inductive treatment with steroid enemas, patients are given an oral aminosalicylate, and topical therapy is tapered. Patients requiring systemic steroids are maintained on an oral aminosalicylate, with or without topical mesalamine.

Extensive Colitis (Pancolitis)

Induction therapies in mild to moderate disease Oral aminosalicylate therapy is the primary therapy for outpatients with extensive mild to moderate colitis; the therapy may be supplemented with topical mesalamine or steroids.[9] The dose of the oral aminosalicylates is more significant than the specific formulation.[15] Response rates up to 80% can be anticipated with 4 to 6 g of sulfasalazine or 2.0 to 4.8 g of a mesalamine formulation. Therapy is continued until clinical remission is achieved (i.e., normal bowel movements without blood or rectal urgency). In the absence of a complete response, the dose of the aminosalicylate should be increased to as much as 4.8 g of mesalamine. An antispasmodic or antidiarrheal preparation may be added to treat abdominal cramping or mild diarrhea.

In the absence of a response or with evidence of worsening, prednisone, 40 to 60 mg/day, is added. Once the patient has achieved clinical remission, generally in 2 to 4 weeks, steroids are tapered according to the time course to improvement. The prednisone dosage can be decreased by approximately 5 mg a week until it is reduced to 20 mg/day. Below 20 mg/day, the tapering schedule is 2.5 to 5 mg every 1 to 2 weeks. Aminosalicylate therapy is continued as steroids are reduced.

AZA and 6-MP are effective steroid-sparing therapies for patients who respond to treatment but are unable to taper steroids completely despite optimal doses of an aminosalicylate.[9] Therapeutic benefits require 3 to 6 months to appear; during this time, steroids are maintained at the lowest dose to prevent recurrence of symptoms. Calcium and vitamin D supplementation is indicated during steroid therapy to prevent metabolic bone disease. Reduced bone density is an indication for additional therapy with a bisphosphonate.[47]

Induction therapies in moderate to severe disease Significant weight loss, fever, disabling extraintestinal manifesta-

tions, frequent nocturnal bowel movements, severe anemia, and progressive symptoms despite outpatient therapy with corticosteroids and aminosalicylates are indications for hospitalization. A low-residue diet with sufficient protein and calories to counter the catabolic influence of active inflammation and steroids minimizes abdominal cramps and bowel movements. Antispasmodics or antidiarrheals are used with caution and with monitoring for worsening symptoms.

Intravenous steroids are indicated for severely ill patients with fever, orthostasis, evidence of dehydration, more than 10 to 12 stools daily, rectal bleeding necessitating transfusion, protein depletion, or evidence of abdominal tenderness or distention.[9] Prompt resuscitative measures should correct fluid and electrolyte imbalances. With active bleeding, transfusions are indicated to maintain the hematocrit above 30%. Anticholinergics, antidiarrheals, and narcotic analgesics are contraindicated to prevent worsening colonic dilatation and masking of peritoneal signs in steroid-treated patients.[8]

An intensive intravenous steroid regimen consists of prednisolone (40 to 60 mg/day), methylprednisolone (32 to 48 mg/day), or hydrocortisone (300 to 400 mg/day) administered in divided doses or as a continuous infusion.[8] Topical steroid enemas (e.g., hydrocortisone, 100 mg) can be administered adjunctly to reduce rectal urgency or tenesmus. Oral aminosalicylates are discontinued because of minor anti-inflammatory effects (compared with high-dose steroids) and potential intolerance; in rare instances, aminosalicylates can worsen colitis.

If the patient's condition does not improve within 5 to 7 days of intensive intravenous steroid therapy, the likelihood of improvement is small,[48] and the patient should be considered a candidate for adjunctive therapy with cyclosporine or for surgery. When vital signs normalize, the hematocrit stabilizes, and bowel movements are formed without blood or urgency on a low-residue diet, the patient can change to an oral therapy. Therapy with an aminosalicylate is resumed, and intravenous steroids are replaced with oral prednisone, 40 mg daily, and tapered.

Intravenous cyclosporine therapy has been an important advance in the treatment of severe UC. The use of cyclosporine should be limited, however, to clinicians who have experience in monitoring immunosuppression.[9,25] Response is anticipated within the first 4 to 5 days; if there is no significant improvement within 1 week, the patient should be referred for surgery.[48] Once clinical remission is achieved, the intravenous regimen is replaced with oral cyclosporine and prednisone. The daily dose of cyclosporine is doubled and administered in two divided doses (e.g., if the patient had been receiving 200 mg/day intravenously, the oral dosing would be 200 mg two times weekly). In most settings, AZA or 6-MP is added to the oral regimen because of the high relapse rate associated with intravenous cyclosporine therapy. Trimethoprim-sulfamethoxazole is given three times weekly as prophylaxis against PCP.

Outpatient monitoring of cyclosporine levels and laboratory studies are repeated weekly for the first month and then at reduced intervals. Steroids are tapered, which generally requires 8 to 12 weeks. After steroids are tapered, cyclosporine is reduced and then discontinued. The patient is maintained on an aminosalicylate and AZA or 6-MP.

Maintenance therapies Maintenance treatment for extensive UC is determined by the intensity of therapy needed to induce remission. If aminosalicylate therapy has been sufficient to induce remission, continuation of the same dosage throughout maintenance therapy is optimal. Patients treated with steroids require a more individualized approach, with the rate of steroid tapering determined by the rapidity of response as maximized doses of an aminosalicylate are continued. Patients receiving AZA or 6-MP are also continued on maximized aminosalicylate therapy. Neither the optimum immunomodulator dose nor the leukopenia requisite has been clarified.[49] The complete blood count should be monitored at least quarterly.

Fulminant Colitis and Toxic Megacolon

Fulminant colitis, with or without colonic dilatation (toxic megacolon), is a medical emergency best managed by an experienced team of gastroenterology specialists and surgeons. Management is similar to the treatment of severe colitis, with several modifications. Patients should receive nothing by mouth until they have clinically improved (i.e., they feel hungry and no longer complain of pain or tenesmus). In the presence of small bowel ileus, a nasogastric tube is indicated, as are maneuvers to reduce colonic distention and allow rectal passage of colonic gas. These maneuvers include rolling the patient from side to side, inserting a rectal tube, or having the patient assume the knee-elbow position. Intravenous steroids are continued, and broad-spectrum antibiotic coverage is added for presumed transmural extension of disease, microperforation, and systemic bacteremia.[8] Cyclosporine therapy is controversial in this setting but has been used in selected cases.

Persistent peritoneal signs and symptoms of deterioration or failure to improve within 24 to 72 hours is an indication for immediate colectomy. Although aggressive medical management is successful for 40% to 50% of patients with fulminant colitis or toxic megacolon, many patients experience complications or resistant disease, including recurrent toxic megacolon.[50]

INDICATIONS FOR SURGERY

UC is cured by proctocolectomy, and quality of life after surgery for UC is excellent. Potential for a surgical cure must be balanced against sustaining morbidity, adverse reactions to therapy, and the risk of neoplasia. Indications for colectomy in UC are either emergent or elective.

Emergent indications include exsanguinating hemorrhage, perforation, and unresponsive fulminant colitis or toxic megacolon. Chronic refractory colitis and significant complications of disease or medical therapy (e.g., hemolytic anemia, pyoderma gangrenosum, or steroid-induced psychosis) can lead to more urgent indications for colectomy.

More often, surgical indications are less acute and allow consultation, preparation, and education of patient and family to optimize timing and minimize physical and emotional consequences. The most common elective indications for surgery are medically intractable disease, poor quality of life, and chronic complications from colitis or medical therapy. Physical debility, psychosocial dysfunction, and intolerable adverse reactions to drugs are not acceptable with the availability of a surgical cure.

SURGICAL ALTERNATIVES

Because UC is confined to the colonic mucosa, proctocolectomy (removal of the colon) with an end ileostomy (formation of a stoma to connect the end of the ileum to the outside of the body) is curative. This procedure is the standard with which all alternatives must be compared. Even in the most urgent cases, proctocolectomy and ileostomy can usually be performed as a single procedure. This operation has the least likelihood of

complications but is compromised by the creation of a permanent stoma. Nevertheless, quality of life after proctocolectomy and ileostomy is usually acceptable.

To avoid permanent stomas, a series of surgical procedures have been developed to remove the proximal colon and strip the rectal mucosa from the distal rectal musculature while sparing the anal sphincter. These sphincter-saving pelvic-pouch procedures afford the opportunity to cure colitis and reestablish the connection between ileum and anus via an anastomosis. An ileal pouch is necessary to provide reservoir function and prevent intolerable diarrhea. These J-, S-, or W-shaped pouches are created by folding the distal ileum and anastomosing the outlet to the anal canal. Depending on the patient's status and the surgeon's discretion, the procedures can be performed in one, two, or three stages.

Quality of life after an ileoanal anastomosis is excellent; most patients report full continence with an average of six unformed (but not urgent) bowel movements daily. Approximately 10% of patients develop small bowel obstructions either between stages or after completion of the surgery.

Treatment of Crohn Disease

As with UC, the therapeutic approach to CD depends on the disease location, severity, complications, and response to previous interventions. The sequential approach to induction and maintenance of remission is advisable for patients with this chronic disease.

TREATMENT OF SPECIFIC CLINICAL MANIFESTATIONS OF CROHN DISEASE

Gastroduodenal Crohn Disease

Gastroduodenal manifestations are rarely the initial presentation of CD. Dyspepsia, epigastric burning, and nausea usually respond to acid-reduction therapy with proton-pump inhibitors. More profound symptoms of nausea or vomiting respond to corticosteroids and subsequently to an immunomodulator for steroid-sparing effects.[51] Gastric outlet obstruction that does not respond to steroids or immunomodulators is an indication for surgical gastrojejunostomy.

Jejunoileitis

Isolated proximal small bowel CD also is uncommon. Patients present with abdominal pain, distention, and diarrhea related to intestinal strictures and small bowel bacterial overgrowth.[10] Diarrhea should be evaluated from a mechanistic standpoint. Malabsorption caused by short bowel or resection is treated with a low-fat diet, whereas small bowel bacterial overgrowth is managed with antibiotics. Patients presenting with prominent pain or small-bowel obstruction are treated with corticosteroids on a short-term basis and then, usually, with AZA or 6-MP. Bowel obstructions that do not respond to short-term steroids require surgical resection or, more commonly, stricturoplasty.

Ileitis, Ileocolitis, and Crohn Colitis

Limited ileal and ileocolonic CD describe the most commonly involved sites; however, these conditions present as a heterogeneous spectrum of symptoms and complications. Therapy should be staged to alleviate the presenting symptoms and maintain long-term well-being while minimizing long-term complications related to the disease or therapy.[7,10]

Mild to moderate disease Anti-inflammatory and symptomatic medications, along with dietary modifications, are provided on an outpatient basis to patients with mild to moderate symptoms of abdominal pain and tenderness; diarrhea; low-grade fever; and weight loss without obstruction, painful mass, or severe malnutrition. Sulfasalazine, 3 to 6 g/day in divided doses, is effective for ileocolonic and colonic CD but not for isolated small bowel disease. Mesalamine, 4 g/day, improves symptoms of small bowel and colonic involvement when the formulation delivers 5-ASA to the involved segments. Sulfasalazine and mesalamine have been shown to be modestly more beneficial than placebo and less beneficial than corticosteroids.[7,10] However, the potential long-term efficacy and absence of side effects make the aminosalicylates a first-line approach despite their limited potency. Therapy should be continued with the inductive dose for as long as the patient continues to respond.

Controlled-release budesonide, 9 mg daily, is an alternative therapy to induce remission in patients with mild to moderate CD confined to the ileum and right colon.[17,20]

Antibiotic therapy with metronidazole, 10 to 20 mg/kg, or ciprofloxacin, 1 g, alone or in combination, is an alternative to aminosalicylates for ileocolonic and colonic CD. Although no long-term trial data are yet available, clinical observations suggest that maintenance therapy is likely to be necessary. Patients receiving long-term metronidazole therapy should be monitored for peripheral neuropathy.

Dietary and nutritional therapy should focus on reduction of symptoms, maintenance or repletion of nutritional deficits, and prevention of long-term complications.[38] Elemental diets are efficacious on a short-term basis but are not practical for most adult patients. Knowledge of the location and complications of the disease, along with surgical history, will direct attention to potential nutrient deficiencies. Calorie and protein requirements are the primary concern. Secondary considerations include maintenance of iron stores and water-soluble vitamins for patients with proximal small bowel disease and maintenance of vitamins A, B$_{12}$, D, and E for those with ileal disease or resection. Calcium and vitamin D supplements are important to minimize metabolic bone disease.

Moderate to severe disease Failure to respond to aminosalicylates or steroids; presentation with fever, significant weight loss (> 10%), abdominal pain accompanied by tenderness but without obstruction; and ability to maintain oral intake can imply moderate to severe ileal and ileocolonic disease.[10] After perforating complications (i.e., abscess) are excluded, corticosteroids are required to induce a clinical remission. Most patients respond to oral steroids (prednisone, 0.5 to 1.0 mg/kg). However, the clinical response usually does not persist after steroid tapering; approximately 70% of patients experience a relapse or become steroid dependent within a year.[52] The initial dose of prednisone is continued until the patient responds completely with resolution of inflammatory symptoms. The dose is then decreased according to the time course to response. Tapering usually can proceed by 5 to 10 mg/wk (to 20 mg/day) and then by 2.5 to 5.0 mg/wk. Calcium and vitamin D supplements should be prescribed, and in the setting of reduced bone density, a bisphosphonate should be considered.[47] Clinical monitoring is continued, with attention paid to relapse of inflammatory symptoms. Persistent noninflammatory symptoms (e.g., nonbloody diarrhea or abdominal cramps) can be treated with dietary modifications, antispasmodic agents, and antidiarrheal agents with no intensification of anti-inflammatory therapy.

Severe disease is defined by symptoms that persist despite administration of oral corticosteroids or by hospitalization because of high fever, cachexia, obstructive symptoms, rebound tenderness, or an abscess.[10] A recent option for CD has been the availability of the chimeric anti-TNF monoclonal antibody, infliximab.[33] A single infusion of 5 mg/kg provides significant improvement for patients who have not responded to aminosalicylates, antibiotics, or steroids. Repeated infusions of the antibody at 8-week intervals prolong improvement and may be necessary on a long-term (indefinite) basis because most patients experience a relapse within 8 to 12 weeks after a single infusion.

Parenteral corticosteroids are indicated for severe manifestations of CD once an abscess has been ruled out. Patients presenting with dehydration or significant anemia require resuscitation with intravenous fluids, electrolytes, or blood transfusion, sometimes in combination. Acute obstructive symptoms without chronic symptoms should be assessed for a possible mechanical cause (e.g., adhesions) rather than an inflammatory narrowing. Parenteral nutritional support is indicated as a supplement for patients unable to tolerate sufficient enteral intake to maintain caloric requirements and is mandatory for patients with profound malnutrition and an inability to eat.

The equivalent of 40 to 60 mg of intravenous prednisolone (e.g., hydrocortisone, 200 to 300 mg, or methylprednisolone, 32 to 45 mg), delivered as an intermittent or continuous infusion, is administered until diarrhea is controlled or the patient is free of pain and able to pass flatus and stool. Subsequently, oral steroids are substituted at an equivalent dose. Failure of intravenous steroid therapy should suggest the need for reevaluation for potential surgical intervention, prolonged TPN and bowel rest, or administration of intravenous cyclosporine or infliximab. Broad-spectrum antibiotics are added for febrile patients, patients with abdominal tenderness, and patients with an inflammatory mass.[10] Antibiotic therapy is continued until defervescence unless a specific pathogen has been identified.

MAINTENANCE THERAPY FOR CROHN DISEASE

Earlier, maintenance therapy for CD was discounted on the basis of negative results from early studies evaluating low-dose sulfasalazine and corticosteroids. It now is apparent that maintenance approaches can reduce clinical relapse when applied in the appropriate clinical situations.[7,10] Steroids are not effective and should not be routinely used as maintenance agents for CD.[20]

The aminosalicylates are useful maintenance agents when continued after inductive therapy but have limited value after steroid-induced remissions.[16] In contrast, there is evidence of steroid-sparing and maintenance benefits from immunomodulators.[23] AZA and 6-MP are effective steroid-sparing agents for patients who cannot otherwise be weaned off steroids. Therapy is initiated with AZA (2 to 2.5 mg/kg) or 6-MP (1 to 1.5 mg/kg), with the dosage adjusted at 2-week intervals on the basis of the white blood cell count (to be maintained above leukopenic levels). As mentioned, AZA and 6-MP may require 3 to 6 months to show efficacy. Continued monitoring of blood counts on a quarterly basis once the patient is off steroids is necessary to prevent unanticipated bone marrow suppression.

INDICATIONS FOR SURGERY

In contrast to UC, CD is not cured by surgery except when the disease is confined to the colon; then, proctocolectomy and end ileostomy are curative. Sphincter-saving procedures are not advocated for patients with CD because of the high likelihood of recurrence of disease after anastomoses. When CD is not confined to the colon, recurrence of CD at the anastomotic site is virtually inevitable.[53] Therefore, surgery for CD is usually reserved for refractory disease or complications. Nevertheless, in view of the potential for excellent quality of life after limited surgery and the increasing capability to reduce or delay recurrence, concerns about recurrence should not necessarily force a decision to defer surgery.[10]

Purulent complications (i.e., abscess) necessitate percutaneous or surgical drainage. In addition, surgery for CD is indicated for intractable hemorrhage, perforation, persistent or recurrent obstruction, and toxic megacolon. The most common indications for surgery are intractable disease, failure of medical therapy, and complications related to treatment (e.g., steroid dependence). Because many of these indications are subjective, the decision requires experienced clinical judgment and cooperative consultation between medical and surgical specialists.

Maintenance Therapy to Delay Postsurgical Relapse

Postsurgical maintenance therapy has been evaluated according to various end-point criteria, including endoscopic evidence of relapse, clinical symptoms, and the need for repeated surgery.[7,53] There is evidence that mesalamine (3 to 4 g/day) can prevent postoperative recurrence,[16] particularly when therapy is initiated shortly after surgery. Postponing chemotherapy for more than 3 months circumvents any benefits. Metronidazole is effective at reducing postoperative recurrence when administered at high doses (20 mg/kg) for 3 months after resection. There are no data regarding lower doses of metronidazole, longer treatment periods, or alternative antibiotics. Recent evidence indicates that 6-MP at a dosage of 50 mg/day reduces evidence of postoperative relapse for at least 2 years after resection. At present, however, it is not possible to make specific recommendations regarding postoperative maintenance on the basis of surgical indications.

Complications

EXTRAINTESTINAL COMPLICATIONS

Extraintestinal complications of IBD can be related to inflammation or to an associated HLA-related autoimmune process. They can also occur as a metabolic consequence of intestinal disease.

Mucocutaneous complications include eye changes of episcleritis or scleritis and most commonly parallel colonic disease activity. Involvement of the anterior or posterior chambers with iritis or uveitis is related to HLA-B27 and follows an independent course from bowel activity. Skin lesions of erythema nodosum and pyoderma gangrenosum usually accompany or herald the onset of colitis and respond to treatment of bowel inflammation.

Musculoskeletal lesions also can be independent of or correlate with intestinal disease activity. Peripheral arthralgia and arthritis commonly involve the hips, knees, ankles, elbows, and wrists in an asymmetrical pattern. The inflammation usually accompanies intestinal disease activity and is almost never deforming, progressive, or associated with rheumatoid nodules. Arthritis of the central spine, ankylosing spondylitis, and sacroiliitis, in contrast, are HLA-B27–associated and progress independently of intestinal disease. Metabolic bone disease is most often related to long-term steroid use and, in patients with CD, can be accelerated by malabsorption or inadequate supplementation of vitamin D or calcium.[54]

There is a spectrum of hepatobiliary involvement in both UC and colonic CD.[55] Inflammation of the intrahepatic and extrahepatic bile ducts may present as a mild, periportal inflammatory infiltrate (pericholangitis or small duct sclerosing cholangitis) that is asymptomatic and nonprogressive and is manifested only as mild elevations of γ-glutamyltransferase (GGT), alkaline phosphatase, and transaminases. However, it may also present as full-blown sclerosing cholangitis with progressive secondary biliary cirrhosis. Hepatic steatosis commonly manifests as a mild elevation of enzymes (e.g., GGT, alkaline phosphatase) in the presence of malnutrition or steroid therapy. Patients with CD who have ileal involvement or have had ileal resections are at increased risk for gallstones caused by reduced enterohepatic circulation of bile salts and elevated biliary cholesterol saturation.

Urinary tract complications are more common in CD than in UC. Kidney stones may be related to dehydration caused by diarrhea or the presence of an ileostomy. In the setting of ileitis or after ileal resections, the mechanism of nephrolithiasis is hyperoxaluria caused by steatorrhea. Normally, oxalate in the diet binds to free calcium in the colonic lumen and is excreted in the feces as calcium oxalate crystals. In patients with steatorrhea, free luminal calcium preferentially binds to fatty acids, creating soaps that are similarly excreted in the feces; free oxalate is absorbed by the colon and excreted by the kidneys in abnormally high amounts; and oxalate complexes with urinary calcium and is excreted as calcium oxalate crystals. Moreover, patients with CD excrete low amounts of urinary citrate, which, under normal circumstances, is a nonspecific solubilizer in the urine.

A 24-hour urine study assessing calcium and oxalate should differentiate hyperoxaluria from calcium oxalate stones caused by idiopathic hypercalciuria. If hyperoxaluria is identified, the treatment is a reduction of fat intake (to reduce steatorrhea) and an increase in calcium supplements.

Hematologic complications of UC and CD include anemia and clotting abnormalities. Anemia is most often related to iron deficiency caused by bleeding. Folic acid deficiency is most often related to concurrent use of sulfasalazine; occasionally, it can be related to inadequate dietary consumption or extensive jejunal disease. Vitamin-B_{12} deficiency can lead to macroscopic anemia in extensive ileal disease or after ileal resection. Hypercoagulability in patients with active IBD is caused by increased production of acute-phase reactants, which increase the risk of venous thromboses. Enteric losses of anticoagulant factors are rarely a consequence of protein-losing enteropathy. In contrast, hypocoagulability may be a complication of vitamin K malabsorption or prolonged antibiotic administration.

Management of Extraintestinal Complications

Extraintestinal manifestations of IBD can be dependent on or independent of intestinal (usually colonic) inflammation. Peripheral arthritis, erythema nodosum, pyoderma gangrenosum, and episcleritis occur in the presence of active disease and require intensification of anti-inflammatory therapy. In some situations, complications can be treated independently as concurrent therapy for intestinal inflammation proceeds. For example, inflamed joints can be drained or injected with steroids, and pyoderma gangrenosum can be treated with a combination of topical and systemic approaches.

Ocular complications should be evaluated by an ophthalmologist to prevent irreversible damage. Erythema nodosum usually responds to aggressive therapy for colitis and should not be treated with NSAIDs. Peripheral articular manifestations of colitis can be treated with acetaminophen and increased doses of sulfasalazine; NSAIDs should be avoided.

In contrast, ankylosing spondylitis, sacroiliitis, iritis, and uveitis are HLA-B27–associated manifestations that, along with primary sclerosing cholangitis, follow a course independent from colitis. Physical therapy is critical for patients with ankylosing spondylitis and sacroiliitis. These central arthropathies may require concurrent immunomodulatory therapy with methotrexate, hydroxychloroquine, or low doses of prednisone.

INTESTINAL COMPLICATIONS

Intestinal complications of IBD include hemorrhage, stricture, fistulas, toxic megacolon, and neoplasia. Chronic blood loss and iron deficiency anemia are common in both UC and CD. Profuse bleeding is uncommon, however, particularly in UC, because of the superficial inflammation that is characteristic of the disease (except in toxic megacolon). In CD, rapid lower gastrointestinal bleeding can occur when deep ulcerations erode into large blood vessels. Strictures also are more common in CD than in UC and are related to transmural inflammation and fibrosis. These strictures remain fixed and can lead to progressive bowel obstruction. In UC, luminal narrowing can be caused by smooth muscle hypertrophy; in this case, it is related to disease activity and is reversible with treatment of acute inflammation. Fixed strictures in UC are almost always dysplastic or malignant. Toxic megacolon is not unique to UC and can occur in infectious colitis and CD.[8]

ADENOCARCINOMA

Adenocarcinoma is a long-term complication of IBD, with features that are distinct from those of sporadic adenocarcinomas.[56] The risk of colonic neoplasia in UC and the risk in CD are similar and are related to the extent and duration of disease, age at onset, stricture formation, and presence of primary sclerosing cholangitis. The risk of dysplasia, a precursor of adenocarcinoma,[56] is not correlated with disease activity; patients with long-standing inactive IBD have the same risk for adenocarcinoma as patients with chronic active inflammation. Dysplasia has been defined on a pathologic basis and has been categorized as indefinite, low grade, or high grade (carcinoma in situ). Identification of dysplasia implies a risk of cancer elsewhere in the colon in up to 50% of patients with high-grade lesions or with low-grade lesions occurring in a raised plaque (dysplasia-associated lesion or mass).[57]

The ability to identify histologic dysplasia in patients with UC offers an opportunity to perform surveillance colonoscopic examinations.[57] After 8 to 10 years, patients with UC should enter a colonoscopic surveillance program according to individual risk factors.[9] Surveillance colonoscopies are recommended at 2- to 3-year intervals for patients with a history of UC for 10 to 20 years and are recommended at 1- to 2-year intervals for patients with a history of UC for more than 20 years. The diagnostic threshold for surveillance is the finding of confirmed low-grade dysplasia (the finding is also sufficient to warrant a recommendation for colectomy). Patients with indefinite dysplasia are treated aggressively to control inflammation, with colonoscopy repeated in 3 to 6 months.

The risk of cancer is related to the location and chronicity of inflammation in CD as well; there is thus a risk of small bowel adenocarcinoma in patients with long-standing small bowel disease.[56] Because of the heterogeneity of location and segmental involvement in CD, however, there are no standardized guidelines for surveillance. In the absence of guidelines, the paradigm of colonoscopic surveillance for UC can be applied to colonic CD. Formation of strictures in patients with CD may interfere with complete colonoscopic surveillance, however.

Inflammatory Bowel Diseases and Pregnancy

Although fertility is usually normal in male and female patients with IBD, there is an inverse correlation between disease activity and libido and a correlation between disease activity and menstrual irregularities. Reversible sperm abnormalities and folate malabsorption are unique complications related to sulfasalazine.

Women with active IBD have an increased risk of early miscarriage. When disease activity is controlled, however, the course and outcome of pregnancy do not differ substantially from those of the general population. The best means of ensuring normal fetal outcome is for conception to occur when the disease is under control, for disease activity to be aggressively treated during pregnancy, and for the health of the mother to be maintained. Aminosalicylates, steroids, and immunomodulators are safe during pregnancy and lactation[58] and are indicated when necessary to maintain maternal well-being. Because of the risk posed by an IBD flare, neither acute treatment nor maintenance therapy should be withdrawn during or after pregnancy. Attention to the mother's nutritional status is essential throughout pregnancy and during the increased nutritional demands of lactation. Neonates delivered by women on high doses of steroids should be monitored for adrenal suppression.

Prognosis and Conclusion

The diagnosis and management of IBD challenge the experience and perseverance of the clinician to guide patients through chronic illness. It is important to recognize the concerns, perceptions, and emotions of patients and family members confronted with a medically incurable, socially embarrassing, and potentially disfiguring condition. In the absence of a known etiology or cure, medical therapy is usually effective, and surgical techniques have improved to the point that longevity and quality of life can be preserved. The life expectancy of patients with nonfulminant IBD does not differ from that of the general population.

With patience, empathy, and optimism, clinicians can do much to help patients and their families balance their concerns and dispel the common and often troubling misconceptions of psychopathology surrounding these diseases.

Additional Information

Additional sources of information and support regarding IBD are available through national organizations such as the Crohn's & Colitis Foundation of America (http://www.ccfa.org), the Crohn's and Colitis Foundation of Canada (http://www.ccfc.ca), the American College of Gastroenterology (http://www.acg.gi.org), the American Gastroenterological Association (http://www.gastro.org), and the National Institute of Diabetes and Digestive and Kidney Diseases (http://www.niddk.nih.gov).

References

1. Fiocchi C: Inflammatory bowel disease: etiology and pathogenesis. Gastroenterology 115:182, 1998

2. Sartor RB: Review article: role of the enteric microflora in the pathogenesis of intestinal inflammation and arthritis. Aliment Pharmacol Ther 11(suppl 3):17, 1997

3. Schreiber S, Hampe J: Genomics and inflammatory bowel disease. Curr Opin Gastroenterol 16:297, 1999

4. Rubin DT, Hanauer SB: Smoking and inflammatory bowel disease. Eur J Gastroenterol Hepatol 12:855, 2000

5. Targan SR: The utility of ANCA and ASCA in inflammatory bowel disease. Inflamm Bowel Dis 5:61, 1999

6. MacDermott RP: Lack of current clinical value of serological testing in the evaluation of patients with IBD. Inflamm Bowel Dis 5:64, 1999

7. Hanauer SB: Review articles: drug therapy: inflammatory bowel disease. N Engl J Med 334:841, 1996

8. Stein RB, Hanauer SB: Life-threatening complications of IBD: how to handle fulminant colitis and toxic megacolon. J Crit Illness 13:518, 1998

9. Kornbluth A, Sachar DB: Ulcerative colitis practice guidelines in adults: American College of Gastroenterology, Practice Parameters Committee. Am J Gastroenterol 92:204, 1997

10. Hanauer SB, Meyers S: Management of Crohn's disease in adults. Am J Gastroenterol 92:559, 1997

11. Farmer RG, Easley KA, Rankin GB: Clinical patterns, natural history, and progression of ulcerative colitis: a long-term follow-up of 1116 patients. Dig Dis Sci 38:1137, 1993

12. Irvine EJ: Quality of life issues in patients with inflammatory bowel disease. Am J Gastroenterol 92(12 suppl):18S, 1997

13. Miner PB: Factors influencing the relapse of patients with inflammatory bowel disease. Am J Gastroenterol 92(12 suppl):1S, 1997

14. Sutherland L, Roth D, Beck P, et al: Oral 5-aminosalicylic acid for maintaining remission in ulcerative colitis. Cochrane Database Syst Rev 2, 1999

15. Sutherland L, Roth D, Beck P, et al: Oral 5-aminosalicylic acid for inducing remission in ulcerative colitis. Cochrane Database Syst Rev 2, 1999

16. Camma C, Giunta M, Rosselli M, et al: Mesalamine in the maintenance treatment of Crohn's disease: a meta-analysis adjusted for confounding variables. Gastroenterology 113:1465, 1997

17. Wikberg M, Ulmius J, Ragnarsson G: Review article: targeted drug delivery in treatment of intestinal diseases. Aliment Pharmacol Ther 11(suppl 3):109, 1997

18. Walker AM, Szneke P, Bianchim LA, et al: 5-Aminosalicylates, sulfasalazine, steroid use, and complications in patients with ulcerative colitis. Am J Gastroenterol 92:816, 1997

19. Cohen RD, Woseth DM, Thisted RA, et al: A meta-analysis and overview of the literature on treatment options for left-sided ulcerative colitis and ulcerative proctitis. Am J Gastroenterol 95:1263, 2000

20. Steinhart AH, Ewe K, Griffiths AM, et al: Corticosteroids for maintaining remission of Crohn's disease. Cochrane Database Syst Rev 2, 1999

21. Sandborn WJ: A review of immune modifier therapy for inflammatory bowel disease: azathioprine, 6-mercaptopurine, cyclosporine, and methotrexate. Am J Gastroenterol 91:423, 1996

22. Ramsey-Goldman R, Schilling E: Immunosuppressive drug use during pregnancy. Rheum Dis Clin North Am 23:149, 1997

23. Pearson DC, May GR, Fick G, et al: Azathioprine for maintaining remission of Crohn's disease. Cochrane Database Syst Rev 2, 1999

24. Sandborn W, Sutherland L, Pearson D, et al: Azathioprine or 6-mercaptopurine for inducing remission of Crohn's disease. Cochrane Database Syst Rev 2, 1999

25. Kornbluth A, Present DH, Lichtiger S, et al: Cyclosporin for severe ulcerative colitis: a user's guide. Am J Gastroenterol 92:1424, 1997

26. Egan LJ, Sandborn WJ: Methotrexate for inflammatory bowel disease: pharmacology and preliminary results. Mayo Clin Proc 71:69, 1996

27. Feagan BG, Rochon J, Fedorak RN, et al: Methotrexate for the treatment of Crohn's disease. The North American Crohn's Study Group Investigators. N Engl J Med 332:292, 1995

28. Feagan BG, Fedorak RN, Irvine EJ, et al: A comparison of methotrexate with placebo for the maintenance of remission in Crohn's disease. N Engl J Med 342:1627, 2000

29. Sandborn W, McLeod R, Jewell D: Pharmacotherapy for inducing and maintaining remission in pouchitis. Cochrane Database Syst Rev 2, 2000

30. Colombel JF, Lemann M, Cassagnou M, et al: A controlled trial comparing ciprofloxacin with mesalazine for the treatment of active Crohn's disease. Groupe d'Etudes Therapeutiques des Affections Inflammatoires Digestives (GETAID). Am J Gastroenterol 94:674, 1999

31. Greenbloom SL, Steinhart AH, Greenberg GR: Combination ciprofloxacin and metronidazole for active Crohn's disease. Can J Gastroenterol 12:53, 1998

32. Sands BE: Biologic therapy for inflammatory bowel disease. Inflamm Bowel Dis 3:95, 1997

33. Targan SR, Hanauer SB, van Deventer SJ, et al: A short-term study of chimeric monoclonal antibody cA2 to tumor necrosis factor alpha for Crohn's disease. Crohn's Disease cA2 Study Group. N Engl J Med 337:1029, 1997

34. Bennink R, Peeters M, Van den Maegdenbergh V, et al: Evaluation of small-bowel transit for solid and liquid test meal in healthy men and women. Eur J Nucl Med 26:1560, 1999

35. Present DH: Review article: the efficacy of infliximab in Crohn's disease: healing of fistulae. Aliment Pharmacol Ther 13(suppl 4):23, 1999

36. Present DH, Rutgeerts P, Targan S, et al: Infliximab for the treatment of fistulas in patients with Crohn's disease. N Engl J Med 340:1398, 1999

37. Korzenik JR: IBD: a vascular disorder? the case for heparin therapy. Inflamm Bowel Dis 3:87, 1997

38. Hunter JO: Nutritional factors in inflammatory bowel disease. Eur J Gastroenterol Hepatol 10:235, 1998

39. Belluzzi A, Brignola C, Campieri M, et al: Effect of an enteric-coated fish-oil preparation on relapses in Crohn's disease. N Engl J Med 334:1557, 1996

40. Hilsden RJ, Scott CM, Verhoef MJ: Complementary medicine use by patients with inflammatory bowel disease. Am J Gastroenterol 93:697, 1998

41. Urayama S, Chang EB: Mechanisms and treatment of diarrhea in inflammatory bowel diseases. Inflamm Bowel Dis 3:114, 1997

42. Hamilton FA: Non-narcotic analgesics: renal and gastrointestinal considerations: introduction. Am J Med 105:1S, 1998

43. Marshall JK, Irvine EJ: Rectal corticosteroids versus alternative treatments in ulcerative colitis: a meta-analysis. Gut 40:775, 1997

44. Gionchetti P, Rizzello F, Venturi A, et al: Comparison of oral with rectal mesalazine in the treatment of ulcerative proctitis. Dis Colon Rectum 41:93, 1998

45. Safdi M, DeMicco M, Sninsky C, et al: A double-blind comparison of oral versus rectal mesalamine versus combination therapy in the treatment of distal ulcerative colitis. Am J Gastroenterol 92:1867, 1997

46. d'Albasio G, Pacini F, Camari E, et al: Combined therapy with 5-aminosalicylic acid tablets and enemas for maintaining remission in ulcerative colitis: a randomized double-blind study. Am J Gastroenterol 92:1143, 1997

47. Ziegler R, Kasperk C: Glucocorticoid-induced osteoporosis: prevention and treatment. Steroids 63:344, 1998

48. Travis SP, Farrant JM, Nolan DJ, et al: Predicting outcome in severe ulcerative colitis. Gut 38:905, 1996

49. Sandborn WJ: Azathioprine: state of the art in inflammatory bowel disease. Scand J Gastroenterol Suppl 225:92, 1998

50. Sheth SG, LaMont JT: Toxic megacolon. Lancet 351:509, 1998

51. Wagtmans MJ, Verspaget HW, Lamers CB, et al: Clinical aspects of Crohn's disease of the upper gastrointestinal tract: a comparison with distal Crohn's disease. Am J Gastroenterol 92:1467, 1997

52. Munkholm P, Langholz E, Davidsen M, et al: Frequency of glucocorticoid resistance and dependency in Crohn's disease. Gut 35:360, 1994

53. Achkar JP, Hanauer SB: Medical therapy to reduce postoperative Crohn's disease recurrence. Am J Gastroenterol 95:1139, 2000

54. Andreassen H, Rungby J, Dahlerup JF, et al: Inflammatory bowel disease and osteoporosis. Scand J Gastroenterol 32:1247, 1997

55. Balan V, LaRusso NF: Hepatobiliary disease in inflammatory bowel disease. Gastroenterol Clin North Am 24:647, 1995

56. Ekbom A: Risk factors and distinguishing features of cancer in IBD. Inflamm Bowel Dis 4:235, 1998

57. Bernstein CN: Challenges in designing a randomized trial of surveillance colonoscopy in IBD. Inflamm Bowel Dis 4:132, 1998

58. Korelitz BI: Inflammatory bowel disease and pregnancy. Gastroenterol Clin North Am 27:213, 1998

Acknowledgment

Figure 4   Tom Moore.

59 Diverticulosis, Diverticulitis, and Appendicitis

William V. Harford, Jr., M.D.

Colonic Diverticulosis and Diverticulitis

Colonic diverticula are herniations of colonic mucosa and submucosa through the muscularis propria. They occur where perforating arteries traverse the circular muscle layer, in parallel rows between the mesenteric and antimesenteric taenia. In Western countries, diverticula involve predominantly the left colon. The sigmoid colon is involved either alone or with proximal segments in 95% of cases. Right-sided diverticula are more common in the Orient, including Japan, than in the West.[1]

Of patients with known diverticulosis, only 10% to 25% will develop acute diverticulitis. The severity of acute diverticulitis varies greatly. Most cases of acute diverticulitis are mild and uncomplicated. Fewer than 20% of patients require hospitalization.[2]

EPIDEMIOLOGY

Diverticulosis

There are no population-based studies of the prevalence of diverticulosis. About 1% of the United States population reported having diverticulosis in the 1983–1987 National Health Interview Survey (NHIS). Women were two to three times more likely than men to report having diverticulosis, and whites were more likely to report having this disorder than African Americans. The prevalence of self-reported diverticulosis increased markedly with age, from 0.1% at 45 years of age or younger to 4.4% at 75 years of age or older. Unrecognized diverticulosis is more common than known diverticulosis. It is estimated that 10% to 20% of individuals older than 50 years have diverticulosis.[3]

Diverticulitis

The epidemiology of diverticulitis is identical to that of diverticulosis.

PATHOGENESIS

Diverticulosis

Reduced colonic diameter and reduced wall compliance may account for diverticulosis. Diverticulosis is common in countries where a low-fiber diet is prevalent. A low-fiber diet reduces stool volume and colonic diameter, particularly in the sigmoid colon. Reduced colonic diameter allows the formation of closed segments during colonic contractions, thereby increasing intraluminal pressure. Although studies in Western countries have not shown a difference in fiber intake between individuals with diverticulosis and those without, animal studies support a correlation.[4] Patients with diverticulosis have an age-related increase in elastin deposition and collagen cross-linking.[5] This leads to decreased colonic wall compliance.[6] Intraluminal pressure is thus higher for any colonic diameter than in patients with normal compliance. The same changes cause shortening of taenia and bunching of circular muscle or myochosis, a corrugation and thickening of the wall of the sigmoid colon. Myochosis narrows the lumen, predisposing to segmentation and high pressures during contractions.

Diverticulitis

Only mucosa and submucosa separate the lumen of diverticula from the colonic serosa. Diverticulitis may result from abrasion of mucosa by inspissated stool, causing inflammation and perforation. Contained perforation may lead to peridiverticulitis, phlegmon, or abscess. The inflammatory process may involve adjacent organs, such as the bladder, and cause a fistula. Repeated episodes of diverticulitis may result in colonic fibrosis, stricture, and obstruction. Free perforation occurs less commonly. It leads to fecal spillage and diffuse peritonitis.

ASYMPTOMATIC OR MINIMALLY SYMPTOMATIC DIVERTICULOSIS

Diverticulosis is asymptomatic or minimally symptomatic in about 80% of cases. Diverticula are most often found incidentally during investigation of another condition. About 85% of those with self-reported diverticulosis in the NHIS survey reported no limitation caused by the condition. Patients who are asymptomatic at the time of diagnosis are unlikely to develop complications from diverticulosis. In the First National Health and Nutrition Examination Survey (NHANES I) Epidemiologic Follow-up Study, a cohort of physicians with asymptomatic diverticulosis was followed for a 10-year period. The probability of hospitalization for diverticular disease was less than 1% in those patients who were 25 to 44 years of age at the beginning of the follow-up period; it was about 5% in those who were 65 to 74 years of age.[3]

Diagnosis

Asymptomatic or minimally symptomatic diverticulosis is usually discovered by barium enema or fiberoptic endoscopy performed for colorectal cancer screening or for investigation of an unrelated medical problem.

Differential Diagnosis

Diverticular disease and irritable bowel syndrome (IBS) are both common clinical conditions; both may be associated with lower abdominal pain and abnormal bowel habits. There is no evidence that they share a common pathophysiology or that IBS precedes diverticular disease. It is unlikely that diverticulosis alone (without diverticulitis) causes abdominal pain and abnormal bowel habits. Some patients with very mild diverticulitis may present with pain but no objective evidence of inflammation. Lower abdominal pain and abnormal bowel habits attributed to diverticulosis are more often the result of coexistent IBS. Other considerations include inflammatory bowel disease and, in older patients, ischemic colitis or colorectal cancer. The presence of diverticulosis does not alter the clinical course of IBS.[7]

Prophylaxis and Treatment

In patients with asymptomatic diverticulosis, increased fiber intake from fruits and vegetables reduces the risk of symptoms and complications.[8] Although bran supplementation may alleviate constipation, it has not been shown to reduce abdominal pain. There is no evidence that anticholinergics or opiates are effective for minimally symptomatic diverticulosis. There is no justification for colonic resection in such patients.

ACUTE DIVERTICULITIS

Diagnosis

Clinical manifestations Patients with mild diverticulitis have limited inflammation in the area of the involved diverticulum (peridiverticulitis). They present with left-sided lower abdominal pain and localized tenderness, low-grade fever, anorexia, and nausea without vomiting. Colonic inflammation may cause either diarrhea or constipation. An inflammatory mass adjacent to the bladder may lead to dysuria. Patients with more severe diverticulitis usually have a phlegmon or abscess. Diverticular abscess is usually contained within the pericolic fat, mesentery, or pelvis but may also extend out of the pelvis. Patients with a phlegmon or abscess are likely to have systemic toxicity, high fever, severe localized abdominal tenderness, and leukocytosis. The phlegmon or abscess may be appreciated on physical examination as a palpable mass. Rupture of a diverticular abscess results in purulent peritonitis with diffuse abdominal tenderness. In rare cases, diverticulitis leads to a large free perforation with fecal soiling of the abdominal cavity. Feculent peritonitis causes severe acute generalized peritonitis and sepsis. Diverticulitis in areas other than the sigmoid colon is uncommon. It may have an atypical presentation. Right-sided colonic diverticulitis is usually clinically indistinguishable from appendicitis.[9] Diverticulitis may cause fistula formation, most commonly from the sigmoid colon to the bladder. Repeated episodes of diverticulitis with fibrosis can cause colonic stricture. After one episode of diverticulitis, 30% to 50% of patients have subsequent episodes, and 20% have a subsequent episode of complicated diverticulitis. After a second episode of diverticulitis, the risk of an episode of complicated diverticulitis rises to 60%.[10] Overt lower gastrointestinal bleeding is rarely associated with acute diverticulitis. Other causes of bleeding must be excluded in patients with diverticulitis who present with overt bleeding or who have positive results on fecal occult blood testing.

Differential diagnosis A number of other conditions may mimic acute diverticulitis [see Table 1].

Chronic diverticular disease is sometimes associated with patchy mucosal hemorrhage, congestion, and granularity in the sigmoid colon, as well as an inflammatory infiltrate on microscopic examination. These changes may mimic Crohn colitis, ulcerative colitis, or ischemic colitis. However, so-called diverticular colitis is limited to areas of diverticulosis.[11] Mucosal inflammation and erosions in the area of the inflamed diverticulum (paradiverticulitis) have been found in some patients.[12]

Evaluation When acute diverticulitis is suspected, the objectives of diagnostic tests are to exclude other important conditions [see Differential Diagnosis, below], to confirm the diagnosis of diverticulitis, to determine whether complications have occurred, and to plan treatment. Leukocytosis is usually present in patients with acute diverticulitis. The urine may contain a modest number of white cells or red cells. Recurrent or polymicrobial urinary tract infections suggest the possibility of a colovesical fistula. Plain abdominal x-rays are most useful in excluding other abdominal conditions, such as intestinal obstruction. Occasionally, an inflammatory mass with gas may be noted, confirming the presence of an abscess. Free air in the abdominal cavity is unusual in diverticulitis.

If the patient has symptoms and signs of mild, uncomplicated diverticulitis and responds promptly to medical treatment, a wa-

Table 1 Differential Diagnosis of Appendicitis

General population	Women of childbearing age
Mesenteric adenitis	Pelvic inflammatory disease
Crohn disease	Rupture of ovarian follicle or cyst
Meckel diverticulitis	Ruptured ectopic pregnancy
Infectious colitis or ileitis	Ovarian torsion
Small bowel obstruction	Middle-aged to elderly patients
Omental torsion	Diverticulitis
Perforated peptic ulcer	Ischemic colitis
Acute cholecystitis	Perforated cancer of right colon
Acute pancreatitis	
Pneumonia	Young children
Urinary tract infection	Intussusception

ter-soluble contrast enema can be performed safely. The diagnosis of diverticulitis is confirmed by the presence of diverticula, in combination with colonic spasm, lumenal narrowing, or mucosal irregularity. If diverticula are not seen, the diagnosis must be reassessed. A barium enema study is contraindicated in patients with acute diverticulitis because of the risk of peritoneal contamination if a perforation is present, but water-soluble contrast does not carry the same risk.[13]

In patients with evidence of severe or complicated acute diverticulitis who require hospitalization, abdominal computed tomography is the most useful study for early evaluation. Rapid helical CT scanning techniques have made CT evaluation easier and more practical. The colon should be filled with contrast for optimal results. This can be accomplished by oral ingestion of water-soluble contrast or by a gentle water-soluble contrast enema. Abdominal CT is a useful method for screening for a wide variety of other abdominal conditions. It allows confirmation of the diagnosis, identification of complications, and planning of treatment. Diverticula are often seen as 5 to 10 mm collections of gas or contrast that protrude from the wall of the colon. Symmetrical thickening of the colonic wall may be noted. In diverticulitis, phlegmon is marked by streaky enhancement of pericolonic or perirectal soft tissue and the mesentery [see Figure 1]. Perforation and fistula may be visualized by air or contrast. Abscess is seen as one or more discrete fluid collections. If the abscess communicates with the colonic lumen, contrast may enter the abscess cavity. CT readily

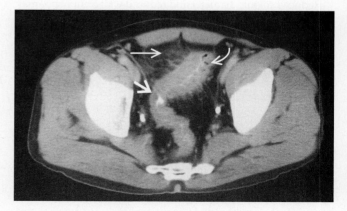

Figure 1 **CT diverticulitis. The wall of the sigmoid colon is thickened (broad arrow). Air is seen within a diverticulum (curved arrow). Streaky enhancement of pericolis fat (horizontal arrow) is caused by inflammation.**

detects remote abscess. When abscess is detected, the feasibility of CT-guided drainage can be determined.[13-17]

Diverticula are echogenic and produce acoustic shadowing on sonography. On graded compression sonography, the colonic wall in diverticulitis is thickened, noncompressible, and hypoechoic. The involved segment is hypoperistaltic. Phlegmon causes irregular enhancement of pericolic soft tissue, whereas an abscess appears as a fluid collection, within which gas is readily appreciated if present. When an abscess is found, CT should be performed to evaluate the potential for radiographic drainage.[13,18] Pelvic and abdominal ultrasonography is particularly useful in women in whom the differential diagnosis includes gynecologic conditions.

Fiberoptic examination is contraindicated in patients with suspected acute diverticulitis because of the risk of worsening a contained perforation by air insufflation. However, patients being treated for acute diverticulitis should have an elective examination with either colonoscopy or fiberoptic sigmoidoscopy and a barium enema study when the acute episode has resolved in order to exclude colon cancer or inflammatory bowel disease.[19]

Treatment

Mild diverticulitis In cases of mild diverticulitis, a trial of outpatient treatment is warranted. The patient should be placed on a liquid diet and oral antibiotics. The antibiotic regimen should provide coverage against gram-negative and anaerobic bacteria. Amoxicillin–clavulanic acid at a dosage of 875 mg/125 mg twice daily is acceptable monotherapy. An example of suitable combination therapy is double-strength trimethoprim-sulfamethoxazole administered twice daily (or a quinolone, such as ciprofloxacin, 500 mg once daily), combined with 500 mg of metronidazole administered twice daily.[20] If the patient improves within 48 to 72 hours, oral antibiotics should be continued for 7 to 14 days. A normal diet can be gradually resumed. If the diagnosis is in question, either a barium enema can be administered or colonoscopy can be performed in 2 to 6 weeks or performed sooner if it is clear that the patient is improving. Once the acute episode has resolved, patients with diverticulosis are generally advised to follow a diet high in fiber or fiber supplements.[19]

Severe or complicated diverticulitis Patients should be hospitalized if there are signs of severe or complicated diverticulitis, such as vomiting, systemic toxicity, temperature over 101° F (38.3° C), an abdominal mass, or significant abdominal tenderness, or if they fail to respond within 2 to 3 days to outpatient treatment. Hospitalized patients should be fasted and given intravenous fluids and antibiotics. The antibiotic regimen must be effective against both gram-negative aerobic bacteria and gram-negative anaerobic bacteria; a variety of such regimens are available. For example, either ampicillin-sulbactam (Unasyn) (1.5 to 3.0 g every 6 hours) or piperacillin-tazobactam (Zosyn) (3.375 g every 6 hours) would be acceptable monotherapy. For combination therapy, a cephalosporin, such as cefotetan (1 g every 12 hours), could be combined with gentamicin (5.0 to 7.5 mg/kg in a single daily dose if there is normal renal function). Clindamycin (400 to 900 mg every 8 hours) could be substituted for the cephalosporin in penicillin-allergic patients.[20] Another suitable combination regimen would be cefepime (Maxipime) (2 g I.V. every 12 hours) combined with metronidazole (Flagyl) (15 mg/kg I.V. as a loading dose, followed by 7.5 mg/kg I.V. every 6 hours). A surgical consultation should be obtained on admission. CT scanning should be considered early in the hospitalization. If a phlegmon or small ab-

scess (< 3 cm) is found, antibiotic treatment alone may suffice. If a single large, accessible abscess is found, CT-guided percutaneous drainage is feasible.[17] Antibiotic treatment and percutaneous abscess drainage often allow control of infection in complicated diverticulitis. Surgery can then be performed electively. Control of infection and preoperative bowel cleansing improve the chances for a single-stage resection and reanastomosis. Multiple abscesses or a large abscess not accessible to drainage requires early surgery. Hospitalized patients failing to respond to I.V. antibiotics within 48 to 72 hours should also be considered for early surgery. Urgent surgery is indicated for patients with evidence of free rupture of a diverticular abscess or a large perforation with fecal spillage. About 20% to 30% of patients hospitalized for the first time with acute diverticulitis require either elective or urgent surgery.[21]

Surgical treatment The optimal surgical treatment of acute diverticulitis includes resection of the involved segment at the initial operation whenever this is technically feasible. Leaving the diseased colon in place and performing only a diverting colostomy is associated with a greater frequency of complications than is primary resection. After resection, the rectal segment can be closed (Hartmann procedure) and a descending colostomy created. Elective reanastomosis is performed 3 months later. However, in about 50% of patients, reanastomosis will be contraindicated, usually because of comorbidities; in these patients, the colostomy will remain in place.[22] Patients should be prepared for this possibility before surgery. If the inflammatory process is not severe, primary reanastomosis at the time of initial surgery is not associated with increased complications.[23] This avoids a colostomy and a second operation.

Laparoscopic colonic resection for diverticulitis can be considered in patients who do not present with purulent or fecal peritonitis and in patients whose abscesses have been drained, provided no gross abnormalities are found during diagnostic laparoscopy.[24]

Factors considered in the recommendation of elective surgery for diverticulitis are the general health of the patient, the number and severity of episodes, and the degree to which symptoms resolve between episodes. Elective surgical resection for diverticular disease is usually recommended after one episode of complicated diverticulitis or after two or more episodes of uncomplicated diverticulitis. The majority of patients who present with complicated diverticulitis will experience recurrent complications if managed medically.[10] There is a 50% risk of recurrence after a second episode of even uncomplicated diverticulitis. Elective surgery has been recommended after a single episode of diverticulitis in men younger than 40 years because the risks of complications and recurrence appear to be greater in such individuals.[19,25-28] Before a patient undergoes elective surgery, a barium enema should be administered to define the extent of diverticulosis. An algorithm for the evaluation and treatment of acute diverticulitis is presented [see Figure 2].

DIVERTICULAR DISEASE IN SPECIAL PATIENT GROUPS

Immunocompromised patients, such as those on corticosteroids or those who have undergone organ transplantation, may not manifest the usual signs of diverticulitis. The severity of diverticulitis may be underestimated in these patients; consequently, the threshold for early diagnostic evaluation should be low. Surgery should be considered early on when complicated disease is found. Several studies have suggested that men younger than 40 years are more likely than older individuals to have complicat-

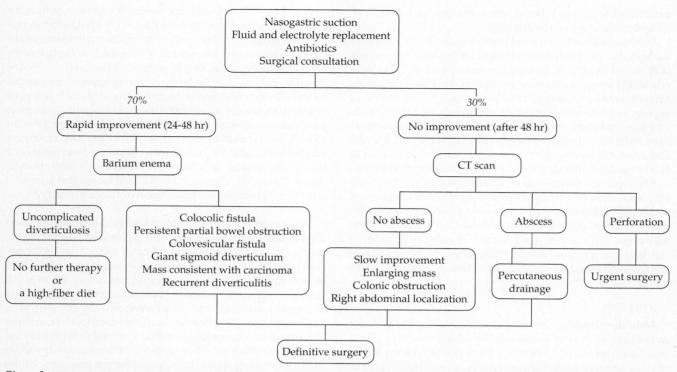

Figure 2   **The initial approach to all patients with signs and symptoms of acute diverticulitis is supportive medical therapy and a surgical consultation. If rapid improvement occurs, a barium enema x-ray study is performed to determine whether complications of diverticulosis or another condition requiring surgical therapy are present. A lack of response after 48 hours necessitates use of an abdominal CT scan to search for abscess or perforation.**

ed diverticulitis on the first episode and are more likely to have recurrent diverticulitis (see above). Patients taking nonsteroidal anti-inflammatory drugs (NSAIDs) may be at increased risk for complications of bleeding or perforation.[29]

COMPLICATIONS OF DIVERTICULAR DISEASE

Fistula

Fistula is the presenting complication in 10% to 15% of patients who require surgery for diverticular disease. There is often no history of acute diverticulitis. Patients may present with symptoms related primarily to the organ involved with the fistula. Colovesical fistulae account for about 50% to 65% of diverticular fistulae.[30] Conversely, diverticular disease is the most common cause of colovesical fistulae, followed by colon cancer and Crohn disease. Colovesical fistulas are much less common in women than in men, presumably because the uterus is interposed between the sigmoid colon and the bladder. Patients with bladder fistulas usually present with recurrent polymicrobial urinary infections, pneumaturia, or both. Fistulas may also involve other parts of the colon, the small bowel, the uterus, or the vagina. Colocutaneous fistulas are unusual and generally occur after surgery for diverticulitis.[31]

Colovesical fistulas are difficult to visualize. CT scanning may be the single most useful study to perform, even though the actual fistulas are rarely visualized directly. However, CT is sensitive for the detection of air in the bladder. This finding is virtually diagnostic of an enterovesicular fistula unless a catheter has been inserted into the bladder previously. Bladder wall thickening adjacent to an area of diverticulitis supports the diagnosis.[32] Cystoscopy often reveals focal mucosal inflammation in the area of the fistula, and contrast cystography may opacify the fistula.[33] A

barium enema study often fails to opacify a colovesical fistula, although secondary changes of diverticulitis are often noted. Colonoscopy is necessary to exclude colon cancer and inflammatory bowel disease. CT, cystoscopy, barium enema, and colonoscopy are complementary studies for the evaluation of suspected colovesical fistula.[32] Patients with a fistula caused by diverticulitis should have elective surgical resection of the involved segment of colon when the acute inflammatory process has been controlled. In colovesical fistulas, the adherent colon can usually be dissected off the bladder and the involved bladder oversewn, rather than resected.[34]

Colonic Stricture

Acute obstruction during an episode of diverticulitis is often self-limited and may be caused by colonic edema. Secondary ileus may mimic obstruction. Chronic colonic stricture is an uncommon presentation of diverticulitis. It usually occurs after repeated episodes of diverticulitis but may be the initial manifestation. A diverticular stricture is often difficult to distinguish from a malignant stricture. Diverticulosis and colon cancer are common and can occur simultaneously. Colonoscopy with biopsy is the best method to determine the cause of a colonic stricture. Examination of the stricture may be limited even with colonoscopy, and surgical resection may be necessary.

Diverticular Bleeding

Diverticular bleeding is a less frequent complication of diverticulosis than of diverticulitis. It is difficult to estimate what percentage of cases of major lower GI bleeding are diverticular. Estimates have ranged from 15% to 56%.[35-39] In many cases, the cause is presumed to be diverticular when no other cause is found.

Pathogenesis Diverticula form where the medium-sized perforating arteries penetrate the muscularis propria to enter the submucosa. Pathologic examination has revealed evidence of chronic injury to the internal elastic lamina and media of these arteries adjacent to the diverticula. This presumably predisposes to arterial rupture into the lumen of the diverticulum. Diverticular bleeding is rarely associated with acute diverticulitis.

Clinical manifestations Diverticular bleeding is usually sudden and painless. Typically, moderate to large amounts of bright-red blood, clots, or maroon stool are passed. Bleeding right-sided diverticula may occasionally lead to melena. Bleeding stops spontaneously in 70% to 80% of cases.[40,41]

Differential diagnosis Lower GI bleeding (occult bleeding in particular) should not be attributed to diverticulosis unless other causes have been excluded. The most common causes of lower GI bleeding in adults are diverticulosis, inflammatory bowel disease, neoplasm, and benign anorectal disease.[42]

Evaluation Practice guidelines for the evaluation and management of lower GI bleeding have been published.[41] An algorithm is presented as part of this chapter [see Figure 2]. The first priority in treating lower GI bleeding is volume restoration with intravenous fluids and blood. During resuscitation, a directed history is taken and a physical examination is performed. Anoscopy and proctoscopy are performed to exclude an anorectal source. A nasogastric aspirate should be obtained because about 10% to 15% of cases of major lower GI bleeding are actually from an upper GI source.[36,43] Lack of blood in the nasogastric aspirate is not conclusive proof of a lower GI source. Bleeding from an upper GI source may have stopped, and residual blood may have been evacuated from the stomach. Blood from a duodenal source may not reflux into the stomach. Some clinicians perform an upper GI endoscopy before colonoscopy even if the nasogastric aspirate is negative for blood, particularly for evaluation of apparent major lower GI bleeding.

Many clinicians consider colonoscopy to be the most useful initial study for the evaluation of patients presenting with major lower GI bleeding of unknown cause.[44] Lower GI bleeding is usually intermittent and often stops before hospital admission or shortly thereafter. Adequate colonic purging followed by colonoscopy is almost always possible even in spite of moderate active lower GI bleeding.[36] Stigmata of diverticular bleeding are found at most in 20% of cases.[23,44,45] However, in cases in which active bleeding or a clot is found, endoscopic therapy can be performed.[44] A presumptive diagnosis of diverticular bleeding is made when diverticula are found and other causes are excluded [see Differential Diagnosis, above]. Colonoscopy serves to determine the distribution of diverticula, which is important if colonic resection becomes necessary.

Technetium-99m–labeled red cell scintigraphy is another tool for the evaluation of acute lower GI bleeding. An aliquot of autologous red cells is labeled in vitro with technetium-99m pertechnetate (using a commercially available kit) and then injected. After injection, imaging is performed continuously for 60 to 120 minutes. The dynamic scans are viewed in a computer-generated cinematic format. Continuous scanning improves the probability of detecting intermittent bleeding.[46] The radioactive label retains activity for more than 24 hours. Thus, if the scan is not positive initially, it can be repeated at any time during the first day if there are indications of recurrent bleeding. If a delayed scan is positive, injection of a second dose of labeled red cells can provide more information. A scan is considered positive if there is a focus of increased activity that changes in location and intensity over time [see Figure 3]. Labeled red cell scanning is very sensitive and can theoretically detect bleeding rates of 0.5 ml a minute or more. Continuous scanning also allows determination of the pattern of movement of the tracer over time, which can aid in approximate localization. Localization to the small bowel, right colon, or left colon is possible. Reports of the ability of scanning to accurately localize the site of bleeding have been inconsistent, most likely because of differences in scanning technique.[46-49] Incorrect localization can be caused by retrograde peristalsis, and it is not advisable to base the decision to perform surgery solely on the results of scanning.[43] False positive readings may occur with vascular neo-

<table>
<tr><td>a</td><td>b</td></tr>
</table>

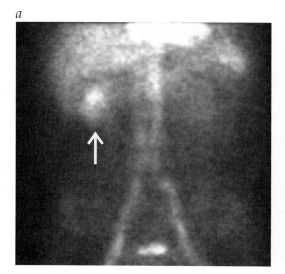 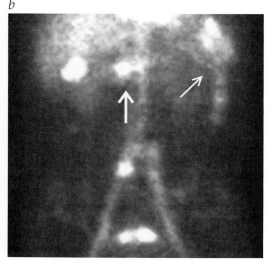

Figure 3 (*a*) Technetium-99m red cell scanning shows increased tracer activity in the area of the hepatic flexure (arrow). (*b*) Later, tracer activity has progressed to the transverse colon (broad arrow) as well as the splenic flexure and descending colon (small arrow), confirming that the right colon is the source of the bleeding.

plasms, inflammatory conditions, vascular grafts, varices, splenosis, and bladder or penile activity. Scanning sheds light only on the activity and location of bleeding, not on the cause of bleeding. Colonoscopy is still necessary to determine the presence of diverticula and to exclude other potential colonic sources of bleeding. Once diverticula have been established as the probable cause of bleeding, scanning has a role in the detection of recurrent bleeding. In patients who have diverticula throughout the colon, scanning may help localize the current bleeding site to the right or left side. Occasionally, patients who appear to be bleeding as a result of diverticular disease are actually bleeding from the small bowel. A positive scan may thus forestall an inappropriate colonic resection. A positive scan also provides prognostic information; patients with positive scans are much more likely to require surgery than those with negative scans.[48]

Visceral angiography may be useful in persistent moderate to severe lower GI bleeding, particularly when the site of bleeding has not been determined by colonoscopy and upper GI endoscopy or when colonoscopy is not feasible. Angiography can accurately locate the site of bleeding in patients with a positive bleeding scan. If active bleeding is detected and localized, it may then be treated with intra-arterial vasopressin infusion. Rebleeding occurs in 25% of patients when the vasopressin infusion is stopped. Even temporary control may provide time to stabilize the patient and prepare for elective surgery.[41,47] Embolization of a bleeding artery has been reported, but it is associated with a substantial risk of intestinal infarction, particularly if followed by vasopressin infusion.[47] Bowel or myocardial ischemia and other complications inherent to contrast arteriography may complicate both vasopressin infusion and embolization.

Treatment

About 20% of patients hospitalized for diverticular bleeding require surgery during that hospitalization.[40] The risk of recurrent diverticular bleeding after the first episode is about 10% after 2 years and 25% after 4 years.[35] The risk is higher after a second episode. Elective surgery is usually recommended after two or more episodes of bleeding. If diverticula are limited to the left side of the colon, left hemicolectomy is appropriate. The decision regarding the extent of resection is more difficult when diverticula are distributed throughout the colon. If all previous episodes of diverticular bleeding have been localized to either the right or left side by scintigraphy or angiography, one alternative is to perform a corresponding hemicolectomy. The risk of recurrent bleeding from diverticula in the remaining colon is not known. Another option is a subtotal colectomy. Occasionally, persistent or recurrent severe lower GI bleeding cannot be localized. Blind segmental resection is associated with an unacceptable recurrence rate; subtotal colectomy is the favored procedure.[37]

Appendicitis

EPIDEMIOLOGY

The incidence of appendicitis in the United States declined from 2.5/1,000 persons per year in 1940 to 1/1,000 persons per year in 1990. In England, the overall incidence of appendicitis declined from 1.8/1,000 persons per year in 1975 to 1.2/1,000 persons per year in 1994.[50] The lifetime risk of appendectomy is about 9% for males and 7% for females. Although appendicitis rarely occurs in infants, it increases in frequency between 2 and 4 years of age, reaches a peak between 10 and 20 years of age, and decreases after that. About 80% of cases occur before 45 years of age. Never-

theless, there is a steady low incidence in older individuals. The mortality associated with acute appendicitis declined between 1945 and 1960, coincident with advances in antibiotic treatment. In 1990, the mortality associated with acute uncomplicated appendicitis was approximately equal to the mortality associated with general anesthesia. However, the mortality associated with gangrenous appendicitis is about 0.5%, and the mortality associated with perforated appendicitis is 5%. Most deaths from acute appendicitis occur in individuals older than 65 years.[51]

PATHOGENESIS

The appendix in adults is a tubular structure 4 to 25 cm long arising from the medial posterior wall of the cecum several centimeters below the ileocecal valve. Its location in the peritoneal cavity varies. Atypical locations, such as the pelvis, retrocecal area, or right upper quadrant, may cause atypical clinical presentations.

Appendicitis is generally caused by obstruction of the lumen of the appendix, followed by infection. The appendix has abundant lymphoid tissue. Appendicitis increases in frequency during the period of lymphoid hyperplasia in childhood. During periods of childhood enteric infection, lymphoid tissue may obstruct the appendiceal lumen. About one third of cases of appendicitis are associated with obstruction by fecaliths. Foreign bodies, tumor (e.g., carcinoid or cecal adenocarcinoma), barium, and adhesions may also cause obstruction. With obstruction, bacterial overgrowth occurs. Mucus accumulates in the lumen proximal to the obstruction, and intraluminal pressure increases. Impairment of lymphatic and venous drainage leads to mucosal ulceration, bacterial invasion, transmural inflammation, and ischemia. Continued inflammation and ischemia, if left untreated, may lead to gangrenous appendicitis, perforation, or both. Perforation may be contained, causing a phlegmon or abscess. Free perforation causes generalized peritonitis.

DIAGNOSIS

Clinical Manifestations

Classic presentation Appendicitis usually causes a distinctive sequence of symptoms and signs. More than 90% of patients with appendicitis complain of pain. In the classic sequence, the pain is initially caused by obstruction of the appendiceal lumen. The pain of appendicitis has the qualities of midgut visceral pain and is referred to the periumbilical or epigastric areas. It may be cramping or aching but is often vague. Within 12 to 24 hours, inflammation usually becomes transmural, involving the adjacent parietal peritoneum. Pain then becomes somatic in quality: sharper and more localized to the right lower quadrant. At this time, patients may note exacerbation of pain by coughing, sneezing, or movement.

Unfortunately, this classic presentation often does not occur. Patients may present initially with right lower quadrant pain. Anorexia is present in 80% to 90% of patients. Prominent vomiting is unusual and suggests the possibility of another diagnosis, such as gastroenteritis or small bowel obstruction. Fever is usually mild. High fever or rigors suggest perforation. Tenderness in the right lower quadrant can be elicited in more than 90% of patients. Proximity of the inflammatory process to the right psoas muscle produces the psoas sign: pain when the patient raises the right leg against resistance or, alternatively, pain when the physician passively extends the right hip with the patient lying on the left side. Local hyperesthesia of the skin in the right lower quadrant may be noted. With worsening of the inflammatory process, voluntary guarding progresses to involuntary muscle rigidity. Free perforation leads to diffuse abdominal tenderness and rigidity. An abdominal mass suggests phlegmon or abscess formation.

Atypical presentation Atypical location of the appendix leads to atypical clinical presentations. An inflamed retrocecal appendix is relatively shielded from the parietal peritoneum. Pain may be less severe and abdominal tenderness less pronounced. The characteristic shift in pain location to the right lower quadrant may be delayed. A pelvic appendix may produce symptoms related to inflammation of the bladder or rectum, such as dysuria or tenesmus. In such cases, tenderness may be best elicited on pelvic or rectal examination. Intestinal malrotation and third-trimester pregnancy displaces the appendix toward the right upper quadrant, a condition that may be confused with cholecystitis or perforated peptic ulcer.

Appendicitis Presentation in Special Patient Groups

The diagnosis of appendicitis is difficult in certain groups of patients. Young children often fail to describe their symptoms clearly. They may present with only lethargy, irritability, and anorexia.[52] In the elderly, the inflammatory reaction may be reduced; pain may be vague, and there may be less fever or abdominal tenderness.[53] Consideration of other diagnoses, such as diverticulitis, may delay surgery. The incidence of perforation can be close to 20% in the elderly and in small children, owing in part to delayed diagnosis.[54] In women of childbearing age, gynecologic conditions and pregnancy make diagnosis difficult.[55,56] In one study, appendicitis was found to occur in one of 766 pregnancies. In this study, fetal loss occurred in 33% of first-trimester cases and 14% of second-trimester cases. The preoperative diagnosis was correct in 75% of cases.[57]

Diagnosis may also be difficult in immunosuppressed patients. In AIDS, symptoms may be typical, but concerns about a multiplicity of other diagnoses may delay surgery.[58] Patients on corticosteroids often have attenuated symptoms, leading to delay in presentation and a high incidence of complications.

There is evidence that appendicitis may resolve spontaneously and recur. Occasionally, patients presenting with symptoms of acute appendicitis have a history of similar episodes that resolved without treatment. Appendixes examined at autopsy or after being removed incidentally at surgery sometimes show fibrosis and obliteration of a portion of the lumen, suggesting previous appendicitis.[59,60]

Differential Diagnosis

The differential diagnosis of appendicitis is broad and varies with sex and age [see Table 1].

Evaluation of Suspected Appendicitis

History and physical examination It is standard practice to base the decision to operate for presumed appendicitis primarily on the history and physical examination. If the diagnosis is not clear at presentation, repeat physical examination within a few hours may clarify matters.

Laboratory tests There are no laboratory studies specific for appendicitis. The total white cell count, the differential count, or both are abnormal in more than 90% of cases, but the decision to perform surgery should not be delayed if the white cell count is not elevated. Urinalysis may show a few white cells or red cells. In addition to a complete blood count and urinalysis, plain x-rays

of the chest and abdomen are obtained routinely. These serve the purpose of excluding other conditions rather than confirming the diagnosis of appendicitis.

In women of childbearing age, a pregnancy test is mandatory. In many cases, no further diagnostic studies are done, because waiting for other tests may delay surgery and increase the risk of perforation. The clinical trade-off for minimizing delay and risk of perforation is a substantial proportion of so-called negative appendectomies, ranging from 15% to as high as 40% in certain groups, such as young women.[55] In certain groups of patients, the use of other diagnostic tests may be useful in reducing the proportion of negative appendectomies.[61]

Laboratory tests and clinical scoring systems have generally not been found to improve preoperative diagnostic accuracy, although a recent report suggests that a negative C-reactive protein test result has a high negative predictive value and should prompt the consideration of another diagnosis.[62,63]

Sonography Transabdominal sonography and transvaginal sonography are useful in excluding a gynecologic cause of symptoms in pregnant women and nonpregnant women of childbearing age.[55,64] Sonography has also been found to be useful in children, particularly in doubtful cases. On graded compression sonography, the inflamed appendix is a noncompressible, aperistaltic tubular structure greater than 6 mm in diameter in the right lower quadrant. It has a target appearance, and the lumen is filled with anechoic or hyperechoic material. An appendicolith may be visualized in up to 30% of cases. Pericecal inflammation or phlegmon is seen as prominent fat, and abscess is seen as loculated fluid. In experienced hands, the sensitivity and specificity of graded compression sonography for the diagnosis of appendicitis are 80% to 90%.[61,65,66] Despite abdominal tenderness, most patients find the examination tolerable if performed gently. Sonography is widely available, fast, safe, and inexpensive. Marked peritonitis or abdominal gas may compromise the examination. Sonography is not as accurate as CT for the evaluation of phlegmon or abscess.[66]

Laparoscopy Like sonography, laparoscopy may be useful in women of childbearing age when gynecologic conditions cannot be excluded. An additional advantage to laparoscopy is that if uncomplicated appendicitis is confirmed, the appendix can often be removed laparoscopically. At laparoscopy, an appendix that is in the early stages of appendicitis (i.e., without serosal inflammation) may be mistaken for a normal appendix.[67-69]

Computed tomography A number of recent studies suggest that the early use of CT scanning can improve diagnostic accuracy in cases of suspected appendicitis. As mentioned above, rapid scanning techniques have made CT readily available and practical, so much so that it can even be employed in the emergency department. A prospective study found that routine use of appendiceal CT in patients suspected of having acute appendicitis markedly reduced both the number of unnecessary appendectomies and delays before necessary appendectomies. The accuracy of CT scanning for the diagnosis of appendicitis was 98% in this study. This approach was also found to be cost-effective, but it requires the ready availability of helical CT scanning in the emergency department and radiologists familiar with the technique.[70] In other studies, CT has been found to have an accuracy of about 95% for the diagnosis of appendicitis.[15,71,72] CT is helpful when an appendiceal abscess is suspected. It is also useful when the diagnosis is unclear, as in elderly patients in whom diverticulitis or

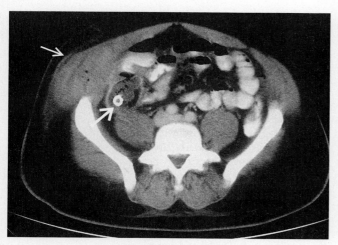

Figure 4   **CT of appendicitis. A calcified appendicolith is noted within a complex abscess containing fluid and air (broad arrow). The abscess involves the soft tissues of the abdominal wall (small arrow).**

perforated colon cancer are important considerations. CT scanning for appendicitis is best performed using thin-collimation helical scanning. The terminal ileum and cecum must be opacified with contrast administered by mouth, by rectum, or both.

The diagnosis of appendicitis is established when pericecal inflammatory changes, phlegmon, or abscess is seen with either an appendicolith or an abnormal appendix. In appendicitis, the appendix is enlarged to greater than 6 mm in diameter and fails to fill with contrast. If intravenous contrast has been given, the inflamed appendix will also show enhancement.[47] CT is useful for the evaluation of the degree and extent of periappendiceal inflammation. Inflammation may cause thickening of the adjacent cecum or ileum. Streakiness of periappendiceal fat is seen with phlegmon. Loculated fluid and, sometimes, gas bubbles or an air-fluid level are seen with abscess [*see Figure 4*]. CT provides information about the size, location, and number of abscesses, as well as the feasibility of percutaneous drainage under radiologic guidance.[73]

Barium enema   In acute appendicitis, the appendix fails to fill on barium enema. This finding is more valuable in children than in adults, as the appendix fails to fill in 15% to 20% of normal adults. Partial filling of the appendix is often difficult to distinguish from complete filling, given the marked anatomic variations in the length of the appendix. Appendicitis may produce a mass effect or inflammatory changes in the adjacent cecum or ileum that can be appreciated by barium enema, but CT provides much more information than barium enema in this regard. Barium enema may be helpful in the evaluation of chronic or recurrent right lower quadrant abdominal conditions that mimic so-called chronic appendicitis, such as Crohn disease.

TREATMENT

The treatment of appendicitis is prompt appendectomy. Preoperative preparation consists of intravenous volume repletion and antibiotics. For simple appendicitis, one dose of a broad-spectrum antibiotic given before surgery and one dose given postoperatively is sufficient. Either ampicillin-sulbactam or a cephalosporin, such as cefotetan, would be appropriate in doses previously mentioned for diverticulitis or adjusted as appropriate for children.[20]

There is no gold standard for the antibiotic treatment of perforated appendicitis. A variety of regimens are effective and are similar to those recommended for complicated diverticulitis (see above).[20,74,75] If phlegmon or abscess is confirmed, antibiotics are continued for 7 to 14 days postoperatively. Patients with free, unconfined perforation should have saline abdominal lavage during surgery. A prolonged ileus should be anticipated.

Some patients with a contained perforation can be managed by interval appendectomy after treatment with antibiotics or percutaneous radiologically guided drainage. The information obtained from preoperative CT or sonography is useful in planning therapy. If imaging shows a phlegmon or small abscess and the patient responds to antibiotic treatment within 48 hours, appendectomy may be postponed for 6 weeks and performed after the inflammatory process has subsided. If the abscess is large but well circumscribed and accessible, CT-guided drainage may be successful. The catheter is left in the abscess until drainage is minimal.[73] Interval appendectomy can then be performed in 6 weeks. However, if a patient with a contained perforation does not respond promptly to antibiotic treatment or drainage, surgery should not be delayed. Catheter drainage is not possible if imaging shows a poorly defined or multilocular abscess or if the abscess is not accessible to percutaneous drainage.

There is no clear consensus regarding the relative merits of laparoscopic versus open appendectomy. Laparoscopy is useful in the evaluation and management of suspected appendicitis in young women. Patients return to normal activities more promptly after laparoscopic appendectomy than after open appendectomy, but there are no other clear-cut advantages, particularly in men.[76,77]

If a patient is operated on for suspected appendicitis and the appendix is found to be normal at surgery, it should be removed to prevent future confusion. The cecum and terminal ileum should be examined for evidence of Crohn disease or other acute inflammatory bowel disease, for tumor, or for Meckel diverticulitis. Lymph nodes in the area should be inspected for evidence of mesenteric adenitis and biopsies should be performed if the lymph nodes are abnormal. The gallbladder and duodenum should be palpated. If necessary, the incision should be extended to permit wider exposure. Before closing, the surgeon must feel confident that the cause of the clinical presentation has been determined and that there is no other acute abdominal condition.

COMPLICATIONS

Complications occur in less than 5% of cases of simple appendicitis but can be anticipated in 30% to 50% of cases of appendicitis after perforation. The most common complications are wound infections, intra-abdominal abscess, intestinal obstruction, and prolonged ileus. Postoperative abscesses are heralded by recurrent malaise, anorexia, and fever and are best evaluated by CT.

Incidental appendectomy, which is performed during surgery for another cause, may be justified in persons younger than 30 years if the primary surgery would not be compromised by the procedure. Appendectomy does not increase morbidity when it is performed under these circumstances.[78]

References

1. Nakada I, Ubukata H, Goto Y, et al: Diverticular disease of the colon at a regional general hospital in Japan. Dis Colon Rectum 38:755, 1995

2. Schechter S, Mulvey J, Eisenstat TE: Management of uncomplicated acute diverticulitis. Dis Colon Rectum 42:470, 1999

3. Mendeloff AI, Everhart JE: Diverticular disease of the colon. Digestive Diseases in the United States: Epidemiology and Impact. Everhart JE, Ed. National Institutes of Health, National Institute of Diabetes and Digestive and Kidney Diseases, Washington, DC, 1994, p 551

4. Fisher N, Berry CS, Fearn T: Cereal dietary fiber consumption and diverticular disease: a lifespan study in rats. Am J Clin Nutr 43:788, 1985

5. Wess L, Eastwood MA, Wess TJ, et al: Cross linking of collagen is increased in colonic diverticulosis. Gut 37:94, 1995

6. Whiteway J, Morson BC: Elastosis in diverticular disease of the sigmoid colon. Gut 26:258, 1985

7. Otte JJ, Larsen L, Andersen JR: Irritable bowel syndrome and symptomatic diverticular disease—different diseases? Am J Gastroenterol 81:529, 1986

8. Aldoori WH, Giovannucci EL, Rockett HR, et al: A prospective study of dietary fiber types and symptomatic diverticular disease in men. J Nutr 128:714, 1998

9. Lo CY, Chu KW: Acute diverticulitis of the right colon. Am J Surg 171:244, 1996

10. Farmakis N, Tudor RG, Keighley MR: The 5-year natural history of complicated diverticular disease. Br J Surg 91:733, 1994

11. Shepherd NA: Diverticular disease and chronic idiopathic inflammatory bowel disease: associations and masquerades. Gut 38:801, 1996

12. Ohyama T, Sakurai Y, Ito M, et al: Clinical features of paradiverticulitis. Dig Dis Sci 43:1521, 1998

13. McKee RF, Deignan RW, Krukowski ZH: Radiological investigation in acute diverticulitis. Br J Surg 80:560, 1993

14. Ambrosetti P, Robert J, Witzig JA, et al: Prognostic factors from computed tomography in acute left colonic diverticulitis. Br J Surg 79:117, 1992

15. Rao PM, Rhea JT, Novelline RA: Helical CT of appendicitis and diverticulitis. Radiol Clin North Am 37:895, 1999

16. Birnbaum BA, Balthazar EJ: CT of appendicitis and diverticulitis. Radiol Clin North Am 32:885, 1994

17. Hachigian MP, Honickman S, Eisenstat TE, et al: Computed tomography in the initial management of acute left-sided diverticulitis. Dis Colon Rectum 35:1123, 1992

18. Zielke A, Hasse C, Nies C, et al: Prospective evaluation of ultrasonography in acute colonic diverticulitis. Br J Surg 84:385, 1997

19. Roberts P, Abel M, Rosen L, et al: Practice parameters for sigmoid diverticulitis. The Standards Task Force of the American Society of Colon and Rectal Surgeons. Dis Colon Rectum 38:125, 1995

20. The Sanford Guide® to Antimicrobial Therapy, 30th ed. Antimicrobial Therapy, Inc., Hyde Park, Vermont, 2000, p 14

21. Practice parameters for sigmoid diverticulitis. The Standards Task Force of the American Society of Colon and Rectal Surgeons. Dis Colon Rectum 38:126, 1995

22. Navarra G, Occhionorelli S, Marcello D, et al: Gasless video-assisted reversal of Hartmann's procedure. Surg Endosc 9:687, 1995

23. Wedell J, Banzhaf G, Chaoui R, et al: Surgical management of complicated colonic diverticulitis. Br J Surg 84:380, 1997

24. Kohler L, Sauerland S, Neugebauer E: Diagnosis and treatment of diverticular disease: results of a consensus development conference. The Scientific Committee of the European Association for Endoscopic Surgery. Surg Endosc 13:430, 1999

25. Cunningham MA, Davis JW, Kaups KL: Medical versus surgical management of diverticulitis in patients under age 40. Am J Surg 174:733, 1997

26. Spivak H, Weinrauch S, Harvey JC, et al: Acute colonic diverticulitis in the young. Dis Colon Rectum 40:570, 1997

27. Ambrosetti P, Robert JH, Witzig JA, et al: Acute left colonic diverticulitis: a prospective analysis of 226 consecutive cases. Surgery 115:546, 1994

28. Schauer PR, Ramos R, Ghiatas AA: Virulent diverticular disease in young obese men. Am J Surg 164:443, 1992

29. Faucheron JL: Toxicity of non-steroidal anti-inflammatory drugs in the large bowel. Eur J Gastroenterol Hepatol 11:389, 1999

30. Woods RJ, Lavery IC, Fazio VW, et al: Internal fistulas in diverticular disease. Dis Colon Rectum 31:591, 1988

31. Lavery IC: Colonic fistulas. Surg Clin North Am 76:1183, 1996

32. Jarrett TW, Vaughan ED Jr: Accuracy of computerized tomography in the diagnosis of colovesical fistula secondary to diverticular disease. J Urol 153:44, 1995

33. Kirsh GM, Hampel N, Shuck JM, et al: Diagnosis and management of vesicoenteric fistulas. Surg Gynecol Obstet 173:91, 1991

34. Wilson RG, Smith AN, Macintyre IM: Complications of diverticular disease and non-steroidal anti-inflammatory drugs: a prospective study. Br J Surg 77:1103, 1990

35. Longstreth GF: Epidemiology and outcome of patients hospitalized with acute lower gastrointestinal hemorrhage: a population-based study. Am J Gastroenterol 92:419, 1997

36. Jensen DM, Machicado GA: Colonoscopy for diagnosis and treatment of severe lower gastrointestinal bleeding: routine outcomes and cost analysis. Gastrointest Endosc Clin North Am 7:477, 1997

37. Vernava AM III, Moore BA, Longo WE, et al: Lower gastrointestinal bleeding. Dis Colon Rectum 40:846, 1997

38. Peura DA, Lanza FL, Gostout CJ, et al: The American College of Gastroenterology Bleeding Registry: preliminary findings. Am J Gastroenterol 92:924, 1997

39. Bramley PN, Masson JW, McKnight G, et al: The role of an open-access bleeding unit in the management of colonic haemorrhage: a 2-year prospective study. Scand J Gastroenterol 31:769, 1996

40. Bokhari M, Vernava AM, Ure T, et al: Diverticular hemorrhage in the elderly: is it well tolerated? Dis Colon Rectum 39:191, 1996

41. Zuccaro G Jr: Management of the adult patient with acute lower gastrointestinal bleeding. Am J Gastroenterol 93:1202, 1998

42. Zuckerman GR, Prakash C: Acute lower intestinal bleeding. Part II: etiology, therapy, and outcomes. Gastrointest Endosc 49:228, 1999

43. Billingham RP: The conundrum of lower gastrointestinal bleeding. Surg Clin North Am 77:241, 1997

44. Jensen DM, Machicado GA, Jutabha R, et al: Urgent colonoscopy for the diagnosis and treatment of severe diverticular hemorrhage. N Engl J Med 342:78, 2000

45. Foutch PG, Zimmerman K: Diverticular bleeding and the pigmented protuberance (sentinel clot): clinical implications, histopathological correlation, and results of endoscopic intervention. Am J Gastroenterol 91:2589, 1996

46. Maurer AH: Gastrointestinal bleeding and cine-scintigraphy. Semin Nucl Med 26:43, 1996

47. Zuckerman DA, Bocchini TP, Birnbaum EH: Massive hemorrhage in the lower gastrointestinal tract in adults: diagnostic imaging and intervention. AJR Am J Roentgenol 161:703, 1993

48. Suzman MS, Talmor M, Jennis R, et al: Accurate localization and surgical management of active lower gastrointestinal hemorrhage with technetium-labeled erythrocyte scintigraphy. Ann Surg 224:29, 1996

49. Bentley DE, Richardson JD: The role of tagged red blood cell imaging in the localization of gastrointestinal bleeding. Arch Surg 126:821, 1991

50. Williams NM, Jackson D, Everson NW, et al: Is the incidence of acute appendicitis really falling? Ann R Coll Surg Engl 80:122, 1998

51. Everhart JE, Mendelloff AI: Acute Appendicitis. Digestive Diseases in the United States: Epidemiology and Impact, 1st ed. Everhart JE, Ed. National Institutes of Health, National Institute of Diabetes and Digestive and Kidney Diseases. Washington, DC, 1994, p 457

52. Mason JD: The evaluation of acute abdominal pain in children. Emerg Med Clin North Am 14:629, 1996

53. Franz MG, Norman J, Fabri PJ: Increased morbidity of appendicitis with advancing age. Am Surg 61:40, 1995

54. Korner H, Sondenaa K, Soreide JA, et al: Incidence of acute nonperforated and perforated appendicitis: age-specific and sex-specific analysis. World J Surg 21:313, 1997

55. Rothrock SG, Green SM, Dobson M, et al: Misdiagnosis of appendicitis in nonpregnant women of childbearing age. J Emerg Med 13:1, 1995

56. Fallon WF, Newman JS, Fallon GL, et al: The surgical management of intra-abdominal inflammatory conditions during pregnancy. Surg Clin North Am 75:1, 1995

57. Andersen B, Nielsen TF: Appendicitis in pregnancy: diagnosis, management and complications. Acta Obstet Gynecol Scand 78:758, 1999

58. Savioz D, Lironi A, Zurbuchen P, et al: Acute right iliac fossa pain in acquired immunodeficiency: a comparison between patients with and without acquired immune deficiency syndrome. Br J Surg 83:644, 1996

59. Barber MD, McLaren J, Rainey JB: Recurrent appendicitis. Br J Surg 84:110, 1997

60. Babb RR, Trollope ML: Recurrent appendicitis: uncommon, but it does occur. Postgrad Med 106:135, 1999

61. Ramachandran P, Sivit CJ, Newman KD, et al: Ultrasonography as an adjunct in the diagnosis of acute appendicitis: a 4-year experience. J Pediatr Surg 31:164, 1996

62. Ohmann C, Yang Q, Franke C: Diagnostic scores for acute appendicitis. Abdominal Pain Study Group. Eur J Surg 161:273, 1995

63. Asfar S, Safar H, Khoursheed M, et al: Would measurement of C-reactive protein reduce the rate of negative exploration for acute appendicitis? J R Coll Surg Edinb 45:21, 2000

64. Barloon TJ, Brown BP, Abu-Yousef MM, et al: Sonography of acute appendicitis in pregnancy. Abdom Imaging 20:149, 1995

65. Orr RK, Porter D, Hartman D: Ultrasonography to evaluate adults for appendicitis: decision making based on meta-analysis and probabilistic reasoning. Acad Emerg Med 2:644, 1995

66. Puylaert JB: Imaging and intervention in patients with acute right lower quadrant disease. Baillieres Clin Gastroenterol 9:37, 1995

67. Taylor EW, Kennedy CA, Dunham RH, et al: Diagnostic laparoscopy in women with acute abdominal pain. Surg Laparosc Endosc 5:125, 1995

68. Borgstein PJ, Gordijn RV, Eijsbouts QA, et al: Acute appendicitis—a clear-cut case in men, a guessing game in young women: a prospective study of the role of laparoscopy. Surg Endosc 11:923, 1997

69. Barrat C, Catheline JM, Rizk N, et al: Does laparoscopy reduce the incidence of unnecessary appendectomies? Surg Laparosc Endosc 9:27, 1999

70. Rao PM, Rhea JT, Novelline RA, et al: Effect of computed tomography of the appendix on treatment of patients and use of hospital resources. N Engl J Med 338:141, 1998

71. Rao PM, Rhea JT, Novelline RA, et al: Helical CT combined with contrast material administered only through the colon for imaging of suspected appendicitis. AJR Am J Roentgenol 169:1275, 1997

72. Stroman DL, Bayouth CV, Kuhn JA, et al: The role of computed tomography in the diagnosis of acute appendicitis. Am J Surg 178:485, 1999

73. Jeffrey RB Jr, Federle MP, Tolentino CS: Periappendiceal inflammatory masses: CT-directed management and clinical outcome in 70 patients. Radiology 167:13, 1988

74. Allo MD, Bennion RS, Kathir K, et al: Ticarcillin/clavulanate versus imipenem/cilastatin for the treatment of infections associated with gangrenous and perforated appendicitis. Am Surg 65:99, 1999

75. Cifci AO, Tanyel FC, Buyukpamukcu N, et al: Comparative trial of four antibiotic combinations for perforated appendicitis in children. Eur J Surg 163:591, 1997

76. Mutter D, Vix M, Bui A, et al: Laparoscopy not recommended for routine appendectomy in men: results of a prospective randomized study. Surgery 120:71, 1996

77. Fingerhut A, Millat B, Borrie F: Laparoscopic versus open appendectomy: time to decide. World J Surg 23:835, 1999

78. Fisher KS, Ross DS: Guidelines for therapeutic decision in incidental appendectomy. Surg Gynecol Obstet 171:95, 1990

60 Diseases Producing Malabsorption and Maldigestion

Charles M. Mansbach II, M.D.

Definition

Malabsorption classically means the impaired absorption of fat (steatorrhea), because measuring fat absorption is the best indicator of the normality of the overall process of nutrient absorption. Under certain conditions, however, fat absorption may be normal but other specific substances may be poorly absorbed, such as iron, calcium, bile salts, or, in certain hereditary conditions, specific amino acids, disaccharides, or monosaccharides.

Overview of Diseases Producing Malabsorption

ETIOLOGY

Generally, there are three possible causes of fat malabsorption: small bowel disease, liver or biliary tract disease, and pancreatic exocrine insufficiency [see Table 1].

Small Bowel Disease

Small bowel disease can result in moderate amounts of fat in the stool (7 to 30 g/day on a diet containing 100 g of fat). Patients with small bowel disease may leak protein (protein-losing enteropathy) through a diseased intestinal mucosa, which results in a reduced serum albumin concentration. Deficiencies of fat-soluble vitamins (i.e., vitamins A, D, E, and K) may be present in small bowel disease. Patients may malabsorb vitamin B_{12} because of a very diseased or previously resected (usually over 60 cm) terminal ileum. Folic acid may also be malabsorbed, and hypocalcemia and hypomagnesemia may also be present.

Liver or Biliary Tract Disease

Patients with liver or biliary tract disease usually have only small increases in fat in the stool (7 to 15 g/day) and may also malabsorb fat-soluble vitamins. The association of cholestatic liver disease, especially primary biliary cirrhosis, with osteoporosis is well known. Osteoporosis may be the presenting symptom of the liver disease. Vitamin K deficiency, as shown by a prolonged prothrombin time, may also occur. Administration of vitamin K corrects the clotting defect in cases where the extent of the liver disease is not severe enough to impede clotting factor synthesis.

Pancreatic Exocrine Insufficiency

Patients with pancreatic exocrine insufficiency may have up to 80 g of fat/day in the stool. That they absorb fat at all is the result of the action of gastric lipases. Gastric lipase is present in the chief cells of the human stomach[1] and is thought to account for any lipid absorbed in the setting of chronic pancreatitis as exemplified by cystic fibrosis. Indeed, in cystic fibrosis, an increase in gastric lipase has been reported.[2]

CLINICAL MANIFESTATIONS

The symptoms of malabsorption are protean. In the most obvious case, the patient complains of weight loss despite a good appetite. In these cases, there is a clear change in the quality of the stool and usually an increase in stool number. The consistency of the stool softens, and in the presence of excess fat, the stool becomes more malodorous and is difficult to flush down the toilet. Oil drops or a lipid sheen may appear on the water. Excess gas in the stool causes the stool to float.[3]

Depending on other dietary constituents that are malabsorbed, patients may experience a distended abdomen, borborygmi, abdominal cramps (lactose intolerance), easy bruising (vitamin K deficiency), osteopenia or tetany (vitamin D deficiency and calcium malabsorption), iron deficiency, or night blindness (vitamin A deficiency). The most challenging cases are those in which the question of malabsorption is not raised because of lack of change in the quality of the stools.

The diarrhea of malabsorption is classified as an osmotic diarrhea and usually stops during fasting. In fat malabsorption, the diarrhea is caused not only by the excessive osmotically active particles but also by fatty acids, which stimulate cyclic adenosine monophosphate (cAMP)–dependent Cl^- secretion.

Specific physical findings of various diseases may accompany the malabsorptive state and assist in making the diagnosis. For example, the skin changes of scleroderma or dermatitis herpetiformis may be present. Signs of diabetic neuropathy may be disclosed. Although thyrotoxicosis may be associated with excessive fat in the stool, patients with thyrotoxicosis usually eat gluttonously but absorb a normal percentage of dietary fat eaten (95%) and therefore do not malabsorb in the true sense.

TESTS FOR SUSPECTED MALABSORPTION

The tests for malabsorption involve determining whether there is excessive fecal fat excretion [see Table 2]. Protein is produced in large quantities by the digestive tract, especially the pancreas, making creatorrhea difficult to interpret. Malabsorbed carbohydrate delivered to the colon may be metabolized by colonic bacteria to short-chain fatty acids, which are in part absorbed by the colon. Thus, the quantitative measurement of car-

---

Table 1 Causes of Malabsorptive Syndromes

Diseases of the small intestine	Diseases of the pancreas
Gluten-sensitive enteropathy	Chronic pancreatitis
Tropical sprue	Cystic fibrosis
Collagenous sprue	Cancer
Eosinophilic enteritis	
Radiation enteritis	*Diseases of the liver and biliary tract*
Amyloidosis	Cirrhosis/parenchymal liver disease
Mastocytosis	Intrahepatic cholestasis syndrome
Abetalipoproteinemia	Cholestasis due to extrahepatic obstruction
Whipple disease	
Intestinal lymphangiectasia	*Combined or multiple defects in digestion and absorption*
Intestinal lymphoma	Hyperthyroidism
Ischemic bowel disease	Diabetes mellitus
Giardia lamblia infection	Carcinoid syndrome
AIDS	Zollinger-Ellison syndrome
Short bowel syndrome	Postgastrectomy (Billroth II type)
Ileal resection	
Ileitis (e.g., Crohn disease)	

Table 2 Tests of Digestive-Absorptive Function

	Characteristics	*Clinical Use*
Fecal fat analysis		
Qualitative	Simple microscopic study for increase in fat globules	A good screening test for moderate increase in stool fat, but quantitative fecal fat analysis is preferable
Quantitative	Chemical analysis for fat excretion during a 72 hr period by titration with NaOH; most sensitive test for malassimilation of fat; normal is < 6 g/day; does not distinguish between small intestine, pancreatic, or luminal abnormalities	The most important test to identify maldigestion or malabsorption; indicated in all patients suspected of having malassimilation
Xylose absorption	As a pentose not requiring luminal or intestinal surface digestion, xylose allows assessment of small intestine function; normally, > 4 g/5 hr is excreted in urine after ingestion of 25 g; plasma xylose should be 10–20 mg/dl/1.73 m² of body surface area at 60–75 min	Indicated whenever quantitative fecal fat is abnormal; not as sensitive as fat analysis but localizes the abnormality to the small intestine
Small intestine x-ray	Allows analysis of continuity of small intestine and identification of diverticula or alteration of mucosa; diseased pancreas may impinge on duodenum	Indicated when quantitative fecal fat excretion is increased
Small intestine peroral biopsy	Permits direct histologic examination of mucosa; characteristic alterations occur in several diseases producing malabsorption	Indicated when fecal fat excretion is increased, particularly if the xylose test or small intestine x-ray is abnormal; a portion of biopsy may be assayed for disaccharidases
Bile acid breath test	In small intestine bacterial overgrowth or ileal disease that produces malabsorption, ^{14}C–glycocholic acid (5 μCi) will be deconjugated, metabolized, and excreted via the lungs as $^{14}CO_2$	Indicated in patients with documented steatorrhea caused by suspected bacterial overgrowth or ileal dysfunction
Bentiromide test	The peptide bond in this nonabsorbable arylamine is cleaved specifically by intraluminal chymotrypsin to yield PABA, which is then readily absorbed and excreted by the intestine	Indicated when fecal fat excretion is increased; less sensitive than quantitative fat analysis but, when positive, establishes insufficiency of intraduodenal pancreatic digestive enzyme levels

bohydrate absorption is inaccurate, although a fall in stool pH occurs, which is indicative of excessive amounts of the short-chain fatty acids that are excreted under these conditions.

Measurement of Fecal Fat

Fecal fat can be measured qualitatively and quantitatively. The qualitative measurement of fecal fat using Sudan II staining has been shown to be surprisingly accurate,[4] especially if clinically significant amounts of fat are being excreted. As with many qualitative tests, however, the skill of the observer is crucial to success.

The quantitative measurement of fecal fat is the benchmark by which all other tests are ranked. It is important to remember that the test cannot be performed unless the patient is able to eat at least 80 g, preferably 100 g, of fat a day.

Xylose Absorption Test

The absorptive surface area of the intestine is measured by the ability of the patient to absorb sugar xylose. Unlike glucose, xylose is not actively absorbed by the intestine but is absorbed by the slower process of passive diffusion. In the xylose absorption test, 25 g of xylose is given by mouth and the urine is collected for 5 hours. The normal urinary excretion of xylose is greater than 4 g over 5 hours. For an adequate urinary flow to be ensured, the patient should drink 500 ml of water after drinking the xylose. This intake should result in a urine volume of at least 300 ml during the collection period. Xylose excretion can be falsely low in patients with reduced renal function or in patients with ascites in which the xylose is diluted in the ascitic fluid. To avoid falsely low results, it is advisable to measure the concentration of xylose in blood [*see Table 2*]. Malabsorbed xylose reaches the colon and can be metabolized by the resident bacteria to hydrogen. Hydrogen may be quantitated in the breath; this test is reported to be as accurate as the measurement of xylose in the serum or urine.

Imaging Studies

A plain film or ultrasonogram of the abdomen is usually not helpful in most cases of malabsorption. However, 30% of cases of chronic pancreatitis have visible calcifications on an abdominal plain film. Detection of pancreatic calcification can be increased if computed tomography or ultrasonography is used. CT or ultrasonography also can identify dilatated pancreatic ducts, another characteristic sign of chronic pancreatitis. Endoscopic retrograde pancreatography (ERP) can also be helpful when ductular changes indicative of chronic pancreatitis are seen [*see Chapter 68*].

Radiographic studies of the small intestine after oral ingestion of barium can aid in the diagnosis of several abnormalities. The presence of diverticula of the small intestine or of impaired peristalsis, as seen in scleroderma or idiopathic intestinal dysmotility, can be an indicator of bacterial overgrowth. A careful examination of the terminal ileum can identify Crohn disease. Stricturing may be identified in some patients with radiation injury or injury caused by nonsteroidal anti-inflammatory drugs. Hypoalbuminemia affecting the small intestine may lead to the so-called stack-of-coins sign.

Small Bowel Biopsy

An experienced pathologist can be helpful in supporting the diagnoses of gluten-sensitive enteropathy (with or without dermatitis herpetiformis), hypogammaglobulinemic sprue, tropical sprue, Whipple disease, *Mycobacterium avium* complex disease, stasis syndrome, amyloidosis, and intestinal lymphangiectasia.

Assessment of Pancreatic Exocrine Function

More than 90% of pancreatic exocrine function needs to be destroyed before symptomatic malabsorption results [*see Chapter 68*].[5] The most sensitive test of pancreatic exocrine function requires the passage of a double-lumen tube.[6] Cholecystokinin (CCK) or secretin is administered intravenously, and gastric and duodenal secretions are collected separately. However, secretin became unavailable in the United States when the manufacturer discontinued production in 1999. If CCK is given, lipase or trypsin activity is determined using appropriate substrates. When secretin is administered, duodenal fluid volume and bicarbonate concentration are measured.

The noninvasive bentiromide test is based on the action of trypsin on bentiromide to yield aminobenzoic acid (PABA) and benzoyl-tyrosine [see Figure 1]. PABA is readily absorbed by the intestine and excreted into the urine. In healthy persons, when 500 mg of bentiromide is ingested, 57% or more of the PABA appears in the urine within 6 hours. In patients with chronic pancreatitis, the amount of PABA excreted is significantly less, averaging 42%. Using the 57% excretion as a cutoff, the sensitivity is 67% to 80% and the specificity is 95%.[7] PABA may also be measured in the plasma 120 minutes after ingestion of bentiromide, which may enhance the sensitivity of the test.[8] Plasma measurements are helpful in cases of impaired renal excretion, which may be seen in the elderly. PABA is identified colorimetrically, and thus, other arylamines can interfere with its determination (e.g., acetaminophen, lidocaine, procainamide, sulfonamides, and thiazide diuretics).[9] In cases in which intestinal absorption is impaired, such as with sprue, the absorption of released PABA may be reduced, leading to a falsely low urinary recovery. Unfortunately, the bentiromide test becomes positive only when the pancreatic gland is more than 90% destroyed. Nevertheless, in considering the workup of a patient with steatorrhea, the test may be useful because it takes an equal amount of glandular destruction to generate steatorrhea.

Although the vast majority of pancreatic proteases and lipases are stored in zymogen granules and are released from the apical portion of the pancreatic exocrine cell into the pancreatic duct, a small percentage leaks into the interstitium of the gland, is carried into the circulation, and can be measured (i.e., by the serum trypsinogen assay). Because the activation peptide of trypsin is not yet released and any active trypsin is quickly bound by α_1-antitrypsin, the free-circulating form of trypsin is trypsinogen. In patients who have chronic pancreatitis with exocrine insufficiency, the serum concentration of trypsinogen is lower than in healthy persons (2 to 18 ng/ml, compared with 29 to 79 ng/ml in healthy persons).[10] A low serum trypsinogen level appears to have a high degree of specificity for chronic pancreatitis but only modest sensitivity.

BILE ACID ABSORPTION TESTS

Bile acids are synthesized from cholesterol in the liver and require conjugation by either glycine or taurine before they are excreted into the intestine via the common bile duct. The bile acid conjugates solubilize the products of triacylglycerol hydrolysis into complex micelles, which facilitate the rapid absorption of dietary lipid. Bile acids are not absorbed in the proximal intestine with dietary lipid but in the distal ileum. The bile acid pool recirculates six times a day. About 95% of bile acids are reabsorbed and recirculate in the enterohepatic circulation each day; approximately 0.5 g of bile acids appears in the stool daily, which equals the hepatic synthetic rate under steady-state conditions. If bile acids are not adequately absorbed, diarrhea results (choleretic enteropathy). In the complete absence of bile salts, fatty acids are less efficiently absorbed, with up to 25% to 50% of ingested lipid appearing in the stool. In patients with idiopathic diarrhea or with diarrhea after ileal resection ($\geq$ 30 cm), the malabsorption of bile acids is an etiologic possibility. Also, children who have unexplained diarrhea may have a congenital defect of the sodium-dependent bile salt transporter in the terminal ileum.[11]

To test for the presence of bile acid malabsorption, two methods are available, although not widely. The first is the ^{14}C-glycocholic acid breath test, and the second is the selenium-75–labeled homocholic acid–taurine (^{75}SeHCAT) absorption test. In the former test [see Figure 2], a trace amount of ^{14}C-glycocholic acid is given by mouth. Many bacteria are capable of hydrolyzing the amide bond and releasing the ^{14}C-glycine; either it is absorbed and ^{14}CO$_2$ is produced in the liver or it is further metabolized in the intestinal lumen to ^{14}CO$_2$. In either event, the ^{14}CO$_2$ appears in the breath in measurable amounts. The percentage of the ingested dose excreted in the breath increases if the intestinal lumen contains more bacteria than normal or if an excess of bile acids is delivered to the colon (ileal dysfunction). A gastric antisecretory drug may also increase the resident population of bacteria in the intestine to a level that results in an abnormal breath test.[12] The usefulness of this test as an indicator of bile acid malabsorption is therefore limited. The ^{75}SeHCAT test has more potential clinical usefulness because of its strong correlation with cholate excretion and the ease of measurement of ^{75}Se retention by the whole-body gamma camera. Normal persons retain greater than 19% of an orally administered dose of ^{75}Se after 7 days, whereas patients with significant ileal dysfunction or resection retain less than 12%.[13]

Now that the human sodium-dependent bile acid transporter has been cloned, congenital defects are being discovered that lead to bile acid malabsorption resulting in diarrhea.[11] Such defects may be the cause of primary bile acid malabsorption.

Small Bowel Diseases Producing Malabsorption

GLUTEN-SENSITIVE ENTEROPATHY

Gluten-sensitive enteropathy (GSE) was once called celiac disease in children and idiopathic or nontropical sprue in

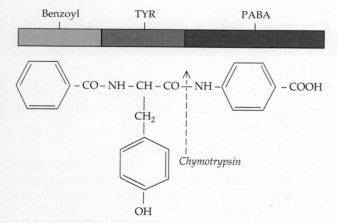

Figure 1 Cleavage of the bentiromide molecule by the intraduodenal enzyme chymotrypsin yields two fragments, benzoyl-tyrosine and aminobenzoic acid (PABA). Bentiromide is composed of benzoyl (light blue), tyrosine (TYR) (blue), and PABA (dark blue). The released PABA is absorbed across the intestine and excreted in significant quantities in the urine. Absence of chymotrypsin, as a result of pancreatic disease or duct obstruction, will result in failure of release, absorption, and urinary excretion of PABA.

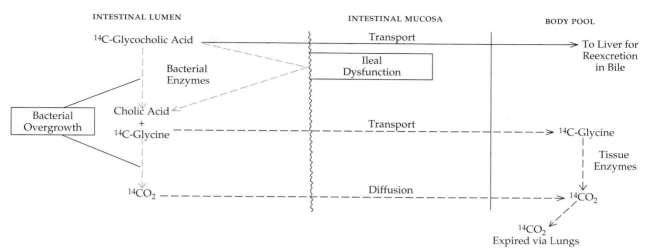

INTESTINAL LUMEN   INTESTINAL MUCOSA   BODY POOL

Figure 2   In the bile acid breath test, a small dose of ^{14}C–glycocholic acid is ingested and its fate determined by measurement of $^{14}CO_2$ excretion in breath. In a normal person, little of the ^{14}C–glycocholic acid is metabolized for excretion in breath because it passes intact to the ileum for absorption and return to the enterohepatic circulation. If there is either intestinal bacterial overgrowth or ileal dysfunction, however, bacterial enzymes will deconjugate the bile acid (broken blue lines), releasing cholic acid and ^{14}C-glycine. The radioactive glycine may be transported across the intestinal mucosa (upper broken gray line) and subsequently degraded to $^{14}CO_2$ by tissue enzymes; alternatively, the ^{14}C-glycine may be metabolized within the intestinal lumen to $^{14}CO_2$, which then diffuses (lower broken gray line) into the circulation and is carried to the lungs. Consequently, $^{14}CO_2$ excretion is 10 times greater in either intestinal bacterial overgrowth or ileal dysfunction than it is in the normal state.

adults. In 1960, it was recognized that the diseases were the same, caused by the major wheat protein gluten and, more specifically, its alcohol-soluble component, gliadin.[14]

Genetic and Etiologic Factors

GSE is less common in the United States than in Western Europe. GSE is associated with haplotypes HLA-DQ2 (DQA1*501, DQB1* 201) and HLA-DQ8 (DQA1*031, DQB1*302). In sets of monozygotic twins, the majority of the opposite twins from the incidence case do not have GSE. This condition leads to the belief that there is another, unknown (nongenetic) factor that is important in disease causation.   The epitope of gliadin that interacts with T cells to presumably initiate the disease process has been localized to a 17-amino-acid peptide (57–73) that has been partially deaminated by transglutaminase.[15]

Pathogenesis

The causes of steatorrhea in GSE are many. CCK cells are either reduced in number or so defective that the amount of CCK present in the duodenal mucosa is greatly reduced.[14] This CCK deficiency leads to a reduced amount of pancreatic lipase and bile acids delivered to the intestinal lumen in response to dietary lipid. The intestinal crypt cells are the major fluid-secreting cells of the intestine, via their cAMP-dependent Cl⁻ secretion with attendant water secretion. In GSE, the cryptal portion of the villous complex is greatly expanded, leading to increased water secretion. Because the villous tip cells, which normally absorb the water, are diseased and reduced in number, water and electrolyte absorption is not as effective as normal, and the intestine becomes secretory.[14] Thus, the concentration of bile acids in the intestinal lumen is reduced below that expected simply from the impaired CCK release. The ability of bile acids to solubilize the products of lipolysis depends on the presence of bile salts at a concentration greater than their critical micellar concentration (CMC) of 1.4 mM.[16] Normally, the intestine has a postprandial bile salt concentration of 10 mM.[17]

The brush borders at the surface of mature enterocytes are severely affected in GSE. Further, the villous structures are flattened. These two conditions lead to a severely reduced surface area that limits lipid absorption. The amount of reduction in surface area can be estimated by the D-xylose absorption test. The enterocytes that are at the surface of the intestine are not as mature as normal enterocytes, because their turnover rate is greatly increased, which probably results in a reduced capacity to process absorbed lipid.

Diagnosis

Clinical manifestations   Although GSE may start in childhood and respond to gluten withdrawal, children with the disease undergo a remission in their teenage years even if they ingest a diet containing gluten. As adults, these patients, 25% or more of whom were symptomatic in childhood, may present with a variety of complaints: usually, weight loss, fatigue, abdominal cramps, distention, bloating, and diarrhea (steatorrhea) are prominent, although there may be no loss of appetite. In some patients, the disease is insidious in onset and the symptoms are mild. It is only after these patients have been treated that they realize, in retrospect, how ill they were. In population studies in which the presence of disease was determined by intestinal biopsy, people with conditions that warranted a biopsy were often asymptomatic but sometimes of shorter stature than unaffected siblings. Because nothing specifically leads to the diagnosis, especially in the absence of clinically evident steatorrhea, the realization that the patient has GSE may be delayed. This problem is most likely to occur with patients who do not have steatorrhea but do have osteoporosis, easy bruising as a result of vitamin K deficiency, or unexplained iron deficiency anemia.

Laboratory tests   In a patient in whom the suspicion of GSE is high—such as a first-degree relative of a known GSE patient; a patient who has a history of a childhood disease that

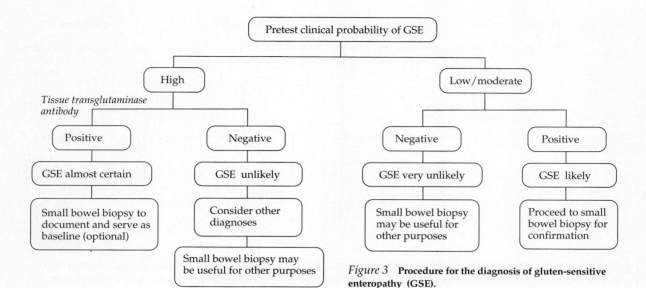

Figure 3 **Procedure for the diagnosis of gluten-sensitive enteropathy (GSE).**

caused diarrhea, was evaluated by a specialist, and was treated with a special diet; or a patient with malabsorption who is not an alcoholic and does not have another obvious reason for malabsorbing fat—a positive tissue transglutaminase antibody test makes the diagnosis almost certain [*see Figure 3*].[18] Alternatively, the diagnosis might rest on small bowel biopsy findings [*see Figure 4*]. Classic features include partial or complete villous atrophy, abnormal-appearing enterocytes at the villous tips, an increase in intraepithelial lymphocytes, a lamina propria infiltrate consisting predominantly of lymphocytes and macrophages, an increase in the size of the crypts both vertically and horizontally, and an increase in the number of mitotic figures.[14] These features, although typical, are not pathognomonic. For the diagnosis to be definitive, the patient must respond to dietary therapy. Symptomatic improvement can be expected in 80% of patients within 1 month, but histologic improvement lags behind considerably. Another 10% of patients do not respond until 2 months, and the remainder may take up to 2 years. Even under the strictest dietary control, the biopsy findings might not return to normal. Most often, the patient remains under good control because of the symptomatic improvement while on the diet, but many patients will

eventually either test whether they are cured or be in a situation that forces them to commit a dietary indiscretion. This lapse inevitably results in recurrence of symptoms, further securing the diagnosis.

Another helpful test is the identification of an antiendomysial antibody. This antibody is present in up to 95% of cases and is rarely present in control subjects.[19] Other tests of malabsorption, such as the D-xylose absorption test or stool fat studies, may be abnormal. Low clotting factors, the presence of anemia caused by folate or iron deficiency, or osteoporosis may also be present. None of these conditions are specific for GSE, however.

Treatment

The treatment of GSE is a strict gluten-exclusion diet—no wheat, rye, or barley. Oats are thought to be safe but are usually avoided during the early stage, when the clinical response to the diet is being judged. Keeping the patient on the diet is sometimes difficult because many foods have hidden gluten content. Maintaining a gluten-exclusion diet is important because intestinal lymphomas are more likely to develop in patients who do not.[20] Support groups, such as those organized by the Celiac Society of America, can be helpful, especially when the disease is

a

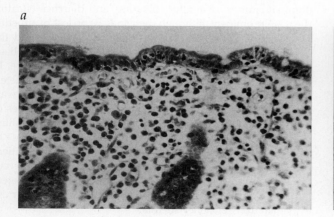

b

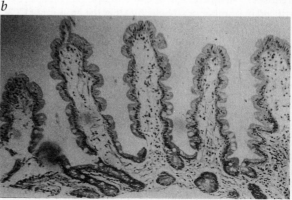

Figure 4 **Biopsy specimen from the small intestine of a patient with untreated celiac sprue (*a*) demonstrates a flat surface with plasmocytic infiltration of the subepithelial region (magnified 400 times). In contrast, a biopsy sample taken from a patient with pancreatic exocrine insufficiency (*b*) is indistinguishable from a normal specimen and shows tall, scalloped villi and minimal subepithelial mononuclear infiltration (magnified 100 times).**

newly diagnosed. Information such as what to look for on package labels and interesting recipes can be very instrumental in helping the patient maintain the gluten-exclusion diet. During the trial period, beer, ale, and whiskey, which may contain enough gluten to sensitize the patient, should not be consumed. After the dietary response is clear, these drinks may be tried, if desired, to determine whether the patient is sensitive. Other products that are not usually thought of as containing gluten, but often do, are ice cream, communion wafers, and even some drugs (as a filler). Despite the restrictions, many dietary options are open to the patient, including certain breakfast cereals, milk, cheese, eggs, meat, chicken, fish, chocolate, and products made from corn, rice, or potato flour.

If the patient does not respond, the most likely reason is that the patient is not accurately following the diet. In such cases, it is helpful to have a dietitian carefully go over the patient's dietary history.[14] Less often, the patient will have an intestinal stasis syndrome or pancreatic insufficiency. When these subsidiary problems are diagnosed and successfully treated, the patient usually shows a response to the diet.

OTHER SPRUELIKE DISORDERS

Dermatitis Herpetiformis and GSE

Many patients with dermatitis herpetiformis will have GSE.[21] The intensely pruritic, blistering lesions appear on the knees, elbows, shoulders, and buttocks [see Chapter 30]. Skin biopsies of dermatitis herpetiformis lesions have characteristic immunoglobulin A (IgA) deposits. On a gluten-exclusion diet, both the dermatologic and the intestinal lesions improve, indicating a linkage between the two. However, the skin lesions respond to dapsone treatment and the intestinal lesions do not, which indicates that there are differences between the two diseases as well.

Tropical Sprue

Tropical sprue is a malabsorptive illness that appears in certain areas of the world, especially the tropics, among both the indigenous populations and tourists. In two carefully studied populations, 5% to 13% of North Americans living in Puerto Rico for 6 months or longer experienced symptoms of tropical sprue. Expatriates from the United States who return from the tropics or other areas endemic for tropical sprue may experience symptoms of tropical sprue more than 10 years after their return.[22] Peace Corps volunteers from the United States who spent time in Pakistan had demonstrable small bowel lesions and functional abnormalities that reverted to normal over several months after returning home.[23] Indians and Pakistanis living in the United States may take a longer time (up to 4 years) to excrete normal amounts of xylose.[24] Exactly what causes these changes in the small bowel is not clear, but the tropical sprue syndrome is thought to be caused by one or more species of coliform bacteria, such as Klebsiella species,[25] which colonize the upper intestinal tract.

Diagnosis The symptoms of tropical sprue differ from those of GSE. Weight loss caused mostly by anorexia is very prominent, as is diarrhea. A sore tongue (70% of patients), pedal edema (25% of patients), folate and vitamin B_{12} deficiency (75% to 100% of patients), or an abnormal result on the Schilling test (96% to 100% of patients) is much more common in tropical sprue than in nontropical sprue.[25] The symptoms can be quite se-

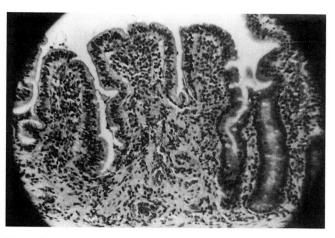

Figure 5 In a biopsy specimen from the small intestine of a patient with tropical sprue, villi are broadened and shortened and the crypts are deepened; these changes yield a villus-to-crypt ratio of 1:1 (magnified 100 times).

vere, sometimes leading to death in endemic areas. However, the prognosis, in general, is excellent for patients either remaining in the tropics or returning to the United States.

The diagnosis of tropical sprue is made by performing a small bowel biopsy in patients with a compatible clinical presentation and travel history. Villi are leaflike or blunt, and the lamina propria are packed with inflammatory cells [see Figure 5]. Thin villous structures are seen in North Americans and Europeans [see Figure 4]. In considering this disease, it should be noted that normal intestinal biopsy results in residents of endemic areas or in tourists who do not stay in mainstream hotels in endemic areas would be classified as abnormal in persons living in the United States or Europe.

Treatment Treatment of tropical sprue should begin with folic acid (5 mg/day).[25] This therapy is associated with rapid improvement in appetite, and it eliminates most of the clinical symptoms. In patients with a short duration of symptoms (less than 4 months), folate given for 6 months to 1 year may suffice. For patients with a longer duration of symptoms (more than 4 months), antibiotics, such as tetracycline (2 g/day for 1 year), should be added. Most patients returning to the United States gain weight quickly even if the results of absorption tests or intestinal biopsies are not normalized.

Collagenous Sprue

Collagenous sprue is a rare, devastating disease in which there is a layer of collagen underneath the enterocytes of the small bowel. The relation of collagenous sprue to collagenous colitis is unclear, but the basic histologic feature of subepithelial collagen deposition is the same. The origin of collagenous colitis is unknown, but it develops in approximately half the patients who have refractory celiac disease (those unresponsive to the gluten-exclusion diet).[26] Although it is known that type 6 collagen is deposited in the more commonly diagnosed collagenous colitis, the type of collagen laid down in the small bowel in collagenous sprue is unknown. In collagenous colitis, the symptoms (primarily diarrhea) are usually modest, but in collagenous sprue, symptoms are more severe and include obvious malabsorption. This severity of symptoms is probably caused by the diffusion barrier presented by the collagen, which prevents nutrients from diffusing either into the portal capillaries or into the lymphatics.

Diagnosis The diagnosis of collagenous sprue is made by the classic histologic picture of villous atrophy and subepithelial collagen deposition. If the diagnosis is missed, however, and the patient is thought to have GSE on the basis of the flat villous structure, the patient will usually not be responsive to the gluten-free diet.

Treatment Therapy for collagenous sprue is uncertain. The most common problem is the osmotic diarrhea caused by the gross malabsorptive state induced by the disease process. In this event, the patient is treated as if he or she had the short bowel syndrome. Some patients respond to steroid therapy. A few respond to steroids and a gluten-exclusion diet, with the patient's improved condition eventually making it possible to taper the steroid dosage.[27]

Hypogammaglobulinemic Sprue

The gastrointestinal tract is the largest lymphoid organ in the body. The environment to which this immune system is exposed is filled with foreign antigens that must be sorted, identified, and, if necessary, reacted to. Thus, it is not surprising that intestinal dysfunction may develop in patients who are immune deficient, particularly those with IgA deficiency, because IgA is the most important immunoglobulin of the intestine. Some patients who have one of the hypogammaglobulinemic syndromes may experience malabsorption.[28] Patients with IgA deficiency also usually have a history of recurrent respiratory infections,[28] which further distinguishes them from patients who have gluten-sensitive enteropathy. The most common cause of malabsorption seen in this condition is giardiasis.

Diagnosis The diagnosis is suspected if the patient has signs and symptoms of malabsorption and low levels of serum immunoglobulins, especially IgA. Intestinal biopsy specimens lack plasma cells and thus are easily distinguishable from those of patients with gluten-sensitive enteropathy, in which plasma cell types are abundant. Plasma cells are readily seen in normal biopsy specimens as well. *Giardia lamblia* organisms may also be present in hypogammaglobulinemic sprue.

Treatment Frequently, the intestinal symptoms improve if metronidazole is given at 750 mg/day for 10 days to treat giardiasis.

MALABSORPTION SECONDARY TO MASSIVE SMALL BOWEL RESECTION

Massive small bowel resection is used to treat various diseases, including mesenteric ischemia, volvulus, and Crohn disease. Because the intestine requires a certain surface area over which absorption can occur, reducing the area below a critical value results in malabsorption. Depending on the amount of bowel resected, the results can range from mildly inconvenient to catastrophic. Retention of the ileocecal valve lessens symptoms. The ileum responds to jejunal resection by hyperplasia much more effectively than the jejunum responds to an ileal resection. There are also specialized mechanisms present in the ileum that are not available to the jejunum, such as bile salt and vitamin B transporters. The maintenance of an adequate bile acid pool is important for fat absorption because the reduced absorptive surface area in patients who have undergone bowel resection makes

it necessary for fat absorption to be as efficient as possible. Alternatively, the ileum can perform most of the functions of the jejunum except for folic acid, Ca^{2+}, and Fe^{2+} absorption. However, these can be replenished by appropriate medication.

Diagnosis The diagnosis is made by history of bowel resection in combination with clinical manifestations of the short bowel syndrome such as diarrhea, steatorrhea, weight loss, trace-element deficiencies, hyponatremia, and hypokalemia.

Treatment Treatment in these patients is dependent on what part of the bowel and how much bowel have been resected. Protein requires the greatest surface area for absorption.[29] Thus, achieving adequate assimilation may become problematic, despite the water-solubility of proteins and their hydrolytic products. Vitamins and minerals also need to be added to any therapeutic regimen, depending on what part of the bowel is missing. Treatment can include eating multiple small meals each day, eating quickly absorbed foods such as canned caloric supplements, having food finely chopped or ground, and eating foods containing medium-chain triglycerides, which can be absorbed in the absence of bile salts.[29] Foods rich in polyunsaturated fatty acids, such as vegetable oils, are more easily absorbed than meats, which have more saturated fat. Finally, completely hydrolyzed dietary supplements are rapidly absorbed. To slow bowel transit, diphenoxylate-atropine, loperamide, or deodorized tincture of opium can be used effectively. An alternative method is to have the patient drink a small amount of safflower oil just before a meal. The lipid quickly goes to the ileum (if present), the colon, or both[30] and elaborates peptide YY (PYY),[31] which is the putative ileal break, slowing gastric emptying. Having patients try different diets will often enable them to ingest food orally rather than receive total parenteral nutrition (TPN), which is less desired.

RADIATION ENTERITIS

Injury of the intestine is an all too common result of delivery of ionizing radiation as oncologic treatment. Injury to the small bowel is more common if the patient has had previous abdominal surgery, which may restrict the movement of the small bowel. The terminal ileum may become involved during pelvic irradiation.

WHIPPLE DISEASE

Whipple disease is a rare wasting disease caused by the bacterium *Tropheryma whippelii*.[32] Accurate diagnosis is imperative because mortality approaches 100% without antibiotic treatment.

Diagnosis

Clinical manifestations Classically, the disease begins in a middle-aged male with a nondeforming arthritis that usually starts years before the onset of the intestinal symptoms. Other complaints include fever, abdominal distention, diarrhea, weight loss, lymphadenopathy, hyperpigmentation of the skin, and steatorrhea.[33] Many patients express the HLA-B27 isotype. Occasionally, intestinal symptoms are absent, even in some patients with central nervous system involvement.[34] In a well-documented but unusual case, intestinal involvement was not identified, even after extensive biopsies in two laboratories, despite the fact that the patient otherwise had typical symptoms of the disease.[35]

Laboratory tests The recognition of Whipple disease in patients without intestinal symptoms or involvement by the disease is increasing with the advent of polymerase chain reaction (PCR) techniques that identify the unique 16S ribosomal RNA of *T. whippelii*[36] The diagnosis rests on identifying the classic periodic acid–Schiff (PAS)–positive macrophages, which contain sickle-form particles.[33] By far the most common site of biopsy that yields positive results is the intestine. The histologic lesion shows distended villi (clubbed villi) with the foamy, PAS-positive macrophages and lymphatic dilatation. A flat villous surface can be seen in extreme cases. These findings need to be differentiated in the appropriate clinical setting from those of *M. avium* complex disease, in which PAS-positive macrophages are also found. A stain for acid-fast bacilli should differentiate between them. Central nervous system involvement, occasionally associated with typical macrophages in the cerebrospinal fluid and substantiated by the more sensitive PCR technique, may be present in the absence of neurologic symptoms.[37] Occasionally, a brain biopsy is required, which can be guided by magnetic resonance imaging. Cardiac and pulmonary involvement may also be found.[38]

Treatment Because the disease is so uncommon, a well-defined treatment plan is difficult to establish. The originally proposed treatment was penicillin (250 mg q.i.d.) and streptomycin (1 g I.M.) for 2 weeks, followed by tetracycline (1 g) for 1 year. Typically today, trimethoprim-sulfamethoxazole (one double-strength tablet b.i.d.) is given for 1 year. All antimicrobial agents are used in customary doses.

Although the intestinal and systemic symptoms respond readily to either treatment, the major concern is treatment of CNS manifestations. Usually, in those patients who do not have CNS involvement initially, CNS symptoms appear a year or more after treatment of the systemic and intestinal symptoms. A progressive dementia may be seen, but the pathognomonic signs of CNS disease, when present, are oculomasticatory myorhythmia and oculofacial-skeletal myorhythmia.[39] Antibiotics that cross the blood-brain barrier are therefore required. Interestingly, the short period of penicillin-streptomycin administration is enough to block CNS symptoms, whereas even long-term trimethoprim-sulfamethoxazole therapy occasionally may not prevent CNS manifestations of Whipple disease.[40] Tetracycline alone does not eradicate CNS disease and should not be given by itself, even though it is effective in treating the intestinal and systemic symptoms. An important aspect to keep in mind is that in 50% of patients, the CSF may contain Whipple disease macrophages or PCR-positive material even in the absence of CNS symptoms.[37] Once CNS involvement occurs, treatment is usually not helpful, although with treatment, some improvement may be noted and the disease may not progress.

IMMUNOPROLIFERATIVE SMALL INTESTINAL DISEASE

Immunoproliferative small intestinal disease (IPSID), previously known as primary intestinal lymphoma, is a condition in which the lamina propria of the small bowel is intensely infiltrated with lymphocytes and the overlying enterocytes are normal morphologically [*see Figure 6*]. In a series of Chinese patients, six of 45 patients with intestinal lymphoma had this condition.[41] These patients presented with severe malabsorption. Among patients without IPSID, 65% had abdominal pain, weight loss, abdominal masses, obstruction, and perforation. IPSID is associated with α heavy chains (from IgA), with paraprotein present in the serum, urine, or jejunal fluid. The disease is rare in developed nations and more common in underprivileged populations, primarily in persons in the second and third decades of

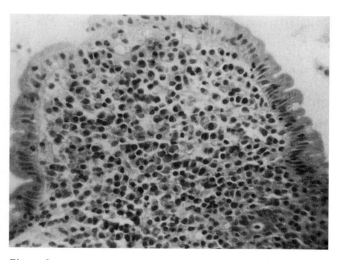

Figure 6 **Small intestinal biopsy specimen from a patient with primary intestinal lymphoma shows a single broadened villus (magnified 400 times). The epithelium is composed of normal columnar cells, but the lamina propria is packed with plasma cells and other mononuclear cells. Surgical biopsies in this patient revealed evidence of generalized subepithelial histiocytic lymphoma.**

life, with a male predominance. It is a B cell disorder involving the mucosa-associated lymphoid tissue (MALT). Duodenography shows thickened folds and many nodular elevations without ulceration. The diagnosis may be made by small bowel biopsy in 85% of cases.[42] Early in the course of the disease, the condition appears to be treatable with antibiotics. If allowed to progress, however, it may develop into more aggressive forms of lymphoma.[43]

INTESTINAL LYMPHANGIECTASIA

Intestinal lymphangiectasia is often a congenital condition in which deformed lymphatics impair the transport of chylomicrons from the enterocytes to the mesenteric lymph duct. A similar pathophysiologic picture is acquired in certain cases of intestinal lymphomas, granulomatous enteritis, tuberculous enteritis, or Whipple disease in which normal lymphatic drainage is blocked.

Diagnosis

The blockage of lymphatic drainage may result in chylous ascites, chyluria, or chylometrorrhea.[44] Protein-losing enteropathy and lymphopenia are prominent features. Modest steatorrhea is also present, with fat excretion commonly reaching 20 g/day. In the congenital form of the disease, lymphedema of the legs or of one leg and one arm is seen. With endoscopic examination, white villi, white nodules, and submucosal elevations may be noted.[45] The white appearance of the mucosa is undoubtedly caused by retained chylomicron triacylglycerol. Double-contrast barium x-ray examination shows smooth nodular protrusions and thick mucosal folds without ulceration.[46] On histologic examination, dilated lymphatics with club-shaped villi are seen, sometimes in asymptomatic patients, in whom outcome is benign.

Treatment

Treatment is directed toward any identified causative process. In patients with the congenital condition, in whom improvement of the lymphatics is not expected, a low-fat diet supplemented with medium-chain triglycerides is usually helpful. Surgery can be used to remove isolated areas of lymphatic dysfunction if these areas can be identified or to anastomose a lymph duct to the venous system. Sometimes a peritoneovenous (LeVeen) shunt is helpful.

ABETALIPOPROTEINEMIA

In the rare congenital condition of abetalipoproteinemia, postprandial chylomicronemia does not develop in patients, because they are unable to adequately couple apolipoprotein B to the developing chylomicron. Because lipid and lipid-soluble vitamins are transported from the intestine in chylomicrons, the consequent reduction in lipid and lipid-soluble vitamin absorption results in symptomatic steatorrhea, neurologic abnormalities, a variant of retinitis pigmentosa, and spiculated red cells. In contrast to earlier theories about the etiology of this disease, these patients have the normally transcribed apolipoprotein B mRNA from which the protein is adequately translated. Nevertheless, apolipoprotein B is not secreted from the intestinal cell. The defect in this condition is in various mutations in the gene that encodes the microsomal triglyceride transport protein.[47] This chaperonlike protein translocates the apolipoprotein across the membrane of the endoplasmic reticulum.[48] Without this step, the apolipoprotein is degraded by cytosolic and microsomal peptidases. The result of this defect is that both the intestine and the liver are unable to produce and secrete their triacylglycerol-rich lipoproteins, chylomicrons, and very low density lipoproteins. Because chylomicrons cannot transport the fat out of the enterocyte, it is presumed, but not proved, that the 80% of the lipid that is absorbed is absorbed via the portal vein.[49]

Diagnosis

In addition to having intestinal symptoms, patients with abetalipoproteinemia have severe neurologic problems. These neurologic problems may be caused in part by essential fatty acid deficiency and in part by either the impaired delivery of lipid to nerves or an interference with the local synthesis of lipids. The result is a demyelinating condition resulting in a sensory ataxia caused by the loss of position and vibratory sensations. The symptoms are similar to but less severe than those of Friedreich ataxia.[50] Patients may have muscle weakness and athetoid movements. Patients also experience retinitis pigmentosa, usually with mild loss of visual acuity but preservation of central vision. In addition to the neurologic abnormalities, patients have acanthocytes in their blood. Acanthocytes are spiculated red cells that have a near-normal life span but that demonstrate an increased susceptibility to mechanical trauma on in vitro testing.

These patients have low plasma triacylglycerol and cholesterol levels. On histologic examination, the enterocytes are seen to be laden with fat. Despite this phenotype, the amount of steatorrhea is modest (about 20 g/day).

Abetalipoproteinemia is usually discovered in childhood because patients with the disease fail to thrive and have steatorrhea. In adults, the disease can be recognized by the combination of neurologic and ophthalmologic findings, the red cell morphology, the very low levels of plasma lipids, and the modest steatorrhea. On small bowel biopsy, the enterocytes are seen to be stuffed with lipid even after an overnight fast, indicating that the absorbed lipid cannot exit the enterocytes.[51]

Treatment

Treatment should include vitamin E as well as the other fat-soluble vitamins and medium-chain triglycerides to reduce the steatorrhea, if required.

EOSINOPHILIC GASTROENTERITIS

Eosinophilic gastroenteritis is a rare disease that is characterized by the presence of eosinophilic infiltration of one or more portions of the gastrointestinal tract, anywhere from the esophagus to the colon, in conjunction with gastrointestinal symptoms. No identifiable cause of the eosinophilic infiltrate, such as parasitic infestation, is present. Many patients have an underlying allergic diathesis (e.g., hay fever, asthma, atopic dermatitis, or drug allergies).

It is not known why eosinophils congregate in the GI tract in this condition, but evidence suggests that eosinophils, once activated, can produce cytokines that self-perpetuate the accumulation of additional eosinophils. These cytokines are interleukin-3 (IL-3), IL-5, and granulocyte-macrophage colony-stimulating factor (GM-CSF), which have been identified in eosinophils of patients but not in control subjects with irritable bowel syndrome. Local production of these cytokines is suggested by the finding that serum levels of IL-5 are normal in patients with eosinophilic gastroenteritis, in contrast to patients with the hypereosinophilic syndrome, who have increased levels of IL-5 in their blood.[52]

Diagnosis

Although eosinophils are a normal constituent of the GI tract, in this instance the eosinophils appear more numerous than normal and are more invasive. For example, eosinophilic invasion of the crypts in the small intestine is a hallmark of this condition. A peripheral eosinophilia is often seen but is not always present.

Eosinophilic gastroenteritis can be divided into two basic forms: a tumorous mass of eosinophils producing a granulomatous-type lesion and a more diffusely infiltrative form. In the former case, the lesions are most often in the distal stomach, which may produce obstructive symptoms, or the masses may be found in the more proximal stomach, small bowel, or colon. When lesions are in the small bowel or colon, the condition needs to be differentiated from a lymphoma or Crohn disease.[53] In the case of diffuse disease involving the small bowel, the infiltration can be mucosal, with symptoms of protein-losing enteropathy or malabsorption. If the infiltration is primarily in the muscle layers of the intestine, obstructive symptoms are common. Finally, the disease may be found in the subserosal area of the intestine, with resultant eosinophilic ascites.[54]

Treatment

Most patients respond to conservative measures and steroids. Surgery should be avoided unless it is needed to relieve persistent or small bowel obstruction.

Prednisone, 40 mg orally every morning and tapered slowly over 2 weeks, is the most effective therapy for patients with obstructive symptoms and ascites. If high-dose steroids are needed to maintain remission, azathioprine can be added for its steroid-sparing effect.

Diet elimination therapy may be beneficial in patients with mucosal layer involvement.

CROHN DISEASE

Crohn disease, a stenosing, fistulizing disease of the intestine, may impair intestinal absorption by at least two mechanisms, ileal dysfunction and the stasis syndrome [see Stasis (Bacterial Overgrowth) Syndrome, below]. In the case of either ileal resection or severe ileal involvement with Crohn disease, the ileum cannot absorb bile salts normally. In that event, postprandial bile salt deficiency occurs in the upper intestine; this condition may become more severe the later in the day a meal is eaten.[55] Postprandial bile salt deficiency occurs despite the liver's response to bile acid loss from the enterohepatic circulation, which is to increase bile acid synthesis. The increase in bile salt synthesis is not adequate, because each time the gallbladder contracts in response to a meal, most of the bile salt pool is lost to the colon[56] if significant amounts of the ileum have been resected. Thus, the liver does not have time to generate enough replacement bile salts for the complete absorption of the meal just eaten or the next one. The colonic perfusion of bile acids may result in diarrhea. This condition has been termed choleretic enteropathy and may occur when more than 30 cm of the terminal ileum is resected. The excess fluid in the colon is caused by cAMP-driven Cl^- secretion, specifically by the dihydroxylated bile acids chenodeoxycholate and deoxycholate, not trihydroxylated cholic acid.[57]

Diagnosis

The loss of bile acids to the colon and thus to the enterohepatic circulation can be associated with no or minimal steatorrhea.[58]

With more extensive (100 cm or greater) ileal resection, however, the diarrhea is caused not only by bile acids but also by malabsorbed fatty acids (steatorrhea).[59] Thus, the diarrhea associated with Crohn disease may be caused not by active disease but rather by the results of ileal resection. This scenario is suggested by the finding that the diarrhea occurs when the patient first eats after surgery, a time when disease activity may be low secondary to active disease resection, or by the fact that the patient had no or minimal diarrhea before surgery, with diarrhea becoming more prominent afterward.

Because of the stenosis present in some patients with Crohn disease, the stasis syndrome can develop [see Stasis (Bacterial Overgrowth) Syndrome, below].

Treatment

When the diarrhea is caused by bile acid loss, the treatment is cholestyramine (4 g a.c. and h.s.).[59] This resin preferentially binds the dihydroxylated bile acids, reducing their aqueous concentration and reducing their proportion in the total bile acid pool. Both effects are beneficial. In the case of larger ileal resections in which steatorrhea is prominent, cholestyramine may actually provoke more diarrhea and malabsorption because it reduces the aqueous bile acid concentration in the upper intestine when taken before meals. In this case, medium-chain fatty acids are used as a replacement for the long-chain fatty acids. The results of this strategy are often not as good as desired. Vitamin B_{12} absorption should also be evaluated in all patients with ileal resection, and if absorption is found to be abnormal, vitamin B_{12} should be given parenterally.

Some patients with severe Crohn disease undergo extensive intestinal resection, resulting effectively in short bowel syndrome. Similarly, patients who have numerous enteroenteric fistulas also have symptoms of short bowel syndrome because the fistulas cause the chyme to bypass large sections of the small intestine. Both types of patients should be treated as if they had short bowel syndrome.

STASIS (BACTERIAL OVERGROWTH) SYNDROME

The stasis (bacterial overgrowth) syndrome occurs when intestinal stasis leads to the opportunity for bacteria to proliferate locally. This condition has a multiplicity of causes. The most prominent causes are diabetes, scleroderma, intestinal diverticulosis, afferent loop of a gastrojejunostomy, and intestinal obstruction caused by strictures, adhesions, or cancer. These disorders may be present years before the development of symptoms.

Symptoms may appear in an otherwise stable patient because of the administration of a proton pump inhibitor that reduces gastric acid production, allowing gastric and small bowel overgrowth, or the administration of an opiate that further reduces intestinal motility.

Intestinal dysfunction in the stasis syndrome is probably caused by bacterial glycosidases that hydrolyze the carbohydrate moieties that form the extensive glycosylation of the apical brush-border proteins.[60] Although bile acid deconjugation occurs in the stasis syndrome, which may theoretically lead to impaired solubilization of the products of triglyceride hydrolysis, studies have shown that in fact the fatty acid concentration in the aqueous phase of postprandial intestinal content is normal.[61] Electron micrographs, however, show that there is damage to the enterocytes, in that absorbed lipid collects in the endoplasmic reticulum and does not progress normally to the Golgi apparatus.[61]

Diagnosis

Clinical manifestations Symptoms of the stasis syndrome are similar to those of other malabsorptive states and include steatorrhea and anemia. The patient may have vitamin B_{12} deficiency, which has several causes, including binding of the vitamin to bacteria[62] and bacterial metabolism of the vitamin to metabolically ineffective metabolites. Folic acid levels are usually high secondary to bacterial production of folate.[63] Serum albumin levels may be low secondary to protein-losing enteropathy and remain low for months after adequate treatment. The diagnosis is usually made in a patient with malabsorption in the appropriate clinical setting. Intestinal (usually jejunal) diverticulosis is usually unsuspected until a small bowel x-ray is performed.

Laboratory tests Establishing the diagnosis of the stasis syndrome is not simple. The most accurate way is to pass an aspiration tube into the intestine. The fluid must be quantitatively cultured both aerobically and anaerobically. In most cases, more than 10^5 anaerobes will be found. Alternatively, the noninvasive hydrogen breath test may be used. A high resting hydrogen level or a quick increase in the breath hydrogen in response to a fermentable substrate, such as glucose or lactulose, can be used. Another breath test is the 1 g (^{14}C)-D-xylose test, in which the breath $^{14}CO_2$ is measured.

Treatment

The first choice of treatment for the stasis syndrome is surgical correction of defects, such as an afferent loop that is harboring bacteria, or a jejunocolic fistula. If the surgery option is not available, then recurrent dosing of an antibiotic is required. Tetracycline, at a dosage of 1 to 2 g/day for a 7- to 10-day course, gives good results, or another antibiotic that is active against anaerobic bacteria may be used (e.g., trimethroprim-sulfamethoxazole, one double-strength tablet b.i.d.). The patient will need to be re-treated if clinical symptoms reappear, or the patient can receive treatment for 1 week every month.

AMYLOIDOSIS

The intestine is often involved in patients with systemic amyloidosis, especially if they have polyneuropathy. In patients older than 85 years, 36% have intestinal involvement with amyloidosis,[64] although most are asymptomatic. Endoscopically, mucosal erosion, friability, or polypoid protrusions can be seen.[65] The diagnosis is made by either full-thickness or peroral intestinal biopsies. If a peroral biopsy is performed, it must be deep enough to have arteries visible, so that amyloid, if present, can be demonstrated. Congo red–stained arterioles that become apple green under polarized light confirm the diagnosis. Small bowel follow-through x-rays may show swollen intestinal plicae, possibly with separated loops of bowel. If steatorrhea is present, it may be the result either of bacterial overgrowth caused by intestinal dysmotility or of impaired bile acid absorption.[66] No specific effective therapy is available. If bacterial overgrowth is present, then appropriate antibiotics should be given.

SYSTEMIC MASTOCYTOSIS

In this rare condition, the skin (99% of cases), bones (9%), liver (12%), spleen (11%), lymph nodes, and GI tract are involved with proliferating mast cells. Diarrhea or abdominal pain or both (23% of cases), peptic ulceration (4%), and itching and flushing (36%) may be seen. Headache, fatigue, and malaise are seen in 12% of cases. There may also be cognitive dysfunction. Eosinophilia is seen in 12% to 50% of cases.[57] Many of these manifestations of the disease are secondary to histamine, which is released from the mast cells. Histamine release may be precipitated by alcohol, aspirin, narcotics, and nonsteroidal anti-inflammatory drugs, causing episodic disturbances of flushing, diarrhea, abdominal pain, and hypotension that may progress to syncope.[67]

Excess histamine is excreted into the urine in excess in approximately 75% of patients, making this test useful for diagnostic purposes.[67] The urinary excretion of a metabolite of prostaglandin D_2 from mast cells may be an even better test.[68] X-ray studies of the small intestine may show thickened folds or nodulation. These findings are not diagnostic but may point to a diseased small bowel.

Histamine-mediated overproduction of gastric acid may lead to peptic ulceration. In that event, H_2 blockers or proton pump inhibitors are effective in controlling symptoms. In the skin, urticaria pigmentosa may be effectively treated with H_1 receptor antagonists such as diphenhydramine (25 µg every 6 to 8 hours). If diarrhea persists, cromolyn sodium may be given at a dosage of 100 mg orally four times a day.

Parasitic Infestations

Hookworm and *G. lamblia* infections can cause mild malabsorption that is rarely clinically important. Eradication of the parasites cures the absorptive defect. These issues are discussed more fully elsewhere [*see Chapter 38*].

Chronic Pancreatitis with Exocrine Insufficiency

Most chronic pancreatitis is caused by alcoholism. In rare cases, the disease is inherited. Patients experience weight loss resulting from malabsorption of food. Malabsorption caused by pancreatitis is discussed elsewhere [*see Chapter 68*].

Combined or Multiple Defects in Digestion and Absorption

POSTGASTRECTOMY STEATORRHEA

One of the consequences of gastric surgery is steatorrhea, primarily in patients who have the Billroth II gastric resection with a gastrojejunostomy. In this operation, the antrum and a variable portion of the body of the stomach are resected, the stomach is sutured closed, and a gastrojejunostomy is created. Thus, food

bypasses the duodenum and most proximal jejunum, the sites of maximal cholecystokinin and secretin concentrations and the active sites for folate calcium and iron absorption. Approximately one half of patients who have undergone the Billroth II procedure have steatorrhea of 10 to 15 g of fat/day. This condition is thought to result from food entering the jejunum without the hormone-sensitive sites in the duodenum receiving the appropriate signals for hormone release. Thus, the optimal admixing of the chyme with pancreatic enzymes and bile acids does not occur. Consequently, the afferent loop, which drains the duodenum and proximal jejunum, may become blocked or atonic and harbor bacteria. The stasis syndrome may occur if enough bacteria are present. Because of their small stomachs, the affected patients cannot eat as much as they previously could. This decrease in food consumption, in combination with steatorrhea, causes many patients who undergo the Billroth II procedure to stabilize at a lower weight than they were before surgery. Osteopenia and iron deficiency anemia are also found. Constant small amounts of blood loss from the gastric ostomy site contribute to the iron-deficient state, which is the most common form of anemia. Folate deficiency secondary to the inability to generate absorbable monoglutamyl folate from nonabsorbable heptaglutamyl folate (the common form of folate found in the diet) is also found.[69] Least commonly seen is vitamin B_{12} deficiency caused by hypochlorhydria and resection of intrinsic factor–containing gastric parietal cells. Treatment of the steatorrhea is usually not necessary, because it is not clinically significant. Iron, calcium, or vitamin B_{12} and folic acid must be replaced as indicated. If the patient has early satiety, multiple small meals may be efficacious.

Symptoms of GSE may develop in patients after gastric surgery.[70] It is likely that these patients had clinically silent GSE before the operation. The operation itself causes modest steatorrhea (10 to 15 g fat/day) in 50% of cases, even in patients whose intestine is otherwise normal. In the compensated GSE patient, however, surgery is enough to cause clinical symptomatology. Therefore, if postgastrectomy patients exhibit excessive steatorrhea, an evaluation for GSE is warranted. Inflammatory bowel disease that develops in patients after gastrectomy may likewise be an indication of the presence of previously silent GSE.[71]

DIABETES MELLITUS AND MALABSORPTION

Diarrhea, a common complication of diabetes, has multiple causes[72] and may result in malabsorption [*see Chapter 61*]. The most common causes are bacterial overgrowth, caused by the autonomic dysfunction present in this condition with attendant intestinal stasis, and gluten-sensitive enteropathy. With the use of antiendomysial antibodies as a screen, gluten-sensitive enteropathy has been found in three of 47 diabetic patients (6%), a much higher incidence than would be expected by chance.[73]

References

1. Moreau H, Gargouri Y, Bernadal A, et al: Etude biochemique et physiologique des lipases préduodéales d'origines animale et humaine. Revue Française des Corps Gras 35:169, 1988

2. Roulet M, Weber A, Roy C: Perspectives in Cystic Fibrosis. Canada Cystic Fibrosis Foundation, Toronto, 1980, p 172

3. Levitt MD, Duane WC: Floating stools: fatus versus fat. N Engl J Med 286:973, 1972

4. Drummy GD, Benson JA Jr, Jones CM: Microscopical examination of the stool for steatorrhea. N Engl J Med 264:85, 1961

5. DiMagno EP, Go VLW, Summerskill WHJ: Relation between pancreatic enzyme outputs and malabsorption in severe pancreatic insufficiency. N Engl J Med 288:813, 1973

6. Dreiling DA, Janowitz HD: The measurement of pancreatic secretory function. The Exocrine Pancreas. De Reuck AVS, Cameron MP, Eds. Ciba Foundation Symposium. Little, Brown & Co, New York, 1961, p 225

7. Kato H, Nakao A, Kishimoto W, et al: ^{13}C-labeled trioctanoin breath test for exocrine pancreatic function test in patients after pancreatoduodenectomy. Am J Gastroenterol 88:64, 1993

8. Lang C: Value of serum PABA as a pancreatic function test. Gut 25:508, 1984

9. Bando N, Ogawa T, Tsuji H: Enzymatic method for selective determination of 4 aminobenzoic acid in urine. Clin Chem 36:1937, 1990

10. Jacobson DG, Curlington C, Connery K, et al: Trypsin-like immunoreactivity as a test for pancreatic insufficiency. N Engl J Med 310:1307, 1984

11. Oelkers P, Kirby LC, Heubi JE, et al: Primary bile acid malabsorption caused by mutations in the ileal sodium-dependent bile acid transporter gene. J Clin Invest 99:1880, 1997

12. Shindo K, Yamazaki R, Koide K, et al: Alteration of bile acid metabolism by cimetidine in healthy humans. J Investig Med 44:462, 1996

13. Nyhlin H, Merrick MV, Eastwood MA, et al: Evaluation of ileal function using 23-selena-25-homotaurocholate, a γ-labeled conjugated bile acid. Gastroenterology 84:63, 1983

14. Make M, Collin P: Coeliac disease. Lancet 349:1755, 1997

15. Anderson RP, Degano P, Godkin AJ, et al: In vivo antigen challenge in celiac disease identifies a single transglutaminase-modified peptide as the dominant α-gliadin T-cell epitope. Nat Med 6:337, 2000

16. Hofmann AF: The function of bile salts in fat absorption. Biochem J 89:57, 1963

17. Mansbach CM II, Cohen RS, Leff PB: Isolation and properties of the mixed micelles present in intestinal content during fat digestion in man. J Clin Invest 56:781, 1975

18. Dieterich W, Laag E, Schöpper H, et al: Autoantibodies to tissue transglutaminase as predictors of coeliac disease. Gastroenterology 115:1317, 1998

19. Volta V, Molinaro N, deFranceschi L, et al: IgA antiendomysial antibodies on human umbilical cord tissue for celiac disease screening. Dig Dis Sci 40:1902, 1995

20. Holmes GKT, Prior P, Lane MR, et al: Malignancy in coeliac disease: effect of a gluten-free diet. Gut 30:333, 1989

21. Gawkrodger DJ, Vestey JP, O'Mahouny S: Dermatitis herpetiformis and established coeliac disease. Br J Dermatol 129:694, 1993

22. Klipstein FA, Falaiye JM: Tropical sprue in expatriates from the tropics living in the continental United States. Medicine (Baltimore) 48:475, 1969

23. Lindenbaum J, Gerson CD, Kent TH: Recovery of small intestinal structure and function after residence in the tropics: I. Studies in Peace Corps. Volunteers. Ann Intern Med 74:218, 1971

24. Gerson CD, Kent TH, Saha JR, et al: Recovery of small intestinal structure and function after residence in the tropics: II. Studies in Indians and Parkistanis living in New York City. Ann Intern Med 75:41, 1971

25. Haghighi P, Wolf PL: Tropical sprue and subclinical enteropathy: a vision for the nineties. Crit Rev Clin Lab Sci 34:313, 1997

26. Robert ME, Ament ME, Weinstein WM: The histologic spectrum and clinical outcome of refractory and unclassified sprue. Am J Surg Pathol 24:676, 2000

27. McCashland TM, Donovan JP, Strobach RS, et al: Collagenous enterocolitis: a manifestation of gluten-sensitive enteropathy. J Clin Gastroenterol 15:45, 1992

28. Hermaszewski RA, Webster AD: Primary hypogammaglobulinaemia: a survey of clinical manifestations and complications. Q J Med 86:31, 1993

29. Ladefoged K, Hessov I, Jarnum S: Nutrition in short-bowel syndrome. Scand J Gastroenterol 216(suppl):122, 1996

30. Lin HC, Zhao X-T, Wang L: Fat absorption is not complete by midgut but is dependent on load of fat. Am J Physiol 271(1 pt 1):G62, 1996

31. Lin HC, Zhao X-T, Wong H: Fat-induced ileal brake in the dog depends on peptide YY. Gastroenterology 110:1491, 1996

32. Redman DA, Schmidt TM, McDermott RP, et al: Identification of the uncultured bacillus of Whipple's disease. N Engl J Med 327:393, 1992

33. Durand DV, Lecomte C, Cathebras P, et al: Whipple disease: clinical review of 52 cases. The SNFMI Research Group on Whipple Disease. Medicine (Baltimore) 76:170, 1997

34. Dobbins WO III: HLA antigens in Whipple's disease. Arthritis Rheum 30:102, 1987

35. Mansbach CM II, Shelburne J, Stevens RD, et al: Lymph node bacilliform bodies morphologically resembling those of Whipple's disease in a patient without intestinal involvement. Ann Intern Med 89:64, 1978

36. Swartz MN: Whipple's disease—past, present and future. N Engl J Med 342:648, 2000

37. von Herbay A, Ditton H-J, Schumacher F, et al: Whipple's disease: staging and monitoring by cytology and polymerase chain reaction analysis of cerebrospinal fluid. Gastroenterology 113:434, 1997

38. Kelly CA, Egan M, Rawlinson J: Whipple's disease presenting with lung involvement. Thorax 51:343, 1996

39. Louis ED, Lynch T, Kaufmann P, et al: Diagnostic guidelines in central nervous system Whipple's disease. J Ann Neurol 40:561, 1996

40. Feurle GE, Marth T: An evaluation of antimicrobial treatment for Whipple's disease: tetracycline versus trimethoprim-sulfamethoxazole. Dig Dis Sci 39:1642, 1994

41. Shih LY, Liaw SJ, Dunn P, et al: Primary small-intestinal lymphomas in Taiwan: immunoproliferative small-intestinal disease and nonimmunoproliferative small-intestinal disease. J Clin Oncol 12:1375, 1994

42. Halphen M, Najjar T, Jaafoura H, et al: Diagnostic value of upper intestinal fiber endoscopy in primary small intestinal lymphoma: a prospective study by the Tunisian-French Intestinal Lymphoma Group. Cancer 58:2140, 1986

43. Khojasteh A, Haghighi P: Immunoproliferative small intestinal disease: portrait of a potentially preventable cancer from the Third World. Am J Med 89:483, 1990

44. Fox C, Lucani G: Disorders of the intestinal mesenteric lymphatic system. Lymphology 26:61, 1993

45. Aoyagi K, Iida M, Yao T, et al: Characteristic endoscopic features of intestinal lymphangiectasia: correlation with histological findings. Hepatogastroenterology 44:133, 1997

46. Aoyagi K, Iida M, Yao T, et al: Intestinal lymphangiectasia: value of double-contrast radiographic study. Clin Radiol 49:814, 1994

47. Sharp D, Blinderman L, Combs KA, et al: Cloning and gene defects in microsomal triglyceride transfer protein associated with abetalipoproteinaemia. Nature 365:65, 1993

48. Gordon DA, Jamil H, Gregg RE, et al: Inhibition of the microsomal triglyceride transfer protein blocks the step of apolipoprotein B lipoprotein assembly but not the addition of bulk core lipids in the second step. J Biol Chem 271:33047, 1996

49. Mansbach CM II, Dowell RF, Pritchett D: Portal transport of absorbed lipids in the rat. Am J Physiol 261:G530, 1991

50. Isselbacher KJ, Scheig R, Plotkin GR, et al: Congenital β-lipoprotein deficiency: an hereditary disorder involving a defect in the absorption and transport of lipids. Medicine (Baltimore) 43:347, 1964

51. Ways PO, Parmentier CM, Kayden HJ, et al: Studies on the absorptive defect for triglyceride in abetalipoproteinemia. J Clin Invest 46:35, 1967

52. Desreumaux P, Blogot F, Seguy D, et al: Interleukin 3, granulocyte-macrophage colony-stimulating factor, and interleukin 5 in eosinophilic gastroenteritis. Gastroenterology 110:768, 1996

53. Salmon PR, Paulley JW: Eosinophilic granuloma of the gastrointestinal tract. Gut 8:8, 1967

54. Klein NC, Hargrove RL, Sleisenger MH, et al: Eosinophilic gastroenteritis. Medicine (Baltimore) 49:299, 1970

55. Van Deest BW, Fordtran JS, Morawski SG, et al: Bile salt and micellar fat concentration in proximal small bowel contents of ileectomy patients. J Clin Invest 47:1314, 1968

56. Low-Beer TS, Wilkins RM, Lack L, et al: Effect of one meal on enterohepatic circulation of bile salts. Gastroenterology 67:490, 1974

57. Merhjian HS, Phillips SF, Hofmann AF: Colonic secretion of water and electrolytes induced by bile acids: perfusion studies in man. J Clin Invest 50:1569, 1971

58. Mansbach CM II, Newton DF, Stevens RD: Fat digestion in patients with bile acid malabsorption but minimal steatorrhea. Dig Dis Sci 25:353, 1980

59. Hofmann AF, Poley JR: Role of bile acid malabsorption in pathogenesis of diarrhea and steatorrhea in patients with ileal resection: I. Response to cholestyramine or replacement of dietary long chain triglyceride by medium chain triglyceride. Gastroenterology 62:918, 1972

60. Riepe S, Goldstein J, Alpers DH: Effect of secreted *Bacteroides* proteases on human intestinal brush border hydrolases. J Clin Invest 66:314, 1980

61. Ament ME, Shimoda SS, Saunders DR, et al: Pathogenesis of steatorrhea in three cases of small intestinal stasis syndrome. Gastroenterology 63:728, 1972

62. Gianella RA, Broitman SA, Zamcheck N: Vitamin B_{12} uptake by intestinal microorganisms: mechanisms and relevance to syndromes of bacterial overgrowth. J Clin Invest 50:1100, 1971

63. Hoffbrand AV, Tabaqchali S, Booth CC, et al: Small intestinal bacterial flora and folate status in gastrointestinal disease. Gut 12:27, 1971

64. Rocken C, Saeger W, Linke RP: Gastrointestinal amyloid deposits in old age: report of 110 consecutive autopsical patients and 98 retrospective bioptic specimens. Pathol Res Pract 190:641, 1994

65. Tada S, Iida M, Yao KK, et al: Endoscopic features in amyloidosis of the small intestine: clinical and morphologic differences between chemical types of amyloid protein. Gastrointest Endosc 40:45, 1994

66. Suhr O, Danielsson A, Steen L: Bile acid malabsorption caused by gastrointestinal motility dysfunction? An investigation of gastrointestinal disturbances in familial amyloidosis with polyneuropathy. Scand J Gastroenterol 27:201, 1992

67. Golkar L, Bernhard JD: Mastocytosis. Lancet 349:1379, 1997

68. Morrow JD, Guzzo C, Lazarus G, et al: Improved diagnosis of mastocytosis by measurements of the major urinary metabolite of prostaglandin D2. J Invest Dermatol 104:937, 1995

69. Rosenberg IH: Folate absorption and malabsorption. N Engl J Med 293:1303, 1975

70. Bai J, Moran C, Martinez C: Celiac sprue after surgery of the upper gastrointestinal tract: report of 10 patients with special attention to diagnosis, clinical behavior, and follow-up. J Clin Gastroenterol 13:521, 1991

71. Kitis G, Holmes GTK, Cooper BT: Association of coeliac disease and inflammatory bowel disease. Gut 21:636, 1980

72. Valdovinos MA, Camilleri M, Zimmerman BR: Chronic diarrhea in diabetes mellitus: mechanisms and an approach to diagnosis and treatment. Mayo Clin Proc 68:691, 1993

73. Rensch MJ, Merenich JA, Lieberman M, et al: Gluten-sensitive enteropathy in patients with insulin-dependent diabetes mellitus. Ann Intern Med 124:564, 1996

Acknowledgments

Figure 1   Janet Betries.

Figure 2   Dana Burns-Pizer.

61 Diarrheal Diseases

Lawrence R. Schiller, M.D.

Definition and Epidemiology

The word diarrhea is derived from the Greek words for "flowing through." For most persons, diarrhea means the frequent passage of loose stools.[1] This definition includes two major components: loose stool consistency (pourable stools) and increased stool frequency (more than two bowel movements daily). Physicians often include a third component: increased stool weight (> 200 g/24 hr), but patients are poor estimators of stool output. In addition, some patients report diarrhea when they have fecal incontinence, even if stools are solid; every patient complaining of diarrhea should be asked about fecal incontinence.

Diarrhea is a universal human experience. Most persons have had acute infectious diarrhea at some time during their lives. The incidence of acute diarrhea is roughly 5% to 7% annually.[2] Infectious diarrhea is associated with contaminated food and water; it is typically spread via fecal-oral transmission. Chronic diarrhea (lasting > 4 weeks) is also common, with a prevalence of approximately 5% in the United States.[3] It is less likely to be caused by infection and is more likely to be a symptom of other disorders.

Pathophysiology and Classification

Diarrhea results from excess water in the stool.[4] To understand the pathophysiology of diarrhea, it is necessary to understand how water is transported across the mucosa of the gastrointestinal tract. Water moves in response to osmotic gradients established by the absorption of salts (mainly sodium chloride, but also potassium and bicarbonate salts) and nutrients (e.g., monosaccharides, amino acids, and fatty acids). Salts and nutrients move both passively, in response to electrochemical gradients across the mucosa, and actively, in response to molecular pumps located in the enterocyte membranes.[5]

Each day, a typical person ingests about 2 L of fluid and produces 7 to 8 L of secretions (i.e., saliva, gastric juice, bile, pancreatic juice, and succus entericus). Thus, a total volume of 9 to 10 L enters the upper intestine daily. Most of the water is absorbed in the jejunum, along with nutrients. Absorption of residual nutrients and salts in the ileum results in a reduction of the volume of luminal contents entering the colon to only 1 to 1.5 L, a 90% reduction in the volume of fluid entering the intestine each day. The colonic mucosa can absorb salt against large electrochemical gradients and can reclaim 90% of the fluid passing the ileocecal valve each day, making the overall efficiency of small bowel and colonic water absorption about 99%.

Diarrhea develops if the overall efficiency of absorption declines by as little as 1%. This can occur under the following circumstances: the rate of intestinal nutrient and salt absorption decreases; net electrolyte secretion develops (an unusual circumstance except with severe diarrhea such as the diarrhea associated with cholera, in which stool output can exceed 10 L/day); transit through the intestine speeds up, thereby limiting the time available for absorption; or poorly absorbable substances are ingested and increase intraluminal osmotic activity, causing the retention of water within the intestine (osmotic diarrhea).[6]

Common problems that primarily cause a reduction in the rate of intestinal nutrient and salt absorption include mucosal diseases, such as celiac disease; inflammatory diseases that disrupt the integrity of the intestinal mucosa (e.g., Crohn disease); and infections with pathogens that produce toxins that affect enterocyte function.

Isolated acceleration of transit is a poorly recognized mechanism of diarrhea, although diarrhea was historically attributed to it. Some patients with so-called functional diarrhea have rapid intestinal transit, which is likely to be important in the pathogenesis of their condition. Many patients with chronic idiopathic diarrhea have normal rates of fluid and electrolyte absorption when measured under perfusion conditions during which motility effects are neutralized, suggesting that motility must be playing a role in the pathogenesis of their diarrhea under ordinary circumstances.[7] Accelerated transit is also a major factor in diarrhea associated with some endocrine disorders (e.g., hyperthyroidism, carcinoid syndrome, or other peptide-secreting tumors).

Poorly absorbed substances that can induce osmotic diarrhea include lactose in lactase-deficient individuals. Osmotic diarrhea can also occur with ingestion of sufficient quantities of other poorly absorbed carbohydrates (e.g., fructose and the sugar alcohols mannitol and sorbitol) and ions such as magnesium, phosphate, and sulfate.

Mechanisms that reduce the overall efficiency of absorption may coexist in various disease states. For instance, in celiac disease, loss of intestinal villi results in reduced salt and water absorption, as well as reduced nutrient absorption. Thus, increased stool water in this condition results from both a reduced rate of electrolyte absorption and the increased intraluminal osmotic activity of poorly absorbed substances. Transit may accelerate in many diarrheal states because of stimulation of peristalsis by increased intraluminal volumes.

FECAL OSMOTIC GAP

As the rate of intestinal salt absorption decreases, the concentration of salts in stool rises to the point where it approaches plasma osmolality (290 mOsm/kg), the osmolality that intestinal contents maintain beyond the proximal jejunum. If the rate of salt absorption is unimpaired but nutrients are malabsorbed or poorly absorbable substances are ingested, fecal salt concentrations decrease because most of the available osmotic space is occupied by the poorly absorbed substance. This is the basis for the calculation of the fecal osmotic gap [*see Figure 1*].[8] In this calculation, the contribution of electrolytes to stool osmolality is estimated by doubling the concentration of sodium and potassium (the predominant cations in stool water) to account for unmeasured anions (mostly fatty acid anions, bicarbonate, or chloride). This value is then subtracted from 290 mOsm/kg (the putative osmolality of gut contents) to determine the contribution of nonelectrolytes to fecal osmolality. When electrolytes constitute most of luminal osmolality, the calculated fecal osmotic gap will be low (< 50 mOsm/kg). When poorly absorbable substances are present, the fecal osmotic gap will be large (> 100 mOsm/kg). Watery diarrhea with a low fecal os-

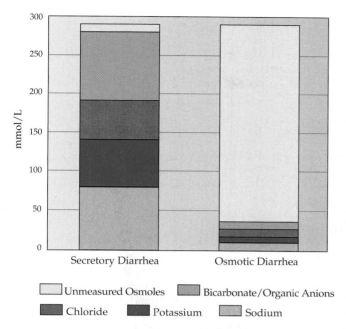

Figure 1 **Fecal electrolyte concentrations in secretory diarrhea (left column) and in osmotic diarrhea (right column). Note that most of the fecal osmolality can be attributed to fecal electrolytes in secretory diarrhea, whereas most of the osmolality in osmotic diarrhea results from the unmeasured (nonelectrolyte) osmoles. Calculation of the fecal osmotic gap allows an estimate of the contribution of unmeasured osmoles to fecal osmolality.**[59]

motic gap is classified as secretory diarrhea; diarrhea with a large fecal osmotic gap is classified as osmotic diarrhea. These categories are most helpful in the evaluation of patients with chronic diarrhea.

CLASSIFICATION OF DIARRHEA

For clinical purposes, diarrhea can be classified as either acute (duration < 4 weeks) or chronic (duration > 4 weeks). Chronic diarrhea is further categorized as watery, inflammatory, or fatty, based on the characteristics of the stools.[3] This classification allows the physician to direct evaluation and management more effectively, because diarrheal diseases can be distinguished by the duration of illness and type of stools produced.

Acute Diarrhea

Most acute diarrheas (those lasting < 4 weeks) are caused by infections and are self-limiting. Most are caused by viruses (e.g., adenovirus, Norwalk agent, rotavirus), but some are caused by bacteria (e.g., *Campylobacter, Salmonella, Shigella, Escherichia coli*) and others by protozoa (e.g., *Giardia lamblia, Entamoeba histolytica*) [*see Table 1*].[2]

The epidemiology of acute infectious diarrhea depends on the circumstances of infection and where one contracts the infection. For example, a history of recent travel, particularly to developing countries, makes a diagnosis of traveler's diarrhea likely. Previous antibiotic use or residence in an institution where antibiotic use is common (e.g., hospitals, nursing homes) are risk factors for *Clostridium difficile* infection. Children in day care facilities and their contacts, persons engaging in promiscuous sexual activity, and users of illicit intravenous drugs are all at enhanced risk for contracting infectious diarrhea. Consump-

tion of potentially contaminated food and drink is another risk factor for infectious diarrhea. With the globalization of commerce and mass processing of food, esoteric infections from overseas and large outbreaks of food-borne diarrhea have become more common.

Pathogenic infections cause diarrhea by one of four mechanisms: (1) enterotoxins that subvert the regulatory mechanisms of enterocytes, (2) cytotoxins that destroy enterocytes, (3) adherence to the mucosa by organisms (so-called enteroadherent organisms) that alter enterocyte function as a result of physical proximity to the mucosa, and (4) invasion of the mucosa by organisms that provoke an inflammatory response by the immune system.[9] In general, patients with cytotoxin-mediated diarrheas and those with invasive organisms experience more toxicity and have more abdominal pain than patients with enterotoxin-mediated diarrhea or enteroadherent infections.

Another mechanism for acute diarrhea is ingestion of a preformed toxin.[10] Several species of bacteria, such as *Staphylococcus aureus, C. perfringens,* and *Bacillus cereus,* can produce toxins that produce so-called food poisoning (i.e., vomiting and diarrhea) within 4 hours of ingestion. In such cases, the bacteria do not need to establish an intraluminal infection; ingestion of the toxin alone can produce the disease. Symptoms subside after the toxin is cleared, usually by the next day; evidence of toxicity (e.g., fever) is minimal.

Other potential causes of acute diarrhea include food allergies and medication reactions. Food allergies are rarely recognized as causes of diarrhea in adults unless the diarrhea is associated with urticaria or other allergic symptoms. Medications often produce diarrhea as a side effect; this association is typically appreciated by the patient because of the temporal relation between drug ingestion and diarrhea.

Finally, acute diarrhea may represent the initial stages of chronic diarrhea. This is significant because acute and chronic diarrhea have very different sets of causes. However, patients with chronic diarrhea often do not seek help during the initial weeks of their illness unless the diarrhea is severe or complicated by dehydration, symptomatic electrolyte disorders, or fever.

DIAGNOSIS

A careful medical history is the key to the diagnosis of diarrhea. The acuity and severity of the diarrheal process should be determined. Frequency of defecation is the easiest parameter for patients to describe, but frequency does not necessarily correlate with stool weight, which is a more meaningful measure of the physiologic impact of diarrhea. Manifestations of dehydration or of volume depletion, such as orthostasis, thirst, decreased urine output, and weakness, suggest voluminous diarrhea. Acute weight loss can also be a guide to the severity of diarrhea; voluminous diarrhea produces substantial weight loss if rehydration efforts are suboptimal.

Stool characteristics are also quite important. The presence of blood or pus suggests possible inflammatory diarrhea, such as that from colitis or enteroinvasive bacteria. Watery stools are more in keeping with a secretory process. The relationship of defecation to meals or fasting and the occurrence of nocturnal diarrhea, fecal urgency, or incontinence are other points of potential significance. Urgency and incontinence do not necessarily indicate voluminous diarrhea; more often they reflect independent defects in continence mechanisms. Additional symptoms that should be noted include abdominal pain or cramps; flatulence, abdominal bloating or distention; and fever. A list of all prescrip-

Table 1   Selected Infectious Diarrheas

Organism	Vehicle	Mechanism	Classic Characteristics	Complications
Campylobacter	Food (poultry); animal-to-person	Invasion; inflammation	Watery or bloody diarrhea; ileitis and/or colitis, ulceration	Guillain-Barré syndrome; reactive arthritis
Salmonella	Food (poultry, eggs, seafood); animal-to-person	Invasion; inflammation	Gastroenteritis, ileitis, colitis; enteric fever (S. typhi)	Endovascular infection; osteomyelitis; sepsis
Shigella	Food (poultry); day care centers	Cytotoxin; inflammation	Two phases: enteritis (fever, cramps, diarrhea), followed by colitis (ulcers, inflammation)	Seizures, encephalopathy; reactive arthritis
E. coli O157:H7	Food (beef); fruit juices	Cytotoxin	Hemorrhagic colitis	Hemolytic-uremic syndrome
Enteroinvasive E. coli	Food (various); water	Invasion; inflammation	Colitis	Fever, sepsis
Enterotoxigenic E. coli	Food (various); water	Enterotoxin	Watery diarrhea	Dehydration, shock
Enteropathogenic and enteroadherent E. coli	Food (various); water	Contact with brush border	Watery diarrhea; may be prolonged	Dehydration
Vibrio cholerae	Water, seafood	Enterotoxin	Voluminous watery diarrhea	Dehydration, shock
Clostridium difficile	Person-to-person	Cytotoxin	Nosocomial infection; antibiotic-associated diarrhea; toxicity	Toxic megacolon; protein-losing enteropathy
Aeromonas, Plesiomonas	Water	Enterotoxin	Watery diarrhea; may be prolonged	
Yersinia	Raw milk	Invasion; inflammation	Acute diarrhea or chronic ileo-colitis-like Crohn disease	Reactive arthritis, extraintestinal infection, Guillain-Barré syndrome
Bacillus cereus	Fried rice	Exotoxin	Acute gastroenteritis	Fulminant liver failure
Staphylococcus	Fatty foods	Exotoxin	Acute gastroenteritis	
Clostridium perfringens	Fatty foods	Exotoxin	Acute gastroenteritis	
Viruses	Person-to-person; water	Inflammation; ?toxins	Acute gastroenteritis; watery diarrhea	
Giardia	Person-to-person; animal-to-person; water; day care	Contact	Watery diarrhea, dyspepsia	
Cryptosporidium	Water; day care; animal-to-person	Contact	Watery diarrhea, may be prolonged; epidemics	
Cyclospora	Imported fruit	Inflammation	Watery diarrhea, flatulence, pain, fatigue; may be prolonged	
Entamoeba histolytica	Person-to-person	Invasion; inflammation	Variable: asymptomatic to dysentery; may mimic irritable bowel syndrome, inflammatory bowel disease	Liver abscess
Strongyloides	Larvae invade skin	Invasion; inflammation	Abdominal pain and diarrhea	Hyperinfection in immunosuppressed hosts

tion, over-the-counter, and herbal medications should be compiled, and previous surgeries or radiation therapy should be discussed. The patient's diet should be scrutinized, and epidemiologic features—such as diarrhea in family members or other contacts, recent travel, water source, occupation, sexual activity, and illicit drug use—should be investigated.

Physical Examination

The physical examination is more useful for judging the severity of diarrhea than for determining its cause. Volume sta-

tus should be assessed by looking for orthostatic change in blood pressure and pulse. Fever and other signs of toxicity should be recorded. A careful abdominal examination should be done, with emphasis on the activity of bowel sounds and the presence of distention or tenderness.

Laboratory Testing

Extensive laboratory testing is not necessary for most patients with acute diarrhea; it should be reserved for those with toxicity, dehydration, or persistence of diarrhea for longer than would be

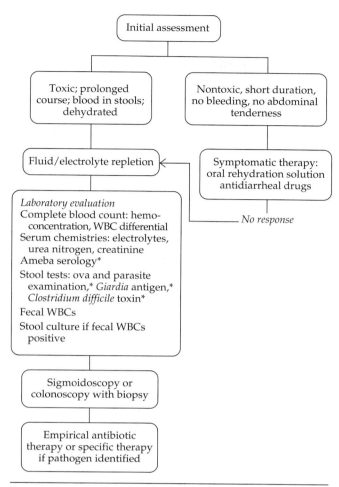

Initial assessment

↓

Toxic; prolonged course; blood in stools; dehydrated

Nontoxic, short duration, no bleeding, no abdominal tenderness

↓

Fluid/electrolyte repletion ← Symptomatic therapy: oral rehydration solution antidiarrheal drugs

— No response

Laboratory evaluation
Complete blood count: hemo-concentration, WBC differential
Serum chemistries: electrolytes, urea nitrogen, creatinine
Ameba serology*
Stool tests: ova and parasite examination,* *Giardia* antigen,* *Clostridium difficile* toxin*
Fecal WBCs
Stool culture if fecal WBCs positive

↓

Sigmoidoscopy or colonoscopy with biopsy

↓

Empirical antibiotic therapy or specific therapy if pathogen identified

*In appropriate epidemiologic circumstances.

Figure 2   **Initial evaluation of acute diarrhea.**[60]

expected, given its probable cause [*see Figure 2*]. In such patients, a complete blood count should be obtained to assess for hemo-concentration, anemia, or leukocytosis. Patients with viral diarrheas typically have normal white blood cell (WBC) counts and differentials, although lymphocytosis may be seen. Invasive bacterial infections typically produce leukocytosis with many immature WBCs, but salmonellosis can induce leukopenia. Serum electrolyte, blood urea nitrogen (BUN), and serum creatinine measurements can define the metabolic impact of diarrhea, which includes hypokalemia, hyponatremia, hyperchloremic acidosis, hypomagnesemia, and prerenal azotemia.

Stool testing is of value in patients with blood in the stool, dehydrating diarrhea, prolonged diarrhea, or dysentery and in patients who present during an outbreak of diarrhea. Stool cultures are sensitive and specific, but they are expensive. Some experts recommend obtaining cultures only in patients who have leukocytes (or the leukocyte marker lactoferrin) in the stool, because the yield of pathogenic bacteria will be higher in that group.[11] Others dispute this.[12] Laboratories routinely test for *Salmonella*, *Shigella*, *Campylobacter*, and *E. coli* serotype O157:H7. Special cultures for tuberculosis, *Yersinia*, *Aeromonas*, or *Plesiomonas* may need to be requested in appropriate circumstances. Examination of stool for ova and parasites has variable utility, depending on the pretest probability of these infections. For ex-

ample, such testing might be very useful in a day care worker with diarrhea, but it would be of little help in a patient with hospital-acquired diarrhea. Enzyme-linked immunosorbent assay (ELISA) stool testing for giardiasis and serologic testing for amebiasis are more accurate tests for those specific infections in most settings. Patients treated with antibiotics in the 3 months preceding onset of diarrhea and those who develop diarrhea in institutional settings should have a stool sample analyzed for *C. difficile* toxin.

In patients who are toxic, in those who have blood in their stools, or in those who have persistent acute diarrhea, sigmoidoscopy or colonoscopy should be considered. In most patients without rectal bleeding, sigmoidoscopy is probably adequate as an initial evaluation, because most patients with colitis will have involvement of the left side of their colons. In patients with bleeding or those with AIDS, colonoscopy is preferable because some opportunistic infections and lymphomas are seen only in the right colon.[13] Mucosal biopsies should be performed in either case, particularly if the colon is grossly inflamed, because the pathologist can readily distinguish self-limited colitis from chronic ulcerative colitis early in the course of the disease.[14] Abdominal x-rays or computed tomography should be obtained in toxic patients to confirm a diagnosis of colitis, to determine its extent, and to look for evidence of ileus or megacolon.

TREATMENT

Nonspecific Therapy

Because most cases of acute diarrhea are self-limited, most patients do not need specific therapy. Instead, judicious replacement of fluid and electrolyte losses is sufficient. This can be accomplished by intravenous fluids or oral rehydration solutions. Oral rehydration solutions are based on the concept that nutrient absorption accelerates the absorption of sodium and fluid by the jejunum.[15] Initially, rehydration formulas used glucose as the absorbable nutrient, but recent work has shown that cereal-based oral rehydration solutions can be more efficient. Oral rehydration solution does not reduce fecal losses (it may actually increase stool output) but, instead, increases net fluid and electrolyte absorption. These solutions cannot be used if vomiting precludes ingestion; intravenous rehydration must be used in those situations. Sports drinks (e.g., Gatorade) are designed to offset fluid and electrolyte losses from sweating and do not contain sufficient sodium to replace fecal losses. Solutions that more closely approximate World Health Organization rehydration solution are now commercially available (e.g., Rehydralyte, Resol, Ricalyte).

Diet   Most patients seek advice about altering their diets when suffering from diarrhea. Other than the provision of adequate water and salt, no specific instructions are needed. Some physicians routinely restrict dairy products in patients with diarrhea on the theory that these patients may have temporary lactase deficiency. This need not be done unless there is clinical evidence of lactose intolerance (e.g., exacerbation of diarrhea or flatus with ingestion of dairy products).

Antibiotics   Empirical antibiotic therapy for acute diarrhea may be appropriate under certain circumstances (e.g., in travelers with diarrhea, during local outbreaks of bacterial or protozoal diarrhea, or in patients who are frail or toxic). However, experts discourage the routine use of empirical antibiotic therapy because of its lack of demonstrable efficacy in many infections and because of concerns about precipitating complications, such as hemolytic-uremic syndrome in patients with *E. coli* serotype O157:H7.[16] A recent meta-analysis suggests that this latter point is not supported by the literature.[17] When indicated, fluoroquinolones or trimethoprim-sulfamethoxazole are commonly used for empirical therapy.

Nonspecific antidiarrheal agents, such as opiates, can reduce stool frequency and stool weight, and they may reduce associated symptoms, such as abdominal cramps.[18] Concerns about slowing the clearance of pathogens from the intestine by reducing peristalsis largely have not been borne out. Intraluminal agents, such as bismuth subsalicylate (Pepto-Bismol) and adsorbants (e.g., kaolin) are also sometimes used [*see Table 2*].

Therapy for Specific Infections and Syndromes

Campylobacter A frequent cause of acute ileocolitis in the United States,[19] *Campylobacter* infection is usually acquired by eating undercooked chicken; it has an incubation period of up to 1 week. Ulceration of the colonic mucosa and bloody diarrhea may occur with this infection. Antibiotics, such as erythromycin or perhaps a fluoroquinolone (although fluoroquinolone resistance is increasingly reported with *Campylobacter* species), shorten the course of the illness if given within the first few days of symptoms.

Salmonella enteritidis and *S. cholerasuis* These nontyphoidal *Salmonella* species are spread via contaminated food or water and cause acute gastroenteritis, ileocolitis, or colitis characterized by watery diarrhea.[20] Antibiotic therapy with a fluoroquinolone, trimethoprim-sulfamethoxazole, or ampicillin should be reserved for severely ill patients or patients with compromised immunity (e.g., infants, the elderly, pregnant women, and AIDS patients).[21]

Salmonella typhi This organism causes typhoid fever, a form of enteric fever.[22] The propensity of *S. typhi* to produce bacteremia distinguishes it from other enteric pathogens. When the infection is limited to the intestine of an otherwise healthy person, no specific therapy is indicated, because antibiotics may paradoxically prolong excretion of the organism and increase relapses. When the infection becomes systemic and the patient is very ill, therapy is necessary, especially if the organism produces a metastatic endovascular infection. Fluoroquinolones are most often used. The diagnosis of a carrier state is is made when stool cultures are found to be positive for a period longer than 1 year.

Shigella *Shigella* species are invasive organisms, but they also produce an enterotoxin that reduces water and electrolyte absorption.[23] Shigellosis commonly causes a watery diarrhea initially (this watery diarrhea is most likely related to the *Shigella* enterotoxin). This is followed by a bloody diarrhea, which results from colitis produced by invasion of the colonic mucosa. Treatment with a fluoroquinolone is recommended for most patients with shigellosis.

E. coli serotype O157:H7 This organism has become a common cause of food-borne infection in the United States.[24] It produces toxins similar to those produced by *Shigella*.[25] Infection with this organism causes a hemorrhagic segmental colitis. The disease often occurs in large outbreaks from contamination of widely distributed foods, such as hamburger meat. Patients can become quite ill; hemolytic-uremic syndrome is a well-recognized complication. Antibiotics do not seem to improve the course of the illness and may be associated with the development of hemolytic-uremic syndrome in children, although this is controversial.[16,17]

Clostridium difficile *C. difficile* has become the most common cause of nosocomial diarrhea in many institutions.[26] In nonhospitalized adults, carriage rates for this organism are low, but it is spread easily from person to person by spores. Suppression of the normal bacterial flora of the colon by antibiotic therapy can result in the overgrowth of *C. difficile*, if it is present. In institutional settings, the organism can be distributed efficiently to a large pool of susceptible patients by health care workers who do not wash their hands. The disease produced can range from a simple, self-limited diarrhea to a fulminant colitis.

Treatment for 2 weeks with metronidazole, 250 mg four times daily, or vancomycin, 125 to 500 mg four times daily, is effective against *C. difficile*. Relapses occur in up to 25% of patients, however, probably because of residual spores. Ingestion of probiotic bacteria or the nonpathogenic yeast *Saccharomyces boulardii* may reduce relapse rates. In most instances of relapse, longer periods of antibiotic therapy are indicated.

Other nosocomial diarrheas Noninfectious causes of nosocomial diarrhea include medications—particularly elixirs that contain sorbitol or mannitol as noncaloric sweeteners and cancer chemotherapeutic drugs—enteral feeding, and paradoxical diarrhea in patients with fecal impaction. Infections with organisms other than *C. difficile* also occur in institutions, particularly extended-stay facilities. An important cohort of hospital patients that may develop infectious diarrhea are those who are immunocompromised by diseases such as AIDS, or by drugs used to prevent transplant rejection or to treat inflammatory diseases. These patients are often infected with opportunistic

Table 2 Nonspecific Treatment of Diarrhea

Category	Treatment	Typical Adult Dose
Rehydration	Intravenous fluid	1–5 L/24 hr
	Oral rehydration solution	1–5 L/24 hr
Intraluminal agents	Adsorbents (kaolin-pectin)	15–60 ml q.i.d
	Bismuth subsalicylate	30 ml q.i.d.
	Texture modifiers (psyllium)	18–30 g/24 hr
Drugs that inhibit transit	*Opiates*	
	Deodorized tincture of opium (10 mg morphine/ml)	5–20 drops q.i.d.
	Paregoric (0.4 mg morphine/ml)	5–10 ml q.i.d.
	Morphine sulfate (20 mg/ml)	2–10 drops q.i.d.
	Codeine phosphate or sulfate	15–60 mg q.i.d.
	Diphenoxylate with atropine	1–2 tablets q.i.d.
	Difenoxin with atropine	1–2 tablets q.i.d.
	Loperamide (2 mg)	1–2 tablets q.i.d.
	Others	
	Clonidine	0.1–0.3 mg t.i.d.
	Octreotide injection	50–200 mg t.i.d.

Table 3 Major Causes of Chronic Diarrhea

Osmotic diarrhea
  Osmotic laxative abuse
    Mg^{2+}, SO_4^{2-}, PO_4^{3-}, lactulose, mannitol, sorbitol, PEG
  Carbohydrate malabsorption
    Lactose, fructose, others
Fatty diarrhea
  Malabsorption syndromes
    Mucosal diseases
    Short bowel syndrome
    Postresection diarrhea
    Small bowel bacterial overgrowth
    Mesenteric ischemia
  Maldigestion
    Pancreatic insufficiency
    Reduced luminal bile acid
Inflammatory diarrhea
  Inflammatory bowel disease
    Ulcerative colitis
    Crohn disease
    Diverticulitis
    Ulcerative jejunoileitis
  Infections
    Invasive bacterial infection
    Clostridium, E. coli, tuberculosis, others

Ulcerating viral infection
  Cytomegalovirus
  Herpes simplex
Invasive parasites
  Amebiasis
  Strongyloides
Ischemic colitis
Radiation enterocolitis
Neoplasia
  Carcinoma of the colon
  Lymphoma
Secretory diarrhea
  Congenital chloridorrhea
  Chronic infections
  Inflammatory bowel disease
    Ulcerative colitis
    Crohn disease (ileum)
    Microscopic colitis
      Lymphocytic colitis
      Collagenous colitis
    Diverticulitis
  Drugs and poisons
    Stimulant laxative abuse

Disordered regulation
  Postvagotomy
  Postsympathectomy
  Diabetic neuropathy
  Irritable bowel syndrome
Ileal bile acid malabsorption
Endocrine diarrhea
  Hyperthyroidism
  Addison disease
Neuroendocrine tumors
  Gastrinoma
  VIPoma
  Somatostatinoma
  Mastocytosis
  Carcinoid syndrome
  Medullary carcinoma of the thyroid
Other neoplasia
  Colon carcinoma
  Lymphoma
  Villous adenoma
Idiopathic secretory diarrhea
  Epidemic (Brainerd)
  Sporadic

pathogens, including viruses (e.g., cytomegalovirus, herpesvirus), bacteria (e.g., *Mycobacterium avium* complex), and parasites (e.g., *Cryptosporidium* species, *Strongyloides* species).[27] In addition, bone marrow transplant recipients may develop acute diarrhea from graft versus host disease.

Parasites Acute diarrhea in noninstitutionalized patients can be from parasitic infection.[28] The likelihood of parasitic disease as a cause of acute diarrhea is profoundly influenced by geography and epidemiologic features. For example, giardiasis is a common infection in some areas but not others, probably because of variability in the effectiveness of water treatment. Ingestion of as few as a dozen cysts of *G. lamblia* may result in an infection. This accounts for the frequency of person-to-person transmission of this disease. ELISA for *Giardia* antigen is superior to microscopic inspection of stool (so-called ova and parasites testing) for the detection of giardiasis. Therapy with metronidazole is effective in most patients, but reinfection can occur.

Amebiasis is also common in some areas. Persons with amebiasis may be asymptomatic or extremely ill from spread of infection to other organs, such as the liver. Diagnosis is typically made by microscopic examination of fresh stools, but ELISA shows promise in distinguishing the pathogenic species *E. histolytica* from nonpathogenic amebae. The colonoscopic appearance of amebiasis often is distinctive, and the organism can be identified in colonic biopsy specimens.

Other parasites that may cause acute diarrhea include *Cryptosporidium, Isospora, Cyclospora,* and *Strongyloides* species, as well as *Trichuris trichiura* (whipworm). Special tests that may be necessary to identify these parasites include concentration of stool samples, acid-fast stains of stool, and mucosal biopsy. If these organisms are suspected, consultation with the laboratory staff allows use of the proper diagnostic tests.

Chronic Diarrhea

CLASSIFICATION

In contrast to acute diarrhea, in which infection is the overwhelmingly likely cause of illness, chronic diarrhea has an extensive and daunting list of possible causes [see *Table 3*].[3] The simplest approach to diagnosis is to classify chronic diarrhea by the characteristics of the stools. Three categories of chronic diarrhea are recognized: watery, inflammatory, and fatty. Watery diarrheas can be subdivided further into osmotic and secretory diarrheas on the basis of stool analysis.

WATERY DIARRHEAS

Osmotic Diarrheas

Osmotic diarrheas result from the ingestion of an osmotically active, poorly absorbable substance that necessitates the retention of water within the gut lumen to maintain isosmolar conditions.[29] In practical terms, osmotic diarrheas are caused by ingestion of osmotic laxatives (magnesium, phosphate, and sulfate salts; sugar analogs, such as lactulose; sugar alcohols, such as mannitol or sorbitol; and polyethylene glycol) and carbohydrate malabsorption. The ingestion of osmotic laxatives may be purposeful (i.e., laxative abuse) or accidental, as when excess magnesium is ingested as part of a mineral supplement or multivitamin tablet. Carbohydrate malabsorption is most often the result of acquired lactase deficiency (a normal development after adolescence) or mucosal disease, such as celiac sprue, that interferes with nutrient absorption.

Secretory Diarrheas

Secretory diarrhea has a much larger differential diagnosis than osmotic diarrhea [see *Table 3*].

Congenital chloridorrhea Rarely, congenital absence of a transporter mechanism results in diarrhea. This is the case in congenital chloridorrhea, in which the chloride-bicarbonate exchanger in the ileum is not active.[30] Under such conditions, chloride becomes poorly absorbable in the distal bowel and obligates intraluminal water retention.

Chronic infections Some bacterial infections can last long enough to produce chronic secretory diarrhea.[31] These include *Aeromonas* and *Pleisiomonas* species, enteropathogenic *E. coli*, *C. difficile*, *M. tuberculosis*, and *Yersinia enterocolitica*. A special situation is small bowel bacterial overgrowth syndrome, in which structural problems, such as jejunal diverticulosis, or motility problems, such as those seen in scleroderma, result in proliferation of bacteria in the jejunum.[32] Although this bacterial overgrowth disrupts digestive processes and may produce fatty diarrhea, it also may reduce water and salt absorption, producing secretory diarrhea. Infection with parasites, such as *G. lamblia*, *E. histolytica*, and *Cryptosporidium*, also can produce chronic diarrhea.[33]

Inflammatory bowel disease Typically, inflammatory bowel diseases (e.g., ulcerative colitis, Crohn disease) produce inflammatory diarrhea, with blood and pus in the stool (see below). Watery diarrhea can occur, however, especially when the distal colon is not involved. One form of inflammatory bowel disease that typically produces a watery diarrhea is microscopic colitis syndrome (lymphocytic colitis and collagenous colitis), in which the mucosa is inflamed but not ulcerated.[34] Although diverticulitis usually presents as an acute illness, some patients who have smoldering diverticulitis with relatively low-grade inflammation (and, in some cases, low-grade obstruction) will present with chronic secretory diarrhea, which is probably mediated by inflammation-linked cytokines. Vasculitis and systemic inflammatory diseases may also be associated with secretory diarrhea.

Drugs Drug therapy is a key cause of secretory diarrhea. Many drugs cause diarrhea as a side effect. These include antibiotics; cardiovascular agents, such as beta-adrenergic antagonists, digitalis, and quinidine; cancer chemotherapy; nonsteroidal anti-inflammatory drugs (NSAIDs); and colchicine. Thus, in taking the history of a patient with chronic diarrhea, it is critical to formulate a detailed drug list, including over-the-counter and alternative medications. A special category of drug-induced secretory diarrhea is surreptitious ingestion of stimulant laxatives.

Other causes Disordered motility or regulation can produce secretory diarrhea.[35] Secretory diarrhea associated with disordered motility can occur in patients who have undergone vagotomy or sympathectomy, patients with autonomic neuropathy from diabetes or amyloidosis, and probably patients with irritable bowel syndrome.[36] In the United States, irritable bowel syndrome is the most commonly diagnosed cause of chronic diarrhea. This diagnosis is often incorrect, however, and may delay appropriate treatment.

Malabsorption of bile acid in the ileum occurs in many diarrheal diseases as a result of ileal disease or resection and may be secondary to other processes, such as vagotomy, cholecystectomy, or rapid transit past the ileum. In a relatively small number of patients, idiopathic bile acid malabsorption is a cause of diarrhea.[37]

Endocrine causes of secretory diarrhea include hyperthyroidism, Addison disease, and a group of rare tumors of the endocrine cells of the gut, including gastrinomas, carcinoid tumors, vasoactive intestinal polypeptide–secreting tumors, somatostatinomas, and medullary carcinoma of the thyroid.[38] These tumors produce peptides and other mediators that affect intestinal mucosal and muscle function and thereby lead to diarrhea. In most cases, rapid intestinal transit seems to be the major mechanism producing diarrhea, although this remains controversial.[39]

Other tumors that produce secretory diarrhea include colon cancer (through an uncertain mechanism), villous adenoma of the rectum, lymphoma, and mastocytosis. Mastocytosis (and probably some lymphomas) produce diarrhea through the release of histamine or other mediators that affect gut function. Infiltration of the mucosa by mast cells or lymphoid cells also may play a role in some cases.

Secretory diarrhea can also be idiopathic.[40] Idiopathic secretory diarrhea occurs in both sporadic and epidemic forms and may be caused by an as-yet unidentified infection.

INFLAMMATORY DIARRHEAS

Inflammatory diarrheas are characterized by the presence of blood and pus in the stools, which usually occurs as a result of ulceration of the mucosa. Inflammatory bowel diseases, such as Crohn disease and ulcerative colitis, are in this category. Some patients with diverticulitis and diarrhea may have blood and pus in the stool, as do patients with the rare condition ulcerative jejunoileitis. Ulcerating infectious diseases may also produce inflammatory diarrhea. These include pseudomembranous colitis from *C. difficile* infection; invasive bacterial infections, such as tuberculosis and yersiniosis; ulcerating viral infections, such as those caused by cytomegalovirus or herpesvirus; and invasive parasitic infections, such as amebiasis and *Strongyloides*. Inflammatory diarrhea also may be seen with ischemic colitis and radiation colitis, as well as colon cancer and lymphoma.

FATTY DIARRHEAS

Fatty diarrhea may result from fat malabsorption in mucosal diseases, such as celiac disease or Whipple disease; short bowel syndrome secondary to extensive surgical resection of the small intestine; small bowel bacterial overgrowth syndrome; and mesenteric ischemia. Fatty diarrhea also may be the consequence of maldigestion of fat caused by pancreatic exocrine deficiency or inadequate luminal bile acid concentration.

DIAGNOSIS

An accurate medical history is even more important for patients with chronic diarrhea than for those with acute diarrhea. In addition to all the issues that should be discussed with patients who have acute diarrhea [see Acute Diarrhea, *above*], the history of patients with chronic diarrhea should include long-term trends in body weight, current appetite and food intake, a review of previous medical problems and surgeries, potential secondary gains from illness, previous evaluations and treatments of diarrhea, and a detailed review of systems to look for clues to systemic illnesses [see Table 4].

A principal diagnostic distinction in chronic diarrhea is between diarrhea associated with irritable bowel syndrome and diarrhea associated with other functional or organic problems. Irritable bowel syndrome is characterized by abdominal pain

Table 4   Steps in the Evaluation and Classification of Chronic Diarrhea[3]

Step	Elements	Findings/Considerations
History	Onset	Congenital, abrupt, gradual
	Pattern	Continuous, intermittent
	Duration	—
	Epidemiologic features	Travel, food, water
	Stool characteristics	Watery, bloody, fatty
	Fecal incontinence	—
	Abdominal pain	Occurs in inflammatory bowel disease, irritable bowel syndrome, ischemia
	Weight loss	May be severe in malabsorption or neoplasm
	Aggravating factors	Diet, stress
	Mitigating factors	Diet, over-the-counter drugs, prescription drugs
	Previous medical evaluation	—
	Iatrogenic diarrhea	From drugs, radiation, surgery
	Factitious diarrhea	Laxatives; may be surreptitious
	Systemic disease	Diarrhea may complicate hyperthyroidism, diabetes mellitus, collagen vascular disease, tumor syndromes, AIDS, immunoglobulin deficiencies
Routine laboratory tests	CBC	Anemia, leukocytosis
	Serum chemistry	Fluid/electrolyte status, nutritional status, serum protein/globulin
Stool analysis	Weight	—
	Electrolytes	For calculating fecal osmotic gap
	pH	Acid stools suggest carbohydrate malabsorption
	Stool leukocytes	Found in inflammatory diarrhea
	Fat output	Can be assessed by Sudan stain or quantitatively
	Laxative screen	
Categorization	Watery diarrhea (secretory or osmotic)	—
	Inflammatory diarrhea	
	Fatty diarrhea	

associated with defecation and an altered bowel habit.[41] Variable stool consistency and intermittent constipation are common. Painless diarrhea was once considered a type of irritable bowel syndrome but is no longer; other causes of diarrhea should be sought in such cases.

Physical Examination

The physical examination may provide clues to the cause of chronic diarrhea. Characteristic skin changes may be seen in mastocytosis, glucagonoma, Addison disease, amyloidosis, carcinoid syndrome, Degos disease, and celiac disease. Amyloidosis may produce orthostatic hypotension and hepatosplenomegaly. Thyroid nodules or signs of hyperthyroidism may suggest medullary carcinoma of the thyroid, Graves disease, or other diseases that cause hyperthyroidism. Carcinoid syndrome may produce hepatosplenomegaly, edema, and a right-sided heart murmur in addition to flushing. Arthritis may be a clue to inflammatory bowel disease, Whipple disease, and some enteric infections. Lymphadenopathy could be present in patients with AIDS or lymphoma. The absence of peripheral arterial pulses or the presence of bruits suggests the possibility of mesenteric vascular disease. Rectal examination may disclose defective anal sphincter or pelvic floor muscle function, which could produce fecal incontinence. The physical findings that reflect the severity of diarrhea should also be recorded [*see* Acute Diarrhea, *above*].

Laboratory Tests

As in acute diarrhea, routine laboratory testing is indicated to help determine the severity of chronic diarrhea [*see* Acute Diarrhea, *above*]. Unlike acute diarrhea, in which stool analysis is typically not used, stool analysis plays a key role in the assessment of chronic diarrhea by allowing categorization of the type of diarrhea, thereby limiting the number of conditions to be considered.[3] The stool analysis can be obtained through either a random sample or a timed collection. The value of a timed collection is that it allows the physician to quantitate stool output accurately. However, stool analysis obtained through a random sample still can provide many diagnostic clues.

Stool characteristics to measure include sodium and potassium concentrations, osmolality, and pH. Measurement of stool electrolyte concentrations allows calculation of the fecal osmotic gap [*see* Fecal Osmotic Gap, *above*]. This can be used to determine whether watery diarrhea is osmotic or secretory. Measurement of actual stool osmolality is of value only in detecting samples that have been contaminated (unintentionally or deliberately) with water or dilute urine and therefore have an osmolality less than 290 mOsm/kg. Stool osmolality rises rapidly in vitro because of bacterial fermentation, so the actual measurement should not be used to calculate the fecal osmotic gap. The pH of stool water can indicate whether or not carbohydrate malabsorption is present. Carbohydrates (or sugar alcohols) that are not absorbed in the small bowel and so reach the bacterial flora of the colon are fermented into short-chain fatty acids that reduce fecal pH, usually to less than 6. Thus, acid stools suggest carbohydrate malabsorption.[8]

Other helpful tests include fecal occult blood testing and examination of stool for leukocytes (or a surrogate chemical test, such as fecal lactoferrin concentration), which can be used to identify an inflammatory diarrhea. Fatty diarrhea can be identi-

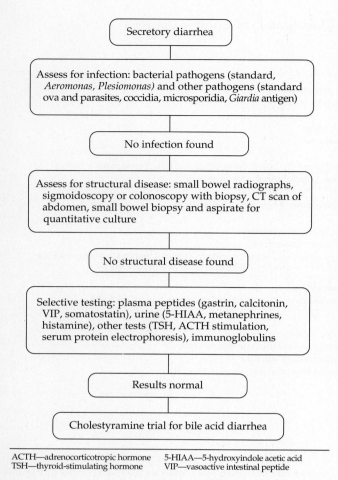

ACTH—adrenocorticotropic hormone   5-HIAA—5-hydroxyindole acetic acid
TSH—thyroid-stimulating hormone   VIP—vasoactive intestinal peptide

Figure 3   **Evaluation of chronic secretory diarrhea.[3] Every test does not need to be done for every patient.**

fied by measurement of stool fat, although careful interpretation of the results is sometimes necessary [*see* Steatorrhea, *below*].

When appropriate, a laxative screen should be obtained. Measurement of laxatives by chemical or chromatographic methods can detect surreptitious laxative ingestion.

Completion of the stool analysis allows the clinician to characterize chronic diarrhea as watery (whether secretory or osmotic), inflammatory, or fatty. The subsequent evaluation depends on this categorization.

Evaluation of Watery Secretory Diarrhea

Secretory diarrhea has a broad differential diagnosis, so a thorough evaluation is needed [*see Figure 3*].

Stool testing   Infection should be excluded by stool culture for bacteria, stool assay for *C. difficile* toxin, and other stool tests for parasites, including ELISA for giardiasis. Biopsies of the small bowel or colon may be necessary to find the pathogens, especially in patients with AIDS or other immunodeficiencies. Quantitative culture of small bowel aspirate is the best test for detecting small bowel bacterial overgrowth.

Imaging and endoscopic tests   Structural diseases (e.g., short bowel syndrome or fistula, mucosal diseases, inflammatory bowel disease, and tumors) should be sought by radiographic and endoscopic testing. Small bowel radiography re-

mains important in these patients. CT scans can detect small bowel and colonic disease, as well as problems extrinsic to the gut that may cause diarrhea, such as endocrine tumors. Inspection of the colonic mucosa by colonoscopy or sigmoidoscopy is essential in patients with secretory diarrhea, both to evaluate for gross changes and to obtain biopsy specimens to look for evidence of microscopic colitis syndrome. Biopsies should be performed even if the gross appearance of the colon is normal, because of the prevalence of microscopic colitis syndrome in patients with chronic watery diarrhea (see below). A long endoscope that can reach the jejunum to obtain biopsy specimens and aspirates is a valuable adjunct when other studies are unrevealing. The role of capsule endoscopy in the evaluation of patients with chronic diarrhea is uncertain, and it does not allow for biopsy of abnormalities that are seen.

Serum peptide measurement   Because diarrheagenic endocrine tumors are very rare, the measurement of serum peptides (e.g., gastrin, vasoactive intestinal polypeptide, calcitonin, and glucagon) or urinary secretagogue metabolites (e.g., 5-hydroxyindoleacetic acid or metanephrine) should be restricted to patients with symptoms consistent with tumor syndromes or those in whom a diagnosis remains elusive after initial testing.[42] More common endocrine problems, such as diabetes, hyperthyroidism, or Addison disease, should be excluded with appropriate blood tests.

Bile acid absorption measurement   Ileal resection or ileal disease can result in the escape of sufficient bile acid into the colon to increase luminal bile acid concentrations above 3 to 5 mmol. At those concentrations, bile acids reduce colonic mucosal water and electrolyte absorption; alternatively, they may stimulate secretion, resulting in increased stool water. In most circumstances, bile acid malabsorption can be inferred from a history of ileal resection or disease. More controversial is the concept that bile acid malabsorption occurring in the absence of ileal resection or obvious ileal disease is responsible for idiopathic secretory diarrhea.[43] Although bile acid malabsorption can be documented in many of these patients, administration of bile acid–binding resins does not always mitigate diarrhea in those patients, casting doubts on bile acid malabsorption as a cause of their diarrhea.[37] Therefore, in patients with secretory diarrhea that appears to be idiopathic, it is more practical to give a therapeutic trial of bile acid–binding resins than to measure bile acid malabsorption directly.

Evaluation of Watery Osmotic Diarrhea

The differential diagnosis of osmotic diarrhea is more limited than that of secretory diarrhea, so the evaluation is simpler [*see Figure 4*]. If stool water has low electrolyte concentrations (and therefore a high fecal osmotic gap), some other substance is taking up the osmotic space and is holding water in the lumen. In practice, this substance is usually ingested magnesium or malabsorbed carbohydrates.

Fecal magnesium   Magnesium can be measured accurately in stool water. Excretion of more than 15 mmol (30 mEq) daily or a concentration of greater than 45 mmol/L (90 mEq/L) in a random stool sample strongly suggests magnesium-induced diarrhea.[44] This may be intentional (surreptitious laxative ingestion) or accidental (use of magnesium-containing antacids or mineral supplements).

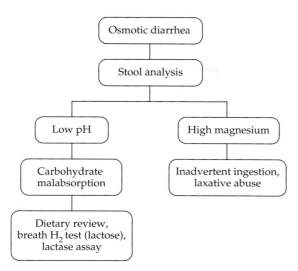

Figure 4 **Evaluation of chronic osmotic diarrhea.³ Every test does not need to be done for every patient.**

Carbohydrate absorption Carbohydrate malabsorption can occur from ingestion of poorly absorbable carbohydrates, such as lactose in a person with lactase deficiency, or from reduced carbohydrate absorption as a result of small bowel mucosal disease. In addition to lactose, common causes of osmotic diarrhea include excessive ingestion of fructose (often used as a sweetener in commercial food products), ingestion of poorly absorbed sugar alcohols (such as mannitol and sorbitol, which are used as low-calorie sweeteners), and use of inhibitors of carbohydrate absorption, such as acarbose. Because malabsorbed carbohydrate is rapidly fermented by colonic bacteria, gas and bloating are frequent symptoms in these patients. Diagnosis is made on the basis of a finding of low stool pH (typically less than 6) and a thorough dietary history.

Evaluation of Chronic Inflammatory Diarrhea

Patients with WBCs or blood in the stool are classified as having inflammatory diarrhea. Causes may include inflammatory bowel disease, infections, ischemia, radiation enteritis, and neoplasia [*see Table 3*]. Sometimes these conditions produce a watery, secretory diarrhea without blood or pus in the stool, so they must be considered in the evaluation of patients with nonbloody diarrhea.

Imaging and endoscopic tests Evaluation should start with radiographic and endoscopic tests to look for structural problems [*see Figure 5*]. Sigmoidoscopy or colonoscopy should be considered first, because colitis is a common cause of inflammatory diarrhea. Biopsies should be performed to properly categorize colitis. CT has proved useful in many of these patients because of its ability to visualize inflammatory changes in the small bowel and colon and to identify complications of inflammation, such as abscess.

Infections that may produce chronic diarrhea, such as *C. difficile*, cytomegalovirus, amebiasis, and tuberculosis, need to be excluded by culture, biopsy, or serologic testing. It is important to realize that infection may complicate the courses of established disorders, such as ulcerative colitis or Crohn disease. Patients with AIDS need an especially careful search for opportunistic infections (see below).

Evaluation of Chronic Fatty Diarrhea

Steatorrhea Excessive fat in the stools implies a problem with fat solubilization, digestion, or absorption in the small intestine [*see Figure 6*]. Steatorrhea is usually defined as stool fat output of more than 7 g/24 hr or more than 9% of daily intake. These criteria may not be valid in patients with diarrhea, however, because voluminous stools per se can increase fat excretion. In one study, artificially induced diarrhea produced mild steatorrhea of up to 14 g/24 hr in 35% of normal persons.⁴⁵ Thus, in patients with diarrhea, fecal fat excretion of 7 to 14 g/24 hr has a low specificity for defective fat absorption. The threshold for diagnosing steatorrhea also should be corrected for fat intake, because some patients with diarrhea have anorexia and some patients with steatorrhea have hyperphagia. When possible, fat intake should be estimated from diet diaries maintained during the collection period. Finally, measurement of fat excretion can be compromised by ingestion of poorly absorbed fat substitutes, such as olestra.

Qualitative estimation of fat excretion by Sudan stain of a fecal smear can be used when a timed collection or quantitative analysis is not possible. Semiquantitative methods employing assessment of the number and size of fat globules correlate well with quantitative analysis of fat excretion.

The fecal fat concentration may provide a clue to the etiology of steatorrhea. The major causes of steatorrhea are mucosal diseases (e.g., celiac disease), pancreatic exocrine insufficiency (e.g., chronic pancreatitis), and lack of bile acids (e.g., advanced biliary cirrhosis). Mucosal diseases are often associated with reduced fluid and electrolyte absorption; as a result, fat is diluted by unabsorbed water. Furthermore, in mucosal disease, fat still can be digested to fatty acids, which can inhibit water absorption in the colon. In contrast, diseases that alter fat solubilization or digestion typically do not alter mucosal water and electrolyte absorption; as a result, unabsorbed fat is disbursed in a smaller stool volume. Fecal fat concentrations of greater than 9.5 g/100 g strongly suggest pancreatic or biliary steatorrhea.⁴⁶

Imaging and endoscopic tests If the cause of steatorrhea is not obvious from the patient's history and the results of fecal fat assessment, the next step is evaluation of the absorptive surface of the small intestine by endoscopic, histologic, and radiographic tests. During endoscopy, small bowel biopsy specimens should be obtained for histologic analysis, and small

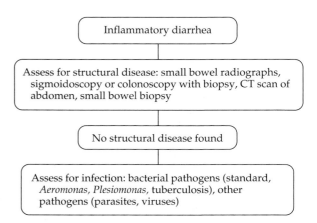

Figure 5 **Evaluation of chronic inflammatory diarrhea.³ Every test does not need to be done for every patient.**

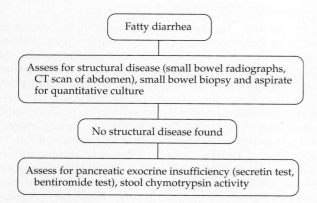

Figure 6 **Evaluation of chronic fatty diarrhea.[3] Every test does not need to be done for every patient.**

bowel contents should be aspirated for quantitative culture to assess for small bowel bacterial overgrowth. Indirect tests, such as measurement of antigliadin, endomysial (antireticulin) antibodies, or tissue transglutaminase antibodies for the diagnosis of celiac disease or breath tests for bacterial overgrowth, have not displaced endoscopic testing as the gold standard for diagnosis of these conditions. These tests may, however, be useful in some cases. Small bowel radiography and CT are valuable adjuncts for structural assessment in these patients.

If the absorptive surface is normal, attention should shift to luminal problems with fat solubilization or digestion. Testing for pancreatic exocrine insufficiency is rarely done, because of unwillingness to use duodenal intubation tests. Indirect tests, such as the bentiromide test and measurement of stool chymotrypsin activity, have limited sensitivity and specificity. The best test for pancreatic exocrine insufficiency may be a therapeutic trial of pancreatic enzyme supplementation. If this is done, a large dose of enzymes should be administered and fat excretion should be measured to assess the response to therapy. Likewise, testing for the adequacy of the solubilization of fat by bile salts is rarely done. If necessary, duodenal bile salt concentration can be measured.

TREATMENT

Nonspecific Therapy

Nonspecific therapy is used for patients with chronic diarrhea in three situations: (1) as a temporizing or initial therapy before diagnostic testing, (2) after diagnostic testing has failed to result in a diagnosis, and (3) when a diagnosis has been made but no specific treatment is available or specific treatment fails.[18]

Antibiotic therapy Antibiotics are less useful in chronic diarrhea than in acute diarrhea because bacterial infection is less likely to be the cause of chronic diarrhea. Nevertheless, many clinicians try an empirical course of metronidazole or a fluoroquinolone before starting an extensive evaluation.

Symptomatic therapy with antidiarrheal drugs is often required in patients with chronic diarrhea. Loperamide or diphenoxylate with atropine can be tried initially [*see Table 2*]. In patients with chronic diarrhea, routine dosing (e.g., two tablets before each meal or at bedtime) is more effective than as-needed dosing after passing loose stools. More potent opiates, such as codeine, opium, or morphine, are underutilized in patients who do not respond to loperamide or diphenoxylate with at-

ropine. Although these are controlled substances because of the possibility of abuse, abuse is unlikely in closely monitored patients with chronic diarrhea. Dosing should be started at a low level (e.g., codeine, 30 mg q.i.d.; deodorized tincture of opium, 3 drops q.i.d.; or morphine, 2 mg q.i.d.) and titrated up gradually to an effective dose. Stool-modifying agents, such as psyllium, can alter stool consistency but do not reduce stool weight. They may be of special help in patients with coexisting fecal incontinence.

Treatment of Selected Specific Diseases and Syndromes

Osmotic diarrhea Osmotic diarrhea should abate with fasting or elimination of the offending agent from the diet. This response may be incomplete if other diarrhea-producing mechanisms are still active, such as short bowel syndrome or diseases of small bowel mucosa.

Irritable bowel syndrome and functional diarrhea Patients with chronic diarrhea in whom no other etiology is established are commonly diagnosed with irritable bowel syndrome or functional diarrhea. Irritable bowel syndrome is characterized chiefly by abdominal pain that is associated with altered bowel function, including constipation, diarrhea, or alternating diarrhea and constipation.[41] A diagnosis of functional diarrhea is made when patients do not have prominent abdominal pain and have no evidence of other specific causes for diarrhea. Obviously, these diagnoses are reliable only if a thorough evaluation has been done to exclude other causes of diarrhea. For example, most cases of diarrhea from malabsorption of bile acid or carbohydrates are characterized as functional diarrhea or irritable bowel syndrome because specific testing for those disorders is not done. Thus, careful consideration of alternative diagnoses should precede a diagnosis of irritable bowel syndrome or functional diarrhea in patients with chronic diarrhea.

Nevertheless, there are certain clues to the diagnosis of irritable bowel syndrome or functional diarrhea that should be sought by the physician. Features that suggest a diagnosis of irritable bowel syndrome include a long history of diarrhea, dating back to adolescence or young adulthood; passage of mucus; and exacerbation of symptoms with stress. Historical points that argue against irritable bowel syndrome include recent onset of diarrhea, especially in older patients; nocturnal diarrhea; weight loss; blood in stools; voluminous stools (> 400 g/24 hr); and blood tests indicating anemia, leukocytosis, or low serum albumin concentration or a high erythrocyte sedimentation rate.

The treatment of irritable bowel syndrome is discussed in detail elsewhere [*see Chapter 62*].

Microscopic colitis syndrome This disorder, which subsumes the diagnoses of lymphocytic colitis and collagenous colitis, is a frequent cause of chronic diarrhea.[34] Microscopic colitis syndrome is characterized by chronic watery diarrhea and microscopic evidence of mucosal inflammation in the presence of normal gross colonoscopic findings. Histologic findings in both lymphocytic colitis and collagenous colitis include intraepithelial lymphocytic infiltration and chronic inflammation in the lamina propria without crypt destruction. Collagenous colitis and lymphocytic colitis are distinguished by the presence or absence of a thickened subepithelial collagen layer.

The cause of microscopic colitis syndrome is uncertain. It is associated with many autoimmune disorders and immunologically mediated diseases, such as celiac disease, which suggests that immune dysregulation is important. Bacterial antigens within the colonic lumen may play a role as well. NSAIDs have been implicated in some reports.

Women are more likely than men to have collagenous colitis; lymphocytic colitis occurs equally in men and women. Diarrhea is of moderate severity (typically, 500 to 1,000 g/24 hr) and is characteristically secretory in nature because it results from the failure of the colonic mucosa to absorb water and salt. Diagnosis is made by obtaining biopsy material from normal-appearing mucosa during sigmoidoscopy or colonoscopy.

Treatment options include bismuth subsalicylate, budesonide, 5-aminosalicylate drugs, prednisone, and azathioprine.[34] Bile acid–binding drugs also have been reported to be successful in reducing diarrhea.[47] Microscopic colitis can have a remitting and relapsing course, and symptomatic therapy with opiate antidiarrheal drugs may be all that is needed. There is no evidence that microscopic colitis is a risk factor for colon carcinoma; no surveillance program is currently recommended.

Laxative abuse Although rarely suspected, laxative abuse occurs regularly in four groups of patients: (1) those with anorexia or bulimia, (2) those who obtain secondary gain from illness (e.g., disability payments or attention from relatives), (3) those with Munchausen syndrome, and (4) those who are dependent on others for health care and who are poisoned by their caregivers (caregivers who do this are usually motivated by the desire to demonstrate their devotion to the patients).[48] Physicians need to consider surreptitious laxative abuse in patients who confound diagnosis and who are in one of those categories.

Detection of laxative abuse requires a high index of suspicion. Clues include the presence of hypokalemia in a patient who is able to eat (suggesting stimulant laxative abuse or concurrent ingestion of diuretics), melanosis coli (brownish pigmentation in the colonic mucosa resulting from ingestion of anthraquinone laxatives) in a patient being evaluated for chronic diarrhea, or a large fecal osmotic gap (seen with magnesium ingestion). Most laxatives can be detected in stool water by chemical techniques. Adulteration of stool by added water or hypotonic urine is evidenced by low stool osmolality (< 250 mOsm/kg). The addition of hypertonic urine is evidenced by impossibly high stool osmolality (> 600 mOsm/kg) and the presence of a negative fecal osmotic gap resulting from high urine sodium or potassium concentrations. Negative fecal osmotic gaps may also be calculated in patients ingesting laxatives containing phosphate or sulfate.

Before confronting patients with the diagnosis of laxative abuse, testing should be confirmed on another stool specimen, and appropriate psychiatric consultation should be available, because some of these patients become suicidal when confronted, and all of them need counseling. In cases of laxative poisoning by a caregiver, legal proceedings need to be instituted to separate the patient from the caregiver. Outcome studies in laxative abuse patients are few. One study suggested that nearly half of the patients sought further medical attention elsewhere for chronic diarrhea.[49]

Postsurgical diarrhea Diarrhea can occur after several different kinds of operations. Peptic ulcer surgery is less common than it used to be, but new kinds of gastric operations, such as gastric bypass for obesity, produce similar complications. Dumping syndrome is the term used to describe a condition characterized by postprandial flushing, hypotension, diarrhea, and hypoglycemia.[50] This syndrome results from unregulated gastric emptying, osmotic shifts of fluid into the gut, and the rapid release of peptide hormones from the small intestine. Dumping syndrome can occur after vagotomy (intentional or accidental), pyloroplasty, gastrojejunostomy, and gastric resection. It can be treated with dietary modifications, antidiarrheal drugs [see Table 2], and injection of the somatostatin analog octreotide. Gastric surgery may also predispose patients to bacterial overgrowth in the small intestine, abnormally rapid intestinal transit, bile acid malabsorption, and pancreatic exocrine insufficiency from inadequate stimulation of the pancreas.

Bowel resection can result in loss of surface area sufficient to impair absorption of nutrients or water and salt. Lesser degrees of resection can result in diarrhea if an area of specialized function is removed.[51] For example, resection of the terminal ileum and right colon reduces bile acid absorption and the ability to absorb sodium against a large electrochemical gradient; these defects cannot be overcome by other areas of the intestine. With time, intestinal adaptation can overcome impaired electrolyte absorption, but intestinal adaptation cannot reverse loss of these specialized functions.

Ileostomy diarrhea is said to occur when stoma output exceeds 1,000 ml/24 hr. It may be caused by loss of absorptive surface area if a substantial length of bowel has been resected; it may also result from stomal stenosis, partial bowel obstruction, bacterial overgrowth, recurrent bowel disease, medications, or intraperitoneal infection.[52] A special situation occurs in patients with ulcerative colitis who have had an ileoanal anastomosis with creation of an ileal reservoir pouch. These patients may develop inflammation of the pouch (so-called pouchitis) from bacterial overgrowth or recurrent inflammatory bowel disease.[53] Pouchitis can be treated with antibiotics such as metronidazole, anti-inflammatory drugs such as mesalamine, or ingestion of probiotic bacteria. Ordinary ileostomy diarrhea can be treated successfully with antidiarrheal opiate drugs.

Postcholecystectomy diarrhea occurs in as many as 20% of patients. It may be delayed in onset, and it is rarely severe. Diarrhea may occur as a result of ileal bile acid malabsorption at night, when the migrating motor complex may sweep bile acid past the absorptive sites in the terminal ileum, but some cases may have other causes.[54] Postcholecystectomy diarrhea is best treated with bile acid–binding agents given at bedtime. Opiate antidiarrheal drugs may be needed in refractory cases.

Diabetic diarrhea Up to 30% of patients with long-standing diabetes mellitus may experience chronic diarrhea.[55] This diarrhea has been attributed to autonomic neuropathy and dysregulation of motility, but definite evidence of neuropathy is not always evident. If steatorrhea is present, three conditions that occur with increased prevalence in diabetic patients should be considered: (1) small bowel bacterial overgrowth, (2) pancreatic exocrine insufficiency, and (3) celiac disease. Other causes that need to be considered include medications, such as acarbose, and ingestion of so-called dietetic foods containing sugar alcohols (e.g., sorbitol or mannitol).

When watery diarrhea is present, treatment with clonidine, an alpha$_2$-adrenergic agonist drug, may have special value. When clonidine cannot be tolerated because of its hypotensive effect or when it does not work, opiate antidiarrheal drugs may be effective. Fecal incontinence from diabetic sensorimotor neuropathy may complicate diarrhea; this form of diarrhea is important to diagnose, because therapies to mitigate incontinence, such as biofeedback training, may have a dramatic effect on quality of life.[56]

Diarrhea in patients with AIDS   Diarrhea in AIDS patients is likely to result from opportunistic infections or lymphoma. A careful search for the cause of diarrhea can lead to targeted therapy that may cure the diarrhea.[57] Colonoscopy is preferable to sigmoidoscopy because it allows visualization and biopsy of the right colon and ileum, which are often the sites of infection. It is possible that HIV-1 may directly produce diarrhea (so-called AIDS enteropathy), but in most cases, a specific infection can be identified.

Idiopathic secretory diarrhea   The diagnosis of idiopathic secretory diarrhea can be made after an exhaustive evaluation fails to reveal a cause of chronic secretory diarrhea. This condition often begins suddenly in previously normal persons and is distinguished from acute secretory diarrhea by its persistence beyond 4 weeks. It occurs in two forms, epidemic and sporadic.

Epidemic idiopathic secretory diarrhea occurs in outbreaks that are seemingly related to contaminated food or water.[58] The initial report of this disorder described an epidemic of chronic diarrhea in Brainerd, Minnesota, and the condition has consequently become known as Brainerd diarrhea. Several outbreaks have been described in detail since the initial epidemic, and although the epidemiology suggests an infectious cause, no organism has been isolated.

Sporadic idiopathic secretory diarrhea affects patients in an identical fashion as the epidemic form, but it does not seem to be acquired easily by family members or others.[40] Many patients describe a history of travel to local lakes or recreational sites, but they are the only members of their parties that become ill.

Both forms of idiopathic secretory diarrhea begin abruptly and reach maximum intensity shortly thereafter. Fever is unusual. Weight loss of up to 20 lb characteristically occurs in the first few months of the illness but does not become progressive thereafter. Empirical trials of antibiotics and bile acid–binding drugs are ineffective, but nonspecific opiate antidiarrheal drugs provide some relief. Idiopathic secretory diarrhea is self-limited and usually disappears within 2 years of onset. The resolution of diarrhea is gradual, occurring over 2 to 3 months.

Diarrhea of obscure origin   This condition is said to be present when chronic diarrhea has evaded diagnosis in spite of an evaluation for structural problems. Patients are often referred to centers interested in diarrheal diseases, where a specific cause for their diarrhea is often identified. Common diagnoses in these patients include fecal incontinence, drug-induced diarrhea, surreptitious laxative ingestion, microscopic colitis syndrome, bile acid–induced diarrhea, pancreatic exocrine insufficiency, carbohydrate malabsorption, sporadic chronic idiopathic secretory diarrhea, and, rarely, endocrine tumors. Most of these conditions can be recognized through a careful history, an appropriate index of suspicion, proper testing, or a well-conducted therapeutic trial. Failure to make a diagnosis is usually the result of not thinking through the differential diagnosis of chronic diarrhea and not appreciating the evidence at hand.

References

1. Talley NJ, Weaver AL, Zinsmeister AR, et al: Self-reported diarrhea: what does it mean? Am J Gastroenterol 89:1160, 1994

2. Dupont HL: Guidelines on acute infectious diarrhea in adults. Am J Gastroenterol 92:1962, 1997

3. Fine KD, Schiller LR: AGA technical review on the evaluation and management of chronic diarrhea. Gastroenterology 116:1464, 1999

4. Wenzl HH, Fine KD, Schiller LR, et al: Determinants of decreased fecal consistency in patients with diarrhea. Gastroenterology 108:1729, 1995

5. Sellin JH: Intestinal electrolyte absorption and secretion. Gastrointestinal and Liver Disease Pathophysiology/Diagnosis/Management, 7th ed. Feldman M, Friedman LS, Sleisenger MH, Eds. WB Saunders Co, Philadelphia, 2002, p 1693

6. Schiller LR, Sellin JH: Diarrhea. Gastrointestinal and Liver Disease: Pathophysiology/Diagnosis/Management, 7th ed. Feldman M, Friedman LS, Sleisenger MH, Eds. WB Saunders Co, Philadelphia, 2002, p 131

7. Fordtran JS: Pathophysiology of chronic diarrhoea: insights derived from intestinal perfusion studies in 31 patients. Clin Gastroenterol 15:477, 1986

8. Eherer AJ, Fordtran JS: Fecal osmotic gap and pH in experimental diarrhea of various causes. Gastroenterology 103:545, 1992

9. Vazquez-Torres A, Fang FC: Cellular routes of invasion by enteropathogens. Curr Opin Microbiol 3:54, 2000

10. Crane JK: Preformed bacterial toxins. Clin Lab Med 19:583, 1999

11. Silletti RP, Lee G, Ailey E: Role of stool screening tests in the diagnosis of inflammatory bacterial enteritis and in selection of specimens likely to yield invasive enteric pathogens. J Clin Microbiol 34:1161, 1996

12. Savola KL, Baron EJ, Tompkins LS, et al: Fecal leukocyte stain has diagnostic value for outpatients but not inpatients. J Clin Microbiol 39:266, 2001

13. Bini EJ, Cohen J: Diagnostic yield and cost-effectiveness of endoscopy in chronic human immunodeficiency virus–related diarrhea. Gastrointest Endosc 48:354, 1998

14. Surawicz CM, Haggitt RC, Husseman M, et al: Mucosal biopsy diagnosis of colitis: acute, self-limited colitis and idiopathic inflammatory bowel disease. Gastroenterology 107:755, 1994

15. Desjeux JF, Briend A, Butzner JD: Oral rehydration solution in the year 2000: pathophysiology, efficacy and effectiveness. Baillieres Clin Gastroenterol 11:509, 1997

16. Wong CS, Jelacic S, Habeeb RL, et al: The risk of the hemolytic-uremic syndrome after antibiotic treatment of Escherichia coli O157:H7 infections. N Engl J Med 342:1930, 2000

17. Safdar N, Said A, Gangnon RE, et al: Risk of hemolytic-uremic syndrome after antibiotic treatment of Escherichia coli O157:H7 enteritis: a meta-analysis. JAMA 288:1014, 2002

18. Schiller LR: Review article: antidiarrhoeal pharmacology and therapeutics. Aliment Pharmacol Ther 9:87, 1995

19. Allos BM: Campylobacter jejuni infections: update on emerging issues and trends. Clin Infect Dis 32:1201, 2001

20. Edwards BH: Salmonella and Shigella species. Clin Lab Med 19:469, 1999

21. Oldfield EC 3rd, Wallace MR: The role of antibiotics in the treatment of infectious diarrhea. Gastroenterol Clin North Am 30:817, 2001

22. House D, Bishop A, Parry C, et al: Typhoid fever: pathogenesis and disease. Curr Opin Infect Dis 14:573, 2001

23. Sandvig K: Shiga toxins. Toxicon 39:1629, 2001

24. Tarr PI, Neill MA: Escherichia coli O157:H7. Gastroenterol Clin North Am 30:735, 2001

25. Nakao H, Takeda T: Escherichia coli Shiga toxin. J Nat Toxins 9:299, 2000

26. Moyenuddin M, Williamson JC, Ohl CA: Clostridium difficile–associated diarrhea: current strategies for diagnosis and therapy. Curr Gastroenterol Rep 4:279, 2002

27. Monkemuller KE, Wilcox CM: Investigation of diarrhea in AIDS. Can J Gastroenterol 14:933, 2000

28. Schuster H, Chiodini PL: Parasitic infections of the intestine. Curr Opin Infect Dis 14:587, 2001

29. Hammer HF, Santa Ana CA, Schiller LR, et al: Studies of osmotic diarrhea induced in normal subjects by ingestion of polyethylene glycol and lactulose. J Clin Invest 84:1056, 1989

30. Aichbichler BW, Zerr CH, Santa Ana CA, et al: Proton-pump inhibition of gastric chloride secretion in congenital chloridorrhea. N Engl J Med 336:106, 1997

31. Lee SD, Surawicz CM: Infectious causes of chronic diarrhea. Gastroenterol Clin North Am 30:679, 2001

32. Attar A, Flourie B, Rambaud JC, et al: Antibiotic efficacy in small intestinal bacterial overgrowth-related chronic diarrhea: a crossover, randomized trial. Gastroenterology 117:794, 1999

33. Thielman NM, Guerrant RL: Persistent diarrhea in the returned traveler. Infect Dis Clin North Am 12:489, 1998

34. Schiller LR: Microscopic colitis syndrome: lymphocytic colitis and collagenous colitis. Semin Gastrointest Dis 10:145, 1999

35. Sellin JH, Hart R: Glucose malabsorption associated with rapid intestinal transit. Am J Gastroenterol 87:584, 1992

36. Camilleri M: Motor function in irritable bowel syndrome. Can J Gastroenterol 13(suppl A):8A, 1999

37. Schiller LR, Bilhartz LE, Santa Ana CA, et al: Comparison of endogenous and radiolabeled bile acid excretion in patients with idiopathic chronic diarrhea. Gastroenterology 98:1036, 1990

38. Jensen RT: Overview of chronic diarrhea caused by functional neuroendocrine neoplasms. Semin Gastrointest Dis 10:156, 1999

39. Von der Ohe MR, Camilleri M, Kvols LK, et al: Motor dysfunction of the small bowel and colon in patients with the carcinoid syndrome and diarrhea. N Engl J Med 329:1073, 1993

40. Afzalpurkar RG, Schiller LR, Little KH, et al: The self-limited nature of chronic idiopathic diarrhea. N Engl J Med 327:1849, 1992

41. Thompson WG, Longstreth GF, Drossman DA, et al: Functional bowel disorders and functional abdominal pain. Gut 45(suppl 2):II43, 1999

42. Schiller LR, Rivera LM, Santangelo WC, et al: Diagnostic value of fasting plasma peptide concentrations in patients with chronic diarrhea. Dig Dis Sci 39:2216, 1994

43. Brydon WG, Nyhlin H, Eastwood MA, et al: Serum 7 α-hydroxy-4-cholesten-3-one and selenohomocholyltaurine (SeHCAT) whole body retention in the assessment of bile acid induced diarrhoea. Eur J Gastroenterol Hepatol 8:117, 1996

44. Fine KD, Santa Ana CA, Fordtran JS: Diagnosis of magnesium-induced diarrhea. N Engl J Med 324:1012, 1991

45. Fine KD, Fordtran JS: The effect of diarrhea on fecal fat excretion. Gastroenterology 102:1936, 1992

46. Bo-Linn GW, Fordtran JS: Fecal fat concentration in patients with steatorrhea. Gastroenterology 87:319, 1984

47. Ung K-A, Gillberg R, Kilander A, et al: Role of bile acids and bile acid binding agents in patients with collagenous colitis. Gut 46:170, 2000

48. Ewe K, Karbach U: Factitious diarrhoea. Clin Gastroenterol 15:723, 1986

49. Slugg PH, Carey WD: Clinical features and follow-up of surreptitious laxative users. Cleveland Clin Q 51:167, 1984

50. Hasler WL: Dumping syndrome. Curr Treat Options Gastroenterol 5:139, 2002

51. Arrambide KA, Santa Ana CA, Schiller LR, et al: Loss of absorptive capacity for sodium chloride as a cause of diarrhea following partial ileal and right colon resection. Dig Dis Sci 34:193, 1989

52. Metcalf AM, Phillips SF: Ileostomy diarrhoea. Clin Gastroenterol 15:705, 1986

53. Heuschen UA, Allemeyer EH, Hinz U, et al: Diagnosing pouchitis: comparative validation of two scoring systems in routine follow-up. Dis Colon Rectum 45:776, 2002

54. Sauter GH, Moussavian AC, Meyer G, et al: Bowel habits and bile acid malabsorption in the months after cholecystectomy. Am J Gastroenterol 97:1732, 2002

55. Saslow SB, Camilleri M: Diabetic diarrhea. Semin Gastrointest Dis 6:187, 1995

56. Wald A: Incontinence and anorectal dysfunction in patients with diabetes mellitus. Eur J Gastroenterol Hepatol 7:737, 1995

57. Cohen J, West AB, Bini EJ: Infectious diarrhea in human immunodeficiency virus. Gastroenterol Clin North Am 30:637, 2001

58. Mintz ED, Weber JT, Guris D, et al: An outbreak of Brainerd diarrhea among travelers to the Galapagos Islands. J Infect Dis 177:1041, 1998

59. Schiller LR: Chronic diarrhea. GI/Liver Secrets, 2nd ed. McNally PR, Ed. Hanley & Belfus, Philadelphia, 2002, p 411

60. Schiller LR: Diarrhea. Med Clin North Am 84:1259, 2000

62 Gastrointestinal Motility Disorders

Michael Camilleri, M.D.

Motility disorders of the stomach, small intestine, and colon are characterized by the acute, recurrent, or chronic presentation of symptoms of stasis or rapid transit in the absence of mucosal disease or any obstruction within the lumen of the gut.[1]

The most common syndromes associated with disorders of motility are nonulcer dyspepsia,[2] irritable bowel syndrome (IBS), functional constipation,[3] and outlet obstruction to defecation (evacuation disorders)[4]; the prevalence of gastroparesis and chronic intestinal pseudo-obstruction[1] is far lower. These disorders result from impaired neurologic or muscular control of the gut or from incoordination of defecation dynamics. Motility disorders are sometimes caused by a process that influences the extrinsic autonomic nerves that supply the gut. Other disorders infiltrate the GI smooth muscle and extraintestinal organs, particularly the urinary bladder.[1]

Physiology

GASTRIC, SMALL BOWEL, AND COLONIC MOTILITY

GI motor functions are characterized by distinct patterns of contractile activity in the fasting and postprandial periods. The fasting period is characterized by a cyclic motor phenomenon called the interdigestive migrating motor complex [*see Figure 1*]. In healthy people, it occurs approximately once every 60 to 90 minutes and comprises a period of quiescence (phase I), a period of intermittent pressure activity (phase II), and an activity front, during which the stomach and small intestine contract at their highest frequency (phase III). These contraction frequencies reach three a minute in the stomach and 11 or 12 a minute in the proximal small intestine. The interdigestive activity front migrates a variable distance down the small intestine; there is a gradient in the frequency of contractions during phase III, from 11 or 12 a minute in the duodenum to as low as five a minute in the ileum. The distal small intestine also demonstrates another characteristic motor pattern—a propagated prolonged contraction, or power contraction, that serves to empty residue from the ileum to the colon in bolus transfers.

In the postprandial period, the fasting cyclic activity of the stomach and small intestine is replaced by irregular, fairly frequent contractions in those regions of the stomach and small bowel that come in contact with food [*see Figure 1*]. The caloric content of the meal is the major determinant of the duration of this so-called fed pattern. The maximum frequency of contractions is below that noted during phase III of the interdigestive migrating motor complex. After meals, segments of the small intestine that are not exposed to digesta may still show the interdigestive complex. Thus, there may be simultaneous patterns of interdigestive activity in the distal small bowel at a time when the proximal small bowel is in contact with intraluminal digesta and is responding with the irregular contractile activity that characterizes the fed pattern.

Solid and liquid food empty from the stomach at different rates. Liquids empty from the stomach in an exponential manner. For nonnutrient liquids, the healthy stomach tends to empty liquids with a half-emptying time of 20 minutes or less. On the other hand, solids are initially retained selectively within the stomach until particles have been triturated to a size smaller than 2 mm, at which point they can be emptied in a linear fashion from the stomach. Thus, the gastric emptying of solids consists of an initial lag period, followed by a more linear postlag gastric-emptying phase. The small intestine transports solids and liq-

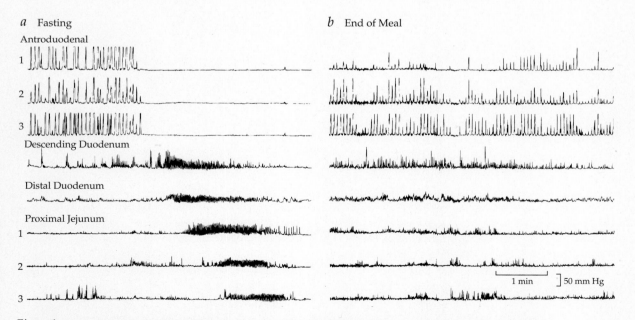

a Fasting

Antroduodenal

b End of Meal

1 min   50 mm Hg

Figure 1 Normal gastrointestinal motility. Note the normal interdigestive migrating motor complex during the fasting phase (*a*) and the irregular but persistent antral and intestinal phasic pressure activity in the fed phase (*b*).[57]

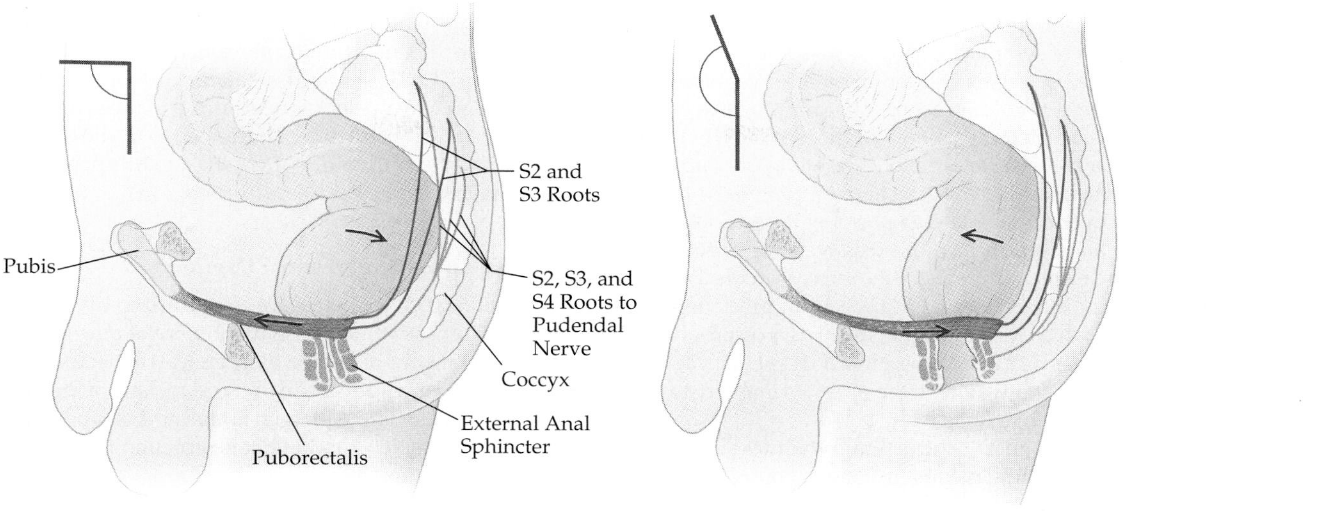

Figure 2 Normal defecation requires relaxation of the puborectalis and external anal sphincter, straightening of the rectoanal angle, and an increase in intraluminal pressure, usually induced by the Valsalva maneuver. Defecation may be obstructed if any of these functions is impaired.[58]

uids at approximately the same rate. Because there is a separation of the two phases in the stomach, it is clear that liquids may arrive in the colon before the head of the solid phase of the meal. Ileal emptying of chyme is characterized by bolus transfers.

Another important function of the stomach is the initial relaxation response that occurs after the ingestion of food. This response, also called accommodation, is mediated by the vagus nerves and involves the activation of intrinsic nitrergic inhibitory nerves in the wall of the stomach. Failure of gastric accommodation results in symptoms such as early fullness, satiety, and bloating and may contribute to nausea, indigestion (dyspepsia), or discomfort postprandially.[5,6]

The colon serves as a reservoir to facilitate absorption of fluids, electrolytes, and short-chain fatty acids produced by bacterial metabolism of unabsorbed carbohydrates. This reservoir function is centered predominantly in the ascending and transverse colonic regions. The descending colon functions as a conduit for the relatively rapid transit of feces to the sigmoid colon, which acts as a second reservoir. Emptying of the sigmoid colon is largely under volitional control. The defecatory process requires the Valsalva maneuver to raise intra-abdominal pressure, which is transmitted to the rectal contents, and relaxation of the puborectalis (or pelvic floor) and external anal sphincter,[4] which necessitates a coordinated series of functions [*see Figure 2*]. This facilitates the opening or straightening of the rectoanal angle and expulsion of stool. The control and function of contractions in the colon are not fully understood; some irregular contractions serve to mix its contents, whereas high-amplitude propagated contractions (HAPCs), which occur on average four to six times a day, are sometimes associated with mass movement of colonic residue and lead to defecation. After meals of at least 500 kcal, there is a greater propensity for HAPCs to develop and for the tone (background state of contractility) of the colon to increase and lead to bowel movements in the first 2 hours after meals.[7]

CONTROL OF GI MOTOR AND SENSORY FUNCTIONS

Motor function of the gut depends on the contraction of the smooth muscle cells and their integration and modulation by enteric and extrinsic nerves.[1] Smooth muscle contraction results

from fluxes of ions that alter the electrical potential of the cell membrane. The enteric nervous system—approximately 100 million (10^8) neurons organized in ganglionated plexi (submucosal and myenteric being the predominant plexi)—is organized in intricate excitatory and inhibitory programmed circuits [*see Figure 3*]. These circuits play essential roles in controlling peristalsis and the migrating motor complex. Among the enteric plexi, there are also interstitial cells of Cajal, which are thought to serve as pacemakers. Enteric nerves are also important in mediating sensation from the gut. Visceral sensation, as with somatic sensation, is mediated by A-delta fibers (which respond to short, sharp stimuli) and polymodal C-unmyelinated fibers (which tend to respond to more prolonged stimuli). The latter nerves mediate pain as well as the autonomic and emotional responses that are commonly noted in patients with functional GI diseases.[8]

Extrinsic neural control is subdivided into the craniosacral parasympathetic outflow and the thoracolumbar sympathetic supply. The cranial outflow is predominantly through the vagus nerve, which supplies neural control from the stomach down to the right side of the colon, and the sacral parasympathetic supply, which provides neural control to the left colon and, through ascending intracolonic fibers, the more proximal regions of the colon. Parasympathetic supply is excitatory to nonsphincteric muscle. Sympathetic fibers to the GI tract arise from levels T5 to L1 of the intermediolateral column of the spinal cord. Sympathetic fibers are stimulatory to sphincteric muscle and relaxatory to nonsphincteric muscle. The prevertebral sympathetic ganglia integrate afferent impulses from the gut and sympathetic supply from the central nervous system. Derangement of any of these intrinsic or extrinsic control mechanisms may lead to altered gut motor function [*see* Gastroparesis and Chronic Intestinal Pseudo-obstruction, *below*].[1]

Structural Diseases and Their Effects on GI Motility

Disturbances of gastric and proximal small bowel motility are frequently observed in symptomatic patients after gastric surgery. Uncoordinated phasic pressure waves occur in the Roux limb after Roux-en-Y partial gastrectomy.[9] In these patients, the vagotomized gastric remnant may also contribute to the development of symptoms, because relaxation and contraction of the gastric remnant are deranged after vagotomy and partial gastric resection. In practice, pharmacologic agents are generally ineffective in this situation; further resection of the gastric remnant may relieve the symptoms resulting from upper gut stasis in about two thirds of these patients.[10]

Another frequently encountered postoperative disorder is the postfundoplication syndrome. An excessively tight repair of hiatal hernia may result in dysphagia; the increase in the use of laparoscopic fundoplication has led to a greater appreciation of the frequency with which this procedure results in postprandial upper abdominal pain, gas, bloating, and a dyspeptic condition that seems further aggravated by the patient's inability to belch as a result of the effective wrap.[11]

In subacute mechanical obstruction, proximal small bowel manometry shows simultaneous prolonged contractions separated by periods of quiescence. This pattern was shown to have a positive predictive value of 80%,[12] and patients showing this pattern should undergo further careful assessment with enteroclysis, laparoscopy, or laparotomy to exclude obstruction. The increased availability and experience of laparoscopic surgeons have led to less need for motility tests to diagnose mechanical obstruction.

Small bowel fistulas, diverticula, and postsurgical blind loops are all associated with bacterial overgrowth, but the pathogenic sequence is not always clear. Experimentally, bacterial toxins induce migrating action potential complexes in the rabbit ileum, as well as abnormal motility, rapid transit through the small bowel, diarrhea, and steatorrhea. It has also been suggested that multiple jejunal diverticula may result from abnormal neuromuscular function.[13]

Volvulus of the stomach, small bowel loops, cecum, and sigmoid colon may present as acute or subacute symptoms caused by mechanical obstruction. These need to be differentiated from conditions that primarily affect the motor apparatus, such as gastroparesis and pseudo-obstruction.

Functional Gastrointestinal Disorders

Functional GI disorders are characterized by disturbances of motor or sensory functions in the absence of mucosal or structural abnormality or of known biochemical or metabolic disorders. These syndromes affect one or more regions of the GI tract and include functional dysphagia, nonulcer dyspepsia,[2] IBS,[3] slow-transit constipation,[4] and outlet obstruction to defecation[4] (also termed evacuation disorders).

Functional GI disorders share common pathogenetic features, including abnormal motility, heightened visceral sensation, and psychosocial disturbance.[2,3] In some patients, these syndromes are preceded by an episode of gastroenteritis. The abnormal motility may be characterized by rapid or slow transit of food or residue through the bowel or abnormal gastric relaxation to accommodate the meal.[5,6] Abnormal contractile patterns have been described, but more important, patients perceive a sensation of excessive gut contractions.[8] In patients with these conditions, there is frequently evidence of psychological comorbidity, such as anxiety, depression, or obsessive-compulsive disorder.[3] These factors appear to influence the decision of patients to consult their physicians.

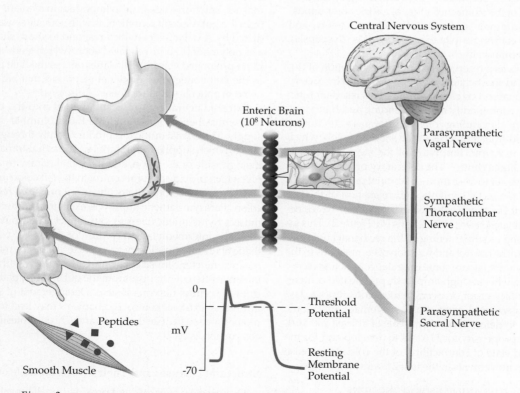

Figure 3 **Control of gut motility. Interactions between extrinsic neural pathways and the intrinsic nervous system (enteric brain) modulate contractions of gastrointestinal smooth muscle. Peptide-receptor interactions alter muscle membrane potentials by stimulating bidirectional ion fluxes. In turn, membrane characteristics dictate whether or not the muscle cell contracts.**[59]

NONULCER DYSPEPSIA

Dyspepsia (from the Greek term for bad digestion) that is not caused by ulcers is characterized by upper abdominal symptoms in the postprandial period, such as nausea, vomiting, pain, bloating, anorexia, and early satiety. It affects about 20% of the population of the United States.

Pathogenesis

Factors other than altered gastric emptying, increased gastric sensitivity, and psychosocial distress may contribute to the development of nonulcer dyspepsia, but the pathogenesis remains unclear. A subgroup of patients may suffer nonerosive reflux esophagitis; others may have *Helicobacter pylori* gastritis. The role *H. pylori* infection plays in dyspepsia is uncertain, but current epidemiologic evidence and the results of eradication studies do not support a causal relationship.[14,15] Dyspepsia is also associated with impaired gastric relaxation or accommodation.[5,6]

Diagnosis

The history usually provides information on the specific symptoms or the spectrum of symptoms experienced by the patient. However, the symptoms have little discriminative value for predicting the physiologic alterations in an individual patient. Studies have suggested that the presence of postprandial fullness or satiation soon after starting the meal may be indicative of delayed gastric emptying and reduced gastric accommodation, respectively.[5,6,16] Moreover, weight loss of more than 5 kg is more frequent in patients with reduced gastric accommodation.[5] However, weight loss should not be dismissed on the basis of being a functional alteration; it mandates performance of endoscopy to exclude ulceration or cancer. The physical examination is usually normal. On rare occasions, there may be a succussion splash in the epigastrium from the retention of food in the stomach. An epigastric mass, hepatomegaly, or supraclavicular lymphadenopathy may suggest that the dyspepsia is the result of malignancy.

In the presence of alarm features such as dysphagia, bleeding, or weight loss in association with dyspepsia, it is essential to exclude mucosal diseases, such as ulcer or cancer.[2] Cancer may still be present, however, even when these alarm features are absent. Patients are reassured by a negative endoscopic examination.

In most cases, the underlying cause of dyspepsia will not be obvious from the history and physical examination. For new-onset dyspepsia, endoscopy and testing for *H. pylori* infection are generally recommended.

The presence of heartburn suggests a component of gastroesophageal reflux. Reflux needs to be differentiated from rumination,[17] which results in the effortless regurgitation of undigested food within 30 minutes after oral ingestion; rumination occurs with virtually every meal and is not associated with nausea. The symptoms that appear to be most closely related to impaired gastric relaxation or accommodation are early satiety and weight loss.[5] This impairment of accommodation may also contribute to hypersensitivity of the stomach of such patients to intraluminal stimuli. There is great interest in identifying ways to demonstrate this hypersensitivity before therapy is initiated, because such knowledge would have a bearing on choice of therapy. Tests in which the patient drinks water or a nutrient beverage have been devised to evaluate the maximal tolerated volume and the symptoms of fullness, satiety, bloating, nausea, and pain at a defined period after ingestion (typically 30 minutes).[5,18,19] These tests are noninvasive and inexpensive, and they have been

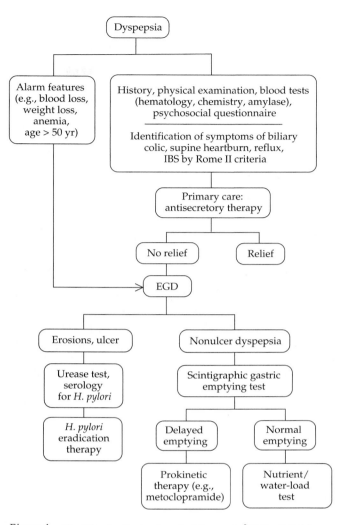

Figure 4 **Algorithm for the treatment of dyspepsia.[2] (IBS—irritable bowel syndrome; EGD—esophagogastroduodenoscopy)**

introduced into clinical practice in some centers. However, they do not necessarily differentiate disturbances in the accommodation response from hypersensitivity per se. Until recently, measurement of accommodation required the placement of an intragastric balloon to measure fasting and postprandial volumes.[5] Recently, a novel imaging approach was developed to measure accommodation noninvasively by use of single-photon emission computed tomography.[6]

Simple, cost-effective tests for mucosal disease, gastric emptying,[20-22] and gastric accommodation[6] provide a rational alternative to the use of sequential empirical trials for identifying the mechanism causing dyspepsia[2] [*see Figure 4*].

Treatment

In clinical practice, dyspepsia is often treated with acid-suppressing regimens consisting of proton pump inhibitors or H_2 receptor antagonists, though the evidence in favor of this approach is limited, and of all patients treated, a cure is achieved in less than one in 10.[23] Temporary acid suppression with a proton pump inhibitor or an H_2 receptor agonist may delay diagnosis of cancer.[24]

In cases of dyspepsia associated with *H. pylori* infection, eradication of the *H. pylori* infection results in resolution of the syndrome in only a small minority of patients[25,26]; the current consensus is that in the absence of erosions or ulcers, eradication of *H. pylori* is not indicated for treatment of dyspepsia,[13] though it is usually treated anyway because of concern with development of atrophy or gastric cancer in the long term.[27]

IRRITABLE BOWEL SYNDROME

Diagnosis

Clinical features IBS is characterized by abdominal pain and alteration in bowel movements. The pain is often worse after eating (experienced by about 30% of patients), is usually located in the lower quadrants or hypogastrium, and is aggravated before and relieved after a bowel movement. Bowel function is disturbed with either diarrhea (increased frequency or stools of loose consistency) or constipation (decreased frequency, abnormally hard stools, need to strain to complete bowel evacuation). Most patients also experience abdominal bloating, and some have a sense of incomplete rectal evacuation or pass mucus with stools. These symptoms constitute the Manning criteria or the Rome criteria[3] and are helpful in diagnosing IBS.

The sense of incomplete evacuation may also suggest a component of outlet obstruction to defecation or increased rectal sensitivity.[4] In clinical practice, the diarrhea may present as either of two variants: (1) loose to watery stools often associated with borborygmi, abdominal cramps, and a borderline-high 24-hour stool weight (i.e., 200 to 300 g/day) or (2) small, pelletlike, repetitive stools that are misinterpreted as diarrhea. Constipation may

be reflected in a reduction in the frequency of bowel movements (fewer than three a week), in incomplete rectal evacuation, or in the need for excessive straining.

The rectal examination is important in excluding anorectal or pelvic floor spasms that obstruct defecation.

IBS may be associated with lactose intolerance and colonic diverticulosis in some patients. It is unclear whether the associated conditions actually contribute to the clinical syndrome. Some patients who manifest clinical features of IBS have celiac disease; the proportion of IBS patients with celiac disease is unclear from the literature.[28] The effect of the exclusion of gluten on IBS symptoms in these patients has not been evaluated.

Laboratory tests The diagnosis of IBS is facilitated by recognition of the symptom complex described above. However, it is a diagnosis of exclusion, requiring selected tests to exclude organic disease, such as stool examination for ova, parasites, and occult blood; blood tests; serologic testing for celiac disease; flexible sigmoidoscopy; and, in patients older than 45 years, barium colon x-ray or colonoscopy [see Figure 5].

Treatment

Constipation in patients with IBS responds to treatment with fiber or simple laxatives, including osmotic agents[29,30]; psychotherapy may also be beneficial.[31] The serotonin (5-HT$_3$) antagonist alosetron was found to provide adequate relief of pain, improved stool frequency, decreased urgency, and consistency for many patients whose predominant bowel disturbance was diar-

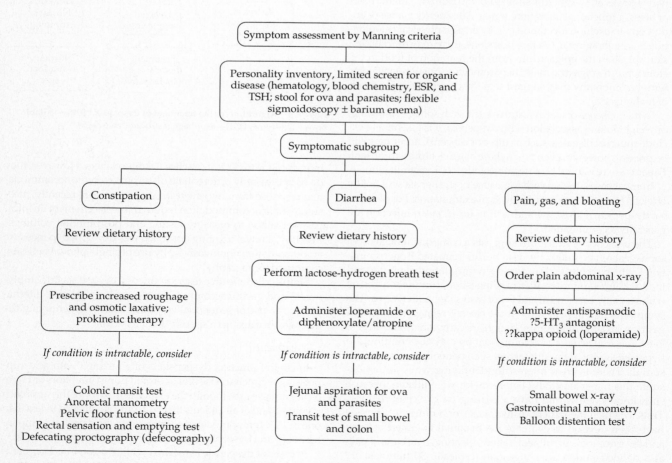

Figure 5 **Algorithm for irritable bowel syndrome.**[60] **(ESR—erythrocyte sedimentation rate; TSH—thyroid stimulating hormone)**

rhea.[32] The medication was withdrawn from the market, but it is possible that it will be reintroduced for specific indications. Other compounds in the same class (e.g., cilansetron) are undergoing trials. Other serotoninergic agents that activate the 5-HT$_4$ receptor may be approved for the treatment of constipation-predominant IBS.[33-35] IBS patients tend to use complementary and alternative medicine (CAM) more frequently than patients with organic bowel diseases. IBS patients who used CAM also were found to have significantly poorer quality-of-life scores for emotional and social factors than patients who did not use CAM.[36] Physicians need to be aware of this, both with regard to the potential for adverse interactions and as an indication of emotional unease in these patients.

SLOW-TRANSIT CONSTIPATION

Slow-transit constipation[4] is a motility disorder of the colon that results in prolonged transit.

Diagnosis

The diagnosis of slow-transit constipation should be made only after exclusion of mucosal diseases, such as tumors and strictures. It is most conveniently diagnosed by assessing mean colonic transit time through use of abdominal radiography and radiopaque markers. There are two commonly used variations of this method. The first type involves ingestion of 24 radiopaque markers in a soluble medication capsule on 4 successive days; plain abdominal radiography is performed on day 5. The number of markers in the colon approximates the mean colonic transit time in hours (normal: < 72 hours). The second variation requires that the patient ingest 20 markers on day 1; an abdominal x-ray is obtained on day 5. Normally, there should be fewer than five markers remaining in the colon. In all patients with delayed colonic transit, the possibility of outlet obstruction to defecation or a pangastrointestinal motility disorder must be ruled out.

Treatment

Treatment of slow-transit constipation consists of increasing dietary bulk or fiber and administering osmotic laxatives (e.g., magnesium salts when not contraindicated) and stimulant laxatives or colonic prokinetic agents.

A more severe variant of slow-transit constipation is colonic inertia. In this disorder, the colon fails to produce a motor response to physiologic stimuli, such as a meal, or to pharmacologic stimulation, as would occur, for example, after administration of neostigmine, 0.5 mg I.M., or intraluminal bisacodyl, 2 to 4 mg.

OUTLET OBSTRUCTION TO DEFECATION

Outlet obstruction to defecation (evacuation disorders) occurs when defecation dynamics [see Figure 2] function poorly and the patient is unable to expel stool.[4]

Diagnosis

The patient may present with constipation or the inability to have spontaneous and complete bowel movements; bloating; and left-sided abdominal pain. The syndrome may thus mimic IBS and is commonly associated with it. A careful clinical history is useful in identifying failure of evacuation; specifically, patients may experience the need for digital disimpaction of the rectum or digital pressure on the posterior wall of the vagina or the perineum to expel stool. Enemas may not be emptied. The rectal examination identifies an immobile perineum during the process

of straining and a tight, unyielding puborectalis sling muscle abutting the rectum posteriorly. This tight pelvic floor persists during attempts to evacuate. In rare instances, the anal sphincter itself is spastic or the entire perineum balloons or herniates down as a result of years of straining or of multiple childbirths, which weaken the ligaments and muscles that normally support the pelvic floor and rectoanal angle.

Treatment

Occasionally, outlet obstruction is caused by an anatomic defect such as a rectocele or rectal internal mucosal prolapse; these are amenable to surgical correction. A spastic pelvic floor or spastic anal sphincter muscles usually respond to biofeedback and muscle relaxation exercises. Some patients with outlet obstruction to defecation have a profound psychological disorder or a history of abuse that requires identification and subsequent therapy.

Gastroparesis and Chronic Intestinal Pseudo-obstruction

PATHOGENESIS

Although several etiologic factors are involved in the development of gastric or small bowel motility disturbances [see Table 1], these can generally be grouped as disorders of the extrinsic nervous system, the enteric nervous system (including the interstitial cells of Cajal or intestinal pacemakers), or smooth muscle.[1]

Extrinsic Neuropathic Disorders

Extrinsic neuropathic processes include vagotomy, diabetes, amyloidosis, and a paraneoplastic syndrome usually associated with small cell carcinoma of the lung. Another common neuropathic problem in clinical practice is the effect of medications such as anticholinergics on neural control.

Enteric or Intrinsic Neuropathic Disorders

Disorders of the enteric nervous system are usually the result of a degenerative, immune, or inflammatory process.[37] The etiology can only rarely be ascertained in these disturbances; gastroparesis and pseudo-obstruction may be caused by viruses (including rotavirus, Norwalk virus, cytomegalovirus, and Epstein-Barr virus) or degenerative disorders associated with infiltration of the myenteric plexus with inflammatory cells [see Figure 6], including eosinophils. Idiopathic chronic intestinal pseudo-obstruction is a condition in which there is no disturbance of the extrinsic neural control and no underlying etiology for the enteric nervous system abnormality.

Full-thickness biopsies of the intestine may be required to evaluate the myenteric plexus[37] and interstitial cells of Cajal.[38] Regrettably, other than resection of the affected region (e.g., colectomy in slow-transit constipation), there are few therapeutic regimens that can be proposed on the basis of the information from the biopsy. The benefits of biopsy need to be weighed against the risk of complications associated with full-thickness intestinal biopsy, which include adhesion formation, with the potential for mechanical obstruction superimposed on episodes of pseudo-obstruction.

Smooth Muscle Disorders

Disturbances of smooth muscle may result in significant disorders of gastric emptying and small bowel transit as well as, occasionally, colonic transit. These disturbances include systemic sclerosis and amyloidosis. Dermatomyositis, dystrophia myotonica, and metabolic muscle disorders such as mitochondrial

Table 1 Classification of Gastroparesis and Chronic Intestinal Pseudo-obstruction

Type	*Myopathic*	*Neuropathic*	*Comments*
Familial	Familial visceral myopathies (auto-somal dominant or recessive)	Familial visceral neuropathies, von Recklinghausen disease	Rare, often present in neonatal period or childhood; neurofibromata may also cause mechanical obstruction
Sporadic			
Infiltrative	Progressive systemic sclerosis	Early progressive systemic sclerosis	Manometry essential to differentiate patho-physiology (neuropathic vs myopathic)
	Amyloidosis	Amyloidosis	
General neurologic disease	Myotonic and other dystrophies	Diabetes, porphyria, spinal cord tran-section, dysautonomias, multiple sclerosis, brain stem tumor	For review, see reference 1
Infectious	—	Chagas disease, Norwalk virus, cytomegalovirus, Epstein-Barr virus	Nonspecific postviral causes appear to be common
Drug-induced	—	Tricyclic antidepressants, narcotics, anticholinergics, antihypertensives, vincristine	Adverse effects of medications to be excluded in all patients
Neoplastic	—	Paraneoplastic (small cell lung cancer, carcinoid lung tumors)	May require computed tomography to exclude tumor if chest x-ray is negative
Idiopathic	Sporadic hollow visceral myopathy	Chronic idiopathic intestinal pseudo-obstruction	Variable manifestations and severity

myopathy are seen infrequently and are suggested by the presence of ptosis, external ocular paralysis, acidosis, and peripheral neuromyopathy.[39] Hollow visceral myopathy may occur either sporadically or, rarely, in families. Motility disturbances may be the result of metabolic disorders such as hypothyroidism and hyperparathyroidism, but patients with these disorders more commonly present with constipation.

DIAGNOSIS

Clinical Features

The clinical features of gastroparesis and chronic intestinal pseudo-obstruction are similar and include nausea, vomiting, early satiety, abdominal discomfort, distention, bloating, and anorexia. In patients in whom stasis and vomiting are significant problems, there may be considerable weight loss, and disturbances of mineral and vitamin stores may result. The severity of the motility problem often manifests itself most clearly in the degree of nutritional and electrolyte depletion. Disturbances of bowel movements, such as diarrhea and constipation, indicate that the motility disorder is more extensive than gastroparesis. Significant vomiting may be complicated by aspiration pneumonia or Mallory-Weiss tears, which may result in acute GI hemorrhage. When patients have a more generalized motility disorder, there may also be symptoms referable to abnormal swallowing or delayed colonic transit.

a

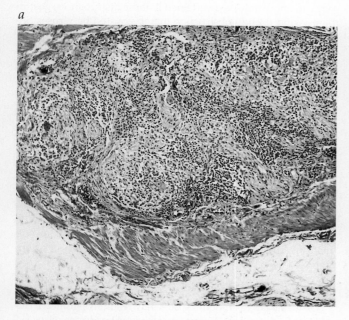

b

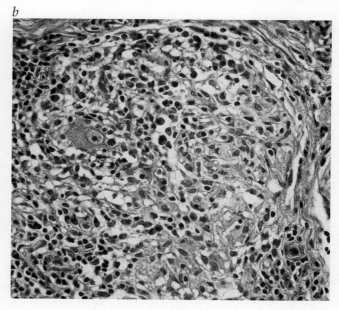

Figure 6 **Mononuclear infiltration in the gastric enteric plexus from a patient with small cell lung cancer and a paraneoplastic gastroparesis. The portion of the plexus rich in ganglion cells was expanded, but no necrosis was observed. Intact nerve fiber bundles can be seen (*a*) (original magnification: ×100). High-power view of the same field (*b*) shows mature small lymphocytes and abundant plasma cells. Although neurons are decreased in number, a normal-appearing ganglion cell can be seen just above the center of the image (original magnification: ×400).[61]**

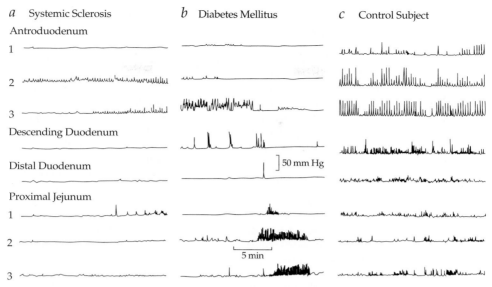

Figure 7 **Postprandial manometric profiles of patients with small bowel dysmotility caused by myopathy (*a*) and neuropathy (*b*), compared with a healthy control subject (*c*).**

Family history and medication history are essential to identify underlying etiologic factors such as diabetes mellitus that may result in gastric or small bowel motor disorders. A careful review of systems will help reveal an underlying collagen vascular disease (e.g., scleroderma) or disturbances of extrinsic neural control that also may be affecting the abdominal viscera. Such symptoms include orthostatic dizziness; difficulties with erection or ejaculation; recurrent urinary tract infections; dry mouth, eyes, or vagina; difficulties with visual accommodation in bright lights; and absence of sweating.

On physical examination, the presence of a succussion splash is usually indicative of a region of stasis within the GI tract, typically the stomach. The hands and mouth may show signs of Raynaud phenomenon or scleroderma. Testing of pupillary responses (to light and accommodation), blood pressure in the lying and standing positions, general features of a peripheral neuropathy, and external ocular movements can identify patients with an associated neurologic disturbance, such as those with a long history (usually longer than 10 years) of diabetes mellitus or oculogastrointestinal dystrophy.

The conditions to be differentiated are mechanical obstruction—which may occur because of peptic stricture or Crohn disease in the small intestine—functional GI disorders, and eating disorders such as anorexia nervosa and rumination syndrome. The degree of impairment of gastric emptying in eating disorders is relatively minor compared with diabetic and postvagotomy gastric stasis. Rumination syndrome is characterized by postprandial, effortless regurgitation of undigested food within 30 minutes after virtually every meal. This condition occurs in mentally challenged children (e.g., those with Down syndrome), and it is also being increasingly recognized in adolescents and adults of normal intelligence.[17] It is treatable by behavioral modification, including diaphragmatic breathing in the postprandial period.

Neonatal pseudo-obstruction rarely occurs alone; it is more often found in association with other anomalies requiring surgical correction, including gastroschisis, duodenal atresia, or megacystis. Prokinetic medications are usually ineffective, and many patients require parenteral nutrition and bowel decompression, including gastrostomies or enterostomies.[40]

Laboratory Tests

A motility disorder of the stomach or small bowel should be suspected whenever large volumes are aspirated from the stomach, particularly after an overnight fast, or when undigested solid food or large volumes of liquids are observed during an esophagogastroduodenoscopy. Barium studies rarely identify the etiology of the motor disorder except in small bowel systemic sclerosis, which is characterized by megaduodenum and packed valvulae conniventes in the small intestine. Barium x-ray, however, serves the important function of excluding mechanical obstruction. The diagnosis of a gastric or small bowel motility disorder, therefore, depends on a careful history and confirmation by transit tests.

The emptying of solids provides the best way to distinguish between healthy and disease states. If the patient's history includes an obvious etiologic factor, such as long-standing diabetes mellitus, it is usually unnecessary to pursue further investigations. When the cause of the gastric or small bowel transit disorder is unclear and the patient does not respond to treatment with a prokinetic agent, referral to a specialized center for autonomic tests and upper GI manometry may be needed [*see Figure 7*]. Transit tests, which can now be performed relatively simply and inexpensively,[20-22] enable good discrimination between healthy and disease states. The two most widely available approaches are the carbon-13 breath tests and scintigraphy with scans taken immediately after ingestion of the radiolabeled meal, as well as 1, 2, 4, and 6 hours later.[20] Manometry is generally available only in specialized centers; it may identify a myopathic or neuropathic disorder or an unsuspected mechanical obstruction resulting from simultaneous prolonged contractions at several levels of the intestine.[12]

In patients presenting with diarrhea, it is important to assess nutritional status (essential element and vitamin levels) and to exclude bacterial overgrowth by culture of small bowel aspirates. It is also important to exclude celiac sprue by small bowel biopsies. Bacterial overgrowth is relatively uncommon in neuropathic disorders but is more often found in myopathic conditions, such as scleroderma, that are more often associated with bowel dilatation.

TREATMENT

Four questions should be considered in the management of each patient. First, is the presentation acute or chronic? Second, is there evidence of a systemic disorder indicative of a neuropathy or myopathy? Third, what is the patient's state of hydration and nutrition? Fourth, which regions of the digestive tract are affected? The principal methods of management include correction of dehydration and nutritional deficiencies, the use of prokinetic and antiemetic medications [see Table 2], suppression of bacterial overgrowth, decompression of dilated segments, and surgery.[41]

Correction of Dehydration and Nutritional Deficiencies

Correction of dehydration and electrolyte and nutritional depletion is particularly important during acute exacerbations of gastroparesis or chronic intestinal pseudo-obstruction syndromes. Nutritional support should be tailored to the severity of the deficiencies of trace elements and dietary constituents in each patient. Dietary measures include the use of low-fiber and low-fat caloric supplements that contain iron, folate, calcium, and vitamins D, K, and B_{12}. Patients who have more severe symptoms, such as severe diabetic gastroparesis or severe myopathic pseudo-obstruction, may need parenteral or enteral nutrition supplementation.[31] For patients in whom supplementation of nutrition may be required for more than 3 months, it is usually best to place the enteral feeding tube via laparoscopy or minilaparotomy to secure the location of the tube in the intestine. Although severely affected patients may need parenteral nutrition, many patients continue to tolerate some oral feeding.

Prokinetic Therapy

Prokinetic medications (e.g., metoclopramide, 10 to 20 mg up to four times a day) are often used for the treatment of neuromuscular motility disorders.[41] Unfortunately, there is little evidence that they are effective in myopathic disturbances. Domperidone, a D_2 dopamine antagonist with antiemetic properties, relieves symptoms of diabetic gastroparesis,[42] but it is not approved for use in the United States.

Erythromycin, a macrolide antibiotic that stimulates motilin receptors partly through a cholinergic mechanism, results in the dumping of nondigestible and digestible solids from the stomach. Erythromycin lactobionate at a dosage of 3 to 6 mg/kg every 8 hours clears bezoars from the stomach in patients with diabetic gastroparesis.[43,44] The effect of oral erythromycin appears to be restricted by tachyphylaxis; there is little evidence that continued therapy is effective beyond 2 weeks, and GI upset may develop in some patients.[44]

Before its withdrawal in 2000, cisapride, a substituted benzamide that acts as a serotonin agonist, was used to treat altered motility, such as impaired gastric emptying, in patients with both gastroparesis and chronic intestinal pseudo-obstruction.[41]

Metoclopramide, with its antinausea and indirect cholinomimetic actions, is the current drug of choice for the treatment of motility disorders, though evidence for its efficacy is limited. Neuropsychiatric side effects such as dystonias are not infrequent, and rare cases of tardive dyskinesia have been reported. The usual dosage is 10 mg four times a day. Metoclopramide is also available for parenteral use; the usual dose is 10 mg I.M. or I.V. It should be used with caution, and a test dose (1 to 2 mg) is often used to exclude dystonic reactions resulting from an idiosyncratic reaction.

The peripheral dopaminergic antagonist domperidone has been shown to be efficacious in diabetic gastroparesis;[45] its efficacy is generally similar to that of metoclopramide. This agent suppresses emesis at the chemoreceptor trigger zone, which is outside the blood-brain barrier. Domperidone is not approved in the United States. The usual dosage is 30 to 80 mg/day in three or four divided doses. Novel prokinetics that are currently undergoing trial include the partial or full 5-HT$_4$ agonists such as tegaserod, levosulpiride, renzapride, and mosapride. Tegaserod accelerates gastric and small bowel transit in healthy persons[46] and small bowel transit in patients with constipation-predomi-

Table 2 Medications Used in the Treatment of Gastrointestinal Motility Disorders

Drug	Dose	Efficacy Rating	Comments
Gastroparesis			
Prokinetics			
Metoclopramide I.M. or p.o	10 mg t.i.d. + h.s.	Moderate	Central side effects; no evidence of efficacy below stomach level
Domperidone, p.o	10–30 mg t.i.d. + h.s.	Moderate	Not approved
Erythromycin I.V. or p.o.	40–200 mg t.i.d.	First choice if I.V. agent needed	Oral administration results in abdominal side effects after 2 wk
Cisapride p.o	10 mg t.i.d. + h.s.	Greater	Limited access because of drug interactions and potential for cardiac dysrhythmia
Octreotide s.c.	25–50 mg h.s.	Modest	For induction of MMCs to avoid bacterial overgrowth; if given with meals, retards transit
Antiemetics			
Prochlorperazine	5–12.5 mg p.r.n.	Significant for adult emesis	I.M., p.o., or rectal suppository
5-HT$_3$ antagonists (e.g., ondansetron)	0.15 mg/kg I.V. or p.o.	Modest	Less effective for dysmotility than for chemotherapy-induced emesis
Dumping, Diarrhea, or Short Bowel			
Octreotide	25 μg t.i.d., a.c.	Moderate	Adjunct to total parenteral nutrition and fluid replacement; prescribe multidraw vial; store in refrigerator
Irritable Bowel Syndrome Diarrhea			
Loperamide	2 mg up to 6 mg/day	First choice	No benefit for pain; very effective for diarrhea

5-HT$_3$ — serotonin   MMCs — mucosal mast cells

nant irritable bowel syndrome.[47] It is chemically different from the benzamides and does not cause cardiac dysrhythmias.[35]

Octreotide, a cyclized octapeptide analogue of somatostatin, has been shown to induce activity fronts (phase III of the migrating motor complex) in the small intestine.[48] In an open trial, octreotide appeared to alleviate symptoms in patients with small bowel scleroderma who received the drug for up to 3 weeks.[49] However, it is unclear whether small bowel transit really improves with use of octreotide. In healthy persons, low doses of octreotide markedly retard small bowel transit.[50] Its therapeutic efficacy needs to be further assessed in clinical trials.

Symptomatic Relief

Standard antiemetics can be used for symptom relief. The more expensive 5-HT_3 antagonists (e.g., ondansetron) have not been proved to be of greater benefit than the less expensive antiemetic agents. Some patients have significant pain; if pain is associated with gut dilatation, decompression may be needed (see below). In the absence of dilatation, narcotics should be avoided, because these agents may aggravate the motility disorder. Parenteral ketorolac may be useful during acute exacerbations of pain.

Antibacterial Therapy

Bacterial overgrowth must be suppressed in infected patients with pseudo-obstruction. A common practice is to use a different antibiotic for 7 to 10 days each month to avoid development of bacterial resistance, although no trials have been performed to study this approach. Typical antibiotics used are doxycycline (100 mg b.i.d.), metronidazole (500 mg t.i.d.), ciprofloxacin (500 mg b.i.d.), or double-strength trimethoprim-sulfamethoxazole (two tablets b.i.d.). These measures usually result in significant symptomatic relief in those patients with diarrhea and steatorrhea.

Decompression

Decompression is rarely necessary in patients with chronic intestinal pseudo-obstruction and should be restricted to patients with severe motility disorders who are being cared for at tertiary care centers. Venting enterostomy creates a means to relieve abdominal distention and bloating and has been shown to significantly reduce the frequency of nasogastric intubations or hospitalizations for acute exacerbations in patients with severe intestinal pseudo-obstruction that require central parenteral nutrition.[40] Access to the small intestine may also provide a way to deliver nutrients by the enteral route. Enteral tubes are available that facilitate both aspiration and feeding with the same apparatus.

Electrical Stimulation and Gastric Pacing

Electrical stimulation and gastric pacing is an evolving treatment option for patients who do not respond to standard medical therapy[51]; however, the evidence for efficacy of electrical stimulation is controversial, and the mechanism for relieving symptoms is unknown.

Surgical Treatment

Surgical treatment should be considered whenever the motility disorder is localized to a portion of the gut that can be resected. In clinical practice, the two most common surgical therapies are (1) colectomy and ileoproctostomy for intractable symptoms associated with slow-transit constipation, colonic inertia, or pseudo-obstruction and (2) completion gastrectomy for patients with stasis syndrome after gastric surgery.[40] The role of small bowel

transplantation in patients with pseudo-obstruction is unclear. Successful transplants have been performed in children with pseudo-obstruction,[52] but the experience in adults is limited.[52]

PROGNOSIS

The prognosis depends on the severity of the case. Patients with suspected postviral gastroparesis appear to have a good overall prognosis, with restoration of nutrition and reduction of symptoms within 2 years. On the other hand, patients with myopathic and dilated bowel have persistent symptoms, are more prone to develop bacterial overgrowth, and usually require long-term parenteral nutrition, which carries inherent morbidity. Between these extremes are patients with mild to moderately severe motility disorders who have recurrent or chronic symptoms. These patients can usually be managed as outpatients with dietary supplementation to maintain nutrition (including liquid formula supplements) and medications (e.g., prokinetics or antiemetics) and decompression to relieve symptoms.

Dumping Syndrome and Accelerated Gastric Emptying

Rapid gastric emptying results from impaired relaxation of the stomach upon ingestion of food. Postprandial intragastric pressure is relatively high and results in active propulsion of liquid foods from the stomach. A high caloric (usually carbohydrate) content of the liquid phase of the meal evokes a rapid insulin response with secondary hypoglycemia. These patients may also have impaired antral contractility and gastric stasis of solids, which may paradoxically result in a clinical picture of both gastroparesis (for solids) and dumping (for liquids). Typically, these conditions follow truncal vagotomy and gastric drainage procedures; with the use of more selective vagotomies in the treatment of peptic ulceration, it is likely that the prevalence of these problems may decrease. The most useful means of assessment is a dual-phase (solid and liquid) radioisotopic gastric emptying test.

Management of dumping[53] includes patient education (particularly regarding the avoidance of high-nutrient liquid drinks) and, possibly, the addition of guar gum or pectin to retard liquid emptying. If these measures are ineffective, pharmacologic approaches, such as use of subcutaneous octreotide (50 to 100 mg) 15 minutes before meals, decreases many of the vasomotor symptoms and also retards gastric emptying and small bowel transit, thereby relieving associated hypoglycemia and diarrhea.[54,55]

Rapid-Transit Dysmotilities of the Small Bowel

Rapid transit through the small bowel is a minor component of IBS in some patients.[4] However, it is a major component of other diseases and results in a significant loss of fluid and osmotically active solutes that overwhelm colonic capacitance and reabsorptive capacity and result in severe diarrhea. Examples include postvagotomy diarrhea, short bowel syndrome, diabetic diarrhea, and carcinoid diarrhea.[56] These disturbances of small bowel transit can best be identified by use of scintigraphy or, if scintigraphy is not available, by use of the lactulose-hydrogen breath test.

The objectives of treatment are restoration of hydration and nutrition and retardation of small bowel transit. Dietary interventions include avoidance of hyperosmolar drinks (e.g., virtually all soft drinks), use of iso-osmolar or hypo-osmolar rehydration solutions, and reduction of the fat content in the diet to around 50 g a day to avoid delivery of unabsorbed fat to the colon (where their metabolites are cathartic). Correction of nutritional deficiencies (commonly, calcium, magnesium, potassium, and water- and fat-soluble vitamins) is often required.

Pharmacotherapy should be delivered in a stepwise fashion. First, an opioid agent in high dosage (e.g., loperamide, 4 mg) is given one-half hour before each meal and at bedtime to suppress the small bowel transit and colonic response to feeding. Next, verapamil (40 mg b.i.d.) or clonidine (0.1 to 0.2 mg orally or by patch) should be given, and if these are ineffective or produce unacceptable side effects (usually hypotension), subcutaneous octreotide, starting at 50 µg before meals, should be prescribed.[54] Patients with less than 1 m of residual small bowel may be unable to sustain fluid and electrolyte homeostasis without parenteral support. However, it is almost invariably possible to maintain patients with more than 1 m of residual small bowel with oral nutrition, pharmacotherapy, and supplements.

References

1. Camilleri M, Bharucha AE: Gastrointestinal dysfunction in neurologic disease. Semin Neurol 16:203, 1996

2. Camilleri M: Nonulcer dyspepsia: a look into the future. Mayo Clin Proc 71:614, 1996

3. Drossman DA, Whitehead WE, Camilleri M: Irritable bowel syndrome: a technical review for practical guideline development. Gastroenterology 112:2120, 1997

4. Camilleri M, Thompson WG, Fleshman JW, et al: Clinical management of intractable constipation. Ann Intern Med 121:520, 1994

5. Tack J, Piessevaux H, Coulie B, et al: Role of impaired gastric accommodation to a meal in functional dyspepsia. Gastroenterology 115:1346, 1998

6. Kim DY, Delgado-Aros S, Camilleri M, et al: Noninvasive measurement of gastric accommodation in patients with idiopathic nonulcer dyspepsia. Am J Gastroenterol 96:3099, 2001

7. Camilleri M, Ford MJ: Review article: colonic sensorimotor physiology in health, and its alteration in constipation and diarrhoeal disorders. Aliment Pharmacol Ther 12:287, 1998

8. Camilleri M, Saslow SB, Bharucha AE: Gastrointestinal sensation: mechanisms and relation to functional gastrointestinal disorders. Gastroenterol Clin North Am 25:247, 1996

9. Miedema BW, Kelly KA, Camilleri M, et al: Human gastric and jejunal transit and motility after Roux gastrojejunostomy. Gastroenterology 103:1133, 1992

10. Karlstrom L, Kelly KA: Roux-Y gastrectomy for chronic gastric atony. Am J Surg 157:44, 1989

11. Wijnhoven BP, Salet GA, Roelofs JM, et al: Function of the proximal stomach after Nissen fundoplication. Br J Surg 85:267, 1998

12. Frank JW, Sarr MG, Camilleri M: Use of gastroduodenal manometry to differentiate mechanical and functional intestinal obstruction: an analysis of clinical outcome. Am J Gastroenterol 89:339, 1994

13. Krishnamurthy S, Kelly MM, Rohrmann CA, et al: Jejunal diverticulosis: a heterogenous disorder caused by a variety of abnormalities of smooth muscle or myenteric plexus. Gastroenterology 85:538, 1983

14. Danesh J, Lawrence M, Murphy M, et al: Systematic review of the epidemiological evidence on Helicobacter pylori infection and nonulcer or uninvestigated dyspepsia. Arch Intern Med 160:1192, 2000

15. Laine L, Schoenfeld P, Fennerty MB: Therapy for Helicobacter pylori in patients with nonulcer dyspepsia: a meta-analysis of randomized, controlled trials. Ann Intern Med 134:361, 2001

16. Stanghellini V, Tosetti C, Paternico A, et al: Predominant symptoms identify different subgroups in functional dyspepsia. Am J Gastroenterol 94:2080, 1999

17. O'Brien MD, Bruce BK, Camilleri M: Rumination syndrome: clinical features rather than manometric diagnosis. Gastroenterology 108:1024, 1995

18. Boeckxstaens GE, Hirsch DP, van den Elzen BD, et al: Impaired drinking capacity in patients with functional dyspepsia: relationship with proximal stomach function. Gastroenterology 121:1054, 2001

19. Chial HJ, Camilleri C, Delgado-Aros S, et al: A nutrient drink test to assess maximum tolerated volume and postprandial symptoms: effects of gender, body mass index and age in health. Neurogastroenterol Motil (in press)

20. Thomforde GM, Camilleri M, Phillips SF, et al: Evaluation of an inexpensive screening scintigraphic test of gastric emptying. J Nucl Med 36:93, 1995

21. Ghoos YF, Maes BD, Geypens BJ, et al: Measurement of gastric emptying rate of solids by means of a carbon-labeled octanoic acid breath test. Gastroenterology 104:1640, 1993

22. Viramontes BE, Kim DY, Camilleri M, et al: Validation of a stable isotope gastric emptying test for normal, accelerated or delayed gastric emptying. Neurogastroenterol Mot 13:567, 2001

23. Delaney BC, Innes MA, Deeks J, et al: Initial management strategies for dyspepsia. Cochrane Database Syst Rev (3):CD001961, 2001

24. Bramble MG, Suvakovic Z, Hungin AS: Detection of upper gastrointestinal cancer in patients taking antisecretory therapy prior to gastroscopy. Gut 46:464, 2000

25. McColl K, Murray L, El-Omar E, et al: Symptomatic benefit from eradicating Helicobacter pylori infection in patients with nonulcer dyspepsia. N Engl J Med 339:1869, 1998

26. Blum AL, Talley NJ, O'Morain C, et al: Lack of effect of treating Helicobacter pylori infection in patients with nonulcer dyspepsia. Omeprazole Plus Clarithromycin and Amoxicillin Effect One Year after Treatment (OCAY) Study Group. N Engl J Med 339:1875, 1998

27. Uemura N, Okamoto S, Yamamoto S, et al: Helicobacter pylori infection and the development of gastric cancer. N Engl J Med 345:784, 2001

28. Sanders DS, Carter MJ, Hurlstone DP, et al: Association of adult coeliac disease with irritable bowel syndrome: a case-control study in patients fulfilling ROME II criteria referred to secondary care. Lancet 358:1504, 2001

29. Tramonte SM, Brand MB, Mulrow CD, et al: The treatment of chronic constipation in adults: a systematic review. J Gen Intern Med 12:15, 1997

30. Voderholzer WA, Schatke W, Muhldorfer BE, et al: Clinical response to dietary fiber treatment of chronic constipation. Am J Gastroenterol 92:95, 1997

31. Guthrie E, Creed F, Dawson D, et al: A controlled trial of psychological treatment for the irritable bowel syndrome. Gastroenterology 100:450, 1991

32. Camilleri M, Northcutt AR, Kong S, et al: Efficacy and safety of alosetron in women with irritable bowel syndrome: a randomised, placebo-controlled trial. Lancet 355:1035, 2000

33. Müller-Lissner SA, Fumagalli I, Bardhan KD, et al: Tegaserod, a 5-HT$_4$ receptor partial agonist, relieves symptoms in irritable bowel syndrome patients with abdominal pain, bloating and constipation. Aliment Pharmacol Ther 15:1655, 2001

34. Camilleri M: Management of the irritable bowel syndrome. Gastroenterology 120:652, 2001

35. Camilleri M: Review article: tegaserod. Aliment Pharmacol Ther 15:277, 2001

36. Langmead L, Chitnis M, Rampton DS: Use of complementary therapies by patients with IBD may indicate psychological distress. Inflamm Bowel Dis 8:174, 2002

37. Singaram C, SenGupta A: Histopathology of the enteric neuropathies: from silver staining to immunohistochemistry. Gastroenterol Clin North Am 25:183, 1996

38. He CL, Burgart L, Wang L, et al: Decreased interstitial cell of Cajal volume in patients with slow-transit constipation. Gastroenterology 118:14, 2000

39. Mueller LA, Camilleri M, Emslie-Smith AM: Mitochondrial neurogastrointestinal encephalomyopathy: manometric and diagnostic features. Gastroenterology 116:959, 1999

40. Murr MM, Sarr MG, Camilleri M: The surgeon's role in the treatment of chronic intestinal pseudo-obstruction. Am J Gastroenterol 90:2147, 1995

41. Camilleri M: Appraisal of medium- and long-term treatment of gastroparesis and chronic intestinal dysmotility. Am J Gastroenterol 89:1769, 1994

42. Soykan I, Sarosiek I, McCallum RW: The effect of chronic oral domperidone therapy on gastrointestinal symptoms, gastric emptying, and quality of life in patients with gastroparesis. Am J Gastroenterol 92:976, 1997

43. Janssens J, Peeters TL, Vantrappen G, et al: Improvement in gastric emptying in diabetic gastroparesis by erythromycin: preliminary studies. N Engl J Med 322:1028, 1990

44. Richards RD, Davenport K, McCallum RW: The treatment of idiopathic and diabetic gastroparesis with acute intravenous and chronic oral erythromycin. Am J Gastroenterol 88:203, 1993

45. Patterson D, Abell T, Rothstein R, et al: A double-blind multicenter comparison of domperidone and metoclopramide in the treatment of diabetic patients with symptoms of gastroparesis. Am J Gastroenterol 94:1230, 1999

46. Degen L, Matzinger D, Merz M, et al: Tegaserod, a 5-HT4 receptor partial agonist, accelerates gastric emptying and gastrointestinal transit in healthy male subjects. Aliment Pharmacol Ther 15:1745, 2001

47. Prather CM, Camilleri M, Zinsmeister AR, et al: Tegaserod accelerates orocecal transit in patients with constipation-predominant irritable bowel syndrome. Gastroenterology 118:463, 2000

48. Haruma K, Wiste JA, Camilleri M: Effect of octreotide on gastrointestinal pressure profiles in health and in functional and organic gastrointestinal disorders. Gut 35:1064, 1994

49. Soudah HC, Hasler WL, Owyang C: Effect of octreotide on intestinal motility and bacterial overgrowth in scleroderma. N Engl J Med 325:1461, 1991

50. von der Ohe MR, Camilleri M, Thomforde GM, et al: Differential regional effects of octreotide on human gastrointestinal motor function. Gut 36:743, 1995

51. WAVESS Study Group: Gastric electrical stimulation for gastroparesis: a multi-center double blind cross over study by the WAVESS study group (abstr). Gastroenterology 118:2060, 2000

52. Sigurdsson L, Reyes J, Kocoshis SA, et al: Intestinal transplantation in children with chronic intestinal pseudo-obstruction. Gut 45:570, 1999

53. Hasler WL: Dumping syndrome. Curr Ther Options Gastroenterology 5:139, 2002

54. Farthing MJ: Octreotide in dumping and short bowel syndromes. Digestion 54:47, 1993

55. Vecht J, Lamers CB, Masclee AA: Long-term results of octreotide-therapy in severe dumping syndrome. Clin Endocrinol 51:619, 1999

56. von der Ohe M, Camilleri M, Kvols LK, et al: Motor dysfunction of the small bowel and colon in patients with the carcinoid syndrome and diarrhea. N Engl J Med 329:1073, 1993

57. Malagelada JR, Camilleri M, Stanghellini V: Manometric Diagnosis of Gastrointestinal Motility Disorders. Thieme Medical Publishers, New York, 1986

58. Camilleri M: Four patients with intractable constipation. Gastrointestinal Diseases Today 2:7, 1993

59. Camilleri M, Phillips SF: Disorders of small intestinal motility. Motility Disorders. Gastroenterology Clinics of North America, Vol 18, No. 2. Ouyang A, Ed. WB Saunders Co, Philadelphia, 1989, p 405

60. Camilleri M, Prather CM: The irritable bowel syndrome: mechanisms and a practical approach to management. Ann Intern Med 116:1001, 1992

61. Lennon VA, Sas DF, Busk MF, et al: Enteric neuronal autoantibodies in pseudoobstruction with small-cell lung carcinoma. Gastroenterology 100:137, 1991

Acknowledgments

I wish to thank Mrs. Cindy Stanislav for her excellent secretarial assistance with the manuscript.

Figures 2 and 3   Tom Moore.

63 Gastrointestinal Bleeding

Harvey S. Young, M.D.

Gastrointestinal bleeding is a common problem in the United States, accounting for more than 300,000 hospital admissions a year.[1-4] The incidence of bleeding increases with increasing age. Most cases originate from an upper GI source.

Clinical Manifestations and Differential Diagnosis

Patients with acute GI hemorrhage experience symptoms and signs of hypotension if the blood loss is 1,500 ml or more (or about 25% of the total blood volume), particularly if the loss has occurred within minutes to a few hours. Impaired vision and light-headedness usually occur when the systolic blood pressure falls below 100 mm Hg and the pulse rate is greater than 100 beats/min. Such symptoms are particularly apparent when patients rise from the sitting or recumbent position. Early signs also include a sense of uneasiness or anxiety; cold, sweaty extremities; and syncope when the patient is in an upright position. Patients frequently report that they have passed very dark or black stools hours or a day or two before a hypotensive episode. Although the passage of black stools usually indicates that bleeding has occurred from a site above the level of the cecum, the degree of blackening also depends on the length of time the blood remains in the gut. It is well known, for example, that a cecal lesion such as carcinoma can produce melena and that very rapidly bleeding peptic ulcers may lead to the passage of grossly bloody or mahogany-colored stools.

A history of epigastric pain that precedes the passage of black stools by 1 to 2 weeks suggests peptic ulcer disease. Weight loss, anorexia, and chronic anemia may antedate acute bleeding from gastric carcinoma. Recurrent retching just before hematemesis may be reported by more than half of the patients with a Mallory-Weiss tear at the esophagogastric junction. Painless hematochezia is usually associated with bleeding from colonic diverticula, angiodysplasia, or tumors.

If bleeding is moderate, physical examination may disclose no abnormalities. Brisk hemorrhage usually causes apprehension, tachycardia, and orthostatic hypotension, and the extremities become cool and moist. Ascites and the stigmas of liver disease (e.g., spider angiomas and palmar erythema) may be seen in patients with variceal bleeding. Mucous membrane, cutaneous, or other bleeding may reflect impaired procoagulant synthesis by a diseased liver or the presence of other hemostatic disorders. Bowel sounds are usually hyperactive because of the presence of blood. An ileus may indicate that intestinal infarction has occurred.

Approach to Acute Gastrointestinal Bleeding

Most GI bleeding is self-limited; as a result, almost all patients (80% to 90%) who are treated conservatively cease bleeding within 24 to 48 hours. However, prompt and appropriate fluid replacement is essential to prevent complications from acute hypovolemia. Careful attention should be given to identifying the few patients who are likely to continue bleeding or to experience recurrent bleeding after admission (e.g., patients with portal hypertension who may have bled from varices) so that appropriate diagnostic and therapeutic plans can be formulated.

Laboratory Analysis

Most patients with symptoms of hypotension have a hematocrit of less than 30%. However, the hematocrit may be normal early in the course of massive acute arterial or variceal bleeding because of insufficient time for equilibration of plasma volume. In upper GI bleeding, the blood urea nitrogen (BUN) level is usually greater than 40 mg/dl because of the absorbed nitrogen load from blood in the small intestine. Colonic bleeding does not usually lead to a rise in the BUN level. Because the serum creatinine level is usually normal in GI bleeding, the ratio of the BUN level to the serum creatinine level may be particularly useful in localizing the source of bleeding to the upper or lower GI tract. The BUN-to–creatinine concentration ratio is almost always greater than 25 in upper GI bleeding and less than 25 (mean, about 15) in colonic bleeding.

SUPPORTIVE THERAPY

Immediate attention should be given to assessing the degree of hypovolemia. Although the blood pressure and pulse rate may be normal when the patient is reclining, a pulse rate increase of 10 to 20 beats/min and a decrease in systolic pressure of 10 to 20 mm Hg when the patient sits upright suggest that a significant loss of blood has occurred.

Intravenous fluid replacement should begin immediately through a large-bore catheter. Thereafter, it is usually advisable to install a central venous catheter so that fluids and blood can be administered rapidly; the catheter can also be used to monitor the central venous pressure. A nasogastric tube is used to obtain gastric aspirate for differentiating between upper and lower GI bleeding. If upper GI bleeding is present, the stomach is then lavaged in preparation for endoscopy. Blood replacement is usually required if the patient's vital signs suggest hypovolemia and the hematocrit is less than 30%. It is advisable to give isotonic saline and then to administer red blood cells. Dilutional thrombocytopenia may ensue after massive transfusion. Replacement of platelets or other blood components may be required [*see Chapter 95*].

Upper Gastrointestinal Bleeding

Peptic ulcer is the most common cause of upper GI bleeding; erosive gastritis and esophageal lesions, such as erosive esophagitis and varices, are also significant causes of hemorrhage [*see Table 1*].[5]

DIAGNOSTIC PROCEDURES

Endoscopy is the diagnostic procedure of choice in patients with upper GI bleeding. Endoscopy can be accomplished rapidly, and it usually yields the correct diagnosis with relatively low morbidity. Endoscopy should be performed once the patient is stabilized. In patients with no debilitating comorbid conditions and no significant hemodynamic compromise, early endoscopy can be useful in assessing the risk of recurrent bleeding. This information can affect the management plan and lead to a significant reduction in length of hospital stay.[6,7] For example, patients with varices or an actively bleeding ulcer are at high risk for recurrent bleeding and require hospitalization. In contrast, patients with an ulcer with a clean base and no evidence of recent

Table 1 Causes of Gastrointestinal Bleeding[5,52]

Causes	Patients (%)
Upper GI Bleeding	
Peptic ulcer	
Duodenal ulcer	36
Gastric ulcer	24
Duodenal and gastric ulcers	1
Mucosal erosive disease	
Gastritis	6
Duodenitis	2
Gastroduodenitis	3
Esophagitis	4
Esophageal varices	6
Mallory-Weiss tear	3
Malignancy	2
Others	5
Unknown	8
Lower GI Bleeding	
Colonic diverticulosis	41.6
Colorectal malignancy	9.1
Ischemic colitis	8.7
Acute colitis, unknown cause	5.0
Hemorrhoids	4.6
Postpolypectomy hemorrhage	4.1
Colonic angiodysplasia	2.7
Crohn's disease	2.3
Others	10.1
Unknown	11.9

bleeding are at low risk of rebleeding and can be managed as outpatients, provided they have no comorbid conditions. Up to 25% of patients presenting with acute GI bleeding meet these guidelines and may be treated as outpatients.[3]

Patients who bleed continuously or massively despite supportive therapy should undergo emergency endoscopy to identify the site of the lesion and to aid in formulating definitive therapy [*see Figure 1*]. Urgent endoscopy is particularly useful when the major clinical diagnosis being considered is a disease such as varices or peptic ulcer, for which specific endoscopic or surgical therapy is likely to halt the blood loss. Before endoscopy is performed in these emergency settings, endotracheal intubation should be considered to prevent aspiration during the procedure.

If no blood is seen in the stomach or duodenum with endoscopy, despite brisk blood loss in stools, or if hemorrhage is so massive that the bleeding site cannot be located, the lesion can be detected with selective mesenteric arteriography in a high percentage of patients.[8] This technique is successful, however, only when bleeding is from a discrete site and occurs at a rate of at least 0.5 ml/min. After the catheter has been positioned in the mesenteric artery and the bleeding site has been defined, vasopressin can be administered intra-arterially through the indwelling catheter. Alternatively, the artery can be embolized with particulate agents. Intra-arterial infusion of vasopressin is effective in controlling the bleeding, at least temporarily.

PHARMACOLOGIC THERAPY

Despite the ability of acid neutralization to prevent clot lysis by gastric juices in vitro, administration of antacid or I.V. infusion of H_2 receptor blockers does not lower the incidence of recurrent bleeding in patients with bleeding peptic ulcers. It is

possible that these regimens do not lower the gastric acidity enough. Proton pump inhibitors such as omeprazole can produce near-total acid suppression. In a randomized, controlled trial, oral omeprazole significantly reduced the risk of rebleeding and the need for surgery in patients with a visible vessel or clot at their ulcer base.[9] In preliminary studies, I.V. omeprazole (which is not yet available for clinical use) was found to be useful in preventing recurrent bleeding and in decreasing transfusion requirement in patients with average risk of rebleeding.[4]

The hormone vasopressin causes splanchnic vasoconstriction that leads to a reduction in portal pressure. Meta-analysis of controlled trials shows that vasopressin is efficacious in stopping acute variceal bleeding.[10] However, almost 50% of treated patients develop cardiovascular side effects. Glypressin (2 mg I.V. every 4 hours for 48 hours), a synthetic analogue of vasopressin, offers the same efficacy but has fewer side effects and is associated with a reduction in mortality in patients with acute variceal bleeding.[10]

Somatostatin or its long-acting synthetic analogue, octreotide, has emerged as the drug of choice for acute treatment of upper GI variceal bleeding. Somatostatin reduces splanchnic blood flow, inhibits acid secretion, and does not have systemic side effects. Somatostatin (250 µg I.V. bolus, followed by 48-hour to 72-hour infusion at 250 µg/hr) or octreotide (100 µg I.V. bolus, followed by 24-hour to 48-hour infusion at 25 µg/hr) is comparable to vasopressin or glypressin in stopping acute variceal bleeding and in preventing early rebleeding.[10,11] The addition of octreotide to emergency sclerotherapy further reduces the blood transfusion requirement.[12]

Meta-analysis of studies using somatostatin or octreotide suggests that these drugs lead to a modest reduction in the risk of continued bleeding from bleeding peptic ulcers.[13]

ENDOSCOPIC THERAPY

Several endoscopic techniques can provide effective low-morbidity therapy for certain lesions. Clinical trials indicate that acute bleeding from peptic ulcers, esophageal varices, and angiodysplastic lesions can be controlled by one or more therapeutic endoscopic techniques. About 10% to 25% of patients with acute upper GI bleeding will require endoscopic therapy for hemostasis.[1,5] For patients with bleeding peptic ulcers, endoscopic coagulation therapy is indicated only when active bleeding is seen during endoscopy or when a visible vessel (i.e., a red, blue, or black protuberance in the ulcer bed, representing a sentinel clot over a disrupted artery) is found in the ulcer base. An ulcer with an actively bleeding vessel or a nonbleeding visible vessel is associated with a 50% to 80% rebleeding rate; the rebleeding rate for an ulcer with a clean base is 5%.[14]

Several studies have shown that the neodymium:yttrium-aluminum-garnet (Nd:YAG) laser can achieve immediate hemostasis in bleeding ulcers, and it prevents rebleeding.[15] These studies also indicate a trend toward reducing the number of blood transfusions, decreasing the need for emergency surgery, and lowering mortality. Nd:YAG laser therapy has been shown to reduce the blood transfusion requirement in patients with chronic bleeding from vascular ectasias in the GI tract.[16] Perforation or exacerbation of bleeding by the laser may occur in about 1% of patients. However, because of poor portability, technical difficulties in using the instrument, and expense, the Nd:YAG laser has mostly been replaced by newer and less expensive techniques for endoscopic hemostasis (see below).

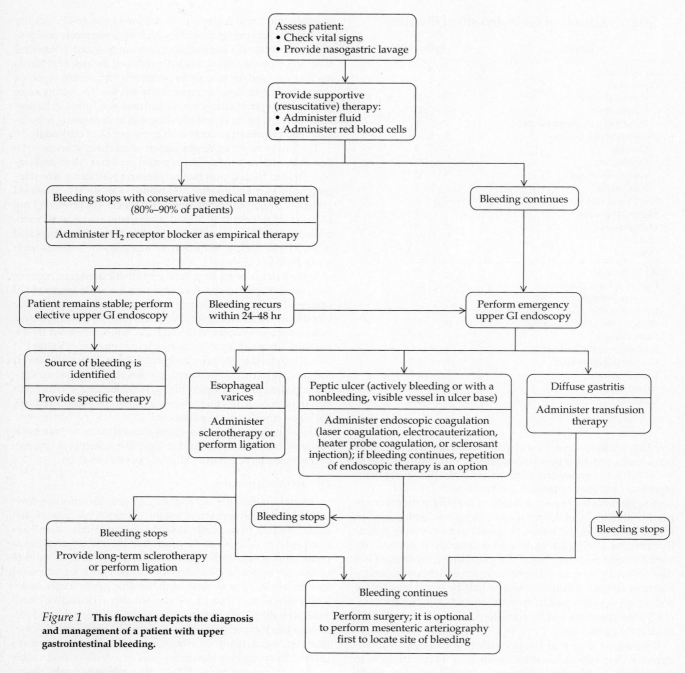

Figure 1 **This flowchart depicts the diagnosis and management of a patient with upper gastrointestinal bleeding.**

Nonvariceal Bleeding

Thermotherapy   Two thermotherapeutic endoscopic modalities have become standard tools in the treatment of upper GI bleeding. The multipolar probe electrocoagulates tissue by the flow of current between six different electrodes on the tip of the probe [*see Figure 2*]. The heater probe coagulates tissue with a high local temperature. Both of these probes require only a compact, portable electric generator. Controlled studies have demonstrated the efficacy of these two thermal devices in controlling bleeding and in reducing the need for blood transfusion and surgery.[14,17]

The argon plasma coagulator is another commercially available device that produces tissue coagulation by delivering a desiccating high-frequency alternating current using ionized argon gas. As with lasers, it does not require tissue contact to achieve coagulation. However, the argon plasma coagulator is significantly less expensive and more portable than lasers. Preliminary studies have shown that this device has an efficacy and safety profile similar to that of the multipolar probe and heater probe.[18]

Injection therapy   Endoscopic injection of epinephrine or a sclerosant, such as ethanol or polidocanol, into a bleeding ulcer has been shown to be efficacious for acute hemostasis. Local compression of the bleeding vessel by the injected solution may be one of the mechanisms of hemostasis.[19] Several controlled studies have shown that the efficacy of injection therapy is comparable to that of the multipolar probe and heater probe.[4,14] Preliminary studies suggest that injection therapy using compounds such as thrombin and fibrin alone or in combi-

a

b

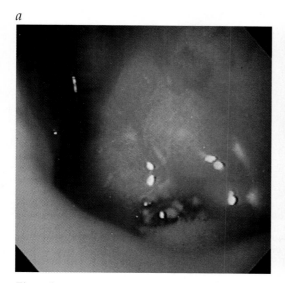
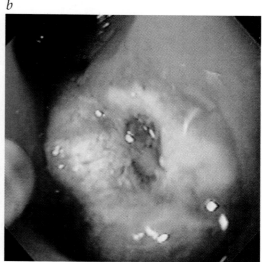

Figure 2 A bleeding vessel, here seen adjacent to a duodenal ulcer (*a*), can be controlled by electrocoagulation with a bipolar probe (*b*). The probe is seen in the lower left corner.

nation with epinephrine may further decrease the rebleeding rate.[4,18] These observations await confirmation.

Injection therapy is the least expensive of these techniques and technically the easiest. Many endoscopists add the application of thermotherapy or the injection of sclerosing agents after the initial epinephrine injection. However, whether these combined therapies offer additional advantages is still unclear.[4,14,20]

Efficacy of therapies All the endoscopic therapies described above have similar efficacy for acute hemostasis and prevention of rebleeding. Perhaps because of the small number of patients studied, most controlled trials of endoscopic therapies for bleeding ulcers have not demonstrated a reduction in overall mortality. However, two meta-analyses have indicated that such therapies offer a 30% to 60% reduction in mortality.[14] Endoscopic therapies cause perforation in 0.5% of treated pa-

tients and induce further bleeding that requires surgical therapy in 0.3%.[14] Ulcer healing is not impaired by endoscopic treatments.[14] Patients who are taking anticoagulants can also be safely treated by these endoscopic methods.[21]

Variceal Bleeding

Sclerotherapy Until recently, sclerotherapy was the treatment of choice for variceal bleeding. Several compounds, such as sodium morrhuate, sodium tetradecyl sulfate, and ethanolamine oleate, are currently used in the United States as variceal sclerosing agents. They are injected into or around the variceal channels with a 25-gauge needle through the endoscope's biopsy channel [*see Figure 3*].

Emergency sclerotherapy was effective in controlling the acute bleeding episode in 74% to 91% of patients with bleeding esophageal varices, whereas balloon tamponade was effective

a

b

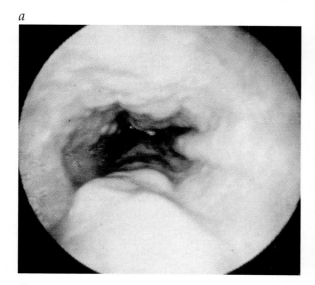
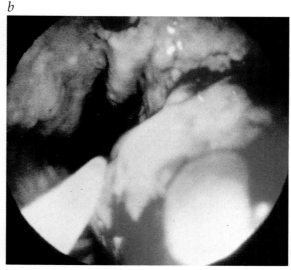

Figure 3 Endoscopic sclerotherapy is an effective method of controlling variceal bleeding. A large, grade 4 esophageal varix (*a*) is injected with an agent that achieves hemostasis. After the injection needle is withdrawn from the varix (*b*), some back-bleeding occurs. The injected varix is slightly larger than it was before injection. The puncture site is seen just adjacent to the tip of the needle.

a

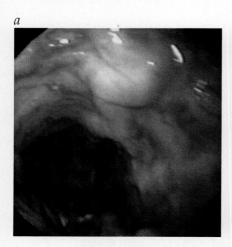

b

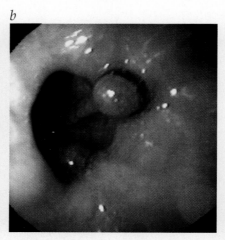

c

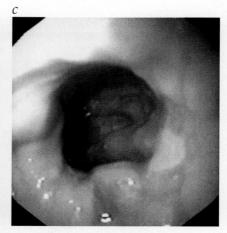

Figure 4 (*a*) **Endoscopy of the upper gastrointestinal tract reveals esophageal varices. (*b*) Rubber-band ligation has been performed on two varices. (*c*) A shallow ulcer is visible at a ligation site 2 weeks after the procedure.**

in only 42% to 55%.[10] Also, the magnitude and frequency of rebleeding were lower when sclerotherapy was compared with tamponade or medical therapy alone.[10] However, sclerotherapy is not effective for treating bleeding gastric varices unless they are located within 2 cm below the gastroesophageal junction.

A short course of sclerotherapy with two or three treatment sessions in the few days after the initial bleeding incident will not improve the long-term survival of patients with bleeding esophageal varices.[10] In patients presenting with severe liver disease, both sclerotherapy and emergency shunt surgery are associated with an acute mortality of about 50%.[22] The long-term efficacy of sclerotherapy will not be apparent until all the variceal channels are obliterated. It usually takes four to six outpatient sclerotherapy sessions during a period of approximately 3 months to achieve this goal. Several controlled trials have reported a significant reduction in recurrent variceal bleeding in patients who underwent long-term sclerotherapy (rebleeding rate, 30% to 40%), compared with those who were followed medically (rebleeding rate, 60% to 75%).[10] The effect of sclerotherapy on the long-term survival of patients with varices is controversial. Meta-analysis of all the reported controlled trial data suggests that sclerotherapy may improve survival in the treated patients by 25%.[10]

About half of patients may experience transient dysphagia, substernal chest pain, and fever in the first 48 hours after endoscopic sclerotherapy.[23] Superficial ulcerations at the injection sites probably occur in all patients undergoing sclerotherapy. This result reflects the natural course of the therapy, which induces fibrosis at the injection sites. However, deep ulceration with necrosis and significant hemorrhage from these ulcers may occur in about 10% of patients.[23] Esophageal perforation immediately after the procedure is rare with use of the flexible fiberoptic endoscope but may occur in 2% to 4% of patients with use of the rigid endoscope.[24] Delayed perforation from transmural necrosis has been reported, but the actual incidence of this complication is unknown.[23]

Strictures at the injection sites, which usually respond to simple dilatation, develop in about 15% of patients. Very rare complications include pericarditis, clinically significant pleural effusion, acute respiratory distress syndrome, brain abscess, and spinal artery occlusion. Overall, clinically significant complications occur in 10% to 15% of patients undergoing sclero-

therapy. This rate compares favorably with the rate of complications associated with decompressive shunt surgery in patients with bleeding esophageal varices.

Endoscopic variceal ligation Ligation of bleeding esophageal variceal channels by a rubber banding device applied through an endoscope is the first-line endoscopic therapy for the condition. The current commercially available variceal ligator consists of a housing cylinder that can be mounted on the tip of most flexible endoscopes. Inside the housing cylinder is a banding cylinder with one to six rubber O rings preloaded on its distal end.[25] During the ligation process, the target variceal channel is drawn into the ligator's chamber by means of suction through the endoscope. The rubber O ring is then released and ensnares the variceal pedicle [*see Figure 4*].

For actively bleeding variceal channels, ligations are started at or near the bleeding sites. For nonbleeding varices, the process should be started at the gastroesophageal junction and should proceed cephalad. For most small varices, one ligation at the distal esophagus is adequate. For larger varices, a second ligation is needed within a few centimeters above the first ligation site. An average of five to 10 ligations are usually performed in the initial session, with progressively decreasing numbers in later sessions. Follow-up ligation sessions are repeated weekly until the varices are obliterated. Three to four treatment sessions are usually required.[26,27]

Hemostasis by rubber-band ligation is achieved initially by strangulation of the variceal channel [*see Figure 4b*]. The banded varix will thrombose and slough off in 3 to 7 days, leaving a shallow ulcer [*see Figure 4c*]. The ulcer heals in 2 to 3 weeks.[28] The initial hemostasis rate achieved by ligation is comparable to the rate achieved by sclerotherapy.[26] Meta-analysis, however, suggests that compared with sclerotherapy, variceal ligation reduces the rebleeding rate, the mortality from bleeding, and the overall mortality.[26] On average, fewer treatment sessions are needed to obliterate the varices by ligation than by sclerotherapy.

Clinically significant complications of variceal ligation therapy occur in only 2% to 3% of cases—significantly lower than the 10% to 15% associated with sclerotherapy. A number of local esophageal complications associated with ligation have been described. Transient substernal discomfort of 24 to 48 hours' duration has been reported by most patients. Large but shallow

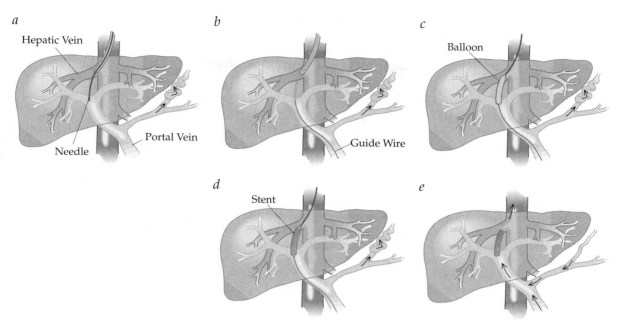

Figure 5 **This figure depicts, in order, the steps involved in the transjugular intrahepatic portosystemic shunt placement procedure. (*a*) A modified transseptal needle is advanced from a hepatic vein into a portal vein via an angiographic catheter inserted through the jugular vein. (Arrows indicate hepatofugal flow in an enlarged coronary vein.) (*b*) A guide wire is advanced through the needle into the portal vein. (*c*) An 8 mm angioplasty balloon is advanced over the guide wire and expanded across the hepatic parenchymal tract. (*d*) A Wallstent, mounted on a delivery catheter, is expanded to bridge the hepatic and portal veins. (*e*) The stent serves as an intrahepatic shunt from the portal vein to the hepatic vein. With return to hepatopetal flow, the coronary vein becomes smaller.[71]**

ulcerations at the ligation sites are a natural result of the therapy.[29] However, because the injury to the esophageal wall at the ligation site spares the muscularis, transmural ulceration and stricture formation after variceal ligation are rare. Esophageal stricture developed in only 2% of the first 100 patients studied and in none of the patients in later controlled trials.[26] Only one case of bleeding from a deep ulcer induced by ligation has been reported.[30] Transient esophageal obstruction caused by the banded variceal pedicle or by spasm may also occur.[31]

The new multiband ligator eliminates the need for an overtube, which can injure the esophagus.[32] Transient bacteremia, aspiration pneumonia, and bacterial peritonitis occur in about 2% to 10% of patients undergoing variceal ligation. This complication rate may also be lower than that associated with sclerotherapy.[26,33] Mortality directly related to variceal ligation therapy is about 0.2%.[26]

Efficacy of therapies Variceal ligation appears to be as efficacious as sclerotherapy in controlling active esophageal variceal bleeding. The technique is superior to sclerotherapy in the prevention of recurrent variceal bleeding and in survival. The low procedure-related complication rate is an additional benefit. Addition of low-dose sclerotherapy to ligation offers no additional benefit to ligation alone and causes more complications.[34,35]

Transjugular intrahepatic portosystemic shunt Another technique in stopping variceal bleeding involves placement of a self-expanding metal mesh stent between the hepatic vein and a branch of the portal vein via angiographic catheters inserted through the right jugular vein [*see Figure 5*]. In centers that have a medical staff experienced in using this procedure, transjugular intrahepatic portosystemic shunts (TIPS) have

been placed in patients with a wide variety of liver diseases to control variceal bleeding. In one large uncontrolled study, the technical success rate of TIPS was 96%, and the mean procedure time was 2.5 hours. Reduction of portal hypertension occurred immediately after stent placement. Variceal bleeding was controlled in 88% of patients; in addition, ascites significantly abated in about 70% of patients.[36] There was no immediate mortality directly related to the procedure.

In a mean follow-up of 2.2 years, the cumulative survival rate was 60% at 1 year and 51% at 2 years.[37] Occlusion of the stent developed in 31% of patients at 1 year and in 47% at 2 years. Stent occlusion led to a rebleeding rate of 26% at 1 year and 32% at 2 years. Percutaneous shunt revision was successful in 95% of the rebleeding patients. Onset or exacerbation of encephalopathy occurred in 18% of patients, most of whom were treated successfully with lactulose. Rare and nonfatal procedure-related complications of TIPS include intraperitoneal hemorrhage, hemobilia, sepsis, transient renal failure, and myocardial infarction.

These results have been substantiated by several other studies.[38,39] TIPS can salvage patients with acute variceal bleeding in whom emergency sclerotherapy failed.[40] Several randomized trials have reported the superiority of TIPS over sclerotherapy or band ligation in preventing rebleeding.[41-43] However, the rate of encephalopathy is significantly higher in patients treated with TIPS than in patients treated with the endoscopic methods. There is no difference in the long-term survival of patients treated by TIPS and of those treated by endoscopic means. Unlike sclerotherapy and variceal ligation, TIPS can effectively control bleeding from gastric varices and portal hypertensive gastropathy. Because of its beneficial effects on ascites, renal function, and nutrition, TIPS has become an important therapy for patients with variceal bleeding who are awaiting liver transplantation.

SURGICAL CONSULTATION AND THERAPY

Surgical consultation should be obtained early. When the surgeon and the physician follow the course of the patient's condition, no time is lost in making the joint decision that is required if surgical treatment becomes necessary.

Surgical therapy in patients with nonvariceal upper GI bleeding is reserved for patients who lose more than six units of blood in 24 hours despite optimal support and in whom appropriate therapeutic endoscopy is unsuccessful. About 20% of patients with nonvariceal upper GI bleeding may develop recurrent bleeding despite endoscopic therapy.[14] Despite a slightly higher risk of perforation, a second session of endoscopic therapy may stop the bleeding in half of these patients.[14] Surgery is therefore needed in only about 10% of patients who originally require endoscopic therapy. For a small bleeding ulcer, simple oversewing or resection of the ulcer is adequate. Traditional ulcer surgery is not necessary, because most peptic ulcers are associated with *Helicobacter pylori* infection, and eradication of the infection effectively reduces ulcer recurrence and rebleeding.[44,45] More extensive gastrectomy is reserved for large bleeding ulcers or diffuse hemorrhagic gastritis.[46]

Surgical portacaval shunt for patients with variceal bleeding is associated with a high hemostasis rate, but it is also associated with high acute morbidity and mortality. Surgical shunt is no better than sclerotherapy for patients with variceal bleeding due to advanced cirrhosis.[14] For patients who fail emergency sclerotherapy, TIPS is probably the salvage procedure of choice when compared with other surgical options.[40,47]

PROGNOSIS

Although the age-adjusted mortality from GI bleeding is lower than in the past,[48] the overall mortality (5% to 14%) remains unchanged.[2,47,48] This lack of improvement in overall mortality is partly the result of an increase in the number of elderly patients presenting with acute GI bleeding and significant comorbid conditions. For patients younger than 60 years who have no underlying malignancy or organ failure, the mortality can be less than 1%.[48] However, very elderly patients, patients with variceal bleeding, patients with malignancy, and patients who develop bleeding after hospitalization for other comorbid diseases may have acute mortality of over 30%.[2,47,48] Multisystem organ failure, rather than exsanguination, is the usual cause of death in these patients.[2,47]

Bleeding in the Small Intestine

Bleeding from sites between the distal duodenum and the lower ileum is uncommon but may be indolent and difficult to localize. Angiodysplasia is the major cause; Meckel's diverticulum and benign tumors also contribute. These lesions may be localized by arteriography or computed tomography, by exploratory surgery with intraoperative enteroscopy, or, occasionally, by barium contrast x-ray of the small intestine.[49]

Other techniques used to localize a bleeding site or a potentially bleeding lesion, especially when the bleeding is relatively slow, are red blood cell scintigraphy and intestinal intubation with a small-diameter plastic tube fitted with a terminal weight. During intubation, the patient is fed a liquid diet, and the tube is aspirated hourly as it is propelled by peristalsis through the small intestine. When gross blood is first identified, the tube can be secured by being taped to the face of the patient; a Gastrografin x-ray contrast study is performed to localize the bleeding lesion before surgery. Small bowel endoscopy with either a push enteroscope or a sonde enteroscope may be able to identify bleeding lesions of the small bowel in one third of patients with chronic GI bleeding of obscure origin [*see Figure 6*].[50] Cauterization of angiodysplasia in the small intestine may reduce long-term blood transfusion requirements.[51]

Lower Gastrointestinal Bleeding

Bleeding from the colon accounts for 10% to 20% of all cases of GI bleeding[2,52] and primarily affects elderly patients.

The most common cause of lower GI bleeding is diverticulosis.[52] Other causes are colorectal malignancy, ischemic colitis, hemorrhoids, inflammatory bowel disease, infectious colitis, and angiodysplasia [*see Table 1*].[52-54]

Lower GI bleeding usually presents as the passage of red blood and clots. Its presentation may be very abrupt. In addition

a

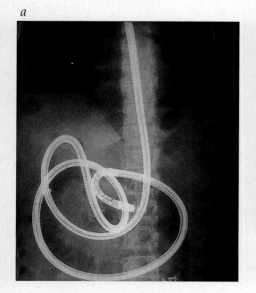

b

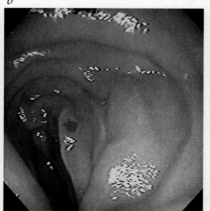

c

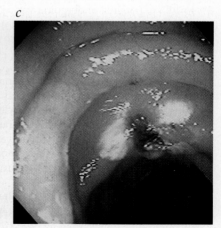

Figure 6 (*a*) Placement of a push enteroscope for small bowel endoscopy is seen on an abdominal x-ray. The push enteroscope allows examination of the jejunum up to 100 cm beyond the ligament of Treitz. (*b*) Small bowel endoscopy reveals a jejunal arteriovenous malformation (AVM). (*c*) The jejunal AVM is seen after coagulation therapy.

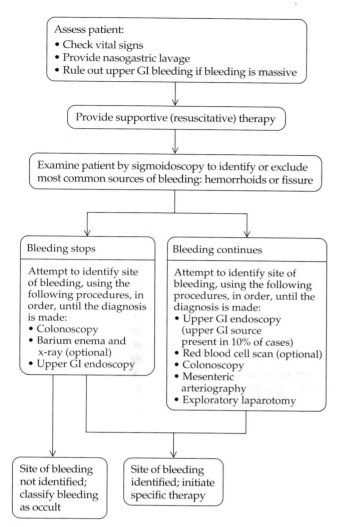

```
Assess patient:
• Check vital signs
• Provide nasogastric lavage
• Rule out upper GI bleeding if bleeding is massive
                    ↓
Provide supportive (resuscitative) therapy
                    ↓
Examine patient by sigmoidoscopy to identify or exclude
most common sources of bleeding: hemorrhoids or fissure
```

Bleeding stops

Attempt to identify site of bleeding, using the following procedures, in order, until the diagnosis is made:
• Colonoscopy
• Barium enema and x-ray (optional)
• Upper GI endoscopy

Bleeding continues

Attempt to identify site of bleeding, using the following procedures, in order, until the diagnosis is made:
• Upper GI endoscopy (upper GI source present in 10% of cases)
• Red blood cell scan (optional)
• Colonoscopy
• Mesenteric arteriography
• Exploratory laparotomy

Site of bleeding not identified; classify bleeding as occult

Site of bleeding identified; initiate specific therapy

Figure 7 **This flowchart depicts the diagnosis of a patient with lower gastrointestinal bleeding.**

to the same supportive therapy as that used for upper GI bleeding, anoscopy and sigmoidoscopy should be done as soon as the patient is stabilized, to exclude anorectal lesions [*see Figure 7*]. Colonoscopy can be performed only after the bowel has been purged with polyethylene glycol solution.[53,54] The diagnostic yield of colonoscopy is high, and up to 70% of detected lesions can be treated endoscopically.[53] If the bleeding is persistent and brisk, angiography and possible embolic therapy may be attempted.[8,52] The accuracy of radionuclide scanning is controversial.[8] Recent developments in continuous dynamic imaging and the commercial availability of a method of in vitro red cell labeling have led to improvements in the quality and accuracy of radionuclide scanning.[55] However, results of large prospective trials evaluating the sensitivity and specificity of the new radionuclide scanning technique have not been reported.

Unlike patients with upper GI bleeding, a significant proportion of patients with lower GI bleeding—up to 15%—may need surgical therapy. The average acute mortality of patients with lower GI bleeding is only about 5% but increases fivefold if bleeding develops after hospitalization for other underlying diseases. Most patients with lower GI bleeding are elderly, a factor contributing to a long-term mortality of about 20% in one study; recurrent bleeding occurred in 25% of patients with

diverticulosis in this study period.[52] However, none of the deaths was due to lower GI bleeding.

Occult Gastrointestinal Bleeding

Occult GI bleeding may present either as unexplained iron deficiency anemia or as intermittent positive results on chemical testing for blood in stool samples (i.e., the Hemoccult test). The lesions that cause occult GI bleeding are the same as those that cause overt GI hemorrhage, varying in incidence around the world.[56] In the United States, peptic ulcer disease and colonic neoplasm are the leading causes of occult GI bleeding. In a prospective study of 100 patients with iron deficiency anemia, 36 were found to have bleeding sites in the upper GI tract, and 25 had bleeding sites in the colon; one patient had lesions in both the upper and the lower GI tracts.[57] Enteroclysis was unable to identify bleeding lesions in the small intestine when upper GI endoscopy and colonoscopy were negative. Regardless of the Hemoccult test results, patients' site-specific symptoms were found to precede abnormalities in the corresponding segment of the intestine.[57] In asymptomatic patients, there was an equal probability of finding lesions in the upper and lower GI tract. Other studies suggested that patients' symptoms are not useful in determining the site of the bleeding.[58,59] All of these studies reported that concomitant bleeding sites in the upper and lower GI tracts are rare.[57-59] Therefore, in the evaluation of symptomatic patients, the choice of upper endoscopy or colonoscopy as the initial evaluation need not be made randomly but can be guided by the patients' symptoms. If a bleeding lesion is found on initial endoscopy, no further evaluation is needed. It may not be necessary to use both upper endoscopy and colonoscopy in all patients; however, for patients at high risk for colon cancer, colonoscopy should always be performed.

For asymptomatic patients, colonoscopy may be used as the initial examination for excluding the possibility of a colonic neoplasm. If the initial endoscopic examination does not reveal the bleeding site, endoscopic evaluation of the remaining bowel segment should be performed. Identification of a lesion at any step of this procedure should be followed by appropriate medical or surgical therapy. If the bleeding source is still not identified after upper GI endoscopy and colonoscopy, several less invasive procedures should be considered. A small bowel enteroclysis study should be performed to rule out rare tumors in the small intestine. Small bowel endoscopy may identify bleeding lesions in 33% of patients with a negative upper GI endoscopy and colonoscopy [*see* Bleeding in the Small Intestine, *above*]. For patients who require transfusions and in whom the source of bleeding is not identified on endoscopy, mesenteric arteriography is the next investigative step. If arteriography fails to reveal the bleeding site, exploratory laparotomy with intraoperative enteroscopy should be performed.

Prevention of Gastrointestinal Bleeding

The reported efficacy of nasogastric infusion of antacid or sucralfate and of I.V. administration of H_2 receptor blockers in the prevention of GI bleeding in critically ill patients has led to generalized use of such prophylactic therapies in the intensive care unit.[60] However, the risk of upper GI bleeding in ICU patients has decreased substantially over the past decade independent of the use of prophylactic therapy.[61] Routine use of prophylactic therapy for the prevention of upper GI bleeding may not be justified in all ICU patients. Besides head injuries and burns that cover more than 30% of the patient's body surface area, two major risk factors for GI bleeding in ICU patients have been identified: (1) respiratory failure that requires mechanical ventilator support and (2) coagulopathy.[61] In a large randomized trial, an intravenous H_2 receptor blocker significantly reduced the rate of clinically important GI bleeding in high-risk patients who required mechanical ventilator support.[62] This study confirmed the value of H_2 receptor blockers reported in previous trials.[60] However, this study showed that sucralfate was inferior to an H_2 receptor blocker in preventing GI bleeding in these patients. There were no significant differences in the rates of ventilator-associated pneumonia, the duration of ICU stay, or mortality.

Patients on long-term nonsteroidal anti-inflammatory drug therapy have a high incidence of gastroduodenal ulcers and bleeding. Misoprostol and high-dose famotidine (40 mg twice daily) and omeprazole (20 mg daily) reduce GI complications in these patients [63-66] [see Chapter 87]. Omeprazole therapy is probably the easiest to follow and the best tolerated for these patients. However, it remains unclear whether prophylactic treatment prevents GI bleeding in these patients.

Prevention of peptic ulcer recurrence and bleeding can be achieved by eradication of H. pylori[44,45] [see Chapter 87]. This short-term therapy probably has a higher patient compliance rate than long-term maintenance therapy with ranitidine, which can also prevent the recurrence of bleeding in patients who have bled from duodenal ulcers.[67]

Reduction in recurrent variceal bleeding can be achieved by means of sclerotherapy, variceal ligation, or TIPS [see Upper Gastrointestinal Bleeding, Endoscopic Therapy, above]. Propranolol, given in a dose that reduces the heart rate by 25%, may also be a beneficial therapy in patients with rebleeding varices.[68]

In patients with varices that have never bled, prophylactic shunt placement or sclerotherapy is of no benefit in preventing a first variceal bleed.[10] Preliminary studies suggest that variceal ligation may be effective in this setting.[69,70] At present, propranolol appears to be the only efficacious prophylactic therapy for patients who have not had bleeding varices. Patients with large varices who are at high risk for bleeding may be started on propranolol therapy.[10]

Additional Information

New information on GI bleeding and endoscopy is posted periodically on the Web sites of the American Gastroenterological Association (http://www.gastro.org/), the American College of Gastroenterology (http://www.acg.gi.org/), and the American Society for Gastrointestinal Endoscopy (http://www.asge.org/).

References

1. Yavorski RT, Wong RK, Maydonovitch C, et al: Analysis of 3,294 cases of upper gastrointestinal bleeding in military medical facilities. Am J Gastroenterol 90:568, 1995

2. Friedman LS, Martin P: The problem of gastrointestinal bleeding. Gastroenterol Clin North Am 22:717, 1993

3. Longstreth GF, Feitelberg SP: Outpatient care of selected patients with acute nonvariceal upper gastrointestinal haemorrhage. Lancet 345:108, 1995

4. Rollhauser C, Fleischer DE: Nonvariceal upper gastrointestinal bleeding: an update. Endoscopy 29:91, 1997

5. Longstreth GF: Epidemiology of hospitalization for acute upper gastrointestinal hemorrhage: a population-based study. Am J Gastroenterol 90:206, 1995

6. Rockall TA, Logan RFA, Devlin HB, et al: Selection of patients for early discharge or outpatient care after acute upper gastrointestinal haemorrhage. Lancet 347:1138, 1996

7. Hay JA, Maldonado L, Weingarten SR, et al: Prospective evaluation of a clinical guideline recommending hospital length of stay in upper gastrointestinal tract hemorrhage. JAMA 278:2151, 1997

8. Shapiro MJ: The role of the radiologist in the management of gastrointestinal bleeding. Gastroenterol Clin North Am 23:123, 1994

9. Khuroo MS, Yattoo GN, Javid G, et al: A comparison of omeprazole and placebo for bleeding peptic ulcer. N Engl J Med 336:1054, 1997

10. D'Amico G, Pagliaro L, Bosch J: The treatment of portal hypertension: a meta-analytic review. Hepatology 22:332, 1995

11. Feu F, del Arbol LR, Bañares R, et al: Double-blind randomized controlled trial comparing terlipressin and somatostatin for acute variceal hemorrhage. Gastroenterology 111:1291, 1996

12. Besson I, Ingrand P, Person B, et al: Sclerotherapy with or without octreotide for acute variceal bleeding. N Engl J Med 333:555, 1995

13. Imperiale TF, Birgisson S: Somatostatin or octreotide compared with H_2 antagonists and placebo in the management of acute nonvariceal upper gastrointestinal hemorrhage: a meta-analysis. Ann Intern Med 127:1062, 1997

14. Laine L, Peterson WL: Bleeding peptic ulcer. N Engl J Med 331:717, 1994

15. Swain CP: Laser therapy for gastrointestinal bleeding. Gastrointest Endosc Clin N Am 7:611, 1997

16. Liberski SM, McGarrity TJ, Hartle RJ, et al: The watermelon stomach: long-term outcome in patients treated with Nd:YAG laser therapy. Gastrointest Endosc 40:584, 1994

17. Kumar P, Fleischer DE: Thermal therapy for gastrointestinal bleeding. Gastrointest Endosc Clin N Am 7:593, 1997

18. Soehendra N, Bohnacker S, Binmoeller KF: Nonvariceal upper gastrointestinal bleeding: new and alternative hemostatic techniques. Gastrointest Endosc Clin N Am 7:641, 1997

19. Lai KH, Peng SN, Guo WS, et al: Endoscopic injection for the treatment of bleeding ulcers: local tamponade or drug effect? Endoscopy 26:338, 1994

20. Lin H-J, Perng C-L, Lee S-D: Is sclerosant injection mandatory after an epinephrine injection for arrest of peptic ulcer haemorrhage? A prospective, randomised, comparative study. Gut 34:1182, 1993

21. Choudari CP, Rajgopal C, Palmer KR: Acute gastrointestinal haemorrhage in anticoagulated patients: diagnoses and response to endoscopic treatment. Gut 35:464, 1994

22. Cello JP, Grendell JH, Crass RA, et al: Endoscopic sclerotherapy versus portacaval shunt in patients with severe cirrhosis and acute variceal hemorrhage. N Engl J Med 316:11, 1987

23. Schuman BM, Beckman JW, Tedesco FJ, et al: Complications of endoscopic injection sclerotherapy: a review. Am J Gastroenterol 82:823, 1987

24. Bornman PC, Kahn D, Terblanche J, et al: Rigid versus fiberoptic endoscopic injection sclerotherapy: a prospective randomized controlled trial in patients with bleeding varices. Ann Surg 208:175, 1988

25. Saeed ZA: The Saeed six-shooter: a prospective study of a new endoscopic multiple rubber-band ligator for the treatment of varices. Endoscopy 28:559, 1996

26. Laine L, Cook D: Endoscopic ligation compared with sclerotherapy for treatment of esophageal variceal bleeding. Ann Intern Med 123:280, 1995

27. Stiegmann GV, Goff JS, Michaletz-Onody PA, et al: Endoscopic sclerotherapy as compared with endoscopic ligation for bleeding esophageal varices. N Engl J Med 326:1527, 1992

28. Marks RD, Arnold MD, Baron TH: Gross and microscopic findings in the human esophagus after esophageal variceal band ligation: a postmortem analysis. Am J Gastroenterol 88:272, 1993

29. Young MF, Sanowski RA, Rasche R: Comparison and characterization of ulcerations induced by endoscopic ligation of esophageal varices versus endoscopic sclerotherapy. Gastrointest Endosc 39:119, 1993

30. Johnson PA, Campbell DR, Antonson CW, et al: Complications associated with endoscopic band ligation of esophageal varices. Gastrointest Endosc 39:181, 1993

31. Stiegmann GV: Endoscopic ligation: now and the future. Gastrointest Endosc 39:203, 1993

32. Dennert B, Ramirez FC, Sanowski RA: A prospective evaluation of the endoscopic spectrum of overtube-related esophageal mucosal injury. Gastrointest Endosc 45:134, 1997

33. Lo G-H, Lai K-H, Shen M-T, et al: A comparison of the incidence of transient bacteremia and infectious sequelae after sclerotherapy and rubber band ligation of bleeding esophageal varices. Gastrointest Endosc 40:675, 1994

34. Laine L, Stein C, Sharma V: Randomized comparison of ligation versus ligation plus sclerotherapy in patients with bleeding esophageal varices. Gastroenterology 110:529, 1996

35. Saeed ZA, Stiegmann GV, Ramirez FC, et al: Endoscopic variceal ligation is superior to combined ligation and sclerotherapy for esophageal varices: a multicenter prospective randomized trial. Hepatology 25:71, 1997

36. LaBerge JM, Ring EJ, Gordon RL, et al: Creation of transjugular intrahepatic portosystemic shunts with the Wallstent endoprosthesis: results in 100 patients. Radiology 187:413, 1993

37. LaBerge JM, Somberg KA, Lake JR, et al: Two-year outcome following intrahepatic transjugular portosystemic shunt for variceal bleeding: results in 90 patients. Gastroenterology 108:1143, 1995

38. Rössle M, Haag K, Ochs A, et al: The transjugular intrahepatic portosystemic stent-shunt procedure for variceal bleeding. N Engl J Med 330:165, 1994

39. Stanley AJ, Redhead DN, Hayes PC: Review article: update on the role of transjugular intrahepatic portosystemic stent-shunt (TIPSS) in the management of complications of portal hypertension. Aliment Pharmacol Ther 11:261, 1997

40. Sanyal AJ, Freedman AM, Luketic VA, et al: Transjugular intrahepatic portosystemic

shunts for patients with active variceal hemorrhage unresponsive to sclerotherapy. Gastroenterology 111:138, 1996

41. Sanyal AJ, Freedman AM, Luketic VA, et al: Transjugular intrahepatic portosystemic shunts compared with endoscopic sclerotherapy for the prevention of recurrent variceal hemorrhage: a randomized, controlled trial. Ann Intern Med 126:849, 1997

42. Rössle M, Deibert P, Haag K, et al: Randomised trial of transjugular-intrahepatic-portosystemic shunt versus endoscopy plus propranolol for prevention of variceal rebleeding. Lancet 349:1043, 1997

43. Jalan R, Forrest EH, Stanley AJ, et al: A randomized trial comparing transjugular intrahepatic portosystemic stent–shunt with variceal band ligation in the prevention of rebleeding from esophageal varices. Hepatology 26:1115, 1997

44. Santander C, Grávalos RG, Gómez-Cedenilla A, et al: Antimicrobial therapy for *Helicobacter pylori* infection versus long-term maintenance antisecretion treatment in the prevention of recurrent hemorrhage from peptic ulcer: prospective nonrandomized trial on 125 patients. Am J Gastroenterol 91:1549, 1996

45. Riemann JF, Schilling D, Schauwecker P, et al: Cure with omeprazole plus amoxicillin versus long-term ranitidine therapy in *Helicobacter pylori*–associated peptic ulcer bleeding. Gastrointest Endosc 46:299, 1997

46. Chung CS: Surgery and gastrointestinal bleeding. Gastrointest Endosc Clin N Am 7:687, 1997

47. Jalan R, John TJ, Redhead DN, et al: A comparative study of emergency transjugular intrahepatic portosystemic stent–shunt and esophageal transection in the management of uncontrolled variceal hemorrhage. Am J Gastroenterol 90:1932, 1995

48. Rockall TA, Logan RFA, Devlin HB, et al: Incidence of and mortality from acute upper gastrointestinal haemorrhage in the United Kingdom. BMJ 311:222, 1995

49. Lewis BS: Small intestinal bleeding. Gastroenterol Clin North Am 23:67, 1994

50. Berner JS, Mauer K, Lewis BS: Push and sonde enteroscopy for the diagnosis of obscure gastrointestinal bleeding. Am J Gastroenterol 89:2139, 1994

51. Askin MP, Lewis BS: Push enteroscopic cauterization: long-term follow-up of 83 patients with bleeding small intestinal angiodysplasia. Gastrointest Endosc 43:580, 1996

52. Longstreth GF: Epidemiology and outcome of patients hospitalized with acute lower gastrointestinal hemorrhage: a population-based study. Am J Gastroenterol 92:419, 1997

53. Richter JM, Christensen MR, Kaplan LM, et al: Effectiveness of current technology in the diagnosis and management of lower gastrointestinal hemorrhage. Gastrointest Endosc 41:93, 1995

54. Jensen DM, Machicado GA: Colonoscopy for diagnosis and treatment of severe lower gastrointestinal bleeding: routine outcomes and cost analysis. Gastrointest Endosc Clin N Am 7:477, 1997

55. Maurer AH: Gastrointestinal bleeding and cine-scintigraphy. Semin Nucl Med 26:43, 1996

56. Richter JM: Occult gastrointestinal bleeding. Gastroenterol Clin North Am 23:53, 1994

57. Rockey DC, Cello JP: Evaluation of the gastrointestinal tract in patients with iron-deficiency anemia. N Engl J Med 329:1691, 1993

58. Zuckerman G, Benitez J: A prospective study of bidirectional endoscopy (colonoscopy and upper endoscopy) in the evaluation of patients with occult gastrointestinal bleeding. Am J Gastroenterol 87:62, 1992

59. McIntyre AS, Long RG: Prospective survey of investigations in outpatients referred with iron deficiency anaemia. Gut 34:1102, 1993

60. Cook DJ, Reeve BK, Guyatt GH, et al: Stress ulcer prophylaxis in critically ill patients: resolving discordant meta-analyses. JAMA 275:308, 1996

61. Cook DJ, Fuller HD, Guyatt GH, et al: Risk factors for gastrointestinal bleeding in critically ill patients. N Engl J Med 330:377, 1994

62. Cook D, Guyatt G, Marshall J, et al: A comparison of sucralfate and ranitidine for the prevention of upper gastrointestinal bleeding in patients requiring mechanical ventilation. N Engl J Med 338:791, 1998

63. Taha AS, Hudson N, Hawkey CJ, et al: Famotidine for the prevention of gastric and duodenal ulcers caused by nonsteroidal antiinflammatory drugs. N Engl J Med 334:1435, 1996

64. Hudson N, Taha AS, Russel RI, et al: Famotidine for healing and maintenance in nonsteroidal anti-inflammatory drug-associated gastroduodenal ulceration. Gastroenterology 112:1817, 1997

65. Yeomans ND, Tulassay Z, Juhasz L, et al: A comparison of omeprazole with ranitidine for ulcers associated with nonsteroidal anti-inflammatory drugs. N Engl J Med 338:719, 1998

66. Hawkey CJ, Karrasch JA, Szczepanski L, et al: Omeprazole compared with misoprostol for ulcers associated with nonsteroidal anti-inflammatory drugs. N Engl J Med 338:727, 1998

67. Jensen DM, Cheng S, Kovacs TOG, et al: A controlled study of ranitidine for the prevention of recurrent hemorrhage from duodenal ulcer. N Engl J Med 330:382, 1994

68. Burroughs AK, Panagou E: Pharmacological therapy for portal hypertension: rationale and results. Semin Gastrointest Dis 6:148, 1995

69. Lay CS, Tsai YT, Teg CY, et al: Endoscopic variceal ligation in prophylaxis of first variceal bleeding in cirrhotic patients with high-risk esophageal varices. Hepatology 25:1346, 1997

70. Sarin SK, Guptan RK, Jain AK, et al: A randomized controlled trial of endoscopic variceal band ligation for primary prophylaxis of variceal bleeding. Eur J Gastroenterol Hepatol 8: 337, 1996

71. Zemel G, Katzen BT, Becker GJ, et al: Percutaneous transjugular portosystemic shunt. JAMA 266:390, 1991

Acknowledgments

Figure 1   Janet Betries.
Figure 7   Talar Agasyan.

64 Acute Viral Hepatitis

Emmet B. Keeffe, M.D.

Most cases of acute hepatitis are caused by one of the hepatotrophic viruses, but drug-induced hepatitis and hepatitis that is secondary to other viruses may at times mimic typical acute viral hepatitis. Classic acute viral hepatitis is caused by one of five etiologic agents: hepatitis A virus (HAV), hepatitis B virus (HBV), hepatitis C virus (HCV), hepatitis D virus (HDV), or hepatitis E virus (HEV).[1,2] In the United States in 1999, 59% of reported cases of acute viral hepatitis were caused by HAV infection and 26.5% by HBV infection; 14.5% were classified as non-A, non-B hepatitis or were unspecified.[3] HDV infection (delta hepatitis) occurs either as a superinfection in chronic HBV carriers or as a coinfection during acute HBV infection. HEV infection occurs predominantly outside the United States, but a few cases have been reported in travelers returning to the United States. All five viruses can cause acute hepatitis, but only three—HBV, HCV, and HDV—can lead to chronic infection. A new hepatitis virus, hepatitis G virus (HGV), has been identified but does not appear to be pathogenic, nor does it account for those cases that have been termed non-A–E viral hepatitis, as some investigators originally suggested. Finally, a number of viruses that cause systemic illnesses may also affect the liver—for example, cytomegalovirus (CMV) and Epstein-Barr virus (EBV).

All five types of viral hepatitis are similar and cannot be distinguished reliably by clinical features or routine laboratory tests. Infection either may occur asymptomatically or may be associated with nonspecific flulike symptoms; some patients experience jaundice. The characteristic laboratory abnormality in acute hepatitis is an elevated aminotransferase level, typically greater than 300 IU/L and, occasionally, 1,000 to 3,000 IU/L. The specific etiology of viral hepatitis is determined by serologic testing [*see Table 1*].

Classification and Pathology

HEPATITIS A VIRUS

HAV is a picornavirus similar to poliovirus and rhinovirus.[4] HAV was initially discovered in stool but has also been found in the serum of patients with acute HAV infection and in the cytoplasm of liver cells and bile of animals infected with HAV.[5] It is a nonenveloped, positive-stranded RNA virus that has at least seven genotypes but only one serotype.[4] The antigenic compositions of HAV throughout the world are remarkably similar, which explains the global efficacy of immune globulin and of hepatitis A vaccine. IgM antibody to HAV is detectable at the onset of clinical illness and usually disappears within 60 to 120 days. IgG antibody reaches a high titer during convalescence, persists indefinitely, and confers immunity.

HEPATITIS B VIRUS

HBV, the only member of the family Hepadnaviridae that infects humans, has a diameter of 42 nm and consists of a 28 nm core surrounded by a protein coat; the core contains protein, circular double-stranded DNA, and DNA polymerase [*see Figure 1*].[6] Immunofluorescent antibody studies have detected HBV in the nuclei of infected liver cells. The core moves through the nuclear membrane into the cytoplasm, where it acquires its surface coat. HBV is found in the serum of almost all patients early in the course of acute HBV infection.

Two additional particles appear in the liver cell cytoplasm and serum of patients with HBV: a 22 nm–diameter sphere and a rod-shaped filament of the same diameter. These particles are found at the onset of jaundice in nearly all patients with acute HBV infection. The surface coat of the hepatitis B virion and the spheres and filaments are composed of pre-S1, pre-S2, and S polypeptides, in both glycosylated and unglycosylated forms. The S polypeptide is the major hepatitis B surface antigen (HBsAg).

Although there is only one major serotype of HBV, HBsAg has five major subtype determinants, termed *a, d, y, w,* and *r,* which are primarily of epidemiologic interest. All HBsAg-positive sera contain determinant *a;* determinants *d* and *y* are mutually exclusive, as are *w* and *r.* Hence, four subtype patterns are possible: *adw, ayw, adr,* and *ayr.* The first three subtype patterns occur frequently; *ayr* is rare. Many studies have attempted to correlate subtype with clinical course. It appears, however, that the subtypes are associated with different geographic distributions of HBV rather than with different degrees of virulence. Subtype *adw* is most common in the Americas and Europe; *adr* prevails in most of the Far East.

HBV can be classified into seven genotypes (A to G) on the basis of an intergroup divergence of 8% or more in the complete nucleotide sequence.[7,8] Genotypes A (serotype *adw*) and D (*ayw*) are most common in the United States and Europe; genotypes B (*adw*) and C (*adr*) are most frequent in China and Southeast Asia.[9] There are also several variations or mutations in the nucleotide sequence of HBV. Core promoter and precore variants produce HBV virions that do not produce hepatitis B e antigen (HBeAg). These variants are most commonly seen in patients with genotypes B, C, and D. These differences in genotypes and the presence or absence of variants may account for variations in clinical manifestations of chronic HBV infection in the United States and other parts of the world.

HEPATITIS C VIRUS

HCV is a single-stranded, positive-sense RNA virus that is 9.4 kb in length and accounts for most cases of non-A, non-B hepatitis.[10,11] It is most closely related to the pestiviruses and flaviviruses and is believed to be a distinct genus in the Flaviviridae family.

Table 1 Serologic Diagnosis of Acute Viral Hepatitis

Disease	Serology	Comments
Hepatitis A	IgM anti-HAV	Reasonably specific
Hepatitis B	HBsAg IgM anti-HBc	May be negative late Indicates acute hepatitis
Hepatitis C	Anti-HCV HCV RNA	Appears late Appears early
Hepatitis D	HBsAg and anti-HDV + IgM anti-HBc – IgM anti-HBc	Anti-HDV may appear late Coinfection Superinfection
Hepatitis E	Anti-HEV	Not licensed in the United States

HAV—hepatitis A virus HBc—hepatitis B virus core HBsAg—hepatitis B surface antigen HCV—hepatitis C virus HDV—hepatitis D virus HEV—hepatitis E virus

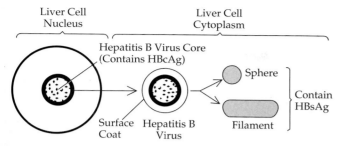

Figure 1 **The hepatitis B virus exists in the cytoplasm of parenchymal liver cells of persons with hepatitis B and constitutes the infective virus. The core of this particle is found in the nucleus of parenchymal cells (left), but as it passes through the cytoplasm, it acquires a surface coat (middle). The core contains hepatitis B core antigen (HBcAg). Spheres and filaments, also in the cytoplasm (right), appear to be excess surface coat material. They are the main source of hepatitis B surface antigen (HBsAg) in serum.**

Structural proteins are encoded at the 5′ end, which is highly conserved [*see Figure 2*]. Further downstream are the HCV core protein, the envelope proteins, and the four nonstructural proteins located at the 3′ end. On the basis of nucleic acid sequence analysis, at least six major genotypes and various subtypes have been identified worldwide. The HCV genotypes are divided into types (1, 2, 3, etc.) and more closely related subtypes (1a, 1b, 2a, etc.). Specific HCV genotypes exhibit different degrees of responsiveness to interferon therapy (e.g., genotypes 2 and 3 respond better to interferon therapy than does genotype 1). In the United States, genotype 1 is the most common, accounting for 70% to 80% of cases; genotype 2 accounts for about 15% of cases, and genotype 3 accounts for 5%. Other genotypes appear to be uncommon in the United States. Coinfection with more than one genotype may occur, particularly in patients with hemophilia or in other patient groups who have been repeatedly exposed to HCV. Quasispecies of HCV also exist. This genetic heterogeneity develops with a longer duration of infection; it may be associated with a poorer response to interferon therapy.

HEPATITIS D VIRUS

HDV, or delta agent, is a single-stranded, circular, negative-polarity, defective RNA virus that requires HBV for its expression.[12] HDV is smaller than any known animal virus and resembles certain plant viruses known as viroids. It circulates in the blood in association with hepatitis D antigen, and the RNA genome has an external coat composed of HBsAg. Although hepatitis D antigen, HDV RNA, and IgM anti–hepatitis D virus (anti-HDV) can be found in the plasma of infected persons, the only commercially available serologic marker for this infection is the total IgG antibody to hepatitis D virus antigen (anti-HDV). When anti-HDV is present in serum, markers of the HBV replication, such as HBeAg and HBV DNA, are usually absent. Although HDV infection is present worldwide, it is most prevalent in Mediterranean countries, the Middle East, and northern Africa. The virus is responsible for epidemics of fulminant hepatitis in South America. HDV infections are uncommon in the United States and northern Europe, except in I.V. drug abusers and persons frequently exposed to blood products. HDV is also uncommon in Southeast Asia and China, areas where HBV is common. Successful vaccination against HBV will prevent HDV infection.

HEPATITIS E VIRUS

HEV is a single-stranded, positive-sense RNA virus of approximately 7.5 kb that causes enterically transmitted non-A, non-B hepatitis.[13] The diagnosis of HEV infection can be made by serologic identification of anti-HEV antibodies (not yet commercially available in the United States). HEV has also been identified in the stool of patients with acute HEV infection through use of immune electron microscopy. Strain variation in HEV has been noted in different parts of the world (e.g., the HEV [B or Burma] and HEV [M or Mexico] strains have only 76% sequence similarity), but there is only one serotype. Acute HEV infection is observed in developing countries; sporadic cases in the United States have been diagnosed in travelers returning from endemic areas.

HEPATITIS F AND G VIRUSES

Between 5% and 20% of cases of acute and chronic hepatitis are not caused by the five known hepatitis viruses and have been presumed to be caused by non-A–E agents. A virus identified in stool extracts from French patients with non-A–E hepatitis was tentatively called the hepatitis F virus (HFV),[14] but the existence of this virus has not been confirmed and is doubtful. HGV was identified as a coinfection in patients with HCV infection and also in persons with non-A–E hepatitis.[15] HGV is an RNA virus closely related to but distinct from HCV. HGV appears to be similar to a GB virus (GBV).[16] Two viruses, GBV-A and GBV-B, are probably nonhuman viruses that are contaminants of serially passed human serum in tamarins. A third virus, GBV-C, is a human virus that is a closely related genotype of HGV. HGV (GBV-C) does not appear to be pathogenic or an independent cause of acute or chronic hepatitis.[17]

Epidemiology

It is particularly important to consider the epidemiology of types A, B, C, D, and E hepatitis and the special tests that may

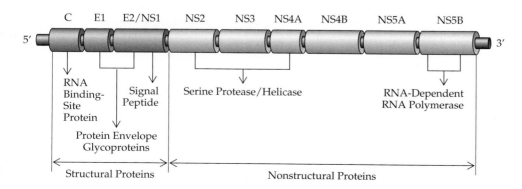

Figure 2 **The hepatitis C virus genome consists of a single, long, open reading frame. The three structural proteins (the RNA binding-site protein [C, core protein] and two envelope glycoproteins [E1 and E2]) are encoded on the 5′ end, and the nonstructural proteins (protease, helicase, and RNA-dependent RNA polymerase [NS2, NS3/NS4A, and NS5B]) are encoded on the 3′ end.**

Table 2 Features of Type A, Type B, Type C, Type D, and Type E Acute Viral Hepatitis

	Type A	Type B	Type C	Type D	Type E
Mode of transmission	Fecal-oral, sewage-contaminated shellfish	Percutaneous, sexual	Percutaneous and community	Percutaneous	Fecal-oral
Incubation period (days)	20–37 (15–49)*	60–110 (25–160)*	35–70 (21–84)*	Appears to be comparable to type B	10–56
Results of serum antigen and antibody tests	Development of IgM antibody early and IgG antibody in convalescence	Antigen (HBsAg) and antibody (anti-HBc) appear early and persist in carriers	Anti-HCV appears in 6 wk to 9 mo	Anti-HDV appears late and may be short-lived	IgM antibody usually detected within 26 days of jaundice; IgG antibody persists indefinitely
Immunity	45% of the U.S. population has hepatitis A antibodies in serum and is probably immune	5%–15% of the population has anti-HBs	Unknown	Patients immune to hepatitis B are also protected against hepatitis D	Unknown
Prevalence	Seen with increasing frequency in adults	Increasing in the United States	80%–90% of post-transfusion hepatitis; 12%–25% of sporadic acute hepatitis	Unusual in the United States but common in I.V. drug abusers	Rare in the United States
Course	Does not progress to chronic liver disease	Chronic liver disease develops in 1%–5% of adults and 80%–90% of children	Chronic liver disease develops in 85%	> 95% resolution of delta coinfection with acute hepatitis B; chronic infection common if delta superinfection is present in chronic hepatitis B carrier	Does not progress to chronic liver disease
Prevention of the disease after exposure	Pooled γ-globulin (0.02 ml/kg) decreases the occurrence of clinical disease 7- to 8-fold	Hepatitis B immune globulin and hepatitis B vaccine prevent clinical disease in adults and the carrier state in infants	The efficacy of pooled γ-globulin is uncertain	Unknown	Uncertain
Mortality	0%–0.2% with fulminant hepatitis	0.3%–1.5%	Uncertain; may approximate rate for type B	2%–20% for acute icteric hepatitis	1%–2%; may be as high as 10%–15% in pregnant women

*Usual range, with outside limits given in parentheses.

permit their differentiation, because their prognoses are considerably different [*see Tables 1 and 2*].[1,2]

HEPATITIS A VIRUS

In HAV infection, virus is shed in the stool 14 to 21 days before the onset of jaundice. Although patients may continue shedding virus for the first 1 to 2 weeks of clinical illness, they are usually no longer infectious 21 days after the illness has begun. However, virus may be detected in the stool again if the patient experiences a relapse of the acute illness. HAV is transmitted via food that has been contaminated by feces-soiled hands of infected persons. The disease is quite contagious; transmission in families is common, and several large point-source epidemics have been reported.[18] Outbreaks of HAV infection have been reported in day care centers, with young children being the most commonly infected.[19] Employees of the day care centers and household contacts and close relatives of the infected children contracted the disease with alarming frequency. Ingestion of sewage-contaminated shellfish has resulted in several epidemics of HAV,[20] as has contamination of raw produce, as in the recent outbreak of HAV infection associated with green onions.[21] The disease is sexually transmitted in men who have sex with men.[22,23] HAV is also common in I.V. drug abusers, but the method of transmission is uncertain. Viremia is present from 1 to 25 days before the onset of symptoms, but transmission by serum or blood products seldom occurs. Patients with HAV develop immunity to the disease—approximately one third of the population of the United States have serum antibodies to HAV. There is no known human or nonhuman reservoir of HAV.

HEPATITIS B VIRUS

HBV is transmitted primarily through percutaneous inoculation of infected serum or blood products. HBsAg and HBV DNA are found in a wide variety of bodily secretions, but the importance of these factors in the spread of HBV is unknown. The most common mode of transmission in men who have sex with men may be by oral or genital contact with asymptomatic bleeding lesions in the rectal mucosa. HBV may also be transmitted to the fetus during pregnancy. An appreciable segment of the population has serum antibodies to HBsAg (anti-HBs). Prevalence of anti-HBs varies among subpopulations: middle-class whites have a 5% prevalence; middle-class African Americans, 12%; Chinese Americans, 37%; and white homosexual men, 48%. This antibody confers immunity to HBV.

HEPATITIS C VIRUS

Before the advent of tests that could screen for HCV and thus help eliminate this virus from the blood supply, HCV caused most cases of posttransfusion hepatitis.[24] Since that time, the rate of HCV transmission by transfusion has declined, and the risk of posttransfusion HCV infection is estimated to be between 0.01% and 0.001% per unit transfused.[25] HCV is responsible for more than 80% of non-A, non-B hepatitis.

HCV is transmitted by parenteral means (e.g., transfusions, I.V. drug use, or occupational exposure to blood or blood products).[26] The risk of transmission from a single needle-stick accident averages 1.8% in prospective studies (range, 0% to 7%).[25] It is estimated that the risk of sexual transmission of HCV in monogamous couples is about 5%, well below the risk of sexual transmission of HBV (about 30%) or HIV (about 10% to 15%). However, the rate of HCV infection is higher in persons who have frequent sexual contact with numerous partners, and in this setting, the risk is higher for female partners of men with anti-HCV.[27] Most studies, particularly those from the United States, have failed to demonstrate any serologic or virologic evidence of HCV transmission to nonsexual partners within households. Perinatal transmission of HCV infection is unusual, except in babies born to mothers with very high levels of HCV RNA, such as mothers with concomitant HIV infection. The risk of perinatal transmission is estimated to be between 5% and 6%. There appears to be no increase in HCV infection in breast-fed babies. In summary, barrier precautions are not recommended for monogamous partners, but persons with multiple sexual partners should practice safe sex and use latex condoms. An additional commonsense precaution is to avoid shared percutaneous exposures, such as razors and toothbrushes. Finally, there is no reason to advise against pregnancy for a woman with HCV infection, because the rate of perinatal infection is low.

Recipients of organs from donors who have antibodies to HCV have a high probability of becoming infected.[28] Transplantation of an organ from an infected donor is controversial.

HEPATITIS D AND E VIRUSES

HDV occurs only in patients with HBV and is transmitted percutaneously. Simultaneous infection with HBV and HDV may produce a more severe acute hepatitis than that caused by HBV alone.[12]

HEV is a common cause of large epidemics of acute viral hepatitis in developing countries. It characteristically affects adults and may be associated with an unusually high mortality in pregnant women.[13] Epidemics have occurred in rural Mexico, with a high attack rate and with jaundice occurring in more than 5% of the local popoulation. HEV infection has also been found in immigrants to the United States and in travelers to Mexico and the Indian subcontinent.[29]

Table 3 Incidence of Symptoms in Acute Viral Hepatitis

Symptom	Percentage of Patients
Dark urine	94
Fatigue	91
Anorexia	90
Nausea	87
Fever	76
Emesis	71
Headache	70
Abdominal discomfort	65
Light stools	52
Myalgia	52
Drowsiness	49
Irritability	43
Itching	42
Diarrhea	25
Arthralgia	21

Diagnosis

CLINICAL MANIFESTATIONS

The onset of viral hepatitis may be gradual or sudden. The symptoms are protean [see Table 3].[12] The most common early symptoms are fatigue, lassitude, drowsiness, anorexia, nausea, and dark urine. Dehydration may result from repeated vomiting. Low-grade fever is common; shaking chills are rare. Frank pain may occur in the right upper quadrant, but vague, generalized abdominal discomfort is more common. Itching may occur but is seldom severe. Diarrhea occurs in some cases. About half of patients have myalgias or arthralgias, and some have acute arthritis with local pain, redness, swelling, and effusions. Joint symptoms are usually associated with HBV and HEV infections. Many of these early symptoms abate when jaundice develops or shortly thereafter. In the case of severe hepatitis, which is unusual, confusion, stupor, or even coma may develop. Fetor hepaticus and asterixis are usually present in these patients.

PHYSICAL EXAMINATION

The sclerae and skin may be icteric. The liver is often enlarged and tender. The spleen is palpable in about 10% of patients. Asterixis, marked peripheral edema, or ascites implies that the disease is unusually severe and suggests a poor prognosis.

LABORATORY TESTS

General Laboratory Findings

Most patients have mild anemia and relative lymphocytosis. The leukocyte count is usually normal but may be greater than $12,000/mm^3$. The serum bilirubin level generally does not exceed 15 to 20 mg/dl; levels greater than 30 mg/dl imply severe disease or associated hemolysis. Serum aspartate aminotransferase (AST) and serum alanine aminotransferase (ALT) levels rise 7 to 14 days before the onset of jaundice and begin to fall shortly after jaundice occurs. The degree of aminotransferase elevation does not necessarily parallel severity, but levels less than 500 IU/L usually reflect mild illness.

The alkaline phosphatase level is slightly increased but may be markedly elevated in the few patients in whom prominent cholestasis develops later in the course of acute illness. Serum γ-globulin levels are normal or slightly elevated; concentrations greater than 3 g/dl suggest chronic active hepatitis rather than acute viral hepatitis. The serum albumin level and prothrombin time reflect the liver cells' synthetic capacity and are depressed in patients with severe, acute viral hepatitis.

Serologic and Virologic Assays

Serologic assays are used to identify each type of viral hepatitis [see Table 1].

Hepatitis A virus The IgM antibody to HAV (IgM anti-HAV) appears early and is quite specific for acute HAV infection. It typically persists for an average of 3 months and is then replaced by the IgG anti-HAV, which lasts throughout life and confers immunity to future infection.

Hepatitis B virus A number of serologic tests are useful to physicians who are caring for patients with acute HBV infection [see Table 4]. HBsAg is present on the surface of the hepatitis B virion and in the circulation as spheres and filaments [see Figure 1]. It appears in the serum of infected persons as early as 1 to 2

Table 4   Tests for Hepatitis B Virus Infection

Symbol	Characteristics
HBsAg	Hepatitis B surface antigen; present in surface coat of the hepatitis B virus and in the 22 nm diameter filaments and spheres; purified surface antigen expressed in yeast cells is used in the recombinant hepatitis B vaccines
Anti-HBs	Antibody to HBsAg; present during convalescent phase of acute hepatitis B infection and after successful hepatitis B vaccination; hepatitis B immune globulin derived from serum with high anti-HBs titers is effective in preventing clinical hepatitis B infection
Anti-HBc	Antibody to the hepatitis B virus core; present in all patients with any form of hepatitis B infection; presence of this antibody in the sera is evidence that the patient has been infected in the past or is currently infected with the hepatitis B virus
IgM anti-HBc	Antibody to the hepatitis B core antigen; present in high titers in patients with acute hepatitis B; may be the only marker of acute infection when HBsAg is no longer detectable
Anti-HDV	Antibody to hepatitis D; serologic marker of coinfection or superinfection by hepatitis D of patients with hepatitis B
HBeAg	A soluble protein derived from the hepatitis B virus core; reflects presence in the blood of circulating hepatitis B virus; sera positive for this antigen are highly infectious
Anti-HBe	Anti-HBe appears weeks to months after HBeAg (and the circulating hepatitis B virus) is no longer detectable in the blood; sera positive for this antibody are substantially less infectious

weeks after parenteral injection of infectious virus and may persist for months. If HBsAg remains in the serum of an infected person for 6 months after an episode of acute HBV infection, it will probably persist indefinitely. The antibody to HBsAg usually appears in the blood 2 to 4 months after an attack of acute HBV infection that resolves—in most cases, after HBsAg is no longer detectable. Antibody to the core antigen (anti-HBc) appears promptly in the blood of infected persons and persists indefinitely. High titers of IgM anti-HBc are found in patients with acute disease and may be the only marker of acute HBV infection if HBsAg is no longer detectable. Detection of HBeAg, a soluble protein derived from the core particle, correlates with the presence of HBV DNA and indicates that the HBV is actively replicating. Serum that is positive for HBeAg is highly infectious. A pregnant woman who is positive for HBsAg is much more likely to transmit HBV to her offspring if her blood also contains HBeAg or HBV DNA. The detection of antibody to HBeAg (anti-HBe) in association with the absence of HBV DNA is evidence that viral replication is minimal and the blood is substantially less infectious.

Hepatitis C virus   Detection of antibodies to HCV (anti-HCV) remains the most practical way to diagnose acute and chronic HCV infection.[30,31] In 1992, a second-generation anti-HCV enzyme-linked immunosorbent assay (ELISA) replaced the original assay. The second-generation assay employs several viral antigens, making it more sensitive and specific than the first-generation test. The most commonly used supplemental assay for specificity is the second-generation recombinant immunoblot assay (RIBA-2), which incorporates four antigens as separate bands. Reaction of

two or more of the four bands is considered a positive RIBA-2 test result; reaction of only one band is indeterminate. Third-generation ELISAs and RIBAs have been developed and should soon be available in the United States.

The detection of serum HCV RNA can be used to establish viremia and has been widely employed in the management of chronic HCV infection.[30,31] The diagnosis of acute HCV infection can also be established early, before the appearance of anti-HCV, by the use of HCV RNA assays. Assays for serum HCV RNA have recently become standardized, and serum HCV RNA can be detected by both qualitative and quantitative assays. The results of a quantitative HCV RNA assay may be useful in predicting the subsequent response to interferon therapy; patients with lower levels of viremia respond better than those with higher levels. Finally, in patients with normal serum aminotransferase levels in whom the results of RIBA-2 are positive for anti-HCV, the presence or absence of serum HCV RNA can distinguish between active infection with viremia and recovery from previous HCV infection.

Hepatitis D and E viruses   HDV infection is diagnosed by the detection of anti-HDV with HBsAg. Patients with acute HDV infection will have HBsAg with IgM anti-HBc along with anti-HDV (i.e., coinfection), whereas patients with chronic HBV infection who are superinfected with HDV will have a negative IgM anti-HBc. HEV is diagnosed by the detection of antibodies to HEV (anti-HEV). Anti-HEV is found in acute and convalescent serum from patients with acute HEV infection. This assay has yet to be licensed in the United States.

Liver Biopsy

Liver biopsy is not usually performed in patients with acute viral hepatitis, because serologic tests are generally diagnostic. Spotty necrosis of liver cells and an inflammatory cell reaction that consists primarily of lymphocytes and histiocytes are the typical histologic findings. Acidophils (dying liver cells) and bile plugs are common. Biopsy performed late in the course of the disease reveals prominent evidence of hepatic cell regeneration (rosette formation and multinucleated cells) and pigment-filled histiocytes. Although usually more marked in the pericentral areas, the inflammatory reaction and cell necrosis appear throughout the parenchyma. In severe hepatitis, necrotic zones link portal areas to one another or to central areas, or they may involve whole lobules (bridging necrosis). The portal tracts contain a mild to moderate mononuclear cell inflammatory reaction, and the limiting plate, which demarcates portal areas from parenchymal cells, may be disrupted.

CLINICAL COURSE

Hepatitis typically produces symptoms for 1 to 2 weeks before the onset of dark urine and jaundice. As icterus deepens, appetite begins to return and malaise lessens. The serum bilirubin level rises for 10 to 14 days and then declines over 2 to 4 weeks. Aminotransferase levels usually begin to decline just before peak jaundice occurs and fall quite rapidly thereafter. The patient often feels much better by the time bilirubin levels have begun to decline. Usually, the clinical course is uneventful and recovery is complete, with liver function returning to normal.

In a small percentage of patients, the clinical course is atypical. Acute viral hepatitis may be protracted in elderly patients or in those infected with either HBV or HCV; the disease may last several months, and full recovery may not occur for a year. Between

6% and 15% of patients with acute viral hepatitis will have recurrent symptoms and worsening of liver function before recovery from the initial attack is complete. This relapse is usually milder than the original attack and is short-lived. In a few patients, the disease has an acute fulminant course leading to hepatic coma and even death. These events appear to be more common in pregnant women infected with HEV. HCV appears to be an unusual cause of fulminant disease.[32] In some countries, a mutant form of HBV that is incapable of encoding for e antigen is associated with fulminant disease.[9] Often, no virus can be identified, leading to speculation that other viruses may be involved—either mutant viruses or as yet unidentified viruses. Some patients do not recover completely from the initial attack, and chronic hepatitis develops. Chronic hepatitis does not occur after HAV or HEV infection. It ensues in 1% to 5% of cases of acute HBV infection and 85% of cases of acute HCV infection.[1,2]

A study in Italy has found that carriers of HBsAg who are symptom-free and whose liver function tests are normal have an excellent prognosis. In this study, the risk of hepatocellular carcinoma was low over the mean follow-up period of about 11 years.[33] The natural history of HCV infection is still being studied. The general view is that chronic HCV infection usually progresses but does so slowly over many decades.[26,34] In two histologic studies of the natural history of chronic HCV infection that resulted from blood transfusion, the times to the presence of chronic HCV infection averaged 12 years; to the presence of cirrhosis, 21 years, and to the presence of hepatocellular carcinoma, 29 years.[35,36] Both of these studies reported experiences from tertiary liver centers, however, which may have introduced referral bias. More recent studies have suggested that chronic HCV infection is more benign than originally reported and is associated with a low rate of cirrhosis.[37-40] In a large, prospective study of 568 patients with posttransfusion non-A, non-B hepatitis (mostly HCV) who were followed for an average of 18 years, there was no increase in mortality from all causes, but there was a small increase in the number of deaths related to liver disease.[39] Another large, cross-sectional study from Europe of 2,235 patients with chronic HCV infection found that the median time from infection to cirrhosis was 30 years,[40] which is about 10 years longer than the 21-year interval from infection to cirrhosis reported earlier from tertiary liver centers.[35,36] Analysis of liver biopsy specimens showed that the rate of fibrosis progression was not normally distributed, with approximately one third of persons progressing to cirrhosis in less than 20 years and another third not appearing to progress to cirrhosis for at least 50 years. Factors associated with an increase in the rate of fibrosis progression were age at which infection occurred (> 40 years of age), daily alcohol use (> 50 g), and male gender. The role of heavy alcohol abuse in exacerbating the risk of cirrhosis has been confirmed.[41] Once cirrhosis develops in patients with chronic HCV infection, the 10-year rates of decompensation of cirrhosis and development of hepatocellular carcinoma are 29% (3.9% yearly) and 14% (1.4% yearly), respectively.[42] Chronic HBV infection also predisposes the infected person to the development of primary hepatocellular carcinoma, perhaps through the integration of viral DNA into the genome of the host's hepatocytes.[43]

Unusual and sometimes fatal complications of acute viral hepatitis include aplastic anemia, hemolytic anemia, hypoglycemia, and polyarteritis. The risk appears to be higher if infection occurs at a very early age or if chronic liver disease is also present.

Differential Diagnosis

At the time of initial presentation with symptoms and elevated aminotransferase levels, before the results of serologic tests are known, it is worthwhile to consider the differential diagnosis of acute viral hepatitis.

EPSTEIN-BARR VIRUS

EBV, a herpesvirus, usually produces mild hepatitis associated with nausea and vomiting; jaundice occurs in only 10% to 20% of patients.[44] Serum aminotransferase levels are moderately elevated (300 to 500 IU/L). In most instances, the hepatitis is part of the typical clinical syndrome of infectious mononucleosis. In rare instances, hepatic dysfunction is severe and proves to be fatal, particularly in immunodeficient patients.[45] The virus appears to be transmitted during oral-oral contact through infected saliva and may be transmitted parenterally; the incubation period is about 28 days. A rise in titer of specific fluorescent antibodies to EBV or detection and quantitation of viral levels confirm the diagnosis.

CYTOMEGALOVIRUS

CMV, which is also a member of the herpesvirus group, is ubiquitous. About 80% of adults have serum complement-fixation reactivity for CMV. This virus can also produce a disease similar to infectious mononucleosis but without adenopathy or tonsillopharyngeal involvement.[46] Liver involvement may mimic that of the more common forms of viral hepatitis, but it is usually mild and does not progress to chronic liver disease. Diagnosis requires inoculation of an appropriate tissue culture with blood to demonstrate viremia. Polymerase chain reaction to assess quantitative viral loads is the best test and is becoming more widely used.

OTHER VIRUSES

Acute hepatitis caused by herpes simplex virus or varicella-zoster virus, usually accompanied by typical skin lesions, has occurred in immunocompromised patients.

DRUG-INDUCED HEPATITIS

Hundreds of drugs can cause hepatitis that may be indistinguishable from acute viral hepatitis.[47] These idiosyncratic drug reactions are infrequent, unpredictable, and not dose dependent. Clinical onset usually occurs within 2 to 6 weeks after therapy is started but may occur on the first day that the drug is administered or not until 6 months later. The disease may progress despite withdrawal of the drug; failure to withdraw the drug promptly may result in death.

One well-documented drug reaction is the hepatic necrosis that occurs in one in 9,000 to 10,000 patients given halothane. The hepatitis is often fatal and is more common in overweight women or in persons exposed a second time to the anesthetic. Fever, malaise, and elevated aminotransferase levels develop 1 to 12 days after initial exposure to the drug. Onset may be sooner after multiple exposures; the average delay is 3 days. Signs of hepatic necrosis include marked eosinophilia, marked elevation of serum aminotransferase and bilirubin levels, reduced serum albumin levels, and a prolonged prothrombin time. Other common drugs that cause hepatitis are isoniazid, methyldopa, phenytoin, and the sulfonamides. Because most drugs will injure the liver on rare occasions, hepatitis that develops shortly after initiation of a new medication should suggest a drug reaction. The treatment of choice is discontinuance of the medication.

Idiosyncratic drug reactions differ from hepatitis that results from drug overdose. Drug reactions of the latter type are rare because a clear potential for hepatotoxicity usually precludes release of the drug. Acetaminophen, however, is an exception: more than 25 g orally, usually in a suicide attempt, will cause profound hepatocellular necrosis in most persons.[48] Cell injury occurs because the liver produces a toxic metabolite that is usually rendered harmless by conjugation with glutathione. When the drug dose is high, hepatic glutathione stores are depleted and the toxic metabolite accumulates and destroys liver cells. Oral N-acetylcysteine, given in a loading dose of 140 mg/kg followed by 70 mg/kg every 4 hours for a total of 18 doses, reduces hepatotoxicity and mortality in cases of acetaminophen overdose.[49] The drug is most effective when given within 8 hours after the overdose but appears to have some effect as long as 24 hours after the ingestion of acetaminophen. Maximal medical support during the 1- to 2-week illness is mandatory. Acetaminophen can also cause severe hepatotoxicity when taken in ordinary doses if hepatic glutathione stores are low as a result of alcoholism with malnutrition (the so-called Tylenol-alcohol syndrome). The beneficial role of N-acetylcysteine in this clinical setting is less certain.

Treatment

Many treatments have been recommended for acute viral hepatitis, but it is unlikely that any of them alters the course of the disease. When the patient feels ill, it seems reasonable to reduce physical activity to a tolerable level. For some patients, bed rest may be indicated during the initial phase of illness. Once the patient feels better, there is no reason to restrict activity. Two large, controlled studies of young servicemen with viral hepatitis have shown convincingly that even heavy physical exercise in the recovery period does not result in more frequent relapse or chronic disease.[50,51]

Patients should be encouraged to eat whatever they can; there is no evidence that a low-fat diet is beneficial. At times, nausea and vomiting are so severe that hospitalization and intravenous fluid and electrolyte replacement become necessary. Abstention from alcohol is advised during the acute phase, although alcohol has not been shown to adversely affect the course of viral hepatitis.

Acute HCV infection is usually silent and thus not commonly seen in clinical practice. However, meta-analyses of published studies of interferon therapy for acute HCV infection support its efficacy in this setting.[52,53] It is generally recommended that standard doses of interferon (e.g., 3 million units of interferon alfa-2b three times a week) be administered for 3 to 6 months, which, in comparison with no therapy, increases the likelihood of sustained biochemical (normal ALT levels) and virologic (undetectable HCV RNA) responses.

Many forms of treatment have been recommended for the patient with severe acute viral hepatitis who becomes encephalopathic, but no regimen is clearly effective. In controlled clinical trials, corticosteroids,[54-57] cimetidine,[58] hyperimmune γ-globulin,[59] and exchange transfusions[60] had no effect on the course of acute hepatitis. Although no controlled trials have been completed, liver transplantation improves survival in patients with acute severe viral hepatitis and stage IV hepatic encephalopathy.[61]

Therapy for encephalopathic patients should be supportive, with evaluation for liver transplantation. Bacterial infections should be treated with suitable antibiotics. Bleeding warrants the administration of appropriate clotting factors (fresh frozen plasma, platelets, or both) and transfusions. Clotting abnormalities without bleeding do not justify massive transfusions of fresh frozen plasma, because congestive heart failure can result. Encephalopathy should be treated with oral lactulose (30 ml every 4 hours), although there is little evidence that acute encephalopathy responds to treatment.

Antiviral therapy is available for chronic HBV and chronic HCV infections [see Chapter 65].

Prevention

Prevention of viral hepatitis entails avoidance of exposure to the virus, passive immunization with globulin products, and active immunization with specific vaccines.

PASSIVE IMMUNIZATION

Immune globulin is prepared from human plasma; when given intramuscularly, it decreases the clinical attack rate for HAV by sevenfold to eightfold. The official recommendation of the U.S. Public Health Service is to administer 0.02 ml/kg to contacts as soon as possible after exposure to a confirmed case of HAV infection.[62] Administration more than 2 weeks after exposure is not protective. The usual dose for adults is 2.0 ml; for children weighing up to 25 kg (55 lb), 0.5 ml; and for children between 25 and 50 kg (110 lb), 1.0 ml. Immune globulin should be given to all persons who share a household, hospital room, or dormitory room with an HAV patient. It should also be given to staff and children in day care centers where cases of HAV infection have been identified. When a food handler with acute HAV infection has been identified, immune globulin should be given to coworkers and considered for patrons of the eating establishment if they can be identified and treated within 2 weeks after exposure. Immune globulin need not be given to all contacts at work or school unless there is clear evidence of spread. Classmates and neighborhood children who play together frequently, however, probably should be immunized. Travelers to developing countries are at risk of acquiring HAV, particularly those who plan to visit extensively or to reside in areas with poor sanitation [see Chapter 7]. A single dose of 0.02 ml/kg of immune globulin will be protective for as long as 2 months; a dose of 0.06 ml/kg will be protective for 5 months.[62]

Immune globulin contains anti-HBs at low titer (approximately 1:100 by radioimmunoassay), whereas HBV immune globulin has an anti-HBs titer of greater than 1:100,000. When the source is known to be HBsAg positive, persons exposed (by percutaneous or mucous membrane routes) should be given HBV immune globulin (0.06 ml/kg) and HBV vaccine within 24 hours.[63,64] When the HBsAg status of the source is unknown, the first dose of HBV vaccine should be given promptly and the series completed as recommended. If the source is subsequently found to be HBsAg positive, HBV immune globulin (0.06 ml/kg) should be administered, provided that it can be given within 7 days after exposure. Infants who are born to HBsAg-positive mothers should receive 0.5 ml of HBV immune globulin intramuscularly and 0.5 ml of HBV vaccine intramuscularly at another site within 12 hours after birth.

Prophylaxis against HCV infection with γ-globulin is more problematic. Its effect in household or casual contacts and after a needle-stick injury is unknown. The value of immune globulin in the prevention of HEV infection is also uncertain.

ACTIVE IMMUNIZATION

Two HBV vaccines that are produced by recombinant DNA techniques are available (Recombivax HB, Merck & Co., and Engerix-B, SmithKline Beecham Biologicals) [see Table 5].[63,64] Both

Table 5 Administration Schedules and Dosing of Hepatitis B Vaccines[63,64]

Patients	Schedule	Engerix-B	Recombivax HB
Infants			
HBsAg-negative mother	0–2, 1–4, and 6–18 mo	10 µg/0.5 ml	2.5 µg/0.5 ml
HBsAg-positive mother	At birth,* 1–2 mo, and 6 mo	10 µg/0.5 ml	5.0 µg/0.5 ml
Children and adolescents (0–19 yr)	0, 1–2, and 4–6 mo	10 µg/0.5 ml	5.0 µg/0.5 ml
Alternative two-dose regimen for adolescents (11–15 yr)	0 and 4–6 mo	—	10 µg/1.0 ml
Adults (≥ 20 yr)	0, 1–2, and 4–6 mo	20 µg/1.0 ml	10 µg/1.0 ml
Immunocompromised adults (hemodialysis)	0, 1, and 6 mo	40 µg/2.0 ml	40 µg/1.0 ml

*Immunization should occur within 12 hr with hepatitis B immune globulin.
HBsAg—hepatitis B surface antigen

vaccines are highly effective in inducing antibody to HBV and preventing HBV infection in infants, children, and adults. The recommendations of the Centers for Disease Control and Prevention for the use of HBV vaccine are outlined [*see Table 6*].

The vaccines are given in three I.M. doses into the deltoid muscle in young children and adults and into the anterolateral thigh muscle in infants and neonates. A suboptimal response has been observed when the vaccine was injected into the buttocks.[65] The second dose is given 1 month after the first; the third dose is usually given 6 months after the first. For healthy adults, depending on the vaccine preparation, each dose should contain 10 or 20 µg of HBsAg; for patients undergoing hemodialysis and for other immunosuppressed patients, each dose should contain 40 µg; and for infants and children younger than 10 years, each dose should contain 2.5 to 10 µg. The vaccine should be given to groups at substantial risk for HBV infection: hospital staff and other health care workers with frequent exposure to blood products, clients and staff of institutions for the mentally retarded, hemodialysis patients, homosexually active males, users of I.V. drugs, recipients of certain blood products, contacts of HBV carriers, infants born to HBsAg-positive mothers, special high-risk populations (e.g., emigrants from areas with highly endemic disease), and prisoners. It should be strongly considered for travelers who plan to reside in areas with high levels of endemic HBV infection.

Approximately 3% to 4% of healthy people have little or no antibody response to the vaccine. They appear to lack an immune response gene in the major histocompatibility complex that accounts for the ability to mount a normal antibody response to HBsAg.[66] Repeat vaccination induces a protective level of antibody in less than 50% of such people.[67] Those who do not respond to vaccine and who later become infected with HBV do not have an unusual clinical course.

After successful vaccination, titers of antibody to HBsAg begin to decline, and in 5 years, 20% to 30% of patients lack protective levels.[68] These persons will respond immediately to a booster dose of vaccine, but the need for routine booster vaccination has not been determined.[69] HBV infection may develop in a few persons when the antibody titer falls to low levels, but the infection is invariably asymptomatic and is usually identified only by the development of antibody to the core antigen. Thus, several countries and certain individuals have a policy of administering a booster injection to certain risk groups if the anti-HBs level falls below 10 mIU/ml.[70]

Vaccine is useless in HBV carriers, and it is unnecessary for those already immune to HBV; however, it has no ill effects on these groups. Therefore, the decision to screen people for susceptibility to HBV infection before vaccination is primarily based on the relative costs of the two procedures. In general, if the expected prevalence of immune persons in a particular population is high (> 20%) and the cost of screening is low (< $30 a person), screening should be done. However, it is difficult to decide which antibody (anti-HBs or anti-HBc) should be used. Anti-HBc provides definitive proof of HBV infection, but it does not discriminate between HBV carriers and noncarriers. Anti-HBs is usually not present in HBsAg carriers, but even when anti-HBs is present in the general population, it may not indicate immunity to HBV infection. Several studies have identified persons who have low serum titers of anti-HBs but who do not have anti-HBc.[71,72] This low-titer anti-HBs is predominantly of the IgM type and may not be immunoprotective.[72,73] Thus, if anti-HBs is used as the screening test, only a titer of 10 radioimmunoassay sample ratio units or higher or a positive enzyme immunoassay should be considered evidence of immunity.

Several different approaches to the development of active immunization against HAV have been attempted. A successful approach has been the preparation of inactivated HAV vaccines [*see Table 7*]. Other approaches to vaccine development, including a live attenuated and recombinant vaccine, have been slower in development because of a number of technical problems.

A large, randomized, double-blind efficacy trial demonstrating protection against HAV infection was carried out in Thailand.[74] A total of 40,119 children 1 to 16 years of age received Hav-

---

Table 6 **Recommendations for Use of Hepatitis B Vaccine**[63,64]

Routine immunization
  All infants and previously unvaccinated children and adolescents 1–18 years of age

Persons at increased risk for HBV infection
  Persons with multiple sexual partners
  Sexual partners or household contacts of HBsAg-positive persons
  Men who have sex with men
  Injecting drug users
  Travelers to regions of high HBV endemicity
  Persons with occupational exposure to blood or body fluids
  Clients and staff of institutions for developmentally disabled persons
  Patients with chronic renal failure
  Patients receiving clotting factor concentrates

HBsAg—hepatitis B surface antigen   HBV—hepatitis B virus

Table 7 Administration Schedules and Dosing of Hepatitis A Vaccines

Vaccine	Patients	Dosage	Schedule (months)
Havrix	Children (2–18 yr) Adolescents and adults (> 18 yr)	720 ELU/0.5 ml 1,440 ELU/1.0 ml	0, 6–12 0, 6–12
VAQTA	Children (2–17 yr) Adolescents and adults (> 17 yr)	25 U/0.5 ml 50 U/1.0 ml	0, 6–18 0, 6

ELU—enzyme-linked immunosorbent assay unit

rix or a control HBV vaccine (Engerix-B) at 0, 1, and 12 months. Patients were crossed over to the alternative vaccine at 18 months. Side effects were minor. The efficacy of the HAV vaccine was 94% before the month-12 booster injection and 99% after it. In an earlier trial, researchers evaluated a different inactivated HAV vaccine.[75] They studied 1,037 children in upstate New York and also found that this HAV vaccine was safe and 100% effective in preventing HAV infection 50 to 137 days after administration of a single dose. These studies led to the licensing of a second HAV vaccine, VAQTA (Merck & Co.). Both Havrix and VAQTA are administered to adults in an initial 1 ml dose I.M. followed by a booster in 6 to 18 months.

Compared with the short-term protection afforded by immune globulin, inactivated HAV vaccine will probably induce protection lasting from 5 to 10 years and perhaps much longer.[76] In the United States, the overall incidence of HAV infection has decreased, leading to a higher proportion of adults who are susceptible. Older individuals are known to experience a more severe clinical course, and thus, the costs of HAV infection in the United States remain substantial.[77] These facts underline the importance of ensuring compliance with the current recommendations for HAV vaccination.[62] The vaccine will be particularly useful in preventing HAV infection in persons at high risk for the disease, such as travelers and immigrants to highly endemic regions. The risk of symptomatic HAV infection in travelers staying in Western-style accommodations in high-risk countries is three per 1,000

persons per month.[78] Backpackers or travelers in areas with poor hygienic conditions have a higher risk (20 per 1,000 persons per month). In unprotected travelers from the United States, the incidence of HAV infection is 10 to 100 times that of typhoid fever and 1,000 times that of cholera. Other persons at risk for HAV infection are listed [*see Table 8*].[62] Finally, patients with chronic liver disease may experience a more severe illness with acute HAV infection.[79,80] HAV vaccination has been shown to be safe and effective in patients with chronic viral liver disease.[81]

References

1. Ryder SD, Beckingham IJ: ABC of diseases of liver, pancreas, and biliary system: acute hepatitis. BMJ 322:151, 2001

2. Younossi ZM: Viral hepatitis guide for practicing physicians. Cleveland Clinic of Medicine. Cleve Clin J Med 67(suppl 1):SI6, 2000

3. Summary of notifiable diseases, United States, 1999. MMWR Morb Mortal Wkly Rep 48:1, 2001

4. Yokosuka O: Molecular biology of hepatitis A virus: significance of various substitutions in the hepatitis A virus genome. J Gastroenterol Hepatol 15(suppl):D91, 2000

5. Feinstone SM, Kapikian AZ, Purcell RH: Hepatitis A: detection by immune electron microscopy of a viruslike antigen associated with acute illness. Science 182:1026, 1973

6. Lee WM: Hepatitis B virus infection. N Engl J Med 337:1733, 1997

7. Norder H, Courouce AM, Magnius LO: Complete genomes, phylogenetic relatedness, and structural proteins of six strains of the hepatitis B virus, four of which represent two new genotypes. Virology 198:489, 1994

8. Stuyver L, De Gendt S, Van Geyt C, et al: A new genotype of hepatitis B virus: complete genome and phylogenetic relatedness. J Gen Virol 81(pt 1):67, 2000

9. Lok AS, Heathcote EJ, Hoofnagle JH: Management of hepatitis B: 2000—summary of a workshop. Gastroenterology 120:1828, 2001

10. Choo QL, Kuo G, Weiner AJ, et al: Isolation of a cDNA clone derived from a blood-borne non-A, non-B viral hepatitis genome. Science 244:359, 1989

11. Bukh J, Miller RH, Purcell RH: Genetic heterogeneity of hepatitis C virus: quasispecies and genotypes. Semin Liver Dis 15:41, 1995

12. Hadziyannis SJ: Review: hepatitis delta. J Gastroenterol Hepatol 12:289, 1997

13. Krawczynski K, Aggarwal R, Kamili S: Hepatitis E. Infect Dis Clin North Am 14:669, 2000

14. Deka N, Sharma MD, Mukerjee R: Isolation of the novel agent from human stool samples that is associated with sporadic non-A, non-B hepatitis. J Virol 68:7810, 1994

15. Linnen J, Wages J Jr, Zhang-Keck ZY, et al: Molecular cloning and disease association of hepatitis G virus: a transfusion-transmissible agent. Science 271:505, 1996

16. Simons JN, Leary TP, Dawson GJ, et al: Isolation of novel virus-like sequences associated with human hepatitis. Nat Med 1:564, 1995

17. Cheung RC, Keeffe EB, Greenberg HB: Hepatitis G virus: is it a hepatitis virus? West J Med 167:23, 1997

18. Hutin YJ, Pool V, Cramer EH, et al: A multistate, foodborne outbreak of hepatitis A. National Hepatitis A Investigation Team. N Engl J Med 340:595, 1999

19. Staes CJ, Schlenker TL, Risk I, et al: Sources of infection among persons with acute hepatitis A and no identified risk factors during a sustained community-wide outbreak. Pediatrics 106:E54, 2000

20. Ruddy SJ, Johnson RF, Mosley JW, et al: An epidemic of clam-associated hepatitis. JAMA 208:649, 1969

21. Dentinger CM, Bower WA, Nainan OV, et al: An outbreak of hepatitis A associated with green onions. J Infect Dis 183:1273, 2001

22. Corey L, Holmes KK: Sexual transmission of hepatitis A in homosexual men: incidence and mechanism. N Engl J Med 302:435, 1980

23. Katz MH, Hsu L, Wong E, et al: Seroprevalence of and risk factors for hepatitis A infection among young homosexual and bisexual men. J Infect Dis 175:1225, 1997

24. Kuo G, Choo Q-L, Alter HJ, et al: An assay for circulating antibodies to a major etiologic virus of human non-A, non-B hepatitis. Science 244:362, 1989

25. Alter MJ: Epidemiology of hepatitis C. Hepatology 26(suppl 1):62S, 1997

26. Liang TJ, Rehermann B, Seeff LB, et al: Pathogenesis, natural history, treatment, and prevention of hepatitis C. Ann Intern Med 132:296, 2000

Table 8 Recommendations for
Use of Hepatitis A Vaccine[62]

Routine immunization

  Children living in areas where rates of HAV infection are at least twice the national average (i.e., ≥ 20 cases per 100,000 population); vaccination should also be considered for children in areas where rates are greater than the national average, which is 10–20 cases per 100,000 population

Persons at increased risk for HAV infection

  Persons traveling to or working in countries with high or intermediate HAV endemicity, such as Mexico, the Caribbean, Southeast Asia, South and Central America, and Africa

  Men who have sex with men

  Illegal drug users

  Individuals who work with HAV-infected primates or with HAV in research laboratories

  Persons with clotting factor disorders

  Outbreaks in communities with high or intermediate rates of HAV infection

Persons at increased risk for more severe disease

  Persons with chronic liver disease

HAV—hepatitis A virus

27. Dienstag JL: Sexual and perinatal transmission of hepatitis C. Hepatology 26(suppl 1): 66S, 1997

28. Pereira BJ, Wright TL, Schmid CH, et al: A controlled study of hepatitis C transmission by organ transplantation. The New England Organ Bank Hepatitis C Study Group. Lancet 345:484, 1995

29. Hepatitis E among U.S. travelers, 1989–1992. MMWR Morb Mortal Wkly Rep 42:1, 1993

30. Gretch DR: Diagnostic tests for hepatitis C. Hepatology 26(suppl 1):43S, 1997

31. Lok ASF, Gunaratnam NT: Diagnosis of hepatitis C. Hepatology 26(suppl 1):48S, 1997

32. Hoofnagle JH: Hepatitis C: the clinical spectrum of disease. Hepatology 26(suppl 1): 15S, 1997

33. de Franchis R, Meucci G, Vecchi M, et al: The natural history of asymptomatic hepatitis B surface antigen carriers. Ann Intern Med 118:191, 1993

34. Seeff LB: Natural history of hepatitis C. Hepatology 26(suppl 1):21S, 1997

35. Kiyosawa K, Sodeyama T, Tanaka E, et al: Interrelationship of blood transfusion, non-A, non-B hepatitis and hepatocellular carcinoma: analysis by detection of antibody to hepatitis C virus. Hepatology 12:671, 1990

36. Tong MJ, el-Farra NS, Reikes AR, et al: Clinical outcomes after transfusion-associated hepatitis C. N Engl J Med 332:1463, 1995

37. Wiese M, Berr F, Lafrenz M, et al: Low frequency of cirrhosis in a hepatitis C (genotype 1b) single-source outbreak in Germany: a 20-year multicenter study. Hepatology 32: 91, 2000

38. Rodger AJ, Roberts S, Lanigan A, et al: Assessment of long-term outcomes of community-acquired hepatitis C infection in a cohort with sera stored from 1971 to 1975. Hepatology 32:582, 2000

39. Seeff LB, Buskell-Bales Z, Wright EC, et al: Long-term mortality after transfusion-associated non-A, non-B hepatitis. The National Heart, Lung, and Blood Institute Study Group. N Engl J Med 327:1906, 1992

40. Poynard T, Bedossa P, Opolon P: Natural history of liver fibrosis progression in patients with chronic hepatitis C. The OBSVIRC, METAVIR, CLINIVIR, and DOSVIRC groups. Lancet 349:825, 1997

41. Harris DR, Gonin R, Alter HJ, et al: The relationship of acute transfusion-associated hepatitis to the development of cirrhosis in the presence of alcohol abuse. Ann Intern Med 134:120, 2001

42. Fattovich G, Giustina G, Degos F, et al: Morbidity and mortality in compensated cirrhosis type C: a retrospective follow-up study of 384 patients. Gastroenterology 112:463, 1997

43. Martin P: Hepatocellular carcinoma: risk factors and natural history. Liver Transpl Surg 4(5 suppl 1):S87, 1998

44. Schiff GM: Hepatitis caused by viruses other than hepatitis A, hepatitis B, and non-A, non-B hepatitis viruses. Diseases of the Liver, 7th ed. Schiff L, Schiff ER, eds. JB Lippincott Co, Philadelphia, 1993, p 578

45. Markin RS, Linder J, Zuerlein K, et al: Hepatitis in fatal infectious mononucleosis. Gastroenterology 93:1210, 1987

46. Weller TH: The cytomegaloviruses: ubiquitous agents with protean clinical manifestations. I. N Engl J Med 285:203, 1971

47. Farrell GC: Drug-induced hepatic injury. J Gastroenterol Hepatol 12:S242, 1997

48. Makin AJ, Wendon J, Williams R: A 7-year experience of severe acetaminophen-induced hepatotoxicity (1987–1993). Gastroenterology 109:1907, 1995

49. Smilkstein MJ, Knapp GL, Kulig KW, et al: Efficacy of oral N-acetylcysteine in the treatment of acetaminophen overdose: analysis of the National Multicenter Study (1976 to 1985). N Engl J Med 319:1557, 1988

50. Chalmers TC, Eckhardt RD, Reynolds WE, et al: The treatment of acute infectious hepatitis: controlled studies of the effects of diet, rest, and physical reconditioning on the acute course of the disease and on the incidence of relapses and residual abnormalities. J Clin Invest 34:1163, 1955

51. Repsher LH, Freebern RK: Effects of early and vigorous exercise on recovery from infectious hepatitis. N Engl J Med 281:1393, 1969

52. Quin JW: Interferon therapy for acute hepatitis C viral infection: a review by meta-analysis. Aust N Z J Med 27:611, 1997

53. Orland JR, Wright TL, Cooper S: Acute hepatitis C. Hepatology 33:321, 2001

54. Gregory PB, Knauer CM, Kempson RL, et al: Steroid therapy in severe viral hepatitis: a double-blind, randomized trial of methyl-prednisolone versus placebo. N Engl J Med 294:681, 1976

55. Redeker AG, Schweitzer IL, Yamahiro HS: Randomization of corticosteroid therapy in fulminant hepatitis (letter). N Engl J Med 294:728, 1976

56. A double-blinded, randomized trial of hydrocortisone in acute hepatic failure (abstr). Acute Hepatic Failure Study Group. Gastroenterology 76:1297, 1979

57. Ware AJ, Cuthbert JA, Shorey J, et al: A prospective trial of steroid therapy in severe viral hepatitis. Gastroenterology 80:219, 1981

58. MacDougall BRD, Bailey RJ, Williams R: H_2-receptor antagonists and antacids in the prevention of acute gastrointestinal hemorrhage in fulminant hepatic failure. Lancet 1:617, 1977

59. Failure of specific immunotherapy in fulminant type B hepatitis. Acute Hepatic Failure Study Group. Ann Intern Med 86:272, 1977

60. Redeker AG, Yamahiro HS: Controlled trial of exchange-transfusion therapy in fulminant hepatitis. Lancet 1:3, 1973

61. Wall W, Adams PC: Liver transplantation for fulminant hepatic failure: North American experience. Liver Transplant Surg 1:178, 1995

62. Prevention of hepatitis A through active or passive immunization: recommendations of the Advisory Committee on Immunization Practices (ACIP). MMWR Morb Mortal Wkly Rep 48(RR-12):1, 1999

63. Hepatitis B virus: a comprehensive strategy for eliminating transmission in the United States through universal childhood vaccination: Recommendations of the Immunization Practices Committee (ACIP). MMWR Morb Mortal Wkly Rep 40(RR-13):1, 1991

64. Update: recommendations to prevent hepatitis B virus transmission—United States. MMWR Morb Mortal Wkly Rep 48:33, 1999

65. Suboptimal response to hepatitis B vaccine given by injection into the buttock. MMWR Morb Mortal Wkly Rep 34:105, 1985

66. Alper CA, Kruskall MS, Marcus-Bagley D, et al: Genetic prediction of nonresponse to hepatitis B vaccine. N Engl J Med 321:708, 1989

67. Weissman JY, Tsuchiyose MM, Tong MJ, et al: Lack of response to recombinant hepatitis B vaccine in nonresponders to the plasma vaccine. JAMA 260:1734, 1988

68. Wainwright RB, McMahon BJ, Bulkow LR, et al: Duration of immunogenicity and efficacy of hepatitis B vaccine in a Yupik Eskimo population. JAMA 261:2362, 1989

69. Horowitz MM, Ershler WB, McKinney WP, et al: Duration of immunity after hepatitis B vaccination: efficacy of low-dose booster vaccine. Ann Intern Med 108:185, 1988

70. Are booster immunisations needed for lifelong hepatitis B immunity? European Consensus Group on Hepatitis B Immunity. Lancet 355:561, 2000

71. Perrillo RP, Parker ML, Campbell C, et al: Prevaccination screening of medical and dental students: should low levels of antibody to hepatitis B surface antigen preclude vaccination? JAMA 250:2481, 1983

72. Kessler HA, Harris AA, Payne JA, et al: Antibodies to hepatitis B surface antigen as the sole hepatitis B marker in hospital personnel. Ann Intern Med 103:21, 1985

73. Werner BG, Dienstag JL, Kuter BJ, et al: Isolated antibody to hepatitis B surface antigen and response to hepatitis B vaccination. Ann Intern Med 103:201, 1985

74. Innis BL, Snitbhan R, Kunasol P, et al: Protection against hepatitis A by an inactivated vaccine. JAMA 271:1328, 1994

75. Werzberger A, Mensch B, Kuter B, et al: A controlled trial of formalin-inactivated hepatitis A vaccine in healthy children. N Engl J Med 327:453, 1992

76. Lemon SM: Inactivated hepatitis A vaccines (editorial). JAMA 271:1363, 1994

77. Berge JJ, Drennan DP, Jacobs RJ, et al: The cost of hepatitis A infections in American adolescents and adults in 1997. Hepatology 31:469, 2000

78. Steffen R, Kane MA, Shapiro CN, et al: Epidemiology and prevention of hepatitis A in travelers. JAMA 272:885, 1994

79. Keeffe EB: Is hepatitis A more severe in patients with chronic hepatitis B and other chronic liver diseases? Am J Gastroenterol 90:201, 1995

80. Vento S, Garofano T, Renzini C, et al: Fulminant hepatitis associated with hepatitis A virus superinfection in patients with chronic hepatitis C. N Engl J Med 338:286, 1998

81. Keeffe EB, Iwarson S, McMahon BJ, et al: Safety and immunogenicity of hepatitis A vaccine in patients with chronic liver disease. Hepatology 27:881, 1998

Acknowledgments

Figure 1   Alan D. Iselin.

Figure 2   Seward Hung.

65 Chronic Hepatitis

Emmet B. Keeffe, M.D.

Definition

Chronic hepatitis is a broad clinical and pathologic syndrome that encompasses an etiologically diverse group of diseases characterized by long-term elevation of liver chemistries and the finding of hepatic inflammation on liver biopsy.[1] Chronic hepatitis is generally defined as disease that has lasted for 6 months or longer; in many cases, however, the diagnosis can be established earlier.

Etiology

The most important groups of diseases that cause chronic hepatitis are autoimmune hepatitis (previously called autoimmune chronic active hepatitis) and chronic viral hepatitis, which is caused by infection with hepatitis B virus (HBV), with or without coinfection with hepatitis D virus (HDV), or by infection with hepatitis C virus (HCV) [*see Table 1*]. Less commonly, chronic hepatitis is cryptogenic or caused by drugs, Wilson disease, α_1-antitrypsin deficiency, or early-stage primary biliary cirrhosis or primary sclerosing cholangitis. Over the past several years, international working groups have substantially modified the terminology of chronic hepatitis to reflect an etiologic basis rather than a pathologic basis.[1]

Approach to Chronic Hepatitis

DIAGNOSIS

Clinical Manifestations

Clinical manifestations of chronic hepatitis are diverse, ranging from asymptomatic stable disease characterized by mildly elevated aminotransferase levels (the usual pattern seen in the early stages of chronic viral hepatitis) to severe, rapidly progressive illness with fulminant hepatic failure. The most common symptoms of chronic hepatitis are fatigue, malaise, and mild abdominal pain. Patients with mild forms of chronic hepatitis are usually asymptomatic or have minimal symptoms with no stigmas of chronic liver disease on physical examination. In more advanced cases, the symptoms and signs of chronic hepatitis include anorexia, jaundice, spider angiomas, palmar erythema, ascites, edema, hepatomegaly, and encephalopathy. Pruritus is unusual, unless the patient has primary biliary cirrhosis or primary sclerosing cholangitis. A small number of patients with autoimmune hepatitis have an acute fulminant course and are critically ill at initial presentation. Extrahepatic manifestations of chronic hepatitis are common and include arthralgias, arthritis, glomerulonephritis, skin rashes, amenorrhea, acne, hirsutism, and thyroiditis.

Table 1 Summary of the Types, Diagnosis, and Treatment of Chronic Hepatitis

Type	Diagnosis	Treatment
Chronic viral hepatitis		
Chronic hepatitis B	(+) HBsAg, (–) IgM anti-HBc	
Active replication	(+) HBeAg, (+) HBV DNA	Interferon alfa-2b, lamivudine
Low replication	(+) Anti-HBe, (–) HBV DNA	Supportive therapy
Chronic hepatitis C	(+) Anti-HCV (second-generation ELISA or RIBA), (+) HCV RNA	Interferon alfa-2b plus ribavirin, interferon monotherapy
Chronic hepatitis D	(+) HBsAg, (+) anti-HDV	Interferon alfa-2b
Autoimmune hepatitis		
Type 1 (classic)	(+) ANA, (+) ASMA	Corticosteroids, azathioprine
Type 2	(+) Anti-LKM1,* (–) ANA, (–) ASMA	
Type 2a	(–) Anti-HCV, (–) anti-GOR, (+) anti-LKM1 (high titer)	Corticosteroids, azathioprine
Type 2b	(+) Anti-HCV, (+) anti-GOR, (+) anti-LKM1 (low titer)	Uncertain
Type 3	(+) Anti-SLA, (+) anti-LP, (–) ANA, (±) ASMA, (±) AMA	Corticosteroids, azathioprine
Cryptogenic hepatitis		
?Autoimmune	(+) Hyperglobulinemia; (+) HLA-B8 or HLA-A1, -B8, and -DR3; (–) autoimmune markers	Consider trial of corticosteroids, azathioprine
?Viral†	Biopsy shows so-called viral features; globulins are normal; (–) autoimmune markers and HLA associations; other causes of liver disease are excluded	Supportive therapy
Unclassified	(–) Clinical, immunoserologic, and histologic clues for autoimmune or viral hepatitis; other causes of liver disease are excluded	Supportive therapy

*Anti-LKM1 was called anti-LKM before LKM2 (associated with tienilic acid) and LKM3 (associated with hepatitis D) were identified.
†The role of a non-A through -E hepatitis agent (hepatitis F or G) remains speculative.
(+)—present (–)—absent (±)—present or absent AMA—antimitochondrial antibody ANA—antinuclear antibody anti-GOR—antibody to GOR protein anti-HBc—antibody to hepatitis B core antigen anti-HBe—antibody to HBeAg anti-HCV—antibody to HCV anti-HDV—antibody to hepatitis D virus anti-LKM—antibody to liver/kidney microsome anti-LKM1—antibody to liver/kidney microsome type 1 anti-LP—antibody to liver/pancreas antigen anti-SLA—antibody to soluble liver antigen ASMA—anti-smooth muscle antibody ELISA—enzyme-linked immunosorbent assay HBeAg—hepatitis B e antigen HBsAg—hepatitis B surface antigen HBV—hepatitis B virus HCV—hepatitis C virus LKM2—liver/kidney microsome type 2 LKM3—liver/kidney microsome type 3 RIBA—recombinant immunoblot assay

Routine Laboratory Tests

The serum alanine aminotransferase (ALT) and aspartate aminotransferase (AST) levels are usually elevated in patients with chronic hepatitis, although a small number of patients with histologic chronic hepatitis have transiently normal aminotransferase levels. Even a mild elevation of aminotransferase levels (5 to 10 IU/L higher than the upper limit of normal) should lead the physician to consider the presence of chronic hepatitis. Elevations of more than 400 IU/L are common in cases of untreated autoimmune hepatitis and severe chronic viral hepatitis. Substantial increases in the aminotransferase levels herald an exacerbation of disease. The serum bilirubin level is usually normal (0.0 to 1.0 mg/dl) in chronic viral hepatitis but is higher than 3 mg/dl in patients with moderately severe autoimmune hepatitis. A characteristic feature of autoimmune hepatitis, but not of chronic viral hepatitis, is an increased γ-globulin level (> 1.6 g/dl), which may be markedly increased (3 to 7 g/dl). In the most severe forms of chronic hepatitis, hepatic synthetic function is impaired; this condition is demonstrated by a low serum albumin level and prolongation of the prothrombin time.

Imaging studies of the abdomen show variable degrees of hepatomegaly with or without splenomegaly; irregularity of liver density or contour; and evidence of portal hypertension with ascites, an increased number of portal collateral vessels, or both.

Liver Biopsy

The specific etiology of chronic hepatitis can usually be determined by clinical evaluation combined with immunologic and serologic testing, but liver biopsy helps confirm certain diagnoses (e.g., Wilson disease or α_1-antitrypsin deficiency) and establish histologic grading and staging. It has been proposed that the etiologic terminology be supplemented by a histologic description of the grade of inflammatory activity and of the stage of fibrosis or cirrhosis. Thus, the diagnosis of chronic hepatitis in a given patient might be autoimmune hepatitis (etiology) with severe activity (grade) and cirrhosis (stage).

The grade and stage of chronic hepatitis can be assessed with various semiquantitative scoring systems.[1,2] In the histology activity index, also known as the Knodell score, the grades of inflammation range from 0 to 18, and the stages of fibrosis range from 0 to 4. This scoring system is often used in clinical research studies, but other scoring systems are more commonly applied in routine practice.[2] The most popular scoring system for chronic hepatitis generates two scores from 1 to 4—one for the degree of inflammation and the other for the degree of fibrosis [see Table 2]. The various numerical scoring systems have been critically important in research, particularly in treatment trials, and are now often used by pathologists in the routine interpretation of liver biopsy specimens from patients with chronic hepatitis. However, it is also important that the final evaluation of a liver biopsy specimen from a patient with chronic hepatitis include descriptive terminology characterizing the etiology, grade, and stage of disease.

DIFFERENTIAL DIAGNOSIS

Primary Biliary Cirrhosis

Primary biliary cirrhosis may be indistinguishable from chronic hepatitis on liver biopsy. Characteristic hyperpigmentation, pruritus, marked elevation of serum alkaline phos-

Table 2　Grades of Inflammation and Stages of Fibrosis on Liver Biopsies

Grade/Stage	Grade of Inflammation	Stage of Fibrosis
1	Minimal	Portal
2	Mild	Periportal
3	Moderate	Bridging
4	Severe	Cirrhosis

Table 3　Types of Autoimmune Hepatitis

Type	ANA	ASMA	Anti-LKM1	Anti-SLA	Anti-HCV
Type 1	+	+	–	–	–
Type 2	–	–	+	–	±
Type 3*	–	±	–	+	–

*Not formally recognized and least well established.

phatase, and high titers of antimitochondrial antibody (AMA) (> 1:160) are helpful in making the differential diagnosis.

Primary Sclerosing Cholangitis

Primary sclerosing cholangitis can sometimes mimic chronic hepatitis. Prominent elevations of the serum alkaline phosphatase level and accompanying inflammatory bowel disease will, in most cases, distinguish this disorder from chronic hepatitis. The definitive diagnosis is made by endoscopic retrograde cholangiography.

Drug-Induced Chronic Hepatitis

Drug-induced chronic hepatitis constitutes a small but important category of chronic hepatitis.[3] Methyldopa, trazodone, and isoniazid are well-recognized causes. In addition, cases have occasionally been reported after therapy with sulfonamides, propylthiouracil, nitrofurantoin, acetaminophen, aspirin, and dantrolene; other drugs are also likely to be implicated. Thus, it is reasonable to discontinue as many medications as possible when chronic hepatitis is first diagnosed. If a patient's hepatitis is drug related, liver function abnormalities and the clinical course of disease frequently improve after the causative agent has been withdrawn.

Wilson Disease

When neurologic abnormalities are absent, Wilson disease mimics chronic hepatitis. It is critical to establish the diagnosis of Wilson disease, because specific treatment with penicillamine, trientine, or zinc is available. Measurement of the hepatic copper content in a needle biopsy specimen is definitive. If a biopsy specimen is not available, the serum ceruloplasmin and 24-hour urinary copper levels should be obtained and slit-lamp examination for Kayser-Fleischer rings performed in all patients younger than 35 years for whom the cause of chronic hepatitis remains obscure after the usual testing. If the results of all three tests are normal, Wilson disease is virtually excluded.

α_1-Antitrypsin Deficiency

α_1-Antitrypsin deficiency is associated with mildly active progressive liver disease, which evolves into cirrhosis. Liver disease associated with α_1-antitrypsin deficiency can be distinguished from chronic hepatitis by a reduced α_1-globulin level on protein electrophoresis, by results of specific serum assays for α_1-antitrypsin, and by inclusions in the liver parenchyma that are positive on periodic acid–Schiff testing.

Autoimmune Hepatitis

The wide spectrum of clinical and immunoserologic manifestations of autoimmune hepatitis has led investigators to characterize types of the disease[4,5] [*see Tables 1 and 3*]. Three types have been described, but only types 1 and 2 have sufficiently distinct features to warrant formal recognition. Whether patients with type 3 autoimmune hepatitis are truly a distinct subpopulation remains uncertain.

TYPE 1 AUTOIMMUNE HEPATITIS

Type 1, or classic, autoimmune hepatitis is the most common form of the disease in the United States.[4,5] It is characterized by hypergammaglobulinemia; the presence of antinuclear antibody (ANA), anti–smooth muscle antibody (ASMA), or both; and a bimodal age at onset (adolescence and around late middle age).

In type 1 autoimmune hepatitis, aminotransferase levels are three to 10 times higher than normal, and the α-globulin level is increased more than twofold. The presentation may be acute or subacute but is more commonly chronic. Other autoimmune diseases may be present concurrently, and associations between type 1 autoimmune hepatitis and the presence of human leukocyte antigen profiles have been identified.

Liver biopsy is a useful prognostic tool because patients with portal or mild periportal hepatitis have a benign course, whereas those with bridging or multilobular necrosis or cirrhosis are at high risk for progressive liver disease.

Patients with severe disease who are treated with corticosteroids have a 10-year survival rate of 60% to 70%, whereas untreated patients have a survival rate of less than 30%.

TYPE 2 AUTOIMMUNE HEPATITIS

Type 2 autoimmune hepatitis [*see Tables 1 and 3*] is characterized by the absence of ANA and ASMA and by the presence of antibody to liver/kidney microsome type 1 (anti-LKM1).[4,5] The target antigen of type 2 autoimmune hepatitis is P-450 IID6.[6] Anti-LKM1 and AMA reactivity may be difficult to distinguish on immunofluorescence, especially in cases of strong reactivity, and patients with anti-LKM1 may be falsely positive for AMA, which suggests the incorrect diagnosis of primary biliary cirrhosis.

Type 2 autoimmune hepatitis appears to be much less common than type 1 and has been observed primarily in Europe. It appears to be predominant in children and is frequently associated with other autoimmune diseases.

The onset of type 2 autoimmune hepatitis is often acute and may be associated with liver failure, and there is a propensity for the disease to progress rapidly to cirrhosis.

TYPE 3 AUTOIMMUNE HEPATITIS

Type 3 autoimmune hepatitis is the most recently encountered and least established type of autoimmune hepatitis.[4,5] It is characterized by the presence of antibody to a soluble liver antigen (anti-SLA), to a recently characterized liver/pancreas antigen (anti-LP), or to both. Approximately one third of patients also are positive for ASMA, AMA, or both. The presence of anti-SLA or anti-LP antibody identifies this small group of patients with autoimmune hepatitis and serves to distinguish them from patients who have chronic hepatitis of an indeterminate viral cause or an unclassified, truly cryptogenic variety of disease.

DIFFERENTIAL DIAGNOSIS

Occasionally, physicians have difficulty distinguishing between type 1 or 2 autoimmune hepatitis and chronic hepatitis C. The distinction is important because autoimmune hepatitis responds to immunosuppressive drugs but may be exacerbated by treatment with interferon. Enzyme-linked immunosorbent assay (ELISA) for antibody to HCV (anti-HCV) may be reactive in patients with untreated type 1 autoimmune hepatitis, but HCV infection can be excluded in nearly all of these patients by the findings of a negative result for anti-HCV on second-generation recombinant immunoblot assay (RIBA) and absent serum HCV RNA. The false positive anti-HCV test result is associated with the hypergammaglobulinemia of autoimmune disease. The distinction between chronic hepatitis C and type 1 autoimmune hepatitis may be further confused by the finding that ANA is present in some patients with HCV infection; however, the ANA titer in patients with chronic hepatitis C is typically lower (i.e., $\leq 1:160$), and significant hypergammaglobulinemia is not present. Although it has been speculated that HCV infection might induce the development of autoimmune markers or disease, this hypothesis remains unproved.

More of a problem is the observation that anti-LKM1 is found in some patients with chronic HCV infection, which causes diagnostic confusion between type 2 autoimmune hepatitis and chronic hepatitis C.[6] Worldwide, the prevalence of markers of HCV infection in patients with detectable anti-LKM1 varies widely—from 0% to more than 80%. Conversely, the prevalence of anti-LKM1 in patients with chronic hepatitis C varies from 0% to 5%. Anti-LKM1–positive, anti-HCV–positive serum reacts significantly less often with P-450 IID6, the target of anti-LKM1, than does anti-LKM1–positive, anti-HCV–negative serum. In particular, serum from patients with type 2 autoimmune hepatitis reacts with a linear epitope contained within P-450 IID6, whereas serum from patients with HCV markers and anti-LKM1 does not. Moreover, anti-GOR, an antibody to GOR protein found in patients with HCV infection, is frequently present in anti-LKM1–positive patients who are positive for anti-HCV but is absent in those who are negative for anti-HCV. Thus, in some patients, HCV seems to induce autoimmunity to both GOR and LKM1.

Table 4 Differences between the Subtypes of Type 2 Autoimmune Hepatitis

Parameter	Type 2a	Type 2b
Age	Younger	Older
Sex	Female > male	Male > female
Anti-LKM1	High titer	Low titer
Anti-HCV	–	+
Anti-GOR	–	+
Disease	Active	Less active
Immunosuppressive therapy	Effective	Less effective

These findings support the division of type 2 autoimmune hepatitis into two subtypes [see Tables 1 and 4].

TREATMENT

Immunosuppressive Therapy

Most patients who have the clinical, biochemical, and histologic features of type 1 autoimmune hepatitis should be treated with corticosteroids.[2,4] Patients with type 2a or type 3 autoimmune hepatitis are treated in a similar fashion. The usual regimen consists of prednisone (15 to 20 mg/day). Although 10% to 20% of patients do not show improvement with this regimen, some show improvement with higher corticosteroid dosages (approximately 60 mg/day). A combination of prednisone at a lower dosage (5 to 10 mg/day) and azathioprine (50 to 100 mg/day) may be given to patients who experience intolerable side effects from prednisone. Azathioprine alone will not induce remission, but long-term therapy is effective in maintaining remission and sparing the use of corticosteroids.[7]

Clinical, biochemical, and histologic remission occurs in 65% of patients within 18 months to 2 years after treatment. In general, symptoms are reduced within 3 months, liver chemistry test results improve within 3 to 6 months, and histologic resolution occurs within 18 months to 2 years. The presence of serum autoimmune markers, such as ANA, does not appreciably influence the initial response to corticosteroids in patients with autoimmune hepatitis.

Cessation of immunosuppressive treatment It is difficult to determine when treatment should be discontinued. One approach is to discontinue drugs when clinical symptoms have subsided, serum aminotransferase levels have stabilized to less than twice normal, and active hepatic cell necrosis is no longer apparent on liver biopsy. Once the decision to discontinue treatment has been made, the drug or drugs should be slowly tapered over 6 to 12 months. Despite every precaution, relapse occurs within 3 to 6 months in 20% to 86% of patients.[4] Relapse is less likely if biopsy shows that the inflammatory activity has completely resolved and the histologic appearance of the liver is normal. Sustained remission (> 5 years) may be achieved in 20% of patients who are treated with immunosuppressive drugs. A subset of patients with autoimmune hepatitis have severe symptoms on presentation and prominent markers of a presumed autoimmune process (i.e., a high autoantibody titer in the blood, marked elevations of γ-globulin levels, and many portal plasma cells on liver biopsy); these patients uniformly suffer relapses after withdrawal of corticosteroid therapy. Withdrawal of therapy in this subset of patients should be carried out only with extreme caution, or long-term therapy should be maintained.

Complications of treatment Corticosteroid treatment is not without risk. Obesity, cushingoid facies, acne, or striae develop within 2 years in at least 80% of patients. When treatment is continued for longer than 18 months, one or more severe complications (e.g., diabetes, hypertension, cataracts, psychosis, infections, or osteoporosis with vertebral collapse) develop in more than 50% of patients. The risk of complications increases with the duration of treatment. In addition, azathioprine may cause severe bone marrow depression or pancreatitis.

Contraindications for treatment Not all patients with pre-sumed autoimmune hepatitis should be treated with immunosuppressive drugs.[2,4] Treatment of elderly patients should be considered very carefully because serious side effects are likely to occur. Patients with advanced cirrhosis and relatively modest abnormalities in serum aminotransferase levels (< 100 IU/L) are also not good candidates; in such patients, severe fibrosis does not resolve, the sequelae of portal hypertension cannot be prevented, and the hepatitis component (against which the anti-inflammatory effect of the corticosteroids is most effective) is not marked. Finally, the benefit of treatment of asymptomatic patients is also questionable. These patients already function normally, their disease appears to progress slowly, and the risk associated with long-term therapy is substantial.

Overlap Syndromes

Overlapping syndromes of autoimmune hepatitis and either primary biliary cirrhosis or primary sclerosing cholangitis have been recognized but are uncommon.[8] The term autoimmune cholangitis has been proposed to characterize patients with biochemical or histologic cholestasis that resembles primary biliary cirrhosis; however, these patients are negative for AMA and have a normal IgM level but have high titers of ANA and an elevated IgG level. Results of cholangiography are normal. These patients respond less well to corticosteroids and seldom experience a remission. Patients with features of both autoimmune hepatitis and primary sclerosing cholangitis also respond poorly to corticosteroids, whereas patients with overlapping features of autoimmune hepatitis and primary biliary cirrhosis respond to corticosteroids in a manner similar to that of patients with only autoimmune hepatitis.

Chronic Hepatitis B

EPIDEMIOLOGY

Chronic hepatitis B is a major global health care problem: 5% of the world's population, or approximately 300 million persons, are chronic carriers.[9] In the United States, 300,000 new cases of acute disease are reported to the Centers for Disease Control and Prevention (CDC) each year; 5% of these patients, or 15,000 persons, become new chronic carriers. The prevalence of hepatitis B surface antigen (HBsAg) carriers in the United States is 0.2% to 0.5% of the general population; approximately 1.25 million persons have chronic HBV infection. However, carrier rates five to 10 times higher have been identified among certain groups, including Asian Americans, persons who have received multiple blood transfusions or hemodialysis, intravenous drug users, homosexual men, and patients with AIDS. In addition, carrier rates of 5% to 20% have been recognized in certain populations in some states, such as Alaska and Hawaii.

DIAGNOSIS

Chronic hepatitis B can be reliably diagnosed with serologic testing [see Table 1]. In patients with chronic HBV infection, HBsAg remains detectable for more than 6 months. After 6 months, HBsAg clears spontaneously in 1% to 2% of patients each year. Persons who continue to test positive for HBsAg, are asymptomatic, and have normal aminotransferase levels are termed HBsAg carriers. Other chronically infected, HBsAg-positive individuals may have clinical or laboratory evidence of chronic hepatic disease (i.e., elevated aminotransferase levels) and are given a diagnosis of chronic hepatitis B.

NATURAL HISTORY

Chronic HBV infection can be divided into two phases. The first phase is a highly infectious, active replicative phase characterized by high levels of circulating virions; the presence of circulating HBV DNA, DNA polymerase, and hepatitis B e antigen (HBeAg); and the presence of free, episomal DNA in hepatocytes. The second phase is a minimally infectious, low replicative phase characterized by few circulating virions; undetectable levels of circulating HBV DNA, DNA polymerase, and HBeAg; the presence of circulating antibody to HBeAg (anti-HBe); and the presence of integrated HBV DNA in hepatocytes.

Age at the time of initial HBV infection is the major determinant of chronicity. Although as many as 90% of infected neonates become carriers, the carrier rate falls with increasing age at the time of infection, so that only 3% to 5% of newly infected adults fail to clear HBsAg. Another important risk factor for chronicity is the presence of intrinsic or iatrogenic immunosuppression. Gender is also a well-established but poorly understood determinant of chronicity; women are more likely than men to clear HBsAg. As a result, men predominate in all populations of HBsAg carriers.

In some patients with chronic HBV infection who have lost previous markers of HBV replication (e.g., HBV DNA and HBeAg), biochemical, clinical, and histologic exacerbations that mimic acute hepatitis have been noted. These exacerbations, termed reactivation, appear spontaneously but also have been reported in oncology patients after withdrawal of chemotherapy. Reactivation appears to be a consequence of increased HBV replication because HBV DNA, DNA polymerase, and HBeAg usually reappear in the serum concurrently with elevation of the ALT level.

Persistent HBV infection is an important risk factor for the development of hepatocellular carcinoma, the most prevalent nondermatologic carcinoma in the world. In Taiwan, the relative risk of hepatocellular carcinoma is about 200 times higher in carriers of HBV than in noncarriers.[9] In addition, very high risk areas for hepatocellular carcinoma have been identified in sub-Saharan Africa and Asia, where a strong correlation between hepatocellular carcinoma rates and HBV carrier rates has been recognized. Several lines of evidence suggest that the use of screening tests, including ultrasonography and serum α-fetoprotein, may be useful in the early diagnosis of hepatocellular carcinoma, which can then be treated.[10]

TREATMENT

The ultimate goal of treatment of chronic hepatitis B is to eradicate HBV infection and prevent the development of cirrhosis or hepatocellular carcinoma.[9,11] Although currently available therapies, such as interferon and lamivudine, have not been proved to achieve these goals, they can suppress HBV replication and lead to improvement in the clinical, biochemical, and histologic features of chronic hepatitis B.

Interferon Therapy

A large number of trials have demonstrated the efficacy of interferon alfa-2b in the treatment of HBV DNA–positive, HBeAg-positive chronic hepatitis B.[11,12] The dosage is 30 to 35 million U/wk (subcutaneously or intramuscularly for 4

months) given as 5 million U/day or 10 million units three times weekly.[9,11] Treatment results in loss of HBV replication (loss of HBeAg and HBV DNA) in 40% of patients and loss of HBsAg in approximately 10%.

Predictors of a response to interferon include an HBV DNA level of lower than 100 pg/ml, an ALT level higher than 200 IU/L, a short duration of infection, heterosexual orientation, and female gender. Studies show that after several years, as many as 60% of patients who responded to interferon lose HBsAg, and many of these persons develop antibody to HBsAg (anti-HBs).[13]

Fortunately, relapse with reappearance of HBeAg is very unusual. In a meta-analysis of interferon trials, loss of viral markers of replication and normalization of the ALT level occurred about 20% more often in treated patients than in control subjects.[14] Moreover, interferon has also been shown to prolong life and lower treatment costs for patients with chronic hepatitis B who have detectable HBeAg.[15]

It should be noted that interferon is considerably less effective in Chinese patients with chronic hepatitis B than in white patients, with sustained loss of HBeAg occurring in only 15% of Chinese patients.[16] However, Chinese patients with an elevated ALT level have a response rate similar to that of whites, whereas Chinese patients with a normal ALT level (and probable immune tolerance to HBV) respond poorly.[17]

Most patients who have anti-HBe have inactive liver disease and are therefore unlikely to benefit from interferon. An exception, however, is the subgroup of anti-HBe–positive patients who harbor a precore mutant, recognized by the absence of HBeAg but the presence of HBV DNA in high concentrations. These patients experience a good response to interferon, although the relapse rate is high.[18]

Finally, patients with mildly decompensated cirrhosis can be treated with low, titrated doses of interferon. One third of such patients will respond and have a sustained loss of HBV DNA and HBeAg that is associated with resolution of the symptoms of cirrhosis.[19] These patients must be monitored closely, however, because bacterial infections and exacerbation of hepatitis are common, serious complications.

Interferon and corticosteroid combination therapy Because studies found that corticosteroid withdrawal was frequently associated with a flare in liver disease and spontaneous clearance of HBeAg, trials were initiated to evaluate the role of a short course of corticosteroids in enhancing the effectiveness of interferon in patients with chronic HBV infection. The majority of studies have shown no difference between use of corticosteroid priming followed by interferon and use of interferon alone in the treatment of patients with chronic hepatitis B.[9,11] Therefore, the combination of prednisone and interferon is generally not used, although this combination may increase HBeAg loss in patients who have a low ALT level (< 100 IU/L).

Side effects of interferon therapy Interferon commonly causes side effects, but they are usually manageable. Among these effects are influenzalike symptoms (fever, myalgia, arthralgia, and headache), hematologic toxicity (granulocytopenia, leukopenia, and thrombocytopenia), systemic symptoms (fatigue and hair loss), neurologic signs (decreased concentration, depression, and irritability), and immune system disorders (development of autoantibodies, thyroid disease, or other autoimmune diseases).

Contraindications to interferon therapy Patients with a history of hypersensitivity to interferon, decompensated cirrhosis, immunosuppression associated with organ transplantation, active autoimmune disease, or significant psychiatric disease, including depression, should not receive treatment.

Lamivudine Therapy

Lamivudine, a nucleoside analogue that inhibits viral DNA synthesis, was approved in late 1998 for the treatment of chronic hepatitis B. A dose of 100 mg/day achieves maximal suppression of HBV DNA. Lamivudine is readily absorbed from the gastrointestinal tract and may be taken with or without food. Lamivudine is cleared mainly in urine, and thus, dose adjustments are required for patients with significant renal failure.

In three placebo-controlled studies, improved liver histology occurred in a significantly higher percentage of patients given lamivudine than patients who received placebo.[20-22] Improvements in liver histology were similar in treatment-naive patients, relapsers, and nonresponders to prior interferon therapy, and the improvements occurred independently of HBeAg seroconversion.[23,24] Serum HBV DNA levels fell rapidly and remained at least 94% below baseline values, and serum ALT levels also decreased during therapy, with 50% of patients achieving and maintaining normal ALT levels after 2 years of therapy. Patients receiving lamivudine for 1 year experienced a 17% to 33% rate of loss of HBeAg. It is generally thought that patients who achieve HBeAg seroconversion (loss of HBeAg and HBV DNA, with development of anti-HBe) can discontinue lamivudine therapy. Relapse appears to occur in 15% to 20% of patients, but more data are needed to define the durability of HBeAg seroconversion.

The efficacy of lamivudine therapy after 1 year is similar to that of interferon therapy after 4 to 6 months. However, the cumulative HBeAg seroconversion rate is higher in patients who had elevated baseline ALT levels before treatment, and the seroconversion rate increases progressively with additional years of lamivudine therapy. In 58 patients treated for 3 years with lamivudine, the cumulative HBeAg seroconversion rate increased from 22% after 1 year of therapy to 27% after 2 years and to 40% after 3 years.[25,26] Within this group, 38% of patients with pretreatment ALT levels greater than twice the upper limit of normal experienced HBeAg seroconversion after 1 year of therapy, with the rate increasing to 42% after 2 years and to 65% after 3 years.

The serum levels of ALT and HBV DNA return to pretreatment levels if lamivudine is discontinued before HbeAg loss or seroconversion is achieved. Some patients may experience serum ALT levels that are transiently higher after treatment than before treatment, as do patients who receive interferon. Generally, no adverse effects have been associated with these elevations, although there are rare reports of severe flares of hepatitis B.

Lamivudine and interferon combination therapy Lamivudine and interferon alfa-2b in combination should theoretically have synergistic effects against HBV. Unfortunately, this combination failed to show greater efficacy than either drug used alone.[27]

Complications of lamivudine therapy Variant strains of HBV that demonstrate changes near the YMDD motif (the amino acid sequence tyrosine-methionine-aspartate-aspartate) may appear after 6 to 8 months of lamivudine therapy. YMDD variants of HBV occur in 27% to 32% of patients after 1 year of therapy.[20-22,27] The median serum ALT and HBV DNA levels were lower than pretreatment levels in patients who developed YMDD variants, but these improvements were not as significant as those in patients who maintained the wild-type HBV. In spite of developing HBV variants, liver histology after 1 year of therapy was still better in patients who received lamivudine than in patients who received placebo. Because the variant HBV is less replication-efficient, it is generally recommended that lamivudine therapy be continued. If therapy is stopped, the wild-type HBV returns and may be associated with a flare of chronic hepatitis B.

Lamivudine and end-stage liver disease Lamivudine may play a role in patients with chronic hepatitis B who have end-stage liver disease, according to preliminary evidence of stabilization and improvement of biochemical and clinical features as well as occasional deferral of the need for liver transplantation.[28,29] Lamivudine therapy may serve as a bridge to transplantation for patients with decompensated cirrhosis while they await a donor liver.

Liver Transplantation

Liver transplantation can be performed for liver failure associated with chronic hepatitis B, but HBV infects the allograft in 80% to 100% of cases (if antiviral prophylaxis is not given), and long-term survival is only 45% to 50% (compared with 80% to 85% in transplant patients with other types of cirrhosis).[29] The HBV reinfection often is accelerated and progresses to cirrhosis. As a result, most transplant centers now implement prophylactic antiviral strategies to reduce reinfection. Two such strategies are (1) the intraoperative, immediately postoperative, and long-term administration of high-dose hepatitis B immune globulin (HBIG) (to maintain an anti-HBs level > 100 to 200 mIU/ml over the long term) and (2) the short-term administration of HBIG with lamivudine, with later discontinuance of HBIG.[29,30] A number of trials using these prophylaxis strategies against HBV reinfection suggest that the reinfection rate can be reduced to 10% to 20% and that 1-year and 3-year survival rates are improved.

Chronic Hepatitis D

Hepatitis D (delta hepatitis) appears to respond at least temporarily to high doses of interferon alfa (9 million units three times a week for 48 weeks).[31] In one study, aminotransferase levels returned to normal in 71% of patients; in 50% of these patients, aminotransferase levels were still normal an average of 39 months later.[31] However, the clearance of HDV RNA from the serum that occurred immediately after treatment was not sustained; HDV RNA was found in the serum of all treated patients at long-term follow-up. Lamivudine is not effective in patients with delta coinfection.[32]

Chronic Hepatitis C

EPIDEMIOLOGY

Approximately 30,000 new cases of acute HCV infection are reported annually to the CDC. Of these patients, at least 85% develop chronic HCV infection.[33] Approximately 4 million persons in the United States (1.8%) have been infected with HCV, and 74% of these individuals (1.4% of the population) are viremic.[34] The high chronicity rate of HCV infection makes chronic hepatitis C a much more prevalent disease than chronic hepatitis B (0.2% to 0.5% of the general population).

DIAGNOSIS

The diagnosis of chronic hepatitis C is typically made by the finding of persistently or intermittently elevated aminotransferase levels in association with reactive anti-HCV on second-generation ELISA.[33] Samples from a small percentage of patients with chronic HCV infection are nonreactive on ELISA but are reactive for anti-HCV on second-generation RIBA or show detectable serum HCV RNA. Chronic hepatitis C is often silent; half of infected patients are asymptomatic. In addition, 20% to 30% of patients who test positive for anti-HCV and are viremic with detectable HCV RNA have persistently normal aminotransferase levels. Liver biopsies demonstrate the full spectrum of disease severity, ranging from mild portal tract inflammation to cirrhosis. Histologic features such as bile duct damage, lymphoid follicles or aggregates, and large droplets of fat are suggestive of chronic hepatitis C.

NATURAL HISTORY

After the onset of acute HCV infection, the infection resolves in 15% to 30% of patients and there is a loss of HCV RNA, although anti-HCV remains detectable. The natural history of chronic hepatitis C appears to typically span several decades.[34] In general, liver disease progresses insidiously, and cirrhosis may not develop for 2 or more decades. The natural history may be more prolonged when HCV infection occurs earlier in life. In a Japanese study, the mean interval from blood transfusion to development of chronic hepatitis was 10 years; to development of cirrhosis, 21 years; and to development of hepatocellular carcinoma (a late risk factor), 29 years.[35] Similar results were found in a population of patients seen in a referral liver center in the United States: the mean interval from transfusion to cirrhosis was 21 years; and for progression to hepatocellular carcinoma, the mean interval was 28 years.[36] In contrast to these reported outcomes, an analysis of post-transfusion studies in the United States found that over 18 years of follow-up, the survival rate of patients who developed non-A, non-B hepatitis after blood transfusion was no different from the survival rate of control subjects who did not develop hepatitis after transfusion.[37] However, mortality in the patients who had posttransfusion hepatitis was significantly more often caused by liver disease than by other forms of disease. In a large cross-sectional European study designed to study the natural progression of hepatic fibrosis in patients with chronic hepatitis C, the median interval from the presumed time of infection to cirrhosis, identified by liver biopsy, was 30 years.[38] The rate of progression to fibrosis and cirrhosis was not normally distributed; findings suggested at least three populations of patients: rapid fibrosers (median time to cirrhosis < 30 years), intermediate fibrosers, and slow fibrosers (no progression to cirrhosis, or at least 50 years from infection to cirrhosis). Three independent factors were associated with an increased rate of progression to cirrhosis: age older than 40 years at the time of infection, daily alcohol consumption of 50 g or more, and male gender.

TREATMENT

Many subtypes of interferon have been evaluated for their effectiveness in treating chronic hepatitis C, including inter-

Table 5   Factors Associated with Favorable Responses to Interferon and Ribavirin in Chronic Hepatitis C

Genotypes 2 and 3
Low baseline serum HCV RNA level (< 2–3 × 10⁶ copies/ml)
Absence of stage 3 or 4 fibrosis
White or Asian (versus African or Hispanic)
Short duration of infection
Female gender
Age younger than 40 years

feron alfa-2b, interferon alfa-2a, interferon alfacon-1 (consensus interferon), and interferon alfa-n1; these interferons appear to be relatively similar with respect to their therapeutic indices. On the basis of recent studies, interferon monotherapy has been superseded by interferon and ribavirin combination therapy.

Interferon and Ribavirin Combination Therapy

Beginning in late 1998, the combination of interferon alfa-2b and ribavirin became the standard therapy for chronic HCV infection in patients with no contraindications. Ribavirin (1,000 to 1,200 mg daily in two divided doses) combined with interferon alfa-2b (3 MU three times weekly) for 6 months was found to provide significantly better biochemical and virologic sustained response rates than interferon used alone.[39,40] Approximately 40% of patients treated for 1 year with combination therapy had sustained virologic response 6 months after the end of treatment.

The 1998 studies of interferon and ribavirin combination therapy[39,40] showed important differences in the outcome based on genotype; that is, approximately 30% of patients with genotype 1 and approximately 65% with genotype 2 or 3 had sustained virologic responses. In addition, patients with genotype 1 had higher rates of sustained virologic response with 48 weeks of combination therapy than with 24 weeks of therapy, whereas patients with other genotypes achieved no additional benefit beyond 24 weeks of therapy.[32,40] These studies have led to the practice of administering therapy for 12 months to patients with genotype 1 but for only 6 months to those with genotype 2 or 3. Factors in addition to genotype are known to predict the likelihood of successful therapy with ribavirin and interferon [*see Table 5*].

Side effects of combination therapy   Side effects are common with interferon and ribavirin combination therapy and may necessitate discontinuance of therapy in 10% to 15% of patients. The major side effect of ribavirin is a dose-dependent hemolytic anemia, which is reversible and usually stabilizes after 6 weeks of treatment.[39,40] If severe anemia develops, treatment must be discontinued. Ribavirin is teratogenic; therefore, pregnancy must be avoided.

Combination therapy should be used cautiously in patients with depression, because interferon can exacerbate depression. These patients can often be managed with antidepressants, with or without reduction in interferon dosage.

Patients with preexisting anemia usually cannot tolerate the degree of hemolysis that occurs with ribavirin therapy, which can be dangerous. Moreover, patients with significant

Table 6 Contraindications to Therapy
with Interferon and Ribavirin
in Chronic Hepatitis C

Severe psychiatric illness
Cardiovascular disease
Seizure disorder
Poorly controlled diabetes mellitus
Autoimmune diseases
Hemoglobin < 12 g/dl in women and < 13 g/dl in men
White blood cell count < 1,500/μl
Platelet count < 100,000/μl
Pregnant or unable to practice contraception
Normal aminotransferase levels
Decompensated cirrhosis

cardiovascular disease are particularly at risk should severe anemia develop during therapy. Patients with chronic hepatitis C and comorbid conditions preventing the use of ribavirin can be treated with interferon monotherapy. Contraindications to combination therapy are summarized [see Table 6].

Sustained response to combination therapy The persistence of a biochemical (normal ALT) or virologic (undetectable HCV RNA) response for 6 months or more after cessation of therapy is the operational definition of a sustained response. In two studies of patients who had an initial posttreatment 6-month sustained response, including a mean 4-year follow-up study of 80 patients and a 10-year follow-up study of five patients, long-term virologic sustained response rates were 96% and 100%, respectively.[41,42] In addition, there was improvement of liver histology, including evidence of regression of hepatic fibrosis in noncirrhotic patients. These studies suggest that some patients may indeed be cured of chronic hepatitis C and that a mortality benefit should be expected if cirrhosis, with its risk of hepatocellular carcinoma, can be prevented.

Treatment after Relapse

Relapse after a course of therapy is defined by an elevated ALT level, which was normal during treatment, and detectable levels of HCV RNA, which were undetectable during treatment. Re-treatment using standard interferon monotherapy is ineffective, but an extended 12-month course of interferon alfa-2b or interferon alfacon-1 resulted in sustained response rates of 32% and 58%, respectively.[43,44] Re-treatment with interferon and ribavirin combination therapy is more commonly employed and gave sustained response rates of 24% to 95%, depending on viral genotype.[45]

Management Options after Nonresponse to Therapy

Nonresponse to antiviral therapy is defined as persistently elevated ALT levels, detectable serum HCV RNA levels, or both during therapy. A variant of nonresponse called breakthrough is characterized by an initial decrease of ALT levels into the normal range or the disappearance of HCV RNA, with subsequent elevation of ALT or reappearance of HCV RNA while the patient is still being treated. In nonresponse or breakthrough patients given interferon alfa-2b initially, re-treatment with interferon alfacon-1 yielded sustained virologic response rates of 13% to

27%.[44,46] There is some evidence that histologic improvement may occur with longer therapy despite nonresponse after 6 months of treatment, thus implying that indefinite low-dose interferon maintenance therapy may be beneficial.[47] Recent trials even demonstrate that interferon therapy may delay or prevent decompensation from cirrhosis and the development of hepatocellular carcinoma, particularly in patients who show a sustained response.[48] Finally, studies have demonstrated that sustained virologic response rates to interferon monotherapy are lower in African Americans than in whites.[49]

Emerging Treatment Options

A number of future options may become available for the treatment of chronic hepatitis C over the next several years.[50] The most promising new treatment soon to be licensed is pegylated interferon. Polyethylene glycol (PEG) is a water-soluble polymer that can be covalently linked to proteins such as interferon, which markedly increases the half-life, resulting in sustained serum levels and allowing once-weekly administration.

Two PEG interferons have been studied: the branched 40 kd PEG interferon alfa-2a (Pegasys) and the linear 12 kd PEG interferon alfa-2b (PEG-Intron).[51,52] Phase 2 studies revealed that the appropriate dosage of PEG interferon alfa-2a was 180 μg once weekly, resulting, after 48 weeks of therapy, in a sustained virologic response rate of 36% in noncirrhotic patients and 30% in cirrhotic patients. A large study of 531 treatment-naive patients who were given PEG interferon alfa-2a or standard interferon alfa-2a for 48 weeks showed a sustained virologic response rate of 39% with PEG interferon alfa-2a versus 19% with standard interferon alfa-2a.[51] In an international study of PEG interferon alfa-2b given once weekly versus interferon alfa-2b given three times weekly for 48 weeks in 1,219 patients with untreated chronic hepatitis C,[52] the sustained virologic response rates were 25% with PEG interferon alfa-2b, 1.0 μg/kg, and 23% with PEG interferon alfa-2b, 1.5 μg/kg, versus 12% with interferon alfa-2b. Thus, PEG interferons achieve sustained virologic response rates that are approximately twice that achieved with standard interferons (39% versus 19% with PEG interferon alfa-2a, and 23% and 25% versus 12% with PEG interferon alfa-2b). In both studies, patients with genotype 1 and higher viral loads had reduced response rates.

Both PEG interferons were tolerated as well as the standard interferons, with discontinuance rates ranging from 6% to 11% in all treatment groups. It is likely that the efficacy of the PEG interferons will be enhanced by the addition of ribavirin to treatment regimens, and sustained virologic response rates may approach 50%.

The results of ongoing large studies of combination therapy with PEG interferon alfa-2a or PEG interferon alfa-2b and ribavirin are under way and will likely lead to a new standard therapy of combination pegylated interferon and ribavirin in 2001.

Liver Transplantation

Chronic hepatitis C with liver failure is the most common indication for liver transplantation.[53] Although hepatitis C virus reinfects the allograft in nearly 100% of cases, the subsequent illness is usually mild, and only a small percentage of cases progress to cirrhosis with liver failure. Some patients may acquire hepatitis C virus infection as a result of liver transplantation, either from the donor organ or from the associated blood transfusions.

References

1. Desmet VJ, Gerber M, Hoofnagle JH, et al: Classification of chronic hepatitis: diagnosis, grading and staging. Hepatology 19:1513, 1994

2. Brunt EM: Grading and staging the histopathological lesions of chronic hepatitis: the Knodell histology activity index and beyond. Hepatology 31:241, 2000

3. Zimmerman HJ, Ishak KG: General aspects of drug-induced liver disease. Gastroenterol Clin North Am 24:739, 1995

4. Czaja AJ: Autoimmune hepatitis: evolving concepts and treatment strategies. Dig Dis Sci 40:435, 1995

5. Krawitt EL: Autoimmune hepatitis. N Engl J Med 334:897, 1996

6. Magrin S, Craxi A, Fabiano C, et al: Hepatitis C virus replication in "autoimmune" chronic hepatitis. J Hepatol 13:364, 1991

7. Johnson PJ, McFarlane IG, Williams R: Azathioprine for long-term maintenance of remission in autoimmune hepatitis. N Engl J Med 333:958, 1995

8. Czaja AJ: Frequency and nature of the variant syndromes of autoimmune liver disease. Hepatology 28:360, 1998

9. Lee WM: Hepatitis B virus infection. N Engl J Med 337:1733, 1997

10. McMahon BJ, Bulkow L, Harpster A, et al: Screening for hepatocellular carcinoma in Alaska natives infected with chronic hepatitis B: a 16-year population-based study. Hepatology 32:842, 2000

11. Hoofnagle JH, Di Bisceglie AM: The treatment of chronic viral hepatitis. N Engl J Med 336:347, 1997

12. Perrillo RP, Schiff ER, Davis GL, et al: A randomized, controlled trial of interferon alfa-2b alone and after prednisone withdrawal for the treatment of chronic hepatitis B. N Engl J Med 323:295, 1990

13. Korenman J, Baker B, Waggoner J, et al: Long-term remission of chronic hepatitis B after alpha-interferon therapy. Ann Intern Med 114:629, 1991

14. Wong DKH, Cheung AM, O'Rourke K, et al: Effect of alpha-interferon treatment in patients with hepatitis B e antigen–positive chronic hepatitis B. Ann Intern Med 119:312, 1993

15. Wong JB, Koff RS, Tinè F, et al: Cost-effectiveness of interferon-alpha 2b treatment for hepatitis B e antigen–positive chronic hepatitis B. Ann Intern Med 122:664, 1995

16. Lok ASF, Lai C-L, Wu P-C, et al: Long-term follow-up in a randomised controlled trial of recombinant α_2-interferon in Chinese patients with chronic hepatitis B infection. Lancet 2:298, 1988

17. Lok ASF, Wu P-C, Lai C-L, et al: A controlled trial of interferon with or without prednisone priming for chronic hepatitis B. Gastroenterology 102:2091, 1992

18. Pastore G, Santantonio T, Milella M, et al: Anti-HBe–positive chronic hepatitis B with HBV-DNA in the serum response to a 6-month course of lymphoblastoid interferon. J Hepatol 14:221, 1992

19. Hoofnagle JH, Di Bisceglie AM, Waggoner JG, et al: Interferon alfa for patients with clinically apparent cirrhosis due to chronic hepatitis B. Gastroenterology 104:1116, 1993

20. Lai CL, Chien RN, Leung NW, et al: A one-year trial of lamivudine for chronic hepatitis B: Asia Hepatitis Lamivudine Study Group. N Engl J Med 339:61, 1998

21. Dienstag JL, Schiff ER, Wright TL, et al: Lamivudine as initial treatment for chronic hepatitis B in the United States. N Engl J Med 341:1256, 1999

22. Schiff E, Karayalein S, Grimm I: A placebo controlled study of lamivudine and interferon alpha-2b in patients with chronic hepatitis B who previously failed interferon therapy (abstr). Hepatology 28:388A, 1998

23. Honkoop P, de Man RA, Zondervan PE, et al: Histological improvement in patients with chronic hepatitis B virus infection treated with lamivudine. Liver 17:103, 1997

24. Suzuki Y, Kumada H, Ikeda K, et al: Histological changes in liver biopsies after one year of lamivudine treatment in patients with chronic hepatitis B infection. J Hepatol 30:743, 1999

25. Leung N, Lai C, Chang T: Three year lamivudine therapy in chronic HBV (abstr). J Hepatol 30(suppl 1):59, 1999

26. Chang T, Lai C, Liaw Y: Enhanced HBeAg seroconversion rates in Chinese patients on lamivudine (abstr). Hepatology 28:420A, 1999

27. Schalm SW, Heathcote J, Cianciara J, et al: Lamivudine and alpha interferon combination treatment of patients with chronic hepatitis B infection: a randomized trial. Gut 46:562, 2000

28. Villeneuve JP, Condreay LD, Willems B, et al: Lamivudine treatment for decompensated cirrhosis resulting from chronic hepatitis B. Hepatology 31:207, 2000

29. Keeffe EB: End-stage liver disease and liver transplantation: role of lamivudine therapy in patients with chronic hepatitis B. J Med Virol 61:403, 2000

30. Samuel D, Muller R, Alexander G, et al: Liver transplantation in European patients with the hepatitis B surface antigen. N Engl J Med 329:1842, 1993

31. Farci P, Mandas A, Cioana A, et al: Treatment of chronic hepatitis D with interferon alfa-2a. N Engl J Med 330:88, 1994

32. Lau DR, Doo E, Park Y, et al: Lamivudine for chronic delta hepatitis. Hepatology 30:546, 1999

33. Liang TJ, Rehermann B, Seeff LB, et al: Pathogenesis, natural history, treatment, and prevention of hepatitis C. Ann Intern Med 132:296, 2000

34. Alter MJ, Kruszon-Moran D, Nainan OV, et al: The prevalence of hepatitis C virus infection in the United States, 1998 through 1994. N Engl J Med 341:556, 1999

35. Kiyosawa K, Sodeyama T, Tanaka E, et al: Interrelationship of blood transfusion, non-A, non-B hepatitis and hepatocellular carcinoma: analysis by detection of antibody to hepatitis C virus. Hepatology 12:671, 1990

36. Tong MJ, El-Farra NS, Reikes AR, et al: Clinical outcomes after transfusion-associated hepatitis C. N Engl J Med 332:1463, 1995

37. Seeff LB, Buskell-Bales Z, Wright EC, et al: Long-term mortality after transfusion-associated non-A, non-B hepatitis. N Engl J Med 327:1906, 1992

38. Poynard T, Bedossa P, Opolon P, et al: Natural history of liver fibrosis progression in patients with chronic hepatitis C. Lancet 349:825, 1997

39. Poynard T, Marcellin P, Lee SS, et al: Randomised trial of interferon alpha-2b plus ribavirin for 48 weeks or for 24 weeks versus interferon alpha-2b plus placebo for 48 weeks for treatment of chronic infection with hepatitis C virus: International Hepatitis Interventional Therapy Group (IHIT). Lancet 352:1426, 1998

40. McHutchison JG, Gordon SC, Schiff ER, et al: Interferon alfa-2b alone or in combination with ribavirin as initial treatment for chronic hepatitis C: Hepatitis Interventional Therapy Group. N Engl J Med 339:1485, 1998

41. Marcellin P, Boyer N, Gervais A, et al: Long-term histologic improvement and loss of detectable intrahepatic HCV RNA in patients with chronic hepatitis C and sustained response to interferon-alpha therapy. Ann Intern Med 127:875, 1997

42. Lau DTY, Kleiner DE, Ghany MG, et al: 10-Year follow-up after interferon-alpha therapy for chronic hepatitis C. Hepatology 28:1121, 1998

43. Payen JL, Izopet J, Galindo-Migeot V, et al: Better efficacy of a 12-month interferon alfa-2b retreatment in patients with chronic hepatitis C relapsing after a 6-month treatment: a multicenter, controlled, randomized trial: le Groupe d'Étude et de Traitement du Virus de l'Hepatite C (Get.Vhc). Hepatology 28:1680, 1998

44. Heathcote EJ, Keeffe EB, Lee SS, et al: Re-treatment of chronic hepatitis C with consensus interferon. Hepatology 27:1136, 1998

45. Davis GL: Combination therapy with interferon alfa and ribavirin as retreatment of interferon relapse in chronic hepatitis C. Semin Liver Dis 19:49, 1999

46. Heathcote EJ, James S, Mullen KD, et al: Chronic hepatitis C virus patients with breakthroughs during interferon treatment can successfully be retreated with consensus interferon: the Consensus Interferon Study Group. Hepatology 30:562, 1999

47. Shiffman ML, Hofmann CM, Contos MJ, et al: A randomized, controlled trial of maintenance interferon therapy for patients with chronic hepatitis C virus and persistent viremia. Gastroenterology 117:1164, 1999

48. Yoshida H, Shiratori Y, Moriyama M, et al: Interferon therapy reduces the risk for hepatocellular carcinoma: national surveillance program of cirrhotic and noncirrhotic patients with chronic hepatitis C in Japan: IHIT Study Group: inhibition of hepatocarcinogenesis by interferon therapy. Ann Intern Med 131:174, 1999

49. Reddy KR, Hoofnagle JH, Tong MJ, et al: Racial differences in responses to therapy with interferon in chronic hepatitis C. Hepatology 30:787, 1999

50. Davis GL, Nelson DR, Reyes GR: Future options for the management of hepatitis C. Semin Liver Dis 19:103, 1999

51. Zeuzem S, Feinman SV, Rasenack J, et al: Evaluation of the safety and efficacy of once-weekly PEG/interferon alfa-2a (PEGASYS™) for chronic hepatitis C: a multinational, randomized study (abstr). J Hepatol 32(suppl 2):29, 2000

52. Trepo C, Lindsay K, Niederau C, et al: Pegylated interferon alfa-2b (PEG-Intron) monotherapy is superior to interferon alfa-2b (Intron A) for the treatment of chronic hepatitis C. J Hepatol 32(suppl 2):29, 2000

53. Berenguer M, Wright TL: Hepatitis C and liver transplantation. Gut 45:159, 1999

66 Cirrhosis of the Liver

Emmet B. Keeffe, M.D.

Cirrhosis is the sequela of a wide variety of chronic, progressive liver diseases. Cirrhosis is present when these processes have so scarred the liver that its normal architecture is disrupted and regenerating nodules of parenchyma appear. The pattern of scarring seldom permits determination of the specific etiology, but associated histologic features may point to the cause. A specific diagnosis generally requires a combination of history, physical findings, laboratory tests, and identification of characteristic histologic features.

In the United States, excessive alcohol intake and chronic hepatitis C are the most common causes of cirrhosis. In other parts of the world, particularly in Asian countries, chronic hepatitis B and hepatitis C are the dominant causes of cirrhosis [*see* Chapter 65].

Approach to the Patient with Suspected Cirrhosis

PRESENTING SYMPTOMS

Fatigue and malaise are common in all forms of cirrhosis, but these nonspecific symptoms are found in almost all acute and chronic liver diseases. Characteristic but nondiagnostic physical findings of cirrhosis include palmar erythema and spider nevi. Other typical findings include gynecomastia, testicular atrophy, and evidence of portal hypertension (splenomegaly, ascites, and prominence of the veins of the abdominal wall). Other physical abnormalities, such as Dupuytren contracture, xanthelasma, xanthomas, Kayser-Fleischer rings, a bronze discoloration of the skin, and hyperpigmentation, are found in specific forms of cirrhosis. The cirrhotic liver is usually large, and the left lobe is often palpable below the xiphoid process. Only a patient in the advanced inactive stage of disease exhibits a small and shrunken liver.

DIAGNOSTIC EVALUATION

Percutaneous liver biopsy can unequivocally establish the presence of cirrhosis. However, cirrhosis can be inferred by the presence of splenomegaly, ascites, spider angiomas on physical examination, or findings of cirrhosis and portal hypertension on imaging studies in patients with underlying chronic liver disease. Liver biopsy can be performed safely when there is no history of unusual bleeding after surgery or dental work and when tests for coagulation yield normal or only mildly abnormal results. Reasonable guidelines include an international normalized ratio (INR) for prothrombin time no greater than 1.5, a partial thromboplastin time of no more than 10 seconds beyond the control value, and a platelet count of at least 50,000/mm³. Other relative contraindications to biopsy include lack of patient cooperation or the presence of ascites or right lower lobe pneumonia. If coagulation abnormalities cannot be corrected or if moderate to severe ascites is present, an adequate amount of tissue for biopsy can be safely obtained using the transjugular, or transvenous, approach.[1]

Marked distortion of hepatic architecture, with regenerative nodules surrounded by scar tissue, provides definitive evidence of cirrhosis. Liver biopsy also helps identify the cause of cirrhosis. In particular, bile duct invasion and destruction with associated granulomas suggest the presence of primary biliary cirrhosis; excess iron in bile duct cells and liver cells points to hereditary hemochromatosis; and Mallory hyalin associated with polymorpho-

nuclear cell reaction usually indicates alcoholic liver disease.

A decreased serum albumin level and a prolonged prothrombin time are characteristic of cirrhosis. Other serum chemistries, such as elevated aminotransferase and alkaline phosphatase levels, are often abnormal. Computed tomography, magnetic resonance imaging, or hepatic ultrasonography with Doppler flow studies may reveal findings consistent with cirrhosis. These findings may include splenomegaly, ascites, an irregular liver surface, increased echogenicity and reversal of portal blood flow, and intra-abdominal varices. In addition, upper endoscopy often establishes the presence of esophagogastric varices.

Specific Forms of Cirrhosis

ALCOHOLIC CIRRHOSIS

Synonyms for alcoholic cirrhosis include portal, Laënnec, nutritional, and micronodular cirrhosis. Because alcohol produces a direct toxic effect on the liver in animals, alcoholic cirrhosis is the most appropriate term.[2]

Etiology

Alcoholic liver disease, including alcoholic cirrhosis, is directly attributable to chronic ingestion of large quantities of alcohol. Alcoholic cirrhosis may develop in women after less alcohol consumption than is necessary to cause cirrhosis in men. Daily alcohol consumption of approximately 50 g, or three or four drinks (one drink = 12 oz of beer, 5 oz of wine, or 1.5 oz of 80-proof liquor), for 10 to 15 years is associated with alcoholic liver disease in women, whereas 80 g, or five or six drinks a day, is associated with alcoholic cirrhosis in men.[3] Its development does not require concomitant malnutrition, although this condition is almost invariably present. Malnutrition undoubtedly reflects a substitution of alcohol for normal dietary calories. All persons who drink heavily experience a bland fatty infiltration, which is reversible when alcohol ingestion ceases. Although the development of alcoholic cirrhosis usually requires more than 10 years of heavy drinking, the disease can develop more rapidly. Alcoholic cirrhosis typically progresses as a result of repeated bouts of clinical and subclinical alcoholic hepatitis. Alcoholic hepatitis, another manifestation of alcoholic liver disease and a frequent precursor to alcoholic cirrhosis, refers to the pathologic Mallory stain findings of alcoholic hyalin surrounded by polymorphonuclear cell inflammation [*see* Figure 1]. These necrotic lesions are accompanied by collagen formation and are typically found in a pericentral location.

Diagnosis

Clinical features Physical examination usually shows the liver to be enlarged—sometimes to a marked degree. Hepatomegaly reflects inflammation, fatty infiltration, and extensive scar formation. The typical histologic picture consists of a weblike scar that separates liver cell cords and surrounds small nodules of liver cells [*see* Figure 2].

An acute clinical syndrome is manifested in only a minority of patients in whom alcoholic hepatitis can be histopathologically demonstrated. Patients with this syndrome, which warrants immediate hospitalization, have a temperature of 38° C (100.4° F) or higher, right upper quadrant pain and tenderness, an enlarged liver, leukocytosis, and jaundice. Not all features are necessarily evident. In patients with severe disease, mortality ranges from 10% to 40%. Some patients with alcoholic hepatitis demonstrated by biopsy do not have cirrhosis, and in half of these patients, the liver returns to normal after cessation of alcohol consumption; cirrhosis develops in the remainder.

Laboratory tests   In patients with decompensated alcoholic cirrhosis, the serum bilirubin level is elevated, often markedly (20 to 40 mg/dl). The serum aspartate aminotransferase (AST) level is usually elevated, perhaps to as high as 200 to 300 IU/L. Characteristically, the AST level is more abnormal than the alanine aminotransferase (ALT) level. Reversal of this relation or the presence of aminotransferase levels above 300 IU/L suggests that the diagnosis may not be alcoholic liver disease. The alkaline phosphatase level is often moderately elevated. Reduction of the serum albumin level to below 3.5 g/dl and prolongation of the prothrombin time are common.

Treatment

The only established therapy for patients with alcoholic liver disease is to stop drinking alcohol. Patients with alcoholic cirrhosis who continue to drink seem to have a poorer prognosis than those who stop. The 5-year survival rate for patients who drink is less than 40% but may reach 60% to 70% if abstinence is maintained.[4] Although pessimism abounds, as many as 30% of patients with alcoholic liver disease may succeed in abstaining completely.[4] Thus, the emphasis in treatment should be to support patients' efforts to stop drinking. Various rehabilitation units, peer support groups, and psychotherapeutic techniques are available [see Chapter 206].

Nutritional support   The marked nutritional deficiencies noted in many patients with alcoholic cirrhosis have led most physicians to recommend nutritional support during the acute illness. A large cooperative study evaluated the role of an enteral food supplement in decompensated alcoholic liver disease.[5] The investigators demonstrated a direct relation between caloric intake and survival and found that vigorous nutritional support enhanced survival, particularly in severely malnourished patients.

Glucocorticoid treatment   Although there have been several studies of glucocorticoid treatment in patients with decompensated alcoholic liver disease, no convincing and consistent proof of efficacy has emerged, except in the subgroup of patients with severe alcoholic hepatitis and hepatic encephalopathy.[6] However, only a few such patients qualify for glucocorticoid treatment, because patients with active gastrointestinal bleeding, infection, or renal insufficiency should not be treated. The usual treatment regimen is either prednisone or prednisolone, 40 mg daily for 4 weeks, followed by tapering of therapy over 1 to 2 weeks. Although propylthiouracil and colchicine have both been used in patients with alcoholic liver disease, the evidence warranting their use is not conclusive. Therefore, therapy for alcoholic cirrhosis is generally supportive and is aimed at improving nutrition, encouraging abstinence, and treating complications.

PRIMARY BILIARY CIRRHOSIS

Primary biliary cirrhosis most often occurs in women between 30 and 50 years of age.[7] The presence of serum autoantibodies, an association with other autoimmune diseases, and the resemblance of the bile duct lesions in primary biliary cirrhosis to those seen in chronic graft versus host disease suggest that immune mechanisms play an important role in the pathogenesis of this disorder. Studies have also shown that primary biliary cirrhosis is associated with the HLA-DR8 haplotype, suggesting a genetic predisposition to the disease.[8]

Diagnosis

Clinical features   Presenting complaints in patients with primary biliary cirrhosis are fatigue and generalized pruritus. Jaundice may not develop until 5 to 10 years after the onset of pruritus and systemic symptoms. Some patients experience bone pain, multiple fractures, and vertebral collapse. The usual cause of primary biliary cirrhosis is osteoporosis, which occurs in 20% to 30% of patients. Less commonly, osteomalacia is also present. Factors

a
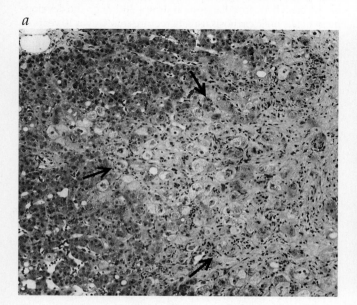

b
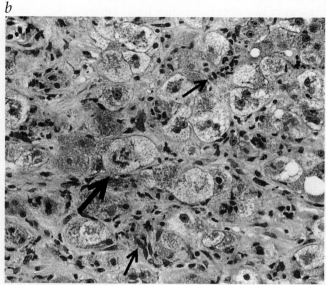

Figure 1   (*a*) Liver biopsy specimen from a 34-year-old man with a 7-year history of heavy alcohol consumption demonstrates a zone of fibrosis, ballooning liver cells, and inflammation (arrows). (*b*) Higher magnification of the specimen reveals typical alcoholic hyalin (thick arrow) and a polymorphonuclear cell inflammatory reaction (thin arrows), which are features of alcoholic hepatitis.

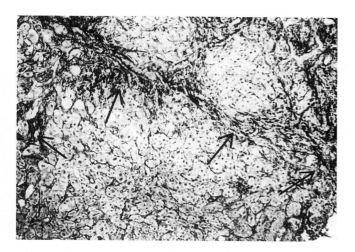

Figure 2   Alcoholic cirrhosis in the liver of a 58-year-old man produces distortion with scar tissue (arrows) that spreads through the parenchyma and outlines small regenerating nodules.

that give rise to the bone abnormalities include malabsorption of calcium and phosphate, altered vitamin D metabolism, cholestyramine therapy, and poor nutrition. Physical examination often reveals xanthelasma, xanthomas, hepatosplenomegaly, hyperpigmentation, and excoriation of the skin [*see Figure 3*]. If the disease is advanced, scleral icterus, ascites, and edema will also be present.

Laboratory tests   Typical laboratory findings of primary biliary cirrhosis include an elevated alkaline phosphatase level (usually > 300 IU/L and often > 700 IU/L), a serum cholesterol level above 300 mg/dl, an elevated IgM level, and antimitochondrial antibody detectable at high titer (in 90% to 95% of patients).

A moderate number of patients with primary biliary cirrhosis have concomitant disease, such as renal tubular acidosis, scleroderma, CREST syndrome (calcinosis, Raynaud phenomenon, esophageal dysmotility, sclerodactyly, and telangiectasia), or Sjögren syndrome.

Primary biliary cirrhosis may have clinical and laboratory features similar to those of cirrhosis secondary to chronic biliary tract disease. Indeed, carcinoma of the pancreas or biliary tree, common duct stones, postoperative bile duct stricture, and primary sclerosing cholangitis or pericholangitis secondary to inflammatory bowel disease may all mimic some of the labora-

tory and histologic features of primary biliary cirrhosis. There is seldom a need, however, to directly visualize the biliary tree in patients who display the typical clinical, laboratory, and histologic features of primary biliary cirrhosis.

Liver biopsy   Liver biopsy may reveal bile duct destruction with lymphocytic-plasmacytic infiltration of portal areas, periportal granuloma formation, and portal scarring with linking of portal tracts [*see Figure 4*]. Ductular proliferation is common. When scarring is extensive, nodule formation, often with retention of the central veins, can be found. Bile stasis is usually periportal and indicates advanced disease.

Treatment

The management of primary biliary cirrhosis includes ursodiol therapy and nonspecific treatment of pruritus, malabsorption, bone disease, and portal hypertension.[9]

Specific treatment   Ursodiol, a hydrophilic bile acid, has been given to patients with primary biliary cirrhosis on the premise that altering the composition of the endogenous bile acid pool may prove beneficial by reducing the concentration of potentially toxic endogenous hydrophobic bile acids. In one large placebo-controlled trial, 2 years of treatment with ursodiol at a dosage of 13 to 15 mg/kg daily resulted in clinical, biochemical, and histologic improvement; decreased need for liver transplantation; and increased survival.[10] These favorable results were confirmed by two additional large trials—a Canadian multicenter trial[11] and a Mayo Clinic trial[12]—which showed trends toward increased survival and decreased need for liver transplantation in the ursodiol treatment group. Most patients are given ursodiol because it appears to be effective, is safe, and may relieve pruritus. In a small pilot study, methotrexate appeared to be of benefit in patients with primary biliary cirrhosis, but therapy was associated with a number of side effects, including bone marrow suppression and pulmonary toxicity.[13] In a 2-year study of the use of methotrexate in combination with ursodiol, no benefit was noted over the use of ursodiol alone, and methotrexate toxicity was substantial.[14] General use of methotrexate is not warranted until its efficacy and safety profile is further studied.

Corticosteroids, azathioprine, penicillamine, cyclosporine, and colchicines have been used to treat patients with primary biliary cirrhosis. Corticosteroids do not alter the course of the disease, and they accelerate the onset of osteoporosis. Azathioprine, cy-

a

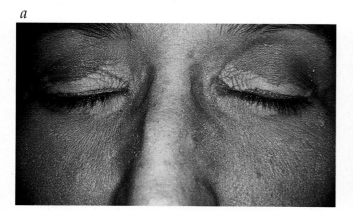

b

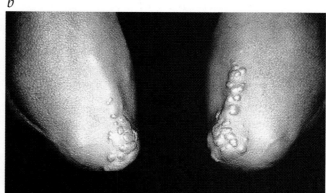

Figure 3   This patient with advanced primary biliary cirrhosis demonstrates some characteristic signs of the disease: (*a*) xanthelasma, a common finding, and (*b*) xanthomas, which are prominent on the elbows.

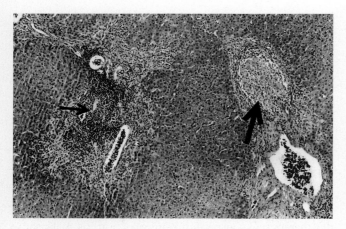

Figure 4 **Dense portal inflammatory reaction (thin arrow) and portal granulomas (thick arrow) characterize primary biliary cirrhosis affecting the liver of a 29-year-old woman who underwent a cholecystectomy.**

closporine, and penicillamine are not used for therapy. Two randomized clinical trials evaluated the efficacy of colchicine therapy at a dosage of 0.6 mg twice daily.[15,16] Colchicine improved the results of liver tests but without improvement in symptoms or histology. There was the suggestion that survival was enhanced. However, a long-term follow-up of one of the randomized colchicine trials did not confirm a survival benefit.[17] Colchicine produced only minor side effects, which were easily controlled by dose reduction in these studies.

Nonspecific treatment Nonspecific therapy is directed at relieving symptoms during the slow but relentless course of the disease. The anion exchange resin cholestyramine may help alleviate pruritus. The usual dosage is 4 g given orally three times a day. Some patients find relief at a lower dosage, although others require up to 16 to 20 g/day. Cholestyramine is often poorly tolerated but may be more palatable when taken with meals or mixed in applesauce or juice. Rifampin (300 to 450 mg/day in divided doses)[18] and ultraviolet light therapy may prove helpful in some patients with severe pruritus. Antihistamines seldom prove efficacious, but their sedative effects may allow a patient to sleep despite continuing pruritus.

Malabsorption of fat-soluble vitamins in rough proportion to the degree of cholestasis occurs in patients with primary biliary cirrhosis. Fat-soluble vitamin supplements are thus recommended for patients with low serum levels. The usual treatment includes oral vitamin K (5 mg/day), a water-soluble form of vitamin A (10,000 to 25,000 U/day), vitamin D in the form of either 25-dihydroxyvitamin D_3 [25-(OH)D_3] (calcifediol) (50 µg/day) or 1,25-dihydroxyvitamin D_3 [1,25-(OH)$_2D_3$] (calcitriol) (0.5 to 1.0 µg/day), supplemental calcium (1.5 g/day), and vitamin E (400 to 1,000 U/day). Serum calcium levels should be monitored during the first few months of vitamin D and calcium therapy.

Prognosis

The prognosis varies, but the clinical course is generally indolent. Major hepatic dysfunction usually does not occur until very late. The median survival time is about 10 years.

HEMOCHROMATOSIS

Hepatic iron overload may be primary (most often caused by hereditary hemochromatosis) or secondary (related to transfusional iron loading, ineffective erythropoiesis, or end-stage liver disease—particularly alcoholic liver disease, chronic hepatitis C, and nonalcoholic steatohepatitis).[19] Patients with these chronic liver diseases may have abnormal iron study results and elevated serum ferritin levels, but hepatic iron concentration measured from a liver biopsy specimen is most often normal or only slightly elevated.

Hereditary hemochromatosis is characterized by the deposition of large amounts of iron in the liver parenchymal cells [*see Figure 5*]. The accumulation leads to periportal cell destruction and hepatic scarring, culminating in cirrhosis. The disease occurs 10 times more often in males than in females. Symptoms generally appear between 40 and 60 years of age in men or after menopause in women. Occasionally, the disease is manifested at a much earlier age.

Etiology and Genetics

Hereditary hemochromatosis is inherited as an autosomal recessive defect that affects approximately one in 300 persons.[19,20] The heterozygote carrier rate is estimated to be one in 10 to 12 of the white population. Heterozygotes may show some abnormalities of iron storage, but clinical disease does not develop under normal circumstances. In 1996, a candidate gene, termed HFE, was discovered; it encodes for a major histocompatibility complex class I–like molecule and requires β_2-microglobulin for normal presentation on the cell surface.[21] Two missense mutations have been identified in the HFE gene: one results in a change of cysteine at position 282 to tyrosine (Cys282Tyr), and the second results in a change in histidine at position 63 to aspartate (His63Asp). Mutation in the homozygous form is present in 85% to 90% of patients with phenotypic hemochromatosis.

Iron deposits in the pancreas and heart muscle lead to dysfunction of these organs. When the symptoms of hepatic dysfunction first appear, about half of patients have diabetes mellitus, 15% have congestive heart failure or arrhythmias, and a significant minority have stiffness and joint pain. Impotence, apparently related to pituitary dysfunction, is also common.

Diagnosis

Clinical features In advanced disease, bronze discoloration of the skin secondary to deposition of both melanin and iron appears. The liver is moderately enlarged; splenomegaly is noted in about half of patients. When disease is less advanced, the skin may have normal color, and the liver may be barely palpable. Signs of portal hypertension eventually develop in most cases. Primary liver cell cancer occurs in about 15% to 20% of patients.

Laboratory tests Laboratory analysis reveals an increase in serum iron associated with an 80% to 90% saturation of serum transferrin (15% to 47% saturation is normal). Serum ferritin is usually elevated as well. An elevated mean linear attenuation coefficient (CT number) on CT scanning of the liver may signal the presence of increased hepatic iron stores.[22] MRI may also demonstrate iron overload in hereditary hemochromatosis.[23] Mild elevations of serum aminotransferase and alkaline phosphatase levels are not uncommon, but jaundice is unusual. The serum albumin level and the prothrombin time remain in the normal range until late in the course.

Serum iron concentration and total iron-binding capacity can be used to screen populations for hemochromatosis.[24] A fasting transferrin saturation of 62% or higher in men (and perhaps 50%

in women) identifies a high proportion of patients who are homozygous for hemochromatosis. The serum ferritin concentration has not proved to be an effective screening tool, because too few homozygous individuals have elevated levels before clinical disease develops. Identifying a homozygous individual warrants investigating his or her siblings, because 25% of siblings are expected to be homozygous for the disease as well.

An elevated serum iron or serum ferritin level is not diagnostic, because these values can be raised in a wide variety of liver diseases marked by hepatic cell death. An elevated serum iron or ferritin level is not uncommon in decompensated alcoholic liver disease, acute viral hepatitis, or chronic active hepatitis. The widely accepted criteria for the diagnosis of iron overload caused by hereditary hemochromatosis include 4 g or more of iron removed by phlebotomy (16 units of blood) before the onset of iron-limited erythropoiesis or at least one of the following results derived from liver biopsy: grade 3 or 4 stainable iron in hepatocytes, hepatic iron concentration greater than 80 μmol (4,500 μg) per gram of dry weight of liver tissue, and a hepatic iron index (hepatic iron concentration in μmol divided by age in years) greater than 1.9. The identification of specific mutations in the *HFE* gene of patients with hemochromatosis has permitted the introduction of genetic testing in the clinical setting. Most patients of northern European descent with classic phenotypic hereditary hemochromatosis are homozygous for C282Y or, less commonly, are heterozygous for compound C282Y/H63D.

Liver biopsy The characteristic finding on liver biopsy is a heavy deposit of hemosiderin granules in hepatocytes and bile duct cells. Fibrosis may range from minimal to well-established cirrhosis. At times, hereditary hemochromatosis is difficult to distinguish from cirrhosis with secondary iron overload. A preponderance of parenchymal iron relative to the amount of scar tissue and the presence of iron in the bile duct cells characterize hereditary hemochromatosis. Iron overload secondary to underlying cirrhosis is usually associated with advanced cirrhosis, relatively less stainable iron, and absence of iron in the bile ducts. When excess hepatic iron derives from an exogenous source, such as a series of massive transfusions for chronic hemolytic anemia, iron is prominent in the Kupffer cells. When the morphologic features of the liver biopsy do not clearly distinguish

between hereditary hemochromatosis and secondary iron overload, quantitative analysis of the hepatic iron content may prove helpful.[25] Patients with hemochromatosis typically have quantitative hepatic iron values ranging from 200 to 800 μmol/g dry weight (normal, < 35 μmol/g), whereas patients with alcoholic siderosis have hepatic iron content ranging from 40 to 100 μmol/g. Another useful diagnostic test for hemochromatosis is calculation of the hepatic iron index; this value is usually greater than 2 in homozygotes and less than 2 in patients with alcoholic siderosis. Finally, tissue obtained from the heart, pancreas, or skin of patients with hemochromatosis shows heavy infiltration of stainable iron.

Treatment

Early detection and treatment of patients with hereditary hemochromatosis is essential. The usual therapy is removal of the excess iron by weekly phlebotomy. Because each pint of blood contains 250 mg of iron, removal of 1 pint of blood a week will deplete the iron stores in most patients with hemochromatosis in 1 to 2 years. Therapy aims for persistently low serum iron and ferritin levels, which reflect absence of stainable iron on liver biopsy. Subsequent phlebotomies can be performed every 3 to 4 months to prevent reaccumulation of iron. If patients are identified before cirrhosis develops and total body iron depletion is successfully accomplished, life expectancy approaches normal.[26] Treated patients who have cirrhosis do better than untreated patients but remain at risk for primary liver cell cancer years after successful iron depletion. Failure to deplete iron stores after 18 months of treatment is a poor prognostic sign. Signs of liver and cardiac disease abate in 70% of treated patients, but endocrine abnormalities and arthropathy are improved in only 20% of those treated.

Repeated phlebotomies are obviously impractical in managing iron overload that results from the therapy for hemolytic anemia. In such patients, deferoxamine, administered subcutaneously at a dosage of 1 to 3 g over 12 hours, produces an average urinary iron loss of 50 mg each day. The addition of ascorbic acid, 500 mg/day orally, may double the rate of urinary iron excretion.

WILSON DISEASE

Wilson disease, or hepatolenticular degeneration, is an autosomal recessive disorder found in about one in 30,000 to 50,000 persons, with a gene frequency of 1:90 to 1:150.[27]

a *b*

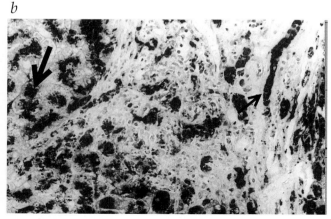

Figure 5 (*a*) A percutaneous liver biopsy specimen was taken from a 30-year-old woman with hepatosplenomegaly and amenorrhea of 6 months' duration. Pigment both in hepatic parenchymal cells (thick arrow) and in bile duct cells (thin arrow) is apparent. (*b*) Higher-magnification iron stain of the specimen confirms that the pigment is iron both in parenchymal cells (thick arrow) and in bile duct cells (thin arrow). The woman, who also had hemochromatosis, required removal of 72 units of blood over 1.5 years to render her liver free of excess iron.

Etiology and Genetics

The genetic defect for Wilson disease is located on chromosome 13, where disease-specific mutations in a gene that codes for a copper-binding P-type adenosine triphosphatase protein have been identified. In this disorder, the excretion of copper into the bile appears to be defective, leading to an accumulation of excess copper in most body tissues. The incorporation of copper into ceruloplasmin is also impaired.

Diagnosis

Clinical features By 15 years of age, affected persons have usually experienced symptoms caused by either neurologic or hepatic dysfunction. Although Wilson disease occasionally presents for the first time in persons as old as 30 years, this late an onset is the distinct exception. In about 40% of patients, the first manifestations of the disease are symptoms related to hepatic dysfunction.[28] The hepatic disease is usually a chronic disorder manifested by fatigue, jaundice, spider nevi, ascites, edema, splenomegaly, and variceal hemorrhage. Associated hemolytic anemia is a clue to the diagnosis. Occasionally, the liver disease mimics severe acute hepatitis and progresses to death in a few days to weeks. Neurologic symptoms include tremors, rigidity, gait disturbances and clumsiness, slurring of speech, and personality changes.

The pathognomonic sign is the Kayser-Fleischer ring, a thin, brown crescent of pigmentation at the periphery of the cornea. Although this feature is usually circumferential, it may be located only superiorly and inferiorly. Early in the disease, a slit-lamp examination may be required to identify the telltale ring. It may be particularly difficult to detect on routine eye examination in brown-eyed patients.

Laboratory tests On first examination, at least 50% of patients have hepatosplenomegaly and moderate liver function abnormality. Two distinguishing laboratory findings are depression or absence of serum ceruloplasmin and an increase of urinary copper levels from a normal value of less than 50 mg/day to as high as 1,000 mg/day. In a small percentage of patients with Wilson disease, serum ceruloplasmin or urinary copper levels may be normal, and Kayser-Fleischer rings may be absent. Hence, it is wise to evaluate all three of these factors because it is likely that at least one will be abnormal. In problematic cases, finding excess urinary copper after the administration of 1,000 mg of penicillamine may also help establish the diagnosis.[29] If doubt persists, the ultimate standard is an increase in hepatic tissue copper concentration; however, this finding is conclusive only if the patient does not have long-standing cholestasis, which can also increase the hepatic copper concentration.

Treatment

Treatment of Wilson disease requires the administration of either trientine or penicillamine, chelating agents that bind copper and promote the urinary excretion of 1,000 to 3,000 mg of copper a day. The usual dosage for either drug is 1 g/day. Clinical improvement generally parallels depletion of the tissue copper buildup. Trientine has become the preferred drug because penicillamine therapy is associated with significant side effects—most commonly, nausea and abdominal discomfort immediately after taking the medication. More serious side effects of penicillamine include leukopenia and thrombocytopenia, which may, in a rare case, lead to aplastic anemia. A small percentage of patients experience the nephrotic syndrome. All patients with Wilson disease should be followed closely with routine urinalyses and blood counts, particularly during the first few months of therapy. Because penicillamine is a pyridoxine antagonist, 50 mg of pyridoxine should be given once a week. If trientine and penicillamine cannot be tolerated, oral zinc therapy should be considered. Elemental zinc may be administered in the form of zinc acetate in three divided doses on an empty stomach for a total daily dose of 150 mg. Zinc therapy increases fecal copper loss and induces a negative copper balance in patients with Wilson disease.[30] The onset of action is delayed, however, and the long-term efficacy of zinc therapy is unknown.

α_1-ANTITRYPSIN DEFICIENCY

Homozygous α_1-antitrypsin deficiency is associated with a rare syndrome of progressive cirrhosis.[31,32] Although originally described in children with juvenile cirrhosis, the combination of α_1-antitrypsin deficiency and cirrhosis has been reported in adults. Adult patients usually have accompanying emphysema. The diagnosis of α_1-antitrypsin deficiency should always be considered in cases in which the cirrhosis does not have an obvious antecedent.

On first presentation, most patients have moderate hepatomegaly and mild abnormality of liver function. Absence of α_1-antitrypsin globulin on protein electrophoresis makes the diagnosis very likely. Specific measurements of α_1-antitrypsin levels in the

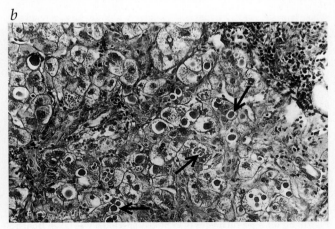

a   *b*

Figure 6 (*a*) Nodules of liver tissue surrounded by scar tissue—a feature of cirrhosis—are seen in a surgical liver biopsy specimen from a 67-year-old man with emphysema and mild hepatomegaly. (*b*) In a higher-magnification view of the specimen, multiple, round, hepatic cell inclusion bodies (arrows) are distinctive for α_1-antitrypsin globulin deficiency.

blood confirm the diagnosis. Genetic variants have been found, reflecting the existence of more than 75 different alleles for the gene that controls production of α_1-antitrypsin. Protease inhibitor type ZZ (PiZZ) is the genotype generally associated with cirrhosis and emphysema. An amino acid substitution in the Z variant protein allows the α_1-antitrypsin protein molecules to polymerize within the liver cell, thereby impairing excretion of the protein from the liver. Characteristic periodic acid–Schiff positive (diastase-resistant) inclusion bodies containing abnormal α_1-antitrypsin globulin can be seen in the hepatocytes [see Figure 6]. Individuals carrying a single PiZ allele may also be at risk for cirrhosis and liver failure.[33] A significant proportion of patients homozygous for PiZZ who also have chronic liver disease show evidence of hepatitis B or hepatitis C infection.[34]

The most important treatment for α_1-antitrypsin deficiency is avoidance of cigarette smoking, which markedly accelerates coexistent lung disease. There is no specific treatment for liver disease associated with α_1-antitrypsin deficiency, and thus, therapy is supportive and includes avoidance of alcohol. Augmentation therapy to increase the circulating levels of α_1-antitrypsin is used to treat emphysema but not liver disease in patients with α_1-antitrypsin deficiency. Patients with end-stage liver disease and liver failure caused by α_1-antitrypsin deficiency are candidates for liver transplantation, and long-term survival is excellent.

NONALCOHOLIC FATTY LIVER DISEASE

Nonalcoholic fatty liver disease (NAFLD) is a relatively common liver disease that was first described in the 1980s.[35,36] NAFLD is believed to be part of a spectrum ranging from simple fatty liver to nonalcoholic steatohepatitis (NASH) with minimal fibrosis to cirrhosis. NAFLD has been reported to occur in 1% to 9% of patients undergoing liver biopsy, with the greatest prevalence in patients 40 to 49 years of age. Common risk factors for NAFLD include obesity, diabetes mellitus, and lipid abnormalities [see Table 1]. Other common factors associated with NASH include total parenteral nutrition, hypobetalipoproteinemia , certain drugs, and jejunoileal bypass for morbid obesity. Hepatic steatosis occurs in 70% of patients who are 10% over ideal weight, in up to 100% of patients who are morbidly obese, and in 33% of patients with type 2 (non–insulin-dependent) diabetes mellitus. The pathogenesis of NASH remains uncertain, but the increased delivery of free fatty acids to the liver and the formation of free radicals is believed to be potentially important.

Increased hepatic fat accumulation occurred in virtually all patients during the period of rapid weight loss after jejunoileal bypass surgery, an operation that is no longer performed.[37] Progressive liver disease that is indistinguishable from alcoholic cirrhosis develops in a small number of patients. The liver is usually enlarged, and hepatic function gradually deteriorates.[38] The cause of this catastrophic complication is unknown. Although scattered reports indicate improvement of liver function after parenteral hyperalimentation, the only certain treatment of progressive liver disease is reanastomosis of the bowel or takedown of the gastroplasty. If this procedure is not done promptly, the liver disease may prove fatal.

Diagnosis

Clinical features Patients with simple fatty liver and NASH are typically asymptomatic, in contrast to patients with alcoholic hepatitis, who are nearly always symptomatic. The most common symptoms are constitutional and nonspecific, such as

Table 1 Conditions Associated with Nonalcoholic Fatty Liver Disease

Type of Disorder	Associated Conditions and Risk Factors
Nutritional abnormalities	Obesity* Total parenteral nutrition Rapid weight loss
Metabolic diseases	Diabetes mellitus* Hypertriglyceridemia* Abetalipoproteinemia Hypobetalipoproteinemia Weber-Christian disease Limb lipodystrophy
Drug Effects	Estrogens Corticosteroids Amiodarone
Surgery	Jejunoileal bypass Extensive small bowel loss Gastroplasty

*Most frequently associated.

fatigue, weakness, and malaise. Right upper quadrant pain or fullness is a less frequent complaint. On physical examination, hepatomegaly is common but may be difficult to detect because of obesity. The presence of other signs of chronic liver disease, such as spider angiomas, jaundice, or ascites, points to the presence of cirrhosis.

Laboratory tests There are no specific laboratory findings that unequivocally lead to the diagnosis of steatosis or NASH. Serum AST and ALT levels are commonly elevated, and the serum alkaline phosphatase level can be elevated up to twice the normal level. Viral, autoimmune, and genetic causes of liver disease must be excluded. Imaging techniques cannot distinguish between simple fatty liver and NASH, although the presence of steatosis in the absence of other causes of liver disease can allow a reasonable, presumptive diagnosis of NAFLD.

Liver biopsy The diagnosis of NAFLD requires liver biopsy, which shows the characteristic findings of fatty change, lobular inflammation, hepatocellular injury, and Mallory stained hyaline, with or without fibrosis [see Table 2]. Simple fatty liver is characterized histologically by hepatic steatosis without inflammation, ballooning degeneration, necrosis, fibrosis, or cirrhosis. The diagnosis of NAFLD can be established only when alcohol abuse (> 20 g/day) is convincingly excluded. The role of liver biopsy to diagnose NAFLD in routine clinical practice is debated, and most clinicians do not recommend it. Arguments against liver biopsy include the generally good prognosis for most patients with NAFLD, lack of an effective therapy, and the risks and costs associated with liver biopsy. Liver biopsy may be warranted to exclude alternative causes of elevated aminotransferase levels, determine the degree of fibrosis, and estimate a prognosis.

Treatment

No therapy has clearly been proved effective for treatment of NAFLD.[35,36] Treatment, therefore, has been directed toward the correction of risk factors for NAFLD (i.e., decreased delivery of fatty acids to the liver and use of drugs that are potentially hep-

Table 2 Histologic Features of Nonalcoholic Fatty Liver Disease

Condition*	Features
Steatosis	Macrovesicular Mild to severe Primarily zone 3

Steatohepatitis	Inflammation
	  Usually mild, lobular, and mixed mononuclear and neutrophilic
	Hepatocyte degeneration
	  Mallory hyaline

Fibrosis	Initially pericellular Cirrhosis in 10% to 15% of patients

*The typical disease spectrum is steatosis → steatohepatitis → steatohepatitis with fibrosis → cirrhosis.

atoprotective). Both gradual and sustained weight loss, exercise, and control of diabetes constitute a standard approach, with use of lipid-lowering agents as needed to control hypertriglyceridemia. Fatty liver can resolve with aggressive weight loss, even when cirrhosis is present. Of the various substances believed to be hepatoprotective, ursodeoxycholic acid and vitamin E have been studied the most. The long-term effects of these therapies remain uncertain. Cirrhosis with end-stage liver disease secondary to NASH may eventuate in liver transplantation, and NASH can recur after liver transplantation.

Prognosis

The prognosis for patients with simple fatty liver is benign. Those with NASH have a 10% to 50% risk of advanced fibrosis or cirrhosis. Older age, obesity, and the presence of diabetes mellitus may be associated with the presence of fibrosis in patients with NASH.

MISCELLANEOUS CIRRHOSES

Chronic exposure to arsenic, methotrexate, or excessive amounts of vitamin A can lead to cirrhosis. Cirrhosis after schistosome infestation is unusual in the United States but is seen in other parts of the world, such as the Far East and Egypt. Cirrhosis can follow a long-term biliary tract disease, such as primary sclerosing cholangitis, and it is a rare complication of sarcoid liver disease. Cardiac cirrhosis has become rare because the introduction of prosthetic valve replacements has allowed correction of valvular disorders. The disease arises after years or even decades of severe right-sided heart failure or tricuspid insufficiency. Some patients with Budd-Chiari syndrome (hepatic vein thrombosis) may survive the acute illness and acquire a histologic picture resembling that of cardiac cirrhosis.[39] In addition, various childhood diseases (which occasionally first occur in adulthood) can eventuate in cirrhosis. The most common of these disorders are cystic fibrosis, glycogen storage disease, biliary atresia, and congenital hepatic fibrosis.

Complications of Cirrhosis

VARICES

Bleeding varices constitute one of the most serious complications of cirrhosis. Mortality during the acute episode may reach 60% to 70%.[40-42] Many factors associated with decompensated cirrhosis augment this high risk, including general debility, co-

agulation defects, and hepatic encephalopathy; the size of the varix is also correlated with the risk of bleeding. Recurrent bleeding, common within the first 2 weeks of the initial episode, also contributes to the high mortality. If the patient survives longer than 6 weeks, the risk of recurrent bleeding drops sharply and approaches that of cirrhotic patients who have never bled. Bleeding esophageal varices are most reliably identified by upper gastrointestinal endoscopy [see Figure 7].

Treatment of Acute Variceal Bleeding

Endoscopic therapy Endoscopic therapy with variceal banding or sclerotherapy is the treatment of choice for the immediate control of esophageal variceal bleeding [see Chapter 63]. Banding or sclerotherapy is also effective in the long-term control of recurrent esophageal variceal hemorrhage, but the effect on survival remains uncertain.[40-42] Esophageal ligation is similar to the banding of hemorrhoids, but it is performed with a modified endoscope. In a meta-analysis of published trials, variceal ligation obliterated varices more rapidly than sclerotherapy and was as effective as sclerotherapy in controlling bleeding with less frequent side effects.[43] Ligation is now considered the endoscopic treatment of choice for patients with esophageal variceal bleeding. In addition, a redesigned endoscope that can deliver several rubber bands after intubation of the esophagus obviates multiple insertions of the scope through an overtube, which was associated with several cases of esophageal perforation. Complications of variceal sclerotherapy are common; these include retrosternal pain, esophageal ulceration, hemorrhage, pleural effusion, and esophageal stricture and perforation. Bleeding from gastric varices is less common in patients with cirrhosis but more difficult to treat effectively, except with surgery.

If variceal bleeding persists or recurs and is life-threatening, insertion of a Sengstaken-Blakemore or Minnesota tube will stop the bleeding, at least temporarily, in more than 90% of patients. This treatment, which is associated with significant morbidity, is fortunately seldom required.

Pharmacologic therapy Intra-arterial vasopressin does not improve overall survival, and its administration requires specialized angiographic expertise that is not widely available. Vasopressin administered intravenously in a continuous drip is of doubtful efficacy in patients with actively bleeding esophageal varices. When vasopressin is used, adjunctive therapy with nitroglycerin should be administered to minimize side effects, particularly tissue ischemia.[44] The intravenous infusion of somatostatin or its analogue, octreotide (50 μg/hr), is more effective than vasopressin and has a lower risk of side effects; it is now the standard pharmacologic therapy used for acute variceal bleeding.[45] Octreotide is usually used with endoscopic therapy and is continued for 24 to 72 hours after the bleeding stops.

Treatment of Recurrent Variceal Bleeding

Transjugular intrahepatic portosystemic shunt The placement of a transjugular intrahepatic portosystemic shunt (TIPS) is rapidly becoming an accepted technique for the treatment of bleeding esophageal varices refractory to endoscopic therapy.[46] This procedure creates a shunt but avoids the complications of major surgery. The initial enthusiasm surrounding the introduction of TIPS has been tempered by recognition of the complications of encephalopathy, which develops in 10% to 30% of patients and is refractory to medical therapy in approximately 5%, and shunt stenosis or occlusion, which develops in 30% to 50% of patients at 12 months. It seems reasonable to restrict this form of treatment to centers with experienced staff and to patients who are poor surgical candidates, are refractory to endoscopic therapy, or have bleeding from gastric rather than esophageal varices.

A number of trials have compared TIPS with endoscopic therapy (either sclerotherapy or banding) after initial control of hemorrhage in patients with Child class A or B cirrhosis; several tentative conclusions can be drawn from these studies.[46] Mortality associated with TIPS is not significantly different from that associated with endoscopic treatment. TIPS is superior to endoscopic therapy in the prevention of variceal rebleeding (19% versus 47%). TIPS may be particularly attractive for patients in whom compliance with follow-up endoscopy is in doubt. However, one must accept the increased risk of hepatic encephalopathy after TIPS (34%, versus 18% after endoscopic therapy). TIPS is less attractive for patients with advanced chronic liver disease and Child class C cirrhosis with poor synthetic function. The survival of patients after TIPS can be predicted by the Mayo Clinic end-stage liver disease score, which includes the following four variables: serum bilirubin, serum creatinine, INR for prothrombin time, and cause of the underlying liver disease.[47] The long-term utility of TIPS must also be evaluated in context of shunt stenosis or occlusion, which is a management problem after TIPS. Thus, for esophageal variceal bleeding, TIPS cannot be recommended as the first-choice treatment for prevention of variceal rebleeding.

Surgical portosystemic shunt   Recurrent or continued bleeding may indicate a need for a surgical portosystemic shunt. This major operation carries a mortality of approximately 40% when performed on an emergency basis.[48] If bleeding can be stopped and shunt surgery performed electively, mortality declines substantially. Although portosystemic shunting procedures do not appear to prolong survival, they do prevent subsequent bleeding. The major problem after surgery is intractable hepatic encephalopathy and hepatic failure. The preferred shunt procedure is the one with which the surgeon is most experienced. A distal splenorenal shunt with concomitant gastroesophageal devascularization selectively decompresses esophageal varices while maintaining mesenteric blood flow to the liver. In most but not all studies, use of the distal splenorenal shunt reduced the incidence of severe encephalopathy as a late complication after surgery, compared with conventional shunts. The procedure is technically difficult; time will reveal if it possesses any long-term advantages.

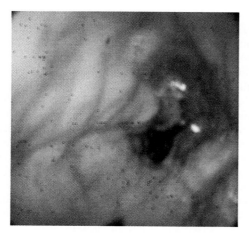

Figure 7   **Endoscopy reveals large, tortuous esophageal varices that have a characteristic bluish color.**

Medical treatment   Propranolol produces a sustained reduction in portal pressure in patients with cirrhosis and may be expected to prevent bleeding from esophageal varices.[49] One study noted a dramatic reduction in episodes of rebleeding and improved 2-year survival when propranolol was given in a sufficient dosage to reduce the resting heart rate by 25%. However, another study found no decrease in variceal hemorrhage with a similar regimen and further reported that the beta blockade induced by propranolol complicated the resuscitation of bleeding patients. Propranolol appears to be less effective than sclerotherapy in preventing rebleeding from esophageal varices.

Prophylactic Treatment for Variceal Bleeding

Because the first episode of variceal bleeding can result in significant morbidity and mortality, there has been considerable interest in the prophylactic treatment of esophageal varices in persons who have never bled. Prophylactic portosystemic shunts decrease rebleeding but do not enhance survival. Prophylactic sclerotherapy has been studied in several centers with mixed results. In the largest study, which was restricted to alcoholic patients, this approach proved harmful.[50] The experience with the beta-adrenergic antagonists propranolol and nadolol has been somewhat more encouraging because the drugs appear both to prevent the first episode of bleeding and to reduce mortality associated with bleeding in patients who have moderate or large esophageal varices.[51] If a patient known to have large varices is well motivated and tolerates the medication, beta-adrenergic antagonists may be considered. Isosorbide-5-mononitrate, a long-acting nitrate, may also help prevent the first variceal hemorrhage.[52]

ASCITES

Diagnosis

Ascites, a common sequela of many forms of cirrhosis, is usually detected by finding shifting dullness or a fluid wave on physical examination of the abdomen.[53] Occasionally, ascites presents as a right-sided pleural effusion. Portal hypertension, decreased serum albumin with consequent loss of oncotic force within the vascular and interstitial spaces, and renal retention of sodium and water contribute to ascites formation.

Although infectious, pancreatic, or neoplastic causes of ascites are infrequent, they should not be overlooked, because therapy and prognosis differ for each condition. To exclude such possible causes, a small amount of ascitic fluid should be removed from the abdominal cavity using a narrow-gauge needle. The gross appearance of the fluid may suggest an unusual etiology. For instance, cloudy fluid implies an infection; bloody fluid, a tumor; and milky fluid, lymphatic obstruction. Routine laboratory studies of the fluid should include white cell and differential cell counts, protein and albumin determinations, and culture. In ascites caused by cirrhosis, the serum-ascites albumin gradient is greater than 1.1, the total protein is less than 2.5 g/dl, the total white cell count is less than 300/mm^3, the proportion of granulocytes is less than 30%, and cultures are negative. Approximately 5% of patients with ascites attributable to cirrhosis have ascitic fluid that has a total protein concentration greater than 2.5 g/dl.

Treatment

Initial treatment   The treatment of uncomplicated ascites in patients with cirrhosis is straightforward.[53,54] First, any medications that inhibit prostaglandin synthesis, such as aspirin or nonsteroidal anti-inflammatory drugs, should be discontinued because they decrease the glomerular filtration rate, reduce sodium excretion, and blunt the natriuretic response to diuretics. After such agents have been withdrawn, sodium and water restriction should be instituted. Although extreme sodium and water restriction can be accomplished in the hospital, it is not usually necessary, nor will it be maintained once the patient goes home. A diet in which sodium is restricted to 2 g and water is restricted to 2,000 ml daily is often well tolerated.

Medical treatment   If dietary restriction and bed rest do not induce diuresis, the medication of choice is spironolactone. Seventy-five percent of hospitalized patients with ascites obtain relief with spironolactone alone. Because spironolactone inhibits the action of aldosterone, it tends to prevent the renal excretion of potassium, which is desirable for patients with cirrhosis. For this reason, however, use of spironolactone is not advisable for patients with renal insufficiency. In addition, patients taking spironolactone should avoid potassium chloride salt substitutes. Long-term use of spironolactone produces gynecomastia in 20% to 30% of patients.

Spironolactone is given in an initial dosage of 100 mg daily, which is increased to 200 mg daily if diuresis has not ensued after 2 to 3 days of treatment. Although spironolactone can be increased to 400 mg/day or more, the drug is less well tolerated at these higher dosages. Therefore, if diuresis has not occurred at 200 mg daily, it is preferable to add furosemide in one 40 mg dose in the morning to the 200 mg daily dose of spironolactone. The furosemide dose may then be increased each day by 40 mg increments (administered in one dose) until diuresis ensues. Most patients begin to respond before daily dosages reach 120 to 160 mg of furosemide and 200 mg of spironolactone. The aim is to use the lowest possible dosages.

The maximum diuresis of ascitic fluid should not exceed 1,000 ml/day. For that reason, daily weight loss in cirrhotic patients should not exceed 1 to 2 lb. A more rapid diuresis, particularly in patients with little or no peripheral edema, leads to dangerous diminution of intravascular and intracellular fluid volumes and to azotemia.

Complications of diuretic treatment include severe electrolyte abnormalities, encephalopathy, azotemia, and dehydration. Complications are most common when diuresis has been rapid or when diuretic medication has been continued after the patient has been clinically judged free of excess body fluid.

Paracentesis   Large-volume paracentesis has become popular in the treatment of patients with ascites. In one study, paracentesis of 4 to 6 L/day was accomplished safely and resulted in shorter hospital stays and fewer complications than conventional diuretic therapy. Patients usually welcome paracentesis because it relieves considerable discomfort. It also provides the physician with the ascitic fluid necessary for diagnostic purposes. Subsequent work has shown that the administration of 6 to 8 g/L of intravenous albumin after 5 L or more prevents renal insufficiency and hyponatremia induced by paracentesis.

In about 5% of patients, ascites do not respond to the usual dosages of conventional diuretic medication, or diuresis is achieved only at the expense of renal function. In these patients, insertion of the LeVeen peritoneovenous shunt has been considered. The shunt routes ascitic fluid subcutaneously from the peritoneal cavity to the internal jugular vein via a one-way valve. Compared with medical therapy alone, the peritoneovenous shunt results in speedier resolution of the ascites. However, placement of the shunt does not alter survival. Because most patients continue to require diuretics, although at lower doses, the shunt may produce benefit by increasing renal blood flow. Serious complications of the shunt include bacterial infection of the peritoneum, disseminated intravascular coagulation, and rupture of esophageal varices. Because of these complications, the peritoneovenous shunt is seldom used.

Treatment of refractory ascites   Refractory ascites can also be effectively managed by placement of a TIPS.[55] The majority of patients still require diuretic therapy, albeit at reduced dosages. The value of TIPS compared with repeated large-volume paracentesis for the management of refractory ascites awaits further study. However, TIPS is effective in the treatment of hepatic hydrothorax, which often accompanies refractory ascites.

SPONTANEOUS BACTERIAL PERITONITIS

Spontaneous bacterial peritonitis (SBP) develops in 10% to 25% of cirrhotic patients followed prospectively for at least a year.[56] The cirrhosis is usually advanced and active, as manifested by hepatic encephalopathy, esophageal varices, and jaundice. The incidence of SBP is substantially higher in patients with ascitic fluid protein levels below 1.0 g/dl and serum bilirubin levels above 2.5 mg/dl. These findings could explain the increased risk of ascitic fluid infection, because the antibacterial activity of the ascitic fluid, as measured by opsonic activity, is proportional to the level of ascitic fluid protein. The exact pathogenesis is unknown. Presumably, hematogenous seeding of the ascitic fluid, which functions as an ideal bacterial culture medium, serves as a major route of infection. Cirrhosis undoubtedly facilitates the process by allowing enteric organisms to enter the bloodstream via the portosystemic collaterals, thus bypassing the major reticuloendothelial system in the liver.

Diagnosis

Clinical features   The typical attack of SBP is heralded by fever, peripheral leukocytosis, abdominal pain, hypoactive or absent bowel sounds, and rebound tenderness. Most patients do not demonstrate all these symptoms, and some have none. Hence, ascitic fluid should be analyzed whenever the condition of a patient with cirrhosis suddenly deteriorates.

Laboratory tests   The ascitic fluid is often turbid because of leukocytosis and bacterial growth. Leukocyte cell counts greater than 1,000/mm³ consisting of more than 85% granulocytes are common. Almost all patients have ascitic fluid cell counts greater than 300/mm³; more than half of these are polymorphonuclear cells. However, not all patients with ascitic fluid leukocytosis have SBP. In practice, it is wise to treat patients with antibiotics when the clinical picture is suggestive and the ascitic fluid contains more than 500 white blood cells/mm³. The ultimate criterion for infection is demonstration of organisms either by Gram stain of the fluid (one fourth of cases) or by culture. To maximize detection of the responsible infectious organisms, 5 ml of ascitic fluid should be injected at bedside into both aerobic and anaerobic blood culture bottles. Two thirds of the causative organisms are enteric; *Escherichia coli* and *Klebsiella* species are the most common agents. *Pneumococcus* and *Streptococcus* organisms are responsible for as many as 20% of cases. In nearly half of cases, blood cultures are positive for the same organism found in the ascitic fluid.

Treatment

Cefotaxime administered intravenously at a dosage of 2 g every 6 hours is an appropriate initial treatment for an episode of SBP[57]; in patients with renal insufficiency, the dosage is adjusted downward. On this regimen, 75% to 80% of treated episodes resolve. A few episodes resolve after a change in the antibiotic regimen. However, 20% to 25% of patients die before the infection resolves. Therapy is equally effective whether given for 5 days or 10 days.[58] Patients should be monitored closely and ascitic fluid checked at least once (e.g., after 48 hours) to ensure that the infection is being effectively treated. Despite optimal therapy, 40% to 60% of patients with SBP die. Half of the deaths are a direct result of the peritonitis; the other half succumb to other complications of their severe liver disease. Long-term oral therapy with norfloxacin (400 mg/day) or ciprofloxacin (750 mg once a week) reduces the incidence of recurrent spontaneous bacterial peritonitis attributable to aerobic gram-negative bacteria and should be considered in patients at high risk for recurrence.[59,60]

HEPATORENAL SYNDROME

The hepatorenal syndrome is defined as a functional renal failure associated with well-established and usually decompensated cirrhosis [see Chapter 162]. When the hepatorenal syndrome develops, the outcome is usually fatal.[61]

The pathogenesis of the hepatorenal syndrome is uncertain, but reduced renal blood flow and glomerular filtration rate may precede overt renal failure by several months. Paradoxically, these alterations occur in association with increased plasma volume. An increase in blood flow to the renal medulla at the expense of the cortex (intrarenal shunting) occurs as well. Because many patients have associated hypotension and respond poorly to pressor agents, false neurotransmitters have been implicated in the pathogenesis of the hepatorenal syndrome.

Diagnosis

The typical patient is deeply jaundiced; is obviously moribund; and exhibits tense ascites, hypoalbuminemia and hypoprothrombinemia, and encephalopathy. As liver disease progresses, urine volume and sodium excretion fall, and serum creatinine and blood urea nitrogen (BUN) levels increase before death. In this setting, renal failure is incidental to the overwhelming liver disease. In perhaps 10% to 20% of patients, however, liver disease may be reasonably stable, and progressive renal failure represents the major threat to the patient's life.

Treatment

Although many diseases can affect the liver and kidney in tandem, the patient's history, oliguria, marked sodium retention, and presence of severe liver disease usually reduce the diagnostic possibilities to two: hepatorenal syndrome and prerenal azotemia. Because these two causes of renal failure are indistinguishable by common laboratory tests and physical signs, it is imperative that patients be initially treated as though they had prerenal azotemia. Diuretic medication should be discontinued, any blood loss replaced, and the plasma expanded with saline or glucose solutions. These steps should be taken carefully while the central venous pressure is being monitored, and they should be halted if diuresis does not commence when central venous pressure has been raised. Once the presence of prerenal azotemia has been excluded by these measures, treatment of the hepatorenal syndrome should be supportive and conservative. Spontaneous reversion of the syndrome, though infrequent, occurs when the liver disease begins to improve.

Reversion of the hepatorenal syndrome after insertion of a peritoneovenous shunt has been reported. The shunt may be considered in the small percentage of patients with prominent renal failure. Life-threatening complications, however, would not be unusual in these patients. Emergency portacaval shunt, corticosteroids, phenoxybenzamine, metaraminol, and methyldopa have all been used without major benefit. Hepatorenal syndrome typically resolves after liver transplantation.

HEPATIC ENCEPHALOPATHY

Hepatic encephalopathy can be roughly classified into four stages. The first stage consists of agitation without accompanying physical findings. Patients in this stage often receive sedatives that promptly deepen the encephalopathy. In the second stage, the patient is moderately obtunded but still responsive, and asterixis can be elicited. In the third stage, the patient is stuporous and barely responsive. In the fourth stage, the patient sinks into deep coma. Asterixis may be absent in the third and fourth stages.

Etiology

The cause of hepatic encephalopathy is undoubtedly multifactorial. Elevated concentrations of blood ammonia, short-chain fatty acids, false neurotransmitters, and certain amino acids have all been implicated in the genesis of this syndrome.[62] In addition, a circulating substance that has properties similar to those of benzodiazepine agonists and that can potentiate the action of γ-aminobutyric acid may be present in liver failure, contributing to the syndrome of hepatic encephalopathy. Some patients with hepatic encephalopathy appear to respond to the administration of a benzodiazepine receptor antagonist,[63] supporting the hypothesis that a benzodiazepine-like substance may play a role in this disorder. Both the shunting of blood around the liver, as a consequence of portal hypertension, and poor function of the diseased liver contribute to the pathogenesis. In addition, the central nervous system of the patient with cirrhosis appears to be sensitive to sedative effects of endogenous products and exogenous medications.

In most instances of hepatic encephalopathy, a precipitating cause can be identified. Initiating events include gastrointestinal bleeding, electrolyte abnormalities (e.g., hyponatremia and acid-base disorders), hypoxia, CO_2 retention, infection, constipation, and the injudicious use of diuretics, sedatives, or other medications. In a few patients, refractory chronic encephalopathy may develop, often as a consequence of portosystemic shunting or TIPS.

Diagnosis

The diagnosis of hepatic encephalopathy depends on documentation of mental obtundation, asterixis, and fetor hepaticus.[64] Fetor hepaticus is an offensive, mixed feculent-fruity odor of the breath. Asterixis, the irregular flexion of the extremities, is most easily elicited by asking a patient to hold his or her arms horizontally with hands extended at the wrist. The flapping motion caused by intermittent loss of extensor tone clearly marks hepatic encephalopathy, although asterixis may also develop in patients with uremia or severe pulmonary disease. Slowing or flattening of waves on an electroencephalogram verifies encephalopathy.

Treatment

The most important aspect of therapy is removal or correction of precipitating causes. The medication chart should be scrupulously searched for sedatives, which should be discontinued.

Once these measures have been undertaken, standard therapy for hepatic encephalopathy includes dietary protein restriction to reduce production of endogenous nitrogenous substances, such as ammonia, and administration of lactulose. The usual approach restricts dietary protein to 40 to 60 g/day. Long-term restriction to much less than 60 g/day results in protein malnutrition.

The drug of choice is lactulose, a disaccharide that travels undigested to the colon, where it undergoes bacterial degradation to two- and three-carbon acids that reduce the intraluminal pH level and produce diarrhea. The usual dosage is 30 ml three or four times a day. The mechanism of action of lactulose is uncertain. Apparently, the reduced stool pH level causes ammonia to be protonated to its ionic form (NH_4), which is poorly absorbed and is excreted in the stool.

Lactulose has proved to be as effective as neomycin in the treatment of chronic or recurrent hepatic encephalopathy. Approximately 80% of patients respond to one of these drugs.[65] In certain patients, neomycin may be effective when lactulose is not. The usual dosage of neomycin is 500 mg or 1 g given orally every 6 hours. Although neomycin is poorly absorbed from the intestine, ototoxicity and renal damage have occurred. Because lactulose is less toxic than neomycin, it should be tried first. Although it may appear theoretically that neomycin would interfere with lactulose, evidence indicates that the two drugs may act synergistically. Lactulose and neomycin are effective for patients with chronic or recurrent encephalopathy, but the benefit is less certain for those with the encephalopathy that accompanies acute overwhelming hepatic disease. Metronidazole, 250 mg three or four times a day, can be used as an alternative to neomycin, but long-term therapy may be associated with neurotoxicity.

MALNUTRITION

Almost all patients with advanced liver disease have varying degrees of protein-calorie malnutrition. Severe malnutrition contributes to salt and water retention, defective immune response, and delayed recovery of liver function. A nutritional assessment should be done for all patients with advanced liver disease, and nutritional supplements should be provided when necessary. Nutritional supplementation can be accomplished by the addition of standard enteral formulas to the diet; in some critically ill patients, nutritional supplementation needs to be provided parenterally. There is little evidence that formulas enriched with branched-chain amino acids have any advantage over standard amino acid formulas, and they are considerably more expensive. These supplements are well tolerated, whether given orally or parenterally. The expected result is a more rapid return to positive nitrogen balance and improved liver function. No convincing improvement in survival has been demonstrated.[66]

MISCELLANEOUS COMPLICATIONS

The incidence of gallstones is increased in patients with cirrhosis, possibly because of the elevated bilirubin load generated by chronic hemolytic anemia and hypersplenism. Hence, the possibility of a common duct stone should be considered in patients with cirrhosis and jaundice. Peptic ulcer occurs more commonly in patients with cirrhosis than in the general population. The diagnosis should be considered if abdominal pain or upper gastrointestinal bleeding develops. Hypoxia is frequent in patients with advanced cirrhosis, and oxygen tension (PO_2) values of 60 to 70 mm Hg are not uncommon. Ascites impairs ventilation, and pulmonary angiomas may be responsible for right-to-left shunting of blood. Because many cirrhotic pa-

tients both drink and smoke, chronic obstructive pulmonary disease often complicates the picture. Primary liver cell cancer develops in 5% to 20% of patients with cirrhosis. If left untreated, the disease follows a rapidly progressive course [*see Chapter 196*].

Liver Transplantation

The widespread availability of liver transplantation has substantially improved the prognosis for almost all forms of end-stage liver disease.[67,68] Because 1-year and 5-year survival rates after transplantation approach 90% and 80%, respectively, at several centers, this form of treatment is widely accepted. Patients who have advanced cirrhosis with the onset of complications are candidates for liver transplantation. Clinical, biochemical, psychosocial, and financial information is reviewed to determine whether global selection criteria are met. There are a number of clinical and biochemical indications for liver transplantation [*see Chapter 69*]. Generally accepted absolute contraindications to liver transplantation include seropositivity for HIV, extrahepatic malignancy, active untreated sepsis, advanced cardiopulmonary disease, and active alcoholism or substance abuse. The major restriction of liver transplantation is the limited supply of donor organs. Approximately 4,500 people underwent liver transplantation in the United States in 1998 and 1999, though more than 15,000 were approved and on the waiting list.

References

1. McAfee JH, Keeffe EB, Lee RG, et al: Transjugular liver biopsy. Hepatology 15:726, 1992

2. Diehl AM: Alcoholic liver disease: natural history. Liver Transpl Surg 3:206, 1997

3. Lieber CS: Medical disorders of alcoholism. N Engl J Med 333:1058, 1995

4. Powell WJ Jr, Klatskin G: Duration of survival in patients with Laënnec's cirrhosis: influence of alcohol withdrawal and possible effects of recent changes in general management of the disease. Am J Med 44:406, 1968

5. Mendenhall CL, Moritz TE, Roselle GA, et al: A study of oral nutritional support with oxandrolone in malnourished patients with alcoholic hepatitis: results of a Department of Veterans Affairs cooperative study. Hepatology 17:564, 1993

6. Imperiale TF, McCullough AJ: Do corticosteroids reduce mortality from alcoholic hepatitis? a meta-analysis of the randomized trials. Ann Intern Med 113:299, 1990

7. Kaplan MM: Primary biliary cirrhosis. N Engl J Med 335:1570, 1996

8. Underhill J, Donaldson P, Bray G, et al: Susceptibility to primary biliary cirrhosis is associated with the HLA-DR8-DQB1*0402 haplotype. Hepatology 16:1404, 1992

9. Heathcote EJ: Management of primary biliary cirrhosis: the American Association for the Study of Liver Diseases practice guidelines. Hepatology 31:1005, 2000

10. Poupon RE, Poupon R, Balkau B, et al: Ursodiol for the long-term treatment of primary biliary cirrhosis. N Engl J Med 330:1342, 1994

11. Heathcote EJ, Cauch-Dudek K, Walker V, et al: The Canadian multicenter double-blind randomized controlled trial of ursodeoxycholic acid in primary biliary cirrhosis. Hepatology 19:1149, 1994

12. Lindor KD, Dickson ER, Baldus WP, et al: Ursodeoxycholic acid in the treatment of primary biliary cirrhosis. Gastroenterology 106:1284, 1994

13. Kaplan MM, Knox TA: Treatment of primary biliary cirrhosis with low-dose weekly methotrexate. Gastroenterology 101:1332, 1991

14. Lindor KD, Dickson ER, Jorgensen RA, et al: The combination of ursodeoxycholic acid and methotrexate for patients with primary biliary cirrhosis: the results of a pilot study. Hepatology 22:1158, 1995

15. Kaplan MM, Alling DW, Zimmerman HJ, et al: A prospective trial of colchicine for primary biliary cirrhosis. N Engl J Med 315:1448, 1986

16. Bodenheimer H Jr, Schaffner F, Pezzullo J: Evaluation of colchicine therapy in primary biliary cirrhosis. Gastroenterology 95:124, 1988

17. Zifroni A, Schaffner F: Long-term follow-up of patients with primary biliary cirrhosis on colchicine therapy. Hepatology 14:990, 1991

18. Ghent CN, Carruthers SG: Treatment of pruritus in primary biliary cirrhosis with rifampin: results of a double-blind, crossover, randomized trial. Gastroenterology 94:488, 1988

19. Bacon BR: Iron overload states. Clin Liver Dis 2:63, 1998

20. Bacon BR, Powell LW, Adams PC, et al: Molecular medicine and hemochromatosis: at the crossroads. Gastroenterology 116:193, 1999

21. Feder JN, Gnirke A, Thomas W, et al: A novel MHC class I-like gene is mutated in pa-

tients with hereditary haemochromatosis. Nat Genet 13:399, 1996

22. Howard JM, Ghent CN, Carey LS, et al: Diagnostic efficacy of hepatic computed tomography in the detection of body iron overload. Gastroenterology 84:209, 1983

23. Johnson CD: Magnetic resonance imaging of the liver: current clinical applications. Mayo Clin Proc 68:147, 1993

24. Edwards CQ, Griffen LM, Goldgar D, et al: Prevalence of hemochromatosis among 11,065 presumably healthy blood donors. N Engl J Med 318:1355, 1988

25. Ludwig J, Batts KP, Moyer TP, et al: Liver biopsy diagnosis of homozygous hemochromatosis: a diagnostic algorithm. Mayo Clin Proc 68:263, 1993

26. Niederau C, Fischer R, Sonnenberg A, et al: Survival and causes of death in cirrhotic and in noncirrhotic patients with primary hemochromatosis. N Engl J Med 313:1256, 1985

27. Ferenci P: Wilson's disease. Clin Liver Dis 2:31, 1998

28. Walshe JM: Wilson's disease presenting with features of hepatic dysfunction: a clinical analysis of eighty-seven patients. Q J Med 70:253, 1989

29. Martins da Costa C, Baldwin D, Portmann B, et al: Value of urinary copper excretion after penicillamine challenge in the diagnosis of Wilson's disease. Hepatology 15:609, 1992

30. Brewer GJ, Hill GM, Prasad AS, et al: Oral zinc therapy for Wilson's disease. Ann Intern Med 99:314, 1983

31. Perlmutter DH: Alpha-1-antitrypsin deficiency. Semin Liver Dis 18:217, 1998

32. Eriksson S: Alpha$_1$-antitrypsin deficiency. J Hepatol 30:34, 1999

33. Graziadei IW, Joseph JJ, Wiesner RH, et al: Increased risk of chronic liver failure in adults with heterozygous α_1-antitrypsin deficiency. Hepatology 28:1058, 1998

34. Propst T, Propst A, Dietze O, et al: High prevalence of viral infection in adults with homozygous and heterozygous alpha$_1$-antitrypsin deficiency and chronic liver disease. Ann Intern Med 117:641, 1992

35. Kumar KS, Malet PF: Nonalcoholic steatohepatitis. Mayo Clin Proc 75:733, 2000

36. Matteoni CA, Younossi ZM, Gramlich T, et al: Nonalcoholic fatty liver disease: a spectrum of clinical and pathological severity. Gastroenterology 116:1413, 1999

37. Holzbach RT, Wieland RG, Lieber CS, et al: Hepatic lipid in morbid obesity: assessment at and subsequent to jejunoileal bypass. N Engl J Med 290:296, 1974

38. Andrassy RJ, Haff RC, Lobritz RW: Liver failure after jejunoileal shunt. Arch Surg 110:332, 1975

39. Dilawari JB, Bambery P, Chawla Y, et al: Hepatic outflow obstruction (Budd-Chiari syndrome): experience with 177 patients and a review of the literature. Medicine (Baltimore) 73:21, 1994

40. Stanley AJ, Hayes PC: Portal hypertension and variceal hemorrhage. Lancet 350:1235, 1997

41. Menon KVN, Kamath PS: Managing the complications of cirrhosis. Mayo Clin Proc 75:501, 2000

42. Bosch J, Garcia-Pagan JC: Complications of cirrhosis: I. portal hypertension. J Hepatol 32(suppl 1):141, 2000

43. Laine L, Cook D: Endoscopic ligation compared with sclerotherapy for treatment of esophageal variceal bleeding: a meta-analysis. Ann Intern Med 123:280, 1995

44. D'Amico G, Pagliaro L, Bosch J: The treatment of portal hypertension: a meta-analytic review. Hepatology 22:332, 1995

45. Imperiale TF, Teran JC, McCullough AJ: A meta-analysis of somatostatin versus vasopressin in the management of acute esophageal variceal hemorrhage. Gastroenterology 109:1289, 1995

46. Burroughs AK, Patch D: Transjugular intrahepatic portosystemic shunt. Semin Liver Dis 19:457, 1999

47. Malinchoc M, Kamath PS, Gordon FD, et al: A model to predict poor survival in patients undergoing transjugular intrahepatic portosystemic shunt. Hepatology 31:864, 2000

48. Iannitti DA, Henderson JM: The role of surgery in the treatment of portal hypertension. Clin Liver Dis 1:99, 1997

49. Grace ND, Bhattacharya K: Pharmacologic therapy of portal hypertension and variceal hemorrhage. Clin Liver Dis 1:59, 1997

50. Prophylactic sclerotherapy for esophageal varices in men with alcoholic liver disease: a randomized, single-blind, multicenter clinical trial: the Veterans Affairs Cooperative Variceal Sclerotherapy Group. N Engl J Med 324:1779, 1991

51. Poynard T, Cales P, Pasta L, et al: Beta-adrenergic-antagonist drugs in the prevention of gastrointestinal bleeding in patients with cirrhosis and esophageal varices: an analysis of data and prognostic factors in 589 patients from four randomized clinical trials: Franco-Italian Multicenter Study Group. N Engl J Med 324:1532, 1991

52. Angelico M, Carli L, Piat C, et al: Isosorbide-5-mononitrate versus propranolol in the prevention of first bleeding in cirrhosis. Gastroenterology 104:1460, 1993

53. Reynolds TB: Ascites. Clin Liver Dis 4:151, 2000

54. Runyon BA: Management of adult patients with ascites caused by cirrhosis. Hepatology 27:264, 1998

55. Rössle M, Ochs A, Gülberg V, et al: A comparison of paracentesis and transjugular intrahepatic portosystemic shunting in patients with ascites. N Engl J Med 342:1701, 2000

56. Andreu M, Sola R, Sitges-Serra A, et al: Risk factors for spontaneous bacterial peritonitis in cirrhotic patients with ascites. Gastroenterology 104:1133, 1993

57. Toledo C, Salmeron JM, Rimola A, et al: Spontaneous bacterial peritonitis in cirrhosis: predictive factors of infection resolution and survival in patients treated with cefotaxime. Hepatology 17:251, 1993

58. Runyon BA, McHutchison JG, Antillon MR, et al: Short-course versus long-course antibiotic treatment of spontaneous bacterial peritonitis: a randomized controlled study of 100 patients. Gastroenterology 100:1737, 1991

59. Gines P, Rimola A, Planas R, et al: Norfloxacin prevents spontaneous bacterial peritonitis recurrence in cirrhosis: results of a double-blind, placebo-controlled trial. Hepatology 12:716, 1990

60. Rolachon A, Cordier L, Bacq Y, et al: Ciprofloxacin and long-term prevention of spontaneous bacterial peritonitis: results of a prospective controlled trial. Hepatology 22:1171, 1995

61. Arroyo V, Ginès P, Gerbes AL, et al: Definition and diagnostic criteria of refractory ascites and hepatorenal syndrome in cirrhosis. International Ascites Club. Hepatology 23:164, 1996

62. Fraser CL, Arieff AI: Hepatic encephalopathy. N Engl J Med 313:865, 1985

63. Pomier-Layrargues G, Giguere JF, Lavoie J, et al: Flumazenil in cirrhotic patients in hepatic coma: a randomized double-blind placebo-controlled crossover trial. Hepatology 19:32, 1994

64. Keeffe EB: Hepatic encephalopathy. Consultations in Gastroenterology. Snape WJ Jr, Ed. WB Saunders Co, Philadelphia, 1996, p 653

65. Conn HO, Leevy CM, Vlahcevic ZR, et al: Comparison of lactulose and neomycin in the treatment of chronic portal-systemic encephalopathy: a double-blind controlled trial. Gastroenterology 72:573, 1977

66. Nompleggi DJ, Bonkovsky HL: Nutritional supplementation in chronic liver disease: an analytical review. Hepatology 19:518, 1994

67. Seaberg EC, Belle SH, Beringer KC, et al: Liver transplantation in the United States from 1987-1998: updated results from the Pitt-UNOS liver transplant registry. Clinical Transplants 1998. Cecka JM, Terasaki PI, Eds. UCLA Tissue Typing Laboratory, Los Angeles, 1999, p 17

68. Keeffe EB: Selection of patients for liver transplantation. Transplantation of the Liver, 3rd ed. Maddrey WC, Schiff ER, Sorrell MF, Eds. Lippincott Williams & Wilkins, Philadelphia, 2001, p 5

Acknowledgment

Figure 7 Radiograph courtesy of Malcolm Anderson, M.D., Department of Radiology, Stanford University School of Medicine.

67 Gallstones and Biliary Tract Disease

Aijaz Ahmed, M.D., and Emmet B. Keeffe, M.D.

Cholelithiasis and biliary tract diseases constitute a major health problem in the United States.[1,2] The prevalence of gallstones increases with age in all racial groups; increased body weight, rapid weight loss, pregnancy, alcoholic cirrhosis, and a family history of gallstone disease also appear to be risk factors.[3-5]

Incidence and Prevalence of Gallstones

In one epidemiologic study of persons 30 years of age and older, new gallstones were found to develop in 2.2% of men and 2.9% of women over a 5-year period.[3] In the United States, gallstones occur in approximately 10% of persons older than 40 years, but the prevalence is significantly higher in women, increasing to 20% to 25% in women older than 50 years. Fortunately, only 20% to 30% of gallstones are symptomatic, with biliary colic being the most common symptom. A recent report from the Third National Health and Nutrition Examination Survey (NHANES III) stated that an estimated 6.3 million men and 14.2 million women 20 to 74 years of age had gallbladder disease.[6]

Gallstone Formation

Two principal types of stone, the cholesterol stone and the pigment stone, form in the gallbladder and biliary tract. The cholesterol stone is composed mainly of cholesterol (> 50% of the stone) and comprises multiple layers of cholesterol crystals and mucin glycoproteins. Mixed gallstones contain 20% to 50% cholesterol. The pigment stone contains a wide variety of organic and inorganic components, including calcium bilirubinate (40% to 50% of dry weight). In Europe and the United States, 90% of gallstones are of the cholesterol or mixed type; the remainder are pigment gallstones. Multiple risk factors for cholesterol and pigment gallstone formation have been identified [see Table 1].

PIGMENT GALLSTONE FORMATION

The pathogenesis of pigment gallstones is not completely understood.[7] Black pigment stones are most often seen in patients with cirrhosis or hemolytic anemia and are found predominantly in the gallbladder. Brown pigment stones, which are common in Asians, are the most common stone to appear de novo in the bile duct and are associated with biliary tract infection. Pigment stones, in contrast to cholesterol stones, are often radiopaque and can be seen on plain abdominal x-rays.

CHOLESTEROL GALLSTONE FORMATION

Cholesterol is a minor but clinically significant component of bile. The other components of bile are bile salts, phospholipids, conjugated bilirubin, fatty acids, water, electrolytes, and other organic and inorganic substances. Cholesterol is a hydrophobic molecule that is relatively insoluble in water and precipitates unless it is maintained in solution by bile salts. Bile salt molecules possess hydrophilic (water-soluble) and hydrophobic (fat-soluble) regions that maintain cholesterol in a soluble state.

When bile salt molecules in water reach concentrations of 2 to 4 mM, they form spherical complexes called micelles; the concentration at which micelles form is known as the critical micellar concentration (CMC). In micelles, the negatively charged hydrophilic ends of the molecules face outward, toward the water, and the uncharged hydrophobic regions face the center of the sphere, toward one another. Cholesterol molecules are enclosed in the hydrophobic interiors.

A pure bile salt micelle must comprise at least 50 molecules to enclose a single molecule of cholesterol. The intercalation of phospholipids, principally lecithin, between bile salt molecules improves the efficiency with which micelles solubilize cholesterol. Such a mixed micelle [see Figure 1], which is the type that exists in bile, needs only seven bile salt molecules to solubilize one cholesterol molecule. Free bile salt molecules exist in equilibrium with mixed micelles in a water solution. The combined molar concentration of bile salt and phospholipid is about 11 times that of cholesterol.

Cholesterol gallstone formation is potentiated by hepatic secretion of bile containing excess cholesterol relative to the concentration of bile salt.[1,4] This occurs most often because of an increase in the biliary concentration of cholesterol but may also result from decreased bile acid secretion in certain disease states. Excess cholesterol is solubilized in micelles and in vesicles composed of phospholipid bilayers. Cholesterol crystal formation seems to occur at the surface of these vesicles.

In addition to supersaturated bile, nucleation of crystals and gallbladder stasis are also important factors in gallstone formation. Microscopic crystals initially precipitate from a supersaturated bile in a process called nucleation, which is influenced by several pronucleating and antinucleating proteins.[1,4] Protein mucins, which are secreted by the gallbladder, and calcium are crucial promoters of the nucleation process. Prostaglandins stimulate the synthesis and secretion of mucins. Antinucleating factors, such as certain apolipoproteins, have been less well studied. Gallbladder stasis, with concentration and acidification of bile, is also an important factor in gallstone formation,

Table 1 Risk Factors for Cholesterol and Pigment Gallstone Formation

Cholesterol Gallstones	Pigment Gallstones
Increasing age	Increasing age
Female gender	Chronic hemolysis
Obesity	Alcoholic liver disease
Rapid weight loss	Biliary infection
Native-American heritage	Hyperalimentation (gallbladder stasis)
Hyperalimentation (gallbladder stasis)	Duodenal diverticulum
Elevated triglyceride levels	Truncal vagotomy
Medications (e.g., fibric acid derivatives, estrogens, octreotide)	Primary biliary cirrhosis
Ileal disease, resection, or bypass	

promoting the growth of cholesterol crystals into stones. Cholesterol stones rarely recur in patients after cholecystectomy.

Biliary sludge (or microlithiasis) is a term that is often applied to cholesterol crystals of sufficient number to be visualized on ultrasonography.[5] Biliary sludge is a mix of mucus, cholesterol monohydrate microcrystals, and calcium bilirubinate granules and is believed to be the precursor of most gallstones.[4,5] Gallbladder sludge and gallstones often form during pregnancy and in patients receiving parenteral nutrition; it is also associated with rapid weight loss.[1,4,5,8-10] Bile sludge has been shown to precipitate biliary colic, acute cholecystitis, or pancreatitis and should be regarded as part of the spectrum of gallstone disease. Common bile duct stones (choledocholithiasis) may form de novo in bile ducts (so-called primary, constituting 5% of bile duct stones) or migrate from the gallbladder to the biliary tract (secondary choledocholithiasis, constituting 95% of bile duct stones). Stones in the biliary tract usually have the same composition as those in the gallbladder, although some are softer and are brownish in color. The brown color is a result of deposition of calcium bilirubinate and other calcium salts as a result of bacterial deconjugation of bilirubin and hydrolysis of phospholipids. Choledocholithiasis is more common in Asian populations, owing to the increased prevalence of parasitic infections of the biliary tree (e.g., clonorchiasis, fascioliasis, and ascariasis).

Cholecystitis and Cholelithiasis

Patients who have stones in the gallbladder or the biliary tree display syndromes that range from acute disease to chronic symptomatic or silent disease. Most gallbladder stones remain silent throughout a person's lifetime. Diagnosis is further complicated by the fact that, with the exception of biliary colic, most symptoms of gallstones are not specific for gallstone disease.[11] At any stage of disease, obstruction of the cystic duct or common bile duct by a gallstone that has passed from the gallbladder may cause pain, with or without acute inflammation.

The most common symptom of gallstones is biliary colic—a misnomer, because the pain is steady and not colicky. The pain of biliary colic is caused by functional spasm of the cystic duct obstructed by a stone, whereas the pain of acute cholecystitis is caused by inflammation of the gallbladder wall.[1,2] Biliary colic often develops without any precipitating events. Typically, the pain is localized to the epigastrium, has a sudden onset, and increases rapidly in intensity to a plateau that can last as long as 3 hours before subsiding. Some patients describe the pain as excruciating or lancinating, whereas others describe it as a deep ache or cramp. The pain may radiate to the interscapular region or to the right shoulder, and it may be associated with nausea or vomiting. The pain is less frequently located in the left upper quadrant, precordium, or lower abdomen. Pain lasting longer than 6 hours or pain that is associated with fever suggests acute cholecystitis. Gastrointestinal symptoms, such as dyspepsia, heartburn, bloating, and fatty food intolerance, are common whether or not gallstones are present. Thus, the diagnosis of biliary colic is based on clinical judgment. Once an episode of biliary colic has occurred, repeated attacks of pain are common.

ACUTE CHOLECYSTITIS

Obstruction of the cystic duct by an impacted gallstone produces acute inflammation of the gallbladder. Cholelithiasis is

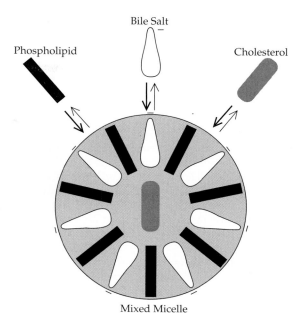

Figure 1 Cholesterol is solubilized in bile by the formation of mixed micelles that consist predominantly of bile salt and phospholipid. Micelles form when the concentration of bile salts in water is between 2 and 4 mM, the so-called critical micellar concentration (CMC). The negatively charged hydrophilic region of the bile salt molecule faces outward into the water phase, whereas the uncharged hydrophobic region is directed inward. These three components—bile salts, phospholipids, and cholesterol—exist in equilibrium between the free state and micelle constituents. At the CMC for bile salts, the equilibrium shifts strongly in the direction of the micelle. If bile salt concentrations are insufficient, the hydrophobic cholesterol molecules will precipitate to form a nidus for a gallstone.

present in 90% to 95% of patients with acute cholecystitis, and most patients have had previous attacks of biliary colic. Acute cholecystitis may present as an acalculous cholecystitis in 5% to 10% of patients. It is predominantly noted in older men who are critically ill following major surgery, severe trauma, or extensive burn injury.[12] Rarely, acute cholecystitis can result from a specific infection, such as that caused by *Salmonella* species. *Salmonella* organisms can also colonize the gallbladder epithelium without inflammation (carrier state). Cytomegalovirus and cryptosporidia can infect the biliary system, resulting in cholecystitis or cholangitis in immunocompromised patients, such as those with AIDS or those who have undergone bone marrow transplantation.

Diagnosis

Clinical manifestations Clinical features of acute cholecystitis include anorexia, nausea, vomiting, fever with temperatures of 38° to 39° C (100.4° to 102.2° F), severe abdominal pain that is initially localized to the epigastrium, and right upper quadrant tenderness. The pain typically lasts longer than 6 hours. Up to 15% of patients notice dark urine and scleral icterus. Most patients with jaundice have stones in the common bile duct at the time of surgery. Patients are ill for several days to a week before the acute attack completely subsides.

Physical examination Physical examination often reveals right upper quadrant subcostal tenderness and pain on inspiration, often with inspiratory arrest (the Murphy sign). The pain may spread to other areas of the abdomen. The gallbladder may be palpable, especially at the time of the first attack, before fibrosis has reduced its distensibility. Tenderness, guarding, and rebound pain in the area of an inflamed gallbladder are important findings. Generalized rebound tenderness in a patient who has been ill for several days may reflect a perforation; localized tenderness may indicate secondary pancreatitis or an abscess in the area of the gallbladder.

Laboratory evaluation Laboratory tests frequently reveal leukocytosis (leukocytes usually number 12,000 to 15,000/mm³). Serum bilirubin and alkaline phosphatase levels are elevated in 30% to 50% of patients. The serum amylase level is frequently increased even in the absence of clinically evident pancreatitis. An alanine aminotransferase level more than 2.5 times above normal is a reliable indicator of gallstone-induced pancreatitis.

Imaging studies Ultrasonography is the diagnostic procedure of choice for a patient with suspected gallstones and acute cholecystitis.[1,2,13] A meta-analysis revealed that ultrasonography has a sensitivity of 88% to 90% and a specificity of 97% to 98% for the diagnosis of gallstones greater than 2 mm in size.[14] Gallbladder ultrasonography should ideally be preceded by an 8-hour fast, because gallstones are best visualized in a distended, bile-filled gallbladder. In addition to detecting gallstones, ultrasonography can be used to identify other causes of right upper quadrant pain, such as hepatic abscess or malignancy, and it may reveal biliary duct obstruction. However, specific evidence of acute cholecystitis (i.e., the presence of pericholecystic fluid, edema of the gallbladder wall, or both) is found infrequently. Occasionally, a "sonographic Murphy sign" will be elicited when the ultrasound probe is positioned below the right costal margin.

Cholescintigraphy is the best method of confirming the clinical diagnosis of acute cholecystitis.[14] This procedure, which takes only 60 to 90 minutes, involves the intravenous injection of technetium-99m–labeled hepatoiminodiacetic acid (HIDA, or lidofenin), which is selectively excreted into the biliary tree and enters the gallbladder. In the presence of acute cholecystitis, radiolabeled material enters the common bile duct and duodenum but not the gallbladder. Meta-analysis confirms that radionuclide scanning is the most accurate method of diagnosing acute cholecystitis.[14] Occasionally, the scan gives false positive results in patients who have alcoholic liver disease or who are fasting or receiving total parenteral nutrition; however, false negative results are rare. Radionuclide scanning may not be useful for patients with deep jaundice, because the labeled agent fails to enter the biliary tree.

Direct examination of bile is more sensitive than ultrasonography in the diagnosis of biliary sludge. Ideally, cholecystokinin-induced gallbladder bile, rather than hepatic and ductal bile, should be obtained to maximize sensitivity for detecting sludge or microlithiasis. Bile must be centrifuged and examined under polarizing or light microscopy for detection of crystals. Bile sample is obtained during endoscopic retrograde cholangiopancreatography (ERCP) by aspiration through a catheter.

Plain abdominal x-rays are much less useful than cholescintigraphy or ultrasonography, because only 15% to 20% of stones are radiopaque; oral cholecystography is also less useful and is now rarely performed because it requires 24 to 48 hours to perform and is less accurate than ultrasonography.

Differential Diagnosis

The differential diagnosis of acute cholecystitis includes a number of diseases that are characterized by severe epigastric symptoms and transient abnormal results on liver function testing.

Severe acute viral hepatitis or alcoholic hepatitis may be associated with moderately severe right upper quadrant pain, fever, and leukocytosis. A history of acute alcoholism, the finding of a very large liver, or very high aminotransferase levels should help distinguish one of these diagnoses from acute cholecystitis.

A patient with a penetrating or perforating ulcer may have severe epigastric pain and usually has a history of ulcer; free air may be evident on a plain abdominal x-ray if the ulcer has perforated. Early in its course, acute appendicitis may produce symptoms similar to those of acute cholecystitis, particularly if the appendix is retrocecal or the cecum is malpositioned in the subhepatic area. Acute pyelonephritis of the right kidney may produce anterior pain similar to the pain that occurs with acute cholecystitis. Pneumonia or infarction of the right lung may also cause abdominal symptoms.

Acute pancreatitis may be nearly impossible to distinguish from acute cholecystitis. Patients with either disorder may exhibit moderate signs on physical examination, with tenderness or localized rebound pain in the epigastrium; serum amylase and lipase levels can be high in either condition, but the higher these enzyme levels are, the more likely it is that pancreatitis is present. Cholelithiasis occasionally causes pancreatitis,[15] which further complicates the diagnosis. At times, only the clinical course distinguishes pancreatitis from cholecystitis.

Treatment

Medical therapy Patients with a clinical diagnosis of acute cholecystitis should not be fed and should be given intravenous fluids and electrolytes. It is usually necessary to give a narcotic analgesic such as morphine or meperidine to alleviate severe pain. Febrile patients who have leukocytosis or bandemia (elevated circulating band forms) should be given a broad-spectrum antibiotic, such as a third-generation cephalosporin or, for broader coverage against *Enterococcus*, ampicillin-sulbactam or piperacillin-tazobactam. The usual course is one of gradual improvement for several days. Persistence of severe symptoms may indicate pericholecystic abscess formation or perforation.

Surgery The timing of surgery is controversial, although the weight of opinion favors semiurgent cholecystectomy after the patient's condition has been optimized.[16] Laparoscopic cholecystectomy has almost completely replaced the once-standard open cholecystectomy procedure.[6,17] In skilled hands, the laparoscopic procedure carries approximately the same risk as open cholecystectomy, but there is much less postoperative pain, and the convalescence period is much shorter.[18] In addition, laparoscopic cholecystectomy can be safely performed in patients with compensated cirrhosis of Child-Pugh class A.[19] Laparoscopic cholecystectomy is more expensive than minilaparotomy cholecystectomy, chiefly because of the higher cost of supplies.[20]

In about 5% of patients, the laparoscopic cholecystectomy has to be converted to open cholecystectomy, primarily because inflammation obscures the anatomy. The complication rate of laparoscopic cholecystectomy is approximately 5%, which is comparable to the rate reported for conventional cholecystectomy. Complications of laparoscopic cholecystectomy are more common when the surgeon is inexperienced.[21] Although mortality appears to be lower for laparoscopic cholecystectomy than for open cholecystectomy, the total number of cholecystectomy-related deaths has not decreased over the years, because more procedures are being done.[22-24] This suggests that the benefits of laparoscopic cholecystectomy have expanded the indications for cholecystectomy.

Cholangiography can be performed during laparoscopic biliary surgery. However, because patients with acute cholecystitis may have common duct stones, the physician should consider preoperative ERCP in patients with suspected choledocholithiasis (e.g., those patients with jaundice or a dilated common bile duct, as seen on ultrasound).[25] Common duct stones can be removed endoscopically. If endoscopic common duct stone removal is not possible, the operative procedure of choice is open cholecystectomy with common bile duct exploration and stone removal.

Prompt performance of laparoscopic cholecystectomy in acute cholecystitis is important because the increasing inflammatory changes that occur over time have been implicated in bile duct injury; these changes may necessitate converting the procedure to an open cholecystectomy.[18,26]

Some patients (e.g., those with septic shock, peritonitis, severe pancreatitis, portal hypertension, or marked clotting disorders or those in the third trimester of pregnancy) are not candidates for laparoscopic cholecystectomy. These patients should generally undergo either open cholecystectomy, if their condition permits, or simple cholecystostomy. Cholecystostomy involves extracting the stones and draining the biliary tree through a catheter left in the gallbladder. Cholangiography can be carried out later through this drainage catheter. More than 50% of patients who undergo cholecystostomy have another episode of biliary tract disease within 5 years. Future elective gallbladder removal is advisable for virtually all patients. A report suggests that simple ultrasound-guided percutaneous puncture and aspiration of the gallbladder may be as effective as open cholecystostomy in critically ill patients with acute cholecystitis.[27]

Surgery is contraindicated for some patients because of the presence of other serious medical problems. In these cases, conservative medical therapy, including the use of antibiotics, may be the only possible approach for the acute attack.

Complications

The major complications of acute cholecystitis are related to severe inflammation and necrosis of gallbladder tissue.[28] Jaundice in the absence of choledocholithiasis can be noted in 15% of patients with acute cholecystitis; the stone impacted in the cystic duct results in edema and swelling, leading to extrinsic compression of the common hepatic duct, the common bile duct, or both (Mirizzi syndrome).

Localized perforation and abscess Localized perforation and abscess formation are commonly found in patients who have severe symptoms that persist for many days. Such patients usually show localized right upper quadrant tenderness and rebound pain. Free perforation occurs in 1% to 2% of patients with acute cholecystitis and is associated with a mortality of 30%. A delay in the diagnosis of acute cholecystitis can result in a distended gallbladder with clear mucoid fluid (hydrops of the gallbladder).

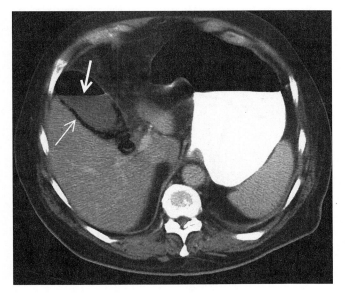

Figure 2 CT scan from an elderly man with nausea and abdominal pain following an acute myocardial infarction, angioplasty, and stent placement. The scan shows air in the wall of the gallbladder and an air-fluid level within the gallbladder, diagnostic of emphysematous cholecystitis. The patient was treated with antibiotics and a percutaneous cholecystostomy tube; laparoscopic cholecystectomy was planned in a few months.

Empyema Empyema of the gallbladder occurs in 2% to 3% of patients with acute cholecystitis.[29] Typically, abdominal pain is severe and lasts for more than 7 days. The physical examination is not distinctive. Mortality approaches 25%; death often occurs as a result of septicemia.

Emphysematous cholecystitis Emphysematous cholecystitis, which has a higher morbidity than uncomplicated acute cholecystitis, is usually caused by gas-forming bacteria, such as *Clostridium perfringens* and other clostridia, *Escherichia coli,* or anaerobic streptococci. Patients who have such infections are often very ill, and 20% also have diabetes or are compromised by coexisting conditions. Emphysematous cholecystitis occurs three times more often in men than in women. Many cases of this type of cholecystitis are not associated with cholelithiasis. A plain abdominal x-ray or CT scan frequently reveals gas within the gallbladder [*see Figure 2*].

Cholecystenteric fistula Another possible complication of acute cholecystitis is a cholecystenteric fistula, in which the gallbladder is connected either to the duodenum or the hepatic flexure of the colon. In rare cases, the gallbladder communicates directly with the stomach or jejunum. A large gallstone (> 2.5 cm in diameter) will erode through the gallbladder wall into the duodenum. Subsequently, the stone may become impacted at the terminal ileum, causing small bowel obstruction, or in the duodenal bulb, resulting in gastric outlet obstruction (Bouveret syndrome). Treatment of cholecystenteric fistula usually consists of one-stage cholecystectomy, exploration of the common bile duct, closure of the fistula, and extraction of the impacted stone.

Gallstones and malignancy Gallstones are present in 80% of patients with gallbladder cancer, although it is not clear

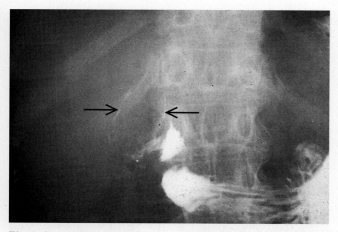

Figure 3 **Radiograph of the right upper abdominal quadrant during upper GI barium study showing a calcified wall of the gallbladder ("porcelain" gallbladder), indicating chronic cholecystitis and a high risk of gallbladder cancer.**

whether gallstones themselves are the causal factor. A palpable gallbladder is usually found in malignant obstruction of the common bile duct (Courvoisier's law) and is uncommon with obstruction from gallstones.

CHRONIC CHOLECYSTITIS

Chronic cholelithiasis is usually accompanied by evidence of chronic cholecystitis. The wall of the gallbladder is often thickened, fibrotic, and rigid, and the gallbladder is thus prevented from contracting and expanding normally. This condition may arise from a series of attacks of acute cholecystitis, from chronic mechanical irritation by calculi, or from both. The gallbladder wall may calcify and appear as the so-called porcelain gallbladder on plain abdominal x-ray [*see Figure 3*].

Diagnosis

Clinical manifestations It is difficult to attribute any symptom to chronic cholecystitis per se. Complaints of flatulence, heartburn, and nonspecific postprandial distress are common in patients with chronic cholecystitis, but such symptoms are also common in patients with no evidence of gallbladder disease. It is possible, however, to elicit a history of discrete attacks of abdominal pain resembling those of acute cholecystitis.

Physical examination Findings on physical examination are usually normal unless the patient is experiencing an acute attack of cholecystitis. The gallbladder is rarely palpable, because the scarring associated with chronic cholecystitis prevents expansion.

Laboratory evaluation Results of routine laboratory tests are usually normal; occasionally, the serum alkaline phosphatase level is modestly elevated.

Imaging studies Ultrasonography is the procedure of choice for the diagnosis of chronic gallbladder disease. In 90% to 95% of cases of cholelithiasis, ultrasonography demonstrates the echo of the calculus and the acoustic shadow behind the calculus [*see Figure 4*]. When the ultrasonogram is nondiagnostic, oral cholecystography may still be used to evaluate a

patient with suspected gallbladder disease. If a double dose of the oral contrast agent fails to cause gallbladder opacification, cholelithiasis and chronic cholecystitis are almost certainly present. Cholescintigraphy [*see* Acute Cholecystitis, *above*] is not helpful in diagnosing chronic cholelithiasis or chronic cholecystitis.

ERCP may reveal gallstones in the gallbladder of patients who have biliary tract pain and whose oral cholecystograms and gallbladder ultrasonograms are normal. In one study, small gallstones were found with ERCP in 29 of 206 such patients (14%); the presence of these stones was confirmed during surgery.[30] CT or MRI may also detect gallstones, but these techniques are unlikely to demonstrate stones not detected by ultrasonography.

Additional tests Duodenal drainage may be useful for establishing a diagnosis of gallstones.[31] This test entails checking the duodenal sediment for cholesterol crystals and calcium bilirubinate granules. Typical cholesterol crystals resemble a rectangular windowpane with one corner cut off. Bilirubinate granules are yellow-brown and amorphous. False positive test results may occur in patients with liver disease.

Treatment

Surgery Elective cholecystectomy is indicated for patients who have symptomatic gallstones and chronic cholecystitis. Recurrent pain is to be expected in these patients if cholecystectomy is not performed. As many as 50% of patients with surgically untreated symptomatic gallstones experience serious complications within 20 years of initial onset of symptoms.[32]

It is occasionally difficult to determine whether abdominal symptoms are secondary to documented gallbladder disease. A history of typical recurrent pain makes this determination easier. In certain cases, elective cholecystectomy is performed as a last diagnostic procedure when a thorough search for other causes of abdominal symptoms has proved negative. All too often, the symptoms recur postoperatively.

Oral dissolution therapy Ursodiol (ursodeoxycholic acid), administered orally for 6 to 12 months, results in the dissolu-

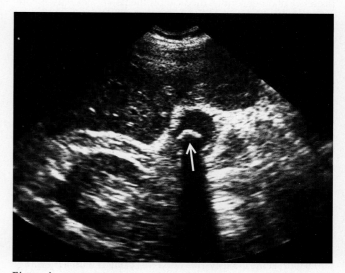

Figure 4 **Ultrasound of the gallbladder showing, in the center of the image, a stone within the gallbladder with a triangular area of acoustic attenuation ("shadowing") behind the gallstone.**

tion of 60% to 90% of susceptible stones. However, this drug is effective only in patients with floating cholesterol stones and a functioning gallbladder, making this treatment applicable to perhaps 15% of patients with symptomatic stones. Moreover, in patients who can benefit from ursodiol, half the stones recur after therapy ceases. Low-dose, long-term therapy with ursodiol may help prevent this recurrence, but such therapy is effective only in patients younger than 50 years.[33] Ursodiol has few side effects. Infusing methyl *tert*-butyl ether through a transhepatic catheter directly into the gallbladder can rapidly dissolve cholesterol stones.[34] The rapid infusion and removal of this ether, which remains liquid at body temperature, results in the dissolution of most cholesterol gallstones within 4 to 31 hours. Dissolution therapy has limited value except in patients who are poor candidates for surgery.

Extracorporeal biliary lithotripsy Stones in the gallbladder or common bile duct have been successfully fragmented using extracorporeal biliary lithotripsy (i.e., shock waves), a technique widely employed for the nonsurgical fragmentation of kidney stones.[35-37] Patients are carefully positioned and monitored so that the shock waves are targeted at the gallstones. Almost all stones show some fragmentation after treatment, but the resultant fragments are smaller than 5 mm in diameter in fewer than half of treated patients.[36] The administration of ursodiol after fragmentation of stones has been associated with an increase in the percentage of patients who are free of gallbladder stones 6 months after lithotripsy.[35,36] In one study, 21% of patients who received 10 to 12 mg/kg of ursodiol daily for 6 months after lithotripsy were free of gallbladder stones; in contrast, of patients who received placebo for 6 months, only 9% were free of stones.[36] Stone fragments in the common bile duct may pass spontaneously after endoscopic sphincterotomy or can be extracted with a Dormia basket. The side effects of lithotripsy are generally not serious and include biliary pain, pancreatitis, and hematuria. Given the widespread availability of laparoscopic cholecystectomy, the usefulness of lithotripsy is now limited. The patients most likely to benefit are the elderly with radiolucent, solitary gallstones less than 30 mm in diameter.[37]

ASYMPTOMATIC CHOLELITHIASIS

Most gallstones are asymptomatic. In one prospective study, gallstones or evidence of previous cholecystectomy was present in 291 of 1,701 persons (17.1%) who were examined post mortem.[38] Of these 291 persons, only 31 had undergone cholecystectomy, presumably because of symptomatic disease. Ten deaths were directly attributable to the gallstones; four of these deaths occurred after cholecystectomy.

Natural History

Silent gallstones seldom lead to problems. In a long-term follow-up study of asymptomatic patients, the cumulative risk of the development of symptoms was 10% at 5 years, 15% at 10 years, and 18% at 15 years or later.[39] Nineteen percent of patients who experienced symptoms (2.5% of the entire group) subsequently developed acute cholecystitis or pancreatitis. No patients died of gallbladder disease during a mean follow-up period of more than 10 years. The results of this study support a conservative, nonsurgical approach to the patient with truly silent gallstones.

Diagnosis

Asymptomatic gallstones are usually identified incidentally with abdominal or pelvic ultrasonography performed for other diagnostic purposes, such as the evaluation of gynecologic symptoms or findings on physical examination.

Treatment

Patients who have asymptomatic gallstones should generally be managed conservatively. Cholecystectomy is generally not indicated. Exceptions may be made for patients at increased risk for gallbladder cancer, such as Pima Indians, persons with calcified gallbladders (porcelain gallbladder), those with very large gallstones (> 3 cm), and patients with an associated gallbladder polyp greater than 10 mm in diameter.[40] If an asymptomatic patient subsequently experiences two or more attacks of abdominal pain typical of gallbladder disease, cholecystectomy should be performed to avoid the later development of serious and sometimes fatal complications. Surgery is not always necessary after the first episode, because as many as 30% of such patients experience no further pain.

In the past, prophylactic cholecystectomy was recommended for diabetic patients who had asymptomatic gallstones; anecdotal reports suggested that such patients did poorly when cholecystectomy was performed as an emergency procedure. However, two well-controlled retrospective studies of patients undergoing surgery for acute cholecystitis and a decision analysis showed that diabetes was not an independent risk factor of operative mortality or serious postoperative complications, and prophylactic cholecystectomy resulted in a shortened life span.[41,42] Thus, prophylactic cholecystectomy cannot be recommended for patients with diabetes.

CHOLEDOCHOLITHIASIS

Choledocholithiasis, a condition in which a stone lodges in the common bile duct after passage from the gallbladder through the cystic duct, develops secondary to chronic cholelithiasis in 15% to 20% of patients.[1,2,43] Stones usually lodge at the point of insertion of the duct into the ampulla of Vater. Primary (de novo) common bile duct stones are more common in Asian populations than in the Western world. Asians are predisposed to primary common bile duct stones because of the increased prevalence of flukes and parasitic infections (clonorchiasis, fascioliasis, ascariasis). Periampullary diverticuli and advancing age are risk factors for choledocholithiasis.

Diagnosis

Clinical manifestations Choledocholithiasis may be complicated by cholangitis, characterized by the triad of fever with shaking chills, jaundice, and right upper quadrant colicky pain. Pain may be severe, have a rapid onset, and last 15 to 60 minutes. It is usually accompanied by nausea and vomiting.

Sometimes, patients with choledocholithiasis present with only jaundice. A history of pain suggestive of cholecystitis or biliary colic may be the only other initial clue that common duct stones are present. Not all stones obstruct the duct; some move up and down the biliary tree, some cause acute (biliary) pancreatitis, and some pass via the common bile duct into the duodenum.

Physical examination Findings on physical examination may resemble those of acute cholecystitis. Often, the findings are less marked, and guarding is moderate in the midepigastri-

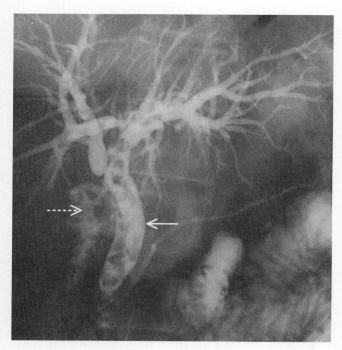

Figure 5 **Endoscopic retrograde cholangiopancreatography reveals abnormalities in a patient with gallstones. Multiple radiolucent areas establish the diagnosis of stones in the gallbladder (broken arrow) and common bile duct (solid arrow).**

um or right upper quadrant. Sometimes, no abnormalities are noted. Hepatomegaly may be found when common bile duct obstruction has been present for some time.

Laboratory evaluation   Laboratory test results are usually abnormal; both serum bilirubin and alkaline phosphatase levels rise markedly and abruptly. However, when the stones do not obstruct the duct, the serum bilirubin level may rise only slightly or not at all, whereas the alkaline phosphatase level is substantially elevated. Aminotransferase levels are typically only modestly elevated. In rare instances, they exceed 1,000 IU/L, rising and falling rapidly early in the course of bile duct obstruction.

Elevated serum bilirubin and alkaline phosphatase levels are associated with cholestasis of many causes, not just biliary tract stones. Thus, more definitive procedures must be undertaken to determine whether stones are present.

Imaging studies   Although ultrasonography is the gold standard for the diagnosis of stones in the gallbladder, it is less sensitive in choledocholithiasis and may detect only 50% of common bile duct stones.[44,45] However, ultrasonography can often reveal a dilated common bile duct and biliary tree. The dilatation may be missed, however, particularly when extensive bowel gas is present. Using 6 mm as the upper limit of normal for the diameter of the common bile duct, the sensitivity of ultrasonography for choledocholithiasis, with assessment based on duct dilatation, is only 76%. Standard CT is no more sensitive or specific than ultrasonography. Cholescintigraphy may show common bile duct obstruction, particularly when symptoms are of recent onset and the likelihood of parenchymal liver disease is low. None of these three procedures, however, reliably delineates the site of obstruction or the location of common bile duct stones.

Two techniques allow direct visualization of the biliary tree. ERCP allows radiographic visualization of the biliary tree in 85% to 95% of cases [*see Figure 5*] and provides both diagnostic capabilities and the option of therapeutic intervention.[46,47] For these reasons, ERCP is the test of choice for the diagnosis and treatment of choledocholithiasis. Percutaneous transhepatic cholangiography (PTC) involves the use of a small-bore needle, which makes it possible to enter even nondilated ducts.[48] The success rate of PTC in patients with dilated ducts is close to 100%; nondilated ducts are entered successfully about 70% of the time. The complication rates for both PTC and ERCP approach 5%, but death is rare. ERCP has replaced PTC as the technique of choice.

An alternative diagnostic procedure for the diagnosis of choledocholithiasis is MR cholangiography.[49,50] MR cholangiography provides good-quality images, is noninvasive, and does not have the potential complications of ERCP or PTC [*see Figure 6*].

Direct visualization of the biliary tree is not warranted in all patients with cholestasis. If the clinical evaluation indicates that the likelihood of biliary tract disease is small, a normal ultrasonogram should preclude invasive workup of the biliary tree. When biliary tract disease is considered likely or is the only treatable alternative, direct visualization of the ducts must be undertaken.

Differential Diagnosis

Acute obstruction of the common bile duct by a stone may clinically resemble ureterolithiasis because of the similarities in location and severity of pain. Liver function tests easily distinguish the two conditions.

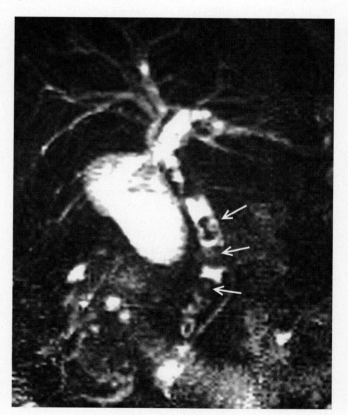

Figure 6   **This magnetic resonance cholangiopancreatogram shows multiple gallstones (arrows) in the common bile duct (choledocholithiasis).**

Acute inflammation of the head of the pancreas may produce temporary obstruction of the common bile duct. Diagnosis of pancreatic head inflammation can usually be made on the basis of an ultrasound study or CT scan. Also, ERCP helps distinguish pancreatitis from choledocholithiasis. Definitive diagnosis may not be possible until the patient has undergone several days of treatment with nasogastric suction, which would allow the pancreatic edema to subside.

Persons with acute myocardial infarction can experience abdominal pain that mimics that of biliary tract disease. Patients with viral or toxic hepatitis may have intrahepatic cholestasis, but these patients usually do not have severe abdominal pain.

Acute intermittent porphyria can cause severe abdominal pain but does not result in strikingly elevated serum alkaline phosphatase or bilirubin levels. A large hepatic abscess or enlarged nodes located in the porta hepatis may obstruct major bile ducts. Carcinomas can develop at the bifurcation of the common bile duct. In such cases, the history is usually one of chronic vague right upper quadrant discomfort rather than sudden severe colic.

Treatment

Endoscopic sphincterotomy should be the initial treatment for the patient with choledocholithiasis. In one large study, sphincterotomy was successful in 97.5% of patients with common bile duct stones, although more than one attempt was necessary in some patients. The overall rate of clearance of bile duct stones was 84.5%. The remaining patients required either surgery or permanent placement of a biliary endoprosthesis. The overall complication rate was 6.9%, and the complications included bleeding, cholangitis, pancreatitis, and perforation. The 30-day procedure-related mortality was 0.6%.[51] Follow-up studies have shown a low rate of recurrence of biliary duct problems and a low incidence of papillary stenosis.[52] Operative exploration of the common duct should be reserved for the few patients in whom endoscopic sphincterotomy is unsuccessful. Laparoscopic removal of biliary stones may be an alternative to preoperative ERCP.[53,54]

Sphincterotomy is also the treatment of choice for patients with retained bile duct stones after gallbladder or biliary tract surgery. If sphincterotomy fails and if the patient has a T tube in place, instrumental extraction through the mature T-tube tract may be successful. If nonsurgical treatments fail, surgical exploration of the biliary tree is indicated.

In one study, patients with acute biliary pancreatitis were shown to benefit from endoscopic sphincterotomy early in the clinical course[55]; in another study, no benefit was found.[56]

Chronic Biliary Tract Disease

A small percentage of patients with chronic cholelithiasis and its complications or other chronic diseases of the biliary ducts experience associated chronic inflammation or a stricturing process in the biliary tree. The usual cause of chronic inflammation of the biliary tree is partial or complete obstruction of the biliary ducts.

DIAGNOSTIC AND MANAGEMENT OVERVIEW

Patients with chronic inflammation of the biliary tree may complain of fatigue, intermittent chills and fever, anorexia, and, at times, weight loss. Physical examination is likely to re-

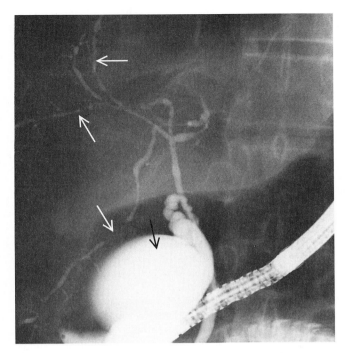

Figure 7   **This cholangiogram, obtained during endoscopic retrograde cholangiopancreatography, shows a normal gallbladder (black arrow) and a narrowed biliary tree with many areas of segmental stenosis (white arrows), diagnostic of primary sclerosing cholangitis.**

veal little, although generalized excoriations of the skin related to marked pruritus may be seen.

Laboratory tests often reveal chronically elevated serum alkaline phosphatase levels and increased levels of serum 5′-nucleotidase, leucine aminopeptidase, and γ-glutamyl transpeptidase. When shaking chills and fever develop, serum alkaline phosphatase levels may rise further, and transient jaundice may occur. Direct visualization of the biliary tree is important in determining whether the symptoms and signs result from an anatomic defect that can be corrected by endoscopic therapy or surgery. Use of ERCP usually leads to identification of the obstructive site. Patients with discrete lesions can be treated endoscopically or by surgical decompression. When surgical correction is delayed too long or cannot be performed, the chronic inflammation becomes irreversible and secondary biliary cirrhosis develops.

Chronic inflammation of the biliary tree occurs in a wide variety of duct diseases. These include common duct stricture, recurrent choledocholithiasis, primary sclerosing cholangitis, choledochal cyst, recurrent pyogenic cholangitis, and pancreatic or biliary duct cancer.

SPECIFIC PRESENTATIONS

Common Bile Duct Stricture

Benign and malignant strictures have similar morphologic appearance, as imaged by ERCP. Thus, epithelial sampling of all biliary strictures is necessary. A variety of techniques are available for epithelial sampling of biliary strictures, including brush cytology, fine-needle aspiration, endoscopic pinch forceps biopsy, and aspiration brush biopsy. The sensitivity of brush cytology is as high as 70% for the diagnosis of a malignant stricture of the bile duct; specificity is as high as 100%. Simple bile aspiration alone is not as reliable. New methods, such as measurement of tumor markers in bile and pancreatic juice or the use of polymerase chain reaction, have shown promising results in differentiating benign from malignant biliary disease in a number of preliminary studies. Common bile duct stricture, which may result from biliary tract surgery, can be treated endoscopically with balloon dilation or with the placement of an endoprosthesis. If either of these treatments is unsuccessful, surgical intervention may prove beneficial for selected patients.

Primary Sclerosing Cholangitis

Primary sclerosing cholangitis is a disease of unknown etiology that is characterized by an irregular inflammatory fibrosis of both the intrahepatic and the extrahepatic bile ducts [see Figure 7].[57] It typically occurs in men 20 to 50 years of age who have one or more of the following symptoms: jaundice, pruritus, nonspecific pain, fever, and weight loss. Chronic ulcerative colitis is present or will develop in three quarters of patients. Liver function tests show cholestatic abnormalities. The 8-year survival of asymptomatic patients is about 80%, and the survival of symptomatic patients is about 50%. Most studies reporting the effects of ursodiol therapy show an improvement in the biochemical markers of cholestasis, but a recent randomized, controlled trial that included close to 100 patients showed no survival benefit.[58] Endoscopic treatment of major ductal strictures may also improve liver function test results and reduce the number of episodes of cholangitis.[59] A combined therapeutic approach employing stricture dilation and ursodiol appears beneficial in selected patients.[60] The incidence of cholangiocarcinoma in patients with primary sclerosing cholangitis is as high as 30%, and there is an increased risk of gallbladder cancer and pancreatic cancer.[61,62] A substantial number of patients with primary sclerosing cholangitis may have undetected cholangiocarcinoma at the time of liver transplantation.

Pyogenic Cholangitis

Repeated attacks of fever, chills, abdominal pain, and jaundice characterize recurrent pyogenic cholangitis. The illness is commonly seen in East Asia and sometimes in immigrants to the United States. Although the exact etiology is unclear, it is known that the parasites Opisthorchis sinensis and Ascaris lumbricoides are commonly found in the stools of affected patients. Treatment consists of antibiotics and operative improvement of biliary drainage, but results are often unsuccessful.

Choledochal Cyst

Biliary cystic disease includes choledochal cyst disease and the less common gallbladder cysts and cystic duct cysts.[63] Choledochal cyst is an ectasia of the common bile duct that may present in late childhood or in adult life as obstructive jaundice. Choledochal cysts may involve any segment of the bile duct and are categorized according to the classification proposed by Todani and colleagues [see Table 2]. An abnormal pancreatobiliary duct junction is more common in patients with choledochal cysts and could expose the bile ducts to pancreatic juices and abnormally high pressures. The etiology, natural history, and management of the choledochal cyst vary with its type. Type I cysts are the most common, accounting for 40% to 60% of all cases, followed by type IV. Types II, III and V are rare.

Diagnosis The classic clinical presentation of type I, II, and IV choledochal cyst disease includes a triad of abdominal pain, mass, and jaundice. However, the typical presentation often includes only one or two of these findings. Fever is also a common presenting symptom. Patients with type III disease often present with recurrent biliary pain or pancreatitis, whereas patients with type V disease usually present with recurrent cholangitis and liver abscesses, pain, and fever. Type V disease is further classified into two subtypes. In the simple type, also known as Caroli disease, cyst formations are limited to the larger intrahepatic bile ducts and patients do not develop portal hypertension or cirrhosis. In the periportal fibrosis type, also known as Caroli syndrome, hepatic fibrosis, cirrhosis, and portal hypertension develop. Caroli syndrome is more common than Caroli disease.

Treatment The initial management of patients with choledochal cysts depends on the age of the patient, the presentation, and the type of the cyst. For example, children with a palpable choledochal cyst should undergo elective surgery; acute suppurative cholangitis should be managed with broad-spectrum antibiotics and endoscopic/percutaneous biliary decompression; and severe biliary pancreatitis might require ERCP followed by resection of the cyst.[64] Patients with extrahepatic bile duct cysts have an increased incidence of an anomalous pancreaticobiliary junction. Identification of the pancreatic duct insertion by a preoperative ERCP is critical in planning the surgical management. Type I and IVB choledochal cysts, which are completely extrahepatic, should be excised and reconstructed using Roux-en-Y jejunal anastomosis [see Table 2]. The preferred approach for type III cysts varies with the presentation. In general, endoscopic sphincterotomy will usually suffice for biliary and pancreatic symptoms, whereas resection will be required for duodenal obstruction. Cholecystectomy must be

Table 2 Modified Classification System for Choledochal Cysts and Surgical Procedure of Choice

Classification	Type	Procedure of Choice
Type I A	Choledochal cyst	Roux-en-Y hepaticojejunostomy
Type I B	Segmented choledochal dilatation	
Type I C	Diffuse or cylindrical duct dilatation	
Type II	Extrahepatic duct diverticulum	Excision of diverticulum
Type III	Choledochocele	Endoscopic sphincterotomy
Type IVA	Multiple intrahepatic and extrahepatic duct cysts	Roux-en-Y hepaticojejunostomy
Type IVB	Multiple extrahepatic duct cysts	
Type V	Intrahepatic duct cysts (Caroli disease and Caroli syndrome)	Hepatic resection, liver transplantation

*All patients with choledochal cysts must undergo cholecystectomy to decrease the risk of malignancy, with the possible exception of patients with type III cysts. For the much rarer gallbladder and cystic duct cysts, treatment is cholecystectomy.

Table 3 Clinical Classification System for Biliary-Specific Abdominal Pain Associated with SOD*

Criteria

A. Typical biliary-type pain
B. Elevated liver enzyme levels (AST, alkaline phosphatase, or both more than two times normal on at least two occasions)
C. Delayed drainage of contrast injection during ERCP (> 45 min)
D. Dilated common bile duct (> 12 mm)

Classification Based on above Criteria

Biliary type I: criteria A through D are present; SOD is present in 80%–90% of patients
Biliary type II : criterion A plus one or two other criteria are present; SOD is present in 50% of patients
Biliary type III: only criterion A is present; SOD is uncommon

---

*A similar classification for SOD and pancreatic-type abdominal pain exists but is not included in this table.
AST — aspartate aminotransferase   ERCP — endoscopic retrograde cholangiopancreatography   SOD — sphincter of Oddi dysfunction

---

performed in all patients to reduce the risk of cancer; the only possible exception to this is patients with type III cysts. Some patients with type IVA and V cysts will require liver resection for unilateral disease or liver transplantation for bilateral disease if severe recurrent sepsis or end-stage liver disease develops. The short- and long-term outcome from early surgical resection of choledochal cysts is excellent. However, patients with biliary cystic disease with cholangiocarcinoma or gallbladder cancer on presentation usually have a poor prognosis. The complications of choledochal cyst disease include gallstones, acute cholecystitis, pancreatitis, recurrent cholangitis, cholangiocarcinoma, and carcinoma of the gallbladder. Rarer complications include cirrhosis, portal hypertension, portal vein thrombosis, spontaneous cyst rupture, and pancreatic cancer.

Sphincter of Oddi Dysfunction

A syndrome of chronic abdominal pain after cholecystomy with features of partial common duct obstruction has been attributed to dysfunction of the sphincter of Oddi.[65] Sphincter of Oddi dysfunction (SOD) is an acquired condition resulting from partial obstruction of the sphincter of Oddi because of sphincter stenosis or dyskinesia. A classification of SOD is shown [see Table 3].

Diagnosis   ERCP is most useful to exclude the presence of other pancreatobiliary diseases, to measure the sphincter pressure, and to ablate the sphincter if an abnormally high pressure is found. SOD is most accurately diagnosed by manometry of the sphincter itself. A basal sphincter of Oddi pressure greater than 40 mm Hg is diagnostic. SOD may also cause biliary pain. In the absence of manometry, other less reliable, noninvasive tests may also indicate the presence of SOD. These include a provocation test using morphine (or neostigmine), which produces biliary pain and enzyme elevation; ultrasound evaluation of dilatation and emptying of the common bile duct after secretin stimulation; or the kinetics of ductal emptying studied by scintigraphy.

Sphincter of Oddi manometry is not required to confirm the diagnosis in biliary type I SOD. However, patients with biliary

type II SOD should undergo sphincter of Oddi manometry because only 50% of patients in this group have SOD [see Table 3]. In biliary type II SOD, only patients whose SOD is confirmed by sphincter of Oddi manometry should undergo endoscopic sphincterotomy. Sphincter of Oddi manometry, endoscopic sphincterotomy, or both have low efficacy in patients with biliary type III SOD.

Treatment   Over 90% of patients with biliary type I SOD will have a favorable response to endoscopic sphincterotomy. The sphincter of Oddi has three parts: the sphincter choledochus, the sphincter pancreaticus, and the common sphincter. Sphincterotomy may be performed in any part or parts of the sphincter. Air in the bile duct (pneumobilia) is a normal finding after an endoscopic sphincterotomy.[66] Other therapies for SOD, such as a low-fat diet, pharmacotherapy (analgesics, nitrates, calcium channel blockers, anticholinergics), other endoscopic therapies (balloon dilation, injection of botulinum toxin, temporary stent placement), and surgical sphincteroplasty have not gained popularity.

References

1. Johnston DE, Kaplan MM: Pathogenesis and treatment of gallstones. N Engl J Med 328:412, 1993
2. Ahmed A, Cheung RC, Keeffe EB: Management of gallstones and their complications. Am Fam Physician 61:1673, 2000
3. Jensen KH, Jorgensen T: Incidence of gallstones in a Danish population. Gastroenterology 100:790, 1991
4. Donovan JM: Physical and metabolic factors in gallstone pathogenesis. Gastroenterol Clin North Am 28:75, 1999
5. Ko CW, Sekijima JH, Lee SP: Biliary sludge. Ann Intern Med 130:301, 1999
6. Everhart JE, Khare M, Hill M, et al: Prevalence and ethnic differences in gallbladder disease in the United States. Gastroenterology 117:632, 1999
7. Trotman BW: Pigment gallstone disease. Gastroenterol Clin North Am 20:111, 1991
8. Yang H, Petersen GM, Roth M-P, et al: Risk factors for gallstone formation during rapid loss of weight. Dig Dis Sci 37:912, 1992
9. Davis A, Katz VL, Cox R: Gallbladder disease in pregnancy. J Reprod Med 40:759, 1995
10. Quigley EM, Marsh MN, Shaffer JL, et al: Hepatobiliary complications of total parenteral nutrition. Gastroenterology 104:286, 1993
11. Berger MY, van der Velden JJ, Lijmer JG, et al: Abdominal symptoms: do they predict gallstones? A systematic review. Scand J Gastroenterol 35:70, 2000
12. Frazee RC, Nagorney DM, Mucha P Jr: Acute acalculous cholecystitis. Mayo Clin Proc 64:163, 1989
13. Bortoff GA, Chen MY, Ott DJ, et al: Gallbladder stones: imaging and intervention. Radiographics 20:751, 2000
14. Shea JA, Berlin JA, Escarce JJ, et al: Revised estimates of diagnostic test sensitivity and specificity in suspected biliary tract disease. Arch Intern Med 154:2573, 1994
15. Soetikno RM, Carr-Locke DL: Endoscopic management of acute gallstone pancreatitis. Gastrointest Endosc Clin North Am 8:1, 1998
16. Tait N, Little JM: The treatment of gall stones. BMJ 311:99, 1995
17. A prospective analysis of 1518 laparoscopic cholecystectomies. The Southern Surgeons Club. N Engl J Med 324:1073, 1991
18. Zacks SL, Sandler RS, Rutledge R, et al: A population-based cohort study comparing laparoscopic cholecystectomy and open cholecystectomy. Am J Gastroenterol 97:226, 2002
19. Poggio JL, Rowland CM, Gores GJ, et al: A comparison of laparoscopic and open cholecystectomy in patients with compensated cirrhosis and symptomatic gallstone disease. Surgery 127:405, 2000
20. McMahon AJ, Russell IT, Baxter JN, et al: Laparoscopic versus minilaparotomy cholecystectomy: a randomised trial. Lancet 343:135, 1994
21. See WA, Cooper CS, Fisher RJ: Predictors of laparoscopic complications after formal training in laparoscopic surgery. JAMA 270:2689, 1993
22. Legorreta AP, Silber JH, Costantino GN, et al: Increased cholecystectomy rate after the introduction of laparoscopic cholecystectomy. JAMA 270:1429, 1993
23. Steiner CA, Bass EB, Talamini MA, et al: Surgical rates and operative mortality for open and laparoscopic cholecystectomy in Maryland. N Engl J Med 330:403, 1994
24. Escarce JJ, Chen W, Schwartz JS: Falling cholecystectomy thresholds since the introduction of laparoscopic cholecystectomy. JAMA 273:1581, 1995
25. Aliperti G, Edmundowicz SA, Soper NJ, et al: Combined endoscopic sphincterotomy and laparoscopic cholecystectomy in patients with choledocholithiasis and cholecystolithiasis. Ann Intern Med 115:783, 1991

26. Wiesen SM, Unger SW, Barkin JS: Laparoscopic cholecystectomy: the procedure of choice for acute cholecystitis. Am J Gastroenterol 88:334, 1993

27. Verbanck JJ, Demol JW, Ghillebert GL, et al: Ultrasound-guided puncture of the gallbladder for acute cholecystitis. Lancet 341:1132, 1993

28. Abou-Saif A, Al-Kawas FH: Complications of gallstone disease: Mirizzi syndrome, cholecystocholedochal fistula, and gallstone ileus. Am J Gastroenterol 97:249, 2002

29. Thornton JR, Heaton KW, Espiner HJ, et al: Empyema of the gall bladder: reappraisal of a neglected disease. Gut 24:1183, 1983

30. Venu RP, Geenen JE, Toouli J, et al: Endoscopic retrograde cholangiopancreatography: diagnosis of cholelithiasis in patients with normal gallbladder x-ray and ultrasound studies. JAMA 249:758, 1983

31. Delchier JC, Benfredj P, Preaux AM, et al: The usefulness of microscopic bile examination in patients with suspected microlithiasis: a prospective evaluation. Hepatology 6:118, 1986

32. Wenckert A, Robertson B: The natural course of gallstone disease: eleven-year review of 781 nonoperated cases. Gastroenterology 50:376, 1966

33. Villanova N, Bazzoli F, Taroni F, et al: Gallstone recurrence after successful oral bile acid treatment: a 12-year follow-up study and evaluation of long-term postdissolution treatment. Gastroenterology 97:726, 1989

34. Thistle JL, May GR, Bender CE, et al: Dissolution of cholesterol gallbladder stones by methyl tert-butyl ether administered by percutaneous transhepatic catheter. N Engl J Med 320:633, 1989

35. Tsumita R, Sugiura N, Abe A, et al: Long-term evaluation of extracorporeal shockwave lithotripsy for cholesterol gallstones. J Gastroenterol Hepatol 16:93, 2001

36. Schoenfield LJ, Berci G, Carnovale RL, et al: The effect of ursodiol on the efficacy and safety of extracorporeal shock-wave lithotripsy of gallstones: the Dornier National Biliary Lithotripsy Study. N Engl J Med 323:1239, 1990

37. Mulagha E, Fromm H: Extracorporeal shock wave lithotripsy of gallstones revisited: current status and future promises. J Gastroenterol Hepatol 15:239, 2000

38. Godrey PJ, Bates T, Harrison M, et al: Gall stones and mortality: a study of all gall stone related deaths in a single health district. Gut 25:1029, 1984

39. Gracie WA, Ransohoff DF: The natural history of silent gallstones: the innocent gallstone is not a myth. N Engl J Med 307:798, 1982

40. Guidelines for the treatment of gallstones. American College of Physicians. Ann Intern Med 119:620, 1993

41. Ransohoff DF, Miller GL, Forsythe SB, et al: Outcome of acute cholecystitis in patients with diabetes mellitus. Ann Intern Med 106:829, 1987

42. Friedman LS, Roberts MS, Brett AS, et al: Management of asymptomatic gallstones in the diabetic patient: a decision analysis. Ann Intern Med 109:931, 1988

43. Frossard JL, Hadengue A, Amouyal G, et al: Choledocholithiasis: a prospective study of spontaneous common bile duct stone migration. Gastrointest Endosc 51:175, 2000

44. Houdart R, Perniceni T, Darne B, et al: Predicting common bile duct lithiasis: determination and prospective validation of a model predicting low risk. Am J Surg 170:38, 1995

45. Lichtenbaum RA, McMullen HF, Newman RM: Preoperative abdominal ultrasound may be misleading in risk stratification for presence of common bile duct abnormalities. Surg Endosc 14:254, 2000

46. Prat F, Amouyal G, Amouyal P, et al: Prospective controlled study of endoscopic ultrasound and endoscopic retrograde cholangiography in patients with suspected common-bile duct stones. Lancet 347:75, 1996

47. Ramesh H: A balanced approach to choledocholithiasis. Surg Endosc 15:1494, 2001

48. Mueller PR, van Sonnenberg E, Simeone JF, et al: Fine-needle transhepatic cholangiography. Ann Intern Med 97:567, 1982

49. Calvo MM, Bujanda L, Calderon A, et al: Role of magnetic resonance cholangiopancreatography in patients with suspected choledocholithiasis. Mayo Clin Proc 77:422, 2002

50. Demartines N, Eisner L, Schnabel K, et al: Evaluation of magnetic resonance cholangiography in the management of bile duct stones. Arch Surg 135:148, 2000

51. Vaira D, D'Anna L, Ainley C, et al: Endoscopic sphincterotomy in 1000 consecutive patients. Lancet 2:431, 1989

52. Hawes RH, Cotton PB, Vallon AG: Follow-up 6 to 11 years after duodenoscopic sphincterotomy for stones in patients with prior cholecystectomy. Gastroenterology 98:1008, 1990

53. Hawasli A, Lloyd L, Cacucci B: Management of choledocholithiasis in the era of laparoscopic surgery. Am Surg 66:425, 2000

54. Ponsky JL, Heniford BT, Gersin K: Choledocholithiasis: evolving intraoperative strategies. Am Surg 66:262, 2000

55. Fan ST, Lai EC, Mok FP, et al: Early treatment of acute biliary pancreatitis by endoscopic papillotomy. N Engl J Med 328:228, 1993

56. Folsch UR, Nitsche R, Lüdtke R, et al: Early ERCP and papillotomy compared with conservative treatment for acute biliary pancreatitis. The German Study Group on Acute Biliary Pancreatitis. N Engl J Med 336:237, 1997

57. Angulo P, Lindor KD: Primary sclerosing cholangitis. Hepatology 30:325, 1999

58. Lindor KD: Ursodiol for primary sclerosing cholangitis. Mayo Primary Sclerosing Cholangitis-Ursodeoxycholic Acid Study Group. N Engl J Med 336:691, 1997

59. Johnson GK, Geenen JE, Venu RP, et al: Endoscopic treatment of biliary tract strictures in sclerosing cholangitis: a larger series and recommendations for treatment. Gastrointest Endosc 37:38, 1991

60. Stiehl A, Rudolph G, Sauer P, et al: Efficacy of ursodeoxycholic acid treatment and endoscopic dilation of major duct stenoses in primary sclerosing cholangitis: an 8-year prospective study. J Hepatol 26:560, 1997

61. Buckles DC, Lindor KD, Larusso NF, et al: In primary sclerosing cholangitis, gallbladder polyps are frequently malignant. Am J Gastroenterol 97:1138, 2002

62. Bergquist A, Ekbom A, Olsson R, et al: Hepatic and extrahepatic malignancies in primary sclerosing cholangitis. J Hepatol 36:321, 2002

63. Liu CL, Fan ST, Lo CM, et al: Choledochal cysts in adults. Arch Surg 137:465, 2002

64. Postema RR, Hazebroek FW: Choledochal cysts in children: a review of 28 years of treatment in a Dutch children's hospital. Eur J Surg 165:1159, 1999

65. Geenen JE, Hogan WJ, Dodds WJ, et al: The efficacy of endoscopic sphincterotomy after cholecystectomy in patients with sphincter-of-Oddi dysfunction. N Engl J Med 320:82, 1989

66. Craig AG, Toouli J: Sphincterotomy for biliary sphincter of Oddi dysfunction. Cochrane Database Syst Rev (3):CD001509, 2001

Acknowledgments

Figure 1   Alan Iselin.

Figure 2   Courtesy of Laura Thomas, M.D., and Mark Feldman, M.D.

Figures 3 and 4   Courtesy of Mark Feldman, M.D.

Figures 5 and 7   Courtesy of Malcolm F. Anderson, M.D.

Figure 6   Courtesy of David Riepe, M.D.

68 Diseases of the Pancreas

J. Steven Burdick, M.D.

Acute Pancreatitis

DEFINITION

Acute pancreatitis is an inflammation of the pancreas with variable involvement of other regional tissues or remote organ systems. Clinically, pancreatitis is classified as mild or severe. Severe pancreatitis is associated with organ failure or local complications, including abscesses or pseudocysts. Pathologic findings can range from interstitial pancreatitis to necrotic pancreatitis. In interstitial pancreatitis, there is edematous change with preservation of the underlying pancreatic parenchymal architecture. Necrotic pancreatitis is associated with cellular death and loss of the pancreatic parenchymal architecture. Necrosis occurs in severe pancreatitis and is found in 20% to 30% of the 185,000 new cases of acute pancreatis diagnosed each year in the United States.[1]

EPIDEMIOLOGY

Population-based studies worldwide have reported a doubling or tripling in the incidence of acute pancreatitis since the 1970s.[2] Incidences currently range from 73 to 750 per million population, with an average mortality of 9%.[2-4] Significant differences in outcome have been noted between interstitial pancreatitis and necrotizing pancreatitis. Interstitial pancreatitis, the more common type, is associated with death in less than 1% of cases. However, 25% of cases of acute pancreatitis are severe and associated with histologic changes of necrotizing pancreatitis.[5] The 30% incidence of death in this subgroup results primarily from infections and respiratory failure. Despite advances in the management of patients in intensive care units, mortality from acute pancreatitis has remained unchanged over the past decade.

ETIOLOGY

Gallstones and alcohol abuse are etiologic factors in 57.8% to 86.8% of cases of acute pancreatitis.[3,6,7] Gallstones are thought to cause pancreatitis by transient obstruction of the pancreatic duct, with small stones causing obstruction more often than large ones. However, the specific initial event that causes pancreatic inflammation is still unknown. Gallstones may cause recurrent episodes of acute pancreatitis but rarely cause chronic pancreatitis.

Most patients presenting with a first episode of acute alcoholic pancreatitis already have permanent functional damage to the pancreas.[8] Typically, chronic pancreatitis develops, although nonprogressive recurrent acute pancreatitis secondary to alcohol abuse has been described.[9] Although acute alcoholic pancreatitis is usually associated with chronic alcohol ingestion, it can also occur with binge drinking.[9]

In approximately 30% of patients with acute pancreatitis, the etiology of the disease is idiopathic. Studies suggest that occult microlithiasis (biliary sludge) may be the cause of pancreatitis in up to 75% of these patients.[10,11] The diagnosis is made by examination of bile collected by either duodenal drainage or endoscopic retrograde cholangiopancreatography (ERCP) for crystals. Certain other conditions may cause pancreatitis by obstruction of the pancreatic duct, including ampullary or pancreatic tumors, choledochocele, foreign bodies, and pancreas

divisum. Pancreas divisum, the most common congenital anomaly of the pancreas, occurs when the ventral pancreas and the dorsal pancreas fail to fuse during embryogenesis. Pancreas divisum is identified in 5% to 10% of patients undergoing ERCP. Whether it represents a risk factor for acute pancreatitis remains controversial.[12]

A potential structural cause is identified by ERCP in about one third of patients with idiopathic acute pancreatitis.[13] If pressure measurements of the sphincter of Oddi are incorporated into ERCP, an elevated sphincter pressure is present in one in seven patients.[14] Either abnormal sphincter of Oddi manometry findings or abnormal ERCP findings are present in close to 40% of patients with idiopathic pancreatitis. Whether a stenotic or high-pressure sphincter of Oddi is a cause or a result of pancreatitis is controversial. For example, some patients with hereditary pancreatitis have sphincter stenosis that benefits from sphincterotomy,[15] which suggests that sphincter stenosis may be a secondary result.

Mutations of the *CFTR* (cystic fibrosis transmembrane conductance regulatory) gene have recently been linked to idiopathic pancreatitis.[16] Patients with idiopathic acute pancreatitis more often have an abnormal *CFTR* allele, detected by genetic testing, than does the general population, and patients with idiopathic chronic pancreatitis have such mutations two to three times more often than the general population.[16,17] There are a number of other causes of idiopathic acute pancreatitis, but most are rarely encountered [*see Table 1*].

PATHOPHYSIOLOGY

Pancreatitis is thought to result when inactive (precursor) pancreatic proteolytic enzymes, such as trypsinogen, are activated within the pancreas. Trypsinogen normally remains inactive until it reaches the lumen of the duodenum, where duodenal enterokinase cleaves a peptide fragment. This cleaved peptide is activated trypsin. The normal pancreas has a series

Table 1 Rare Causes of Acute Pancreatitis[123]

Cause	Comment
Hypertriglyceridemia	Familial or acquired; triglyceridemia > 1,000 mg/dl
Hypercalcemia	Hyperparathyroidism (1%–2% of cases); vitamin D excess; other causes of high calcium levels
Drugs	Azathioprine; 6-mercaptopurine (6-MP); 2′,3′-dideoxyinosine (ddI); usually benign
Toxins	Organophosphate insecticides; scorpion bites (Central and South America); methanol
Trauma	Blunt or penetrating; ERCP; surgery
Peptic ulcer	Penetrating duodenal or gastric ulcer
Vasculitis	Systemic lupus erythematosus; polyarteritis nodosa; mixed connective tissue disease
Infections	Viral (mumps, HIV); worms (*Ascaris, Strongyloides, Clonorchis*); fungal or bacterial

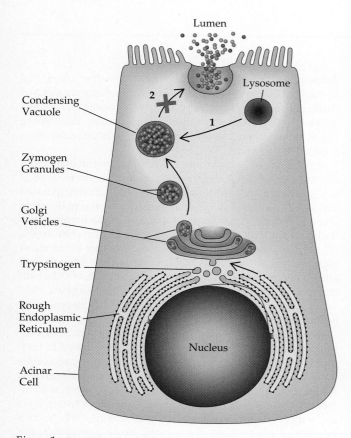

Lumen

Lysosome

Condensing
Vacuole

2

1

Zymogen
Granules

Golgi
Vesicles

Trypsinogen

Rough
Endoplasmic
Reticulum

Nucleus

Acinar
Cell

Figure 1 **Possible pathophysiologic mechanisms of acute pancreatitis include blockade of secretion and fusion of zymogens and lysosomes into a condensing vacuole.**[124] **(1—premature activation with lysosome/zymogen fusion; 2—secretory blockade)**

of mechanisms that protect against premature activation of trypsin within the pancreas, including the separation of lysosomes and zymogen granules containing trypsinogen, synthesis of pancreatic trypsin inhibitors, regulation of intracellular calcium levels and pH, and an arginine residue 117 (R-117) failsafe autolysis site.[18] In pancreatitis, trypsinogen activation occurs within a cytosolic vacuole containing digestive enzymes and cathepsin B, and after activation, trypsin is released into the cytosol. However, the initiating event remains unclear.

Two theories have been proposed to explain these findings. According to one theory, activation of digestive enzymes is initiated by lysosomal hydrolases acting on trypsinogen after fusion of the zymogen granules and lysosomes. The second theory suggests that activation within the normal secretory pathway occurs as a consequence of secretory blockage downstream. A unifying feature of both mechanisms is the colocalization of digestive zymogens with lysosomal hydrolases, resulting in activation of the zymogens [*see Figure 1*].

Mutations in the trypsinogen gene are also associated with premature activation of trypsinogen. Trypsinogen activation within the pancreas normally undergoes hydrolysis at the R-117 position, followed by the reduction of a disulfide bond and separation of two globular domains. This separation inactivates trypsin, protecting the pancreas from autodigestion, and represents a protective mechanism against premature protease activation. A hereditary form of pancreatitis has been linked with the T cell receptor chain (*TCRb*) gene locus on chromosome

7q35. An arginine-to-histidine substitution (*HP1*) was identified at R-117 in four families [19] However, this mutation is not found universally in patients with hereditary pancreatitis. A second mutation (*HP2*), involving an arginine-to-isoleucine substitution at position 21, also has been identified.[15] These mutations prevent hydrolysis and separation of activated trypsin, which renders patients susceptible to recurrent pancreatitis.

The *CFTR* gene regulates the chloride flow through a cyclic adenosine monophosphate–dependent channel and normally promotes the dilution and alkalization of pancreatic juice. The pancreas is very susceptible to decreased *CFTR* function. Mutations in this gene may lead to ductal obstruction, damage to the acinar cell, or impairment of ion transport.

Once pancreatitis is initiated, systemic effects may occur, especially if pancreatitis is severe. The multiorgan system failure (MOF) associated with pancreatitis is similar to MOF in other conditions, including sepsis, major burns, and trauma. The progression from a local event (pancreatitis) to systemic complications (MOF) has been linked to the production of cytokines. Activated pancreatic enzymes per se are not capable of inducing pulmonary disease in rats when given intravenously. However, ascitic fluid collected from rats with pancreatitis, when given intravenously, induces acute respiratory distress syndrome (ARDS).[20] Levels of interleukin-1 (IL-1) and tumor necrosis factor messenger RNA (TNF mRNA) are markedly elevated after intravenous administration of pancreatic ascites.[21] ARDS is aborted in knockout mice lacking IL-1 or TNF receptors.

The mechanism responsible for initiating the cytokine cascade in pancreatitis is incompletely understood. Macrophages are believed to be the most important source of cytokines, as acute inflammation precedes the recruitment of immune-specific T and B cells.[22] A variety of other mediators are released, including platelet-activating factor, prostanoids, complement, and bradykinin. Serum levels of IL-6 and IL-8 correlate with the severity of pancreatitis.[22-25] Clinical trials involving an antagonist to platelet-activating factor have shown promise. Reductions in MOF and pseudocyst formation were noted, although survival benefit was found only in a subgroup of patients who received treatment within 48 hours of onset of pancreatitis.[26,27]

DIAGNOSIS

Clinical Manifestations

At least 95% of patients with acute pancreatitis complain of midepigastric pain, often excruciating, which usually radiates to the back. The pain is nonfluctuating and may last for many hours or even days, usually compelling the patient to seek medical evaluation. About 75% to 85% of patients experience nausea and vomiting. Fever develops in more than half of the patients, although there is usually no demonstrable infection, and shock occurs in nearly half of the patients who have fever. Obtundation and psychosis may be initial presenting symptoms but can also develop in the course of severe pancreatitis. The change in mental status may be caused by pancreatitis alone, but more commonly, it is caused by delirium tremens associated with alcohol withdrawal.

At presentation, the patient is acutely ill, with severe pain and a temperature of about 38° C (100.4° F). Many patients find that sitting and leaning forward relieves the pain, apparently because retroperitoneal structures are involved. Breathing may be painful if pleural effusion and pleuritis are present. There may be signs of shock, with a rapid heartbeat and cool, moist extremities. The abdomen is frequently distended, and bowel sounds are decreased or absent because of a secondary ileus. Physical examination, however, usually reveals a soft abdomen or only mild voluntary guarding. In severe pancreatitis, the pain may be excruciating, with marked guarding and even rebound tenderness. A bluish-brown discoloration of the flank (Turner sign) and of the periumbilical area (Cullen sign) indicates retroperitoneal hemorrhage (hemorrhagic pancreatitis). Occasionally, severe pancreatitis leads to hyperglycemia and diabetic coma. A mass may be palpated, indicating the presence of a pseudocyst or an inflammatory mass. Because hypocalcemia may develop, the patient should be observed for signs of tetany, although frank tetany is rare. In a minority of patients, mild jaundice develops as a result of common bile duct compression by the edematous pancreatic head. Fat necrosis may result in painful subcutaneous nodules. The clinical signs are thus nondiagnostic, and pancreatitis should be considered in patients with significant abdominal pain or shock without another cause.

Laboratory Tests

Pancreatitis is typically associated with a serum amylase level of at least two to three times normal (sensitivity, 87% to 96%).[28] However, the severity of pancreatitis is not a function of the serum amylase level; patients with alcoholic pancreatitis often have lower levels. Elevations in serum amylase may occur in diabetes, renal insufficiency, pancreatic and nonpancreatic tumors, and intra-abdominal processes, including bowel infarction, bowel obstruction, and appendicitis. A normal serum amylase level, on the other hand, does not rule out a diagnosis of acute pancreatitis. If a patient presents several days after the onset of an acute episode, the serum amylase level can be normal because the half-life of amylase in serum is only about 10 hours. If the patient has a pleural effusion or ascites associated with pancreatitis, needle aspiration will usually reveal a markedly high amylase content. Peritoneal or pleural fluid in other diseases (e.g., perforated peptic ulcer, ischemic bowel disease, and malignancy) may have a high amylase concentration, but its absence strongly militates against a diagnosis of acute pancreatitis.

An elevated serum lipase level is more specific for pancreatitis but is slightly less sensitive than total serum amylase. Hyperlipasemia can be useful in differentiating pancreatitis from other causes of hyperamylasemia, because the pancreas is the predominant source of lipase. Renal clearance of lipase is a few days slower than that of amylase; consequently, the measurement of serum lipase is especially useful in diagnosing pancreatitis in patients who present later in the course of their illness, when the serum amylase level has returned to normal. However, both hyperlipasemia and hyperamylasemia may be present in renal failure and conditions associated with injured bowel mucosa. Although newer lipase assay methods are more specific, a minor elevation of the serum lipase level is quite nonspecific; the serum lipase level must be three times the normal level to confirm the diagnosis of pancreatitis.[29]

Urinary trypsinogen is an alternative to serum amylase and lipase for the diagnosis of acute pancreatitis. A small amount of trypsinogen escapes from the pancreas into the blood. Circulating trypsinogen is filtered at the glomeruli, and reabsorption occurs at the renal tubules. However, in pancreatitis, tubular reabsorption of trypsinogen is impaired, and isoenzyme trypsinogen-2 appears in the urine. In one study, a urinary dipstick for trypsinogen-2 had greater than 90% sensitivity and specificity in acute pancreatitis.[30]

Imaging Tests

A plain film of the abdomen can aid in distinguishing pancreatitis from the possibility of bowel perforation by identifying free air in the abdomen. An uncommon but fairly reliable sign of pancreatitis on a plain abdominal x-ray is the colon cutoff sign, which is an abrupt termination of a gaseous transverse colon at the splenic flexure. Because the transverse mesocolon is attached to the anterior surface of the pancreas, pancreatic inflammation may cause spasm of the colon, resulting in occlusion in this region. Enhancement of the perirenal fat caused by retroperitoneal inflammation in pancreatitis may produce a radiolucent halo around the margin of the left kidney on a plain abdominal film.

Upper gastrointestinal radiographs are not indicated in acute pancreatitis but are sometimes obtained to evaluate abdominal pain. Such films may reveal an enlarged duodenal loop, which occurs in both forms of pancreatitis. In chronic pancreatitis, pseudocyst formation causes extrinsic compression of the duodenum. In acute pancreatitis, the duodenal mucosal folds tend to widen and angulate as a result of inflammation and encroachment by the inflamed pancreatic head.

Ultrasonography is recommended in the initial evaluation to exclude gallstone pancreatitis and is more sensitive than computed tomography for the diagnosis of gallstones.[31] It also may provide information regarding the severity of pancreatitis or demonstrate changes associated with chronic pancreatitis. However, approximately 30% to 40% of ultrasound examinations in patients with pancreatitis are inadequate because of interference with visualization of the pancreas by bowel gas.

CT is the best noninvasive tool to document the range of morphologic changes in acute pancreatitis. In mild pancreatitis, the pancreas occasionally can appear entirely normal.[32] Changes that may be seen include pancreatic enlargement, inflammatory stranding (hazy and streaky changes in the peripancreatic region), fluid accumulation, and hypodense areas within the pancreas. Rapid intravenous injection of a bolus of a contrast agent during dynamic CT can further clarify hypodense areas and reveal necrosis in nonenhancing areas. The finding of pancreatic necrosis is associated with an increased risk of complications and death. Infected pancreatic necrosis is of particular concern because surgical drainage is frequently required. A dynamic CT scan cannot differentiate infected pancreatic necrosis from sterile necrosis. Therefore, a CT-guided fine-needle aspiration of the pancreas for microbiologic study is necessary to make this distinction, and the method is safe and accurate.[33] A classification of pancreatitis according to CT findings correlates well with the severity of the disease and prognosis[34,35] [see Table 2 and Figure 2].

Advances in and increased use of CT have been helpful in

Table 2 Balthazar-Ranson Grading System of Pancreatitis Using CT Scan[124]

Grade	Finding
A	Normal pancreas appearance
B	Enlargement of pancreas
C	Inflammatory stranding
D*	Single fluid collection
E*	Multiple fluid collections

*Grades D and E are associated with increased risk of death and abscess.

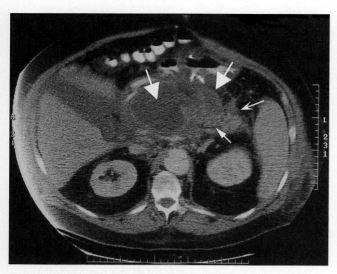

Figure 2 **Intravenous contrast–enhanced CT image of severe pancreatitis. The lowermost triangular arrow indicates enhancing area in tail of pancreas. The top left triangular arrow indicates nonenhancing area of the head and genu of the pancreas, which corresponds to necrosis. The top right triangular arrow and the notched arrow delineate a fluid collection and inflammatory stranding, respectively.**

defining peripancreatic complications in the course of severe acute pancreatitis. Accumulation of pancreatic fluid and inflammatory exudate in the pancreatic bed and along the fascial planes occurs in as many as 50% of patients. Pseudocyst formation, however, occurs in only 10% to 15% of patients with acute pancreatitis [*see* Pseudocysts, *below*].

DIFFERENTIAL DIAGNOSIS

The differential diagnosis of acute pancreatitis should include the diseases that cause severe abdominal pain and those that cause a marked increase in serum amylase levels. These include perforated duodenal or gastric ulcer, acute cholecystitis, mesenteric ischemia, myocardial infarction, and pneumonia.

Macroamylasemia, a condition in which the serum amylase level can range from normal to 10 times normal, may be discovered during an evaluation for intermittent abdominal pain. This rare condition accounts for 0.5% of hyperamylasemia cases in the general population and may be responsible for up to 20% of all cases of chronic unexplained hyperamylasemia.[36] Macroamylase is formed by the binding of normal amylase to a group of heterogeneous glycoproteins, resulting in a high-molecular-weight complex. Because this complex is not filtered by the glomeruli, the amylase-to-creatinine clearance ratio is markedly reduced. Also, the serum lipase level is normal in patients with macroamylasemia. These two tests will establish the diagnosis of macroamylasemia; further radiologic evaluation is unnecessary.

PREDICTORS OF SEVERE PANCREATITIS

The variable presentations of pancreatitis and the subjective criteria for predicting severity of disease can lead to confusion over appropriate care. Ranson and coworkers[37] developed prognostic scoring systems for biliary and alcoholic etiologies of acute pancreatitis on the basis of variables correlated with morbidity and mortality [*see* Table 3]. Wilson and associates[38] proposed a simplified system, which has been validated with different etiologies of pancreatitis. Scores of 3 or higher, according to either Ranson or Imrie criteria, indicate severe pancreatitis. A

Ranson score of 3 is associated with a mortality of 10% to 20%, and a score of 6 is associated with a mortality of 50%. When a score of 3 is used as the cutoff point, both scoring systems seem to have a higher sensitivity (63% to 72%) but a lower specificity (76% to 84%) than scores achieved by clinical assessment.

A significant disadvantage of the Ranson and Imrie scoring systems is the inability to provide objective monitoring after the initial 48 hours. The APACHE-II (Acute Physiology and Chronic Health Evaluation II) scoring system, which is effective in recognizing delayed onset of disease, has been validated for pancreatitis; the APACHE score is based on a total of points derived from physiologic, Glasgow Coma score, age, and chronic health variables [*see* Table 4].[38]

APACHE-II scores have been compared with Ranson, Imrie, and Simplified Acute Physiologic (SAP) scores; Medical Research Council (MRC) sepsis scores; and clinical assessment. At admission, APACHE-II scores greater than 9 correctly predicted severe attacks in 63% of patients, versus 44% correctly predicted by clinical assessment. Other scoring systems could not achieve a score at admission. APACHE-II scoring continued to be more sensitive than clinical scoring at 24 hours (71% versus 59%), with similar overall accuracy rates (87% versus 88%). APACHE-II scoring was most accurate at 48 hours and correctly predicted outcomes in 88% of attacks, versus 69% for Ranson criteria and 84% for Imrie criteria.

Pathophysiology insights suggest that therapy within 48 hours is necessary to abort the inflammatory cascade of severe pancreatitis and that early recognition of severity is critical. The advantages of an instantaneous scoring system and the ability to use one throughout the patient's hospitalization will lead to increased utilization of the APACHE scoring system.

Clinical factors that correlate with poor outcomes include obese body habitus, organ failure, pleural effusion, and ascites.[39-41]

TREATMENT

Severe pancreatitis is a life-threatening illness that requires significant health care resources. The median length of stay in the hospital for pancreatitis patients is 74 days, at a cost of $29,505 to $45,000. [42,43] Treatment of acute pancreatitis is largely supportive and expectant, except in the case of gallstone pancreatitis. Etiologic factors should be eliminated or treated if possible (e.g., alcohol, drugs, or hyperlipidemia). Supportive care includes use of intravenous fluids and electrolytes, keeping the patient fasting, and use of parenteral analgesics such as meperidine. ERCP, which is generally not necessary for the diagnosis of acute pancreatitis, is relatively contraindicated early in the course of acute pancreatitis because it may exacerbate the disease process. The only two exceptions for early use of ERCP are traumatic pancreatitis and severe gallstone pancreatitis. ERCP may guide surgical therapy in pancreatic trauma by accurate localization of the injury, and endoscopic stent placement has the potential to obviate surgery in some patients.[44] In severe gallstone pancreatitis, ERCP is performed for endoscopic extraction of bile duct stones.

Three prospective, randomized trials have clarified the use of ERCP in gallstone pancreatitis.[45-47] Two trials support the use of ERCP within 24 to 72 hours of admission for patients with severe pancreatitis or cholangitis.[45,46]

Antibiotics

The use of antibiotics is appropriate in suspected cholangitis or necrotizing pancreatitis but not in mild pancreatitis. Outcome data correlated with cost analysis of hospital stay identified infections (infected pancreatic necrosis) as the most frequent cause of death. Selection of antibiotic therapy to treat or prevent pancreatic abscess formation is based on three factors: tissue concentration of antibiotics, organisms, and susceptibility of organisms. Tissue concentrations of antibiotics in patients with pancreatic cancer, acute pancreatitis, and chronic pancreatitis are similar.[48] A so-called efficacy factor was proposed that considered the various organisms involved, pancreatic tissue concentrations of antibiotics, and percentage of inhibited bacteriologic strains for each antibiotic. Imipenem and fluoroquinolones became popular, in view of their respective efficacies.

One study randomized patients with necrotizing pancreatitis (mostly gallstone or alcoholic) to receive imipenem (500 mg I.V. every 8 hours for 14 days) or no antibiotic unless warranted by other clinical conditions. There was less sepsis (pancreatic and nonpancreatic) in the imipenem group but no difference in mortality between the two groups. A second trial evaluated cefuroxime in patients with necrotizing alcoholic pancreatitis.[49] The cefuroxime group had a lower mortality, fewer complications, and fewer urinary tract infections. The length of hospital stay and intensive care unit time also were lower in the antibiotic group, but these differences did not reach significant levels.

The fluoroquinolones appear to have an efficacy factor similar to that of imipenem. However, a controlled trial did not find the two to be equal.[50] The incidences of infected pancreatic necrosis, extrapancreatic infections, and death favored imipenem treatment over the quinolone pefloxacin, and the difference in rates of pancreatic infection was significant.

Translocation of bacteria across the intestinal lumen may have a role in the development of infected pancreatic necrosis. A significant reduction in pancreatic infections, gram-negative infections, and laparotomies occurred with selective decontamination of the gastrointestinal tract.[51]

Antibiotics alone generally are not adequate for the treatment of infected pancreatic necrosis or pancreatic abscess. Surgical consultation is essential. Recent advances in surgical timing and alternative therapies such as percutaneous and endoscopic drainage emphasize the importance of a team approach.[4,52,53]

Nutritional Support

Patients who have severe pancreatitis are expected to have a protracted illness and should receive nutritional support early in their illness. Trials comparing the influence of enteral versus parenteral support in pancreatitis favor enteral feedings.[54,55]

Chronic Pancreatitis

EPIDEMIOLOGY

The prevalence of chronic pancreatitis is estimated to be 0.04% to 5%. In developed countries, 60% to 70% of patients with chronic pancreatitis have a significant ethanol abuse history. An average use of 150 to 175 g of ethanol a day for 6 to 12 years was noted. A high-protein diet may facilitate the alcohol injury. The peak age of incidence is 35 to 45 years, and the disease is most frequently noted in males.[56]

Chronic pancreatitis can be defined as a chronic pancreatic inflammation that results in irreversible pancreatic damage and dysfunction. The clinical course of chronic pancreatitis may consist of recurrent acute attacks or unrelenting progression of symptoms.[57]

Patients with chronic pancreatitis have a reduced life expectancy, with mortality approaching 50% within 20 to 25 years after the diagnosis is made. However, only 15% to 20% of the deaths are directly caused by complications of pancreatitis. Health problems associated with alcohol and tobacco abuse are the major causes of death.[56,58,59] Chronic pancreatitis is associated with an increased risk of pancreatic carcinoma.[60,61]

ETIOLOGY

Common Causes

The major known causes of chronic pancreatitis are alcohol ingestion and malnutrition [see Table 5]. The most common cause of chronic pancreatitis is alcoholism, and in Western countries, chronic alcoholic pancreatitis accounts for 80% to 90% of all cases of chronic pancreatitis. At autopsy, 10% to 20% of alcoholics are found to have had chronic pancreatitis. The risk of this condition is directly proportional to the duration and daily amount of alcohol consumption. In general, it takes 6 to 12 years of heavy alcohol consumption to produce symptomatic chronic pancreatitis; however, the duration required to produce histologic changes is unknown. The quantity of alcohol that must be consumed to produce permanent pathologic changes in the pancreas is also undetermined. Both epidemiologic and laboratory data suggest that a diet high in protein, with high or low fat content, increases the risk of chronic alcoholic pancreatitis.[56] Men are affected five to 10 times more frequently than women. However, the incidence of chronic alcoholic pancreatitis is increasing in women, presumably because of two factors: (1) women are consuming more alcohol, and (2) they absorb alcohol more rapidly than men, making them more susceptible to its effects.[62,63]

Idiopathic chronic pancreatitis is the second most common form of chronic pancreatitis in North America and Europe, accounting for 10% to 20% of all cases. The ages of onset for idiopathic chronic pancreatitis are the late teenage years and after age 50. The predominant symptom for the early onset group is severe abdominal pain, and the characteristic clinical feature for the late-onset group is painless pancreatic insufficiency.[58] A probable distinct subset of patients with idiopathic chronic pancreatitis has been described.[64] These patients all present with pain and increased serum amylase levels in early adulthood. Radiologic examination shows equivocal to minimal pancreatic changes, but pancreatic specimens show chronic inflammatory changes.

Table 3 Ranson Prognostic Scoring System for Pancreatitis

Type	On Admission	Within 48 Hours
Nongallstone pancreatitis	Age > 55 yr WBC count > 16,000/mm^3 Glucose > 200 mg/dl LDH > 350 U/L AST > 250 IU/L	Decrease in Hct > 10 points Increase in BUN > 5 mg/dl Serum calcium < 8 mg/dl P_aO_2 < 60 mm Hg Base deficit > 4 mmol/L Fluid deficit > 6 L
Gallstone pancreatitis	Age > 70 yr WBC count > 18,000/mm^3 Glucose > 220 mg/dl LDH > 400 U/L AST > 500 IU/L	Decrease in Hct > 10 points Increase in BUN > 2 mg/dl Serum calcium < 8 mg/dl Base deficit > 5 mmol/L Fluid deficit > 4 L

AST—aspartate aminotransferase BUN—blood urea nitrogen Hct—hematocrit LDH—lactate dehydrogenase P_aO_2—arterial oxygen tension WBC—white blood cell

Table 4   APACHE-II Severity of Disease Classification System

Physiologic Variable	Physiologic Points								
	Range								
Rectal temperature (°C)	≥ 41°	39.0°–40.9°	—	38.5°–38.9°	36.0°–38.4°	34.0°–35.9°	32.0°–31.9°	30.0°–31.9°	≤ 29.9°
Mean arterial pressure (mm Hg)	≥ 160	130–159	110–129	—	70–109	—	50–69	—	≤ 49
Heart rate (ventricular response)	≥ 180	140–179	110–139	—	70–109	—	55–69	40–54	≥ 39
Respiratory rate (nonventilated or ventilated)	≥ 50	35–49	—	25–34	12–24	10–11	6–9	—	≤ 5
A-aPo$_2$ (mm HG) F$_I$O$_2$ ≥ 0.5 (record A-aPo$_2$)	≥ 500	350–499	200–349	—	< 200	—	—	—	—
F$_I$O$_2$ < 0.5 (record only Pao$_2$)	—	—	—	—	Po$_2$ > 70	Po$_2$ 61–70	—	Po$_2$ 55–60	Po$_2$ < 55
Arterial pH	≥ 7.7	7.6–7.69	—	7.5–7.59	7.33–7.49	—	7.25–7.32	7.15–7.24	< 7.15
Serum sodium (mmol/L)	≥ 180	160–179	155–159	150–154	130–149	—	120–129	111–119	< 110
Serum potassium (mmol/L)	≥ 7.0	6.0–6.9	—	5.5–5.9	3.5–5.4	3.0–3.4	2.5–2.9	—	< 2.5
Serum creatinine (mg/dl)*	≥ 3.5	2.0–3.4	1.5–1.9	—	0.6–1.4	—	< 0.6	—	—
Hematocrit (%)	≥ 60	—	50.0–59.9	46.0–49.9	30.0–45.9	—	20.0–29.9	—	< 20
White blood cell count 1,000/mm^3	≥ 40	—	20.0–39.9	15–19.9	3.0–14.9	—	1.0–2.9	—	< 1
Serum HCO$_3$ (mmol/L)†	≥ 52	41.0–51.9	—	32.0–40.9	22.0–31.9	—	18.0–21.9	14.0–17.9	< 15
Individual variable points	+4	+3	+2	+1	0	+1	+2	+3	+4

Total acute physiology score = sum of the individual variable points for all 12 variables.

Tropical pancreatitis is an important form of chronic pancreatitis worldwide, especially in Indonesia, India, and tropical Africa. The mean age at presentation is 12 years. Brittle diabetes is the usual presenting problem, but a history of recurrent abdominal pain can be elicited from most patients. Tropical pancreatitis almost exclusively affects impoverished people and affects males and females equally. All patients with tropical pancreatitis are malnourished. Disseminated calcification in the pancreas is a dominant feature at presentation, but steatorrhea is uncommon, probably because of the low-fat diets of these patients. The underlying cause of tropical pancreatitis is not entirely clear, but malnutrition is probably a major contributing factor.[65]

Uncommon Causes

Hereditary pancreatitis is a rare but well-described entity.[66-68] It is transmitted in an autosomal dominant pattern with variable penetrance. The involved gene has recently been mapped to chromosome 7q35[69] [see Pathogenesis, below]. Patients usually present with pain at 10 to 12 years of age, but they can also present with pain in adulthood. If the first presentation with pain occurs in adulthood, the disease course is similar to that in nonalcoholic idiopathic chronic pancreatitis. Pancreatic calcification is seen in 50% of patients who have hereditary pancreatitis. Diabetes develops in 10% to 25% and malabsorption in 5% to 45%. An increased risk of adenocarcinoma of the pancreas and other intra-abdominal carcinomas has been observed.

Hyperparathyroidism is another rare cause of chronic pancreatitis. The role of hypercalcemia as the underlying pathogenic factor is still debatable.

Ampullary stenosis, pancreas divisum, and scarring from pancreatic ductal trauma can cause obstructive chronic pancreatitis. Intraductal stones are rarely found in obstructive chronic pancreatitis.

Traumatic pancreatitis is frequently caused by blunt trauma. Because the traumatic event may have occurred many years before the apparent onset of disease, the event may have been forgotten by the patient. Typical types of trauma are steering-wheel injury to the abdomen, a punch to the abdomen, or a fall onto a blunt object. Such an episode may cause a tear of the main pancreatic duct, which may lead to pain weeks later. The development of a pseudocyst is very common.

PATHOGENESIS

Our understanding of the pathogenesis of chronic pancreatitis is derived primarily from studies of alcoholic pancreatitis and remains incomplete. One leading hypothesis suggests that the pathogenesis of alcoholic chronic pancreatitis is distinct from that of acute pancreatitis. This theory proposes that alcohol alters the composition of pancreatic secretions and that a pancreatic juice with a high viscosity and high protein concentration is secreted by acinar cells.[70] Precipitation of these proteins causes protein plugs to form in the interlobular and intralobular ducts. Abnormal processing of lithostathine (formerly known as pancreatic stone protein) and GP2 (a homologue of the protein uromodulin, which is responsible for the formation of renal casts) may be a factor in the precipitation and calcification of these plugs.[71] These calcified protein plugs can obstruct the ductules, causing periductular inflammation and fibrosis. Early in the course of the disease, the main pancreatic duct is normal, but it eventually becomes involved as areas of fibrosis coalesce. However, long-term prospective morphologic studies suggest that alcoholic chronic pancreatitis may be the result of injury caused by recurrent acute pancreatitis.[72]

Table 4 (*continued*)

Glasgow Coma Points		
	Response	*Points*
Eyes open	Spontaneous	+4
	To voice	+3
	To pain	+2
	None	+1
Verbal response	Oriented	+5
	Confused conversation	+4
	Inappropriate words	+3
	Incomprehensible sounds	+2
	None	+1
Best motor response	Obeys commands	+6
	Localizes pain	+5
	Flexion-withdrawal to pain	+4
	Abnormal flexion (decorticate)	+3
	Abnormal extension (decerebrate)	+2
	None/flaccid	+1

Total Glasgow Coma points = 15 – Glasgow Coma score.

Age Points	
Age (yr)	*Points*
< 44	0
45–54	2
55–64	3
65–74	5
≥ 75	6

Chronic Health Points	
Hepatic	Biopsy-proven cirrhosis and documented portal hypertension; past episodes of upper GI bleeding attributed to portal hypertension; or prior episodes of hepatic failure, encephalopathy, or coma
Cardiovascular	New York Heart Association class IV status
Respiratory	Chronic restrictive, obstructive, or vascular disease resulting in severe exercise restriction (e.g., unable to climb stairs or perform household duties) or documented chronic hypoxia, hypercapnia, secondary polycythemia, severe pulmonary hypertension (> 40 mm Hg), or respirator dependency
Renal	Recurring long-term dialysis
Immunocompromised	The patient has received therapy that suppresses resistance to infection (e.g., immunosuppression, chemotherapy, radiation, long-term or recent high-dose steroids) or has a disease that is sufficiently advanced to suppress resistance to infection (e.g., leukemia, lymphoma, or AIDS)
	If the patient has a history of severe organ system insufficiency,[‡] or is immunocompromised,[‡] assign points as follows:
	Nonoperative or emergency postoperative patients, 5 points
	Elective postoperative patients, 2 points

APACHE-II Score = Physiologic points + Glasgow Coma points + Age points + Chronic Health points.
*Double point score for acute renal failure.
[†]Venous; not preferred use if there are no arterial blood gases.
[‡]Organ insufficiency or immunocompromised state must have been evident before hospital admission.
A-aPo$_2$—alveolar-arterial oxygen tension difference   F$_I$O$_2$—fraction of inspired oxygen
P$_a$O$_2$—arterial oxygen tension

DIAGNOSIS

A diagnosis of chronic pancreatitis may be based on pancreatic calcification and a history of chronic alcohol abuse. Evaluation may then target detection of disease complications. Nonalcoholic chronic pancreatitis may be more difficult to diagnose, especially early in the disease course.

Clinical Manifestations

Alcoholic and nonalcoholic chronic pancreatitis have similar clinical features. Most patients have abdominal pain. The pain is epigastric, with radiation to the back, and is often postprandial. Episodes of severe abdominal pain similar to those in acute pancreatitis occur early in the course of both forms of chronic pancreatitis. As the disease becomes established in later years, episodes may persist or recur daily for weeks or months. The abdominal pain may diminish, with progressive loss of pancreatic exocrine function.[56] However, over 50% of patients with well-developed exocrine insufficiency continue to have significant pain.[73] Abstinence from alcohol may or may not influence the clinical course once alcoholic chronic pancreatitis has developed.[56] Chronic pancreatitis may be painless in about 10% to 30% of patients and is more common in patients with late-onset idiopathic chronic pancreatitis.[58]

Both exocrine and endocrine pancreatic insufficiency develop as chronic pancreatitis progresses. Steatorrhea begins when 90% of the pancreas is destroyed. This usually presents 10 years after alcoholic chronic pancreatitis has been diagnosed. Diabetes mellitus will not develop for another 10 years, and ketoacidosis is uncommon. Steatorrhea and diabetes usually take twice as long

to develop in patients with early onset idiopathic chronic pancreatitis as in patients with alcoholic chronic pancreatitis.

Pancreatic calcification develops in over 50% of patients with alcoholic chronic pancreatitis approximately 8 years after the diagnosis is made. However, only 25% of patients with idiopathic chronic pancreatitis will have pancreatic calcification 15 years after the diagnosis is made. In about 10% of patients, obstructive jaundice develops because of stricture formation involving the distal common bile duct. Another common complication is pseudocyst formation, the incidence of which varies in reported series but is probably about 25%. Other less common complications include pancreatic fistulas, splenic vein thrombosis, pancreatic ascites, and pleural effusion.

Early in the course of chronic pancreatitis, the physical examination is usually normal. When chronic pancreatitis is well established, the patient is usually thin or even emaciated and appears to be older than his or her actual age. Tender subcuta-

Table 5 Causes of Chronic Pancreatitis

Chronic pancreatitis	Alcoholism
	Idiopathic
	Malnutrition (tropical pancreatitis)
	Hereditary
	Hyperparathyroidism
Obstructive chronic pancreatitis	Trauma
	Pancreas divisum
	Ampullary stenosis

neous nodules on the abdomen and extremities reflect development of fat necrosis, and a friction rub may be heard over the abdomen at the time of acute inflammation. A venous hum may be noted if the splenic vein is compressed by a pseudocyst. Although excessive alcohol use frequently leads to fatty infiltration of the liver, liver enlargement is usually not seen. Often, even massive pseudocysts cannot be palpated because of the retroperitoneal location.

Routine Laboratory Tests

Routine laboratory tests are usually normal. The patient may have a low serum cholesterol level because of inanition and poor dietary intake. The serum amylase and lipase levels and the renal clearance of amylase are usually normal or close to normal in recurrent episodes of chronic pancreatitis. Once exocrine secretion becomes markedly reduced, to the point that the level of enzymes entering the duodenum is 10% to 20% of normal, gross maldigestion of fat and protein supervenes. Fecal fat excretion may reach 60 to 80 g/day on a diet containing 80 to 100 g of fat (normal excretion is 6 g/day).

Imaging Tests

Abdominal films may demonstrate calcifications in the area of the pancreas. An upper gastrointestinal x-ray series frequently demonstrates widening of the duodenal loop or an extrinsic pressure defect on the greater curvature of the stomach, related to the development of a pancreatic pseudocyst. These are late signs of chronic pancreatitis.

Ultrasound findings associated with chronic pancreatitis include enlargement of the pancreas and an increase in echogenicity. Ultrasonography has a sensitivity of 60% to 70% and a specificity of 80% to 90% in diagnosing chronic pancreatitis. It is particularly useful in identifying a fluid-filled pseudocyst.[56]

CT findings of chronic pancreatitis include calcification, main pancreatic duct dilatation or irregularity, and increased pancreatic size. CT is the most sensitive imaging test to detect calcifications, and it can provide better anatomic detail of pseudocysts than ultrasonography. Overall, CT is 10% to 20% more sensitive than ultrasonography in detecting chronic pancreatitis.[74]

Endoscopic ultrasound (EUS) allows parenchymal and ductal abnormalities to be recognized. Ductal abnormalities include narrowing, dilatation, contour changes, duct wall echogenicity, calculi formation, and side branch dilatation. Parenchymal features include gland size, echogenicity, echogenic foci, cyst formation, and lobular pattern. In one study, a threshold of three or more abnormalities on EUS provided a sensitivity of 80% and a specificity of 86%, except for calculi, which was diagnostic.[75]

Magnetic resonance cholangiopancreatography (MRCP) is a radiologic technique that produces images of the pancreatic and biliary ducts similar to images obtained by ERCP. The principle underlying MRCP is that body fluids have a high signal intensity on T_2-weighted resonance sequences, whereas background tissues generate little signal. Abnormal features in the pancreatic duct that can be visualized with MRCP include dilatation, strictures, calculi, and pseudocysts. ERCP is the most sensitive imaging tool for detecting early changes in the pancreatic ductal system caused by chronic pancreatitis. Pancreatic ductal changes may progress from slight ectasia in secondary ductules to alternating dilatation and stenosis (chain-of-lakes sign) in a main pancreatic duct that becomes filled with calcified stones [see Figure 3]. The ductal appearance has been used to classify chronic pancreatitis into mild, moderate, and advanced forms.[76] Ductal

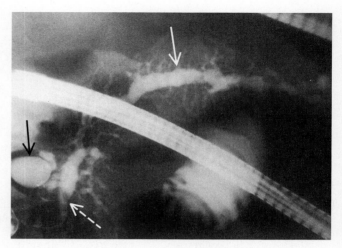

Figure 3 **Endoscopic retrograde cholangiopancreatography in a patient with chronic alcoholic pancreatitis shows two segments of the flexible endoscope, which can be identified by distinct radiolucent cross-markings. After the side-viewing endoscope is passed perorally to the duodenum, a catheter is advanced through a channel within the instrument until it enters the pancreatic duct. The radiopaque contrast material is then injected to allow visualization of the pancreatic ductal system. The pancreatic duct (broken white arrow) shows areas of segmental dilatation marked by widening of the lumen and distortion of the walls of the duct. The small ducts leading to the main pancreatic duct are markedly narrowed. A small pseudocyst (black arrow) containing contrast material is seen near the entrance of the catheter at the ampulla of Vater (solid white arrow). If this pseudocyst were to enlarge, it would probably block the distal main pancreatic duct.**

changes correlate fairly well with deterioration of pancreatic function.[77] However, the earliest impairment of pancreatic secretory function usually precedes ductal changes detected by ERCP.[78] An obviously abnormal pancreatogram is seen in over 80% of patients with chronic alcoholic pancreatitis but in only about 40% of patients with nonalcoholic chronic pancreatitis. In the alcoholic form, pancreatic ductal damage often worsens despite abstinence from alcohol.[79]

Tests of Pancreatic Function

Pancreatic function can be evaluated in three ways: (1) by measuring pancreatic secretions after stimulation by hormones or a test meal; (2) by measuring metabolites of ingested substrates, which provides an indirect estimate of pancreatic enzyme activity; and (3) by measuring pancreatic hormones or enzymes in serum or body secretions. These tests can be categorized into two groups: invasive and noninvasive. Invasive tests require placement of oroduodenal tubes to aspirate pancreatic secretion after the pancreas has been stimulated by intravenous secretin or cholecystokinin (CCK), or both, or by a test meal. Noninvasive tests avoid the discomfort of oroduodenal tube placement. Both invasive and noninvasive tests have been extensively reviewed elsewhere in the literature.[80]

Invasive tests The secretin test is the gold standard of all the pancreatic function tests. Pancreatic secretions are aspirated from the duodenum after the pancreas has been stimulated by intravenous secretin. Bicarbonate secretion is measured in the duodenal aspirate after injection of secretin. The earliest abnormality in chronic pancreatitis is a decrease in bicarbonate secretion; a decrease in volume output occurs later. The sensitivity and specificity of the secretin test for detection of chronic pancreatitis approach 90%. In pancreatic carcinoma, bicarbonate secretion is usually normal, but the volume of fluid secreted decreases because of discrete obstruction of large pancreatic ducts. Addition of CCK to the secretin test does not appear to increase the yield substantially. The major drawbacks of the secretin test are that it is uncomfortable, cumbersome to perform, and not readily available in all centers, partly because supplies of secretin may be scarce. Invasive tests that depend on indirect stimulation of pancreatic secretion by test meals are less specific than the secretin test because they rely on secretion of hormones (e.g., CCK and secretin) from the small intestine to stimulate the pancreas.

Noninvasive tests The most commonly used noninvasive test is based on the ability of chymotrypsin to hydrolyze an oral dose of a synthetic tripeptide, N-benzoyl-L-tyrosyl-p-aminobenzoic acid (NBT-PABA). Para-aminobenzoic acid (PABA), a product of the hydrolysis of NBT-PABA, is absorbed in the small intestine, conjugated in the liver, and excreted in the urine. A diminished serum level or urine level of PABA indicates reduction of pancreatic secretion of chymotrypsin. Many drugs (e.g., acetaminophen, phenacetin, benzocaine, lidocaine, procaine, chloramphenicol, sulfonamides, sulfonylureas, and thiazides) and some food products (e.g., prunes and cranberries) that interfere with PABA measurement, as well as exogenous pancreatic enzymes that contain chymotrypsin, should be avoided for 3 days before the test. The NBT-PABA test is accurate in 80% to 90% of patients with severe pancreatic insufficiency.[81] However, its sensitivity is only about 40% in detecting early chronic pancreatitis.

The pancreolauryl test is a two-day test that measures the urinary fluorescein level after an oral dose of fluorescein dilaurate, a synthetic ester. This compound is digested by pancreatic arylesterase to form fluorescein. The sensitivity and specificity of the pancreolauryl test are similar to those of the NBT-PABA test.[81]

The dual-labeled Schilling test relies on the diminished digestion of the R protein–cobalamin complex in pancreatic insufficiency. Under normal conditions, pancreatic enzymes release cobalamin from R protein, allowing cobalamin to bind to intrinsic factor. R protein–(^{58}Co)cobalamin and intrinsic factor–(^{57}Co)cobalamin are given orally, and a lowered ratio of (^{58}Co)cobalamin to (^{57}Co)cobalamin in the urine indicates pancreatic insufficiency.[82] The dual-labeled Schilling test may have a similar sensitivity but a higher specificity than the NBT-PABA test.[83] However, the accuracy of this test needs further confirmation.

The amino acid consumption test is based on the prompt pancreatic uptake of plasma amino acids for protein synthesis after stimulation by CCK and secretin, leading to a fall in plasma amino acid levels. The accuracy of this test may be equal to that of the secretin test; however, the usefulness of this test in mild to moderate chronic pancreatitis is still controversial.[84-86]

Other noninvasive tests that have been evaluated for pancreatic insufficiency include measurement of serum pancreatic polypeptide, isoamylase, trypsinogen, and fecal chymotrypsin and breath tests to detect carbohydrate and lipid maldigestion. These tests are fairly sensitive in severe pancreatic insufficiency, but their usefulness in mild to moderate chronic pancreatitis is inconsistent.

TREATMENT

Treatment of chronic pancreatitis focuses primarily on managing the patient's pain, malabsorption, diabetes, and other

complications. For obstructive chronic pancreatitis, treatment consists of relief of the obstruction.

Pain

The etiology of pain in chronic pancreatitis is probably multifactorial. Intraductal hypertension, pancreatic parenchymal and neuronal inflammation, pseudocyst formation, and bile duct or duodenal obstruction are contributory factors. For patients with chronic alcoholic pancreatitis, abstinence from alcohol will reduce and may ultimately eliminate pain.[87] However, compliance with abstinence is usually poor. Mild analgesics such as acetaminophen and aspirin should be tried initially for pain control [*see Figure 4*]. A trial of exogenous pancreatic enzymes may be beneficial when mild analgesia fails. This treatment is based on the feedback-inhibition theory, which suggests that

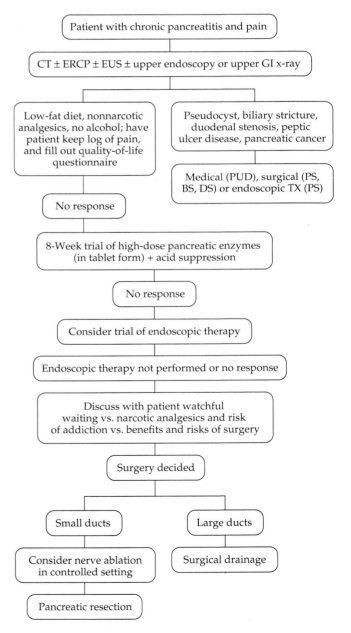

Figure 4 **Algorithm for treatment of pain in chronic pancreatitis.[88]**

protease in the duodenum inhibits CCK release and hence pancreatic secretion and thereby decreases pancreatic pain. Enzyme replacement should be given in the conventional non–enteric-coated form of pancrelipase (e.g., eight tablets Viokase with each meal) because the enteric-coated preparations may not be able to deliver sufficient proteases into the duodenum to suppress CCK secretion. Addition of H_2 receptor blockers may be needed to prevent gastric acid degradation of the enzyme supplement. The role of oral pancreatic enzyme therapy for chronic pancreatitis pain control is unclear. Additional studies to define the effectiveness and subsets of patients who benefit are needed.[88] Frequently, narcotics are required, but they should be used cautiously because addiction to these medications is common.

Recent technical successes in endoscopic placement of stents and extraction of stones from the pancreatic duct have spawned enthusiasm for their use in treatment of chronic pancreatic pain.[89,90] About 50% to 85% of patients at 15 to 25 months have less pain.[88,91-93]

Despite receiving maximal medical therapy, as many as 30% of patients may still have inadequate pain control. In some centers, celiac ganglion block is advocated as the next step, and it provides pain control for 3 to 6 months. Endoscopic ultrasound-guided celiac plexus block may provide pain relief superior to that of a CT-guided block.[88] A repeat block may be as effective as the initial administration; however, patients for whom medical therapy proves unsuccessful may benefit from surgery for pain control. A preoperative ERCP helps define the proper surgical approach. For patients with a diffusely dilated duct, a lateral pancreaticojejunostomy may achieve pain control in 70% to 80% of cases. For patients without a dilated duct, a duodenum-preserving resection of the pancreatic head has been advocated for pain control.[88,94-96] Long-term follow-up studies of these patients are not available.

Pseudocysts

Most pseudocysts are located in the body of the pancreas, the lesser sac of the peritoneal cavity, and the pararenal space. Pseudocyst formation increases with severe and protracted attacks of pancreatitis. Studies suggest that as many as 64% of pseudocysts resolve spontaneously and that the complication rate (infection, bleeding, or perforation) is only 10%.[97] Cysts that last for more than 6 weeks are unlikely to resolve, and complications are more likely to develop in patients with cysts greater than 5 to 6 cm in diameter.

Bleeding from a pseudocyst occurs in 2% to 7% of patients and is associated with a mortality of as high as 35%. Angiographic studies may define the bleeding site and may provide for temporary embolization before definitive surgery. Pseudocysts rupture in 10% to 20% of cases. The associated mortality ranges from 14% to 40% and is higher if a hemorrhage occurs or if the cyst ruptures into the peritoneal cavity.

Concepts in the treatment of pseudocysts are changing. Large pseudocysts do not always require surgery. Studies suggest that the complication rate associated with large cysts that are present longer than 6 weeks is low in patients who are asymptomatic and in patients in whom the cyst is not enlarging.[97] An expectant management with serial CT monitoring may therefore be appropriate for these patients. Symptomatic cysts may be drained surgically, percutaneously with catheters, or endoscopically.

Surgical resection or internal drainage of these cysts is still the definitive therapy. The perioperative mortality is 2.5%, and the complication rate is 7%. The recurrence rate of cysts is 2%. External drainage is associated with a twofold increase in mortality and complications.[98,99]

Percutaneous cyst drainage is a reasonable alternative to surgery, with a success rate of over 95%. The procedure-related mortality, complication rate, and cyst-recurrence rate are comparable to those associated with surgical drainage. However, a pancreatic-cutaneous fistula requiring surgery or endoscopic therapy may form in 10% of patients.[100,101]

Endoscopic gastrocystostomy or duodenocystostomy is safe and efficacious for cysts that are adjacent and adherent to the gastric or proximal duodenal wall.[102] The success rate is about 95%. Cyst recurrence and complications such as infection and bleeding occur in 10% of patients.

Ascites and Pleural Effusion

Pancreatic ascites and pleural effusion are rare complications of chronic pancreatitis, particularly alcoholic pancreatitis. As many as one third of these patients may have the two conditions simultaneously.[103-105] Initial treatment should consist of 2 to 3 weeks of parenteral nutritional support, inhibition of pancreatic secretion with the somatostatin analogue octreotide, and repeated paracentesis or thoracentesis. About 40% to 50% of the ascites and pleural effusions resolve spontaneously.[103-105] Patients who do not respond to conservative management should undergo a perioperative ERCP to try to identify the leakage site before surgical repair. Treatment with somatostatin analogue and endoscopic stent placement has been successful but needs further confirmation.[106,107]

Malabsorption

Steatorrhea and azotorrhea develop when the pancreatic enzyme output is less than 10% of normal. In about 30% of patients with chronic pancreatitis, malabsorption occurs late in the course of the disease. Because a reduction in lipase output usually precedes a reduction in protease output, steatorrhea usually presents earlier than azotorrhea.[108] Steatorrhea may coincide with a decrease in abdominal pain.[109]

The principle of treating steatorrhea is to deliver an adequate concentration of lipase into the duodenum for fat digestion. The estimated requirement is 28,000 IU of lipase delivered over a postprandial 4-hour period.[110] The major difficulty in meeting this dosage requirement has been the degradation of exogenous lipase by gastric acid and pepsin. In most patients, a dosage of eight tablets of Viokase with each meal will significantly reduce but not eliminate steatorrhea. On this regimen, patients usually can maintain their nutritional status and remain relatively asymptomatic. Increasing the dosage of lipase will not decrease steatorrhea any further but will cause a marked increase in bloating and cramps.

Enzymes in enteric-coated microsphere preparations of pancrelipase that are released from the coatings at a pH of 5.5 have had mixed results in clinical tests in treating malabsorption. One of the reasons for failure is that in many patients with chronic pancreatitis, the gastric pH immediately after ingestion of a meal can be greater than 5. The enzymes in the enteric-coated preparations are therefore released prematurely in the stomach. Because these microspheres are too large to be emptied from the stomach rapidly, the released enzyme is inactivated in the acid environment. Microsphere preparations of pancrelipase, such as Creon and Pancrease MT, have a higher lipase content and may resist inactivation in the stomach. Enteric-coated enzyme supplements are more suitable for patients who maintain a pH of no greater than 4 during the entire postprandial period, but these patients cannot easily be identified.

For patients who continue to be symptomatic after receiving

a maximum dosage of enzyme supplement, concomitant bacterial overgrowth should be considered and, if present, treated. If it is not present, adjuvant gastric acid suppression with sodium bicarbonate (650 mg before and after a meal), H_2 receptor blockers, or a proton pump inhibitor should then be instituted. However, agents for acid suppression should be combined only with non–enteric-coated enzyme regimens (e.g., Viokase). Calcium- and magnesium-based antacids are ineffective and make the steatorrhea worse by formation of calcium or magnesium soaps, with fatty acids liberated from triglycerides.

Azotorrhea is easier to treat than steatorrhea because the amount of exogenous protease that escapes gastric degradation is often adequate for protein digestion in the duodenum. If a patient continues to have hypoproteinemia while being treated with an enzyme supplement, other causes of hypoproteinemia, such as liver disease, pancreatic ascites, or protein-losing enteropathy, should be excluded.

Diabetes

Overt diabetes mellitus develops in about 30% to 40% of patients with chronic pancreatitis, caused by loss of insulin-producing beta cells in the islets. The diabetes is usually mild, and ketoacidosis rarely develops, probably because glucagon-producing alpha cells are also lost. Diabetic retinopathy and other diabetic complications may develop.[111]

Pancreatic Disease in Cystic Fibrosis

Physicians are seeing increasing numbers of adult patients with cystic fibrosis. The prognosis for persons with this disorder has improved markedly in recent years, and survival is increasing.[112] About 90% of patients with cystic fibrosis eventually display evidence of pancreatic insufficiency.

Cystic fibrosis is caused by defective chloride conduction across the apical membrane of involved epithelial cells. Chloride conduction becomes defective as a result of a mutation in the CFTR gene [see Chapter 213].[113] More than 200 different CFTR mutations have been detected. Some lead to pancreatic insufficiency, whereas others are associated with adequate pancreatic function. Mutant alleles associated with pancreatic sufficiency seem to have a dominant effect over alleles that cause pancreatic dysfunction. F508, which is the most common mutation and is found in 70% of patients with cystic fibrosis, is associated with pancreatic insufficiency.[114-116] Mutations of the CFTR gene and 5T genotype are associated with chronic pancreatitis without the sinopulmonary disease and the high sweat chloride level diagnostic of cystic fibrosis.

The pathogenetic event leading to pancreatic insufficiency is presumed to be either the partial or the complete occlusion of ductal and saccular structures by inspissated secretions. Pancreatic involvement begins in utero. Mild inflammation may be present, and eventually, atrophy occurs. In most cases, the islet cells are preserved until late in the course of the illness. Early in the disease course, pancreatic insufficiency may be inapparent or mild, but it tends to be progressive. Maldigestion and increased fecal loss of fat and protein result in difficult-to-flush, voluminous stools. Malnutrition and deficiencies of lipid-soluble vitamins, especially vitamin E, may occur. Some patients, especially those with residual pancreatic function, experience abdominal pain caused by attacks of acute pancreatitis. About one third of patients have impaired glucose tolerance; and clinically apparent diabetes mellitus, which is relatively uncommon in children, is becoming increasingly prevalent among adults, in whom its onset is insidious.[112,117, 118] Therapy includes pancreatic enzymes, fat-soluble vitamins, and insulin if necessary.

Liver disease occurs in 20% to 50% of adult patients, although frank biliary cirrhosis is not common.[119] Bile duct abnormalities primarily involve the intrahepatic system, but distal common bile duct strictures can develop.[120] Gallbladder abnormalities are common and include small gallbladder and, in about 10% of patients, the presence of sludge and gallstones. Patients with pancreatic insufficiency are more likely to have gallstones.

Potential gene therapy for pancreatic insufficiency (lipase gene) and cystic fibrosis (CFTR gene) is being investigated.[121,122]

Pancreatic Neoplasms

The major neoplasms of the pancreas are endocrinoma, cystadenoma, cystadenocarcinoma, and, most important, ductal adenocarcinoma. Although many potent diagnostic techniques are available, including ultrasonography, CT scanning, ERCP, and needle biopsy of the pancreas, the prognosis for patients with pancreatic carcinoma remains dismal. Pancreatic carcinoma is discussed under Oncology [see Chapter 196].

References

1. Bradley III EL: A clinically based classification for acute pancreatitis. Arch Surg 128:586, 1993

2. Steinberg W, Tenner S: Acute pancreatitis. N Engl J Med 330:1198, 1994

3. Corfield AP, Cooper MJ, Williamson RCN: Acute pancreatitis: a lethal disease of increasing incidence. Gut 26:724, 1985

4. Baron TH, Morgan DE: Acute necrotizing pancreatitis. N Engl J Med 340:1412, 1999

5. Carr-Locke DL: Endoscopic approaches to acute pancreatitis. ASGE Clinical Update 3:1, 1995

6. Winslet M, Hall C, London NJM, et al: Relation of diagnostic serum amylase levels to aetiology and severity of acute pancreatitis. Gut 33:982, 1992

7. Lankisch PG, Assmus C, Pflichtofer D, et al: Which etiology causes the most severe pancreatitis? Int J Pancreatol 26:55, 1999

8. Singh M, Simsek H: Ethanol and the pancreas: current status. Gastroenterology 98:1051, 1990

9. Steer ML: Classification and pathogenesis of pancreatitis. Surg Clin North Am 69:467, 1989

10. Lee SP, Nicholls JF, Park HZ: Biliary sludge as a cause of acute pancreatitis. N Engl J Med 326:589, 1992

11. Ros E, Navarro S, Bru C, et al: Occult microlithiasis in "idiopathic" acute pancreatitis: prevention of relapses by cholecystectomy or ursodeoxycholic acid therapy. Gastroenterology 101:1701, 1991

12. Carr-Locke DL: Pancreas divisum: the controversy goes on? (editorial). Endoscopy 23:88, 1991

13. Feller ER: Endoscopic retrograde cholangiopancreatography in the diagnosis of unexplained pancreatitis. Arch Intern Med 144:1797, 1984

14. Venu RP, Greene JE, Hogan W, et al: Idiopathic recurrent pancreatitis: an approach to diagnosis and treatment. Dig Dis Sci 34:56, 1989

15. Gorry MC, Gabbaizedeh D, Furey W, et al: Mutations in the cationic trypsinogen gene are associated with recurrent acute and chronic pancreatitis. Gastroenterology 113:1063, 1997

16. Cohn JA, Friedman KJ, Noone PG, et al: Relation between mutations of the cystic fibrosis gene and idiopathic pancreatitis. N Engl J Med 339:653, 1998

17. Sharer N, Schwarz M, Malone G, et al: Mutations of the cystic fibrosis gene in patients with chronic pancreatitis. N Engl J Med 339:645, 1998

18. Whitcomb D: Early trypsinogen activation in acute pancreatitis. Gastroenterology 116:770, 1999

19. Whitcomb DC, Gorry MC, Preston RA, et al: Hereditary pancreatitis is caused by a mutation in the cationic trypsinogen gene. Nat Genet 14:141, 1996

20. Denham W, Yang J, Norman J: Evidence for an unknown component of pancreatic ascites that induces adult respiratory distress syndrome through an interleukin-1 and tumor necrosis factor-dependent mechanism. Surgery 122:295, 1997

21. Denham W, Yang J, Fink G, et al: Gene targeting demonstrates additive detrimental effects of interleukin-1 and tumor necrosis factor during pancreatitis. Gastroenterology 113:1741, 1997

22. Kingsnorth A: Role of cytokines and their inhibitors in acute pancreatitis. Gut 40:1, 1997

23. Heath DI, Cruickshank A, Gudgeon M, et al: Role of interleukin-6 in mediating the acute phase protein response and potential as an early means of severity assessment in acute pancreatitis. Gut 34:41, 1993

24. McCay CJ, Gallagher G, Brooks B, et al: Increased monocyte cytokine production in association with systemic complications in acute pancreatitis. Br J Surg 83:919, 1996

25. Kusske AM, Ronfione AJ, Reber HA, et al: Cytokines and acute pancreatitis. Gastroenterology 110:639, 1996

26. Kingsnorth AN, Galloway SW, Formela LJ, et al: Randomized, double-blind phase II trial of Lexipafant, a platelet-activating factor antagonist in human acute pancreatitis. Br J Surg 82:1414, 1995

27. Early treatment with Lexipafant, a platelet activating factor antagonist reduces mortality in acute pancreatitis: a double blind, randomized placebo controlled study. British Acute Pancreatitis Study Group. Gastroenterology 113:A453, 1997

28. Clavien PA, Robert J, Meyer P, et al: Acute pancreatitis and normoamylasemia: not an uncommon combination. Ann Surg 210:614, 1989

29. Levitt MD, Eckfeldt JH: Diagnosis of acute pancreatitis. The Pancreas: Biology, Pathobiology, and Disease, 2nd ed. Go VLW, DiMagno EP, Gardner JD, et al, Eds. Raven Press, New York, 1993, p 613

30. Kemppainen EA, Hedstrom JI, Puolakkainen PA, et al: Rapid measurement of urinary trypsinogen-2 as a screening test for acute pancreatitis. N Engl J Med 336:1788, 1997

31. Jeffery RB Jr: Sonography in acute pancreatitis. Radiol Clin North Am 27:5, 1989

32. Balthazar EJ: CT diagnosis and staging of acute pancreatitis. Radiol Clin North Am 27:19, 1989

33. Gerzof SG, Banks PA, Robbins A, et al: Early diagnosis of pancreatic infection by computed tomography-guided aspiration. Gastroenterology 93:1315, 1987

34. Johnson CD, Stephens DH, Sarr MG: CT of acute pancreatitis: correlation between lack of contrast enhancement and pancreatic necrosis. AJR Am J Roentgenol 156:93, 1991

35. Hill MC, Huntington DK: Computed tomography and acute pancreatitis. Gastroenterol Clin North Am 19:811, 1990

36. Levitt MD, Ellis CJ, Meier PB: Extrapancreatic origin of chronic unexplained hyperamylasemia. N Engl J Med 302:670, 1980

37. Ranson JHC, Rifkind KM, Roses SF, et al: Prognostic signs and role of operative management in acute pancreatitis. Surg Gynecol Obstet 139:69, 1974

38. Wilson C, Heath DI, Imrie CW: Prediction of outcome I acute pancreatitis: a comparative study of APACHE II clinical assessment and multiple factor scoring systems. Br J Surg 77:1260, 1990

39. Funnell IC, Bornman PC, Weakley SP, et al: Obesity: an important prognostic factor in acute pancreatitis. Br J Surg 80:484, 1993

40. McFadden DW: Organ failure and multiple organ system failure in pancreatitis. Pancreas 6(suppl):S37, 1991

41. Maringhina A, Ciambra M, Patti R, et al: Ascites, pleural, and pericardial effusions in acute pancreatitis: a prospective study of incidence, natural history, and prognostic role. Dig Dis Sci 41:848, 1996

42. Broome AH, Eisen G, Harland RC, et al: Quality of life after treatment for pancreatitis. Ann Surg 223:665, 1996

43. Fenton-Lee D, Imrie CW: Pancreatic necrosis: assessment of outcome related to quality of life and cost of management. Br J Surg 80:1579, 1993

44. Kozarek RA, Ball TJ, Patterson DJ, et al: Endoscopic transpapillary therapy for disrupted pancreatic duct and peripancreatic fluid collections. Gastroenterology 100:1362, 1991

45. Neoptolemos JP, London NJ, Bailey IA, et al: Controlled trial of urgent endoscopic retrograde cholangiopancreatography and endoscopic sphincterotomy versus conservative treatment for acute pancreatitis due to gallstones. Lancet 2:979, 1988

46. Fan ST, Lai ECS, Mok FPT, et al: Early treatment of acute biliary pancreatitis by endoscopic papillotomy. N Engl J Med 328:228, 1993

47. Folsch UR, Nitschie R, Ludtke R, et al: Early ERCP and papillotomy compared with conservative treatment for acute biliary pancreatitis. N Engl J Med 336:237, 1997

48. Buchler M, Malfertheiner P, Frieb H, et al: Human pancreatic tissue concentration of bactericidal antibiotics. Gastroenterology 103:1902, 1992

49. Sainio V, Kemppainen E, Puolakkainen P, et al: Early antibiotic treatment in acute necrotizing pancreatitis. Lancet 346:663, 1995

50. Bassi C, Falconi M, Talamini G, et al: Controlled clinical trial of pefloxacin versus imipenem in severe acute pancreatitis. Gastroenterology 115:1513, 1998

51. Luiten EJT, Hop WCJ, Lange JF, et al: Controlled clinical trial of selective decontamination for the treatment of severe acute pancreatitis. Ann Surg 222:57, 1995

52. Bradley EL III, Allen K: A prospective longitudinal study of observation versus surgical intervention in the management of necrotizing pancreatitis. Am J Surg 161:19, 1991

53. Ranson JHC: The role of surgery in the management of acute pancreatitis. Ann Surg 211:382, 1990

54. Kalfarentzos F, Kehagias J, Kokkinis K, et al: Enteral nutrition is superior to parenteral nutrition in severe acute pancreatitis: results of a randomized prospective trial. Br J Surg 84:1665, 1997

55. Windsor ACJ, Kanwar S, Li AGK, et al: Compared with parenteral nutrition, enteral feeding attenuates the acute phase response and improves disease severity in acute pancreatitis. Gut 42:431, 1998

56. Steer ML, Waxman I, Freedman S: Chronic pancreatitis. N Engl J Med 332:1482, 1995

57. Sarles H, Adler G, Dani R, et al: The pancreatitis classification of Marseilles-Rome 1988. Scand J Gastroenterol 24:641, 1989

58. Layer P, Yamamoto H, Kalthoff L, et al: The different courses of early- and late-onset idiopathic and alcoholic chronic pancreatitis. Gastroenterology 107:1481, 1994

59. Lowenfels AB, Maisonneuve P, Cavallini G, et al: Prognosis of chronic pancreatitis: an international multicenter study. Am J Gastroenterol 89:1467, 1994

60. Lowenfels AB, Maisonneuve P, Cavallini G, et al: Pancreatitis and the risk of pancreatic cancer. N Engl J Med 328:1433, 1993

61. Bansal P, Sonnenberg A: Pancreatitis is a risk factor for pancreatic cancer. Gastroenterology 109:247, 1995

62. Riela A, Zinsmeister AR, Melton LJ, et al: Trends in the incidence and clinical characteristics of chronic pancreatitis. Pancreas 5:727, 1990

63. Frezza M, di Padova C, Pozzato G, et al: High blood alcohol levels in women: the role of decreased gastric alcohol dehydrogenase activity and first-pass metabolism. N Engl J Med 322:95, 1990

64. Walsh TN, Rode J, Theis BA, et al: Minimal change chronic pancreatitis. Gut 33:1566, 1992

65. Pitchumoni CS: "Tropical" or "nutritional" pancreatitis—an update. Pancreatitis: Concepts and Classification. Gyr KE, Singer MV, Sarles H, Eds. Elsevier Science Publishers, Amsterdam, 1984, p 359

66. Konzen KM, Perrault J, Moir C, et al: Long-term follow-up of young patients with chronic hereditary or idiopathic pancreatitis. Mayo Clin Proc 68:449, 1993

67. Moir CR, Konzen KM, Perrault J: Surgical therapy and long-term follow-up of childhood hereditary pancreatitis. J Pediatr Surg 27:282, 1992

68. Miller AR, Nagorney DM, Sarr MG: The surgical spectrum of hereditary pancreatitis in adults. Ann Surg 215:39, 1992

69. Whitcomb DC, Preston RA, Aston CE, et al: A gene for hereditary pancreatitis maps to chromosome 7q35. Gastroenterology 110:1975, 1996

70. Sarles H, Bernard JP, Johnson C: Pathogenesis and epidemiology of chronic pancreatitis. Annu Rev Med 40:453, 1989

71. Freedman SD, Sakamoto K, Venu RP: GP2, the homologue to the renal cast protein uromodulin, is a major component of intraductal plugs in chronic pancreatitis. J Clin Invest 92:83, 1993

72. Ammann RW, Heitz PU, Klöppel G: Course of alcoholic chronic pancreatitis: a prospective clinicomorphological long-term study. Gastroenterology 111: 224, 1996

73. Lankisch PG, Seidensticker F, Lohr-Happe A, et al: The course of pain is the same in alcohol- and nonalcohol-induced chronic pancreatitis. Pancreas 10:338, 1995

74. Thoeni RF, Gorczyca DP: Non-invasive pancreatic imaging in inflammatory diseases. Semin Gastrointest Dis 2:152, 1991

75. Wiersema MJ, Hawes RH, Lehman G, et al: Prospective evaluation of endoscopic ultrasonography and endoscopic retrograde cholangiopancreatography in patients with chronic abdominal pain of suspected pancreatic origin. Endoscopy 25:555, 1993

76. Sarner M, Cotton PB: Classification of pancreatitis. Gut 25:756, 1984

77. Dominguez-Munoz JE, Manes G, Pieramico O, et al: Effect of pancreatic ductal and parenchymal changes on exocrine function in chronic pancreatitis. Pancreas 10:31, 1995

78. Malfertheiner P, Büchler M: Correlation of imaging and function in chronic pancreatitis. Radiol Clin North Am 27:51, 1989

79. Nagata A, Homma T, Tamai K, et al: A study of chronic pancreatitis by serial endoscopic pancreatography. Gastroenterology 81:884, 1981

80. DiMagno EP, Layer P, Clain JE: Chronic pancreatitis. The Pancreas: Biology, Pathobiology, and Disease. Go VLW, DiMagno EP, Gardner JD, et al, Eds. Raven Press, New York, 1993, p 665

81. Lankisch PG, Brauneis J, Otto J, et al: Pancreolauryl and NBT-PABA tests: are serum tests more practicable alternatives to urine tests in the diagnosis of exocrine pancreatic insufficiency? Gastroenterology 90:350, 1986

82. Brugge WR, Goff JS, Allen NC, et al: Development of a dual label Schilling test for pancreatic exocrine function based on the differential absorption of cobalamin bound to intrinsic factor and R protein. Gastroenterology 78:937, 1980

83. Chen WL, Morishita R, Eguchi T, et al: Clinical usefulness of dual-label Schilling test for pancreatic exocrine function. Gastroenterology 96:1337, 1989

84. Domschke S, Heptner G, Kolb S, et al: Decrease in plasma amino acid level after secretin and pancreozymin as an indicator of exocrine pancreatic function. Gastroenterology 90:1031, 1986

85. Gullo L, Pezzilli R, Ventrucci M, et al: Caerulein induced plasma amino acid decrease: a simple, sensitive, and specific test of pancreatic function. Gut 31:926, 1990

86. Maringhini A, Jones JD, Nelson DK, et al: Is plasma amino acid concentration (AA) after CCK-OP an accurate measurement of exocrine pancreatic function? Pancreas 5:721, 1990

87. Trapnell JE: Chronic relapsing pancreatitis: a review of 64 cases. Br J Surg 66:471, 1979

88. Warshaw A, Banks P, Fernandez-Del Castillo C: AGA technical review: treatment of pain in chronic pancreatitis. Gastroenterology 115:765, 1998

89. Kozarek RA, Ball TJ, Patterson DJ: Endoscopic approach to pancreatic duct calculi and obstructive pancreatitis. Am J Gastroenterol 87:600, 1992

90. Delhaye M, Vandermeeren A, Baize M, et al: Extracorporeal shock-wave lithotripsy of pancreatic calculi. Gastroenterology 102:610, 1992

91. Smits ME, Badiga SM, Rauws EAJ, et al: Long-term results of pancreatic stents in chronic pancreatitis. Gastrointest Endosc 42:461, 1995

92. Ponchon T, Bory RM, Hedelius F, et al: Endoscopic stenting for pain relief in chronic pancreatitis: results of a standardized protocol. Gastrointest Endosc 42:452, 1995

93. Dumonceau J-M, Devière J, Le Moine O, et al: Endoscopic pancreatic drainage in chronic pancreatitis associated with ductal stones: long-term results. Gastrointest Endosc 43:547, 1996

94. Bloechle C, Izbicki JR, Knoefel WT, et al: Quality of life in chronic pancreatitis—results after duodenum-preserving resection of the head of the pancreas. Pancreas 11:77, 1995

95. Izbicki JR, Bloechle C, Knoefel WT, et al: Duodenum-preserving resection of the head of the pancreas in chronic pancreatitis: a prospective, randomized trial. Ann Surg 221:350, 1995

96. Buchler MW, Friess H, Muller MW, et al: Randomized trial of duodenum-preserving pancreatic head resection versus pylorus-preserving Whipple in chronic pancreatitis. Am J Surg 169:65, 1995

97. Yeo CJ, Bastidas JA, Lynch-Nyhan A, et al: The natural history of pancreatic pseudocysts documented by computed tomography. Surg Gynecol Obstet 170:411, 1990

98. Vitas GJ, Sarr MG: Selected management of pancreatic pseudocysts: operative versus expectant management. Surgery 111:123, 1992

99. Newell KA, Liu T, Aranha GV, et al: Are cystgastrostomy and cystjejunostomy equivalent operations for pancreatic pseudocysts? Surgery 108:635, 1990

100. Freeny PC, Lewis GP, Traverso LW, et al: Infected pancreatic fluid collections: percutaneous catheter drainage. Radiology 167:431, 1988

101. vanSonnenberg E, Wittich GR, Casola G, et al: Percutaneous drainage of infected and noninfected pancreatic pseudocysts: experience in 101 cases. Radiology 170:757, 1989

102. Cremer M, Devière J, Engelholm L: Endoscopic management of cysts and pseudocysts in chronic pancreatitis: long-term follow-up after 7 years of experience. Gastrointest Endosc 35:1, 1989

103. Sankaran S, Walt AJ: Pancreatic ascites: recognition and management. Arch Surg 111:430, 1976

104. Cameron JL: Chronic pancreatic ascites and pancreatic pleural effusions. Gastroenterology 74:134, 1978

105. Rockey DC, Cello JP: Pancreaticopleural fistula: report of 7 patients and review of the literature. Medicine (Baltimore) 69:332, 1990

106. Pezzilli R, Gullo L, Stefano MD, et al: Treatment of pancreatic ascites with somatostatin. Pancreas 8:120, 1993

107. Kozarek RA, Ball TJ, Patterson DJ, et al: Endoscopic transpapillary therapy for disrupted pancreatic duct and peripancreatic fluid collections. Gastroenterology 100:1362, 1991

108. DiMagno EP, Malagelada JR, Go VLW: Relationship between alcoholism and pancreatic insufficiency. Ann NY Acad Sci 252:200, 1975

109. Ammann RW, Akovbiantz A, Largiader F, et al: Course and outcome of chronic pancreatitis: longitudinal study of a mixed medical-surgical series of 245 patients. Gastroenterology 86:820, 1984

110. DiMagno EP, Go VLW, Summerskill WHJ: Relations between pancreatic enzyme outputs and malabsorption in severe pancreatic insufficiency. N Engl J Med 288:813, 1973

111. Gullo L, Parenti M, Monti L, et al: Diabetic retinopathy in chronic pancreatitis. Gastroenterology 98:1577, 1990

112. Hodson ME: Diabetes mellitus and cystic fibrosis. Baillieres Clin Endocrinol Metab 6:797, 1992

113. Rommens JM, Iannuzzi MC, Kerem B, et al: Identification of the cystic fibrosis gene: chromosome walking and jumping. Science 245:1059, 1989

114. Kerem E, Corey M, Bat-Sheva K, et al: The relation between genotype and phenotype in cystic fibrosis—analysis of the most common mutation (F508). N Engl J Med 323:1517, 1990

115. Correlation between genotype and phenotype in patients with cystic fibrosis. Cystic Fibrosis Genotype-Phenotype Consortium. N Engl J Med 329:1308, 1993

116. Shalon LB, Adelson JW: Cystic fibrosis: gastrointestinal complications and gene therapy. Pediatr Clin North Am 43:157, 1996

117. Moran A, Diem P, Klein DJ, et al: Pancreatic endocrine function in cystic fibrosis. J Pediatr 118:715, 1991

118. De Schepper J, Hachimi-Idrissi S, Smitz J, et al: First-phase insulin release in adult cystic fibrosis patients: correlation with clinical and biological parameters. Horm Res 38:260, 1992

119. De Arce M, O'Brien S, Hegarty J, et al: Deletion F508 and clinical expression of cystic fibrosis–related liver disease. Clin Genet 42:271, 1992

120. O'Brien S, Keogan M, Casey M, et al: Biliary complications of cystic fibrosis. Gut 33:387, 1992

121. Maeda H, Danel C, Crystal RG: Adenovirus-mediated transfer of human lipase complementary DNA to the gallbladder. Gastroenterology 106:1638, 1994

122. Yang Y, Raper SE, Cohn JA, et al: An approach for treating the hepatobiliary disease of cystic fibrosis by somatic gene transfer. Proc Natl Acad Sci USA 90:4601, 1993

123. Steinberg W, Tenner S: Acute pancreatitis. N Engl J Med 330:1198, 1994

124. Steer ML, Meldolesi J: The cell biology of experimental pancreatitis. N Engl J Med 316:144, 1987

Acknowledgment

Figure 1   Seward Hung.

69 Liver and Pancreas Transplantation

Robert L. Carithers, Jr., M.D., and James D. Perkins, M.D

Liver Transplantation

More than 3,500 liver transplantations are performed annually in the United States. Enhancements in surgical technique and the availability of powerful immunosuppressive agents have resulted in steady improvement in patient survival. As a result, liver transplantation has been accepted as the standard of care for patients with severe acute or chronic liver disease who have failed conventional modalities of therapy. The major obstacle to the procedure is the critical shortage of donor organs.

CANDIDATES FOR TRANSPLANTATION

Any patient with acute or chronic liver failure is a potential candidate for liver transplantation; there are a number of common indications [see Table 1].[1]

The methods of evaluating transplantation candidates include echocardiography, color flow Doppler imaging of the portal vein, computed tomographic angiography of the hepatic arterial supply, and a careful evaluation of social factors and support. Echocardiography is useful in assessing left ventricular function and detecting pulmonary hypertension, which is seen in as many as 5% of cirrhotic patients.[2,3] Color flow Doppler studies of the portal vein are used to gauge the integrity of portal vein flow. If portal vein thrombosis is detected, the transplant surgeon can obtain extra donor vessels to bypass the blockade if necessary. CT angiography permits detection of small hepatocellular carcinomas, detection of aberrant arterial blood supply to the liver, and visualization of the splenic artery. Careful evaluation of the patient for any addictive behavior and assessment of the patient's social support system allow the transplant team to plan in advance for any needed services, such as counseling, specialized addiction treatment, housing, transportation, and financial assistance for medications and other expenses.

CONTRAINDICATIONS TO TRANSPLANTATION

Patients with severe neurologic or cardiopulmonary disease cannot withstand the stress of transplantation surgery. Patients with cirrhosis who have severe hypoxia or pulmonary hypertension rarely survive the operation and perioperative period.[4] Other contraindications to transplantation include extrahepatic malignancies, systemic infection, and cholangiocarcinoma. The most common surgical contraindication to liver transplantation is thrombosis of the portal vein and other splanchnic veins to such an extent that no viable portal blood flow can be achieved.[5] Finally, the most frequent contraindications to liver transplantation are ongoing destructive behavior resulting from drug or alcohol addiction and the inability of the patient to comply with the complex medical regimen required after the operation.

TIMING OF TRANSPLANTATION

Determining the optimal timing for liver transplantation can be as important as patient selection. A few simple clinical approaches have proved useful in determining the prognosis of patients with liver disease. These approaches include use of the Child-Turcotte-Pugh (CTP) classification [see Table 2], use of the Mayo model for predicting survival in patients with end-stage liver disease

(MELD), the determination of degree of ascites, and the identification of other complications of cirrhosis.[6,7] For example, only 50% of patients with CTP scores greater than 10 survive 1 year without transplantation, patients with CTP scores of 7 to 9 have an 80% chance of surviving 5 years, and the prognosis is more favorable in patients with CTP scores of 5 to 6 [see Figure 1].[6,8,9] To be placed on the organ donor list for liver transplantation in the United States, patients must have a CTP score of 7 or greater. Patients with CTP scores of 10 or greater or patients with severe complications such as intractable ascites, spontaneous bacterial peritonitis, or hepatorenal syndrome receive a more favorable listing. However, many of these sicker patients do not survive the extended waiting period for a donor organ. Because most patients have to wait 1 to 2 years for a donor organ, it is important that patients be referred for transplantation before advanced liver disease occurs.

The MELD model, which includes the serum bilirubin level, the serum creatinine level, and international normalized ratio (INR) for prothrombin time, also can be used to predict short-term survival in patients with severe liver disease.[7] It has the advantage of simplicity and may prove to be more useful than the CTP scoring system in differentiating the severity of disease in patients with advanced end-stage liver disease, thus allowing the sickest patients earlier access to donor organs.

OPERATIVE PROCEDURES

Most liver transplantations are performed using a whole cadaveric liver placed in the orthotopic position. To increase the overall organ supply and especially to aid young children for whom there is a chronic shortage of donor organs, a cadaveric liver can be divided into parts for more than one recipient [see Figure 2]. The same techniques can be used with living donors, with only part of the liver being removed for transplantation. Living related donor transplantation for children is a well-established procedure.[10] Living related donor transplantation for adults is currently being explored at many transplantation centers.[11]

Table 1 **Common Indications for Liver Transplantation**

Chronic hepatitis	Hemangioendothelioma
Hepatitis C	Alcoholic liver disease
Hepatitis B	Cryptogenic cirrhosis
Autoimmune hepatitis	Miscellaneous conditions
Cholestatic liver disease	Hepatic veno-occlusive disease
Biliary atresia (in children)	Nonalcoholic steatohepatitis
Primary biliary cirrhosis	Tyrosinemia
Sclerosing cholangitis	Crigler-Najjar syndrome
Metabolic diseases	Fulminant hepatic failure
Wilson disease	Hepatitis B
α_1-Antitrypsin deficiency	Hepatitis A
Hemochromatosis	Acetaminophen overdose
Malignancy	Other drug-induced hepatitis
Primary hepatocellular carcinoma	Toxin-induced hepatitis
	Other viral hepatitides

Table 2   Child-Turcotte-Pugh (CTP) Classification*

	Score		
	1	*2*	*3*
Encephalopathy (grade)	None	1–2	3–4
Ascites	Absent	Slight	Moderate
Bilirubin (mg/dl)	1–2	2–3	> 3
Albumin (g/dl)	> 3.5	2.8–3.5	< 2.8
Prothrombin time (seconds prolonged)	1–4	4–6	> 6

*Minimum CTP score, 5 points; maximum CTP score, 15 points. CTP class A: 5 to 6 points. CTP class B: 7 to 9 points. CTP class C: 10 to 15 points.

Liver transplantation is a complex, time-consuming operation that requires three vascular system reconstructions, including hepatic venous drainage to the inferior vena cava, hepatic artery, and portal vein. Biliary reconstruction is usually accomplished using an end-to-end anastomosis of the proximal donor bile duct to the distal recipient duct; however, in recipients with diseased ducts, the donor duct is usually anastomosed to the jejunum using a Roux-en-Y loop.

A number of complications can be anticipated after liver transplantation, including perioperative and surgical complications, immunologic and infectious disorders, and a variety of medical complications.

Perioperative and Surgical Complications

The most serious immediate complication seen after liver transplantation is nonfunction of the transplanted liver, which occurs in 5% to 10% of cases. These patients fail to recover neurologic function, coagulopathy fails to improve spontaneously, and there is progressive jaundice and acidosis. Emergent retransplantation is the only recourse for the patient.

Other important surgical complications encountered after liver transplantation include hepatic artery thrombosis, portal vein thrombosis, and biliary tract complications such as bile leaks and obstruction. Biliary tract complications are the most common; fortunately, most can be managed effectively with endoscopic techniques. Hepatic artery thrombosis is a much more serious complication that can result in the need for retransplantation.

Immunologic Complications (Graft Rejection)

Two types of allograft rejection are seen after liver transplantation. Cellular rejection, which is usually manifested by elevated aminotransferase levels, is most commonly seen 6 to 10 weeks after transplantation. The diagnosis is confirmed by liver biopsy, which reveals cellular invasion of small bile ducts and vascular endothelium. Most patients respond rapidly to increased immunosuppression. Ductopenic rejection is a more indolent process that usually presents as progressive jaundice months to years after transplantation. Liver biopsies reveal gradual disappearance of intrahepatic bile ducts. Most patients with this condition ultimately require retransplantation.

Infectious Complications

Infections remain among the most serious complications encountered after liver transplantation. Many potential pathogens, such as *Pneumocystis carinii* and cytomegalovirus, can usually be prevented with aggressive prophylaxis. In the early postoperative period, the most common pathogens are fungal and nosocomial bacterial infections. Candidiasis and aspergillosis remain the most serious infections encountered after liver transplantation.[12] They often occur in malnourished, critically ill patients and are frequently fatal. After the first few months following surgery, cytomegalovirus infection and recurrent hepatitis B and C virus infections become much more prominent. The emergence of antimicrobial-resistant bacteria, such as methicillin-resistant *Staphylococcus aureus* (MRSA) and vancomycin-resistant *Enterococcus faecium* (VREF), is of growing concern in liver transplant recipients.[13]

Medical Complications and Complications of Immunosuppressive Therapy

A number of immunosuppressive agents are now available for use after solid-organ transplantation. These agents include cyclosporine, tacrolimus, azathioprine, mycophenylate mofetil, sirolimus, and corticosteroids, as well as various polyclonal or monoclonal antilymphocyte preparations.[14] Most liver transplant recipients receive either cyclosporine or tacrolimus in combination with one or more other immunosuppressive agents.

Cyclosporine and tacrolimus are both associated with a number of complications, including renal dysfunction, neurologic toxicity, hypertension, pancreatic injury, and a variety of metabolic abnormalities. Most patients who take cyclosporine and tacrolimus lose 20% to 30% of their renal function within the first year.[15] If blood levels of the drugs are carefully managed, renal function usually stabilizes, with only mild loss of renal function thereafter. Some patients receiving cyclosporine or tacrolimus experience severe neurologic complications, including psychosis, seizures, and apraxia.[16] Many patients who take these drugs complain of headaches, tremors, and severe musculoskeletal pains. Hypertension, which is quite common among patients who take either cyclosporine or tacrolimus, is thought to result from peripheral and renal vasoconstriction.[17] Pancreatic damage with development of type 1 (insulin-dependent) diabetes mellitus is more common after the use of tacrolimus. Patients who take either drug can experience hyperkalemia, hyperuricemia, and elevated cholesterol and triglyceride levels.[18] Cyclosporine, but not tacrolimus, is associated with gingival hyperplasia and excessive hair growth, particularly on the arms and face.

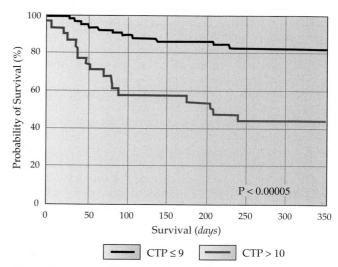

Figure 1   **Graph shows survival of patients awaiting liver transplantation on the basis of the Child-Turcotte-Pugh (CTP) classification.**

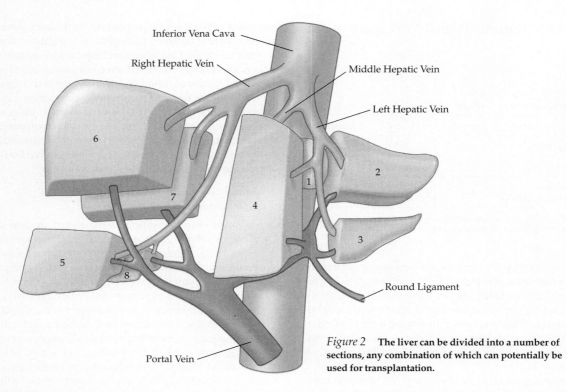

Figure 2 **The liver can be divided into a number of sections, any combination of which can potentially be used for transplantation.**

Azathioprine and mycophenylate mofetil can cause bone marrow depression with leukopenia, thrombocytopenia, and anemia. A number of patients who take mycophenylate mofetil also experience gastrointestinal side effects such as nausea, abdominal pain, and diarrhea. Long-term corticosteroid therapy is associated with obesity, hypertension, glucose intolerance, cataracts, osteoporosis, and hypercholesterolemia. Sirolimus side effects include gastrointestinal symptoms and marked elevations of serum lipids.

Both cyclosporine and tacrolimus are extensively metabolized in the liver, primarily via the cytochrome P-450 IIIA enzyme. As a result, both drugs are prone to numerous drug-drug interactions. The most dramatic examples include interactions with ketoconazole and phenytoin. Ketoconazole inhibits the P-450 IIIA enzyme and can result in marked increases in circulating levels of cyclosporine and tacrolimus. In contrast, phenytoin induces the enzyme, resulting in enhanced metabolism of cyclosporine and tacrolimus and difficulty maintaining adequate circulating levels of both drugs. A number of other commonly used drugs have lesser but important effects on cyclosporine and tacrolimus metabolism. Awareness of these interactions is important in managing patients after transplantation.

Most of the delayed complications seen after liver transplantation are secondary to the long-term use of immunosuppressive drugs. The most common of these complications include renal dysfunction, hypertension, diabetes, hyperkalemia and hyperuricemia, hyperlipidemia, and obesity.[19] Renal dysfunction usually results from the combination of preexisting renal disease and the use of cyclosporine or tacrolimus. In most cases, renal function remains stable for many years; however, some patients experience progressive renal failure and require dialysis or kidney transplantation.[20] Hypertension can usually be effectively managed with the combination of calcium channel blockers and beta blockers. Transient hyperkalemia can be managed effectively with sodium polystyrene sulfonate. If hyperkalemia is sustained, fludrocortisone can be used. Although many patients experience hyperuricemia after liver transplantation, very few experience gout. Treatment of gout is difficult because allopurinol can interfere with azathioprine metabolism, which can result in profound, life-threatening leukopenia, and because nonsteroidal anti-inflammatory drugs often worsen renal function. The necessity for treatment of hyperlipidemia after liver transplantation remains unclear. Obese patients who have undergone liver transplantation need a regular exercise program, limited caloric intake, and reduction or discontinuance of corticosteroids.

Disease-Specific Complications

Certain patients require specific management after liver transplantation because of potential disease-specific complications. For example, progressive liver disease can develop rapidly in patients with hepatitis B and can become fatal within a year after transplantation.[21] However, results of a retrospective study have shown that if patients are treated from the time of transplantation with hepatitis B immune globulin or antiviral therapy, they have an excellent outcome after transplantation, with minimal risk of severe recurrent disease.[22,23]

Patients with chronic hepatitis C who undergo liver transplantation invariably have persistent infection after the operation.[24] However, the long-term survival of these patients approximates that seen in other transplant recipients.[25] Nevertheless, some patients experience rapidly progressive disease with cirrhosis and liver failure within the first few years after liver transplantation. The optimal approach to managing these patients is not clear. However, because chronic liver disease secondary to hepatitis C is the leading indication for liver transplantation, management of these patients will be an issue of increasing importance.

Patients with liver disease caused by sclerosing cholangitis often have associated inflammatory bowel disease. Although the transplant effectively addresses their liver disease, these patients remain at high risk for colon cancer.[26] As a result, they require careful monitoring with colonoscopy and biopsies at least annually. If severe dysplasia is detected, these patients can be effectively treated with colectomy.[27]

OUTCOMES AFTER TRANSPLANTATION

Survival after liver transplantation has improved steadily over the past decade. Most centers now report 1-year survival rates of 85% to 90% and 5-year survival rates of 75% to 80%. The longest survivor after liver transplantation continues to do well 30 years after the operation. The quality of life for most patients after successful transplantation is quite good. Most patients have been able to return to work, and physically active recipients have returned to vigorous endeavors, such as marathon running.

Pancreas Transplantation

Pancreas transplantation, which aims at providing physiologic insulin replacement, is a therapy that reliably achieves euglycemia in patients with type 1 diabetes mellitus. Islet transplantation (en-grafting only the insulin-producing B cells of the pancreas) is an exciting alternative that is still in its clinical infancy.[28]

Since the first vascularized pancreas transplantation in 1966, more than 13,000 have been performed worldwide.[29,30] Approximately 80% of pancreas transplantations have been performed with a kidney transplantation from the same donor (simultaneous pancreas and kidney, or SPK, transplantation), in recipients in whom renal failure is imminent or who are already on dialysis.[30] The remaining transplantations have been performed as a pancreas after kidney (PAK) transplantation in diabetic patients with a previous kidney transplant or as a pancreas transplant alone (PTA) in diabetic patients who have not yet experienced significant renal failure.

The goals of pancreas transplantation are to improve the quality of life for patients with type 1 diabetes mellitus, reverse the

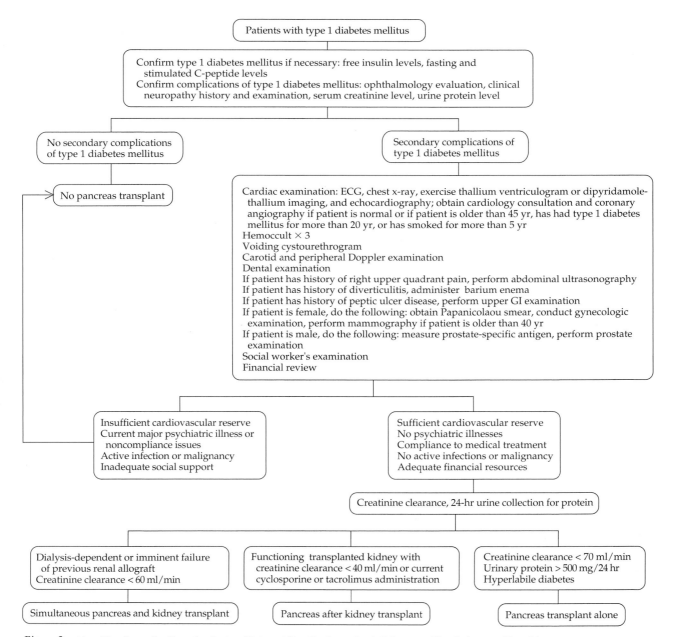

Figure 3 **Algorithm for evaluation of patients with type 1 (insulin-dependent) diabetes mellitus being considered for pancreas transplantation.**

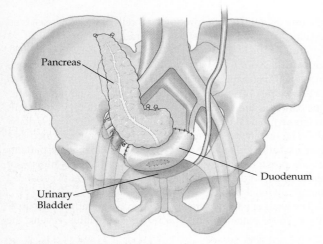

Figure 4 **During the pancreas transplantation procedure, the pancreaticoduodenal graft is anastomosed to the posterolateral aspect of the urinary tract. The arteries and veins of the graft are anastomosed to the common iliac vessels.**

metabolic abnormalities caused by the disease, and prevent the secondary complications of the disease. Despite these lofty goals, postoperative complications and the need for long-term immunosuppression have rendered pancreas transplantation controversial except in a select subpopulation of patients.

CANDIDATES FOR TRANSPLANTATION

During evaluation it is essential to confirm the diagnosis of type 1 diabetes mellitus, to confirm that secondary complications of diabetes are present, to determine the candidate's ability to undergo a major operation, and to rule out any contraindications to the operation.[31] The type of procedure to be performed is determined by the renal functional status of the potential recipient [*see Figure 3*].

CONTRAINDICATIONS FOR TRANSPLANTATION

Patients with insufficient cardiovascular reserve (e.g., recent myocardial infarction), with a left ventricular ejection fraction below 50%, or with coronary angiographic evidence of significant uncorrectable coronary artery disease should not undergo pancreas transplantation[31] [*see Figure 3*]. Excluding patients with current major psychiatric illness or evidence of significant noncompliance prevents avoidable loss of pancreas grafts. In addition, transplantation should not be considered in patients with an active infection or malignancy.

Other contraindications are controversial and depend on the individual transplantation center. Extremity amputations because of vascular disease usually indicate severe generalized vasculopathy and suggest a condition in which pancreas transplantation would not be beneficial. Patients who weigh more than 130% of their ideal body weight often have insulin resistance and, as a result, are not helped by transplantation.[31] Blindness cannot be reversed by pancreas transplantation, but quality of life can be significantly improved. Continued cigarette use often indicates poor compliance in patients who have already been strongly encouraged to stop smoking. Severe neurogenic bladder dysfunction usually predicts a complicated postoperative course and is considered a contraindication at some centers.

OPERATIVE PROCEDURES

The operation includes placement of the pancreas graft, usually in the right lower quadrant with the reconstructed arteries of the pancreas anastomosed to the common iliac artery [*see Figure 4*].[32] To provide drainage for pancreatic exocrine excretions, the duodenum of the graft can be anastomosed either to the mobilized urinary bladder or to the recipient's small bowel.[32,33] The venous drainage of the graft can be anastomosed to the mobilized common iliac vein or to the portal circulation.[32,33] In SPK transplantation, the kidney is placed in the left lower quadrant.

Perioperative Care and Surgical Complications

In the immediate postoperative period, specific care should be directed toward monitoring cardiovascular function.[32] Insulin infusions are generally given for a few days to rest the transplanted islets. Because many patients have some form of diabetic gastropathy, a nasogastric tube is required for 4 to 7 days. A urinary catheter is required for an extended period because of the large area of anastomosis to the bladder and the potential for neurogenic bladder.

Vascular thrombosis, the leading cause of nonimmunologic pancreatic graft failure, occurs in 12% of transplants (5% arterial and 7% venous), usually within the first week after transplantation.[34] With rare exception, salvage of the graft is impossible, and delaying removal of the nonfunctional graft can risk the recipient's life.

Immunologic Complications (Graft Rejection)

Rejection is the leading cause of graft loss after a successful pancreas transplantation procedure.[30] Urinary amylase determinations remain the most useful biochemical parameter for indicating rejection in bladder-drained allografts; however, the gold standard for diagnosis of rejection is histopathologic evaluation of the graft.[35] Rejection can be confirmed histologically because tissue samples of the graft can be obtained by percutaneous biopsies.[35]

*Medical Complications and Complications
of Immunosuppressive Therapy*

Dehydration and metabolic acidosis are the next most common adverse effects that follow bladder-drained pancreas transplantations. There is obligatory loss of pancreatic secretions rich in sodium and bicarbonate into the urinary tract. All transplant recipients must increase their fluid and salt intake, and most require continuous oral bicarbonate supplementation. The dehydration and metabolic acidosis can be avoided by use of enteric-drained pancreas transplants.[33]

Graft pancreatitis, which is also a common side effect, is manifested by hyperamylasemia, abdominal pain, and graft tenderness. Most bladder-drained grafts can be successfully treated with bladder drainage by catheter for a few days, although a few require conversion to enteric drainage.

Tacrolimus has become the mainstay of immunosuppressive therapy for pancreas transplantation, permitting steroid withdrawal in selected patients.[36] Complications associated with immunosuppressive therapy are similar to those associated with hepatic transplantation.

Metabolic Outcomes

Successful pancreas transplantation results in normalization of glucose and hemoglobin A_{1c} levels.[31] Glucose tolerance tests are normal or near normal; however, insulin levels are much higher than normal. The systemic venous drainage of the graft causes elevated plasma levels of insulin, which is known to be a potent regulator of plasma lipoprotein metabolism. As a result, SPK transplant recipients have a favorable lipid profile compared with type 1 diabetes mellitus patients who have kidney transplants.[37]

Diabetic Nephropathy, Retinopathy, Neuropathy, and Vasculopathy

A transplanted pancreas can prevent or reduce the nephropathy that eventually develops in diabetic patients with a kidney graft. Pancreas transplantation also reduces the risk of recurrent diabetic nephropathy in the kidneys of SPK transplant recipients.[38] In contrast, diabetic glomerular lesions are ameliorated by PTA, but reversal requires more than 5 years of normoglycemia.[39]

Pancreas transplantation appears to have a stabilizing effect on retinopathy. In one study, most diabetic patients who received SPK transplants experienced no progression of diabetic retinopathy but did require maintenance laser therapy.[40]

Reestablishment of the euglycemic state by successful pancreas transplantation halts or reverses diabetic neuropathy. In patients who undergo kidney transplantations, the neuropathy initially improves with elimination of uremia but tends to worsen during longer follow-up. In patients who also receive pancreas transplants, the severe and prevalent peripheral neuropathy shows a rapid initial improvement followed by stabilization.[41]

There is no evidence that pancreas transplantation has a beneficial effect on the macroangiopathy of type 1 diabetes mellitus. However, compared with type 1 diabetes mellitus patients who receive kidney transplants, SPK recipients show improvement of diabetic microangiopathy.[40]

OUTCOMES AFTER TRANSPLANTATION

Patient survival exceeds 95% at 1 year and 90% at 3 years. Graft survival (complete insulin independence) exceeds 85% at 1 year and 75% at 3 years.[36] Patients who undergo SPK transplantation have a markedly improved 10-year survival compared with diabetic patients who undergo kidney transplantation alone.[42]

Quality of Life

Quality of life in terms of general health perception, physical ability, and sexual activity is higher for SPK transplant recipients than for patients with type 1 diabetes mellitus who have kidney transplants and is far higher for SPK transplant recipients than for patients who remain on hemodialysis.[43]

References

1. Carithers RL Jr: Liver transplantation: American Association for the Study of Liver Diseases practice guidelines. Liver Transpl 6:122, 2000

2. Kim WR, Krowka MJ, Plevak DJ, et al: Accuracy of Doppler echocardiography in the assessment of pulmonary hypertension in liver transplant candidates. Liver Transpl 6:453, 2000

3. Hadengue A, Benahayoun M, Lebrec D, et al: Pulmonary hypertension complicating portal hypertension: prevalence and relation to splanchnic hemodynamics. Gastroenterology 100:520, 1991

4. Krowka MJ, Plevak DJ, Findlay JY, et al: Pulmonary hemodynamics and perioperative cardiopulmonary-related mortality in patients with portopulmonary hypertension undergoing liver transplantation. Liver Transpl 6:443, 2000

5. Langnas AN, Marujo WC, Stratta RJ, et al: A selective approach to preexisting portal vein thrombosis in patients undergoing liver transplantation. Am J Surg 163:132, 1992

6. Oellerich M, Burdelski M, Lautz H-U, et al: Predictors of one-year pretransplant survival in patients with cirrhosis. Hepatology 14:1029, 1991

7. Malinchoc M, Kamath PS, Gordon FD, et al: A model to predict poor survival in patients undergoing transjugular intrahepatic portosystemic shunts. Hepatology 31:864, 2000

8. Shetty K, Rybicki L, Carey WD: The Child-Pugh classification as a prognostic indicator for survival in primary sclerosing cholangitis. Hepatology 25:1049, 1997

9. Propst A, Propst T, Sangeri G, et al: Prognosis and life expectancy in chronic liver disease. Dig Dis Sci 40:1805, 1995

10. Otte JB, Ville-de-Goyet J, Reding R, et al: Pediatric liver transplantation: from the full-size liver graft to reduced, split, and living related liver transplantation. Pediatr Surg Int 13:308, 1998

11. Marcos A: Right lobe living donor liver transplantation: a review. Liver Transpl 6:3, 2000

12. Rabkin JM, Oroloff SL, Corless CL, et al: Association of fungal infection and increased mortality in liver transplant recipients. Am J Surg 179:426, 2000

13. Singh N: The current management of infectious diseases in the liver transplant recipient. Advances in Liver Transplantation. Clinics in Liver Disease, Vol 2, No 3. Rosen HR, Martin P, Eds. WB Saunders Co, Philadelphia, 2000, p 657

14. Jain A, Khanna A, Molmenti EP, et al: Immunosuppressive therapy. Surg Clin North Am 79:59, 1999

15. Jindal RM, Popescu I: Renal dysfunction associated with liver transplantation. Postgrad Med J 71: 513, 1995

16. Wijdicks EFM, Wiesner RH, Krom RAF: Neurotoxicity in liver transplant recipients with cyclosporine immunosuppression. Neurology 45:1962, 1995

17. Textor SC, Taler SJ, Canzanello VJ: Posttransplantation hypertension related to calcineurin inhibitors. Liver Transpl 6:521, 2000

18. Charco R, Cantarell C, Vargas V, et al: Serum cholesterol changes in long-term survivors of liver transplantation: a comparison between cyclosporine and tacrolimus therapy. Liver Transpl Surg 5:204, 1999

19. Sheiner PA, Magliocca JF, Bodian CA, et al: Long-term medical complications in patients surviving > or = 5 years after liver transplant. Transplantation 69:781, 2000

20. Jain AB, Kashyap R, Rakela J, et al: Primary adult liver transplantation under tacrolimus: more than 90 months actual follow-up survival and adverse events. Liver Transpl Surg 5:144, 1999

21. Todo S, Demetris AJ, Van Thiel DH, et al: Orthotopic liver transplantation for patients with hepatitis B virus-related liver disease. Hepatology 13:619, 1991

22. Samuel D, Muller R, Alexander G, et al: Liver transplantation in European patients with the hepatitis B surface antigen. N Engl J Med 329:1842, 1993

23. Perrillo RP, Kruger M, Sievers T, et al: Posttransplantation: emerging and future therapies. Semin Liver Dis 20(suppl 1):13, 2000

24. Gretch DR, Bacchi CE, Corey L, et al: Persistent hepatitis C virus infection after liver transplantation: clinical and virological features. Hepatology 22:1, 1995

25. Gane EJ, Portman BC, Naoumov NV, et al: Long-term outcome of hepatitis C infection after liver transplantation. N Engl J Med 334:815, 1996

26. Brentnall TA, Haggitt RC, Rabinovitch PS, et al: Risk and natural history of colonic neoplasia in patients with primary sclerosing cholangitis and ulcerative colitis. Gastroenterology 110:331, 1996

27. Goss JA, Shackleton CR, Farmer DG, et al: Orthotopic liver transplantation for primary sclerosing cholangitis: a 12-year single center experience. Ann Surg 225:472, 1997

28. Shapiro AM, Lakey JR, Ryan EA, et al: Islet transplantation in seven patients with type 1 diabetes mellitus using a glucocorticoid-free immunosuppressive regimen. N Engl J Med 343:230, 2000

29. Kelly WD, Lillehei RC, Merkel FK, et al: Allotransplantation of the pancreas and duodenum along with the kidney in diabetic nephropathy. Surgery 61:827, 1967

30. Gruessner AC, Sutherland DE: Analyses of pancreas transplant outcomes for United States cases reported to the United Network for Organ Sharing (UNOS) and non-US cases reported to the International Pancreas Transplant Registry (IPTR). Clin Transpl 51, 1999

31. Stratta RJ, Larsen JL, Cushing K: Pancreas transplantation for diabetes mellitus. Annu Rev Med 46:281, 1995

32. Perkins JD, Fromme GA, Narr BJ, et al: Pancreas transplantation at Mayo: II. Operative and perioperative management. Mayo Clin Proc 65:483, 1990

33. Stratta RJ, Gaber AO, Shokouh-Amiri MH, et al: A prospective comparison of systemic-bladder versus portal-enteric drainage in vascularized pancreas transplantation. Surgery 127:217, 2000

34. Troppmann C, Gruessner AC, Benedetti E, et al: Vascular graft thrombosis after pancreatic transplantation: univariate and multivariate operative and nonoperative risk factor analysis. J Am Coll Surg 182:285, 1996

35. Laftavi MR, Gruessner AC, Bland BJ, et al: Significance of pancreas graft biopsy in detection of rejection. Transplant Proc 30:642, 1998

36. Jordan ML, Shapiro R, Gritsch HA, et al: Long-term results of pancreas transplantation under tacrolimus immunosuppression. Transplantation 67:266, 1999

37. Foger B, Konigsrainer A, Palos G, et al: Effect of pancreas transplantation on lipoprotein lipase, postprandial lipemia, and HDL cholesterol. Transplantation 58:899, 1994

38. Wilczek HE, Jaremko G, Tyden G, et al: Evolution of diabetic nephropathy in kidney grafts. Transplantation 59:51, 1995

39. Fioretto P, Steffes MW, Sutherland DE, et al: Reversal of lesions of diabetic nephropathy after pancreas transplantation. N Engl J Med 339:69, 1998

40. Pearce IA, Ilango B, Sells RA, et al: Stabilisation of diabetic retinopathy following simultaneous pancreas and kidney transplant. Br J Ophthalmol 84:736, 2000

41. Nankivell BJ, Al Harbi IS, Morris J, et al: Recovery of diabetic neuropathy after pancreas transplantation. Transplant Proc 29:658, 1997

42. Tyden G, Tollemar J, Bolinder J: Combined pancreas and kidney transplantation improves survival in patients with end-stage diabetic nephropathy. Clin Transplant 14:505, 2000

43. Esmatjes E, Ricart MJ, Fernandez-Cruz L, et al: Quality of life after successful pancreas-kidney transplantation. Clin Transplant 8:75, 1994

Acknowledgment

Figures 2 and 4 Tom Moore.

70 Enteral and Parenteral Nutrition

Khursheed N. Jeejeebhoy, M.B.B.S., Ph.D.

Definitions

Enteral nutrition is the process of nourishing a patient with a liquid diet of defined composition, usually given through a nasogastric, nasointestinal, gastrostomy, or jejunostomy tube. Parenteral nutrition is the administration of nutrients directly into the bloodstream through a central venous catheter or by peripheral infusion. When the only source of nutrient intake is via the parenteral route, it is called total parenteral nutrition (TPN). The term nutritional support refers to the use of enteral or parenteral nutrition rather than to an oral diet, with or without supplements.

Etiology of Malnutrition

In circumstances in which food is available, malnutrition has three main causes: (1) insufficient intake of food, as a result of conditions such as anorexia, coma, dysphagia, gastric lesions, and psychological factors; (2) heightened metabolic requirements, as may occur in burns, trauma, sepsis, and neoplasia; and (3) intestinal failure, which comprises all conditions that prevent the proper intake, digestion, or absorption of a normal oral diet. Malnutrition from reduced food intake or gastrointestinal failure is most amenable to treatment or prevention with nutritional support. Although nutritional support may overcome some of the effects of trauma, burns, sepsis, or cancer, nutritional support alone may be unable to prevent the development of critical malnutrition in such cases.

Effects of Malnutrition

Even in the absence of disease, malnutrition adversely influences function and survival. A study of Irish hunger strikers found a 30% mortality in strikers who lost 35% to 40% of their body weight.[1] Similarly, in patients with cancer, weight loss of about 30% preceded death.[2] In 12 human volunteers, semistarvation (with a 15% to 20% weight loss over 24 weeks) led to a 60% decrease in function on the basis of a fitness score.[1] Even after 20 weeks of refeeding, the fitness score and handgrip strength in these individuals did not return to normal. Other studies have shown that lack of food intake results in substantial loss of muscle function in addition to loss of body mass.[3] Surgical patients who had weight loss greater than 10% and clinical evidence of dysfunction of two or more organ systems (including skeletal and respiratory muscles) preoperatively had significantly more postoperative complications than did normal patients or those with weight loss but no physiologic dysfunction.[4]

The presence of various diseases compounds the effects of malnutrition. In ill patients, malnutrition results in nutritionally associated complications such as poor wound healing, increased infections, delayed rehabilitation, and increased mortality.

Evidence Regarding Nutritional Support

Well-nourished patients are unlikely to benefit from nutritional support. However, in patients with initial malnutrition and poor function who have continued inability to eat or to absorb ingested food, randomized controlled trials have demonstrated that nutritional support favorably influences outcome by reducing nutritionally associated complications.

PARENTERAL NUTRITION

Three large meta-analyses of parenteral nutrition have given inconsistent results. In a comparison of parenteral nutrition with standard care in 26 trials, Heyland and colleagues[5] found that parenteral nutrition did not influence overall mortality but did reduce complications in malnourished patients. Benefit from TPN was observed in studies performed before 1988, in studies deemed to be of less statistical quality, and in patients who did not receive lipid. These researchers found only six trials of parenteral nutrition in critical illness; in these trials, complications and mortality were significantly higher than in trials done in surgical patients. Another meta-analysis showed that in malnourished patients, standard care, compared with parenteral nutrition, was associated with increased mortality and a trend toward increased infectious complications; in well-nourished patients, infections were more frequent with parenteral nutrition than with standard care or enteral nutrition.[6] These authors speculated that the increased infectious complications in patients on parenteral nutrition were attributable to hyperglycemia. Not all the studies included in this meta-analysis mentioned blood glucose, but of the seven that did, six found both hyperglycemia and increased infectious complications.

Koretz and colleagues[7] have done a technical review and made recommendations to the American Gastroenterological Association about parenteral nutrition. They found that overall, mortality with parenteral nutrition was no lower than mortality with standard care. In contrast to the meta-analysis by Heyland and colleagues,[5] this analysis showed that total complications and length of stay were lower only in studies in which lipid was a component of TPN. Infectious complications were increased with TPN, especially in cancer patients. Benefit from parenteral nutrition was seen only in patients with upper GI cancer, who had significantly fewer complications when given perioperative parenteral nutrition.

ENTERAL NUTRITION

Enteral nutrition has not been compared with standard care in the same systematic way as has parenteral nutrition. However, comparisons of enteral nutrition with parenteral nutrition have consistently shown fewer infectious complications with enteral nutrition than with parenteral nutrition.[6] Data from a large controlled trial in intensive care unit patients showed that keeping blood glucose levels below 127 mg/dl (7 mmol/L) significantly reduced mortality from sepsis-related multisystem organ failure.[8] Hyperglycemia probably was more frequent with parenteral nutrition because patients randomized to parenteral nutrition received more calories than those on enteral nutrition,[9] despite the intent to make both groups isocaloric. None of these studies prove that enteral nutrition is better than standard therapy; rather, they show that enteral nutrition is less likely than parenteral nutrition to cause infection. In a 562-patient trial of enteral nutrition versus TPN that mirrored the conventional practice of nutritional support, Woodcock and colleagues[10] concluded that TPN did not increase sepsis, enteral nutrition delivered less than the target nutritional intake, and procedure-related complications were greater with enteral nutrition.

Determining the Need for Nutritional Support

Unfortunately, for many clinical situations there are no data from randomized, controlled trials to help clinicians determine how to identify patients who are likely to progress to critical weight loss and to determine when to start nutritional support in patients who are at risk. In the absence of reliable data, clinicians have to make decisions about nutritional support at the bedside. Obviously, a previously healthy person who does not eat for 1 or 2 days does not need nutritional support. On the other hand, if inadequate nutritional intake persists for weeks, weight loss will continue; the loss will accelerate if there is added trauma or sepsis; and when loss of body weight exceeds 30%, there is an increased likelihood of death.

The risk of malnutrition can be assessed with a clinical tool called the Subjective Global Assessment (SGA).[11] The SGA, which can be used by physicians, dietitians, or nurses after brief training, is based on a focused history and physical examination that includes the degree and progression of any weight loss, dietary intake, ability to take and absorb food (state of the GI tract), the degree of stress from comorbidity, and functional status.[12] This information is used to classify the patient into one of three groups: A (normally nourished and unlikely to progress to a malnourished state), B (normally nourished but likely to progress to a malnourished state), or C (malnourished and progressing to increasing malnutrition).

The SGA not only provides an assessment of the patient's current nutritional status but also predicts the possible nutritional outcome if nutritional support is not instituted. More important, it allows the clinician to weigh the role of disease severity versus limited nutrient intake as the cause of malnutrition.

Two controlled studies of the SGA have shown that the likelihood of nutritionally associated complications progressively increased from grades A to C. Patients who are classified as SGA C are very likely to develop nutritionally associated complications and therefore should benefit from nutritional support. These studies also found that the SGA grade correlated with other objective measures of nutritional status but was more likely to predict nutritionally associated complications than several of the objective measures taken individually.[13] SGA has been shown to be a valid predictor of nutritionally associated complications in general surgical patients, patients on dialysis, and liver transplant patients. In two large studies, SGA independently identified increased mortality and morbidity from malnutrition, even when the data were adjusted for other factors influencing survival and complications.[14,15]

Nutritional Support in Specific Clinical Conditions

INSUFFICIENT ORAL INTAKE DESPITE A NORMAL GUT

Well-nourished Patients

In general, most patients with serious illness have reduced food intake, partly from the illness itself and partly as a result of iatrogenic factors. Most hospital inpatients eat insufficient food or are prevented from eating. Several studies have indicated that a significant number of hospital patients have signs of malnutrition. Patients likely to have an inadequate intake of food are those with critical illness (e.g., trauma, burns, severe sepsis, respiratory failure); coma and neurologic diseases; or major psychiatric illnesses. Although many hospital patients fit these categories, there are no controlled trials to provide guidelines that can be confidently used to guide nutritional support in such patients and to confirm that nutritional support can reduce the occurrence of nutritionally associated complications. Clinically, it is a common practice to start nutritional support if the period of reduced intake exceeds 7 to 10 days or weight loss exceeds 10%.[16] Unfortunately, this practice has no supporting data except consensus and expert opinion.

Early enteral feeding has been recommended on the basis of a randomized trial in trauma patients who were to undergo a laparotomy and had an abdominal trauma index greater than 15.[17] This subset constituted 20% of all trauma patients admitted during the period of study. These patients, who were well nourished on admission, were randomized to a group who received early (12 to 18 hours after surgery) institution of enteral feeding through a jejunostomy tube inserted at surgery or to a control group in whom TPN was started 5 days after surgery if the patient was not yet on a regular oral diet. There was no difference in overall complications between the groups, but septic complications were significantly lower in the early-fed group (4%, versus 26% in the TPN group). Such data are subject to the criticism that there was no control group receiving standard care. However, there are other reasons to support early feeding. In a randomized trial of postoperative supplemental sip

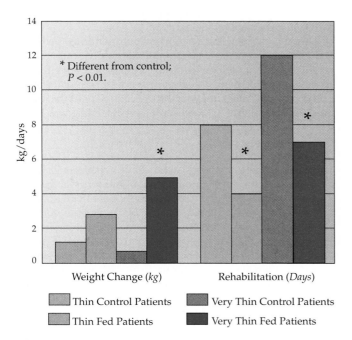

Figure 1 In elderly women with femoral neck fractures, weight increase was greater and rehabilitation time was shorter in those who received overnight supplementary enteral feeding than in control subjects, who were given a normal hospital diet. The effect was evident in thin patients and was particularly marked in very thin patients.[22]

feeding of a liquid formulation, grip strength significantly improved and the occurrence of serious infections was reduced.[18] In a trial of 501 hospitalized elderly patients randomized to oral supplements or a ward diet, Larsson and colleagues[19] showed that irrespective of their initial nutritional status, the supplemented patients had lower mortality, better mobility, and a shorter hospital stay. The difference between ward diet and supplementation was even more pronounced in a secondary analysis of patients with weight loss.

Recommendations The available data suggest that well-nourished patients who are admitted with major trauma should receive enteral nutrition. Elderly patients should receive supplemental feeding or enteral nutrition if they are incapable of eating adequately. However, all hospitalized patients should have their SGA assessed so that possible future outcome without nutritional support can be documented and considered. For example, if a previously healthy patient has a severe head injury and is likely to remain comatose (and therefore unable to eat) for an indefinite period, it is easy to predict that malnutrition will occur in the absence of nutritional support. Such a patient should be started on enteral nutrition. Similarly, major burns, the hypermetabolic state, anorexia, and ileus all result in rapid weight loss unless nutritional support is given. Each case needs to be assessed individually, however. Repeated evaluation of the SGA allows the clinician to determine any impediment to the intake of food, the presence of GI dysfunction, and progressive functional loss and weight loss, which signal the need to start nutritional support.

The purely scientific approach would be to avoid nutritional support in all situations for which proof of benefit from randomized, controlled studies is lacking; however, in patients without adequate oral intake, this approach could in some cases result in starvation and death. The pragmatic approach is to evaluate the patient, using the SGA, and start nutritional support if the clinical evidence shows that otherwise the patient is likely to progress to critical malnutrition.[20]

Malnourished Patients

There are no controlled trials to show that nutritional support will reduce complications in all patients classified as SGA C. However, there are several indirect lines of evidence suggesting that nutritional support in such patients will reduce complications and improve outcome.

A multicenter, randomized, controlled trial undertaken by the Veterans Affairs Total Parenteral Nutrition Cooperative Study Group[21] stratified patients into three nutritional groups. In the group of severely malnourished patients, the rate of major noninfectious complications was significantly lower in patients randomized to TPN than in control subjects (5.3% versus 42.9%). Overall rates of complications and infectious complications in TPN-treated patients in this trial were not different from those in control patients, however.

Other studies have shown that nutritional supplementation can significantly reduce rehabilitation time in patients with hip fractures who had severe weight loss [see Figure 1][22] and that elderly patients with hip fractures, especially those with weight loss, benefit the most from supplemental feeding.[19]

Recommendations Elderly patients, especially those with weight loss, should receive nutritional supplements in the hospital. Despite the lack of data from well-designed controlled trials, patients who are classified as SGA C should be given nutritional support.

SURGERY

In a meta-analysis of perioperative parenteral nutrition, Detsky and colleagues[23] combined the results of 14 randomized or quasi-randomized trials and showed that absolute morbidity was reduced by 5.2% and the relative risk reduction was 20.7%. These differences were not statistically significant, however ($P = 0.21$). Of the 14 studies, only one showed a significant reduction in complication and fatality rates with TPN. These authors concluded that perioperative TPN did not influence outcome. On the other hand, only three of the 14 trials were limited to malnourished patients (who were the most likely to benefit from TPN), so the negative result may simply reflect the fact that the trials were weighted by patients who were unlikely to benefit from nutritional support. In contrast, Twomey[24] concluded that the pooled estimate in malnourished surgical patients shows a 7.1% reduction in morbidity with TPN. In the VA trial,[21] secondary analysis showed that the severely malnourished patients had a reduction in overall morbidity from 47% to 26% with perioperative TPN.

Fan and colleagues[25] conducted a controlled trial of perioperative nutritional support in 124 patients undergoing major hepatic resection for hepatocellular carcinoma. The patients were randomized to parenteral nutrition plus oral diet or to diet only. Patients in the treatment arm received 1.5 g/kg of amino acids, of which 35% were branched-chain amino acids (BCAA), with 30 kcal/kg of a glucose-lipid mixture for energy. Medium-chain triglycerides (MCT) constituted 50% of the lipid infused. The parenteral formulation was given for 14 days. At least 20% of the patients had a preoperative weight loss of greater than 10% and therefore were likely to be malnourished, but 80% did not have weight loss. Overall morbidity, morbidity from sepsis, and diuretic use for ascites all were lower in patients who received nutritional support.

Although the benefits of parenteral nutrition in the perioperative state are controversial, randomized trials of postoperative enteral feeding have shown improved outcome. In hip fracture patients,[22] supplemental feeding of a liquid formula diet reduced recovery time. In general surgical patients,[26] the rate of infectious complications with early enteral feeding was lower than that with nil per os (NPO).

Recommendations

Postoperatively, patients who have undergone major surgery should receive supplemental liquid formula feeding. The data do not support the routine use of parenteral nutrition for perioperative nutritional support, but parenteral nutrition clearly reduces complications in patients undergoing hepatic resection. It is not clear whether standard parenteral formulations will reduce complications in patients undergoing hepatic resection or whether it is necessary to give BCAA or MCT. Patients with hip fracture and weight loss will benefit from enteral feeding. Despite the lack of proven benefit, other severely malnourished patients (i.e., those classified as SGA C) should receive perioperative nutritional support.

SERIOUS COMPROMISE OF BOWEL FUNCTION

In patients with massive small bowel resection (i.e., less than 60 cm remaining), chronic bowel obstruction, extensive bowel disease, severe radiation enteritis, or end jejunostomy in which oral feeding results in uncontrolled fluid and electrolyte losses, parenteral nutrition is needed because oral feeding is very unlikely to provide sufficient nourishment. An economic analysis of such patients showed that provision of parenteral nutrition at home was associated with improved quality of life and was cost-effective.[27] The outlook was especially good for those with chronic intestinal failure from benign disease.[28]

Recommendations

Initially, all patients with a short bowel (see above) need parenteral nutrition. Later, about 30% (especially those with an intact or partially intact colon) can be treated with oral diet and supplements. Enteral nutrition is not necessary in these patients; controlled studies have shown that enteral nutrition was no better than an oral diet in patients with a short bowel and end jejunostomy.[29] Patients with a massive resection can absorb 50% to 60% of an oral diet.[30] By using oral rehydration solution, supplements, and a high-calorie oral diet, about 30% of such patients can reduce or stop home parenteral nutrition. The remaining patients will require supplemental fluid and electrolytes or parenteral nutrition to maintain a normal weight and electrolyte-fluid status.

BOWEL REST

Parenteral Nutrition

Bowel rest is widely used in pancreatitis, intestinal fistulas, and inflammatory bowel disease. The bowel is rested by keeping the patient NPO. Malnutrition is avoided by instituting parenteral nutrition.

Parenteral nutrition is used in pancreatitis because eating often induces pain in such cases. The only controlled trial of parenteral nutrition versus oral diet in patients with mild pancreatitis showed that TPN did not influence recovery.[31] In two trials comparing parenteral nutrition with enteral nutrition in patients with mild or acute pancreatitis, the trial of patients with mild pancreatitis[32] found no difference in septic complications, whereas the trial of patients with severe pancreatitis[33] found less sepsis with enteral nutrition. However, in the latter trial, twice the number of patients on parenteral nutrition were hyperglycemic, a factor known to increase septic complications.[8] Again, these trials do not prove that enteral nutrition is better than standard care.

Parenteral nutrition is useful in patients with intestinal fistulas, in whom eating increases output and fasting reduces output by 30% to 50%. However, there are no controlled trials comparing the effect of bowel rest plus parenteral nutrition with that of oral intake in the healing of fistulas.

In inflammatory bowel disease, bowel rest reduces abdominal discomfort and diarrhea. Controlled trials have not shown that bowel rest aids recovery in these patients, however.[34]

Recommendations Because pancreatitis, intestinal fistulas, and inflammatory bowel disease may prevent the ingestion or absorption of oral nutrients and result in malnutrition, the use of bowel rest and parenteral nutrition is a reasonable strategy in some of these cases, despite the lack of evidence that bowel rest alters the course of the disease. Specifically, enteral or parenteral nutrition should be given to prevent or treat malnutrition when a patient cannot take in or absorb nutrients for 7 to 10 days, when a patient loses nutrients because of a fistula for 7 to 10 days, or when a patient is clearly malnourished (SGA C).

The route of administration selected should be capable of delivering the ideal nutrient intake successfully. For example, enteral nutrition is unlikely to be successful in a patient with a high jejunal fistula who is putting out large volumes of intestinal contents.

Enteral Nutrition in Crohn Disease

Controlled trials in Crohn disease have shown that enteral nutrition reduces the activity of the disease and, in children, promotes growth.[35] However, a recent meta-analysis of eight randomized, controlled trials of 413 patients with Crohn disease showed that enteral nutrition was not as effective as corticosteroids in inducing a remission (odds ratio of enteral nutrition/corticosteroids, 0.35; confidence interval, 0.23–0.53). In addition, there was no difference between elemental and polymeric diets in inducing clinical remission.[36] Regrettably, there are no placebo-controlled trials to show whether enteral nutrition is an effective modality for treatment of active Crohn disease.

Recommendations Enteral nutrition is not a replacement for routine drug treatment of active Crohn disease, but under certain circumstances it has definite benefits. Enteral nutrition is especially useful in promoting growth and reducing disease activity in children with growth failure. In such children, enteral nutrition can be given on a long-term basis at home, along with other treatment to promote growth.

In line with other recommendations for nutritional support, patients with active Crohn disease who are SGA C should be treated with enteral nutrition and other modalities as required. However, if they are SGA C and are unable to tolerate enteral nutrition, parenteral nutrition should be used until they can tolerate adequate nutrition by the oral route. Nutritional support is also necessary when serial SGA determinations show evidence of poor intake and the patient has severe GI symptoms and continued functional impairment that could lead to critical malnutrition. The route used depends on the capacity of the GI tract to absorb nutrients.

CANCER MALNUTRITION

Malnutrition in metastatic cancer has been used as an indication for parenteral nutrition. Controlled trials have failed to substantiate that nutritional support is beneficial in patients with metastatic cancer,[37] however, and in fact have suggested that parenteral nutrition may have adverse effects. On the other hand, parenteral nutrition has been shown to favorably influence graft survival in patients receiving a bone marrow transplant.[38]

Recommendations

In cancer patients, nutritional support with enteral or parenteral nutrition is appropriate for preventing or treating malnutrition that is not caused by the tumor per se. For example, patients whose colon cancer has been eradicated but who suffer from short bowel because of extensive radiation enteritis should respond to parenteral nutrition. Criteria for nutritional support in cancer patients are as follows: (1) there is no evidence of tumor or its progression; (2) the patient has a GI complication, such as radiation enteritis or resection; and (3) as a result of this GI complication, critical malnutrition has occurred or will predictably occur (i.e., the patient is SGA C, or serial evaluation of SGA indicates progression toward SGA C).

The most difficult ethical question concerns the use of parenteral nutrition for patients in whom tumor progression causes intestinal obstruction or cachexia. Parenteral nutrition is being increasingly used for this indication [see Home Parenteral Nutrition, below].

RENAL FAILURE

Because patients with renal disease cannot excrete nitrogen normally, parenteral nutrition in which the source of nitrogen is limited to essential amino acids (EAA) has been used to reduce urea production. A meta-analysis has concluded that parenteral nutrition with EAA does not improve survival to discharge; when the trials were adjusted for quality, there was no effect of EAA.[39]

Recommendations

Patients with renal failure who cannot meet their nutritional requirements by the oral route should be given nutritional support and have fluid, electrolytes, and nitrogenous metabolites removed by dialysis or continuous arteriovenous hemofiltration. Fluid intake is minimized by using enteral nutrition with a calorie density of 2 kcal/ml or parenteral nutrition containing 35% dextrose or 20% lipid as the source of energy. Sodium intake should be restricted to 40 to 70 mmol/day, and other electrolytes should be added if their plasma levels fall. Acidosis should be controlled by appropriate dialysis. Trace elements and vitamin supplements need not be curtailed.

HEPATIC FAILURE AND ALCOHOLIC LIVER DISEASE

The discovery that hepatic encephalopathy is associated with reduced BCAAs and increased aromatic amino acids in plasma has led to the use of parenteral nutrition formulas enriched in BCAAs and reduced in aromatic amino acids. Meta-analysis of trials comparing BCAA-enriched mixtures with standard therapy has shown significant improvement in encephalopathy and, possibly, in short-term mortality.[40] On the other hand, there is no evidence that standard amino acid mixtures or enteral nutrition providing 0.8 to 1 g/kg/day of protein or amino acids has precipitated encephalopathy. In fact, 75 g/day of supplementary amino acids with 400 kcal/day of dextrose improved liver function and was tolerated by patients with severe alcoholic hepatitis.[41]

Recommendations

Patients with hepatic failure who are unable to be on a normal diet need enteral or parenteral nutrition. The protein intake should be about 0.8 to 1 g/kg/day of a high-quality protein or balanced amino acids. Carbohydrates and fat should be given in equal proportions because these patients are carbohydrate intolerant but utilize fat well, and fat infusions increase the levels of BCAA in plasma.[42] Because these patients are sodium and water overloaded, they should receive a total of about 1,500 ml of water daily, and their sodium intake should be restricted to 20 mmol/day. Supplemental potassium, vitamins (A, D, and B complex), and zinc should be given.

Practice of Nutritional Support

GENERAL PRINCIPLES OF NUTRITIONAL CARE

At hospital admission, all patients should be interviewed by a dietitian and have their SGA calculated to determine whether they can be maintained on a normal or modified oral diet (with

---

Table 1 Procedure for Nasogastric or Nasoenteral Tube Placement

1. Explain the procedure to the patient, to obtain cooperation.
2. Seat the patient comfortably at the edge of the bed, sitting upright.
3. Check nostrils for painful lesions and obstruction.
4. Insert stylet into tube and lubricate.
5. Measure approximate length of tube to be passed by the distance between the tip of the nose to the ear and down to the midepigastrium. Add about 25 cm to this distance.
6. Flex neck slightly.
7. Pass tube through an unobstructed nostril. If the patient finds this very uncomfortable, spray nostril with lidocaine 4% topical solution.
8. Ask the patient to swallow water as the tube is passed.
9. If the patient coughs or chokes, withdraw tube into the pharynx and reinsert.
10. Aspirate gastric contents to confirm position of tube.
11. Air may be injected into the tube while auscultating to determine the intragastric location of the tube.
12. For nasogastric feeding, confirm the tube position by x-ray before infusing.
13. For nasoenteral feeding, place the patient in right lateral position and gradually advance tube. Metoclopramide, 10 mg I.V., may be used to propel the tube.
14. If tube has not passed into the bowel by 24 hours, endoscopic or fluoroscopic guidance may be used.

---

supplements) in sufficient quantities or whether nutritional support is indicated and, if so, how urgently. In patients requiring nutritional support, the physician and the dietitian should define nutrient intake, route of administration, and goals. The most important objective is maintenance of uninterrupted nutrient intake, to avoid weeks of starvation followed by the urgent institution of parenteral nutrition to an iatrogenically malnourished patient.

Oral Nutrition

In patients who can eat, close attention to maintenance of oral dietary intake—and use of supplements, where required—should be the standard of care. Enteral nutrition should be considered if it becomes clear that this approach does not permit sufficient intake to meet requirements.

Enteral Nutrition

Enteral nutrition is applicable to all patients, but it should be used with caution in patients with (1) clinically significant gastroesophageal reflux; (2) intestinal obstruction; (3) GI fistula or recent surgical anastomosis, unless the tube can be inserted distal to the area in question or threaded at operation past the area; and (4) cardiovascular instability with shock. Gastric retention is a relative contraindication. In patients who accumulate secretions in the stomach and then aspirate, it may be possible to pass a feeding tube into the small intestine and aspirate the stomach with a second tube. However, in such cases the relative discomfort of two tubes versus parenteral nutrition should be considered. A recent survey showed that patients preferred parenteral nutrition over enteral nutrition.[43]

Short-term enteral access Nasogastric or nasoenteric placement of a feeding tube provides short-term enteral access. The tube should be small bore (9 to 12 French) and 105 to 110 cm long [see Table 1]. These tubes are usually made of Silastic or polyurethane. The latter become very slippery when wet, thus aiding insertion. I prefer intestinal placement of the tube, because controlled trials have shown better achievement of nutrient intake[44] and, possibly, reduced risk of aspiration when the tube is placed beyond the ligament of Treitz.

Long-term feeding The definition of long-term feeding is arbitrary. Children with Crohn disease have been fed for months by teaching them to pass a nasogastric tube each night, receive a nocturnal feeding, and then remove the tube in the morning before going to school. However, in many instances nasal tubes become uncomfortable, and a gastrostomy tube can be placed endoscopically by a gastroenterologist or an interventional radiologist. This method has been shown to be safer and more cost-effective than a surgically placed gastrostomy. There are two methods of percutaneous endoscopic gastrostomy (PEG): the pull (Ponsky-Gauderer) method and the push (Russell) method.

Feeding into the small bowel can be performed after the insertion of a percutaneous endoscopic jejunostomy (PEJ). After the tract of the PEG tube is established, a PEJ tube with two arms can replace the tube. One arm remains in the stomach and can be used to drain this organ; the other arm is advanced under endoscopic guidance through the pylorus into the small intestine. In this way, the stomach can be decompressed, and simultaneously, the patient can be fed into the small bowel.

To eliminate the inconvenience of the bulky feeding tube, patients with long-term gastrostomies can be fitted with a so-called button device, which lies flush with the abdominal wall. Between feedings, a valve in the device closes off access to the stomach; during feedings, the feeding tube is inserted past the valve, permitting access to the stomach.

Parenteral Nutrition

The intravenous route is used as a supplement to oral or enteral nutrition or is used as the sole source of nutrition (TPN) when it becomes clear that the patient is not receiving sufficient nutrients by the other routes. Regular evaluation of SGA should be performed during TPN to ensure that the patient's nutrient requirements are being met.

Short-term parenteral feeding Short-term infusions are best given through a peripherally inserted central catheter (PICC). These catheters are inserted into an arm or forearm vein and advanced into the superior vena cava. PICCs are comfortable and avoid the risks of subclavian puncture or the difficulties of maintaining sterility of the exit sites of jugular catheters. In addition, full TPN with hypertonic mixtures can be given through these catheters without risk of thrombosis. Despite the designation "short term," these catheters can be used for months.

Long-term parenteral feeding Patients with intestinal failure often require parenteral feeding for years. To permit long-term parenteral feeding, an interventional radiologist advances a specially designed catheter through a subcutaneous tunnel via the jugular vein to the superior vena cava. The tip of this catheter should lie just above the right atrium, to avoid thrombotic complications. Near the exit site, within the subcutaneous tunnel, the catheter is surrounded by a Dacron cuff. Fibroblasts will grow into the cuff, sealing and anchoring the skin exit site.

Protein

Protein requirements are met by giving whole proteins, peptides, or amino acids in enteral nutrition and by infusing an amino acid mixture in parenteral nutrition. The goal is to promote nitrogen retention and protein synthesis. Although limiting glucose and lipid (energy) intake will maximize nitrogen retention, dietary protein has an anabolic effect independent of energy intake, and will reduce nitrogen losses when infused alone.[45] Thus, the amount of amino acids given appears to be a very important determinant of nitrogen balance.

About 1 to 1.5 g/kg of ideal body weight of protein or amino acids will be sufficient for most patients with normal renal function. Additional amounts should be added for losses from prior depletion or current hypercatabolism. In patients with hepatic failure, protein intake should be restricted to 0.8 to 1.0 g/kg a day.

Glutamine

Glutamine is an amino acid released by muscle and used by immune cells and enteral cells for energy. In malnutrition and after trauma, muscle glutamine and muscle protein synthesis are reduced. The infusion of glutamine normalizes muscle glutamine and restores protein synthesis.[46] Clinically, bone marrow transplant patients were noted to have fewer episodes of sepsis and a shorter hospital stay if they received a glutamine-supplemented amino acid solution.[47] Because glutamine does not have a long shelf-life in solution, dipeptides containing glutamine have been used as a substitute. Infusion of solutions containing such dipeptides has been found to increase muscle glutamine and improve protein synthesis.[46]

Immunonutrition

Enteral formulations enriched in arginine, omega-3 fatty acids, and glutamine nucleotides are considered to enhance the immune response; treatment with these formulations is referred to as immunonutrition. These formulations vary in composition, but they are distinguished by high (12 to 15 g/L) or low (4 to 6 g/L) arginine content, presence or absence of glutamine and nucleotides, and different concentrations of omega-3 fatty acids. A recent summit on immune-enhancing enteral therapy[48] concluded, on the basis of published literature, that immunonutrition should be given to malnourished patients undergoing elective GI surgery and to trauma patients with an injury severity score of 18 or greater or an abdominal trauma index of 20 or greater. Immunonutrition was also recommended, despite lack of evidence, in patients undergoing head and neck surgery or aortic reconstruction, as well as in patients with severe head injury or burns, and in ventilator-dependent nonseptic patients. It was not recommended for patients with splanchnic hypoperfusion or bowel obstruction distal to the access site or after major upper GI hemorrhage.

A systematic review of immunonutrition by Heyland and colleagues[49] showed that it reduced septic complications but did not reduce mortality. Their analysis of 22 randomized, controlled trials covering 2,419 critically ill or surgical patients indicated that only high-arginine formulations reduced infectious complications and length of stay. These authors concluded that in patients undergoing elective surgery, immunonutrition may reduce complications and reduce length of stay. Pending further studies, however, immunonutrition was not recommended in patients with critical illness. Because many trauma and septic patients may be critically ill, these authors' recommendations are at variance with those of the immunonutrition summit (see above). The finding that benefit is seen only with the formulation containing higher amounts of arginine raises the question whether arginine per se or the higher nitrogen intake is responsible for the benefit.

Energy (Glucose and Lipids)

In healthy persons, basal energy expenditure (BEE), or basal metabolic rate (BMR), in kilocalories a day can be predicted with the Harris-Benedict equation:

$$\text{BEE in males} = 66.5 + (13.8 \times \text{weight in kg})$$
$$+ (5.0 \times \text{height in cm}) - (6.8 \times \text{age in yr})$$

$$\text{BEE in females} = 655.1 + (9.6 \times \text{weight in kg})$$
$$+ (1.8 \times \text{height in cm}) - (4.7 \times \text{age in yr})$$

A calculator to be used for determining BEE according to the Harris-Benedict equation can be found on the Internet, at www-users.med.cornell.edu/~spon/picu/calc/beecalc.htm.

For patients substantially on bed rest, about 30% should be added to the BEE to meet their metabolic requirements. In practice, this calculates as a daily expenditure of about 31 kcal/kg. An expert group has suggested a daily intake of 25 kcal/kg in ICU patients.[50] Therefore, 25 to 30 kcal/kg/day will meet the needs of most patients, except those with burns. Malnutrition reduces the expected BEE by as much as 35%; injury, sepsis, and, especially, burns increase requirements.[51] Baker and colleagues[52] found that in critically sick patients in respiratory failure, the maximal degree of hypermetabolism was about 30%.

Energy requirements during TPN can be met by infusing glucose or lipid emulsions. These nonprotein energy sources enhance nitrogen retention. The most striking increase in nitrogen balance has been found to occur when energy was increased from 0 kcal/kg to 30 kcal/kg of ideal body weight. Increases above that provided only slight improvement. In obese persons, a high-protein formulation with only about 14 kcal/kg/day meets nitrogen requirements[53] and is associated with satisfactory wound healing.[54]

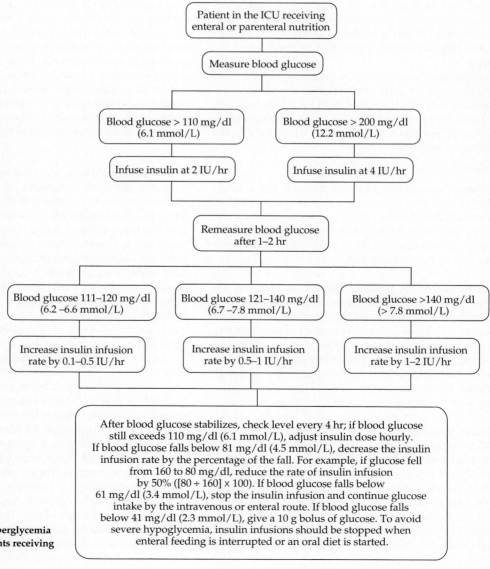

Figure 2 **Controlling hyperglycemia in intensive care unit patients receiving nutritional support.**

Table 2   Daily Electrolyte and Trace Element Requirements for Adults on Total Parenteral Nutrition

Element	Normal	Increased GI Losses	Renal Failure	Comments
Sodium (mmol)	80–120	Meet losses	20–40	Reduce in heart failure
Potassium (mmol)	40—80	80–120	0–20	Correct hypokalemia before starting nutrition
Magnesium (mmol)	5–10	10–20	0–5	Correct hypomagnesemia before starting nutrition
Phosphorus (mmol)	10–15	10–15	0–5	Risk of dangerously low serum levels when feeding patients with severe malnutrition
Zinc (mg)	TPN: 3–4 Enteral: 15–20	TPN: 12–25 Enteral: 50–100	No change	—
Copper (mg)	TPN: 0.25–0.3 Enteral: 2–4	TPN: 0.5–0.7 Enteral: 4–8	No change	Reduce to 0.1 in hepatic failure

Because glucose spares nitrogen in fasting persons, it has been advocated as the main source of energy for parenteral nutrition. However, recent studies have shown that in malnourished patients and septic patients, lipids can promote nitrogen retention and increase total body nitrogen to the same extent as glucose, provided amino acids are given.[55] Fats constitute about 30% of total energy in most enteral formulas. Furthermore, glucose-lipid mixtures facilitate the control of severe hyperglycemia in septic patients with insulin resistance.[50]

Infusion of glucose at rates that exceed energy requirements elevates O_2 consumption, CO_2 production, resting energy expenditure, and urinary norepinephrine excretion. However, the magnitude of increased CO_2 production is small if total calories infused conform to levels recommended for the patient's clinical situation.[51]

The exact amount of lipid to include in the parenteral nutrition regimen is controversial. In a randomized, controlled trial of 512 bone marrow transplant patients receiving TPN, sepsis was no more frequent in patients who received 30% of energy as lipid than in those who received only sufficient lipids to meet essential fatty acid (EFA) needs (6% to 8% of energy intake).[56] In addition, EFA deficiency developed in some of the latter patients, and in some, this small amount of lipid was insufficient to meet energy requirements without induction of hyperglycemia from the glucose component. These authors recommend giving 25% to 30% of energy as long-chain triglycerides (LCTs). In contrast, a study in 57 trauma patients found that TPN with added lipid increased sepsis and hospital stay.[57] It was not clear whether the adverse effect was from the lipid per se or the increased energy intake while on lipid.

Because of their glucose content, both enteral nutrition and TPN enhance the risk of sepsis if the blood glucose level is allowed to rise above 127 mg/dl (7 mmol/L).[8] Therefore, insulin should be infused in patients receiving nutritional support to keep them as close to normoglycemia as possible [*see Figure 2*].

Whereas the major concern with glucose-based formulations is hyperglycemia, the key concern with lipid emulsions is hypertriglyceridemia, which may induce pancreatitis. Lipid particles also reduce gas diffusion in the lungs and inhibit the reticuloendothelial system. Provided that lipid emulsions are infused continuously at a rate that does not exceed 110 mg/kg/hr, hypertriglyceridemia does not occur. When these principles are followed, 30% to 50% of nonprotein calories can be given as fat, especially in glucose-intolerant patients.

Electrolytes, Trace Elements, and Vitamins

In patients receiving nutritional support, levels of electrolytes and trace elements should be adjusted to fit the clinical circumstances [*see Table 2*]. Carbohydrate feeding induces sodium retention, resulting in refeeding edema. In malnourished patients, great care should be taken to prevent salt and water overload.

Body potassium is disproportionately reduced relative to nitrogen in malnourished patients. Positive nitrogen balance does not occur unless potassium, phosphorus, and magnesium are given.[58,59] During enteral and parenteral nutrition, serum phosphorus may drop precipitously and cause dangerous neurologic symptoms.[60]

Micronutrients comprise vitamins and trace elements. The former are complex organic compounds; the latter are inorganic elements. Trace elements important to nutritional support include zinc, copper, chromium, and selenium. Diarrhea increases zinc requirements markedly and copper requirements modestly [*see Table 2*]. Oral chromium requirements have not been precisely determined, but deficiency occurs in patients receiving TPN; in one of my patients, the daily chromium needs were increased to 10 to 20 µg. Patients receiving parenteral nutrition may develop selenium deficiency, with muscle pains and cardiomyopathy. Increased losses of selenium can occur from the GI tract and from wounds. The recommended dose of selenium for stable patients is 40 µg/day. Patients depleted of selenium may require as much a 120 µg/day to regain normal levels.

The current recommendations for vitamins [*see Table 3*] specify the amounts required to maintain normal plasma or blood levels in patients on long-term home parenteral nutrition. There are no clearly defined recommendations for critically sick or septic patients.

HOME PARENTERAL NUTRITION

Patients with intestinal failure from a short bowel, chronic bowel obstruction, radiation enteritis, or untreatable malabsorption can be nourished by parenteral nutrition given at home. Arteriovenous shunts were initially used for long-term venous access in these patients, but success was limited because of clotting or disruption of the shunt. Long-term success has been achieved with a tunneled silicone rubber catheter or an implanted reservoir. Premixed nutrients are infused overnight. The catheter is then disconnected and a heparin lock applied, leaving the patient free to attend to daily activities. We have used home parenteral nutrition for more than 20 years in

Table 3 Recommendations for Vitamins in Adults on Total Parenteral Nutrition

Vitamin	Recommended Daily Dose
A	3,300 IU
D_2	200 IU
E	10 IU
K_1	150 mg
Ascorbate	200 mg
Thiamin	6 mg
Riboflavin	3.6 mg
Pyridoxine	6 mg
Niacin	40 mg
Pantothenate	15 mg
Biotin	60 μg
Folate	600 μg
Cobalamin	5 μg

two patients with total jejunoileal resection; one continues to receive it after 30 years. Survival of patients with short bowel from treatment for Crohn disease or pseudo-obstruction is excellent. Home parenteral nutrition increases quality-adjusted years of life in these patients and is cost-effective. On the other hand, mean survival in AIDS patients or those with metastatic cancer who receive home parenteral nutrition is about 3 months. There is no evidence that home parenteral nutrition prolongs their survival or enhances their quality of life. Trials are urgently required to justify the use of home parenteral nutrition in terminal cancer and AIDS.

Complications of Long-term Home Parenteral Nutrition

At the start of nutritional support, patients are vulnerable to complications related to venous and enteral access and to metabolic complications. Careful and frequent monitoring and adjusting of nutrient intake will prevent these complications. Over the longer term, patients receiving TPN are vulnerable to three organ-specific complications: hepatic disease, bone disease, and gallstones.

Hepatic disease The most serious form of hepatic disease related to TPN is chronic cholestasis with fibrosis. This condition is most common in patients with a very short bowel. The exact cause is unknown, but absorption of endotoxin or alteration in bile salts by bacterial dehydroxylation are possible factors. Successful treatment with metronidazole and with ursodeoxycholic acid has been reported. In some patients, carnitine infusions have corrected cholestasis.

Bone disease Bone loss during long-term TPN is a complex issue. In a prospective longitudinal study, patients were noted to have a high bone turnover before the institution of home parenteral nutrition, but during TPN this changed to osteomalacia and slow bone turnover. This process has been attributed to aluminum toxicity but occurs in its absence[61] and

seems to respond to withdrawal of vitamin D from the TPN formula. In a prospective 4-year study of patients on home parenteral nutrition, withdrawal of vitamin D increased spinal bone mass.[62] On the other hand, patients on home parenteral nutrition can lose bone mass as a result of factors such as active inflammatory bowel disease, corticosteroid therapy, and inactivity. Some clinicians are treating reduced bone mineral density in these patients with intravenous bisphosphonates such as pamidronate and clodronate (the latter is not available in the United States). Although there are no controlled trials of bisphosphonates in patients receiving home parenteral nutrition, there are anecdotal reports of improvement of bone mass with this therapy.

Gallstones The short bowel state results in bile salt deficiency and increased biliary cholesterol secretion. In addition, sludge composed of bilirubin and calcium forms in the gallbladder. Consequently, the incidence of gallstones is high in these patients. These stones are mixed cholesterol and pigment.

References

1. Allison SP: The uses and limitations of nutritional support. Clin Nutr 11:319, 1992

2. DeWys WD, Begg D, Lavin PT: Prognostic effect of weight loss prior to chemotherapy in cancer patients. Am J Med 69:491, 1980

3. Jeejeebhoy KN: Rhoads lecture—1988. Bulk or bounce—the object of nutritional support. JPEN J Parenter Enteral Nutr 12:539, 1988

4. Windsor JA, Hill GL: Weight loss with physiologic impairment: a basic indicator of surgical risk. Ann Surg 207:290, 1988

5. Heyland DK, MacDonald S, Keefe L, et al: Total parenteral nutrition in the critically ill patient: a meta-analysis. JAMA 280:2013, 1998

6. Braunschweig CL, Levy P, Sheean PM, et al: Enteral compared with parenteral nutrition: a meta-analysis. Am J Clin Nutr 74:534, 2001

7. Koretz RL, Lipman TO, Klein S: AGA Technical Review on Parenteral Nutrition. American Gastroenterological Association. Gastroenterology 121:970, 2001

8. van den Berghe G, Wouters P, Weekers F, et al: Intensive insulin therapy in the critically ill patient. N Engl J Med 345:1359, 2001

9. Jeejeebhoy KN: TPN: potion or poison. Am J Clin Nutr 74:160, 2001

10. Woodcock NP, Zeigler D, Palmer MD, et al: Enteral versus parenteral nutrition: a pragmatic study. Nutrition 17:1, 2000

11. Baker J, Detsky AS, Wesson DE, et al: Nutritional assessment: a comparison of clinical judgment and objective measurements. N Engl J Med 306: 969, 1982

12. Detsky AS, McLaughlin JR, Baker JP, et al: What is subjective global assessment of nutritional status? JPEN J Parenter Enteral Nutr 11:8, 1987

13. Detsky AS, Baker JP, O'Rourke K, et al: Predicting nutrition-associated complications for patients undergoing gastrointestinal surgery. JPEN J Parenter Enteral Nutr 11:440, 1987

14. Perman M, Crivelli A, Khoury M: Nutritional prognosis in hospitalized patients. Am J Clin Nutr 75:426S, 2002

15. Pirlich M, Schütz T, Gastell S, et al: Malnutrition affects long-term prognosis in hospitalized patients. Gastroenterology 122(suppl):A636, 2002

16. Guidelines for the use of parenteral and enteral nutrition in adult and pediatric patients. JPEN J Parenter Enteral Nutr 26(1 suppl):1SA, 2002

17. Moore EE, Jones TN: Benefits of immediate jejunostomy feeding after major abdominal trauma: a prospective, randomized study. J Trauma 26:874, 1986

18. Rana SK, Bray J, Menzis-Gow N, et al: Short term benefits of post-operative oral dietary supplements in surgical patients. Clin Nutr 11:337, 1992

19. Larsson J, Unosson M, Ek AC, et al: Effect of dietary supplement on nutritional status and clinical outcome in 501 geriatric patients: a randomized study. Clin Nutr 9:179, 1990

20. Detsky AS: Parenteral nutrition: is it helpful? N Engl J Med 325:573, 1991

21. Perioperative total parenteral nutrition in surgical patients. The Veterans Affairs Total Parenteral Nutrition Cooperative Study Group. N Engl J Med 325:525, 1991

22. Bastow MD, Rawlings J, Allison SP: Benefits of supplementary tube feeding after fractured neck of femur: a randomised controlled trial. BMJ 287:1589, 1983

23. Detsky AS, Baker J, O'Rourke K, et al: Perioperative parenteral nutrition: a meta-analysis. Ann Intern Med 107:195, 1987

24. Twomey PL: Cost-effectiveness of total parenteral nutrition. Clinical Nutrition, Parenteral Nutrition. Rombeau JL, Caldwell MD, Eds. WB Saunders Co, Philadelphia, 1993, p 401

25. Fan S-T, Lo C-M, Lai ECS, et al: Perioperative nutritional support in patients undergoing hepatectomy for hepatocellular carcinoma. N Engl J Med 331:1547, 1994

26. Lewis SJ, Egger M, Sylvester PA, et al: Early enteral feeding versus "nil by mouth" after gastrointestinal surgery: systematic review and meta-analysis of controlled trials. BMJ 323:773, 2001

27. Detsky AS, McLaughlin JR, Abrams HB, et al: A cost-utility analysis of the home parenteral nutrition program at Toronto General Hospital: 1970–1982. JPEN J Parenter Enteral Nutr 10:49, 1986

28. Messing B, Lemann M, Landis P, et al: Prognosis of patients with nonmalignant chronic intestinal failure receiving long-term home parenteral nutrition. Gastroenterology 108:1005, 1995

29. McIntyre PB, Fitchew M, Lennard-Jones JE: Patients with a high jejunostomy do not need a special diet. Gastroenterology 91:25, 1986

30. Woolf GM, Miller C, Kurian V, et al: Diet for patients with a short bowel: high fat or high carbohydrate? Gastroenterology 84:823, 1983

31. Sax HC, Warner BW, Talamini MA, et al: Early total parenteral nutrition in acute pancreatitis: lack of beneficial effects. Am J Surg 153:117, 1987

32. McClave SA, Greene LM, Snider HL, et al: Comparison of the safety of early enteral vs parenteral nutrition in mild acute pancreatitis. JPEN J Parenter Enteral Nutr 21:14, 1997

33. Kalfarentzos F, Kehagias J, Mead N, et al: Enteral nutrition is superior to parenteral nutrition in severe acute pancreatitis: results of a randomized trial. Br J Surg 84:1665, 1997

34. Greenberg GR, Fleming CR, Jeejeebhoy KN, et al: Controlled trial of bowel rest and nutritional support in the management of Crohn's disease. Gut 29:1309, 1988

35. Polk DB, Hattner JAT, Kerner JA: Improved growth and disease activity after intermittent administration of a defined formula diet in children with Crohn's disease. JPEN J Parenter Enteral Nutr 16:499, 1992

36. Griffiths AM, Ohlsson A, Sherman PM, et al: Meta-analysis of enteral nutrition as primary treatment of active Crohn's disease. Gastroenterology 108:1056, 1995

37. McGeer AJ, Detsky AS, O'Rourke K: Parenteral nutrition in cancer patients undergoing chemotherapy: a meta-analysis. Nutrition 6:233, 1990

38. Weisdorf SA, Lysne J, Wind D, et al: Positive effect of prophylactic total parenteral nutrition on long-term outcome of bone marrow transplantation. Transplantation 43:833, 1987

39. Naylor CD, Detsky AS, O'Rourke K, et al: Does treatment with essential amino acids and hypertonic glucose improve survival in acute renal failure? A meta-analysis. Ren Fail 10:141, 1987

40. Naylor CD, O'Rourke K, Detsky AS, et al: Parenteral nutrition with branched-chain amino acids in hepatic encephalopathy: a meta-analysis. Nutrition 6:233, 1989

41. Bonkovsky HL, Fiellin DA, Smith GS, et al: A randomized, controlled trial of treatment of alcoholic hepatitis with parenteral nutrition and oxandrolone. I: Short-term effects on liver function. Am J Gastroenterol 86:1200, 1991

42. Glynn MJ, Powell-Tuck J, Reaveley DA: High lipid parenteral nutrition improves portosystemic encephalopathy. JPEN J Parenter Enteral Nutr 12:457, 1988

43. Scolapio JS, Picco MF, Tarrosa VB: Enteral versus parenteral nutrition: the patient's preference. JPEN J Parenter Enteral Nutr 26:248, 2002

44. Montecalvo MA, Steger KA, Farber HW, et al: Nutritional outcome and pneumonia in critical care patients randomized to gastric versus jejunal tube feedings. Crit Care Med 20:1377, 1992

45. Greenberg GR, Marliss EB, Anderson GH, et al: Protein-sparing therapy in postoperative patients: effects of added hypocaloric glucose or lipid. N Engl J Med 294:1411, 1976

46. Hammarqvist F, Wernerman J, von der Decken A, et al: Alanyl-glutamine counteracts the depletion of free glutamine and the postoperative decline in protein synthesis in skeletal muscle. Ann Surg 212:637, 1990

47. Ziegler TR: Glutamine supplementation in bone marrow transplantation. Br J Nutr 87(suppl 1):S9, 2002

48. Proceedings from Summit on Immune-Enhancing Enteral Therapy. May 25-26, 2000, San Diego, California, USA. JPEN J Parenter Enteral Nutr 25(2 suppl):S1, 2001

49. Heyland DK, Novak F, Drover JW, et al: Should immunonutrition become routine in critically ill patients? JAMA 286:944, 2001

50. Applied nutrition in ICU patients. Consensus statement of the American College of Chest Physicians. Chest 111:769, 1997

51. Allard JP, Pichard C, Hoshino E, et al: Validation of a new formula for calculating the energy requirements of burn patients. JPEN J Parenter Enteral Nutr 14:115, 1990

52. Baker JP, Detsky AS, Stewart S, et al: Randomized trial of total parenteral nutrition in critically ill patients: metabolic effects of varying glucose-lipid ratios as the energy source. Gastroenterology 87:53, 1984

53. Choban PS, Burge JC, Scales D, et al: Hypoenergetic nutrition support in hospitalized obese patients: a simplified method for clinical application. Am J Clin Nutr 66:546, 1997

54. Dickerson RN, Rosato EF, Mullen JL: Net protein anabolism with hypocaloric parenteral nutrition in obese stressed patients. Am J Clin Nutr 44:747, 1986

55. MacFie J, Smith RC, Hill GL: Glucose or fat as a non-protein energy source? A controlled clinical trial in gastroenterological patients requiring intravenous nutrition. Gastroenterology 80:103, 1981

56. Lenssen P, Bruemmer BA, Bowden RA, et al: Intravenous lipid dose and incidence of bacteremia and fungemia in patients undergoing marrow transplantation. Am J Clin Nutr 67:927, 1998

57. Battistella FD, Widergren JT, Anderson JT, et al: A prospective, randomized trial of intravenous fat emulsion administration in trauma victims requiring total parenteral nutrition. J Trauma 43:52, 1997

58. Rudman D, Millikan WJ, Richardson TJ, et al: Elemental balances during intravenous hyperalimentation of underweight adult subjects. J Clin Invest 55:94, 1975

59. Freeman JB, Wittime MF, Stegink LD, et al: Effects of magnesium infusions on magnesium and nitrogen balance during parenteral nutrition. Can J Surg 25:570, 1982

60. Silvis SE, DiBartolomeo AG, Aaker HM: Hypophosphatemia and neurological changes secondary to oral caloric intake: a variant of hyperalimentation syndrome. Am J Gastroenterol 73:215, 1980

61. Karton MA, Rettmer R, Lipkin EW, et al: D-Lactate and metabolic bone disease in patients receiving long-term parenteral nutrition. JPEN J Parenter Enteral Nutr 13:132, 1989

62. Verhage AH, Cheong WK, Allard JP, et al: Vars Research Award. Increase in lumbar spine bone mineral content in patients on long-term parenteral nutrition without vitamin D supplementation. JPEN J Parenter Enteral Nutr 19:431, 1995

GENETICS

71 Genetics for the Clinician

Robb Moses, M.D., and Jone E. Sampson, M.D.

The human genome consists of approximately three billion pairs of nucleotides (bases) that encode about 40,000 genes in a string array consisting of a DNA polymer duplex. The information in the protein-coding genes is converted to functional elements through the copying of base sequences to RNA. RNA may itself be active—heterogeneous ribonucleotide proteins can interact with newly synthesized RNA to regulate structural changes or conformation—or it may be copied to protein. Whereas DNA is a relatively stable molecule, RNA is much less so, and RNA molecules are replaced by other RNA molecules rapidly in the cell. Models of how the genome is packaged within the nucleus, copied, and read by the cell have evolved at the molecular level. Science has also come to recognize how the genome is partitioned during cell division and during the formation of germ cells. At all levels, the information content is protected by mechanisms safeguarding the stability of the genome. Information is transferred out of the genome along two paths: information is transferred within the cell for defined functions specific to cell type (horizontal information transfer) and is transferred from one generation of cells to another through cell division, either for cell multiplication or for reproduction (vertical transfer).

The advances in the past century, from the verification of Mendel's observations[1] to having in hand the essentially complete sequence of the human genome, occurred in bursts in understanding or in technology. During the first 50 years of the 20th century, the principle of inheritance by means of packets of genetic information that were stable and that persisted independently of other units of inheritance from generation to generation was verified in animals and plants, with the fruit fly *Drosophila melanogaster* being a notable organism of study. In the 1940s, DNA was unequivocally shown to be the chemical basis of the gene.[2] Within another dozen years, the structure of DNA at the chemical level was proposed by Watson and Crick.[3] The model had immediate implications for the copying of genes and the mode of transfer of information. During the next 2 decades, the fundamental rules and mechanisms of these processes were determined; these advances relied heavily on the study of bacteria and their viruses, the phages. In the 1970s, three different technological advances catapulted genetics to the point at which the human DNA sequence was determined by century's end. These disparate techniques were as follows: the development of the ability to determine DNA sequence information in a relatively simple and reproducible manner; the ability to move and duplicate isolated segments of DNA; and the evolution of computers with adequate power for storing and comparing large amounts of sequence information. Refinements in these basic advances, coupled with automation, led to the sequencing of the human genome during the last 15 years before the turn of the millennium.

With progress in technology, genetics has become applicable to clinical practice. The physician needs to be responsive to patterns of inheritance suggestive of genetic disease in a family member; the physician should also be aware of diagnostic capabilities for inherited diseases and be able to interpret the results of genetic testing for the patient or refer the patient for counseling. Given the pace of advances and the complexity of techniques, it is important that clinicians have knowledge of resources for patient referral and other relevant information. These resources include the Internet and other resources for technical and medical information and patient referral.

Diagnostic capabilities continue to improve, but therapies based on genetic technologies still lag. Prenatal diagnosis and neonatal screening are already powerful tools for the prevention of disease. However, researchers in genetic medicine are striving to address and develop treatments. New diagnostic powers based on microarray analysis, the hope of gene therapy, and the tailoring of drug therapies to maximize responsiveness and sensitivity for individuals seem feasible.

This chapter addresses basic knowledge of the human genome for the physician, gives reference points for the nongenetic physician, and focuses on the pathophysiology of genetic disease.

Genome Structure and Function

DNA STRUCTURE

Understanding the structure of the DNA duplex led at once to recognition that the polymer strand, composed only of four bases, could encode information in a linear format. DNA is composed of two polymer strands with a sugar-phosphate backbone, with the bases attached to each deoxyribose moiety [*see Figure 1*]. The two strands of DNA are stabilized by the bonding of hydrogen between the bases—the purine adenine (A) pairs with the pyrimidine thymine (T), and the purine guanine (G) pairs with the pyrimidine cytosine (C). The discovery of this was pivotal in modeling the structure of DNA. Alternative forms of pairing can be projected, but the pairings based on the most common structures of the bases and the strongest hydrogen bonds are predominant. The sugar-phosphate backbones of the strands have a chemical polarity, and the strands are antiparallel with respect to the polarity of the bonds between deoxyribose components. The information can be duplicated using each separate strand as a template. The linear code of the four-base alphabet allows enormous potential for information content—each cell contains about 1 m of DNA packaged within it.

DNA REPLICATION

The replication of DNA is a critical step in information storage. Although the structure is suggestive of a model for the replication of DNA, the definition of the apparatus took decades [*see Figure 2*]. Because the information is contained in the sequence of the bases, any change of a base could result in a subsequent change (mutation); mutations may be silent, in which case they do not lead to a change in protein function, or mutations may result in the inactivation of the product of the gene. Cells possess mechanisms to protect against changes in the DNA sequence, although natural variety—an advantage in selection—requires a low rate of change.

The replication machinery is centered on a DNA polymerase. DNA polymerase is an unusual enzyme in that it catalyzes a reaction directed by the base sequence of the strand be-

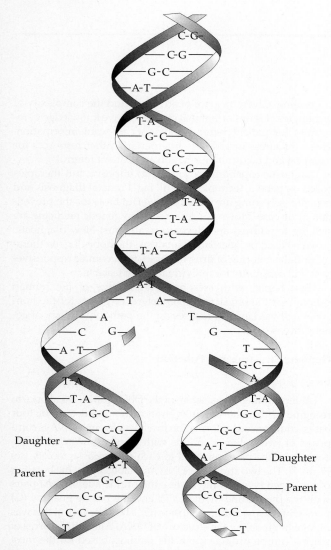

Figure 1 **In replication, the two strands of the parent DNA molecule (gray) separate as the base pairs detach. The daughter strands (blue) form when guanine (G) pairs with cytosine (C) and when adenine (A) pairs with thymine (T). The orientation of the two strands is antiparallel, so the strands grow in opposite directions.**

ing copied; that is, the base inserted into the new strand is directed by the base opposite. The enzyme uses all four bases with equal affinity, and the reaction is determined by the template. DNA polymerases are part of an assembly of proteins termed the replisome. The synthesis of new DNA is faithful; only about one base in 100,000 is a misincorporation. The replisome is actively proofreading the product, an exonuclease, which can remove a mispaired base from the growing end of the DNA strand (all DNA is made only in the 5′ to 3′ direction, based on the convention for the sugar-phosphate backbone). This proofreading by the replisome removes 99% of misincorporations. A last line of defense for integrity of information during replication is the system of mismatch repair. A complex of proteins tracks DNA synthesis, recognizes mismatches in the DNA that occur as a result of misincorporation, and corrects those mismatches. About 99% of mismatches are removed; the overall mistake rate in replication is about one in one billion to 10 billion.

Information is copied from the long-lived DNA molecule to the less stable messenger RNA (mRNA) molecule, which serves to translate the information into proteins. mRNA represents only 1% or so of the RNA in the cell; other categories of RNA synthesize proteins or act as catalytic units in the processing of genetic information. For protein synthesis, the mRNA must be read and the information transferred in a three-base code (codon). This allows for more triplet codons than the 20 amino acids used to build proteins would require. Several of the codons are delegated to terminating protein synthesis, and there is redundancy in the codons for the amino acids.[4]

mRNA is initially transcribed as a long, exact copy of the DNA strand, but posttranslational processing results in retention of the essential information needed for translation to protein. The genome contains introns, which interrupt the coding sequences, the exons. The intron material does not contain information for translation, so it must be removed for translation. This occurs during the RNA processing step, which is regulated by conserved sequences that identify the end and start of the exons [*see Figure 3*], allowing the coding portions to be spliced together. Because the signals that lead to removal are not stringent, it is possible for exons to be occasionally skipped and for splice variants and splice mutations to occur. This gives a great degree of flexibility for the final gene product and allows tissue-specific products.

The primary RNA transcript has other notable features. The 5′ end is capped with a protective methylated base; the 3′ end contains a region rich in pyrimidines and ends in a stretch of A residues, the poly-A region. After processing, the mRNA is transported to the cytoplasm, where translation on the ribosome protein synthesizing machine occurs.

After a protein is made, it may be modified through the attachment of sugars, acetyl groups, phosphates, or other modifying groups. Specific sequences direct the export or subcellular localization of the protein.

CHROMOSOME STRUCTURE AND IDENTIFICATION

The DNA double helix is packaged into the chromosome, a structure recognizable by light microscopy. The packaging is very efficient; the DNA is in the form of supercoils—like a rubber band that is tightly wound until it compacts upon itself. It is then folded into the chromatin assembly by the binding of basic histone proteins. The resulting structure resembles beads on a string, with the DNA wound tightly around a core of histone proteins—two H2A, two H2B, two H3, and two H4 residues—to form the nucleosome. Nucleosomes are spaced approximately 80 bases apart. The DNA structure is further condensed by the addition of other proteins. The DNA in chromatin also may be modified by the addition of methyl groups to certain positions, and the histones may be modified by phosphorylation, acetylation, or the addition of ubiquitin. These modifications to the chromatin are related to the regulation of gene expression.

There are 23 chromosome packages of genes in a cell; two of these chromosomes, X and Y, are the sex chromosomes. In females, there are two X chromosomes; in males, an X and a Y chromosome. The remaining 22 pairs of chromosomes are the autosomes. In the process of cell division, or mitosis, the chromosomes condense and are duplicated, with a complete, new set going to each daughter cell [*see Figure 4*]. In producing germ cells for reproduction, the number of chromosomes is halved to a haploid number of autosomes through the process of meiosis,

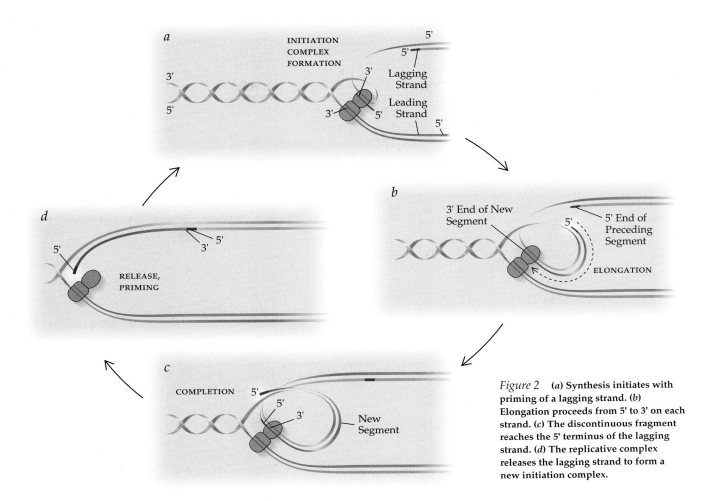

Figure 2 (*a*) **Synthesis initiates with priming of a lagging strand.** (*b*) **Elongation proceeds from 5' to 3' on each strand.** (*c*) **The discontinuous fragment reaches the 5' terminus of the lagging strand.** (*d*) **The replicative complex releases the lagging strand to form a new initiation complex.**

with either an X or a Y chromosome in spermatozoa and an X chromosome in oocytes. Telomeres are special DNA sequences at the ends of chromosomes that maintain integrity at chromosome termini and require telomerase enzyme activity for maintenance of normal length. The chromosomes contain a region of repeated sequence DNA, which is the centromere. This is the portion that anchors the replicated duplexes (chromatids) together at the time of cell division. The centromere is not centrally located; this results in a long arm, termed the q arm, and a short arm, termed the p arm, for petite. There is a standard system of nomenclature for describing the number of chromosomes and recognizable alterations or rearrangements of the chromosomes. For example, the normal male karyotype is listed as 46,XY and the normal female as 46,XX.

Chromosome identification and characterization was much improved by the development of staining or banding techniques. This process involves partial denaturation of the DNA and proteins, followed by staining. The resulting preparations allow identification of up to 800 bands, which may then be evaluated for structural changes. These techniques have led to the recognition of many rearrangements, leading to localization of genes.

Additional staining techniques based on binding to complementary short stretches of DNA tagged with fluorescent probes have been developed. Further development has led to chromogenic stains, which allow the identification of individual chromosomes and of certain regions of the chromosome—for example, the centromere or telomere.

Mutations in Clinical Conditions

Mutations are changes in the sequence of nucleotides within DNA, which may result in an abnormal or deleterious function of the gene product. There are different types of mutations leading to genetic disease. These mutations range in size from single base changes that alter the gene product to the addition or deletion of whole chromosomes. Intermediate structural rearrangements may involve segments that are large enough to be able to be detected microscopically, or they may involve segments that are so small as to require detection by molecular labeling methods. Genetic diseases resulting from single gene mutations are inherited in classic Mendelian fashion, although there is always the possibility of new mutations occurring in individuals with unaffected parents. Several disorders were originally thought to be genetic in nature, but the pedigrees of affected individuals were not consistent with known patterns of Mendelian inheritance. Understanding the mechanisms by which mutations occur in these disorders led to an understanding of other factors that influence disease; such factors include the effect of imprinting on phenotype expression, the role of trinucleotide expansion in genetic diseases, and the role of mitochondrial DNA (mtDNA) mutations in disorders of energy metabolism.

The following discussions describe the roles of the different mechanisms of mutation in genetic conditions seen more commonly in the general population.

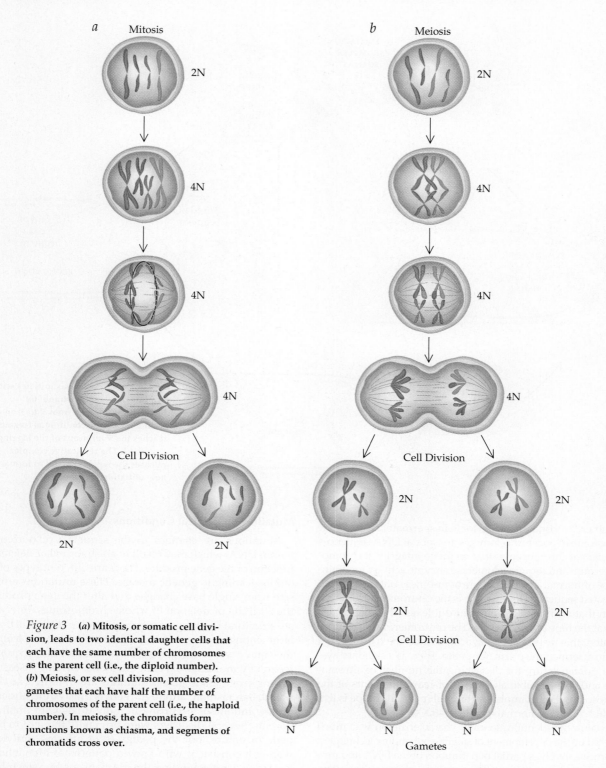

Figure 3 **(a) Mitosis, or somatic cell division, leads to two identical daughter cells that each have the same number of chromosomes as the parent cell (i.e., the diploid number). (b) Meiosis, or sex cell division, produces four gametes that each have half the number of chromosomes of the parent cell (i.e., the haploid number). In meiosis, the chromatids form junctions known as chiasma, and segments of chromatids cross over.**

DISORDERS CAUSED BY AN ABNORMAL NUMBER OF CHROMOSOMES

Our ability to associate clinical disease with detectable changes in genetic material was established in patients who were identified as having an abnormal number of chromosomes, including trisomy 21 and the sex chromosomes. Before the development of techniques for identifying and separating individual chromosomes from cell preparations, these patients were described clinically on the basis of a shared constellation of congenital anomalies and dysmorphic features (i.e., a syndrome). Individuals with Down syndrome have characteristic facial features; they experience hypotonia in infancy, delayed development, and cognitive impairment, as well as a pattern of congenital malformations. With the ability to karyotype individuals, rarer abnormalities of whole chromosomes were detected in dysmorphic stillborn infants or in live-born infants who subsequently died early in infancy (for example, from trisomy 18 or 13 syndrome) and were detected in analyses of first-trimester abortuses, which in general have a 50% rate of chromosome abnormalities.

The gain or loss of an entire chromosome is generally the result of nondisjunction or the missegregation of chromosomes at the time of cell division (i.e., in meiosis or mitosis). This results in one daughter cell having two copies of a particular chromosome and in the other daughter cell having no copy. Fertilization of a germ cell with two copies of a single chromosome results in a zygote trisomic for that chromosome. Three autosomal trisomy syndromes have been described in live-born infants: the syndromes associated with trisomies 13, 18, and 21. Occasionally, trisomies of other autosomes occur, but there is usually a normal cell line present as well (mosaicism). In most cases, this is the result of a postzygotic segregation error in mitosis that occurs early in embryogenesis. Extra chromosomal material is better tolerated than missing material; there are no viable autosomal monosomy syndromes. The lack

of one of the sex chromosomes is deleterious; the lack of a single X chromosome is lethal. Having a single X chromosome without a Y chromosome (Turner syndrome, which is associated with karyotype 45,X) results in a high proportion of fetal wastage. Triploidy and tetraploidy result in abnormal embryogenesis, and a haploid conceptus has never been reported.[5]

The development of techniques for chromosome banding allowed the identification of individual chromosomes by banding pattern rather than merely by size. This enabled the detection of the addition, loss, or rearrangement of large groups of genes by means of changes in chromosome appearance; thus, translocations, inversions, duplications, isochromosomes, and ring or marker chromosomes were described. These changes may or may not have an effect on phenotype, depending on whether there is a net conservation of genetic material, but they can have profound effects on reproductive fitness, affecting the process of chromosome segregation in meiosis. In approxi-

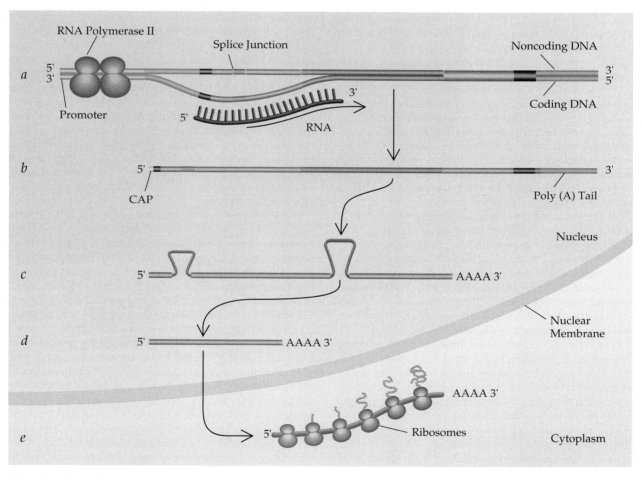

Figure 4 (*a*) The β-globin gene contains three exons (orange) separated by two introns (green). The boundaries between exons and introns are known as splice junctions and contain specific nucleotide sequences that are required for proper joining of the exons. The synthesis of messenger RNA (mRNA) from the β-globin gene proceeds in a 5′ to 3′ direction. The enzyme RNA polymerase II (dark green) binds to a promoter region (light green) located 200 to 300 base pairs in the 5′ direction or located upstream of the point at which mRNA synthesis begins. (*b*) mRNA begins with a 7-methylguanosine residue, referred to as the CAP site, and includes a 5′ untranslated region (light purple), a coding region of exons and introns, and a 3′ untranslated region (light purple). Nearly all mRNAs that encode proteins terminate at their 3′ ends with a string of approximately 200 adenine residues [known as the poly (A) tail], which are added 18 to 20 base pairs downstream from an AAUAAA signal in the 3′ untranslated region. (*c*) After mRNA is synthesized but before it leaves the nucleus, the introns are excised and the exons are spliced together to form mature mRNA (*d*). (*e*) Once the mature mRNA reaches the cytoplasm, it attaches to ribosomes and is translated into protein.

mately 5% of couples with a history of three or more first-trimester losses, one of the partners will be found to have a chromosome abnormality; thus, karyotype analysis is indicated in such persons.[6]

DISORDERS OF PARTIAL CHROMOSOME DELETION

22q11 deletion syndrome is a microdeletion syndrome that is common (occurring in one in 4,000 persons) and unique, in that most cases are de novo, not inherited from an affected individual. Persons with 22q11 deletion syndrome have variable clinical features, including (1) congenital heart disease (occurring in 74% of patients), particularly conotruncal malformations, such as tetralogy of Fallot, interrupted aortic arch, and truncus arteriosus; (2) palatal abnormalities (69%), notably velopharyngeal incompetence, submucosal cleft, and cleft palate; (3) characteristic facial features, including auricular abnormalities, hypoplastic alae nasi with a bulbous nasal tip, prominent nasal root, malar flatness, and hooded eyelids (> 50%); and (4) learning disabilities (70% to 90%).

Before the identification of the 22q11 microdeletion, patients were diagnosed on the basis of clinical features. The condition went under several names, including velocardiofacial syndrome, DiGeorge syndrome, Shprintzen syndrome, CATCH-22 (cardiac defects, abnormal facies, thymic hypoplasia, cleft palate, hypocalcemia), Cayler syndrome, and conotruncal anomaly face syndrome. Velocardiofacial syndrome was originally described as the combination of velopharyngeal incompetence, congenital heart disease, characteristic facial features, and developmental delay. DiGeorge syndrome, which includes the previously mentioned features as well as parathyroid deficiency and immune dysfunction from thymic aplasia or hypoplasia, was thought to be a developmental field defect of the third and fourth pharyngeal pouches.

In 1992, the first report of a microdeletion of chromosome 22 at the 11.2q band was reported; this was subsequently confirmed in other cases. In approximately 15% of cases, a visible deletion can be seen. Deletion 22q11 is diagnosed in individuals with submicroscopic deletions by use of fluorescence in situ hybridization (FISH) using DNA probes from the DiGeorge chromosome region [see Figure 3]. Fewer than 5% of patients with clinical features of deletion 22q11 have normal results on cytogenetic studies and negative results on FISH testing.[7]

The typical deletion encompasses three million base pairs, with smaller deletions of several hundred thousand base pairs reported. However, there is no correlation between the size of the deletion and the expression of the syndrome. It is still unknown whether the syndrome is a contiguous gene syndrome or whether the majority of the phenotype is the result of a single gene deletion that is variably expressed in affected individuals. The broadness of the phenotype and the unification of the various above-mentioned syndromes under the umbrella of deletion 22q11 have created some confusion. All cases of velocardiofacial syndrome, DiGeorge syndrome, Cayler syndrome, and conotruncal anomaly face syndrome that are associated with a deletion at 22q11 represent the same disorder.

The high occurrence of de novo deletions of 22q11 suggests some instability in this region. Because the overwhelming majority of patients have the same deletion in the 3 Mb (megabase) region, this area has been sequenced and carefully examined. This region contains four copies of duplicated sequence or low copy repeats, located nearer to the end points of the region. Each low copy repeat contains one or more dupli-

cated modules, which contain duplicated markers. The presence of these low copy repeats at this typically deleted region suggests that sometimes these areas misalign; during cell division and homologous recombination, this leads to duplication of the region on one chromatid and deletion on the other. The presence of these low copy repeats, therefore, gives us some insight into the mechanisms responsible for the recurrence of this common de novo deletion involving chromosome 22.[8] Repetitive sequences contribute to the inherent instability of some chromosome regions.

DISORDERS OF SINGLE GENE MUTATIONS

Anemia, which is a common clinical problem, is an excellent example of a condition that has many causes, both genetic and environmental. As monogenic disorders, the hemoglobinopathies are varied and complex. Approximately 7% of the world's population are carriers of different inherited disorders of hemoglobin, including structural hemoglobin variants and the thalassemias, which are disorders that result from defective synthesis of the globin chains. Hemoglobin is a tetramer of two pairs of dissimilar globin chains, commonly α-globin and β-globin chains in hemoglobin A (HbA) or α-globin and δ-globin chains in HbA_2. Healthy adults can have a residual amount of HbF (fetal hemoglobin, composed of two α-globin and two γ-globin chains), which is produced during fetal life and then replaced by adult hemoglobin in the first year of life. Since the discovery of a single point mutation that leads to the amino acid substitution of valine for glutamine, resulting in sickle cell anemia, over 700 structural hemoglobin variants have been identified, the most common of which are sickle hemoglobin HbS, HbC, and HbE. The thalassemias are generally classified on the basis of the particular globin chain or chains that are inefficiently synthesized.[9]

β-Thalassemia results from defective β-globin synthesis, which leads to an excess of α-globin chains. Over 200 mutations in β-globin genes have been identified in patients with β-thalassemia. The majority of these are point mutations—the loss of one or two bases that results in the disruption of gene function at the transcriptional, translational, or posttranslational level and in the decreased synthesis of the β-globin chain. Clinically, one would expect the severity of the condition to correlate with the amount of β-globin chain produced, with homozygotes or compound heterozygotes being profoundly anemic and requiring lifelong blood transfusions and heterozygotes having a milder or silent condition. Sibship studies have demonstrated phenotypic diversity in family members with the same genotype. This diversity may be a reflection of the inheritance of mutations in other loci involved in globin synthesis, because mutations for thalassemias and structural hemoglobinopathies occur together at a higher frequency in many populations. Combinations of structural hemoglobinopathies may positively alter the phenotype of thalassemia and reduce the concurrence of α- and β-thalassemia mutations in an individual; the occurrence of this process can vary from individual to individual in families. In addition, there are several mutations in the β-globin gene cluster and in the promoter region of the γ-globin genes that result in the persistence of fetal hemoglobin; such persistence produces a milder phenotype overlaying either a structural hemoglobinopathy or a β-thalassemia. Finally, mutations or polymorphisms in genes involved in bilirubin, iron, and bone metabolism may play a role in the clinical course of the disease in affected individuals.[10]

IMPRINTING DEFECTS

Gregor Mendel reported that the outcomes of reciprocal crosses were independent of the parental origin of a trait. In the late 1980s, however, researchers discovered that the two parental genomes are not equivalent in mammals. In the mouse zygote, the two pronuclei are distinct from one another and can be individually removed from the cell, and a zygote containing two female pronuclei or two male pronuclei can be created (a phenomenon known as uniparental disomy). Early embryonic development in such zygotes is abnormal. Purely female-derived embryos have poorly developed extraembryonic tissues, and purely male-derived embryos demonstrate abnormal embryo development. This phenomenon occurs sporadically in human conception, when a sperm fertilizes an egg without a pronucleus. This causes a doubling of the sperm chromosomes. The resulting diploid conceptus is a hydatidiform mole, which is a mass of extraembryonic membranes without an embryo. In contrast, ovarian dermoid cysts are derived from the spontaneous division of an oocyte; this results in the duplication of the maternal genome.

This phenomenon whereby progeny phenotypes differ according to whether the genetic material is maternal or paternal in origin is called genomic imprinting. This represents an extreme situation wherein the genetic material is derived entirely from one parent. In studying this phenomenon, investigators focused on the chromosomal regions responsible for the genomic imprinting effects observed in mouse embryos. Certain regions of distinct chromosomes were found to produce markedly different phenotypes, depending on whether the two copies were inherited from one parent, resulting in duplication or deficiency of one parental complement. An imprinted allele is one whose expression is changed or silenced as it passes through a particular sex. An allele is paternally imprinted if it is not expressed when it is inherited from the father. It is maternally imprinted if it is not expressed when it is inherited through the mother. Imprinted regions have been identified in both mouse and human chromosomes; alterations in normal imprinting patterns are associated with disorders of growth and development, cell proliferation, and behavior.

It is thought that during gamete formation in mammals, some genes are altered by the methylation of certain cytosine groups in DNA. This process tends to prevent access by transcription machinery to that region of the chromosome for transcription, thus resulting in the "silencing" of that gene or genes. Whatever the process, the imprinting procedure would have to be erased during embryogenesis so that an individual could reimprint its genes according to its own sex during gametogenesis. Demethylation in embryonic cells occurs in the early cleavage divisions. Shortly after implantation, the embryonic somatic cells are methylated again, whereas the germ cells in the developing embryo are methylated later, as they develop in the gonads. An imprinting center on chromosome 15 may play a role in this process.[11]

Prader-Willi syndrome (PWS) and Angelman syndrome (AS) are two clinically distinct genetic diseases associated with deletions of the same region of chromosome 15. These syndromes are characterized by deficiencies in growth and sexual development, behavioral abnormalities, and mental retardation. Major diagnostic criteria for PWS include hypotonia; hyperphagia with resulting obesity; hypogonadism; and developmental delay. Patients with AS may have ataxia; sleep disorders; seizures; and hyperactivity with severe mental retardation. They may exhibit characteristic outbursts of inappropriate laughter.

Approximately 70% of patients with PWS and AS have a de novo 3 to 4 Mb deletion in the q11–q13 region of chromosome 15. Because this region is imprinted, the phenotypes that result from this deletion differ, depending on the allele upon which the deletion occurred. When the deletion occurs on the paternal chromosome, it results in PWS; when it occurs in the maternal copy, it results in AS. This suggests that the normal *PWS* gene is expressed from the paternal chromosome and that the normal *AS* gene is expressed from the maternal chromosome. Most of the remaining cases of PWS are the result of maternal uniparental disomy; paternal uniparental disomy accounts for only 4% of AS cases.[12] In uniparental disomy, an individual inherits both copies of a chromosome from either the mother or the father through a nondisjunction error in meiosis. Again, lack of paternal 15q11–15q13 results in PWS; lack of maternal 15q11–15q13 results in AS. Imprinting defects have been implicated in some individuals with these syndromes.

Defects in a region termed the imprinting center, located within 15q11–15q13, can change the DNA methylation and transcription activity of certain genes that reside in the region. Thus, if there is a mutation in the imprinting center, the process of activation or inactivation of the imprinted region may not occur. Because the different mechanisms are associated with different risks of recurrence, it is recommended that the diagnostic workup begin with a search for a deletion by use of chromosome analysis and FISH; if the results are normal, DNA methylation should be performed. Although the risk of recurrence of a deletion is low, a mutation of the imprinting center is associated with a recurrence risk of 50%.

TRINUCLEOTIDE REPEAT DISORDERS

Several inherited disorders are known to have a worsening phenotype in each subsequent generation of family members affected by the disease.

Fragile X Syndrome, Huntington Disease, and Friedreich Ataxia

In the early 1990s, molecular geneticists discovered a new type of mutation, first in fragile X syndrome and then in a series of inherited neurologic disorders, including myotonic dystrophy, Huntington disease, and Friedreich ataxia. The mutation involves a repeat expansion of a DNA triplet, a trinucleotide repeat in an exon, or an intron of the gene. In patients with these conditions, the normal number of repeats (in an unaffected individual) is expanded. The number of nucleotide repeats can increase in successive generations, causing disease symptoms to appear at an earlier age. The molecular basis of repeat instability is not well understood, but increased severity of the phenotype and earlier age of onset in successive generations (a phenomenon termed anticipation) are generally associated with larger repeat length. The parental origin of the disease allele can also influence expression; for most of these disorders, there is greater risk of repeat expansion with paternal transmission, although in fragile X syndrome and congenital myotonic dystrophy (see below), the maternally transmitted alleles are more prone to expansion, thereby causing more severe phenotypes. Most of the trinucleotide repeat disorders are inherited in an autosomal dominant or X-linked fashion, with the exception of Friedreich ataxia, which is an autosomal recessive disorder [see Table 1].[13]

Table 1 Trinucleotide Repeat Disorders

Disease	Gene Locus/Protein	Repeat	Location
Fragile X syndrome	Xq27.3/FMR-1 protein	CGG	Noncoding
Fragile XE syndrome	Xq28/FMR-2 protein	GCC	Noncoding
Friedreich ataxia	9q13–9q21.1/frataxin	GAA	Noncoding
Myotonic dystrophy 1	19q13/myotonic dystrophy protein kinase	CTG	Noncoding
Myotonic dystrophy 2	3q21	CCTG	Noncoding
Spinobulbar muscular atrophy	Xq13–Xq21/androgen receptor	CAG	Coding
Huntington disease	4p16.3/huntington	CAG	Coding
Dentatorubral-pallidoluysian atrophy	12p13.31/atrophin-1	CAG	Coding
SCA type 1	6p23/ataxin-1	CAG	Coding
SCA type 2	12q24/ataxin-2	CAG	Coding
SCA type 3 (Machado-Joseph disease)	14q32.1/ataxin-3	CAG	Coding
SCA type 6	19p13/α-1A (voltage-dependent calcium channel subunit)	CAG	Coding
SCA type 7	3p12–3p13/ataxin-7	CAG	Coding
SCA type 8	13q12/none identified	CTG	?
SCA type 12	5q31–5q33	CAG	Noncoding

SCA—spinocerebellar ataxia

Myotonic Dystrophy

Myotonic dystrophy is a trinucleotide repeat disorder resulting in multisystem involvement of skeletal and smooth muscle, as well as involvement of the eye, heart, endocrine system, and central nervous system. The disorder represents a continuum of clinical findings; it has been classified for diagnostic purposes into three somewhat overlapping phenotypes: mild, classic, and congenital. Mild myotonic dystrophy is characterized by the development of cataracts in early adulthood and mild myotonia (difficulty relaxing the muscles after contraction). The symptoms may be so subtle that diagnosis is made retrospectively, after the birth of an affected offspring. Classic myotonic dystrophy is characterized by muscle weakness and wasting, myotonia, cataract formation, and cardiac conduction abnormalities that occur in adulthood. The life span of these patients may be somewhat shorter than normal.

Congenital myotonic dystrophy is a disease of the neonate characterized by generalized hypotonia, respiratory insufficiency requiring ventilatory support, and mental retardation if the infant survives to childhood. Individuals have characteristic facial features, which include drooping eyelids, facial weakness resulting in an open-mouthed appearance, and wasting of the muscles in the jaw and neck. The overall incidence of myotonic dystrophy is estimated to be one in 20,000 persons.

The diagnosis of myotonic dystrophy is confirmed by detection of an expansion of the CTG trinucleotide repeat that affects the noncoding regions of two adjacent genes (*DMPK* and *SIX5*) on chromosome 19q13. Normal individuals have a repeat of 37 trinucleotides or fewer. The trinucleotide repeat is located at the 3′ end of the gene (the transcription occurs in the 5′ to 3′ direction), but it is in a part of the gene that is transcribed but not translated into the final protein product. Unaffected individuals have a polymorphic repeat length of 5 to 37 CTG repeats; this repeat length is stable when passed from generation to generation. Stability is disrupted, however, when the number of repeats exceeds 37. When the number exceeds 37, this repeat expansion not only disrupts the function of the gene but also engenders further instability and larger expansions. This ten-dency accounts for the phenomenon of anticipation seen in families with this disorder, in which a mildly affected adult can give birth to a child with the congenital form of the disease. In rare cases, the region will contract, with the CTG repeat being smaller in an offspring. In affected individuals, further expansion can occur during somatic cell division, resulting in mosaicism from tissue to tissue.[14]

The gene product of *DMPK* is a protein kinase. It is expressed in the different organs involved in the disease: skeletal muscle, the heart, the brain, and the testes. The function of the protein is unknown, and it is unclear how the expansion in the untranslated region leads to the phenotype. There is evidence, however, that the mutant *DMPK* transcripts accumulate abnormally in the nuclei and bind to RNA-binding proteins, thus disrupting RNA splicing and metabolism. A second form of myotonic dystrophy has recently been described. This form involves a chromosome 3 trinucleotide repeat, which also results in the accumulation of RNA in cells.[15]

This disorder presents a unique genetic counseling problem. Individuals who are mildly affected have a 50% chance of passing on the expanded allele to their offspring. However, because of the instability of the expanded region, it is impossible to predict the severity of the condition in an affected child. There is a risk of having a child with the severe form of the disease—congenital myotonic dystrophy—only if the mutation is transmitted through the mother. Approximately 20% of the offspring of an affected mother who inherit the mutation manifest the severe form, depending on the size of the expansion in the mother. Although prenatal testing for the expansion is available, often the diagnosis of mild myotonic dystrophy in the mother is established only after the birth of an infant with the congenital form of the disease.

Mitochondrial Inheritance

In general, the inheritance (autosomal dominant, recessive, or X-linked) of a condition can be determined by pedigree analysis of large families. Mechanisms such as imprinting and anticipation affect the expression of mutations, but transmission still abides by classic Mendelian patterns of inheritance. Recently, mutations in mtDNA have been associated with a number of disorders with a unique inheritance pattern, termed maternal transmission. In maternal transmission, a condition affects individuals in each generation, suggesting dominant inheritance. Males and females may be affected, but men never transmit the disorder to their offspring. Women pass the trait on to all of their children, although there is great variability in expression.

Mitochondria are the cellular organelles responsible for the generation of energy in the form of adenosine triphosphate (ATP) through aerobic metabolism. Some mtDNA molecules are encoded in the nuclear genome and are transported out to the mitochondria, but a minority are encoded and synthesized in the mitochondria. mtDNA is a circular, double-stranded structure without introns; it resembles a prokaryotic genome. It contains 16,569 base pairs that encode at least 13 proteins required for oxidative phosphorylation. In addition, it contains the transfer RNA (tRNA) and ribosomal RNA (rRNA) involved in the translation of these proteins in the organelle.

The manner in which mitochondria are passed from one generation to the next accounts for the phenomena of maternal transmission. At the time of fertilization, the sperm sheds its cytoplasm, and only the nuclear DNA enters the egg. Therefore, all mitochondria in the zygote are contributed by the egg cell. However, there are hundreds of copies of mtDNA in each cell. During cell division, each mtDNA replicates, but unlike nuclear DNA, the newly synthesized mitochondria segregate passively to the daughter cells. A mitochondrial mutation arises randomly, and chance segregation leads to an accumulation of mutant mitochondria in a cell. The phenotypic expression of a mutation in mtDNA depends on the relative proportion of normal functioning product above a certain threshold value for manifesting the phenotype. This unpredictability in phenotype from individual to individual is the result of this random segregation of mitochondria; such random segregation of mitochondria is termed heteroplasmy. Additionally, different types of mtDNA mutations are inherited differently; deletions occur only sporadically and are not transmitted from affected females to their offspring. Examples of disorders associated with such deletions are chronic progressive external ophthalmoplegia, Kearns-Sayre syndrome, and Pearson syndrome. Point mutations result in mitochondrial encephalomyopathy with lactic acidosis and strokelike episodes (MELAS), myoclonic epilepsy with ragged-red fibers (MERRF), and neuropathy, ataxia, and retinitis pigmentosa (NARP).[16]

The number of mitochondria per cell is dependent on the energy production in the cell. The brain, retina, and muscle cells have a relatively higher demand for energy than other cell types. Thus, mutations in mtDNA tend to result in disorders with muscle and neurologic dysfunction, such as myopathies, cardiomyopathy, ophthalmoplegia, encephalopathies, and encephalomyopathies. Defects in oxidative phosphorylation should be considered in the differential diagnosis of any patient with unexplained multisystem involvement, including a progressive myopathy or neurologic problem. Although routine laboratory testing in such patients may reveal hypoglycemia, abnormal liver function, or elevated blood lactate levels, muscle biopsy is often necessary to make a diagnosis. The abnormal pathologic appearance of the cellular mitochondria is apparent on electron microscopy and through the use of special staining. Some examples of conditions resulting from mutations in mtDNA are listed [see Table 2]. Defects in oxidative phosphorylation may also result from mutations in nuclear DNA that code for mitochondrial proteins. Diagnosis of these disorders is difficult, and subsequent counseling issues can be complex.

Cancer Genetics

Thus far, we have focused on genetic diseases with specific phenotypes associated with the presence of germline mutations that lead to expression of one or more abnormally functioning proteins. This type of mutation is presumably present in all the cells of an individual from birth, although there can be a degree of mosaicism, depending on the stage of development at which the mutation occurs. Investigation into the control of cell growth has given new insight into genetic changes that occur in both germ cells and somatic cells and that can lead to malignancy. Mutations in three types of genes that regulate cell growth are involved in the development of cancer: tumor suppressor genes, proto-oncogenes, and DNA repair genes. Somatic mutations in these genes may result in unchecked proliferation or clonal expansion of a single cell with subsequent loss of cellular organization; somatic mutations may also confer the ability to metastasize. This process generally requires a number of mutations, because there is an elaborate backup system in place to prevent faulty cell proliferation. Although sporadic mutations arise in individual somatic cells and ultimately play a role in cancer development, the study of familial or inherited cancer syndromes has contributed to our understanding of the genetic changes responsible for the development of some of the more common cancers.

It is perhaps easiest to understand how a germline mutation in a tumor suppressor gene could lead to a predisposition to

Table 2 Disorders Resulting from Mitochondrial Mutations

Disease	Phenotype
Chronic progressive external ophthalmoplegia	Progressive weakness of extraocular muscles; ptosis
Kearns-Sayre syndrome	Progressive external ophthalmoplegia before age 20; pigmentary retinopathy and CSF protein > 1g/L; cerebellar ataxia or heart block
Leber hereditary optic neuropathy	Rapid bilateral optic nerve death resulting in loss of central vision in early adulthood
Mitochondrial encephalopathy with lactic acidosis and strokelike episodes	Strokelike episodes before age 40, seizures, dementia, ragged-red fibers, lactic acidosis
Myoclonic epilepsy with ragged-red fibers	Myoclonus, epilepsy, ataxia, myopathy, sensorineural deafness
Pearson syndrome	Sideroblastic anemia, pancytopenia, pancreatic insufficiency, lactic acidosis
Leigh disease	Neuropathy, ataxia, retinitis pigmentosa, developmental delay, lactic acidemia
Deafness	Progressive sensorineural deafness often induced by aminoglycoside antibiotics

cancer. Such is the case in families with an inherited mutation in *BRCA1* and *BRCA2*. Such individuals have only one functional copy of the gene; a subsequent somatic mutation in the normal copy in a single cell gives rise to a population of cells that have no *BRCA1* or *BRCA2* gene and have therefore lost the tumor suppressor activity that limits cell proliferation. In individuals with a germline mutation in *BRCA1*, the chance of developing breast cancer over one's lifetime is estimated to be 80%; the chance of developing ovarian cancer is 15%. The cancer usually develops at an earlier age than is seen in the general population, and there can be multiple primary sites. Nevertheless, most breast cancer disease is sporadic, and the disease is common enough that family history may be misleading, particularly in a large family. There are algorithms for assessing a patient's risk of developing breast cancer, as well as the risk of carrying a germline mutation. Such risk-assessment algorithms are based on personal health history and family history of breast cancer, ovarian cancer, or both. With regard to family history, important factors include the age of onset in affected individuals and whether there was more than one primary site. Verification of the family member's medical records is imperative.[17]

Proto-oncogenes are recessively acting genes that regulate the cell cycle. Mutant dominant genes, called oncogenes, are usually gain-of-function mutations; the altered products of such mutations cause uncontrolled cell proliferation. Oncogenes were discovered by transformation experiments in tissue culture. In these experiments, normal cells were made into malignant cells by the insertion of a mutant piece of DNA (the oncogene). A number of proto-oncogenes have been located in the human genome, and mutations in them have been implicated in the development of leukemias, lymphomas, breast and ovarian carcinomas, and cancer of the colon, thyroid, lung, and pancreas. Many oncogenes are caused by chromosomal changes that result from breakage and translocations occurring as cell proliferation becomes more disorganized. The so-called Philadelphia chromosome seen in chronic myelogenous leukemia is a translocation between chromosomes 9 and 22. The breakpoint in chromosome 9 occurs in the cellular proto-oncogene *ABL*, which normally codes for a tyrosine kinase that binds to DNA. The breakpoint in chromosome 22 is in a gene called *BCR*, or breakage cluster region, which codes for a serine kinase. The fused *BCR-ABL* gene in the Philadelphia chromosome makes a novel protein, which leads to unregulated proliferation of hematopoietic stem cells and chronic myeloid leukemia.[18]

Although most cases of colorectal cancer are sporadic, there are two more common forms of autosomal, dominantly inherited colorectal cancer, familial adenomatous polyposis (FAP) and hereditary nonpolyposis colorectal cancer, which together account for about 10% of cases of colorectal cancer. FAP is caused by a germline mutation in a tumor suppressor gene, the *APC* gene. Loss of function of the second *APC* allele leads to adenoma formation and progression to cancer through the accumulation of other somatic mutations.

Supporting the concept that accumulated genetic changes underlie the development of neoplasia, the defect in hereditary nonpolyposis colorectal cancer (HNPCC) was found to be in a group of genes that function in DNA mismatch repair. In the course of normal cell division, DNA replication is subject to error, although, as discussed earlier, the fidelity of DNA polymerase is quite good. The mismatch repair genes, of which at least six are known (*MSH2, MSH6, MLH1, MLH3, PMS1,* and

PMS2) function in DNA replication errors resulting from misincorporation. The mismatch repair proteins function as a complex to recognize the deformation in the double helix and to then recruit enzymes to correct the error. Without these proteins, errors are propagated in successive generations of cells. Individuals with a germline mutation in the mismatch repair system, again, may undergo loss of function in the second mismatch repair allele, resulting in the characteristic microsatellite instability (MSI). Microsatellites are repeating DNA sequences of unknown function that are found throughout the genome. These repetitive sequences are more prone to errors in replication. Loss of mismatch repair mechanisms permits expansion of these repeats, as may be demonstrated in tumor specimens. The presence of MSI indicates an increased likelihood of HNPCC, although MSI is seen in 15% of sporadic colorectal cancers. Families with HNPCC have an increased incidence of other types of cancers, including endometrial, ovarian, upper GI, renal, pelvis, and brain cancers.[19]

Human Genome Project

The Human Genome Project was undertaken to determine the sequence of the entire human genome. It is a massive effort that will have major effects on medical research and practice. With the advent of recombinant DNA technology and the development of DNA sequencing, the question arose in the 1980s as to whether the genome might be sequenced. By 1990, the National Institutes of Health had founded a National Institute of Human Genome Research. The projected date of completion of the sequencing of the human genome was 2005; advances in technology, chiefly in terms of sequencing, were incorporated into the time estimate. As it turned out, the genome was for the most part completed by 2000; some 3% to 5% of the genome remained uncertain because of high redundancy.[20,21] However, the remaining sequences are not thought to contain many meaningful coding sequences.

The earlier-than-expected completion was in part the result of a strong organization and cooperation among the centers. Investigators around the world who had linked constructs of DNA sent them to genome centers for sequence determination. The government-sponsored project required that such sequences be made public within a day, thus aiding dissemination of information. A second factor in timely completion was that technology improved even faster than anticipated. A third factor was the cooperative interaction of private industry, which participated under the original NIH rules. A fourth factor contributing to early completion was the competition of private industry using a modified approach to sequence determination. By 1998, 3% of the sequence was actually known. Three years later, more than 95% of the sequence had been determined.

Hybridization, or complementary pairing, of single strands of DNA to each other, allows identification of overlapping DNA fragments by labeling the short fragment and hybridizing to a library. The genome of a person contains regions that vary in a manner specific to that individual. By definition, a variation present in 1% of the population is termed a polymorphism. For the Human Genome Project, the most useful of these turned out to be blocks of CA sequence, which vary in the number of times the dinucleotide is repeated.[22] The repeats serve as signposts in the genome of an individual. As the genome project progressed, these, along with other markers, served to build a map of signposts along the genome.

Amplification of DNA sequences for cloning and for utilization of the markers depended on the polymerase chain reaction technique.[23] If the sequence of a region of DNA is known, then a large amount of the sequence can be cloned and mapped by the use of excess primers, which hybridize to the specific sequence. Usually, the primers are about 20 nucleotides long; this length is sufficient to give adequate specificity in binding. The amplification depends on the repeated denaturing and renaturing of the DNA, so that the excess primers create a site for DNA synthesis in each cycle. With a thermoresistant DNA polymerase, the progress can be automated [see Figure 5].

Another major technical advance facilitating positional cloning and the genome project was the cloning of large blocks of human genome sequence. Stable vectors containing up to 1 Mb of genome sequence were developed using yeast artificial chromosomes.[24] However, these tend to recombine the DNA frequently; bacterial artificial chromosomes (BACs) proved to be more useful for the genome project because they are more stable. As libraries of BACs were made, the assignment of markers to each BAC allowed the development of a map for signposts and the establishment of contiguous sequences (contigs) as subunits of the overall genome. These were frequently verified by cytogenetics with the use of FISH.

As the Human Genome Project developed many markers along the genome, a second technique became feasible—

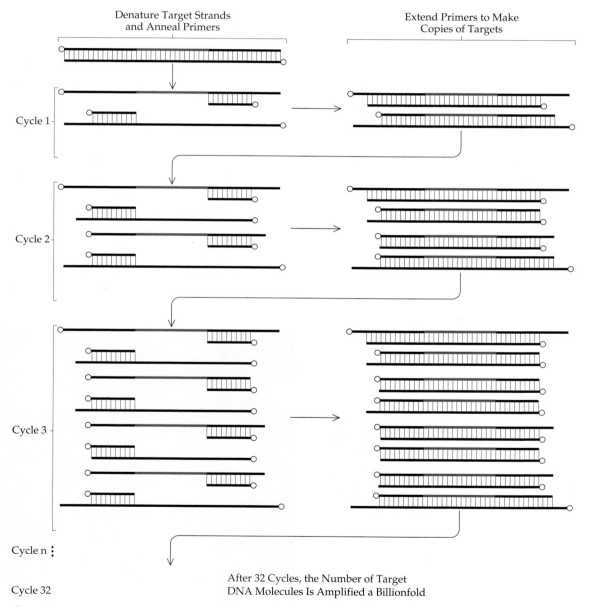

Figure 5 The polymerase chain reaction. The strands in each targeted DNA duplex are separated by heating and then cooled to allow single-stranded oligonucleotide primers that are complementary to the end sequences of the opposite strands to bind to those sequences. DNA polymerase extends the primers (i.e., adds nucleotides), using the target DNA strands as templates. In this way, duplicates of the original DNA strands are produced in each cycle, and the quantity of the target DNA duplex increases exponentially.

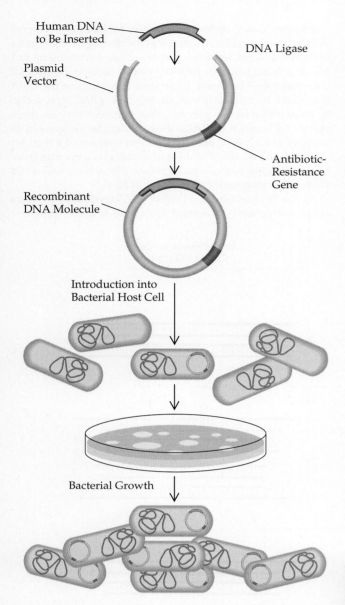

Human DNA to Be Inserted

Plasmid Vector

DNA Ligase

Antibiotic-Resistance Gene

Recombinant DNA Molecule

Introduction into Bacterial Host Cell

Bacterial Growth

Figure 6   **Restriction fragments of human DNA generated by digestion of chromosomal DNA with a restriction endonuclease (e. g., *Eco*RI) can be inserted into a cloning vector, such as an *Escherichia coli* plasmid. The plasmid contains a single recognition site for *Eco*RI and a bacterial gene that confers antibiotic resistance. After EcoRI cuts the plasmid, the fragments of human DNA and the linear plasmid can be covalently joined by the action of the enzyme DNA ligase. The plasmid can replicate within a bacterial host to produce many copies of the DNA fragment, and the bacteria themselves reproduce. The bacteria are grown on plates containing antibiotics to select for those cells that contain copies of the plasmid with the human DNA insert. The human DNA (e.g., a gene) can then be recovered when the harvested plasmid DNA is digested with *Eco*RI.**

shotgun sequencing. In that approach, the genome was sequenced repetitively in small fragments; with appropriate computer algorithms, it was then possible to reconstruct the sequence. This method was aided by the existence of the knowledge of the markers that had already been obtained. Regions of redundancy present problems for the combined methodologies.

Currently, the human genome appears to contain approximately 38,000 genes. In terms of complexity of function, it is thought that protein modification may be the basis for varied activities of gene products. Only about 1% of the genome codes directly for information. About 24% is intronic sequence; the remaining 75% is intergenic. The genes are not distributed at an average frequency but are clustered in gene-rich regions, and there is significant variability among the chromosomes as to gene content per unit length. The human genome contains many retroviruses, or transposable elements, most of which do not appear to be active; however, many can function as mobile genetic elements in the genome. The results emphasize the presence of introns and lead to the question of whether there is additional information encoded in them, other than by the triplet code. For example, do these introns contain topologic or conformational information that is important in gene regulation?

Another remaining difficulty is that we do not understand the rules of genomic "punctuation." With genes embedded in small exons occupying less than 1% of the genome, recognition of the coding regions is difficult. Identification of genes is based on the assumption that genes are expressed and usually converted to mRNA. Because mRNA has a poly-A 3' tail, it is possible to capture portions of messages. These snippets are termed expressed sequence tags; they were used to identify the signposts for genes in the genome project. The portion of DNA coding for the desired sequence was expanded by cloning the DNA into plasmid vectors and then growing these vectors in bacteria [*see Figure 6*]. Cloning depends on restriction enzymes that cut double-stranded DNA at specific sites; recognition is usually based on a sequence of 4 to 8 bases, and the cleavage may produce overhang or blunt termini in the DNA. If the same enzyme is used to cut the plasmid vector, the DNA piece may be joined to the plasmid by ligase enzyme, and the plasmid will thus be able to replicate with the complementary

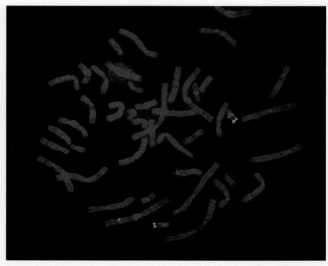

Figure 7   **Fluorescence in situ hybridization (FISH) was performed using the TUPLE1 probe (red) for the VCFS/DGS region at 22q11.2 along with an identifier probe (green) (Vysis, Inc., Downers Grove, Illinois). One homologue has both probe signals (red and green); however, the other homologue has only the identifier signal (green), which indicates that this homologue is deleted.**

DNA (cDNA) insert [*see Figure 7*]. Plasmids were engineered that would exist in the bacterial host cell in groups of several hundred copies each; in this way, the DNA insert was amplified, and such amplifed inserts were relatively easy to rescue for study.

Our knowledge of human genetics and its application to clinical medicine is constantly evolving. We have progressed from inferring inheritance modes by pedigree analysis and from inferring risk to future offspring by probability calculations to molecular testing based on the identification of mutations in a gene or genes involved in a specific disorder. The human genome has been sequenced, but it still must be deciphered as to the genetic bases of the remaining single-gene disorders, the genetic component of multifactorial inheritance conditions, and the function of noncoding DNA. Aided by improvements and advances in molecular technology, scientists will have this task in the 21st century.

FUTURE APPLICATIONS OF GENETICS TO MEDICINE

Scanning the Genome for Risk of Disease

Technology holds the promise of detailed analysis of the genomes of individuals with attention to particular areas. By combining computer-chip design with DNA hybridization techniques, arrays of DNA sequences containing many thousands of specified sequence variations can be made.[13] This will allow searching for disease-specific mutations or associated polymorphisms in a person. However, because it appears that most common diseases have a genetic component but are made manifest on the basis of other factors (multifactorial disease), so-called array analysis offers a new tool. The human genome contains single base variations—single nucleotide polymorphisms (SNPs) that occur at a rate of about one per 1,000 bases; there are close to three million SNPs in the human genome. Of these, perhaps 1% are in exons and can be used to identify disease risk by linkage. As associations with multifactorial disease are made, scanning for markers linked to risk—even though, at the molecular level,

the basis of the risk remains unknown—will allow determination of the apparent risk of multifactorial disease in an individual patient. It is expected that array analysis will prove useful in assessing the risk of diabetes, heart disease, cancers, and other common diseases.

Identifying Drug Responsiveness

A second avenue of use for the complex analysis of individual genomes may come with regard to drug prescription. Associations of drug responsiveness and genome markers will develop. It seems likely that genome variations affect a patient's response to drug therapy and that such variations may thus have a role in drug selection and dosage schedules. Medical practice may thus come to utilize an array analysis for a given drug.

Privacy Issues in Genetics

The testing capabilities and the ability to store and compare sequence data raise ethical concerns. To a large degree, these questions are not new in medicine, but the extent of the knowledge and the possible predictive nature of the information make the issue one of new focus and attention. Collection, storage, and dissemination of an individual's genetic information have become topics for discussion at the state and national level. Already a number of states have revised statutes regarding privacy. The question of privacy in a time of electronic records is in itself a difficult one for health care providers. Access to records is a thorny issue. Added to this are concerns over the availability of health care insurance and life insurance for individuals with a family history of genetic disease. With patient profiles that include a large number of disease-causing sequence alterations now a reality, the problem has only become larger.

Online Resources for Genetic Information

Several Web-based sites for information regarding the genome or genetic diseases are available [*see Sidebar* Selected Internet Resources for Genetic Information].

References

1. Henig RM: The Monk in the Garden. Houghton Mifflin Company, Boston, 2000

2. Avery OT, MacLeod CM, McCarty M: Induction of transformation by a deoxyribonucleic acid fraction isolated from pneumococcus type III. J Exp Med 79:137, 1944

3. Watson JD, Crick FC: Molecular structure of nucleic acids: a structure for deoxyribose nucleic acid. Nature 171:737, 1953

4. Crick F: The genetic code. Sci Am 207:66, 1962

5. Korf BR: Chromosomes and chromosomal abnormalities. Human Genetics: A Problem Based Approach, 2nd ed. Malden MA, Ed. Blackwell Science, Oxford, 2000, p 181

6. Olson SB, Magenis RE: Cytogenetic aspects of recurrent pregnancy loss. Semin Reprod Endocrinol 6:191, 1988

7. McDonald-McGinn DM, Emanuel BS, Zackai EH: 22q11 deletion syndrome, September 1999 http://www.geneclinics.org

8. Shaikh TH, Kurahashi H, Emanuel BS: Evolutionarily conserved low copy repeats (LCRs) in 22q11 mediate deletions, duplications, translocations, and genomic instability: an update and literature review. Genet Med 3:6, 2001

9. Tuzmen S, Schechter AN: Genetic diseases of hemoglobin: diagnostic methods for elucidating β-thalassemia mutations. Blood Rev 15:19, 2001

10. Weatherall DJ: Phenotype-genotype relationships in monogenic disease: lessons from the thalassemias. Nat Rev Genet 2:245, 2001

11. Mange EJ, Mange AP: Complicating factors. Basic Human Genetics, 2nd ed. Sinauer Associates, Inc., Sunderland, Massachusetts, 1999, p 209

12. Falls JG, Pulford DJ, Wylie AA, et al: Genomic imprinting: implications for human disease. Am J Pathol 154:635, 1999

13. Cummings CJ, Zoghbi HY: Trinucleotide repeats: mechanisms and pathophysiology. Annu Rev Genomics Hum Genet 1: 281, 2000

14. Adams C: Myotonic dystrophy, August 2001 http://www.geneclinics.org

15. Alfred J: Myotonic dystrophy comes into focus. Nat Rev Genet 2:736, 2001

16. Chinnery PF, Turnbull DM: Mitochondrial DNA and disease. Lancet 354(suppl 1):SI17, 1999

17. Frank TS: Hereditary cancer syndromes. Arch Pathol Lab Med 125:85, 2000

18. Faderl S, Talpaz M, Estrov Z, et al: The biology of chronic myeloid leukemia. N Engl J Med 341:164, 1999

19. Kinzler KW, Vogelstein B: Lessons from hereditary colorectal cancer. Cell 87:159, 1996

20. Lander ES, Linton LM, Birren B, et al: Initial sequencing and analysis of the human genome. Nature 409:860, 2001

21. Venter JC, Adams MD, Myers EW, et al: The sequence of the human genome. Science 291:1304, 2001

22. Mullis KB: The unusual origin of the polymerase chain reaction. Sci Am 262:56, 1990

23. Botstein D, White RL, Skoltnick M, et al: Construction of a genetic linkage map in man using restriction fragment length polymorphisms. Am J Hum Genet 32:314, 1980

24. Kim UJ, Birren BW, Slepak T, et al: Construction and characterization of a human bacterial artificial chromosome library. Genomics 34:213, 1996

Acknowledgments

Figure 1   George Kelvin.

Figure 2   Seward Hung.

Figures 4, 6, and 7   Dimitry Schidlovsky.

Figure 5   Tom Moore.

72 Genetic Diagnosis and Counseling

Roberta A. Pagon, M.D.

Genetic testing is an increasingly useful cost-effective, sensitive, noninvasive tool that allows clinicians to identify disease in symptomatic persons, predict the probability of disease in asymptomatic at-risk persons, detect carriers of heritable disorders, and diagnose genetic disease in fetuses.

Although genetic tests involve the analysis of DNA, RNA, chromosomes, proteins, and certain metabolites, the most widely used of these tests over the past decade has been DNA-based testing for the diagnosis of heritable disorders and genetic counseling. The effectiveness of genetic tests depends on the technical skill with which they are performed, the clinical skill with which they are interpreted, and the patient's interest in the results. As with all other medical testing, genetic testing is context specific. Before proceeding, the clinician must be able to answer the question, "Why am I testing this patient at this time?"

Genetic testing differs from traditional medical testing in that genetic-test results have recurrence-risk implications for the individual patient and his or her family. A positive genetic test result always raises the consideration of referral for genetic counseling. Genetic testing that is used only for personal decision making does not fit with the model of traditional medical care.

The focus of this chapter is on germline mutations that are present at conception and have phenotypic effects, implications for reproduction, or both. Germline mutations contrast with somatic mutations, which are the basis of certain acquired disorders, such as many cancers. Somatic mutations, with the exception of so-called germline mosaicism in which the mutations affect the gonads, are not heritable and are not discussed in this chapter.

Classification of Genetic Testing

Direct and indirect testing are the two broad categories of DNA-based testing. Direct testing refers to the positive identification of disease-causing genetic alterations that establish a person's genetic status independent of knowledge of family history or a priori risk status. Indirect testing relies on linkage analysis, in which DNA sequences serve as markers to track a gene within a family with at least two affected members. Indirect testing is used when direct DNA analysis is not possible because the gene is not known or because the large number of known mutations precludes positive identification of the specific disease-causing mutation in a given family. Linkage analysis can determine the genetic status of an asymptomatic person only within the context of a highly structured study of family DNA samples and absolute certainty of the correct clinical diagnosis in the family.

In the evaluation of patients and their families, genetic-testing information can be used in a medical-testing paradigm, a genetic-counseling paradigm, or both [*see Table 1*].

Medical-Testing Paradigm

In the medical-testing paradigm, genetic tests provide patients and their physicians with information that directly influences medical care. Issues of sensitivity, specificity, positive predictive value, cost-effectiveness, and recurrence risk are relevant. Sensitivity refers to the probability that a test will be positive in an affected person; specificity refers to the probability that a person with a positive test result has or will develop a specific condition. Diagnostic testing establishes or confirms a diagnosis in a symptomatic person.

DIRECT DNA-BASED DIAGNOSTIC TESTING IN SYMPTOMATIC PERSONS

A direct DNA-based diagnostic test relies on knowledge of the disease-causing genetic alterations and on the ability to detect them in readily obtainable tissue samples, usually blood.

High Sensitivity and Specificity

A test of high sensitivity and specificity detects a specific disease and excludes other diseases with certainty.

Trinucleotide repeat diseases, caused by the presence of an abnormally large number of tandem trinucleotide repeats within a gene, are examples of diseases for which direct DNA-based test-

Table 1 Use of DNA-Based Testing for Certain Inherited Disorders

Disease Name	Medical Paradigm		Genetic Counseling Paradigm		
	Diagnosis	Predictive	Predictive	Carrier Detection	Prenatal Diagnosis
Huntington disease	X		X		X
Friedreich ataxia	X	X	X	X	X
Factor V Leiden	X	X			X
Duchenne muscular dystrophy Becker muscular dystrophy	X		X	X	X
Familial adenomatous polyposis		X			X
Retinoblastoma		X			X
Breast cancer		X	X		X
Cystic fibrosis		X		X	X

Table 2 Trinucleotide Repeat Diseases[1,2]

Disease Name	Type of Repeat	Mode of Inheritance	Normal Alleles*	Permutation (Intermediate) Alleles*	Abnormal Alleles*	Stabilization by Repeat Interruption	Parental Effect	Somatic Mosaicism
X-linked spinal and bulbar muscular atrophy	CAG	XLR	9–33		38–75	No	pat > mat	No
Huntington disease	CAG	AD	9–26	27–35	36–121	No	pat > mat	Yes
Dentatorubral-pallidoluysian atrophy	CAG	AD	3–36		49–88	No	pat > mat	Yes
Spinocerebellar ataxia type 1 (SCA1)	CAG	AD	6–36		39–81	Yes (CAT)	pat > mat	Yes
SCA2	CAG	AD	15–34		34–64	Yes (CAA)	pat = mat	ND
SCA3	CAG	AD	12–40		60–84	No	pat = mat	Yes
SCA6	CAG	AD	4–16		21–30	No	?	ND
SCA7	CAG	AD	6–17		34–200		pat > mat	
SCA8	CTG	AD	16–34		100–250			
SCA12	GAG	AD	6–26		66–78			
Fragile X syndrome locus A	CGG	XLD	< 55	55–220	> 200	Yes (AGG)	mat > pat	Yes
Fragile X syndrome locus E	GCC	XLD	6–35		> 220			
Myotonic dystrophy	CTG	AD	5–27		> 50		mat > pat	
Friedreich ataxia	GAA	AR	8–22		120–1,700			Occasional
Oculopharyngeal muscular dystrophy	GCG	AD	6		8–13		no	no
Oculopharyngeal muscular dystrophy	GCG	AR	6		7		no	no

*Alleles are described by trinucleotide repeat size.
AD—autosomal dominant AR—autosomal recessive mat—maternal ND—no data pat—paternal XLR—X-linked recessive

ing is highly sensitive and specific [*see Table 2*].[1,2] The tests for these disorders measure the repeat size (i.e., number of trinucleotide repeats present). Cost-effectiveness is undisputed because of the straightforward laboratory methodologies used in testing. Because the molecular genetic basis of trinucleotide repeat diseases is known, the disease spectrum for a number of these disorders has been redefined. Establishing the diagnosis requires molecular testing; conversely, the sensitivity and specificity of the test for the disease are 100%. For example, in spinocerebellar ataxia type 3 (Machado-Joseph disease), four overlapping but age-related phenotypes are recognized. The spectrum of clinical involvement ranges from spasticity or predominance of extrapyramidal findings (rigidity, dystonia, or involuntary movements) with cerebellar findings (ataxia or ophthalmoplegia) in young patients to predominance of parkinsonism and neuropathy in patients older than 40 years. The different clinical phenotypes all derive from a mutation in the same gene.[3]

Another example of a spectrum of clinical phenotypes resulting from mutations in the same gene is Friedreich ataxia. In a study that examined the predictive value of the molecular test for Friedreich ataxia (FDRA) in 187 patients with autosomal recessive childhood-onset ataxia,[4] only 60% had findings that were considered typical of FDRA by strict diagnostic criteria. All of the patients with typical findings and 46% of patients with atypical presentations had GAA expansions in the frataxin gene consistent with the diagnosis of FDRA. To accommodate the molecular diagnostic criteria, the phenotypic spectrum of FDRA was broadened to include older age at onset and preservation of deep tendon reflexes.

Although a rough correlation exists between the number of trinucleotide repeats and the severity and age at onset of disease in all of these disorders, the positive predictive value of the number of repeats for these findings is less than 100%. This value is not relevant when the test that measures repeat number is used for diagnosis of symptomatic persons, but it becomes relevant when the test is used for predictive testing and recurrence-risk counseling. Recurrence-risk counseling for trinucleotide repeat disorders depends not only on the usual mendelian genetics but also on the empirical risk of further gene expansion (i.e., increase in length of the trinucleotide repeat) during meiosis. For unknown reasons, expansion can be influenced by the sex of the transmitting parent; for example, further expansion is probable when a mother transmits the expanded allele in fragile X syndrome and myotonic dystrophy and when the father transmits the abnormal allele in Huntington disease, Kennedy disease, dentatorubral-pallidoluysian atrophy, or spinocerebellar ataxia types 1 and 3.[1] The risk of further expansion may depend on the total length of the trinucleotide repeat region and the presence of different stabilizing sequences within or adjacent to the gene.

High Sensitivity, Low Specificity, and Low Positive Predictive Value

A test of high sensitivity detects a disease but does not exclude with certainty other diseases as the cause of the patient's symptoms.

Factor V Leiden mutation analysis, the most commonly ordered genetic test, is an example of a direct DNA-based test that is 100% sensitive, but its specificity and positive predictive value are low. The specific mutation in coagulation factor V, named factor V Leiden, is a glutamine substituted for an arginine at codon 506.[5] By definition, the test that detects this mutation is 100% sensitive. Factor V Leiden causes resistance to activated protein C, a natural anticoagulant that allows extravascular blood to clot while maintaining intravascular fluidity.[5] Epidemiologic data support a predisposition to primary and recurrent venous thromboembolism in factor V Leiden heterozygotes. It is estimated that 5% of whites are heterozygous for factor V Leiden and that approximately 20% of all persons with venous thromboembolism are heterozygous for factor V Leiden.[6] Heterozygotes with the mutation have a 2.4-fold greater risk of recurrent thromboembolism than patients without the mutation. Factor V Leiden is present in more than half of families with a so-called thrombophilic tendency; that is, several family members have deep vein thromboses that are often multiple, early in onset, or without clear risk factors.[7] It is presumed that in these families, other risk factors—some genetic and some environmental—are present.[8,9]

The advisability of screening high-risk populations, such as oral-contraceptive users and pregnant women, for factor V Leiden has been debated by Vandenbroucke and coworkers.[10] These investigators point out that recommendations for management of factor V Leiden heterozygotes have focused on high-risk families for whom the risks for thromboembolism may be substantially different from those in low-risk families.[11] In addition, the discontinuance of oral contraceptives and the use of anticoagulants in pregnancy have substantial risks themselves that may outweigh the risk of thromboembolism.[10] Despite the ease of testing and the high gene prevalence, the low positive-predictive value of factor V Leiden outside of well-defined clinical settings makes interpretation of the test problematic in low-risk persons. Vandenbroucke and coworkers[10] concluded that the clinical situation of the patient and the family members, rather than the presence or absence of a mutation, will dictate the physician's advice.

Low Sensitivity, High Specificity, and High Positive Predictive Value

A test of low sensitivity does not always detect a specific disease, but when the test is positive, identification of disease is certain.

Mutation analysis of leukocyte DNA in the diagnosis of Duchenne muscular dystrophy (DMD) and Becker muscular dystrophy (BMD) is an example of diagnostic direct DNA-based testing in which sensitivity is less than 100% but specificity and positive predictive value are high.[12] In these diseases, allelic heterogeneity reduces the ability to detect all disease-causing mutations, thereby reducing test sensitivity. Allelic heterogeneity (sometimes called mutational heterogeneity) refers to the situation in which more than one disease-causing mutation (allele) at one locus causes a given phenotype. About 70% of males with DMD have a deletion in the dystrophin gene, resulting in a frameshift and no production of the protein dystrophin.[13,14] The detection of an out-of-frame mutation is sufficient to establish the diagnosis of DMD. When no deletion is detected, the diagnostic test is muscle biopsy using immunohistochemical and immuno-electron microscopic techniques to visualize the protein dystrophin in the subsarcolemmal area. The absence of dystrophin is diagnostic of DMD.

BMD is allelic to DMD; that is, the two disorders are caused by different mutations at the same locus. BMD is rarer than DMD, and BMD has a later onset and a milder course than DMD. Deletions of the dystrophin gene also occur in about 85% of males with BMD, but these deletions are in-frame mutations that lead to the production of a truncated protein. Muscle function and prognosis are better for patients with BMD than those with DMD. Muscle biopsy plays the same role in patients

suspected of having BMD who have no discernible dystrophin mutation. In this instance, dystrophin is detectable in the subsarcolemma but is reduced in quantity.

The use of dystrophin testing also exemplifies the positive predictive value of DNA testing through genotype-phenotype correlation of frameshift and in-frame mutations.

Leukocyte DNA analysis costs several hundred dollars, compared with several thousand dollars for an open muscle biopsy, which requires a surgeon, an anesthesiologist, a pathologist, and related staff. Furthermore, recurrence-risk counseling for female relatives of DMD and BMD patients requires that results of mutation analysis on at least one affected male family member be available.

PREDICTIVE TESTING IN ASYMPTOMATIC AT-RISK PERSONS

Predictive testing is used to identify a disease-causing gene alteration in at-risk asymptomatic relatives. Predictive testing is considered presymptomatic when it is certain that all persons who have the altered gene will become symptomatic and is considered predispositional when penetrance of the gene is reduced and less than 100% of persons with the altered gene will be affected.

In asymptomatic at-risk persons, test sensitivity may be less than 100%, but specificity and positive predictive value must be high. Cost-effectiveness of predictive testing is realized by reducing morbidity and mortality in patients at high risk through early detection and treatment and by removing persons who do not have the gene from screening protocols that can be expensive and invasive. The disorders in this category are primarily autosomal dominant cancers [*see Table 3*].[15]

Although presymptomatic testing and predispositional testing are often distinguished, the issues seem to be the same when the test is for a gene associated with a high risk for a disorder that has a low population risk (e.g., retinoblastoma). Mutation analysis may not be required to establish the diagnosis in the proband when the disorder is diagnosed by clinical findings. However, testing of an affected family member is required to determine whether the disease-causing mutation can be identified for the purpose of testing asymptomatic at-risk relatives.

Presymptomatic Testing

Familial adenomatous polyposis (FAP) is an autosomal dominant disorder in which penetrance of the disease-causing gene mutations is 100%. Persons with an *APC* gene mutation develop adenomas in the colorectum starting at around 16 years of age; in these individuals, the number of adenomas increases to hundreds or thousands, and colorectal cancer develops at a mean age of 39 years. The mean age at death is 42 years in those who go untreated. Early diagnosis via presymptomatic testing reduces morbidity and increases life expectancy through im-

Table 3 Autosomal Dominant Cancer Syndromes for Which Genetic Testing Is Available

Von Hippel–Lindau disease	Multiple endocrine neoplasia type 2
Familial adenomatosis polyposis	Multiple endocrine neoplasia type 1
Hereditary nonpolyposis colorectal cancer	Breast cancer
Retinoblastoma	Melanoma

proved surveillance and timely prophylactic colectomy.[16] Testing of the *APC* gene has been shown to be cost-effective when used to identify carriers of the disease-causing *APC* mutation among at-risk relatives of individuals with FAP.[17] However, the currently available in vitro synthesized-protein assay can identify a truncating *APC* gene mutation in about 90% of families that have members with FAP.

Before asymptomatic members of a family are tested, it is preferable for a symptomatic family member to be tested to establish the molecular diagnosis in the family. The results are considered positive when a truncating mutation is identified. Only after an affected member has a positive test result can DNA-based testing be done on asymptomatic, at-risk relatives. In testing at-risk family members, a result is said to be positive when the proband's mutation is found in a family member and is said to be negative when the disease-causing mutation is not present. In such cases, the APC test has a 100% positive predictive value and a 100% negative predictive value for FAP in at-risk relatives. In the 10% of families for whom an *APC* gene mutation cannot be identified in an affected family member, predictive APC testing cannot be used in asymptomatic at-risk relatives. The probability of FAP is calculated by pedigree analysis, although the actual genetic status of each family member is considered indeterminate.

Predispositional Testing

Retinoblastoma is an example of a disorder in which penetrance of disease-causing gene mutations is less than 100%. It is caused by mutations in the *Rb1* gene and can be inherited in an autosomal dominant manner. On average, penetrance of *Rb1* gene mutations is 90% (i.e., 90% of persons with a germline disease-causing gene mutation will develop retinoblastoma). Cost-effectiveness and improved outcome through the use of predispositional gene testing have been demonstrated.[18]

Improved outcome is defined as preserving vision in at-risk persons through early detection and treatment of ocular tumors and reducing morbidity through early detection of nonocular second tumors.[11] Early detection of retinoblastoma, while the tumor is small, allows less aggressive treatments that ablate tumors but preserve vision. Before the availability of molecular genetic testing, recurrence-risk counseling for the parents of a child with retinoblastoma or for an adult with retinoblastoma was empirical and based on a positive or negative family history and the presence of a single tumor or multiple tumors. The surveillance protocol is required whether a child has a 6% risk of retinoblastoma (parent or sibling with unilateral, sporadic retinoblastoma), a 40% risk (parent with bilateral retinoblastoma), or a 90% risk (person known to have a germline *Rb1* mutation).

Sequencing the *Rb1* gene detects mutations in over 80% of patients with bilateral or hereditary retinoblastoma.[19] Although it is both labor intensive and expensive, gene sequencing is required to establish the molecular diagnosis in a proband. Because of extensive allelic heterogeneity, gene sequencing is the gold standard for detection of *Rb1* gene mutations. Thus, an adult proband who has had retinoblastoma can undergo *Rb1* mutation analysis to plan the management of his or her at-risk offspring. When a germline *Rb1* mutation is identified in the proband, the offspring can be tested prenatally or at birth to determine the genetic status and whether there is a need for frequent ophthalmologic examinations. When no mutation is identified in the adult, the risk of recurrence is empirical, and all offspring must be evaluated regularly by an ophthalmologist. Cost-effectiveness results from

removing at-risk children from unnecessary and expensive screening protocols when they test negative for an *Rb1* germline mutation known to be in their family.[20]

Genetic-Counseling Paradigm

In the genetic-counseling paradigm, genetic testing provides persons with genetic information for personal decision making, which may include reproductive planning. Issues of test sensitivity, specificity, positive predictive value, and recurrence risk are relevant as in the medical model, but cost-effectiveness cannot be assessed when testing is used only for personal decision making.

PREDICTIVE TESTING

Predictive testing is used for presymptomatic and predispositional diagnosis of persons at risk for disorders for which no medical interventions exist. Predictive testing for a disorder in an asymptomatic person is appropriate when no medical intervention exists to alter the course of the disorder.

Presymptomatic Diagnosis

Huntington disease is an example of a disorder for which there is no medical intervention. Huntington disease is caused by a CAG trinucleotide repeat expansion in the *HD* gene. When the CAG expansion is greater than 41 repeats, the penetrance is 100%—that is, all individuals with an allele that size will eventually develop Huntington disease. Clarification of genetic status among persons at risk for Huntington disease allows those who have inherited the altered gene and those who have not inherited the altered gene to make informed personal and social decisions. Such decisions may include matters of lifestyle, employment, personal finance, and family planning. Offering genetic testing to persons at risk for an untreatable, debilitating, fatal disorder requires careful forethought. The molecular diagnosis must always be confirmed in a symptomatic relative before testing can be offered to asymptomatic family members at risk. Because no medical intervention can be offered, anticipating and addressing the patient's psycho-emotional needs are paramount. In a position paper, the National Society of Genetic Counselors emphasized that pretest education and genetic counseling are necessary and that posttest follow-up care must be in place at the time of genetic testing.[21] In this instance, informing the patient of normal results requires as much preparation and counseling as the relaying of abnormal results. The pretest counseling with the patient must address the positive predictive value of the test, particularly as relating to age at onset and severity of the disease. Although greater repeat length is usually associated with earlier onset and more severe disease, repeat length is not always a predictor of disease onset or severity. Furthermore, patients with an intermediate number of trinucleotide repeats (36 to 41 CAG repeats) may have an indeterminate genetic risk. Trinucleotide repeat sizes in this range are considered to have reduced penetrance because they can cause disease symptoms but do not always do so within a normal life expectancy.[2] Thus, the patient who has prepared to hear a negative or positive result may be in the same uncertain position after testing as before.

Confidentiality of test results and possible discrimination in employment and health insurance coverage[22] may be issues for an asymptomatic person who has undergone genetic testing. Predictive genetic testing of asymptomatic children in the ge-

Table 4 Carrier Detection through DNA-Based Testing

Cystic fibrosis	Tay-Sachs disease
Phenylketonuria	Carbohydrate-deficient
Congenital adrenal hyperplasia	glycoprotein disease
	β-Thalassemia

netic-counseling paradigm is strongly discouraged because of concerns that children will be inappropriately labeled at a time when they cannot be expected to use this information for personal planning or reproductive decision making.[23]

Predispositional Testing

Predispositional testing for a disorder may not be appropriate when it is associated with a high population risk and when the efficacy of measures to reduce risk in persons with disease-predisposing mutations is unknown. Predispositional testing for breast cancer through mutation analysis of the genes BRCA1 and BRCA2 can be considered in this category because the efficacy of measures to reduce cancer risk for carriers of BRCA1 and BRCA2 cancer-predisposing mutations is unknown.[24] Furthermore, the high prevalence of breast cancer in the general population means that the rigorous screening for early breast cancer identification recommended for all women cannot be relaxed even when an at-risk woman does not have the BRCA1 or BRCA2 cancer-predisposing mutation identified in a relative.

The dilemma posed by the indeterminate role of BRCA1 and BRCA2 molecular genetic testing in reducing morbidity from breast cancer may turn out to be a recurring issue in genetic testing for common diseases. Breast cancer, like such other common disorders as coronary artery disease, diabetes mellitus, and Alzheimer disease, is regarded by geneticists as a complex disorder. Complex disorders have multiple etiologies, including heritable single genes, multiple genes with an additive effect that interact with often undefined environmental influences, and acquired environmental or genetic changes. Single heritable genes may represent a relatively small contribution to the overall incidence and morbidity from common diseases, including breast cancer, which affects one in nine women. Only 5% to 10% of cases of breast cancer are attributed to mutations in single genes, including BRCA1 and BRCA2. For a woman whose relatives have a known BRCA1 mutation but who has tested negative for the mutation known to be in the family, the chance of breast cancer developing is still one in nine. She therefore has the same need for close surveillance as women in the general population. Furthermore, detection of a BRCA1 or BRCA2 mutation may not alter the surveillance protocol for breast cancer that is recommended for all women. The options for breast cancer prevention (e.g., bilateral mastectomy), however, might be considered in a different light for women with a BRCA1 or BRCA2 mutation. Caution has been advised because the positive predictive value of a BRCA1 or BRCA2 mutation for development of breast cancer may not be fully understood and may be biased upward as a result of higher risks and different disease spectra in the high-risk families studied initially. The same issue is raised in factor V Leiden testing.

There are serious issues relating to testing for BRCA1 and BRCA2 mutations, including appropriate pretest counseling for at-risk women,[25] appropriate interpretation of positive and nega-

tive test results, recommendations for surveillance, and consideration of prophylactic mastectomy [see Chapter 195].

CARRIER TESTING

Carrier testing is used primarily to identify carriers of autosomal recessive gene mutations and X-linked recessive gene mutations. There are no health-related issues for carriers of an autosomal recessive gene mutation, because all are expected to be asymptomatic, as are most female carriers of an X-linked recessive gene mutation.

Autosomal Recessive Disorder

In cases of autosomal recessive disorders, testing may be used for diagnosis in a symptomatic person, for evaluation of at-risk asymptomatic persons, and for detection of carriers and affected fetuses. Although the gene causing an autosomal recessive disorder may be well characterized, allelic heterogeneity may reduce the sensitivity of DNA-based testing below levels acceptable for use diagnostically because it may not be technically feasible to identify all possible disease-causing mutations. However, carrier detection and prenatal testing may be possible only through DNA-based testing, providing information for reproductive decision making that would not otherwise be accessible [see Table 4].

Cystic fibrosis (CF) is an example of such an autosomal recessive disorder. Although discovery of disease-causing mutations in the CFTR gene has led to new tests for CF and redefinition of the disease spectrum, the traditional diagnostic criteria for classic CF are still valid.[26] The diagnosis of CF is established when sweat chloride is greater than 60 mEq/L in the presence of one or more characteristic clinical findings (typical gastrointestinal or sinopulmonary disease or obstructive azoospermia) or when there is a family history of the disease. In questionable cases, CFTR mutation analysis can be helpful in establishing the diagnosis; however, genotyping alone rarely establishes the diagnosis of CF. Some persons with two abnormal alleles can have yet another mutation that mitigates the effect of the abnormal allele. Others may have classic CF without a detectable CFTR disease-causing mutation because of allelic heterogeneity. Allelic heterogeneity in CF is extensive, with over 900 known disease-causing mutations. A panel of 25 mutations has been recommended by the American College of Medical Genetics for routine testing in clinical laboratories.[27] Mutation detection rates vary by ethnicity. In white Europeans, 2% of CF patients will have no detectable abnormal alleles and 26% will have only one detectable abnormal allele.

When two disease-causing alleles are identified in the proband, both parents can be tested to determine which parent carries which allele. Then, relatives of the mother can be tested for the presence of her disease-causing allele, and relatives of the father can be tested for the presence of his disease-causing allele. Any relative who is found to be a carrier of a disease-causing allele has the option of having his or her spouse tested with the clinically available panel of 25 common disease-causing alleles. Couples in which both partners are carriers of disease-causing alleles have a 25% chance of having a child who inherits two CFTR disease-causing mutations. When the spouse has no identifiable disease-causing mutations, carrier risk can be calculated using Bayesian analysis.[28]

Although the use of DNA-based testing is sensitive and specific in high-risk families, its use in preconceptual counseling for carrier detection is problematic because of its low sensitivity. DNA-based testing has been discussed extensively, and the American College of Medical Genetics has affirmed its use in the genetic counseling of high-risk persons but says that further study is required before DNA-based testing is instituted as a population-based screening method.[29,30]

X-Linked Recessive Disorders

In X-linked recessive disorders, DNA-based testing may be used to diagnose symptomatic males and the occasional symptomatic female and to detect carrier females and affected male fetuses. As in autosomal recessive disorders, DNA-based testing is often the only option for carrier detection and prenatal testing. Situations that add complexity to carrier testing for X-linked recessive disorders are the high frequency of new gene mutations in a male who is the only affected family member and the possibility of germline mosaicism in the mother of a male who is the only affected family member. New gene mutations are borne by only a single egg or a single sperm. Germline mosaicism is the presence of a mutation in some germline cells (eggs or sperm) that is not found in other germline cells or somatic cells. A female with a germline mosaicism for a gene mutation tests negative for the disease-causing mutation in white blood cells but can bear more than one affected child.

DMD is an example of an X-linked recessive disorder in which these issues must be taken into account in genetic counseling. Carrier detection in DMD can be problematic because a significant number of males with DMD are single cases in a family. The following three equally probable possibilities exist for males with DMD who have a negative family history:

1. The affected boy has a new gene mutation. In this case, his mother does not carry a disease-causing allele, and her female relatives are not at risk to be carriers of the altered allele.
2. The mother carries a new gene mutation, which places her daughters, but not her sisters, at risk to be carriers of the altered allele.
3. The maternal grandmother carries a new gene mutation, which places her daughters at risk to be carriers of the altered allele.

Thus, in families where there is a single case of DMD, recurrence-risk counseling depends on establishing which, if any, of the women are carriers of a disease-causing mutation. The following testing and recurrence-risk counseling paradigm is used.

DNA testing is performed on the male proband with DMD to identify the causative *DMD* mutation. When a dystrophin gene mutation is identified, a blood sample from the proband's mother is tested for the same mutation. If she has the same mutation as her son, she is counseled regarding the 50% risk of sons being affected and 50% risk of daughters being carriers; it is appropriate to test the proband's grandmother for the presence of the same disease-causing mutation. When the proband's mother tests negative for his mutation, two possibilities exist: the son has a new gene mutation or the mother has germline mosaicism, which occurs in about 20% of women in this situation. If the son has a new gene mutation, the mother is not at increased risk of having other affected sons, and other women in the family are not at increased risk of being mutation carriers. If the mother has germline mosaicism, she is at risk of having carrier daughters and additional affected sons. Her sisters, however, are not at risk of being carriers.

When a *DMD* gene mutation is not identified in the affected male, linkage analysis for carrier detection can be performed. Linkage analysis is most effective when there is at least one other affected male in the family on whom DNA samples are available. As in all linkage studies, the DNA markers used in tracking genes cannot determine whether the allele at the locus is normal or abnormal. The linkage study itself cannot detect new gene mutations and can be used only to clarify the genetic status of offspring of women who are known to be carriers of a disease-causing allele.

PRENATAL TESTING

Prenatal testing is used to evaluate a fetus at high risk for a genetic disorder on the basis of family history or to evaluate a fetus at no known increased risk but suspected of having a genetic disorder because of suggestive findings during the pregnancy.

Positive Family History

Testing of fetuses using DNA-based methodologies can be offered to couples at risk of having a child with an autosomal dominant, autosomal recessive, or X-linked disorder for which the specific gene mutation (or mutations) has been identified in the family. Prior genetic evaluation must establish the sensitivity, specificity, and positive predictive value of the tests available, and genetic counseling must be offered to provide the family an opportunity to review their reproductive options. To provide timely information should pregnancy termination be considered, DNA-based testing can be performed on tissues obtained by chorionic villus sampling (CVS) at 9 to 11 weeks' gestation or from amniocentesis at 16 to 18 weeks' gestation.

Findings Suggestive of a Genetic Disorder

Prenatal testing with DNA-based methodologies can be a part of the diagnostic evaluation of a fetus not known to be at increased risk for a genetic disorder that is being evaluated further because of abnormalities detected during routine monitoring of the pregnancy. When such findings are detected early in the pregnancy, DNA-based diagnosis may be undertaken if pregnancy termination is being considered. When findings are not apparent until the third trimester, diagnosis may be initiated for the purpose of perinatal management. For example, ultrasound findings of intestinal obstruction with hyperechoic meconium would warrant *CFTR* mutation analysis. Such testing can be performed on DNA extracted from amniocytes obtained from amniocentesis after 16 weeks' gestation when timing is not an issue or from white cells obtained by percutaneous umbilical blood sampling when results are needed urgently.

Genetic Consultation

Genetic evaluation and genetic counseling are integral to genetic testing. Genetic consultation is as essential to care of the patient with a genetic disorder as the testing itself.[31-33] Genetic evaluation is the process of information gathering on a patient or family with a known or suspected genetic disorder. Genetic counseling is the process of helping patients understand the nature and cause of the inherited disorder and providing them with information that allows them to make informed medical and personal decisions.[31,33,34]

Genetic evaluation involves the gathering of information before a clinic visit and during the initial portion of the usually 1-hour visit. The following information is obtained from the patient or family: the reason for referral; a family history, including first- and second-degree relatives to the consultand; additional directed family history based on the known or suspected diagnosis and information provided by the patient or other family members; medical records of affected relatives; prenatal and perinatal history;

past medical history; and information on growth, development, education, and employment. In addition, family functioning is assessed, potential ethical issues are identified, and a physical examination is performed on the patient and other family members as needed.

Once the gathering of information is complete, genetic counseling is provided. Discussion with the patient or family includes a summary of information obtained; possible diagnosis and degree of certainty on the basis of available information; recommended tests and evaluations necessary to establish the diagnosis or for management of the patient; the sensitivity, specificity, and positive predictive value of such tests; natural history of the disorder, including prognosis; inheritance pattern, including penetrance and expressivity; and recurrence risk for affected and at-risk persons, including reproductive options and options for prenatal diagnosis. Medical management and referrals to appropriate medical specialists are discussed. Psychosocial issues discussed include anticipatory guidance of the patient and family, and availability of community support services, and availability of regional or national disease-specific or umbrella organizations, many of which can be identified through the Genetic Alliance (www.geneticalliance.org). Genetic counseling issues for the extended family are addressed. Geographically dispersed family members are referred to locally available genetic services that can be identified through the GeneTests (www.genetests.org) Genetics Clinic Directory. Clinic visits and genetic-counseling sessions are documented with detailed summaries suitable for distribution to the family and health care providers. Summary letters are often sent to the family. Short-term follow-up is planned for conveying outstanding test results or other information; long-term follow-up at 2- to 5-year intervals is planned for routine management and updating of genetic counseling issues.

Difficulties Encountered in DNA-Based Testing for Inherited Disorders

LACK OF AWARENESS OF TEST AVAILABILITY

For many inherited disorders, molecular genetic testing is not available, because the causative gene (or genes) is not known. In other instances, the gene is known but test sensitivity is less than that of clinical evaluation, and testing is done only in a research context (e.g., Marfan syndrome). Often, the gene is known, and although a clinical test is theoretically possible, clinical laboratories have not offered the test because of the high cost of low-volume, high-complexity tests for rare disorders. In other instances, causative genes are known, testing is available only on a research basis, and clinical test availability is predicted for the near future (e.g., the autosomal dominant hypertrophic cardiomyopathies).[35,36] The rapid transition of testing from research laboratory to clinical practice makes it difficult even for those who are familiar with genetic testing to keep abreast of new developments. For those not familiar with genetic testing and its applications to patient care, the task is even more daunting.[37]

GeneTests is a genetic-testing resource, maintained at the University of Washington and the Children's Hospital and Regional Medical Center, in Seattle, designed to address this lack of awareness of test availability.[38] GeneTests (formerly called Helix) serves as a directory to help health care providers identify clinical and research laboratories offering testing of heritable disorders. As of January 2001, GeneTests contained listings of over 780 diseases for which testing was offered by more than 485 laboratories. Clinical laboratories are defined as those that examine human specimens and report results for the purpose of diagnosis, prevention, or treatment in the care of individual patients and must be licensed by Clinical Laboratory Improvement Amendments.[39]

COMPLEXITY OF TESTING METHODOLOGIES AND MODES OF INHERITANCE

Physicians may not be familiar with the use and limitations of DNA-based tests in patient care. Giardiello and colleagues[32] determined that almost 20% of clinicians ordering *APC* testing for FAP used the wrong testing strategy. These investigators also determined that 34% of clinicians ordering *APC* testing were unable to identify and interpret false negative results. Several genetic concepts that are intrinsic to the correct use of testing may be confusing. These concepts include (1) locus heterogeneity, in which the identical phenotype is caused by mutations at more than one locus (e.g., genes at two different loci are known to cause tuberous sclerosis), which means that negative testing at one locus does not rule out the disease; (2) allelic heterogeneity, in which multiple disease-causing mutations at a locus reduce the sensitivity of molecular testing below an acceptable level for use in diagnosis but not for recurrence-risk counseling; and (3) redefinition of phenotypes on the basis of molecular genetic findings (e.g., trinucleotide repeat diseases, CF, and the dystrophinopathies, including DMD, BMD, and X-linked dilated cardiomyopathy).

GeneClinics (www.geneclinics.org) is an NIH-supported medical genetics knowledge base that is maintained at the University of Washington. It contains current information on the use of genetic testing in diagnosis, management, and genetic counseling for specific inherited disorders. Entries on more than 100 diseases (as of January 2001) provide expert-authored, peer-reviewed information for health care professionals.

CONFUSION BETWEEN TESTING PARADIGMS

The intertwining of diagnostic testing and testing for personal decision making may lead to confusion about such issues as cost-effectiveness, medical necessity, privacy, and discrimination. Just as the application of testing to patient care is context specific, consideration of these social issues is also context specific.

UNDERUTILIZATION OF GENETIC SERVICES

Giardiello and colleagues determined that only 18% of patients undergoing predictive testing for FAP, an autosomal dominant disorder with 100% penetrance and associated with a 100% risk of cancer by 40 years of age, received genetic counseling. A recent survey of 600 primary care physicians in Oregon revealed that 20% of internists did not know whether there were any genetic services for them to consult. Furthermore, most felt they did not need to refer patients for genetic consultation and preferred to offer risk counseling themselves.[40] The need for primary care physicians to understand and use genetic services has been emphasized.[37,41,42] Possible explanations of underutilization of genetic services are the so-called therapeutic gap between diagnosis and prediction of diseases and the ability to treat or prevent them,[43] real or perceived restrictive reimbursement policies of health care payors, and concern for ethical and social issues that would seem to extend genetic testing beyond the purview of traditional medical care.[44] The change in use of some genetic tests from a diagnostic role to a screening role (e.g., factor V Leiden) may shift the emphasis of testing away from evaluation of at-risk family members and genetic counseling to a broader role related to population-based health care.

Conclusion

There can be no doubt that with the continuing progress of the Human Genome Project, the ongoing media enthusiasm for reporting new gene discoveries and other genetic advances, increasing patient access to information (particularly on the Internet), energetic patient advocacy groups, and the likelihood of direct marketing of genetic testing to the public, the thoughtful use of genetic testing will be essential to good medical practice and the appropriate use of genetic counseling will be essential to good patient care.

References

1. La Spada AR: Trinucleotide repeat instability: genetic features and molecular mechanisms. Brain Pathol 7:943, 1997

2. Potter NT, Nance MA: Genetic testing for ataxia in North America. Mol Diagn 5:91, 2000

3. Nance MA: Clinical aspects of CAG repeat diseases. Brain Pathol 7:881, 1997

4. Dürr A, Cossee M, Agid Y, et al: Clinical and genetic abnormalities in patients with Friedreich's ataxia. N Engl J Med 335:1169, 1996

5. Majerus PW: Bad blood by mutation. Nature 369:14, 1994

6. Simioni P, Prandoni P, Lensing AW, et al: Risk for subsequent venous thromboembolic complications in carriers of the prothrombin or the factor V gene mutation with a first episode of deep-vein thrombosis. Blood 96:3329, 2000

7. Briet E, van der Meer FJ, Rosendal FR, et al: The family history and inherited thrombophilia. Br J Haematol 87:348, 1994

8. Simioni P: The molecular genetics of familial venous thrombosis. Baillieres Best Pract Res Clin Haematol 12:479, 1999

9. van Boven HH, Vandenbroucke JP, Briet E, et al: Gene-gene and gene-environment interactions determine risk of thrombosis in families with inherited antithrombin deficiency. Blood 94:2590, 1999

10. Vandenbroucke JP, van der Meer FJM, Helmerhorst FM, et al: Factor V Leiden: should we screen oral contraceptive users and pregnant women? BMJ 313:1127, 1996

11. Lensen RP, Bertina RM, de Ronde H, et al: Venous thrombotic risk in family members of unselected individuals with factor V Leiden. Thromb Haemost 83:817, 2000

12. Reitter B, Goebel HH: Dystrophinopathies. Sem Pediatr Neurol 3:99, 1996

13. Yau SC, Bobrow M, Mathew CG, et al: Accurate diagnosis of carriers of deletions and duplications in Duchenne/Becker muscular dystrophy by fluorescent dosage analysis. J Med Genet 33:550, 1996

14. Yamagishi H, Kato S, Hiraishi T, et al: Identification of carriers of Duchenne/Becker muscular dystrophy by a novel method based on detection of junction fragments in the dystrophin gene. J Med Genet 33:1027, 1996

15. Offit K: Clinical Cancer Genetics: Risk Counseling and Management. Wiley-Liss, New York, 1998

16. Markowitz AJ, Winawer SJ: Screening and surveillance for colorectal cancer. Semin Oncol 26:485,1999

17. Cromwell DM, Moore RD, Brensinger JD, et al: Cost analysis of alternative approaches to colorectal screening in familial adenomatous polyposis. Gastroenterology 114:893, 1998

18. Gallie BL: Predictive testing for retinoblastoma comes of age. Am J Hum Genet 61:279, 1997

19. Lohmann DR: RB1 gene mutations in retinoblastoma. Hum Mutat 14:283, 1999

20. Noorani HZ, Khan HN, Gallie BL, et al: Cost comparison of molecular versus conventional screening of relatives at risk for retinoblastoma. Am J Hum Genet 59:301, 1996

21. McKinnon WC, Baty BJ, Bennett RL, et al: Predisposition genetic testing for late-onset disorders in adults: a position paper of the National Society of Genetic Counselors. JAMA 178:1217, 1997

22. Pokorski RJ: Insurance underwriting in the genetic era. Am J Hum Genet 60:205, 1997

23. Points to consider: ethical, legal, and psychosocial implications of genetic testing in children and adolescents. ASHG/ACMG Report. Am J Hum Genet 57:1233, 1995

24. Burke W, Daly M, Garber J, et al: Recommendations for follow-up care of individuals with an inherited predisposition to cancer: II. BRCA1 and BRCA2. JAMA 277:997, 1997

25. Burke W, Culver JO, Bowen D, et al: Genetic counseling for women with an intermediate family history of breast cancer. Am J Med Genet 90:361, 2000

26. Stern RC: The diagnosis of cystic fibrosis. N Engl J Med 336:487, 1997

27. Statement on genetic testing for cystic fibrosis: recommended core mutation panel for general population carrier screening for cystic fibrosis. (www.faseb.org/genetics/acmg/pol-32.htm)

28. Curnow RN: Carrier risk calculations for recessive diseases when not all the mutant alleles are detectable. Am J Med Genet 52:108, 1994

29. Genetic Testing for Cystic Fibrosis. NIH Consensus Statement 1997, Apr 14–16, 15(4):1 (http://dowland.cit.nih.gov/odp/consensus/cons/106/106_statement.htm)

30. ACMG Statement on Genetic Testing for Cystic Fibrosis. ACMG Consensus Statement 1997, Oct 28

31. Assessing Genetic Risks: Implications for Health and Social Policy. Andrews LB, Fullarton JE, Holtzman NA, et al, Eds. National Academy Press, Washington, DC, 1994

32. Giardiello FM, Brensinger JD, Petersen GM, et al: The use and interpretation of commercial APC gene testing for familial adenomatous polyposis. N Engl J Med 336:823, 1997

33. Marymee K, Dolan CR, Pagon RA, et al: Development of critical elements of genetic evaluation and genetic counseling for genetics professionals and perinatologists in Washington State. J Genetic Counseling 7:133, 1998

34. Schneider KA: Counseling about Cancer: Strategies for Genetic Counselors. Katherine A. Schneider, Boston, Massachusetts, 1994

35. Maron BJ: Hypertrophic cardiomyopathy. Lancet 350:127, 1997

36. Yu B, French JA, Jeremy RW, et al: Counseling issues in familial hypertrophic cardiomyopathy. J Med Genet 35:183, 1998

37. Cotton P: Prognosis, diagnosis, or who knows? Time to learn what gene tests mean. JAMA 273:93, 1995

38. Sikorski R, Peters R: Genomic medicine: Internet resources for medical genetics. JAMA 278:1212, 1997

39. Clinical improvements amendments. Federal Register. February 28, 1992; 57:40

40. Stephenson J: As discoveries unfold, a new urgency to bring genetic literacy to physicians. JAMA 278:1225, 1997

41. Touchette N, Holtzman NA, Davis JG, et al: Toward the 21st Century: Incorporating Genetics into Primary Health Care. Cold Spring Harbor Laboratory Press, 1997

42. Seashore MR, Wappner RS: Genetics in Primary Care & Clinical Medicine. Appleton & Lange, Stamford, Connecticut, 1996

43. Holtzman NA, Watson MS: Promoting safe and effective genetic testing in the United States: final report of the task force on genetic testing. National Institutes of Health/Department of Energy, Sept 1997

44. McCrary SV, Allen B, Moseley R, et al: Ethical and practical implications of the human genome initiative for family medicine. Arch Fam Med 2:1158, 1993

GERIATRICS

73 Assessment of the Geriatric Patient

Helen K. Edelberg, M.D.

The conventional medical approach, which focuses on single diseases and organ systems, does not meet the complex medical and psychosocial needs of many elderly patients. Over the past 20 years, geriatric assessment (GA) has evolved as a way to account for the atypical or nonspecific presentation of illness, the impact of medical comorbidity, and the influence of psychosocial stressors on the health of elderly persons.[1,2]

Different models of GA have been devised, utilizing a variety of settings, personnel, and approaches. Most models also include treatment and follow-up of some kind. Hence, the term assessment is something of a misnomer; these would more accurately be described as evaluation and management programs. Despite their diversity, many GA programs have resulted in improved diagnostic accuracy, functional status, affect, cognition, placement outcomes, and survival. They have also had a beneficial effect on health care utilization, reducing the number of hospital admissions (and readmissions) and institutionalization, as well as total health care costs. A recent multicenter randomized, controlled trial of 1,388 frail elderly persons reported significant reductions in functional decline with inpatient GA and improvements in mental health with outpatient GA, with no increase in costs.[2]

Studies suggest that for a GA program to be successful, it should be targeted to those patients most likely to benefit from the intervention.[3] For all intents and purposes, frail patients (i.e., those 80 years of age and older and those suffering from multiple medical and psychosocial problems) can be considered appropriate candidates for GA programs that focus on rehabilitation or chronic disease management and improved care coordination.[4,5] A number of criteria can be used for the selection of these high-risk elderly patients [see Table 1]. In contrast, GA programs that aim to identify risk factors for functional decline and develop interventions to prevent or delay impairment are more likely to benefit low-risk elderly persons.[6]

Principles of Geriatric Assessment

General features of GA include the following: (1) an interdisciplinary team approach to patient care; (2) a focus on prevention, including the prevention of decline (maintaining functional status); and (3) a feedback loop to promote adherence to recommendations by other health care providers, patients, and caregivers, as well as to promote patient self-efficacy or confidence in the ability to perform specific activities.[7]

TEAM APPROACH

The traditional components or functional domains of GA are physical, cognitive, psychological, and social [see Table 2]. Teams are more effective in assessing these domains and creating an effective care plan than are professionals working alone.[8] The core disciplines of GA are medicine, nursing, and social work. Other professionals—such as a physical, occupational, or speech therapist; a pharmacist; a psychologist; a nutritionist; a dentist; a visiting nurse; a podiatrist; or a member of the clergy—may participate in the GA team or serve as consultants. The composition and structure of the team reflect the treatment goals and resources of the specific setting, whether it is a specialized geriatric ward, consultation service, outpatient clinic, patient's home, or a nursing home.

In general, team leadership rotates, with the key provider of care reporting on the patient's progress. For example, if the major concern is the medical condition of the patient, a physician should lead the team meeting and introduce the team to the patient and family members. To be effective team members, physicians must be knowledgeable about geriatric medicine, familiar with the patient, dedicated to the team process, and have good communication skills. As team members, physicians explain the medical conditions and differential diagnoses that affect care, incorporate the team advice into medical orders, and alert the patient, family members, and caregivers about team decisions.[8] To create, monitor, or revise the care plan, interdisciplinary teams must communicate openly, freely, and regularly. Core team members must collaborate with trust and respect for the contributions of others and coordinate (i.e., delegate, share accountability, and jointly implement) the care plan. Some team members work together at the same site, so communication can be informal and expeditious. Teams should set deadlines for reaching their goals and have regular meetings to discuss team structure, process, and communication. Team effectiveness should be defined by specific goals at the outset and monitored by continuous quality-improvement measures.[8]

When formal teams do not exist, physicians may be able to achieve the benefits of an interdisciplinary approach by assembling informal teams through referrals to other professionals and community-based organizations, such as adult day programs and home care agencies. The Eldercare Locator service (1-800-677-1116), operated by the National Association of Area Agencies on Aging, provides information on and refers callers to local

---

Table 1   Suggested Criteria for Geriatric Assessment

Impairment of activities of daily living
Incontinence
Confusion or dementia
Chronic and disabling illness that prevents patient self-care
Impaired mobility
Malnutrition or weight loss
Falls
Depression
Socioeconomic or family problems
Sensory impairment (e.g., visual or hearing)
Cerebrovascular accident
Prolonged bed rest
Restraints
Pressure sore
Polypharmacy

Table 2   Domains of Geriatric Assessment

Physical health	Illness Incontinence Balance and gait Falls Nutrition Dental Hearing Vision Sexual functioning Polypharmacy Prevention
Mental health	Cognition Depression Anxiety Psychosis
Functioning	Basic activities of daily living Instrumental activities of daily living Advanced activities of daily living
Social support	Caregiver burden Finances Service needs Values and advance directives Communication and emergency support Elder abuse and neglect
Environmental adequacy	Safety Impact of climate

services for elderly persons. Resources are also available on the Internet [*see Table 3*].

FOCUS ON PREVENTION

Primary and secondary prevention for the elderly have become increasingly important as the population has continued increasing in average age and average life expectancy.[9] Because primary care practice guidelines do not always address the specific needs of elderly persons, physicians may be compelled to rely on clinical judgment to modify preexisting recommendations that were designed for middle-aged adults.[10] Assessment categories unique to elderly patients include functional status (e.g., activities of daily living [ADL] and instrumental ADL) [*see Table 4*], sensory perception, and injury prevention.[11] Interventional areas that are common to other age groups but have special implications for elderly patients include immunizations, diet and exercise, and sexuality [*see Table 5*]. Cognitive ability and mental health issues should also be evaluated within the context of the individual patient's social situation—not by screening all patients but by being alert to the occurrence of any change in mental function. The prevalence of undetected, correctable conditions and comorbid diseases is high in elderly persons. The American College of Physicians has advocated incorporating GA into routine medical care for elderly persons, particularly patients 75 years of age and older.[12]

FEEDBACK LOOP

Communication among team members and with patients and caregivers—whether it is face to face or by telephone, e-mail, or fax—is the key to effective GA programs. The team and patient must develop ways to communicate honestly, to prevent the patient from suppressing an opinion and agreeing to every sugges-

tion. For example, patients can help the team to set goals (e.g., advance directives and end-of-life care). They can also discuss drug treatment, rehabilitation, dietary plans, and other forms of therapy. If the team learns that the patient will not take a particular drug or change certain dietary habits, the care plan can be modified accordingly. Caregivers, including family members, may help by identifying realistic and unrealistic expectations on the basis of the patient's habits and lifestyle.[8]

Settings for Geriatric Assessment

GA originated in the inpatient setting, but it has since taken on significance in the outpatient setting and across the continuum of care in integrated delivery systems. It may play a critical role in hospital discharge planning and during the transition from independent living to assisted living or nursing home. Formal GA programs are available on a limited basis only, because of the nationwide shortage of trained geriatricians, and are more likely to be found in large regional or academic medical centers. Local community hospitals, visiting nurse agencies, adult day programs and senior centers may provide some of the resources necessary to provide comprehensive geriatric care, such as social work support, home nursing care and safety evaluations, and physical and occupational therapy.

INPATIENT MODELS

Community Hospital

The benefits of GA at a community rehabilitation hospital were first reported in 1990, in a 1-year randomized, controlled trial involving 155 functionally impaired elderly patients recovering from acute medical or surgical illnesses and considered at

Table 3   Selected Internet Resources for Geriatric Care

Organization	Web Site
Administration on Aging	www.aoa.gov
Aging Network Services	www.agingnets.com
Alzheimer's Association	www.alz.org
American Academy of Home Care Physicians	www.aahcp.org
American Association of Homes and Services for the Aging	www.aahsa.org
American Geriatrics Society	www.americangeriatrics.org
American Hospital Association	www.aha.org
American Medical Directors Association	www.amda.com
American Seniors Housing Association	www.seniorshousing.org
American Society of Consultant Pharmacists	www. ascp.com
Assisted Living Federation of America	www.alfa.org
CareGuide	www.careguide.net
Family Caregiver Alliance	www.caregiver.org
Gerontological Society of America	www.geron.org
Medicare	www.medicare.gov
National Adult Day Services Association	www.ncoa.org/nadsa
National Association for Home Care	ww.nahc.org
National Association of Area Agencies on Aging	www.n4a.org
National Association of Professional Geriatric Care Managers	www.caremanager.org
National Institute on Aging	www.nia.nih.gov
Visiting Nurse Associations of America	www.vnaa.org

Table 4 Activities of Daily Living and Instrumental Activities of Daily Living

Activities of daily living (ADL)	Feeding Dressing Ambulation Toileting Bathing Transfer (from bed to chair) Continence Grooming
Instrumental activities of daily living (IADL)	Using telephone Shopping Food preparation Housekeeping Laundry Travel, use of transportation Managing medications Managing finances

risk for nursing home placement. Compared with usual care, treatment in a GA unit resulted in improved function and decreased risk of nursing home placement. The beneficial effects of inpatient GA on mortality and function appeared greatest for

patients at a moderate rather than high risk of nursing home placement.[13] The researchers of this study also found that improved outcomes from GA required an investment in rehabilitation that was not totally offset by decreased institutional charges in the following year.[14] Since then, less costly and labor-intensive approaches to inpatient GA have been developed and implemented, including limited support from a geriatric nurse practitioner and use of current hospital personnel to educate attending nurses and staff physicians.[15] These options include wards or beds assigned to elderly patients and consultation services dedicated to the care of elderly persons.

Geriatric Acute Care Units

In 1990, the University Hospitals of Cleveland established an Acute Care for Elders (ACE) unit that reengineered the process of caring for elderly patients to improve functional outcomes. This program comprised four key elements: (1) a specially prepared environment (e.g., uncluttered hallways, large clocks and calendars, and handrails); (2) patient-centered care emphasizing independence, including specific protocols for prevention of disability and for rehabilitation; (3) discharge planning with the goal of returning the patient to his or her home; and (4) intensive review of medical care to minimize the adverse effects of procedures and medications. A randomized, controlled trial of 651 acutely ill patients 70 years of age or older demon-

Table 5 Evidence-Based Preventive Services Recommended for the General Population 65 Years of Age and Older[9]

Service	Activity	Frequency	Condition to Detect or Prevent
Screening	Blood pressure	At least annually	Hypertension
	Mammography	Every 2–3 yr	Breast cancer
	Fecal occult blood testing	Annually	Colorectal cancer
	and/or		
	Flexible sigmoidoscopy	Every 3–5 yr	—
	or		
	Colonoscopy	Once	—
	Pap smear	Every 3 yr or less*	Cervical cancer
	Height and weight	At least annually	Obesity, malnutrition
	Alcoholism questionnaire	†	Alcoholism
	Serum lipids in persons with angina, prior MI, DM	Annually	Risk factor for CAD
	Vision testing	Annually	Visual impairment
	Hearing testing	Annually	Hearing loss
Counseling	Low-fat, well-balanced diet	Annually	Obesity, CAD
	Adequate calcium intake	Annually	Osteoporosis
	Physical activity	Annually	Immobility, CAD, osteoporosis
	Injury prevention	Annually	Falls, motor vehicle accidents, burns, other injuries
	Smoking cessation	‡	COPD, many cancers, CAD
	Regular dental visits	Annually	Malnutrition, oral cancers, edentulism
Immunization	Influenza vaccination	Each fall	Influenza
	Pneumococcal vaccination	§	Pneumococcal disease
	Tetanus booster	Every 10 yr	Tetanus
Chemoprophylaxis	Discussion, implementation of HRT in women	¶	Osteoporosis
	Aspirin therapy after MI	Daily	Additional MI, TIA, or stroke

*May stop screening at age 65 if patient had regularly normal smears up to that age; if never tested before age 65, may stop after two normal annual smears.
†Perform at initial visit and whenever problem drinking is suspected.
‡Discuss at every visit of patients who smoke.
§Immunize once at age 65 for immunocompetent patients; revaccinate high-risk immunocompromised patients after 7–10 yr.
¶Discuss at menopause and at least one time after age 65.
CAD—coronary artery disease   COPD—chronic obstructive pulmonary disease   DM—diabetes mellitus   HRT—hormone replacement therapy   MI—myocardial infarction   TIA—transient ischemic attack

Table 6   Checklist for Assessing Environmental Hazards in the Home

House or rooms	Lack of cleanliness Inadequate insulation Inadequate lighting Hot-water temperature not regulated at 110° F Inaccessible entries and exits
Stairs or furniture	Unsafe stairs Steps with sharp or broken edges Pointed, broken, or hanging furniture (e.g., suspended chairs) Wheels on furniture
Bathroom	Absence of handrails or secure railings Absence of skid strips for bathtub Outdated prescription drugs Absence of working toilet or acceptable substitute
Signs of neglect	Old food in refrigerator Unwashed dishes Insufficient supply of food Accumulated clothing or newspapers Other signs of disrepair
Obvious dangers	Loose, frayed, or worn carpets; scatter rugs Loose or waxed flooring Absence of smoke alarm Frayed electrical cords or overloaded outlets Exposed pipes and radiators

strated that at the time of hospital discharge, patients admitted to the ACE unit were better able to perform basic ADL and more likely to return home. However, by 90 days after discharge, the functional status of ACE patients was similar to that of standard care patients.[16] However, the costs to the hospital for ACE unit care were less than those for usual care.[17] A recently published trial of 1,531 community-dwelling patients found that an ACE unit in a community hospital improved the process of care and patient and provider satisfaction without increasing hospital length of stay or costs.[18] Publications such as *The ACE (Acute Care for Elders) Manual: Meeting the Challenge of Providing Quality and Cost-Effective Hospital Care to Older Adults*[19] provide valuable information and practical advice for health care providers interested in establishing an ACE unit at their local hospital.

Geriatric Evaluation and Management Units

In the United States, the Department of Veterans Affairs helped to pioneer inpatient geriatric evaluation and management units (GEMUs), which undertake interdisciplinary diagnosis to improve the health of frail elderly patients. The GEMU team, consisting of a geriatrician, a social worker, and a nurse, follows standard protocols for geriatric evaluation and management, with specific instructions in five areas: (1) complete the history taking and physical examination, including screening for geriatric syndromes such as falls or incontinence; (2) develop a list of problems; (3) assess the patient's functional, cognitive, affective, and nutritional status; (4) evaluate the caregiver's capabilities; and (5) assess the patient's social situation. A care plan is developed on the basis of that evaluation, and the team meets at least twice a week to discuss the plan. Preventive and management services (e.g., physical and occupational therapy, nutrition,

clinical pharmacy) are coordinated to address the problems identified, with a general emphasis on maintaining functional status.[2] Although the Department of Veterans Affairs mandated that every VA facility have a GEMU by 1996, there are at present only 110 GEMUs functioning in the United States.[20] In the United Kingdom, the counterpart to the GEMU, the geriatric day hospital, continues to play a major role in the multidisciplinary assessment and rehabilitation of elderly people, despite limited evidence to support its efficacy.[21]

Inpatient Consultation Services

If GA is performed as a consultation, special care must be taken in transmitting the findings and recommendations to the primary care provider.[6] The transition between the GA team and the primary care physician frequently presents the greatest obstacle to achieving optimal care of the elderly patient.[3] The GA literature depicts a range of consulting services, from single-focus services (addressing delirium, falls, and other geriatric syndromes) to more comprehensive programs. For example, the Hospital Elder Life Program, developed by Inouye and colleagues, employs an interdisciplinary team that works closely with primary nurses. The team includes a geriatric nurse specialist and an elder life specialist. The latter is a team member with a bachelor's degree in human services or a health care–related field who has experience in geriatrics and management; this person is responsible for program operations, interventions, and volunteer coordination. The Elder Life Program is unique in its hospital-wide focus, in providing skilled staff and volunteers to implement interventions, and in targeting practical interventions toward evidence-based risk factors. In elderly persons who are cognitively impaired, sleep deprived, immobile, dehydrated, and vision or hearing impaired, the program has successfully implemented a nonpharmacologic sleep protocol, documented a reduction in incidence delirium, and prevented cognitive and functional decline.[22]

OUTPATIENT MODELS

Primary Care

Outpatient GA programs may be used as an adjunct to or a substitute for routine primary care. A consultative or primary care team—usually consisting of a physician, nurse (or nurse practitioner), and social worker—provides GA services in the ambulatory setting. Whenever appropriate, referrals are made to other providers (e.g., podiatry, neurology, physical therapy). These programs utilize self-administered questionnaires to screen for common conditions in elderly persons. Patients can complete these questionnaires in the waiting room or with the assistance of a trained receptionist.[23] For example, Moore and colleagues developed and tested a 10-minute office-staff administered screening measure to evaluate malnutrition or weight loss, visual impairment, hearing loss, cognitive impairment, urinary incontinence, depression, physical limitations, and reduced leg mobility. In a large randomized, controlled trial, the measure was associated with more frequent detection and assessment of hearing loss but did not appear to affect detection and management of other conditions included in the screen or health status at 6 months.[24]

Preventive medical care may be provided by the medical staff and psychosocial issues addressed by the nurse or social worker. Lachs and colleagues proposed a short, simple approach that primary care providers in office practice can use to routinely screen the functional status of elderly patients. The approach focuses on a limited number of functions that often cause problems for elderly patients but that conventional histories and physical examinations often fail to uncover. The screening instrument, which employs brief questions and easily observed tasks, consists of carefully selected tests of vision, hearing, arm and leg function, urinary incontinence, mental status, instrumental and basic ADL, environmental hazards, and social support systems; and it may be administered by a physician or nurse.[25]

Outpatient GA can benefit caregivers as well as patients. In a randomized trial of 568 high-risk, community-dwelling elderly persons who received outpatient GA or usual care for 6 months, caregivers of participants in the GA group were less than half as likely as the usual-care group (16.7% versus 38.5%)to report increased burden during the 1-year follow-up period.[26] Moreover, participants given outpatient GA were significantly less likely than the usual-care patients to lose functional ability, to experience increased health-related restrictions in their daily activities, to have possible depression, or to use home health care services during the 12 to 18 months after randomization. Mortality, use of most health services, and total Medicare payments did not differ significantly between the two groups. The intervention cost $1,350 a person.[27]

In 1997, Beck and colleagues described another GA model for use in primary care. In this model, elderly patients with high health services utilization and one or more chronic conditions had monthly group visits with their primary care physician and nurse. Visits included health education and prevention measures, along with opportunities for socialization, mutual support, and one-to-one consultations with physicians, when necessary. A 12-month randomized, controlled trial of 321 chronically ill HMO enrollees 65 years of age and older showed that group visits resulted in reduced repeat hospital admissions and emergency care use, reduced cost of care, more effective delivery of certain preventive measures, and increased patient and physician satisfaction.[28]

Veterans Affairs Medical Centers

There is a long-established tradition of GA within the VA system. In a randomized, controlled trial involving 160 frail elderly outpatients that compared ongoing outpatient GA through the VA system with usual care, GA proved significantly more effective in reducing mortality, increasing patient satisfaction, and improving the quality of health and social care. It did not, however, reduce health care utilization or costs.[29] In a recent 2-year randomized, controlled trial, 128 veterans 65 years of age or older were treated with outpatient GA or usual care. GA resulted in greater improvement in perceived health; smaller increases in numbers of clinic visits and impairment in instrumental ADL; improved social activity; and greater improvement in measures of depression, general well-being, life satisfaction, and cognitive status. There were no significant treatment effects in ADL scores, number of hospitalizations, or mortality.[30]

Consultation Services

GA can be a consultative service provided through hospital-based outpatient clinics. In a 12-month multicenter, randomized, controlled trial of outpatient consultative GA versus usual care in 442 elderly patients with a health problem or recent change in health status, outpatient consultative GA led to significantly improved diagnosis of cognitive impairment, depression, and incontinence; to psychological and emotional benefits for patients; and to reduced levels of caregiver stress.[31]

Even a single outpatient GA consultation, coupled with subsequent intervention to improve adherence to consultative recommendations, can be beneficial in elderly patients with identified problems.[32,33] In a 15-month randomized, controlled trial of 363 community-dwelling elderly persons in whom screening identified one or more specific geriatric conditions (falls, urinary incontinence, depressive symptoms, or functional impairment), intervention not only prevented functional and health-related quality-of-life decline but also was cost effective.[32]

In-Home Geriatric Assessment

GA in the home may be provided as part of an ongoing office-based program, as an extension of hospitalization through a post–acute care program,[34-36] or as a freestanding entity.[37] In-home GA includes the assessment of environmental hazards, which can serve an important preventive function [see Table 6].

The physician's role in in-home GA is to serve as a member of an interdisciplinary team composed of nurses, therapists (speech, physical, occupational, and respiratory), social workers, personal care attendants, home medical equipment suppliers, and informal caregivers (e.g., family members and friends).[38] In-home GA is used to establish a baseline, monitor the course of an illness, and evaluate the effects of an intervention. A recent meta-analysis of 18 randomized, controlled trials found that preventive home-visitation programs (based on multidimensional GA that included multiple follow-up home visits) helped prevent nursing home admission and functional decline, particularly in low-risk elderly persons.[39]

INTEGRATED DELIVERY SYSTEMS

GA programs have been developed and implemented by health systems to improve the evaluation and management of older adults. Managed care organizations and other integrated delivery systems have employed registered nurses, nurse practitioners, social workers, or public health workers as care or case managers to follow, organize, and coordinate care for elderly persons.[40,41] Chronic disease management programs incorporate the basic principles of GA in a variety of different settings, including outpatient clinics, senior centers, and home care.[42-44]

Programs of All-Inclusive Care for the Elderly (PACE)

More than 6,000 Medicare nursing home certifiable beneficiaries receive care from PACE, a program designated for expansion under the Balanced Budget Act of 1997.[45] PACE replicates the model of comprehensive, community-based geriatric care pioneered by On Lok. This model enrolls frail elderly persons who meet states' criteria for nursing home care and uses interdisciplinary teams to assess the participants and to deliver care in appropriate settings. Analysis of data from PACE's minimum data set reveals that short-term hospital utilization among PACE participants is lower than that for other older and disabled populations.[46]

Reimbursement

There is currently no explicit Medicare reimbursement mechanism to cover hospital or physician GA services in the United States. Elderly persons can receive GA in the context of hospitalization for acute illness, provided that the assessment does not prolong the hospital length of stay. A number of Diagnostic Related Groups (DRGs) of the Medicare system apply to frail elderly patients and can be used to justify the hospitalization of patients with coexisting conditions who require GA. Documentation of the need for hospitalization is critical.[47] As managed care, PACE receives capitated payment from Medicare and Medicaid on the basis of the rate structure of the Medicare+Choice payment system, adjusted for the comparative frailty of PACE enrollees and other factors deemed to be appropriate by the Secretary of Health and Human Services.

References

1. Fried LP, Storer DJ, King DE, et al: Diagnosis of illness presentation in the elderly. J Am Geriatr Soc 39:117, 1991

2. Cohen HJ, Feussner JR, Weinberger M, et al: A controlled trial of inpatient and outpatient geriatric evaluation and management. N Engl J Med 346:905, 2002

3. Stuck AE, Siu AL, Wieland GD, et al: Comprehensive geriatric assessment: a meta-analysis of controlled trials. Lancet 342:1032, 1993

4. Winograd CH, Gerety MB, Chung M, et al: Screening for frailty: criteria and predictors of outcomes. J Am Geriatr Soc 39:778, 1991

5. Manton KG, Gu X: Changes in the prevalence of chronic disability in the United States black and nonblack population above age 65 from 1982 to 1999. Proc Natl Acad Sci U S A 98:6354, 2001

6. Osterweil D, Brummel-Smith K, Beck JC: Comprehensive Geriatric Assessment. McGraw-Hill Book Co, New York, 2000

7. Holman H, Lorig K: Patients as partners in managing chronic disease: partnership is a prerequisite for effective and efficient health care. BMJ 320:526, 2000

8. Fulmer TT, Hyer K: Geriatric interdisciplinary teams. The Merck Manual of Geriatrics. Beers MH, Berkow R, Eds. Merck & Co, Whitehouse Station, New Jersey, 2000

9. Bloom HG, Edelberg HK: Prevention.Geriatrics Review Syllabus: A Core Curriculum in Geriatric Medicine, Fifth ed. Cobbs EL, Duthie EH, Eds. Kendall/Hunt Publishing Co, Dubuque, Iowa, 2002, p 61

10. Edelberg HK, Wei JY: Primary-care guidelines for community-living older persons. Clin Geriatrics 7:42, 1999

11. U.S. Preventive Services Task Force. Guide to Clinical Preventive Services: Report of the U.S. Preventive Services Task Force. Williams & Wilkins, Baltimore, 1996

12. Comprehensive functional assessment for elderly patients. American College of Physicians Health and Public Policy Committee. Ann Intern Med 109:70, 1988

13. Applegate WB, Miller ST, Graney MJ, et al: A randomized, controlled trial of a geriatric assessment unit in a community rehabilitation hospital. N Engl J Med 322:1572, 1990

14. Applegate WB, Graney MJ, Miller ST, et al: Impact of a geriatric assessment unit on subsequent health care charges. Am J Public Health 81:1302, 1991

15. Cefalu CA, Colbourne G, Duffy M, et al: A university-affiliated community hospital inpatient geriatrics program functioning in an administrative and educational capacity. J Am Geriatr Soc 45:355, 1997

16. Landefeld CS, Palmer RM, Kresevic DM, et al: A randomized trial of care in a hospital medical unit especially designed to improve the functional outcomes of acutely ill older patients. N Engl J Med 332:1338, 1995

17. Covinsky KE, Palmer RM, Kresevic DM, et al: Improving functional outcomes in older patients: lessons from an acute care for elders unit. Jt Comm J Qual Improv 24:63, 1998

18. Counsell SR, Holder CM, Liebenauer LL, et al: Effects of a multicomponent intervention on functional outcomes and process of care in hospitalized older patients: a randomized controlled trial of Acute Care for Elders (ACE) in a community hospital. J Am Geriatr Soc 48:1572, 2000

19. Counsell SR, Holder C, Liebenauer MA, et al: The ACE (Acute Care for Elders) Manual: Meeting the Challenge of Providing Quality and Cost-Effective Hospital Care to Older Adults. Summa Health Systems, Akron, Ohio, 1998

20. Wieland D, Hedrick SC, Rubenstein LZ, et al: Inpatient geriatric evaluation and management units: organization and care patterns in the Department of Veterans Affairs. Gerontologist 34:652, 1994

21. Black DA: The modern geriatric day hospital. Hosp Med 61:539, 2000

22. Inouye SK, Bogardus ST Jr, Baker DI, et al: The Hospital Elder Life Program: a model of care to prevent cognitive and functional decline in older hospitalized patients. J Am Geriatr Soc 48:1697, 2000

23. Wasson JH, Jette AM, Johnson DJ, et al: A replicable and customizable approach to improve ambulatory care and research. J Ambulatory Care Manage 20:17, 1997

24. Moore AA, Siu AL, Partridge JM, et al: A randomized trial of office-based screening for common problems in older persons. Am J Med 102:371, 1997

25. Lachs MS, Feinstein AR, Cooney LM Jr, et al: A simple procedure for general screening for functional disability in elderly patients. Ann Intern Med 112:699, 1990

26. Weuve JL, Boult C, Morishita L: The effects of outpatient geriatric evaluation and management on caregiver burden. Gerontologist 40:429, 2000

27. Boult C, Boult LB, Morishita L, et al: A randomized clinical trial of outpatient geriatric evaluation and management. J Am Geriatr Soc 49:351, 2001

28. Beck A, Scott J, Williams P, et al: A randomized trial of group outpatient visits for chronically ill older HMO members: the Cooperative Health Care Clinic. J Am Geriatr Soc 45:543, 1997

29. Toseland RW, O'Donnell JC, Engelhardt JB, et al: Outpatient geriatric evaluation and management: results of a randomized trial. Med Care 34:624, 1996

30. Burns R, Nichols LO, Martindale-Adams J, et al: Interdisciplinary geriatric primary care evaluation and management: two-year outcomes. J Am Geriatr Soc 48:8, 2000

31. Silverman M, Musa D, Martin DC, et al: Evaluation of outpatient geriatric assessment: a randomized multi-site trial. J Am Geriatr Soc 43:733, 1995

32. Reuben DB, Frank JC, Hirsch SH, et al: A randomized clinical trial of outpatient comprehensive geriatric assessment coupled with an intervention to increase adherence to recommendations. J Am Geriatr Soc 47:269, 1999

33. Keeler EB, Robalino DA, Frank JC, et al: Cost-effectiveness of outpatient geriatric assessment with an intervention to increase adherence. Med Care 37:1199, 1999

34. Naylor MD, Brooten D, Campbell R, et al: Comprehensive discharge planning and home follow-up of hospitalized elders: a randomized clinical trial. JAMA 281:613, 1999

35. Siu AL, Kravitz RL, Keeler E, et al: Postdischarge geriatric assessment of hospitalized frail elderly patients. Arch Intern Med 156:76, 1996

36. Landi F, Gambassi G, Pola R, et al: Impact of integrated home care services on hospital use. J Am Geriatr Soc 47:1430, 1999

37. Rockwood K, Stadnyk K, Carver D, et al: A clinimetric evaluation of specialized geriatric care for rural dwelling, frail older people. J Am Geriatr Soc 48:1080, 2000

38. Eleazer GP: Community-based care. Geriatrics Review Syllabus: A Core Curriculum in Geriatric Medicine, Fifth ed. Cobbs EL, Duthie EH, Eds. Kendall/Hunt Publishing Co, Dubuque, Iowa, 2002, p 61

39. Stuck AE, Egger M, Hammer A, et al: Home visits to prevent nursing home admission and functional decline in elderly people: systematic review and meta-regression analysis. JAMA 287:1022, 2002

40. Marshall BS, Long MJ, Voss J, et al: Case management of the elderly in a health maintenance organization: the implications for program administration under managed care. J Health Manag 44:477, 1999

41. Gagnon AJ, Schein C, McVey L, et al: Randomized controlled trial of nurse case management of frail older people. J Am Geriatr Soc 47:1118, 1999

42. Rich MW, Beckham V, Wittenberg C, et al: A multidisciplinary intervention to prevent the readmission of elderly patients with congestive heart failure. N Engl J Med 333:1190, 1995

43. Leveille SG, Wagner EH, Davis C, et al: Preventing disability and managing chronic illness in frail older adults: a randomized trial of a community-based partnership with primary care. J Am Geriatr Soc 46:1191, 1998

44. Coleman EA, Grothaus LC, Sandhu N, et al: Chronic care clinics: a randomized controlled trial of a new model of primary care for frail older adults. J Am Geriatr Soc 47:775, 1999

45. Temkin-Greener H, Meiners MR, Gruenberg L: PACE and the Medicare+Choice risk-adjusted payment model. Inquiry 38:60, 2001

46. Wieland D, Lamb VL, Sutton SR, et al: Hospitalization in the Program of All-Inclusive Care for the Elderly (PACE): rates, concomitants, and predictors. J Am Geriatr Soc 48:1373, 2000

47. Fillit H: Challenges for acute care geriatric inpatient units under the present Medicare prospective payment system. J Am Geriatr Soc 42:553, 1994

74 Management of Common Clinical Disorders in Geriatric Patients

Robert M. Palmer, M.D.

The process of aging predisposes elderly patients to homeostatic failure, chronic disease, and a loss of independence in the performance of daily activities (functional decline). Consequently, clinical disorders often manifest themselves as geriatric syndromes, which are clinical illnesses that are characterized by numerous etiologies and complex pathophysiology. Common examples of geriatric syndromes are cognitive dysfunction, urinary incontinence, and falls.[1] Geriatric syndromes increase in frequency and clinical importance in advanced age, growing more prevalent in patients older than 75 years. These syndromes are frequently encountered by physicians in ambulatory, hospital, and long-term care settings.

Geriatric syndromes reflect the presence of common chronic conditions in the elderly population. In the United States, an estimated 90 million people live with at least one chronic condition that threatens their independent self-care or compromises the quality of their lives. Rates of chronic conditions are highest among the elderly, 88% of whom have at least one chronic condition.[2] By identifying, evaluating, and treating these common conditions, physicians can help patients regain or maintain a good quality of life.

Delirium

Common causes of cognitive dysfunction in elderly patients are delirium, dementia, and depression. Dementia and depression are discussed elsewhere [see Chapters 173, 175, 176, 184, and 205].

Delirium is an important condition to identify and treat in elderly patients because it can lead to a number of adverse outcomes. Elderly patients with delirium are at risk for future functional decline (a loss of independence in their performance of daily activities), cognitive decline, and mortality.[3] Delirium is also associated with prolonged hospitalization, increased risk of nursing home placement, persistent functional decline, and debilitating complications (e.g., falls, injury, and immobility).

The criteria for delirium caused by a general medical condition include the following: disturbance of consciousness (i.e., reduced awareness of the environment) with reduced ability to focus, sustain, or shift attention; change in cognition (e.g., memory deficit, disorientation, language disturbance) or perceptual disturbance that is not better accounted for by a preexisting, established, or evolving dementia; increased or reduced psychomotor activity; disorganized sleep-wake cycle; acute onset of disturbance (usually hours to days) with fluctuation over the course of the day; and evidence from the history, physical examination, or laboratory findings that the disturbance is caused by an etiologically related general medical condition.[4,5] The cognitive disturbances contribute substantially to problems in identifying and managing delirium.

Medical Illness

Delirium is most often identified in hospitalized patients. It is present in 5% to 15% of older patients at hospital admission for treatment of medical illnesses, and it develops in 5% to 15% of older medical patients during hospitalization.[3] The use of psychoactive drugs and the presence of azotemia, fracture, or abnormal serum sodium levels are independent risk factors for delirium in elderly hospitalized patients.[3] In one study, significant risk factors for delirium in elderly medical patients during hospitalization included severe illness, cognitive impairment, vision impairment, and a high ratio of blood urea nitrogen to creatinine, implying dehydration.[6] In all studies, dementia or cognitive impairment is the single most important risk factor for delirium, perhaps reflecting impaired brain homeostasis in these highly vulnerable patients.[7] The precipitating factors for delirium in hospitalized elderly persons in one study were the use of physical restraints, more than three medications added to the patient's drug regimen, bladder catheterization, and any iatrogenic event (e.g., unintentional injury).[7] These findings establish ways to both identify high-risk patients and prevent incident delirium through appropriate medical, behavioral, and pharmacologic approaches.

Postoperative Delirium

Postoperative delirium occurs in 10% to 15% of older general surgery patients and in 30% to 60% of older patients admitted with hip fractures or who are undergoing knee arthroplasty.[8] The incidence of delirium or other cognitive impairments is not related to the type of anesthesia administered, whether general or epidural.[9] In a large prospective study, postoperative cognitive dysfunction was present in 25.8% of patients 60 years of age and older 1 week after surgery.[10] Although both surgery and anesthesia are factors contributing to the development of both short-term and long-term postoperative cognitive impairment, uncertainty remains about the specific factors that contribute to postoperative delirium. Putative risk factors for postoperative delirium include polypharmacy, the use of preoperative anticholinergic drugs, cognitive impairment, and older age.[8] Other contributing factors might include intraoperative hypoxemia, perioperative hypotension, and postoperative complications.

Among low-risk adult patients undergoing elective noncardiac surgery, postoperative delirium occurred in 9% and was independently correlated with an age of 70 years or older, self-reported alcohol use, poor cognitive status, poor functional status, markedly abnormal preoperative serum sodium level, and thoracic surgery.[11] In these patients, the postoperative use of meperidine and benzodiazepines increased the risk of delirium.[11]

Virtually any acute physical stress can precipitate delirium in elderly patients, particularly those with risk factors [see Table 1]. In medically ill patients, delirium is most commonly associated with acute infections, such as pneumonia and urosepsis; hypoxemia; hypotension; and use of psychoactive medications, such as

Table 1 Prevention and Management of Delirium

	Predisposing or Precipitating Factors	Interventions

Prevention	Psychotropic medications
	  Benzodiazepines
	  Alcohol
	  Anticholinergic agents
	  Opiates
		Avoid or discontinue antihistamines (e.g., diphenhydramine) and benzodiazepines
		Observe for possible alcohol withdrawal
		Titrate doses of opiates to achieve analgesia
		Promote sleep by applying relaxation techniques and keeping hallways quiet at night

	Preexisting cognitive impairment
	  or dementia
	  Alzheimer disease
	  Vascular cognitive impairment
	  Major depressive disorder
		Orient to date, place, caregivers, and upcoming events
		Use psychotropic medications judiciously to treat specific symptoms
		Encourage visits by family members or sitters

	Dehydration
	  High BUN-to-creatinine ratio
	  Hypotension
	  Poor skin turgor
		Prescribe fluids, and monitor intake and discharge
		Utilize intravenous hydration if oral intake is inadequate
		Have nursing staff assist with eating and drinking
		Monitor basic electrolytes

	Severe illness
	  High fever
	  Infection
	  Hypotension
		Diagnose illness quickly and follow with empirical therapy (e.g., intravenous antibiotics for community-acquired pneumonia)
		Optimize hemodynamic status (ensure adequate oxygenation and cardiac output)

	Sensory impairment
	  Vision
	  Hearing
		Utilize visual aids (e.g., corrective lenses, large-print books, diffuse illumination)
		Utilize hearing aids (e.g., portable amplifying devices, cerumen disimpaction)

	Immobility/physical restraint
	  Bed-rest orders
	  Mechanical or chemical restraints
		Ambulate or apply bedside exercises
		Obtain physical therapy consultation for gait assessment and strengthening exercises
		Obtain occupational therapy consultation for functional assessment and adaptive devices

	Interventions	Suggested Guidelines

Management	Medications
	  Neuroleptics
	  Anxiolytics
	  Opiates
		Judiciously use neuroleptics to treat disturbing psychiatric symptoms (e.g., delusions, hallucinations, aggressiveness)
		Administer haloperidol, 0.5–1.0 mg orally or parenterally, every 6–8 hr (higher doses are justified when there is a risk that patient will disrupt life-sustaining therapies)
		Administer risperidone, 0.5–1.0 mg orally daily in divided doses, when long-term neuroleptic therapy is warranted
		Administer lorazepam, 0.5–1.0 mg every 6–8 hr orally or parenterally, to patients with disturbing anxiety (higher doses for benzodiazepine or alcohol withdrawal)
		Control acute pain with morphine sulfate, administered slowly in low initial doses (e.g., start with 2–4 mg parenterally every 3 hr); monitor pain relief with visual analogue scale
		Avoid meperidine

	Nursing care	Keep sitter at bedside Move patient closer to nurses' station Implement preventive measures Educate patient and family about delirium
	Environmental measures	Keep hallways or corridors quiet Dim lights at night Provide recreational activities outside patient's room Reduce clutter in rooms and hallways

BUN—blood urea nitrogen

narcotics, benzodiazepines, and anticholinergic drugs, including drugs with significant anticholinergic activity.[12] The last include many antiarrhythmic agents, tricyclic antidepressants, neuroleptics, gastrointestinal medications, and antihistamines. These agents used in large doses or in combination at therapeutic doses may induce delirium. Antibiotics (e.g., ciprofloxacin), analgesics (e.g., nonsteroidal anti-inflammatory drugs), opiates (e.g., meperidine), and H_2 receptor antagonists (e.g., cimetidine) have been associated with delirium.[13] Other causes of delirium include alcohol and drug intoxication and withdrawal and neurologic illness (e.g., stroke, tumor, or infection).

PATHOPHYSIOLOGY

The pathophysiology of delirium in elderly patients is complex. Patients with risk factors for delirium are regarded as vulnerable on the basis of the hypothetical assumption of limited homeostatic (brain) reserves. The most important unifying hypothesis is that of neurotransmitter disturbances (e.g., acetylcholine or dopamine). The best evidence of neurotransmitter disturbance is found in studies of cholinergic failure. For example, depressed acetylcholine transmission secondary to anticholinergic drugs with central effects can disturb normal cognition.[13] Patients with Alzheimer disease are said to be sensitive to the central anticholinergic effects of various drugs and show improved cognition with cholinesterase inhibitors, which potentiate the effects of acetylcholine. In some conditions, such as hepatic encephalopathy, the presence of delirium correlates with the accumulation of toxic metabolites (e.g., ammonia). Disturbances in the elaboration of cytokines, including interleukin-1 (IL-1) and IL-2, have also been associated with delirium.[14]

DIAGNOSTIC EVALUATION

Clinical Features

The patient with delirium presents with an acute change in mental status and clinical features of disturbed consciousness, impaired cognition, and a fluctuating course. The patient has a reduced ability to focus (i.e., sustain or shift) attention, which is associated with incoherent or tangential speech and disorganized or erratic thought processes. Perceptual disturbances, such as misperceptions, illusions or frank delusions, and hallucinations, are often accompanied by increased psychomotor activity. Most patients with delirium vacillate between hypoalertness and hyperalertness. However, the majority of elderly patients with delirium have a so-called quiet confusion, with fluctuations in behavior and level of cognition throughout the day (e.g., increased confusion in the evening, referred to as sundowning).

Several instruments or scales have been found to have significant likelihood ratios and reasonable specificity for the diagnosis of delirium.[3] Of these tools, confusion assessment is the most often used methodology in clinical studies and is easily applied at the bedside.[3] Confusion assessment allows diagnosis of delirium in patients who have both inattention and evidence of an acute onset of fluctuating course and who have disorganized thinking, altered level of consciousness, or both.

Laboratory Tests

The evaluation of a patient with delirium focuses on a search for the most probable etiologies and the need to treat life-threatening illnesses. Often, the precipitant of delirium is obvious, but careful monitoring is needed to exclude other causes or contributing conditions (e.g., pneumonia accompanied by hypoxemia, electrolyte imbalance, and adverse drug effects). A neuroimaging head scan is rarely useful unless patients have focal neurologic findings. Because infection is so frequently the precipitant of delirium, a complete blood count and chemistry panel should be obtained on all patients when infection cannot be excluded. In select cases, blood and urine cultures are warranted, as are a chest x-ray, an electrocardiogram, arterial blood gas analysis, a lumbar puncture (LP), a computed tomographic scan of the head, and an electroencephalogram. The LP is rarely diagnostic in patients who are not immunocompromised or in patients with no signs that suggest a serious diagnosis (e.g., meningitis). Although the EEG is useful in distinguishing delirium from depression or dementia, it only occasionally suggests a diagnosis (e.g., partial-complex seizure disorder) that could not be established on the basis of clinical findings.[3,14]

DIFFERENTIAL DIAGNOSIS

Delirium is often misdiagnosed as dementia, depression, or functional psychosis. The clinical features of delirium and dementia may overlap, but the findings of inattention and altered level of consciousness and the duration of symptoms usually enable a separation of these two diagnoses [see Table 2]. Psychosis caused by late-onset schizophrenia or major depression is not

Table 2 Differential Features
of Delirium and Dementia

Feature	Delirium	Dementia
Onset	Rapid	Insidious
Duration	Hours to days (transient)	Months to years (persistent)
Attention	Decreased (digit span test ≤ 4 words, distractible, fluctuating)	Usually normal (mild to moderate dementia)
Awareness	Always impaired	Usually normal
Alertness	Fluctuates	Usually normal
Consciousness	Depressed	Normal
Memory	Impaired (varies)	Impaired (recent is better than remote)
Language	Normal or incorrect naming	Aphasia, anomia, paraphasia
Perception	Misperceptions, illusions, hallucinations (common)	Usually normal (or delusions)
Psychomotor activity	Increased, decreased (varies)	Usually normal
Sleep-wake pattern	Disrupted (reversal)	Normal or fragmented

characterized by impaired attention or altered level of consciousness and fluctuating mental status. Although many depressed patients perform poorly on formal tests of cognition, they remain alert and attentive, and they do not display the fluctuating course of delirium. The depressed patient often refuses to complete a mental status test or gives many "I don't know" responses. Likewise, many anxious patients have impaired concentration and may appear inattentive, but they do not have the fluctuating course and altered level of consciousness seen in delirium.

PREVENTION AND MANAGEMENT

Protocols Targeted at Risk Factors

Delirium can be prevented in patients who are at risk for the disorder [see Table 1]. In the Elder Life Program, patients at risk for incident delirium were identified shortly after hospital admission and followed daily with the Confusion Assessment Method.[15] An array of protocols targeted at specific risk factors served to optimize cognitive function (reorientation and therapeutic activities), prevent sleep deprivation (relaxation and noise reduction), avoid immobility (ambulation and exercises), improve vision (visual aids and illumination), improve hearing (hearing devices), and treat dehydration (volume repletion). In 852 patients studied, the incidence of delirium was 9.9% in the intervention group, compared with an incidence of 15% in the usual-care group. The total number of days and number of episodes of delirium were also significantly reduced in the intervention group, but no significant effects were seen on the severity of delirium or on recurrence rates.

Increased Socialization

Other nursing and environmental interventions that are often helpful in the management of delirium include placement of a patient in a room near the nurses' station for greater observation and socialization; social visits with family members, a caregiver, or hired sitter; the avoidance of physical restraints, which can aggravate agitation; and the promotion of normal sleep cycles through noise control and dim lighting at night.

Pharmacotherapy

Pharmacologic interventions are often warranted for patients with specific indications, including bothersome hallucinations and delusions, physical aggression and risk of harm to self or others, or severe personal distress or discomfort. Pharmacologic interventions are often utilized in patients in whom disruption of medical therapy must be avoided, such as those who are critically ill. However, no agents have been approved by the Food and Drug Administration specifically for the treatment of delirium. Definitive clinical trials of the drug therapy for elderly patients with delirium are lacking. As a general recommendation, for patients with bothersome symptoms, haloperidol is the usual drug of choice. It is administered in dosages of 0.5 to 1.0 mg given orally or intramuscularly every 6 to 8 hours. Higher doses may be needed to control agitation when patients require endotracheal intubation or other life-saving procedures.[4] Adverse effects of neuroleptics include extrapyramidal effects, dystonic reactions, and torsade de pointes, which is associated with high doses of intravenous haloperidol.

For treatment of anxiety and sleep disturbance, lorazepam, 0.5 to 1.0 mg given orally or parenterally every 6 to 8 hours, is the usual drug of choice.

Patients with delirium secondary to alcohol or drug withdrawal should be treated with benzodiazepines, although a neuroleptic such as haloperidol or risperidone, 0.5 to 1.0 mg/day given orally, can be used as an adjunct to control the psychotic symptoms. Haloperidol and lorazepam may also be useful in preparing patients for neuroimaging scans or when invasive or supportive therapies are necessary (e.g., insertion of a central line). Adverse effects of benzodiazepines include paradoxical confusion, amnesia, and falls. Novel approaches to the prevention or reversal of delirium (e.g., use of cholinesterase inhibitors) await clinical trials.

Severe pain associated with agitation should be treated parenterally with morphine sulfate in lower than usual adult dosages (e.g., 4 to 6 mg every 3 hours; with lower doses used in very old or frail patients). In general, repeated doses of meperidine should be avoided to prevent the neurotoxic effect of its metabolite, normeperidine.

PROGNOSIS

Treatment of the underlying cause of delirium usually results in rapid improvement, although full resolution of cognitive symptoms can take several days to several months. Functional and cognitive deficits often persist after hospital discharge. In a multicenter cohort study, delirium that occurred in hospitalized elderly patients was associated with an increased risk of nursing home admission and mortality, underscoring the seriousness of the diagnosis of delirium and the need to closely monitor such patients after discharge from the hospital.[5] The persistence of cognitive deficits may be related to underlying conditions, especially dementia.

Urinary Incontinence

Urinary incontinence (UI)—the involuntary loss of urine of sufficient severity to be a social or health problem—is a common, costly, and potentially disabling condition that is never a consequence of normal aging and is always treatable and often curable.[16] Urinary incontinence is a source of social embarrassment for older patients, results in a loss of self-esteem and physical independence, and increases the patient's risk of institution- alization. Furthermore, the direct costs of caring for persons of all ages with urinary incontinence is estimated to be greater than $16 billion annually.[16]

EPIDEMIOLOGY

The prevalence of UI increases from approximately 10% to 15% in women 65 years of age to more than 25% in men and women 85 years of age and older.[16] The prevalence of incontinence approaches 50% in nursing home residents and frail homebound elderly patients. Despite the high prevalence of incontinence in community-dwelling elders, fewer than half consult health care providers about this problem.[17]

RISK FACTORS AND ETIOLOGY

Impaired cognition and physical functioning are strongly associated with urinary incontinence.[16] In addition, medications, fecal impaction, environmental barriers, estrogen depletion in women, and pelvic muscle weakness increase the risk of incontinence.

The most common cause of bladder outlet obstruction in men is prostatic hyperplasia; less common causes are carcinoma and urethral stricture. An underactive or acontractile bladder may result from neurologic diseases such as diabetic neuropathy, spinal cord injury, and idiopathic detrusor underactivity. In women, overflow incontinence occurs as a complication of anti-incontinence operations or severe pelvic organ prolapse. Acute urinary retention (often secondary to medications) is a common cause of overflow incontinence in hospitalized elderly patients.

PATHOPHYSIOLOGY

An understanding of the pathophysiology of UI helps clarify the rationale for the myriad treatments of this common condition. Incontinence results from neurologic or anatomic defects that interfere with normal urinary micturition. The urinary bladder is responsible for the storage and emptying of urine.[18] Lesions that interfere with bladder contraction or emptying will predispose patients to urinary incontinence. Urine storage occurs when the muscular wall (detrusor) relaxes, and micturition occurs when the detrusor contracts. Bladder relaxation and filling are promoted by sympathetic stimulation via the hypogastric plexus (T11-L2), which inhibits parasympathetic tone and augments beta-adrenergic tone. Bladder contraction is initiated through parasympathetic (cholinergic) stimulation via the sacral complex (S2-4) and relaxation of the pelvic floor musculature (external sphincter), which is under control of the somatic (pudendal) nerve. As the urinary bladder fills, contraction of the detrusor muscle is inhibited by closure of the bladder neck under sympathetic tone, somatic innervation of pelvic floor muscles and striated muscles around the urethra, and activation of inhibitory pathways from the brain stem and cerebral (frontal) cortex. Detrusor pressure increases, resulting in involuntary contractions and the subjective sensation of a need to void. During voluntary urination, the increase in detrusor pressure overcomes inhibitory pathways and exceeds urethral resistance.

UI occurs when there is a disruption in this complex and dynamic process. Lesions that interfere with bladder contraction and emptying (e.g., sensory neuropathy) predispose patients to incontinence. Contractions of the detrusor muscle at low bladder filling volumes (detrusor overactivity or instability) may occur in patients with lesions of the central nervous system (e.g., stroke) or with increased sensory stimulation from the bladder, which may be seen in urinary tract infection (UTI) or prostatic hyperplasia. Incompetence of the internal urethral sphincter (e.g., caused by pelvic relaxation or intrinsic sphincter deficiency [ISD]) allows urine to leak from the bladder (stress incontinence) whenever intra-abdominal pressure exceeds urethral resistance.[18] Loss of detrusor contractility (acontractile bladder) or bladder outlet obstruction may result in a distended bladder and leakage of urine (overflow incontinence) with or without a subjective sensation of urinary urgency.

DIAGNOSTIC EVALUATION

Clinical Features

Acute UI UI may present as either an acute (transient) or chronic (established) condition. Acute incontinence typically has a sudden onset and is associated with an acute illness (e.g., infection or delirium) or iatrogenic event (e.g., polypharmacy or restricted mobility). UTI is the most commonly recognized cause of transient incontinence in ambulatory elderly patients. In hospitalized patients, delirium or acute confusion, excessive infusions of intravenous fluids, and metabolic disorders, such as hyperglycemia with glucosuria, will predispose the patient to incontinence. Acute urinary incontinence is also associated with functional impairments such as an inability to toilet quickly enough or a lack of awareness of the need to urinate (e.g., in patients with dementia or acute confusion). Despite the common distinction between acute and chronic causes of incontinence, the two are often difficult to distinguish and often share a similar pathophysiology.

Established UI Four basic types of established UI occur in elderly patients: stress, urge, overflow, and functional incontinence [see Table 3]. UI is often caused by a combination of two or more of the subtypes of incontinence (mixed incontinence). The clinical type and most likely etiology of UI can be determined by a focused medical history and physical examination, a few laboratory studies, and simple office procedures.

Medical History

The medical history, the key to diagnosis, includes a description of the onset, duration, and characteristics of incontinence; the most significant symptoms; the frequency, timing, and quantity of episodes; and the precipitants of incontinence, such as the relationship of incontinence to exercise, previous surgery, or onset of acute diseases. In men, symptoms related to prostatism should be elicited (i.e., nocturia, dysuria, hesitancy, or decreased stream). The patient's bowel habits (e.g., constipation or impaction) and fluid intake should be noted. A written record or diary of incontinent episodes recorded for 7 days (or a continence flow sheet in nursing home residents) provides clues to the etiologies and severity of urinary incontinence.

Physical Examination

The physical examination focuses on diseases affecting genitourinary function. The abdominal examination seeks abdominal masses caused by bladder distention or fecal impaction. The rectal examination evaluates patients for fecal impaction, rectal masses, and abnormalities of the prostate gland in men. The pelvic examination evaluates women for pelvic organ prolapse, genital atrophy, and urethral abnormalities. Neuromuscular examination identifies patients with impaired mobility or diseases of the central nervous system that predispose to urinary incontinence (e.g., stroke, Parkinson disease, or dementia).

Laboratory Tests

The laboratory evaluation of an incontinent elderly patient is driven by the clinical type, frequency, and significance of the incontinence. Patients with acute UI associated with a UTI should first be treated with antibiotics before further urodynamic evaluation. Although many patients with established incontinence have asymptomatic bacteriuria, there is no evidence that treatment of the infection will lead to resolution of the incontinence.[19] A urinalysis will suggest the presence of infection, possible inflammation, or the need for further diagnostic evaluation to rule out tumor or stones (e.g., if the patient has hematuria or pyuria).

In patients with established incontinence, blood tests should measure renal function, electrolytes, blood glucose, and serum calcium (to exclude polyuric conditions that may cause incontinence).

The most useful bedside test of lower urinary tract function is measurement of the postvoiding residual (PVR) urine. Accurate measurement of the PVR is most often accomplished by straight catheterization of the urinary bladder after the patient attempts complete voiding. Pelvic ultrasonography or portable bladder scanning are safe and accurate alternative methods of estimating PVR.[16] A PVR of less than 50 ml of urine is considered normal. A PVR of greater than 150 ml is abnormal even in elderly patients and indicates the need for further urologic evaluation or repeat measurement of PVR. Simple cystometry is able to determine bladder filling capacity, detrusor compliance and contractility, and PVR.

A detailed urodynamic evaluation is sometimes needed to determine the cause and most appropriate treatment of incontinence. Studies are particularly helpful before operative treatments of incontinence. For example, stress UI is diagnosed and categorized according to abdominal leak point pressures.[20] Urodynamic studies are essential for making a definitive diagnosis of urinary obstruction or detrusor hyperactivity with impaired contractility and for determining the type of stress incontinence.

MANAGEMENT

Strategies for the management of UI include behavioral modification techniques, medications, patient and caregiver education, surgical procedures, catheter placement, and incontinence supplies [see Table 3]. The acute onset of UI should be evaluated and treated promptly. UTI, acute urinary retention, stool impaction, and adverse effects of medications (e.g., diuretics) should be excluded. After the initial diagnostic evaluation, most patients should be treated on the basis of the most likely type of incontinence. This empirical approach will lead to successful management of a large percentage of incontinent patients.[21]

Stress Incontinence

For established stress and urge incontinence in female outpatients, behavioral interventions, bladder training, and pelvic muscle exercises are recommended as first-line therapy. Daily repeated pelvic floor exercises will strengthen the voluntary periurethral and perivaginal muscles, augment urethral pressure, and inhibit urinary leakage. Pelvic muscle exercise is assumed to enhance urethral resistance by increasing the strength and endurance of the periurethral and perivaginal muscles and by improving the anatomic support to the bladder neck and proximal urethra.

Typically, pelvic floor exercises are conducted for 10-second intervals several times a day. The effectiveness of these exercises

Table 3 Types, Characteristics, and Treatments of Urinary Incontinence

Types	Characteristics	Treatments		
		Nondrug	Drug	Precautions
Stress	Associated with urethral hypermobility or intrinsic sphincter deficiency (ISD); urinary leakage with an increase in intra-abdominal pressure resulting from coughing, sneezing, or physical exertion; continuous leakage with ISD	*Behavioral:* pelvic muscle exercises (repeated contraction of pelvic muscles); scheduled toileting (urinate at defined intervals), bladder training (interrupt urination, avoid straining) *Surgical:* needle bladder neck suspension for urethral hypermobility; vaginal sling or periurethral (collagen) injections for ISD	Estrogens Conjugated, 0.3–0.625 mg orally daily (plus progestin if uterus is intact) Topical, 0.5–1.0 g/application Alpha-adrenergic agonists Pseudoephedrine, 30–60 mg three times daily	Oral estrogens increase the risk of endometrial cancer, elevated blood pressure, and venous thrombosis Alpha-adrenergic agonists are not FDA approved treatment of stress incontinence; they may increase the risk of stroke, hypertension, headache, and tachycardia
Urge	Urinary urgency and frequency (small to moderate volumes); overactive bladder caused by detrusor instability	Bladder training (scheduled or prompted voiding), pelvic muscle rehabilitation (contraction and relaxation of pelvic muscles), biofeedback (reduction of intensity of uninhibited contractions)	Anticholinergics/bladder relaxants Oxybutynin, 2.5–5.0 mg three times a day (or a single dose at night for nocturia and urgency) Oxybutynin XL, 5–10 mg every day Tolterodine, 1–2 mg twice a day (or a single dose at night for nocturia and urgency) Tolterodine LA, 2–4 mg every day	Common side effects are dry mouth, constipation, and blurred vision; potential risk of increased intraocular pressure, delirium, and tachyarrhythmias
Overflow	Associated with either an acontractile bladder or bladder outlet obstruction (BPH, stricture, or bladder neck constriction); bladder distention with frequent or constant dribbling, with or without urgency	Intermittent or continuous catheter drainage for acontractile bladder Surgical relief of urethral obstruction (prostatectomy) Bladder retraining and scheduled toileting can be attempted after acute urinary retention	Cholinergic agonist Bethanechol, 10–30 mg three times daily (initiate with lower doses) Alpha$_1$-adrenergic antagonists Terazosin, 1–5 mg at night Doxazosin, 1–4 mg at night Tamsulosin, 0.4–0.8 mg at night	Cholinergic agonists should be used judiciously for acontractile bladder; bethanechol may exacerbate bradycardia, hypotension, bronchoconstriction, and peptic ulcer exacerbation Alpha$_1$-adrenergic antagonists should be used only for mild outlet obstruction caused by BPH; possible side effects are postural hypotension, fatigue, and sexual dysfunction
Functional	Associated with inability or unwillingness to perform toileting (physical disability, environmental barriers, or psychiatric illness)	*Behavioral:* toileting schedule and prompted voiding; assisted toileting, bedside commode or urinal; assistive devices to aid ambulation and toileting (canes, walkers, rails, grab bars); discontinue physical restraints; increase exercise *Medical:* absorbent pads and garments; indwelling catheters for severely debilitated patients	Change treatments (reduce diuretic and vasodilator dosages) Treat depression Treat Parkinson disease	Minimize use of drugs that worsen functional impairments (e.g., neuroleptics with extrapyramidal side effects and vasodilators that cause postural hypotension)

Note: Elderly patients frequently have mixed incontinence (urge and stress) and functional impairments that precipitate incontinence. Treatments should not be started until after a basic evaluation is completed to exclude reversible causes of acute incontinence and overflow incontinence. Many frail patients have detrusor hyperactivity with impaired contractility presenting with urinary urgency and small-volume voids.
BPH—benign prostatic hyperplasia   LA—long acting   XL—extended length

depends on patient compliance; benefits may not be seen for several weeks.

Medications play a modest role in the treatment of stress incontinence. Middle-aged women with stress UI and hypoestrogenism may benefit from intravaginal, oral, or transdermal estrogen replacement therapy.[16] Alpha-adrenergic agonists (e.g., phenylpropanolamine [PPA] and pseudoephedrine) are thought to reduce the frequency of stress UI by increasing internal sphincter tone and bladder outflow resistance. These agents, particularly PPA, however, have been associated with an increased risk of stroke.

Surgical options include bladder neck resuspension, or periurethral injections of collagen. The long-term effectiveness of percutaneous needle operations has been disappointing and suggests that conservative approaches should be fully explored before resorting to major operations.[22] Vaginal slings or periurethral injections of collagen are the treatments of choice for patients with intrinsic sphincter deficiency (ISD). In one study, collagen injection therapy for female ISD showed excellent 1-year responses. Of 94 patients, 67.0% achieved continence, 38.3% became dry, and 28.7% became socially continent.[20]

Stress incontinence in elderly men is usually caused by ISD resulting from trauma to the bladder outlet, most commonly secondary to prostatectomy. Stress incontinence caused by ISD may be treated with either periurethral injections or the placement of an artificial sphincter.[16] Success rates with collagen are less impressive in men than in women. However, very high continence rates have been reported in men who had artificial sphincters implanted to treat postprostatectomy incontinence. [23]

Urge Incontinence

Detrusor instability with urge incontinence often responds to behavioral therapies such as scheduled toileting and bladder retraining or to biofeedback in younger and cognitively intact women. Bladder training is assumed to improve cortical inhibition over lower urinary tract functioning and has been used primarily in the treatment of urge incontinence. Cognitively impaired patients also benefit from scheduled toileting (e.g., every 2 hours) or prompted voiding (requesting the caregiver to toilet them). Bladder relaxant medications that also have anticholinergic properties are the most effective drug therapies for urge incontinence. Most commonly, either oxybutynin or tolterodine is used for treating detrusor overactivity.[16] Oxybutynin is short acting and often produces significant side effects of constipation, dry mouth, and occasionally confusion in vulnerable patients. A long-acting preparation of oxybutynin (Ditropan XL) may enhance compliance and reduce the incidence of anticholinergic side effects. [24] Tolterodine appears to cause less constipation and dry mouth than oxybutynin and is available in both short-acting and long-acting forms.[25]

For the frail elderly, behavioral and environmental interventions are most effective in the treatment of urge incontinence. Strategies that maintain or improve mobility may prevent incontinent episodes.[16] Devices, including urinals, bedside commodes, or other external collecting devices may help these patients to achieve continence. Other helpful aids are canes, walkers, or wheelchairs for patients with impaired ambulation; elevated toilet chairs; and the avoidance of physical or chemical restraints that impede the patient's toileting ability. For patients with intractable incontinence, absorbent undergarments or adult diapers are frequently used.

Combined Stress and Urge Incontinence

Because mixed forms of UI are common in women, patients may benefit from both behavioral therapies and medications. One randomized clinical trial contrasted a biofeedback-based behavioral approach with both drug treatment (oxybutynin chloride, 2.5 to 5.0 mg three times daily) and a placebo.[26] Women 55 years of age or older with urge or mixed urge-stress incontinence were assigned to behavioral treatment consisting of anorectal biofeedback while learning to contract their pelvic muscles and keep their abdominal muscles relaxed. At home, the patients did 15 pelvic muscle exercises three times a day, gradually increasing the contractile period. Episodes of incontinence decreased nearly 81% on average with behavioral treatment, which was significantly better than the decreases that occurred with drug treatment (68.5%) or placebo (39%). A toileting schedule may also be effective in combination with behavioral and pharmacologic approaches. Patients should be encouraged to urinate at regular intervals and before physical exertion. Other conservative measures, including vaginal cones, electronic devices, pessaries, or elevating devices can be useful for individual patients, although their long-term effectiveness has not been established.[27]

Overflow Incontinence

Acute overflow incontinence, precipitated by medications (e.g., anticholinergic drugs), anesthesia, or urethral manipulation, may be treated with intermittent urethral catheterization until the acute precipitating event subsides. Patients with incontinence resulting from bladder outlet obstruction (e.g., urethral stricture or tumor) will require either surgical correction or intermittent catheterization. Occasionally, men with prostatic hyperplasia respond to alpha-adrenergic antagonists, which may reduce internal sphincter tone.[28] Intermittent self-catheterization is ideal in patients who have atonic or neurogenic bladders. Long-term indwelling urinary catheterization is usually reserved for patients who cannot be catheterized intermittently because of discomfort or terminal illness. External (condom) catheters for males are used selectively because they often fail and can lead to local skin infection or UTI.

Functional Incontinence

UI is common in patients with neuropsychiatric illnesses, such as delirium, dementia, and depression. Immobile patients may suffer incontinence when they are unable to toilet because of physical illness, restraints, or environmental barriers. If urinary retention with overflow incontinence is excluded, patients with functional incontinence can be managed through exercise, toileting schedules, and assistive devices that enhance toileting ability.

Fecal Incontinence

Fecal incontinence, the involuntary passage of feces, is a common, socially embarrassing, and often incapacitating problem in elderly patients.[29] Fecal incontinence is usually a functional bowel disorder and is most often managed conservatively.[30]

EPIDEMIOLOGY

The prevalence of fecal incontinence increases with aging, occurring in more than 18% of men 80 years of age and older,[31] in 10% of patients in nursing homes, and in 30 % of patients in hospitals.[30] Constipation, the passage of infrequent, hard, or difficult-to-pass stools, is often associated with incontinence, particularly in patients with fecal impactions.

RISK FACTORS AND ETIOLOGY

Common causes of constipation include a diet low in fiber and fluids, dehydration, immobility, and medications.[30]

PATHOPHYSIOLOGY

The process of normal defecation requires the integrity of skeletal and striatal muscles involved in anal sphincter function, cognitive awareness and ability to get to the toilet, and normal function of the pelvic floor muscles and nerves.[30] A disruption of any of these links predisposes the patient to incontinence. Rectal trauma, pudendal nerve injury, autonomic neuropathies, rectal prolapse, hyperosmolar diets, and fecal impaction are common physiologic factors contributing to incontinence.[30] Fecal impaction occurs most often in the distal or rectosigmoid colon. Mucus and fluids are secreted proximal to the impaction and leak around the mass or are passed after therapeutic disimpaction. Medications, especially opiates and anticholinergic agents, are common causes of constipation, impaction, and incontinence. Acute fecal incontinence may be seen in diarrheal states, and intermittent incontinence is often seen in patients with dementia, delirium, pelvic floor denervation, or excessive laxative use.

DIAGNOSTIC EVALUATION

Medical History and Physical Examination

The evaluation of fecal incontinence includes a careful review of the patient's cognitive status, anorectal and neurologic function, and a rectal examination. In hospitalized or institutionalized patients, the diagnosis of a fecal impaction is suggested by the passage of watery stools laden with mucus. This suspicion is confirmed by rectal examination, which generally reveals firm or hard stool in the ampulla, often associated with a patulous rectum. With high impactions, feces may be palpable during abdominal examination or confirmed by x-ray of the abdomen. Mental status examination identifies the patient with dementia or delirium who has lost self-toileting capacity. The absence of anal sphincter tone or anal wink may suggest denervation of the pudendal nerve (S2-4), resulting from a local or spinal cord lesion. The rectal and abdominal examinations also help identify inflammatory diseases or tumors as causes of incontinence.

Laboratory Tests

Diagnostic studies are needed when either the diagnosis or the appropriate management of the incontinent patient remains uncertain. Useful studies include anoscopy or flexible sigmoidoscopy for confirmation of masses or inflammation. Infrequently, anorectal manometry to measure intraluminal pressure, anal endosonography to identify mass lesions, pudendal nerve conduction measurement to diagnose neuropathy, or defecography to define intrinsic lesions are needed to ascertain the cause of fecal incontinence.[32]

PREVENTION AND MANAGEMENT

The prevention of fecal incontinence begins with an assessment of risk factors for fecal impaction and functional incontinence. The most common approaches to the prevention of fecal incontinence and constipation include changes in diet, increased physical activity, the judicious use of laxatives and enemas, and surgical correction in patients with anatomic abnormalities (e.g., rectocele) [see Table 4]. In highly motivated and cognitively normal patients, biofeedback is effective.

Laxatives

Laxatives are prescribed for patients with incontinence resulting from constipation. Stimulant laxatives (e.g., senna and bisacodyl), hyperosmolar laxatives (e.g., sorbitol and lactulose), rectal suppositories (e.g., glycerin and bisacodyl), or enemas (e.g., tap water) are often sufficient to treat constipation. Saline laxatives (e.g., milk of magnesia) can also be used, but hypermagnesemia limits their usefulness in patients with renal insufficiency.[33] Recently, mixed electrolyte solutions containing polyethylene glycol, a major hyperosmolar laxative,[33] have been found effective in relieving fecal impactions. The solution is usually given in large amounts, often 2 to 3 L/day in divided doses. Sodium phosphate solution, 45 ml given orally, is commonly used to prepare patients for colonoscopy but is also effective in treating impactions. It should be avoided in patients with renal insufficiency or hyperphosphatemia.

High-Fiber Diet

Once the impaction is resolved and colonic function is restored, patients should be placed on a high-fiber diet or given fiber supplements (e.g., psyllium or methylcellulose) along with liquids. If constipation is associated with hard stools, fiber and

Table 4 Fecal Incontinence: Prevention and Management

	Intervention	Example
Prevention of Constipation	Physical activity	Aerobic exercises (e.g., walking, water aerobics)
	High-fiber (8–12 g daily) diet* (to induce bulking effects, alter microbial ecology) plus fluids	High-fiber vegetables, bran supplements, psyllium supplement, methylcellulose supplement
	Laxatives (when fiber is ineffective or not tolerated)	Lactulose or sorbitol preferred (osmolar agents); irritant laxatives (for patients intolerant of osmolar agents): bisacodyl, senna; enemas (for patients with colonic dysfunction)
	Avoid constipating medications or use judiciously	Anticholinergic agents; antispasmodics, antiparkinsonian drugs, tricyclic antidepressants, neuroleptics, iron supplements, opiates, calcium channel blockers (verapamil)
Management of Fecal Incontinence	Treatment of fecal impaction†	Enemas: saline, water, sodium phosphate, bisphosphonate; colonic irrigation; high-fiber diet (after disimpaction); oral hyperosmolar solutions
	Treatment of colitis (e.g., from radiation, inflammatory bowel disease)	Medical: soluble fiber supplements, opiates (loperamide)
	Modification of behavior	Biofeedback (motivated, cognitively intact patients), toileting schedule for physically or cognitively impaired patients
	Treatment of anatomic abnormalities	Surgical repair of rectal prolapse or anal sphincter

*Fiber should be avoided until fecal impaction resolves.
†Often, a combination of soluble fiber, hyperosmolar agents, and periodic enemas is needed to prevent impaction in bedridden patients and those with chronic colonic dysfunction (e.g., chronic laxative use, diverticular disease).

fluids should be gradually increased over several weeks to ensure a soft stool.

Suppositories and Enemas

The intermittent use of glycerin or bisacodyl suppositories is warranted if rectosigmoid outlet delay or difficult passage of a soft stool is the primary concern.[33] Patients unable to retain a suppository can be treated with periodic enemas or hyperosmolar solutions.

Falls and Gait Disturbances

Accidental falls, defined as unintentionally coming to rest on the ground, floor, or other lower level, are common and potentially preventable causes of morbidity and mortality in elderly adults.[34] Studies published in the past decade have elucidated the risk factors for falls and have demonstrated the effectiveness of multifactorial interventions to prevent recurrent falls in carefully targeted patients.

Falls are often attributed to host (intrinsic) predisposing or situational risk factors or environmental (extrinsic) predisposing or situational risk factors. For example, predisposing host factors for falls include intrinsic disturbances of balance and gait, and environmental factors include poor lighting and frayed rugs [see Risk Factors, below].

Falls are often classified as syncopal or presyncopal, resulting from cardiac arrhythmias, postural hypertension, or postprandial hypotension.

EPIDEMIOLOGY

Each year, falls occur in about one third of community-dwelling persons older than 65 years and in about half of persons 80 years of age or older. About half of these individuals who fall experience multiple falls. Falls account for serious injuries that include hip fractures and soft tissue trauma and often lead to an older person's loss of functional independence and a fear of falling.[34] Unintentional injury, most often attributed to falls, is the seventh leading cause of death in elderly persons. About 5% of falls by community-dwelling elderly persons result in a fracture. Falling increases the probability of hospitalization, nursing home placement, and death. About half of falls by elderly patients result in soft tissue injuries such as bruises, lacerations, and abrasions. Less common complications are subdural hematomas and cervical fractures. Falls and nonvertebral fractures are also associated with urinary incontinence in women.[35]

About 90% of the annual 250,000 hip fractures that occur in elderly people result from falls. More than half of the survivors of hip fracture are discharged to a nursing home, and half of those remain in a nursing home a year later. After hip fracture, fewer than 30% of patients regain their prefracture level of physical functioning.

Falls are associated with increased health care costs, including an annual hospital cost of $11,042 (in 1996 dollars) per patient.[36] These health care costs reflect neither the personal costs to families and other caregivers at home nor the pain and suffering of the patient, who often remains functionally impaired or disabled by the effects of an injurious fall.[36]

RISK FACTORS

In retrospective studies, risk factors for hip fractures resulting from falls included low bone mineral density, use of long-acting benzodiazepines (e.g., diazepam), vision impairment, reduced mobility and physical independence, and cognitive dysfunction.[37] In prospective studies, significant independent risk factors for falls were sedative use, cognitive impairment, disability of the lower extremities, abnormalities of balance and gait, and foot problems.[38] Falls are a strong predictor of placement in a skilled nursing facility; the risk increases progressively for individuals with one noninjurious fall, multiple noninjurious falls, and at least one injurious fall.[39] In a large cohort study of women older than 65 years, it was found that hip fractures were more common in women with multiple risk factors for falling, a prior history of falls, poor performance on tests of neuromuscular function (e.g., gait speed), and low bone mineral density.[40] About a third of fallers develop a "fear of falling" that is itself predictive of an increasing risk of balance and gait problems, a decline in self-care abilities, and an increased risk of falling.[41] Environmental factors also contribute to the risk of falling. Poor lighting, frayed rugs, loose cords, old and unstable furniture, and uneven surfaces all raise the risk of falling for older patients.

ETIOLOGY

Accidental falls stem from the combination of environmental hazards and the increased susceptibility to falls related to aging or diseases. Accidents, simple slips, and trips are the most common causes of falls occurring in the community-dwelling elderly population and are usually associated with environmental hazards. In nursing home patients, however, environmental factors are the most common immediate cause of falls, followed by weakness, gait or balance disturbances, drop attacks, dizziness or vertigo, and confusion. Less common causes of falls are postural hypotension, syncope, acute illness (e.g., infection), and medications. Gait impairments with falls are associated with lower extremity weakness from deconditioning, stroke, cardiovascular disease (e.g., arrhythmias), and neurologic disease (e.g., Parkinson disease). Dizziness, vertigo, delirium, postural hypotension, visual disorders, alcohol use, and medications (e.g., psychotropic agents) are other causes of falls.[34] Medications associated with falls most notably include those that cause postural hypotension, such as loop diuretics, vasodilators, or adrenergic antagonists, and those with psychotropic properties, such as antidepressants and sedative-hypnotic agents.

PATHOPHYSIOLOGY

The maintenance of normal balance and gait requires the successful integration of sensory (afferent), central nervous (brain and spinal cord), and musculoskeletal systems. A disturbance in sensory input (e.g., peripheral neuropathy), central nervous system functioning (e.g., dementia), or motor function (e.g., arthritis or muscle weakness) will predispose elderly patients to falls. In older patients, the risk of falls increases with the increased number of chronic illnesses. In particular, weakness of the lower extremity muscles, often associated with deconditioning, impairs gait and predisposes the patient to falling even in the face of a minor perturbation. The aging process may also predispose patients to falls by increasing postural sway and reducing adaptive reflexes. Postural stability limits appear to decrease with aging. However, changes in gait such as slowing of walking speed, reduced stride length, and prolonged double support, which are often attributed to the aging process, likely represent adaptations to the fear of falling. In laboratory studies of induced trips during walking, older adults who walked faster or took more or longer steps were more likely to fall after tripping.[42]

DIAGNOSTIC EVALUATION

Patients at risk for falls can be identified through a medical history, physical examination, and a few laboratory studies. A review of risk factors, medications (vasodilators, adrenergic blockers, and psychotropic agents), and screening instruments (vision, mental status, balance, and gait) help identify patients at risk. In the ambulatory setting, a review of the circumstances surrounding the fall, including symptoms before and after the event, provides clues to the likely causes. For example, vertigo may precede loss of balance and a fall; a loss of consciousness preceding the fall suggests a diagnosis of syncope.

Observation of the patient's balance and gait is the most useful aspect of the examination. Performance-based measures have been validated and are predictive of gait and balance impairments. The Timed Get-up-and-Go test is particularly useful, is quickly performed, and appears to be predictive of falling. The test requires a patient to stand up, walk 10 ft, turn, walk back, and sit down. Older adults at risk for falls require more than 20 seconds to complete this task. During the test, postural instability, lower extremity weakness, reduced steppage, increased lateral sway, stride variability, and ataxia can be easily identified. Patients with these impairments are at risk for falling and deserve further diagnostic evaluation.

The further diagnostic evaluation of a patient who has recently fallen is based on the circumstances surrounding the fall and a judgment about the most likely causes. An extensive diagnostic workup is not usually warranted in nonsyncopal falls. However, in the emergency evaluation of an elderly faller, the history of head trauma and the finding of focal neurologic deficits suggests the need for a neuroimaging procedure (e.g., CT scan of the head).

PREVENTION AND MANAGEMENT

Multicomponent Interventions

The effectiveness of interventions [see Table 5] targeted at both intrinsic and environmental risk factors of individuals has been well documented in clinical trials.[43] The most impressive results are seen with multicomponent interventions, particularly those employing exercises targeted at elderly patients with lower extremity weakness or postural instability.[44] In a clinical trial involving community-residing persons 70 years of age or older with risk factors for falling, those who received interventions that included an adjustment of medications, behavioral instructions, and an exercise program (e.g., balance exercises, gait training, and low-intensity resistive exercises) had fewer falls in the subsequent year than did control subjects.[45]

Tai Chi Exercise

Tai Chi exercises to enhance balance and body awareness when combined with balance training may also reduce the rate of falls. A randomized trial of Tai Chi exercise for 15 weeks in 200 persons 70 years of age and older resulted in a 47% decrease in falls after a 4-month follow-up. Fear of falling is reduced as well, which might account for the benefits of exercise rather than improved postural balance.[46,47]

Therapist-Conducted Exercise

In one study, home visits of women 80 years of age and older made by a physiotherapist led to a 41% reduction in self-reported falls in 1 year, a decreased risk of fall with injury, and improved balance.[48,49] The therapist conducted an exercise program designed to increase balance and muscle strength. Benefits persisted for 2 years in compliant patients. Another clinical trial, involving elderly patients who had had a recent fall, included a comprehensive medical examination (visual acuity, balance, cognition, affect, and prescriptions) and assessment of home safety by an occupational therapist. After 1 year, the self-reported incidence of falls decreased by 61%, recurrent falls decreased by 67%, and there was a decreased risk of hospitalization.[50]

Resistive Exercise

Clinical trials provide convincing evidence of the effectiveness of both low-intensity and progressive high-intensity resistive exercise in improving lower-extremity strength. Bands, tubes, pulleys, and weight machines have been used under therapist supervision in these studies.[44] In a clinical trial, an intervention that included progressive-resistance exercise training in residents of a nursing home with a mean age of over 85 years led to significant increases in muscle strength in the legs and increases in gait velocity.[51]

Table 5   Interventions to Reduce the Risk of Falls

Risk Factors	Interventions
Medications 　Use of ≥ 4 medications 　Alcohol reduction 　Use of any benzodiazepine or other sedative-hypnotic agent 　Vasodilators (arterial and venous)	Review medications, and reduce, taper, or discontinue use of alcohol and psychotropics (benzodiazepines and sedative-hypnotics); if necessary, replace with antidepressants (for insomnia, depression, or anxiety) Use nonpharmacologic therapy for sleep disorders (sleep restriction, no long daytime naps, aerobic exercise early in day, utilization of relaxation techniques such as music and massage) Use alternatives to vasodilators (beta blockers and calcium channel blockers)
Postural hypotension 　Drop in systolic blood pressure ≥ 20 mm Hg 　Postural dizziness or light-headedness	Change doses of medications (e.g., loop diuretics, vasodilators) If syncopal or presyncopal, consider workup for autonomic nervous system or hemodynamic causes If venous pooling occurs in legs, try leg pumps, salt repletion, or graded compression stockings
Lower-extremity weakness 　Generalized decreased strength of quadriceps, knee extensors, or flexors 　Deconditioning resulting from recent illness, hospitalization, or immobility	Low-intensity resistive exercises (bands, tubes, pulleys, or weights) under therapist supervision Endurance exercises (walking, biking, or water exercise)
Balance/gait impairment 　Postural instability 　Inability to transfer safely to bathtub or toilet 　Antalgic gait 　Fear of falling	Physical-therapy consultation for gait assessment Prescription of assistive devices (canes, walkers) Training in transfer skills Gait training and balance exercises (e.g., Tai chi) Analgesics for pain relief Environmental alterations (raised toilet seats, commodes, grab bars, and handrails)
Sensory impairments 　Hearing 　Vision	Hearing aids (headset microphones, reduced background noise) Visual aids (corrective lenses, improved illumination of room)
Environmental hazards 　Uneven surfaces 　Frayed rugs 　Loose cords 　Poor lighting 　Uneven steps or stairs	Occupational-therapy consultation (home visit, safety evaluation) Diffuse illumination of rooms Install handrails and grab bars Resurface slippery floors Install ramps Rearrange furniture Remove frayed rugs and cords

Patient Compliance with Osteoporosis Therapy

The association between falls and hip fractures suggests that the prevention or treatment of osteoporosis should reduce the risk of hip fractures [*see Chapter 52*]. Hip protectors have been found to reduce the risk of hip fracture in nursing home patients. A clinical trial confirms the benefit of hip protectors in ambulatory frail elderly patients.[52] The risk of fracture was reduced by 60% with use of the protectors, but compliance was problematic.

Recommended Treatment Plan

Clinicians who are evaluating an elderly patient with a history of falls should begin with a discussion of the circumstances surrounding the fall and determine if the fall was syncopal or nonsyncopal. If the fall was nonsyncopal, the next step is to review the patient's medications, perform a test of mobility such as the Timed Get-up-and-Go test, and evaluate the patient's muscles and joints (especially knees, hips, and ankles) for range of motion, strength, and stability. If the causes of falls remain unclear and the falls occur primarily at home, the clinician should consider a home-safety evaluation. For patients with lower extremity weakness, a referral of the patient to a physical therapist for gait assessment and muscle strengthening is warranted.[34] The referral should request a gait assessment and low-intensity resistive exercises of the lower extremities, including hip and knee extensors. Clinicians should also treat comorbid conditions that increase the risk of injurious falls, notably osteoporosis, drug intoxication, and being underweight.

Immobility

Prolonged bed rest produces many physiologic changes, including decreases in blood volume and cardiac output, orthostatic hypotension, hypoxemia, muscle atrophy and generalized weakness, and decreased muscle oxidative capacity. In hospitalized elderly patients, immobility increases the risks of functional dependency; nursing home placement after discharge; and medical complications, including deep vein thrombosis, urinary incontinence, pressure sores, joint contractures, cardiac deconditioning and muscle weakness, and falls.[53] Multicomponent interventions targeted at elderly hospitalized patients at risk for immobility can improve clinical outcomes.[54]

Pressure Ulcers

Pressure ulcers result in substantial morbidity, increased health care costs, and reduced quality of life for older patients.[55] Pressure ulcers are common in immobilized patients and increase in incidence with increasing age. Ulcers that occur in a hospital or nursing home are potentially preventable. Early stage ulcers should be identified and managed aggressively to prevent their progression to more severe stages. The National Pressure Ulcer Advisory Panel[56] has defined four stages of pressure ulcers:

1. Stage I is nonblanchable erythema of intact skin.
2. Stage II is partial-thickness skin loss involving the epidermis, the dermis, or both.
3. Stage III is extension into subcutaneous tissues to the deep fascia with or without undermining.
4. Stage IV is extension into muscle, bone, or both.

EPIDEMIOLOGY

The prevalence of stage II and greater ulcers among patients in acute care hospitals ranges from 3% to 11%, with an incidence during hospitalization of 1% to 3%. The rate is higher among bedridden patients. The prevalence of pressure ulcers in nursing home residents in one study was 11.3% for stage II, III, or IV pressure ulcers.[57] For residents admitted to the nursing home without pressure ulcers, the incidence was 13.2% at 1 year and increased to 21.6% after 2 years of nursing home stay.[57] About 80% of pressure ulcers in nursing home patients develop over the sacrum or coccyx, hips (femoral trochanter), ischia, and heels.[58]

RISK FACTORS AND ETIOLOGY

Most prospective studies of stage II or greater pressure ulcers in hospitalized patients have implicated impaired mobility, incontinence, undernutrition, and impaired consciousness as significant risk factors for pressure ulcers.[58] In hospitalized patients who are bedridden or chairbound, risk factors include hypoalbuminemia, fecal incontinence, and fractures.[58] A prospective study of hospitalized patients with activity limitation (e.g., bedridden or hip fracture) identified the following five independent predictors of incident pressure ulcers in patients 55 years of age or older: nonblanchable erythema (stage I ulcer), lymphopenia, immobility, dry skin, and decreased body weight.[58] In general, impaired mobility is the most important risk factor for pressure ulcers.

PATHOPHYSIOLOGY

Four factors have been implicated in the pathogenesis of pressure ulcers: pressure, shearing forces, friction, and moisture. Sustained pressure over bony prominences (e.g., for more than 2 hours) results in ischemic damage to muscle and subcutaneous tissues. Shearing forces lower the amount of pressure required to cause damage to the epidermis. Shearing forces are tangential forces that are exerted when a person seated toward the head of the bed slides toward the floor or foot of the bed. Repeated exposures to pressure will cause skin necrosis at lower pressures. The loss of subcutaneous tissue also lowers the threshold for skin breakdown caused by pressure. Friction is the force that results in skin abrasion when a patient is dragged across bedsheets, for instance. Moisture secondary to incontinence or perspiration can result in skin maceration and predispose the patient to pressure ulcers.[58] Any disease process leading to immobility and limited activity levels increases the risk of pressure ulcers. The aging skin predisposes patients to pressure ulcers: it is more susceptible to shearing forces, has decreased vascularity, and, in malnourished patients, decreased subcutaneous fat. Furthermore, patients with cognitive impairment, depression, or spinal cord injury are likely to be immobile or unable to report symptoms of pain and discomfort.

DIAGNOSTIC EVALUATION

Although stage I ulcers are not true ulcerations, their identification and early treatment are critical to prevent progression to stage II, III, or IV. In stage IV ulcers, undermining and sinus tracts may also be present.[58] Full thickness injury is often manifested by eschar, which must be removed before staging can be completed. The most common sites for pressure ulcers in elderly patients include the scapula, iliac crest, sacrum, ischium, trochanter, lateral malleolus, heel, and lateral edge of the foot.[58] Pressure ulcers often present as a skin blister, which evolves to frank ulceration with exudate or plaque eschar over the next few days. The ulcer represents the tip of the iceberg as the ischemic injury extends in a triangular fashion down to subcutaneous tissue. Clinically, this becomes evident as a stage III ulcer as the le-

Table 6 Stages and Usual Treatments for Pressure Ulcers

Stage	Presentation	Usual Treatment
I	Nonblanchable erythema of intact skin; the heralding lesion of skin ulceration	Reduce pressure over ulcer and bony prominence; bedridden patients with sacral, ischial, or back ulcers are repositioned (e.g., side-to-side at 30° angle) at least every 2 hr. For chair-bound patients, use pressure-reducing device (e.g., foam, gel, or air), reposition hourly; treat dry skin with moisturizers (e.g., creams, lotions, ointments, or lubricants); protect skin from moisture; maintain proper positioning, transferring, and turning techniques; provide nutritional support; apply semipermeable polyurethane film (change weekly)
II	Partial-thickness skin loss involving epidermis, dermis, or both; the ulcer is superficial and presents clinically as an abrasion, blister, or shallow crater	Debride devitalized tissue. Medical debridement: cleanse wound with saline; use wet-to-dry saline dressing, thin-film polymer dressing, or hydrocolloid dressing (wet-to-dry saline dressings when exudate is present, wet-to-moist when ulcer base is free of exudate and eschar; change hydrocolloid dressing every 4–7 days [reduces caregiver time]); schedule exercise for patients able to walk Surgical debridement: use scalpel if eschar or advancing cellulitis is evident; use thick foam mattress or air mattress as a support surface
III	Full-thickness skin loss involving damage or necrosis of subcutaneous tissue, which may extend down to but not through underlying fascia; the ulcer presents clinically as a deep crater with or without undermining of adjacent tissue	Intervention for stage II ulcers Medical: use hydrogel or alginate, moist gauze packs (saline), enzymatic debridement (noninfected ulcers), or topical antibiotic (if exudate or nonhealing persists after ≥ 2 wk of optimal care) for 2 wk (gram-negative, gram-positive, anaerobic coverage) Surgical: debride large eschar and devitalized tissue; use air-fluidized bed or low-air-loss bed (for deep, large, or multiple ulcers) as a support surface
IV	Full-thickness skin loss with extensive destruction, tissue necrosis, or damage to muscle, bone, or supporting structures (e.g, tendon or joint capsule)	Interventions for stage II–III ulcers Medical: systemic antibiotics for bacteremia, sepsis, advancing cellulitis, or osteomyelitis; suspect osteomyelitis in patients with deep ulcers that fail to heal with appropriate therapy and in patients with elevated temperature and white blood cell count or abnormal bone scan Surgical: create myocutaneous flap (after debridement) of large (wide) ulcers; use split-thickness skin grafts

sion extends beneath the dermis to involve muscle fascial structures. Sinus tracts in stage IV lesions can be identified by probing the ulcer margin. Pressure ulcers also can become colonized by bacteria, resulting in cellulitis or bacteremia, especially in debilitated or immunocompromised patients.

PREVENTION AND MANAGEMENT

Patients at risk for an ulcer can be identified with the use of the Norton or Braden scales. These scales relate the risk of pressure ulcer to impaired sensory perception, increased skin moisture, decreased physical activity, immobility, poor nutrition, and friction and shearing force.[55]

Basic principles of pressure ulcer management include identification and treatment of known risk factors. For all stages of pressure ulcers, the first step is to reduce pressure. The principles of stage I ulcer management apply to all patients with stage II, III, or IV ulcers [see Table 6].[59] For stage II, III, or IV ulcers, necrotic tissue is eliminated by either medical or surgical debridement. Necrotic tissue is a barrier to epithelialization and serves as a nidus for infection. Adequate dietary intake should be provided to prevent malnutrition, and nutritional deficiencies should be corrected.

Strategies for treating pressure ulcers usually comprise a combination of pressure relief and wound care.[60]

Wound Care

Wound management strategies such as use of wound dressings, debridement techniques, physical therapies, antibiotics, and antiseptics are employed.[59] Occlusive dressings such as transparent films in hydrocolloid dressings improve healing of stage II pressure ulcers. The dressings remain in place for several days and facilitate epithelial migration.[59] A 2-week trial of a topical antibiotic such as silver sulfadiazine can be considered for clean pressure ulcers that are not healing or are continuing to produce exudate after 2 to 4 weeks of optimal management. Povidone-iodine should not be used, because it is toxic to fibroblasts. When necrotic tissue is present, debridement should be performed. Debridement can be accomplished with a sharp blade; by mechanical approaches such as wet-to-dry dressings, hydrotherapy, irrigation, or dextranomers; by enzymatic approaches (collagenase); or by autolytic techniques (synthetic dressing cover).[55,59] Once an ulcer is clean and epithelialization occurs, a moist wound environment should be maintained.

Pressure Relief

Treatment of pressure ulcers may include the use of a pressure-reducing device.[60] Air or foam products may be helpful, but some patients require the use of specialized beds, such as an air-fluidized bed or a low-air-loss bed.[61] Air-fluidized beds contain microspheres of ceramic glass, and warm pressurized air is forced up through the beads, causing them to take on the characteristics of a fluid. Patients float on the beads, with pressure reduced under prominences. Low-air-loss beds consist of large fabric cushions that are constantly inflated with air. The cushions of low-air-loss beds are fitted on a regular hospital bed frame, which is more practical for patient transfers. The use of these beds should be considered when patients have large, multiple, or full-thickness (stage III or IV) pressure ulcers; when an individual has fewer than two turning surfaces free of pressure ulcers; or when a patient has experienced recurrent ulceration and an inability to heal on a static pressure-reducing device.[61] In a clinical trial conducted in three nursing homes, low-air-loss beds provided significantly better healing rates of stage II or greater pressure ulcers than foam mattresses.[62]

Most stage I and stage II pressure ulcers heal within 60 days with the usual optimal therapies. The choice of dressings and debridement techniques has little impact on this good prognosis. In general, a moist saline gauze wound dressing is as effective as the application of hydrogel dressings.[63] The choice of treatment for these ulcers is based on considerations of cost, convenience, and caregiver preferences.

Malnutrition

EPIDEMIOLOGY

In the United States, protein-calorie malnutrition (PCM), also known as protein-energy undernutrition, is uncommon among community-residing elderly persons. In community surveys, however, the prevalence of nutrient-specific malnutrition is greater in people older than 65 years.[64] In the National Health and Nutrition Examination Survey III, median energy intake for elderly adults was below the recommended levels, with higher intakes for whites than for African Americans. Minorities tended to have lower median energy, dietary, and mineral intakes than whites.[64] A survey of patients 65 years of age and older who were admitted to general medicine, orthopedic, general surgery, and neuroscience services revealed that 41% were well nourished, 44% had moderate risk for malnutrition, and 15% were malnourished.[65]

In long-term care, malnutrition has been identified in 50% of residents and is an independent predictor of subsequent mortality. Poor nutritional status and PCM have been associated with altered immunity, impaired wound healing, reduced functional status, increased health care utilization, and increased mortality. Weight loss of 5% or more of usual body weight is associated with increased morbidity and mortality. Illness-related weight loss exceeding 10% of preillness weight is associated with functional abnormalities and poor clinical outcomes.[66]

RISK FACTORS AND ETIOLOGY

Common medical problems contributing to PCM are congestive heart failure, chronic obstructive pulmonary disease, and neoplastic diseases. Gastrointestinal disorders associated with anorexia, malabsorption, or dysphagia and oral disorders (e.g., poor dentition) may also contribute to weight loss and poor nutrition. Less common causes are endocrine disorders, (e.g., thyrotoxicosis or uncontrolled diabetes mellitus). Unintentional weight loss and malnutrition can occur as a syndrome of so-called failure to thrive.[66] Studies of involuntary weight loss and failure to thrive suggest that depression, cognitive impairment (dementia), gastrointestinal disorders (peptic ulcer or motility disorders), and cancer are the most common causes. Often, inflammation caused by infections and catabolic states contribute to the weight loss, hypoalbuminemia, and other serum markers of chronic disease.[66]

Psychosocial factors contribute to the risk of inadequate nutrition in older adults. Many older patients live on fixed incomes, have reduced access to food (social isolation), have poor knowledge of nutrition, or are dependent on others (caretakers or institutions) for food preparation. They may also suffer from depression, bereavement, or dementia. Other contributing factors that affect shopping for and selecting or preparing food are impaired strength, impaired mobility, impaired sensory input, poor dentition, malabsorption, chronic illness, alcohol use, and use of anorexigenic drugs.

PATHOGENESIS

At middle age, there is an increase in body mass and percentage of body fat in both men and women. At 70 years of age and beyond, declines in both lean body mass (sarcopenia) and body fat occur.[67] So-called anorexia of aging has been described that accounts for elderly patients consuming fewer calories, particularly in the form of fat. Factors involved in producing the physiologic anorexia of aging include early satiation, increased postprandial release of cholecystokinin, reduced feedback from physiologic mechanisms that control food intake, and reduced opioid feeding drive.[67]

DIAGNOSTIC EVALUATION

Clinical Features

Major indicators of poor nutritional status include significant weight loss over time (10% or more of body weight in 6 months or involuntary weight loss), significantly low weight for height (20% below desirable weight), serum albumin of less than 3.5 g/dl, change to dependence in two activities of daily living, sustained inappropriate food intake (e.g., excessive alcohol or dietary imbalance), reduction in midarm circumference to less than 10th percentile, decrease in triceps skinfold to less than 10th percentile, and presence of nutrition-related disorders (e.g., osteoporosis, vitamin B_{12} deficiency, folate deficiency).

Laboratory Tests

The serum albumin is generally the most reliable, although nonspecific, indicator of chronic malnutrition. An albumin level below 3.5 g/dl, an unexplained normocytic anemia, and a very low serum cholesterol level (< 160 mg/dl) are compatible with a diagnosis of PCM. Reduced levels of serum transferrin and prealbumin and a low total lymphocyte count also suggest PCM.

PREVENTION AND MANAGEMENT

For healthy older people, a well-balanced diet is recommended and includes adequate amounts of calories, protein and essential amino acids, essential fatty acids, fiber, and complex carbohydrates and sufficient amounts of minerals and vitamins. Patients who are chronically ill, who have recent weight loss resulting from illness or surgery, or who consume an unbalanced diet should be advised to take a multivitamin and mineral supplement daily. Calcium supplementation to ensure a daily consumption of 1 g or more of elemental calcium, along with vitamin D supplementation, is advisable. When treating frail patients, education of the patient and family caregivers is an important step in preventing malnutrition. Patients should take advantage of nutritional programs available in the community, such as Meals on Wheels and Title III nutrition services. A referral to the local office on aging or the Area Agency on Aging will enable the patient to access these services.

Patients with social, physical, and psychological risk factors for malnutrition can be readily identified using screening instruments and a targeted physical examination.[68] The subjective global assessment, a validated measure of nutritional status based on medical history and physical examination findings, accurately classifies patients as severely malnourished, moderately nourished, or well nourished. The subjective global assessment combines elements of the patient's nutrition history (weight loss in previous 6 months) and physical examination (e.g., muscle wasting) to generate a valid and subjective impression of nutritional status.[69] When combined with a review of biochemical indicators of nutritional status, this information should drive the process of further evaluation and treatment of PCM.

Balanced Diet and Nutritional Supplements

A well-balanced diet with calorie-dense foods should be prescribed, along with vitamin and mineral supplements. Powdered breakfast formulas or canned nutritional supplements provide balanced nutrition between meals. Available interventions include frequent meals and snacks, enhanced flavors of favorite foods, protein-calorie supplements, multivitamins, appetite stimulants, and enteral and parenteral nutrition [see Table 7].

Elderly patients who are acutely ill, delirious, or demented are at great risk for oropharyngeal dysphagia and aspiration pneumonia. A swallowing evaluation may help enhance the safety and success of oral feeding.

Although nutritional oral or enteral supplements may improve the outcomes of hospitalization, as demonstrated for patients admitted with hip fractures and pulmonary infections, they are often underutilized in hospitalized patients. A prospective cohort study found that 20% of elderly patients consumed an average daily in-hospital nutrient intake of less than 50% of their calculated maintenance energy requirements. These patients often had orders for nothing by mouth, and canned supplements were often ordered but not consumed by the patients.[70] In a randomized, controlled trial of 88 nursing home patients, an oral supplement was well accepted and resulted in increased daily protein and energy intake, body weight, and nutritional status in most malnourished patients and in those at risk for malnutrition.[71]

Nutritional Support

Nutritional support (nonoral feeding) is considered if prevention or treatment of PCM will improve prognosis or quality of life and if the nutritional requirements cannot be met with oral foods and supplements [see Table 7]. If the gastointestinal tract is functional, enteral nutrition (nasogastric or nasoenteric tubes) is preferred over parenteral nutrition. Percutaneous tube placement is indicated when long-term tube feeding is not anticipated for weeks to months or for patient comfort. Total parenteral nutrition (intravenous feeding) is essential for survival in patients who cannot eat for extended periods of time and who are not candidates for enteral support (e.g., because of bowel obstruction). However, gastrostomy tube feedings are not recommended for patients with severe dementia, given the absence of data to show that tube feedings improve clinical outcomes in such patients.[72]

Correction of Nutrient Deficiencies

Specific nutrient deficiencies result from dietary imbalance, chronic disease, or medications. The most commonly recognized examples are vitamin B_{12} (cobalamin), calcium, and iron deficiencies. Cobalamin deficiency can occur in the absence of classic hematologic or neurologic findings of pernicious anemia. A low serum cobalamin level accompanied by an elevated serum level of methylmalonic acid supports the diagnosis of B_{12} deficiency. Dietary calcium deficiency is common among elderly women. Dietary supplementation is often needed to maintain a daily consumption of 1.2 to 1.5 g of elemental calcium. Vitamin D supplementation, 800 I.U. daily, is often recommended for the treatment of elderly patients who lack sun exposure or have evidence of osteoporosis or osteomalacia. Iron deficiency is more common among the elderly because of long-term internal or external causes of blood loss.

Sensory Impairment

Hearing and visual losses are the most important and common sensory impairments in elderly people. Sensory impairments adversely affect the older patient's physical, cognitive, and social functioning. Among community-dwelling elders, mood and social relationships are particularly affected by vision impairment, and performance of daily activities is strongly reduced by hearing impairment.

HEARING IMPAIRMENT

Epidemiology

In the National Health Interview Survey, about 30% of community-dwelling elderly people reported hearing impairment; about 12% of elderly overall and 30% of those 85 years of age and older considered themselves deaf in at least one ear.[73] Hearing aids were used by 8% of the sample and 16% of those 85

Table 7 Nutritional Support

Route	Patient Characteristics	Nutritional Intervention
Oral	Alert, normal swallowing, mildly to moderately malnourished	High-calorie, high-protein diet; calorie-dense foods (high fat); nutritional supplements between meals
Intravenous fluids	Acutely ill, decreased oral fluid intake, unable to swallow	Glucose solution with electrolytes for ≤ 48 hr as sole nutritional source
Enteral	Oropharyngeal dysphagia, cognitive dysfunction, critically ill (e.g., intubated), or severely malnourished; ability to resume oral feeding within a few weeks (or cyclic use)	Nasoenteric tube feedings (continuous or cyclic) with lactose-free enteral feeding solutions (normal-calorie or normal-calorie, high-nitrogen solutions)
Peripheral parenteral nutrition	Oral and nasoenteric routes temporarily contraindicated (e.g., acute pancreatitis, bowel obstruction)	Peripheral intravenous infusion with isotonic glucose-electrolyte-lipid solution
Total parenteral nutrition	Severely malnourished; hypermetabolic state (e.g., sepsis syndrome); enteral route contraindicated or inadequate	Central intravenous catheter (e.g., in subclavian vein): infusion of high-calorie, hypertonic, balanced (protein, carbohydrate, and amino acid) solutions
Percutaneous endoscopic gastrostomy	Severely malnourished; oropharyngeal dysphagia contraindicates oral feeding (e.g., stroke or advanced dementia) for prolonged time (e.g., ≥ 2 mo) or indefinitely*	Enteral solutions: isotonic or hypertonic (limited by diarrhea; high- or normal-nitrogen formulas)

*Severely demented patients not included.

years of age and older. In community-dwelling people 65 to 74 years of age, about 24% had significant hearing loss (hearing loss with functional impairment); among persons older than 75 years, about 40% had significant hearing impairment. Hearing loss is associated with significant emotional and social dysfunction. Significant hearing loss has been reported in 70% to 90% of nursing home residents.

Etiology

Hearing loss is categorized as sensorineural, conductive, or mixed. Sensorineural hearing loss is caused by cochlear or retrocochlear diseases and is characterized by decreased thresholds for both air and bone conduction. Presbycusis is the most common cause of sensorineural hearing loss in elderly patients. Other causes include ototoxicity from medications (e.g., aminoglycosides and chemotherapeutic agents), infections involving the eighth cranial nerve, and injury caused by vascular events or tumors of the eighth cranial nerve.

Presbycusis is a bilateral, symmetrical cause of hearing loss at high frequencies, especially at frequencies above 2,000 Hz, and is associated with impaired speech discrimination and loudness recruitment. Presbycusis begins in middle age and causes progressive hearing loss. The most severe changes occur in the inner ear, which is responsible for sensitivity, sound, understanding of speech, and maintenance of equilibrium. Signs and symptoms of presbycusis include a history of progressive high-frequency hearing loss and difficulty in understanding speech, especially in noisy environments. The cause of presbycusis remains uncertain.[74] Presbycusis is also associated with an auditory processing disorder, which makes understanding speech more difficult than would be predicted on the basis of loss of peripheral hearing sensitivity.

Conductive hearing loss occurs when there is impairment of sound transmission to the inner ear. Lesions of the external or middle ear may cause conductive hearing loss. Typically, bone-conduction thresholds are better than air-conduction thresholds. The most common causes of conduction hearing loss are cerumen impaction and otosclerosis. Less common causes include tumors and degenerative disorders (e.g., Meniere disease), trauma, vasculitis, and hemorrhagic disorders.[75]

Diagnostic Evaluation

Hearing impairment may be obvious during casual conversation with the patient. Patients with hearing impairments should be first examined for cerumen impaction. Six independent factors for hearing loss can be identified by brief self-reports of patients 55 to 74 years of age. These factors are (1) age 70 years or older, (2) male gender, (3) 12 or more grades of education, (4) having seen a doctor for deafness or hearing loss, (5) inability to hear a whisper across a room, and (6) inability to hear a normal voice across the room.[76] Several office measures of hearing impairment are useful to clinicians. The whisper test can be performed by asking patients to repeat a short list of whispered numbers from an examiner positioned 2 ft behind them. Although a reasonably sensitive measure, the whisper test lacks reproducibility. A more quantitative approach is a handheld otoscope with a built-in audiometer. This device has high sensitivity and specificity but is expensive and requires some skill to be used correctly.

Patients with hearing loss should undergo formal audiologic assessment. The evaluation includes a pure-tone audiogram to document the decibel loss across frequency ranges and to determine whether the loss is sensorineural or mixed.

Management

Management of hearing loss may be surgical, medical, or rehabilitative. Patient education is important with any treatment. The treatment of presbycusis is limited to counseling regarding hearing strategies, emotional support from family members and health care professionals, and the use of hearing aids or various types of assistive listening devices.[77] Surgical approaches are indicated for patients with obstructive lesions of the external auditory canal and remedial causes of conductive hearing loss. Stapedectomy is the most common surgical intervention for otosclerosis. Cochlear implants are of value to patients with profound sensorineural deafness for whom a conventional hearing aid is not feasible.

A change in medical treatments may be indicated for patients who experience sensorineural hearing loss. Serial evaluations of hearing are helpful for patients who are receiving high doses of potentially ototoxic drugs (e.g., anticancer drugs and high-dose loop diuretics).

Most patients with sensorineural or cochlear disease will benefit from aural rehabilitation. Aural rehabilitation includes treatment modalities such as hearing aids, auditory training, and training in lip reading. Styles of hearing aids include behind the ear, in the ear canal, and completely in the canal.[74,75] Hearing aids remain the usual treatment of patients with sensorineural hearing loss. A variety of devices are available, including programmable hearing aids and amplification circuits that reduce distortion. Hearing aids may fit entirely within the external auditory canal or fit over the patient's earlobe. Assistive listening devices include television listening systems, alerting devices, telephone amplifiers, large-area amplification systems, and remote microphone systems. Remote microphone systems with headsets can be purchased at radio supply stores. They are inexpensive, practical, and capable of improving communication with even severely hearing-impaired patients.

To improve communication with a hearing-impaired patient, an attempt should be made to get the listener's attention before speaking, to face the listener directly to afford visual cues, to reduce background noise, to use facial expressions and gestures, to speak slowly and clearly, to speak only slightly louder than normal and not shout, to rephrase the message if the listener does not understand rather than repeating it, to alert the listener to changes in the topic, and to not turn and walk away while talking.

VISION IMPAIRMENT

Age-related changes in vision, especially presbyopia or farsightedness, are common causes of increasing vision impairment. Other important changes that affect vision include reduced pupillary dilatation, which contributes to poor night vision; discoloration of the crystalline lens; and changes in the vitreous fluid, which may produce dots in the visual field. With normal aging, little change occurs in acuity that cannot be corrected or compensated for with ease. Major causes of vision impairment associated with low vision or blindness (i.e., vision worse than 20/200 in either one or both eyes with correction) include cataracts, glaucoma, macular degeneration, and diabetic retinopathy [see Chapter 48].

Epidemiology

In a study of older adults from three communities, the prevalence of functional blindness increased from 1% at 71 to 74 years of age to 17% in those 90 years of age and older. Functional vision impairment increased from 7% in the 71-year-old to 74-year-old age group to 39% in those 90 years of age and older.[78] Racial differences are reflected in patterns of vision loss, with whites being more likely to have age-related macular degeneration and African Americans being more likely to have primary open-angle glaucoma. African Americans have a twofold greater prevalence of blindness and vision impairment than whites; there is no difference in prevalence by gender. In nursing homes, the prevalence of bilateral blindness is 17% and the prevalence of vision impairment (i.e., worse than 20/40 but better than 20/200) is 19%. The prevalence of blindness is 29% in residents 90 years of age and older.[79]

Cataract

A cataract is an opacity of the crystalline lens that may affect visual acuity, contrast sensitivity, and light perception. Senile cataracts are often classified as cortical, subcapsular, or nuclear. Although the prevalence of opacification of the lens increases with aging to nearly 100% of those older than 90 years, functional impairment occurs in only half of people with cataracts. Cortical or cuneiform cataracts present as translucent spokes, flakes, or wedges of opacity around the nucleus. Cortical cataracts progress slowly and may eventually involve the entire cortex of the lens. Subcapsular cataracts are more common in younger patients and are associated with use of corticosteroids. They often appear as irregular granules and crystals with various colors. Nuclear cataracts are the most common in elderly patients; they appear as a yellow or brown discoloration and are associated with increasing myopia and vision deterioration.

Risk factors and etiology   The possible risk factors for cataract include exposure to ultraviolet B radiation, a history of diabetes mellitus, alcohol consumption, cigarette smoking, a vitamin-deficient diet, and corticosteroid use.[80] The prevalence of age-related cataract increases from less than 5% in persons younger than 65 years to 46% in persons 75 to 85 years of age.[80] Cigarette smoking has been shown to be an important independent risk factor for age-related cataract. In a prospective cohort study of nearly 21,000 physicians free of cataract at baseline, the relative risk of age-related cataract in men was reduced 36% in those who were never smokers. Smoking cessation appears to reduce the risk of cataract primarily by limiting total dose-related damage to the lens.[81]

Diagnostic evaluation   Initial symptoms of a cataract include glare and poor contrast sensitivity. Contrast sensitivity is the ability to discern subtle variations in shade. It can be tested through the use of figures that vary in contrast, luminance, and spatial frequency.[82] The glare is caused by excess refraction of light rays penetrating the clouded lenses and is most troublesome in bright sunlight or during night driving. Decreased contrast sensitivity is manifested by difficulty distinguishing field objects in poorly illuminated settings. Near visual acuity is more often reduced in posterior subcapsular cataract, and patients often complain of disabling glare during daytime. Patients with cortical cataract complain of glare with oncoming headlights while driving at night. A nuclear sclerotic cataract affects distance vision more than near vision.[80,82] Nuclear and cortical cataracts have distinct characteristics on examination. Nuclear cataract may be invisible against the red reflex until the cataract is fairly mature. The cataract then appears as a poorly defined central fog. The cortical cataract is typically composed of radially oriented, sharply defined, spokelike opacities.[80]

Management   Symptomatic cataracts are managed surgically. The decision whether to perform cataract surgery is based on the likely degree of visual improvement that will occur and its impact on the quality of life weighed against the risks and cost of surgery. A cataract is considered to be clinically significant if it causes a decrease in visual acuity or function that interferes with the patient's performance of activities of daily living.[82] Most cataract surgery in the United States is performed under regional or local anesthesia in an ambulatory setting. Extracapsular cataract surgery with implantation of a posterior chamber lens implant is the procedure of choice. Phacoemulsification enables the surgeon to emulsify the lens nucleus into small pieces through a very small incision, reducing or eliminating the need to suture the incision.[82] Approximately 95% of patients without other ocular comorbidity who undergo cataract extraction achieve a visual acuity of 20/40 or better.[82]

Glaucoma

Glaucoma is a chronic progressive optic neuropathy characterized by excavation of the optic nerve head and loss of visual field in the midperiphery. Two anatomic classifications of glaucoma are based on whether the angle of the anterior chamber is open or narrow; the more common open-angle glaucoma is a chronic disease, whereas the less common angle-closure glaucoma is usually an acute disease.

Risk factors and etiology   The major risk factor for open-angle glaucoma is thought to be elevation of the intraocular pressure beyond the statistical norm of 21 mm Hg.[83] The high intraocular pressure originates from an increased resistance to drainage of aqueous humor through the trabecular meshwork.[83]

However, many patients with glaucoma have normal-pressure glaucoma with pressures of less than 21 mm Hg.[83] Putative risk factors for open-angle glaucoma include high intraocular pressure, African-American ancestry, positive family history, myopia, and possibly diabetes and systemic hypertension.[83]

Angle-closure glaucoma results from obstruction of aqueous humor flow from the posterior chamber through the pupil into the anterior chamber through the pores of the Schlemm canal. Production of aqueous humor continues, resulting in very high intraocular pressures. The main characteristic of the angle-closure glaucomas is a relative pupillary block with a forward bulging of the iris face, thereby obstructing the aqueous humor flow at the chamber angle.[83] Acute angle-closure glaucoma can be precipitated by the use of dilating eyedrops and is a medical emergency. In contrast, primary open-angle glaucoma is an insidious disease most often discovered during routine examinations.

Diagnostic evaluation   Glaucoma is frequently asymptomatic at the time of diagnosis but can result in progressive loss of visual field and eventual blindness. The diagnosis of glaucoma is based on an eye examination that includes tonometry, gonioscopy (which examines the angle of the anterior chamber), inspection of the optic disk and nerve fiber layer, and visual field testing. With injury to the optic nerve, there is the appearance of cupping of the optic disk with an increase in the cup-to-disk ratio and visual dysfunction in the midperipheral field of vision. As the disease progresses, deterioration of central visual functions, including acuity, becomes evident.

If the optic nerve appears abnormal, visual field testing should be performed with attention to glaucomatous visual field defects.[84] Intraocular pressure is measured by determination of the force required to flatten the central cornea (applanation). Applanation tonometry can be performed with an optical measuring device or an electrical strain gauge.

Management The treatment of glaucoma includes both medical and surgical approaches. Intraocular pressure is reduced either by decreasing the amount of aqueous humor produced by the ciliary body or by increasing its outflow through the trabecular meshwork, through the uveoscleral pathway or through a surgically created path.[84] Medical treatments are targeted at the physiology of intraocular pressure. The cell membranes of the nonpigmented ciliary epithelial cells contain α-adrenoceptors and β-adrenoceptors, carbonic anhydrase, and sodium and potassium activated adenosine triphosphatases (ATPases). By stimulation or inhibition of these enzymes or receptors, the active transport of aqueous humor across the blood-aqueous barrier can be modulated to reduce intraocular pressure.[83]

Topical eyedrops are the most common medical treatment of open-angle glaucoma. Agents either decrease the production of aqueous or increase its outflow and absorption.

Currently used ocular hypotensive agents consist of sympathomimetics, parasympathomimetics (pilocarpine), sympatholytics, carbonic anhydrase inhibitors (including the oral agent acetazolamide), and prostaglandins. The aim of medical treatment is to obtain a target pressure at which progression of visual field defects is halted.[82] Therapy is usually begun with topical beta blockers, provided that the patient has no cardiac or pulmonary disease. The most commonly used topical beta blocker is timolol because of excellent pressure-lowering efficacy, long duration of action, and few ocular side effects. The cardioselective beta blocker betaxolol is less likely to cause systemic side effects but may be less effective in lowering intraocular pressure.[83] Alternative drugs are topical carbonic anhydrase inhibitors (dorzolamide and brinzolamide), prostaglandin analogues (latanoprost), alpha$_2$-adrenergic agonists (brimonidine and apraclonidine), or dipivalyl epinephrine. Latanoprost has become widely used for the treatment of glaucoma but has the unique side effect of increasing iris pigmentation. If treatment with one of these alternative agents also fails to reduce or maintain target pressures or if there is progression of visual field defects, combination therapy is recommended.[83,84]

Surgical therapy for glaucoma includes iridectomy to enhance flow of aqueous in the treatment of angle-closure glaucoma and, for open-angle glaucoma, argon laser therapy to improve outflow through the trabecular meshwork. Surgery for glaucoma is usually reserved for patients in whom target pressures cannot be achieved with medical or laser therapy. Good success rates have been described with argon laser trabeculectomy, but additional surgery is often needed.

Age-Related Macular Degeneration
Age-related macular degeneration (AMD) causes sudden worsening and distortion of central vision, or scotoma, progressing rapidly over weeks or months until scarring is complete and no further vision is lost (legal blindness).[85] AMD impairs central vision that is required for reading, driving, face recognition, and all fine visual tasks. The insidious loss of central vision results in the initial symptoms of reduced visual perception and visual sensitivity to light and to gradual progression to legal blindness despite preservation of peripheral vision.[86]

Risk factors and etiology Epidemiologic studies show a relation between the development of AMD and cigarette smoking and the consumption of dietary carotenoids and vitamins A, C, and E. In a prospective cohort study, women who smoked cigarettes for 65 or more pack-years had a 2.4 times higher risk of AMD than nonsmokers.[87] Similar findings were seen in the Physicians' Health Study, where the relative risk of AMD was 2.5 times greater in men who smoked 20 or more cigarettes daily than in nonsmokers.[88]

Diagnostic evaluation AMD is characterized by the presence of abnormalities in the macular area. These abnormalities include soft drusen, yellow-white deposits of extracellular material containing debris external to the retinal pigment epithelium (RPE), and hyperpigmentation or hypopigmentation (or both) of the RPE. Neurosensory detachment, retinal hemorrhages, and retinal scarring gradually result in decreased visual function of photoreceptors in the central vision.[89] Late maculopathy includes both dry and neovascular AMD. The dry form of AMD is most common and occurs with atrophy of the RPE. Neovascular, or exudative, AMD is characterized by choroidal neovascularization with vascular leakage into subretinal spaces. Recognition of the less common exudative AMD is important because argon laser photocoagulation is effective in reducing loss of visual acuity.[89]

Management There is no effective treatment of the dry form of AMD. Four large clinical trials, however, have found that laser photocoagulation of exudative forms of AMD decreases the rate of severe vision loss and preserves contrast sensitivity.[89] Laser photocoagulation therapy is the only treatment for AMD with proven long-term benefit. However, other therapies have shown promise, including photodynamic therapy (verteporfin), which delays or prevents loss of vision during at least 1 year of follow-up in patients with predominantly classic neovascular lesions.[89] To identify patients who may benefit from laser therapy, home monitoring for symptoms of scotoma or distorted vision is performed with the use of an Amsler grid.[89]

Iatrogenic Illness

Iatrogenic, or physician-induced, illness results from a diagnostic procedure or therapeutic intervention that is not a natural consequence of the patient's disease.[90] Iatrogenic illnesses include complications of drug therapy and of diagnostic or therapeutic procedures, nosocomial infections, fluid and electrolyte disorders, and trauma.[90]

POLYPHARMACY

The most common documented cause of iatrogenic illness is adverse drug reactions, usually associated with polypharmacy.[90] The incidence of adverse drug reactions increases with advancing age and number of chronic diseases requiring drug therapy. The concomitant use of several medications increases the risk of drug interactions, unwanted effects, and adverse reactions. Suboptimal drug prescribing, including the inappropriate use or underuse of medications, is common in older outpatients and inpatients and is associated with significant morbidity.[91] For example, inappropriate drug prescribing in community-residing elders is common, and contraindicated drugs such as amitriptyline, chlorpropamide, or diazepam are still being commonly prescribed.[92]

Age-Related Changes in Drug Metabolism
Many medications should be used with special caution in elderly patients because of age-related changes in drug pharmaco-

kinetics (drug disposition) and pharmacodynamics (target tissue effects).[91] Although drug absorption is not reduced in healthy elderly persons, absorption of medications can be reduced by disease states (e.g., malabsorption) or concomitant administration of drugs that decrease absorption of medications (e.g., antacids). Drug distribution is altered by aging, primarily because of body composition changes, with a decrease in total body water and lean body mass and a relative increase in body fat. Consequently, water-soluble drugs achieve a higher serum concentration, whereas lipid-soluble drugs have a prolonged elimination half-life. This change is especially important in regard to drugs that are lipid soluble and penetrate the blood-brain barrier (e.g., diazepam). Although levels of serum proteins are not significantly affected by aging, many elderly patients have reduced levels of serum albumin resulting from acute or chronic disease or malnutrition. Consequently, displacement of a drug by one that binds very highly to albumin enhances the delivery of that agent to the target site, thereby increasing the risk of an adverse reaction. For example, bleeding (excessive anticoagulation) may occur when patients treated with warfarin are given drugs such as sulfas or phenytoin.

A decrease in hepatic blood flow with usual aging will decrease the rate of metabolism of drugs that undergo a high degree of first-pass extraction (e.g., propranolol). Aging and diseases affect phase I hepatic metabolism, the microsomal enzyme mixed function oxidase system. Active metabolites of drugs that undergo phase I metabolism may prolong the effects of the parent medication (e.g., diazepam). Phase II metabolism, the conjugation of drugs, is not significantly affected by aging. Consequently the elimination of agents that undergo phase II metabolism is unaffected by normal aging.

Drug elimination is mainly influenced by renal function. The age-associated decrease in renal function, which results in decreased creatinine clearance, necessitates lower maintenance doses of renally excreted drugs in elderly patients.

The effect of aging on target-organ responsiveness to medications is less well established. However, decreased beta-receptor sensitivity and increased sensitivity to opiates is well established. Many elderly patients are also more sensitive to the adverse effects of anticholinergic drugs, notably constipation, dry mouth, and delirium.

Diagnostic Evaluation

Because of unpredictable effects of aging on the metabolism of drugs, physicians should suspect an adverse drug reaction whenever any new symptom occurs. Also, blood levels of medications that have narrow therapeutic windows (e.g., aminoglycosides) should be considered.

Prevention and Management

The prevention of iatrogenic illness from inappropriate drug prescribing begins with an understanding of the rational use of medications in elderly patients. Consensus criteria for appropriate drug prescribing offer useful guidelines.[92]

In general, prescribing the fewest medications at the lowest needed dosage is a rational approach to the prevention of iatrogenic illness. Knowing the pharmacology of prescribed drugs and the age-related alterations in drug disposition and tissue sensitivity and using lower than standard doses of most drugs when the therapeutic dose is uncertain should help physicians avoid adverse drug reactions. When prescribing a new medication for an elderly patient, a practical approach is to use the following criteria:

1. Determine whether the drug is lipid or water soluble.
2. Determine whether the drug is highly bound to albumin.
3. Determine whether the drug undergoes cytochrome P-450 metabolism (substrate, inducer, or inhibitor of microsomal enzymes).
4. Determine whether the drug is renally excreted (use lower maintenance doses in older patients and in those with renal insufficiency).

This information can be found by literature searches, a review of newsletters on drug prescribing, or consultation with a pharmacologist or clinical pharmacist.[91]

MEDICAL ERRORS

Medical errors are common in the care of elderly hospitalized patients. These errors often involve incorrect drug dispensing that sometimes causes patient morbidity or mortality. Most medical errors are the result of systems errors in hospitals. Concerns over the reported incidence of medical errors led the Institute of Medicine to release a report advocating dramatic, systemwide changes in hospitals, such as the use of computerized medical information systems and other support systems, to reduce the rate of errors.[93] Computerized medical information systems can improve antibiotic selection, limit the emergence of antibiotic-resistant pathogens, and lessen the risk of adverse drug events.[93]

NOSOCOMIAL INFECTION

Nosocomial pathogens are primarily transmitted through contact with hospital or nursing home personnel. Urinary tract, skin (intravascular), lung, and wound infection are common examples of nosocomial infection.[90] Of growing concern for elderly patients are infections with resistant strains of gram-negative bacilli, methicillin-resistant *Staphylococcus aureus*, and vancomycin-resistant enterococci (VRE). Resistant urinary tract infections are common after prolonged indwelling urinary catheterization.

Risk Factors and Etiology

Factors promoting nosocomial pneumonia include gastric aspiration, spread of pathogens by poorly cleansed hands of medical and nursing personnel, fecal-oral spread of pathogens, and cross-contamination from other patients. Patients with physical debility, prolonged hospitalization, and exposure to broad-spectrum antibiotics are at risk for nosocomial infections.

VRE are likely transmitted from patient to patient by the unwashed hands of health care workers, contaminated medical equipment, or environmental surfaces (e.g., bed rails or blood pressure cuffs). Nosocomial pneumonia results from colonization of the upper respiratory and gastrointestinal tracts and occurs most often in critically ill and ventilator-dependent patients.

Prevention and Management

Nosocomial infection can be prevented by washing hands and cleaning medical equipment (e.g., stethoscopes) between patient contacts, wearing gloves during invasive procedures or contact with wounds or mucous membranes, using aseptic techniques when inserting or changing urinary catheters, isolating infected patients (e.g., in nursing homes), elevating the patient's head (to lessen the risk of aspiration), replacing broad-spectrum antibiotics with narrow-spectrum antibiotics on the basis of bacterial sensitivity reports, and limiting the use of urinary catheters. Prophylactic antimicrobial therapies and routine catheter replacement are not recommended.[90]

Table 8   Long-term Care Options

Site	Patient Characteristics	Comments
Home (independent living, house, apartment)	Independent performance of ADL; stable chronic diseases; adequate social support network	Acute medical illness may require short-term home care (skilled nursing services); home safety evaluation for environmental hazards
Home with formal support services	Needs assistance with performance of ADL (e.g., bathing, dressing); adequate social support network; acute illness or convalescence from hospitalization; requires skilled nursing care or physical therapy	Skilled services covered for limited period by Medicare; custodial services not covered long-term (e.g., home health aid); risk of elder abuse or neglect because of caregiver strain or loss of informal supports (e.g., illness of spouse)
Community services	Physically or cognitively impaired (limits performance of ADL); limited finances; limited informal supports; caregivers need respite (relief from caregiving)	Options: adult day care; nutritional programs (e.g., Meals-on-Wheels); protective services (suspected elder abuse); transportation services; case management services (professionally coordinated); categorized services (e.g., PACE) for eligible patients
Residential care facilities (assisted living, continuing care retirement communities)	Patients for whom independent living is either no longer desired or feasible; retirees, persons able to perform ADL with minimal or no assistance	Assisted living is ideal for demented patients who are too functional for a nursing home but are unable to safely live at home; retirement communities are vertically integrated, permitting residents to move from independent living (apartment) to assisted living or nursing care as needed
Rehabilitation/hospital	Categorical illness (e.g., stroke or hip fracture); able to tolerate physical therapy (e.g., ≥ 3 hr daily); good informal home supports; likely return home	Interdisciplinary care with focus on returning patient to independent living; patients must be able to participate in rehabilitative services and demonstrate potential to improve ambulation and performance of ADL
Skilled nursing facility	Dependence in ADL or ambulation preventing discharge to home; requires skilled nursing care or physical therapy; too impaired for rehabilitation hospital (noncategorical illness, cannot perform therapy for ≥ 3 hr daily); inadequate social supports at home	The choice of skilled nursing facility, home care, or subacute care unit is often an issue of patient choice, disease severity, availability of services (geographic), and family or caregiver availability; limited Medicare coverage for skilled services forces many patients to eventually enter a long-term care facility or return home
Subacute care unit	Similar to patients in skilled nursing care but typically requiring augmented professional services (e.g., hyperalimentation, respiratory care, peripheral intravenous catheters, or increased nursing staff time)	Subacute care units bridge the gap between acute hospitalization and the patient's return home; market forces have encouraged growth of these units (e.g., hospitals reduce patient length of stay and are reimbursed for cost-based skilled nursing care); short-term stay (< 2 mo) is typical
Long-term care facility	Dependent in performance of ADL; unable to return home (temporarily or permanently) to independent living; ineligible for skilled, subacute, or rehabilitative services; inadequate social supports (e.g., lives alone, no caregivers)	Self-pay and Medicaid are usual sources of payment; many states offer a Medicaid waiver program to provide home services to frail patients who would otherwise require nursing home placement
Palliative (hospice) care	Patients with terminal illness (prognosis ≤ 6 mo) (e.g., metastatic cancer or end-stage heart or renal failure)	Provides comfort measures in home (or inpatient unit where available); Medicare covers palliative (comfort-related) not curative (e.g., elective surgery) services; underutilized by patients (delayed recommendation by physician; home hospice services limited compared with skilled nursing care)

ADL—activities of daily living   PACE—Program for All-inclusive Care of Elderly

Long-term Care

Long-term care refers to the provision of comprehensive health care services, including personal health and social services, delivered over an extended period to people with limited functional capacity.

AVAILABLE CARE SERVICES

The spectrum of long-term care ranges from home and social services provided to patients living in the community to residential and long-term care facilities [see Table 8].

In the United States, most elderly persons live in the community. Only 5% at any time are residing in long-term care facilities (i.e., nursing homes). However, the probability of nursing home use increases sharply with age: 25% of those 85 years of age and older reside in nursing homes, and the lifetime risk of entering a nursing home for people who turned 65 years of age in 1990 is estimated at 40%.[94] About 25% of individuals in the United States will spend at least 1 year in a nursing home, with more women than men having total lifetime nursing home use of 5 years or more.[94] The high cost of institutional care and the growing number of frail Americans have provided an impetus to develop less-expensive levels of care (e.g., residential care facilities), ambulatory health centers (e.g., Program for All-inclusive Care of Elderly [PACE]), and community services that will enable the frail elderly patient to remain at home.

ADVANCE DIRECTIVES

Health care institutions are required to ascertain whether patients have advance directives and to include copies of them in the medical record. A living will is an advance directive by which a person specifies the circumstances in which life-sustaining treatment is to be provided or discontinued in the event of terminal illness if the person is unable to communicate with health professionals. A durable power of attorney for health care is an advance directive by which a person designates a proxy to represent his or her wishes if he or she loses decision-making capacity. In discussions with physicians, patients should communicate their wishes for end-of-life care, including cardiopulmonary resuscitation, intensive care (e.g., ventilator support), and nutritional support during acute or end-stage illness.[95]

References

1. Tinetti ME, Inouye SK, Gill TM, et al: Shared risk factors for falls, incontinence, and functional dependence: unifying the approach to geriatric syndromes. JAMA 273:1348, 1995

2. Hoffman C, Rice D, Sung HY: Persons with chronic conditions: their prevalence and costs. JAMA 276:1473, 1996

3. Inouye SK: Delirium in hospitalized older patients. Clin Geriatr Med 14:745, 1998

4. Diagnostic and Statistical Manual of Mental Disorders, 4th ed. American Psychiatric Association, Washington, DC, 1994

5. Meagher DJ: Delirium: optimising management. BMJ 322:144, 2001

6. Inouye SK, Viscoli CM, Horwitz RI, et al: A predictive model for delirium in hospitalized elderly medical patients based on admission characteristics. Ann Intern Med 119:474, 1993

7. Inouye SK, Charpentier PA: Precipitating factors for delirium in hospitalized elderly persons. JAMA 275:852, 1996

8. Dyer CB, Ashton CM, Teasdale TA: Postoperative delirium: a review of 80 primary data-collection studies. Arch Intern Med 155:461, 1995

9. Williams-Russo P, Sharrock NE, Mattis S, et al: Cognitive effects after epidural vs general anesthesia in older adults: a randomized trial. JAMA 274:44, 1995

10. Moller JT, Cluitmans P, Rasmussen LS, et al: Long-term postoperative cognitive dysfunction in the elderly ISPOCD1 study. ISPOCD investigators. International study of post-operative cognitive dysfunction. Lancet 351:857, 1998

11. Marcantonio ER, Goldman L, Mangione CM, et al: A clinical prediction rule for delirium after elective noncardiac surgery. JAMA 271:134, 1994

12. Tune LE: Serum anticholinergic activity levels and delirium in the elderly. Semin Clin Neuropsychiatry 5:149, 2000

13. Brown TM: Drug-induced delirium. Semin Clin Neuropsychiatry 5:113, 2000

14. Trzepacz PT: Delirium: advances in diagnosis, pathophysiology, and treatment. Psychiatr Clin North Am 19:429, 1996

15. Inouye SK, Bogardus ST Jr, Charpentier PA, et al: A multicomponent intervention to prevent delirium in hospitalized older patients. N Engl J Med 340:669, 1999

16. Fantl JA, Newman DK, Colling J, et al: Urinary incontinence in adults: acute and chronic management. Clinical Practice Guideline, No 2. US Department of Health and Human Services, Public Health Service, Agency for Health Care Policy and Research (AHCPR Publication No 96-0682), Rockville, Maryland, March 1996

17. Burgio KL, Ives DG, Locher JL, et al: Treatment seeking for urinary incontinence in older adults. J Am Geriatr Soc 42:208, 1994

18. Chutka DS, Fleming KC, Evans MP, et al: Urinary incontinence in the elderly population. Mayo Clin Proc 71:93, 1996

19. Ouslander JG, Schapira M, Schnelle JF, et al: Does eradicating bacteriuria affect the severity of chronic urinary incontinence in nursing home residents? Ann Intern Med 122:749, 1995

20. Smith DN, Appell RA, Winters JC, et al: Collagen injection therapy for female intrinsic sphincteric deficiency. J Urol 157:1275, 1997

21. Seim A, Sivertsen B, Eriksen BC, et al: Treatment of urinary incontinence in women in general practice: observational study. BMJ 312:1459, 1996

22. Tebyani N, Patel H, Yamaguchi R, et al: Percutaneous needle bladder neck suspension for the treatment of stress urinary incontinence in women: long-term results. J Urol 163:1510, 2000

23. Singh G, Thomas DG: Artificial urinary sphincter in patients with neurogenic bladder dysfunction. Br J Urol 77:252, 1996

24. Gleason DM, Susset J, White C, et al: Evaluation of a new once-daily formulation of oxybutynin for the treatment of urinary urge incontinence. Urology 54:420, 1999

25. Millard R, Tuttle J, Moore K, et al: Clinical efficacy and safety of tolterodine compared to placebo in detrusor overactivity. J Urol 161:1551, 1999

26. Burgio KL, Locher JL, Goode PS, et al: Behavioral vs drug treatment for urge urinary incontinence in older women: a randomized controlled trial. JAMA 280:1995, 1998

27. Thakar R, Stanton S: Regular review: management of urinary incontinence in women. BMJ 321:1326, 2000

28. Johnson TM 2nd, Ouslander JG: Urinary incontinence in the older man. Med Clin North Am 83:1247, 1999

29. Romero Y, Evans JM, Fleming KC, et al: Constipation and fecal incontinence in the elderly population. Mayo Clin Proc 71:81, 1996

30. DeLillo AR, Rose S: Functional bowel disorders in the geriatric patient: constipation, fecal impaction, and fecal incontinence. Am J Gastroenterol 95:901, 2000

31. Camilleri M, Lee JS, Viramontes B: Insights into the pathophysiology and mechanisms of constipation, irritable bowel syndrome, and diverticulosis in older people. J Am Geriatr Soc 48:1142, 2000

32. Soffer EE, Hull T: Fecal incontinence: a practical approach to evaluation and treatment. Am J Gastroenterol 95:1873, 2000

33. Wilson JA: Constipation in the elderly. Clin Geriatr Med 15:499, 1999

34. Palmer R: Falls in elderly patients: predictable and preventable. Cleve Clin J Med 68:303, 2001

35. Brown JS, Vittinghoff E, Wyman JF, et al: Urinary incontinence: does it increase the risk for falls and fractures? Study of the Osteoporotic Fractures Research Group. J Am Geriatr Soc 48:7, 2000

36. Gregg EW, Pereira MA, Caspersen CJ: Physical activity, falls, and fractures among older adults: a review of the epidemiologic evidence. J Am Geriatr Soc 48:883, 2000

37. Tinetti ME, Speechley M, Ginter SF: Risk factors for falls among elderly persons living in the community. N Engl J Med 319:1701, 1988

38. Tinetti ME, Doucett J, Claus E, et al: Risk factors for serious injury during falls by older persons in the community. J Am Geriatr Soc 43:1214, 1995

39. Tinetti ME, Williams CS: Falls, injuries due to falls, and the risk of admission to a nursing home. N Engl J Med 337:1279, 1997

40. Cummings SR, Nevitt MC, Browner WS, et al: Risk factors for hip fracture in white women. N Engl J Med 332:767, 1995

41. Maki BE: Gait changes in older adults: predictors of falls or indicators of fear. J Am Geriatr Soc 45:313, 1997

42. Pavol MJ, Owings TM, Foley KT, et al: Gait characteristics as risk factors for falling from trips induced in older adults. J Gerontol A Biol Sci Med Sci 54:M583, 1999

43. Gillespie LD, Gillespie WJ, Cumming R, et al: Interventions for preventing falls in the elderly. Cochrane Database Syst Rev 2:CD000340, 2000

44. Gardner MM, Robertson MC, Campbell AJ: Exercise in preventing falls and fall related injuries in older people: a review of randomised controlled trials. Br J Sports Med 34:7, 2000

45. Tinetti ME, Baker DI, McAvay G, et al: A multifactorial intervention to reduce the risk of falling among elderly people living in the community. N Engl J Med 331:821, 1994

46. Wolf SL, Barnhart HX, Kutner NG, et al: Reducing frailty and falls in older persons: an investigation of Tai Chi and computerized balance training. Atlanta FICSIT Group. Frailty and Injuries: Cooperative Studies of Intervention Techniques. J Am Geriatr Soc 44:489, 1996

47. Province MA, Hadley EC, Hornbrook MC, et al: The effects of exercise on falls in elderly patients: a preplanned meta-analysis of the FICSIT trials. JAMA 273:1341, 1995

48. Campbell AJ, Robertson MC, Gardner MM, et al: Randomised controlled trial of a general practice programme of home based exercise to prevent falls in elderly women. BMJ 315:1065, 1997

49. Robertson MC, Devlin N, Gardner MM, et al: Effectiveness and economic evaluation of a nurse delivered exercise programme to prevent falls. 1: Randomised control trial. BMJ 322:697, 2001

50. Close J, Elis M, Hooper R, et al: Prevention of Falls in the Elderly Trial (PROFET): a randomised controlled trial. Lancet 353:93, 1999

51. Fiatarone MA, O'Neill EF, Ryan ND, et al: Exercise training and nutritional supplementation for physical frailty in very elderly people. N Engl J Med 330:1769, 1994

52. Kannus P, Parkkari J, Niemi S, et al: Prevention of hip fracture in elderly people with use of a hip protector. N Engl J Med 343:1506, 2000

53. Mahoney JE: Immobility and falls. Clin Geriatr Med 14:699, 1998

54. Inouye SK, Bogardus ST Jr, Baker DI, et al: The Hospital Elder Life Program: a model of care to prevent cognitive and functional decline in older hospitalized patients. Hospital Elder Life Program. J Am Geriatr Soc 48:1697, 2000

55. Bergstrom N, Bennett MA, Carlson CE, et al: Treatment of pressure ulcers. Clinical Practice Guideline, No 15. US Department of Health and Human Services, Public Health Service, Agency for Health Care Policy and Research (AHCPR Publication No 95-0652), Rockville, Maryland, December 1994

56. Pressure ulcers: prevalence, cost and risk assessment: consensus development conference statement. The National Pressure Ulcer Advisory Panel. Decubitus 2:24, 1989

57. Brandeis GH, Morris JN, Nash DJ, et al: The epidemiology and natural history of pressure ulcers in elderly nursing home residents. JAMA 264:2905, 1990

58. Allman RM: Pressure ulcer prevalence, incidence, risk factors, and impact. Clin Geriatr Med 13:421, 1997

59. Orlando PL: Pressure ulcer management in the geriatric patient. Ann Pharmacother 32:1221, 1998

60. Remsburg RE, Bennett RG: Pressure-relieving strategies for preventing and treating pressure sores. Clin Geriatr Med 13:513, 1997

61. Cullum N, Deeks J, Sheldon TA, et al: Beds, mattresses and cushions for pressure sore prevention and treatment. Cochrane Database Sys Rev 2:CD001735, 2000

62. Ferrell BA, Osterweil D, Christenson P: A randomized trial of low-air-loss beds for treatment of pressure ulcers. JAMA 269:494, 1993

63. Thomas DR, Goode PS, LaMaster K, et al: Acemannan hydrogel dressing versus saline dressing for pressure ulcers: a randomized, controlled trial. Adv Wound Care 11:273, 1998

64. Marwick C: NHANES III health data relevant for aging nation. JAMA 277:100, 1997

65. Azad N, Murphy J, Amos SS, et al: Nutrition survey in an elderly population following admission to a tertiary care hospital. CMAJ 161:511, 1999

66. Verdery RB: Clinical evaluation of failure to thrive in older people. Clin Geriatr Med 13:769, 1997

67. Morley JE: Anorexia of aging: physiologic and pathologic. Am J Clin Nutr 66:760, 1997

68. Reuben DB, Greendale GA, Harrison GG: Nutrition screening in older persons. J Am Geriatr Soc 43:415, 1995

69. Covinsky KE, Martin GE, Beyth RJ, et al: The relationship between clinical assessment of nutritional status and adverse outcomes in older hospitalized medical patients. J Am Geriatr Soc 47:532, 1999

70. Sullivan DH, Sun S, Walls RC: Protein-energy undernutrition among elderly hospitalized patients: a prospective study. JAMA 281:2013, 1999

71. Lauque S, Arnaud-Battandier F, Mansourian R, et al: Protein-energy oral supplementation in malnourished nursing-home residents: a controlled trial. Age Ageing 29:51, 2000

72. Finucane TE, Christmas C, Travis K: Tube feeding in patients with advanced dementia: a review of the evidence. JAMA 282:1365, 1999

73. Moss AJ, Parsons VL: Current estimates from the National Health Interview Survey. United States, 1985. Vital Health Stat 10. 160:1, 1986

74. Mansour-Shousher R, Mansour WN: Nonsurgical management of hearing loss. Clin Geriatr Med 15:163, 1999

75. Nadol JB Jr: Hearing loss. N Engl J Med 329:1092, 1993

76. Reuben DB, Walsh K, Moore AA, et al: Hearing loss in community-dwelling older persons: national prevalence data and identification using simple questions. J Am Geriatr Soc 46:1008, 1998

77. Cohn ES: Hearing loss with aging: presbycusis. Clin Geriatr Med 15:145, 1999

78. Salive ME, Guralnik J, Christen W, et al: Functional blindness and visual impairment in older adults from three communities. Ophthalmology 99:1840, 1992

79. Tielsch JM, Javitt JC, Coleman A, et al: The prevalence of blindness and visual impairment among nursing home residents in Baltimore. N Engl J Med 332:1205, 1995

80. Das A: Prevention of visual loss in older adults. Clin Geriatr Med 15:131, 1999

81. Christen WG, Glynn RJ, Ajani UA, et al: Smoking cessation and risk of age-related cataract in men. JAMA 284:713, 2000

82. Valluri S: Gradual painless visual loss: anterior segment causes. Clin Geriatr Med 15:87, 1999

83. Hoyng PF, Van Beek LM: Pharmacological therapy for glaucoma: a review. Drugs 59:411, 2000

84. Alward WL: Medical management of glaucoma. N Engl J Med 339:1298, 1998

85. Bird AC, Bressler NM, Bressler SB, et al: An international classification and grading system for age-related maculopathy and age-related macular degeneration. The International ARM Epidemiological Study Group. Surv Ophthalmol 39:367, 1995

86. Arnold JJ, Sarks SH: Extracts from "clinical evidence": age-related macular degeneration. BMJ 321:741, 2000

87. Seddon JM, Willett WC, Speizer FE, et al: A prospective study of cigarette smoking and age-related macular degeneration in women. JAMA 276:1141, 1996

88. Christen WG, Glynn RJ, Manson JE, et al: A prospective study of cigarette smoking and risk of age-related macular degeneration in men. JAMA 276:1147, 1996

89. Fine SL, Berger JW, Maguire MG, et al: Age-related macular degeneration. N Engl J Med 342:483, 2000

90. Riedinger JL, Robbins LJ: Prevention of iatrogenic illness: adverse drug reactions and nosocomial infections in hospitalized older adults. Clin Geriatr Med 14:681, 1998

91. Hanlon JT, Schmader KE, Ruby CM, et al: Suboptimal prescribing in older inpatients and outpatients. J Am Geriatr Soc 49:200, 2001

92. Beers MH: Explicit criteria for determining potentially inappropriate medication use by the elderly: an update. Arch Intern Med 157:1531, 1997

93. To Err Is Human: Building a Safer Health System. Kohn L, Corrigan J, Donaldson M, Eds. National Academy Press, Washington, DC, 2000

94. Kemper P, Murtaugh CM: Lifetime use of nursing home care. N Engl J Med 324:595, 1991

95. Miller DL, Bolla LR: Patient values: the guide to medical decision making. Clin Geriatr Med 14:813, 1998

75 Rehabilitation of Geriatric Patients

Stephanie Studenski, M.D., M.P.H., and Pamela Woods Duncan, Ph.D., P.T.

The Role of the Generalist in Rehabilitation

The generalist plays a key role in the recovery of function in older patients who have had disabling illnesses. In most health care settings other than formal inpatient rehabilitation units, the primary care physician is the coordinator of medical rehabilitation services. Access to and duration of rehabilitation services are undergoing rapid change as Medicare and managed-care policies become more restrictive. Medicare is currently converting rehabilitation services in the inpatient, postacute, and home settings to prospective payment systems with extensive regulatory and documentation requirements.[1] The primary care physician must be able to assess rehabilitation potential, determine specific patient needs, and match them with the appropriate setting to optimize patient care.

To fulfill this responsibility, the physician must be able to assess the degree of disability, the effect of comorbidity on function, the possibility of recovery, and the indications for specific rehabilitation therapies.[2] Rehabilitation service planning is usually based on a different model of diagnosis and treatment than traditional medical care. The recently revised World Health Organization International Classification of Functioning, Disability and Health (ICIDH-2) can be used to assess the causes of disability, plan treatment approaches, and determine the outcomes of care [*see Figure 1*].[3] In this framework, abnormalities in organ system structure or physiologic function are called impairments. They lead to difficulties with individual activities and participation in society. Environmental factors, such as stairways and crosswalks, and personal factors, such as culture and education, can influence the effect of organ system impairments on activities and participation. Thus, the individual who has recently had a stroke may have impairments of sensory, motor, and language function that cause activity limitations in mobility and self-care. These activity limitations can create problems with work and family roles. The rehabilitation assessment will include evaluation of impairments in body structure and function, activity limitations, and individual participation goals. The treatment plan will include efforts to reverse or modify impairments such as decreased strength and adapt to activity limitations such as difficulty in walking. An evaluation of effectiveness of the service may include measurement of gains in organ functioning, activities, and participation, taking into account environmental and personal factors. The generalist team can also implement early exercise-rehabilitation services during hospitalization for acute illness. This practice has been shown to contribute to improved function.[4]

Stroke

Each year, more than 700,000 people in the United States suffer a stroke. Stroke is the leading cause of long-term major functional limitation. Each year, more money is spent in the rehabilitation of stroke patients than is spent on the rehabilitation of any other patient group. Guidelines for poststroke rehabilitation have been developed by an interdisciplinary panel to offer evidence-based recommendations for assessment, referral, and patient management.[5]

ASSESSMENT

The primary care physician should assess the type of stroke, the extent of neurologic deficits [*see Table 1*], the presence or absence of comorbid conditions, and the patient's prestroke functional status. Stroke guidelines provide extensive recomendations to help assess these features, measure recovery, and determine the benefits of rehabilitation.[6] A compendium of the recommended assessments has been gathered into a so-called stroke toolbox, which can be found on the Internet (www2.kumc.edu/coa).

SELECTING THE BEST SETTING FOR CARE

The setting for rehabilitation should be determined as soon as the patient's neurologic function and medical condition are reasonably stable. The appropriate setting is determined by the presence, severity, and complexity of the patient's functional limitations; cognitive status (especially ability to learn); ability to tolerate up to 3 hours of therapy daily; need for close medical monitoring; and the availability of social support [*see Figure 2*]. Under managed care, stroke rehabilitation is shifting from settings that provide acute rehabilitation to settings that provide subacute care, sometimes with a negative effect on outcome.[7-9]

Organized inpatient multidisciplinary stroke care is defined as care from a team of physicians, nurses, and therapists whose work is coordinated through regular weekly meetings and is dedicated to rehabilitation. A systematic review has shown that organized inpatient multidisciplinary stroke care, compared with conventional inpatient medical care or multidisciplinary care in a different setting, reduces mortality, institutionalization, and dependency. For every 100 patients receiving organized inpatient multidisciplinary stroke rehabilitation, an additional five will return home in an independent state.[10]

Age itself does not influence recovery. Problems such as memory loss, diminished ability to follow instructions, urinary or fecal incontinence, and visuospatial deficits such as unilater-

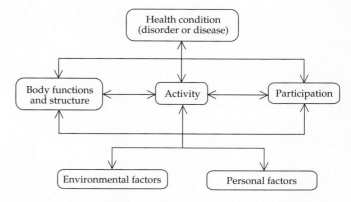

Figure 1   **Current understanding of interactions between the components of ICIDH-2.**[3]

Table 1 Selected Results of the Neurologic Examination of a Patient with Stroke[5]

Type of Deficit	Tests Used	Key Findings	Effect of Persistent Deficit on Rehabilitation
Altered level of consciousness	Repeated observation and testing of responses to external stimuli; Glasgow Coma Scale	Drowsiness, stupor, coma	An altered level of consciousness is a contra-indication to rehabilitation
Cognitive deficits in higher functions, memory, ability to learn	Observation; questions to probe mental functions; standardized screening test	Various degrees and types of deficits	A severe deficit is a contraindication to rehabilitation; a moderate deficit may impede rehabilitation and must be incorporated into the rehabilitation management plan
Motor deficits	Tests of strength and tone in muscles of the upper and lower extremities and face	Various degrees and sites of weakness, incoordination, abnormal movements	Motor deficits are the primary indications for rehabilitation; absence of any voluntary movement is a sign of poor prognosis
Disturbances in balance and coordination	Tests of coordination, sitting, standing, walking	Various degrees and types of deficits	Deficits impede but are not a contraindication to rehabilitation
Somatosensory deficits	Specific tests for sensory modalities (e.g., pain, touch); complex sensory tests	Various degrees and types of deficits	Deficits impede but are not a contraindication to rehabilitation
Disorders of vision	Tests of pupillary responses, ocular motility, optic fundus, visual fields, acuity	Visual loss or field defect; conjugate gaze deficits	Severe visual loss or ocular motility disturbances impede rehabilitation
Unilateral neglect	Observation; description of complex picture by patient; sensory testing	One side of body or external environment is ignored (often clears spontaneously)	Neglect impedes but is not a contraindication to rehabilitation
Speech and language deficits	Observation of spontaneous speech and language use, including language comprehension and, if possible, simple reading and writing skills	Aphasia, dysarthria, apraxia of speech	Severe problems in communication impede rehabilitation; treatment becomes an integral part of rehabilitation
Swallowing disorder (dysphagia)	History; test of ability to swallow liquids and solids; cineradiography with barium swallow	Abnormal swallowing mechanism; aspiration	Dysphagia requires careful attention if aspiration and pneumonia are to be prevented
Affective disorder	History; observation; depression screening test	Symptoms of depression	Depression may impede rehabilitation if it is not treated
Pain	Description of pain by patient; observation of restrictions in range of motion; observation of facial expressions or resistance to movement	Location, severity, and precipitating causes of pain	Pain impedes rehabilitation and may require specific treatment or medication

al neglect (i.e., ignoring one side of the body or failing to be attentive to people and objects on one side of the body) are associated with poorer outcome.[11] The prognosis is also affected by coexisting or associated medical problems, such as delirium and fecal impaction. Simple assessment measures such as the Orpington Prognostic Scale [*see Figure 3*], which contains items for motor function, sensory function, balance, and cognition, can be completed in 5 to 10 minutes and are easily obtained in the first weeks after stroke.[6] The initial Orpington score is a strong predictor of functional status at 3 and 6 months. A score of 2.4 or less, suggesting mild deficits in the first 2 weeks after stroke, is associated with an 80% chance of being independent in personal care and homemaking activities at 6 months, whereas a score of 4.4 or higher, suggesting more severe early deficits, is associated with about a 20% chance of achieving independence in these activities.[12]

KEY ASPECTS OF REHABILITATION

Optimal rehabilitation for stroke starts in the acute care setting. Mobilization and efforts at self-care should be instituted as soon as they are medically feasible. Urinary continence and bladder function programs should be initiated; indwelling catheters should not be used unless they are medically necessary, as in cases of urinary retention or cases involving wounds that must be kept clean. An educational program aimed at informing the patient and the patient's family about

stroke and stroke recovery should be started.

The next stage in rehabilitation is the defining of functional goals on the basis of the patient's own goals, deficits, and potential. Therapies are devised to improve impairments in strength, range of motion, endurance, balance, sensorimotor coordination, and mobility; to facilitate self-care and household maintenance; to relieve pain; and to educate the patient and caregivers on maintaining functional gains. A recent clinical trial comparing an intensive home-based program that included endurance training, strengthening, balance, and upper extremity activities with usual home health care showed greater gains in mobility and neurologic status in the intensive therapy group.[13] High-intensity strength training improves functional performance after stroke.[14] Adaptive devices can help the patient eat, bathe, use the toilet, dress, walk, transfer between the bed and chairs and commode, and engage in leisure activities. Other aspects of treatment include further education and involvement of the patient and family and attention to the emotional and psychological sequelae of stroke.[15,16] Good coordination and communication must be maintained during transitions between rehabilitation settings.

Until recently, there has been little scientific basis for stroke rehabilitation practice. Previously, it was believed that nerve cells were irreplaceable and that their death led inevitably to losses of neurologic function. Recent studies in animal models and in humans demonstrate, however, that after nerve cells die their functions can be taken over by other nerve cells. Thus, after destruction of motor neurons controlling the hand, specific rehabilitation approaches can induce new motor neurons to control hand movement. Neuroplasticity in the adult after neurologic injury has been demonstrated by use of functional magnetic resonance imaging and transcranial magnetic stimulation.[17] The potential for neuroplastic change is revolutionizing approaches to neurologic rehabilitation.[18] Systematic studies of treatment approaches that maximize neural reorganization are under way. One successful approach is based on intensive repetitive practice using rhythm or robot aids for the upper extremity and treadmill training for the lower extremity.[19-23] Another method is to force the use of the damaged extremity by limiting the use of the uninvolved extremity, an approach termed constraint-induced movement therapy.[24]

The potential for neural reorganization is also changing the timing of neurologic rehabilitation. Previously, rehabilitation focused on the immediate poststroke period, because the natural history of recovery suggests that neurologic status plateaus at 6 months after injury. However, recent studies have documented significant gains in function in chronic stroke patients who undergo treatments that focus on repetitive and forced practice.[25-27]

Neuropharmacologic interventions that promote neural reorganization are being studied as a means to enhance neurologic recovery. One area of interest is the use of stimulants such as amphetamines, which have been shown to accelerate motor and sensory recovery in animal models. It is postulated that increased central noradrenergic—rather than serotoninergic or dopaminergic—mechanisms are the neurochemical basis for motor and sensory recovery secondary to treatment with amphetamines. Human studies have been small and have not consistently included a control group, but they have demonstrated enhanced recovery with amphetamines or methylphenidate, with little adverse effect on blood pressure or heart rate in persons with blood pressure under 160/100 at entry.[28-30]

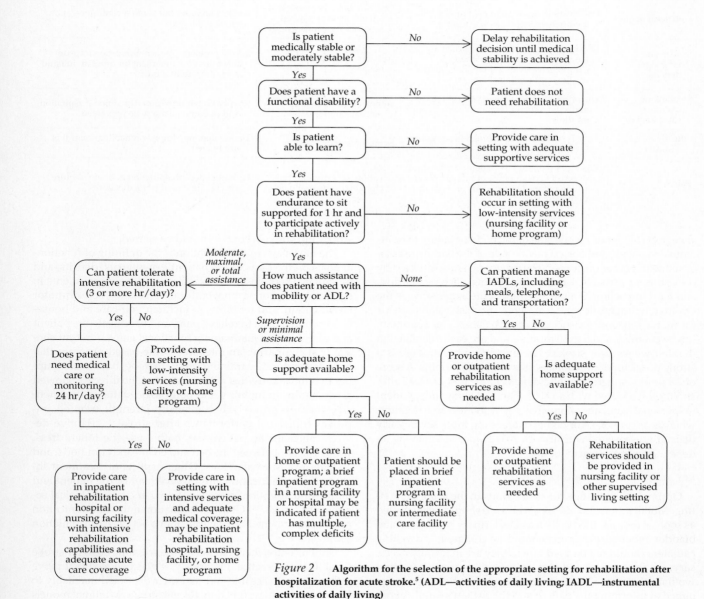

Figure 2   **Algorithm for the selection of the appropriate setting for rehabilitation after hospitalization for acute stroke.[5] (ADL—activities of daily living; IADL—instrumental activities of daily living)**

INSTRUCTIONS: Circle the appropriate response.

A. **Motor deficit in arm**
Lying supine, patient flexes shoulder to 90° and is given resistance.
0.0 = MRC Grade 5   (normal power)
0.4 = MRC Grade 4   (diminished power)
0.8 = MRC Grade 3   (movement against gravity)
1.2 = MRC Grade 1–2 (movement with gravity eliminated or trace)
1.6 = MRC Grade 0   (no movement)

B. **Proprioception (eyes closed)**
Locates affected thumb:
0.0 = Accurately
0.4 = Slight difficulty
0.8 = Finds thumb via arm
1.2 = Unable to find thumb

C. **Balance**
0.0 = Walks 10 ft without help
0.4 = Maintains standing position (unsupported for 1 min)
0.8 = Maintains sitting position
1.2 = No sitting balance

D. **Cognition**
Score 1 point for each correct answer:

_____ 1. Age of patient
_____ 2. Time (to the nearest hour)
          I am going to give you an address, please remember it and
          I will ask you later: *42 West Street*
_____ 3. Name of hospital
_____ 4. Year
_____ 5. Date of birth of patient
_____ 6. Month
_____ 7. Year of the Second World War
_____ 8. Name of the President
_____ 9. Count backwards (20–1)
_____ 10. What is the address I asked you to remember: *42 West Street*

0.0 = Mental test score of 10
0.4 = Mental test score of 8–9
0.8 = Mental test score of 5–7
1.2 = Mental test score of 0–4

TOTAL SCORE:

1.6 + _____ + _____ + _____ + _____ = _____
       Motor   Proprioception   Balance   Cognition

Figure 3   **The Orpington Prognostic Scale is useful for estimating stroke recovery.**[62]

PREVENTING COMPLICATIONS AND FUTURE STROKES

Complications of stroke and other disabling conditions are described [*see Table 2*]. Mobilization of the patient is always preferable to inactivity; when inactivity is inevitable, however, bed exercise and skin care protocols should be instituted. Prevention of deep vein thrombosis during immobilization is a standard component of care after stroke. Low-dose or low-molecular-weight heparin is the preferred treatment, but warfarin, intermittent pneumatic compression, and elastic stockings are acceptable alternatives [*see Chapter 29*].[31]

In patients with a swallowing disorder, long-term enteral feeding and cessation of oral feeding may prevent aspiration; however, this measure is not always effective and has many ethical implications for quality of life. Incontinence may be exacerbated by one or more factors: a mobility problem that prevents the patient from getting to the bathroom, constipation, a urinary tract infection, or drug-induced urinary retention.[32] Stroke can cause an uninhibited bladder, characterized by frequent episodes of urgency and incontinence. Treatment with bladder relaxants may help, but these drugs can worsen confusion.

Seizures can occur at any time after a stroke as a result of the presence of scarred brain tissue, which serves as a focus of irritation. Standard anticonvulsants are indicated. Major depression occurs in at least one third of patients after stroke. The guidelines for poststroke rehabilitation emphasize the need for screening for and treatment of this commonly overlooked complication.[5] Increased socialization, counseling, and medication are appropriate. Cognitive impairment caused by poststroke depression may improve with treatment of the depression.[33] Medications that cause less sedation and fewer anticholinergic side effects, such as most selective serotonin reuptake inhibitors or low-level anticholinergic tricyclic antidepressants such as nortriptyline, are preferred. Methylphenidate, given in the morning and at noon, can reduce apathy and increase motivation early in poststroke rehabilitation and has a rapid onset of effect [see Table 3].

Shoulder pain and dislocation are especially likely in the patient with a flaccid upper extremity, because the joint capsule is normally stabilized by the surrounding muscles. Prevention of dislocation includes supporting the shoulder in a normal position, using a pull sheet rather than the underarm to reposition the patient in bed, and restricting range of motion to 90° of flexion and abduction. Reflex sympathetic dystrophy (chronic regional pain syndrome) occurs in as many as 25% of patients with hemiplegia. Early signs are exquisite cutaneous sensitivity and diffuse swelling of the hands. Treatment includes the use of compression gloves, anti-inflammatory agents, steroids, analgesics, injections for sympathetic nerve blockade, and, most important, aggressive and consistent range-of-motion exercises.[34]

Stroke recurs in 7% to 10% of survivors every year. Screening and intervention to prevent recurrence must be considered in all patients except, perhaps, those with severe brain damage.[35] Carotid endarterectomy may be indicated if stenosis of 70% or more is detected in a vessel that feeds a large area of viable brain tissue. Anticoagulation with warfarin in patients with atrial fibrillation significantly reduces risk of stroke. In one meta-analysis, only one third as many strokes occurred in patients receiving warfarin as occurred in control subjects.[35] Warfarin therapy is the standard of care for patients with atrial fib-

rillation in the absence of an increased risk of bleeding or falls. For an acceptable risk-to-benefit ratio, the international normalized ratio (INR) should be maintained at 2.0 to 3.0. Antiplatelet agents such as aspirin, ticlopidine, clopidogrel, and combinations of aspirin and dipyramidole can be used instead of warfarin. Control of hypertension and hyperlipidemia and smoking cessation reduce the risk of stroke.

Amputation and Peripheral Vascular Disease

SELECTING CANDIDATES FOR PROSTHESES

About 50,000 lower extremity amputations are performed each year in the United States. In the past, most amputations were performed because of trauma; today, as many as 90% are performed because of peripheral vascular disease. Lower extremity ischemia often occurs in the setting of widespread atherosclerosis, which includes cerebrovascular, cardiovascular, and renovascular disease. Patients with diabetes are at increased risk for amputation because of vascular disease, peripheral neuropathy that causes the feet to become insensitive, and an increased vulnerability to infection. Thus, the candidate for amputation is very likely to have potentially disabling comorbid conditions.[16]

Candidates for whom prosthetic rehabilitation is successful generally are ambulatory before undergoing amputation, can bear weight on the contralateral leg, have stabilized medical conditions, and are able to follow the caregiver's instructions. In patients with prostheses, the presence of a natural knee joint significantly reduces the energy cost of walking; therefore,

Table 2   Assessment and Management of Complications of Stroke and Other Disabling Conditions[5]

Complication	Cause	Assessment	Intervention
Pressure sores	Immobility, malnutrition, incontinence	Monitor skin over pressure sites	Mobilize patient; provide protective bedding and pads; keep skin dry; maintain good nutrition and local skin care
Deep vein thrombosis	Inactivity, loss of muscle pump action in calf	Look for swelling and pain in leg; frequently, however, there are no findings	Prevent with low-dose or low-molecular-weight heparin
Swallowing disorders	Cranial nerve dysfunction	Observe swallowing; listen for hoarse, wet voice; perform cineradiography	Reposition patient; alter food consistency; suggest chewing adaptations; switch to enteral feeding
Incontinence	Mobility problems, infection, impaction, drug side effects, urinary retention, outlet obstruction	Assess frequency and volume of incontinent episodes; assess postvoiding residual volume and ability to get to toilet; perform urinalysis and rectal examination; monitor drugs	Treat superimposed problems; institute toileting program; give oxybutynin for uninhibited bladder
Depression	Local brain effects, sensory isolation, situational factors	Administer depression screens	Give antidepressants
Shoulder pain	Loss of muscle tone around the shoulder, poor repositioning technique	Monitor symptoms and shoulder stability	Use careful positioning technique; give analgesics; conduct ROM exercises
Contractures	Increased muscle tone, immobility	Look for brisk DTRs, clonus, reduced ROM of joints	Conduct ROM exercises; use appropriate braces, heat/cold modalities, antispasticity drugs (baclofen), motor point blocks, botulinum injections, serial casting
Deconditioning	Immobility, depression, malnutrition	Test for reduced endurance and orthostatic hypotension; look for lack of motivation and poor exercise tolerance	Mobilize patient; conduct graded exercise program with scheduled rest breaks
Secondary osteoporosis	Dietary factors, smoking, immobility, medication	Test functional status; perform the following laboratory tests: vitamin D level, CBC, TFT, PTH level, 24 hr urine; measure bone mass	Modify diet; begin hormone therapy; conduct weight-bearing exercises and mobilize patient
Obesity	Dietary factors, immobility	> 20% of ideal body weight	Institute aerobic program; modify diet

CBC—complete blood count   DTR—deep tendon reflex   PTH—parathyroid hormone   ROM—range of motion   TFT—thyroid function test

Table 3 Pharmacologic Therapy for Poststroke Depression

Drug Class	Drug Name	Initial Dose	Maintenance Dose	Controlled Trial Evidence in Stroke	Side Effects	Advantages	Comments
Heterocyclics	Nortriptyline	10–25 mg	25–100 mg	Yes	Sedation, orthostasis	Blood levels measurable; goal, 50–150 ng/ml	—
	Desipramine	10 mg	25–100 mg	No	Orthostasis	Less sedation; blood levels measurable; goal, 125–300 ng/ml	—
	Trazodone	25–50 mg	25–200 mg	Yes	Hypotension; sedation	Useful in sleep disturbance	—
Selective serotonin reuptake inhibitors	Fluoxetine	5–10 mg	5–60 mg	No	Nausea; tremor; insomnia	Long half-life	Morning dosing
	Sertraline	25 mg	—	No	Nausea; tremor; insomnia	Few drug interactions; not sedating	Morning dosing
	Citalopram	10 mg	20–40 mg	Yes	Nausea; tremor	Few drug interactions	Morning dosing
	Paroxetine	5–10 mg	5–40 mg	No	Nausea; tremor	Mild sedation	Evening dosing
Stimulants	Methylphenidate	2.5 mg morning and noon	5–30 mg	Yes	Nervousness; insomnia; anorexia	Rapid onset; useful in early period for treatment of apathy	Recommended for short-term use during rehabilitation only; change to other preparation for long-term use

every effort should be made to preserve the joint by performing a below-the-knee procedure, even though this procedure is associated with a higher risk of poor wound healing than above-the-knee amputation. The prognosis for successful prosthetic ambulation is best for patients who undergo unilateral below-the-knee amputation. Patients who undergo a second amputation or those in whom other major disabling conditions develop are most likely to regain the ability to walk if they were able to walk after the initial amputation. Older patients who undergo bilateral above-the-knee amputation rarely learn to walk with prostheses.

KEY ASPECTS OF REHABILITATION

Rehabilitation comprises three phases: preoperative preparation, postoperative wound healing, and prosthetic ambulation. Before undergoing amputation, the patient should be educated about the healing and mobilization process and be prepared for life as an amputee. After surgery, measures that promote proper wound healing should be instituted and the stump prepared for weight bearing and mobilization. Traditionally, weight bearing on the residual limb was discouraged until full healing took place; this sometimes resulted in prolonged inactivity for the patient. This practice is now changing: earlier mobilization using a rigid, removable dressing and sometimes a temporary artificial leg can simultaneously protect the fragile healing tissues and prevent the complications caused by prolonged immobility.[36]

Successful prosthetic ambulation depends on selection of an appropriate device, progressive mobilization, and management of concurrent problems. The permanent prosthesis for an older adult must be lightweight and easy to put on and take off. A comfortable prosthesis fits snugly and has one or more liners, socks, sleeves, or removable attachments. There are many options available for the components (materials, feet, and suspensions) of prostheses. The primary care physician should form a relationship with a reputable prosthetist who can integrate the technical issues involved in designing a prosthesis with the medical and functional status of the older amputee. The prosthetic limb should be adapted to existing comorbidity; for example, patients with congestive heart failure or advanced renal disease often have wide variations in limb edema that must be accommodated by altering the size of the socket and by use of fillers. Progressive mobilization is accomplished by gradually lengthening the period during which the prosthesis is worn and changing the means of external support from parallel bars to walker to cane. Because increasing activity affects diabetes control, salt and water balance, myocardial oxygen demand, and local weight-bearing tissues, the physician should monitor the patient's glucose levels, weight, orthostatic blood pressure, and anginal symptoms, adjusting therapy as needed. The stump must be examined for signs of skin breakdown, edema, and infection.

PREVENTING COMPLICATIONS AND FUTURE AMPUTATIONS

About 25% of patients who undergo unilateral amputation because of peripheral vascular disease and 50% of patients who undergo the procedure because of diabetes will need to have the other leg amputated within 5 years.[37] Care of the contralateral extremity is essential; each amputee should have a program of regular foot care, should check for foot lesions, and should practice control of peripheral vascular disease. Footwear should protect and support the foot. Shoes should be wide at the toe and very roomy and should have cushioned soles or inserts. Many athletic shoes meet these criteria. Mea-

Internet Resources Relevant to Geriatric Rehabilitation

National Stroke Association
www.stroke.org

American Heart Association/American Stroke Association
www.americanheart.org

Stroke Toolbox
www2.kumc.edu/coa

National Institute of Neurological Disorders
www.ninds.nih.gov/health_and_medical/disorders/stroke.htm

Stroke Clubs International
www.strokeclub@aol.com

National Aphasia Association
www.aphasia.org

Falls and hip fracture prevention
www.cdc.gov/health/diseases.htm

Home safety for elders
www.safehomes4elderly.com

NIH Osteoporosis and Related Bone Diseases National Resources Center Falls and Fracture Prevention
www.osteo.org/newsvol2no1.html

Exercise for total hip replacement
www.orthoinfo.aaos.org

Missouri Arthritis Rehabilitation Research and Training Center
www.hsc.missouri.edu/arthritis

Resources for rehabilitation booklets for seniors
www.rfr.org

National Institute of Arthritis and Musculoskeletal and Skin Diseases
www.nih.gov/niams

sures used to control vascular disease include cessation of smoking, control of diabetes, management of cholesterol levels, and a program of exercise of the lower extremity.[38] The role of angioplasty in reducing the need for amputation is unclear.[39]

Hip Fracture

CONSEQUENCES OF HIP FRACTURE

Each year in the United States, hip fracture occurs in about 250,000 persons, of whom 75% are women. Age-adjusted rates of hip fracture are higher in nursing home residents and patients with dementia.

Hip fracture in elderly patients results in increased mortality and loss of functional independence. One-year mortality is 20%.[40] In those who survive, early decline in function is common[21]; up to 50% require temporary nursing home stays. Although most survivors return to their original functional status within 1 year, about 25% still require long-term care.[41]

TYPES OF HIP FRACTURE AND REPAIR

Hip fractures occur at the femoral neck in about one third of cases. Such fractures are likely to disrupt the blood supply to the femoral head, particularly if the fractures are displaced; this in turn may lead to avascular necrosis or nonunion. Nondisplaced fractures of the femoral neck are usually treated by internal fixation with pins or nails, whereas displaced fractures may be treated either by reduction and fixation or by hemiarthroplasty with a prosthetic femoral head. Selected patients with significant underlying bony acetabular disease may benefit from complete hip arthroplasty for displaced fracture of the femoral neck.

Two thirds of hip fractures occur across the trochanter. Intertrochanteric fractures are often associated with significant bleeding into the surrounding soft tissue. Surgical treatment usually consists of open reduction and internal fixation with a variety of mechanisms, such as compression screws or sliding nails.

Preoperative stabilization of concurrent medical problems and early surgical intervention is usually recommended. Complications such as deep vein thrombosis, pneumonia, pressure sores, urinary tract infection, malnutrition, delirium, and deconditioning should be prevented or treated.[42] Delirium has been shown to be an independent predictor of poor outcome at 1 year after injury.[43]

KEY ASPECTS OF REHABILITATION

Rehabilitation should be offered to all patients in the absence of near-terminal conditions or possibly to bedridden patients with end-stage dementia. Such patients may be treated nonsurgically with early mobilization from bed to chair, control of pain, and treatment of complications. Patients with mild to moderate dementia can benefit from rehabilitation after fracture.[44,45]

After hip fracture, the care setting may not influence outcome as much as it does in stroke; in an observational study, settings involving intensive rehabilitation did not achieve better outcomes than subacute programs.[46] Well-defined home-based programs can be effective.[47] Coordinated multidisciplinary approaches to inpatient rehabilitation of older patients have been found to have borderline effectiveness, with about a 10% reduction in combined outcomes such as death or institutionalization.[48] Early intervention with early surgery, minimal narcotic analgesia, intense daily therapy, and multidisciplinary management reduced length of stay without affecting function or survival.[49]

The goal of rehabilitation is to regain prefracture function. Short-term goals include pain control, prevention of medical complications, maintenance of range of motion and muscle strength in other joints, early mobilization, and gradual improvement in the movement of the affected hip. Early mobilization reduces all the complications of immobility, including bedsores, constipation, loss of strength, and risk of thromboembolism. If a prosthetic femoral head is placed by the posterior approach, the risk of dislocation is reduced by the intentional limitation of hip motion to 90° of flexion, with no internal rotation and no adduction. Shortening of the affected leg can occur after fracture, resulting in an abnormal gait, which can be corrected with shoe lifts.

Weight bearing after hip fracture is controversial. Surgical factors and surgeons' preferences affect recommendations. Pain, the hazards of inactivity, and the practical difficulties in limiting weight bearing must also be considered. Early mobilization with unrestricted weight bearing after hip fracture results in mild spontaneous weight shifting and accelerates hospital discharge without adversely affecting healing.[50,51] A synthesis of clinical trials comparing mobilization strategies after hip fracture, including twice-daily physical therapy, treadmill training, neuromuscular stimulation, and early mobilization, found no significant effects on the outcomes assessed.[52]

Pharmacologic approaches to improving rehabilitation outcomes are also being applied in hip fracture. A recent clinical trial of human growth hormone in the immediate postfracture phase demonstrated reduced functional decline and increased rates of return to independent living in the subset of patients older than 75 years.[53] These results have not been replicated.

PREVENTING FUTURE FRACTURES

Efforts should be made to prevent future fractures. Preventive practices include treatment of osteoporosis [*see Chapter 52*], evaluation and management of falling, and instruction on how to avoid injury in the event of a fall.[42] Higher levels of physical activity have been shown to be associated with lower rates of hip fracture in epidemiologic and case-control studies. As yet, no prospective, randomized clinical trials of physical activity as a preventive approach to hip fracture have been carried out. Hip protectors have been shown to significantly reduce the incidence of hip fracture.[54]

Rheumatoid Arthritis

Management of rheumatoid arthritis involves pain relief, preservation of strength and joint function, and prevention of deformities [*see Chapter 112*]. Patients with arthritis can safely participate in exercise programs and often experience relief of pain and of disability as a result.[55]

Arthroplasty

Each year, over 100,000 Americans undergo total hip replacement (THR) and over 50,000 have a total knee replacement (TKR). Joint replacement should be considered in persons with structural damage to the joint who experience pain and loss of function despite nonsurgical management. Most candidates have osteoarthritis, are older than 60 years, and often have multiple other medical conditions.

Surgical interventions for uncontrolled knee pain and mobility limitation include lavage with or without debridement, osteotomy, and knee replacement. Lavage can produce significant temporary relief. Osteotomy is preferred in active persons younger than 60 years. Knee replacement can be total or limited to one compartment. Joint replacement relieves pain and improves function in most patients. Joint replacement in selected persons older than 80 years does not increase complication rates or length of stay and leads to greatly reduced pain and increased function. A retrospective cohort study included only patients who received THR, and thus, it is likely that a high degree of selection bias occurred. Nonetheless, the increasing population of persons older than 80 years who are in good health with stable chronic conditions appear to have a tolerable surgical risk; therefore, age alone should not be used as a criterion for eligibility for THR.[56]

KEY ASPECTS OF REHABILITATION

Hip

Good pain control and anticoagulation with warfarin to prevent thrombosis are the major goals of the immediate THR postoperative period. Weight bearing often begins on the second postoperative day. The rehabilitation program emphasizes progressive range of motion, strengthening, and gait training. Hip abductors, which are often weak as a direct result of surgery, are a focus of the strengthening program. Patients are taught to avoid motions that increase risk of dislocation; such motions include deep squatting and crossing the knees. A raised toilet seat is recommended for use during the first months after surgery to prevent excess hip flexion. The appropriate site and the duration of rehabilitative services are determined on the basis of medical and functional status as well as on the availability of caregivers. Many low-risk patients can be discharged from the acute care hospital within 5 days.[57] Patients at higher risk (i.e., those older than 70 years or those with two or more comorbid conditions) can benefit from inpatient rehabilitation beginning as early as the third postoperative day and can experience faster recovery of mobility and reduced total length of stay.[58]

Knee

Initial goals after TKR are pain control, wound drainage, and joint stabilization. The patient is usually allowed to bear weight with a straight leg by the second postoperative day. Improved range of motion is a critical step in recovery and is often aided by the use of a continuous passive motion (CPM) machine. Early postoperative CPM has been shown to be more effective than physical therapy alone in reducing flexion contracture and shortening length of stay. Therapy with the CPM machine involves a gradually increasing passive range of motion in the operated knee over a period of several days. Good recovery of knee motion is represented by full extension and at least 90° of flexion. Home CPM produced satisfactory range of motion at about half the cost of home physical therapy in a recent clinical trial.[59] Strength training is often deferred for several weeks to promote stable healing of tissues. Isometric and resistive exercise with gradually increasing loads generally can be introduced safely by 8 weeks after surgery. Low-risk TKR patients appear to do well with discharge from acute care on the fourth postoperative day, and high-risk patients benefit from early transfer to intensive rehabilitation.[57,58] Long-term outcomes include significant relief of pain and improved function,[60] although many patients do not achieve levels of strength or mobility comparable to those of age-matched control subjects.[61]

Additional Information

Additional information on topics that are discussed in this chapter can be found at various Internet sites [*see Sidebar* Internet Resources Relevant to Geriatric Rehabilitation].

References

1. Liu K, Gage B, Harvell J, et al: Medicare's post-acute care benefit: background, trends, and issues to be faced. Department of Health and Human Services Assistant Secretary for Planning and Evaluation, Office of Disability, Aging, and Long-Term Care Policy, January 1999

2. Hoenig H, Nusbaum N, Brummel-Smith K: Geriatric rehabilitation: state of the art. J Am Geriatr Soc 45:1371, 1997

3. ICIDH-2. International Classification of Functioning, Disability and Health. Classification, Assessment, Surveys and Terminology Team, World Health Organization, Geneva, Switzerland, December 2000

4. Siebens H, Aronow H, Edwards D, et al: A randomized controlled trial of exercise to improve outcomes of acute hospitalization in older adults. J Am Geriatr Soc 48:1545, 2000

5. Gresham GE, Duncan PW, Stason WB, et al: Post-stroke rehabilitation (Clinical Practice Guideline, No. 16). US Dept of Health and Human Services, Public Health Service, Agency for Health Care Policy and Research (AHCPR Publication No. 95-0662), Rockville, Maryland, May 1995

6. Duncan PW, Lai SM, van Culin V, et al: Development of a comprehensive assessment toolbox for stroke. Clin Geriatr Med 15:885, 1999

7. Kramer AM, Kowalsky JC, Lin M, et al: Outcome and utilization differences for older persons with stroke in HMO and fee-for-service systems. J Am Geriatr Soc 48:726, 2000

8. Kane RL, Chen Q, Finch M, et al: Functional outcomes of posthospital care for stroke and hip fracture patients under Medicare. J Am Geriatr Soc 46:1525, 1998

9. Kane RL, Chen Q, Finch M, et al: The optimal outcomes of post-hospital care under Medicare. Health Serv Res 35:615, 2000

10. Langhorne P, Duncan P: Does the organization of postacute stroke care really matter? Stroke 32:268, 2001

11. Galski T, Bruno RL, Zorowitz R, et al: Predicting length of stay, functional outcome, and aftercare in the rehabilitation of stroke patients: the dominant role of higher-order cognition. Stroke 24:1794, 1993

12. Studenski S, Wallace D, Duncan PW, et al: Predicting stroke recovery: three- and six-month rates of patient-centered functional outcomes based on the Orpington Prognostic Scale. J Am Geriatr Soc 49:308, 2001

13. Duncan P, Richards L, Wallace D, et al: A randomized, controlled pilot study of a home-based exercise program for individuals with mild and moderate stroke. Stroke 29:2055, 1998

14. Weiss A, Suzuki T, Bean J, et al: High intensity strength training improves strength and functional performance after stroke. Am J Phys Med Rehabil 79:369, 2000

15. Evans RL, Hendricks RD, Haselkorn JK, et al: The family's role in stroke rehabilitation: a review of the literature. Am J Phys Med Rehabil 71:135, 1992

16. Downhill JE Jr, Robinson RG: Longitudinal assessment of depression and cognitive impairment following stroke. J Nerv Ment Dis 182:425, 1994

17. Liepert J, Bauder H, Wolfgang HR, et al: Treatment-induced cortical reorganization after stroke in humans. Stroke 31:1210, 2000

18. Cramer SC: Stroke recovery. Lessons from functional MR imaging and other human brain mapping. Phys Med Rehabil Clin N Am 10:875, 1999

19. Feys HM, De Weerdt WJ, Selz BE, et al: Effect of a therapeutic intervention for the hemiplegic upper limb in the acute phase after stroke: a single-blind, randomized controlled clinical trial. Stroke 29:785, 1998

20. Volpe BT, Krebs HI, Hogan N, et al: A novel approach to stroke rehabilitation: robot aided sensorimotor stimulation. Neurology 54:1938, 2000

21. Krebs HI, Hogan N, Volpe BT, et al: Overview of clinical trials with MIT-MANUS: a robot-aided neuro-rehabilitation facility. Technol Health Care 7:419, 1999

22. Visintin M, Barbeau H, Korner-Bitensky N, et al: A new approach to retrain gait in stroke patients through body weight support and treadmill stimulation. Stroke 29:1122, 1998

23. Hesse S, Konrad M, Uhlenbrock D: Treadmill walking with partial body weight support versus floor walking in hemiparetic subjects. Arch Phys Med Rehabil 80:421, 1999

24. Dromerick AW, Edwards DF, Hahn M: Does the application of constraint-induced movement therapy during rehabilitation reduce arm impairment after ischemic stroke? Stroke 31:2984, 2000

25. Taub E, Miller NE, Novack TA, et al: Technique to improve chronic motor deficit after stroke. Arch Phys Med Rehabil 74:347, 1993

26. Whitall J, McCombe Waller S, Silver KH, et al: Repetitive bilateral arm training with rhythmic auditory cueing improves motor function in chronic hemiparetic stroke. Stroke 31:2390, 2000

27. van der Lee JH, Wagenaar RC, Lankhorst GJ, et al: Forced use of the upper extremity in chronic stroke patients: results of a single-blind randomized clinical trial. Stroke 30:2369, 1999

28. Grade C, Redford B, Chrostowski J, et al: Methylphenidate in early poststroke recovery: double-blind, placebo-controlled study. Arch Phys Med Rehabil 79:1047, 1998

29. Goldstein LB: Effects of amphetamines and small related molecules on recovery after stroke in animals and man. Neuropharmacology 39:852, 2000

30. Gladstone DJ, Black SE: Enhancing recovery after stroke with noradrenergic pharmacotherapy: a new frontier? Can J Neurol Sci 27:97, 2000

31. Kamran SI, Downey D, Ruff RL: Pneumatic sequential compression reduces the risk of deep vein thrombosis in stroke patients. Neurology 50:1683, 1998

32. Gelber DA, Good DC, Laven LJ, et al: Causes of urinary incontinence after acute hemispheric stroke. Stroke 24:378, 1993

33. Kimura M, Robinson RG, Kosier JT: Treatment of cognitive impairment after poststroke depression: a double-blind treatment trial. Stroke 31:1482, 2000

34. Stanton-Hicks M, Janig W, Hassenbusch S, et al: Reflex sympathetic dystrophy: changing concepts and taxonomy. Pain 63:127, 1995

35. Matchar DB, McCrory DC, Barnett HJM, et al: Medical treatment for stroke prevention. Ann Intern Med 121:41, 1994

36. Cutson T, Bongiorni D: Rehabilitation of the older lower limb amputee: a brief review. J Am Geriatr Soc 44:1388, 1996

37. Coletta EM: Care of the elderly patient with lower extremity amputation. J Am Board Fam Pract 13:23, 2000

38. Gardner AW, Poehlman ET: Exercise rehabilitation programs for the treatment of claudication pain: a meta-analysis. JAMA 274:975, 1995

39. Tunis SR, Bass EB, Steinberg EP: The use of angioplasty, bypass surgery, and amputation in the management of peripheral vascular disease. N Engl J Med 325:556, 1991

40. Parker MJ, Palmer CR: Prediction of rehabilitation after hip fracture. Age Ageing 24:96, 1995

41. Egol KA, Koval KJ, Zuckerman JD: Functional recovery following hip fracture in the elderly. J Orthop Trauma 11:594, 1997

42. Morrison RS, Chassin MR, Siu AL: The medical consultant's role in caring for patients with hip fracture. Ann Intern Med 128:1010, 1998

43. Dolan MM, Hawkes WG, Zimmerman SI, et al: Delirium on hospital admission in aged hip fracture patients: prediction of mortality and 2-year functional outcomes. J Gerontol A Biol Sci Med Sci 55:M527, 2000

44. Goldstein FC, Strasser DC, Woodard JL, et al: Functional outcome of cognitively impaired hip fracture patients on a geriatric rehabilitation unit. J Am Geriatr Soc 45:35, 1997

45. Huusko TM, Karppi P, Avikainen V, et al: Randomised, clinically controlled trial of intensive geriatric rehabilitation in patients with hip fracture: subgroup analysis of patients with dementia. BMJ 321:1107, 2000

46. Kramer AM, Steiner JF, Schlenker RE, et al: Outcomes and costs after hip fracture and stroke. JAMA 277:396, 1997

47. Tinetti ME, Baker DI, Gottschalk M, et al: Systematic home-based physical and functional therapy for older persons after hip fracture. Arch Phys Med Rehabil 78:1237, 1997

48. Cameron ID, Handoll HH, Finnegan TP, et al: Co-ordinated multidisciplinary approaches for inpatient rehabilitation of older patients with proximal femoral fracture. Cochrane Database Syst Rev 4:CD000106, 2000

49. Swanson CE, Day GA, Yelland CE, et al: The management of elderly patients with femoral fractures: a randomised controlled trial of early intervention versus standard care. Med J Aust 169:515, 1998

50. Koval KJ, Friend KD, Aharonoff GB, et al: Weight bearing after hip fracture: a prospective series of 596 geriatric hip fracture patients. J Orthop Trauma 10:526, 1996

51. Koval KJ, Sala DA, Kummer FJ, et al: Postoperative weight-bearing after a fracture of the femoral neck or an intertrochanteric fracture. J Bone Joint Surg Am 80:352, 1998

52. Parker MJ, Handoll HH, Dynan Y: Mobilisation strategies after hip fracture surgery in adults. Cochrane Database Syst Rev 3:CD001704, 2000

53. Van Der Lely AJ, Lamberts SW, Jauch KW, et al: Use of human GH in elderly patients with accidental hip fracture. Eur J Endocrinol 143:585, 2000

54. Kannus P, Parkkari J, Niemi S, et al: Prevention of hip fracture in elderly people with use of a hip protector. N Engl J Med 343:1506, 2000

55. Ettinger WH Jr: Physical activity, arthritis, and disability in older people. Clin Geriatr Med 14:633, 1998

56. Brander VA, Malhotra S, Jet J, et al: Outcome of hip and knee arthroplasty in persons aged 80 and over. Clin Orthop 345:67, 1997

57. Weingarten S, Riedinger MS, Sandhu M, et al: Can practice guidelines safely reduce hospital length of stay? Results from a multicenter interventional study. Am J Med 105:33, 1998

58. Munin MC, Rudy TE, Glynn NW, et al: Early inpatient rehabilitation after elective hip and knee arthroplasty. JAMA 279:847, 1998

59. Worland RL, Arredondo J, Angles F, et al: Home continuous passive motion machine versus professional physical therapy following total knee replacement. J Arthroplasty 13:784, 1998

60. Hawker G, Wright J, Coyte P, et al: Health-related quality of life after knee replacement. J Bone Joint Surg Am 80:163, 1998

61. Walsh M, Woodhouse LJ, Thomas SG, et al: Physical impairments and functional limitations: a comparison of individuals 1 year after total knee arthroplasty with control subjects. Phys Ther 78:248, 1998

62. Lai S, Duncan PW, Keighley J: Prediction of functional outcome after stroke. Stroke 29:1838, 1998

Acknowledgment

Figure 2 Marcia Kammerer.

GYNECOLOGY AND WOMEN'S HEALTH

76 Amenorrhea

Robert L. Barbieri, M.D.

The menstrual cycle is orchestrated through the interaction of the hypothalamus, pituitary gland, ovaries, and uterus. The hypothalamus secretes gonadotropin-releasing hormone (GnRH), which stimulates the pituitary to secrete luteinizing hormone (LH) and follicle-stimulating hormone (FSH). LH and FSH stimulate follicular growth, ovulation, corpus luteum formation, and the secretion of estradiol and progesterone by the ovaries, which leads to the cyclic growth and shedding of the uterine endometrium. At the endometrial level, the menstrual cycle has three key phases: estradiol stimulates endometrial growth, progesterone induces differentiation of the endometrium, and withdrawal of estradiol and progesterone results in sloughing of the endometrium and menstrual bleeding.

Failure of any part of this process can result in the absence of menstruation. A girl may not start to menstruate when she reaches puberty (primary amenorrhea); or as is far more common, a woman who has been menstruating may have her cycles cease (secondary amenorrhea).

Pathophysiology

The hypothalamus contains approximately 10,000 GnRH-secreting neurons that drive the menstrual cycle by secreting pulses of GnRH. The embryonic precursors of the GnRH neurons develop in the olfactory bulb and migrate to the arcuate and preoptic nuclei. Improper development of the olfactory bulb in early embryogenesis can result in both anosmia and amenorrhea because of the absence of the GnRH neurons (Kallman syndrome).

The main function of the GnRH neurons is to receive neural signals from the brain and transform them into an endocrine output, the pulsatile release of GnRH. This conversion of electrical signal into endocrine output takes place in the arcuate nucleus. To determine the appropriate pulse frequency and amplitude of GnRH secretion, the hypothalamus monitors numerous environmental cues, including body composition, stress, nutritional status, and emotion. From a teleologic perspective, it is inefficient to ovulate and reproduce if the environment is hostile to the nurturing of a newborn.

The hypothalamus is the conductor that sets the tempo for the menstrual cycle. When the hypothalamus secretes GnRH at a low pulse frequency and amplitude, the pituitary gland is not driven to secrete LH and FSH, so the ovary and endometrium become quiescent. This causes amenorrhea. When the hypothalamus secretes GnRH at an abnormally elevated pulse frequency and amplitude, there is an exaggerated secretion of LH, causing the ovary to become androgenic and secrete testosterone. Follicular growth is blocked and no ovulation occurs. This results in the polycystic ovary syndrome (PCOS), which can be associated with oligomenorrhea or amenorrhea.

The pituitary gland is the main link between the brain and ovarian function. Secretion of the gonadotropins LH and FSH by the pituitary gland is not only stimulated by GnRH from the hypothalamus but also modulated by the negative feedback of steroid and protein hormones from the ovaries, especially estradiol, progesterone, and inhibin A and B [*see Figure 1*]. Estradiol

and inhibin A are secreted by growing follicles and the corpus luteum. Inhibin B is secreted by the small antral follicles and growing follicles. Progestersone is secreted by the corpus luteum.

The follicle is the functional unit of the ovary. At puberty, the ovary contains approximately 300,000 follicles, of which only a few hundred will be ovulated in the woman's lifetime. The follicle has three components: an outer shell of thecal cells that respond to LH and secrete the androgen precursor androstenedione; an inner cell mass of granulosa cells that respond to FSH by converting androstenedione to estradiol; and, at the center of the follicle, the oocyte [*see Figure 2*]. Resting fol-

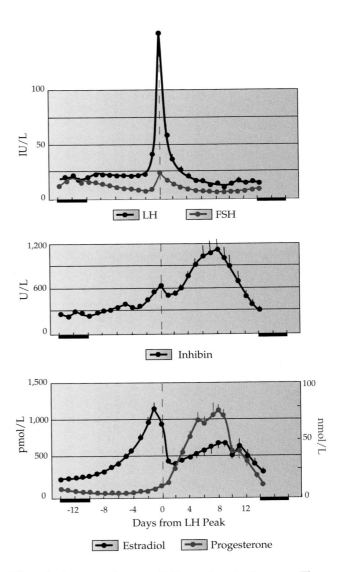

Figure 1 **Interaction between pituitary and ovarian hormones. The surge of luteinizing hormone (LH) and follicle-stimulating hormone (FSH), which prompts ovulation, is followed by an increase in inhibin and progesterone secretion and a decrease in estradiol.**[28]

947

licles are recruited into a cohort of active follicles, only one of which will be destined to ovulate each cycle; the remainder undergo atresia. Under FSH stimulation, granulosa cell numbers increase dramatically, from approximately 10 cells in the primordial follicle to approximately 50 million cells in the preovulatory dominant follicle. The dominant follicle, which is the one destined to ovulate, can be identified early in its development by three characteristics: it has captured large amounts of FSH in its follicular fluid, it has the optimal number of granulosa cells for its size, and it produces much more estradiol than testosterone. Excess stimulation by LH results in an androgen-dominant follicle, which is characterized by thecal cell overactivity and a preference to produce testosterone over estradiol. In PCOS, the ovary contains many androgen-dominant follicles that do not have the potential to ovulate.

The purpose of the menstrual cycle is to generate a single oocyte for fertilization and to prepare the endometrium for implantation. Estradiol stimulates endometrial proliferation, gland formation, and vascular growth in the endometrium. When stimulated by estradiol, the endometrium increases production of its own intracellular estrogen receptors, which augment its response to estradiol; it also produces more progesterone receptors. After ovulation, progesterone causes gland development and differentiation of the endometrium; in addition, glycogen is stored in preparation for embryo implantation. If pregnancy does not occur, the decline in ovarian production of estradiol and progesterone causes vasospasm of the endometrial blood vessels and sloughing of the endometrium, resulting in menstrual bleeding.

Abnormalities in GnRH secretion, LH or FSH secretion, ovarian follicular function, or endometrial function can cause amenorrhea or oligomenorrhea. In a given patient, the differential diagnosis—and hence the evaluation—depends on whether the amenorrhea is secondary or primary.

Secondary Amenorrhea

Secondary, or adult-onset, amenorrhea is present when a woman who had been menstruating has no menses for longer than three of her previous cycles, or 6 months. Determining the cause of secondary amenorrhea starts with measuring serum levels of human chorionic gonadotropin (hCG), prolactin, FSH, and testosterone and calculating the body mass index (BMI) [see Figure 3].

The most common cause of secondary amenorrhea is pregnancy. Pregnancy is best diagnosed by measuring the serum or urine hCG level. The hCG pregnancy test is one of the most accurate in medicine, with a sensitivity and specificity exceeding 99%.

In women who are not pregnant, the most common causes of secondary amenorrhea are as follows: hypothalamic dysfunction (low GnRH pulse frequency, amplitude, or both), pituitary dysfunction (low LH and FSH production), loss of all ovarian follicles (ovarian failure), PCOS, Asherman syndrome (intrauterine adhesions), and thyroid disease [see Table 1].[1]

AMENORRHEA CAUSED BY HYPOTHALAMIC DYSFUNCTION

Low GnRH Secretion

Low BMI, vigorous exercise, psychosocial stress, and nutritional abnormalities decrease GnRH production. This reduces LH and FSH secretion and can cause amenorrhea.

Diagnosis The patient typically has a history of regular vigorous exercise, psychosocial stress, or reduced caloric intake. On physical examination, the BMI is often less than 20 kg/m^2 [see Figure 4]. Serum FSH, prolactin, and testosterone levels are usually reported as normal in women with secondary amenorrhea caused by low GnRH secretion. Women with secondary amenorrhea from hypothalamic hypofunction should be screened for eating disorders; the prevalence of eating disorders in this population is 5% to 10%. Rarely, hypothalamic dysfunction can be caused by structural abnormalities of the hypothalamus, including lymphoma, histiocytosis X, sarcoidosis, and hypothalamic cysts.

The absence of menses in association with hypothalamic hypofunction suggests severe estrogen deficiency, although varying degrees of hypoestrogenism may be present. The severity of the hypoestrogenism can be tested by performing a progestin withdrawal test [see Figure 5].[2] Serum estradiol assays are not sufficiently accurate for this purpose. Women with amenorrhea resulting from hypothalamic hypofunction often have triiodothyronine (T$_3$) levels less than 70 ng/dl, reverse T$_3$ levels greater than 40 ng/dl (similar to those of nutritionally deprived individuals), and elevated levels of cortisol

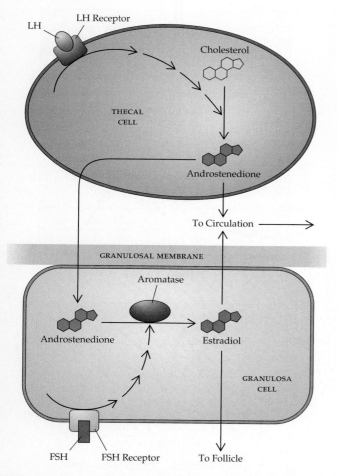

Figure 2   **Relationship between granulosa cells and thecal cells of the ovarian follicle. Luteinizing hormone (LH) stimulates thecal production of androstenedione, which diffuses to the granulosa cells. In the granulosa cells, follicle-stimulating hormone (FSH) stimulates the conversion of androstenedione to estradiol.**[29]

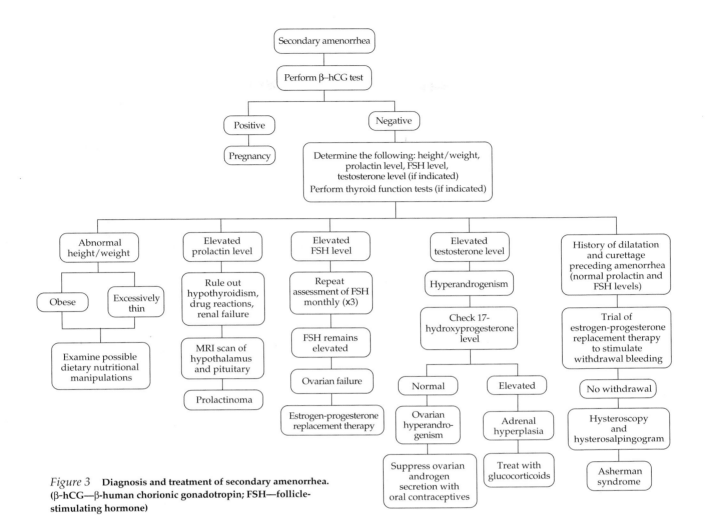

Figure 3 **Diagnosis and treatment of secondary amenorrhea.**
(β-hCG—β-human chorionic gonadotropin; FSH—follicle-stimulating hormone)

secretion (as seen in depressed women or women under significant stress).

Treatment Reversing the underlying cause of hypothalamic hypofunction (reducing psychosocial stress, gaining weight, lowering exercise intensity) often results in resumption of ovulatory menses. However, many women with amenorrhea from low GnRH secretion prefer to maintain the exercise and nutritional regimens that cause the amenorrhea, and those with an eating disorder may not respond to treatment of it. These women are best treated with hormone replacement. Therapeutic choices include oral contraceptives and low-dose hormone replacement, such as a standard combined continuous regimen of conjugated estrogens, 0.625 mg, plus medroxyprogesterone acetate, 2.5 mg, daily. Cyclic hormone replacement may also be used. The use of sustained-release vaginal gel to supply the progesterone component of hormone replacement therapy has been reported.[3] Vitamin D (400 IU/day) and calcium (1,200 to 1,500 mg/day) supplements should be administered to slow the rate of decline in bone mineral density associated with low estrogen levels.

AMENORRHEA CAUSED BY PITUITARY DYSFUNCTION

The most common pituitary diseases that cause secondary amenorrhea are prolactin-secreting pituitary tumors (prolactin-omas), the empty sella syndrome, Sheehan syndrome, and other pituitary tumors, such as those that secrete adrenocorticotropic hormone (ACTH) or growth hormone.

Prolactin-Secreting Pituitary Tumors

Most pituitary tumors are monoclonal, which indicates that they arise from a somatic mutation in a single progenitor cell. In general, pituitary tumors are benign and slow growing.

Diagnosis The most common causes of an elevation in the serum prolactin level are, in order of frequency, advanced pregnancy; the use of psychotropic medications that are dopamine antagonists, such as haloperidol; prolactin-secreting pituitary tumors; hypothyroidism; and renal failure. After excluding those causes, the workup should focus on the pituitary.

A magnetic resonance imaging scan of the hypothalamus and pituitary can confirm the diagnosis of prolactinoma. The MRI is also used to determine whether the diameter of the tumor is less than 10 mm (microprolactinoma) or greater than 10 mm (macroprolactinoma), because this measurement has clinical implications. Finally, the MRI can assess for possible involvement of the sella turcica and the optic chiasm.

If the MRI shows a pituitary tumor, it is important to also measure serum insulinlike growth factor–1 (IGF-1). IGF-1 levels will be elevated in patients whose pituitary tumor secretes

Table 1 The Most Common Causes of Secondary Amenorrhea in Women Who Are Not Pregnant

Organ	Cause	Relative Frequency (%)
Hypothalamus	Abnormalities of height/weight and nutrition	15
	Exercise	10
	Psychosocial stress	10
	Infiltrative disease or tumors of the hypothalamus (sarcoidosis, histiocytosis, craniopharyngioma)	< 0.1
Pituitary	Prolactin-secreting pituitary tumor	17
	Empty sella syndrome	1
	Sheehan syndrome	< 1
	ACTH-secreting tumor (Cushing disease)	< 1
	GH-secreting tumor	< 1
Ovary	Premature ovarian failure	10
	Polycystic ovary syndrome	30
Uterus	Asherman syndrome (intrauterine synechiae)	5
Other	Nonclassical adrenal hyperplasia	< 1
	Thyroid disease	1
	Ovarian tumors	< 1

ACTH—adrenocorticotropic hormone GH—growth hormone

growth hormone; this is a more reliable test than measurement of growth hormone itself.

Treatment In general, microprolactinomas have a benign course and can be managed by the patient's primary care physician. Observational studies indicate that over a period of 4 to 6 years, 95% of microprolactinomas do not increase in size.[4,5] Macroprolactinomas, however, can be associated with significant complications, such as pituitary apoplexy and compression of the optic chiasm, and should be managed by an endocrinologist. The initial treatment of both microprolactinomas and macroprolactinomas should be medical therapy, not surgery.

The two best approaches to management of microprolactinomas in women with amenorrhea are low-dose oral contraceptives and a dopamine agonist (bromocriptine, pergolide, or cabergoline). Both contraceptives and dopamine agonists can initiate regular withdrawal bleeding and prevent osteoporosis. In women with microprolactinomas, treatment with an estrogen-progestin oral contraceptive is safe and is not associated with clinically significant tumor growth.[6]

Women with amenorrhea caused by a prolactinoma who wish to become pregnant should receive treatment with a dopamine agonist to induce ovulation. Dopamine agonists directly suppress prolactin production by the tumor and cause an increase in endogenous GnRH secretion, which stimulates pituitary secretion of LH and FSH and consequently induces follicle development and ovulation. In addition, dopamine agonists decrease the size of prolactin-secreting pituitary tumors.[7,8]

Bromocriptine has been used to induce ovulation in women with hyperprolactinemia for more than 25 years.[9] In one study of 280 women with hyperprolactinemia, bromocriptine normalized the circulating prolactin level in 82% of the women.[10]

The main side effects associated with the use of bromocriptine are nausea, vomiting, and orthostatic hypotension. To minimize these potential side effects, it is recommended that bromocriptine be initiated at a dose of 1.25 mg at bedtime. After 1 week, the dosage can be increased to 1.25 mg twice daily. The dosage can then be increased to 2.5 mg twice daily, a standard dosage that successfully reduces serum prolactin in most women with hyperprolactinemia.[10] Long-acting oral and injectable forms of bromocriptine have been developed,[11,12] but those are not yet available in the United States.

Pergolide, an ergot dopamine agonist, has been approved by the Food and Drug Administration for the treatment of Parkinson disease but not for the treatment of hyperprolactinemia. Unlike bromocriptine, pergolide can be given once a day. Pergolide is the least expensive of the dopamine agonists; its cost is about one sixth that of cabergoline.

Cabergoline is a non-ergot dopamine agonist that is administered once or twice a week and causes less nausea than bromocriptine or pergolide.[13] The FDA-approved dosage of cabergoline is 0.25 mg twice a week. Many clinicians start cabergoline at a dosage of 0.5 mg a week, then increase the dosage to 1 mg once or twice a week, depending on the response of the serum prolactin level (see below). In about 25% of women, the serum prolactin level returns to normal through therapy with cabergoline at a dosage of 1 mg a week; in these patients, the dosage can be reduced to 0.5 mg a week and the serum prolactin level will remain normal. About one half of women who do not respond to bromocriptine treatment will respond to treatment with cabergoline.[14] Many authorities believe that cabergoline is more effective than bromocriptine in treating hyperprolactinemia.[15] In a series of 459 women with hyperprolactinemia and amenorrhea, 83% of the women treated with cabergoline experienced normalization of their prolactin levels, compared with 52% of those treated with bromocriptine.[16] Cabergoline is significantly more expensive than bromocriptine, however.

With dopamine agonist therapy, near-maximal decreases in serum prolactin levels are typically achieved after 4 weeks of treatment. Serum prolactin levels should be measured approximately 1 month after initiating therapy and about 1 month after a change in dose or drug. If the serum prolactin concentration is normal and no side effects have occurred, the initial dose should be continued. If serum prolactin has not decreased to normal and no side effects are present, the dose should be gradually increased. Maximal dosages of the dopamine agonists are as follows: bromocriptine, 5 mg twice daily; pergolide, 0.25 mg once daily; and cabergoline, 1.5 mg two or three times weekly. If the serum prolactin level does not decrease to normal, switching to a different dopamine agonist may be effective. If the patient cannot tolerate the side effects of the dopamine agonist initially prescribed, a different dopamine agonist may be tried. If the patient experiences side effects with all the dopamine agonists, then vaginal administration of bromocriptine can be tried.[17] If all attempts at medical therapy fail, transsphenoidal surgery is indicated. Successful removal of the tumor will result in the normalization of the prolactin secretion level and resumption of ovulatory menses.

After correction of hyperprolactinemia, about 80% of women will ovulate; cumulative pregnancy rates of 80% are commonly observed.[18] Treatment is usually discontinued once a pregnancy is diagnosed. However, in women with a macroprolactinoma,

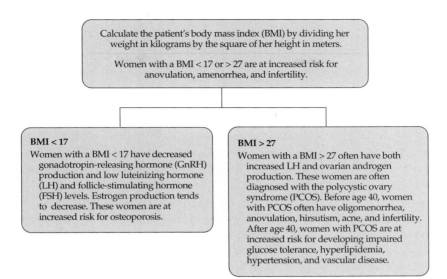

Figure 4   **Relation of body mass index to anovulation.**

therapy should be continued throughout pregnancy to reduce the risk that the tumor will grow and cause neurosurgical complications, such as compression of the optic nerve.

Empty Sella Syndrome

The roof of the pituitary gland (the diaphragm of the sella) is perforated by the pituitary stalk, which connects the hypothalamic median eminence to the pituitary. If the perforation in the diaphragm of the sella is excessively large, the pia mater and accompanying cerebrospinal fluid can herniate into the pituitary fossa. Herniation of this fluid, which is under reasonably high pressure, can produce compression atrophy of the pituitary gland, resulting in hypopituitarism and amenorrhea.

The empty sella syndrome can be diagnosed on the basis of high-resolution MRI or computed tomography of the pituitary. Therapy is directed to the specific replacement of documented hormonal abnormalities.

Sheehan Syndrome

Sheehan syndrome is the onset of hypothalamic and pituitary dysfunction after severe obstetric hemorrhage and maternal hypotension at delivery. During pregnancy, the pituitary volume increases by approximately 100%. The increase in pituitary size and the low-flow, low-pressure nature of the portal circulation may make the pituitary and parts of the hypothalamus susceptible to ischemia brought on by obstetric hemorrhage and hypotension. Worldwide, Sheehan syndrome is the most common cause of hypopituitarism.

Diagnosis   Every possible pattern of pituitary hormone deficiency has been reported in Sheehan syndrome, but growth hormone and prolactin deficiencies are the most common presentations. In a study of 10 African women with Sheehan syndrome, all had both prolactin and growth hormone deficiency, nine had cortisol deficiency, eight had TSH deficiency, seven had LH deficiency, and four had FSH deficiency.[19] Clinical studies have demonstrated that many women with Sheehan syndrome also have mild defects in vasopressin secretion.[20] The best test to diagnose Sheehan syndrome is to administer thyrotropin-releasing hormone (TRH), 100 µg intravenously, and measure prolactin at 0 and 30 minutes. The ratio of prolactin at 30 minutes to prolactin at 0 minutes should be greater than 3.[21] If the ratio is less than 3, the patient should undergo a complete evaluation for panhypopituitarism.

Treatment   Treatment of Sheehan syndrome is with hormone replacement. The particular regimen is based on the patient's pattern of hormone deficiency.

Premature Ovarian Failure

Ovarian failure is the loss of all functional ovarian follicles. Ovarian failure in patients younger than 40 years is termed premature ovarian failure. The causes of premature ovarian failure include genetic abnormalities (e.g., microdeletions of the X chromosome), autoimmune processes (e.g., polyglandular autoimmune disease and myasthenia gravis), chemotherapy (especially with alkylating agents), and pelvic radiotherapy (> 500 cGy to the ovaries).

Diagnosis   Loss of all follicles results in a decrease in estradiol and inhibin B production. In the absence of the negative feedback effect of these two hormones, FSH secretion increases markedly. Therefore, ovarian failure is most accurately diagnosed by measurement of serum FSH. Complete ovarian failure is associated with serum FSH levels greater than 25 U/L. In women with incipient ovarian failure, FSH levels are often between 15 and 25 U/L and can fluctuate.[22] Clinically, women with premature ovarian failure often experience vasomotor symptoms (hot flashes) or vaginal dryness.

Treatment   There are no proven therapies specifically for ovarian failure. Because women with premature ovarian failure (like all women with estrogen deficiency) are at high risk for osteoporosis, they should be treated with estrogen-progestin replacement. Although women with ovarian failure are by definition infertile, they may be able to bear a child through oocyte donation. In this process, a donor egg and sperm from the woman's

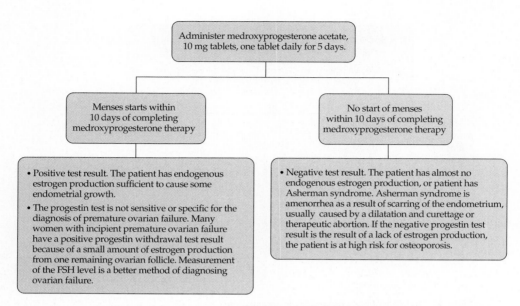

Figure 5 **The progestin withdrawal test. (FSH—follicle-stimulating hormone)**

partner are incubated in vitro. The embryo is then transferred to the woman's uterus, after she undergoes treatment with estrogen and progesterone to mature the endometrium.

Hyperandrogenism and the Polycystic Ovary Syndrome

Hyperandrogenism is marked by clinical evidence of excess androgens, including severe hirsutism, and elevated serum androgen levels. PCOS causes 80% of hyperandrogenism; idiopathic hirsutism causes 15%, and nonclassical adrenal hyperplasia (NCAH) causes 4%. Rare causes, such as androgen-secreting ovarian or adrenal tumors, account for 1% of cases. Idiopathic hirsutism is hirsutism associated with regular menses and therefore is not a cause of amenorrhea. PCOS, NCAH, and androgen-secreting tumors can all cause amenorrhea. Women who have amenorrhea with hyperandrogenism are at increased risk for endometrial carcinoma.

Diagnosis Androgen-secreting tumors are usually associated with circulating testosterone levels greater than 200 ng/dl. In menopausal women, small ovarian hilar cell androgen-secreting tumors can be associated with elevations in the serum testosterone level in the range of 150 to 200 ng/dl. In most women with PCOS, the serum testosterone level ranges from 50 and 200 ng/dl. The 17-hydroxyprogesterone level, when measured at 8:00 A.M., is greater than 4 ng/ml in women with NCAH and is less than 4 ng/ml in women with PCOS. A sonogram that shows multiple small ovarian follicles can support the diagnosis of PCOS.[22]

Treatment Ovarian hyperandrogenism, such as PCOS, is treated by suppression of ovarian androgen secretion with oral contraceptives. Adrenal hyperplasia is treated with glucocorticoids.

Asherman Syndrome (Intrauterine Adhesions)

Asherman syndrome is the presence of intrauterine scar tissue that interferes with normal endometrial growth and shedding. In women with this condition, intrauterine scar tissue usually develops after vigorous curettage of infected endometrium early in pregnancy.

Diagnosis The history is an important clue to Asherman syndrome. For patients whose history is suggestive, a commonly used way to assess endocrine function is to prescribe conjugated estrogens, 2.5 mg for 35 days, plus medroxyprogesterone acetate, 10 mg daily, on days 26 to 35. The estrogen and progestin are then discontinued. Absence of withdrawal bleeding after such a challenge strongly suggests Asherman syn-

Table 2 **The Most Common Causes of Primary Amenorrhea**

Cause	Rate of Occurrence (%)
Gonadal dysgenesis, including 45X (Turner syndrome)	45
Physiologic delay of puberty	20
Müllerian agenesis	15
Obstructed outflow tract: transverse vaginal septum or imperforate hymen	5
Absence of hypothalamic gonadotropin-releasing hormone production (Kallmann syndrome)	5
Anorexia nervosa	2
Hypopituitarism	2
Androgen insensitivity	1
Hyperprolactinemia	1
Adrenal hyperplasia	1
Hypothyroidism	1
Pituitary tumors	1
Craniopharyngioma	1

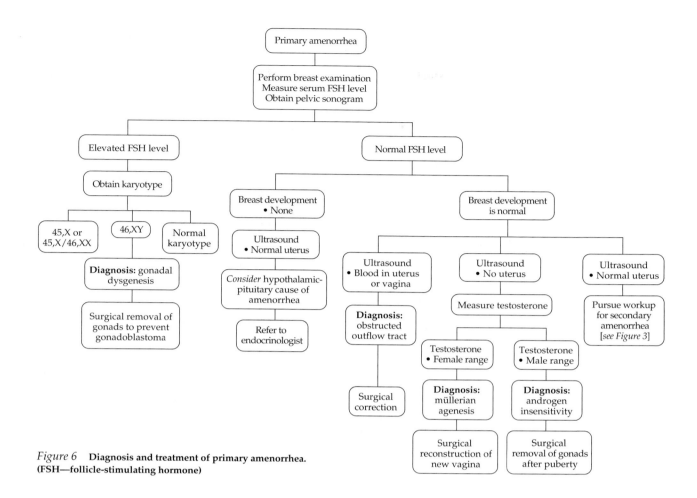

Figure 6 **Diagnosis and treatment of primary amenorrhea. (FSH—follicle-stimulating hormone)**

drome. The diagnosis can be confirmed radiologically by hysterosalpingogram or by direct visualization of the scar tissue with hysteroscopy.

Treatment The treatment of Asherman syndrome involves surgical lysis of the intrauterine adhesions by operative hysteroscopy, followed by stimulation of endometrial growth with estrogen. Some women who become pregnant after treatment experience placental defects such as placenta accreta. This is probably the result of disruption of function of the endometrial stroma by the disease and treatment.

Primary Amenorrhea

Primary amenorrhea is present when the first menses has not occurred by the time a girl reaches 16 years of age. Girls who reach 14 years of age and have no breast development should also undergo a workup similar to that for primary amenorrhea.[23] Primary amenorrhea is usually caused by genetic or congenital disorders and is often associated with developmental problems during puberty.[24] These developmental problems include delayed height and weight gain, delayed breast development, and delayed development of pubic and axillary hair.

In a large case series, the most common causes of primary amenorrhea were found to be gonadal dysgenesis resulting from chromosomal abnormalities such as 45,X, 45,X/46,XX,

and 46,XY (45% of cases); physiologic delay of puberty (20% of cases); müllerian agenesis (15% of cases); transverse vaginal septum or imperforate hymen (5% of cases); absence of hypothalamic GnRH production, such as seen in Kallman syndrome (5% of cases); anorexia nervosa (2% of cases); and hypopituitarism (2% of cases).[25] Less common causes of primary amenorrhea are hyperprolactinemia, hypothyroidism, pituitary tumors, Cushing disease, and craniopharyngiomas [*see Table 2*].

Primary amenorrhea is evaluated by focusing on the serum FSH level; breast development; and the presence of the cervix and uterus, as determined by an imaging study (pelvic sonogram or MRI) [*see Figure 6*].

If the FSH level is elevated, a diagnosis of gonadal dysgenesis can be made in most cases. A karyotype should be obtained in such cases to determine whether a Y chromosome is present. Girls with gonadal dysgenesis and a Y chromosome on the karyotype have a high rate of malignant transformation of the gonad to a dysgerminoma or a gonadoblastoma. In these cases, the ovaries need to be removed surgically.

If the FSH level is normal, then breast development should be assessed, and it should be determined whether a uterus and a cervix are present. If breast development is absent and a uterus is present, the differential diagnosis includes hypothalamic and pituitary causes of amenorrhea; the patient should then be referred to an endocrinologist. If breast development is normal and a uterus is present, the differential diagnosis is the same as that for secondary amenorrhea (see above). However, if the pelvic ultrasound shows not only that the patient has a uterus but that the uterus or vagina is dilated by blood, the diagnosis is a blocked reproductive outflow tract (transverse vaginal septum or imperforate hymen). Surgical relief of the outflow tract is necessary to prevent the development of hematocolpos, hematometria, and endometriosis.[26]

If breast development is present and no uterus is present on ultrasound, then the serum testosterone level should be assessed. If the testosterone level is in the normal range for a girl, the likely diagnosis is müllerian agenesis.[27] Treatment of müllerian agenesis is surgical construction of a new vagina, which should be scheduled for the time when the patient is expected to begin having sexual relations.

In a patient with breast development, no uterus, and a testosterone level that is elevated to the male range, the likely diagnosis is androgen insensitivity. Females with androgen insensitivity usually do not have pubic or axillary hair. Breast development is usually normal because in the absence of a tissue androgen receptor, low levels of estrogen have a markedly stimulating effect. Although the karyotype in these patients is 46,XY, their likelihood of developing a gonadoblastoma is low until after puberty. Removal of the gonads is typically delayed until puberty is complete.

References

1. Reindollar RH, Novak M, Tho SP, et al: Adult-onset amenorrhea: a study of 262 patients. Am J Obstet Gynecol 155:531, 1986

2. Hull MG, Knuth UA, Murray MA, et al: The practical value of the progestogen challenge test, serum oestradiol estimation or clinical examination in assessment of the oestrogen state and response to clomiphene in amenorrhoea. Br J Obstet Gynaecol 86:799, 1979

3. Warren MP, Biller BM, Shangold MM: A new clinical option for hormone replacement therapy in women with secondary amenorrhea: effects of cyclic administration of progesterone from the sustained-release vaginal gel Crinone (4% and 8%) on endometrial morphologic features and withdrawal bleeding. Am J Obstet Gynecol 180:42, 1999

4. Sisam DA, Sheehan JP, Sheeler LR: The natural history of untreated microprolactinoma. Fertil Steril 48:67, 1987

5. Schlechte J, Dolan K, Sherman B, et al: The natural history of untreated hyperprolactinemia. J Clin Endocrinol Metab 68:412, 1989

6. Corenblum B, Donovan L: The safety of physiological estrogen plus progestin replacement therapy and with oral contraceptive therapy in women with pathological hyperprolactinemia. Fertil Steril 59:671, 1993

7. Shimon I, Melmed S: Management of pituitary tumors. Ann Intern Med 129:472, 1998

8. Touraine P, Plu-Bureau G, Beji C, et al: Long-term follow-up of 246 hyperprolactinemic patients. Acta Obstet Gynecol Scand 80:162, 2001

9. Molitch ME: Disorders of prolactin secretion. Endocrinol Metab Clin North Am 30:585, 2001

10. Vance ML, Evans WS, Thorner MO: Drugs five years later: bromocriptine. Ann Intern Med 100:78, 1984

11. Zgliczynski W, Zgliczynski S, Makowska A, et al: New long-acting bromocriptine (Parlodel MR and Parlodel LAR) in the treatment of pituitary tumours with hyperprolactinemia. Endokrynol Pol 43:234, 1992

12. Jamrozik SI, Bennet AP, James-Deidier A, et al: Treatment with long acting repeatable bromocriptine (Parlodel-LAR) in patients with macroprolactinomas: long-term study in 29 patients. J Endocrinol Invest 19:472, 1996

13. Biller BM, Molitch ME, Vance ML, et al: Treatment of prolactin-secreting macroadenomas with the once-weekly dopamine agonist cabergoline. J Clin Endocrinol Metab 81:2338, 1996

14. Verhelst J, Abs R, Maiter D, et al: Cabergoline in the treatment of hyperprolactinemia. J Clin Endocrinol Metab 84:2518, 1999

15. Di Sarno A, Landi ML, Cappabianca P, et al: Resistance to cabergoline as compared with bromocriptine in hyperprolactinemia: prevalence, clinical definition, and therapeutic strategy. J Clin Endocrinol Metab 186:5256, 2001

16. Webster J, Piscitelli MD, Polli A, et al: A comparison of cabergoline and bromocriptine in the treatment of hyperprolactinemic amenorrhea. N Engl J Med 331:904, 1994

17. Ricci G, Giolo E, Nucera G, et al: Pregnancy in hyperprolactinemic infertile women treated with vaginal bromocriptine: report of two cases and review of the literature. Gynecol Obstet Invest 51:266, 2001

18. Crosignani PG: Management of hyperprolactinemia in infertility. J Reprod Med 44(suppl):1116, 1999

19. Jialal I, Maidoo C, Norman RJ, et al: Pituitary function in Sheehan's syndrome. Obstet Gynecol 63:15, 1984

20. Jialal I, Desai RK, Rajput MC: An assessment of posterior pituitary function in patients with Sheehan's syndrome. Clin Endocrinol (Oxf) 27:91, 1987

21. Barbieri RL, Cooper DS, Daniels GH, et al: Prolactin response to thyrotropin-releasing hormone (TRH) in patients with hypothalamic-pituitary disease. Fertil Steril 43:66, 1985

22. Lewis V: Polycystic ovary syndrome: a diagnostic challenge. Obstet Gynecol Clin North Am 28:1, 2001

23. Lee PA, Guo SS, Kulin HE: Age of puberty: data from the United States of America. APMIS 109:81, 2001

24. Pletcher JR, Slap GB: Menstrual disorders: amenorrhea. Pediatr Clin North Am 46:505, 1999

25. Reindollar RH, Byrd JR, McDonough PG: Delayed sexual development: a study of 252 patients. Am J Obstet Gynecol 140:371, 1981

26. Valdes C, Malini S, Malinak LR: Ultrasound evaluation of female genital tract anomalies: a review of 64 cases. Am J Obstet Gynecol 149:285, 1984

27. Buttram VC Jr, Gibbons WE: Müllerian anomalies: a proposed classification. (An analysis of 144 cases.) Fertil Steril 32:40, 1979

28. Roseff SJ, Bangah ML, Kettel LM, et al: Dynamic changes in circulating inhibin levels during the luteal-follicular transition of the human menstrual cycle. J Clin Endocrinol Metab 69:1033, 1989

29. Ryan KJ: The endocrine pattern and control of the ovulatory cycle. Infertility: Male and Female. Insler V, Lunenfeld B, Eds. Churchill Livingstone, New York, 1986

77 Premenstrual Syndrome

Sarah L. Berga, M.D.

Premenstrual syndrome (PMS) is a recurrent constellation of affective and physical symptoms that begin during the luteal phase of the menstrual cycle and resolve completely or almost completely during the follicular phase. The number, severity, and duration of symptoms occur along a spectrum. It is estimated that 20% to 40% of women report premenstrual symptoms during the luteal phase, but only 5% to 10% of women report symptoms severe enough to significantly interfere with their lifestyle. The long-term natural history of PMS is unclear.

The fourth edition of the *Diagnostic and Statistical Manual* of the American Psychiatric Association (DSM-IV) has defined a related syndrome, premenstrual dysphoric disorder (PMDD), to facilitate an accurate psychiatric diagnosis [*see Table 1*].[1] The criteria for PMDD are also used to define research populations so that therapeutic responses can be quantitated and generalized. PMDD is often considered a variant of depression, an impression buttressed by the treatment efficacy of antidepressants, particularly selective serotonin reuptake inhibitors (SSRIs), in women who meet the criteria for PMDD.[2-4]

Pathogenesis

Most evidence suggests that PMS/PMDD is caused by aberrant responses of target tissues, particularly the brain, to normal fluctuations in serum levels of ovarian gonadal steroids.[5-7] The causes of the untoward central nervous system responses are not firmly established[8] [*see Table 2*], but several pathogenic mechanisms are currently being explored. Altered metabolism of progesterone by the CNS may lead to altered CNS reactivity and neurotransmission. Specifically, one of the principal metabolites of progesterone, allopregnanolone, decreases anxi-

ety. Women with PMS show lower levels of allopregnanole during their luteal phase[9]; they may instead produce a predominance of anxiogenic progesterone metabolites.

PMS/PMDD may involve alterations in CNS neurotransmission that cause heightened reactivity to normal excursions in gonadal steroid levels. This exaggerated reactivity may be inherited or acquired. An acquired cause of altered CNS neurotransmission is chronic stress. Chronobiologic disturbances documented in women with PMDD have been interpreted as evidence of an underlying aberration in CNS function.[10] High levels of estrogen or of estrogen and progesterone may elicit or aggravate this underlying brain dysfunction, which would explain why symptoms are greatest during the luteal phase or at ovulation. In women with PMS/PMDD, but not in women without it, the symptom complex can be replicated by exposure to, followed by withdrawal from, exogenous estrogen and progesterone.[11] There is also an association between PMS and dysmenorrhea, further suggesting that PMS is an exaggerated tissue response to normal hormonal changes.

Diagnosis

To warrant medical attention, evaluation, and intervention, premenstrual symptoms must be recurrent and sufficiently severe to interfere with daily work and social activities. To establish the diagnosis of PMS/PMDD, the clinician must confirm that the patient has the characteristic manifestations of the disorder at the appropriate time in her menstrual cycle.

It is also important to identify any concurrent conditions likely to complicate treatment [*see Table 3*]. Many women with PMS/PMDD have a personal or family history of alcoholism. A history of sexual abuse, particularly in childhood or adolescence, may be common in women with severe PMS.[12] This population also has an increased personal and family history of posttraumatic stress disorder, mood disorders, schizophrenia, eating disorders, postpartum depression or psychosis, personality disorders, and anxiety disorders. A positive family history does not necessarily imply an inherited biologic vulnerability, because persistent exposure to dysfunctional family interactions is a chronic stress that can alter underlying CNS function.

Conclusive diagnosis of PMS or PMDD requires the documentation of concordance between symptoms and the luteal or periovulatory phase. The diagnosis of PMS/PMDD cannot be made in an anovulatory patient. Ideally, symptoms and menstrual dates should be followed prospectively to establish synchrony between the luteal phase and increase in symptoms. Two or more cycles and at least five symptoms [*see Table 1*] should be charted before the diagnosis is made. However, with a patient who is suffering severe psychological distress, there may not be time for prospective evaluation. Immediate referral to a psychiatrist may be indicated to prevent suicide or homicide.

If the menstrual cycle is irregular (menstrual cycle is ordinarily between 26 and 30 days) and there is no clear pattern of symptoms, the progesterone level should be measured weekly

---

Table 1 DSM-IV Criteria for Premenstrual Dysphoric Disorder

Symptoms occur in the luteal phase, with prospective confirmation of a 30% increase in symptoms during the luteal phase above the level in the follicular phase

Not an exacerbation of major depression, panic dysthymia, or personality disorder

Marked disturbance in functioning

At least five of the following

Marked lability	headache, joint or muscle pain, bloating, weight gain)
Marked irritability	
Marked anxiety	
Markedly depressed mood	Avoidance of social activities
Decreased interest	Decreased productivity
Lethargy	Increased sensitivity to rejection
Difficulty concentrating	
Food craving	Feeling overwhelmed
Hypersomnia or insomnia	Feeling out of control
Physical symptoms (breast tenderness or swelling,	Increased interpersonal conflict

---

Table 2 Potential Causes of PMS/PMDD

Aberrant responses of target tissues, especially the brain, to normal gonadal steroid exposures mediated by the following:

    Opioid withdrawal
    Serotonergic imbalance
    Entrainment to endogenous cycles
    Chronobiologic disturbance
    Membrane effects of steroids or steroid metabolites
    Genomic effects of steroids
    Variation in steroid metabolism

---

throughout a cycle to determine whether there is a luteal phase. A progesterone concentration greater than 5 ng/ml, or 15 nmol/L, is generally considered evidence that a woman is in the luteal phase and ovulation is impending. No rise in progesterone indicates anovulation, which may be stress induced. These patients may require further evaluation [see Chapter 76]. Symptoms should be charted concurrently with progesterone levels. To meet the criteria for PMS/PMDD, the patient's symptoms should become at least 30% more severe during the luteal phase (or when the progesterone concentration is greater than 5 ng/ml) than they were in the follicular phase.

DIFFERENTIAL DIAGNOSIS

If a patient has regular menses and severe dysmenorrhea but no behavioral symptoms, she should be evaluated for possible endometriosis [see Chapter 84]. As with all psychiatric diagnoses, it is important to exclude organic causes. In PMS/PMDD, it is especially important to exclude thyroid dysfunction (hyperthyroidism or hypothyroidism) and drug abuse or dependence as contributing factors.

Premenstrual changes in hormone levels can exacerbate underlying medical conditions, including migraine, epilepsy, asthma, irritable bowel syndrome, and diabetes mellitus.[13] This is not PMS but may resemble it.

If behavioral symptoms are severe and are present throughout the menstrual cycle and if there is no clear pattern of increase in symptom severity during the luteal phase, another psychiatric diagnosis must be considered. The following psychiatric disorders must be excluded: major depression, panic and anxiety disorders, dysthymia, and personality disorder. Such patients should be referred to a psychiatrist for definitive diagnosis and treatment. The most important condition to exclude is depression.

Treatment

Available therapies for PMS/PMDD range from lifestyle modification to surgery. Sustained improvement in a woman with PMS/PMDD generally requires a combination of modalities. The severity of a patient's symptoms and her response to particular modalities should guide the choice of therapies and the pace of their introduction. Mild cases can be treated with lifestyle modification and nonpharmacologic options; severe cases deserve immediate and aggressive intervention.

NONPHARMACOLOGIC THERAPY

Lifestyle interventions for PMS include institution of good sleep patterns and regular exercise. The patient should reduce or eliminate the use of tobacco, alcohol, and other drugs.

Dietary treatment helps some patients. Calcium supplementation may be beneficial.[14] It has been suggested that diets high in carbohydrates and protein buttress the serotonergic axis.[15] A diet high in tryptophan, a precursor of serotonin, may also be of benefit for mild PMS.[16]

Full-spectrum bright-light therapy given in the evening has been shown to markedly reduce symptoms of PMS/PMDD. Its use can be limited to the luteal phase.[17,18]

Stress management is integral to lifestyle treatment. Biofeedback,[19] massage,[20] and other relaxation methods may be helpful. Education, emotional support, and attention from the physician or therapist are instrumental. However, almost any intervention can be temporarily helpful, as the placebo response is quite high in this disorder.

Some women may wish to treat their PMS with herbal remedies, such as oil of primrose, chaste tree berries, or St. John's wort [see Chapter 8]. The use of herbal medicine and other complementary and alternative measures for PMS/PMDD has not been strongly validated in randomized, controlled trials, however.[21]

Behavioral Therapy

Patients with PMS may benefit from cognitive-behavioral therapy or interpersonal therapy. These are formal, structured psychotherapies designed to help patients institute behavioral changes and address cognitive patterns that sustain maladaptative behavior. Response to treatment may take as long as 6 months, but the effects persist indefinitely. If a patient is having difficulty coping with her symptoms during the early months of psychotherapy, there is no reason not to add pharmacologic treatment. The effects of medication are more rapid in onset than those of psychotherapy, but the effects persist only as long as the patient takes the medication. The model of combined psychotherapy and pharmacotherapy is considered the most effective approach to major depression; it has not been formally tested in PMS/PMDD, but there is no reason to believe it would not work well in this disorder, given the similarities between depression and PMS/PMDD.

Disposition

Benefit from nonpharmacologic interventions should be evident within two menstrual cycles. If the patient has shown no improvement at all during that time, the clinician should move on to pharmacotherapy. Complete recovery is not to be expected, however; that seldom or never occurs, regardless of the therapy chosen. Nevertheless, it is unwise for the clinician to lower the patient's expectations about these modalities, because enthusiasm inspires patients to participate in therapy and enhances the placebo effect. To set the stage for follow-up without lowering expectations, the clinician can tell the patient,

---

Table 3 Pertinent History in PMS/PMDD

Reproductive events	Sleep
Dysmenorrhea	Drug, alcohol, and medication
Psychosocial adjustments and	use
stressors	Endocrine disorders
Diet	Family and personal history
Exercise	of psychiatric disorders

"I want to see how you are doing in 2 months. If you are feeling perfectly fine and don't want to come back in, just give me a call. In case you aren't perfectly fine, though, I would rather see you back."

It is reasonable to wait more than 2 months for a response in a patient who has initiated behavioral therapy in a formal psychiatric setting. On the other hand, with a patient who is in severe psychological distress, 2 months may be too long to wait. The worst-case scenario is that such a patient will interpret a prescription of lifestyle modification and a distant follow-up appointment as a dismissal by her physician and, in the meantime, commit suicide or a homicide or ruin her life in some way. Clinicians who have limited psychiatric expertise or who practice in a stringent managed-care setting that severely restricts follow-up should refer severely distressed patients to a psychiatrist.

Pharmacologic Therapies for Somatic Symptoms

Bromocriptine (2.5 mg/day orally) has been promoted as treatment for breast tenderness. Spironolactone (25 to 50 mg/day orally) has been given to alleviate bloating. Nonsteroidal anti-inflammatory drugs can be effective treatment for dysmenorrhea [see Chapter 78].

Progesterone treatment has been shown to be ineffective for PMS.[22] Oral contraceptives are likely to aggravate rather than attenuate PMS/PMDD symptoms.

Pharmacologic Therapies for Affective Symptoms

Because the pathogenesis of PMS/PMDD probably involves an aberrant CNS response to normal ovarian function, the first-line treatment is to buttress CNS function with antidepressants. The SSRIs fluoxetine and sertraline have been shown to be effective[2-4]; other agents in this class presumably would work but are not as well studied. Although use of SSRIs can be limited to the luteal phase (10 to 14 days), that approach is impractical for many patients, who may have difficulty determining when to start the drug. It is simpler for patients simply to take the medication every day.

Sertraline has a shorter half-life than fluoxetine. The advantage of a shorter half-life is that if the patient experiences unacceptable side effects, the side effects will fade more rapidly once the medication is discontinued. The most prominent side effect of SSRIs in patients with PMS/PMDD—and a common reason for poor compliance with SSRI therapy for the disorder—is sexual dysfunction.[23] Some patients are willing to accept impaired libido as a trade-off for the relief of their symptoms. Buspirone is mildly effective for PMS/PMDD and may be a useful alternative in patients who find the sexual side effects unacceptable.[24] Classified as an atypical antidepressant, buspirone tends to be used for the anxious variety of depression.

Benzodiazepine therapy with alprazolam, taken during the luteal phase, is appropriate for patients whose main symptom is anxiety.[25] However, alprazolam has many more side effects than do SSRIs, even though the dose can be titrated to minimize side effects.

Pharmacologic Interventions That Alter Ovarian Steroid Exposure

Patients with PMS/PMDD who fail to respond adequately to lifestyle modification and SSRI therapy or who refuse or are unable to follow such measures can be treated with go-nadotropin-releasing hormone (GnRH) agonist therapy (e.g., leuprolide, nafarelin, or goserelin).[26-29] GnRH agonists effect a medical oophorectomy. They cannot be continued indefinitely without hormone replacement therapy because of concerns about the long-term deleterious effects of sustained hypoestrogenism. Add-back hormone regimens generally involve continuous exposure to small amounts of both estrogen and progestin,[29] thereby obviating the hormonal changes associated with a menstrual cycle.

There is a variety of hormonal preparations available for add-back regimens. It is usually a good idea to administer the estrogen and progestin separately at first, so that the response to each can be monitored. The progestin dose must be large enough to prevent endometrial hyperplasia but below the threshold for triggering PMS symptoms. Ongoing exposure to even small amounts of progestin (e.g., oral medroxyprogesterone acetate, 2.5 mg daily) may provoke symptoms, however.

The synthetic androgen danazol can be used to temporarily suppress endogenous ovarian function and provide an androgenic environment. However, its side effects may be as problematic as the PMS/PMDD symptoms. The androgenic side effects of danazol include voice changes, hirsutism, and breast regression, all of which may be permanent.

Surgical Therapy

GnRH agonist therapy is expensive, so if a patient is responding very well to a GnRH agonist and has completed her childbearing, oophorectomy and hysterectomy may be a reasonable step. Surgery may also be the therapy of choice for patients who have sustained improvement with GnRH-agonist therapy but experience recurrent symptoms with add-back hormone regimens. Postoperatively, these patients are given hormone replacement therapy with continuous estrogen alone. Continuing SSRI therapy may be indicated.

References

1. American Psychiatric Association: Diagnostic and Statistical Manual of Psychiatric Disorders, 4th ed. United States Department of Health and Human Services, Washington, DC, 1996, p 714

2. Steiner M, Steinberg S, Stewart D, et al: Fluoxetine in the treatment of premenstrual dysphoria. Canadian Fluoxetine/Premenstrual Dysphoria Collaborative Study Group. N Engl J Med 332:1529, 1995

3. Steiner M, Korzekwa M, Lamont J, et al: Intermittent fluoxetine dosing in the treatment of women with premenstrual dysphoria. Psychopharmacol Bull 33:771, 1997

4. Symptomatic improvement of premenstrual dysphoric disorder with sertraline treatment: a randomized controlled trial. Sertraline Premenstrual Dysphoric Collaborative Study Group. JAMA 278:983, 1997

5. Sundstrom I, Andersson A, Nyberg S, et al: Patients with premenstrual syndrome have a different sensitivity to a neuroactive steroid during the menstrual cycle compared to control subjects. Neuroendocrinology 67:126, 1998

6. Rabin DS, Schmidt PJ, Campbell G, et al: Hypothalamic-pituitary-adrenal function in patients with the premenstrual syndrome. J Clin Endocrinol Metab 71:1158, 1990

7. Korzekwa MI, Lamont JA, Steiner M: Late luteal phase dysphoric disorder and the thyroid axis revisited. J Clin Endocrinol Metab 81:2280, 1996

8. Berga SL: Understanding premenstrual syndrome. Lancet 351:465, 1998

9. Rapkin AJ, Morgan M, Goldman L, et al: Progesterone metabolite allopregnanolone in women with premenstrual syndrome. Obstet Gynecol 90:709, 1997

10. Parry BL, Berga SL, Kripke DF, et al: Altered waveform of plasma nocturnal melatonin secretion in premenstrual depression. Arch Gen Psychiatry 47:1139, 1990

11. Schmidt PJ, Nieman LK, Danaceau MA, et al: Differential behavioral effects of gonadal steroids in women with and in those without premenstrual syndrome. N Engl J Med 338:209, 1998

12. Golding JM, Taylor DL, Menard L, et al: Prevalence of sexual abuse history in a sample of women seeking treatment for premenstrual syndrome. J Psychosom Obstet Gynaecol 21:69, 2000

13. Case AM, Reid RL: Menstrual cycle effects on common medical conditions. Compr Ther 27:65, 2001

14. Calcium carbonate and the premenstrual syndrome: effects on premenstrual and menstrual symptoms. Premenstrual Syndrome Study Group. Am J Obstet Gynecol 179:444, 1998

15. Wurtman JJ, Brzezinski A, Wurtman RJ, et al: Effect of nutrient intake on premenstrual depression. Am J Obstet Gynecol 161:1228, 1989

16. Sayegh R, Schiff I, Wurtman J, et al: The effect of a carbohydrate-rich beverage on mood, appetite, and cognitive function in women with premenstrual syndrome. Obstet Gynecol 86:520, 1995

17. Parry BL, Berga SL, Mostofi N, et al: Morning versus evening bright light treatment of late luteal phase dysphoric disorder. Am J Psychiatry 146:1215, 1989

18. Parry BL, Mahan AM, Mostofi N, et al: Light therapy of late luteal phase dysphoric disorder: an extended study. Am J Psychiatry 150:1417, 1993

19. Van Zak DB: Biofeedback treatments for premenstrual and premenstrual affective syndromes. Int J Psychosom 41:53, 1994

20. Hernandez-Reif M, Martinez A, Field T, et al: Premenstrual symptoms are relieved by massage therapy. J Psychosom Obstet Gynaecol 21:9, 2000

21. Stevinson C, Ernst E: Complementary/alternative therapies for premenstrual syndrome: a systematic review of randomized controlled trials. Am J Obstet Gynecol 185:227, 2001

22. Wyatt K, Dimmock P, Jones P, et al: Efficacy of progesterone and progestogens in management of premenstrual syndrome: systematic review. BMJ 323:776, 2001

23. Sundstrom-Poromaa I, Bixo M, Bjorn I, et al: Compliance to antidepressant drug therapy for treatment of premenstrual syndrome. J Psychosom Obstet Gynaecol 21:205, 2000

24. Landen M, Eriksson O, Sundblad C, et al: Compounds with affinity for serotonergic receptors in the treatment of premenstrual dysphoria: a comparison of buspirone, nefazodone and placebo. Psychopharmacology (Berl) 155:292, 2001

25. Freeman EW, Rickels K, Sondheimer SJ, et al: A double-blind trial of oral progesterone, alprazolam, and placebo in treatment of severe premenstrual syndrome. JAMA 274:51, 1995

26. Freeman EW, Sondheimer SJ, Rickels K: Gonadotropin-releasing hormone agonist in the treatment of premenstrual syndrome with and without ongoing dysphoria: a controlled study. Psychopharmacol Bull 33:303, 1997

27. Brown CS, Ling FW, Andersen RN, et al: Efficacy of depot leuprolide in premenstrual syndrome: effect of symptom severity and type in a controlled trial. Obstet Gynecol 84:779, 1994

28. Mezrow G, Shoupe D, Spicer D, et al: Depot leuprolide acetate with estrogen and progestin add-back for long-term treatment of premenstrual syndrome. Fertil Steril 62:932, 1994

29. Mortola JF, Girton L, Fischer U: Successful treatment of severe premenstrual syndrome by combined use of gonadotropin-releasing hormone agonist and estrogen/progestin. J Clin Endocrinol Metab 72:252A, 1991

78 Dysmenorrhea

Alan H. DeCherney, M.D.

Dysmenorrhea—colicky pain in the lower abdomen and pelvis around the time of menses—is a common condition that disturbs the lives and families of the women who suffer from it. Severe pain and discomfort often lead to absenteeism from work or school, resulting in an overall reduction in productivity and enormous economic loss.

Dysmenorrhea can be classified as primary or secondary, depending on its cause. Secondary dysmenorrhea results from a known pathologic process occurring within the pelvis. Primary dysmenorrhea does not have an anatomic cause.

Because many women seek help for this disorder, the physician should be sensitive to the concerns of each patient and provide a treatment that is specific to each patient's needs. The goal of therapy is to enable the patient to resume her daily life without the fear of being disabled by pain.

Primary Dysmenorrhea

The prevalence of primary dysmenorrhea is between 40% and 90%, with an average of 75%. It occurs predominantly in women younger than 25 years.

PATHOGENESIS

Primary dysmenorrhea results from tissue hypoxia and ischemia. An elevation in the basal tone of the uterus, combined with an increase in contraction strength and frequency, leads to vasospasm and a reduction in uterine blood flow.[1] Increased levels of prostaglandin $F_{2\alpha}$ ($PGF_{2\alpha}$), leukotrienes, and vasopressin are responsible for these alterations [*see Figure 1*].[2] It is important to note that this abnormality in prostaglandin production occurs only in endometrial tissue that has been exposed to both estrogen and progesterone.

DIAGNOSIS

Diagnosis of primary dysmenorrhea is based on patient history; results of physical examination are usually normal. Symptoms characteristically begin within 6 to 12 months after menarche, as ovulatory cycles become established. The pain occurs only during ovulatory cycles and lasts about 48 to 72 hours each month. In most patients, the pain starts a few hours before menstruation or at the onset of menstruation.

The degree of pain suffered is variable, but fewer than 15% of women with primary dysmenorrhea have severe pain. Patients with severe pain may also experience other symptoms, such as nausea, vomiting, dizziness, and diarrhea.

TREATMENT

Treatment of primary dysmenorrhea includes nonsteroidal anti-inflammatory drugs (NSAIDs), oral contraceptives, and transcutaneous electrical nerve stimulation (TENS).[3] Other nonpharmacologic approaches that may be effective are the use of a lower abdominal heating pad,[4] supplemental vitamin B_1 (100 mg daily) or magnesium (400 mg daily),[5] and a low-fat vegetarian diet.[6]

NSAIDs inhibit the action of cyclooxygenase and prevent the conversion of arachidonic acid into prostaglandins (PGs). NSAIDs significantly alleviate pain in approximately 75% of patients. The fenamates (e.g., mefenamic acid) are considered the

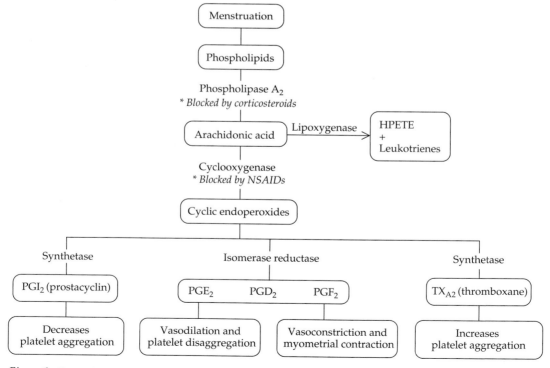

Figure 1 **Prostaglandin synthesis. (HPETE—hydroperoxyeicosatetraenoic acid)**

Table 1 Common Prostaglandin Synthesis Inhibitors

Chemical Group	Derivative	Usual Dosage
Benzoic acid	Acetylsalicylic acid (aspirin)	650 mg p.o. every 4 hr
Fenamates	Mefenamic acid	250 mg p.o. every 6 hr
	Meclofenamate sodium	100 mg p.o., t.i.d., for up to 6 days
Indoleacetic acid	Indomethacin	25–50 mg p.o. every 8 hr
Arylpropionic acid	Ibuprofen	400–800 mg p.o. every 4 hr
	Naproxen	250–500 mg p.o. every 12 hr
	Naproxen sodium	275–550 mg p.o. every 12 hr
Cyclooxygenase-2 (COX-2) inhibitors	Celecoxib	200 mg p.o., b.i.d.
	Rofecoxib	50 mg p.o., q.d.
	Valdecoxib	20 mg p.o., b.i.d.

best choice of NSAIDs because they act as antiprostaglandins, preventing both the production of PGs and the binding of the PG to its receptor [see Table 1].[7,8] Therapy with NSAIDs should be discontinued if adverse side effects occur.[9] Definitive research on the use of cyclooxygenase-2 (COX-2) inhibitors (e.g., celecoxib [Celebrex] or rofecoxib [Vioxx]) in dysmenorrhea has not been completed, but these agents seem promising for this purpose.

If NSAIDs are ineffective or poorly tolerated, the next step is the use of combined estrogen-progestin oral contraceptives. In a normal menstrual cycle, the progesterone level increases after ovulation and steadily decreases during the luteal phase. As the level of progesterone decreases, lysosomal enzymes within the endometrial cells are released, causing an increase in the production of PGs. Oral contraceptives prevent fluctuations of endogenous progesterone levels, reducing the amount of pain and symptoms associated with primary dysmenorrhea.[10] Regular-cycle oral contraceptives are not usually effective for treatment of primary dysmenorrhea; continuous oral contraceptives are preferable. Many patients consider continuous oral contraceptives unnatural but are willing to compromise by taking long-cycle contraceptives, so that they have three or four menses a year [see Chapter 80].

If neither NSAIDs nor oral contraceptives alone alleviate primary dysmenorrhea, the two can be used together. If combination therapy also fails, the patient should be reevaluated and a diagnostic workup initiated for secondary dysmenorrhea.

Secondary Dysmenorrhea

The pain associated with secondary dysmenorrhea is the direct result of a pathologic process. Unlike primary dysmenorrhea, secondary dysmenorrhea varies with regard to the patient's age at onset and the causative condition. Some of the conditions that can cause secondary dysmenorrhea include endometriosis, adenomyosis, pelvic adhesions and infection, pelvic congestion, cervical stenosis, psychological stress, and psychological disturbances.

ENDOMETRIOSIS

Endometriosis is the presence of endometrial glands and stroma outside the uterus [see Chapter 84]. Approximately 7%

of women in the United States suffer from this disorder. Endometriosis causes intra-abdominal hemorrhage, fibrosis, and adhesion formation. Consequently, dyspareunia, infertility, and pelvic pain occur.[11]

The pain usually begins 2 to 3 days before menses and worsens during menstruation. Tender nodules along the uterosacral ligament, a posteriorly fixed uterus, and enlarged cystic ovaries are characteristic findings; however, results of physical examination are often normal. Definitive diagnosis requires direct visualization during laparoscopy, with or without a tissue biopsy.

Treatment may entail either medical intervention or surgery. Oral contraceptives, intramuscular injection of leuprolide acetate depot, oral danazol, or high-dose progestins (oral or intramuscular) are all beneficial in suppressing the endometrial implants and relieving the symptoms of pain.

ADENOMYOSIS

Adenomyosis is the presence of ectopic endometrial glands and stroma in the myometrium of the uterus. Unlike the ectopic glands in endometriosis, the ectopic glands in adenomyosis do not undergo monthly cyclical changes.

Symptoms of adenomyosis classically include dysmenorrhea and menorrhagia (heavy menstrual bleeding). As the disease progresses, so does the dysmenorrhea. On physical examination, the uterus is soft, globular, and uniformly enlarged. Typically, the uterus is tender just before and during menstruation.

Diagnostic aids include pelvic sonography, magnetic resonance imaging, and hysterosalpingography. Unfortunately, most cases go undiagnosed until histologic evaluation is made at the time of a hysterectomy.

Treatment starts with medical suppression of ovarian function and culminates in hysterectomy if symptoms do not abate. Thermal balloon ablation of the endometrium, which is an effective treatment for some patients with dysmenorrhea from other causes,[12] does not work in adenomyosis.

CERVICAL STENOSIS

When menstrual flow is impeded at the level of the internal cervical os, intrauterine pressure increases and pelvic pain occurs. A narrow or stenotic os may be a congenital abnormality or the result of trauma, infection, or surgery.

The diagnosis of cervical stenosis should be considered in women who have a history of hypomenorrhea and severe pelvic pain during menses or if the diameter of the external cervical os is less than 5 mm.

During the physical examination, the physician should attempt to pass a uterine sound into the endometrial cavity. Inability to document a clear passage through the cervical canal warrants further investigation. Diagnostic workup with hysterosalpingography may reveal a narrow cervical canal.

Treatment consists of dilating the cervical canal with laminaria tents or performing a formal dilatation and curettage (D and C) under anesthesia. These procedures have limited therapeutic benefit and need to be repeated frequently. Complete resolution of symptoms typically occurs with pregnancy and vaginal delivery, which therefore is considered the ultimate therapy.

PELVIC INFLAMMATORY DISEASE

Most pelvic infections are caused by Chlamydia, Neisseria gonorrhoeae, and mixed microbial organisms. Pelvic anatomy is often distorted as a consequence of dense adhesion formation. During menstruation, adhesion edema and venous congestion result in severe pelvic pain and discomfort. This pain may eventually become chronic.

Patients at risk for pelvic inflammatory disease (PID) include current or past users of intrauterine devices (IUDs) and women with more than one sexual partner. The workup includes cervical cultures, endometrial biopsy, and pelvic sonography.

Treatment of the dysmenorrhea associated with PID includes NSAIDs for pain management and antibiotics for acute infection. Surgery can be offered to patients with chronic pain and to those with a known tubo-ovarian abscess or hydrosalpinx. Although lysis of adhesions can be performed, results are usually poor because recurrence is high.

PELVIC CONGESTION SYNDROME

Engorgement and thrombosis of the pelvic veins are another cause of dysmenorrhea.[13] The pooling of blood in the pelvic vasculature results in a burning and throbbing pain. The pain is characteristically worse at night and after prolonged periods of standing. Bimanual examination often reveals a uterus that is mildly enlarged and tender to the touch. The diagnosis of pelvic congestion syndrome is made almost exclusively during laparoscopic evaluation.

Although the underlying cause of pain is not well understood, treatment often entails NSAIDs and psychological therapy. New treatment approaches that utilize uterine artery embolization show promising results. Hysterectomy should be reserved for patients who do not respond to other therapeutic modalities.

OTHER CAUSES OF CHRONIC PELVIC PAIN

Secondary dysmenorrhea can also be caused by psychological problems, including stress, tension, and abnormal conditioned behavior. For these patients, resolution of symptoms is best achieved through lifestyle and behavior modification. Chronic pelvic pain, rather than acute pain, is more common among women with psychological disorders.

Patients who have pain for more than 6 months are considered to have chronic pelvic pain. In addition to a gynecologic cause of the pelvic pain, the physician should always consider other causes. The basic workup should include gastrointestinal, urologic, musculoskeletal, and psychological evaluations. Once a diagnosis has been established, treatment should focus on correcting the underlying disorder. Treatment should be initiated with medical therapy. If this fails, more aggressive treatment can be attempted, including presacral neurectomy or a laparoscopic uterine nerve ablation (LUNA) procedure.[14-16]

References

1. Dawood MY: Dysmenorrhea. Clin Obstet Gynecol 26:719, 1983

2. Smith RP: Cyclic pelvic pain and dysmenorrhea. Obstet Gynecol Clin North Am 20:753, 1993

3. Kaplan B, Rabinerson D, Pardo J, et al: Transcutaneous electrical nerve stimulation (TENS) as a pain-relief device in obstetrics and gynecology. Clin Exp Obstet Gynecol 24:123, 1997

4. Akin MD, Weingand KW, Hengehold DA, et al: Continuous low-level topical heat in the treatment of dysmenorrhea. Obstet Gynecol 97:343, 2001

5. Wilson ML, Murphy PA: Herbal and dietary therapies for primary and secondary dysmenorrhoea. Cochrane Database Syst Rev (3):CD002124, 2001

6. Barnard ND, Scialli AR, Hurlock D, et al: Diet and sex-hormone binding globulin, dysmenorrhea, and premenstrual symptoms. Obstet Gynecol 95:245, 2000

7. Owen PR: Prostaglandin synthetase inhibitors in the treatment of primary dysmenorrhea: outcome trials reviewed. Am J Obstet Gynecol 148:96, 1984

8. Rosenwaks Z, Seegar-Jones G: Menstrual pain: its origin and pathogenesis. J Reprod Med 25:207, 1980

9. Brooks P: Use and benefits of nonsteroidal anti-inflammatory drugs. Am J Med 104 (suppl 3A):9S, 1998

10. Crosignani PG, Vegetti W, Biachedi D: Hormonal contraception and ovarian pathology. Eur J Contracept Reprod Health Care 2:207, 1997

11. Fedele L, Bianchi S, Bocciolone L, et al: Pain symptoms associated with endometriosis. Obstet Gynecol 79:767, 1992

12. Ulmsten U, Carstensen H, Falconer C, et al: The safety and efficacy of Meno Treat, a new balloon device for thermal endometrial ablation. Acta Obstet Gynecol Scand 80:52, 2001

13. Cordts PR, Eclavea A, Buckley PJ, et al: Pelvic congestion syndrome: early clinical results after transcatheter ovarian vein embolization. J Vasc Surg 28:862, 1998

14. Polan ML, DeCherney A: Presacral neurectomy for pelvic pain in infertility. Fertil Steril 34:557, 1980

15. Kwok A, Lam A, Ford R: Laparoscopic presacral neurectomy: a review. Obstet Gynecol Surv 56:99, 2001

16. Carter JE: Surgical treatment for chronic pelvic pain. JSLS 2:129, 1998

79 Polycystic Ovary Syndrome

Robert L. Barbieri, M.D.

Polycystic ovary syndrome (PCOS) is defined as hyperandrogenism and reduced frequency of ovulation in the absence of other hyperandrogenic disorders. The clinical manifestations of PCOS in women with hyperandrogenism are cosmetic and reproductive. These patients present with hirsutism, acne, and irregular menstrual periods; ovulation may be infrequent or absent, and infertility can occur.

When assessing a patient with possible PCOS, the physician must rule out other conditions that can produce clinical hyperandrogenism, such as androgen-secreting tumors and nonclassic congenital adrenal hyperplasia. It is also necessary to identify patients whose hirsutism or acne results from increased sensitivity to normal androgen levels.

Epidemiology

PCOS is one of the most common endocrine disorders of women. In three population-based studies, the average prevalence of PCOS in women of reproductive age was reported to be about 6%.[1-3] Among anovulatory women, the prevalence of PCOS is approximately 30%.[4]

Pathophysiology

In women, luteinizing hormone (LH) and adrenocorticotropic hormone (ACTH) normally drive the secretion of androgens by the ovaries and adrenal glands, respectively. PCOS is caused by abnormally increased secretion of LH, insulin, or both. Increased levels of those hormones stimulate the ovarian theca and stroma to produce excess quantities of androgen, including testosterone and androstenedione. Elevated ovarian androgen secretion tends to block the growth of a dominant ovarian follicle. Instead, many small follicles accumulate; these follicles range in size from 4 to 8 mm in diameter. In the absence of a dominant follicle, an LH surge is not triggered, and ovulation does not occur regularly.

About 95% of women with PCOS have elevated levels of LH secretion, and 50% have hyperinsulinemia.[5] Those rates are influenced by body mass and genetics. In a population with a high prevalence of obesity, up to 100% of the women with PCOS will have hyperinsulinemia. Indeed, there may be two major phenotypes of PCOS: (1) lean women with markedly elevated levels of LH secretion and minimal or no insulin resistance and (2) obese women with slightly elevated or normal levels of LH secretion and insulin resistance and with markedly elevated levels of insulin secretion.

Women with PCOS show an abnormal increase in both the amplitude and the frequency of LH pulses in the early follicular phase of the menstrual cycle.[6] The elevated LH pulse frequency suggests an underlying increase in the pulse frequency of gonadotropin-releasing hormone (GnRH) secretion by the hypothalamus; this in turn suggests that PCOS results from a neuroendocrine disorder. The neuroendocrine mechanisms that raise GnRH pulse frequency are poorly characterized but may include alterations in hypothalamic opioid and catecholamine tone.

The insulin resistance in women with PCOS, as in other patients, has many possible causes, including genetic mutations in the insulin receptor and autoantibodies to the insulin receptor. The most common cause, however, is obesity. When pancreatic function is normal, resistance to the action of insulin in the liver, adipose tissue, muscle, and other insulin-sensitive tissues results in a compensatory and chronic hypersecretion of insulin. Laboratory studies suggest that insulin, especially in high concentrations, can stimulate ovarian androgen secretion.[7] Why insulin resistance develops in muscle and fat but not the ovary remains unclear. It is possible that insulin stimulates ovarian androgen secretion indirectly by binding to the insulin-like growth factor–1 receptor in the theca and the stroma.

HIRSUTISM

At birth, all areas of the body except the scalp and eyebrows are covered with vellus hair, which is light colored; individual vellus hairs have a very narrow diameter. Androgens can transform vellus hair into terminal hair, which is dark; individual terminal hairs have a thick diameter. The amount of androgen necessary to stimulate this transformation depends on many factors, including the sensitivity of hair follicles to androgens and the site of the hair follicle on the body. When girls reach puberty, small quantities of adrenal and ovarian androgens stimulate the transformation of vellus hair in the pubic region and axilla into terminal hair. Substantially larger amounts of androgen are required to stimulate the growth of terminal hair in a male-pattern distribution—that is, on the face, chest, and abdomen.

The term hirsutism denotes an increase in terminal hair in a male-pattern distribution. Hirsutism varies considerably by race: it is rare in Asian women, for example, because their hair follicles are relatively insensitive to androgens. In some families, women may inherit heightened sensitivity of the follicles to androgens and therefore may experience a degree of hirsutism at normal levels of circulating androgens.

ACNE

The hair follicle is part of the pilosebaceous unit, which also contains a sweat or sebaceous gland. Androgenic stimulation of the pilosebaceous unit promotes not only hair growth but also the production of sebum. Blockage of the follicle by excessive sebum (in concert with inflammation from free fatty acids produced by bacteria and yeast in the follicle) produces acne. The pilosebaceous unit is both a target organ responsive to androgen stimulation and a site of androgen production and metabolism.[8] Consequently, acne, like hirsutism, reflects both circulating androgen concentrations and genetic makeup.

Diagnosis

In PCOS, hyperandrogenism and oligo-ovulation or anovulation are present, but other hyperandrogenic disorders, such as androgen-secreting tumors and nonclassic adrenal hyperplasia, are absent.

No single feature is pathognomonic for PCOS. The history, physical examination, and laboratory evaluation can all provide evidence that establishes the diagnosis of PCOS and that excludes other conditions associated with those features. Clinical evidence of hyperandrogenism includes hirsutism, acne, and menstrual irregularity. Laboratory evidence of hyperandrogenism includes an elevated total or free serum testosterone concentration [see Table 1].

HISTORY

The history can provide key information in the differential diagnosis of androgen excess (and heightened androgen sensitivity) in women.

Age of Onset

In PCOS, oligomenorrhea, hirsutism, and acne typically begin in the perimenarchal or teenage years. The onset of severe hirsutism in menopause suggests an ovarian neoplasm.

Menstrual History

Patients with PCOS typically experience irregular menstrual cycles starting at menarche. Regular cycles are more consistent with familial or idiopathic hirsutism. A history of initially regular periods followed by onset of oligomenorrhea or amenorrhea and hirsutism with virilization in adult life suggests an androgen-secreting tumor.

Pace of Progression of Hirsutism

In PCOS, hirsutism tends to progress slowly, over many years. Rapid progression to severe hirsutism suggests a virilizing disorder from an androgen-secreting tumor. Patients with androgen-secreting tumors typically report other manifestations of virilization, such as deepening of the voice and secondary amenorrhea. Virilization will be evident on the physical examination (see below).

Family History

Approximately 50% of women with PCOS have a family history of PCOS, type 2 diabetes mellitus, or both. Alternatively, the history may disclose familial hirsutism, which begins at puberty and is accompanied by regular menstrual cycles and normal concentrations of circulating androgens. In the absence of a positive family history, hirsutism that is disproportionate to the patient's racial background and is accompanied by regular periods is considered idiopathic, if laboratory test results are normal (see below).

Medication Use

Some medications appear to cause increased LH secretion and thus promote the development of PCOS. In particular, long-term use of the anticonvulsant valproate is strongly associated with the onset of PCOS.[9]

Cigarette Smoking

Women who smoke have higher concentrations of androstenedione and testosterone than do nonsmoking women.[10] Hence, smoking may contribute to hyperandrogenism.

PHYSICAL EXAMINATION

Hirsutism can be assessed objectively with the Ferriman-Gallwey scoring system [see Figure 1].[11] Along with providing a baseline measurement of hirsutism, this system can also be used to follow the efficacy of treatment.

Various physical findings point to insulin resistance [see Table 2]. Excess weight is a major determinant of insulin resistance and hyperinsulinemia.[12] Relative weight is best assessed by means of the body mass index (BMI), which is calculated by dividing the patient's weight in kilograms by the square of the patient's height in meters. Women with a BMI of greater than 27 (i.e., those who are overweight) are often insulin resistant and usually demonstrate hyperinsulinemia in response to a glucose stimulus. Women with a BMI of greater than 30 (i.e., those who are obese) are almost always insulin resistant. Women with a BMI of less than 22 are unlikely to be insulin resistant unless they have one of a relatively rare group of acquired or inherited lipodystrophic disorders.

Other physical findings that suggest insulin resistance are a waist-to-hip ratio greater than 0.85 and a waist circumference greater than 90 cm (35.5 in). The presence of acanthosis nigricans or achrochordons (skin tags) suggests hyperinsulinemia. The syndrome of hyperandrogenism, insulin resistance, and acanthosis nigricans (HAIR-AN syndrome) is the most severe form of the insulin-resistant phenotype of PCOS.

Unfortunately, the physical findings that are associated with insulin resistance tend to be specific but not sensitive. For example, patients with acanthosis nigricans are almost always in-

Table 1 Characteristics of Common Causes of Androgen Excess

Diagnosis	Cause	Ovulation Status	Testosterone Level	8 A.M. Follicular-Phase 17-Hydroxyprogesterone Level
PCOS	Elevated LH, serum insulin, or both	Anovulation or oligo-ovulation	Elevated (0.75–2 ng/ml)	Normal (< 4 ng/ml)
Idiopathic hirsutism	Elevated production of androgen in the pilosebaceous unit, or a mild form of PCOS	Regular ovulation	Normal (< 0.75 ng/ml)	Normal (< 4 ng/ml)
Adrenal hyperplasia	Decrease in 21-hydroxylase activity because of a gene mutation	Anovulation or oligo-ovulation	Elevated (0.75-2 ng/ml)	Elevated (> 4 ng/ml)
Ovarian or adrenal tumor	Disorder of cell growth	Anovulation	Markedly elevated (> 2 ng/ml)	May be elevated

LH—luteinizing hormone PCOS—polycystic ovary syndrome

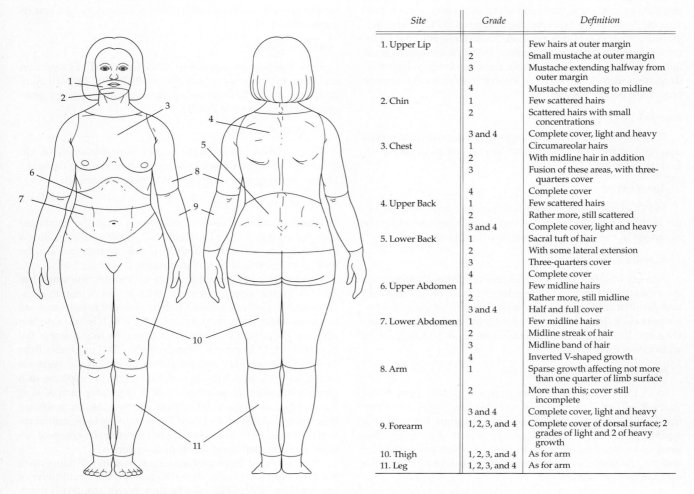

Site	Grade	Definition
1. Upper Lip	1	Few hairs at outer margin
	2	Small mustache at outer margin
	3	Mustache extending halfway from outer margin
	4	Mustache extending to midline
2. Chin	1	Few scattered hairs
	2	Scattered hairs with small concentrations
	3 and 4	Complete cover, light and heavy
3. Chest	1	Circumareolar hairs
	2	With midline hair in addition
	3	Fusion of these areas, with three-quarters cover
	4	Complete cover
4. Upper Back	1	Few scattered hairs
	2	Rather more, still scattered
	3 and 4	Complete cover, light and heavy
5. Lower Back	1	Sacral tuft of hair
	2	With some lateral extension
	3	Three-quarters cover
	4	Complete cover
6. Upper Abdomen	1	Few midline hairs
	2	Rather more, still midline
	3 and 4	Half and full cover
7. Lower Abdomen	1	Few midline hairs
	2	Midline streak of hair
	3	Midline band of hair
	4	Inverted V-shaped growth
8. Arm	1	Sparse growth affecting not more than one quarter of limb surface
	2	More than this; cover still incomplete
	3 and 4	Complete cover, light and heavy
9. Forearm	1, 2, 3, and 4	Complete cover of dorsal surface; 2 grades of light and 2 of heavy growth
10. Thigh	1, 2, 3, and 4	As for arm
11. Leg	1, 2, 3, and 4	As for arm

Figure 1 **Ferriman-Gallwey scoring system for quantitating hirsutism. The 11 sites are graded from 0 (no terminal hair) to 4 (severe hirsutism). Women with a total score greater than 8 are considered hirsute.[11]**

sulin resistant, but many women with insulin resistance do not have acanthosis nigricans.[13] Although the identification of severe insulin resistance on the basis of clinical manifestations may be relatively simple, the detection of mild insulin resistance may be difficult.

A key aspect of the physical examination is a search for signs of virilization, such as clitoromegaly, increased upper body muscle mass, and male pattern baldness. These may indicate the presence of an androgen-secreting tumor.

Women with PCOS have enlarged ovaries, although the ovaries typically are not palpable on pelvic examination. If pelvic examination discloses a large, complex mass, the patient may have an adrenal or ovarian tumor.

LABORATORY TESTS

The goals of the laboratory evaluation of hyperandrogenism are to rule out an adrenal and ovarian tumor, assess the severity of the androgen excess, and determine whether the source of the hyperandrogenism is adrenal or ovarian. Laboratory tests that are the most useful in the evaluation of hyperandrogenism include determination of the total serum testosterone level; determination of the 8 A.M. follicular phase 17-hydroxyprogesterone level; determination of the serum dehydroepiandrosterone sul-

fate (DHEAS) level (if fertility is an issue); and determination of the serum prolactin level (if the patient has amenorrhea).

Testosterone

The serum testosterone concentration provides the best laboratory estimate of the severity of androgen overproduction. Either total or free testosterone can be measured. Total testosterone measurement is performed by all clinical laboratories; these tests are well standardized and are less expensive than free testosterone measurement. However, because the level of sex hormone–binding globulin decreases as testosterone production increases, the total testosterone level does not fully reflect the degree of hyperandrogenism, especially if the overproduction of testosterone is minimal. Many women with mild PCOS have a total testosterone level in the upper end of the normal range. If the total testosterone level is greater than 2 ng/ml (200 ng/dl), the patient probably has ovarian stromal hyperthecosis or an adrenal or ovarian tumor and needs a detailed evaluation, which should include imaging studies of the ovary and adrenal glands.

The free testosterone measurement is more sensitive in detecting mild androgen overproduction. Nevertheless, because the total testosterone adequately identifies women with marked

Table 2 Physical Findings Associated with Insulin Resistance

Body mass index* > 27	Acanthosis nigricans
Waist-to-hip ratio > 0.85	Numerous achrochordons
Waist > 90 cm	(skin tags)

*Calculated by dividing the patient's weight in kilograms by the square of her height in meters.

androgen overproduction who need additional evaluation and because free testosterone is usually more expensive to assay, measurement of free testosterone is not routinely indicated.

17-Hydroxyprogesterone

Approximately 2% of women who present with hyperandrogenism and oligo-ovulation or anovulation have nonclassic adrenal hyperplasia resulting from a 21-hydroxylase deficiency. The prevalence of this congenital disorder varies markedly among different ethnic groups, from below 1% in Hispanic populations to as high as 5% to 8% in Ashkenazi Jewish populations. The decision to screen for the disorder depends on the cost-benefit assessment of detection and the baseline prevalence of the disorder in the patient's ethnic group.

If the 17-hydroxyprogesterone level at 8 A.M. (measured in the follicular phase of the menstrual cycle) is greater than 4 ng/ml, the patient probably has nonclassic adrenal hyperplasia resulting from a 21-hydroxylase deficiency. This diagnosis can be confirmed by a 60-minute ACTH stimulation test. The test utilizes a form of synthetic ACTH (cosyntropin) that contains the first 24 of the 39 amino acids of natural ACTH: 0.25 mg is given intravenously or intramuscularly, and the 17-hydroxyprogesterone level is measured 60 minutes later. A post-ACTH 17-hydroxyprogesterone level greater than 10 ng/ml confirms the diagnosis of nonclassic adrenal hyperplasia resulting from a 21-hydroxylase deficiency.

DHEAS

DHEAS, an androgen prohormone that can be converted to testosterone in the periphery, is secreted almost exclusively by the adrenal glands. The normal DHEAS level in premenopausal women is 0.12 to 5.35 µg/dl. A DHEAS level above 10.70 µg/dl—that is, more than twice the upper limit of normal—should raise concern over a possible adrenal tumor. Many women with PCOS have a DHEAS level in the upper range of normal, for reasons that have not been clearly identified. In infertile women with PCOS whose DHEAS level is greater than 2 µg/ml, the combination of clomiphene and a glucocorticoid may result in higher pregnancy rates than clomiphene alone (see below).

Serum Prolactin

If the patient has amenorrhea, the laboratory workup should include an assessment of the serum prolactin level to rule out a prolactin-secreting pituitary tumor [see Chapter 76]. Many clinicians also routinely measure serum follicle-stimulating hormone (FSH) and thyroid-stimulating hormone (TSH) levels in amenorrheic patients.

Serum Luteinizing Hormone

The measurement of serum LH presents a special problem in the laboratory evaluation of PCOS. In the research setting—using multiple serum LH measurements (every 10 minutes for at least 8 hours) and a precise and reliable LH assay—elevated LH levels can be documented in about 95% of women with PCOS. However, because LH secretion is pulsatile and the standard commercial assays are not as precise as research assays, measurement of LH in clinical practice is of only modest utility. An elevated LH level is reasonably specific for PCOS, provided the sample was not taken during a preovulatory LH surge. A normal LH value does not necessarily exclude PCOS, however, because the test sample may have been drawn when the patient was at the nadir of an LH pulse. Another important point is that as BMI increases, the normal range for LH decreases [see Figure 2].[14] Nomograms that control serum LH for BMI are not widely available.

Pelvic Imaging

Demonstration of polycystic ovaries on pelvic ultrasonography is not essential for the diagnosis of PCOS. Pelvic imaging is indicated only if the ovaries are palpable on physical examination or the total testosterone concentration is greater than 200 mg/dl.

Tests for Detection of Insulin Resistance and Hyperinsulinemia

About 50% of women with PCOS have insulin resistance and hyperinsulinemia. There is no clear consensus on how to detect those conditions. A major problem is that the least resource-intensive laboratory techniques for diagnosing insulin resistance and hyperinsulinemia are specific but not sensitive. Elevation of the fasting serum insulin level or a fasting serum insulin-to-glucose ratio of less than 4.5 is almost always associ-

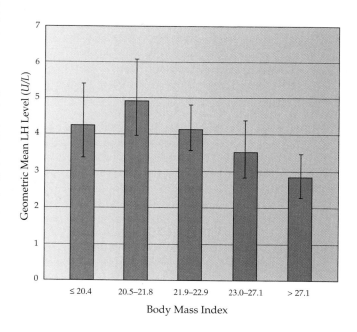

Figure 2 Relationship between body mass index (BMI) and basal luteinizing hormone (LH) levels in women in the follicular phase of the menstrual cycle.[14]

ated with insulin resistance, but many insulin-resistant women do not have fasting hyperinsulinemia. Laboratory techniques that are both specific and sensitive for detecting insulin resistance, such as euglycemic hyperinsulinemic clamp studies, are too complex and expensive for application in general clinical practice. Until both specific and sensitive laboratory tests that can be widely applied in practice become available, clinicians should use clinical findings and, if necessary, simple laboratory tests—such as assessment of fasting insulin levels or assessment of insulin response to an oral glucose challenge—to identify women with insulin resistance. Even nonobese women with PCOS have marked increases in circulating insulin after a glucose challenge [*see Figure 3*].[15]

Differential Diagnosis

IDIOPATHIC HIRSUTISM

Idiopathic hirsutism is defined as hirsutism in a woman with regular, ovulatory menstrual cycles. Women with idiopathic hirsutism have circulating testosterone and androstenedione concentrations at the upper limit of the normal range, but in these patients, such levels are lower than the levels observed in women with PCOS. Women with idiopathic hirsutism often have sisters with PCOS, and they tend to have a lower BMI than the sisters with PCOS.[16,17] Many authorities believe that idiopathic hirsutism is a mild form of PCOS in which hyperandrogenism is present but the disease has not progressed to the point where ovulatory menses have become disrupted. Other authorities believe that idiopathic hirsutism is

the result of overactive skin conversion of weak precursor androgens (e.g., as androstenedione) to potent androgens (e.g., dihydrotestosterone) directly in the pilosebaceous unit. Regardless of the etiology, idiopathic hirsutism is best treated with the same approach as that for hirsutism in women with PCOS (see below).

VIRILIZATION SYNDROMES

Women with the rapid onset of virilization or a serum testosterone level greater than 2 ng/ml (200 ng/dl) should be evaluated for an adrenal or ovarian tumor. Use of magnetic resonance imaging to screen for an adrenal tumor and use of pelvic sonography to screen for an ovarian tumor are helpful.

Adrenal carcinoma presents with the rapid onset of virilization; it is often associated with systemic symptoms such as fatigue, weakness, and weight loss. DHEAS concentration is often greater than 8 µg/ml, and 24-hour urinary 17-ketosteroid excretion is markedly increased, to about 30 mg/dl.

OVARIAN HYPERTHECOSIS

Careful histologic examination of ovaries from women with PCOS often reveals islands of luteinized, steroid-secreting stromal cells (stromal hyperthecosis) in the medullary portion of the ovary that are not associated with follicular structures.[18] Severely hyperthecotic ovaries may contain only a small number of follicles, each 4 to 8 mm in diameter. PCOS patients with more severe hyperinsulinemia seem to be at highest risk for hyperthecosis.

Only a small subset of women with hyperandrogenism have stromal hyperthecosis. The diagnosis should be considered in a

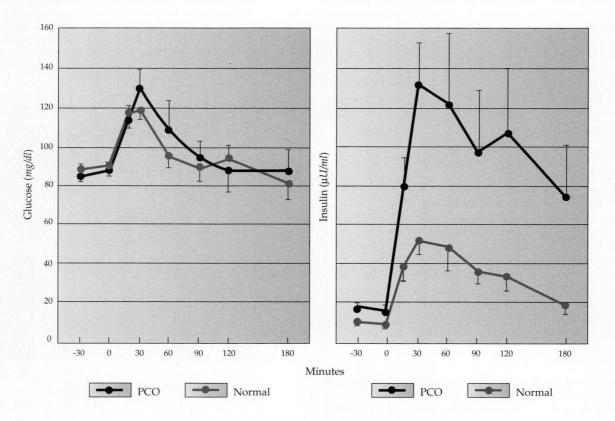

Figure 3   In response to an oral glucose challenge, nonobese women with PCOS experience an exaggerated increase in circulating insulin compared with weight-matched control subjects; the increase persists for over 3 hours.[15]

patient who presents with virilization, a total serum testosterone concentration of greater than 2 ng/ml, a normal LH level, and marked insulin resistance and hyperinsulinemia. Pathologic confirmation of the diagnosis, which requires removal of the ovaries, is not necessary.

Differentiation of ovarian hyperthecosis from PCOS is important because women with ovarian hyperthecosis often do not have significant suppression of circulating testosterone when treated with estrogen-progestin contraceptive alone. Instead, treatment with a GnRH analogue (e.g., leuprolide acetate depot, 3.75 mg intramuscularly every 4 weeks) plus an estrogen-progestin contraceptive often results in the normalization of circulating androgens.[19] A possible interpretation of this observation is that LH must be profoundly suppressed to decrease ovarian androgen production in women with hyperthecotic ovaries. Low-dose estrogen-progestin contraceptives alone do not suppress pituitary LH secretion as completely as they do in combination with a GnRH agonist analogue.

Treatment

Treatment for PCOS may be general—directed at the underlying hormonal imbalance—or specific to a particular manifestation (e.g., hirsutism or infertility) [see Table 3]. PCOS should be treated, because it poses long-term risks of endometrial cancer, diabetes mellitus, and possibly cardiovascular disease.

Regardless of the patient's presenting complaint, treatment of PCOS in a woman who smokes cigarettes includes smoking cessation. Discontinuance of smoking may result in a reduction in circulating androgens; also, smoking is a contraindication to the use of oral contraceptives, which are often prescribed for patients with PCOS.

TREATMENT OF HIRSUTISM

The mainstay of the treatment of hirsutism resulting from androgen excess is the combination of an estrogen-progestin oral contraceptive (used in regular or long cycles) and an antiandrogen. Patients should be advised that response to therapy tends to be slow; for more immediate results, patients may prefer the use of techniques that directly destroy the hair follicle.

Oral Contraceptives

Cyclic estrogen-progestin oral contraceptives produce multiple beneficial effects in patients with PCOS. These effects include the following: (1) decreased LH secretion, which suppresses ovarian androgen production; (2) increased liver production of sex hormone–binding globulin, which decreases free testosterone concentration; (3) decreased adrenal androgen production, through an unidentified pathway; (4) prevention of endometrial hyperplasia; and (5) regular uterine withdrawal bleeding. Of course, oral contraceptives also prevent pregnancy. The choice of agent does not seem important; it appears that any oral contraceptive, regardless of the estrogen dose or the progestin employed, can be effective in the treatment of hirsutism.

By suppressing both ovarian and adrenal androgen production, oral contraceptives decrease the stimulus to terminal hair growth. In patients with hirsutism, therapy with an oral contraceptive first brings a decrease in the diameter of the hair shaft and in the intensity of pigment in the hair—the unwanted hair becomes thinner and lighter in color. With prolonged treatment, the linear rate of hair growth diminishes. Ultimately, the hair follicle becomes senescent. If no new hair follicle starts to grow, the hirsutism then diminishes.

Long-cycle oral contraceptives When oral contraceptives are used in a standard cyclic manner (21 days of active pills followed by 7 days of inactive pills), LH secretion tends to increase during the 7 days in which inactive pills are taken. This stimulates a small rise in ovarian testosterone secretion, which, in turn, can stimulate hair growth. As an alternative, oral contraceptives can be taken in a continuous manner. In the initial treatment of hirsutism caused by PCOS, use of continuous oral contraceptives may be more effective than use of cyclic oral contraceptives for the suppression of LH and androgen production.[20]

Table 3   Treatment of Hirsutism, Anovulatory Infertility, and Endometrial Hyperplasia in Women with PCOS

Presenting Problem	Standard Treatment	Alternative Treatment
Hirsutism	Oral contraceptive plus spironolactone Weight loss	Oral contraceptive used in a long-cycle regimen, plus spironolactone Oral contraceptive plus GnRH analogue Insulin sensitizer, preferably metformin Finasteride
Acne	Oral contraceptive	Topical agents, oral antibiotics
Infertility	Weight loss Clomiphene Metformin plus clomiphene Clomiphene plus glucocorticoids Low-dose FSH injections Low-dose FSH injections plus metformin	Ovarian surgery IVF-ET
Endometrial hyperplasia	Oral contraceptives High-dose progestins	Weight loss

FSH—follicle-stimulating hormone GnRH—gonadotropin-releasing hormone IVF-ET—in vitro fertilization with embryo transfer

Most women with PCOS would like to restore a regular pattern of menses. To accommodate this desire while maximally suppressing LH levels, the clinician can employ the following regimen: the patient takes an active pill daily for 63 days (using the active pills from three packs), then takes inactive pills for 7 days. This long-cycle oral contraceptive regimen may induce regular withdrawal bleeding every other month and produce better suppression of LH and testosterone than oral contraceptives used in monthly cycles.

Antiandrogens

Antiandrogens are a cornerstone of therapy for hirsutism. In a 1-year trial, antiandrogen therapy using cyproterone acetate, 50 mg daily, plus ethinyl estradiol on cycle days 16 through 25, was compared with glucocorticoid suppression with hydrocortisone, 20 mg daily. Although hydrocortisone was more effective at normalizing plasma androgen levels, cyproterone provided superior treatment of hirsutism.[21] This study demonstrated that in established hirsutism, suppressing circulating androgens to normal levels is less important than blocking peripheral androgen action in the pilosebaceous unit.

Cyproterone acetate is not available in the United States. However, spironolactone has proved to be an effective antiandrogen, and its effects on hirsutism are similar to those of cyproterone acetate.[22] Because spironolactone has been used for many decades in the treatment of hirsutism and has an excellent safety profile, it should be considered the first-line agent for this indication in the United States. The usual dosage of spironolactone as an antiandrogen is 100 mg once daily.

The 5α-reductase inhibitor finasteride, which the Food and Drug Administration has approved only for treatment of men with benign prostatic hyperplasia, also reduces hirsutism in women.[23] The dosage of finasteride is 5 mg daily.

The androgen receptor antagonist flutamide (Eulexin) is as effective as spironolactone and finasteride in the treatment of hirsutism, but flutamide has liver toxicity and may cause fulminant liver failure.[24] Although the risk of liver failure with flutamide is small, hirsutism is a benign condition, so treatment regimens must have a high degree of safety.

Spironolactone, finasteride, and flutamide are believed to be human teratogens and may induce abnormal genital tract development in male fetuses. Women taking these agents need to use effective birth control. In addition, spironolactone, finasteride, and flutamide do not protect against endometrial hyperplasia and are not likely to induce regular menstrual cycles. These considerations support the use of an oral contraceptive in combination with an antiandrogen in the treatment of hirsutism in women of reproductive age.

Weight Loss

Numerous studies have demonstrated the benefits of weight loss in hyperandrogenic, insulin-resistant women.[25-27] In these studies, mean weight loss ranging from about 10 to 20 kg has been associated with a decrease in insulin levels and testosterone concentration and with ovulation and subsequent pregnancy in many women.[28-30]

Weight loss is difficult to achieve. A structured program that includes consultation with a nutritionist, encouragement by the physician, a low-calorie diet, and initiation of an exercise program may be the most effective nonsurgical approach in these patients. Surgical methods of weight reduction can be very effective, especially in women whose BMI is greater than 40.

Gonadotropin-Releasing Hormone Agonists

Women with hirsutism who do not respond to treatment with an oral contraceptive plus an antiandrogen can often be successfully treated with a combination of a GnRH agonist (e.g., leuprolide acetate) and an oral contraceptive,[31] with or without an antiandrogen. It is likely that the combination of leuprolide and an oral contraceptive produces greater suppression of LH and androgens than the oral contraceptive alone. Leuprolide is not ordinarily recommended as a first-line therapy for hirsutism because it is expensive (costing approximately $400 a month). Also, when used as a single agent, a GnRH agonist produces profound hypoestrogenism and accelerated bone loss. The addition of an oral contraceptive prevents GnRH agonist–induced hypoestrogenism and vasomotor symptoms and preserves bone density.

Glucocorticoids

Treatment with glucocorticoids may be appropriate in women with ACTH-dependent adrenal androgen overproduction, such as those with nonclassic adrenal hyperplasia resulting from 21-hydroxylase deficiency,[32,33] but it is not appropriate for the treatment of hirsutism in PCOS. A major problem with glucocorticoid therapy is that the complete suppression of ACTH production often requires giving more glucocorticoid than would normally be produced by the adrenal glands. As a result, patients receiving long-term glucocorticoid treatment are at increased risk for iatrogenic Cushing syndrome, osteoporosis, and diabetes mellitus. In addition, the corticotropin-releasing hormone–ACTH–cortisol axis may become so suppressed that the adrenal response to stress is blunted. For those reasons, I avoid using glucocorticoids to treat hirsutism. If the clinician does decide to use glucocorticoid therapy, use of low-dose glucocorticoids (5 or 7.5 mg of prednisone daily) or an alternate-day regimen of glucocorticoids may minimize those risks. Also, because almost all women treated with glucocorticoids gain weight and many develop osteoporosis, the clinician should carefully monitor weight and bone density in these patients.

Ovarian Surgery

Ovarian surgery can be used to decrease the mass of androgen-secreting thecal and stromal tissue. No randomized, controlled trials have been published concerning the benefits and risks of ovarian surgery for hyperandrogenism. In my opinion, the risks of ovarian surgery are greater than the potential benefits for women with hirsutism. I recommend ovarian surgery only for women with PCOS and infertility in whom conservative therapy has failed (see below).

Laser, Electrolysis, and Depilatory Treatment

Techniques that directly destroy the hair follicle are helpful in the treatment of hirsutism. Mechanical techniques include plucking, waxing, and shaving. These methods do not lead to a worsening of hirsutism, as some people believe, but may cause skin irritation. Electrolysis can destroy both the hair and the cells responsible for the growth of the hair, thereby producing a more prolonged beneficial effect than mechanical techniques.

Laser therapy is an evolving technique that is highly effective in the treatment of hirsutism. Multiple case series have been reported using the ruby laser to treat hirsutism. The melanin in the hair is used as a natural chromophore. The energy delivered by the ruby laser causes photothermal damage to the hair and key cells surrounding the hair, which may prevent hair regrowth. In one study, two treatments with the ruby laser resulted in a 50% reduction in hair follicle density.[34] Unwanted side effects of laser treatment of hirsutism include skin hyperpigmentation and hypopigmentation and pitting of the skin surface. Most of these changes resolve spontaneously over 6 months.[35]

A new chemical inhibitor of hair growth is eflornithine 13.9% cream (Vaniqa). Eflornithine irreversibly inhibits the activity of skin ornithine decarboxylase, an enzyme that is necessary for the synthesis of polyamines and hence for hair growth. In clinical studies, which excluded pregnant and nursing women, eflornithine reduced facial hirsutism.[36]

TREATMENT OF ACNE

As with the treatment of hirsutism, the treatment of acne in patients with PCOS begins with an oral contraceptive. Randomized, placebo-controlled clinical trials have demonstrated the benefits of combination estrogen-progestin oral contraceptives for acne after 6 months of treatment.[37, 38] Because norgestrel is more androgenic than gestodene and desogestrel, some authorities recommend, on theoretical grounds, that oral contraceptives containing one of the latter progestins be used to treat acne.

Topical agents and oral antibiotics may also be indicated for acne in women with PCOS [see Chapter 31].

TREATMENT OF ANOVULATION

Ovulation induction in PCOS follows a stepwise approach [see Table 4]. If the BMI is greater than 27, weight loss is an important goal. If normalization of the BMI cannot be achieved, clomiphene citrate is often prescribed because it is relatively inexpensive and has an excellent safety profile. Hyperandrogenic, insulin-resistant women are more likely to fail to ovulate and become pregnant with clomiphene than are women who are not insulin resistant. If both weight loss and clomiphene do not induce ovulation and result in pregnancy, the currently available choices for ovulation induction include insulin-sensitizing agents (for patients with insulin resistance), FSH injec-

tions, ovarian surgery, and in vitro fertilization with embryo transfer (IVF-ET).

Weight Loss

Many women with PCOS are overweight or obese. In such women, weight loss (see above) is associated with a decrease in insulin secretion, a decrease in LH secretion, and a decrease in androgen production. The result is often a resumption of regular ovulation and, in some women, pregnancy.

Clomiphene Citrate

Clomiphene citrate is the most widely used agent for ovulation induction in women with PCOS. The FDA-approved doses for clomiphene are 50 or 100 mg daily for a maximum of 5 days per cycle. After a spontaneous menses or the induction of menses with a progestin withdrawal maneuver (medroxyprogesterone acetate, 10 mg p.o. daily for 5 days), clomiphene (50 mg daily for 5 days) is started on cycle day 3, 4, or 5. In properly selected women, 50% will ovulate through the use of this clomiphene regimen. Another 25% will ovulate if the dose of clomiphene is increased to 100 mg daily. During each cycle, determination of ovulation should be attempted by use of basal body temperature charts, ultrasound monitoring of follicle growth and rupture, or luteal-phase progesterone measurements. Some clinicians use endometrial biopsies to document ovulation in cycles where conception is not attempted. In most women, ovulation occurs approximately 5 to 12 days after the last dose of clomiphene. Measurement of the urinary LH surge is recommended to assist the patient in prospectively determining the periovulatory interval.

Although the FDA has approved maximal clomiphene doses of 100 mg daily, many clinicians have used clomiphene at doses of up to 250 mg daily. Women who fail to ovulate after taking clomiphene in doses of 100 mg daily for 5 days may ovulate if they are treated with clomiphene at doses of 150 mg daily for 5 days. Some authorities advocate use of clomiphene at doses up to 250 mg daily for up to 14 days. As many as 70% of the women who fail to ovulate with doses of 100 mg daily will ovulate with higher doses, but fewer than 30% of those become pregnant. In my opinion, there are few data to support the use of clomiphene at doses greater than 150 mg daily. Women who do not become pregnant at that dose should consider other approaches to ovulation induction (see below).

Clomiphene treatment can be associated with adverse changes in the reproductive tract, including induction of a luteal-phase defect (delay of endometrial maturation) and the creation of a hostile cervical environment from low quantity and quality of cervical mucus. Some clinicians recommend endometrial biopsy in a test cycle of clomiphene treatment to assess whether clomiphene induces luteal-phase deficiency. Many clinicians recommend that a postcoital test be performed during the first clomiphene cycle of treatment to screen for poor cervical mucus properties.

Multiple pregnancy is a well known outcome of clomiphene use. The absolute risk of high-order multiple gestation with clomiphene treatment is low: in a manufacturer's study of 2,369 clomiphene-induced pregnancies, 7% resulted in twins, 0.5% triplets, 0.3% quadruplets, and 0.13% quintuplets. However, because clomiphene is a heavily prescribed medication, the number of triplets resulting from clomiphene is substantial. The rate of spontaneous abortion after clomiphene-induced ovulation

---

Table 4 **A Stepwise Approach to the Induction of Ovulation in Infertile Women with PCOS***

Step 1: if BMI is > 27, weight loss of at least 10%

Step 2: clomiphene

Step 3: if DHEAS > 2 µg/ml (200 µg/dl), clomiphene plus glucocorticoid therapy

Step 4: metformin for 8 to 12 wk

Step 5: metformin plus clomiphene

Step 6: low-dose FSH therapy

Step 7: metformin plus low-dose FSH therapy

Step 8: in vitro fertilization

Step 9: laparoscopic ovarian surgery to reduce ovarian androgen production

*Steps proceed in order of increasing resource intensity.

and pregnancy is approximately 15%. The most common side effects of clomiphene include vasomotor symptoms (20%), adnexal tenderness (5%), nausea (3%), headache (1%), and, rarely, blurring of vision or scotomata. Most clinicians permanently discontinue clomiphene in women who experience visual changes from the drug.

Clomiphene plus Glucocorticoid

Anovulatory women with PCOS whose serum DHEAS concentration is above the midnormal range (2 µg/ml) appear to have reduced ovulation and pregnancy rates when they are treated with clomiphene. Some studies suggest that adding a glucocorticoid (e.g., dexamethasone) to clomiphene improves pregnancy rates in these women.[39]

Insulin Sensitizers

A major advance in reproductive endocrinology is the discovery that insulin sensitizers can induce ovulation in infertile women with oligo-ovulation, hyperandrogenism, and insulin resistance. Insulin sensitizers that have been approved for the treatment of diabetes include metformin, rosiglitazone, and pioglitazone. The insulin sensitizer D-chiro-inositol has been demonstrated to induce ovulation in hyperandrogenic insulin-resistant women, but it is currently available for use in research trials only.[40]

Metformin An oral biguanide antihyperglycemic agent approved for the treatment of type 2 diabetes mellitus, metformin has been evaluated in multiple studies for its ability to induce ovulation in women with hyperandrogenism and insulin resistance.

Metformin decreases blood glucose by inhibiting hepatic glucose production and enhancing peripheral glucose uptake. It increases insulin sensitivity at the postreceptor level and stimulates insulin-mediated glucose disposal. Unlike the sulfonylureas, metformin's mechanism of action does not involve increased insulin secretion.

Metformin increases the number of ovulatory cycles in infertile women with hyperandrogenism and insulin resistance. When used together with clomiphene, metformin significantly increases the rate of ovulation and of pregnancy resulting in live-born singleton births.[41-44] Metformin has also been shown to enhance response to the induction of ovulation with FSH injections in oligo-ovulatory, hyperandrogenic, insulin-resistant women.[45]

Metformin is commonly used at a dosage of 500 mg three times daily. To minimize gastrointestinal side effects, such as nausea, many clinicians start metformin at 500 mg daily for the first week, then increase the dosage to 500 mg twice daily for the second week, and then increase the dosage again to 500 mg three times daily. After the full dosage is reached, some clinicians switch to a regimen of 850 mg twice daily to enhance compliance. Although metformin is not approved for ovulation induction by the FDA, it may be significantly less expensive than FSH injections, ovarian surgery, or IVF-ET and may have fewer serious side effects than these treatments.

The most common side effects associated with metformin are GI disturbances, including diarrhea, nausea, vomiting, and abdominal bloating. In rare cases, metformin treatment has caused fatal lactic acidosis, but most of these patients had some degree of renal insufficiency or were severely hypoxic. Before starting treatment with metformin, it is advisable to confirm that the patient's serum creatinine level is less than 1.4 mg/dl.

If a patient has not ovulated after 5 to 10 weeks of metformin treatment, clomiphene can be added (see above). If the patient becomes pregnant, metformin can be discontinued, although it is a category B drug for pregnant women and has been used by some clinicians to treat diabetes in pregnant women.[46]

Thiazolidinediones The thiazolidinediones increase cellular sensitivity to the effects of insulin. Agents in this category include pioglitazone, rosiglitazone, and troglitazone. Several studies of troglitazone reported a decrease not only in fasting insulin but also in LH and testosterone levels, along with an increase in ovulatory cycles.[47-49] Troglitazone was reported to induce ovulation in obese, infertile women with hyperandrogenism and severe insulin resistance who had previously failed to ovulate when treated with clomiphene.[50] In this study, some women ovulated and became pregnant with troglitazone alone, whereas others responded to troglitazone plus clomiphene.

Troglitazone was removed from the market because of its association with the risk of death from liver failure.[51] The risk was extremely small but measurable, affecting approximately 1 in 50,000 patients treated with the drug. Pioglitazone and rosiglitazone, although now widely used in the treatment of diabetes mellitus, have not been extensively studied for their impact on ovulation. One might reasonably assume that they would offer benefits similar to troglitazone. However, until their efficacy and safety in PCOS is well established, it is probably best to use metformin as the main insulin sensitizer in women with PCOS.

Clomiphene plus Gonadotropin Induction

In women who fail to ovulate after therapy with clomiphene alone, gonadotropin injections can be added to clomiphene treatment to induce ovulation.[52] Typically, the injections are started after clomiphene, 100 to 200 mg daily, has been given for 5 days. The main benefit of this combination is that it tends to reduce the quantity of gonadotropins (an expensive medication) needed to induce ovulation during each cycle, because the rise in endogenous LH and FSH levels induced by clomiphene increases the sensitivity of the follicles to the injected gonadotropins. This regimen has been associated with a 50% decrease in the dosage of gonadotropin required to induce ovulation.[53]

Gonadotropins

The gonadotropins currently available for ovulation induction include (1) FSH produced by recombinant DNA technology and immunopurification and (2) LH plus FSH derived from menopausal urine. The recombinant FSH preparations can be given as subcutaneous injections and are available in ampules of 37.5 or 75 IU. FSH is the primary hormone responsible for follicular recruitment and growth in humans; it can be used as a single agent to induce ovulation in most anovulatory women. Women with PCOS generally do not require exogenous LH to induce follicular development, because their levels of LH secretion are already increased.

In women with PCOS, induction of ovulation with long-term, low-dose FSH treatment appears to result in a high pregnancy rate with a low rate of complications such as high-order multiple gestation and ovarian hyperstimulation.[54] In this approach, 75 units of FSH are given daily for the first 14 days; the dose is then raised by 37.5 units every 7 days until follicular ripening is complete. If FSH treatment fails to result in pregnancy, consideration should be given to the combination of metformin and FSH, ovarian surgery, or IVF-ET.

During gonadotropin induction of ovulation, as many as 20% of patients experience mild to moderate enlargement of the ovaries. Some women treated with gonadotropins develop increased vascular permeability and accumulation of fluid in the peritoneal cavity and pleural space, a condition termed the ovarian hyperstimulation syndrome (OHSS). Clinical manifestations of OHSS include abdominal pain, abdominal distention, nausea, vomiting, diarrhea, and dyspnea. Other physical and laboratory findings of OHSS include weight gain, ovarian enlargement, ascites, pleural effusion, hemoconcentration, electrolyte imbalances, renal dysfunction, and thrombosis.[55] Treatment includes bed rest, maintenance of intravascular volume, prophylaxis against thrombosis, and surgical correction of ovarian torsion.

Before the utilization of repetitive estradiol measurements and sonographic evaluation of the follicular development, OHSS occurred in as many as 5% of women receiving gonadotropin treatment. In recent series that employed intense monitoring with those techniques, the rate of OHSS was approximately 0.5%. OHSS may be more severe and have a longer course if a successful pregnancy occurs. Multiple births occur in approximately 15% of pregnancies that take place after ovulation induction with gonadotropins.

Ovarian Surgery

Many gynecologists recommend that in infertile women with PCOS, ovarian surgery be attempted before FSH injections or IVF-ET. Laparoscopic drilling of the ovary is the most widely studied surgical treatment for ovulation in PCOS; approximately 1,000 cases have been reported, although no controlled studies have been undertaken.[56] These reports demonstrate that surgery to induce ovulation causes a decrease in circulating LH (50% decline) and testosterone (30% decline) and an increase in FSH (30% increase). The pregnancy rate is in the range of 50% at 12 months and 70% at 24 months.

The surgical techniques used for ovarian drilling vary between centers. However, all use a laser or electrosurgery to make multiple millimeter-size punctures in each ovary.[57-59]

In Vitro Fertilization with Embryo Transfer

IVF-ET has recently been demonstrated to be effective in the treatment of infertile women with PCOS who fail to become pregnant with gonadotropin injections.[60] In preliminary reports, IVF-ET treatment of infertile women with PCOS has been associated with a per-cycle pregnancy rate of 0.24 to 0.27.[61,62]

Metabolic Abnormalities Associated with PCOS

DIABETES MELLITUS

Obese women with PCOS may be at high risk for diabetes. In one study, testing in 254 PCOS patients found new-onset diabetes in 7%, most of whom had a BMI greater than 30.[63] Another study showed that by 40 years of age, 10% of women with PCOS will have been diagnosed with diabetes.[64]

It is important to assess for diabetes in an obese infertile woman with PCOS before using an ovulation-inducing agent.

Poorly controlled diabetes is associated with a significantly increased risk of fetal malformations. Sacral agenesis and caudal dysplasia are 400 times more common in the offspring of women with diabetes than in those of women with normal glucose metabolism. Other anomalies associated with diabetes include anencephaly, open spina bifida, renal agenesis, ventricular septal defects, and transposition of the great vessels. Control of diabetes before conception decreases the risk of fetal malformations.

HYPERLIPIDEMIA

Women with PCOS have hyperandrogenism, and obesity and insulin resistance are common. These conditions are often associated with hyperlipidemia. In one study, levels of total cholesterol, low-density lipoprotein (LDL) cholesterol, and triglycerides were higher in obese women with PCOS than in weight-matched control subjects. Elevated LDL levels were the predominant lipid abnormality observed in women with PCOS, independent of obesity.[65] High-density lipoprotein (HDL) cholesterol levels were also higher, however, which could provide some degree of protection against cardiovascular disease. One epidemiologic study that included a 30-year follow-up of women with PCOS found no increase in mortality from cardiovascular disease.[66]

References

1. Knochenhauer ES, Key TJ, Kahsar-Miller M, et al: Prevalence of PCOS in unselected black and white women of the southeastern United States: a prospective study. J Clin Endocrinol Metab 83:3078, 1998

2. Diamanti-Kandarakis E, Kouli CR, Bergiele AT, et al: A survey of the polycystic ovary syndrome in the Greek island of Lesbos: hormonal and metabolic profile. J Clin Endocrinol Metab 84:4006, 1999

3. Asuncion M, Calvo RM, San Millan JL, et al: A prospective study of the prevalence of the polycystic ovary syndrome in unselected Caucasian women from Spain. J Clin Endocrinol Metab 85:4182, 2000

4. Reindollar RH, Novak M, Tho SP, et al: Adult-onset amenorrhea: a study of 262 patients. Am J Obstet Gynecol 155:531, 1986

5. Smith S, Ravnikar VA, Barbieri RL: Androgen and insulin response to an oral glucose challenge in hyperandrogenic women. Fertil Steril 48:72, 1987

6. Waldstreicher J, Santoro NF, Hall JE, et al: Hyperfunction of the hypothalamic-pituitary axis in women with polycystic ovary disease: indirect evidence for partial gonadotroph desensitization. J Clin Endocrinol Metab 66:165, 1988

7. Barbieri RL, Makris A, Randall RW, et al: Insulin stimulates androgen accumulation in incubations of ovarian stroma obtained from women with hyperandrogenism. J Clin Endocrinol Metab 62:904, 1986

8. Pochi PE, Strauss JS: Endocrinologic control of the development and activity of the human sebaceous gland. J Invest Dermatol 62:191, 1974

9. Joffe H, Taylor AE, Hall JE: Polycystic ovarian syndrome: relationship to epilepsy and antiepileptic drug therapy (editorial). J Clin Endocrinol Metab 86:2946, 2001

10. Longcope C, Johnstone CC: Androgen and estrogen dynamics in pre- and postmenopausal women: a comparison between smokers and non-smokers. J Clin Endocrinol Metab 67:379, 1988

11. Ferriman D, Gallwey JD: Clinical assessment of body hair growth in women. J Clin Endocrinol Metab 21:1440, 1961

12. Weyer C, Bogardus C, Mott DM, et al: The natural history of insulin secretory dysfunction and insulin resistance in the pathogenesis of type 2 diabetes mellitus. J Clin Invest 104:787, 1999

13. Dunaif A: Insulin resistance and the polycystic ovary syndrome: mechanism and implications for pathogenesis. Endocrin Rev 18:774, 1997

14. Bohlke K, Cramer D, Barbieri RL: Relation of luteinizing hormone levels to body mass index in premenopausal women. Fertil Steril 69:500, 1998

15. Chang JR, Nakamura RM, Judd HL, et al: Insulin resistance in nonobese patients with polycystic ovarian disease. J Clin Endocrinol Metab 57:356, 1983

16. Glickman SO, Rosenfield L: Androgen metabolism by isolated hairs from women with idiopathic hirsutism is usually normal. J Inv Derm 82:62, 1984

17. Escobar-Morreale HF, Serrano-Gotarredona J, Garcia-Robles R, et al: Mild adrenal and ovarian steroidogenic abnormalities in hirsute women without hyperandrogenism: does idiopathic hirsutism exist? Metabolism 46:902, 1997

18. Hughesdon PE: Morphology and morphogenesis of the Stein Leventhal ovary and of so called hyperthecosis. Obstet Gynecol Surv 37:58, 1982

19. Adashi EY: Potential utility of gonadotropin releasing hormone agonists in the management of ovarian hyperandrogenism. Fertil Steril 53:765, 1990

20. Ruchhoft EA, Elkind-Hirsch KE, Malinak R: Pituitary function is altered during the same cycle in women with polycystic ovary syndrome treated with continuous or cyclic oral contraceptives or a gonadotropin releasing hormone agonist. Fertil Steril 66:54, 1996

21. Spritzer P, Billaud L, Thalabard JC, et al: Cyproterone acetate versus hydrocortisone treatment in late onset adrenal hyperplasia. J Clin Endocrinol Metab 70:642, 1990

22. O'Brien RC, Cooper ME, Murray RML, et al: Comparison of sequential cyproterone acetate/estrogen versus spironolactone plus oral contraceptive in the treatment of hirsutism. J Clin Endocrinol Metab 72:1008, 1991

23. Wong IL, Morris RS, Chang L, et al: A prospective randomized trial comparing finasteride to spironolactone in the treatment of hirsute women. J Clin Endocrinol Metab 80:233, 1995

24. Andrade RJ, Lucena MI, Fernandez MC, et al: Fulminant liver failure associated with flutamide therapy for hirsutism (letter). Lancet 353:983, 1999

25. Bates GW, Whitworth NS: Effect of body weight reduction on plasma androgens in obese infertile women. Fertil Steril 38:406, 1982

26. Pasquali R, Antenucci D, Casimirri F, et al: Clinical and hormonal characteristics of obese and amenorrheic women before and after weight loss. J Clin Endocrinol Metab 8:173, 1989

27. Clark AM, Thornley B, Tomlinson L, et al: Weight loss in obese infertile women results in improvements in reproductive outcome for all forms of fertility treatment. Human Reprod 13:1502, 1998

28. Hollman M, Runnebaum B, Gerhard I: Effects of weight loss on the hormonal profile in obese infertile women. Human Reprod 11:1884, 1996

29. Clark AM, Ledger W, Galletly C, et al: Weight loss results in significant improvement in pregnancy and ovulation rates in anovulatory obese women. Human Reprod 10:2705, 1995

30. Guzick DS, Wing R, Smith D, et al: Endocrine consequences of weight loss in obese, hyperandrogenic, anovulatory women. Fertil Steril 1:598, 1994

31. Elkind-Hirsch KE, Anania C, Mack M, et al: Combination gonadotropin releasing hormone agonist and oral contraceptive therapy improves treatment of hirsute women with ovarian hyperandrogenism. Fertil Steril 63:970, 1995

32. Rittmaster RS, Loriaux DL, Cutler GB: Sensitivity of cortisol and adrenal androgens to dexamethasone suppression in hirsute women. J Clin Endocrinol Metab 81:462, 1985

33. Carmina E, Lobo RA: Ovarian suppression reduces clinical and endocrine expression of late-onset congenital adrenal hyperplasia due to 21-hydroxylase deficiency. Fertil Steril 62:738, 1994

34. Gault DT, Grobbelaar AO, Grover R, et al: The removal of unwanted hair using a ruby laser. Br J Plastic Surg 52:173, 1999

35. Sommer S, Render C, Sheehan-Dare R: Facial hirsutism treated with the normal-mode ruby laser: results of a 12-month follow-up study. J Am Acad Dermatol 41:974, 1999

36. Balfour JA, McClellan K: Topical eflornithine. Am J Clin Dermatol 2:197, 2001

37. Lucky AW, Henderson TA, Olson WH, et al: Effectiveness of norgestimate and ethinyl estradiol in treating moderate acne vulgaris. J Am Acad Dermatol 37:746, 1997

38. Lemay A, DeWailly SD, Grenier R, et al: Attenuation of mild hyperandrogenic activity in postpubertal acne by a triphasic oral contraceptive containing low doses of ethinyl estradiol and d,l-norgestrel. J Clin Endocrinol Metab 71:8, 1990

39. Daly DC, Walters CA, Soto-Albors CE, et al: A randomized study of dexamethasone in ovulation induction with clomiphene citrate. Fertil Steril 41:844, 1984

40. Nestler JE, Jakubowicz DJ, Reamer P, et al: Ovulatory and metabolic effects of D-chiro-inositol in the polycystic ovary syndrome. N Engl J Med 340:1314, 1999

41. Nestler JE, Jakubowicz DJ, Evans WS, et al: Effects of metformin on spontaneous and clomiphene-induced ovulation in the polycystic ovary syndrome. N Engl J Med 338:1876, 1998

42. Vandermolen DT, Ratts VS, Evans WS, et al: Metformin increases the ovulatory rate and pregnancy rate from clomiphene citrate in patients with polycystic ovary syndrome who are resistant to clomiphene citrate alone. Fertil Steril 75:310, 2001

43. Sarlis NJ, Weil SJ, Nelson LM: Administration of metformin to a diabetic woman with extreme hyperandrogenemia of non-tumoral origin: management of infertility and prevention of inadvertent masculinization of a female fetus. J Clin Endocrinol Metab 84:1510, 1999

44. Morin-Papunen LC, Koivunen RM, Ruokonen A, et al: Metformin therapy improves the menstrual pattern with minimal endocrine and metabolic effects in women with polycystic ovary syndrome. Fertil Steril 69:691, 1998

45. DeLeo V, LaMarca A, Ditto A, et al: Effects of metformin on gonadotropin induced ovulation in women with polycystic ovary syndrome. Fertil Steril 72:282, 1999

46. Coetzee EJ, Jackson WU: Metformin in management of pregnant insulin-dependent diabetics. Diabetologia 16:241, 1979

47. Hasegawa I, Murakawa H, Suzuki M, et al: Effect of troglitazone on endocrine and ovulatory performance in women with insulin resistance–related polycystic ovary syndrome. Fertil Steril 71:323, 1999

48. Dunaif A, Scott D, Finegood D, et al: The insulin sensitizing agent troglitazone improves metabolic and reproductive abnormalities in the polycystic ovary syndrome. J Clin Endocrinol Metab 81:3299, 1996

49. Elkind-Hirsch KE, McWilliams RB: Pregnancy after treatment with the insulin sensitizing agent troglitazone in an obese woman with the hyperandrogenic insulin-resistant acanthosis nigricans syndrome. Fertil Steril 71:943, 1999

50. Mitwally MFM, Kuscu N, Yalcinkaya TM: High ovulatory rates with use of troglitazone in clomiphene resistant women with polycystic ovary syndrome. Human Reprod 14:2700, 1999

51. Neuschwander-Tetri BA, Isley WL, Oki JC, et al: Troglitazone induced hepatic failure leading to liver transplantation. Ann Intern Med 130:163, 1999

52. Kistner RW: Sequential use of clomiphene citrate and human menopausal gonadotropin in ovulation induction. Fertil Steril 27:72, 1976

53. Jarrell J, McInnes R, Crooke R: Observations on the combination of clomiphene citrate-hMG-hCG in the management of anovulation. Fertil Steril 35:634, 1981

54. Homburg R, Levy R, Ben Rafael Z: A comparative study of conventional regimens with low dose FSH for ovulation in PCOS. Fertil Steril 63:729, 1995

55. Schenker JG, Weinstein D: Ovarian hyperstimulation syndrome: a current survey. Fertil Steril 30:255, 1978

56. Donesky BW, Adashi EY: Surgically induced ovulation in the polycystic ovary syndrome: wedge resection revisited in the age of laparoscopy. Fertil Steril 63:439, 1995

57. Armar NA, McGarrigle HG, Honour J, et al: Laparoscopic ovarian diathermy in the management of anovulatory infertility in women with polycystic ovaries: endocrine changes and clinical outcome. Fertil Steril 53:45, 1990

58. Gjonnaess H: Polycystic ovarian syndrome treated by ovarian electrocautery through the laparoscope. Fertil Steril 41:20, 1984

59. Sanfillipo JS, Rock JA: Surgery for benign disease of the ovary. TeLinde's Operative Gynecology. Rock JA, Thompson JD, Eds. Lippincott, Williams & Wilkins, Philadelphia, 1997

60. Buyalos RP, Lee CT: Polycystic ovary syndrome: pathophysiology and outcome with in vitro fertilization. Fertil Steril 65:1, 1996

61. Wada I, Matson PL, Troup SA, et al: Assisted conception using buserelin and human menopausal gonadotropins in women with polycystic ovary syndrome. Br J Obstet Gynecol 100:3665, 1993

62. Urman B, Fluker MR, Yuen BH, et al: The outcome of in vitro fertilization and embryo transfer in women with polycystic ovary syndrome failing to conceive after ovulation induction with exogenous gonadotropins. Fertil Steril 57:1269, 1992

63. Legro RS, Kunselman AR, Dodson WC, et al: Prevalence and predictors of risk for type 2 diabetes mellitus and impaired glucose tolerance in polycystic ovary syndrome: a prospective, controlled study in 254 affected women. J Clin Endocrinol Metab 84:165, 1999

64. Ehrmann DA, Cavaghan MK, Barnes RB, et al: Prevalence of impaired glucose tolerance and diabetes in women with PCOS. Diabetes Care 22:141, 1999

65. Legro RS, Kunselman AR, Dunaif A: Prevalence and predictors of dyslipidemia in women with PCOS. Am J Med 111:665, 2001

66. Pierpoint T, McKeigue PM, Isaacs AJ, et al: Mortality of women with polycystic ovary syndrome at long term follow up. J Clin Epidemiol 51:581, 1998

80 Contraception

Sarah L. Berga, M.D.

Contraception means to prevent conception, but in common medical usage, it also refers to methods that prevent implantation. The goal of contraception is to make every child a wanted child. Most methods of contraception (e.g., barrier methods and hormone preparations) also reduce the risk of sexually transmitted diseases (STDs), but intrauterine devices (IUDs) may increase the risk of STDs or their consequences.

Contraceptive methods are generally categorized as reversible [*see Table 1*] or irreversible. Irreversible methods are often referred to as sterilization procedures. Pregnancy termination is not typically regarded as contraception, but the availability of medical methods of abortion has blurred this distinction. Emergency postcoital contraceptive methods are also available.

Most methods of contraception are designed for use by women. Hormonal methods of male contraception are under development, but they are not yet commercially available.[1] In any case, unless such products prove to be almost free of side effects, their acceptance by men is likely to be limited.

Historically, methods to prevent or terminate pregnancy have been subject to intense legal regulation. In the United States, legal regulations vary widely from state to state regarding the provision of services to minors, waiting periods for termination and sterilization, husband and parental consent, reporting of complications and deaths, and restrictions on advance directives by pregnant or potentially pregnant women. Some states also have regulations regarding the type of practitioner or the type of facility in which contraceptive and fertility management procedures can be provided, but no state currently bans the use of reversible contraceptives. Medical insurance coverage for contraception varies widely.

The percentage of women using a contraceptive method rose from 56% in 1982 to 64% in 1995.[2] The most widely used methods in 1995 were female sterilization, combined estrogen and progestin oral contraceptives (COCs), and the male condom. Male condom use is common among unmarried couples; this popularity is due in part to the protection its use affords against certain STDs, particularly HIV infection.

Combined Estrogen-Progestin Contraceptives

COCs are formulated with estrogen (in the form of ethinyl estradiol), in doses ranging from 20 to 35 μg, and a variety of progestins derived from 19-nortestosterone. Individual formulations may have a fixed dose of progestin (monophasic) or may have doses that vary by cycle phase (triphasic). Two preparations contain varying estrogen doses.

EFFICACY AND MECHANISM OF ACTION

Combined estrogen and progestin oral contraceptives are a highly effective method of birth control. Theoretical efficacy is about 99.9%, but the typical efficacy is around 97%.[3] The contraceptive effect of COCs derives principally from the suppression of the hypothalamic release of gonadotropin-releasing hormone (GnRH) and the concomitant suppression of the pituitary release of luteinizing hormone (LH) and follicle-stimulat-

ing hormone (FSH). The decrease in LH reduces ovarian androgen secretion. The suppression of GnRH is primarily caused by the progestin component. Estrogen also independently suppresses FSH at the pituitary level, thereby retarding folliculogenesis.

COCs are progestin dominant. Progestin exposure causes endometrial decidualization and atrophy, rendering the endometrium unfavorable for implantation and thickening of the cervical mucus, thereby blocking the entry of sperm and bacteria into the upper genital tract. There are three generations of progestins. Third-generation progestins, which are theoretically less androgenic, include desogestrel, gestodene, and norgestimate. The clinical superiority of one progestin over any other has not been demonstrated.

REDUCTION OF ANDROGEN EXPOSURE

All COC preparations reduce androgen exposure by two mechanisms: (1) suppression of ovarian androgen production, as a result of the reduction in LH stimulation of the ovarian theca compartment and (2) elevation of the level of sex hormone–binding globulin protein, which binds androgens and thereby lowers the unbound fraction of circulating androgens. COCs reduce facial or androgen-dependent hair growth and acne by reducing the circulating concentrations of androgens available to occupy androgen receptors on the pilosebaceous unit. Although women with polycystic ovary syndrome have elevated GnRH and LH levels, COCs containing 30 to 35 μg of estrogen adequately suppress their androgen secretion.[4]

CONTINUOUS VERSUS CYCLIC COC REGIMENS

Traditional COCs follow a 28-day cycle, with 21 days of active pills and 7 days of placebo pills. The 7-day placebo window permits significant follicular development, and higher estrogen and progestin doses are then needed to inhibit further folliculogenesis and ovulation. Further, if there is a delay in starting the next pill pack, a so-called escape ovulation may result.

In patients taking COCs to effect ovarian suppression for medical purposes, this 28-day cycle may be ineffective. These patients may benefit from a long-cycle regimen—42 to 105 days of active pills, and then 1 week off—or a continuous regimen.

Table 1 Categories of Commercially Available Reversible Contraceptives

Barrier methods	Progestin preparations
Condoms	Oral
Diaphragms	Injectable
Cervical caps	Implantable
Hormonal	Intrauterine devices
Combined estrogen-	
progestin preparations	
Oral	
Vaginal ring	
Transdermal	
Injectable	

For long-cycle regimens, patients use the active pills from several packs; however, a commercial long-cycle preparation that includes 63 days' worth of active pills is under development. The use of continuous COC regimens has not been well studied, but it is common to omit the placebo week in women undergoing hormonal treatment for disorders such as polycystic ovary syndrome or endometriosis, as well as in those who desire amenorrhea or have headaches or other symptoms provoked by estrogen withdrawal during the placebo week. There are several advantages to a continuous approach, including better suppression of ovarian function. Persistent ovarian cysts may be less likely with a continuous regimen than with a cyclic regimen.

Increased breakthrough bleeding is a potential side effect of a continuous regimen as compared with a cyclic regimen. The increase in breakthrough bleeding is attributable partly to the development of fragile endometrial vessels coursing along the surface of the endometrium and partly to impaired local hemostasis.[5] The only near-continuous COC preparation that avoids the increase in breakthrough bleeding while increasing follicular suppression is Mircette, which has 2 placebo days, 5 days of 10 µg estrogen, and 21 days of 20 µg estrogen plus 150 µg desogestrel.[6] One objective of these modifications is to lower overall sex steroid exposure and minimize the unwanted consequences of pill use while minimizing breakthrough bleeding.

NONORAL COMBINED CONTRACEPTIVES

Several combined estrogen-progestin contraceptives that do not use the oral route have recently been developed. All offer the convenience of less-frequent dosing.

The hormonal vaginal contraceptive ring (NuvaRing) was approved by the Food and Drug Administration in October 2001. This product is a flexible polymer ring, about 2 in. in diameter, which the patient inserts in her vagina. The ring releases a continuous low dose of estrogen and etonogestrel. The ring is left in place for 3 weeks, then removed for the week during which the patient will have her menstrual period. Neither patients nor their partners can tell that the ring is in place. Comparison of the vaginal ring with a COC has shown a lower incidence of irregular bleeding and a higher incidence of a normal intended bleeding pattern with the ring.[7]

The transdermal contraceptive patch (Ortho Evra) was approved by the FDA in November 2001. The patch delivers estrogen and norelgestromin over the course of a week. Patches are applied once a week for 3 consecutive weeks to the skin of the buttocks, the abdomen, the upper torso, or the upper outer arm.[8] In general, the efficacy and cycle control provided by the patch are comparable to those of COCs, but the efficacy of the patch may be lower in women who weigh 198 lb (90 kg) or more.[9] The overall rate of patch detachment is about 4%; about 2% of users experience skin irritation at the site of application.

An injectable estrogen-progestin contraceptive (Lunelle) is available in the United States. The preparation, which is given intramuscularly once a month, contains medroxyprogesterone acetate and estradiol cypionate in a timed-release form. In clinical trials, efficacy and patient satisfaction have been comparable to that seen with COCs.[10]

SIDE EFFECTS

A myriad of serious and nuisance side effects are associated with COCs [see Table 2]. Smoking markedly increases the risk of venous thromboembolism. Smoking is a relative contraindication to COC use, particularly in women older than 35 years.[11]

Table 2   **Potential Side Effects of Oral Contraceptives**

Serious side effects	Metabolic changes
	    Decreased insulin action
	    Increase in clotting factors
	    Elevation of triglyceride levels
	    Increase in the metabolic work load
	        of the liver
	    Increase in renin substrate
	Clinical manifestations*
	    Venous thromboembolic events
	    Fatty liver or hepatoma
	    Cholestasis or cholecystitis
	    Diabetes mellitus
	    Hypertension
	    Cardiovascular events
	Exacerbation of depression
	Drug interactions

Nuisance side effects	Mastodynia Reduced libido Reduced vaginal lubrication Increased appetite Weight gain Fatigue Bloating

*These events are rare in healthy women younger than 50 years.

The crucial clinical issue is to convince the woman who smokes to stop smoking rather than deny her access to an acceptable form of contraception. For nonsmokers who take COCs containing 35 µg or less of estrogen, the risk of nonfatal venous thromboembolism is approximately one half that of pregnancy (60 per 100,000 women) but greater than that observed in healthy women who do not take oral contraceptives (5 per 100,000 women). The alleged excess mortality from venous thromboembolism attributable to third-generation progestins as compared with other progestins is less than two per million women per year.[12] However, women with familial thrombophilia caused by factor V Leiden or prothrombin mutation 20210A have a greatly increased risk of venous thromboembolism when using any oral contraceptive[13] [see Chapter 94]. In white women, the carrier rate of factor V Leiden is approximately 3% and that of prothrombin mutation 20210A is less than 2%, so screening has not been routinely advised.[14] Also, there are other known causes of thrombophilia, but not all the thrombophilias can be detected.

COCs may decrease insulin action, an effect that has been attributed to the progestin component. The use of COCs does not increase the risk of diabetes mellitus in women who do not have other risk factors for the disease. However, in a nonrandomized clinical trial that followed Latin-American women with gestational diabetes for 7.5 years post partum, the rate of development of diabetes mellitus was 8.7% for those given nonhormonal contraception, 10.4% for those who used COCs, and 26.5% for those who used progestin-only pills. Life-table analysis showed an increase in diabetes mellitus within 2 years in the progestin-only group.[15] Given these considerations, it is prudent to avoid prescribing any progestin-only form of contraception in women predisposed to diabetes mellitus or in frankly diabetic women. Fortunately, COC use by insulin-dependent diabetic women does not increase the risk of diabetic retinopathy or nephropathy.[16]

COCs have a negligible effect on the overall risk of cancer.[17] Among women who take oral contraceptives for 8 years, the estimated increase in the number of cases of cancer is 125 per 100,000 for cervical cancer and 41 per 100,000 for liver cancer; those increases are offset, however, by decreases in endometrial cancer and ovarian cancer [see Benefits, below].[17] Oral contraceptive use does not appear to increase the risk of breast cancer significantly—regardless of the dose, duration of use, or age at use—even in women with a family history of breast cancer.[18] However, the effect of oral contraceptive use on risk of breast cancer in carriers of BRCA1 and BRCA2 has not been defined.

Exposure to high doses of estrogen or progestin may provoke depression and mood disturbances, but this effect is limited to women with an underlying diathesis.[19] It is not known whether oral contraceptive use increases the lifetime risk of depression or hastens its onset in women so predisposed.

Progestins have mineralocorticoid activity that results in the retention of up to 2 lb of water in sensitive women. The progestins also increase plasma renin activity; in predisposed women, hypertension may result.

Oral contraceptive use can cause drug interactions by increasing liver production of proteins that bind other drugs, by inhibiting oxidative metabolism in the liver by the P-450 and P-448 cytochrome systems, and by competing for or accelerating conjugation. Conversely, drugs that stimulate the hepatic microsomal system, such as oral antifungal agents or rifampin, may decrease plasma levels of contraceptive steroid and lead to unintended pregnancy. Antibiotics such as ampicillin, tetracyclines, and metronidazole do not interfere with COC efficacy.

CONTRAINDICATIONS

There are specific contraindications to oral contraceptives [see Table 3]. Lactating women should probably not take COCs. Women with hypertension, epilepsy, depression, hepatitis, gallbladder disease, migraine, or premenstrual syndrome (PMS) need to be carefully monitored. Fibroids are not a contraindication to COC use.

BENEFITS

Women use oral contraceptives primarily for birth control. If side effects are tolerable, they are pleased to gain the other benefits [see Table 4]. Women generally appreciate the lighter and predictable menses. The option of long cycles or continuous use to schedule or skip bleeding episodes is a major advantage for any busy woman, particularly one who travels or spends time outdoors. Other women use oral contraceptives to treat an

---

Table 3 Contraindications to Oral Contraceptives

Active liver or gallbladder disease
Medically significant hypertriglyceridemia
Active or past venous thromboembolic events
Atherosclerotic heart disease
Undiagnosed vaginal bleeding
Estrogen-dependent neoplasia
    Breast cancer
    Endometrial cancer
Symptomatic mitral valve prolapse
Smoking after 35 years of age

Table 4 Potential Benefits of Oral Contraceptives

Reduced risk of the following disorders:
    Ectopic pregnancy
    Benign breast disease
    Anemia
    Ovarian cysts and cancer
    Endometrial cancer
Lighter and predictable menses
Reduction or elimination of dysmenorrhea
Bone accretion

---

underlying disorder, such as polycystic ovary syndrome, dysmenorrhea, endometriosis, or idiopathic hirsutism. In general, the same benefits accrue.

One of the major benefits of COC use is bone accretion. One study showed that as little as 10 μg of estrogen was bone sparing in women older than 40 years, and 5 μg of estrogen plus 1 mg of norethindrone caused bone accretion.[20] Women who are hyperandrogenic but eumenorrheic have greater bone mass than do hyperandrogenic women who are oligomenorrheic. The latter have slightly higher bone mass than eumenorrheic, nonhirsute women. Women with polycystic ovary syndrome or idiopathic hirsutism who take oral contraceptives will have a decrement in endogenous androgen exposure, but COC use in this setting is expected to be bone sparing. Women with hypothalamic hypogonadism, particularly those with an eating disorder, have underlying metabolic disturbances that render their bones less responsive to exogenous steroid exposure. These women may continue to lose or not accrue bone even if they use COCs.

Long-term use of COCs reduces the incidence of endometrial cancer and ovarian cancer. Among women who take oral contraceptives for 8 years, it is estimated that there will be 197 fewer cases of endometrial cancer per 100,000 users and 193 fewer cases of ovarian cancer per 100,000 users.[17] Newer COCs, which contain 20 μg of estrogen, appear to provide identical risk reduction for ovarian cancer as did older formulations, which contained 50 μg or more of estrogen.[21] A recent study showed that oral contraceptives also markedly reduce the risk of ovarian cancer in carriers of BRCA1 and BRCA2 mutations (who are at increased risk for ovarian cancer and premenopausal breast cancer). The longer the duration of use, the greater is the protection from ovarian cancer.[22]

Progestin-Only Contraceptives

EFFICACY AND MECHANISM OF ACTION

Two progestin-only contraceptives are commercially available. Norplant is composed of Silastic rods impregnated with the progestin levonorgestrel. The new Norplant system contains only two rods. A single-rod system will soon be available. The rods are inserted subdermally, generally in the upper arm. Diffusion of levonorgestrel through the wall of each capsule provides a continuous low dose of progestin for at least 5 years. The progestin modestly inhibits the hypothalamic-pituitary-ovarian axis to block ovulation; it also induces endometrial shedding, making implantation unlikely, and thickens cervical mucus, thereby retarding the entry of sperm and bacteria to the upper genital tract. The birth-control efficacy is greater than 99.9%.

Depot medroxyprogesterone acetate (DMPA) is an aqueous suspension of 150 mg designed to be given intramuscularly every 3 months. The birth-control efficacy is greater than 99%.

SIDE EFFECTS

Subdermal and injectable progestins have side effects [see Table 5]. The principal side effect is breakthrough bleeding caused by the development of fragile endometrial vessels and local derangement of hemostatic mechanisms as a result of excess progestin exposure relative to estrogen exposure.[5] The breakthrough bleeding may respond to the administration of an estrogen such as transdermal estradiol. Progestin implants and injections are relatively contraindicated in women with past or active depression or other psychiatric disorders [see Table 6]. There is some suggestion that progestin-only contraceptives are more mood destabilizing than COCs. The long-term effect on bone accretion depends on the extent of ovarian suppression and its attendant decline in estradiol secretion and on the age of the patient. Younger patients who have not attained peak bone mass may be more adversely affected. Levonorgestrel may be more bone sparing than DMPA. Progestin-only contraceptives have been found to increase the risk of diabetes mellitus in Latin-American women who have had gestational diabetes (see above).[15] This may be partly caused by the lack of estrogen, which is an insulin sensitizer. The long-term cardiovascular risks are largely unknown, but in some experimental settings, synthetic progestins provoke vasoconstriction, an effect not seen with progesterone. A recent epidemiologic analysis from the World Health Organization (WHO) found no excess risk of cardiovascular disease with either combined or progestin-only methods other than an increased risk of stroke in hypertensive women who were given the progestin-only contraceptives.[23]

Another common side effect of progestin-only contraceptives is delay in return of menses. DMPA is given at 90-day intervals, but patients who discontinue this method may not experience immediate return of menses because of variability in the metabolism of the depot form and variable sensitivity of the hypothalamic GnRH pulse generator to low levels of progestin.

Intrauterine Devices

IUDs interfere with sperm migration, fertilization, ovum transport, and implantation, presumably by causing a sterile salpingitis, endometritis, or both. The birth-control efficacy is greater than 97%.

One of the principal benefits of IUDs is that they provide a nonhormonal method of birth control. They are ideal for women who have completed childbearing and who desire a

---

Table 5 Potential Side Effects of Injectable and Implantable Progestin Contraceptives

Breakthrough bleeding	Mastodynia
Headaches	Acne
Mood changes	Bone loss
Weight gain	

Table 6 Contraindications to Injectable and Implantable Progestin Contraceptives

Active liver disease	Active thromboembolic disease
Diabetes mellitus	Active cardiovascular disease
Unexplained vaginal bleeding	Depression
Breast cancer	Other psychiatric disorders

---

low-maintenance, reversible method of contraception. IUDs are also relatively economical.

Two IUDs are currently available: the Copper T 380A, which lasts 10 years, and the 5-year, levonorgestrel-releasing Mirena. With the copper IUD, both the inert plastic device and the copper contribute to the spermicidal effect and prevention of implantation. With the progestin-containing IUD, part of the efficacy is attributed to the effects of the progestin on the endometrium that retard implantation.[24]

The main side effect associated with IUD use is pelvic inflammatory disease (PID). Most of the increased risk of PID occurs in the first 3 weeks after insertion. Women with more than one sexual partner who are at risk for contracting gonorrhea and chlamydial infection also are at increased risk for PID. Patient selection, rigorous aseptic insertion technique, and screening for STDs may minimize this risk. Routine antibiotic prophylaxis during insertion may not be necessary.[25] Uterine perforation is a rare insertion risk. Dysmenorrhea and menorrhagia have been reported with the copper IUD, whereas decreased menstrual flow, dysmenorrhea, and increased risk of ectopic pregnancy have been reported with the progesterone-releasing IUD.

The primary contraindication to IUD use is a history of PID. Nulligravidity is a relative contraindication. Sexual monogamy should be emphasized as a means of minimizing the risk of STDs and PID.

Barrier Methods

Male and female barrier contraceptives are available. When used correctly, the male condom protects against pregnancy and STDs. The theoretical efficacy of barrier methods for birth control is 98%, but the actual efficacy is about 88%. The efficacy gap results from inconsistent use and condom breakage. The female condom is more difficult to use and has not gained popularity. The diaphragm and cervical cap do not protect against STDs as effectively as condoms. When they are used with spermicides, the birth-control efficacy of diaphragms and cervical caps is theoretically 94%; in practice, however, the efficacy is about 82%. Both cervical caps and diaphragms require fitting and a prescription. They also require user training and diligence. Instructions on their use are provided in the products' package inserts. Spermicides may independently decrease the risk of STDs. When used alone, spermicides have a birth-control efficacy of about 79%.[3] Spermicides that also have antimicrobial activity are in development.

Allergic reactions to latex and hypersensitivity to spermicides occur. Diaphragm use may increase the risk of urinary tract infections because the rim presses against the symphysis pubis and urethra, which may cause incomplete emptying of the bladder.

The main contraindication to barrier methods is lack of user motivation and hypersensitivity to spermicides or allergy to latex. The primary benefits of condoms are that they are available without prescription, inexpensive, relatively easy to use, nonhormonal, and protective against STDs. Other barrier methods are only slightly more difficult to use but require fitting and a prescription, so the need for birth control must be anticipated.

Periodic Abstinence

Periodic abstinence, or natural family planning, depends on recognition of the periovulatory window and avoidance of sexual intercourse during that window. As such, it requires that a woman have highly regular menstrual cycles and that both partners be motivated to avoid intercourse when the woman is fertile. There are several methods of detecting the fertile window, including avoiding intercourse on days 9 to 14 of a 28-day cycle, monitoring cervical mucus and body temperature, and monitoring salivary estradiol levels.

Successful use of fertility-awareness methods for birth control requires not only dedication but education. Family health centers, family planning centers, and church-affiliated centers may offer courses on this subject. Information is available on the Internet at sites such as http://my.webmd.com/encyclopedia/article/1819.51010.

Mastering the concepts of menstrual-cycle physiology can be empowering, and couples can use this information to plan a pregnancy as well as to avoid it. There are no known contraindications. There are no religious prohibitions against periodic abstinence, so it is theoretically available to all women who have predictable cycles.

Periodic abstinence can be frustrating, however, and it is less reliable than other forms of contraception, with an estimated efficacy of 80%. Several factors can interfere with fertility awareness. Even women who usually have very regular cycles may occasionally have a cycle that deviates from normal. Vaginitis may obscure the recognition of midcycle mucus. Fever may mimic the progesterone-induced rise in body temperature that normally indicates the onset of the luteal phase, thereby falsely signaling that the fertile period has passed.

Sterilization

Sterilization procedures generally entail occlusion or ligation of the fallopian tubes in women or the vas deferens in men. The birth-control efficacy of sterilization procedures is greater than 99%; they are meant to be permanent. Reversal procedures are available, but the reversibility of tubal ligation or vasectomy is not guaranteed. Sterilization procedures may fail if the fallopian tube is not properly identified or if it recannulates. Vasectomy failures primarily result from not waiting a sufficient length of time after the procedure before having unprotected sexual intercourse. In women, sterilization procedures can be done post partum, but interval procedures are safer and more effective. Interval procedures employ laparoscopy, with or without general anesthesia. The fallopian tubes are either fulgurated or banded.

Patients may experience feelings of regret after a tubal ligation or vasectomy. Appropriate counseling can minimize this emotional side effect. There is no concrete evidence that vasectomy causes heart disease or prostate cancer. A recent review of tubal ligation found no evidence of increased rates of premenstrual distress, menorrhagia, dysmenorrhea, or menstrual irregularities in women 30 years of age or older who had undergone interval tubal ligation.[26]

The main contraindication to sterilization is ambivalence. In addition, women who undergo laparoscopic procedures must be suitable surgical candidates. The main benefit of sterilization is its permanence. Because sterilization is a one-time procedure with high efficacy, it is highly cost-effective in appropriately selected candidates. Tubal ligation may decrease the risk of PID and ovarian cancer.

Emergency Contraception

Postcoital contraception aims to desynchronize endometrial development and prevent implantation. Various methods have been proposed.[27] They include high doses of COCs taken within 72 hours after intercourse; levonorgestrel taken within 72 hours after intercourse; high doses of estrogen; danazol; mifepristone, as a single 600 mg dose; and insertion of a copper IUD up to 5 days after ovulation. The contraceptive efficacy of mifepristone or IUDs is at least 99%. One study compared a treatment consisting of 100 μg of estrogen plus 0.5 mg of levonorgestrel taken twice, 12 hours apart, with a treatment consisting of levonorgestrel, 0.75 mg, taken twice, 12 hours apart.[28] Both treatments were taken within 72 hours after intercourse. Levonorgestrel alone had an efficacy of 85% and was associated with fewer side effects than the combined therapy, which had an efficacy of 57%. The efficacy of levonorgestrel taken within 24 hours after intercourse was greater than 99%. This would appear to be the treatment of choice because it is inexpensive, widely available, well tolerated, and highly effective. A recent Scottish study also suggested that women given a single emergency contraceptive kit used it correctly without experiencing significant side effects, and they had a lower unintended pregnancy rate.[29] Given the safety and efficacy of emergency contraception, many physicians strongly advocate that it be made available over the counter.[30] Patient information on emergency contraception is available on the Internet at http://ec.princeton.edu.

Choosing a Contraceptive Method

There is no perfect contraceptive; all may fail, and all have drawbacks and side effects. Age, motivation, marital status, partner attitude, perceived risk of pregnancy, frequency of intercourse, medical conditions, costs, cultural considerations, and religious beliefs affect the choice of contraceptive methods. The patient's or couple's medical history and preferences must guide the selection of a contraceptive [see Table 7]. Patients should be encouraged to revise their choice on the basis of side effects and changing circumstances.

Patients should be advised to inform the physician of new symptoms before discontinuing a contraceptive method. The physician must remain sensitive to the patient's concerns. Even if a symptom sounds trivial from a medical perspective, it may alarm the patient and cause her to discontinue the method.

The role of condoms and other contraceptives in the reduction of STD transmission must be emphasized so that patients can choose properly from among the available options. Emergency contraception should be discussed and offered to those not seeking long-term contraception.

REVERSIBLE METHOD DESIRED

The first decision point in the choice of a reversible contraceptive method hinges on whether the patient has more than one sexual partner or is in a long-term monogamous relationship. If

Table 7 Contraceptive Characteristics
Affecting Choice[29]

Characteristic	Method
High efficacy	Combined oral contraceptives Intrauterine devices Depot medroxyprogesterone acetate Subdermal progestin implants
Limited or no systemic side effects	Barriers Spermicides Periodic abstinence
Minimal effort	Intrauterine devices Subdermal progestin implants Depot medroxyprogesterone acetate
Low cost	Male condom Spermicides Combined oral contraceptives
Nonprescription	Male condom Spermicides Periodic abstinence
No religious prohibitions	Periodic abstinence
Protection against sexually transmitted diseases Cervical gonorrhea and chlamydial infection Salpingitis HIV infection	 Barriers Barriers, hormone contraceptives Male and female latex condoms
Other health benefits	Hormone contraceptives
Minimal risk to future fertility	Hormone contraceptives Barriers Periodic abstinence

the patient has more than one sexual partner, condoms with or without hormonal contraception should be recommended. User reluctance and lack of familiarity are the main limitations to condom use. Condoms are ideal for unplanned intercourse.

For healthy women, the ancillary health benefits of combined estrogen-progestin contraceptives should be emphasized. These include a reduced risk of ovarian and endometrial cancer and preservation or accretion of bone mass. The option of using combined hormonal contraceptives to regulate menstrual timing should be discussed as a means of aiding compliance.

COCs, particularly the generic brands, are relatively inexpensive—in the range of $10 to $20 a month. COCs work best if taken daily, and some women find it difficult to remember to do so; they may prefer a vaginal ring, transdermal patch, or injectable contraceptive. Women who do not take the pills reliably will have increased rates of pregnancy and side effects, such as breakthrough bleeding. They should be counseled to use a barrier method or spermicide if they miss two consecutive pills or if they start the next package of pills after a hiatus of 8 or more days. In healthy nonsmokers without predisposing medical conditions, the pill is a safe and highly efficacious method of contraception that can be used in women up to 50 years of age. In women who are approaching menopause, COC use not only provides effective contraception but also can regularize menstrual cycles, relieve vasomotor symptoms, and stabilize bone mass.[31]

Women with epilepsy may need to have their antiseizure medications adjusted when they start oral contraceptive therapy. Not all the newer antiseizure drugs interact with oral contraceptives, however,[32] so patients need to be evaluated on a case-by-case basis. Consultation with a pharmacist may be useful.

Follow-up is important in women who choose hormonal contraceptives. Blood pressure should be measured around 3 months after the start of COCs and annually thereafter. If hypertension results, it is prudent to discontinue COCs. Women using hormonal contraception who develop a severe, unremitting headache should be evaluated for possible stroke and cerebral thrombosis.

With prolonged use of COCs—even on a cyclic regimen—some women develop endometrial atrophy and amenorrhea. Once pregnancy has been excluded, it is prudent to recommend a long-cycle or a continuous regimen or one with a shortened placebo window.

It is prudent for women who develop serious mood disturbances to discontinue COCs. Women with active or past PMS and depression, including postpartum depression, should be advised about the potential for negative mood effects associated with COCs.

Switching to a lower-dosage regimen may reduce nuisance side effects. Physically smaller women or women who metabolize synthetic sex steroids slowly (such as women of Asian descent) should start with a 20 μg pill. Although most women do well on 20 μg pills, there may be a slight increase in breakthrough bleeding with some formulations. The benefit is fewer estrogen-dependent side effects, such as breast tenderness or nausea. Women with a history of headaches may do better on the lowest dose given in a continuous or nearly continuous (Mircette) regimen.

If a patient has a low risk of depression, PMS, and osteoporosis, Norplant or DMPA may be an appropriate method of contraception. The patient must desire extended protection and be willing to undergo the insertion procedure or an injection. Subdermal implants and DMPA are relatively expensive.

The DMPA cannot be removed if a patient experiences adverse effects, and continuance rates are low with DMPA. Insertion of subdermal implants requires training and skill. If adverse effects occur with subdermal implants, a surgical procedure is required for their removal. Removal is often more difficult than introduction because of scarring around the capsules. In appropriate patients, however, subdermal implants provide a long-term, low-maintenance birth-control method.

IUDs, barrier methods, or periodic abstinence may be considered if the patient is not a candidate for hormone contraception and is in a long-term monogamous relationship.

Prospective users of IUDs must be made aware of the attendant risks and benefits. To make an informed decision, users need to understand the risks and potential consequences of PID.

Diaphragms and cervical caps are ideal for highly motivated users who desire a nonhormonal method of birth control. Spermicides increase the efficacy of all barrier methods of contraception but also increase cost and bother. Use of barrier methods is increased by public health education and by suggestion that the barrier method be incorporated into foreplay.

Women who report vaginal pruritus, irritation, inflammation, pain, or discharge associated with the use of a barrier method may have a latex allergy or hypersensitivity to spermicide. Latex allergies are particularly common in health care workers, many of whom are women. Formal allergy testing can be done to detect latex allergy, but current tests are not highly reliable. Latex allergy can provoke life-threatening anaphylaxis. Although most spermicides contain nonoxynol-9 as the active contraceptive ingredient, the other constituents may vary. Therefore, it may be possible to minimize irritation by switching to a different preparation. Men may also report allergies to latex or hypersensitivity to spermicides. Latex is preferred for condoms and barrier methods because it is impermeable to HIV.

NONREVERSIBLE METHOD DESIRED

All potential reversible and permanent options must be reviewed before a sterilization procedure is chosen. In general, if a couple seeks sterilization, a vasectomy is recommended because it is safer and less expensive than a laparoscopic tubal ligation. Postpartum tubal ligation is the most risky, least effective, and most likely to cause regret.

Laparoscopic tubal ligation is expensive and must be performed by a skilled surgeon in an appropriate setting, so availability may be limited by cost or access to an appropriate physician. Many states require mandatory waiting periods. Some require spousal consent. Counseling is the cornerstone of success.

References

1. Anawalt BD, Amory JK: Male hormonal contraceptives. Expert Opin Pharmacother 2:1389, 2001

2. Piccinino LJ, Mosher WD: Trends in contraceptive use in the United States: 1982–1995. Fam Plann Perspect 30:4, 1998

3. Trussell J, Hatcher RA, Cates W Jr, et al: A guide to interpreting contraceptive efficacy studies. Obstet Gynecol 76:558, 1990

4. Daniels TL, Berga SL: Resistance of gonadotropin releasing hormone drive to sex steroid-induced suppression in hyperandrogenic anovulation. J Clin Endocrinol Metab 82:4179, 1997

5. Runic R, Schatz F, Krey L, et al: Alterations in endometrial stromal cell tissue factor protein and messenger ribonucleic acid expression in patients experiencing abnormal uterine bleeding while using Norplant-2 contraception. J Clin Endocrinol Metab 82:1983, 1997

6. Killick SR, Fitzgerald C, Davis A: Ovarian activity in women taking an oral contraceptive containing 20 microgram ethinyl estradiol and 150 microgram desogestrel: effects of low estrogen doses during the hormone-free interval. Am J Obstet Gynecol 179:S18, 1998

7. Bjarnadottir RI, Tuppurainen M, Killick SR: Comparison of cycle control with a combined contraceptive vaginal ring and oral levonorgestrel/ethinyl estradiol. Am J Obstet Gynecol 186:389, 2002

8. Burkman RT: The transdermal contraceptive patch: a new approach to hormonal contraception. Int J Fertil Womens Med 47:69, 2002

9. Zieman M, Guillebaud J, Weisberg E, et al: Contraceptive efficacy and cycle control with the Ortho Evra/Evra transdermal system: the analysis of pooled data. Fertil Steril 77(2 suppl 2):S13, 2002

10. Kaunitz AM: Lunelle monthly injectable contraceptive: an effective, safe, and convenient new birth control option. Arch Gynecol Obstet 265:119, 2001

11. Farley TM, Collins J, Schlesselman JJ: Hormonal contraception and risk of cardiovascular disease: an international perspective. Contraception 57:211, 1998

12. Hampton N, Kubba A: Contraception: a slow train gathers speed. Lancet 352 (suppl 4):SIV3, 1998

13. Martinelli I, Sacchi E, Landi G, et al: High risk of cerebral-vein thrombosis in carriers of a prothrombin-gene mutation and in users of oral contraceptives. N Engl J Med 338:1793, 1998

14. Bertina RM, Rosendaal FR: Venous thrombosis: the interaction of genes and environment. N Engl J Med 338:1840, 1998

15. Kjos SL, Peters RK, Xiang A, et al: Contraception and the risk of type 2 diabetes mellitus in Latina women with prior gestational diabetes mellitus. JAMA 280:533, 1998

16. Garg SK, Chase HP, Marshall G, et al: Oral contraceptives and renal and retinal complications in young women with insulin-dependent diabetes mellitus. JAMA 271:1099, 1994

17. Schlesselman JJ: Net effect of oral contraceptive use on the risk of cancer in women in the United States. Obstet Gynecol 85:793, 1995

18. Marchbanks PA, McDonald JA, Wilson HG, et al: Oral contraceptives and the risk of breast cancer. N Engl J Med 346:2025, 2002

19. Schmidt PJ, Nieman LK, Danaceau MA, et al: Differential behavioral effects of gonadal steroids in women with and in those without premenstrual syndrome. N Engl J Med 338:209, 1998

20. Speroff L, Rowan J, Symons J, et al: The comparative effect on bone density, endometrium, and lipids of continuous hormones as replacement therapy (CHART study): a randomized controlled trial. JAMA 276:1430, 1996

21. Risk of ovarian cancer in relation to estrogen and progestin dose and use characteristics of oral contraceptives. SHARE Study Group. Steroid Hormones and Reproductions. Am J Epidemiol 152:233, 2000

22. Oral contraceptives and risk of hereditary ovarian cancer. Hereditary Ovarian Cancer Clinical Study Group. N Engl J Med 339:424, 1998

23. Cardiovascular disease and use of oral and injectable progestogen-only contraceptives and combined injectable contraceptives: results of an international, multicenter, case-control study. World Health Organization Collaborative Study of Cardiovascular Disease and Steroid Hormone Contraception. Contraception 57:315, 1998

24. Kaunitz AM: Reappearance of the intrauterine device: a "user-friendly" contraceptive. Int J Fertil Womens Med 42:120, 1997

25. Walsh T, Grimes D, Frezieres R, et al: Randomised controlled trial of prophylactic antibiotics before insertion of intrauterine devices. IUD Study Group. Lancet 351:1005, 1998

26. Gentile GP, Kaufinan SC, Helbig DW: Is there any evidence for a post-tubal sterilization syndrome? Fertil Steril 69:179, 1998

27. Glasier A: Emergency postcoital contraception. N Engl J Med 337:1058, 1997

28. Randomised controlled trial of levonorgestrel versus the Yuzpe regimen of combined oral contraceptives for emergency contraception. Task Force on Postovulatory Methods of Fertility Regulation. Lancet 352:428, 1998

29. Glasier A, Baird D: The effects of self-administering emergency contraception. N Engl J Med 339:1, 1998

30. Grimes DA, Raymond EG, Jones BS: Emergency contraception over-the-counter: the medical and legal imperatives. Obstet Gynecol 98:151, 2001

31. Kaunitz AM: Oral contraceptive use in perimenopause. Am J Obstet Gynecol 185 (2 suppl):S32, 2001

32. Hachad H, Ragueneau-Majlessi I, Levy RH: New antiepileptic drugs: review on drug interactions. Ther Drug Monit 24:91, 2002

81 Infertility

Alan H. DeCherney, M.D.

Infertility is defined as the inability to conceive after 1 or more years of regular coital activity without contraception. Fecundity is the statistical probability of achieving a pregnancy (resulting in a live birth) within 1 month (one menstrual cycle) of unprotected sexual intercourse. Monthly fecundity for a fertile couple ranges from 20% to 35% [*see Table 1*].[1] Within 1 year, more than 85% of all couples trying to conceive will achieve a pregnancy.

The incidence of infertility has been increasing over the past 3 decades. It is estimated that nearly 10% of all couples in the United States have disorders associated with infertility. As a result, about 2.5 million couples seek advice for treatment each year in the United States.[2,3]

The practitioner needs to approach the infertile couple in a rational and organized manner. After the initial evaluation, all the reproductive factors should be assessed and a treatment plan proposed that addresses the risk,[4] benefit, and cost[5] to the couple [*see Figures 1 and 2*]. Couples who go through this process and have little or no success may experience severe emotional and psychological distress. For this reason, patients should be counseled about the probability of their achieving a pregnancy before embarking on this potentially expensive treatment course, and psychological counseling during treatment may be valuable.[6]

Evaluation and Treatment of the Infertile Couple

During the first encounter, both partners should be interviewed. The physician should take note of each partner's age, duration of infertility, past pregnancies, past surgeries, frequency of coital activity, and problems encountered during intercourse (e.g., dyspareunia, impotence, anorgasmia, and lack of libido). All potential problems that are revealed during the initial examination should be addressed and treated accordingly. The initial evaluation should also cover other conditions that can affect fertility rates in women. Obese and sedentary women are at higher risk for infertility,[7] because obesity promotes anovulation. Cigarette smoking[8] and long-term use of nonsteroidal anti-inflammatory drugs (NSAIDs)[9] can contribute to infertility. These effects are most noticeable at the extremes (i.e., marked obesity, heavy smoking, or high NSAID doses).

AGE

A woman's reproductive capability decreases with advancing age. After women reach 30 years of age, pregnancy rates decrease.[10] By 40 years of age, a woman's monthly fecundity is less than 5%.[11] Poor oocyte quality is the predominant factor responsible for this decline in pregnancy rate.

Male fertility also diminishes with age. Sperm quality declines, and the frequency of ejaculation decreases as men grow older. Nearly 50% of the infertility experienced by couples older than 40 years is caused by problems associated with advancing age.[12] Therefore, age is an independent risk factor that is instrumental in determining a couple's chance of achieving a successful pregnancy.

The duration of infertility may be just as important a risk factor as the age of the couple. The longer the duration of infertility, the lower is the probability of achieving a successful pregnancy.

MALE INFERTILITY

Infertility in the male partner is the primary cause of infertility in approximately 35% of couples who seek help.[10] Any previous testicular injury, infection, surgery, radiation, or chemotherapy should be documented during the initial history. The physical examination should focus on penile and testicular anomalies (e.g., hypospadia, cryptorchidism, and varicoceles). If any such anomaly is present, the patient should be referred to a urologist for evaluation and treatment.

After the initial physical examination, a semen analysis should be performed. The specimen is collected after 48 hours of abstinence from coital activity and evaluated no more than 1 hour after collection.[13] If any parameters are abnormal [*see Table 2*], two additional semen analyses should be performed 2 weeks apart. Persistent abnormalities may warrant urologic evaluation and workup for diabetes mellitus, prolactin elevation, and chromosomal abnormalities.

Other tests that can be performed are the sperm penetration assay and the immunobead-binding assay. These tests can detect abnormalities in sperm penetration and motility, respectively, but may not indicate the true nature of a patient's problem.

If the results of the semen tests are normal and the female partner's evaluation appears normal, a diagnosis of unexplained infertility is appropriate [*see Unexplained Infertility, below*].

Idiopathic oligospermia is the most common cause of infertility in men. Although there is no cure for this problem, treatment may include in vitro fertilization (IVF) with microinjection of sperm into egg (intracytoplasmic sperm injection [ICSI]) [*see Table 3*]. In severe cases of infertility, this technique can achieve fertilization rates as high as 65%.[14]

FEMALE INFERTILITY

Tubal and Pelvic Factors

Nearly 35% of the infertility experienced by couples and 40% of the infertility in women is of pelvic origin. Uterine, tubal, and other pelvic abnormalities are responsible for this type of infertility. The practitioner should elicit information regarding any history of sexually transmitted diseases, pelvic inflammatory disease, appendicitis with rupture, pelvic tuberculosis, or adnexal surgery. Many patients with tubal or pelvic damage have a history that includes a previous diagnosis of endometriosis, ectopic pregnancy, or submucous myomas. Al-

Table 1 Fecundity of Normal Couples over Time

Time (Months)	Couples Achieving Pregnancy (%)
1	20–36
3	57
6	72
12	85
24	93

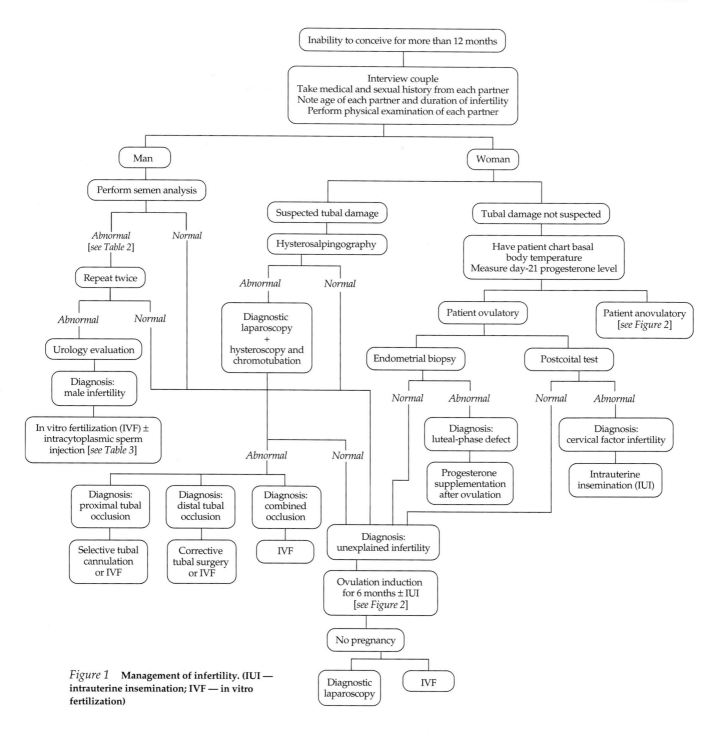

Figure 1 **Management of infertility. (IUI —**
intrauterine insemination; IVF — in vitro
fertilization)

though uterine myomas seldom cause infertility, they may cause recurrent early pregnancy loss and preterm labor.

Hysterosalpingography (HSG) is one of the initial diagnostic tests used to evaluate uterine, tubal, and pelvic abnormalities. This test is performed during the early proliferative phase, after the cessation of menstrual flow (cycle day 5 to 10). HSG can help identify abnormalities of uterine filling caused by submucous myomas, polyps, uterine synechiae (adhesions), and congenital malformations.

Tubal patency should be evaluated at the time of HSG. A delayed set of radiographs can detect pelvic adhesions and other pelvic abnormalities that prevent the release of contrast material into the pelvis. Once the site of blockage (which may be proximal or distal) has been identified, it can be dealt with accordingly.[15] Patients who are known to be anovulatory may forgo an initial HSG. If ovulation induction is successfully attempted for at least four consecutive cycles and conception does not occur, however, HSG should be performed.

HSG should never be performed on a woman with acute salpingitis, a tender pelvic mass, or allergy to iodine. Women with a known contraindication are better evaluated directly by laparoscopy. Patients who undergo HSG should receive prophylactic treatment for chlamydial infection; oral doxycycline, 100 mg twice daily for 7 days, is effective.

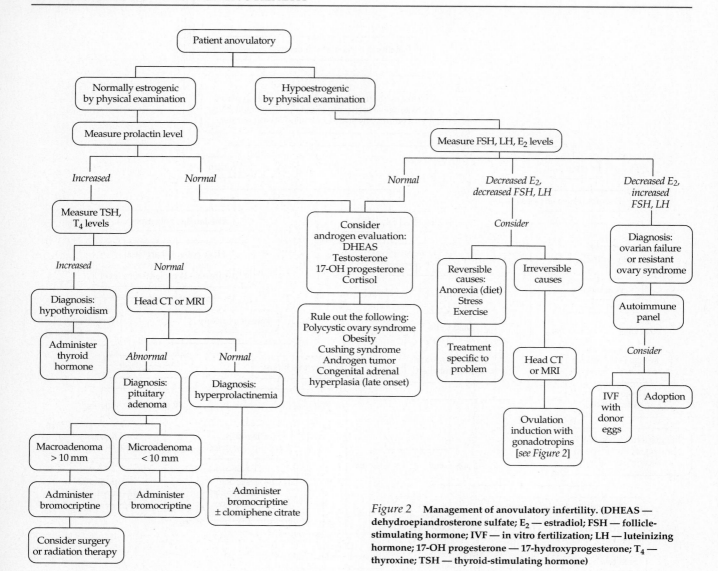

Figure 2 **Management of anovulatory infertility. (DHEAS — dehydroepiandrosterone sulfate; E$_2$ — estradiol; FSH — follicle-stimulating hormone; IVF — in vitro fertilization; LH — luteinizing hormone; 17-OH progesterone — 17-hydroxyprogesterone; T$_4$ — thyroxine; TSH — thyroid-stimulating hormone)**

Laparoscopy with chromotubation (intrauterine injection of colored liquid [indigo carmine] to confirm tubal patency) is indicated for patients with abnormal findings on HSG and for patients with unexplained infertility. This procedure may be omitted from the diagnostic workup if IVF is the main focus of treatment. However, surgical resection of the diseased tube should be considered for patients who are diagnosed with a hydrosalpinx on the basis of HSG or laparoscopy. Studies indicate that the mere presence of a hydrosalpinx can adversely affect embryo implantation and the success of IVF.[16]

If the laparoscopy and chromotubation reveal tubal occlusion, surgery may be indicated. Isolated proximal or distal tubal occlusions may be treated by various surgical techniques. However, combined proximal and distal occlusions are not well corrected with surgery, and IVF should be recommended as the treatment of choice to achieve pregnancy in these patients. Age is also important when deciding between tubal surgery and IVF. Older couples should be encouraged to have IVF rather than tubal surgery because the probability of their achieving a pregnancy is higher with IVF.

Cervical Factors

Abnormal cervical mucus is the recognized cause of infertil-

ity in 5% to 10% of couples trying to conceive. The postcoital test provides information regarding both the quality of the cervical mucus and its interaction with sperm. This test is performed on cycle day 11 to 13 (24 to 48 hours before ovulation); the male partner must abstain from ejaculation for 48 hours before testing. The cervical mucus is examined 2 to 8 hours after intercourse. The consistency of the cervical mucus is examined and the number of motile sperm per high-power field (hpf) is

Table 2   Semen Analysis Parameters

Parameter	Normal Value
Volume of semen	≥ 2.0 ml
pH	7.2–8.0
Sperm concentration	$\geq 20 \times 10^6$ spermatozoa/ml
Total sperm count	$\geq 40 \times 10^6$ spermatozoa/ejaculate
Motility	$\geq 50\%$ with forward progression
	$\geq 25\%$ with rapid progression
Morphology	$\geq 30\%$ with normal forms
Vitality	$\geq 75\%$ or more living
White blood cell count	$\leq 1 \times 10^6$/ml

Table 3 In Vitro Fertilization

Step 1 Stimulation of ovulation with injectable gonadotropins. Monitoring of follicular development with vaginal ultrasound.
When mean follicle diameter is ≥ 15 mm, ovulation is triggered with hCG administered intramuscularly.

Step 2 Collection of eggs 34 to 36 hours after hCG injection.

Step 3 Collection of sperm on day of ovum capture or obtain frozen sample.

Step 4 Laboratory (in vitro) incubation of egg(s) with sperm for fertilization and embryo growth.
If sperm are of poor quality, fertilization is facilitated by microinjection (ICSI) of sperm into egg.

Step 5 Transfer of embryo to uterus 3 to 5 days after oocyte aspiration.
Administration of progesterone in oil, 50 to 100 mg/day I.M., or vaginal progesterone suppositories.

Step 6 14-day wait for pregnancy or menstruation.
Measure β-hCG.

hCG—human chorionic gonadotropin   ICSI—intracytoplasmic sperm injection

---

determined. Normal mucus is acellular, clear, thin, and elastic; the mucus should stretch approximately 8 to 10 cm when placed on a glass slide and pulled. This elasticity of the cervical mucus is known as spinnbarkeit. The mucus should also contain at least 5 to 10 progressively motile sperm/hpf.

Cervical mucus that is of poor quality (i.e., thick and nonelastic) will demonstrate a globular rather than a fernlike pattern after drying on a microscope slide. Absent or poor-quality cervical mucus may reflect either inaccurate timing of the test or an abnormality in mucus production. Cervical trauma and infection have been implicated as antecedents to abnormal mucus production.

Sperm that are both shaky and immotile on microscopic inspection are found in the cervical mucus of women who produce antisperm antibodies. When all the sperm from a postcoital test are found to be immotile, the patient should be asked whether lubricants or spermicides were used during coitus.

Intrauterine insemination (IUI) is the treatment of choice for those patients with cervical factor infertility.[17] This procedure bypasses the cervix and allows the physician to place washed sperm directly into the endometrial cavity.[18]

Ovulatory Factors

Ovulatory dysfunction is the cause of 15% of the infertility detected in couples and 40% of the infertility found in women. Anovulation and oligo-ovulation account for most menstrual abnormalities. Shortened menstrual cycles and luteal phase defects are less common causes of ovulatory dysfunction.

A patient's ovulatory status can be determined by several techniques. The cheapest and least invasive technique is to have the patient chart her basal body temperature (BBT). When done correctly, charting can aid the clinician by providing indirect evidence of ovulation. A biphasic temperature curve (i.e., an elevated temperature for at least 11 to 16 days) is an indication that ovulation probably occurred. The patient's own assessment of premenstrual molimina further strengthens the indirect evidence of ovulation.

Measurement of the progesterone level on day 21 of the menstrual cycle also provides an indirect assessment of ovulatory status. This method is less time-consuming than BBT

charting. Progesterone values of more than 15 ng/ml are consistent with ovulation. A value of less than 5 ng/ml may indicate that ovulation has not occurred. Because progesterone is secreted in a pulsatile manner, only elevated values of progesterone are diagnostically useful. Levels between 5 and 15 ng/ml probably indicate ovulation but give insufficient information regarding the adequacy of the luteal phase.

Of all menstrual cycles in normally menstruating women, 5% to 30% involve a luteinized unruptured follicle. Although ovulatory symptoms and elevated progesterone levels occur during these cycles, an oocyte is not released and fertilization is impossible. Thus, the predictive value of indirect measures of ovulatory status is limited.

An endometrial biopsy can be performed on cycle days 23 to 26. This test can assess both the ovulatory status of the patient and the adequacy of the luteal phase. A luteal phase defect is defined as a lag in the histologic development of the endometrium by 2 or more days when compared with the cycle day of sampling. This defect in the luteal phase is presumably caused by inadequate progesterone secretion from the corpus luteum.

Treatment has entailed prolonging the luteal phase by administering progesterone either intramuscularly or intravaginally. The benefit of this approach, however, has not been substantiated.

Anovulation

Measurement of the prolactin level should be done during the initial evaluation of patients who are believed to be anovulatory [see Figure 2].[19] Elevated prolactin levels have a negative feedback effect on the hypothalamus, preventing the pulsatile release of gonadotropin-releasing hormone (GnRH). This, in turn, prevents secretion of follicle-stimulating hormone (FSH) and luteinizing hormone (LH) from the anterior pituitary. Consequently, follicular development and ovulation do not occur.

Hyperprolactinemia is responsible for 15% of all ovulatory disturbances.[20] If the patient has an elevated prolactin level, with or without galactorrhea, the thyroid-stimulating hormone (TSH) level should be measured to rule out primary or secondary hypothyroidism. If the TSH level is normal, a computed tomography scan or magnetic resonance image of the head should be obtained to determine whether the patient has a prolactinoma. Of import is that prolactin levels may also be elevated as a result of the use of specific medications. Pharmacologic agents that deplete dopamine reserves (i.e., antidepressants, antipsychotics, and other psychotropic agents) may also result in hyperprolactinemia and anovulation.

If the CT or MRI findings are abnormal or reveal a pituitary adenoma, the patient should be treated with oral bromocriptine, starting at a dosage of 2.5 to 5 mg daily, or oral cabergoline, 0.25 mg twice weekly [see Chapter 76]. These medications should be titrated until prolactin levels return to normal. When prolactin levels are normalized, restoration of ovulatory function should occur.[21] Patients with symptomatic macroadenomas may require ablative therapy with either surgery or radiation if medical therapy does not reduce the size of the tumor or if symptoms associated with the tumor persist or worsen.

Patients with hyperprolactinemia and oligomenorrhea (except those with primary and secondary hypothyroidism, who require thyroid hormone replacement) should be treated with bromocriptine only if they are bothered by symptoms (i.e., galactorrhea) or desire fertility. If a patient remains anovulatory despite treatment with bromocriptine, oral clomiphene citrate, starting at a dosage of 50 mg daily for 5 days, can be added as an adjunctive therapy to stimulate ovulation.

If, at the time of initial examination, the patient is determined to be hypoestrogenic (i.e., she has an atrophic vagina and perineum and reports hot flashes and lack of lubrication during coital activity), the clinician should obtain serum levels of FSH, LH, and estradiol (E$_2$). These values will identify patients with hypogonadotropic hypogonadism and those with ovarian failure. Patients with hypogonadotropic hypogonadism should be evaluated with a GnRH-stimulation test to determine whether the problem is reversible.

Special attention should be given to anovulatory women who have normal levels of estrogen and prolactin and who have signs of hyperandrogenism and virilization. In these patients, measurements should be made of dehydroepiandrosterone sulfate (DHEAS), total testosterone, 17-hydroxyprogesterone, and 8 A.M. free urine cortisol levels. These tests will help to identify those patients who have polycystic ovary syndrome (PCOS), ovarian and adrenal neoplasms, congenital adrenal hyperplasia, or Cushing syndrome [see Chapter 79].

Patients with PCOS that is associated with elevated insulin or glucose levels who wish to conceive may benefit from a combined regimen of oral metformin, 850 mg twice daily, and clomiphene citrate. Studies have shown that women treated with this combination have a higher rate of ovulation than those treated with clomiphene citrate alone.[22] Hirsutism and acne should not be treated medically during ovulatory induction cycles.

Elevated levels of both FSH and E$_2$ on cycle day 3 signify a decrease in ovarian reserve (i.e., a decrease in the total number of follicles present for maturation and ovulation). The diagnosis of premature ovarian failure is reserved for women who are younger than 40 years and have gonadotropin (FSH and LH) levels in the menopausal range.

Depending on the incipient age of ovarian failure, a complete autoimmune profile and possibly a genetic karyotype should be considered to establish a diagnosis.[23] Women with an autoimmune disorder are at increased risk for developing multiple organ failure and should be screened annually. These women should be counseled to consider IVF with donor eggs or adoption.

UNEXPLAINED INFERTILITY

The incidence of unexplained infertility is estimated to be between 15% and 20%. Couples who do not receive treatment have a monthly fecundity of 3% and a cumulative 3-year pregnancy rate of 60%. However, when a couple has experienced long-standing infertility (> 3 years) and the female partner is older than 35 years, the probability of achieving a pregnancy is markedly reduced.[24]

The treatment for couples with unexplained infertility includes inducement of superovulation with either clomiphene citrate or gonadotropins[25,26] and IUI or one of the assisted reproductive technologies (e.g., IVF, gamete intrafallopian transfer, and zygote intrafallopian transfer).[27] IUI with ovulation induction using gonadotropins produces higher pregnancy rates for couples with male-factor or unexplained infertility than does either procedure performed alone.[17]

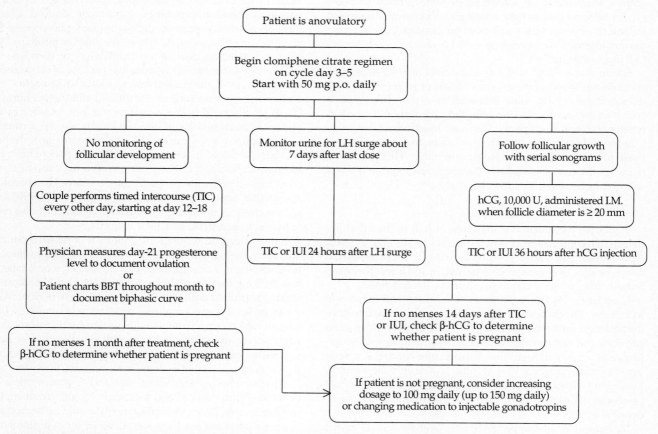

Figure 3 Ovulation induction with clomiphene citrate. (BBT — basal body temperature; hCG — human chorionic gonadotropin; IUI — intrauterine insemination; TIC — timed intercourse)

Ovulation Induction with Clomiphene Citrate

To induce ovulation in a woman who has been determined to be anovulatory, clomiphene citrate, 50 mg orally daily, is begun on cycle day 3 to 5 and is continued for a total of 5 days [*see Figure 3*]. The couple and the physician must decide whether to add IUI to the ovulation induction regimen or have the couple perform timed sexual intercourse.

The couple and physician must also decide whether to monitor follicular development and timing for intercourse or IUI and, if so, whether to use a low-, moderate-, or high-technology method for monitoring. Low-technology monitoring entails charting the BBT. A moderate level of monitoring by the patient can be achieved with an LH kit. The kit enables urinary detection of the LH surge, which usually occurs about 7 days after the last dose of clomiphene citrate. High-technology monitoring entails serial vaginal sonography, with administration of human chorionic gonadotropin (hCG) to trigger ovulation when appropriate; hCG is given in a dose of 10,000 units intramuscularly when the follicle diameter is at least 20 mm.

If the clinician is not monitoring follicular development, the couple is directed to perform timed intercourse every other day, starting on cycle days 12 to 18. Timed intercourse or IUI should begin 24 hours after urinary detection of the LH surge or 36 hours after the administration of hCG. One study has shown that in couples with anovulatory, male, or unexplained infertility, clinical pregnancy rates with IUI and clomiphene citrate did not depend on the method used to establish the timing for IUI.[28] Thus, if cost is a consideration for the couple, urinary LH testing may lower the expense by reducing the number of patient visits and eliminating the midcycle ultrasound.

If menses does not begin 14 days after timed intercourse or IUI, the hCG level should be checked to determine whether the patient is pregnant. If the patient is not pregnant but did ovulate, as evidenced by an elevation in the progesterone level on day 21 or a biphasic BBT chart, she should undergo another stimulation cycle with the same dosage of clomiphene citrate. This method can be repeated for as long as 6 months. If pregnancy is not achieved by that time, the use of injectable gonadotropins to stimulate ovulation should be considered [*see Chapter 79*].

It is important for the clinician to realize that the incidence of multiple gestations (e.g., twins) is nearly 8% in patients taking clomiphene citrate and as high as 35% in patients who use injectable gonadotropins.[17] Therefore, extreme caution and judgment should be exercised with these medications.

For patients who do not ovulate with the initial 50 mg/day dosage of clomiphene citrate (as determined on the basis of a low day-21 progesterone level or a monophasic BBT chart), the dose can be increased to 100 or 150 mg daily. If ovulation still does not occur with the higher dosage, ovulation induction with gonadotropins should be employed.[29]

References

1. Guttmacher AF: Factors affecting normal expectancy of conception. JAMA 161:855, 1956
2. Chandra A, Mosher WD: The demography of infertility and the use of medical care for infertility. Study Design and Statistics for Infertility Research 64:781, 1994
3. Stephen EH, Chandra A: Use of infertility services in the United States: 1995. Fam Plann Perspect 32:132, 2000
4. Schover LR, Thomas AJ, Falcone T: Attitudes about genetic risk of couples undergoing in-vitro fertilization. Hum Reprod 13:862, 1998
5. Van Voorhis BJ, Stovall DW, Allen BD, et al: Cost-effective treatment of the infertile couple. Fertil Steril 70:995, 1998
6. Kainz K: The role of the psychologist in the evaluation and treatment of infertility. Womens Health Issues 11:481, 2001
7. Rich-Edwards JW, Spiegelman D, Garland M, et al: Physical activity, body mass index, and ovulatory disorder infertility. Epidemiology 13:184, 2002
8. Delayed conception and active and passive smoking. The Avon Longitudinal Study of Pregnancy and Childhood Study Team. Fertil Steril 74:725, 2000
9. Mendonca LL, Khamashta MA, Nelson-Piercy C, et al: Non-steroidal anti-inflammatory drugs as a possible cause for reversible infertility. Rheumatology (Oxford) 39:880, 2000
10. Collins JA, Crosignani PG: Unexplained infertility: a review of diagnosis, prognosis, treatment efficacy and management. Int J Gynaecol Obstet 39:267, 1992
11. Menken J, Trussel J, Larsen U: Age and infertility. Science 233:1389, 1986
12. van Kooij RJ, Looman CW, Habbema JD, et al: Age-dependent decrease in embryo implantation rate after in vitro fertilization. Fertil Steril 66:769, 1996
13. World Health Organization: WHO Laboratory Manual for the Examination of Human Semen and Semen-Cervical Mucus Interaction, 3rd ed. Cambridge University Press, New York, 1992
14. Hlinka D, Herman M, Vesela J, et al: A modified method of intracytoplasmic sperm injection without the use of polyvinylpyrrolidone. Hum Reprod 13:1922, 1998
15. Penzias AS, DeCherney AH: Is there ever a role for tubal surgery? Am J Obstet Gynecol 174:1218, 1996
16. Murray DL, Sagoskin AW, Widra EA, et al: The adverse effect of hydrosalpinges on in vitro fertilization pregnancy rates and the benefit of surgical correction. Fertil Steril 69:41, 1998
17. Guzick DS, Carson SA, Coutifaris C, et al: Efficacy of superovulation and intrauterine insemination in the treatment of infertility. National Cooperative Reproductive Medicine Network. N Engl J Med 340:177, 1999
18. Keck C, Gerber-Schafer C, Wilhelm C, et al: Intrauterine insemination for treatment of male infertility. Int J Androl 20(suppl 3):55, 1997
19. Cunnah D, Besser M: Management of prolactinomas. Clin Endocrinol 34:231, 1991
20. Colao A, Annunziato L, Lombardi G: Treatment of prolactinomas. Ann Med 30:452, 1998
21. Shimon I, Melmed S: Management of pituitary tumors. Ann Intern Med 129:472, 1998
22. Nestler JE, Jakubowicz DJ, Evans WS, et al: Effects of metformin on spontaneous and clomiphene-induced ovulation in the polycystic ovary syndrome. N Engl J Med 338:1876, 1998
23. Conway GS, Kaltsas G, Patel A, et al: Characterization of idiopathic premature ovarian failure. Fertil Steril 65:337, 1996
24. Guzick DS, Sullivan MW, Adamson GD, et al: Efficacy of treatment for unexplained infertility. Fertil Steril 70:207, 1998
25. Kousta E, White DM, Franks S: Modern use of clomiphene citrate in induction of ovulation. Hum Reprod Update 3:359, 1997
26. Rust LA, Isreal R, Mishell DR Jr: An individualized graduated therapeutic regimen of clomiphene citrate. Am J Obstet Gynecol 120:785, 1974
27. Dodson WC, Haney AF: Controlled ovarian hyperstimulation and intrauterine insemination for treatment of infertility. Fertil Steril 55:457, 1991
28. Deaton JL, Clark RR, Pittaway DE: Clomiphene citrate ovulation induction in combination with a timed intrauterine insemination: the value of urinary luteinizing hormone versus human chorionic gonadotropin timing. Fertil Steril 68:43, 1997
29. ACOG Practice Bulletin. Clinical management guidelines for obstetrician-gynecologists number 34, February 2002. Management of infertility caused by ovulatory dysfunction. American College of Obstetricians and Gynecologists. ACOG Committee on Practice Bulletins–Gynecology. Obstet Gynecol 99:347, 2002

Alan H. DeCherney, M.D.

Ectopic Pregnancy

Ectopic pregnancy is the implantation of an embryo outside the endometrial cavity (i.e., lining of the uterus). The embryo may be implanted in the fallopian tubes, ovaries, abdomen, or cervix. More than 95% of ectopic pregnancies occur in the fallopian tubes, with nearly 80% of ectopic pregnancies occurring in the ampullary portion of the fallopian tube.

Ectopic pregnancies comprise approximately 2% of all reported pregnancies in the United States. If left untreated, ectopic pregnancy can result in rupture of the fallopian tube, which can lead to hemorrhagic shock and death. For that reason, ectopic pregnancy is a major cause of morbidity and mortality in women of reproductive age. It is the third leading cause of maternal mortality and is responsible for nearly 9% of all pregnancy-related deaths.[1] Between 1970 and 1992, the incidence of ectopic pregnancy increased sixfold, which is consistent with the increased prevalence of important risk factors for ectopic pregnancy (see below).[2]

Improvements in diagnostic skills have enabled physicians to treat ectopic pregnancies at an earlier gestational age and by more conservative approaches. Therefore, it is imperative that the primary care physician be able to diagnose and intervene as early as possible to reduce the incidence of irreversible tubal damage and the risk of future infertility [see Figure 1].[3]

DIAGNOSIS

Clinical Manifestations

The principal diagnostic task in ectopic pregnancy is distinguishing it from intrauterine pregnancy or threatened abortion. The symptoms of an ectopic pregnancy [see Table 1] vary with its location and the rate of its growth. Nearly all women with ectopic pregnancies complain of a colicky abdominal pain that is vague in location. As the pregnancy grows, capillaries are broken and blood spills into the abdominal cavity. The blood that fills the intraperitoneal cavity causes irritation of the left hemidiaphragm, resulting in left shoulder pain; the liver occupies the space directly under the right hemidiaphragm and prevents the blood from reaching the right hemidiaphragm. Almost one quarter of the patients with ruptured ectopic pregnancies have left shoulder pain.

Amenorrhea, the second most common symptom, occurs in more than 75% of patients. The duration of amenorrhea depends on the site of implantation and usually lasts 6 to 8 weeks before the onset of other symptoms.

Vaginal bleeding is also common and may occur a few days to weeks before the patient's initial visit. The pattern of bleeding is most often described as spotting and usually is preceded by the onset and worsening of abdominal pain.

Other symptoms, which occur less frequently, are dizziness, fainting, nausea, vomiting, other signs of pregnancy, the urge to defecate, and passage of tissue through the vagina.

History and Physical Examination

At the initial visit, the patient's medical history should be taken. Patients in whom ectopic pregnancy is suspected often have a history of infertility, pelvic inflammatory disease, endometriosis, or tubal damage [see Table 2]. In rare cases, ectopic pregnancy can occur in patients who have undergone tubal sterilization, even many years after the procedure.[4] If the diagnosis of ectopic pregnancy is suspected, a pregnancy test should be performed (e.g., measurement of the human chorionic gonadotropin [hCG] level in urine). The urine hCG test is extremely sensitive; false negative results are very rare.

Patients who have a negative urine hCG test result should be evaluated for other gynecologic problems, including ovarian torsion, a ruptured ovarian cyst, and pelvic inflammatory disease. Gastrointestinal disorders and possible surgical conditions (e.g., appendicitis) should also be investigated.

If the urine hCG test result is positive, a physical examination should be performed and a pelvic sonogram obtained.[5] The physician should assess the degree of abdominal and pelvic pain experienced by the patient and try to elicit signs of peritonitis, which could indicate rupture of an ectopic pregnancy.

Inspection of the patient's cervix with a speculum can help distinguish ectopic pregnancy from spontaneous or threatened abortion. If the cervical os is open, fetal tissue should be observed at the internal cervical os; the diagnosis of an inevitable abortion or incomplete abortion should be made, and a dilatation and curettage (D&C) should be performed. If the cervical os is closed, the examiner should determine both the amount of blood present in the vagina and the amount emanating from the external cervical os. Most women with ectopic pregnancies do not experience heavy vaginal bleeding and have only a light bloody vaginal discharge. In the case of threatened or complete abortion, the patient should be instructed to have pelvic rest and bed rest until the symptoms resolve.

Laboratory Testing

A pelvic sonogram should be obtained to document whether an intrauterine pregnancy (IUP) or extrauterine pregnancy (EUP) exists. The sonographer should focus attention on the uterus, the adnexa, and the cul-de-sac. The endometrium should be inspected, and the presence of a gestational sac and fetal pole should be verified. Attempts should be made to observe the fetal heartbeat to help distinguish normal from abnormal pregnancies. If nothing is present in the uterus, the adnexa should be inspected. If a gestational sac and fetal pole are identified outside the uterus, the diagnosis of an EUP should be made. The ectopic pregnancy can then be treated by medical or surgical means [see Treatment, *below*].

If no IUP or EUP can be documented on sonography, further laboratory evaluation should be pursued. The evaluation should include measurement of the serum β-hCG level, a complete blood count (CBC), and measurement of the prothrombin time (PT) or partial thromboplastin time (PTT). A progesterone assay is optional (see below). A β-hCG value of 1,500 mIU/ml occurs

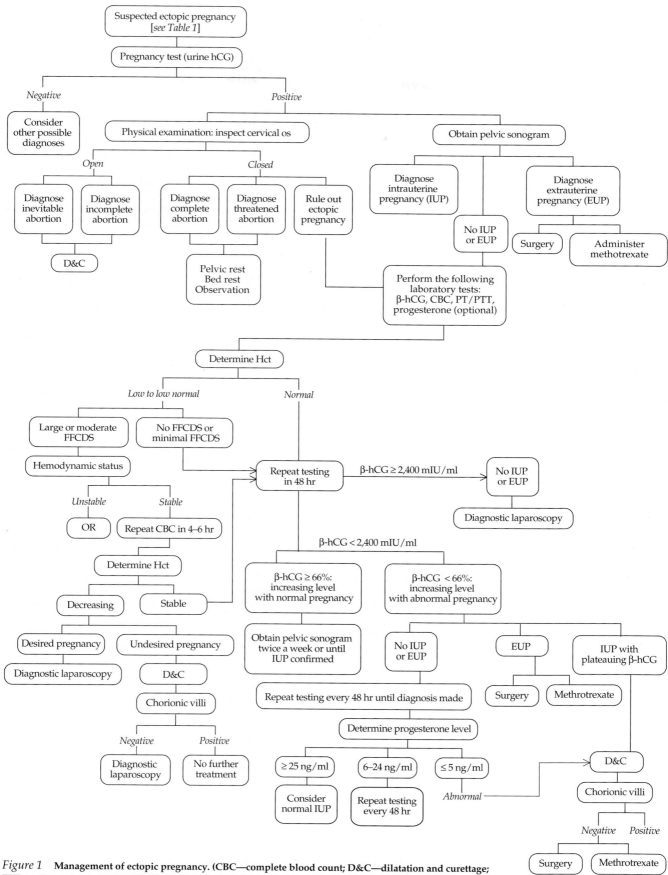

Figure 1   **Management of ectopic pregnancy. (CBC—complete blood count; D&C—dilatation and curettage; EUP—extrauterine pregnancy; FFCDS—free fluid in the cul-de-sac; hCG—human chorionic gonadotropin; Hct—hematocrit; IUP—intrauterine pregnancy; PT—prothrombin time; PTT—partial thromboplastin time)**

Table 1   Signs and Symptoms of Ectopic Pregnancy

Abdominal pain
Amenorrhea
Vaginal bleeding
Dizziness and fainting
Other symptoms of pregnancy

Table 2   Patient History Consistent with Suspected Ectopic Pregnancy

Prior ectopic pregnancy
History of infertility
Past infection with *Chlamydia* or *Neisseria gonorrhoeae* or history of pelvic inflammatory disease
Past or present use of an intrauterine device (IUD)
Current pregnancy conceived with in vitro fertilization (IVF)
History of endometriosis
Current pregnancy conceived while taking oral contraceptives

around the time a normal IUP first becomes visible on pelvic sonography. If no IUP is observed and the β-hCG value is 2,400 mIU/ml or higher, an ectopic pregnancy should be suspected.

A baseline hematocrit, along with sonographic evaluation of the patient's cul-de-sac, will provide insight for prognosis and possible treatment options. Free fluid in the cul-de-sac may be blood; this finding increases the likelihood of ectopic pregnancy.[6] Patients with aborting ectopic and early nonruptured ectopic pregnancies may present with blood in the cul-de-sac. If the patient has a normal hematocrit and minimal to no free fluid in the cul-de-sac, repeating pelvic sonography and measurements of the β-hCG level and a CBC in 48 hours is recommended. Patients with low to low-normal hematocrits in conjunction with mild to moderate amounts of free fluid in the cul de sac need further evaluation, including a repeat CBC.

If a moderate to large amount of free fluid is found in the cul-de-sac, blood pressure needs to be checked immediately. If the blood pressure is unstable, the patient should be taken to the operating room for an exploratory laparotomy and transfusion with packed red blood cells and crystalloids to replenish intravascular losses.

Some patients require hospitalization for confirmation of hemodynamic stability. The CBC should be repeated within 4 to 6 hours in patients who are hemodynamically stable. If the hematocrit remains stable, the laboratory tests and sonographic evaluation should be repeated within 48 hours (see below).

Patients with decreasing hematocrits should be evaluated with either a D&C or diagnostic laparoscopy, depending on their desire to maintain the pregnancy. When a D&C is performed for removal of fetal tissue, histology of the removed tissue should show chorionic villi. If no villi are obtained, an ectopic pregnancy should be suspected.

Repeat hCG levels   The doubling time of the β-hCG level in early pregnancies ranges from 48 to 72 hours. A rise in the β-hCG level of at least 66% in 2 days is generally indicative of a

normal IUP. Patients who have normal doubling values of their β-hCG level on repeat evaluation should be followed up in 1 week with a repeat sonogram to confirm a pregnancy in utero.[7]

An abnormally rising β-hCG level (< 66% higher than original values) should be further investigated. Correlation with a repeat sonogram and hematocrit will help guide the clinician to the correct diagnosis and treatment. Although the presence of an ectopic pregnancy should be suspected, an abnormally developing IUP cannot be ruled out. Treatment should be decided not on the basis of only two β-hCG values but, rather, on the entire clinical picture. An abnormally rising β-hCG level that is not substantiated by other laboratory or radiographic evidence should not be treated as an ectopic pregnancy. Surgical or medical treatment of these patients should be considered only when the diagnosis is confirmed and an EUP is documented.

Serum progesterone level   Progesterone values can help the clinician determine the viability of a pregnancy, but only in rare instances can they reveal an ectopic pregnancy.[8] A progesterone level of greater than 25 ng/ml is associated with a normal IUP in nearly 97% of cases. Values of less than 5 ng/ml are associated with abnormal pregnancies, and values between 5 and 25 ng/ml are indeterminate. The usefulness of the progesterone assay is limited because more than 85% of the values obtained are between 5 and 25 ng/ml. Furthermore, most centers are unable to process this test in a timely fashion, with results being unavailable for review and interpretation on the same day that the sample is drawn.

TREATMENT

Ectopic pregnancy can be treated medically or surgically. The choice of treatment should be tailored to the patient's clinical circumstances and preferences.[9,10]

Medical Therapy

Methotrexate should be considered as the primary modality of treatment in all patients who meet the criteria for medical therapy [see Table 3].[11,12] Methotrexate is an antimetabolite that interferes with the conversion of dihydrofolic acid to tetrahydrofolic acid, inhibiting DNA synthesis and cell division and thereby terminating the pregnancy. Because methotrexate may, in rare cases, produce hepatotoxicity or bone marrow suppression, baseline liver function tests (LFTs) and a CBC, along with a β-hCG level, must

Table 3   Criteria and Contraindications for Methotrexate Treatment

Criteria
Patient is diagnosed with ectopic pregnancy
Patient is reliable and expected to comply with regimen
Patient is hemodynamically stable
The ectopic pregnancy is no greater than 3.5 to 4 cm in diameter
Contraindications
Absolute
   Hepatic dysfunction
   Moderate to severe anemia
Relative
   Human chorionic gonadotropin concentration ≥ 10,000 mIU/ml
   Fetal cardiac activity detected with sonography

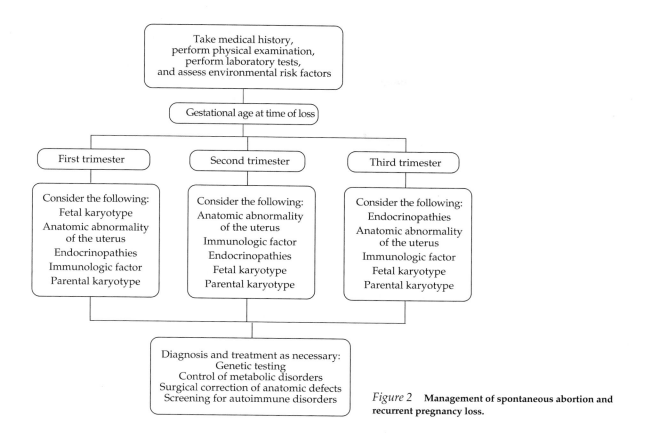

Figure 2 **Management of spontaneous abortion and recurrent pregnancy loss.**

be done in all patients being considered for methotrexate therapy. LFTs and CBCs must be monitored during treatment with repeated doses of methotrexate, and methotrexate should be discontinued if test results become abnormal.

Methotrexate therapy can be given by local injection into the area of the ectopic pregnancy, which requires ultrasound or laparoscopic guidance, or by intramuscular injection as a single-dose or multiple-dose regimen. The multiple-dose regimen is rarely used today, unless the patient fails to respond to the single-dose regimen. The multiple-dose regimen includes citrovorum rescue to protect maternal cells. In the single-dose regimen, 50 mg/m² of methotrexate is given and baseline studies are repeated on day 3 or 4. If the β-hCG level decreases by less than 15%, the treatment can be repeated in 1 week. Of the patients who receive methotrexate, 64% are cured with a single dose.[13] An additional 14% require two or three doses. This gives an overall cure rate of 78%. Patients who are cured with methotrexate have fertility rates equivalent to those of patients who are treated surgically. Unfortunately, 20% of the patients whose ectopic pregnancy is treated pharmacologically will ultimately require surgical intervention.

Surgical Therapy

Surgical modalities for ectopic pregnancy include laparoscopy and laparotomy [*see Figure 1*]. Laparoscopy with conservative tubal therapy (salpingostomy or salpingotomy) is the preferred surgical method in hemodynamically stable patients, for the following reasons: (1) Less intraoperative blood loss occurs, (2) less postoperative analgesia is required, (3) the hospital stay is shorter, and (4) the cost savings per patient is greater. After laparoscopy, β-hCG levels should be

measured serially until they decrease to nonpregnant levels. If the β-hCG level plateaus, increases, or does not decrease more than 15% in 48 hours, treatment with methotrexate or salpingectomy is required.

In the past, laparotomy and radical tubal surgery (salpingectomy) was recommended for hemodynamically unstable patients. Because of improvements in anesthesia and cardiovascular monitoring, together with advances in laparoscopic surgical skills and experience, operative laparoscopy can now be justified for surgical treatment of ectopic pregnancy even in women with hemodynamic instability.[14] Serial measurement of β-hCG levels is not required after salpingectomy.

Fertility after surgery is not a function of the surgical method employed. Rather, future fertility in these cases depends on three patient factors. The first is a history of infertility; patients with prior infertility have a fourfold lower pregnancy rate than patients without. The second is the status of the contralateral fallopian tube. The third is the extent of adhesions involving the ipsilateral tube.

Spontaneous Abortions

A spontaneous abortion is defined as the spontaneous termination of a pregnancy before 20 weeks' gestation (from the onset of the last menstrual period) or the loss of a pregnancy with a fetal weight of less than 500 g. All pregnancy losses that occur later than 20 weeks' gestational age are termed miscarriages.

Spontaneous abortions occur in about 15% to 20% of all known pregnancies.[15] It has been estimated that more than 50% of all conceptions end in spontaneous abortion. This rate is higher than previous estimates, because spontaneous abortions often

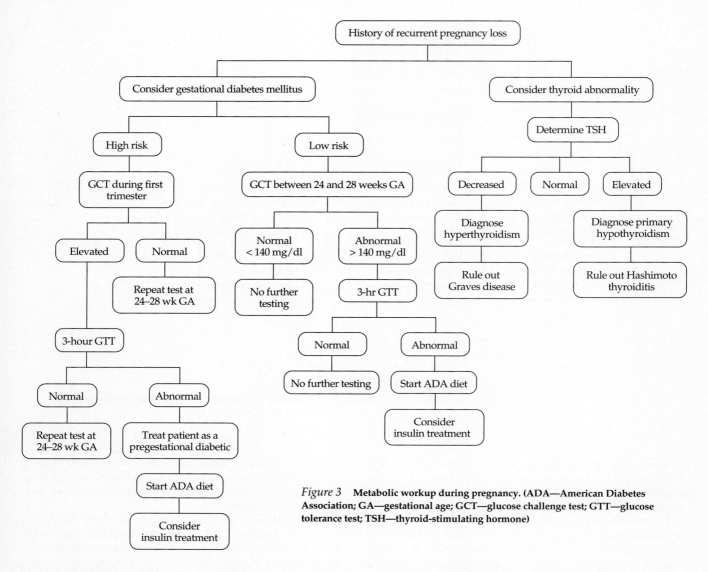

Figure 3 **Metabolic workup during pregnancy. (ADA—American Diabetes Association; GA—gestational age; GCT—glucose challenge test; GTT—glucose tolerance test; TSH—thyroid-stimulating hormone)**

occur around the time of expected menses and are not recognized as abortions.

Traditionally, women who had three or more consecutive pregnancy losses were designated habitual aborters, and it was considered likely that they would continue to have frequent spontaneous abortions. It is now known, however, that in women who have two or more consecutive losses and no history of a live birth, the maximum likelihood that a subsequent pregnancy will result in spontaneous abortion is only about 45%. Women who have at least one live birth before three or more losses have an abortion frequency of less than 30%.[16]

Factors responsible for pregnancy termination vary from one trimester to the next. A strong correlation exists between the gestational age at which the loss occurs and its cause. Therefore, it is important to recognize these potential risks and begin treatment when necessary [*see Figure 2*].

DETERMINING CAUSE OF SPONTANEOUS ABORTION

When a spontaneous abortion has occurred, the physician must investigate the possible causes. A medical history should be taken, possible environmental risk factors should be assessed, and laboratory tests for common infections should be performed.

Depending on whether the abortion occurred during the first, second, or third trimester, the likelihood of genetic, anatomic, or endocrinologic causes varies (see below).

Infections

Organisms that can cause spontaneous abortions include *Ureaplasma, Chlamydia, Listeria,* mycoplasmas, and the TORCH (toxoplasmosis, other [e.g., hepatitis B] rubella, cytomegalovirus, herpes) organisms. Diagnosis is made by cultures of blood or amniotic fluid. Treatments may include antibiotics, γ-globulins, or vaccinations.

Environmental Factors

Cigarette smoking, alcohol consumption, and caffeine consumption can cause spontaneous abortion. The greater the number of cigarettes smoked in a day, the greater the risk of fetal loss. Cleaning solvents and anesthetic gases have been linked to fetal wastage. It is important that pregnant women take precautions and limit their exposure to these agents.

Genetic Factors

Chromosomal abnormalities are responsible for more than 70% of all first-trimester abortions.[17] Aneuploidy problems predominate, with trisomies as a whole constituting the largest group (nearly 50%). Monosomy X (Turner syndrome) is the single most common chromosomal abnormality, accounting for nearly 25% of spontaneous abortions. Maternal nondisjunction during metaphase I is the most common cause of trisomies. It is estimated that only 30% of second-trimester losses and 3% of third-trimester losses are the result of chromosomal defects.

Balanced translocations are the most commonly transmitted parental chromosomal abnormalities responsible for recurrent losses. Thus, genetic testing should be done in couples who have experienced recurrent spontaneous abortion, to determine whether either partner is a carrier. Genetic testing is often done on spontaneously aborted fetuses.

Endocrine Factors

Patients with uncontrolled diabetes mellitus or thyroid disease have an increased risk of fetal demise and spontaneous abortion. Workup for an endocrine disorder should be considered for all patients with recurrent pregnancy losses. Any history or physical examination that is suspect for a metabolic problem should prompt the physician to investigate immediately.

Second- and third-trimester losses are more often the result of a maternal endocrine abnormality. Recognition and control of the metabolic disturbance are the goals of treatment [see Figure 3]. Initial screening begins with a 1-hour glucose challenge test (GCT). This test should be performed in all pregnant women between 24 and 28 weeks' gestational age. A 3-hour glucose tolerance test (GTT) is performed only in women with abnormal GCT values. Evaluation for a thyroid abnormality should be performed at the first prenatal visit. Determining the thyroid-stimulating hormone (TSH) level will distinguish women who have a suspected thyroid dysfunction from those who are euthyroid.[18,19]

Luteal-phase defect is another factor thought to be responsible for early pregnancy loss. Women with this problem characteristically have abnormally shortened secretory phases (< 10 days) or an endometrial lining that is not in phase with the presumed day of the menstrual cycle. An endometrial biopsy that is 2 or more days out of phase with the menstrual cycle is considered diagnostic. Treatment entails the use of progesterone suppositories (25 mg twice daily) to support the luteal phase. However, the benefit of this treatment regimen has not been substantiated.

Anatomic Abnormalities

Uterine cavity malformations are responsible for nearly 15% of recurrent pregnancy losses. Most of these losses occur in the second and third trimesters. Uterine septa are most commonly associated with recurrent abortions. Other causes are submucous myomas, intrauterine adhesions, congenital abnormalities, and cervical incompetence.

A pelvic sonogram and hysterosalpingogram are useful for establishing an initial diagnosis. A magnetic resonance image of the pelvis or a combined laparoscopy and hysteroscopy may be needed for further examination of the uterus. Treatment entails surgical correction of the anatomic defect.

Immunologic Factors

Autoimmune disorders have also been associated with pregnancy losses.[20] These losses commonly occur in the second and third trimesters. Approximately 30% of patients with recurrent pregnancy losses test positive for antinuclear antibodies. Antiphospholipid antibodies, lupus anticoagulants, anticardiolipin antibodies, anti–SS-A (Ro), and anti–SS-B (La) have also been implicated as risk factors. Diagnosis is made by screening the patient for common autoimmune disorders [see Chapter 114].

References

1. Atrash HK, Friede A, Hogue CJ: Ectopic pregnancy mortality in the United States, 1970-1983. Obstet Gynecol 70:817, 1987

2. Ectopic pregnancy—United States, 1990–1992. MMWR Morb Mortal Wkly Rep 44:46, 1995

3. Stovall TG, Ling FW, Carson SA, et al: Nonsurgical diagnosis and treatment of tubal pregnancy. Fertil Steril 54:537, 1990

4. The risk of ectopic pregnancy after tubal sterilization. U.S. Collaborative Review of Sterilization Working Group. N Engl J Med 336:762, 1997

5. Gracia CR, Barnhart KT: Diagnosing ectopic pregnancy: decision analysis comparing six strategies. Obstet Gynecol 97:464, 2001

6. Dart R, McLean SA, Dart L: Isolated fluid in the cul-de-sac: how well does it predict ectopic pregnancy? Am J Emerg Med 20:1, 2002

7. Kador N, Romero R: Serial human chorionic gonadotropin measurements in ectopic pregnancy. Am J Obstet Gynecol 158:1239, 1988

8. Stovall TG, Ling FW, Cope BJ, et al: Preventing ruptured ectopic pregnancy with a single serum progesterone. Am J Obstet Gynecol 160:1425, 1989

9. Yao M, Tulandi T: Current status of surgical and nonsurgical management of ectopic pregnancy. Fertil Steril 67:421, 1997

10. Stovall T, Ling FW, Buster JE: Outpatient chemotherapy of unruptured ectopic pregnancy. Fertil Steril 51:435, 1989

11. Stovall TG, Ling FW, Gray LA, et al: Methotrexate treatment of unruptured ectopic pregnancy: a report of 100 cases. Obstet Gynecol 77:749, 1991

12. Carson SA, Buster JE: Ectopic pregnancy. N Engl J Med 329:1174, 1993

13. Stovall TG, Ling FW, Cope BJ, et al: Single-dose methotrexate for treatment of ectopic pregnancy. Obstet Gynecol 77:754, 1991

14. Sagiv R, Debby A, Sadan O, et al: Laparoscopic surgery for extrauterine pregnancy in hemodynamically unstable patients. J Am Assoc Gynecol Laparosc 8:529, 2001

15. Wilcox AJ, Weinberg CR, O'Connor JF, et al: Incidence of early loss of pregnancy. N Engl J Med 319:189, 1988

16. Harger JH, Archer DF, Marchese SG, et al: Etiology of recurrent pregnancy losses and outcome of subsequent pregnancies. Obstet Gynecol 62:574, 1983

17. Byrne J, Warburton D, Kline J, et al: Morphology of early fetal deaths and their chromosomal characteristics. Teratology 32:297, 1985

18. Kjos SL, Buchanan TA: Gestational diabetes mellitus. N Engl J Med 342:896, 2000

19. ACOG Practice Bulletin. Thyroid disease in pregnancy. Obstet Gynecol 98(5 pt 1):879, 2001

20. Coulam CB: Immunologic tests in the evaluation of reproductive disorders: a critical review. Am J Obstet Gynecol 167:1844, 1992

83 Medical Problems in Pregnancy

John T. Repke, M.D., and Robert L. Barbieri, M.D.

Thanks to modern medicine, many women whose fertility—or even survival—would once have been compromised by disease are able to conceive and carry a child to term. Consequently, many more pregnancies require skilled medical management than in the past.

A variety of physiologic adaptations take place over the course of pregnancy. For example, blood volume increases by as much as 50%, resulting in a mild dilutional anemia. Cardiac output rises in compensation. Placental secretion of hormones, such as placental lactogen, promotes maternal insulin resistance; glucose is shunted to the fetus, and the mother uses ketones and triglycerides to meet her metabolic needs.

To achieve favorable outcomes in pregnancy, the clinician needs to understand how pregnancy may change the management of preexisting disease (e.g., hypertension) or result in the development of new disease (e.g., preeclampsia). Because the outcome of pregnancy is often influenced by maternal status in the initial weeks, counseling and management are best done before conception. Because pregnancy is often unplanned, these considerations should be part of the medical management in any woman of reproductive age.

Teratogens

Concerns about teratogenesis are important and warranted. The perceived risk is often greater than the actual risk, however. Female patients of reproductive age should be made aware of the teratogenic potential of the medications they are taking [*see Table 1*]. In patients who are planning to become pregnant, the clinician needs to discuss teratogenicity versus efficacy, because inadequately controlled disease may be dangerous for mother and fetus alike.

Hypertensive Disorders

Hypertension in pregnancy can be difficult to classify and, on occasion, may be difficult to manage. The hypertensive disorders of pregnancy have been divided into three categories: chronic hypertension, preeclampsia, and gestational hypertension.

CHRONIC HYPERTENSION

Chronic hypertension is defined as hypertension that predates pregnancy or is diagnosed in the first half of pregnancy. Chronic hypertension can be classified as either essential (idiopathic) or secondary. Essential hypertension accounts for 90% of all cases. Secondary hypertension may be the result of underlying renal disease, connective tissue disease, endocrine disease, genetic predisposition, or other cardiovascular disease.

Epidemiology

From 1% to 5% of pregnancies in the United States are complicated by chronic hypertension. The incidence varies somewhat by race and age. African-American women are affected more often than women of other races. In women who are older than 30 years, the rate is about 5%, whereas in women who are 20 to 29 years of age, the rate is approximately 1%.

Diagnosis

Ideally, chronic hypertension is diagnosed before the patient becomes pregnant. The National High Blood Pressure Working Group on High Blood Pressure in Pregnancy has established criteria for making this diagnosis [*see Table 2*].[1] This diagnosis is best made before 20 weeks' gestation, lest the disorder be confused with either early-onset preeclampsia or gestational hypertension.

Initial laboratory evaluation should include a complete blood count, determination of serum creatinine and blood urea nitrogen (BUN) levels, and urinalysis. Quantification of urinary protein excretion and calculation of creatinine clearance are also recommended to establish baseline renal function. If indicated, a complete metabolic panel may be included to screen for elevations in liver enzymes, uric acid, and hyperlipidemia.[2] The liver enzyme and uric acid measurements will serve as a baseline to guide later assessment for superimposed preeclampsia, in which case these values will tend to rise; hyperlipidemia may provide an indication of cardiac risk. Also, in patients older than 40 years—especially those who have had hypertension for more than 10 years—an electrocardiogram is worthwhile because of the possibility of ischemic heart disease.[2] In women at very high risk, prepregnancy exercise tolerance testing may also be recommended.

Treatment

Chronic hypertension is most effectively managed before conception. Evaluation of risk status, disease severity, and medication regimens will allow the clinician to better inform

---

Table 1 **Selected Drugs with Suspected or Known Teratogenic Potential**[49]

Alcohol	Phenytoin
Aminopterin	Quinolones
Androgens	Retinoids and derivatives
Angiotensin-converting enzyme inhibitors	Tetracycline
	Thalidomide
Carbamazepine	Trimethadione/
Cocaine	paramethadione
Lithium	Valproic acid
Methotrexate	Warfarin

Table 2 **Diagnostic Criteria for Chronic Hypertension in Pregnancy**

Mild: Systolic blood pressure > 139 mm Hg
and
Diastolic blood pressure > 89 mm Hg

Severe: Systolic blood pressure > 179 mm Hg
or
Diastolic blood pressure > 109 mm Hg

Onset before 20 weeks' gestation

Use of antihypertensive medication before pregnancy

Postpartum persistence of hypertension

the patient about the risks of pregnancy to herself and to the fetus. Also, uncontrolled severe hypertension at the time of conception is associated with a much higher rate of first-trimester pregnancy loss, preeclampsia, fetal growth restriction, and abruptio placentae.

The treatment of chronic hypertension during pregnancy depends to a large degree on disease severity. Mild to moderate chronic hypertension does not require pharmacotherapy, because drug treatment does not seem to improve maternal and fetal/neonatal outcomes in such cases.[3,4] Pharmacotherapy is indicated when systolic blood pressures persist above 179 mm Hg or when diastolic blood pressures persist above 109 mm Hg.[5] In so-called high-risk hypertensive patients (e.g., those with severe hypertension before pregnancy, diabetes, underlying cardiac disease, or retinopathy), treatment is recommended for diastolic pressures that persist above 90 mm Hg.[6] There are a number of agents from which to choose when treating chronic hypertension during pregnancy.

α-Methyldopa Long used in obstetrics, α-methyldopa has an established record of efficacy and safety and is widely regarded as the agent of choice for nonacute oral antihypertensive therapy in this setting.[5] Dosing generally begins at 250 mg twice a day and may be increased to a maximum of 1 g four times a day.

Beta blockers Labetalol, a combination alpha blocker and beta blocker, is effective for managing hypertension during pregnancy and may also be used for acute blood pressure lowering when indicated. There have been reports of fetal growth restriction with labetalol, as there have been with all beta blockers, and although this is not a contraindication to the use of these agents, close surveillance of fetal growth should be done in patients who receive them.[7] Labetalol may be started at a dosage of 100 mg twice a day; the dosage may be increased to a maximum of 400 mg every 4 hours. The beta blockers metoprolol and atenolol have been successfully used in pregnancy, although atenolol should be used with great care in pregnant patients because of its association with fetal growth restriction.

Nifedipine The usual dosage of this calcium channel blocker in pregnant women is 10 to 30 mg three times a day.[5] It is not clear whether long-acting preparations are as effective in pregnant patients as they are in nonpregnant patients.

Angiotensin inhibitors The use of angiotensin-converting enzyme (ACE) inhibitors in the second and third trimester has been associated with fetal hypocalvaria, oligohydramnios, fetal renal failure, and neonatal death. It is recommended that ACE inhibitors and angiotensin receptor blockers not be used during pregnancy.[8,9]

Maternal and Fetal Risks

Chronic hypertension can result in adverse pregnancy outcomes for both mother and fetus. Maternal risks include superimposed preeclampsia and abruptio placentae.[10] Uncontrolled hypertension can also result in maternal stroke. Fetal risks include growth restriction, prematurity (usually secondary to superimposed preeclampsia in the mother), and an overall increase in the risk of fetal and neonatal death. Experts are not in agreement on how best to monitor pregnancies complicated by chronic hypertension. However, most recommend regular ultrasonographic evaluation of fetal growth as well as weekly as-

sessment of the fetus using nonstress testing and biophysical profile determination. Such assessment should begin at 26 to 34 weeks, depending on the risk status of the mother and fetus.[5,11] Hospitalization is required for all patients in whom the control of blood pressure is difficult. Patients with chronic hypertension should be delivered by 40 weeks' gestation. Successful vaginal delivery may be expected in the majority of patients with chronic hypertension, although the rate of cesarean section is higher in this population. The long-term prognosis for mother and fetus is generally excellent, provided that maternal end-organ damage and fetal complications arising from growth restriction and prematurity can be avoided.

PREECLAMPSIA

Preeclampsia is defined as hypertension, proteinuria, and pathologic edema, occurring after the 20th week of gestation. It is a multiorgan disease that affects blood pressure, vascular permeability, vascular reactivity, coagulation, and platelet function.

Epidemiology

Preeclampsia affects approximately 5% to 7% of all pregnancies. There does not seem to be a predisposition by race, although some variants of preeclampsia may show racial predilection. Risk factors include nulliparity, extremes of maternal age (younger than 15 or older than 35 years), and obesity. Additional risk factors for preeclampsia include chronic hypertension, multiple gestation, underlying renal disease, a history of preeclampsia with a previous pregnancy, type 1 (insulin-dependent) diabetes mellitus, and carriage of the angiotensinogen gene mutation *T235*. Less clear associations are with thrombophilias such as factor V Leiden, the prothrombin gene mutation, and antiphospholipid antibodies.[12,13]

Pathogenesis

Although the etiology of preeclampsia remains unknown, disordered trophoblast invasion and endothelial cell injury appear to be central to development of clinical disease.[14] The cause of the injury is the subject of speculation but probably involves oxygen free radical formation, ischemia, and microthrombosis. Several strategies addressing each of these putative mechanisms have been developed in the hope of preventing this disorder, but thus far results have been disappointing.

Diagnosis and Treatment

Clinically, the onset of preeclampsia is typically marked by acute fluid retention, which presents as edema of the face or hands (as opposed to the lower-extremity edema that characteristically develops in the second and third trimesters). Diagnostic criteria for preeclampsia include blood pressure greater than 140/90 mm Hg on at least two occasions separated by at least 6 hours and proteinuria of 300 mg or more on a 24-hour urine test. Severe preeclampsia causes a variety of other clinical and laboratory abnormalities, including central nervous system dysfunction, pulmonary edema, and thrombocytopenia [see Table 3].

Once the diagnosis of preeclampsia is made, a plan for management and possible delivery is required. To date, delivery of the fetus and placenta is the only known cure for preeclampsia. Essential features of a management strategy include minimizing maternal risks of preeclampsia, particularly stroke. Additionally, the risks of prematurity must be weighed against the risks to the mother of continuing the pregnancy. In mild preeclampsia, expectant management may continue to term if

---

Table 3   Diagnostic Criteria for
Severe Preeclampsia*

Blood pressure > 160 mm Hg (systolic) or > 110 mm Hg (diastolic)
   on two or more occasions separated by at least 6 hours while
   patient is at rest
Proteinuria in the nephrotic range (> 5 g in a 24-hour specimen)
Oliguria (output < 500 ml in 24 hours)
Visual disturbances
Pulmonary edema
Epigastric or right upper quadrant pain
Elevated transaminase levels
Thrombocytopenia
Fetal growth restriction

---

* Presumes that criteria for preeclampsia have been met.

---

mother and fetus are well.[5] In severe preeclampsia, premature delivery is necessary, but expectant management may be considered until 32 to 34 weeks' gestation, provided that blood pressure can be controlled, liver and kidney function remain stable, and coagulation remains normal. Close surveillance in a tertiary setting is essential for the expectant management of patients with severe preeclampsia.[5,15]

In addition to careful control of blood pressure, liberal utilization of magnesium sulfate is recommended for preventing disease progression to eclampsia, which is defined as a tonic-clonic grand mal seizure in a patient with preeclampsia without underlying neurologic disease. Although the value of magnesium sulfate in the management of preeclampsia has been a source of controversy for decades, several recent large clinical trials have demonstrated the efficacy of this approach.[16]

Complications

The major complications from preeclampsia are end-organ damage in the mother and the risks associated with prematurity in the fetus. Antenatal corticosteroids are used in the management of these cases to accelerate fetal lung development and reduce the incidence of CNS bleeding and necrotizing enterocolitis. Careful control of blood pressure and judicious fluid management will minimize the risks of adverse sequelae in the mother. Maternal death from preeclampsia is most often secondary to stroke or pulmonary edema. The risk of stroke is especially high in patients with a variant of severe preeclampsia known as the HELLP syndrome, which comprises hemolysis, elevated liver enzyme levels, and low platelet counts. As with other cases of severe preeclampsia, imminent delivery is advised in cases of HELLP syndrome.

Prognosis

In general, the prognosis for women with preeclampsia is excellent. A single episode of preeclampsia does not seem to pose long-term health risks to the mother. More than one episode of preeclampsia is, however, associated with an increased risk of the development of chronic hypertension later in life. Recurrence of preeclampsia in subsequent pregnancies ranges from 15% to 65%. The earlier preeclampsia occurs in gestation, and the more severe it is, the more likely that it will recur in a subsequent pregnancy. This information may be helpful in counseling patients with respect to future pregnancy risk.

GESTATIONAL HYPERTENSION

Gestational hypertension is defined as hypertension diagnosed in the last half of pregnancy that is not chronic hypertension and is not preeclampsia. It is probably the least problematic of the three forms of hypertension seen in pregnancy. The treatment guidelines for gestational hypertension are the same as those for chronic hypertension (see above). However, gestational hypertension is usually mild; in most cases, blood pressure does not become high enough to require treatment.

Diabetes Mellitus

In the past, diabetes management in pregnancy focused on gestational diabetes. Until the advent of insulin therapy, most patients with type 1 (insulin-dependent) diabetes mellitus were infertile or did not live to reproductive age; until recently, onset of type 2 (non–insulin-dependent) diabetes mellitus most often occurred after a woman's reproductive years. Now, pregnancy is commonplace in women with type 1 diabetes, and type 2 diabetes is becoming epidemic in adolescents.[17]

TYPE 1 DIABETES

Poorly controlled type 1 diabetes is associated with increased rates of spontaneous abortion, congenital abnormalities, and other adverse pregnancy outcomes. For that reason, preconception counseling and diagnostic screening is preferred. Optimizing glycemic control and overall health before establishment of pregnancy will improve the likelihood of a normal outcome.

Preconception evaluation in patients with type 1 diabetes should include an evaluation of renal function, an ophthalmologic examination, and, depending on age and blood pressure status, a cardiac evaluation. Screening for evidence of hyperlipidemia may also be warranted, although treatment during pregnancy is not recommended.

The need for insulin shifts during pregnancy and postpartum: typically, insulin needs decrease early in pregnancy, increase later in pregnancy (to as much as three times the nonpregnant dose), then decrease markedly after delivery. Consequently, pregnancy in women with type 1 diabetes is best managed by a clinician familiar with insulin management and the complications of pregnancy that occur with increased frequency in this group of patients.

Because neural tube defects and cardiac anomalies occur more frequently in pregnancy associated with type 1 diabetes, second-trimester ultrasonography is recommended to screen for congenital anomalies. Complications developing later in pregnancy in this population include fetal growth restriction, abruptio placentae, and preeclampsia (among others). Therefore, fetal surveillance consisting of nonstress testing and ultrasound biophysical assessment of the fetus is also recommended, beginning in the third trimester.[18] In patients with well-controlled diabetes, delivery at term is permitted, provided the results of fetal testing have been reassuring, the maternal condition is stable, and fetal growth has remained normal.

TYPE 2 DIABETES

When a patient with type 2 diabetes becomes pregnant, standard practice is to treat with diet only, if possible. Patients should check their blood sugar level regularly; if fasting levels exceed 140 mg/dl, insulin therapy is indicated.

Insulin-sensitizing agents are not approved for use in pregnancy by the Food and Drug Administration. Metformin is a pregnancy category B drug; there is a growing body of evidence that metformin is safe in pregnant women, but this evidence is still preliminary, so this drug typically is discontinued if the patient becomes pregnant. The thiazolidinediones—pioglitazone and rosiglitazone—are category C drugs. Because their safety in pregnancy has not yet been confirmed, these agents also are typically discontinued in pregnancy. Because of their efficacy, however, and because the original agent in this class, troglitazone, was found to be safe in pregnancy, some endocrinologists use thiazolidinediones during pregnancy in selected cases.

ACE inhibitors are widely used in patients with type 2 diabetes to treat hypertension and maintain renal function. Because of their teratogenic effects, however, these agents are contraindicated in pregnancy [see Angiotensin Inhibitors, above]. When pregnancy is planned, withdrawal of ACE-inhibitor treatment can be arranged before conception. With unplanned pregnancy, the ACE inhibitor should be stopped as soon as pregnancy is confirmed. The patient can be reassured that the adverse effects of ACE inhibitors are seen with their use later in pregnancy.

Poorly controlled type 2 diabetes places the fetus at risk for macrosomia; consequently, the likelihood of delivery by cesarean section is increased. Birth injury and metabolic disturbances may also afflict the macrosomic newborn. Unfortunately, avoidance of macrosomia is frequently an elusive goal. Careful and regular evaluation of fetal size and growth will help minimize complications caused by macrosomia.

Prematurity is another complication of diabetes, because early delivery is sometimes necessitated by deteriorating maternal or fetal condition or superimposition of another disease process, such as severe preeclampsia. After adjusting for congenital anomalies, prematurity is the leading cause of death among infants of diabetic mothers. Maternal prognosis tends to be more favorable if pregnancy was negotiated without complication. Pregnancy in diabetic patients with renal disease may have long-term adverse effects on renal function, although the data are inconclusive. In diabetic patients with hypertension, blood pressure should be more aggressively controlled to protect renal function as much as possible.

GESTATIONAL DIABETES

In otherwise normoglycemic pregnant women, gestational diabetes is usually diagnosed in the second or early third trimester of pregnancy. The diagnosis of gestational diabetes may be a marker for increased risk of developing type 2 diabetes later in life.[19]

The diagnosis of gestational diabetes is most often made on the basis of a two-step screening procedure. There is controversy as to whether universal screening is superior to screening on the basis of risk factors, but universal screening appears to be the predominant practice at this time.[20]

Universal screening for gestational diabetes is performed at 24 to 28 weeks' gestation. In patients considered to be at very high risk or in whom glucose intolerance is suspected, screening may be carried out earlier in the pregnancy.

Screening for gestational diabetes utilizes a glucose challenge test, which consists of giving an oral 50 g glucose load and obtaining a blood glucose determination at 60 minutes. A value of less than 140 mg/dl (7.8 mmol/L) is considered normal.[19] A value exceeding 140 mg/dl warrants a 3-hour glucose tolerance test with 100 g oral glucose [see Table 4].[21,22] Two abnor-

Table 4 Normal Results for 3-Hour Glucose Tolerance Testing

Time	Normal Maximum Values
Pretest (fasting)	105 mg/dl (5.8 mmol/L)
1 hr	190 mg/dl (10.5 mmol/L)
2 hr	165 mg/dl (9.1 mmol/L)
3 hr	145 mg/dl (8.0 mmol/L)

mal values on the 3-hour glucose tolerance test constitute a diagnosis of gestational diabetes.

Treatment of gestational diabetes is with diet, if possible. Maintenance of fasting blood glucose levels below 105 mg/dl and of 2-hour postprandial levels below 120 mg/dl is ideal.[23] If fasting blood glucose levels exceed 140 mg/dl, insulin therapy is indicated.

In general, no special evaluation of other organ systems is required for diet-controlled gestational diabetic patients. Performance of these evaluations before pregnancy will allow the best opportunity for thorough follow-up and will allow for optimal counseling of the patient with respect to risks of pregnancy.

Fetal surveillance in gestational diabetic patients is somewhat less clearly defined than it is for patients with type 1 diabetes.[19] In diet-controlled gestational diabetes, fetal surveillance may not be needed, although initiation of nonstress testing at 38 weeks is commonly done. If other risk factors exist, however—such as hypertension, macrosomia, preeclampsia, or growth restriction—then fetal testing should be done. If evidence of fetal distress is detected, consideration should be given to initiating delivery.

The prognosis for patients with gestational diabetes is, in general, excellent. Because of the increased risk of developing type 2 diabetes later in life, it is particularly important for these patients to avoid obesity and maintain a regimen of regular exercise. Although postpartum follow-up testing for diabetes has been advocated, long-term studies to confirm the benefits of this approach have not been reported.[19] However, such testing may be indicated on the basis of other risk factors (e.g., obesity or ethnicity).

Thyroid Disease

Thyroid disease can be present before pregnancy, or it can manifest itself during pregnancy.[24] In either case, the disease must be distinguished from the changes in the thyroid and its function that normally occur during pregnancy.

In women who live in iodine-deficient areas, the thyroid enlarges in size during pregnancy.[25] In all pregnant women, thyroxine-binding globulin levels increase as a result of increased estrogen levels; consequently, blood levels of total triiodothyronine (T_3) and thyroxine (T_4) rise. Levels of free T_4 and thyroid-stimulating hormone (TSH) remain in the normal range, although free T_4 levels increase transiently in the first trimester and then drop to low-normal values.[25]

Hypothyroidism in pregnancy is associated with hypertension and premature labor.[26] Some children born to women whose TSH level was mildly elevated during pregnancy have been found to have lower scores on tests of neuropsychological development.[27]

The goal of treatment is to maintain TSH in the normal range, which may require a higher dose of T_4 than before pregnancy. In one study, the mean replacement dose needed to maintain TSH in the normal range rose from 100 μg before pregnancy to 150 μg during pregnancy.[28]

Hyperthyroidism occurs in 0.2% of pregnancies. Diagnosis of mild cases can be complicated by the fact that many of the physiologic changes of pregnancy mimic the milder manifestations of the disease. Mild to moderate hyperthyroidism in pregnancy generally poses little risk, but severe disease can cause spontaneous abortion or premature labor, and thyroid storm can be fatal.

Management of hyperthyroidism during pregnancy is typically most difficult in the first trimester and easiest in the third trimester. The treatment of choice is propylthiouracil, which should be given in the lowest dose possible to maintain the free T_4 level in the high-normal range. Propylthiouracil crosses the placenta, but to a lesser degree than methimazole, and is associated with a lower incidence of fetal aplasia cutis than is methimazole. Aplasia cutis is a localized failure of skin development, often occurring on the scalp. Instead of skin and hair, there is a thin, translucent membrane that can become ulcerated and covered by granulation tissue. Supplemental treatment with beta blockers and potassium iodide may be indicated in refractory cases. Use of radioactive iodine (for either scanning or treatment) is absolutely contraindicated during pregnancy because of its effects on the fetal thyroid.

Thromboembolism

Thromboembolism is the leading cause of maternal mortality in the United States.[29] The major elements of thrombosis are described by the classic triad of Virchow, which comprises stasis, local injury or trauma to the vessel wall, and hypercoagulability. Both hypercoagulability and a tendency toward stasis (especially in late pregnancy, as the expanding uterus compromises venous return from the lower extremities) are part of the normal physiologic changes of pregnancy. The risk of thromboembolism is further increased in patients who have an underlying predisposition to development of a thromboembolic event [see Chapter 94]. The most commonly identified inherited predisposition to thromboembolism is resistance to activated protein C, or the so-called factor V Leiden mutation.[30] Far less commonly implicated are disorders of protein C, protein S, antithrombin III, and plasminogen; the prothrombin gene (G20210A) mutation is also implicated. Antiphospholipid antibody syndrome and methylenetetrahydrofolate reductase (C677T) deficiency have also been associated with increased risk of thromboembolism. Dislodgement of a thrombus resulting in thromboembolism (usually pulmonary) often produces no symptoms. Symptomatic thromboembolism is a medical emergency.

DIAGNOSIS

The most common symptom of pulmonary thromboembolism is dyspnea. However, dyspnea is common in normal pregnancy, because as the uterus grows, it forces the diaphragm higher into the chest cavity, reducing the residual volume of the lungs and resulting in an increased respiratory rate. Therefore, careful clinical assessment is essential. The laboratory and radiologic evaluation for pulmonary embolism in pregnancy is essentially identical to that of the nonpregnant patient [see Chapter 29]. The standard tests in pregnancy are screening for deep vein thrombosis with Doppler ultrasound

of the lower extremities and follow-up spiral chest CT if the screening test is positive or if there is a high clinical suspicion of pulmonary embolism (the CT beams are sufficiently focused that shielding of the uterus is unnecessary, although shielding does no harm).

TREATMENT

The management of thromboembolism in the pregnant patient is essentially the same as that in the nonpregnant patient. Aggressive treatment is essential. In general, treatment with either unfractionated or low-molecular-weight heparin is acceptable. A number of administration protocols are available for either approach.[31] Warfarin is generally avoided, because it is teratogenic in the first trimester and can interfere with fetal and neonatal coagulation, owing to the fact that it freely crosses the placenta. Therapy is continued for the duration of pregnancy, with conversion to warfarin in the postpartum period; warfarin is not contraindicated in breast-feeding women. Cessation of heparin just before delivery is preferred, if scheduled delivery is possible.

COMPLICATIONS AND PROGNOSIS

Vascular insufficiency and death are the major complications of thromboembolic disease. Cardiovascular collapse from pulmonary embolism is the most common cause of death. Recurrent thromboembolism requiring surgical intervention with filter placement in the inferior vena cava is also a complication, especially for younger women, in whom the long-term consequences of filter placement may be less understood.

Thorough evaluation for underlying disorders (genetic or acquired) is essential to better assess long-term prognosis. However, if such evaluations are negative and the clot resolves completely, the prognosis is excellent. Support of the pregnancy through the critical phase of thromboembolism is essential, and premature delivery may be required because of maternal instability or a deteriorating fetal status secondary to poor maternal oxygenation.

Valvular Heart Disease

Valvular heart disease is the most common cardiac problem complicating pregnancy. Preconception counseling and management is based on whether the valvular heart disease is congenital or acquired. Congenital cardiac disease in the mother, with the exception of a few known mendelian disorders that affect the heart, is thought to be genetically multifactorial. Therefore, there is an increased risk of the fetus being affected (2% to 5%); genetic counseling and screening for such patients is appropriate. Fetal echocardiography is an effective tool and will usually identify major cardiac anomalies prenatally, allowing appropriate delivery preparations to be arranged.

Acquired heart disease can pose specific risks for the mother with respect to her ability to tolerate a pregnancy. One study showed a marked increase in maternal morbidity—including congestive heart failure and arrhythmias—but only rare mortality; higher morbidity and unfavorable fetal outcome were seen mostly in patients with moderate or severe mitral or aortic stenosis.[32]

MITRAL STENOSIS

Mitral stenosis is the valvular lesion most likely to result in maternal decompensation and death during pregnancy. Long-standing mitral stenosis may lead to pulmonary hypertension, which may cause sudden death, especially if pregnancy is complicated by sudden hypovolemia, as might occur with intrapartum or postpartum hemorrhage. Persistent tachycardia, which may develop in patients with severe mitral stenosis, can lead to inadequate ventricular filling times and consequent rate-related congestive heart failure.

In severe cases of mitral stenosis, balloon valvulotomy may be accomplished during pregnancy. Otherwise, management focuses on labor and delivery.

If pulmonary hypertension has been identified, labor and delivery is best carried out in a setting in which intensive care services and pulmonary artery catheterization are available. In general, vaginal delivery is less hemodynamically stressful than cesarean section. During labor, careful attention must be paid to management of pain and fluid volume to minimize fluctuations in blood pressure and heart rate.

MITRAL REGURGITATION AND AORTIC REGURGITATION

The decreased systemic vascular resistance that occurs in normal pregnancy tends to minimize the effects of mitral and aortic regurgitation, so these lesions are generally well tolerated during pregnancy. Mitral valve prolapse, unless severe or accompanied by other disturbances of cardiac rhythm, is generally well tolerated during pregnancy.

AORTIC STENOSIS

In general, aortic stenosis is well tolerated during pregnancy. Moderate to severe cases may be managed with limitation of activity. As with mitral stenosis, balloon valvuloplasty may be accomplished during pregnancy, if necessary.

ARTIFICIAL HEART VALVES

Women with mechanical heart valves are advised to avoid pregnancy, but management of pregnancy in these patients is certainly possible. Attention to coagulation status and cardiac function is essential. Although warfarin is the usual anticoagulant of choice for patients with mechanical heart valves, its use during pregnancy is probably not justified, because of the risks it poses to the fetus.[31,33,34] Heparin anticoagulation is generally preferred, with brief discontinuance during labor and delivery, rapid reinstitution postpartum, and conversion back to warfarin as soon as possible. Anticoagulation aside, pregnancy in women with cadaveric or porcine replacement valves who have normal cardiac function and are otherwise in good health may be managed according to routine obstetric protocol.

Cardiomyopathy

In rare cases, idiopathic dilated cardiomyopathy may develop late in pregnancy or in the early postpartum months [see

---

Chapter 26]. Patients present with dyspnea and other manifestations of heart failure. Treatment for this condition is largely the same as that for heart failure. Outcomes range from spontaneous resolution to death; heart transplant may be lifesaving in severe cases.

Infections

BACTERIAL INFECTIONS

Urinary Tract Infection

After bacterial vaginosis, urinary tract infections are the most common bacterial infections in pregnant women. Screening for asymptomatic bacteriuria should be done at the initial prenatal visit in all pregnant women. Asymptomatic bacteriuria is more common during pregnancy; if left untreated, it may progress to symptomatic urinary tract infection. It is estimated that 75% of cases of pyelonephritis in pregnancy are the result of untreated asymptomatic bacteriuria. Pyelonephritis in pregnancy is associated with an increased risk of preterm delivery.

Group B Streptococcus

Carriage of group B Streptococcus (GBS) at the time of vaginal delivery places the newborn at increased risk for developing acute GBS disease. To minimize this potentially devastating outcome, intrapartum treatment is given to patients at high risk for GBS [see Table 5]. All other women are screened at 35 to 37 weeks' gestation and treated if GBS is found. Penicillin G is the drug of choice for maternal intrapartum treatment. Ampicillin may also be used. Clindamycin is recommended in penicillin-allergic patients.[35]

VIRAL INFECTIONS

HIV

One of the success stories of the past decade has been the ability to reduce vertical transmission of HIV from 25% to less than 1%. These results have been accomplished by increasing our understanding about viral load; utilizing antiviral therapies, particularly intrapartum zidovudine (AZT); and more liberally utilizing cesarean section before the onset of labor.[36] All women should be offered HIV screening as part of prenatal care; in many states, such screening is required. Management of these cases in consultation with an infectious disease specialist will further optimize outcome. There is no evidence that pregnancy significantly alters the course of HIV disease, nor is there evidence that well-managed HIV disease significantly alters the course of pregnancy. Breast-feeding is not recommended in HIV-positive women.

Cytomegalovirus

Cytomegalovirus (CMV) is the most common cause of congenital viral infection in the United States.[37] Approximately 50% to 90% of women of childbearing age will already have developed antibodies to CMV; reactivation of infection is fortunately a very rare cause of congenital infection. Most cases of congenital CMV are secondary to primary maternal infection during pregnancy. There is no established effective therapy for fetal CMV, and it is not currently possible to predict which exposed fetuses will sustain significant sequelae from in utero infection.

Although screening for antibodies to CMV is not recommended as part of routine prenatal care, primary CMV infec-

---

Table 5 Obstetric Risk Factors for Early-Onset Neonatal Group B Streptococcus (GBS) Infection

GBS bacteriuria during pregnancy
Previous delivery of infant with GBS infection
Gestational age < 37 weeks at time of labor onset
Membrane rupture > 18 hours
Intrapartum temperature ≥ 38° C (100.4° F)

tion should be suspected in pregnant patients who develop a mononucleosis-like syndrome with high fever, fatigue, malaise, myalgias, headache, and splenomegaly. The diagnosis of CMV should be aggressively pursued in such cases, to permit appropriate counseling and presentation of options for further diagnosis and management.[38]

Herpes Simplex Virus

Herpes simplex virus (HSV) may be acquired before or during pregnancy. Recurrent genital herpes infection poses risks to the newborn. To prevent transmission of HSV during the birth process, cesarean section is recommended if there is evidence of active disease or if there is a strong suggestion of a preactivation prodrome, either at the time of presentation in labor or near the expected date of delivery. Use of acyclovir during the last 4 weeks of gestation in women who developed their primary infection during pregnancy may reduce the risk of clinical recurrence, but whether this practice confers protection of the neonate has not been established.[39] Disseminated neonatal herpes infection is often fatal, and many survivors have serious neurologic sequelae.

Parvovirus

Infection during pregnancy with human parvovirus B19 rarely results in fetal hydrops secondary to cardiac failure from the profound anemia that develops from fetal erythroid aplasia. Determination of maternal immune status may be indicated if the patient has been exposed to a child with erythema infectiosum (fifth disease), which is caused by parvovirus B19. Close fetal surveillance with ultrasound may be warranted if the pregnancy is in the second or third trimester. Occasionally, intervention and intrauterine transfusion are required. Fortunately, most cases do not require this level of intervention.

PARASITIC INFECTION

Toxoplasmosis

In the United States, nearly 70% of women of childbearing age are susceptible to infection with toxoplasmosis.[40] Unfortunately, acute toxoplasmosis in immunocompetent persons is difficult to detect because most cases are asymptomatic. In symptomatic patients, the most common manifestation is cervical lymphadenopathy; a minority of symptomatic patients have generalized lymphadenopathy, sometimes accompanied by a flulike syndrome.

Most cases of primary toxoplasmosis are contracted through the ingestion of undercooked meat, but contact with contaminated feces, particularly cat feces, has also been identified as a source of infection. Congenital toxoplasmosis may be diagnosed via amniocentesis or cordocentesis, though the latter test is definitive. If pregnancy termination is not possible or is not desired, intravascular fetal treatment (provided by a specialist in obstetric infection or infectious disease) may reduce the risk of severe neonatal infection. Routine prenatal screening is not recommended.[37]

Asthma

Asthma may improve, worsen, or remain stable during pregnancy. Well-controlled asthma appears to have no adverse effects on pregnancy outcome, but poorly controlled asthma is associated with a variety of adverse effects on both mother and fetus.[41] The goal of therapy is prevention of hypoxia. In general, pregnant patients are candidates for the same therapy as nonpregnant patients [see Chapter 212]. Beta agonists, theophylline derivatives, glucocorticoids, and cromolyn may all be used as needed. There are insufficient data on the safety and efficacy of leukotriene antagonists to support their use during pregnancy.

Management should include patient education and utilization of at-home peak expiratory flow rate monitoring. Because asthma has implications for both mother and fetus, more liberal use of in-hospital evaluation and management may be warranted.

Alcohol and Tobacco Use

It has been estimated that 15% of cases of low birth weight may be attributed to cigarette smoking.[42] Adverse antepartum effects of smoking include uteroplacental insufficiency and preterm delivery. Although it is unclear whether smoking increases the risk of preterm labor, prematurity is increased secondary to increases in placenta previa, abruptio placentae, and preterm premature rupture of membranes. Smoking has also been associated with intrauterine fetal demise[43] and increased risks of placenta previa, abruptio placentae, impaired cognitive development, and sudden infant death syndrome. Smoking cessation during pregnancy is possible and should be encouraged. Nicotine replacement therapy is commonly prescribed as an aid to smoking cessation in pregnant women.[44] Large-scale trials of the safety and efficacy of nicotine replacement therapy in pregnancy have not been done; nicotine is a category D drug, but of course smoking delivers not only nicotine but a variety of other documented reproductive toxins as well.[45] Adjunctive use of bupropion for smoking cessation during pregnancy has not been well studied, but safety studies of bupropion use in pregnancy have shown no risk in humans (category B).

Alcohol is a known teratogen. Despite this fact and the determination that there is no safe lower limit of alcohol consumption during pregnancy, drinking in pregnant women increased between 1991 and 1995 in the United States.[46,47] Data on the effects of alcohol use during pregnancy have been inconsistent with respect to specific risks, such as spontaneous miscarriage, and neurobehavioral disorders, such as attention deficit disorder. More conclusive is the association of maternal alcohol use with the development of fetal alcohol syndrome (FAS). Manifestations of FAS include growth deficiency (intrauterine and postnatal), low intelligence, fine-motor dysfunction, and a range of craniofacial, skeletal, cardiac, and other abnormalities. There is evidence that the risk of fetal alcohol syndrome increases as alcohol consumption increases. Mild to moderate alcohol use may not result in the complete syndrome but may result in infants being born with varying degrees of affliction, or so-called fetal alcohol effects. The effects of alcohol use limited to the first trimester are less well characterized.[48]

References

1. National High Blood Pressure Education Program Working Group on High Blood Pressure in Pregnancy. Am J Obstet Gynecol 163:1691, 1990

2. The sixth report of the Joint National Committee on prevention, detection, evaluation and treatment of high blood pressure. Arch Intern Med 157:2413, 1997

3. Sibai BM, Mabie WC, Shamsa F, et al: A comparison of no medication versus methyldopa or labetalol in chronic hypertension during pregnancy. Am J Obstet Gynecol 162:960, 1990

4. Sibai BM: Treatment of hypertension in pregnant women. N Engl J Med 335:257, 1996

5. Report of the National High Blood Pressure Education Program Working Group on High Blood Pressure in Pregnancy. Am J Obstet Gynecol 183:S1, 2000

6. ACOG Practice Bulletin. Chronic hypertension in pregnancy. ACOG Committee on Practice Bulletins. Obstet Gynecol 98:S177, 2001

7. Magee LA, Elran E, Bull SB, et al: Risks and benefits of beta-receptor blockers for pregnancy hypertension: an overview of randomized trials. Eur J Obstet Gynecol Reprod Biol 88:15, 2000

8. Briggs GG, Freeman RK, Yaffe SJ: Drugs in Pregnancy and Lactation: A Reference Guide to Fetal and Neonatal Risk, 5th ed. Williams & Wilkins, Baltimore, 1998

9. Postmarketing surveillance for angiotensin-converting enzyme inhibitor use during the first trimester of pregnancy—United States, Canada, and Israel, 1987–1995. MMWR Morb Mortal Wkly Rep 46:240, 1997

10. Ananth CV, Smulian JC, Vintzileos AM: Incidence of placental abruption in relation to cigarette smoking and hypertensive disorders during pregnancy: a meta-analysis of observational studies. Obstet Gynecol 93:622, 1999

11. Management of chronic hypertension during pregnancy. Agency for Health Care Research and Quality. Evidence Report/Technology Assessment No.14. AHRQ Publication No.00-E011. Rockville, Maryland, 2000

12. Walker JJ: Pre-eclampsia. Lancet 356:1260, 2000

13. Morgan T, Craven C, Lalouel JM, et al: Angiotensinogen Thr235 variant is associated with abnormal physiologic change of the uterine spiral arteries in first trimester deciduas. Am J Obstet Gynecol 180:95, 1999

14. Madazli R, Budak E, Calay Z, et al: Correlation between placental bed biopsy findings, vascular cell adhesion molecule and fibronectin levels in pre-eclampsia. Br J Obstet Gynaecol 107:514, 2000

15. Sibai BM, Mercer BM, Schiff E, et al: Aggressive versus expectant management of severe preeclampsia at 28–32 weeks gestation: a randomized controlled trial. Am J Obstet Gynecol 171:818, 1994

16. Do women with pre-eclampsia, and their babies, benefit from magnesium sulphate? The Magpie Trial: a randomized placebo-controlled trial. The Magpie Trial Collaboration Group. Lancet 359:1877, 2002

17. Rosenbloom AL, Joe JR, Young RS, et al: Emerging epidemic of type 2 diabetes in youth. Diabetes Care 22:345, 1999

18. Antepartum Fetal Surveillance. ACOG Practice Bulletin 9:1, 1999
http://www.acog.com/publications/educational_bulletins/pb009.htm

19. ACOG Practice Bulletin. Clinical management guidelines for obstetrician-gynecologists. Number 30, September 2001. Gestational diabetes. Obstet Gynecol 98:525, 2001

20. Weeks JW, Major CA, deVeciana M, et al: Gestational diabetes: does the presence of risk factors influence perinatal outcome? Am J Obstet Gynecol 171:1003, 1994

21. Classification and diagnosis of diabetes mellitus and other categories of glucose intolerance. National Diabetes Data Group. Diabetes 28:1039, 1979

22. Report of the Expert Committee on the Diagnosis and Classification of Diabetes Mellitus. Diabetes Care 23:S4, 2000

23. Huddleston JF, Cramer MK, Vroon DH: A rationale for omitting two hour postprandial glucose determinations in gestational diabetes. Am J Obstet Gynecol 169:257, 1993

24. ACOG Practice Bulletin. Clinical management guidelines for obstetrician-gynecologists. Number 37, August 2002. Thyroid disease in pregnancy. Obstet Gynecol 100:387, 2002

25. Berghout A, Wiersinga W: Thyroid size and thyroid function during pregnancy: an analysis. Eur J Endocrinol 138:536, 1998

26. Bishnoi A, Sachmechi I: Thyroid disease during pregnancy. Am Fam Physician 53:215, 1996

27. Haddow JE, Palomaki GE, Allen WC, et al: Maternal thyroid deficiency during pregnancy and subsequent neuropsychological development of the child. N Engl J Med 341:549, 1999

28. Mandel SJ, Larsen PR, Seely EW, et al: Increased need for thyroxine during pregnancy in women with primary hypothyroidism. N Engl J Med 323:91, 1990

29. Berg CJ, Atrash HK, Koonin LM, et al: Pregnancy related mortality in the United States, 1987–1990. Obstet Gynecol 88:161, 1996

30. Grandone E, Margaglione M, Colaizzo D, et al: Genetic susceptibility to pregnancy related venous thromboembolism: roles of factor V Leiden, prothrombin G20210A, and methylenetetrahydrofolate reductase C677T mutations. Am J Obstet Gynecol 179:1324, 1998

31. Thromboembolism in Pregnancy. ACOG Practice Bulletin 19:1, 2000
http://www.acog.com/publications/educational_bulletins/pb019.htm

32. Hameed A, Karaalp IS, Tummula PP, et al: The effect of valvular heart disease on maternal and fetal outcome of pregnancy. J Am Coll Cardiol 37:893, 2001

33. Chan WS, Anand S, Ginsberg JS: Anticoagulation of pregnant women with mechanical heart valves. Arch Intern Med 160:191, 2000

34. Salazar E, Izaguirre R, Verdejo J, et al: Failure of adjusted doses of subcutaneous heparin to prevent thromboembolic phenomena in pregnant patients with mechanical cardiac valve prostheses. J Am Coll Cardiol 27:1698, 1996

35. ACOG committee opinion. Prevention of early-onset group B streptococcal disease in newborns. Number 173—June 1996. Committee on Obstetric Practice. American College of Obstetrics and Gynecologists. Int J Gynaecol Obstet 54:197, 1996

36. The mode of delivery and the risk of vertical transmission of human immunodeficiency virus type I: a meta-analysis of 15 prospective cohort studies. The International Perinatal HIV Group. N Engl J Med 340:977, 1999

37. ACOG practice bulletin. Perinatal viral and parasitic infections. Number 20, September 2000. American College of Obstetrics and Gynecologists. Int J Gynaecol Obstet 76:95, 2002

38. Grangeot-Keros L, Simon B, Audibert F, et al: Should we routinely screen for cytomegalovirus antibody during pregnancy? Intervirology 41:158, 1998

39. Brockelhurst P, Kinghorn G, Carney O, et al: A randomized placebo controlled trial of suppressive acyclovir in late pregnancy in women with recurrent genital herpes infection. Br J Obstet Gynecol 105:275, 1998

40. Sever JL, Ellenberg JH, Ley AC, et al: Toxoplasmosis: maternal and pediatric findings in 23,000 pregnancies. Pediatrics 82:181, 1988

41. Schatz M: Interrelationships between asthma and pregnancy: a literature review. J Allergy Clin Immunol 103(2 pt 2):S330, 1999

42. Lindsay CA, Thomas AJ, Catalano PM: The effect of smoking tobacco on neonatal body composition. Am J Obstet Gynecol 177:1124, 1997

43. Schellscheidt J, Jorch G, Menke J: Effects of heavy maternal smoking on intrauterine growth patterns in sudden infant death victims and surviving infants. Eur J Pediatr 157:246, 1998

44. Oncken CA, Pbert L, Ockene JK, et al: Nicotine replacement prescription practices of obstetric and pediatric clinicians. Obstet Gynecol 96:261, 2000

45. Dempsey DA, Benowitz NL: Risks and benefits of nicotine to aid smoking cessation in pregnancy. Drug Saf 24:277, 2001

46. Update: trends in fetal alcohol syndrome—United States, 1979–1993. MMWR Morb Mortal Wkly Rep 44:249, 1995

47. Alcohol and other drug-related birth defects awareness week—May 11–17, 1997. MMWR Morb Mortal Wkly Rep 46:345, 1997

48. Polygenis D, Wharton S, Malmberg C, et al: Moderate alcohol consumption during pregnancy and the incidence of fetal malformation: a meta-analysis. Neurotoxicol Teratol 20:61, 1998

49. ACOG educational bulletin. Teratology. Number 236, April 1997. American College of Obstetricians and Gynecologists. Int J Gynaecol Obstet 57:319, 1997

84 Endometriosis

Robert L. Barbieri, M.D.

Definition and Pathophysiology

Endometriosis is a condition in which tissue resembling endometrial glands or stroma occurs outside the uterus. Endometriosis lesions are most often found in the pelvis. Common sites are the peritoneal surfaces posterior to the uterus; the ovary; the peritoneal surfaces anterior to the uterus; the bowel; the bladder; and the appendix. Rarely, endometriosis lesions occur at sites outside the pelvis, such as the respiratory diaphragm.

Endometriosis lesions are heterogeneous, ranging from 1 mm superficial peritoneal lesions to 4 cm deeply invasive lesions in the rectovaginal septum. Ovarian lesions of endometriosis can grow to 4 to 10 cm in size, necessitating surgical resection. Endometriosis lesions undergo cycles of growth and bleeding in tandem with the menstrual cycle. Intraperitoneal bleeding from the lesions elicits an inflammatory response in the pelvis that is associated with pain and infertility.

Epidemiology

Many authorities believe that approximately 5% of women between 15 and 45 years of age have endometriosis.[1] The precise incidence is difficult to determine because there is no inexpensive, highly reliable method for diagnosing endometriosis. The current gold standard for the diagnosis of endometriosis is surgical visualization of endometriosis lesions, usually by laparoscopy, and so (as with any disease that requires expensive and invasive procedures for diagnosis) a significant number of cases may be missed.[2] Collection of definitive data would require selecting a random sample of women and performing laparoscopy on them to determine whether they have endometriosis; understandably, no such study has been done.

Endometriosis is rare before menarche and after menopause, when estrogen production is low. Most cases of endometriosis are diagnosed in women in their 20s who have never had a child. Full-term pregnancy and delivery appear to markedly reduce the risk of developing endometriosis. Multiple full-term pregnancies further reduce the risk. Long periods of amenorrhea (for example, the amenorrhea of athletes) is associated with a reduced risk of endometriosis, as is aerobic exercise for more than 7 hours a week.

Pathogenesis

The pathogenesis of endometriosis lesions involves mechanical, hormonal, immunologic, and genetic factors. The prominence of particular factors may vary from case to case; indeed, it is possible that endometriosis comprises several different diseases with a common clinical outcome.

MECHANICAL FACTORS

In women with a normal uterus, 99.9% of menstrual blood flow occurs in an antegrade direction—that is, from the endometrium through the cervix and into the vagina. Numerous clinical observations as well as experiments in laboratory animals indicate that anatomic changes, such as cervical stenosis, that hinder antegrade flow are associated with an increased risk of endometriosis. In women with cervical stenosis, the relative obstruction at the level of the cervix causes blood to flow from the uterus back through the fallopian tubes and into the peritoneal cavity. This retrograde menstrual flow contains blood, growth factors, and viable bits of endometrial tissue. The greater the amount of retrograde blood flow, the higher the risk of endometriosis. For example, about 80% of women with congenital cervical stenosis and a functioning endometrium will develop endometriosis. Epidemiologic studies suggest that more prolonged menstrual flow (> 8 days) and more frequent menses (cycle length < 27 days) are also associated with an increased risk of endometriosis.[3]

HORMONAL FACTORS

Steroid hormones control the growth and function of endometriosis lesions. Estradiol stimulates growth, and androgens cause atrophy of endometriosis lesions [see Table 1]. High doses of progestins induce terminal differentiation in endometriosis lesions, a process called pseudodecidualization. Once endometriosis tissue undergoes pseudodecidualization, it can no longer grow. The reason pregnancy reduces the risk of endometriosis is probably that the extremely high progesterone levels that occur in pregnancy cause pseudodecidualization of endometriosis lesions.

Organochlorine chemicals (e.g., dioxin) can disrupt steroid metabolism; exposure to these pollutants has been proposed as a factor in the development of endometriosis. In animal models, dioxin has been found to increase the incidence and severity of endometriosis,[4] possibly by interfering with the action of progesterone,[5] but the effect in humans has yet to be confirmed.

Table 1 Effects of Different Steroids on Endometrium and Endometriosis Lesions

Steroid	Effect on Endometrium	Effect on Endometriosis Lesions
Estrogen	Growth	Growth
Androgen	Atrophy	Atrophy
Progesterone at physiologic concentrations	Differentiation and secretory changes	No effect on lesions that have no progesterone receptors; differentiation and secretory changes in lesions with progesterone receptors
Progesterone at high concentrations	Decidualization	Pseudodecidualization (a terminal differentiation step)

IMMUNOLOGIC FACTORS

Numerous studies indicate that in women with endometriosis, the pelvic peritoneal environment is immunologically abnormal, with increased concentrations of white blood cells, cytokines, and growth factors. Indeed, elevated levels of cytokines—specifically, tumor necrosis factor–α in peritoneal fluid and interleukin-6 in serum—have been proposed as a potential diagnostic marker for endometriosis.[6] One group of researchers has found an increased incidence of autoimmune disease in women with endometriosis—a finding that supports the concept that immunologic abnormalities play a role in the development of endometriosis.[7]

Some authorities believe that in women with endometriosis, a primary immunologic abnormality prevents the clearance, from the peritoneal environment, of the endometrial tissue fragments deposited by retrograde menstruation.[8] This postulated primary alteration in the immune response allegedly contributes to the development of endometriosis. Other authorities believe that the observed peritoneal immunologic changes are not a cause of endometriosis but a consequence of it: the endometriosis lesions produce a chronic pelvic inflammation, which leads to an increase of immune cells in the peritoneal fluid. Interestingly, factors secreted by these immune cells appear to promote angiogenesis and cause endometriosis lesions to grow. It is likely that there is cross-talk between the immune system and endometriosis lesions: endometriosis lesions cause inflammation, inducing immune cells to enter the peritoneal environment; in turn, immune cells secrete factors that can stimulate the growth of endometriosis lesions.

GENETIC ABNORMALITIES

The risk of endometriosis is approximately doubled in first-degree relatives of women with endometriosis.[9] The heritable aspects of endometriosis may involve alterations in the immune response that predispose women to ectopic transplantation and survival of endometrial tissue.

Ovarian endometriosis cysts (endometriomas) are monoclonal and appear to arise from a somatic mutation in a precursor cell, although those mutations have not been characterized.[10] This finding suggests that a small number of genes play a central role in the pathogenesis of endometriosis.

ENDOMETRIOSIS AND INFERTILITY

An association between endometriosis and infertility in women has long been noted,[11] and many possible mechanisms for the infertility have been identified. Nevertheless, the hypothesis that endometriosis decreases fertility has not been definitively proved by consistent data from rigorous studies.

In advanced endometriosis, infertility can have an anatomic cause: adhesions interfere with the release of the ovum from the ovary and its uptake into the fallopian tube. Although women with early-stage endometriosis often have reduced fertility, a causal link between the endometriosis and the infertility is not clear.

Abnormalities in peritoneal, tubal, and endometrial function caused by endometriosis may inhibit fertility, especially in women with early-stage disease.[11] Numerous investigators have reported peritoneal abnormalities in women with endometriosis, including an increased volume of peritoneal fluid[12] and increased concentrations of activated macrophages,[13] prostaglandin, interleukin-1, tumor necrosis factor, and proteases.[14] Peri-

toneal fluid from women with advanced endometriosis appears to inhibit sperm function, thereby possibly reducing fertility.[15]

A few investigators have reported that women with endometriosis may have increased levels of antiendometrial antibodies, which may impair endometrial function.[16,17] Some women with early-stage endometriosis have luteal phase dysfunction,[18] abnormal follicle growth,[19] multiple premature luteinizing hormone surges,[20] and luteinized unruptured follicle syndrome.

Intrauterine endometrium may be abnormal in women with endometriosis, which suggests the possibility of a so-called field defect in the müllerian tract. Significant suppression of β_3 integrin has been reported in the endometrium of women with early-stage endometriosis.[21] This decrease in β_3 integrin expression may be associated with an impaired interaction of the embryo with the endometrium. In addition, elevated levels of the müllerian antigen CA-125 have been found on endometrial biopsies taken during the luteal phase of the menstrual cycle from women with advanced endometriosis[22] and in the menstrual discharge of women with endometriosis.[23]

Diagnosis

Although endometriosis is a common disorder, it remains remarkably difficult to diagnose. In one cohort study, women with endometriosis reported that, on average, 4 years elapsed between their first presentation with symptoms caused by endometriosis and their diagnosis.

CLINICAL PRESENTATION

Women with endometriosis typically present because of chronic pelvic pain or infertility. Other possible symptoms include secondary dysmenorrhea, dyspareunia, pain with bowel movements (dyschezia), and pelvic pain not associated with menses. The rare cases of diaphragmatic endometriosis have been associated with chest pain at the onset of menstruation.[24]

PHYSICAL EXAMINATION

In most women with endometriosis, the physical examination is normal. However, certain findings on physical examination suggest the presence of endometriosis. These include tender, thickened, or nodular uterosacral ligaments and fixed adnexal masses. A retroverted, fixed uterus suggests involvement of the cul-de-sac with endometriosis.

The uterosacral ligaments connect the base of the uterus to the sacrum. Nodularity of the ligaments is evident on bimanual pelvic examination as pea-sized nodules palpable at 4 o'clock and 8 o'clock at the base of the cervix. These nodules most often are implants of endometriosis.

Two less common physical findings in endometriosis are cervical stenosis[25] and lateral displacement of the cervix. Lateral displacement of the cervix occurs when one uterosacral ligament becomes severely involved with endometriosis, shortens as a result of scarring, and pulls the cervix to the side.[26]

NONINVASIVE LABORATORY TESTS

A complete blood count, urinalysis, and endocervical cultures for gonococci and *Chlamydia* should be performed to rule out infectious causes of pelvic pain in women. Results of all these tests will be normal in women with endometriosis. In most women with endometriosis, the pelvic sonogram is normal, but other conditions, such as uterine leiomyomas, will be evident on sonography. Although many conditions can cause adnexal masses, including dermoids (mature teratomas), serous and mucinous cysts, and hemorrhagic corpora lutea, endometriomas have classic characteristics on ultrasound, which aids in their diagnosis.

SURGICAL STAGING

The current gold standard for the diagnosis of endometriosis is the surgical visualization of lesions, usually by laparoscopy. The normal peritoneal surface is smooth and glistening, like the inner surface of the oral mucosa. Classic endometriosis lesions are often black, purple, or red and measure 1 to 5 mm in diameter; they stud the surface of the peritoneum. Atypical endometriosis lesions are often translucent or yellow, and they may take the form of either flat plaques or vesicles.

Unfortunately, surgeons vary considerably in their ability to detect endometriosis lesions reliably. One study reported pathologic confirmation rates of visually diagnosed endometriosis at 42%, 65%, and 76% for three different surgeons.[27]

Endometriosis is staged surgically using the American Society of Reproductive Medicine staging system. This system divides the disease into four stages: stage I, minimal; stage II, mild; stage III, moderate; and stage IV, severe. As with detection, however, staging is not always performed consistently. Studies of intersurgeon and intrasurgeon variability in the staging of endometriosis report low reproducibility and a kappa coefficient in the range of 0.28.[28]

HISTOLOGIC DIAGNOSIS

Biopsy and histologic analysis of lesions found on laparoscopy may enable more reliable diagnosis of endometriosis than does visual inspection alone. The criteria for histologic diagnosis of endometriosis include the presence of one of the following components: (1) both endometrial glands and stroma; (2) glandular epithelium with hemosiderin; or (3) endometrial stroma–like tissue with hemosiderin. One weakness of histologic diagnosis for endometriosis is that diagnostic criteria vary among pathologists.[29,30] Furthermore, no study has demonstrated high interobserver reproducibility in the histologic diagnosis of endometriosis.

CLINICAL DIAGNOSIS

An innovative approach to the diagnosis of endometriosis is to use a combination of history, physical examination, and noninvasive laboratory testing.[31] This approach is called clinical diagnosis.

DIFFERENTIAL DIAGNOSIS

Pelvic Pain

Chronic pelvic pain, defined as the presence of pain below the umbilicus for more than 6 months, is a common gynecologic problem. In one study of primary care practices that included 284,162 women 12 to 70 years of age, the reported prevalence of chronic pelvic pain was 3.8%.[32] Along with endometriosis, other common gynecologic causes of chronic pelvic pain include chronic pelvic inflammatory disease, adenomyosis, and uterine leiomyomata. Nongynecologic diseases such as irritable bowel syndrome and fibromyalgia, as well as psychiatric diseases such as somatization, may also contribute to chronic pelvic pain. In populations in which the prevalence of sexually transmitted diseases is low, endometriosis is the most common cause of chronic pelvic pain. In three large studies, 70% to 80% of women with chronic pelvic pain had endometriosis as the cause.[31,33,34]

Infertility

Endometriosis is considered to be responsible for 8% of all cases of infertility. The most common causes of infertility, accounting for about 75% of cases, are ovulatory disorders, tubal disease, and semen abnormalities. Miscellaneous factors, such as cervical or immunologic abnormalities and uterine synechiae, cause 2% of cases; 15% are unexplained.[35-37]

Treatment of Pelvic Pain

Interventions that reduce estradiol production are the most reliable way to cause atrophy of endometriosis lesions and are the most effective in treating pain symptoms. A variety of hormonal and surgical interventions are available for this purpose. Most authorities recommend a stepwise approach to the use of these interventions [see Table 2].

Table 2 Stepwise Treatment of Pelvic Pain

Step	Description	Recommendation
1	Thorough history and physical examination	Detailed history and physical examination forms for evaluating pelvic pain are available on the Internet at www.pelvicpain.org
2	Noninvasive laboratory testing	Pelvic ultrasound, complete blood count, urinalysis, endocervical cultures for gonococci and *Chlamydia*
3	Empirical therapy	Oral contraceptive plus nonsteroidal anti-inflammatory medication
4	Surgical diagnostic procedure	Laparoscopy to determine the cause of pain if empirical therapy does not result in sufficient relief of pain
5	GnRH agonist therapy	For regimens, see Table 3
6	GnRH agonist therapy plus steroid add-back	Consider for reduction of GnRH agonist side effects; for regimens, see Table 4
7	Progestin-only treatment	If GnRH agonists cannot be tolerated because of side effects; for regimens, see Table 5

GnRH—gonadotropin-releasing hormone

HORMONAL TREATMENT FOR RELIEF OF PAIN

Randomized clinical trials have demonstrated that combination estrogen-progestin oral contraceptives, gonadotropin-releasing hormone (GnRH) agonist analogues, danazol, and progestins are all effective in relieving pelvic pain caused by endometriosis. GnRH agonist analogues are the most effective; combination estrogen-progestin oral contraceptives are the least expensive.

Combination Estrogen-Progestin Oral Contraceptives

Oral contraceptives are sometimes effective in the treatment of pelvic pain caused by endometriosis because progestins can block the growth of endometrium and endometriosis lesions. Although estrogen stimulates the growth of endometriosis lesions, modern oral contraceptives are progestin dominant and contain low doses of estrogen.

In the United States, almost all women with chronic pelvic pain are initially treated empirically with a combination of cyclic oral contraceptives and nonsteroidal anti-inflammatory drugs (NSAIDS), such as ibuprofen. In contrast, in some European countries, the standard practice is to perform laparoscopy on women with chronic pelvic pain to determine the cause of the pain before starting hormonal treatment. In one randomized study, women with endometriosis who had not previously undergone hormonal treatment were randomized to receive treatment with either low-dose cyclic oral contraceptives or a GnRH agonist analogue. Both groups experienced significant improvement in pelvic pain and dysmenorrhea. However, the group treated with GnRH agonists had better relief of dyspareunia.[38]

Oral contraceptives can be used in monthly cycles or long-cycle regimens. If a regimen of oral contraceptives taken in monthly cycles does not relieve the pain, many physicians will try a regimen of long-cycle oral contraceptives. In long-cycle regimens, the active pills are taken for 42 to 105 days in a row; no pills are taken for a period of 1 week between cycles.

If oral contraceptives and NSAIDs fail to relieve chronic pelvic pain, most physicians recommend laparoscopy to definitively determine whether endometriosis is present.

GnRH Agonist Analogues

Several GnRH agonists have been approved for use in endometriosis [see Table 3]. These agents are analogues of the native decapeptide GnRH, with substitutions in amino acids 6 and 10. The introduction of D-amino acids at position 6 of native GnRH produces GnRH analogues that are resistant to degradation by endopeptidases and have long half-lives, high affinity for the GnRH receptor, and long receptor occupancy.

Paradoxically, initial treatment with a GnRH agonist analogue stimulates the secretion of luteinizing hormone (LH) and follicle-stimulating hormone (FSH). Prolonged treatment, however, suppresses gonadotropin secretion through the cellular processes of downregulation and desensitization. The suppression of secretion is greater for LH than for FSH. The suppression of pituitary gonadotropin secretion results in suppression of ovarian follicle growth and a 95% decrease in estrogen production. In women treated with many GnRH analogues, the circulating estradiol concentration is suppressed to about 15 pg/ml, which is in the range observed in menopausal women. In essence, this therapy constitutes a reversible medical oophorectomy.

Numerous clinical trials have demonstrated that approximately 85% of women with endometriosis and pelvic pain who are treated with GnRH agonist analogues experience relief of

Table 3 GnRH Agonists Approved for the Treatment of Endometriosis*

GnRH Agonist	Dose
Leuprolide acetate depot	3.75 mg I.M. every 4 wk
Goserelin acetate	3.6 mg subcutaneous implant every 4 wk
Nafarelin acetate	200 µg twice daily as a nasal spray

*Note: In the United States, GnRH agonist therapy is approved for 6 mo as single-agent therapy and for 1 yr when used in combination with a steroid add-back.

their pain. In one placebo-controlled trial, treatment with a GnRH agonist resulted in better relief of pelvic pain than the administration of placebo (85% and 30%, respectively).[39]

GnRH Agonist Analogues plus Steroid Add-Back

GnRH agonist treatment is associated with hypoestrogenic side effects such as vasomotor symptoms (hot flashes), decreased libido, dry vagina, and decreased bone density. Recent trials have demonstrated that use of a steroid (either high-dose progestin or very low dose estrogen) in so-called add-back therapy can minimize these side effects. GnRH agonist treatment combined with low-dose steroid add-back causes atrophy of endometriosis lesions and improves pelvic pain while minimizing hypoestrogenic vasomotor symptoms and bone loss. In one clinical trial, women with endometriosis and chronic pelvic pain were randomized to four different hormone treatment groups: GnRH agonist alone, GnRH agonist plus progestin only (norethindrone, 5 mg daily), GnRH agonist plus low-dose estrogen-progestin (conjugated equine estrogen, 0.625 mg daily, plus norethindrone acetate, 5 mg daily), or GnRH agonist plus high-dose estrogen plus progestin (conjugated equine estrogen, 1.25 mg daily, plus norethindrone acetate, 5 mg daily). All women were treated with the GnRH agonist leuprolide acetate, given in a depot injection of 3.75 mg I.M. every 4 weeks for 1 year. The rate of treatment discontinuance because of continuing pain was significantly higher in the group that received the combination of GnRH agonist and high-dose estrogen than in any of the other treatment groups.[40] The high-dose estrogen probably stimulated continuing function of the endometriosis implants. Consequently, treatment with a combination of GnRH agonist and high-dose estrogen is not recommended for most women with endometriosis and pelvic pain. The women in the three other groups experienced similar decreases in their pelvic pain, suggesting that all three regimens are effective. Bone density de-

Table 4 Steroid Hormone Regimens for Pelvic Pain from Endometriosis

Regimen	Comments
Transdermal estradiol patch, 25 µg daily, plus medroxyprogesterone acetate, 2.5 mg daily[27]	Does not completely prevent bone loss; achieves estradiol concentration in the range of 30 pg/ml
Norethindrone acetate, 5 mg daily[26]	A high dose of progestin; may be associated with symptoms such as bloating and mood changes
Conjugated equine estrogen, 0.625 mg daily, plus norethindrone, 5 mg daily[26]	Preserves bone density and markedly reduces vasomotor symptoms

creased significantly in the women who received the GnRH agonist alone. Bone density was preserved in the groups that were treated with a combination of a GnRH agonist and steroid add-back therapy, and vasomotor symptoms were significantly reduced. This study and others suggest that an optimal treatment of pelvic pain from endometriosis may involve the use of GnRH agonists to suppress ovarian estrogen production, followed by add-back therapy with low doses of estrogen-progestin or progestin alone [see Table 4].

Endometriosis lesions grow when serum estradiol concentration is in the premenopausal range (30 to 300 pg/ml), and they regress when estradiol levels are in the menopausal range (< 20 pg/ml). An important clinical question is, What concentration of estradiol will minimize the growth of endometriosis implants but not cause severe hypoestrogenic side effects? Treatments that achieve estradiol levels in the range of 20 to 30 pg/ml are associated with amenorrhea and regression of endometriosis lesions. In addition, these treatments are associated with fewer side effects than treatments that target estradiol levels to less than 20 pg/ml.[41]

Danazol

The first hormonal treatment of endometriosis was the intramuscular administration of testosterone. High-dose parenteral testosterone therapy was demonstrated to cause regression in endometriosis lesions. Unfortunately, many women became virilized by this treatment. Androgen treatment of endometriosis was resurrected after the development of synthetic oral androgens, such as danazol, which had attenuated androgen properties.[42]

Randomized clinical trials that have directly compared danazol and the GnRH agonists have demonstrated that both treatments improve pelvic pain in approximately 85% of treated women.[43] The side effects of these two treatments are very different. The main side effects of the GnRH agonists are those associated with hypoestrogenism (see above). The main side effects of danazol are weight gain (on average, approximately 4 kg at doses of 800 mg/day), muscle cramps, decrease in breast size, oily skin, and hirsutism.[44] In the United States, these side effects have limited the use of danazol for the treatment of endometriosis.[45] Many of the side effects of danazol are dose dependent. Doses of 50, 100, and 200 mg daily can be effective in relieving pelvic pain caused by endometriosis and are associated with less severe side effects than daily doses of 400 or 800 mg. Doses of danazol of less than 400 mg/day do not reliably suppress ovulation. Danazol crosses the placenta and is a known teratogen, so patients who are taking low doses of danazol must use a reliable method of contraception.

Progestins

High-dose synthetic progestins have been demonstrated to be effective in the treatment of pelvic pain in women with endometriosis [see Table 5]. These agents have multiple mechanisms of action: (1) suppression of LH and FSH secretion, which suppresses estradiol production; (2) direct antiestrogenic effects on endometriosis lesions; and (3) induction of pseudodecidualization. A problem with progestin treatment is that many women gain weight or experience symptoms typical of the premenstrual period, such as mood changes and bloating.

SURGICAL TREATMENT

Surgical treatment of endometriosis is termed either conservative or definitive. In conservative surgery, all the pelvic or-

Table 5 Progestins Effective for Single-Agent Treatment of Endometriosis

Progestin	Dose
Norethindrone acetate	5 mg p.o. daily
Medroxyprogesterone acetate	50 mg p.o. daily; 150 mg I.M. every 90 days
Norgestrel	0.075 mg p.o. daily

gans are preserved; in definitive surgery, both ovaries are removed.

Conservative Surgery

Conservative endometriosis surgery is best accomplished by laparoscopy because postoperative recovery is very rapid, with discharge usually occurring within 1 day. Most surgeons utilize sharp excision to remove endometriosis lesions, electrosurgery to ablate endometriosis lesions, or a combination of the two methods. In one clinical trial, women with pelvic pain caused by endometriosis were randomized to undergo diagnostic laparoscopy and aspiration of peritoneal fluid or to undergo conservative surgery with laparoscopy and resection or ablation of endometriosis lesions. Six months after surgery, 63% of the women treated with surgical resection of endometriosis lesions reported relief of pain, whereas 23% of those treated with diagnostic laparoscopy without surgical resection reported pain relief.[46]

Conservative surgery typically fails to provide permanent relief of endometriosis, however. Within 2 years after surgical treatment, pain recurs in most women with endometriosis.[47] Also, surgical treatment may result in pelvic adhesions, which can become a primary cause of continuing pelvic pain.

Definitive Surgery

Definitive surgery for endometriosis involves removal of both ovaries. Typically, the uterus is removed as well; indeed, in the United States, endometriosis is second only to uterine fibroids as a reason for performing hysterectomy. Many large cohort studies report that about 90% of women with endometriosis and pelvic pain experience long-term relief of their pain through bilateral oophorectomy.[48,49]

After bilateral oophorectomy for endometriosis, patients are typically started on low-dose estrogen replacement. Low-dose estrogen therapy prevents vasomotor symptoms and osteoporosis; pelvic pain usually does not recur.

SURGICAL EXCISION OF OVARIAN MASSES

Endometriomas require surgical excision if they are causing pain or are enlarging. Large ovarian cysts may be the result of ovarian cancer. Surgical removal of the cyst allows a definitive diagnosis of the cause of the cyst to be made. A randomized clinical trial demonstrated that surgical removal of endometriomas resulted in better long-term results than simple aspiration and fenestration of the cyst.[50]

Treatment of Infertility

EARLY-STAGE ENDOMETRIOSIS AND INFERTILITY

Women with minimal or mild (stage I or II) endometriosis and infertility have a baseline fecundity of approximately 0.03

Table 6 Stepwise Treatment of Infertility in Early-Stage Endometriosis

Step	Description	Recommendation
1	Identify and treat all reversible causes of infertility	Proper timing of coitus in relation to ovulation Optimal coital frequency Cessation of cigarette smoking Optimal body mass index Reduce consumption of alcohol and caffeine
2	Laparosocopic surgery to resect endometriosis and remove adhesions	Attempt to restore pelvic anatomy to normal
3	Ovarian stimulation with clomiphene plus intrauterine insemination	Insemination timed to the day before and day of ovulation
4	Ovarian stimulation with gonadotropin injections plus intrauterine insemination	Insemination timed to the day before and day of ovulation; because of increased risk of twin, triplet, and quadruplet pregnancy, some clinicians prefer to skip step 4 and move directly to step 5
5	In vitro fertilization and embryo transfer	—

(3% per cycle, compared with 20% to 36% in normal couples). Numerous randomized studies have demonstrated that a stepwise approach to treatment can increase pregnancy rates in women with early-stage endometriosis [*see Table 6*].

Treatment of Infertility from Other Causes

The first step in the management of early-stage endometriosis and infertility is to identify and treat all reversible causes of infertility in the couple. Many couples have multiple causes of their infertility (e.g., endometriosis in the female partner and a low sperm count in the male partner).

Laparoscopic Surgery

If other causes of infertility have been addressed but the woman is still unable to conceive, the next step is to consider a laparoscopic surgical procedure to ablate or excise endometriosis implants and adhesions and to attempt to restore the pelvis to normal. In one randomized, prospective trial, diagnostic laparoscopy alone was compared with diagnostic laparoscopy combined with surgical resection or ablation of endometriosis in 341 women with early-stage endometriosis. During 36 weeks of post-operative follow-up, fecundity was 0.024 in the diagnosis-only group and 0.047 in the surgically treated group; cumulative pregnancy rates during follow-up were 18% and 31%, respectively.[51]

Intrauterine Insemination

Women who fail to become pregnant after laparoscopic surgery can be treated with intrauterine insemination (IUI) in combination with either clomiphene or gonadotropin injections. Clomiphene is far less expensive than gonadotropins; therefore it is generally used first. These methods are designed to cause multifollicle development and multiple ovulation. In addition, IUI places a large number of motile sperm high in the reproductive tract. Thus, the spermatazoa do not have to travel through the vagina, cervix, and lower portion of the uterus. Both of these methods have been demonstrated to improve pregnancy rates in women with early-stage endometriosis. In one randomized study in 40 women with early-stage endometriosis, fecundity was 0.045 (4.5% per cycle pregnancy rate) in the group that received no treatment and 0.15 in the group treated with three cycles of gonadotropin injections in combination with IUI.[52] Similar findings have been reported by other groups.[53-56]

Table 7 Stepwise Treatment of Infertility in Advanced Endometriosis

Step	Description	Recommendation
1	Identify and treat all reversible causes of infertility	Proper timing of coitus in relation to ovulation Optimal coital frequency Cessation of cigarette smoking Optimal body mass index Reduce consumption of alcohol and caffeine
2	Surgery to resect endometriosis and remove adhesions	Attempt to restore pelvic anatomy to normal
3	Ovarian stimulation with clomiphene plus intrauterine insemination	Insemination timed to the day before and day of ovulation; limited to patients with patent fallopian tubes and no dense ovarian adhesions
4	Ovarian stimulation with gonadotropin injections plus intrauterine insemination	Insemination timed to the day before and day of ovulation; limited to patients with patent fallopian tubes and no dense ovarian adhesions; because of increased risk of twin, triplet, or quadruplet pregnancy, some clinicians prefer to skip step 4 and move directly to step 5
5	In vitro fertilization and embryo transfer	—

Many authorities believe that the per-cycle pregnancy rate drops significantly after three or four cycles of clomiphene or gonadotropin injections in combination with IUI. Consequently, after three cycles of such treatment, the clinician should review with the couple the advantages of proceeding to the next step, which is in vitro fertilization (IVF) with embryo transfer.[57]

In Vitro Fertilization

There are no prospective, large-scale, randomized trials that demonstrate the efficacy of IVF in the treatment of infertility caused by endometriosis. However, the use of IVF in women with endometriosis and infertility routinely results in treatment-cycle pregnancy rates of approximately 0.30, a 10-fold increase over the baseline fecundity seen in such women.[58-60] It should be noted, however, that the outcome of IVF is highly influenced by the woman's age: women younger than 37 years have much better success with IVF than do women older than 37 years.

ADVANCED ENDOMETRIOSIS AND INFERTILITY

In women with moderate or severe endometriosis and infertility, a stepwise approach to treatment is warranted [see Table 7].

The first step, as in the treatment of early-stage endometriosis, is to identify and correct all other reversible causes of infertility.

Surgical Treatment

The second step is to perform surgical resection for ovarian endometriosis, peritoneal endometriosis, and pelvic adhesions to restore pelvic anatomy and function. There are no randomized, prospective studies that demonstrate the efficacy of surgery in the treatment of advanced endometriosis. However, most authorities believe that surgery improves fertility in these women. One retrospective analysis reviewed the outcome in 130 infertile women with endometriosis who were treated with expectant management, conservative surgery, or expectant management followed by surgery. Although no significant difference was noted between expectant management and surgery in women with mild or moderate endometriosis, women with severe endometriosis appeared to benefit from surgery. Of the 32 women with advanced endometriosis who were observed over 231 months of cumulative follow-up, none became pregnant. Of the 34 women with advanced endometriosis who underwent conservative surgery, 10 became pregnant during 702 cumulative months of follow-up.[61] Similar results have been reported in a meta-analysis of the impact of surgery on fertility in women with endometriosis.[62] These studies suggest that expectant management is not warranted in the treatment of infertility associated with advanced endometriosis and that surgical treatment may improve fecundity.

Pregnancy rates are highest in the 6 to 18 months after the surgical procedure. Additional surgical procedures have not been shown to be effective in increasing fecundity[63]; therefore, if pregnancy does not occur after the first surgery, the clinician should usually move on to intrauterine insemination. Physicians should carefully weigh the limited benefits of second and third operative procedures to enhance fertility against the potential risks of major surgery.

Intrauterine Insemination

Clomiphene or gonadotropin injections in combination with IUI are used empirically in patients with advanced endometri-

osis and infertility. Most of the clinical trials that have tested these modalities have focused on women with early-stage endometriosis (see above). However, many authorities believe that the benefits of these measures probably extend to women with advanced disease. In patients with severe pelvic adhesions, clinicians may choose to move directly from surgery to in vitro fertilization. Clomiphene or gonadotropins in combination with IUI should not be recommended for women with tubal blockage or dense ovarian adhesions.

In Vitro Fertilization

There are no large, randomized, controlled clinical trials that definitively demonstrate that IVF increases pregnancy rates in women with advanced endometriosis. In one small study involving 21 women with endometriosis and infertility, none of the six women randomized to undergo expectant management became pregnant, whereas five of the 15 women who were treated with IVF became pregnant.[64] Because of the small sample size, however, this study did not have sufficient statistical power to detect true differences between the two groups. One analysis of various infertility treatments demonstrated that for infertile women with advanced endometriosis, rapid progression through the steps to IVF is the most cost-effective treatment approach.[65] In the United States, the median projected cost per IVF cycle in 2001 was $9,226.[66] The cost of having a child with IVF is within the range of the cost of adopting a child. Furthermore, over the past decade, IVF success rates have increased.[67]

IVF is less successful in women with advanced endometriosis who have previously undergone bilateral ovarian surgery; after unilateral oophorectomy and a contralateral ovarian cystectomy, ovarian stimulation is often ineffective, and the pregnancy rate is low. Reduced pregnancy rates for women with advanced endometriosis (compared with women who have early-stage endometriosis or tubal factor infertility) may be the result of a premature depletion of the ovarian follicle pool,[68] abnormal folliculogenesis,[69] or reduced fertilization potential of oocytes.[70]

References

1. Houston DE, Noller KL, Melton LJ, et al: Incidence of pelvic endometriosis in Rochester, Minnesota, 1970–1979. Am J Epidemiol 125:959, 1987

2. Holt VL, Weiss NS: Recommendations for the design of epidemiologic studies of endometriosis. Epidemiology 11:654, 2000

3. Cramer DW, Wilson E, Stillman RJ, et al: The relation of endometriosis to menstrual characteristics, smoking and exercise. JAMA 225:1904, 1986

4. Birnbaum LS, Cummings AM: Dioxins and endometriosis: a plausible hypothesis. Environ Health Perspect 110:15, 2002

5. Bruner-Tran KL, Rier SE, Eisenberg E, et al: The potential role of environmental toxins in the pathophysiology of endometriosis. Gynecol Obstet Invest 48(suppl 1):45, 1999

6. Bedaiwy MA, Falcone T, Sharma RK, et al: Prediction of endometriosis with serum and peritoneal fluid markers: a prospective controlled trial. Hum Reprod 17:426, 2002

7. Sinaii N, Cleary SD, Ballweg ML, et al: Autoimmune and related disease among women with endometriosis: a survey analysis. Fertil Steril 77(suppl 1):S7, 2002

8. Gazvani R, Templeton A: New considerations for the pathogenesis of endometriosis. Int J Gynaecol Obstet 76:117, 2002

9. Simpson JL, Elias S, Malinak LR, et al: Heritable aspects of endometriosis. Am J Obstet Gynecol 137:327, 1980

10. Jimbo J, Hitami Y, Yoshikawa H, et al: Evidence for monoclonal expansion of epithelial cells in ovarian endometrial cysts. Am J Pathol 150:1173, 1997

11. Barbieri RL, Missmer S: Endometriosis and infertility: a cause-effect relationship? Ann N Y Acad Sci 955:23, 2002

12. Haney AF, Muscato JJ, Weinberg JB: Peritoneal fluid cell populations in infertility patients. Fertil Steril 41:122, 1984

13. Halme J, Becker S, Haskill S: Altered maturation and function of peritoneal macrophages: possible role in the pathogenesis of endometriosis. Am J Obstet Gynecol 156:783, 1987

14. Fakih H, Baggett B, Holtz G: Interleukin-1: a possible role in the infertility associated with endometriosis. Fertil Steril 47:213, 1987

15. Oral E, Arici A, Olive DL, et al: Peritoneal fluid from women with moderate or se-

vere endometriosis inhibits sperm motility: the role of seminal fluid components. Fertil Steril 66:787, 1996

16. Badawy SZ, Cuenca V, Stitzel A: Autoimmune phenomena in infertile patients with endometriosis. Obstet Gynecol 63:271, 1984

17. Weed JC, Aquembourg PC: Endometriosis: can it produce an autoimmune response resulting in infertility? Clin Obstet Gynecol 23:885, 1980

18. Cheesman KL, Cheesman SD, Chatterton RT: Alterations in progesterone metabolism and luteal function in infertile women with endometriosis. Fertil Steril 29:270, 1978

19. Wardle PG, McLaughlin EA, McDermott A: Endometriosis and ovulatory disorder: reduced fertilization in vitro compared with tubal and unexplained infertility. Lancet 2:236, 1985

20. Polan ML, Totora M, Caldwell BV, et al: Abnormal ovarian cycles as diagnosed by ultrasound and serum estradiol levels. Fertil Steril 37:342, 1982

21. Lessey BA, Castlebaum AJ, Sawin SW, et al: Aberrant integrin expression in the endometrium of women with endometriosis. J Clin Endocrinol Metab 79:643, 1994

22. McBean JH, Brumsted JR: In vitro CA-125 secretion from women with advanced endometriosis. Fertil Steril 59:89, 1993

23. Takahashi K, Nagata H, Musa AA, et al: Clinical usefulness of CA-125 levels in the menstrual discharge of women with endometriosis. Fertil Steril 54:360, 1990

24. Redwine DB: Diaphragmatic endometriosis: diagnosis, surgical management, and long-term results of treatment. Fertil Steril 77:288, 2002

25. Barbieri RL: Stenosis of the external cervical os: an association with endometriosis in women with chronic pelvic pain. Fertil Steril 70:571, 1998

26. Propst AM, Storti K, Barbieri RL: Lateral cervical displacement: an association with endometriosis. Fertil Steril 70:568, 1998

27. Pardanani S, Barbieri RL: The gold standard for the surgical diagnosis of endometriosis: visual findings or biopsy results. J Gynecol Tech 4:121, 1998

28. Hornstein MD, Friedman AJ, Gleason RE, et al: The reproducibility of the revised American Fertility Society classification of endometriosis. Fertil Steril 59:1015, 1993

29. Jansen RS, Russell P: Non-pigmented endometriosis: clinical, laparoscopic and pathologic definitions. Am J Obstet Gynecol 155:1154, 1986

30. Blaustein A: Pelvic endometriosis. Blaustein's Pathology of the Genital Tract, 2nd ed. Blaustein A, Ed. Springer-Verlag, New York, 1982, p 464

31. Randomized controlled trial of depot leuprolide in patients with chronic pelvic pain and clinically suspected endometriosis. Pelvic Pain Study Group. Obstet Gynecol 93:51, 1999

32. Zondervan KT, Yudkin PL, Vessey MP, et al: Prevalence and incidence of chronic pelvic pain in primary care: evidence from a national general practice database. Br J Obstet Gynaecol 106:1149, 1999

33. Carter JE: Combined hysteroscopy and laparoscopic findings in patients with chronic pelvic pain. J Am Assoc Gynecol Laparoscopy 2:43, 1994

34. Koninckx PR, Lessafre E, Meuleman C, et al: Suggestive evidence that pelvic endometriosis is a progressive disease, whereas deeply infiltrating endometriosis is associated with pelvic pain. Fertil Steril 55:759, 1991

35. Collins JA, Crosignani PG: Unexplained infertility: a review of diagnosis, prognosis, treatment efficacy and management. Int J Gynaecol Obstet 39:267, 1992

36. Templeton AA, Penney GC: The incidence, characteristics, and prognosis of patients whose infertility is unexplained. Fertil Steril 37:175, 1982

37. Guzick DS, Grefenstette I, Baffone K, et al: Infertility evaluation in fertile women: a model for assessing the efficacy of infertility testing. Hum Reprod 9:2306, 1994

38. Vercellini P, Trespidi L, Colombo A, et al: A gonadotropin-releasing hormone agonist versus a low-dose oral contraceptive for pelvic pain associated with endometriosis. Fertil Steril 60:75, 1993

39. Lupron depot (leuprolide acetate for depot suspension) in the treatment of endometriosis: a randomized, placebo-controlled, double-blind study. Lupron Study Group. Fertil Steril 54:419, 1990

40. Leuprolide acetate depot and hormonal add-back in endometriosis: a 12-month study. Lupron Add-Back Study Group. Obstet Gynecol 91:16, 1998

41. Howell R, Edmonds D, Dowsett M, et al: Gonadotropin releasing hormone analogue plus hormone replacement therapy for the treatment of endometriosis: a randomized clinical trial. Fertil Steril 64:474, 1995

42. Barbieri RL, Ryan KJ: Danazol: endocrine pharmacology and therapeutic applications. Am J Obstet Gynecol 141:453, 1981

43. Henzl MR, Corson SL, Moghissi K, et al: Administration of nasal nafarelin as compared with oral danazol for endometriosis. N Engl J Med 318:485, 1988

44. Barbieri RL, Evans S, Kistner RW: Danazol in the treatment of endometriosis: analysis of 100 cases with a 4-year follow-up. Fertil Steril 37:737, 1982

45. Selak V, Farquhar C, Prentice A, et al: Danazol for pelvic pain associated with endometriosis. Cochrane Database Syst Rev (2):CD000068, 2002

46. Sutton CJ, Ewen SP, Jacobs SA, et al: Laser laparoscopic surgery in the treatment of ovarian endometriosis. J Am Assoc Gynecol Laparoscopy 4:319, 1997

47. Hornstein MD, Hemmings R, Yuzpe AA, et al: Use of nafarelin versus placebo after reductive laparoscopic surgery for endometriosis. Fertil Steril 68:860, 1997

48. Ranney B: Endometriosis. 3. Complete operations. Reasons, sequelae, treatment. Am J Obstet Gynecol 109:1137, 1971

49. Hickman TN, Namnoum AB, Hinton EL, et al: Timing of estrogen replacement following hysterectomy with oophorectomy for endometriosis. Obstet Gynecol 91:673, 1998

50. Beretta P, Franci M, Ghezzi F, et al: Randomized clinical trial of two laparoscopic treatments of endometriomas: cystectomy versus drainage and coagulation. Fertil Steril 70:1176, 1998

51. Laparoscopic surgery in infertile women with minimal or mild endometriosis. The Canadian Collaborative Group on Endometriosis. N Engl J Med 337:217, 1997

52. Fedele L, Bianchi S, Marchini M, et al: Superovulation with human menopausal gonadotropins in the treatment of infertility associated with minimal or mild endometriosis. Fertil Steril 58:28, 1992

53. Tummon IS, Asher LJ, Martin JS, et al: Randomized controlled trial of superovulation and insemination for infertility associated with minimal or mild endometriosis. Fertil Steril 68:8, 1997

54. Nulsen JC, Walsh S, Dumez S, et al: A randomized and longitudinal study of human menopausal gonadotropin with intrauterine insemination in the treatment of infertility. Obstet Gynecol 82:780, 1993

55. Chaffkin LM, Nulsen JC, Luciano AA, et al: A comparative analysis of the cycle fecundity rates associated with combined human menopausal gonadotropin and intrauterine insemination versus either hMG or IUI alone. Fertil Steril 55:252, 1991

56. Guzick DS, Carson SA, Coutifaris C, et al: Efficacy of superovulation and intrauterine insemination in the treatment of infertility. N Engl J Med 340:177, 1999

57. Isaksson R, Tiitinen A: Superovulation with combined insemination or timed intercourse in the treatment of couples with unexplained infertility and minimal endometriosis. Acta Obstet Gynecol Scand 76:550, 1997

58. Olivenenes F, Feldberg D, Liu HC, et al: Endometriosis: a stage by stage analysis: role for in vitro fertilization. Fertil Steril 64:392, 1995

59. Oehninger S, Acosta AA, Kreiner D, et al: In vitro fertilization and embryo transfer: an established and successful therapy for endometriosis. J In Vitro Fertilization and Embryo Transfer 5:249, 1988

60. Chillik CF, Acosta AA, Garcia JE, et al: The role of in vitro fertilization in infertile patients with endometriosis. Fertil Steril 44:56, 1985

61. Olive DL, Lee KL: Analysis of sequential treatment protocols for endometriosis-associated infertility. Am J Obstet Gynecol 154:613, 1986

62. Adamson GD, Pasta DJ: Surgical treatment of endometriosis-associated infertility: meta-analysis compared with survival analysis. Am J Obstet Gynecol 171:1404, 1994

63. Pagidas K, Falcone T, Hemmings R, et al: Comparison of reoperation for moderate and severe endometriosis-related infertility with in vitro fertilization-embryo transfer. Fertil Steril 65:791, 1996

64. Soliman S, Daya S, Collins J: A randomized trial of in vitro fertilization versus conventional treatment for infertility. Fertil Steril 59:1239, 1993

65. Phillips Z, Barraza-Llorens M, Posnett J: Evaluation of the relative cost-effectiveness of treatments for infertility in the UK. Human Reproduction 15:95, 2000

66. Collins J: Cost-effectiveness of in vitro fertilization. Semin Reprod Med 19:279, 2001

67. Cramer DW, Liberman RF, Powers DR, et al: Recent trends in assisted reproductive techniques and associated outcomes. Obstet Gynecol 95:61, 2000

68. Hornstein MD, Barbieri RL, McShane PM: The effects of previous ovarian surgery on the follicular response to ovulation induction in an in vitro fertilization program. J Reprod Med 34:277, 1989

69. Toya M, Saito H, Ohta N, et al: Moderate and severe endometriosis is associated with alterations in the cell cycle of granulose cells in patients undergoing in vitro fertilization and embryo transfer. Fertil Steril 73:344, 2000

70. Pal L, Shifren JL, Isaacson KB, et al: Impact of varying stages of endometriosis on the outcome of in vitro fertilization—embryo transfer. J Assisted Reproduction and Genetics 15:27, 1998

85 Urinary Incontinence and the Overactive Bladder

Robert L. Barbieri, M.D.

The involuntary loss of urine is an extremely common problem in women—more common than Alzheimer disease or osteoporosis. Urinary incontinence affects approximately 15% of women younger than 65 years, 25% of women older than 65 years, and 50% of women who are nursing home residents.[1,2] It is underdiagnosed and undertreated; patients may fail to report it, and physicians may fail to address it.[3]

Pathogenesis

The normal pattern of urinary voiding requires the interaction of the central nervous system, the sacral parasympathetic and thoracolumbar sympathetic systems, the bladder muscle (detrusor muscle), the urinary sphincter muscle, and the mechanical support of the pelvic fascia. In the resting state, urine collects in the bladder, the bladder muscle is quiescent, and the tone of the urinary sphincter muscle is high, ensuring that urine remains in the bladder. Urination is initiated when signals from the CNS induce the bladder muscle to contract and the urethral sphincter muscle to relax. At the completion of voiding, the bladder muscle relaxes and the urethral sphincter contracts. A key feature of the urinary system is that in the normal resting state, the urethral pressure is greater than the pressure in the bladder. Reversal of that differential—whether from a rise in bladder pressure, a decrease in urethral pressure, or both—will result in incontinence.

Urinary Incontinence in the Nongeriatric Population

In the nongeriatric population, the five main causes of urinary incontinence are (1) loss of fascial support of the urethra (stress incontinence), (2) an overactive bladder muscle (detrusor instability), (3) intrinsic sphincter deficiency, (4) neuropathies, and (5) urinary tract fistulas. Many women with incontinence have both stress incontinence and bladder muscle overactivity. In a study of 303 women with urinary incontinence, 43% were diagnosed as having stress incontinence, 21% as having bladder muscle overactivity, and 36% as having both disorders.[4] In some women, the stress incontinence is predominant, with bladder muscle overactivity playing less of a role; in other women, the bladder muscle overactivity is predominant, and there is less of a contribution from stress incontinence. Race may be a factor: African-American women have lower rates of stress incontinence than Hispanic and white women but have higher rates of detrusor instability.[5]

The initial approach to urinary incontinence should include a history; physical examination; and laboratory tests, including a urinalysis and urine culture. In the history, the patient should be asked to describe the episodes of incontinence. Women with stress incontinence typically report urinary leakage with events that increase intra-abdominal pressure—for example, coughing, laughing, sneezing, and the lifting of heavy weights. Women with detrusor instability often report a sudden and intense urge to void that occurs just before the loss of urine. Symptoms such as frequency, nocturia, hesitancy, and terminal dribbling are not specific to incontinence from any one cause.

A voiding diary is a reliable method to establish the severity of urinary incontinence. In the voiding diary, the patient reports the time of continent and incontinent voids, the volume of continent voids, and any events that precipitate incontinence. To facilitate measurement of continent voids, patients can be given a graduated plastic receptacle (a so-called hat) to place on their toilet seat at home.

In the history, the physician should assess for substances that may contribute to incontinence. Caffeine, which is both a diuretic and a bladder irritant, may worsen incontinence in some cases. Other possible dietary bladder irritants include alcohol, citrus or other highly acidic fruit, tomatoes, spicy foods, dairy products, and sugar. Alpha blockers and some muscle relaxants (e.g., dantrolene) can exacerbate incontinence by relaxing the urinary sphincter.

The assessment should include a complete review of the patient's obstetric history, including the number of deliveries, their route, and any complications. Details of any abdominal or pelvic surgery should also be obtained.

The physical examination should include inspection of the vagina for mucosal atrophy and herniation of the pelvic structures.

Urinalysis and culture are necessary to screen for urinary tract infection or glucosuria. If those conditions are found, they should be treated before one proceeds with further evaluation of urinary incontinence. Curing the urinary tract infection or controlling the diabetes may correct the urinary incontinence in such cases.

Additional initial tests for incontinence include a clinical stress test and measurement of postvoid residual urinary volume. One approach to these two tests is to ask the patient to void and then catheterize the bladder to determine the postvoid residual urinary volume. If the postvoid residual volume is more than 200 ml, the physician should assess for a neurogenic process or a bladder outflow obstruction. Using the same catheter, 300 ml of fluid (sterile water or sterile saline) at body temperature can be instilled into the bladder. The patient is then asked to cough while in the supine and upright positions. Immediate leakage of urine with the cough is diagnostic of stress incontinence.

URODYNAMIC TESTING WITH MULTICHANNEL EQUIPMENT

Urodynamic testing with multichannel pressure recording devices is the gold standard for identifying both stress incontinence and bladder overactivity. In this procedure, the intravesical pressure is directly measured by means of a bladder catheter, and intra-abdominal pressure is measured by use of a vaginal or rectal probe. Subtracting intra-abdominal pressure from intravesical pressure yields the true detrusor pressure. A separate channel in the bladder catheter allows fluid to be instilled into the bladder [see Figure 1].

Urodynamic testing is not necessary for every incontinent patient. Although widely available, the testing is expensive and time consuming. Some clinicians prefer to forgo urody-

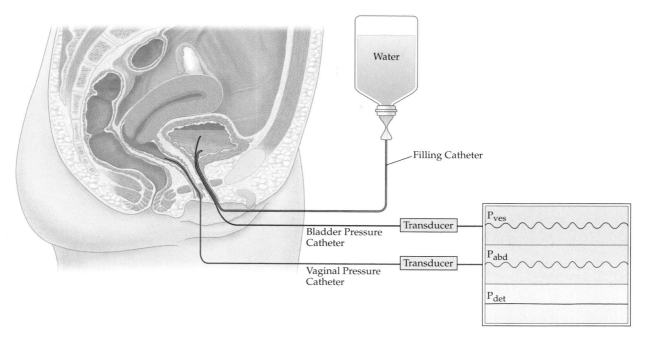

Figure 1   **Subtracted cystometry. Intra-abdominal pressure (Pabd) is measured with an intravaginal or intrarectal pressure catheter. Bladder pressure (Pves) is measured with an intravesical catheter. Subtraction of Pabd from Pves yields the true detrusor pressure (Pdet). Fluid can be instilled into the bladder through a separate channel in the intravesical channel. Bladder contractions that occur as the bladder is filling and that the patient is unable to completely suppress indicate detrusor instability.**

namic testing and treat on the basis of clinical diagnosis, whereas others (especially urogynecologists) use the testing routinely.

STRESS INCONTINENCE

Stress incontinence refers to a sudden involuntary loss of urine, usually secondary to a sudden increase in intra-abdominal pressure, in the absence of a bladder contraction. Intra-abdominal pressure can increase as a result of coughing, sneezing, running, climbing stairs, standing, or lifting heavy weights.

Normally, the pelvic fascia holds the urethral sphincter in an intra-abdominal position; consequently, any increase in intra-abdominal pressure is transmitted equally to the urethra and bladder, and the urethral sphincter remains closed. Damage to the pelvic fascia, laxity in the pelvic ligaments, and partial pelvic muscle tears and denervation—all common sequelae of childbirth—can cause the urethra to drop below the pelvic floor. If intra-abdominal pressure then increases suddenly, the pressure will be transmitted primarily to the bladder; bladder pressure will then exceed urethral pressure, the urethral sphincter will open involuntarily, and urine will spill.

Diagnosis

If the history suggests stress incontinence, the vaginal walls should be examined for laxity of the pelvic structures. Possible underlying abnormalities in stress incontinence include cystocele (a hernia of the bladder into the anterior vaginal wall), rectocele (a hernia of the rectum into the posterior vaginal wall), enterocele (a hernia of the small bowel into the posterior apex of the vaginal wall), and uterine prolapse (a hernia of the uterus into the lower portion of the vagina).

Treatment

If the physical examination reveals the cervix at the vaginal opening (uterine prolapse) or a cystocele, rectocele, or enterocele at the vaginal opening, the patient should be referred to a gynecologist or urogynecologist for surgical repair. If the physical examination reveals no significant herniations, a nonsurgical approach can be recommended.

Nonsurgical treatment   The nonsurgical approach to the treatment of stress incontinence includes exercises to strengthen the pelvic floor musculature (Kegel exercises) and electrical stimulation of the pelvic muscles. The Kegel exercise is the voluntary contraction of the pubococcygeal muscles in sets of 10 contractions, five to 10 times daily. Contraction of the pubococcygeal muscle can be taught by asking the patient to stop her stream of urine while voiding. This requires contraction of pelvic muscles and relaxation of the abdominal muscles. Many patients have difficulty isolating the correct muscles and may benefit from instruction sheets on performing the exercises; one source for such instructional material is http://www.niddk.nih.gov/health/urolog/uibcw/exerc/exerc.htm.

Kegel exercises alleviate the symptoms in about 70% of women with stress incontinence.[6] Improvement in continence may not become apparent for 6 to 12 weeks, but once attained, the benefits may be maintained for years.[7]

Vaginal cones can also be used to teach women to contract pelvic floor muscles without contracting the abdominal muscles.[8] Vaginal cones come in sets of five cones, each of a different weight [*see Figure 2*]. Depending on the manufacturer, the cones may be all the same size or may decrease in diameter as they increase in weight. The patient inserts the lightest cone

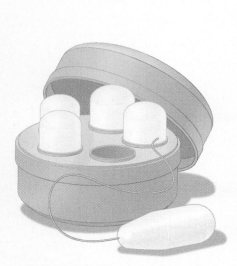
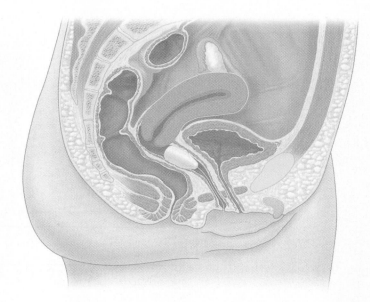

Figure 2   **Vaginal cones. Women with stress incontinence can use vaginal cones to learn how to contract their pelvic floor muscles. The cones come in sets of graduated weight and are shaped like a tampon, with a string to facilitate removal from the vagina (*a*). The patient inserts the cone (*b*) and keeps it in her vagina for 15 minutes. Successively heavier cones are used as the pelvic floor muscles increase in strength.**

into the vagina and uses the pelvic floor muscles to hold the cone in the vagina while walking. Once those muscles can hold the cone in place for at least 15 minutes, the patient progresses to the next heavier cone. For some women, the cones are superior to Kegel exercises for strengthening the pelvic floor musculature. As with the Kegel exercises, patients may not experience benefit for a number of weeks.

An alternative to Kegel exercises and vaginal cones is to electrically stimulate the paravaginal musculature. An approved device for strengthening the pelvic musculature consists of a probe that is placed in the vagina twice daily for 15 to 30 minutes. The probe stimulates the afferent fibers of the pudendal nerve, contracting the muscles of the pelvic floor and periurethral muscles. This stimulation strengthens the muscles that maintain the urethral pressure profile.

Estrogen therapy has been suggested for women with atrophic vaginitis and stress incontinence. Estrogen has not been documented to improve symptoms of stress incontinence,[9,10] but some researchers have speculated that topical estrogen may be effective even if oral estrogen is not[11]; and the combination of estrogen and pelvic floor exercises has been found to be more effective than exercises alone.[12] In one study, imipramine, 25 mg three times a day, produced significant improvement or cure in 60% of patients with stress incontinence.[13]

Surgical treatment   If nonsurgical measures fail, the patient with stress incontinence should be referred to a urogynecologist for further evaluation. Incontinence surgery is very effective in the treatment of stress incontinence. In women older than 65 years, incontinence surgery has an overall mortality of less than 0.3%,[14] and surgery for stress incontinence has high cure rates.[15]

The current state-of-the art surgical procedure for stress incontinence is the tension-free vaginal tape procedure.[16] This procedure can be performed on an outpatient basis using local or regional anesthesia and conscious sedation. In this technique, a strip of polypropylene mesh (the tape) is used to create a urethral sling. The tape is inserted under the wall of the vagina, beneath the midurethra, and the ends of the tape are passed retropubically up to two small incisions on the lower abdomen near the superior border of the pubic hair. The tape is elevated just enough to eliminate urine leakage with coughing. It stays in place without sutures because of its Velcro-like surface, and it is further anchored by postoperative fibrosis. The tape allows increases in intra-abdominal pressure to be efficiently transmitted to the urethra, preventing loss of urine. In one study of women with stress incontinence, the tension-free vaginal tape procedure resulted in cure in about 85% of patients.[17] Other bladder neck suspension procedures for stress incontinence include the Burch colposuspension and the Raz needle vaginal suspension.

DETRUSOR INSTABILITY—OVERACTIVE BLADDER MUSCLE

Detrusor instability is defined as spontaneous or provoked bladder contractions during the filling phase of cystometry that cannot be completely suppressed by a neurologically normal patient.[18] A problem with this definition is that it requires an invasive test, cystometry, for the diagnosis. Some authorities prefer the term overactive bladder muscle to describe the condition. In the nonvoiding state, the bladder muscle should not contract spontaneously. Spontaneous contractions of the bladder muscle can raise the bladder pressure above that of the urethral sphincter, resulting in the involuntary loss of urine. Bladder muscle from women with detrusor instability is more sensitive to electrical and acetylcholine stimulation than is bladder muscle from healthy women.[19]

Detrusor hyperreflexia is defined as an overactive bladder muscle caused by a neurologic disorder, such as multiple sclerosis, Parkinson disease, cerebrovascular disease, or spinal cord injury. As many as 80% of women with multiple sclerosis have detrusor hyperreflexia.[20]

Diagnosis

Women with detrusor instability typically complain of urinary urgency (a desire to urinate immediately), urinary frequency (a need to urinate every half hour or hour), urge incontinence, and nocturia. A severe urge to void followed by incontinence at rest is common. Incontinent episodes typically involve the loss of large amounts of urine. Women who void 10 or more times a day often have detrusor instability. Physical examination discloses no specific findings in women with overactive bladder. However, because stress incontinence and overactive bladder can coexist, the physical findings associated with stress incontinence may be observed in women with overactive bladder muscle.

Treatment

Bladder retraining and acetylcholine blockade are the two most effective approaches to the treatment of overactive bladder. Surgery is not recommended for women with bladder overactivity.

Bladder retraining   The goal of bladder retraining is to elicit behavioral changes that will lead to an increase in bladder capacity and will prolong the interval between episodes of voiding. At the beginning of bladder retraining, the patient is asked to urinate approximately once every hour. No nighttime schedule is recommended. As training progresses, the woman is asked to void once every 90 minutes, then once every 2 hours. Millard and Oldenburg reported that bladder retraining alleviated symptoms in as many as 75% of women with overactive bladder.[21] Biofeedback using a vaginal or anorectal probe may help some women better control urge incontinence.[22] Many physical therapy programs teach bladder retraining and biofeedback techniques.

Behavioral treatment may be as effective as drug treatment for many women with bladder overactivity. In one trial, behavioral therapy resulted in an 86% improvement in incontinent episodes, versus a 69% improvement with oxybutynin.[23]

Drug therapy   Detrusor muscle stimulation is mediated by cholinergic fibers. Anticholinergic agents [see Table 1] can decrease detrusor muscle activity, reduce the urge to void, and result in improvement in women with urge incontinence. Traditional anticholinergic agents, such as oxybutynin, block detrusor muscle stimulation, but they also block cholinergic effects in the salivary glands, causing dry mouth. The typical dose of immediate-release oxybutynin is 2.5 or 5 mg three or four times a day. Contraindications to oxybutynin include narrow-angle glaucoma and cardiac arrhythmia. A new, extended-release formulation of oxybutynin (starting dose, 5 mg once daily, titrated to 20 to 30 mg once daily) appears to have fewer side effects, such as dry mouth, than the original rapid-acting formulation of the drug.[24] In a prospective, randomized, controlled trial, extended-release oxybutynin proved significantly more effective than tolterodine in improving incontinence and urinary frequency.[25]

Tolterodine, one of a new class of anticholinergic agents, has anticholinergic effects on the bladder but has little effect on the salivary glands. In one study, the mean number of incontinence episodes was reduced by 47% in women treated with tolterodine (2 mg twice daily), compared with 17% in women treated with placebo.[26] For young women, a dosage of 2 mg twice daily is usually effective in reducing the frequency of voiding. For older women, dosages of tolterodine as low as 1 mg daily may control the problem of frequent voiding.

Although alpha blockers are not often used for treating overactive bladder in women, these agents have a modulating effect on bladder smooth muscle. One prospective study found doxazosin [see Table 1], 2 mg at bedtime, to be effective in women with urinary frequency and urgency.[27]

INTRINSIC SPHINCTER DEFICIENCY

Intrinsic sphincter deficiency (ISD) is a form of urinary incontinence caused by the failure of the urethra to close completely. Urethral dysfunction in these patients results from mucosal and muscular atrophy and denervation. Postoperative scarring of the urethra can also cause ISD. Urinary leakage in ISD is often continual and can occur without an increase in intra-abdominal pressure. Surgical treatments for ISD include sling procedures, such as the tension-free vaginal tape procedure, or the periurethral injection of bulking agents, such as glutaraldehyde cross-linked bovine collagen (Contigen)[28] or carbon beads suspended in gel (Durasphere)[29] [see Figure 3]. Short-term success rates with injectable agents are very high, but long-term durability remains in question.[30]

Table 1   Drugs Used in the Treatment of Overactive Bladder

Class	Agent (Brand Name)	Dosage	Cost	Comment
Anticholinergic agents	Oxybutynin	2.5–5 mg, t.i.d.–q.i.d	5 mg t.i.d.: $10–19.99/mo	Dry mouth a common side effect
	Oxybutynin, extended release (Ditropan XL)	5–30 mg q.d.	5 mg: $100.99/mo 10 mg: $107.99/mo	Dry mouth a common side effect
	Tolterodine (Detrol)	1 mg q.d.–2 mg b.i.d.	2 mg b.i.d.: $70–79.99/mo	Lower dose often effective in older women
	Tolterodine, extended release (Detrol LA)	2–4 mg q.d.	2 mg: $100.99/mo	—
Alpha blocker	Doxazosin (Cardura)	2 mg h.s.	2 mg q.d.: $20—29.99/mo	—

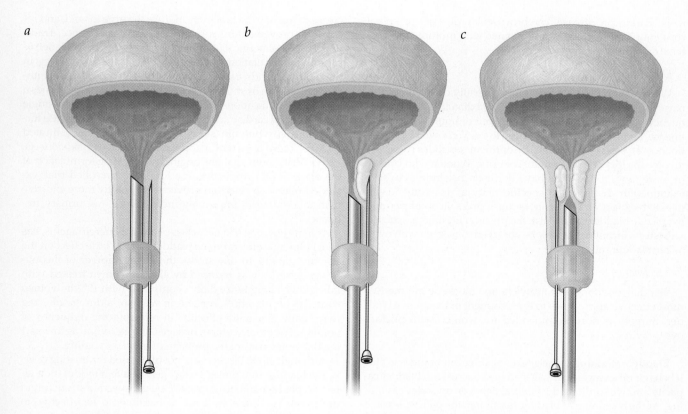

Figure 3   **Injection of bulking agents to treat intrinsic sphincter deficiency. The needle is advanced to the proximal urethra just below the bladder neck (*a*), and the bulking agent is then injected (*b*). Injection of the agent bilaterally closes off the proximal urethra (*c*).**

OVERFLOW INCONTINENCE

Rarely, neurologic problems that result in denervation of the detrusor muscle can lead to overfilling of the bladder and so-called overflow incontinence. Overdistention of the bladder can also be caused by outflow obstruction. Pharmacologic contributors to overflow incontinence include calcium channel blockers, which can relax the detrusor muscle, and alpha agonists, which can increase urethral resistance. Denervation of the detrusor muscle leading to overflow incontinence can result from cerebrovascular accidents, multiple sclerosis, spinal cord injury, cauda equina tumors, diabetes, and pelvic nerve damage during surgery.

A simple way to test the status of the sacral nerves is to look for the anal wink reflex. If the perianal region is lightly stroked with the wooden end of a cotton-tipped applicator, the anal sphincter should contract. Presence of this reflex suggests that the sacral dermatomes S2, S3, and S4 are intact. If an anal wink is not present, a complete neurologic evaluation is warranted.

URINARY TRACT FISTULAS

Fistulas between the bladder and vagina are a rare cause of incontinence. Most urinary tract fistulas occur after a pelvic surgical procedure, such as cesarean section, surgical vaginal delivery (e.g., involving repair of severe lacerations or forceps use), hysterectomy, or bladder surgery. Spontaneous fistulas are uncommon. Incontinence resulting from fistulas usually involves chronic, continuous leakage of urine.

In many cases, fistulas between the bladder and vagina can be observed on speculum examination of the vagina. Small fistulas can be detected by giving the patient a dose of oral pyridium and placing a tampon in the vagina. If the tampon turns orange after 2 hours, a fistula between the urinary tract and vagina is likely.

Urinary Incontinence in the Geriatric Population

As many as half of the women in nursing homes have urinary incontinence. Aging is associated with decreased urethral pressure and increased involuntary detrusor contractility, which increase the risk of symptomatic bladder overactivity. In addition, in the elderly, urine production increases during the night. Resnick has suggested the mnemonic DIAPPERS for the evaluation of incontinence in the geriatric population.[31] This mnemonic summarizes the most common causes of incontinence in the elderly: delirium, infection, atrophic urethritis, pharmaceuticals that interfere with bladder and urethral function, psychiatric causes (depression), excess urinary output, restricted mobility, and stool impaction. Treatment of these problems can often significantly alleviate the incontinence.

The incontinent woman with cognitive impairment often responds well to prompted voiding. One program of prompted voiding requires that the woman be asked every 2 hours if she would like to void. If she responds in the affirmative, she is escorted to the toilet.

References

1. Milsom I, Ekelund P, Molander U, et al: The influence of age, parity, oral contraception, hysterectomy and menopause on the prevalence of urinary incontinence in women. J Urol 149:1459, 1993

2. Ouslander JG, Schnelle JF: Incontinence in the nursing home. Ann Intern Med 122:438, 1995

3. Stoddart H, Donovan J, Whitley E, et al: Urinary incontinence in older people in the community: a neglected problem? Br J Gen Pract 51:548, 2001

4. Walter S, Olesen KP: Urinary incontinence and genital prolapse in the female: clinical, urodynamic and radiological examinations. Br J Obstet Gynaecol 89:393, 1982

5. Duong TH, Korn AP: A comparison of urinary incontinence among African American, Asian, Hispanic, and white women. Am J Obstet Gynecol 184:1083, 2001

6. Tchou DC, Adams C, Varner RE, et al: Pelvic-floor musculature exercises in treatment of anatomical urinary stress incontinence. Phys Ther 68:652, 1988

7. Bo K, Talseth T: Long-term effect of pelvic floor muscle exercise 5 years after cessation of organized training. Obstet Gynecol 87:261, 1996

8. Peattie AB, Plevnik S, Stanton SL: Vaginal cones: a conservative method of treating genuine stress incontinence. Br J Obstet Gynecol 95:1049, 1988

9. Fantl JA, Bump RC, Robinson D, et al: Efficacy of estrogen supplementation in the treatment of urinary incontinence. Obstet Gynecol 88:745, 1996

10. Grady D, Brown JS, Vittinghoff E, et al: Postmenopausal hormones and incontinence: the heart and estrogen/progestin replacement study. Obstet Gynecol 97:116, 2001

11. Ouslander JG, Greendale GA, Uman G, et al: Effects of oral estrogen and progestin on the lower urinary tract among female nursing home residents. J Am Geriatr 49:803, 2001

12. Ishiko O, Hirai K, Sumi T, et al: Hormone replacement therapy plus pelvic floor muscle exercise for postmenopausal stress incontinence: a randomized, controlled trial. J Reprod Med 46:213, 2001

13. Lin HH, Sheu BC, Lo MC, et al: Comparison of treatment outcomes for imipramine for female genuine stress incontinence. Br J Obstet Gynecol 106:1089, 1999

14. Sultana CJ, Campbell JW, Pisanelli WS, et al: Morbidity and mortality of incontinence surgery in elderly women: an analysis of Medicare data. Am J Obstet Gynecol 176:344, 1997

15. Leach GE, Dmochowski RR, Appell RA, et al: Female Stress Urinary Incontinence Clinical Guidelines Panel summary report on surgical management of female stress urinary incontinence. J Urol 158:875, 1997

16. Bezerra CA, Bruschini H: Suburethral sling operations for urinary incontinence in women (Cochrane Review). Cochrane Database Syst Rev 3:CD001754, 2001

17. Ulmsten U, Johnson P, Rezapour M: A three year follow up of tension free vaginal tape for surgical treatment of female stress urinary incontinence. Br J Obstet Gynecol 106:345, 1999

18. Abrams P, Blaivas JG, Stanton SL, et al: The standardization of terminology of lower urinary tract function. Scan J Urol Nephrol Suppl 114:5, 1988

19. Kinder RB, Mundy AR: Pathophysiology of idiopathic detrusor instability and detrusor hyperreflexia: an in vivo study of human detrusor muscle. Br J Urol 60:509, 1987

20. Blaivas JG, Bhimani G, Labib KB: Vesicourethral dysfunction in multiple sclerosis. J Urol 122:342, 1979

21. Millard RJ, Oldenburg BF: The symptomatic, urodynamic and psychodynamic results of bladder re-education programs. J Urol 130:715, 1983

22. Burgio KL, Engel BT: Biofeedback-assisted behavioral training for elderly men and women. J Am Geriatr Soc 38:338, 1990

23. Burgio KL, Locher JL, Goode PS, et al: Behavioral versus drug treatment for urge urinary incontinence in older women: a randomized controlled trial JAMA 280:1995, 1998

24. Anderson RU, Mobley D, Blank B, et al: Once-daily controlled versus immediate release oxybutynin chloride for urge urinary incontinence. J Urol 161:1809, 1999

25. Prospective randomized controlled trial of extended-release oxybutynin chloride and tolterodine tartrate in the treatment of overactive bladder: results of the OBJECT Study. Overactive Bladder: Judging Effective Control and Treatment Study Group. Mayo Clin Proc 76:358, 2001

26. Abrams P, Freeman R, Anderstrom C, et al: Tolterodine, a new antimuscarinic agent: as effective but better tolerated than oxybutynin in patients with an overactive bladder. Br J Urology 81:801, 1998

27. Serels S, Stein M: Prospective study comparing hyoscyamine, doxazosin, and combination therapy for the treatment of urgency and frequency in women. Neurourol Urodyn 17:31, 1998

28. Nataluk EA, Assimos DG, Kroovand RL: Collagen injections for treatment of urinary incontinence secondary to intrinsic sphincter deficiency. J Endourol 9:403, 1995

29. Lightner D, Calvosa C, Andersen R, et al: A new injectable bulking agent for treatment of stress urinary incontinence: results of a multicenter, randomized, controlled, double-blind study of Durasphere. Urology 58:12, 2001

30. Herschorn S: Current status of injectable agents for female stress urinary incontinence. Can J Urol 8:1281, 2001

31. Resnick NM: Geriatric incontinence. Urol Clin North Am 23:55, 1976

Acknowledgment

Figures 1 through 3   Tom Moore.

HEMATOLOGY

86 Approach to Hematologic Disorders

David C. Dale, M.D.

The circulating blood sustains life by transporting oxygen and essential nutrients, removing waste, and delivering the humoral and cellular factors necessary for host defenses. Platelets and coagulation factors, together with vascular endothelial cells, maintain the integrity of the circulatory compartment. Hematology deals with the normal functions and disorders of the formed elements in the blood (i.e., erythrocytes, leukocytes, and platelets) and the plasma factors governing hemostasis. Some hematologic disorders such as anemia, leukocytosis, and internal bleeding are quite common, usually occurring secondary to infectious, inflammatory, nutritional, and malignant diseases. Other disorders, including the hematologic malignancies, are far less common. This chapter presents the general principles for understanding the hematopoietic system [*see other chapters under Hematology for a more detailed description of pathophysiology of hematologic diseases and their treatment*].

Hematopoiesis

Hematopoiesis begins in the fetal yolk sac and later occurs predominantly in the liver and the spleen. Recent studies demonstrate that islands of hematopoiesis develop in these tissues from hemangioblasts, which are the common progenitors for both hematopoietic and endothelial cells.[1] These islands then involute as the marrow becomes the primary site for blood cell formation by the seventh month of fetal development.[2] Barring serious damage, such as that which occurs with myelofibrosis or radiation injury, the bone marrow remains the site of blood cell formation throughout the rest of life. In childhood, there is active hematopoiesis in the marrow spaces of the central axial skeleton (i.e., ribs, vertebrae, and pelvis) and the extremities, extending to the wrists, ankles, and the calvaria. With normal growth and development, hematopoiesis gradually withdraws from the periphery. This change is reversible, however; distal marrow extension can result from intensive stimulation, as occurs with severe hemolytic anemias, long-term administration of hematopoietic growth factors, and hematologic malignancies. The term medullary hematopoiesis refers to the production of blood cells in the bone marrow; the term extramedullary hematopoiesis indicates blood cell production outside the marrow in the spleen, liver, and other locations.

ORGANIZATION OF HEMATOPOIETIC TISSUES

In its normal state, the medullary space in which hematopoietic cells develop contains, normally, many adipocytes and has a rich vascular supply [*see Figure 1*].[3] Vascular endothelial cells, marrow fibroblasts, and stromal cells are important sources of the matrix proteins that provide structure to the marrow space; these cells also produce the hematopoietic growth factors and chemokines that regulate blood cell production.[4,5] The vascular endothelial cells also form an important barrier that keeps immature cells in the marrow and permits mature hematopoietic elements to enter the blood. The abundant adipocytes may influence hematopoiesis by serving as a localized energy source, by synthesizing growth factors, and by affecting the metabolism of androgens and estrogens.[6] Marrow macrophages remove effete or apoptotic cells and clear the blood of foreign materials when it enters the marrow. Osteo-

blasts and osteoclasts maintain and remodel the surrounding cancellous bone and the calcified lattice, which crisscrosses the marrow space.[3]

The thymus, lymph nodes, mucosa-associated lymphatic tissues (MALT), and the spleen have multiple hematopoietic functions. Early in development, they are major sites of hematopoiesis. In adulthood, they are principally sites of lymphocyte development, processing of antigens, development of effector T cells, and antibody production. In leukemia and the myeloproliferative disorders, the size and cellular architecture of these tissues are deranged, leading to many of the clinical manifestations of these two disorders.

Hematopoietic Stem Cells

All cells of the hematopoietic system are derived from common precursor cells, the hematopoietic stem cells.[7] These cells are difficult to identify, in part because they normally represent only about 0.05% of marrow cells. Through self-renewal, this population is maintained at a constant level.[8] Through the use of monoclonal antibodies that recognize specific cell surface molecules expressed selectively on developing hematopoietic cells and other specialized techniques, the stem cells can now be separated from other marrow cells. With these methods, very primitive hematopoietic stem cells have been found to be positive for c-kit and thy-1 but negative for CD34, CD38, CD33, and HLA-DR.[8] For clinical purposes, CD34+ progenitor cell populations, which contain stem cells and some more mature cells, are often used for hematopoietic stem cell transplantation[9] [*see Chapter 96*].

Stem cells give rise to daughter cells, which undergo irreversible commitment to differentiation along various hematopoietic cell lineages [*see Figure 2*].[10] Many aspects of the earliest steps in this differentiation process are not well understood. With lineage commitment, however, differentiation, maturation, and release of cells to the blood come under the control of well-defined hematopoietic growth factors. These growth factors have overlapping activities for the early phases of differentiation.[11] Later in development, some growth factors are lineage specific, meaning that they govern the maturation and deployment of single lineages. Erythropoietin (EPO), thrombopoietin (TPO), granulocyte colony-stimulating factor (G-CSF), and macrophage colony-stimulating factor (M-CSF) are the best-characterized lineage-specific factors.

Hematopoietic Growth Factors

The hematopoietic growth factors, also referred to as hematopoietic cytokines, are a family of glycoproteins produced in the bone marrow by endothelial cells, stromal cells, fibroblasts, macrophages, and lymphocytes; they are also produced at distant sites, from which they are transported to the marrow through the blood [*see Table 1*]. The naming of these factors is somewhat confusing. Erythropoietin and thrombopoietin derive part of their names from the Greek word *poiesis,* meaning "to make." The colony-stimulating factors were first recognized because of their capacity to stimulate early hematopoietic cells to grow into clusters and large colonies in tissue culture systems. The term interleukin denotes factors that are produced by leukocytes and that affect other leukocytes. This is a large family of factors that predomi-

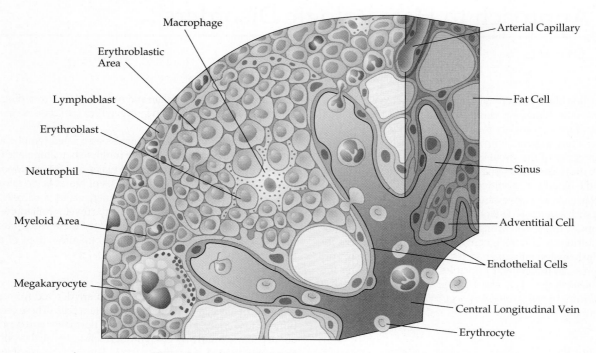

Macrophage

Erythroblastic Area

Lymphoblast

Erythroblast

Neutrophil

Myeloid Area

Megakaryocyte

Arterial Capillary

Fat Cell

Sinus

Adventitial Cell

Endothelial Cells

Central Longitudinal Vein

Erythrocyte

Figure 1   **The architecture of the bone marrow showing the various types of cells.**

nantly governs lymphocytopoiesis, but many members also have broad effects on other lineages. The discovery of new growth factors and of the biologic consequences of deficiencies or excesses of these factors continues to evolve rapidly.

Hematopoietic cells have distinctive patterns of expression of growth factor receptors, and the patterns evolve as the cells differentiate [*see Figure 2*].[11,12] Each growth factor binds only to its specific receptor.[12] It is now known that some growth factors share components of the receptor (e.g., interleukin-3 [IL-3], IL-5, and granulocyte-macrophage colony-stimulating factor [GM-CSF] share a common β chain of their receptor); specificity comes from other unique or private components of the receptor. Binding of the ligand to the receptor leads to a conformational change, activation of intracellular kinases, and, ultimately, the triggering of cell proliferation.[13,14] For some growth factors, these pathways are well defined; for others, the pathways are still unclear [*see Figure 3*].

Hematopoietic growth factors not only stimulate cell proliferation but also prolong cell survival; that is, they have anti-apoptotic effects.[15] For some lineages, such as neutrophils and monocytes, growth factor receptors occur on fully mature cells; exposure of these cells to the factors primes the cells for an enhanced responsiveness to bacteria or other stimulators of their metabolic activity. Thus, for cells of the neutrophil lineage, the growth factors G-CSF and GM-CSF can stimulate early hematopoietic cell proliferation, increase the number of cells produced by the marrow, prolong the life span of these cells, and augment cell functions.[16]

Erythropoietin

The peritubular interstitial cells located in the inner cortex and outer medulla of the kidney are the primary site for erythropoietin production.[17] In response to hypoxia, transcription of the erythropoietin gene in these cells increases, resulting in increased secretion of erythropoietin. The protein is then transported through the blood to the marrow to stimulate erythropoiesis. With renal failure, erythropoietin production is severely impaired. In infections and many chronic inflammatory conditions, the erythropoietin response is blunted, and erythropoietin levels are low.[18]

Erythropoietin is a glycosylated protein that modulates erythropoiesis by affecting several steps in red cell development. The most primitive identifiable erythroid cells, the burst-forming unit–erythroid cells (BFU-E), are relatively insensitive to erythropoietin. More mature cells, the colony-forming unit–erythroid cells (CFU-E), are very sensitive. Erythropoietin treatment prolongs survival of erythroid precursors, shortens the time between cell divisions, and increases the number of cells produced from individual precursors.[19]

Erythropoietin can be administered intravenously or subcutaneously for the treatment of anemia caused by inadequate endogenous production of erythropoietin.[20] Treatment is maximally effective when the marrow has a generous supply of iron and other nutrients, such as cobalamin and folic acid. For patients with renal failure, who have very low erythropoietin levels, the starting dosage is 50 to 100 units S.C. three times a week. The most easily monitored immediate effect of increased endogenous or exogenous erythropoietin is an increase in the blood reticulocyte count. Normally, as red cell precursors mature, the cells extrude their nucleus at the normal blast stage. The resulting reticulocytes, identified by the supravital stain of their residual ribosomes, persist for about 3 days in the marrow and 1 day in the blood. Erythropoietin shortens the transit time through the marrow, leading to an increase in the number and proportion of blood reticulocytes within a few days.

In some conditions, particularly chronic inflammatory disease, the effectiveness of erythropoietin can be predicted from measurement of the serum erythropoietin level by immunoassay.[17,18] It is often cost-effective to measure the level before initiating treatment in patients with anemia attributable to suppressed erythropoietin production, such as patients with HIV infection, cancer, and chronic inflammatory diseases.[21] Several studies have shown

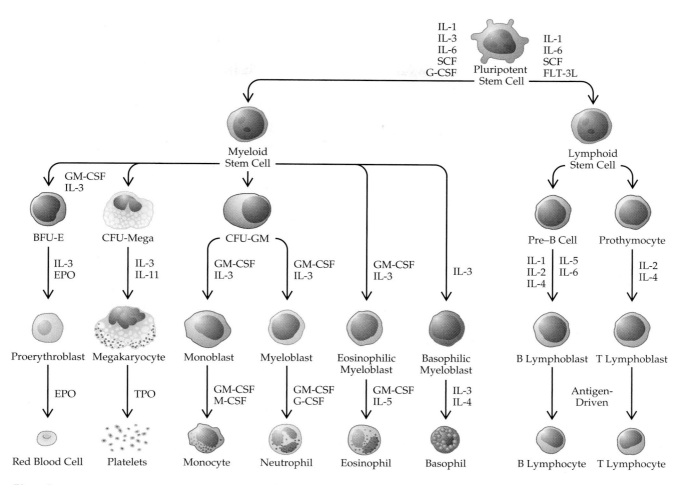

Figure 2   **The pattern for development of various types of blood cells in the bone marrow. (BFU-E—burst-forming unit–erythroid; CFU-GM— colony-forming unit–granulocyte-macrophage; CFU-mega—colony-forming unit–megakaryocyte; EPO—erythropoietin; EPOR—surface compo- nent of the erythropoietin receptor; FLT-3L—fms-like tyrosine kinase 3 ligand; G-CSF—granulocyte colony-stimulating factor; GM-CSF—granu- locyte-macrophage colony-stimulating factor; IL—interleukin; M-CSF—macrophage colony-stimulating factor; TPO—thrombopoietin; SCF—stem cell factor)**

that erythropoietin treatment decreases the severity of anemia and improves the quality of life for these patients.[22]

Thrombopoietin

The development of megakaryocytes from hematopoietic stem cells and the level of platelets in the blood are governed by thrombopoietin.[23] Thrombopoietin is produced primarily by the liver and is similar to erythropoietin in structure. Plasma throm- bopoietin levels are inversely related to the blood platelet count.[24] Deficiencies of thrombopoietin cause thrombocytopenia, and ex- cesses in thrombopoietin cause thrombocytosis. Recombinant human thrombopoietin is being studied for use in the treatment of thrombocytopenia of diverse causes; thrombopoietin is not yet approved for clinical use.

Granulocyte Colony-Stimulating Factor

G-CSF is a glycosylated protein produced by monocytes, mac- rophages, fibroblasts, stromal cells, and endothelial cells through- out the body.[25] It stimulates the growth and differentiation of neu- trophils both in vitro and in vivo. G-CSF levels are normally very low or undetectable but increase with bacterial infections or after administration of bacterial endotoxin.[16] G-CSF (the synthesized form is known as filgrastim or lenograstim) administration caus-

es a dose-dependent increase in the blood neutrophil count in healthy persons. Studies in animals have shown that G-CSF defi- ciency causes neutropenia.[26] As with erythropoietin, administra- tion of G-CSF leads to an acceleration in the development of neu- trophils in the bone marrow, with the neutrophils shifting at an earlier stage than normal from the marrow to the blood.[27]

G-CSF is approved for treatment of neutropenia after cancer chemotherapy, for acceleration of neutrophil recovery after bone marrow transplantation, for mobilization of hematopoietic pro- genitor cells from the marrow to the blood in hematopoietic trans- plantation, and for treatment of severe chronic neutropenia. The usual dosage is 5 µg/kg S.C. daily, but higher doses are used to mobilize progenitor cells, and lower doses are used for long-term treatment of neutropenia. Side effects are principally musculo- skeletal pain and headaches during the period of rapid marrow expansion soon after therapy is initiated. Other side effects are uncommon.

Granulocyte-Macrophage Colony-Stimulating Factor

GM-CSF is a glycosylated protein produced by many types of cells, including T cells.[28] GM-CSF stimulates formation of neutro- phils, monocytes, and eosinophils and may also enhance the growth of early cells of other lineages. In contrast to G-CSF, GM-

CSF levels generally do not increase with infections or acute inflammatory conditions,[29] and neutropenia does not result from deficiencies of GM-CSF.[30] The marrow effects of G-CSF and GM-CSF are similar, but GM-CSF is less potent in elevating the blood neutrophil count.[31] GM-CSF (the synthesized form is known as sargramostim or molgramostim) is approved in the United States for acceleration of marrow recovery after bone marrow transplantation or chemotherapy and for mobilization of progenitor cells from the marrow. The usual dosage is 250 µg/m²/day S.C. Its side effects include bone and musculoskeletal pain, myalgias, and injection-site reactions.

Interleukin-11

IL-11 (oprelvekin) is a pleiotropic cytokine that is expressed by and active in many tissues.[32] IL-11 acts synergistically with other growth factors, including thrombopoietin, to stimulate megakaryocyte development and platelet formation. It is approved for use in the prevention of severe thrombocytopenia and for patients who need platelet transfusions after chemotherapy. The usual dosage is 50 µg/kg/day S.C. Its side effects include edema, tachycardia, and dyspnea.

Other Growth Factors

Several other hematopoietic growth factors have potential clinical uses. IL-3 acts at an early phase in hematopoiesis to stimulate cell proliferation but has relatively little effect on peripheral counts. IL-3 has been molecularly coupled to other growth factors, including GM-CSF, G-CSF, and TPO, to produce hybrid molecules

Table 1   Hematopoietic Growth Factors

Factor	Other Names	Cell Source	Chromosome Location	Function
EPO	Erythropoietin	Juxtaglomerular cells	7q	Stimulates erythrocyte formation and release from marrow
TPO	Thrombopoietin; megakaryocyte growth and development factor (MGDF)	Hepatocytes, renal and endothelial cells, fibroblasts	3q27	Stimulates megakaryocyte proliferation and platelet formation
G-CSF	Granulocyte colony-stimulating factor; filgrastim; lenograstim	Endothelial cells, monocytes, fibroblasts	17q11.2-q21	Stimulates formation and function of neutrophils
GM-CSF	Granulocyte-macrophage colony-stimulating factor	T cells, monocytes, fibroblasts	5q23-q31	Stimulates formation and function of neutrophils, monocytes, and eosinophils
M-CSF	Macrophage colony-stimulating factor; colony stimulating factor–1 (CSF-1)	Endothelial cells, macrophages, fibroblasts	5q33.1	Stimulates monocyte formation and function
IL-1α and IL-1β	Interleukin-1α and -1β, endogenous pyrogen hemopoietin-1	Monocytes, keratinocytes, endothelial cells	2q13	Proliferation of T cells, B cells, and other cells; induces fever and catabolism
IL-2	T cell growth factor	T cells (CD4⁺, CD8⁺), large granular lymphocytes (natural killer, or NK, cells)	4q	T cell proliferation, antitumor and antimicrobial effects
IL-3	Multi–colony stimulating factor; mast cell growth factor	Activated T cells; large granular lymphocytes (NK cells)	5q23-q31	Proliferation of early hematopoietic cells
IL-4	B cell growth factor; T cell growth factor II; mast cell growth factor II	T cells	5q23-q31	Proliferation of B cells and T cells; enhances cytotoxic activities
IL-5	Eosinophil differentiation factor; eosinophil colony-stimulating factor	T cells	5q23.3-q32	Stimulates eosinophil formation; stimulates T cell and B cell functions
IL-6	B cell stimulatory factor II; hepatocyte stimulatory factor	Monocytes, tumor cells, B cells and T cells, fibroblasts, endothelial cells	7p	Stimulates and inhibits cell growth; promotes B cell differentiation
IL-7	Lymphopoietin 1; pre–B cell growth factor	Lymphoid tissues and cell lines	8q12-q13	Growth factor for B cells and T cells
IL-11	Plasmacytoma stimulating factor	Fibroblasts, trophoblasts, cancer cell lines	19q13.3-q13.4	Stimulates proliferation of early hematopoietic cells; induces acute-phase protein synthesis
IL-12	Natural killer cell stimulating factor	Macrophages, B cells	5q31-q33; 3p12-q13.2	Stimulates T cell expansion and interferon-gamma; synergistically promotes early hematopoietic cell proliferation
LIF	Leukemia inhibitory factor	Monocytes and lymphocytes; stomal cells	22q	Stimulates hematopoietic cell differentiation
SCF	Stem cell factor; kit ligand; steel factor	Endothelial cells; hepatocytes	4q11-q20	Stimulates proliferation of early hematopoietic cells and mast cells
FLT-3 ligand	fms-like tyrosine kinase 3; STK-1	T cells, stromal cells, and fibroblasts	19q13.3	Stimulates early hematopoietic cell differentiation; increases blood dendrite cells

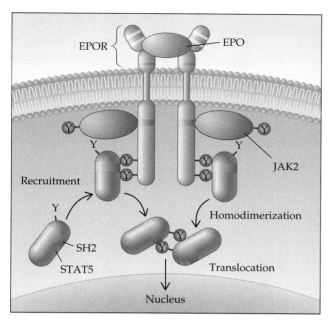

Figure 3   **A model of how hematopoietic growth factors interact with their receptors to initiate cell proliferation. (EPO—erythropoietin; JAK2—Janus kinase 2; SH2—Src homology 2; STAT5—signal transducer and activator of transcription 5)**

that are under investigation. Stem cell factor (SCF)[33,34] and fms-like tyrosine kinase 3 (FLT-3) ligand[35] are other early-acting factors under investigation. M-CSF is a selective factor for monocytes and macrophage formation.[36,37] IL-5 is a similar selective factor for the generation of eosinophils.[38]

It is presumed that normally, hematopoietic cell formation is governed by combinations of factors, released in a cascade, that closely coordinate the development of these cells. The details of how this process occurs, however, are not yet clear. Numerous laboratory and clinical studies have investigated combinations of factors, but the therapeutic benefit of using multiple growth factors is not yet proved.

DYNAMICS OF HEMATOPOIESIS

In the marrow, blood cells develop in two phases, the proliferative and the maturational phases. During cell proliferation, the precursors of blood cells normally undergo cell division at intervals of about 18 to 24 hours. In the maturational phase, cell division ceases, but final features are added before the cells enter the blood. During this phase, erythrocytes normally lose all their nuclear material, acquire their biconcave shape, and develop their final content of enzymes necessary for maintaining the biconcave shape and resisting destruction by oxidative stress. Normally, it takes 7 to 10 days for erythrocytes to develop from their early precursors, but this process can be accelerated by erythropoietin therapy.[39]

Neutrophils acquire most of their granules (known as the primary, secondary, and tertiary granules), which are necessary for their microbicidal activities, during the proliferative phase.[40] During maturation, their nuclear chromatin condenses, the glycogen content of the cytoplasm increases, and the surface properties governing the circulation, adherence, and migration to tissues are added. Neutrophils reach a fully mature state in the marrow before they are released into the blood. These mature marrow cells are called the marrow neutrophil reserve. Quantitatively, this neu-

trophil pool is substantially larger—probably five to 10 times larger—than the total circulating supply of neutrophils. Normally, it takes 10 to 14 days for blood neutrophils to develop from early precursors, but this process is accelerated in the presence of infections and by treatment with G-CSF or GM-CSF [*see Chapter 91*].

Platelets form from the cytoplasm of megakaryocytes, which are also derived from hematopoietic stem cells.[23] Megakaryocytes undergo reduplication of their nuclear chromatin without cell division, which results in the production of extremely large cells. Platelets form from the breaking apart of the cytoplasm of the fully mature megakaryocytes. When marrow damage occurs from chemotherapeutic agents and after hematopoietic transplantation, the megakaryocytes are often the slowest cells to recover, and thrombocytopenia is often the last cytopenia to resolve.

There are important differences in the dynamics or kinetics of erythrocytes, platelets, and leukocytes in the blood. For instance, neutrophils have a blood half-life of only 6 to 8 hours; essentially, a new blood population of neutrophils is formed every 24 hours.[40] Erythrocytes last the longest by far: the normal life span is about 100 days.[39] These differences partially account for why neutrophils and their precursors are the predominant marrow cells, whereas in the blood, erythrocytes far outnumber neutrophils. Similarly, the short half-life and high turnover rate of neutrophils account for why neutropenia is the most frequent hematologic consequence when bone marrow is damaged by drugs or radiation. Finally, transfusion of erythrocytes and platelets is feasible because of their relatively long life span, whereas the short life span of neutrophils has greatly impeded efforts to develop neutrophil transfusion therapy.

Clinical Manifestations of Hematologic Disorders

The symptoms and signs of hematologic diseases are also common manifestations of diseases that primarily affect other organ systems. Because of its simplicity and low cost, a complete blood cell count (CBC) enables the clinician to easily consider whether the hematopoietic system is involved. The following signs and symptoms are frequent indications for performing a CBC.

Weakness, fatigue, and pallor   Weakness, fatigue, and pallor are common complaints of patients with anemia of recent onset, such as anemia caused by recent blood loss or acute hemolysis. Anemia that develops gradually, particularly in inactive persons, may cause only fatigue, or it may go unnoticed. Pallor is recognized by examining the conjunctiva, mucous membranes, nail beds, and palmar creases.

Pain   Pain, particularly bone pain, is an important marker of hematologic disease. It occurs with marrow expansion in myeloproliferative disorders, particularly in acute leukemia and other diseases in which there is rapid cell growth in the marrow, such as the lymphomas, myeloma, or invading carcinomas. Symptoms caused by these disorders are mimicked by marrow expansion in response to treatment with hematopoietic growth factors. In sickle cell disease, severe bone pain and pain in many other tissues occur with vascular obstruction and infarction caused by blockage of blood flow by the buildup of abnormal cells.

Fatigue, pharyngitis, and fever   Fatigue, pharyngitis, and fever are a frequently observed sequence in patients with acutely developing neutropenia, occurring as an idiosyncratic or toxic reaction to many drugs. In cases of severe neutropenia, cough and respiratory symptoms, perianal pain and tenderness, or acute abdominal pain often occurs and necessitates immediate medical assessment.

Mouth ulcers, gingivitis, and cervical adenopathy Mouth ulcers, gingivitis, and cervical adenopathy are common problems of patients with chronic neutropenia. Gingivitis is a serious problem often leading to periodontal disease and tooth loss.

Lymphadenopathy and splenomegaly Lymphadenopathy and splenomegaly are common presentations of infectious, inflammatory, and hematologic diseases, particularly the lymphomas and leukemias. These findings sometimes occur without symptoms, but often, fatigue and intermittent fever (i.e., Pel-Ebstein fever) occur. In contrast to acute infectious diseases leading to lymphadenopathy, in most hematologic disorders the lymph nodes and spleen are nontender, with a soft to rubbery consistency.

Bleeding Bleeding occurs as a consequence of thrombocytopenia, deficiencies of coagulation factors, or both. Thrombocytopenia usually presents as petechial bleeding that is first observed in the lower extremities. Coagulation factor deficiencies more often cause bleeding into the gastrointestinal tract or joints. Intracranial bleeding, however, can occur with a deficiency of platelets or coagulation factors and can be catastrophic.

Thrombosis Thrombosis can be either venous or arterial. With venous thrombosis, swelling, tenderness, and pain beyond the obstruction usually occur, and embolization to the lungs is a frequent concern. Venous thrombosis usually occurs after inactivity or obstruction of venous flow or with imbalances of coagulation factors. On the other hand, arterial thrombosis usually occurs because of abnormalities of the arterial wall from atherosclerosis or acute vascular injury, as in thrombotic thrombocytopenic purpura, or from thrombocytosis in the myeloproliferative disorders.

Laboratory Evaluation

The following basic tests are widely used to diagnose hematologic disorders.

Complete blood cell counts CBCs are routinely performed in most laboratories through the use of an electronic particle counter, which determines the total white blood cell and platelet counts and calculates the hematocrit and hemoglobin from the erythrocyte count and the dimensions of the red cells. Abnormalities in the CBC are described in other Hematology chapters [*see also Appendix A*].

Peripheral blood smears Peripheral blood smears usually stain with Wright stain. When examined by light microscopy, they reveal the size and shape of blood cells, which allows an estimate to be made of the amount of hemoglobin in erythrocytes. Differential leukocyte counts, enumerating the number of neutrophils, monocytes, lymphocytes, eosinophils, and basophils, are made by manually counting cells on the blood smears or by using an automated cell counter [*see Appendix A*]. The morphology of the leukocytes often provides a clue for the diagnosis of leukemia and for recognizing some disorders of leukocytes that lead to susceptibility to infections [*see Chapter 91*].

Reticulocyte counts Reticulocyte counts are useful for evaluating the marrow response to anemia [*see Appendix A*]. Normally, during their first 24 to 36 hours in the circulation, young red cells contain residual ribosomal RNA, which precipitates with certain dyes such as methylene blue. An increase in the proportion or absolute number of reticulocytes occurs a few days after significant blood loss or in response to red blood cell destruction in hemolytic anemias. Low reticulocyte counts in chronic anemia suggest either an endogenous erythropoietin deficiency or a marrow abnormality.

Bone marrow examination Hematopoietic cells of the bone marrow can be removed by aspiration or by needle biopsy. In adults, the best site is the posterior iliac crest, with the patient in a prone position [*see Figure 4*]. Under special circumstances and in children, other sites can be used, such as the anterior iliac crest, the sternum, or the long bones. With local anesthesia and sterile technique, the patient experiences only transient pain. Bleeding or infection at the injection site is quite uncommon. The aspirate yields cells for morphologic examination, and differential counts reveal the ratio of myeloid cells to erythroid cells (M:E ratio) [*see Appendix A*]. A biopsy reveals the cellularity of the marrow at the site sampled. Biopsies are particularly useful for examination of the marrow for infiltrative cells (e.g., in lymphomas or carcinomas involving the marrow) and for diagnosing leukemia, charac-

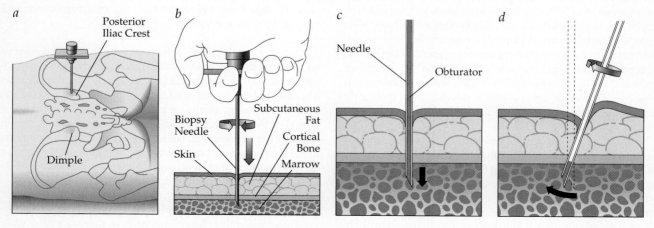

Figure 4 **Bone marrow aspirate and biopsy procedure. (*a*) The posterior iliac crest is the usual site for sampling; (*b*) the needle is placed through the skin to the marrow space; (*c*) the marrow sample is aspirated; and (*d*) the biopsy sample is carefully removed.**

terized by the marrow's being so densely packed with cells that none of the bone marrow can be aspirated. Biopsies take longer for interpretation because they must be decalcified and stained before examination.

Imaging Studies

Radionuclide scanning (e.g., using technetium-99m) reveals the extent of the hematopoietic tissue in the marrow because the phagocytic cells of the marrow take up the radiolabeled particles. Marrow scanning is sometimes used to determine the extensiveness of the hematopoietic tissue; more often, it is useful in determining whether there are localized areas of increased uptake resulting from infection or a malignancy that has metastasized to the marrow. Computed tomography and ultrasonography are useful in determining the size of lymph nodes and spleen, but they are not particularly useful for marrow examination. The marrow is seen well with magnetic resonance imaging. This technique is principally used to look for infiltrative processes in the marrow space, such as occur in malignancies and infections.

References

1. Robertson S, Kennedy M, Keller G: Hematopoietic commitment during embryogenesis. Ann NY Acad Sci 872:9, 1999
2. Tavassoli M: Embryonic and fetal hemopoiesis: an overview. Blood Cells 1:269, 1991
3. Verfaillie CM: Anatomy and physiology of hematopoiesis in hematology: Basic Principles and Practice, 3rd ed. Hoffman R, Benz EJ, Shattil SJ, et al, Eds. Churchill Livingstone, New York, 2000, p 139
4. Ogawa M, Matsunaga T: Humoral regulation of hematopoietic stem cells. Ann N Y Acad Sci 872:17, 1999
5. Broxmeyer HE, Kim CH: Regulation of hematopoiesis in a sea of chemokine family members with a plethora of redundant activities. Exp Hematol 27:1113, 1999
6. Gimble JM, Robinson CE, Wu X, et al: The function of adipocytes in the bone marrow stroma: an update. Bone 19:421, 1996
7. Weissman IL: Stem cells: units of development, units of regeneration, and units in evolution. Cell 100:157, 2000
8. Williams DA: Stem cell model of hematopoiesis. Hematology: Basic Principles and Practice, 3rd ed. Hoffman R, Benz EJ Jr, Shattil SJ, et al, Eds. Churchill Livingstone, New York, 2000, p 126
9. Civin CI, Almeida-Porada G, Lee MJ, et al: Sustained, retransplantable, multilineage engraftment of highly purified adult human bone marrow stem cells in vivo. Blood 88:4102, 1996
10. Metcalf D: Lineage commitment and maturation in hematopoietic cells: the case for extrinsic regulation. Blood 92:345, 1998
11. D'Andrea AD: Hematopoietic growth factors and the regulation of differentiative decisions. Curr Opin Cell Biol 6:804, 1994
12. Drachman JG, Kaushansky K: Structure and function of the cytokine receptor superfamily. Curr Opin Hematol 2:22, 1995
13. Avalos BR: Molecular analysis of the granulocyte colony-stimulating factor receptor. Blood 88:761, 1996
14. Dong F, Larner AC: Activation of Akt kinase by granulocyte colony-stimulating factor (G-CSF): evidence for the role of a tyrosine kinase activity distinct from the Janus kinases. Blood 95:1656, 2000
15. Yoshida Y, Anzai N, Kawabata H: Apoptosis in normal and neoplastic hematopoiesis. Crit Rev Oncol Hematol 22:1, 1996
16. Dale DC, Liles WC, Summer WR, et al: Review: granulocyte colony-stimulating factor—role and relationships in infectious disease. J Infect Dis 172:1061, 1995
17. Spivak JL: The biology and clinical applications of recombinant erythropoietin. Semin Oncol 25(3 suppl 7):7, 1998
18. Means RT Jr: Advances in the anemia of chronic disease. Int J Hematol 70:7, 1999
19. Spivak JL, Ferris DK, Fisher J, et al: Cell cycle–specific behavior of erythropoietin. Exp Hematol 24:141, 1996
20. Adamson JW, Eschbach JW: Erythropoietin for end-stage renal disease. N Engl J Med 339:625, 1998
21. Henry DH, Spivak JL: Clinical use of erythropoietin. Curr Opin Hematol 2:118, 1995
22. Cremieux PY, Finkelstein SN, Berndt ER, et al: Cost effectiveness, quality-adjusted life-years and supportive care: recombinant human erythropoietin as a treatment of cancer-associated anaemia. Pharmacoeconomics 16:459, 1999
23. Kaushansky K: Thrombopoietin. N Engl J Med 339:746, 1998
24. Verbeek W, Faulhaber M, Griesinger F, et al: Measurement of thrombopoietic levels: clinical and biological relationships. Curr Opin Hematol 7:143, 2000
25. Welte K, Gabrilove J, Bronchud MH, et al: Filgrastim (r-metHuG-CSF): the first 10 years. Blood 88:1907, 1996
26. Lieschke GJ, Grail D, Hodgson G, et al: Mice lacking granulocyte colony-stimulating factor have chronic neutropenia, granulocyte and macrophage progenitor cell deficiency, and impaired neutrophil mobilization. Blood 84:1737, 1994
27. Price TH, Chatta GS, Dale DC: Effect of recombinant granulocyte colony-stimulating factor on neutrophil kinetics in normal and elderly humans. Blood 88:335, 1996
28. Kwon EM, Sakamoto KM: The molecular mechanism of action of granulocyte-macrophage colony-stimulating factor. J Investig Med 44:442, 1996
29. Cebon J, Layton JE, Maher D, et al: Endogenous haemopoietic growth factors in neutropenia and infection. Br J Haematol 86:265, 1994
30. Stanley E, Lieschke GJ, Grail D, et al: Granulocyte/macrophage colony-stimulating factor–deficient mice show no major perturbation of hematopoiesis but develop a characteristic pulmonary pathology. Proc Natl Acad Sci USA 91:5592, 1994
31. Dale DC, Liles WC, Llewellyn C, et al: Effects of granulocyte-macrophage colony-stimulating factor (GM-CSF) on neutrophil kinetics and function in normal human volunteers. Am J Hematol 57:7, 1998
32. Du X, Williams DA: Interleukin-11: Review of molecular, cell biology, and clinical use. Blood 89:3897, 1997
33. McNiece IK, Briddell RA: Stem cell factor. J Leukoc Biol 58:14, 1995
34. Facon T, Harousseau JL, Maloisel F, et al: Stem cell factor in combination with filgrastim after chemotherapy improves peripheral blood progenitor cell yield and reduces apheresis requirements in multiple myeloma patients: a randomized, controlled trial. Blood 94:1218, 1999
35. Shurin MR, Esche C, Lotze MT: FLT3: receptor and ligand: biology and potential clinical application. Cytokine Growth Factor Rev 9:37, 1998
36. Bourette RP, Rohrschneider LR: Early events in M-CSF receptor signaling. Growth Factors 17:155, 2000
37. Kuhara T, Uchida K, Yamaguchi H: Therapeutic efficacy of human macrophage colony-stimulating factor, used alone and in combination with antifungal agents, in systemic Candida albicans infection. Antimicrob Agents Chemother 44:19, 2000
38. Gleich GJ: Mechanisms of eosinophil-associated inflammation. J Allergy Clin Immunol 105:651, 2000
39. Adamson J: Erythropoietin, iron metabolism, and red blood cell production. Semin Hematol 33:5, 1996
40. Skubitz KM: Neutrophilic leukocytes. Wintrobe's Clinical Hematology, 10th ed. Lee GR, Foerster J, Lukens J, et al, Eds. Lippincott Williams & Wilkins, Philadelphia, 1999, p 300

Acknowledgment

Figures 1 through 4   Seward Hung.

87 Red Blood Cell Function and Disorders of Iron Metabolism

Gary M. Brittenham, M.D.

Red Blood Cell Function

The primary functions of the red blood cell, or erythrocyte, are the transport of oxygen (O_2) from the lungs to peripheral tissues for utilization and the transport of carbon dioxide (CO_2) from tissues to the lungs for excretion.[1] The mature erythrocyte dedicates more than 95% of its intracellular protein, as hemoglobin, to this task. Hemoglobin, the oxygen transport molecule, binds oxygen molecules at the high oxygen tensions of the pulmonary alveoli and releases oxygen molecules at low oxygen tensions to peripheral tissues. Hemoglobin also acts as a carrier of nitric oxide (NO), a potent vasorelaxant that is released during arteriovenous transit, increasing blood flow and therefore O_2 transport in hypoxic tissue.[2,3]

The erythrocyte has a biconcave, discoid shape, which optimizes passage of the cell through the circulatory system and permits apposition of erythrocytes and parenchymal cells across the thin endothelium of capillaries, facilitating exchange of oxygen and carbon dioxide. Without erythrocytes, blood plasma can carry only about 5 ml O_2/L; with erythrocytes containing normal hemoglobin, whole blood can transport about 200 ml O_2/L.

STRUCTURE OF HEMOGLOBIN

Hemoglobin is composed of two pairs of dissimilar globin chains, with a heme group, ferroprotoporphyrin IX, bound covalently at a specific site in each chain.[4] The tetramer forms a spherical molecule with a molecular weight of 64,400. The major adult hemoglobin, hemoglobin A, is formed from a pair of α chains

(each containing 141 amino acids) and a pair of β chains (each containing 146 amino acids) and is written as $\alpha_2\beta_2$ [*see Figure 1*].

The configuration of hemoglobin shifts with oxygenation and deoxygenation. The deoxy configuration of hemoglobin is stabilized through the binding of protons and 2,3-diphosphoglycerate (2,3-DPG), a highly charged anion. With oxygenation of one subunit, these bonds are sequentially broken, and the resulting change in tertiary structure increases oxygen affinity of the remaining unliganded subunits. This phenomenon is termed cooperativity or heme-heme interaction.[5] As oxygen is released in the tissues, a reversal of this process decreases oxygen affinity, facilitating the release of oxygen. Conformational changes also contribute to the decrease in oxygen affinity with decreasing pH.[1,4] This effect, called the Bohr effect, is physiologically beneficial both in the lungs, where elimination of carbon dioxide raises the pH, enhancing oxygen affinity and uptake, and in tissues, where carbon dioxide uptake decreases the pH, lowering oxygen affinity and facilitating oxygen release.

FACTORS AFFECTING HEMOGLOBIN'S CAPACITY TO CARRY OXYGEN

Oxygen-Hemoglobin Dissociation Curve

The oxygen-hemoglobin dissociation curve [*see Figure 2*] is a plot of the equilibriums between oxygen and hemoglobin at various oxygen tensions (Po_2).[1,5] At sea level and at a partial pressure of oxygen of about 90 mm Hg, hemoglobin is 97% saturated in

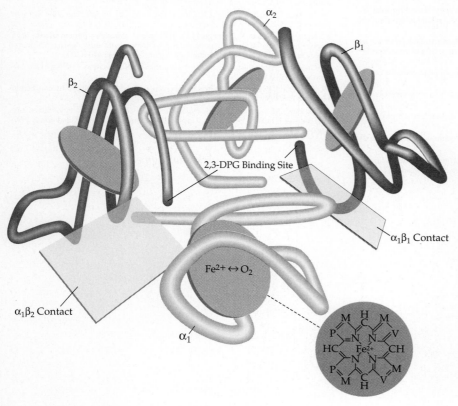

Figure 1 **A model of the hemoglobin molecule shows the relative alignment of the α chains (light gray) and β chains (dark gray). 2,3-Diphosphoglycerate (2,3-DPG), a glycolytic intermediate binds in the central cavity of the hemoglobin and stabilizes the deoxygenated form by cross-linking the β chains, thus reducing the oxygen affinity of hemoglobin. Note that the α and β chains are in contact at two points. On oxygenation, movement of the iron atom into the plane of the heme group (colored disks) apparently triggers other structural changes in the α and β subunits as the molecule assumes the oxygenated conformation. Sliding occurs at the $\alpha_1\beta_2$ interface, and the spacing between the two β chains is reduced in oxyhemoglobin. In detail showing the structure of heme, M is methyl, V is vinyl, and P is propionic acid.**

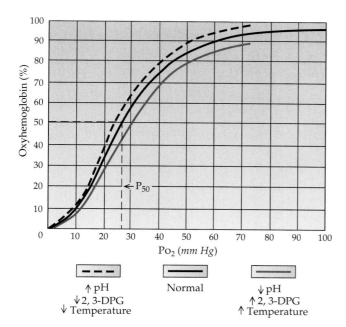

Figure 2 **The normal oxygen-hemoglobin dissociation curve (solid black line) is shifted by changes in temperature, pH, and the intracellular concentration of 2,3-DPG. P_{50} stands for 50% oxygen saturation; Po_2 stands for oxygen tension.**

the lungs. After unloading oxygen to tissues, at a Po_2 of about 40 mm Hg in mixed venous blood, the hemoglobin saturation is about 75%. The P_{50}, the partial pressure of oxygen at which hemoglobin is half saturated, is a useful measure of the oxygen affinity of hemoglobin: the higher the affinity, the lower the P_{50}. Under normal physiologic conditions (i.e., a temperature of 37° C [98.6° F], pH of 7.40, 2,3-DPG of 5 mmol/L, and carbon dioxide tension [Pco_2] of 40 mm Hg), the P_{50} of normal adult blood is 26 ± 1 mm Hg. The P_{50} is decreased (shifted to the left on the oxygen-hemoglobin dissociation curve) by increasing pH, decreasing 2,3-DPG, or decreasing temperature.[1,4]

Effects of 2,3-Diphosphoglycerate

The glycolytic intermediate 2,3-DPG, which is present in mature erythrocytes at approximately the same intracellular concentration as hemoglobin, is the most important allosteric regulator of oxygen affinity. With acute hypoxia, 2,3-DPG concentrations increase within hours, which shifts the oxygen-hemoglobin dissociation curve to the right. The increase in the 2,3-DPG concentration promotes delivery of oxygen to tissues but also impedes the acquisition of oxygen in the lungs. Short-term adaptation to hypoxic stress may be helped if the supply of oxygen is plentiful and the cardiopulmonary reserve robust. At high altitude, with the cardiovascular system unable to effectively meet increased circulatory demands, or in other pathologic circumstances, increased amounts of 2,3-DPG may be counterproductive.[1]

OXYGEN TRANSPORT

Several other physiologic factors function in an integrated manner to provide an adequate supply of oxygen, including blood volume, blood viscosity, pulmonary and cardiac function, and regional blood flow.[4] The concentration of circulating red blood cells depends on the production of erythropoietin by the kidney and the erythropoietic response of the erythroid marrow. Hemoglobin transport of nitric oxide, which binds to both heme iron and globin, helps match regional blood flow and oxygen requirements.[2,3] In peripheral tissues, for example, the erythrocyte releases nitric oxide, which relaxes the microvasculature, improves blood flow, and enhances oxygen delivery.[3]

CARBON DIOXIDE TRANSPORT

After delivering oxygen, hemoglobin binds carbon dioxide. Most of the carbon dioxide from tissue capillaries is transported to the lungs as bicarbonate, with about 10% carried as a carbamino complex reversibly bound to N-terminal amino groups of the globin chains.[4] Deoxyhemoglobin has a higher binding affinity for carbon dioxide than does oxyhemoglobin, facilitating unloading of carbon dioxide from tissues and pulmonary excretion.[1]

Iron Metabolism

Remarkable progress has been made in understanding disorders of iron metabolism and in improving the diagnosis and management of both iron deficiency and iron overload. Iron is used to transport and store oxygen, to carry electrons, to catalyze reactions in oxidative metabolism, and to sustain cellular growth and proliferation. With iron deficiency, the body is unable to produce sufficient amounts of heme, other iron-porphyrin complexes, metalloenzymes, and other iron-containing compounds to sustain normal functions. With iron overload, injurious reactions can occur that result in progressive and eventually lethal damage to vital organs.

MOLECULAR BASIS OF IRON METABOLISM

A variety of proteins are involved in the absorption, transport, utilization, and storage of iron [*see Figure 3*].

Transferrin and Apotransferrin

Transferrin carries iron to developing red cells and other cells in the body, especially growing or proliferating cells.[6] Apotransferrin, transferrin without attached iron, is a bilobular single-chain glycoprotein with two similar lobes at the N-terminus and the carboxyl(C)-terminus. Because a single ferric ion can be bound by each lobe, four forms of this molecule exist: (1) apotransferrin, (2) monoferric transferrin, with an atom of iron bound to the N-terminal lobe ($Fe_N Tf$), (3) monoferric transferrin, with an atom of iron bound to the C-terminal lobe ($Fe_C Tf$), and (4) diferric transferrin ($Fe_2 Tf$). In humans, the hepatocyte is the source of almost all the circulating apotransferrin. After delivering iron to cells, apotransferrin is promptly returned to the plasma to again function as an iron transporter.[6] The transferrin saturation is the proportion of the available iron-binding sites on transferrin that are occupied by iron atoms, expressed as a percentage.

Transferrin Receptor

Transferrin receptors are found on the surface membrane of all nucleated cells and provide the only physiologic route of entry for transferrin-bound iron. The number of transferrin receptors expressed on the cell surface is the predominant determinant of the iron supply for the cell. Accordingly, the number of transferrin receptors is highest in cells from the erythroid marrow, the liver, and the placenta.[7] The transferrin receptor helps free iron from transferrin for use in the cell.[8] Structurally, the transferrin receptor consists of two identical glycoprotein transmembrane subunits linked by a disulfide bond. Each subunit can bind a molecule of transferrin, so the transferrin receptor can accept two molecules of transferrin. The efficiency with which the transferrin receptor

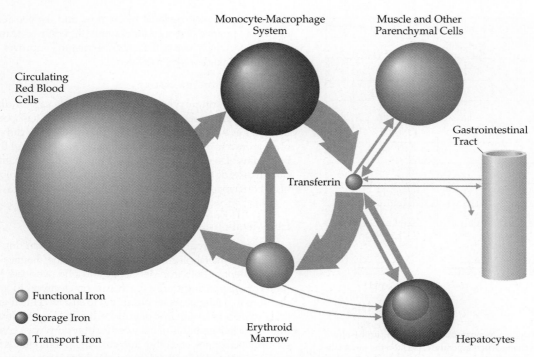

Circulating Red Blood Cells

Monocyte-Macrophage System

Muscle and Other Parenchymal Cells

Gastrointestinal Tract

Transferrin

○ Functional Iron

○ Storage Iron

○ Transport Iron

Erythroid Marrow

Hepatocytes

Figure 3 **Body iron supply and storage. The figure shows a schematic representation of the routes of iron movement in the adult. The area of each circle is proportional to the amount of iron contained in the compartment, and the width of each arrow is proportional to the daily flow of iron from one compartment to another. The major portion of iron is found in the erythron as hemoglobin iron (28 mg/kg in women; 32 mg/kg in men) dedicated to oxygen transport and delivery. Small amounts of erythron iron (< 1 mg/kg) are also present in heme and nonheme enzymes in developing red blood cells. The remainder of functional iron is found as myoglobin iron (4 mg/kg in women; 5 mg/kg in men) in muscle and as iron-containing and iron-dependent enzymes (1 to 2 mg/kg) throughout the cells of the body. Small amounts of iron are deposited within ferritin in erythroid cells, but most storage iron (5 to 6 mg/kg in women; 10 to 12 mg/kg in men) is held in reserve by hepatocytes and macrophages in the liver, bone marrow, spleen, and muscle. The small fraction of transport iron (about 0.2 mg/kg) in the plasma and extracellular fluid is bound to the protein transferrin, which carries iron to meet tissue needs throughout the body.[27]**

can deliver transferrin-bound iron depends on the iron content of transferrin. Thus, the dimeric receptor can provide entry to four atoms of iron if each transferrin is diferric or entry to two atoms of iron if each transferrin molecule is monoferric.

Ferritin

Almost all cells contain the protein ferritin, which functions both as a safe storage site for iron and as a readily accessible reserve for iron that has been acquired by the cell in excess of its immediate metabolic needs. As a consequence, the greatest amounts of ferritin are found in cells dedicated to iron storage (i.e., macrophages and hepatocytes) and in cells with the highest iron requirements for the synthesis of iron-containing compounds (i.e., developing erythroid cells). Hepatic ferritin has a half-life of about 60 hours.[9]

Apoferritin, which is ferritin without attached iron, is a spherical shell with a molecular weight of 440,000. Each molecule can store as many as 4,500 atoms of iron in the interior in a ferric hydroxyphosphate polynuclear core.[9] Apoferritin is composed of 24 oblong subunits that are designated as H (heavy) and L (light). Ferritin molecules with a greater proportion of H subunits seem to be more active in iron metabolism; ferritin molecules with a greater abundance of L subunits apparently are used for the longer-term storage of iron.[9]

Iron Regulatory Proteins

Iron regulatory proteins IRP-1 and IRP-2 permit iron to self-regulate its intracellular availability [*see Figure 4*]. They function by binding to iron-responsive elements (IREs) in messenger RNA (mRNA).[10,11] Functional IREs are found in the 3′ untranslated region (UTR) of mRNA for transferrin and in the 5′ untranslated region of the mRNAs for ferritin, the erythroid-specific form of δ-aminolevulinic acid synthase (eALAS), and mitochondrial aconitase.

Divalent Metal Transporter–1

DMT1,[12] previously called either the divalent cation transporter–1 (DCT1) or the natural resistance-associated macrophage protein–2 (Nramp2),[13] moves iron from the lumen of the gastrointestinal tract into the upper intestinal absorptive cell (enterocyte). This intestinal iron transporter, located on the apical surface of the duodenal enterocyte, is a plasma membrane glycoprotein with 12 putative membrane-spanning domains and a broad substrate range that includes not only Fe^{2+} but also Zn^{2+}, Mn^{2+}, Co^{2+}, Cd^{2+}, Cu^{2+}, Ni^{2+}, and Pb^{2+} [*see Figure 5*].[12] DMT1 is also present in the endosomal vesicles of hematopoietic precursors, macrophages, and other cells and mediates the passage of iron from transferrin within the endosome to the cytoplasm of the cell for utilization or storage.[14,15]

Hephaestin

Hephaestin is a newly identified transmembrane-bound ceruloplasmin homologue with a perinuclear localization within the intestinal enterocyte.[16] This multicopper protein seems to be necessary for the exit of iron from the intestinal enterocyte into the systemic circulation. The homology with ceruloplasmin suggests

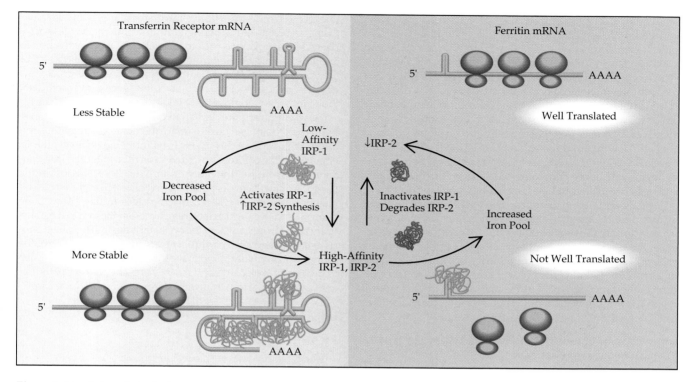

Figure 4 **Regulation of transferrin receptor and ferritin expression by the iron regulatory proteins IRP-1 and IRP-2.**

that hephaestin functions as an intracellular ferroxidase, but the exact mechanism of action has not been determined.

HFE

HFE, the protein that is defective in most patients with hereditary hemochromatosis (see below), is structurally similar to major histocompatibility complex (MHC) class I proteins.[17] The exact role of HFE in iron metabolism and the means whereby mutations in HFE result in the increased iron absorption found in hereditary hemochromatosis are still unknown, but a number of potentially relevant observations have been made. For example, newly synthesized HFE forms a 1:1 complex with β_2-microglobulin, which can in turn form a stable complex with the transferrin receptor and apparently decrease the affinity of the transferrin receptor for transferrin.[18-20] Also, HFE is abundantly expressed in the crypt cells of the duodenal mucosa,[21] and some evidence suggests that levels of HFE and DMT1 are reciprocally related in intestinal cells.[22]

Ceruloplasmin

Ceruloplasmin is an α_2-serum glycoprotein and multicopper oxidase that transports 95% of the copper found in plasma; each molecule can bind up to six atoms of copper. Persons with hereditary deficiency of ceruloplasmin develop a form of iron overload (see below),[23] indicating that it has a role in human iron metabolism, but the exact functions of this protein are unknown. Recent studies have suggested that ceruloplasmin increases transferrin-independent cellular iron uptake, a role that may partly depend on the ability of this protein to catalyze the conversion of ferrous to ferric iron.[24]

SFT (Stimulator of Fe Transport)

An apparent stimulator of iron transport, SFT has been identified. This protein seems to increase cellular iron uptake, but its exact role and interrelations with other proteins of iron metabolism are uncertain.[25]

CELLULAR IRON SUPPLY AND STORAGE

Transferrin, transferrin receptor, and ferritin function together in the provision of iron for the cell [*see Figure 4*].[8] Initially, two molecules of transferrin (monoferric or diferric) bind to a transferrin receptor on the cell surface; HFE may have a role in determining the affinity of the transferrin receptor for transferrin.[19] The iron-transferrin–transferrin receptor–HFE complex then aggregates with other complexes in a clathrin-coated pit, which is subsequently translocated to the interior of the cell as a coated vesi-

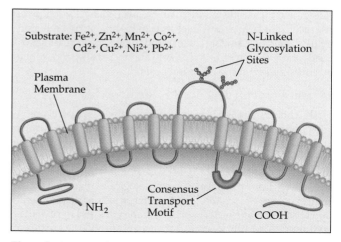

Figure 5 **The divalent metal transporter–1 (DMT1) is the intestinal iron transporter that moves iron from the intestinal lumen into the intestinal absorptive cell and from within the endosome in erythroid and other cells into the cytoplasm.**

cle. After the clathrin is stripped away, the uncoated vesicle fuses with other vesicles to form a multivesicular endosome. The endosome is then acidified to a pH of about 5.6 by a proton pump while traveling into the cell interior. With the fall in pH, the transferrin receptor undergoes conformational changes that help free iron from the monoferric or diferric transferrin.[8] The dissociated iron is then transported across the endosomal membrane via DMT1 for utilization in the synthesis of iron-containing compounds or for storage in cytoplasmic ferritin.[14] In the endosome at an acidic pH, the iron-free apotransferrin binds avidly to the transferrin receptor,[8] and the complex is then carried back to the cell membrane in the endosome. Conversely, the high-affinity binding between HFE and the transferrin receptor is lost at acidic pH levels.[20] Although some endosomes detour through the Golgi apparatus for resialylation and other overhaul, most endosomes proceed directly to the cell surface and fuse with the cell membrane. The apotransferrin–transferrin receptor complex is exposed to the plasma pH of 7.4, which results in the loss of affinity of apotransferrin for the transferrin receptor. The apotransferrin then reenters the circulating pool in the plasma, and the transferrin receptor, now apparently tightly bound by HFE, again becomes available for the binding of iron-bearing transferrin.

REGULATION OF CELLULAR IRON UPTAKE AND STORAGE BY THE IRON REGULATORY PROTEINS

In a coordinated manner, IRPs orchestrate the intracellular uptake and storage of iron by translational control of the synthesis of transferrin receptor and ferritin [see Figure 4].[10,11] IRP-1 and IRP-2 respond similarly to changes in intracellular iron availability, although they respond through different regulatory routes. Transferrin receptor synthesis is regulated by controlling the stability of cytoplasmic transferrin receptor mRNA, whereas ferritin synthesis is regulated by controlling translation of ferritin mRNA without changing the amount of ferritin mRNA in the cytoplasm. As a result, changes in the amount of the IRPs have opposite effects on the production of transferrin receptor and ferritin. If intracellular iron levels fall, the amount of high-affinity IRPs is increased. The increase in high-affinity IRPs bound to IREs in the 3' UTR of transferrin receptor mRNA stabilizes the mRNA, augmenting transferrin receptor protein production and increasing intracellular iron availability. The binding of IRPs to the 5' UTR of ferritin mRNA brings ferritin protein synthesis to a halt, thereby decreasing iron storage and increasing intracellular iron availability. By contrast, a rise in the intracellular iron level reduces the amount of high-affinity IRPs, thereby reducing cellular iron uptake by decreasing synthesis of transferrin receptor protein and increasing iron storage by enhancing synthesis of ferritin protein.

PATTERNS OF IRON BALANCE AND METABOLISM

The concentration of iron in the human body is carefully regulated and normally maintained at about 40 mg Fe/kg in women and about 50 mg Fe/kg in men.[26,27] Iron balance is the result of the difference between the amount of iron taken up by the body and the amount lost [see Figure 3]. Because humans are unable to excrete excess iron, iron balance is physiologically regulated by the control of iron absorption. The two major factors that influence iron absorption are the level of body iron stores and the extent of erythropoiesis.[28] If iron stores increase, absorption decreases; if stores decrease, absorption increases. Absorption increases with increased erythropoietic activity, especially with ineffective erythropoiesis. The predominant pathway of internal iron flux [see Figure 3] is a unidirectional flow from plasma transferrin to the erythron

(the erythron comprises the totality of circulating erythrocytes and their precursors in the bone marrow) to the monocyte-macrophage system and then back to transferrin.[26,27] Most of the iron in the body is located in the erythron. The erythron uses about 80% of the iron passing through the transferrin compartment each day. Under normal physiologic conditions, this process is very efficient; less than 0.05% of the total body iron is acquired or lost each day.

The erythron acquires iron from transferrin via a specific transferrin receptor located on the surface membrane of immature erythroid cells. Most of this iron is used for hemoglobin synthesis. Small quantities of iron are stored in ferritin, enter the iron-containing enzymes of immature erythroid cells, or are lost in the products of ineffective erythropoiesis. Senescent erythrocytes are phagocytized by specialized macrophages in the spleen, bone marrow, and liver, which then return most of the iron to the transferrin compartment, where the cycle starts again. The phagocytosis of flawed and aged erythrocytes accounts for almost all of the storage iron normally found in the macrophages of the liver, bone marrow, and spleen. By contrast, the parenchymal cells of the liver may either take iron from or give iron to plasma transferrin.

Iron Deficiency

DEFINITIONS

Iron is required not only to restore physiologic losses and meet the needs for growth and pregnancy but also to replace pathologic losses. Iron deficiency designates conditions in which the body iron is decreased because of a sustained increase in iron requirements over iron supply.[28]

The daily physiologic iron loss in the adult male is just under 1.0 mg/day; in normal menstruating women, iron loss is about 1.5 mg/day.[26] Sequential stages of decreases in body iron can be identified [see Figure 6 and Table 1]. A decrease in iron stores without a change in the amounts of functional iron compounds is designated as reduced iron stores. When iron stores are exhausted, patients may be described as having iron depletion. Further decrements in the level of body iron result in limited production of hemoglobin and other iron-containing functional compounds; this stage is termed iron-deficient erythropoiesis. Still further decreases in body iron produce iron deficiency anemia. Worldwide, iron deficiency is the most common cause of anemia.[29]

EPIDEMIOLOGY

Almost one third of the world population of about six billion is believed to be anemic, and iron deficiency anemia is thought to account for or contribute to the anemia in at least 500 million people.

ETIOLOGY

Blood loss is the most common cause of increased iron requirements that lead to iron deficiency [see Table 2].[29] In men and postmenopausal women, iron deficiency is almost always the result of gastrointestinal blood loss. In menstruating women, genitourinary blood loss often accounts for increased iron requirements. Oral contraceptives often decrease menstrual blood loss, but intrauterine devices tend to increase menstrual bleeding. Other causes of genitourinary bleeding and respiratory tract bleeding can also increase iron requirements [see Table 2]. For blood donors, each donation results in the loss of 200 to 250 mg of iron. During periods of growth in infancy, childhood, and adolescence, iron requirements may outstrip the supply of iron available from diet and stores.[30] Pregnancy increases the need for iron and, without supplemental iron, causes the net loss of the equivalent of about 1,200

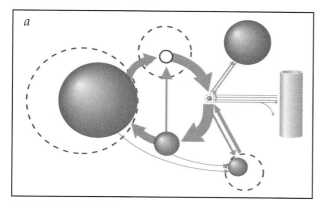

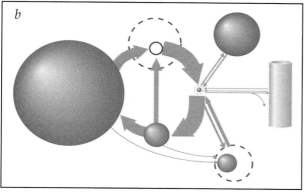

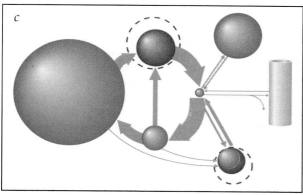

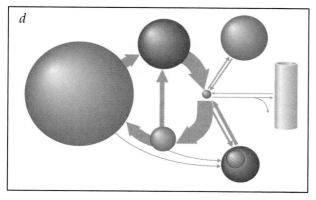

Figure 6 Continuum of changes in iron stores and distribution of iron in the presence of increased or decreased body iron content. The patterns shown are those developing in the absence of complicating factors, such as infection, inflammation, liver disease, malignancy, ascorbate deficiency, and other disorders. [*See Figure 3 for identification of the iron compartments.*] (*a*) Iron deficiency anemia. (*b*) Iron stores depletion. (*c*) Reduced iron stores. (*d*) Normal iron stores.

to 1,500 ml of blood.[30] After delivery, breast-feeding increases iron requirements by about 0.5 to 1.0 mg a day.

An insufficient supply of iron may contribute to the development of iron deficiency. In infants and women with high iron requirements, diets containing inadequate amounts of bioavailable iron may increase the risk of iron deficiency. For older children, men, and postmenopausal women, a poor supply of dietary iron is almost never the only factor responsible for iron deficiency; therefore, other etiologic factors must be sought, especially blood loss. Impaired absorption of iron is an uncommon cause of iron deficiency. In some patients, intestinal malabsorption of iron is only one aspect of more generalized malabsorption [*see Table 2*]. Gastric surgery, especially partial or total gastric resection or gastroenterostomy for bypass of the duodenum, may result in iron deficiency. Although absorption of dietary iron may be poor, therapeutic iron salts are usually well absorbed, and the iron deficiency can be readily corrected.

The risk of iron deficiency is especially high when iron requirements are increased and the supply of iron is inadequate. For example, infants who are fed cow's milk often become iron deficient because of the combination of increased iron losses from cow's milk–induced gastrointestinal bleeding and the small amounts of bioavailable iron in cow's milk.[30] Women with high iron requirements resulting from menstruation often consume diets that have little bioavailable iron and contain inhibitors of iron absorption, such as calcium.

DIAGNOSIS

Clinical Manifestations

Clinically, patients with iron deficiency may be asymptomatic and recognized only because of abnormal results of laboratory tests.[29] Other patients may come to medical attention because of the manifestations of the underlying disorder that produced iron deficiency, but they may have no other findings related to the iron deficiency. Still other patients may present with the signs and symptoms common to all anemias, such as weakness, dizziness, easy fatigability, pallor, irritability, and other indefinite and nonspecific complaints. Iron deficiency may also be associated with signs and symptoms that are unrelated to anemia, such as angular stomatitis, glossitis, postcricoid esophageal stricture or web, and gastric atrophy. Finally, some patients present with one or more of the limited number of signs and symptoms thought to be highly specific for iron deficiency—blue sclerae, koilonychia, and pagophagia. Pagophagia, or pica with ice, is thought to be a highly specific symptom of iron deficiency and disappears shortly after iron therapy is begun.[29] Other types of pica may accompany iron deficiency, but none is as specific a symptom as pagophagia. The nonhematologic consequences of a lack of iron are diminished exercise tolerance and work performance and impaired immunity and resistance to infection. In children, iron deficiency adversely affects growth, motor development, behavior, and cognitive function; these abnormalities may not be reversible with later treatment.[30,31]

Laboratory Tests

Iron deficiency anemia is the only microcytic hypochromic anemia associated with absent iron stores. In other microcytic hypochromic disorders, marrow iron stores are normal or increased. Indirect measures of body iron can be used to identify a characteristic sequence of changes that occur as body iron decreases from the iron-replete normal levels to levels found in iron deficiency anemia [*see Figure 6 and Table 1*]. Measurement of the

Table 1 Changes in Iron Stores and Distribution with Increased or Decreased Body Iron Content

Condition	Marrow Iron (0–6+)	Liver Iron (µmol/g, dry weight)	Plasma Ferritin (µg/L)	Plasma Transferrin Receptor (mg/L)	Plasma Iron (µg/dl)	Transferrin Saturation (%)	Protoporphyrin (µg/dl Red Blood Cells)	Red Blood Cells
Iron deficiency anemia [see Figure 6a]	0	< 3.0	< 12	10	< 40	< 10	150	Microcytic, hypochromic
Iron stores depletion [see Figure 6b]	0 to trace amounts	3.0	< 20	5.5	< 115	< 30	30	Normal
Reduced iron stores [see Figure 6c]	1+	< 10.0	< 25	5.5	< 115	30	30	Normal
Normal [see Figure 6d]	2–3+	15.0 ± 5.0	100 ± 60	5.5 ± 1.5	115 ± 50	35 ± 15	30	Normal
Increased iron stores, HLA-linked hemochromatosis	2–3+	100	1,000*	5.5	> 150	> 60	30	Normal
Increased iron stores; transfusional iron overload	4+	20	1,000	5.5	> 150	> 50	30	Normal
Massive iron overload, HLA-linked hemochromatosis	3–4+	500	4,000*	5.5	200	> 60	30	Normal
Massive iron overload; transfusional iron overload	6+	300	4,000	5.5	200	> 90	30	Normal

*May be normal in some patients.

plasma ferritin concentration is the most useful test for the detection of iron deficiency, because plasma ferritin concentrations decrease as body iron stores decline.[29] A plasma ferritin concentration below 12 µg/L is virtually diagnostic of absent iron stores. In contrast, a normal plasma ferritin concentration does not confirm the presence of storage iron, because plasma ferritin may be increased independently of body iron by infection, inflammation, liver disease, malignancy, and other conditions. Because the plasma transferrin receptor concentration seems to be unaffected by these conditions, determination of this value provides a means of distinguishing between the anemia of iron deficiency and the anemia associated with chronic inflammatory disorders.[32] The plasma transferrin saturation is decreased in both iron deficiency and infectious and inflammatory states and is of little practical assistance in distinguishing between these conditions. Although bone marrow examination is seldom performed solely for the assessment of iron status, the diagnosis of iron deficiency can almost always be verified by direct assessment of marrow iron stores. If no iron stores are present, the diagnosis of iron deficiency is established; if hemosiderin (an intracellular granule that stores iron-containing molecules) is found, iron deficiency is excluded. In addition, with iron deficiency, marrow sideroblasts will be absent or present in low numbers (less than 10% of the number of normoblasts). A therapeutic trial of iron may also be an effective means of establishing the diagnosis of iron deficiency.

TREATMENT

Therapy for iron deficiency anemia should both correct the hemoglobin deficit and replace storage iron. For almost all patients, oral iron is the treatment of choice.[29] Oral iron therapy is effective, safe, and inexpensive. Because of the risk of local and systemic adverse reactions, parenteral iron should be used only in the small number of patients who cannot absorb or tolerate oral iron or who have iron requirements that cannot be met by oral therapy because of chronic, uncontrollable bleeding. In severe iron deficiency anemia, red cell transfusions are needed in rare instances to prevent cardiac or cerebral ischemia. Red cell transfusions may also be necessary for patients whose chronic rate of iron loss exceeds the rate of replacement possible with parenteral therapy. Although most patients take oral iron without difficulty, 10% to 20% experience side effects related to iron, most commonly gastrointestinal complaints.

Iron deficiency can almost always be treated effectively, with oral and parenteral therapy yielding similar results [see Sidebar, Iron Replacement Therapy].[29] Alleviation of symptoms often occurs within the first few days of treatment. With uncomplicated iron deficiency, the initial hematologic response—a mild reticulocytosis—usually begins within 3 to 5 days after the start of therapy, reaches a maximum within 8 to 10 days, and declines thereafter. After the first week, the hemoglobin concentration begins to increase and is usually normal within 6 weeks. Microcytosis may not completely resolve for as long as 4 months. If the iron deficiency is treated with oral iron at a dosage of 200 mg/day or less, the plasma ferritin concentration remains below 12 µg/L until the anemia is corrected and then gradually rises as storage iron is replenished. If the response to iron therapy is not complete and characteristic, review and reevaluation of the patient is mandatory. One of the most common problems is mistaking the anemia of chronic disease for the anemia of iron deficiency. Recovery may be retarded by coexistent disorders, including other nutritional deficiencies; liver or kidney disease; infectious, inflammatory, or malignant disorders; or continued occult blood loss. If the patient is treated with oral iron, the form and dosage of iron used should be reviewed, compliance evaluated, and the possibility of malabsorption considered.

Iron Overload

Iron overload arises from a sustained increase in iron supply over iron requirements and causes a characteristic pattern of changes in functional, transport, and storage iron [see Figure 6 and Table 1]. The amount of body iron is normally controlled by regulation of dietary iron absorption. Iron overload develops with conditions that modify or circumvent the regulation of intestinal

Table 2 Causes of Iron Deficiency

INCREASED IRON REQUIREMENTS

Blood loss

Gastrointestinal tract

Hemorrhagic lesions (e.g., hiatal hernia, esophageal varices, gastritis, duodenitis, peptic ulcer, cholelithiasis, intrahepatic bleeding, inflammatory bowel disease, diverticulosis, hemorrhoids, or adenomatous polyp)

Occult gastrointestinal malignancy

Chronic ingestion of drugs (e.g., alcohol, salicylates, steroids, and nonsteroidal anti-inflammatory drugs)

Helminthic infections (e.g., hookworm, *Schistosoma mansoni*, *S. japonicum*, or severe *Trichuris trichiura*)

Other (e.g., vascular purpura with scurvy, aberrant pancreas, Meckel diverticulum, hereditary hemorrhagic telangiectasia, other vascular ectasia of the bowel, or colonic polyposis)

Genitourinary tract

Menstrual blood loss

Other (e.g., uterine malignancies or fibroids, stones, infarction, infection with *S. haematobium*, inflammatory disease, malignancy of the urinary tract, or chronic hemoglobinuria or hemosiderinuria resulting from paroxysmal nocturnal hemoglobinuria or chronic intravascular hemolysis)

Respiratory tract

Chronic recurrent hemoptysis

Idiopathic pulmonary siderosis

Goodpasture syndrome

Blood donation

Growth

Infants, premature infants

Children

Adolescents

Pregnancy and lactation

INADEQUATE IRON SUPPLY

Diets with insufficient amounts of bioavailable iron

Impaired absorption of iron

Intestinal malabsorption (e.g., steatorrhea, sprue, celiac disease, diffuse enteritis, atrophic gastritis with achlorhydria, or pica)

Gastric surgery

---

iron absorption [*see Table 3*]. Because humans have no physiologic means of eliminating excess iron, any persistent increase in intake may eventually result in iron overload. Regardless of the cause of the accumulation of excess iron, when the extent of iron loading exceeds the ability of the body to safely sequester the surplus iron, a potentially lethal pattern of tissue damage develops. The precise features of the pathologic consequences of iron overload are a result, in part, of the magnitude of the body iron burden; the rate at which the increase in body iron has occurred; the specific distribution of the excess iron between storage sites in macrophages and, potentially more harmful, deposits in parenchymal cells; and the coexistence of conditions that may ameliorate (e.g., ascorbate deficiency) or worsen (e.g., alcohol use or hepatitis) the outcome. The most common consequences of iron overload are liver disease, pancreatic disease associated with diabetes mellitus, endocrine disorders associated with gonadal insufficiency, cardiac dysfunction, arthropathy, and, occasionally, neurologic and psychological abnormalities.

Increased iron absorption may develop because of abnormal control of iron absorption from a diet containing normal amounts of bioavailable iron, such as in hereditary hemochromatosis, or from a diet with such an overabundance of bioavailable iron that the normal means of regulation is overridden, such as in African

dietary iron overload. Iron-loading anemias are a heterogeneous group of disorders that may be acquired or inherited and have in common pronounced erythroid hyperplasia with marked ineffective erythropoiesis. Iron overload can also result from transfusion (see below).

HEREDITARY HEMOCHROMATOSIS

Epidemiology

Hereditary hemochromatosis, an autosomal recessive disease, is the most common genetic disorder in persons of northern European descent. In the United States, as much as 10% of the population is heterozygous for this condition; the homozygous state is believed to affect as much as 0.5% of the population, but it is greatly underdiagnosed.[33]

Etiology/Genetics

The discovery of the gene responsible for most cases of hereditary hemochromatosis has revolutionized both the understanding and the diagnosis of this disorder.[17] A defect in the HFE protein results in an abnormality in the control of iron absorption, which causes an inappropriate increase in iron uptake and a progressive buildup of body iron. Initially, the iron overload has a predominantly parenchymal pattern of deposition, first accumulating in hepatocytes; subsequently, the iron builds up in the pancreas, heart, and other organs.[34] Characteristically, macrophage iron in the bone marrow may be normal or even decreased despite severe parenchymal iron deposition [*see Figure 6 and Table 1*].

Missense mutations in the HFE gene are responsible for about 85% of cases of hereditary hemochromatosis in the United States; in other areas of the world, the percentage ranges from about 60% to 100%.[35] In one study, the most prevalent mutation (homozygous in 83% of patients) was a Cys282Tyr substitution; a second mutation, His63Asp, was enriched in patients who were compound heterozygotes for the Cys282Tyr substitution.[17] Recently, a third mutation, Ser65Cys, was identified.[36] It is important to note that in the United States, 10% to 15% of patients with primary iron overload have none of these three mutations, but they are clinically indistinguishable from patients who do have one of these mutations. The Cys282Tyr mutation disrupts the binding of HFE to β_2-microglobulin, which almost completely prevents the association of the mutant HFE and the transferrin receptor[19]; the effects of the His63Asp and Ser65Cys mutations are less well characterized. The available data suggest that the pathogenesis of hereditary hemochromatosis may be related to a disturbance of the transferrin–transferrin receptor pathway, but the exact mechanism whereby this change increases dietary iron absorption is uncertain.

Clinical manifestations In homozygotes who present with hereditary hemochromatosis in middle age or later, the classic tetrad of clinical signs is liver disease, diabetes mellitus, skin pigmentation, and gonadal failure.[37-39] Cardiac failure develops in about 10% to 15% of untreated homozygotes. Body iron stores have usually increased from the normal amount of 1 g or less to 15 to 20 g or more by the time symptoms of parenchymal damage occur, usually in middle or late life.[38] Additional increases in body iron may be fatal, although some patients are able to tolerate a total iron accumulation of as much as 40 to 50 g. Environmental factors, including dietary iron content, blood loss, and alcohol use, may greatly influence the rate and severity of organ damage. In heterozygotes, hereditary hemochromatosis is incompletely ex-

Iron Replacement Therapy

ORAL IRON THERAPY

Indication

Treatment of choice for iron deficiency anemia

Initial therapy to correct iron deficiency anemia

Ferrous iron salt (e.g., ferrous sulfate) given separately from meals in two or three divided doses; for example, ferrous sulfate tablets, 325 mg three times a day, or ferrous gluconate tablets, 300 mg two or three times a day

Continued therapy to replace iron stores

Ferrous iron salt given as a single daily dose of approximately 60 mg of elemental iron until the plasma ferritin concentration is > 50 µg/L (often requires 6 mo or more of treatment)

Management of side effects

Gastrointestinal side effects are the most common (10%–20% of patients) and usually can be managed symptomatically by (1) giving iron with or immediately after meals, (2) reducing the amount of iron in each dose, or (3) reducing the dose frequency to once daily

PARENTERAL IRON THERAPY

Indications

Chronic, uncontrollable blood loss producing iron needs that cannot be met by oral iron therapy

Malabsorption of iron

Intolerance of oral iron despite repeated modifications in dosage regimen

Risks

Immediate, life-threatening anaphylactic reactions

Delayed but severe serum sickness–like reactions with fever, urticaria, adenopathy, myalgias, and arthralgias

Exacerbation of rheumatoid arthritis and related conditions

Local reactions with intramuscular iron (skin staining, muscle necrosis, phlebitis, and persistent pain at injection site)

Precautions

Iron dextran is the only currently available parenteral preparation; a 0.5 ml test dose is to be given at least 1 hr before every intramuscular or intravenous injection of iron dextran, but the value of this precaution is limited because anaphylaxis is not dose dependent and can occur with the test dose

Administration and dosage

Parenteral iron may be administered either intramuscularly (limited to 2 ml or 100 mg of iron per injection) or intravenously (as an undiluted injection, as a total-dose infusion, or as an additive to total parenteral nutrition); because of the risks of therapy, recommendations of the manufacturers and recent-study recommendations for treatment should be reviewed carefully before parenteral iron is given

tary hemochromatosis who have HFE mutations varies from 60% to 100% in different populations.[33] In addition, a number of persons who are homozygous for the Cys282Tyr mutation but without iron overload have been identified.[37,42,43] The number of patients in the United States who are not homozygous for the Cys282Tyr mutation but who meet the clinical criteria for hereditary hemochromatosis is so large that reliance on genetic testing alone would miss many affected individuals. A more practical approach is initial screening for iron overload with phenotypic testing.[37,33]

In pedigree studies, genotyping should replace HLA typing in the assessment of siblings of a Cys282Tyr homozygote. In addition, genotyping the spouse of a Cys282Tyr homozygote is a cost-efficient strategy that leads to a more selective investigation of children for the hemochromatosis gene.[42]

Studies have recently suggested that initial screening for hereditary hemochromatosis should still rely on transferrin saturation, followed by testing for the Cys282Tyr mutation in patients with a transferrin saturation greater than 40% and, for Cys282Tyr homozygotes who are identified, assessment of iron burden by serum ferritin or liver biopsy.[37,44] In patients with liver disease and suspected iron overload, genotypic screening may identify Cys282Tyr homozygotes who would otherwise be missed.[45] Liver biopsy permits a definitive diagnosis of hereditary hemochromatosis regardless of genotype.[34,46]

Evaluation should include quantitative determination of the nonheme iron concentration, histochemical evaluation of the pattern of iron deposition, and pathologic assessment of tissue injury. Calculation of the hepatic iron index (the hepatic iron concentration [expressed as µmol Fe/g of liver, dry weight] divided by the age of the patient [expressed in years]) may be helpful in distinguishing homozygotes for hereditary hemochromatosis from heterozygotes or from patients with increased body iron associated with chronic (usually alcoholic) liver disease.[37] Liver biopsy is particularly useful in assessing the extent of hepatic injury and detecting the development of fibrosis or cirrhosis.

pressed; about 25% of such persons have minor increases in body iron stores to a total of not more than 4 to 5 g but do not develop other manifestations of the disease.[37,38]

Screening and diagnostic tests Because early detection and treatment can prevent disease manifestations, routine screening for hemochromatosis is recommended for all patients.[40] Measurements of the plasma iron concentration, transferrin saturation, and plasma ferritin concentration provide the best means of screening patients for hereditary hemochromatosis, although it should be recognized that the plasma ferritin concentration may be normal in a small number of patients with hereditary hemochromatosis.[41] Genotyping can be used as a confirmatory test in a patient that is suspected of having hemochromatosis clinically or who has an elevated transferrin saturation, serum ferritin level, or both.

The characterization of the HFE gene mutations was rapidly followed by the development of a diagnostic genotypic test.[35] The exact diagnostic role of this test partly depends on the population being examined, because the percentage of patients with heredi-

Table 3 Causes of Iron Overload

Increased iron absorption

Hereditary (HLA-linked) hemochromatosis

Iron-loading anemias (refractory anemias with hypercellular erythroid marrow)

Chronic liver disease (cirrhosis, portacaval shunt)

Porphyria cutanea tarda

Familial apoceruloplasmin deficiency

Congenital defects (atransferrinemia and other disorders)

African dietary iron overload*

Medicinal iron ingestion (?)

Parenteral iron overload

Transfusional iron overload

Inadvertent iron overload from therapeutic injections

Perinatal iron overload

Hereditary tyrosinemia

Cerebrohepatorenal syndrome

Perinatal hemochromatosis

Focal sequestration of iron

Idiopathic pulmonary hemosiderosis

Renal hemosiderosis

Hallervorden-Spatz disease

*May have genetic component.

Treatment

The treatment of choice for hereditary hemochromatosis is phlebotomy to reduce and maintain the body iron at normal or near-normal levels. In patients with hereditary hemochromatosis who develop cardiac failure, the use of both phlebotomy and chelation therapy has been suggested. Phlebotomy therapy should be started as soon as the diagnosis of the homozygous state for hereditary hemochromatosis has been established; postponement only increases the risk of organ damage from iron overload. The phlebotomy program should remove 500 ml of blood (containing 200 to 250 mg of iron) once weekly or, for heavily loaded patients, twice weekly, until the patient is iron deficient. Before each phlebotomy, the hematocrit or hemoglobin concentration should be measured. Initially, the hematocrit and hemoglobin will decline by about 10% of their initial values but may then rise as the rate of erythropoiesis increases to match the demands of phlebotomy. Measurements of plasma ferritin, iron, and transferrin saturation should be done regularly to follow the progress of iron removal. As iron is removed, the plasma ferritin concentration will decrease progressively, but the plasma iron concentration and transferrin saturation will remain raised until iron stores are almost exhausted. Finally, when all the storage iron has been removed, the ferritin concentration will fall to less than 12 µg/L, the plasma iron concentration and transferrin saturation will drop, and the hemoglobin concentration will decrease to less than 10 g/dl for 2 weeks without further phlebotomy. In patients with hereditary hemochromatosis, prolonged treatment is often needed. For example, if the initial body iron burden is 25 g, complete removal of the iron burden with weekly phlebotomy may require 2 years or more. After the iron load has been completely removed, a lifelong program of maintenance phlebotomy is required to prevent reaccumulation of the iron burden. Typically, phlebotomy of 500 ml of blood every 3 to 4 months is needed. The goal of maintenance phlebotomy should be to maintain a normal transferrin saturation with a plasma ferritin concentration of less than about 50 µg/L. If phlebotomy therapy removes the iron load before the development of diabetes mellitus or cirrhosis, the patient's life expectancy is normal.[47] If cirrhosis develops, however, the risk of hepatocellular carcinoma is increased by more than 200-fold. In hereditary hemochromatosis, hepatomas develop almost exclusively in patients with hepatic cirrhosis and are the ultimate cause of death in 20% to 30% of these patients, even after successful removal of the iron burden. Phlebotomy therapy is almost always indicated for patients with hereditary hemochromatosis, even when cirrhosis or organ damage is already present, because further progression of the disease can be stopped and alleviation of some organ dysfunction is possible.

IRON-LOADING ANEMIAS

In patients with iron-loading anemias, severe iron overload may develop as a result of increased gastrointestinal iron absorption.[48] Any red cell transfusions these patients receive will contribute to the iron loading. The iron-loading anemias include congenital dyserythropoietic anemia, pyruvate kinase deficiency, thalassemia major (Cooley anemia) and thalassemia intermedia, hemoglobin E–β-thalassemia, a variety of forms of sideroblastic anemia, some myelodysplastic anemia, and other anemic disorders in which the incorporation of iron into hemoglobin is impaired.[48] Because the extent of ineffective erythropoiesis, not the severity of the anemia, seems to determine the rate of iron loading, severe iron overload may develop in patients with only slight or mild anemia. The clinical manifestations and pathology that may develop in patients with iron-loading anemias are similar to those seen in hereditary hemochromatosis, including liver disease, diabetes mellitus, endocrine disorders, and cardiac dysfunction.

OTHER FORMS OF IRON OVERLOAD RESULTING FROM INCREASED ABSORPTION

Some patients with chronic liver disease, including those with alcoholic cirrhosis and those with portacaval shunting, may experience minor or modest degrees of iron loading as a result of increased dietary iron absorption.[48] The mechanisms responsible for the increased gastrointestinal iron uptake have not been identified, although ineffective erythropoiesis and hyperferremia associated with alcohol-induced folate and sideroblastic abnormalities have been proposed as etiologic factors. Body iron stores are increased only to a minor degree, typically to 2 to 4 g. The pattern of iron deposition is predominantly in Kupffer cells, rather than in hepatocytes, as in hereditary hemochromatosis. The distinction between the iron overload in patients with chronic liver disease and that in homozygotes for hereditary hemochromatosis can almost always be made by quantitative iron determination on a sample of liver obtained by biopsy and calculation of the hepatic iron index.

Symptomatic patients with porphyria cutanea tarda, a hepatic porphyria, usually have a modest increase in body iron that almost always is the result of increased gastrointestinal absorption.[48] Aceruloplasminemia has been recognized as an autosomal recessive disorder of iron metabolism that leads to iron accumulation in both the liver and the brain, and presents as a neurologic disorder in later life.[23] Other rare congenital defects associated with iron overload have been recognized. For example, in patients with atransferrinemia, transferrin is virtually absent.[48] Gastrointestinal iron absorption is increased, but because the physiologic means for iron transport are absent, almost none of the absorbed iron can be taken up by developing erythroid cells. Instead, iron accumulates in the liver, pancreas, heart, thyroid, and kidneys, and almost none of the iron is deposited in the bone marrow or spleen. African dietary iron overload has been described in at least nine countries in sub-Saharan Africa in association with greatly increased dietary iron intake from a fermented maize beverage home-brewed in steel drums.[49] Iron burdens may be as great as those found in hereditary hemochromatosis, and liver disease (with cirrhosis and hepatoma), pancreatic disease (with diabetes mellitus), endocrine disorders, and cardiac dysfunction may develop. Although increased dietary iron intake was long considered the sole cause of the increased iron absorption in this disorder, pedigree analysis has suggested that a genetic component may be involved and may be common in populations of African ancestry.[49] In the United States, severe iron overload has been documented in patients of African ancestry,[50] but its relation to African dietary iron overload is still under investigation. Medicinal iron ingestion can undoubtedly contribute to the body iron burden of patients with iron-loading disorders, but the extent to which orally administered iron can increase the body iron stores of normal individuals remains uncertain. Although some case reports have described iron accumulation in patients who have taken medicinal iron for long periods, the potential involvement of an unrecognized allele for hereditary hemochromatosis in these individuals cannot be excluded.

TRANSFUSIONAL AND OTHER PARENTERAL IRON OVERLOAD

Etiology and Diagnosis

An adequate transfusion program can sustain life in patients with severe chronic refractory anemia, but transfusion therapy alone produces a progressive accumulation of the iron contained in transfused red cells.[51] Iron accumulation from transfusion initially occurs predominantly in macrophage sites, followed by redistribution to parenchymal tissues [*see Figure 6*]. In patients with severe congenital anemias, such as thalassemia major and the Blackfan-Diamond syndrome, regular transfusions can prevent death from anemia in infancy and permit normal growth and development during childhood. Acquired transfusion-dependent anemias, such as aplastic anemia, pure red cell aplasia, hypoplastic or myelodysplastic disorders, and other disorders, may cause the development of marked iron overload. If the transfusion-dependent anemia includes erythroid hyperplasia with ineffective erythropoiesis, increased gastrointestinal iron absorption may add to the iron loading. In such cases, dietary iron uptake may be minimized by suppression of erythropoiesis with an adequate transfusion program. Although not transfusion-dependent, patients with sickling disorders, such as sickle cell anemia and sickle cell–β-thalassemia, may acquire a considerable iron load from chronic transfusions for the prevention of stroke,[52] painful crises, and other recurrent complications. Because humans lack a physiologic means of eliminating excess iron, iron contained in transfused red cells progressively accumulates and eventually damages the liver, heart, pancreas, and other organs; death usually occurs from cardiac failure. In younger patients, the iron burden results in growth failure and, in adolescence, delayed or absent sexual maturation. Parenteral medicinal iron may needlessly add to the iron burden in patients with refractory microcytic anemias who are misdiagnosed as iron deficient.

Treatment

About 200 to 250 mg of iron is added to the body iron load with each unit of transfused red cells. Most transfusion-dependent patients require 200 to 300 ml/kg/yr of blood; for example, a 70 kg adult requires about two to three units of blood every 3 to 4 weeks, adding about 6 to 10 g of iron a year. The severity of iron toxicity seems to be related to the magnitude of the body iron burden. Almost all patients who have been treated with transfusion alone and have received 100 or more units of blood (about 20 to 25 g of iron) have developed cardiac iron deposits, often in association with signs of hepatic, pancreatic, and endocrine damage.[51] For patients who are transfusion dependent or severely anemic, the only means available to circumvent the physiologic limitation that prevents the elimination of accumulated iron is treatment with a chelating agent capable of complexing with iron and permitting its excretion. The only iron-chelating agent now available for clinical use is a bacterial siderophore first introduced 3 decades ago, deferoxamine B, a trihydroxamic acid produced by *Streptomyces pilosus*. Clinical trials with deferoxamine have now documented the effectiveness of iron chelation as a therapeutic approach to iron overload, demonstrating that regular iron chelation can decrease the body iron burden, alleviate organ dysfunction, and improve survival.[51,53] Although various toxic side effects can occur, especially with intensive therapy, deferoxamine has been a remarkably safe drug, even with near-lifelong use in some patients.

Iron chelation therapy should be started early to prevent the accumulation of toxic amounts of iron in vulnerable tissues and to maintain body iron stores at concentrations associated with a low risk of early death and clinical complications. The longer chelation therapy is delayed, the greater the risk of iron toxicity. Because deferoxamine is poorly absorbed after oral administration and rapidly eliminated from the circulation, deferoxamine must be given by slow subcutaneous or intravenous infusion over 9 to 12 hours each day at least 5 days a week to be optimally useful in the treatment of patients with transfusional iron overload. In patients with thalassemia major and other congenital refractory anemias who have been transfusion dependent from early infancy, chelation therapy is best started after about 10 to 20 transfusions, usually when the patient is 3 or 4 years of age. Deferoxamine is administered by slow subcutaneous infusion at a dosage not exceeding 25 mg/kg/day to minimize the risk of growth retardation.[51] In older patients and adults with acquired refractory anemias who require regular transfusion and in patients with sickle cell disease who are chronically transfused for prevention of complications, early therapy also seems prudent, beginning after transfusion of 10 to 20 units of blood. The usual dose of deferoxamine in these older patients is not more than 50 mg/kg/day, given over 9 to 12 hours by slow subcutaneous infusion at least 5 days a week. In some patients who are unable to tolerate the local pain and discomfort of subcutaneous infusion or who need rapid reduction of high body iron burdens, deferoxamine may be administered intravenously through implantable venous access ports.[51] Compliance with these near-daily regimens of prolonged subcutaneous or intravenous infusions may be difficult, and lack of compliance is the chief obstacle to effective iron chelation therapy. Administration of ascorbic acid can enhance deferoxamine-induced iron excretion but carries the risk of an internal redistribution of iron from relatively benign storage sites in macrophages to a potentially toxic pool in parenchymal cells. Although the evidence is anecdotal, large doses of ascorbic acid should be regarded as hazardous in patients with iron overload. Although deferoxamine is a generally safe and nontoxic drug in the iron-loaded patient, systemic complications have been reported,[51] including allergic anaphylactoid reactions, infectious complications, visual abnormalities and auditory dysfunction, and growth retardation. As a result, regular evaluation for drug toxicity should be included in the management of any patient receiving deferoxamine, including annual audiograms, retinal examination, and assessment of growth in children and adolescents. The risk of many of these complications may be minimized by adjusting the deferoxamine dose to the magnitude of the body iron load. Orally active chelating agents and new formulations of deferoxamine are under development,[51,54] but none is available for clinical use.

ADDITIONAL FORMS OF IRON OVERLOAD

Perinatal iron overload has been recognized in association with some rare metabolic abnormalities of the neonate, including hereditary tyrosinemia (hypermethioninemia); the cerebrohepatorenal syndrome, or Zellweger syndrome; and perinatal hemochromatosis, also known as neonatal hemochromatosis or neonatal iron storage disease. Focal sequestration of iron in other rare disorders produces various patterns of localized iron deposition in idiopathic pulmonary hemosiderosis, in renal hemosiderosis, and in the Hallervorden-Spatz disease.[48] Hyperferritinemia with autosomal dominant congenital cataract is a newly recognized disorder of iron metabolism,[55] in which affected family members present with early onset, bilateral nuclear cataracts and moderately elevated plasma ferritin concentrations (about 1,000 to 2,500 µg/L); the two conditions are coinherited as an autosomal dominant trait. The body iron is normal in these patients, but overload is often suspected because of the elevated plasma ferritin concentrations.

References

1. Hsia CC: Respiratory function of hemoglobin. N Engl J Med 338:239-247, 1998
2. Jia L, Bonaventura C, Bonaventura J, et al: S-nitrosohaemoglobin: a dynamic activity of

blood involved in vascular control. Nature 380:221, 1996

3. Stamler JS, Jia L, Eu JP, et al: Blood flow regulation by S-nitrosohemoglobin in the physiological oxygen gradient. Science 276:2034, 1997

4. Bunn HF, Forget BF: Hemoglobin: Molecular, Genetic and Clinical Aspects. WB Saunders Co, Philadelphia, 1986

5. Perutz MF, Wilkinson AJ, Paoli M, et al: The stereochemical mechanism of the cooperative effects in hemoglobin revisited. Annu Rev Biophys Biomol Struct 27:1, 1998

6. Ponka P, Beaumont C, Richardson DR: Function and regulation of transferrin and ferritin. Semin Hematol 35:35, 1998

7. Levy JE, Jin O, Fujiwara Y, et al: Transferrin receptor is necessary for development of erythrocytes and the nervous system. Nat Genet 21:396, 1999

8. Aisen P: Transferrin, the transferrin receptor, and the uptake of iron by cells. Met Ions Biol Syst 35:585, 1998

9. Harrison PM, Arosio P: The ferritins: molecular properties, iron storage function and cellular regulation. Biochim Biophys Acta 1275:161, 1996

10. Hentze MW, Kuhn LC: Molecular control of vertebrate iron metabolism: mRNA-based regulatory circuits operated by iron, nitric oxide, and oxidative stress. Proc Natl Acad Sci USA 93:8175, 1996

11. Rouault T, Klausner R: Regulation of iron metabolism in eukaryotes. Curr Top Cell Regul 35:1, 1997

12. Gunshin H, Mackenzie B, Berger UV, et al: Cloning and characterization of a mammalian proton-coupled metal-ion transporter. Nature 388:482, 1997

13. Fleming MD, Trenor CC 3rd, Su MA, et al: Microcytic anaemia mice have a mutation in Nramp2, a candidate iron transporter gene. Nat Genet 16:383, 1997

14. Fleming MD, Romano MA, Su MA, et al: Nramp2 is mutated in the anemic Belgrade (b) rat: evidence of a role for Nramp2 in endosomal iron transport. Proc Natl Acad Sci USA 95:1148, 1998

15. Gruenheid S, Canonne-Hergaux F, Gauthier S, et al: The iron transport protein NRAMP2 is an integral membrane glycoprotein that colocalizes with transferrin in recycling endosomes. J Exp Med 189:831, 1999

16. Vulpe CD, Kuo YM, Murphy TL, et al: Hephaestin, a ceruloplasmin homologue implicated in intestinal iron transport, is defective in the sla mouse. Nat Genet 21:195, 1999

17. Feder JN, Gnirke A, Thomas W, et al: A novel MHC class I-like gene is mutated in patients with hereditary haemochromatosis. Nat Genet 13:399, 1996

18. Feder JN, Tsuchihashi Z, Irrinki A, et al: The hemochromatosis founder mutation in HLA-H disrupts beta$_2$-microglobulin interaction and cell surface expression. J Biol Chem 272:14025, 1997

19. Feder JN, Penny DM, Irrinki A, et al: The hemochromatosis gene product complexes with the transferrin receptor and lowers its affinity for ligand binding. Proc Natl Acad Sci USA 95:1472, 1998

20. Lebron JA, Bennett MJ, Vaughn DE, et al: Crystal structure of the hemochromatosis protein HFE and characterization of its interaction with transferrin receptor. Cell 93:111, 1998

21. Waheed A, Parkkila S, Saarnio J, et al: Association of HFE protein with transferrin receptor in crypt enterocytes of human duodenum. Proc Natl Acad Sci USA 96:1579, 1999

22. Han O, Fleet JC, Wood RJ: Reciprocal regulation of HFE and Nramp2 gene expression by iron in human intestinal cells. J Nutr 129:98, 1999

23. Harris ZL, Takahashi Y, Miyajima H, et al: Aceruloplasminemia: molecular characterization of this disorder of iron metabolism. Proc Natl Acad Sci USA 92:2539, 1995

24. Attieh ZK, Mukhopadhyay CK, Seshadri V, et al: Ceruloplasmin ferroxidase activity stimulates cellular iron uptake by a trivalent cation-specific transport mechanism. J Biol Chem 274:1116, 1999

25. Yu J, Wessling-Resnick M: Structural and functional analysis of SFT, a stimulator of Fe Transport. J Biol Chem 273:21380, 1998

26. Bothwell TH, Charlton RW, Cook JD, et al: Iron Metabolism in Man. Blackwell Scientific Publications, Oxford, England, 1979

27. Brittenham GM: Iron in the red cell cycle. Iron Metabolism in Health and Disease. Brock J, Pippard M, Halliday J, et al, eds. Academic Press, London, 1994, p 31

28. Finch C: Regulators of iron balance in humans. Blood 84:1697, 1994

29. Cook JD: Iron-deficiency anaemia. Baillieres Clin Haematol 7:787, 1994

30. Recommendations to prevent and control iron deficiency in the United States. MMWR Morb Mortal Wkly Rep 47(RR-3):1, 1998

31. de Andraca I, Castillo M, Walter T: Psychomotor development and behavior in iron-deficient anemic infants. Nutr Rev 55:125, 1997

32. Cook JD, Baynes RD, Skikne BS: The physiological significance of circulating transferrin receptors. Adv Exp Med Biol 352:119, 1994

33. Cogswell ME, McDonnell SM, Khoury MJ, et al: Iron overload, public health, and genetics: evaluating the evidence for hemochromatosis screening. Ann Intern Med 129:971, 1998

34. Edwards CQ, Griffen LM, Ajioka RS, et al: Screening for hemochromatosis: phenotype versus genotype. Semin Hematol 35:72, 1998

35. Burke W, Thomson E, Khoury MJ, et al: Hereditary hemochromatosis: gene discovery and its implications for population-based screening. JAMA 280:172, 1998

36. Mura C, Raguenes O, Ferec C: HFE mutations analysis in 711 hemochromatosis probands: evidence for S65C implication in mild form of hemochromatosis. Blood 93:2502, 1999

37. Crawford DH, Jazwinska EC, Cullen LM, et al: Expression of HLA-linked hemochromatosis in subjects homozygous or heterozygous for the C282Y mutation. Gastroenterology 114:1003, 1998

38. Niederau C, Stremmel W, Strohmeyer GW: Clinical spectrum and management of haemochromatosis. Baillieres Clin Haematol 7:881, 1994

39. Adams PC, Deugnier Y, Moirand R, et al: The relationship between iron overload, clinical symptoms, and age in 410 patients with genetic hemochromatosis. Hepatology 25:162, 1997

40. Phatuk PD, Guzman G, Woll JE, et al: Cost-effectiveness of screening for hereditary hemochromatosis. Arch Intern Med 154:769, 1994

41. Feller ER, Pout A, Wands JR, et al: Familial hemochromatosis: physiologic studies in the precirrhotic stage of the disease. N Engl J Med 296:1422, 1977

42. Adams PC, Chakrabarti S: Genotypic/phenotypic correlations in genetic hemochromatosis: evolution of diagnostic criteria. Gastroenterology 114:319, 1998

43. Brissot P, Moirand R, Jouanolle AM, et al: A genotypic study of 217 unrelated probands diagnosed as "genetic hemochromatosis" on "classical" phenotypic criteria. J Hepatol 30:588, 1999

44. Olynyk JK: Hereditary haemochromatosis: diagnosis and management in the gene era. Liver 19:73, 1999

45. Bacon BR, Olynyk JK, Brunt EM, et al: HFE genotype in patients with hemochromatosis and other liver diseases. Ann Intern Med 130:953, 1999

46. Angelucci E, Baronciani D, Lucarelli G, et al: Needle liver biopsy in thalassaemia: analyses of diagnostic accuracy and safety in 1184 consecutive biopsies. Br J Haematol 89:757, 1995

47. Niederau C, Fischer R, Purschel A, et al: Long-term survival in patients with hereditary hemochromatosis. Gastroenterology 110:1107, 1996

48. Bottomley SS: Secondary iron overload disorders. Semin Hematol 35:77, 1998

49. Moyo VM, Mandishona E, Hasstedt SJ, et al: Evidence of genetic transmission in African iron overload. Blood 91:1076, 1998

50. Wurapa RK, Gordeuk VR, Brittenham GM, et al: Primary iron overload in African Americans. Am J Med 101:9, 1996

51. Olivieri NF, Brittenham GM: Iron-chelating therapy and the treatment of thalassemia. Blood 89:739, 1997

52. Adams RJ, McKie VC, Hsu L, et al: Prevention of a first stroke by transfusions in children with sickle cell anemia and abnormal results on transcranial Doppler ultrasonography. N Engl J Med 339:5, 1998

53. Brittenham GM, Griffith PM, Nienhuis AW, et al: Efficacy of deferoxamine in preventing complications of iron overload in patients with thalassemia major. N Engl J Med 331:567, 1994

54. Bergeron RJ, Wiegand J, Brittenham GM: HBED: the continuing development of a potential alternative to deferoxamine for iron-chelating therapy. Blood 93:370, 1999

55. Beaumont C, Leneuve P, Devaux I, et al: Mutation in the iron responsive element of the L ferritin mRNA in a family with dominant hyperferritinaemia and cataract. Nat Genet 11:444, 1995

Acknowledgments

Figures 1 and 6   Seward Hung.

Figure 2   Marcia Kammerer.

Figure 3   Seward Hung.

Figures 4 and 5   Dimitry Schidlovsky.

88 Anemia: Production Defects

Stanley L. Schrier, M.D.

Classification of Production Defects

Red blood cell production defects cause anemia that is marked by a low absolute reticulocyte count. Examination of the peripheral blood count and the bone marrow aids in classifying these disorders. The marrow characteristically shows one of the following:

1. A normal ratio of myeloid cells to erythroid cells (M:E ratio), normal overall cellularity, and a normal pattern of erythroid maturation.
2. Virtual absence of normal bone marrow elements caused by aplasia (absence of marrow cells) or by replacement of normal marrow elements by fibrosis, solid tumors, granulomas, or leukemia.
3. Erythroid hyperplasia with increased cellularity. Because of defects of erythroid maturation, there is ineffective erythropoiesis or intramedullary hemolysis. Erythroid precursors die in the marrow, and few cells reach the periphery.

Production Defects Associated with Apparently Normal Bone Marrow

ANEMIA OF CHRONIC DISEASE

Definition

The anemia of chronic disease occurs secondary to neoplastic, infectious, and inflammatory diseases and other chronic illnesses, including liver disorders, congestive heart failure, and diabetes mellitus.[1,2] Hematocrit values usually range from 27% to 35%, although 20% of patients have hematocrit values below 25%.[2]

Pathophysiology

The anemia of chronic disease usually results from a combination of slightly shortened red blood cell survival, the sequestration of iron in the reticuloendothelial system, and erythropoietin levels that are less than expected for the degree of anemia.[1,2] Red blood cells usually have a normal morphologic appearance, although they may occasionally be mildly hypochromic and microcytic. The serum iron and transferrin levels are low, and iron saturation is frequently as low as 15%.[1,2] The serum ferritin level is usually normal or elevated.[2,3] All these changes can be induced by the inflammatory cytokines (e.g., interleukin-1 [IL-1]; tumor necrosis factor–α; interferons alfa, beta, and gamma; and perhaps transforming growth factor–β).[4] Under experimental conditions, these cytokines reduce erythropoietin production, cause hypoferremia, increase serum ferritin levels, impair erythropoiesis, and block release of iron from reticuloendothelial cells.[5]

Diagnosis

Mild anemia, with normal or elevated levels of leukocytes and platelets, in a patient with a chronic illness suggests the diagnosis of anemia of chronic disease. This normocytic or hypochromic and microcytic anemia is easily misdiagnosed as iron deficiency anemia, thalassemia trait, or a sideroblastic anemia. If the diagnosis is uncertain after careful examination of the blood smear, measurement of the serum ferritin level and a bone marrow examination that includes an iron stain are the most useful tests for making the differential diagnosis [see Table 1 and Figure 1]. In some cases, there is more than one cause of the anemia, and thorough examination of the patient may be required to establish the primary cause. For example, a patient who has anemia of chronic disease resulting from carcinoma of the colon may also be iron deficient because of intestinal bleeding. HIV infection produces complex hematologic effects, including Coombs-positive autoimmune hemolytic anemia, but it also causes anemia of chronic disease in the majority of patients with AIDS.[6]

Treatment

Identifying and treating the primary disease is the most important part of managing the anemia of chronic disease. Oral or parenteral iron administration is usually not helpful. Erythropoietin is the standard treatment for patients with anemia of

Table 1 Differential Diagnosis of Hypochromic Anemias

	Anemia of Chronic Disorders	Iron Deficiency Anemia	Thalassemia Trait	Sideroblastic Anemias
Smear	Usually normochromic, normocytic but can be mildly hypochromic, microcytic	Varies with the degree of the anemia [see Chapter 87]	Hypochromia, target cells, microcytes, basophilic stippling	May be similar to that of the thalassemia trait
Serum iron level	Low	Low	Normal	High
Iron-binding capacity	Low	High	Normal	Normal
Percent saturation	5–16	0–16	Normal (20–40)	60–90
Serum ferritin level	Normal or high	Low	Normal	High
Marrow iron in RE cells	+ + to + + +	0	+ + to + + +	+ + + +
Marrow iron in sideroblasts	0	0	+ + to + + +	+ + + + with ringed sideroblasts
Marrow erythroid precursors	Normal	Generally normal; cytoplasm may be scanty	Usually mild erythroid hyperplasia	Intense erythroid hyperplasia with dyserythropoiesis

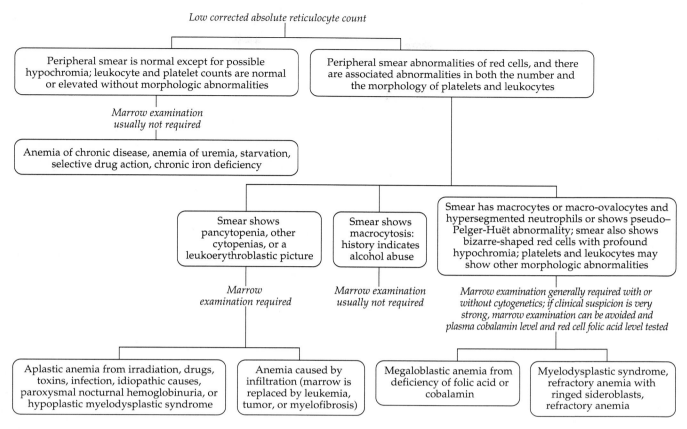

Figure 1 **Flowchart shows steps in the diagnosis of anemia caused by production defects. This type of anemia is suggested by a low corrected reticulocyte count or the finding of associated leukocyte or platelet abnormalities on the peripheral blood smear.**

chronic disease. For many patients, administration of pharmacologic doses of erythropoietin corrects the anemia of chronic disease by overriding the defect in erythropoietin production. It is useful to obtain a baseline measurement of the plasma erythropoietin level, because a response to erythropoietin is unlikely in patients whose endogenous levels are above 500 mU/ml. Erythropoietin responses have been reported in patients with rheumatoid arthritis,[7] AIDS,[8] inflammatory bowel disease,[9,10] and cancer.[11] To respond optimally, the patient must have adequate available iron stores (i.e., normal or elevated ferritin level or marrow iron stain) [*see Chapter 86*]. A common program is to start the patient on 100 to 150 U/kg subcutaneously three times weekly; if the hemoglobin level does not rise in 6 to 8 weeks, the dosage is increased to 300 U/kg three times weekly,[11] or daily injections are administered. If the hemoglobin level does not rise after 12 weeks, erythropoietin should be discontinued. Some physicians give a single subcutaneous dose of 40,000 units of erythropoietin weekly, but few data show this to be an equally effective schedule.[12]

ANEMIA IN SEVERE RENAL DISEASE

Pathophysiology and Etiology

The predominant cause of anemia in renal disease is a deficiency of erythropoietin production by the diseased kidneys. If underlying inflammatory renal disease is present, there may be a component of anemia of chronic disease.[13] Anorexia and poor iron intake, frequent blood sampling, and loss of erythrocytes during hemodialysis may produce iron deficiency. Folic acid de-

ficiency, hypersplenism, and secondary hyperparathyroidism with marrow fibrosis[4] may also promote anemia.

Aluminum toxicity can also cause an anemia in hemodialysis patients. This anemia was initially identified in patients who had so-called dialysis dementia. Very high plasma aluminum levels probably result from aluminum contamination of the dialysis fluid or gastrointestinal absorption of the aluminum gels taken to bind dietary phosphates. In vitro experiments have shown that aluminum inhibits the growth of the erythroid precursors colony-forming unit–erythroid (CFU-E) and burst-forming unit–erythroid (BFU-E).[14]

Diagnosis

The blood smear should be examined for erythrocyte fragmentation or echinocytosis to exclude other causes of the anemia. The presence of Heinz bodies suggests that oxidative hemolysis has occurred, perhaps caused by oxidants in the hemodialysis fluid.

Treatment

Erythropoietin is the standard treatment for anemic patients with renal disease. Erythropoietin therapy can eliminate the transfusion requirement for patients on hemodialysis and in patients with progressive renal disease who do not yet require hemodialysis. Such treatment significantly improves their quality of life.[15] Side effects, such as hyperkalemia and hypertension, occur infrequently. It is customary to start therapy with 50 U/kg of erythropoietin three times weekly, either intravenously or subcutaneously, and to increase the dosage as necessary to bring the hemoglobin level to the desired value. Parenteral iron supplementation improves the response. ImFed (a form of iron dextran) can be given intramuscularly or intravenously at doses ranging from 100 to 500 mg, with an anticipated frequency of reaction of 4.7%. Ferrlecit (a form of sodium ferric gluconate) can be infused intravenously (125 mg over 1 hour), with the occasional occurrence of hypotension and rash.[12] In a study of patients with anemia caused by aluminum toxicity, treatment with I.V. deferoxamine (30 mg/kg I.V. at the end of each dialysis session) produced substantial improvement.[16]

ANEMIA SECONDARY TO OTHER CONDITIONS

Alcohol Abuse

Excessive alcohol ingestion—either acute or chronic—has profound hematologic effects.[17] Ingestion of about 80 g of alcohol (one bottle of wine, six pints of beer, or one-third bottle of whiskey) daily may produce macrocytosis,[18] vacuolization of proerythroblasts, thrombocytopenia,[19] a sharp drop in serum folic acid levels, and a rise in serum iron levels; it may also impair the reticulocyte response to administered folic acid in a patient known to be folic acid deficient. Acute alcohol ingestion itself does not produce a sideroblastic or megaloblastic anemia.[17] Megaloblasts, macroovalocytes, and hypersegmented polymorphonuclear neutrophils (PMNs) usually appear when concomitant folic acid deficiency is present. Chronic alcohol abuse often results in folic acid or iron deficiency, severe liver disease, GI bleeding, hypersplenism, and the anemia of chronic disease.

Starvation

Starvation resulting from anorexia nervosa or protein deficiency can cause anemia and even pancytopenia. Hemolysis may also be present [see Figure 2]. The bone marrow biopsy is hypocellular, with a characteristic gelatinous background material consisting of acid mucopolysaccharides. The anemia can occur despite normal folic acid and cobalamin (vitamin B_{12}) levels and can be corrected with proper nutrition.

Immunotherapy

Immunotherapy for cancer using IL-2, either alone or in combination with lymphokine-activated killer (LAK) cells, produces several hematologic effects, the most serious of which is transfusion-dependent anemia. It is thought that IL-2 suppresses hematopoiesis, perhaps by causing the release of interferon gamma, a known inhibitor of hematopoiesis. Other hematologic effects produced by IL-2 and LAK cells include thrombocytopenia, lymphopenia, and eosinophilia.[20]

Chloramphenicol and Other Toxins

Chloramphenicol produces sporadic or idiosyncratic aplastic anemia [see Aplastic Anemia, below] and regularly causes dose-dependent, reversible erythroid suppression.[21] Arsenic can produce anemia by interfering with red blood cell production. Leukopenia and thrombocytopenia, as well as a peripheral neuropathy, can also result from arsenic exposure. The bone marrow cellularity may be increased, decreased, or normal.

Hypothyroidism

Hypothyroidism impairs erythrocyte production. The presence of macrocytosis in a hypothyroid patient suggests concomitant dietary folic acid deficiency or pernicious anemia.

Panhypopituitarism

The mild anemia that is associated with severe panhypopituitarism can be corrected by replacement of adrenal, thyroid, and gonadal hormones; the enhancing effect of androgens on the action of erythropoietin is well known.

Aging

The hemoglobin levels, red blood cell indices, and leukocyte and platelet counts of healthy older people are similar to those of younger adults; this finding was confirmed in a study of patients who were 84 years of age or older.[22] Thus, a workup is required when anemia occurs in such older patients.

Production Defects Associated with Marrow Aplasia or Replacement

The combination of anemia and neutropenia or thrombocytopenia or the combination of all three of these abnormalities (i.e., pancytopenia) usually indicates that the hematopoietic marrow is

a

b

c

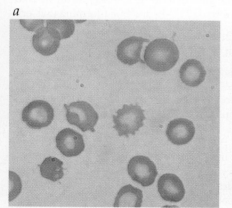
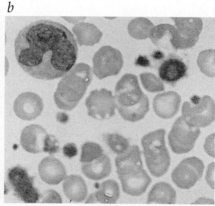
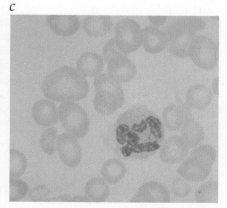

Figure 2 The peripheral smear changes seen in severe liver disease or starvation (*a*) include distinct variation in size and shape of red blood cells; both sharply spiculed cells (spur cells) and scalloped erythrocytes are prominent. The leukoerythroblastic blood smear (*b*) indicates marrow replacement with extramedullary hematopoiesis. It is characterized by variation in the size and shape of red blood cells, by the presence of nucleated red blood cells in the peripheral blood, by giant platelets, and by immaturity in the myeloid series. In folic acid or cobalamin deficiency (*c*), the smear is characterized by variation in erythrocyte size and by distinct macrocytosis. Occasionally, fish-tailed erythrocytes are present, along with hypersegmented neutrophils.

damaged. If the marrow cavity is infiltrated but pluripotent stem cells are intact, extramedullary hematopoiesis will often develop in the organs of fetal hematopoiesis (i.e., spleen, liver, and distal bones).

Pancytopenia can be congenital or acquired. The finding of combined cytopenias or of immature cells in the blood (myelocytes, metamyelocytes, and erythroblasts)—that is, a leukoerythroblastic blood smear—suggests extramedullary hematopoiesis [*see Figure 2*]. These findings are an indication for bone marrow aspiration and biopsy.

APLASTIC ANEMIA

Definition

Pancytopenia (i.e., anemia, neutropenia, and thrombocytopenia) and aplastic marrow on biopsy examination [*see Figure 3*] establish a working diagnosis of aplastic anemia. The biopsy specimen must not be taken from a marrow site that has been irradiated. Severe aplastic anemia (SAA) is defined by (1) marrow of less than 25% normal cellularity, or marrow of less than 50% normal cellularity in which fewer than 30% of the cells are hematopoietic, and (2) two out of three abnormal peripheral blood values (absolute reticulocyte count less than 40,000/μl, absolute neutrophil count [ANC] less than 500 μl, or platelet level less than 20,000/μl). These criteria have been criticized as being relatively insensitive. Some investigators prefer to identify a cohort of patients with very severe aplastic anemia (VSAA) as those who had an ANC less than 200/μl.[23]

Etiology

Aplastic anemia has a number of causes [*see Table 2*], although in many cases the exact cause cannot be determined.

Ionizing irradiation and chemotherapeutic drugs that are used in the management of malignant and immunologic disorders have the capacity to destroy hematopoietic stem cells. With careful dosing and scheduling, recovery is expected. Certain drugs, such as chloramphenicol, produce marrow aplasia that is not dose dependent. Gold therapy and the inhalation of organic solvent vapors (e.g., benzene or glue) can also cause fatal marrow failure.

In 2% to 10% of hepatitis patients, severe aplasia occurs 2 to 3 months after a seemingly typical case of acute disease, usually in young men. Often, the hepatitis has no obvious cause, and tests for hepatitis A, B, and C are negative.[24] There is a high incidence of aplastic anemia after liver transplantation in patients with severe non-A, non-B hepatitis.[25]

Several lines of evidence support the possibility that immune disorders can lead to aplasia. Marrow aplasia occurs in graft versus host disease (GVHD).[26] Immunosuppressive preconditioning improves the chances of successful transplantation of syngeneic marrow into patients with aplastic anemia,[27] and immunosuppressive therapy has been used successfully to treat idiopathic aplastic anemia.[26,27] The blood of some patients with aplastic anemia appears to contain suppressor T cells that suppress the growth of the committed progenitor cells known as colony-forming unit–granulocyte-macrophage (CFU-GM). The suppressor T cells may act by producing interferon gamma.[27] The result of these complex immune mechanisms involving suppressor T cells is a profound decrease in primitive hematopoietic cells as measured by both the long-term culture–initiating cell (LTC-IC) assay and the ability to form secondary colonies from the colonies surviving 5 weeks of marrow culture.[28]

Aplasia can also be part of a prodrome to hairy-cell leukemia [*see Chapter 203*], acute lymphoblastic leukemia [*see Chapter 202*], or, in rare cases, acute myeloid leukemia, or it can develop in the course of myelodysplasia [*see Chapter 202*].

Diagnosis

The diagnosis of aplastic anemia requires a marrow aspirate and biopsy [*see Figure 3*] as well as a thorough history of drug exposures, infections, and especially symptoms suggesting viral illnesses and serologic test results for hepatitis, infectious mononucleosis, HIV, and parvovirus [*see Figure 4*]. Measurement of red cell CD59 is helpful in the diagnosis of paroxysmal nocturnal hemoglobinuria.

It is also important to determine the severity of aplastic anemia. Severe cases are associated with a very low rate of spontaneous remission and a mortality of 70% within 1 year. In contrast, 80% of patients who have milder forms of aplastic anemia survive for 1 year.[23]

Differential Diagnosis

Hypersplenism can produce pancytopenia by splenic sequestration and then removal of all three cell lines in diseases such as chronic lymphocytic leukemia, systemic lupus erythematosus, and congestive splenomegaly. In these diseases, however, the marrow is not aplastic but rather shows hyperplasia of the involved cell lines.

Treatment of Mild Aplastic Anemia

Treatment of milder forms of aplastic anemia involves removing the offending agent and providing supportive therapy, primarily transfusion therapy, anticipating that the remaining pluripotent stem cells will repopulate the marrow.

Platelet transfusion Thrombocytopenia is often a major problem associated with aplastic anemia. It should be managed by platelet transfusion as needed to control or prevent bleeding.

a

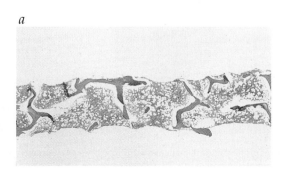

b

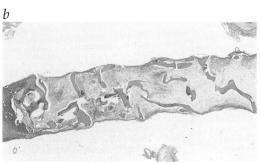

Figure 3 Shown are (*a*) biopsy of normal bone marrow and (*b*) biopsy of bone marrow from a patient with aplastic anemia showing almost complete aplasia.

Table 2 Causes of Aplastic Anemia

IRRADIATION

DRUGS

Agents whose use regularly causes myelosuppression
Alkylating agents: melphalan, cyclophosphamide, chlorambucil, busulfan
Antimetabolites: azathioprine, 6-mercaptopurine, hydroxyurea, methotrexate
Other antitumor agents: daunorubicin, doxorubicin, carmustine, lomustine, amsacrine

Agents whose use occasionally causes myelosuppression
Chloramphenicol, gold compounds, arsenic, sulfonamides, mephenytoin, trimethadione, phenylbutazone, quinacrine, indomethacin, diclofenac, felbamate

TOXINS
Benzene, glue vapors

INFECTIONS
Non-A, non-B, non-C hepatitis, infectious mononucleosis, parvovirus infection (attacks erythroid precursors), HIV

MALIGNANT DISEASES
Hairy-cell leukemia, acute lymphocytic leukemia, acute myeloid leukemia (rarely), myelodysplastic syndromes

CLONAL DISORDERS
Paroxysmal nocturnal hemoglobinuria

IMMUNE-MEDIATED APLASIA
Eosinophilic fasciitis

INHERITED DISORDERS
Fanconi anemia

PREGNANCY

Usually, a threshold of 10,000 platelets/μl is used for transfusion, but conservative treatment is best, and as few transfusions as possible are given. Extensive platelet replacement may result in allosensitization to platelets and may complicate future allogeneic bone marrow transplantation. Red blood cell transfusions are given as required to control the symptoms and signs of anemia.

Hematopoietic growth factor therapy Granulocyte colony-stimulating factor (G-CSF) and granulocyte-macrophage colony-stimulating factor (GM-CSF) have been given to patients to raise the absolute neutrophil count and help combat infection. They are usually ineffective when used alone, because of the severe deficiency in precursor cells, which are the target for the actions of G-CSF and GM-CSF.[29] It is generally preferable to proceed to definitive treatment: immunosuppressive therapy or preferably allogeneic bone marrow transplantation if a matched sibling donor is available [*see Chapter 96*].[30]

Gold therapy Because gold may cause aplastic anemia by its toxic effect on stem cells, I.V. acetylcysteine and dimercaprol have been used as chelating agents. The suggestion that gold mediates an immunologic attack on stem cells has led to trials of immunosuppressive therapy consisting of antithymocyte globulin (ATG) and high-dose glucocorticoids in patients with gold-induced aplasia.[31]

Immunosuppression Three forms of immunosuppression have been shown to produce partial remission in aplastic anemia.[29,30,32] ATG produced sustained remission in about half of the patients in a randomized trial.[30] High-dose corticosteroids improved blood counts in about 40% of treated patients, and cyclosporine was also shown to be beneficial.[30] (Androgens such as oxymetholone may have a role in the treatment of severe aplastic anemia but are not given alone.[29,32])

Although each of these agents can be used individually or consecutively in the treatment of aplastic anemia, a controlled study suggests that results are better when all three are used simultaneously.[29,30] The combination of ATG, a corticosteroid, and cyclosporine resulted in an actuarial survival of 62% at 36 months. The first signs of response occurred at about 4 weeks; the median time to remission was 60 to 82 days.[30]

One recommendation, based on the usual availability of horse ATG in the United States,[29,30] is to administer horse ATG at a dosage of 40 mg/kg/day in 500 ml of saline for 4 days over a period of 4 to 5 hours through an I.V. line equipped with a microaggregate in-line filter. The toxic side effect of ATG is serum sickness, which can usually be controlled with corticosteroids. Prednisone (60 to 100 mg/day) is given orally in divided doses, or methylprednisolone (40 mg) is added to the infusion bottle, and the dose can be increased to 1 mg/kg/day. Corticosteroid therapy is adjusted to control serum sickness, but it can usually be tapered after 2 weeks and stopped after 30 days. Because ATG can lower platelet counts, platelet transfusions are given as needed to maintain the platelet count at more than 20,000 μl.

Cyclosporine (10 to 12 mg/kg/day) is given orally in two divided doses, with the aim of achieving whole blood trough levels of 500 to 800 ng/ml or a serum level of 100 to 200 ng/ml. After 29 days, the cyclosporine dosage can be tapered for a trough whole blood level of 200 to 500 ng/ml.[29,30] The cyclosporine is continued for at least 6 months. Cyclosporine can cause hypertension, renal toxicity, hypomagnesemia, vitiligo, tremors, hypertrichosis, susceptibility to *Pneumocystis carinii* pneumonia (PCP), and gingival hyperplasia.[29,30] In one study, 300 mg of aerosolized pentamidine was given every 4 weeks as PCP prophylaxis.[30]

In another study, G-CSF (5 μg/kg/day) was given subcutaneously for the first 90 days, along with I.V. methylprednisolone (2 mg/kg/day on days 1 through 5, followed by 1 mg/kg/day on days 6 through 10, and tapered off in 30 days), with good results.[33]

In contrast to patients who undergo allogeneic bone marrow transplantation, patients who respond to immunosuppressive therapy are not actually cured. Many of these patients continue to have moderate cytopenia[34]; 20% to 36% experience relapses of aplastic anemia,[29,30,34] and as many as 20% to 36% eventually devel-

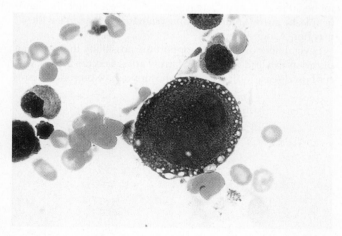

Figure 4 **Giant pronormoblast, evident on this marrow smear, strongly suggests a diagnosis of parvovirus infection.**

Table 3 Causes of Acquired Pure Red Cell Aplasia

Primary

Associated with thymoma in 10%–15% of cases[44]

Idiopathic causes

Secondary

Neoplasia: chronic lymphocytic leukemia, chronic myeloid leukemia, Hodgkin and non-Hodgkin lymphomas; large granular lymphocytic proliferative disorders; prodrome to myelodysplastic syndromes[44]

Systemic lupus erythematosus or rheumatoid arthritis

Associated with pregnancy

Associated with autoimmune hemolytic anemia

Drugs: those most commonly associated are phenytoin, chlorpropamide, zidovudine,[50] trimethoprim-sulfamethoxazole, isoniazid[44]

Multiple endocrine gland insufficiency

Primary amyloidosis

Infections: infectious mononucleosis, viral hepatitis, parvovirus infection, HIV[44]

ABO-incompatible bone marrow transplantation

---

op clonal disorders, such as paroxysmal nocturnal hemoglobinuria, myelodysplastic syndrome, and acute leukemia.[29,30] Patients also are at increased risk for the development of solid tumors after treatment of aplastic anemia, but the risk is the same for patients who underwent immunosuppressive therapy as it is for those who underwent allogeneic bone marrow transplantation.[35] More than 50% of patients who have relapses of aplastic anemia after initially responding to immunosuppressive therapy may respond to a second course of therapy.[29,30] For unresponsive patients, a trial of rabbit ATG may work. The rabbit ATG (3.5 mg/kg/day diluted in saline and infused over 6 to 8 hours for 5 consecutive days)[36] is given along with cyclosporine (5 mg/kg/day p.o. on days 1 through 180, then tapered) and G-CSF (5 µg/kg/day on days 1 through 90).

An intriguing report concerns 10 patients with severe aplastic anemia who were treated with high-dose I.V. cyclophosphamide (45 mg/kg/day) for 4 consecutive days.[37] Some patients also received cyclosporine. Only one course of I.V. cyclophosphamide was given. Seven of 10 patients had a complete hematologic response, and six were still alive after a median follow-up of 10.8 years (range, 7.3 to 17.8 years). This approach clearly needs to be tested and evaluated.

Treatment of Severe Aplastic Anemia

The choice of appropriate therapy for patients with SAA is influenced by age and disease severity. The European Group for Blood and Marrow Transplantation reported on the results of immunosuppressive therapy in 810 patients subdivided into three age-groups: younger than 49, 50 through 59, and older than 60. The 5-year survival rates for those with SAA were 86%, 72%, and 54%, respectively; for those with VSAA, the comparable rates were 49%, 40%, and 21%.[38] Older patients had more bleeding and infections.

Patients younger than 20 years Allogeneic bone marrow transplantation should be performed in patients younger than 20 years if a matched sibling donor is available. Although there are risks, including chronic GVHD and organ dysfunction caused by the conditioning program,[29] 50% to 80% of patients may be cured; the incidence of later clonal disorders is very low.[32] Allogeneic

bone marrow transplantation along with conditioning programs consisting of cyclophosphamide and ATG produced an actuarial survival rate of 69% after 15 years.[32] Patients younger than 20 years who do not have a matched sibling donor should receive immunosuppressive therapy until the results with matched unrelated donors improves. Allogeneic transplantation from a matched unrelated donor has produced a 2-year survival rate of only 29% because of severe GVHD.[29]

Patients between 20 and 45 years of age Patients between 20 and 45 years of age who are in excellent health and have a fully matched sibling donor may be able to tolerate GVHD and thus benefit from the curative potential of an allogeneic bone marrow transplant. Some experts propose that allogeneic bone marrow transplantation should be considered for this age-group,[32] particularly because newer conditioning programs seem to be capable of reducing the severity of GVHD.[32,39]

Patients older than 45 years It is thought that the impact of GVHD is too severe for patients older than 45 years and that these patients should receive immunosuppressive therapy.[29,32]

ACQUIRED PURE RED CELL APLASIA

Definition

In adults, pure red cell aplasia (PRCA) is an acquired disorder. The anemia is severe (hematocrit usually less than 20%), reticulocytopenia is profound (often 0%), and marrow erythroid precursors are virtually absent. Marrow myeloid and megakaryocytic elements are preserved, however, and the peripheral platelet and white blood cell counts are also normal.

Pathophysiology

In PRCA, erythropoiesis is thought to be inhibited primarily by immune mechanisms, including autoantibody-mediated and T cell–mediated suppression of erythroid progenitors, usually at a stage after the CFU-E stage of erythroid differentiation and before formation of proerythroblasts. T cells, particularly of the large granular lymphocyte (T-LGL) class, may be involved in the suppression of erythropoiesis, and in some cases, there is evidence that the suppression is caused by clonal T cells.[40] Autoantibody inhibition of erythropoietin has also been described, but it is quite uncommon.[41] Two other mechanisms probably cause PRCA: (1) a specific attack on erythroid precursors by the parvovirus B19 (one report indicated that 14% of cases were caused by this virus[42]) and (2) an underlying hematopoietic clonal abnormality that may be a prodrome to myelodysplastic syndrome.[41]

Etiology

PRCA may be caused by a variety of processes, including neoplasia, autoimmune disorders, drugs, and infections [see Table 3].

The association of PRCA with LGL proliferation and leukemia is increasingly being recognized. The routine use of T cell receptor gene rearrangement studies in one series showed that nine of 14 patients had a clonal LGL disorder.[43] Presumably, these LGL cells directly mediate inhibition of erythropoiesis.[42,43] In perhaps as many as 20% of cases, PRCA may be a prodrome to the myelodysplastic syndromes or acute myeloid leukemia.[42,44]

Erythroblastopenia also occurs in a small percentage of patients who have autoimmune hemolytic anemia [see Chapter 89] and may be caused by autoantibody attack on maturing normoblasts.

The treatment of HIV infection with zidovudine (AZT) produces, in virtually all patients, an anemia that is usually marked by significant macrocytosis.[45] Moderate erythroid hypoplasia is the usual cause of this anemia, which can progress to PRCA.

Parvovirus infection is the cause of the transient aplastic crises that occur in patients who have severe hemolytic disorders. The marrow in patients with such disorders must compensate for the peripheral hemolysis by increasing its production up to sevenfold and thus typically shows an intense erythroid hyperplasia. Although parvovirus can affect all precursor cells, the red cell precursors are the most profoundly affected.[42]

PRCA can complicate ABO-incompatible allogeneic bone marrow transplantation; the recipient's serum continues to express anti-A or anti-B isohemagglutinins against donor A or B antigen expressed on the surface of erythroid progenitors.[44] With PRCA of pregnancy, antibodies against BFU-E usually disappear after delivery, coinciding with clinical remission.[46]

Diagnosis

After the marrow aspirate and biopsy, the workup to diagnose PRCA usually includes computed tomography of the chest to evaluate the possibility of thymoma, immunophenotypic analysis of circulating blood or marrow lymphocytes to identify LGL proliferation, marrow cytogenetics to evaluate the possibility of myelodysplastic syndromes, and antibody tests for parvovirus.[42] A diagnostic hallmark of parvovirus infection is the appearance of giant pronormoblasts in the marrow [see Figure 4]. The distinction between PRCA associated with the myelodysplastic syndromes and acute myeloid leukemia may be difficult to determine at the time of diagnosis unless a typical myelodysplastic cytogenetic abnormality is detected during a bone marrow examination.

Treatment

Treatment of PRCA depends on the identified cause. Offending drugs should be stopped. If a thymoma is present, it should be removed surgically[44]; this procedure leads to improvement in about one third of such patients.[44] When surgery is impossible, one should consider a course of prednisone combined with octreotide, a somatostatin analogue that binds to thymomas and may inhibit the function of thymic immune cells.[47]

When red cell aplasia is not attributable to thymoma, LGL syndrome, or leukemia, therapy can begin with the administration of 60 mg of oral prednisone daily in divided doses; this regimen should be continued for 1 to 3 months.[42] If a patient fails to respond, as indicated by a rise in the reticulocyte count, cyclophosphamide or azathioprine should be added at a dosage of 2 to 3 mg/kg/day orally. Patients with marrow cytogenetic abnormalities suggestive of myelodysplastic syndrome respond poorly.[42,43] Some patients who are refractory to other forms of therapy have responded well to I.V. IgG (0.4 g/kg/day for 5 days).[48]

Patients with LGL proliferation as the underlying cause respond well to cyclophosphamide.[43,49] Usually, low doses of cyclophosphamide (50 to 100 mg/day p.o.) for 3 to 6 months suffice to produce remission, which is sometimes associated with disappearance of LGL proliferation.[43,50] Patients who respond poorly usually respond to oral cyclosporine.[43,50] Cyclosporine (12 mg/kg/day) has been shown to produce responses of approximately 65%, even in patients who did not respond to corticosteroids, plasmapheresis, cyclophosphamide, or azathioprine therapy.[44,51]

For patients in whom parvovirus infection is the cause of PRCA, I.V. IgG works well; the standard dosage is 0.4 g/kg/day for 5 days.[42] For AIDS patients with parvovirus infection and PRCA, I.V. IgG may have to be continued.[50] Recovery from the transient crises of parvovirus infection occurs spontaneously in 1 to 2 weeks after onset of the infection.

ATG therapy for patients with refractory PRCA is similar to that for patients with aplastic anemia (40 mg/kg/day I.V. for 4 days).[44] In very refractory cases, allogeneic bone marrow transplantation can be effective.[52]

Production Defects Associated with Marrow Erythroid Hyperplasia and Ineffective Erythropoiesis

DEFINITION

Anemia with a low reticulocyte count may occur despite intense marrow erythroid hyperplasia. This paradoxical situation is the hallmark of ineffective erythropoiesis or intramedullary hemolysis. Generalized erythroid impairment may be present, or specific subpopulations of erythroid precursors may be involved. Some of these subpopulations escape death in the marrow, but their progeny are so severely damaged that they are rapidly removed from the circulation, thus giving the picture of peripheral hemolysis. Other signs of ineffective erythropoiesis include jaundice, a very high serum lactic dehydrogenase level, and 75% to 90% saturation of serum iron-binding capacity. The classic ferrokinetic picture shows rapid plasma iron clearance, which indicates intense erythroid precursor activity. The delivery of labeled red blood cells to the peripheral circulation, however, is dramatically reduced, which suggests that the precursors are being destroyed by intramedullary hemolysis.

The differential diagnosis includes megaloblastic anemias, sideroblastic anemias, thalassemia [see Chapter 89], myelodysplastic syndromes [see Chapter 202], and agnogenic myeloid metaplasia [see Chapter 204].

MEGALOBLASTIC ANEMIAS

Etiology

Megaloblastic anemias are caused by cobalamin or folic acid deficiency, by drugs that interfere with the synthesis of DNA or with the absorption or metabolism of cobalamin, and by genetic disorders that interfere with DNA metabolism or with the absorption or distribution of cobalamin.

Pathophysiology

Megaloblastic erythropoiesis is characterized by defective DNA synthesis and arrest at the G_2 phase, with impaired maturation and a buildup of cells that do not synthesize DNA and that contain anomalous DNA. This condition leads to asynchronous maturation between the nucleus and cytoplasm.[53] RNA production and protein synthesis continue; thus, larger cells, or megaloblasts, are produced. Ineffective erythropoiesis results, and there is disagreement about the presence of increased apoptosis.[54,55] It is presumed that similar defects in DNA synthesis characterize the mucosal abnormalities of the stomach and tongue. In the granulocytic line, the presence of giant metamyelocytes represents ineffective granulopoiesis.[53]

The role of folic acid and cobalamin The interactions between folic acid and cobalamin are critical in the metabolism of single carbon units, mainly methylene and formyl analogues, which have a key role in the synthesis of DNA and purines [see

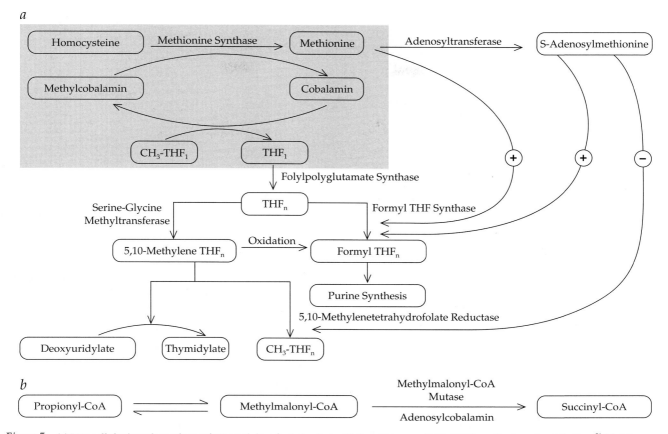

Figure 5 (*a*) **Intracellular interdependent cofactor activity of cobalamin and folic acid is essential in DNA synthesis and metabolism.**[56] (*b*) **Adenosylcobalamin is a cofactor in the synthesis of succinyl–coenzyme A from methylmalonyl–coenzyme A.**[56] **(CoA—coenzyme A)**

Figure 5a].[56] There are two major coenzymes of cobalamin, adenosylcobalamin and methylcobalamin. Adenosylcobalamin is the coenzyme for methylmalonyl–coenzyme A mutase, which catalyzes a step in the catabolism of propionic acid [*see Figure 5b*].[56] Methylcobalamin is the coenzyme for methionine synthase, which functions as a methyltransferase in the reaction that converts 5-methyltetrahydrofolate (CH_3-THF_1) to tetrahydrofolate (THF_1) [*see Figure 5a*].[56] Cobalamin and folic acid [*see Figure 6*] combine in the methionine synthase reaction [*see Figure 5a*], in which the methyl group of CH_3-THF_1 is transferred to cobalamin to form methylcobalamin. Methylcobalamin then transfers its methyl group to homocysteine to form methionine. The monoglutamated tetrahydrofolate (THF_1), which is formed by this reaction, is polyglutamated by the enzyme folylpolyglutamate synthase, and a methylene group is added to it by the serine-glycine methyltransferase to form 5,10-methylene THF_n. 5,10-Methylene THF_n provides its methylene to convert deoxyuridylate to thymidylate, a key step in DNA synthesis. 5,10-Methylene THF_n can also be directly converted to CH_3-THF_n by the enzyme 5,10-methylene tetrahydrofolate reductase, thereby making its methyl group available. Formyl THF_n (also called leucovorin, folinic acid, or citrovorum factor) has an important role in purine synthesis and DNA metabolism. It can be generated by oxidation of 5,10-methylene THF_n or directly from THF_n by the enzyme formyl THF synthase, with methionine providing the formate group [*see Figure 5a*].[56] When cobalamin is deficient, CH_3-THF_1 cannot transfer its methyl group to cobalamin; therefore, THF_1 is not free to be polyglutamated by folylpolyglutamate synthase [*see Figure 5a*]. The polyglutamated form is required for synthesis of either 5,10-methylene THF_n or formyl THF_n; thus, DNA synthesis and purine synthesis are blocked. This hypothesis, the methylfolate trap hypothesis, is supported by the finding of increased levels of CH_3-THF_1 in the plasma of cobalamin-deficient patients. An alternative explanation is the formate starvation hypothesis, wherein cobalamin deficiency impairs methionine generation, which there-

Figure 6 **Folic acid functions as a coenzyme in single-carbon transfer reactions. It is not physiologically active until it is reduced at positions 5, 6, 7, and 8 to tetrahydrofolate (THF). Single-carbon groups (R) such as methyl analogues and formate are added at either position 5 or position 10, or they may bridge from 5 to 10, as shown. There may be several glutamates attached in sequence (R_1), which convert the monoglutamate to the polyglutamate form. Enzymes of the intestinal mucosa split polyglutamates back to monoglutamate, whereas liver enzymes add glutamate to tetrahydrofolate or to other reduced folic acids.**

fore cannot provide the methyl groups needed by the enzyme formyl THF_n synthase to produce formyl THF_n.

Exposure to nitrous oxide (N_2O) anesthesia for as little as 6 hours produces marrow megaloblastosis; long-term exposure to N_2O can cause neuropathy similar to that seen in patients with severe cobalamin deficiency. The serum folic acid level rises quickly, and methionine levels fall because N_2O inactivates methionine synthase.[57] This observation supports the importance of methionine metabolism in the megaloblastosis of cobalamin and folic acid deficiency.

Other aspects of folic acid and cobalamin metabolism   Neither folic acid nor cobalamin is produced by humans in adequate amounts; both must be absorbed from food. Cobalamin, in particular, is derived from microbial sources and is ingested in the form of meat or eggs.

Most of the dietary folic acid is in the polyglutamate form and is absorbed at the intestinal mucosa. Absorption of radioactively labeled folic acid approaches 80% of a 200 μg dose.[53,56] The serum folic acid level appears to be maintained by folic acid absorbed from food. Enterohepatic circulation of folic acid has been observed in which folic acid passing into the bile and small intestine is quantitatively reabsorbed. In an animal model, ethanol administration blocks the entry of folic acid into the bile. This effect could account, in part, for the sharp fall in the serum folic acid level seen 8 hours after alcohol consumption. A similar fall in serum folic acid level follows phenytoin ingestion. The daily requirement of cobalamin is about 1 μg, and the amount usually provided by the Western diet, which is rich in animal products, is about 5 to 15 μg.[58]

R proteins are a class of cobalamin-binding glycoproteins found in saliva and gastric juice; they are produced by granulocytes and other tissues. Intrinsic factor (IF) is a 45 kd glycoprotein, secreted by gastric parietal cells, that is highly specific for unaltered cobalamin. The R protein–cobalamin complex does not bind to ileal receptors and thus is not absorbed. In the stomach, cobalamin binds preferentially to R proteins rather than to IF[53,56,58]; thus, it is the physiologically inactive R protein–cobalamin complex that is discharged into the duodenum. In the duodenum and small intestine, however, the pancreatic proteases along with pepsin degrade the R proteins, freeing cobalamin and allowing it to bind to IF. Thus, gastric atrophy and pancreatic insufficiency contribute to cobalamin malabsorption.[56,58] The IF-cobalamin complex, in the presence of Ca^{2+} and at a pH level greater than 5.4, binds specifically to a limited number of sites on the microvilli of mucosal cells in the terminal portion of the ileum, where absorption takes place [see Figure 7].[56,58]

In the plasma, most of the cobalamin is bound to the physiologically unimportant R proteins, transcobalamins I and III (TC-I and TC-III), which are about 70% saturated with cobalamin.[59] The physiologically important transport protein is transcobalamin II (TC-II), which has considerable specificity for cobalamin and is only 5% to 10% saturated with cobalamin. Receptors for the TC-II–cobalamin complex are present on many cell membranes. TC-II binds about 90% of a newly injected dose of cobalamin; and the complex is rapidly cleared, with a half-life of 6 to 9 minutes.[58,59] In persons with congenital TC-II deficiency, which results in severe megaloblastic anemia, both plasma cobalamin transport and cobalamin absorption are impaired. Impaired cobalamin absorption implies that TC-II has a role within the ileal enterocyte, where cobalamin is transferred from IF to TC-II.

The elevation of cobalamin levels seen in patients with chronic granulocytic leukemia or significant granulocytosis is caused by

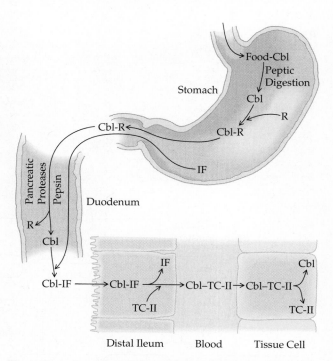

Figure 7   **Cobalamin assimilation. Dietary cobalamin (Cbl) enters the stomach and binds to R protein. This physiologically inactive complex enters the duodenum. In the small intestine, pancreatic enzymes and pepsin digest the R protein, and Cbl binds to intrinsic factor (IF). The Cbl-IF complex passes through the intestine until it reaches receptors on the microvilli of mucosal cells in the distal ileum. The Cbl is then transferred to transcobalamin II (TC-II), which circulates in the blood until it binds to receptors on cells in the body and is internalized.**

increases in TC-I and, to a lesser extent, TC-III, which are produced in granulocytes.

Diagnostic Approach to Megaloblastic Anemias

Signs of ineffective erythropoiesis include jaundice, a very high level of serum lactic dehydrogenase, and 75% to 90% saturation of serum iron-binding capacity. The classic ferrokinetic picture shows rapid plasma iron clearance, indicating intense erythroid precursor activity; but delivery of labeled red blood cells to the peripheral circulation is dramatically reduced, suggesting that the precursors are being destroyed by intramedullary hemolysis.

The peripheral smear shows macro-ovalocytes, fish-tailed red blood cells, hypersegmented neutrophils, and, occasionally, nucleated red blood cells [see Figure 2]. The finding that a single polymorphonuclear neutrophil has six lobes or that 5% of PMNs have five lobes constitutes strong evidence of megaloblastic anemia. In severe cases, granulocytopenia as well as thrombocytopenia is present. Examination of the bone marrow reveals megaloblastic erythroid hyperplasia and giant metamyelocytes.[53] If concurrent severe iron deficiency is present, the full morphologic expression of megaloblastosis is blocked, although the giant metamyelocytes in the marrow and hypersegmented PMNs in the peripheral blood are not affected.

MEGALOBLASTIC ANEMIA CAUSED BY COBALAMIN DEFICIENCY (PERNICIOUS ANEMIA)

Diagnosis

Clinical manifestations   In addition to macrocytic and megaloblastic anemia, the patient with cobalamin deficiency may have atrophy of the lingual papillae and glossitis. Neuropathy is the presenting feature in about 12% of patients with cobalamin (vitamin B$_{12}$) deficiency without concomitant anemia.[60] Patients with severe cobalamin deficiency initially complain of paresthesia. The sense of touch and temperature sensitivity may be minimally impaired. Memory impairment and depression may be prominent.[60] The disease may progress, involving the dorsal columns, causing ataxia and weakness. The physical examination reveals a broad-base gait, Romberg sign, slowed reflexes, and loss of sense of position and feeling of vibration (especially when tested with a 256 Hz tuning fork). If the disorder is not detected and treated, the lateral columns become involved, resulting in weakness, spasticity, inability to walk, sustained clonus, hyperreflexia, and Babinski sign. Because the peripheral nerves as well as the dorsal and lateral columns are involved, these neurologic manifestations are sometimes termed subacute combined degeneration or subacute combined system disease.

Cobalamin deficiency appears to be the cause of various neuropsychiatric disorders, with such symptoms as paresthesia, ataxia, limb weakness, gait disturbance, memory defects, hallucinations, and personality and mood changes.[59] These symptoms, however, cannot be easily accounted for by the type of spinal cord lesions that occur in patients with cobalamin deficiency.

Investigators have tried to determine whether a defect in methionine synthesis or an abnormality in propionic acid metabolism accounts for the neuropathy associated with cobalamin deficiency [see Figure 5b], but the exact mechanism remains obscure. However, two observations point to impairment of methionine synthase as the cause of the neuropathy. First, the administration of N$_2$O to monkeys produces a neuropathy that is blocked by simultaneous treatment with methionine. Second, a patient with a congenital impairment of methionine synthase activity was reported to have a neuropathy characterized by abnormal gait, numbness, and paresthesias.[53,60]

Laboratory tests Macrocytosis (mean corpuscular volume [MCV] greater than 100 fl) that may not be apparent on examination of the peripheral smear is easily detected when red blood cell counts are made with an electronic particle counter. Plasma cobalamin levels and red blood cell folic acid levels should probably be measured if the MCV is greater than 100 fl. If performed, a bone marrow aspirate and biopsy typically reveal enormous megaloblastic erythroid hyperplasia with giant metamyelocytes.[53] The hypercellularity can be so dramatic and megaloblasts so immature that clinicians still sometimes make the erroneous diagnosis of leukemia.[53,61]

The standard approach to determining the cause of proven cobalamin deficiency relies on the Schilling test, which measures the absorption of cobalamin labeled with cobalt-57 (^{57}Co). After 1 μg of radioactively labeled cobalamin is given orally, 1,000 μg of unlabeled cobalamin is given parenterally. The parenteral dose saturates transcobalamins I, II, and III, so that a significant portion of the absorbed material is flushed and excreted in the urine. If the amount of ^{57}Co-labeled cobalamin measured in an accurately collected 24-hour urine sample is less than 10% of the dose that was administered orally, cobalamin absorption is poor.

One can repeat the Schilling test, adding supplementary oral intrinsic factor. For pernicious anemia, addition of IF should correct the poor cobalamin absorption, unless the supplementary IF is not fully active, the patient secretes antibodies to IF, or the patient is taking drugs that interfere with cobalamin absorption. Prolonged cobalamin deficiency impairs ileal uptake, which may

affect test results. Therefore, the Schilling test with IF is best done after the patient has had several weeks of cobalamin therapy.

There are increasing numbers of reports of patients with proven pernicious anemia who have low or borderline serum cobalamin levels but normal Schilling test results. As the gastric atrophic lesion of pernicious anemia progresses, the ability to produce acid-pepsin is lost before all IF activity disappears. Thus, the ability to cleave the R protein–cobalamin complex, freeing cobalamin to bind to IF, is impaired. However, there may be sufficient IF to bind the free oral cobalamin administered in the Schilling test and therefore yield a normal value. Malabsorption of cobalamin can be demonstrated by means of a food Schilling test, which is not available clinically. This test is performed with eggs from chickens that have been injected with radioactive cobalamin[62] and indicates whether there is insufficient acid-pepsin to split the cobalamin-enzyme complex and release free cobalamin to be bound by IF. If pernicious anemia is strongly suspected in a patient whose Schilling test result is apparently normal, other steps should be taken to confirm the diagnosis, including examination of the blood cell morphology, measurement of the anti-IF antibody or the serum levels of homocysteine and methylmalonic acid, or performance of a therapeutic trial with parenterally administered cobalamin.

It is important to remember that macrocytosis can be caused by other conditions, including folic acid deficiency, liver disease, alcohol abuse, reticulocytosis, and ingestion of drugs such as antimetabolites, alkylating agents, and zidovudine.[45,63] The macrocytosis of megaloblastic anemia may be masked by conditions that can produce hypochromic and microcytic erythrocytes; thalassemia is one such condition. This possibility should be considered particularly in patients of African descent, among whom there is a high incidence of α-thalassemia (about 30%). Concurrent α-thalassemia may minimize the macrocytosis of pernicious anemia.[63] Anemia of chronic disease, or anemia resulting from blood loss and iron deficiency, can also reduce the degree of macrocytosis but will not affect the hypersegmentation of neutrophils. In one study, iron deficiency was discovered in 20% of 121 patients with pernicious anemia[64]; in another study, 19% of patients with pernicious anemia were not anemic, and 33% did not have macrocytosis.[65]

Falsely low serum cobalamin levels occur during pregnancy and in folic acid deficiency states.[63] In the past, a decline in the serum cobalamin level was usually not considered important unless the value was very low (i.e., < 150 pg/ml). It has become clear, however, that patients with serum cobalamin levels as high as 250 pg/ml and perhaps higher may have cobalamin deficiency.[63,65,66] Fortunately, the finding of macro-ovalocytes or hypersegmented PMNs on the peripheral smear remains a sensitive indicator for the presence of cobalamin deficiency.

Differential Diagnosis

After the presence of macrocytosis and a reduced cobalamin level have been determined, the cause of these conditions must be ascertained [see Table 4]. The incidence of gastric cancer, gastric carcinoid tumors, esophageal cancer,[67] and perhaps colorectal cancer[68] is higher in patients with pernicious anemia than in control subjects. Pernicious anemia occurs in association with other autoimmune disorders. In one study, autoimmune thyroid disorders were observed in 24% of 162 patients with pernicious anemia.[69] Thus, clinical evaluation of thyroid status should be included in the diagnostic assessment for pernicious anemia.

Pernicious anemia appears to involve autoimmune phenomena, namely autoimmune gastritis and two types of anti-IF anti-

Table 4 Causes of Cobalamin Deficiency

Inadequate Diet
  Strict vegetarianism

Inadequate Absorption
  Gastric abnormalities that produce deficient or defective
      intrinsic factor
    Pernicious anemia
    Total gastrectomy
    Gastritis
  Small bowel disease
    Ileal resection or bypass
    Blind loop syndrome with abnormal gut flora
    Malabsorption
    Tropical sprue
    Crohn disease
  Pancreatic insufficiency

Interference with Cobalamin Absorption
  Drugs
    Neomycin
    Biguanides
    Colchicine
    Ethanol
    Aminosalicylic acid
    Omeprazole
  Fish tapeworm competing for cobalamin

Degradation of Cobalamin Coenzymes
  N_2O anesthesia

Rare Congenital Disorders
  Transcobalamin II deficiency
  Defective intrinsic factor production

bodies. One of these antibodies blocks attachment of cobalamin to IF, and the other blocks attachment of the IF-cobalamin complex to ileal receptors.[70] Clinically, highly specific anti-IF antibodies are found in about 70% of patients with pernicious anemia.

There are other causes of cobalamin deficiency. In vegetarians, especially vegans, profound nutritional megaloblastic anemia can develop as a result of very low cobalamin intake. Deficiencies of folic acid and iron have also been observed in vegans.[71] Infants of vegan mothers can become severely cobalamin deficient, particularly when they are breast-fed.[59] Cobalamin deficiency is surprisingly common in less well developed countries where people are not strict vegans.[59] The incidence is particularly high in pregnant women and in preschool children.[59]

Gastric surgery in which the IF, pepsin, and acid-secreting components are removed often results in cobalamin deficiency (it occurred in 31% of patients in one study[72]). Patients who have undergone gastric surgery should be regularly screened by measurements of plasma cobalamin or homocysteine levels and supplemented with lifelong cobalamin therapy if the levels are low.[72]

Pancreatic insufficiency can result in malabsorption of cobalamin if the damaged pancreas does not produce enough trypsin and chymotrypsin for digesting the R protein–cobalamin complex and freeing the vitamin to form the complex with IF [*see Figure 7*].

Treatment

Specific replacement should be started promptly after the diagnosis has been made and serum samples have been taken to determine cobalamin levels. Patients who have a low serum cobalamin level and macrocytic anemia should undergo a trial of parenteral cobalamin therapy. The diagnosis of cobalamin defi-

ciency is confirmed if cobalamin therapy produces a reticulocytosis in 3 to 4 days that is associated with a rise in the hemoglobin level and a fall in the MCV. To supplement this approach, the deoxyuridine (dU) suppression test is used in some centers to identify patients with cobalamin deficiency. This test, which is not generally available, has been used to investigate megaloblastic anemia and has provided much of the current information about the roles of cobalamin and folic acid. When normal marrow cells are preincubated with cold dU, the subsequent incorporation of ³H-thymidine into DNA is markedly reduced. This reduction occurs because normal marrow cells convert dU to deoxyuridylate, which is then methylated to thymidylate [*see Figure 5a*], which in turn becomes deoxythymidine triphosphate (dTTP), a substrate for DNA synthesis. Thus, preincubation with dU markedly expands the normal cellular pool of dTTP, so that the conversion of ³H-thymidine into DNA is diluted and reduced. In cobalamin- and folic acid–deficient marrow cells, however, the deficiency interferes with the methylation of dU to thymidylate [*see Figure 5a*], so that preincubation with dU does not suppress ³H-thymidine incorporation into DNA.[53]

If the patient has symptoms of severe anemia, packed red blood cells can be transfused; the transfusion should be administered very slowly to avoid precipitating or aggravating congestive heart failure. This circumstance is one of the few in which a single-unit transfusion may be justified, because it may produce a 25% increase in oxygen-carrying capacity. A large dose of cobalamin should be given because the retention of parenterally administered cobalamin is poor but variable; the vitamin is inexpensive and has no harmful side effects. The reticulocyte response begins in 4 to 6 days, and the granulocyte count, if low, begins to increase at the same time. The hypersegmentation of PMNs disappears after 10 to 14 days, which suggests that in the megaloblastic anemias, granulopoiesis is affected by cobalamin deficiency at two different steps: (1) the lobe number of the PMNs is determined, and (2) granulocytes mature and leave the marrow.[53] Weekly dosages of 1,000 μg of parenteral cobalamin for 6 weeks should be followed by parenteral dosages of 1,000 μg monthly for life. The standard parenteral preparation is cyanocobalamin. For pancreatic insufficiency, cobalamin can be given parenterally or pancreatic enzymes can be administered orally. Specific therapy must be designed for patients with intestinal forms of malabsorption.

Because a small amount of cobalamin is absorbed even in the absence of IF and because only 1 μg/day is required, oral cobalamin has proved adequate for replacement in patients with pernicious anemia; freeing the patient from monthly injections (2,000 μg/day p.o. is recommended).[73]

MEGALOBLASTIC ANEMIA CAUSED BY FOLIC ACID DEFICIENCY

Definition

Patients with megaloblastic anemia who do not have glossitis, a family history of pernicious anemia, or the neurologic features described for cobalamin deficiency may have folic acid deficiency. Tests to determine folic acid deficiency vary in their accuracy. Serum folic acid levels are less reliable than red blood cell folic acid levels. A serum folic acid level less than 2 ng/ml is consistent with folic acid deficiency, as is a red blood cell folic acid level less than 150 ng/ml.

Diagnosis

A meticulous dietary history is important because food faddism, poor dietary intake, and alcoholism are the usual causes of

Table 5 Causes of Folic Acid Deficiency

Mechanism	Cause
Absolutely inadequate intake	Alcoholism Nutritional deficiencies
Relatively inadequate intake (resulting from increased folic acid requirements)	Pregnancy Severe hemolysis Chronic hemodialysis or peritoneal dialysis
Inadequate absorption	Tropical sprue Gluten-sensitive enteropathy (nontropical sprue) Crohn disease Lymphoma or amyloidosis of small bowel Diabetic enteropathy Intestinal resections or diversions
Drug-induced interference with folic acid metabolism	Action of dihydrofolate reductase blocked by methotrexate, trimethoprim, pyrimethamine Reduced folate absorption and tissue folate depletion caused by sulfasalazine Interference of unknown mechanism caused by phenytoin, ethanol, antituberculosis drugs, ?oral contraceptives

severe folic acid deficiency [see Table 5]. Ingestion of ethanol by well-nourished individuals does not produce megaloblastosis, but in patients with borderline folic acid stores, ethanol can lower serum folic acid levels and block the reticulocyte response to folic acid administration. Alcohol may block release of folic acid from tissues to the serum.

Megaloblastic anemia occurring as a consequence of drug administration or pregnancy is likely to be caused by folic acid deficiency. Because the combination of folic acid and iron deficiency is common, full expression of megaloblastosis is often blocked, and the patient will have a dimorphic anemia rather than the easily identifiable macro-ovalocytosis. Hypersegmentation of PMNs persists.[53,74] A thermolabile variant of the enzyme 5,10-methylenetetrahydrofolate reductase, C677T, has been discovered that causes a relative enzyme deficiency. About 5% to 10% of the general population are homozygous for this variant. The enzyme deficiency interferes with the recycling of 5,10-methylene THF_n to methyl THF_n, which in turn provides the methyl group for the conversion of homocysteine to methionine. Not surprisingly, the homocysteine levels in affected patients rise, and they may develop a hypercoagulable state [see Chapter 94]. Both pregnant and nonpregnant women who are homozygous for the C677T mutation have significantly lower red blood cell folic acid levels.[75] These women may be susceptible to cardiovascular disease and stroke and may bear children with neural tube defects.[75,76]

The serum folic acid level decreases within 2 weeks after dietary folic acid ingestion completely ceases. Therefore, many hospitalized patients have low serum folic acid levels without real tissue folic acid deprivation. In evaluating patients for folic acid deficiency, values for the levels of serum folic acid, serum cobalamin, and red blood cell folic acid must be obtained. The red blood cell folic acid level reflects tissue stores[74] but may be reduced in patients with severe cobalamin deficiency. In isolated cases, the serum folic acid level of cobalamin-deficient patients is usually normal or elevated (the methylfolate trap). Severe, long-standing cobalamin deficiency leads to anorexia and GI disturbances, which may cause dietary folic acid deficiency. As a result, both

serum cobalamin and folic acid levels are low, producing a double-deficiency state. When the diagnosis of folic acid deficiency has been established, other diagnostic procedures must be performed to pinpoint the causes of the deficiency. When it is difficult but necessary to distinguish the megaloblastosis of cobalamin deficiency from that of folic acid deficiency, measurements of the serum methylmalonic acid and homocysteine levels are helpful. In cobalamin deficiency, both the methylmalonic acid and homocysteine levels are elevated, whereas in folic acid deficiency, only the homocysteine level is elevated [see Figure 5].[74]

Treatment

Standard therapy for folic acid deficiency is 1 mg/day orally. The response, manifested by reticulocytosis in 4 to 6 days, loss of megaloblastosis, and the return of normal blood counts, confirms the diagnosis of folic acid deficiency. Neutrophil hypersegmentation disappears only after 10 to 14 days, however.[53] Patients with megaloblastosis and severe bone marrow depression secondary to administration of drugs that block dihydrofolate reductase, such as pyrimethamine and methotrexate, may be treated with folinic acid. In the case of toxicity after single large doses of methotrexate, a single equivalent dose of I.M. folinic acid (i.e., milligram for milligram) will suffice. For toxicity after chronic pyrimethamine therapy, 1 to 5 mg of folinic acid daily can be given without blocking the antimalarial effects of pyrimethamine. Megaloblastosis caused by anticonvulsant therapy can be treated with 1 mg of folic acid daily. Supplementation during pregnancy is advised and may also be useful for patients who have severe chronic hemolysis.

In most patients (i.e., those who do not require a large amount of folic acid because of conditions such as hemolysis or pregnancy), a hematologic response occurs after administration of 200 μg of folic acid daily. The increased demand of folic acid during pregnancy requires administration of about 200 to 300 μg/day.[77] Furthermore, folic acid supplementation seems to prevent fetal neural tube defects.[78] Such neural tube defects may occur in the embryo or very early in gestation—even before the pregnancy is confirmed.[79,80] Therefore, it is recommended that women of childbearing age or those who plan to become pregnant receive about 400 μg of folic acid a day. Women who are homozygous for the C677T mutation should also take folic acid supplements. Staple foods such as flour and cereal grains can be fortified with folic acid. Concern has been expressed, however, that folic acid supplementation may mask the megaloblastosis of pernicious anemia, causing the development of severe neuropathy rather than anemia.[79]

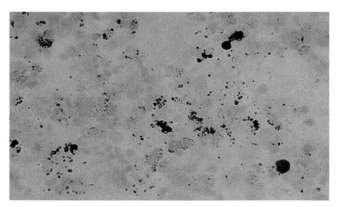

Figure 8 Prussian blue stain shows ringed sideroblasts in the bone marrow of a patient who has idiopathic sideroblastic anemia.

Table 6 Sideroblastic Anemias

Type	Disorders
Hereditary variant, probably benign	Sex-linked disorders, autosomal disorders
Acquired variant, probably benign	Mitochondrial DNA deletions (Pearson syndrome)
Probably benign variant	Induced by drugs (e.g., isoniazid or other antituberculosis drugs) or by lead intoxication; alcoholic sideroblastosis; pyridoxine-responsive anemia
Clonal disorder (myelodysplastic syndrome)	Refractory anemia with ringed sideroblasts, acquired idiopathic sideroblastic anemia

If the cause of megaloblastosis is not clearly related to abnormalities of cobalamin or folic acid metabolism, other causes of impaired DNA synthesis should be sought. Many of the antineoplastic and immunosuppressive agents that interfere with DNA synthesis also produce megaloblastosis; these include fluorouracil, hydroxyurea, mercaptopurine, thioguanine, cytarabine, and azathioprine.

SIDEROBLASTIC ANEMIAS

Definition

The sideroblastic anemias are a heterogeneous group of disorders characterized by anemia, ringed sideroblasts in the marrow, and ineffective erythropoiesis. There are hereditary and acquired forms; the latter are subdivided into benign and malignant variants, particularly the form of myelodysplastic syndrome called refractory anemia with ringed sideroblasts. Other than alcohol and drugs (e.g., isoniazid), the causes of these diseases are largely unknown.

Pathophysiology

Abnormalities of heme synthesis are probably the most frequent cause of sideroblastic anemia. Molecular defects of the enzyme 5-aminolevulinate synthase have been described as the cause of this abnormality.[80,81] This enzyme initiates the heme synthetic pathway, and its impairment profoundly affects heme synthesis. In other cases, there are major deletions in mitochondrial DNA. Iron enters erythroid precursors, but because heme synthesis is impaired, the iron cannot be incorporated into heme and accumulates on the cristae of mitochondria.[80]

Diagnosis

Patients usually have refractory anemia. The diagnosis of sideroblastic anemia is established by reticulocytopenia; the presence of ringed sideroblasts (bone marrow normoblasts with heavy incrustations of nonferritin iron on the mitochondria) [see Figure 8]; saturation of serum iron-binding capacity (usually approaching 80%); elevation of the serum lactate dehydrogenase level; and a bizarre peripheral blood smear with hypochromia, distorted red blood cells, and basophilic stippling.[82,83] Cytogenetic study of the bone marrow may reveal one of the typical patterns seen in the myelodysplastic syndromes. The sideroblastic anemias can be classified into four groupings [see Table 6].

Treatment

For prognostic purposes, it is important to decide whether the patient has a benign or malignant form of sideroblastic anemia. It is also important to recognize reversible forms of sideroblastic anemia (e.g., those caused by alcoholism, folic acid deficiency, and drugs such as isoniazid and chloramphenicol) and to discontinue any potentially offending agents.

Indicators of myelodysplasia include granulocytopenia, thrombocytopenia, dysplastic marrow granulopoiesis, bilobed megakaryocytes, and typical cytogenetic abnormalities. In rare cases, patients have a reticulocyte and hemoglobin response to pyridoxine (200 to 600 mg/day), with or without folic acid.[84]

References

1. Means RT Jr, Krantz SB: Progress in understanding the pathogenesis of the anemia of chronic disease. Blood 80:1639, 1992

2. Cash JM, Sears DA: The anemia of chronic disease: spectrum of associated diseases in a series of unselected hospitalized patients. Am J Med 87:638, 1989

3. Means RT Jr: Pathogenesis of the anemia of chronic disease: a cytokine-mediated anemia. Stem Cells 13:32, 1995

4. Lacombe C: Resistance to erythropoietin. N Engl J Med 334:660, 1996

5. Voulgari PV, Kolios G, Papadopoulos GK, et al: Role of cytokines in the pathogenesis of anemia of chronic disease in rheumatoid arthritis. Clin Immunol 92:153, 1999

6. Weiss G: Iron and anemia of chronic disease. Kidney Int 55(suppl 69):12, 1999

7. Pincus T, Olsen NJ, Russell IJ, et al: Multicenter study of recombinant human erythropoietin in correction of anemia in rheumatoid arthritis. Am J Med 89:161, 1990

8. Henry DH, Beall GN, Benson CA, et al: Recombinant human erythropoietin in the treatment of anemia associated with human immunodeficiency virus (HIV) infection and zidovudine therapy. Ann Intern Med 117:739, 1992

9. Dowlati A, R'Zik S, Fillet G, et al: Anaemia of lung cancer is due to impaired erythroid marrow response to erythropoietin stimulation as well as relative inadequacy of erythropoietin production. Br J Haematol 97:297, 1997

10. Schreiber S, Howaldt S, Schnoor M, et al: Recombinant erythropoietin for the treatment of anemia in inflammatory bowel disease. N Engl J Med 334:619, 1996

11. Ludwig H, Fritz E, Leitgeb C, et al: Prediction of response to erythropoietin treatment in chronic anemia of cancer. Blood 84:1056, 1994

12. Goodnough LT, Skikne B, Brugnara C: Erythropoietin, iron, and erythropoiesis. Blood 96:823, 2000

13. Allen DA, Breen C, Yaqoob MM, et al: Inhibition of CFU-E colony formation in uremic patients with inflammatory disease: role of IFN-γ and TNF-α. J Invest Med 47:204, 1999

14. Mladenovic J: Aluminum inhibits erythropoiesis in vitro. J Clin Invest 81:1661, 1988

15. Eschbach JW, Egrie JC, Downing MR, et al: Correction of the anemia of end-stage renal disease with recombinant human erythropoietin: results of a combined phase I and II clinical trial. N Engl J Med 316:73, 1987

16. Altmann P, Plowman D, Marsh F, et al: Aluminum chelation therapy in dialysis patients: evidence for inhibition of haemoglobin synthesis by low levels of aluminum. Lancet 1:1012, 1988

17. Coleman N, Herbert V: Hematologic complications of alcoholism: overview. Semin Hematol 17:164, 1980

18. Lindenbaum J: Folate and vitamin B₁₂ deficiencies in alcoholism. Semin Hematol 17:119, 1980

19. Conrad ME, Barton JC: Anemia and iron kinetics in alcoholism. Semin Hematol 17:149, 1980

20. Ettinghausen SE, Moore JG, White DE, et al: Hematologic effects of immunotherapy with lymphokine-activated killer cells and recombinant interleukin-2 in cancer patients. Blood 69:1654, 1987

21. Yunis AA: Chloramphenicol-induced bone marrow suppression. Semin Hematol 10:225, 1973

22. Baldwin JG Jr: Hematopoietic function in the elderly. Arch Intern Med 148:2544, 1988

23. Bacigalupo A, Hows J, Gluckman E, et al: Bone marrow transplantation (BMT) versus immunosuppression for the treatment of severe aplastic anaemia (SAA): a report of the EBMT SAA working party. Br J Haematol 70:177, 1988

24. Brown KE, Tisdale J, Barrett AJ, et al: Hepatitis-associated aplastic anemia. N Engl J Med 336:1059, 1997

25. Tzakis AG, Arditi M, Whitington PF, et al: Aplastic anemia complicating orthotopic liver transplantation for non-A, non-B hepatitis. N Engl J Med 319:393, 1988

26. Young NS: Autoimmunity and its treatment in aplastic anemia. Ann Intern Med 126:166, 1997

27. Young NS, Maciejewski J: The pathophysiology of acquired aplastic anemia. N Engl J Med 336:1365, 1997

28. Maciejewski JP, Selleri C, Sato T, et al: A severe and consistent deficit in marrow and circulating primitive hematopoietic cells (long-term culture-initiating cells) in acquired aplastic anemia. Blood 88:1983, 1996

29. Young NS, Barrett AJ: The treatment of severe acquired aplastic anemia. Blood 85:3367, 1996

30. Rosenfeld SJ, Kimball J, Vining D, et al: Intensive immunosuppression with antithymocyte globulin and cyclosporine as treatment for severe acquired aplastic anemia. Blood 85:3058, 1995

31. Doney K, Storb R, Buckner CD, et al: Treatment of gold-induced aplastic anaemia with immunosuppressive therapy. Br J Haematol 68:469, 1988

32. Doney K, Leisenring W, Storb R, et al: Primary treatment of acquired aplastic anemia: outcomes with bone marrow transplantation and immunosuppressive therapy. Ann Intern Med 126:107, 1997

33. Bacigalupo A, Bruno B, Saracco P, et al: Antilymphocyte globulin, cyclosporine, prednisolone, and granulocyte colony-stimulating factor for severe aplastic anemia: an update of the GITMO/EBMT study on 100 patients. Blood 95:1931, 2000

34. Frickhoffen N, Kaltwasser JP, Schrezenmeier H, et al: Treatment of aplastic anemia with antilymphocyte globulin and methylprednisolone with or without cyclosporine. N Engl J Med 324:1297, 1991

35. Socié G, Henry-Amar M, Bacigalupo A, et al: Malignant tumors occurring after treatment of aplastic anemia. N Engl J Med 329:1152, 1993

36. Di Bona E, Rodeghiero B, Bruno A, et al: Rabbit antithymocyte globulin (r-ATG) plus cyclosporine and granulocyte colony stimulating factor is an effective treatment for aplastic anaemia patients unresponsive to a first course of intensive immunosuppressive therapy. Br J Haematol 107:330, 1999

37. Brodsky RW, Sensenbrenner LL, Jones RJ: Complete remission in severe aplastic anemia after high-dose cyclophosphamide without bone marrow transplantation. Blood 87:491, 1996

38. Tichelli A, Socie G, Henry-Amar M, et al; Effectiveness of immunosuppressive therapy in older patients with aplastic anemia. Ann Intern Med 130:193, 1999

39. Paquette RL, Tebyani N, Frane M, et al: Long-term outcome of aplastic anemia in adults treated with antithymocyte globulin: comparison with bone marrow transplantation. Blood 85:283, 1995

40. Maung ZT, Norden J, Middleton PG, et al: Pure red cell aplasia: further evidence of T cell clonal disorder. Br J Haematol 87:189, 1994

41. Casadevall N, Dufuy E, Molho-Sabatier P, et al: Brief report: autoantibodies against erythropoietin in a patient with pure red-cell aplasia. N Engl J Med 334:630, 1996

42. Charles RJ, Sabo KM, Kidd PG, et al: The pathophysiology of pure red cell aplasia: implications for therapy. Blood 87:4831, 1996

43. Lacy MQ, Kurtin PJ, Tefferi A: Pure red cell aplasia: association with large granular lymphocyte leukemia and the prognostic value of cytogenetic abnormalities. Blood 87:3000, 1996

44. Marmont AM: Therapy of pure red cell aplasia. Semin Hematol 28:285, 1991

45. Walker RE, Parker RI, Kovacs JA, et al: Anemia and erythropoiesis in patients with the acquired immunodeficiency syndrome (AIDS) and Kaposi sarcoma treated with zidovudine. Ann Intern Med 108:372, 1988

46. Baker RI, Manoharan A, De Luca E, et al: Pure red cell aplasia of pregnancy: a distinct clinical entity. Br J Haematol 85:619, 1993

47. Palmieri G, Lastoria S, Colao A, et al: Successful treatment of a patient with thymoma and pure red-cell aplasia with octreotide and prednisone. N Engl J Med 336:263, 1997

48. McGuire WA, Yang HH, Bruno E, et al: Treatment of antibody-mediated pure red-cell aplasia with high-dose intravenous gamma globulin. N Engl J Med 317:1004, 1987

49. Yamada O, Mizoguchi H, Oshimi K: Cyclophosphamide therapy for pure red cell aplasia associated with granular lymphocyte-proliferative disorders. Br J Haematol 97:392, 1997

50. Ramratnam B, Gollerkeri A, Schiffman FJ, et al: Management of persistent B19 parvovirus infection in AIDS. Br J Haematol 91:90, 1995

51. Means RT Jr, Dessypris EN, Krantz SB, et al: Treatment of refractory pure red cell aplasia with cyclosporine A: disappearance of IgG inhibitor associated with clinical response. Br J Haematol 78:114, 1991

52. Miller BU, Tichelli A, Passweg JR, et al: Successful treatment of refractory acquired pure red cell aplasia (PRCA) by allogeneic bone marrow transplantation. Bone Marrow Transplant 23:1205, 1999

53. Wickramasinghe S: Morphology biology and biochemistry of cobalamin- and folate-deficient bone marrow cells. Baillieres Clin Haematol 8:441, 1995

54. Koury MJ, Horne DW: Apoptosis mediates and thymidine prevents erythroblast destruction in folate deficiency anemia. Proc Natl Acad Sci U S A 91:4067, 1994

55. Igram CF, Davidoff AN, Marais E, et al: Evaluation of DNA analysis for evidence of apoptosis in megaloblastic anaemia. Br J Haematol 96:576, 1997

56. Tefferi A, Pruthi RK: The biochemical basis of cobalamin deficiency. Mayo Clin Proc 69:181, 1994

57. Skacel PO, Hewlett AM, Lewis JD, et al: Studies on the haemopoietic toxicity of nitrous oxide in man. Br J Haematol 53:189, 1983

58. Pruthi RK, Tefferi A: Pernicious anemia revisited. Mayo Clin Proc 69:144, 1994

59. Allen LH: Vitamin B_{12} metabolism and status during pregnancy, lactation and infancy. Adv Exp Med Biol 352:173, 1996

60. Weir DG, Scott JM: The biochemical basis of the neuropathy in cobalamin deficiency. Baillieres Clin Haematol 8:479, 1995

61. Dokal IS, Cox TM, Galton DAG: Vitamin B_{12} and folate deficiency presenting as leukaemia. BMJ 300:1263, 1990

62. Carmel R, Sinow RM, Siegel ME, et al: Food cobalamin malabsorption occurs frequently in patients with unexplained low serum cobalamin levels. Arch Intern Med 148:1715, 1988

63. Chanarin I, Metz J: Diagnosis of cobalamin deficiency: the old and the new. Br J Haematol 97:695, 1997

64. Carmel R, Weiner JM, Johnson CS: Iron deficiency occurs frequently in patients with pernicious anemia. JAMA 257:1081, 1987

65. Carmel R: Pernicious anemia: the expected findings of very low serum cobalamin levels, anemia, and macrocytosis are often lacking. Arch Intern Med 148:1712, 1988

66. Green R: Screening for vitamin B_{12} deficiency: caveat emptor. Ann Intern Med 124:509, 1996

67. Hsing AW, Hansson L-E, McLaughlin JK, et al: Pernicious anemia and subsequent cancer. Cancer 71:745, 1993

68. Talley NJ, Chute CG, Larson DE, et al: Risk for colorectal adenocarcinoma in pernicious anemia: a population-based cohort study. Ann Intern Med 111:738, 1989

69. Carmel R, Spencer CA: Clinical and subclinical thyroid disorders associated with pernicious anemia: observations on abnormal thyroid-stimulating hormone levels and on a possible association of blood group O with hyperthyroidism. Arch Intern Med 142:1465, 1982

70. Guéant JL, Safi A, Aimone-Gastin I, et al: Autoantibodies in pernicious anemia type I patients recognize sequence 251-256 in human intrinsic factor. Proc Assoc Am Physicians 109:462, 1997

71. Pippard MJ: Megaloblastic anaemia: geography and diagnosis. Lancet 334:6, 1994

72. Sumner AE, Chin MM, Abrahm JL, et al: Elevated methylmalonic acid and total homocysteine levels show high prevalence of vitamin B_{12} deficiency after gastric surgery. Ann Intern Med 124:469, 1996

73. Kuzminski AM, Del Giacco EJ, Allen RH, et al: Effective treatment of cobalamin deficiency with oral cobalamin. Blood 92:1191, 1998

74. Amose RJ, Dawson DW, Fish DI, et al: Guidelines on the investigation and diagnosis of cobalamin and folate deficiencies. Clin Lab Haematol 16:101, 1994

75. Molloy AM, Daly S, Mills JL, et al: Thermolabile variant of 5,10-methylenetetrahydrofolate reductase associated with low red-cell folates: implications for folate intake recommendations. Lancet 349:1591, 1997

76. Wilcken DE: MTHFR 677CT mutation, folate intake, neural-tube defect, and risk of cardiovascular disease. Lancet 350:603, 1997

77. McPartlin J, Halligan A, Scott JM, et al: Accelerated folate breakdown in pregnancy. Lancet 341:148, 1993

78. Wald NJ, Bower C: Folic acid, pernicious anaemia, and prevention of neural tube defects. Lancet 343:307, 1994

79. Carmel R: Subtle cobalamin deficiency. Ann Intern Med 124:338, 1996

80. Cotter PD, May A, Li L, et al: Four new mutations in the erythroid-specific 5-aminolevulinate synthase (ALAS2) gene causing X-linked sideroblastic anemia: increased pyridoxine responsiveness after removal of iron overload by phlebotomy and coinheritance of hereditary hemochromatosis. Blood 93:1757, 1999

81. Nakajima O, Takahashi S, Harigae H, et al: Heme deficiency in erythroid lineage causes differentiation arrest and cytoplasmic iron overload. EMBO J 18:6282, 1999

82. Bottomley SS, Healy HM, Brandenburg MA, et al: 5-Aminolevulinate synthase in sideroblastic anemias: mRNA and enzyme activity levels in bone marrow cells. Am J Hematol 41:76, 1992

83. Bottomley SS, May BK, Cox TC, et al: Molecular defects of erythroid 5-aminolevulinate synthase in X-linked sideroblastic anemia. J Bioenerg Biomembr 27:161, 1995

84. Cotter PD, May A, Fitzsimons EJ, et al: Late-onset X-linked sideroblastic anemia: missense mutations in the erythroid-aminolevulinate synthase (ALAS2) gene in two pyridoxine-responsive patients initially diagnosed with acquired refractory anemia and ringed sideroblasts. J Clin Invest 96:2090, 1995

Acknowledgments

Figures 1 and 6   Talar Agasyan.
Figure 5   Alan D. Iselin.
Figure 7   Tom Moore.

89 Hemoglobinopathies and Hemolytic Anemias

Stanley L. Schrier, M.D.

Alteration of the erythrocyte membrane is the final stage in the pathway leading to hemolysis. Membrane alteration usually signals the reticuloendothelial macrophages to remove the damaged red cell from the circulation. In extraordinary circumstances, however, the damage to the membrane is so great that the intracellular contents, including hemoglobin, are liberated into the plasma. This chapter describes structural and functional features of normal erythrocytes and diseases involving membrane architecture, red cell proteins, and extracorpuscular factors that can lead to shortened red cell survival.

Development, Structure, and Physiology of the Erythrocyte

Erythroid precursor cells undergo four or five cell divisions in the bone marrow and then extrude their nuclei and become reticulocytes. As these enucleate cells mature, hemoglobin synthesis decreases. The cells lose most of their transferrin receptors and enter the peripheral blood; they survive in the circulation for about 4 months.

As they move through the circulation, erythrocytes must withstand severe mechanical and metabolic stresses, deform to traverse capillaries with diameters half their own, resist high shearing forces across the cardiac valves, survive repeated episodes of stasis-induced acidemia and substrate depletion, and avoid removal by the macrophages of the reticuloendothelial system. They must also maintain an internal environment that protects hemoglobin from oxidative attack and sustain the optimum concentration of 2,3-diphosphoglycerate (2,3-DPG) needed for hemoglobin function.

HEMOGLOBIN

The normal adult red cell contains three forms of hemoglobin (Hb): HbA (96%), HbA_2 (2% to 3%), and HbF (< 2%). Normal HbA ($\alpha_2\beta_2$) is composed of two α chains, coded by four genes on chromosome 16, and two β chains, coded on chromosome 11. HbA_2 is composed of two α chains and two δ chains ($\alpha_2\delta_2$), and fetal hemoglobin (HbF) is composed of two α chains and two γ chains ($\alpha_2\gamma_2$). The genes for the β, α, and δ chains are closely linked to one another on chromosome 11. The extraordinarily high concentration of hemoglobin in the red cell—33 to 35 g/dl (the mean corpuscular hemoglobin concentration, or MCHC)—produces a viscous solution intracellularly.

NONHEMOGLOBIN CYTOSOL

Erythrocytes principally utilize glucose to maintain the reducing power that protects the cell against oxidative attack, to generate the 2,3-DPG required to modulate the function of hemoglobin, and to control the salt and thus the water content of the red cell by the actions of adenosine triphosphate (ATP) and the transport adenosine triphosphatases (ATPases) [see Table 1]. The water and the hemoglobin content of the red cell determine the mean corpuscular volume (MCV) and the MCHC.

PLASMA MEMBRANE

The red cell normally has a discoid shape with a diameter of 7 to 8 μm, an MCV of 85 to 90 femtoliters (fl) (1 fl = 10^{-15} L), and a surface area of 140 μm^2 [see Figure 1]. Its unique shape enables it to squeeze through capillaries as narrow as 3 μm in diameter.

Lipids (phospholipids and cholesterol) account for 50% of the weight of the surface membrane. The phospholipids are distributed asymmetrically in the bilayer; the positively charged phospholipids, sphingomyelin and phosphatidylcholine, are in the outer half of the bilayer, and the relatively negatively charged aminophospholipids, phosphatidylserine and phosphatidylethanolamine, occur predominantly in the inner half of the bilayer. This asymmetry of the phospholipid bilayer permits small charged molecules to be selectively intercalated in and cause expansion of either the outer or inner half of the bilayer, producing echinocytes or stomatocytes [see Figure 1].

The red cell membrane proteins are classified on the basis of their mobility on sodium dodecyl sulfate-polyacrylamide gel electrophoresis (SDS-PAGE). Integral proteins interact with and span the hydrophobic phospholipid bilayer [see Figure 2]. The

Table 1 Erythrocyte Metabolism

Pathway	Product	Functions of Metabolic Products
Glycolysis by Embden-Meyerhof pathway	ATP	Serves as a substrate for all kinase reactions, for the ATPase-linked sodium-potassium pump, for the ATPase-linked calcium efflux pump, and for other ATPases of the RBC membrane, including aminophospholipid translocase Maintains deformable state of RBC membrane
	2,3-DPG	Interacts with deoxyhemoglobin, shifting equilibrium to favor unloading of O_2 from oxyhemoglobin Acts as an intracellular anion that cannot cross the RBC membrane
	NADH	Acts as a substrate for a methemoglobin reductase, enabling it to reduce methemoglobin (Fe^{3+}) to hemoglobin (Fe^{2+})
Pentose phosphate pathway (hexose monophosphate shunt)	NADPH	Serves as a substrate for another methemoglobin reductase in methemoglobin reduction (a fail-safe mechanism) Serves as a coenzyme for glutathione reductase in reduction of oxidized glutathione; reduced glutathione (GSH) protects RBC against oxidative denaturation

ATP—adenosine triphosphate   2,3-DPG—2,3-diphosphoglycerate   NADH—reduced nicotinamide-adenine dinucleotide   NADPH—reduced nicotinamide-adenine dinucleotide phosphate

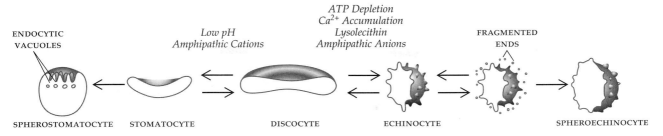

Figure 1 The normal erythrocyte, or discocyte, undergoes shape changes in response to conditions created by treatment with certain agents. Most changes are reversible if inducing agents are removed before the permanent loss of membrane material.

major integral proteins of the erythrocyte membrane are the glycophorins (which contain most of the membrane sialic acid and carry the MNSs blood group antigens) and band 3, which is the anion and bicarbonate transporter.

The peripheral proteins are all found at the cytosol face of the membrane. Bands 1 (α) and 2 (β) of spectrin, a peripheral protein, interact to form a heterodimer; two of these heterodimers then link to form a heterotetramer, the predominant form of spectrin. By themselves, the heterotetramers contribute little to stability, but when they are cross-linked by oligomers of band 5, or actin, in an interaction that is vastly enhanced by band 4.1, the result is the tough but resilient cytoskeleton.

The peripheral cytoskeleton is connected to the integral proteins by band 2.1 (ankyrin), which links spectrin to band 3 [*see Figure 2*]. One of the glycophorins, glycophorin C, also is linked to band 4.1. Peripheral membrane proteins, which are present in smaller amounts, include adducin, tropomyosin, and dematin—all of which may support the functions of the membrane skeleton.[1,2]

The membrane carbohydrates contribute to the external negative charge of the membrane and function partly as blood group antigens. Some of these glycolipids associate with phosphatidylinositol to form a glycolipid anchor, called the glycosylphosphatidylinositol (GPI) anchor [*see Figure 3*]. These GPI anchors provide the membrane-anchoring site for several classes of proteins, such as decay-accelerating factor (DAF, or CD55) and membrane inhibitor of reactive lysis (MIRL, or CD59), which serve to control complement action [*see Paroxysmal Nocturnal Hemoglobinuria, below*].[3]

CONTROL OF HYDRATION AND VOLUME

Control of red cell volume has considerable pathophysiologic importance because the water and cation contents of red cells determine intracellular viscosity and the ratio of surface area to volume. The Na^+ and K^+ content is determined by passive diffusion and by active transport, primarily through the Na^+,K^+-ATPase. The major intracellular anion is Cl^-; it enters the red cell with high permeability through band 3, the major anion exchanger (also called AE1, or anion exchanger–1). The K^+-Cl^- cotransporter drives the K^+-Cl^- gradient and is activated by red cell swelling and low intracellular pH, causing a net

Figure 2 Band 3, the anion transport channel (orange), and the other integral proteins glycophorin A (not shown), glycophorin B (not shown), and glycophorin C (green) span the red cell membrane. Branching external carbohydrate side chains are attached to these proteins. The hydrophilic, polar heads of the phospholipid molecules that make up the bilayer are oriented toward the cell surface, whereas the hydrophobic fatty acid side chains are directed toward the interior of the bilayer. Cholesterol is intercalated between the fatty acid chains. Band 3 binds hemoglobin and glyceraldehyde-3-phosphate dehydrogenase on its cytosol surface. Spectrin (yellow), actin (red), tropomyosin (blue), and band 4.1 (light green) form a latticework on the inner membrane surface. The spectrin heterodimers associate to form heterotetramers. The lower figure depicts the hexagonal cytoskeletal lattice on the inner membrane surface. Band 2.1 (ankyrin) links the integral protein band 3 to the peripheral cytoskeleton through the β chain of spectrin. Additional linkage is provided by glycophorin C and band 4.1.

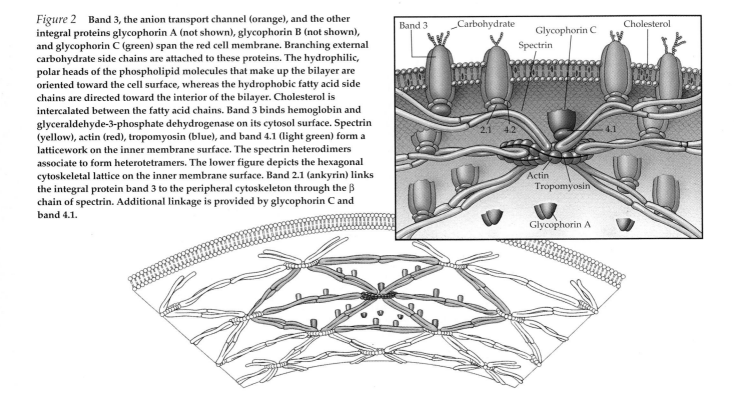

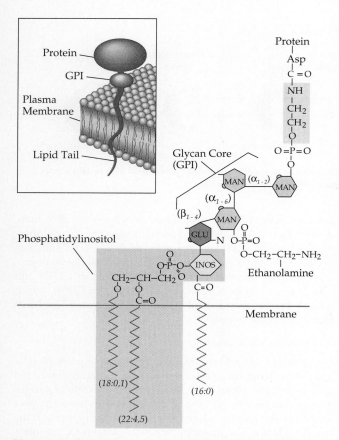

Figure 3 Detailed diagram of the glycosyl-phosphatidylinositol (GPI) molecule, which provides an anchor for a large number of proteins that have important biologic functions at membrane surfaces.

loss of K^+ and Cl^-. The Ca^{2+}-ATPase actively pumps Ca^{2+} out of the red cell, making the free cytosolic Ca^{2+} content less than 0.1 μM—four orders of magnitude lower than the plasma concentration of 1 mM. The Gardos channel, which is a Ca^{2+}-activated K^+ efflux channel, plays an important role in volume regulation. Water enters and exits through a water channel called CHIP 28 (28 kd channel-forming integral membrane protein) or aquaporin. Other important intracellular anions are 2,3-DPG and hemoglobin, neither of which penetrates the cell membrane. When the concentration of free cytosolic Ca^{2+} rises to levels even as low as 0.3 μM, the channel is activated and results in a net loss of K^+. If such a loss is not corrected, the affected red cell becomes dehydrated.[4]

SHAPE CHANGES

ATP depletion, calcium ion accumulation, or treatment with lysolecithin or with anionic amphipathic compounds transforms the normal erythrocyte, or discocyte, into an echinocyte—a crenated spiculated cell sometimes called a burr cell [*see Figure 1*]. Calcium, acting either alone or in concert with the calcium-binding protein calmodulin, can effect the echinocytic shape change. If the echinocytic process persists, fragmentation or budding of the tips of the echinocyte leads to loss of membrane components, particularly of band 3 and phospholipids. This results in loss of surface area, a reduction in the ratio of surface area to volume, and the formation of poorly deformable spheroechinocytes.

PRINCIPLES OF BLOOD FLOW

The major determinants of blood flow are the hematocrit; the plasma concentration of proteins such as fibrinogen and immunoglobulins, which influence the degree of rouleau formation or aggregation; red cell deformability; the caliber of blood vessels; and the shear rate (the ratio of flow rate to tube radius). At the low shear rates that exist in postcapillary venules, the red cells tend to clump in asymmetrical masses, with a consequent increase in blood viscosity and resistance to flow.

CELL AGING AND DEATH

In the bone marrow, the developing reticulocyte progressively loses its residual RNA over a 4-day period after nuclear extrusion. At the conclusion of this stage, the reticulocyte can no longer engage in protein synthesis. The active K^+-Cl^- cotransporter functions to reduce cell volume. With membrane protein assembly complete, the resulting mature cell enters the circulation and survives for a period of 100 to 120 days.[5] Erythrocyte death is an age-dependent phenomenon and may be related to mechanical and chemical stresses the cell encounters in the circulation. As the erythrocyte ages, it loses water and its surface area diminishes. The ratio of surface area to volume decreases and the mean corpuscular hemoglobin concentration increases, impairing cell deformability. In addition, decreased enzymatic activity lowers the cell's ability to withstand metabolic stress. Aging may be manifested by changes at the erythrocyte's surface, such as a decrease in the density or type of surface charge or the appearance of a senescence neoantigen, perhaps clustered band 3 [*see Figure 2*], that binds specific immunoglobulins and complement components.[6] By such changes, the age-worn erythrocyte signals its incapacity to the reticuloendothelial system, triggering removal by macrophages.

Under physiologic conditions, slightly less than 1% of the cells are destroyed each day and are replaced by a virtually identical number of new cells. Each day, a 70 kg (154 lb) man with a blood volume of about 5 L destroys and replaces about 50 ml of whole blood, which contains approximately 22 ml of packed erythrocytes. Inasmuch as one third of each erythrocyte is hemoglobin, the replacement of these cells requires the synthesis of about 7 g of hemoglobin each day. Normal adult bone marrow can readily increase its erythroid output fivefold. After extensive and prolonged anemic stress, erythroid production can be raised by as much as seven or eight times. The supply of iron, however, places an important limit on red cell replacement: three fourths of the iron used in the synthesis of cells in 1 day comes from cells that were destroyed on the previous day.

General Features of Hemolytic Anemias

The severity of anemia is determined both by the rate of red cell destruction and by the marrow's capacity to increase erythroid production. When a person has a healthy marrow, erythrocyte survival time can be reduced from 120 days to 20 days without inducing anemia or jaundice; however, a substantial reticulocytosis will be present in such cases.

Most forms of hemolysis are extravascular; the damaged cell signals its changed status to the reticuloendothelial system via its membrane and is removed. In unusual circumstances in which damage to the erythrocyte is devastating—as in some forms of complement-mediated lysis—or in circumstances in which the reticuloendothelial system cannot cope with the burden of damaged cells, intravascular lysis develops and leads to hemoglobinemia.

Hemoglobin released to the plasma is degraded to $\alpha\beta$ dimers, which bind to haptoglobin. The hemoglobin-haptoglobin complexes are removed by the reticuloendothelial system. When the haptoglobin-binding capacity is exceeded, $\alpha\beta$ dimers pass into the glomerular filtrate. Some of the $\alpha\beta$ dimers are excreted into the urine directly, producing hemoglobinuria, whereas others are taken up by renal tubule cells. Iron-containing renal tubule cells may be excreted for several days after an episode of intravascular hemolysis. Hemosiderinuria can be identified with Prussian blue stain. Free plasma hemoglobin can dissociate into globin and hemin. Hemin may bind to hemopexin and may reach the renal tubule cells in that form, or it may bind to plasma albumin, producing methemalbuminemia.

Intravascular hemolysis is an example of dramatic erythrocyte destruction and may thus produce severe anemia acutely. In addition, erythrocytic membrane particles released into the plasma may act as potent stimuli for disseminated intravascular coagulation.

When hemolysis is chronic, pigment stones often develop in the gallbladder. When a patient compensating for a marked increase in hemolysis has an infection that sharply impairs marrow erythroid activity,[7] the hemoglobin level may fall dramatically—a condition called aplastic crisis. Acute severe hemolysis is also a cause of acute renal failure [see Chapter 162], and acute intravascular hemolysis is a cause of disseminated intravascular coagulation.

Causes of hemolysis may be classified as either extracorpuscular or intracorpuscular. The intracorpuscular causes, which are essentially erythrocyte defects, comprise membrane abnormalities, metabolic disturbances, and disorders of hemoglobin structure or biosynthesis. Extracorpuscular causes represent abnormal elements within the patient's vascular bed that attack and destroy normal erythrocytes. Because erythrocytes with intracorpuscular defects that cause hemolysis are intrinsically abnormal, when they are transfused into normal recipients, their survival time is characteristically short. Of the intracorpuscular defects, only one disorder, paroxysmal nocturnal hemoglobinuria, is not hereditary.

Erythrocyte Membrane Defects

DISORDERS OF SALT AND WATER METABOLISM

Hydrocytosis (Hereditary Stomatocytosis)

Hydrocytosis is a hereditary disorder that usually presents early in life as partly compensated hemolytic anemia; occasionally, the spleen is palpable. The MCV is usually elevated. The peripheral smear shows stomatocytes [see Figure 4]. Passive flux of both Na^+ and K^+ increases greatly. The Na^+,K^+-ATPase is overwhelmed; the cation concentration and thus the water content of the red cell increase, accounting for the increase in MCV and the decrease in the ratio of surface area to volume. Stomatocytes appear to adhere more avidly than normal red cells, a finding that may account for the reported increase in thromboembolic events.[8] Splenectomy may lead to improvement in the anemia. Other therapies may eventually prove useful. The vaso-occlusive events were controlled in one patient by long-term red cell transfusion and in another by therapy with pentoxifylline.[8]

Xerocytosis

Xerocytosis, another hereditary hemolytic disorder, is characterized by a membrane defect that leads to loss of cations and to cellular dehydration. Patients present with variably compensated

hemolysis. Splenomegaly is not a prominent feature. The peripheral smear is variable, showing target cells, stomatocytes, echinocytes, or so-called hemoglobin puddling (i.e., hemoglobin collected around the circumference of the cell). MCHC is increased. Dehydration of erythrocytes occurs because the K^+ leak exceeds the Na^+ influx, possibly as a result of an overactive K^+-Cl^- cotransporter. Because these rigid cells are removed in many parts of the reticuloendothelial system, splenectomy is of little benefit.[9]

PROTEIN ABNORMALITIES

Hereditary Elliptocytosis

There are perhaps 250 to 500 cases of hereditary elliptocytosis per million population.[10] Three morphologic variants are seen: (1) common hereditary elliptocytosis, (2) spherocytic hereditary elliptocytosis, and (3) stomatocytic hereditary elliptocytosis.[10] Most patients with common hereditary elliptocytosis are heterozygous for this autosomal dominant disorder and have only elliptical red cells or, at worst, compensated hemolysis. Homozygotes for the disorder may have severe uncompensated hemolytic anemia.

Under applied shear stress, discocytes assume an elliptical shape; when the stress is removed, the cell normally recoils to its discoid shape. It has been hypothesized that membrane defects in hereditary elliptocytosis interfere with normal recoil. The membrane defect appears to be a lesion in the membrane cytoskeleton, usually involving spectrin. In most patients, the spectrin heterodimers do not self-associate normally to form tetramers or oligomers [see Figure 2]. Other defects involve band 4.1 or the interaction between ankyrin and band 3. Red cell membranes from patients with hereditary elliptocytosis are almost invariably mechanically fragile.

The diagnosis is made in patients with extravascular intracorpuscular hemolysis with elliptocytes. Elliptocytosis can also be seen in severe iron deficiency, myeloproliferative and myelodysplastic disorders, and, occasionally, cobalamin and folate deficiencies.[10] Results of the osmotic fragility test are usually normal. Splenectomy has been useful in patients with severe common hereditary elliptocytosis.

Hereditary Pyropoikilocytosis

The syndrome of hereditary (autosomal recessive) pyropoikilocytosis, a variant of hereditary elliptocytosis, causes severe hemolysis in young children. It is caused by an abnormal α or β spectrin mutation. The blood smear shows extreme microcytosis and extraordinary variation in the size and shape of erythrocytes [see Figure 4]. Splenectomy may reduce the rate of hemolysis.

Hereditary Spherocytosis

Hereditary spherocytosis is usually inherited as an autosomal dominant trait and affects about 220 per million people worldwide. A rare autosomal recessive variant of hereditary spherocytosis has been described.

Because of a loss of surface membrane, red cells assume a microspherocytic shape and thus cannot deform sufficiently to pass through the splenic vasculature; splenic trapping of red cells, hemolysis, and compensatory increase in red cell production result. The underlying membrane defects lead to budding of membrane vesicles under conditions of metabolic depletion. These membrane vesicles are enriched in phospholipids from the bilayer along with associated transmembrane proteins [see Figure 2]. The underlying molecular lesions appear to consist of deficiencies of spectrin, spectrin-ankyrin, band 3, and band 4.2.[10,11]

a   b   c

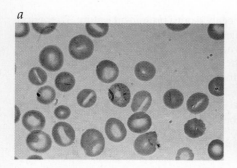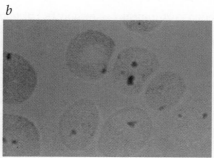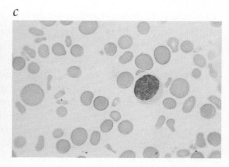

Figure 4   **Stomatocytes are identified by slitlike areas of central pallor (*a*); the smear also shows microspherocytes, which are a more advanced stage of stomatocytosis. On scanning electron microscopy or examination of wet preparations, the microspherocytes are shown to be stomatocytes. Microspherocytes are seen in hereditary spherocytosis and in autoimmune hemolytic anemia, as well as in other conditions characterized by relatively selective loss of membrane material or increase in cell volume. Supravital stain of erythrocytes (*b*) shows single and multiple blue-staining Heinz bodies within counterstained erythrocytes. Phase microscopy can also be used to demonstrate Heinz bodies. Elliptocytes are visualized in a smear from a patient with hereditary elliptocytosis (*c*).**

About 25% of patients with hereditary spherocytosis have completely compensated hemolysis without anemia; their disorder is diagnosed only when a concomitant condition, such as infection or pregnancy, increases the rate of hemolysis or reduces the marrow's compensatory capacity. In other patients, mild anemia, pigmented gallstones, leg ulcers, and splenic rupture may develop. Aplastic crises may be precipitated by ordinary respiratory tract infections, especially by parvovirus infection.[7]

This diagnosis is suggested by a predominance of microspherocytes on the peripheral smear [*see Figure 4b*], an MCHC of 35 g/dl or greater, reticulocytosis, mild jaundice, splenomegaly, and a positive family history. Confirmation of the diagnosis is made by a 24-hour incubated osmotic fragility test. A negative Coombs test and a family history positive for hereditary spherocytosis rule against a diagnosis of acquired autoimmune hemolytic anemia. Splenectomy eradicates clinical manifestations of the disorder, including aplastic crises.

PAROXYSMAL NOCTURNAL HEMOGLOBINURIA

Paroxysmal nocturnal hemoglobinuria (PNH) is a clonal disorder of hematopoiesis caused by a deficiency of the membrane-anchoring protein phosphatidylinositol glycan class A [*see Figure 3*]. PNH arises through a somatic mutation in marrow stem cells[12]; the resulting mature hematopoietic cells are usually chimeric. The gene *PIG-A* maps to the short arm of the X chromosome.[12]

Normal human erythrocytes, and probably platelets and neutrophils, modulate complement attack by at least three GPI membrane-bound proteins: DAF (CD55), C8-binding protein (C8BP), and MIRL (CD59). In the absence of the GPI anchor, all of the proteins that use this membrane anchor will be variably deficient in the blood cells of persons with PNH.[13] Because the defective synthesis of GPI affects all hematopoietic cells, patients with PNH may have variable degrees of anemia, neutropenia, or thrombocytopenia, or they may have complete bone marrow failure.[14]

Diagnosis

Classically, acute episodes of intravascular hemolysis are superimposed on a background of chronic hemolysis. The patient typically notes hemoglobinuria on voiding after sleep.[15,16] Recurrent venous occlusions lead to pulmonary embolism and hepatic and mesenteric vein thrombosis, possibly resulting from release of procoagulant microparticles derived from platelets.[17] Occasionally, PNH patients with thrombosis are mistakenly thought to have psychosomatic disorders because they complain of recur-

rent severe and undiagnosed pain in the abdomen and back. In these cases, the associated anemia and hemolysis may be very mild, and episodes of hemolysis do not necessarily correlate with bouts of pain.

A diagnosis of PNH should be considered in any patient with chronic or episodic hemolysis. The diagnosis should also be considered for patients with recurrent venous thromboembolism, particularly if the thrombus occurs in a site such as the inferior vena cava or the portal mesenteric system or if it produces Budd-Chiari syndrome. Evidence of intravascular hemolysis such as hemoglobinemia, reduced serum haptoglobin, increased serum methemalbumin, hemoglobinuria, or hemosiderinuria suggests the diagnosis. The association of marrow hypoplasia with hemolysis is an important clue. The erythrocytes' morphology is usually normal. Diagnosis is made by specific tests based on fluorescence-activated cell sorter (FACS) analysis using antibodies that quantitatively assess DAF (CD55) and MIRL (CD59) on the erythrocyte or on the leukocyte surface.[18]

Treatment

In PNH, the anemia is occasionally so severe (hemoglobin level < 8 g/dl) that the patient needs transfusions regularly[16]; therefore, the choice of transfusion component is critical. It is believed that infusion of blood products containing complement may enhance hemolysis. Infusion of donor white cells (which are ordinarily present in a unit of packed red cells) into an HLA-immunized recipient may provide the antigen-antibody reaction that activates complement by the classical pathway. In such a case, the use of special leukocyte-poor units may be helpful [*see Chapter 95*].

A trial of prednisone (e.g., 60 mg a day with rapid tapering or 20 to 60 mg every other day) may reduce transfusion requirements and may be helpful in alleviating the anemia. Splenectomy is of very questionable benefit. Surgery is risky in patients with PNH because stasis and trauma accentuate hemolysis and venous occlusion. If surgery is to be performed, prophylactic anticoagulation with warfarin in the perioperative period should be considered.

Patients with PNH are frequently iron deficient. The simple administration of iron to correct this defect, however, often aggravates hemolysis because iron therapy produces a cohort of new cells, many of which are susceptible to complement-mediated lysis. Transfusion before iron therapy may help circumvent this problem because it will decrease the erythropoietic stimulus to the marrow.

Thrombocytopenia due to poor platelet production may necessitate platelet transfusions [*see Chapter 95*].[15] Budd-Chiari syndrome and inferior vena cava thrombosis must be diagnosed and treated quickly with heparin, followed by long-term administration of warfarin. If heparinization is ineffective, thrombolytic therapy (e.g., streptokinase) may be used. In a case of Budd-Chiari syndrome,[19] thrombolysis was achieved through administration of systemic streptokinase in a loading dose of 250,000 units I.V. for 30 minutes, followed by a maintenance dose of 100,000 U/hr I.V. In a similar circumstance, urokinase was administered in a bolus of 250,000 units for 40 minutes followed by 250,000 units by continuous I.V. infusion for 12 hours. Children and adolescents with aplastic anemia complicating PNH should be considered for allogeneic bone marrow transplantation.[16,20]

Prognosis

A study of 80 patients with PNH indicated that median survival was 10 years.[15] The cause of PNH-related death was thrombocytopenia, PNH hemolysis, thromboses, or PNH-associated aplastic anemia [*see Chapter 88*]. Of interest is that 15% of patients underwent spontaneous remission. In this study, the venous thromboembolism recurred in unusual and life-endangering sites, such as the hepatic vein (Budd-Chiari syndrome), the inferior vena cava, the cerebral and mesenteric veins, and the lung (pulmonary embolism).[15] Aplasia occurred in five of the 80 patients. In rare instances, prolonged and severe iron loss may occur as a result of chronic hemosiderinuria, producing iron deficiency; some patients develop transfusion-associated hemochromatosis.[16]

Acute myeloid leukemia has been found to develop during the course of PNH. In one series, the incidence was only three of 80 cases; in another series, of 220 patients, the incidence of myelodysplastic syndromes was 5% and the incidence of acute leukemia was 1%.[16]

Abnormalities of Erythrocyte Metabolism

DEFECTIVE REDUCING POWER

The reducing power of the erythrocyte is provided by reduced glutathione (GSH) and the reduced coenzymes nicotinamide adenine dinucleotide (NADH) and nicotinamide-adenine dinucleotide phosphate (NADPH) [*see Table 1*]. When erythrocytic stores of these materials are inadequate, hemoglobin and membrane-associated proteins can be oxidized, leading to the production of Heinz bodies, which consist predominantly of oxidative degradation products of hemoglobin. Such bodies can be seen either with phase-contrast microscopy or with ordinary light microscopy after staining with methyl violet [*see Figure 4b*]. Erythrocytes containing Heinz bodies are rigid and are therefore selectively removed by the reticuloendothelial system.

Defective Glutathione Synthesis

Deficiencies of certain enzymes involved in GSH synthesis lead to oxidative attacks on erythrocytes and to hemolysis [*see Figure 5*]. Several reports have described families whose members show almost negligible GSH synthesis and have hemolysis associated with the production of Heinz bodies. Glutathione peroxidase deficiency apparently contributes to hemolysis in newborn infants.

GLUCOSE-6-PHOSPHATE DEHYDROGENASE DEFICIENCY

Glucose-6-phosphate dehydrogenase (G6PD) is the first enzyme in the pentose phosphate pathway, or hexose monophosphate shunt. It catalyzes the conversion of $NADP^+$ to NADPH, a powerful reducing agent. NADPH is a cofactor for glutathione reductase and thus plays a role in protecting the cell against oxidative attack. Red cells deficient in G6PD are therefore susceptible to oxidation and hemolysis.[21,22]

G6PD deficiency is one of the most common disorders in the world; approximately 10% of male blacks in the United States are affected, as are large numbers of black Africans and some inhabitants of the Mediterranean littoral. Presumably, the disorder once conferred some selective advantage against endemic malaria, but the mechanism of this effect is conjectural.

The gene for G6PD is on the X chromosome at band q28; males carry only one gene for this enzyme; thus, those affected by the disorder are hemizygous. Females are affected much less frequently because they would have to carry two defective *G6PD* genes to show clinical disease of the same severity as that in males. However, expression of a defective *G6PD* gene is not completely masked in heterozygous women; in fact, such women exhibit highly variable G6PD enzyme activity. According to the X-inactivation, or Lyon-Beutler, hypothesis,[22] females heterozygous at the X-linked locus for the gene that codes for G6PD have two cell lines: one that contains an active X chromosome with a gene for normal G6PD and another that contains an active X chromosome with a gene for deficient G6PD. Chance partly determines the relative proportions of the two cell lines, which in turn control the clinical severity of the defect.

Classification

There are three clinical classes of G6PD deficiency: class I, which is the uncommon chronic congenital nonspherocytic hemolytic anemia; class II, in which the enzyme deficiency is severe but hemolysis tends to be episodic; and class III, the most common variant, in which the enzyme deficiency is moderate and hemolysis is caused by oxidant attack. The severity of the hemolysis and the anemia is directly related to the magnitude of the enzyme deficiency, which is determined by the half-life of the enzyme. The normal G6PD half-life is 62 days; in class III G6PD deficiency, the enzyme has a half-life of 13 days; and in class II deficiency, G6PD has a half-life of several hours. The cloning and sequencing of the *G6PD* gene have clarified a very complex literature that had described more than 300 variants of G6PD deficiency.[22]

Etiology

Hemolysis occurs in persons with class III G6PD deficiency after exposure to a drug or substance that produces an oxidant stress. Ingestion of or exposure to fava beans may cause a devastating intravascular hemolysis (known as favism) in G6PD-deficient patients, but it usually occurs only in those with the Mediterranean variant of class II deficiency. Fava beans contain isouramil and divicine, two strong reducing agents that may also attack the membrane and reduce its normal barrier to Ca^{2+} entry.[21] Elevated Ca^{2+} levels and intracellular oxidation then reduce the level of red cell proteases that ordinarily protect against the accumulation of oxidized products of hemoglobin. Oxidant attack on membrane thiols leads to oxidation of membrane proteins. This produces a rigid cell, with hemoglobin confined to one part of the cytosol and the other part of the cytosol appearing as a clear ghost (i.e., the classic bite, hemiblister, or cross-bonded cell) [*see Figure 6*]. These membrane defects cause extravascular and intravascular hemolysis.[21] Severe infections, diabetic ketoacidosis, and renal failure also reportedly trigger hemolysis.

Diagnosis

Hemolytic anemia characterized by the appearance of bite cells and Heinz bodies after administration of certain drugs suggests the possibility of G6PD deficiency [*see Table 2*]. Dapsone, which is capable of inducing oxidant-type hemolysis, has increasingly come into use as prophylaxis for *Pneumocystis carinii* pneumonia in patients infected with HIV [*see Chapter 133*].

Therefore, it is important to screen potential users of dapsone for G6PD deficiency with the standard enzymatic tests [*see Table 2*].

Other disorders to be considered in the differential diagnosis of oxidative hemolysis include unstable hemoglobinopathy, hemoglobin M disease, and deficiencies of other enzymes essential to glutathione metabolism. A G6PD screening test or direct en-

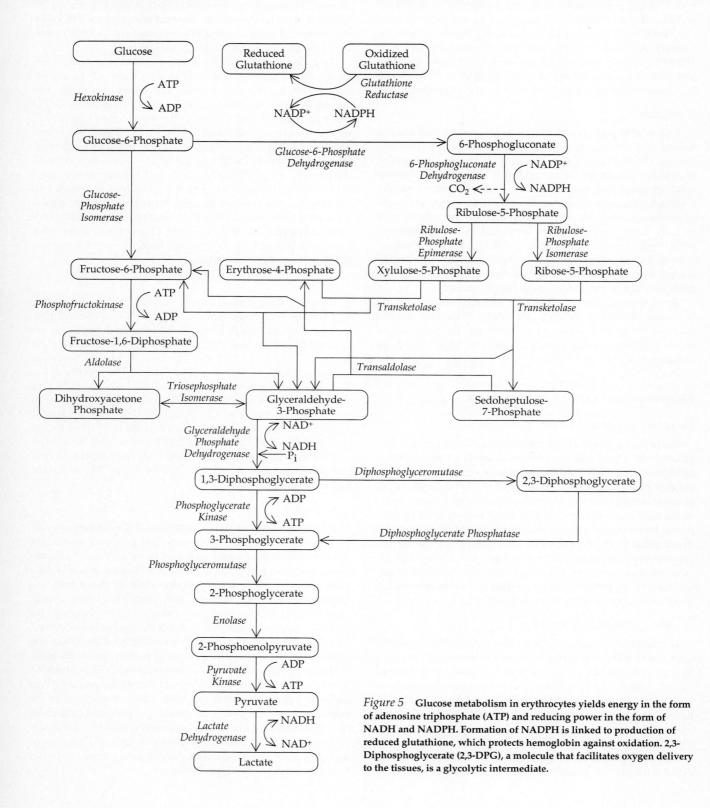

Figure 5 **Glucose metabolism in erythrocytes yields energy in the form of adenosine triphosphate (ATP) and reducing power in the form of NADH and NADPH. Formation of NADPH is linked to production of reduced glutathione, which protects hemoglobin against oxidation. 2,3-Diphosphoglycerate (2,3-DPG), a molecule that facilitates oxygen delivery to the tissues, is a glycolytic intermediate.**

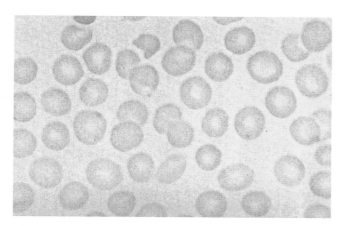

Figure 6   Bite, hemiblister, or cross-bonded cells are indicative of oxidative attack leading to oxidative hemolysis.

zyme assay usually resolves the question. Patients with A-type G6PD (class III) deficiency and brisk reticulocytosis, however, may have a near-normal G6PD level. In such cases, it is best to repeat the tests when the reticulocyte count returns to normal.

Treatment

Avoidance of drugs that may produce hemolysis is critical in management. Acute favism requires circulatory support, maintenance of good renal blood flow, and transfusions with erythrocytes that are not G6PD deficient. The physician must also be alert to the possible onset of disseminated intravascular coagulation.

DEFECTS IN GLYCOLYSIS

The series of reactions constituting the glycolytic pathway [*see Figure 5*] generates several products, such as ATP, that have various essential functions in erythrocyte metabolism [*see Table 1*]. Defects involve the major glycolytic pathway (Embden-Meyerhof pathway) and generally interfere with ATP production.

Pyruvate kinase (PK) catalyzes the formation of pyruvate, a reaction associated with ATP synthesis. After G6PD deficiency, PK deficiency (autosomal recessive) is the second most common hereditary enzymopathy. Hemolysis, mild jaundice, and occasionally palpable splenomegaly are the presenting problems. The peripheral smear usually reveals normal red cells, but in a few cases, the red cells show extreme spiculation. Aplastic crises may occur.[7]

Congenital nonspherocytic hemolysis raises the possibility of PK deficiency. An enzyme assay establishes the diagnosis. Splenectomy should be considered for patients who require transfusions.

Glucose-6-phosphate isomerase deficiency is the third most common enzymopathy that leads to hemolysis. Other enzymopathies are quite rare. Screening tests and specific assays are available for deficiencies of such enzymes as hexokinase, phosphofructokinase, triose phosphate isomerase, phosphoglycerate kinase, and aldolase.

DEFECTS IN NUCLEOTIDE METABOLISM

In hemolytic anemia associated with pyrimidine 5'-nucleotidase deficiency, coarse basophilic stippling persists in mature erythrocytes, presumably because the enzyme deficiency prevents degradation of reticulocyte RNA. This accumulation results in expansion of the total red cell nucleotide pool to a level five times normal. Pyrimidine nucleotides accumulate, and ade-

nine nucleotides are decreased. Glycolysis is impaired by an undetermined mechanism.

Disorders Involving Hemoglobin

CLASSIFICATION OF THE HEMOGLOBINOPATHIES

The clinically important hemoglobinopathies are classified into five categories on the basis of the underlying defect. The defects are as follows:

1. Hemoglobin tends to gel or crystallize (e.g., sickle cell anemia or hemoglobin C disease).
2. Hemoglobin is unstable (e.g., the congenital Heinz body anemias).
3. Hemoglobin has abnormal oxygen-binding properties (e.g., the disorder caused by hemoglobin Chesapeake).
4. Hemoglobin is readily oxidized to methemoglobin (e.g., methemoglobinemia).
5. Hemoglobin chains are synthesized at unequal rates (e.g., the thalassemias).

SICKLE CELL DISEASE

Sickle Cell Anemia

Definition   Sickle cell anemia is an autosomal recessive disease caused by the substitution of the amino acid valine for glutamine at the sixth position of the β-hemoglobin chain, which results in the production of HbS. The red cells of individuals with sickle trait (HbAS) have an HbS concentration of less than 50%; frequently, the level is as low as 30%. With rare exceptions, sickle trait is asymptomatic.

Epidemiology   From 8% to 10% of African Americans and a lesser percentage of persons with eastern Mediterranean, Indian, or Saudi Arabian ancestry have the HbS gene. Disease develops in persons who are homozygous for the sickle gene *(HbSS)*, where 70% to 98% of hemoglobin is of the S type. About 0.2% of African Americans have sickle cell anemia. The geographic coincidence of the sickle gene and endemic falciparum malaria suggests that sickle heterozygosity confers a protective advantage against malaria.[23]

Restriction endonuclease analyses indicate that the sickle gene mutation probably arose spontaneously in at least five geogra-

Table 2   Drugs That Produce Hemolysis in G6PD-Deficient Patients

Class	Example
Antimalarials	Primaquine Chloroquine
Sulfonamides	Sulfamethoxazole Sulfapyridine
Sulfones	Dapsone
Analgesics	Acetanilid Phenacetin Acetylsalicylic acid (10 g/day)
Nitrofurans	Nitrofurantoin Furazolidone
Water-soluble vitamin K derivatives	Menadiol

a 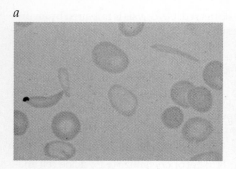   *b* 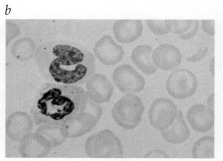   *c*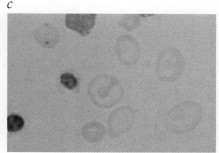

Figure 7   Sickle cell anemia is characterized by markedly distorted sickle cells, including elongated forms (*a*). Target cells (*b*) are seen in a variety of conditions, including hypochromia caused by iron deficiency, hemoglobinopathies such as HbC variants and the thalassemias, and liver disease. Cooley anemia (*c*), or β-thalassemia major, is indicated by profound hypochromia, targeting, variation in size and shape of erythrocytes, and the presence of nucleated red cells.

phic locations. These variations are called Senegal, Benin, Central African Republic (or Bantu), Saudi-Asian, Cameroon, and Indian (which may be the same as the Saudi-Asian variant). These variants are important clinically because some variants are associated with higher output of γ-globin chains (and thus higher HbF levels); others are associated more often with the gene for α-thalassemia-2 [*see* The Thalassemias, *below*]. Either of these associations may alleviate some aspects of the sickling process.[23]

Pathophysiology   Two major clinical features characterize sickle cell anemia: (1) chronic hemolysis and (2) acute, episodic vaso-occlusive crises that cause organ failure and account for most of the morbidity and mortality associated with the disease.

In chronic hemolysis, HbS liganded to oxygen or carbon monoxide shows near-normal solubility. When the molecule gives up its oxygen and changes to the deoxy S form, however, its solubility decreases. In an environment with reduced oxygen, HbS polymerizes into long tubelike fibers that induce erythrocytic sickling.[24]

The deoxyhemoglobin S polymer is in equilibrium with surrounding soluble molecules of deoxyhemoglobin S. An increase in the concentration of HbS, a decrease in pH, or an increase in the concentration of 2,3-DPG tends to stabilize the deoxy S form and enhances gelation.[24] In addition, sickled erythrocytes retain the K^+-Cl^- cotransport function and have sufficient intracellular calcium to activate the Gardos efflux channel[25] [*see* Control of Hydration and Volume, *above*]. These two mechanisms act together to produce a population of very dense sickled erythrocytes with MCHCs ranging up to 50 g/dl.[25] HbF inhibits polymerization because the glutamine residue at position 87 on the γ chain blocks lateral contact of the sickle fiber.[25] Therefore, patients with high HbF values, such as those with the Saudi-Asian variant of sickle cell anemia, have milder disease.[23] When hypoxemia and the MCHC reach a critical level, polymerization occurs after a variable delay[25]; this delay represents the period during which the deoxyhemoglobin S tetramers are slowly associating to form a nucleus. When the nucleus reaches a critical size, rapid and almost explosive gelation occurs. Free deoxyhemoglobin S tetramers rapidly attach to the nucleus to produce the long tubelike fibers that align to form parallel tubelike structures that distort the cell and produce the sickle shape [*see* Figure 7].

Most cells in the venous circulation are not sickled. However, sickling will occur if the delay time to polymerization is shortened to less than 1 second or if red cells become trapped in the microcirculation. Some red cells contain polymerized sickle hemoglobin even in the arterial circulation.

The extreme sensitivity of sickling to local environment has caused attention to be focused on cellular factors. The extreme

hyperosmolality of the renal medulla (1,200 mOsm) dehydrates red cells and raises the MCHC. Consequently, sickling sufficient to abolish the renal medullary concentrating ability may occur even in patients who have only the sickle trait. Sickle red cells also have a greater tendency to adhere to endothelial cells than do normal red cells.[26] There is some disorganization of the membrane phospholipid bilayer, with phosphatidylserine moving to the outer leaflet, possibly enhancing the thromboembolic manifestations of sickle disease.[27] In sickle cell anemia, there also appears to be an increase in circulating endothelial cells, which abnormally express tissue factor and may provide an additional basis for thromboembolism.[28]

Another manifestation of membrane damage in sickle cells is the irreversibly sickled cell, which retains its sickle shape even when reoxygenated.[29] These poorly deformable red cells are directly derived from a subpopulation of reticulocytes that are low in HbF[30] and are removed predominantly in the reticuloendothelial system. The rapid removal of these young cells results in chronic extravascular hemolysis.

Sickle Crisis and Ischemic Infarction

Sickle crisis is a potentially life-threatening complication of sickle disease. The initiating event in the sickle crisis is not known, nor is it clear why some patients have severe crises and others do not. Risk factors predisposing to painful crises include a hemoglobin level greater than 8.5 g/dl, pregnancy, cold weather, and a high reticulocyte count. Conversely, the low hematocrit in sickle cell anemia reduces blood viscosity and is protective. Sickle cell patients also characteristically have a high plasma fibrinogen level, which enhances the aggregation of already rigid erythrocytes and increases viscosity, particularly at the low shear rates encountered in the microcirculation.[31]

Clusters of increasingly rigid sickle cells will occlude the microvasculature in the following circumstances: (1) the pH falls or deoxygenation increases or the MCHC rises; (2) nitric oxide production decreases; (3) microvascular disease is present; or (4) capillary transit time is prolonged. Thrombosis may also play a role in sickle occlusion. Blockage leads to ischemic infarction, the release of inflammatory cytokines, and an amplifying sequence of stasis-induced occlusion, which may progress to sickle crisis. Portal circulations in which oxygen tension is low, such as those in the liver or the kidney, are at particular risk for occlusion.

DIAGNOSIS OF SICKLE CELL DISEASE

In the past, the diagnosis of sickle cell anemia was usually made in childhood; the affected child was seen to have limitation in exercise tolerance, shortness of breath, tachycardia, frequent severe infections, and episodes of very painful dactylitis. More recently, the identification of an affected family member has led to family screening. In California and other states, every fetal cord blood sample is examined by high-performance liquid chromatography. Rarely, the disorder is diagnosed in adult life, occasionally during a first pregnancy, when prenatal screening reveals anemia. The general symptoms are limited exercise tolerance, exertional dyspnea, painful crises, bouts of jaundice, and even biliary colic.

The clinical appearance of the patient and a blood smear showing sickled cells, holly leaf cells, and erythrocytes with Howell-Jolly bodies are fairly suggestive of sickle cell anemia. Howell-Jolly bodies represent cytoplasmic remnants of nuclear chromatin that are normally removed by the pitting action of the spleen. Platelet and white cell counts are usually high. Unless an aplastic crisis is in progress, causing a virtual absence of normoblasts, the marrow shows erythroid hyperplasia. Diagnosis is confirmed by doing a sickle prep: a drop of blood is incubated with fresh 2% sodium metabisulfite, and the proportion of sickle cells is measured immediately and then 1 hour later. Commercial testing sets such as Sickledex rely on the relative insolubility of HbS in 1.0 M phosphate buffers to make the diagnosis. The most definitive test for sickle cell anemia, however, is hemoglobin electrophoresis, which indicates the relative percentages of HbS and HbF. All of these tests are also useful in screening family members for sickle cell trait. Patients who are heterozygous for both the HbS gene and the β-thalassemia gene may appear to be homozygous for HbS. Other varieties of sickling hemoglobin are observed very infrequently. DNA-based methods can also be used to pinpoint the specific genetic abnormality and to identify the subpopulations from which the patients descended.[23]

For example, persons with sickle cell anemia and α-thalassemia have higher hemoglobin levels, lower reticulocyte counts, a lower MCHC, a lower MCV, and less dense red cells than persons who have sickle cell anemia alone. Such patients may have increased life expectancy and perhaps a different pattern of manifestations of veno-occlusive complications.[32] The combination of G6PD deficiency and sickle cell anemia has neither beneficial nor harmful effects.[33]

Primary Therapies for Sickle Cell Disease

Reduction of hemolysis Until recently, treatment focused on management of sickle crises. Currently, there are several approaches designed to more fundamentally alter the conseqences of sickle disease. Standard conservative management of sickle crisis consists of appropriate examination followed by rest, hydration, and analgesia. In demonstrably acidotic patients, mild alkalinization should be induced by administration of a bicarbonate solution, which is prepared by addition of an ampule of sodium bicarbonate to 1 L of either 5% dextrose in water or half-normal saline. The bicarbonate solution should be infused at a rate of 5 to 7 ml/kg/hr for the first 4 hours and then at a rate of 4 ml/kg/hr for the next 20 hours. The role of O_2 administration in patients with normal arterial oxygen tension (P_aO_2) and no cardiopulmonary problems is untested.

Pain management Pain [see Chapter 173] is the major concern for 10% to 20% of patients with sickle cell anemia. Avascular necrosis of bone marrow produces excruciating pain that can last as long as 8 to 10 days. The need for pain relief sometimes results in habituation or addiction. Because there are few objective ways to monitor the sickle crisis, the physician may not know

whether a demand for narcotics is a manifestation of drug-seeking behavior.

The patient with sickle cell anemia should be provided with oral analgesics for use at home in an attempt to abort the pain crisis at its onset. Nonsteroidal anti-inflammatory drugs (NSAIDs), such as naproxen (500 mg p.o.) and ketorolac (10 mg), can be used initially. If NSAIDs alone are not sufficient, they can be followed by a narcotic-analgesic combination, such as hydrocodone and acetaminophen or oxycodone and aspirin. The use of adjuvants such as diphenhydramine (50 mg p.o.) or lorazepam (1 to 2 mg p.o.) may calm the patient and perhaps antagonize the actions of released histamine.[34] If these measures, perhaps repeated every 6 hours, do not control the pain, the patient usually requires parenteral treatment. Care from the patient's regular physicians is far preferable to reliance on unfamiliar providers in emergency rooms.[34] The patient needs rapid evaluation for possible infection, acute chest syndrome, bone infarction, and other complications, and the pain should be treated either with 10 mg of intravenous morphine along with 50 mg of intramuscular diphenhydramine every 2 hours or with 4 mg of intramuscular hydromorphone along with 50 mg of intramuscular diphenhydramine every 2 hours. If there is no pain relief or there is inadequate pain relief 30 minutes after the first dose, 50% of the initial dose of opiates can be administered, with close monitoring of the respiratory rate, particularly if it approaches 10 respirations a minute. Some units have used patient-controlled analgesia with good results. It is important to continue to administer parenteral analgesia at regular intervals to provide increased doses for breakthrough pain. The patient will probably need a laxative and may need an antiemetic, such as prochlorperazine (10 mg p.o. or I.M). If the patient responds, home therapy with oral controlled-release morphine, such as MS Contin, is usually effective. If pain continues for more than 8 to 12 hours, the patient will probably need to be hospitalized to receive extended therapy with increased doses of analgesia and parenteral fluids and observation.[34]

Measures to alter the pathophysiology of sickle cell anemia
A clearer understanding of the kinetics of sickling suggests some future prospects for the therapy of sickle cell anemia. Decreasing the MCHC should diminish gelation. One approach being tested attempts to block the Ca^{2+}-dependent K^+ efflux (Gardos channel) [see Control of Hydration and Volume, above].[35] A compound tested in a sickle mouse model shows promise in preventing red cell dehydration.[35,36]

Therapies to interfere with sickling are being actively pursued. The presence of 20% to 30% HbF in sickle red cells delays gelation by a factor of 103 to 104, and therefore, a mechanism that would switch on the genes that control fetal hemoglobin synthesis and that would thus lessen the severity of sickle disease appears feasible.[37,38] Hydroxyurea produces an increase in F reticulocyte and HbF levels. In a phase III trial, hydroxyurea was administered at a starting dosage of 15 mg/kg/day; patients treated with hydroxyurea had fewer painful crises, fewer admissions for crisis, and fewer episodes of acute chest syndrome and required fewer transfusions than patients given a placebo.[39] There was no effect on stroke; however, after 8 years of follow-up, there was a clear reduction in mortality of 40%.[40] The beneficial effect accrued after about 8 weeks of therapy and was accompanied by an increase in MCV and an increase in the proportion of F cells; in addition, there was a decrease in neutrophils and a decrease in sickle RBC adhesion to endothelial cells.[41] Trials are also being conducted with butyrate, which can increase γ-chain production, thereby increasing HbF levels and interfering with gelation.[42,43] Demethylating agents such as 5-azacytidine and decitabine can also increase HbF to therapeutically useful levels. Because sickle cells adhere abnormally to the endothelium, attempts have been made to block adhesion; thus far, these efforts have not proved useful.

Inflammatory cytokines appear to play an important role in the sickle crisis, as evidenced by the fact that a predictor of success in hydroxyurea therapy is a decrease in the white cell count.[40,41] Other investigators are studying the possible vasodilatory role of nitric oxide.

Sibling-donor allogeneic bone marrow transplantation can result in cure or can lead to a substitution of sickle trait for sickle cell anemia. In 22 carefully selected patients, primarily those with stroke or recurrent episodes of acute chest syndrome, bone marrow transplantation resulted in apparent cure in 15 patients; there were two fatalities (9%), and the remaining five patients had complications such as graft failure.[44]

The role of long-term transfusion therapy Long-term transfusion therapy has been found to prevent stroke.[45] Some investigators have shown that preventive transfusions reduce or eliminate pain crisis, episodes of acute chest syndrome, bacterial infection, and hospitalization.[46,47] Other clinicians, however, warn against the dangers of iron overload,[48,49] transfusion hepatitis, problems with venous access, and red cell alloimmunization.[50] Further studies may identify appropriate roles for chronic transfusion therapy.

Prognosis in Sickle Cell Disease

A major study of almost 4,000 patients has provided new information regarding life expectancy and causes of death in patients with sickle cell disease.[37] Whereas it was once assumed that most patients with sickle cell anemia would die by 20 years of age, it is now clear that the median age of death is 42 years for men and 48 years for women. This life expectancy is 25 to 30 years less than that of the general African-American population. Of the identified causes of death, only 18% were the result of organ failure—predominantly renal disease, congestive heart failure, or the consequences of chronic strokes. Thirty-three percent of patients died during acute pain crises, frequently associated with the acute chest syndrome and less often associated with stroke. The presence of α-thalassemia had no measurable effect. Predictors of poor outcome were a white cell count greater than 15,000/μl; a low HbF level; and organ involvement manifested by renal disease, acute chest syndrome, and neurologic events.

Complications and Their Management

Skeletal problems Aseptic necrosis (osteonecrosis) of the femoral head occurs in about 10% of patients, particularly those who also have α-thalassemia. Arthroplasty has been relatively ineffective, partly because of the presence of adjacent hard bone, which interferes with the placement of the prosthesis, and because of the increased risk of infection.[51]

Cardiopulmonary problems Cardiac complications associated with anemia are the result of a large increase in cardiac output. There is chamber enlargement, cardiomegaly, left ventricular hypertrophy, and flow murmurs.[52] Acute myocardial infarction has occurred in relatively young adults who do not have coronary disease.[53]

Acute pulmonary complications are a major cause of morbidity and mortality; such complications include local infection, vascular occlusions in the pulmonary vessels (both in situ thrombo-

sis and embolism), and pulmonary fat embolism from ischemic marrow fat necrosis.[54] In a study of 1,722 episodes of acute chest syndrome in 939 patients, adults in the study were found to be afebrile but had shortness of breath, chills, and pain in the chest and in at least one extremity.[55] Physical examination frequently showed no abnormal chest findings. The P_aO_2 was low, averaging 71 mm Hg (25% were below 60 mm Hg). The death rate in adults was 4.3%; death was preceded by a lower hemoglobin value, a higher white cell count, and multilobe involvement. Autopsy of 16 cases showed that nine patients had pulmonary embolism and fat emboli and possibly 20% had bacterial infections. Thoracic vertebral bone infarctions contributed substantially to the pain.[50]

Usually, therapy should include incentive spirometry,[50] search for infection and treatment with antimicrobials, cautious use of analgesia, aggressive fluid replacement, and consideration of bronchoalveolar lavage to identify microbial infection or the fat-laden macrophages of fat emboli. Meticulous monitoring is required and includes repeat measurement of oxygenation and transfusions when clinically necessary. One of the most important benefits of hydroxyurea therapy is its ability to reduce the frequency of acute chest syndrome.[39,56] Children may also need supplementary penicillin prophylaxis.[57] Because routine use of pneumococcal vaccine has lowered the incidence of pneumococcal pneumonia in patients with sickle cell anemia, *Haemophilus influenzae* is now responsible for a relatively higher percentage of pneumonia cases among these patients; the choice of antibiotics should reflect this change.

Hepatobiliary disease Cholelithiasis is a complication that occurs in 30% to 70% of patients, some of whom exhibit signs and symptoms of cholecystitis.[58] There is conflicting data regarding frequency of cholecystitis or obstruction of the common bile duct. In one study of 77 patients known to have had gallstones for 1 to 10 years, only five underwent cholecystectomy.[59] Another study found that of 604 procedures in patients with sickle cell anemia, 40% were for cholecystitis and cholelithiasis.[58] Patients who were given transfusions to a level of hemoglobin of 10 g/dl before surgery did better perioperatively.[58] If cholecystectomy is to be done, one should wait until the painful crisis is over, and the procedure should be done laparoscopically.[58]

Hepatic complications include congestive hepatopathy secondary to heart failure and viral hepatitis from frequent transfusions. Sickling in the liver can also produce hepatopathy. Often, serum bilirubin levels exceed 30 mg/dl in intrahepatic cholestasis, and coagulation abnormalities may lead to hemorrhagic complications and death.

Renal and urologic complications Water loss as a result of an inability to concentrate urine may enhance the sickling process. The extremely hypertonic milieu of the renal medulla induces severe sickling and destruction of the vasa recta. Hematuria and papillary necrosis ensue. These complications are also observed in patients with sickle trait and in those who have sickle cell–hemoglobin C disease. The defect in renal concentrating ability appears to depend on the amount of HbS polymer contained in cells and is thus less severe in patients who also have α-thalassemia variants.[60]

Complications include renal tubular acidosis, hyperkalemia, and proteinuria. Treatment with enalapril reduces proteinuria, suggesting the presence of a component of glomerular capillary hypertension.[61] Renal failure, with accompanying worsening of anemia, contributes to the death of about one fifth of patients older than 40 years who have homozygous sickle disease.

Priapism is an extraordinarily painful complication of sickle cell anemia and may result in impotence. I recommend red cell exchange transfusion when conservative measures fail to produce improvement within 24 hours.

Neurologic disorders   Neurologic complications of sickle cell disease include stroke, subarachnoid hemorrhage, and isolated functional losses that suggest a focal occlusion. The pathogenesis of occlusion of the large cerebral arteries is probably different from that of the microvascular occlusive events that occur in hypoxic capillary beds. The underlying defect is probably damage to the vascular endothelium, followed by extensive intimal proliferation and then probably thrombosis of the damaged vascular bed.[32] A recent multi-institutional study of 4,082 patients revealed a 4% to 5% cerebrovascular accident (CVA) prevalence and an incidence of 0.61 per 100 patient-years.[62] Of the CVAs, 54% were infarcts, 34% were hemorrhagic in nature, 11% were transient ischemic attacks (TIAs), and 1% had both infarctive and hemorrhagic features. Of the patients who survived, the recurrence rate of CVA was 14%. Mortality was 11%, and virtually all patients who died had hemorrhagic CVAs.

In a prospective study in which transcranial Doppler ultrasonography was used to pinpoint children at risk for stroke, treatment with standard care or transfusion therapy (to reduce the HbS concentration to < 30%) resulted in 10 CVAs and one intracerebral hematoma in the 65 control subjects, whereas the transfusion group had only 1 CVA (P < 0.002). The trial was terminated early.[45] The success of this trial raises many serious issues about the necessity of ultrasonographic devices for successful management; the optimum duration of transfusion therapy; the inevitable consequences of transfusional hemochromatosis [see β-Thalassemia major (Cooley anemia), below] and the necessity for ethnically matched blood to minimize allotransfusion reaction; the willingness of patients and families to accept transfusion therapy; and the role of allogeneic bone marrow transplantation as a potential alternative.[45,63]

Ocular complications   The major ocular problems associated with sickle cell anemia are retinopathy, vitreous hemorrhage, and neovascularization. Annual ophthalmologic evaluations are recommended. The efficacy of laser photocoagulation in treating sickle-induced ocular changes is currently being investigated.

Dermatologic complications   Poorly healing leg ulcers can be an important cause of morbidity in patients with sickle cell anemia. The degree of anemia does not seem to correlate with the presence or severity of these ulcers, but incompetence of venous valves and the resulting venous insufficiency have been associated with ulceration.[64] Standard management includes debridement, control of local infection, use of wet-dry dressings, and possibly red cell transfusion. The use of granulocyte-macrophage colony-stimulating factor (GM-CSF), either injected perilesionally or added topically to the wound, enhances healing, perhaps by stimulating the local growth of macrophages.[65] Several sorts of application have been used, but the more successful applications involve the subcutaneous injection of 100 μg of GM-CSF in each of four sites circumferentially around the ulcer at a distance of 5 mm from its edge (resulting in a total dose of 400 μg in the wound). In some circumstances, one treatment sufficed, whereas in others, weekly treatments were necessary for up to 4 to 12 weeks. This therapy has not been approved by the Food and Drug Administration.

Aplastic crisis   Aplastic crisis rapidly lowers hemoglobin and hematocrit levels and produces reticulocytopenia, as it does in any chronic hemolytic state. Parvovirus has been found to cause aplastic crisis,[7] as has bone marrow necrosis.[66]

Susceptibility to infections   Patients with sickle cell anemia are hyposplenic and exhibit complement system abnormalities. Deficient serum opsonizing activity for *Salmonella* organisms may confer an increased susceptibility to those infections, including osteomyelitis.

Possible complications of general anesthesia   The hypoxemia and vascular stasis that may occur during general anesthesia enhance sickling and may lead to a sickle crisis in the postoperative period. In an analysis of almost 4,000 patients, 12 deaths were associated with 1,079 procedures. There were more complications after regional anesthesia than after general anesthesia.[67] A simple transfusion program to raise the hemoglobin level to 10 g/dl was as effective as more aggressive preoperative programs in reducing the rate of complications.[68]

Pregnancy and contraception   The dangers of pregnancy for women with sickle disease include pulmonary problems, increased incidence of urinary tract infection, hematuria, preeclampsia, and maternal death. Presumably, pelvic hypoxemia and the vascular overload associated with pregnancy lead to enhanced sickling, with its attendant complications. Vaso-occlusion in the placenta may account for fetal death and low birth weight.

Experienced clinicians differ in their approach to the pregnant patient with sickle disease. Some advocate only meticulous conservative care, whereas others recommend prophylactic transfusions. A controlled study has indicated that there is no advantage to the use of prophylactic transfusions.[69]

Chorionic villus sampling (which can provide DNA for analysis in the first trimester of pregnancy), DNA amplification techniques, and probes that identify the specific nucleotide change of sickle cell anemia can give a relatively safe and very reliable prenatal diagnosis.[70] Oral contraceptives may also pose a special hazard to women with sickle cell anemia, because they have been associated with a slight increase in the incidence of stroke, venous thromboembolism, and myocardial infarction. However, the emerging evidence that daily use of oral contraceptives containing less than 50 mg of synthetic estrogens is relatively safe suggests that patients with sickle disease can take such medication with reasonable confidence. The use of the Norplant implantable contraceptive device is another alternative for some patients. In any event, pregnancy or abortion in sickle disease carries significant risk.[69]

Genetic Counseling

A key element to be considered in the provision of genetic counseling to patients with sickle trait or sickle disease is the significant morbidity in affected children and adults. Couples with sickle disease or sickle trait may want to have children despite the associated fetal and maternal risks. There are about 4,000 to 5,000 such pregnancies in the United States each year.[70] In one study, 286 of 445 pregnancies (64%) in mothers with sickle cell anemia proceeded to delivery. There was a resultant increase in fetal loss; 21% of the infants were small and thus would be expected to require additional care, which the mother might have difficulty providing. In this study, there was one maternal death caused by sickle cell disease[71] [see Genetic Counseling and Prenatal Diagnosis, below].

SICKLE VARIANTS

Sickle Trait

Generally, patients with sickle trait are well and lead normal, healthy lives. A few complications occur: hyposthenuria, renal hematuria, and, during pregnancy, bacteriuria and pyelonephritis. Splenic infarction occurs under conditions of hypoxia; it also occurs at high altitudes, predominantly in nonblack persons who have sickle cell anemia.

Sickle trait has been identified as a major risk factor for sudden death during basic training in the military[72]; death has resulted from unexplained cardiac arrest, heatstroke, heat stress, or rhabdomyolysis. Increasing age has been correlated with an increased risk of sudden death. However, these events have occurred under extreme conditions: very strenuous physical activity, usually in untrained persons, occasionally at high altitudes or in extreme heat. Usually, persons with sickle trait who are accustomed to physical activity do not have an increased risk of sudden death. For example, African-American football players with sickle trait do not have a higher incidence of sudden death than other players.[73]

Therapeutic options for renal hematuria include the administration of diuretics, parenteral bicarbonate, transfusions, or ε-aminocaproic acid.

Sickle Cell–β-Thalassemia

When combined with sickle trait, a defect in the β-thalassemia gene produces a disease very similar to sickle cell anemia. The β-thalassemia gene reduces the rate of synthesis of the β^A chain, resulting in a predominance of β^S in patients with sickle trait. The patient's red cells contain varying amounts of HbS, HbA, HbA_2, and HbF. The disease is severe when only a small amount of HbA is present, but it is milder if HbA constitutes 25% or more of the total hemoglobin and less HbS is produced.

Diagnosis is based on an elevated level of HbA_2 or HbF, or both, on hemoglobin electrophoresis and a positive family history of thalassemia and the sickle gene. A study of 55 Greek patients treated with hydroxyurea showed distinct clinical improvement.[74,75]

Sickle Cell–Hemoglobin C Disease

In sickle cell–hemoglobin C (HbSC) disease, almost equal amounts of HbS and HbC are formed. Between 1% and 2% of hemoglobin is HbF, and small amounts of HbA_2 are also present; however, HbA is absent. The red cells are microcytic, and the very high MCHC facilitates the crystallization and aggregation of HbC.[76]

As many as 30% to 50% of patients with this disorder are not anemic and have only modest reticulocytosis. Patients may not be identified until the disorder manifests itself in the form of a vaso-occlusive crisis during surgery, pregnancy, or a medical emergency.[76] Splenomegaly, proliferative retinopathy, and aseptic necrosis of long bones also occur. The peripheral smear [see Figure 7] shows irreversibly sickled cells in addition to target cells, stomatocytes, and erythrocytes, with eccentric hemoglobin depositions probably representing HbC aggregates or crystals. Diagnosis is confirmed by hemoglobin electrophoresis.[76]

Management is the same as that for sickle cell anemia. In a small study, hydroxyurea at a dosage of 1,000 mg/day was given to six patients with HbSC disease; this regimen resulted in an increase in MCV, a decrease in so-called stress reticulocytes, an increase in hemoglobin, and probably a reduction in cell density. Although not definitive, this small study suggests that hydroxyurea benefits patients with HbSC disease.[77] Life expectancy for patients with HbSC disease is almost 20 years greater than that for patients with HbSS disease.[37]

OTHER HEMOGLOBINOPATHIES

Hemoglobin C Disease

The HbC molecule is $\alpha_2\beta_2^{6glu\rightarrow lys}$; the gene mutation probably originated at a single site in Burkina Faso, in West Africa.[76] The presence of this hemoglobin produces almost no illness in the heterozygous state but causes mild compensated hemolysis and palpable splenomegaly in the homozygous state.

The relative insolubility of HbC is responsible for the pathologic changes associated with its presence. HbC probably interacts with the K^+-Cl^- cotransporter, which keeps it active, whereas the K^+-Cl^- cotransporter normally shuts off in red cells after the reticulocyte stage. The result is a loss of K^+, cellular dehydration with elevated MCHC, and then aggregation and crystallization of the poorly soluble HbC.[76] The relative insolubility of HbC causes erythrocytes to become rigid and thereby subject to fragmentation and to loss of membrane material, resulting in the microspherocytes seen on a peripheral blood smear [see Figure 4].

Target cells, an important morphologic finding, constitute about 80% of the erythrocytes. HbC crystals are in the oxyhemoglobin state and dissolve when the red cells are deoxygenated, probably accounting for the absence of vaso-occlusive episodes.

Diagnosis of hemoglobin C disease is based on blood-smear findings and the absence of evidence of either iron deficiency or thalassemia; the diagnosis is confirmed by hemoglobin electrophoresis. No therapy is required.

Hemoglobin E Disease

In hemoglobin E disease, lysine is substituted for glutamic acid at position 26 of the β-globin chain. Hemoglobin E trait is found predominantly in Southeast Asia. It has come to clinical attention in the United States as a result of the influx of Southeast Asians, in whom the incidence of this trait is about 10%.

HbE is oxidatively unstable because the mutation occurs at the $\alpha_1\beta_1$ contact site. The decreased content of β^E is the result of decreased production of β^E messenger RNA (mRNA) and production of unstable β^E mRNA.

Patients heterozygous for HbE have normal hemoglobin values, microcytosis, and no splenomegaly. Electrophoresis reveals that 70% of the hemoglobin is HbA, 25% is HbE, and the remainder is HbA_2 or HbF. On electrophoresis, HbE runs with HbA_2 and may be reported as HbA_2 by inexperienced laboratories. The clue is that HbA_2 never accounts for more than 8% of the total hemoglobin. A laboratory report of an HbA_2 level of 25% should prompt a review of the data.

Patients homozygous for HbE have mild anemia, with a hemoglobin level of about 12 to 13 g/dl, a low mean corpuscular volume, and an elevated red cell count but no reticulocytosis; they exhibit microcytes and target cells. Electrophoresis shows only HbE. Chronic hemolysis does not occur. Oxidant drugs such as dapsone should be avoided in both heterozygotes and homozygotes.

A serious clinical problem occurs when a patient is doubly heterozygous for HbE and β-thalassemia trait. Such patients present with β-thalassemia intermedia, characterized by severe anemia and splenomegaly (see below). These patients occasionally require transfusions of blood and even allogeneic bone marrow transplantation.[78]

Unstable Hemoglobinopathies

Many individual variants make up the unstable hemoglobinopathies. The hemoglobin instabilities stem from amino acid substitutions that deprive the molecule of its heme group, alter the heme pocket, loosen the link between its α and β chains, or weaken the subunit structure [*see Chapter 86*]. The result is disruption and precipitation of hemoglobin, particularly when it is subjected to oxidant attack. Precipitated hemoglobin forms Heinz bodies, which are observed even in persons heterozygous for the unstable hemoglobin variant. Because of the deleterious effects of Heinz bodies on the erythrocyte and its membrane, significant hemolysis can occur even in the heterozygous state.

Diagnosis of an unstable hemoglobinopathy is suggested by the presence of a partly compensated chronic nonspherocytic hemolysis. Heinz bodies are observed in the erythrocytes of patients who have undergone splenectomy. Erythrocytes from patients who have not undergone splenectomy demonstrate Heinz bodies on incubation with brilliant cresyl blue dye. The differential diagnosis of a hemoglobinopathy includes G6PD deficiency; this disorder can usually be ruled out by direct assay for the enzyme.

Management includes avoidance of oxidant drugs. Splenectomy may be considered when hemolysis is severe and inadequately compensated.

Hemoglobin with Abnormal Oxygen Affinity

The presence of hemoglobin with increased oxygen affinity should be considered in the differential diagnosis of unexplained erythrocytosis, particularly if there is a familial association [*see Chapter 90*]. Hemoglobin electrophoresis may reveal the disorder, but in suspected cases, measurement of the oxyhemoglobin dissociation curve [*see Chapter 86*] is preferable as a basis for diagnosis. Hemoglobin Chesapeake and hemoglobin Rainier are examples of forms with particularly increased oxygen affinity.

The rare instances of hemoglobin with low oxygen affinity, such as hemoglobin Kansas, represent mutations. Patients with low-oxygen-affinity hemoglobinopathy are sometimes cyanotic because of enhanced oxygen unloading.

Methemoglobinemia

Methemoglobin is an oxidation product of hemoglobin in which iron is in the ferric form; thus, the molecule cannot bind oxygen reversibly. Ordinarily, 1% of hemoglobin is in the ferric state. Between 0.5% and 3% of deoxyhemoglobin is normally spontaneously oxidized to methemoglobin every day. The normal reducing power of erythrocytes [*see Table 1*] maintains the balance between oxidation and reduction. The enzyme system that reduces 95% of methemoglobin to hemoglobin involves two proteins, NADH-cytochrome b_5 reductase and cytochrome b_5, and also requires NADH. (NADH is generated by glyceraldehyde phosphate dehydrogenase [*see Figure 5*].) As the name suggests, NADH-cytochrome b_5 reductase, a flavin-containing enzyme, uses NADH to reduce cytochrome b_5. Reduced cytochrome b_5 then reduces methemoglobin.[79,80] Novel mutations in the affected gene have been described.[81]

Most often, methemoglobinemia is acquired by ingestion of or exposure to oxidants that oxidize Fe^{+2} so fast that the reducing systems are overwhelmed [*see* Mechanism of Oxidative Attack, *below*].

There are two congenital forms of methemoglobinemia. In the hereditary enzymopenic form of methemoglobinemia, patients are homozygous or doubly heterozygous for a deficiency of NADH-cytochrome b_5 reductase. These patients appear blue even when only about 10% of their hemoglobin is in the form of methemoglobin, but they are not sick and easily tolerate methemoglobin levels of 25% or more. In contrast, the presence of about 5 g/dl of reduced, deoxygenated hemoglobin produces cyanosis. Patients with this form of methemoglobinemia do not

exhibit hemolysis and generally do not require treatment. Assay of NADH-cytochrome b_5 reductase, done by a special laboratory, can establish the diagnosis. If desired, methylene blue at a dosage of 100 to 300 mg/day orally can be used, but it may produce urinary discomfort.[79] Methylene blue transfers electrons from NADPH to methemoglobin.

The other hereditary form of methemoglobinemia is caused by HbM, of which there are five rare variants. Each of these variants contains an amino acid substitution in the heme pocket, which allows stable bonds to be formed between the heme iron and the amino acid side chains. These bonds keep hemoglobin in the Fe^{3+} form—a form that is unable to bind oxygen and is inaccessible to the reducing enzymes. The disorder is seen only in heterozygotes; about 30% of hemoglobin is abnormal, as detected by electrophoresis. Cyanosis is noted at birth. Hemolysis is minimal, and therapy is not needed.

THE THALASSEMIAS

The thalassemias have a worldwide distribution; in many regions, they are responsible for major medical, social, and economic perturbations. Throughout the world, the regions in which the thalassemias occur are contiguous with regions endemic for malaria, indicating that the heterozygous forms of thalassemia provide protection against malaria.[82] The techniques of molecular biology have helped elucidate the pathophysiology of these syndromes.[82] The improved understanding of the molecular basis of these diseases has enabled investigators to make unambiguous antenatal diagnoses. Using these data, expectant parents can make thoughtful, informed choices regarding the outcome of pregnancies in which the fetus is severely affected.

Pathophysiology

In a healthy person, the synthesis of α and β chains is meticulously coordinated in producing adult HbA ($\alpha_2\beta_2$). In contrast, patients with thalassemia usually demonstrate imbalanced synthesis of normal globin chains. Occasionally, however, thalassemia-like syndromes can result from diminished production of a structurally abnormal chain.[83] Because one of the globin chains is present in reduced amounts, the unpaired chain accumulates in the developing erythroid precursor cell, and toxicity results [*see Figure 8*]. Consequently, erythroid cells die in the marrow, giving rise to a classic form of ineffective erythropoiesis [*see Chapter 88*], and affected erythrocytes undergo hemolysis in the peripheral blood.

The β-thalassemias are characterized by diminished production of β-globin chains, causing unmatched β-globin chains to accumulate and aggregate. These aggregates of α chains precipitate, causing decreased ATP synthesis, potassium leak, and reduced amounts of surface sialic acid; the affected erythrocytes are misshapen and relatively rigid. The membrane Ca^{2+} barrier is breached, allowing Ca^{2+} to enter. These α-globin aggregates also appear to keep the K^+-Cl^- cotransporter functioning; as a result, in severe forms of β-thalassemia, dehydration of varying degree is seen.[84] These destructive alterations of the membrane, which can be detected by macrophages, may in part be caused by local oxidation that is triggered by membrane accumulation of hemichromes; hemichromes cause aggregation of band 3 [*see Figure 2*], to which IgG antibodies and complement are bound.[85] Abnormal accumulations of α chains probably account for the accelerated apoptosis and ineffective erythropoiesis seen in marrow erythroid precursors.[85] The overall decrease in hemoglobin synthesis per cell accounts for the observed hypochromia and target cell formation.

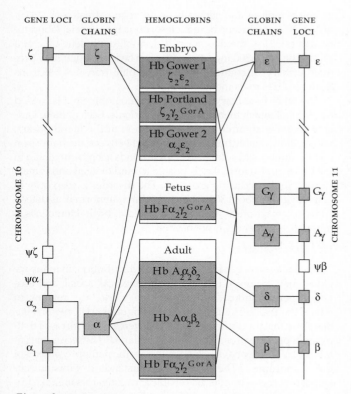

Figure 8 The genes encoding the α and non-α chains that come together to form the hemoglobin tetramer lie on chromosomes 16 and 11, respectively. The α genes are present at duplicated loci. Six distinct species of normal hemoglobin have been described. Three of these hemoglobins are synthesized only during embryonic stages of development (Hb Gower 1, Hb Portland, and Hb Gower 2). HbF predominates during fetal development, and a small amount continues to be synthesized in adult life. HbA and HbA₂ constitute the major forms of adult hemoglobin. Different hemoglobin genes are activated at various stages of development. In the embryo, ζ chains combine with ε chains to yield Hb Gower 1 and with γ chains to form Hb Portland; α and ε chains are linked to form Hb Gower 2. There are two varieties of γ chains that are derived from separate loci and that differ in a single amino acid; $^{G}\gamma$ contains glycine at position 136, whereas $^{A}\gamma$ contains alanine at this position. The genes coding for the two other non-α chains, β and δ, which are required for the synthesis of adult hemoglobins, are switched on late in fetal development. The factors regulating this precisely coordinated sequence of changes in hemoglobin production are poorly understood; some evidence suggests that DNA segments intervening between the various hemoglobin genes may control the relative rates of synthesis of the adjacent gene products.

Patients with α-thalassemia demonstrate accumulations of excess β chains that, if present in sufficient amounts, form β_4 tetramers (HbH) [*see Figure 8*]. Such tetramers have high oxygen affinity and are unstable, aggregating in the presence of oxidative stresses such as infection. β-Globin aggregates also become attached to the erythrocyte's membrane skeleton, but they produce lesions different from those produced by α-globin aggregates. In the severe α-thalassemias, ineffective erythropoiesis is less prominent[85]; rather, destruction of peripheral red cells is the critical characteristic. Red cells in severe α-thalassemia are rigid, but in contrast to those in severe β-thalassemia, the membranes in severe α-thalassemia are more stable than normal. Also in contrast to β-thalassemia, the red cells in severe α-thalassemia are uniformly overhydrated.[84]

Both α-thalassemia and β-thalassemia are characterized by variable degrees of anemia. This variation is attributable to varying degrees of ineffective erythropoiesis and hemolysis.[85] When the anemia is severe, the associated hypoxia induces a vigorous compensatory erythropoiesis, leading to expansion of the marrow cavity, osteopenia, and enlargement of reticuloendothelial organs; tumors may arise at sites of extramedullary erythropoietic activity. Destruction of erythroblasts and erythrocytes may predispose to cholelithiasis and obstructive jaundice. Patients with the more severe forms of thalassemia require regular transfusions, which may eventually generate iron overload and such consequences as cardiomyopathy, hepatopathy, and endocrinopathy [*see Chapter 87*].

Molecular Genetics

Defects that lead to imbalanced chain synthesis include gene deletion, abnormalities in transcription and translation [*see Chapter 71*], and instability of the mRNA directing globin synthesis or of the globin itself. The genes controlling the synthesis of the α and non-α chains of hemoglobin are located on chromosomes 11 and 16 [*see Figure 8*].

During the embryonic phase, ζ chains [*see Figure 8*] substitute for α chains, but during fetal, neonatal, and adult life, no substitutes exist for the α chain of hemoglobin, a fact that has important clinical implications.[86] In contrast, both δ and γ chains supplement the normal β chain of adult life, and the γ chains (of which there are two variants, differing in only a single amino acid) can serve as the non-α chains in fetal and neonatal life.[87]

Diagnostic Approach to Thalassemia

The HbF and HbA₂ measurements that aid in the diagnosis of the β-thalassemias are readily available from clinical laboratories. In contrast, the tests required to diagnose the α-thalassemias are quite sophisticated and are performed only in institutions specifically engaged in thalassemia research. The diagnostic tools used to assess patients suspected of having α-thalassemia include clinical history, smear evaluation, calculation of indices, brilliant cresyl blue staining, and family studies. In practice, α-thalassemia trait is diagnosed on the basis of a finding of microcytosis in an iron-replete patient who has normal HbA₂ and HbF levels.

The diagnosis of either α- or β-thalassemia should be suspected when the MCV is less than 75 fl and the red cell count is greater than 5 million cells/μl. A patient with these two findings has an 85% chance of having a thalassemia syndrome.[88] In one study, diagnosis of thalassemia was not considered in about half of the patients with the disease.

β-Thalassemia

The deficient synthesis of β-globin characteristic of β-thalassemia leads to accumulation of unmatched α chains. This decrease in β-chain synthesis can be a consequence of abnormal nuclear processing of mRNA transcripts, premature termination of translation, or gene deletion. A diagnostically significant development in β-thalassemia is the partial compensatory increase of the δ and γ chains that yields elevated levels of HbA₂ ($\alpha_2\delta_2$) and HbF ($\alpha_2\gamma_2$), respectively [*see Figure 8*]. The β-thalassemia variants produce three clinical syndromes: β-thalassemia major, β-thalassemia minor, and thalassemia intermedia.

β-Thalassemia major (Cooley anemia) β-Thalassemia major is usually a homozygous or doubly heterozygous condition; both parents of an affected individual carry a β-thalassemia trait. In β⁰-

thalassemia, the most severe variant, no β chains are synthesized; only HbF and HbA_2 are found. β^+-Thalassemia is somewhat less severe. It is characterized by small amounts of β chains and small quantities of HbA in addition to HbF and HbA_2. δβ-Thalassemia is yet milder; it is caused by deletion of the δ-globin and β-globin genes. This mutation prohibits production of HbA_2 and HbA, permitting synthesis of fetal hemoglobin alone.

β-Thalassemia major is characterized by severe anemia that appears in the first year of life. It is associated with jaundice, hepatosplenomegaly, expansion of the erythroid marrow with secondary body changes (including retarded growth), and an increased susceptibility to infection.

Diagnosis is not difficult; no other condition closely resembles Cooley anemia. The peripheral smear shows nucleated red cells, distorted hypochromic erythrocytes, and basophilic stippling, which represents aggregates of ribosomal RNA [see Figure 7]. Supravital staining reveals accumulations of excess unmatched α chains.

Management consists of aggressive transfusion aimed at maintaining a hemoglobin level of about 12 g/dl, thus preventing such complications as congestive heart failure, fluid overload, and skeletal deformity. Splenectomy is usually necessary to enhance survival of the patient's own red cells as well as transfused red cells.[89] Vaccination with pneumococcal vaccine is indicated because of the risk of pneumococcal sepsis after splenectomy.

Long-term transfusions eventually generate iron overload, which if untreated leads to death from cardiac hemochromatosis during adolescence. Iron overload should be managed prophylactically by infusion of subcutaneous deferoxamine, an iron chelator, before iron buildup occurs. Subcutaneous deferoxamine at a dosage of 50 mg/kg/day can effect iron losses of 50 to 200 mg/day but only if infused continuously over 8 to 12 hours.[90] Such therapy not only prevents left ventricular dysfunction but also reverses already established abnormalities.[91] The beneficial effects of iron chelation have improved the prognosis for persons with Cooley anemia[91]: it is no longer inevitable that patients die in their 20s of arrhythmia and left ventricular failure. With current deferoxamine therapy, 61% of patients born before 1976 have had no cardiovascular disease. Compliant patients whose ferritin levels are mostly below 2,500 ng/ml have a survival rate of 91% after 15 years.[92] The oral iron chelator deferiprone was compared with parenteral desferoxamine and was found to provide inadequate control of iron load as measured by pretreatment and posttreatment levels of iron in liver biopsy specimens.[93] However, it is recommended that the deferiprone not be discarded until further data are available.[94]

Bone marrow transplantation has been performed with HLA-matched sibling donors. More than 1,000 patients have now undergone allogeneic bone marrow transplantation from sibling donors who either were normal or had β-thalassemia trait.[95] Some patients with hemoglobin E β-thalassemia have a phenotype fully as severe as β-thalassemia major and require the same therapy, including allogeneic bone marrow transplantation.[78] Experience with cord blood transplantation is more limited.[96] Depending on the condition of the patient at the time of transplantation, the rate of transplantation-related mortality was 5% to 19%, with a cure rate of 54% to 90%.[97] Other approaches to the treatment of severe β-thalassemia are still experimental.[42,98,99]

β-Thalassemia minor (β-thalassemia trait) Patients with β-thalassemia minor are usually heterozygous for a β-globin mutation and have either mild or no anemia. The peripheral smear shows distinct hypochromia and microcytosis with basophilic stippling. Splenomegaly is occasionally found.

The HbA_2 level is elevated above 5% in 90% of patients, and the HbF level is raised above 2% in 50% of patients. This increase in fetal hemoglobin occurs in varying proportions per red cell (a phenomenon known as heterocellular distribution), as shown by the Kleihauer-Betke stain. Patients with higher HbF levels have less severe anemia. Heterozygotes for δβ-thalassemia produce increased amounts of HbF but only normal amounts of HbA_2.

Iron deficiency anemia should be excluded from the differential diagnosis of β-thalassemia trait [see Chapter 87]. Generally, it is easy to distinguish the two disorders. Both are associated with hypochromia and microcytosis, but iron deficiency produces hypoproliferation of red cells, whereas β-thalassemia minor causes only a minimal reduction in their number. At a hemoglobin level of 9 g/dl, an iron-deficient patient has a red cell count of about 3 million cells/μl, whereas a patient with β-thalassemia trait has a red cell count of about 5 million cells/μl. If the diagnosis remains in doubt, measurement of the serum iron and iron-binding capacity or of the serum ferritin level can be used to distinguish these disorders. It is important to remember, however, that a patient with thalassemia trait may also be iron deficient as a consequence of vaginal bleeding, gastrointestinal bleeding, or both.

Thalassemia intermedia As the term implies, thalassemia intermedia is characterized by clinical manifestations of moderate severity. Patients with this syndrome have distinct anemia, with hemoglobin levels as low as 6 to 7 g/dl; they exhibit variable degrees of hepatosplenomegaly, but they usually do not require regular transfusions. During infections or other erythropoietic insults, however, transfusions may be needed transiently. In two small clinical trials, isobutyramide was found to be of benefit.[100,101]

β-Thalassemia–like variants The hemoglobinopathy associated with hemoglobin Lepore represents another β-thalassemia variant. Patients who are homozygous for this disorder present with Cooley anemia or thalassemia intermedia, and their red cells contain only hemoglobin Lepore and HbF.[83]

Hereditary persistence of fetal hemoglobin The red cells of patients heterozygous for hereditary persistence of fetal hemoglobin (HPFH) contain about 50% of HbF, whereas homozygotes have 100% of HbF. It had been supposed that patients with HPFH were well and had minimal or no anemia, but some clinical variants of HPFH associated with distinct anemia have been described.

α-Thalassemia

Two major differences serve to distinguish the α-globin gene from the β-globin gene. First, there are no fetal, neonatal, or adult substitutes for the α-globin genes; second, there are only two β-globin genes but four α-globin genes—two α-globin genes on each chromosome 17 [see Figure 8]. The normal α-globin genotype is designated αα/αα. Patients who carry the α-thalassemia-1 variant exhibit a deletion of two α-chain genes from the same chromosome and thus have the --/ or α^0 haplotype; this deletion is common among Asian patients. Patients who have the α-thalassemia-2 variant have lost one α gene on one chromosome and show the -α/ or α^+ haplotype. Although this mutation is particularly frequent among blacks, it is also observed in Asian and Mediterranean populations. Five clinically distinct syndromes have been recognized among patients who carry different genotypes for the α-globin genes: hemoglobin Barts or hydrops fetalis (--/--); hemoglobin H disease (--/-α); heterozygous α-thalassemia-1 (--/αα); homozygous α-thalassemia-2 (-α/-α); and the silent carrier syndrome (-α/αα).

Hemoglobin Barts Children with hemoglobin Barts syndrome are homozygous for α-thalassemia-1 (--/--) and therefore produce no α chains. The unmatched γ chains form γ$_4$ tetramers (hemoglobin Barts). All infants with this condition are born hydropic. The parents are usually heterozygous for α-thalassemia-1 (--/αα).

Hemoglobin H disease The clinical picture of hemoglobin H disease is that of variable hemolytic anemia occurring in patients of Asian, Middle Eastern, or Mediterranean origin. HbH, which precipitates on staining with brilliant cresyl blue, can usually be detected in the patient's freshly drawn red cells. The molecular mechanisms may involve deletion of three α genes, as would be the case if the patient were doubly heterozygous for α-thalassemia-1 (--/) and α-thalassemia-2 (-α/), yielding a --/-α genotype. Splenomegaly is common. Patients usually do not require regular transfusions, but transient red cell support may be necessary when the patient has infection or experiences other oxidative stresses that lead to the precipitation of the unstable HbH and enhanced hemolysis.

Heterozygous α-thalassemia Heterozygous α-thalassemia-1 (--/αα), a common genotype among Asians, causes mild or no anemia; rather, it engenders distinctly hypochromic, microcytic red cells. Patients homozygous for α-thalassemia-2 (-α/-α), a common genotype among blacks, lack two α genes; the clinical manifestations of patients with this genotype resemble those of patients heterozygous for α-thalassemia-1. The heterozygous state for α-thalassemia-2 (-α/αα) is clinically undetectable and thus represents the silent carrier syndrome.

α-Thalassemia–like syndrome Hemoglobin constant spring (hemoglobin CS) is a structurally abnormal hemoglobin common in some Asian populations. The α-globin gene contains a mutation in the termination codon, resulting in the synthesis of an α-globin that contains an additional 31 amino acids. Patients heterozygous for this defect have a clinical picture similar to that of a patient homozygous for α-thalassemia-2. Patients homozygous for hemoglobin CS tend to have slightly more severe clinical manifestations than patients heterozygous for α-thalassemia-1. In patients who are doubly heterozygous for α-thalassemia-1 and alpha CS (--/αCS α) and who have HbH/HbCS, disease is slightly more severe than in those with hemoglobin H disease.[85]

Genetic Counseling and Prenatal Diagnosis

Parents who have had a stillborn hydropic infant or a child with Cooley anemia are justifiably reluctant to repeat the experience. Adults from thalassemia families who know themselves to be heterozygous for thalassemia are often eager to receive genetic counseling when starting their own families. Genetic counseling entails screening prospective parents on the basis of routine diagnostic tests and family studies. In addition, advances in molecular genetics can now provide accurate, unambiguous prenatal diagnoses of the thalassemias. In the first trimester, chorionic villus sampling combined with the use of polymorphic DNA markers and synthetic oligonucleotide probes can provide the definitive diagnosis in about 80% of cases of β-thalassemia [see Chapter 71].[102,103] Indeed, the incidence of births of infants with

thalassemia major has fallen in several parts of the world. Different ethnic groups respond differently to genetic counseling.

Extracorpuscular Defects

Erythrocytes can be damaged through trauma or by antibodies, drugs, abnormally functioning organs, and toxins. These causes for an extracorpuscular defect should be considered whenever hemolysis develops in a patient who has a negative personal or family history of anemia.

MECHANICAL INJURY: MICROANGIOPATHIC HEMOLYSIS

Microangiopathic hemolysis is characterized by the appearance of bizarre, fragmented erythrocytes (e.g., schistocytes, or helmet cells) on a peripheral smear and by signs of intravascular and extravascular hemolysis.

Pathophysiology

The normal erythrocyte can withstand considerable elongation and twisting, but it disintegrates when subjected to strong stretching or shearing forces. Stresses of this magnitude have been observed to occur in jets produced by deformed aortic valves, by arteriovenous shunts, by ventricular septal defects, or by the older valvular prostheses.

Localized intravascular coagulation, in which fibrin strands bridge the arteriolar lumen, is thought to occur in arterioles supplying inflamed or neoplastic tissues. Fibrin strands lop off fragments of red cells, whose membranes promptly reseal. Some of the erythrocyte contents leak out, however, producing varying degrees of intravascular hemolysis. The distorted red cells are then removed by the reticuloendothelial system.

Diagnosis

Hemolysis in conjunction with typical blood smear findings indicates the diagnosis of microangiopathic hemolysis [see Figure 7]. If the angiopathy is extensive, thrombocytopenia and disseminated intravascular coagulation develop. Causes include hemodynamic jets, vasculitis,[104] giant hemangiomas, thrombotic thrombocytopenic purpura, metastatic cancer,[105] certain infections (especially meningococcemia and rickettsial diseases and including the hantavirus), hemolytic-uremic syndrome, disseminated intravascular coagulation, drugs (cocaine, cyclosporine, mitomycin, and tacrolimus [FK506]), and even subclavian catheters.[105,106]

Treatment

In treating microangiopathic hemolysis, primary attention must be focused on the underlying disease. Patients may become iron deficient and require iron therapy. Supplementation of depleted folate stores may stimulate erythropoiesis. In rare cases, anemia caused by an old prosthetic aortic valve may be severe enough to warrant valve replacement. Plasmapheresis provides effective therapy for thrombotic thrombocytopenic purpura [see Chapter 95].

March hemoglobinuria March hemoglobinuria, a disorder that somewhat resembles microangiopathic hemolysis, usually occurs in young persons after prolonged marching or running or playing on bongo drums. The severe and repetitive trauma to the feet or hands is thought to destroy red cells circulating in the vessels of the soles and palms. The patient notices red urine that clears in 1 day or less after the activity. Transient hemoglobinemia and hemoglobinuria without anemia, smear abnormalities, or reticulocytosis confirm the diagnosis. The use of padded shoes and avoidance of paved surfaces may prevent recurrences in persons who continue running.

IMMUNE HEMOLYSIS

General Mechanisms

A classic, well-delineated example of immune (not autoimmune) hemolysis involves fetomaternal incompatibility at Rh locus D, in which the D-negative mother, after contact with D-positive erythrocytes, may produce an IgG anti-D antibody; the antibody crosses the placenta and attacks and destroys fetal erythrocytes. The fetus becomes jaundiced and has spherocytic erythrocytes.

The fetal red cells, now coated with maternal IgG anti-D antibody, attach to fetal macrophages and monocytes that contain receptors for the Fc portion of these IgG molecules. Macrophagic digestion of portions of the erythrocytic membrane leads to the loss of considerable surface area. The resulting rigid spherocyte returns to the circulation and becomes trapped in the fetal reticuloendothelial system, particularly in the spleen. Hemolysis results. The IgG antibody is maximally active at 37° C; it generally cannot extensively activate the complement pathway, and it cannot agglutinate attacked red cells suspended in saline.

The direct Coombs antiglobulin test [see Figure 9] is used clinically to detect IgG coating of red cells. This test is negative in the mother, because her erythrocytes lack D antigen and thus are not coated with anti-D antibody. The indirect Coombs test [see Figure 9], which detects the presence of free serum antibody that reacts with red cells, is positive for the mother's serum because she has circulating anti-D antibody. In the fetus, in contrast, the direct Coombs test is strongly positive because the fetus's red cells, which express D antigen, are coated with maternal anti-D antibody. The results of the fetus's indirect Coombs test may be positive or negative, depending on the amount of anti-D antibody that has been transferred by the mother, the avidity of the anti-D antibody for fetal D-positive red cells, and the availability of D antigen sites on fetal red cells.

These antibodies are described as warm (maximum activity at 37° C, usually IgG1 or IgG3) or cold (maximum activity at 5° C, usually IgM). Antibodies have also been classified as complete (i.e., capable of agglutinating saline-suspended red cells) and incomplete (i.e., incapable of agglutinating saline-suspended red cells), and their detection requires the use of techniques such as the direct Coombs antiglobulin test [see Figure 9] or enzyme treatment of red cells.[107] Warm autoantibodies are usually incomplete, whereas cold agglutinins, being IgM, are usually complete.[108]

Autoimmune Hemolytic Anemia

Autoimmune hemolytic anemia is generally an acute disorder characterized by extravascular hemolysis. Intravascular hemolysis in this condition is rare and indicates that an extremely rapid rate of erythrocyte destruction is occurring or that the extravascular removal mechanisms have been overwhelmed.

Pathophysiology In autoimmune hemolytic anemia, for reasons that are unclear, autoantibodies form and are directed against central components of the erythrocyte (e.g., Rh antigen, Kell antigen,[107] glycophorin A).[109] Alternatively, the patient's red cells are sensitized with both an IgG antibody and a complement component, usually C3d. In other circumstances, however, it appears that complement is fixed to the red cell surface by an IgM antibody that is subsequently washed away. Occasionally, the red cells may exhibit only complement components, and no IgG can be detected by the Coombs test. Complement fixation in such cases may be explained by the continued presence of IgG at a level below that detectable in the usual direct antiglobulin test; alternatively, a complement-fixing IgG or IgM had been attached to the cell earlier but was eluted in the testing procedure.[108]

The severity of hemolysis correlates with the number and class of IgG molecules attached to the red cell surface. Antibody-coated red cells attach to the macrophages' receptors (FcRI, FcRII, or FcRIII) by the antibody's Fc portion [see Chapter 98]. The firm binding of red cells to these macrophage receptors is then followed either by removal of a portion of the red cell membrane, which results in the production of a spherocyte or by phagocytosis of the entire red cell.[107] Relatively low levels of IgG1 attachment to red cells produce a positive result on direct Coombs antiglobulin testing without evidence of hemolysis (approximately 1,000 molecules per red cell), whereas much higher levels of IgG1 autoantibody per red cell are associated with frank hemolysis.[107] The combined presence of IgG and complement components may enhance the severity of hemolysis.

Erythrocytes sensitized to IgG alone are usually removed in the spleen, whereas red cells sensitized to IgG plus complement or to complement alone are generally destroyed in the liver, because hepatic Kupffer cells carry receptors specific for complement component C3b.

Differential diagnosis Both an idiopathic variety of autoimmune hemolytic anemia and a variety that occurs secondary to other disorders have been described. Such primary disorders include systemic lupus erythematosus, non-Hodgkin lymphoma (especially chronic lymphocytic leukemia), Hodgkin disease, cancer, myeloma, dermoid cyst, HIV infection, angioimmunoblastic lymphadenopathy with dysproteinemia, and chronic ulcerative colitis.

Diagnosis Patient presentations vary markedly, from asymptomatic to severe. A person may be found to have a positive Coombs test result when undergoing blood bank or blood donation screening. Such persons can usually be shown to have complement or the combination of complement and IgG (usually IgG1 or IgG4) on their red cells, but they are generally not undergoing hemolysis. By contrast, an acute hemolytic episode can lower the hematocrit from 45% to 15% in 2 days. With this extreme presentation, severe fatigue and cardiorespiratory symptoms will develop together with jaundice, lymphadenopathy, and hepatosplenomegaly.

In severe cases, the blood smear shows macrocytosis, polychromatophilia, variable spherocytosis, and autoagglutination of red cells. The platelet count is also often depressed (Evans syndrome), and there may be leukopenia. One third of patients may have reticulocytopenia at presentation[110] because the reticulocyte response may take a few days to develop. The direct Coombs test will be positive. Any or all of these findings may be absent in mild disease.

Whether complement, IgG, or both are present on red cells should be determined by the use of Coombs reagents that are specifically directed against IgG or complement components. Occasionally, an autoimmune hemolytic anemia is suspected, but the direct Coombs test is repeatedly negative; in such cases, the level of autoantibody may be below the level of detectability for very active autoantibodies, such as subclass IgG3 autoantibodies, or the autoantibody may be IgA or IgM.[107]

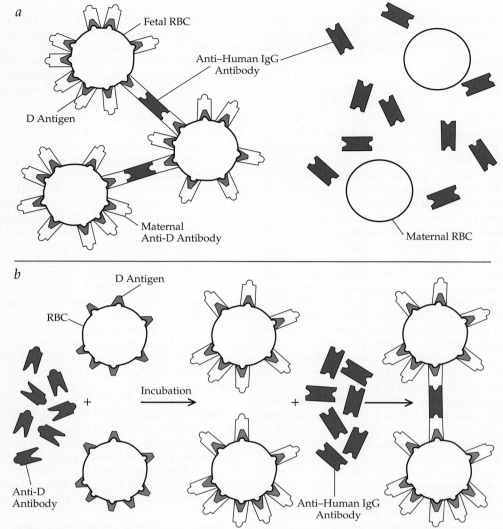

a

Fetal RBC

Anti–Human IgG
Antibody

D Antigen

Maternal
Anti-D Antibody

Maternal RBC

b

D Antigen

RBC

Incubation

Anti-D
Antibody

Anti–Human IgG
Antibody

Figure 9   **The Coombs test detects the presence of human antibodies or complement components on erythrocytes or the presence of antibodies in serum. The test is useful in diagnosing Rh hemolytic disease of the newborn, autoimmune hemolysis, or potential hemolytic transfusion reactions. The figure illustrates Rh hemolytic disease of the newborn.**

In the direct Coombs test (*a*), fetal erythrocytes (RBCs) are shown with D antigen attached to their surfaces. Maternal anti-D antibody binds to the fetal erythrocytes at the D antigen sites in utero. Coombs antiserum, which contains antibody to human IgG, binds to the anti-D antibody on a sample of washed fetal erythrocytes, causing them to clump (a positive reaction). Washed maternal erythrocytes, having no D antigen, will have no attached anti-D antibody and are therefore not clumped by Coombs serum (a negative reaction).

In the indirect Coombs test (*b*), maternal or fetal serum is added to the red cells of another person or to panels of erythrocytes of known antigenic specificity; Coombs antiserum is then added. Clumping in this case occurs only if the test serum, such as the maternal serum, contains anti-D antibody and if the red cells chosen have the D antigen.

The direct Coombs test is used to detect immunoglobulin molecules already attached to erythrocytes, such as those found on the fetal erythrocytes in Rh hemolytic disease of the newborn or in autoimmune hemolytic anemia. Therefore, the test is done on the patient's thoroughly washed erythrocytes. The indirect Coombs test is used for determining whether specific antibodies are present in a serum sample, and it is performed on the patient's serum.

Patients with evidence of hemolytic anemia should be screened for autoimmune diseases (e.g., systemic lupus erythematosus) and other forms of hemolysis, such as paroxysmal nocturnal hemoglobinuria, cold agglutinin disease, and paroxysmal cold hemoglobinuria.

Treatment   Treatment of clinically affected patients is directed at decreasing autoantibody production and reducing the macro-phagic attack on the red cells. Initial therapy usually consists of 60 to 100 mg of prednisone a day, given in divided doses. This approach usually produces a slow decrease in antibody coating of red cells and is thought to interfere with phagocytic attack on coated erythrocytes. A good response to corticosteroid use—indicated by a rise in the reticulocyte count and an improvement in hemoglobin and hematocrit—may be apparent within 1 or 2 days. Supplementation with 1 mg of folic acid a day is recommended.

After the initial response to therapy, which is usually satisfactory, the hemoglobin level and reticulocyte count may return to normal. The Coombs test is then repeated to determine whether the response has become weaker; if so, the prednisone dosage is tapered cautiously. Approximately 20% of patients remain well indefinitely, but the majority suffer from a chronic, treacherous disease that can produce sudden relapses with abrupt anemia. The prednisone should be titrated in accordance with the hemoglobin level, the reticulocyte count (elevation indicates continued hemolysis), and the direct Coombs titer; and alternate-day therapy should be considered to minimize steroid side effects. If patients do not respond to standard prednisone therapy, high-dose dexamethasone (e.g., 40 mg/day p.o. for 4 consecutive days in 28-day cycles[111]) may be effective.

If the corticosteroid dose required for long-term therapy produces significant morbidity, one can proceed empirically either to splenectomy or to the use of immunosuppressive agents. Measurements of splenic sequestration of chromium-51 (^{51}Cr)-labeled erythrocytes do not reliably indicate the benefits of splenectomy. Splenectomy rarely results in extended remission but is valuable as a prednisone-sparing measure. After splenectomy, low-dose prednisone (5 to 10 mg/day) may stabilize the hemoglobin concentration.

The immunosuppressive agent azathioprine or cyclophosphamide can be used as an alternative to splenectomy. There is no reliable evidence, however, to support the use of one of the agents over the other. For patients with very aggressive disease, cyclosporine has been used successfully.[112] Azathioprine should be started at a dosage of 100 to 200 mg a day; the peripheral blood count should be monitored with a view toward preventing reticulocytopenia or neutropenia. Cyclophosphamide is started at a dosage of 100 to 200 mg a day, with monitoring of blood counts and urine; however, because cyclophosphamide can cause therapy-related acute myeloid leukemia or myelodysplastic syndrome, its use should be limited [see Chapter 204].

Azathioprine or cyclophosphamide doses have to be adjusted to reduce the white cell count to about 3,000/mm^3. Improvement usually comes in 3 to 4 weeks. When a response occurs, the prednisone dose can be reduced and the hemoglobin level, reticulocyte count, and Coombs titer monitored to determine the minimally required therapy. For patients with very refractory disease, therapy with I.V. cyclophosphamide at doses used for allogeneic bone marrow transplantation has been tried. This approach is clearly myelotoxic, and its usefulness awaits further confirmation. High-dose I.V. IgG has been used to treat autoimmune hemolytic anemia. In one report, only one third of patients had a transient response, and doses larger than those used in idiopathic thrombocytopenic purpura (i.e., 1.0 g/kg/day for 5 days) were required.[113,114]

Patients with symptomatic anemia require a red cell transfusion, but often, the blood bank reports an incompatibility. Many blood banks regularly perform a direct Coombs antiglobulin test on the recipient's red cells. A patient who has free antibodies in the serum will exhibit very extensive and broad reactivity against donor panels of red cells and will usually produce an incompatible major cross-match when tested with the antiglobulin reagent. If transfusions are needed to support cardiorespiratory and central nervous system functions, immediate consultation with the transfusion medicine service is recommended.[108] An important caveat is that no patient should be allowed to die because the blood bank does not have a perfectly compatible unit of red cells. If transfusion is clinically indicated, the physician should administer the best units of blood that are available, because it has been shown that these patients can tolerate even imperfectly matched red cells.[115]

Drug-Related Immune Hemolysis

Drug-initiated immune hemolysis is often indistinguishable from autoimmune hemolytic anemia. There are two variants—the hapten type and the hemolysis that results from alteration of a membrane antigen.[116]

Hapten type   Drugs such as the penicillins and the cephalosporins bind firmly to the erythrocyte membrane. In rare circumstances in which massive dosages of the drug (e.g., more than 10 million units of penicillin a day) are required, the protein-bound drug may act as a hapten and elicit an immune response. An IgG antibody that appears to be directed against the drug–red cell complex is produced[117,118]; this leads to a positive result on direct Coombs testing with the anti-IgG reagent and a negative result with the anti-C3d reagent. When the offending drug is stopped, hemolysis ends in a few days. In contrast, the drug may also be bound loosely to produce a neoantigen that generates the immune response.[116] In this circumstance, the result of direct Coombs testing with the anti-C3d reagent is usually positive, and the result of testing with the anti-IgG reagent may be negative.

If the patient's serum is tested against normal cells (i.e., the indirect Coombs test is used), no reaction occurs unless the offending drug and a source of complement are first added to the normal red cells. Stopping or switching the drug is effective in eliminating the hemolysis because the antibody is usually very specific.

Alteration of a membrane antigen   Some drugs may alter a membrane antigen, thereby stimulating the production of IgG antibodies that cross-react with the native antigen. Methyldopa is the classic example of a drug that causes autoimmune hemolytic anemia. Other examples are levodopa, mefenamic acid, and procainamide. Drug administration leads to a positive direct Coombs test with anti-IgG reagents in 15% to 20% of treated patients, but hemolysis occurs in fewer than 1%. The eluted antibody is seen to be a classic IgG autoantibody directed against Rh components. The mechanism of hemolysis is identical to that of autoimmune hemolytic anemia.[119]

The NSAID diclofenac sodium has been reported to cause a devastating acute hemolytic anemia, with evidence of intravascular and extravascular hemolysis accompanied occasionally by shock, organ failure, and even disseminated intravascular coagulation (DIC).[120] Patients develop both red cell autoantibodies and drug-dependent antibodies. It is thought that diclofenac sodium binds to the surface of red cells, forming neoantigens that lead to the generation of true autoantibodies as well as drug-dependent antibodies. The direct Combs test is positive with both the IgG and the C3d reagents. Additional antibody reactivity occurs with the addition of diclofenac sodium metabolites obtained from the urine of patients treated with the drug. Therapy consists of recognizing the cause, stopping the diclofenac sodium, and supporting the patient for several days until the process stops.[120]

Delayed Hemolysis of Transfused Erythrocytes

Blood is usually typed only for ABO and Rh-D antigens, but other antigens are also present on red cells. Thus, a patient who receives extensive transfusions over 1 to 2 weeks may develop an antibody response to one or more of these other antigens. Kell, Duffy, Kidd, and Rh antigens other than D are the usual offenders. When the patient with antibodies receives red cells expressing these antigens, an acute self-limited hemolysis, usually extravascular, may ensue. Clues are a history of transfusion, spherocytosis on peripheral smear, positive direct Coombs test, and the recent appearance of an antibody in the patient's serum (positive indirect Coombs test). Usually, no therapy is required, but further transfusions should be cross-matched with the patient's serum [see Chapter 95]. Similar problems arise with transplantation of bone marrow and other tissue.[121]

Cold Agglutinin Disease

Cold agglutinin disease has several variants. One rare variant affects young adults and usually occurs after infection with Mycoplasma pneumoniae or infectious mononucleosis; however, several cases of this variant have been reported in association with chronic falciparum malaria. A more common variant affects persons about 60 years of age and may present as idiopathic cold agglutinin disease, as a prodrome to a lymphoproliferative or an immunoproliferative disorder, or in association with an already established lymphoproliferative disorder.[122]

Pathophysiology Serologically, cold agglutinin disease is characterized by the presence of high titers of IgM agglutinins (> 1:1,000 and usually > 1:10,000) in serum. These antibodies are maximally active at 4° C, are capable of activating the complement sequence, and are directed against the polysaccharide antigens. Presumably, IgM reacts with erythrocytes circulating in the cooled blood of the nose, ears, and shins, where it fixes complement and then dissociates from the red cells when they reach warmer areas of the body.

In the postinfectious variety of this disorder, IgM cold agglutinin is oligoclonal and short-lived. Conversely, the IgM is monoclonal in chronic idiopathic cold agglutinin disease or in cases associated with Waldenstrom macroglobulinemia, chronic lymphocytic leukemia, or other lymphomas. IgM predominantly contains λ light chains in patients with chronic idiopathic cold agglutinin disease or Waldenstrom macroglobulinemia; in patients with lymphoma, however, the IgM mainly contains κ light chains. Occasionally, the IgM cold agglutinin is detectable as an M protein spike on serum protein electrophoresis [see Chapter 203].

In the post-Mycoplasma variant, the mycoplasmas appear to bind to the red cell surface at the Ii antigen site. This receptor-ligand interaction results in the presentation of the I antigen in an immunogenic form.[123] Listeria monocytogenes contains the I antigen,[122] further supporting the idea that some infectious agents stimulate the naturally occurring cold agglutinins as well as cause the postinfectious cold agglutinin disease.

Diagnosis The clinical syndrome of cold agglutinin disease is quite variable. Patients occasionally show only low titers of cold agglutinins and have no other symptoms or have a history of recent pneumonia. In patients with warm-and-cold autoimmune hemolytic anemia, the associated hemolysis tends to be severe and chronic. The red cells of these patients are coated with IgG and complement components, whereas their serum contains a relatively low titer of cold agglutinin that acts at 30° C and perhaps even at temperatures up to 37° C.

The diagnosis is suggested by hemolytic anemia with acral signs and symptoms. It may be difficult to draw blood, and the red cells may visibly agglutinate in a cold syringe and on the blood smear. The automated blood cell counters may count the agglutinated red cells as single cells and thus report absurdly high values for the MCV and MCHC. Usually, the laboratory detects a broadly active cold agglutinin. The direct Coombs test is positive with anticomplement reagents but infrequently positive with anti-IgG.

Findings that support the diagnosis of idiopathic cold agglutinin disease include a high IgM cold agglutinin titer with broad thermal reactivity[107] and I specificity (reacting with erythrocytes from adults but not with cord erythrocytes), pure κ light-chain composition, occasionally an absolute serum IgM elevation, and an M protein pattern on serum protein electrophoresis. Investigation should be directed at discovering a possible lymphoma or other underlying disorder in these patients. Conversely, post-Mycoplasma and post–infectious mononucleosis cold agglutinins are polyclonal. The post–infectious mononucleosis antibody is usually directed against i antigens (cord red cells).

Treatment The post-Mycoplasma or the post–infectious mononucleosis variant is usually mild and self-limited and requires no specific management. Patients with the idiopathic variety who have acral symptoms must change their way of life, either by moving to a warmer climate or by keeping their ears, nose, hands, and feet covered during cold weather. In severely anemic patients, transfusions with packed red cells may be required; in such patients, careful cross-matching and warming of the blood is necessary to minimize cold agglutination.

Splenectomy and corticosteroids are generally of no benefit in controlling hemolysis associated with cold agglutinin disease. Presumably, complement-coated cells are removed to a substantial degree by hepatic rather than splenic macrophages, and the cells that produce IgM are relatively insensitive to the effects of corticosteroids. Occasionally, however, high doses of corticosteroids (e.g., 100 mg of prednisone a day) have resulted in a reduction in the hemolytic rate in patients with relatively low titers of cold agglutinins. In the relatively rare variant caused by IgG cold agglutinins, corticosteroids and splenectomy may be of benefit. Use of penicillamine or other reducing agents containing sulfhydryl groups produces no benefit. Good responses are occasionally obtained by the use of chlorambucil at a dosage of 4 to 6 mg/day. Exchange transfusion and plasmapheresis appear to be logical therapies for acute disease, but further clinical studies are needed to evaluate these techniques. Interferon alfa, at a dosage of 3 million U/m² three times weekly, was reported to produce an impressive drop in cold agglutinin titer, with a decrease in serum IgM monoclonal protein and in acral symptoms over a 1-month period.[107]

Paroxysmal Cold Hemoglobinuria

Patients with the rare disorder of paroxysmal cold hemoglobinuria have cold-induced signs and symptoms of intravascular hemolysis. The hemolysis is associated with the presence of an IgG serum antibody that is directed against the red cell's P system. The IgG antibody is best demonstrated by the Donath-Landsteiner test; the serum is mixed either with the patient's own blood cells or with blood cells from a normal person. The mixture is chilled to 4° C. If the IgG antibody associated with this disorder is present, hemolysis occurs after warming to 37° C. In the past, paroxysmal cold hemoglobinuria was usually seen as a complication of syphilis, but it has recently been observed in association with viral infections and non-Hodgkin lymphoma.[124]

HYPERSPLENISM

Hypersplenic disorders constitute a diverse group of clinical conditions sharing the common features of splenomegaly and hemolysis. Splenic enlargement and hemolysis occur in many disorders, including hepatic cirrhosis with congestive splenomegaly, Gaucher disease, lymphoma, connective tissue disorders, Felty syndrome, sarcoidosis, tuberculosis, and other infectious diseases.

Pathophysiology

The spleen's unique structure accounts for several of the pathophysiologic features of hypersplenism. Splenic arterioles have a few direct branches leading to the sinusoids, but most of the terminal arterioles open into the splenic cords. Blood cells pass from the cords to the pulp through slits in the sinus walls; the slits have dimensions of about 1 by 3 μm.[125] Blood cells must squeeze through the longitudinal spaces, which are lined with reticular fibers, and between adventitial cells that are located outside the sinus. Macrophages and endothelial cells line the inside of the sinus. Repeated intimate contact occurs between blood cells and these macrophages.

Blood flow in the spleen is slow. The erythrocyte's pH and oxygen tension (PO_2) levels fall, glucose is consumed, and the cell's metabolism is impaired. The hematocrit may increase, further elevating viscosity and resistance to flow. As a consequence, the blood cells are exposed to metabolic and mechanical stresses in the presence of macrophages and other leukocytes that can recognize cell membrane damage. As erythrocytes age, phagocytes remove defective surface areas, transforming the biconcave erythrocytes into rigid spherocytes or red cell fragments; these particles are later trapped and removed by the reticuloendothelial system. A big spleen has a greater than normal blood flow and exposes an unusually large proportion of blood cells to its culling activities. Thus, the problem in hypersplenism is essentially a quantitative one. A vicious circle may evolve in patients undergoing hemolysis because hemolysis itself may cause splenomegaly.

Diagnosis

If the spleen is not palpable but the clinical situation is strongly suggestive of splenomegaly, ultrasonography or CT scanning may prove useful. Because blood cells other than erythrocytes are affected by a large spleen, the patient may be pancytopenic. Unless the underlying disease specifically involves the bone marrow, the marrow of patients with hypersplenism is generally hyperplastic because of rapid regeneration of all affected cell lines. The peripheral blood smear is not diagnostic of hypersplenism.

Treatment

If hypersplenism is producing clinically significant complications and if therapy for the patient's primary disease does not shrink the spleen, splenectomy may be necessary. Anemia, however, is not necessarily attributable to hypersplenism, irrespective of the size of the spleen. Hemodilution is another possible mechanism. Patients with massive splenomegaly who have very low hematocrit and hemoglobin values may have a normal red cell mass as assessed with the ^{51}Cr technique. Massive splenomegaly often is associated with an increase in plasma volume that results in extraordinary hemodilution. Moreover, greatly enlarged spleens may contain a pool of erythrocytes that constitutes as much as 25% of the total red cell mass—in contrast to normal spleens, which have no such red cell pool. In patients with splenomegaly who have a true decrease in red cell mass, the underlying disease may act to reduce red cell production by suppressing erythropoietin production rather than by accelerating destruction. Therefore, it is prudent to determine red cell mass before making the diagnosis of hypersplenism.

Mechanism of Oxidative Attack

Dapsone, sulfasalazine, phenacetin, sodium perchlorate, nitroglycerin, phenazopyridine, primaquine,[79] paraquat, and vitamin K analogues can insert themselves into the oxygen-binding cleft of hemoglobin. By this action, such agents can generate oxidizing free radicals, such as superoxide, hydroxyl free radical, and peroxide. If the erythrocyte's protective reducing mechanisms are overwhelmed [see Table 1], hemoglobin is oxidized to form Heinz bodies and methemoglobin. Sulfhemoglobin is also produced by oxidative attack. The molecule contains a sulfur atom in the porphyrin ring, which gives it a blue-green color. The source of the sulfur atom is not clear, but the presence of sulfur in the heme ring makes it a poor oxygen transporter.[126] The red cell membrane may also suffer from oxidative attack. Damaged cells are removed in the reticuloendothelial system. Hemolysis is usually, but not invariably, extravascular, and Heinz bodies can be seen on a specially stained blood smear. The smear may also show the bite, hemiblister, or cross-bonded cells typical of oxidative attack on erythrocytes [see Figure 6]. Severe oxidative damage apparently causes hemoglobin to puddle at one side of the red cell, leaving a plasma membrane–enclosed hemighost in the remainder. Such hemighosts can be detected in the peripheral blood. Severe oxidative destruction is associated with increased methemoglobin levels and a decrease in red cell levels of GSH. The methemoglobin level is elevated. (As little as 1.5 g/dl of methemoglobin or 0.5 g/dl of sulfhemoglobin can produce the physical finding of cyanosis. By contrast, 5 g/dl of reduced deoxyhemoglobin is required to produce comparable cyanosis.[79])

Nitrites can oxidize hemoglobin to methemoglobin. Consequently, the recreational use of butyl and isobutyl nitrites as stimulants, psychedelics, and aphrodisiacs has led to clinical problems. When inhaled in usual amounts, these agents may produce a mild to modest increase in methemoglobin, raising its concentration from the normal level of 1% to 2% to as much as 20%. More extensive inhalation or ingestion of these agents has induced severe methemoglobinemia, characterized by methemoglobin levels approaching 62%. Because methemoglobin does not carry oxygen, these high levels are accompanied by manifestations of tissue hypoxia such as headache, shortness of breath, lethargy, and stupor. Physical examination shows tachycardia, postural hypotension, and cyanosis; the venous blood is purple-brown.[127] If untreated, it is likely to be fatal.

Diagnosis Diagnosis is based on a history of exposure to an oxidant drug or other toxin, together with characteristic peripheral blood smear findings and elevated methemoglobin measurements.

Treatment Treatment should restore normal methemoglobin levels. Management starts with the identification and withdrawal of the offending agent. Patients with severe methemoglobinemia should be treated immediately with 1 to 2 mg/kg of methylene blue; the agent is infused intravenously in a 1 g/dl solution over a 5-minute period. In the presence of the red cell enzyme NADPH-methemoglobin reductase and adequate amounts of the electron donor NADPH [see Table 1], methylene blue is rapidly reduced to leukomethylene blue. This product in turn quickly reduces methemoglobin to hemoglobin. Cyanosis is thereby reversed, and the patient should turn pink immediately after the infusion. Several hours later, however, the patient may again become cyanotic, presumably because nitrates released from tissues reenter the peripheral blood at that time. Readministration of methylene blue at a dosage of 1 mg/kg intravenously over a 5-minute period should restore normal hemoglobin levels.

Successful methylene blue therapy requires adequate supplies of NADPH. Patients who have abnormalities of the pentose phosphate pathway [see Figure 5] such as G6PD deficiency will not respond to this approach and should receive emergency exchange transfusions.[127]

Patients with very high levels of methemoglobin (at least 60%) or those whose smears contain many hemighosts should undergo exchange transfusion, perhaps with hemodialysis.[79,127]

Other Forms of Drug-Induced Hemolysis

Lead exposure results in hypertensive encephalopathy, neuropathy, and hemolytic anemia characterized by coarse basophilic stippling in red cells. The mechanism of lead-induced hemolysis is complex because the metal has several actions: it blocks heme synthesis, thus causing a buildup of red cell protoporphyrin; it produces a deficiency of pyrimidine 5'-nucleotidase[128]; and it attacks erythrocyte membrane phospholipids, producing potassium leak and interfering with Na^+,K^+-ATPase activity.

Diagnosis Screening for lead poisoning entails measuring the free erythrocyte protoporphyrin level (sometimes called the zinc protoporphyrin level), which is elevated because lead blocks the last step in heme synthesis. The diagnosis is confirmed by measuring blood and urine lead levels.

Treatment After the exposure to lead is stopped, use of a chelating agent such as edetate calcium disodium ($CaNa_2EDTA$) may be considered. Treatment is started with 0.5 to 1.0 g of I.V. $CaNa_2EDTA$, given over a period of 6 to 8 hours; the compound is given daily for 5 days.

After this initial course, 0.5 g of $CaNa_2EDTA$ is given as an intravenous bolus or intramuscular injection every 2 days for 2 weeks, during which time the urine lead levels are monitored. An alternative to continuation of $CaNa_2EDTA$ after the initial 5-day course is treatment with oral penicillamine as follows: 1 g a day is given for the first 7 days; the drug is withheld for the next 7 days; and during the final 7 days of the regimen, the dosage of 1 g a day is resumed and the urine lead level is measured at the end of the final day. Another study recommends giving 500 mg of penicillamine a day and continuing this dosage for 60 days after the patient has become asymptomatic.[129]

VENOMS AND PHYSICAL AGENTS AS CAUSES OF HEMOLYSIS

Enzymatic Attack on Erythrocytes

Classic examples of attacking enzymes are the snake-venom or clostridial lecithinases (e.g., phospholipase C). Such enzymes attack the phospholipids of the membrane bilayer and produce red cell fragmentation, spherocytosis, and intravascular and extravascular hemolysis. Disseminated intravascular coagulation and shock may occur. Prompt recognition and management of the primary disorder is critical, as is supportive therapy.

Physical Causes of Hemolysis

Freshwater drowning and accidental I.V. administration of sterile water can cause intravascular hemolysis by osmotic lysis. In such cases, red cells swell and become spheroidal. Saltwater drowning can induce hemolysis by desiccating red cells. Burns cause temperature-mediated denaturation of erythrocyte membrane polypeptides, resulting in hemolysis.

Infectious Diseases Causing Hemolysis

Infections produce hemolysis by several mechanisms. Infection with *M. pneumoniae* and infectious mononucleosis can cause cold agglutinin hemolysis. Infection with *H. influenzae* type b can cause hemolysis; the major virulence factor of *H. influenzae*, polyribose ribosyl phosphate (PRRP), allows the organism to escape phagocytosis. When PRRP is released into the circulation, it binds to red cells. The binding of anti-PRRP antibodies then leads to complement-dependent hemolysis.[130] Patients infected with HIV or cytomegalovirus (CMV) may have autoimmune hemolytic anemia (see above).[131]

Clostridial sepsis can be devastating; the appearance of free plasma hemoglobin or hemoglobinurea should suggest this often fatal infection. *Clostridium* species are capable of sudden, explosive growth; they can release many enzymes, including phospholipases and proteases, that digest red cells, producing intravascular hemolysis.

Some infections can cause splenomegaly and hypersplenic hemolysis. Meningococcemia or overwhelming gram-negative septicemia often produces DIC and microangiopathic hemolysis.

Some infectious agents, such as *Plasmodium*, which causes malaria, directly parasitize and destroy red cells. Autologous, nonparasitized red cells are also cleared faster than usual.[132] This finding suggests that the reticuloendothelial system is hyperactive during malaria. The diagnosis is made by pathognomonic blood smear [see Chapter 156].

Babesiosis caused by a parasite that invades red cells and that is transmitted from its rodent reservoir by the same ixodid tick that carries Lyme disease and human granulocytic ehrlichiosis is being more frequently diagnosed, particularly in the New England area. Immunocompromised persons, such as those with HIV, are more likely to have chronic and severe infections. The diagnosis has been made on peripheral blood smears, but newer polymerase chain reaction methods are more sensitive.[133]

HEMOLYSIS ASSOCIATED WITH LIVER DISEASE

Several mechanisms, including hemolysis, may produce anemia in patients with liver disease. The inflammatory aspect of an underlying disease (as in viral hepatitis) may lead to a production defect. Alcohol ingestion blocks red cell production [see Chapter 96]. Folate malnutrition in a patient with alcoholic cirrhosis may result in classic megaloblastic ineffective erythropoiesis. Alcoholic gastritis may cause serious bleeding. Iron stores may become depleted in destitute alcoholic persons who sell their blood too frequently. The cirrhotic patient may have congestive splenomegaly with hypersplenic hemolysis. Macrocytes (with or without B_{12} or folate deficiency) and target cells (caused by cholesterol elevation) are also common findings.

Echinocytosis, Acanthocytosis, and Spur Cell Anemia

In patients with liver disease, echinocytosis is a very common finding when red cells are examined in wet preparation or by scanning electron microscopy, although standard dried films infrequently show such echinocytes.[134] When normal red cells are incubated in plasma from patients with echinocytosis, the cells quickly become echinocytic.

Echinocytes may undergo a further shape change, to irregularly spiculated red cells or spur cells (acanthocytes). Acanthocytosis, or spur cell hemolysis, is caused by alterations in the red cell membrane lipids, with a decrease in phospholipid synthesis resulting in a decreased ratio of phospholipids to cholesterol.[135] These membrane changes will shorten erythrocyte survival.

OTHER CAUSES OF HEMOLYSIS

Copper Accumulation

In rare instances, Wilson disease, a metabolic disorder associated with excessive copper deposition, is first detected during a coincident episode of dramatic, acute hemolysis. The release of free copper into the serum and its subsequent entry into red cells are thought to be the underlying hemolytic mechanism. In addition to affecting hexokinase levels, the intracellular copper appears to cause formation of oxygen radicals that react with and oxidize membrane components. Although no successful therapeutic intervention has been reported, penicillamine can be given at a dosage of 2 to 4 g once a day orally to reduce the free copper level. The administration of 1,000 to 2,000 IU of vitamin E (α-tocopherol) a day for several days may also be helpful if oxidative attack is an important factor.

Cardiopulmonary Bypass

After cardiopulmonary bypass, transient leukopenia may develop in some patients. This leukopenia is thought to be caused by activation of the complement pathway, leading to the generation of C3a and C5a [see Chapter 100]. Free plasma hemoglobin also increases after cardiopulmonary bypass; it appears to be associated with hemolysis caused by deposition of the C5b-C9 attack complex on the red cell surface.[136]

References

1. Liu S-C, Derick LH: Molecular anatomy of the red blood cell membrane skeleton: structure-function relationships. Semin Hematol 29:231, 1992

2. Cohen CM, Gascard P: Regulation and post-translational modification of erythrocyte membrane and membrane-skeletal proteins. Semin Hematol 29:244, 1992

3. Schwartz RS: PIG-A: the target gene in paroxysmal nocturnal hemoglobinuria (editorial). N Engl J Med 330:283, 1994

4. Canessa M: Red cell volume-related ion transport systems in hemoglobinopathies. Hematol Oncol Clin North Am 5:495, 1991

5. Hanspal M, Palek J: Biogenesis of normal and abnormal red blood cell membrane skeleton. Semin Hematol 29:305, 1992

6. Turrini F, Mannu F, Arese P, et al: Characterization of the autologous antibodies that opsonize erythrocytes with clustered integral membrane proteins. Blood 81:3146, 1993

7. Potter CG, Potter AC, Hatton CSR, et al: Variation of erythroid and myeloid precursors in the marrow and peripheral blood of volunteer subjects infected with human parvovirus (B19). J Clin Invest 79:1486, 1987

8. Smith BD, Segel GB: Abnormal erythrocyte endothelial adherence in hereditary stomatocytosis. Blood 89:3451, 1997

9. Vives Corrons JL, Besson I, Aymerich M, et al: Hereditary xerocytosis: a report of six unrelated Spanish families with leaky red cell syndrome and increased heat stability of the erythrocyte membrane. Br J Haematol 90:817, 1995

10. Palek J, Jarolim P: Clinical expression and laboratory detection of red blood cell membrane protein mutations. Semin Hematol 30:249, 1993

11. Dhermy D, Galand C, Bournier O, et al: Heterogenous band 3 deficiency in hereditary spherocytosis related to different band 3 gene defects. Br J Haematol 98:32, 1997

12. Rosse WF: Hematopoiesis and the defect in paroxysmal hemoglobinuria. J Clin Invest 100:953, 1997

13. Ohashi H, Hotta T, Ichikawa A, et al: Peripheral blood cells are predominantly chimeric of affected and normal cells in patients with paroxysmal nocturnal hemoglobinuria: simultaneous investigation on clonality and expression of glycophosphatidylinositol-anchored proteins. Blood 83:853, 1994

14. Rosti V: The molecular basis of paroxysmal nocturnal hemoglobinuria. Haematologica 85:82, 2000

15. Hillmen P, Lewis SM, Bessler M, et al: Natural history of paroxysmal nocturnal hemoglobinuria. N Engl J Med 333:1253, 1995

16. Socie G, Marie J-Y, de Gramont A, et al: Paroxysmal nocturnal haemoglobinuria: long-term follow-up and prognostic factors. Lancet 348:573, 1996

17. Hugel B, Socié G, Vu T, et al: Elevated levels of circulating procoagulant micropar-

ticles in patients with paroxysmal nocturnal hemoglobinuria and aplastic anemia. Blood 93:3451, 1999

18. Hall SE, Rosse WF: The use of monoclonal antibodies and flow cytometry in the diagnosis of paroxysmal nocturnal hemoglobinuria. Blood 87:5332, 1996

19. Sholar PW, Bell WR: Thrombolytic therapy for inferior vena cava thrombosis in paroxysmal nocturnal hemoglobinuria. Ann Intern Med 103:539, 1985

20. Saso R, Marsh J, Cevreska L, et al: Bone marrow transplants for paroxysmal nocturnal haemoglobinuria. Br J Haematol 104:392, 1999

21. Arese P, De Flora A: Pathophysiology of hemolysis in glucose-6-phosphate dehydrogenase deficiency. Semin Hematol 27:1, 1990

22. Beutler E: G6PD deficiency. Blood 84:3613, 1994

23. Nagel RL, Ranney HM: Genetic epidemiology of structural mutations of the beta-globin gene. Semin Hematol 27:342, 1990

24. Rodgers GP, Noguchi CT, Schecter AN: Sickle cell anemia. Scientific American Science & Medicine 1:48, 1994

25. Bunn HF: Pathogenesis and treatment of sickle cell disease. N Engl J Med 337:762, 1997

26. Hebbel RP: Adhesive interactions of sickle erythrocytes with endothelium. J Clin Invest 99:2561, 1997

27. Kuypers FA, Lewis RA, Hua M, et al: Detection of altered membrane phospholipid asymmetry in subpopulations of human red blood cells using fluorescently labeled annexin V. Blood 87:1179, 1996

28. Solovey A, Gui L, Key NS, et al: Tissue factor expression by endothelial cells in sickle cell anemia. J Clin Invest 101:1899, 1998

29. Hebbel RP: Beyond hemoglobin polymerization: the red blood cell membrane and sickle disease pathophysiology. Blood 77:214, 1991

30. Bookchin RM, Ortiz OE, Lew VL: Evidence for a direct reticulocyte origin of dense red cells in sickle cell anemia. J Clin Invest 87:113, 1991

31. Singhal A, Doherty JF, Raynes JG: Is there an acute-phase response in steady-state sickle cell disease? Lancet 341:651, 1993

32. Francis RB, Johnson CS: Vascular occlusion in sickle cell disease: current concepts and unanswered questions. Blood 77:1405, 1991

33. Steinberg MH, West MS, Gallagher D, et al: Effects of glucose-6-phosphate dehydrogenase deficiency upon sickle cell anemia. Blood 71:748, 1988

34. Ballas SK: Neurobiology and treatment of pain. Sickle Cell Disease: Basic Principles and Clinical Practice. Embury SH, Hebbel RP, Mohandas N, et al, Eds. Raven Press, New York, 1994, p 745

35. Brugnara C, de Franceschi L, Alper SL: Inhibition of Ca^{2+}-dependent K^+ transport and cell dehydration in sickle erythrocytes by clotrimazole and other imidazole derivatives. J Clin Invest 92:520, 1993

36. Bennekou P, de Franceschi L, Pedersen O, et al: Treatment with NS3623, a novel Cl^- conductance blocker, ameliorates erythrocyte dehydration in transgenic SAD mice: a possible new therapeutic approach for sickle cell disease. Blood 97:1451, 2001

37. Platt OS, Brambilla DJ, Rosse WF, et al: Mortality in sickle cell disease: life expectancy and risk factors for early death. N Engl J Med 330:1639, 1994

38. Bunn HF: Induction of fetal hemoglobin in sickle cell disease. Blood 93:1787, 1999

39. Charache S, Terrin ML, Moore RD, et al: Effect of hydroxyurea on the frequency of painful crises in sickle cell anemia. N Engl J Med 332:1317, 1995

40. Steinberg MH, Barton F, Castro O, et al: Hydroxyurea (HU) is associated with reduced mortality in adults with sickle cell anemia (abstr). J Am Soc Hematol 96:485a, 2000

41. Bridges KR, Barabino GD, Brugnara C, et al: A multiparameter analysis of sickle erythrocytes in patients undergoing hydroxyurea therapy. Blood 88:4701, 1996

42. Perrine SP, Ginder GD, Faller DV, et al: A short-term trial of butyrate to stimulate fetal-globin-gene expression in the β-globin disorders. N Engl J Med 328:81, 1993

43. Atweh GF, Sutton M, Nassif I, et al: Sustained induction of fetal hemoglobin by pulse butyrate therapy in sickle cell disease. Blood 93:1790, 1999

44. Walters MC, Patience M, Leisenring W, et al: Bone marrow transplantation for sickle cell disease. N Engl J Med 335:369, 1996

45. Adams RJ, McKie VC, Hsu L, et al: Prevention of a first stroke by transfusions in children with sickle cell anemia and abnormal results on transcranial Doppler ultrasonography. N Engl J Med 339:5, 1998

46. Vichinsky EP: Understanding the morbidity of sickle cell disease (correspondence). Br J Haematol 99:974, 1997

47. Ohene-Frempong K: Indications for red cell transfusion in sickle cell disease. Semin Hematol 38(1 suppl 1):5, 2001

48. Olivieri NF: Progression of iron overload in sickle cell disease. Semin Hematol 38(1 suppl 1):57, 2001

49. Cohen AR, Martin MB: Iron chelation therapy in sickle cell disease. Semin Hematol 38(1 suppl 1):69, 2001

50. Bellet PS, Kalinyak KA, Shukla R, et al: Incentive spirometry to prevent acute pulmonary complications in sickle cell diseases. N Engl J Med 333:699, 1995

51. Milner PF, Kraus AP, Sebes JI, et al: Sickle cell disease as a cause of osteonecrosis of the femoral head. N Engl J Med 325:1476, 1991

52. Koate P: Cardiovascular pathology in sickle cell anemia. Bull Acad Natl Med 175:1055, 1991

53. Norris S, Johnson CS, Haywood LJ: Sickle cell anemia: does myocardial ischemia occur during crisis? J Natl Med Assoc 83:209, 1991

54. Vichinsky E, Williams R, Das M, et al: Pulmonary fat embolism: a distinct cause of severe acute chest syndrome in sickle cell anemia. Blood 83:3107, 1994

55. Vichinsky EP, Styles LA, Colangelo LH, et al: Acute chest syndrome in sickle cell disease: clinical presentation and course. Blood 89:1787, 1997

56. Styles LA, Schalkwijk CG, Aarsman AJ, et al: Phospholipase A$_2$ levels in acute chest syndrome of sickle cell disease. Blood 87: 2573, 1996

57. Gaston MH, Verter JI, Woods G, et al: Prophylaxis with oral penicillin in children with sickle cell anemia: a randomized trial. N Engl J Med 314:1593, 1986

58. Haberkern CM, Neumayr LD, Orringer EP, et al: Cholecystectomy in sickle cell anemia patients: perioperative outcome of 364 cases from national preoperative transfusion study. Blood 89:1533, 1997

59. Serjeant GR: Sickle-cell disease. Lancet 350:725, 1997

60. Gupta AK, Kirchner KA, Nicholson R, et al: Effects of α-thalassemia and sickle polymerization tendency on the urine-concentrating defect of individuals with sickle cell trait. J Clin Invest 88:1963, 1991

61. Falk RJ, Scheinman J, Phillips G, et al: Prevalence and pathologic features of sickle cell nephropathy and response to inhibition of angiotensin-converting enzyme. N Engl J Med 326:910, 1992

62. Ohene-Frempong K, Weiner SJ, Sleeper LA, et al: Cerebrovascular accidents in sickle cell disease: rates and risk factors. Blood 91:288, 1998

63. Cohen AR: Sickle cell disease: new treatments, new questions. N Engl J Med 339:42, 1998

64. Mohan JS, Vigilance JE, Marshall JM, et al: Abnormal venous function in patients with homozygous sickle cell (SS) disease and chronic leg ulcers. Clin Sci (Colch) 98:667, 2000

65. Groves RW, Schmidt-Lucke JA: Recombinant human GM-CSF in the treatment of poorly healing wounds. Adv Skin Wound Care 13:107, 2000

66. Serjeant GR, Serjeant BE, Thomas PW, et al: Human parvovirus infection in homozygous sickle cell disease. Lancet 341:1237, 1993

67. Koshy M, Weiner SJ, Miller ST, et al: Surgery and anesthesia in sickle cell disease. Blood 86:3676, 1995

68. Vichinsky EP, Haberkern CM, Neumayr L, et al: A comparison of conservative and aggressive transfusion regimens in the perioperative management of sickle cell disease. N Engl J Med 333:206, 1995

69. Koshy M, Burd L: Management of pregnancy in sickle cell syndromes. Hematol Oncol Clin North Am 5:585, 1991

70. Embury SH: Prenatal diagnosis. Sickle Cell Disease: Basic Principles and Clinical Practice. Embury SH, Hebbel RP, Mohandas N, et al, Eds. Raven Press, New York, 1994, p 485

71. Smith JA, Espeland M, Bellevue R, et al: Pregnancy in sickle cell disease: experience of the Cooperative Study of Sickle Cell Disease. Obstet Gynecol 87:199, 1996

72. Kark JA, Posey DM, Schumacher HR, et al: Sickle-cell trait as a risk factor for sudden death in physical training. N Engl J Med 317:781, 1987

73. Sullivan LW: The risks of sickle-cell trait: caution and common sense. N Engl J Med 317:830, 1987

74. Loukopoulos D, Voskaridou E, Kalotychou V, et al: Reduction of the clinical severity of sickle cell/beta-thalassemia with hydroxyurea: the experience of a single center in Greece. Blood Cells Mol Dis 26:453, 2000

75. Rogers ZR: Hydroxyurea therapy for diverse pediatric populations with sickle cell disease. Semin Hematol 34(3 suppl 3):42, 1997

76. Nagel RL, Lawrence C: The distinct pathobiology of sickle cell–hemoglobin C disease. Hematol Oncol Clin North Am 5:433, 1991

77. Steinberg MH, Nagel RL, Brugnara C: Cellular effects of hydroxyurea in Hb SC disease. Br J Haematol 98:838, 1997

78. Rees DC, Styles L, Vichinsky EP, et al: The hemoglobin E syndromes. Ann NY Acad Sci 850:334, 1998

79. Jaffe ER: Methemoglobinemia in the differential diagnosis of cyanosis. Hosp Pract (Off Ed) 20:92, 1985

80. Charache S: Methemoglobinemia-sleuthing for a new cause (editorial). N Engl J Med 314:776, 1986

81. Manabe J, Arya R, Sumimoto H, et al: Two novel mutations in the reduced nicotinamide adenine dinucleotide (NADH)-cytochrome b5 reductase gene of a patient with generalized type, hereditary methemoglobinemia. Blood 88:3208, 1996

82. Weatherall DJ, Clegg JB: Thalassemia: a global public health problem. Nat Med 2:847, 1996

83. Adams JG III, Coleman MB: Structural hemoglobin variants that produce the phenotype of thalassemia. Semin Hematol 27:229, 1990

84. Schrier SL: Thalassemia: pathophysiology of red cell changes. Annu Rev Med 45:211, 1994

85. Pootrakul P, Sirankapracha P, Hemsorach S, et al: A correlation of erythrokinetics, ineffective erythropoiesis, and erythroid precursor apoptosis in Thai patients with thalassemia. Blood 96:2606, 2000

86. Chui DHK, Waye JS: Hydrops fetalis caused by α-thalassemia: an emerging health care problem. Blood 91:2213, 1998

87. Sadelain M: Genetic treatment of the haemoglobinopathies: recombinations and new combinations. Br J Haematol 98:247, 1997

88. Hansen RM, Hanson G, Anderson T: Failure to suspect and diagnose thalassemic syndromes: interpretation of RBC indices by the nonhematologist. Arch Intern Med 145: 93, 1985

89. Piomelli S: The management of patients with Cooley's anemia: transfusions and splenectomy. Semin Hematol 32:262, 1995

90. Hoffbrand AV: Oral iron chelation. Semin Hematol 33:1, 1996

91. Brittenham GM, Griffith PM, Nienhuis AW, et al: Efficacy of deferoxamine in preventing complications of iron overload in patients with thalassemia major. N Engl J Med 331:567, 1994

92. Olivieri NF, Nathan DG, MacMillan JH, et al: Survival in medically treated patients with homozygous β-thalassemia. N Engl J Med 331:574, 1994

93. Olivieri NF, Brittenham GM, McLaren CE, et al: Long-term safety and effectiveness of iron-chelation therapy with deferiprone for thalassemia major. N Engl J Med 339:417, 1998

94. Kowdley KV, Kaplan MM: Iron-chelation therapy with oral deferiprone: toxicity or lack of efficacy (editorial). N Engl J Med 339:468, 1998

95. Winterbourne CC: Oxidative denaturation in congenital hemolytic anemias: the unstable hemoglobins. Semin Haematol 27:41, 1990

96. Issaragrisil S, Visuthisakchai S, Suvatte V, et al: Brief report: transplantation of cord-blood stem cells into a patient with severe thalassemia. N Engl J Med 332:367, 1995

97. Lucarelli G, Galimberti M, Giardini C, et al: Bone marrow transplantation in thalassemia. Ann NY Acad Sci 850:270, 1998

98. Sher GD, Ginder GD, Little J, et al: Extended therapy with intravenous arginine butyrate in patients with β-hemoglobinopathies. N Engl J Med 332:1606, 1995

99. Olivieri NF: Reactivation of fetal hemoglobin in patients with β -thalassemia. Semin Hematol 33:24, 1996

100. Domenica Cappellini M, Graziadei G, Ciceri L, et al: Oral isobutyramide therapy in patients with thalassemia intermedia: results of a phase II open study. Blood Cells Mol Dis 26:105, 2000

101. Reich S, Buhrer C, Henze G, et al: Oral isobutyramide reduces transfusion requirements in some patients with homozygous beta-thalassemia. Blood 96:3357, 2000

102. Kazazian HH Jr: The thalassemia syndromes: molecular basis and prenatal diagnosis in 1990. Semin Hematol 27:209, 1990

103. Dover GJ, Valle D: Therapy for β -thalassemia: a paradigm for the treatment of genetic disorders. N Engl J Med 331:609, 1994

104. Ross CN, Reuter H, Scott D, et al: Microangiopathic haemolytic anaemia and systemic vasculitis. Br J Rheumatol 35:377, 1996

105. Rytting M, Worth L, Jaffe N: Hemolytic disorders associated with cancer. Hematol Oncol Clin North Am 10:365, 1996

106. Mach-Pascual S, Samii K, Beris P, et al: Microangiopathic hemolytic anemia complicating FK 506 (tacrolimus) therapy. Am J Hematol 52:310, 1996

107. Engelfriet CP, Overbeeke MAM, von dem Borne AEGK: Autoimmune hemolytic anemia. Semin Hematol 29:3, 1992

108. Jefferies LC: Transfusion therapy in autoimmune hemolytic anemia. Hematol Oncol Clin North Am 8:1087, 1994

109. Leddy JP, Falany JL, Kissel GE, et al: Erythrocyte membrane proteins reactive with human (warm-reacting) anti-red cell autoantibodies. J Clin Invest 91:1672, 1993

110. Liesveld JL, Rowe JM, Lichtman MA: Variability of the erythropoietic response in autoimmune hemolytic anemia: analysis of 109 cases. Blood 69:820, 1987

111. Meyer O, Stahl D, Beckhove P, et al: Pulsed high-dose dexamethasone in chronic autoimmune haemolytic anaemia of warm type. Br J Haematol 98:860, 1997

112. Emilia G, Messora C, Longo G, et al: Long-term salvage treatment by cyclosporin in refractory autoimmune haematological disorders. Br J Haematol 93:341, 1996

113. Collins PW, Newland AC: Treatment modalities of autoimmune blood disorders. Semin Hematol 29:64, 1992

114. Flores G, Cunningham-Rundles C, Newland AC, et al: Efficacy of intravenous immunoglobulin in the treatment of autoimmune hemolytic anemia: results in 73 patients. Am J Hematol 44:237, 1993

115. Salama A, Berghofer H, Mueller-Eckhardt C: Red blood cell transfusion in warm-type autoimmune haemolytic anaemia. Lancet 340:1515, 1992

116. Salama A, Mueller-Eckhardt C: Immune-mediated blood cell dyscrasias related to drugs. Semin Hematol 29:54, 1992

117. Garratty G: Immune cytopenia associated with antibiotics. Transfus Med Rev 7:255, 1993

118. Kopicky JA, Packman CH: The mechanisms of sulfonylurea-induced immune hemolysis: case report and review of the literature. Am J Hematol 23:283, 1986

119. Petz LD: Drug-induced autoimmune hemolytic anemia. Transfus Med Rev 7:242, 1993

120. Salama A, Kroll H, Wittmann G, et al: Diclofenac-induced immune haemolytic anaemia: simultaneous occurrence of red blood cell autoantibodies and drug-dependent antibodies. Br J Haematol 95:640, 1996

121. Ramsey G: Red cell antibodies arising from solid organ transplants. Transfusion 31:76, 1991

122. Silberstein LE: B-cell origin of cold agglutinins. Adv Exp Med Biol 347:193, 1994

123. Loomes LM, Uemura K, Childs RA, et al: Erythrocyte receptors for Mycoplasma pneumoniae are sialylated oligosaccharides of Ii antigen type. Nature 307:560, 1984

124. Sharara AI, Hillsley RE, Wax TD, et al: Paroxysmal cold hemoglobinuria associated with non-Hodgkin's lymphoma. South Med J 87:397, 1994

125. Rosse WF: The spleen as a filter. N Engl J Med 317:704, 1987

126. Lu HC, Shih RD, Marcus S, et al: Pseudomethemoglobinemia: a case and review of sulfhemoglobinemia. Arch Pediatr Adolesc Med 152:803, 1998

127. Coleman MD, Coleman NA: Drug-induced methaemoglobinaemia: treatment issues. Drug Saf 14:394, 1996

128. Valentine WN, Paglia DE, Fink K, et al: Lead poisoning: association with hemolyt-

ic anemia, basophilic stippling, erythrocyte pyrimidine 5'-nucleotidase deficiency, and intraerythrocytic accumulation of pyrimidines. J Clin Invest 58:926, 1976

129. Carton JA, Maradona JA, Arribas JM: Acute-subacute lead poisoning: clinical findings and comparative study of diagnostic tests. Arch Intern Med 147:697, 1987

130. Shurin SB, Anderson P, Zollinger J, et al: Pathophysiology of hemolysis in infections with *Hemophilus influenzae* type b. J Clin Invest 77:1340, 1986

131. van Spronsen DJ, Breed WPM: Cytomegalovirus-induced thrombocytopenia and haemolysis in an immunocompetent adult. Br J Haematol 92:218, 1996

132. Looareesuwan S, Merry AH, Phillips RE, et al: Reduced erythrocyte survival following clearance of malarial parasitaemia in Thai patients. Br J Haematol 67:473, 1987

133. Krause PJ, Spielman A, Telford SR III, et al: Persistent parasitemia after acute babesiosis. N Engl J Med 339:160, 1998

134. Owen JS, Brown DJC, Harry DS, et al: Erythrocyte echinocytosis in liver disease. J Clin Invest 76:2275, 1985

135. Allen DW, Manning N: Cholesterol-loading of membranes of normal erythrocytes inhibits phospholipid repair and arachidonoyl-CoA:1-palmitoyl-sn-glycero-3-phosphocholine acyl transferase: a model of spur cell anemia. Blood 87:3489, 1996

136. Salama A, Hugo F, Heinrich D, et al: Deposition of terminal C5b-complement complexes on erythrocytes and leukocytes during cardiopulmonary bypass. N Engl J Med 318:408, 1988

Virginia C. Broudy, M.D.

Classification of the Polycythemias

Polycythemia, also called erythrocytosis, is an increase in the number of circulating red blood cells per volume of blood, as reflected by an elevated hematocrit or hemoglobin level. The three major categories of polycythemia are (1) relative polycythemia, (2) secondary polycythemia, and (3) primary polycythemia, or polycythemia vera.

In relative polycythemia, the red cell mass is normal but the plasma volume is decreased. Secondary polycythemia is caused by an elevated erythropoietin level. Polycythemia vera is a neoplastic stem cell disorder characterized by an autonomous overproduction of red blood cells and, often, of white blood cells and platelets.

Initial Evaluation

Patients are often asymptomatic, and the elevated hemoglobin or hematocrit level is usually discovered accidentally. When such an increase is found, it should be promptly evaluated to determine its cause [*see Figure 1*]. Any family history of polycythemia and results of any previous hematocrit determinations should be obtained. History and physical examination findings suggestive of congenital heart disease, severe chronic obstructive pulmonary disease (COPD), or sleep apnea syndrome should be sought, and the presence or absence of splenomegaly should be determined. The results of the complete blood count, including the platelet count and white blood cell differential, should be critically reviewed for abnormalities. Findings of leukocytosis, thrombocytosis, an occasional circulating immature white blood cell, or increased basophils are suggestive of polycythemia vera and argue against secondary causes of erythrocytosis.

A man or woman with a hematocrit level of 60% or higher or 57% or higher, respectively, virtually always has a true increase in red blood cell mass (i.e., primary or secondary polycythemia). If the patient's hematocrit is below these values but above normal, a red blood cell mass study should be done.[1] To perform this study, a sample of the patient's red blood cells is labeled with radioactive chromium (^{51}Cr) ex vivo and injected back into the patient. A second blood sample is then obtained to quantitate the concentration of ^{51}Cr-labeled red blood cells among the unlabeled red blood cells. In parallel, the patient is given an injection of albumin labeled with radioactive iodine (^{125}I) to measure the plasma volume. The results of the ^{51}Cr-labeled red blood cell mass determination identify the patient as having either relative polycythemia because of a plasma volume contraction or true (i.e., primary or secondary) polycythemia because of increased red blood cell mass. Once a relative or an absolute increase in red blood cell mass is documented, an exact diagnosis should be determined [*see Figure 1*].

Relative Polycythemia

Patients with relative polycythemia (Gaisböck syndrome) are often obese, hypertensive men who may also be heavy smokers[2]; they often are 45 to 55 years of age—a decade younger than the typical age for polycythemia vera patients [*see* Polycythemia Vera, *below*]. It has been estimated that 0.5% to 0.7% of the healthy male population in the United States have relative polycythemia. Diuretic use for treatment of hypertension may exacerbate the deficit in plasma volume, and smoking-induced high carboxyhemoglobin levels or hypoxemia may also play a role.

Relative polycythemia is usually mild (hematocrit lower than 55%). In patients with a hematocrit lower than 60%, this diagnosis should be considered, and red blood cell mass and plasma volume should be measured [*see Figure 1*] to avoid an extensive and ultimately frustrating workup for other causes of polycythemia. Patients with relative polycythemia fall into two major groups: (1) those with normal red blood cell mass and clearly decreased plasma volume and (2) those with red blood cell mass and plasma volume at the upper and lower range of normal, respectively. Behavior modification (e.g., an exercise regimen and smoking cessation) is recommended for these patients. Hematocrit returns to normal over time in approximately one third of patients.

Secondary Polycythemia

Secondary polycythemia occurs when erythropoietin production is increased because of chronic tissue hypoxia. Causes of tissue hypoxia include life at high altitude, high-affinity hemoglobin, cardiopulmonary disease, obesity-hypoventilation syndrome, obstructive sleep apnea, and high serum levels of carboxyhemoglobin. Polycythemia also occurs in some renal and hepatic disorders, in rare genetic disorders, and from treatment with androgens or erythropoietin.

POLYCYTHEMIA CAUSED BY APPROPRIATE INCREASES IN ERYTHROPOIETIN PRODUCTION

Life at High Altitude

Initial human adaptation to high altitude includes increased respiratory rate, cardiac output, and level of 2,3-bisphosphoglycerate to facilitate oxygen unloading from hemoglobin to the tissues [*see Figure 2*]. Within 6 to 24 hours after a person has ascended to a high altitude, erythropoietin levels increase, resulting in reticulocytosis within 24 to 48 hours. Over several days, serum erythropoietin levels return to normal, but the increase in hematocrit is sustained. In addition to the increase in red cell mass, a modest decrease in plasma volume occurs. A patient's travel history should be taken to determine the likelihood of high-altitude effect and possibly avoid an extensive workup.

High-Affinity Hemoglobin

High-affinity hemoglobin is caused by an amino acid substitution in either the α chain or, more commonly, the β chain of globin that impedes the normal conformational change during oxygen loading and unloading. This condition results in impaired ability to release oxygen in the tissues, causing tissue hypoxia and increased erythropoietin production. More than 40 mutations causing high-affinity hemoglobin have been described. They are

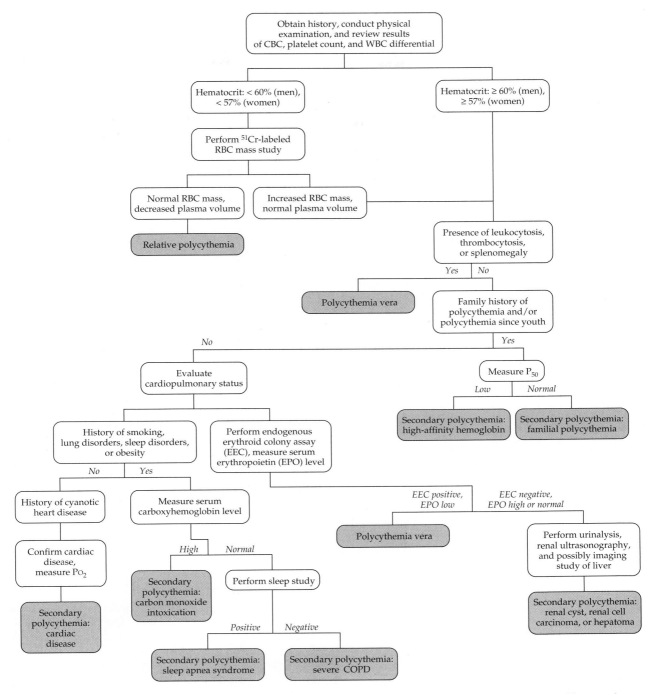

Figure 1   **This flowchart depicts an approach to the evaluation of a patient with polycythemia, as evidenced by an elevated hematocrit or hemoglobin level on routine complete blood count. (CBC—complete blood cell count; COPD—chronic obstructive pulmonary disease; EEC—endogenous erythroid colony; EPO—erythropoietin; RBC—red blood cell count; WBC—white blood cell count)**

usually familial and are inherited in an autosomal dominant manner but are occasionally the result of spontaneous mutation. A record review should show evidence of lifelong polycythemia. The hematocrit of patients is usually less than 60%, and the white blood cell and platelet counts are normal. The partial pressure of oxygen at which hemoglobin is 50% saturated (P_{50}) should be measured; it is reduced in patients with high-affinity hemoglobin [*see Figure 2*]. Hemoglobin electrophoresis is usually not helpful, because many of the mutations that result in high-affini-

ty hemoglobin are electrophoretically silent. Patients with high-affinity hemoglobin usually have no symptoms of hyperviscosity and require no therapy.

Cardiopulmonary Disease

Polycythemia caused by cardiopulmonary defects (e.g., Eisenmenger complex, univentricular heart, and tetralogy of Fallot) results from failure to load oxygen onto hemoglobin adequately in the lungs.[3,4] The hematocrit may range from 60% to 75% and cause profound symptoms of hyperviscosity, including headache, dizziness, visual disturbances, fatigue, paresthesias, and decreased mental acuity. Some adults with cyanotic congenital heart disease have decompensated erythrocytosis, which is characterized by unstable, rising hematocrit and symptomatic hyperviscosity; these patients may benefit from phlebotomy.[4] Other adults with cyanotic congenital heart disease have compensated erythrocytosis, in which a stable (though elevated) hematocrit is maintained without overt symptoms of hyperviscosity; these patients do not require phlebotomy.[4] A practical approach is to cautiously phlebotomize patients who have a hematocrit higher than 60% to 65% and symptoms of hyperviscosity.[4] The extent of phlebotomy should be guided by the patient's symptoms. Acute dehydration, which exacerbates polycythemia, should be excluded from the diagnosis before phlebotomy is performed, and the volume of blood withdrawn should be replaced with isotonic saline. Iron deficiency should be avoided by the use of oral iron therapy if necessary because severe iron deficiency may alter red blood cell rheology and increase the risk of stroke.[5]

Severe COPD can be associated with polycythemia, although the clinical features of COPD usually predominate. In patients who continue to smoke, both hypoxemia and elevated carboxyhemoglobin levels may contribute to the development of polycythemia. Reduction of hematocrit in patients with significant polycythemia caused by COPD results in increased cerebral blood flow, relief from hyperviscosity symptoms of dizziness and headache, and dramatic improvement in mental alertness. In a study of seven patients with severe COPD and pulmonary hypertension, serial phlebotomy reduced pulmonary artery pressure and improved exercise capacity.[6]

Obesity-Hypoventilation Syndrome

Obesity-hypoventilation syndrome is also known as pickwickian syndrome in reference to Charles Dickens' astute description of the obese coachboy who had excessive daytime sleepiness. Patients with this syndrome are usually obese (i.e., they are more than 120% of ideal body weight) and have hypoxemia and hypercapnia, in part because of a blunted ventilatory response to these stimuli.[7] Some of these patients also have a component of nocturnal obstructive sleep apnea. Hypoxemia provides the stimulus for increased erythropoietin production and polycythemia. Other clinical features associated with obesity-hypoventilation syndrome are daytime hypersomnolence and cor pulmonale.

Management of this condition includes weight loss and progesterone therapy to stimulate the central respiratory drive [*see Chapter 216*].

Obstructive Sleep Apnea

Sleep apnea syndrome is estimated to occur in 4% and 2% of middle-aged men and women, respectively. Recurrent episodes of upper airway collapse during sleep obstruct air movement, resulting in intermittent nocturnal hypoxemia. Patients may have a history of loud snoring, alternating with periods of silence lasting 10 seconds to 1 minute, followed by gasping sounds. Fragmented sleep results in excessive daytime sleepiness and impaired work performance and may increase the risk of motor vehicle accidents.[8] Hematocrit may be modestly increased in patients with severe obstructive sleep apnea, and this syndrome should be considered in patients with unexplained polycythemia. Nocturnal polysomnography can establish the diagnosis.

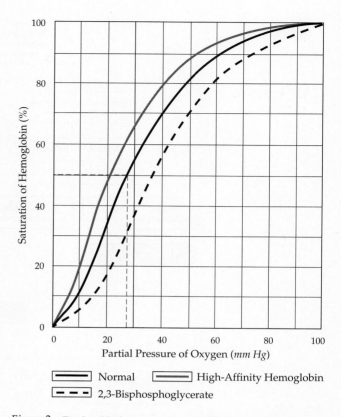

Figure 2   Depicted is the oxygen-hemoglobin dissociation curve (solid black line). The partial pressure of oxygen at which hemoglobin is 50% saturated (P_{50}) is normally 27 mm Hg (broken blue lines). The presence of high-affinity hemoglobin shifts the curve to the left, reflecting impaired oxygen unloading in the tissues (solid blue line). An increase in the level of 2,3-bisphosphoglycerate—a feature of adaptation to high altitude—shifts the curve to the right, reflecting increased oxygen unloading in the tissues (broken black line).

Management of this condition may include weight loss, nasal continuous positive airway pressure, and surgery[9] [*see Chapters 187 and 216*].

High Carboxyhemoglobin Levels

Long-term exposure to carbon monoxide results in chronic high carboxyhemoglobin levels [*see Chapter 13*]. Carbon monoxide binds to hemoglobin with an affinity 210 times greater than that of oxygen, decreasing the quantity of hemoglobin available for oxygen transport. Carbon monoxide binding also increases the affinity of the remaining heme groups for oxygen, shifting the oxygen-hemoglobin dissociation curve to the left [*see Figure 2*] and impairing unloading of oxygen in the tissues. By these mechanisms, long-term carbon monoxide exposure can cause polycythemia. Cigarette and cigar smokers and persons with long-term occupational exposure to automobile exhaust in poorly ventilated areas (e.g., tollbooth operators, underground-garage attendants, and truck loaders) are at risk.

Symptoms may include subtle neuropsychiatric abnormalities and exacerbation of angina (likely as a result of impaired myocardial oxygen delivery). The diagnosis can be established by measuring the percentage of carboxyhemoglobin in the blood. Because the half-life of carboxyhemoglobin is approximately 4 hours, the test should be done late in the day, when the patient has smoked the usual number of cigarettes or spent several hours in the work

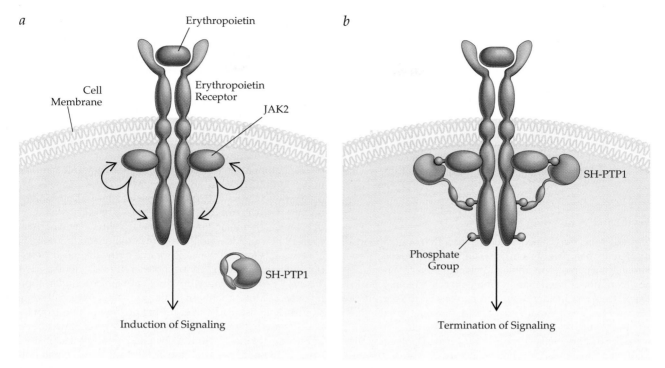

Figure 3 (*a*) **Binding of erythropoietin to the erythropoietin receptor on an erythroid progenitor cell triggers association and activation of the protein-tyrosine kinase JAK2 and the initiation of signal transduction, stimulating growth of the erythroid progenitor cell. (*b*) Binding of the protein-tyrosine phosphatase SH-PTP1 results in dephosphorylation of JAK2 and termination of signal transduction.**

environment. Polycythemic smokers usually have both elevated red blood cell mass and decreased plasma volume.

The most effective therapy is smoking cessation; abnormal blood and plasma levels revert to normal within 3 months.

POLYCYTHEMIA CAUSED BY RENAL AND HEPATIC DISORDERS

Polycythemias arise when erythropoietin production is increased because of renal or, less often, hepatic disorders. In adults, approximately 90% of erythropoietin production occurs in the kidney and 10% in the liver. The precise molecular mechanisms are not yet fully understood. However, it is known that an oxygen-binding heme protein in the kidney senses tissue hypoxia, which results in enhanced erythropoietin production by peritubular interstitial cells of the kidney. Because of the intricate regulation of erythropoietin production in the kidney, distortion of renal anatomy can result in polycythemia. Case reports document that renal cysts, hydronephrosis, focal glomerulonephritis, and Bartter syndrome can cause polycythemia. After renal transplantation, approximately 20% of patients have transient or persistent polycythemia and may require phlebotomy or angiotensin-converting enzyme inhibitors. In addition, primary malignancies of the kidney or liver can cause polycythemia. Polycythemia develops in approximately 3% of patients with renal cell carcinoma. Erythropoietin production by primary renal cell carcinoma and hepatoma tissues is the likely cause of polycythemia in these patients. In rare instances, focal nodular hyperplasia of the liver, hemangiomas of the liver or cerebellum, uterine fibroids, adrenal adenomas, and pheochromocytomas have been reported to cause polycythemia.

FAMILIAL POLYCYTHEMIA

In autosomal dominant polycythemia, affected members of families have erythrocytosis that remains stable over time; they do not experience leukocytosis or thrombocytosis and are not at increased risk for acute myelogenous leukemia. Abnormalities in the erythropoietin receptor or in the regulation of erythropoietin production have been identified in some of these families.[10-12]

Erythropoietin initiates its biologic effects by binding to a specific receptor that is found on the surface of erythroid progenitor cells, precursor cells, and certain other types of cells. Binding triggers a cascade of events, including activation of the protein-tyrosine kinase JAK2 [*see Figure 3*]. Tyrosine phosphorylation of the erythropoietin receptor creates docking sites for other signal transduction molecules and for the protein-tyrosine phosphatase SH-PTP1, which dephosphorylates JAK2 and terminates signal transduction. In one large Finnish family with polycythemia, a point mutation in the erythropoietin receptor affecting SH-PTP1 rendered the erythroid progenitor cells hypersensitive to erythropoietin. Interestingly, one member of this family who had a hematocrit of 60% won three gold medals in cross-country skiing at the 1964 Winter Olympics. Most mutations in the erythropoietin receptor identified to date result in deletion of the carboxyl terminus negative regulatory region of the receptor.[11,12] In other patients with familial polycythemia, abnormalities in transcriptional regulation of the erythropoietin gene may be found.[13] A high frequency of familial polycythemia is found in the Chuvash region of Russia.[14] Affected members of these families have high levels of erythropoietin, and initial studies suggest that Chuvash polycythemia may be caused by an abnormality in the renal oxygen-sensing mechanism.[14]

POLYCYTHEMIA CAUSED BY DRUG USE

Androgens (e.g., testosterone) can cause polycythemia by stimulating erythropoietin production.[15] The elevated hematocrit is usually mild and returns to normal 2 to 3 months after discontinuance of anabolic steroid use. Since recombinant human erythropoietin has become available, concern has been raised that competitive athletes involved in endurance sports, such as bicycle racing, cross-country skiing, and long-distance running, might surreptitiously self-inject this drug to improve athletic performance.[16] Phlebotomy followed by blood doping is known to improve performance in runners and skiers. A similar increase in hematocrit can be achieved with erythropoietin injections. The unmonitored increase in red blood cell production may cause significant polycythemia, which, when coupled with exercise-induced dehydration, can result in tragic consequences. There is speculation that the sudden death of a number of competitive bicyclists between 1987 and 1990 was related to erythropoietin abuse.[16]

Polycythemia Vera

Polycythemia vera is a neoplastic disorder that originates in a pluripotent hematopoietic stem cell. The annual incidence is approximately 10 persons per million. Polycythemia vera is slightly more common in men than in women (male-to-female ratio, 1.2:1) and peaks in incidence among persons 50 to 75 years of age.[17] However, approximately 5% of cases are diagnosed in patients younger than 40 years.[17]

In the 1950s and 1960s, a group of untreated polycythemia vera patients had a mean survival of approximately 18 months; most deaths were caused by stroke. Today, however, the median survival of treated patients is approximately 10 to 15 years. Because polycythemia vera is most often diagnosed in patients in their 60s and 70s, the resultant life span may not differ from that of an age-matched control population. A study of young polycythemia vera patients (younger than 40 years) showed that more than 70% survived 15 years after diagnosis.

PATHOPHYSIOLOGY

In a healthy adult, hematopoiesis is polyclonal in that the circulating peripheral blood cells are derived from a multitude of hematopoietic stem cells [see Chapter 86]. In patients with polycythemia vera, however, many or all of the circulating red blood cells, white blood cells, and platelets are derived from one neoplastic hematopoietic stem cell.

Polycythemia vera is one of a group of related stem cell disorders termed myeloproliferative disorders, all of which are clonal

---

Table 1 Criteria for the Diagnosis of Polycythemia Vera[30]

Major Criteria*

1. Elevated red cell mass (> 25% above mean normal predicted value)
2. Absence of cause of secondary polycythemia
3. Splenomegaly
4. Clonal chromosomal abnormality

Minor Criteria*

1. Thrombocytosis (platelet count > 400,000/mm³)
2. Neutrophil leukocytosis (neutrophils > 10,000/mm³)
3. Positive endogenous erythroid colony assay or low serum erythropoietin level

*Polycythemia vera is diagnosed if any of the following criteria are met: major criteria 1, 2, and 3; major criteria 1, 2, and 4; or major criteria 1 and 2 and two minor criteria.

---

in origin. Myeloproliferative disorders also include chronic myeloid leukemia (CML), essential thrombocythemia, and agnogenic myeloid metaplasia [see Chapter 204]. The dominant features of CML are dramatic leukocytosis, presence of the Philadelphia chromosome, and certain evolution to acute myeloid leukemia (AML) or acute lymphocytic leukemia. Essential thrombocythemia is distinguished by predominant thrombocytosis, without erythrocytosis or the cytogenetic abnormality of CML. Agnogenic myeloid metaplasia is characterized by massive splenomegaly accompanied by bone marrow fibrosis, anemia, and a leukoerythroblastic peripheral blood smear.

The pathophysiology of polycythemia vera is incompletely understood.[18] In healthy adults, erythroid progenitor cells do not proliferate in the absence of exogenous erythropoietin. However, erythroid progenitor cells from patients with polycythemia vera develop into hemoglobinized colonies in vitro even when erythropoietin is not added to the serum-containing cultures.[19] These observations formed the basis for one of the diagnostic tests for polycythemia vera, the endogenous erythroid colony assay [see Table 1].[19] Endogenous erythroid colonies can be found in approximately 97% of patients with polycythemia vera. Subsequent studies demonstrated that erythroid progenitor cells from these patients are hypersensitive to the growth-promoting effects of multiple cytokines, including insulinlike growth factor–1.[20] Because of these findings and the fact that multiple hematopoietic lineages can be involved in polycythemia vera, it is unlikely that a mutation in the receptor for one of the late-acting cytokines (e.g., erythropoietin) could explain the pathophysiology of polycythemia vera. Sequence analysis shows that the erythropoietin receptor is structurally intact in polycythemia vera patients. The receptor for thrombopoietin, Mpl, is expressed on stem cells, progenitor cells, and some mature cells, and some studies[21,22] indicate that the levels of Mpl expression on megakaryocytes and platelets from patients with polycythemia vera are lower than on normal megakaryocytes and platelets. This finding is perhaps the result of a defect in posttranslational processing of the receptor.[21,22] However, other studies have found variable Mpl expression in patients with polycythemia vera[23] and low levels of Mpl in another myeloproliferative disorder, essential thrombocythemia.[24] Thus, at present, tests for Mpl expression on platelets or megakaryocytes cannot reliably identify patients with polycythemia vera. Polycythemia vera erythroid cells overexpress an inhibitor of apoptosis, Bcl-x, which may enhance their survival and thus contribute to the development of erythrocytosis.[25] Additionally, subtraction hybridization has identified a novel gene, PRV-1, that is highly expressed in neutrophils from polycythemia vera patients but not in neutrophils from patients with other myeloproliferative disorders or from healthy control subjects.[26] The role of PRV-1 in the pathogenesis and, potentially, the diagnosis of polycythemia vera are under investigation.

DIAGNOSIS

The natural history of polycythemia vera includes a latent and relatively asymptomatic prothrombotic phase[17]; an overt proliferative phase, during which the red blood cell mass expands [see Table 1] and the patient may have hyperviscosity or hypermetabolic symptoms [see Table 2] or thrombosis; and a so-called spent phase (i.e., postpolycythemic myeloid metaplasia), which is characterized by a decline in red blood cell production and development of anemia, leukopenia, thrombocytopenia, marrow fibrosis, and progressive hepatosplenomegaly. Myeloid metaplasia eventually develops in about 20% of patients. AML is a naturally oc-

Table 2 Symptoms in Patients
with Polycythemia Vera[49]

Symptom	Incidence (%)
Headache	48
Weakness	47
Pruritus	43
Dizziness	43
Excessive sweating	33
Visual symptoms	31
Weight loss	29
Paresthesias	29
Dyspnea	26
Joint symptoms	26
Epigastric distress	24

curring complication of polycythemia vera that develops in approximately 1% to 2% of patients treated with phlebotomy alone; it is also a complication of certain treatments themselves [*see* Complications, *below*].

Clinical Features

Although certain symptoms are common to all polycythemias, other symptoms are more specific for polycythemia vera [*see Table 2*]. Many polycythemic patients have headache or vague cognitive changes, including memory changes and inability to perform rapid mental calculations. Weakness and dizziness are common nonspecific symptoms. Pruritus after a hot shower or bath is more specific for polycythemia vera and may be very troubling. Less commonly, polycythemia vera patients have hypermetabolic symptoms, including fever, weight loss, and excessive sweating. Erythromelalgia, episodic severe burning pain, and erythema in the fingers or toes are caused by digital ischemia and are highly suggestive of a myeloproliferative disorder.[27] Approximately 20% of patients with polycythemia vera have had a premonitory arterial or venous thrombotic event.[17] Patients may also be asymptomatic.

Physical Examination Findings

Physical examination usually shows facial plethora, which is common to all patients with true (i.e., primary or secondary) polycythemia. Splenomegaly is found in 70% of patients with polycythemia vera; the cause is extramedullary hematopoiesis along with splenic congestion with red blood cells. Hepatomegaly is found in 40% of polycythemia vera patients; it may also be caused by extramedullary hematopoiesis or, on occasion, by Budd-Chiari syndrome.[28]

Laboratory Findings

The complete blood count of patients presenting with polycythemia vera usually shows an elevated hematocrit. A hematocrit value of 60% or higher in men or 57% or higher in women is virtually diagnostic of primary or secondary polycythemia.[29] However, because of the high prevalence of gastrointestinal blood loss in polycythemia vera patients, some present with a normal hematocrit level. Mean corpuscular volume of red blood cells may be reduced, reflecting iron deficiency. Leukocytosis is found in approximately 45% of patients. Peripheral blood smear may show modest basophilia and occasional circulating immature white blood cells, including myelocytes and metamyelocytes. Approximately 65% of patients with polycythemia vera have thrombocy-

tosis. The major differential diagnosis in the patient with a normal hematocrit, thrombocytosis, and low mean corpuscular volume is iron deficiency polycythemia vera, essential thrombocythemia, or thrombocytosis caused by the iron deficiency itself. If the patient is iron-replete, the likely diagnosis is essential thrombocythemia. Thrombocytosis resulting from iron deficiency usually responds to iron repletion therapy.

Other laboratory findings include an elevated uric acid level in 30% to 50% of polycythemia vera patients, caused by the chronically increased production and destruction of red blood cells. The leukocyte alkaline phosphatase (LAP) score is elevated in 70% of patients with polycythemia vera; in patients with CML, the LAP score is reduced.

The serum erythropoietin level is often reduced as a result of feedback mechanisms [*see Figure 4*]. However, values for the serum erythropoietin level in polycythemia vera patients can be within the normal range.[30] In one study of 80 patients with polycythemia vera, the mean serum erythropoietin levels were 0.5 U/L in newly diagnosed patients, 2.5 U/L in patients treated with phlebotomy alone, and 7 to 11 U/L in patients treated with various myelosuppressive agents.[31] Thus, prior therapy may influence the serum erythropoietin value.

Bone marrow evaluation may be helpful in looking for a marker of clonality, such as deletion of the long arm of chromosome 20. Bone marrow findings include increased cellularity, increased megakaryocytes, and low iron stores. Reticulin fibers may also be increased.[32]

Cytogenetic abnormalities are found at diagnosis in approximately 20% of patients with polycythemia vera and commonly include trisomy 8, trisomy 9, and deletion of the long arm of chromosome 20. Presence of cytogenetic abnormalities at diagnosis does not identify patients at greater risk for AML or those whose condition may progress to myeloid metaplasia.

TREATMENT

Consensus has not occurred regarding the best treatment approach for polycythemia vera, and new multi-institutional clinical trials comparing interferon alfa and hydroxyurea are needed. Therapy must be tailored to each patient and must consider the patient's age and risk profile for thrombosis and the inherent risks of each treatment strategy.

Phlebotomy

For most patients, initial treatment should include phlebotomy. Generally, 500 ml of blood is removed once or twice a week until the target hematocrit value of less than 45% is achieved. Thereafter, intermittent phlebotomy can maintain the hematocrit between 40% and 45%. By lowering the hematocrit, phlebotomy may also improve cognitive impairment.[33]

Iron deficiency develops in many patients after phlebotomy, limiting the patient's ability to produce red blood cells and thus decreasing the frequency of phlebotomy. The patient must be instructed not to take iron-containing multivitamins. Iron-containing multivitamins will replenish their iron stores and increase the frequency of phlebotomy. Controversy remains as to whether severely hypochromic, microcytic, iron-deficient red blood cells exhibit altered rheologic behavior that increases blood viscosity and perhaps slightly increases the risk of thrombosis. For this reason, it is probably wise to avoid severe iron deficiency as reflected by inducing severe microcytosis (mean corpuscular volume < 65 fl). On occasion, for patients with severe symptoms attributable to iron deficiency (e.g., pica, glossitis, and exercise-induced muscle

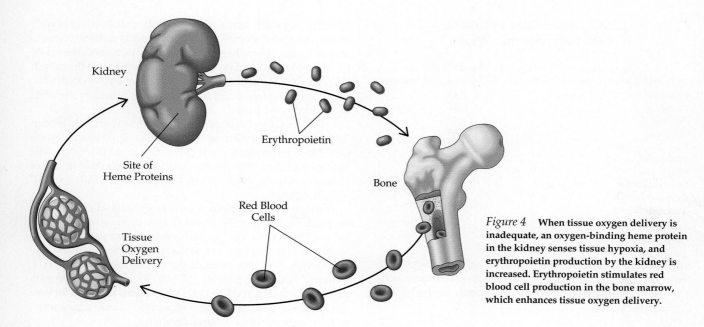

Figure 4 **When tissue oxygen delivery is inadequate, an oxygen-binding heme protein in the kidney senses tissue hypoxia, and erythropoietin production by the kidney is increased. Erythropoietin stimulates red blood cell production in the bone marrow, which enhances tissue oxygen delivery.**

fatigue), it may be best to give replacement iron and increase the frequency of phlebotomy as necessary. For most patients, however, modest iron deficiency is a desirable consequence of phlebotomy because it helps maintain the hematocrit in the target range. Most patients initially treated with phlebotomy alone eventually require myelosuppressive therapy. Of 104 patients treated with phlebotomy, 50% required another form of treatment within 5 years and 90% within 10 years.[34]

Myelosuppressive Agents

Patients deemed at increased risk for thrombosis (e.g., those older than 70 years, those who have had a thrombotic event, and those who require a high-maintenance phlebotomy) are probably best treated with a myelosuppressive agent (e.g., hydroxyurea)[30,35] in addition to phlebotomy. It has been demonstrated that hydroxyurea (usually 500 mg to 1.5 g orally daily) and phlebotomy can effectively control the hematocrit in most patients with polycythemia vera[30,35] and that the risk of thrombosis is lower with this therapy than with phlebotomy alone.

Hydroxyurea is an oral agent that is generally well tolerated. However, its use requires frequent monitoring of the complete blood count to avoid excessive myelosuppression, and some patients treated with hydroxyurea experience painful leg ulcers.[36] Controversy exists as to whether hydroxyurea increases the risk of AML. However, two reports show a 5% to 6% incidence of AML in hydroxyurea-treated patients versus 1% to 2% in patients treated with phlebotomy alone.[30,35] The yearly cost of hydroxyurea therapy (on the basis of a dose of 1 g/day) is approximately $1,000.

Busulfan, an alkylating agent, is an alternative orally active myelosuppressive drug with a risk of AML possibly similar to that in patients treated with radioactive phosphorus (^{32}P). The long-term side effects of busulfan include the risk of pulmonary fibrosis and risk of damage to hematopoietic stem cells, which may result in long-term marrow suppression. Because of its toxicity profile, busulfan is usually reserved for patients who do not respond to hydroxyurea.

Intermittent treatment with ^{32}P (2.3 mCi/m^2 I.V. every 3 to 6 months as needed to control the hematocrit; maximum dose, 5 mCi) generally results in smooth control of the hematocrit, does not require frequent monitoring, and is very convenient for patients.[34,37] However, treatment with ^{32}P increases the risk of AML. Therapy with ^{32}P may be appropriate for elderly polycythemia vera patients. The cost of one dose of ^{32}P is $2,600.

Compared with patients treated with a myelosuppressive agent, patients managed by phlebotomy alone have an increased risk of thrombosis during the first 3 years after treatment begins.[30,35] For this reason, treatment with aspirin (300 mg three times a day) plus dipyridamole (75 mg three times a day) in addition to phlebotomy was studied to determine whether this regimen would decrease the risk of thrombosis compared with treatment with ^{32}P. Addition of aspirin at this relatively high dosage did not prevent thrombosis and increased the risk of significant gastrointestinal bleeding. Thus, aspirin at this dosage cannot be recommended as initial therapy for polycythemia vera, although lower doses of aspirin appear to be safe.[38]

Anagrelide is an orally active vasodilator that inhibits megakaryocyte maturation, thus decreasing the platelet count. In a study of more than 900 patients with thrombocytosis caused by a myeloproliferative disorder, anagrelide was found to reduce the platelet count in 80%, usually within 2 weeks.[39] A retrospective study of patients with the myeloproliferative disorder essential thrombocythemia showed that anagrelide was well tolerated over a 10-year period but that thrombotic events continued to occur in patients whose platelets remained above 400,000/µl.[40] No thrombotic events were observed in patients whose platelets were maintained in the normal range. Anagrelide is costly (approximately $10,300 a year for a total daily dose of 2.5 mg) and has a number of side effects, including headache, palpitations, diarrhea, fluid retention, and anemia. An advantage is that anagrelide has not been shown to increase the risk of AML. Anagrelide may be most useful in polycythemia vera patients who require a supplemental agent for optimal control of thrombocytosis; and if anagrelide is used, the goal should be to reduce the platelet count to normal.

Interferon alfa

Interferon alfa is a parenterally administered agent that can induce cytogenetic remission in some patients with CML. Because polycythemia vera, like CML, is a clonal myeloproliferative disorder, it was postulated that interferon alfa might also cause regression of the polycythemia vera neoplastic clone. Studies of patients who have been treated with interferon alfa for up to 6 years have shown that interferon alfa given three times a week can effectively control the hematocrit level and platelet count and reduce spleen size.[41,42] No thrombotic events were diagnosed in the patients treated with interferon alfa, in contrast to the high incidence of thrombosis in polycythemia vera patients treated with phlebotomy alone. Because only a small fraction of polycythemia vera patients have a cytogenetic abnormality, it is less clear what effect interferon alfa has on the neoplastic clone. Side effects of interferon alfa include prominent flulike symptoms that may abate after the first 1 to 2 months of therapy; approximately 20% of patients discontinue interferon alfa because of side effects.[42] Other problems include slow onset of action (months) and high cost (approximately $4,500 a year for 3 million units S.C. three times a week). However, if interferon alfa can be demonstrated to induce regression of the neoplastic clone or to impede progression to myeloid metaplasia, its benefits may outweigh these disadvantages.

Allogeneic Stem Cell Transplantation

Only a few patients with polycythemia vera have undergone myeloablative therapy and allogeneic stem cell transplantation. This highly investigational approach might be considered for a young patient with early evidence of marrow fibrosis.[43] Nonmyeloablative stem cell transplantation is also under investigation.

COMPLICATIONS

The postoperative period is a particularly risky time for patients with uncontrolled polycythemia vera (hematocrit higher than 52% at time of surgery). Many patients experience a postoperative complication, most often bleeding or thrombosis. The complication rate could be minimized by achieving good hematocrit control for at least 4 months before elective surgery.

Thrombosis

Thrombosis is the most common complication of polycythemia vera.[17,44] Several features of polycythemia vera likely contribute to this high incidence. The hematocrit value is directly related to risk of thrombosis: as hematocrit increases, cerebral blood flow declines, and incidence of thrombotic complications rises. This association between the hematocrit and risk of thrombosis forms the basis for a key recommendation regarding treatment of polycythemia vera: the hematocrit must be kept lower than 45% to decrease the risk of thrombosis. The platelets are derived from a neoplastic clone and may not function normally, which can result in either thrombosis or clinical bleeding. Bruising, epistaxis, and gastrointestinal bleeding are common.

In the initial clinical trial conducted by the Polycythemia Vera Study Group (PVSG), 431 patients were randomly assigned to treatment with phlebotomy alone, ^{32}P, or chlorambucil to keep the hematocrit level lower than 45%. In an update of this trial, 34% of patients had experienced thrombosis.[45] Polycythemia vera patients are at increased risk for both arterial thrombosis and venous thrombosis[17,44] [see Table 3]. Common clinical problems include stroke, myocardial infarction, deep vein thrombosis in the legs, transient ischemic attacks, and peripheral arterial occlusion. Patients often note exacerbation of angina as their hematocrit increases.

Hepatic vein thrombosis may occur, resulting in Budd-Chiari syndrome. In a study of 22 patients with Budd-Chiari syndrome,

Table 3 Arterial and Venous Thrombotic Events in 1,213 Polycythemia Vera Patients[17]

Event	Number
Arterial thrombosis	**145**
Myocardial infarction	55
Ischemic stroke	36
Transient ischemic attack	39
Peripheral arterial thrombosis	15
Venous thrombosis or embolism	**87**
Deep vein thrombosis	35
Superficial thrombophlebitis	37
Venous thrombosis, unknown site	15
Unknown	**22**
Total	**254**

10 (45%) had endogenous erythroid colonies, and their hepatic vein thrombosis may have been caused by an underlying myeloproliferative disorder; only two of these patients had overt polycythemia vera.[28] However, the low incidence of Budd-Chiari syndrome during the many years of follow-up of the first PVSG study argues against its being a frequent complication of polycythemia vera.

Polycythemia vera patients who have an acute thrombotic event and thrombocytosis should undergo plateletpheresis to rapidly reduce the platelet count to normal. They should then start myelosuppressive therapy (e.g., hydroxyurea) to maintain the platelet count within the normal range, even though no clear relation between high platelet count and risk of thrombosis has been established. If the patient has no history of excessive bleeding, addition of an agent that inhibits platelet function (e.g., aspirin, 81 mg/day) should also be considered. Patients with mucosal bleeding and thrombocytosis should be given a myelosuppressive agent to reduce the platelet count to normal.

Acute Myeloid Leukemia

One of the most feared complications of polycythemia vera is evolution to AML. Incidence of AML in polycythemia vera patients managed by phlebotomy alone is approximately 1% to 2%, a 100-fold increase over the incidence in an adult population of comparable age.[30] Treatment with chlorambucil or ^{32}P is associated with increased risk of AML. In one study, the onset of AML in the chlorambucil-treated patients was early; most cases occurred less than 5 years after the start of therapy, and AML eventually developed in 17% of the patients.[30] In patients who received ^{32}P, onset of AML was relatively late; most cases occurred 6 to 10 years after initiation of therapy, with a cumulative incidence of 10.9%.[30] Evolution to myelodysplasia may occur in some polycythemia vera patients, and a series of case reports suggests that myelosuppressive therapy may increase this risk as well. Treatment with either chlorambucil or ^{32}P was also associated with increased risk of nonhematopoietic malignancy.

If polycythemia vera evolves into AML, the chance of achieving durable, complete remission with standard induction chemotherapy is very low. Frank discussion of the therapeutic options, including the risks and benefits of induction chemotherapy versus supportive care, is warranted with these patients, who are often elderly and may have significant comorbid conditions [see Chapter 202].

Gout and Nephrolithiasis

Because of hyperuricemia, patients with polycythemia vera are at increased risk for gout or nephrolithiasis [*see Chapters 118 and 168*].

Myeloid Metaplasia

Approximately 20% of polycythemia vera patients experience postpolycythemic myeloid metaplasia, or the so-called spent phase of the myeloproliferative disorders.[37,46] Myeloid metaplasia is characterized by insidious replacement of the marrow space with reticulin fibrosis and gradual movement of hematopoiesis from the marrow into the spleen, liver, and occasionally other organs. The spleen and liver progressively enlarge and may become massive. Patients become progressively pancytopenic, in part because these organs provide a less nurturing niche for hematopoiesis and likely in part because of abnormalities intrinsic to the hematopoietic stem cells themselves. Teardrop red blood cells and a plethora of early myeloid cells are found in the circulation, giving rise to the leukoerythroblastic peripheral smear characteristic of myeloid metaplasia. Patients with myeloid metaplasia may have splenic pain and infarction because of massive splenomegaly and may experience early satiety, resulting in weight loss. Fibrosis in the marrow of patients with myeloid metaplasia is not part of the neoplastic clone; rather, it is reactive and may be induced by cytokines, such as platelet-derived growth factor, released by the abnormal megakaryocytes. Survival of patients with myeloid metaplasia is only about 3 years.

Treatment of myeloid metaplasia includes supportive care, with transfusions as needed, and judicious administration of hydroxyurea or busulfan to decrease spleen size. Splenectomy can be considered for the patient who has massive splenomegaly with weight loss caused by early satiety, pain from splenic infarction, or thrombocytopenia exacerbated by sequestration of platelets in a massively enlarged spleen. Splenectomy is a major undertaking in these patients and is usually followed by progressive hepatomegaly.[47] There is no convincing evidence at present that regression of marrow fibrosis can be achieved with hydroxyurea, ^{32}P, or interferon alfa.[32] Current research protocols are examining the use of allogeneic stem cell transplantation for treatment of myeloid metaplasia.[48]

Hypermetabolism and Pruritus

Hypermetabolic symptoms (e.g., chills, sweating, and fever not caused by infection) and pruritus often respond to hydroxyurea, interferon alfa,[41] or other myelosuppressive agents. For a patient with pruritus, avoidance of inciting events (e.g., hot showers) and the use of H_1 and H_2 receptor blockers can also be helpful.

References

1. Pearson TC, Guthrie DL, Simpson J, et al: Interpretation of measured red cell mass and plasma volume in adults: expert panel on radionuclides of the International Council for Standardization in Haematology. Br J Haematol 89:748, 1995

2. Messinezy M, Pearson TC: Apparent polycythaemia: diagnosis, pathogenesis and management. Eur J Haematol 51:125, 1993

3. Vongpatanasin W, Brickner ME, Hillis LD, et al: The Eisenmenger syndrome in adults. Ann Intern Med 128:745, 1998

4. Thorne SA: Management of polycythaemia in adults with cyanotic congenital heart disease. Heart 79:315, 1998

5. Ammash N, Warnes CA: Cerebrovascular events in adult patients with cyanotic congenital heart disease. J Am Coll Cardiol 28:768, 1996

6. Borst MM, Leschke M, König U, et al: Repetitive hemodilution in chronic obstructive pulmonary disease and pulmonary hypertension: effects on pulmonary hemodynamics, gas exchange, and exercise capacity. Respiration 66:225, 1999

7. Martin TJ, Sanders MH: Chronic alveolar hypoventilation: a review for the clinician. Sleep 18:617, 1995

8. Teran-Santos J, Jimenez-Gomez A, Cordero-Guevara J: The association between sleep apnea and the risk of traffic accidents. N Engl J Med 340:847, 1999

9. McNicholas WT: Obstructive sleep apnea syndrome: who should be treated? Sleep 23(suppl 4):S187, 2000

10. de la Chapelle A, Traskelin AL, Juvonen E: Truncated erythropoietin receptor causes dominantly inherited benign human erythrocytosis. Proc Natl Acad Sci U S A 90:4495, 1993

11. Arcasoy MO, Degar BA, Harris KW, et al: Familial erythrocytosis associated with a short deletion in the erythropoietin receptor. Blood 89:4628, 1997

12. Gregg XT, Prchal JT: Erythropoietin receptor mutations and human disease. Semin Hematol 34:70, 1997

13. Ebert BL, Bunn HF: Regulation of the erythropoietin gene. Blood 94:1864, 1999

14. Sergeyeva A, Gordeuk VR, Tokarev YN, et al: Congenital polycythemia in Chuvashia. Blood 89:2148, 1997

15. Besa EC: Hematologic effects of androgens revisited: an alternative therapy in various hematologic conditions. Semin Hematol 31:134, 1994

16. Gareau R, Audran M, Barnes R, et al: Erythropoietin abuse in athletes (letter). Nature 380:113, 1996

17. Polycythemia vera: the natural history of 1213 patients followed for 20 years: Gruppo Italiano Studio Policitemia. Ann Intern Med 123:656, 1995

18. Pahl HL: Towards a molecular understanding of polycythemia rubra vera. Eur J Biochem 267:3395, 2000

19. Shih LY, Lee CT, See LC, et al: In vitro culture growth of erythroid progenitors and serum erythropoietin assay in the differential diagnosis of polycythaemia. Eur J Clin Invest 28:569, 1998

20. Correa PN, Eskinazi D, Axelrad AA: Circulating erythroid progenitors in polycythemia vera are hypersensitive to insulin-like growth factor-1 in vitro: studies in an improved serum-free medium. Blood 83:99, 1994

21. Moliterno AR, Hankins WD, Spivak JL: Impaired expression of the thrombopoietin receptor by platelets from patients with polycythemia vera. N Engl J Med 338:572, 1998

22. Moliterno AR, Spivak JL: Posttranslational processing of the thrombopoietin receptor is impaired in polycythemia vera. Blood 94:2555, 1999

23. LeBlanc K, Andersson P, Samuelsson J: Marked heterogeneity in protein levels and functional integrity of the thrombopoietin receptor c-Mpl in polycythaemia vera. Br J Haematol 108:80, 2000

24. Horikawa Y, Matsumura I, Hashimoto K, et al: Markedly reduced expression of platelet c-Mpl receptor in essential thrombocythemia. Blood 90:4031, 1997

25. Silva M, Richard C, Benito A, et al: Expression of Bcl-x in erythroid precursors from patients with polycythemia vera. N Engl J Med 338:564, 1998

26. Temerinac S, Klippel S, Strunck E, et al: Cloning of PRV-1, a novel member of the uPAR receptor superfamily, which is overexpressed in polycythemia rubra vera. Blood 95:2569, 2000

27. Van Genderen PJ, Michiels JJ: Erythromelalgia: a pathognomonic microvascular thrombotic complication in essential thrombocythemia and polycythemia vera. Semin Thromb Hemost 23:357, 1997

28. Hirshberg B, Shouval D, Fibach E, et al: Flow cytometric analysis of autonomous growth of erythroid precursors in liquid culture detects occult polycythemia vera in the Budd-Chiari syndrome. J Hepatol 32:574, 2000

29. Pearson TC: Evaluation of diagnostic criteria in polycythemia vera. Semin Hematol 38(suppl 2):21, 2001

30. Fruchtman SM, Mack K, Kaplan ME, et al: From efficacy to safety: a polycythemia vera study group report on hydroxyurea in patients with polycythemia vera. Semin Hematol 34:17, 1997

31. Andreasson B, Carneskog J, Lindstedt G, et al: Plasma erythropoietin concentrations in polycythaemia vera with special reference to myelosuppressive therapy. Leuk Lymphoma 37:189, 2000

32. Kreft A, Nolde C, Busche G, et al: Polycythaemia vera: bone marrow histopathology under treatment with interferon, hydroxyurea and busulphan. Eur J Haematol 64:32, 2000

33. Di Pollina L, Mulligan R, Van der Linden A, et al: Cognitive impairment in polycythemia vera: partial reversibility upon lowering of the hematocrit. Eur Neurol 44:57, 2000

34. Najean Y, Rain J-D: The very long-term evolution of polycythemia vera: an analysis of 318 patients initially treated by phlebotomy or 32P between 1969 and 1981. Semin Hematol 34:6, 1997

35. Tatarsky I, Sharon R: Management of polycythemia vera with hydroxyurea. Semin Hematol 34:24, 1997

36. Best PJ, Daoud MS, Pittelkow MR, et al: Hydroxyurea-induced leg ulceration in 14 patients. Ann Intern Med 128:29, 1998

37. Najean Y, Rain J-D: Treatment of polycythemia vera: use of 32P alone or in combination with maintenance therapy using hydroxyurea in 461 patients greater than 65 years of age. Blood 89:2319, 1997

38. Low-dose aspirin in polycythaemia vera: a pilot study: Gruppo Italiano Studio Policitemia (GISP). Br J Haematol 97:453, 1997

39. Petitt RM, Silverstein MN, Petrone ME: Anagrelide for control of thrombocythemia in polycythemia and other myeloproliferative disorders. Semin Hematol 34:51, 1997

40. Storen EC, Tefferi A: Long-term use of anagrelide in young patients with essential thrombocythemia. Blood 97:863, 2001

41. Silver RT: Interferon alfa: effects of long-term treatment for polycythemia vera. Semin Hematol 34:40, 1997

42. Lengfelder E, Berger U, Hehlmann R: Interferon α in the treatment of polycythemia vera. Ann Hematol 79:103, 2000

43. Anderson JE, Sale G, Appelbaum FR, et al: Allogeneic marrow transplantation for primary myelofibrosis and myelofibrosis secondary to polycythaemia vera or essential thrombocytosis. Br J Haematol 98:1010, 1997

44. Brodmann S, Passweg JR, Gratwohl A, et al: Myeloproliferative disorders: complications, survival and causes of death. Ann Hematol 79:312, 2000

45. Berk PD, Wasserman LR, Fruchtman SM, et al: Treatment of polycythemia vera: a summary of clinical trials conducted by the Polycythemia Vera Study Group. Polycythemia Vera and the Myeloproliferative Disorders. Wasserman LR, Berk PD, Berlin NI, Eds. WB Saunders Co, Philadelphia, 1995, p 166

46. Tefferi A: Myelofibrosis with myeloid metaplasia. N Engl J Med 342:1255, 2000

47. Tefferi A, Mesa RA, Nagorney DM, et al: Splenectomy in myelofibrosis with myeloid metaplasia: a single-institution experience with 223 patients. Blood 95:2226, 2000

48. Guardiola P, Anderson JE, Bandini G, et al: Allogeneic stem cell transplantation for agnogenic myeloid metaplasia: a European Group for Blood and Marrow Transplantation, Société Francaise de Greffe de Moelle, Gruppo Italiano per il Trapianto del Midollo Osseo, and Fred Hutchinson Cancer Research Center Collaborative Study. Blood 93:2831, 1999

49. Berlin NI: Diagnosis and classification of the polycythemias. Semin Hematol 12:339, 1975

Acknowledgments

Figures 1 and 2   Marcia Kammerer.

Figures 3 and 4   Jared Schneidman.

David C. Dale, M.D.

Leukocytes, or white blood cells, protect the body against infections and participate in many types of immunologic and inflammatory responses. There are two main types of leukocytes: lymphocytes, which are responsible for antibody production and cell-mediated immunity, and phagocytes, which are responsible for the ingestion and killing of microorganisms. Neutrophils, monocytes, macrophages, and eosinophils are all phagocytes [see Figure 1]. Leukocytes interact with one another and modulate immune responses through the release of cytokines (interleukins and growth factors), enzymes, and vasoactive substances. This chapter covers the diagnosis of disorders of neutrophils, monocytes, and eosinophils and the treatment of neutropenia; the functions and disorders of lymphocytes are discussed elsewhere [see Immunology, Allergy, and Rheumatology].

The White Blood Cell Count

The total white blood cell (WBC) count and differential count are often the first studies performed in evaluating a patient with a suspected infection or with susceptibility to infections. Many laboratories use automated cell-counting techniques, which are now quite reliable.[1] The normal WBC ranges from 4,300 to 10,000/mm³, with a median of 7,000/mm³ [see Table 1]. A differential count gives the percentage for each type of leukocyte. The absolute count is determined by multiplying the total WBC by this percentage (e.g., WBC × percent neutrophils = absolute neutrophil count). Because the blood level of each type of leukocyte is separately regulated, it is always better to use the absolute count rather than the percentage in assessing abnormalities.

Indications of the Presence of a Phagocytic Cell Disorder

Because the phagocytes, particularly neutrophils, represent the first line of defense against invading microorganisms, disorders in the number or function of these cells often result in an increased susceptibility to infection. A quantitative or qualitative disorder of phagocytic cells should be suspected when a patient has an increased number of bacterial or fungal infections, increasingly severe infections, or infections with unusual organisms.

Neutrophil Physiology

NEUTROPHIL PRODUCTION

Neutrophils are derived from the common stem cell, which also gives rise to erythrocytes, platelets, and other leukocytes. The proliferation and differentiation of the neutrophil precursors are governed by a family of regulatory cytokines. For example, granulocyte-macrophage colony-stimulating factor (GM-CSF) stimulates progenitor cells to differentiate into neutrophils, eosinophils, and monocyte-macrophages. Granulocyte colony-stimulating factor (G-CSF) more selectively stimulates progenitor cells to differentiate into neutrophils [see Figure 2].[2] G-CSF and GM-CSF also affect the rate of neutrophil formation, the release of these cells into the blood, and their functions in the blood and tissues.[3,4]

The life cycle of the neutrophil consists of bone marrow, blood, and tissue phases. Neutrophil production in the bone marrow takes approximately 10 to 14 days, and the bone marrow pro-

duces approximately 1×10^9 neutrophils/kg/day.[5] Most of the body's neutrophil pool exists in the bone marrow. The mitotic compartment, which contains about 20% of the total neutrophil pool, consists of myeloblasts (the earliest morphologically recognizable precursors), promyelocytes, and myelocytes. The postmitotic pool or maturation compartment—the metamyelocytes, bands, and mature neutrophils—contains about 70% of the body's neutrophils. The marrow neutrophils and bands are sometimes called the storage compartment or marrow reserve. As neutrophils mature, they develop the capacity to enter the blood through increasing deformability and through changes in the adhesion proteins on their surface membranes. Entry into the blood involves complex and as yet poorly understood interactions of the mature cells and the endothelial cells of the marrow sinusoids. Stimulation of neutrophil release from the marrow with G-CSF, GM-CSF, corticosteroids, or endotoxin administration can result in a doubling or tripling of the blood neutrophil count within 3 to 5 hours. The peripheral blood contains fewer than 10% of the body's neutrophils. In the blood, the neutrophils are divided approximately evenly between the circulating pool and the marginating pool; these pools are in dynamic equilibrium. Cells in the marginating pool can be swept rapidly (within minutes) into the circulation by endogenous or exogenous epinephrine or as a result of exercise or any cause of rapid increase in cardiac output. This response, called demargination, can double the blood neutrophil count very rapidly and is also quickly reversible. The blood half-life of the neutrophils is approximately 6 to 10 hours. Neutrophils leave the blood and enter the tissues by migrating between endothelial cells and penetrating the capillary basement membrane. It is now believed that neutrophils that are not engaged in an extravascular inflammatory process die by apoptosis in the marrow or blood.[6]

NEUTROPHIL STRUCTURE

As neutrophil precursors mature, condensation and segmentation of nuclear chromatin occurs. Mature cells have no nucleoli, few mitochondria, and very little endoplasmic reticulum. The cytoplasm is filled with granules and glycogen. The primary granules, which appear at the myeloblast and promyelocyte stages, contain myeloperoxidase (MPO) proteases, defensins, and other antibacterial substances.[7] Secondary granules, produced primarily during the myelocyte stage, predominate in mature cells. They contain collagenase, lactoferrin, lysozyme, vitamin B_{12}–binding protein, and several other proteins. Small tertiary granules are also found in mature neutrophils. Neutrophils also may have cytoplasmic vesicles containing lactases, alkaline phosphatases, and components of NADPH oxidase.

The cytoskeleton of the neutrophil is composed of microtubules and microfilaments that are critical for phagocytic shape and movement, including migration through the vascular endothelium.[8] The microfilaments, which consist primarily of actin polymers, are dispersed throughout the cytoplasm.[9]

The surface of the neutrophil is replete with deep folds and ruffles. On the neutrophil surface, there are numerous receptors, including receptors for immunoglobulins (e.g., FcγRII [CD32], FcγRIII [CD16]), complement (e.g., CR3 [CD11b18], CR1 [CD35]),

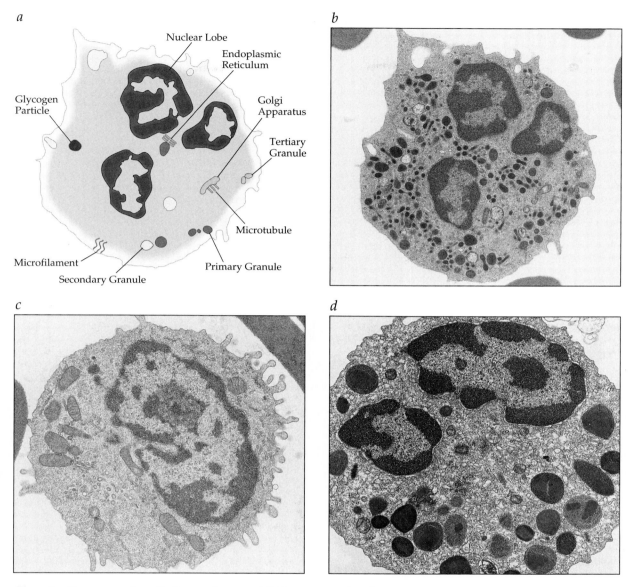

Figure 1 Shown are a schematic diagram of a neutrophil (*a*), a corresponding electron micrograph of a neutrophil (*b*), and electron micrographs of a monocyte (*c*) and an eosinophil (*d*).

chemokines, the colony-stimulating factors G-CSF and GM-CSF, Fas, tumor necrosis factor receptor (TNF-R), and the apoptosis-related receptors.

NEUTROPHIL FUNCTION

The major function of neutrophils is to respond rapidly to microbial invasion to kill the invaders. This response has several distinct steps—adherence, migration, recognition, phagocytosis (or ingestion), degranulation, oxidative metabolism, and bacterial killing [*see Figure 3*]. Susceptibility to infection results from abnormalities in any one or a combination of these processes.

Adherence

For neutrophils to move to an inflammatory site, they must first adhere to a capillary wall.[10] Loose adherence is facilitated by L-selectins, such as sialyl-Lewis^x (sLe^x), on the neutrophil and E-selectin and P-selectin on capillary endothelial cells [*see Figure 4*]. Bacterial invasion increases local selectin expression and neu-

trophil accumulation. Other neutrophil surface proteins, called β_2 integrins, facilitate firmer adhesion to endothelial cells and interact with actin and myosin to initiate movement of neutrophils to the tissue.[11] The three proteins in this family have a common β subunit (CD18) and a different α subunit (CD11a, CD11b, or CD11c). There is generally increased expression of these proteins (e.g., CD 11b/C18) on neutrophils in response to inflammation.[10] Concomitantly, there is increased expression of the intracellular adherence molecules (ICAMs) on the endothelial cells, with a net result of increased localization of neutrophils at the inflammatory focus.

Chemotaxis

Chemotaxis, the directed movement of cells, occurs when neutrophils detect a chemoattractant at low concentrations and move up the concentration gradient toward its source, which is usually a site in the extravascular spaces. Well-characterized stimulators of neutrophil chemotaxis are the complement proteins c3a and c5a, interleukin 8 (IL-8), and a family of small peptides, the che-

Table 1 Normal Leukocyte Values in Peripheral Blood

Cell Type	Cells/mm³*		Percentage of Total Differential Count
	Median	Range	
All leukocytes (white blood cells)	7,000	4,300–10,000	100
Total neutrophils	4,000	1,800–7,200	55
Band neutrophils	500	100–2,000	10
Segmented neutrophils	3,500	1,000–6,000	45
Lymphocytes	2,500	1,500–4,000	36
Monocytes	450	200–900	6
Eosinophils	150	0–700	2
Basophils	30	0–150	1

*To calculate the number of cells/L, multiply by 10^6.

mokines.[12] The trafficking of neutrophils is unidirectional; they do not return to the circulation.

Recognition and Phagocytosis

At the site of inflammation, neutrophils utilize their immunoglobulin and complement receptors to recognize bacteria and other particles coated or opsonized by immunoglobulins or complement [*see Chapters 98 and 100*]. Inflammation stimulates neutrophils to express increased numbers of the high-affinity IgG receptor FcγRI (CD64).[13] As the neutrophil internalizes a particle, a phagocytic vesicle, or phagosome, develops around it. This process stimulates degranulation and activates a burst of oxidative metabolism.

Degranulation

When the neutrophil is activated, the granule membranes come in contact with the plasma membranes surrounding the phago-some. The membranes fuse, which leads to the release of granule proteins into the phagosome and to the reorganization of the components of the critical NADPH oxidase system.[14]

Oxidative Metabolism and Bacterial Killing

Resting granulocytes are primarily anaerobic cells that rely on anaerobic glycolysis for adenosine triphosphate (ATP) production. Although chemotaxis, ingestion, and degranulation require some energy, they also proceed quite well anaerobically. However, bacterial killing generally is associated with a rapid increase (within seconds) in oxygen use. This respiratory burst occurs as a result of the activation of an NADPH oxidase.[15] Before activation, the components of the oxidase are located separately in the plasma and granule membranes and in the cytosol. The membranes contain two components, gp91phox and p22phox. The cytosol contains a p47 protein, a p67 protein, and some other proteins. When the neutrophil is activated, the cytosolic proteins first

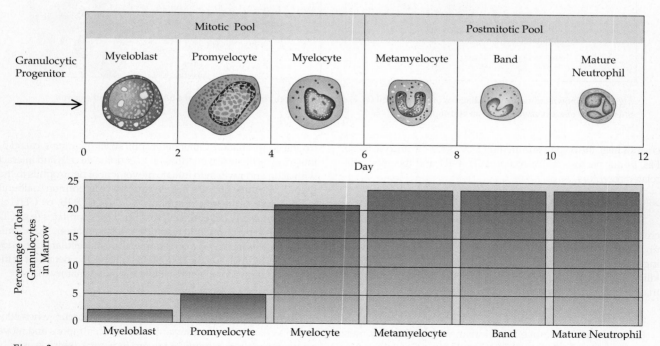

Figure 2 **The process of neutrophil maturation begins in the bone marrow (top). After about 12 days, approximately 10% of the mature neutrophils are released into the peripheral blood, where they have a half-life of approximately 6 to 10 hours. Eventually, the neutrophils migrate into the tissues by diapedesis. The percentage of neutrophils at each stage of development (bottom) ranges from about 2% at the myoblast stage to almost 25% at the mature neutrophil stage.**

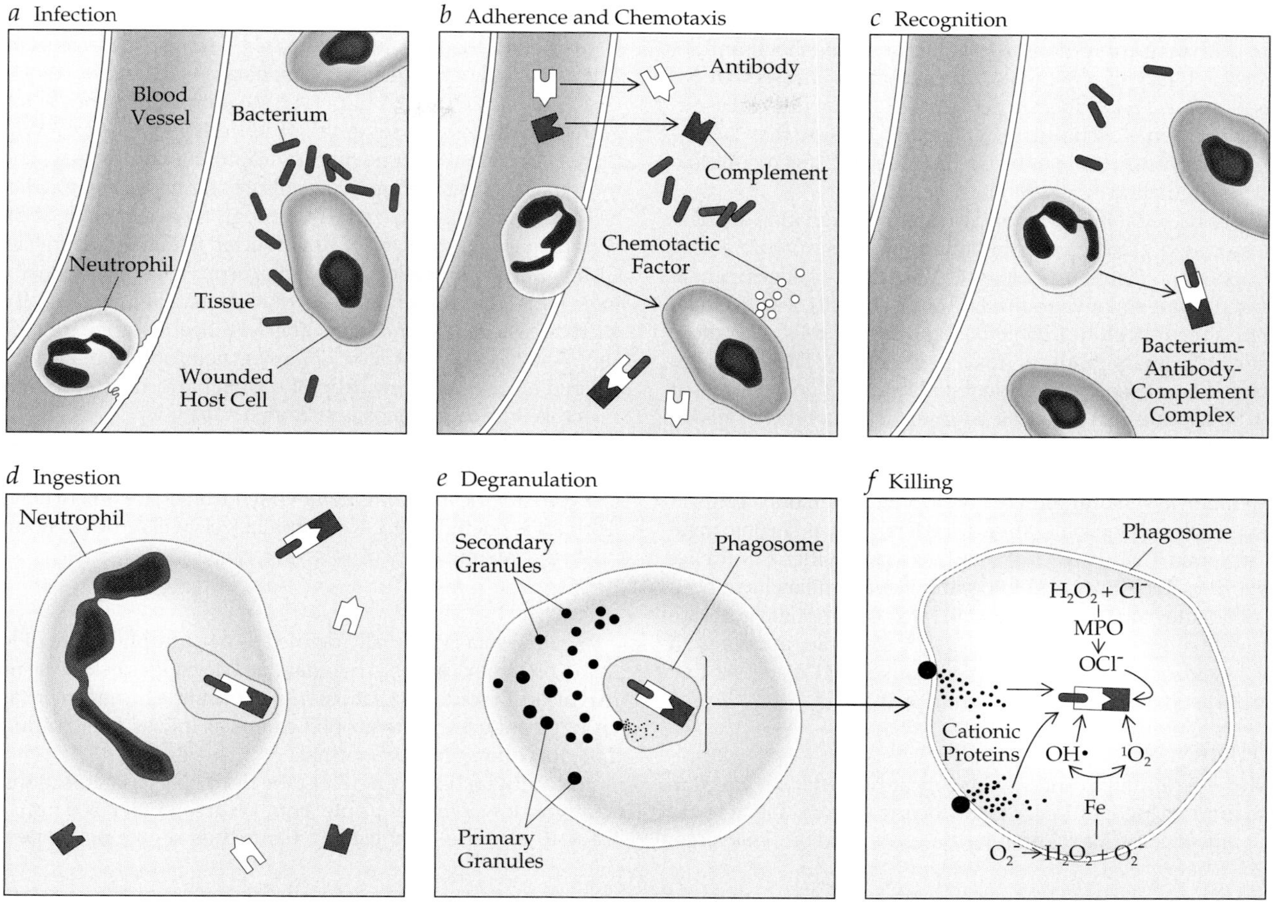

a Infection

Blood
Vessel
Bacterium

Neutrophil

Tissue

Wounded
Host Cell

b Adherence and Chemotaxis

Antibody

Complement

Chemotactic
Factor

c Recognition

Bacterium-
Antibody-
Complement
Complex

d Ingestion

Neutrophil

e Degranulation

Secondary
Granules

Phagosome

Primary
Granules

f Killing

Phagosome

$H_2O_2 + Cl^-$

MPO

OCl^-

Cationic
Proteins $OH\cdot$ $^1O_2$

Fe

$O_2^- \rightarrow H_2O_2 + O_2^-$

Figure 3   The neutrophil response to bacterial invasion involves several stages. A bacterium infects a host cell and injures it (*a*). Bacterial products, antibodies, and complement cause the release of chemotactic factors, which activate a neutrophil in the adjacent blood vessel. The neutrophil adheres to the vessel wall and undergoes chemotaxis and diapedesis into tissue (*b*) to follow the chemoattractants to their sites of generation or expression. The neutrophil recognizes (*c*) and ingests (*d*) the bacterium-antibody-complement complex, forming a phagosome. The neutrophil then undergoes degranulation, a process in which granule membranes fuse with the plasma membrane (*e*). Degranulation releases various enzymes and enhances oxidative metabolism, the products of which are bactericidal (*f*). For example, hydrogen peroxide (H_2O_2), produced from superoxide (O_2^-) can interact with O_2^- in the presence of iron (Fe) to produce hydroxyl radicals ($OH\cdot$) and singlet oxygen ($^1O_2$), both of which are highly toxic to bacteria. In addition, H_2O_2 and chloride (Cl^-) combine in the presence of the myeloperoxidase (MPO) released in the phagosome to produce hypochlorite (OCl^-), which is also bactericidal.

associate and then combine with the membrane components to produce the complete NADPH oxidase. NADPH oxidase can reduce oxygen by one electron to superoxide O_2^-; in the process, NADPH is converted to $NADP^+$. The NADPH is then regenerated through the hexose monophosphate shunt. Dismutation of the superoxide in the presence of superoxide dismutase produces hydrogen peroxide (H_2O_2), which can then be converted to hydroxyl radical ($OH\cdot$); H_2O_2, O_2^-, and $OH\cdot$ are highly toxic. In addition, within the phagocyte vacuole, hydrogen peroxide and chloride (Cl^-) can combine in the presence of myeloperoxidase to produce hypochlorous acid (HOCl), which is bactericidal.[16] These products of the respiratory burst can also be released from the activated neutrophil and subsequently damage the surrounding cells and tissues.

Responses to and Production of Cytokines

The growth factors that affect neutrophil production, such as G-CSF and GM-CSF, also influence neutrophil function.[17] These cytokines upregulate stimulus-dependent NADPH oxidase ac-

tivity and can enhance bactericidal and fungicidal activities. Although neutrophils contain very few ribosomes, they can respond to bacterial stimuli by synthesizing and secreting proinflammatory cytokines such as interleukin-1 (IL-1), IL-6, and tumor necrosis factor–α (TNF-α).[18]

Disorders of Neutrophil Number

NEUTROPHILIA

Neutrophilia, or granulocytosis, is usually defined as a neutrophil count greater than 10,000/mm[3].

Etiology

Neutrophilia most often occurs secondary to inflammation, stress, or corticosteroid therapy. Cigarette smoking commonly causes neutrophilia as a result of inflammation in the airways and lungs. Malignancies, hemolytic anemia, and lithium therapy are less common causes. Neutrophilia is also associated with splenectomy. Extreme neutrophilia (i.e., neutrophil counts of more than 30,000 to 50,000/mm³), often called a leukemoid reaction, occurs with severe infections, sepsis, hemorrhagic shock, and severe tissue injury of any cause. Neutrophilia is also seen in patients with leukocyte adhesion deficiency (LAD), a rare disease in which neutrophils accumulate in the blood because they lack either the integrin CD11b18 or the selectin sLe^x (CD15s) required to leave the circulation.[19]

Serious bacterial infections and chronic inflammation are usually associated with changes in both the number of circulating neutrophils and their morphology. Characteristic changes include increased numbers of young cells (bands), of cells with residual endoplasmic reticulum (Döhle bodies), and of cells with more prominent primary granules (toxic granulation). These changes are probably caused by the endogenous production of G-CSF or GM-CSF and are also seen with administration of these growth factors.

Primary neutrophilia (i.e., neutrophilia attributed to defects in proliferation and maturation of neutrophil precursors) occurs in patients with myeloproliferative disorders, such as chronic myeloid leukemia (CML) [*see Chapter 204*] and polycythemia vera [*see Chapter 90*]. Hereditary and idiopathic neutrophilias have been described; they are benign and quite rare. Neutrophilia is associated with congenital abnormalities. For example, infants with Down syndrome can have transient leukemoid reactions that must be distinguished from congenital leukemia.[20]

Diagnosis

When neutrophilia cannot be readily attributed to an infection or inflammatory condition or to glucocorticosteroid therapy, the possibility of a myeloproliferative disease should be considered.

The presence of splenomegaly, metamyelocytes, and myelocytes in the blood, together with increased basophils or eosinophils and a low leukocyte alkaline phosphatase (LAP) score, suggests CML [*see Chapter 204*]. A high LAP score or the presence of toxic granulations usually suggests an underlying infection. When there is uncertainty, bone marrow aspiration and biopsy, chromosomal analysis, and marrow cultures for bacteria (e.g., *Salmonella, Brucella, Mycobacterium,* and fungi) are warranted. The results of these tests will enable the clinician to make a diagnosis of CML (or another myeloproliferative disorder), a granulomatous infection, inflammatory disease, or metastatic malignancy. If no such cause can be found in an otherwise healthy-appearing person, a diagnosis of idiopathic or familial neutrophilia may be considered and repeated neutrophil counts performed at monthly intervals until the diagnosis is clarified.

Treatment

Except for the myeloproliferative syndromes, treatment of neutrophilia is not indicated. Neutrophil levels will return to normal when the inflammatory process is resolved.

NEUTROPENIA

Neutropenia is generally defined as a neutrophil count of less than 1,800/mm³, which is two standard deviations below the normal mean. In some populations (e.g., Africans, African Americans, and Yemenite Jews), neutrophil counts as low as 1,000/mm³, or 1.0×10^9/L, are probably normal.[21,22]

In otherwise healthy persons, the risk of bacterial infections is relatively low if the neutrophil count is greater than 500 mm³, or 0.5×10^9/L—the level usually defined as severe neutropenia.

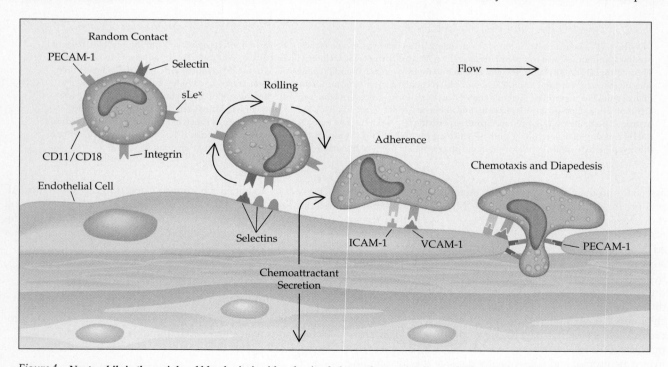

Figure 4 Neutrophils in the peripheral blood exist in either the circulating or the marginating pool. The marginated neutrophils roll along a vessel wall, where their surface carbohydrates interact with selectins on the endothelial cells. After activation by chemotactic agents, the neutrophils change shape and change the affinity of their integrin molecules for endothelial cell intercellular adhesion molecules. The neutrophils then crawl and undergo diapedesis by interacting with platelet–endothelial cell adhesion molecules on the endothelial surface and by liberating hydrolases that permit passage of the neutrophils through the capillary basement membrane. (PECAM-1—platelet–endothelial cell adhesion molecule–1; sLe^x—sialyl-Lewis^x carbohydrate; ICAM-1—intercellular adhesion molecule–1; VCAM-1—vascular cell adhesion molecule–1)

Table 2   Drugs Associated with Neutropenia

ANALGESICS	ANTICONVULSANTS	ANTITHYROID DRUGS	PHENOTHIAZINES
Aminopyrine	Phenytoin	Methimazole	Chlorpromazine
Dipyrone	Primidone	Methylthiouracil	Methylpromazine
	Trimethadione	Potassium perchlorate	Prochlorperazine
ANTIBIOTICS		Propylthiouracil	Promazine
Cephalosporins	ANTIHISTAMINES		Thioridazine
Chloramphenicol	Brompheniramine	CARDIOVASCULAR AGENTS	Trifluoperazine
Clindamycin	Cimetidine	Captopril	Trimeprazine
Doxycycline	Ranitidine	Diazoxide	
Flucytosine	Thenalidine	Hydralazine	SEDATIVES AND
Gentamicin	Tripelennamine	Methyldopa	NEUROPHARMACOLOGIC
Griseofulvin		Pindolol	AGENTS
Isoniazid	ANTI-INFLAMMATORY AGENTS	Procainamide	Chlordiazepoxide
Lincomycin	Fenoprofen	Propranolol	Clozapine
Metronidazole	Gold salts	Quinidine	Desipramine
Nitrofurantoin	Ibuprofen		Diazepam
Penicillins	Indomethacin	DIURETICS	Imipramine
Rifampin	Phenylbutazone	Acetazolamide	Meprobamate
Streptomycin		Bumetanide	Metoclopramide
Sulfonamides	ANTIMALARIALS	Chlorothiazide	
Vancomycin	Amodiaquine	Chlorthalidone	MISCELLANEOUS AGENTS
	Dapsone	Hydrochlorothiazide	Allopurinol
ANTICONVULSANTS	Hydroxychloroquine	Methazolamide	Colchicine
Carbamazepine	Pyrimethamine	Spironolactone	Ethanol
Ethosuximide	Quinine		Levamisole
Mephenytoin		HYPOGLYCEMIC AGENTS	Levodopa
	ANTITHYROID DRUGS	Chlorpropamide	Penicillamine
	Carbimazole	Tolbutamide	

The risk of infection, however, is greater when neutropenia develops after myelotoxic chemotherapy or when there are other abnormalities in a patient's host defenses. These conditions include lymphocytopenia, monocytopenia, hypogammaglobulinemia, HIV infection, disruptive mucosal or cutaneous barriers, and the administration of corticosteroids. Patients with neutropenia are at higher risk for infection by those pathogenic organisms that normally colonize body surfaces, particularly the skin, the oropharynx, and the GI tract. Thus, infections from staphylococci occur in neutropenic patients after breaks in the skin. Infection by mixtures of aerobic and anaerobic organisms of the oropharynx frequently causes gingivitis, pharyngitis, and sinusitis with neutropenia. Gram-negative bacilli often invade the blood from the GI tract in these patients. Antibiotic therapy, particularly therapy involving broad-spectrum antibiotics and protracted treatments, leads to colonization by resistant bacteria and to fungal infections.[23,24]

Neutropenia results from primary abnormalities of cell formation in congenital disorders and in the myeloid malignancies, as well as from secondary causes such as drug therapy, infections, and immunologic disorders, including autoimmune diseases. Neutropenia arises from secondary causes far more often than from primary disorders of cell formation.

Etiology

Drug-induced neutropenia   In aggregate, drug reactions are probably the most common cause of neutropenia in adults [*see Table 2*].[25] Many cancer chemotherapy drugs, some of which are also used as cytotoxic immunosuppressive agents (e.g., cyclophosphamide, methotrexate, and azathioprine), predictably cause dose-dependent neutropenia. The use of these agents requires careful attention to medical history, dosages, treatment schedules, and serial neutrophil counts to avoid serious and life-threatening toxicity. Other drugs cause neutropenia idiosyncrati-

cally. Many of these reactions probably occur because drugs can act as immunogens or as haptens, causing immunologic injury to neutrophils and their precursors. Other mechanisms of drug-induced neutropenia may involve direct toxicity of marrow cells in susceptible persons.[26] Most patients recover from drug-induced neutropenia; the time for recovery can vary from 2 days to 2 weeks or more.

Infection-associated neutropenia   Viral infections often cause mild neutropenia, especially in children. Such infections include measles and other viral exanthems, infectious mononucleosis, hepatitis, and HIV infection. The mechanisms are diverse. For example, in HIV infection, possible mechanisms include infections of the hematopoietic precursor cells and the marrow stromal cells, which lead to decreased production; induction of autoantibodies, which leads to accelerated turnover of mature neutrophils; and accelerated apoptosis of mature cells.[27] HIV-associated neutropenia generally develops late in AIDS and is often compounded by the use of antiviral agents (e.g., zidovudine, ganciclovir), antibiotics (e.g., sulfonamides), or the presence of hematologic malignancies (e.g., lymphoma, Kaposi sarcoma).[28] With other viral infections, the neutropenia is usually mild and without serious consequences. In rare instances, infectious mononucleosis causes severe hypoplasia, which has more severe consequences.[29] Neutropenia and anemia are common features of human parvovirus B19 infection.[30]

With severe bacterial infections, neutropenia occurs as a consequence of endotoxemia, which results in rapid neutrophil mobilization and turnover, especially in patients with a marrow reserve that is impaired because of previous chemotherapy, other drugs, or alcohol.[31] In this setting, neutropenia generally portends a grave prognosis. Neutropenia occurs in parasitic infections associated with splenomegaly, such as kala-azar and acute malaria, presumably as a result of splenic trapping of the cells.

Autoimmune and idiopathic neutropenia Autoimmune neutropenia occurs as an isolated phenomenon or secondary to other autoimmune disorders. In patients with Evans syndrome, it is associated with immune thrombocytopenia and hemolytic anemia.[32] Characteristically, the bone marrow cellularity is normal or increased, with a relative decrease in the number of cells in the late stages of the neutrophil pathway and an increase in blood monocytes. The diagnosis of autoimmune neutropenia requires specific antineutrophil antibody tests.[33] Because these tests are not widely available,[34] it is often difficult to distinguish autoimmune neutropenia from cases otherwise categorized as idiopathic neutropenia. Neutropenia with antineutrophil antibodies also occurs in systemic lupus erythematosus,[35,36] Sjögren syndrome,[37] rheumatoid arthritis,[38] and Felty syndrome (i.e., rheumatoid arthritis, splenomegaly, and neutropenia).[39,40]

Patients with rheumatoid arthritis and neutropenia often have clonal expansion of large granular lymphocytes (usually CD2+, CD3+, CD8+, and CD57+ cells), which may impair neutrophil production by excessive Fas ligand production.[41] The marrow typically shows increased lymphocytes with reduced neutrophils in the later stages of development. In most patients, the lymphocytosis is clonal and may evolve very gradually into a lymphoid malignancy.[42]

In sarcoidosis, cirrhosis, and congestive splenomegaly of diverse causes, neutropenia and thrombocytopenia often occur concomitantly, presumably because of splenic sequestration. In most instances, the neutropenia is mild and without recognizable consequences.

Other secondary causes of neutropenia Neonates can have neutropenia because of transplacental transfer of maternal IgG antibodies to the FcγRIII (CD16) isotype (previously called NA-1 or NA-2) that is inherited from the infant's father.[43] This abnormality is transient, usually lasting less than 3 months. Transient neutropenia also can occur in an infant as a result of transplacental transfer of other antibodies (e.g., transfer of IgG) from a mother with autoimmune neutropenia. The causes of other forms of benign neutropenia in children and adults are often difficult to establish; these forms of neutropenia may be either autoimmune or of unknown cause.[32,33] Pure white cell aplasia is a rare acquired condition characterized by a complete absence of myeloid precursors.[44] Pure white cell aplasia may be associated with a thymoma; if so, the aplasia may respond on removal of the thymoma. The short-term consequences of all these conditions depend primarily upon the level of blood neutrophils and the proliferative response of the marrow when inflammation or infections occur.

Primary forms of neutropenia There are a number of congenital and inherited causes of neutropenia [see Table 3].

Diagnosis

Neutropenia is easily diagnosed by performing a white blood cell count and differential count. When severe neutropenia occurs after cancer chemotherapy, either from immunosuppressive drugs or as an idiosyncratic reaction to other drugs, the patient is often febrile and acutely ill, a condition often referred to as acute febrile neutropenia. In this circumstance, attention is immediately focused on determining whether the patient has an infection and on instituting empirical antibiotic therapy. Hematologic studies (e.g., bone marrow examination) are generally not necessary, because the neutropenia will resolve if the inciting cause has been eliminated.

Table 3 Intrinsic Disorders of Neutrophils That Cause Neutropenia

Disorder	Inheritance	Clinical Features	Diagnosis	Treatment
Severe congenital neutropenia (also known as infantile genetic agranulocytosis and Kostmann syndrome)	AR, S	From birth, upper respiratory, lung, liver, and skin infections; mild anemia; thrombocytosis; a normal immune system; possible development of leukemia	Selective, severe neutropenia; marrow promyelocytes but few more mature cells; marrow eosinophils; normal chromosomes; possible G-CSF receptor defect	G-CSF (effective in most cases); bone marrow transplantation; prophylactic antibiotics
Congenital neutropenia (also known as benign congenital or childhood neutropenia)	AD, AR, S	Similar to but less severe than severe congenital neutropenia; may be asymptomatic	Similar to but less severe than severe congenital neutropenia	G-CSF, but treatment is usually unnecessary
Myelokathexis	AD, S	Recurrent infections; severe leukopenia and neutropenia	Marrow cellularity normal with maturing, often binucleate neutrophils	G-CSF
Cyclic neutropenia (also known as cyclic hematopoiesis)	AD, S	Regular oscillations of blood cell counts, most prominently of neutrophil and monocyte counts	Serial CBCs show severe neutropenia that recurs regularly, usually every 21 days	G-CSF
Shwachman-Diamond syndrome	AR	Neutropenia with pancreatic insufficiency and sometimes with anemia or thrombocytopenia	Neutropenia with malabsorption caused by pancreatic enzyme deficiency; tests for cystic fibrosis negative	G-CSF; pancreatic enzymes
Chédiak-Higashi syndrome	AR, S	Recurrent infections; partial albinism; lymphoproliferative syndrome; neutropenia; thrombocytopenia	Giant cytoplasmic granules; defective neutrophil migration and bacterial killing	Antibiotics; vitamin C; bone marrow transplantation
Reticular dysgenesis and congenital immunodeficiency syndromes with neutropenia	AR, S	From birth, severe infections with severe leukopenia	Neutropenia; hypogammaglobulinemia; T cell and B cell deficiencies	Bone marrow transplantation; immunoglobulin therapy; G-CSF for neutropenia
Dyskeratosis congenita	AR	Severe infections; skin hyperpigmentation; dystrophic nails; leukoplakia	Skin changes associated with severe neutropenia	Prophylactic antibiotics

AD—autosomal dominant AR—autosomal recessive CBC—complete blood count G-CSF—granulocyte colony-stimulating factor S—sporadic cases

Table 4 Guidelines for Management and Prevention of Febrile Neutropenia[45]

Management

Take careful history and conduct thorough physical examination of the patient

Examine patient carefully for portal for bacterial or fungal infections

Culture blood and other appropriate body fluids

Start antibiotics immediately

Monotherapy (e.g., ceftazidime or imipenem) or duotherapy (e.g., an aminoglycoside, such as gentamicin, with a β-lactam drug that is effective against *Pseudomonas,* such as piperacillin

Add vancomycin if there is a significant risk of gram-positive sepsis

Adjust antibiotic therapy after 3 days, depending on the results of cultures and the patient's clinical status

Switch low-risk patients to oral therapy

Continue broad-spectrum therapy for severely ill patients*

Consider antifungal treatments

Consider colony-stimulating factors as an adjunct to antibiotics for febrile neutropenia in severely ill, high-risk patients†

Prevention

Primary prophylaxis with G-CSF reduces incidence of febrile neutropenia by ~50% when the risk of febrile neutropenia is ~40%‡

Use G-CSF or GM-CSF as a preventive strategy for patients who have had their treatment reduced or experienced a delay in treatment because of an episode of febrile neutropenia or a prolonged period of neutropenia

Consider reducing the intensity of chemotherapy

Note: further information can be found at the following Web sites: www.idsociety.org, www.asco.org, and www.guidelines.gov.
*Resolution of illness generally follows resolution of neutropenia.
†For most patients with febrile neutropenia, CSF therapy has no proven benefit.
‡Administration of G-CSF or GM-CSF is not routinely indicated in previously untreated patients.
G-CSF—granulocyte colony-stimulating factor   GM-CSF—granulocyte-macrophage colony-stimulating factor

Initial evaluation of patients with chronic neutropenia should include a careful family history and review of the incidence and severity of infections, including oral ulcers, gingivitis, cellulitis, and more serious problems. A complete blood count will reveal whether the neutropenia is isolated or associated with other hematologic abnormalities. Medications should be discontinued if they can be implicated as causes of the neutropenia. A bone marrow biopsy and aspirate are indicated if there is any question of myelodysplasia or a hematologic malignancy. Serologic testing for infectious mononucleosis, hepatitis, and HIV is often warranted, as is measurement of antinuclear antibodies and rheumatoid factor titers. Broader immunologic assessments (i.e., lymphocyte subtypes and immunoglobulin levels) are warranted if the history suggests a susceptibility to infections by viruses, parasites, or bacteria, and they are also used to detect clonal proliferation of lymphocytes and to diagnose the large granular lymphocyte syndrome.[42] Neutrophil mobilization with corticosteroids and demargination tests with epinephrine are rarely helpful.

Treatment

Evidence-based guidelines for management and prevention of acute febrile neutropenia associated with cancer chemotherapy have been developed by the Infectious Disease Society of America (www.idsociety.org) and the American Society of Clin-

ical Oncology (www.asco.org). Other guidelines are also available (www.guideline.gov) [*see Table 4*]. In general, acute management of severe, idiosyncratic, drug-induced neutropenia should be similarly managed.[45]

Treatments for chronic neutropenia vary with the severity of neutropenia and the pattern of susceptibility to infection. With few exceptions, use of corticosteroids, γ-globulin injections, androgens, and splenectomy is rarely helpful. When these patients have a suspected infection, short-term, broad-spectrum antibiotic therapy is indicated, usually initiated after culture of blood and other body fluids for bacteria. Long-term antibiotic therapy is of unproven benefit in preventing infections, and it carries the risk of colonization by antibiotic-resistant organisms. The neutropenia in Felty syndrome often responds to splenectomy as well as to weekly doses of methotrexate.[46,47] G-CSF, usually in doses of 1 to 5 μg/kg/day, is of proven benefit for the treatment of congenital, idiopathic, and cyclic neutropenia and hastens the recovery of marrow from neutropenia after cancer chemotherapy.[48] G-CSF and GM-CSF have been widely used to treat other forms of chronic neutropenia, including the neutropenia associated with HIV infection.[28,49]

Disorders of Neutrophil Function

In patients who have recurrent, severe, or unusual infections but who have a normal number of neutrophils, the presence of a neutrophil function disorder must be considered. Neutrophil function disorders are caused by defects in neutrophil adherence, chemotaxis, degranulation, or oxidative metabolism [*see Table 5*].

The evaluation of patients with confirmed, recurrent, or unusual infections is first to review the family history and then to examine the patient [*see Figure 5*]. A complete blood count and examination of the granulocytes in a blood smear can show neutrophilia or neutropenia, specific granule deficiency, or giant granules such as those that occur in Chédiak-Higashi syndrome. In children, if significant normocytic anemia is present, glucose-6-phosphate dehydrogenase (G6PD) deficiency or glutathione synthetase deficiency should be considered.[50] Evaluation of immunoglobulin levels (IgG, IgM, IgA, and IgE) and complement levels (C3 and CH₅₀) are also potentially helpful, especially if there is a pattern of infection by encapsulated bacteria or unusual organisms [*see Chapter 100*]. After these considerations, neutrophil function should be evaluated with the nitroblue tetrazolium (NBT) test, superoxide production assays, and chemotactic assays. The NBT test and superoxide assays can determine whether a patient has chronic granulomatous disease (CGD), severe G6PD deficiency, or a glutathione pathway disorder[19]; chemotactic assays can be used to confirm the diagnosis of Chédiak-Higashi syndrome and acquired chemotactic defects.[51] Leukocyte adhesion deficiency types I and II are diagnosed by flow cytometry.[19] If the results of all of these tests are normal, ingestion assays using the patient's serum and cells and staining for MPO may be helpful. In this manner, all of the known neutrophil function abnormalities can be diagnosed, often with the aid of specialty consultations and a research laboratory.

Monocytes and Macrophage Physiology

Monocytes and macrophages play critical roles in homeostasis and in host defense mechanisms. Monocytes and macrophages perform tissue maintenance functions, such as clearance of particles—including bacteria—from the blood and removal of old red blood cells. They process antigens by interacting with T cells and B cells and are essential for containment of mycobacterial, parasitic, fungal, and viral infections.

MONOCYTE-MACROPHAGE DEVELOPMENT

Monocytes develop from hematopoietic progenitor cells in the bone marrow. Once the progenitor cells are committed to a monocyte lineage, they develop morphologically into monoblasts, then promonocytes, and then monocytes. The cytokines responsible for final commitment of these cells to the monocyte lineages are probably macrophage colony-stimulating factor (M-CSF) and GM-CSF.[52]

MONOCYTE-MACROPHAGE FUNCTION

The tissue mononuclear phagocyte system comprises monocytes, tissue and alveolar macrophages, Kupffer cells, osteoclasts, peritoneal and splenic macrophages, dendritic cells, and Langerhans cells. In addition to having phagocytic capabilities, monocytes and macrophages play a role in many aspects of the immune response.

With the exception of the alveolar macrophages, which are uniquely dependent on aerobic metabolism for energy production, monocytes and macrophages are facultative anaerobes. Phagocytosis by monocytes and macrophages is associated with an oxidative burst and stimulation of the hexose monophosphate shunt. Adhesion, chemotaxis, and activation are similar for monocytes and neutrophils, although macrophages are better than neutrophils at phagocytosis and perform chemotaxis less rapidly and efficiently. Macrophages are also capable of oxygen-independent bactericidal activity that may depend on lytic activity. Furthermore, stimulated macrophages are capable of producing nitric oxide.[53] Macrophages are capable of secreting many cytokines, growth factors, and acute-phase reactants.

Monocytes and macrophages present antigen to T cells in association with major histocompatibility complex (MHC) class II molecules. This association occurs within the lysosomes of a mononuclear cell before the MHC class II molecules are expressed on the cell surface [see Chapter 99]. Monocytes and macrophages are involved in antibody-dependent and antibody-independent cell-mediated cytotoxicity. The cytotoxicity involves oxidative metabolism, the production of nitric oxide and cytokines, and the secretion of cytotoxic mediators.

Macrophages play a key role in metabolizing high-molecular-weight proteins, glycoproteins, and other material and are intimately involved in the destruction of senescent and killed cells. They also are required for angiogenesis and wound healing and are able to induce neovascularization and endothelial cell proliferation.

Disorders of Monocytes and Macrophages

HISTIOCYTIC SYNDROMES

Histiocytic syndromes are a group of malignant and nonmalignant disorders in which the macrophages and dendritic (Langerhans) cells are the principal cells of abnormality.[54] The malignant disorders include acute monocytic leukemia; malignant histiocytosis, also called histiocytic medullary reticulosis [see Chapter 202]; and true histiocytic lymphoma.[55] The nonmalignant disorders include the Langerhans cell histiocytosis (LCH) syndromes and the hemophagocytic syndromes, such as sinus histiocytosis with massive lymphadenopathy, familial hemophagocytic lymphohistiocytosis (FHL), and infection-associated hemophagocytic syndrome (IAHS).

Table 5 Selected Disorders of Neutrophil Function

	Disorder	Inheritance	Clinical Features	Diagnosis	Treatment
Adherence Defects	Leukocyte adhesion deficiency I	AR	Neutrophilia with recurrent severe infections; failure of pus formation; delayed umbilical cord separation	Decreased neutrophil adherence and migration; CD11/CD18 deficiency	Bone marrow transplantation; antibiotics
	Leukocyte adhesion deficiency II	S, possibly AR	Neutrophilia with recurrent infections	Neutrophils lack surface sLe^x and have deficient adherence	Bone marrow transplantation; antibiotics
	Actin polymerization defect	AR, S	Recurrent severe infections	Defective neutrophil migration and ingestion of bacteria	Bone marrow transplantation; antibiotics
Granule Defects	Chédiak-Higashi syndrome	AR, S	Recurrent infections; partial albinism; lymphoproliferative syndrome; neutropenia; thrombocytopenia	Giant cytoplasmic granules; defective neutrophil migration and bacterial killing	Antibiotics; vitamin C; bone marrow transplantation
	Specific granule deficiency	S, possibly AR	Recurrent infections, especially sinopulmonary and skin infections	Absence of specific (secondary) granules in neutrophils; abnormal neutrophil migration and respiratory burst	Antibiotics
Respiratory Burst Defects	Chronic granulomatous disease	AR or X-linked	Recurrent skin, pulmonary, and liver abscesses	Severely defective respiratory burst; NBT test; abnormality in one of four subunits of NADPH oxidase	Interferon gamma; antibiotics
	Glucose-6-phosphate dehydrogenase deficiency	X-linked	Recurrent bacterial infections; hemolytic anemia	Reduced levels of glucose-6-phosphate dehydrogenase	Antibiotics
	Myeloperoxidase deficiency	AR	Mild, if any, susceptibility to infection	Reduced levels of myeloperoxidase	Generally none indicated

AR—autosomal recessive   NBT—nitroblue tetrazolium   S—sporadic cases   sLe^x—sialyl-Lewis^x

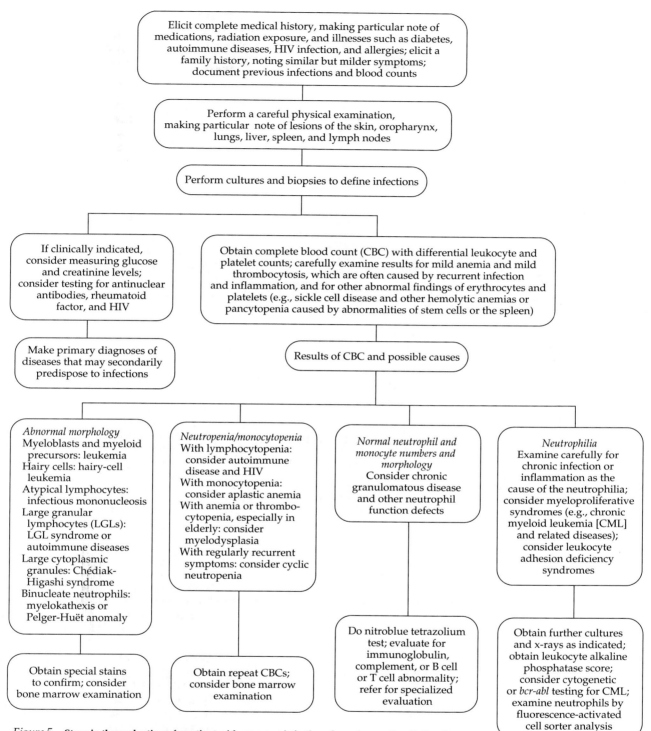

Figure 5 **Steps in the evaluation of a patient with recurrent infections for a phagocytic cell disorder.**

Langerhans Cell Histiocytosis Syndromes

Classically, the LCH syndromes comprise solitary eosinophilic granuloma, multifocal eosinophilic granuloma, Hand-Schüller-Christian disease, and Letterer-Siwe disease.[56] These disorders predominantly affect infants and young children but have also been seen in young adults. Because the LCH syndromes represent a continuum of disease that frequently cannot be broken down into these rigid and arbitrary designations, other classification systems that relate to age at diagnosis, extent of disease, and presence of organ dysfunction have been developed.[57] The signs and symptoms of the LCH syndromes depend on the organs involved.[58] The bones, skin, teeth, gingival tissue, ears, endocrine organs, lungs, liver, spleen, lymph nodes, and bone marrow can all be involved and become dysfunctional as a result of cellular infiltration. Diabetes insipidus is also common.

Both solitary and multifocal eosinophilic granuloma are found predominantly in older children and young adults. On presentation, patients with solitary lesions may have an inability to bear weight, or they may have tender swelling caused by tissue infiltrates that overlie a sharply marginated bony lesion. Hand-Schüller-Christian disease, generally a multifocal condition, occurs in children 2 to 5 years of age and manifests as bony defects with exophthalmos caused by a tumor mass in the orbital cavity. The rarest and most severe form of LCH is Letterer-Siwe disease, which typically occurs in infants younger than 2 years. Presenting symptoms include scaly, pruritic rashes; lymphadenopathy; and hepatosplenomegaly. Diagnosis is made by demonstration of either electron-dense granules in Langerhans cells (Birbeck granules) on electron microscopy or CD1 antigen on immunostaining.[57,58]

Treatment of local LCH is sometimes unnecessary; when it is necessary, surgery or local radiation therapy can be curative.[53,54] LCH syndromes respond to chemotherapeutic agents, including vinblastine, methotrexate, 6-mercaptopurine, etoposide, or 2-chlorodeoxyadenosine (cladribine).

Sinus Histiocytosis with Massive Lymphadenopathy

Sinus histiocytosis with massive lymphadenopathy or Rosai-Dorfman disease is characterized clinically as a benign, frequently chronic, painless, massive lymphadenopathy that usually involves the cervical nodes and less frequently involves the axillary, hilar, peritracheal, or inguinal nodes.[59] Extranodal disease in the respiratory tract, bones, orbits, skin, liver, and kidneys is present in almost 30% of patients.[60] The disease is usually benign, but significant morbidity and even death may result if massive tissue invasion of the liver, kidneys, lungs, and other critical structures occurs. Patients are usually of African descent, and the incidence of this disease is highest in Africa and the West Indies.

The affected lymph nodes show marked sinusoidal dilatation and follicular hyperplasia with proliferation of foamy histiocytes and multinucleated giant cells in the sinuses. The etiology of this disorder is unknown and may be related to abnormal immune regulation. Attempts at treatment should be reserved for special circumstances that are potentially life threatening. Surgery, irradiation, corticosteroids, vinblastine, and cyclophosphamide have all been administered with varying degrees of success.

Familial Hemophagocytic Lymphohistiocytosis

FHL is a rapidly fatal inherited disorder that is characterized by fever, pancytopenia, hepatic dysfunction, and activated macrophages, which overproduce inflammatory cytokines.[61] Studies suggest that the disease locus is at 9q21.3-22 and 10q21-22, but the molecular defect is not yet known.[62] Most cases are recognized in young children with hepatic necrosis. Bone marrow transplantation is currently the best therapy.[63]

Infection-Associated Hemophagocytic Syndrome

IAHS is often seen in persons who are immunocompromised as a consequence of underlying viral or bacterial infection or immunosuppressive therapy. Pathologically, the diseases are very similar to the other histocytic syndromes. If the infection can be cured, the condition may resolve.

LYSOSOMAL STORAGE DISEASES

Monocytes and macrophages play a role in tissue remodeling and the removal of senescent cellular debris, and lysosomes are the organelles that perform these functions; therefore, enzymatic abnormalities that involve lysosomal constituents result in disorders of storage that are related to macrophage function. These disorders, usually diagnosed in early childhood, include the mucopolysaccharidoses, the glycoproteinoses, the sphingolipidoses,

and the neutral lipid storage diseases [see Table 6]. Enzymatic defects have been described for most of these disorders, and diagnosis depends on demonstrating the enzymatic abnormality in macrophages or histiocytes. Most of these defects result from point mutations or genetic rearrangements at a single locus of the gene that codes for a single lysosomal hydrolase.

The two types of therapy for lysosomal storage diseases that are currently available are cellular transplantation and enzyme therapy. Gaucher disease was formerly treated with bone marrow transplantation, but it is currently treated with alglucerase, an α-mannosyl–terminated glucocerebrosidase.[64] Bone marrow transplantation for the other lysosomal storage diseases is investigational and has yielded mixed results.[65]

Eosinophil Physiology

Eosinophils can enhance or suppress acute inflammatory reactions and mediate responses to helminthic infection, allergy, and certain tumors.[66] Like neutrophils, eosinophils are capable of phagocytosis, but eosinophils are primarily secretory cells. Most of the functions they perform require the release of granule contents or reactive oxygen species. The eosinophils respond to unique chemotactic agents and growth factors that permit their accumulation at sites of inflammation.

EOSINOPHIL STRUCTURE

The granules of eosinophils contain strongly basic proteins and stain intensely with acid dyes. They have a striking and unique appearance on electron microscopy [see Figure 1]. The granules consist of an electron-dense core surrounded by a relatively radiolucent matrix; eosinophil peroxidase is active in the matrix. The dense core has a crystalloid structure and contains eosinophil cationic proteins (ECPs), major basic proteins (MBPs), and eosinophil-derived neurotoxins. MBPs and ECPs are capable of inflicting considerable damage to parasites such as schistosomula by binding to and disrupting their cell membranes. In addition, MBPs enhance the adherence of eosinophils and neutrophils to schistosomula.[67]

EOSINOPHIL FUNCTION

Eosinophils respond to a variety of chemotactic factors that enable them to enter tissues and carry out their functions. Some chemokines and chemotactic factors, such as C5a, N-formylmethionyl–containing peptides, and leukotriene B$_4$, stimulate both eosinophils and neutrophils. Several chemotactic stimuli, however, are highly specific for eosinophils. Among these eosinophil-specific stimuli are platelet-activating factor (PAF), eosinophil chemotactic factor of anaphylaxis, and a variety of parasite-derived factors. Responses to PAF, one of the most potent activators of normal eosinophils, include chemotaxis, adherence, enhanced binding of IgE, production of superoxide, release of granule proteins, and synthesis of prostanoids.

Both the production and activation of eosinophils are affected by GM-CSF, IL-5, and IL-3. IL-5 appears to be critical for eosinophil production and deployment.[68] Exposure to low doses of IL-5 also specifically primes eosinophils for later actions by other stimulants. Once activated, the eosinophils have enhanced generation of reactive oxygen species, enhanced glucose utilization and transport, increased oxygen consumption, a reduced cell surface charge, and activation of acid phosphatases in specific granules.

Eosinophils enhance the immune response to helminths. They perform this function by binding to the surface of both larval and

Table 6 Lysosomal Storage Diseases

Disease	Common Name	Enzymatic Defect	Organs and Tissues Involved	Stored Material
Mucopolysaccharidoses (MPS)				
MPS IH	Hurler syndrome	L-Iduronidase	Liver, spleen, brain, heart, cornea, bone (mild and severe variants)	Dermatan sulfate, heparan sulfate
MPS II	Hunter syndrome	Iduronate-2-sulfatase	Liver, spleen, brain, heart, bone	Dermatan sulfate, heparan sulfate
MPS III	Sanfilippo A syndrome	Heparan N-sulfatase	Brain, liver, spleen, heart, bone	Heparan sulfate
	Sanfilippo B syndrome	α-N-Acetylglucosaminidase	Brain, liver, spleen, heart, bone	Heparan sulfate
MPS IV	Morquio A syndrome	N-Acetylgalactosamine-6-sulfatase	Bone, cornea	Keratan sulfate, chondroitin 6-sulfate
	Morquio B syndrome	β-Galactosidase	Bone, cornea	Keratan sulfate
MPS VI	Maroteaux-Lamy syndrome	N-Acetylgalactosamine-4-sulfatase	Bone, cornea, liver, spleen, heart (moderate and severe variants)	Dermatan sulfate
MPS VII	Sly syndrome	β-Glucuronidase	Brain, liver, spleen, bone, coronary arteries	Dermatan sulfate, heparan sulfate, chondroitin 4-sulfate, chondroitin 6-sulfate
Glycoproteinoses				
Mannosidosis	—	Lysosomal α-mannosidase	Brain, liver, spleen, bone (several variants)	Mannose-rich oligosaccharides
Fucosidosis	—	Glycoprotein α-fucosidase	Brain, liver, spleen, heart, skin (several variants)	Fucose-containing oligosaccharides
Aspartylglucosaminuria	—	Aspartylglucosaminidase	Brain, liver, spleen, bone, heart	Aspartylglucosamine-containing peptides
Sialidosis	—	Glycoprotein neuraminidase (sialidase)	Brain, liver, spleen, bone, retina (several variants)	Sialylated glycopeptides
Galactosialidosis	—	Protector protein deficiency, combined neuraminidase (sialidase) and β-galactosidase deficiency	Brain, liver, spleen, bone (several variants)	GM_1 ganglioside, sialylated glycopeptides
Mucolipidosis II	I-cell disease	N-Acetylglucosamine-1-phosphotransferase	Brain, bone, connective tissue	Glycoproteins, glycolipids
Mucolipidosis III	Pseudo-Hurler polydystrophy	N-Acetylglucosamine-1-phosphotransferase	Brain, bone, connective tissue	Glycoproteins, glycolipids
Sphingolipidoses				
Gaucher disease	Gaucher disease type 1 (nonneuronopathic)	Acid β-glucosidase, glucocerebrosidase	Liver, spleen, bone, bone marrow (highly variable phenotype)	Glucosylceramide
	Gaucher disease type 2 (acute neuronopathic)	Acid β-glucosidase, glucocerebrosidase	Brain, brain stem, liver, spleen, bone marrow, lungs	Glucosylceramide, glucosylsphingosine
	Gaucher disease type 3 (subacute neuronopathic)	Acid β-glucosidase, glucocerebrosidase	Brain, liver, spleen, bone marrow, lungs (variable phenotype)	Glucosylceramide, glucosylsphingosine

(continued)

adult forms, by damaging target cells through oxygen-dependent mechanisms that are similar to those of neutrophils, and by damaging cell surfaces by releasing granule proteins such as MBP and ECP.[69] Although the release of these proteins similarly damages tumor cells, the interaction between eosinophils and tumor cells is less well understood. The presence of eosinophilia in patients with Hodgkin disease appears to be a function of the production of IL-5 by Reed-Sternberg cells.[70] Eosinophils contribute to the fibrosis of the nodular sclerosis type of Hodgkin disease by producing transforming growth factor–β1.[71]

Disorders of Eosinophil Number

EOSINOPHILIA

Evaluation of the patient with eosinophilia (eosinophil count > 700/mm³) is difficult because the causes of this disorder are multiple and diverse.[72] Common causes of secondary eosinophilia include allergic disorders, infections caused by parasites and other organisms, dermatologic diseases, pulmonary diseases, collagen vascular disease, neoplasms, and immunodeficiency diseases. There are also myriad uncommon causes, such as eosinophilic gastroenteritis, inflammatory bowel disease, chronic active hepatitis, pancreatitis, and hypopituitarism.

HYPEREOSINOPHILIC SYNDROME

The term hypereosinophilic syndrome (HES) is often used for patients with chronic eosinophilia of unknown cause.[72] The criteria used to diagnose HES are an unexplained eosinophil count of greater than 1,500/mm³ for longer than 6 months and signs or symptoms of infiltration of eosinophils into tissues. This condition may be the result of production of excessive IL-5 by an abnormal clone of T cells.[73]

The clinical features of HES are rash, fever, cough, dyspnea, diarrhea, and peripheral neuropathy. Patients may have chronic congestive heart failure, valvular abnormalities, and distinctive, fibrous, biventricular endocardial thickening with mural thrombi.[73] The blood smear of a patient with HES usually reveals normal mature eosinophils of typical morphology; however, the presence

Table 6   (continued)

Disease	Common Name	Enzymatic Defect	Organs and Tissues Involved	Stored Material
Metachromatic leukodystrophy (MLD)	Infantile MLD	Arylsulfatase A	Brain, peripheral nerves	Sulfatide
	Juvenile MLD	Arylsulfatase A	Brain, peripheral nerves	Sulfatide
	Adult MLD	Arylsulfatase A	Brain, peripheral nerves	Sulfatide
		Saposin B deficiency	Brain, peripheral nerves	Sulfatide
	Pseudodeficiency	Partial arylsulfatase A	Normal	None
Multiple sulfatase deficiency	—	Unknown primary defect, multiple lysosomal and nonlysosomal sulfatase deficiencies	Brain, liver, spleen, bone	Sulfatide, dermatan sulfate, heparan sulfate
Gangliosidoses				
GM_2 gangliosidoses	Infantile Tay-Sachs disease (TSD)	Hexosaminidase A (α chain)	Brain	GM_2 ganglioside
	Juvenile TSD	Hexosaminidase A (α chain)	Brain	GM_2 ganglioside
	Adult TSD	Hexosaminidase A (α chain)	Brain	GM_2 ganglioside
	Activator deficiency	GM_2 activator	Brain	GM_2 ganglioside
	Sandhoff disease	Hexosaminidase B and A (β chain)	Brain, liver, spleen, bone	GM_2 ganglioside, globoside
GM_1 gangliosidoses	Landing disease	β-Galactosidase	Brain, liver, spleen, bone	GM_1 ganglioside, keratan sulfate
Neutral sphingo-lipidoses				
Fabry disease	—	α–Galactosidase A	Kidney, vascular endothelial system, heart, central nervous system vessels	Globotriaosylceramide
Schindler disease	—	α-N-Acetylgalactosaminidase	Brain (probably several variants)	N-Acetylgalactosamine–linked oligosaccharides
Krabbe disease	—	Galactocerebrosidase	Brain	Galactocerebroside
Niemann-Pick disease	Niemann-Pick A disease (infantile)	Sphingomyelinase	Brain, liver, spleen, lungs	Sphingomyelin
	Niemann-Pick B disease (late-onset)	Sphingomyelinase	Liver, spleen, lungs	Sphingomyelin
Neutral lipid storage diseases				
Wolman disease	—	Lysosomal acid lipase	Liver, spleen, adrenal glands, bone marrow	Cholesteryl esters, triglycerides
Cholesterol ester storage disease	—	Lysosomal acid lipase	Liver, spleen, blood vessels	Cholesteryl esters
Farber disease	—	Ceramidase	Brain, joints, tendons, skin, liver	Ceramide

of hypogranulation and cytoplasmic vacuoles has been reported.[74] The total leukocyte count is typically 10,000 to 30,000/mm³, 30% to 70% of which are eosinophils. The bone marrow is generally hypercellular, with eosinophils constituting 25% to 75% of the marrow elements.

HES can usually be distinguished from malignant disorders associated with eosinophilia, such as acute or chronic eosinophilic leukemias.[75] Allergic reactions must also be excluded; the exclusion of such a reaction is usually based on the history, physical examination, and review of current medications. Because many drugs may generate an allergic reaction accompanied by eosinophilia, all nonessential medication should be discontinued before the patient is evaluated.

Parasitic infections, most commonly with such tissue-invasive helminths as filariae and *Strongyloides*, *Trichinella*, *Schistosoma*, and *Toxocara* species, frequently present with eosinophilia. To eliminate parasitosis as the cause of eosinophilia, multiple stool samples and a small bowel aspirate are recommended, particularly in patients who are at particular risk for infection (e.g., those who frequently travel, those who are exposed to animals, and those who have immunodeficiencies). If these test results are negative, serologic assays, radiologic tests, and peripheral blood and bone marrow smears should be performed to exclude the pres-

ence of connective tissue diseases, occult lymphoproliferative syndromes and solid tumors, and hematologic malignancies, respectively. In patients with possible cardiac involvement, an echocardiogram should be performed.

Therapy is directed toward lowering the eosinophil count and correcting specific symptoms. If symptoms involving the lungs or the heart are present, prednisone at a dosage of 1 mg/kg/day should be given for 2 weeks, followed by 1 mg/kg every other day for 3 months or longer. If this treatment fails or if an alternative is necessary to avoid steroid side effects, hydroxyurea at a dosage of 0.5 to 1.5 g/day should be given to lower the WBC count to less than 10,000/mm³ and the eosinophil count to less than 5,000/mm³. Alternative agents include interferon alfa, cyclosporine, and etoposide.

Basophil and Mast Cell Physiology

Basophils and mast cells are important in immediate hypersensitivity reactions, asthma, urticaria, allergic rhinitis, and anaphylaxis.[76] They are derived from a common hematopoietic progenitor cell in the bone marrow and are stimulated by soluble mediators, primarily IgE, to release granule contents and arachidonic acid metabolites from their plasma membranes.

Table 7   Causes of Lymphocytosis

Lymphoproliferative disorders (primary lymphocytosis)
   Leukemia
      Acute lymphocytic leukemia
      Chronic lymphocytic leukemia
      Hairy-cell leukemia
      Large granular lymphocyte leukemia
   Lymphoma
   Monoclonal B cell lymphocytosis

Reactive (secondary) lymphocytosis
   Viral infection (most likely with EBV, CMV, HIV, HSV, VZV,
      rubella, adenovirus, or hepatitis virus)
   Toxoplasmosis
   Pertussis
   Stress
      Acute
         Cardiovascular collapse
         Septic shock
         Sickle cell crisis
         Status epilepticus
         Trauma
         Surgery
         Drugs
         Hypersensitivity
      Chronic
         Autoimmune disorders
         Cancer
         Hyposplenism
         Sarcoidosis
         Cigarette smoking

CMV—cytomegalovirus EBV—Epstein-Barr virus HSV—herpes simplex virus VZV—varicella-zoster virus

The cytoplasmic granules of both basophils and mast cells contain sulfated glycosaminoglycans; in normal basophils, the sulfated glycosaminoglycans are predominantly heparin.[77] The sulfated glycosaminoglycans are the granule contents that are primarily responsible for the intense staining of the basophil. Most, if not all, of the circulating histamine in the body is synthesized by the basophil and stored within its granules. Degranulation causes the release of histamine, which mediates many immediate hypersensitivity effects and which, because it is a potent eosinophil chemoattractant, draws eosinophils to the site of degranulation. Other substances that are released on basophil degranulation include additional eosinophil chemotactic factors and a variety of arachidonic acid metabolites, the most important of which is leukotriene C_4. In addition, the cell membranes of basophils contain high-affinity IgE receptors, the number of which tends to be increased in allergic persons [see Chapter 106].

Disorders of Basophil Number

BASOPHILIA

Basophilia (basophil count >150/mm^3) is seen in myeloproliferative disorders, such as CML, polycythemia vera, and myeloid metaplasia; after splenectomy; in some hemolytic anemias; and in Hodgkin disease. The basophil count can also be increased in patients with ulcerative colitis or varicella infection. Although basophils and mast cells are involved in immediate hypersensitivity reactions and basophils are often seen in areas of contact dermatitis, basophilia is not seen in patients with these disorders.

Disorders of Lymphocytes

LYMPHOCYTOSIS

Lymphocytosis in adults is defined as an absolute lymphocyte count greater than 4,000/mm^3. However, it must be kept in mind that lymphocyte counts in children are higher than in adults and may be as high as 20,000/mm^3 in the first year of life. The blood film of any patient with lymphocytosis should be carefully examined to determine the morphology and diversity of the lymphocytes (e.g., reactive lymphocytes, large granular lymphocytes, blasts, or smudge cells).

Lymphocytosis can be either primary or secondary. Primary lymphocytosis, often called lymphoproliferative disease, is caused by dysregulation in the production of lymphocytes. The primary lymphocytoses include the leukemias (such as chronic lymphocytic leukemia, acute lymphocytic leukemia, hairy-cell leukemia, and large granular lymphocyte leukemia), the lymphomas, and monoclonal B cell lymphocytosis [see Table 7].

The reactive, or secondary, lymphocytoses are conditions that involve absolute increases in lymphocytes caused by physiologic or pathophysiologic responses to infection, inflammation, toxins, cytokines, or unknown agents. The most common cause of reactive lymphocytosis is viral infection; Epstein-Barr virus, cytomegalovirus, herpes simplex virus, varicella-zoster virus, rubella, HTLV-1, HIV, adenovirus, or one of the hepatitis viruses is frequently responsible. Other pathogens that produce lymphocytosis are *Toxoplasma gondii* and, in children, *Bordetella pertussis* (which causes the lymphocyte count to rise to as high as 70,000/mm^3). Lymphocytosis is also associated with stress and consequent release of epinephrine, such as that seen in patients with cardiovascular collapse, septic shock, sickle cell crisis, status epilepticus, or trauma and with major surgery, drug reactions, and hypersensi-

Table 8   Causes of Lymphocytopenia

Inherited
   Congenital immunodeficiency diseases
      Severe combined immunodeficiency
         Adenosine deaminase deficiency
         Purine-nucleoside phosphorylase deficiency
         Reticular dysgenesis
      Ataxia-telangiectasia
      Wiskott-Aldrich syndrome
      Cartilage-hair hypoplasia
   Idiopathic CD4$^+$ T lymphocytopenia

Acquired
   Infection
      Viral (e.g., with HIV, a hepatitis virus, influenza virus, or
         respiratory syncytial virus)
      Bacterial (e.g., typhoid fever, pneumonia, sepsis, or
         tuberculosis)
   Aplastic anemia
   Autoimmune diseases
   Hodgkin disease
   Sarcoidosis
   Renal failure
   Protein-losing enteropathies
   Chylous ascites
   Zinc deficiency
   Chronic alcohol ingestion
   Immunosuppressive agents (e.g., antithymocyte globulin,
      corticosteroids, chemotherapeutic agents, and radiation)

tivity. Persistent lymphocytosis may be seen in patients with autoimmune disorders, sarcoidosis, hyposplenism, and cancer and in those who are long-term cigarette smokers.

LYMPHOCYTOPENIA

Lymphocytopenia is defined as a total lymphocyte count less than $1,000/mm^3$. Because in adults 80% of lymphocytes are T cells, most cases of lymphocytopenia are caused by a reduction in the T cell count. The mechanisms of lymphocytopenia are often unknown, and the causes are usually differentiated as either inherited or acquired.

Inherited lymphocytopenias are usually caused by congenital immunodeficiency diseases. These diseases include severe combined immunodeficiency (e.g., adenosine deaminase deficiency, purine-nucleoside phosphorylase deficiency, and reticular dysgenesis), ataxia-telangiectasia, Wiskott-Aldrich syndrome, and cartilage-hair hypoplasia [see Table 8]. In addition, some persons have idiopathic $CD4^+$ T cell lymphocytopenia.

Acquired lymphocytopenia can be seen in patients with viral infections, such as HIV infection, hepatitis, influenza, and respiratory syncytial virus infection; in patients with certain bacterial infections, such as typhoid fever, pneumonia, sepsis, and tuberculosis; and in patients with aplastic anemia, autoimmune diseases, Hodgkin disease, sarcoidosis, renal failure, protein-losing enteropathies, and chylous ascites. Zinc deficiency and long-term alcohol ingestion are also associated with lymphocytopenia. Finally, immunosuppressive agents, such as antithymocyte globulin, corticosteroids, chemotherapeutic agents, and radiation, also produce lymphocytopenia.

References

1. Atwater S, Corash L: Advances in leukocyte differential and peripheral blood stem cell enumeration. Curr Opin Hematol 3:71, 1996

2. Root RK, Dale DC: Granulocyte colony-stimulating factor and granulocyte-macrophage colony-stimulating factor; comparisons and potential for use in treatment of infections in nonneutropenic patients. J Infect Dis 179:S342, 1999

3. Price TH, Chatta GS, Dale DC: Effect of recombinant granulocyte colony-stimulating factor on neutrophil kinetics in normal young and elderly humans. Blood 88:335, 1996

4. Dale DC, Liles WC, Llewellyn C, et al: Effects of granulocyte-macrophage colony-stimulating factor (GM-CSF) on neutrophil kinetics and function in normal human volunteers. Am J Hematol 57:7, 1998

5. Dancey JT, Deubelbeiss KA, Harker LA, et al: Neutrophil kinetics in man. J Clin Invest 58:705, 1976

6. Homburg CH, Roos D: Apoptosis of neutrophils. Curr Opin Hematol 3:94, 1996

7. Gullberg U, Bengtsson N, Bulow E, et al: Processing and targeting of granule proteins in human neutrophils. J Immunol Methods 232:201, 1999

8. Gautam N, Herwald H, Hedqvist P, et al: Signaling via beta (2) integrins triggers neutrophil-dependent alteration in endothelial barrier function. J Exp Med 191:1829, 2000

9. Torres M, Coates TD: Function of the cytoskeleton in human neutrophils and methods for evaluation. J Immunol Method 232:89, 1999

10. Dransfield I: Granulocyte adhesion molecules—structure/function relationships. Semin Cell Biol 6:337, 1995

11. Anderson SI, Hotchin NA, Nah GB: Role of the cytoskeleton in rapid activation of CD11b/CD18 function and its subsequent downregulation in neutrophils. J Cell Sci 113:2737, 2000

12. Murdoch C, Finn A: Chemokine receptors and their role in inflammation and infectious diseases. Blood 95:3032, 2000

13. McKenzie SE, Schreiber AD: Fc gamma receptors in phagocytes. Curr Opin Hematol 5:16, 1998

14. Vaissiere C, Le Cabec V, Maridonneau-Parini I: NADPH oxidase is functionally assembled in specific granules during activation of human neutrophils. J Leukoc Biol 65:629, 1999

15. Nauseef WM: The NADPH-dependent oxidase of phagocytes. Proc Assoc Am Physicians 111:373, 1999

16. Klebanoff SJ: Myeloperoxidase. Proc Assoc Am Physicians 111:383, 1999

17. Pitrak DL: Effects of granulocyte colony-stimulating factor and granulocyte-macrophage colony-stimulating factor on the bactericidal function of neutrophils. Curr Opin Hematol 3:183, 1997

18. Dale DC, Liles WC, Summer W, et al: Review: granulocyte colony-stimulating factor role and relationships in infectious diseases. J Infect Dis 172:1061, 1995

19. Malech HL, Nauseef WM: Primary inherited defects in neutrophil function: etiology and treatment. Semin Hematol 34:279, 1997

20. Creutzig U, Ritter J, Vormoor J, et al: Myelodysplasia and acute myelogenous leukemia in Down's syndrome: a report of 40 children of the AML-BFM Study Group. Leukemia 10:1677, 1996

21. Bain BJ, Phillips D, Thomson K, et al: Investigation of the effect of marathon running on leukocyte counts of subjects of different ethnic origins: relevance to the aetology of ethnic neutropenia. Br J Haematol 108:483, 2000

22. Weingarten MA, Pottick-Schwartz EA, Brauner A: The epidemiology of benign leukopenia in Yemenite Jews. Isr J Med Sci 29:297, 1993

23. Marie JP, Vekhoff A, Pico JL, et al: Neutropenic infections: a review of the French Febrile Aplasia Study Group trials in 608 febrile neutropenic patients. J Antimicrob Chemother 41(suppl D):57, 1998

24. Zinner SH: Changing epidemiology of infections in patients with neutropenia and cancer: emphasis on gram-positive and resistant bacteria. Clin Infect Dis 29:490, 1999

25. van der Klauw MM, Wilson JH, Stricker BH: Drug-associated agranulocytosis: 20 years of reporting in the Netherlands (1974–1994). Am J Hematol 57:206, 1998

26. Guest I, Uetrecht J: Drugs that induce neutropenia/agranulocytosis may target specific components of the stromal cell extracellular matrix. Med Hypotheses 53:145, 1999

27. Pitrak DL, Tsai HC, Mullane KM, et al: Accelerated neutrophil apoptosis in the acquired immunodeficiency syndrome. J Clin Invest 98:2714, 1996

28. Kuritzkes DR: Neutropenia, neutrophil dysfunction, and bacterial infection in patients with human immunodeficiency virus disease: the role of granulocyte colony-stimulating factor. Clin Infect Dis 30:256, 2000

29. Levy M, Kelly JP, Kaufman DW, et al: Risk of agranulocytosis and aplastic anemia in relation to history of infectious mononucleosis: a report from the International Agranulocytosis and Aplastic Anemia Study. Ann Hematol 67:187, 1993

30. Brown KE, Young NS: Parvovirus B19 in human disease. Annu Rev Med 48:59, 1997

31. Mammen EF: The haematological manifestations of sepsis. J Antimicrob Chemother 41(suppl A):17, 1998

32. Dale DC: Immune and idiopathic neutropenia. Curr Opin Hematol 5:33, 1998

33. Bux J, Behrens G, Jaeger G, et al: Diagnosis and clinical course of autoimmune neutropenia in infancy: analysis of 240 cases. Blood 91:181, 1998

34. Bux J, Chapman J: Report on the second international granulocyte serology workshop. Transfusion 37:977, 1997

35. Keeling DM, Isenberg DA: Haematological manifestations of systemic lupus erythematosus. Blood Rev 7:199, 1993

36. Kurien BT, Newland J, Paczkowski C, et al: Association of neutropenia in systemic lupus erythematosus (SLE) with anti-Ro and binding of an immunologically cross-reactive neutrophil membrane antigen. Clin Exp Immunol 120:209, 2000

37. Ramakrishna R, Chaudhuri K, Sturgess A, et al: Haematological manifestations of primary Sjögren's syndrome: a clinicopathological study. Q J Med 83:547, 1992

38. Campion G, Maddison PJ, Goulding N, et al: The Felty syndrome: a case-matched study of clinical manifestations and outcome, serologic features, and immunogenetic associations. Medicine (Baltimore) 69:69, 1990

39. Rosenstein ED, Kramer N: Felty's and pseudo-Felty's syndromes. Semin Arthritis Rheum 21:129, 1991

40. Ditzel HJ, Masaki Y, Nielsen H, et al: Cloning and expression of a novel human antibody-antigen pair associated with Felty's syndrome. Proc Natl Acad Sci USA 97:9234, 2000

41. Liu JH, Wei S, Lamy T, et al: Chronic neutropenia mediated by fas ligand. Blood 95:3219, 2000

42. Lamy T, Loughran TP: Large granular lymphocyte leukemia. Cancer Control 5:25, 1998

43. Huizinga TW, Kuijpers RW, Kleijer M, et al: Maternal genomic neutrophil FcRIII deficiency leading to neonatal isoimmune neutropenia. Blood 76:1927, 1990

44. Marinone G, Roncoli B, Marinone MG Jr: Pure white cell aplasia. Semin Hematol 28:298, 1991

45. Beauchesne MF, Shalansky SJ: Nonchemotherapy drug-induced agranulocytosis: a review of 118 patients treated with colony-stimulating factors. Pharmacotherapy 19:299, 1999

46. Rashba EJ, Rowe JM, Packman CH: Treatment of the neutropenia of the Felty syndrome. Blood Rev 10:177, 1996

47. Hellmich B, Schnabel A, Gross WL: Treatment of severe neutropenia due to Felty's syndrome or systemic lupus erythematosus with granulocyte colony-stimulating factor. Semin Arthritis Rheum 29:82, 1999

48. Dale DC, Bonilla MA, Davis MW, et al: A randomized controlled phase III trial of recombinant human granulocyte colony-stimulating factor (filgrastim) for treatment of severe chronic neutropenia. Blood 181:2496, 1993

49. Kuritzkes DR, Parenti D, Ward DJ, et al: Filgrastim prevents severe neutropenia and reduces infective morbidity in patients with advanced HIV infection: results of a randomized, multicenter, controlled trial. G-CSF 930101 Study Group. AIDS 12:65, 1998

50. Ardati KO, Bajakian KM, Tabbara KS: Effect of glucose-6-phosphate dehydrogenase deficiency on neutrophil function. Acta Haematol 97:211, 1997

51. Wilkinson PC: Defects of leukocyte locomotion and chemotaxis: prospects, assays, and lessons from Chédiak-Higashi neutrophils. Eur J Clin Invest 23:690, 1993

52. Takahashi K, Naito M, Takeya M: Development and heterogeneity of macrophages and their related cells through their differentiation pathways. Pathol Int 46:473, 1996

53. MacMicking J, Xie QW, Nathan C: Nitric oxide and macrophage function. Annu Rev Immunol 15:323, 1997

54. Favara BE, Feller AC, Pauli M, et al: Contemporary classification of histiocytic disor-

ders. The WHO committee on histiocytic/reticulum cell proliferations. Reclassification Working Group of the Histiocyte Society. Med Pediatr Oncol 29:157, 1997

55. Mongkonsritragoon W, Li CY, Phyliky RL: True malignant histiocytosis. Mayo Clin Proc 73:520, 1998

56. Ladisch S: Langerhans cell histiocytosis. Curr Opin Hematol 5:54, 1998

57. Lieberman PH, Jones CR, Steinman RM, et al: Langerhans cell (eosinophilic) granulomatosis: a clinicopathologic study encompassing 50 years. Am J Surg Pathol 20:519, 1996

58. Vassallo R, Ryu JH, Colby TV, et al: Pulmonary Langerhans'-cell histiocytosis. N Engl J Med 342:1969, 2000

59. Cabone A, Passannante A, Gloghini A, et al: Review of sinus histiocytosis with massive lymphadenopathy (Rosai-Dorfman disease) of head and neck. Ann Otol Rhinol Laryngol 108:1095, 1999

60. Veinot JP, Eidus L, Jabi M: Soft tissue Rosai Dorfman disease mimicking inflammatory pseudotumor: a diagnostic pitfall. Pathology 30:14, 1998

61. Ishii E, Ohga S, Tanimura M, et al: Clinical and epidemiologic studies of familial hemophagocytic lymphohistiocytosis in Japan. Japan LCH Study Group. Med Pediatr Oncol 30:276, 1998

62. Graham GE, Graham LM, Bridge PJ, et al: Further evidence for genetic heterogeneity in familial hemophagocytic lymphohistiocytosis. Pediatr Res 48:227, 2000

63. Imashuku S, Hibi S, Todo S, et al: Allogeneic hematopoietic stem cell transplantation for patient hemophagocytic syndrome (HPS) in Japan. Bone Marrow Transplant 23:569, 1999

64. Beutler E: Enzyme replacement therapy for Gaucher's disease. Baillieres Clin Haematol 10:751, 1997

65. O'Marcaigh AS, Cowan MJ: Bone marrow transplantation for inherited diseases. Curr Opin Oncol 9:126, 1997

66. Martin LB, Kita H, Leiferman KM, et al: Eosinophils in allergy: role in disease, degranulation, and cytokines. Int Arch Allergy Immunol 109:207, 1996

67. Gleich GJ: Mechanisms of eosinophil-associated inflammation. J Allergy Clin Immunol 105:651, 2000

68. Karlen S, DeBoer ML, Lipscombe RJ, et al: Biological and molecular characteristics of interleukin-5 and its receptor. Int Rev Immunol 16:227, 1998

69. Trottein F, Nutten S, Papin JP, et al: Role of adhesion molecules of the selectin-carbohydrate families in antibody-dependent cell-mediated cytotoxicity to schistosome targets. J Immunol 159:804, 1997

70. Samoszuk M, Nansen L: Detection of interleukin-5 messenger RNA in Reed-Sternberg cells of Hodgkin's disease with eosinophilia. Blood 75:13, 1990

71. Kadin M, Butmarc J, Elovic A, et al: Eosinophils are the major source of transforming growth factor–beta 1 in nodular sclerosing Hodgkin's disease. Am J Pathol 142:11, 1993

72. Rothenberg ME: Eosinophilia. N Engl J Med 338:1592, 1998

73. Simon HU, Plotz SG, Dummer R, et al: Abnormal clones of T cells producing interleukin-5 in idiopathic eosinophilia. N Engl J Med 341:1112, 1999

74. Brito-Babapulle F: Clonal eosinophilic disorders and the hypereosinophilic syndrome. Blood Rev 11:129, 1997

75. Barin BJ: Hypereosinophilia. Curr Opin Hematol 7:21, 2000

76. Dvorak AM: Cell biology of the basophil. Int Rev Cytol 180:87, 1998

77. Galli SJ, Hammel I: Mast cell and basophil development. Curr Opin Hematol 1:33, 1994

Acknowledgments

Figure 1   Tom Moore. Electron micrographs courtesy of Dr. E. Chi, University of Washington School of Medicine, Seattle.

Figure 3   Tom Moore.

Lawrence L. K. Leung, M.D.

Hemostasis, the process of blood clot formation, is a coordinated series of responses to vessel injury. It requires the allied activity of platelets, the clotting cascade, blood flow and shear, endothelial cells, and fibrinolysis.

Platelet Plug Formation

Platelets are activated at the site of vascular injury to form a plug to stop bleeding. Physiologic platelet stimuli include adenosine diphosphate (ADP), epinephrine, thrombin, and collagen. ADP and epinephrine are relatively weak platelet stimulators; thrombin and collagen are strong agonists. Thrombin activation is mediated by G protein–coupled protease-activated receptors (PAR),[1] specifically PAR-1 and PAR-4. Thrombin cleaves the external domain of the PAR to initiate transmembrane signaling [*see Figure 1*].[2] There are also specific receptors for ADP, epinephrine, and collagen.

Platelet activation involves four distinct processes: adhesion (deposition of platelets on subendothelial matrix); aggregation (cohesion of platelets); secretion (release of platelet granule proteins); and procoagulant activity (enhancement of thrombin generation) [*see Figure 2*].

ADHESION

Platelet adhesion is primarily mediated by the binding of platelet surface receptor glycoprotein (GP) Ib-IX-V complex to the adhesive protein von Willebrand factor (vWF) in the subendothelial matrix.[3] Deficiency of GPIb-IX-V complex or vWF leads to two congenital bleeding disorders, Bernard-Soulier disease and von Willebrand disease, respectively [*see Chapter 93*]. Other adhesive interactions (e.g., binding of platelet collagen receptor GPIa-IIa to collagen fibrils in the matrix) also contribute to platelet adhesion.[4]

AGGREGATION

Platelet aggregation involves binding of fibrinogen to the platelet fibrinogen receptor (i.e., the GPIIb-IIIa complex). GPIb-IIIa (also termed $\alpha IIb\beta3$) is a member of a superfamily of adhesive protein receptors, called integrins, which are found in many different cell types. It is the most abundant receptor on the platelet surface. GPIIb-IIIa does not bind fibrinogen on nonstimulated platelets. After platelet stimulation, GPIIb-IIIa undergoes a conformational change and is converted from a low-affinity fibrinogen receptor to a high-affinity receptor in a process termed inside-out signaling. Fibrinogen, a divalent molecule, serves to bridge the activated platelets [*see Figure 3*]. The cytosolic portion of the activated GPIIb-IIIa complex binds to the platelet cytoskeleton and can mediate platelet spreading and clot retraction (in a process termed outside-in signaling).[5] Congenital deficiency of GPIIb-IIIa or fibrinogen leads to Glanzmann thrombasthenia and afibrinogenemia. The GPIIb-IIIa–fibrinogen pathway is the final common course for platelet aggregation. Blockade of this pathway is the basis of an important class of antiplatelet drugs.

PROTEIN SECRETION

After stimulation, platelet granules release ADP and serotonin, which stimulate and recruit additional platelets; adhesive proteins such as fibronectin and thrombospondin, which reinforce and stabilize platelet aggregates; factor V, a component of the clotting cascade; thromboxane, which stimulates vasoconstriction; and growth factors such as platelet-derived growth factor (PDGF), which stimulate proliferation of smooth muscle cells and mediate tissue repair. PDGF may also contribute to the development of atherosclerosis and reocclusion after coronary angioplasty.

PROCOAGULATION

Platelet procoagulation involves the assembly of the enzyme complexes of the clotting cascade on the platelet surface. It is an

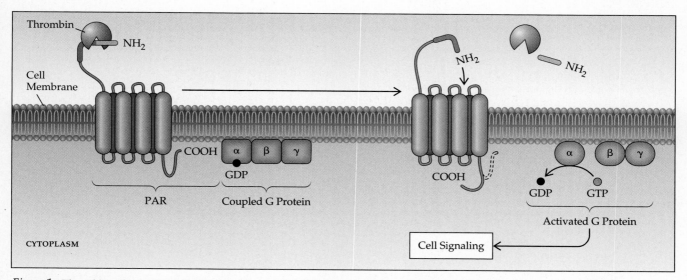

Figure 1 Thrombin activation is mediated by G protein–coupled protease-activated receptor (PAR). Thrombin cleaves the NH2-terminal exodomain of the PAR, exposing a new NH2 terminus, which then serves as a tethered ligand to bind intramolecularly to the body of the receptor to initiate transmembrane signaling.

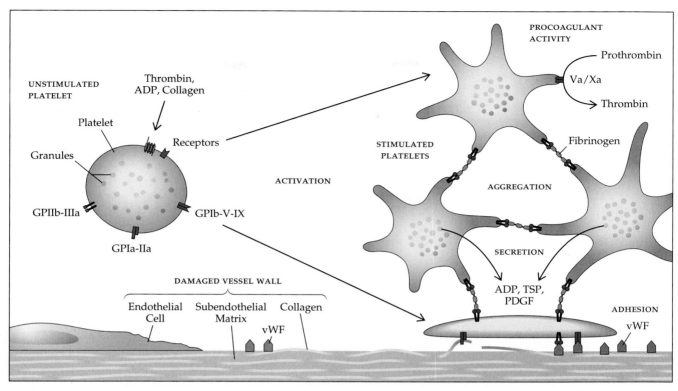

Figure 2   **After platelets are activated, they undergo significant morphologic changes, producing elongated pseudopods. They also become extremely adhesive. The functional response of activated platelets involves four distinct processes: adhesion (deposition of platelets on subendothelial matrix); aggregation (cohesion of platelets); secretion (release of platelet granule proteins); and procoagulant activity (enhancement of thrombin generation).**

important example of the close inter-relationship between platelet activation and the activation of the clotting cascade.

Clotting Cascade

The central feature of the clotting cascade is the sequential activation of a series of proenzymes (zymogens) to enzymes, ultimately generating fibrin and reinforcing the platelet plug. Another key feature, amplification, ensures rapid response for effective hemostasis but demands tight regulation to prevent untoward thrombosis.

The clotting cascade is usually depicted as comprising intrinsic and extrinsic pathways [*see Figure 4*]. The intrinsic pathway is initiated by the exposure of blood to a negatively charged surface (e.g., glass), whereas the extrinsic pathway is activated by tissue factor or thromboplastin. Both pathways converge on the activation of factor X, which then activates prothrombin (factor II) to thrombin, the final enzyme of the clotting cascade.

Although this classic view of the clotting cascade has been useful in the interpretation of clotting times, it is not completely accurate. Patients who are severely deficient in factor XII—as well as many patients deficient in factor XI— do not bleed clinically, which indicates that the initiation part of the intrinsic pathway (the contact phase) is not important in vivo. It is now established that generation or exposure of tissue factor at the wound site is the primary physiologic event that initiates clotting [*see Figure 4*].[6] Tissue factor functions as a cofactor that is absolutely required by factor VII/factor VIIa to initiate clotting. Factor VIIa activates factor

X directly and indirectly via the activation of factor IX. This dual pathway of factor X activation is necessary apparently because of the limited amount of tissue factor generated in vivo and the presence of the tissue factor pathway inhibitor (see below), which, when complexed with factor Xa, inhibits the tissue factor/factor VIIa complex.

All of the procoagulants are synthesized in the liver except vWF, which is synthesized in megakaryocytes and endothelial cells. The vitamin K–dependent procoagulants are prothrombin, factor VII, factor IX, and factor X; and the vitamin K–dependent anticoagulants are protein C and protein S. For each of these factors, the yielding of γ-carboxyglutamic acid residues by vitamin K–dependent carboxylation of glutamic acid residues acts as a recognition signal that guides the posttranslational modification of the protein required for biologic activity.[7]

INTERACTION BETWEEN ACTIVATED PLATELETS AND THE CLOTTING CASCADE

There is an extremely close interaction between the clotting cascade and activated platelet surface in vivo. When platelets are activated, anionic lipids become exposed on the platelet surface, and factor V (stored in platelet granules) is released and bound on the anionic lipids. The factor V on the platelet surface is activated to factor Va and acts as an assembly site for the binding of factor Xa (enzyme) and prothrombin (substrate) known as the prothrombinase complex. At the assembly site, thrombin generation by the prothrombinase complex is approximately 300,000 times more efficient than thrombin generation by fluid-phase factor Xa and prothrombin alone, and the platelet plug keeps the thrombin localized. Factor Xa bound on factor Va is also relatively protected from inhibition by circulating inhibitors such as antithrombin III (see below). Similar enzyme complex assembly applies to the activation of factor X by factor VIIIa (cofactor) and factor IXa (the intrinsic tenase). The result of these processes is efficient amplification and localization of clotting.

Control Mechanisms

Coagulation is modulated by a number of mechanisms: dilution of procoagulants in flowing blood; removal of activated factors through the reticuloendothelial system, especially in the liver; and control by natural antithrombotic pathways. At least six separate and distinct control systems modulate each phase of hemostasis and protect against thrombosis, vascular inflammation, and tissue damage [*see Table 1*]. Antithrombin III, protein C, protein S, and TFPI collectively regulate the clotting cascade; prostacyclin and nitric oxide modulate vascular and platelet reactivity; and fibrinolysis removes the fibrin clot.

ANTITHROMBIN III — HEPARAN SULFATE SYSTEM

Antithrombin III (AT-III) is a circulating plasma protease inhibitor. It inhibits thrombin and factor Xa, the two key enzymes in the clotting cascade. AT-III also inhibits activated factor XII and factor XI. In the absence of the glycosaminoglycan heparin, AT-III inhibits thrombin and factor Xa relatively slowly (complete inhibition requires a few minutes). When present, heparin binds to a discrete binding site on AT-III that causes a conformational change in AT-III, which then inhibits thrombin instantaneously and irreversibly. This augmentation of the inhibition of thrombin and factor Xa is the basis for the therapeutic use of heparin as an anticoagulant. Heparan sulfate proteoglycans on the luminal surface of endothelial cells appear to activate AT-III in a manner similar to that of heparin [*see Figure 5*].[8]

Thus, the endothelial surface is normally coated with a layer of AT-III that is already activated by the endogenous heparan sulfate. Because 1 ml of blood can be exposed to as much as 5,000 cm² of endothelial surface, the AT-III–heparan sulfate system is poised to rapidly inactivate any thrombin in the general circulation.

PROTEIN C AND PROTEIN S — THROMBOMODULIN SYSTEM

Thrombomodulin is an integral membrane protein found on the luminal surface of the vascular endothelium in the microcirculation. Thrombin undergoes a conformational change when it binds to thrombomodulin, resulting in a remarkable switch in its substrate specificities: it no longer clots fibrinogen or activates platelets [*see Figure 6*]. On the other hand, it acquires the ability to activate protein C in plasma.[9] A distinct endothelial receptor for protein C has been found that enhances the activation of protein C by the thrombin-thrombomodulin complex.[10] Activated protein C degrades factor Va and factor VIIIa, the two cofactors responsible for the assembly of the prothrombinase and intrinsic tenase complex in the clotting cascade. Protein S serves as a cofactor for activated protein C. Deficiencies of AT-III, protein C, and protein S are important causes of a hypercoagulable state.

Protein C and protein S both show some structural similarity to the vitamin K–dependent clotting factors (prothrombin, factor VII, factor IX, and factor X). Protein S circulates in two forms: a free form, in which it is active as an anticoagulant, and a bound, inactive form, in which it is complexed to C4b-binding protein of the complement system. C4b-binding protein acts as an acute-phase reactant. The resultant increase in inflammatory states reduces the activity of free protein S, enhancing the likelihood of thrombosis.

TISSUE FACTOR PATHWAY INHIBITOR

Tissue factor pathway inhibitor (TFPI) is a circulating plasma protease inhibitor that is synthesized by the microvascular endothelium. Unlike AT-III, TFPI has a very low plasma concentration. TFPI inhibits factor Xa. The TFPI/factor Xa complex becomes an effective inhibitor of tissue factor/factor VIIa, thus mediating feedback inhibition of tissue factor/factor VIIa [*see Figure 7*]. Animal studies have shown that depletion of the endogenous

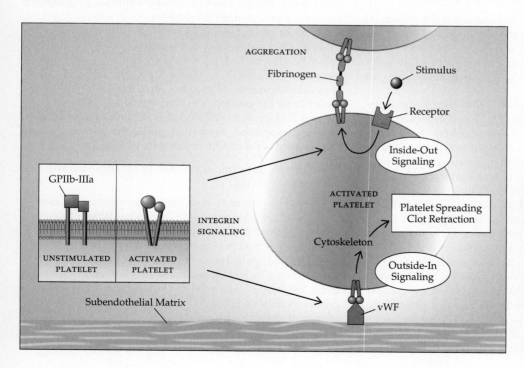

Figure 3 **Platelet aggregation involves binding of the divalent molecule fibrinogen to the platelet fibrinogen receptor (the GPIIb-IIIa complex). After platelet stimulation, GPIIb-IIIa is converted from a low-affinity fibrinogen receptor to a high-affinity receptor (inside-out signaling). The cytosolic portion of the activated GPIIb-IIIa complex can mediate platelet spreading and clot retraction (outside-in signaling).**

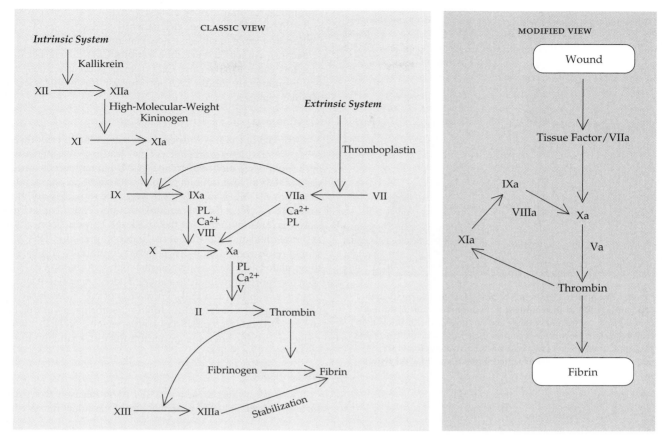

CLASSIC VIEW

Intrinsic System

MODIFIED VIEW

Figure 4 In the classic view of the clotting cascade (*left*), the intrinsic pathway is initiated by the exposure of blood to a negatively charged surface (e.g., glass) and the extrinsic pathway is activated by tissue factor or thromboplastin. In the modified view (*right*), generation or exposure of tissue factor at the wound site is the primary physiologic event that initiates clotting.

TFPI will sensitize the animals to the development of disseminated intravascular coagulation induced by tissue factor or endotoxin.[11]

TFPI is primarily synthesized by the microvascular endothelium. Approximately 20% of TFPI circulates in plasma associated with lipoproteins; the majority remains associated with the endothelial surface, apparently bound to the cell-surface glycosaminoglycans. Plasma level of TFPI is greatly increased after intravenous administration of heparin. This release of endothelial TFPI may contribute to the antithrombotic efficacy of heparin and low-molecular-weight heparin. Recombinant TFPI is now in early clinical trials.[12]

PROSTACYCLIN

Upon cell perturbation, the fatty acid arachidonic acid is released from cell membrane phospholipids by phospholipase A_2.

Table 1 Natural Antithrombotic Mechanisms of Endothelial Cells

Regulation of clotting cascade	Tissue factor pathway inhibitor Antithrombin III Protein C/Protein S
Modulation of vessel and platelet activity	Prostacyclin Nitric oxide
Removal of fibrin clot	Fibrinolysis

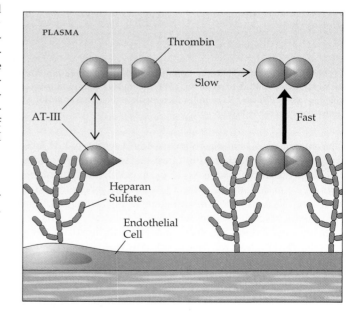

Figure 5 In the absence of heparan sulfate (HS), antithrombin III (AT-III) inhibits thrombin slowly. When HS is present, it binds to a specific site on AT-III that causes a conformational change in AT-III, allowing it to reach the active site of thrombin and inhibit the enzyme instantaneously. HS also binds to a specific site on thrombin, positioning it for optimal inhibition by AT-III.

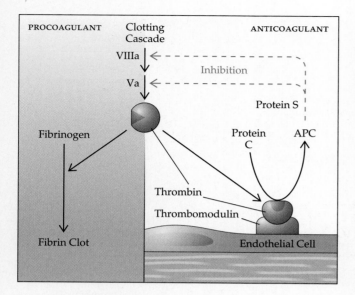

Figure 6 The protein C/protein S pathway is complementary to the AT-III pathway. When thrombin binds to thrombomodulin, thrombin undergoes a conformational change and no longer clots fibrinogen or activates platelets. However, it acquires the ability to activate protein C in plasma. Protein S serves as a cofactor for activated protein C. Activated protein C degrades activated factors V and VIII, the two cofactors in the clotting cascade.

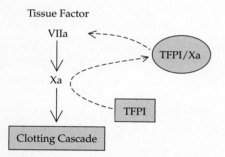

Figure 7 Tissue factor pathway inhibitor (TFPI) binds to and inhibits factor Xa. After binding to factor Xa, TFPI undergoes a conformational change. The TFPI/factor Xa complex then mediates feedback inhibition of tissue factor/factor VIIa.

The enzyme prostaglandin endoperoxide H synthase–1 (PGHS-1) converts arachidonic acid into prostaglandin endoperoxides and finally to thromboxane A_2 (TXA_2) in platelets and prostacyclin (PGI_2) in endothelial cells. TXA_2 and PGI_2 have opposite functions. TXA_2 is a potent stimulator of platelet aggregation and causes vasoconstriction, whereas PGI_2 inhibits platelet aggregation and induces vasodilatation. PGI_2 functions by activating adenylate cyclase, which leads to an increase in intracellular cyclic adenosine monophosphate (cAMP) [*see Figure 8*].

Cyclooxygenase-1 and Cyclooxygenase-2

Cyclooxygenase-1 (COX-1) is the constitutive isoform of PGHS. Recently, an inducible isoform of PGHS, cyclooxygenase-2 (COX-2), has been characterized. COX-2 is undetectable in most tissues. However, it can be rapidly induced in response to growth factors, endotoxins, and cytokines in endothelial cells and monocytes (although not in platelets).[13] Aspirin acetylates and irreversibly inhibits both COX-1 and COX-2. Other non-

steroidal anti-inflammatory drugs (NSAIDs) also inhibit COX-1 and COX-2, although not permanently. Selective COX-2 inhibitors are now available as a new generation of NSAIDs.[14]

Because aspirin irreversibly inhibits COX-1 and because platelets cannot make new COX-1, brief exposure to aspirin will permanently inhibit TXA_2 production for the life span of affected platelets.

NITRIC OXIDE

Nitric oxide (NO) is formed from L-arginine in endothelial cells. NO stimulates guanylate cyclase, leading to an increase in cyclic guanosine monophosphate (cGMP) in target cells; causes vasodilatation; and inhibits platelet adhesion and aggregation [*see Figure 8*].[15] NO is rapidly destroyed by hemoglobin and thus functions as a local (i.e., paracrine) hormone. Intravenous infusion of an arginine analogue that blocks NO production leads to an immediate and substantial rise in blood pressure. This phenomenon suggests that NO is released continually and basally to regulate vascular tone (in contrast to the production of PGI_2, which is more stimulus-responsive). There is significant synergism between NO and PGI_2. Formation of NO is catalyzed by NO synthases, which exist in different isoforms in various tissues. In addition to regulating vascular events, NO has a wide range of biologic effects (e.g., neurotransmittal function in the central nervous system).

FIBRINOLYSIS

Tissue plasminogen activator (t-PA) is released from perturbed endothelial cells near the site of vascular injury. t-PA

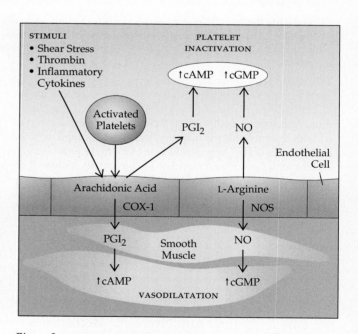

Figure 8 Significant synergism exists between nitric oxide (NO) and prostacyclin (PGI2), leading to platelet inactivation and vasodilatation. The enzyme prostaglandin endoperoxide H synthase–1 (PGHS-1) converts arachidonic acid into PGI2 in endothelial cells. PGI2 activates adenylate cyclase, which leads to an increase in intracellular cyclic adenosine monophosphate (cAMP), inhibiting platelet aggregation and inducing vasodilatation. NO, formed from l-arginine, stimulates production of cyclic guanosine monophosphate (cGMP). Cyclooxygenase-1 (COX-1) is the constitutive isoform of PGHS; NO formation is catalyzed by NO synthases (NOS).

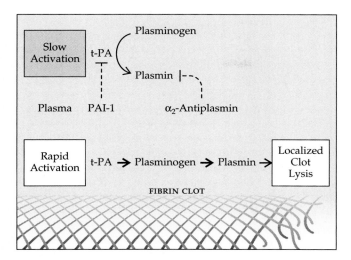

Figure 9 **Tissue-type plasminogen activator (t-PA), released from perturbed endothelial cells near an injured blood vessel, converts plasminogen to plasmin. Free plasmin is rapidly inactivated by plasma α2-antiplasmin; plasmin bound to the fibrin clot is protected from inactivation.**

converts plasminogen to plasmin. Analogously to the AT-III interaction with thrombin, which is accelerated in the presence of endothelial cell surface heparan sulfate, generation of plasmin takes place optimally on a surface (in this case, the fibrin clot). Both t-PA and plasminogen bind to fibrin (via recognition of lysine residues), which facilitates plasmin generation and localized fibrinolysis [*see Figure 9*].

Plasmin cleaves the polymerized fibrin strand at multiple sites and releases fibrin degradation products. One of the major fibrin degradation products is D-dimer, which consists of two D domains from adjacent fibrin monomers that have been crosslinked by activated factor XIII [*see Figure 10*]. Plasmin has a broad substrate specificity and, in addition to fibrin, cleaves fibrinogen and a variety of plasma proteins and clotting factors. Plasmin bound on the fibrin clot is protected from inactivation, whereas plasmin released into the circulation is rapidly inactivated by plasma α2-antiplasmin. Thus, localized fibrinolysis is achieved but nonspecific plasmin degradation of plasma proteins is prevented. In rare cases, patients have bleeding problems caused by a congenital deficiency in α2-antiplasmin.

Urokinase is the second physiologic plasminogen activator. It is present in high concentration in the urine. Although t-PA is largely responsible for initiating intravascular fibrinolysis, urokinase is the major activator of fibrinolysis in the extravascular compartment. Urokinase is secreted by many cell types in the form of prourokinase, also termed single-chain urokinase-type plasminogen activator (scu-PA). Prourokinase is converted to urokinase by plasmin. Urokinase lacks fibrin specificity in converting plasminogen to plasmin, whereas prourokinase displays such specificity.

The major physiologic inhibitor of t-PA and urokinase plasminogen activator (u-PA) is plasminogen activator inhibitor–1 (PAI-1).[16] Substantial amounts of PAI-1 are found in platelets. PAI-1 is also released from endothelial cells. PAI-1 deficiency is associated with bleeding diathesis, usually related to trauma or surgery.[17] A second inhibitor, PAI-2, is normally secreted by monocytes. During pregnancy, PAI-2 levels are greatly increased because of synthesis by the placenta. The biologic importance of PAI-2 remains to be established.

Thrombin-Activatable Fibrinolysis Inhibitor

Plasma carboxypeptidase is a newly recognized thrombin-activatable fibrinolysis inhibitor (TAFI) [*see Figure 11*].[18,19] TAFI is the second known physiologic substrate for the thrombin-thrombomodulin complex. One may envisage that after the initial fibrin clot is formed by thrombin at the site of a vascular wound, thrombin binds to thrombomodulin on the nearby intact endothelial surface. The thrombomodulin-bound thrombin leads to the generation of activated protein C, which dampens the clotting cascade and prevents excessive thrombin generation. At the same time, the thrombomodulin-bound thrombin activates TAFI, thus slowing down the lysis of the existing clot. It remains to be demonstrated whether TAFI deficiency leads to bleeding and whether excessive TAFI activity leads to thrombosis.

Overview of Blood Coagulation

The clotting cascade is initiated by the exposure of tissue factor at a vascular wound, which leads to the generation of thrombin and the deposition of a fibrin clot [*see Figure 12*]. Simultaneously, the damaged endothelium releases t-PA, which converts plasminogen to plasmin, which then lyses the clot. Both pathways are regulated: TF/factor VIIa is regulated by the TFPI/factor Xa complex, and thrombin is regulated by protein C and protein S. Similarly, the activity of t-PA is regulated by PAI-1. Thrombin and plasmin are under the control of their respective inhibitors, AT-III and α2-antiplasmin. When these two pathways work in coordinated symmetry, a clot is laid down to stop bleeding, and clot lysis and tissue remodeling follow. Diminished thrombin generation (as in factor VIII deficiency) or enhanced plasmin production (as in α2-antiplasmin deficiency) causes hemorrhage [*see Chapter 93*]. Conversely, excessive production of thrombin (as in AT-III or protein C deficiency) leads to thrombosis [*see Chapter 94*].

Heterogeneity of Endothelial Cells and Vascular Bed–Specific Hemostasis

Although the endothelium is generally considered to be a distinct, homogeneous organ system, there are significant differences between arterial, venous, and capillary endothelial cells in terms of morphology and disease susceptibility. Recent studies have shown distinct sets of proteins that mark the arterial and venous endothelial cells from the earliest stages of angiogenesis. Ephrin-B2, an Eph family transmembrane ligand, marks arterial but not venous endothelial cells. Conversely, Eph-B4, a receptor tyrosine kinase for ephrin-B2, marks veins but not arteries.[20]

It is also likely that endothelia from different vascular beds are not identical.[21] For example, the high endothelium in the postcapillary venules of lymph nodes and Peyer patches regulates the circulation of lymphocytes from blood to lymphatics and peripheral tissues. Specific adhesive protein receptors and matrix proteins are highly expressed in these high endothelial venules. The specialized endothelium representing the blood-brain barrier is another example.

These differences between arterial and venous endothelial cells and the vascular bed– specific endothelium may partly account for their different susceptibilities to thrombosis. For example, whereas AT-III and protein C deficiencies are usually associated with deep vein thrombosis of the lower extremities, thrombosis of portal and hepatic veins is frequently associated with myeloproliferative diseases.[22] In both conditions, the underlying defect is a systemic hypercoagulable state, and yet there is a clear predisposition of thrombosis to specific vascular beds. Thus, clinical thrombosis is attributable to an imbalance between systemic prothrombotic stimuli and local antithrombotic mechanisms [*see Chapter 94*].

Platelet Production and Thrombopoietin

Platelets are derived from megakaryocytes, which arise from pluripotent myeloid stem cells. Platelet production is controlled by a thrombopoietin that is involved in the final maturation of the megakaryocyte. Thrombopoietin, also referred to as c-Mpl lig-

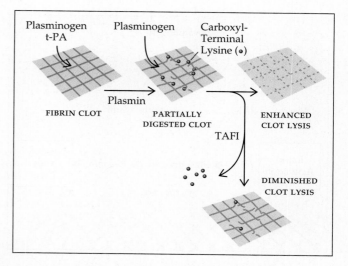

Figure 11   **Plasma carboxypeptidase is a thrombin-activatable fibrinolysis inhibitor (TAFI). When fibrin is degraded by plasmin, new carboxyl-terminal lysines are exposed in the partially digested clot. These lysines provide additional sites for plasminogen incorporation and activation in the clot, setting up a positive feedback loop in clot lysis. Thrombin activates carboxypeptidase-B in plasma, which removes the exposed carboxyl-terminal lysines and prevents further plasminogen incorporation into the clot.**

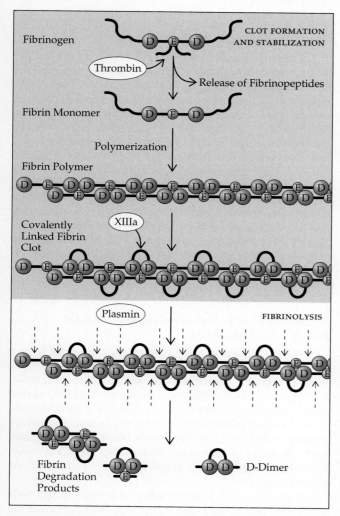

Figure 10   **The transformation of fibrinogen to fibrin is initiated by thrombin cleavage of fibrinopeptides A and B from the E domains of fibrinogen to form fibrin monomer. The cleavage apparently changes the overall negative charge of the E domain to a positive charge. This change in charge permits the spontaneous polymerization of fibrin monomers, because the positively charged E domain assembles with the negatively charged D domains of other monomers. The polymer is initially joined by hydrogen bonds. Thrombin activates factor XIII, which catalyzes the formation of covalent bonds between adjacent D domains in the fibrin polymer. Plasmin cleaves the polymerized fibrin strand at multiple sites and releases fibrin degradation products, including D-dimer.**

and, has multiple actions in megakaryocyte development.[23] It shares some structural homology with erythropoietin and is produced principally by the liver. It increases the size and number of megakaryocytes, stimulates the expression of platelet-specific markers, and is a potent megakaryocyte colony-stimulating factor. Although thrombopoietin is clearly a key factor, stem cell factor (also called kit ligand), interleukin-3 (IL-3), IL-6, and IL-11 all play contributory roles in controlling megakaryocytopoiesis.

Megakaryocytes undergo endomitosis, in which nuclear divisions occur without cell division and are followed by nuclear fusion, to yield a cell with a chromosomal content of 8n, 16n, or 32n. The megakaryocyte cytoplasm then changes into a series of thin, cylindrical strands that eventually fragment into small pieces of megakaryocytes, called proplatelets, that are released into the circulation. Megakaryocyte volume correlates with ploidy and cytoplasmic maturity; the largest megakaryocytes produce the greatest number of platelets. Large platelets called megathrombocytes are seen in the peripheral blood in thrombocytopenic states, especially in idiopathic thrombocytopenic purpura [*see Chapter 93*]. These megathrombocytes probably are young proplatelets and account for the increase in mean platelet volume that occurs during response to or recovery from acute thrombocytopenia.

Platelets entering the circulation survive about 8.5 to 10 days and have a half-life of about 4 days. Approximately 30% to 40% of the platelets are present in a splenic pool that can freely exchange with the circulation. When the need for platelets arises, production can increase sevenfold to eightfold. Because there is no marrow pool of platelets waiting to be released, increasing requirements for platelets may require a few days. Platelets have receptors for thrombopoietin and remove it from plasma, and the platelet mass functions as a major thrombopoietin regulator.[24] In states of megakaryocyte hypoplasia and thrombocytopenia, little thrombopoietin is metabolized and plasma thrombopoietin level rises, leading to increased megakaryocyte

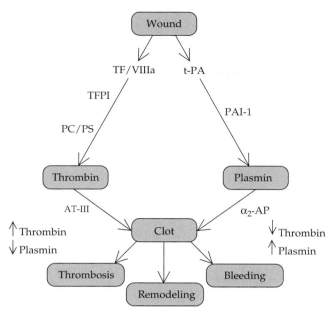

Figure 12 **Exposure of tissue factor at a vascular wound initiates the clotting cascade. Generation of thrombin and deposition of a fibrin clot occur simultaneously with release of t-PA from the damaged epithelium and conversion of plasminogen to plasmin. Plasmin then lyses the clot. When these two pathways work in coordinated symmetry, a clot is laid down to stop bleeding, and clot lysis and remodeling follow. (α2-AP—α2-antiplasmin; AT-III—antithrombin III; PAI-1—plasminogen activator inhibitor–1; PC/PS—protein C/protein S; TF—tissue factor; TFPI—tissue factor pathway inhibitor; t-PA—tissue-type plasminogen activator)**

and platelet production. In the setting of thrombocytosis, thrombopoietin metabolism increases, lowering the plasma thrombopoietin level and decreasing platelet production.

Coagulation Tests and Their Use

TESTS OF COAGULATION CASCADE

Most coagulation tests measure the time required for fibrin from plasma to form strands, which can be detected by either optical or electrical devices. Prolongation may represent a low factor concentration, inactive factor or factors, or the presence of inhibitors.

Partial thromboplastin time (PTT) The PTT, sometimes termed the activated PTT (aPTT), tests the intrinsic coagulation system. A negatively charged surface (e.g., kaolin or silica), followed by cephalin, is added to whole plasma to activate factors XII and XI. The PTT is most sensitive to abnormalities and deficiencies in the sequence of the coagulation cascade before factor X activation. The PTT is also quite sensitive to the action of heparin. It is used to monitor and adjust anticoagulant therapy with regular heparin, but not low-molecular-weight heparins.

Prothrombin time (PT) The PT is a test of the extrinsic system. It detects deficiencies in fibrinogen, factor II (prothrombin), factor V, factor VII, and factor X. Tissue factor is added to whole plasma, leading to fibrin formation, normally in 9 to 12 seconds. Results are usually reported using the international normalized ratio (INR). The INR is calculated by using the following equation:

$$INR = (Log\ patient\ PT\ /\ Log\ control\ PT)^C$$

where C represents the international sensitivity index (ISI). In this way, the thromboplastin used in an individual laboratory, with its specific ISI, is calibrated against a standard reference thromboplastin, and the PT is reported as an INR.[25] The presence of a lupus anticoagulant may also interfere with the PT.[26]

Dilute Russell viper venom time (DRVVT) The Russell viper venom contains an enzyme that activates factor X; therefore, the DRVVT measures the common pathway of the clotting cascade. It is sensitive to the presence of a lupuslike anticoagulant that inhibits the phospholipid-dependent prothrombinase complex.

Thrombin time (TT) The TT is used to test abnormalities of the conversion of fibrinogen to fibrin. It can be prolonged because of hypofibrinogenemia, abnormal fibrinogen (dysfibrinogen), or the presence of inhibitors (e.g., fibrin degradation products) that interfere with fibrin polymerization. The clinical factors commonly associated with prolonged TT are severe liver disease, disseminated intravascular coagulation, and heparin therapy.

Reptilase time (RT) Reptilase is a thrombinlike enzyme that converts fibrinogen to fibrin. RT is prolonged under conditions similar to those for prolonged TT, with one significant difference: reptilase is not inhibited by the AT-III–heparin complex. Therefore, RT is not prolonged by heparin. A long thrombin time and normal RT suggest a heparin effect.

Fibrinopeptide A (FPA) Thrombin activates fibrinogen by splitting off two molecules each of the fibrinopeptides A and B, leaving one molecule of the fibrin monomer. Measurement of FPA in the blood can be used as an index of thrombin activity in vivo. Because the clotting cascade can be activated during the blood sample collection, however, precautions are required in the measurement and interpretation of FPA levels.

Fibrinogen Fibrinogen level in plasma can be measured either antigenically or more commonly by clotting assays. The results are reported in mg/dl.

D-dimer and fibrin-fibrinogen degradation products (FDP) FDP and fibrin-fibrinogen split products (FSP) result from plasmin degradation of fibrinogen and fibrin clot [*see Figure 9*]. D-dimer is released by the plasmin-mediated degradation of fully polymerized fibrin. Plasmin cleavage of fibrinogen or soluble fibrin monomer does not yield the D-dimer. Thus, elevated D-dimer is a specific measure of intravascular fibrin deposition and plasmin degradation characteristic of disseminated intravascular coagulation. The D-dimer test has largely replaced the FSP test.

Factor XIII Factor XIII is the only clotting factor whose activity is not assessed in PT or PTT because the end point for both tests is the formation of fibrin polymers, irrespective of whether these polymers are cross-linked covalently by activated factor XIII. Factor XIII deficiency may be suspected in an infant who has significant bleeding after circumcision or, more rarely, in an adult patient who has unexplained bleeding.

Plasminogen and α2-antiplasmin The activation of the plasminogen-plasmin system can be inferred from the findings of a long TT, a low plasma fibrinogen level, and an elevated D-dimer level. Another crude test used to measure plasminogen-plasmin activation is the euglobulin lysis time. The sensitivity and specificity of this test is not well defined, however. During extensive thrombosis and fibrinolysis, both plasminogen and α_2-antiplasmin (the physiologic inhibitor of plasmin) are consumed. The direct measurement of plasma levels of plasminogen and α_2-antiplasmin is sometimes useful to assess the extent of fibrinolysis and the requirement for replenishment of these plasma proteins using fresh frozen plasma.

TESTS OF PLATELETS AND OF PLATELET FUNCTION

Peripheral blood smear evaluation This examination provides quick, definitive information to confirm or question a platelet count. Normally, there are eight to 12 platelets per high-power field (1,000x magnification), corresponding to a normal platelet count of 150,000 to 300,000/μl. The smear also shows platelet granularity and whether megathrombocytes are present.

Bleeding time This test primarily measures platelet function. A spring-loaded device is used to make a standard skin incision on the forearm. Usually, the bleeding time is normal at platelet counts greater than 100,000/μl and prolonged below this level. A prolonged bleeding time with platelets greater than 100,000/μl suggests impaired function. The bleeding time is difficult to standardize, and a normal bleeding time does not predict the safety of surgical procedures or accurately predict hemorrhage.[27] It should not be used as a general screening test in a preoperative setting. It may be useful for screening a patient for von Willebrand disease or certain platelet function disorders.

Platelet aggregometry Platelet aggregometers are photometric devices for recording the transmission of light through a suspension of platelets. When platelets aggregate, light passes through the suspension more readily. To test aggregation, dilute concentrations of platelet agonists (e.g., ADP, epinephrine, collagen, and ristocetin) are added to citrated platelet-rich plasma. With the weak agonists, such as ADP and epinephrine, the initial primary wave of aggregation is followed by a secondary wave. The secondary wave reflects the induction of the platelet release reaction, in which platelet granule contents are released to augment further platelet aggregation. A suboptimal secondary wave is seen with platelet storage pool defects in which either platelet granule content is diminished or its release activity is impaired. The latter is commonly associated with aspirin intake or uremia-related thrombocytopathy. Patients with von Willebrand disease will have a suboptimal platelet aggregation response to ristocetin but a normal response to the other agonists.

TESTS OF INHIBITORS OF HEMOSTASIS

Mixing studies A prolonged clotting time (e.g., PTT of 60 seconds [normal, 28 to 30 seconds]) can be caused by either a clotting factor deficiency or an inhibitor. An inhibitor is generally an antibody directed against a specific clotting factor or against a phospholipid-protein complex, the so-called lupus anticoagulant [see Chapter 94]. In a mixing study, one volume of a patient's plasma is mixed with an equal volume of normal plasma. The resulting mixture will provide at least 50% of a deficient factor and correct the abnormality. If the problem is caused by an inhibitor, the resulting plasma mixture still has a prolonged clotting time. A mixing study should always be done when a prolonged clotting time is noted.

Antithrombin III Bioassays and immunoassays are available for assessing AT-III activity. Two types of assays are necessary, because patients may have normal levels of AT-III on immunologic tests but abnormal levels on functional assays.

Protein C and protein S Functional and immunologic methods are available. Because protein C and protein S are vitamin K dependent, their measurement can be problematic in patients taking warfarin. It is best to measure protein C or protein S when the patient has been off warfarin for 3 to 4 weeks.

References

1. Coughlin SR: How thrombin 'talks' to cells: molecular mechanisms and roles in vivo. Arterioscler Thromb Vasc Biol 18:514, 1998
2. Kahn ML, Zheng YW, Huang W, et al: A dual thrombin receptor system for platelet activation. Nature 394:690, 1998
3. Clemetson KJ: Platelet GPIb-V-IX complex. Thromb Haemost 78:266, 1997
4. Sixma JJ, Zanten HV, Huizinga EG, et al: Platelet adhesion to collagen: an update. Thromb Haemost 78:434, 1997
5. Shattil SS, Kashiwagi H, Pampori N: Integrin signaling: the platelet paradigm. Blood 91:2645, 1998
6. Rapaport SI, Rao LVM: The tissue factor pathway: how it has become a "prima ballerina". Thromb Haemost 74:7, 1995
7. Furie B, Bouchard BA, Furie BC: Vitamin K-dependent biosynthesis of γ-carboxyglutamic acid. Blood 93:1798, 1999
8. Marcum JA, McKenney JB, Rosenberg RD: Acceleration of thrombin-antithrombin complex formation in rat hindquarters via heparinlike molecules bound to the endothelium. J Clin Invest 74:341, 1986
9. Esmon CT: The roles of protein C and thrombomodulin in the regulation of blood coagulation. J Biol Chem 264:4743, 1989
10. Esmon CT, Ding W, Yasuhiro K, et al: The protein C pathway: new insights. Thromb Haemost 78:70, 1997
11. Morten S, Bendz B: Tissue factor pathway inhibitor: clinical deficiency states. Thromb Haemost 78:467, 1997
12. Bajaj MS, Bajaj SP: Tissue factor pathway inhibitor: potential therapeutic applications. Thromb Haemost 78:471, 1997
13. Smith WL, Garavito RM, DeWitt DL: Prostaglandin endoperoxide H synthases (cyclooxygenases)-1 and -2. J Biol Chem 271:33157, 1996
14. Hawkey CJ: COX-2 inhibitors. Lancet 353:307, 1999
15. Moncada S, Higgs A: The L-arginine–nitric oxide pathway. N Engl J Med 329:2002, 1993
16. Van Meijer M, Pannekoek H: Structure of plasminogen activator inhibitor 1 (PAI-1) and its function in fibrinolysis: an update. Fibrinolysis 9:263, 1995
17. Fay WP, Parker AC, Condrey LR, et al: Human plasminogen activator inhibitor-1 (PAI-1) deficiency: characterization of a large kindred with a null mutation in the PAI-1 gene. Blood 90:204, 1997
18. Bajzar L, Morser J, Nesheim M: TAFI, or plasma procarboxypeptidase B, couples coagulation and fibrinolytic cascades through the thrombin-thrombomodulin complex. J Biol Chem 271:16603, 1996
19. Broze GJ, Higuchi DA: Coagulation-dependent inhibition of fibrinolysis: role of carboxypeptidase-U and the premature lysis of clots from hemophilic plasma. Blood 88:3815, 1996
20. Wang HU, Chen ZF, Anderson DJ: Molecular distinction and angiogenic interaction between embryonic arteries and veins revealed by ephrin-B2 and its receptor Eph-B4. Cell 93:741, 1998
21. Garlanda C, Dejana E: Heterogeneity of endothelial cells: specific markers. Arterioscler Thromb Vasc Biol 17:1193, 1997
22. Dilawari JB, Bambery P, Chawla Y, et al: Hepatic outflow obstruction (Budd-Chiari syndrome): experience with 177 patients and a review of the literature. Medicine (Baltimore) 73:21, 1994
23. Kaushansky K: Thrombopoietin. N Engl J Med 339:746, 1998
24. Kuter DJ, Rosenberg RD: The reciprocal relationship of thrombopoietin (c-Mpl ligand) to changes in the platelet mass during busulfan-induced thrombocytopenia in the rabbit. Blood 85:2720, 1995
25. Hirsh J, Dalen JE, Anderson DR, et al: Oral anticoagulants: mechanism of action, clinical effectiveness, and optimal therapeutic range. Chest 114(suppl):445S, 1998
26. Moll S, Ortel TL: Monitoring warfarin therapy in patients with lupus anticoagulants. Ann Intern Med 127:177, 1997
27. The bleeding time (editorial). Lancet 337:1447, 1991

Acknowledgments

Figures 1, 2, 3, 5, 6, and 8 through 11   Seward Hung.
Figures 4, 7, and 12   Marcia Kammerer.

93 Hemorrhagic Disorders

Lawrence L. K. Leung, M.D.

Approach to Patients with Hemorrhagic Disorders

Whereas many healthy people consider their bleeding and bruising excessive, patients with underlying von Willebrand disease, the most common hereditary bleeding disorder, often fail to identify their bleeding symptoms.[1] Therefore, it is necessary to ask for specific information from patients about bleeding and bruising (Is the patient easily bruised? What is the size of the bruises? If the patient has had surgery, were blood transfusions needed?). If the patient had a wisdom tooth extracted, were return visits required for packing, suturing, or transfusion? The patient should be questioned about drug use (including intravenous drug abuse), sexual activity, anemia, transfusions, recurrent infections, connective tissue diseases, malignancies, and immunocompromised states.

The type of bleeding is informative. Active bleeding can be caused by a localized anatomic lesion or an underlying bleeding diathesis. Mucosal bleeding, with recurrent epistaxis, gum bleeding, ecchymoses, and menorrhagia, is suggestive of von Willebrand disease or other platelet disorders. Deep-tissue bleeding (e.g., hemarthrosis and painful muscle hematomas) is more commonly seen in hemophilia and clotting factor deficiencies. Patients with clotting factor deficiencies may have delayed bleeding, presumably because the initial platelet thrombus provides immediate hemostasis but is not properly stabilized by the fibrin clot.

Aspirin can partially impair platelet function and trigger bleeding symptoms in a patient with mild underlying von Willebrand disease. Because several hundred drug formulations contain aspirin (often with no indication of aspirin content in the product name), identification of aspirin as the cause of a hemorrhagic disorder can be difficult.

Thrombocytopenia

Thrombocytopenia, a decreased platelet count, may be caused by abnormal platelet production, accelerated platelet removal resulting from immunologic or nonimmunologic mechanisms, sequestration of platelets in the spleen, or combinations of these disorders.

The hallmark of thrombocytopenia is nonpalpable petechiae, which reflect bleeding probably from capillaries or postcapillary venules. Petechiae usually are only a few millimeters in diameter and occur at sites of increased intravascular pressure, such as over the lower extremities and on the oral mucosa, and at sites constricted by certain types of clothing, such as brassiere straps. Purpura, more extensive subcutaneous bleeding, may occur with a confluence of petechial lesions. Palpable purpura indicates an additional component of vascular inflammation and suggests underlying systemic vasculitis, such as cryoglobulinemia. Thrombocytopenia also leads to mucosal bleeding; deep-tissue bleeding is less common.

There is no clearly demarcated level of platelets above which patients can be considered safe. In general, a platelet count greater than 20,000/µl is considered safe; platelet counts of 10,000/µl or below may be tolerated in nonsurgical patients [*see Chapter 95*]. Patients with idiopathic thrombocytopenic purpura bleed less at a given platelet level than patients with aplastic anemia. Presumably, the larger, younger platelets are more effective in hemostasis. The risk of intracranial hemorrhage usually directs therapy.

Elderly patients and patients with coexistent illnesses bleed more than young patients and patients with thrombocytopenia alone. An associated disorder, such as liver dysfunction or connective tissue disease, increases the risk of serious bleeding.

In the initial laboratory evaluation, the complete blood count will establish whether the thrombocytopenia is an isolated finding or associated with anemia or leukopenia. If thrombocytopenia is an isolated finding, the physician should confirm the platelet count by repeating the complete blood count. A falsely low platelet count can be the result of in vitro platelet clumping caused by the presence of cold-dependent or ethylenediamenetetraacetic acid–dependent agglutinins. Examination of the blood smear and a repeat platelet count in a citrated or heparin-anticoagulated blood sample will resolve this problem.[2]

The peripheral smear may reveal morphologic abnormalities in platelets and indicate the presence of polychromatophilia, neutropenia, lymphopenia, spherocytosis, blasts, or fragmented microangiopathic erythrocytes. The mean platelet volume, as determined by automated blood cell counters, may provide an additional clue to the cause of the thrombocytopenia. Low platelet volumes (< 6.4 femtoliters) suggest poor production, whereas larger volumes suggest rapid platelet regeneration or dysplastic platelet production.

PLATELET PRODUCTION DEFECTS

Diagnosis

A marrow aspiration with biopsy is critical for diagnosis of thrombocytopenia. The finding of a hypoplastic marrow in which the total cellularity is reduced with a concomitant decrease in megakaryocytes implies aplastic or hypoplastic anemia. The first presumption of a cause in these cases is drug toxicity. A marrow that is fibrosed or infiltrated with leukemic or other malignant cells represents the syndrome of pancytopenia from infiltrated marrow.

A marrow aspirate and biopsy sample showing normal cellularity and normal maturation of the erythroid and myeloid precursors, with decreased numbers of apparently normal megakaryocytes, suggests that the patient has ingested a drug, such as ethanol, that specifically affects the megakaryocytic progenitor cells.[3] Ethanol also produces ineffective megakaryopoiesis. In vitamin B_{12} deficiency and folate deficiency, all three marrow cell lines are affected. The marrow smear shows many large hyperlobated megakaryocytes. Some myeloproliferative disorders are characterized by ineffective megakaryopoiesis with bizarre binucleate megakaryocytes.

When accelerated removal appears to be the cause of the patient's thrombocytopenia, a rapid differential diagnosis should be made [*see Table 1*]. A bone marrow aspirate and biopsy will be very helpful. Usually, thrombocytopenia with an abundance of normal megakaryocytes in the marrow is the result of accelerated platelet removal.[4] Normally, platelets survive for 10 days and have a half-life of about 4 days; in accelerated-removal states, such as idiopathic thrombocytopenic purpura, the platelet half-life may be as short as 30 to 60 minutes. The platelet count will then reflect the balance between accelerated platelet removal and compensatory megakaryopoiesis.

Platelet survival studies are not generally available and are not usually necessary to determine whether accelerated platelet

Table 1   Causes of Thrombocytopenia

Type	Disorder	Cause
Platelet production defect	Marrow aplasia or hypoplasia, pancytopenia	Radiation, cytotoxic drugs, idiopathic
	Marrow infiltration, pancytopenia	Cancer (leukemia, lymphoma), fibrosis
	Selective impairment of platelet production	Drugs (ethanol, gold, trimethoprim-sulfamethoxazole, sulfonamides, thiazides, phenylbutazone); infections (childhood rubella, HIV)
	Ineffective megakaryopoiesis	Vitamin B_{12} deficiency, folic acid deficiency, myelodysplastic syndrome, alcohol abuse
Accelerated platelet removal	Immune destruction	Autoantibodies (idiopathic thrombocytopenic purpura, systemic lupus erythematosus, lymphoproliferative disease); proven drug antibodies (quinidine, quinine, heparin, GPIIb-IIIa antagonists); infections (infectious mononucleosis, HIV, gram-negative septicemia, malaria); suspected drug antibodies (thiazide diuretics, acetaminophen, cimetidine, aminosalicylic acid); posttransfusion purpura
	Nonimmunologic removal	Disseminated intravascular coagulation, preeclampsia, vasculitis, thrombotic thrombocytopenic purpura, hemolytic-uremic syndrome, HELLP syndrome, severe bleeding, platelet washout after massive transfusion, giant hemangioma, gram-negative septicemia
	Hypersplenism	Enlarged spleen from various causes

HELLP—hemolysis, elevated liver enzymes, low platelet count

removal is occurring. Infusion of random-donor platelets can be used as a diagnostic and therapeutic procedure. When accelerated platelet removal is responsible for the thrombocytopenia, transfusion with six platelet packs only slightly elevates the platelet count, which then returns to baseline values in less than 24 hours. This therapeutic test becomes unreliable, however, if the patient has been previously alloimmunized by blood or platelet transfusions or by multiple pregnancies.

Treatment

If a drug is the suspected cause of the thrombocytopenia, it should be discontinued. Specific replacement is required for deficiencies of vitamin B_{12} and folate. When the thrombocytopenia is causing significant bleeding, platelet transfusion will be required until the situation resolves [*see Chapter 95*].

Recombinant thrombopoietin is in clinical trials. Interleukin-11 (IL-11), which plays a contributory role in megakaryopoiesis, has been shown to be efficacious in reducing the need for platelet transfusion after chemotherapy[5] and has approval by the Food and Drug Administration for secondary prophylaxis against thrombocytopenia after chemotherapy.

ACCELERATED PLATELET REMOVAL DUE TO IMMUNE DESTRUCTION

Idiopathic Thrombocytopenic Purpura

Pathophysiology   Idiopathic thrombocytopenic purpura (ITP) is an autoimmune disorder characterized by rapid platelet destruction; antibodies against the patient's own platelets are present. These autoantibodies bind to specific proteins on the platelet surface, and the antibody-coated platelets are removed by the reticuloendothelial system, especially in the spleen. The immunoglobulin on the platelet membrane is usually IgG (most commonly of the subclass IgG_1). This immunoglobulin is frequently directed against the platelet glycoprotein (GP) IIb-IIIa, the receptor complex that mediates fibrinogen binding and platelet aggregation. Less frequently, the immunoglobulin is directed against the GPIb complex.[6] The marrow may respond to

the thrombocytopenia by increasing platelet production. In some cases, the marrow response is suboptimal probably because the antiplatelet antibodies also react with megakaryocyte cell surface antigens. The platelets produced in ITP are usually large and functional, which may account for the clinical observation that most patients with ITP do not have significant clinical bleeding.

Clinical features   ITP typically appears in young women, but in some communities, the prevalence of ITP in young women has been superseded by its occurrence in men who are seropositive for HIV infection. Predisposing diseases and contributing factors may also include infectious mononucleosis and other acute viral illnesses, Graves disease, and Hashimoto thyroiditis,[7] as well as anticardiolipin antibody syndrome and antiphospholipid antibody syndrome.[8] For ITP patients who have antiphospholipid antibody, the outcomes, courses, and response to therapy do not differ from those of other ITP patients.

The onset of ITP is usually insidious. History and physical examination are usually negative except for the presence of petechiae, most commonly in the lower extremities. Clinical bleeding is usually mild, consisting of purpura, epistaxis, gingival bleeding, and menorrhagia. Blood blisters (wet purpura) in the mouth indicate the presence of severe thrombocytopenia. Retinal hemorrhages are uncommon. The spleen is usually not palpable. The presence of a palpable spleen raises the possibility of systemic lupus erythematosus (SLE), lymphoma, infectious mononucleosis, or hypersplenism from underlying chronic liver disease.

Laboratory evaluation   The peripheral smear is usually normal; the few platelets that are present are large and well granulated. The presence of hypochromia suggests iron deficiency from chronic blood loss; spherocytes raise the possibility of associated autoimmune hemolysis (Evans syndrome); and red blood cell fragments (schistocytes) suggest a disease such as disseminated intravascular coagulation (DIC), thrombotic thrombocytopenic purpura (TTP), or hemolytic-uremic syndrome (HUS). The marrow shows abundant megakaryocytes, many of which are small; erythroid and myeloid precursors remain normal. Results of tests for SLE are negative. Platelet-associated IgG (PA-IgG) levels are elevated; however, because platelets normally contain IgG in their α-granules, PA-IgG does not distinguish between antiplatelet antibodies, immune complexes deposited on platelet surface, and antibodies released from the platelet granules and bound on its surface. Therefore, tests for PA-IgG are not useful in the diagnosis of ITP.[9]

Differential diagnosis The differential diagnosis of ITP includes a falsely low platelet count resulting from ethylenediamenetetraacetic acid–dependent or cold-dependent agglutinins that cause in vitro platelet clumping (diagnosed by reexamination of the platelet count in citrated or heparin-anticoagulated blood sample); the gestational thrombocytopenia of pregnancy (usually a mild problem that is not associated with increased bleeding risk); myelodysplastic syndrome (usually associated with anemia and leukopenia); and underlying lymphoproliferative disease.

Course and prognosis ITP is a relatively benign disorder that has a mortality of approximately 1% to 5%; most deaths in adult cases result from intracranial bleeding. Acute ITP is usually confined to children and young adults and is frequently preceded by a viral illness. Permanent spontaneous remission occurs in less than 3 months. Chronic ITP, the usual adult variety, refers to disease that persists for more than 3 months. Although spontaneous remissions and relapses do occur in chronic ITP, long-term spontaneous remissions are uncommon. On the other hand, the long-term prognosis of ITP is benign, even in refractory cases, when these patients are managed properly.[10]

Treatment The treatment of ITP depends on the age of the patient; disease severity; whether petechiae are present alone or with moderate or severe mucosal or central nervous system bleeding; and whether the patient is pregnant.[11]

The American Society of Hematology has released an evidence-based practice guideline for the management of ITP,[9] which can be summarized as follows:

1. Patients with platelet counts above 50,000/μl do not routinely require treatment.
2. Treatment is indicated in patients with platelet counts below 20,000 to 30,000/μl and in patients with platelet counts below 50,000/μl and significant mucosal bleeding or risk factors for bleeding (e.g., hypertension, peptic ulcer disease, or a vigorous lifestyle).
3. Patients with platelet counts below 20,000/μl need not be hospitalized if they are asymptomatic or if they have only mild purpura.

Patients with asymptomatic mild or moderate thrombocytopenia (i.e., platelet count > 50,000/μl) do not require active therapy. They may be followed and simply alerted to report any mucosal bleeding or crops of new petechiae. Avoidance of aspirin and other nonsteroidal anti-inflammatory drugs (NSAIDs) is strongly advised.

For patients with moderate mucosal bleeding, therapy is begun with prednisone at a dosage of 60 to 100 mg/day in divided doses. Corticosteroids interfere with the macrophage attack on platelets and eventually reduce the amount of antiplatelet antibody produced by splenic and marrow lymphoid cells. Unless bleeding is severe, the patient need not be hospitalized. Heavy physical activity, particularly any activity that involves the Val-salva maneuver, should be avoided so as not to increase intracranial pressure. The avoidance of aspirin and other NSAIDs should be emphasized. If required, red blood cell transfusions can be given; however, it is rarely necessary to transfuse platelets in such cases.

The platelet count usually rises several days to 2 to 3 weeks after the start of therapy. When the platelet count reaches normal levels, the prednisone dose can be tapered over a 3- to 4-week period. Although complete long-term remissions with prednisone alone have been reported, sustained complete response after therapy occurs in fewer than 10% of patients.

Splenectomy is indicated if platelet counts remain below 30,000/μl after 4 to 6 weeks of steroid therapy or when the platelet count begins to fall again after the tapering of steroid. The procedure produces long-standing remission in about 65% of patients with ITP. It is best to resume oral corticosteroid therapy before splenectomy so that the patient will have a platelet count of at least 30,000 to 50,000/μl at the time of surgery. Alternatively, if the patient is not responsive to steroid therapy, intravenous immune globulin (IVIG) may be administered at a dosage of 1g/kg/day for 2 days or 0.4 g/kg/day for 5 days a few days before surgery. IVIG will produce a transient increase in the platelet count in the majority of patients, but it is a very expensive therapy. The platelet count usually begins to rise on the first postoperative day, often overshooting normal values by the second week. Pneumococcal, *Haemophilus influenzae*, and meningococcal vaccines should be administered 1 to 2 weeks before surgery.

If the patient is elderly or frail and hence may not survive splenectomy, the disease may be controlled by administration of the minimum amount of corticosteroids required to raise the platelet count to 30,000 to 50,000/μl, a level above which severe bleeding rarely occurs. Because patients with ITP who are classified as therapeutic failures generally do well clinically, the role of such potentially dangerous agents as cyclophosphamide and azathioprine in the management of such cases should be evaluated on a case-by-case basis.

Severe mucosal or CNS bleeding is a true medical emergency requiring hospitalization. Red cells are transfused as required, and prednisone is administered immediately, beginning with a 100 mg dose and then continuing at a level of 25 mg every 6 hours. IVIG should be administered at a dosage of 0.4 g/kg/day for 5 days or 1 g/kg/day for 2 days, and transfusion with 8 to 10 U of random-donor platelets should be carried out when the infusion of the first dose of IVIG, usually given over approximately 60 minutes, is complete. The platelet transfusion after the infusion of IVIG produces a greater and more durable increase in the platelet count. Side effects include generalized aches, headache, flushing, fever, and chills. When severe uterine bleeding occurs, a single 25 mg dose of conjugated estrogen can be administered intravenously to control the hemorrhage. It should be emphasized that the benefit of IVIG is usually transitory and lasts only a few days. Plans for splenectomy should follow this emergency therapy.

The mechanism of action of IVIG is not completely understood. It may produce reticuloendothelial blockade by blocking the IgG-Fc sites on the monocyte-macrophages. Highly specific anti-idiotype antibodies may also block the binding of platelet autoantibodies to the platelet GPIIb-IIIa antigen.[12] Studies indicate that the catabolic rate of IgG is mediated by a new receptor for the Fc component of IgG, termed FcRn (neonatal Fc receptor, so named because it was initially identified in neonatal intestinal epithelium), on the vascular endothelial cells. Normally, IgG, but not IgM, that enters the cell through the process of pinocytosis is protected from catabolic breakdown by binding to the FcRn. After the administration of high-dose IVIG, this receptor is presumably saturated, permitting the degradation of the pathologic antibody to occur in proportion to its concentration in plasma.[13]

Refractory Idiopathic Thrombocytopenic Purpura

A patient who remains severely thrombocytopenic after splenectomy and corticosteroid therapy or who goes into remission but later experiences a relapse and fails to respond to high doses of prednisone is said to have refractory ITP. Because serious hemorrhage is uncommon with platelet counts above 30,000/µl, it is often prudent to accept an incomplete response and not proceed to more toxic forms of management. Immunosuppressive agents are generally the mainstay of therapy at this stage. However, it should be emphasized that there are no large randomized studies to address this difficult problem and that generally these patients should be referred to a hematologist.

There are several major treatment alternatives for refractory patients. Azathioprine (100 to 150 mg/day orally) or, alternatively, cyclophosphamide (100 to 150 mg/day orally) plus prednisone (40 to 60 mg/day orally), can be given, with weekly monitoring of complete blood count and platelet count. Prednisone may be tapered and azathioprine or cyclophosphamide adjusted to avoid severe leukopenia. A frequent mistake is to discontinue the therapeutic trial prematurely. Both azathioprine and cyclophosphamide are myelosuppressive and should be given in sufficient dosages to cause a mild leukopenia, with a white blood cell count of approximately 3,000/µl, and both have been associated with development of myelodysplastic syndrome and acute myeloid leukemia. After 1 month, alternate-day prednisone therapy should be considered to avoid steroid side effects.

Another alternative is antibody therapy with intermittent courses of IVIG at the dosage schedules described above. The cost of this therapy and the usual short-lived response to it make it an unattractive choice. Anti-D antibody has been administered to Rh+(D+) patients with ITP on the theory that the antibody-coated red blood cells would block Fc receptors on macrophages and prevent the accelerated removal of platelets. Other therapeutic options include vincristine, vinblastine,[14] danazol,[15] high-dose dexamethasone, cyclosporine, interferon alfa, and plasmapheresis.

In the refractory splenectomized patient, it is important to check for the continued presence of Howell-Jolly bodies and the possibility of an accessory spleen. The disappearance of Howell-Jolly bodies suggests the presence of a remaining accessory spleen or a regenerated spleen.

Patients with clinically significant thrombocytopenic bleeding can also benefit from fibrinolysis inhibitor ε-aminocaproic acid (EACA). EACA can be given at 2 to 3 g orally four times daily until hemostasis is achieved.

HIV-Related Idiopathic Thrombocytopenic Purpura

GPIIIa, a linear peptide in the platelet membrane, has been identified as a major antigenic determinant for anti-GPIIIa antiplatelet antibody in HIV-1–related ITP.[16] In patients with HIV infection, platelets also contain increased amounts of IgG, IgM, complement, and immune complexes. Platelet survival is moderately short and platelet production is impaired, especially at the later stage of the disease.[17]

The use of immunosuppressive agents in HIV-infected patients is hazardous. If the drop in the platelet count is modest, no therapy is needed. When the thrombocytopenia is severe, a short course of prednisone can be administered, followed by splenectomy.

Acute thrombocytopenic hemorrhage in HIV-associated ITP may be managed by the administration of high-dose IVIG, similar to management in other ITPs. Chronic HIV-associated ITP may respond to oral zidovudine (AZT) or other antiviral therapies [see Chapter 133]. Anti-D antibody, dapsone, and interferon have also been used with some success.[18-20] Patients who refuse splenectomy or who are thought to be poor surgical candidates may respond to low-dose splenic irradiation.[21]

Idiopathic Thrombocytopenic Purpura in Pregnancy

Platelet counts as low as 70,000/µl occur in 5% of healthy pregnant women. When thrombocytopenia is observed for the first time during pregnancy, the differential diagnosis must include preeclampsia [see Table 1]. If other diagnoses can be excluded, the diagnosis is gestational thrombocytopenia, or incidental thrombocytopenia of pregnancy, and requires no management.[22] If the diagnosis of ITP is made, however, the therapeutic choices are limited because splenectomy may cause spontaneous abortion and immunosuppressive agents may damage the developing fetus. Therefore, therapy is usually limited to corticosteroids or IVIG. Corticosteroids increase the risk of preeclampsia and gestational diabetes. In cases of severe thrombocytopenic hemorrhage, however, all of the available therapies should be used to protect the life and well-being of the mother.

Because the antiplatelet autoantibody in ITP has broad specificity and is almost always an IgG, it can cross the placenta and produce thrombocytopenia in the fetus. During a vaginal delivery, the pressure applied to the head of a thrombocytopenic fetus may induce an intracranial hemorrhage. Concern about this occurrence had led many experts to recommend early cesarean sections in women with a history of ITP or active disease. Although cesarean sections may help minimize fetal morbidity, they can cause significant bleeding in the thrombocytopenic mother. No area of hematology has produced more differences of opinion than the management of ITP during delivery, because of the potential danger to the fetus as well as to the mother.

A large prospective surveillance study has shown that measurement of maternal antiplatelet antibody is of no clinical utility. A mother with a history of ITP who has a normal platelet count can deliver a thrombocytopenic neonate (two of 15 births, or 13%). The overall incidence of thrombocytopenic neonates in women with ITP is quite low (four of 46 births, or 9%).[22] No intracranial hemorrhages were observed in the study. In the six most severely thrombocytopenic neonates (platelet counts below 20,000/µl), the disorder was caused not by ITP in pregnancy but by the syndrome of neonatal alloimmune thrombocytopenia.[23] Nevertheless, this issue remains highly charged, with some experienced investigators recommending percutaneous umbilical blood sampling in women with platelet counts below 70,000/µl and cesarean section if the fetal platelet count is below 50,000/µl.

Thrombocytopenic Purpura with Lymphomas and Systemic Lupus Erythematosus

Patients with SLE, Hodgkin disease, or non-Hodgkin lymphoma can present with a clinical picture identical to that seen in ITP. The diagnostic approach and therapy are the same as in ITP. Splenomegaly with splenic sequestration, marrow infiltration with malignant cells, and recent antineoplastic or immunosuppressive therapy should be excluded. Patients with SLE or lymphoma may have Evans syndrome, in which ITP is associated with autoimmune hemolytic anemia. The management of Evans syndrome is the same as that of ITP and autoimmune hemolytic anemia.

Posttransfusion Purpura

Posttransfusion purpura (PTP) is characterized by acute onset of severe thrombocytopenia, often below 10,000/µl, accompanied by clinical bleeding. It may occur from 2 to 10 days after a transfusion of whole blood, packed red blood cells, or platelet-containing components. Almost all of the affected patients are multiparous women. Such disorders as septic thrombocytopenia, DIC, and heparin-induced thrombocytopenia must be considered in the differential diagnosis. The thrombocytopenia usually lasts for about 4 weeks. Because platelet transfusions are usually futile and sometimes precipitate severe systemic responses, they should be avoided if possible.

The pathophysiology of PTP is not completely understood. In most cases, the patient has been exposed to platelet alloantigens during pregnancy or as a result of a transfusion. Most patients with this disorder have antibodies to the platelet antigen PLA-1 (also termed HPA-1a), an antigen that is present on GPIIIa on the platelet surface. In the United States, approximately 98% of the white population, 99% of the African-American population, and 99% of the Asian-American population are homozygous for PLA-1. Patients in whom PTP develops are usually PLA-1 negative and PLA-2 (HPA-1b) positive. The patient has been sensitized to the PLA-1 antigen, most frequently during pregnancy, and reexposure to PLA-1 platelets during red cell transfusion leads to an anamnestic response and the destruction of the foreign platelets. It is an apparent paradox that alloantibody directed against an antigen present on foreign platelets results in destruction of the patient's autologous platelets, which do not express the PLA-1 antigen. There is evidence suggesting that the PLA-1 antigen becomes soluble and attaches to the PLA-1 negative platelets. Alternatively, exposure to foreign platelets may induce the formation of a true autoantibody against the endogenous platelets. The PLA-1/PLA-2 polymorphism accounts for 80% to 90% of PTP.

Confirmation of the diagnosis requires serologic studies demonstrating the presence of anti–PLA-1 antibody and a homozygous PLA-2 genotype. Several rapid platelet genotyping techniques based on the polymerase chain reaction have been developed.

There are no controlled clinical trials evaluating therapy for PTP because of the limited number of cases. Reports indicate that IVIG, used at doses similar to those used in the treatment of ITP, is efficacious in about 80% of cases. Another option is plasmapheresis, which appears to be as efficacious as IVIG but more cumbersome. High doses of corticosteroid is also effective, although this treatment is not as consistently effective as IVIG.[24]

Drug-Induced Immune Platelet Destruction

Drug-induced immune platelet destruction is indistinguishable from ITP. The bone marrow shows abundant megakaryocytes, and special laboratories can detect the presence of antidrug antibodies.

Quinidine and quinine purpura The pathogenic antibodies in cases of quinidine and quinine purpura develop as early as 12 days after exposure to the offending agent. In most cases, drug-dependent antibodies to platelet surface GPIb-IX have been identified in patients' sera.[25] The antibodies are drug dependent because they bind to the platelets only in the presence of quinine or quinidine. Presumably, the binding of the drugs to these platelet surface glycoproteins induces new antigenic sites on the proteins that are recognized by the antibodies.

The agent (quinidine or quinine) should be withdrawn in such cases. Neither corticosteroid therapy nor emergency splenectomy is of documented benefit in purpura induced by these agents. Plasmapheresis to remove the drug and antibodies would appear to be a logical treatment, but there are no systematic studies of its effectiveness. Transfused platelets are removed as rapidly as the recipient's own platelets. Nevertheless, platelet transfusion may be attempted to control life-threatening bleeding. Treatment with prednisone and IVIG in a dose similar to that used in ITP is recommended.

A quinine-induced thrombocytopenia that is closely followed by the development of HUS has been recognized. Quinine-dependent antibodies to platelets, as well as to endothelial cells, have been found in patients' sera.[26] Even the small amount of quinine in tonic water seems to be sufficient to trigger recurrent bouts of the syndrome. Other drugs that may occasionally produce drug-dependent thrombocytopenia include dipyridamole and trimethoprim-sulfamethoxazole.[27]

Heparin-induced thrombocytopenia Heparin-induced thrombocytopenia (HIT) is a frequent cause of drug-induced thrombocytopenia in hospitalized patients. Despite the presence of modest to moderate thrombocytopenia, HIT is rarely associated with bleeding but is associated with significant and sometimes fatal thrombosis [see Chapter 94].

Gold-induced thrombocytopenia Gold salt therapy for rheumatoid arthritis produces thrombocytopenia in 1% to 3% of patients. There is no evidence of a drug-antidrug antibody reaction as exists for quinidine and quinine thrombocytopenia. The condition is characterized by increased marrow megakaryocytes, shortened platelet survival, and, infrequently, antiplatelet antibodies. Most patients respond to therapy with 60 mg of prednisone daily. The usefulness of dimercaprol as a gold-chelating agent has not been established. Patients who are not responding to corticosteroid therapy appear to benefit from splenectomy.

Cocaine-associated thrombocytopenia An ITP-like syndrome has been reported in intravenous cocaine users. These individuals responded to an approach similar to that employed in ITP.[28]

Thrombocytopenia caused by platelet glycoprotein IIb-IIIa receptor antagonists Three parenteral GPIIb-IIIa antagonists—abciximab (ReoPro), eptifibatide (Integrilin), and tirofiban (Aggrastat)—have been approved for use in the treatment of acute coronary syndrome and as adjunctive therapy in coronary angioplasty. Meta-analysis of clinical trials with GPIIb-IIIa antagonists suggests that the parenteral administration of a GPIIb-IIIa antagonist increases the likelihood of thrombocytopenia (platelet count below 100,000/µl) by approximately 50% (overall risk, 1.48), as compared with placebo, with an incidence of approximately one to two cases per 100 patients treated.[29] The inclusion of heparin had no apparent additive effect. The development of thrombocytopenia can be acute (i.e., within 24 hours of exposure to the drug) or delayed (i.e., up to 14 days after the initiation of long-term therapy). Acute profound thrombocytopenia, with platelet counts below 20,000/µl, has been observed in 0.3% to 0.7% of patients receiving abciximab.[30]

The most likely mechanism of thrombocytopenia appears to be autoimmune mediated. Presumably, preexisting anti–GPIIb-IIIa autoantibodies are present in these patients, and after the administration of the anti–GPIIb-IIIa antagonist, the binding of the drug to GPIIb-IIIa induces conformational changes in GPIIb-IIIa such that new epitopes are exposed that are recognized by the autoantibodies. These actions would explain the acute onset of profound thrombocytopenia. The incidence of anti–GPIIb-IIIa antibodies that will bind to autologous platelets in the presence of GPIIb-IIIa antagonists has been estimated to be approximately 1% in selected patient populations.[31]

When thrombocytopenia develops, with platelet counts below 100,000/μl, the GPIIb-IIIa antagonist and any other potential offending medications (e.g., heparin) should be discontinued immediately. Depending on the platelet count, it may not be advisable to discontinue antiplatelet agents such as aspirin, ticlopidine, or clopidogrel (Plavix), because patients with this disorder are at high risk for acute coronary artery or stent thrombosis. If the platelet count drops below 10,000/μl, strong consideration should be given to platelet transfusion. In general, only one single-platelet transfusion is sufficient. There are anecdotal reports of acute coronary thrombosis associated with platelet transfusion in this setting when the platelet count climbs over 50,000/μl and the patient is off all antiplatelet agents. Thus, antiplatelet agents may need to be reinstituted. In most cases, the platelet count returns to normal within 4 days, although it may take up to 2 weeks in the case of abciximab. It is recommended that a platelet count be obtained in all patients within 2 to 4 hours after the initiation of an intravenous GPIIb-IIIa antagonist and within 24 hours of ingestion of an oral GPIIb-IIIa inhibitor.

Thrombocytopenia caused by metabolites of naproxen and acetaminophen Five patients experienced thrombocytopenia after taking naproxen and acetaminophen. In each case, antibodies that reacted with normal platelets in the presence of a known drug metabolite of naproxen or acetaminophen were identified.[32] Therefore, the sensitizing agents are drug metabolites that formed in vivo.

ACCELERATED REMOVAL OF PLATELETS BY
NONIMMUNOLOGIC MECHANISMS

There are several nonimmunologic causes for thrombocytopenia. Blood vessel wall injury with increased thrombin generation and increased platelet activation and consumption occurs in several of these conditions.

Thrombotic Thrombocytopenic Purpura and Adult Hemolytic-Uremic Syndrome

TTP and HUS encompass a group of clinical syndromes in which a primary event damages the endothelia of small vessels, leading to widespread platelet-fibrin thrombi deposition in the small arteries and arterioles and capillaries. Thrombotic microangiopathy is a distinct feature of both TTP and HUS.

Clinical features and diagnosis The five major manifestations (pentad) of TTP are (1) severe microangiopathic hemolytic anemia associated with a very high serum lactic dehydrogenase (LDH) level and a blood smear showing the characteristic schistocytes and helmet cells; (2) moderate to severe thrombocytopenia with increased marrow megakaryocytes, which indicates intravascular platelet activation and consumption; (3) fever, which is occasionally quite high; (4) CNS signs and symptoms that can be quite mild initially with transient agitation, headache, and disorientation but sometimes progress explosively to hemiparesis, aphasia, seizures, focal deficits, coma, and death; and (5) renal disease, which is usually mild and produces moderate elevations of

serum creatinine and urine protein. It should be emphasized that many patients do not present with all these signs and symptoms.

The adult form of HUS is a similar condition. Common features of TTP and HUS include microangiopathic hemolytic anemia, thrombocytopenia, and the presence of platelet fibrin thrombi in the small vessels. Renal involvement is uniformly severe in HUS, whereas CNS disease is less prominent than in TTP. There is a distinct form of HUS that occurs in approximately 15% of children after gastrointestinal infection with *Escherichia coli*, usually serotype 0157:H7. These patients present with bloody diarrhea and hemorrhagic colitis. *E. coli* 0157:H7 or other strains elaborate verotoxins (also called Shiga toxins) that bind to specific receptors on the endothelial surface, causing cell damage and even cell death.[33] Studies show that verotoxin-1 (VT-1) can induce the upregulation of various prothrombotic and proinflammatory adhesive molecules on endothelial cells.[34] The microvascular endothelial cells are particularly susceptible because they have a high expression of VT-1 receptors, which may explain the propensity for thrombosis in the microcirculation. Antibiotic treatment of children with *E. coli* 0157:H7 infection increases rather than decreases the risk of HUS, presumably because it causes the release of verotoxins from injured bacteria in the intestine, making the toxins more available for absorption. Thus, routine treatment with antibiotics is not recommended.[35]

Differential diagnosis Both TTP and HUS must be differentiated from SLE and from Evans syndrome. Microangiopathic hemolysis, neutrophilic leukocytosis, and a negative direct Coombs test (direct antiglobulin test) strongly suggest TTP or HUS. Coagulation tests usually reveal no significant abnormalities (i.e., no evidence of DIC); serum LDH is usually elevated. A marrow biopsy is generally not required but may show the characteristic, but not pathognomonic, platelet-fibrin hyaline thrombi in small arteries and arterioles.

Etiology TTP/HUS occurs spontaneously and is also associated with pregnancy, cancer, bone marrow transplantation, autoimmune diseases, and various drugs. In pregnancy, it resembles severe preeclampsia. In the postpartum period, the CNS manifestations may initially be confused with postpartum depression, with tragic results. Cases have been reported after a normal delivery and with abruptio placentae and preeclampsia.

Several drugs appear to cause TTP/HUS. These include chemotherapeutic drugs (e.g., mitomycin C, bleomycin, and cisplatin), immunosuppressive agents (e.g., cyclosporine and FK506), the antiplatelet agent ticlopidine, oral contraceptives, and quinine. For ticlopidine, the incidence is very low (0.02%) and the majority of cases occur after 2 to 4 weeks of therapy. However, the condition is difficult to predict. In one study, overall mortality in ticlopidine-induced TTP/HUS was 21%, with all deaths occurring in patients not treated with plasmapheresis.[36] Such findings underscore the importance of a high index of suspicion and the prompt institution of plasmapheresis. Anecdotal cases of TTP/HUS associated with clopidogrel, which is related to ticlopidine, have also been reported.[37]

Pathophysiology Two mechanisms have been proposed to account for TTP/HUS. One hypothesis postulates the presence of a circulating platelet activating factor that stimulates platelets causing extensive intravascular platelet aggregation. The second hypothesis suggests that the primary insult is extensive arteriolar endothelial damage. Platelet activation, adherence, occlusion, and fibrin strand formation then lead to thrombocytopenia and microangiopathic hemolysis. There are data to support both hypotheses.

Many investigators have observed that abnormally large multimers of von Willebrand factor (vWF) are present in patients with chronic relapsing TTP.[38,39] These abnormal vWF multimers may have enhanced binding affinity to platelets and may contribute to the development of microvascular thrombosis. They accumulate because of a defect in the normal processing of vWF multimers, thus predisposing the patient to thrombosis. In support of this hypothesis, the vWF-cleaving protease has been purified.[40,41] This enzyme is a new member of the ADAMTS (a disintegrin and metalloprotease with thrombospondin type 1 motif) family of metalloprotease that binds to zinc and calcium and is synthesized in the liver as a proenzyme (zymogen). It is then activated by proteolytic cleavage. There are multiple variants of this enzyme generated by alternative splicing of the messenger RNA, which may be of physiologic significance.[42]

A decrease in the vWF-cleaving protease activity in chronic relapsing TTP was initially described by two groups.[38,39] This decrease has been confirmed and extended.[43,44] In a prospective study of 111 adult patients with thrombotic microangiopathies, a decrease in vWF-cleaving protease activity was found in 59 of 66 TTP patients (89%) and in 6 of 45 HUS patients (13%).[43] In this study, the TTP/HUS was considered either idiopathic or secondary, associated with clinical factors that include neoplasia, immunologic disorders, bacterial or viral infections, bone marrow transplantation, and drugs. In a second study, reduced protease activity was found in only 9 of 20 patients with TTP.[44] Furthermore, a deficiency or decrease in the vWF-cleaving protease activity is not specific for TTP, because it was also found in patients with other thrombocytopenic disorders, including some patients with ITP, DIC, SLE, and leukemia, many of whom did not have evidence of microangiopathy.[44]

The two groups who originally reported the decrease in vWF-cleaving protease activity in chronic relapsing TTP described the isolation of inhibitory antibodies from the patient plasma.[38,39] This development has also been confirmed in the recent prospective study.[43] A protease inhibitor was found in 47% of the TTP patients but not in the HUS patients. In the majority of cases, the inhibitor was not detectable when the patients were in remission.

Thus, evidence strongly suggests that a deficiency or decrease in the vWF-cleaving metalloprotease plays a major role in the pathogenesis of TTP but not HUS, suggesting that these two clinical entities may differ in pathophysiology. In the acquired form of TTP, this difference may be related to the presence of an inhibitory antibody. In the much rarer familial form, it may be the result of a constitutive enzyme deficiency. Plasma exchange could remove the abnormally large vWF multimers and the inhibitory antibodies in the patient's plasma, as well as replenish the protease.

However, it should be noted that normal vWF-cleaving protease activity is also observed in some patients with TTP. There is no apparent relation between protease activity and disease severity.[44] It is also likely that the abnormally large vWF multimers are not sufficient to account for the pathogenesis of TTP. Large multimers can be detected in the plasma of patients with relapsing TTP when these patients enter clinical remission.[39] In one well-studied case of chronic relapsing TTP, normalization of the abnormal vWF multimers failed to increase the platelet count

and induce clinical remission.[45] Extensive damage or activation of endothelial cells, perhaps in the setting of infection, pregnancy, or exposure to certain drugs, causes them to release the largest vWF multimers, which, as a result of defective processing, may cause platelet aggregation and microvascular thrombosis. With the identification of the vWF-cleaving metalloprotease, specific assays for this enzyme should be available to help clarify these issues.

Treatment Prompt institution of plasma exchange with fresh frozen plasma is the treatment of choice for TTP/HUS. In a large randomized trial by the Canadian Apheresis Group, intensive plasma exchange was more effective than plasma infusion in terms of patient survival (78% versus 63%).[46] In that study, 1.5 times the calculated plasma volume was removed and replaced with fresh frozen plasma during each of the first 3 days of therapy and then one plasma volume a day thereafter for a minimum of 7 days. Some investigators obtained good results with a daily single-volume exchange instead of 1.5-volume exchange.[47] It is reasonable to start with a daily single-volume exchange if the patient is clinically relatively stable, with moderate thrombocytopenia and no significant neurologic impairment. However, if the clinical situation worsens, more intensive double-volume plasma exchange (5,000 to 6,000 ml/day, or approximately 80 ml/kg/day) is indicated. Because vWF multimers are present in cryoprecipitate, cryosupernatant (i.e., fresh frozen plasma from which cryoprecipitate has been removed) can be substituted as replacement fluid when a patient is not responding to routine plasma exchange. One uncontrolled study showed increased benefit from this preparation as compared with fresh frozen plasma.[48] Once therapeutic benefit has been achieved (as measured by restoration of normal CNS function, by rising platelet counts, and by falling LDH levels), the intensity and frequency of plasma exchange can be reduced to single-volume exchanges, first three times weekly and then twice weekly.

Although the importance of prompt plasma exchange has been established, the use of corticosteroids,[49] aspirin, and dipyridamole has not been tested in prospective clinical trials. Because pheresis tends to lower the platelet count in a patient who is already thrombocytopenic, the problem of platelet transfusion arises. Some investigators have observed that platelet infusion may lead to exacerbation of TTP,[50] whereas others use platelet transfusions as required.

Microangiopathy may persist for weeks or months after all other evidence of disease has subsided. In a large follow-up study of TTP patients, about one third of those who entered remission relapsed during a 10-year period, and about one in 10 experienced other serious medical problems. Therefore, careful follow-up is required.[51]

Splenectomy has been highly recommended by several experienced clinicians,[52] and I have had some success with this approach. However, there have also been several failures that were complicated by the effects of splenectomy in an already difficult clinical situation. Thus, I do not routinely employ splenectomy in patients with TTP. The same modalities employed in TTP have also been used in HUS, along with hemodialysis for renal failure and medical management for hypertension.

Thrombocytopenia Induced by Infection

Severe viral, bacterial, fungal, and parasitic infection can produce DIC and, consequently, thrombocytopenia [see Chapter 94];

however, mechanisms other than DIC may also cause infection-associated thrombocytopenia.

Viral infections Viral infections such as dengue fever and congenital rubella can directly damage the megakaryocytes. Varicella can cause a form of thrombocytopenia that has the characteristics of an immune reaction: increased numbers of megakaryocytes, no evidence of DIC, and the presence of PA-IgG or platelet-associated IgM. Usually, no therapy is required. The acute thrombocytopenia in infectious mononucleosis is probably immune mediated, as shown by the increase in marrow megakaryocytes, the rise in PA-IgG, and the favorable response to corticosteroids. At times, the thrombocytopenia is severe, but as noted, it responds to corticosteroids.

Bacterial septicemia Patients who have severe gram-negative septicemia and platelet counts lower than 50,000/μl usually have evidence of DIC. However, many patients who have both gram-negative and gram-positive septicemia and platelet counts between 50,000 and 150,000/μl have no signs of DIC. An immunologic mechanism may be involved in these cases because the PA-IgG levels are often elevated, and the degree of elevation correlates with the severity of the thrombocytopenia. The elevated PA-IgG may represent immune complexes deposited on the platelet surface rather than antiplatelet autoantibodies. The key to controlling the thrombocytopenia is establishing appropriate therapy for the infection. If DIC is present, it should be managed with careful control of hypotension and blood volume.

If clinically significant thrombocytopenia that has not been caused by DIC is present, platelet transfusion should be given as required to prevent hemorrhage.

Protozoan infection Thrombocytopenia is common in malaria, although DIC is rare. Platelet survival is short, and elevated PA-IgG has been found to be elevated. The IgG antibody appears to bind to malarial antigens adsorbed to the platelet surface.[53]

Thrombocytopenia during Pregnancy and Peripartum Period

Mild thrombocytopenia with platelet counts as low as 70,000/μl occurs in 5% to 8% of pregnant women (gestational thrombocytopenia). It has no clinical significance, but it must be distinguished from ITP, pregnancy-associated TTP, and preeclampsia.

In addition to having hypertension, proteinuria, and evidence of pathologic changes in the kidneys, liver, CNS, and placenta, approximately 15% of patients with preeclampsia have moderate thrombocytopenia. Only a minority of patients with preeclampsia and thrombocytopenia demonstrate laboratory evidence of DIC. The megakaryocyte number is increased, and platelet survival is somewhat shortened. Some patients with preeclampsia and thrombocytopenia also have microangiopathic hemolysis, which suggests that damaged vessels containing fibrin strands are destroying red blood cells and platelets. Intense vasospasm that causes endothelial damage and leads to platelet activation, adherence, and destruction may also play a role. The clinical picture may be indistinguishable from TTP, in which case it should be managed as TTP. Otherwise, management consists of prenatal care for preeclampsia and efforts to detect thrombocytopenia as early as possible.

HELLP syndrome The HELLP syndrome refers to a disorder that occurs during pregnancy and is characterized by hemolysis, elevated levels of liver enzymes, and a low platelet count. It probably represents an extremely severe form of preeclampsia. At some point between the 23rd and 39th week of pregnancy, affected patients present with thrombocytopenia marked by a platelet count of less than 100,000/μl, microangiopathic hemolysis, abnormal liver function tests, and, occasionally, hypertension.[54] The results of the standard coagulation tests for DIC are normal, although there may be some elevation in the level of fibrin degradation products and depression of the antithrombin III (AT-III) levels. Patients with the HELLP syndrome are often severely ill, with circulatory, respiratory, and renal failure; postpartum hemorrhage; intrahepatic hemorrhage; and seizures. The disorder is treated by terminating the pregnancy, usually by delivery, and by providing meticulous supportive care. In a large series of patients with HELLP, the nadir of thrombocytopenia occurs 1 to 2 days after delivery.[55] Persistent thrombocytopenia with microangiopathy, or the presence of organ failure, suggests postpartum TTP/HUS, and plasma exchange therapy should be considered.

Thrombocytopenia in Hypothermia

Thrombocytopenia caused by the hypothermia induced during cardiac surgery can occasionally occur. Hypothermia in elderly persons apparently can also cause thrombocytopenia; platelet levels as low as 30,000/μl have been reported.[56] The mechanisms proposed to account for the thrombocytopenia include DIC and hepatic and splenic sequestration. After the patient's body temperature has been restored to normal, the platelet count spontaneously returns to normal levels over a period of 1 to 2 weeks.

Platelet Washout and Vascular Bed Abnormalities

Perioperative platelet washout formerly was a frequent cause of nonimmune thrombocytopenia. Patients who have brisk bleeding during surgery and are then transfused with more than 10 U of stored whole blood experience thrombocytopenia. In effect, the patients have undergone an exchange transfusion with blood that contained nonviable platelets. The platelet count is low; the prothrombin time (PT), partial thromboplastin time (PTT), and thrombin time (TT) are normal [see Chapter 92]. Therefore, the platelet count should be monitored in patients who are receiving massive transfusions (e.g., 10 U of red blood cells or whole blood). If the level falls below 100,000/μl and the patient is undergoing surgery or another hemostatic challenge, platelets should be administered.

Platelets may also be removed by an abnormal vascular bed. In giant hemangiomas, there is sluggish blood flow through improperly endothelialized channels. These surfaces may produce low-grade DIC.

Platelet Sequestration

The third major mechanism of thrombocytopenia is platelet sequestration. Platelet counts of 40,000 to 80,000/μl are common in patients with marked splenomegaly. Clinically significant hemorrhage rarely occurs unless a coexistent hemorrhagic disorder is present. Management is directed toward the primary disease. Splenectomy is rarely necessary.

Platelet Function Disorders

The clue to the existence of a platelet function defect is the finding of clinical hemorrhage in the presence of a prolonged bleeding time and a platelet count higher than 100,000/μl. Petechiae are rare. Platelet morphology and tests of platelet function may be abnormal [see Table 2].

Table 2 Classification of Platelet Function Disorders

Type	Characteristic	Cause
Congenital	Membrane abnormalities	Bernard-Soulier disease (GPIb-IX-V defect, impaired adhesion); Glanzmann thrombasthenia (GPIIb-IIIa defect, impaired aggregation)
	Granule abnormalities	Gray platelet syndrome (absent or impaired α-granule release, impaired aggregation); dense granule deficiency (absent or impaired dense granule release, impaired aggregation)
	Deficiency of a plasma factor	von Willebrand disease (deficiency or abnormality of von Willebrand factor, impaired adhesion); afibrinogenemia (deficiency of fibrinogen, impaired aggregation)
Acquired	Production of abnormal platelets	Myeloproliferative disease (essential thrombocytopenia, chronic myelogenous leukemia, polycythemia vera, myelofibrosis, acute myelogenous leukemia); myelodysplasia
	Dysfunction of normal platelets	Systemic disease (uremia, liver disease, paraproteinemias, disseminated intravascular coagulation); drugs (aspirin and other nonsteroidal anti-inflammatory drugs, ticlopidine, clopidogrel, GPIIb-IIIa antagonists, dextran, antibiotics [penicillin, carbenicillin, moxalactam], psychotropic drugs)

HEREDITARY ABNORMALITIES OF PLATELET FUNCTION

Platelet Membrane Disorders

Bernard-Soulier syndrome is a rare autosomal recessive disease characterized by giant platelets, a prolonged bleeding time, moderate thrombocytopenia, and risk of fatal hemorrhage. The defect, an absence of platelet GPIb-IX-V complex (the major vWF binding site of the platelet), causes impaired platelet adhesion to wound surfaces. Ristocetin-induced platelet agglutination is abnormal and not corrected by the addition of normal plasma containing vWF. Acute hemorrhage is treated by platelet transfusions.

Glanzmann thrombasthenia is a rare autosomal recessive disorder in which platelet morphology and the platelet count are normal but the bleeding time is long. Because the critically important GPIIb-IIIa complex that forms the platelet binding site for fibrinogen is absent, the platelets do not undergo aggregation after stimulation by adenosine diphosphate (ADP), thrombin, or collagen. Ristocetin-induced agglutination, however, is normal. Treatment is platelet transfusions when necessary.

Platelet Granule Disorders

Patients with the gray platelet syndrome, a rare disorder, have mucosal bleeding, ecchymoses, and petechiae. Moderate thrombocytopenia is present, and the bleeding time is prolonged. The platelets are larger than normal and appear agranular because of the absence of α-granules. Because the α-granule contents are severely reduced, platelet adhesion and platelet-supported coagulation are deficient. Platelet aggregation with collagen is abnormal. Bleeding episodes should be treated by infusion of normal platelets.

Another rare disorder, the dense granule deficiency syndrome, is characterized by mucosal bleeding associated with a normal platelet count, normal platelet morphology, and variable prolongation of the bleeding time. Platelet aggregation with ADP and collagen are abnormal. The decrease in the dense granular contents of ADP impairs ADP-mediated events. Hemorrhage is treated by platelet transfusion.

1-Desamino-8-D-arginine vasopressin (DDAVP or desmopressin) is an alternative therapy for patients with primary platelet disorders requiring surgery.

ACQUIRED ABNORMALITIES OF PLATELET FUNCTION

Myeloproliferative Diseases and Associated Platelet Abnormalities

Platelet function abnormalities occur in the myeloproliferative diseases: chronic myeloid leukemia, polycythemia vera, essen-

tial thrombocythemia, and acute leukemia. The platelet count in chronic myeloproliferative disorders is often very high, but the bleeding time may be prolonged, and clinical bleeding may appear as mucosal hemorrhage and hematomas. The abnormality resembles an acquired storage-pool defect. Megakaryocytes often are abnormal with separated nuclei; the peripheral blood platelets are large and may be degranulated. Management of acute hemorrhage consists of transfusion of normal platelets to bring the level of normal platelets up to 50,000/μl. Aspirin and other NSAIDs should be avoided.

Uremia and Associated Platelet Abnormalities

A prolonged bleeding time associated with clinical bleeding despite a normal platelet count has been well documented in uremia. The identity of the inhibitory substance in uremic plasma that causes this thrombocytopathy is still unclear. DDAVP (0.3 μg/kg in 50 ml of saline over a 30-minute period) is effective in controlling uremic bleeding for about 4 to 6 hours. DDAVP infusion produces an increase in plasma vWF activity and particularly in the larger multimers of vWF, which may enhance platelet adhesion.

The hematocrit should be maintained above 30% in bleeding uremic patients because the bleeding time is prolonged when the hematocrit falls below 26%.[57] Bleeding may also be controlled by the use of conjugated estrogens. Conjugated estrogen (Premarin) given orally (50 mg/day) or intravenously (0.6 mg/kg/day) for 4 to 5 days shortens the bleeding time by approximately 50% for about 2 weeks.[58] The advantage of conjugated estrogens over DDAVP is the longer duration of their beneficial effect on platelet function, but they have a more delayed onset of action. The two drugs can be used concomitantly.

Liver Disease and Associated Platelet Abnormalities

In addition to hypersplenism and defective procoagulant synthesis, there is evidence that low-grade DIC occurs continually in severe liver disease. Impaired clearance of fibrin degradation products may further contribute to high plasma levels of fibrin-fibrinogen degradation products. These products interfere with platelet function and fibrin polymerization, and their level correlates with clinical hemorrhage in severe hepatic cirrhosis. Therapy for this condition must be directed against the primary disease.

Effects of Macroglobulinemia and Other Dysproteinemias on Platelet Function

The presence of high concentrations of viscous proteins produces complicated effects on the entire hemostatic mechanism.

The proteins appear to coat platelets and interfere with adhesion and perhaps with aggregation. Management is directed at the primary disease, but if hyperviscosity and bleeding are significant, prompt plasmapheresis may be required to lower the level of abnormal protein and to correct the bleeding disorder.

Drug-Induced Platelet Disorders

Aspirin and other nonsteroidal anti-inflammatory drugs In normal persons, ingestion of 0.6 g of aspirin prolongs the template bleeding time by 2 to 3 minutes. The platelets are irreversibly affected. Thromboxane A2 (TXA2) is a potent inducer of platelet release and aggregation [see Chapter 92]. Aspirin acetylates and irreversibly inhibits cyclooxygenase-1 (COX-1) and blocks the subsequent generation of thromboxane. Some apparently normal persons display marked sensitivity to the action of aspirin, so that their bleeding times are very much prolonged and they have clinically significant bleeding, particularly during or after surgery or trauma. These patients may have a mild form of von Willebrand disease or storage pool disease, and their mild bleeding diathesis becomes exacerbated by aspirin's antiplatelet effect.

Uremic patients are especially sensitive to bleeding induced by aspirin. A small dose of aspirin does not prolong the bleeding time of normal persons but produces a significant prolongation, often as much as 15 minutes, in uremic patients. The combination of alcohol and aspirin is also dangerous because of aspirin's ability to prolong the bleeding time.

Aspirin-induced bleeding is diagnosed by determining the existence of an acquired platelet function defect (a platelet count above 100,000/μl, abnormal platelet aggregation test results, and no prior bleeding history) and finding evidence of aspirin ingestion. Because some 300 compounds on the market contain aspirin, a negative history should be supplemented either by determining a serum salicylate level or by detecting an abnormal collagen aggregation pattern that reverts to normal in 7 days (the typical pattern of aspirin ingestion).

If bleeding is significant, it can be managed by platelet transfusion. Because inhibition of platelet COX-1 by aspirin is irreversible, the hemostatic compromise may last for 4 to 5 days after the aspirin has been discontinued. If the patient needs analgesia, acetaminophen or codeine can be used because neither affects platelet function. If the patient requires anti-inflammatory drugs, as in the therapy of rheumatoid arthritis, cyclooxygenase-2 (COX-2) inhibitors, which do not affect platelet function, can be used.

Alcohol In addition to producing thrombocytopenia by suppressing platelet production, alcohol consumption can cause platelet function defects.[59] In vitro studies have shown that alcohol impairs platelet aggregation and TXA2 release. Platelet function returns to normal after 2 to 3 weeks of abstinence.

Dextrans The 40,000-molecular-weight form of dextran is readily excreted, but 70,000-molecular-weight dextran may persist in the circulation for 3 days and interfere with platelet

---

Table 3   Selected Platelet-Modifying Agents[118]

Anesthetics
 General
  Halothane
 Local
  Butacaine
  Cocaine
  Cyclaine
  Dibucaine
  Procaine
  Tetracaine
Antibiotics (β-lactam)
 Cephalosporins
  Cefazolin
  Cefotaxime
  Cefoxitin
  Cephalothin
  Moxalactam
 Penicillins
  Ampicillin
  Apalcillin
  Azlocillin
  Carbenicillin
  Methicillin
  Mezlocillin
  Nafcillin
  Penicillin G
  Piperacillin
  Sulbenicillin

Temocillin
Ticarcillin
Antibiotics (other)
 Nitrofurantoin
Anticoagulants
 Heparin
Antihistamines
 Chlorpheniramine
 Diphenhydramine
 Mepyramine
Cardiovascular drugs
 Diltiazem
 Isosorbide dinitrate
 Nifedipine
 Nitroglycerin
 Nitroprusside
 Propranolol
 Quinidine
 Verapamil
Drugs that increase platelet
  cAMP concentration
 Dipyridamole*
 Iloprost
 Prostacyclin
Fibrinolytic agents
Foods and food additives
 Ajoene

Chinese black tree fungus
Cloves
Cumin
Ethanol
Omega-3 fatty acids
Onion extract
Turmeric
Glycoprotein IIb-IIIa
  antagonists
 Abciximab
 Eptifibatide
 Lamifiban
 Tirofiban
Narcotics
 Heroin
Nonsteroidal anti-inflammatory
  drugs
 Aspirin*
 Diflunisal
 Ibuprofen
 Indomethacin
 Meclofenamic acid
 Mefenamic acid
 Naproxen
 Phenylbutazone
 Piroxicam
 Sulfinpyrazone*
 Sulindac

Tolmetin
Oncologic drugs
 BCNU
 Daunorubicin
 Mithramycin
Plasma expanders
 Dextrans
 Hydroxyethyl starch
Psychotropic drugs
 Phenothiazines
  Chlorpromazine
  Promethazine
  Trifluoperazine
 Tricyclic antidepressants
  Amitriptyline
  Imipramine
  Nortriptyline
Miscellaneous agents
 Clofibrate
 Clopidogrel
 Ketanserin
 Radiographic contrast
  agents
  Conray-60
  Renografin-76
  Renovist II
 Ticlopidine*

*Used as a therapeutic antithrombotic agent.
BCNU—bischloronitrosourea (carmustine)   cAMP—cyclic adenosine monophosphate

surface action. Management involves support until the dextran is excreted. Transfused platelets are affected by the dextran in plasma.

Antibiotics   Carbenicillin and ticarcillin can inhibit platelet aggregation and contribute to a bleeding disorder, as can massive doses of penicillin. Massive doses of penicillin impair collagen-induced and ristocetin-induced platelet aggregation. Moxalactam, a third-generation cephalosporin, also causes a platelet function disorder. The clinical situation is most important when an acquired platelet function defect develops in a pancytopenic patient being treated for septicemia. Changing the antibiotics usually corrects this problem.

Miscellaneous agents   A wide variety of other agents can modify platelet function [*see Table 3*].[60]

Thrombocytosis and Thrombocythemia

DIAGNOSIS

A platelet count higher than 500,000/µl is referred to as reactive thrombocytosis. In reactive thrombocytosis, tests of platelet function (including platelet aggregation studies) are generally normal, and patients do not experience increased incidence of hemorrhage or thromboembolism even when the platelet count exceeds 1 million/µl.

Elevated platelet counts (often 1 million to 3 million/µl or more) also occur in chronic myeloid leukemia, agnogenic myeloid metaplasia with myelofibrosis, polycythemia vera, and essential thrombocythemia. In the diagnosis of essential thrombocythemia, the platelet count is higher than 600,000/µl and other causes of thrombocytosis (e.g., another myeloproliferative disorder or reactive thrombocytosis) have been excluded.

In myeloproliferative disorders, tests of platelet function are frequently abnormal [*see Platelet Function Disorders, above*]. Some patients with myeloproliferative disorders appear to show an enhanced propensity for hemorrhage and thromboembolism. Neither platelet number nor measurements of platelet function predict the degree of thrombosis or hemorrhage.

Clinically, the hemorrhagic signs include mucosal (particularly gastrointestinal) bleeding, hematomas, and ecchymoses. There may be splenic vein thrombosis, portal or mesenteric vein thrombosis, and recurrent deep vein thrombosis with or without pulmonary embolism. Arterial thrombosis is less common.

TREATMENT

Patients with essential thrombocythemia and polycythemia vera may have debilitating erythromelalgia (burning and itching of the fingers and toes) that can progress to ischemic acrocyanosis.[61] This symptom complex appears to be caused by occlusion and inflammation of arterioles by platelet aggregates. Aspirin or indomethacin produces relief within hours. Aspirin given at a dosage of 325 mg daily can produce lasting benefit.

Hemorrhage and thrombosis are uncommon events even with platelet counts of 1 million/µl. In a patient with essential thrombocythemia who has clinically significant hemorrhage or thrombosis, good control of the platelet count can be achieved with oral hydroxyurea (15 mg/kg/day) with adjustments in the dosage as needed to lower the platelet count. Hydroxyurea therapy requires careful monitoring of the blood count; thus far, hydroxyurea therapy does not appear to increase the risk of a second

Table 4   Classification of the Vascular Purpuras

Type	Causes
Direct damage to the endothelium	Infections: rickettsioses, infections associated with endotoxin production Toxins: snake venoms ?Immune complex diseases
Damage to supporting structures that decreases the mechanical strength of the microvasculature	Scurvy Amyloidosis Hereditary connective tissue disorders: Ehlers-Danlos syndrome, Marfan syndrome, pseudoxanthoma elasticum Hereditary hemorrhagic telangiectasia Senile purpura Adrenal cortisol excess
Leukocytoclastic vasculitis	Rheumatic diseases: systemic lupus erythematosus, polyarteritis nodosa, Wegener granulomatosis Idiopathic immune complex diseases: Waldenström macroglobulinemia, cryoglobulinemia, hepatitis B, Henoch-Schönlein purpura, drug-induced disease (e.g., by sulfonamides)
Damage to the microvasculature by emboli	Fat embolization Cholesterol embolization Thrombosis Leukostasis Septic and bland emboli from heart valves: subacute bacterial endocarditis (SBE)

malignant disorder. Newer therapies for thrombocythemia include the use of anagrelide, a powerful platelet-lowering agent.[62]

Vascular Purpuras

Vascular purpuras are a heterogeneous group of disorders [*see Table 4*] that are characterized by cutaneous hemorrhage, occasionally associated with mucosal bleeding. The leakage occurs from terminal arterioles, capillaries, and postcapillary venules. The results of tests of platelet number and function and tests of procoagulant function are normal.

HEREDITARY HEMORRHAGIC TELANGIECTASIA

Hereditary hemorrhagic telangiectasia (HHT) is transmitted as an autosomal dominant trait and is manifested most commonly as epistaxis or gastrointestinal bleeding.[63] Recent linkage analyses have identified at least three HHT loci, including the genes for endoglin and activinlike receptor kinase. Both proteins are expressed on vascular endothelial cells and may function as receptors for transforming growth factor–β (TGF-β). TGF-β plays a complex role in coordinating responses between endothelial cells and the extracellular matrix, and mutations in the genes for endoglin and activinlike receptor kinase lead to the development of abnormal blood vessels and arteriovenous channels.[64]

Physical examination reveals telangiectasias on finger pads, buccal mucosa, the tongue, and lip borders. Coagulation tests are generally normal. The pulmonary arteriovenous malformations that occur in some patients may produce dyspnea, hemoptysis, low arterial oxygen tension (P_aO_2), and secondary erythremia. The diagnosis can be confirmed by pulmonary angiography. If the shunts are large and clinically significant, they can be treated by balloon embolotherapy.[65] Paradoxical embolus with stroke can occur in patients with HHT who have pulmonary arteriovenous shunts and malformations.

Management of recurrent epistaxis often involves devising methods for obtaining nasal tamponade. Gastrointestinal bleeding is managed by the use of iron preparations when possible.

SCURVY

Vitamin C is required for the normal metabolism of collagen, folate, and perhaps iron. The patient with scurvy suffers primarily from impaired collagen synthesis. The lack of proper collagen support for the microvasculature leads to perifollicular hemorrhages, bleeding gums, and even deep tissue hematomas. Presumably, similar collagen defects lead to the so-called corkscrew hair and hyperkeratosis associated with this disorder.[66] The characteristic clinical picture in a malnourished person suggests the diagnosis. Plasma or buffy coat levels of ascorbic acid are low, and other vitamin deficiencies are usually present as well. Effective therapy consists of 1 g of ascorbic acid daily in divided doses.

CORTICOSTEROID EXCESS

Corticosteroid excess, whether from endogenous or exogenous causes, produces cutaneous hemorrhages, probably because of corticosteroid-induced catabolism of protein in vascular supportive tissues.

AMYLOIDOSIS

Amyloidosis can present with subcutaneous ecchymoses that have a predilection for the neck and upper chest. Biopsy of the site shows the amyloid, which by its infiltration may weaken the vessel walls or interfere with surface activation of platelets, procoagulants, or both. In patients with primary systemic amyloidosis, especially when accompanied by a huge amyloid spleen, the amyloid can in very rare instances adsorb enough factor X to cause profound factor X deficiency and clinical bleeding.

LEUKOCYTOCLASTIC VASCULITIS

The purpuric lesions in patients with leukocytoclastic vasculitis may be raised (palpable purpura). On biopsy, these lesions may show mast cell degranulation and, when stained appropriately, immune complex deposition. Presumably, the immune complexes provide the chemotactic stimulation that leads to the congregation of neutrophils. Damage to the microvasculature is caused by the complement attack complex and by the release of the contents of the neutrophil granules. This inflammatory component produces the palpable purpura.

SENILE PURPURA

Patients with senile purpura have cutaneous hemorrhages on the dorsum of the hand, the wrist, and the upper arms and occasionally on the calves. Serious bleeding does not occur; no treatment is required. Presumably, this condition represents an age-dependent deterioration of the vascular supportive tissue.

DAMAGE TO THE MICROVASCULATURE DUE TO EMBOLI

DIC and TTP can cause localized vaso-occlusions leading to microvascular damage and leakage of red blood cells. Similar damage can be caused by emboli that arise from infected heart valves. Fat embolism may complicate fractures of the long bones and pelvis. The syndrome consists of fever, confusion, and petechiae or purpura, or both, over the neck, chest, face, and axillae. Cholesterol embolism can also cause petechiae, usually over the lower extremities. It typically occurs in a patient with severe atherosclerosis who has recently undergone an invasive procedure involving the abdominal aorta or renal arteries. Biopsy of the purpura shows cholesterol crystals when an appropriate stain is used.

Hereditary Coagulation Disorders

The coagulation disorders appear clinically as either spontaneous hemorrhage or excessive hemorrhage after trauma or surgery. The history usually indicates whether the disorder is congenital or acquired. The hereditary disorders are characterized by appearance in early life and by the presence of a single abnormality that can account for the entire clinical picture.

VON WILLEBRAND DISEASE

Pathophysiology

von Willebrand disease, the most common hereditary bleeding disorder, is caused by a deficient or defective plasma vWF. The gene encoding vWF is on chromosome 12. vWF has specific domains for binding clotting factor VIII, heparin, collagen, platelet GPIb, and platelet GPIIb-IIIa. These domains relate directly to the following functions of vWF: (1) its action as a carrier molecule for factor VIII:C, in which it protects the clotting factor from proteolysis and substantially prolongs its plasma half-life; (2) its promotion of primary platelet adhesion at high wall shear rates by linking platelets via their GPIb-IX-V receptor to subendothelial tissues at the wound site; and (3) its support of platelet aggregation by linking platelets via their GPIIb-IIIa receptors.[67] The vWF circulates as multimers that range in size from 0.5 million daltons (the dimer) to 20 million daltons. Even larger noncirculating multimers are present in endothelial cells, where they are stored in the Weibel-Palade bodies. The vWF is released either into the circulation or abluminally, where it attaches to subendothelial collagen. Platelet α-granules also contain vWF, which is released when platelets are activated. The vWF multimers that are 12 million daltons or larger are probably the most effective in supporting platelet adhesion.

Laboratory Evaluation

The many variant forms of von Willebrand disease differ in their clinical manifestations, laboratory abnormalities, and required therapies. Therefore, specific tests are needed to identify the type of disease and its severity. Testing begins with an activated PTT (aPTT) and a platelet count [see Chapter 92]. Because vWF is a carrier protein for factor VIII, the aPTT is prolonged when the vWF level is low. The platelet count is usually, but not invariably, normal. Bleeding time is generally prolonged but not sufficiently reliable to be used for diagnosis. The diagnosis depends then on necessary factor VIII and vWF levels. There are two caveats concerning the tests for von Willebrand disease: (1) laboratory testing is notoriously variable and (2) the patient's blood group affects the vWF level—that is, patients with blood group O have lower vWF levels than those with blood group A, B, or AB, by as much as 30%.[68]

The vWF level is measured by immunologic methods. The result is usually reported as a percentage of normal vWF antigen (factor VIIIR:Ag). Because vWF circulates in physiologically important multimeric forms, it is sometimes helpful to determine the multimeric composition of the vWF in the patient's plasma. The functional capabilities of vWF are tested by the ris-

Table 5 Classification and Differentiation of von Willebrand Disease

	Type 1	Type 2A	Type 2B	Type 2M	Type 2N	Type 3	Pseudo–von Willebrand Disease
Inheritance	Autosomal dominant	Autosomal dominant	Autosomal dominant	Autosomal dominant	Autosomal dominant	Autosomal recessive	Autosomal dominant
Incidence	~75%	~20%	~5%	Rare	Rare	Uncommon	Uncommon
Cause	Deficiency of normal vWF	Abnormal vWF	Abnormal vWF	Abnormal vWF	Abnormal vWF	Severe deficiency of vWF	Abnormal platelet membrane
Template bleeding time	N or ↑	↑	↑	↑	N or ↑	↑↑	N or ↑
Factor VIII assay	↓	N or ↓	N or ↓	N or ↓	↓↓	↓↓	N or ↓
vWF antigen	↓	Variable	Variable	Variable	N	↓↓	Variable
Ristocetin cofactor (RIPA)	↓	↓	↑	↓	N	↓↓	↑
Plasma vWF multimer analysis	N	Only low-molecular-weight forms present	Only low- and intermediate-molecular-weight forms present	N	N	Variable	Only low- and intermediate-molecular-weight forms present

N—normal ↓—decreased ↑—increased vWF—von Willebrand factor

tocetin-induced platelet aggregation test. Ristocetin is added to a patient's platelet-rich plasma, where it causes vWF to bind to platelets via the GPIb-IX-V receptor, leading to platelet activation and aggregation. In some laboratories, formalin-fixed platelets are used and agglutination of fixed platelets after the addition of ristocetin is measured. A new automated platelet function test utilizing a platelet function analyzer (PFA-100) has been developed. Citrated whole blood is aspirated through a capillary tube under high shear onto a membrane coated with collagen in which a central aperture is made. Platelets are activated by either ADP or epinephrine. The closure time is a measure of platelet-vWF interaction. It has been shown to be a good screening test for vWD.[69]

Clinical Variants

The current classification scheme for variants of von Willebrand disease comprises three major groups: type 1 is a partial quantitative deficiency of vWF, type 2 is a qualitative abnormality of vWF, and type 3 is a severe and virtually total quantitative deficiency of vWF [see Table 5].[70]

Type 1 Type 1 von Willebrand disease is the most common form (75% of cases). It is generally an autosomal dominant trait that usually appears in the heterozygous form. Patients with classic type 1 von Willebrand disease have a lifelong history of mild to moderate bleeding, typically from mucosal surfaces. They may be unaware of a bleeding disorder until they undergo surgery or experience trauma, when bleeding may be severe. vWF antigen, factor VIII, and the ristocetin cofactor levels are all decreased. The rare homozygous or double heterozygous form (type 3 von Willebrand disease) is characterized by severe hemorrhage, a long PTT, and factor VIII levels of less than 5%.

Type 2 Type 2 von Willebrand disease is characterized by qualitative abnormalities of vWF and a variable decrease in vWF antigen, factor VIII, and ristocetin cofactor. In type 2A, the largest

multimers are absent. In type 2B, multimers bind excessively to platelets because of a gain-of-function mutation. In type 2M, the abnormal vWF does not bind to GPIb-IX-V; in type 2N, the binding site of vWF for factor VIII is mutated.

Pseudo–von Willebrand disease A platelet form of von Willebrand disease, which is termed pseudo–von Willebrand disease, has been described in which an abnormal GPIb is present on platelets, causing excessive binding of normal plasma vWF to unstimulated platelets.

Treatment

Mild or moderate types 1 and 2 DDAVP is effective in the management of traumatic bleeding and before surgery in some patients with mild or moderate type 1 and type 2A von Willebrand disease. The intravenous administration of DDAVP at a dosage of 0.3 mg/kg over a 15- to 30-minute period causes the release of vWF from endothelial cell stores. The peak response usually occurs in 30 to 60 minutes and persists for up to 4 to 6 hours. Subcutaneous administration of DDAVP has also been reported to be effective.[71] Repeated DDAVP administrations over a 24-hour period are ineffective; tachyphylaxis follows depletion of the endothelial vWF store. A nasal DDAVP spray (300 µg) can be used in the ambulatory treatment of patients with von Willebrand disease, both for the management of bleeding episodes and as preparation for minor surgery.[72] The side effects of intravenous DDAVP are generally mild, including significant water retention and, rarely, thrombosis. Myocardial infarction has been reported. Because of the variability of response to DDAVP, a patient should be give a trial infusion of DDAVP before undergoing a planned procedure to determine whether the patient has an adequate response. EACA, 3 g four times daily orally for 3 to 7 days, is also useful for dental procedures and minor bleeding events. Aspirin must be avoided.

Moderate and severe types 2 and 3 Patients with type 3 von Willebrand disease and with types 2A and 2B, which are more severe than type 3, generally require replacement therapy with Humate-P, a pasteurized intermediate-purity factor VIII concentrate that has a substantial amount of large vWF multimers, or with cryoprecipitate infusion containing vWF, factor VIII, and fibrinogen. Cryoprecipitate is generally not recommended unless the risk of viral contamination can be avoided by testing or treatment. Transfusion of normal platelets can also be attempted on the grounds that platelet vWF can be hemostatically effective.[73]

Treatment during pregnancy Treatment is generally not needed during pregnancy in women with von Willebrand disease. The plasma vWF level rises during the second and third trimesters but falls rapidly after delivery. Late hemorrhage may occur 2 to 3 weeks post partum.[74] DDAVP is not used before delivery because of the concern that it may initiate contractions. Patients with type 2B von Willebrand disease may have worsening thrombocytopenia during pregnancy because of the increase of abnormal vWF in plasma.[75]

HEMOPHILIA A

Hemophilia A affects one in 10,000 males and is characterized by a deficient or defective clotting factor VIII. The factor VIII gene, which is located on chromosome X at Xq28, is among the largest known human genes, spanning 186 kb and containing 26 exons. It encodes a protein of about 300,000 daltons, which circulates in plasma at very low concentrations, and is normally bound to and protected by vWF. The primary source of factor VIII production is unknown, but the liver must be a significant source because hemophilia A can be corrected by liver transplantation.

Because the gene for factor VIII coagulant activity is carried on the X chromosome, the disease is manifested in hemizygous males. All of the daughters of a hemophiliac male will be carriers, whereas half of the sons of a mother who carries the hemophilia trait will be hemophiliacs and half of her daughters will be carriers. Families appear to be affected to varying degrees, depending on the specific nature of the genetic defect.

The clinical severity of hemophilia A correlates well with the measured levels of factor VIII coagulant activity. In general, factor VIII levels below 1% are associated with severe hemorrhagic symptoms, levels between 1% and 5% with moderate hemophilia, and levels between 5% and 25% with mild hemophilia [see Table 6].

Approximately one third of hemophilia A patients represent new mutations and have a negative family history. More than 300 abnormal factor VIII genes have been found. The abnormalities, which include point mutations, gene insertions, and gene deletions, result in either deficient factor VIII production or the generation of a functionally defective factor VIII. Interestingly, an inversion within intron 22 of the factor VIII gene, which results in a truncated and unstable factor VIII protein, is found in approximately 45% of all severely affected hemophilia A patients (factor VIII levels below 1%).[76]

Diagnosis

Diagnosis is made on the basis of the clinical picture, family history (positive in two thirds of cases), and the factor VIII coagulant activity level. In most cases, the type of bleeding history and a classic family history rule out von Willebrand disease (which, unlike hemophilia A, is autosomally transmitted). Accurate DNA analysis for the common intron 22 inversion is now available in DNA testing laboratories. This test provides molecular diagnosis in approximately 45% of patients with severe he-

Table 6 **Correlation of Factor VIII Coagulant Activity Level with Bleeding Patterns in Hemophilia**

Plasma Factor VIII Level	Bleeding Pattern
< 1%	Severe, presentation in first year of life, bleeding with circumcision, spontaneous hemarthrosis and deep-tissue bleeding
1%–5%	Moderate, presentation in childhood, bleeding after trauma, spontaneous hemarthrosis rare
5%–25%	Mild; may be present in childhood; bleeding after trauma, surgery, or dental extraction
25%–50%	May be undetected, may present in adulthood with bleeding after major trauma or surgery

mophilia. However, it should not be ordered in patients with mild or moderate hemophilia.

Treatment

General principles The psychosocial aspects of hemophilia are complex. A child is often absent from school, is prone to crippling deformities, and runs a risk of drug addiction because of severe pain. Parents are understandably deeply concerned and sometimes troubled by guilt. Treatment should address these issues as well as the specific coagulation problem.

Factor VIII replacement Factor VIII concentrates are effective in controlling spontaneous and traumatic hemorrhage. Cryoprecipitate, tested or treated to prevent hepatitis viruses and HIV, remains the mainstay of care. The potential of contamination has stimulated efforts to develop concentrated, virus-free preparations. A number of such preparations are now available, and the problem is to balance cost against presumed benefit. Highly pure factor VIII preparations (e.g., Monoclate-P and Hemofil M) are made by using monoclonal antibodies and affinity chromatography. Factor VIII gene has been cloned, and two forms of full-length recombinant factor VIII (Recombinate and Kogenate) have been on the market for several years; formal studies as well as extensive clinical experience indicate that they are safe and efficacious.[77,78] A second-generation, B-domain–deleted recombinant factor VIII has also been developed, and it was found to be effective and well tolerated in an open-label, multicenter trial.[79] The new recombinant factor VIII has the advantage of considerably higher specific activity, and the final formulation is stable without added human serum albumin, thus further reducing the potential risk of transmission of human infectious agents.

Dental prophylaxis is critically important to reduce the need for dental surgery. Aspirin must be avoided. Revaccination against hepatitis B virus also should be considered.

Genetic counseling should be part of the management program. Because of the difficult life severe hemophiliacs lead, a woman may opt to terminate pregnancy if she is certain of her carrier status or if she knows that her fetus is affected. There are several strategies for detecting carriers. In women who are carriers, factor VIII levels are typically about half of normal, whereas vWF levels are normal. The ratio of factor VIII to vWF for carriers is thus 0.5[80]; however, the error rate for this test is 10% to 17%. A more accurate genetic diagnosis for carriers can be made by a linkage approach. This approach is based on restriction fragment length polymorphisms (RFLPs) within the factor VIII gene. Analysis of the affected male will establish the pattern for the X chromosome carrying the hemophilia allele, without knowledge of the precise mutation. There are a large number of intragenic polymorphisms that allow the two copies of factor VIII genes in an at-risk female potential carrier to be distinguished, identifying her carrier state with high accuracy.

These molecular probes for RFLPs are now being used to determine the status of the fetus. Tissue can be obtained by amniocentesis or chorionic villus sampling.

Management of acute hemorrhage   Deep tissue bleeding, hemarthrosis, and hematuria are the common forms of clinical bleeding in hemophilia A. Acute threats to life are posed by retroperitoneal hemorrhage; bleeding of the mouth, tongue, or neck that impairs the airway; and intracranial hemorrhage. Both ultrasonography and computed tomography can be used to identify retroperitoneal and intramuscular hematomas.

Principles of replacement therapy   A plasma procoagulant level of 100% means that there is one unit of procoagulant per milliliter of plasma. Most persons have 40 ml of plasma per kilogram of body weight. Thus, from a determination of a patient's plasma volume and procoagulant level, the required amount of factor VIII replacement can be calculated. For example, in the case of a 60 kg boy who has an uncomplicated hemarthrosis of the knee and a baseline factor VIII of less than 1%, raising the factor VIII level to about 25% (0.25 U/ml) for 2 to 3 days should suffice. This patient has a plasma volume of 60 kg × 40 ml/kg, or 2,400 ml; he will need 0.25 U/ml × 2,400 ml, or 600 U of factor VIII, as an initial bolus. Another method of estimation is based on the following effect: the infusion of 1 U of factor VIII per kg increases factor VIII levels by 2%. Thus, dividing the desired level of factor VIII increase by 2 will give the number of U/kg required. In the example cited, 25% of factor VIII will require 12.5 U/kg, or 750 U, of factor VIII replacement.

The biologic half-life of factor VIII is approximately 12 hours; the dose can be repeated every 12 to 24 hours as long as needed to control the hemorrhage. In patients with hemarthrosis, the factor VIII level should be maintained for 2 to 3 days.

Elective surgery and dental extraction   Dental work should be performed by a dentist who is experienced in the treatment of hemophiliacs. Before dental extraction, factor VIII is administered to raise the level to approximately 50%. The fibrinolytic inhibitor EACA is started the night before surgery at a loading dose of 3 g orally and continued at 2 to 3 g three to four times daily for 7 to 10 days after the dental work has been completed. Usually, further administration of factor VIII is not required.

Before elective surgery, the factor VIII level should be raised to 50% to 100% (0.5 to 1.0 U/ml) and then maintained above 50% for the next 10 to 14 days. Maintaining a higher concentration of factor VIII does not reduce the frequency of hemorrhage.[81]

DDAVP can be used to treat acute traumatic hemorrhage in patients with mild to moderate hemophilia and even to prepare such patients for minor surgery. DDAVP, which causes the release of vWF from endothelial cell stores, cannot be used repeatedly over many days, because such stores become depleted. DDAVP is infused at a dosage of 0.3 μg/kg in 50 ml of saline over 15 to 30 minutes and produces a prompt increase in factor VIII. The biologic half-life of the released factor VIII is 11 to 12 hours.

Management of an inhibitor   Inhibitors tend to occur in more severely affected patients, who tend to receive the greatest number of factor VIII concentrates. In a recent single-center study of 431 patients over 3 decades, approximately 10% of patients with severe hemophilia A had an inhibitor (about a third were children younger than 10 years).[82] Not all inhibitors produce clinical problems. Assays for factor VIII inhibitors should be performed at regular intervals in all patients who have severe hemophilia.

Hemorrhage in a patient with an inhibitor can be life threatening. In a patient who has an inhibitor titer of less than 5 Bethesda units and who is not a vigorous antibody responder, a large amount of factor VIII concentrate should be administered in an attempt to overwhelm the antibody. Alternative therapies are porcine factor VIII (Hyate:C), prothrombin complex concentrates (e.g., Konyne and Proplex) to circumvent the factor VIII deficiency,[83,84] and activated prothrombin complex concentrates, such as Autoplex and FEIBA.

Recombinant activated factor VII (rFVIIa) has been found to be safe and efficacious in 70% to 85% of more than 1,500 bleeding episodes in hemophilia patients with inhibitors.[85,86] Recombinant factor VIIa may compete against the normal plasma unactivated factor VII for tissue factor binding and thus enhance thrombin generation at the bleeding site.[87] In addition, high-dose rFVIIa may bind to activated platelets and activate factors IX and X on the platelet surface in the absence of tissue factor.[88]

High-dose intravenous IgG has been used to treat nonhemophiliacs with acquired factor VIII inhibitors, but it is usually not efficacious in hemophiliacs with inhibitors.

OTHER HEREDITARY HEMORRHAGIC DISORDERS

Factor IX Deficiency (Hemophilia B)

Factor IX deficiency (hemophilia B, or Christmas disease) is an X-linked disorder that is clinically indistinguishable from hemophilia A. The factor IX gene is on the X chromosome and produces a protein of 56 kd that, like other vitamin K–dependent factors, has a region rich in γ-carboxylated glutamic acids. Presumably, calcium ion bridges link this region to the activated platelet cell surface, where factor IXa interacts with factor VIIIa to form a membrane-associated complex that efficiently converts factor X to factor Xa (intrinsic tenase) [*see Chapter 92*]. A large number of insertions, rearrangements, and deletions have been detected in the factor IX gene, and the hemophilia B syndrome is very heterogeneous.[89]

Diagnosis   Diagnosis requires a factor IX assay. The management principles are the same as those for hemophilia A. Factor IX is replaced with fresh frozen plasma or with prothrombin complex concentrates. One of the newer factor IX concentrates (Mononine) has been sterilized and displays excellent specific activity and a desirable biologic half-life of 18 to 34 hours. Recombinant factor IX is also commercially available.

Treatment   The level of factor IX needed to control hemostasis in patients with hemophilia B is somewhat lower than the level of factor VIII required for the treatment of hemophilia A—about 0.15 to 0.20 U/ml for the former and 0.30 to 0.50 U/ml for the latter. Factor IX is a smaller molecule than factor VIII and is distributed in the albumin space. In making replacement calculations, it is assumed that administration of 1 U/kg of factor IX will increase the plasma level by 1%, or by 0.01 U/ml. Factor IX has a biphasic half-life, and plasma levels of this factor can be maintained by infusing the concentrate every 24 hours during an acute bleeding episode in a patient with hemophilia B. Gene cloning techniques can now detect the factor IX deficiency carrier state and permit accurate genetic counseling.

Sustained correction of a bleeding disorder in hemophilia B mice has been demonstrated by the gene therapy approach,[90] and clinical trials of factor IX in both hemophilia A and hemophilia B have been initiated. Different gene transfer approaches are used, including ex vivo transduction and transfection, retroviral vector, and adeno-associated virus. The collective interim results indicate that the current approaches and doses are safe and that low levels of factor VIII and factor IX expression are detected.[91]

Factor VII Deficiency

Occasionally, preoperative screening tests reveal that a patient has a mildly prolonged PT in the absence of liver disease, poor diet, or antibiotic administration. Some of these patients can be shown to be heterozygous for factor VII deficiency states, as confirmed by family testing and by measuring the factor VII antigen level in plasma. Therapy is not required unless major surgery is contemplated, in which case factor VII can be supplied in the form of fresh frozen plasma. Clinical bleeding in these patients is quite variable, ranging from nonexistent to severe. Less often, factor VII deficiency has been reported to be associated with thrombosis.[92]

Fibrinolytic Abnormalities

Two uncommon congenital hemorrhagic disorders have been ascribed to abnormalities of fibrinolysis. Deficiency of α_2-antiplasmin, the major plasmin inhibitor, has led to uncontrolled plasmin activity with consequent hemorrhage. Enhanced fibrinolytic activity with occasional clinical bleeding has also been linked to deficiency of plasminogen activator–1 (PAI-1), the physiologic inhibitor of tissue plasminogen activator (t-PA) and urokinase.[93] Treatment of both types of fibrinolytic abnormalities consists of the antifibrinolytic agents, tranexamic acid, or EACA, which block the binding of plasminogen and plasmin with fibrin.

Acquired Hemorrhagic Disorders

In addition to the hereditary coagulation disorders, several acquired disorders have also been identified that can lead to generalized hemorrhage.

VITAMIN K DEFICIENCY

A vitamin K–dependent carboxylase in the liver synthesizes γ-carboxyglutamic acid, which is required for the biologic function of prothrombin and factors VII, IX, and X. In the absence of vitamin K, an abnormal prothrombin that lacks γ-carboxyglutamic residues is synthesized. Specific immunoassays performed in patients with vitamin K deficiency reveal a sharp decrease in normal prothrombin and a concomitant increase in the abnormal des-γ-carboxyprothrombin. The same molecular derangement occurs with factors VII, IX, and X.[94]

Clinical Features and Diagnosis

Deficiency of vitamin K, which decreases prothrombin and factors VII, IX, and X, occurs in severe malnutrition, intestinal malabsorption, and obstructive jaundice. In obstructive jaundice, bile salts, which are necessary for the emulsification and absorption of the fat-soluble vitamins (vitamins A, D, E, and K), cannot enter the intestine. Chronic ingestion of oral antibiotics suppresses vita-

min K production by intestinal organisms. The effect is especially marked in patients who, because of their illness, are unable to consume a full, nourishing diet. Mucosal bleeding and ecchymoses occur if the procoagulant levels fall below 10% to 15% of normal.

Treatment

Therapy with phytonadione (10 to 25 mg/day orally) for 2 to 3 days, or parenteral phytonadione in obstructive jaundice, usually reverses the abnormality in about 6 to 24 hours. If there is severe bleeding, fresh frozen plasma (approximately 3 U) restores procoagulant levels rapidly [see Principles of Replacement Therapy, above].

DRUG-INDUCED HEMORRHAGE

Warfarin-Induced Hemorrhage

Warfarin overdose or potentiation of its action by other drugs can cause very severe bleeding. The PT is prolonged, and mucosal bleeding, gastrointestinal bleeding, or ecchymosis is the usual pattern. If hemorrhage is significant, treatment to restore procoagulant levels to 30% of normal must be started with fresh frozen plasma. If there is no urgency, oral phytonadione may be given. Surreptitious warfarin use can be identified by a serum warfarin assay, which is available at special laboratories. It should be noted that some of the long-acting vitamin K antagonists that are used as rodenticides (superwarfarins) may lead to prolonged bleeding symptoms after factitious or accidental ingestion of these compounds. The synthesis of vitamin K–dependent clotting factors can be impaired for months after the initial exposure. Repeated administration of fresh frozen plasma, supplemented by massive doses of oral vitamin K_1 (100 to 150 mg/day), may be required to control bleeding symptoms.

Heparin-Induced Hemorrhage

Heparin overdose may not be obvious. It causes subcutaneous hemorrhages and deep tissue hematomas. The PTT, PT, and TT are vastly prolonged, but the reptilase time (RT) is normal. Intravenous protamine administration at a dosage of 1 mg/100 U of administered heparin terminates the disorder. Because the half-life of protamine is shorter than that of heparin, a heparin rebound may occur, necessitating a second administration of protamine. Low-molecular-weight heparin (LMWH) preparations cause as much bleeding as standard unfractionated heparin. The ability of protamine to reverse the actions of these LMWH preparations is highly specific for each compound. For example, protamine does not completely reverse the actions of enoxaparin.

Hemorrhage Caused by Thrombolytic Therapy

Thrombolytic therapy is now used for acute myocardial infarction and for some cases of pulmonary embolism. The complications of thrombolytic therapy are essentially all hemorrhagic. In general, bleeding has been confined to relatively trivial oozing at vascular invasion sites, but subdural hematomas, cerebral infarction, and intracranial bleeding have also occurred. The thrombolytic agents, even those designed to be relatively fibrin specific, occasionally cause a significant systemic lytic state, with low levels of fibrinogen, factor V, and factor VIII. Furthermore, the generation of fibrinogen degradation products in turn interferes with the formation of a firm clot and with platelet function.

If thrombolytic therapy is suspected as the cause of bleeding in a particular patient, blood should be drawn quickly for an aPTT, a TT, an RT, and a fibrinogen level. If thrombolytic thera-

Table 7 Causes of Disseminated Intravascular Coagulation (DIC)

Events that initiate DIC
- Septicemia
- Cancer procoagulants (Trousseau syndrome)
- Acute promyelocytic leukemia
- Crush injury, complicated surgery
- Severe intracranial hemorrhage
- Retained conception products, abruptio placentae, amniotic fluid embolism
- Eclampsia, preeclampsia
- Major ABO blood mismatch, hemolytic transfusion reaction
- Burn injuries
- Heatstroke
- Malignant hypertension
- Extensive pump-oxygenation (repair of aortic aneurysm)
- Giant hemangioma (Kasabach-Merritt syndrome)
- Severe vasculitis

Events that complicate and propagate DIC
- Shock
- Complement pathway activation

py is the cause, the aPTT is prolonged, the fibrinogen level is usually below 50 mg/dl, and the TT and RT are both prolonged (as a result of the fibrin degradation products and decreased plasma fibrinogen).

The disorder is treated with cryoprecipitate (to raise the fibrinogen level to approximately 100 mg/dl), approximately 2 U of fresh frozen plasma (which can be increased to up to 6 U as needed to replace factor V and other procoagulants), and approximately 6 U of platelet concentrates. If these measures do not stop the bleeding, the use of a specific antifibrinolytic agent such as EACA should be considered. EACA is given as a 5 g bolus I.V. over 30 to 60 minutes and then in a dosage of 1 g/hr by continuous I.V. infusion.[95]

DYSPROTEINEMIAS

The abnormal proteins associated with myeloma and macroglobulinemia can interfere with platelet function and cause clinical bleeding. These proteins can cause abnormalities in the coagulation tests as well. Both IgG and IgA myeloma proteins can cause prolonged TTs by interfering with the fibrin polymerization process. Less commonly, they may interact with specific clotting factors. Management is directed at the primary disease. Generally, these paraproteins do not cause clinically significant bleeding. If bleeding occurs, plasmapheresis rapidly corrects the defects by abruptly lowering the level of abnormal protein.

DISSEMINATED INTRAVASCULAR COAGULATION

Pathophysiology

Many different circumstances can cause DIC [see Table 7]. In each case, massive activation of the clotting cascade overwhelms the natural antithrombotic mechanisms, giving rise to uncontrolled thrombin generation. This condition results in thromboses in the arterial and venous beds, leading to ischemic infarction and necrosis that intensify the damage, release tissue factor, and further activate the clotting cascade. Massive coagulation depletes clotting factors and platelets, giving rise to consumption coagulopathy and bleeding. Tissue damage and the deposi-

tion of fibrin result in the release and activation of plasminogen activators and the generation of plasmin in amounts that overwhelm its inhibitor, α_2-antiplasmin. Plasmin degrades fibrinogen, prothrombin, and factors V and VIII and produces fibrin-fibrinogen degradation products. These substances interfere with normal fibrin polymerization and impair platelet function by binding to the platelet surface GPIIb-IIIa fibrinogen receptor. These fibrin-fibrinogen degradation products thus function as circulating anticoagulant and antiplatelet agents, exacerbating the consumption coagulopathy, and play a significant role in the bleeding diathesis [see Figure 1].

Endotoxin released during gram-negative septicemia enhances the expression of tissue factor, thereby accelerating procoagulant activation while suppressing thrombomodulin expression. These actions downregulate the protein C/protein S system, further promoting the tendency to DIC.[96] In patients with solitary or multiple hemangiomas associated with thrombocytopenia (Kasabach-Merritt syndrome), DIC is presumably initiated by prolonged contact of abnormal endothelial surface with blood in areas of vascular stasis. Platelets and fibrinogen are consumed in these hemangiomas, where fibrinolysis appears to be enhanced,[97] and such consumption can lead to hemorrhage. Certain snakebites can also produce DIC; several mechanisms have been identified. For example, Russell viper venom contains a protease that directly activates factor X and can produce almost instantaneous defibrination.

Clinical Consequences

The consequences of DIC depend on its cause and the rapidity with which the initiating event is propagated. If the activation occurs slowly, an excess of procoagulants is produced, predisposing to thrombosis. At the same time, as long as the liver can compensate for the consumption of clotting factors and the bone

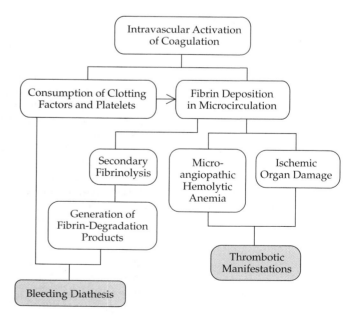

Figure 1 In compensated disseminated intravascular coagulation (DIC), such as that which occurs in Trousseau syndrome, thrombotic manifestations predominate in the clinical presentation. In decompensated DIC, however, fibrin-fibrinogen degradation products exacerbate the consumption coagulopathy and play a significant role in the bleeding diathesis.

marrow maintains an adequate platelet output, the bleeding diathesis will not be clinically apparent. The clinical situation consists of primarily thrombotic manifestations, which can be both venous thrombosis and arterial thrombosis [see Chapter 94]. Venous thromboses commonly involve deep vein thrombosis in the extremities or superficial migratory thrombophlebitis. Patients can also experience arterial thrombosis, leading to digital ischemia, renal infarction, or stroke. Arterial ischemia can in part be the result of emboli that originate from fibrin clots in the mitral valve, a condition termed nonbacterial thrombotic endocarditis, or marantic endocarditis. This condition is sometimes known as compensated, or chronic, DIC and accounts for Trousseau syndrome[98] (a chronic DIC caused by an underlying malignancy, most frequently pancreatic or other gastrointestinal cancer). The cancer cells may produce either tissue factor or another procoagulant that activates the clotting system.

If the reaction is brisk and explosive, the clinical picture is dominated by intravascular coagulation; depletion of platelets, fibrinogen, prothrombin, and factors V and VIII; and the production by plasmin action of fibrin degradation products, which further interfere with hemostasis. The clinical consequence is a profound systemic bleeding diathesis, with blood oozing from wound sites, intravenous lines, and catheters, as well as bleeding into deep tissues. The intravascular fibrin strands produce microangiopathic hemolytic anemia.

Diagnosis

Microangiopathic red blood cells on smear and a moderate to severe thrombocytopenia suggest the diagnosis. A number of laboratory abnormalities are present in DIC, depending on the stage of the DIC. Because of clotting factor depletion, the PTT and PT are prolonged and the fibrinogen level is low. Because fibrin degradation products interfere with fibrin polymerization, the TT and RT are also prolonged. The level of fibrin degradation products, as measured by the D-dimer level, is elevated. Plasma plasminogen, protein C, and α_2-antiplasmin levels are also low because of consumption; however, these measurements are generally not required. In the case of compensated DIC, most of these parameters can be normal except for the elevation of the D-dimer level, which indicates the presence of intravascular cross-linked fibrin deposition and fibrinolysis. Sometimes, the fibrinogen level can even be high because fibrinogen is an acute-phase reactant. When the DIC becomes decompensated, consumption coagulation predominates and the other laboratory abnormalities listed above are present. Repetition at regular intervals of the coagulation tests listed earlier, especially the platelet count, fibrinogen, and D-dimer levels, is critical. These tests provide a kinetic parameter that greatly aids in the assessment of the severity of the DIC and the choice of appropriate management.

Treatment

In one study, recombinant human activated protein C (aPC) was shown to significantly reduce mortality in patients with severe sepsis (mortality was 30.8% in patients given placebo versus 24.7% in patients given aPC).[99] Although aPC is associated with an increased risk of bleeding, it appears to be an effective agent in the treatment of severe DIC in sepsis. aPC has not yet been approved by the Food and Drug Administration.

Currently, management must be directed at the primary disease to switch off the initiating event. This approach may involve chemotherapeutic treatment of an underlying tumor, administration of antibiotics and surgical drainage of an abscess, or emptying the uterus when complications of pregnancy have been the inciting cause. Hemodynamic support is essential. The use of antifibrinolytic agents such as EACA or aprotinin is contraindicated. Despite its bleeding complications, DIC is a severe hypercoagulable state, and these agents block the fibrinolytic system and may exacerbate its thrombotic complications. The administration of blood products, such as platelets, fresh frozen plasma, or cryoprecipitate, may add fuel to the fire and worsen the consumption coagulopathy. However, if clinical bleeding becomes significant, it is prudent to give vigorous blood product support.

The use of heparin in acute DIC is not established. Although heparin, by activating AT-III, is effective in inhibiting thrombin and therefore should be efficacious in the treatment of DIC, its use is generally limited to situations of chronic or compensated DIC. Heparin, given subcutaneously, is effective in the treatment of venous thrombosis in patients with Trousseau syndrome. Another situation in which heparin may be considered is at the beginning of induction chemotherapy, when an explosive release of thromboplastic materials associated with the lysis of the tumor cells is anticipated. For example, judicious use of heparin can ameliorate the marked exacerbation of DIC frequently associated with the use of chemotherapy in the treatment of acute promyelocytic leukemia. In this situation, if the patient presents with significant DIC even before chemotherapy, low-dose heparin (in the range of 300 U/hr by continuous infusion) may dampen the DIC as demonstrated by lowering the D-dimer and raising the plasma fibrinogen level. However, with the advent of all-trans retinoic acid in the initial treatment of acute promyelocytic leukemia, the use of heparin is generally not required. In the case of decompensated DIC, in which bleeding is the major clinical manifestation, heparin may significantly exacerbate the bleeding and its use is generally not indicated. Recently, the use of high-dose AT-III infusion has been advocated in this situation, but its efficacy has not been established by randomized studies.[100,101]

Management of the DIC associated with solitary or multiple hemangiomas presents particular problems. When the hemangiomas are localized, they can be excised; occasionally, they show a good response to local irradiation. Attempts to control the DIC using heparin, corticosteroids, aspirin, sulfinpyrazone, estrogens, and dipyridamole have not been successful. The key to successful management of DIC associated with certain snakebites is identification of the snake and prompt administration of appropriate antivenin.

ACQUIRED HEMOPHILIA AND OTHER DISORDERS OF CIRCULATING INHIBITORS

In addition to the circulating alloantibody inhibitors seen in severe hemophilias A and B, clinical hemorrhage is occasionally caused by circulating inhibitors directed against specific clotting factors that seem to appear spontaneously. Because acquired autoantibody to factor VIII, which gives rise to the clinical picture of acquired hemophilia, is the most common of these circulating inhibitors, it will be described here in some detail, but many of the principles also apply to other inhibitors.

Autoantibodies to factor VIII are usually IgGa and frequently IgG4 and thus do not fix complement. They are usually directed against the functionally important A2 and C2 domains[102] on factor VIII. About half of the patients with an acquired factor VIII inhibitor have no identifiable associated disorder, but many different disease states have been identified in the remainder. Such associated conditions include autoimmune disorders such as

SLE, lymphoproliferative disorders, plasma cell malignancies, drug reactions (e.g., reaction to penicillin), the postpartum state, and skin disorders.[103]

Diagnosis

Patients with an acquired factor VIII inhibitor commonly present with new-onset mucosal hemorrhages, hematomas, and ecchymoses, along with a negative bleeding history. Typically, this disorder occurs in an elderly patient or in a young woman during pregnancy or in the postpartum period. The laboratory hallmark of an acquired inhibitor to a clotting factor is a prolonged clotting time that is not corrected by mixing equal parts of the patient's plasma with normal plasma. In the case of factor VIII inhibitor, the PTT is prolonged and the PT and TT are normal. The antibody binds to factor VIII with complex kinetics such that the inhibitory effect becomes apparent only after prolonged incubation. Therefore, if an acquired factor VIII inhibitor is suspected, mixing studies should be performed after 5-minute and 60-minute incubations. The diagnosis can be confirmed by demonstration of a very low factor VIII level when other clotting factor levels are normal.

Treatment

The hemorrhage may be clinically life threatening. Attempts at replacement are usually not successful, because the inhibitor inactivates the exogenous factor VIII. Occasionally, if the inhibitor has a low titer, massive factor VIII replacement can overwhelm the inhibitor. However, this treatment may trigger a significant anamnestic response in the antibody level, which complicates further management. Immunosuppressive therapy with a combination of cyclophosphamide (given either as a monthly intravenous pulse therapy or orally on a daily basis) and prednisone has been successful in most cases.[104,105] The inhibitor usually becomes undetectable after three to four monthly cycles of chemotherapy. In the case of severe or life-threatening hemorrhage in which there is not sufficient time to try to reduce the level of inhibitor, porcine factor VIII can be administered because the autoantibody usually displays low cross-reactivity.

The other alternative therapy for acute bleeding is the administration of procoagulant complexes, which may bypass the inhibitor block by providing large amounts of factor X and factor VII.[106] Other therapeutic options include plasmapheresis and high-dose intravenous IgG, although the response rate for IVIG appears to be quite low.[107] Recombinant activated factor VII (90 µg/kg given as an I.V. bolus every 2 to 3 hours) has been used successfully in patients with this condition.

ACQUIRED VON WILLEBRAND DISEASE

Diagnosis

Acquired von Willebrand disease is being recognized.[108] Patients, generally in their 50s and 60s and without past history or family history of bleeding, present with mucocutaneous-type bleeding, and the workup is consistent with von Willebrand disease. It frequently occurs in the setting of underlying lymphoproliferative, myeloproliferative, or cardiovascular disease and is associated with a small monoclonal gammopathy on serum protein electrophoresis. The plasma antibody to vWF is functional in a minority of cases, as demonstrated by inhibition of vWF in a functional assay by mixing studies.[109] However, most cases involve nonneutralizing antibodies to vWF, which can be demonstrated by enzyme-linked immunologic assay. Presumably, the antibody binds to vWF and causes its rapid clearance, leading to a low plasma vWF level. Nonimmune mechanisms (e.g., adsorption of vWF onto tumor cells) have also been described. Multimeric analysis of plasma vWF typically shows a decrease in the high-molecular-weight multimers.

Treatment

DDAVP is useful in correcting the bleeding diathesis in about one third of cases. High-dose intravenous IgG (1 g/kg I.V. daily for 1 to 2 days) generally gives a good temporary response, with an increase in the vWF level and a shortening of the PTT, lasting from a few days to 2 weeks. If the patient has a defined lymphoproliferative, myeloproliferative, or autoimmune disease, the underlying disease should be treated. However, the response to immunosuppressive therapy with cyclophosphamide and prednisone is generally not as favorable as the response in the case of acquired factor VIII inhibitor.

HEMORRHAGE CAUSED BY SEVERE LIVER DISEASE

Patients with severe liver disease may suffer life-threatening hemorrhages. The most frequent are esophageal and gastrointestinal hemorrhage related to varices, gastritis, or peptic ulcer. There may also be bleeding from biopsy sites and during and after surgery. Mucosal and soft tissue bleeding may occur but generally are not the dominant bleeding problem.

The coagulopathy of severe liver disease is complex and not well delineated. Because the liver is the major site of synthesis for all the clotting factors, decreased levels of multiple clotting factors are observed, including fibrinogen, prothrombin, factor V, and factor VII; factor VIII is excepted, presumably because it is an acute-phase reactant. An increased level of abnormal fibrinogen with reduced clotting capability is also observed in patients with cirrhosis.[110] In addition, there is reduced clearance of activated clotting factors by the liver. DIC appears to occur commonly in patients with cirrhosis[111] (presumably because of triggering of the clotting cascade by hepatic tissue damage), but its precise role in both acute fulminant hepatitis and chronic liver disease has not been firmly established. Platelet survival is shortened, and platelet splenic sequestration is increased, but platelet function is generally maintained. There is also evidence of hyperfibrinolysis, but its contribution to the overall hemostatic defect is uncertain. The liver also synthesizes most of the natural anticoagulant proteins. AT-III, protein C, and protein S levels are decreased. The best screening tests for this disorder include the PT, PTT, platelet count, fibrinogen level, and D-dimer level. Specific assays that may guide therapy include factor V, factor VII, and AT-III. Replacement for active bleeding is accomplished by administering fresh frozen plasma, cryoprecipitates, and platelets as required. Prothrombin-complex concentrates are not recommended, because they do not replenish all the deficient clotting factors and may exacerbate the DIC. In general, although the multiple hemostatic defects contribute to the bleeding diathesis in severe liver disease, hemodynamic and anatomic factors are the primary determinants in this situation.

PRIMARY FIBRINOLYSIS

Cases of generalized primary fibrinolysis are rare. Many of the early reports of primary fibrinolysis probably represented secondary fibrinolysis associated with DIC. Postprostatectomy hematuria may constitute a true example of hemorrhage caused

Table 8 Differential Diagnosis of Postoperative Hemorrhage

Dilutional thrombocytopenia caused by massive transfusion
Acquired platelet function defect after cardiopulmonary bypass
Inadequate heparin neutralization
Disseminated intravascular coagulation
Coagulopathy caused by shock liver
Acquired antithrombin and anti–factor V inhibitors after exposure to fibrin glue
Heparin-induced thrombocytopenia
Thrombocytopenia caused by GPIIb-IIIa inhibitors (e.g., abciximab)
Hyperfibrinolysis after prostate surgery
Undiagnosed von Willebrand disease or hemophilia
Thrombocytopenia caused by posttransfusion purpura
False abnormalities in coagulation test results

by localized fibrinolysis. The high concentration of urokinase in the urine in this condition causes plasminogen to be converted to plasmin with resulting clot lysis. If other causes of persistent postoperative hematuria can be ruled out, the condition can be treated with oral or intravenous EACA. Local instillation of EACA by urethral catheter is also effective.

BLEEDING AFTER CARDIOPULMONARY BYPASS

Patients who undergo heart surgery with cardiopulmonary bypass sometimes experience intraoperative and postoperative bleeding in the absence of significant procoagulant consumption or heparin overdose. Thrombocytopenia may occur from heparin or platelet consumption during bypass. A significant acquired platelet function disorder may develop in some patients, perhaps caused by contact between the platelets and the oxygenator apparatus, but the exact nature of the defect remains controversial.[112] In addition to the release of platelet α-granule contents, activation of fibrinolysis may occur together with modest clotting factor depletion.[113] The hemorrhage in such cases generally responds to platelet transfusions. The use of DDAVP in this setting has been reported to reduce postoperative blood loss; however, a meta-analysis of 17 clinical trials showed only a modest beneficial effect.[114]

The protease inhibitor aprotinin has also been tested in patients undergoing cardiopulmonary bypass on the basis that some of the bleeding is caused by enhanced proteolysis of clotting factors and platelet membrane proteins triggered by the procedure and the oxygenator. Aprotonin appears to be superior to EACA and DDAVP in reducing blood loss and blood transfusion requirement.[115] Aprotonin should be reserved for patients who are likely to require blood transfusion, especially those undergoing second operations and those with preexisting hemostatic defects. Preoperative testing of hemostasis appears not to be useful.

During bypass surgery, patients are sometimes exposed to topical thrombin (fibrin glue), which is used for local hemostasis control. Generally, bovine thrombin and trace amounts of other clotting factors to which patients may develop antibodies are used in these preparations. The antibodies against bovine thrombin cause a prolongation of the TT but are innocuous in themselves. However, potentially serious complications arise when the antibodies cross-react with human thrombin. Some patients develop antibodies against bovine factor V that cross-react with

human factor V and may lead to clinical bleeding.[116,117] Mixing studies utilizing the patient's plasma and normal plasma will reveal the presence of the inhibitors, and the measurement of the appropriate factor levels will allow the correct diagnosis to be made. Sometimes, plasmapheresis is required to control the acute bleeding.

EVALUATION OF POSTOPERATIVE BLEEDING

Serious hemorrhage during or after surgery is a complicated clinical problem requiring rapid diagnosis and prompt intervention. The first question is whether the bleeding has a local anatomic cause (e.g., unligated vessel) or is the result of a systemic hemostatic failure. If the patient is bleeding only in the operative area, it would suggest a local anatomic cause, such as an unligated bleeding vessel. The patient's bleeding history, especially with the results of prior surgical procedures, is extremely useful, but the available history may be inadequate or incomplete. A revealing clue to a systemic malfunction is bleeding at multiple sites, particularly areas other than the surgical wound. Bleeding around a catheter, from venipuncture sites, and from venous cutdowns is highly indicative of a hemorrhagic disorder. Rapid assessment of the total clinical setting is imperative. The following questions should be addressed:

- Does the patient have underlying renal, hepatic, or malignant disease?
- Has the surgery required pump bypass techniques or the induction of hypothermia, or has the patient been in shock or been hypothermic?
- How many units of blood and blood products have been given and over what period of time?
- Were baseline screening procoagulant tests obtained before surgery, and is the patient's frozen plasma still available?

The differential diagnosis of postoperative hemorrhage should include a number of bleeding disorders [*see Table 8*].

Prompt resolution requires a panel of coagulation tests—including PTT, PT, TT, fibrinogen assay, and D-dimer—a platelet count, and a well-stained blood smear for evaluation of platelet morphology. This battery of tests should be performed immediately. More specialized studies can be obtained if there is evidence of a specific disorder.

References

1. Ginsburg D: Molecular genetics of von Willebrand disease. Thromb Haemost 82:585, 1999

2. George JN, el-Harake MA, Raskob GE: Chronic idiopathic thrombocytopenic purpura. N Engl J Med 331:1207, 1994

3. Gewirtz AM, Hoffman R: Transitory hypomegakaryocytic thrombocytopenia: aetiological association with ethanol abuse and implications regarding regulation of human megakaryocytopoiesis. Br J Haematol 62:333, 1986

4. Hirsh J, Dalen JE, Anderson DR, et al: Oral anticoagulants: mechanism of action, clinical effectiveness, and optimal therapeutic range. Chest 114:445S, 1998

5. Tepler I, Elias L, Smith JW II, et al: A randomized placebo-controlled trial of recombinant human interleukin-11 in cancer patients with severe thrombocytopenia due to chemotherapy. Blood 87:3607, 1996

6. He R, Reid DM, Jones CE, et al: Spectrum of Ig classes, specificities, and titers of serum antiglycoproteins in chronic idiopathic thrombocytopenic purpura. Blood 83:1024, 1994

7. Hofbauer LC, Heufelder AE: Coagulation disorders in thyroid diseases. Eur J Endocrinol 136:1, 1997

8. Stasi R, Stipa E, Masi M, et al: Prevalence and clinical significance of elevated antiphospholipid antibodies in patients with idiopathic thrombocytopenic purpura. Blood 84:4203, 1994

9. George JN, Woolf SH, Raskob GE, et al: Idiopathic thrombocytopenic purpura: a practice guideline developed by explicit methods for the American Society of Hematology. Blood 88:3, 1996

10. Stasi R, Stipa E, Masi M, et al: Long term observation of 208 adults with chronic idiopathic thrombocytopenic purpura. Am J Med 98:436, 1995

11. Cortelazzo S, Finazzi G, Buelli M, et al: High risk of severe bleeding in aged patients with chronic idiopathic thrombocytopenic purpura. Blood 77:31, 1991

12. Berchtold P, Dale GL, Tani P, et al: Inhibition of autoantibody binding to platelet glycoprotein IIb/IIIa by anti-idiotypic antibodies in intravenous gammaglobulin. Blood 74:2414, 1989

13. Yu Z, Lennon VA: Mechanism of intravenous immune globulin therapy in antibody-mediated autoimmune diseases. N Engl J Med 340:227, 1999

14. Facon T, Caulier MT, Wattel E, et al: A randomized trial comparing vinblastine in slow infusion and by bolus I.V. injection in idiopathic thrombocytopenic purpura: a report on 42 patients. Br J Haematol 86:678, 1994

15. Laveder F, Marcolongo R, Zamboni S: Thrombocytopenic purpura following treatment with danazol. Br J Haematol 90:970, 1995

16. Nardi MA, Liu L-X, Karpatkin S: GPIIIa-(49-66) is a major pathophysiologically relevant antigenic determinant for anti-platelet GPIIIa of HIV-1-related immunologic thrombocytopenia. Proc Natl Acad Sci USA 94:7589, 1997

17. Najean Y, Rabin JD: The mechanism of thrombocytopenia in patients with HIV infection. J Lab Clin Med 123:415, 1994

18. Scaradavou A, Woo B, Woloski BMR, et al: Intravenous anti-D treatment of immune thrombocytopenic purpura: experience in 272 patients. Blood 89:2689, 1997

19. Durand JM, Lefevre P, Hovette P, et al: Dapsone for thrombocytopenic purpura related to human immunodeficiency virus infection. Am J Med 90:675, 1991

20. Marroni M, Gresele P, Landonio G, et al: Interferon-α is effective in the treatment of HIV-1-related, severe, zidovudine-resistant thrombocytopenia. Ann Intern Med 121:423, 1994

21. Needleman SW, Sorace J, Poussin-Rosillo H, et al: Low-dose splenic irradiation in the treatment of autoimmune thrombocytopenia in HIV-infected patients. Ann Intern Med 116:310, 1992

22. Burrows RF, Kelton JG: Fetal thrombocytopenia and its relation to maternal thrombocytopenia. N Engl J Med 329:1463, 1993

23. Flug F, Karpatkin M, Karpatkin S: Should all pregnant women be tested for their PLA (Zw, HPA-1) phenotype? Br J Haematol 86:1, 1994

24. McCrae KR, Herman JH: Posttransfusion purpura: two unusual cases and a literature review. Am J Hematol 52:205, 1996

25. Burgess JK, Lopez JA, Berndt MC, et al: Quinine-dependent antibodies bind a restricted set of epitopes on the glycoprotein Ib-IX complex: characterization of the epitopes. Blood 92:2366, 1998

26. Glynne P, Salama A, Chaudhry A, et al: Quinine-induced immune thrombocytopenic purpura followed by hemolytic uremic syndrome. Am J Kidney Dis 33:133, 1999

27. Kaufman DW, Kelly JP, Johannes CB, et al: Acute thrombocytopenic purpura in relation to the use of drugs. Blood 82:2714, 1993

28. Burday MJ, Martin SE: Cocaine-associated thrombocytopenia. Am J Med 91:656, 1992

29. Giugliano RP, Hyatt RR Jr: Thrombocytopenia with GPIIb/IIIa inhibitors: a meta-analysis. JACC 31:185A, 1998

30. Berkowitz SD, Harrington RA, Rund MM, et al: Acute profound thrombocytopenia after c7E3 Fab (abciximab) therapy. Circulation 95:809, 1997

31. Bednar B, Bednar RA, Cook JJ, et al: Drug-dependent antibodies against glycoprotein IIb/IIIa induce thrombocytopenia. Circulation 94(suppl):99, 1996

32. Bougie D, Aster R: Immune thrombocytopenia resulting from sensitivity to metabolites of naproxen and acetaminophen. Blood 97:3846, 2001

33. Boyce TG, Swerdlow DL, Griffin PM: Escherichia coli 0157:H7 and the hemolytic-uremic syndrome. N Engl J Med 333:364, 1995

34. Morigi M, Galbusera M, Binda E, et al: Verotoxin-1–induced up-regulation of adhesive molecules renders microvascular endothelial cells thrombogenic at high shear stress. Blood 98:1828, 2001

35. Wong CS, Jelacic S, Habeeb RL, et al: The risk of the hemolytic-uremic syndrome after antibiotic treatment of Escherichia coli O157:H7 infections. N Engl J Med 342:1930, 2000

36. Steinhubl SR, Tan WA, Foody JM, et al: Incidence and clinical course of thrombotic thrombocytopenic purpura due to ticlopidine following coronary stenting. EPISTENT investigators: evaluation of platelet IIb/IIIa inhibitor for stenting. JAMA 281:806, 1999

37. Bennett CL, Connors JM, Carwile JM, et al: Thrombotic thrombocytopenic purpura associated with clopidogrel. N Engl J Med 342:1773, 2000

38. Moake JL: Moschcowitz, multimers, and metalloprotease. N Engl J Med 339:1629, 1998

39. Rock G, Kelton JG, Shumak KH, et al: Laboratory abnormalities in thrombotic thrombocytopenic purpura. Canadian Apheresis Group. Br J Haematol 103:1031, 1998

40. Gerritsen HE, Robles R, Lammle B, et al: Partial amino acid sequence of purified von Willebrand factor-cleaving protease. Blood 98:1654, 2001

41. Fujikawa K, Suzuki H, McMullen B, et al: Purification of human von Willebrand factor-cleaving protease and its identification as a new member of the metalloproteinase family. Blood 98:1662, 2001

42. Zheng X, Chung D, Takayama TK, et al: Structure of von Willebrand factor cleaving protease (ADAMTS13), a metalloprotease involved in thrombotic thrombocytopenia. J Biol Chem September 13, 2001[epub]

43. Veyradier A, Obert B, Houllier A, et al: Specific von Willebrand factor-cleaving protease in thrombotic microangiopathies: a study of 111 cases. Blood 98:1765, 2001

44. Moore JC, Hayward CP, Warkentin TE, et al: Decreased von Willebrand factor protease activity associated with thrombocytopenic disorders. Blood 98:1842, 2001

45. Tsai HM: Physiologic cleavage of von Willebrand factor by a plasma protease is dependent on its conformation and requires calcium ion. Blood 87:4235, 1996

46. Rock G, Shumak KH, Buskard NA, et al: Comparison of plasma exchange with plasma infusion in the treatment of thrombotic thrombocytopenic purpura. Canadian Apheresis Study Group. N Engl J Med 325:393, 1991

47. George JN, Gilcher RO, Smith JW, et al: Thrombotic thrombocytopenic purpura-hemolytic uremic syndrome: diagnosis and management. J Clin Apheresis 13:120, 1998

48. Rock G, Shumak KH, Sutton DM, et al: Cryosupernatant as replacement fluid for plasma exchange in thrombotic thrombocytopenic purpura. Members of the Canadian Apheresis Group. Br J Haematol 94:383, 1996

49. Bell WR, Braine HG, Ness PM, et al: Improved survival in thrombotic thrombocytopenic purpura-hemolytic uremic syndrome: clinical experience in 108 patients. N Engl J Med 325:398, 1991

50. Harkness DR, Byrnes JJ, Lian EC-Y: Hazard of platelet transfusion in thrombotic thrombocytopenic purpura. JAMA 246:1931, 1981

51. Shumak KH, Rock G, Nair RC, et al: Late relapses in patients successfully treated for thrombotic thrombocytopenic purpura. Ann Intern Med 122:569, 1995

52. Onundarson PT, Rowe JM, Heal JM, et al: Response to plasma exchange and splenectomy in thrombotic thrombocytopenic purpura: a 10-year experience at a single institution. Arch Intern Med 152:791, 1992

53. Mohanty D, Marwaha N, Ghosh K, et al: Functional and ultrastructural changes of platelets in malarial infection. Trans R Soc Trop Med Hyg 82:369, 1988

54. Van Dam PA, Renier M, Baekelandt M, et al: Disseminated intravascular coagulation and the syndrome of hemolysis, elevated liver enzymes, and low platelets in severe preeclampsia. Obstet Gynecol 73:97, 1989

55. Martin JN Jr, Blake PG, Perry KG Jr, et al: The natural history of HELLP syndrome: patterns of disease progression and regression. Am J Obstet Gynecol 164:1500, 1991

56. Easterbrook PJ, Davis HP: Thrombocytopenia in hypothermia: a common but poorly recognized complication. Br Med J 291:23, 1985

57. Weigert AL, Schafer AI: Uremic bleeding: pathogenesis and therapy. Am J Med Sci 316:94, 1998

58. Mannucci PM: Hemostatic drugs. N Engl J Med 339:245, 1998

59. Lacoste L, Hung J, Lam JY: Acute and delayed antithrombotic effects of alcohol in humans. Am J Cardiol 87:82, 2001

60. George JN, Shattil SJ: The clinical importance of acquired abnormalities of platelet function. N Engl J Med 324:27, 1991

61. Layzer RB: Hot feet: erythromelalgia and related disorders. J Child Neurol 16:199, 2001

62. Anagrelide, a therapy for thrombocythemic states: experience in 577 patients. Anagrelide Study Group. Am J Med 92:69, 1992

63. Haitjema T, Westermann CJJ, Overtoom TTC, et al: Hereditary haemorrhagic telangiectasia (Osler-Weber-Rendu syndrome): new insights into pathogenesis, complications, and treatment. Arch Intern Med 156:714, 1996

64. Shovlin CL: Molecular defects in rare bleeding disorders: hereditary haemorrhagic telangiectasia. Thromb Haemost 78:145, 1997

65. White RI Jr, Lynch-Nyhan A, Terry P, et al: Pulmonary arteriovenous malformation: techniques and long-term outcome of embolotherapy. Radiology 169:663, 1988

66. Hirschmann JV, Raugi GJ: Adult scurvy. J Am Acad Dermatol 41:895, 1999

67. Clemetson KJ: Platelet GPIb-V-IX complex. Thromb Haemost 78:266, 1997

68. Triplett DA: Laboratory diagnosis of von Willebrand's disease. Mayo Clin Proc 66:832, 1991

69. Fressinaud E, Veyradier A, Truchaud F, et al: Screening for von Willebrand disease with a new analyzer using high shear stress: a study of 60 cases. Blood 91:1325, 1998

70. Sadler JE, Gralnick HR: A new classification for von Willebrand's disease. Blood 84:676, 1994

71. Sutor AH: DDAVP is not a panacea for children with bleeding disorders. Br J Haematol 108:217, 2000

72. Rose EH, Aledort LM: Nasal spray desmopressin (DDAVP) for mild hemophilia A and von Willebrand disease. Ann Intern Med 114:563, 1991

73. Castillo R, Monteagudo J, Escolar G, et al: Hemostatic effects of normal platelet transfusion in severe von Willebrand's disease patients. Blood 77:1901, 1991

74. Ito M, Yoshimura K, Toyoda N, et al: Pregnancy and delivery in patients with von Willebrand's disease. J Obstet Gynaecol Res 23:37, 1997

75. Rick ME, Williams SB, Sacher RA, et al: Thrombocytopenia associated with pregnancy in a patient with type IIb von Willebrand's disease. Blood 69:786, 1987

76. Antonarakis SE, Rossiter JP, Young M, et al: Factor VIII inversions in severe hemophilia A: results of an international consortium study. Blood 86:2206, 1995

77. Bray GL, Gomperts ED, Courter S, et al: The Recombinate Study Group: a multicenter study of recombinant factor VIII (Recombinate): safety, efficacy, and inhibitor risk in previously untreated patients with hemophilia A. Blood 83:2428, 1994

78. Seremetis S, Lusher JM, Abildgaard CF, et al: Human recombinant DNA-derived antihemophilic factor (factor VIII) in the treatment of hemophilia A: conclusions of a 5-year study of home therapy. The KOGENATE Study Group. Haemophilia 5:9, 1999

79. Courter SG, Bedrosian CL: Clinical evaluation of B-domain deleted recombinant factor VIII in previously untreated patients. Semin Hematol 38(suppl 4):52, 2001

80. Green PP, Mannucci PM, Briet E, et al: Carrier detection in hemophilia A: a cooperative international study: II. The efficacy of a universal discriminant. Blood 67:1560, 1986

81. Rochat C, McFadyen ML, Schwyzer R, et al: Continuous infusion of intermediate-

purity factor VIII in haemophilia A patients undergoing elective surgery. Haemophilia 5:181, 1999

82. Yee TT, Pasi KJ, Lilley PA, et al: Factor VIII inhibitors in haemophiliacs: a single-center experience over 34 years, 1964–97. Br J Haematol 104:909, 1999

83. Hough RE, Hampton KK, Preston FE, et al: Recombinant VIIa concentrate in the management of bleeding following prothrombin complex concentrate-related myocardial infarction in patients with haemophilia and inhibitors. Br J Haematol 111:974, 2000

84. Lusher JM: Controlled clinical trials with prothrombin complex concentrates. Prog Clin Biol Res 150:277, 1984

85. Hedner U, Glazer S, Falch J: Recombinant activated factor VII in the treatment of bleeding episodes in patients with inherited and acquired bleeding disorders. Transfusion Med Rev 7:78, 1993

86. Negrier C, Lienhart A: Overall experience with NovoSeven. Blood Coagul Fibrinolysis 11 (suppl 1):S19, 2000

87. van't Veer C, Golden NJ, Mann KG: Inhibition of thrombin generation by the zymogen factor VII: implications for the treatment of hemophilia A by factor VIIa. Blood 95:1330, 2000

88. Monroe DM, Hoffman M, Allen GA, et al: The factor VII–platelet interplay: effectiveness of recombinant factor VIIa in the treatment of bleeding in severe thrombocytopathia. Semin Thromb Hemost 26:373, 2000

89. Roberts HR, Eberst ME: Current management of hemophilia B. Hematol Oncol Clin North Am 7:1269, 1993

90. Wang L, Takabe K, Bidlingmaier SM, et al: Sustained correction of bleeding disorder in hemophilia B mice by gene therapy. Proc Natl Acad Sci USA 30:3906, 1999

91. White GC II: Gene therapy in hemophilia: clinical trials update. Thromb Haemost 86:172, 2001

92. Cooper DN, Millar DS, Wacey A, et al: Inherited factor VII deficiency: molecular genetics and pathophysiology. Thromb Haemost 78:151, 1997

93. Fay WP, Parker AC, Condrey LR, et al: Human plasminogen activator inhibitor-1 (PAI-I) deficiency: characterization of a large kindred with a null mutation in the PAI-1 gene. Blood 90:204, 1997

94. Furie B, Furie BC: Molecular and cellular biology of blood coagulation. N Engl J Med 326:800, 1992

95. Sane DC, Califf RM, Topol EJ, et al: Bleeding during thrombolytic therapy for acute myocardial infarction: mechanisms and management. Ann Intern Med 111:1010, 1989

96. Esmon CT, Fukudome K, Mather T, et al: Inflammation, sepsis, and coagulation. Haematologica 84:254, 1999

97. Hall GW: Kasabach-Merritt syndrome: pathogenesis and management. Br J Haematol 112:851, 2001

98. Rickles FR, Levine MN, Edwards RL: Hemostatic alterations in cancer patients. Cancer Metastasis Rev 11:237, 1992

99. Bernard GR, Vincent JL, Laterre PF, et al: Efficacy and safety of recombinant human activated protein C for severe sepsis. N Engl J Med 344:699, 2001

100. Jochum M: Influence of high-dose antithrombin concentrate therapy on the release of cellular proteases, cytokines, and soluble adhesion molecules in acute inflammation. Semin Hematol 32:14, 1995

101. Fourrier F, Chopin C, Huart JJ, et al: Double-blind, placebo-controlled trial of antithrombin III concentrates in septic shock with disseminated intravascular coagulation. Chest 104:882, 1993

102. Scandella DH, Nakai H, Felch M, et al: In hemophilia A and autoantibody inhibitor patients: the factor VII A2 domain and light chain are most immunogenic. Thromb Res 101:377, 2001

103. Ludlam CA, Morrison AE, Kessler C: Treatment of acquired hemophilia. Sem Hematol 31:16, 1994

104. Lian C-Y, Larcada AF, Chiu AY-Z: Combination immunosuppressive therapy after factor VIII inhibitor. Ann Intern Med 110:774, 1989

105. Shaffer LG, Phillips MD: Successful treatment of acquired hemophilia with oral immunosuppressive therapy. Ann Intern Med 127:206, 1997

106. Morrison AE, Ludlam CA, Kessler C: Use of porcine factor VIII in the treatment of patients with acquired hemophilia. Blood 81:1513, 1993

107. Crenier L, Ducobu J, des Grottes JM, et al: Low response to high-dose intravenous immunoglobulin in the treatment of acquired factor VIII inhibitor. Br J Haematol 95:750, 1996

108. Federici AB, Rand JH, Bucciarelli P: Acquired von Willebrand syndrome: data from an international registry. Thromb Haemost 84:345, 2000

109. Mohri H, Motomura S, Kanamori H, et al: Clinical significance of inhibitors in acquired von Willebrand syndrome. Blood 91:3623, 1998

110. Francis JL, Armstrong DJ: Acquired dysfibrinogenemia in liver disease. J Clin Pathol 35:667, 1982

111. Stein SF, Harker LA: Kinetic and functional studies of platelets, fibrinogen, and plasminogen in patients with hepatic cirrhosis. J Lab Clin Med 99:217, 1986

112. Kestin AS, Valeri CR, Khuri SF, et al: The platelet function defect of cardiopulmonary bypass. Blood 82:107, 1993

113. Bolan CD, Alving BM: Pharmacologic agents in the management of bleeding disorders. Transfusion 30:541, 1990

114. Cattaneo M, Harris AS, Stromberg U, et al: The effect of desmopressin on reducing blood loss in cardiac surgery: a meta-analysis of double-blind, placebo-controlled trials. Thromb Haemost 74:1064, 1995

115. Fremes SE, Wong BI, Lee E, et al: Metaanalysis of prophylactic drug treatment in the prevention of postoperative bleeding. Ann Thorac Surg 58:1580, 1994

116. Zehnder JL, Leung LL: Development of antibodies to thrombin and factor V with recurrent bleeding in a patient exposed to topical bovine thrombin. Blood 76:2011, 1990

117. Berruyer M, Amiral J, French P, et al: Immunization by bovine thrombin used with fibrin glue during cardiovascular operations. J Thorac Cardiovasc Surg 105:892, 1993

118. George J: Hemostasis and thrombosis. Hematology: Basic Principles and Practice, 3rd ed. Hoffman R, Benz EJ Jr, Shattil SJ, Eds. Churchill Livingstone, Philadelphia, 1999, p 1928

94 Thrombotic Disorders

Lawrence L. K. Leung, M.D.

Thrombosis is more than excessive blood clotting; it also involves vascular inflammation. Virchow's classic triad identifies three major elements in the pathophysiology of thrombosis: endothelial injury, decrease in blood flow, and imbalance between procoagulant and anticoagulant factors.

Endothelial cells can be activated or injured by a variety of stimuli, including mechanical trauma, endotoxins and cytokines, proteases, inflammatory mediators, immune complex deposition, oxygen radicals, and hypoxia. Each of these stimuli affects multiple facets of endothelial cell function, ultimately changing the cell from its natural antithrombotic state to a prothrombotic one.

The vascular endothelium, in its unique location in the vessel wall, is capable of sensing and responding to the different mechanical forces in the blood circulation. The shear stress caused by the friction from blood flow seems to be particularly important in modulating endothelial functions. In areas of linear flow, the blood moves in ordered laminar patterns in a regular pulsatile fashion. Such a steady, laminar blood flow apparently promotes an antithrombotic endothelial phenotype. In areas of disrupted flow, such as at vascular bifurcations or stenoses, the endothelium may be exposed to significant changes in shear gradients, and the cells may become activated and prothrombotic.

Imbalance between procoagulant and anticoagulant factors can be hereditary or acquired [see Table 1]. Some clotting factors, such as factor VIII and fibrinogen, are acute-phase reactants: their plasma levels increase significantly with acute inflammation, possibly conferring a transient prothrombotic state. Some hereditary deficiencies of anticoagulant proteins, such as factor V Leiden and antithrombin III (AT-III), are associated with recurrent thrombosis; these are among the best understood clinical hypercoagulable states.

Although the hypercoagulable state is systemic, thrombosis occurs locally (e.g., in the lower extremities). The clinical outcome likely reflects a complex interaction between the systemic prothrombotic predisposition and local hemostatic control mechanisms specific to the vascular bed.

Assessment of Patients with Thrombotic Disorders

PRIMARY CLINICAL ISSUES IN THROMBOTIC DISORDERS

Important questions in the assessment of thrombosis include the following: (1) How likely is it that the thrombosis is caused by an underlying hypercoagulable state? (2) How extensive a workup is indicated? (3) When should the workup be done? Answers to these questions come from a consideration of the patient's age at the time of the first thrombosis; presence or absence of a provoking factor; family history and past medical history of response to situations associated with high risk of thrombosis; and the site, type, and severity of the thrombosis.

Age of Onset of First Thrombosis

In a recent retrospective study involving 150 families with an inherited predisposition to recurrent thrombosis (thrombophilia), the mean age at the time of the first thrombosis was 35 to 40 years. However, the first episode of thrombosis can occur as early as the second decade of life if the patient has more than one hereditary risk factor.[1]

Presence or Absence of a Provoking Factor

Common triggers of thrombosis are surgery, trauma, pregnancy, malignancy, prolonged immobilization, and infection. Malignancy or infection can be clinically overt or subclinical. Those circumstances can provoke thrombosis even in persons with a normal coagulation system, and they often uncover a thrombophilia that had been clinically silent.[1] However, sometimes no provoking factors can be identified. Such a spontaneous, idiopathic thrombosis, especially when it occurs in a young person, strongly suggests an underlying hereditary hypercoagulable state.

If thrombosis develops in a patient who has had previous pregnancies or surgeries (especially orthopedic procedures) without any thrombotic complications, an acquired hypercoagulable state should be considered. Likely conditions in such cases are antiphospholipid antibody syndrome or Trousseau syndrome (see below).

Table 1 Inherited and Acquired
Hypercoagulable States

Inherited
   Resistance to activated protein C/factor V Leiden
   Prothrombin gene mutation 20210A
   Antithrombin III deficiency
   Protein C deficiency
   Protein S deficiency
   Hyperhomocysteinemia

Acquired
   Antiphospholipid antibody syndrome
   Hypercoagulable state associated with physiologic or thrombogenic stimuli:
      Advancing age
      Oral contraceptives
      Pregnancy
      Surgery
      Trauma
   Hypercoagulable state associated with other clinical conditions:
      Malignancy—Trousseau syndrome
      Heparin-induced thrombocytopenia with thrombosis
      Nephrotic syndrome
      Hyperviscosity (polycythemia vera, Waldenström macroglobinemia, multiple myeloma)
      Myeloproliferative disorders (polycythemia vera, essential thrombocytopenia)
      Paroxysmal nocturnal hemoglobinuria
      Sickle cell anemia

Rare or Not Well Established
   Dysfibrinogenemia
   Hypoplasminogenemia, dysplasminogenemia
   Abnormal thrombomodulin
   Factor XII deficiency
   Elevated factor VII, factor VIII, fibrinogen, lipoprotein(a), plasminogen activator inhibitor–1

Family History

Clinical thrombosis before 50 years of age in a first-degree family member strongly suggests a hereditary thrombotic disorder. However, a negative family history does not exclude a hereditary condition. Clinical thrombosis is frequently the culmination of multiple thrombogenic risk factors, only one of which may be hereditary and irreversible. In patients with symptomatic thrombosis and well-documented hereditary hypercoagulable states, it is not uncommon to find other family members with the same deficiency but no clinical thrombosis.

Recurrent Thrombosis

A patient who experiences recurrent thrombosis likely has a hypercoagulable state (hereditary or acquired). However, if a patient who initially presented with deep vein thrombosis (DVT) in a lower extremity returns with symptoms involving the same leg, the problem may be postphlebitic syndrome rather than recurrent thrombosis. Acute exacerbation of the postphlebitic syndrome, with its increased leg edema and pain, can be difficult to distinguish from recurrent acute DVT. As an anticipatory measure, it is sometimes useful to obtain a repeat Doppler study of the lower extremity after resolution of an acute episode of DVT; the repeat scan can provide a baseline for future comparison.

Site of Thrombosis

Most commonly, thromboses involve the deep veins of the lower extremities. Thrombosis at an atypical site, such as the

---

Table 3   Clinical Features That Suggest Thrombophilia

Age at onset of first thrombosis < 50 yr
No identifiable risk factor
Positive family history
Recurrent thrombosis
Atypical site of thrombosis

---

hepatic, mesenteric, or cerebral veins (or skin necrosis after warfarin administration), increases the likelihood of an underlying hypercoagulable state. Spontaneous axillary vein thrombosis may also indicate the presence of an underlying hypercoagulable state, but this association is controversial.[1-3]

Recurrent thrombosis at arterial sites has a differential diagnosis—and therefore a workup—that is quite different from that for recurrent venous thrombosis [see Table 2]. Most of the common hereditary hypercoagulable states (e.g., AT-III deficiency or factor V Leiden) are associated with venous thromboses, such as DVT in the lower extremities. They are seldom associated with arterial thromboses, such as transient ischemic attack, stroke, digital ischemia, and myocardial infarction. A few hypercoagulable states, such as the antiphospholipid syndrome and hyperhomocysteinemia, are associated with both types of thrombosis.

The Hypercoagulable Workup

Extent of the workup   On the basis of the above clinical considerations, one may estimate the likelihood of an underlying thrombophilia in a given patient with thrombosis [see Table 3]. Because studies of cost-effectiveness and outcomes are not available, it is difficult to list strict practice guidelines regarding the extent of the hypercoagulable workup. In general, however, if the likelihood of an underlying hypercoagulable state is high, an extensive workup is warranted.

A limited workup is appropriate for mild to moderate DVT of the lower extremities with an obvious provoking factor. For example, in a young woman who experiences DVT in the superficial femoral vein while on an oral contraceptive, evaluation of factor V Leiden, prothrombin mutation 20210A, AT-III, protein C, protein S, homocysteine, anticardiolipin antibodies, and lupus anticoagulant may be sufficient. On the other hand, an acquired hypercoagulable state should be considered in an elderly patient with a spontaneous DVT and no history of previous thrombosis. Diagnostic possibilities in such cases would include antiphospholipid antibody syndrome, acquired AT-III deficiency (if the patient has evidence of nephrotic syndrome), or Trousseau syndrome.

In a patient in whom thrombophilia is strongly suspected on the basis of clinical history, such as recurrent thrombosis or thrombosis at atypical sites, one may argue that a workup for an underlying hypercoagulable state is unnecessary because the result will not alter the management of the case. However, the identification of any underlying risk factors will improve the understanding of the disease for both the patient and the treating physician; and it will guide the counseling of the patient, especially regarding the need for screening of related family members. In the case of hyperhomocysteinemia and elevated lipoprotein(a), identification of risk factors will permit the use of specific therapies (see below).

Table 2   Screening Tests for Patients with Suspected Hypercoagulable State

Underlying State	Laboratory Evaluation

Venous thrombosis	Resistance to activated protein C
	  Factor V Leiden (genetic test)
	  Clotting assay (unnecessary if the genetic test for factor V Leiden is positive)
	Prothrombin mutation 20210A (genetic test)
	Antithrombin III (functional assay)
	Protein C (functional assay)
	Protein S
	  Functional assay
	  Antigenic assay for free protein S

Arterial thrombosis	Antibodies associated with heparin-induced thrombocytopenia* Chronic disseminated intravascular coagulation (Trousseau syndrome)* Lipoprotein(a)

Venous thrombosis and/or arterial thrombosis	Plasma homocysteine
	  Fasting level
	  Level after methionine loading (if thrombophilia is strongly suspected)
	Antiphospholipid antibody
	  Clotting assays for lupuslike anticoagulant
	  ELISA for anticardiolipin antibodies IgG and IgM
	Dysfibrinogenemia (if thrombophilia is strongly suspected)
	  Functional assay for fibrinogen level
	  Thrombin time, reptilase time

*In appropriate clinical settings.
ELISA—enzyme-linked immunosorbent assay

Timing of the workup The clinician needs to know not only what tests to order but when to order them. In acute thrombosis, many inhibitors of the clotting cascade (e.g., AT-III and protein C) are consumed. Immediately after the episode, their plasma levels may be decreased, even in patients who do not have a hereditary deficiency. Usually it is best to postpone measurement of these inhibitors until the acute thrombotic episode is completely resolved, preferably a few weeks after termination of oral anticoagulation therapy. Tests for specific genotypes (e.g., factor V Leiden) can be performed at any time, however. Antiphospholipid antibody tests should be done at the time of diagnosis, because the presence of these antibodies will affect anticoagulation therapy.

Frequency and Relative Risk of Venous Thromboembolism

The frequency of various hypercoagulable states in unselected patients who present with venous thrombosis ranges from 1% to 25% [see Table 4]. It should be recognized that these thrombophilias do not confer equivalent thrombotic risk. Factor V Leiden and prothrombin mutation 20210A, the two most prevalent risk factors, confer only a modest increase in relative risk of thrombosis, approximately threefold to sevenfold above normal. Moderate hyperhomocysteinemia, another common risk factor, also carries a modest increase in risk. Heterozygous deficiencies of AT-III, protein C, and protein S are generally considered more significant risk factors than factor V Leiden. AT-III deficiency and the antiphospholipid antibody syndrome are probably the greatest risk factors. The recurrence rate in patients with antiphospholipid antibody syndrome is as high as 50% to 70% in some studies.

Patients with symptomatic thrombosis frequently have more than one risk factor, which may have a synergistic effect in increasing the thrombosis risk. For example, patients with factor V Leiden who use oral contraceptives have a risk of venous thromboembolism that is 35-fold higher than that in the general population.

Hereditary Hypercoagulable States

ANTITHROMBIN III DEFICIENCY

Epidemiology

The frequency of symptomatic inherited AT-III deficiency in the general population has been estimated to be approximately 1 per 2,000 people.[4] The deficiency is transmitted in an autosomal dominant pattern. Homozygous AT-III deficiency has not been reported, presumably because the condition is incompatible with normal fetal development.

There are two types of inherited AT-III deficiency. Type I is quantitative, as measured by antigenic and functional assays. A large number of molecular mutations have been characterized in type I AT-III deficiency, including partial gene deletions and single nucleotide substitutions that cause nonsense or missense mutations leading to premature stop signals in the protein-translation process.

Type II deficiency is qualitative; plasma levels of AT-III antigen are normal. The underlying defect is generally a single nucleotide change that causes missense mutations, giving rise to a dysfunctional protein.

In rare cases, AT-III deficiency is acquired. This condition may occur after administration of intravenous heparin for more than 3 days or after asparaginase therapy. It may also de-

Table 4 Frequency and Relative Risk of Venous Thrombosis in Selected Hypercoagulable States*

Condition	Relative Risk†	Frequency‡
Antithrombin III deficiency	High	1%–2%
Protein C deficiency	High	3%–4%
Protein S deficiency	High	2%–3%
Factor V Leiden	Modest	20%–25%
Prothrombin mutation 20210A	Modest	10%
Hyperhomocysteinemia	Modest	10%
Oral contraceptive use	Modest	NA

*The incidence of venous thromboembolism in the normal population is estimated to be 0.008% a year (0.03% a year in patients who take oral contraceptives).
†Modest risk is defined as an approximate 2.5-fold to fivefold increase in thromboembolism, on the basis of data from the Leiden Thrombophilia Study[144]; high risk is defined as an approximate threefold to fourfold increase over that for factor V Leiden.[1]
‡In unselected patients with venous thromboembolism.

velop in patients with disseminated intravascular coagulation (DIC), severe liver disease, or the nephrotic syndrome.

Pathophysiology

AT-III inactivates factor Xa and thrombin by forming a stable stoichiometric complex with each of them. AT-III is present in sufficient amounts in plasma to inactivate all the thrombin formed in a given plasma volume, but it does so slowly unless it is activated by endothelial cell surface heparan sulfate or by administered heparin [see Chapter 93]. Patients with hereditary AT-III deficiency have evidence of continuous factor X activation and thrombin generation (as supported by elevated plasma levels of prothrombin fragment F1.2) even when they are clinically asymptomatic.

Clinical Presentation

Patients with AT-III deficiency show an increased incidence of venous thrombosis, usually triggered by a prothrombotic stimulus such as surgery, infection, immobilization, or trauma. This association suggests that the superimposition of a prothrombotic stimulus on an underlying subclinical hypercoagulable state leads to clinical thrombosis.

Typical clinical presentations are DVT of the legs, pulmonary embolism, and occasionally mesenteric vein thrombosis. There is no convincing evidence to suggest that AT-III deficiency increases the risk of arterial thrombosis.[5]

Affected patients usually have a family history of recurrent thromboses, generally beginning in youth and often associated with surgery or trauma. Pregnancy and the use of oral contraceptives also increase the risk of thromboses in AT-III–deficient patients. The tendency to thrombosis increases with advancing age: by age 50, only 10% of AT-III–deficient patients are free of symptoms.

Diagnosis

The AT-III level should be determined by a functional assay rather than an antigenic assay, so that both type I and type II deficiency can be evaluated. Patients with AT-III deficiency have a surprisingly modest reduction in the protein: values measured by both bioassay and immunoassay range from 25% to 60% of normal in type I disease.

Treatment

Study of a large AT-III–deficient kindred indicates that long-term anticoagulant prophylaxis is not warranted in asymptomatic carriers of this deficiency.[6] Asymptomatic carriers should receive prophylactic anticoagulation only in situations known to increase the risk of thrombogenesis, such as abdominal surgery.[6] Once such patients have experienced a thrombotic event, however, they probably require lifelong warfarin therapy. Warfarin is the mainstay of long-term therapy for patients with AT-III deficiency and recurrent thromboembolism.

Acute episodes of thrombosis must be treated with heparin. Because AT-III deficiency may render heparin relatively ineffective, the physician should be alert to heparin resistance. In patients receiving unfractionated heparin, resistance is manifested by minimal prolongation of the partial thromboplastin time (PTT) despite the administration of therapeutic doses. If low-molecular-weight heparin (LMWH) is used, as is commonly the case, the level of anti–factor Xa (anti-FXa) should be checked to ensure that a therapeutic antithrombotic effect is achieved [see Chapter 92].

If heparin resistance occurs despite increased doses of heparin, heparin plus purified AT-III concentrates or fresh frozen plasma should be given. AT-III has a half-life of about 60 hours. These preparations can be used to carry an AT-III–deficient patient through surgery or delivery and should bring the AT-III level up to nearly 100%, depending on the patient's baseline AT-III level. The AT-III level should be checked and the infusion repeated at 24-hour intervals to maintain a normal AT-III level for 5 to 7 days after delivery or surgery.

Pregnancy in an AT-III–deficient patient is difficult to manage. Because warfarin may cause fetal malformations and neonatal hemorrhage, patients should be treated with full-dose regular heparin or LMWH; those receiving LMWH should be switched to regular heparin 1 to 2 weeks before delivery so that rapid reversal of anticoagulation, if necessary, can be more easily attained. If a therapeutic effect cannot be achieved (as measured by PTT with regular heparin or anti-FXa level with LMWH), an AT-III infusion can be given.[7] Generally, this is not necessary. Anticoagulation should be promptly reinstituted after delivery.

PROTEIN C AND PROTEIN S DEFICIENCY

Pathophysiology and Clinical Presentation

Deficiency or defect in protein C or protein S results in a loss of ability to inactivate excess factor VIIIa and factor Va, the two major cofactors that regulate amplification of the clotting cascade. Protein C levels are low in patients with DIC and liver disease, probably because the activation of hemostasis consumes this factor [see Chapter 93].

Homozygous protein C deficiency causes lethal thrombosis in infancy. Heterozygous protein C deficiency probably occurs with a prevalence of 1 per 200 to 300 in the general population. Clinical expression of heterozygous deficiency varies: many of these individuals, as well as persons with low-normal protein C levels from other causes, do not experience thrombosis.[8] Some patients with heterozygous deficiency, however, exhibit a definite tendency toward venous thrombosis even though their protein C levels are 40% to 50% of normal. This phenotypic variability suggests multiple gene interactions and supports the hypothesis that clinical thrombosis in these patients may result from a combination of protein C deficiency and one or more other prothrombotic mutations.[9] Cerebral venous thrombosis presumably accounts for cases of cerebral hemorrhagic infarction that occur in young adults with protein C deficiency.

Deficiency of protein S also leads to venous thrombosis, including mesenteric vein thrombosis. Pregnancy and the use of oral contraceptives lower the protein S level, which may account for some cases of thromboembolism that occur under such circumstances.[10] Acquired protein S deficiency also occurs in patients with the nephrotic syndrome, who lose protein S in urine.[11] Case reports have associated protein S deficiency with warfarin-induced skin necrosis.[12] The pathophysiology for this phenomenon is obscure; protein S has a much longer half-life than protein C (approximately 60 hours for protein S versus 6 hours for protein C), so protein S should not be affected by warfarin in a similar fashion.

Diagnosis

Functional and antigenic assays for protein C and protein S are now available in most coagulation laboratories. Functional assays are preferable for diagnosis. It is important to measure free protein S because some patients who have low free protein S levels have normal or borderline total protein S levels. Coagulation assays for protein C and protein S can give falsely low values in patients with factor V Leiden.[13]

Treatment

Warfarin is the treatment of choice for preventing thrombosis, even though it lowers protein C levels still further. Because the half-life of protein C is only 6 to 7 hours, much shorter than that of prothrombin and factor X, a period of enhanced hypercoagulability follows initiation of warfarin therapy in patients with protein C deficiency. Heparin should be given along with warfarin during the initiation of anticoagulation; it can be withdrawn afterward. Warfarin-induced skin necrosis is a rare complication of anticoagulation therapy.

FACTOR V LEIDEN

Epidemiology

Factor V Leiden refers to a defect caused by a mutated form of factor V (first identified by researchers in Leiden, The Netherlands) that is resistant to the anticoagulant effects of activated protein C (APC). The defect is transmitted as an autosomal dominant trait. Approximately 5% of the general white population is heterozygous for factor V Leiden; the defect is almost absent in other ethnic groups.[14] Factor V Leiden is now considered the most common hereditary hypercoagulable state. Its prevalence in patients with thrombophilia is as high as 20% to 50%.[15] In a large cohort study of unselected patients with a first episode of symptomatic DVT, factor V Leiden was found in 16% of patients.[16] In women who have thrombosis while taking oral contraceptives, the frequency of factor V Leiden is about 23%.[17] The relative risk of DVT in a patient with homozygous factor V Leiden mutation (estimated incidence, 0.5% to 1% a year) is approximately 80-fold higher than in a normal person.[18] The risk of thrombosis in carriers of factor V Leiden is estimated to be fourfold to eightfold higher than in noncarriers; the relative risk increases to more than 30-fold when factor V Leiden is combined with oral contraceptive use. The absolute risk of thrombosis, however, is low.[19] Association of factor V Leiden with deficiencies of protein C, protein S, or AT-III has been reported in some families.[20-22] Overall, although factor V Leiden is highly prevalent, it is a relatively weak risk factor for thrombosis.

Approximately 5% of cases associated with inherited resistance to APC are attributable to other mutations and defects.[23-25] Conditions such as factor VIII elevation, pregnancy, oral contraceptive use, and lupus anticoagulation may result in APC resistance.[26] APC resistance that is not caused by factor V Leiden may be a risk factor for stroke [27,28] and venous thrombosis.[29,30] The overall risk of venous thrombosis from APC resistance is similar to or less than that posed by factor V Leiden.[31]

Pathophysiology

Resistance to the anticoagulant effects of APC is caused by a specific mutation in factor V (factor V Leiden or factor V R506Q) that results from a single nucleotide substitution that leads to the replacement of arginine with glutamine at position 506.[31] Arginine 506 is located at one of the two major APC cleavage sites of activated factor V. Activated factor V Leiden expresses normal procoagulant activity, but its degradation by APC is approximately 10 times slower than that of normal acti-

vated factor V (factor Va). This slowing leads to increased thrombin generation.[32] In addition, recent evidence suggests that factor V (but not factor Va), together with protein S, serves as a cofactor of APC in the inhibition of the factor VIIIa/factor IXa complex and that factor V Leiden has a poor APC cofactor function [*see Figure 1*].

Clinical Presentation

Clinical manifestations of factor V Leiden are similar to those of deficiencies of AT-III, protein C, and protein S—mainly, venous thrombosis. However, the first thrombotic manifestation in factor V Leiden often occurs later than in the other hereditary thrombophilic states. Approximately 25% of apparently healthy men older than 60 years who experience a first episode of venous thrombosis are carriers of factor V Leiden.[33] There are conflicting data on whether factor V Leiden is associated with an increased risk of recurrent deep vein thrombosis. Several studies reported a slightly enhanced recurrence risk (twofold to fourfold), but a more recent study showed that the risk of recurrence is similar to that in persons without the mutation. [16,34]

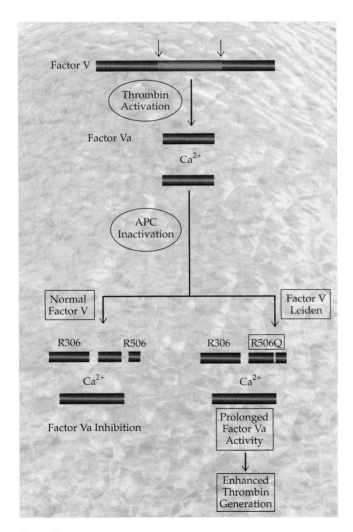 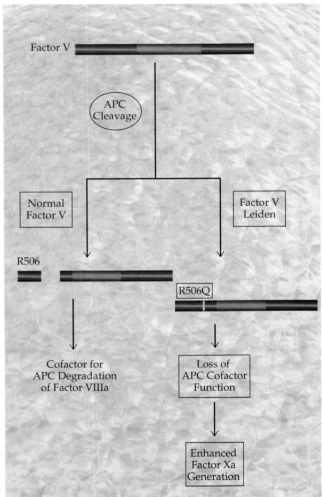

Figure 1 Degradation of factor V Leiden by activated protein C (APC) is significantly slower than that of normal activated factor V (factor Va), which leads to enhanced thrombin generation (*left*). Recent evidence suggests that normal factor V, together with protein S, serves as a cofactor of APC in the inhibition of factor VIIIa (*right*). This APC cofactor function of factor V requires the cleavage of factor V by APC at arginine 506; therefore, factor V Leiden has a poor cofactor function.

Diagnosis

Factor V Leiden can be identified rapidly and precisely with simple DNA-based tests. These tests allow the diagnosis to be made in patients receiving anticoagulation therapy with warfarin and in those who have coexisting antiphospholipid antibodies. Because factor V Leiden is not the sole cause of APC resistance, it may be worthwhile to pursue the diagnosis with an APC resistance test in selected cases.

Treatment

Management of factor V Leiden is similar to that of AT-III, protein C, and protein S deficiencies. Patients with a first episode of venous thrombosis should receive anticoagulation therapy for 6 months. Thereafter, they should be given prophylactic anticoagulation therapy in situations known to provoke thrombosis. Long-term anticoagulation should be considered in patients with recurrent thrombosis.[35]

Young women known to be factor V Leiden carriers should avoid the use of oral contraceptives, which increases the relative risk of thrombosis (although the risk remains low in terms of absolute incidence). The optimal treatment of carriers during pregnancy has not been established. The rate of venous thromboembolism is low, about 2% without thrombosis prophylaxis.[19] My practice is not to use thrombosis prophylaxis routinely, but I will consider postpartum prophylaxis, especially when the family history of thrombosis is strong. Routine screening of family members of patients with factor V Leiden is not cost-effective.[36]

PROTHROMBIN GENE MUTATION 20210A

A G-to-A mutation at nucleotide position 20210 in the 3' untranslated region of the prothrombin gene is associated with an increased incidence of venous thrombosis. The prevalence of the mutation in healthy persons is about 2.3%. Like factor V Leiden, this mutation is very rare in Asians and Africans. Unlike factor V Leiden, it is more common in southern Europeans than in northern Europeans.[37] The relative risk of thrombosis in persons with this mutation is 2.8, which is similar to the relative risk in those with factor V Leiden.[38] The mutation can be found in up to 18% of patients with thrombosis and family histories of thrombosis. The most common presentation is DVT of the lower extremities. Recent prospective studies have not shown an increased risk of recurrent DVT in patients with this mutation.[39] However, carriers who are heterozygous for both factor V Leiden and the prothrombin mutation have a higher risk of recurrent thrombosis.[34] The combination of oral contraceptive use and the prothrombin gene mutation is associated with an approximately 150-fold increase in cerebral vein thrombosis in young women.[40]

HYPERHOMOCYSTEINEMIA

Epidemiology

Hyperhomocysteinemia can be divided into three classes: severe (homocysteine plasma concentration > 100 μmol/L), moderate (25 to 100 μmol/L), or mild (16 to 24 μmol/L). Severe hyperhomocysteinemia is usually caused by a homozygous deficiency of the enzyme cystathionine β-synthase. Affected persons have severe mental retardation, ectopic lens, skeletal abnormalities, and severe early-onset arterial and venous thrombotic disease.[36]

Mild or moderate hyperhomocysteinemia results from either hereditary or acquired defects in the homocysteine metabolic pathway. Heterozygous deficiency in cystathionine β-synthase is quite common in the general population, with a frequency of 0.3% to 1.4%.[41] A defect in the remethylation pathway is commonly caused by a thermolabile mutant of the methylenetetrahydrofolate reductase (MTHFR) enzyme whose activity is approximately 50% of normal; the homozygous state has a prevalence of 5% in the general population.[42] However, the homozygous form of the MTHFR thermolabile enzyme isoform is not clinically relevant in patients whose diet includes adequate folate.

Common causes of acquired hyperhomocysteinemia are deficiencies of dietary cobalamin, folate, or pyridoxine (the essential cofactors for the homocysteine metabolic pathway). A recent prospective study showed that mild hyperhomocysteinemia is quite common in the elderly, despite normal serum vitamin concentrations.[43]

Mild to moderate hyperhomocysteinemia is associated with cerebrovascular disease, coronary artery disease, and peripheral vascular disease in persons younger than 55 years and with carotid artery stenosis in the elderly.[44,45] It is found in 10% of patients with a first episode of DVT.[46] In a recent prospective study, a graded relationship was found between elevated plasma homocysteine levels and mortality in patients with coronary artery disease.[47]

Pathophysiology

Normally, homocysteine is derived from methionine by a transmethylation process. Homocysteine can then be remethylated to methionine by two pathways or can be converted to cysteine by transsulfuration [see Figure 2]. One remethylation pathway is catalyzed by methionine synthase, with the methyl group donated by 5-methyltetrahydrofolate and with cobalamin (vitamin B_{12}) acting as a cofactor. The other remethylation pathway involves betaine as a methyl donor. In the transsulfuration process, homocysteine is first converted to cystathionine, catalyzed by the enzyme cystathionine β-synthase, with pyridoxine acting as a cofactor.

Homocysteine is a highly reactive amino acid containing a free sulfhydryl group. It can promote oxidation of low-density lipoprotein (LDL) cholesterol and presumably is toxic to vascular endothelium.[48,49] It may also inhibit thrombomodulin expression and protein C activation and suppress endothelial heparan sulfate expression; both of these effects lead to hypercoagulability.[50,51] Recently, homocysteine was shown to enhance the binding of lipoprotein(a) (an atherogenic lipoprotein) to fibrin, which may provide a link between hyperhomocysteinemia, thrombosis, and premature atherosclerosis [see Lipoprotein(a), below].[52] The vascular damage caused by high homocysteine levels leads to arterial and venous thrombosis and, perhaps, accelerated atherosclerosis.

Clinical Presentation

Severe hyperhomocysteinemia should be suspected in patients with the characteristic phenotype (see above). Mild to moderate hyperhomocysteinemia should be suspected in cases of arterial and venous thrombotic disease—including cerebrovascular disease, peripheral artery disease, and DVT—especially in young persons.

Diagnosis

Plasma homocysteine exists in free and protein-bound forms and is generally measured and reported as total plasma

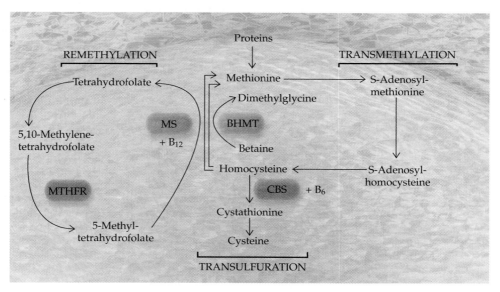

Figure 2   Homocysteine's intracellular metabolism occurs through remethylation to methionine or transsulfuration to cysteine.[140] (BHMT—betaine-homocysteine methyltransferase; CBS—cystathionine–β-synthase; MS—methionine synthase; MTHFR—5,10-methylenetetrahydrofolate reductase)

homocysteine (normal range, 6 to 15 µmol/L). Diagnosis of hyperhomocysteinemia is usually made by measuring plasma homocysteine after an overnight fast. However, because as many as 40% of patients with hyperhomocysteinemia may have a normal fasting level, a methionine-loading test should be considered when indicated.[53] In this test, oral L-methionine (100 mg/kg) is given after an overnight fast and blood samples are taken 4, 6, or 8 hours later for measurement of the plasma homocysteine level. The 90th percentiles for 4-hour and 6-hour levels are 41.3 µmol/L and 58.8 µmol/L, respectively.[53,54] The 95th percentile for the 8-hour level is 35.8 µmol/L for women and 38.9 µmol/L for men.[55] Plasma folate and vitamin B_{12} levels should also be measured to exclude hyperhomocysteinemia caused by folate or B_{12} deficiencies. DNA genotyping for the MTHFR enzyme is also available in commercial laboratories.

Treatment

Daily oral pyridoxine (250 mg) and folic acid (5 mg) brings the elevated homocysteine levels down to normal in most cases.[56] Patients who have vitamin B_{12} deficiency should be given B_{12} supplements. Repeat measurement of plasma homocysteine levels (generally done 1 month after starting supplementation) may be prudent to ensure that the pyridoxine and folate treatment is working. Betaine (3 g p.o., b.i.d.) is sometimes effective in patients with hyperhomocysteinemia that is resistant to pyridoxine and folate. Whether correction of the hyperhomocysteinemia by these measures leads to clinical benefit is currently unknown.

LIPOPROTEIN(A)

Lipoprotein(a) [Lp(a)] is an independent risk factor for thrombosis of the coronary arteries.[57] A recent prospective case-control study associated elevated plasma Lp(a) levels with an approximately threefold increase in risk of coronary artery disease in men.[58] The association between high Lp(a) and ischemic stroke in young adults is controversial.[59,60] Distributions of Lp(a) are skewed in the general population—especially among whites, in whom the median is 3.7 mg/dl but the mean is 6.9 mg/dl.[61] The 95th percentile for plasma Lp(a) is estimated to be in the 25 to 30 mg/dl range.

The Lp(a) class of lipoproteins is formed by the assembly of LDL particles and apoprotein(a), a protein that has some structural similarities to plasminogen (specifically, in the kringle domains) and competes with plasminogen for the endothelial cell binding site, thereby displacing plasminogen and downregulating plasmin generation at the endothelial cell surface.[62] High plasma concentrations of Lp(a) may therefore suppress the endothelial fibrinolytic response. Lp(a) is found in the intima of human atherosclerotic vessels, and transgenic mice expressing human Lp(a) develop extensive atherosclerosis.[63] Measurement of Lp(a) levels can now be done in commercial laboratories and should be considered in young patients with arterial thrombosis. Elevated LDL cholesterol levels appear to elicit or exacerbate the risk factors associated with high Lp(a), and therefore, diet, exercise, and standard pharmacologic approaches should be used in patients with high LDL cholesterol levels.[64] In small studies, niacin at high doses (2 to 4 g p.o. daily) and tamoxifen (20 mg daily) have lowered elevated Lp(a) levels by 30% to 40%.[65,66] High doses of niacin are frequently associated with facial flushing and headaches. These unpleasant side effects can be ameliorated by starting niacin at a low dose (e.g., 300 mg daily) and then increasing the dose incrementally over time or through the use of extended-release niacin. Liver function should be checked periodically.

DYSFIBRINOGENEMIA

Approximately 300 abnormal fibrinogens (dysfibrinogens) have been reported, and about 85 structural defects have been identified in dysfibrinogenemia. These are most commonly characterized by functional defects of fibrinopeptide A release and fibrin polymerization and less commonly by defective plasminogen binding and activation. About half of the fibrinogen mutations are not associated with any clinical symptoms. Mild bleeding or recurrent thrombosis occurs in about equal numbers in the remaining mutations.[67] In rare cases, patients experience both bleeding and thrombosis. Acquired dysfibrinogenemia may complicate hepatocellular carcinoma or chronic liver disease. Evaluation in a general laboratory usually shows a discrepancy between antigenic and functional levels of fibrinogen, because most patients with dysfibrinogens have suboptimal clotting function, with prolonged thrombin time (TT) and reptilase time (RT). The abnormal fibrinogens form fibrin clots that are resistant to clot lysis. Precise identification of the structural defect requires substantial effort in a research laboratory. Management of recurrent thrombosis caused by dysfibrinogenemia is the same as in other patients with thrombophilia.

DYSPLASMINOGEN AND ABNORMAL FIBRINOLYSIS

In rare cases, abnormal plasminogens (dysplasminogens), which are defective in their activation to plasmin, are associated with thrombosis. Patients with such a disorder have a low plasma plasminogen level on functional assays.[68] Increased levels of plasminogen activator inhibitor–1 (PAI-1) and decreased plasma fibrinolytic activity have been reported in patients with preeclampsia.[69] Acquired impairment of fibrinolytic activity may be associated with postoperative thrombosis.[70] However, more studies are required to establish the role of abnormal fibrinolysis in recurrent clinical thrombosis.[71] Antigenic assays for tissue plasminogen activator (t-PA) and PAI-1 are available in some commercial laboratories, but specific functional assays are available only in research laboratories.

ELEVATED FIBRINOGEN, FACTOR VII, AND FACTOR VIII LEVELS

A high plasma fibrinogen level is an independent risk factor for coronary artery disease.[72] An elevated factor VII level has also been associated with the development of heart disease.[73] A factor VIII level above the 90th percentile of normal is associated with an approximately fivefold increased risk of a first episode of DVT.[74,75] It also increases the risk of recurrence.[76] Additional studies are required to establish the clinical utility of measuring these parameters in patients with thrombosis.

Acquired Hypercoagulable States

ANTIPHOSPHOLIPID ANTIBODY SYNDROME

The antiphospholipid antibody syndrome is caused by autoantibodies to proteins associated with negatively charged phospholipids. The terms antiphospholipid and anticardiolipin are used synonymously. Lupus anticoagulant refers to an inhibitor that was first identified in patients with systemic lupus erythematosus. Its appearance correlates with a false positive Wassermann reaction for syphilis. Many patients who have this inhibitor do not have lupus, and it is sometimes called lupuslike anticoagulant.

Epidemiology

Antiphospholipid antibody syndrome occurs secondary to systemic lupus erythematosus and, less commonly, to rheumatoid arthritis, temporal arteritis, and other connective tissue disorders. It is also associated with HIV-1 and hepatitis C infections, lymphoproliferative diseases, and certain drugs (e.g., phenothiazine and procainamide). When no risk factor can be identified, the syndrome is regarded as primary.

Pathophysiology

The two most common protein targets for the antiphospholipid antibodies appear to be β_2-glycoprotein I (β_2-GPI) and prothrombin. β_2-GPI is a plasma protein that binds anionic phospholipids with high affinity. It has weak anticoagulant function in vitro. β_2-GPI can induce cardiolipin from its usual bilaminar form to a hexagonal form that is highly immunogenic.[77] The anticardiolipin antibody enzyme-linked immunosorbent assay (ELISA) usually detects antibodies directed against the cardiolipin/β_2-GPI complex. Lupus anticoagulant antibodies have been purified that specifically react with prothrombin but not thrombin. These purified antibodies can enhance the binding of prothrombin to the cultured endothelial cell surface.[78] Other protein-phospholipid targets may also be involved. Antiphosphatidylethanolamine antibodies are found in many patients with antiphospholipid antibody syndrome, and some of these antibodies inhibit activated protein C function.[79] Antibodies to heparin and heparan sulfate, which inhibit the heparin-dependent neutralization of thrombin by AT-III, have been found.[80] On the basis of this heterogeneity of antiphospholipid antibodies, it seems likely that multiple mechanisms are involved in the pathogenesis of thrombosis in this syndrome.

Clinical Presentation

Thrombotic events occur in approximately 30% of patients with antiphospholipid antibodies (overall incidence, 2.5 events per 100 patient-years).[81] Venous thrombosis occurs in approximately two thirds of patients and arterial thrombosis in approximately one third [see Chapter 114].

Diagnosis

The diagnosis of antiphospholipid antibody syndrome should be considered in any patient who presents with an idiopathic arterial or venous thrombosis. The diagnosis is

Table 5 Proposed Clinical and Laboratory Criteria for the Antiphospholipid Antibody Syndrome[93]

Clinical features	Pregnancy morbidity (any of the following):
	  More than one unexplained fetal death at greater than 10 wk
	  Delivery at less than 34 wk, with severe pregnancy-induced hypertension
	  Three or more pregnancy losses at less than 10 wk
	Thrombosis:
	  Venous (superficial thrombophlebitis; deep vein thrombosis; pulmonary embolism; cerebral and retinal vein thrombosis; renal, splanchnic, and mesenteric vein thrombosis)
	  Arterial (ischemic cerebral infarction, transient cerebral ischemia, amaurosis fugax, migraine, carotid and vertebrobasilar artery thrombosis, aortic arch syndrome, peripheral arterial thrombosis and embolism, renal and mesenteric artery thrombosis, livedo reticularis)

Laboratory features	Lupuslike anticoagulant:
	  Activated partial thromboplastin time, dilute Russell viper venom time, kaolin clotting time, tissue thromboplastin inhibition test
	Anticardiolipin antibodies (either of the following):
	  IgG anticardiolipin antibodies (> 20 GPL)
	  IgM anticardiolipin antibodies (> 20 MPL)

GPL—IgG phospholipid units   MPL—IgM phospholipid units

Table 6 Classification of Antiphospholipid Antibodies[145]

Autoimmune Causes
Primary (do not fulfill criteria for systemic lupus erythematosus)
Secondary (fulfill criteria for systemic lupus erythematosus or other connective tissue diseases)
Drug-induced (e.g., phenothiazines, quinidine, quinine, synthetic penicillins, hydralazine)

Alloimmune Causes
Infections (viral, bacterial, fungal)
Malignancies (e.g., hairy-cell leukemia, lymphoproliferative disease)

confirmed by the presence of anticardiolipin antibodies on ELISA (see above) or lupus anticoagulant on clotting assays.

The general criteria for the diagnosis of lupus anticoagulant are (1) prolongation of at least one phospholipid-dependent clotting assay, (2) proof, by mixing studies, that the prolongation is caused by an inhibitor and not a clotting factor deficiency, and (3) confirmation that the inhibitor is phospholipid dependent [*see Table 5*]. The clotting tests commonly used are activated PTT (aPTT) and dilute Russell viper venom time (RVVT). The reagents in aPTT are variably sensitive to the lupus anticoagulant and are influenced by concentrations of some plasma clotting factors (e.g., factor VIII). Therefore, the sensitivity of this test is not high, and at least one other clotting test should be carried out. Dilute RVVT is much more sensitive than aPTT but is a manual test and not generally available. Other tests, such as kaolin clotting time and the tissue thromboplastin inhibition test, are useful when available. The presence of an inhibitor necessitates a mixing study to demonstrate lack of correction with normal plasma. Correction of the prolongation by addition of phospholipid in the form of platelet lysates or as hexagonal-phase phospholipid will confirm the diagnosis. Clotting factor assays can be carried out in equivocal cases. A lupus anticoagulant will cause functional deficiency of several phospholipid-dependent clotting factors, not just one particular factor.

Anticardiolipin antibodies are reported as IgG (in IgG phospholipid [GPL] units) and IgM (in IgM phospholipid [MPL] units). The prevalence of elevated anticardiolipin IgG and IgM antibodies in normal populations is approximately 5%, with less than 2% remaining abnormal upon repeated testing.[82] High titers of anticardiolipin IgG antibodies (> 33 GPL) are associated with an approximately fivefold increase in overall thrombotic risk.[81,83] The importance of low titers of IgG antibodies (< 20 GPL), isolated IgM antibodies, and IgA antibodies has not been established.[84,85] Both functional and antigenic assays should be ordered in the evaluation of a patient because these two assays do not completely overlap.

Certain infections and drug exposures may lead to a transient appearance of antiphospholipid antibodies, which disappear after the resolution of infection or discontinuance of the drug [*see Table 6*]. Therefore, laboratory tests should be repeated at least once (6 weeks after the first tests) to confirm the diagnosis. Conversely, approximately 20% of patients with low titers of anticardiolipin IgG antibodies will have higher titers upon repeat testing. Retesting is also warranted in patients with new or recurrent thrombosis.[84]

Treatment

The current therapeutic recommendations for antiphospholipid antibody syndrome are mostly based on observational studies that support an association between antiphospholipid antibodies and thrombosis, particularly recurrent thrombosis.[81-85] In the acute treatment of DVT in patients with antiphospholipid antibody syndrome, monitoring the effect of regular heparin can be problematic because lupus anticoagulant prolongs the aPTT. The use of LMWH circumvents this problem because LMWH does not require dose titration and monitoring. The patient should be treated with LMWH and warfarin in the usual fashion, with an overlap of at least 5 days before discontinuing LMWH.

Retrospective analysis shows that patients with the antiphospholipid antibody syndrome and a history of thrombosis have a high recurrence rate of thrombosis (in the range of 50% to 70%) if they are not given intensive warfarin therapy.[86,87] The site of the first thrombotic event (i.e., arterial or venous) tends to predict the site of the recurrent event.[87] High-intensity warfarin treatment with the international normalized ratio (INR) targeted to greater than 3.0 gives the best results, although it is associated with a significant risk of bleeding. Aspirin provides no additional benefit and increases the bleeding risk.[88] It is my practice to maintain the INR at 3.0 to 3.5 in such patients. However, because of the increased risk of bleeding, some experienced clinicians use an INR of 2.5 while awaiting prospective trial results.[89]

The optimal duration of oral anticoagulation therapy for antiphospholipid antibody syndrome is not fully established. Recurrent venous thrombosis or ischemic stroke usually justifies long-term warfarin. In a patient with a first episode of DVT who is found to have antiphospholipid antibodies, warfarin therapy is indicated for at least 6 months and perhaps for life.[90] The severity of the specific thrombotic episode, the coexistence of any reversible thrombotic risk factors, and the risks of long-term oral anticoagulation therapy should also be considered. It should be noted that the lupus anticoagulant may occasionally increase the prothrombin time (PT) and, in turn, the INR, thus posing a problem for the monitoring of warfarin therapy.[91] When PT and INR increase, use of a lupus anticoagulant-insensitive thromboplastin reagent is helpful.

In asymptomatic patients with anticardiolipin antibodies or lupus anticoagulant but no history of thrombosis, anticoagulation is not required.

Pregnancy Loss in Antiphospholipid Antibody Syndrome

Several prospective studies confirm an association between recurrent miscarriages and antiphospholipid antibodies. The antibodies presumably cause pregnancy loss by promoting placental thrombosis.[92] Antiphospholipid antibodies should be measured in patients with a history of unexplained second- or third-trimester loss, fetal demise, early-onset severe preeclampsia, and intrauterine growth retardation.[93] In contrast, antiphospholipid antibodies are not associated with sporadic early pregnancy loss,[94] which is frequently the result of genetic abnormalities in the fetus. The relationship of antiphospholipid antibodies with infertility is uncertain at present.

The management of pregnant women with antiphospholipid antibody syndrome is difficult because of the syndrome's association with thrombosis and the increased risk of bleeding with antithrombotic therapy. In a recent prospective, randomized, placebo-controlled trial, a combination of prednisone and aspirin was demonstrated to be ineffective in promoting live birth; in fact, it increased the risk of prematurity.[95] On the other hand, two recent prospective trials demonstrated that heparin and low-dose aspirin (81 mg a day) provide a significantly better pregnancy outcome than low-dose aspirin alone, with viable infants being delivered in 70% to 80% of cases.[96,97] Furthermore, low-dose heparin (given initially as 5,000 units subcutaneously twice daily and adjusted to maintain the aPTT within the upper limits of the normal range) seems to be as effective as higher-dose heparin combined with low-dose aspirin.[98] Treatment should begin as soon as pregnancy is confirmed. LMWH is preferable to regular heparin for long-term use because LMWH can be given once or twice daily and may reduce the risk of osteopenia and heparin-induced thrombocytopenia (see below). In a recent study, enoxaparin (40 mg once daily) and aspirin (100 mg daily) were given from week 12 of gestation until 6 weeks postpartum with good results.[99]

HEPARIN-INDUCED THROMBOCYTOPENIA AND THROMBOSIS

Epidemiology

Heparin-induced thrombocytopenia (HIT) is a relatively common antibody-mediated drug reaction, occurring in about 1% of patients receiving porcine heparin and 5% of patients receiving bovine heparin.[100] The incidence of HIT is much lower in patients treated with LMWH. In a subset of patients, HIT progresses to a potentially fatal disorder characterized by venous and arterial thrombosis. Interestingly, both the frequency of HIT antibody formation and the clinical manifestations of HIT vary considerably in different patient populations. The incidence of HIT antibody formation is much higher after cardiac surgery than after orthopedic surgery (50% versus 15%); however, the incidence of clinically significant postoperative HIT appears to be lower in cardiac surgical patients than in orthopedic patients, in whom the incidence is 5%.[101,102]

Pathophysiology

The pathogenesis of HIT is attributable to the presence of an IgG antibody that recognizes a complex of heparin and platelet factor 4 (PF4) [see Figure 3].[103] PF4 is a cationic protein found in platelet α-granules, which, when released, binds to the negatively charged heparin molecule with high affinity. The IgG antibody binds to the PF4-heparin complex on platelet membranes, forming a ternary complex that in turn binds to the platelet membrane FcgRII receptor. This binding activates the platelets, leading to further release of PF4 and formation of PF4-heparin complex. The immune complex–coated platelets are cleared rapidly by the reticuloendothelial system, giving rise to thrombocytopenia. The thrombotic complications in HIT are caused by activation of platelets by the immune complex, which leads to the formation of platelet microparticles and enhanced thrombin generation.[104] PF4 also binds to heparinlike sulfated glycosaminoglycans (e.g., heparan sulfate) on the endothelial cell surface. In vitro evidence indicates that the antibody in HIT is able to bind to endothelial cells. The cells may then become activated, giving rise to thrombosis.[105] Given that only a minority of patients who form HIT antibodies experience clinical HIT,[102] the induction of HIT antibodies and the development of thrombocytopenia and subsequent thrombosis should be regarded as a continuum. Concomitant thrombotic risk factors probably play a major role in determining the clinical progression and manifestations of HIT.

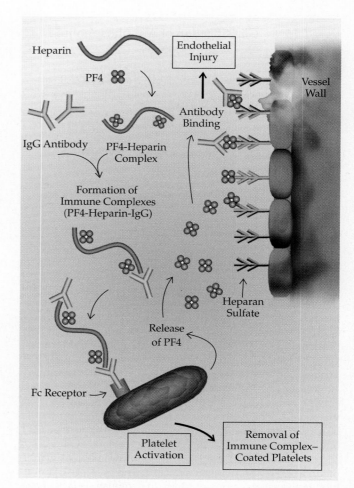

Figure 3 In a proposed explanation for heparin-induced thrombocytopenia, IgG antibodies recognize platelet factor 4 (PF4)–heparin complexes. The resulting PF4-heparin-IgG immune complexes bind to Fc receptors on circulating platelets. Fc-mediated platelet activation releases PF4 from α-granules in platelets, establishing a cycle of platelet activation and formation of prothrombotic platelet microparticles. Removal of immune complex–coated platelets by the reticuloendothelial system results in thrombocytopenia. PF4 also binds to heparan sulfate on the surface of endothelial cells, leading to immune-mediated injury, thrombosis, and disseminated intravascular coagulation.[143]

Clinical Presentation

HIT typically develops 5 to 10 days after the initiation of heparin therapy. However, in patients who received heparin within the previous 100 days and are being re-treated, the onset can be rapid—within hours after starting heparin.[106] Conversely, onset of HIT may not occur until as long as 19 days after stopping heparin therapy.[107] This delayed-onset HIT appears to be associated with a higher titer of IgG antibodies against the PF4-heparin complex.

HIT is generally defined as a platelet count below $150 \times 10^9/L$, or a drop in the platelet count by more than 50% from the postoperative peak, occurring 5 to 14 days after starting heparin. The mean platelet count in HIT is about $60 \times 10^9/L$. Severe thrombocytopenia, with platelet counts below $20 \times 10^9/L$, occurs in fewer than 10% of patients; in 10% to 15% of patients, despite the 50% drop from peak levels, the platelet count nadir is above $150 \times 10^9/L$.[102]

The risk of HIT-associated thrombosis was once thought to be quite small; however, it is now recognized that thrombosis occurs in about one third to one half of patients with HIT, with venous thrombosis more frequent than arterial thrombosis.[104] Thrombosis can occur at any platelet count, even a very low one.

DVT, with or without pulmonary embolism, is the most common event leading to the diagnosis of HIT. The disorder may be further complicated by limb gangrene, especially in the setting of warfarin treatment without concomitant alternative anticoagulant coverage (see below). Cerebral vein thrombosis and adrenal hemorrhagic necrosis are uncommon but well-documented complications of HIT, and early diagnosis and urgent therapy can be lifesaving. Arterial thrombosis may manifest as limb ischemia, stroke, myocardial infarction, and, less commonly, mesenteric thrombosis and renal artery thrombosis. Some patients have laboratory findings that support a diagnosis of DIC. Heparin-induced skin lesions may occur at heparin injection sites and range from painful erythematous papules to extensive dermal necrosis.[108]

Unlike antibodies induced by quinine, quinidine, or sulfonamides, which can persist for years, heparin-induced antibodies appear to be quite transient. They fall to undetectable levels at a median of 50 to 85 days, depending on the assay performed.[106]

Diagnosis

The most widely used assay in the diagnosis of HIT is heparin-induced platelet aggregation in the presence of the patient's serum. However, the sensitivity of this test can be as low as 50%.[109] Sometimes, the patient's serum can cause spontaneous aggregation of donor platelets in the absence of heparin, most likely caused by the presence of immune complexes unrelated to HIT, which makes proper interpretation of the test result impossible. ELISAs have been developed to detect antibodies that are reactive to the PF4-heparin complex, and these are now commercially available. These ELISAs have a higher sensitivity than the platelet aggregation assay and can be more easily performed in a general clinical diagnostic laboratory. Because HIT can be complicated by serious thrombotic problems, however, diagnosis of HIT should be based primarily on appropriate clinical findings and management begun while laboratory confirmation is awaited.

Treatment

Management of HIT consists of stopping heparin immediately and starting alternative anticoagulation therapy. It is important to discontinue all types of heparin: there are anecdotal reports of HIT caused by trace amounts of heparin used in heparin flushes of intravascular lines.

If the patient has mild thrombocytopenia alone without any evidence of thrombosis, it may be reasonable just to discontinue heparin and follow the patient closely without alternative anticoagulation therapy. It is my practice, however, to treat the underlying hypercoagulable state with an alternative anticoagulant. This aggressive approach is supported by a recent retrospective cohort study in which thrombosis developed within 30 days of heparin cessation in approximately half of patients who initially had no clinical symptoms from their HIT.[100]

HIT may develop in patients who were receiving heparin for preexisting thrombosis and are in the process of being switched over to warfarin. If the patient has been on warfarin for 4 or 5 days and the INR has reached an adequate therapeutic range, the clinician may rely on warfarin alone and monitor the patient carefully. However, if the patient has been on warfarin for less than 4 days or has evidence of a thrombotic complication from the HIT, an alternative anticoagulant should be used in addition to warfarin.

Alternative anticoagulant agents include danaparoid, hirudin, lepirudin, and argatroban. Although LMWH is much less immunogenic than standard heparin in causing HIT,[104] it cannot be used as a safe substitute when a patient develops HIT caused by standard heparin. LMWH and standard heparin have extensive cross-reactivity (> 90%) in terms of antibody recognition. LMWH is not an appropriate choice in patients with HIT.

Danaparoid is an anticoagulant approved for DVT prophylaxis. The drug can be used off label in patients with HIT. It is a low-molecular-weight heparinoid composed of heparan sulfate, dermatan sulfate, and chondroitin sulfate. The anticoagulant effect of danaparoid is mediated by a combination of AT-III, heparin cofactor II, and an undefined endothelial cellular mechanism that acts to make danaparoid a more selective factor Xa inhibitor than LMWH. Danaparoid has a ratio of anti-FXa to antithrombin activity of 28 to 1, which is about 10 times higher than the ratio with LMWH. Danaparoid is monitored by anti-FXa assay, not aPTT, and has low cross-reactivity (approximately 10%) to the antibody in HIT in vitro.[110] The anti-Xa level is maintained between 0.5 and 0.8 U/ml.

Danaparoid is effective in treating acute DVT and HIT (at a dose of 2,000 anti-Xa units in an I.V. bolus, followed by 2,000 units S.C., b.i.d.).[111] It has also been used successfully in pregnant women with HIT.[112] Potential disadvantages of danaparoid are its high cost and long half-life (25 hours) and that it has no antidote. Bleeding that occurs after administration of danaparoid can be difficult to reverse. Like LMWH, danaparoid is cleared renally; anti-Xa levels should be monitored in patients with renal insufficiency.

Hirudin, a 65-amino-acid protein originally extracted from the salivary gland of the medicinal leech (*Hirudo medicinalis*), is a potent direct thrombin inhibitor. Hirudin binds directly to thrombin's active site, independently of AT-III. It is not neutralized by PF4. Hirudin's anticoagulant function is monitored by aPTT.

Lepirudin is a recombinant form of hirudin that is approved for treatment of HIT. In two prospective clinical trials, use of lepirudin reduced serious thrombotic complications to about 20% (compared with a rate of about 40% in historical control subjects).[112,113] Lepirudin was given by intravenous bolus (0.4 mg/kg) followed by continuous infusion at 0.15 mg/kg/hr for 2 to 10 days, as indicated. The dose was adjusted to maintain a target aPTT 1.5 to 3 times normal. Patients experienced an increase of minor bleeding (from puncture sites, epistaxis, and hematuria) but no intracranial bleeding. Of note, 40% of patients developed antihirudin antibody. These are not neutralizing antibodies and may actually enhance the drug's potency, perhaps by delaying its clearance—another reason to monitor aPTT levels. Judging from cardiology intervention trials, bleeding risk would be substantially increased with concomitant use of thrombolytics; therefore, it is not advisable to use the agents in combination. There is no effective antidote for lepirudin, but lepirudin has a much shorter half-life than danaparoid (approximately 1.3 hours versus 25 hours). Like danaparoid, lepirudin is cleared by the kidneys and its dose needs to be adjusted carefully, on the basis of creatinine clearance values.

Argatroban, a synthetic direct thrombin inhibitor, was recently approved for prophylaxis or treatment of thrombosis in patients with HIT. It is given by continuous intravenous infusion of 2 mg/kg/min to maintain an aPTT of 1.5 to 3 times baseline (not to exceed 100 seconds or 10 mg/kg/min). In one study, argatroban reduced the serious thrombotic complications of HIT by about 50%, as compared with historical controls, with a major bleeding rate of about 7%.[114] Its half-life is only 40 to 50 minutes. In contrast to danaparoid and lepirudin, argatroban is cleared by the liver and therefore can be used more easily in patients with renal insufficiency. It does not have a specific antidote, and bleeding complications need to be watched for carefully.

Patients who have HIT without associated thrombotic complications should be treated with one of the alternative anticoagulants until the platelet count has returned to normal, which generally takes only 4 to 5 days. In those who require prolonged anticoagulation—whether because they have other indications for anticoagulation or they have had thrombotic complications from HIT—warfarin is used for long-term treatment. Warfarin should be started only after the patient has received adequate anticoagulation therapy with one of the alternative anticoagulants. The two agents should be used concurrently for at least 5 days before the alternative anticoagulant is discontinued. Both lepirudin and argatroban may increase prothrombin time and INR, thus interfering with warfarin dose adjustments. The prothrombin time should be rechecked 6 hours after the discontinuance of lepirudin or argatroban to ensure that an INR of 2 to 3 has been achieved. For patients who have had HIT-associated thrombosis, warfarin therapy for 3 months should be adequate.

Some patients with serologically confirmed HIT may, at some point in the future, require surgery that involves cardiopulmonary bypass. There are anecdotal case reports of use of recombinant hirudin, argatroban, or danaparoid in that situation.[113,115,116] Given the transient nature of the heparin-induced antibodies, subsequent reuse of heparin is theoretically reasonable, and indeed a limited number of patients have been given heparin again after the disappearance of heparin-induced antibodies without any significant clinical sequelae.[117,106] Nevertheless, the use of heparin in this situation should be restricted to patients with a compelling indication for it, such as cardiac or vascular surgery, and only after the absence of detectable heparin-dependent antibodies has been confirmed by a sensitive assay, such as a PF4-heparin ELISA. Also, since reexposure to heparin may elicit a recurrence of heparin-dependent antibodies, heparin should be used only during the procedure itself and as an alternative anticoagulant for postoperative antithrombotic prophylaxis or therapy.

MALIGNANCY—TROUSSEAU SYNDROME

Epidemiology

Some patients with cancer—especially those with occult solid tumors of the pancreas, ovary, liver, brain, colon, lung, or breast—may experience spontaneous venous thrombosis of the upper and lower extremities, or Trousseau syndrome. These patients also have an increased propensity toward recurrent arterial thrombosis and thromboembolism.[118] In a prospective study of patients who presented with idiopathic symptomatic DVT, cancer was diagnosed in approximately 8% of patients during a 2-year follow-up (odds ratio, 2.3). In patients with recurrent thrombosis, the incidence of cancer was even higher (17%; odds ratio, 4.3).[119]

Pathophysiology

The underlying cause of Trousseau syndrome is a chronic, compensated form of DIC [see Chapter 93]. The activated procoagulants generated in DIC enhance thrombosis. Immunochemical staining of sections from tumors commonly associated with Trousseau syndrome often reveals tissue factor on the tumor surface.[120,121] A cancer procoagulant, identified as a cysteine protease, has been purified from some adenocarcinomas and leukemic cells that can activate the clotting cascade by directly activating factor X.[122,123] Interaction of the tumor cells with monocytes, platelets, and endothelial cells may also generate inflammatory cytokines and induce endothelial and monocytic procoagulant activities, further exacerbating the thrombosis.

Clinical Presentation

Venous thrombosis in Trousseau syndrome usually manifests as migratory superficial thrombophlebitis or DVT of the lower extremities. The recurrent arterial thrombosis in these patients arises from a nonbacterial thrombotic endocarditis in which sterile fibrin is deposited in the mitral valve. The fibrin clot may embolize to cause digital ischemia, transient ischemic attacks, and stroke.

Diagnosis

Coagulation studies in Trousseau syndrome show evidence of chronic, low-grade DIC (i.e., slightly low or even high fibrinogen and platelet levels and high levels of D-dimer). The PT and PTT are generally not prolonged. Overt DIC in such patients is uncommon.

How aggressively should one pursue the diagnosis of an underlying cancer in patients with idiopathic DVT? Research has not yet demonstrated the benefit and cost-effectiveness of an extensive screening approach.[124] In a recent large cohort study, cancer diagnoses after a primary thrombotic event were highest during the first 6 months of follow-up and declined rapidly to normal levels after the first year. Moreover, 40% of the patients who were diagnosed with cancer in the first year had distant metastases at the time of the diagnosis. It is unclear whether an earlier diagnosis after the thrombotic event would have changed the outcome in these patients. The researchers concluded that an aggressive search for a hidden underlying cancer in such patients is not warranted.[125]

At present, it is prudent to perform a careful history, physical examination, chest x-ray, routine blood counts, and chemistries. Some experts have also recommended multiple tests for fecal occult blood, prostate-specific antigen tests in men, and mammography and pelvic ultrasonography in women.[126,127] Careful follow-up examination and tests should be done as indicated by the initial evaluation.[128]

Treatment

The key to management of Trousseau syndrome is diagnosis and treatment of the underlying tumor. Unfortunately, tumors often manifest explosively in patients with Trousseau syndrome and may not respond to the usual therapies. Warfarin, used at the conventional therapeutic INR of 2 to 3, is often not effective in managing thrombosis in these patients. Patients with Trousseau syndrome usually require long-term administration of full-dose heparin (either unfractionated heparin or LMWH). If a patient is receiving chemotherapy for the underlying cancer, an exacerbation of the DIC associated with tumor lysis should be anticipated. An increase in the dose of heparin may be required.

THROMBOTIC REACTIONS TO ESTROGENS

Oral contraceptives increase the risk of thromboembolic disease approximately fourfold.[129] Recent epidemiologic studies indicate that contraceptives containing a third-generation progestin (e.g., desogestrel) carry a twofold greater risk of thrombosis than those with a second-generation drug (levonorgestrel).[130] For that reason, the preferred choice for first-time users of oral contraceptives is a compound containing a second-generation drug (e.g., Alesse, Levlite, Levora, Nordette, Triphasil, Trivora). The risk of venous thromboembolism disappears when the drugs are discontinued.

In postmenopausal women, estrogen replacement increases the risk of venous thromboembolism about threefold. The absolute risk is low, however—it is estimated at approximately 3.2 per 10,000 patient-years. Therefore, estrogen replacement is not contraindicated in patients who are interested in its potential to prevent osteoporosis and coronary artery disease.[131,132] However, a recent clinical trial showed that patients with a previous history of DVT or pulmonary embolism are at increased risk of recurrence and therefore should avoid hormonal replacement therapy if possible.[133]

The association between estrogen use and thromboembolic disease remains unexplained.[134] Estrogen treatment is known to produce changes in the plasma levels of many proteins involved in coagulation and fibrinolysis, including decreases in protein S and AT-III and increases in plasminogen. The changes are generally quite modest, however, and are not thought to account for the increased risk of thrombosis.

Management of Venous Thromboembolism

The acute management of an initial episode of DVT or pulmonary embolism in patients with proven or presumed underlying risk factors for thrombosis is the same as for other patients: heparin and then warfarin [see Chapter 29].

Warfarin therapy usually should be continued for 3 to 6 months. In a prospective study of oral anticoagulation therapy in patients with a first episode of venous thromboembolism, 6 weeks of therapy was adequate for patients with temporary, reversible risk factors for thrombosis (e.g., surgery, trauma, temporary immobilization, or use of oral contraceptives). On the other hand, 6 months of oral anticoagulation therapy was clearly superior for patients with idiopathic venous thromboembolism (who are presumed to have intrinsic risk factors).[135] The recurrence rate was quite high, however—approximately 12% at 2 years. On the basis of this evidence, at least 6 months of oral anticoagulation therapy is indicated in a patient with a first episode of idiopathic DVT or pulmonary embolism.

Further management should depend on results of the hypercoagulable workup (see above). A risk assessment for other predisposing factors will also be relevant.

Three prospective studies have evaluated the risks and benefits of long-term treatment of venous thromboembolism. In one study, patients were randomly assigned to either 6 months or an indefinite duration of oral anticoagulation therapy after a second episode of DVT or pulmonary embolism.[136] By study design, patients with AT-III, protein C, and protein S deficiencies were excluded. After 4 years of follow-up, the group assigned to

6 months of therapy had a much higher recurrence rate (20.7%) than the continuing-therapy group (2.6%). Not surprisingly, there was increased major bleeding in the continuous-therapy group (8.6% versus 2.7% in the 6-month therapy group), with an annual incidence of major bleeding of 2.4% a year.

In another study, patients with a first episode of idiopathic venous thromboembolism were randomly assigned to either placebo or 2 years of oral anticoagulation therapy after completion of 3 months of oral anticoagulation therapy.[137] The recurrence rate per patient-year was approximately 27% in the placebo group and 1.3% in the warfarin group. The warfarin group had major bleeding at a rate of 3.8% per patient-year. When the risk factors for recurrence were analyzed, neither factor V Leiden nor prothrombin mutation 20210A had any significant effect. Only lupus anticoagulant was significantly associated with recurrence.[137] These results demonstrate that 3 months of oral anticoagulation therapy is inadequate in patients with idiopathic venous thromboembolism.

More recently, a prospective, randomized trial compared 3 months with 1 year of oral anticoagulation in patients with a first episode of idiopathic DVT, with long-term follow-up.[138] As in the previous studies, patients assigned to continued warfarin therapy had a significantly lower recurrence rate than the placebo group (0.7% versus 8.3%), along with a slightly increased (3%) nonfatal major bleeding risk. However, after the discontinuance of warfarin at 1 year, recurrence of thromboembolic events increased; by 3 years, there was no longer any difference between the two groups (about a 16% recurrence rate in each). The data strongly suggest that although continued warfarin therapy will prevent recurrence of thromboembolic events (albeit at the cost of an increased risk of bleeding), the clinical benefit is not maintained after the discontinuance of oral anticoagulation.

Table 7 General Guidelines for Management of Patients with Venous Thromboembolism

Recurrence Risk	Management
High Recurrent idiopathic thrombosis One life-threatening thrombosis One spontaneous thrombosis at an unusual site (e.g., mesenteric or cerebral thrombosis) One spontaneous thrombosis associated with antiphospholipid antibody syndrome One thrombosis with two permanent risk factors One thrombosis with Trousseau syndrome	Lifelong oral anticoagulation therapy: INR 2.0 to 3.0 in all cases except antiphospholipid syndrome (INR, 3.0 to 3.5)
Medium One thrombosis with one permanent risk factor (except Trousseau syndrome) Idiopathic thrombosis with no identifiable risk factor Asymptomatic with one permanent risk factor	6 mo of oral anticoagulation therapy after first episode of thrombosis; vigorous prophylaxis in high-risk situations
Low One thrombosis with reversible risk factor	6 wk of oral anticoagulation therapy after first episode of thrombosis; vigorous prophylaxis in high-risk situations

INR—international normalized ratio

Therefore, the optimal duration of long-term oral anticoagulation therapy for patients with thromboembolism remains undefined; at present, this is best addressed individually, on the basis of an estimation of the risk of recurrence [*see Table 7*].[139,140] Before undertaking long-term anticoagulation therapy in a high-risk patient, the clinician must take the patient's risk of bleeding into account.

Of note, none of the published studies shows a significant difference in mortality between patients who receive long-term therapy and those who receive short-term therapy. There is also no evidence to suggest that prophylactic anticoagulation therapy improves overall survival. In historical studies, families with deficiencies of AT-III and protein C show no higher mortality than the general population displays.[141,142] Current clinical trials are studying the use of full-dose oral anticoagulation therapy for an extended period of time followed by an indefinite period of low-dose anticoagulation therapy. The results of these studies will help to define the optimal long-term treatment for patients who are at high risk for recurrence of thromboembolism.

References

1. Martinelli I, Mannucci PM, De Stefano V, et al: Different risks of thrombosis in four coagulation defects associated with inherited thrombophilia: a study of 150 families. Blood 92:2353, 1998

2. Martinelli I, Cattaneo M, Panzeri D, et al: Risk factors for deep venous thrombosis of the upper extremities. Ann Intern Med 126:707, 1997

3. Prandoni P, Polistena P, Bernardi E, et al: Upper-extremity deep vein thrombosis: risk factors, diagnosis, and complications. Arch Intern Med 157:57, 1997

4. Abilgaard U: Antithrombin and related inhibitors of coagulation. Recent Advances in Blood Coagulation. Poller L, Ed. Churchill Livingstone, Edinburgh, Scotland, 1981, p 151

5. De Stefano V, Leone G, Mastrangelo S, et al: Clinical manifestations and management of inherited thrombophilia: retrospective analysis and follow-up after diagnosis of 238 patients with congenital deficiency of antithrombin III, protein C, protein S. Thromb Haemost 72:352, 1994

6. Demers C, Ginsberg JS, Hirsh J, et al: Thrombosis in antithrombin-III-deficient persons: report of a large kindred and literature review. Ann Intern Med 116:754, 1992

7. Menache D, O'Malley JP, Schorr JB, et al: Evaluation of the safety, recovery, half-life, and clinical efficacy of antithrombin III (human) in patients with hereditary antithrombin III deficiency. Blood 75:33, 1990

8. Miletich J, Sherman L, Broze G Jr: Absence of thrombosis in subjects with heterozygous protein C deficiency. N Engl J Med 317:991, 1987

9. Miletich JP, Prescott SM, White R, et al: Inherited predisposition to thrombosis. Cell 72:477, 1993

10. Boerger LM, Morris PC, Thurnau GR, et al: Oral contraceptives and gender affect protein S status. Blood 69:692, 1987

11. Vigano-D'Angelo S, D'Angelo A, Kaufman CE Jr, et al: Protein S deficiency occurs in the nephrotic syndrome. Ann Intern Med 107:42, 1987

12. Sallah S, Abdallah JM, Gagnon GA: Recurrent warfarin-induced skin necrosis in kindreds with protein-S deficiency. Haemostasis 28:25, 1998

13. Faioni EM, Franchi F, Asti D, et al: Resistance to activated protein C in nine thrombophilic families: interference in a protein S functional assay. Thromb Haemost 70:1067, 1993

14. Rees DC, Cox M, Clegg JB: World distribution of factor V Leiden. Lancet 346:1133, 1995

15. Svensson PJ, Dahlback B: Resistance to activated protein C as a basis for venous thrombosis. N Engl J Med 330:517, 1994

16. Simioni P, Prandoni P, Lensing AWA, et al: The risk of recurrent venous thromboembolism in patients with an Arg506 Gln mutation in the gene for factor V (factor V Leiden). N Engl J Med 336:399, 1997

17. Vandenbroucke JP, Koster T, Briet E, et al: Increased risk of venous thrombosis in oral-contraceptive users who are carriers of factor V Leiden mutation. Lancet 344:1453, 1994

18. Rosendaal FR, Koster T, Vandenbroucke JP, et al: High-risk of thrombosis in patients homozygous for factor V Leiden (APC-resistance). Blood 85:1504, 1995

19. Middeldorp S, Henkens CMA, Koopman MMW, et al: The incidence of venous thromboembolism in family members of patients with factor V Leiden mutation and venous thrombosis. Ann Intern Med 128:15, 1998

20. Koeleman BPC, Reitsma PH, Allaart RC, et al: Activated protein C resistance as an additional risk factor for thrombosis in protein C–deficient families. Blood 84:1031, 1994

21. Zoller B, Berntsdotter A, Garcia de Frutos P, et al: Resistance to activated protein C resistance as an additional genetic risk factor in hereditary deficiency of protein S. Blood 85:3518, 1995

22. van Boven HH, Reitsma PH, Rosendaal FR, et al: Factor V Leiden (FV R506Q) in families with inherited antithrombin deficiency. Thromb Haemost 75:417, 1996

23. Williamson D, Brown K, Luddington R, et al: Factor V Cambridge: a new mutation (Arg306→Thr) associated with resistance to activated protein C. Blood 91:1140, 1998

24. Chan WP, Lee CK, Kwong YL, et al: A novel mutation of Arg306 of factor V gene in Hong Kong Chinese. Blood 91:1135, 1998

25. Zoller B, Svensson PJ, He X, et al: Identification of the same factor V gene mutation in 47 out of 50 thrombosis-prone families with inherited resistance to activated protein C. J Clin Invest 94:2521, 1994

26. Bertina RM: Laboratory diagnosis of resistance to activated protein C (APC-resistance). Thromb Haemost 78:478, 1997

27. van der Bom JG, Bots ML, Haverkate F, et al: Reduced response to protein C is associated with increased risk for cerebral vascular disease. Ann Intern Med 125:265, 1996

28. Fisher M, Fernandez JA, Ameriso SF, et al: Activated protein C resistance in ischemic stroke not due to factor V arginine506→glutamine mutation. Stroke 27:1163, 1996

29. Rodeghiero F, Tosetto A: Activated protein C resistance and factor V Leiden mutation are independent risk factors for venous thromboembolism. Ann Intern Med 130:643, 1999

30. de Visser MCH, Rosendaal FR, Bertina RM: A reduced sensitivity to activated protein C in the absence of factor V Leiden increases the risk of venous thrombosis. Blood 93:1271, 1999

31. Bertina RM, Koeleman BPC, Koster T, et al: Mutation in blood coagulation factor V associated with resistance to activated protein C. Nature 369:64, 1994

32. Kalafatis M, Bertina RM, Rand MD, et al: Characterization of the molecular defect in factor V R506Q. J Biol Chem 270:4053, 1995

33. Ridker PM, Hennekens CH, Lindpaintner K, et al: Mutation in the gene coding for coagulation factor V and the risk for myocardial infarction, stroke, and venous thrombosis in apparently healthy men. N Engl J Med 332:912, 1995

34. De Stefano V, Martinelli I, Mannucci PM, et al: The risk of recurrent deep venous thrombosis among heterozygous carriers of both factor V Leiden and the G20210A prothrombin mutation. N Engl J Med 341:801, 1999

35. Dahlback B: Resistance to activated protein C caused by the factor V R506Q mutation is a common risk factor for venous thrombosis. Thromb Haemost 78:483, 1997

36. Middeldorp S, Meinardi JR, Koopman MM, et al: A prospective study of asymptomatic carriers of the factor V Leiden mutation to determine the incidence of venous thromboembolism. Ann Intern Med 135:322, 2001

37. Rosendaal FR, Doggen CJ, Zivelin A, et al: Geographic distribution of the 20210 G to A prothrombin variant. Thromb Haemost 79:706, 1998

38. Poort SR, Rosendaal FR, Reitsma PH, et al: A common genetic variation in the 3'-untranslated region of the prothrombin gene is associated with elevated plasma prothrombin levels and an increase in venous thrombosis. Blood 88:3698, 1996

39. The risk of recurrent venous thromboembolism in carriers and non-carriers of the G1691A allele in the coagulation factor V gene and the G20210A allele in the prothrombin gene. DURAC Trial Study Group. Duration of Anticoagulation. Thromb Haemost 81:684, 1999

40. Martinelli I, Sacchi E, Landi G, et al: High risk of cerebral-vein thrombosis in carriers of a prothrombin-gene mutation and in users of oral contraceptives. N Engl J Med 338:1793, 1998

41. Mudd SH, Levy HL, Skovby F: Disorders of transulfuration. The Metabolic Basis of Inherited Disease. Scriver CR, Beaudet AL, Sly WS, et al, Eds. McGraw-Hill, New York, 1989, p 693

42. Malinow MR: Homocyst(e)ine and arterial occlusive diseases. J Intern Med 236:603, 1994

43. Naurath HJ, Joosten E, Riezier R, et al: Effects of vitamin B12, folate, and vitamin B6 supplements in elderly people with normal serum vitamin concentrations. Lancet 346:85, 1995

44. Clarke R, Daly L, Robinson K, et al: Hyperhomocysteinemia: an independent risk factor for vascular disease. N Engl J Med 324:1149, 1991

45. Selhub J, Jacques PF, Bostom AG, et al: Association between plasma homocysteine concentrations and extracranial carotid-artery stenosis. N Engl J Med 332:286, 1995

46. Den Heijer M, Koster T, Blom HJ, et al: Hyperhomocysteinemia as a risk factor for deep-vein thrombosis. N Engl J Med 334:759, 1996

47. Nygard O, Nordrehaug JE, Refsum H, et al: Plasma homocysteine levels and mortality in patients with coronary artery disease. N Engl J Med 337:230, 1997

48. Harker LA, Harlan JM, Ross R: Effect of sulfinpyrazone on homocysteine-induced endothelial injury and arteriosclerosis in baboons. Circ Res 53:731, 1983

49. Starkebaum G, Harlan JM: Endothelial cell injury due to copper-catalyzed hydrogen peroxide generation from homocysteine. J Clin Invest 77:1370, 1986

50. Lentz SR, Sadler JE: Inhibition of thrombomodulin surface expression and protein C activation by the thrombogenic agent homocysteine. J Clin Invest 88:1906, 1991

51. Nishinaga M, Ozawa T, Shimada K: Homocysteine, a thrombogenic agent, suppresses anticoagulant heparan sulfate expression in cultured porcine aortic endothelial cells. J Clin Invest 92:1281, 1993

52. Harpel PC, Chang VT, Borth W: Homocysteine and other sulfhydryl compounds enhance the binding of lipoprotein(a) to fibrin: a potential biochemical link between thrombosis, atherogenesis, and sulfhydryl compound metabolism. Proc Natl Acad Sci USA 89:10193, 1992

53. Bostom AG, Jacques PF, Nadeau MR, et al: Post-methionine load hyperhomocysteinemia in persons with normal fasting total plasma homocysteine: initial results from The NHLBI Family Heart Study. Arteriosclerosis 116:147, 1995

54. Den Heijer M, Blom HJ, Gerrits WBJ, et al: Is hyperhomocysteinemia a risk factor for recurrent venous thrombosis? Lancet 345:882, 1995

55. Fermo I, D'Angelo SV, Paroni R, et al: Prevalence of moderate hyperhomocysteinemia in patients with early-onset venous and arterial occlusive disease. Ann Intern Med 123: 747, 1995

56. Franken DG, Boers GHJ, Blom HJ, et al: Treatment of mild hyperhomocysteinemia in vascular disease patients. Arterioscler Thromb Vasc Biol 14:465, 1994

57. Bostom A, Cupples A, Jenner J, et al: Elevated plasma lipoprotein(a) and coronary heart disease in men aged 55 years and younger. JAMA 276:544, 1996

58. Wild SH, Fortmann SP, Marcovina SM: A prospective case-control study of lipoprotein(a) levels and Apo(a) size and risk of coronary heart disease in Stanford Five-City Project participants. Arterioscler Thromb Vasc Biol 17:239, 1997

59. Nagayama M, Shinohara Y, Nagayama T: Lipoprotein(a) and ischemic cerebrovascular disease in young adults. Stroke 25:74, 1994

60. Ridker PM, Stampfer MJ, Hennekens CH: Plasma concentration of lipoprotein(a) and the risk of future stroke. JAMA 273:1269, 1995

61. Marcovina SM, Albers JJ, Jacobs DR Jr, et al: Lipoprotein(a) concentrations and apolipoprotein(a) phenotypes in Caucasians and African-Americans. The CARDIA study. Arterioscler Thromb 13:1037, 1993

62. Hajjar KA, Gavish D, Breslow JL, et al: Lipoprotein (a) modulation of endothelial cell surface fibrinolysis and its potential role in atherosclerosis. Nature 339:303, 1989

63. Callow MJ, Verstuyft J, Tangirala R, et al: Atherogenesis in transgenic mice with human apolipoprotein B and lipoprotein(a). J Clin Invest 96:1639, 1995

64. Maher VM, Brown BG, Marcovina SM, et al: Effects of lowering elevated LDL cholesterol on the cardiovascular risk of lipoprotein(a). JAMA 274:1771, 1995

65. Gurakar A, Hoeg JM, Kostner G, et al: Levels of lipoprotein(a) decline with neomycin and niacin treatment. Atherosclerosis 57:293, 1985

66. Shewmon DA, Stock JL, Rosen CJ, et al: Tamoxifen and estrogen lower circulating lipoprotein(a) concentrations in healthy postmenopausal women. Arterioscler Thromb 14:1586, 1994

67. Martinez J: Congenital dysfibrinogenemia. Curr Opin Hematol 4:357, 1997

68. Aoki N, Moroi M, Sakata Y, et al: Abnormal plasminogen: a hereditary molecular abnormality found in a patient with recurrent thrombosis. J Clin Invest 61:1186, 1978

69. Estelles A, Gilabert J, Aznar J, et al: Changes in the plasma levels of type 1 and type 2 plasminogen activators in normal pregnancy and in patients with severe preeclampsia. Blood 74:1332, 1989

70. Prins MH, Hirsh J: A critical review of the evidence supporting a relationship between impaired fibrinolytic activity and venous thromboembolism. Arch Intern Med 151:1721, 1991

71. Wiman B: Plasminogen activator inhibitor-1 (PAI-1) in plasma: its role in thrombotic disease. Thromb Haemost 74:71, 1995

72. Meade TW: Fibrinogen in ischemic heart disease. Eur Heart J 16(suppl):31, 1995

73. Meade TW, Mellows S, Brozovic M, et al: Haemostatic function and ischaemic heart disease: principal results of the Northwick Park Heart Study. Lancet 2:533, 1986

74. Koster T, Blann AD, Briet E, et al: Role of clotting factor VIII in effect of von Willebrand factor on occurrence of deep-vein thrombosis. Lancet 345:152, 1995

75. O'Donnell J, Tuddenham EGD, Manning R, et al: High prevalence of elevated factor VIII levels in patients referred for thrombophilia screening: role of increased synthesis and relationship to the acute phase reaction. Thromb Haemost 77:825, 1997

76. Kyrle PA, Minar E, Hirschl M, et al: High plasma levels of factor VIII and the risk of recurrent venous thromboembolism. N Engl J Med 343:457, 2000

77. Rauch J, Janoff AS: Role of antibodies in understanding the interactions between anti-phospholipid antibodies and phospholipids. Phospholipid-Binding Antibodies. N Harris, T Exner, GRV Hughes, et al, Eds. CRC Press, Boca Raton, Florida, 1991, p 108

78. Rao LVM, Hoang AD, Rapaport SI: Mechanisms and effects of the binding of lupus anticoagulant IgG and prothrombin to surface phospholipid. Blood 88:4173, 1996

79. Smirnov MD, Triplett DT, Comp PC, et al: On the role of phosphatidylethanolamine in the inhibition of activated protein C activity by antiphospholipid antibodies. J Clin Invest 95:309, 1995

80. Shibata S, Harpel PC, Gharavi A, et al: Autoantibodies to heparin from patients with antiphospholipid antibody syndrome inhibit formation of antithrombin III–thrombin complexes. Blood 83:2532, 1994

81. Finazzi G, Brancaccio V, Ciavarella N, et al: Natural history and risk factors for thrombosis in 360 patients with antiphospholipid antibodies: a four-year prospective study from the Italian registry. Am J Med 100:530, 1996

82. Vila P, Hernandez MC, Lopez-Fernadez MF, et al: Prevalence, follow-up and clinical significance of the anticardiolipin antibodies in normal subjects. Thromb Haemost 72:209, 1994

83. Ginsburg KS, Liang MH, Newcomer L, et al: Anticardiolipin antibodies and the risk for ischemic stroke and venous thrombosis. Ann Intern Med 117:997, 1992

84. Silver RM, Porter TF, van Leeuween I, et al: Anticardiolipin antibodies: clinical consequences of "low titers." Obstet Gynecol 87:494, 1996

85. Selva-O'Callaghan A, Ordi-Ros J, Monegal-Ferran F, et al: IgA anticardiolipin antibodies: relation with other antiphospholipid antibodies and clinical significance. Thromb Haemost 79:282, 1998

86. Khamashta MA, Cuardrado MJ, Mujic F, et al: The management of thrombosis in the antiphospholipid-antibody syndrome. N Engl J Med 332:993, 1995

87. Rosove MH, Brewer MC: Antiphospholipid thrombosis: clinical course after the first thrombotic event in 70 patients. Ann Intern Med 117:303, 1992

88. Palareti G, Leali N, Coccheri S, et al: Bleeding complications of oral anticoagulant treatment: an inception-cohort, prospective collaborative study (ISCOAT). Lancet 348:423, 1996

89. Greaves M: Antiphospholipid antibodies and thrombosis. Lancet 353:1348, 1999

90. Kearon C, Gent M, Hirsh J, et al: A comparison of three months of anticoagulation with extended anticoagulation for a first episode of idiopathic venous thromboembolism. N Engl J Med 340:901, 1999

91. Moll S, Ortel TL: Monitoring warfarin therapy in patients with lupus anticoagulants. Ann Intern Med 127:177, 1997

92. Rand JH, Wu X-X, Andree HAM, et al: Pregnancy loss in the antiphospholipid-antibody syndrome—a possible thrombogenic mechanism. N Engl J Med 337:154, 1997

93. Kutteh WH, Rote NS, Silver R: Antiphospholipid antibodies and reproduction: the antiphospholipid antibody syndrome. Am J Reprod Immunol 41:133, 1999

94. Infante-Rivard C, David M, Gauthier R, et al: Lupus anticoagulants, anticardiolipin antibodies, and fetal loss: a case-controlled study. N Engl J Med 325:1063, 1991

95. Laskin CA, Bombardier C, Hannah ME, et al: Prednisone and aspirin in women with autoantibodies and unexplained recurrent fetal loss. N Engl J Med 337:148, 1997

96. Kutteh WH: Antiphospholipid antibody–associated recurrent pregnancy loss: treatment with heparin and low-dose aspirin is superior to low-dose aspirin alone. Am J Obstet Gynecol 174:1584, 1996

97. Rai R, Cohen H, Dave M, et al: Randomized, controlled trial of aspirin and aspirin plus heparin in pregnant women with recurrent miscarriage asssociated with phospholipid antibodies. BMJ 314:253, 1997

98. Kutteh WH, Ermel LD: A clinical trial for the treatment of antiphospholipid antibody–associated recurrent pregnancy loss with lower dose heparin and aspirin. Am J Reprod Immunol 35:402, 1996

99. Eldor A: Thrombophilia, thrombosis and pregnancy. Thromb Haemost 86:104, 2001

100. Warkentin TE: Heparin-induced thrombocytopenia: a ten-year retrospective. Ann Rev Med 50:129, 1999

101. Bauer TL, Arepally G, Konkle BA, et al: Prevalence of heparin-associated antibodies without thrombosis in patients undergoing cardiopulmonary bypass surgery. Circulation 95:1242, 1997

102. Warkentin TE: Heparin-induced thrombocytopenia: a clinicopathologic syndrome. Thromb Haemost 82:439, 1999

103. Amiral J, Bridey F, Dreyfus M, et al: Platelet factor 4 complexed to heparin is the target for antibodies generated in heparin-induced thrombocytopenia. Thromb Haemost 68:95, 1992

104. Warkentin TE, Levine MN, Hirsh J, et al: Heparin-induced thrombocytopenia in patients treated with low-molecular-weight heparin or unfractionated heparin. N Engl J Med 332:1330, 1995

105. Visentin GP, Ford SE, Scott JP, et al: Antibodies from patients with heparin-induced thrombocytopenia/thrombosis are specific for platelet factor 4 complexed with heparin or bound to endothelial cells. J Clin Invest 93:81, 1994

106. Warkentin TE, Kelton JG: Temporal aspects of heparin-induced thrombocytopenia. N Engl J Med 344:1286, 2001

107. Warkentin TE, Kelton JG. Delayed-onset heparin-induced thrombocytopenia and thrombosis. Ann Intern Med 135:502, 2001

108. Sallah S, Thomas DP, Roberts HR: Warfarin and heparin-induced skin necrosis and the purple toe syndrome: infrequent complications of anticoagulant treatment. Thromb Haemost 78:785, 1997

109. Greinacher A, Amiral J, Dummel V, et al: Laboratory diagnosis of heparin-associated thrombocytopenia and comparison of platelet aggregation test, and platelet factor 4/heparin enzyme linked immunosorbent assay. Transfusion 34:381, 1994

110. Magnani HN: Orgaran (danaparoid sodium) use in the syndrome of heparin-induced thrombocytopenia. Platelets 8:74, 1997

111. de Valk HW, Banga JD, Wester JWJ, et al: Comparing subcutaneous danaparoid with intravenous unfractionated heparin for the treatment of venous thromboembolism. Ann Intern Med 123:1, 1995

112. Greinacher A, Volpol H, Potzsch B: Recombinant hirudin in the treatment of patients with heparin-induced thrombocytopenia (HIT). Blood 88(suppl):281a, 1996

113. Schiele F, Vuillemenot A, Kramarz P, et al: Use of recombinant hirudin as antithrombotic treatment in patients with heparin-induced thrombocytopenia. Am J Hematol 50:20, 1995

114. Lewis BE, Wallis DE, Berkowitz SD, et al: Argatroban anticoagulant therapy in patients with heparin-induced thrombocytopenia. Circulation 103:1838, 2001

115. Matsuo T, Yamada T, Yamanashi T, et al. Anticoagulant therapy with MD805 of a hemodialysis patient with heparin-induced thrombocytopenia. Thromb Res 58:663, 1990

116. Gillis S, Merin G, Zahger D, et al: Danaparoid for cardiopulmonary bypass in patients with previous heparin-induced thrombocytopenia. Br J Haematol 98:657, 1997

117. Potzsch B, Klovekorn WP, Madlener K: Use of heparin during cardiopulmonary bypass in patients with a history of heparin-induced thrombocytopenia. N Engl J Med 343:515, 2000

118. Callander N, Rapaport SI: Trousseau's syndrome. West J Med 158:364, 1993

119. Prandoni P, Lensing AWA, Buller HR, et al: Deep-vein thrombosis and the incidence of subsequent symptomatic cancer. N Engl J Med 327:1128, 1992

120. Callander NS, Varki N, Rao LVM: Immunohistochemical identification of tissue factor in solid tumors. Cancer 70:1194, 1992

121. Contrino J, Hair G, Kreutzer DL, Rickles FR: In situ detection of tissue factor in vascular endothelial cells: correlation with malignant phenotype of human breast disease. Nat Med 2:209, 1996

122. Falanga A, Gordon SG: Isolation and characterization of cancer procoagulant: a cysteine proteinase from malignant tissue. Biochemistry 24:5558, 1985

123. Falanga A, Consonni R, Marchetti M, et al: Cancer procoagulant and tissue factor are differentially modulated by all-trans-retinoic acid in acute promyelocytic leukemic cells. Blood 92:143, 1998

124. Prins MH, Hettiarachchi RJK, Lensing AWA, et al: Newly diagnosed malignancy in patients with venous thromboembolism: search or wait and see? Thromb Haemost 78:121, 1997

125. Sorensen HT, Mellemkjaer L, Steffensen FH, et al: The risk of a diagnosis of cancer after primary deep venous thrombosis or pulmonary embolism. N Engl J Med 338:1169, 1998

126. Silverstein RL, Nachman RL: Cancer and clotting: Trousseau's warning. N Engl J Med 327:1163, 1992

127. Buller H, Ten Cate JW: Primary venous thromboembolism and cancer screening. N Engl J Med 338:1221, 1998

128. Cornuz J, Pearson SD, Creager MA, et al: Importance of findings on the initial evaluation for cancer in patients with symptomatic idiopathic deep venous thrombosis. Ann Intern Med 125:785, 1996

129. Vandenbroucke JP, Koster T, Briet E, et al: Increased risk of venous thrombosis in oral-contraceptive users who are carriers of factor V Leiden mutation. Lancet 344:1453, 1994

130. Helmerhorst FM, Bloemenkamp KWM, Rosendaal FR, et al: Oral contraceptives and thrombotic disease: risk of venous thromboembolism. Thromb Haemost 78:327, 1997

131. Jick H, Derby LE, Myers MW, et al: Risk of hospital admission for idiopathic venous thromboembolism among users of postmenopausal oestrogens. Lancet 348:981, 1996

132. Daly E, Vessey MP, Hawkins MM, et al: Risk of venous thromboembolism in users of hormone replacement therapy. Lancet 348:977, 1996

133. Hoibraaten E, Qvigstad E, Arnesen H, et al: Increased risk of recurrent venous thromboembolism during hormone replacement therapy—results of the randomized, double-blind, placebo-controlled estrogen in venous thromboembolism trial (EVTET). Thromb Haemost 84:961, 2000

134. Vandenbroucke JP, Rosing J, Bloemenkamp KW, et al: Oral contraceptives and the risk of venous thrombosis. N Engl J Med 344:1527, 2001

135. Schulman S, Rhedin AS, Lindmarker P, et al: A comparison of six weeks with six months of oral anticoagulant therapy after a first episode of venous thromboembolism. N Engl J Med 332:1661, 1995

136. Schulman S, Granqvist S, Holmstrom M, et al: The duration of oral anticoagulant therapy after a second episode of venous thromboembolism. N Engl J Med 336:393, 1997

137. Kearon C, Gent M, Hirsh J, et al: A comparison of three months of anticoagulation with extended anticoagulation for a first episode of idiopathic venous thromboembolism. N Engl J Med 340:901, 1999

138. Three months versus one year of oral anticoagulant therapy for idiopathic deep venous thrombosis. Warfarin Optimal Duration Italian Trial Investigators. N Engl J Med 345:165, 2001

139. Bauer KA: Management of patients with hereditary defects predisposing to thrombosis including pregnant women. Thromb Haemost 74:94, 1995

140. De Stefano V, Finazzi G, Mannucci PM: Inherited thrombophilia: pathogenesis, clinical syndromes, and management. Blood 87:3531, 1996

141. Rosendaal FR, Heijboer H, Briet E, et al: Mortality in hereditary antithrombin-III deficiency: 1830 to 1989. Lancet 337:260, 1991

142. Allaart CF, Rosendaal FR, Noteboom WM, et al: Survival in families with hereditary protein C deficiency, 1820 to 1993. BMJ 311:910, 1995

143. Aster RH: Heparin-induced thrombocytopenia and thrombosis. N Engl J Med 332:1374, 1995

144. Koster T, Rosendaal FR, de Ronde H, et al: Venous thrombosis due to poor anticoagulant response to activated protein C: Leiden Thrombophilia Study. Lancet 342:1503, 1993

145. Triplett DA: Protean clinical presentation of antiphospholipid-protein antibodies (APA). Thromb Haemost 74:329, 1995

Acknowledgment

Figures 1 through 3   Dr. Rajeev Doshi.

95 Transfusion Therapy

W. Hallowell Churchill, M.D.

Transfusion medicine has developed rapidly owing to several key discoveries and technical advances. These include the discovery of blood group antigens and the understanding of the host immune response to these antigens, the development of methods of anticoagulation and storage of blood, and the creation of plastic bags that allow sterile fractionation of whole blood into components. More recently, the potential of blood to act as an agent of disease transmission has heavily shaped both the donation process and transfusion practice.[1]

Decisions about whether to transfuse must involve weighing the benefits against the risks. This chapter provides a basis for these decisions, including indications for blood-component use, complications of transfusion therapy, and methods of reducing risks during the collection, processing, and preparation of blood components.

Blood Donation

The donation process for either whole blood or special products, such as single-donor platelets (SDPs) obtained by apheresis, is designed to protect both the donor and the recipient. For example, persons weighing less than 110 lb (49.9 kg) have too small a blood volume to donate blood safely. Donors taking drugs that would impair recovery to a vasovagal donor reaction are excluded for reasons of donor safety. Safety of recipients is promoted by excluding donors who are at risk for viral or bacterial infections or who are taking medications that could cause recipient reactions or impair the function of donated blood products.

AUTOLOGOUS AND DIRECTED DONATION

Autologous donations and directed donations are two strategies adopted by patients seeking to minimize their real or perceived risk of infection from blood products.

Autologous Donation

In autologous donation, patients first deposit their own blood and then receive that blood when they need it for transfusion therapy. This eliminates the infectious and sensitization risks associated with allogeneic blood. Absolute contraindications to autologous donation are tight aortic stenosis, unstable angina, and active bacterial infection.[2] Low hemoglobin levels and poor venous access frequently limit the number of units that can be collected. With the increasing safety of allogeneic blood, the rationale for autologous donation may ultimately depend more on the importance of the possible modulation of recipient immune function associated with allogeneic transfusion and less on avoidance of blood-borne infections.

Directed Donation

Directed donation is donation for a specific recipient. It usually involves donations made by friends or family members of the intended recipient. It is based on the assumption that transfusions involving donors selected by the recipient carry lower risk of infections than transfusions involving donors from the general population. However, a study comparing markers for hepatitis and HIV infection found that the prevalence of positive test results for exposure to these diseases was the same in directed donors and volunteer first-time donors.[3] This finding undermines the rationale for most directed donations, except in cases in which a donor serves as the only source of blood products, thereby reducing the recipient's risk from exposure to multiple donors. This last form of directed donation is most appropriate for neonatal transfusions, in which one of the biologic parents often serves as the sole donor.[4]

SCREENING PROCEDURES

The combination of improved donor selection and postdonation testing has greatly decreased the risk of infection from allogeneic blood [*see Table 1*]. Predonation donor screening to identify clinical and lifestyle characteristics associated with higher incidences of infection has produced the biggest decrease in the risk of transfusion-transmitted disease. Postdonation testing is also essential in identifying donors likely to transmit blood-borne infections who are missed in the initial screening process.

POSTDONATION TESTING

Screening for Hepatitis Viruses

Hepatitis C Specific screening for hepatitis C began in 1990 with the availability of a single antigen-based enzyme-linked immunosorbent assay (ELISA). This assay, together with second- and third-generation assays and their associated confirmatory assays, has reduced the per unit risk of hepatitis C virus (HCV) transmission to about 0.001%.[5-7] Before these tests were available, the risk per unit was about 4%. Improved specific testing for hepatitis C has eliminated the need for nonspecific surrogate tests, such as tests for elevations of alanine aminotransferase (ALT) levels and the detection of antibody to hepatitis B virus (HBV) core antigen. Testing for antibody to HBV core antigen is still being used, to detect recently infected donors who lack measurable circulating HBV antigen.

The epidemiology of HCV is still poorly understood. Approximately 20% to 25% of persons found to be HCV positive have no known risk factors.[8] Sexual transmission occurs with enough frequency to warrant evaluation of partners and appropriate use of methods of barrier protection.[9] Heterosexual transmission of HCV may be asymptomatic.[10] Thus, blood-borne HCV infection

Table 1 **Risk of Infection from Blood Products***

Virus	Risk
Human immunodeficiency virus type 1 (HIV-1)[†]	1 in 660,000
Human immunodeficiency virus type 2 (HIV-2)	Unknown
Human T cell lymphotropic virus type I/type II (HTLV-I/II)[‡]	1 in 641,000
Hepatitis B	1 in 63,000
Hepatitis C	< 1 in 103,000

*Risk is estimated per transfused product.
[†]p24 antigen testing and HIV antibody testing.
[‡]Approximately 50% are HTLV-II.

could result from the use of blood from a donor who has been infected via sexual contact but who has not yet developed detectable antibodies. This justifies the exclusion of donors who are known to be sexual partners of HCV-infected persons. Donors found to be ELISA positive for HCV are permanently deferred. The importance of supplemental tests, such as the second-generation and third-generation recombinant immunoblot assays (RIBA-2, RIBA-3), is well established. Donors with positive supplemental test results are likely to have a chronic HCV infection and require further clinical evaluation.[11] Donors with negative supplemental test results probably had false positive screening results and may be eligible for reentry into the allogeneic donor pool after 6 months.[12] The infection status of donors with indeterminate supplemental results is best resolved by testing for HCV RNA; donors with only a single band on the most sensitive supplemental test (RIBA-3) have a less than 4% chance of having circulating HCV RNA.[13]

Within the past year, gene amplification methodologies for detecting HCV RNA have become available on an investigational basis.[14] These methodologies directly detect the presence of virus before antibody development. It is hoped that these tests will further reduce HCV in the blood supply.

Hepatitis B Transmission of other forms of hepatitis by blood products is extremely rare. Modern testing methods and the elimination of the practice of compensating whole blood donors have reduced HBV infections to about one in 63,000 units transfused.[7]

Hepatitis A The viremic phase of hepatitis A, before symptoms develop, lasts about 17 days in humans. This may explain why hepatitis A transmission from single-donor products is extremely rare compared with transmission through pooled products, such as factor concentrates.[15]

Hepatitis D Hepatitis D is a defective virus that requires HBV to produce fulminating hepatitis; it is a concern only for patients already infected with HBV.

Hepatitis G The recently discovered flavivirus hepatitis G virus is present in about 4.5% of normal donors; it is transmitted from mother to infant, sexually, and by blood.[16] Hepatitis G RNA is removed after the recipient develops antibodies; hepatitis G RNA has not been linked to any form of hepatitis in children or adults. Hepatitis G virus is an example of a blood-borne virus without defined pathogenicity; the costs associated with both testing and donor exclusions are likely to preclude any attempt to remove it from the blood supply.

Screening for Retroviruses

All blood products are screened for HIV-1, HIV-2, human T cell lymphotropic virus type I (HTLV-I), and HTLV type II (HTLV-II). Data obtained nationally from American Red Cross donors indicate that excluding high-risk donors and postdonation testing for HIV-1 and HIV-2 antibodies have reduced the infection risk from two per 100 transfusions to about two per million transfusions.[17]

To have predictive value, the ELISA screening test for HIV must be confirmed by Western blot assay. Studies based on the polymerase chain reaction (PCR), culture data, and donor lookback studies all indicate that donors with negative or indeterminate Western blot results are seldom, if ever, HIV positive.[18] A fol-

low-up study of donors who were ELISA positive and whose Western blot results were indeterminate demonstrated that positive ELISA results persisted in about 45% of cases. Of these, 84% still had indeterminate Western blot results, but none were shown to be HIV positive by PCR.[19] There have been occasional false positive results of Western blot assays in low-risk donors.[20] The possibility of a false positive result should be remembered when one is counseling low-risk donors who have had unexplained positive results on Western blot testing; these false positive results must always be confirmed by careful clinical follow-up.

The prevalence of HTLV-I and HTLV-II in donors in the United States is about 0.03%; about two thirds of these patients have HTLV-II. Several longitudinal studies have defined the clinical consequences of HTLV-I/II infection.[21-23] These studies are useful in advising donors who have had positive or indeterminate test results. In a prospective, longitudinal study comparing seropositive blood donors with seronegative blood donors, both viruses were associated with an increase in the incidence of some infectious diseases. No cases of adult T cell leukemia or lymphoma were identified; myelopathies, though rare, were associated with both HTLV types.[21] The risk of HTLV-I/II transmission by blood products is one per 641,000 persons.[7] As with HIV, laboratory studies and epidemiologic investigations of HTLV-I/II indicate that patients with positive screening-test results and negative or indeterminate supplemental-test results are unlikely to have clinical sequelae, and that the positive results are most likely false positives.[24]

False Positive Test Results during Donor Screening

The causes of false positive test results for HCV and retroviruses are poorly understood. Flu vaccines administered in 1992 were associated with an increase in false positive results for these viruses.[25] However, the proteins responsible for cross-reactivity have not yet been identified. Tests for low-prevalence infections, even tests with excellent specificity and sensitivity, will always be associated with a substantial proportion of false positive results. Consequently, test characteristics, as well as culture and PCR results, can provide reassurance for donors who are not at risk but who have had positive screening-test results and negative or indeterminate confirmatory-test results. As PCR technology improves, it will probably become the most reliable means of establishing whether a positive result represents infection or is a false positive result.

Pretransfusion Testing

ANTIGEN PHENOTYPING

Blood recipients are routinely tested to establish their ABO phenotype and Rh type. Establishing ABO type is essential because isoagglutinins (antibodies) against A or B antigens not present on a person's red cells are acquired during the first 2 years of life. These IgM antibodies will cause an immediate hemolytic reaction if ABO-incompatible red cells are transfused.

The terminal carbohydrate on these antigens determines specificity in the ABO system, with type A being associated with N-acetylgalactosamine and type B being associated with a terminal galactose. Persons with type O lack both of these terminal sugars. These residues are added by a glycosyltransferase, which may be either nonfunctional or absent in type O persons. Yamamoto and colleagues[26] used molecular techniques to prove that glycosyltransferase in type O persons is very similar to the transferase in type A persons. The type O glycosyltransferase is

Table 2 ABO Typing

Blood Type	Erythrocytes plus Anti-A Serum	Erythrocytes plus Anti-B Serum	Antibodies in Patient's Serum
A	+	0	Anti-B antibodies
B	0	+	Anti-A antibodies
AB	+	+	No antibodies
O	0	0	Anti-A and anti-B antibodies

+—agglutination   0—no agglutination

nonfunctional because of a single base deletion that produces a frameshift and a downstream stop codon.

All methods of ABO typing depend on demonstrating that the antigens found on the red cells are consistent with the expected isoagglutinins [see Table 2]. Molecular methods to determine ABO genotype are available.[27] Typing for the D antigen specificity in the Rh system is done because of the potency of this antigen as an immunogen. Antibodies to the D antigen are the most important cause of isoimmune hemolytic disease of newborns. Rh antigens are membrane glycolipids or glycoproteins. Antibodies against antigens of this class, which includes the Rh, Duffy, Kell, Kidd, and Lutheran systems, will usually cause shortened red cell survival. In contrast to antigens with carbohydrate-mediated specificity, glycolipid and glycoprotein antigens do not stimulate antibody formation unless the transfusion recipient was previously exposed to allogeneic red cells either from transfusion or from fetal red cells during pregnancy or delivery.

D antigen typing is also done using agglutination techniques. In some cases, less antigenic forms of the D antigen, called D^u, require an antiglobulin reagent to enhance detection. Structural studies of the complementary DNA associated with the major Rh antigens (D, Cc, and Ee) have provided probes for direct genotyping.[28] Molecular methods can now be used for prenatal determination of Rh type.[29] These methods have revealed that most Rh-negative persons lack the D gene and that some persons with the D^u phenotype have mosaic D genes because of exchange with some of the exons of the CcEe gene.[30]

Because the genotypes of many of the clinically relevant red cell antigens are now known, it should now be possible to predict red cell phenotype by DNA analysis. Reid and colleagues[31] were able to correctly predict the red cell phenotype in 60 multitransfused patients by DNA analysis of each patient's white blood cells. This approach, although not yet generally available, will be useful for recently transfused patients, for whom circulating allogeneic red cells complicate antigen phenotyping.

SCREENING FOR ANTIBODIES

In addition to identifying patient ABO and D red cell phenotypes, serum must be screened for red cell–specific antibodies, which can cause serious reactions with transfused red cells. Screening is done by testing serum against indicator type O red cells displaying all the clinically important red cell antigens. Positive reactions are detected by adding an antiglobulin reagent (Coombs reagent) to the incubated mixture of type O red cells after it has been washed free of serum. Any observed agglutination is from the reaction of the antiglobulin reagent with antibody adsorbed on the surface of the indicator red cells [see Chapter 89]. Agglutination of the indicator red cells indi-

cates the presence of other antibodies, which require identification. The absence of agglutination excludes all antibodies except those against antigens so rare that they are not displayed on the indicator red cells.

Use of type-specific blood removes the risk of ABO incompatibility. There is, however, a residual risk of an immunologic reaction from the antibodies to other red cell antigens; such antibodies are present in about 3% to 5% of a random population and 10% to 15% of persons recently transfused or of women with a history of pregnancy. Screening for antibodies reduces the chance of a reaction by more than 100-fold, to about 0.06%. Performing a full crossmatch, in which the recipient's serum is tested against the red cells actually being transfused, is of negligible additional benefit, because it excludes only technical errors and the rare antibody not detected by the screening. Therefore, a full crossmatch is performed only for persons already known to have made antibodies, because such persons are more likely to form additional antibodies if they are further stimulated by red cell transfusion.

Because of the stimulating effect of allogeneic red cells, patients who wish to receive allogeneic therapy and who have undergone a transfusion or have become pregnant within the past 3 months must have a new blood specimen tested for antibodies every 3 days. There is no consensus concerning how long the interval should be between patient specimen collection and use of the specimen in pretransfusion testing for patients not recently exposed to red cells. Commonly, specimens are accepted up to 2 weeks before the date for use. However, a recent study showed that no new antibodies appeared in paired specimens collected up to 1 year apart, suggesting that a longer acceptance interval may be possible.[32]

Blood Components

Most blood donations undergo a fractionation process that allows each component to be used for specific indications. Whole blood can be fractionated into red cells (which contain most of the leukocytes), platelet concentrates (which contain some leukocytes), and plasma [see Table 3]. Plasma can be further subdivided into coagulation components and albumin. Each whole blood unit can potentially support many recipients and clinical needs, maximizing use of each donation.

After 24 hours' storage, whole blood contains no active platelets, and after 2 days, it is deficient in factors V and VIII. Therefore, except for some autologous blood programs that use whole blood rather than packed red cells, use of whole blood has now been almost completely supplanted by therapy employing specific blood components.

RED BLOOD CELLS

The anticoagulant used determines the shelf life of red cells [see Table 3]. Citrate-phosphate-dextrose (CPD) with the addition of adenine (CPDA-1) increases storage time from 28 days to 35 days. Most red cells are now stored in CPD to which extra nutrients have been added; the final product, Adsol, increases storage time to 42 days. Adsol contains about 100 ml of additional saline, making the hematocrit of red cells stored in Adsol 55% rather than 70%. If necessary, the saline can be removed before the product is issued.

To prevent transfusion reactions or to delay the onset of alloimmunization, red cells are further processed by leukocyte reduction (see below) or washing to remove plasma proteins. Current filter technology can reduce white cell counts to less than 5 ×

Table 3 Characteristics of Blood Products and Indications for Use

Product (One Unit)	Volume, Hematocrit (HCT), or Cell Count	White Cell Count	Shelf Life	Donors per Unit	Storage Outside Blood Bank	Indication
Whole blood (WB)	450 ± 45 ml	$3-5 \times 10^9$	Adsol = 42 days CPDA-1 = 35 days CPD = 28 days	1	2°–6° C	Massive transfusion if available; exchange transfusions in newborns younger than 3 days
Red cells	If Adsol used: vol = 350 ml, HCT = 55 If CPD used: vol = 250 ml, HCT = 70	$1-2 \times 10^9$	Same as WB	1	Same as WB	To increase oxygen-carrying capacity; to maintain volume and oxygen-carrying capacity when bleeding
Platelet concentrates (PCs)	40 ml, 5×10^{10}	$2-6 \times 10^7$	5 days	1/U; given as pool of 5–6 U	Room temperature	To increase platelets in a bleeding patient whose platelet count is < 100,000; to increase platelets for procedure when platelet count is < 50,000; to increase platelets prophylactically in a nonbleeding patient whose platelet count is < 10,000; to support patient refractory to SDPs when bleeding and HLA or crossmatched platelets are not available
Single-donor platelets	200–250 ml, 3×10^{11}	Depends on method of collection	5 days	1	Room temperature	Same as PCs except that this product is preferred because of fewer donor exposures
Fresh frozen plasma (FFP)	200–250 ml	$< 1 \times 10^5$	1 yr; 24 hr when thawed	1	2°–6° C	Replacement of multiple coagulation factor/deficiency from bleeding or disseminated intravascular coagulation; reversal of warfarin therapy; factor XI deficiency unless factor XI concentrates are available; treatment of thrombotic thrombocytopenic purpura
Cryoprecipitate	10–20 ml; pool of 10 U ~ 200 ml	$< 1 \times 10^5$	1 yr; 24 hr when thawed	1/U; given as pool of 10 U	2°–6° C wet ice	Replacement of fibrinogen when acutely depleted or when patient cannot tolerate volume load of equivalent amount of FFP (1 pool of cryoprecipitate = 4 FFP); fibrin glue (usually only 1 unit); replacement of von Willebrand factor if concentrate is not available; replacement of factor XIII; replacement for qualitatively abnormal fibrinogen

Adsol—CPD with extra nutrients   CPDA-1—citrate phosphate dextrose (CPD) with adenine

10^6 cells per unit, a concentration sufficient to reduce febrile transfusion reactions and delay alloimmunization and platelet refractoriness. Washed red cells have less than 0.5 ml of residual plasma per unit. This degree of plasma depletion is usually effective in treating allergic transfusion reactions. Leukocyte filtration and the washing of red cells to remove plasma usually shorten the product shelf life to 24 hours. This shortening of shelf life occurs because these procedures require breaking the seal on the plastic bag that contains the red cells, thereby increasing the risk of bacterial contamination. Leukocyte reduction can be accomplished during collection, immediately after collection in the blood bank, or at the bedside during product infusion. Prestorage or laboratory filtration is preferred to bedside filtration.[33]

Freezing is an alternative method for storing red cells. Red cells can be kept in a cryoprotectant (usually glycerol) for 10 years. Freezing is therefore ideal for storing rare units or autologous units from persons with rare blood types, for whom it is difficult to find compatible allogeneic red cells. When a unit is at the end of its liquid storage shelf life, the cells can be rejuvenated with fresh media and nutrients; they can then be frozen and stored. To be used, frozen red cells must be thawed and the glycerol removed, so preparation time for this product is longer than for products stored in the liquid state. Thawed, deglycerolized red cells generally must be transfused within 24 hours.

PLATELETS

Platelets can be provided either as platelet concentrates from a number of blood donors or from a single donor. SDPs are collected by a continuous apheresis process that removes platelets and returns all other blood components. Platelet concentrates are usually transfused as a pool of four to six concentrates; in this way, the number of platelets transfused is about the same in one platelet concentrate from multiple donors as in one SDP concentrate. The advantage of SDP therapy is the reduced risk of blood-borne infection and antigen exposure, because the product is from one donor rather than four to six; disadvantages are a longer collection time, greater cost, and often limited supply. The potential advantages of each of these products were summarized in a recent review.[34] ABO Rh–compatible platelets should be used when possible, because studies have shown significantly better therapeutic results from compatible transfusions.[35]

PLASMA

Fresh plasma, frozen within 8 hours of collection (FFP), contains all the procoagulants at normal plasma concentrations. After thawing, it can be kept for 24 hours at 2° to 6° C with 3 to 4 mg/ml of fibrinogen and 1 IU/ml of all the other coagulation components.

Solvent/detergent-treated plasma (S/D plasma) is a recent alternative to FFP. It is prepared from a pool of 2,500 donors that is treated with the solvent tri-*n*-butyl phosphate and the detergent Triton-X. This procedure reliably inactivates lipid-coated viruses. After the solvent and detergent are removed, the plasma is screened for hepatitis A virus and parvovirus B19 and then undergoes filtration to remove viruses, bacteria, and residual white cells. It is then packaged in 200 ml aliquots for transfusion. The main advantage of S/D plasma is that it minimizes the risks from lipid-coated pathogens for patients who would require a large amount of FFP.[36] Small observational studies of patients with liver disease, patients who had undergone liver transplantation, or both have shown S/D plasma to be as effective as FFP.[37] It may also be effective in treating thrombotic thrombocytopenic purpura (TTP), but more studies are needed to confirm this. The main disadvantage of S/D plasma is that it is a pooled product and therefore its use carries a greater risk of introducing new, unrecognized pathogens into the blood supply. Although most coagulation components are unaffected by this process, some, such as antiplasmin, antitrypsin, protein S, and high-molecular-weight von Willebrand factor are inactivated.[38] S/D plasma is also significantly more costly than FFP. The indications for use of S/D plasma are still being defined. The available information clearly shows that this product has other important modifications besides inactivation of lipid-coated viruses. It may be that its use will be restricted to patients requiring large volumes of plasma, but more clinical studies are required to settle this and other issues.

Cryoprecipitate consists of the cryoproteins recovered from FFP when it is rapidly frozen and then allowed to thaw at 2° to 6° C. These cryoproteins include fibrinogen, factor VIII, von Willebrand factor, factor XIII, and fibronectin. About 40% of the components in FFP are recovered. The cryoproteins are suspended in a small amount of plasma that contains ABO isoagglutinin at the concentration found in normal plasma. A pool of 10 units of cryoprecipitate (each derived from one unit of FFP) contains an amount of fibrinogen equivalent to four units of FFP but in one fourth to one fifth the volume. Consequently, a cryoprecipitate pool permits more rapid replacement of fibrinogen than FFP but has the disadvantage of more donor exposures. After the cryoprecipitate is removed from FFP, the residual product is known as cryopoor plasma. Once frozen, cryopoor plasma has the same shelf life as FFP.

Transfusion of Red Cells

INDICATIONS FOR ALLOGENEIC TRANSFUSION

Acute Blood Loss

The decision to use red cells depends on the etiology and duration of the anemia, its rate of change, and assessment of the patient's ability to compensate for the diminished capacity to carry oxygen that results from the decrease in red cell mass. Management of acute anemia caused by bleeding or operative blood loss will differ from management of chronic anemia to which the patient has adapted. However, the question underlying any red cell transfusion is whether there is sufficient oxygen delivery to tissues for current needs.

Compensatory mechanisms during acute blood loss include adrenergic response leading to constriction of venous beds with improved venous return; increased stroke volume, tachycardia, or both; and increased peripheral resistance with eventual redistribution of blood flow to essential organs. Also contributing to the maintenance of intravascular volume is the shifting of fluid to the intravascular space; this shifting occurs relatively rapidly from extravascular space and more slowly from intracellular to extravascular space.[39]

A decrease in blood volume has distinct effects on oxygen delivery, depending on the volume of blood lost and the functioning of the compensatory cardiovascular responses. Restoration of intravascular volume, usually with crystalloid, ensures adequate perfusion of peripheral tissue and is the first treatment goal for a patient with acute blood loss. Whether red cell transfusion is required depends on the extent of blood loss and the presence of comorbid conditions that may limit host response to the blood loss. The American College of Surgeons has correlated blood loss with clinical findings. Loss of up to 15% of total blood volume usually has little effect; this amount is the maximum permitted in normal blood donation. A class II hemorrhage (15% to 30% loss) results in tachycardia, decreased pulse pressure, and, possibly, restlessness. A class III hemorrhage (30% to 40% loss) leads to obvious signs of hypovolemia; mental status often remains normal. Red cell transfusion is usually indicated when blood loss exceeds 30% in a patient without other significant comorbid conditions. However, the presence of serious cardiac, peripheral vascular, or pulmonary disease can lower this threshold. For example, anemic patients with significant coronary artery disease are more likely to have serious postoperative myocardial complications.

The 1988 National Institutes of Health Consensus Development Conference on Perioperative Red Cell Transfusion concluded that the decision to transfuse is a clinical one and that otherwise healthy patients with hemoglobin levels of 10 g/dl seldom need transfusion, whereas those with a hemoglobin count of less than 7 g/dl frequently require transfusions.[40] Transfusion decisions for patients in intermediate ranges depend on associated conditions, particularly cardiopulmonary functioning and the presence of significant vascular disease. The American College of Physicians emphasized the importance of clinical symptoms once intravascular volume has been restored and recommended no transfusion in the absence of symptoms, even for patients with clinical evidence of vascular disease.[41] This guideline must be applied with caution to anesthetized patients who have significant vascular disease. Such patients may have cardiac or cerebral ischemia without changes in heart rate or blood pressure.[39]

The threshold for red cell transfusion was recently evaluated in two randomized, controlled trials. In one study, patients undergoing coronary artery bypass who received transfusions of less than 8 g/dl of hemoglobin had the same outcomes as control patients who received transfusions of less than 9 g/dl of hemoglobin.[42] In the other trial, the outcomes of critical care patients who received transfusions of less than 7 g/dl of hemoglobin were compared with outcomes of patients who received less than 10 g/dl.[43] Enrollment in this study was limited to patients who were euvolemic at entry and whose hemoglobin levels were from 7 to 9 g/dl; patients who had undergone routine cardiac procedures or who were actively bleeding upon entry to the intensive care unit were excluded. There was no statistical difference in 30-day mortality for these two groups. Indeed, among two subgroups—patients 54 years of age or younger and patients whose illness was less severe, as defined by standardized clinical criteria—Kaplan-Meier survival estimates were significantly better in the group receiving less than 7 g/dl. These results are provocative but must be interpreted cautiously. The enrollment criteria may have biased the findings and call into question the applicability of these findings to other settings. However, these results do suggest that more restrictive transfusion policies may be safely adopted for selected patients.

Chronic Anemia

In the chronically anemic patient, an increase in red cell 2,3-diphosphoglycerate leads to a shift in the oxygen dissociation curve and improved delivery of oxygen to tissues. This adaptation augments the mechanisms for improved oxygen delivery described above. Indications for transfusion depend on clinical assessment of the adequacy of oxygen delivery and are also guided by the etiology of the anemia. If the anemia can be reversed with iron, folic acid, or vitamin B_{12}, transfusion therapy is indicated only in the presence of clinical findings that cannot be tolerated while endogenous red cell mass is being regenerated. Patients with chronic renal disease are typically deficient in erythropoietin. Replacement exogenous erythropoietin therapy [*see Chapter 88*] often corrects this and obviates the need for transfusion. Patients with anemia that is a result of chronic disease such as rheumatoid arthritis, malignancy, or AIDS may also respond to erythropoietin.[44]

INDICATIONS FOR AUTOLOGOUS TRANSFUSION

Whether the criteria for autologous transfusion should be the same as that for allogeneic transfusion remains unresolved. Although the risk associated with autologous blood is less than that associated with allogeneic blood, it is not zero. Errors in labeling, storage, and processing can still occur. For these reasons, many argue that uniform standards based on oxygen delivery should apply, regardless of the blood source. Others, citing the reduced risk, advocate returning most or all of the predeposited units to the patient. There is no clinical evidence that either transfusion policy is associated with better or worse patient outcomes.[45]

Intraoperative and postoperative blood salvage can also help limit allogeneic blood use. Blood salvage is employed in procedures associated with the shedding of large volumes of blood; it involves returning concentrated red cells to the patient after those cells have been washed. Preoperative isovolemic hemodilution is a process in which blood collected immediately before surgery is returned as needed postoperatively. This strategy has been shown to be a cost-effective alternative to preoperative autologous donation in radical prostatectomy.[46] Preoperative isovolemic hemodilution would be particularly useful if an oxygen-carrying blood substitute were available to replace the autologous blood that is removed. Until it is clear that the cardiovascular risks associated with acute hemodilution do not outweigh the risks associated with allogeneic blood, this approach should be considered with caution.

Table 4 Indications for Transfusion of Platelets

Platelet count < 10,000 in asymptomatic patients

Platelet count < 15,000; transfuse if there is coagulation disorder or minor bleeding

Platelet count > 20,000; transfuse if major bleeding or for procedure

---

Transfusion of Platelets

In general, the decision to transfuse platelets rests on the answers to two questions: (1) Is the thrombocytopenia the result of underproduction or increased consumption of platelets? and (2) Do the existing platelets function normally?

INDICATIONS FOR TRANSFUSION

Low Platelet Count

Thrombocytopenia can result from decreased production caused by marrow hypoplasia or from increased consumption caused by such conditions as idiopathic thrombocytopenic purpura (ITP). In a patient with ITP, the surviving platelets are larger and younger and function better than would be expected given the platelet count; platelet transfusion is largely avoided or minimized for such a patient. In contrast, with hypoplasia, platelet function is more severely impaired, and the risk of bleeding is relatively higher. Thus, the decision to transfuse patients who have hypoproliferative thrombocytopenia is generally based on their platelet count and is initiated prophylactically when the count drops below a certain threshold.

Studies have shown that the prevalence of bleeding increases significantly below a threshold of about 10,000 platelets/µl in otherwise asymptomatic patients. The desire to avoid allogeneic donor exposure, cost concerns, and increasing platelet demand have encouraged the use of transfusion policies similar to the policy proposed by Wandt and colleagues [*see Table 4*].[47]

Nonfunctioning Platelets

Platelet function is the second criterion for the transfusion of platelets. Transfusion is appropriate in a bleeding patient whose platelet count is adequate and whose platelets are nonfunctional as a result of medications such as aspirin or nonsteroidal anti-inflammatory drugs or as a result of bypass surgery. In a bleeding patient, if platelet dysfunction is from inherited or acquired defects, transfusion is indicated to provide a minimum number of normal platelets. Platelet function is abnormal in uremic patients, and definitive treatment requires correction of the uremia. Some studies suggest that interventions that increase von Willebrand factor levels, such as 1-desamino-8-D-arginine vasopressin, conjugated estrogen, or cryoprecipitate, may favorably influence platelet function in uremia.[48,49]

CONTRAINDICATIONS TO PLATELET TRANSFUSION

Proper investigation of the causes of thrombocytopenia will identify clinical situations in which platelets should be withheld because they will contribute to evolution of the illness. These disorders include thrombotic microangiopathies such as TTP, hemolytic-uremic syndrome, and the HELLP syndrome (hemolysis, elevated liver enzymes, and a low platelet count). Posttransfusion purpura is usually unresponsive to platelet transfusion but may respond to plasma exchange or intravenous immunoglobulin (IVIG). Patients with autoimmune thrombocytopenia (e.g., ITP) will not be harmed by platelet transfusion, but they will not respond to the therapy.

RESPONSE TO PLATELET TRANSFUSIONS

Both platelet and host factors influence the response to platelet transfusions. Length of in vitro storage, storage temperature, adequacy of oxygenation, and extent of pretransfusion manipulation all influence in vivo survival. Important host factors that influence survival are temperature, splenomegaly, ABO compatibility, and immune status.

When a patient with no adverse host factors receives appropriately stored fresh platelets, one should expect about 10,000 platelets per unit (5.5×10^{10} platelets) to be transfused. This applies both to pooled platelet concentrates and to SDPs, so either product should yield an increment per unit of about 60,000 platelets/μl in an unsensitized 75 kg (165 lb) recipient. The posttransfusion count is usually obtained after 1 hour but can be obtained as early as 10 minutes after transfusion. A patient is considered refractory to platelet transfusions when the 1-hour posttransfusion increment is less than 10,000 platelets/μl after the patient is given 3×10^{11} platelets.

PLATELET TRANSFUSIONS IN A REFRACTORY PATIENT

Platelets have platelet-specific antigens, HLA antigens, and blood group antigens. Immune response to any of these antigens can contribute to platelet unresponsiveness. Platelet surfaces have only class I HLA antigens, of which only HLA-A and HLA-B are clinically important. Polymorphic antigens are found in association with each of the major platelet proteins: PI$^{A1/A2}$ and Pen on glycoprotein IIIa, Bak system on glycoprotein IIb, and Br and Ko on glycoproteins Ia and Ib. Each of these antigen groups has been associated with isoimmune neonatal thrombocytopenia. The prevalence of antibodies to platelet-specific antigens is increased for patients sensitized to HLA antibodies; therefore, antibodies to both sets of epitopes may contribute to refractoriness in patients who fail to respond to HLA-matched platelets.[50]

Treatment of a patient refractory to platelet transfusions involves addressing nonimmune causes (e.g., fever, sepsis, bleeding, and disseminated intravascular coagulation [DIC]) and providing recently collected ABO-compatible products. If these strategies fail, minimization of the effects of HLA antibodies or platelet antigens through HLA typing, platelet crossmatching, or both is indicated.[51] Selecting platelets matched at the HLA-A and HLA-B loci may improve responsiveness in about half of patients with positive HLA antibody screens. Unless contraindicated because of transplant considerations, an empirical trial of donations from family members may also be helpful.

In one study undertaken to determine the best method of treating refractory patients, platelet selection by crossmatching was compared with selection by HLA criteria. Selection by crossmatching was equivalent to HLA selection and yielded results better than those for the HLA matches.[52] Another study found that crossmatched platelets provided equivalent platelet increments that were independent of the grade of HLA match.[53] Although these results are promising, the effectiveness of selection either by HLA and crossmatching or by crossmatching alone is often limited by nonimmune host factors. Additionally, these techniques are not yet routinely available.

Modifying the effects of alloimmunization is difficult. IVIG can improve platelet increments but not platelet survival. A recent analysis of IVIG therapy found that about 50% of alloimmunized patients appeared to benefit from such therapy.[51] Plasma exchange is of limited value because it is difficult to remove IgG antibodies. In some patients, the lymphocytotoxic antibodies responsible for refractoriness may regress over time, so it is important to periodically retest for HLA antibodies. If the HLA antibody screen becomes negative, a trial of non–HLA-matched platelets is warranted.

All in all, the best strategy is prevention, which can be achieved by avoiding unnecessary transfusions and using only leukocyte-depleted products. A randomized, prospective trial of how best to prevent alloimmunization of newly diagnosed patients with acute myeloid leukemia showed equivalent rates of alloimmunization and platelet refractoriness for filtered platelet concentrates, filtered SDPs, and ultraviolet B–irradiated platelets.[54] However, leukocyte reduction did not prevent secondary immune responses in patients already sensitized through either pregnancy or transfusion.[55]

Transfusion of Fresh Frozen Plasma and Plasma Derivatives

FRESH FROZEN PLASMA

Despite a paucity of indications for FFP use, roughly two million units are transfused annually[56] [see Table 3]. FFP is most appropriate for replacing the multiple coagulation deficiencies that result from massive transfusion, liver disease, warfarin toxicity, or acute or chronic DIC. In addition, it can be used to treat thrombotic microangiopathies and specific factor deficiencies when factor concentrates are not available. After one blood volume exchange using only red cells, plasma components are diluted to about 40% of their original concentration; after two blood volume exchanges, plasma components are diluted to 15%. Prothrombin time (PT) and partial thromboplastin time (PTT) become prolonged when coagulation components are lower than 30%, but abnormal bleeding from dilution usually does not occur until these values are less than 17% of normal. Microvascular bleeding associated with a PT and PTT greater than 1.5 times normal is an indication for use of FFP.[57] Whether FFP replacement is needed when PT and PTT are over 1.5 times normal but not associated with bleeding is less clear-cut; paracentesis and thoracentesis did not cause increased bleeding in patients with PT and PTT that were up to twice normal values.[58]

The FFP dose depends on whether or not a consumptive process is being treated in addition to hemodilution. For hemodilution, 15 ml/kg will usually be sufficient. However, if consumption is present, the dose is best guided by the effect of treatment on PT and PTT. If fibrinogen is lower than 80 mg/dl, cryoprecipitate may be required to rapidly increase fibrinogen. However, four units of FFP can be used in most cases to provide the same amount of fibrinogen as one pool of cryoprecipitate. Urgent reversal of the effects of warfarin can usually be accomplished with about 3 to 5 ml/kg of FFP.

Factor XI concentrates, which still have some thrombogenic potential, are available but not yet licensed in the United States.[59] Therefore, FFP is the method of choice for factor XI deficiency. FFP is no longer used to replace antithrombin III, because a purified concentrate is available.[60]

Thrombotic microangiopathies [see Chapter 93] are treated with either FFP transfusions or, more often, plasma exchange with either FFP or cryopoor plasma.[61] Studies suggest that cryopoor plasma may be an alternative to FFP in the treatment of TTP.[62] The dose of either product is usually equal to a plasma volume exchange of 1.0 to 1.5, which is carried out daily until clinical improvement occurs.

FACTOR VIII CONCENTRATES

Since 1980, new methods of heat sterilization, solvent/detergent treatment, and immunoaffinity purification have yielded an array of factor concentrates that are highly purified and unable to transmit HIV and HCV. Measuring HCV RNA in factor

VIII concentrates by reverse transcription and PCR validates the effectiveness of viral inactivation; HCV RNA was present in 100% of products before treatment but was undetectable after treatment. Besides reducing the risk of infection, use of high-purity factor VIII concentrates may be associated with better preservation of patients' cell-mediated immunity.

Four factor VIII preparations (Humate-P, Koāte-HP, Alphanate, and Profilate OSD) are also rich in von Willebrand factor and can be used to treat von Willebrand disease. They have the major advantage of being free of the risks of infection associated with cryoprecipitate. A recombinant factor VIII product that is cloned from two different cell lines expressing factor VIII seems to be therapeutically equivalent to highly purified preparations.[63] These advances in safety and purity, especially in the case of the recombinant factor VIII, have increased the cost per unit fivefold to 10-fold. Recombinant products are used primarily for newly diagnosed patients with hemophilia who have not been exposed to plasma products. Because of the additional costs, benefits over and above those of highly purified plasma products will have to be demonstrated before recombinant products are widely used.

The possibility that a nonhuman source of factor VIII would be useful in the treatment of patients with acquired factor VIII inhibitors led to the development of a highly purified porcine factor VIII concentrate. This was shown to be effective for patients whose anti–factor VIII antibody does not cross-react with the porcine product.[64] About one third of patients develop antibodies to the porcine product, which limits its usefulness for repeat treatments.

FACTOR IX CONCENTRATES

Factor IX complex concentrates contain about equal amounts of the vitamin K–dependent factors II, VII, IX, and X. These preparations are available in several degrees of purity, but all have the disadvantage of being thrombogenic when used for extended periods or in patients with liver disease. The highly purified factor IX, prepared by immunoaffinity chromatography, is free of this complication and is the product of choice in treating factor IX deficiency.[65] Factor IX complex concentrates, especially the less pure products, which have more activated contaminants, have been used to bypass the need for factor VIII in selected patients with hemophilia A and acquired antibody inhibitors. This provides an alternative for patients who do not respond to porcine factor VIII [see Chapter 93].

Transfusion of Granulocytes

Studies have shown granulocyte transfusion to be effective in the treatment of neutropenic patients. Transfusion of granulocytes in doses in the range of 8.3×10^{10} can be obtained by apheresis of donors who have been pretreated with granulocyte colony-stimulating factor (G-CSF) and a single dose of dexamethasone. Granulocyte transfusions at these dose levels have been shown to produce measurable sustained increments in neutrophils, even into the normal range. The indications and clinical benefits of granulocyte transfusion at these higher dose levels are still being determined. Randomized trials are required to fully define the clinical efficacy of granulocyte transfusions. After collection, granulocytes must be stored at room temperature and irradiated to prevent transfusion-associated graft versus host disease. Crossmatching should be performed to ensure compatibility.[66]

Transfusion of Immune Globulin

Many human immune globulin preparations are available. Immune serum globulin, administered intramuscularly, is used to treat chronic immunodeficiency disease, as prophylaxis against hepatitis A, and for prevention or alleviation of measles. For hepatitis A prophylaxis, a traveler who will spend less than 3 months in an endemic area should receive 0.02 ml/kg of immune serum globulin. Hepatitis B immune globulin is used for postexposure prophylaxis against HBV infection [see Chapter 5]. It is prepared from plasma with high titers of antibody to hepatitis B surface antigen. $Rh_o(D)$ immune globulin is used to prevent the development of anti-Rh_o (anti-D) antibodies in Rh-negative women who have just given birth, undergone amniocentesis, or aborted, if the biological father is thought to be Rh positive.

Intravenous administration of human immune globulin promptly elevates circulating IgG levels and is preferable to intramuscular administration. Several preparations of IVIG are available to treat chronic immunodeficiency disease.[67] The intravenous dosage for such deficiency syndromes is 0.2 g/kg a month but can be raised to 0.3 g/kg a month or the agent can be given more often if needed.

The most common side effects of IVIG therapy—headache, nausea, and fever—usually respond to symptomatic treatment and reduction of the infusion rate. Rarer and potentially more severe side effects are cardiac and cerebral embolus, anaphylactic reaction, hemolysis from anti-A and anti-B antibodies, and acute renal failure. Renal failure has been attributed to osmotic nephrosis caused by the high sucrose concentration in many IgG preparations.[68,69] In one study, aseptic meningitis was shown to be the most common of the serious side effects, with a frequency of 11% (95% confidence interval = 4% to 23%); patients with a history of migraine had a significantly higher incidence of aseptic meningitis.[70] Aseptic meningitis usually occurs within 24 hours of administration and does not respond to a reduction of the infusion rate. Patients may be required to stay in the hospital for symptomatic treatment; if further treatment is needed, changing the lot or preparation of IVIG may alleviate this side effect. Current manufacturing practices eliminate HCV from IVIG preparations.

Transfusion of Stem Cells

Stem cell transplantation, initially pioneered for use in leukemia, is used to treat a number of life-threatening, malignant, hereditary, and immunologic disorders [see Chapter 96].

Complications of Transfusions

HEMOLYTIC TRANSFUSION REACTIONS

Hemolytic transfusion reactions are classified as immediate or delayed, depending on their pathophysiology. Immediate hemolytic reactions are the result of a preexisting antibody in the recipient that was not detected during pretransfusion testing. Delayed hemolytic reactions are the result of an anamnestic response to an antigen to which the recipient is already sensitized. The renewed antigenic stimulation in a person already primed by previous antigenic exposure results in recrudescence of antibody to levels that can cause hemolysis. This is in contrast to an immune response during primary sensitization, which seldom causes hemolysis because antibody levels develop at a much slower rate.

Patients with sickle cell disease are more likely than others to become alloimmunized and to have delayed hemolytic transfusion reactions, which often occur in association with recrudescence of an occlusive pain crisis. These reactions are occasionally associated with severe hemolysis involving autologous as well as allogeneic red cells. The cause of these episodes is unknown but has been attributed to so-called bystander hemolysis associated with abnormal function of CD59 (MIRL, membrane inhibitor of reactive lysis), transfusion-associated marrow suppression, or both.[71]

Diagnosis of Hemolytic Reactions

The pathophysiologic differences between immediate and delayed hemolytic transfusion reactions account for some of their differences in clinical findings. Fever is a common sign associated with both immediate and delayed hemolytic transfusion reactions.

Clinical evidence of hemolysis is likely to be more severe in immediate hemolytic reactions and may include back pain, pain along the vein into which the blood is being transfused, change in vital signs, evidence of acute renal failure, and signs of developing DIC. These findings are probably caused by immune complexes activating the complement and kinin systems, by the direct effects of red cell stroma on kidney function, and possibly by the release of such inflammatory cytokines as interleukin-1β (IL-1β), IL-6, and tumor necrosis factor (TNF).[72]

In delayed hemolytic reactions, hemolysis with hemoglobinemia and hematuria (sometimes associated with renal failure) also occurs, but it is less common and generally less severe. In many delayed hemolytic transfusion reactions, the only clinical findings may be a newly positive Coombs test result, the appearance of a new antibody against red cell antigens not present on the recipient's red cells, or both. When hemolysis is absent, these reactions are sometimes called delayed serologic transfusion reactions. At the Mayo Clinic, two surveys sought to identify the relative incidence of both kinds of delayed transfusion reactions. The most recent survey, covering the period from 1993 to 1998, revealed a relative increase in delayed serologic transfusion reactions and an associated decrease in delayed hemolytic reactions, with overall increases in the incidence of these reactions. The earlier survey, which covered the period from 1980 to 1992, revealed an association between delayed transfusion reactions and the presence of antibodies to Jk[a] and Fy[a] or antibodies with multiple specificity; this association was not found in the later survey. These changes probably result from improved systems for identifying clinically significant nonhemolytic antibodies.[73]

In some cases, antiglobulin testing may yield positive results after all the transfused cells have been cleared, often with only complement being detected on the red cells. This finding has been attributed to autoimmune hemolysis after the delayed transfusion reaction.

Treatment of Hemolytic Reactions

As soon as a hemolytic transfusion reaction is suspected, the transfusion should be immediately discontinued. The diagnosis can be confirmed or excluded by sending the remaining blood product, together with a freshly drawn posttransfusion specimen, to the blood bank. The blood bank rechecks all records, confirms the patient's type and antibody screen, checks for evidence of hemoglobin in the plasma, and rechecks the crossmatch and antiglobulin test results. These tests will confirm or disprove the diagnosis and identify the antibody causing the immediate hemolytic reaction, when present. Until these studies have been completed, any further blood products can be given only with the approval of the blood bank's medical director.

The side effects of an acute hemolytic transfusion reaction can be managed by supporting renal blood flow with furosemide and supporting tubular urine flow with mannitol; treating shock, if required, with pressors; and giving platelets and FFP as needed to control coagulopathy if DIC develops. Intravenous steroids may be useful. Until the antibody causing the immune hemolysis is identified, only type O red cells and AB plasma can be used. Once the identification is made, red cells negative for the appropriate antigens can be transfused.

Management of delayed transfusion reactions is simpler because of the slower tempo at which these reactions develop. The diagnosis requires demonstrating that a new antibody against red cell antigens has been identified and searching for clinical evidence of hemolysis. Treatment requires replacement with the appropriate antigen-negative blood products. Acute renal failure and DIC are unlikely but would be managed as described for immediate hemolytic reactions. The severe, atypical delayed transfusion reactions sometimes found in patients with sickle cell disease may require steroids as well as transfusion support.

Prevention of Hemolytic Reactions

Prevention of immediate and delayed hemolytic transfusion reactions depends on recognizing their respective proximate causes. Immediate hemolytic reactions are usually caused by technical errors made during the procurement or processing of blood specimens, during pretransfusion testing, or during product infusion. In a review of transfusion-related deaths reported to the Food and Drug Administration between 1976 and 1985, approximately 50% were caused by errors that led to transfusion of ABO-incompatible blood.[74] Prevention of immediate transfusion reactions can best be accomplished by following protocols for obtaining specimens from patients in adequate time before transfusion and checking to see that blood products are appropriate for the intended recipient.

Delayed transfusion reactions are the result of an anamnestic response of antibodies from a previous transfusion (or pregnancy) that are not present in detectable levels at the time the specimen is crossmatched. A careful transfusion history can best prevent delayed hemolytic reactions. Many patients will know whether there were difficulties involving blood obtained for transfusion. If a patient has a history of difficulty with crossmatches, the blood bank can obtain the details from the institution responsible for the previous transfusion. A proper transfusion history can uncover patients likely to have antibodies that the blood bank would not detect. For example, antibodies to Jk[a] and Fy[a] are characteristically hard to identify because they are quick to rise on stimulation and fall equally rapidly, making later detection difficult.

FEBRILE TRANSFUSION REACTIONS

Nonhemolytic febrile transfusion reactions occur in 1% to 2% of all transfusions and are more likely to occur after platelet transfusions. Until recently, febrile transfusion reactions were attributed to recipient antibody reactions against donor leukocytes and HLA antigens on donor leukocytes in the transfused product. Cytokines produced during storage may also contribute to these reactions.[72] These conclusions are based on observations that platelet products associated with transfusion reactions have higher levels of such inflammatory cytokines as IL-1β, TNF, IL-6, and IL-8 in the supernatant than are found in platelets that do not cause febrile transfusion reactions.[75]

Diagnosis of Febrile Reactions

Febrile reactions are characterized by the development of fever during transfusion or within 5 hours after transfusion. These reactions may be limited to an increase in body temperature of 1° to 2° F but are often associated with chills and rigors.

The differential diagnosis for a patient undergoing a non-hemolytic febrile transfusion reaction should always include unrecognized sepsis. When febrile reaction is suspected, immediate management consists of discontinuing the transfusion, obtaining appropriate cultures, and returning the product to the blood bank. The blood bank obtains cultures from the product and verifies that there have not been any errors in its preparation. The probability that a febrile transfusion reaction has occurred is influenced by the type of product, the number of white cells contained therein, and the transfusion history of the recipient. Febrile reactions to products that have few or no white cells, such as deglycerolized red cells or FFP, are unusual. Unmodified whole blood and red cells contain between 1×10^9 and 3×10^9 white cells and are much more likely to cause febrile reactions. In the case of platelets, reactions can be from cytokines made during in vitro storage or from bacterial contamination.

Treatment of Febrile Transfusion Reactions

Febrile transfusion reactions are usually self-limited and respond to symptomatic management with antipyretics. However, symptoms may be of sufficient magnitude to require the use of 50 to 75 mg of meperidine by intravenous bolus. Leukocyte-depleted products are indicated for patients who have had two or more febrile transfusion reactions to prevent further occurrences.

Prevention of Febrile Reactions

Newer designs of filters for leukocyte reduction should decrease the white cell content to below the threshold for febrile transfusion reactions. Because inflammatory cytokines may be involved in febrile transfusion reactions, methods are being implemented to accomplish leukocyte reduction either during collection or after collection but before storage. A study compared the incidence of febrile transfusion reactions from products that had undergone leukocyte reduction before storage and the incidence of reactions to products that had undergone reduction at the bedside. The study found significantly fewer febrile reactions in patients receiving prestorage leukocyte-depleted products; there was no difference in the number of allergic reactions.[76]

Prestorage leukocyte reduction is particularly important for platelets because platelets are stored at room temperature and accumulate significantly more cytokines than do red cells, which are refrigerated. Febrile transfusion reactions are also more likely with older products. In one study, platelets that were used after they had been in storage for 3 days or less were found to cause significantly fewer febrile transfusion reactions than platelets that were used after longer storage periods.[77] Unfortunately, testing for infectious diseases often takes 2 to 3 days, during which time the product cannot be used. It is therefore impractical to rely on younger products to reduce the risk of febrile transfusion reactions. Other benefits of leukocyte reduction are prevention of HLA alloimmunization; prevention of transmission of leukocyte-bound viruses such as cytomegalovirus (CMV), Epstein-Barr virus, HTLV-I, and HTLV-II; and possibly reduction of immune modulation.[78]

Whether these advantages justify leukocyte reduction for all blood products is currently a topic of debate; it is likely to be settled soon in favor of universal leukocyte reduction by mandate from the Food and Drug Administration.[78] Managing patients who continue to have febrile reactions after receiving leukocyte-depleted products is a clinical problem for which there are no clear solutions. In addition to premedication with steroids, use of HLA-matched products for patients demonstrated to have HLA antibodies may be helpful. Occasionally, use of washed products is beneficial.

TRANSFUSION-RELATED ACUTE LUNG INJURY

Transfusion-related acute lung injury (TRALI) usually presents as bilateral pulmonary infiltrates within 4 hours of transfusion.[79] The clinical and radiographic picture is that of normal-pressure acute respiratory distress syndrome (ARDS), so the differential diagnosis is sufficiently broad to make the possible causal role of transfusion often go unnoticed. TRALI is thought to usually result from interaction between granulocytes and antibodies in the lung, leading to endothelium injury, alveolar exudation, and the clinical findings of ARDS. However, not all cases can be explained by the presence of HLA or granulocyte antibodies. Another model has been proposed in which TRALI is initiated when patients receive infusions of biologically active lipids in certain clinical settings (e.g., recent surgery, massive transfusion, cytokine therapy, or infection).[80] In this two-event model, mediators that arise from sepsis, surgery, or trauma "prime" neutrophils. The primed neutrophils adhere to pulmonary endothelium and are activated by a second event such as exposure to lipids from blood products. This model is based on clinical findings and observations in a rat lung model.[81,82] Diagnosing TRALI depends on excluding cardiac and other causes of ARDS. It is important because most patients will respond to conservative management, with improvement within 24 hours after initiation of therapy. Demonstration of antileukocyte antibodies helps confirm the diagnosis, but their absence does not exclude TRALI in the appropriate clinical setting.

ALLERGIC TRANSFUSION REACTIONS

Allergic transfusion reactions are more common than febrile nonhemolytic transfusion reactions, occurring in 3% to 4% of transfusions. Allergic transfusion reactions usually present as pruritus and urticaria. A small percentage of patients have anaphylactoid symptoms, including wheezing, bronchospasm, and, occasionally, true anaphylaxis.[83] The reactions have been thought to be caused by immune response to plasma proteins. However, a recent study suggested that increased levels of RANTES (regulated on activation, normal T cell expressed and secreted), a proinflammatory chemokine, might be the cause of allergic reactions in platelets.[84] RANTES is stored in platelet alpha granules and accumulates during in vitro storage. This is an intriguing hypothesis because this mediator is known to affect eosinophil and basophil function.

In most cases, symptoms of allergic reactions are local and do not require discontinuing the transfusion if they are controlled with antihistamines. There is, however, no means as yet to identify the rare patient who will respond with anaphylaxis.[83] It is known that IgA deficiency is associated with an increased likelihood of anaphylaxis, but many patients who are IgA deficient never have any difficulty.

For most patients with urticaria, which seldom progresses to anaphylaxis, management is symptomatic. However, patients known to be IgA deficient should receive cells that have been washed so as to remove plasma. When plasma products are required, they should be administered in a facility equipped to manage anaphylactic reactions. Using IgA-deficient plasma can minimize the risk, but such plasma is difficult to obtain and may require drawing from a rare donor pool, testing family members, or both.

ATYPICAL REACTIONS

Occasionally, reactions occur that have characteristics that do not fit the categories already defined yet clearly seem related to blood transfusion. These have been mainly severe hypotensive reactions after platelet infusions. These reactions lack allergic features and are associated with blood product infusions through a negatively charged leukocyte reduction filter. They often occur in patients who are receiving angiotensin-converting enzyme (ACE) inhibitors. A recent study suggests that such reactions may be caused by excessive accumulation of des-Arg9-bradykinin. This metabolite of bradykinin is known to be vasoactive and to be metabolized by ACE.[85] Clinical observations suggest that atypical hypotensive reactions are more likely to occur in patients receiving ACE inhibitors during plasma exchange, hemodialysis, low-density lipoprotein apheresis, IgG affinity column apheresis, and desensitization immunotherapy. These findings have led to the suggestion that ACE inhibitors should be withheld for 24 hours before administration of any of these procedures. These reactions are sufficiently rare that it may be adequate to apply this restriction prospectively only in patients who have already experienced one of these reactions.[86]

TRANSFUSION-ASSOCIATED GRAFT VERSUS HOST DISEASE

The diagnosis of transfusion-associated graft versus host disease (TA-GVHD) should be considered in any patient who presents with fever, skin rash, pancytopenia, and diarrhea and who has abnormal results on liver function tests after transfusion.[87] Neonates present with signs and symptoms similar to those of adults, but fever and rash develop later in neonates than in adults (the median time to presentation of fever in adults is 10 days; in neonates, it is 28 days, with the rash appearing 1 to 2 days later).[88] TA-GVHD is a much-feared consequence of transfusion therapy because mortality approaches 100%.[87] It results from transfusing immunocompetent lymphocytes into a recipient who is unable to reject the allogeneic cells. Reaction of the transfused lymphocytes with host antigens leads to the multiple manifestations of TA-GVHD.

Prevention of TA-GVHD rests on identifying potentially susceptible transfusion recipients. Patients who are at significant risk for TA-GVHD include premature infants receiving large doses of allogeneic lymphocytes, patients with congenital defects in cellular immunity or immunity resulting from illness or chemotherapy, and patients who are unable to reject infused cells because of shared antigens with the allogeneic lymphocytes. Patients undergoing autologous or allogeneic bone marrow transplantation are particularly at risk. Many case reports document the association of Hodgkin disease with TA-GVHD, which occurs presumably as a result of acquired defects in T cell immunity. The intensive chemotherapy used to treat leukemia, high-grade lymphomas, and solid tumors may also

---

Table 5 Patients for Whom Irradiated Blood Products Are Recommended

Fetuses and neonates
Patients with congenital immunodeficiency
Allogeneic and autologous bone marrow transplantation patients
Recipients of some solid-organ transplants*
Patients with hematologic malignancies†
Patients with nonhematologic malignancies, especially if undergoing intensive chemotherapy‡
Recipients who may share haplotypes with donor§

*No consensus, but most agree that heart, liver, and lung recipients should receive irradiated products, whereas recipients of renal allografts do not require irradiated blood.
†Patients with low-grade lymphomas and leukemias in remission may not require irradiated products. Applying restriction to all lymphoma and leukemia patients avoids mistakes.
‡Except for immunosuppression from intensive chemotherapy, there is no consensus.
§Donors in this group include directed donors and first- and second-degree relatives.

---

set the stage for TA-GVHD. However, no cases have been identified in AIDS patients. One hypothesis explaining this surprising finding is that the HIV-mediated injury to $CD4^+$ T cells blocks the development of TA-GVHD.[89]

Patients who are at risk for TA-GVHD as a result of receiving transfusions from a donor who is homozygous for a shared haplotype are the hardest to identify a priori. Donor lymphocytes cannot be rejected by the recipient but can respond to the nonshared recipient haplotype. This mechanism probably accounts for the majority of cases of TA-GVHD. The chance of receiving haplotype-homozygous blood from an unrelated donor varies in different populations. In Japan, the risk for adults may be as high as 1 in 874; it is estimated to be 1 in 102 in neonates because of the practice of using fresh whole blood from family members.[88] In France, the risk is estimated to be 1 in 16,835. In the United States, the risk for the white population is thought to be about 1 in 7,147.[90] These risks increase when first-degree relatives are donors.

Once patients at risk are identified [*see Table 5*], pretreatment of all transfused products with gamma radiation is indicated. On the basis of in vitro studies, the current recommended dose is 2,500 cGy, which does not affect red cell function or platelet survival if it is administered immediately before transfusion.[91] However, irradiated red cells stored for 42 days show significant increases in plasma potassium and hemoglobin and a small but significantly decreased survival. Consequently, recommended storage after irradiation is only 28 days; most institutions prefer to irradiate immediately before product release when possible. Platelets have normal storage survival 5 days after irradiation and can be irradiated at regional centers before distribution. Leukocyte reduction may provide some protection against TA-GVHD, which is related to the dose of lymphocytes. However, filtration alone is not preventive and must never be used as a substitute for gamma irradiation. Because of the risk associated with a one-way HLA match, blood bank standards require that family members' blood and blood of directed donors be irradiated.

Treatment of TA-GVHD is ineffective, but one case report suggests that cyclosporine in combination with anti-CD3 monoclonal antibody (OKT3) may be successful.[92]

BACTERIAL AND PROTOZOAN INFECTIONS

Platelets are associated with the majority of transfusion-related sepsis cases because the platelets are stored at room temperature.[93] Controlling this problem requires improved disinfection of skin, better detection of subclinical infection, and the development of methods for storage at lower temperatures. If sepsis is suspected in patients who have been given red cells, one should consider the possibility of *Yersinia enterocolitica* infection.[94] This organism can grow in the cold, iron-rich environment provided by stored red cells. When such infections occur, the blood is almost always at least 2 weeks old; this period corresponds to the time needed for the usually small initial inoculum to reach clinically significant amounts. Malaria infections have been almost completely eliminated by predonation screening. *Trypanosoma cruzi* can be a chronic parasitic infection; the incidence of blood-borne transmission has increased to the point that pretransfusion testing for it may soon be needed. Spirochetes cannot be transmitted by products that have been stored longer than 80 hours and are no longer considered a clinically significant blood-borne infection.

CYTOMEGALOVIRUS INFECTION

CMV is a common blood-borne infection of no clinical consequence to healthy, immunocompetent recipients, but it can be a severe problem for patients with either acquired or congenital immunodeficiency [*see Table 6*]. Judged on the basis of screening for antibody to CMV, more than 40% of healthy donors may have the potential to transmit CMV.

There are two approaches to the prevention of CMV transmission. The first is to use CMV antibody–negative products. The second, more practical approach is to use leukocyte-reduced products, because CMV is transmitted only by leukocytes. On the basis of a prospective, randomized study of more than 500 transplant patients, products that have undergone leukocyte reduction to the current standard of fewer than 5×10^6 leukocytes per milliliter are considered to be as effective as seronegative products in preventing CMV infection.[95] It is unclear which product provides the best protection against transfusion-associated CMV infection.[96] Direct comparisons between seroconversion rates after transfusion of prestorage leukocyte-depleted products and seroconversion rates after transfusion of CMV-negative products are required to settle this issue.

IMMUNE MODULATION AS A RESULT OF TRANSFUSION

Evidence that transfusions result in modulation of host immunity has come from studies of transplantation, cancer recurrence, and posttransfusion infection rates. The effect was first observed in cadaver kidney transplantation; patient survival was enhanced by increased transfusions. Although this benefit is less important since the introduction of cyclosporine, Opelz and colleagues[97] found improved cadaver graft survival in transfused recipients whose immunosuppression regimen included cyclosporine.

The hypothesis that this effect is related to infused white cells has been supported by studies in animal models and by clinical observations of tumor recurrence and posttransfusion infection rates. Bordin and colleagues[98] have shown in a rabbit animal model that the number of pulmonary metastases is enhanced by allogeneic blood transfusions but not by blood from syngeneic littermates. This effect of allogeneic blood is abrogated by prestorage leukocyte reduction but not by poststorage reduction. Randomized clinical studies of posttransfusion infec-

---

Table 6 Patients for Whom Cytomegalovirus-Negative Blood Products Are Recommended

Neonates, especially if weight is less than 1,200 g

Pregnant women, as a means of preventing primary intrauterine infections

Recipients of solid-organ transplants, especially when the recipient and the organ donor are both CMV negative

Patients with severe combined immunodeficiency

---

tion and cancer recurrence have produced conflicting results.[99] One trial showed a better response with prestorage or poststorage leukocyte reduction than with buffy-coat–depleted red cells in cardiac surgery.[100] In patients who underwent hip and knee surgery, those who received autologous blood transfusions or no transfusions had fewer infections than those who received allogeneic buffy-coat–depleted blood transfusions. Multivariate analysis confirmed that allogeneic blood is an independent risk factor for infection.[101] The conflicting data concerning the magnitude and clinical relevance of transfusion-induced immunomodulation need to be resolved. If leukocyte reduction is shown to reduce posttransfusion infections and cancer recurrence, the argument for universal leukocyte reduction of cellular blood products, which is already strong, would become irrefutable. Until this matter is settled, the possible immunomodulatory effects of blood transfusion are another important reason to avoid allogeneic blood transfusion whenever possible.

Apheresis

Apheresis therapy is the converse of transfusion therapy; it entails treating disease by removing plasma, specific antibodies, or cells. It has been tried in a broad spectrum of diseases [*see Table 7*]. Therapeutic apheresis has real risks and may provide little benefit. It is usually an acute intervention that is only transiently effective, unless the underlying problem is being treated effectively. Consequently, it is important to identify criteria for stopping as well as initiating treatment.

INDICATIONS FOR APHERESIS THERAPY

Neurologic Diseases

Neurologic diseases whose pathogenesis may be antibody mediated are now the most common indications for plasma exchange. Myasthenia gravis occurs when antibodies to acetylcholine receptors cause abnormal neuromuscular transmission. Reductions in these antibody titers from plasma exchange are associated with clinical improvement. A randomized trial compared the use of plasma exchange with the use of IVIG therapy in the treatment of myasthenia gravis; the investigators noted a trend toward better results with plasma exchange, but this trend was not statistically significant.[102] Similar findings were reported from much larger studies of Guillain-Barré syndrome, which is thought to be caused by antibodies to myelin. Two large series comparing plasma exchange with current best therapy showed more rapid improvement with the addition of plasma exchange.[103] Randomized comparisons of plasma exchange and IVIG in the treatment of Guillain-Barré syndrome have shown these approaches to be equivalent; no additional benefit from using both therapies was shown.[104,105]

Chronic inflammatory demyelinating polyneuropathy (CIDP) is an autoimmune disorder that causes proximal and distal weakness; it has a progressive or relapsing course and is sometimes associated with monoclonal gammopathies. CIDP responds to plasma exchange except in patients with distal weakness and associated IgM monoclonal gammopathies[106,107]; such patients respond poorly to all modalities of therapy.[108,109] IVIG therapy and plasma exchange have been shown to be comparably effective in CIDP.[109]

The use of plasma exchange in multiple sclerosis remains controversial. Meta-analysis of six controlled trials of plasma exchange provided some evidence of benefit, but the authors concluded that the subgroups of patients likely to benefit needed further definition.[110] A recent randomized study of plasma exchange in patients with acute inflammatory demyelinating central nervous system disease showed a significant benefit from the therapy. However, patients continued to have problems with relapse.[111]

Hematologic Diseases

Leukocyte exchange The hematologic diseases that require apheresis are those associated with obstruction of vascular flow by cells or the blockage of flow by proteins as a result of viscosity or cryoprecipitation; antibody-mediated diseases that lead to destruction of the formed elements of the blood; and thrombotic microangiopathies.

Leukostasis is a function of cell number and cell type. Myeloblasts are more likely to cause stasis than are an equivalent number of lymphocytes in a patient with chronic lymphocytic leukemia. Unless pulmonary or cerebral leukostasis is severe enough to cause progression in clinical findings, hydroxyurea treatment usually decreases the cell count sufficiently within 24 hours. However, when clinical findings demand improvement within 4 to 8 hours, leukapheresis is the treatment of choice.

Red cell exchange Red cell exchange has been used to treat acute chest crises, stroke, and priapism, and it is sometimes used to prepare patients with sickle cell disease for surgery. In these patients, the indications for red cell exchange, versus simple transfusion, are poorly defined. For example, in a recent analysis of causes and outcomes in acute chest syndrome, simple transfusions were used instead of red cell exchange in about two thirds

of patients.[112] Many believe that red cell exchanges should be reserved for patients with progressive pulmonary disease or for those who fail to respond to transfusions. Use of Rh and Kell antigen–compatible red cells reduces the incidence of alloimmunization from 7% to 1%[113] and should be standard practice. Red cell exchange leads to less iron accumulation than transfusion therapy, which is an advantage in the treatment of patients with sickle cell disease who require long-term therapy, such as those who have a history of stroke.[114]

Plasma exchange The concentration of paraprotein influences plasma protein viscosity, as does its heavy-chain class. IgM is the largest plasma protein and is nearly 100% intravascular; it is most likely to cause hyperviscosity. IgA and IgG3 are more likely to aggregate and are associated with hyperviscosity more often than other IgG subclasses. As in leukostasis, the choice between plasma exchange and chemotherapy is guided mainly by the clinical symptoms and their rate of progression. Plasma exchange can lower viscosity within hours, whereas most chemotherapy requires days. Acute-onset renal failure caused by myeloma proteins can be improved by lowering the plasma concentration of paraprotein, but more data are needed for this to be considered an established indication.[115]

Despite the role that antibody and immune complexes play in hematologic cytopenia, there are no well-controlled studies supporting the use of plasma exchange. The available case reports usually describe the role of plasma exchange as being that of backup after failure of more established therapies. FFP or cryopoor plasma is used in replacement therapy for thrombotic microangiopathies. Case reports suggest that patients with severe preeclampsia, HELLP syndrome, or both may benefit from plasma exchange with FFP replacement if they fail to improve after delivery.[116]

Antibody-Mediated Renal, Muscular, and Cutaneous Diseases

Despite promising reports from case studies, controlled trials of patients with pemphigus vulgaris,[117] polymyositis,[118] dermatomyositis,[118] and Goodpasture syndrome[119] have raised doubts concerning the value of plasma exchange, although plasma exchange appears valuable in stopping pulmonary hemorrhage in Goodpasture syndrome.[119]

Table 7 Indications for Plasma Exchange

Indications Based on Randomized Trials	Indications Based on Consensus and on Case Reports	Possible Indications
Guillain-Barré syndrome	Myasthenia gravis	Pemphigus vulgaris
Chronic inflammatory polyneuropathy	Hyperviscosity	Goodpasture syndrome
Peripheral neuropathy associated with MGUS	Hemolytic-uremic syndrome	Autoimmune hemolytic anemia
Thrombotic thrombocytopenic purpura	Persistent HELLP syndrome	Antibody to coagulation factors
	Posttransfusion purpura	Idiopathic thrombocytopenic purpura
	Lupus nephritis	Cold agglutinin disease
	Cryoglobulinemia	
	Vasculitis	
	Familial hypercholesterolemia	

HELLP—hemolysis, elevated liver enzymes, and low platelet count   MGUS—monoclonal gammopathy of unknown significance

Immune Complex Diseases

The only indication for plasma exchange in rheumatoid arthritis and systemic lupus erythematosus is severe vasculitis that does not respond to other therapies.

Metabolic Diseases

Plasma exchange and selective removal of low-density lipoproteins (LDLs) have both been used to treat familial hypercholesterolemia [*see Chapter 54*]. Selective removal of LDLs can be accomplished by immunoadsorption, heparin precipitation, or dextran sulfate cellulose absorption, whereas plasma exchange also causes significant reduction of high-density lipoproteins.

COMPLICATIONS OF PLASMA EXCHANGE

The complications of plasma exchange are best divided into problems related to apheresis machines and problems related to venous access, type of replacement fluids, and anticoagulant. Apheresis machines accomplish cell and plasma separation by either centrifugation or membrane filtration. All systems monitor air and access pressure, so air emboli are eliminated and access problems are promptly recognized. Excess transmembrane pressure may cause red cell hemolysis, which leads to increased hemoglobin in the separated plasma. The majority of complications associated with plasma exchange result from the replacement fluid and anticoagulant used. Plasma removed by exchange is commonly replaced with 5% albumin, which carries no risk of infection and does not increase the citrate return but does dilute coagulation factors, causing mild coagulopathy for 24 to 48 hours. On an every-other-day treatment schedule, the coagulation abnormalities are usually not clinically significant, but they may require placing the patient on a daily treatment schedule. Use of FFP avoids dilutional coagulopathy but increases risks of blood-borne infection and allergic reactions. Peripheral venous access is often inadequate to maintain the required flow rates of 45 to 80 ml/min, necessitating central venous access with a large, double-lumen catheter; life-threatening or fatal complications from central catheter placement have been reported.[120] Catheter malfunction should always be considered when a patient shows clinical evidence of hypovolemia, shock, or both while undergoing plasma exchange. The majority of complications, however, are side effects of the citrate anticoagulant. These can include paresthesias, abdominal cramps, and, in rare instances, cardiac arrhythmias or seizures. Citrate toxicity is usually managed easily by slowing the return rate and providing extra calcium, either orally or sometimes intravenously. Patients with renal failure who receive large amounts of citrate may develop a profound metabolic alkalosis.[121]

Future Prospects for Transfusion Therapy

The evolution of transfusion practice has been a steady progression from whole blood to fractionated products designed for specific therapies. The search for a practical replacement for red cells that would allow stable storage, provide adequate oxygen delivery, and be free of significant toxins has been long and filled with substantial obstacles. Hemoglobin-based substitutes are most promising, but they still have major problems with purification, adequate oxygen unloading, and potential toxicity. Perfluorocarbons improve oxygen delivery by increasing solubility in plasma. The effectiveness of these compounds is limited by their poor solubility in plasma and the require-

ment for high oxygen tension. Because of these considerations, Fluosol-DA is licensed only for oxygen delivery during coronary angioplasty when the balloon is inflated. In the case of coagulation components, a recombinant factor VIII is already available, but the extent of its use is limited because of the relative efficacy and much improved safety of the highly purified products derived from human plasma.

A major change in transfusion practice may evolve from the availability of cytokines that can modify endogenous production. Erythropoietin has changed the treatment of anemia from chronic renal disease, so that many dialysis patients no longer require transfusions. Erythropoietin also can facilitate patients' self-banking their blood for anticipated surgical needs. The availability of myeloid growth factors has contributed substantially to the development of methods for collection, and potentially mobilizing leukocytes with growth factors may increase the effectiveness of granulocyte transfusions. Thrombopoietin may in time be used to enhance platelet apheresis collections. The immunomodulatory effects of blood transfusion are in the early stages of description. It may be that a better understanding of the mechanisms underlying immunomodulation will permit using these effects to therapeutic advantage, such as to induce tolerance to an organ graft or to downregulate antibody production.

Evaluation of the clinical gains versus the risks and costs of transfusion practice has not been done as widely in transfusion medicine as it has in other medical specialties. An analysis of the newly available S/D plasma showed that the benefit of eliminating lipid-coated viruses from plasma products was incurred at a huge expenditure when the additional costs, the potential increased risk from blood-borne pathogens from a pooled product, and the minimal safety gains were considered. The cost per quality-adjusted life-year was found to be one of the highest in the literature.[122] Yet the search for a risk-free blood supply continues, with ever-decreasing increments in benefit as the safety of blood products increases.

Even in an era of accelerating change, certain aspects of transfusion medicine will remain constant. The blood donor remains a kingpin who cannot be replaced by recombinant methodology. Transfusion practice has improved in safety, but there will always be residual risks. Each transfusion will always require careful assessment of whether the risks to the recipient of the transfusion will exceed the risks of going without.

References

1. Williams AE, Thomson RA, Schreiber GB, et al: Estimates of infectious disease risk factors in US blood donors. JAMA 277:967, 1997

2. Thomas MJG, Gillon J, Desmond MJ: Consensus Conference on Autologous Transfusion: preoperative autologous donation. Transfusion 36:633, 1996

3. Starkey JM, MacPherson JL, Bolgiano DC, et al: Markers for transfusion-transmitted disease in different groups of blood donors. JAMA 262:3452, 1989

4. Strauss RG, Burmeister LF, Johnson K, et al: Randomized trial assessing the feasibility and safety of biologic parents as RBC donors for their preterm infants. Transfusion 40:450, 2000

5. Kleinman S, Alter H, Busch M, et al: Increased detection of hepatitis C virus (HCV)-infected blood donors by a multiple-antigen HCV enzyme immunoassay. Transfusion 32:805, 1992

6. Epstein J: Hepatitis C virus lookback: emerging science and public policy (editorial). Transfusion 40:3, 2000

7. Schreiber GB, Busch MP, Kleinman SH, et al: Risk of transfusion-transmitted viral infections. The Retrovirus Epidemiology Donor Study. N Engl J Med 334:1685, 1996

8. Centers for Disease Control and Prevention: Recommendations for prevention and control of hepatitis C virus (HCV) infection and HCV-related chronic disease. MMWR Morb Mortal Wkly Rep 47:RR-19, 1998

9. Akahane Y, Kojuma M, Sugai Y, et al: Hepatitis C virus infection in spouses of patients with type C chronic liver disease. Ann Intern Med 120:748, 1994

10. Capelli C, Prati D, Bosoni P, et al: Sexual transmission of hepatitis C virus to a repeat blood donor. Transfusion 37:436, 1997

11. Fried MW: Diagnostic testing for hepatitis C: practical considerations. Am J Med 107:31S, 1999

12. Epstein JS: Clarification of the use of unlicensed anti-HCV supplemental test results in regard to donor notification. FDA memorandum, August 19, 1993

13. Lemaire JM, Courouce AM, Defer C, et al: HCV RNA in blood donors with isolated reactivities by third-generation PCR. Transfusion 40:867, 2000

14. Gallarda JL, Dragon E: Blood screening by nucleic acid amplification technology: current issues, future challenges. Mol Diagn 5:11, 2000

15. Bower WA, Nainan OV, Han X, et al: Duration of viremia in hepatitis A virus infection. J Infect Dis 182:12, 2000

16. Lefrére JJ, Sender A, Mercier B, et al: High rate of GB virus type C/HGV transmission from mother to infant: possible implications for the prevalence of infection in blood donors. Transfusion 40:602, 2000

17. Lackritz EM, Satten GA, Aberle-Grasse J, et al: Estimated risk of transmission of the human immunodeficiency virus by screened blood in the United States. N Engl J Med 333:1712, 1995

18. Jackson JB, Hanson MR, Johnson GM, et al: Long-term follow-up of blood donors with indeterminate human immunodeficiency virus type 1 results on Western blot. Transfusion 35:98, 1995

19. Busch MP, Kleinman SG, Williams AE, et al: Frequency of human immunodeficiency virus (HIV) infection among contemporary anti-HIV-1 and anti-HIV-1/2 supplemental test-indeterminate blood donors. Transfusion 36:37, 1996

20. Sayre KR, Dodd RY, Tegtmeier G, et al: False-positive human immunodeficiency virus type 1 Western blot tests in noninfected blood donors. Transfusion 36:45, 1996

21. Murphy EL, Glynn SA, Fridey J, et al: Increased prevalence of infectious diseases and other adverse outcomes in human T lymphotropic virus types I- and II-infected donors. J Infect Dis 176:1468, 1997

22. Marsh BJ: Infectious complications of human T cell leukemia/lymphoma virus type I infections. Clin Infect Dis 23:138, 1996

23. Murphy EL, Fridey J, Smith JW, et al: HTLV-associated myelopathy in a cohort of HTLV-I and HTLV-II infected blood donors. The REDS investigators. Neurology 48:315, 1997

24. Busch MP, Switzer WM, Murphy EL, et al: Absence of evidence of infection with divergent primate T-lymphotropic viruses in United States blood donors who have seroindeterminate HTLV test results. Transfusion 40:443, 2000

25. Zaran BS, Hibbard AJ, Becker G, et al: False-positive serologic tests for human T-cell lymphotropic virus type I among blood donors following influenza vaccination, 1992. MMWR Morb Mortal Wkly Rep 42:173, 1993

26. Yamamoto FI, Clausen H, White T, et al: Molecular genetic basis of the histo-blood group ABO system. Nature 345:229, 1990

27. Mifsud NA, Haddad AP, Condon JA: ABO genotyping by polymerase chain reaction–restriction fragment length polymorphism. Immunohematology 12:143, 1996

28. Issit PD, Telen MJ: D, weak D (Dᵘ), and partial D: the molecular story unfolds (editorial). Transfusion 36:97, 1996

29. Bennett PR, Le Van Kim C, Colin Y, et al: Prenatal determination of fetal RhD type by DNA amplification. N Engl J Med 329:607, 1993

30. Wagner FF, Gassner C, Muller TH, et al: Three molecular structures cause rhesus D category VI phenotypes with distinct immunohematologic features. Blood 92:2157, 1998

31. Reid ME, Rios M, Powell VI, et al: DNA from blood samples can be used to genotype patients who have recently received a transfusion. Transfusion 40:48, 2000

32. Marrosszeky S, McDonald J, Sutherland H, et al: Suitability of preadmission blood samples for pretransfusion testing in elective surgery. Transfusion 37:910, 1997

33. Popovsky MA: Quality of blood components filtered before storage and at the bedside: implications for transfusion practice. Transfusion 36:470, 1996

34. Chambers LA, Herman JH: Considerations in the selection of a platelet component: apheresis versus whole blood derived. Transfus Med Rev 13:331, 1999

35. Heal JM, Rowe JM, McMican A, et al: The role of ABO matching in platelet transfusion. Eur J Haematol 50:110, 1993

36. Solheom BG, Rollag H, Svennevig JL, et al: Viral safety of solvent/detergent-treated plasma. Transfusion 40:84, 2000

37. Williamson LM, Llewelyn CA, Fisher NC, et al: A randomized trial of solvent/detergent-treated plasma and standard fresh-frozen plasma in the coagulopathy of liver disease and liver transplantation. Transfusion 39:1227, 1999

38. Mast AE, Stadanlick JE, Lockett JM, et al: Solvent/detergent-treated plasma had decreased antitrypsin activity and absent antiplasmin activity. Blood 94:3922, 1999

39. Practice guidelines for blood component therapy: a report by the American Society of Anesthesiologists Task Force on Blood Component Therapy. Anesthesiology 84:732, 1996

40. Preoperative red cell transfusion. Office of Medical Applications of Research, National Institutes of Health. JAMA 260:2700, 1988

41. Practice strategies for elective red blood cell transfusion. American College of Physicians. Ann Intern Med 116:403, 1992

42. Bracey AW, Radovancevic R, Riggs SA, et al: Lowering the hemoglobin threshold for transfusion in coronary artery bypass procedures: effect on patient outcome. Transfusion 39:1070, 1999

43. Hebert PC, Wells G, Blajchman MA, et al: A multicenter, randomized, controlled clinical trial of transfusion requirements in critical care. N Engl J Med 340:409, 1999

44. Cazzola M, Mercuriali F, Brugnara C: Use of recombinant human erythropoietin outside the setting of uremia. Blood 89:4248, 1997

45. Churchill WH, McGurk S, Chapman RH, et al: The Collaborative Hospital Transfusion Study: variations in the use of autologous blood account for hospital differences in red cell use during primary hip and knee surgery. Transfusion 38:530, 1998

46. Monk TG, Goodnough LT, Birkmeyer JD, et al: Acute normovolemic hemodilution is a cost-effective alternative to preoperative autologous blood donation by patients undergoing radical retropubic prostatectomy. Transfusion 35:559, 1995

47. Wandt H, Frank M, Ehniger G, et al: Safety and cost effectiveness of a 10×10^9/L trigger for prophylactic platelet transfusions compared with the traditional 20×10^9/L trigger: a prospective comparative trial in 105 patients with acute myeloid leukemia. Blood 91:3601, 1998

48. Janson PA, Jubelirer SJ, Weinstein MJ, et al: Treatment of the bleeding tendency in uremia with cryoprecipitate. N Engl J Med 303:1318, 1980

49. Shemin D, Elnour M, Amarantes B, et al: Oral estrogens decrease bleeding time and improve clinical bleeding in patients with renal failure. Am J Med 89:436, 1990

50. Kickler T, Kennedy SD, Braine HG: Alloimmunization to platelet-specific antigens on glycoproteins IIb-IIIa and Ib/IX in multiply transfused thrombocytopenic patients. Transfusion 30:622, 1990

51. Delaflor-Weiss E, Mintz PD: The evaluation and management of platelet refractoriness and alloimmunization. Transf Med Rev 14:180, 2000

52. Moroff G, Garratty G, Heal JM: Selection of platelets for refractory patients by HLA matching and prospective crossmatching. Transfusion 32:633, 1992

53. Friedberg RC, Donnelly SF, Mintz PD: Independent roles for platelet crossmatching and HLA in the selection of platelets for alloimmunized patients. Transfusion 34:215, 1994

54. Leukocyte reduction and ultraviolet irradiation of platelets to prevent alloimmunization and refractoriness to platelet transfusions. The Trial to Reduce Alloimmunization to Platelets Study Group. N Engl J Med 337:1861, 1997

55. Novotny VM, van Doorn R, Witvliet MD, et al: Occurrence of allogeneic HLA and non-HLA antibodies after transfusion of prestorage filtered platelets and red blood cells: a prospective study. Blood 85:1736, 1995

56. Wallace EL, Churchill WH, Surgenor DM, et al: Collection and transfusion of blood and blood components in the United States, 1994. Transfusion 38:625, 1998

57. Practice parameters for the use of fresh-frozen plasma, cryoprecipitate, and platelets. Administration Practice Guidelines Development Task Force of the College of American Pathologists. JAMA 271:777, 1994

58. McVay PA, Toy PT: Lack of increased bleeding after paracentesis and thoracentesis in patients with mild coagulation abnormalities. Transfusion 31:164, 1991

59. Mannucci PM, Bauer KA, Santagostino E, et al: Activation of the coagulation cascade after infusion of a factor XI concentrate in congenitally deficient patients. Blood 84:1314, 1994

60. Lechner K, Kyrle PA: Antithrombin III concentrates—are they clinically useful? Thromb Haemost 73:340, 1995

61. George JN: How I treat patients with thrombotic thrombocytopenic purpura–hemolytic uremia syndrome. Blood 96:1223, 2000

62. Rock G, Sutton DM, Nair RC: Cryosupernatant as replacement fluid for plasma exchange in thrombotic thrombocytopenic purpura. Members of the Canadian Apheresis Group. Br J Haematol 94:383, 1996

63. Schwartz RS, Abildgaard CF, Aledort LM, et al: Human recombinant DNA–derived antihemophilic factor (factor VIII) in the treatment of hemophilia A. N Engl J Med 323:1800, 1990

64. Brettler DB, Forsberg AD, Levine PH, et al: The use of porcine factor VIII concentrate (Hyate:C) in the treatment of patients with inhibitor antibodies to factor VIII: a multicenter US experience. Arch Intern Med 149:1381, 1989

65. Thompson AR: Factor IX concentrates for clinical use. Semin Thromb Hemost 19:25, 1993

66. Price TH: The current prospects for neutrophil transfusions for the treatment of granulocytopenic infected patients. Transfus Med Rev 14:2, 2000

67. Brugnara C, Churchill WH: Plasma component therapy. Thrombosis and Hemorrhage, 2nd ed. Loscalzo J, Schafer AI, Eds. Williams & Wilkins, Baltimore, 1998, p 1135

68. Ahsan N, Weigand LA, Abendroth CS, et al: Acute renal failure following immunoglobulin therapy. Am J Nephrol 16:532, 1996

69. Renal insufficiency and failure associated with immune globulin intravenous therapy—United States, 1985–1998. MMWR Morb Mortal Wkly Rep 48:518, 1999

70. Sekul EA, Cupler EJ, Dalakas MC: Aseptic meningitis associated with high-dose intravenous immunoglobulin therapy: frequency and risk factors. Ann Intern Med 121:259, 1994

71. Garratty G: Severe reactions associated with transfusion of patients with sickle cell disease. Transfusion 37:357, 1997

72. Davenport RD, Kunkel SL: Cytokine roles in hemolytic and nonhemolytic transfusion reactions. Transfus Med Rev 8:157, 1994

73. Pineda AA, Vamvakas EC, Gorden LD, et al: Trends in the incidence of delayed hemolytic and delayed serologic transfusion reactions. Transfusion 39:1097, 1999

74. Sazama K: Reports of 355 transfusion-associated deaths: 1976 through 1985. Transfusion 30:583, 1990

75. Heddle NM, Klama L, Singer J: The role of plasma from platelet concentrates in transfusion reactions. N Engl J Med 331:625, 1994

76. Federowicz I, Barrett BB, Andersen JW, et al: Characterization of reactions after transfusion of cellular blood components that are white cell reduced before storage. Transfusion 36:21, 1996

77. Kelley DL, Mangini J, Lopez-Plaza I, et al: The utility of ≤ 3-day-old whole-blood platelets in reducing the incidence of febrile nonhemolytic transfusion reactions. Transfusion 40:439, 2000

78. Dzik S, Aubuchon J, Jeffries L, et al: Leukocyte reduction of blood components: public policy and new technology. Transfus Med Rev 14:34, 2000

79. Popovsky MA, Chaplin HC Jr, Moore SB: Transfusion-related acute lung injury: a neglected, serious complication of hemotherapy. Transfusion 32:589, 1992

80. Silliman CC, Paterson AJ, Dickey WO, et al: The association of biologically active lipids with the development of transfusion-related acute lung injury: a retrospective study. Transfusion 37:719, 1997

81. Silliman CC: Transfusion-related acute lung injury. Transfus Med Rev 13:177, 1999

82. Silliman CC, Voelkel NF, Allard JD, et al: Plasma and lipids from stored packed red blood cells cause acute lung injury in an animal model. J Clin Invest 101:1458, 1998

83. Sandler SG, Mallory D, Malamut D, et al: Hemagglutination assays for the diagnosis and prevention of IgA anaphylactic transfusion reactions. Transfus Med Rev 9:1, 1995

84. Klüter H, Bubel S, Kirchner H, et al: Febrile and allergic transfusion reactions after the transfusion of white cell–poor platelet preparations. Transfusion 39:1179, 1999

85. Cyr M, Hume HA, Champagne M, et al: Anomaly of the des-Arg9-bradykinin metabolism associated with severe hypotensive reactions during blood transfusions: a preliminary study. Transfusion 39:1084, 1999

86. Owen HG, Brecher ME: Atypical reactions associated with use of angiotensin-converting enzyme inhibitors and apheresis. Transfusion 34:891, 1994

87. Ohto H, Anderson KC: Survey of transfusion-associated graft-versus-host disease in immunocompetent recipients. Transfus Med Rev 10:31, 1996

88. Ohto H, Anderson KC: Posttransfusion graft-versus-host disease in Japanese newborns. Transfusion 36:117, 1996

89. Ammann AJ: Hypothesis: absence of graft-versus-host disease in AIDS is a consequence of HIV-1 infection of CD4+ T cells. J Acquir Immune Defic Syndr 6:1224, 1993

90. Ohto H, Yasuda H, Noguchi M: Risk of transfusion-associated graft-versus-host disease as a result of directed donation from relatives (letter). Transfusion 32:691, 1992

91. Morof FG, Luban NLC: The irradiation of blood and blood components to prevent graft-versus-host disease: technical issues and guidelines. Transfus Med Rev 11:15, 1997

92. Yasukawa M, Shinozaki F, Hato T, et al: Successful treatment of transfusion-associated graft-versus-host disease. Br J Haematol 86:831, 1994

93. McDonald CP, Hartley S, Orchard K, et al: Fatal Clostridium perfringens sepsis from a pooled platelet transfusion. Transfusion 37:259, 1997

94. Centers for Disease Control and Prevention: Red blood cell transfusions contaminated with Yersinia enterocolitica: United States, 1991–1996, and initiation of a national study to detect bacteria-associated transfusion reaction. MMWR Morb Mortal Wkly Rep 46:553, 1997

95. Bowden RA, Slichter SJ, Sayers M, et al: A comparison of filtered leukocyte-reduced and cytomegalovirus (CMV) seronegative blood products for the prevention of transfusion-associated CMV infection after marrow transplant. Blood 86:3598, 1995

96. Preiksaitis JK: The cytomegalovirus "safe" blood product: is leukoreduction equivalent to antibody screening? Transfus Med Rev 14:112, 2000

97. Opelz G, Vanrenterghem Y, Kirste G, et al: Prospective evaluation of pretransplant blood transfusions in cadaver kidney recipients. Transplantation 63:964, 1997

98. Bordin JO, Bardossy L, Blajchman MA: Growth enhancement of established tumors by allogeneic blood transfusion in experimental animals and its amelioration by leukodepletion: the importance of the timing of the leukodepletion. Blood 84:344, 1998

99. Vamvakas EC, Blajchman MA: Prestorage versus poststorage white cell reduction for the prevention of the deleterious immunomodulatory effects of allogeneic blood transfusion. Transfus Med Rev 14:23, 2000

100. van de Watering LM, Hermans J, Houbiers JG, et al: Beneficial effect of leukocyte depletion of transfused blood on post-operative complications in patients undergoing cardiac surgery: a randomized clinical trial. Circulation 97:562, 1998

101. Innerhofer P, Walleczek C, Luz G, et al: Transfusion of buffy coat-depleted blood components and risk of postoperative infection in orthopedic patients. Transfusion 39:625, 1999

102. Gajdos P, Chevret S, Clair B, et al: Clinical trial of plasma exchange and high-dose intravenous immunoglobulin in myasthenia gravis. Myasthenia Gravis Clinical Study Group. Ann Neurol 41:789, 1997

103. Plasma exchange in Guillain-Barré syndrome: one-year follow-up. French Cooperative Group on Plasma Exchange in Guillain-Barré Syndrome. Ann Neurol 32:94, 1992

104. Randomised trial of plasma exchange, intravenous immunoglobulin, and combined treatments in Guillain-Barré syndrome. Plasma Exchange/Sandoglobulin Guillain-Barré Syndrome Trial Group. Lancet 349:225, 1997

105. van der Meché FG, Schmitz PI: A randomized trial comparing intravenous immune globulin and plasma exchange in Guillain-Barré syndrome. The Dutch Guillain-Barré Study Group. N Engl J Med 326:1123, 1992

106. Dyck PJ, Low PA, Windebank AJ, et al: Plasma exchange in polyneuropathy associated with monoclonal gammopathy of undetermined significance. N Engl J Med 325:1482, 1991

107. Hahn AF, Bolton CF, Pillay N, et al: Plasma-exchange therapy in chronic inflammatory demyelinating polyneuropathy: a double-blind, sham-controlled, cross-over study. Brain 119:1055, 1996

108. Katz JS, Saperstein DS, Gronseth G, et al: Distal acquired demyelinating symmetric neuropathy. Neurology 54:615, 2000

109. Dyck PJ, Litchy WJ, Kratz KM, et al: A plasma exchange versus immune globulin infusion in chronic inflammatory demyelinating polyradiculoneuropathy. Ann Neurol 36:838, 1994

110. Vamvakas EC, Pineda AA, Weinshenker BG: Meta-analysis of clinical studies of the efficacy of plasma exchange in the treatment of chronic progressive multiple sclerosis. J Clin Apheresis 10:163, 1995

111. Weinshenker BG, O'Brien PC, Petterson TM, et al: A randomized trial of plasma exchange in acute central nervous system inflammatory demyelinating disease. Ann Neurol 46:878, 1999

112. Vichinsky EP, Neumayr LD, Earles AN, et al: Causes and outcomes of the acute chest syndrome in sickle cell disease. N Engl J Med 342:1855, 2000

113. Vichinsky EP, Earles AN, Johnson RA, et al: Alloimmunization in sickle cell anemia and transfusion of racially unmatched blood. N Engl J Med 322:1617, 1990

114. Hilliard L, Williams B, et al: Erythrocytapheresis limits iron accumulation in chronically transfused sickle cell patients. Am J Hematol 59:28, 1998

115. Zucchelli P, Pasquali S, Cagnoli L, et al: Controlled plasma exchange trial in acute renal failure due to multiple myeloma. Kidney Int 33:1175, 1988

116. Martin JN, Files FC, Blake PG: Plasma exchange for preeclampsia: I. Postpartum use for persistently severe preeclampsia-eclampsia with HELLP syndrome. Am J Obstet Gynecol 162:126, 1990

117. Guillaume JC, Roujeau JC, Morel P, et al: Controlled study of plasma exchange in pemphigus. Arch Dermatol 124:1659, 1988

118. Miller FW, Leitman SF, Cronin ME, et al: Controlled trial of plasma exchange and leukapheresis in polymyositis and dermatomyositis. N Engl J Med 326:1380, 1992

119. Johnson JP, Moore J Jr, Austin HA III, et al: Therapy of anti-glomerular basement membrane antibody disease: analysis of prognostic significance of clinical, pathologic and treatment factors. Medicine (Baltimore) 64:219, 1985

120. Rizvi MA, Vesely JN, Chandler GL, et al: Complications of plasma exchange in 71 consecutive patients treated for clinically suspected thrombotic thrombocytopenic purpura–hemolytic-uremic syndrome. Transfusion 40:869, 2000

121. Pearl RG, Rosenthal MM: Metabolic alkalosis due to plasmapheresis. Am J Med 79:391, 1985

122. Aubuchon JP, Birkmeyer JD: Safety and cost-effectiveness of solvent-detergent-treated plasma: in search of a zero-risk blood supply. JAMA 272:1210, 1994

96 Hematopoietic Stem Cell Transplantation

Frederick R. Appelbaum, M.D.

Because hematopoietic stem cells can be collected from the peripheral blood, bone marrow, and umbilical cord blood, the term bone marrow transplantation is being replaced by the more inclusive term hematopoietic stem cell transplantation. With transplantation, an abnormal but nonmalignant lymphohematopoietic system can be replaced with a healthy one, making transplantation an effective therapy for a variety of nonmalignant diseases (e.g., severe combined immunodeficiency disease [SCID], Wiskott-Aldrich syndrome, aplastic anemia, thalassemia, sickle cell anemia, and Gaucher disease). In addition, hematopoietic transplantation is used to treat a variety of malignancies because it allows administration of higher and potentially more effective doses of chemotherapy and radiotherapy that would otherwise cause unacceptable myelosuppression. Allogeneic transplantation also confers its own antitumor effects beyond those of chemoradiotherapy. Worldwide, an estimated 47,000 patients underwent hematopoietic stem cell transplantation in 1997.[1]

The Hematopoietic Stem Cell

Three features of the lymphohematopoietic system make transplantation feasible: its regeneration capacity, the homing of stem cells to sites for survival and proliferation, and the ability of stem cells to survive cryopreservation. In mice, a single hematopoietic stem cell can reconstitute a lethally irradiated recipient.[2] In humans, transplantation of considerably less than 10% of a donor's marrow regularly results in complete and sustained replacement of the recipient's entire lymphohematopoietic system, including red cells, platelets, granulocytes, T cells, and B cells, as well as pulmonary alveolar macrophages, Kupffer cells of the liver, osteoblasts, Langerhans cells of the skin, and microglial cells of the brain [*see Chapter 86*].

The mechanisms of homing are not entirely understood, but a remarkably high percentage of transplanted primitive hematopoietic cells are retained in the marrow shortly after intravenous injection. Cell adhesion molecules on marrow endothelial cells, termed selectins, which bind to carbohydrate-based ligands on early hematopoietic cells, may be responsible.

Finally, with relatively simple cryopreservation techniques, stem cells survive freezing and thawing with little, if any, damage.

The human hematopoietic stem cell expresses distinctive surface antigens. One of these, the CD34 antigen, is expressed on only 1% to 5% of normal adult bone marrow cells, but when marrow is cultured in vitro, virtually all colonies derive from the CD34+ population. Successful transplantation in humans can be carried out using only positively selected CD34+ cells. Over 90% of CD34+ cells also express CD38, but the 10% that are CD34+ and CD38– are the population best able to support long-term hematopoiesis in vitro and are thus considered a more primitive population. The most primitive subset of these cells stain poorly with Rh123, a mitochondrial dye. These cells also lack known markers of B cell or T cell lineage and are therefore said to be lineage negative.

Types of Hematopoietic Stem Cell Transplantation

Hematopoietic stem cell transplantation can be categorized according to the relation between the donor and the recipient and according to the anatomic source of the stem cell. Hematopoietic stem cells for transplantation may be syngeneic, allogeneic, or autologous.

SYNGENEIC TRANSPLANTATION

Identical twins are the best possible donors of stem cells. When syngeneic donors are used, neither graft rejection nor graft versus host disease (GVHD) will develop in the recipient. Syngenicity is easily established by DNA typing, using one of two techniques—either restriction fragment length polymorphisms or variable nucleotide tandem repeats. Only about one in 100 patients undergoing transplantation will have an identical twin.

ALLOGENEIC TRANSPLANTATION

Allogeneic transplantation is more complicated than syngeneic or autologous transplantation (see below) because of immunologic differences between donor and host. With hematopoietic stem cell transplantation, in which the immune system of the patient is provided by the graft, the clinical concerns are not only with the prevention of graft rejection by host cells surviving the pretransplant preparative regimen but also with the prevention of donor cells from causing immune-mediated injury to the patient (i.e., GVHD).

Immunologic reactivity between donor and host is largely mediated by immunocompetent cells that react with human leukocyte antigens (HLAs), which are encoded by genes of the major histocompatibility complex [*see Chapter 101*]. HLA molecules bind antigenic peptides and present them to T cells, an important step in the initiation of an immune response [*see Chapter 98*]. If two persons do not share the same HLA antigens, T cells taken from one person will react vigorously to the mismatched HLA molecules on the surface of the cells from the other. These are reactions against so-called major HLA determinants. Even when two persons who are not identical twins have identical HLA types, the antigenic peptides presented by the HLA antigens will differ, triggering a response against so-called minor HLA determinants.

The genes encoding HLA class I and class II antigens are tightly linked and tend to be inherited together as haplotypes with low recombination frequencies. For any given patient, there is a 25% probability that any one sibling has inherited the same paternal and maternal haplotype, making the siblings identical with regard to HLA genotype. Given that the average number of children per family in the United States is slightly more than two, the average chance that a patient has an HLA-matched sibling is approximately 35%. The formula for calculating the probability that a patient has an HLA-identical sibling is $1 - (0.75)^n$, where n equals the number of siblings.

Allogeneic transplantation has been performed using HLA-identical sibling donors, other matched and mismatched family member donors, and matched unrelated donors. The best results have been achieved with HLA-identical sibling donors.

With transplantation from family member donors who are identical for one haplotype but mismatched for a single locus (i.e., HLA-A, HLA-B, or HLA-D) on the other haplotype, the survival rate is nearly equal to that with HLA-identical donors, although there is a higher incidence of GVHD.[3] Transplants using family member donors mismatched for two or more loci have worse results—a higher incidence of GVHD and graft rejection and a lower probability of survival.[3]

Because of the highly polymorphic nature of HLA antigens, the probability that two unrelated persons will match is extremely low. Matched unrelated donor transplantation was first performed in the late 1970s. The broader application of this technique was made feasible by the formation of the National Marrow Donor Program in 1987. Since then, the number of unrelated-donor transplantations has rapidly increased [see Figure 1]. Currently, more than three million healthy persons have volunteered to serve as marrow donors in the United States alone, making the odds of finding an unrelated donor matched for HLA-A, HLA-B, and HLA-D approximately 50%. On average, it takes about 4 months from the time a search is initiated to identify a donor and begin transplantation. In 1999, approximately 1,600 unrelated-donor transplantations were performed in the United States. Initial results suggested that GVHD is more common and long-term cure rates are slightly worse with the use of matched unrelated donors than with the use of matched family member donors.[4]

AUTOLOGOUS TRANSPLANTATION

Autologous transplantation entails removal, cryopreservation, and later reinfusion of stem cells to reestablish hematopoietic function after the administration of high-dose chemotherapy or chemoradiotherapy. When compared with allogeneic transplantation, autologous transplantation has the advantage of avoiding GVHD and associated complications; disadvantages are that the autologous cells lack a graft versus tumor effect and may contain viable tumor cells. Removal of tumor cells by use of antibodies to tumor-specific antigens together with complement, toxins, or immunomagnetic beads is very efficient, reducing the number of tumor cells 1,000-fold to 10,000-fold.[5] Other methods of purifying stem cells that are currently under investigation are antibody adherence and flow techniques that would select normal hematopoietic stem cells while leaving tumor cells behind; in vitro treatment of the autologous cells with selective chemotherapeutic agents; and in vitro culturing to selectively grow hematopoietic cells. Although gene-marking studies have definitively demonstrated that remaining tumor cells can contribute to relapse,[6] it remains unknown which, if any, of the above-mentioned techniques can prevent relapse. Further, many of the techniques result in delayed hematologic and immunologic recovery after transplantation. Several retrospective analyses suggest that in vitro marrow treatment might be effective in acute myeloid leukemia (AML) and B cell non-Hodgkin lymphoma, but sufficiently large prospective, controlled studies have not been published.[5]

PERIPHERAL BLOOD STEM CELL TRANSPLANTATION

Hematopoietic stem cells normally circulate in the peripheral blood, albeit at very low numbers. Experiments in animal models have shown that at least 10 times more mononuclear cells are needed to rescue animals from lethal total body irradiation when the cells are collected from peripheral blood rather than from marrow of untreated animals. Initial attempts to use

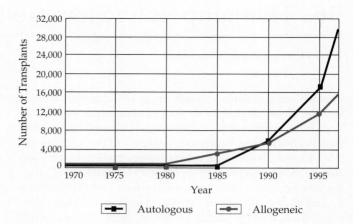

Figure 1 Depicted are the estimated total numbers of allogeneic and autologous hematopoietic stem cell transplantations performed worldwide from 1970 to 1997, according to estimates of the International Bone Marrow Transplant Registry. The number of allogeneic transplantations has increased rapidly since the formation of the National Marrow Donor Program in 1987.

peripheral blood stem cells as a source of hematopoietic grafts were complicated by the large number of collections (phereses) required—often seven or more—and by slow engraftment. Subsequently, it was shown that a marked increase in the number of hematopoietic progenitors in the blood, measured either as hematopoietic colony-forming units or as CD34+ cells, occurs during recovery from previous chemotherapy or shortly after exposure to hematopoietic growth factors.[7,8] This led to studies of the use of peripheral blood stem cells as a substitute for marrow. These studies were initially conducted in the autologous setting because peripheral blood stem cell collections contain a large number of T cells, which could induce GVHD if the collections were used for allogeneic transplantation. In the autologous setting, cells sufficient in number to achieve engraftment

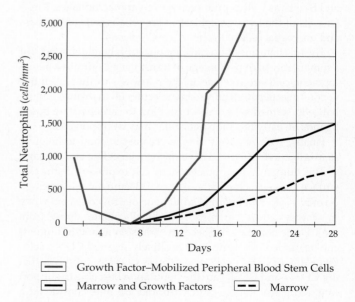

Figure 2 Shown are the typical patterns of myeloid recovery after hematopoietic stem cell transplantation using marrow alone, marrow plus posttransplant myeloid growth factors, and growth factor–mobilized peripheral blood stem cells.

can usually be collected with one to three leukaphereses of 4 hours' duration after treatment of the patient with granulocyte colony-stimulating factor (G-CSF) or granulocyte-macrophage colony-stimulating factor (GM-CSF). If more than 2.5 million CD34+ cells/kg are infused, recovery to 500 granulocytes/mm^3 by 12 days after transplantation and recovery to 20,000 platelets/mm^3 by 14 days after transplantation almost always occur.[9] This rate of recovery is significantly faster than with autologous marrow [see Figure 2]. It is not yet known whether peripheral blood stem cells are more likely or less likely than marrow to be contaminated with transplantable tumor cells.

Peripheral blood stem cells have also been used for allogeneic transplantation. Initial studies with G-CSF–mobilized peripheral blood stem cells from HLA-identical matched donors suggest they engraft more rapidly, and the incidence of acute GVHD does not appear greater than would be expected with marrow despite the transplantation of at least 10 times more mature T cells.[10] Recently conducted randomized trials confirm that the use of peripheral blood stem cells accelerates engraftment without increasing the incidence of acute GVHD. Although the incidence of chronic GVHD may be somewhat higher with peripheral blood stem cells, the incidence of tumor recurrence appears to be less.[11]

UMBILICAL CORD BLOOD TRANSPLANTATION

Umbilical cord blood is rich in CD34+ cells, and these cells can thus serve as an alternative source of stem cells. The first human umbilical cord blood transplantations were performed in the late 1980s for patients with Fanconi anemia. In a series of 44 children treated with cord blood from siblings, the speed of myeloid engraftment was similar to that seen with marrow transplantation, but platelet recovery was slower.[12] The incidence of GVHD was 6%, which was low; this probably reflected both the young ages of the recipients and the fact that umbilical cord blood is relatively devoid of mature T cells. Subsequently, several studies were undertaken that entailed banking unrelated umbilical cord blood and using it for subsequent transplantation.[13] A summary of the first 272 unrelated cord blood transplants facilitated by the New York Blood Center's program reported engraftment in approximately 90% of patients, but the time to engraftment was significantly prolonged—24 days for neutrophils and 72 days for platelets. A close relation was found between the number of nucleated cord blood cells infused and the incidence and speed of engraftment. The overall incidence of acute GVHD of grades II, III, and IV was 40%.

Transplantation Procedure

PREPARATIVE REGIMENS

A preparative regimen is administered before hematopoietic stem cells are transplanted. The purpose of this regimen is to eliminate the abnormal or malignant cells causing disease and to suppress the immune system sufficiently to avoid graft rejection. The appropriate regimen for any particular patient is determined by the disease to be treated, the age and health of the patient, and the source of the stem cells to be grafted.

At one extreme, patients undergoing transplantation for the treatment of SCID with stem cells from an HLA-matched sibling require no preparative regimen because there are no abnormal cells to eliminate (the disease being caused by a lack of normal cells) and because the patients' immune systems are al-ready sufficiently suppressed to avoid graft rejection. Patients with aplastic anemia lack a normal hematopoietic system but are sufficiently immunocompetent to reject allogeneic marrow if no immunosuppression is given. In this setting, treatment with high-dose cyclophosphamide plus antithymocyte globulin is sufficiently immunosuppressive to ensure engraftment as long as the donor is an HLA-identical sibling. When the transplant is from an unrelated donor, greater immunosuppression is required; thus, total body irradiation is often added. When transplantation is used to treat diseases characterized by an abnormal but nonmalignant population of cells, such as thalassemia and sickle cell anemia, the preparative regimen must eliminate the abnormal population and suppress the patient's immune system. To accomplish this, high-dose busulfan is often added to cyclophosphamide in the preparative regimen.

In developing preparative regimens for transplantation to treat malignancies, most investigators have focused on the use of agents that are highly active against the malignancy being treated and whose dominant dose-limiting toxicity in the nontransplant setting is myelosuppression. Thus, the therapies most commonly used are alkylating agents (e.g., cyclophosphamide, busulfan, thiotepa, melphalan, carmustine), etoposide, cytarabine, and total body irradiation.

Although high-dose preparative regimens are typically used when transplantations are performed to treat malignancies, the realization that some of the antitumor effects of transplantation are mediated by an allogeneic graft versus tumor effect has led investigators to ask whether less intensive, nonablative regimens might be effective and less toxic. Allogeneic engraftment can be reliably achieved using lower-dose regimens that combine fludarabine with busulfan, cyclophosphamide, or total body irradiation; complete responses have been achieved in a variety of malignancies with this approach. The appropriate role of nonablative transplants is currently undefined.[14]

STEM CELL COLLECTION AND INFUSION

Marrow is usually obtained from the donor's anterior and posterior iliac crests with the donor under spinal or general anesthesia. A total marrow volume equivalent to 10 to 15 ml/kg is withdrawn, with each aspiration site limited to 3 to 5 ml of marrow to avoid excessive dilution with peripheral blood. The heparinized marrow is filtered through 0.3 mm and 0.2 mm screens to remove bone spicules and fat. The marrow may require further in vitro treatment to remove other cells, such as donor red cells to avoid a hemolytic transfusion reaction in the setting of ABO incompatibility; donor T cells to avoid GVHD; and tumor cells from autologous marrow (see above). The risks of marrow donation are small: in one series, there were six serious but nonfatal complications out of 1,220 consecutive marrow donations.

Peripheral blood stem cells are usually collected by use of continuous flow apheresis from donors previously treated with hematopoietic growth factor alone or, in the case of autologous transplantation, after chemotherapy plus treatment with growth factors. Attempts are made to collect a minimum of 5×10^6 CD34+ cells/kg; there is consistent rapid engraftment with this dose.[9]

Marrow and peripheral blood stem cell infusions are usually well tolerated, though patients sometime develop fever, cough, or mild shortness of breath. Slowing the infusion usually alleviates these symptoms.

ENGRAFTMENT

The rate of engraftment depends on the source of the stem cells, the choice of prophylaxis against GVHD, and whether hematopoietic growth factors are used. The most rapid engraftment is seen with peripheral blood stem cells; recovery to granulocyte counts of 100 cells/mm^3 usually occurs by day 10 and counts of 500 cells/mm^3 by day 12. If marrow or umbilical cord blood is used, the granulocyte count usually reaches 100 cells/mm^3 by about day 16 and 500 cells/mm^3 by day 22. The rate of myeloid recovery can be accelerated by 4 to 6 days with the use of G-CSF or GM-CSF after marrow transplantation, but posttransplant growth factors have less of an effect when mobilized peripheral blood is the source of transplanted stem cells [*see Figure 2*].[15] The use of methotrexate after allogeneic transplantation delays recovery by an average of 4 days. Platelet recovery generally occurs shortly after granulocyte recovery.

Complications of Transplantation

EARLY DIRECT TOXICITIES OF THE PREPARATIVE REGIMEN

Pretransplant preparative regimens are associated with a substantial array of toxicities, which vary considerably depending on the specific regimen used. For example, after the standard cyclophosphamide–total body irradiation regimen, nausea, vomiting, and mild skin erythema develop immediately in almost all patients. Occasionally, hemorrhagic cystitis is seen despite bladder irrigation or therapy with a sulfhydryl compound (MESNA); in rare instances (fewer than 2% of cases), acute hemorrhagic carditis develops. Oral mucositis inevitably develops about 5 to 7 days after transplantation, usually requiring narcotic analgesia. Patient-controlled analgesia provides the greatest patient satisfaction and, surprisingly, results in a lower cumulative dose of narcotics. By 10 days after transplantation, complete alopecia and profound granulocy-

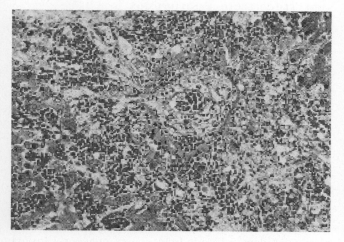

Figure 3   Photomicrograph of a liver biopsy stained with Trichrome shows the typical changes of veno-occlusive disease of the liver. A sublobular vein is outlined by dense, blue connective tissue in the outer adventitial layer. There is marked narrowing of the lumen of the vein by a widened and edematous subendothelial zone containing trapped red cells and loose extracellular matrix. The hepatocyte cords surrounding the vein are necrotic, and the intervening sinusoids are hemorrhagic. Deposition of coagulants in the sinusoids and in the subendothelial zone of the vein obstructs outflow of blood from the liver, producing sinusoidal hypertension and hepatomegaly.

topenia have developed in most patients.

Veno-occlusive disease of the liver is a serious complication of high-dose chemoradiotherapy; it develops in approximately 10% to 20% of patients.[16] Veno-occlusive disease of the liver, characterized by the development of ascites, tender hepatomegaly, jaundice, and fluid retention, may occur at any time during the first month after transplantation; the peak incidence occurs at around day 16. Histologic features of veno-occlusive disease of the liver include concentric narrowing or fibrous obliteration of terminal hepatic venules and sublobular veins and necrosis of zone 3 hepatocytes [*see Figure 3*]. Predisposing factors are pretransplant hepatitis of any cause and the use of more intensive conditioning regimens. Although the precise sequence of events leading to the clinical presentation of veno-occlusive disease is unknown, direct cytotoxic injury to hepatic venular and sinusoidal endothelium occurs early on, with subsequent deposition of fibrin and the development of a local hypercoagulable state. Direct cytotoxic injury to zone 3 hepatocytes is a contributing factor. Approximately 30% of patients who develop veno-occlusive disease of the liver die as a result of the disease, with progressive hepatic failure leading to a terminal hepatorenal syndrome. Antithrombotic and thrombolytic agents, including prostaglandin E^1 and tissue plasminogen activator, with or without heparin, have been evaluated as treatment. These therapies have been associated with significant toxicities, and randomized trials demonstrating efficacy are lacking. It has been reported that defibrotide, a polydeoxyribonucleotide, may benefit patients with veno-occlusive disease.[17]

Most pneumonias that occur after transplantation are caused by microbial agents, but idiopathic interstitial pneumonia, which is probably caused by direct toxicity of intensive chemoradiotherapy to the lung, occurs in 5% to 10% of patients.[18] Biopsies reveal some cases to be characterized by diffuse alveolar damage, whereas other cases have a more clearly interstitial component. Treatment with high-dose glucocorticoids is often attempted, but randomized trials evaluating their efficacy have not been performed.

LATE DIRECT TOXICITIES OF THE PREPARATIVE REGIMEN

Direct complications of chemoradiotherapy seen late after transplantation are a decreased growth rate in children and a delay in the development of secondary sex characteristics. Most children will have a deficiency in growth factor and should undergo replacement therapy. Ovarian failure develops in most postpubertal women. Azoospermia develops in most men. Aseptic osteonecrosis occurs in as many as 10% of transplant patients, particularly in those with chronic GVHD, necessitating corticosteroid treatment. Similarly, cataracts develop in 10% to 20% of patients; the risk is higher in patients who take steroids to treat chronic GVHD.

Patients treated with high-dose chemoradiotherapy and hematopoietic stem cell transplantation are at increased risk for the development of secondary malignancies.[19,20] The risk is highest among patients receiving T cell–depleted marrow and among those who receive multiple cycles of highly immunosuppressive drugs after transplantation to treat GVHD; in these cases, a high incidence of Epstein-Barr virus–associated lymphoproliferative disease is seen. A smaller increase is seen in the incidence of solid tumors after transplantation, with a 2.9% 10-year cumulative rate. The actuarial incidence of myelodysplasia after autologous transplantation for non-Hodgkin lymphoma and Hodgkin disease may be as high as 10%.[21]

GRAFT FAILURE

Although complete and sustained engraftment is the general rule after transplantation, in some cases marrow function does not return; and in other cases, after temporary engraftment, marrow function is lost. Graft failure after autologous transplantation can result from marrow damage before harvesting, during ex vivo treatment, during storage, or after exposure to myelotoxic agents after transplantation.[22] Infections with cytomegalovirus (CMV) or human herpesvirus type 6 may also result in poor marrow function. Graft failure after allogeneic transplantation may be the result of graft rejection and is more common after conditioning regimens that are less immunosuppressive, in recipients of T cell–depleted marrow, and in recipients of HLA-mismatched marrow.

The treatment of graft failure begins with removal of all potentially myelosuppressive agents. A reasonable second step is to attempt a short trial of a myeloid growth factor (GM-CSF or G-CSF); 40% to 50% of patients respond.[23] Identification of persistent host lymphocytes in peripheral blood or marrow of the patient suggests immunologic rejection. These patients should receive further immunosuppression before a second transplant is performed. Several studies have reported successful second transplants after a regimen of cyclophosphamide plus antithymocyte globulin or a regimen of anti-CD3 antibody plus high-dose steroids.

GRAFT VERSUS HOST DISEASE

When allogeneic T cells that are transferred with the graft or that develop from it react with targets of the genetically different host, GVHD results [see Chapter 98].[24] GVHD that develops within the first 3 months after transplantation is categorized as acute and is characterized by an erythematous maculopapular skin rash that, unlike many rashes, often manifests on the palms and soles [see Chapter 36]. Acute GVHD is also characterized by persistent anorexia or diarrhea, or both, and by liver disease, evidenced by increased levels of bilirubin, alanine and aspartate aminotransferases, and alkaline phosphatase. Also characteristic of acute GVHD is epithelial damage to the skin, liver, and intestines [see Figure 4]. Skin, liver, and endoscopic intestinal biopsies are the usual methods of establishing a diagnosis. The epidermis and hair follicles are damaged, small bile ducts show segmental disruption, and destruction of intestinal crypts results in mucosal ulceration. Clinical staging of acute GVHD is determined by the extent of involvement of skin, liver, and gut [see Table 1]. The incidence of acute GVHD increases in older patients, in recipients of mismatched marrow, and in patients unable to receive full doses of the drugs used to prevent GVHD.[25]

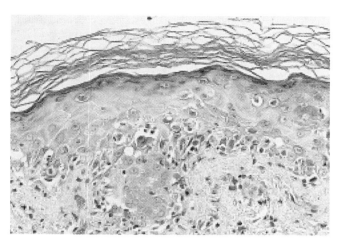

Figure 4 This photomicrograph of a skin biopsy stained with hematoxylin and eosin demonstrates the features of acute graft versus host disease of the skin. Both intercellular edema (spongiosis) and intracellular edema (reticular degeneration) of the lower epidermis are evident. Mononuclear cells are scattered throughout the epidermal area along with many bodies that have undergone apoptosis, including dead epidermal cells with hypereosinophilic cytoplasm and dense basophilic pyknotic nuclei. The inflammatory process has produced incontinence of melanin pigment into the papillary dermis as well as coarse intraepidermal blocks of melanin, leading to hyperpigmentation. Because the apoptosis and basal layer damage are extensive, the epidermis will become grossly scaly and will possibly slough.

Two general approaches are used to prevent acute GVHD: use of immunosuppressive agents during the early posttransplant period and removal of T cells from the transplanted cell population. Methotrexate alone and cyclosporine alone are equally effective as prophylaxis, but their use in combination is more effective. Prednisone, FK 506 (tacrolimus), and trimetrexate have also been used in various combinations. Removal of T cells from the allogeneic marrow is effective in preventing acute GVHD, but in most circumstances, it has been associated with an increased incidence of graft rejection and leukemic relapse. Accordingly, several potential therapies are now under study, including partial T cell depletion and complete T cell depletion followed by the reintroduction of a fraction of the T cells. Once acute GVHD develops, it can be treated with glucocorticoids, antithymocyte globulin, and monoclonal antibodies targeted against T cells or their receptors.

GVHD that develops or persists 3 months or more after transplantation is termed chronic GVHD. Chronic GVHD has features in common with collagen vascular diseases, including

Table 1 Clinical Staging of Acute Graft versus Host Disease*

Stage	Skin Changes	Liver	Gut
I	Maculopapular rash < 25% body surface	Bilirubin 2–3 mg/dl	Diarrhea 500–1,000 ml/day
II	Maculopapular rash 25%–30% body surface	Bilirubin 3–6 mg/dl	Diarrhea 1,000–1,500 ml/day
III	Generalized erythroderma	Bilirubin 6–15 mg/dl	Diarrhea > 1,500 ml/day
IV	Desquamation and bullae	Bilirubin > 15 mg/dl	Pain and ileus

*Overall severity ranges from mild skin involvement (stage I) to severe multiorgan involvement, usually with a fatal outcome (stage IV).

a malar rash, sclerodermatous changes, sicca syndrome, arthritis, obliterative bronchiolitis, and, in some cases, bile duct degeneration and cholestasis. Chronic GVHD develops in 20% to 40% of patients, more often in older patients and in those who previously had acute GVHD.[26] Prednisone, cyclosporine, or the two in combination is the usual treatment; in some studies, azathioprine or thalidomide was useful.[27] In most patients, chronic GVHD eventually resolves and immunosuppressive therapy can be withdrawn, but 1 to 3 years of treatment may be required. Patients with chronic GVHD who are on immunosuppressive therapy are susceptible to bacterial infections and should receive prophylactic antibiotics.

INFECTIOUS DISEASES

During the first 2 to 3 weeks after transplantation, all patients are severely granulocytopenic. Fever develops in most, and about one third have a positive blood culture. Febrile granulocytopenic patients should be treated with broad-spectrum antibiotics; in many centers, once patients become granulocytopenic, antibiotics are initiated to prevent septicemia. The prophylactic administration of fluconazole reduces the incidence of Candida albicans infection.[28] The treatment of patients who remain febrile despite antibiotic and antifungal therapy is a difficult challenge; in such cases, therapy is guided by individual aspects of the patient's condition and by the institution's experience. At most centers, therapy proceeds with the addition of amphotericin B to the patient's regimen.[29] Granulocyte transfusions can be effective in treating specific infections, particularly now that donors can be treated with G-CSF before donation to greatly increase the number of granulocytes that can be collected and transfused.[30] There is no established role, however, for prophylactic granulocyte transfusions. Laminar airflow isolation can reduce the incidence of infection but has no impact on survival in transplant patients treated for malignancy. With current methods of supportive care, the risk of death from an infectious cause during the period of granulocytopenia is less than 5%.

In the past, CMV infection frequently occurred after transplantation, particularly among recipients of allogeneic marrow. More recently, it has been shown that primary CMV infection can be prevented in CMV-seronegative patients by the use of CMV-seronegative blood products. In CMV-seropositive patients, treatment with ganciclovir as soon as virus excretion is evident can diminish the incidence of CMV-associated disease and death, but in some patients CMV disease develops before or at the same time as viral excretion is noted. Ganciclovir prophylaxis beginning at the time of engraftment can prevent the development of CMV infection in most patients, but ganciclovir causes significant marrow suppression in at least 10% of patients.[31] Currently at most centers, after transplantation, peripheral blood is monitored for the development of CMV antigenemia, and prophylaxis with ganciclovir is initiated only if and when patients test positive for the presence of CMV antigen. Foscarnet is effective for patients who develop CMV antigenemia or infection despite ganciclovir therapy or for patients who cannot tolerate ganciclovir.

Herpes simplex virus infection, when not prevented, contributes to the severity of early oral mucositis and esophagitis. However, the prophylactic use of acyclovir at a dosage of 250 mg/m² I.V. every 8 hours can prevent herpes simplex virus reactivation in almost all seropositive patients.

Pneumocystis carinii once caused pneumonia in 5% to 10% of patients after transplantation, but now this complication can be prevented in virtually all patients by first treating the patient with oral trimethoprim-sulfamethoxazole for 1 week before transplantation and then resuming treatment 2 days a week once engraftment occurs. Desensitization should be attempted in patients with allergic reactions to trimethoprim-sulfamethoxazole, because neither dapsone nor I.V. pentamidine is as effective as trimethoprim-sulfamethoxazole in preventing P. carinii infection.

More than 3 months after transplantation, patients are still at risk for varicella-zoster virus infections and, if they have chronic GVHD, for recurrent bacterial infections. Varicella-zoster virus infection usually manifests initially as localized disease (i.e., herpes zoster, or shingles), but it can disseminate; disseminated infection is often fatal if left untreated. Thus, patients with localized varicella-zoster virus infection should be treated with acyclovir to prevent dissemination. Many centers now routinely place all allogeneic transplant recipients on prophylactic acyclovir therapy for the first year after transplantation.

Hematopoietic Stem Cell Transplantation for Specific Diseases

TREATMENT OF IMMUNODEFICIENCY STATES

The widest experience in treating immunodeficiency with hematopoietic stem cell transplantation has been in the treatment of SCID.[32] When current techniques of supportive care are used, the expected outcome of transplantation from an HLA-identical donor is excellent, with a better than 90% probability of long-term survival [see Table 2]. In patients without matched donors, transplantation from a haplotype-mismatched parent results in engraftment and survival longer than 2 years in 50% to 70% of patients. The experience in the treatment of Wiskott-Aldrich syndrome and other immunodeficiency states is limited. Cures have been noted in more than half of patients, with the best results seen in patients who undergo transplantation when they are younger than 5 years.

TREATMENT OF NONMALIGNANT DISEASES OF HEMATOPOIESIS

Aplastic Anemia

Transplantation from matched siblings after a preparative regimen of high-dose cyclophosphamide and antithymocyte globulin, together with the use of methotrexate and cyclosporine for GVHD prophylaxis, is a very effective regimen for patients with aplastic anemia. Current results suggest a cure rate greater than 90% [see Table 2].[33] Results with mismatched or unrelated matched donors are considerably worse; therefore, patients with aplastic anemia who are without sibling donors are often given a trial of immunosuppressive therapy before transplantation.

Thalassemia

Marrow transplantation from an HLA-identical sibling after a preparative regimen of busulfan and cyclophosphamide can cure from 70% to 90% of patients with thalassemia major [see Table 2]. The best results have been obtained in patients who undergo transplantation before they develop hepatomegaly or portal fibrosis and who have been given adequate iron chelation therapy. In one study, among 121 such patients, the proba-

Table 2 Disease-Free Survival after Hematopoietic Stem Cell Transplantation

Disease	Five-Year Disease-Free Survival (%)
Chronic myeloid leukemia	
Chronic phase	60–70
Accelerated phase	30–40
Blastic phase	15–20
Acute myeloid leukemia	
First remission	40–70
Second remission	30
Chronic lymphocytic leukemia	50
Acute lymphocytic leukemia	30–50
Multiple myeloma	35
Non-Hodgkin lymphoma	
After first relapse, chemosensitive tumors	40–50
Hodgkin disease	
First treatment after standard treatment	40–70
Advanced disease	15–30
Myelodysplastic syndromes	45
Severe aplastic anemia	> 90
Thalassemia major	70–90
Fanconi anemia	50–70
Sickle cell disease	50–90
Severe combined immunodeficiency disease	90
Breast cancer (stage IV disease)	10–30

bilities of survival and disease-free survival 5 years after transplantation were 95% and 90%, respectively.[34] Prolonged survival can also be achieved with aggressive chelation therapy, but transplantation remains the only curative treatment. Fewer than 30% of patients with thalassemia have an HLA-identical sibling. Selection of alternative donors of hematopoietic stem cells (i.e., unrelated persons or HLA-nonidentical family members) has been aided by the establishment of worldwide donor registries, by improvements in the methods of controlling GVHD, and by prevention of fungal and cytomegalovirus infection.

Sickle Cell Anemia

Experience in transplantation for sickle cell disease is small but growing. In a European study of 100 patients with sickle cell disease who received transplants from HLA-matched siblings, the survival rate at 2 years was 90%, and disease-free survival was 79%.[35] In an American study of 22 patients, similar rates of 91% and 73%, respectively, were reported.[36]

Other Nonmalignant Diseases

Hematopoietic stem cell transplantation has been used successfully to treat a variety of other nonmalignant but nonetheless fatal diseases. Included in this group are congenital disorders of white cells, including Kostmann syndrome, chronic granulomatous disease, neutrophil actin defects, leukocyte adhesion deficiency, and Chédiak-Higashi syndrome. Congenital anemias, including Fanconi anemia and Blackfan-Diamond anemia, are likewise treatable with hematopoietic stem cell transplantation.[37,38] Osteopetrosis is a rare inherited disorder caused by an inability of the osteoclast to resorb bone. Because the osteoclast is a specialized macrophage derived from the marrow, it follows that this disease can be treated with marrow transplantation. A final category of treatable nonmalignant diseases are storage diseases caused by enzymatic deficiencies, including Maroteaux-Lamy syndrome, metachromatic leukodystrophy, Gaucher disease, Hurler syndrome, and Hunter syndrome. Transplantation for these disorders has not been universally successful, but treatment early in the disease course, before irreversible end-organ damage occurs, increases the chance for a successful outcome. Studies have recently been done on the use of transplantation in the treatment of severe autoimmune disorders. These studies are based on the demonstration that transplantation can cure autoimmune diseases in some animal models and on the observation that some patients with coexistent hematologic malignancies and autoimmune disorders have been cured of both with transplantation.

TREATMENT OF MALIGNANT DISEASES

Acute Myeloid Leukemia

Allogeneic marrow transplantation cures 15% to 20% of patients with AML who fail induction therapy and, indeed, is the only form of therapy that can cure such patients.[39] Thus, all patients 55 years of age or younger with newly diagnosed AML should have their HLA type determined, as should their families, soon after diagnosis to enable transplantation for those who fail induction therapy. Allogeneic transplantation can cure approximately 30% of patients in second remission and 35% of patients in untreated first relapse—situations that are clear indications for the procedure, because these results are superior to those achieved without transplantation.[40,41] The best results with allogeneic transplantation for AML are obtained in patients undergoing transplantation in first remission, in whom a cure rate of 40% to 70% is reported [see Table 2].

In 14 prospective studies, the cure rate with marrow transplantation for patients with HLA-matched siblings ranged from 40% to 64%, whereas the cure rate for chemotherapy for patients without HLA-matched siblings ranged from 19% to 24%, suggesting that allogeneic transplantation is the preferred form of postremission therapy for younger patients with AML and a matched sibling.[42-44] However, important advances have been made in both chemotherapy and transplantation since many of these studies were conducted. Further, it remains untested whether transplantation in first remission is superior to a regimen of initial chemotherapy followed by transplantation as salvage therapy.

In several phase II studies, autologous transplantation for patients with AML in first and second remission yielded results not dissimilar to those achieved with allogeneic transplantation. In general, relapse rates after autologous transplantation have been substantially higher than those seen with allogeneic transplantation, but the mortality from transplant-related complications has been lower. Several large trials compared allogeneic transplantation, autologous transplantation, and aggressive chemotherapy as postremission therapy for patients with AML in first remission. The European Organization for Research and Treatment of Cancer compared these therapies in 333 patients with AML in first remission and found the rate of disease-free survival at 4 years to be 54% with allogeneic transplantation, 49% with autologous transplantation, and 30% with continued chemotherapy.[45] In a recent update of a similarly designed American Intergroup study, the estimated rate of survival at 5 years was 52% with allogeneic transplantation, 42% with autologous transplantation, and 39% with chemotherapy.[46] In a study from the United Kingdom Medical Research Council, patients with AML in first remission who had been treated with three cycles of postremission therapy were randomized either to receive no further therapy or to undergo autologous transplantation in first remission.[47] The group who underwent transplantation had a lower relapse rate, and the rates of disease-free survival and overall survival were improved.

Acute Lymphocytic Leukemia

As with AML, allogeneic transplantation can cure 15% to 20% of patients with acute lymphocytic leukemia (ALL) who fail induction therapy or in whom chemotherapy-resistant disease develops; thus, these patients are candidates for the procedure. The results of transplantation for patients in second remission are better, with cure rates of 30% to 50% [see Table 2]. However, further intensive chemotherapy also can cure some patients who suffered initial relapse. This is particularly true for children who experience relapse more than 18 months after initial induction chemotherapy. A study comparing the use of allogeneic transplantation in 255 children with the use of chemotherapy in an equal number of children found the rate of disease-free survival at 5 years to be 40% in transplant patients and 17% in chemotherapy patients. The relative benefits of transplantation were similar for children with short and long initial remissions. Thus, allogeneic transplantation can be recommended for all patients with ALL in second complete remission who have appropriate donors.[48]

Allogeneic transplantation for ALL in first remission results in long-term disease-free survival in 40% to 70% of adult patients. In a retrospective study comparing these results with those achieved with chemotherapy, no clear advantage could be found for either approach.[49] In the largest prospective, randomized study published to date (involving 572 patients), the 3-year disease-free survival rate for those undergoing allogeneic transplantation was 43%; for those undergoing autologous transplantation, 39%; and for those receiving continued chemotherapy, 32%.[50] Some categories of patients, such as those with Philadelphia chromosome–positive ALL, would probably benefit from transplantation in first remission.[51] Studies comparing allogeneic transplantation with autologous transplantation in ALL patients have consistently shown a substantially higher relapse rate with autologous transplantation but a somewhat higher rate of death from complications with allogeneic transplantation. On balance, most investigators recommend use of allogeneic marrow when an appropriate donor is available.

Myelodysplastic Syndromes

The myelodysplastic syndromes are generally considered to be incurable except with marrow transplantation. In some patients, the myelodysplastic syndromes have a relatively indolent course, and transplantation can be safely withheld until the disease progresses. However, once significant granulocytopenia (fewer than 1,000 cells/mm³) or thrombocytopenia (fewer than 40,000 cells/mm³) develops or the proportion of blast cells in the marrow exceeds 5%, transplantation should be seriously considered, because without transplantation, the expected survival time is short. When an HLA-matched sibling is available to serve as a donor, the chance of long-term survival with transplantation is roughly 45%, with better results being obtained in younger patients and in those who receive transplants earlier in the course of their disease.[52] No role has been established for autologous transplantation in the myelodysplastic syndromes, but this is a current focus of research.

Chronic Myeloid Leukemia

Allogeneic and syngeneic marrow transplantation are the only forms of therapy known to cure chronic myeloid leukemia (CML). Five-year disease-free survival rates are 15% to 20% for patients who undergo transplantation in blast crisis, 30% to 40% for patients who undergo transplantation during the accelerated phase, and 60% to 70% for patients who undergo transplantation during the chronic phase [see Table 2].

Time from diagnosis influences the outcome of transplantation during the chronic phase. The best results are obtained in patients who receive transplants within 1 year of diagnosis; progressively worse results are seen the longer the procedure is delayed.[53] Previous exposure to busulfan is an adverse risk factor for transplantation.[53] Thus, patients younger than 55 years with HLA-matched siblings should probably undergo transplantation as soon as possible after diagnosis, and the use of busulfan during the chronic phase should be avoided. A small number of patients between 55 and 65 years of age with CML have undergone transplantation, with results not significantly worse than those seen in younger patients.[54]

Although the initial experience with the use of unrelateddonor transplantation in chronic myeloid leukemia was substantially worse than the experience with matched-sibling transplantation, more recent results at some centers demonstrate a 70% probability of disease-free survival at 3 years.[55]

Autologous transplantation for the treatment of CML is increasingly being studied. At present, there are no data to suggest that this technique can lead to long-term cures. There is, however, some suggestion that autologous transplantation may slow the rate of disease progression.[56]

Chronic Lymphocytic Leukemia

Use of marrow transplantation in chronic lymphocytic leukemia (CLL) has received only limited attention, probably because of the indolent nature of the disease and its propensity to occur in older patients. Among the small number of patients receiving allogeneic transplantation, complete remissions were achieved in many, and approximately half remained disease free, though follow-up has been short.[57,58] However, the transplant-related mortality in this group of patients has been substantial. The number of patients treated with autologous transplantation is even smaller, and their follow-up is shorter.[58] Complete remissions have been achieved, some of which appear to be sustained. Further study is needed to determine whether transplantation significantly improves long-term outcome in CLL.

Non-Hodgkin Lymphoma

Patients with disseminated intermediate or high-grade non-Hodgkin lymphoma who fail conventional therapy can seldom be cured without transplantation. High-dose therapy followed by autologous or allogeneic marrow transplantation can cure a substantial portion of such patients. A number of studies have documented cure rates of 40% to 50% in patients who receive transplants after an initial relapse and whose tumors remain sensitive to chemotherapy [see Table 2].[59] In one randomized study of 216 patients, the 5-year disease-free survival rate for patients who underwent autologous transplantation for chemosensitive disease was 46%, compared with 12% in the chemotherapy group (P = 0.001). Cure rates decrease substantially once the disease becomes resistant to conventional-dose chemotherapy.[59] A poor performance status and large tumor bulk are additional adverse risk factors. As in other diseases, patients who receive transplants of allogeneic marrow have a lower relapse rate but a higher risk of nonrelapse mortality than patients who receive transplants of autologous marrow.[60]

For most categories of intermediate- and high-grade non-Hodgkin lymphoma, the outcomes for allogeneic and autologous transplantation appear roughly similar, though an advantage has been suggested for the use of allogeneic transplantation for patients with lymphoblastic lymphoma. The role of transplantation for patients in first remission is unsettled. Among the randomized studies so far performed, some have found a significant benefit, some have found no benefit, and others have found a benefit only for the subgroup of patients with high-intermediate–risk or high-risk disease.[61,62]

Autologous marrow transplantation has also been studied in patients with low-grade disease. The probabilities of survival at 3 years after transplantation have averaged 83% for patients who undergo transplantation in first remission, 65% for patients in first relapse or second remission, and 50% for patients with more advanced disease. Whether these results are superior to what could be achieved with therapies that do not involve transplantation has not been demonstrated in prospective, randomized trials. Further, late relapses have been seen after autologous transplantation, raising questions about the possibility of cure, but studies of allogeneic transplantation for this group showed long-term disease-free survival in some patients.

Hodgkin Disease

The results of transplantation for Hodgkin disease mimic those for non-Hodgkin lymphoma. A substantial portion of patients who failed first-line chemotherapy for Hodgkin disease can be cured with salvage transplantation. Results of treatment for recurrent Hodgkin disease are better when transplantation is performed in patients who have chemotherapy-sensitive disease with minimal tumor bulk and a good performance status. In this setting, cure rates of 40% to 70% have been reported [see Table 2]. As with non-Hodgkin lymphoma, lower relapse rates but higher nonrelapse mortality are seen with the use of allogeneic stem cells than with the use of autologous stem cells.[63] There is currently no established role for transplantation for patients in first remission, though pilot studies in patients with high-risk disease are being performed.

Multiple Myeloma

Allogeneic marrow transplantation has been used to treat patients with multiple myeloma. Overall survival rates for patients in whom first-line therapy failed averaged 35% at 5 years after allogeneic transplantation [see Table 2]. An important finding is that there appears to be a plateau in the rate of disease-free survival, suggesting that some of these patients were cured, but transplant-associated complications were substantial and

occurred more frequently than in most other hematologic malignancies.[64]

Autologous transplantation is also being studied. There is less evidence that this approach can lead to long-term cure, at least with current techniques. However, when employed before patients have resistant disease, autologous transplantation can result in a substantial reduction in tumor burden and, in many cases, at least temporary complete remissions. In one large randomized study, autologous transplantation performed shortly after patients achieved a complete remission led to significantly longer disease-free survival and greater overall survival than further conventional chemotherapy.[65]

Other Hematologic Malignancies

Long-term survival has been documented after allogeneic marrow transplantation for patients with hairy-cell leukemia, myelofibrosis, and various myeloproliferative syndromes, but the number of patients reported in any one disease category is small.

Breast Cancer

In women with stage IV breast cancer, high-dose chemotherapy followed by autologous transplantation results in a higher rate of complete remission than standard-dose chemotherapy. Studies of a large number of patients have reported disease-free survival at 5 years to be 10% to 30% [see Table 2].[66] In patients who underwent transplantation for stage IV disease, the highest rates of progression-free survival (32%) were seen in patients who received transplants after they had achieved a complete response to conventional chemotherapy; lower rates were seen in patients with partially responding disease (13%) or progressive disease (7%). Although these results appear to be superior to those achieved with standard-dose chemotherapy, longer follow-up and the completion of randomized trials are needed to determine whether patients who achieved complete response are cured and whether this percentage of patients is truly higher than that seen with standard-dose chemotherapy. On the basis of these initial high response rates, high-dose chemotherapy followed by autologous transplantation has been increasingly studied in patients with earlier-stage disease. Pooled registry results show a 42% 3-year disease-free survival for patients who received transplants for inflammatory breast cancer and a 74% 3-year disease-free survival for women with high-risk (> 10 nodes) stage II disease. Randomized trials are in progress that will test whether autologous transplantation leads to improved cure rates for women with high-risk disease.

Testicular Cancer

Although standard-dose chemotherapy for testicular cancer is very effective, conventional regimens fail in 30% to 40% of patients. High-dose chemotherapy with autologous marrow support has resulted in a 2-year disease-free survival of approximately 20% in patients with advanced recurrent disease—a rate seemingly better than that achieved with conventional approaches.[67]

Other Solid Tumors

The utility of high-dose chemotherapy with autologous stem cell support for several other solid tumors, including ovarian cancer, small cell lung cancer, neuroblastoma, and pediatric sarcomas, is being studied. As in virtually all other situations, best results occur in patients with limited tumor bulk in whom the tumor remains sensitive to conventional-dose chemotherapy. Randomized trials evaluating the usefulness of transplantation in these settings have not been reported.

Treatment of Posttransplant Relapse

Patients with malignancies who experience relapse after autologous transplantation occasionally respond to further conventional-dose chemotherapy, particularly when the interval from transplantation to relapse is long. There are more options available to the patient who experiences relapse after allogeneic transplantation. Patients with CML frequently respond to interferon therapy, and other patients occasionally respond to withdrawal of immunosuppression. Patients who experience relapse after allogeneic transplantation sometimes respond to nonirradiated donor lymphocyte infusions. In a summary of 258 patients reported by a European registry, complete responses were seen in 75% of patients with CML, 38% with myelodysplasia, 24% with AML, and 15% with myeloma.[68] Responses were seldom seen in ALL. The major complications of posttransplant donor lymphocyte infusions have been GVHD and myelosuppression, both of which can be severe or fatal. Starting the transfusion with a low cell dose and then gradually increasing the dose can lessen the risk of severe toxicity. A second marrow transplantation can occasionally be effective, particularly in younger patients and in patients who experience a longer interval from first transplant to relapse and who do not have advanced disease.

References

1. Horowitz MM, Rowlings PA: An update from the International Bone Marrow Transplant Registry and the Autologous Blood and Marrow Transplant Registry on current activity in hematopoietic stem cell transplantation. Curr Opin Hematol 4:395, 1997

2. Spangrude GJ, Heimfeld S, Weissman IL: Purification and characterization of mouse hematopoietic stem cells. Science 241:58, 1988

3. Anasetti C, Amos D, Beatty PG, et al: Effect of HLA compatibility on engraftment of bone marrow transplants in patients with leukemia or lymphoma. N Engl J Med 320:197, 1989

4. Kernan NA, Bartsch G, Ash RC, et al: Analysis of 462 transplantations from unrelated donors facilitated by the National Marrow Donor Program. N Engl J Med 328:593, 1993

5. Gribben JG, Freedman AS, Neuberg D, et al: Immunologic purging of marrow assessed by PCR before autologous bone marrow transplantation for B-cell lymphoma. N Engl J Med 325:1525, 1991

6. Brenner MK, Rill DR, Moen RC, et al: Gene-marking to trace origin of relapse after autologous bone-marrow transplantation. Lancet 341:85, 1993

7. Richman CM, Weiner RS, Yankee RA: Increase in circulating stem cells following chemotherapy in man. Blood 47:1031, 1976

8. Socinski MA, Cannistra SA, Elias A, et al: Granulocyte-macrophage colony stimulating factor expands the circulating haemopoietic progenitor cell compartment in man. Lancet 1:1194, 1988

9. Bensinger WI, Longin K, Appelbaum F, et al: Peripheral blood stem cells (PBSCs) collected after recombinant granulocyte colony stimulating factor (rhG-CSF): an analysis of factors correlating with the tempo of engraftment after transplantation. Br J Haematol 87:825, 1994

10. Bensinger WI, Weaver CH, Appelbaum FR, et al: Transplantation of allogeneic peripheral blood stem cells mobilized by recombinant human granulocyte colony-stimulating factor. Blood 85:1655, 1995

11. Bensinger WI, Martin P, Storer B, et al: A prospective, randomized trial of transplantation of marrow vs. peripheral blood stem cells from HLA-identical siblings in patients treated for hematologic malignancies. N Engl J Med (in press)

12. Wagner JE, Kernan NA, Steinbuch M, et al: Allogeneic sibling umbilical-cord-blood transplantation in children with malignant and non-malignant disease. Lancet 346:214, 1995

13. Kurtzberg L, Laughlin M, Graham ML, et al: Placental blood as a source of hematopoietic stem cells for transplantation into unrelated recipients. N Engl J Med 335:157, 1996

14. Khouri IF, Keating M, Korbling M, et al: Transplant-lite: induction of graft-versus-malignancy using fludarabine-based nonablative chemotherapy and allogeneic blood progenitor-cell transplantation as treatment for lymphoid malignancies. J Clin Oncol 16:2817, 1998

15. Nemunaitis J, Rabinowe SN, Singer JW, et al: Recombinant granulocyte-macrophage colony-stimulating factor after autologous bone marrow transplantation for lymphoid cancer. N Engl J Med 324:1773, 1991

16. Bearman SI: The syndrome of hepatic veno-occlusive disease after marrow transplantation. Blood 85:3005, 1995

17. Richardson PG, Elias AD, Krishnan A, et al: Treatment of severe veno-occlusive disease with defibrotide: compassionate use results in response without significant toxicity in a high-risk population. Blood 92:737, 1998

18. Crawford SW, Hackman RC: Clinical course of idiopathic pneumonia after marrow transplantation. Am Rev Respir Dis 147:1393, 1993

19. Deeg HJ, Socie G, Schoch G, et al: Malignancies after marrow transplantation for aplastic anemia and Fanconi's anemia: a joint Seattle and Paris analysis of results in 700 patients. Blood 87:386, 1996

20. Curtis RE, Rowlings PA, Deeg HJ, et al: Solid cancers after bone marrow transplantation. N Engl J Med 336:897, 1997

21. Stone RM, Neuberg D, Soiffer R, et al: Myelodysplastic syndrome as a late complication following autologous bone marrow transplantation for non-Hodgkin's lymphoma. J Clin Oncol 12:2535, 1994

22. Rabinowe SN, Neuberg D, Bierman PJ, et al: Long-term follow-up of a phase III study of recombinant human granulocyte-macrophage colony-stimulating factor after autologous bone marrow transplantation for lymphoid malignancies. Blood 81:1903, 1993

23. Nemunaitis J, Singer JW, Buckner CD, et al: Use of recombinant human granulocyte-macrophage colony-stimulating factor in graft failure after bone marrow transplantation. Blood 76:245, 1990

24. Ferrara JLM, Deeg HJ: Graft-versus-host disease. N Engl J Med 324:667, 1991

25. Nash RA, Pepe MS, Storb R, et al: Acute graft-versus-host disease: analysis of risk factors after allogeneic marrow transplantation and prophylaxis with cyclosporine and methotrexate. Blood 80:1838, 1992

26. Atkinson K, Horowitz MM, Gale RP, et al: Risk factors for chronic graft-versus-host disease after HLA-identical sibling bone marrow transplantation. Blood 75:2459, 1990

27. Vogelsang GB, Farmer ER, Hess AD, et al: Thalidomide for the treatment of chronic graft-versus-host disease. N Engl J Med 326:1055, 1992

28. Goodman JL, Winston DJ, Greenfield RA, et al: A controlled trial of fluconazole to prevent fungal infections in patients undergoing bone marrow transplantation. N Engl J Med 326:845, 1992

29. Pizzo PA: Management of fever in patients with cancer and treatment-induced neutropenia. N Engl J Med 328:1323, 1993

30. Bensinger WI, Price TH, Dale DC, et al: The effects of daily recombinant human granulocyte colony-stimulating factor administration on normal granulocyte donors undergoing leukapheresis. Blood 81:1883, 1993

31. Goodrich JM, Bowden RA, Fisher L, et al: Ganciclovir prophylaxis to prevent cytomegalovirus disease after allogeneic marrow transplant. Ann Intern Med 118:173, 1993

32. Fischer A, Landais P, Friedrich W, et al: European experience of bone-marrow transplantation for severe combined immunodeficiency. Lancet 336:850, 1990

33. Storb R, Etzioni R, Anasetti C, et al: Cyclophosphamide combined with antithymocyte globulin in preparation for allogeneic marrow transplants in patients with aplastic anemia. Blood 84:941, 1994

34. Lucarelli G, Galimberti M, Polchi P, et al: Marrow transplantation in patients with thalassemia responsive to iron chelation therapy. N Engl J Med 329:840, 1993

35. Vermylen C, Cornu G: Bone marrow transplantation in sickle cell anemia: the European experience. Am J Pediatr Hematol Oncol 16:18, 1994

36. Walters MC, Patience M, Leisenring W, et al: Bone marrow transplantation for sickle cell anaemia. N Engl J Med 335:369, 1996

37. Guardiola P, Pasquini R, Dokal I, et al: Outcome of 69 allogeneic stem cell transplantations for Fanconi anemia using HLA-matched unrelated donors: a study on behalf of the European Group for Blood and Marrow Transplantation. Blood 95:422, 2000

38. MacMillan ML, Auerbach AD, Davies SM, et al: Haematopoietic cell transplantation in patients with Fanconi anaemia using alternate donors: results of a total body irradiation dose escalation trial. Br J Haematol 109:121, 2000

39. Biggs JC, Horowitz MM, Gale RP, et al: Bone marrow transplants may cure patients with acute leukemia never achieving remission with chemotherapy. Blood 80:1090, 1992

40. Clift RA, Buckner CD, Appelbaum FR, et al: Allogeneic marrow transplantation during untreated first relapse of acute myeloid leukemia. J Clin Oncol 10:1723, 1992

41. Gale RP, Horowitz MM, Rees JKH, et al: Chemotherapy versus transplants for acute myelogenous leukemia in second remission. Leukemia 10:13, 1996

42. Nesbit ME Jr, Buckley JD, Feig SA, et al: Chemotherapy for induction of remission of childhood acute myeloid leukemia followed by marrow transplantation or multiagent chemotherapy: a report from the children's cancer group. J Clin Oncol 12:127, 1994

43. Archimbaud E, Thomas X, Michallet M, et al: Prospective genetically randomized comparison between intensive postinduction chemotherapy and bone marrow transplantation in adults with newly diagnosed acute myeloid leukemia. J Clin Oncol 12:262, 1994

44. Hewlett J, Kopecky JK, Head D, et al: A prospective evaluation of the roles of allogeneic marrow transplantation and low-dose monthly maintenance chemotherapy in the treatment of adult acute myelogenous leukemia (AML): a Southwest Oncology Group study. Leukemia 9:562, 1995

45. Zittoun RA, Mandelli F, Wellemze R, et al: Autologous or allogeneic bone marrow transplantation compared with intensive chemotherapy in acute myelogenous leu-

kemia. N Engl J Med 332:217, 1995

46. Cassileth PA, Harrington D, Appelbaum FR, et al: A comparison of chemotherapy versus autologous bone marrow transplantation versus allogeneic bone marrow transplantation in first remission of adult acute myeloid leukemia: an intergroup study (E3489). N Engl J Med 339:1649, 1998

47. Burnett AK, Goldstone AH, Stevens RM, et al: Randomised comparison of addition of autologous bone-marrow transplantation to intensive chemotherapy for acute myeloid leukaemia in first remission: results of MRC AML 10 trial. Lancet 351:700, 1998

48. Barrett AJ, Horowitz MM, Pollock BH, et al: Bone marrow transplants from HLA-identical siblings as compared with chemotherapy for children with acute lymphoblastic leukemia in a second remission. N Engl J Med 19:1253, 1994

49. Horowitz MM, Messerer D, Hoelzer D, et al: Chemotherapy compared with bone marrow transplantation for adults with acute lymphoblastic leukemia in first remission. Ann Intern Med 115:13, 1991

50. Fiere D, Lepage E, Sebban C, et al: Adult acute lymphoblastic leukemia: a multicentric randomized trial testing bone marrow transplantation as postremission therapy. J Clin Oncol 11:1990, 1993

51. Barrett AJ, Horowitz MM, Ash RC, et al: Bone marrow transplantation for Philadelphia chromosome–positive acute lymphoblastic leukemia. Blood 79:3067, 1992

52. Appelbaum FR, Anderson JE: Allogeneic bone marrow transplantation for myelodysplastic syndrome: outcomes analysis according to IPSS score. Leukemia 12(suppl 1): S25, 1998

53. Goldman JM, Szydlo R, Horowitz MM, et al: Choice of pretransplant treatment and timing of transplants for chronic myelogenous leukemia in chronic phase. Blood 82:2235, 1993

54. Clift RA, Appelbaum FR, Thomas ED: Treatment of chronic myeloid leukemia by marrow transplantation (editorial). Blood 82:1954, 1993

55. Hansen JA, Gooley TA, Martin PJ, et al: Unrelated donor marrow transplants for patients with chronic myeloid leukemia in chronic phase. N Engl J Med 338:962, 1998

56. McGlave PB, De Fabritiis P, Deisseroth A, et al: Autologous transplants for chronic myelogenous leukaemia: results from eight transplant groups. Lancet 343:1486, 1994

57. Michallet M, Archimbaud E, Bandini G, et al: HLA-identical sibling bone marrow transplantation in younger patients with chronic lymphocytic leukemia: European Group for Blood and Marrow Transplantation and the International Bone Marrow Transplant Registry. Ann Intern Med 124:311, 1996

58. Rabinowe SN, Soiffer RJ, Gribben JG, et al: Autologous and allogeneic bone marrow transplantation for poor prognosis patients with B-cell chronic lymphocytic

leukemia. Blood 82:1366, 1993

59. Philip T, Guglielmi C, Hagenbeek A, et al: Autologous bone marrow transplantation as compared with salvage chemotherapy in relapses of chemotherapy-sensitive non-Hodgkin's lymphoma. N Engl J Med 333:1540, 1995

60. Chopra R, Goldstone AH, Pearce R, et al: Autologous versus allogeneic bone marrow transplantation for non-Hodgkin's lymphoma: a case-controlled analysis of the European Bone Marrow Transplant Group Registry data. J Clin Oncol 10:1690, 1992

61. Haioun C, Lepage E, Gisselbrecht C, et al: Benefit of autologous bone marrow transplantation over sequential chemotherapy in poor-risk aggressive non-Hodgkin's lymphoma: updated results of the prospective study LNH87-2. J Clin Oncol 15:1131, 1997

62. Gianni AM, Bregni M, Siena S, et al: High-dose chemotherapy and autologous bone marrow transplantation compared with MACOP-B in aggressive B-cell lymphoma. N Engl J Med 336:1290, 1997

63. Anderson JE, Litzow MR, Appelbaum FR, et al: Allogeneic, syngeneic, and autologous marrow transplantation for Hodgkin's disease: the 21-year Seattle experience. J Clin Oncol 11:2342, 1993

64. Gahrton G, Tura S, Ljungman P, et al: Allogeneic bone marrow transplantation in multiple myeloma. N Engl J Med 325:1267, 1991

65. Attal M, Harousseau JL, Stoppa AM, et al: A prospective, randomized trial of autologous bone marrow transplantation and chemotherapy in multiple myeloma. N Engl J Med 335:91, 1996

66. Antman K, Rowlings P, Vaughn W, et al: High-dose chemotherapy with autologous hematopoietic stem cell support for breast cancer in North America. J Clin Oncol 15:1870, 1997

67. Broun ER, Nichols CR, Kneebone P, et al: Long-term outcome of patients with relapsed and refractory germ cell tumors treated with high-dose chemotherapy and autologous bone marrow rescue. Ann Intern Med 117:124, 1992

68. Kolb HJ, Schattenberg A, Goldman JM, et al: Graft-versus-leukemia effect of donor lymphocyte transfusions in marrow grafted patients. Blood 86:2041, 1995

Acknowledgments

Figures 1 and 2   Marcia Kammerer.

Figures 3 and 4   Courtesy of the Fred Hutchinson Cancer Research Center.

This work was supported in part by grants CA-18029, CA-47748, and CA-26386 from the National Institutes of Health, U.S. Department of Health and Human Services.

IMMUNOLOGY, ALLERGY, AND RHEUMATOLOGY

97 Organs and Cells of the Immune System

John R. David, M.D., and Cox Terhorst, Ph.D.

The Characteristics of the Immune System

The immune system mediates the individual's relationship with the environment. Immunity involves innate, or natural, responses and acquired, or specific, responses. The essential difference between the two types of immunity is the means by which microorganisms are recognized. In innate immunity, carbohydrates, primarily, that are unique to infectious organisms are recognized by cell surface receptors on macrophages and natural killer (NK) cells or by the complement system. In acquired immunity, lymphocytes use very specific antigen receptors to recognize infectious agents. Once a normal individual has had an infection such as smallpox or measles, the immune system recognizes it and prevents its recurrence. In addition, the immune system has the remarkable capacity to discriminate between antigens, even if their structures are closely related.

Lymphocytes

There are two major groups of lymphocytes, the T cells (also called thymus-dependent lymphocytes, or T lymphocytes) and the B cells (also called bone marrow–derived lymphocytes, or B lymphocytes) [*see Figure 1*]. Neither T cells nor B cells constitute a homogeneous population of cells; each group comprises a number of subgroups that can be differentiated by their surface markers and by their function. In addition, there is a heterogeneous group of lymphocytes that comprises neither T cells nor B cells. The binding of monoclonal antibodies to surface markers is currently the most specific technique used to identify the major subsets of these cells.

T CELLS

All mature T cells and medullary thymocytes express CD2 and CD3. CD4 is expressed on 50% to 65% of peripheral T cells, and CD8 is found on 25% to 35% of peripheral T cells. Although CD4 and CD8 are expressed together on stage II thymocytes, only one or the other is expressed on the complementary subsets of mature T cells (CD4+ and CD8+ T cells). CD4+ T cells recognize antigen when it is presented in association with MHC class II molecules (HLA-D antigens); CD8+ T cells recognize antigen in the context of MHC class I molecules (HLA-A, HLA-B, and HLA-C antigens).

CD4+ helper T cells can be further differentiated into Th1 and Th2 cells on the basis of the lymphokines they produce.[1,2] Th1 cells produce IL-2 and interferon gamma, which are important for cell-mediated immunity. Th2 cells produce IL-4, IL-5, IL-6, IL-10, and IL-13, which are critical for antibody production. The lymphokines that are produced by each of these cell types also influence the other cell type. The interferon gamma produced by Th1 cells can inhibit the function of Th2 cells, whereas IL-10, which is produced by Th2 cells (as well as by monocytes, macrophages, and B cells), can inhibit the function of Th1 cells.

It is of note that the CD4 on helper T cells acts as a coreceptor for HIV, together with a chemokine receptor. CCR5—a CC (cysteine-cysteine) or β-chemokine receptor for RANTES (regulated on activation, normal T cell expressed and secreted),

macrophage inflammatory protein–1α (MIP-1α), and MIP-1β—is the coreceptor for early HIV isolates. One percent of whites are homozygous for a defect in this receptor and are resistant to HIV infection. CCR5 is also on macrophages. The T cell–specific α-chemokine receptor CCR4, which is a receptor for stromal cell–derived factor–1 (SDF-1), is involved in infections of late HIV isolates.[3-5]

B CELLS

B cells are the immunoglobulin-producing cells of the immune system that can be identified by the presence of immunoglobulin on their surface. These surface membrane immunoglobulin–positive (SmIg+) cells constitute 5% to 15% of the peripheral blood lymphocytes [*see Figure 1*]. The majority of B cells have both IgM and IgD on their surface; about one quarter of all B cells have only IgM or IgD on their surface. One percent of B cells exhibit IgG or IgA. T cells and B cells make up 80% to 95% of the peripheral blood lymphocytes. The remaining lymphocytes in the peripheral blood are a heterogeneous population of cells.

On the surface of B cells is complement receptor 2 (CR2), which binds C3d, C3dg, and iC3b. B cells also possess receptors for the Epstein-Barr virus and for the Fc portion of IgG. CD20, a 35 kd phosphoprotein found on the surface of B cells, is a commonly used B cell marker. Some alloantigens are found on the B cell surface but are absent on T cells. Some precursors of B cells lack SmIg but have these alloantigens.

It is important to remember that immunoglobulins produced by B cells can attach passively to the surface membranes of non–B cells. For example, cells with Fc receptors bind immunoglobulin complexes; furthermore, fluorescent antibodies to immunoglobulins, which are often used to identify SmIg+ cells,

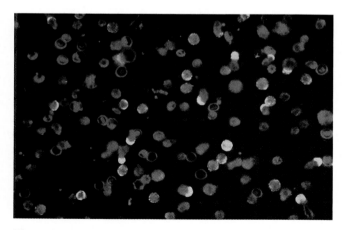

Figure 1 **Immunoglobulins can be demonstrated on the surface of lymphocytes by immunofluorescence microscopy; these lymphocytes are designated as cells that are positive for surface membrane immunoglobulin (SmIg+). The immunofluorescence pattern is patchy in some cells, whereas in others, the stain is localized to one pole of the cell in a process called capping. The lymphocytes shown here are from mouse spleen.**

can also bind to Fc receptors. In addition, autoantibodies to T cells will increase the number of SmIg$^+$ cells that are mistaken for B cells. Such antilymphocyte antibodies have been found in a number of diseases, including systemic lupus erythematosus, infectious mononucleosis, atypical pneumonia, rheumatoid arthritis, and various lymphoproliferative disorders.

A subset of B cells, called B1 cells, develop early and have a very long life.[6] B1 cell progenitors are found in fetal liver and in embryonic omentum but not in adult bone marrow. B1 cells that express CD5 on their surface are referred to as B1a, and B1 cells that lack CD5 are called B1b. B1 cells are frequently associated with autoantibody production. They also produce copious amounts of IL-10.

PLASMA CELLS

Under the influence of antigen, T cells, and accessory cells, B cells differentiate into plasma cells, the mature antibody-producing cells. These cells are larger than lymphocytes and are characterized by an eccentric round nucleus with coarse heterochromatin arranged in a cartwheel pattern. Plasma cells have a highly basophilic cytoplasm and a well-developed endoplasmic reticulum, often organized in parallel concentric layers. Plasma cells may be distended with granular material, which consists of the antibody they are producing [*see Figure 2*]. Sometimes, one or more of the endoplasmic cisterns are distended by large inclusions called Russell bodies. These bodies are aggregates of incompletely formed immunoglobulin molecules. Plasma cells no longer bear surface immunoglobulin. They are also end cells, which means they do not divide. The immature precursors of plasma cells, the plasmablasts, are difficult to distinguish from lymphoblasts and large lymphocytes. Plasma cells are not normally found in the peripheral blood.

NATURAL KILLER CELLS

Natural killer cells are large granular lymphocytes that lack the TCR-CD3 complex characteristic of T cells and the SmIg characteristic of B cells. In vitro, they can kill a number of tumor cells and virus-infected cells in a nonspecific manner; that is, they do not require previous sensitization or the presence of antibody to be cytotoxic. The granules contain pore-forming proteins that can mediate cell lysis. NK cells do not have memory and do not show MHC restriction. The precise precursor of NK cells is not known, but it is thought to be different from the thymic stem cell (the precursor of T cells) and from the pro–B cell (the precursor of B cells). IL-12 stimulates NK cells to proliferate and to produce interferon gamma, which is important in many immune reactions.[7,8]

NK cells have a number of surface markers, including CD56, a 140 kd glycoprotein that is also called NKH1; CD2, which is also present on T cells; and CD16, an Fc receptor. CD16 is associated with the ζ chain of the TCR-CD3 complex. This chain is involved in the signal transduction that is triggered by antibodies binding to CD16, which leads to activation of the cell.

A major breakthrough has been the identification of NK receptors for MHC class I molecules by means of clones of NK-CD3$^-$ cells. These receptors differ in their molecular weights and show allelic specificity for all three major human class I molecules encoded by HLA-A, HLA-B, and HLA-C. The receptors differ from TCRs in that they do not undergo gene rearrangement and therefore have less diversity.[9] Like the TCRs, the 13 receptors that have been cloned are single-chain transmembrane proteins belonging to the immunoglobulin gene su-

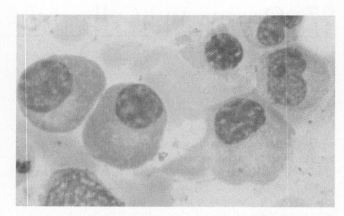

Figure 2 **Plasma cells are the antibody-producing cells of the immune system. They differentiate from B cells; are 6 to 20 μm in diameter; and have an eccentric nucleus, a highly basophilic cytoplasm, and a prominent, clear juxtanuclear area that contains the Golgi apparatus and the diplosome.**

perfamily. They bind to self-MHC class 1 molecules and inhibit the NK cytotoxic response and therefore are termed killer inhibitory receptors. On the other hand, there are other receptors on the NK cell belonging to the same gene superfamily that activate the NK cell when ligating to MHC class I molecules and are termed activator receptors. It is thought that alterations of the self-MHC class I molecules, by either virus or malignant transformation, may prevent recognition of the deficient self-marker by the NK cell killer inhibitor receptors and allow the cell to kill the target.[9]

A population of non–MHC-restricted cytotoxic T cells can lyse some of the same target cells that NK cells can lyse. These cytotoxic T cells have a surface marker that can be detected by anti-CD56 but not by anti-CD16. In addition, they express the TCR-CD3 complex.[10]

A small proportion of null cells in the blood are myeloid precursors and precursors of immature T cells and B cells.

MONOCYTES AND MACROPHAGES

Monocytes belong to the mononuclear phagocytic system, previously called the reticuloendothelial system. They are large mononuclear cells that constitute 3% to 8% of the peripheral blood leukocytes. Their cytoplasm is much more abundant than that of the lymphocytes. Usually, their nucleus is eccentric and either oval or kidney shaped [*see Figure 3*]. Lysosomes filled with degradative enzymes appear as small vacuoles in the cytoplasm. Monocytes originate from promonocytes, which are rapidly dividing precursors in the bone marrow. When the mature cells enter the peripheral blood, they are called monocytes; when they leave the blood and infiltrate tissues, they undergo additional changes and are then known as macrophages.

Macrophages, as one of the cell types that present processed antigen to lymphocytes, play an important role in the induction of the immune response. They act as effector cells, attacking microorganisms and neoplastic cells and removing foreign material.

Macrophages contain receptors for antibody and complement, which enhances their ability to phagocytose organisms that are coated with these substances. The antibody receptors are for the Fc portion of IgG1 and the Fc portion of IgG3. There is also a receptor for the Fc portion of IgE. There are two complement receptors: CR1 and CR3. CR1 has a high affinity for

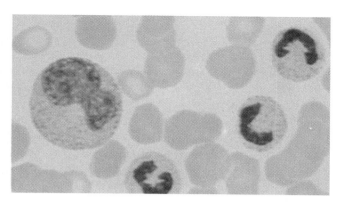

Figure 3   **A monocyte (large cell at left), which can reach 17 μm in diameter, has abundant basophilic cytoplasm and a large eccentric nucleus.**

the complement component C3b and a lower affinity for iC3b and C4b. CR3, which is also called MAC-1, interacts with iC3b as well as with certain carbohydrate molecules, including carbohydrate-containing antigens of the protozoan *Leishmania*.

A small amount of MHC class II antigen is present on monocytes; the expression of MHC class II molecules is greatly increased when macrophages are activated. Macrophages can be activated by a number of cytokines, including interferon gamma, granulocyte-macrophage colony-stimulating factor (GM-CSF),

macrophage-activating factor (MAF), and migration inhibitory factor (MIF) [*see Chapter 99*]. Cytokines such as IL-4 and TGF-β antagonize this activation. The antigen Mo3e, a 50 kd protein, is a urokinase receptor. This antigen has been detected by a monoclonal antibody, and it appears to be specific for activated macrophages; Mo3e is not found on other hematopoietic cells.[11]

Macrophages produce an enormous number of soluble substances that are important in the immune response and in the process of inflammation.[12] These substances include enzymes such as plasminogen activating factor and elastase; growth factors such as GM-CSF; cytokines such as IL-1, IL-6, IL-10, IL-12, and TNF-α; factors that are critical for combating microorganisms, such as oxygen metabolites and nitric oxide; complement components for the classical and the alternative pathway; MIPs; and factors that promote tissue repair, such as fibroblast growth factor (FGF).

Lymphoid Organs and Lymphocyte Traffic

The immune system consists of a number of lymphoid organs, including the thymus, lymph nodes, spleen, and tonsils; aggregates of lymphoid tissue in nonlymphoid organs, such as Peyer's patches in the gut; clusters of lymphoid cells dispersed throughout the connective and epithelial tissues of the body, as well as throughout the bone marrow and blood; and a variety of individual cells that travel from the various lymphoid or-

Figure 4   **Lineages of cells of the immune system and of blood cells all begin with the stem cell. Stem cells that differentiate to generate B cells reside in the bone marrow, and those that produce T cells migrate from the bone marrow to the thymus. T cell maturation involves the progressive expression of selected cell surface markers and the activation of various genes, including α, β, γ, and δ genes that code for the chains that make up the αβ and γδ T cell receptors (TCRs).**

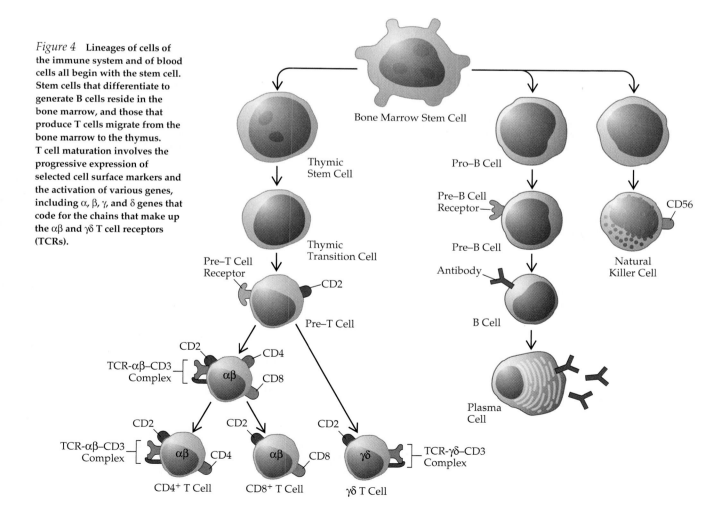

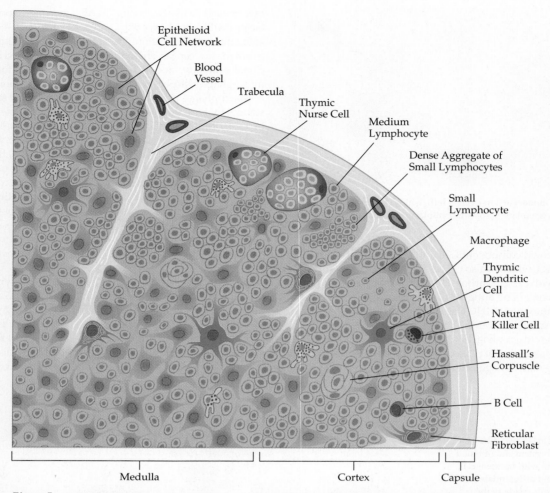

Figure 5 **Many lobules make up the thymus gland. Most of the lymphocytes in the cortex are immature, rapidly dividing cells that can readily be destroyed by cortisone. During maturation, they move to the medulla, where they become immunocompetent and resistant to cortisone. From there, they migrate to the secondary lymphoid organs, including the lymph nodes and the spleen. Cell division and maturation are influenced by the epithelial cells; dense aggregates of these cells form bodies known as Hassall's corpuscles.**

gans to the rest of the body. A number of other cells, including monocytes, macrophages, granulocytes (e.g., neutrophils, eosinophils, basophils, and mast cells), and platelets, play important accessory roles in the immune system [*see Figure 4*].

THE THYMUS

The thymus, which originates in the embryo from the third and fourth pharyngeal pouches, lies in the anterior mediastinum and consists of many lobules, each containing a cortex and a medulla [*see Figure 5*].

Bone marrow–derived pre–T cells enter the thymus. Their daughter cells can express the TCR-CD3 complex (TCR is T cell receptor; CD stands for cluster of differentiation) and subsequently acquire the potential to react with different peptides bound to the major histocompatibility complex (MHC). These thymocytes are then involved in a process of negative or positive selection. Only a small percentage of positively selected thymocytes, the majority of which are self-MHC restricted (*see* Self and Nonself, *below*), migrate to the medulla and then move into the peripheral lymphoid system.

Two to 3 days after the stem cells enter the thymus, the lymphocytes migrate through the wall of the postcapillary venules

of the medulla; they then enter the bloodstream and home in on the lymphoid system's peripheral organs. Once there, the lymphocytes leave the bloodstream, again through the postcapillary venules, and enter the thymus-dependent regions of the peripheral lymphoid system; the inner cortex of the lymph nodes; the periarterial sheaths of the spleen; and the intranodular areas in Peyer's patches, the tonsils, and the appendix. Some T cells in the intestinal mucosa (intraepithelial lymphocytes) may not derive from the thymus but differentiate in situ.

If the thymus is absent at birth, the patient has lymphocytopenia, with a marked depletion or an absence of T cells. The thymus-dependent areas of the peripheral lymphoid system are also devoid of lymphocytes. There is marked impairment of cell-mediated immunity, and antibody responses that require cooperation from T cells (except the IgM response) are severely impaired.

The thymus involutes with age, which may explain the development of immune system deficiencies in elderly persons.

Current evidence indicates that in humans, stem cells differentiate into B cells in the bone marrow [*see Figure 4*] and in the peripheral lymphoid organs themselves.

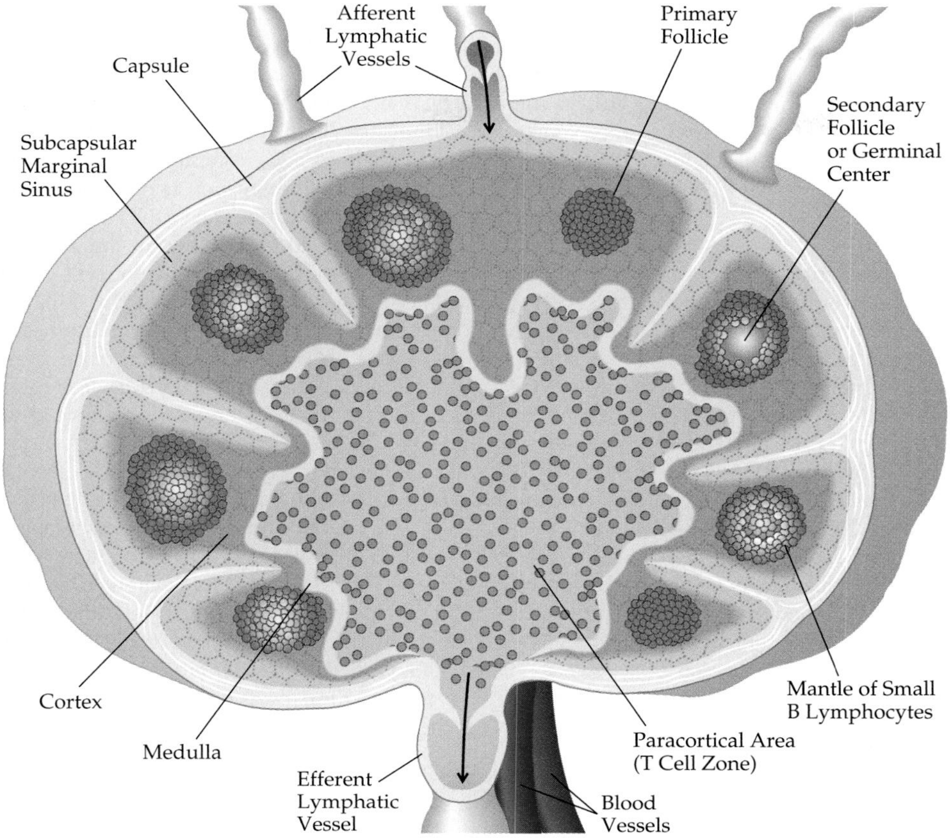

Figure 6 **Wandering cells and macromolecules that have penetrated the lymphatic capillaries in surrounding tissues enter the lymph nodes via afferent lymphatic vessels. In the lymph nodes, these assorted cells and molecules are exposed to a battery of immune system cells. T cells are found mostly in the paracortical areas, whereas B cells are concentrated in and around the germinal centers in the cortex. Plasma cells are found predominantly in the medulla, and macrophages are distributed throughout the lymph node sinuses. The presence of antigen bound to macrophages stimulates proliferation of lymphocytes in the lymph nodes.**

Labels on figure: Capsule; Subcapsular Marginal Sinus; Afferent Lymphatic Vessels; Primary Follicle; Secondary Follicle or Germinal Center; Cortex; Medulla; Efferent Lymphatic Vessel; Blood Vessels; Paracortical Area (T Cell Zone); Mantle of Small B Lymphocytes

LYMPH NODES

The major site of initial T cell activation is the lymph node, where blood-borne lymphocytes and lymph-borne antigen, soluble mediators, and cells converge [*see Figure 6*]. The afferent lymphatics carrying lymph and cells to the node enter in the subcapsular region and percolate into the subcapsular sinus. Lymph and cells leave through the efferent lymphatics in the hilum.

The infrastructure of the lymph node is an extensive reticular network where antigen-presenting cells (APCs) and T cells meet and interact. For example, dendritic cells in the skin pick up antigen and travel through the lymphatics to the draining lymph node. The cells then migrate through the floor of the subcapsular sinus of the lymph node, through the interfollicular regions, and settle in the reticular network of the paracortex as interdigitating dendritic cells (IDCs). T cells from the blood migrate through specialized postcapillary venules, known as high endothelial venules (HEVs), and migrate along the same reticular network, where they come in contact with the numerous antigen-presenting IDCs.[13]

The germinal centers contain B cells and distinctive follicular dendritic cells (FDCs), which are not derived from the bone marrow and can retain antigen-antibody complexes for a long time. Active germinal centers are surrounded by a mantle of B cells (follicular mantle cells) that express IgD on their surface and can mature into plasma cells that produce IgM antibodies only. The B cells in the germinal center (centrocytes) undergo class switching to produce the other isotypes, such as IgG, IgA, and IgE. The B cells with high-affinity antibody on their surfaces are thought to be selected by binding to the antigen-retaining FDCs. The B cells that are not selected die by apoptosis (programmed cell death). The most mature B cell, the memory cell, is also found in the germinal center and can develop into plasma cells producing all the isotypes.

Bone marrow–derived dendritic cells, found in the paracortical areas of the lymph node, play a crucial role in initiating T cell–dependent immune responses.[14] These cells are also found as immature cells in nonlymphoid organs, especially in the epidermis (where they are called Langerhans cells). They phagocytose and process antigens, and they express surface MHC class II, Fc, and mannose receptors. Inflammatory cytokines, such as interleukin-1β (IL-1β) and tumor necrosis factor–α (TNF-α), promote the migration of the dendritic cells via afferent lymphatics to the lymph nodes, where they mature; lose their ability to phagocytose; and express critical costimulatory molecules CD80 (B7-1) and CD86 (B7-2), giving the dendritic cells the ability to present antigen to T cells. Immature dendritic cells are also found in lymph nodes, where they can phagocytize antigen coming in via the afferent lymphatics and then mature into APCs.

THE SPLEEN

In the spleen, the lymphocytes are concentrated in the white pulp that surrounds the central arterioles [*see Figure 7*].

OTHER LYMPHOID TISSUE

Lymphocytes are also found in various other locations. Gut-associated lymphoid tissue includes Peyer's patches and the appendix. These gut-associated lymphoid tissues contain regions with concentrations of T cells or B cells similar to those found in germinal centers. Specialized epithelial cells termed M cells are thought to have a unique ability to take up and present antigen to the adjacent lymphocytes.[15] M cells are found close to Peyer's patches. Other lymphocytes in the intestine are the lamina propria lymphocytes (LPLs), found in the villi, and the intraepithelial lymphocytes (IELs), found between epithelial cells. Migration and adherence of LPLs are in part dictated by integrins and selectins. Mucosa-associated lymphoid cells are also found in the respiratory tract and genitourinary tract but not in recognized inductive structures.

LYMPHOCYTE CIRCULATION

There are three major types of lymphocyte circulation: (1) the seeding of the stem cells from the fetal liver or bone marrow to the primary lymphoid organs and the subsequent differentiation and distribution of these cells to the peripheral lymphoid system, (2) the recirculation of lymphocytes from blood to lymph to blood, and (3) the distribution of effector cells to particular parts of the body. Lymphocytes circulate continuously from blood to tissues and back to the blood. However, the trafficking of naive lymphocytes (CD45RA) is different from that of activated effector or memory cells (CD45RO). Naive lymphocytes recirculate through the secondary lymphoid tissues, such as the lymph nodes, spleen, tonsils, and Peyer's patches, to special microenvironments where they encounter antigen, cytokines, and other cells leading to their activation. In contrast, activated effector or memory cells can also traffic to extralymphoid sites in various tissues, such as skin and intestinal lamina propria.[16]

Lymphocyte homing is controlled by the expression of various receptors on the cell surface and counterreceptors on the vascular endothelium [*see Figure 8*]. To stop the flow of cells in the vessels, initial primary adhesion is made between lymphocyte receptors on the cells' microvilli, such as L-selectin, and the counterreceptor on the endothelium, such as peripheral lymph node addressin (PNAd). If this initial interaction is not followed by subsequent interactions, a protease will cleave the L-selectin, releasing the cell.[17] Other cell receptors will allow attachment to endothelial E-selectin and P-selectin. Subsequently, the cells can attach and roll using integrin-Ig surface receptors such as α4β7 and α4β1, which bind to endothelial mucosal addressin cell adhesion molecule–1 (MAdCAM-1) and vascular cell adhesion molecule–1 (VCAM-1), respectively. These interactions can lead to stable arrest involving a receptor that triggers adhesion through intracellular signaling by a guanosine triphosphate (GTP) binding protein. Cooperation between receptor interactions is essential because the initial interaction with L-selectin may be too weak to induce the LFA-1/ICAM-1 (leukocyte-function–associated antigen–1/intercellular adhesion molecule–1) stable interaction and therefore requires the α4β7/MAdCAM-1 interaction. In contrast, when tissues display high levels of receptor L-selectin, contact and rolling mediated by L-selectin may be sufficient to allow LFA-1–mediated stable arrest. Cytokines produced during inflammation can up-regulate the expression of adhesion receptors and thus enhance the infiltration of cells into the site.

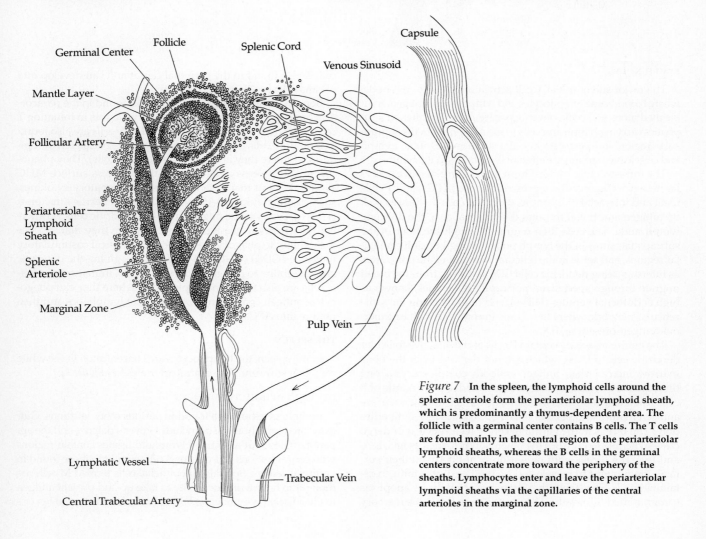

Figure 7 In the spleen, the lymphoid cells around the splenic arteriole form the periarteriolar lymphoid sheath, which is predominantly a thymus-dependent area. The follicle with a germinal center contains B cells. The T cells are found mainly in the central region of the periarteriolar lymphoid sheaths, whereas the B cells in the germinal centers concentrate more toward the periphery of the sheaths. Lymphocytes enter and leave the periarteriolar lymphoid sheaths via the capillaries of the central arterioles in the marginal zone.

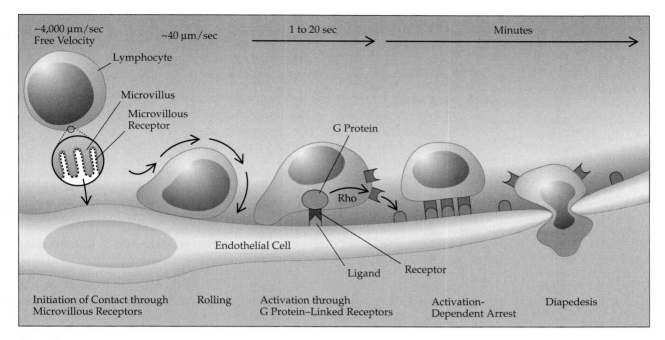

Figure 8 **The multistep model of lymphocyte–endothelial cell recognition and recruitment of lymphocytes from the blood. The velocities shown are from observations of lymphocytes in the Peyer's patch high endothelial venule: velocities may differ in other vascular beds.**

Variations on these mechanisms are thought to channel subsets of lymphocytes to the various microenvironments in the lymph node, such as the germinal centers, the paracortical areas, and the T zone, where cells, antigen, and soluble factors lead to particular immunologic responses. These microenvironments are further regulated by various cytokines, such as transforming growth factor–β1 (TGF-β1), which can up-regulate integrins and mediate B cell binding to APCs. Cytokines such as IL-2 and IL-10, and especially the many chemokines generated by inflammatory processes, also regulate lymphocyte adhesion receptors such as CD44, and other cytokines influence lymphocyte activity as they traverse the tissues.

Immunologic Memory and Specificity

The ability of T cells and antibodies produced by B cells to discriminate among antigens is governed by two independent sets of variable region genes, referred to as V (variable), D (diversity), and J (joining) region genes. Rearrangement of the DNA sequences of these genes occurs as T cells and B cells mature; additional somatic mutation occurs in B cells. The resulting few hundred V, D, and J region genes code for immunoglobulins (antibodies) and TCRs, which can discriminate between a billion different antigenic specificities. Each lymphocyte has a surface receptor that recognizes a single antigenic determinant, or epitope. B cell receptors recognize native antigens. After B cells interact with an antigen, they proliferate and differentiate into memory cells and plasma cells for the production of antibodies.

Before being recognized by T cells, an antigen is taken up by an APC (e.g., a dendritic cell or a macrophage), which breaks up the antigen into small peptide fragments. In the APC, certain peptide fragments or epitopes are taken up by MHC class II molecules and carried to the surface of the APC. The requirement that the antigen be presented in association with an MHC molecule is referred to as MHC restriction. Thus, TCRs do not recognize native antigen, only processed parts of it [*see*

Chapter 98]. After T cells interact with an antigen, they proliferate and differentiate into memory cells. They also become regulators of the production of antibodies by B cells and the cell-mediated effector responses of other T cells.

AMPLIFICATION

Characteristic of the immune response is its ability to increase the number of antigen-specific lymphocytes after an antigenic stimulus occurs; therefore, subsequent exposure to the same antigen results in a faster and a greater response (i.e., the anamnestic response). The basis for this enhanced response is the proliferation of antigen-specific lymphocytes and the production of memory cells after lymphocytes interact with an antigen. These responses are mediated through production of cytokines by lymphocytes and other cells [*see Chapter 99*]. Immune response mechanisms are also amplified through the release of mediator substances from antibody-coated mast cells and basophils, the activation of complement proteins [*see Chapter 100*], and the expression of integrin molecules on cells. Altered vascular permeability, the expression of receptors for leukocytes on endothelial cells, and the release of chemotactic factors through these secondary mechanisms attract a host of other cell types to the reaction. These cells greatly contribute to the resulting inflammation by aiding the phagocytic process and the disposal of foreign antigens.

ANAMNESTIC RESPONSE

A group of B cells, the memory cells, enhance the immune response to previously encountered antigens in what is known as the secondary immune response, the anamnestic response, or the booster response. These memory B cells undergo somatic mutation in the variable regions of their immunoglobulin genes. When this somatic mutation occurs in the lymph node germinal centers that contain antigens bound to follicular dendritic cells, it leads to the selection of memory B cells that have high-affinity receptors for the antigens.

SELF AND NONSELF

It is important that the immune response be able to distinguish between self and nonself. If it were not able to distinguish between the two, T cells and antibodies would constantly be attacking autologous cells and tissue components. In the 1950s, Sir Frank Macfarlane Burnet first proposed that in the prenatal state, the interaction of self-antigens with antigen-specific lymphocytes leads to the elimination of self-reactive lymphocytes[18] and immunologic tolerance. When immunologic tolerance breaks down, the antibodies and sensitized (antigen-reactive) cells that are directed against self-antigens cause autoimmune diseases [*see Chapter 104*].[19]

GENETIC CONTROL

The immune responses are controlled by three large gene families: (1) the genes coding for the variable elements of the immunoglobulins, (2) the genes coding for the TCRs, and (3) the genes coding for the MHC antigens [*see Chapter 98*]. In each person, there are an enormous number of genes coding for the variable elements of the immunoglobulins and TCRs, allowing specific recognition of millions of antigens. However, the extreme variability of the MHC applies to the population as a whole; there are only a few variations in any individual.

The genes that control the production of the MHC antigens (also referred to as histocompatibility antigens, or HLA antigens, in humans) are located very close to one another on chromosome 6. HLA antigens identify autologous cells as self and differentiate them from the cells of other individuals. The *Ir* gene in mice and the *HLA* gene in humans constitute part of the MHC, which plays a crucial role in the immune response. The nature of the MHC explains why some individuals may not respond to certain antigens. For example, although TCRs recognize epitopes that are bound to MHC molecules, some antigen peptides may not fit into the groove of the particular MHC molecule of an individual. Thus, the appropriate T cell type will not react to that epitope, and the individual will not be able to mount an immune response against it.

T CELL RECEPTOR GENE REARRANGEMENT

The genes that code for TCRs are rearranged, and the V, J, D, and C (constant) gene segments come together to form two types of TCR, each consisting of two chains. Each type of TCR is associated with a particular specificity [*see Chapter 98*]. The genes that encode the γ and the δ chains are rearranged to form the TCR-γδ; then the genes that encode the α and β chains are rearranged to form the TCR-αβ. After gene rearrangement occurs, the TCR is expressed on the surface of the T cell, together with the CD3 proteins. At about the same time as gene rearrangement occurs, several important accessory molecules, including CD4, CD8, CD2, and CD3, are expressed.[20,21] Relatively few T cells develop into CD4⁻CD8⁻ TCR-γδ cells, whose function is still not well understood. Most T cells become TCR-αβ cells that first express both CD4 and CD8 and that subsequently, after positive selection, become either CD4⁺,CD8⁻ TCR-αβ (helper) cells or CD4⁻,CD8⁺ TCR-αβ cells (exhibiting cytotoxic functions, suppressor functions, or both). CD4⁺ and CD8⁺ mature thymocytes express high levels of TCR-CD3 complex [*see Chapter 98*].

POSITIVE SELECTION

Positive selection is controlled by epithelial cells of the thymic cortex and dedicated APCs, such as macrophages, dendritic cells, and interdigitating cells. Many of these stromal cells are located in the corticomedullary junction.[22] Because T cells can react to antigens only in association with self-MHC, only T

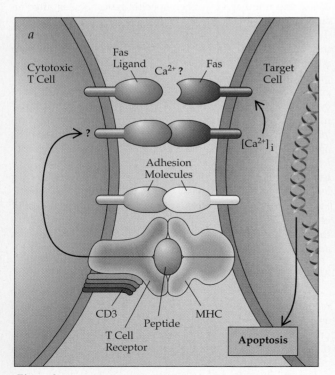
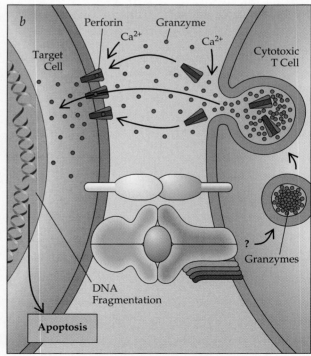

Figure 9 Cytotoxic T cells recognize surface markers on cells that are to be destroyed. (*a*) Apoptosis is triggered by the cytotoxic T cell through nonsecretory Fas–Fas ligand interaction. (*b*) Apoptosis is triggered by the cytotoxic T cell by means of secretory mechanisms initiated by perforin and granzymes.

cells with a TCR that can bind to self-MHC are selected. When these cells react with self-MHC on thymic stromal cells, CD4+,CD8+ TCR-αβ cells that bind to MHC class II molecules become CD4+ and CD8−, down-regulating the CD8 and up-regulating the TCR-CD3 complex. Conversely, the CD4+,CD8+ cells that bind to MHC class I molecules down-regulate the CD4 and become CD4−,CD8+ TCR-αβ cells. In this manner, self-MHC–restricted CD4+ TCR-αβ cells and CD8+ TCR-αβ cells are selected. It is presumed that T cells that bind even weakly to MHC molecules with the help of the CD4 or CD8 ligand will be able to bind more strongly to APCs; thus, foreign antigens need not be present for positive selection. Most T cells do not interact with self-MHC and undergo programmed cell death, or apoptosis.

NEGATIVE SELECTION

The process of negative selection eliminates T cells that have a TCR with a strong affinity for self-antigens. If they were not removed, such T cells could cause serious autoimmune disease. There are many self-antigens on thymic epithelial cells, and studies show that certain self-antigens can be presented by various APCs in the thymus, such as macrophages and dendritic cells. It is possible that negative selection for some self-antigens occurs when the T cells move to the peripheral lymphoid system after leaving the thymus. This high-affinity interaction between the self-antigen presented by the MHC and the TCR on immature T cells presumably triggers cell death. In contrast, an interaction between an MHC-presented antigen and the TCR on mature T cells leads to cell activation. Whether or how γδ TCRs are positively or negatively selected is unknown.

APOPTOSIS

Apoptosis plays a critical role in the development and function of the lymphoid system. Apoptotic signals acting on the cell membrane lead to cell blebbing, cell shrinking, and nuclear chromatin condensation and cleaving, and within minutes to hours, the cell is destroyed and cleared by macrophages.

The main receptors on lymphoid cells for apoptosis are the Fas (CD95/APO-1), triggered by Fas ligand,[23] and the tumor necrosis factor receptor–1 (TNFR-1), triggered by TNF-α and lymphotoxin-α. The lymphotoxin-β receptor can also be involved. Of note, the TNFR-1 also can trigger pathways that lead to activation of nuclear factor κB (NF-κB), which protects against apoptosis,[24,25] and Jun N-terminal kinase (JNK), which activates genes and is not involved in apoptosis. These responses are mediated through separate pathways.[26]

The signals for apoptosis eventually act on a family of cysteine proteases similar to the IL-1β converting enzyme (ICE), the prototype that acts on the cytokine precursor IL-1β, converting it to the active cytokine. ICE-related proteases activate other proteases, which then act on a number of substrates and in turn lead to apoptosis.

Cytotoxic T cells also use the Fas and TNFR-1 apoptotic pathways to destroy target cells. In addition to this nonsecretory pathway, cytotoxic T cells can mediate apoptosis in their target cell by a secretory pathway using perforins, which facilitate the entry of cytotoxic proteases such as granzyme A and B into the target cell [*see Figure 9*]. Granzyme B has been shown to activate CPP32, the precursor of the protease responsible for cleaving poly(ADP-ribose) polymerase.[27] Apoptosis can also be induced in B cells and T cells by corticosteroids. One of the mechanisms by which corticosteroid induces apoptosis is by

increasing the expression of type 3 inositol 1,4,5-trisphosphate receptor (IP₃R3) on the plasma membrane.[28] IP₃R3 allows the increase in intracellular calcium that facilitates apoptosis of T and B cells.

References

1. Mosmann TR, Coffman RL: Heterogeneity of cytokine secretion patterns and functions of helper T cells. Adv Immunol 46:111, 1989

2. Romagnani S: Human T_H1 and T_H2 subsets: doubt no more. Immunol Today 12:256, 1991

3. Feng Y, Broder CC, Kennedy PE, et al: HIV-1 entry cofactor: functional cDNA cloning of a seven-transmembrane, G protein–coupled receptor. Science 272:872, 1996

4. Choe H, Farzan M, Sun Y, et al: The β-chemokine receptors CCR3 and CCR5 facilitate infection by primary HIV-1 isolates. Cell 85:1135, 1996

5. Doranz BJ, Rucker J, Yi Y, et al: A dual-tropic primary HIV-1 isolate that uses fusin and the β-chemokine receptors CKR-5, CKR-3, and CKR-2 as fusion cofactors. Cell 85:1149, 1996

6. Qin XF, Schwers S, Yu W, et al: Secondary V(D)J recombination in B-1 cells. Nature 397:355, 1999

7. Wolf SF, Temple PA, Kobayashi M, et al: Cloning of cDNA for natural killer cell stimulatory factor, a heterodimeric cytokine with multiple biologic effects on T and natural killer cells. J Immunol 146:3074, 1991

8. Williams NS, Klem J, Puzanov IJ, et al: Natural killer cell differentiation: insights from knockout and transgenic mouse models and in vitro systems. Immunol Rev 165:47, 1998

9. Rolstad B, Naper C, Vaage JT: Natural killer (NK) cell recognition of MHC class I molecules. The Immunologist 4:165, 1996

10. Lanier LL, Le AM, Cwirla S, et al: Antigenic, functional, and molecular genetic studies of human natural killer cells and cytotoxic T lymphocytes not restricted by the major histocompatibility complex. Fed Proc 45:2823, 1986

11. Todd RF III, Liu DY: Mononuclear phagocyte activation: activation-associated antigens. Fed Proc 45:2829, 1986

12. Auger MJ, Ross JA: The biology of the macrophage. The Macrophage. Lewis CE, McGee JO'D, Eds. Oxford University Press, Oxford, England, 1992, p 1

13. Gretz JE, Kaldjian EP, Anderson AO, et al: Sophisticated strategies for information encounter in the lymph node: the reticular network as a conduit of soluble information and a highway for cell traffic. J Immunol 157:495, 1996

14. Austyn JM: New insights into the mobilization of phagocytic activity of dendritic cells. J Exp Med 183:1287, 1996

15. Neutra MR, Frey A, Kraehenbuhl J-P: Epithelial M cells: gateways for mucosal infection and immunization. Cell 86:345, 1996

16. Watson SR, Bradley LM: The recirculation of naive and memory lymphocytes. Cell Adhes Commun 6:105, 1998

17. Steeber DA, Tang ML, Zhang XQ, et al: Efficient lymphocyte migration across high endothelial venules of mouse Peyer's patches requires overlapping expression of L-selectin and beta 7 integrin. J Immunol 161:6638, 1998

18. Burnet M: The Clonal Selection Theory of Acquired Immunity. Cambridge University Press, London, 1959

19. Ring GH, Lakkis FG: Breakdown of self-tolerance and pathogenesis of autoimmunity. Semin Nephrol 19:25, 1999

20. Knapp W, Dörken B, Gilks WR, et al, Eds: Leukocyte Typing IV: White Cell Differentiation Antigens. Oxford University Press, Oxford, England, 1989

21. Schlossman SF, Boumsell L, Gilks W, et al: Update: CD antigens 1993. J Immunol 152:1, 1994

22. Cosgrove D, Chan SH, Waltzinger C, et al: The thymic compartment responsible for positive selection of CD4+ T cells. Int Immunol 4:707, 1992

23. Fraser A, Evan G: A license to kill. Cell 85:781, 1996

24. Beg AA, Baltimore D: An essential role for NF-κB in preventing TNF-α–induced cell death. Science 274:782, 1996

25. Van Antwerp DJ, Marting SJ, Kafri T, et al: Suppression of TNF-α–induced apoptosis by NF-κB. Science 274:787, 1996

26. Lui Z-g, Hsu H, Goeddel DV, et al: Dissection of TNF receptor 1 effector functions: JNK activation is not linked to apoptosis while NF-kB activation prevents cell death. Cell 87:565, 1996

27. Darmon AJ, Nicholson DW, Bleackley RD: Activation of the apoptotic protease CPP32 by cytotoxic T-cell–derived granzyme B. Nature 377:446, 1995

28. Khan AA, Soloski MJ, Sharp AH, et al: Lymphocyte apoptosis: mediation by increased type 3 inositol 1, 4, 5-trisphosphate receptor. Science 273:503, 1996

Acknowledgments

Figure 1   Courtesy of Dr. Curtis B. Wilson, Scripps Clinic and Research Foundation.

Figures 2 and 3   Courtesy of Dr. Arthur T. Skarin, Harvard Medical School and Dana-Farber Cancer Institute.

Figures 4, 5, 6, 8, and 9   Seward Hung.

Figure 7   Carol Donner.

Cox Terhorst, Ph.D., and John R. David, M.D.

Antigens

An antigen is any substance capable of generating an immune response; that is, antigens react with T cells and B cells to induce the formation of antibodies and sensitize lymphocytes and then react with those antibodies and cells once they are formed. The first antigens to be studied were various microorganisms and foreign proteins, and it remains true that proteins are almost universally antigenic. The basis for the general immunogenicity of proteins is not known, but it is probably related to their unique and stable configurations. Given the appropriate conditions, a wide range of molecules can effect an immune response, and in abnormal situations, the body will even mount an immune response against self-antigens [*see Chapter 104*].

Polysaccharides can induce antibody formation when coupled to proteins, and some purified polysaccharides are themselves effective antigens. One such example is purified pneumococcal polysaccharide, which can be used as a vaccine against the particular strain of pneumococci from which the polysaccharide is obtained. It has been shown that human antibodies to polysaccharides are mainly of the IgG class, but lesser amounts of IgM and IgA can also be detected [*see* Classification of Immunoglobulins, *below*]. Although most antigens are macromolecules, some small molecules can also be antigenic. Antibodies to DNA or RNA occur in patients with systemic lupus erythematosus, Crohn's disease, or amyotrophic lateral sclerosis.

ANTIGEN RECOGNITION

Antigens are recognized not only by antibodies but also by antigen-specific B cell receptors (BCRs) [*see* B cell receptors, *below*] and T cell receptors (TCRs) [*see* T Cell Receptors, *below*], which are located on the extracellular surfaces of B cells and T cells, respectively. In general, TCRs and immunoglobulins recognize different antigenic determinants.

Two distinct types of TCR exist: TCR-αβ and TCR-γδ. The several types of T cells each have different mechanisms for recognizing antigens [*see Chapter 99*]. For example, T cells bearing TCR-αβ recognize antigens that have been processed by antigen-presenting cells (APCs) to become peptide fragments bound to major histocompatibility complex (MHC) class I or class II molecules on the surface of the APCs. In contrast, T cells bearing TCR-γδ appear not to require antigen presentation by MHC molecules. Helper T cells recognize only peptide fragments bound to MHC class II molecules, whereas cytotoxic T cells recognize processed viral antigens presented by both MHC class I and MHC class II molecules on the surface of virus-infected cells. Pure lipids from mycobacteria can be presented as antigen to TCR-αβ by CD1 molecules rather than by MHC class I or class II molecules.

ADJUVANTS

Adjuvants are substances capable of increasing the immunogenicity of antigens and are critical in the production of vaccines. Many microbial products have been used as adjuvants,[1] including substances from *Mycobacterium tuberculosis*, bacillus Calmette-Guérin (BCG), *Corynebacterium parvum*, *Brucella abortus*, and *Bordetella pertussis*, as well as toxoids from *Vibrio cholerae* and *Clostrid-*

ium tetani. Adjuvants have also been derived from vaccinia virus and other poxviruses, BCG, and *Salmonella*, each transfected with genes for an antigen of interest. Others have come from lipopolysaccharide derivatives, such as monophosphoryl lipid A. Freund's complete adjuvant, which consists of dead mycobacteria in oil emulsified with an antigen in aqueous solution, is now used infrequently because it generally causes a strong local inflammatory reaction. Other adjuvants are extracts from the soap bark tree (*Quillaja saponaria*), polymers (e.g., inulin), peptide complexes, and a number of cytokines. Interleukin-12 (IL-12), for instance, appears to act as a strong promoter of cell-mediated immune reactions in mice.[2] The aluminum salt alum is approved for general use as an adjuvant in humans.

Antibodies

Antibodies are a heterogeneous group of serum proteins called immunoglobulins. Immunoglobulins are secreted by differentiated B cells called plasma cells. According to Sir Francis MacFarlane Burnett's clonal selection theory, a single plasma cell produces only one specific antibody. This theory is aptly illustrated by the disease multiple myeloma, in which malignant proliferation of plasma cells occurs in bone marrow. The multiple myeloma plasma cell produces an abnormal monoclonal immunoglobulin called myeloma protein. Its homogeneity is clearly visible with electrophoresis: a single dense band results. Certain antibodies that are produced in response to highly homogeneous antigens, such as streptococcal polysaccharide, may also be homogeneous.

Immunoglobulin monomers are made up of two identical heavy chains and two identical light chains [*see Figure 1a*]. Each light chain is attached to a heavy chain by disulfide (S—S) bonds, and the heavy chains are also attached to each other by one or more S—S bridges. Amino acid sequences in both heavy and light chains are divided into regions that are either constant or variable [*see Figure 1b*]; in addition, each variable region contains sequences that are hypervariable.

CLASSIFICATION OF IMMUNOGLOBULINS

There are five broad classes of immunoglobulins, and each class contains a specific heavy chain: IgG contains two γ chains; IgM, two μ chains; IgA, two α chains; IgD, two δ chains; and IgE, two ε chains [*see Table 1*]. There are also two types of light chains, κ and λ, which can be differentiated antigenically. One form of IgM, the secreted form, is a pentamer [*see Figure 2*]. The monomeric form of IgM is expressed on the extracellular surface of B cells. IgA exists as a monomer or a dimer. The polymeric forms of IgM and IgA have an additional J (joining) chain that facilitates polymerization.

IgG IgG is the major immunoglobulin in the serum, where it exists as a monomer. IgG has a half-life in the blood of approximately 23 days. It is the main antibody raised after antigenic challenge. There are four subclasses of IgG—IgG1, IgG2, IgG3, and IgG4—each different in structure and biologic properties. For example, only IgG1 and IgG3 bind the first component of comple-

a

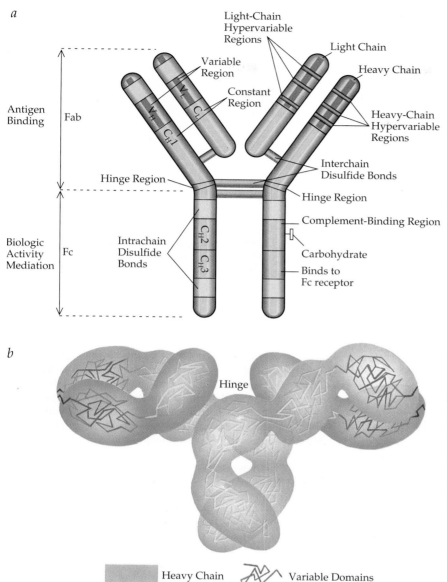

Antigen Binding — Fab

Biologic Activity Mediation — Fc

Light-Chain Hypervariable Regions

Variable Region

Constant Region

Light Chain

Heavy Chain

Heavy-Chain Hypervariable Regions

Interchain Disulfide Bonds

Hinge Region

Hinge Region

Complement-Binding Region

Intrachain Disulfide Bonds

Carbohydrate

Binds to Fc receptor

V_L C_L V_H C_H1 C_H2 C_H3

b

Hinge

Heavy Chain

Light Chain

Variable Domains

Constant Domains

Figure 1 (*a*) **The immunoglobulin molecule is a Y-shaped protein made up of four polypeptide chains. Two heavy chains (blue) are joined to two light chains (green) by disulfide bonds. Blue squares represent intrachain S—S bonds; blue bars indicate interchain S—S bonds. The heavy chains extend from the stem of the Y into the arm; the two light chains are confined to the arms. Each polypeptide has regions whose amino acid sequences are constant (white and yellow) and variable (red). The variable regions also contain hypervariable regions. All antibodies of a given type have the same constant regions, but the variable regions differ from one clone of a B cell to another. The heavy- and light-chain variable regions fold to create an antigen-binding site. (*b*) Schematic model of the domain structure of an antibody molecule. The domains have a characteristic folding pattern, which is also seen in the T cell receptor and proteins of the major histocompatibility complex.**[18]

ment and adhere to monocytes. The antibodies that coat microorganisms and render them more susceptible to phagocytosis (i.e., opsonization) are of the IgG class. IgG antibodies can also neutralize viruses and toxins such as diphtheria toxin. Although the fetus does not produce this class of immunoglobulin, IgG readily crosses the placenta; therefore, any IgG antibodies found in the newborn are from the mother.

Clinically, IgG has been used successfully for reconstituting the immunity of patients with agammaglobulinemia and for preventing hemolytic disease in the newborn. Women with the Rh-negative blood group who bear a fetus with Rh1-positive red blood cells are sensitized at the first delivery by Rh1-positive red blood cells from the fetus. The mother then produces anti-Rh1 IgG antibodies that will cross the placenta during subsequent pregnancies; these antibodies react with fetal red blood cells, causing hemolytic disease. Erythroblastosis fetalis can be prevented by injecting IgG rich in anti–Rh-positive antibodies (RhoGAM) into the Rh1-negative mother at the time of delivery or abortion. These antibodies presumably combine with any fetal Rh1-positive red blood cells present and prevent them from immunizing the mother.

IgG can be split into three fragments by the proteolytic enzyme papain [*see Figure 1a*]. Two of the fragments are similar and are called Fab; the third is called Fc. The Fc portion is responsible for the biologic activity of the various immunoglobulins; among other things, the Fc portion controls the ability of immunoglobulins to bind to cells, fix complement, and traverse the placenta. Another proteolytic enzyme, pepsin, splits the IgG molecule behind the S—S bonds that bridge the heavy chains, leaving one large fragment, F(ab′)$_2$, which is able to bind and precipitate antigen because of its bivalency and capacity to form a lattice.

IgA IgA is the predominant immunoglobulin in secretions, where it is usually found as a dimer and is released as such by local plasma cells. Monomeric IgA constitutes 15% of the serum immunoglobulins. In the serum, it has a half-life of 5 to 6 days. There are two subclasses of IgA—IgA1 and IgA2. The IgA dimer com-

Table 1 Physical, Chemical, and Biologic Properties of Human Immunoglobulins

Property	IgG	IgA	IgM	IgD	IgE
Sedimentation constant	7S	7S monomer 11S dimer	19S	7S	8S
Molecular weight $\times 10^{-3}$	160	170–340	970	184	188
Mean concentration in serum (mg/dl)	1,250	280	120	0.3–30.0	0.002–0.200
Percentage of carbohydrate	3	8	12	13	12
Light chains	κ, λ	κ, λ	κ, λ	κ, λ	κ, λ
Heavy chains (subgroups)	γ1, γ2, γ3, γ4	α1, α2	μ	δ	ε
J chain	No	In dimer	Yes	No	No
Half-life in serum (days)	23	6	5	3	2.5
Localization	Serum, amniotic fluid	Serum, secretions, colostrum, saliva, tears, GI tract	Serum	Serum	Serum

bines with the secretory piece, which is a polypeptide chain produced by local epithelial cells. In this form, IgA is quite resistant to proteolytic digestion. Unlike serum IgA, IgA combined with the secretory piece can undergo active transport across the mucosal epithelium by endocytosis [*see Figure 3*].

IgA is present in saliva, tears, and colostrum. It also occurs in the respiratory and gastrointestinal tracts, in the vagina, and in the prostate. The increased levels of antibodies to dietary antigens that are found in persons with IgA deficiency suggest that the IgA class of immunoglobulin normally limits the absorption of such antigens.

IgA may play an important role in local immunity by neutralizing viruses and by combining with viruses and bacteria, thereby preventing their adherence to mucosal surfaces. Although IgA does not bind complement, it can activate the alternative complement pathway [*see Chapter 100*]. One of the complement components generated by this pathway, C3b, can aid in the opsonization of bacteria, enhancing their uptake and killing by phagocytes.

IgM Most B cells have monomeric IgM on their surface. However, IgM exists primarily as a pentamer and is found mainly in the serum, where it makes up 10% of the immunoglobulins. In the immune response, IgM is the first immunoglobulin raised in response to antigen stimulation. Cells that produce IgM or their precursors do not become memory cells, so that a second challenge with antigen produces no more IgM antibody than the first stimulus. Because the IgM response to antigen is short-lived, the presence of such a response may also be helpful in establishing the diagnosis of a particular infection. The fetus makes IgM antibodies to certain microorganisms, which can be helpful in the diagnosis of fetal toxoplasmosis, rubella, or syphilis. Not all fetuses infected by these organisms, however, produce such antibodies.

As a pentamer, IgM is highly efficient at fixing complement. Molecule for molecule, IgM is 20 times as effective as IgG in agglutinating bacteria and red blood cells and 1,000 times as active in bactericidal reactions. Isohemagglutinins, such as anti-A and anti-B, are of the IgM class. Waldenström's macroglobulinemia is a disease characterized by the monoclonal production of IgM.

IgD IgD, which is a monomer, occurs in the serum in trace amounts. It is found in relatively high concentrations in umbilical cord blood. Most of the B cells of umbilical cord blood have IgD on their surface, and most adult B cells have both IgM and IgD on their surface. Plasma cells that produce IgD have been found in the tonsils and adenoids, although they are very rare in other lymphoid tissues.

IgE IgE is present in trace amounts in the serum, constituting only 0.004% of the immunoglobulins. It is the heat-labile antibody (formerly referred to as reagin) that plays a primary role in immediate hypersensitivity—namely, the immune reaction in hay fever, extrinsic asthma, wheal-and-flare reactions, and anaphylaxis. IgE binds tightly to mast cells and basophils. When these IgE-coated cells interact with specific antigens, termed allergens, they release potent mediators of immediate hypersensitivity, including histamine, slow-reacting substance of anaphylaxis (SRS-A), and an eosinophilic chemotactic factor. Levels of IgE are higher than normal in persons with atopic dermatitis, and the level of IgE antibody specific for a particular allergen is also elevated, correlating with the susceptibility of the individual. In patients with allergies, specific IgE antibodies are detected by means of a radioimmunoassay called the radioallergosorbent test, or RAST.

IgE binds to the mast cell or basophil by its Fc portion; heating the antibody destroys its cell-binding ability. Plasma cells that produce IgE are found in the tonsils and adenoids and on the mucosa of the respiratory and GI tracts. Distinct receptors for IgE are found on the surface of mast cells, B cells, T cells, macrophages, and eosinophils.

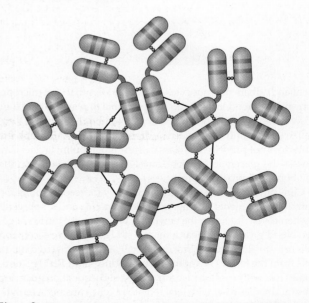

Figure 2 **The pentamer structure of the secreted form of IgM. Bars indicate interchain disulfide bonds. The IgM pentamer is stabilized by an associated J chain (not shown).**[19-21]

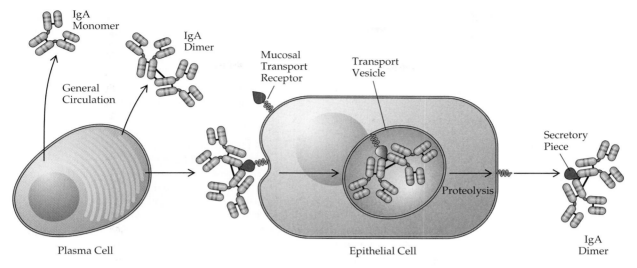

Figure 3   Plasma cells secrete IgA molecules into the general circulation as either monomers or dimers. The circulating dimer can combine with a mucosal transport receptor on the surface of an epithelial cell. As the antibody-receptor complex is transported through the cell, the receptor is cleaved. The portion of the receptor that remains attached to the antibody dimer is called the secretory piece. The secretory piece is joined to the constant region of IgA by disulfide bonds. The mucosal transport receptor contains five immunoglobulin-like domains and is anchored in the membrane by a proteolytically labile segment.[22]

The exact function of IgE is unknown. Certainly, the manifestations of immediate hypersensitivity, such as hay fever and extrinsic asthma, do not appear to serve any useful purpose for the person affected or for the species in general. Therefore, the observation that IgE levels are sometimes elevated in persons living in the tropics, and especially in those afflicted with helminthic parasites, was greeted by immunologists as a possible indication that IgE plays a protective role against parasites. The mediators released could affect the parasite either directly or by producing an increase in vascular permeability and releasing eosinophilic chemotactic factor, which may lead to the accumulation of other necessary antibodies (e.g., IgG) and cells to attack the parasite. In this context, it is of interest that eosinophils can mediate IgG-dependent damage to schistosomula (the larval form of the parasite *Schistosoma mansoni*). In addition, parasite-specific IgE immune complexes can induce a macrophage-mediated cytotoxic response to schistosomulum organisms.

Antigenic Differences of Immunoglobulins

Immunoglobulins have three types of serologic, or antigenic, determinants: isotypic, allotypic, and idiotypic.

Isotypic determinants   Isotypic determinants distinguish between the constant regions of the various classes and subclasses of heavy chains and light chains; they represent the different constant-region genes [*see Table 1*]. For example, there are four IgG heavy-chain isotypes: γ_1, γ_2, γ_3, and γ_4, representing the subclasses IgG1, IgG2, IgG3, and IgG4, respectively. There is only one κ light-chain isotype and one λ light-chain isotype.

Allotypic determinants   Allotypic determinants distinguish between immunoglobulins of a particular isotype; they represent different alleles of immunoglobulin genes and therefore are genetically determined according to mendelian laws in a manner similar to the way that the ABO blood groups are determined. The γ heavy-chain molecules of a person can have a number of different allotypic markers; there are no known allotypic markers for the μ, δ, and ε heavy chains or for the λ light chain. The γ heavy chains

have more than 20 different allotypic markers, which are collectively termed Gm. In addition, κ light chains contain a set of at least three allotypic markers, collectively called Km.

Idiotypic determinants   An idiotope is defined as a single antigenic determinant on the hypervariable region of an antibody. An idiotype is the antigenic character of the variable region of an antibody. Idiotypic determinants distinguish one immunoglobulin from another of the same allotype.

Genetic Source of Antibody Diversity

The carboxyl-terminal halves of all κ light chains have almost identical amino acid sequences; this portion of the molecule is therefore called the constant, or C, domain. The amino-terminal half has a variable sequence of amino acids and is known as the variable, or V, domain [*see Figure 1*]. The first 110 amino acids of the amino-terminal portion of the λ light chain and the heavy chain are also variable. The remaining 75% of the heavy chain is constant and contains three homologous regions.

Within the variable regions, three areas—referred to as the hypervariable, or complementarity-determining, regions—show great variation; these areas correspond to the antigen-binding site of the antibody [*see Figure 4*]. X-ray analysis has shown that immunoglobulin molecules are built up from compact globular units connected by short segments of more or less linear polypeptide chains [*see Figure 1*]. As expected, the hypervariable regions are located at the interface between immunoglobulin and antigen.

The most intriguing aspect of the genetic control of immunoglobulin synthesis is the diversity of the product: plasma cells can make antibodies that react with an indefinite number of different antigenic sites. How can DNA code for such a large number of antigens, many of which have only recently (on the evolutionary time scale) come into existence?

VDJ RECOMBINATION

In all cells, DNA for the κ light chain codes for more than 300 variable (V) regions, five joining (J) regions, and one constant (C) region. The V and J regions are separated from the C region by an intervening stretch of DNA. Thus, in the so-called germline configuration, DNA encodes the information for at least 1,500 different combinations of V and J regions; in other words, at least 1,500 different κ light chains are possible.

The emergence of individual plasma cell lines is the result of somatic recombination in the DNA and RNA splicing [*see Figure 5*]. As the pre–B cell differentiates into a plasma cell, rearrangements and deletions in the DNA bring one of the V genes, chosen at random, adjacent to one of the J genes. This V-J unit and the remaining J regions are separated from the C gene by a short length of DNA. In the next step, the DNA is transcribed to nuclear RNA, and the stage is set for a second event.

This event begins when an enzyme cleaves the nuclear RNA to produce messenger RNA (mRNA). In a process called RNA splicing, the segment that separates the V-J unit from the C region is removed, along with any superfluous J segments. The remaining V-J-C segment is now translated into one of the 1,500 κ light-chain proteins. Actually, the number of possible proteins is higher because the joining of any V region to a J region can involve one of a variety of base pairs at the recombination site.

Variability in the heavy chain makes an important contribution to the specificity of an antibody and also results from somatic recombination and RNA splicing. The germline configuration of the DNA carries instructions for several hundred different heavy-chain V genes, six J genes, 10 to 20 diversity (D) genes, and nine C genes (these C genes code for the heavy-chain classes: IgM, IgD, IgG1, IgG2, IgG3, IgG4, IgA1, IgA2, and IgE). DNA deletion, transcription to nuclear RNA, and RNA splicing produce the final V-D-J-C sequence in the mRNA that is translated by ribosomes to a heavy-chain protein. This assembly process produces more than 18,000 possible varieties of heavy-chain proteins (antibody specificity does not vary with class, so the nine C genes do not enter into the calculation).

The combination of more than 1,500 light-chain varieties with the 18,000 heavy-chain varieties yields more than 27 million different kinds of antibodies with different antigen-binding sites. In addition, somatic mutation occurs, particularly during affinity maturation, and the rate of somatic mutation is relatively high (one base pair per 1,000 cell divisions). Therefore, the potential number of specific antibodies in one person is indefinite.

Although some of the mechanisms of V-D-J rearrangement are unique to B cells (and T cells, as synthesis of TCRs occurs by a similar mechanism [*see* T Cell Receptors, *below*]), the general mechanisms of DNA repair are also engaged.[3] Two genes involved in V-D-J rearrangement in B cells are the recombination-activating genes *rag1* and *rag2*.[4-6] Disruption of the *rag1* or *rag2* gene causes a block in B cell development before the transition from pro–B cell to pre–B cell, as found in patients with severe combined immunodeficiency syndrome or Omenn syndrome.[7] Disruption of the surface IgM gene, the J region of the heavy chain, or the J region of the κ light chain leads to a similar block in B cell development.

ALLELIC EXCLUSION

In each individual B cell, only one of the chromosomes undergoes complete V-D-J recombination leading to expression of heavy and light chains. A mechanism exists that prevents the other chromosome from being rearranged and therefore expressed in the same cell. This is called allelic exclusion. It prevents a B cell from expressing two entirely different immunoglobulins or BCRs. A similar mechanism operates during synthesis of TCRs in T cells [*see* T Cell Receptors, *below*].

Primary and Secondary Antibody Responses

When antigen is first introduced into the body, a primary response occurs that is characterized by a lag phase that lasts several days and during which no antibody is detected. Increasing amounts of IgM antibody appear in the serum, usually reaching a peak level after 7 days. After 6 to 7 days, IgG antibody is also detected. The IgM titer begins to wane before the maximal IgG titer is reached, about 10 to 14 days after the antigen is introduced. An-

a

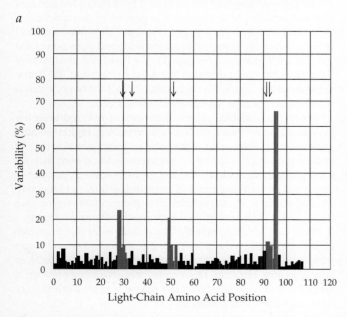

b

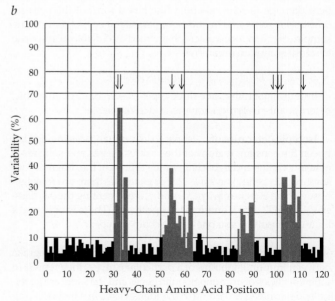

Figure 4 In affinity-labeling experiments, hapten is linked irreversibly to an immunoglobulin. After digestion and amino acid sequencing, it can be seen that the hapten-antibody binding site (arrows) coincides with the hypervariable regions (blue bars) of both light chains (*a*) and heavy chains (*b*) of the antibody. The ability of immunoglobulins to respond specifically to large numbers of antigens may be explained by the presence of these hypervariable amino acid sequences at the binding site.[23-25]

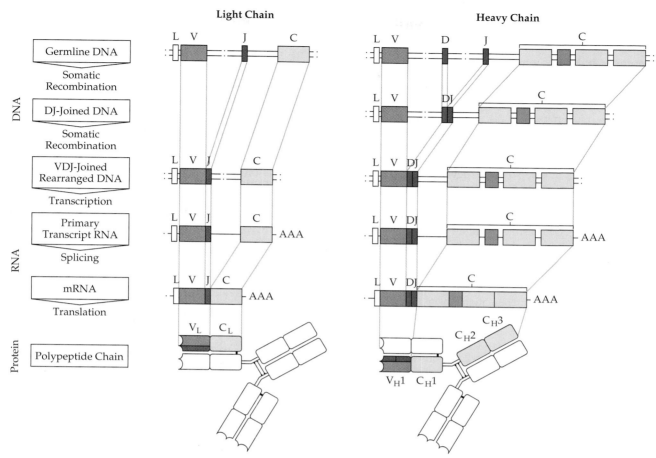

Light Chain　　**Heavy Chain**

Figure 5　Variable-region genes are constructed from gene segments. Light-chain variable genes are constructed from two segments (center panel). A variable (V) and a joining (J) gene segment in the genomic DNA are joined to form a complete light-chain variable-gene–region gene. The constant region is encoded in a separate exon and is joined to the variable-region gene by RNA splicing of the light-chain message to remove the L to V and the J to C introns. Immunoglobulin chains are extracellular proteins, and the V gene segment is preceded by an exon encoding a leader peptide (L), which directs the protein into the cell's secretory pathways and is then cleaved. Heavy-chain variable regions are constructed from three gene segments (right panel). First the diversity (D) and J gene segments join, then the V gene segment joins to the combined DJ sequence, all at the genomic DNA level. The heavy-chain constant-region sequences are encoded in several exons: note the separate exon encoding the hinge domain (purple). The constant-region exons together with the L sequence are spliced to the variable-domain sequence during processing of the heavy-chain gene RNA transcript. Posttranslational alterations remove the L sequence and attach carbohydrate moieties.[26]

tibody titers then decrease, and very little antibody is detected 4 to 5 weeks after a single dose of antigen.

If the antigen is encountered a second time, a secondary response (also called an anamnestic or booster response) occurs because of the existence of memory B cells. Both IgM and IgG titers rise exponentially, without the lag phase seen in the primary response. Whereas the peak IgM level during the secondary response may be the same as or slightly higher than the peak IgM level during the primary response, the IgG peak level during the secondary response is much greater and lasts longer than the peak level during the primary response. This variation in response is an apt illustration of immunologic memory and is caused by a proliferation of antigen-specific B cells and helper T cells during the primary response. The characteristics of the primary and secondary responses explain the need for booster injections in immunization programs.

AFFINITY MATURATION

The binding properties of antibodies change with time by a process termed affinity maturation that involves somatic muta-

tion and selection. After the first stimulation, the antibodies have greater and greater affinity for the antigen as time progresses, and increasingly stable antigen-antibody complexes are formed. In addition, the antibody becomes less specific and cross-reactions with related antigens increase. The lessening specificity reflects the fact that cross-reactions were previously too weak to detect; they become apparent as antibody develops greater affinity for antigen.

IMMUNOGLOBULIN CLASS SWITCHING

The genes that code for the IgM and IgD heavy chains (the μ and δ genes, respectively) play a critical role in the primary immune response. Whereas IgM antibodies are unable to act in the many tissues of the human body, IgG and IgA serve functions in the peripheral immune system. Class switching means that the same variable region can be transferred from the heavy chain of IgM to one of the other antibody heavy chains. In the switch from IgM to IgG production that constitutes the booster response, constant-region genes are deleted before the DNA is transcribed to RNA [*see Figure 6*].[7,8] If the cell switches to production of IgG3, for example, the genes for μ and δ are deleted [*see Figure 7*]. After transcription, RNA splicing produces an mRNA with the sequence V-D-J-C$_{\gamma3}$, which is translated into protein.

Immunoglobulin Receptors

B CELL RECEPTORS

In addition to being secreted, immunoglobulins are also be expressed on the surface of B cells, where they act as antigen receptors.[9] These cell surface membrane immunoglobulins (SmIgs) differ from secreted immunoglobulins in that they have a transmembrane domain and are monomeric. The first SmIg a B cell expresses is IgM; at a later stage of B cell development, IgD is coexpressed. SmIgs do not travel to the cell surface by themselves; the process requires formation of a complex consisting of the immunoglobulin and two polypeptide chains called Igα and Igβ, which takes place in the endoplasmic reticulum [see Figure 8a]. The resultant BCR binds antigen; this drives the B cell to maturation. Stimulation by the helper T cell activates the B cell, causing it to differentiate into a plasma or memory cell that produces secretory antibody specific for the antigen encountered. Igα and Igβ are not expressed after terminal differentiation. The mature plasma cell ceases to express SmIgs, although it may retain the SmIg mRNA.

BCRs play important roles in regulation of the immune response. B cell responses to antigen can become anergic, thus providing a control mechanism for B cell responses and antibody production. A precursor of the BCR expressed on the surface of pre–B cells is thought to control allelic conclusion. In addition, BCRs interplay with Fc receptors.

FC RECEPTORS

Fc receptors bind the Fc portion of an immunoglobulin; they are expressed on a multitude of cells, including mast cells, macrophages, eosinophils, and tumor cells. Fc receptors are composed of a family of molecules. The Fc receptor for IgE (FcεRI) is the model for all Fc receptors and consists of three polypeptide chains, designated α, β, and γ. FcεRI mediates signal transduction in the mast cell when IgE binds to the receptor. FcεRIα is the binding site for the Fc portion of IgE. FcεRIβ is a transmembrane molecule that connects FcεRIα with FcεRIγ, the chain responsible for recruiting signal transduction molecules.[10,11] FcRIIβ1, another Fc receptor that is expressed on B cells, provides a negative feedback signal to the BCR, which leads to the termination of humoral immune responses.[12]

Engineered Antibodies

LYMPHOCYTE HYBRIDOMA

The development of the lymphocyte hybridoma, a product of cell fusion, has had a revolutionary impact on immunology and clinical medicine. B lymphocyte hybridomas are the means by which extraordinarily high titers of very specific, pure antibodies can be produced for experimental purposes. The B lymphocyte

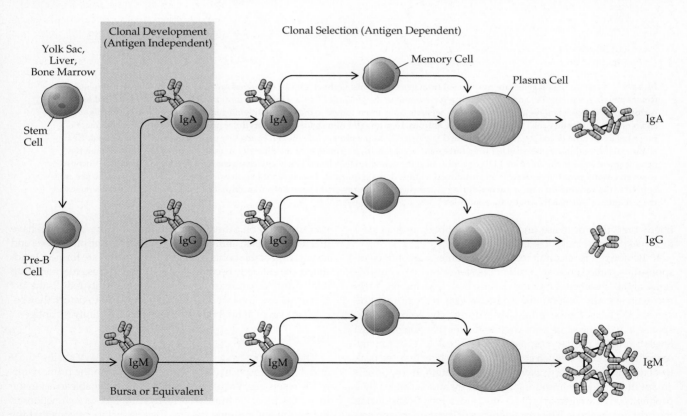

Figure 6 Stem cells formed in the yolk sac, liver, or bone marrow (left) migrate to the lymph nodes and spleen, where the individual pre–B cell lines undergo clonal development independent of antigen stimulation. The various B cell types are differentiated by the particular immunoglobulin they produce (IgA, IgG, or IgM). Most cells initially produce IgM, but some of these later switch to IgG or IgA production; it is not known whether cells that produce IgG can switch to production of IgA (center). Once the B cells are released into the circulation and reach the peripheral lymphoid tissues, they are capable, if stimulated by antigen, of differentiating into plasma cells that can produce antibody specific for the particular antigen encountered. Other cells of the same clone become memory cells (right) with the ability to respond with appropriate antibody if the antigen is encountered again.[27]

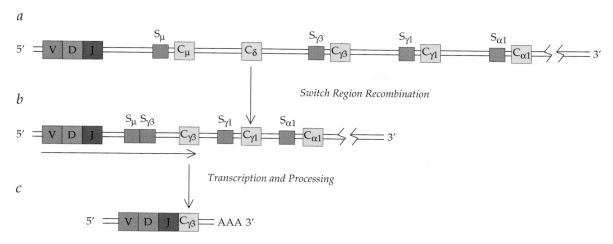

Figure 7 In the booster response, a plasma cell switches from IgM production to IgG production, a process called class switching. In this hypothetical model of heavy-chain class switching to $C_{\gamma3}$, the heavy-chain C-region exon clusters (yellow) and the switch regions (light green) are indicated (*a*). The switch region is a stretch of DNA that directs the deletion events. In this model, recombination of the switch regions S_{μ} and $S_{\gamma3}$ and the deletion of the intervening DNA occur first to produce a DNA sequence in which the gene for $C_{\gamma3}$ has been brought into close proximity to the V-D-J segment (*b*). Further processing and transcription of this DNA yields the messenger RNA (mRNA) encoding IgG3 (*c*).

hybridoma, as developed by Köhler and Milstein,[13] is the product of the fusion of a mouse myeloma cell and a lymphocyte from the spleen of a mouse immunized with a specific antigen. The hybrids can be cloned and selected for specific antibody production.

HUMAN MONOCLONAL ANTIBODIES

Several methods of generating human monoclonal antibodies exist. One method entails taking the complementary DNA cod-

ing for a mouse monoclonal antibody and systematically replacing the mouse sequences with human sequences. DNA cassettes containing sequences for the constant regions of human heavy and light chains replace the mouse DNA sequences of the variable regions by means of various types of mutagenesis, leaving the hypervariable regions intact. A disadvantage of this method is that the affinity may be altered.

Another method of humanizing mouse monoclonal antibod-

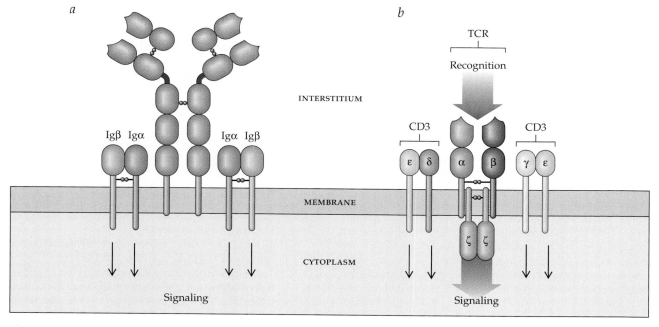

Figure 8 (*a*) Cell surface membrane immunoglobulins form a complex with the proteins Igα and Igβ. Igα and Igβ are linked by disulfide bonds, but the exact stoichiometry is unknown. The exact ratio of these two proteins to each immunoglobulin molecule is also unknown. (*b*) The TCR-CD3 complex is shown. A T cell receptor for antigens is composed of six distinct polypeptide chains. Two of the chains, α and β, are the disulfide-bonded chains of the heterodimer TCR that binds to antigen. The four other chains—γ, δ, and two ε chains—are collectively called CD3. CD3 associates with TCR and transports it to the T cell surface. When antigen binds to the TCR, CD3, along with a homodimer of ζ chains, sends a signal to the nucleus, via intracellular signaling pathways. Specific genes are then transcribed, and cytokines, chemokines, and other immunodulatory molecules are produced that mediate the antigen-specific immune response.

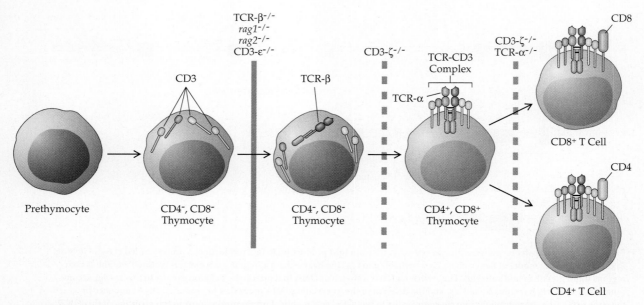

Figure 9 The developmental pathway of the T cell has been confirmed through both spontaneous and engineered mutations of T cell receptors (TCRs) in mice. The thymocytes of mice in which the *rag1*, *rag2*, or other genes governing the TCR-β locus were disrupted by gene targeting procedures (-/-) showed a block in development (first bar) at the early CD4⁻, CD8⁻ thymocyte stage; they failed to go on to express TCR-β. Mice in which the CD3ζ gene was disrupted expressed TCR-β, but further development was blocked (second bar). The TCR-CD3 complex, including the TCR-α chain, is expressed on the cell surface membrane of the CD4⁺,CD8⁺ thymocytes, but further development was blocked in mice in which genes governing CD3ζ and TCR-α were disrupted (third bar). The block in development of CD3ζ is partial, and some cells go on to become single positive. If none of the genes are disrupted, the thymocytes will proceed to the process of positive or negative selection and, if positively selected, will go on to become either CD4⁺ T cells or CD8⁺ T cells.[28]

ies entails making a transgenic mouse containing large segments of human DNA, including several variable regions and all the human constant regions.[14] Because this mouse still has its own immunoglobulin regions, it is bred with a mouse in which there has been a targeted disruption of the mouse J region of the Ig heavy-chain and κ light-chain genes. The progeny of this breeding can then be injected with any antigen, and humanized monoclonal antibodies will be produced. Because the transgenic mouse contains a limited number of human variable regions, the potency of these antibodies depends on the natural somatic mutation and affinity maturation that occurs in the mouse.

A third method of generating human monoclonal antibodies entails constructing expression libraries of human variable regions either in bacteria or in bacteriophages. In theory, all the variable regions can be cloned. The antibody can be expressed on the surface of the bacterium or bacteriophage and selected by affinity to the antigen of interest.

Monoclonal antibodies are being used in many therapies. For instance, humanized monoclonal antibodies to tumor necrosis factor–α (TNF-α) have been used successfully in the treatment of Crohn's disease. In other applications, monoclonal antibodies are used to remove T cells and tumor cells before bone marrow transplantation and during acute transplant rejection. Other potential uses of monoclonal antibodies are the production of anti-IgE antibodies and anti–hormone receptors to prevent allergy and modulate endocrine abnormalities, respectively.

T Cell Receptors

Unlike the immunoglobulin receptors on B cells, which recognize free antigens, TCRs recognize antigens only in conjunction with autologous major histocompatibility complex antigens, which are usually on the surface of a macrophage, although they may

also be on the surface of a B cell, dendritic cell, or endothelial cell. The CD4⁺ helper T cells (as well as the few CD4⁺ cytotoxic T cells) require MHC class II molecules, and the CD8⁺ cytotoxic T cells require MHC class I molecules [*see Chapter 101*]. This phenomenon is referred to as MHC restriction. The ability of T cells to recognize these self–MHC molecules is determined during development in the thymus before the lymphocytes are exposed to antigen [*see Chapter 97*].

The molecules that make up the TCR and the genes that encode these molecules have been isolated and cloned. The TCR is composed of six distinct polypeptides known as the TCR-CD3 complex.[15-17] From 85% to 95% of normal peripheral blood lymphocytes carry TCR-αβ; only 5% to 15% carry TCR-γδ. The antigen-recognizing portion of the TCR-αβ complex consists of two glycosylated polypeptide chains, termed TCR-α and TCR-β, that are linked by disulfide bonds to form a heterodimer. The corresponding polypeptide chains in the TCR-γδ complex consist of TCR-γ and TCR-δ. The TCR-α, TCR-β, TCR-γ, and TCR-δ chains each contain variable and constant portions that are analogous to those of immunoglobulin molecules.

TCR-αβ and TCR-γδ heterodimers are closely associated with the CD3 proteins CD3γ, CD3δ, CD3ε, and CD3ζ [*see Figure 8b*]. The CD3 proteins are present on all peripheral blood T cells and on 90% of thymocytes. Expressions of the CD3 and the TCR complexes on the cell surface are mutually dependent: neither complex is observed on the surface of the T cell without the other. Structural and functional data suggest that the activities of the TCR are distributed among the subunits of the TCR-CD3 complex: the TCR polypeptides (α, β, γ, and δ) bind to antigen and MHC gene products, and the CD3 proteins transduce the binding signal to the cytoplasm of the T cell, which results in activation of T cell functions.

By the use of mice containing spontaneous and engineered

mutations of various genes of TCRs, the development pathway of the T cell has been confirmed [*see Figure 9*]. The organization of the genes that encode the human TCR-α, -β, -γ, and -δ chains is analogous to that of the immunoglobulin heavy-chain genes: there are V, D, and J segments, which are flanked by recognition sequences that mediate site-specific recombination [*see Antibodies, above*]. Thus, the diversity of TCRs is generated by many of the same mechanisms that are used by B cells for the production of immunoglobulins. T cells and B cells may in fact use the same recombination enzyme, or recombinase.

The genomic sequences that encode the TCR-β chain contain two very similar constant-region genes, $C\beta_1$ and $C\beta_2$, each of which is associated with a cluster of six or seven J genes and a single D gene. There are at least 70 Vβ genes that are associated with the two Cβ genes. These variable regions are distinct from the immunoglobulin variable regions. Rearrangement of the β-chain gene segments can lead to the production of approximately 3,600 different β chains.

The TCR-α genes are arranged differently. A single Cα gene is preceded by a very large stretch of DNA containing at least 50 distinct J genes. A Dα gene segment has not been demonstrated directly. Some Vα genes are organized as families of related genes. Rearrangement of the α-chain gene segments can account for approximately 2,500 different polypeptides. No somatic mutation has been detected in TCRs. Thus, 10^7 TCR-αβs can be formed. The genes for CD3γ, CD3δ, CD3ε, and CD3ζ are transcribed in all T cells; however, they do not undergo rearrangement.

References

1. Furlong ST, David JR: Adjuvants. Therapeutic Immunology. Austen KF, Burakoff SJ, Rosen FS, Eds. Blackwell Scientific Publications, Cambridge, 1996

2. Afonso LC, Scharton TM, Vieira LQ, et al: The adjuvant effect of interleukin-12 in a vaccine against *Leishmania major*. Science 263:235, 1994

3. Frank KM, Sekiguchi JM, Seidl KJ, et al: Late embryonic lethality and impaired V(D)J recombination in mice lacking DNA ligase IV. Nature 396:173, 1998

4. Oettinger MA, Schatz DG, Gorka C, et al: RAG-1 and RAG-2, adjacent genes that synergistically activate V(D)J recombination. Science 248:1517, 1990

5. Hofker MH, Walter MA, Cox DW: Complete physical map of the human immunoglobulin heavy chain constant region gene complex. Proc Natl Acad Sci USA 86:5567, 1989

6. Seidl KJ, Manis JP, Bottaro A, et al: Position-dependent inhibition of class-switch recombination by PGK-neor cassettes inserted into the immunoglobulin heavy chain constant region locus. Proc Natl Acad Sci USA 96:3000, 1999

7. Villa A, Santagata S, Bozzi F, et al: Partial V(D)J recombination activity leads to Omenn syndrome. Cell 93:885, 1998

8. Rolink A, Melchers F, Andersson J: The SCID but not the RAG-2 gene product is required for S mu-S epsilon heavy chain class switching. Immunity 5:319, 1996

9. Kurosaki T: Genetic analysis of B cell antigen receptor signaling. Annu Rev Immunol 17:555, 1999

10. Kinet JP: The high-affinity IgE receptor (Fc epsilon RI): from physiology to pathology. Annu Rev Immunol 17:931, 1999

11. Metzger H: It's spring, and thoughts turn to…allergies. Cell 97:287, 1999

12. Scharenberg AM, Kinet JP: PtdIns-3,4,5-P3: a regulatory nexus between tyrosine kinases and sustained calcium signals. Cell 94:5, 1998

13. Köhler G, Milstein C: Continuous cultures of fused cells secreting antibody of predefined specificity. Nature 256:495, 1975

14. Lonberg N, Taylor LD, Harding FA, et al: Antigen-specific human antibodies from mice comprising four distinct genetic modifications. Nature 368:856, 1994

15. Terhorst C, Spits H, Staal F: T lymphocyte signal transduction. Molecular Immunology. Hames BD, Glover DM, Eds. IRL Press, Washington, DC, 1995, p 237

16. Garcia KC, Teyton L, Wilson IA: Structural basis of T cell recognition. Annu Rev Immunol 17:369, 1999

17. Davis MM, Boniface JJ, Reich Z, et al: Ligand recognition by alpha beta T cell receptors. Annu Rev Immunol 16:523, 1998

18. Tonegawa S: The molecules of the immune system. Sci Am 253(4):122, 1985

19. Gally JA: Structure of Immunoglobulins. The Antigens. Sela M, Ed. Academic Press, New York, 1973

20. Frangione B: Immunogenetics and Immunodeficiency, 2nd ed. Medical and Technical Publishing Co, London, 1975

21. Kabat EA: Structural Concepts in Immunology and Immunochemistry, 2nd ed. Holt, Rinehart & Winston, New York, 1976

22. Underdown BJ, Schiff JM: Immunoglobulin A: strategic defense initiative at the mucosal surface. Annu Rev Immunol 4:389, 1986

23. Cohn M, Blomberg B, Geckeler W, et al: First order considerations analyzing the generator of diversity. The Immune System: Genes, Receptors, Signals. Sercarz EE, Williamson AR, Fox CF, Eds. Academic Press, New York, 1974

24. Kabat EA, Bilovsky H, Wu TT: Data Compiled by the Prophet Computer System of the National Institutes of Health (unpublished)

25. Wu TT, Kabat EA: An analysis of the sequences of Bence Jones proteins and myeloma light chains and their implications for antibody complementarity. J Exp Med 132:211, 1970

26. Janeway CA Jr, Travers P: Immunology. The Immune System in Health and Disease, 3rd ed. Current Biology Ltd, London, 1997

27. Cooper M, Lawton AR III: The development of the immune system. Sci Am 231(5):50, 1974

28. Mombaerts P, Iacomini J, Johnson RS, et al: RAG-1–deficient mice have no mature B and T lymphocytes. Cell 68:869, 1992

Acknowledgments

Figure 1A   Talar Agasyan.

Figure 1B   Dana Burns-Pizer. Computer graphic model by A. J. Olson, Ph.D. © 1985 Research Institute of Scripps Clinic. Used by permission.

Figures 2, 3, 6, 8, and 9   Seward Hung.

Figure 4   Albert Miller.

Figure 5   Seward Hung.

Figure 7   Dana Burns-Pizer.

99 Immune Response Mechanisms

John R. David, M.D., and Cox Terhorst, Ph.D.

The immune response is defined by the principles of self/non-self discrimination, specificity, and memory [*see Chapter 97*]. On exposure to a pathogen or another source of antigens, macrophages and dendritic cells initiate a response that stimulates the migration of T and B cells to the inflammatory sites and to the draining lymph nodes. Antigens are concentrated in macrophages and dendritic cells, and there the antigens are processed into peptides. These antigen-presenting cells (APCs) then present the processed antigens on their extracellular surface in a complex with class I or II major histocompatibility complex (MHC) molecules.

The critical first step of the antigen-specific immune response is the recognition and binding of the antigenic peptide–MHC molecule complex on the surface of APCs by the $\alpha\beta$ T cell receptor (TCR) on the surface of CD4$^+$ and CD8$^+$ helper T cells [*see Chapter 97*]. This event is relayed to the helper T cell nucleus by a cascade of cytoplasmic signaling molecules. In the nucleus, activation of specific transcription factors stimulates expression of the genes that encode soluble factors, or cytokines, that mediate the immune response.

Activated CD4$^+$ $\alpha\beta$ T cells secrete cytokines that induce antigen-stimulated B cells to differentiate into antibody-secreting plasma cells (humoral response) and cause CD8$^+$ T cells to differentiate into cytolytic effectors (cell-mediated response). In addition, T cells and B cells are induced to expand and control the initial infection and to produce memory cells for long-term acquired immunity.

T Cell Responses to Antigen

The diversity of the variable regions in TCRs facilitates highly specific responses to antigens [*see Chapter 98*]. The prototypical T cells, $\alpha\beta$ T cells, have a TCR made up of α and β chains, which are expressed in association with the CD3 [*see Chapter 98*]. A subset of peripheral T cells, $\gamma\delta$ T cells, have a TCR made up of γ and δ chains. The $\gamma\delta$ T cells appear not to require antigen presentation by MHC molecules.

T CELL RECEPTORS RECOGNIZE ANTIGEN-MHC COMPLEXES

The gene products that constitute the MHC form an integral membrane glycoprotein complex that binds antigenic peptide within an APC and transports it to the cell surface for interaction with T cells [*see* Antigen Processing, *below*].[1] An extensive polymorphism exists in the MHC (i.e., a large number of alleles per locus); within the human population, however, each individual expresses only a small number of different MHC molecules. To ensure an adequate immune response against a large number of non–self-antigens, each MHC molecule must be able to bind a large number of different peptides.

MHC class I molecules consist of an α heavy chain and a β2-microglobulin (β_2M) light chain, whereas MHC class II molecules consist of α and β chains of nearly the same size. The two classes of molecules have a similar structure: two immunoglobulin-like domains and a peptide-binding site formed by an eight-stranded β-pleated sheet and two α-helical regions [*see Chapter 101*]. Whereas MHC class I molecules bind only smaller peptides of defined lengths (eight to 11 amino acids), MHC class II molecules bind longer peptides with no apparent restriction on peptide length.

An interesting finding is that certain peptides bind only to specific alleles of either MHC class I or MHC class II molecules. Thus, persons who lack a particular allele would not develop an immune response to the associated peptide.

The peptides that bind to MHC class I molecules are bound at their amino and carboxyl termini by a network of hydrogen bonds to conserved amino acid residues in the peptide-binding site of the MHC class I molecule. Binding of peptides to MHC class II molecules is a little different because these peptides tend to be larger and of arbitrary lengths. The main chain of the peptide is secured along much of its length by hydrogen bonds to conserved amino acid residues positioned throughout the peptide-binding site.

The differences in peptide binding between MHC class I and MHC class II molecules result from small structural dissimilarities within the relatively fixed framework of the peptide-binding site and probably also from fundamental differences in the mechanism of peptide processing, which takes place in the endoplasmic reticulum (ER) for MHC class I molecules and in the endosomes and lysosomes for MHC class II molecules.

Antigen Processing

FORMATION OF ANTIGEN-MHC COMPLEXES

Class I Endogenous Pathway

Antigen processing associated with MHC class I molecules essentially entails three steps: (1) generation of antigenic peptides in the cytosol of the APC, (2) transport of the peptides into the ER, and (3) assembly of the peptide–MHC class I complexes. The completed complexes then migrate through the Golgi apparatus to the cell surface and fuse to the plasma membrane for presentation on the extracellular surface [*see Figure 1a*].

Antigenic proteins—endogenous host nuclear and cytosolic proteins as well as proteins introduced by intracellular pathogens (e.g., viral proteins)—are first tagged by ubiquitin conjugation before undergoing proteolytic degradation in proteasomes. A large multisubunit endoprotease, the proteosome, is the principal non-lysosomal protein-degrading machine and is found in the nucleus and cytoplasm of all eukaryotic cells. In addition to generating antigenic peptides, proteasomes rid the cell of excess synthesized proteins.

To reach the peptide-binding site of the MHC class I molecule in the lumen of the ER, peptides are translocated across the ER lipid bilayer by an adenosine triphosphate (ATP)–driven peptide pump system consisting of the proteins TAP1 and TAP2 (TAP refers to transporter-associated protein). A third component, called tapasin (TAP-A), is involved in the association of the class I molecule with TAP and in the assembly of the peptide–MHC class I molecule complex.[2] The assembly of the class I α heavy chain and the β_2M light chain in the ER requires the presence of peptide. If the peptide-$\alpha\beta_2$M complex does not form, MHC class I molecules do not travel to the cell surface and are degraded in the lumen of the ER.

Class II Exogenous Pathway

The assembly of antigenic peptide–MHC class II molecule complexes requires four steps: (1) uptake of exogenous antigens by

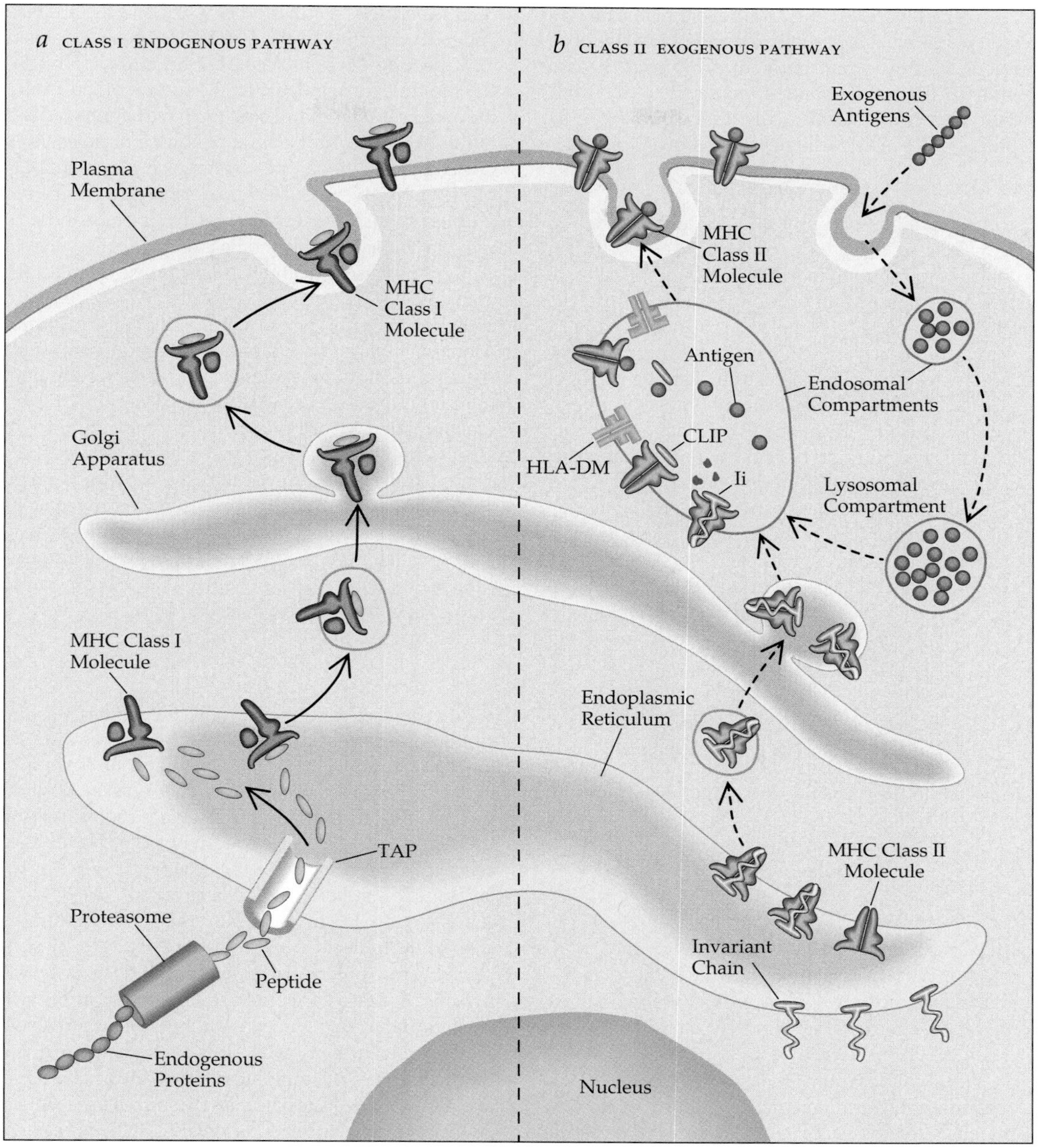

Figure 1 **The pathways for formation of antigenic peptide–MHC molecule complexes on antigen-presenting cells. (*a*) In the MHC class I molecule pathway, endogenous proteins are broken down by proteasomes into smaller peptides. In the endoplasmic reticulum (ER), an antigenic peptide binds to the peptide binding site in an MHC class I molecule. The peptide-MHC complex then migrates through the Golgi apparatus to the cell surface. (*b*) In the MHC class II molecule pathway, the α and β subunits of the MHC class II molecule bind to the invariant chain (Ii) in the ER. Ii is partially degraded in an endosomal compartment. The portion of Ii that occupies the antigenic peptide binding site on the MHC class II molecule (called CLIP) is removed with the help of HLA-DM, freeing the molecule for binding processed antigen. Once antigenic peptide has bound to an MHC class II molecule, the complex migrates to the cell surface.**

proteolytic vesicles (endosomes, lysosomes, and, possibly, undefined endosomal subcompartments) in the APC, (2) proteolytic degradation of proteins in the endosome, (3) assembly of MHC class II molecules in the ER and migration of these molecules through the Golgi apparatus to the endosomes, and (4) assembly of the peptide–MHC class II complexes in the endosome. After the peptides are bound to MHC class II molecules, the endosome containing these complexes migrates to the cell surface and fuses to the plasma membrane [*see Figure 1b*]. Of note is that partially

unfolded antigenic proteins can bind to MHC class II molecules before undergoing proteolytic degradation. This may explain why the length of peptides bound to MHC class II molecules is highly variable.

Two critical proteins control peptide–MHC class II molecule interactions: the invariant chain (Ii) and the gene product HLA-DM. Ii plays a major role in the assembly and intracellular transport of MHC class II molecules and peptide selection. Ii blocks the peptide-binding site during assembly of the α and β subunits of

MHC class II molecules in the ER, thereby preventing the binding of ER-processed peptides. Ii is partially degraded in an endosomal compartment, leaving a small fragment termed class II–associated Ii peptide (CLIP) in the peptide-binding site of the MHC class II molecule. Removal of CLIP catalyzes the binding of the antigenic peptides.[3,4] HLA-DM facilitates the removal of CLIP.

ALTERNATIVE ANTIGEN-PRESENTING COMPLEXES

A third group of antigen-presenting molecules are the nonpolymorphic MHC class I–like β_2M-associated proteins, which include the products of the nonpolymorphic *CD1* genes. CD1 molecules bind lipid and glycolipid antigens for presentation to a wide variety of T cells. For example, CD1 molecules present glycolipids from *Mycobacterium tuberculosis* to $\alpha\beta$ T cells that do not carry CD4 or CD8.[5] This example of nonprotein, microbial antigen recognition suggests that $\alpha\beta$ T cells recognize a broader range of antigens than was once thought. CD1-restricted T cells have frequently been found to be autoreactive and have been implicated in such autoimmune diseases as type 1 (insulin-dependent) diabetes mellitus and lupus erythematosus. It has been suggested that they are involved at the early innate phase of these immune responses.[6]

Another method of antigen presentation involves MHC class II molecules and superantigens, a class of immunostimulatory proteins derived from microbial agents (e.g., viral proteins and toxins produced by *Staphylococcus aureus* that cause toxic-shock syndrome and food poisoning). Superantigens bind to MHC class II molecules outside the conventional antigen-binding site and stimulate T cells.[7] For example, the intact bacterial superantigen *S. aureus* enterotoxin B binds to the α_1 domain of the α subunit of the human MHC class II molecule HLA-DR1, creating a novel TCR-binding site adjacent to the conventional antigen-MHC binding site [*see Chapter 101*]. Different MHC class II alleles have distinct binding constants for superantigens; thus, superantigens can activate distinct segments of the T cell repertoire.

PROFESSIONAL ANTIGEN-PRESENTING CELLS

Whereas MHC class I molecules are expressed on the surface of all eukaryotic cells, MHC class II molecules have a restricted tissue distribution. In fact, certain cells—including B cells, dendritic cells, macrophages, Langerhans cells, and endothelial cells—are termed professional APCs because they present antigenic peptide with MHC class II molecules more efficiently than other APCs.[8] This efficiency is primarily attributed to their ability to process endocytosed antigens. Professional APCs also interact with T cells more efficiently because they have several cell surface markers that bind to costimulatory molecules on the surface of T cells (see below). The most potent APCs are dendritic cells, which present antigen only on maturation and migration to the lymph nodes. This maturation process is triggered by the uptake of antigen.

MECHANISMS OF ANTIGEN PRESENTATION TO T CELLS

T cell recognition of antigen proceeds in two distinct stages: a nonspecific cell-cell adhesion step between a T cell clone expressing one type of $\alpha\beta$ TCR and an APC, followed by a specific interaction between the TCR and the antigen-MHC complex. This process highlights two fundamental properties of T cells: their ability to migrate throughout the body and adhere to many types of cells and their great specificity for particular antigens.

APCs simultaneously process many peptide antigens and thus express on their cell surfaces a large number of different antigen-MHC complexes. Only a small number of these complexes can be recognized by a given $\alpha\beta$ T cell clone. Through cell-cell adhesion, T cells screen APCs; adhesion is aborted in the absence of specific antigen recognition by the TCR and is intensified when the correct TCR–peptide–MHC molecule contact is made. On adhesion, TCR-CD3 complexes aggregate on the surface of the T cell and bind to the antigen-MHC complexes that have aggregated on the surface of the APC. Downregulation of adhesion molecules permits cell detachment. In the absence of antigen recognition, TCR-CD3 complexes are unable to cluster and detachment occurs immediately.

Interactions between a helper T cell clone and an APC or between a cytotoxic T cell and its target cell follow the same general pattern. Because the binding constant between the TCR and the antigen-MHC complex is low, only a very small number of the complexes initially engage with specific TCRs in an area of cell-cell contact established by adhesion. Subsequently, TCR-CD3 complexes and MHC molecules bearing the correct antigenic peptide migrate into the T cell–APC contact region. This establishes a high local density of TCRs, which promotes antigen binding and T cell activation. The existence of these clustered TCRs has been demonstrated using confocal microscopy and tagged monoclonal antibodies in studies of the interface between a helper T cell clone and an antigen-specific APC.[9] In addition, clusters of TCRs can be visualized using fluorescence-tagged tetramers of antigen-MHC complexes.[10] This novel technique has permitted incisive studies of epitope-specific T cell responses to infections with Epstein-Barr virus or HIV.[11]

COSTIMULATORY MOLECULES

Aberrant activation of the TCR can initiate disastrous immune responses, such as those seen in autoimmune diseases and other immunopathologies. Thus, recognition of antigen by the TCR and subsequent signal transduction events are positively or negatively regulated by other T cell surface molecules [*see Figure 2*].[12] Costimulatory molecules are involved in both adhesion and T cell signal transduction and play a major role in the coordination and kinetic regulation of T cell activation.

CD4 and CD8 molecules are TCR coreceptors that interact with MHC molecules on the surface of APCs. This interaction is probably instrumental in generating CD4+ and CD8+ T cells in the thymus. Because CD4 and CD8 are both part of the TCR-MHC clusters and are associated with the protein tyrosine kinase Lck, they directly influence TCR-initiated signal transduction (see below). Other key costimulators are the adhesion molecules CD2 and CD11/CD18. The natural APC surface–bound ligand for CD2 is CD58, whereas the ligands for CD11/CD18 are intercellular adhesion molecule–1 (ICAM-1, also designated CD54), the complement component iC3b, and extracellular matrix proteins.

CD28 and CTLA-4 provide the most important second signal, initiating a pathway of signal transduction that is different from and often independent of the pathway mediated by the TCR-CD3 complex. CD28 is a cell surface glycoprotein expressed on essentially all CD4+ and most CD8+ T cells. CD28 binds to B7-1 (CD80), which is expressed in low densities on APCs (although its expression can be upregulated). Binding of CD28 to B7-1 or to a second counterstructure, B7-2 (CD86), leads to costimulatory signal transduction and consequent T cell activation and proliferation. In contrast, expression of CTLA-4, which is homologous to CD28, is upregulated after T cell activation. Binding of CTLA-4 to B7-1 or B7-2 delivers an inhibitory signal that leads to downregulation of T cell proliferation. Of note is that research entailing manipulation of CD28/CTLA-4 interactions with their natural ligands has produced novel results in transplantation and tumor therapy settings and may have potential in the treatment of such diseases as

a

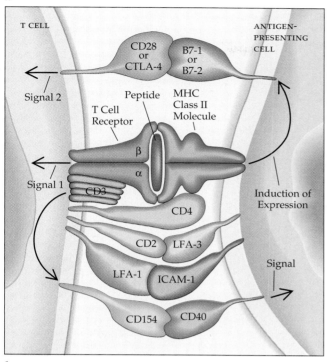

b

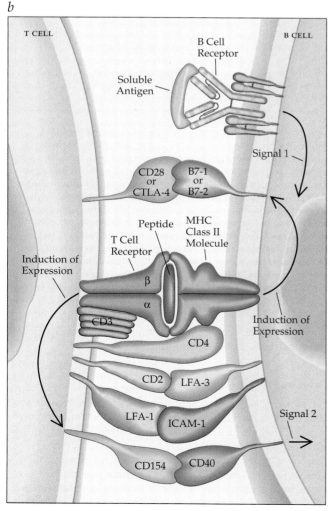

arthritis, multiple sclerosis, and asthma and in protection against HIV infection.[13]

The costimulatory molecule CD27 is expressed on T cell activation and acts synergistically with TCR-associated activation to induce T cell proliferation. CD27 on T cells is a member of the tumor necrosis factor receptor (TNFR) family, whereas its ligand, CD70, which is found on activated T and B cells, is a member of the TNF family.

Another member of the TNFR family, Fas (also called APO-1 and CD95), has been implicated in both positive and negative signaling events through interaction with the Fas ligand (CD95L) that is expressed on cytolytic effectors. The ligation of Fas on T cells to CD95L typically causes its programmed cell death (i.e., apoptosis; see below). However, ligation of Fas to an anti-Fas monoclonal antibody has shown that Fas can function as a costimulatory molecule for TCR-CD3 activation. Thus, a single molecule can have different signaling outcomes at different stages of T cell development.

T Cell Signal Transduction on Antigen Recognition

In response to antigen recognition, resting T cells undergo a complex series of events known as T cell activation.[14,15] The extracellular event—recognition and binding of TCRs to antigen-MHC complexes and of costimulatory molecules to their appropriate ligands—is followed by an intracellular cascade of biochemical events (i.e., signal transduction) that ultimately reaches specific genes in the nucleus. The specific production of cytokines, chemokines, and other immunomodulatory molecules leads to cell proliferation, differentiation, and expression of unique effector functions.

Most of the biochemical events that occur immediately after engagement of the TCR with the antigen-MHC complex have been defined [*see Figure 3*]. The first step is recruitment of one of two principal Srk family protein tyrosine kinases, Lck and Fyn, to the CD3 elements (CD3-γ, CD3-δ, CD3-ε, and CD3-ζ) of the TCR-CD3 complex. These enzymes phosphorylate specific tyrosine residues in the so-called immunoreceptor tyrosine-based activation motif (ITAM) sequences found on the CD3 cytoplasmic tails. The level of CD3-ζ phosphorylation depends on the avidity between the antigen-MHC complex and the αβ TCR.[16,17]

A cycle of tyrosine phosphorylation and dephosphorylation

Figure 2 (*a*) Two signals are necessary for activation of an antigen-specific T cell by an antigen-presenting cell (APC). Signal 1 is initiated by the interaction between the antigen bound to a class II major histocompatibility complex (MHC) and the T cell receptor (TCR) and its coreceptor (in this example, CD4). The costimulatory molecules B7-1 and B7-2 are transiently expressed on the surface of so-called professional APCs and are presumed to be inducible by signaling from the antigen-MHC complex. Thus, signal 2 is initiated by the binding of CD28 on the T cell to B7-1 or B7-2. CTLA-4, which is homologous to CD28, is upregulated after T cell activation.

(*b*) Activation of B cells can occur with either helper T cells or soluble antigen. Binding of soluble antigen to the B cell receptor, a cell surface immunoglobulin associated with Igα and Igβ, can lead to B cell proliferation or apoptosis. Alternatively, B cells can process antigen for presentation to TCRs on T cells. Binding of antigen-MHC complex to the TCR induces expression of the CD40 ligand (CD154) on the T cell surface, which in turn induces expression of CD40 on the B cell surface. This results in B cell proliferation and is indispensable for immunoglobulin class switching and probably for somatic mutation. CD154 signaling also plays an important role in the maturation of dendritic cells. (ICAM-1—intercellular adhesion molecule–1; LFA—leukocyte-function–associated antigen)

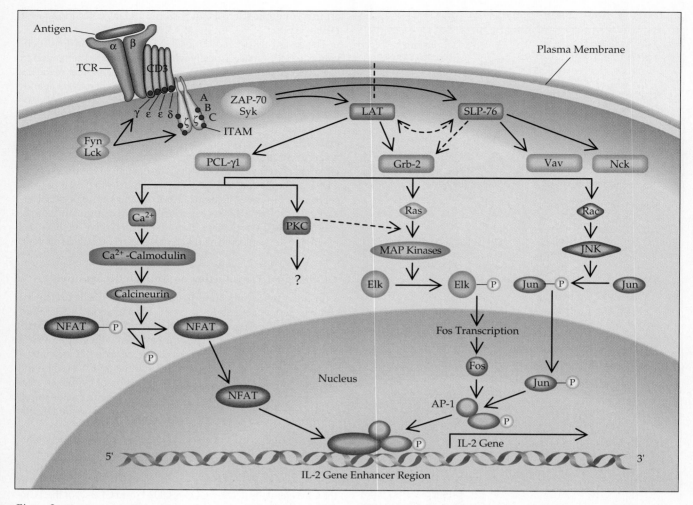

Figure 3   The downstream signaling pathways induced after TCR stimulation are shown. Phosphorylation of the cytoplasmic tails of the CD3-γ, CD3-δ, CD3-ε, and CD3-ζ by the Src kinase Fyn or Lck recruits the kinase Syk or ZAP-70, which relays the signal of TCR binding through tyrosine phosphorylation of two adapter proteins, LAT and SLP-76. Nck is an adapter protein associated with SLP-76. These adapter proteins act on components of classic signal transduction pathways, including phospholipase C-γ1 (PLC-γ1), growth factor receptor–bound protein–2 (Grb-2, a protein-linking receptor tyrosine kinase), the p85 subunit of phosphatidylinositol 3–kinase (PI-3 kinase), and possibly Vav (a guanosine triphosphate/guanosine diphosphate [GTP/GDP] exchange factor for Rho-family GTPases, including Ras and Rac). Activation of PLC-γ causes the release of diacylglycerol, which in turn activates protein kinase C (PKC). PKC is involved in initiating the cascade of other serine-threonine kinases, including Raf-1, mitogen-activated protein (MAP) kinase and MAP kinase kinase (MEK). The central signal transduction molecule Ras appears to be involved in late events after PKC activation. The Ras and Rac pathways and the serine–threonine kinase pathways are coupled; they activate early genes, such as *jun* and *fos*. The Ca²⁺ generated by PLC-γ1 activates another downstream cascade, the calcineurin pathway. Calcineurin, a serine-threonine phosphatase, is a calcium- and calmodulin-dependent enzyme involved in induction of transcription factor NFAT (nuclear factor for activated T cells). PI-3 kinase is a ubiquitous enzyme in the mitogenic signaling and apoptotic pathways of both receptor and nonreceptor protein tyrosine kinases. These various signaling pathways converge by delivering a distinct set of transcription factors, including Jun, Elk, NFAT, Fos, and AP-1 (all DNA-binding proteins), to the promoter region of the *IL-2* gene, stimulating expression of the gene and production of IL-2.

regulates antigen-induced T cell activation. Dephosphorylation and prevention of tyrosine phosphorylation are carried out by tyrosine phosphatases (e.g., CD45) and the Src-inactivator Csk, respectively. Csk has been shown to inhibit TCR-induced cytokine gene activation by its phosphorylation of the negative regulatory sites in Lck and Fyn, causing these two enzymes to be inactivated.

After phosphorylation of docking sites in the cytoplasmic tails of the CD3s, one of two membrane-localized protein tyrosine kinases, Syk or ZAP-70, is recruited into the complex. These kinases activate cytoplasmic signaling proteins, which induce the activation of transcription factors that control the expression of genes mediating T cell effector function (e.g., the gene for the cytokine interleukin-2 [IL-2]) [*see Figure 3*]. Thus, the exquisitely T cell

clone–specific TCR connects, via a number of intermediate molecules, with universal signal transduction pathways.

Cytokines and T Cell Subsets

Cytokines, a diverse group of proteins produced by a number of different cell types, are critical in the regulation of immune responses. They are also important in the differentiation of cell systems. In general, cytokines are not stored in cells but are synthesized on appropriate stimulation. The resultant messenger RNA (mRNA) is short-lived. In some cases, the active cytokine is released from an inactive precursor by proteolysis. After secretion, cytokines usually act locally by binding to receptors on cell surfaces. Cytokines may act on many different cells, and different cytokines may have similar activities. Cytokine receptors are often composed of the same protein chains. For instance, the cytokine receptors IL-2R, IL-4R, IL-7R, IL-9R, IL-13R, and IL-15R have the γ chain in common. Most cytokines form a network that regulates the activation of cells and the production of other cytokines.[18] Through binding to receptors on cell surfaces, cytokines exert their effects by activating intracellular signaling mechanisms, which lead to expression of particular genes (e.g., genes for themselves or other cytokines). The principal intracellular cytokine signal transducers are the Jak (Janus kinase) protein tyrosine kinases and the STAT (signal transducers and activators of transcription) family of transcription factors.

HELPER T CELLS

Cytokines play a major role in T cell development and regulation. Indeed, the two helper T cell subsets, Th1 and Th2, are defined by the cytokines they produce [see Chapter 97]. Th1 and Th2 cells play key roles in determining the balance between two immunologic outcomes: host resistance and immunopathology.[19] Th1 responses are potentially effective in the eradication of infectious agents, but when a Th1-dominated response is poorly effective or too prolonged, host damage may result. Th2 responses are primarily involved in allergic reactions, antibody production, and antibody class switching. They can limit potentially harmful Th1-mediated responses and may be part of the suppressor mechanism for exaggerated or inappropriate Th1 responses.[20]

Each of the two helper T cell subsets inhibits the development and function of the other. Interferon gamma produced by Th1 cells inhibits the development and function of Th2 cells. In contrast, IL-4 and IL-10 produced by Th2 cells inhibit the development and function of Th1 cells. IL-4 acts partly by downregulating the expression of the IL-12 receptor, IL-12Rβ, which is upregulated by interferon gamma [see Figure 4]. IL-12 enhances cell function because it is a potent growth factor for natural killer (NK) cells, which also produce interferon gamma. The fact that Th2 cells inhibit Th1 immune responses and that Th1 cells inhibit Th2 antibody-mediating responses can probably be attributed to the fact that both subsets also induce inflammation, which must be regulated [see Cytokines and Inflammation, below].

Studies of the immune response to Schistosoma parasites have shown that a surface carbohydrate, lacto-N-fucopentaose–III (LNFP-III) can switch a Th1-protective cell-mediated response to a Th2 response mediated primarily by antibody.[21] LNFP-III stimulates the expansion of B_1 cells and causes them to secrete large amounts of IL-10. Acting through macrophages, IL-10 inhibits Th1 cells and favors the Th2 response. IL-12 blocks the expansion of B_1 cells by the carbohydrate. This phenomenon has important implications for immunity to many organisms because this carbohydrate, which contains Lewis^x, is present on other parasites and on cancer cells. The microorganism or cancer cell might use this carbohydrate to inhibit the host's protective cell-mediated immune response. Carbohydrates might also inhibit Th1-controlled autoimmune diseases.

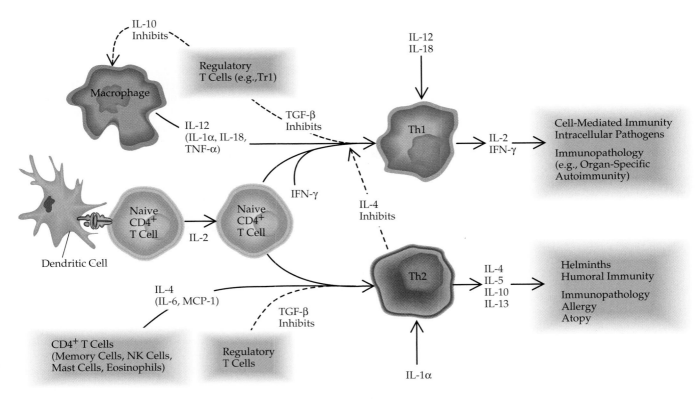

Figure 4 Regulation of helper T cell responses. In response to IL-12 and cofactors such as IL-18 and IL-1α, naive CD4$^+$ T cells can develop into Th1 cells responsible for cell-mediated immunity; differentiation is dependent on interferon gamma (IFN-γ). Th1 cells produce IFN-γ and IL-2. Th1 responses are directly antagonized by IL-4 and indirectly by IL-10, as it inhibits production of IL-12 and IL-18 by macrophages. Th2 cells, which are responsible for inducing antibody production by B cells and allergic responses, depend on IL-4 for differentiation from naive CD4$^+$ T cells. Th2 cells produce IL-4, IL-5, IL-10, and IL-13. TGF-β can inhibit both Th1 and Th2 development. (MCP—monocyte chemoattractant protein; TGF—transforming growth factor)

MEMORY T CELLS

On reexposure to an antigen, memory cells mediate a more rapid and stronger immune response than naive T cells. Compared with naive T cells, memory cells respond differently and have a different pattern of surface markers. CD45RO is a marker found on memory cells. Memory cells secrete a full range of cytokines and may show the same polarization as Th1 and Th2 cells.[12] The requirements for proliferation and cytokine production in memory cells are not as strict as for naive T cells, but optimum responses require costimulation.[22] Memory T cells selectively migrate (home) to specific nonlymphoid tissues such as gut, skin, and lung. Those that home to the gut have specialized integrins (adhesion molecules) on their surface called $\alpha4\beta7$ that mediate this migration [see Chapter 97]. Memory cells appear to persist in the absence of antigenic stimulation as nondividing cells. Reencounter with an antigen can expand the population to a stable, higher level; competition from another antigen can decrease the population.[22]

T REGULATORY CELLS

Chronic activation of human CD4+ T cells in the presence of IL-10 gives rise to a subset of antigen-specific CD4+ T cell clones with low proliferative capacity that produce high levels of IL-10, low levels of IL-2, and no IL-4. These T cells, called T regulatory cells (Tr1), suppress the proliferation of CD4+ T cells in response to antigen, which suppresses antigen-specific immune responses and actively downregulates a pathologic immune response.[23]

Cytokines and Inflammation

PROINFLAMMATORY CYTOKINES

Tumor Necrosis Factor–α

Cytokines are critically involved in inflammation. TNF-α, a major proinflammatory cytokine, is one of the most abundant substances produced by macrophages after stimulation with interferon gamma, migration inhibitory factor (MIF), or bacterial lipopolysaccharide (LPS). TNF-α is also produced by activated T cells, NK cells, and mast cells.

The inflammatory response begins with the expression of the adhesion molecules ICAM-1, vascular cell adhesion molecule–1 (VCAM-1), and E-selectin (ELAM-1) on vascular endothelial cells. These molecules promote the adhesion of neutrophils, monocytes, and lymphocytes to the vessel wall, from which they extravasate into the tissues [see Chapter 97]. At low concentrations, TNF-α enhances the protective inflammatory response, activating and enhancing the function of various leukocytes, including neutrophils, macrophages, and eosinophils. This can further stimulate the production of cytokines by macrophages, including TNF-α itself, IL-1, IL-6, and a variety of chemotactic cytokines [see Chemokines, below]. TNF-α enhances expression of MHC class I molecules, potentiates cytotoxic T cell–induced cell lysis, functions as an endogenous pyrogen (i.e., TNF-α induces fever, along with IL-1 and IL-6, by direct and indirect actions on the brain), activates the clotting system and the production of acute-phase proteins by the liver, and can cause immunodeficiency through suppression of the bone marrow. TNF-α also causes cachexia when present for prolonged periods.

TNF-α plays a primary role in the host response to gram-negative bacteria, the source of endotoxin and LPS. LPS causes the release of MIF, which in turn enhances TNF-α production by macrophages. At low concentrations of LPS, TNF-α mediates a protective response. At high concentrations of LPS, however, TNF-α mediates disseminated intravascular coagulation—part of what is known as the Shwartzman reaction—and death from shock.

Protective immunity to certain intracellular organisms, such as *Leishmania*, is enhanced by TNF-α, and TNF-α has potent antiviral activity. However, many of the symptoms of malaria, especially of cerebral malaria, and some symptoms of HIV infection may be mediated by TNF-α. Antibody to TNF-α has been approved for treatment of Crohn's disease [see Chapter 58].[24]

Lymphotoxin

Produced exclusively by activated T cells (Th1 cells), lymphotoxin has many of the same biologic properties as TNF-α and is also referred to as TNF-β. Like TNF-α, lymphotoxin lyses tumor cells but not normal cells, activates neutrophils, and increases vascular adhesion and extravasation of leukocytes. The effects of lymphotoxin are mediated when lymphotoxin binds to another protein, lymphotoxin-β, to form a complex. It utilizes the same cell receptor as TNF-α. In addition, lymphotoxin plays a role in the development of lymphoid tissue.

Interleukin-1 and Interleukin-6

IL-1 is produced mainly by monocytes and macrophages but also by other cells, such as epithelial and endothelial cells. It is an endogenous pyrogen, and many of its functions are similar to those of TNF-α. It induces the production of additional IL-1 and of IL-6 from macrophages and induces glucocorticoid synthesis and the release of prostaglandin, collagenase, and acute-phase proteins. IL-1 increases the expression of surface molecules on endothelial cells, leading to adhesion of leukocytes and coagulation, and stimulates the production of macrophage chemokines that in turn activate neutrophils. IL-1 differs from TNF-α in that it does not produce necrosis of tumors or tissue injury, increase expression of MHC, or, by itself, mediate the Shwartzman reaction.

Macrophages produce an IL-1 receptor antagonist (IL-1rα) that is structurally similar to IL-1 and binds to the IL-1 receptor but is inactive. IL-1rα, along with the IL-1 receptors shed from activated cells, inhibits IL-1 and thus acts as a regulator. Such natural inhibitors to IL-1 are being investigated as potential agents for clinical use to counteract certain inflammatory processes.

IL-6 is induced by IL-1 and TNF-α from macrophages and in turn inhibits macrophage production of IL-1 and TNF-α. IL-6 acts on hepatic cells to produce acute-phase proteins, such as fibrinogen, α_2-macroglobulin, and serum amyloid A protein. This cytokine can also inhibit macrophage activation.

Interferon Gamma

Interferon gamma, produced by T cells and NK cells, is the primary macrophage-activating factor (MAF) and is thus a potent cytokine in cell-mediated immunity. Activated macrophages produce many cytokines and chemokines intimately involved in inflammation, including TNF-α, IL-1, IL-6, and MIF. Other MAFs include granulocyte-macrophage colony-stimulating factor (GM-CSF) and MIF. IL-1 and TNF-α have weak MAF activity. IL-12 stimulates NK cells to produce greater amounts of interferon gamma, enhancing interferon gamma–dependent reactions. On its own and by enhancing the effects of TNF-α, interferon gamma causes the expression of adhesion molecules on the surface of vascular endothelial cells, leading to T cell adhesion and extravasation.

The proinflammatory effects of interferon gamma are countered by transforming growth factor–β (TGF-β) and IL-10, which inhibit macrophage activation. Interferon gamma has been used successfully to treat chronic granulomatous disease and drug-resistant visceral leishmaniasis.[25]

Migration Inhibitory Factor

MIF was the first discovered T cell cytokine produced after the stimulation of sensitized T cells with specific antigen. It derives its name from the fact that it inhibits the random migration of macrophages. MIF acts as an endogenous hormone that counterregulates glucocorticoid action.[26] Macrophages and T cells release MIF in response to glucocorticoids and other proinflammatory stimuli. MIF then overrides the immunosuppressive effects of steroids on macrophage and T cell cytokine production.[26]

The gene for MIF is a delayed early gene expressed in many different tissues.[27] Large amounts of the gene are found in macrophages and pituitary cells. Indeed, LPS stimulates the release of MIF by the pituitary. When given to mice, MIF greatly enhances the lethality of LPS; conversely, anti-MIF antibodies completely reverse the lethality of LPS.[28] Recombinant MIF has been shown to activate macrophages to kill *Leishmania* and stimulate macrophages to produce TNF-α and nitric oxide. Mice lacking the gene for MIF show enhanced resistance to the lethal effects of high doses of LPS and *S. aureus* enterotoxin B as well as to *Pseudomonas aeruginosa*, but they are susceptible to *Leishmania*.[29]

Of note is that anti-MIF therapies are under development. The goal is to increase the immunosuppressive and anti-inflammatory properties of endogenously released glucocorticoids, thereby reducing the need for steroid therapy in a variety of autoimmune and inflammatory conditions.[26]

INTERLEUKIN-5

IL-5 mainly affects eosinophil recruitment and activation. IL-5 is produced by Th2 cells and activated mast cells and stimulates the growth and differentiation of eosinophils. Eosinophils are activated by IL-5, TNF-α, and an eosinophil cytotoxicity–enhancing factor derived from monocytes. Activated eosinophils produce tissue damage in allergic states and kill helminthic parasites.

ANTI-INFLAMMATORY CYTOKINES

Interleukin-4 and Interleukin-13

IL-4 stimulates the expression of VCAM on endothelial cells, leading to the binding of eosinophils, lymphocytes, neutrophils, and monocytes and their subsequent extravasation. However, IL-4 also acts as an anti-inflammatory cytokine, inhibiting activated macrophages and diminishing the production of TNF-α and nitric oxide.

IL-13 has the ability to take over some of the functions of IL-4. Both interleukins induce IgE synthesis in B cells and differentiation of T cells to Th2 cells and can suppress inflammatory processes induced by Th1 cells. IL-4 and IL-13 mediate their effects through binding to receptors on target cells (IL-4R and IL-13R, respectively) and activating intracellular signal transduction through Jak kinases and the transcription factor STAT6, which mediates transcription of IL-4 responsive genes. These cytokines also act on macrophages to suppress a number of proinflammatory cytokines, chemokines, and hematopoietic growth factors, including IL-1, IL-8, TNF-α, macrophage inflammatory protein–1α (MIP-1α), and GM-CSF. This results in the downregulation of Fc receptors on macrophages and inhibition of antibody-dependent cell-mediated cytotoxicity (ADCC) and nitric oxide production.

Activated mast cells and basophils produce additional IL-4. Of interest is that mutated IL-4 can inhibit IgE synthesis by IL-4 and IL-13 and may prove useful in treating some allergic states.

Transforming Growth Factor–β

TGF-β is produced by a variety of cells, including platelets, lymphocytes, activated macrophages, and placenta cells. It is an important anti-inflammatory cytokine because it inhibits macrophage activation and the maturation of cytotoxic T cells and thus controls the effects of many cytokines.

Interleukin-10

IL-10 is produced by CD4+ and CD8+ T cells, B cells, macrophages, activated mast cells, and keratinocytes. Although usually associated with activity of Th2 cells, IL-10 can also be produced by Th1 cells. IL-10 suppresses lymphocyte responses by downregulating macrophage cytokines—including IL-1, TNF-α, IL-6, IL-8, GM-CSF, and granulocyte colony-stimulating factor (G-CSF)—and inhibiting nitric oxide production.

Chemokines

Chemokines are a superfamily of low-molecular-weight cytokines that mediate the directional migration of leukocytes during normal and inflammatory processes.[30] They play an important role in attracting granulocytes into sites of inflammation. There are four distinct families of chemokines that are distinguished on the basis of the position of their first two conserved cysteine residues: CXC (the first two cysteines are separated by one amino acid), CC, C, and CX3C. The receptors for chemokines are all integral membrane G-protein coupled receptors, which constitute one of the largest classes of signaling molecules.

CXC chemokines predominantly activate neutrophils.[31] This family includes IL-8, β-thromboglobulin (β-TG), gro-α, gro-β, gro-γ, and platelet factor 4. They are usually produced by monocytes; some are produced by other cells, including T cells, endothelial cells, and platelets. IL-8 induces expression of neutrophil-binding integrins on endothelial cells, resulting in the rapid accumulation of neutrophils in tissues. The chemokine gro (growth-related gene product) also stimulates neutrophil accumulation as well as the release of lysosomal enzymes that contribute to the local inflammatory response. Platelet factor 4 and β-TG are released from aggregated platelets and stimulate fibroblasts, which are required for repair at sites of hemorrhage or thrombosis.

The CC chemokines activate T cells, monocytes, and eosinophils. This family includes RANTES (regulated on activation, normal T cell expressed and secreted), macrophage chemotactic and activating factor (MCAF), MIP-1α, and MIP-1β. CC chemokines are produced by activated T cells and monocytes. RANTES is a potent attractant for memory T cells (but not for naive T cells) and also attracts monocytes. MCAF acts exclusively on monocytes, attracting them, activating them, and regulating the expression of integrins on their surface. MIP-1α and MIP-1β attract only monocytes. The CC chemokines eotaxin, eotaxin-2, and monocyte chemoattractant protein-4 (MCP-4) predominantly activate eosinophils.[31]

Chemokine receptors play an important role as coreceptors for HIV. The virus first interacts with CD4 on T cells but requires a coreceptor to penetrate the cell membrane. The CC chemokine receptor–5 (CCR5) that mediates activation of T cells and macrophages is the major coreceptor for some HIV-1 strains. The natural ligands for CCR5 include RANTES, MIP-1α, and MIP-1β.[32] The CXC chemokine receptor–4 (CXCR4) appears to be important in late-stage HIV infection.[33]

B Cell Responses to Antigen

When a B cell receptor (BCR) binds soluble antigen, one of two events takes place: apoptosis or proliferation and further maturation of B cells. The signals for these processes are generated intracellularly by Igα and Igβ. These proteins are associated with BCRs in the way that CD3 proteins are associated with TCRs. Igα and Igβ recruit signal transduction molecules in a manner similar to that of the TCR-CD3 complex—namely, in two waves of protein tyrosine kinases, the first wave consisting of Lyn, Fyn, and Btk and the second wave consisting of Syk. Some of the same proteins involved in T cell activation are then recruited (e.g., PI-3 kinase, Vav, Ras, Raf-1, MEK, PLC-β, and PLC-γ). The pathway for activating B cells is similar but not identical to that for activating T cells.

Relatively little is known about the signaling that takes place in B cells when they have presented an antigen to a helper T cell that recognizes it. T cell–B cell interaction can also lead to either apoptosis or proliferation of B cells. With T cell help, however, proliferation results in the generation of several different classes of B cells.

B CELL SUBSETS

Follicular Mantle Cells

Follicular mantle cells express IgD (IgD$^+$,CD38$^-$) on their surface and can mature into plasma cells that produce IgM antibodies only. These cells produce IgMs that display extensive heterogeneity, but the cells do not undergo somatic mutation to generate even larger numbers of heterogeneous antibody molecules.

Centrocytes

The process leading to somatic mutation occurs in the centrocytes, which are IgD$^-$,CD38$^+$ B cells that have undergone class switching to produce IgG. The maturation step from IgD$^+$,CD38$^-$ B cells to IgD$^-$,CD38$^+$ B cells depends on cell-cell contact with antigen-specific T cells and cytokines. IL-4 in particular is of great importance for the events that lead to class switching.

Memory B Cells

The most mature B cell, the memory cell, does not express IgD or CD38 but is distinguished by other cell surface markers and by its location within the germinal center. Memory cells can also develop into plasma cells producing IgM, IgG, IgA, and IgE. In general, the generation of plasma cells from memory B cells is independent of T cell help.

T CELL–B CELL INTERACTIONS

CD40 is a cell surface receptor belonging to the TNFR family that was first identified on B cells. The natural ligand for CD40, CD40L (also called CD154), is a T cell surface type 2 glycoprotein related to TNF. Transient CD40L expression on the surface of T cells is induced by TCR binding to antigen-MHC complex and by binding of B7 to CD28 or CTLA-4. CD40-CD40L binding stimulates B cell immunoglobulin class switching. This was best demonstrated by elucidation of the molecular defect in a genetic immunodeficiency termed hyper-IgM syndrome. A mutation in the gene encoding CD40L is responsible for the defective antibody class switching in this syndrome. T cell–independent B cell responses and responses induced by anti-CD40 are unaffected by this mutation. Thus, T cell help for B cell activation is primarily directed through the CD40-CD40L costimulatory pathway. Persons with hyper-IgM syndrome are susceptible to pathogens that produce AIDS-like opportunistic infections—normally dealt with by T cells—underscoring the role of CD40L costimulation in normal T cell activation. Absence of CD40L has a more dramatic effect on Ig class switching than does an absence of T cells. Thus, it seems that CD40L may be expressed on cells other than T cells that could induce immunoglobulin class switching in B cells through the ligation of CD40.

Effector Mechanisms in Cell-Mediated Immunity

Cell-mediated immunity encompasses the killing of invading microorganisms, such as bacteria, viruses, fungi, and parasites; the destruction of tumor cells; the rejection of tissue grafts; and injury to tissues in various disease states, including autoimmunity. Cell-mediated immune reactions can also be induced by contact with antigens, such as those found in poison ivy and numerous drugs. Drugs are more likely to provoke cell-mediated reactions when applied topically than when given systemically.

Most cell-mediated immune reactions involve initial interaction between sensitized T cells and antigens on presenting cells. This reaction can trigger several effector pathways, including activation of cytotoxic T cells, stimulation of T cell production of cytokines that activate macrophages and promote the proliferation of NK cells, and production of antibodies involved in antibody-dependent cell-mediated cytotoxicity by NK cells and other cell types. Although cell-mediated immune reactions other than ADCC do not require the presence of antibody or complement, they can be modified by these humoral factors. Subsequent events require cooperation between different subsets of T cells; the reactions involved are controlled by various cytokines.

The mechanisms of cell-mediated immunity involving T cell–macrophage interactions can be both protective (leading to the killing of invading microorganisms) and harmful (leading to inflammation and tissue destruction). Sometimes, the two go hand in hand; in tuberculosis, for example, both the killing of tubercle bacilli and the production of cavities in the lungs are consequences of T cell–macrophage interactions.

APOPTOSIS

Cytotoxic T cells and NK cells are the body's primary defense against viral-infected and tumorigenic cells. These killer cells induce target cell death by two mechanisms. The classic mechanism is granule-mediated apoptosis. A second mechanism is receptor-mediated apoptosis. In response to binding of the ligand expressed on the killer cell, cell surface receptors aggregate on the target cell, which leads to the recruitment of cytoplasmic proteins to the receptors and transduction of a death signal to the target cell.[34]

Cytotoxic T Cells

Cytotoxic T cells are antigen-specific effector cells that are important in resisting infectious agents, especially viruses present in cells other than macrophages; in killing tumors; and in allograft rejection. Most cytotoxic T cells are CD8$^+$ T cells that recognize antigen presented by MHC class I molecules, although a considerable number of CD4$^+$ T cells have the capability to kill target cells.

A Mg^{2+}-dependent cytotoxic T cell–target cell adhesion phase is followed by a Ca^{2+}-dependent phase that leads to the delivery of cytotoxic chemicals to the target cell. The cytotoxic T cell then dissociates from the target cell; death proceeds in the absence of the cytotoxic T cell, which recycles to attack another target cell. If the cytotoxic T cell adheres to a cell that does not carry the correct antigenic peptide–MHC molecule combination, no cytotoxic chemicals are released and the cells dissociate more rapidly.

Cytotoxic T cells develop granules that contain cytotoxic molecules, including perforins (proteins that produce holes or pores in a cell's surface membrane), serine proteases (granzyme A and granzyme B), and serine esterases. Of these, perforins are the most important, as has been shown in mice in which the gene encoding peforin has been deleted. A second killing mechanism involves the Fas ligand on the cytotoxic T cell and Fas on the target cell. This is the only mechanism of killing available to perforin[null] mice, and it is used preferentially—but not exclusively—in CD4[+] cytotoxic T cells.

In response to viruses, a large number of virus-specific cytotoxic T cells are produced. This is most dramatically shown during the initial responses to B cells infected with Epstein-Barr virus. It has been found that cytotoxic T cell clones specific for some antigen-MHC complexes are extremely abundant, constituting approximately 50% of all cytotoxic T cells.[11] When the cytotoxic T cell response diminishes, these abundant T cell clones are probably removed through apoptotic mechanisms.

Natural Killer Cells

NK cells are the cytolytic effectors of the innate immune system [see Chapter 97]. IL-12 is a potent inducer of activation and proliferation of NK cells; interferon gamma and IL-2 also activate these cells. IL-2 enhances the tumoricidal capacity of NK cells that leads to development of lymphokine-activated killer (LAK) cells. NK cells can also secrete interferon gamma, which acts in an autoactive manner to enhance NK cell activity. TNF-α appears to counteract the development of NK cells induced by IL-12.

The receptor-mediated attachment of NK cells to the target cell occurs in a Ca^{2+}-independent step. Once the NK cells are activated, however, they require Ca^{2+} ions for lysis. Cytolysis is initiated when the NK cells orient their granules toward the target cell and release perforins and proteolytic enzymes; the mechanism of action is similar to that of cytotoxic T cells. Killing by NK cells, in contrast to killing by cytotoxic T cells, however, is not blocked by anti-CD3 or anti-CD8 monoclonal antibodies but by antibodies to the adhesion molecule LFA-1.

NK cells are also subject to receptor-mediated inhibition of effector function.[35] Killer inhibitory signals are transduced by receptors on NK cells that detect MHC class I molecules on target cells. On ligand binding to the inhibitory receptor, phosphorylation of immunoreceptor tyrosine-based inhibition motif (ITIM) sequences occurs, providing a substrate for the binding of protein tyrosine phosphatases SHP-1 and SHP-2. These phosphatases mediate the cytoplasmic transduction of a negative signal that results in the inhibition of cytotoxicity and cytokine expression. Killer inhibitory receptors are also found on the surface of some cytotoxic T cells, indicating that cytotoxic T cell responses can also be affected by members of the inhibitory receptor superfamily.[35,36]

Additional Information

An extensive list of CD antigen designations has been posted on the World Wide Web. The URL for this list is www.cx.unibe.ch/dkf6/immunology/info/cd_table.htm. Illustrations of the known structures of cytokines, as determined by x-ray crystallography or multidimensional nuclear magnetic spectroscopy, can also be viewed on the World Wide Web. The URL for this site is www.psynix.co.uk/cytweb/cyt_strucs/struc_class.html.

References

1. Davis MM, Boniface JJ, Reich Z, et al: Ligand recognition by alpha beta T cell receptors. Annu Rev Immunol 16:523, 1998
2. Li S, Paulsson KM, Sjogren HO, et al: Peptide-bound major histocompatibility complex class I molecules with tapasin before dissociation from transporter associated with peptide processing. J Biol Chem 274:8649, 1999
3. Ploegh HL: Viral strategies of immune evasion. Science 280:248, 1998
4. Barrera CA, Almanza RJ, Ogra PL, et al: The role of the invariant chain in mucosal immunity. Int Arch Allergy Immunol 117:85, 1998
5. Beckman EM, Porcelli SA, Morita CT, et al: Recognition of a lipid antigen by CD1-restricted alpha beta+ T cells. Nature 372:691, 1994
6. Park SH, Chiu YH, Jayawardena J, et al: Innate and adaptive functions of the CD1 pathway of antigen presentation. Semin Immunol 10:391, 1998
7. Jardetzky TS, Brown JH, Gorga JC, et al.: Three-dimensional structure of a human class II histocompatibility molecule complexed with superantigen. Nature 368:711, 1994
8. Banchereau J, Steinman RM: Dendritic cells and the control of immunity. Nature 392:245, 1998
9. Viola A, Schroeder S, Sakakibara Y, et al: T lymphocyte costimulation mediated by reorganization of membrane microdomains. Science 283:680, 1999
10. Altman JD, Moss PAH, Goulder PJR, et al: Phenotypic analysis of antigen-specific T lymphocytes. Science 274:94, 1996
11. McMichael AJ, O'Callaghan CA: A new look at T cells. J Exp Med 187:1367, 1998
12. Van Parijs L, Abbas AK: Homeostasis and self-tolerance in the immune system: turning lymphocytes off. Science 280:243, 1998
13. Ward SG: The complexities of CD28 and CTLA-4 signalling: PI3K and beyond. Arch Immunol Ther Exp (Warsz) 47:69, 1999
14. Bolen JB, Brugge JS: Leukocyte protein tyrosine kinases: potential targets for drug discovery. Annu Rev Immunol 15:371, 1997
15. Rao A, Luo C, Hogan PG: Transcription factors of the NFAT family: regulation and function. Annu Rev Immunol 15:707, 1997
16. Kersh GJ, Kersh EN, Fremont DH, et al: High- and low-potency ligands with similar affinities for the TCR: the importance of kinetics in TCR signaling. Immunity 9:817, 1998
17. Itoh Y, Hemmer B, Martin R, et al: Serial TCR engagement and down-modulation by peptide: MHC molecule ligands: relationship to the quality of individual TCR signaling events. J Immunol 162:2073, 1999
18. O'Garra A: Cytokines induce the development of functionally heterogeneous T helper cell subsets. Immunity 8:275, 1998
19. Sher A, Gazinelli RT, Jankovic D, et al: Cytokines as determinants of disease and disease interactions. Braz J Med Biol Res 31:85, 1998
20. Granger DN: Cell adhesion and migration: II. Leukocyte-endothelial cell adhesion in the digestive system. Am J Physiol 275:G982, 1997
21. Velupillai P, Harn DA: Oligosaccharide-specific induction of interleukin 10 production by B220+ cells from schistosome-infected mice: a mechanism for regulation of CD4+ T-cell subsets. Proc Natl Acad Sci USA 91:18, 1994
22. Dutton RW, Bradley LM, Swain SL: T cell memory. Annu Rev Immunol 16:201, 1998
23. Groux H, O'Garra A, Bigler M, et al: A CD4+ T-cell subset inhibits antigen-specific T-cell responses and prevents colitis. Nature 389:737, 1997
24. Baert FJ, Rutgeerts PR: Anti-TNF strategies in Crohn's disease: mechanisms, clinical effects, indications. Int J Colorectal Dis 14:47, 1999
25. Locksley RM, Fowell DJ, Shinkai K, et al: Development of CD4+ effector T cells and susceptibility to infectious diseases. Adv Exp Med Biol 452:45, 1998
26. Bucala R: Neuroimmunomodulation by macrophage migration inhibitory factor (MIF). Ann NY Acad Sci 840:74, 1998
27. Lanahan A, Williams JB, Sanders LK, et al: Growth factor-induced delayed early response genes. Mol Cell Biol 12:3919, 1992
28. Bernhagen J, Calandra T, Mitchell RA, et al: MIF is a pituitary-derived cytokine that potentiates lethal endotoxaemia. Nature 365:756, 1993
29. Bozza M, Satoskar AR, Lin G, et al: Targeted disruption of migration inhibitory factor gene reveals its critical role in sepsis. J Exp Med 189:341, 1999
30. Baggiolini M, Dewald B, Moser B: Human chemokines: an update. Annu Rev Immunol 15:675, 1997
31. Petering H, Gotze O, Kimmig D, et al: The biologic role of interleukin-8: functional analysis and expression of CXCR1 and CXCR2 on human eosinophils. Blood 93:694, 1999
32. Olbrich H, Proudfoot AE, Opperman M: Chemokine-induced phosphorylation of CC chemokine receptor 5 (CCR5). J Leukoc Biol 65:281, 1999
33. Choe H: Chemokine receptors in HIV-1 and SIV infection. Arch Pharm Res 21:634, 1998
34. Darmon AJ, Bleackley RC: Proteases and cell-mediated cytotoxicity. Crit Rev Immunol 18:255, 1998
35. Lanier LL: NK cell receptors. Annu Rev Immunol 16:359, 1998
36. Bruhns P, Marchetti P, Fridman WH, et al: Differential roles of N- and C-terminal immunoreceptor tyrosine-based inhibition motifs during inhibition of cell activation by killer cell inhibitory receptors. J Immunol 162:3168, 1999

Acknowledgment

Figures 1 through 4   Dimitry Schidlovsky.

100 Disorders of the Complement System

Douglas Fearon, M.D., and John R. David, M.D.

Components of the Complement System

The complement system, which is composed of 18 plasma proteins, is the principal humoral effector of immunologically induced inflammation [*see Table 1*]. It plays a crucial role both in immunologically induced and nonspecific resistance to infections and in the pathogenesis of tissue injury. The products of complement activation regulate a number of biologic events, including the release of mediators from mast cells, which increases vascular permeability. Activated complement components also promote smooth muscle contraction; the chemotaxis of neutrophils, mononuclear cells, and eosinophils; and phagocytosis by immune adherence. Other effects of complement activation are solubilization of immune complexes, cell membrane lysis, neutralization of viruses, and the killing of certain types of bacteria.

Complement activation can be initiated by either of two pathways: the classical and the alternative.[1] Although both pathways culminate in the formation of enzymes that activate the same critical component, C3, each pathway appears to have a distinct role in protecting the body, either against autoimmune disease or against infection. People who have genetic deficiencies of components of the classical pathway are predisposed to immune complex–mediated diseases, whereas people with deficiencies of the components of the alternative pathway are predisposed to certain bacterial infections. The roles of the two pathways are related to the mechanisms by which they are activated: the classical pathway is activated by antibody in the form of antigen-antibody complexes, whereas the alternative pathway is activated by bacteria in the presence or even in the absence of antibody.

The complement components of the pathway activated by antibody, as well as those of the terminal sequence, which lyses cells, are designated C1 through C9. Components of the alternative, or properdin, pathway are given letters—that is, properdin is P and factor B is B. A bar over a component, as in C$\overline{1}$, indicates that it has been activated. The cleavage products are given lowercase-letter suffixes—for example, C3 → C3a + C3b. When a component or fragment becomes inactive, an i prefix or suffix is added, as in iC3b or Bbi.

The components of the two pathways participate in a cascade of limited proteolytic reactions. The cleavage of a peptide bond in an inactive precursor molecule liberates a minor fragment, which may itself have specific biologic activities, and a major fragment. The major fragment may participate in further proteolytic activity or may complex with and modify the specificity of a previously formed protease, which leads to cleavage of the next protein in the sequence. Some reactions of the terminal lytic sequence, which results in formation of the membrane attack complex, involve protein-protein complexes without causing cleavage of peptide bonds.

Both the classical pathway and the alternative pathway lead to the cleavage of C3. This important proteolytic step initiates a common terminal sequence that generates most of the biologic activities of the complement system. In addition, components of the alternative pathway play an important part in amplifying complement activity [*see Figure 1*].

The complement system, once fired, is controlled by a number of proteins. In addition, the enzymes that cleave and activate C3 and C5, C3 convertase and C5 convertase, respectively, undergo rapid natural decay.

The Classical Pathway

IgM, IgG1, IgG2, and IgG3 bound to antigens can trigger the classical complement pathway. Because IgM is a pentamer (and thus has five binding sites per molecule), a single IgM molecule is sufficient to activate the first complement component, C1. In contrast, two adjacent molecules of IgG are required to activate C1. Thus, triggering by IgG is less efficient than triggering by IgM.

C1 is composed of three proteins, or subcomponents, termed C1q, C1r$_2$, and C1s$_2$; C1q is formed of 18 polypeptide chains, whereas the other two proteins are polypeptide dimers. Each subcomponent has a unique function: C1q binds to immunoglobulin, C1r$_2$ activates C1s$_2$, and C1s$_2$ activates C4 [*see Figure 2*]. The structure of C1q resembles that of six tulips intertwined at the stems. The blossomlike structures are the globular portions of the molecule, which bind to the Fc region of IgM or IgG and give C1q a potential valence of six. The stemlike structures resemble collagen and provide the sites of interaction of C1q with C1r$_2$ and C1s$_2$. C1r$_2$ and C1s$_2$ are serine proteases that are converted from their precursors to active forms by proteolytic reactions; C1r$_2$ is activated autocatalytically, and C1s$_2$ is activated by C$\overline{1}$r$_2$. Autocatalytic activation of C1r$_2$ is usually prevented by C1 inhibitor (C$\overline{1}$ INH). However, when C1q has bound to immunoglobulin that is bound to antigen, access of C$\overline{1}$ INH to C1r$_2$ is prevented, and autoactivation occurs. C$\overline{1}$s$_2$ is also subject to inhibition by C$\overline{1}$ INH, which limits the number of C4 and C2 molecules that this subcomponent can activate [*see Figure 1*].

Activated C1, the first enzyme of the classical pathway, cleaves C4 into a small fragment (C4a) and a large fragment (C4b). This proteolytic reaction exposes a site on the large fragment that allows C4b to bind covalently to cell membranes. A

Table 1 Physiochemical Characteristics of Complement System Proteins

Protein	Approximate Molecular Weight (daltons)	Serum Concentration (µg/ml)
Classical pathway and effector sequence		
C1q	390,000	70
C1r	95,000	35
C1s	87,000	35
C4	209,000	430
C2	117,000	30
C3	190,000	1,200
C5	206,000	75
C6	128,000	60
C7	120,000	55
C8	163,000	80
C9	79,000	160
Alternative pathway of activation and amplification		
P (properdin)	223,000	25
D	25,000	2
B	100,000	240
Control proteins		
C$\overline{1}$ INH	105,000	180
I (C3b INA)	90,000	50
H (β1H)	150,000	520
C4–binding protein	1,200,000	250

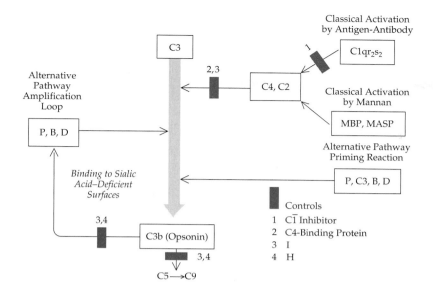

Figure 1 **Complement activation by the classical and alternative pathways involves cleavage of the centrally important C3 protein. Activation via the classical pathway requires components $C1qr_2s_2$, C4, and C2 and is down-regulated by $C\overline{1}$ inhibitor, C4-bp, and I. Alternative pathway activation occurs when C3b generated by the priming reaction binds to a cell surface deficient in sialic acid. C3 bound to such a surface is resistant to the regulatory effects of H and I and initiates the amplification loop. C3b also confers C5 cleaving activity on both the classical and the amplification C3 convertases, thereby permitting activation of the terminal components through C9. (MBP—mannose-binding protein; MASP—MBP-associated serine protease)**

single $C\overline{1}$ generates many C4a and C4b fragments. High concentrations of C4a can cause mast cells to secrete histamine. $C\overline{1}$ also cleaves C2; this cleavage yields a large fragment (C2a) that binds to C4b in the presence of Mg^{2+}, forming the second new enzyme, $C\overline{4b2a}$ (or simply $C\overline{42}$). This enzyme, which is termed C3 convertase because it cleaves C3, has a proteolytic site on the C2a fragment. The activity of this C3 convertase is abolished by the combined effects of C4-binding protein (C4-bp) and I (formerly termed C3b INA). C4-bp binds to C4b and displaces C2a, rendering C2a inactive (C2ai). Factor I proteolytically cleaves C4b into its C4c and C4d fragments.

An additional means by which certain microorganisms, such as yeast, can activate the classical pathway in persons lacking specific antibody involves a family of proteins termed collectins.[2] One of these collectins, mannose-binding protein (MBP), interacts with the MBP-associated serine proteases (MASPs) to form a complex functionally and structurally homologous to C1 complex. MBP binds to mannan-containing carbohydrates, which are especially abundant on yeast, and triggers activation of the MASPs, which interact with C4 and C2 to generate C4b2a.

The convertase $C\overline{42}$ acts by cleaving C3 into two parts [*see Figure 2*]. The small fragment (C3a), which is released into the fluid phase, is a peptide that can release mediators from mast cells; it is active at very low concentrations. The large fragment (C3b) can bind covalently to membranes. If it binds adjacent to the $C\overline{42}$, it modifies the specificity of the enzyme, allowing it to act on C5. The $C\overline{42}$ modified by C3b is called the C5 convertase. In addition, C3b bound to the cell surface induces immune adherence—that is, it facilitates the binding of the C3b-coated cell to phagocytes that have C3b receptors, thereby enhancing phagocytosis. C3b is inactivated by I in the presence of H (formerly termed β1H).

The C5 convertase, $C\overline{423b}$, cleaves C5 into a small fragment, C5a, and a large fragment, C5b [*see Figure 2*]. C5a has properties similar to those of C3a and is chemotactic for leukocytes. C5b binds C6, and the C5b6 formed in this manner can bind C7 either while fixed to the C5 convertase or in the fluid phase. The complex C5b67 can detach from the C5 convertase and attach to the membrane at another site [*see Figure 2*]. Furthermore, it can attach to membranes of nonsensitized cells, a process known as reactive lysis, which extends the cytolytic effects of complement to so-called innocent-bystander cells. If C5b67 does not attach to a membrane, it becomes C5i67, which is lytically inactive.

When the C5b67 complex enters the membrane, it binds one molecule of C8, causing some damage to the cell membrane and allowing ions to flow in [*see Figure 2*]. This complex now binds up to six molecules of C9, inducing rapid lysis [*see Figure 2 and Figure 3*]. If this sequence occurs on a gram-negative bacterium, the bacterium will be killed by the terminal attack complex.

The chain of events from the binding of C1q to the binding of C9 and the lysis of the cell involves many proteins, but only two new enzymatic complexes, $C\overline{1}$ and $C\overline{4b2a}$, are generated. The latter enzymatic complex is modified in the presence of C3b to form the C5 convertase. The rest of the cascade of events involves protein-protein interactions.

The Alternative Pathway

The incubation of fresh serum with a variety of bacteria, yeast, certain parasites, heterologous mammalian cells, virally infected homologous cells, or insoluble immune complexes will induce cleavage of C3 and activate the terminal complement sequence. This system of triggering complement activation has been termed the alternative pathway [*see Figure 4*]. Because this pathway does not require antibody, it may play a critical role in the initial nonimmunologic defense against infection.

Two types of C3 convertase—priming and amplification—are formed. Priming C3 convertase is formed in the fluid phase by the interaction between C3, in which the thioester has been hydrolyzed, B, and D. This enzyme, C3Bb, then activates C3 to generate C3b, which attaches covalently to nearby cell surfaces. If the C3b is protected from inactivation by I and H, it remains available to interact with B and D to form C3b,Bb. This enzyme is termed the amplification C3 convertase because its product, C3b, can feedback to form additional enzyme. The convertase is stabilized by the binding of P and destabilized by the binding of H, which releases Bb.

The essential difference between surfaces that activate the alternative pathway and those that do not is that the former protect C3b from inactivation by I and H. Although there may be several chemical characteristics that contribute to protection, one that has been identified is the absence of sialic acid. Because most prokaryotes lack an ability to synthesize sialic acid, many microbial cell surfaces activate the alternative pathway. Not surprisingly, human parasites such as *Leishmania major* and *Trypanoso-*

ma cruzi have evolved several strategies for evading recognition by the alternative pathway, including synthesis of glycoproteins containing sialic acid, rapid degradation of bound C3b, and synthesis of a protein that competes with B for binding to C3b.[3-5]

Host cells are protected from the effects of complement activation by at least three membrane proteins: decay-accelerating factor (DAF), membrane cofactor protein (MCP), and CD59. DAF and MCP each interacts with cell-bound C4b and C3b and prevents activation of the classical and alternative pathways. CD59 inhibits the binding of C9 to the C5b678 complex, which prevents formation of the C5b-C9 attack complex.

Both DAF and CD59 are anchored in the lipid bilayer by glycolipid tails. This structure may facilitate rapid lateral diffusion of these proteins and thereby allow individual molecules to protect large areas of membrane. A deficiency in these two proteins causes the increased sensitivity of erythrocytes to cell-mediated lysis that is characteristic of paroxysmal nocturnal hemoglobinuria, an acquired abnormality affecting clonally related hematopoietic cells. Paroxysmal nocturnal hemoglobinuria is now known to be caused by a somatic mutation in hematopoietic stem cells of the *PIG-A* gene on the X chromosome.[6] The product of the *PIG-A* gene is active in the biosynthesis of the gly-

cophosphatidylinositol (GPI) anchor of membrane proteins. Thus, the cellular progeny of the affected clones lack DAF and CD59, the two GPI-anchored membrane proteins that protect cells from complement attack [*see Chapter 89*].

Some patients with membranoproliferative glomerulonephritis and most patients with partial lipodystrophy with or without glomerulonephritis demonstrate an unusual mechanism of antibody-mediated activation of the alternative pathway. These patients exhibit a serum complement profile indicative of alternative pathway activation—that is, low levels of C3 and normal concentrations of C1, C4, and C2. Their sera also contain an IgG autoantibody, termed C3 nephritic factor, that is specific for antigenic determinants expressed by the amplification C3 convertase. One molecule of C3 nephritic factor binds one of C3b,Bb, creating a stable trimolecular enzyme. Thus stabilized, the amplification C3 convertase can resist H-mediated dissociation of the Bb subunit and fire the terminal complement sequence.

The Biologic Activity of the Complement System

The proteolytic fragments of the complement factors, especially C5a, play important roles in acute inflammation. C5a, by

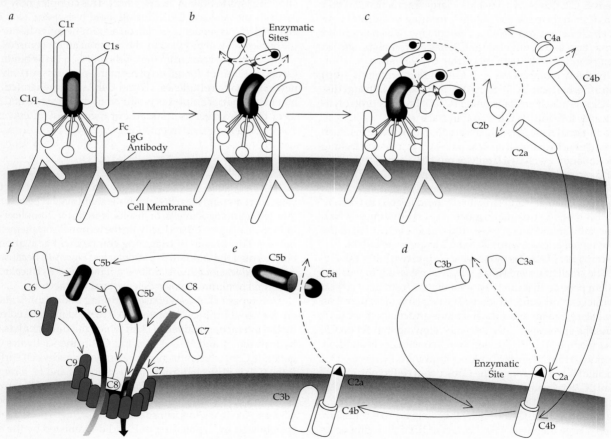

Figure 2 (*a*) At the start of the classical complement activation pathway, antibodies bind to the antigen, and complement C1 subunits C1q, C1r$_2$, and C1s$_2$ bind to two adjacent antibodies. (*b*) Binding alters the configuration of the C1q subunit, which in turn produces conformational changes in C1r$_2$ and exposes a proteolytic site on one C1r molecule. Consequently, a single peptide bond is cleaved in each of the C1r molecules, and two C1r enzymatic sites are generated. (*c*) The enzymatic sites act on C1s$_2$, exposing two more sites. The C1s$_2$ cleaves complement components C4 and C2. (*d*) The C4b fragment attaches to the cell membrane. C2a then binds to C4b, producing C4b2a (C3 convertase), which cleaves C3. (*e*) C3b attaches to the cell membrane close to the C3 convertase, altering the specificity of the enzymatic site on the C2a moiety. Altered C3 convertase becomes C5 convertase and splits C5. (*f*) C5b binds to C6 and C7 and attaches to the cell surface. C8 and C9 combine with C5b67. Insertion of this late complex into the cell membrane permits a rapid flux of ions (thick arrows) that ultimately leads to cell lysis.

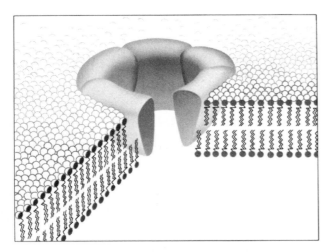

Figure 3 **The complex of the five late-acting complement components (C5b, C6, C7, C8, and C9) forms a circular channel that traverses the lipid bilayer, which permits the flow of water, ions, and smaller proteins and results in lysis of the cell.**

binding to specific receptors, provides the signal for neutrophils, monocytes, and other leukocytes to migrate to the site of complement activation. Binding of C5a increases the number of receptors on monocytes and neutrophils that recognize other factors, including C3b and iC3b. C5a and C3a stimulate tissue mast cells to release histamine and other mediators of inflammation, which assist the movement of neutrophils across the endothelium. C3e, a fragment of C3b, increases the number of neutrophils in peripheral blood that are available for recruitment to sites of complement activation by promoting the release of these cells from bone marrow and marginated pools.

The activities of these complement fragments are usually beneficial when they are associated with defense against microbial infection. However, these actions can be detrimental when they are associated with excessive local or systemic complement activation. For example, certain types of dialysis membranes activate the alternative pathway and generate large amounts of C5a, leading to the formation of leukocyte aggregates that are transiently trapped in the pulmonary capillary bed. Overproduction of C5a and trapping of leukocyte aggregates may also contribute to the pulmonary endothelial damage that occurs in patients with the acute respiratory distress syndrome. Another example is seen in patients with burns, who exhibit extended activation of the complement system by

the injured tissue; neutrophils are activated systemically by the overproduction of C5a. The beneficial effects of C3 depletion in animal models of acute myocardial infarction probably result from the lack of C5a production and diminished infiltration of ischemic myocardium by neutrophils.

The receptors for C3b, C3dg, and iC3b are termed complement receptors 1, 2, and 3 (CR1, CR2, and CR3), respectively [*see Table 2*]. These receptors are important because the C3 fragments with which they interact are bound to the targets of complement activation, such as bacteria or immune complexes. For example, CR1 and CR3 enhance the ability of neutrophils, eosinophils, and monocytes to phagocytize bacteria that are coated with C3b and iC3b. The binding of C5a increases the concentration of CR1 and CR3. Increased expression of CR3 also promotes the adherence of neutrophils to endothelial cells, an essential primary step in the localization of neutrophils at the site of complement activation. The critical role of CR3 is demonstrated by patients with an inherited deficiency of CR3, who experience repeated bacterial infections because the ability of neutrophils to accumulate at the site of infection is impaired.

CR1 also allows erythrocytes to bind to circulating immune complexes that are bound to C3b and thereby prevents these complexes from diffusing into tissues. The binding of C3b to CR1 leads to formation of C3dg, which is transferred to CR2. CR2 associates with CD19, a membrane protein of B cells that decreases the number of antigen receptors that must be ligated for cellular activation to occur.[7] The consequence of these reactions is a heightened antibody response to low doses of antigen. It is of interest that CR2 on B cells serves as the receptor for Epstein-Barr virus (EBV), mediating infection and immortalization. (EBV is associated with Burkitt's lymphoma in Africa and with nasopharyngeal carcinoma [*see Chapter 148*].) The primary role of CR2 in the pathogenesis of EBV infection is demonstrated by the finding that murine L cells that have been transfected with complementary DNA (cDNA) for human CR2 are susceptible to EBV infection.

Two biologic effects of complement do not involve specific membrane receptors: cytolysis of target cells by the insertion of the C5b-C9 complex into the cell membrane and maintenance of the solubility of antigen-antibody complexes. The former mechanism represents one way in which complement contributes to host defense, whereas the latter reaction may be important for preventing immune complex disease; both mechanisms require an intact classical pathway. In any inflammatory disease in which there are large amounts of antigen-antibody complexes, complement activation via the classical pathway occurs,

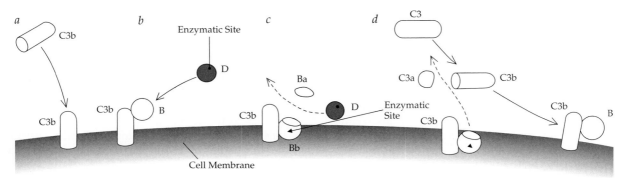

Figure 4 (*a*) **The alternative, or properdin, pathway is triggered when complement component C3b, generated from C3 by the priming convertase, attaches to a sialic acid–deficient surface. (*b and c*) Component B then attaches to C3b and is activated by a serine protease, D, to form the amplification convertase C3b,Bb. (*d*) The enzymatic site on Bb cleaves more C3, generating additional C3b, which attaches to the membrane.**

Table 2 Cellular Distribution and
Function of Complement Receptors

Receptor	Cell Type	Function
C3a	Mast cell	Secretion
C5a	Mast cell	Secretion
	Neutrophil Monocyte Eosinophil	Chemotaxis, respiratory burst, adherence, increased expression of CR1 and CR3, secretion of secondary granules
CR1 (C3b, CD35)	Neutrophil Monocyte Eosinophil	Phagocytosis of C3b-coated particles
	Erythrocyte	Clearance of C3b-coated immune complexes
	B cell	Generates ligand for CR2
	Glomerular podocyte	Unknown
CR2 (C3dg, CD21)	B cell	Associates with CD19, proliferation, receptor for Epstein-Barr virus
	Follicular dendritic cell	Possibly antigen presentation
CR3 (iC3b, CD11b/18)	Neutrophil Monocyte Eosinophil	Adhesion to and phagocytosis of iC3b-coated particles
	Large granular lymphocyte	Enhanced cytolysis of targets of natural killer cells

leading to the generation of complement cleavage fragments, such as C3adesArg and C3dg, and consumptive deficiencies of certain of the complement proteins, mainly C1q, C4, and C3. Representative diseases in which classical pathway activation is observed are systemic lupus erythematosus (SLE), synovial fluid in rheumatoid arthritis (or serum of such patients when disease is associated with systemic vasculitis), and acute post-streptococcal glomerulonephritis. The diagnosis of excessive complement activation is made by assaying elevations of C3adesArg, for example, and depressions of either C4 or C3. If elevated levels of C3adesArg are found in association with lower serum levels of C3 but not C4, consideration should be given to the possibility of relatively selective activation of the alternative pathway, as in patients with C3 nephritic factor. Diseases in which the immunologic reaction is entirely cell mediated are not associated with evidence of complement activation.

In rare instances, evaluation of a patient with SLE will uncover the inherited absence of one of the components of the classical pathway, C1q, C1r, C1s, C4, or C2.[8] In these instances, the hemolytic assays of complement function will be zero, which is almost never observed with acquired complement deficiencies. The mechanism by which these deficiencies cause autoimmunity is not known, although it may relate to the clearance of immune complexes by erythrocyte-associated CR1.

The complement system, whether triggered by the classical or the alternative pathway, comprises a series of reactions that are vital to the body's defense. This series of reactions first produces an increase in vascular permeability, permitting more complement components and antibody to penetrate the reaction site and amplify the activation process. Activated complement C5a then attracts effector cells, such as neutrophils and monocytes; C3b, by binding to the foreign antigen-antibody complex, further facilitates the phagocytic process. Some organisms and cells are lysed directly. Like the humoral antibody-mediated and cell-mediated systems, however, the complement system is a double-edged sword: it can enhance the body's resistance to infection, but it can also cause tissue injury.

Inherited Deficiencies of the Complement System

Deficiences of complement proteins may be inherited [*see* Table 3] or acquired secondary to overactivation of the complement system. Of 15 inherited abnormalities of complement proteins that have been described, 14 are associated with disease.

HEREDITARY ANGIOEDEMA

Hereditary angioedema (HAE) results from a deficiency in C1̄ INH and is transmitted in an autosomal dominant manner; patients who are heterozygous for the C1̄ INH defect manifest the disease. Serum from patients with the disease contains only five to 30 percent of the normal amount of C1̄ INH. The disorder is characterized by recurrent attacks of nonpitting edema that involve the skin and the gastrointestinal and respiratory tracts; a typical attack lasts from 48 to 72 hours. Laryngeal edema, the most dangerous manifestation, can lead to respiratory obstruction and death. Edema of the jejunum causes severe abdominal cramps and bilious vomiting, whereas colonic involvement produces watery diarrhea. The edema is not painful, nor is it accompanied by redness of the skin or itching.

Attacks may occur in the absence of an obvious initiating cause, or they may be induced by tissue trauma (e.g., that produced by dental extraction). C1̄ INH levels drop even further during an attack, and C1̄s appears in the serum. The C4 level is depressed even between attacks, and the levels of both C4 and C2, the substrates for C1̄s, are markedly diminished during acute attacks; the levels of other complement components, however, are generally normal. A vasoactive peptide that increases local vascular permeability is generated during attacks and is responsible for the edema. The vasoactive peptide has not been identified, although some investigators have suggested that it is derived from the breakdown of C2 by plasmin and C1̄s. C1̄ INH also normally inhibits activated Hageman factor and kallikrein, and thus, the regulation of these enzymes may be impaired in patients with C1̄ INH deficiency. Because these two enzymes are involved in the kinin-forming system, it has been proposed by other investigators that bradykinin, a product of the kallikrein-mediated cleavage of kininogen, is the vasopermeability factor.

Prophylaxis against attacks of angioedema has been achieved by the administration of compounds such as ε-aminocaproic acid and tranexamic acid, which inhibit the conversion of plasminogen to plasmin. These drugs, however, do not alter the plasma levels of C1̄ INH or C4, and the mechanism by which they prevent attacks is not known. Anabolic steroids with attenuated androgenic effects, such as danazol and stanozolol, stimulate the synthesis of normal C1̄ INH in patients with C1̄ INH deficiency and thus are now preferred for prophylaxis. By raising the levels of inhibitor, these agents provide more effective regulation of C1̄ and produce a secondary increase in the plasma concentration of C4. Use of attenuated androgens for long periods requires consideration of their side effects, which include impairment of growth rate in children, masculinization in women, and hepatic dysfunction. Therefore, it is critical to establish the lowest effective dose of these agents. Such a dose, however, may represent a compromise between disease suppression and adverse effects. Establishing the lowest effective dosage is particularly important in women of childbearing age. The use of anabolic steroids in pregnant women and in children is not recommended.

No therapy is available to interrupt ongoing attacks of HAE. Remedies have been tried, but because attacks are self-limited, the efficacy of the remedies is not clear. Plasma transfusions can reportedly arrest an attack, although such therapy might also

Table 3 Diseases Associated with
Inherited Complement Deficiencies[3]

Deficient Component	Number of Reported Cases	Associated Diseases
C1	31	Autoimmune diseases, SLE-like syndromes
C4	20	Autoimmune diseases, SLE-like syndromes
C2	109	Autoimmune diseases, SLE-like syndromes
C3	20	Bacterial infections; mild glomerulonephritis
C5	28	Gram-negative coccal infections
C6	76	Gram-negative coccal infections
C7	67	Gram-negative coccal infections
C8	68	Gram-negative coccal infections
C9	18	Gram-negative coccal infections
Properdin	70	Gram-negative coccal infections
Factor I	17	Bacterial infections
Factor H	13	Bacterial infections
Factor D	3	Bacterial infections
C4–binding protein	3	—
C1 INH	>100	Hereditary angioedema

SLE—systemic lupus erythematosus

be hazardous because additional substrate—that is, C4 and C2—is present in the plasma. The hazards of transfusion therapy may be circumvented by the use of partially purified $C\overline{1}$ INH, but this compound is not generally available. Intraoperative and postoperative attacks of angioedema in patients with $C\overline{1}$ INH deficiency have been suppressed by giving high doses of stanozolol for several days before surgery.

SUSCEPTIBILITY TO BACTERIAL INFECTIONS

People with homozygous deficiency of C3 or of factor I, the C3b inactivator, suffer repeated pyogenic infections with gram-negative and gram-positive organisms. When the control protein I is absent from the plasma, the amplification C3 convertase, C3b,Bb, is inadequately regulated. Consequently, C3 and B undergo persistent hypercatabolism, thereby leading to C3 deficiency. The association between recurrent pyogenic infection and C3 deficiency makes clear the central role of C3 in maintaining normal host defenses. C3 is required for the opsonization of foreign organisms: the C3b fragment generated from C3 by C3 convertase acts as a ligand for attaching such agents to neutrophils and macrophages. Interruption of complement activation at the C3 step also prevents the bactericidal reaction of the C5b–C9 complex and the generation of C5a chemotactic factor, which would otherwise localize leukocytes to the infection site.

Persons with homozygous deficiencies of properdin, C5, C6, C7, or C8 appear to be unusually susceptible to systemic *Neisseria* infections involving gonococci or meningococci. This observation indicates that opsonization mediated by the alternative pathway and bacteriolysis by the C5b-C9 complex are important factors in resistance to these organisms. Immunization of a properdin-deficient person with meningococcal polysaccharide induced the production of antimeningococcal antibody and corrected the bactericidal defect of the serum, presumably by recruiting the classical pathway of complement activation.[9]

ASSOCIATION WITH RHEUMATIC DISEASES

Individuals who have inherited deficiencies of components of the classical activation pathway—that is, C1, C2, and C4—do not generally exhibit impaired host resistance to bacterial infection. This finding indicates that C3 activation by the alternative pathway is usually sufficient for host defense. People with deficiencies of classical complement components, however, do manifest an increased incidence of rheumatic disease. This finding suggests that the classical activation pathway, which can interact directly with antibody, may play a role in augmenting the clearance of immune complexes; it also suggests that impairment of this function by a complement deficiency state predisposes to rheumatic disease.

There is some evidence, however, supporting another explanation for the association between deficiencies of classical complement components and rheumatic disorders. This hypothesis suggests that a silent or null gene for a classical complement component is in linkage disequilibrium with certain alleles of genes that are located in the major histocompatibility complex and that control immune responsiveness (*Ir* genes). It further postulates that the association between these *Ir* genes and rheumatic disease is primary and that the association with the complement allele is secondary. Evidence supporting such a secondary association includes the observation that the frequency of HLA-DR2, as well as that of homozygous and heterozygous C2 deficiency, is increased in patients with SLE. The greater frequency of HLA-DR2 in SLE and the fact that heterozygous C2 deficiency has only a marginal effect on complement function suggest that the HLA-D association is the significant pathogenic factor. A similar explanation may account for the association of rheumatic disease with C4 deficiency.

An observation that apparently does not fit with this hypothesis is the finding that rheumatic diseases are also associated with deficiencies of complement components that are not encoded in the major histocompatibility region. Deficiencies of the complement components C1r, C1s, and $C\overline{1}$ INH would fall into this category. The association of rheumatic disease with these abnormalities may be the result of a selection bias attributable to the kind of population screened for complement deficiency—that is, patients with rheumatic disorders may undergo such screening more frequently than an average population. Alternatively, the association may be real, which would indicate that impaired clearance of immune complexes alone is capable of increasing susceptibility to rheumatic disease.

References

1. Müller-Eberhard HJ: Molecular organization and function of the complement system. Annu Rev Biochem 57:321, 1988

2. Hoppe HJ, Reid KB: Collectins-soluble proteins containing collagenous regions and lectin domains and their roles in innate immunity. Protein Sci 3:1143, 1994

3. Figueroa JE, Densen P: Infectious diseases associated with complement deficiencies. Clin Microbiol Rev 4:359, 1991

4. Frank MM: The mechanism by which microorganisms avoid complement attack. Curr Opin Immunol 4:14, 1992

5. Tomlinson S: Complement defense mechanisms. Curr Opin Immunol 5:83, 1993

6. Takeda J, Miyata T, Kawagoe K, et al: Deficiency of the GPI anchor caused by a somatic mutation of the *PIG-A* gene in paroxysmal nocturnal hemoglobinuria. Cell 73:703, 1993

7. Fearon DT, Carter RH: The CD19/CR2/TAPA-1 complex of B lymphocytes: linking natural to acquired immunity. Annu Rev Immunol 13:127, 1993

8. Colten HR, Rosen FS: Complement deficiencies. Annu Rev Immunol 10:809, 1992

9. Densen P, Weiler JM, Griffis JM, et al: Familial properdin deficiency and fatal meningococcemia: correction of the bactericidal defect by vaccination. N Engl J Med 316: 922, 1987

Acknowledgments

Figures 1, 2, and 4   George V. Kelvin.

Figure 3   George V. Kelvin. Adapted from "The Complement System," by M. M. Mayer, in *Scientific American* 229(November):54, 1973. © 1973 Scientific American, Inc. All rights reserved.

101 Histocompatibility Antigens and Immune Response Genes

Charles B. Carpenter, M.D.

Structure and Antigens of the Major Histocompatibility Complex

Studies of transplantation of tumors and grafts in mice gave rise to the science of immunogenetics. If an inbred strain A mouse were given a skin graft from a strain B mouse, the A mouse would reject the B graft. Mouse A would make antibodies that could kill cells from mouse B (in the presence of complement). The membrane antigens recognized by such antibodies are encoded by genes at closely linked loci on chromosome 17, in a region designated *H-2*. This chromosomal region, analogous forms of which encode strong transplantation antigens in other mammals, is called the major histocompatibility complex (MHC).

In humans, antibodies to MHC-encoded antigens are found in sera from multiparous women and from recipients of multiple blood transfusions. Such sera agglutinate or lyse leukocytes from some persons but not others. The MHC in humans is specified by the logo HLA and comprises several loci on the short arm of chromosome 6 [*see Figure 1*].

There are two structural types of MHC molecules, class I and class II. The molecules of both classes are active in antigen recognition and help focus immune defenses during invasions from the microbial world. They are also engaged in the communication that occurs between cells during the immune response. MHC molecules act by binding potential antigens in the form of peptide fragments that have been processed in antigen-presenting cells. Clonally determined antigen receptors on T cells then recognize and bind to specific peptide-MHC complexes, setting into motion the appropriate immune response. Segments of MHC molecules show sequence homologies with immunoglobulins, T cell antigen receptors, and T cell interaction molecules such as CD4 and CD8, suggesting that all these molecules have a common evolutionary ancestry.

ANTIGENS OF THE MAJOR HISTOCOMPATIBILITY COMPLEX

Traditionally, the term MHC antigen has been applied to the product of a genetic locus that displays polymorphism in a specific population. The sequence and structure of molecules bearing MHC antigens have been extensively elucidated, and it has been determined that the polymorphic, or antigenic, portions of MHC molecules are quite small. In fact, the polymorphic portions frequently comprise only one to four amino acid substitutions encoded in regions of DNA nucleotide sequence hypervariability. A specific configuration in an MHC molecule resulting from the particular substitutions of amino acids is called an epitope.

MHC Class I Antigens

MHC class I antigens consist of two polypeptide chains held together noncovalently. One chain is heavy and glycosylated (44 kd) and determines antigenic specificity. The extracellular portion of this class I heavy chain is divided into three domains, designated α_1, α_2, and α_3. The other chain is a small protein (11.5 kd) known as β_2-microglobulin [*see Figure 2*]. In mice, class I antigens are encoded by genes at loci designated *H-2K* and *H-2D*, as well as at several other loci.

In humans, class I heavy chains are the gene products of three MHC loci, designated *HLA-A*, *HLA-B*, and *HLA-C*. There are many alleles for each locus; therefore, considerable polymorphism exists [*see Table 1*]. β_2-Microglobulin is encoded

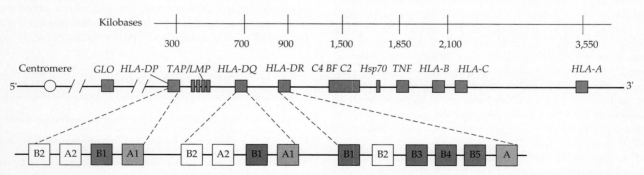

Figure 1 The best-characterized loci of the human major histocompatibility complex (MHC), located in the *HLA* region of the short arm of chromosome 6, are depicted. Distances are shown in recombination units (centimorgans), as determined by crossover frequencies in family studies, and in kilobases, as determined by sequence analysis of fragments produced by DNases having defined cleavage sites. MHC class II molecules are encoded in the *HLA-DP*, *HLA-DQ*, and *HLA-DR* genes, and MHC class I molecules are encoded by *HLA-B*, *HLA-C*, and *HLA-A* genes. A cluster of closely linked complement genes—*C4*, *BF*, and *C2*—lies in the center of the region. There are two structural genes for *C4*, interspersed with two genes for the adrenal enzyme 21-hydroxylase. Next is the heat shock protein gene, *Hsp70*, followed by the tumor necrosis factor (TNF) genes, *A* and *B*. The orientation of the complement cluster and the *TNF* cluster has not been established, but an expanded view of this area could be depicted as— (C4–210HA–C4B–210HB–BF–C2)–(HSP70)–(TNFA–TNFB)—. *GLO* is a marker gene for the enzyme glyoxylase. An expansion of the class II region is in the lower portion of the figure. Each class II molecule is a heterodimer of an α and a β chain, which are encoded in the *A* and *B* genes, respectively. Pseudogenes, which are not expressed on the cell surface, are shown in white boxes. *HLA-DP* and *HLA-DQ* have one expressed heterodimer, A1B1; *HLA-DR* has only one A chain but nine genes for B chains (four are shown in the figure). The principal expressed heterodimers for *HLA-DR* are AB1, AB3, AB4, and AB5. In the region between *HLA-DP* and *HLA-DQ* lie the closely linked *TAP1*, *TAP2*, *LMP2*, and *LMP7* genes. The *TAP* genes encode peptide transporters, whereas the *LMP* genes encode proteosomes that fragment proteins into peptides. This cytoplasmic system is believed to be responsible for production and delivery of peptides to MHC class I molecules before their movement to the cell surface.

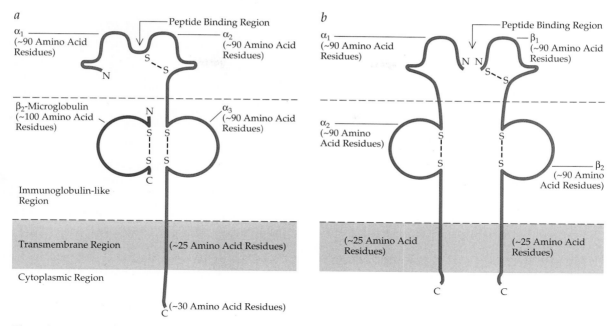

Figure 2 **MHC molecules are of two structural types with very similar peptide binding sites on the membrane distal surface.
(*a*) MHC class I molecules consist of heavy chains made up of three polypeptide domains (α_1, α_2, α_3) and a noncovalently associated light chain, β_2-microglobulin. (*b*) MHC class II molecules are heterodimers of α and β chains with a very similar overall structure and peptide binding surface. N is the amino terminus; C is the carboxyl terminus; and S–S represents an intrachain disulfide bond.[21]**

by a gene on chromosome 15. Both the β_2-microglobulin and the α_3 domain of the heavy glycosylated chain of MHC class I antigens demonstrate considerable structural similarity to the constant region of the heavy chain of IgG (C_H3).

MHC class I molecules have been crystallized and their structure has been determined by x-ray diffraction to a resolution of 3.5 Å [*see Figure 3*].[1] It was found that two of the heavy-chain domains, α_1 and α_2, are located at the membrane-distal portion of the heavy chain and form a groove along the top surface of the molecule. The sides of the groove are composed of α helices from the α_1 and α_2 domains, and the base is composed of eight antiparallel β-pleated sheets from these domains. The hypervariable (antigenic) regions are found mostly

along the sides of the groove, but there is variability in the β-pleated sheet region as well. The rest of the molecule shows minimal variability in relation to other molecules of the same *HLA* locus. In the crystals studied, the groove, which faces away from the cell membrane and is approximately 25 Å long and 10 Å wide, contains material representing processed antigen (i.e., peptide fragments). When peptides eluted from purified class I molecules are sequenced, they show patterns of amino acids, called motifs, that bind to particular sets of HLA class I molecules.[2] These findings helped confirm the hypothesis that MHC molecules bind and present processed antigens to responding T cells and that the T cell receptor (TCR) recognizes foreign antigen as a peptide in the context of self-antigen;

Table 1   Antigens of the HLA System*

	Genes	Number of Alleles (DNA Sequencing)	Number of Antigens (Serologic Polymorphism)
Class I	HLA-A	50	39
	HLA-B	97	46
	HLA-C	34	15
	HLA-E	4	0
	HLA-G	4	0
Class II	HLA-DRA	2	0
	HLA-DRB1	106	14[†]
	DRB3	4	1
	DRB4	5	1
	DRB5	5	1
	HLA-DQA1	15	0
	DQB1	26	7
	HLA-DPA1	8	0
	DPB1	59	6

*Principal expressed genes for which sequences are known.
†Thirty-three Dw alleles are defined by in vitro T cell proliferation responses. They are determined by class II differences, with contributing epitopes in various combinations on *DRB1, DRB3, DRB4, DRB5, DQA1,* and *DQB1.*

a

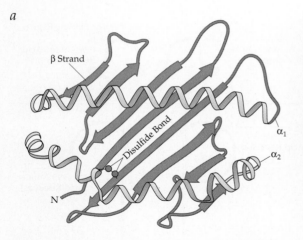

b

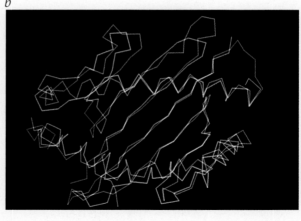

c

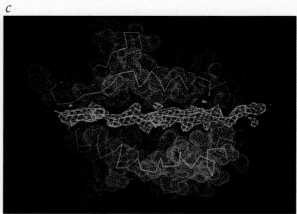

Figure 3 (*a*) Top view of α_1 and α_2 domains of HLA-A2, showing the surface that faces away from the cell membrane, reveals a groove in which peptides are bound for presentation to T cells. The groove has a base composed of eight β strands. The disulfide bond shown in Figure 2 connects the first β strand of α_2 to the α_2 helix. The amino terminus (N) marks the beginning of the α_1 domain. Polymorphism is found both along the edges of the helices and in the base. (*b*) A crystallogram of the core structure of MHC class II HLA-DR1 (blue), superimposed on MHC class I HLA-A2 (red), shows the overall similarity of their peptide binding sites.[3] (*c*) A crystallogram of peptides bound to crystalline DR1 shows the surface as it is probably exhibited to T cells. The α_1 helix is on top, the β_1 domain is on the bottom, and the amino terminus is at the bottom left. Red indicates the electron density of the collection of endogenous bound peptides, and blue indicates the van der Waals surface of DR1.[3]

that is, it binds to a surface composed of both MHC and a bound peptide.

MHC class I antigens can be expressed on all cell types, except erythrocytes and trophoblasts, and can be detected by staining with labeled antibodies. Striated muscle cells and liver parenchymal cells are normally negative for class I antigens (i.e., they lack class I molecules or express only a low density of class I molecules), but in inflammatory states, these cells may become strongly positive for class I antigens.

MHC Class II Antigens

Some antibodies, elicited by immunizations with histoincompatible cells, react with a limited variety of cells, most notably B cells, monocytes, dendritic cells, and activated T cells. Normally, these cells are the only ones found to bear MHC class II antigens. As is the case with class I antigens, however, inflammatory states cause many tissues to express class II antigens.

Each MHC class II antigen consists of two membrane-inserted glycosylated polypeptides, designated α (34 kd) and β (28 kd), which are bound together noncovalently [*see Figure 2*]. The extracellular portion of the α chain is divided into two domains, designated α_1 and α_2; the extracellular portion of the β chain is also divided into two domains, β_1 and β_2. In mice, MHC class II antigens are encoded by a gene region designated by the letter I. In humans, class II antigens are encoded by the *HLA-D* gene region, which is divided into at least three subregions: *HLA-DP*, *HLA-DQ*, and *HLA-DR* [*see Figure 1*].

Crystallographic studies indicate that MHC class II molecules have a structure similar to that of MHC class I molecules,

with the α_1 and β_1 domains forming a groove in which β-pleated sheets form the base and α helices form the sides [*see Figure 3*].[3] As in MHC class I molecules, the hypervariable (antigenic) regions of MHC class II molecules are located primarily along the groove, which again indicates a molecular basis for corecognition by the TCR of foreign antigen and self-MHC.

In inbred mice, immune responses to immunization with synthetic peptides were found to be significantly influenced by so-called *H-2*–linked immune response genes. Subsequent work established that these genes were, in fact, encoding MHC class II molecules. Mice have genes for two sets of class II molecules: one set at the *I-A* locus (containing genes for A_α and A_β subunits) and the other at the *I-E* locus (encoding E_α, E_β, and E_{β_2} subunits). The subdivision of the mouse class II region has been established by studies in congenic mice, which are bred to be genetically identical except in portions of the major histocompatibility complex. It is possible to breed mice with identical *K* and *D* (class I) alleles but with differences in the class II regions. By cross-immunization, antibodies are raised to various antigens encoded in the *A* and *E* loci of the class II region.

In humans, similar antigens can be identified by the use of sera from multiparous women that react predominantly with B cells. A serum is first exposed to platelets from a pool of many individuals because platelets contain MHC class I, but not MHC class II, antigens and thus will adsorb antibodies to class I antigens, leaving antibodies to class II antigens in the serum. The naming of genes from the *HLA-D* region is now based on knowledge of the biochemistry of expressed antigens and on a growing database of DNA nucleotide sequences. The gene encoding the HLA-DR α chain, for example, is called *DRA*. Similarly, the closely linked genes encoding the β chains have been named *DRB1* (encoding the β chains for DR1 through DR18), *DRB3* (encoding the β chain for DR52), *DRB4* (encoding the β chain for DR53), and *DRB5* (encoding the β chain for DR51). Because *DRB2* expresses no protein product, it is termed a pseudogene. Each of the HLA-DR β chains associates with the common nonpolymorphic HLA-DRA α chain to form functional class II HLA-DR molecules. Because DRA α chains are always the same, the difference in *HLA-DR* antigenic alleles is accounted for by variations in the genes encoding the DR β chains. The *HLA-DQ* locus contains the genes *DQA1*, *DQB1*, *DQA2*, and *DQB2*. *DQA2* and *DQB2* are pseudogenes, whereas the products of *DQA1* and *DQB1*—that is, the α and β chains of HLA-DQ—are both polymorphic. *HLA-DP* gene organization is similar to that of *HLA-DQ* [*see Figure 1*].

Sequence Analysis and HLA Nomenclature

Most alleles of the *HLA* system can be identified by restriction fragment length polymorphism (RFLP) analysis, a technique that entails electrophoresis of DNA fragments after the DNA has been digested by various restriction endonucleases.[4] The polymerase chain reaction provides a more convenient and accurate method of typing *HLA* alleles than RFLP analysis. In this procedure, oligonucleotide primers specific for certain loci (e.g., *DRB1*, *DQA1*) are used to promote selective amplification of DNA segments that include the variable coding regions for specific alleles. The amplified DNA is then hybridized to oligonucleotide probes to detect the presence of a specific sequence.[5] The PCR method has the advantage of requiring very small numbers of cells; with further modifications, it should be able to provide results as rapidly as standard serologic tests.

Information about DNA sequences is now so extensive that *HLA* alleles are officially defined by their sequences, rather than by serologic patterns. The structural basis for the specificity of alloreactivity is being clarified as new data accumulate. Several new alleles have been identified by sequence analysis but have not yet been serologically defined [*see Table 1*]. Amino acid differences may occur at several sites on the α helix or β strands [*see Figure 3*]. Although there are three to five areas on an HLA molecule that are most likely to vary (so-called hypervariable regions), only one or two amino acid substitutions may be sufficient to produce a serologic difference. Sequencing is also providing insight into the basis of *HLA-Dw* polymorphisms, which have been classically defined only by reactivity in the mixed lymphocyte reaction in tissue culture (see below).

In the HLA nomenclature, the convention is to show first the locus, followed by an asterisk and a four-digit number. The first two digits are the allele number, and the last two digits indicate a unique sequence for variants. For example, the four most common *HLA-A2* variants are now designated as *A*0201*, *A*0202*, *A*0203*, and *A*0204*. Only unique sequences fit within the new nomenclature. Another example is provided by *DR2*, which is the parent antigen for the *DR15* and *DR16* serologic splits. It is now known that there are four *DRB1* chains for *DR2*. In the nomenclature based on nucleotide sequences, *DR2* is written as *DRB1*1501*, *DRB1*1502*, *DRB1*1601*, or *DRB1*1602*. The 01 and 02 splits account for four previously known *HLA-Dw* specificities: *Dw2*, *Dw12*, *Dw21*, and *Dw22*, respectively. There are many examples of cellular (i.e., *HLA-Dw*) and serologic correlations with *HLA-A*, *HLA-B*, *HLA-C*, *DRB1*, *DRB3*, *DRB4*, *DRB5*, *DQA1*, *DQB2*, and *DPB1* sequences, but not all sequences are definable by serologic typing techniques.[6]

Frequency of Different HLA Alleles

Two terms, haplotype and linkage disequilibrium, describe important associations between MHC genes. Haplotype refers to the set of genes on any one chromosome. Every individual has two haplotypes of the MHC, one from each parent. Each haplotype has a particular set of antigens determined by the *HLA-A*, *HLA-B*, *HLA-C*, *HLA-DR*, and other loci.

The second term, linkage disequilibrium, refers to the observation that some HLA antigens coincide within a single haplotype much more frequently than expected. If discrete genes were distributed independently throughout the population, the frequency at which any two linked antigens encoded at different loci would occur within a haplotype would simply be the product of their frequency in the population. However, the HLA-A1 antigen and the HLA-B8 antigen are associated six to 21 times more often than is predicted by their gene frequency. Such linkage disequilibrium may occur because not enough evolutionary time has elapsed for the genes governing the antigens to be normally distributed or because such an association results in a selective advantage to the individual. Recombination, or crossover, takes place during meiosis and occurs about 1.5% of the time between MHC class I and MHC class II loci [*see Figure 1*]. Over many generations, such recombination leads to an equilibrium of linked alleles in a population unless selective pressures favor survival of certain haplotypes. A hypothetical example of such selection would be the survival of individuals bearing *HLA* haplotypes that confer resistance to epidemics, such as smallpox and plague. Racial differences are reflected in marked variations in the frequencies of certain HLA antigens and haplotypes. Fewer, though often striking, examples of such differences are also observed in various ethnic groups.

Role of MHC in Immune Response

THE MIXED LYMPHOCYTE REACTION

When lymphocytes from one individual are cultured with those from another, the cells are stimulated to divide. This division, which can be measured from the rate of uptake of ^{3}H-thymidine into the DNA of the cells, is called the mixed lymphocyte reaction (MLR). By preventing the division of one of the sets of cells by treatment with mitomycin or irradiation, it is possible to study the antigens on the membrane of the treated cells that stimulate this proliferative response. In mice, class II molecules encoded at the *I-A* and *I-E* loci carry the MLR antigens. In humans, after the *HLA-DR*, *HLA-DP*, and *HLA-DQ* class II loci were serologically defined, it was found that *HLA-DR* antigenic determinants appear to be most influential in evoking a primary MLR. HLA-DQ antigens play a lesser role, and HLA-DP antigens do not appear to be involved in the primary MLR. However, responding lymphocytes that have been primed by previous exposure to HLA-DQ or HLA-DP antigens proliferate vigorously when reexposed to the same antigen in a secondary MLR. Therefore, T cells behave as if they were already immune to another individual's HLA-DR, suggesting that peptide presentation by DR molecules is most likely to result in immunity.

ANTIGEN PROCESSING AND PRESENTATION

The breakdown of protein molecules into peptide fragments is an important part of the process by which antigens are presented to T cells and other immune effector cells. MHC molecules come to the cell surface with peptides already bound. Proteins are first degraded internally, and the peptide fragments are bound to MHC class I and MHC class II molecules within the cell. Class I molecules are expressed on virtually all tissues. Virally infected cells are recognized principally by class I–restricted T cells, usually those with a cytotoxic function. In contrast, class II–directed T cells are restricted to antigen-presenting cells of the immune system (i.e., B cells, macrophages, dendritic cells, or Langerhans cells) that are principally concerned with defense against external infectious agents. Because class II–positive cells also carry class I molecules, they may act as antigen-presenting cells for both endogenous and exogenous proteins.

Exogenous and endogenous antigens reach the cell surface by different pathways.[7] Exogenous proteins are taken up into endosomes or lysosomes, where they are catabolized. Peptides from exogenous proteins are generally bound to MHC class II molecules, and the class II–peptide complexes are then brought to the surface for presentation to T cells. Peptides from endogenous proteins (e.g., secretory proteins or products of viral infection) appear to be complexed in the endoplasmic reticulum to MHC class I molecules. Genes also located in the MHC region, called *LMP*, encode proteins that are responsible for breaking down proteins into small peptides (eight to 10 amino acids long); closely linked *TAP* genes encode chaperones that transport peptides across intracellular membranes [*see Figure 1*].[8] This system delivers peptides of intracytoplasmic origin to newly formed class I molecules. As previously noted, certain peptide sequence motifs are known to be characteristic of peptides eluted from purified molecules of a given MHC allele. These findings indicate that the allelic sequence differences at the margins of the peptide binding groove determine which peptide sequences will bind. Class I–bound peptides are usually nine amino acids long, with residues at particular locations that have similar charge or hydrophobicity (e.g., at positions 1, 3, and 9)[2,9] for different groups of *HLA* alleles. In addition, a number of synthetic peptides representing immunogenic portions of infectious agents or other foreign proteins also align on similar common motifs. Peptides eluted from purified HLA-DR class II molecules are variable in length up to 25 residues and have a minimal length of 13 to 14 amino acids.[10] The motifs for DR1 represent a positively charged residue at position 1, a hydrogen bond donor at position 6, and hydrophobic residue at position 10. In the future, it may be possible to predict the affinity of binding a given sequence for each MHC molecule.

CLONAL SELECTION OF T CELLS

The corecognition of MHC and peptide fragments of an antigen bound in the groove of the class I or II molecules appears to require that the binding surface of the TCR and the binding surface formed by MHC plus peptide be attached at multiple points [*see Chapter 98*]. Each T cell clone is specific for the self-MHC plus peptide complex and generally does not have sufficient affinity for MHC or peptide to bind to either component alone. There is extensive evidence that the development of the T cell repertoire in the thymus begins during the fetal period and continues well into adult life as new precursor cells from the bone marrow mature in the thymus. In this process, many potential clones are destroyed and others are selected to mature. The selected T cell clones then leave to populate the rest of the body.[11]

The MHC of the host plays a major role in selection: T cell clones that are strongly autoreactive to self-MHC molecules are eliminated, leaving clones with weak affinity to self-MHC to survive. Because the surviving clones have a large variety of T

cell receptor rearrangements [*see Chapter 98*], the necessary repertoire of T cell clones that can recognize self-MHC plus peptide remains. The successful crystallization of a complex consisting of a human TCR, its viral peptide, and the HLA-A2 molecule that binds it has revealed the configuration and extent of the binding surface between the TCR and the MHC plus peptide surface.[12] The axis of the TCR is diagonal to that of the MHC helices, and it covers a large portion of both α helices and the peptide between them [*see Figure 4*]. Although the extensive MHC polymorphisms increase the likelihood that a particular peptide fragment will be bound so that it can be recognized by T cells, a given individual has a small repertoire of such MHC binding sites compared with the rich combinatorial possibilities in the TCR gene complex. The inheritance of multiple *HLA* loci from two parents, however, increases the potential for recognizing a greater number of different self-MHC plus peptide complexes and therefore increases the likelihood that at least some individuals will survive a given infection.

The alloresponse, which is the immune response mounted against another individual's cells, is a special case. Except for direct activation of T cell subsets with bacterial superantigens (e.g., staphylococcal exotoxins), the in vitro proliferation of T cells in the MLR is the most vigorous antigen-specific response known because it does not require the priming that is needed to induce proliferation to microbial antigens. Transplantation is, of course, an experimental and clinical artifact and would not have been encountered during evolution; only pregnancy has the potential for exposing the cells of one individual to those of another having different *HLA* haplotypes. The allobarrier could have made pregnancy difficult or impossible during evolution except for the presence of several imperfectly defined mechanisms at the placental level that protect the fetus from rejection. The existence of such mechanisms suggests that the need for MHC polymorphisms is most important and requires special protection at the the maternal-fetal interface.

Alloreactive T cells are known to either indirectly perceive allo-MHC peptides presented on self-MHC molecules or directly recognize intact allo-MHC molecules that hold a self-peptide.[13] Because a number of peptides derived from endogenous proteins presumably occupy MHC binding sites at all times, such self-peptides need not be polymorphic or unique to an in-

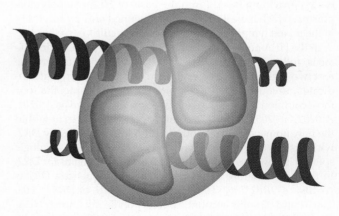

Figure 4 **The T cell receptor binds diagonally across the helical regions of MHC class I and class II molecules, covering the bound peptide. Shown is the overall footprint of the α and β chains of the T cell receptor. Each chain has three hypervariable regions that recognize the variable portions of the MHC and its bound peptide.**[12]

dividual. The functional significance of the indirect as well as the direct pathways in transplantation is under active investigation, as it has been shown experimentally that immunization with synthetic allopeptides alone can cause accelerated graft rejection,[14] whereas administration of such peptides by the oral or intrathymic route can increase tolerance for alloantigens.[15]

GENERATION OF CYTOTOXIC T CELL

The MLR leading to the generation of cytotoxic T cells requires two distinct types of responding T cells. The process begins with the stimulating cell—a B cell, dendritic cell, or monocyte—which has both MHC class I and MHC class II molecules on its surface. The class II molecule stimulates subsets of responding T cells to proliferate and become helper T cells. This subset is marked by the CD4 antigen. The class I molecule sensitizes a second subset of T cells, which become cytotoxic T cells if stimulated by the proliferating helper T cells. One of these stimulatory signals is mediated by the lymphokine interleukin-2. This second T cell subset is marked by the CD8 antigen. Cytotoxic T cells that develop against cells that differ only in their class II antigens bear the CD4 marker. The two stimuli—the one that induces helper T cell proliferation and the one that sensitizes T cells to become cytotoxic—can be delivered by different cells [see Table 2]. This type of cell interaction and cooperation is thought to mirror in vivo events that lead to graft rejection by cytotoxic T cells, showing why it is desirable to have both class I antigen and class II antigen compatibility between donor and recipient cells.

It was formerly thought that CD4+ T cells were simply helper lymphocytes and that CD8+ T cells were either cytotoxic or suppressor lymphocytes, but these functional divisions do not appear to be clear-cut. Ongoing molecular studies indicate that the CD4 surface molecule is closely associated with the TCR and guides interaction between T cells and antigen-presenting cells by binding to a nonpolymorphic region of MHC class II molecules [see Chapter 98]. Similarly, the CD8 molecule binds to MHC class I molecules on antigen-presenting cells. CD4 and CD8 molecules also increase the strength with which the TCR complex binds to the antigen-MHC complex. In addition, these surface molecules participate in signaling activation of the adherent T cell. Regarding suppressor functions, evidence suggests that CD4+ T cells induce CD8+ suppressor T cells, but the relation between the CD4 and CD8 surface molecules and MHC molecules in regulatory cells has yet to be elucidated.

Immune Response Genes

As previously mentioned, many lines of evidence indicate that MHC class II molecules are the expressed products of immune response (Ir) genes; in other words, immune responsiveness can be a direct function of antigen presentation. If an antigen fragment is not bound to a class II molecule, an individual's immune system is unable to recognize it. Certain diseases in animals—including virally induced forms of leukemia, mammary tumors, and lymphocytic choriomeningitis—have been linked to class II genes of the MHC. However, the ability of specific HLA antigens to confer susceptibility to clinically important infectious agents has rarely been suggested (see below). It is likely that evolution has resulted in selection of MHC alleles that are capable of binding at least some portions of antigenic molecules on infectious agents. In addition, the duplication of class II genes with expression of HLA-DR, HLA-DQ, and HLA-DP sets of molecules increases the likelihood that a

Table 2 Cell-Mediated Lympholysis in a Mixed Culture

Lymphocyte Antigens Matched between Responder and Stimulator Cells*		Mixed Lymphocyte Culture Reaction	Cell-Mediated Lympholysis
Class II	Class I		
Yes	Yes	No	No
No	No	Yes	Yes
No	Yes	Yes	No[†]
Yes	No	No	No
{ Yes	No }[‡]	Yes	Yes
No	Yes }		

*The stimulator cells that induce proliferation of the responder T cells in the mixed lymphocyte culture reaction also serve as the targets for the cytotoxic cells that develop from the responder population (as measured by the cell-mediated lympholysis assay).
[†]Low numbers of cytotoxic T cells may develop against class II antigens.
[‡]Stimulator cells from two individuals are mixed with responder cells from a single individual.

response can be initiated in a given case. In particular, polymorphisms on both α and β chains of HLA-DQ and HLA-DP provide considerable variation in binding configurations, especially when α/β dimers are composed of chains inherited from both parents; for example, $\alpha_{mother}/\beta_{father}$ may provide a peptide binding molecule not present in either parent. There are also many non-MHC influences on immune responsiveness; none of these have yet been well characterized clinically.

Studies in humans have also suggested the ability of the MHC to suppress immunologic responses to environmental agents, such as streptococcal infection, schistosomiasis, and leprosy, as well as antigens from cedar pollen and hepatitis B vaccine. Thus, it has been postulated that immune suppressor (Is) genes may be responsible. As is the case with Ir genes, the MHC class II region has been implicated. For example, the in vitro IgE response to cedar pollen antigen is suppressed by T cells of individuals bearing HLA-DQ3,[16] but the mechanisms of such T cell–mediated suppression are ill defined.

COMPLEMENT FACTOR GENES

Several complement proteins are encoded by genes that are linked to the MHC. These proteins include C2 and factor B (BF), which are closely linked and also similar in structure, suggesting gene duplication. In addition, two loci for C4 (C4A and C4B) are closely linked to C2 and BF. The C2 deficiency associated with systemic lupus erythematosus is associated with the HLA-A25, B18 haplotype. Indeed, extended haplotypes in which the same HLA-B, HLA-DR, HLA-DQ, and complement types are found among apparently unrelated persons with the same disease have been described. These circumstances could result from a mutation occurring in a common ancestor. Alternatively, there may be selective pressures to keep in close proximity genes that produce proteins that act together.

NONIMMUNOLOGIC FUNCTIONS OF MHC GENES

MHC genes are possibly also important in a variety of nonimmunologic cell-cell interactions. In 1976, a study showed that a male mouse presented with two H-2 congenic females in estrus would often choose to mate with females of an H-2 type different from his own. Further experiments showed that the male discriminated H-2 by sense of smell. The advantage most apparent in this example of opposites attracting is that the heterozygosity of genes in the *H-2* region, especially of Ir genes, ensures a wider range of immune defenses for the hybrid progeny of such matings. There is no evidence that humans can sense HLA antigens, however. Although MHC-controlled surface antigens may also play an important role in organogenesis and differentiation, there is contrary evidence for this hypothesis from studies of mice that completely lack surface MHC expression.

Disease and the Major Histocompatibility Complex

HLA-ASSOCIATED DISEASE

Many diseases have been associated with certain MHC antigens [*see Table 3*].[17] Such associations per se show only that the MHC molecules, or some other genes closely linked in the *HLA* region, have an influence on initiation or expression of disease. A relative risk of 5, for example, means only that there is a fivefold increase in the likelihood of disease in an individual with a particular HLA antigen, compared with someone who does not have that antigen. It indicates nothing about the frequency of the disease itself, which may be rare or common. One explanation for such associations is that the disease in question is related to a deficiency in the immune response to a particular causative organism. There is increasing evidence, however, that organ-spe-

cific, HLA-associated diseases—such as insulin-dependent diabetes mellitus (IDDM), multiple sclerosis, Graves' disease, the glomerulonephritides, celiac disease, ankylosing spondylitis, and rheumatoid arthritis—have a major component of autoimmunity.

In animal models in which appropriate breeding studies have been done, it has been demonstrated that autoimmune states depend on five to 15 randomly segregating genes, one of which is in the MHC. Polygenic etiology of human autoimmunity is very likely, but the HLA components may be useful targets for intervention, particularly in diseases in which HLA presentation of an immunogenic self-peptide is a key event.[18] Also, with the development of inflammation, de novo expression of HLA class II molecules on tissue cells may provide the immune stimulus for perpetuation of the autoimmune process. For example, patients with thyroiditis show aberrant expression of HLA-DR on thyroid cells, providing a possible mechanism by which thyroid antigen could be presented to T cells.

There has been progress in discerning which diseases may be directly related to immunogenic peptide presentation. Analysis of the sequences of genes encoding MHC class II molecules from patients with IDDM suggests that inheritance of particular *HLA* alleles is important in determining susceptibility to this disease, which may involve a T cell–mediated autoimmune response to pancreatic islet antigens. Resistance to IDDM is strongly associ-

Table 3   Diseases Showing Positive HLA Antigen Association(s)[22]

	Disease	HLA Antigen	Relative Risk*		Disease	HLA Antigen	Relative Risk*
Rheumatic	Ankylosing spondylitis	B27	69.1	*Endocrine*	Insulin-dependent diabetes mellitus (juvenile diabetes mellitus)	DR4	3.6
	Reiter's syndrome	B27	37.0			DR3	4.8
	Acute anterior uveitis	B27	8.2			DR2	0.2
	Reactive arthritis (*Yersinia, Salmonella,* gonococcus)	B27	18.0			BfF1[†]	15.0
	Psoriatic arthritis, central	B27	10.7		Graves' disease	B8	2.5
		B38	9.1			DR3	3.7
	Psoriatic arthritis, peripheral	B27	2.0		Graves' disease (Japanese)	B35	4.4
		B38	6.5		Addison's disease	Dw3	10.5
	Juvenile rheumatoid arthritis	B27	3.9		Subacute thyroiditis (de Quervain)	B35	13.7
	Juvenile rheumatoid arthritis, pauciarticular	DR5	3.3		Hashimoto's thyroiditis	DR5	3.2
	Rheumatoid arthritis	Dw4/DR4	3.8		Congenital adrenal hyperplasia	Bw47	15.4
	Sjögren's syndrome	Dw3	5.7	*Neurologic*	Myasthenia gravis (without thymoma)	B8	3.3
	Systemic lupus erythematosus	DR3	2.6		Multiple sclerosis	Dw2/DR2	6.0
Gastro-intestinal	Gluten-sensitive enteropathy	DR3	11.6		Manic-depressive disorder	B16	2.3
	Chronic active hepatitis	DR3	6.8		Narcolepsy	DR2	130.0
	Ulcerative colitis	B5	3.8		Schizophrenia	A28	2.3
	IgA deficiency	DR3	13.0	*Renal*	Idiopathic membranous glomerulo-nephritis	DR3	5.7
Hematologic	Idiopathic hemochromatosis	A3	6.7		Goodpasture's syndrome (anti-GBM)	DR2	15.9
		B14	2.7		Minimal change disease (steroid responsive)	DR7	4.2
		A3, B14	90.0		IgA nephropathy (French, Japanese)	DR4	3.1
	Pernicious anemia	DR5	5.4		Gold/penicillamine nephropathy	DR3	14.0
	Hodgkin's disease (white)	DP3	2.0		Polycystic kidney disease	B5	2.6
Skin	Dermatitis herpetiformis	DR3	17.3	*Infections*	Tuberculoid leprosy (Oriental)	B8	6.8
	Psoriasis vulgaris	Cw6	7.5		Paralytic polio	B16	4.3
	Psoriasis vulgaris (Japanese)	Cw6	8.5		Low vs high response to vaccinia virus	Cw3	12.7
	Pemphigus vulgaris (Jewish)	DR4	14.6				
		A26	4.8				
	Behçet's disease (white)	B5	3.8				
	Behçet's disease (Japanese)	B51	12.4				

*Relative risk = $\dfrac{(\% \text{ antigen-positive patients})\,(\% \text{ antigen-negative control subjects})}{(\% \text{ antigen-negative patients})\,(\% \text{ antigen-positive control subjects})}$

[†]BfF1 is an allele of the complement system that is HLA-linked but is not an antigen.

ated with the presence of aspartate at position 57 of the HLA-DQB β chain.[19] In individuals with the *HLA-DR2* haplotype, for example, the relative risk for IDDM drops to 0.2 [*see Table 3*]. *HLA-DR2* is in linkage disequilibrium with *HLA-DQB* β alleles, such as *DQB1*0602*, encoding aspartate at position 57. In contrast, when aspartate is not present at position 57, particularly in individuals with the *HLA-DR3* or *HLA-DR4* haplotype, there is an increased risk of IDDM. Amino acid residue 57 on the HLA-DQB β chain would lie toward one end of the groove; aspartate at that position may influence binding of a peptide to this class II molecule, causing reduction of helper T cell responses or activation of suppressor T cell responses to pancreatic islet antigens. Many studies among ethnic groups have shown that the greatest susceptibility to IDDM is related to *HLA-DQ*. The DQA/DQB heterodimer DQA1*0301/DQB1*0201 is associated with the highest risk. What is of interest here is that this heterodimer is uncommon, except in individuals who have inherited the *DQA* gene from one parent and *DQB* from the other. Whereas *DQA1*0301* and *DQB1*0201*, usually found with *DR4* and *DR3* haplotypes, respectively, separately increase the risk for IDDM, together they provide the highest risk of disease. As noted in a previous section, the formation of a heterodimer from the products of genes inherited from both parents does occur with the HLA-DQ molecule. The hypothesis is that this peptide binding site will be most effective in the presentation of pancreatic islet autoantigen. Definition of the binding motifs of this site may provide a clue to the antigen. There are additional and independent effects of *HLA-DR*—particularly the *DR4* alleles, some of which enhance and others suppress the IDDM risk. Amino acid differences in the hypervariable regions of MHC class II molecules have also been associated with such autoimmune disorders as pemphigus vulgaris and rheumatoid arthritis.

The association of narcolepsy with *HLA-DR2* (*DRB1*1501*) is more than 90%, but the highest association is with *HLA-DQA1*0102/DQB1*0602*.[19] The HLA effect is dominant, not recessive, and there is no indication of an immunologic defect in affected individuals. An abnormality in a peptide neurotransmitter or its receptor has been postulated, but the relation to the *HLA-D*–region genes is unknown.

Between 80% and 90% of celiac disease is associated with *HLA DQA1*0501/DQB1*0201*.[20] The peptide binding groove of this molecule is known to bind a peptide of wheat protein gliadin—a potentiating, if not the etiologic, factor in this disease.

Although an HLA molecule may determine specificity to a particular autoantigen, it is possible that genes that control other factors (e.g., the production of antigen receptors, specific subsets of regulatory cells, or helper and suppressor molecules) are responsible for a general tendency to an abnormal immune response. Additional study of the peculiar role of the HLA system in autoimmunity may well reveal mechanisms of autoimmune disease that are currently unknown.

HLA-LINKED DISEASE

A few diseases are clearly linked to specific *HLA* haplotypes in families, sometimes having common alleles in the general population and inherited as autosomal recessive defects. One example is congenital adrenal hyperplasia [*see Chapter 49*], an autosomal recessive defect involving the enzyme 21-hydroxylase that results in failure to synthesize cortisol and in overproduction of androgenic hormones. This condition may be associated with the *HLA-B47, BFF, DR7* haplotype. Similarly, idio-

pathic hemochromatosis is an autosomal recessive disorder of excessive dietary iron absorption [*see Chapter 87*] that is associated with the *HLA-A3, B14* haplotype. Hodgkin's disease in families also shows a strong *HLA*-linked recessive pattern. Because association with particular *HLA* alleles is weak [*see Table 3*], there may have been a common mutation occurring in several founders.

References

1. Bjorkman PJ, Saper MA, Samraoui B, et al: Structure of the human class I histocompatibility antigen, HLA-A2. Nature 329:506, 1987
2. Sidney J, Grey HM, Kubo RT, et al: Practical, biochemical and evolutionary implications of the discovery of HLA class I supermotifs. Immunol Today 17:261, 1996
3. Brown JH, Jardetzky TS, Gorga JC, et al: Three-dimensional structure of the human class II histocompatibility antigen HLA-DR1. Nature 364:33, 1993
4. Mytilineos J, Scherer S, Opelz G: Comparison of RFLP-DR beta and serological HLA-DR typing in 1500 individuals. Transplantation 50:870, 1990
5. Mytilineos J, Lemoert M, Middleton D, et al: HLA class I typing of 215 "HLA-A,-B,-DR zero mismatched" kidney transplants. Tissue Antigens 50:355, 1997
6. Bodmer JG, Marsh SGE, Albert ED, et al: Nomenclature for factors of the HLA system, 1996. Genetic Diversity of HLA: Functional and Medical Implication, Vol 1. Charron D, Ed. EDK, Paris, 1997, p 505
7. Harding CV, Unanue ER: Cellular mechanisms of antigen processing and the function of class I and II major histocompatibility complex molecules. Cell Regulation 1:499, 1990
8. Powis SH, Tonks S, Mockridge I, et al: Alleles and haplotypes of the MHC-encoded ABC transporters TAP1 and TAP2. Immunogenetics 37:373, 1993
9. Hunt DF, Michel H, Dickinson TA, et al: Peptides presented to the immune system by the murine class II major histocompatibility complex molecule I-A^d. Science 256:1817, 1992
10. Chicz RM, Urban RG, Gorga JC, et al: Specificity and promiscuity among naturally processed peptides bound to HLA-DR alleles. J Exp Med 178:27, 1993
11. Von Boehmer H: Positive selection of lymphocytes. Cell 76:219, 1994
12. Garboczi DN, Ghosh P, Utz U, et al: Structure of the complex between human T-cell receptor, viral peptide and HLA-A2. Nature 384:134, 1996
13. Sayegh MH, Watschinger B, Carpenter CB: Mechanisms of T cell recognition of alloantigen: the role of peptides. Transplantation 57:1295, 1994
14. Fangmann J, Dalchau R, Fabre JW: Rejection of skin allografts by indirect allorecognition of donor class I major histocompatibility complex peptides. J Exp Med 175:1521, 1992
15. Sayegh MH, Khoury SJ, Hancock WW, et al: Induction of immunity and oral tolerance by polymorphic class II major histocompatibility complex allopeptides in the rat. Proc Natl Acad Sci USA 89:7762, 1992
16. Matsushita S, Muto M, Suemura M, et al: HLA linked nonresponsiveness to *Cryptomeria japonica* pollen antigen: I. Nonresponsiveness is mediated by antigen-specific suppressor T cells. J Immunol 138:109, 1987
17. Thorsby E: HLA-associated disease susceptibility: which genes are involved? The Immunologist 3:51, 1995
18. Todd JA, Acha-Orbea, Bell JI, et al: A molecular basis for MHC class II–associated autoimmunity. Science 240:1003, 1988
19. Thorsby E: HLA-associated diseases. A summary of the 12th International Histocompatibility Workshop component. Genetic Diversity of HLA: Functional and Medical Implication, Vol 2. Charron D, Ed. EDK, Paris, 1997, p 91
20. Sollid LM, Marjussen G, Ek J, et al: Evidence for a primary association of celiac disease to a particular HLA-DQ α/β heterodimer. J Exp Med 169:345, 1989
21. Abbas AK, Lichtman AH, Pober JS: The major histocompatibility complex. Cellular and Molecular Immunology, 2nd ed. WB Saunders Co, Philadelphia, 1994, p 96
22. Carpenter CB: The major histocompatibility gene complex. Harrison's Principles of Internal Medicine, 11th ed. Braunwald E, Isselbacher KJ, Petersdorf RG, et al, Eds. McGraw-Hill Book Co, New York, 1987, p 341

Acknowledgments

Figure 1   Laura Brown.
Figures 2 and 3A   Tom Moore.
Figure 4   Dimitry Schidlovsky.

Reviews

Eckels D: Alloreactivity: allogeneic presentation of endogenous peptides or direct recognition of MHC polymorphism. Tissue Antigens 35:35, 1990

Germain RN: MHC-dependent antigen processing and peptide presentation: providing ligands for T lymphocyte activation. Cell 76:287, 1994

Nossal GJV: Negative selection of lymphocytes. Cell 76:229, 1994

Carpenter CB: HLA class I DNA typing in organ transplantation. Tissue Antigens 50:322, 1997

Erlich HA, Gyllensten UB: Shared epitopes among HLA class II alleles: gene conversion, common ancestry and balancing selection. Immunol Today 12:411, 1991

Sayegh MH, Carpenter CB. Role of indirect allorecognition in allograft rejection. Int Rev Immunol 13:221, 1996

102 Immunogenetics of Disease

Edgar L. Milford, M.D., and Charles B. Carpenter, M.D.

Differences in genetic makeup from individual to individual have long been recognized to have physiologic consequences in both health and disease. The recent ability to do high-throughput sequencing of genes has revealed that many genes have variants that are present in a significant proportion of the population. Inherited variants of specific genes, either alone or in combination with other genes, may confer a differential risk of disease or of rejection of transplanted tissue.

Genetic Polymorphism

The fundamental basis of genetic polymorphism in a population is variation of the nucleotide sequence of DNA at homologous locations in the genome. These differences in sequence can result from mutations involving a single nucleotide or from deletions or insertions of variable numbers of contiguous nucleotides. Each of these variants presumably occurred in a single ancestor in the distant past. Most new mutations are extinguished through random genetic drift and never become established in the population at any significant frequency. When the gene frequency of a mutation becomes established at more than 1% to 2%, it is often given the more dignified appellation of allele.

Allelic variants can occur anywhere in the genome. Some are found within coding regions of genes, and others are located in introns or gene regulatory regions. However, still others are found in areas that are not closely linked to any known expressed gene.

EQUILIBRIUM, DISEQUILIBRIUM, GENOTYPES, AND HAPLOTYPES

There can be multiple polymorphic nucleotide positions in or near an expressed gene on the same chromosome. In such cases, it is desirable to know whether specific variants at each of the polymorphic positions are independent of the variants at the other positions. If examination of a population shows that the variants at the different positions occur independently of one another, the system is said to be in Hardy-Weinberg equilibrium.[1] If certain variants at one of the positions are statistically associated with specific variants at another of the linked positions, the system is said to exhibit linkage disequilibrium.[1]

Hardy-Weinberg equilibrium can be reestablished over many generations through recombination events. The closer the polymorphic loci are to each other on the chromosome, the less likelihood there is of a recombination and the more likely it is for the specific alleles at the two linked loci to be inherited en bloc as a haplotype. For example, if there are two polymorphic positions within a gene, each of which has two alleles, a given individual will have up to four definable alleles. These alleles are inherited as two parental haplotypes, each of which carries one allele from each of the two loci. Most methods used to type individuals cannot organize the genotype into haplotypes without additional information. The common assays simply define the genotype at each of the two polymorphic positions. Extensive population studies permit sophisticated maximum-likelihood estimates of haplotype frequencies within the population.[2] These studies, combined with confirmatory cloning and sequencing studies of individual DNA strands, often reveal that some theoretically possible haplotypes never occur, whereas others can be assumed when a specific allele is present (because of linkage disequilibrium) [*see Figure 1*]. The ability to deduce haplotypes provides a much higher degree of specificity to the analysis of genetic polymorphism, because the haplotype more accurately defines a larger inherited region of DNA.

TYPES OF GENETIC POLYMORPHISM

Single-nucleotide polymorphisms (SNPs) are allelic variants that have been generated as the result of conversion of one nucleotide to another at a homologous position. When present within a coding region (exon) of a gene, the expressed product may or may not have a single amino acid difference, depending on the resulting codon change. In some cases, the change can lead to either a nonsense codon or a stop codon, which halts the transcription process and results in the production of a truncated peptide. SNPs that are located in regulatory regions of an expressed gene can alter the transcription efficiency of that gene but not the protein sequence [*see Figure 2*].

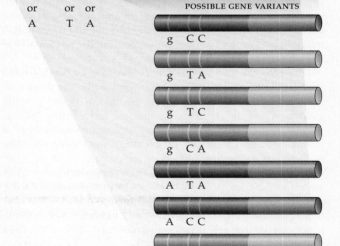

Variants of the Interleukin-10 Gene

Figure 1 **Single-nucleotide variants occur at positions −1082, −819, and −592 in the promoter region of the interleukin-10 (IL-10) gene. Although eight variants are theoretically possible, only three of these potential IL-10 variants (in purple) are actually observed in large population studies. This is a consequence of strong linkage disequilibrium between the variants at those three positions.**

Deletion or insertion mutants have also been found in functional genes, sometimes at frequencies that merit their inclusion as alleles. Again, the consequence of a deletion depends on the precise location of the deletion; whether it produces a nonsense frameshift; and whether it alters the function of the expressed product. Angiotensin-converting enzyme (ACE) represents a gene that has a deletion variant in which a 278-base-pair segment of intron 16 is excised. This deletion variant is associated with increased ACE levels.

Another class of allelic variance in association with a particular gene is short tandem repeat (STR) polymorphism. Short sequences of two to four base pairs at a given location can be duplicated back-to-back a specific number of times and inherited as a genetic variant. Because such variation would usually result in a nonsense codon, these STRs are almost always located in noncoding regions. The interferon gamma (IFN-γ) gene has such an STR within intron 1, in which the (CA) dinucleotide motif is repeated a variable number of times. The allele with $(CA)_{12}$—that is, with 12 repeats of the CA motif—is associated with high IFN-γ production [see Figure 3].

METHODS OF DETECTION OF GENETIC POLYMORPHISM

DNA-based genotyping methods are rapid, accurate, and economical. SNPs can easily be detected, with a high degree of specificity and sensitivity. The assays depend on amplification of the polymorphic locus in question to produce sensitivity in the setting of a background of sample genomic DNA. Specificity is ensured by using tailored oligonucleotides that are complementary to the DNA sequence of the allele one wants to detect.

One strategy for typing is to use polymerase chain reaction to amplify a segment of DNA that includes the polymorphic position and a moderate amount of flanking DNA on both the 3' and 5' sides of the polymorphic position. This is done with primers that are complementary to conserved sequences in either side of the desired segment to be amplified. This yields an amplicon of known size that contains inherited alleles and is present in an amount that can be tested for the presence of specific alleles without significant interference from genomic DNA. The amplicon can then be probed, using a set of fluoresceinated or radiolabeled oligonucleotides, each of which is complementary to the DNA sequence of one of the possible alleles. This method is often referred to as site-specific oligonucleotide probe (SSOP) testing.

TGF-β1 Gene Polymorphisms

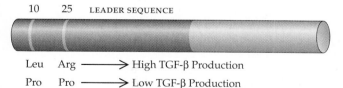

Figure 2   **Single-nucleotide polymorphisms have been identified in the gene for transforming growth factor–β1 (TGF-β1). Each polymorphism involves two alleles in the leader sequence of the gene. These biallelic nucleotide substitutions produce codon changes that result in alternative amino acids. Leu10 is in linkage disequilibrium with Arg25, and Pro10 is in linkage disequilibrium with Pro25. The Leu10Arg25 variant is associated with high TGF-β1 production, whereas the Pro10Pro25 variant is associated with lower production. This may be the consequence of different efficiency of posttranslational modification for the two variants, which differ only in the leader amino acid sequence.**

IFN-γ Gene Variants and Expression

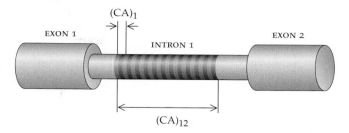

Figure 3   **Illustration of a short tandem repeat (STR) polymorphism within intron 1 of the interferon gamma (IFN-γ) gene. STR polymorphisms in this intron differ according to the number of repetitions of the cytosine-arginine (CA) motif. The allelic variant with 12 tandem repeats [(CA_{12})] is associated with higher IFN-γ production.**

Another strategy for SNP typing, which does not require two steps, is called site-specific priming (SSP). This method takes advantage of the fact that the 3' terminal base of a primer is where DNA synthesis commences during each cycle of PCR. For synthesis to proceed, the 3' base must be closely bonded to its complementary base on the template DNA. Therefore, the terminal 3' base of the primer can be used to render the PCR reaction itself exquisitely sensitive to the identity of the base that is on the template. For detection of SNPs, one can craft a set of PCR primers that are complementary to the alleles to be detected, with the terminal 3' base of one of the primers located at the polymorphic position. The second PCR primer is usually complementary to a conserved segment of DNA and positioned to yield a product of a convenient size. If an allele is present, use of the appropriate set of primers will produce an amplicon. The amplicon can be separated from genomic DNA by simple agarose gel electrophoresis and identified by ethidium bromide staining under ultraviolet light, and the expected size can be confirmed.

Both SSOP and SSP can be modified to detect deletion or insertion variants. With SSP, using primers that flank the deletions or insertions, amplicons of characteristic sizes are produced. SSOP can confirm the presence or absence of the deletions or insertions through the use of probes that include the junctions of the deleted or inserted regions.

RELEVANCE OF GENETIC POLYMORPHISM IN HUMANS

Historically, polymorphisms in several genetic systems have been recognized as a barrier to transfusion and transplantation. The ABO blood group antigens were among the earliest genetically determined glycoproteins that exhibited mendelian inheritance and had biologic relevance in humans.[3] Mismatch for the ABO antigens is a risk factor not only for transfusion reactions but also for solid-organ transplantation because of the prominent expression of these antigens on the vascular endothelium.

The major histocompatibility complex (MHC)—so called because of its prominent role in rejection of allogeneic tissue—is a primary barrier to transplantation of solid organs, tissue, and hematopoietic stem cells. This closely linked cluster of highly polymorphic genes, grouped on the short arm of chromosome 6, encodes cell surface molecules (human leukocyte antigens [HLA]). The normal role of the MHC is presentation of endogenous and exogenous peptide antigen fragments to T cells, thereby initiating an immune response against the molecule (or pathogenic organism) from which the peptide was derived.[4] The extreme variability of molecular structure in the MHC antigens permits a wide range of different peptides to be presented by autologous human antigen-presenting cells, although some persons may have a specific repertoire of MHC antigens that do not present certain antigens effectively. The focused immunogenicity of MHC molecules and the variability of these molecules from person to person render them prominent targets for the immune response in the context of solid-organ and bone marrow transplantation. In cases in which live allogeneic cells are the target of the immune response, the apparent target is the nonself MHC molecule itself. Freedom from rejection and, in the case of bone marrow transplantation, graft versus host disease (GVHD) is improved with HLA matching of donor and recipient.

Innate and Adaptive Responses

It has become abundantly clear that the selective (adaptive) immunologic response, which is important in organ transplantation, tissue transplantation, and defense against certain microorganisms, is closely associated with the innate cellular and humoral pathways of nonspecific tissue injury, inflammation, hypoxia, and healing. Macrophages, for example, play a central role in the response to hypoxia, trauma, bacterial invasion, and inflammation caused by exogenous toxins, but they are also important in the processing and presentation of antigen to the specific immune system. Natural killer (NK) cells, which constitute approximately 10% of human mononuclear cells, are thought to be important mediators of innate immunity. Their cytolytic activity is regulated by inhibitory receptors, called killer immunoglobulin-like receptors (KIRs).[5] Class I MHC molecules are ligands for the KIRs—in particular, genetically determined epitopes on HLA-B and HLA-C molecules that have limited polymorphism.[5] In bone marrow transplantation, recipients who present the appropriate class I ligands to donor NK cells will downregulate the NK response. This is thought to decrease both GVHD and graft versus tumor activity.

Humans also have innate humoral immunity against a number of glycoprotein antigens. This so-called natural antibody is thought to have protective effects against a wide range of bacterial products. At the same time, the humoral immune system is able to mount a robust adaptive response to an astonishingly broad spectrum of specific antigens, if challenged to do so. The genes responsible for the adaptive immune response are highly polymorphic, but they are found only in specific subsets of T cells with antigen receptor genes that are rearranged during thymic development and in B cells that undergo somatic mutation in response to antigenic challenge. Specific germline variant alleles of the T cell receptor for antigen (before somatic mutation) are also associated with differential susceptibility to a number of immunologically mediated conditions, including renal allograft rejection and several rheumatic diseases, such as rheumatoid arthritis.[6]

Other Polymorphic Genes Involved in Organ and Tissue Injury

Variants of genes can influence organ and tissue physiology, directly induce diseases, or render the person more susceptible or resistant to a pathologic state. Variants that directly induce a profound disease state are usually rare in the population, because the disease may cause death before the person can reproduce. Variants or mutations that cause severe early disease are not discussed in this chapter. Polymorphic variants of loci that have a more subtle effect on disease susceptibility are more likely to become established in the population at frequencies of 1% or more (i.e., to become alleles). Several patterns can be appreciated with these alleles. Variant alleles may exhibit a gene-dose effect, with heterozygotes having an intermediate influence, between that of the normal genotype (the so-called wild type) and the homozygous variant genotype. In other cases, a variant allele appears to have a dominant influence; presumably, these variants are able to achieve significant frequency in the population because the condition they produce does not substantially decrease reproduction. The disease phenotype that is a measurable physiologic consequence of a particular genotype may be a downstream effect that depends on multiple influences, including the genotype in question, interaction with other genes, and environmental exposure.

Loci that encode cytokines, chemokine receptors, costimulatory molecules, and components of physiologically important pathways such as the angiotensin system are all concrete examples in which genetic polymorphism influences pathophysiology. These examples can be used to highlight some ways in which determination of individual genotype can assist in assessing risk of disease.

Cytokines and chemokines are secreted proteins and glycoproteins that act as important signaling devices in both the innate and the adaptive responses. They serve variously as chemoattractants and as inducers or suppressors of leukocyte, endothelial cell, platelet, fibroblast, and myocyte function. They have a particularly notable effect on cells that bear the appropriate receptors. Cytokines and chemokines often represent a common pathway that links the classical immune pathway and other pathways of tissue injury and repair, such as those involved in ischemia, trauma, and toxic damage.[7]

Costimulatory molecules such as CTLA-4 are expressed on the cell membranes of T cells and serve as ligands for complementary molecules on antigen-presenting cells [see Chapter 104]. The engagement of costimulatory molecules with their ligands can augment or suppress the magnitude of the immune response induced by the recognition of antigen via the T cell receptor.[8,9] Soluble CTLA-4 has been used to block antigen-dependent T cell activation by competitive blockade of normal cell membrane–bound interaction.

Functional Consequences of Specific Genetic Variants

CYTOKINE POLYMORPHISMS

Variants in the genes that govern the production of cytokines such as interleukin-10 (IL-10), tumor necrosis factor–α (TNF-α), and transforming growth factor–β (TGF-β) can help determine whether a person has high or low levels of these cytokines.[10] The cytokine network is thought to play an important role both in rejection of allografts and in tolerance,[11] and a number of clinical effects of these polymorphisms in cytokine genes have now been described [see Tables 1 and 2].

TGF-β has two well-studied dimorphic positions within the leader sequence of the gene [see Figure 2]. These polymorphisms are in linkage disequilibrium; only two variants of the TGF-β gene have been described, rather than the four theoretically possible combinatorial variants. TGF-β is considered to be

Table 1   Cytokine Genetic Polymorphisms and Their Pathophysiologic Effects[9,31-59]

Locus	Position	Genotype	Pathophysiologic Effect
CTLA4	Microsatellite	Allele 3 and allele 4	Increased rejection, liver/kidney transplants
IFN-γ	Microsatellite	Allele 2 (12 CA repeat)	Increased production
IFN-γ	Microsatellite	Allele 2 (12 CA repeat)	Increased production
IFN-γ	Microsatellite	Allele 2 (12 CA repeat)	Increased acute rejection, kidney transplants
IFN-γ	Microsatellite	Allele 3 homozygotes	Increased GVHD, bone marrow transplant patients
IFN-γ	T+874A	T allele	Increased production
IL-10	-1082A	A allele	Low producer
IL-10	-1082A	A/A homozygotes	Increased frequency in Wegener granulomatosus
IL-10	-1064	Low producer	Increased GVHD, bone marrow transplant patients
IL-10	-1082, -819, -592	Low producer	Increased rejection, pediatric heart transplant patients
IL-10	-1064	High producer	Increased graft survival, renal transplants
IL-10	-1082A	High producer	Increased rejection, if high TNF genotype
IL-10	-1082A	High producer	Increased rejection episodes, renal transplants
IL-10	-1082A	Recipient high; donor low	Increased rejection, renal transplants
IL-4	-590T	Recipient and donor low	Decreased rejection, renal transplants
IL-6	-174C	G allele	Increased acute GVHD, bone marrow transplants
TGF-β1	Arg25Pro	A/A homozygotes	Increased production
TGF-β1	Arg25Pro	Arg	Increased in patients with fibrotic lung disease
TGF-β1	Arg25Pro	A/A homozygotes	Progression of renal insufficiency, heart transplant patients
TGF-β1	Arg25Pro	A/A homozygotes	Decreased gingival hyperplasia with cyclosporine
TGF-β1	Arg25Pro	A/A homozygotes	Increased coronary vasculopathy, heart transplants
TGF-β1	Arg25Pro	Arg	No correlation with renal transplant rejection
TGF-β1	Leu10Pro	Leu	Progression of renal insufficiency, heart transplant patients
TGF-β1	Leu10Pro	L/L homozygotes	Decreased renal dysfunction, heart transplant patients
TGF-β1	Leu10Pro	Pro	Association with dilated cardiomyopathy
TGF-β1	Leu10Pro	Pro/Pro	Increased gingival hyperplasia with cyclosporine
TNF-α	-308A	High A/A or A/G	Increased rejection and creatinine, renal transplants
TNF-α	-308A	High A/A or A/G	Increased GVHD and mortality, bone marrow transplant patients
TNF-α	-308A	High A/A or A/G	Increased rejection, renal transplants
TNF-α	-308A	Low producer	Decreased acute rejection, pediatric heart transplants
TNF-α	-308A	A allele	Sixfold to sevenfold higher production
TNF-α	-308A	A allele	Risk factor renal transplants, if HLA-DR mismatch
TNF-α	-308A	A allele	Increased rejection, pediatric heart transplants
TNF-α	-308A	A allele	Increased frequency in primary sclerosing cholangitis
TNF-α	-308A	A allele	Increased mortality, heart transplant patients
TNF-α	-308A	A allele	Increased rejection, renal transplants
TNF-α	-308A	A allele	Increased hepatitis C recurrence after liver transplants
TNF-α	-308A	A allele	Decreased plasma TNF levels
TNF-α	-308A	A/A homozygotes	Increased rejection, liver transplants
TNF-α	-308A	A/A homozygotes	Increased acute rejection, liver transplants
TNF-α	Microsatellite	High producer	Increased rejection, cardiac transplants (low IL-10 subset)
TNF-α	Microsatellite	High producer	Increased acute GVHD, bone marrow transplant patients
TNF-α	Microsatellite	a9	Increased in rejection, renal transplants, in patients with HLA-B35
TNF-α	Microsatellite	d3/d3 homozygotes	Increased GVHD grade III/IV
TNF-α	Microsatellite	d4	Decreased in rejection, renal transplants, in patients with HLA-B44
TNF-α	NcoI	Low recipient	Increased infection, renal transplants
TNF-α	-308A	A allele	Nonischemic cardiac dysfunction

Note: Some of these gene variants appear to have paradoxical effects, depending on the investigator and the assay system.
GVHD—graft versus host disease   IFN—interferon   IL—interleukin   TGF—transforming growth factor   TNF—tumor necrosis factor

a major mediator of fibrosis in kidney and lung allografts.[12,13] Specific variants of the TGF gene that result in high production of TGF-β (so-called high-producer genotypes) are associated with poor outcome in lung transplants: 98% of patients with chronic rejection are homozygous for the high-producer TGF-β genotype represented by Leu at position 10 and Arg at position 25. Moreover, fibrosis develops in the lung grafts of 93% of those with homozygous high-producer TGF-β genotype but only in 7% of those with heterozygous (high/low) producer genotype.[12] TGF-β also mediates the gingival hypertrophy induced by the immunosuppressive agent cyclosporine. In-

creased gingival hypertrophy has been reported in patients with the low-producer TGF-β genotype, represented by Pro at both position 10 and position 25. Because the two variants differ only in the leader amino acid sequence, the different production levels may be the consequence of different efficiency of posttranslational modification.

ANGIOTENSIN SYSTEM POLYMORPHISMS

The renin-angiotensin system is a metabolic-hormonal pathway that plays a critical role in blood pressure homeostasis and salt and water balance. In the renin-angiotensin pathway, the

Table 2   Renin-Angiotensin System and Chemokine Polymorphism and Pathophysiology[26,60-72]

Locus	Position	Genotype	Pathophysiologic Effect
ACE	Deletion variant	I/I or I/D	Favorable function trend, pediatric renal transplants
ACE	Deletion variant	D	Favorable renal function, bone marrow transplant patients
ACE	Deletion variant	D/D homozygotes	Favorable renal function, renal transplants
ACE	Deletion variant	D	Increased cardiac allograft vascular disease
ACE	Deletion variant	D/D homozygotes	Increased risk of renal failure, pediatric kidney transplants
ACE	Deletion variant	D/D homozygotes	Inreased risk of renal failure, high-risk renal transplants
ACE	Deletion variant	D	Increased frequency in systemic lupus erythematosus
ACE	Function	Function	ACE inhibitor suppresses IL-12, IFN-γ
ACE	Deletion variant	D/D homozygotes	Increased ACE levels
ACE	Deletion variant	D/D homozygotes	Increased blood pressure with salt administration
ACE	Deletion	D	Increased risk of renal dysfunction, renal transplants
AGT	Met235Thr	Met vs Thr	No function association, pediatric renal transplants
AGT	G → A,-6	A/A	Increased risk of renal dysfunction, renal transplants
AT1	A1166C	A vs C	No function association, pediatric renal transplants
AT1	Function	Function	Activation of NF-κB via IL-12 and IFN-γ
AT1	A1166C	C	Increased blood pressure, renal transplant patients
CCR2	V64I	I	Less acute rejection, renal transplants
CCR2	Expression	Expression	High expression in renal transplants during rejection
CCR5	A59029G	A/A homozygotes	Less acute rejection, renal transplants
CCR5	Expression	Expression	High expression in renal transplants during rejection
CXCR3	Expression	Expression	High expression in heart biopsy infiltrates

Note: Some of the gene variants appear to have paradoxical effects, depending on the investigator and the assay system.
ACE—angiotensin-converting enzyme   IFN—interferon   IL—interleukin

prohormone angiotensinogen (AGT) is converted to angiotensin I by renin. Angiotensin-converting enzyme then catalyzes the conversion of angiotensin I to angiotensin II [*see Figure 4*]. Angiotensin II is one of the most potent vasoconstrictive human hormones. In addition, angiotensin II has indirect inflammatory and fibrotic effects, which are distinct from its physiologic vasoconstrictive role. These indirect effects appear to be mediated by cytokines. Angiotensin II promotes the secretion of a number of inflammatory cytokines, including TGF-β, platelet-derived growth factor (PDGF), fibroblast growth factor (FGF), IL-6, IL-12, TNF-α, and IFN-γ.[14-17] There are two receptors for angiotensin II, type 1 (AT1) and type 2 (AT2). AT1 receptors mediate the major vasoconstrictive activity of angiotensin II but also appear to be involved in angiotensin II–dependent augmentation of immune activation and stimulation of TGF-β production. The AT2 receptors are implicated in remodeling; may promote angiotensin II–dependent apoptosis; and have some functions that oppose the AT1 receptor, including vasodilation and increased production of nitric oxide.[18,19]

Several of the genes encoding members of the renin-angiotensin pathway exhibit polymorphisms that influence function. Genomic variants of the genes encoding AGT, ACE, AT1, and AT2 have been described.[20] There is evidence that the AGT(A/A) and ACE(D/D) variants result in increased angiotensin II activity; in turn, the angiotensin II can interact differentially with receptors of different genotypes and influence ultimate pathophysiology. A deletion variant of the ACE gene (D14091-14378) and a single-nucleotide polymorphic variant of the AGT gene (G → A, -6) are correlated with increased peripheral ACE activity and AGT levels, respectively.[21,22] Both genotypes confer increased susceptibility to hypertension, and ACE(D14091-14378) also worsens ischemic heart disease and progression of intrinsic renal insufficiency [*see Table 2*].[23] An analysis of ACE polymorphism in diabetes revealed that the ACE(D) allele is highly associated with diabetic nephropathy.[24]

Of the different classes of white blood cells, T cells contain the highest level of ACE, approximately 28-fold more than

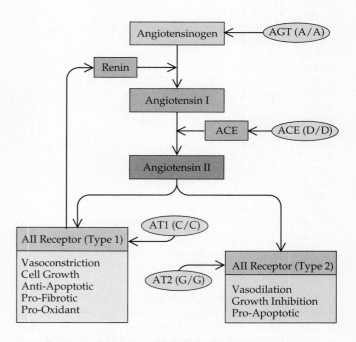

Figure 4   **The renin-angiotensin system is illustrated, along with proven variants of genes responsible for its components. The variant genes indicated are thought to result in a quantitative increase in function in the system. The final hormone, angiotensin II (AII), has a variety of vasoactive, inflammatory, or anti-inflammatory effects, which appear to be dependent on the receptor that is engaged. (ACE—angiotensin-converting enzyme; AGT—angiotensinogen; AT1—angiotensin type 1 receptor; AT2—angiotensin type 2 receptor)**

Polymorphisms in Chemokine Genes

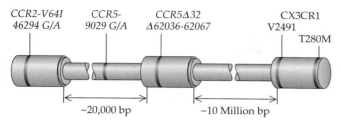

Figure 5 Locations of chemokine receptor genes and variant positions associated with those genes are shown. The CCR2, CCR5, and CX3CR1 genes are located on the same chromosome. CX3CR1 has two variable positions within the coding region. The location of the deletion variant of CCR5 and the location of the G-to-A variant of CCR5 in the 5' promoter region of the gene are illustrated. The CCR2 gene has a G-to-A variant located within the coding region.

monocytes. Indeed, immunologically competent T cells appear to be the major cell type expressing ACE in blood.[25] The ACE expression can vary up to 100-fold during the differentiation of T cells. Monocytes express angiotensin II, the final product of the angiotensin synthetic pathway. Monocyte angiotensin II appears to mediate recruitment of inflammatory cells during renal damage through the synthesis of monocyte chemoattractant protein-1.[26]

A variant of the AT2 gene (A → G, 1332) has been associated with congenital anomalies of the kidney and urinary tract. These developmental abnormalities are preceded by delayed apoptosis of undifferentiated mesenchymal cells surrounding the urinary tract during key ontogenic events.[27] In kidney transplant recipients, specific variants of the ACE and AGT genes are correlated with poor clinical outcomes. Renal transplant patients who have either the ACE(D14091-14378) or the AGT homozygous (G → A, -6)/(G → A, -6) variant have poorer renal transplant function at 3 years, as well as more rapid progression of transplant failure, defined as an increase of serum creatinine levels over time. Diastolic blood pressure in these patients was also significantly higher as a function of the AT1(A → C, 1166) C gene dose. The pathophysiologic reasons for the association between specific angiotensin system gene polymorphisms and renal transplant outcomes are not well understood. Further work is needed to reveal the degree to which this association is a function of hypertensive organ damage or modulation of the immunologic response mediated by angiotensin.

CHEMOKINE RECEPTOR POLYMORPHISMS

Chemokines are molecules with a variety of functions, some of which influence the recruitment of inflammatory cells to sites of injury. Three of the genes encoding chemokine receptors are located on one chromosome. CCR2 and CCR5 are located within 20,000 base pairs of each other; CX3CR1 is located 10 million base pairs away from CCR5 [*see Figure 5*].

The leukocyte chemokine receptor CCR5 is expressed on monocytes, as well as on helper T cells involved in augmentation of the immune response (T_{H1} subset)[28] [*see Chapter 105*]. CCR5 is a coreceptor for entry of HIV-1 into macrophages. CCR5 binds the inflammatory chemokines RANTES (regulated on activation, normal T cell expressed and repeated), macrophage inflammatory protein (MIP)-1α, and MIP-1β, whereas CCR2 and CX3CR1 are receptors for the chemokines monocyte chemoattractant protein (MCP)-1 and fractalkine, re-

spectively. Antagonists of CCR5, such as met-RANTES, prolong renal allograft survival in MHC-incompatible mice. Furthermore, prolonged heart transplant survival is achieved if the recipient is a homozygous CCR2 or CCR5 knockout. In humans, a 32-base-pair deletion of the CCR5 gene (CCR5 Δ32) renders the gene nonfunctional. There is also a polymorphic single-nucleotide variant of CCR5, CCR5-9029(G → A), which is located in the promoter region of the gene. The G variant is associated with defective transcription. Gene variants of some of these chemokine receptors have been associated with different rates of HIV disease progression.[29] The CCR5 Δ32 variant is associated with lower incidence and severity of asthma and rheumatoid arthritis.[30] Patients with homozygosity for CX3CR1-V2491I(G → A), CX3CR1-T280M(C → T), and CCR5-9029(G → A) have higher HIV progression rates. In contrast, patients with CCR2V64I(G → A) and CCR5(Δ32) exhibit slower progression of HIV, presumably because of reduced binding of the virus to target cells.

In renal transplant patients, the A/A homozygous genotype of the CCR59029(A → G) polymorphic locus is associated with significantly lower incidence of acute rejection episodes in the first posttransplant year. Although this could be explained by a protective effect of A/A homozygosity, it might instead be from a dominant detrimental effect of the G variant, given that both A/G heterozygotes and G/G homozygotes have been found to have similarly high rejection frequencies, which were twice that of patients with A/A genotype.[14]

Practical Applications of Genotyping Polymorphisms

The genetic polymorphisms discussed in this chapter represent but examples of the many inherited variants of physiologically important genes that influence susceptibility to disease. These variants can act alone, in conjunction with variants at other loci, or through interaction with environmental factors to increase or decrease disease incidence or severity. The cytokine genes, chemokine genes, and genes of the renin-angiotensin system are important modulators of the immune response and, in the case of the renin-angiotensin axis, of hypertension and vascular disease. Knowledge of a patient's genotype may assist physicians in assessing prior risk of a pathophysiologic outcome and in tailoring therapy. Clinical trials may, in some cases, be better interpreted by knowledge of participant genotypes, because certain genotypes may impart differential incidence of disease and responsiveness to pharmacologic agents.

References

1. Kaessmann H, Zollner S, Gustafsson AC, et al: Extensive linkage disequilibrium in small human populations in Eurasia. Am J Hum Genet 70:673, 2002

2. Mori M, Beatty PG, Graves M, et al: HLA gene and haplotype frequencies in the North American population: the National Marrow Donor Program Donor Registry. Transplantation 64: 1017, 1997

3. Rydberg L: ABO-incompatibility in solid organ transplantation. Transfus Med 11:325, 2001

4. Rudolph MG, Wilson IA: The specificity of TCR/pMHC interaction. Curr Opin Immunol 14:52, 2002

5. Vilches C, Parham P: KIR: diverse, rapidly evolving receptors of innate and adaptive immunity. Annu Rev Immunol 20:217, 2002

6. VanderBorght A, Geusens P, Vandevyver C, et al: Skewed T-cell receptor variable gene usage in the synovium of early and chronic rheumatoid arthritis patients and persistence of clonally expanded T cells in a chronic patient. Rheumatology (Oxford) 39:1189, 2000

7. Goddard S, Williams A, Morland C, et al: Differential expression of chemokines and chemokine receptors shapes the inflammatory response in rejecting human liver trans-

plants. Transplantation 72:1957, 2001

8. Onodera K, Chandraker A, Schaub M, et al: CD28-B7 T cell costimulatory blockade by CTLA4Ig in sensitized rat recipients: induction of transplantation tolerance in association with depressed cell-mediated and humoral immune responses. J Immunol 159:1711, 1997

9. Slavcheva E, Albanis E, Jiao Q, et al: Cytotoxic T-lymphocyte antigen 4 gene polymorphisms and susceptibility to acute allograft rejection. Transplantation 72:935, 2001

10. Rudwaleit M, Siegert S, Yin Z, et al: Low T cell production of TNFalpha and IFNgamma in ankylosing spondylitis: its relation to HLA-B27 and influence of the TNF-308 gene polymorphism. Ann Rheum Dis 60:36, 2001

11. Suthanthiran M: The importance of genetic polymorphisms in renal transplantation. Curr Opin Urol 10:71, 2000

12. El-Gamel A, Awad MR, Hasleton PS, et al: Transforming growth factor-beta (TGF-beta1) genotype and lung allograft fibrosis. J Heart Lung Transplant 18:517, 1999

13. Freedman BI, Yu H, Spray BJ, et al: Genetic linkage analysis of growth factor loci and end-stage renal disease in African Americans. Kidney Int 51:819, 1997

14. Klahr S, Morrissey J: Angiotensin II and gene expression in the kidney. Am J Kidney Dis 31:171, 1998

15. Guo G, Morrissey J, McCracken R, et al: Contributions of angiotensin II and tumor necrosis factor-alpha to the development of renal fibrosis. Am J Physiol Renal Physiol 280:F777, 2001

16. Moriyama T, Fujibayashi M, Fujiwara Y, et al: Angiotensin II stimulates interleukin-6 release from cultured mouse mesangial cells. J Am Soc Nephrol 6:95:101, 1995

17. Khalil A, Tullus K, Bakhiet M, et al: Angiotensin II type 1 receptor antagonist (losartan) down-regulates transforming growth factor-beta in experimental acute pyelonephritis. J Urol 164:186, 2000

18. Cigola E, Kajstura J, Li B, et al: Angiotensin II activates programmed myocyte cell death in vitro. Exp Cell Res 231:363, 1997

19. Yamada T, Horiuchi M, Dzau VJ: Angiotensin II type 2 receptor mediates programmed cell death. Proc Natl Acad Sci U S A 93:156, 1996

20. Abdi R, Tran TB, Sahagun-Ruiz A, et al: Chemokine receptor polymorphism and risk of acute rejection in human renal transplantation. J Am Soc Nephrol 13:754, 2002

21. Ruprecht B, Schurmann M, Ziegenhagen MW, et al: [Corrected normal values for serum ACE by genotyping the deletion-/insertion-polymorphism of the ACE gene.] Pneumologie 55:326, 2001

22. Bloem LJ, Manatunga AK, Tewksbury DA, et al: The serum angiotensinogen concentration and variants of the angiotensinogen gene in white and black children. J Clin Invest 95:948, 1995

23. Petrovic D, Zorc M, Kanic V, et al: Interaction between gene polymorphisms of renin-angiotensin system and metabolic risk factors in premature myocardial infarction. Angiology 52:247, 2001

24. Solini A, Dalla Vestra M, Saller A, et al: The angiotensin-converting enzyme DD genotype is associated with glomerulopathy lesions in type 2 diabetes. Diabetes 51:251, 2002

25. Costerousse O, Allegrini J, Lopez M, et al: Angiotensin I–converting enzyme in human circulating mononuclear cells: genetic polymorphism of expression in T-lymphocytes. Biochem J 290:33, 1993

26. Ruiz-Ortega M, Lorenzo O, Egido J: Angiotensin III increases MCP-1 and activates NF-kappaB and AP-1 in cultured mesangial and mononuclear cells. Kidney Int 57:2285, 2000

27. Pope JC 4th, Brock JW 3rd, Adams MC, et al: How they begin and how they end: classic and new theories for the development and deterioration of congenital anomalies of the kidney and urinary tract, CAKUT. J Am Soc Nephrol 10:2018, 1999

28. Reynes J, Portales P, Segondy M, et al: CD4 T cell surface CCR5 density as a host factor in HIV-1 disease progression. AIDS 15:1627, 2001

29. Tang J, Shelton B, Makhatadze NJ, et al: Distribution of chemokine receptor CCR2 and CCR5 genotypes and their relative contribution to human immunodeficiency virus type 1 (HIV-1) seroconversion, early HIV-1 RNA concentration in plasma, and later disease progression. J Virol 76:662, 2002

30. Mitchell TJ, Walley AJ, Pease JE, et al: Delta 32 deletion of CCR5 gene and association with asthma or atopy. Lancet 356:1491, 2000

31. Pravica V, Perrey C, Stevens A, et al: A single nucleotide polymorphism in the first intron of the human IFN-gamma gene: absolute correlation with a polymorphic CA microsatellite marker of high IFN-gamma production. Hum Immunol 61:863, 2000

32. Asderakis A, Sankaran D, Dyer P, et al: Association of polymorphisms in the human interferon-gamma and interleukin-10 gene with acute and chronic kidney transplant outcome: the cytokine effect on transplantation. Transplantation 71:674, 2001

33. Cavet J, Dickinson AM, Norden J, et al: Interferon-gamma and interleukin-6 gene polymorphisms associate with graft-versus-host disease in HLA-matched sibling bone marrow transplantation. Blood 98:1594, 2001

34. Pravica VP, Borreiro LF, Hutchinson IV: Genetic regulation of interferon-gamma production. Biochem Soc Trans 25:176S, 1997

35. Agarwal P, Oldenburg MC, Czarneski JE, et al: Comparison study for identifying promoter allelic polymorphism in interleukin 10 and tumor necrosis factor alpha genes. Diagn Mol Pathol 9:158, 2000

36. Murakozy G, Gaede KI, Ruprecht B, et al: Gene polymorphisms of immunoregulatory cytokines and angiotensin-converting enzyme in Wegener's granulomatosis. J Mol Med 79:665, 2001

37. Cavet J, Middleton PG, Segall M, et al: Recipient tumor necrosis factor-alpha and interleukin-10 gene polymorphisms associate with early mortality and acute graft-versus-host disease severity in HLA-matched sibling bone marrow transplants. Blood 94:3941, 1999

38. Awad MR, Webber S, Boyle G, et al: The effect of cytokine gene polymorphisms on pediatric heart allograft outcome. J Heart Lung Transplant 20:625, 2001

39. Pelletier R, Pravica V, Perrey C, et al: Evidence for a genetic predisposition towards acute rejection after kidney and simultaneous kidney-pancreas transplantation. Transplantation 70:674, 2000

40. Sankaran D, Asderakis A, Ashraf S, et al: Cytokine gene polymorphisms predict acute graft rejection following renal transplantation. Kidney Int 56:281, 1999

41. Poole KL, Gibbs PJ, Evans PR, et al: Influence of patient and donor cytokine genotypes on renal allograft rejection: evidence from a single centre study. Transpl Immunol 8:259, 2001

42. Awad MR, El-Gamel A, Hasleton P, et al: Genotypic variation in the transforming growth factor-beta1 gene: association with transforming growth factor-beta1 production, fibrotic lung disease, and graft fibrosis after lung transplantation. Transplantation 66:1014, 1998

43. Shahbazi M, Fryer AA, Pravica V, et al: Vascular endothelial growth factor gene polymorphisms are associated with acute renal allograft rejection. J Am Soc Nephrol 13:260, 2002

44. Linden GJ, Haworth SE, Maxwell AP, et al: The influence of transforming growth factor-beta1 gene polymorphisms on the severity of gingival overgrowth associated with concomitant use of cyclosporin A and a calcium channel blocker. J Periodontol 72:808, 2001

45. Densem CG, Hutchinson IV, Cooper A, et al: Polymorphism of the transforming growth factor-beta 1 gene correlates with the development of coronary vasculopathy following cardiac transplantation. J Heart Lung Transplant 19:551, 2000

46. Baan CC, Balk AH, Holweg CT, et al: Renal failure after clinical heart transplantation is associated with the TGF-beta 1 codon 10 gene polymorphism. J Heart Lung Transplant 19:866, 2000

47. Holweg CT, Baan CC, Niesters HG, et al: TGF-beta1 gene polymorphisms in patients with end-stage heart failure. J Heart Lung Transplant 20:979, 2001

48. Poli F, Boschiero L, Giannoni F, et al: Tumour necrosis factor-alpha gene polymorphism: implications in kidney transplantation. Cytokine 12:1778, 2000

49. Hahn AB, Kasten-Jolly JC, Constantino DM, et al: TNF-alpha, IL-6, IFN-gamma, and IL-10 gene expression polymorphisms and the IL-4 receptor alpha-chain variant Q576R: effects on renal allograft outcome. Transplantation 72:660, 2001

50. Bathgate AJ, Pravica V, Perrey C, et al: Polymorphisms in tumour necrosis factor alpha, interleukin-10 and transforming growth factor beta1 genes and end-stage liver disease. Eur J Gastroenterol Hepatol 12:1329, 2000

51. Azzawi M, Hasleton PS, Turner DM, et al: Tumor necrosis factor-alpha gene polymorphism and death due to acute cellular rejection in a subgroup of heart transplant recipients. Hum Immunol 62:140, 2001

52. Rosen HR, Lentz JJ, Rose SL, et al: Donor polymorphism of tumor necrosis factor gene: relationship with variable severity of hepatitis C recurrence after liver transplantation. Transplantation 68:1898, 1999

53. Abdallah AN, Cucchi-Mouillot P, Biteau N, et al: Analysis of the polymorphism of the tumour necrosis factor (TNF) gene and promoter and of circulating TNF-alpha levels in heart-transplant patients suffering or not suffering from severe rejection. Eur J Immunogenet 26:249, 1999

54. Bathgate AJ, Pravica V, Perrey C, et al: The effect of polymorphisms in tumor necrosis factor-alpha, interleukin-10, and transforming growth factor-beta1 genes in acute hepatic allograft rejection. Transplantation 69:1514, 2000

55. Turner D, Grant SC, Yonan N, et al: Cytokine gene polymorphism and heart transplant rejection. Transplantation 64:776, 1997

56. Asano H, Kobayashi T, Uchida K, et al: Significance of tumor necrosis factor microsatellite polymorphism in renal transplantation. Tissue Antigens 50:484, 1997

57. Middleton PG, Taylor PR, Jackson G, et al: Cytokine gene polymorphisms associating with severe acute graft-versus-host disease in HLA-identical sibling transplants. Blood 92:3943, 1998

58. Sahoo S, Kang S, Supran S, et al: Tumor necrosis factor genetic polymorphisms correlate with infections after renal transplantation. Transplantation 69:880, 2000

59. Densem CG, Hutchinson IV, Yonan N, et al: Tumour necrosis factor alpha gene polymorphism: a predisposing factor to non-ischaemic myocardial dysfunction? Heart 87:153, 2002

60. Filler G, Yang F, Martin A, et al: Renin angiotensin system gene polymorphisms in pediatric renal transplant recipients. Pediatr Transplant 5:166, 2001

61. Juckett MB, Cohen EP, Keever-Taylor CA, et al: Loss of renal function following bone marrow transplantation: an analysis of angiotensin converting enzyme D/I polymorphism and other clinical risk factors. Bone Marrow Transplant 27:451, 2001

62. Viklicky O, Hubacek JA, Pitha J, et al: ACE gene polymorphism and long-term renal graft function. Clin Biochem 34:87, 2001

63. Pethig K, Heublein B, Hoffmann A, et al: ACE-gene polymorphism is associated with the development of allograft vascular disease in heart transplant recipients. J Heart Lung Transplant 19:1175, 2000

64. Barocci S, Ginevri F, Valente U, et al: Correlation between angiotensin-converting enzyme gene insertion/deletion polymorphism and kidney graft long-term outcome in pediatric recipients: a single-center analysis. Transplantation 67:534, 1999

65. Broekroelofs J, Stegeman CA, Navis G, et al: Risk factors for long-term renal survival after renal transplantation: a role for angiotensin-converting enzyme (insertion/deletion) polymorphism? J Am Soc Nephrol 9:2075, 1998

66. Pullmann R Jr, Lukac J, Skerenova M, et al: Association between systemic lupus erythematosus and insertion/deletion polymorphism of the angiotensin converting enzyme (ACE) gene. Clin Exp Rheumatol 17:593, 1999

67. Constantinescu CS, Goodman DB, Ventura ES: Captopril and lisinopril suppress production of interleukin-12 by human peripheral blood mononuclear cells. Immunol Lett 62:25, 1998

68. Poch E, Gonzalez D, Giner V, et al: Molecular basis of salt sensitivity in human hypertension: evaluation of renin-angiotensin-aldosterone system gene polymorphisms. Hypertension 38:1204, 2001

69. Abdi R, Tran TB, Zee R, et al: Angiotensin gene polymorphism as a determinant of posttransplantation renal dysfunction and hypertension. Transplantation 72:726, 2001

70. Kranzhofer R, Browatzki M, Schmidt J, et al: Angiotensin II activates the proinflammatory transcription factor nuclear factor-kappaB in human monocytes. Biochem Biophys Res Commun 257:826, 1999

71. Segerer S, Cui Y, Eitner F, et al: Expression of chemokines and chemokine receptors during human renal transplant rejection. Am J Kidney Dis 37:518, 2001

72. Melter M, Exeni A, Reinders ME, et al: Expression of the chemokine receptor CXCR3 and its ligand IP-10 during human cardiac allograft rejection. Circulation 104:2558, 2001

Acknowledgment

Figures 1 through 5   Seward Hung.

103 Deficiencies in Immunoglobulins and Cell-Mediated Immunity

Fred S. Rosen, M.D.

Immunoglobulin Deficiency Syndromes

Insufficient production of one or more kinds of antibodies characterizes the immunoglobulin deficiency syndromes [*see Table 1*].[1,2] Patients with these deficiencies are subject to recurrent pyogenic infections, such as otitis media, sinusitis, and pneumonia. Repeated episodes of pneumonia can lead to chronic obstructive pulmonary disease. For many of these deficiencies, the genetic basis has now been defined. The primary care physician's role in these disorders is to suspect the diagnosis under the appropriate clinical circumstances—often, unusual susceptibility to certain infections in a patient with a family history of the same—and to order the preliminary laboratory studies. Definitive diagnosis and management is typically the responsibility of the immunologist. Control of the infections to which these patients are susceptible is principally managed by the intravenous administration of large doses of γ-globulin.

X-LINKED AGAMMAGLOBULINEMIA

X-linked agammaglobulinemia, also known as congenital agammaglobulinemia or Bruton disease, was the first immunodeficiency disorder to be described, in 1952.

Genetics and Pathogenesis

The gene responsible for X-linked agammaglobulinemia is located on the long arm of the X chromosome (Xq21.33–q22).[3-5] This gene, termed *btk*, is a member of the *src* family of oncogenes and encodes a unique tyrosine kinase.[4-8] It probably plays a critical role in the maturation of B cells: pre–B cells are present in normal numbers in the bone marrow of males with X-linked agammaglobulinemia, but they do not develop into mature B cells.[2] Because the genes governing the structure of immunoglobulins are on autosomal chromosomes, the mechanism of the disorder must also involve a defect in a regulatory gene.

In patients with X-linked agammaglobulinemia, the lymphoid organs are characterized by a lack of germinal follicles, B cells, and plasma cells. On bone marrow studies, pre–B cells (which contain immunoglobulin μ heavy chains in their cytoplasm and therefore can be identified by immunofluorescence staining with antiserum to the μ chain) are present in normal numbers.

Diagnosis

Clinical manifestations Because infants are born with IgG from their mother in their blood, boys who have X-linked agammaglobulinemia do not start to show the effects of the disorder

Table 1 Primary Specific Immunodeficiencies Involving Antibodies

Designation	Usual Phenotypic Expression		Presumed Level of Basic Cellular Defect	Known or Presumed Pathogenetic Mechanism	Inheritance
	Antibody Deficiencies	Cellular Abnormalities			
X-linked agammaglobulinemia	All immunoglobulins	↓ B cells	Pre–B cells	Mutations in the gene for Bruton's X-linked tyrosinase (*btk*)	X-linked
Common variable immunodeficiency	All immunoglobulins	Faulty B cell maturation	Immaturity of B cells	↓ Helper T cell function Intrinsic B cell defect Underproduction of B cells Autoantibodies to B cells	Unknown
Selective IgA deficiency	IgA	↓ IgA plasma cells ± ↑ IgA⁺ B cells	Terminal differentiation of IgA⁺ B cells impaired	Unknown	Usually unknown (autosomal recessive more common than autosomal dominant); frequent in families of patients with common variable immunodeficiency
Ig deficiencies, with increased IgM	IgG, IgA, and IgE	↓ IgG and IgA plasma cells ↑ IgM and IgD plasma cells ± ↑ IgM⁺ B cells	Failure of immunoglobulin class switching	X-linked form: mutations in the gene for the CD40 ligand Autosomal recessive form: activation-induced cytidine deaminase	X-linked, autosomal recessive, or unknown
Selective deficiency of IgG subclasses	One or more IgG isotypes	↓ Plasma cells ± ↓ T cells	Unknown	Unknown	Unknown
κ-Chain deficiency	IgG(κ)	↓ κ⁺ B cells	Unknown	Point mutation at 2p11	Autosomal recessive
Transient hypogammaglobulinemia of infancy	IgG and IgA	↓ Plasma cells B cells normal	Impaired terminal differentiation of B cells	↓ Helper T cells	Frequent in heterozygous individuals in families with various severe combined immunodeficiencies

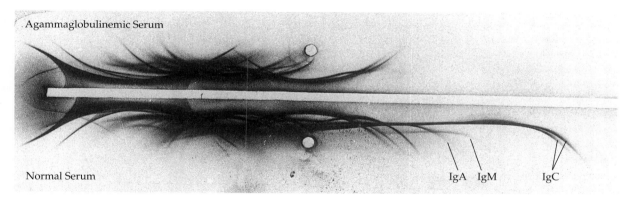

Figure 1 **When an immunoelectrophoretic pattern of agammaglobulinemic serum is compared with a normal serum pattern, the absence of IgA, IgM, and IgG—characteristic of the disorder—is clearly demonstrated.**

until 6 to 15 months of age. They then demonstrate unusual susceptibility to infections by pyogenic organisms (e.g., otitis media, sinusitis, and pneumonia from *Haemophilus influenzae*, pneumococci, streptococci, staphylococci, and meningococci). Those infections are more frequent and more severe in boys with X-linked agammaglobulinemia than in normal children, and recurrent infection by the same organism is common. Frequently, the infections are slow to respond to antibiotics. Recurrent pulmonary infections often lead to bronchiectasis and pulmonary insufficiency. Affected males have normal resistance to the common viral diseases, fungi, and most gram-negative organisms, but some have developed polio after receiving oral polio vaccine. About one third of patients have symptoms that resemble rheumatoid arthritis, including swollen and painful joints. A severe late complication is a fatal syndrome similar to dermatomyositis but with central neurologic involvement, as well. This syndrome is gradual in onset, usually starting in the second or third decade of life. In several patients with this syndrome, echoviruses have been cultured from the blood, stool, and cerebrospinal fluid.[9]

Laboratory testing Diagnosis begins with measuring the serum level of each class of immunoglobulin [*see Figure 1*]. Patients with X-linked agammaglobulinemia usually have less than 100 mg/dl of IgG (normal levels are 614 to 1,295 mg/dl), and they have levels of IgA, IgM, IgD, and IgE that are extremely low or undetectable. Such findings should prompt referral of the patient to an immunologist.

In patients with X-linked agammaglobulinemia, analysis of white blood cells by flow cytometry reveals a lack of B cells. These patients are unable to mount an antibody response to antigen challenge, such as routine diphtheria-pertussis-tetanus (DPT) or *H. influenzae* vaccination, and they cannot neutralize the toxin in a Schick test (intradermal injection of diphtheria toxin). In contrast, cell-mediated immune functions, such as delayed hypersensitivity–mediated skin reactions and graft rejection, are essentially normal, and the T cells respond in vitro to phytohemagglutinin and produce lymphokines normally.

Screening All subsequent male offspring of the mother or maternal aunts of a patient with X-linked agammaglobulinemia should be screened for mutations of the *btk* gene. Because the defect is limited to B cells, female carriers of the gene can be detected by analysis of X-chromosome inactivation in B cells.[10,11] In female carriers, pre–B cells in which the X chromosome bearing

the normal gene has been inactivated will not develop into B cells; therefore, all mature B cells will bear an active X chromosome containing only the normal gene.

Treatment

Preparations of 5% or 10% γ-globulin solution are now used as replacement therapy for agammaglobulinemia. Parents can be reassured that these preparations pose no risk of transmitting HIV or other viral infection. Intravenous administration of these preparations is well tolerated; large doses can be given without discomfort or pain. Infants do not require permanent intravenous access.

Dosages of γ-globulin are adjusted according to the patient's health. The minimal effective dosage of intravenous γ-globulin is 300 mg/kg a month; however, higher doses, such as 500 mg/kg a month, are usually optimal.[12] Dividing the monthly dosage of γ-globulin and administering it at 1-week or 2-week intervals is preferable, because it maintains higher immunoglobulin levels. The γ-globulin is infused at a rate of 3 ml/min or slower. Side effects may include headache, shaking chills, flank pain, fever, and hypotension. These can be ameliorated by giving an antihistamine or methylprednisolone before the infusion.

Bacterial infections in patients with X-linked agammaglobulinemia require vigorous antibiotic treatment. Antibiotics should be given in prolonged courses (e.g., 2 weeks) at full doses.

Prognosis The prognosis is very good for patients whose condition is diagnosed and treated early. A recent study of 31 patients with X-linked agammaglobulinemia found that early and prolonged γ-globulin replacement therapy is effective in preventing bacterial infections and pulmonary insufficiency. Viral infections still developed, however, and one patient died of enteroviral meningoencephalopathy.[13]

COMMON VARIABLE IMMUNODEFICIENCY

Common variable immunodeficiency (CVID) is so called because it accounts for over 50% of cases of immunodeficiency and because patients present with variable clinical manifestations and somewhat inconsistent laboratory findings; disease course varies, as well.

Etiology and Pathogenesis

The cause of CVID is unknown. CVID does not appear to be genetically transmitted—apparently the germ cells are not involved—although some family clusters have been seen. CVID affects males and females equally.

A variety of pathogenetic mechanisms underlie CVID.[2] These include (1) B cells that do not respond to stimulatory signals from T cells, (2) B cells that can synthesize but cannot secrete immunoglobulins, (3) the absence of helper T cells (required for normal B cell function), and (4) the presence of autoantibodies to B cells. In a few cases of CVID, B cells cannot be detected. All patients show markedly low serum levels of all immunoglobulins.

Diagnosis

Clinical manifestations Onset of CVID can occur at any age, but it usually occurs after puberty. Patients have the same heightened vulnerability to infections as those with X-linked agammaglobulinemia; also, there is chronic involvement of the sinuses and respiratory tract.

CVID is associated with several autoimmune diseases, such as rheumatoid arthritis, idiopathic thrombocytopenia, hemolytic anemia, neutropenia, and, predominantly, pernicious anemia. Infectious diarrhea and malabsorption syndrome are common. CVID is also associated with severe malabsorption syndrome caused by gluten-sensitive enteropathy. It is unclear whether CVID is a cause or an effect of these disorders. Chronic lung disease that produces bronchiectasis is common in CVID; this condition should be differentiated from cystic fibrosis, chronic allergy, and α_1-antitrypsin deficiency. In contrast to X-linked agammaglobulinemia, CVID is often marked by considerable enlargement of regional lymph nodes and splenomegaly.

Laboratory tests IgG levels in patients with CVID are generally lower than 250 mg/dl, and other immunoglobulins are also markedly decreased. B cells are usually present, but they do not mature normally into plasma cells, which synthesize and secrete immunoglobulins. Tests of cell-mediated immunity also demonstrate defects.

Lymphoid hyperplasia may occur in the gut of patients with CVID. This can be visualized by barium contrast x-ray of the upper GI tract, which is indicated in CVID patients with GI symptoms.

Treatment

Treatment of CVID is essentially the same as that of X-linked agammaglobulinemia: replacement γ-globulin therapy and vigorous use of antibiotics during acute infections. Diarrhea in these patients is frequently caused by *Giardia lamblia* infection, which can be rapidly controlled with quinacrine hydrochloride or metronidazole.[11] Special care must be taken if steroids are used as therapy for the associated autoimmune diseases, because these agents may heighten susceptibility to infection.

Prognosis

Patients with CVID can have a normal life span. Women with the disease can carry a normal pregnancy to term and have normal babies. Although those babies will lack maternal IgG and the passive immunity it confers in the first months of life, they do well without treatment with γ-globulin.

SELECTIVE IMMUNOGLOBULIN DEFICIENCIES

Selective IgA Deficiency

Epidemiology Selective IgA deficiency is one of the most common immunodeficiencies in whites, occurring in one in 600

to 800 persons in this population. It does not occur in Africans and almost never occurs in Asians.

Genetics and pathogenesis The genetics of IgA deficiency are unclear. Data on inheritance are conflicting, with some suggesting autosomal dominant inheritance and others suggesting autosomal recessive inheritance.

A few patients lacking serum IgA have secretory IgA, and some patients have monomeric IgM in their secretions. B cells bearing surface IgA are present, indicating that the defect is probably in the terminal differentiation of IgA-secreting cells. In vitro, IgA-bearing cells can be stimulated by mitogens to produce IgA.[14]

Diagnosis Many patients with IgA deficiency are surprisingly healthy. Nevertheless, IgA deficiency is associated with many clinical syndromes. Patients most often come to medical attention because of recurrent sinus and pulmonary infection by bacteria and viruses. These patients also show a higher incidence of autoimmune, GI, allergic, connective tissue, and malignant diseases. Some patients with IgA deficiency produce antibodies to bovine proteins, suggesting that IgA in the gut normally helps prevent absorption of foreign antigens. IgA deficiency is found in about 70% of patients with ataxia-telangiectasia (see below).

The serum IgA level is less than 5 mg/dl (normal, 60 to 309 mg/dl). Other immunoglobulin levels are normal. Although patients with IgA deficiency usually also have defects in T cell function, most of these patients have normal cell-mediated immunity.

Treatment There is currently no satisfactory means of supplying adequate levels of IgA. Sinus and pulmonary infections in IgA-deficient patients are treated by standard means.

Complications In extremely rare instances, patients with IgA deficiency produce IgE antibodies to IgA and will have anaphylactic reactions when given immunoglobulin.[15] Immunoglobulin replacement therapy should be avoided in such patients; blood transfusion can also precipitate an anaphylactic reaction. Patients who require blood should receive red cells from an IgA-deficient donor because anaphylactic reactions may occur even if the red blood cells are washed three times.

Immunoglobulin Deficiency with Elevated IgM

The combination of markedly elevated IgM levels and deficiency of other immunoglobulins is termed the hyper-IgM syndrome. The IgM in these patients is heterogeneous; thus, it is polyclonal and does not emerge from malignant cells.

In 70% of hyper-IgM cases, the syndrome is X-linked; in the remainder, it is autosomal recessive and affects both males and females. The X-linked form of the hyper-IgM syndrome results from a genetic defect in the CD40 ligand, which is found on the surface of activated T cells.[16-18] Normally, this ligand interacts with the CD40 molecule on the B cell surface, inducing isotype switching. The autosomal recessive form of the hyper-IgM syndrome results from a genetic defect in an enzyme called activation-induced cytidine deaminase (AID).[19] This enzyme is involved in RNA editing, but its precise role in immunoglobulin class switching is unknown.

Diagnosis Patients with hyper-IgM syndrome show increased susceptibility to infection similar to that seen in X-linked agammaglobulinemia (see above). Immunoglobulin assays show an elevated level of IgM (350 to 1,000 mg/dl); the IgD level may also be elevated. IgA is usually undetectable, and the IgG level is normally less than 100 mg/dl. Many plasma cells, as well as lymphocytoid and plasmacytoid cells structurally similar to those of Waldenström macroglobulinemia, are seen in the gut, lymphoid organs, and blood. These plasma cells stain with fluorescein-labeled antibodies to IgM. In the X-linked form of hyper-IgM syndrome, lymph nodes are small and contain no germinal centers. In AID deficiency, lymph nodes are enlarged and contain germinal centers. Lymph node biopsy is not usually obtained for clinical diagnosis, however.

Treatment Treatment for hyper-IgM syndrome is the same as that for X-linked agammaglobulinemia (see above).

Selective Deficiencies of IgM or the Subclasses of IgG

Selective IgM deficiency is rare. This deficiency may precede the onset of CVID. Patients with selective deficiencies of the IgG subclasses have a decrease in total IgG, the degree of which depends on the subclass involved. The decrease is most profound in the case of IgG1 deficiency because almost three quarters of IgG molecules belong to this subclass. Some patients with IgG deficiency are unable to mount an antibody response to certain antigens. Patients with IgG2 deficiency are especially prone to infection by bacteria with a large amount of surface polysaccharide, such as pneumococci and *H. influenzae*. The diagnosis is confirmed by quantitation of the IgG subclasses and administration of a polysaccharide-antigen vaccine (typically, pneumococcal vaccine); patients with IgG deficiency will fail to produce antibodies in response to vaccination. Patients with selective deficiencies of the IgG subclasses respond to intravenously administered γ-globulin.

Deficiencies of Cell-Mediated Immunity

Extreme susceptibility to opportunistic infection is the most important clinical feature of deficiencies of cell-mediated immunity, or T cell deficiencies. Such deficiencies, which manifest as impairment in delayed hypersensitivity, may be inherited or may be secondary to another disorder [*see Table 2*]. The ac-

---

Table 2 Conditions Associated with Impaired Delayed Hypersensitivity

Primary deficiencies of cell-mediated immunity [*see Table 3*]

Chromosomal abnormalities: Bloom syndrome, Down syndrome, Fanconi syndrome

Infections: HIV (AIDS), lepromatous leprosy, Epstein-Barr virus (X-linked lymphoproliferative syndrome), chronic mucocutaneous candidiasis, secondary syphilis, and many other viral and parasitic diseases

Neoplasms: thymoma, Hodgkin disease and other lymphomas, any advanced malignant disease

Connective tissue diseases: systemic lupus erythematosus, advanced rheumatoid arthritis

Physical agents: burns, x-irradiation

Other conditions: sarcoidosis, malnutrition, aging, inflammatory bowel disease, intestinal lymphangiectasia

Iatrogenic causes: chemotherapy, postsurgery, x-irradiation therapy

---

quired immunodeficiency syndrome is discussed elsewhere [*see Chapter 133*].

In general, patients with T cell deficiencies have more frequent and more severe infections than do patients who have pure B cell deficiencies [*see Table 3*].[2] Patients with deficiencies of cell-mediated immunity cannot cope with a number of ordinarily innocuous organisms, such as *Candida albicans* and *Pneumocystis carinii*, and are especially susceptible to enteric bacteria, viruses, and fungi. Live attenuated vaccines are dangerous in these patients: vaccination for smallpox or administration of bacillus Calmette-Guérin (BCG) has led to rapid death.

Determining the defects of cell-mediated immunity requires testing in a specialized immunology laboratory. An extensive array of tests is available at such laboratories [*see Table 4*]. The choice of tests and the order in which they are performed depend on the particular case.

CONGENITAL THYMIC HYPOPLASIA

Pathogenesis

Congenital thymic hypoplasia (DiGeorge syndrome) results from the lack of normal development of the third and fourth brachial, or pharyngeal, pouches, which leads to abnormality in the great vessels and to the absence of the thymus and the parathyroids. Congenital thymic hypoplasia is not inherited; rather, it is thought to result from an intrauterine accident occurring before the eighth week of pregnancy. The absence of the thymus leads to deficiency in cell-mediated immunity.

Diagnosis

Clinical manifestations Patients with congenital thymic hypoplasia have distinctive facial features, including low-set ears, a shortened philtrum, and ocular hypertelorism. Hypocalcemia from associated parathyroid deficiency is a universal finding and often results in neonatal tetany. There can be a right-sided aortic arch or tetralogy of Fallot or many other cardiac malformations.

Laboratory tests The T cell defect in children with congenital thymic hypoplasia varies from mild to profound. Severely affected children do not exhibit delayed hypersensitivity reactions; their lymphocytes do not respond to mitogens or antigens in vitro, nor do they produce lymphokines. The lymph nodes lack paracortical lymphocytes. Plasma cells are present, however, and immunoglobulin levels are normal. Although patients with congenital thymic hypoplasia produce specific antibodies when they are immunized with various antigens, the antibody response is not quite normal, because secondary responses are lacking.

As the patient ages, T cell function improves; and usually by the time the child is 5 years of age, skin testing reveals no abnormality in cell-mediated immunity. However, the abnormal T cell phenotype—as indicated by a higher than normal ratio of CD4[+] to CD8[+] T cells—persists for life. Karyotyping reveals microdeletions at chromosome 22q11 in approximately 90% of patients.

Treatment

Thymus transplantation should be undertaken in those infants with congenital thymic hypoplasia who experience frequent infections. Transplantation of fetal thymus results in rapid acquisition of normal T cell function, which is thought to be secondary to production of a thymic hormone secreted by the thymic epithelium. Rejection appears not to be a problem.

Table 3   Classification of Primary Specific Immunodeficiencies Involving Cell-Mediated Immunity

Designation	Usual Phenotypic Expression		Presumed Level of Basic Cellular Defect	Known or Presumed Pathogenetic Mechanism	Inheritance	Main Associated Features
	Functional Deficiencies	Cellular Abnormalities				
Congenital thymic hypoplasia (DiGeorge syndrome)	CMI, impaired antibody	↓ T cells	Thymocytes	Embryopathy of third and fourth pharyngeal pouch areas	Usually not familial	Hypoparathyroidism Abnormal facies Cardiovascular abnormalities
Severe combined immunodeficiency	CMI, antibody	- T cells, + B cells	LSC	Mutation in γ chain of IL-2R, IL-4R, IL-7R, IL-11R, IL-15R, *JAK3*, or IL-7 receptor α chain	X-linked or autosomal recessive	—
		- T cells, - B cells		Mutation in *RAG1* or *RAG2*	Autosomal recessive	
Adenosine deaminase (ADA) deficiency	CMI, antibody	↓ T cells, ± B cells	LSC or early T cells	Metabolic effects of ADA deficiency	Autosomal recessive	—
Purine nucleoside phosphorylase (PNP) deficiency	CMI ± antibody	↓ T cells	T cells	Metabolic effects of PNP deficiency	Autosomal recessive	Hypoplastic anemia
Reticular dysgenesis	CMI, antibody, phagocytes	↓ T cells, ↓ B cells, ↓ phagocytes	HSC	Unknown	Autosomal recessive	Neutropenia
Wiskott-Aldrich syndrome	Antibody to certain antigens (mainly polysaccharides), CMI (progressive)	↓ T cells, ↑ B cells (progressive)	HSC	Mutations in *WASP* gene	X-linked	Thrombocytopenia Eczema Lymphoreticular cancers
Immunodeficiency with ataxia-telangiectasia	CMI, antibody (partial)	↓ T cells, ↓ plasma cells (mainly those cells producing IgA, IgE, ± IgG)	Defective check-points in T and B cell division	Mutations in *ATM* gene	Autosomal recessive	Cerebellar ataxia Telangiectasia Chromosomal abnormalities Raised serum α-feto-protein levels
MHC class II deficiency	CMI ± antibody	None	T cells, B cells, and antigen-presenting cells	Defects of promoter proteins	Autosomal recessive	Intestinal malabsorption
CD3 deficiency	CMI	None	T cells	Mutations in CD3-ε or CD3-γ	Autosomal recessive	—
CD8 deficiency	CMI	↓ CD8⁺ T cells, normal number of CD4⁺ cells	Early T cells	Mutations in *ZAP* genes	Autosomal recessive	—

CMI—cell-mediated immunity   HSC—hematopoietic stem cell   LSC—lymphocytic stem cell

SEVERE COMBINED IMMUNODEFICIENCY

Severe combined immunodeficiency disease (SCID) is characterized by marked depletion of cells that mediate both humoral and cellular immunity—B cells and T cells, respectively. SCID is fatal if left untreated.

Several variants of SCID have been identified. They are designated as T⁻B⁻ or T⁻B⁺, depending on whether B cells are normal or increased (B⁺) or absent (B⁻). In addition to the extent of B cell involvement, the variants also differ in the site of the basic cellular defect, the pathogenetic mechanism, and the mode of inheritance [*see* Table 3].

Genetics and Pathogenesis

T⁻B⁺ SCID may be transmitted as either an X-linked or an autosomal recessive trait. The specific genetic defect responsible for the X-linked form of T⁻B⁺ SCID results from mutations in the γ chain of the interleukin-2 receptor (IL-2R),[20] whose gene is localized to the long arm of the X chromosome at Xq13.[21] This γ chain is also found in the receptors for IL-4, IL-7, IL-11, and IL-15.[22] Engagement of the IL-7 receptor by IL-7 is required for T cell maturation, so precursor T cells in these patients do not mature.

When any of those receptors, or IL-2R, are engaged by its ligands, a cytoplasmic tyrosine kinase (Janus-family tyrosine kinase, or JAK3) bound to the γ chain is activated. The gene encoding JAK3 is on an autosome, not the X chromosome. Thus, autosomal recessive T⁻B⁺ SCID is caused by mutations in the *JAK3* gene.[23,24]

T⁻B⁻ SCID is inherited in an autosomal recessive manner. About half of the cases are caused by a deficiency in the enzyme adenosine deaminase (ADA),[25] and another large fraction results from mutations in the recombination-activating genes *RAG-1* and *RAG-2*.[26] These recombinase enzymes are required for the gene rearrangements that occur before T cell receptor or immunoglobulin synthesis. Other patients with autosomal recessive T⁻B⁻ SCID lack the enzyme purine nucleoside phosphorylase (PNP).[27]

ADA deficiency leads to an accumulation of adenosine, adenosine triphosphate (ATP), and deoxy-ATP (dATP). It has

Table 4 Laboratory Tests Used to Determine Deficiencies of Cell-Mediated Immunity

Skin test: 24- to 48-hr reaction to *Candida, Trichophyton*, PPD

Response to nonspecific mitogens: phytohemagglutinin, concanavalin A, pokeweed mitogen

Response to specific mitogens: diphtheria, tetanus, *Candida*

Response to alloantigens: mixed lymphocyte reaction

When responses to alloantigens and nonspecific and specific mitogens are negative: repeat tests while stimulating cells with IL-2

Enumerate T cells with monoclonal antibody to CD3, with or without a cell sorter

Enumerate T cell subsets with monoclonal antibody to CD4 for helper T cells and with monoclonal antibody to CD8

Enumerate T cells positive for Ia (class II) antigens (which measures the number of activated T cells)

Quantitate IL-2 receptors with monoclonal antibody TAC

Quantitate IL-2 and interferon-gamma synthesis

Enumerate NK cells with monoclonal antibodies Leu-7 and Leu-11

Assay NK cell activity using cell line K-562

Assay cytotoxic T cell activity using cell lines of cloned T cells

Enumerate monocytes with monoclonal antibody Mo-1

Assay for IL-1 production by stimulated monocytes

Determine serum level of anti–T cell antibodies

Determine if antibody to HIV is present

HLA typing

Assay erythrocytes for adenosine deaminase and purine nucleoside phosphorylase activity

Detect thymus shadow on x-ray

Note: All patients with defects in cell-mediated immunity should receive all tests listed, except the last three, for optimal examination. The last three tests are for patients suspected of having severe combined immunodeficiency or congenital thymic hypoplasia. HLA typing is needed for prospective recipients of bone marrow transplants.
IL-1—interleukin-1 IL-2—interleukin-2 NK—natural killer
PPD—purified protein derivative of tuberculin

been shown that dATP poisons ribonucleotide reductase, an enzyme required for DNA synthesis. Thus, lymphocytes lacking ADA cannot divide until the dATP overload is decreased or removed. In a similar manner, lymphocytes that lack PNP accumulate guanosine, guanosine triphosphate (GTP), and deoxy-GTP, causing metabolic abnormalities that resemble those seen in ADA deficiency. SCID caused by ADA or PNP deficiency can be diagnosed prenatally by amniocentesis because fibroblasts in the amniotic fluid also show the enzymatic defect.

CD8 deficiency is a rare form of SCID that results from mutations in the *ZAP-70* gene.[28,29] ZAP-70 is a tyrosine kinase that binds to the CD3 chain and is involved in signal transduction from the T cell receptor (the TCR-CD3 complex). CD8+ T cells fail to mature, and mature CD4+ T cells fail to function as a result of the mutations in *ZAP-70*.

Another variant of SCID is reticular dysgenesis, a severe combined immunodeficiency with a generalized granulocyte deficiency. Newborns with this disease lack granulocytes in the blood and bone marrow and die of infection within the first few days of life.

Diagnosis

Clinical manifestations Chronic pulmonary infections, diarrhea, moniliasis, and failure to thrive are the most common manifestations of SCID. The lymph nodes are small to absent despite chronic infections, which usually begin at 3 to 6 months of age.

Laboratory tests Complete blood counts show a low number

of lymphocytes. There is absence of a thymic shadow on chest x-ray. (Autopsy in fatal cases has revealed an embryonic thymus that resembles the thymus at 6 weeks of gestation, before invasion with lymphocytes.) Tests for cutaneous delayed hypersensitivity and contact sensitization and in vitro assays of blood lymphocytes are negative, demonstrating the absence of T cells, a phytohemagglutinin response, and lymphokine production. Antibody levels are usually low, although occasionally the IgM level is normal; and sometimes, a myeloma component is seen.

Treatment

Hundreds of cases of SCID have been successfully treated by transplantation of bone marrow cells.[30] By 3 to 8 months after receiving the bone marrow, these patients show normal delayed hypersensitivity and T cell function and are no longer abnormally susceptible to infection.

Immunologic reconstitution with bone marrow cells should be attempted only in specialized centers where comprehensive histocompatibility typing and intensive 24-hour care can be given. If the donor and the recipient are not exceedingly well matched, fatal graft versus host disease (GVHD) will ensue. Even an HLA-mismatched blood transfusion can produce fatal GVHD in such patients: the patient is immunocompromised and thus cannot reject the injected cells, but the histoincompatible cells that have been administered recognize the patient's cells as foreign and react against them.

The manifestations of GVHD include fever, diarrhea, depression of the bone marrow, splenomegaly, and an erythematous rash on the face, trunk, and extremities. The reaction eventually leads to death. GVHD can be avoided by irradiating the blood before transfusion.

It is possible to establish grafts of half-matched (haploidentical) parental marrow in infants with SCID. GVHD can be avoided in those cases if the parental marrow is depleted of T cells before transplantation by passage over lectin columns or by treatment with anti–T cell monoclonal antibody plus complement.

Patients with ADA deficiency have also been treated successfully with infusions of purified adenosine deaminase modified with polyethylene glycol. The ADA gene has been cloned and inserted into a retroviral vector.[31] In a few ADA-deficient children, this vector has been transfected into peripheral blood lymphocytes, which were then reinfused. This gene therapy procedure has corrected the immunodeficiency in these patients, although it must be repeated periodically.[32] Successful gene therapy has also been carried out in X-linked SCID by transducing a Maloney virus vector bearing the gene for the common γ chain into bone marrow cells. Sustained responses have been reported in four of these patients: T cell number and function normalized in these patients, as did B cell function, and infusions of γ globulin were no longer required.[33]

WISKOTT-ALDRICH SYNDROME

An X-linked recessive disease, Wiskott-Aldrich syndrome (WAS), results from a mutation that has been mapped to the Xp11.3–p11.22 region of the X chromosome. The *WAS* gene has been cloned.[34,35]

The lymphoid system of a patient with WAS appears anatomically intact at birth. Starting in the first months of life, however, there is a decrease in T cells in the paracortical areas of the lymph nodes and a polyclonal expansion of B cells. The T cells in these patients respond poorly to mitogens. The protein encoded by the *WAS* gene appears to be involved in signal transduction that leads to reorganization of the cytoskeleton when lymphocytes are stimulated, which results in defective collaboration between T cells and B cells. Lymphocytes have a markedly abnormal appearance when visualized by scanning electron microscopy. Platelets are abnormally small and few in number.[36] Certain missense mutations in the *WAS* gene lead to a mild disease called X-linked thrombocytopenia.[37]

Diagnosis

Clinical manifestations WAS is characterized by eczema, easy bruising, increased susceptibility to infection (both pyogenic and opportunistic), and bloody diarrhea. These manifestations appear in the first months of life. An increased incidence of hematopoietic malignancies is seen, starting in the second or third decade of life.

Laboratory testing Patients with WAS have normal levels of IgG, high levels of IgE and IgA, and low levels of IgM. Severe thrombocytopenia is universal. Tests of cell-mediated immunity [*see Table 4*] show a variety of abnormalities: WAS patients lack isohemagglutinins and are unable to make antibodies to polysaccharides. They respond to some protein antigens but not to others; in addition, they may exhibit anergy and may not display positive results to skin tests for the usual bacterial or fungal antigens.

Treatment

WAS patients have been treated with marrow transplantation after receiving irradiation or busulfan and antilymphocyte serum to destroy residual lymphocytes; they have then shown normal immune and platelet functions. In WAS patients who do not receive a bone marrow transplant and who experience severe bleeding from thrombocytopenia, splenectomy may be considerably beneficial.[38]

IMMUNOLOGIC DEFICIENCY WITH ATAXIA-TELANGIECTASIA

Ataxia-telangiectasia (A-T) is a disease associated with defects in cell-mediated immunity and with immunoglobulin deficiencies. It is inherited as an autosomal recessive trait. The gene for A-T (*ATM* for A-T mutated) maps to the chromosomal region 11q22.3.[39,40] Normally, the gene appears to function in repair of breaks in double-stranded DNA. Patients with A-T have a disorder of the cell-cycle checkpoint pathway that results in an extreme hypersensitivity to ionizing radiation. Consequently, frequent chromosomal breaks, inversions, and translocations are observed. Postmortem examination may disclose abnormalities in the thymus, which is small and deficient in lymphocytes. There also may be an abnormality in lymph node structure.

Diagnosis

Clinical manifestations A-T presents as a progressive neurologic disease that begins in early childhood. It is characterized by cerebellar ataxia, starting at 18 months of age, followed by increasing tremor and deterioration of mental function. By 5 years of age, progressive telangiectasia is seen in the vessels of the bulbar conjunctiva and is later visible on the skin. The immune deficiencies in these patients leads to recurrent sinus and bronchial infections and subsequent bronchiectasis. An unusually high incidence of lymphoid malignant disorders has been reported in patients with A-T.[41]

Laboratory testing About 70% of patients with A-T have a severe deficiency in IgA. On tests of cell-mediated immunity [*see Table 4*], some A-T patients are anergic and fail to show delayed hypersensitivity responses to common microbial antigens. They may also have abnormal in vitro cell-mediated immune responses and may tolerate allografts.

Treatment and Prognosis

No satisfactory treatment for A-T is currently available. Persons with A-T who survive into their second decade may fail to mature sexually. A-T patients usually die of lymphoid malignancies or other causes by the end of their second decade.

References

1. Rosen FS, Wedgwood RJ, Eibl M, et al: Primary immunodeficiency diseases: report of a WHO Scientific Group. Clin Exp Immunol 109(suppl 1):1, 1997

2. Rosen FS, Cooper MD, Wedgwood RJP: The primary immunodeficiencies. N Engl J Med 333:431, 1995

3. Kwan SP, Terwilliger J, Parmley R, et al: Identification of a closely linked DNA marker, DXS178, to further refine the X-linked agammaglobulinemia locus. Genomics 6:238, 1990

4. Vetrie D, Vorechovsky I, Sideras P, et al: The gene involved in X-linked agammaglobulinaemia is a member of the src family of protein-tyrosine kinases. Nature 361:226, 1993

5. Tsukada S, Saffran DC, Rawlings DJ, et al: Deficient expression of a B cell cytoplasmic tyrosine kinase in human X-linked agammaglobulinemia. Cell 72:279, 1993

6. Hagemann TL, Chen Y, Rosen FS, et al: Genomic organization of the Btk gene and exon scanning for mutations with X-linked agammaglobulinemia. Hum Mol Genet 3:1743, 1994

7. Zhu Q, Zhang M, Winkelstein J, et al: Unique mutations of Bruton's tyrosine kinase in fourteen unrelated X-linked agammaglobulinemia families. Hum Mol Genet 3:1899, 1994

8. Conley ME, Fitch-Hilgenberg ME, Cleveland GL, et al: Screening of genomic DNA to identify mutations in the gene for tyrosine kinase. Hum Mol Genet 3:1751, 1994

9. Misbah SA: Chronic enteroviral meningoencephalitis in agammaglobulinemia: case report and literature review. J Clin Immunol 12:266, 1992

10. Fearon ER, Winkelstein JA, Civin CI, et al: Carrier detection in X-linked agammaglobulinemia by analysis of X-chromosome inactivation. N Engl J Med 316:427, 1987

11. Conley ME, Brown P, Pickard AR, et al: Expression of the gene defect in X-linked agammaglobulinemia. N Engl J Med 315:564, 1986

12. Buckley RH, Schiff RI: The use of intravenous immune globulin in immunodeficiency diseases. N Engl J Med 325:110, 1991

13. Quartier P, Debre M, De Blic J, et al: Early and prolonged intravenous immunoglobulin replacement therapy in childhood agammaglobulinemia: a retrospective survey of 31 patients. J Pediatr 134:589, 1999

14. Conley ME, Cooper MD: Immature IgA B cells in IgA-deficient patients. N Engl J Med 305:495, 1981

15. Burks AW, Sampson HA, Buckley RH: Anaphylactic reactions after gamma globulin administration in patients with hypogammaglobulinemia: detection of IgE antibodies to IgA. N Engl J Med 314:560, 1986

16. Fuleihan R, Ramesh N, Loh R, et al: Defective expression of the CD40 ligand in X chromosome-linked immunoglobulin deficiency with normal or elevated IgM. Proc Natl Acad Sci USA 90:2170, 1993

17. Korthauer U, Graf D, Mages HW, et al: Defective expression of T-cell CD40 ligand causes X-linked immunodeficiency with hyper-IgM. Nature 361:539, 1993

18. Mayer L, Kwan S-P, Thompson C, et al: Evidence for a defect in "switch" T cells in patients with immunodeficiency and hyperimmunoglobulin M. N Engl J Med 314:409, 1986

19. Revy P, Muto T, Levy Y, et al: Activation-induced deaminase (AID) deficiency causes the autosomal recessive form of the hyper-IgM syndrome (HIGM2). Cell 102:565, 2000

20. Noguchi M, Yi H, Rosenblatt HM, et al: Interleukin 2 receptor γ chain mutation results in X-linked severe combined immunodeficiency in humans. Cell 73:147, 1993

21. Puck JM, Conley ME, Bailey LC: Refinements of linkage of human severe combined immunodeficiency (SCDX1) to polymorphic markers in Xq13. Am J Hum Genet 53:176, 1993

22. Puel A, Ziegler SF, Buckley RH, et al: Defective IL7R expression in T(-)B(+)NK(+) severe combined immunodeficiency. Nat Genet 20:394, 1998

23. Macchi P, Villa A, Gillani S, et al: Mutations of Jak 3 gene in patients with autosomal recessive combined immune deficiency (SCID). Nature 377:65, 1995

24. Russell SM, Tayebi N, Nakajima H, et al: Mutation of Jak3 in a patient with SCID: essential role of Jak3 in lymphoid development. Science 270:797, 1995

25. Hirschhorn R: Adenosine deaminase deficiency. Immunodefic Rev 2:175, 1990

26. Schwarz K, Gauss GH, Ludwig L, et al: RAG mutations in human B cell-negative SCID. Science 274:97, 1996

27. Markert ML: Purine nucleoside phosphorylase deficiency. Immunodef Rev 3:45, 1991

28. Arpaia E, Shahar M, Dadi H, et al: Defective T cell receptor signaling and CD8+ thy-

mocyte selection in humans lacking Zap-70 kinase. Cell 76:947, 1994

29. Chan AC, Kadlecek TA, Elder ME, et al: ZAP-70 deficiency in autosomal recessive form of severe combined immunodeficiency. Science 264:1599, 1994

30. Buckley RH, Schiff RI, Schiff SE, et al: Human severe combined immunodeficiency: genetic, phenotypic, and functional diversity in one hundred eight infants. J Pediatrics 130:378, 1997

31. Williams DA, Lemischka IR, Nathan DG, et al: Introduction of new genetic material into pluripotent hematopoietic stem cells of the mouse. Nature 310:476, 1984

32. Blaese RN, Culver KW, Miller AD, et al: T-lymphocyte-directed gene therapy for ADA deficiency SCID: initial trial results after 4 years. Science 270:470, 1995

33. Hacein-Bey-Abina S, Le Deist F, Carlier F, et al: Sustained correction of X-linked severe combined immunodeficiency by ex vivo gene therapy. N Engl J Med 346:1185, 2002

34. Derry JMJ, Ochs HD, Francke U: Isolation of a novel gene mutated in Wiskott-Aldrich syndrome. Cell 78:635, 1994

35. Kwan S-P, Hagemann T, Radke BE, et al: Identification of mutations in the gene responsible for the Wiskott-Aldrich syndrome and characterization of a polymorphic dinucleotide repeat at the DXS 6940 locus adjacent to the disease gene. Proc Natl Acad Sci USA 92:4706, 1995

36. Remold-O'Donnell E, Rosen FS, Kenney DM: Defects in Wiskott-Aldrich syndrome blood cells. Blood 87:2621, 1996

37. Villa A, Notarangelo L, Macchi P, et al: X-linked thrombocytopenia and Wiskott-Aldrich syndrome are allelic diseases with mutations in the WASP gene. Nat Genet 9:414, 1995

38. Mullen CA, Anderson KD, Blaese RM: Splenectomy and/or bone marrow transplantation in the management of Wiskott-Aldrich syndrome: long term follow-up of 62 cases. Blood 82:2961, 1993

39. Gatti RA, Berkel I, Boder E, et al: Localization of an ataxia-telangiectasia gene to chromosome 11q22-23. Nature 336:577, 1988

40. Savitsky K, Barshira A, Gilad S, et al: A single ataxia telangiectasia gene with a product similar to PI-3 kinase. Science 268:1749, 1995

41. Swift M: Genetic aspects of ataxia-telangiectasia. Immunodefic Rev 2:67, 1990

104 Immunologic Tolerance and Autoimmunity

Paul Anderson, M.D., Ph.D.

A central concept of immunology is that autoimmune reactions are injurious to the host. Around 1900, Paul Ehrlich postulated that the immune system acquires a state of tolerance to self-antigens; as a corollary, he proposed that the breakdown of tolerance would lead to self-destruction, a condition he described as "horror autotoxicus."[1] Subsequent work by mid–20th-century researchers such as Ray Owen,[2] Macfarlane Burnet,[3] and Peter Medawar[4] established the basic mechanism for the development of immunologic tolerance. In recent years, many important advances have been made in our understanding of tolerance at the molecular and cellular level. These advances are beginning to transform the clinical management of autoimmune diseases and may lead to therapies that prevent rejection of transplanted organs.

Tolerance

Tolerance is defined as a state of immunologic unresponsiveness to antigens, whether self or foreign. Antigens are recognized by specific receptors expressed on the surface of T cells and B cells. Binding of an antigen to the receptor can either activate or inhibit these immune effector cells. The molecular and cellular factors that determine whether receptor ligation induces immunity or tolerance are beginning to be unraveled.

MECHANISMS OF TOLERANCE

Tolerance results from one of three inhibitory influences on T and B cells: (1) clonal deletion, in which antigenic recognition leads to the activation-induced death of specific lymphocytes; (2) clonal anergy, in which lymphocytes are not killed but are rendered unresponsive to the recognized antigen; and (3) T cell–mediated suppression, in which regulatory T cells actively inhibit an immune response to an antigen. Several factors help determine which of those responses will occur.

Immature lymphocytes are more susceptible to induction of tolerance than are mature lymphocytes. Tolerance can be induced in immature lymphocytes either centrally or in the periphery. Central tolerance is acquired when immature lymphocytes encounter antigens in the organs that generate these cells: the thymus (T cells) and the bone marrow (B cells).

T cells recognize antigens that have been processed into peptides and presented in a complex with major histocompatibility complex (MHC) molecules (self-MHC–peptide complexes). Consequently, immature T cells must be screened for their ability to recognize self-MHC. This screening takes place in the thymus gland. T cells bearing receptors that recognize self-MHC are subjected to the processes of positive and negative selection [*see Figure 1*].[5] Positive selection occurs when T cells bearing receptors with a moderate affinity for self-MHC–peptide complexes receive survival and maturation signals after receptor ligation. Once these cells mature, they are exported to the periphery. Negative selection occurs when T cells bearing receptors with a high affinity for self-MHC–peptide complexes undergo activation-induced death. The thymus gland is capable of presenting many self-antigens that are normally expressed outside of the thymus or during restricted developmental stages.[6] This allows the elimination of most T cells bearing high-affinity receptors for self-MHC–peptide complexes and plays a major role in preventing autoimmunity in peripheral organs.

Because positive selection allows the maturation of T cells bearing receptors capable of low-affinity interactions with self-MHC–peptide complexes, potentially self-reactive T cells are normally found in peripheral lymphoid organs. Peripheral tolerance prevents these cells from inducing autoimmune disease.

Peripheral tolerance is achieved in one of three ways.[7,8] Perhaps the most common mechanism is the failure of T cells bearing low-affinity receptors to recognize self-antigen in the periphery. In this situation, the potentially self-reactive T cell is not activated and remains functionally naive. These cells are functional, however, as is shown by the fact that they can be activated by immunization with self-antigen delivered in the presence of immune adjuvants (e.g., complete Freund adjuvant, which contains microbial products that strongly activate the immune system at many levels). Failure to respond to self-antigen may simply reflect a receptor-binding affinity that is below the threshold for T cell activation.

T cells bearing receptors with high affinity for a self-antigen can remain in an unactivated state if that self-antigen is sequestered from immune effector cells. An example of an antigen that is sequestered from the immune system is myelin basic protein. Because T cells do not normally circulate through the

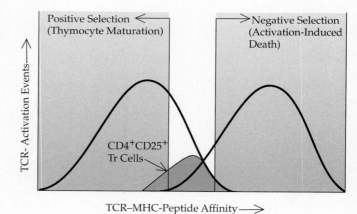

Figure 1 In the thymus, tolerance is induced through positive and negative selection of immature T cells. The fate of a particular T cell depends on the affinity of its receptor (TCR) for complexes of major histocompatibility complex (MHC) and self-peptides. After ligation, T cells whose receptors have low affinity for self-MCH–peptide complexes receive survival and maturation signals and are exported to the periphery (positive selection); T cells with high affinity undergo activation-induced death (negative selection).

$CD4^+$ regulatory T cells (Tr) that express CD25 have intermediate affinity for self-MCH–peptide complexes. This subpopulation of T cells matures in the thymus gland; suppression of their activation takes place in the periphery.

central nervous system, potentially self-reactive cells can persist in an unactivated state in the periphery. Similarly, pancreatic islet cells are normally sequestered from the immune system. In transgenic mice, recombinant proteins expressed on pancreatic islet cells are ignored by high-affinity T cells specific for the recombinant protein. This appears to result from the failure of naive T cells to contact islet cells in the absence of inflammation. In contrast, T cells do become activated in an antigen-specific manner in transgenic mice that express the same recombinant protein in hepatocytes. It therefore appears that circulating lymphocytes contact different tissues in different ways.

A second mechanism of peripheral tolerance involves the elimination of self-reactive T cells by apoptosis. This process is analogous to clonal deletion in the thymus. An example of peripheral deletion is the ability of superantigens (bacterial proteins that bridge selected T cell receptors and selected MHC molecules in an antigen-nonspecific manner) to induce the activation and subsequent death of T cells.[9] Whether peripheral deletion plays an important role in tolerance to self-antigens is not known, however.

A third mechanism of peripheral tolerance involves the acquisition of anergy after ligation of the T cell receptor complex.[10] This antigen-nonresponsive state can be induced in several distinct ways. The most extensively characterized mechanism of anergy induction occurs when the T cell receptor is ligated in the absence of costimulation. In the classic studies of Schwartz and colleagues, T cell clones that were activated by MHC-peptide complexes incorporated into artificial lipid bilayers were rendered nonresponsive to subsequent challenge with peptide-pulsed antigen-presenting cells (APCs).[11] It was subsequently shown that once a T cell has bound with an antigen, the cell requires a so-called second signal delivered by one or more costimulatory molecules to be primed for an immune response. T cells express several surface molecules that can transmit this second signal. These costimulatory receptors are engaged by ligands expressed on the surface of APCs. T cells that are activated in the absence of costimulation acquire defects in the transcriptional control pathways that allow the production of interleukin-2 (IL-2), an important T cell autocrine growth factor.[10] In vitro anergy can often be overcome by supplying exogenous IL-2 to anergic T cells.

Costimulatory signals can be delivered to T cells by soluble factors or cell-surface molecules expressed on APCs. The most potent costimulatory signals are delivered when CD28,[12-14] CD154, or both[15] are ligated on the surface of T cells [see Figure 2]. Blockade of costimulatory signals by monoclonal antibodies or recombinant receptor antagonists confers potent immunosuppression and allows the acceptance of skin, cardiac, and pancreatic allografts in rodents.[16] Simultaneous blockade of both the CD28 and CD154 pathways is significantly more immunosuppressive than blockade of a single costimulatory pathway. The ligand for CD154 is CD40, a protein expressed on the surface of activated B cells, dendritic cells, and macrophages. The ligands for CD28 (B7-1, B7-2, and related proteins) are expressed on the surface of APCs, such as dendritic cells, monocytes, and B cells. Their expression is induced when APCs are activated in the course of microbial infection. This property heightens the immune response in the setting of perceived danger (i.e., microbial infection). B7-1 and B7-2 have overlapping immunostimulatory roles: mice lacking either protein are only partially deficient in generating an immune response to foreign antigen.[14,17]

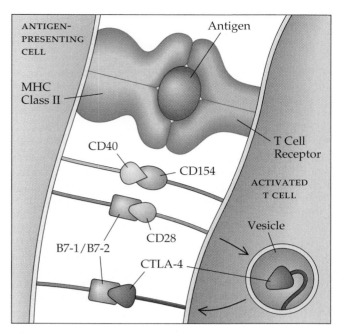

Figure 2 Activation of T cells begins when the T cell receptor binds with a complex of an MHC molecule and a peptide expressed on the surface of an antigen-presenting cell (APC). Activation is completed by a second signal generated by the ligation of costimulatory molecules expressed on the cell surface of the APC. B7-1/B7-2 interacts with CD28 on the T cell, and CD40 interacts with CD154.

In unactivated T cells, CTLA-4 (a relative of CD28) is a component of intracellular vesicles. After CD28 ligation, CTLA-4 moves to the cell surface and binds with B7-1/B7-2, generating negative signals that turn off the immune response.

Ligation of CD28 induces the expression of CTLA-4, a structurally related protein that turns off activated T cells.[12,17] By this mechanism, the activated T cell initiates a program that will ensure its elimination at the conclusion of the immune response. Compared with CD28, CTLA-4 has a higher affinity for B7-1 and B7-2.[17] The importance of the negative regulatory influence of CTLA-4 is dramatically observed in CTLA-4–null mice. These animals develop a fatal lymphoproliferative syndrome from the uncontrolled activation of self-reactive T cells.[18]

Given the central importance of CD28-B7 interactions in T cell activation and the ability of costimulatory blockade to prevent allograft rejection, it was surprising to discover that NOD mice (a strain that develops spontaneous diabetes) that also lack either CD28 alone or both B7-1 and B7-2 have more severe diabetes.[19] This paradoxical result appears to reflect the role of CD28-B7 interactions in promoting tolerance to self-antigens. CD28-B7 interactions are required for the maturation of a distinct class of regulatory T cells that help maintain peripheral tolerance. These regulatory T cells (Tr) are included in a subpopulation (5% to 15%) of peripheral blood CD4+ T cells that express CD25, a subunit of the IL-2 receptor.[20,21] The selective removal of CD4+ and CD25+ T cells from BALB/c mice results in the development of T cell–mediated autoimmune thyroiditis, gastritis, and diabetes. The CD4+ and CD25+ Tr cells that mature in the thymus gland bear receptors that have an intermediate affinity for self-MHC–peptide complexes [see Figure 1]. In the periphery, antigen exposure confers the ability to suppress the activation of CD4+ and CD25+ T cells in an antigen-independent, cell contact–dependent manner. Although these cells secrete IL-10, a potent anti-inflammatory cytokine, their suppressive activity is cytokine independent. CD4+ and CD25+ T cells can suppress graft versus host disease in allotransplants, and they can prevent autoimmune disease in several different animal models.[21] Consequently, these cells probably play an essential role in maintaining peripheral tolerance to self-antigens.

Autoimmunity

Despite the multiple and redundant mechanisms that exist to ensure immunologic tolerance to self, autoimmune phenomena are relatively common. In some cases, autoimmune responses accompany a normal immune response to a microbial pathogen. Thus, the appearance of rheumatoid factor (anti-immunoglobulin antibodies) in the serum of patients with bacterial endocarditis is relatively common. In general, these autoantibodies are not pathogenic. Their appearance probably results from antigen-nonspecific activation of T cells and B cells bearing low-affinity receptors for self-antigens that are normally held in check by mechanisms of peripheral tolerance. The ability of bacterial products (e.g., lipopolysaccharide) to function as immune adjuvants appears to overcome these repressive influences.

MOLECULAR MIMICRY

In rare cases, the normal immune response to a specific microbial peptide can trigger immunity to a related self-peptide, a phenomenon known as molecular mimicry.[22] The classic example of molecular mimicry is rheumatic heart disease, which results from antistreptococcal antibodies that cross-react with myocardial antigens. The molecular identity of the cross-reactive peptide antigens in rheumatic heart disease is not known.

A more fully characterized example of molecular mimicry may underlie Lyme arthritis. During the immune response to the tick-borne spirochete *Borrelia burgdorferi*, the human leukocyte antigen (HLA) DRB1*0401 activates T cells specific for a nine-amino-acid peptide derived from the spirochete's outer-surface protein A ($Osp_{A165-173}$). Some of these T cells can also recognize a self-peptide derived from leukocyte function–associated antigen–1α (LFA-$1\alpha_{332-340}$), a protein that is highly expressed on inflammatory cells infiltrating the infected synovium. This autoimmune response has been proposed to promote a syndrome of inflammatory arthritis that, in some patients, persists long after the pathogen has been eliminated. The relative importance of the autoimmune T cell response to LFA-$1\alpha_{332-340}$ in the pathogenesis of chronic Lyme arthritis remains to be determined, however.

FAILURE OF TOLERANCE

Self-tolerance requires the elimination, during thymic ontogeny, of T cells bearing receptors with high affinity for self-MHC–peptide complexes. It is likely that defects in the expression or presentation of self-antigens in the thymus gland will be found to contribute to some forms of human autoimmune disease. Similarly, failure to eliminate thymic T cells bearing high-affinity receptors for self-antigen (i.e., negative selection) is likely to contribute to some forms of human autoimmune disease. Although defective negative selection has been reported to contribute to the autoimmune diathesis observed in the NOD mouse,[23] defects in central tolerance have not yet been identified in patients with autoimmune disease.

T cells bearing high-affinity receptors for self-antigen that escape negative selection will normally be held in check by mechanisms of peripheral tolerance. Consequently, defects in central tolerance are unlikely to result in autoimmune disease unless there are also defects in peripheral tolerance. Molecular and cellular defects that promote the bypass of tolerance to self-antigens in the periphery are beginning to be identified. Progress has been made in both the genetic basis for autoimmune susceptibility and the identification and characterization of specific autoantigens that are targeted by the immune response.

IDENTIFICATION OF AUTOANTIGENS

A common feature of autoimmune diseases is the appearance of autoantibodies in the serum. In some cases, these autoantibodies are directly pathogenic: the clinical syndrome is produced when the antibody binds to its target antigen. The molecular pathogenesis of these autoimmune conditions can be determined with some precision. Unfortunately, the molecular defects that allow the bypass of tolerance to the disease-inducing autoantigen are less well understood.

Pathogenic Autoantibodies

Myasthenia gravis Nearly all patients with myasthenia gravis have autoantibodies to acetylcholine receptors (ACRs) on skeletal muscle. However, the degree of neuromuscular blockade seen in this disease does not always parallel the serum levels of anti-ACR antibodies. The antibodies are polyclonal and bind to several distinct epitopes on the ACR. Although these antibodies inhibit ACR function, they rarely block the acetylcholine binding site. The supposition that these anti-ACR antibodies have direct pathogenic effects is supported by the fact that injection of ACR antibodies can induce myasthenic weakness in animals and that plasmapheresis is an effective treatment in some patients. Some patients with myasthenia gravis have a coincident thymoma, and thymectomy can be an effective treatment in those patients,[24] suggesting that defects in thymic selection of maturing T cells may play a role in the autoimmune response to the ACR.

Pemphigus Pemphigus vulgaris and bullous pemphigoid are autoimmune skin diseases characterized by the presence of serum autoantibodies that react with adhesion molecules found at the dermoepidermal basement membrane zone. One of the target antigens is desmoglein 3, a desmosomal adhesion molecule. Several lines of evidence support a pathogenic role for these autoantibodies. First, antidesmosomal antibodies are consistently present in patients with pemphigus, levels of those antibodies correlate with disease activity, and the removal of the antibodies by plasmapheresis results in improvement of symptoms. Second, serum from patients with pemphigus vulgaris causes pemphiguslike lesions in mice. Third, newborns of mothers with pemphigus have transient disease resulting from transplacental transmission of maternal antibody.

Autoimmune endocrinopathies Autoantibodies reactive with hormone receptors can contribute to endocrine disorders. High levels of antibody reactive with the peripheral insulin receptor can result in insulin-dependent diabetes mellitus. Paradoxically, low levels of antibody may stimulate the insulin receptor by mimicking insulin, resulting in hypoglycemia.

Autoimmune disease of the thyroid is associated with antibodies directed toward three antigens: microsomal thyroid peroxidase, thyroglobulin, and the thyroid receptor for thyroid-stimulating hormone (TSH). Antibodies to the TSH receptor may mimic the action of TSH, thereby resulting in Graves disease. Another apparent autoimmune disease of the thyroid, Hashimoto thyroiditis, is associated with antibodies to the TSH receptor, but their pathogenic role in this disease is unclear. Less commonly, antibodies to the TSH receptor may block the action of TSH and cause hypothyroidism. A pathogenic role for the other two classes of antithyroid autoantibodies has not been established.

Antiphospholipid syndrome   The antiphospholipid syndrome (APS) consists of recurrent thrombosis, fetal loss, and thrombocytopenia in association with antibodies to cardiolipin or other negatively charged phospholipids, along with abnormalities of certain clotting tests, referred to as the lupus anticoagulant. APS can be primary or secondary; secondary APS is usually associated with systemic lupus erythematosus (SLE) or its variants. The antiphospholipid antibodies do not bind to phospholipids alone but to a complex of phospholipids and the plasma proteins β_2-glycoprotein I and prothrombin. These antibodies induce the expression of adhesion molecules on endothelial cells that promote the binding of monocytes and platelets as the first step in a thrombotic cascade.

Nonpathogenic Autoantibodies

Autoantibodies reactive with intracellular targets can serve as markers of specific autoimmune diseases. For example, antibodies reactive with citrullinated peptides are specific markers of rheumatoid arthritis, antibodies reactive with the mitochondrial enzyme 2-oxo acid dehydrogenase are specific markers of primary biliary cirrhosis, and antibodies reactive with the Smith small nuclear ribonucleoprotein (snRNP) complex are specific markers of SLE. Although these autoantibodies are unlikely to be pathogenic, their presence is highly correlated with specific autoimmune diseases. An understanding of the process that promotes the disease-specific bypass of tolerance to a selected antigen is likely to shed light on the pathogenic mechanism underlying individual autoimmune syndromes. An important insight into the mechanism by which tolerance is abrogated in an antigen-specific manner came with the realization that the targets of many autoantibodies found in the serum of patients with autoimmune disease are proteins that are modified in cells undergoing apoptotic cell death [*see Table 1*].[25] During apoptosis, myriad intracellular proteins, nucleic acids, and lipids are subjected to enzymatic and nonenzymatic modification. These modifications include protease cleavage, phosphorylation, transglutamination, ubiquitination, citrullination, and isoaspartylation.[25] It has been proposed that these modifications create neo-epitopes to which the immune system has not been tolerized.

Although proteins that are modified during apoptosis are preferred targets of the autoantibodies found in the serum of patients with autoimmune disease, it is clear that apoptosis per se is not sufficient to break tolerance to these self proteins. Apoptosis is a ubiquitious process, yet most people do not develop autoimmune disease. Apparently, the necessary additional element is delay in the execution of the apoptotic program or the clearance of the apoptotic cell. This phenomenon has been demonstrated in mice that lack the first component of complement. C1q functions as an opsonin that binds to apoptotic cells and promotes their clearance by professional phagocytes (neutrophils and macrophages). In the absence of C1, the clearance of apoptotic corpses is delayed. Delayed clearance of apoptotic cells somehow increases their immunogenicity.[26]

A similar phenomenon occurs when the execution of the apoptotic program is delayed. For example, influenza virus–induced apoptosis in macrophages has been shown to increase the immunogenicity of viral proteins.[27] This phenomenon requires the phagocytosis of infected macrophages by dendritic cells. By a process of cross-priming, the dendritic cell can then present antigens derived from the infected macrophage in a highly efficient manner. Because influenza virus encodes several genes that function to inhibit apoptosis (e.g., NS1), virus-induced apoptosis requires many hours to complete. During this delay, the virus replicates within the infected cell, and the virus-infected cell expresses stress-response proteins (heat shock proteins [HSPs]), including HSP70 and HSP90. These HSPs function as natural adjuvants that can deliver peptides to class I MHC molecules expressed by APCs.[28] The generation of modified peptides and the induction of HSPs may account for the increased immunogenicity of apoptotic cells and the generation of autoantibodies reactive with proteins that are modified during apoptotic cell death.

This model suggests that the autoantibodies that serve as markers of specific autoimmune diseases are generated when the target cell undergoes delayed or aberrant apoptosis. This implies that the primary insult to the target tissue is produced by a stimulus that induces aberrant cell death and modification of the specific autoantigen. Such a process may be initiated by specific environmental factors (e.g., viruses, toxins, or ultraviolet radiation).

GENETICS OF AUTOIMMUNITY

Systemic autoimmunity is a multigenic trait that is significantly influenced by environmental factors. The concordance rate for SLE in monozgotic twins is only 30%, indicating that both genetic and environmental factors contribute to disease onset. The specific genes that promote autoimmunity can be identified in two ways. Most of the genes currently known to promote autoimmunity have been discovered using case-control association methodologies.[29] These studies have linked the expression of specific HLA haplotypes to specific autoimmune diseases. In a similar fashion, case-control studies have linked defects in both classical pathway complement components (C1q, C2, and C4) and Fc receptor alleles to the development of SLE. More recently, genetic linkage analysis has been applied to families in which two or more members have SLE, in an attempt to identify disease-susceptibility loci. These studies have identified six different chromosomal loci with significant linkage to human SLE.[29] It is likely that future studies will identify a cohort of genes that, alone or in combination, contribute to the autoimmune diathesis.

In keeping with the hypothesis that aberrant apoptosis can promote autoimmunity, several genes that are known to regulate apoptotic cell death have been implicated in the onset of autoimmune disease. The autoimmune syndromes that result from defects in a family of death receptors and their ligands are instructive examples. Specific members of this family (e.g., Fas and tumor necrosis factor type I [TNF RI]) are required for the clonal elimination of activated T cells after an immune response to microbial infection. Mice lacking either Fas or its ligand develop lymphadenopathy and splenomegaly from the accumulation of previously activated T cells. In some genetic back-

Table 1 Autoantigens from Proteins Modified during Apoptosis in Autoimmune Disease

Disease	Antigen	Modification
Myositis	Mi-2, tRNA synthase	Granzyme B cleavage
Rheumatoid arthritis	Fibrin	Deimination
Scleroderma	CENP-B, Ku-70, topoisomerase-I, U1-70K	Caspase/granzyme cleavage
Sjögren syndrome	α-Fodrin	Caspase cleavage
Systemic lupus erythematosus	Fibrillarin, histone H3, hnRNPs, Ku-70, nuclear lamins, nucleolin, PARP, U1-70K, vimentin	Caspase/granzyme cleavage
	SR proteins	Phosphorylation
	Actin, histone H2B, troponin, tubulin	Transglutamination
	Topoisomerase-II, histone H2A	Ubiquitination
	PARP	ADP-ribosylation

ADP—adenosine diphosphate   CENP-B—centromere protein B   hnRNP—heterogeneous nuclear ribonucleoprotein
PARP—poly (ADP-ribose) polymerase   tRNA—transfer RNA

grounds (e.g., strain MRL), but not in others (e.g., strain BALB/c), failure to eliminate activated T cells results in an autoimmune disease that resembles SLE. Thus, the absence of Fas or Fas ligand (FasL) promotes the phenotypic expression of an autoimmune diathesis that is intrinsic to the MRL strain (a genetic phenomenon known as epistasis). Although defects in Fas or FasL are not linked to autoimmunity in patients with SLE, mutations in either Fas or FasL produce the autoimmune lymphoproliferative syndrome (ALPS), an autosomal dominant condition characterized by lymphadenopathy, splenomegaly, and autoantibody production.[30,31] ALPS is also caused by mutations in caspase-10, a component of the effector arm of the apoptotic death program. Thus, ALPS is an autoimmune disease that results from defective execution of an apoptotic program in activated T cells.

Genome-wide linkage mapping has identified mutations in NOD2 as an etiologic factor in familial Crohn disease, an autoimmune inflammatory process that targets the intestinal mucosa.[32] Although the specific function of NOD2 is not known, it encodes a caspase recruitment domain (CARD) that is found in several protein components of the apoptotic death machinery (e.g., Apaf-1). NOD1, a relative of NOD2, has been reported to bind to apoptotic signaling molecules and activate apoptotic caspases. It remains to be determined whether NOD2 subverts the apoptotic signaling cascade in intestinal epithelial cells.

ORGAN-SPECIFIC VERSUS SYSTEMIC AUTOIMMUNITY

For many years, organ-specific immunity was thought to result from the activation of lymphocytes bearing receptors specific for a tissue-restricted antigen. In rare cases of molecular mimicry, this may be the case. However, recent results in studies of autoimmune disease with animal models, as well as studies of hereditary autoimmune syndromes, suggest that the target of an autoimmune attack can shift from one tissue to another in response to defined or undefined genetic modifiers. For example, persons with an underlying autoimmune diathesis produced by mutations in the autoimmune regulator (AIRE), a nucleic acid–binding protein expressed in thymic epithelial and dendritic cells, develop various combinations of autoimmune thyroiditis, parathyroid disease, and type 1 (insulin-de-

pendent) diabetes.[33] Although the factors that determine which tissues become targets of autoimmune attack have not been identified, the fact that different tissues are affected in different persons suggests that unique, tissue-specific autoantigens may not be the primary triggers of disease.

The concept that organ-specific autoimmunity need not be driven by a tissue-specific autoantigen is supported by observations made in two different animal models of autoimmunity. In NOD mice whose MHC locus has been replaced with that of another strain, autoimmune thyroiditis develops instead of diabetes.[19] This result suggests that the NOD strain harbors an autoimmune diathesis that can manifest itself as different types of organ-specific autoimmunity. In support of this concept, NOD mice lacking the costimulatory molecule B7-2 develop autoimmune peripheral neuropathy, rather than diabetes.[19] Although the mechanism by which individual tissues are selected for immune attack is not known, these results strongly suggest that factors other than tissue-restricted autoantigens can be the primary determinant of organ-specific autoimmune disease.

Another instructive example of organ-specific autoimmunity that arises in the absence of a defined, tissue-restricted autoantigenic trigger is the inflammatory arthritis that develops in the F1 progeny of K/B×NOD mice.[34] The K/B strain expresses a transgenic T cell receptor that recognizes a self-peptide derived from glucose-6-phosphate isomerase (GPI) presented in the context of Ag7, a class II MHC molecule from the NOD strain. In K/B×NOD mice, T cells bearing the transgene provide help for B cells encoding immunoglobulins that bind to GPI. GPI is an enzyme expressed in all cells, yet anti-GPI antibodies somehow provoke a symmetrical, inflammatory arthritis involving diarthrodial joints in these mice. Although the mechanism by which anti-GPI antibodies provoke arthritis is not fully understood, this model illustrates the potential for an immune response directed at a ubiquitous antigen to trigger organ-specific autoimmunity.

One way in which organ-specific autoimmunity can be induced in the absence of a tissue-specific autoantigen is by the pathologic overexpression of inflammatory cytokines.[35] Thus, overexpression of tumor necrosis factor–α (TNF-α) in transgenic mice is sufficient to induce a symmetrical polyarthritis that resembles rheumatoid arthritis.[36] This appears to result from the ability of TNF-α to initiate an inflammatory cytokine cascade within the cells that make up the synovium. The importance of TNF-α in the pathogenesis of rheumatoid arthritis has been dramatically validated by the clinical efficacy of TNF blockers such as infliximab and etanercept[37] [*see Chapter 112*]. In an analogous fashion, BAFF/Blys, a TNF-α–related protein that promotes the survival and differentiation of B cells, has been proposed to participate in the induction of SLE-like autoimmune syndromes.[38,39] Transgenic mice engineered to overexpress BAFF/Blys develop hypergammaglobulinemia and autoimmune symptoms because of the survival of autoreactive B cells that would normally be deleted from the B cell repertoire. These observations suggest that neutralization of TNF family members may play an important role in the treatment of selected autoimmune diseases.

References

1. Ehrlich P, Morgenroth J: On haemolysis: third communication. Berlin Klin Wochenschr 37:453, 1900

2. Owen R: Immunogenetic consequences of vascular anastomosis between bovine twins. Science 102:400, 1945

3. Burnet F: Clonal selection theory: a modification of Jerne's theory of antibody production using the concept of clonal selection. Aust J Sci 20:67, 1957

4. Billingham R, Brent L, Medawar P: Actively acquired tolerance of foreign cells. Nature 172:603, 1953

5. Nossal GJ: Negative selection of lymphocytes. Cell 76:229, 1994

6. Heath V, Mason D, Ramirez F, et al: Homeostatic mechanisms in the control of autoimmunity. Semin Immunol 9:375, 1997

7. Fazekas de St. Groth B: DCs and peripheral T cell tolerance. Semin Immunol 13:311, 2001

8. Steinman RM, Nussenzweig MC: Avoiding horror autotoxicus: the importance of dendritic cells in peripheral T cell tolerance. Proc Natl Acad Sci USA 99:351, 2002

9. Sundberg EJ, Li Y, Mariuzza RA: So many ways of getting in the way: diversity in the molecular architecture of superantigen-dependent T-cell signaling complexes. Curr Opin Immunol 14:36, 2002

10. Lechler R, Chai JG, Marelli-Berg F, et al: T-cell anergy and peripheral T-cell tolerance. Philos Trans R Soc Lond B Biol Sci 356:625, 2001

11. Quill H, Schwartz R: Stimulation of normal inducer T cell clones with antigen presented by purified Ia molecules in planar lipid membranes. J Immunol 138:3704, 1987

12. Chambers CA, Kuhns MS, Egen JG, et al: CTLA-4-mediated inhibition in regulation of T cell responses: mechanisms and manipulation in tumor immunotherapy. Annu Rev Immunol 19:565, 2001

13. Chambers CA: The expanding world of co-stimulation: the two-signal model revisited. Trends Immunol 22:217, 2001

14. Salomon B, Bluestone JA: Complexities of CD28/B7: CTLA-4 costimulatory pathways in autoimmunity and transplantation. Annu Rev Immunol 19:225, 2001

15. Kirk A, Blair P, Tadaki D, et al: The role of CD154 in organ transplant rejection and acceptance. Philos Trans R Soc Lond B Biol Sci 356:691, 2001

16. Yu X, Carpenter P, Anasetti C: Advances in transplantation tolerance. Lancet 357:1959, 2001

17. Sharpe AH, Freeman GJ: The B7-CD28 superfamily. Nature Rev Immunol 2:116, 2002

18. Tivol E, Borriello F, Schweitzer A, et al: Loss of CTLA-4 leads to massive lymphoproliferation and fatal multiorgan tissue destruction, revealing a critical negative regulatory role of CTLA-4. Immunity 3:541, 1995

19. Lesage S, Goodnow C: Organ-specific autoimmune disease: a deficiency of tolerogenic stimulation. J Exp Med 194:F31, 2001

20. Maloy KJ, Powrie F: Regulatory T cells in the control of immune pathology. Nat Immunol 2:816, 2001

21. Shevach EM: Certified professionals: CD4(+)CD25(+) suppressor T cells. J Exp Med 193:F41, 2001

22. Benoist C, Mathis D: Autoimmunity provoked by infection: How good is the case for T cell epitope mimicry? Nature Immunol 2:797, 2001

23. Kishimoto H, Sprent J: A defect in central tolerance in NOD mice. Nature Immunol 2:1025, 2001

24. Vincent A, Palace J, Hilton-Jones D: Myasthenia gravis. Lancet 357:2122, 2001

25. Utz P, Gensler T, Anderson P: Death, autoantigen modifications, and tolerance. Arthritis Research 2:101, 2000

26. Botto M, Dell'Agnola C, Bygrave A, et al: Homozygous C1q deficiency causes glomerulonephritis associated with multiple apoptotic bodies. Nat Genetics 19:56, 1998

27. Albert M, Sauter B, Bhardwaj N: Dendritic cells acquire antigen from apoptotic cells and induce class I–restricted CTLs. Nature 392:86, 1998

28. Srivastava P: Roles of heat-shock proteins in innate and adaptive immunity. Nature Rev Immunol 2:185, 2002

29. Wakeland EK, Liu K, Graham RR, et al: Delineating the genetic basis of systemic lupus erythematosus. Immunity 15:397, 2001

30. Fleisher T, Puck J, Strober W, et al: The autoimmune lymphoproliferative syndrome: a disorder of human lymphocyte apoptosis. Clin Rev Allergy Immunol 20:109, 2001

31. Fleisher TA, Straus SE, Bleesing JJ: A genetic disorder of lymphocyte apoptosis involving the fas pathway: the autoimmune lymphoproliferative syndrome. Curr Allergy Asthma Rep 1:534, 2001

32. Beutler B: Autoimmunity and apoptosis: the Crohn's connection. Immunity 15:5, 2001

33. Aaltonen J, Bjorses P: Cloning of the APECED gene provides new insight into human autoimmunity. Ann Med 31:111, 1999

34. Ji H, Ohmura K, Mahmood U, et al: Arthritis critically dependent on innate immune system players. Immunity 16:157, 2002

35. O'Shea JJ, Ma A, Lipsky P: Cytokines and autoimmunity. Nature Rev Immunol 2:37, 2002

36. Kollias G, Douni E, Kassiotis G, et al: On the role of TNF and receptors in models of multiorgan failure, rheumatoid arthritis, multiple sclerosis and inflammatory bowel disease. Immunol Rev 169:175, 1999

37. Feldmann M, Maini R: Anti-TNF therapy of rheumatoid arthritis. Annu Rev Immunol 19:163, 2001

38. Laabi Y, Egle A, Strasser A: TNF cytokine family: more BAFF-ling complexities. Curr Immunol 11:R1013, 2001

39. Do RK, Chen-Kiang S: Mechanism of BLyS action in B cell immunity. Cytokine Growth Factor Rev 13:19, 2002

Acknowledgment

Figure 2   Seward Hung.

105 Allergic Response

Pamela J. Daffern, M.D., and Lawrence B. Schwartz, M.D., Ph.D.

Definition of Allergic Response

The word anaphylaxis was coined in 1902 by Charles Richet, in order to contrast the condition with prophylaxis. Richet described anaphylaxis as "the peculiar attribute which certain poisons possess of increasing instead of diminishing the sensitivity of an organism to their action...."[1] One hundred years later, we understand anaphylaxis as the extreme of a spectrum of events mediated by immunoglobulin E (IgE). Persons with IgE-mediated disorders have a genetic propensity to form IgE antibodies against otherwise innocuous environmental antigens (allergens); this propensity is termed atopy (from the Greek *atopos*, meaning "out of place"). In atopic persons, IgE mediates a wide range of reactions, including dermatitis, rhinitis, asthma, urticaria, angioedema, and anaphylaxis.

Confusion arises over the misapplication of the term allergy to describe any untoward reaction to food or medications or to perceived environmental exposures. This confusion is further complicated by the fact that both IgE-mediated and non–IgE-mediated forms of rhinitis, asthma, and atopic dermatitis occur, often in the same person.

In the nonatopic person, exposure to allergen results in immunologic tolerance or neglect, whereas in atopic persons, exposure results in sensitization. On reexposure to the allergen, atopic persons mount an immunologically mediated inflammatory response in the target organ. Other environmental factors—such as tobacco smoke, air pollution, respiratory virus infection, and lack of exposure to certain microbes in childhood—may also promote an allergic inflammatory response.

Epidemiology of Atopic Disorders

Up to 30% of the United States population may be affected by allergic rhinoconjunctivitis, asthma, or atopic dermatitis. This high incidence of atopic disease may reflect societal factors. Fetal development takes place in an intrauterine environment that favors atopic sensitization[2]; the maternal immune system suppresses cell-mediated immune responses in order to prevent rejection of the fetus. Thus, the neonate may enter the world with T cells that are already primed by common environmental and food allergens that have crossed the placenta. It has been proposed that microbial exposure and infections during infancy shift the immune response away from the allergic pattern to a protective immune response.[3] Specifically, after macrophages or dendritic cells ingest microbes, T cells produce cytokines that promote non-IgE responses by B cells. Therefore, the increasing prevalence of atopic disorders in countries that have adopted a Western lifestyle, including overuse of antibiotics, has been attributed to a lack of microbial antigen stimulation.

Humoral and Cellular Mechanisms of Allergic Inflammation Associated with Immediate Hypersensitivity

ANTIGEN-PRESENTING CELLS AND SENSITIZATION

All persons encounter environmental antigens that are capable of inducing an allergic response. Soluble antigens, such as allergens, undergo endocytosis by professional antigen-presenting cells (APCs), which include dendritic cells, such as epidermal Langerhans cells; macrophages; and B cells.[4] However, only dendritic cells and Langerhans cells are able to prime naive T cells and thus are responsible for the sensitization phase.[5,6] Once primary sensitization has been achieved, monocytes and B cells amplify the process. B cells bind allergen through immunoglobulin receptors specific for the allergen, as opposed to nonspecific endocytic pathways used by other APCs. The internalization of antigen results in two processes. The first is general activation of the APC: this includes upregulation of major histocompatibility complex (MHC) and accessory molecules. The second process is fusion of the endocytic vesicle with lysosomes, which results in the formation of specialized antigen-processing vesicles in which antigens are hydrolyzed into protein fragments. The linear peptides that result are incorporated into the antigen-binding groove of a class II human lymphocyte antigen (HLA) molecule during its transport to the cell surface.

In general, APCs will co-express a heterogeneous assortment of allergen-derived peptides and HLA class II molecules on their surface. The efficiency with which processed allergen peptides bind to the HLA class II molecules presumably depends on variations in the HLA loci; these variations are genetically determined. The binding efficiency in turn influences the predisposition of the person to develop allergy to or tolerance of a particular antigen. The APC loaded with processed antigen/HLA class II complexes presents this complex to CD4+,CD8– helper T cells. The genetically determined binding efficiency of an HLA-derived molecule to an antigen also may influence how T cells develop when exposed to that complex.[7] In addition, the quantity of interleukin-12 (IL-12) produced by APCs also influences the type of T cell response.[5]

T CELLS AND MEDIATION OF ALLERGIC INFLAMMATION

The helper T cell response is influenced not only by APCs but also by the age of the person and by the amount, type, duration, and route of allergen exposure.[7,8] Also, the cytokine milieu during lymphocyte differentiation determines the type of effector function of the helper T cell [*see Table 1*].

For example, bacterial DNA sequences have immunostimulatory regions containing deoxycytidine-phosphate-deoxyguanosine (CpG) repeats. CpG repeats are recognized as foreign by pattern recognition receptors called Toll-like receptor-9 (TLR-9) on APCs.[9,10] These CpG repeats stimulate macrophages and dendritic cells to secrete inflammatory cytokines, including IL-12 and IL-18. These cytokines then induce T cells and natural killer (NK) cells to produce interferon gamma (IFN-γ), a cytokine known to promote nonallergic, protective responses.

Table 1 Cytokines Involved in IgE-Mediated Allergic Inflammation

Cytokine	Source	Function
IL-3	T_{H2} cells,* mast cells, basophils, eosinophils	Promotes granulocyte and macrophage maturation; eosinophil activation and survival
IL-4	T_{H2} cells,* mast cells, basophils	Promotes differentiation of T_{H0} to T_{H2} cells; antagonizes differentiation of T_{H0} to T_{H1} cells; IgE isotype switching
IL-5	T_{H2} cells,* mast cells, eosinophils	Promotes eosinophil development, activation, and survival
IL-13	T_{H2} cells,* mast cells, basophils	IgE isotype switching, eosinophil activation
GM-CSF	T_{H2} cells and activated macrophages,* endothelial and epithelial cells	Promotes granulocyte and macrophage maturation, eosinophil activation, and survival
TNF-α	Monocytes/macrophages,* mast cells	Promotes chemotaxis and activation of leukocytes and vascular endothelium

*Major source.

GM-CSF—granulocyte-macrophage colony-stimulating factor   IL—interleukin   TNF—tumor necrosis factor

This pattern of response by helper T cells is termed a T_{H1} response, because it is associated with differentiation of naive helper T (T_{H0}) cells into mature T_{H1} cells. Similarly, the helper T cells of persons without atopy respond to presentation of potentially allergenic peptides by ignoring them or by producing IFN-γ and directing the production of allergen-specific IgG1 and IgG4 antibodies.[11]

In contrast, helper T cells of atopic persons respond to processed aeroallergens by forming IL-4, IL-5, and IL-13 and by directing the production of allergen-specific IgE antibodies. This type of helper T cell response is termed a T_{H2} response. IL-4 and IL-13 share a number of functions, because both cytokines signal through the IL-4Rα/IL-13Rα heterodimer.[12] However, only IL-4 is able to induce the differentiation of T_{H0} cells to T_{H2} cells and to antagonize the differentiation of T_{H0} cells to T_{H1} cells, resulting in IgE-mediated allergic inflammation. In contrast, both IL-12 and IFN-γ induce the differentiation to T_{H1} cells; T_{H2} cell differentiation is inhibited by IFN-γ. Differentiation to T_{H1} cells results in cell-mediated immunity and inflammation.[13] Therefore, the differentiation of T_{H0} cells to either T_{H1} cells or T_{H2} cells appears to be the crucial event that determines which type of immune response will follow.

GENETICS AND THE DEVELOPMENT OF ATOPY

Research has begun to identify specific genetic variants that contribute to the development of the atopic state. For example, a mutation of the IL-12R beta$_2$-chain gene has recently been shown to impair signaling through IL-12. Because IL-12 is a potent inducer of IFN-γ production and because IFN-γ downregulates IgE production (see above), this mutation results in increased IgE production in atopic persons.[14] Polymorphisms in the gene for STAT-6, a transcription factor selectively regulated by IL-4 and IL-13 (cytokines that upregulate IgE production), have also been described.[15] These genetic variations in STAT-6 also appear to be associated with a predisposition to atopy. Finally, an asthma gene (*ADAM-33*) associated with bronchial hyperresponsiveness but not atopy was recently defined by genetic-linkage analysis of affected sibling pairs. The *ADAM-33* gene product, a membrane metalloprotease, may function to modulate the response to cytokines in the lung by solubilizing cytokine membrane receptors, but its precise role still needs to be determined.[16] Like other allergies, however, asthma involves environmental factors. For example, the predisposition to asthma is modified by the presence of allergens and endotoxins.[17]

IgE SYNTHESIS

Once allergen is processed by APCs and presented to T_{H2} cells, a specific sequence of events must follow for IgE production by B cells to occur [*see Figure 1*]. The switch from IgM or IgG production to IgE production by B cells occurs in the genome and requires two signals.[18] The first signal is delivered through the IL-4Rα chain by either IL-4 or IL-13.[12] Signaling through these cytokine receptors initiates transcription from the germline promoter site of the constant portion of the heavy chain of IgE. The IgE heavy-chain gene is located downstream of the IgG and IgM heavy-chain genes and replaces IgG or IgM on the immunoglobulin molecule. The second signal is delivered through activation of the cluster differentiation 40 (CD40) receptor on B cells.[19] Signaling through CD40 activates the recombinases necessary to remove the upstream IgG or IgM heavy-chain constant region and replace it with the corresponding region of IgE. This process switches the type of antibody being produced without altering its antigenic specificity. Stimulation of B cells through CD40 also stimulates growth, differentiation, and survival of these cells.[20]

The ligand for CD40 (CD154, CD40L) is expressed not only on T cells but also on mast cells and basophils. Importantly, all of these cells also secrete IL-4, IL-13, or both, and therefore could potentially play a role in directing B cell production of IgE. However, it seems likely that T cells are responsible for initiating the switch to antigen-specific IgE production. Mast cells and basophils may then amplify deviation of immune responses toward IgE production after the primary IgE sensitization has occurred.[19] It seems likely that binding to CD40 on B cells by mast cells and basophils would enhance polyclonal (i.e., not antigen-dependent or specific) IgE production by B cells, because mast cells and basophils are not dedicated APCs. IgE antibody secreted by B cells circulates briefly, having a serum half-life of 2 to 3 days, before binding to IgE receptors.

IgE RECEPTORS AND REGULATION OF IgE

Receptors for IgE (FcϵR) are expressed on various cells.[21] The high-affinity receptor for IgE, FcϵRI, has two forms that differ by the presence or absence of a beta chain. The beta chain is present in the high-affinity receptor found on mast cells and basophils.[19] The presence of the beta chain amplifies the cellular signaling that occurs when IgE bound to FcϵRI is cross-linked by allergen. Its presence also increases the amount of IgE receptor on the surfaces of mast cells and basophils by up to sixfold.[22]

Levels of FcεRI on the surface of basophils have been shown to correlate with serum IgE levels in various IgE-associated diseases.[23,24] The high-affinity receptor lacking the beta chain is also expressed on monocytes, Langerhans cells, dendritic cells (i.e., APCs other than B cells), activated eosinophils, and epithelial cells.

The low-affinity IgE receptor, FcεRII, bears structural homology to C-type lectins, but not to FcεRI. (Lectin receptors recognize pathogens and also function as adhesion receptors and signaling molecules.) FcεRII, also known as CD23, is expressed on B and T cells, monocytes, eosinophils, and platelets.[25] CD23 expression is increased by IL-4 and IL-13, and increased CD23 expression would presumably facilitate allergen uptake and presentation to T cells by APCs.[26] Furthermore, B cells from allergic asthmatic patients exposed to allergen have increased CD23 expression.[27] Whether allergic inflammation is initiated when IgE is bound to FcεRII is not clear. However, the solubilized form of CD23 may play a regulatory role in IgE synthesis.[26,28]

When a sensitized individual is exposed to allergen, the allergen binds to IgE receptors on mast cells and basophils. If multivalent, the allergen will cross-link a critical number of cell-bound IgE receptors, leading to cellular activation, secretion of media-tors, and production of the symptoms characteristic of early-phase allergic responses.[28]

Clearly, treatment that interferes with IgE activation of mast cells and basophils may be beneficial. Omalizumab, a recombinant, humanized monoclonal antibody directed against the Fcε portion of IgE, has recently been developed.[29] Important features of this anti-IgE molecule are (1) it does not bind IgE already attached to FcεRI, and therefore does not cause anaphylaxis; (2) it does not activate complement; and (3) it has a much longer half-life than IgE. In phase III trials, omalizumab was administered by subcutaneous injections given every 2 or 4 weeks to patients with allergic rhinitis or with allergic asthma of varying severity.[30,31] All studies showed dramatic reductions in free IgE levels that were dependent on omalizumab dose as well as baseline IgE levels.[32] As levels of serum IgE decreased, so did surface expression of FcεRI on basophils. Moreover, the posttreatment level of free IgE directly correlated with reduced symptom scores, reduced use of rescue medication, and improved quality of life. For asthma, significant reductions in asthma exacerbations, in hospitalizations for asthma, and in the dose of inhaled or oral steroids were also found. A recent phase II trial of omalizumab in peanut-sensitive children showed a decreased sensitivity to oral peanut challenges.

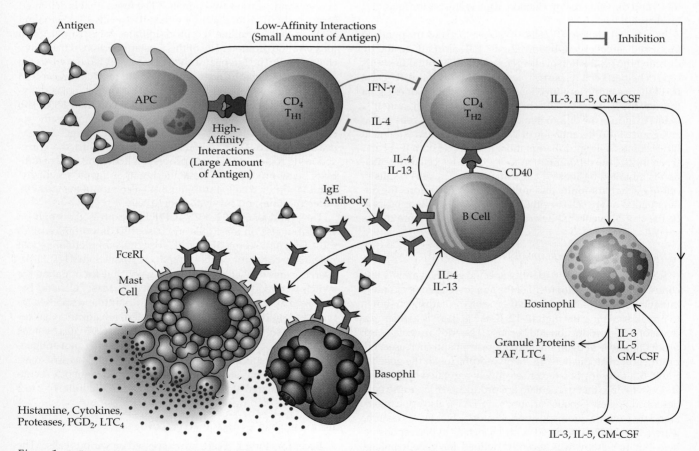

Figure 1 Inflammatory mechanisms in allergic inflammation. Antigen is taken up by antigen-presenting cells (APCs), processed, and then presented to CD4+ helper T cells (T_H). The strength of interactions between APCs and helper T cells and the quantity of antigen present determine the type of T cell response. Production of interferon gamma (IFN-γ) during T_H1 responses downregulates T_H2 responses, whereas interleukin-4 (IL-4) production by T_H2 inhibits T_H1 responses. IL-4 is also critical for switching B cell antibody production to IgE. Signaling through cluster differentiation 40 (CD40) on the B cell is also required for IgE production. Other T_H2 cytokines, such as IL-3, IL-5, and granulocyte-macrophage colony-stimulating factor (GM-CSF) lead to eosinophil (Eos) and basophil (Baso) production and activation. IgE binds to high-affinity receptors on basophils and mast cells (FcεRI); cross-linking by allergen initiates mediator release. (CpG—deoxycytidine-phosphate-deoxyguanosine; LTC₄—leukotriene C₄; PAF—platelet-activating factor; PGD₂—prostaglandin D₂)

DEVELOPMENT AND ACTIVATION OF EOSINOPHILS

Eosinophils share a common origin with basophils: a single bone-marrow–derived myeloid progenitor cell has the capacity to give rise to a mixed colony of eosinophils and basophils or to pure colonies of either cell type.[33] A common origin for eosinophils and basophils is further supported by the presence of Charcot-Leyden crystal (CLC) protein and major basic protein (MBP) in both cell types. Eosinophil development is uniquely dependent on the presence of IL-5, a cytokine whose chief source is the T_{H2} helper cell.[34] Along with IL-5, other T cell cytokines—IL-3 and granulocyte-macrophage colony-stimulating factor (GM-CSF)—promote maturation, activation, and prolonged survival of eosinophils.[33] However, only IL-5 potently stimulates the bone marrow to produce eosinophils. In vitro, a low dose of IL-3 favors the development of basophils from progenitors, whereas a high dose of IL-3 favors the development of eosinophils. In contrast, other cytokines may inhibit the growth of eosinophil progenitors. Transforming growth factor–β (TGF-β) contributes to eosinophil apoptosis in vitro and influences progenitor development toward the basophil pathway.[35] IFN-α inhibits progenitor cells in vitro and has been used for treatment of certain patients with eosinophilia refractory to treatment with prednisone.[36]

Eosinophils dwell primarily in tissue. Circulating eosinophils have a short half-life and represent only about 1% of the total number of eosinophils in the body. Epithelial surfaces of mucosal tissues that are exposed to the external environment are heavily inhabited by eosinophils, whereas other tissues are normally devoid of eosinophils.[33] The epithelial tissues of the respiratory tract produce GM-CSF, which is capable of prolonging eosinophil survival in vitro for up to 14 days.

Cell Surface Receptors

Two overlapping populations of circulating eosinophils are thought to represent differing states of eosinophil activation.[37] Nonallergic individuals have greater numbers of eosinophils of normal density and fewer numbers of low-density activated eosinophils. The reverse is true for patients with disorders leading to eosinophilia. This heterogeneity suggests that priming of eosinophils by various cytokines may lead to changes in expression of surface receptors and mediator release [see Table 2]. For example, both high-affinity receptors (FcεRI) and low-affinity receptors (FcεRII) for IgE have been found on peripheral blood eosinophils from patients with hypereosinophilic syndrome. However, eosinophils derived from normal donors or from patients with allergy fail to stain with a panel of monoclonal antibodies directed against IgE receptors.[38] Similar differences have been observed for IgG receptors (FcγR) on eosinophils. Freshly isolated eosinophils express FcγRIIb, a low-affinity IgG receptor that may inhibit mediator release when cross-linked.[34] Both FcγRI and FcγRIII can be induced on eosinophils in vitro when these cells are cultured with IFN-γ, which, in contrast to FcγRIIb, may result in activation. Sera from patients with hay fever contain allergen-specific IgG1 and IgG3, which cause eosinophils to degranulate in vitro in an allergen-dependent manner.[39] Surface receptors for IgA are also present on eosinophils and provide a potent stimulus for release of granule proteins in vitro. The presence of secretory IgA (sIgA) together with eosinophils at mucosal surfaces suggests that IgA-dependent activation also occurs in vivo.[40]

Receptors for complement (C3a and C5a); the lipid mediators platelet-activating factor (PAF), leukotriene C_4 (LTC_4), and LTB_4; and numerous cytokines and chemokines bind to and activate

Table 2 Receptors on Eosinophils	
IgE receptors	Lipid-mediator receptors
FcεRI (high affinity)	Leukotriene (LT) receptors
FcεRII (low affinity)	LTC_4
IgA receptor	LTB_4
Complement receptors	Platelet-activating factor (PAF)
C3a	Chemokine receptors
C5a	CCR3
	Others

eosinophils.[33,34] Chemokines of the C-C family play an important chemotactic role for eosinophils. Chemokines of this large family have adjacent cysteine residues (C-C) and have the same receptors. A particular C-C chemokine receptor, CCR3, is found abundantly on eosinophils but not on neutrophils.[41] CCR3 binds at least four chemokines that play crucial roles in the homing of eosinophils to epithelial tissues and that activate eosinophils to release mediators. Another mechanism, which leads to preferential accumulation of eosinophils rather than neutrophils at sites of allergic inflammation, relates to differences in expression of surface adhesion molecules. Eosinophils and neutrophils share several selectins and integrins that initiate the rolling of circulating cells along the endothelium, as well as the subsequent firm adhesion, diapedesis, and transmigration of these cells through the vessel wall. However, eosinophils—but not neutrophils—express an integrin, very late antigen (VLA)-4, whose ligand on endothelial cells (VCAM-1) is upregulated by IL-4 and IL-13, cytokines that are present during T_{H2} responses; consequently, these cytokines promote adherence of eosinophils, but not neutrophils, to endothelium.[42]

Mediators

An array of inflammatory mediators are produced when eosinophils are activated. Preformed mediators are stored in granules and rapidly released once eosinophils are activated. Major basic protein (MBP) is the principal constituent of the granule proteins.[43] Other granule proteins include eosinophil peroxidase (EPO), eosinophil-derived neurotoxin (EDN), and eosinophil cationic protein (ECP). MBP, ECP, and EPO have been shown to damage parasites in vitro; in patients with eosinophil-associated diseases, these proteins are present in high concentrations that can cause toxicity to autologous cells and tissues. Unfortunately, MBP and EPO cause ciliostasis and detachment of respiratory epithelial cells in vitro, and they may contribute to epithelial damage and inflammation in allergic respiratory disorders.[43] However, in one study, treatment of asthmatic patients with anti–IL-5 monoclonal antibody resulted in the selective elimination of eosinophils from the airway, but airway hyperreactivity or the airway response to inhaled allergen were not affected. This leaves open the question of the precise role that eosinophils play in the pathogenesis of atopic asthma.[44] Proteases present in the eosinophils may contribute to airway damage by degrading collagen.[45]

Lipid mediators are rapidly generated by eosinophils after appropriate stimulation. PAF production may lead to activation of platelets, neutrophils, and smooth muscle cells, and thereby induce bronchoconstriction and amplify inflammation. The major eicosanoid product of eosinophils is LTC_4, from which LTD_4 and LTE_4 are derived. These sulfidopeptides are extremely potent at contracting airway smooth muscle, stimulating mucus produc-

a

b

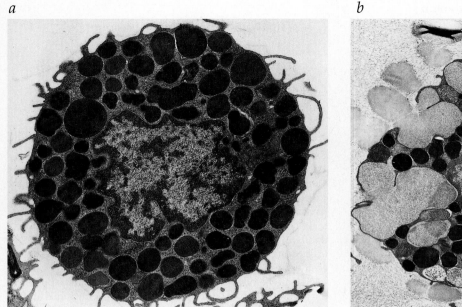
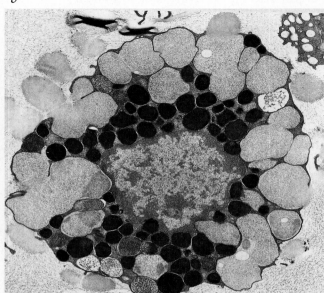

Figure 2 (*a*) **Before introduction of antigen, a sensitized mast cell contains many osmotic granules.** (*b*) **Sixty seconds after treatment with antigen, the peripheral granules have enlarged, neighboring granules have fused, and expulsion of granules from the mast cell has begun.**

tion, causing capillary leakage, and promoting chemotaxis of eosinophils.

Numerous cytokines have been identified as potential eosinophil products. Some may function in an autocrine or paracrine manner to activate or prime eosinophils. Others enhance eosinophil development and survival. In addition, eosinophils produce cytokines that regulate immune responses. However, eosinophils elaborate a considerably smaller quantity of cytokines than do lymphocytes. Therefore, the importance of the eosinophil-derived cytokines to allergic inflammation is unclear. Some cytokines that have been demonstrated in vitro have been confirmed in vivo by identifying the protein product in eosinophils infiltrating affected tissues. For example, eosinophils from nasal polyp tissue stain for TGF-β1 and could contribute to the structural pathology.[46] Exposure of allergic patients to allergen revealed eosinophils in nasal mucosal tissues that stain for IL-5 protein; however, much larger contributions of IL-5 are anticipated from T cells in the same tissue.[47]

MAST CELLS AND BASOPHILS AS EFFECTORS OF THE ALLERGIC RESPONSE

Microscopy of mast cells and basophils reveals intensely staining metachromatic granules [*see Figure 2*]. Other common features shared by these cells include the presence of high-affinity receptors for IgE, the release of histamine after cross-linking of the FcεRI by allergen, and common intracellular signaling pathways.[48] There are also numerous differences between the two cell types. Basophils generally complete their maturation in the bone marrow, circulate in the blood, and then are recruited to sites of inflammation.[49] Mast cells that complete their maturation in the bone marrow appear to remain there, whereas those found in peripheral tissues develop from progenitor cells that seed these tissues. Mature mast cells in peripheral tissues may reside there for many months, retaining antigen-specific IgE for periods that exceed the lifespan of IgE in the circulation. Mast cells are strategically distributed in tissues or at mucosal surfaces that interface with the external environment; they are also in proximity to blood vessels and nerves.[50]

All mast cells contain tryptase in their granules; its release is characteristic of mast cell degranulation. However, several additional features further distinguish two types of mast cells [*see Figure 3*].[51] Mast cells of the T type (MC$_T$ cells) are normally the predominant type of mast cell found in the mucosa of the small intestine and in the alveolar wall and epithelium of the respiratory tract. MC$_T$ cells are identified morphologically by a scroll-rich granule structure; they contain tryptase but not chymase, cathepsin G, or mast cell carboxypeptidase. The numbers of MC$_T$ cells in respiratory epithelium are increased in allergic airway inflammation, making them more accessible to inhaled allergens. In a study in asthmatics, increased mast cells predominantly of the MC$_{TC}$ type were localized to the airway smooth muscles but were not present in control subjects or in patients with eosinophilic bronchitis.[52]

In contrast, the MC$_{TC}$ type of mast cell is the dominant type of mast cell in the dermis, conjunctiva, blood vessel walls, and small-intestinal submucosa. Morphologically, MC$_{TC}$ cells display a lattice/grating, scroll-poor granule structure. In addition to tryptase, TC-type mast cells contain chymase, cathepsin G, and mast cell carboxypeptidase. The development of both mast cell types requires stem cell factor (SCF), the ligand for the Kit (tyrosine kinase) receptor. Factors that regulate the recruitment, development, or survival of one mast cell type over the other are not known. Lineage-committing growth factors such as GM-CSF may divert hematopoietic progenitor cells that are capable of forming mast cells when exposed to SCF alone to non–mast cell lineages.[53]

Mediators

Mast cells and basophils form histamine by decarboxylation of histidine. They then store the histamine in their granules. Degranulation releases the histamine, which then interacts with histamine receptors on various tissues. Histamine induces smooth-

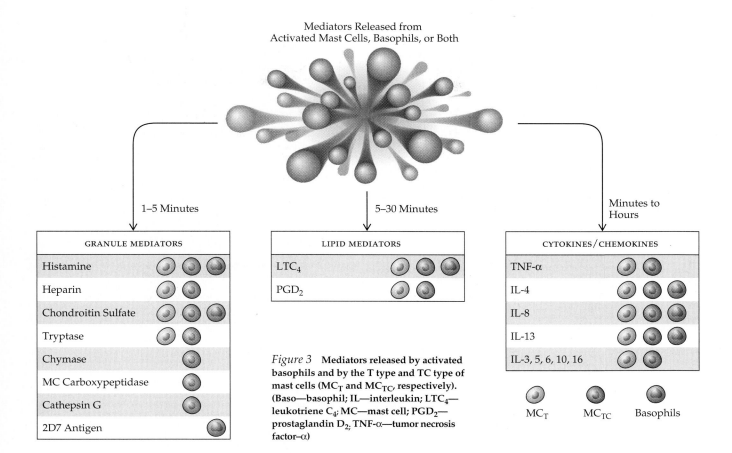

Figure 3 **Mediators released by activated basophils and by the T type and TC type of mast cells (MC$_T$ and MC$_{TC}$, respectively). (Baso—basophil; IL—interleukin; LTC$_4$—leukotriene C$_4$; MC—mast cell; PGD$_2$—prostaglandin D$_2$; TNF-α—tumor necrosis factor–α)**

muscle contraction, increases mucous secretion in the airway, and stimulates nerve fibers. In addition, it enhances vascular permeability and dilates blood vessels, which results in hypotension if a critical number of cells degranulate. Chondroitin sulfates are proteoglycans that are present in the granules of both basophils and mast cells; heparin proteoglycan is stored exclusively in all mast-cell secretory granules. Both chondroitin sulfate and heparin proteoglycans play a role in packaging of histamine, proteases, and carboxypeptidases in the granules.[54] Heparin is also involved in the processing of chymase and tryptase to catalytically active enzymes. Neutralization of the acidic granule pH during degranulation facilitates the dissociation of histamine from the protease-proteoglycan macromolecular complex.[55] Consequently, histamine appears in the serum within minutes of induction of systemic anaphylaxis by allergen-dependent cross-linking of IgE on mast cells and basophils. Not surprisingly, peak plasma levels of histamine occur 5 minutes after insect-sting–induced anaphylaxis begins and decline to baseline within 20 minutes. Because they are relatively transient, these elevations in histamine levels in plasma are difficult to utilize for the clinical determination of anaphylaxis as a cause of hypotension. However, tryptase diffuses into, and is removed from, the circulation more slowly than histamine. Tryptase levels peak in the circulation 15 minutes to 2 hours after mast-cell degranulation and decline with a half-life of about 2 hours. Peak levels during insect-sting–induced anaphylaxis correlate closely to the drop in mean arterial blood pressure, which is an important measure of clinical severity. For that reason, serum or plasma tryptase levels have recently been recognized as a clinically useful marker for the diagnosis of systemic anaphylaxis.[55]

Prostaglandin D$_2$ (PGD$_2$) is a newly synthesized cyclooxygenase product of arachidonic acid produced by MC$_T$ and MC$_{TC}$ cells, but not by basophils. PGD$_2$ causes airway smooth muscle to contract, blood vessels to dilate, and platelets to remain unaggregated. In one study of patients with systemic mastocytosis and recurrent episodes of cardiovascular collapse that did not respond to antihistamines, therapeutic success was achieved with cyclooxgenase inhibition that diminished PGD$_2$ production.[56] LTC$_4$ is produced by both mast cells and basophils, as well as by eosinophils, and it is a potent mediator of airway smooth muscle contraction and mucus secretion. Effects of LTC$_4$ are blocked by 5-lipoxygenase inhibition and by leukotriene receptor antagonists.

Mast cells secrete a diverse array of cytokines, including TNF-α, GM-CSF, SCF, and interleukins 3, 4, 5, 6, 10, 13, and 16.[50] TNF-α can reside preformed in mast cell granules and is also synthesized and secreted after mast cell activation. TNF-α causes chemotaxis and activation of many leukocytes, as well as activation of vascular endothelium. IL-4 and IL-13 are central to T$_{H2}$ differentiation, IgE isotype switching, and induction of the adhesion receptors VCAM-1 on endothelium and VLA-4 on eosinophils. Basophils do not synthesize TNF-α and generally produce fewer cytokines than do mast cells. However, activated basophils synthesize more IL-4 and IL-13 on a per-cell basis than any other cell type. In tissues with allergic inflammation that are challenged with allergen, basophils appear to be the predominant source of antigen-specific production of IL-4 and IL-13.[49]

As with eosinophils, a subpopulation of low-density (so-called hypodense) basophils can be detected in peripheral blood samples. This subpopulation is more sensitive to the effects of glucocorticoids than the higher-density basophils. However, functional differences in the hypodense basophils have not been characterized, as they have for eosinophils. Recently, basophil-specific markers have been developed.[57] The monoclonal antibodies named 2D7 and BB1 detect basophil-specific antigens in secretory granules and should prove useful for more precise assessment of basophil involvement in human allergic diseases. For example, substantial numbers of basophils can now be detected in skin and respiratory tissues during the late-phase response to an allergen challenge, and these cells account for a major portion of the IL-4–containing cells in such tissues. Basophils appear to be similar to eosinophils in expression of numerous cytokines and chemokine receptors, including CCR3. Exposure of basophils to most CC chemokines leads to histamine release.

References

1. Richet C: Anaphylaxis. The University Press, Liverpool, 1913

2. Prescott SL, Macaubas C, Holt BJ, et al: Transplacental priming of the human immune system to environmental allergens: universal skewing of initial T cell responses toward the Th2 cytokine profile. J Immunol 160:4730, 1998

3. Bjorksten B: The intrauterine and postnatal environments. J Allergy Clin Immunol 104:1119, 1999

4. Klein J, Sato A: The HLA system: first of two parts. N Engl J Med 343:702, 2000

5. Langenkamp A, Messi M, Lanzavecchia A, et al: Kinetics of dendritic cell activation: impact on priming of Th1, Th2 and nonpolarized T cells. Nat Immunol 1:311, 2000

6. Palucka K, Banchereau J: Dendritic cells: a link between innate and adaptive immunity. J Clin Immunol 19:12, 1999

7. Klein J, Sato A: The HLA system: second of two parts. N Engl J Med 343:782, 2000

8. Rogers PR, Croft M: Peptide dose, affinity, and time of differentiation can contribute to the Th1/Th2 cytokine balance. J Immunol 163:1205, 1999

9. Wild JS, Sur S: CpG oligonucleotide modulation of allergic inflammation. Allergy 56:365, 2001

10. Tighe H, Corr M, Roman M, et al: Gene vaccination: plasmid DNA is more than just a blueprint. Immunol Today 19:89, 1998

11. Kay AB: Allergy and allergic diseases: first of two parts. N Engl J Med 344:30, 2001

12. Wills-Karp M, Luyimbazi J, Xu X, et al: Interleukin-13: central mediator of allergic asthma. Science 282:2258, 1998

13. Till S, Durham S, Dickason R, et al: IL-13 production by allergen-stimulated T cells is increased in allergic disease and associated with IL-5 but not IFN-gamma expression. Immunology 91:53, 1997

14. Kondo N, Matsui E, Kaneko H, et al: Reduced interferon-gamma production and mutations of the interleukin-12 receptor beta (2) chain gene in atopic subjects. Int Arch Allergy Immunol 124:117, 2001

15. Tamura K, Arakawa H, Suzuki M, et al: Novel dinucleotide repeat polymorphism in the first exon of the STAT-6 gene is associated with allergic diseases. Clin Exp Allergy 31:1509, 2001

16. Van Eerdewegh P, Little RD, Dupuis J, et al: Association of the ADAM33 gene with asthma and bronchial hyperresponsiveness. Nature 418:426, 2002

17. Gehring U, Bischof W, Fahlbusch B, et al: House dust endotoxin and allergic sensitization in children. Am J Respir Crit Care Med 166:939, 2002

18. Busse WW, Lemanske RF Jr: Asthma. N Engl J Med 344:350, 2001

19. Bacharier LB, Geha RS: Molecular mechanisms of IgE regulation. J Allergy Clin Immunol 105:S547, 2000

20. Doyle IS, Hollmann CA, Crispe IN, et al: Specific blockade by CD54 and MHC II of CD40-mediated signaling for B cell proliferation and survival. Exp Cell Res 265:312, 2001

21. Kinet JP: The high-affinity IgE receptor (Fc epsilon RI): from physiology to pathology. Annu Rev Immunol 17:931, 1999

22. Donnadieu E, Jouvin MH, Kinet JP: A second amplifier function for the allergy-associated Fc(epsilon)RI-beta subunit. Immunity 12:515, 2000

23. Saini SS, MacGlashan DWJ, Sterbinsky SA, et al: Down-regulation of human basophil IgE and Fc epsilon RI alpha surface densities and mediator release by anti-IgE infusions is reversible in vitro and in vivo. J Immunol 162:5624, 1999

24. Saini SS, Richardson JJ, Wofsy C, et al: Expression and modulation of Fc epsilon RI-alpha and Fc epsilon RIbeta in human blood basophils. J Allergy Clin Immunol 107:832, 2001

25. Squire CM, Studer EJ, Lees A, et al: Antigen presentation is enhanced by targeting antigen to the Fc epsilon RII by antigen-anti-Fc epsilon RII conjugates. J Immunol 152:4388, 1994

26. Kisselgof AB, Oettgen HC: The expression of murine B cell CD23, in vivo, is regulated by its ligand, IgE. Int Immunol 10:1377, 1998

27. Bonnefoy JY, Lecoanet-Henchoz S, Aubry JP, et al: CD23 and B-cell activation. Curr Opin Immunol 7:355, 1995

28. Pearlman DS: Pathophysiology of the inflammatory response. J Allergy Clin Immunol 104:S132, 1999

29. Presta LG, Lahr SJ, Shields RL, et al: Humanization of an antibody directed against IgE. J Immunol 151:2623, 1993

30. Milgrom H, Fick RB Jr, Su JQ, et al: Treatment of allergic asthma with monoclonal anti-IgE antibody. rhuMAb-E25 Study Group. N Engl J Med 341:1966, 1999

31. Adelroth E, Rak S, Haahtela T, et al: Recombinant humanized mAB-E25, an anti-IgE mAb, in birch pollen-induced seasonal allergic rhinitis. J Allergy Clin Immunol 106:253, 2000

32. Johansson SG, Haahtela T, O'Byrne PM: Omalizumab and the immune system: an overview of preclinical and clinical data. Ann Allergy Asthma Immunol 89:132, 2002

33. Gleich GJ: Mechanisms of eosinophil-associated inflammation. J Allergy Clin Immunol 105:651, 2000

34. Rothenberg ME: Eosinophilia. N Engl J Med 338:1592, 1998

35. Atsuta J, Fujisawa T, Iguchi K, et al: Inhibitory effect of transforming growth factor beta 1 on cytokine-enhanced eosinophil survival and degranulation. Int Arch Allergy Immunol 108:31, 1995

36. Gratzl S, Palca A, Schmitz M, et al: Treatment with IFN-alpha in corticosteroid-unresponsive asthma. J Allergy Clin Immunol 105:1035, 2000

37. Fukuda T, Dunnette SL, Reed CE, et al: Increased numbers of hypodense eosinophils in the blood of patients with bronchial asthma. Am Rev Respir Dis 132:981, 1985

38. Smith SJ, Ying S, Meng Q, et al: Blood eosinophils from atopic donors express messenger RNA for the alpha, beta, and gamma subunits of the high-affinity IgE receptor (Fc epsilon RI) and intracellular, but not cell surface, alpha subunit protein. J Allergy Clin Immunol 105:309, 2000

39. Kaneko M, Swanson MC, Gleich GJ, et al: Allergen-specific IgG1 and IgG3 through Fc gamma RII induce eosinophil degranulation. J Clin Invest 95:2813, 1995

40. Abu-Ghazaleh RI, Fugisawa T, Mestecky J, et al: IgA-induced eosinophil degranulation. J Immunol 142:2393, 1989

41. Heath H, Qin S, Rao P, et al: Chemokine receptor usage by human eosinophils: the importance of CCR3 demonstrated using an antagonistic monoclonal antibody. J Clin Invest 99:178, 1997

42. Schleimer RP, Sterbinsky SA, Kaiser J, et al: IL-4 induces adherence of human eosinophils and basophils but not neutrophils to endothelium: association with expression of VCAM-1. J Immunol 148:1086, 1992

43. Gleich GJ, Adolphson MS, Leiferman KM: Annual Reviews of Medicine: Selected Topics in Clinical Sciences. Creger WP, Coggins CH, Hancock EW, Eds. Annual Reviews, Inc., Palo Alto, California, 1993, p 85

44. Leckie MJ, ten Brinke A, Khan J, et al: Effects of an interleukin-5 blocking monoclonal antibody on eosinophils, airway hyper-responsiveness, and the late asthmatic response. Lancet 356:2144, 2000

45. Mallya SK, Hall JE, Lee HM, et al: Interaction of matrix metalloproteinases with serine protease inhibitors: new potential roles for matrix metalloproteinase inhibitors. Ann NY Acad Sci 732:303, 1994

46. Bachert C, Gevaert P, Holtappels G, et al: Nasal polyposis: from cytokines to growth. Am J Rhinol 14:279, 2000

47. Lee CH, Lee KS, Rhee CS, et al: Distribution of RANTES and interleukin-5 in allergic nasal mucosa and nasal polyps. Ann Otol Rhinol Laryngol 108:594, 1999

48. Holgate ST: The role of mast cells and basophils in inflammation. Clin Exp Allergy 30:28, 2000

49. Bochner BS: Systemic activation of basophils and eosinophils: markers and consequences. J Allergy Clin Immunol 106:S292, 2000

50. Williams CM, Galli SJ: The diverse potential effector and immunoregulatory roles of mast cells in allergic disease. J Allergy Clin Immunol 105:847, 2000

51. Gurish MF, Austen KF: The diverse roles of mast cells. J Exp Med 194:71, 2001

52. Brightling CE, Bradding P, Symon FA, et al: Mast-cell infiltration of airway smooth muscle in asthma. N Engl J Med 346:1699, 2002

53. Mekori YA, Metcalfe DD: Mast cell–T cell interactions. J Allergy Clin Immunol 104:517, 1999

54. Galli SJ: Mast cells and basophils. Curr Opin Hematol 7:32, 2000

55. Schwartz LB, Irani AM: Serum tryptase and the laboratory diagnosis of systemic mastocytosis. Hematol Oncol Clin North Am 14:641, 2000

56. Roberts LJ 2nd, Sweetman BJ, Lewis RA, et al: Increased production of prostaglandin D2 in patients with systemic mastocytosis. N Engl J Med 303:1400, 1980

57. Kepley CL, Craig SS, Schwartz LB: Identification and partial characterization of a unique marker for human basophils. J Immunol 154:6548, 1995

Acknowledgment

Figures 1 and 3   Seward Hung.

Mitchell H. Grayson, M.D., *and Phillip Korenblat,* M.D.

By definition, allergy is an untoward physiologic event mediated by immune mechanisms, usually involving the interaction of an allergen with the allergic antibody, IgE. Common illnesses mediated in this manner include allergic asthma and rhinitis, Hymenoptera hypersensitivity, and certain other causes of anaphylaxis. In addition, a significant proportion of drug, food, and skin reactions are allergic in origin.

Allergic diseases in general, and asthma in particular, have been increasing in prevalence in high-income societies.[1] Although there are undoubtedly many reasons for this increase, one is described in the so-called hygiene hypothesis, which posits that greater exposure to infectious agents (and bacterial endotoxins in particular) early in life reduces the likelihood of subsequent allergy.[2] This hypothesis acknowledges an etiologic role for both genetic and environmental factors in allergy: a child with a hereditary predisposition to atopy is more likely to develop clinical allergy if raised in a relatively aseptic environment.

History

In allergic illnesses, the importance of a careful and thorough medical history cannot be overstated. The clinician must dissect the allergic reaction to understand the nature of the event and identify the antigen that was responsible for the reaction. Formal diagnosis of allergy has three elements: characterization of the allergic reaction, correlation with antigen exposure, and demonstration of IgE specific for the suspected allergen. The history is essential for the first two elements, and for practical purposes, the history can sometimes obviate the third element.

The history should begin with a review of the patient's symptoms and their temporal pattern. If the presenting symptoms include wheezing, the clinician should remember the time-honored statement that all that wheezes is not asthma. Furthermore, all that is asthma is not allergy [see Chapter 212].

The presenting symptoms must match the set of features that characterize the suspected allergic illness. For example, patients with perennial allergic rhinitis typically present with sneezing, rhinorrhea, nasal itching, and nasal congestion. Postnasal drainage is not the only symptom of this disease, so postnasal drainage alone—even with evidence of antigen exposure and the presence of specific IgE antibodies—would not support the diagnosis of allergic rhinitis.

A central aspect of the history is to establish a link between the time and site of exposure to the presumed allergen and the development of allergic symptoms. Seasonal allergic events are often so characteristic that the diagnosis can be made solely on the basis of the presenting symptoms and their correlation with environmental exposure to the allergen; laboratory evidence may not be needed for the diagnosis. Similarly, symptoms that develop immediately after exposure to animals or their dander often do not need additional supporting evidence for diagnosis.

In the United States, the presence of airborne pollen may vary both temporally and geographically.[3] In general, early spring is accompanied by tree pollen, and late spring, by grass pollen. Ragweed and other weed pollens are prevalent in the fall, usually until the first hard frost. Mold spores can be found indoors year-round, except in very dry areas. Outdoor mold spores peak during the summer and fall months, and they diminish when snow covers the landscape [see Table 1].

Illnesses such as asthma or rhinitis that occur on a perennial basis, if allergic, should correlate with environmental exposure to a perennial allergen (e.g., dust mites, indoor mold spores, animal dander, or cockroach antigen). Such exposure most often takes place in the household, but the possibility of exposure to allergens in the workplace should not be forgotten.

Allergic reactions to ingested substances typically include skin eruptions, abdominal discomfort, or respiratory symptoms. Severe and life-endangering reactions involving the cardiovascular or respiratory system, or both, may also occur. The list of ingested substances said to cause allergic reactions is seemingly endless. However, foods (particularly peanuts, tree nuts, shellfish, and seeded fruits) and medications are the most common triggers of this type of allergic reaction. Again, the history is essential to establishing a particular substance as the probable cause of an allergic reaction.

The family history is important. Allergic predisposition is genetically mediated, so patients with allergies often report that family members have similar problems. However, in a patient who has both a personal and a family history of angioedema, the disorder may be inherited but not allergic: hereditary angioedema results from the absence of the C1 esterase inhibitor.

Physical Examination

The physical examination of a patient with a suspected allergic illness requires an in-depth focus on the involved organ system or systems. In atopic dermatitis, the skin findings may include patches of lesions that are pruritic, erythematous, papular, scaling, crusting, vesicular, or lichenified—qualities that may occur alone or in combination [see Figure 1]. Lesions are usually characterized by periodic exacerbations, and it is important to examine these lesions for pyogenic infections.

The distribution of allergic dermatitis lesions varies with the age of the patient. In infants, the dermatitis begins to appear by

---

Table 1 Inhaled Aeroallergens That Cause Rhinitis, Conjunctivitis, and Asthma

Pollens (tree, grass, and weed pollens)
Dust mites (*Dermatophagoides* species)
Animal proteins (cat, dog, horse, guinea pig, gerbil, and rat proteins)
Fungal spores (*Alternaria, Aspergillus, Penicillium,* and *Cladosporium* species)
High-molecular-weight organic compounds derived from plants, bacteria, and insects
Low-molecular-weight inorganic and organic chemicals

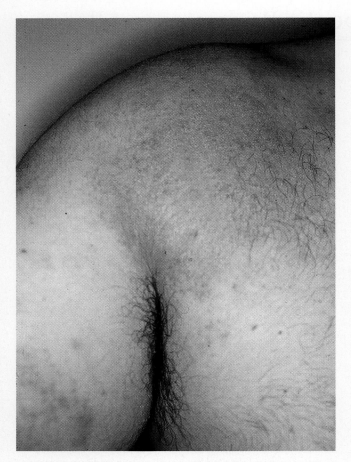

Figure 1 **Atopic dermatitis is characterized by patches of lesions that may be pruritic, erythematous, papular, scaling, crusting, vesicular, or lichenified.**

the sixth to eighth week of life. At this age, the eruptions ordinarily involve the scalp, face (especially the cheeks), ears, and extensor surfaces of the extremities. The trunk, buttocks, and anogenital regions may also be involved. The dermatitis may continue into childhood, or it may first develop at about 2 years of age. Dermatitis in childhood is often found in the antecubital and popliteal fossa, on the neck, and at the flexor and extensor areas of the wrist. In adolescents and adults, the lesions frequently involve the neck and the flexural areas but may occur anywhere on the skin.[4]

Typical urticarial lesions are pruritic, transient (individual lesions resolve within 24 hours), erythematous, and raised; they comprise a wheal with a surrounding erythematous flare. Urticaria can be confused with skin lesions of vasculitis. The presence of hemorrhage or a lesion that lasts longer than 24 hours should raise the specter of urticarial vasculitis. Skin biopsy may be required to differentiate urticarialike lesions.

The hallmarks of allergic rhinoconjunctivitis are bilateral erythema and edema of the conjunctiva, watery ocular discharge, and, often, mild periorbital edema.[5] Allergic shiners (bluish discoloration just below the eye orbits) may be observed. Patients with allergic rhinitis may also have an extra fold in the lower eyelids (Dennie-Morgan lines). On the exterior portion of the nose, a so-called allergic crease may be present, which results from continued upward rubbing of the tip of the nose (the so-called allergic salute). Examination of the nasal cavity often re-

veals watery secretions and edematous, bluish nasal turbinates that partially occlude the nasal passages [*see Chapter 107*]. Translucent nasal polyps may be observed, but these are not necessarily a hallmark of allergy; they can be seen in both allergic and nonallergic patients.

The chest examination often may reveal no abnormalities. However, a methodical examination is warranted. The clinician should observe specifically for cyanosis and the use of accessory muscles for respiration. In addition, auscultation for a prolonged expiratory respiratory phase or inspiratory and expiratory wheezing is indicated. If wheezing is present, it is important to confirm that the sounds emanate from the lungs and not the trachea. All too often, extrathoracic obstruction is missed on the physical examination.

Assays of IgE

Because allergic diseases result from the interaction of an allergen with specific IgE, analysis for specific IgE in a patient with clinical allergy is a major diagnostic consideration. Specific IgE can be identified both by in vivo methods (skin testing) and in vitro methods (radioallergosorbent testing [RAST]).[6]

SKIN TESTING

Epicutaneous Testing

The most rapid and sensitive test for allergy is skin testing. This in vivo method depends on mast cell–bound or basophil-bound IgE specific for the allergen being tested. Because a positive test requires degranulation of mast cells or basophils and subsequent histamine release, antihistamines will interfere with the outcome. In general, patients should discontinue antihistamines 1 week before skin testing, although certain antihistamines can be discontinued 3 days beforehand [*see Table 2*]. Corticosteroids do not inhibit this immediate-phase response, and hence, their use is not a contraindication for skin testing.

Skin testing should be performed by a qualified allergist. Initial testing is performed by pricking the epidermis with a small amount of the specific allergen. In patients with IgE specific for the allergen, a wheal-and-flare response will develop at the site within 20 minutes. The areas of edema and erythema are then measured. The results are often reported as wheal size over flare size (both in millimeters) or, alternatively, identified on a scale of 1 to 4+. This scale compares the skin response to an antigen with the response to a skin prick with histamine, which is used as a positive control. Because some patients develop hives in re-

Table 2   Time before Skin Testing to Stop Antihistamines*

Antihistamine (Trade Name)	Days
Azelastine	7
Cetirizine (Zyrtec)	7
Chlorpheniramine	3
Desloratadine (Clarinex)	7
Diphenhydramine	3
Fexofenadine (Allegra)	7
Loratadine (Claritin)	7

*Note: Other medications (e.g., tricyclic antidepressants) may also have antihistaminic activity.

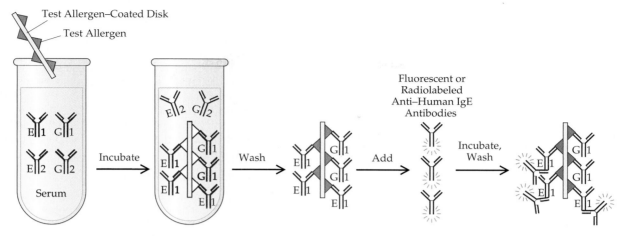

Figure 2   The radioallergosorbent test (RAST). A solid-phase disk coated with the test allergen is incubated with the patient's serum. IgE and IgG antibodies to the test allergen (E1 and G1, respectively) will bind with the allergens on the disk, whereas IgE and IgG antibodies to other allergens (E2 and G2, respectively) will remain free in the serum. After the free antibodies have been washed off, the disk is incubated with antibodies against human IgE that have been labeled with a radioactive or a fluorescent tracer. The tagged anti–human IgE antibodies will then bind IgE attached to the disk; a second washing then removes any unbound tagged antibody. The level of radioactivity or fluorescence is then proportional to the amount of specific IgE against the antigen (E1). IgG against the antigen (G1) does not react with the tagged antibody and therefore is not counted in this test.

sponse to any strong pressure on the skin (dermatographism), a negative control using saline is also used.

Intradermal Testing

If the results of epicutaneous skin testing are negative but the patient's symptoms strongly suggest an allergic etiology, intradermal testing can be performed. This involves injecting 0.02 ml of a dilute allergen solution (usually a 1:100 or 1:1,000 dilution of the concentrated extract) into the dermis. As with epicutaneous testing, the skin is observed for the development of a wheal and flare within 20 minutes. Grading of the results is the same as for epicutaneous testing.

Intradermal testing has a higher sensitivity but a lower specificity than epicutaneous testing. This means that intradermal testing produces more false positives but fewer false negatives than epicutaneous testing.

Intradermal testing exposes the body to a significant antigen load and, therefore, poses a higher risk of a systemic reaction. For that reason, intradermal testing is contraindicated in patients who have not had a prior negative result on epicutaneous testing. It is not surprising that five of the six skin-testing fatalities reported from 1945 to 1987 occurred in patients who underwent intradermal testing without previous epicutaneous testing.[7] Food allergens should never be used for intradermal testing, because they are associated with increased irritant responses. Furthermore, some foods (e.g., peanuts and shellfish) are such potent antigens that they could provoke severe systemic reactions if injected intracutaneously.

Inaccurate or incorrect skin-testing results can occur for a variety of reasons. For example, the use of low-potency extracts can lead to false negative results, as can certain patient factors, such as (1) age (wheals are small in infants, increase until age 50, and then decline), (2) race (whites produce smaller wheals than African Americans[8]), and (3) antihistamine use (including drugs with antihistaminic properties, such as tricyclic antidepressants). In addition, skin-testing results depend on vascular leak; medications such as adrenergic agents can inhibit this response, lead-

ing to false negatives. False positives most often result because of irritant reactions, dermatographism, or a nonspecific reaction from a nearby strong reaction (a so-called bystander reaction).

RADIOALLERGOSORBENT TESTING

RAST and other in vitro tests measure the concentration of nonspecific and allergen-specific IgE in the patient's serum. Because these tests do not depend on IgE-mediated histamine release for their interpretation, they are not adversely affected by the use of antihistamines and other medications (except for anti-IgE, omalizumab [see below]). Although there are circumstances in which high levels of nonspecific IgE can be found, determination of nonspecific IgE is generally of little value, because IgE concentrations vary substantially and there is significant overlap between patients with atopic disease and patients with nonatopic disease. However, the determination of allergen-specific IgE can be useful, especially in patients in whom skin testing cannot be performed (e.g., because of skin disease or inability to stop using antihistamines).

RAST is the most common method of determining allergen-specific IgE in the serum [*see Figure 2*]. This test involves adding the patient's serum to a solid phase (usually a disk) coated with the allergen to be tested. Antibodies in the patient's serum that are specific for the allergen will bind to the solid phase. After the disk is washed, to remove the unbound allergen, antibodies against human IgE that have been tagged with either a radioactive isotope or a fluorescent marker are added. The disk is then washed again, to remove unbound tagged IgE. The level of radiation or fluorescence that is present after washing the disk is directly proportional to the quantity of allergen-specific IgE in the patient's serum. Comparing these values with those obtained by known standards allows for the determination of allergen-specific IgE.

Although RAST results generally correlate with allergic sensitivity, RAST is more likely than skin testing to produce false positive results. As such, the sensitivity of RAST is lower than that of

---

Table 3 Environmental Control
for Allergy Management

General measures
   Eliminate irritants, especially cigarette smoke, from home
   Keep relative humidity at 45% or less by using air conditioners
      and dehumidifiers
Specific measures
   Pollens: use air conditioner and keep windows of house and car
      closed; during peak pollen season, avoid outside activities
   Molds: outdoor molds can be excluded by keeping windows
      closed; use exhaust fan in bathroom and kitchen to keep
      humidity at 50% or less
   Dust mites: cover mattresses, box spring, and pillows with
      impermeable cases; all bedding should be washed in hot
      water (> 130° F) once a week; use synthetic pillows; if
      possible, remove carpet; keep the humidity at 45% or less
   Feathers: replace feather pillow with Dacron (washable) pillow
      and wash regularly
   Pets: remove the pet from the home; if the patient does not
      agree to remove the pet, the pet should not be permitted in
      the bedroom; in addition, to decrease antigen shedding, the
      pet should be bathed once a week

---

skin testing. Therefore, skin testing is still the preferred method of identifying the allergens to which a person is sensitive.

INTERPRETATION OF IgE TEST RESULTS

Regardless of the modality used to test for IgE, all results must be correlated with the clinical findings. Only tests whose results fit with the patient's symptoms should be considered relevant for explaining those specific symptoms. In other words, a positive result is useful for therapeutic intervention only if the patient has symptoms when exposed to the allergen, and a negative test is useful only if the patient has no symptoms on exposure to the allergen. An example would be a patient who has a positive skin test to a tree pollen yet has no symptoms in the spring but instead has symptoms in the fall, in a region devoid of tree pollen at that time of the year. Even if tests for weeds and molds were negative, this seasonality of symptoms would still suggest that a fall pollen or untested mold spore is to blame for the symptoms rather than trees, as the testing would suggest. A positive skin test in the absence of exposure or symptoms, however, does not mean that the patient will not develop symptoms to the antigen at some time in the future. In general, the clinician should use the clinical history to guide all testing modalities, rather than using the testing to try to identify unknown triggers.

Treatment

ENVIRONMENTAL CONTROL

The most effective therapeutic intervention for atopic disease is removal of the offending allergen or allergens from the patient's environment [*see Table 3*]. For example, environmental control for a patient who is allergic to dust mites would include encasing the pillows and mattress in dust-mite–proof covers, washing all bedding in hot (> 130° F) water weekly, and lowering the ambient humidity in the house to below 45%. For pet-allergic patients, the pet should be removed from the household or, at a minimum, should be kept out of the bedroom at all times. Pollen-sensitive individuals will benefit from staying in air-conditioned environments during the time of year when the offending pollen is prevalent.

PHARMACOLOGIC AGENTS

Although environmental control measures constitute the primary treatment for atopic disease, such interventions are sometimes either impossible to carry out or do not fully resolve the disease. This is the point at which pharmacotherapy should be added. The medications used in allergic disease are targeted to various components of the allergic cascade [*see Figure 3*]. These medications include antihistamines and decongestants, long-acting and short-acting bronchodilators, corticosteroids (both topical and systemic), leukotriene receptor antagonists, and cromolyn or nedocromil sodium.

Antihistamines and Decongestants

Antihistamines block the action of histamine at its receptor.[9] Although there are at least four histamine receptors, most allergic symptoms have been attributed to the H_1 receptor. Symptoms mediated by histamine include pruritus, nasal itching, conjunctivitis, and the wheal-and-flare response.

H_1 receptor antagonists can be divided into two broad categories on the basis of their ability to cross the blood-brain barrier and cause sedation. The classic antihistamines, which cause more sedation, include over-the-counter drugs such as diphenhydramine and chlorpheniramine, as well as prescription medications such as cyproheptadine and hydroxyzine. These medications are strong antihistamines, but their usefulness is limited by their central nervous system side effects. Of particular significance is that CNS effects have been shown to last beyond the sedative effects of these medications, leading to decreased reaction time. Therefore, the recommended choice for long-term therapy is a second-generation or third-generation (active metabolite) antihistamine, which will produce minimal sedation. Examples of such agents include cetirizine (Zyrtec), fexofenadine (Allegra), and loratadine (Claritin) and its metabolite desloratadine (Clarinex). Also available as a nasal spray is azelastine (Astelin), which has both antihistaminic and mast cell–stabilizing properties. In the United States, these medications are currently available by prescription only; however, a Food and Drug Administration panel recently recommended that they be changed to over-the-counter status.[10] It is anticipated that this will happen in the next several years.

Antihistamines do not have a significant effect on nasal congestion. For intermittent congestion, a systemic decongestant may be used. Since phenylpropanolamine (PPA) was taken off the market because of its association with increased frequency of strokes, pseudoephedrine has been the only systemic decongestant available in the United States. Nevertheless, although decongestants provide some relief of the sensation of nasal fullness, they do not alter the underlying etiology.

Bronchodilators

Both short-acting and long-acting bronchodilators are available for treatment of asthma. Short-acting bronchodilators relieve bronchoconstriction but have no effect on the underlying inflammatory process, whereas long-acting bronchodilators not only provide symptomatic relief of bronchoconstriction but also may have slight anti-inflammatory properties. Unfortunately, over time there is loss of potency of bronchodilators when they are used alone (subsensitivity). This loss of potency does not occur, however, when bronchodilators are combined with an inhaled corticosteroid. Given the lack of sufficient anti-inflammatory activity and the subsensitivity of bronchodilators, most authorities recommend using these medications in combination with an inhaled corticosteroid rather than as monotherapy.[11,12]

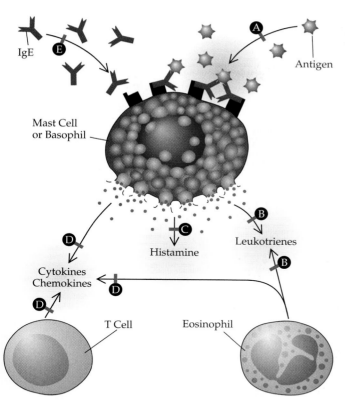

Figure 3 **Mechanisms of action of medications used in allergic diseases. Environmental control (A) minimizes exposure to the antigen to which the patient has specific IgE. If the antigen is present, it binds with specific IgE; cross-linking of the antigen-bound IgE on the surface of a mast cell or basophil starts the allergic cascade, with release of leukotrienes, histamine, cytokines, and chemokines. Leukotriene antagonists (B) block the action of leukotrienes; antihistamines compete with histamine at H_1 receptors; corticosteroids (D) inhibit the production of inflammatory cytokines and chemokines. Anti-IgE therapy (e.g., omalizumab) (E) works by directly reducing the amount of IgE in the body. It is unclear at which sites immunotherapy and cromolyn and nedocromil sodium exert their anti-inflammatory action.**

Corticosteroids

Topical corticosteroids are capable of potent anti-inflammatory effects and are the mainstay of allergic therapy. These medications, inhaled for asthma or taken intranasally for rhinitis, have the ability to abrogate the inflammatory response and interfere with multiple aspects of the allergic cascade. However, unlike antihistamines, which provide rapid relief (within 1 to 2 hours), topical corticosteroids may require 3 to 5 days of therapy before full relief is realized. In rhinitis, steroids can relieve the congestion and raise the threshold for the development of symptoms to allergen exposure.[13,14] Corticosteroids work by inhibiting the production of inflammatory cytokines and chemokines, thus reducing the inflammation and cellular recruitment to sites of disease. These medications play a major role in the treatment of allergic disease.

Oral steroids are quite potent at resolving and preventing most allergic disease. The mechanism of action is felt to be similar to that of topical corticosteroids—that is, by inhibition of cytokines and reduction of edema. Unfortunately, the usefulness of chronic systemic corticosteroid use is limited by the potentially devastating side effects of these agents, including weight gain, abnormal fat deposition, adrenal suppression, cataracts, type 2

(non–insulin-dependent) diabetes mellitus, and osteoporosis. Although these side effects are possible with topical corticosteroid use, they are not usually a major problem. In general, oral corticosteroids are prescribed only for short bursts (< 2 weeks). Longer courses are reserved for patients whose condition has been refractory to all other standard therapies.

Cromolyn and Nedocromil Sodium

Cromolyn and nedocromil sodium are indicated for asthma and allergic rhinitis. These medications have mild anti-inflammatory properties without any significant side effects. Their exact mechanism of action remains unknown.

Leukotriene Antagonists

Leukotriene antagonists (either receptor antagonists or 5-lipoxygenase [5-LO] inhibitors) also have anti-inflammatory properties.[15] Leukotrienes are found at sites of allergic inflammation. Although corticosteroids affect many other inflammatory pathways, they do not seem to have a clinically significant impact on the generation and release of leukotrienes. These molecules are capable of inducing further inflammation by causing the release of additional mediators, as well as the recruitment of inflammatory cells to sites of allergic disease. Consequently, leukotriene antagonists are used in the treatment of asthma as well as allergic rhinitis.[16]

IMMUNOTHERAPY

Immunotherapy, or allergy shots, involves injecting increasing doses of the offending antigen or antigens in an attempt to turn off the specific allergic response. Clinical trials have shown that immunotherapy is successful in treating allergic rhinitis with or without associated asthma.[17,18]

An immunotherapy extract is prepared on the basis of skin-testing results. The patient then receives increasing doses subcutaneously on a weekly or twice-weekly schedule for about 5 months. After this so-called build-up phase, the patient is maintained on a stable dose that is administered weekly to monthly for several years. Usually, patients achieve maximal benefit after being on the maintenance dose for 1 year. The duration of treatment is still under investigation; therefore, the discontinuance of immunotherapy must be determined on an individual basis.

Immunotherapy is usually reserved for those patients in whom environmental and pharmacologic interventions have been less than fully successful. The only patients for whom immunotherapy is almost always indicated are those who have systemic symptoms from venom (Hymenoptera) allergy. Immunotherapy is often indicated for allergic rhinitis or asthma that is clearly associated with sensitivity to specific allergens.[19] It is also used in children, as some data suggest that early treatment of allergic rhinitis with immunotherapy may prevent the subsequent development of asthma.[20] Because of the small but real risk of anaphylaxis, immunotherapy should be given only in a medical office or in another carefully screened location, where personnel and supplies are readily available to treat reactions. Similarly, patients with severe asthma should not be given immunotherapy because of the risk of developing even worse bronchospasm.

Standard immunotherapy (also known as conventional high-dose immunotherapy) should not be confused with other invalidated and inappropriate methods of immunotherapy. These techniques, which should be avoided, include skin-titration testing and treatment (the Rinkel method), subcutaneous provocation and neutralization, and sublingual provocation.[6]

ANTI-IgE THERAPY

The allergic response requires the presence of IgE. A new therapeutic modality that likely soon will be available in the United States is omalizumab, a humanized anti-IgE monoclonal antibody that is administered subcutaneously on a biweekly to monthly schedule and can reduce serum IgE to undetectable levels. This molecule is the hypervariable region from a mouse antibody against human IgE that is genetically grafted onto a human IgG molecule—hence the term humanized. Clinically, omalizumab has been shown to significantly reduce symptom scores in patients with allergic rhinitis, as well as to relieve symptoms and improve airway function in patients with moderate to severe asthma.[21-23] This medication has the ability to block the allergic cascade at its initiation and has not been associated with significant side effects. How it will be used in clinical practice remains to be seen. It is anticipated that omalizumab will be given FDA approval by early 2003.

References

1. Woolcock AJ, Peat JK: Evidence for the increase in asthma worldwide. Ciba Found Symp 206:122,1997

2. Martinez FD: The coming-of-age of the hygiene hypothesis. Respir Res 2:129, 2001

3. Lewis WH, Vinay P, Zenger VE: Airborne and Allergic Pollen of North America. Johns Hopkins University Press, Baltimore, 1983

4. Korenblat PE, Wedner HJ: Allergy, theory and practice, 2nd ed. WB Saunders Co, Philadelphia, 1992, p 210

5. Naclerio R, Solomon W: Rhinitis and inhalant allergens. JAMA 278:1842, 1997

6. Practice parameters for allergy diagnostic testing. Joint Task Force on Practice Parameters for the Diagnosis and Treatment of Asthma. The American Academy of Allergy, Asthma and Immunology and the American College of Allergy, Asthma and Immunology. Ann Allergy Asthma Immunol 75:543, 1995

7. Lockey RF, Benedict LM, Turkeltaub PC, et al: Fatalities from immunotherapy and skin testing. J Allergy Clin Immunol 79:660, 1987

8. Van Niekerk CH, Prinsloo AE: Effect of skin pigmentation on the response to intradermal histamine. Int Arch Allergy Appl Immunol 76:73, 1985

9. Day J: Pros and cons of the use of antihistamines in managing allergic rhinitis. J Allergy Clin Immunol 103:S395, 1999

10. Rollins G: FDA panel recommends OTC status for second-generation antihistamines. Ann Allergy Asthma Immunol 87:3, 2001

11. Sears MR: Asthma treatment: inhaled beta-agonists. Can Respir J 5(suppl A):54A, 1998

12. Taylor DR, Sears MR, Cockcroft DW: The beta-agonist controversy. Med Clin North Am 80:719, 1996

13. Corren J: Intranasal corticosteroids for allergic rhinitis: how do different agents compare? J Allergy Clin Immunol 104:S144, 1999

14. O'Byrne PM: Inhaled corticosteroids in asthma: importance of early intervention. Inhaled Glucocorticoids in Asthma: Mechanisms and Clinical Actions. Schleimer RP, Busse WW, O'Byrne P, Eds. Marcel Dekker, New York, 1996, p 493

15. O'Byrne PM, Israel E, Drazen JM: Antileukotrienes in the treatment of asthma. Ann Intern Med 127:472, 1997

16. Grayson MH, Bochner BS: New concepts in the pathogenesis and treatment of allergic asthma. Mt Sinai J Med 65:246, 1998

17. Dykewicz MS, Fineman S, Skoner DP, et al: Diagnosis and management of rhinitis: complete guidelines of the Joint Task Force on Practice Parameters in Allergy, Asthma and Immunology. American Academy of Allergy, Asthma, and Immunology. Ann Allergy Asthma Immunol 81:478, 1998

18. Abramson MJ, Puy RM, Weiner JJ: Is allergen immunotherapy effective in asthma? A meta-analysis of randomized controlled trials. Am J Respir Crit Care Med 151:969, 1995

19. Bousquet J, Lockey R, Malling HJ: Allergen immunotherapy: therapeutic vaccines for allergic diseases. A WHO position paper. J Allergy Clin Immunol 102:558, 1998

20. Jacobsen L: Preventive aspects of immunotherapy: prevention for children at risk of developing asthma. Ann Allergy Asthma Immunol 87(suppl):43, 2001

21. Busse WW: Anti-immunoglobulin E (omalizumab) therapy in allergic asthma. Am J Respir Crit Care Med 164:S12, 2001

22. Casale TB: Anti-immunoglobulin E (omalizumab) therapy in seasonal allergic rhinitis. Am J Respir Crit Care Med 164:S18, 2001

23. Casale TB, Condemi J, LaForce C, et al: Effect of omalizumab on symptoms of seasonal allergic rhinitis: a randomized controlled trial. JAMA 286:2956, 2001

Acknowledgments

Figure 1   Mark G. Lebwohl, M.D.

Figure 2   Tom Moore.

Figure 3   Seward Hung.

107 Allergic Rhinitis, Conjunctivitis, and Sinusitis

Raymond G. Slavin, M.D.

Allergic rhinitis, allergic conjunctivitis, and sinusitis are closely related disorders. Allergic rhinitis and conjunctivitis share the same causes and pathophysiology; sinusitis typically occurs as a complication of allergic rhinitis.

Allergic Rhinitis

Allergic rhinitis is an allergic inflammatory response in the nose. It can be classified as seasonal or perennial, depending on the allergens triggering the reaction.

EPIDEMIOLOGY

Allergic rhinitis is the most common atopic disorder in the United States. It affects about 39 million Americans—an estimated 16% of the population—with an equal distribution between males and females.[1] The prevalence of allergic rhinitis varies by age: 32% of patients are 17 years of age or younger, 43% are 18 to 44 years of age, 17% are 45 to 64, and only 8% are 65 years of age or older. The costs of treating allergic rhinitis (and the indirect costs of the disorder, such as lowered productivity and time lost from work or school) are substantial. In 1996, the direct health care cost of treating the combined entity of allergic rhinitis and allergic conjunctivitis was close to $2 billion.[2]

ETIOLOGY AND PATHOPHYSIOLOGY

The airborne allergens responsible for allergic rhinitis can be divided into seasonal (trees, grass, weeds, and mold) and nonseasonal or perennial (dust mites, pets, and insects).[3] These soluble aeroallergens land on the nasal mucosa, are processed by antigen-presenting cells, and are then presented to helper T cells. In genetically predisposed persons, this interaction promotes generation and release of cytokines that induce B cells to produce antigen-specific IgE. The IgE attaches to receptors on mast cells and basophils, and the patient is thereby sensitized. On subsequent exposure, the allergen bridges IgE molecules, resulting in release of mediators, most notably histamine.[4] Histamine causes increased epithelial permeability, vasodilatation, and stimulation of a parasympathetic reflex. As a result, acetylcholine is released, resulting in marked hypersecretion of mucus and increased blood flow. Activation of centers in the central nervous system results in sneezing.

DIAGNOSIS

Clinical Manifestations

Symptoms of allergic rhinitis may include paroxysms of sneezing, nasal congestion, clear rhinorrhea, and itching of the nose and palate. Distinct temporal patterns of symptom production may aid diagnosis. For example, seasonal allergic rhinitis symptoms typically appear during a specific time of the year when aeroallergens are abundant in the outside air. Symptoms of rhinitis that occur whenever the patient is exposed to a pet with fur suggest IgE-mediated sensitivity to that species.[5]

Physical Examination

A patient with allergic rhinitis may appear uncomfortable, exhibiting mouth breathing. Children in particular may have so-called allergic shiners (dark rings under the eyes). Allergic shiners develop because the edematous nasal tissue compresses the veins that drain the eyes, leading to pooling of blood under the orbits. On the bridge of the nose, a so-called allergic crease may be present—a result of continued upward rubbing of the tip of the nose (the so-called allergic salute). On nasal examination, the mucosa typically appears pale and swollen, with a bluish-gray hue when the mucosal edema is severe [*see Figure 1*].

Laboratory Testing

Although a careful history is the most important step toward the diagnosis of allergic disease, skin testing may be useful in pinpointing the offending allergen [*see Chapter 106*]. The simplicity, ease and rapidity of performance, low cost, and high sensitivity of skin tests make them preferable to in vitro testing.[6]

DIFFERENTIAL DIAGNOSIS

The two nasal conditions most commonly confused with allergic rhinitis are infectious rhinitis and perennial nonallergic rhinitis (vasomotor rhinitis). Infectious rhinitis is characterized by constitutional symptoms and purulent rhinorrhea. A nasal smear shows a preponderance of neutrophils, whereas in allergic rhinitis, eosinophils predominate. Perennial nonallergic rhinitis is more frequent in women and is precipitated by such nonspecific factors as changes in temperature, humidity, and barometric pressure; strong odors; alcohol; and cigarette smoke. Nasal congestion frequently shifts from side to side and is often alleviated by exercise.[7]

TREATMENT

Therapy for allergic rhinitis comprises three elements. First, the patient should minimize contact with the allergen (environmental control). The second is pharmacotherapy. The third element, immunotherapy, is reserved for selected patients. To-

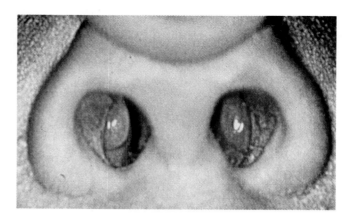

Figure 1 **The nasal mucosa of a patient with allergic rhinitis typically appears pale and swollen. If the edema is severe, the mucosa may have a bluish-gray hue.**

gether, these treatments ensure an excellent prognosis for allergic rhinitis.

Environmental Control

Reducing or completely avoiding the offending allergen is a vital part of allergy management [see Chapter 106]. In the case of seasonal allergies, keeping the doors and windows closed and the air conditioning on will reduce the aeroallergen burden manyfold.[8] Measures to avoid dust mites should focus on the patient's bedroom and include encasing the mattress, box spring, and pillows in occlusive covers; weekly washing of bedding in water at 130° F or hotter; dehumidification to less than 50%; and removal of reservoirs, such as carpeting. Removal of pets is the optimal approach for pet-sensitive patients. If the patient will not part with the pet, weekly washing of the animal will reduce airborne levels of its allergen.[9] Also, patients with allergic rhinitis appear to be more sensitive to nonspecific irritants, such as cigarette smoke.[10]

Pharmacotherapy

Oral antihistamines are effective in reducing itching, sneezing, and rhinorrhea from allergic rhinitis. A major limitation of the first-generation (classic) antihistamines has been sedation. The second-generation antihistamines—cetirizine (Zyrtec), fexofenadine (Allegra), and loratadine (Claritin) and its metabolite desloratadine (Clarinex)—produce significantly less sedation. In patients with nasal congestion, an antihistamine-decongestant combination can be used.[11] An intranasal antihistamine spray, azelastine (Astelin), has also been proven to be efficacious.

The most effective medications for controlling symptoms of allergic rhinitis are nasally inhaled corticosteroids.[12] They include beclomethasone (Vancenase), budesonide (Rhinocort), flunisolide (Nasarel), fluticasone (Flonase), mometasone (Nasonex), and triamcinolone (Nasacort). These agents are generally not associated with significant systemic side effects. Local side effects (e.g., irritation and a burning sensation) are minimized if patients are instructed to direct the spray toward the ear and away from the septum.

Leukotriene receptor antagonists have been considered as a component of combination therapy for allergic rhinitis, but recent studies have not been encouraging, and these agents are not approved for this use. Similarly, cromolyn sodium is not nearly as effective as nasal steroids, and it is inconvenient in that it must be taken four times a day.

On the horizon is the use of anti-IgE therapy for allergic rhinitis. Omalizumab—a recombinant, humanized, monoclonal antibody—has been shown to significantly reduce serum IgE and to have beneficial effects on allergic rhinitis.[13]

Immunotherapy

Allergen immunotherapy is highly effective in controlling symptoms of allergic rhinitis. It should be considered in patients with severe symptoms not controlled by other treatment modalities and in those with comorbid conditions such as asthma. Immunotherapy may prevent worsening of asthma and possibly prevent its development.[14]

COMPLICATIONS

There is good evidence that poorly managed allergic rhinitis can result in otitis media[15] and sinusitis.[16] Rhinitis and asthma frequently coexist. More than that, rhinitis appears to be a risk factor for development of asthma,[17] and treatment of rhinitis can improve coexisting asthma.[18] Prevention of asthma is an especially important goal in patients with a family history of asthma or atopic disease and early sensitization to aeroallergens.[19]

Allergic Conjunctivitis

Allergic conjunctivitis is the ocular counterpart of allergic rhinitis, and the two often occur together. Approximately 70% of patients with allergic conjunctivitis have an associated atopic disease, such as allergic rhinitis, asthma, or atopic dermatitis.

EPIDEMIOLOGY

Seasonal and perennial allergic conjunctivitis are the most prevalent forms of ocular allergy. The incidence ranges from 5% to 22% of the population, depending on the area studied.[20]

ETIOLOGY AND PATHOGENESIS

Allergic conjunctivitis is triggered by the same aeroallergens and results from the same pathophysiologic processes as allergic rhinitis (see above).

DIAGNOSIS

Clinical Manifestations

Patients present with itching of the eyes, accompanied by tearing and a burning sensation. The reaction is usually bilateral, although unilateral conjunctivitis may occur in a patient who has had direct hand-to-eye contact with an allergen such as dog or cat dander.

Physical Examination

The periocular tissues are usually swollen and reddened. The conjunctiva is injected, with mild to moderate chemosis, and there is a ropy mucous discharge in the tear film.

Laboratory Tests

Although examination of the ocular discharge in allergic conjunctivitis typically reveals large numbers of eosinophils, this test is almost never done. Instead, allergic conjunctivitis is generally diagnosed clinically. As with allergic rhinitis, skin testing may be performed to identify the offending allergen or allergens (see above).

DIFFERENTIAL DIAGNOSIS

The eye condition most likely to be confused with allergic conjunctivitis is infectious conjunctivitis (viral or bacterial). Patients with infectious conjunctivitis complain of matting of the eyelids, with a clear to mucopurulent ocular discharge. The conjunctiva is deeply red and although a burning sensation is common, itching is not as profound as in allergic conjunctivitis.

TREATMENT

Allergic conjunctivitis results from the same allergens as allergic rhinitis. Hence, environmental control measures and immunotherapy for this disorder are the same as for allergic rhinitis (see above).

Pharmacotherapy

Drug treatment for allergic conjunctivitis typically begins with an over-the-counter antihistamine-decongestant combination such as antazoline-naphazoline (Vasocon-A) or pheniramine-naphazoline (Naphcon-A).[20] The next line of therapy is a selective H₁ receptor antihistamine, a category that includes ketotifen (Zaditor), levocabastine (Livostin), and olopatadine (Patanol).[20] Ketotifen and olopatadine have mast cell–stabilizing properties. An additional therapeutic option is a nonsteroidal anti-inflammatory agent such as ketorolac (Acular).[21] For the most severe cases of allergic conjunctivitis, the clinician may consider giving corticosteroid eyedrops—loteprednol etabonate (Lotemax) or rimexolone (Vexol)—for 2 to 3 weeks. Long-term use of these agents has been associated with the development of glaucoma, cataracts, and secondary infection and hence should be managed by an ophthalmologist.

Sinusitis

It has been suggested that the term rhinosinusitis may be more accurate than sinusitis, for the following reasons: (1) rhinitis typically precedes sinusitis, (2) sinusitis without rhinitis is rare, (3) the mucosae of the nose and sinuses are contiguous, and (4) symptoms of nasal obstruction and nasal discharge are prominent in sinusitis.[22]

Rhinosinusitis is classified as acute, recurrent acute, subacute, and chronic. Acute sinusitis is defined as inflammation of the sinuses for less than 8 weeks in adults and less than 12 weeks in children. Subacute sinusitis is the development and manifestation of minimal to moderate signs of sinus inflammation without an overt upper respiratory tract infection (URI) or abrupt onset of symptoms. Chronic sinusitis is defined as persistent sinus inflammation for more than 8 to 12 weeks. An operational definition of chronic sinusitis is persistent inflammation, documented with imaging techniques, continuing for at least 4 weeks after initiation of appropriate medical therapy in the absence of an intervening acute episode.

EPIDEMIOLOGY

Rhinosinusitis is the most frequently reported chronic disease in the United States, affecting 14.7% of the population. It accounts for 11.6 million physician office visits a year and is the fifth most common reason for antibiotic use.[23]

In one study of patients with rhinosinusitis, a 36-item health survey showed significant worsening in several domains, including bodily pain, general health, vitality, and social functioning. Comparison with other chronic diseases (e.g., chronic obstructive pulmonary disease, heart failure, angina, and back pain) revealed significantly worse bodily pain and social functioning in patients with sinusitis.[24]

PATHOGENESIS

The paranasal sinuses are composed of the ethmoid, frontal, maxillary, and sphenoid sinuses [see Figure 2]. Microorganisms, pollutants, irritants, and other foreign particles that escape the filtering apparatus of the nose are trapped in the mucus of the sinuses. The steady beating of the cilia that line the sinuses moves mucus out of the sinuses and into the nasal passages via the drainage ostia. This ongoing clearance of the sinuses is important for maintaining health.

The key factors that predispose a person to rhinosinusitis are local [see Table 1]. The most common of these are viral URIs and allergic rhinitis. Edema of the nasal mucosa (which is character-

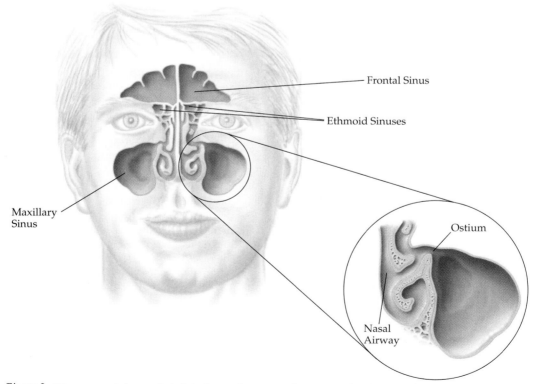

Figure 2 **The paranasal sinuses drain into the nasal passages via narrow ostia. The ostium through which the maxillary sinus drains is on the superior medial wall of the sinus, and hence the maxillary sinuses drain against the force of gravity. Edema of the nasal mucosa from allergic rhinitis can obstruct the ostia, and the resulting accumulation of mucus within the sinuses promotes bacterial infection.**

Table 1 Factors Predisposing to Sinusitis

Upper respiratory infection

Allergic rhinitis

Anatomic variants
  Septal deviation
  Haller cells (infraorbital ethmoid cells)

Hypertrophied adenoids

Nasal polyps, chronic mucosal thickening

Nasal or sinus tumors

Foreign bodies

Cigarette smoke

Swimming and diving; barotraumas

Rhinitis medicamentosa

Cocaine abuse

Nasal intubation

Periapical abscess in a protruding tooth

Dental extraction or injections

istic of acute infectious or allergic rhinitis) results in obstruction of the ostia, decreased ciliary action in the paranasal sinuses, and increased mucus volume and viscosity. The subsequent accumulation of mucus in the sinus provides an environment for secondary bacterial infection and the conversion of mucus to mucopus.

Cultures from both adults and children with acute sinusitis grow predominantly aerobic organisms, with the heaviest yield being *Streptococcus pneumoniae*, *Haemophilus influenzae*, and *Moraxella* (formerly *Branhamella*) *catarrhalis*. Although the role of viruses and bacteria in causing acute infectious sinusitis is well established, the role of microbial infection in chronic sinus disease is much less clear. It was once believed that anaerobic organisms were responsible for chronic sinusitis, but aerobes have now been implicated as the major cause. Alternatively, chronic inflammation rather than infection may be the underlying factor in many patients with chronic sinusitis.[25]

DIAGNOSIS

Clinical Manifestations and Physical Examination

Acute sinusitis The most important clinical clue to the diagnosis of acute sinusitis is the failure of symptoms to resolve after a typical cold. The previously clear nasal discharge becomes yellow or green. Fever persists and chills may develop. Pain is often felt in the cheek, or it may be referred to the forehead. The discomfort is often worse on bending over or straining. If the ostium of the maxillary sinus is blocked, pain may be severe and felt in the teeth.

On physical examination, thick, purulent, green or deep-yellow secretions are seen in the nose on the side of the diseased sinus. Because the maxillary sinus is most frequently involved, purulent secretions will be seen most often in the middle meatus, which is the drainage site of the maxillary sinus [*see Chapter 124*]. The middle meatus may be hidden by the middle turbinate, so it may be necessary to shrink the turbinate with a topical decongestant. Once this is accomplished, the nose (particularly the middle meatus) can be examined thoroughly not only for pus but also for underlying problems, such as nasal septal deviation, spurs, and polyps. Frequently, a streak of pus is visible along the lateral wall of the oropharynx. When the diagnosis of sinusitis is in doubt, referring the patient to an otolaryngologist for fiberoptic nasopharyngoscopy can be helpful, because this technique affords a better opportunity for visualization of the drainage ostia of infected sinuses.

Chronic sinusitis If mucopus is not evacuated, acute sinusitis may enter a subacute or chronic phase. Chronic maxillary sinusitis may exist alone, but it is usually associated with

chronic ethmoid and frontal sinusitis. The lack of pain or systemic symptoms make chronic sinusitis difficult to diagnose on history alone. A patient may complain of dull pressure in the face or head. Chronic sinusitis generally presents as persistent, sometimes unilateral nasal stuffiness, hyposmia, purulent nasal and postnasal secretions, sore throat, fetid breath, and malaise. The secretions often pool in the hypopharynx at night, and the patient complains of increasing postnasal drainage with resultant cough and sometimes wheezing. On physical examination, a patient with chronic sinusitis may display an edematous and hyperemic nasal mucosa bathed in mucopus.

Nasal Smear and Sinus Culture

Nasal culture does not give an adequate picture of the organisms responsible for sinusitis. Microscopic examination of nasal secretions, however, may be of great diagnostic value. In instances of sinusitis, one sees sheets of polymorphonuclear neutrophils and bacteria. This is unlike viral URIs (in which polymorphonuclear neutrophils are scanty) or allergic rhinitis (in which a high percentage of eosinophils may be seen). Antral puncture provides a true specimen of the microbiology of the sinus cavity and is generally performed by an otolaryngologist when it is important to determine the pathogen (e.g., if fungal infection is suspected).[26]

Radiology

Two imaging modalities are used for the diagnosis of sinusitis: plain x-rays and computed tomography. In adults, plain films of the sinuses that show mucosal thickening greater than 8 mm, an air-fluid level, or opacification have been shown to correlate with positive bacterial cultures on antral punctures. In children older than 1 year, abnormal findings on maxillary sinus radiographs are generally related to inflammation of the upper airway. Crying has not been shown to be a cause of abnormalities on sinus radiographs in these children.[27]

The diagnostic value of plain films is controversial. Some authorities advise against ordering plain radiographic studies, particularly for diagnosing chronic sinusitis. Conventional radiographs can depict changes of acute sinusitis in maxillary, ethmoid, frontal, and sphenoid sinuses but cannot delineate the status of individual ethmoid air cells or the ostiomeatal complex, nor can they accurately show the extent of inflammatory disease in affected patients. For these reasons, CT is the radiographic modality of choice for examining the paranasal sinuses. Coronal CT scans demonstrate the ostiomeatal complex and detect subtle disease that is not shown on plain films. In the past, the cost of CT scanning was prohibitive, but through improved technology and the use of limited slices, the price has been reduced to the point where it is quite close to that of plain films in most centers. A limited four-slice coronal CT scan of the sinuses provides much more information than plain films do, and compared with full CT, four-slice coronal CT provides the increased information at a much reduced radiation dose and cost.[28]

Transillumination and ultrasonography are used in the diagnosis of sinusitis. Both are subject to great error, however, and cannot be recommended at the present time.

Ancillary Laboratory Tests

Other laboratory tests may have to be considered in some cases of treatment-resistant sinusitis. Underlying allergy can be determined by appropriate skin testing after a careful history has identified likely allergens. Immunologic testing may be indicated, because patients with refractory sinusitis may have immune dysfunction.[29] Associated immunodeficiency is diagnosed by serum immunoglobulin levels and by antibody responses to specific antigens such as pneumococci, diphtheria, and tetanus. Other considerations in medically resistant sinusitis include cystic fibrosis, fungal infection, and anatomic abnormalities.

DIFFERENTIAL DIAGNOSIS

The condition most often misdiagnosed as rhinosinusitis is a viral URI, which is the most important predisposing cause of acute rhinosinusitis. One is probably dealing with rhinosinusitis if URI symptoms do not resolve in 3 to 6 days, if the secretions (particularly postnasal secretions) turn yellow or green and persist throughout the day, and if the patient notes fullness of the head and discomfort in the face and teeth.

TREATMENT

The antibiotic of choice for treatment of acute sinusitis is ampicillin or amoxicillin. An appropriate dosage of amoxicillin for acute sinusitis in an adult is 875 mg twice a day for 10 to 14 days. In patients with penicillin sensitivity, trimethoprim-sulfamethoxazole (one double-strength tablet twice daily) is an adequate alternative. More and more cases of β-lactamase–producing organisms are being reported. In penicillin-resistant sinusitis, recommended antibiotics include amoxicillin with clavulanic acid (Augmentin) and the quinolones (e.g., levofloxacin [Levaquin]). Antibiotic treatment for chronic sinusitis should be continued for at least 2 weeks. If the patient reports feeling better by the last day of the regimen but still has purulent nasal discharge, the antibiotic can be continued for another 5 to 7 days.

Ancillary treatments for sinusitis, including oral decongestants and mucus thinners, have been advocated, but there are no controlled studies showing their effectiveness. However, the use of intranasal corticosteroids along with antibiotic therapy has been shown to provide significant clinical improvement over antibiotic use alone.[30]

In some cases of chronic resistant sinusitis, surgical treatment must be considered. A wide array of surgical procedures are available, but functional endoscopic sinus surgery (FESS) has emerged as the technique of choice.[31]

COMPLICATIONS

Complications of sinusitis have decreased in incidence since the introduction of antibiotics. The complications most commonly encountered are cellulitis, abscess, and cavernous sinus thrombosis (all involving the orbit); epidural or subdural abscess; mucocele formation; and osteomyelitis.[32] It is evident in both children[33] and adults[34] not only that there is an association between sinusitis and asthma but also that sinusitis is an important trigger for asthma. In a patient who has both sinusitis and asthma, the asthma will be difficult to manage until the sinusitis is brought under control by either medical or surgical means.

PROGNOSIS

The prognosis for patients with sinusitis should be excellent if the diagnosis is made accurately and promptly and an appropriate antibiotic is administered for a sufficient period of time.

References

1. Malone DC, Lawson KA, Smith DN, et al: A cost of illness study of allergic rhinitis in the United States. J Allergy Clin Immunol 99:22, 1997
2. Ray NF, Baraniuk JN, Thamer M, et al: Direct expenditures for the treatment of allergic rhinoconjunctivitis in 1996. J Allergy Clin Immunol 103:401, 1999
3. Badhwar AK, Druce HM: Allergic rhinitis. Med Clin North Am 76:789, 1992
4. Naclerio RM: Allergic rhinitis. N Engl J Med 325:860, 1991
5. Norman PS: Allergic rhinitis. J Allergy Clin Immunol 75:531, 1985
6. Dykewicz MS, Fineman S: Executive Summary of Joint Task Force Practice Parameters on diagnosis and management of rhinitis. Ann Allergy Asthma Immunol 81:463, 1998
7. Zieger RS: Allergic and non-allergic rhinitis: classification and pathogenesis (pts 1 and 2). Am J Rhinol 3:21, 113, 1989
8. Nelson HS, Hirsch SR, Ohman JL, et al: Recommendations for the use of residential air-cleaning devices in the treatment of allergic respiratory disease. J Allergy Clin Immunol 82:661, 1988
9. Patel NJ, Bush RK: Role of environmental allergens in rhinitis. Immunol Allergy Clin North Am 20:323, 2000
10. Effect of passive smoking on respiratory symptoms, bronchial responsiveness, lung function, and total serum IgE in the European Community Respiratory Health Survey: a cross-sectional study. European Community Respiratory Health Survey. Lancet 358:2103, 2001
11. Corren J: Allergic rhinitis: treating the adult. J Allergy Clin Immunol 105:S610, 2000
12. Kaszuba SM, Baroody FM, deTineo M, et al: Superiority of an intranasal corticosteroid compared with an oral antihistamine in the as-needed treatment of seasonal allergic rhinitis. Arch Intern Med 161:2581, 2001
13. Casale TB, Condemi J, LaForce C, et al: Effect of omalizumab on symptoms of seasonal allergic rhinitis: a randomized controlled trial. JAMA 286:2956, 2001
14. Durham SR, Walker JM, Varga EM, et al: Long term clinical efficacy of grass pollen immunotherapy. N Engl J Med 341:468, 1999
15. Rachelefsky GS: National guidelines needed to manage rhinitis and prevent complications. Ann Allergy Asthma Immunol 82:296, 1999
16. Shapiro GG: The role of nasal airway obstruction in sinus disease and facial development. J Allergy Clin Immunol 82:935, 1988
17. Settipane RJ, Hagy GW, Settipane GA: Long-term risk factors for developing asthma and allergic rhinitis: a 23-year follow-up study of college students. Allergy Proc 15:21, 1994
18. Simons FER: Allergic rhinobronchitis: the asthma-allergic rhinitis link. J Allergy Clin Immunol 104:534, 1999
19. What are the candidate groups for pharmacotherapeutic intervention to prevent asthma? ETAC Study Group. Pediatr Allergy Immunol 11 (suppl 13):41, 2000
20. Bielory L: Allergic and immunologic disorders of the eye. Allergy: Principles and Practice, 5th ed. Middleton E Jr, Reed CE, Ellis EF, et al, Eds. Mosby Year Book, St. Louis, 1998, p 1,148
21. Berdy GJ, Abelson MB: Antihistamines and mast cell stabilizers in allergic ocular disease. Principles and Practice of Ophthalmology. Albert DM, Jacobrec FA, Eds. WB Saunders Co, Philadelphia, 2000, p 306
22. Kaliner MA, Osguthorpe JD, Fireman P: Sinusitis: bench to bedside. J Allergy Clin Immunol 99:S829, 1997
23. Benson V, Marons MA: Current estimates from the National Health Interview Survey, 1993. National Center for Health Statistics. Vital Health Statistics 10:182, 1993
24. Gliklich RE, Metson R: The health impact of chronic sinusitis in patients seeking otolaryngic care. Otolaryngol Head Neck Surg 113:104, 1995
25. Wald ER, Byers C, Guerra N, et al: Subacute sinusitis in children. J Pediatr 115:28, 1989
26. Evans FO Jr, Sydnor JB, Moore WE, et al: Sinusitis of the maxillary antrum. N Engl J Med 293:735, 1975
27. Kovatch AL, Wald ER, Ledesma-Medina J, et al: Maxillary sinus radiographs in children with nonrespiratory complaints. Pediatrics 73:306, 1984
28. Wippold FJ II, Levitt RG, Evens RG, et al: Limited coronal CT: an alternative screening examination for sinonasal inflammatory disease. Allergy Proc 16:165, 1995
29. Chee L, Graham SM, Carothers DG, et al: Immune dysfunction in refractory sinusitis in a tertiary care setting. Laryngoscope 111:233, 2001
30. Meltzer EO, Charous BL, Busse WW, et al: Added relief in the treatment of acute recurrent sinusitis with adjunctive mometasone furoate nasal spray. J Allergy Clin Immunol 106:630, 2000
31. Kennedy DW: Functional endoscopic sinus surgery technique. Arch Otolaryngol 111:643, 1985
32. Sheffield RW, Cassisi NJ, Karlan MS: Complications of sinusitis: what to watch for. Postgrad Med 63:93, 1978
33. Rachelefsky GS, Katz RM, Siegal SC: Chronic sinus disease with associated reactive airway disease in children. Pediatrics 73:526, 1984
34. Slavin RG: Relationship of nasal disease and sinusitis to bronchial asthma. Ann Allergy 49:76, 1982

Acknowledgment

Figure 2   Alice Y. Chen.

108 Urticaria, Angioedema, and Anaphylaxis

Vincent S. Beltrani, M.D.

Urticaria (hives), angioedema, and anaphylaxis are the prototypical manifestations of mast cell activation. The common denominator in these conditions is the release of potent inflammatory mediators from activated mast cells[1] [*see Chapter 105*]. Urticaria and angioedema are effected primarily by activation of cutaneous mast cells, which are preferentially located around capillaries, lymphatics, appendages, and nerves in the skin. Massive activation of mast cells in the intestinal tract, respiratory tract, and central nervous system produces the multisystemic, potentially catastrophic symptom complex of anaphylaxis.

Although the three conditions have common features and may occur in various combinations, they are more easily understood when discussed individually.

Urticaria

Urticaria is a cutaneous eruption that consists of erythematous, pruritic wheals. Although urticaria is typically transient, it can be persistent, with lesions occurring for weeks to months.

EPIDEMIOLOGY

Urticaria is a common problem, with 15% to 23% of the general population experiencing at least one episode in their lifetime.[2,3] The precise prevalence of urticaria may never be known. Many patients experience transient episodes of hives and do not report them to a health care provider because of their readily identifiable cause, inconsequential nature, and spontaneous resolution. If the papular urticaria that develops after an arthropod bite is included in the spectrum of urticarial lesions, urticaria must be considered a virtually universal human experience.

ETIOLOGY

Injecting histamine into the skin will produce the so-called triple response of Lewis—a prototypical hive. This response comprises the following: (1) erythema, the clinical manifestation of vasodilatation; (2) a wheal, the result of vascular leakage; and (3) pruritus, caused by activation of dendritic itch receptors on nonmyelinated C fibers (neurons) in the epidermis [*see Table 1*]. A fourth feature of intradermally injected histamine is its spontaneous dissipation within 1 hour. Urticaria lasting longer than 1 hour is not caused solely by histamine. Multiple inflammatory mediators have been identified in the effluent of urticarial lesions, and some of these vasoactive mediators (e.g., prostaglandin D_2 and platelet-activating factor) have produced urticaria—with and without pruritus—lasting longer than 1 hour when injected subcutaneously.

PATHOGENESIS

Because histamine plays a leading role in the pathogenesis of urticaria, tracing the source and mechanism of histamine release is the key to understanding urticarial lesions. Most of the body's histamine is stored in tissue mast cells; much smaller amounts are present in basophils and CNS neurons. Mast cells at different anatomic locations, and even at a single site, can vary substantially in mediator content, sensitivity to agents that induce activation, quantity of mediator released, and response to pharmacologic agents.[1] Agents having the ability to initiate the release of mediators from mast cells are called secretagogues. There is debate regarding whether the number of cutaneous mast cells in patients with persistent urticaria increases[4] or remains unchanged.[5] However, it has been generally agreed that these cells have a lower threshold for mediator release. Thus, a more appropriate label for chronic or idiopathic urticaria would be twitchy mast cell syndrome.

A practical categorization of urticaria is a three-part classification based on the etiology and mechanism of mast cell degranulation [*see Table 2*]. The first category comprises cases with an identifiable cause; the second, idiopathic cases; and the third, mastocytosis. Mastocytosis encompasses a wide spectrum of clinical conditions, characterized by a localized or diffuse increase in mast cells in the skin or internal organs. Most cases of mastocytosis are transient, which suggests that this disorder represents a hyperplastic response to abnormal stimuli rather than a true neoplastic process.

DIAGNOSIS

The diagnosis of urticaria is made almost exclusively from an appropriate, complete history. The history should include questions about substances or circumstances that may trigger the urticaria; the clinical features of the urticaria, including its duration, the presence and degree of pruritus, and whether the urticaria is localized or generalized; underlying illnesses; any previous diagnostic procedures or therapy for the condition; and family history of urticaria. A personal or family history of atopy should also be noted. Although the occurrence of urticaria with identifiable triggers is increased in atopic patients, whether the incidence of atopic disease is higher in patients with idiopathic urticaria remains debatable.[6,7]

Many patients presenting with IgE-induced urticaria can identify the cause of their generalized, very pruritic, explosive hives. By merely avoiding that trigger, they remain symptom

Table 1 Pathologic Changes in Urticaria and Their Associated Mediators

Symptom	Pathologic Event	Mediators
Wheal	Vascular permeability	Histamine (H_1) Prostaglandin D_2 Platelet activating factor Bradykinin Leukotrienes C4, D4, E4
Flare	Vasodilatation	Histamine (H_1) Prostaglandin D_2 Platelet activating factor Bradykinin Leukotrienes C4, D4, E4
Pruritus	Sensory nerve stimulation	Histamine (H_1)

Table 2 Classification of Urticarial Lesions
Identifiable cause
Immunologic
Nonimmunologic (e.g., cyclooxygenase pathway, opiates)
Physical urticaria
Aquagenic urticaria
Cholinergic urticaria
Cold urticaria
Contact urticaria (e.g., jellyfish, nettles)
Delayed pressure
Dermatographism
Solar urticaria
Vibratory urticaria
Nonidentifiable cause (idiopathic)
Persistent — occurring almost daily
Episodic — recurrent, with days of no hives between episodes
Associated with an underlying disease
Anaphylaxis (IgE-induced)
Anaphylactoid (non–IgE-induced)
Bullous pemphigoid
Erythema multiforme
Leukocytoclastic vasculitis
Serum sickness (via immune complexes)
Systemic lupus erythematosus
Viral syndrome (via immune complexes)
Mastocytosis
Mastocytoma
Urticaria pigmentosa
Diffuse cutaneous mastocytosis
Telangiectasia macularis eruptiva perstans (TMEP)
Systemic mastocytosis

free. These patients are at greater risk of developing fatal anaphylactic reactions, with or without urticaria.

Common Triggers of Urticaria

Before concluding that urticaria is idiopathic, the clinician must complete a systematic review of possible mast cell secretagogues. These include immunologic and nonimmunologic activators, as well as some whose mechanism is unknown [*see Table 3*].

Drugs Drugs are probably the most easily recognized of the identifiable causes of urticaria because the symptoms usually appear within 36 hours of administration of the drug.[8] The penicillins, aspirin and other nonsteroidal anti-inflammatory drugs (NSAIDs), and sulfa drugs are most commonly involved, but virtually any drug may elicit urticaria. When urticaria develops within 1 to 2 weeks after initiation of therapy with a drug that is known to cause urticaria, that drug must be suspected.

Drugs can cause urticaria via immunologic and nonimmunologic mechanisms. The best understood mechanism involves drug-specific IgE antibodies. These IgE-induced reactions typically arise within 2 weeks after a drug is started, are not dose-related, occur from seconds to minutes after administration of the drug, and may herald an anaphylactic episode [*see Figure 1*].[8] Non-IgE reactions to drugs (e.g., aspirin or other NSAIDs, opioids, and vancomycin) can occur on first exposure or from hours to days after ingestion, are dose related, and may herald an anaphylactoid reaction.[9]

Although urticarial reactions to aspirin and other NSAIDs

are rarely induced through IgE, they occur most frequently in atopic persons.[10] Angioedema, with or without urticaria, is the most common symptom of NSAID hypersensitivity. Respiratory symptoms are not more likely to occur in patients who develop an urticarial reaction from an NSAID. Some cyclooxygenase-2 (COX-2) inhibitors, especially rofecoxib, are relatively safe in patients who experience urticaria or angioedema from standard NSAIDs.[11] Patients whose history suggests a non-IgE drug reaction should not undergo routine skin testing and radioallergosorbent testing (RAST) [*see Chapter 106*].

Drug-specific IgE antibodies can be detected by skin testing, but penicillin is the only antibiotic for which reliable skin-test reagents have been developed. Standardized antigens for penicillin include penicilloyl-poly-L-lysine (penicilloyl polylysine), which is considered the major determinant and is commercially available, and several investigational minor determinants. With these reagents, numerous studies have documented the presence of penicillin-specific IgE antibodies in patients who have experienced penicillin-induced urticaria. In contrast, IgE antibodies to other antibiotics have not been demonstrated routinely in patients who have experienced an antibiotic-induced urticaria. Although it is possible that these reactions are not IgE mediated, it is more likely that the IgE antibodies have not been detected because the patients had antibodies directed against a drug metabolite not used in the testing.[12] Consequently, the diagnostic test for confirming drugs (other than the penicillins) as an identifiable cause of an individual's urticaria is to carefully rechallenge the patient, under direct medical su-

Table 3 Mast Cell Secretagogues

Immunologic activators (act on receptors)	IgE antigens (e.g., foods, drugs, latex)
	IgG directed against IgE (autoimmunity)
	Anti-FcεRI (IgE receptor) antibodies
	Lectins (e.g., strawberries, conconavalin A)
	Neuropeptides (e.g., substance P, somatostatin)
	Complement activators (C3a, C5a)
	Radiocontrast media
	Blood products
	Cytokines
	IL-1, IL-3, IL-6
	Granulocyte-macrophage colony-stimulating factor
	Histamine-releasing factors (HRF)
	c-*kit* ligand
Nonimmunologic activators	Ionophores (opiates, adrenocorticotropic hormone [ACTH], compound 48/80)
	Arachidonic acid metabolic pathway inhibition (nonsteroidal anti-inflammatory drugs)
	Direct effect on cell
	Opiates (e.g., morphine, codeine)
	Radiocontrast media
	Peptides
	Jellyfish, lobster, eosinophil major basic protein (EMB), polymyxin B, defensins
	Irradiation
	Dextran
	Physical contact (pressure, light, water)
Mechanism unknown	Alcohol, amphetamine, bradykinin, ciprofloxacin, papaverine, rifampin, thiamine, thiopental, tolazoline, vancomycin

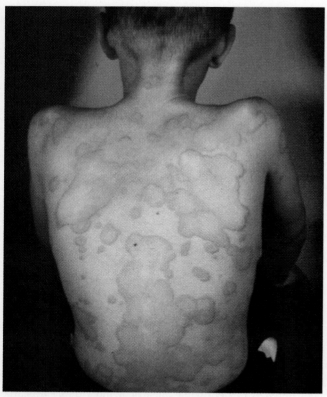

Figure 1 Generalized, symmetrical, very pruritic urticaria appeared within 10 minutes of an intramuscular injection of penicillin G in this boy. The reaction is polymorphic, with papular urticaria evolving to larger, evanescent urticarial plaques that appear annular because of central clearing. The patient in this photograph subsequently demonstrated a positive prick test to the penicillin allergen penicilloyl polylysine.

pervision, several weeks after the original episode has resolved. In practice, this is rarely done unless the drug in question is absolutely required to treat a disease.

Foods Foods and additives are the second most easily recognized IgE-induced trigger. Symptoms usually appear within 1 hour after ingestion, and in 80% of these cases, GI symptoms (e.g., cramps, diarrhea, and nausea and vomiting) also occur. Respiratory or, less frequently, cardiovascular symptoms may also accompany or precede cutaneous reactions.[13]

Foods are a common cause of urticaria.[14,15] Although studies of different populations of patients with urticaria provide estimates of the prevalence of food-induced urticaria, prevalence in the general population is unknown. Determining prevalence is complicated by the fact that even in patients with histories of adverse reactions to foods, only about 60% or fewer have reproducible reaction to foods.[16]

Urticarial reactions to foods may result from exposure by ingestion, injection, contact, or inhalation. Eggs, peanuts, milk, nuts, soy, wheat, fish, and shellfish are the foods most often implicated in allergic reactions, but IgE-mediated reactions to numerous other foods and to contaminating substances in foods, such as molds or antibiotics, have been reported.[17] Certain foods, such as egg white, strawberries, and shellfish, have been shown to contain substances that liberate histamine directly through a nonimmunologic mechanism.[18] Urticaria can also result from the ingestion of foods that contain large amounts of histamine, either naturally or as a result of spoilage (e.g., scombroidosis) [*see Chapter 13*].

Some children who experience urticaria after exposure to certain foods such as milk, eggs, soy, or wheat early in life may later tolerate these foods without difficulty. Loss of sensitivity to foods such as peanuts,[19] nuts, or fish may occur less frequently.[20]

The diagnostic tools available to determine whether foods play a role in the production of urticaria in a patient include the history, physical examination, skin testing or RAST, diet and symptom diaries, elimination diets, and food challenges. Although slightly less sensitive than skin-prick test, RASTs for specific IgE antibodies are more widely available; they require only a serum sample and are performed by commercial laboratories, and therefore, they are practical in most primary care practices. As with skin tests, a negative result is very reliable in ruling out an IgE-mediated reaction to a particular food, but a positive result has low specificity.[21] Many patients have positive skin tests and RASTs to several members of a botanical or animal species, indicating immunologic cross-reactivity, but very few patients have symptomatic intrabotanical or intraspecies cross-reactivity. The practice of avoiding all foods within a botanical family when one member is suspected of provoking allergic symptoms generally appears to be unwarranted.[21]

Occupational and hobby exposures Contact urticarial reactions are seen in certain occupational situations, such as health care workers (latex induced) and food handlers (shellfish). Atopic individuals are at a higher risk of developing these immediate-type contact reactions, which may present as pruritus, urticaria, or anaphylaxis.

Latex or natural-rubber latex hypersensitivity is a fairly common identifiable IgE-induced cause of urticaria [*see Chapter 35*]. These patients may experience localized urticaria at the contact area, generalized urticaria with angioedema, or urticaria with systemic involvement (including anaphylaxis). The diagnosis is made from a history of exposure and confirmed by a skin-prick test or RAST.

Systemic illness Urticaria occurs in a variety of autoimmune and infectious diseases. Urticaria is rarely the sole symptom of an underlying disease, however. If the history and physical examination do not suggest an underlying problem, routine laboratory testing is not indicated.

Generalized, urticarial lesions that persist for longer than 24 hours or that burn or sting more than they itch may be a manifestation of rheumatoid arthritis, systemic lupus erythematosus, or other rheumatic disease. Lesions associated with rheumatic illness usually do not blanch on diascopy and may leave ecchymosis and eventually hyperpigmentation. Patients who present in this manner should be assessed for rheumatic disease [*see Chapter 111*].

Approximately 5% to 10% of patients with chronic urticaria have been reported to have antithyroid antibodies but are clinically and biochemically euthyroid.[22,23] For that reason, autoimmune thyroid serologic studies have been recommended for patients with chronic urticaria.[24] There is only anecdotal evidence that treating these patients with exogenous thyroid hormone leads to significant improvement of their urticaria, however.[25,26]

Changes in mast cell reactivity apparently can be part of the immune response to infection. Urticaria reportedly can be a feature of streptococcal pharyngitis, otitis media, infectious mononucleosis, and hepatitis (a slightly higher incidence of hepatitis C antibodies has been reported in patients with urticaria, but whether there is a causal relationship is questionable). Pathogens reportedly associated with urticaria include coxsackievirus, *Mycoplasma*, fungi, and *Candida*. A causative relationship of urticaria with *Helicobacter pylori* has not been confirmed.[27,28] Extensive searches for occult focal infections (e.g., sinusitis) as the cause of urticaria are consistently unsuccessful.[29]

A number of parasitic infestations produce transient urticaria.[30] The urticaria in these patients usually appears from the second to the sixth week of infestation. Random examinations of stool for ova and parasites rarely, if ever, prove positive in patients with urticaria who do not have typical symptoms of parasitic infestation.

Psychological factors Emotional stress can influence mast cell and IgE activity, resulting in the release of vasoactive mediators and exacerbations of chronic urticaria.[31] However, there is no good evidence that psychological factors by themselves can cause urticaria, so urticaria without an identifiable cause should not be dismissed as a psychosomatic illness.

Neoplasms Lymphomas and carcinomas may promote urticaria (paraneoplastic syndrome), but urticaria in patients with neoplasms is usually coincidental. In most cases, the malignancy is known; current evidence does not warrant routinely subjecting patients with unexplained urticaria to an exhaustive evaluation for an occult neoplasm.

Chronic urticaria may occur as part of Schnitzler syndrome, which also includes a monoclonal IgM gammopathy, intermittent fever, joint or bone pain, lymphadenopathy, leukocytosis, and an elevated erythrocyte sedimentation rate (ESR). In 15% of cases, Schnitzler syndrome evolves to lymphoplasmocytic malignancy.[32]

Genetic factors Several of the physical urticarias can be familial. Examples include urticaria induced by cold, heat, light, water, and vibration (see below), as well as urticaria associated with erythropoietic protoporphyria. The Muckle-Wells syndrome is a form of familial urticaria associated with deafness and amyloidosis.[33]

Localized Urticaria

Papular urticaria, some of the physical urticarias, and contact urticaria are the entities to consider when urticaria is restricted to a limited area of the body. Dermatographism, cold urticaria, delayed pressure urticaria, solar urticaria, and aquagenic urticaria are localized wheals produced by specific physical stimuli (i.e., stroking of the skin, cold, sustained pressure, ultraviolet light, and water, respectively).

Papular urticaria Papular urticaria consists of 4 to 8 mm wheals or firm papules, often in grouped clusters and especially on areas of exposed skin. Papular urticaria that is very pruritic, persists longer than typical hives, and is located on exposed parts of the body is often caused by insect bites (fleas, bedbugs, scabies, and other mites). The pattern of the eruption corresponds to the biting habits of the offending insect (e.g., mosquito bites often comprise three quasilinear lesions—referred to as breakfast, lunch, and supper), and the seasonal occurrence corresponds to the peak prevalence of that insect. IgE and IgG antibodies against mosquito antigens have been detected in human sera,[34] but there have been no reported cases of

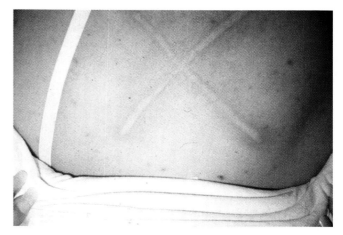

Figure 2   **Dermatographism elicited by gentle stroking of the skin of the back.**

anaphylaxis or death associated with hypersensitivity to mosquitoes. Arthropod bites are the only known cause of bulla on papular urticaria. Papular urticaria persists for 2 to 10 days and may leave postinflammatory hyperpigmentation. Occasionally, healed lesions may recrudesce when fresh crops appear.[35]

Dermatographism Firm stroking of the skin may elicit a wheal and erythema in 5% of a healthy population, but only in a minority of these persons does it also cause any pruritus (so-called symptomatic dermatographism) [*see Figure 2*]. The etiology of dermatographism is uncertain, but passive transfer tests are sometimes positive. Dermatographism (Darier sign) is a common finding in patients with idiopathic urticaria and may be associated with other conditions. For example, dermatographism can be elicited in more than 90% of patients with mastocytosis.[36] Confirmation of mastocytosis always requires biopsy, however. The elicitation of symptomatic dermatographism in patients with urticaria supports the use of both H_1 and H_2 receptor antagonists, which may more effectively reduce wheal size and duration of urticaria.[37]

Delayed pressure urticaria Urticaria that results from localized, continuous (4 to 6 hours) pressure is seen most often in patients with persistent urticaria without an identifiable cause.[38] It may be associated with systemic complaints such as myalgias, arthralgias, and fever. It responds best to aspirin or NSAIDs and poorly to antihistamines.

Cold urticaria The lesions of cold urticaria develop 5 to 30 minutes after exposure to cold and can be caused by wind, bathing, contact, or eating cold foods or drinking cold liquids.[39] Although the urticaria may appear during the period of exposure, more often it develops upon rewarming of the skin. The urticaria usually lasts approximately 30 minutes and resolves spontaneously.

Cold urticaria is often idiopathic and acquired. Patients with these lesions usually have a positive response to an ice-cube–challenge test.[40] Rare forms of acquired cold urticaria include delayed, localized, and reflex cold urticaria. In delayed cold urticaria, lesions develop several hours after exposure; localized cold urticaria lesions occur only at sites of injections or bites; and reflex cold urticaria lesions present as widespread whealing in response to a fall in core body temperature.

Much rarer than acquired forms of cold urticaria is familial cold urticaria. In this autosomal dominant disorder, lesions appear 30 minutes after exposure to generalized cooling, rather than to local application of cold, and may persist for up to 48 hours.

Solar urticaria Solar urticaria is a rare idiopathic disorder in which erythema heralds a pruritic wheal that appears within 5 minutes after exposure to a specific wavelength of light and dissipates within 15 minutes to 3 hours after onset [*see Figure 3*].[41,42] Solar urticaria is usually provoked by light in the visible spectrum, although the specific wavelength that leads to mast cell degranulation may vary from patient to patient. The severity of the reaction depends on the duration of the exposure, the intensity of the irradiation, and the light spectrum.[43] These reactions are believed to result from the development of an antigenic photoproduct, which then triggers an IgE-mediated response. Patients should usually be referred to an allergist or dermatologist for provocative testing.

Aquagenic urticaria Urticaria that appears 2 to 30 minutes after water immersion, regardless of its temperature or source (seawater or tap water) has been reported in a few patients.[44] These pruritic, follicular, cholinergic-like wheals can be reproduced by applying wet compresses to the patient's back for at least 30 minutes. It is believed that aquagenic urticaria occurs when sensitized mast cells are activated by a water-soluble antigen that diffuses through the epidermis, causing the release of acetylcholine and histamine.

Vibratory urticaria Urticaria that follows massage and vigorous toweling has been described in a single family.[45]

Contact urticaria Immediate contact reactions can appear on normal or eczematous skin within minutes to an hour after exposure. The reaction then will disappear within a few hours. Itching, tingling, or burning accompanied by erythema are the mildest form of contact reactions. They are often caused by cosmetics, fruits, and vegetables. Generalized urticaria after a local contact is a rare phenomenon, but it can occur with some allergens.[46]

Contact reactions may have either immunologic or nonimmunologic mechanisms. Immunologic mechanisms require

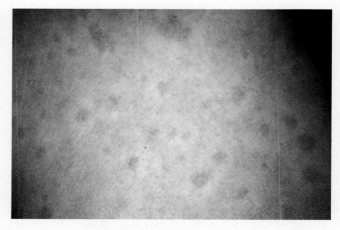

Figure 4   Lesions of generalized urticaria tend to be symmetrical and sometimes have a halo of pallor surrounding the wheal.

prior sensitization to the causative agent. The respiratory and gastrointestinal tracts are typically the routes of sensitization, but sensitization to natural latex and some foods may occur through the skin. The substances causing immunologic immediate contact reactions are usually proteins. Foods most commonly involved are fish, shellfish, and wheat flour. Most cases of protein contact dermatitis develop after the person has handled food products for a protracted period. Symptoms usually appear within 30 minutes after direct cutaneous contact with the offending agent.[47] Specific IgE antibodies against the causative allergen can be found by skin testing or RAST.

Most immediate contact reactions are nonimmunologic and occur without previous sensitization. These reactions remain localized. The pathophysiology of nonimmunologic immediate contact reactions has not been established, but it may involve direct influence on dermal vessel walls or a non-IgE release of inflammatory mediators. A list of chemicals that cause occupational allergic contact dermatitis can be found on the Internet at http://www.haz-map.com/allergic.htm.

Generalized Urticaria

The clinical features and natural history of generalized urticaria are as varied and unpredictable as the etiology. Generalized lesions tend to be numerous and symmetrical. Characteristically, they are intensely pruritic, especially at onset. Except for cholinergic papular urticaria, little information about the etiology can be obtained from the morphology. Individual lesions fade completely within 24 hours. Occasionally a halo of pallor surrounds the wheal [*see Figure 4*].

Cholinergic urticaria The lesions of cholinergic urticaria are highly distinctive, consisting of 2 to 3 mm scattered papular wheals surrounded by large, erythematous flares. These lesions are extremely pruritic, and they may affect the entire body but often spare the palms, soles, and axilla.[48] Precipitating stimuli include exercise, warm temperature, ingestion of hot or spicy foods, and possibly emotional stress. The condition often remits within several years but can last for more than 30 years. The diagnosis can be made by provocation with exercise or a hot bath. Cholinergic urticaria can be aborted by the prompt application of cold water or ice to the skin, and a refractory period of up to 24 hours can be induced by a hot bath.

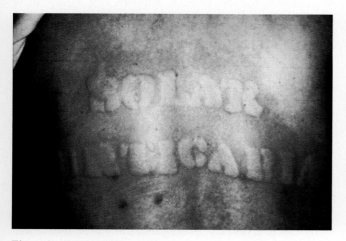

Figure 3   **Solar urticaria.**

Table 4 H$_1$ Antihistamines Available for Treatment of Urticaria

Chemical Group	Agents	Antihistaminic Activity	Sedation	Anticholinergic Activity	Cost
Ethanolamine derivatives	Diphenhydramine	+	++/+++	++	$
	Clemastine	+	++	+	$
Ethylenediamine derivatives	Tripelennamine (PBZ)	++	+	+	$
Piperidine derivatives	Azatadine	+	+	+	$$
	Cyproheptadine	+/++	+/++	+	$
	Fexofenadine (Allegra)*	++/+++	0	0	$$$
	Loratadine (Claritin)*	+/++	0	0	$$$$
Piperazine derivatives	Hydroxyzine	+++	++	+	$
	Cetirizine (Zyrtec)	+++	+/0	0/+	$$$$
Propylamine derivatives	Acrivastine	++	0/+	0	$$$
	Brompheniramine	+	+	+	$
	Chlorpheniramine	+/++	+	+	$
	Dexchlorpheniramine	+/++	+	+	$$
Phenothiazine derivatives	Promethazine	++/+++	+++	++	$
	Trimeprazine	++	+/++	++	$
Tricyclic antidepressants	Doxepin	+++++	+++	+++	$
	Amitriptyline	+++++	+++/++++	+++	$

*Considered second-generation antihistamines, which are nonsedating (Zyrtec less so) and have other anti-inflammatory properties besides being antihistaminic.

Physical Examination

Recognition of urticaria does not usually present a problem. Unfortunately, except for the contact and physical urticarias, the examination does not facilitate identification of the cause. Episodes of angioedema occur in half the patients presenting with persistent urticaria. The individual swellings of angioedema always last longer than an individual hive and are almost always nonpruritic.

Laboratory Evaluation

The use of laboratory tests in patients with urticaria should be directed toward confirmation of diagnoses suggested by the history and physical examination. Routine laboratory testing should not be performed, because it has consistently proved disappointing for the identification of an etiology. A skin biopsy is indicated if the diagnosis of urticaria is in question. A biopsy should be performed on any urticaria that lasts more than 24 hours, is only mildly pruritic or nonpruritic, is associated with vesicles or bullae, or does not respond to appropriate therapy. The subtleties of the histologic variances demand interpretation by a dermatopathologist.

TREATMENT

Eliminating or avoiding the triggers of mast cell activation is the basis of treatment for urticaria. However, this strategy may be impractical in patients with persistent idiopathic urticaria, which usually has multiple triggers. Any underlying disease should be treated. Idiopathic urticaria is managed symptomatically. Fortunately, the hyperreactive state in patients with idiopathic urticaria eventually resolves spontaneously.

H$_1$ Receptor Antagonists

When used appropriately, antihistamines can offer significant relief to most patients with urticaria. The more the skin lesions resemble the triple response of Lewis, the better they respond to antihistamine treatment. Urticarial vasculitis and delayed pressure urticaria are resistant to antihistamines. Antihistamines compete with histamine for H$_1$ receptor sites on effector cells and thereby prevent, but do not reverse, responses mediated by histamine alone. There are eight recognized chemical groups of H$_1$ receptor antihistamines; all effectively compete for H$_1$ receptor sites [see Table 4]. Among these groups are tricyclic antidepressants, which also have potent antihistaminic activity.

The choice of antihistamine is based on its effectiveness, frequency of administration, and side-effect profile. The dose of the agent selected should be increased to tolerance; if adequate relief is not achieved at the maximal tolerated dose, a drug from another group can be added. Patients do not all respond in the same way to agents from each group. Most of the so-called first-generation (sedative) antihistamines are virtually equivalent in effectiveness, with the major differences being the degree of sedation or anticholinergic effects. Activation of H$_1$ receptors in the brain is responsible for alertness; inhibiting these sites with antihistamines results in sedation. Second-generation (nonsedating) antihistamines tend not to cause drowsiness, because they cross the blood-brain barrier poorly.[49] Many patients find the itching and urticaria to be most troublesome in the evening and at night, so a useful strategy is to combine sedating antihistamines given at bedtime with nonsedating antihistamines during the day. This combination is effective, promotes compliance, and is economical. Tachyphylaxis has not been noted with H$_1$ receptor antagonists.

Because other mediators besides histamine are involved in urticaria, antihistamines are not a panacea. Also, none of the antihistamines have the ability to displace histamine from the H$_1$ receptor site, so the best clinical results are attained when the antihistamines occupy those receptors before the arrival of histamine; hence, round-the-clock dosing is necessary for patients with persistent symptoms.

An effective cocktail for persistent urticaria is fexofenadine (180 mg) or loratidine (10 mg) in the early morning and cetirizine (10 to 20 mg) in the early evening. If this is insufficient, the tricyclic antidepressant doxepin, 10 to 50 mg, can be added at bedtime. (A single dose of doxepin suppresses the histamine-induced wheal and flare for 4 to 6 days.[50]) This cocktail controls symptoms in more than three quarters of patients with persistent urticaria. Prednisone, 0.5 to 1.0 mg/kg/day, should be used only for patients with refractory idiopathic urticaria or with urticarial vasculitis. The goal of treatment should not be to attain a hive-free status but, rather, to minimize compromise of the patient's quality of life from both the disease and its treatment.

In urticaria with an identifiable cause, antihistamines are discontinued once the substance is gone from the body. In persistent urticaria, antihistamines can be sequentially discontinued when patients have been completely free of hives for at least 96 hours. At that point, the morning dose of nonsedating antihistamines can be discontinued. If the patient is still symptom free after another 96 hours, the doxepin dosage can begin to be reduced and, lastly, the cetirizine can be discontinued.

H_2 Receptor Antagonists

Human skin has H_2 receptors as well as H_1 receptors. H_2 receptors are present on the cutaneous arterioles, and their activation can result in vasodilatation (noted as flushing). For that reason, combining H_2 antagonists with H_1 antagonists can be helpful in patients who have prominent flushing, dermatographism, or angioedema.[51] The available evidence does not justify the routine addition of H_2 antagonists to H_1 antagonists in patients with persistent urticaria or urticarial vasculitis.

Beta Agonists

Beta agonists increase intracellular levels of cyclic adenosine monophosphate (cAMP), thereby reducing mediator release by mast cells and promoting vasoconstriction of cutaneous vasculature. Any explosive, generalized urticaria demands the subcutaneous administration of 0.2 ml of aqueous epinephrine 1:1000 (which has combined alpha-agonist and beta-agonist properties), in addition to H_1 antagonists and H_2 antagonists (e.g., doxepin, 10 mg). This is the treatment of choice for anaphylaxis (see below).

Oral beta agonists have been tried for chronic urticaria and angioedema in conjunction with H_1 antagonists and H_2 antagonists. Terbutaline (2.5 to 5.0 mg q.i.d.) deserves a trial in patients not responding to standard treatment. Some studies have demonstrated efficacy, and others have found none.[52,53]

Corticosteroids

Because corticosteroids do not inhibit cutaneous mast cell degranulation, they have no effect on acute urticaria. However, these agents are often used in patients with persistent urticaria whose symptoms are disabling and unresponsive to maximum standard therapy.[54] In these cases, steroids are given in a pulse dose to break the cycle of a resistant episode. The recommended starting dosage of prednisone for persistent urticaria is 0.5 to 1.0 mg/kg/day. This dosage should not be reduced until the patient shows definite clinical improvement.

A protocol for steroid therapy for patients with persistent urticaria has been recommended by the Parameters of Care Committee of the American Academy of Allergy, Asthma and Immunology.[55] Daily steroids are recommended only during the first 1 or 2 weeks for patients with persistent urticaria who have had no relief for a protracted period. The goal is then to utilize an alternate-day regimen with a gradually decreasing dosage over a period of months. Patients should be started on a daily dose of prednisone, 0.5 to 1.0 mg/kg (while continuing the maximum antihistamine regimen). If the symptoms become tolerable, the prednisone dose is decreased by 5 mg every 1 to 3 days until 25 mg a day is reached. The patient's progress is then reassessed every 1 to 2 weeks. Once the patient's condition stabilizes, the dose is decreased by 2.5 to 5 mg every 2 to 3 weeks. When the lowest dose is reached, alternate-day therapy may be tried. Usually, the alternate-day dose is 1.5 times the daily dose. Should some rebound occur on the off day, the alternate-day treatment can be given in divided doses (at 8 A.M. and at 5 P.M.). Once a maintenance dose is reached, the dose of prednisone should be reduced by 1 mg every 1 to 2 weeks.

Other Agents

There are recent reports of success using the anabolic steroid stanozolol for chronic urticaria,[56] aquagenic urticaria,[57] familial cold urticaria,[58] and cholinergic urticaria. Nifedipine, 20 mg three times daily, has been reported effective for chronic urticaria.[59] This treatment deserves further evaluation. Patients with chronic urticaria are advised to avoid aspirin and all NSAIDs, yet there are anecdotal reports of patients with urticaria who benefit from these drugs. Indomethacin has been used successfully in the management of urticarial vasculitis.[60]

Cyclosporine has proved effective in some cases of chronic idiopathic urticaria refractory to antihistamines, as well as in urticarial vasculitis and solar urticaria.[61] Doses used are 2.5 to 6 mg/kg daily. Higher doses can cause elevation in the blood urea nitrogen (BUN) and serum creatinine levels, but these have returned to normal on discontinuance of the drug.

Leukotriene antagonists have been combined with antihistamines for the management of allergic rhinitis and have been noted to be more effective than the antihistamine alone. Therefore, many allergists have tried this combination for urticaria, with some anecdotal success. There is nothing in the literature to support its use, however, and in my experience, the use of a leukotriene antagonist with an antihistamine offers no advantage for persistent urticaria without angioedema.

PROGNOSIS

Except for IgE-induced urticaria, which may progress to fatal anaphylaxis, the prognosis for the other urticarias is benign, although prolonged episodes of these disorders can be extremely bothersome. To date, there is no evidence that the natural history of any of the urticarial syndromes, whether induced by an identifiable cause or idiopathic, is influenced by treatment. Almost all cases of persistent urticaria eventually resolve, however; even the majority of cases of IgE-induced urticarias (especially those without anaphylaxis) are rarely permanent. Chronic urticaria tends to last longer in elderly persons than in younger ones. Studies of chronic (persistent) idiopathic urticaria have found that with or without treatment, 50% of cases will resolve within 6 to 12 months of onset; 20%, within 12 to 36 months; and another 20%, within 36 to 60 months. Less than 2% of cases persist for 25 years or longer. Over 50% of patients will have at least one recurrence.[62] Interestingly, although anaphylactic or anaphylactoid reactions have been noted in patients with identifiable causes of urticaria, there have been no reports of these reactions ever occurring in patients with persistent urticaria without an identifiable cause. More than 50% of patients with idiopathic urticaria can be made comfortable with appropriate antihistamine therapy. Immunosuppression with corticosteroid dependence occurs in fewer than 5% of patients.

Angioedema

Angioedema is an episodic, asymmetrical, nonpitting swelling of loose tissue (usually skin) [*see Figure 5*]. It is usually nonerythematous and nonpruritic, and it may be painless. Angioedema rarely lasts less than 2 hours, and it frequently persists for 24 hours or longer. It may occur together with urticaria. Angioedema involving the face can be disfiguring during its course. Laryngeal swelling from angioedema may compromise the airway, leading to stridor and even asphyxiation. Gastrointestinal involvement can cause crampy abdominal pain, followed by watery diarrhea. Most cases of angioedema are a reaction to a food or a drug, but some episodes have no identifiable trigger. There are both hereditary and acquired forms of angioedema.

EPIDEMIOLOGY

It is estimated that approximately 10% of the population will experience at least one episode of angioedema.[63] Angioedema occurs episodically in 50% of patients with urticaria. Of patients who have angioedema as their primary disorder, approximately 20% will also experience episodes of urticaria.[64]

ETIOLOGY

Angioedema can be induced by a variety of mechanisms, including IgE, inhibition of the cyclooxygenase pathway of arachidonic acid metabolism, activation of the kinin-forming system, and activation of complement. In some patients, none of these mechanisms can be identified; these cases are labeled idiopathic.

IgE

IgE-induced angioedema resembles IgE allergy and is typically provoked by foods or drugs. It tends to occur in atopic persons and can be confirmed by prick skin testing or RAST.

Cyclooxygenase Inhibition

There is increasing evidence that the inhibition of the enzyme cyclooxygenase causes the de novo release of leukotrienes, an inflammatory mediator derived from arachidonic acid, in response to injury. Of particular interest in the skin is leukotriene B_4, which can induce neutrophil chemotaxis and increase vascular permeability.[65] Aspirin and other NSAIDs directly inhibit the ability of cyclooxygenase to decrease the formation of prostaglandins and thromboxanes, but not leukotrienes, from arachidonic acid. Angioedema (with or without urticaria) may occur in 100% of patients with hypersensitivity to aspirin or other NSAIDs.[11] Interestingly, not all patients who are hypersensitive to aspirin react to other NSAIDs,[66] and in one study, only 3% of patients sensitive to both aspirin and other NSAIDs reacted to the COX-2 inhibitor rofecoxib.[67]

Activation of the Kinin-Forming System

Bradykinin increases vascular permeability. Angiotensin-converting enzyme (ACE) inhibitors inhibit the kininase enzymes required for degradation of bradykinin, and the resulting elevation in bradykinin levels may lead to angioedema.[68] Angioedema has been reported in approximately 0.1% to

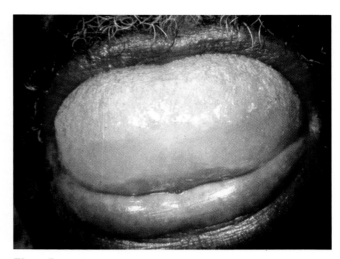

Figure 5 Angioedema of the tongue is evident in this photograph of a 54-year-old man. This episode, the patient's fifth, was unresponsive to epinephrine, antihistamines, and prednisone; his sixth episode required intubation for 92 hours, after which the angioedema resolved spontaneously.

0.5% of patients who take ACE inhibitors.[69] However, because these agents are so widely used, ACE inhibitor–induced angioedema is relatively common.

Angiotensin II receptor blockers (ARBs), such as losartan and valsartan, do not increase bradykinin levels. Nevertheless, rare instances of angioedema have been reported with the use of ARBs.[70]

Complement Activation

Increased susceptibility to angioedema can result from either an inherited defect in C1-esterase inhibitor (C1-INH) activity or an acquired deficiency of C1-INH. The inherited form of the disease, known as hereditary angioedema, is rare. There are two principal types of hereditary angioedema: type 1, which accounts for 80% to 85% of cases and is caused by decreased production of C1-INH, and type 2, in which normal or elevated amounts of functionally deficient C1-INH are produced.[71] A third, very rare form of hereditary angioedema that may be X-linked has recently been described in women.[72]

Acquired angioedema results from increased metabolism or destruction of C1-INH. Two types of acquired angioedema have been described. Type 1, which is caused by excessive activation of complement and subsequent consumption of C1-INH, typically occurs in patients with rheumatologic disorders and B cell lymphoproliferative diseases. Patients with type 2 produce autoantibodies against C1-INH, leading to its inactivation.[73,74]

PATHOGENESIS

Angioedema is consistently described as a variant of urticaria in which the subcutaneous tissues, rather than the dermis, are mainly involved. However, unlike urticaria, which seems to be mediated primarily by histamine, angioedema seems to be mediated primarily by bradykinin and leukotrienes. Anecdotal evidence indicates that although urticaria can be elicited with a histamine prick or intradermal injection, the injection of histamine deeper in the dermis does not produce angioedema. On the other hand, there are patients whose angioedema will dissipate with the administration of antihistamines (especially the combination of H_1 and H_2 receptor antagonists).[75] These observations suggest that several vasoactive mediators are capable of producing angioedema.

Unfortunately, angioedema is almost never biopsied, so there are no documented pathologic descriptions of the disorder. The histopathology is always included with urticaria, and its morphology seems to be assumed. Teleologically, the vasodilatation and vascular leakage occur deeper in the skin, and the specific cellular infiltrate, if any, remains uncertain.

DIAGNOSIS

Diagnosis of angioedema is usually straightforward. Cellulitis, edematous states, trauma (stings), and fasciitis occasionally are considerations in the differential diagnosis. Insights into causes and mechanisms of induction are derived primarily from the history.

The history in a patient with angioedema—especially one who has had repeated episodes—should include the following questions: (1) Is the angioedema always, sometimes, or never associated with urticaria? (2) Is the swelling pruritic? (3) Are there accompanying gastrointestinal symptoms (e.g., pain, nausea and vomiting, or diarrhea)? (4) Is the patient taking any medications? (5) Can the patient identify any apparent triggers for the angioedema?

Patients with IgE-induced angioedema are most likely to present with concomitant urticaria. This form of angioedema may be pruritic and may progress to an anaphylactic reaction. Typically, IgE-induced angioedema occurs within 30 minutes after contact with the IgE antigen. It is most likely to occur in atopic patients. Gastrointestinal symptoms may occur but are uncommon. IgE-induced angioedema often occurs as a drug reaction, with β-lactam antibiotics being the most common trigger.

Cyclooxygenase inhibitors (i.e., aspirin or other NSAIDs) are more apt to cause nonpruritic angioedema. NSAID-induced angioedema is occasionally accompanied by urticaria.

Angioedema induced by ACE inhibitors is nonpruritic and rarely occurs with urticaria. No sex predominance has been noted in patients without gastrointestinal tract involvement, but all patients with GI involvement have been women.[76]

Complement-activated angioedema is never pruritic and is not accompanied by urticaria. In 20% to 25% of patients with hereditary angioedema, there is no family history of the disease (these cases may represent new mutations).[77] Therefore, a positive family history of hereditary angioedema is not a prerequisite for the consideration of this disorder in the differential diagnosis when typical symptoms are present. Symptoms of hereditary angioedema are usually mild or nonexistent during childhood, typically first manifesting during the second decade of life. Acquired angioedema usually develops during or after the fourth decade of life.

Hereditary and acquired angioedema have similar clinical presentations. Episodes can occur without provocation, but some episodes may be associated with trauma, medical procedures, emotional stress, menstruation, oral contraceptive use, infections, or the use of medications such as ACE inhibitors.[71] Manifestations include marked edema of the skin and lining of hollow visceral organs. GI tract involvement results in varying degrees of intestinal obstruction, with severe abdominal pain, nausea, and vomiting. Despite the absence of fever and leukocytosis, these cases are often mistaken for an acute abdomen, which occasionally leads to unnecessary surgical exploration of the abdomen. Typically, the attacks last about 2 to 5 days before resolving spontaneously.

Laboratory Tests

IgE-induced drug reactions are readily identifiable with skin-prick tests or RAST. In complement-activated angioedema, a low level of the complement component C4 is a constant finding and therefore represents a sensitive screening test. A normal level, especially during an attack, rules out both hereditary and acquired angioedema. In patients with suspected complement-activated angioedema, confirmation of the diagnosis can be obtained by measuring antigenic levels of C1-INH, which are low in 85% of patients, or functional levels, which are low in 100% of patients. Hereditary forms of complement-activated angioedema can be distinguished from acquired forms by measurement of C1q complement—levels of which are normal in hereditary forms but decreased in acquired forms.

TREATMENT

Discontinuance of the causative agent is an obvious initial step in angioedema. Emergency measures are necessary to secure the airway if there is airway obstruction by a swollen tongue, uvula, or epiglottis. Monitoring the airway in these patients until the angioedema resolves is imperative. Subcutaneous epinephrine should be given and is helpful in most types of angioedema, except those associated with low levels of C1-INH. Aerosolized epinephrine sprayed on the swollen mucous membrane may at times be helpful.

Antihistamines (both H_1 and H_2 receptor antagonists) are indicated for IgE-induced angioedema (see above). Idiopathic angioedema has been split into those presentations that respond to antihistamine therapy and those that do not.[78] Doxepin (see above) should be given to all patients with idiopathic angioedema, but results are often disappointing if this agent is administered without epinephrine. Leukotriene inhibitors counteract the vasodilation produced by leukotrienes and can reduce the edema.

Intramuscular or intravenous glucocorticoids (prednisone, 0.5 to 1 mg/kg/day, or methylprednisolone, 0.4 to 0.8 mg/kg/day) can be used as adjunctive treatment. However, the anti-inflammatory action of these agents does not affect the underlying cause of the inflammation, and they require hours to take effect. Injectable C1-INH concentrate has been developed and is effective in treating patients with hereditary angioedema,[79] but it is difficult to obtain.

To prevent future episodes of angioedema, patients should avoid identified triggers. ACE inhibitors are contraindicated in patients with idiopathic or C1-INH deficiency, and ARBs should be used only with extreme caution. Patients with idiopathic angioedema should undergo an annual general medical evaluation to identify any underlying occult disease.

Anaphylaxis

Anaphylaxis is an explosive, massive activation of mast cells, with release of their inflammatory mediators in the skin, respiratory tract, and circulatory system resulting in urticaria, wheezing, and hypotension.

The term anaphylaxis has been restricted to IgE-mediated mast cell and basophil activation. Anaphylactoid reactions, although similar in presentation, result from non–IgE-dependent mechanisms and are less likely to have a fatal outcome.[80] For practical purposes, however, it does not matter whether the patient is having true anaphylaxis or an anaphylactoid reaction, because the clinical manifestations and the treatment of these two types of reactions are identical.

EPIDEMIOLOGY

The authors of all epidemiologic reports regarding anaphylaxis believe the incidence to be underestimated because of failure to report or recognize every episode. A Dutch study estimated that only 4% to 8% of anaphylactic reactions were reported.[81] From the combined results of reported series, several significant conclusions can be drawn: First, the occurrence of atopy in anaphylaxis patients can be as high as 53%.[82] Second, the incidence of females predisposed to anaphylactic episodes can be as high as 61%.[83] Third, when the cause of anaphylaxis is found, food and drugs head the list, with peanuts and shellfish being the most common offending foods and NSAIDs and antibiotics being the most common drug offenders.[84] Fourth, cutaneous symptoms are by far the most common manifestation.[85] Fifth, the risk of anaphylaxis in hospitalized patients is reported to be 196 per million population, with the risk being highest in women and in persons younger than 30 years.[86]

ETIOLOGY

A number of substances are known to cause anaphylactic and anaphylactoid reactions [see Table 5]. IgE-mediated anaphylaxis is caused by agents that act as haptens (e.g., β-lactam antibiotics) or by complete antigens (e.g., venoms, foods, allergen extracts). Anaphylatoxins (C3a and C5a) often mediate reactions to human plasma and blood products. The nonimmunologic mast cell activators include radiocontrast media, opiates, and some muscle relaxants. Other anaphylactoid-inducing agents include those agents that modulate arachidonic acid metabolism (i.e., aspirin and other NSAIDs). In a number of cases, the mechanism that leads to anaphylactic or anaphylactoid reactions is unknown (i.e., idiopathic, exercise, and cold urticaria or cholinergic urticaria with anaphylaxis; mastocytosis; and some drug-induced reactions).[87] Patients with idiopathic persistent urticaria or episodic urticaria do not experience anaphylaxis.

PATHOGENESIS

Any of the mast cell secretagogues [see Table 3] have the potential to induce an anaphylactic or anaphylactoid reaction. Activation of the mast cell through the FcεRI receptor by an antigen releases the greatest amount of histamine. The physiologic responses to the release of inflammatory mediators include smooth-muscle spasm in the bronchi and GI tract, vasodilatation, increased vascular permeability, and stimulation of nociceptor nerve endings.

DIAGNOSIS

The classic symptoms of anaphylaxis include flushing, urticaria, angioedema, pruritus, bronchospasm, and abdominal cramping with nausea, vomiting, and diarrhea. Hypotension and shock can result from intravascular volume loss, vasodilatation, and myocardial dysfunction. Symptoms usually begin within 5 to 30 minutes after the causative agent is introduced into the body and within 2 hours after it is ingested. The shorter the latent period, the more ominous the prognosis. In rare cases, symptoms can be delayed in onset for several hours. These are called late reactions. The biphasic reaction, which includes both immediate and late reactions, tends not to be recognized and therefore is more likely to result in a fatal outcome. Least common is the protracted reaction, in which the immediate reaction persists for hours.

Table 5 Estimated Incidence or Prevalence of Acute Anaphylactic Reactions[91]

Cause	Incidence/Prevalence
General cause	1 per 2,700 hospitalized patients
Insect sting	0.4%–0.8% of United States population
Radiocontrast medium	1 per 1,000–14,000 procedures
Penicillin (fatal outcome)	1.0–7.5 per million treatments
General anesthesia	1 per 300 inductions
Hemodialysis	1 per 1,000–5,000 sessions
Immunotherapy (severe reactions)	0.1 per million injections

Table 6 Grading System for Anaphylaxis

Group	Clinical Manifestations
I	Pruritus, flushing, urticaria, or angioedema
II	Pruritus, flushing, urticaria, or angioedema Nausea, dyspnea, tachycardia, or hypotension
III	Pruritus, flushing, urticaria, or angioedema Nausea, dyspnea, tachycardia, or hypotension Bronchospasm and shock
IV	Respiratory arrest Cardiac arrest Other manifestations may be present

Clinical Manifestations

At the onset of anaphylaxis, patients often initially experience a sense of impending doom, accompanied by generalized pruritus and flushing. Almost all patients with anaphylaxis present with cutaneous manifestations that include pruritus, flushing, urticaria, or angioedema.

Anaphylaxis is graded by its clinical presentation [see Table 6]. Cases with signs and symptoms limited to the skin are designated as group I. Group II comprises cutaneous manifestations plus nausea, dyspnea, tachycardia, or hypotension; group III includes all the manifestations of groups I and II plus bronchospasm and true shock. Group IV consists of respiratory arrest, cardiac arrest, or both, with or without other manifestations.

Physical Examination

Cutaneous involvement Flushing, urticaria, and angioedema have been reported in 88% to 100% of patients experiencing anaphylaxis. Pruritus, especially of the scalp, soft palate, palms, soles, and anogenital areas, usually heralds an impending anaphylactic or anaphylactoid reaction or may be the only cutaneous signs of the episode. Conjunctival pruritus, injection, and edema are not unusual.

Respiratory involvement Nasal congestion (occurring in up to 56% of patients), rhinorrhea (16%), laryngeal edema, dyspnea (47%), bronchospasm (24% to 47%), cough, and hoarseness may all be part of the anaphylaxis syndrome.

Cardiovascular involvement Tachycardia and hypotension are common cardiovascular manifestations of anaphylaxis. Uncommon findings include bradycardia (6%), angina (6%), syncope, palpitations, and cardiac arrest (2% to 14%).

Gastrointestinal involvement GI symptoms, including nausea, vomiting, diarrhea, abdominal cramps, and bloating occur in 30% of patients with anaphylaxis.

Neurologic involvement Dizziness or syncope (33%), headache (up to 15%), and seizures (1.5%) may be among the presenting symptoms of anaphylaxis.

Laboratory Evaluation

Anaphylaxis is a clinical diagnosis. Laboratory studies are rarely helpful. Postmortem testing may help clarify the diagnosis in cases of so-called sudden death or in patients who are dead on arrival at the emergency department.

If a patient is seen shortly after an episode, plasma histamine, urinary histamine, or serum tryptase may be helpful in confirming the diagnosis. Plasma histamine levels rise within 10 minutes, but they fall again within 1 hour. Serum β-tryptase levels peak by 1 hour and may remain elevated for as long as 5 hours. However, a negative histamine and tryptase study does not completely rule out the diagnosis of anaphylaxis. Skin testing and RAST for the causative agent (e.g., food, Hymenoptera venom, latex, or drug), if indicated, should be performed 4 to 6 weeks after the episode for greatest sensitivity.

TREATMENT IN THE FIELD

The essential steps in the treatment of anaphylaxis are (1) prevention, (2) recognition, (3) prompt therapy, and (4) early transport to an emergency care facility.

Prevention

Prevention depends on recognition of persons at risk. Use of oral rather than parenteral medications should always be considered in patients at high risk for anaphylaxis. This includes patients with atopy or those with a possible history of allergic reactions to drugs. If drugs are administered parenterally, such patients should remain in a medically supervised area for at least 30 minutes afterward. Patients with known food or drug allergies must read labels to avoid the foods or drugs to which they are allergic. Severely food-allergic patients must be especially careful when dining out and may wish to avoid eating in restaurants altogether. Patients with a history of anaphylactic reaction to Hymenoptera venom should be given information on avoiding future stings and should be referred to an allergist for consideration of venom immunotherapy [see Chapter 110]. Patients with a history of anaphylaxis should always carry an epinephrine autoinjector (Epi-Pen).

Recognition

Immediate diagnosis of a developing reaction is imperative. Because of the risk of respiratory and cardiovascular collapse, the patient's airway, breathing, and circulation (the so-called emergency ABCs) must be rapidly assessed.

Prompt Initiation of Therapy

Anaphylaxis can rarely be overtreated. Treatment must be expeditious and appropriate. A protocol and supplies for prompt treatment should be in place at every medical office or facility. A protocol for diagnosis and management of anaphy-laxis has been developed by the Joint Task Force on Practice Parameters.[88] The supplies should include oxygen, aqueous epinephrine, injectable antihistamines, intravenous or intramuscular glucocorticoids, oropharyngeal airways, and I.V. fluids. If the clinical assessment even suggests an anaphylactic reaction, it is best to call 911 and initiate therapy.

Whenever possible, decrease the absorption of the antigen. With insect bites and stings on an extremity, for example, apply a tourniquet above the injection site to block venous return and remove the insect stinger. Inject epinephrine (1:1000) locally.

Give supplemental oxygen, 6 to 8 L/min, and administer epinephrine (1:1000) subcutaneously or intramuscularly. The epinephrine dose is 0.2 to 0.5 mg in adults and 0.01 mg/kg in children. If the patient is in cardiopulmonary arrest, epinephrine (1:10,000) should be administered intravenously, in a dose of 0.1 to 1.0 mg for adults and 0.001 to 0.002 mg in children. Patients and their caregivers should recognize that more than one dose of epinephrine may be required.[89]

Intravenous H_1 antihistamines (e.g., diphenhydramine, 50 mg) and H_2 antihistamines (e.g., ranitidine, 50 mg, or cimetidine, 300 mg) should be given. If the patient can swallow, H_2 antihistamines can be given orally. Bronchospasm may be treated with aerosolized beta-adrenergic agonists (albuterol). Severe bronchospasm may require endotracheal intubation or cricothyrotomy. Respiratory failure can occur with or without upper airway compromise. Persistent hypoperfusion and ischemia may lead to myocardial infarction, cerebral ischemia, or renal failure.

Once the acute reaction is under control, systemic corticosteroids (e.g., hydrocortisone sodium phosphate, 100 mg every 2 to 4 hours) may be administered. The patient can be transferred to the emergency department.

PROGNOSIS

Most patients experience only a single episode of anaphylaxis,[82] but some patients have three or more episodes.[90] Death from anaphylaxis is uncommon. Complications are also unusual; most patients recover completely. However, respiratory failure from severe bronchospasm or laryngeal edema can cause hypoxia, which if prolonged could lead to brain injury. Hypotension and hypoxia may lead to cardiac ischemia or arrhythmias.

References

1. Galli SJ: New concepts about the mast cell. N Engl J Med 328:257, 1993

2. Doutre M: Physiopathology of urticaria. Eur J Dermatol 9:601, 1999

3. Longley J, Duffy TP, Kohn S: The mast cell and mast cell disease. J Am Acad Dermatol 32:545, 1995

4. Haas N, Toppe E, Henz BM: Microscopic morphology of different types of urticaria. Arch Dermatol 134:41, 1998

5. Bedard PM, Brunet C, Pelletier G, et al: Increased compound 48/80 induced local histamine release from nonlesional skin of patients with chronic urticaria. J Allergy Clin Immunol 78:1121, 1986

6. Kaplan AP: Urticaria and angioedema. Allergy: Principles & Practice, 5th ed. Middleton E, Reed CE, Ellis EF, et al, Eds. Mosby, St Louis, 1998, p 1104

7. Plumb J, Norlin C, Young PC: Exposures and outcomes of children with urticaria seen in a pediatric practice-based research network: a case-control study. Arch Pediatr Adolesc Med 155:1017, 2000

8. Shipley D, Ormerod AD: Drug-induced urticaria: recognition and treatment. Am J Clin Dermatol 2:151, 2001

9. Bircher AJ: Drug-induced urticaria and angioedema caused by non-IgE mediated pathomechanisms. Eur J Dermatol 9:657, 1999

10. Sanchez-Borges M, Capriles-Hulett A: Atopy is a risk factor for non-steroidal anti-inflammatory drug sensitivity. Ann Allergy Asthma Immunol 84:101, 2000

11. Sanchez Borges M, Capriles-Hulett A, Caballero-Fonseca F, et al: Tolerability to new COX-2 inhibitors in NSAID-sensitive patients with cutaneous reactions. Ann Allergy Asthma Immunol 87:201, 2001

12. Gruchalla RS, Beltrani VS: Drug-induced cutaneous reactions. Allergic Skin Disease. Leung DYM, Greaves MW, Eds. Marcel Dekker, New York, 2000, p 318

13. Sampson HA: Food allergy. Part 2: diagnosis and management. J Allergy Clin Immunol 103:981, 1999

14. Sehgal VN, Rege VL: An interrogative study of 158 urticaria patients. Ann Allergy 31:279, 1973

15. Eggesbo M, Halvorsen R, Tambs K, et al: Prevalence of parentally perceived adverse reaction to food in young children. Pediatr Allergy Immunol 10:122, 1999

16. Bock SA, Sampson HA, Atkins FM, et al: Double-blind, placebo-controlled food challenge as an office procedure: a manual. J Allergy Clin Immunol 82:986, 1988

17. Rockwell WJ: Reactions to molds in foods. Food allergy: a practical approach to diagnosis and management. Chiaramonte LT, Schneider AT, Lifshitz F, Eds. Marcel Dekker, New York, 1988, p 153

18. Anderson JA: Milestones marking the knowledge of adverse reactions to food in the decade of the 1980s. Ann Allergy 72:143, 1994

19. Spergel JM, Beausoleil JL, Pawlowski NA: Resolution of childhood peanut allergy. Ann Allergy Asthma Immunol 85:435, 2000

20. Bock SA: Natural history of severe reactions to foods in young children. J Pediatr 107:676, 1985

21. Sicherer SH, Sampson HA: Food hypersensitivity and atopic dermatitis: pathophysiology, epidemiology, diagnosis, and management. J Allergy Clin Immunol 104:S114, 1999

22. Leznoff A, Sussman GL: Syndrome of idiopathic chronic urticaria and angioedema with thyroid auto-immunity: a study of 90 patients. J Allergy Clin Immunol 84:66, 1989

23. Turktas I, Gokcora N, Demirsoy S, et al: The association of chronic urticaria and angioedema with autoimmune thyroididitis. Int J Dermatol 36:187, 1997

24. Zauli D, Delonardi G, Foderaro S, et al: Thyroid autoimmunity in chronic urticaria. Allergy Asthma Proc 22:93, 2001

25. Rumbyrt JS, Katz JL, Schocket AL: Resolution of chronic urticaria in patients with thyroid autoimmunity. J Allergy Clin Immunol 96:901, 1995

26. Heymann WR: Chronic urticaria and angioedema associated with thyroid autoimmunity: review and therapeutic implications. J Am Acad Dermatol 40:229, 1999

27. Liutu M, Kalimo K, Uksila J, et al: Etiologic aspects of chronic urticaria. Int J Dermatol 37:515, 1998

28. Schnyder B, Helbling A, Pichler WJ: Chronic idiopathic urticaria: natural course and association with Helicobacter pylori infection. Int Arch Allergy Immunol 119:60, 1999

29. Nelson H: Routine sinus roentgenograms and chronic urticaria. JAMA 251:1680, 1984

30. deGentile L, Grandiere-Perez L, Chabasse D: Urticaria and parasites. Allergy Immunol (Paris) 31:288, 1999

31. Picardi A, Abeni D: Stressful life events and skin diseases: disentangling evidence from myth. Psychother Psychosom 70:118, 2001

32. Lipsker D, Veran Y, Grunenberger F, et al: The Schnitzler syndrome: four new cases and review of the literature. Medicine (Baltimore) 80:37, 2001

33. Muckle TJ: The 'Muckle-Wells' syndrome. Br J Dermatol 100:87, 1979

34. Demain JG, Taylor TM: Reactions to stinging and biting arthropods. Cutaneous Allergy. Charlesworth EN, Ed. Blackwell Science Publications, Cambridge, England, 1996, p 299

35. Stibich AS, Schwartz RA: Papular urticaria. Cutis 68:89, 2001

36. Tharp MD, Longley BJ Jr: Mastocytosis. Dermatol Clin 19:679, 2001

37. Kobza-Black A: Management of urticaria. Clin Exp Dermatol 27:328, 2002

38. Sibbald RB: Physical urticaria. Dermatol Clinics North Am 4:57, 1984

39. Wanderer AA: Cold urticaria syndromes: historical background, diagnostic classification, clinical and laboratory characteristics, pathogenesis, and management. J Allergy Clin Immunol 85:965, 1990

40. Neittaanmaki H: Cold urticaria: clinical findings in 220 patients. J Am Acad Dermatol 13:636, 1985

41. Monfrecola G, Masturzo E, Riccardo AM, et al: Solar urticaria: a report of 57 cases. Am J Contact Dermat 11:89, 2000

42. Uetsu N, Miyauchi-Hashimoto H, Okamoto H, et al. The clinical and photobiological characteristics of solar urticaria in 40 patients. Br J Dermatol 142:32, 2000.

43. Ryckaert S, Roelandts R: Solar urticaria. Arch Dermatol 134:71, 1998

44. Luong KV, Nguyen LT: Aquagenic urticaria: report of a case and review of the literature. Ann Allergy Asthma Immunol 80:483, 1998

45. Paterson R, Mellies CJ, Blankenship ML, et al: Vibratory angioedema: a hereditary type of physical hypersensitivity. J Allergy Clin Immunol 50:174, 1972

46. Lahti A: Immediate contact reactions. Curr Probl Dermatol 22:17, 1995

47. Hjorth N, Ree-Peterson J: Occupational protein contact dermatitis in foodhandlers. Contact Derm 2:28, 1976

48. Hirschmann JV, Lawlor F, et al: Cholinergic urticaria. Arch Dermatol 123:462, 1987

49. Lee EE, Maibach HI: Treatment of urticaria: an evidence-based evaluation of antihistamines. Am J Clin Dermatol 2:27, 2001

50. Goldsobel AB, Rohr AS, Siefel SC, et al: Efficacy of doxepin in the treatment of chronic idiopathic urticaria. J Allergy Clin Immunol 78:867, 1986

51. Mansfield LE, Smith JA, Nelson HS: Greater inhibition of dermographia with combination of H1 and H2 antagonists. Ann Allergy 50:264, 1983

52. Kennes B, De Maubeuge J, Delespesse G: Treatment of chronic urticaria with a beta2-adrenergic stimulant. Clin Allergy 7:35, 1977

53. Spangler DL, Vanderpool GE, Carroll MS, et al: Terbutaline in the treatment of chronic urticaria. Ann Allergy 45:246, 1980

54. Kaplan AP: Clinical practice: chronic urticaria and angioedema. N Engl J Med 346:175, 2002

55. The diagnosis and management of urticaria: a practice parameter. Part I: acute urticaria/angioedema; part II: chronic urticaria/angioedema. Joint Task Force on Practice Parameters. Ann Allergy Asthma Immunol 85:521, 2000

56. Parsad D, Pandhi R, Juneja A: Stanozolol in chronic urticaria: a double-blind, placebo controlled trial. J Dermatol 28:299, 2001

57. Fearfield LA, Gazzard B, Bunker CB: Aquagenic urticaria in HIV virus infection treated with stanozolol. Br J Dermatol 137:620, 1997

58. Omerud AD, Smart L, Reid TM, Milford-Ward A: Familial cold urticaria: investigation of a family and response to stanozolol. Arch Dermatol 129:34, 1993

59. Bressler RB, Sowell K, Huston DP: Therapy of chronic idiopathic urticaria with nifedipine: demonstration of beneficial effect in a double blinded, placebo controlled cross-over trial. J Allergy Clin Immunol 83:756, 1989

60. Millins JL, Randle HW, Solley GO, et al: The therapeutic response of urticarial vasculitis to indomethacin. J Am Acad Dermatol 3:349, 1980

61. Grattan CE, O'Donnell BF, Francis DM, et al: Randomized double-blind study of cyclosporin in chronic `idiopathic' urticaria. Br J Dermatol 143:365, 2000

62. Beltrani VS: An overview of chronic urticaria. Clin Rev Allergy Immunol 23:147, 2002

63. Hedner T, Samuelsson O, Lunde H, et al: Angioedema in relation to treatment with angiotensin converting enzyme inhibitors. Br Med J 304:941, 1992

64. Champion RH: Urticaria and angio-edema: a review of 554 patients. Br J Dermatol 81:588, 1969

65. Henig NR, Henderson WR Jr: Anti-leukotriene agents in the treatment of asthma. Current Review of Allergic Diseases. Kaliner MA, Ed. Current Medicine, Philadelphia, 2000, p 71

66. Quiralte J, Bianco C, Castillo R, et al: Intolerance to nonsteroidal anti-inflammatory drugs: results of controlled drug challenges in 98 patients. J Allergy Clin Immunol 98:678, 1996

67. Kelkar PS, Butterfield JH, Teaford HG: Urticaria and angioedema from cyclooxygenase-2 inhibitors. J Rheumatol 28:2553, 2001

68. Agostini A, Cicardi M, Cugno M, et al: Angioedema due to angiotensin-converting enzyme inhibitors. Immunopharmacology 15:21, 1999

69. Hedner T, Samuelsson O, Lunde H, et al: Angioedema in relation to treatment with angiotensin converting enzyme inhibitors. BMJ 304:941, 1992

70. Rodgers JE, Patterson JH: Angiotensin II receptor blockers: clinical relevance and therapeutic role. Am J Health Syst Pharm 58:671, 2001

71. Nzeako UC, Frigas E, Tremaine WJ: Hereditary angioedema: a broad review for clinicians. Arch Intern Med 161:2417, 2001

72. Bork K, Barnstedt SE, Koch P, et al: Hereditary angioedema with normal C1-inhibitor activity in women. Lancet 356:213, 2000

73. Laurent J, Guinnepain MT: Angioedema associated with C1 inhibitor deficiency. Clin Rev Allergy Immunol 17:513, 1999

74. Jackson J, Sims RB, Whelan A, et al: An IgG autoantibody which inactivates C1-inhibitor. Nature 323:722, 1986

75. Black AK, Greaves MW: Antihistamines in urticaria and angioedema. Clin Allergy Immunol 17:249, 2002

76. Chase MP, Fiarman GS, Scholz FJ, et al: Angioedema of the small bowel due to an angiotensin-converting enzyme inhibitor. J Clin Gastroenterol 31:254, 2000

77. Agostini A, Ciccardi M: Hereditary and acquired C-1 inhibitor deficiency: biological and clinical characteristics in 235 patients. Medicine (Baltimore) 71:206, 1992

78. Cicardi M, Bergamaschini L, Zingale LC, et al: Idiopathic nonhistaminergic angioedema. Am J Med 106:650, 1999

79. Bork K, Barnstedt SE: Treatment of 193 episodes of laryngeal edema with C1 inhibitor concentrate in patients with hereditary angioedema. Arch Intern Med 161:714, 2001

80. Luskin AT, Luskin SS: Anaphylaxis and anaphylactoid reactions: diagnosis and management. Am J Ther 3:515, 1996

81. Van der Klauw MM, Stricker BHCH, Herings RMC, et al: A population-based case-cohort study of drug-induced anaphylaxis. Br J Clin Pharmacol 35:400, 1993

82. Yokum MW, Butterfield J, Klein J, et al: Epidemiology of anaphylaxis in Olmsted County, a population-based study. J Allergy Clin Immunol 104:452, 1999

83. Yocum MW, Khan DA: Assessment of patients who have experienced anaphylaxis: a 3-year survey. Mayo Clin Proc 69:16, 1994

84. Kemp SF, Lockey RF, Wolf BL, Lieberman P: Anaphylaxis: a review of 266 cases. Arch Intern Med 155:1749, 1995

85. Perez C, Tejedor MA, Hoz A, et al: Anaphylaxis: a review of 182 patients (abstr). J Allergy Clin Immunol 95:368, 1995

86. Kaufman DW: An epidemiologic study of severe anaphylactic and anaphylactoid reactions among hospital patients: methods and overall risks—abstract from report from the International Collaborative Study of Severe Anaphylaxis. Epidemiology 9:141, 1998

87. Boxer M, Greenberger PA, Patterson R: Clinical summary and course of idiopathic anaphylaxis in 73 patients. Arch Intern Med 147:26, 1987

88. The diagnosis and management of anaphylaxis. Joint Task Force on Practice Parameters, American Academy of Allergy, Asthma and Immunology, American College of Allergy, Asthma and Immunology, and the Joint Council of Allergy, Asthma and Immunology. J Allergy Clin Immunol 101:S465, 1998

89. Korenblat P, Lundie MJ, Dankner RE, et al: A retrospective study of epinephrine administration for anaphylaxis: How many doses are needed? Allergy Asthma Proc 20:383, 1999

90. Weiler JM: Anaphylaxis in the general population: a frequent and occasionally fatal disorder that is under-recognized. J Allergy Clin Immunol 104:271, 1999

91. Sim TC: Anaphylaxis. How to manage and prevent this medical emergency. Postgrad Med 92:277, 1992

109 Food and Drug Allergies

Dennis J. Beer, M.D., and Ross E. Rocklin, M.D.

Allergic reactions to foods or drugs are among the most common and readily recognized forms of allergic response. However, many adverse reactions to food or drugs are not immunologically mediated. Appropriate management may hinge on this distinction.

Food Allergy

Food allergy or hypersensitivity results from an IgE-mediated reaction to a food or food additive.[1,2] The risk of development of IgE-mediated food allergy appears to be significantly greater in persons in whom the process of acetylation proceeds slowly. Speed of acetylation is mediated genetically.[3]

When a sensitized person ingests food that contains the offending allergen, gastrointestinal mast cells coated with IgE specific for the allergen degranulate and release mediators; these mediators induce local changes in vasopermeability, stimulate mucus production, increase muscle contraction, stimulate pain fibers, and recruit inflammatory cells.

Shellfish, nuts, peanuts, eggs, and dairy products are the foods that most commonly cause severe anaphylaxis; peanuts are the most frequent cause of fatal anaphylaxis. Both children and adults with allergies to certain foods may develop tolerance to these foods over time, although this is less likely with peanuts, nuts, and seafood.[4] Allergy to peanuts that is associated with anaphylaxis is not outgrown, but some peanut-allergic children who do not have a history of anaphylaxis may develop tolerance.[5] Persons who are allergic to peanuts should be made aware that this food is often a hidden additive in cookies, pastries, egg rolls, chili, cooking oil, and candy.

CLINICAL MANIFESTATIONS

The clinical expression of food allergy is influenced by the age of the patient, the quality and quantity of food ingested, and the type and extent of associated medical problems. Edema and pruritus of the lips, oral mucosa, and pharynx occur when the food comes in contact with the oropharynx. Such reactions are transient and are not necessarily followed by other symptoms. Entry of the offending food into the stomach and intestine may result in nausea, cramping pain, abdominal distention, vomiting, flatulence, and diarrhea. Food allergy can also be expressed as urticaria, angioedema, asthma, and rhinoconjunctivitis. Systemic anaphylaxis can occur within minutes but occasionally may take hours to manifest.

Symptoms generally develop within minutes to 2 hours after ingesting the food allergen. In unusual cases, systemic reactions can be provoked by exposure to food allergens without ingestion of the food (e.g., by inhalation, skin contact, or mucous membrane contact).[6] A food suspected of being an allergen may fail to consistently cause allergic reactions because of variability in the amount consumed; the simultaneous ingestion of other foods, which may delay digestion; and the manner in which the food is prepared. For instance, although the ingestion of fresh fruits or vegetables may be associated with pruritus and angioedema of the lips, tongue, palate, and throat,

the ingestion of cooked varieties of the same fruits or vegetables often produces no noxious symptoms. Similarly, if the skin of an offending fruit or vegetable is removed before it is eaten, allergic symptoms may not occur.

DIAGNOSIS

The diagnosis of IgE-mediated food allergy is established by the clinical history, results of selective immediate hypersensitivity skin testing or radioallergosorbant testing (RAST), complete elimination of the suspected food allergen from the diet for 2 weeks to determine whether symptoms resolve, and double-blind, placebo-controlled food challenges.[7]

IgE to specific food groups can be demonstrated by skin tests or RAST. False positive skin tests occur, but false negative results are unlikely if the tests are performed correctly. Thus, the best use of skin testing appears to be to support a clinical impression that one or more foods are capable of causing IgE-mediated reactions in a given person.

Using an elimination diet is helpful if it is not clear whether ingestion of a specific food causes the symptoms. The likelihood of establishing a diagnosis by use of elimination diets is greater when fewer foods are responsible for the symptoms. Offending foods that are identified in this way should be eliminated from the diet permanently. If removal of one or several foods from the diet does not eliminate symptoms, initiation of a severely limited diet is warranted. Extensive elimination diets should include lamb and rice because these foods seldom cause allergic reactions. Failure of such a diet to eliminate symptoms

---

Table 1 Differential Diagnosis of Food Hypersensitivity

Additives and contaminants
  Dyes (e.g., tartrazine)
  Flavorings and preservatives: nitrites and nitrates, monosodium glutamate, sulfites (e.g., sodium metabisulfite), sodium benzoate
  Toxins: botulinum toxin, mushroom toxins, saxitoxin (found in shellfish), ciguatoxin (found in fish)
  Insect body parts
  Molds

Gastrointestinal diseases
  Structural abnormalities: hiatal hernia, obstruction
  Enzyme deficiencies: lactase deficiency, glucose-6-phosphate dehydrogenase deficiency, galactosemia, favism
  Malignant diseases
  Peptic ulcer
  Cholelithiasis

Miscellaneous diseases: collagen vascular diseases, endocrine disorders, parasitic diseases (e.g., amebiasis, roundworm), cystic fibrosis

Pharmacologic agents: caffeine, histamine, tyramine, phenylethylamine, alcohol

Psychological reactions

indicates that the symptoms are not caused by food.

If the correlation between specific foods and symptoms remains unclear, oral challenge with a suspected food may be used for diagnosis; however, oral challenge should be avoided when the suspected food is associated with a history of anaphylaxis. Furthermore, no food challenge is without risk of side effects, and the patient must be made aware of this fact. Such procedures should be done only under the supervision of an allergist.[8] Ideally, food challenges should be double-blind and placebo-controlled; such challenges are considered the gold standard for in vivo diagnosis of allergy to a specific food.[9]

It is important to distinguish IgE-mediated food allergy from other food reactions[10] [see Table 1]. In some cases, the reaction may not be to the food itself but to additives or contaminants (e.g., dyes, preservatives, insect parts, or mold). In patients with gastrointestinal symptoms, GI disease must be excluded. Pain relieved by a bowel movement or the presence of abdominal bloating suggests irritable bowel syndrome rather than food allergy.[11]

TREATMENT

Treatment of food allergy is primarily preventive. Breast-feeding should be encouraged because it prevents early exposure of the immature GI system of an infant to foreign milk and soy proteins. There is as yet no evidence that immunotherapy or oral desensitization is beneficial. Future therapeutic possibilities include DNA-based vaccination, which animal studies suggest may be effective in reversing anaphylactic hypersensitivity to food.[12] A long-term elimination diet must be designed to provide optimal nutrition while completely eliminating the offending foods. Such diets should be designed in conjunction with a nutritionist. The development of GI symptoms after inadvertent food ingestion is usually treated with antihistamines.[13,14] Patients with a history of anaphylaxis after ingestion of certain foods should be provided with an epinephrine autoinjector (Epi-Pen) so that they can self-administer the drug in an emergency; these patients should also have antihistamines available at all times. An identification tag that states the patient's food sensitivity is also recommended.

Drug Allergy

Allergic reactions to drugs constitute only 6% of adverse drug reactions; the majority of adverse drug reactions occur through nonimmunologic or unknown mechanisms. Allergic reactions require previous exposure to the drug, so that sensitization can take place; once the patient is sensitized, reactions can be precipitated by small doses of the drug. Drug allergy must be distinguished from drug intolerance, an undesirable pharmacologic effect that may occur at low concentrations, and from idiosyncratic reactions, which result from biochemical alterations in the metabolism of a drug. An idiosyncratic reaction is independent of the dose, does not require previous exposure, and is not a pharmacologic effect of the drug.[15]

Host factors that increase the risk of allergic drug reactions include adult age, female gender, concurrent infections, and HIV infection.[16,17] Patients with cystic fibrosis also have a high rate of drug reactions, which cannot be fully explained by their repetitive exposure to multiple medications. It is a common misconception that atopic persons are at higher risk for serious drug reactions. In fact, atopic and nonatopic patients show the same incidence of reactivity to penicillin on skin testing.

The β-lactam family of antibiotics, most notably penicillin and penicillin derivatives, accounts for most allergic reactions to drugs and 97% of the deaths caused each year by anaphylactic drug reactions. Between 1% and 5% of patients who receive penicillin have an allergic reaction.[18] Other agents that can cause allergic reactions include sulfa-containing antibiotics, streptomycin, aspirin, local anesthetics, opiates, hormones, heparin, protamine, streptokinase, radiocontrast media, diagnostic reagents such as sulfobromophthalein and Congo red, dehydrocholic acid, dextran, vitamins, tetracycline, and organic iodine.[15]

CLINICAL MANIFESTATIONS

Drug reactions can be immediate, accelerated, or delayed. Immediate reactions include anaphylaxis, which occurs more commonly with parenteral administration; symptoms usually appear minutes after injection of the offending drug. Oral administration can occasionally produce anaphylaxis; such cases may have a prolonged course because of gradual absorption of the drug. Initial symptoms are generalized pruritus associated with skin hyperemia, angioedema, laryngeal edema, and swelling of the eyelids. These manifestations may be followed by a decrease in the plasma volume, which results in hypotension, vascular collapse, and shock.

Accelerated reactions occur within 72 hours after administration of the drug. These reactions include urticaria and angioedema. Delayed reactions occur 72 hours or more after administration. One of the most common clinical manifestations of drug allergy is the development of a mild systemic illness, similar to serum sickness, that is characterized by urticarial eruptions, arthralgias or arthritis, lymphadenopathy, and fever. These symptoms begin 6 to 12 days after the administration of a drug and may take several days to a week to subside after cessation of the drug. Drug-induced fever can occur alone or in combination with the symptoms described and usually develops during the second week of treatment.

Delayed reactions involving morbilliform or maculopapular rash may develop after exposure to amoxicillin or penicillin. These are thought to involve a T cell–mediated immune mechanism.[18] In contrast, the rash that develops in 3% to 8% of patients receiving ampicillin is thought to be nonallergic in nature. Patients who experience typical ampicillin rashes, which are characterized by maculopapular erythema with minimal irritation or pruritus, need not necessarily discontinue the ampicillin and are not at higher risk for future intolerance to ampicillin or other β-lactam antibiotics.[19]

A syndrome of allergy to multiple antibiotics of different chemical families has been described. Its origin is uncertain. Risk factors include female sex, a history of multiple antibiotic reactions, and intolerance to nonsteroidal anti-inflammatory drugs.[20]

DIAGNOSIS

Drug allergy is primarily a clinical diagnosis, based on a detailed history and the physician's knowledge of which drugs are most likely to provoke allergic reactions.[21] One or more of the following observations suggest an allergic drug reaction: the reaction does not correspond to the known pharmacologic action of the drug; it can be elicited by minute doses of the drug; it occurs days after the initial administration of the drug; it includes symptoms that are generally associated with allergy; it reappears on challenge with the drug, with progressive shortening of the latency period before symptoms appear; and similar reactions are observed with structurally similar drugs.

The detection of IgE directed against a suspected drug is useful in establishing an immunologic basis for the symptoms; the presence of antibodies of other classes that react with the drug or a cell-mediated immune response does not necessarily correlate with symptoms.

Although many in vitro assays can detect sensitivity to a drug, none are clinically reliable. In contrast, skin tests for specific drugs such as penicillin and its derivatives have diagnostic and predictive value. The reagents for the penicillin skin test include penicilloyl polylysine, which is a synthetic penicillin derivative that is used to measure sensitivity to the major antigenic determinant, and modified forms of benzyl penicillin G, which can help identify sensitivity to minor antigenic determinants. Because of the risk of life-threatening reactions, it is important to avoid skin testing in patients with a history of exfoliative dermatitis or bullous skin lesions (e.g., Stevens-Johnson syndrome or toxic epidermal necrolysis) associated with use of penicillin. Patients with a family history of penicillin allergy, but no personal history of it, are not at increased risk for penicillin allergy and do not require skin testing.

Patients with a positive skin test are at risk for an immediate hypersensitivity reaction to penicillin; those with a negative skin test are unlikely to have a serious immediate hypersensitivity reaction.[22,23] Skin testing for most other drugs is unreliable because correlation between a positive test and clinical conditions is lacking.

TREATMENT

If a drug is suspected of causing a drug allergy, administration should be stopped. Symptoms should subside within 1 or 2 days, although they may take a week to disappear. In severe cases, the drug may be eliminated faster by the administration of large amounts of fluids, diuretics, or laxatives. If anaphylaxis is present, treatment should be instituted immediately. Corticosteroids have been useful for Arthus-type reactions, such as serum sickness and polyarteritis, as well as for manifestations of delayed hypersensitivity (e.g., maculopapular rash). Large daily doses of prednisone (40 to 60 mg) can be administered for several days and then stopped without the dose being tapered.

If a drug that has caused an allergic reaction must be used, the patient can be desensitized first; the drug can then be safely administered.[24,25] Intravenous or oral desensitization should be carried out only by qualified personnel in a hospital, where immediate treatment can be instituted if a reaction should occur. Once desensitization is achieved, the drug must be continued or desensitization may be lost, requiring repeat desensitization before the drug can be given again.

References

1. Sampson HA, Metcalfe DD: Food allergies. JAMA 268:2840, 1992
2. Leung AK: Food allergy: a clinical approach. Adv Pediatr 45:145, 1998
3. Gawronska-Szklarz B, Pawlik A, Czaja-Bulsa G, et al: Genotype of N-acetyltransferase 2 (NAT2) polymorphism in children with immunoglobulin E-mediated food allergy. Clin Pharmacol Ther 69:372, 2001
4. Burks W: Current understanding of food allergy. Ann N Y Acad Sci 964:1, 2002
5. Spergel JM, Beausoleil JL, Pawlowski NA: Resolution of childhood peanut allergy. Ann Allergy Asthma Immunol 85:473, 2000
6. Bahna SL: Unusual presentations of food allergy. Ann Allergy Asthma Immunol 86:414, 2001
7. Sicherer SH: Food allergy. Lancet 360:701, 2002
8. Bock SA, Sampson HA, Atkins FM, et al: Double-blind placebo-controlled food challenge procedures as an office procedure: a manual. J Allergy Clin Immunol 82:986, 1986
9. Helm RM: Food allergy: in-vivo diagnostics including challenge. Curr Opin Allergy Clin Immunol 1:255, 2001
10. Sampson HA: Differential diagnosis in adverse reactions to foods. J Allergy Clin Immunol 78:212, 1986
11. Neri M, Laterza F, Howell S, et al: Symptoms discriminate irritable bowel syndrome from organic gastrointestinal diseases and food allergy. Eur J Gastroenterol Hepatol 12:981, 2000
12. Nguyen MD, Cinman N, Yen J, et al: DNA-based vaccination for the treatment of food allergy. Allergy 56(suppl 67):127, 2001
13. Sogn DD: Medications and their use in the treatment of adverse reactions to foods. J Allergy Clin Immunol 78:238, 1986
14. Pastorello EA, Stocchi L, Pravettoni V, et al: Role of the elimination diet in adults with food allergy. J Allergy Clin Immunol 84:475, 1989
15. Weiss ME: Drug allergy. Med Clin North Am 76:857, 1992
16. Demoly P, Bousquet J: Drug allergy diagnosis work up. Allergy 57(suppl 72):37, 2002
17. Pirmohamed M, Park BK: HIV and drug allergy. Curr Opin Allergy Clin Immunol 1:311, 2001
18. Schnyder B, Pichler WJ: Skin and laboratory tests in amoxicillin- and penicillin-induced morbilliform skin eruption. Clin Exp Allergy 30:590, 2000
19. Adcock BB, Rodman DP: Ampicillin-specific rashes. Arch Fam Med 5:301, 1996
20. Asero R: Detection of patients with multiple drug allergy syndrome by elective tolerance tests. Ann Allergy Asthma Immunol 80:185, 1998
21. Primeau MN, Adkinson NF Jr: Recent advances in the diagnosis of drug allergy. Curr Opin Allergy Clin Immunol 1:337, 2001
22. Idsoe O, Guthe T, Willcox RR, et al: Nature and extent of penicillin side-reactions, with particular reference to fatalities from anaphylactic shock. Bull World Health Organ 38:159, 1968
23. Sullivan TJ, Wedner HJ, Shatz GS, et al: Skin testing to detect penicillin allergy. J Allergy Clin Immunol 68:171, 1981
24. Sullivan TJ, Yecies LD, Shatz GS, et al: Desensitization of patients allergic to penicillin using orally administered beta-lactam antibiotics. J Allergy Clin Immunol 69:275, 1982
25. Weiss ME, Adkinson NF Jr: Immediate hypersensitivity reactions to penicillin and related antibiotics. Clin Allergy 18:515, 1988

110 Allergic Reactions to Hymenoptera

David B. K. Golden, M.D.

Allergic reactions to insect venom primarily occur as a result of stings by insects of the order Hymenoptera. Allergic swelling can occur at the site of the insect sting, but only rarely does anaphylaxis result. Nonallergic reactions to insect venom have also been reported; these include nephropathy, central and peripheral neurologic syndromes, idiopathic thrombocytopenic purpura, and rhabdomyolysis. These are toxic reactions and are not IgE mediated. Allergic reactions to stings manifest themselves as either late-phase local inflammation (severe prolonged swelling) or systemic responses (e.g., anaphylaxis).

Epidemiology

Allergic reactions to Hymenoptera stings have been reported in persons of all ages. The reactions may be preceded by a number of uneventful stings. Systemic allergic reactions are reported in up to 1% of children and 3% of adults, although allergic antibodies to Hymenoptera venoms can be detected in 17% to 26% of adults.[1] The frequency of large local allergic reactions is uncertain but is estimated to be about 10% in adults. Fatal allergic reactions to insect stings may occur at any age but are most common in adults older than 45 years.[2] Half of those persons in whom a fatal reaction occurred had no previous history of allergy to insect stings; the other half had previous reactions but failed to take adequate preventive measures. In the United States, at least 40 deaths occur each year as the result of insect stings; other sting fatalities may go unrecognized. In many cases of unexplained sudden death, postmortem blood samples show the presence of both Hymenoptera venom–specific IgE antibodies and elevated serum tryptase levels, indicating the true cause of the fatal reactions.[3] For 50 years, whole body extracts were used as standard treatment for immunotherapy; such use was based on a lack of knowledge of the natural history of anaphylaxis.[4] We now recognize that the risk of an anaphylactic reaction to a sting varies in accordance with the history of previous stings and is correlated with the results of venom skin tests or radioallergosorbent tests (RAST). The risk declines gradually with time [*see Table 1*]. In high-risk patients, the risk of reaction is 50% to 70%; other persons with a history of insect-sting allergy are at much lower risk. Most affected children have only cutaneous systemic reactions, with no respiratory or vascular symptoms, and have less than a 10% risk of a systemic reaction to a subsequent sting.[5] The risk is also less than 10% in adults or children who have experienced only large local reactions to stings. Furthermore, the allergy is self-limited in many cases. The risk of reaction falls from 50% initially to 33% after 3 to 5 years; the risk is 20% to 25% if more than 10 years have passed since the reaction.[6] However, in some individuals, the risk of anaphylaxis persists for decades, even with no intervening stings.

Etiology

Hymenoptera allergy is directed against the allergenic proteins in the venoms of the stinging insects. Three families of Hymenoptera are important causes of allergy. The bees (honeybees, bumblebees) and vespids (yellow jackets, hornets, wasps) are the best known [*see Figures 1 and 2*]. Imported fire ants (*Solenopsis* species) are a rapidly increasing public health hazard in the Southeast and South Central United States, especially on the Gulf Coast [*see Figure 3*].[7] Honeybee stings are more common in agricultural areas. Yellow jackets are the most frequent culprits in the northern areas of North America and Europe, whereas paper wasps (*Polistes* species) are more commonly implicated along the Gulf Coast in the United States and the Mediterranean Coast in Europe.

Knowledge of the behavior of these insects can be helpful in evaluating the history of affected patients. Honeybees are relatively docile and rarely sting or swarm unless provoked. Stings usually occur as a result of garden exposures or from going barefoot outdoors. The barbed stinger of the honeybee remains in the skin, causing the death of the honeybee. Africanized honeybees (killer bees) are more aggressive and are now present in the southern United States.[8] Although an Africanized honeybee is no different from a domestic honeybee with regard to anatomy or venom, Africanized honeybees have a tendency to swarm with little provocation and to sting in large numbers. A large number of stings can cause massive envenomation; the resulting toxic reactions have been fatal to livestock and humans. Bumblebees sting infrequently, but a few cases of systemic reactions have been reported.

Yellow jackets usually nest underground or in the cracks of buildings or wooden ties or logs used in residential landscaping, whereas hornets generally build their nests in shrubs and trees. Paper wasps build an open nest with visible cells; nests are often found on the eaves or windowsills of a home. Yellow jackets are scavengers; they are commonly found around food at picnics and in orchards, trash cans, and dumpsters. They are highly aggressive and will sting quite readily. Wasps are less aggressive but will sting readily when disturbed. The vespid stinger usually has finer barbs than the stinger of the bee and does not commonly remain in the skin.

Fire ants have stingers, and it is the sting rather than the bite that causes the allergic reaction. Fire ants are widespread in the

Table 1 Risk of Systemic Reactions and Clinical Recommendations Based on Reaction to Previous Stings and Results of the Venom Skin Test or RAST

Reaction to Previous Sting	Skin Test or RAST	Risk of Systemic Reaction	Clinical Recommendation
None	Positive	10%–20%	Avoidance
Large local	Positive	5%–10%	Avoidance
Cutaneous systemic	Positive, child	1%–10%	Avoidance
	Positive, adult	10%–20%	Venom immunotherapy
Anaphylaxis	Positive	30%–60%	Venom immunotherapy
	Negative	5%–10%	Repeat skin test/RAST

RAST—radioallergosorbent test

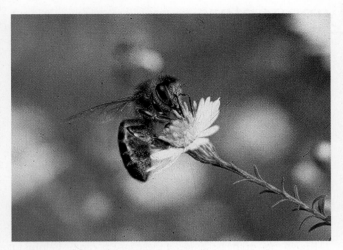

Figure 1   **The honeybee (*Apis mellifera*).**

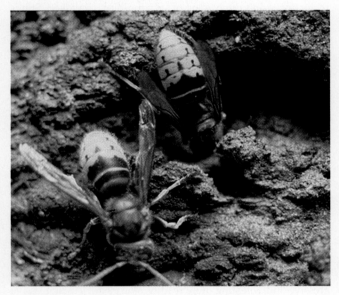

Figure 2   **The European hornet (*Vespa crabro germana*) was introduced into the United States in the mid-19th century. In the United States, its habitat includes most of the eastern United States, Louisiana, and the Dakotas. Although it is a woodland species, its nests can be found in barns, attics, hollow walls, birdhouses, and abandoned beehives.**

Pathogenesis

The pathogenesis of Hymenoptera allergy is the same as that of other forms of anaphylaxis. An initial encounter with a sting in genetically susceptible individuals causes the production of IgE antibodies to the venom allergens. The IgE antibodies become affixed to tissue mast cells and circulating basophils, which thus become armed for response to a later encounter with the same allergen. A subsequent sting can cause cross-linking of these allergic antibodies, leading to the release of mediators (e.g., histamine, leukotrienes, and cytokines) that cause the clinical manifestations of the allergic reaction. There is an association between conditions involving abnormal mast cell number or function and insect-sting anaphylaxis. The allergic reactions to stings are more severe in patients with elevated baseline serum tryptase levels or mastocytosis, and there is a higher incidence of treatment failures and relapse after treatment in these patients.[10-12]

Diagnosis

CLINICAL MANIFESTATIONS

Allergic reactions to insect stings may cause local allergic inflammation or the full spectrum of manifestations of anaphylaxis. Large local reactions are late-phase allergic reactions. Progressive swelling begins 6 to 12 hours after the sting, reaching peak size in 24 to 48 hours and resolving in 5 to 10 days. Large local reactions are usually defined as being greater than 6 in. in diameter; they can be massive in size and cause considerable pain. On the extremities, inflammatory lymphangitic streaks occur toward the axillary or inguinal nodes; these streaks are mistaken for signs of infection. Systemic reactions most commonly cause cutaneous signs and symptoms, including generalized flushing, pruritus, urticaria, and angioedema. Other typical manifestations are respiratory (e.g., throat or chest tightness, dyspnea, wheezing) or circulatory (e.g., light-headedness or unconsciousness). Less common signs of anaphylaxis include gastrointestinal or uterine cramps, cardiac arrhythmias (e.g., tachycardia or, occasionally, bradycardia), and coronary vasospasm.

In children, systemic reactions to stings usually cause only cutaneous symptoms (e.g., urticaria or angioedema). Respiratory symptoms are less common, and circulatory manifestations are infrequent. Systemic reactions usually follow a predictable and individual pattern in each patient, with worsening of the reaction occurring in less than 10% of cases.[13] Affected individuals

southeastern United States; in many areas, stings are very frequent, with up to 50% of the population being stung each year. Fire ants build nests in the shape of large mounds; these nests are common in residential and coastal areas. In most cases of fire-ant stings, multiple ants each administer multiple stings, which cause minimal pain. The unique lesions form sterile pustules that can become infected if excoriated [*see Figure 4*].

The allergic sensitivity is directed against proteins in the venoms (but not in the saliva or bodies) of the stinging insects.[9] Honeybee venom contains unique allergens, whereas the vespid venoms cross-react extensively with one another and contain essentially the same allergens. The venom of *Polistes* wasps is less cross-reactive than that of the other vespids. Only 50% of patients who are allergic to yellow-jacket venom experience reactions to wasp venom. The allergenic proteins in fire-ant venom are unique.

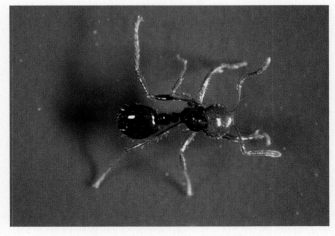

Figure 3   **Red imported fire ant (*Solenopsis invicta*).**

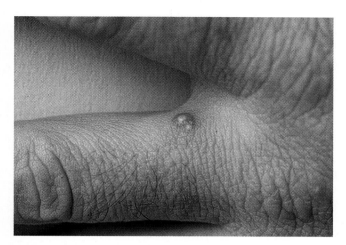

Figure 4 **Appearance of a pustule resulting from the sting of a fire ant. This photograph was taken 24 hours after the patient was stung.**

commonly do not seek medical attention and usually fail to report having sting reactions unless they are asked.

The diagnosis of insect-sting allergy rests on a history of allergic reactivity, because venom-specific IgE antibodies can be detected in many normal individuals. The positive venom skin test provides confirmation of the allergic nature of the sting reaction and helps define allergenic specificity. The history is most important and should be reviewed in detail with respect to the nature, number, and timing of stings in the past; the time course of the reaction; and all associated symptoms and treatments. The family history, atopic history, and general medical history are also of interest. It is also helpful to know of any medications the patient took before the reaction occurred, as well as any medications the patient is currently using.

PHYSICAL EXAMINATION

It is most important to measure the vital signs, including air flow, when there is dyspnea and to document cutaneous signs. Some patients have symptoms, such as dizziness and dyspnea, that do not correspond to the objective signs (e.g., blood pressure, peak expiratory flow rate) and may be the result of anxiety, panic, and hyperventilation. Any history suggestive of systemic allergic reaction must be taken seriously.

DIAGNOSTIC TESTS

The diagnosis of insect-venom allergy can be confirmed by skin tests or serologic tests (RAST) using Hymenoptera venoms. Both methods are useful, and they are often complementary in the diagnostic evaluation of affected patients. Both methods require specific experience and training to prevent false interpretations.

Intradermal skin tests using serial dilutions of the five Hymenoptera venom protein extracts is the recommended procedure. In the case of fire-ant sensitivity, whole body extracts of imported fire ants give reasonable diagnostic sensitivity and specificity. For Hymenoptera venom testing, intradermal tests are performed with venom concentrations ranging from 0.001 to 1.0 μg/ml to find the minimal concentration that yields a positive result as compared with a negative diluent control (e.g., human serum albumin saline) and a positive histamine control. Scratch tests with a value of 0.01 μg/ml may be used initially for patients with a history of very severe reactions.

The diagnosis of insect-sting allergy by detection of allergen-specific IgE antibodies in serum (typically by RAST) is a method of high potential but variable performance.[14] An elevation in the level of venom-specific IgE is certainly diagnostic; but the test is often qualitative and poorly standardized, and it yields negative results in at least 15% to 20% of patients whose skin-test results are positive.

In the majority of patients who have a definite history of insect-venom reactions, skin-test results are clearly positive; in a few such patients, the results are clearly negative. Negative skin-test results in a patient with a history of insect-venom reactions may represent the loss of sensitivity, but it is important to test for venom-specific IgE antibodies in the serum (e.g., by use of RAST).[15] The venom skin test may be repeated after several months. A few cases of sting anaphylaxis are non–IgE mediated and may be related to subclinical mastocytosis or simply toxic mast cell hyperreleasability.[11] It is important to note that the degree of skin-test sensitivity does not correlate reliably with the degree of sting reaction. The strongest skin tests often occur in patients who have had only large local reactions, and some patients who have had near-fatal anaphylactic shock show only weak sensitivity on skin testing or RAST. Because of cross-reactivity, skin tests are positive to all three of the common vespid venoms (yellow jacket, yellow hornet, white-faced hornet) in 95% of patients allergic to vespid venom. More than half of patients sensitive to yellow-jacket venom also have positive reactions to testing for sensitivity to *Polistes* wasp venom. It is possible to determine whether the patient has a specific or a cross-reactive sensitivity to wasp venom using a RAST-inhibition test in specialized laboratories.[16]

Differential Diagnosis

Although the diagnosis of insect-sting allergy is relatively straightforward, the history and diagnostic tests can be misleading in some cases. Local swelling may be the result of nonallergic inflammation, but infection is very uncommon and would likely occur many days after the sting. Local cutaneous signs should not be mistaken for systemic eruption. Symptoms of dyspnea, chest discomfort, and dizziness can be the result of hyperventilation associated with anxiety. Patients with asthma who receive a sting may have asthmatic symptoms that are difficult to distinguish from an allergic reaction. Approximately 1% of patients with a history of allergic reactions to insect stings experience an abnormal release of mediator by mast cells or basophils, as demonstrated by elevated baseline serum tryptase levels. Some of these patients have a form of mastocytosis.[12]

Treatment

ACUTE TREATMENT

The treatment of the acute systemic allergic reaction is the same as that of other causes of anaphylaxis. The treatment of choice is epinephrine by intramuscular injection.[17] The recommended dose is 0.3 to 0.5 mg (0.3 to 0.5 ml in a solution of 1:1,000 weight in volume [w/v]) for adults, and 0.01 mg/kg for children. Delay in the use of epinephrine has contributed to fatal reactions. Some individuals with anaphylactic shock are resistant to epinephrine. Patients taking beta blockers can also be resistant to the effects of epinephrine. In some cases, anaphylaxis is prolonged or recurrent for 6 to 24 hours and may require intensive medical care.[18] All patients with anaphylaxis should have full emergency medical attention and observation for 6 hours or longer.

Large local reactions may require a burst of corticosteroid medication, which is most effective if started within 2 hours of the sting. After an initial dose of 40 to 60 mg, the dose is tapered rapidly over 3 to 5 days.

PREVENTIVE TREATMENT

General Measures

Patients who are discharged from emergency care after suffering anaphylaxis must receive information on the risk of future reactions. They should also be advised to receive allergy consultation, and they should be given information about prevention and the need for an epinephrine kit. The affected individual should avoid bushes and gardens, as well as food and drink that are most likely to attract insects. Drinks, especially in cans, bottles, and straws, can be an unsuspected source of a sting to the tongue or throat. Epinephrine autoinjectors are available for adults and children (Epi-Pen and Epi-Pen Jr., Dey Labs, Napa, California). The age at which a patient should be prescribed an adult-strength autoinjector, rather than a pediatric autoinjector, is uncertain; use of the adult-strength injector may be considered when the child attains a weight of 25 kg.[19] All patients should understand that use of an epinephrine kit is not a substitute for emergency medical attention.

Venom Immunotherapy

Patient selection Current indications for venom immunotherapy are a history of previous systemic allergic reaction to a sting and a positive venom skin test.[20-22] The patients at highest risk are those with a recent history of anaphylaxis and positive skin-test results; in such patients, the risk of a systemic reaction to a subsequent sting is approximately 50%. Children and adults with a history of large local reactions are at low risk for a systemic reaction (< 10%),[23] as are children whose systemic reactions are limited to cutaneous signs and symptoms.[5] In these low-risk persons, venom immunotherapy is not required, but some patients will still request treatment because of their fear of reaction or because of frequent exposure. There are some cases of progressively worsening reactions in adults, so all adults with systemic reactions are advised to undergo venom immunotherapy. There is no test that accurately predicts which patients will progress to more severe reactions and which will not.

Initial therapy Initial venom immunotherapy can be completed with a regimen of eight weekly injections or a traditional regimen lasting for 4 to 6 months.[20-22] Rush immunotherapy, typically administered over a period of 2 to 3 days, has been reported to be as safe and effective as the usual regimens.[24,25] The recommended maintenance dose is 100 μg of each of the venoms for which a positive result was seen on skin testing. Standard therapy is 85% to 98% effective in completely preventing systemic allergic reactions, but some patients require higher doses for full protection.[26] The same dose has been recommended for children 3 years of age and older, even though their immune response to venom immunotherapy is twice that of adults.

Adverse reactions Venom immunotherapy causes reactions no more frequently than inhalant allergen immunotherapy.[27] Systemic symptoms occur in 10% to 15% of patients during the initial weeks of treatment, regardless of the regimen used.

Most reactions are mild, and fewer than half of the reactions require epinephrine. In unusual cases, there can be repeated problems with systemic reactions to injections. Large local reactions are common but are not predictive of systemic reactions to subsequent injections. All patients must achieve the full 100 μg dose to have optimal clinical protection.

Maintenance and monitoring After reaching the full dose, the same dose is repeated at 4-week intervals for at least 1 year. The dosing interval may then be increased to once every 6 to 8 weeks over several years of treatment. Therapeutic efficacy can be confirmed serologically, but use of only some assays for venom-specific IgG antibodies has correlated strongly with clinical protection.[28] Venom skin tests or RASTs are repeated periodically—usually every 2 to 3 years—to determine whether there has been a significant decline in venom-specific IgE.[29] The results of skin testing generally remain unchanged during the first 2 to 3 years but show a significant decline after 4 to 6 years.[6] Fewer than 20% of patients have negative skin-test results after 5 years, but 50% to 60% have negative results after 7 to 10 years.[30]

Duration The package inserts for the commercial venom immunotherapy products available in the United States recommend indefinite immunotherapy. However, the published practice parameters reflect more recent experience and recommendations.[22,29] In most patients, skin-test results and RAST results remain positive after 5 to 10 years of treatment. Studies of several hundred adults and children show that even when skin tests remain positive, venom immunotherapy can usually be stopped after 5 years.[29] Observation of patients for 5 to 10 years after completing a 5- to 8-year course of venom treatment has shown a 5% to 10% risk of systemic symptoms after any sting but only a 2% risk of a reaction requiring epinephrine treatment.[31] Patients who have a higher frequency of relapse include those receiving honeybee-venom therapy, those with a history of very severe pretreatment sting reactions, and those who have had a systemic reaction to a sting or an injection during the period of venom immunotherapy.[21] Several studies have shown that 5 years of therapy is superior to 3 years for suppression of the IgE response and for longer-lasting remission.[32,33] Some patients prefer to continue venom treatment for their continued sense of security.

References

1. Golden DK, Marsh DG, Kagey-Sobotka A, et al: Epidemiology of insect venom sensitivity. JAMA 262:240, 1989

2. Barnard JH: Studies of 400 Hymenoptera sting deaths in the United States. J Allergy Clin Immunol 52:259, 1973

3. Schwartz HJ, Sutheimer C, Gauerke B, et al: Venom-specific IgE antibodies in postmortem sera from victims of sudden unexpected death. J Allergy Clin Immunol 73:189, 1984

4. Golden DB, Langlois J, Valentine MD, et al: Treatment failures with whole-body extract therapy of insect sting allergy. JAMA 246:2460, 1981

5. Valentine MD, Schuberth KC, Kagey-Sobotka A, et al: The value of immunotherapy with venom in children with allergy to insect stings. N Engl J Med 323:1601, 1990

6. Reisman RE: Natural history of insect sting allergy: relationship of severity of symptoms of initial sting anaphylaxis to re-sting reactions. J Allergy Clin Immunol 90:335, 1992

7. Stafford CT: Hypersensitivity to fire ant venom. Ann Allergy Asthma Immunol 77:87, 1996

8. Schumacher MJ, Egen NB: Significance of Africanized bees for public health: a review. Arch Intern Med 155:2038, 1995

9. King TP, Spangfort MD: Structure and biology of stinging insect venom allergens. Int Arch Allergy Immunol 123:99, 2000

10. Ludolph-Hauser D, Rueff F, Fries C, et al: Constitutively raised serum concentrations of mast-cell tryptase and severe anaphylactic reactions to Hymenoptera stings.

Lancet 357:361, 2001

11. Fricker M, Helbling A, Schwartz L, et al: Hymenoptera sting anaphylaxis and urticaria pigmentosa: clinical findings and results of venom immunotherapy in ten patients. J Allergy Clin Immunol 100:11, 1997

12. Oude Elberink J, de Monchy J, Kors JW, et al: Fatal anaphylaxis after a yellow jacket sting, despite venom immunotherapy, in two patients with mastocytosis. J Allergy Clin Immunol 99:153, 1997

13. van der Linden PG, Hack CE, Struyvenberg A, et al: Insect-sting challenge in 324 subjects with a previous anaphylactic reaction: current criteria for insect-venom hypersensitivity do not predict the occurrence and the severity of anaphylaxis. J Allergy Clin Immunol 94:151, 1994

14. Hamilton RG: Responsibility for quality IgE antibody results rests ultimately with the referring physician. Ann Allergy Asthma Immunol 86:353, 2001

15. Golden DB, Kagey-Sobotka A, Norman PS, et al: Insect sting allergy with negative venom skin test responses. J Allergy Clin Immunol 107:897, 2001

16. Hamilton RH, Wisenauer JA, Golden DB, et al: Selection of Hymenoptera venoms for immunotherapy on the basis of patient's IgE antibody cross-reactivity. J Allergy Clin Immunol 92:651, 1993

17. Simons FE, Gu X, Simons KJ: Epinephrine absorption in adults: intramuscular versus subcutaneous injection. J Allergy Clin Immunol 108:871, 2001

18. Lockey RF, Turkeltaub PC, Baird-Warren IA, et al: The Hymenoptera venom study I, 1979–1982: demographic and history-sting data. J Allergy Clin Immunol 82:370, 1988

19. Simons FE, Peterson S, Black CD: Epinephrine dispensing for the out-of-hospital treatment of anaphylaxis in infants and children: a population-based study. Ann Allergy Asthma Immunol 86:622, 2001

20. Golden DB, Schwartz HJ: Guidelines for venom immunotherapy. J Allergy Clin Immunol 77:727, 1986

21. Muller U, Mosbech H: Position paper: immunotherapy with Hymenoptera venoms. Allergy 48:37, 1993

22. Portnoy JM, Moffitt JE, Golden DB, et al: Stinging insect hypersensitivity: a practice parameter. J Allergy Clin Immunol 103:963, 1999

23. Mauriello PM, Barde SH, Georgitis JW, et al: Natural history of large local reactions from stinging insects. J Allergy Clin Immunol 74:494, 1984

24. Bernstein JA, Kagen SL, Bernstein DI, et al: Rapid venom immunotherapy is safe for routine use in the treatment of patients with Hymenoptera anaphylaxis. Ann Allergy 73:423, 1994

25. Tankersley MS, Walker RL, Butler WK, et al: Safety and efficacy of an imported fire ant rush immunotherapy protocol with and without prophylactic treatment. J Allergy Clin Immunol 109:556, 2002

26. Rueff F, Wenderoth A, Przybilla B: Patients still reacting to a sting challenge while receiving conventional Hymenoptera venom immunotherapy are protected by increased venom doses. J Allergy Clin Immunol 108:1027, 2001

27. Lockey RF, Turkeltaub PC, Olive ES, et al: The Hymenoptera venom study: III. Safety of venom immunotherapy. J Allergy Clin Immunol 86:775, 1990

28. Golden DB, Lawrence ID, Hamilton RH, et al: Clinical correlation of the venom-specific IgG antibody level during maintenance venom immunotherapy. J Allergy Clin Immunol 90:386, 1992

29. Graft DF, Golden DK, Resiman RE, et al: The discontinuation of Hymenoptera venom immunotherapy. Report from the Committee on Insects. J Allergy Clin Immunol 101:573, 1998

30. Golden DB, Kwiterovich KA, Kagey-Sobotka A, et al: Discontinuing venom immunotherapy: extended observations. J Allergy Clin Immunol 101:298, 1998

31. Golden DB, Kagey-Sobotka A, Lichtenstein LM: Survey of patients after discontinuing venom immunotherapy. J Allergy Clin Immunol 105:385, 2000

32. Keating MU, Kagey-Sobotka A, Hamilton RG, et al: Clinical and immunologic follow-up of patients who stop venom immunotherapy. J Allergy Clin Immunol 88:339, 1991

33. Lerch E, Muller U: Long-term protection after stopping venom immunotherapy: results of re-stings in 200 patients. J Allergy Clin Immunol 101:606, 1998

Acknowledgments

The photographs in Figures 1 and 2 are by Stephen B. Bambara; the photographs in Figures 3 and 4 are by James Baker, Ph.D. All photographs are courtesy of the North Carolina State University Department of Entomology.

111　Introduction to the Rheumatic Diseases

Shaun Ruddy, M.D.

About 43 million Americans (16%) had some form of arthritis in 1997.[1] By 2020, an estimated 59 million people (18.2%) will be affected; it is estimated that there will be approximately 21 million cases of osteoarthritis, 3.7 million cases of fibromyalgia syndrome, and 2.1 million cases of rheumatoid arthritis.[2] Arthritis and musculoskeletal disorders are the leading causes of disability in persons 18 to 65 years of age, and it is a common cause of disability related to employment. One in seven patients who visit a physician's office has a complaint regarding the musculoskeletal system.[3] Although most of those patients have benign, self-limited conditions that respond to simple remedies, some patients have serious, complex problems for which timely intervention may be crucial for a successful outcome.

Diagnosis of the rheumatic diseases primarily relies on the history and physical examination.[4,5] Expensive laboratory and imaging studies are usually of little use; most have low sensitivity and specificity, and their findings are seldom definitively diagnostic. For example, the serum level of uric acid, a substance intimately involved in the pathogenesis of gout, is of little use in diagnosing gouty arthritis. Twenty percent of patients with gout have normal uric acid levels (false negative results), and most persons with elevated levels will never have gouty arthritis (false positive results) [*see Chapter 118*]. Wide-ranging and expensive investigations often lead to the wrong conclusions. The dearth of useful laboratory aids to diagnose rheumatic disease makes the clinical skills of the physician very important and the diagnosis of such disease an exciting undertaking.

History

A careful and detailed history is the most important part of the evaluation of a patient with arthritis. It focuses the subsequent physical examination and laboratory studies. In addition to the patient's age, sex, and race, the location of the pain, which includes both the distribution of affected joints and the point of origin of the pain (i.e., whether it arises from a joint or surrounding structures), should be elicited [*see Table 1*]. Symmetrical involvement of the small joints of the hands and feet but not the distal interphalangeal joints suggests rheumatoid arthritis. In contrast, distal interphalangeal involvement often occurs in psoriatic arthritis. Bony overgrowth with distal interphalangeal involvement suggests osteoarthritis. Asymmetrical involvement of the large joints accompanied by back pain in a young man is characteristic of spondyloarthropathy. The sudden onset of severe pain in the great toe is a feature of gout (podagra).

Knowing the nature of the pain helps the physician determine whether the disease is inflammatory or noninflammatory [*see Table 1*]. The date of onset and the temporal course of the pain should also be elicited [*see Figure 1*]. The new involvement of joints that had not previously been affected in a patient with joint involvement is common in rheumatoid arthritis and systemic lupus erythematosus (SLE). Migratory polyarthritis, in which one affected joint becomes asymptomatic as another becomes painful, occurs in gonococcal arthritis, Reiter syndrome, and acute rheumatic fever. Intermittent arthritis, in which asymptomatic intervals are punctuated by acute flares, is common in crystal-induced arthritis.

RHEUMATOLOGIC EMERGENCIES

Although rheumatologic emergencies seldom occur, failure to recognize any of a few important symptoms or signs [*see Table 2*] may result in permanent disability or death; thus, the initial contact with the patient requires being alert for these conditions.[5] If a rheumatologic emergency is suspected, prompt initiation of appropriate diagnostic testing and treatment is essential.

After emergencies have been excluded, the approach to diagnosis need not be rushed. Although patients often come to the office with the preconceived notion that they have arthritis and expect quick diagnostic confirmation and treatment, they often must be observed for some time before the diagnosis can be made. Considerable patience and tact may be required in communicating this need to the patient. He or she should be informed that an uncertain diagnosis at presentation is usually a good prognostic sign; the prognosis for patients with clear-cut, easily diagnosed disease is often poor. Temporizing with an indefinite diagnosis—for example, knee pain of uncertain etiology—is better than prematurely classifying a patient's musculoskeletal complaints into a particular diagnostic category. The nosology of the rheumatic diseases is incomplete, and new diseases continue to be recognized (most recently, Lyme disease and eosinophilia-myalgia syndrome). In at least 10% of patients, a diagnosis cannot be made with certainty.

LOCATION OF PAIN

Patients are often not precise in identifying the location of musculoskeletal pain; it helps to ask them to put their hands on the place that hurts. A patient who complains of pain in the hip may point to one of three areas: the inguinal ligament and anterior thigh, suggesting involvement of the true hip joint; the lateral hip girdle, characteristic of trochanteric bursitis; or the buttock, consistent with sacroiliac joint disease or radiation of back pain along the sciatic nerve. During the physical examination, detailed attention to the location of pain helps identify the structures affected. If a specific structure cannot be identified, the pain may be referred from elsewhere. Pain described as diffuse or poorly localized may suggest a serious systemic disease, such as polymyositis, but more commonly is a manifestation of fibromyalgia or a related pain syndrome.

Table 1　Common Rheumatic Diseases

	Intra-articular	Extra-articular
Inflammatory	Rheumatoid arthritis Systemic lupus erythematosus Septic arthritis Gout Pseudogout Spondyloarthropathy	Tendinitis Bursitis Polymyositis Vasculitis
Noninflammatory	Osteoarthritis	Fibromyalgia

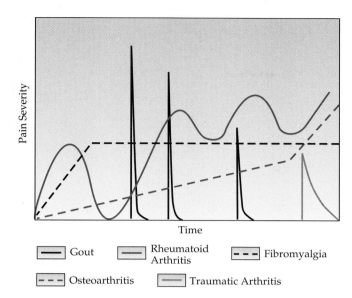

Gout   Rheumatoid Arthritis   - - - Fibromyalgia

- - - Osteoarthritis   Traumatic Arthritis

Figure 1   **Variations in the temporal course and severity of pain in the rheumatic diseases. The pain of rheumatoid arthritis may vary in intensity over time. The pain of osteoarthritis tends to be slowly progressive until late in the course of disease, when it may become very severe. The pain of fibromyalgia remains constant. Gout has an intermittent course of high-intensity pain flares. Traumatic arthritis improves more slowly than gout.[4]**

CHARACTER OF PAIN

Pain that arises from joints and that is dull, alleviated by rest, and worsened by weight bearing or movement of the joint suggests joint damage such as occurs in osteoarthritis. Pain that is more intense, is accompanied by swelling, and is present when the patient is at rest or pain that awakens the patient at night suggests an inflammatory process such as rheumatoid arthritis.

Table 2   Symptoms and Signs of Rheumatologic Emergencies[5]

Symptom or Sign	*Condition*
History of significant trauma	Fracture, compartmental syndrome, rhabdomyolysis
Systemic symptoms (fever, weight loss)	Infection (septic arthritis, osteomyelitis, endocarditis, necrotizing fasciitis)
Weakness	
Focal	Radiculopathy, entrapment neuropathy, compartmental syndrome, motor neuron disease, mononeuritis multiplex
Global or progressive	Spinal cord compression, myelopathy, transverse myelitis, myositis, response to toxin
Neurogenic pain (burning, numbness, paresthesias)	Radiculopathy, entrapment neuropathy
Point tenderness	Fracture
Red, hot, swollen joint	Septic arthritis, gout, pseudogout
Asymmetrical painful, swollen leg	Deep vein thrombosis
Diffuse shoulder and hip pain, headache in elderly patient	Temporal arteritis
Bowel or bladder dysfunction	Cauda equina syndrome

Inflammation also causes stiffness after prolonged immobility— the so-called gelling phenomenon, which may last longer than 30 minutes. Patients who have inflammatory joint pain caused by rheumatoid arthritis or SLE typically have significant morning stiffness that lasts as long as several hours and that improves as the day goes on—or at least until they are overwhelmed by the deep fatigue that also accompanies these diseases. The duration of morning stiffness is a rough measure of the activity of the inflammatory disease. Patients who have the noninflammatory joint pain that characterizes osteoarthritis, tendinitis, or bursitis describe focal morning pain that lasts for a few minutes; they are most uncomfortable at the end of the day, after prolonged activity. Shooting, burning, or so-called pins-and-needles discomfort is usually neurogenic.

Symptoms of giving way or locking in a weight-bearing joint generally suggest a mechanical process, such as a cartilage or ligament tear or a loose body within the joint. Locking may also occur when soft tissue inflammation impairs mobility, as when triggering of a finger is caused by a nodule in a flexor tendon as a result of tenosynovitis.

WEAKNESS

A complaint of weakness may reflect one of several disease processes. In patients with focal loss of muscle power in a specific region, indicated by complaints such as "I can't raise my arm," the obvious possibilities include a neurologic lesion; local muscle atrophy; failure of a musculoskeletal unit, such as a ruptured tendon or torn muscle; or weakness secondary to joint pain. A patient who says, "I feel weak all over," should be asked to distinguish true muscle weakness (i.e., loss of power or endurance) from a more generalized sense of asthenia, malaise, or fatigue. The patient with true muscle weakness has difficulty starting or maintaining an activity that requires muscle strength, such as arising from a chair, getting out of bed, or walking up stairs. Physical examination usually confirms the muscular nature of such problems, with the proximal musculature being most affected in myopathies and the distal muscles involved in neuropathies. If the examination shows no objective weakness or other neurologic abnormalities, such as loss of deep tendon reflexes, the patient's report of weakness probably corresponds to asthenia, fatigue, and loss of sense of well-being. If this occurs together with other constitutional symptoms such as anorexia, weight loss, and low-grade fever, it may indicate an active systemic rheumatic disease such as rheumatoid arthritis or SLE. If the asthenia and fatigue are not accompanied by objective constitutional symptoms, fibromyalgia is more likely.

PSYCHOSOCIAL AND ENVIRONMENTAL FACTORS

After pain, loss of function is of the greatest concern to the patient, making the functional assessment an important part of the history. Exploring this area often affords the physician insights into the way the patient views the disease and what the patient expects. Simple questions asked by the physician may include the following: How has your disease affected you? What can you not do now that you could do before? and What can you not do that you would like to do? Patients with significant functional impairment should be asked more detailed questions about routine activities of daily living. Explicit questions about sexual function may uncover problems that the patient might otherwise hesitate to describe. The sexual history also identifies risk factors for sexually transmitted joint diseases, such as gonococcal arthritis, Reiter syndrome, and HIV-associated arthropathy. A vocational history may identify specific tasks that exacerbate the disease and need modification; it may also indicate whether the patient is likely to be exposed to ticks carrying Lyme disease. The history of use of devices such as a cane or crutches and information as to when the patient began using them is helpful in assessing the temporal course of the disease. Claims for workers' compensation or disability or other pending litigation should also be noted.

FAMILY HISTORY

Many rheumatic diseases have strong familial predispositions. Ankylosing spondylitis is the most well known, but other autoimmune diseases such as rheumatoid arthritis and SLE also have a genetic basis, as do gout and, to a lesser extent, pseudogout.

REVIEW OF SYSTEMS

Once a specific disease is suspected, the patient should be questioned about the presence of other systemic features of the disease. These features include conjunctivitis, iritis, or other eye problems; hair loss; skin rash or photosensitivity; nasopharyngeal infection or mouth ulcers; thyroid problems; chest pain or pleurisy; abdominal pain or diarrhea; urethral or vaginal discharge; kidney stones; symptoms of Raynaud phenomenon; and numbness or paresthesias.

Physical Examination

GENERAL EXAMINATION

By the time the history is finished, the clinician should have formulated some diagnostic hypotheses that can be used to guide the physical exam. If a patient's complaints are localized and the history elicits no suggestion of a more generalized process, the examination may be limited to the region involved. When systemic symptoms are present, a complete and detailed examination is required. Asymmetrical joint disease and inflammatory back pain raise the possibility of psoriatic arthritis and spondylitis, in which case the physician should very carefully inspect the skin for a patch of psoriasis of which the patient may be unaware. In the sexually active patient with asymmetrical involvement of large joints and a history of conjunctivitis, detailed examination of the genitalia for the lesions of Reiter syndrome should be performed. The patient with complaints of sinus trouble, arthritis, and hemoptysis should undergo thorough scrutiny of the nasopharynx and sinuses for the lesions of Wegener granulomatosis. Other important findings are iritis or conjunctivitis, nodules, pericardial or pleural rubs, hepatic or splenic enlargement, lymphadenopathy, and neurologic abnormalities.

JOINT EXAMINATION

By looking at and palpating the joints, the physician can identify the precise anatomic structures that are the source of the patient's pain and decide whether the pain is caused by inflammation. A goal of the examination is to reproduce the patient's pain, either by motion of the joint or by palpation. Frank redness of the skin overlying a joint is unusual; however, increased temperature, best detected by palpation with the backs of the fingers, is not unusual and, when present, indicates inflammation. Apparent swelling may be caused by periarticular edema, an effusion in the joint, synovial proliferation, or bony overgrowth; in all cases, it indicates organic disease. Palpation for tenderness may re-

Table 3 Factors That Influence ESR[6]

Factors That Increase ESR	Factors That Decrease ESR
Advancing age	Congestive heart failure
Female sex	Sickle cell disease
Pregnancy	Altered erythrocyte shape
Hypercholesterolemia	(e.g., anisocytosis, spherocytosis, acanthosis, microcytosis)
B cell neoplasm (e.g., myeloma, macroglobulinemia, cryoglobulinemia)	Polycythemia
	Extreme leukocytosis
	Cachexia
Renal failure	Hypofibrinogenemia
	Cryoglobulinemia

ESR—erythrocyte sedimentation rate

veal whether the problem lies within the joint or is discretely localized to an overlying bursa or tendon sheath. The finding of fine crepitus with motion of the structure corresponds to the grinding of subchondral bone, denuded of articular cartilage, against opposing bone. Coarser (so-called creaking) crepitus is associated with the fibrinous tendinitis that occurs in scleroderma or traumatic tendinitis. When the examiner is able to move the joint through a passive range of motion that exceeds the active range of motion accomplished voluntarily by the patient, failure of a musculoskeletal unit (e.g., rupture of the rotator cuff in the shoulder) or a neurologic deficit should be suspected. Examination of the spine is the most neglected part of the musculoskeletal examination, probably because it entails moving the patient from the sitting position through the supine and prone positions and then to the standing position. Patients with findings suggestive of a lumbar radiculopathy should have detailed testing of the motor, sensory, and reflex systems in the legs. An experienced physician can perform a complete musculoskeletal examination in less than 10 minutes.

Laboratory Studies

THE ACUTE-PHASE RESPONSE

The cellular response to inflammation or tissue injury elaborates cytokines such as interleukin-1 (IL-1), IL-6, and tumor necrosis factor, which have profound effects on the hepatic synthesis of plasma proteins.[6] Concentrations of C-reactive protein (CRP) increase as much as 100-fold within 1 or 2 days after tissue damage; parallel increases in serum amyloid A protein occur. Slower and less marked increases occur in coagulation proteins such as fibrinogen and prothrombin, most of the complement components, normal plasma protease inhibitors, and transport proteins such as ferritin and haptoglobin. Corresponding decreases occur in serum transferrin and albumin, accounting for the low serum iron and albumin levels that accompany inflammatory diseases.

The erythrocyte sedimentation rate (ESR) is the time-honored test used to detect the acute-phase response.[7] The increased rate of fall of the column of erythrocytes is caused by stacking of the cells into rouleaux, induced mainly by increases in the highly asymmetrical fibrinogen molecule; the increased levels of immunoglobulins seen in chronic inflammatory conditions also favor rouleaux formation. The ESR is influenced by many extraneous factors [*see Table 3*], the most important of which is age. The upper limit of normal for men is obtained by dividing the age in years by 2; for women, it is obtained by adding 10 to the age in years and then dividing that number by 2. The CRP level is measured by immunoassay and is not influenced by most of the extraneous factors that affect the ESR. It also increases more rapidly than the ESR, which may take several days to increase. The ESR and CRP tests are nonspecific: ESR and CRP levels may be elevated in a number of inflammatory conditions, such as malignancy, chronic infection, pneumonia, and acute myocardial infarction. They are most useful in excluding significant inflammatory disease. For example, in a patient with diffuse pain and tenderness at trigger points, suggesting fibromyalgia, a normal ESR value supports this diagnosis; an ESR of 90 mm/hr dictates close scrutiny for other diseases. If the patient with these symptoms is older than 60 years, polymyalgia rheumatica and temporal arteritis are the primary possibilities. The acute-phase tests are also moderately useful in distinguishing inflammatory from noninflammatory

arthritis and in monitoring the course of an inflammatory disease such as rheumatoid arthritis or polymyalgia rheumatica.

IMMUNOLOGIC TESTS

As a class, immunologic tests have low specificity and only moderate sensitivity. They are also more expensive and less reproducible than most other clinical laboratory tests. They should never be used as screening tests; their greatest utility occurs when the pretest probability of disease is high. The misuse of immunologic tests frequently confounds the diagnosis. Two common examples of unnecessary rheumatology referrals are the octogenarian with arthritis of the knees or shoulders who tests positive for rheumatoid factor (unnecessary because positivity in healthy persons increases with age, and osteoarthritis of these joints is common in octogenarians) and the young woman with fatigue, diffuse pains, and a positive, usually low-titer, antinu-

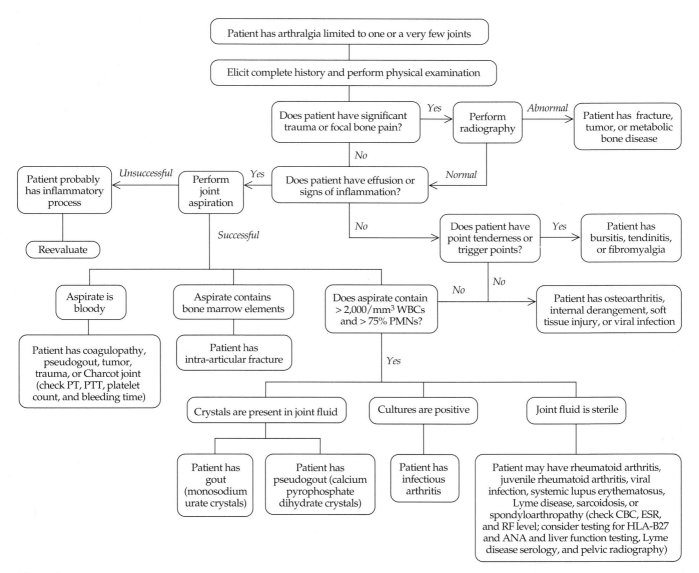

Figure 2   The initial approach to the patient with symptoms of monoarticular disease. Most cases can be diagnosed on the basis of the history and physical examination. The cultures referred to in the figure are a synovial fluid culture as well as cervical, urethral, pharyngeal, and rectal evaluations for gonococci and *Chlamydia* species, when infection with these organisms is suspected.[5] (ANA—antinuclear antibody; CBC—complete blood count; ESR—erythrocyte sedimentation rate; PMNs—polymorphonuclear neutrophils; PT—prothrombin time; PTT—partial thromboplastin time; RF—rheumatoid factor; WBCs—white blood cells)

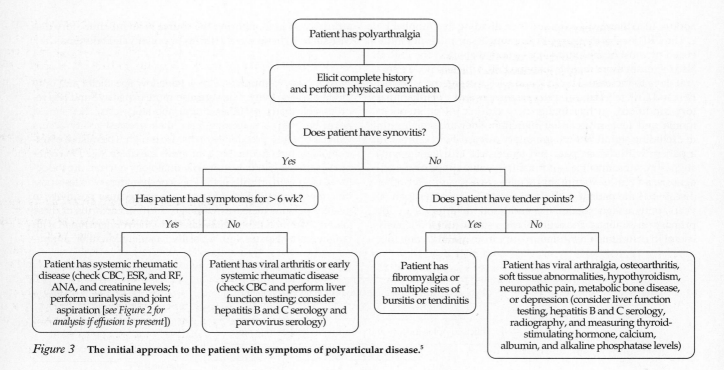

Figure 3 **The initial approach to the patient with symptoms of polyarticular disease.**[5]

clear antibody test (unnecessary because low titers of antinuclear antibody are found in as many as 32% of young women[8]; the patient probably has depression or fibromyalgia). The use of so-called arthritis panels, in which many serologic tests are bundled together, increases the likelihood of an abnormal result in a patient without rheumatic disease and should be avoided. Highly specific (and expensive) tests, such as those for antineutrophil cytoplasmic antibody, Lyme disease serology, HLA-B27, antiphospholipid antibody, and antibodies against individual nuclear constituents, should be performed only when the pretest probability of a particular disease is high. In one study of patients with swelling of at least one joint, the rheumatoid factor test had a sensitivity of 65% and a specificity of 87% for the diagnosis of arthritis.[9] At disease onset, a positive test result for rheumatoid factor is predictive of increased severity, as assessed by radiographic evidence of erosions.[10]

SYNOVIAL FLUID ANALYSIS

Examination of synovial fluid is perhaps the most important diagnostic test in rheumatology. It gives the physician one of the few opportunities available for the precise diagnosis of rheumatic disease and permits immediate initiation of specific and effective therapy. In addition, aspiration of synovial fluid is a low-risk procedure: the frequency of iatrogenic infection is less than one in 10,000. Joint aspiration should be performed with aseptic technique as part of the evaluation of every case of acute monoarthritis.

Analysis of the synovial fluid includes a white blood cell count and differential, appropriate cultures and stains for microorganisms, and polarized-light microscopy. The white blood cell count in the synovial fluid is useful in distinguishing inflammatory from noninflammatory arthritis: levels greater than $2,000/mm^3$ are consistent with inflammation. Patients with crystal-induced arthritis usually have counts in excess of $30,000/mm^3$. The reliability of the examination of fluid for crystals by polarized-light microscopy depends very much on the laboratory do-

ing the test. The finding of monosodium urate or calcium pyrophosphate dihydrate crystals on polarized-light microscopy is pathognomonic for gout and pseudogout, respectively; the absence of crystals does not exclude these diagnoses. Gram stain and culture may be diagnostic of infection. If patients with established arthritis have fever and an apparent flare, joint infection should be excluded by joint aspiration because septic arthritis occurs more frequently in such patients.

Imaging

The findings on radiography are unlikely to be abnormal in most patients with acute arthritis, mechanical back pain, tendinitis, or bursitis; radiography should not be used in these cases. For patients with established arthritis, such as rheumatoid arthritis, it takes longer than 6 months for radiographic abnormalities such as joint space narrowing and marginal erosions to appear. In patients with osteoarthritis, radiography may be useful in assessing the extent of joint damage, but the correlation between its findings and the patient's symptoms is surprisingly poor.

Table 4 **Differential Diagnosis of Diffuse Aches and Pains**

Benign postviral syndromes
Postexertional syndromes
Fibromyalgia
Polymyalgia rheumatica
Temporal arteritis
Hypothyroidism
Metabolic bone disease
Hypophosphatemia
Atypical onset of systemic rheumatic disease (e.g., rheumatoid arthritis, systemic lupus erythematosus)

Plain radiography is most useful in patients with significant trauma that suggests the possibility of fracture, in those who experience a sudden loss of function (e.g., an inability to bear weight), in those with symptoms that do not improve despite appropriate treatment, and in those with a suspected infection or neoplastic disease. Computed radiography and digital imaging improves the quality of plain radiographs, makes long-distance transmission easy, and eliminates the problem of the lost radiograph. When it is likely that a fracture is present, special views may be required; repeat imaging 7 to 10 days later may detect callus formation at a previously unrecognized fracture site. In patients with chronic disease, repeat radiography is useful in assessing the progress of disease or the necessity of surgical intervention.

Although computed tomography, magnetic resonance imaging, and radionuclide bone scanning are powerful techniques for obtaining information about bones and joints, they should be used only when their results will be used to make important diagnostic or therapeutic decisions. As is true for plain radiography, myelography, and even autopsy, MRI of the spine often reveals abnormalities in people who do not have back pain. In one study, only 36% of patients free of back pain had normal findings on MRI of the lumbar spine.[11] Bone scans are useful in detecting osteomyelitis, stress fractures, and metastases to bone.

Initial Approach to the Patient

MONOARTICULAR DISEASE

Patients with symptoms that involve one or, at most, a few joints may have posttraumatic syndromes, bursitis, tendinitis, septic arthritis, crystal-induced inflammation (gout or pseudogout), or an atypical presentation of a systemic arthritis such as rheumatoid arthritis [see Figure 2]. Arthralgia, in which pain arises from structures surrounding the joint, must be distinguished from arthritis, in which there is evidence of frank involvement of the joint itself. Monoarticular arthritis should be considered to have an infectious etiology until proved otherwise. Prompt aspiration and examination of synovial fluid are usually indicated.

POLYARTICULAR DISEASE

In contrast to monoarticular disease, which often requires an aggressive and invasive diagnostic approach, arthritis involving numerous joints usually requires a more gradual and expectant strategy. There is less urgency in arriving at the diagnosis, and observation for 6 weeks or more may be required. During this period, it is unwise to alarm the patient unnecessarily by musing about the possibility that he or she has a particular systemic rheumatic disease; a wait-and-see attitude is more appropriate. Eventually, most patients with polyarthralgia will prove not to have a systemic rheumatic disease but to have a more benign condition [see Figure 3].

DIFFUSE ACHES AND PAINS

Most patients with diffuse aches and pains have a benign, self-limited illness of unknown cause that improves after 1 or 2 weeks of observation. The history often identifies antecedent viral infection or exertional stress as a precipitating factor. Another substantial number of patients prove to have fibromyalgia, which is suggested by an inability to precisely locate the anatomic origins of the pain on physical examination and by the finding of tender trigger points. A hemogram and measurements of the ESR or CRP, thyroid-stimulating hormone, creatine kinase (if weakness is an issue), calcium, and phosphate levels are usually sufficient to exclude other diseases [see Table 4].

Prognosis

Patients who present with complaints of joint pain often express the opinion, "Nothing can be done for my arthritis—I'll just have to learn to live with it." One of the most important things the physician can do during the initial contact is to correct this misconception. Most kinds of arthritis can be managed quite effectively, and the patient must understand that treatment greatly improves the condition of most patients with arthritis. Even for the most severe diseases, such as rheumatoid arthritis, very effective treatments have been available for 20 years, such that the long-term outcome has distinctly improved.[12,13] New treatments with biologic agents that block the inflammatory cytokines TNF-α and IL-1 are very effective, have a rapid onset of action, and prevent radiographic progression of the disease.[14,15] Educating the patient about the effectiveness of treatment is the first step toward a successful outcome.

References

1. Prevalence of arthritis—United States, 1997. MMWR Morb Mortal Wkly Rep 50:334, 2001
2. Lawrence RC, Helmick CG, Arnett FC, et al: Estimates of the prevalence of arthritis and selected musculoskeletal disorders in the United States. Arthritis Rheum 41:778, 1998
3. Schappert SM: Ambulatory care visits to physician offices, hospital outpatient departments, and emergency departments: United States, 1997. Vital Health Stat [13] 143:1, 1999
4. Liang MH, Roberts WN, Robb-Nicholson C, et al: Sorting out musculoskeletal complaints. Rheumatology: Problems in Primary Care. Medical Economics Books, Oradell, New Jersey, 1990, p 3
5. American College of Rheumatology Ad Hoc Committee on Clinical Guidelines: Guidelines for the initial evaluation of the adult patient with acute musculoskeletal symptoms. Arthritis Rheum 39:1, 1996
6. Gabay C, Kushner I: Acute-phase proteins and other systemic responses to inflammation. N Engl J Med 340:448, 1999
7. Sox HC Jr, Liang MH: The erythrocyte sedimentation rate: guidelines for rational use. Ann Intern Med 104:515, 1986
8. Tan EM, Feltkamp TE, Smolen JS, et al: Range of antinuclear antibodies in "healthy" individuals. Arthritis Rheum 40:1601, 1997
9. Saraux A, Berthelot JM, Chales G, et al: Value of laboratory tests in early prediction of rheumatoid arthritis. Arthritis Rheum 47:155, 2002
10. Bukhari M, Lunt M, Harrison BJ, et al: Rheumatoid factor is the major predictor of increasing severity of radiographic erosions in rheumatoid arthritis: results from the Norfolk Arthritis Register Study, a large inception cohort. Arthritis Rheum 46:906, 2002
11. Jensen MC, Brant-Zawadzki MN, Obuchowski N, et al: Magnetic resonance imaging of the lumbar spine in people without back pain. N Engl J Med 331:69, 1994
12. Fries JF, Williams CA, Morfeld D, et al: Reduction in long-term disability in patients with rheumatoid arthritis by disease-modifying antirheumatic drug–based treatment strategies. Arthritis Rheum 39:616, 1996
13. O'Dell JR, Haire CE, Erikson N, et al: Treatment of rheumatoid arthritis with methotrexate alone, sulfasalazine and hydroxychloroquine, or a combination of all three medications. N Engl J Med 334:1287, 1996
14. Kremer JM: Rational use of new and existing disease-modifying agents in rheumatoid arthritis. Ann Intern Med 134:695, 2001
15. Cohen S, Hurd E, Cush J, et al: Treatment of rheumatoid arthritis with anakinra, a recombinant human interleukin-1 receptor antagonist, in combination with methotrexate: results of a twenty-four-week, multicenter, randomized, double-blind, placebo-controlled trial. Arthritis Rheum 46:614, 2002

Acknowledgment

Figures 1 through 3   Marcia Kammerer.

112 Rheumatoid Arthritis

Gary S. Firestein, M.D.

Rheumatoid arthritis (RA) is the most common chronic inflammatory arthritis and affects about 1% of adults; it is two to three times more prevalent in women than in men. RA may begin as early as infancy, but onset usually occurs in the fifth or sixth decade. There are no specific laboratory tests for RA; diagnosis depends on a constellation of signs and symptoms that can be supported by serology and radiographs. Involvement of the small joints of the hands and feet is often the key to the diagnosis. Specific clinical criteria have evolved [*see Table 1*], but in practice, diagnosis is established by careful observation of the pattern of disease activity over time.

Immunogenetics

Genetic makeup plays a critical role in susceptibility to RA. Identical twins show 30% to 50% concordance for the disease; first-degree relatives of patients with RA have about a twofold to threefold increased incidence. Study of the major histocompatibility complex (MHC) has identified a shared epitope on the β chains of certain HLA-DR haplotypes in RA patients. This susceptibility epitope is associated with the third hypervariable region of DR β chains, which contains amino acids 70 through 74 (glutamine-leucine-arginine-alanine-alanine, also known as QKRAA) found in DRB1*0401, DRB1*0404, and other immunologically distinct alleles.[1] This sequence is common to most RA patients, although the disease develops in only a small fraction of those with the epitope.

Susceptibility to RA is likely polygenic; for instance, certain immunoglobulin genotypes and, perhaps, genetic differences in the galactosylation of immunoglobulin may be predisposing factors. Further studies have identified associations with microsatellite alleles of cytokines. Tumor necrosis factor (TNF) alleles are in linkage disequilibrium with the DR β gene and may be independent risk factors for RA.[2] In addition, a polymorphism of the interleukin-1α (IL-1α) gene is associated with juvenile RA.[3] Studies of IL-10 promoter polymorphisms have been variable, although on balance, there does not appear to be an association between a specific polymorphism and susceptibility to RA.

Etiology

It is unlikely that a single etiologic factor accounts for all cases of adult RA. A pathogenic organism is often assumed to be responsible, but despite some suggestive data, no conclusive evidence implicates bacteria or mycoplasmas. Viruslike particles have been isolated from synovial effusions in RA,[4] and some RA patients exhibit evidence of a recent parvovirus B19 infection.[5] The potential role of parvovirus B19 is controversial. Whereas some studies have not shown any correlation between RA and serologic evidence of previous infection or presence of *B19* genes in synovial tissue, one study demonstrated parvovirus B19 proteins by immunohistochemistry and potentially infectious virus particles in RA synovium.[6] Recent data suggest that B19 can infect cultured synovial fibroblasts and increase invasion into cartilage matrix.[7]

Other viruses that have been isolated from synovial fluid include rubella and Epstein-Barr virus (EBV). Sera from most RA patients contain greater amounts of antibodies to various EBV-derived antigens than normal sera. Suppression of EBV infection by lymphocytes from RA patients is impaired, possibly because T cells mount an insufficient response with low levels of interferon gamma. Although EBV infection is probably not the initial event in RA, it may contribute to persistent immunologic stimulation by acting as a polyclonal activator of B cells, thereby augmenting the production of autoantibodies.

Lymphocytes from some RA patients respond to a region of EBV glycoprotein gp110 that contains the same QKRAA sequence as the susceptibility epitope on DR β chains.[8] Thus, molecular mimicry may lead to autoimmunity in certain EBV-infected individuals. Other xenoproteins, most notably *Escherichia coli* DNA J protein, also contain QKRAA and may contribute to a response against self-MHC.[9] Although many patients undergo an autoimmune response to type II collagen, this response is nonspecific and may be of secondary etiologic significance.

Retroviruses could also serve as infectious causes of RA-like diseases. Synovial human T cell lymphotropic virus type I (HTLV-I) infection is associated with chronic arthritis, and in vitro transduction of synoviocytes with the HTLV-I *tax* gene leads to increased growth.[10] Retrovirus-like particles have been observed in some synovial samples, and expression of zinc-finger proteins associated with retroviral infections offers some support.[11]

Although autoimmunity occurs in patients with RA, it may not be responsible for initiation of the disease. An alternative hypothesis ascribes the initiation of disease to the activation of innate immunity in the synovium of susceptible persons.[12] This process, which involves primitive pattern-recognition receptors on macrophages, dendritic cells, mast cells, and neutrophils, leads to nonspecific articular inflammation. A local immune response then occurs as the synovium permits the influx of lymphocytes, which, in the appropriate cytokine milieu, recognize a variety of xenoantigens and autoantigens. In this scenario, no single etiologic agent is required. Instead, nonspecific inflammation in a patient with a particular gene set can lead to local responses directed at many articular antigens.

Pathogenesis

SYNOVIAL HISTOPATHOLOGY AND INVASION

The synovial tissue in RA becomes markedly hyperplastic, with redundant folds, frondlike villi, and edema. In the earliest stages, blood vessel proliferation and endothelial damage are prominent. Hyperplasia of the synovial intimal lining (the region in direct contact with synovial fluid) can occur, although the sublining inflammatory infiltrate can be mild. As the chronic phase begins, intimal lining hyperplasia becomes more prominent, increasing up to fivefold from the normal thickness of one or two cell layers [*see Figure 1*]. Synovial lining hyperplasia is caused, in part, by local proliferation of the fibroblast-like type B synoviocytes and migration of new macrophage-like type A synoviocytes from bone marrow and blood into the joint. The rate of cell death also determines tissue cellularity. Many cells of the intimal lining contain damaged DNA that

Table 1   American Rheumatism Association Criteria
for the Classification of Rheumatoid Arthritis[91]

Criteria

Morning stiffness: morning stiffness in and around the joints lasting at least 1 hr before maximal improvement

Arthritis of three or more joint areas: at least three joint areas have simultaneously had soft tissue swelling or fluid (not bony overgrowth alone) observed by a physician; the 14 possible joint areas (right and left) are proximal interphalangeal (PIP), metacarpophalangeal (MCP), wrist, elbow, knee, ankle, and metatarsophalangeal (MTP) joints

Arthritis of hand joints: at least one joint area swollen as above in wrist, MCP, or PIP joint

Symmetrical arthritis: simultaneous involvement of the same joint areas (as in arthritis of three or more joint areas, above) on both sides of the body (bilateral involvement of PIP, MCP, or MTP joints is acceptable without absolute symmetry)

Rheumatoid nodules: subcutaneous nodules over bony prominences or extensor surfaces or in juxta-articular regions that are observed by a physician

Serum rheumatoid factor: demonstration of abnormal amounts of serum rheumatoid factor by any method that has been positive in fewer than 5% of normal control subjects

Radiographic changes: radiographic changes typical of rheumatoid arthritis on posteroanterior hand and wrist x-rays, which must include erosions or unequivocal bony decalcification localized to or most marked adjacent to the involved joints (osteoarthritis changes alone do not qualify)

Exclusions

The presence of any of the following excludes the diagnosis of rheumatoid arthritis:

Typical rash of systemic lupus erythematosus (SLE)

High concentration of lupus erythematosus cells (four or more in two smears); because of the frequent finding of LE cells in patients with clinically typical rheumatoid arthritis, however, it is suggested that such patients be listed separately

Histologic evidence of polyarteritis nodosa with segmented necrosis of arteries associated with nodular leukocytic infiltration extending perivascularly, including many eosinophils

Persistent muscle swelling of dermatomyositis or weakness of neck, trunk, and pharyngeal muscles

Definite scleroderma (not limited to the fingers)

A clinical picture characteristic of rheumatic fever with migratory joint involvement and evidence of endocarditis, especially if accompanied by subcutaneous nodules, erythema marginatum, or chorea (an elevated antistreptolysin titer will not rule out the diagnosis of rheumatoid arthritis)

A clinical picture characteristic of gouty arthritis with acute attacks of swelling, redness, and pain in one or more joints, especially if responsive to colchicine

Tophi

A clinical picture characteristic of acute infectious arthritis of bacterial or viral origin with an acute focus of infection or a close association with a disease of known infectious origin; chills; fever; acute joint involvement, usually initially migratory (especially if organisms are present in the joint fluid or there is a response to antibiotic therapy)

Tubercle bacilli in joints or histologic evidence of joint tuberculosis

A clinical picture characteristic of reactive arthritis with urethritis and conjunctivitis associated with acute joint involvement, usually initially migratory

A clinical picture characteristic of the shoulder-hand syndrome with unilateral involvement of shoulder and hand and diffuse swelling of the hand, followed by atrophy and contractures

A clinical picture characteristic of hypertrophic osteoarthropathy with clubbing of fingers or hypertrophic periostitis, or both, along the shafts of the long bones, especially if an intrapulmonary lesion is present

A clinical picture characteristic of neuroarthropathy with condensation and destruction of bones of involved joints and associated neurologic findings

Homogentisic acid in the urine grossly detectable by alkalinization

Histologic evidence of sarcoid or a positive Kveim test

Multiple myeloma evidenced by marked increase in plasma cells in the bone marrow or by Bence Jones protein in the urine

Characteristic skin lesions of erythema nodosum

Leukemia or lymphoma with characteristic cells in peripheral blood, bone marrow, or tissues

A clinical picture characteristic of ankylosing spondylitis, psoriasis, ulcerative colitis, or regional enteritis

Note: for classification purposes, a patient is said to have rheumatoid arthritis if he or she has satisfied at least four of the above seven criteria. The first four must be present for at least 6 wk. Patients with two clinical diagnoses are not excluded. Designation as classic, definite, or probable rheumatoid arthritis is *not* to be made.

normally leads to apoptosis (programmed cell death), but relatively few cells complete this process.[13] RA synovial cells possibly have defective apoptosis that contributes to hyperplasia.

In chronic RA, inflammatory cells, including T cells, B cells, macrophages, and plasma cells, accumulate in the sublining region. Lymphocytes can organize into discrete aggregates, although diffuse mononuclear cell infiltration or relatively acellular fibrous tissue can also be present. The majority of T cells are CD4+ memory cells with small nuclei and scant cytoplasm. Although the cells are functionally quiescent, many express surface antigens that suggest previous activation. An increased number of blood vessels remains a prominent finding in the chronic phase. Capillary morphometry studies suggest that the capillary network is more disorganized than normal, and the tissue bulk outstrips the proliferation of blood vessels.

Rheumatoid synovitis is usually accompanied by increased synovial effusions. The white blood cell count in synovial fluid in active RA is about 10,000/mm³ (about 70% neutrophils). In contrast to the synovium, there are more CD8+ T cells than CD4+ T cells in synovial effusions. Total WBC counts sometimes exceed 50,000/mm³ and include 90% to 95% polymorphonuclear leukocytes. The polymorphonuclear leukocytes are drawn into the joint fluid along a gradient formed by chemotactic substances that include leukotriene B4, platelet-activating factor, the C5a fragment of complement, and chemokines such as IL-8. Lymphocytes, macrophages, and shed lining cells are also seen in synovial fluid. Surprisingly, very few neutrophils are present in RA synovium even though they are abundant in the effusions.

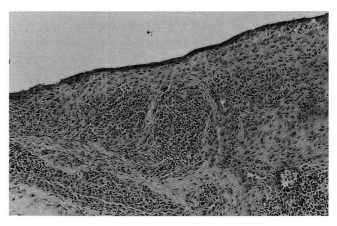

Figure 1   **Section of a proliferative synovium from a patient with classic rheumatoid arthritis reveals synovial lining hyperplasia and a sublining lymphocyte infiltration and aggregation.**

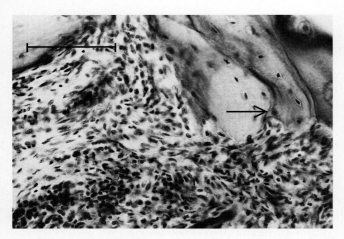

Figure 2 **At the junction between a proliferative inflamed rheumatoid synovium and the bone, scalloped regions of erosion can be seen (arrow). Section is stained with hematoxylin and eosin (bar scale = 100 μm).**

Pannus, the invasive region of synovium that erodes into cartilage and bone [*see Figure 2*], contains macrophages and primitive mesenchymal cells but very few lymphocytes. It is not clear whether these mesenchymal cells are related to type B synoviocytes, but morphologic and functional studies suggest that pannus-derived fibroblasts (pannocytes) have distinctive characteristics (e.g., very high expression of vascular cell adhesion molecule–1).[14] Mesenchymal stem cells have also been described in RA synovial tissue; these cells express distinct surface proteins (e.g., bone morphogenic protein receptors and endoglin) and can migrate into the synovium directly through pores in the bone or through the circulating blood.[15]

Damage to bone and cartilage by synovial tissue and pannus is mediated by several families of enzymes, including serine proteases and cathepsins. The most damaging enzymes are the metalloproteinases (e.g., collagenase, stromelysin, and gelatinase) and cathepsins (especially cathepsin K), which can degrade the major structural proteins in the joint. Cytokines such as IL-1 and TNF-α are potent inducers of metalloproteinase gene expression. Although protease inhibitors, like tissue inhibitors of metalloproteinases, are expressed by the rheumatoid synovial lining, the balance between proteases and inhibitors appears to favor the former in RA.[16] Chondrocytes in the cartilage, synoviocytes in pannus, and osteoclasts in the bone are the primary sources of proteases. The receptor activator of nuclear factor κB (RANK) and the RANK ligand (RANKL) together play a critical role in local osteoclast activation and bone destruction; the RANKL/RANK system is counterbalanced by the natural inhibitor osteoprotegerin (OPG). In animal models of arthritis, administration of OPG markedly decreases bone destruction, even though inflammation is unaffected.[17]

Destruction of extracellular matrix by rheumatoid synovium mesenchymal cells may occur either as a result of a normal response to the inflammatory cytokine milieu or as a result of abnormal synoviocyte function.[18] Evidence of partial transformation of RA synoviocytes, including adhesion-independent growth and loss of contact inhibition in vitro, suggests that immunosuppression may slow but not necessarily halt joint destruction. Cultured RA synoviocytes that have been coimplanted with cartilage explants into mice with severe combined immunodeficiency disease invade the cartilage matrix, whereas osteoarthritis synoviocytes and normal dermal fibroblasts do not.[19] Somatic mutations in the genes encoding key regulatory proteins, such as the *p53* tumor-suppressor gene, may contribute to the transformed phenotype of synoviocytes.[20] Such mutations are likely caused by the high local concentration of oxidants in the rheumatoid joint. Hence, the invasive component of rheumatoid synovitis potentially functions as an autonomous cytokine-independent tissue that erodes into cartilage.

CELLULAR IMMUNITY

Attempts to identify an etiologic agent by determining the proliferative response of synovial T cells to specific antigens have been relatively unrewarding. Articular T cells are often less responsive than peripheral blood cells. For instance, the proliferation of lymphocytes in synovial fluid in response to mitogens or recall antigens (e.g., tetanus toxoid) is significantly lower than the proliferation of blood T cells. Production of cytokines (e.g., interferon gamma and IL-2) by synovial fluid T cells in vitro is also low after stimulation by nonspecific mitogens. The mechanism of defective T cell responses in RA appears to be related to abnormal intracellular redox balance, which interferes with transduction of the T cell receptor signal.[21] Mycobacterial antigens and the 60 kd heat shock protein appear to be exceptions in that lymphocyte proliferation in response to these antigens is greater in cells from rheumatoid effusions than in blood cells. However, this response is not specific to RA and is even more prominent in reactive arthritis.

Immune dysregulation has been observed in peripheral blood T cells in patients with RA, especially with EBV infection. The deficient T cell response can be correlated with disease activity, but it also occurs in patients with other forms of arthritis. A more specific defect is observed in the autologous mixed lymphocyte reaction, in which T cells proliferate and produce cytokines in response to MHC class II antigens expressed on autologous antigen-presenting cells. Autoimmune responses directed toward joint-specific antigens can contribute to synovitis. In addition to type II collagen, which is localized to hyaline cartilage, other articular antigens have been implicated. For instance, T cell immunity directed against heat shock proteins, cartilage protein gp39, cartilage link protein, and proteoglycans have been variably implicated in RA. Many of these antigens can induce arthritis in mice or rats when the animals are immunized with the antigen in combination with complete Freund adjuvant. An unusual T cell phenotype (CD4+, CD28−) has been noted in the synovial tissue of patients with RA that might possess functions of both innate and adaptive immunity.[22]

HUMORAL IMMUNITY

Rheumatoid Factors

Rheumatoid factors are immunoglobulins with antibody specificity for the Fc region of IgG. The tests usually employed in clinical diagnosis (latex fixation, sensitized sheep red blood cell agglutination, nephelometry, and enzyme-linked immunosorbent assay) detect only IgM rheumatoid factors. The tests are positive in up to 90% of patients with classic RA, depending on the method used. Although patients with classic RA may have negative test results, a high-titer positive result indicates a poor prognosis—an unremitting course and a greater degree of joint damage.

Rheumatoid factor is not a specific finding for RA. Significant titers are found in patients with related diseases (e.g., systemic lupus erythematosus [SLE], progressive systemic sclerosis, and dermatomyositis) and in patients with nonrheumatic chronic inflammatory disorders and infections. Healthy elderly persons, particularly women, often have positive test results. Rheumatoid factor may be a feature of the early immune response to many proteins, facilitating antigen clearance by macrophages.

IgM rheumatoid factor is most commonly detected; IgG and, less frequently, IgA rheumatoid factors are also sometimes found. The presence of IgG rheumatoid factor is associated with a higher rate of systemic complications (e.g., necrotizing vasculitis).[23] Rheumatoid factors in RA may result from somatic mutation in response to an antigen-driven immune response.[24] Rheumatoid factor can be synthesized by B cells and plasma cells that infiltrate the synovium in RA patients, including some seronegative patients.

Other autoantibodies also have a role in RA, including antibodies directed at joint-specific antigens such as gp39, RA33, and p205.[25] Antibodies to glucose-6-phosphate isomerase (GPI), a ubiquitous antigen, can cause arthritis in mice and have also been detected in patients with RA and other inflammatory arthropathies.[26] Anti-GPI antibodies appear to localize in the joints and activate complement, perhaps because GPI can adhere to articular cartilage. The relative contribution of autoantibodies to RA as either a primary or a secondary phenomenon is still uncertain.

Complement Activation

Interaction of rheumatoid factors with normal IgG activates complement and thereby starts a chain of events that includes production of anaphylatoxins and chemotactic factors. Polymorphonuclear leukocytes then engulf the rheumatoid factor–IgG–complement complexes and release lysosomal enzymes and other products. Complexes of IgG rheumatoid factor with IgG and complement components are readily detected in the synovium, synovial fluid, and extra-articular lesions. Although the synovium is a rich source of complement production, the levels in rheumatoid synovial fluid are low because of local consumption. Deposits of immunoglobulin and complement have been identified in avascular cartilage and other collagenous tissues of rheumatoid joints and may play a role in the formation of the destructive lesion of RA. These deposits, which are highly specific for RA, may be an attractant for the invasive pannus.

Cytokines

Early studies suggested an unrestricted abundance of cytokines in the rheumatoid joint. However, later experiments demonstrated a relative paucity of many T cell–derived cytokines, including IL-2, IL-4, and TNF-β.[27] One exception is the recently described IL-17, which can regulate cartilage metabolism and may be produced by CD4+ T cells in the joint.[28] T cells can also potentially contribute to macrophage and synoviocyte activation by inducing metalloproteinase gene expression via direct cell-cell contact.

T helper cells can be divided into subsets that mediate distinct functions of the immune system. T helper type 1 (Th1) cells produce interferon gamma and IL-2 but not IL-4, IL-5, or IL-10; T helper type 2 (Th2) cells produce the opposite cytokine profile. Th1 overactivity predominates in most animal models of autoimmunity, whereas Th2 cytokines mediate disease suppression.[29] The small amounts of T cell cytokines that can be detected in RA are biased toward the Th1 phenotype, including

IL-17. In contrast, Th2 cytokines (especially IL-4) are virtually absent from the joint. Some IL-10 is present but is derived mainly from macrophages, and the amount is not sufficient to suppress Th1 cytokine production.[30] The relative lack of suppressive Th2 cytokines may contribute to the pathogenesis of rheumatoid synovitis. Levels of other suppressive cytokines, such as the natural IL-1 receptor antagonist (IL-1ra), are also low in RA joint tissues.[31]

Macrophage- and fibroblast-derived cytokines (e.g., IL-1, IL-6, TNF-a, and granulocyte-macrophage colony-stimulating factor [GM-CSF]) are abundantly expressed in the rheumatoid joint.[32] Although many of these cytokines are involved in the pathogenesis of RA, TNF-α and IL-1 are major pathogenic factors: both can induce synoviocyte proliferation, collagenase production, and prostaglandin release; overexpression can induce arthritis in animal models. IL-15 is produced by macrophages but shares many activities of the T cell–derived cytokine IL-2. It increases the ability of T cells to induce TNF-α production by macrophages through an antigen-independent mechanism that involves cell-cell contact.[33] IL-18 is also present in the RA joint and can bias T cell responses toward Th1 or directly activate macrophages to produce proinflammatory mediators.[34] Cytokine networks can potentially establish paracrine or autocrine networks that can perpetuate arthritis long after the etiologic agent has been cleared. Recent studies suggest that anticytokine therapy (including therapy with IL-1, TNF-α, and IL-6) is effective in severe RA and demonstrates the importance of fibroblast and macrophage products in chronic synovitis.

Diagnosis

CLINICAL FEATURES

The onset of RA in adults may be either acute or insidious. In the latter case, systemic manifestations may precede overt symptoms of arthritis by months. In some patients, external events (e.g., major infections, surgical procedures, trauma, or childbirth) precede the clinical onset. How these events relate to pathogenesis is unknown. Small joints of the hands and feet are usually involved at the outset, although large joints (e.g., knees and ankles) are sometimes affected first. In about 10% of cases, monoarthritis of a large joint can presage progression to polyarticular RA.

An insidious onset followed by progression to polyarticular involvement is the most common course. Most patients experience some degree of joint stiffness, especially in the morning after awakening, which may accompany or precede joint swelling or pain. These symptoms are hallmarks of disease activity and help distinguish RA from noninflammatory diseases such as osteoarthritis. However, joint stiffness and swelling are not specific for RA and can occur with other types of inflammatory arthritis. RA patients frequently complain of morning stiffness that lasts more than 30 minutes (often up to several hours).

Examination of the joints reveals varying degrees of swelling, warmth over the involved joint, tenderness to palpation, and limitation of active and passive range of motion. Swelling may be caused by thickening, edema, and increased vascularity of the synovium; by synovial effusions; or by combinations of these factors. In small joints, such as metacarpophalangeal joints, effusions may be difficult to detect: the presence of synovial thickening causes loss of the landmarks and can obscure the peaks and valleys formed by the joints. In large joints, especially the knees, effusions are usually easy to

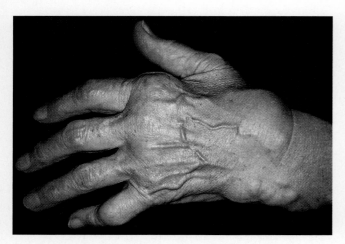

Figure 3   **The hand and wrist are common sites of synovitis in rheumatoid arthritis. Marked swelling in the wrist and metacarpophalangeal joints is caused by synovial proliferation. Modest ulnar deviation of the fingers is also present.**

demonstrate. Unlike acute inflammatory arthritides (e.g., gout or septic arthritis), RA tends not to cause marked erythema, and swelling usually does not extend far beyond the articulation. In elderly patients, the most prominent manifestation may be diffuse swelling of the hands accompanied by aching and marked stiffness in the absence of erythema. This can be difficult to distinguish from polymyalgia rheumatica, especially in patients lacking rheumatoid factor.

Classically, RA is symmetrical. When RA is progressive and unremitting, nearly every peripheral joint may eventually be affected, although the thoracic and lumbar spine are usually spared. This clinical presentation is observed in perhaps 10% of patients. In about 75%, the disease waxes and wanes over a period of years. In the remaining patients, complete remissions may be achieved with no evidence of inflammation. Remissions may be only partial, with mild clinical disease persisting despite clear improvement. When the course is progressive, the periods of remission may become shorter, and less impressive decreases in symptoms and findings may occur.

A relatively favorable course with long remissions tends to be associated with age less than 40 years, acute onset restricted to a few large joints, disease duration less than 1 year, and negative test results for rheumatoid factor. Conversely, an unfavorable prognosis is often associated with insidious onset, constitutional symptoms (e.g., weight loss, low-grade fever, and profound fatigue), rapid appearance of rheumatoid nodules, and high titers of rheumatoid factor. Homozygosity for the QKRAA sequence in the HLA-DR locus is also associated with more severe disease with extra-articular manifestations. The duration and intensity of inflammation correlates with long-term disability, and there is a significant relationship between persistent elevations in the level of C-reactive protein and poor outcome. The appearance of bone erosions early in the course of disease also portends a worse prognosis.

Pregnancy often relieves the symptoms of RA in the second or third trimester through a poorly clarified mechanism. One possible explanation is that the placenta produces large amounts of the suppressive cytokine IL-10. The risk of developing RA appears to be lower in women who have been pregnant. The effect of oral contraceptives on disease susceptibility is controversial; the effect, if any, is probably small.[35] In long-

term studies, multiple pregnancies or the use of oral contraceptives did not significantly alter the course of RA.[36]

Mortality is higher in RA patients than in the normal population. For the most part, RA patients die of the same causes as the general public, albeit earlier. In severe RA, mortality can approach that of severe congestive heart failure or Hodgkin disease, thereby justifying aggressive early management. Cardiovascular disease accounts for about 40% to 45% of deaths in RA patients; cancer, about 15%; and infection, about 10%. The inflammatory response, especially when associated with an increase in C-reactive protein and the use of proatherogenic treatments such as corticosteroids, correlates with an increased incidence of coronary artery disease.[37] The incidence of lymphoproliferative diseases is increased in patients with RA; non-Hodgkin lymphoma, leukemia, multiple myeloma, and Hodgkin disease account for most excess malignancies.

Specific Joint Disease

Hands and wrists   Involvement of the hands and wrists is the most characteristic finding. Swelling and tenderness are usually noted first at the metacarpophalangeal and proximal interphalangeal joints [*see Figure 3*]. Fusiform swelling at the proximal interphalangeal joints is typical. Distal interphalangeal joints are usually spared. Grip strength is decreased because of pain and mechanical derangement. Flexor tenosynovitis is common; progressive flexion limitation prevents the making of a fist.

Depending on the site and severity of the rheumatoid lesions, varying degrees of ulnar deviation and subluxation at the metacarpophalangeal joints result. These deformities are, in large part, caused by inflammation and radial deviation at the wrist. As the wrist abnormalities progress, the extensor tendons apply torque across the metacarpophalangeal joints and tend to pull the digits into the classic ulnar deviation position. Other changes in the phalanges include (1) hyperextension at the proximal interphalangeal joint and flexion at the distal interphalangeal joint (so-called swan-neck deformity) and (2) flexion at the proximal interphalangeal joint and extension at the distal interphalangeal joint (boutonnière deformity). Several deformities also affect the thumb and interfere with grasp and pinch. In extreme instances, the fingers are markedly deformed and flail as a result of destruction of cartilage and bone.

In early RA, relatively symptomless swelling of the dorsum of the wrist may be noted. Most often, the wrist is painful and is the source of functional limitations (e.g., inability to remove the lid from a jar). At the volar aspect, median nerve compression caused by synovial expansion can produce carpal tunnel syndrome. On the dorsal surface, synovial proliferation may erode and rupture the extensor tendons of the fingers, rendering the patient unable to extend the fingers actively at the metacarpophalangeal joints. Decreased dorsiflexion and plantar flexion of the wrist caused by fusion of carpal bones is common in severe disease. Volar subluxation and radial deviation are also common deformities; the ulnar styloid is often one of the first sites of bone erosion.

Elbows and shoulders   Synovitis of the elbow joint and inflammation and nodules in the olecranon bursa are frequent in established RA [*see Figure 4*]. Mild flexion contractures occur early; late in the disease, they cause functional disability, especially when associated with decreased shoulder abduction and rotation. Pain with decreased range of motion is commonly

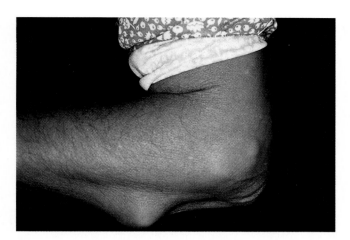

Figure 4   **Rheumatoid nodules commonly form near the extensor surface of the elbow. They can be fixed to the underlying periosteum or can be freely mobile.**

caused by synovitis of the glenohumeral joint; occasionally, large anterior effusions are evident. Shoulder pain commonly causes difficulty sleeping at night and functional disability. In chronic RA, the joint space becomes contracted, and rupture of the rotator cuff is very common. On physical examination, true glenohumeral joint arthritis can usually be distinguished from acromioclavicular pain, rotator cuff tendinitis, and subdeltoid bursitis.

Hips   The hip is affected later than most other joints. In osteoarthritis, the femoral head tends to migrate superiorly in the acetabulum, but in RA, symmetrical destruction of cartilage leads to axial migration. End-stage rheumatoid disease with typical cartilage loss produces acetabular protrusion of the femoral head [*see Figure 5*].

Knees   Knee arthritis is common and is occasionally a primary manifestation in early RA. Swelling and thickening of the synovium and effusions are usually simple to detect; arthrocentesis readily provides synovial fluid for analysis. Occasionally, large effusions expand into the suprapatellar pouch. Atrophy of muscles around the knee, especially the quadriceps, and resultant weakness can be detected early. Persistent synovitis eventually limits walking because of cartilage destruction, ligament laxity, joint instability, and contractures.

Baker cysts of the popliteal space are lined with synovial membrane and usually communicate with the cavity of the knee joint. The high pressure generated during knee flexion may be propagated posteriorly and cause rupture or dissection of these cysts. Calf swelling, pain, and erythema result, mimicking thrombophlebitis. Rupture of cysts is not specific to RA, occurring in other forms of inflammatory synovitis as well. Diagnosis of popliteal cysts can be confirmed by ultrasonography or arthrography. Generally, treatment of the cyst is directed toward the underlying knee synovitis. Corticosteroid injections are usually directed into the knee rather than into the cyst.

Ankles and feet   Inflammation of the ankle joints and of the small joints of the feet is common. Pain on flexion and extension is a result of tibiotalar arthritis, whereas pain on inversion and eversion is caused by subtalar disease. The metatarsophalangeal joints are sites of early synovitis, which causes pain in the ball of the foot on weight bearing [*see Figure 6*]. Lat-

er in the disease, there is subluxation with protrusion of the metatarsal heads, hallux valgus, and collapse of the arch.

Cervical spine   Joints of the thoracic, lumbar, and sacral spine are relatively unaffected in adult RA, but cervical spine disease is frequent and may result in severe pain or neurologic complications.[38] The lesion that has received the most attention is atlantoaxial subluxation and consequent separation at the atlanto-odontoid articulation [*see Figure 7*]. This deformity is best seen on lateral roentgenograms obtained with the neck flexed, so that the separation of the anterior margin of the odontoid process from the posterior margin of the anterior arch of the atlas can exceed 3 mm. When the separation is severe, the odontoid process may protrude into the foramen magnum and exert pressure on the spinal cord, causing paresthesia or even muscle weakness in the arms and hands. Often, the odontoid process itself is eroded, which minimizes pressure complications but produces instability. Prophylactic surgery to correct subluxation is usually not recommended because of the high morbidity and mortality associated with the procedure. Surgical fixation is indicated in the presence of neurologic signs and symptoms related to spinal cord compression. If the patient requires other surgical procedures, the anesthesiologist should be alerted to the presence of atlantoaxial subluxation to minimize complications of intubation.

Other cervical spine lesions are also seen, including subluxation at multiple levels, erosions at end plates or apophyseal joints, or fusion at these joints. Management of cervical spine pain in the absence of significant subluxation can be frustrat-

a

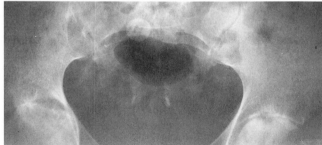

b

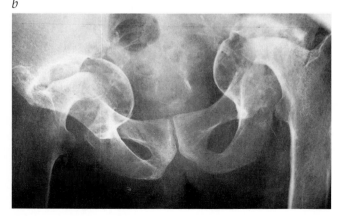

Figure 5   **(*a*) A pelvic roentgenogram of a patient with classic seropositive rheumatoid arthritis was taken early in the course of the disease. (*b*) Another roentgenogram taken 4 years later demonstrates marked acetabular protrusion and resorption of the femoral heads, both of which are characteristic of the disease.**

ing. Traction can be gently applied, but one must always be cognizant of instability. Soft collars can provide some temporary relief, but if used excessively, they can exacerbate the problem by weakening the cervical muscles.

Other joints   Synovitis of the temporomandibular joints may produce pain on chewing and limit jaw motion. If the joint is sufficiently destroyed, posterior subluxation of the jaw may cause a receding chin. Sternoclavicular arthritis is uncommon but occurs in patients with widespread arthritis. In acute cricoarytenoid arthritis, hoarseness and pain on swallowing may accompany tenderness over the larynx.

Extra-articular Manifestations

RA is a systemic disease, even though it characteristically affects structures in and around the joints. Its systemic manifestations include mild fever, anorexia, weight loss, fatigue, and muscular weakness. Specific organ involvement usually occurs in the context of severe RA, with high titers of rheumatoid factor and nodule formation.

Rheumatoid nodules   Rheumatoid nodules are the most common extra-articular manifestation, occurring in about 15% of patients. Almost all patients in whom nodules develop are seropositive for rheumatoid factor and have erosive disease [*see Figure 8*]. Nodules are usually subcutaneous and often are found in areas exposed to pressure—for example, over the extensor surfaces of the forearm, the olecranon bursa, the knuckles, the ischial regions, the Achilles tendon, and the bridge of the nose (if glasses are worn). They also occur in viscera. Rheumatoid nodules are firm and are either freely movable or attached to connective tissue (e.g., periosteum or tendons). They range from a few millimeters to more than 2 cm in diameter and often occur in clusters. Nodules typically have a rubbery or gritty feel and can

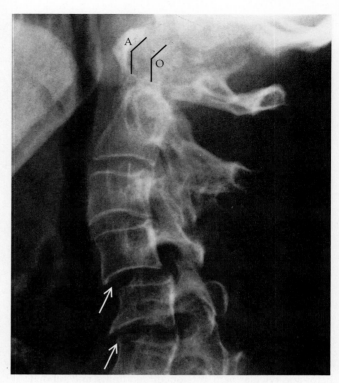

Figure 7   The anterior edge of the odontoid process (O) is abnormally separated from the posterior margin of the arch of the atlas (A) in this lateral roentgenogram of the cervical spine of a patient with rheumatoid arthritis. Subluxations of the lower cervical vertebral bodies (arrows) are also visible.

be indistinguishable from gouty tophi on physical examination. The lesion contains a center of fibrinoid necrosis (a mixture of fibrin and other proteins, such as degraded collagen) surrounded by a zone of histiocytes, which tend to be arranged radially. Lymphocytes and plasma cells form an outer layer. The pathogenesis of nodules is likely similar to that of synovitis, with early vascular involvement and local cytokine production.

There is no specific therapy for nodules other than treatment of the underlying arthritis. Surgical removal is often ineffective

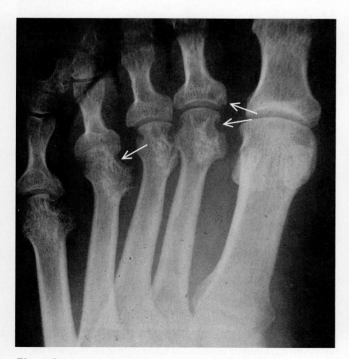

Figure 6   Erosions (arrows) are visible in the metatarsal heads and in some of the phalanges in this roentgenogram of the foot of a patient with classic seropositive rheumatoid arthritis.

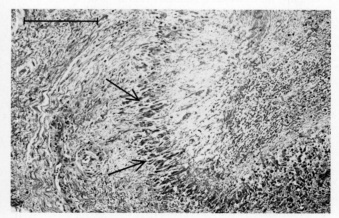

Figure 8   A typical rheumatoid nodule contains an area of fibrinoid necrosis (center) surrounded by palisading histiocytes (arrows). At the periphery are round cells (predominantly lymphocytes). Stain is hematoxylin and eosin (bar scale = 300 μm).

because nodules can return; it is generally reserved for severe functional impairment or obvious cosmetic problems. The appearance of fresh crops of nodules can indicate active disease. In some cases, exuberant nodule production (rheumatoid nodulosis) is a complication of methotrexate therapy. Rheumatoid nodules are not specific to RA, occurring in other connective tissue diseases (e.g., SLE) or in isolation (e.g., granuloma annulare).

Eyes The sicca syndrome, which is part of Sjögren syndrome, is the most frequent ocular manifestation of RA. Symptoms include sensations of grittiness, accumulation of dried mucoid material (especially in the morning immediately after waking up), and decreased tear production. The relative paucity of tears is demonstrated by decreased wetting of a filter paper strip in a Schirmer test. The dryness is not limited to the eyes and involves other exocrine glands, including those in the nose, the mouth, the rectum, and the vagina. Marked enlargement of lacrimal and salivary glands can occur in severe cases, although this is more common in primary Sjögren syndrome than in RA.

The genetic basis of RA with dry eyes is different from that of primary Sjögren syndrome, which is associated with HLA-DR3 antigen rather than HLA-DR4 antigen.[39] Patients with the primary syndrome without joint inflammation have a greater frequency of recurrent parotitis, Raynaud phenomenon, purpura, lymphadenopathy, myositis, and renal involvement. In all patients with sicca syndrome, lacrimal and salivary glands are characterized histologically by lymphocyte infiltration and distortion of ductal structures. Patients with Sjögren syndrome often have high titers of anti-Ro antibody (also called anti–SS-A). Biopsy of minor salivary glands in the lip can help establish the diagnosis.

Scleritis is painful and may lead to perforation of the sclera and blindness. Episcleritis is common and can often be managed with topical corticosteroids. Matrix loss around the limbus and corneal melting may also lead to perforation. Uveitis and iritis occur no more often in adults with RA than in control populations.

Lungs The most common form of lung involvement is pleurisy with effusions.[40] Evidence of pleuritis is often found at postmortem examination, but symptomatic pleurisy occurs in fewer than 10% of patients. Clinical features include gradual onset and variable degrees of pain and dyspnea. The effusions generally have protein concentrations greater than 3 to 4 g/dl as well as glucose concentrations lower than 30 mg/dl, which have been ascribed to a primary defect in glucose transport. The leukocyte count is rarely higher than 5,000/mm^3 and is dominated by lymphocytes. The lactate dehydrogenase level is often markedly elevated; occasionally, the lipid content is also high. Complement levels are usually low, and rheumatoid factors are present. Pleural biopsy usually reveals nonspecific fibrosis or granulomas. The pleural effusions usually resolve spontaneously within months. Occasionally, repeated aspirations are required to relieve dyspnea; if effusions are troublesome, instillations of glucocorticoids are useful.

Rheumatoid nodules occur in the pulmonary parenchyma as well as on the pleural surface. They range in size from just detectable to several centimeters in diameter. They may be single or multiple and, at times, cavitate. Such nodules can be difficult to distinguish radiologically from tuberculous or malignant lesions and often require further evaluation, including biopsy.

Progressive, symptomatic interstitial pulmonary fibrosis that produces coughing and dyspnea in conjunction with radi-

ographic changes of a diffuse reticular pattern (i.e., honeycomb lung) is usually associated with high titers of rheumatoid factor. The lesion is histologically indistinguishable from idiopathic pulmonary fibrosis. Chest radiographs show pleural thickening, nodules, diffuse or patchy infiltrates, and a restrictive ventilatory defect that is characterized by a decreased CO diffusion rate. These abnormalities are often associated with cigarette smoking, other extra-articular manifestations, and active disease. Bronchiolitis obliterans, an unusual form of airway obstruction that usually has a viral or toxic etiology, may also develop.

Heart Cardiac involvement is common but rarely symptomatic. Echocardiographic evidence of pericardial effusion or thickening has been found in about one third of patients studied.[41] Autopsy findings include rheumatoid nodules, healed or active pericarditis, myocarditis, endocarditis, and valvular fibrosis.

Symptomatic pericarditis is most frequent in patients with severe seropositive disease. Overt manifestations include chest pain, friction rub, and associated pleural effusions. The pericardial effusions resemble the pleural effusions in RA. Cardiac tamponade is rare, as is constrictive pericarditis.

Rheumatoid nodules and inflammation in the valves and the conduction system may cause conduction disturbances, including complete heart block. Aortic regurgitation secondary to aortitis and dilation of the aortic root may lead to congestive heart failure.

Blood Mild anemia of chronic disease is characteristic of active RA, although the hemoglobin level is usually greater than 10 mg/dl. Nonsteroidal anti-inflammatory drugs (NSAIDs) often cause GI blood loss, leading to iron deficiency. Although its levels are not reduced in RA, administration of erythropoietin alleviates anemia.[42]

The constellation of RA with splenomegaly and leukopenia is known as Felty syndrome.[43] The mean serum leukocyte count in such patients is usually 1,500 to 2,000/mm^3, and the mean granulocyte count is 500 to 1,000/mm^3. Severe thrombocytopenia is uncommon. Infections, particularly of the skin, the perianal region, and the lungs, are frequent and are usually caused by common organisms. Other findings in Felty syndrome include hepatomegaly, lymphadenopathy, and chronic cutaneous ulcerations.

The neutropenia is the result of excessive vascular margination of leukocytes, increased peripheral destruction of leukocytes caused by IgG and IgM antigranulocyte antibodies,[44] and the inhibitory effects of T cells on granulopoiesis. Some cases of Felty syndrome are associated with oligoclonal or monoclonal expansion of large granular lymphocytes in the blood and represent a form of chronic leukemia.[45] Splenectomy usually produces an increase in the leukocyte count, but this increase is sustained in only 30% of patients. Lithium chloride may alleviate the neutropenia, as may treatment of active arthritis with disease-modifying drugs such as methotrexate.[46] Treatment with recombinant colony-stimulating factors, such as granulocyte colony-stimulating factor (G-CSF), can increase peripheral granulocyte counts in patients with Felty syndrome. The drug must be given for extended periods because discontinuance leads to relapse.

Neuromuscular involvement Weakness of muscles adjacent to joints with active synovitis is common. The most common neuropathy is median nerve compression caused by synovitis of the wrist. Entrapment of the ulnar nerve at the elbow or branches of the sural nerve in the tarsal tunnel also occurs.

Mononeuritis multiplex is seen in patients who have severe disease with necrotizing vasculitis and, frequently, deposits of immune complexes in the walls of the blood vessels supplying the involved nerves.[47] In milder cases, only segmental demyelination without vascular abnormalities may be found. Aseptic meningitis resulting from a hypersensitivity reaction to NSAIDs has been reported.[48]

Blood vessels Vasculitis in small synovial vessels is a hallmark of early RA, but more widespread vascular inflammation of medium-sized muscular arteries also occurs in older men with advanced disease, rheumatoid nodules, and high titers of rheumatoid factor. The involvement of larger vessels is distinct from small vessel disease; such involvement includes leukocytoclastic vasculitis or nail-fold infarcts. The course and prognosis of systemic rheumatoid vasculitis are similar to those of polyarteritis nodosa. Clinically, patients with rheumatoid vasculitis demonstrate polyneuropathy (mononeuritis multiplex), skin ulcerations, purpura, and cutaneous infarctions (sometimes progressing to gangrene). Manifestations of visceral ischemia, including bowel perforations, myocardial infarctions, and cerebral infarctions, are also common. Treatment usually requires high-dose corticosteroid or cyclophosphamide treatment, or both, and still may not be effective. This feared complication has become quite rare, perhaps because of improved therapy for the underlying disease.

Other systems Apart from gastric and duodenal lesions caused by NSAIDs, GI complications are rare in RA. Rheumatoid nodules may involve the pharynx and esophagus. Mild elevations of liver enzymes are common and are usually drug related. Other hepatic abnormalities, particularly elevations in serum alkaline phosphatase and 5'-nucleotidase levels, occur in Sjögren syndrome. These hepatobiliary lesions are ascribed to immune responses to cross-reacting salivary and biliary antigens. Hepatitis C infection is also associated with development of the sicca syndrome.[49] RA rarely causes specific renal lesions; NSAIDs and amyloid are more often responsible.

IMAGING FEATURES

Because early joint pathology in RA is confined to the synovium, standard radiographs are often not useful. Periarticular osteopenia of the metacarpophalangeal joints and proximal interphalangeal joints in the hand can be evident within months of onset. Joint space narrowing, caused by the loss of articular cartilage, indicates irreversible damage to such cartilage; RA must be active for at least 6 months for such damage to occur. Arthroscopic visualization of articular cartilage (e.g., in the knee) identifies damage to cartilage considerably earlier, but such findings have no value in the management of RA. Subchondral sclerosis is a feature of osteoarthritis but not of RA. Prominent periostitis with new bone formation is much more common in psoriatic arthritis or reactive arthritis syndrome.

Radiographically visualized bone erosions are best seen at the margins of the joint, where the synovium is reflected near the attachment of the capsule. The bone in this region (the so-called "bare area") is not protected by a layer of cartilage and is directly attacked by the invading synovium and osteoclasts. The erosions associated with RA may be difficult to distinguish

from those of gout: the latter tend to have sharper borders and overhanging edges of bone, whereas the former are usually small and irregularly shaped. Cystlike radiolucencies may be seen in larger joints. Entire portions of bone adjacent to the joints, such as the metacarpal ends and the ulnar styloid process, may be resorbed. Cartilage destruction caused by RA tends to be evenly distributed within a joint. For instance, both the medial and the lateral compartments of the knee joint are narrowed in RA, whereas the medial compartment is more often affected in osteoarthritis. Progression of erosions takes time in RA; it is rarely necessary to repeat radiographs more often than every 12 months. Damage that is radiographically evident often occurs during the first 2 to 5 years and can progress inexorably in the absence of treatment.

MRI can distinguish synovial pannus from cartilage and synovial fluid and thus can detect pannus as it invades joint structures. The use of intravenous contrast materials, such as gadolinium, permits accurate assessment of synovial invasion and volume. MRI has replaced arthrography for the investigation of large joints, such as the knees.[50] The use of MRI to monitor response to therapy is still experimental because of a lack of uniform standards for judging damage. Although most erosions persist or progress, up to one quarter of them heal spontaneously.[51] Because of the lack of standardization, plain radiographs remain the gold standard for following disease progression.

LABORATORY EVALUATION

A mild normochromic, normocytic anemia and an elevated platelet count are usually present in patients with RA. The leukocyte count is generally normal, although neutropenia occurs in association with splenomegaly in Felty syndrome. The erythrocyte sedimentation rate (ESR) and the C-reactive protein level are usually elevated in active RA and are useful in monitoring disease activity and response to therapy. Results of serum chemistry studies are normal, although the use of either NSAIDs or methotrexate can lead to elevations in liver enzyme levels. Urinalysis is generally normal.

About 80% to 85% of patients with RA are seropositive for rheumatoid factor. If seropositivity develops, it usually does so before the end of the first year of disease. From 1% to 5% of healthy persons test positive for rheumatoid factor, with the higher percentage noted in the elderly. Many chronic inflammatory conditions besides RA are associated with positive rheumatoid factor test results, although the titers are usually lower.

Other serologic tests commonly used to diagnose rheumatic diseases are of limited value in RA. Antinuclear antibodies (ANA) are often present in low titer. If anti-DNA antibodies are detected, they are almost always directed against single-stranded DNA rather than native double-stranded DNA. Antibodies to the antigens associated with Sjögren syndrome (SS-A and SS-B) may be positive. Serum complement levels are normal in uncomplicated RA; hypocomplementemia suggests systemic rheumatoid vasculitis. Serologic tests for viruses may help identify patients with postrubella arthritis or parvovirus B19 infection. Hepatitis B and C serologies can also provide useful information, because these infections can cause a self-limited symmetrical polyarthritis that mimics RA.

Analysis of synovial fluid provides supportive data but is rarely diagnostic. Synovial fluid in RA usually appears straw colored and mildly turbid. Bits of fibrin and, occasionally, small fronds of synovium may be aspirated. Leukocyte counts range from 2,000 to 20,000/mm³. On differential counts, most of the cells (50% to 80%) are neutrophils; the remainder are lymphocytes (mainly T cells) and monocytes. The synovial fluid glucose level is usually normal, which distinguishes RA from acute infection. Synovial fluid complement levels are usually low in inflamed rheumatoid joints despite abundant production of complement proteins by synovium. Tests for rheumatoid factor, antinuclear antibodies, total protein, or lactate dehydrogenase in synovial fluid are not clinically useful. Synovial biopsies, either blind or arthroscopically directed, can be used in clinical trials to assess response to therapy. However, their utility for differential diagnosis or in predicting response to therapy remains limited.

Differential Diagnosis

The onset and course of RA can be highly variable, and the lack of a specific biologic marker makes diagnosis difficult. Prolonged observation and the integration of clinical and laboratory data that meet established criteria are often required.

Diagnostic criteria have been formulated by the American College of Rheumatology [see Table 1]. Conditions mimicking RA should be ruled out, if possible. Patients with other rheumatic diseases often have a symmetrical polyarticular arthritis resembling RA. The presence of high-titer ANA and anti–double-stranded DNA, a low serum complement level, and major organ system involvement (especially nephritis) are clues to the diagnosis of SLE. Careful physical examination often helps the clinician distinguish other rheumatic diseases. Elderly persons with polymyalgia rheumatica can present with peripheral synovitis, although prominent proximal muscle stiffness and a very high ESR (often higher than 80 to 100 mm/hr) are useful differential findings. Viral arthritis mediated by immune complex deposition, as in hepatitis B or rubella, often has the same distribution as RA but is transient.

Metabolic disorders such as gout and calcium pyrophosphate deposition arthropathies can mimic RA. Radiographs may indicate characteristic gouty erosions or chondrocalcinosis. The finding of crystals in synovial fluid distinguishes these disorders from RA. Septic arthritis is also relatively easy to identify through clinical examination and evaluation of synovial fluid.

Seronegative spondyloarthropathies can present a diagnostic challenge when they exhibit peripheral polyarticular disease. They can generally be distinguished by the lack of symmetry, the distribution of affected joints (usually, lower extremities are affected more than upper, and large joints more than small), the absence of rheumatoid factor, the presence of proliferative bone changes on radiographs, and characteristic skin lesions. However, in some cases, psoriatic arthritis has a clinical picture almost identical to that of RA.

Morning stiffness and involvement of the wrist and metacarpophalangeal joints are uncommon in osteoarthritis, which typically affects the weight-bearing joints and the distal interphalangeal joints. Patients with osteoarthritis usually are seronegative for rheumatoid factor and lack marginal erosions. Synovial effusions are noninflammatory, with a WBC lower than 2,000/mm³ and a predominance of mononuclear cells.

Rheumatoid joints are more susceptible to bacterial infection than normal joints, and superimposed sepsis may not be readily apparent. The usual signs (e.g., localized erythema, increased pain, and limitation of motion) may be difficult to distinguish from the underlying rheumatoid synovitis or may be suppressed by antirheumatic therapy. Multiple joints may be infected simultaneously; the diagnosis requires arthrocentesis and culture [see Chapter 130].

Table 2 Comparison of Various Antirheumatic Treatments

Drug	Response Rate; Onset of Action	Magnitude of Efficacy (0 to ++++)	Major Toxicities	Dosage
Anakinra	30%; 1–3 mo	+ to ++	Injection site reactions, infection	100 mg/day S.C.
Azathioprine	30%–50%; 2–3 mo	++	Hematologic, immunosuppression, cholestasis	100–150 mg/day
Cyclosporine	30%; 2–3 mo	++	Renal (irreversible), hypertension, hypertrichosis, immunosuppression	2.5–5.0 mg/kg/day
Etanercept	50%–70%; 2–4 wk	+++	Injection-site reaction, ?immune surveillance	25 mg S.C. twice a week
Gold	30%; 3–6 mo	++	Skin rash, hematologic, renal	5.0 mg/wk I.M. × 6 mo
Hydroxychloroquine	30%–50%; 2–6 mo	++	Retinopathy, myopathy, hyperpigmentation	200 mg b.i.d.
Infliximab	50%–70%; 2–4 wk	+++	Increased infection	3 mg/kg I.V. q. 8 wk
Leflunomide	50%; 2–3 mo	++	Liver, teratogen, gastrointestinal, skin rash	100 mg/day × 3, then 20 mg/day
Methotrexate	> 70%; 6–8 wk	+++	Liver (fibrosis, elevated enzymes), hematologic, oral ulcers	7.5–15 mg/wk
NSAIDs	> 75%; < 2 wk	+	Gastric erosion, renal	Varied
Prednisone	> 90%; < 1 wk	+++	Skin atrophy, cataracts, osteoporosis, avascular necrosis	5.0–7.5 mg/day
Sulfasalazine	> 30%; 2–3 mo	++	Dyspepsia, hemolysis in glucose-6-phosphate dehydrogenase deficiency	1 g b.i.d. or t.i.d.

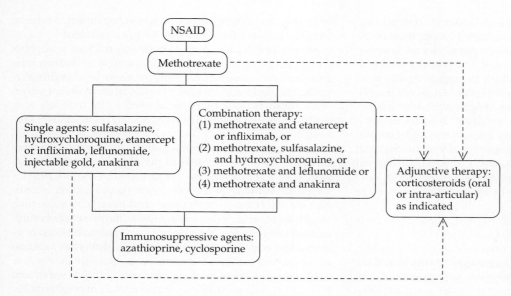

Figure 9 **Proposed algorithm for pharmacologic management of rheumatoid arthritis. The solid lines indicate the standard management options, and the broken lines indicate stages at which adjunctive therapy may be introduced. Most patients require rapid advancement from nonsteroidal anti-inflammatory drugs to a second-line agent, most often methotrexate.**

Management

Optimal management requires an awareness of the variable course of the disorder. Statistical predictions about outcome can be made from clinical features and laboratory abnormalities, but remissions and exacerbations are common, and the risks associated with drugs and surgery must be viewed in the light of this uncertainty. The patient should be aware of the risks both of taking a drug and of not taking it. Active synovitis that persists for a year or more after the onset of RA results in irreversible cartilage damage, joint destruction, and increased mortality. Thus, every effort should be made to suppress the synovitis by pharmacologic methods during the early months.

No specific climate or diet alters the course of RA. Alternative therapies, including cartilage extracts, rarely have more than a placebo effect. The power of placebo effects should not be underestimated in these circumstances; most arthritis and pain studies demonstrate a "therapeutic" response in 20% to 30% of patients who receive placebo. Glucosamine and chondroitin sulfate have been studied in osteoarthritis, but few data support their use in RA. In addition to conveying to the patient an understanding of the disease, management involves efforts to relieve pain and discomfort, preserve strength and joint function, prevent deformities, and attend to systemic complications. Surgical intervention is important not only for replacing destroyed joints but also, at times, for restoring function or preventing further damage.

DRUG THERAPY

Drugs are used for analgesia, to control inflammation, and to alter the natural history of disease. With some currently available agents, only empirical data support their use, and their mechanism of action is unknown. In formal studies of individual drug therapies, systematic measurements are taken of the number of inflamed joints, the extent of swelling, and the range of joint motion. Laboratory measurements (e.g., ESR and hematocrit value) and assessments of subjective features (e.g., pain and morning stiffness) are also made. The information is then assessed globally. Some objective and subjective improvement is usually observed with any agent; placebo effects may be striking [*see Table 2*].

General Recommendations

The appropriate management of RA is rapidly evolving; previous treatment algorithms based on a gradual escalation of treatment (i.e., the traditional pyramid approach) have been replaced by more aggressive treatment approaches.[52] The change has been fomented by a variety of factors, including the following: (1) active RA significantly decreases the life span of affected individuals; (2) active inflammation is associated with increased morbidity and mortality; (3) more effective therapy is available; and (4) the advent of combination therapy and new drugs has had a clear effect on the natural history of disease. No single algorithm can capture the complexity of RA management today because of the extensive pharmacopoeia, although broad guidelines can be given [*see Figure 9*].

Most patients require rapid advancement from NSAIDs to a second-line agent, most often methotrexate. Because symptoms of RA will not be adequately controlled in 70% of patients by methotrexate alone, the clinician is usually faced with the choice of either "add-on" therapy or testing a series of single agents (e.g, sulfasalazine, antimalarials, leflunomide, a TNF inhibitor, or gold). In the United States, most rheumatologists prefer to increase the methotrexate dosage rapidly to 20 to 25 mg/wk and then add another agent within 2 to 3 months if necessary. The physician tolerance for active disease is much less today than in the past; morning stiffness lasting longer than 30 minutes, continued pain, or evidence of active synovitis on physical examination is an indication for advancing therapy even if the patient has experienced significant improvement on methotrexate. Typically, one would add either a TNF inhibitor, leflunomide, or a sulfasalazine (with or without hydroxychloroquine). Care must be exercised, especially with combinations of methotrexate and leflunomide, because of hepatotoxicity. In some cases, clinicians experiment with several combinations to find the correct cocktail for an individual patient.

Few data demonstrate the superiority of one combination of drugs over another, although there is an increasing bias toward use of TNF inhibitors early in management.[53] Prednisone is generally reserved for patients requiring adjunctive "bridge" therapy because such patients cannot perform activities of daily living while various single-drug and combination therapies are being evaluated. The most recent addition to the armamentarium, the IL-1 inhibitor anakinra, is modestly effective; it is usually reserved for patients who do not respond to combinations of methotrexate and TNF inhibitors.[54]

Alternative algorithms have also been proposed for the management of RA. Some data suggest that early management with triple therapy (e.g, sulfasalazine, hydroxychloroquine, and methotrexate) is very effective.[55] Other options include early high-dose corticosteroid treatment with a tapering dose over several months in combination with methotrexate and sulfasalazine. In such protocols, patients tend to improve quite rapidly because of the steroid. This form of early aggressive treatment appears to have a persistent effect with less radiographically evident joint damage, even after corticosteroids or one of the other agents has been discontinued.[56] However, it is very difficult to assess the efficacy of second-line drugs if prednisone is added early in the course of treatment.

Although the number of cases of treatment-resistant disease is decreasing, a fraction are recalcitrant to all of the aforementioned drugs. Immunosuppressive agents such as azathioprine or cyclosporine can be used, although the therapeutic ratio is narrow. Experimental approaches can also be considered with appropriate oversight from institutional review boards.

Nonsteroidal Anti-inflammatory Drugs

The use of aspirin for RA has decreased substantially because of the availability of newer NSAIDs. Nonacetylated salicylate compounds, such as choline salicylate and choline magnesium trisalicylate, produce less gastric irritation than aspirin but are more expensive and exert less anti-inflammatory effect.

Other NSAIDs are probably no more effective than aspirin but may have certain advantages (e.g., fewer GI effects, better pharmacokinetics, and, usually, fewer pills to be taken daily, which may enhance compliance). The prostaglandin analogue misoprostol, proton pump inhibitors, and, to a lesser extent, H_2 receptor blockers can suppress the GI toxicity of NSAIDs[57] and should be considered for patients who take a nonselective cyclooxygenase inhibitor but have a history of duodenal ulcer or gastritis.[58] Helicobacter pylori infection, use of salicylates, and use of NSAIDs are likely independent risk factors for peptic ulceration.[59]

Pharmacokinetics aside, there are a few pharmacologic differences between the various NSAIDs. Sulindac may have less renal toxicity than other NSAIDs, but the clinical relevance is not certain. Most currently available NSAIDs nonselectively block both the constitutively expressed cyclooxygenase COX-1 and the inducible cyclooxygenase COX-2, although the relative selectivity for COX-2 can be favorable with some compounds (e.g., meloxicam and diclofenac). Physicians generally should be familiar with a limited number of these agents, and therapy should be individualized. Selective COX-2 inhibitors (e.g., celecoxib and rofecoxib) are also effective anti-inflammatory and analgesic agents.[60] They have fewer GI side effects than nonselective COX inhibitors. In addition, they do not block platelet function and may be used in some situations in which traditional NSAIDs may be contraindicated. Both selective and nonselective agents, however, can alter renal blood flow and glomerular filtration rate. Celecoxib is administered in a dosage of 100 to 200 mg orally once or twice daily, whereas rofecoxib is usually given in a once-daily oral dosage of 12.5 to 25 mg. Although safety issues have arisen regarding cardiovascular risk factors and selective COX-2 inhibitors, the question of safety remains unresolved.[61]

Advancement from NSAIDs to second-line agents is recommended if (1) symptoms have not improved sufficiently after a short trial of NSAIDs, (2) the patient has aggressive seropositive disease, or (3) there is radiographic evidence of erosions or joint destruction. The trend today is for more aggressive treatment, and the majority of patients require additional pharmacotherapy.

Methotrexate

Methotrexate is one of the most effective second-line drugs. Methotrexate not only alleviates the signs and symptoms of RA but also decreases the ESR and raises the hematocrit value.[62] It probably also slows the rate of bone erosion in RA, perhaps by decreasing expression of destructive enzymes such as collagenase in synovium.[63]

Methotrexate is given in weekly oral doses, beginning at 7.5 mg and, if necessary, increasing to 15 mg over 2 to 3 months. Response to therapy is usually relatively rapid, with improvement occurring in 6 to 8 weeks. If no response is observed, the dose can be increased to 20 to 25 mg/wk [see Figure 9]. Over 70% of patients have a response to methotrexate, and half remain on the drug for at least 5 years. Efficacy remains excellent even after years of use.[64] Complete remissions are uncommon, although patients' sense of well-being is often dramatically improved.

Inflammation usually reappears within weeks after discontinuance. Monitoring of hematologic and liver parameters every 4 to 8 weeks is required. The primary action of methotrexate is anti-inflammatory at the doses used in RA, although immunosuppression resulting in Pneumocystis pneumonia has been reported. Improved survival as a result of a reduction in cardiovascular mortality has been reported in patients treated with methotrexate.[65]

Risk factors for toxicity include alcoholism, diabetes, obesity, advanced age, and renal disease. The major concern is hepatic fibrosis, although marrow toxicity and sterility are also important side effects. Methotrexate is a potent teratogen and should not be used in women of childbearing age unless they are using a reliable form of contraception. Idiosyncratic interstitial lung disease can develop even at low doses. Other adverse reactions to methotrexate include nausea, stomatitis, leukopenia, diarrhea, and elevations of serum aminotransferase levels. Some of these toxicities (especially oral ulcers) can be minimized by prophylactic administration of folic acid, 1 mg/day.[66] Hepatotoxicity leading to clinically significant fibrosis or cirrhosis is exceedingly uncommon; accordingly, most centers have abandoned routine monitoring with liver biopsies.[67] A biopsy should be performed if a patient develops persistent abnormalities in blood tests for liver enzymes that do not promptly resolve with discontinuance. Other medications that interfere with folate metabolism (e.g., trimethoprim) should be used with caution in patients taking methotrexate.

Leflunomide

Leflunomide is an effective antirheumatic agent that blocks the pyrimidine synthesis required for stimulated lymphocytes to proliferate. In vitro, it inhibits mitogen-stimulated proliferation of both B cells and T cells. Randomized, controlled trials have demonstrated that leflunomide is approximately as effective as methotrexate in the treatment of active RA.[68] Because the half-life of leflunomide is 2 weeks, loading doses are necessary to achieve therapeutic blood levels promptly. A loading dose of 100 mg/day for 3 days is followed by daily dosing with 20 mg/day. Adverse effects include diarrhea, liver toxicity, rash, oral ulcers, and reversible hair loss. Periodic monitoring of liver enzymes is required. In animal studies, leflunomide has been associated with birth defects; thus, this agent should not be used by pregnant women or women of childbearing age who are not using a reliable form of contraception. Leflunomide can be used in combination with methotrexate, although the initial dose of leflunomide is half the usual dose, and patients must be followed very carefully for hepatotoxicity.[69] In addition to clinical efficacy, leflunomide slows radiographic progression of RA.[70]

Antimalarial Drugs and Sulfasalazine as Single and Combination Agents

The antimalarial drug hydroxychloroquine is useful as early second-line therapy for RA.[71] Its response rate is lower than that of methotrexate, and less improvement is seen; however, its relative safety makes it an ideal choice for patients with mild early disease or as an additive agent in combination therapy. Adverse reactions to antimalarials occur, particularly retinopathy that may lead to an irreversible decrease in vision; this reaction is rare and can be minimized with regular ophthalmologic examinations.

Sulfasalazine is also useful.[72] It is effective in at least 30% of patients at a dosage of 2 to 3 g/day in divided doses. Only moderate side effects have been reported, especially GI upset. Sulfasalazine is well tolerated; over 30% of patients continue to take it for at least 5 years.[73]

A significant percentage of RA patients do not experience satisfactory symptomatic relief with a single disease-modifying antirheumatic drug. This lack of response has led clinical investigators to study combination regimens,[74] but most of the studies performed have been poorly controlled. A prospective study examining azathioprine and methotrexate alone and in combination demonstrated safety but no additive benefits.[75] A 2-year study showed that a combination of methotrexate, sulfasalazine, and hydroxychloroquine is more effective than any of the agents alone.[76]

Gold Salts

Injectable gold salts decrease inflammation and increase the likelihood of remission. Gold was once the primary second-line agent, but its relatively modest efficacy and high side-effect profile, coupled with the increased use of methotrexate and anticytokine therapy, have led to a dramatic decrease in its use. Although the mechanism of action of gold compounds has not been fully explained, it appears that these compounds alter the function of mononuclear phagocytes at the inflammatory site. Treatment usually consists of intramuscular administration of a compound such as gold sodium thiomalate in a test dose of 10 mg, followed by a single 25 mg dose 1 week later and then by 50 mg once weekly for 20 weeks. If the response is satisfactory at this point, the compound can be given every other week for another several months and monthly thereafter for an indefinite period. When a good response occurs, it is usually within the first 6 months; if there is no response after 20 doses, further doses are unlikely to be helpful. The response rate to gold is about 30%, although toxicity and lack of efficacy result in discontinuance in almost 90% of patients within 5 years. Major adverse side effects involve hematologic, renal, and dermatologic reactions. Oral gold preparations appear to be less toxic than injectable ones but are less effective.

Anticytokine Therapy

Interference with the function of TNF-α, either by soluble receptor blockade or by giving monoclonal antibody, is effective in treating RA.[77] By itself, the soluble 75 kd TNF receptor has a very short biologic half-life. Recombinant technology was used to engineer the fusion of the receptor to the Fc portion of the immunoglobulin molecule (etanercept), greatly prolonging the half-life and making twice-weekly subcutaneous injections feasible. The fusion protein is entirely human in origin, and antibody formation against it is minimal. Etanercept has been approved for use in the United States (25 mg S.C. twice a week) and has been shown to be beneficial in patients who have only a partial response to methotrexate used either in combination therapy or as monotherapy.[78] The fusion protein is also effective in children with RA.

The human-mouse chimeric monoclonal antibody infliximab has also been approved for use in adults with RA, although this agent must be used in combination with methotrexate. This combination appears to permit long-term use of infliximab with less formation of neutralizing antibodies.[79] Infliximab is administered by intravenous infusion, with a recommended dose of 3 to 10 mg/kg every 8 weeks. As with etanercept, the drug must be used with care in the presence of infections. Adalimumab, a fully human monoclonal antibody, has demonstrated efficacy similar to that of infliximab in RA and can be administered either subcutaneously or intravenously.

The clinical response to TNF inhibitors can be dramatic, and an improved sense of well-being can occur within days. Typically, patients who respond to TNF inhibitors will notice decreased pain and stiffness after a few weeks of therapy. About two thirds of patients have at least 20% improvement in the number of swollen and tender joints, and half of these patients will have more than 50% improvement. Concomitant with decreased symptoms, serum and synovial cytokine levels decrease, and peripheral blood markers of inflammation (i.e., ESR and C-reactive protein) decline. Although the clinical effect occurs sooner with the TNF inhibitors, a significant benefit over methotrexate has not been demonstrated after 3 months.[78] There are subtle differences in the pharmacology of the two TNF inhibitors. Etanercept binds both TNF-α and TNF-β, whereas the monoclonal antibodies have a greater affinity for the TNF-α ligand and binds only to TNF-α. However, the clinical impact of this difference is not clear, and the response rates are similar. In addition to providing symptomatic improvement, TNF inhibitors prevent or slow bone and cartilage destruction in RA. Perhaps most intriguing is the observation that radiographic progression is prevented even in patients who do not have clinical improvement after treatment with infliximab. This observation could have important implications for the widespread clinical use of these agents if long-term studies confirm these findings. For now, however, these agents are generally used only after an adequate trial of methotrexate.

Because TNF is important in host defense and possibly in tumor surveillance, impairment of these functions in treated patients could contribute to increased risk of infection and even cancer. The most common adverse reaction to etanercept is local inflammation at the injection site, although serious bacterial and mycobacterial infections have also been observed with TNF inhibitors.[80] Hence, these agents should be used with caution in patients with active infections. Before therapy with an anti-TNF agent is initiated, a skin test should be performed and a chest x-ray obtained to rule out tuberculosis; prophylactic treatment with isoniazid should be initiated if indicated. More intriguing is the induction of antinuclear and anti-DNA antibodies and, in a few cases, frank SLE in some RA patients treated with anti–TNF-α therapy. Long-term studies of larger numbers of patients are required to assess these problems, although very few serious side effects have been noted in patients treated for up to 3 years with etanercept. However, demyelinating syndromes and aplastic anemia have been noted in a small number of patients receiving TNF inhibitors. Because these agents appear to exacerbate multiple sclerosis, the association with the former may be based on a protective role for TNF-α in the central nervous system.[81]

The natural inhibitor to IL-1, IL-1ra (anakinra), demonstrates modest anti-inflammatory activity in RA.[82] Anakinra also appears to have disease-modifying activity, evidenced by a decrease in radiographic progression. Anakinra is administered subcutaneously (100 mg) by daily injection, either alone or in combination with methotrexate.[83] The most common side effect is injection-site reaction, although an increased incidence of infections has also been reported. Use of anakinra in combination with TNF inhibitors may markedly increase infectious complications; therefore, such combinations should be avoided until further studies clarify the risks and benefits. Anakinra has been approved for use in the United States.

Antibodies to the IL-6 receptor also may be effective, and suppressive cytokines such as IL-4 and IL-11 are under investigation. A preliminary study using IL-10 to treat RA did not show significant alterations in synovial histology, synovial cytokine production, or clinical disease activity.[84] Many other approaches, including use of anti–IL-12 antibodies, IL-18 binding proteins, and inhibitors of specialized chemoattractant cytokines called chemokines, are also under investigation.

Glucocorticoids

Glucocorticoids are some of the most potent anti-inflammatory agents available. When used systemically, they decrease joint swelling, pain, and morning stiffness and improve ability to function. Unfortunately, the dosages necessary to maintain such improvement are usually high enough to be associated with long-term side effects (e.g., osteoporosis, osteonecrosis, increased susceptibility to infection, cataracts, myopathy, and poor wound healing). Alternate-day therapy usually cannot be used to reduce these side effects, because RA patients are usually symptomatic on the off days. The conventional wisdom is that glucocorticoids neither alter the course of the disease nor affect the ultimate degree of damage to joints or other structures; however, some evidence indicates that low-dose prednisolone given early in RA can slow the rate of radiographic progression.[85] Although there is considerable difference of opinion regarding the most appropriate use of steroids in RA, they are typically employed as "bridge" therapy for severe disease while awaiting a therapeutic response from other second-line agents. Systemic glucocorticoids, however, even in these low dosages, are associated with accelerated bone loss. Estrogen replacement and supplemental calcium and vitamin D (given as calcitriol) can be given to postmenopausal women who require daily prednisone therapy, even in low doses.[86] Dual-energy x-ray absorptiometry (DEXA) scans should be used to monitor bone mineral density, and bisphosphonates should be used to treat or prevent osteoporosis in susceptible patients.

Intra-articular glucocorticoids are also useful in limited flares. Administration of such agents requires careful aseptic technique. The procedure involves injection of a local anesthetic agent (e.g., lidocaine) and an insoluble glucocorticoid preparation (e.g., triamcinolone hexacetonide, 20 to 40 mg) into a large joint; smaller amounts (5 to 10 mg) may be injected into small joints, bursae, and tendon sheaths. These local injections usually result in relief of pain and inflammation within days and do not often produce serious side effects. The risk of infection is probably about one in 10,000 procedures. The beneficial effects may last for weeks or months (on average, about 3 to 6 months), but repeated injections may result in increased cartilage destruction, osteonecrosis, and tendon rupture. Thus, intra-articular glucocorticoids are only occasionally useful in relieving inflammation in one or two joints that are particularly symptomatic.

Immunosuppressive Agents

Alkylating agents, particularly cyclophosphamide, and antimetabolites such as azathioprine have been used in patients with severe progressive disease who have not responded to the measures already described. These drugs decrease inflammation and possibly reduce the frequency of new joint erosions. Cyclophosphamide is also effective in controlling rheumatoid vasculitis in some patients. Hematologic toxicity and GI toxicity can be severe; hemorrhagic cystitis is a disturbing complication of oral cyclophosphamide therapy. Azathioprine is safer but has only modest efficacy. The additional potential hazard of inducing neoplasias and chromosomal abnormalities also restricts the usefulness of these agents.

Cyclosporine is a more focused immunosuppressive drug than azathioprine or cyclophosphamide because it targets T cells; it has been used extensively in allograft rejection. Hypertension and decreased creatinine clearance are common side effects, generally related to the cumulative dose. In RA, cyclosporine at a dosage of 2.5 to 5.0 mg/kg/day is an alternative to cyclophosphamide or azathioprine in patients who need immunosuppressive therapy, provided patients are closely monitored for renal toxicity.[87] Despite its potent immunosuppressive effects, a minority of patients have a meaningful clinical response to cyclosporine.

Other Therapies

Minocycline appears to provide benefit in some studies, although the improvement is modest and not always reproducible.[88] Its mechanism of action is unclear and may be related to the ability of tetracycline analogues to inhibit metalloproteinases. Current research into therapies for RA includes trials of recombinant products and humanized monoclonal antibodies. Some of these preparations showed promising results in early open studies, only to fail in controlled trials. This is especially true of antibodies directed against T cell markers (e.g., CD4).[89] Other novel therapies have had mixed success. Attempts to induce tolerance by oral administration of type II collagen or cartilage protein gp39 have not provided significant benefit. A diet supplemented with fish oils, which contain omega-3 fatty acids, reduces synthesis of inflammatory arachidonate metabolites and may be a useful adjuvant therapy for selected patients.[90]

The Food and Drug Administration has approved a *Staphylococcus* protein A immunoadsorption column (Prosorba) for a 12-week course of outpatient apheresis treatment in RA patients who do not respond to or cannot tolerate treatment with disease-modifying antirheumatic drugs. Clinical efficacy needs to be verified by larger controlled trials. The mechanism of action of the immunoadsorption column in RA is not yet known, nor is the duration of efficacy after completion of treatment.

PHYSICAL THERAPY

Hospitalization is occasionally helpful in management, although this approach in an era of managed care and cost constraints is not feasible. Removing the patient from a stressful home environment and instituting a program of rest combined with physical therapy are of great value. Splinting inflamed joints may decrease synovitis.

Physical therapy has a role in the management of RA, although data supporting its ability to change outcome are lacking. Passive range-of-motion exercises help prevent contractures. Isometric exercises build up muscle strength without subjecting inflamed joints to excessive wear, and isotonic exercises further increase muscle strength and help preserve function. Most physical measures, such as whirlpools, heated wax, ultrasonography, and diathermy, make patients feel better during the procedure and perhaps for a short time afterward but offer no significant long-term functional, anti-inflammatory, or disease-modifying benefit; consequently, many patients eventually become disillusioned with them. It is important for patients to maintain an active life, and guidance from physical therapists with range-of-motion exercises and aerobic training is useful. Swimming or other water exercises are especially useful aerobic stresses that minimize the load on the lower extremities.

SURGERY

Indications for surgical intervention include intractable pain and impaired function. Eroded cartilage, ruptured ligaments, and progressive destruction of bone can lead to severe functional derangement that is amenable only to surgical correction. Besides helping restore function to weight-bearing joints, surgery may also restore function in severely deformed hands. In a joint such as the wrist, dorsal synovectomy may prevent extensor tendon ruptures. Although proliferative synovitis often recurs after synovectomy, it may take 1 or 2 years to return and may be less intense than it was initially. Surgery is also useful for removing frayed menisci and other loose bodies that interfere with joint function. In the hands and wrists, operations on periarticular structures (e.g., repair of capsules and replacement of tendons) may restore appearance and function; release of carpal tunnel compression usually relieves pressure on the median nerve. Arthroscopic surgery to remove cartilaginous fragments and to perform a partial synovectomy may be useful when a large, accessible joint (e.g., the knee) is involved with proliferative synovitis.

If gross deformity and joint destruction have occurred, more definitive procedures may be required. In some joints, such as the wrist and ankle, function may be improved by stabilizing the joint through fusion, albeit at the cost of loss of motion. For destroyed joints, total replacement may be necessary. Hip prostheses provide a stable, pain-free joint with a good range of motion in more than 90% of patients. Metal-to-plastic prostheses are also useful in reconstruction of knee, elbow, and shoulder joints. Joint replacement procedures involve a relatively high risk of thromboembolism, but serious infections are rare. Loosening of the components has been observed within several years in as many as 20% of patients.

References

1. Nepom GT, Byers P, Seyfried C, et al: HLA genes associated with rheumatoid arthritis: identification of susceptibility alleles using specific oligonucleotide probes. Arthritis Rheum 32:15, 1989

2. Cvetkovic JT, Wallberg-Jonsson S, Stegmayr B, et al: Susceptibility for and clinical manifestations of rheumatoid arthritis are associated with polymorphisms of the TNF-alpha, IL-1beta, and IL-1Ra genes. J Rheumatol 29:212, 2002

3. McDowell TL, Symons JA, Ploski R, et al: A genetic association between juvenile rheumatoid arthritis and a novel interleukin-1 alpha polymorphism. Arthritis Rheum 38:221, 1995

4. Stransky G, Vernon J, Aicher WK, et al: Virus-like particles in synovial fluids from patients with rheumatoid arthritis. Br J Rheumatol 32:1044, 1993

5. Stahl HD, Pfeiffer R, Von Salis-Soglio G, et al: Parvovirus B19-associated mono- and oligoarticular arthritis may evolve into a chronic inflammatory arthropathy fulfilling criteria for rheumatoid arthritis or spondylarthropathy. Clin Rheumatol 19:510, 2000

6. Takahashi Y, Murai C, Shibata S, et al: Human parvovirus B19 as a causative agent for rheumatoid arthritis. Proc Natl Acad Sci USA 95:8227, 1998

7. Ray NB, Nieva DR, Seftor EA, et al: Induction of an invasive phenotype by human parvovirus B19 in normal human synovial fibroblasts. Arthritis Rheum 44:1582, 2001

8. Albani S, Carson DA: A multistep molecular mimicry hypothesis for the pathogenesis of rheumatoid arthritis. Immunol Today 17:466, 1996

9. Auger I, Roudier J: A function for the QKRAA amino acid motif: mediating binding of DnaJ to DnaK: implications for the association of rheumatoid arthritis with HLA-DR4. J Clin Invest 99:1818, 1997

10. Nakajima T, Aono H, Hasunuma T, et al: Overgrowth of human synovial cells driven by the human T cell leukemia virus type I tax gene. J Clin Invest 92:186, 1993

11. Aicher WK, Heer AH, Trabandt A, et al: Overexpression of zinc-finger transcription factor Z-225/Egr-1 in synoviocytes from rheumatoid arthritis patients. J Immunol 152:5940, 1994

12. Firestein GS, Zvaifler NJ: How important are T cells in chronic rheumatoid synovitis? II. T cell-independent mechanisms from beginning to end. Arthritis Rheum 46:298, 2002

13. Firestein GS, Yeo M, Zvaifler NJ: Apoptosis in rheumatoid arthritis synovium. J Clin Invest 96:1631, 1995

14. Zvaifler NJ, Firestein GS: Pannus and pannocytes: alternative models of joint destruction in rheumatoid arthritis. Arthritis Rheum 37:783, 1994

15. Corr M, Zvaifler NJ: Mesenchymal precursor cells. Ann Rheum Dis 61:3, 2002

16. Mengshol JA, Mix KS, Brinckerhoff CE: Matrix metalloproteinases as therapeutic targets in arthritic diseases: bull's-eye or missing the mark? Arthritis Rheum 46:13, 2002

17. Gravallese EM, Goldring SR: Cellular mechanisms and the role of cytokines in bone erosions in rheumatoid arthritis. Arthritis Rheum 43:2143, 2000

18. Firestein GS: Invasive fibroblast-like synoviocytes in rheumatoid arthritis: passive responders or transformed aggressors? Arthritis Rheum 39:1781, 1996

19. Muller-Ladner U, Kriegsmann J, Franklin BN, et al: Synovial fibroblasts of patients with rheumatoid arthritis attach to and invade normal human cartilage when engrafted into SCID mice. Am J Pathol 149:1607, 1996

20. Tak PP, Zvaifler NJ, Green DR, et al: Rheumatoid arthritis and p53: how oxidative stress might alter the course of inflammatory diseases. Immunol Today 21:78, 2000

21. Gringhuis SI, Leow A, Papendrecht-Van Der Voort EA, et al: Displacement of linker for activation of T cells from the plasma membrane due to redox balance alterations results in hyporesponsiveness of synovial fluid T lymphocytes in rheumatoid arthritis. J Immunol 164:2170, 2000

22. Warrington KJ, Takemura S, Goronzy JJ, et al: CD4+,CD28− T cells in rheumatoid arthritis patients combine features of the innate and adaptive immune systems. Arthritis Rheum 44:13, 2001

23. Wollheim FA: Predictors of joint damage in rheumatoid arthritis. APMIS 104:81, 1996

24. Ermel RW, Kenny TP, Chen PP, et al: Molecular analysis of rheumatoid factors derived from rheumatoid synovium suggests an antigen-driven response in inflamed joints. Arthritis Rheum 36:380, 1993

25. Goldbach-Mansky R, Lee J, McCoy A, et al: Rheumatoid arthritis associated autoantibodies in patients with synovitis of recent onset. Arthritis Res 2:236, 2000

26. Benoist C, Mathis D: Autoimmunity provoked by infection: how good is the case for T cell epitope mimicry? Nat Immunol 2:797, 2001

27. Firestein GS, Zvaifler NJ: How important are T cells in chronic rheumatoid synovitis? Arthritis Rheum 33:768, 1990

28. Chabaud M, Lubberts E, Joosten L, et al: IL-17 derived from juxta-articular bone and synovium contributes to joint degradation in rheumatoid arthritis. Arthritis Res 3:168, 2001

29. Liblau RS, Singer SM, McDevitt HO: Th1 and Th2 CD4+ T cells in the pathogenesis of organ-specific autoimmune diseases. Immunol Today 16:34, 1995

30. Katsikis KD, Chu CQ, Brennan FM, et al: Immunoregulatory role of interleukin 10 in rheumatoid arthritis. J Exp Med 179:1517, 1994

31. Firestein GS, Boyle D, Yu C, et al: Synovial interleukin-1 receptor antagonist and interleukin-1 balance in rheumatoid arthritis. Arthritis Rheum 37:644, 1994

32. Firestein GS, Alvaro-Gracia JM, Maki R: Quantitative analysis of cytokine gene expression in rheumatoid arthritis. J Immunol 144:3347, 1990

33. McInnes IB, Leung BP, Sturrock RD, et al: Interleukin-15 mediates T cell-dependent regulation of tumor necrosis factor-alpha production in rheumatoid arthritis. Nat Med 3:189, 1997

34. Gracie JA, Forsey RJ, Chan WL, et al: A proinflammatory role for IL-18 in rheumatoid arthritis. J Clin Invest 104:1393, 1999

35. Brennan P, Bankhead C, Silman A, et al: Oral contraceptives and rheumatoid arthritis: results from a primary care-based incident case-control study. Semin Arthritis Rheum 26:817, 1997

36. Drossaers-Bakker KW, Zwinderman AH, van Zeben D, et al: Pregnancy and oral contraceptive use do not significantly influence outcome in long term rheumatoid arthritis. Ann Rheum Dis 61:405, 2002

37. Weyand CM, Goronzy JJ, Liuzzo G, et al: T-cell immunity in acute coronary syndromes. Mayo Clin Proc 76:1011, 2001

38. Kauppi M, Sakaguchi M, Konttinen YT, et al: Pathogenetic mechanism and prevalence of the stable atlantoaxial subluxation in rheumatoid arthritis. J Rheumatol 23:831, 1996

39. Foster H, Stephenson A, Walker D, et al: Linkage studies of HLA and primary Sjögren's syndrome in multicase families. Arthritis Rheum 36:473, 1993

40. Helmers R, Galvin J, Hunninghake GW: Pulmonary manifestations associated with rheumatoid arthritis. Chest 100:235, 1991

41. MacDonald WJ, Crawford MH, Klippel JH, et al: Echocardiographic assessment of cardiac structure and function in patients with rheumatoid arthritis. Am J Med 63:890, 1977

42. Peeters HR, Jongen-Lavrencic M, Vreugdenhil G, et al: Effect of recombinant human erythropoietin on anaemia and disease activity in patients with rheumatoid arthritis and anaemia of chronic disease: a randomised placebo controlled double blind 52 weeks clinical trial. Ann Rheum Dis 55:739, 1996

43. Sienknecht CW, Urowitz MB, Pruzanski W, et al: Felty's syndrome: clinical and serological analysis of 34 cases. Ann Rheum Dis 36:500, 1977

44. Hartman KR: Anti-neutrophil antibodies of the immunoglobulin M class in autoimmune neutropenia. Am J Med Sci 308:102, 1994

45. Starkebaum G, Loughran TP Jr, Gaur LK, et al: Immunogenetic similarities between patients with Felty's syndrome and those with clonal expansions of large granular lymphocytes in rheumatoid arthritis. Arthritis Rheum 40:624, 1997

46. Rashba EJ, Rowe JM, Packman CH: Treatment of the neutropenia of Felty syndrome. Blood Rev 10:177, 1996

47. Puechal X, Said G, Hilliquin P, et al: Peripheral neuropathy with necrotizing vasculitis in rheumatoid arthritis: a clinicopathologic and prognostic study of thirty-two patients. Arthritis Rheum 38:1618, 1995

48. Davis BJ, Thompson J, Peimann A, et al: Drug-induced aseptic meningitis caused by two medications. Neurology 44:984, 1994

49. Jorgensen C, Legouffe MC, Perney P, et al: Sicca syndrome associated with hepatitis C virus infection. Arthritis Rheum 39:1166, 1996

50. Poleksic L, Musikic P, Zdravkovic D, et al: MRI evaluation of the knee in rheumatoid arthritis. Br J Rheumatol 35(suppl 3):36, 1996

51. McQueen FM, Benton N, Crabbe J, et al: What is the fate of erosions in early rheumatoid arthritis? Tracking individual lesions using x rays and magnetic resonance imaging over the first two years of disease. Ann Rheum Dis 60:859, 2001

52. Guidelines for the management of rheumatoid arthritis: 2002 update. Arthritis Rheum 46:328, 2002

53. Furst DE, Breedveld FC, Burmester GR, et al: Updated consensus statement on tumour necrosis factor blocking agents for the treatment of rheumatoid arthritis (May 2000). Ann Rheum Dis 59(suppl 1):i1, 2000

54. Jiang Y, Genant HK, Watt I, et al: A multicenter, double-blind, dose-ranging, randomized, placebo-controlled study of recombinant human interleukin-1 receptor antagonist in patients with rheumatoid arthritis: radiologic progression and correlation of Genant and Larsen scores. Arthritis Rheum 43:1001, 2000

55. Neva MH, Kauppi MJ, Kautiainen H, et al: Combination drug therapy retards the development of rheumatoid atlantoaxial subluxations. Arthritis Rheum 43:2397, 2000

56. Landewe RB, Boers M, Verhoeven AC, et al: COBRA combination therapy in patients with early rheumatoid arthritis: long-term structural benefits of a brief intervention. Arthritis Rheum 46:347, 2002

57. Raskin JB, White RH, Jackson JE, et al: Misoprostol dosage in the prevention of nonsteroidal anti-inflammatory drug-induced gastric and duodenal ulcers: a comparison of three regimens. Ann Intern Med 123:344, 1995

58. Gabriel SE, Jaakkimainen RL, Bombardier C: The cost-effectiveness of misoprostol for nonsteroidal antiinflammatory drug–associated adverse gastrointestinal events. Arthritis Rheum 36:447, 1993

59. Furst DE: Are there differences among nonsteroidal antiinflammatory drugs? Comparing acetylated salicylates, nonacetylated salicylates, and nonacetylated nonsteroidal antiinflammatory drugs. Arthritis Rheum 37:1, 1994

60. Hinz B, Brune K: Cyclooxygenase-2: 10 years later. J Pharmacol Exp Ther 300:367, 2002

61. Mukherjee D, Nissen SE, Topol EJ: Risk of cardiovascular events associated with selective COX-2 inhibitors. JAMA 286:954, 2001

62. Alarcon GS: Methotrexate use in rheumatoid arthritis: a clinician's perspective. Immunopharmacology 47:259, 2000

63. Lopez-Mendez A, Daniel WW, Reading JC, et al: Radiographic assessment of disease progression in rheumatoid arthritis patients enrolled in the cooperative systematic studies of the rheumatic diseases program randomized clinical trial of methotrexate, auranofin, or a combination of the two. Arthritis Rheum 36:1364, 1993

64. Weinblatt ME, Kaplan H, Germain BF, et al: Methotrexate in rheumatoid arthritis: a five-year prospective multicenter study. Arthritis Rheum 37:1492, 1994

65. Choi HK, Hernan MA, Seeger JD, et al: Methotrexate and mortality in patients with rheumatoid arthritis: a prospective study. Lancet 359:1173, 2002

66. Morgan SL, Baggott JE, Vaughn WH, et al: Supplementation with folic acid during methotrexate therapy for rheumatoid arthritis: a double-blind, placebo-controlled trial. Ann Intern Med 121:833, 1994

67. Erickson AR, Reddy V, Vogelgesang SA, et al: Usefulness of the American College of Rheumatology recommendations for liver biopsy in methotrexate-treated rheumatoid arthritis patients. Arthritis Rheum 38:1115, 1995

68. Mladenovic V, Domljan Z, Rozman B, et al: Safety and effectiveness of leflunomide in the treatment of patients with active rheumatoid arthritis: results of a randomized, placebo-controlled, phase II study. Arthritis Rheum 38:1595, 1995

69. Weinblatt ME, Kremer JM, Coblyn JS, et al: Pharmacokinetics, safety, and efficacy of combination treatment with methotrexate and leflunomide in patients with active rheumatoid arthritis. Arthritis Rheum 42:1322, 1999

70. Sharp JT, Strand V, Leung H, et al: Treatment with leflunomide slows radiographic progression of rheumatoid arthritis: results from three randomized controlled trials of leflunomide in patients with active rheumatoid arthritis. Leflunomide Rheumatoid Arthritis Investigators Group. Arthritis Rheum 43:495, 2000

71. Conaghan PG, Brooks P: Disease-modifying antirheumatic drugs, including methotrexate, sulfasalazine, gold, antimalarials, and D-penicillamine. Curr Opin Rheumatol 5:276, 1993

72. Rains CP, Noble S, Faulds D: Sulfasalazine: a review of its pharmacological properties and therapeutic efficacy in the treatment of rheumatoid arthritis. Drugs 50:137, 1995

73. McEntegart A, Porter D, Capell HA, et al: Sulfasalazine has a better efficacy/toxicity profile than auranofin—evidence from a 5 year prospective, randomized, trial. J Rheumatol 23:1887, 1996

74. Paulus HE: History of combination therapy of rheumatoid arthritis. J Rheumatol Suppl 44:38, 1996

75. Willkens RF, Sharp JT, Stablein D, et al: Comparison of azathioprine, methotrexate, and the combination of the two in the treatment of rheumatoid arthritis: a forty-eight-week controlled clinical trial with radiologic outcome assessment. Arthritis Rheum 38:1799, 1995

76. O'Dell JR, Haire CE, Erikson N, et al: Treatment of rheumatoid arthritis with methotrexate alone, sulfasalazine and hydroxychloroquine, or a combination of all three medications. N Engl J Med 334:1287, 1996

77. Moreland LW, Baumgartner SW, Schiff MH: Treatment of rheumatoid arthritis with a recombinant human tumor necrosis factor receptor (p75) fusion protein. N Engl J Med 337:141, 1997

78. Weinblatt ME, Kremer JM, Bankhurst AD, et al: A trial of etanercept, a recombinant tumor necrosis factor receptor:Fc fusion protein, in patients with rheumatoid arthritis receiving methotrexate. N Engl J Med 340:253, 1999

79. Maini R, St Clair EW, Breedveld F, et al: Infliximab (chimeric anti-tumour necrosis factor alpha monoclonal antibody) versus placebo in rheumatoid arthritis patients receiving concomitant methotrexate: a randomised phase III trial. ATTRACT Study Group. Lancet 354:1932, 1999

80. Keane J, Gershon S, Wise RP, et al: Tuberculosis associated with infliximab, a tumor necrosis factor alpha-neutralizing agent. N Engl J Med 345:1098, 2001

81. Mohan N, Edwards ET, Cupps TR, et al: Demyelination occurring during anti-tumor necrosis factor alpha therapy for inflammatory arthritides. Arthritis Rheum 44:2862, 2001

82. Bresnihan B, Alvaro-Gracia JM, Cobby M, et al: Treatment of rheumatoid arthritis with recombinant human interleukin-1 receptor antagonist. Arthritis Rheum 41:2196, 1998

83. Cohen S, Hurd E, Cush J, et al: Treatment of rheumatoid arthritis with anakinra, a recombinant human interleukin-1 receptor antagonist, in combination with methotrexate: results of a twenty-four-week, multicenter, randomized, double-blind, placebo-controlled trial. Arthritis Rheum 46:614, 2002

84. Smeets TJ, Kraan MC, Versendaal J, et al: Analysis of serial synovial biopsies in patients with rheumatoid arthritis: description of a control group without clinical improvement after treatment with interleukin 10 or placebo. J Rheumatol 26:2089, 1999

85. Kirwan JR: The effect of glucocorticoids on joint destruction in rheumatoid arthritis. The Arthritis and Rheumatism Council Low-Dose Glucocorticoid Study Group. N Engl J Med 333:142, 1995

86. American College of Rheumatology Task Force on Osteoporosis Guidelines: Recommendations for the prevention and treatment of glucocorticoid-induced osteoporosis. Arthritis Rheum 39:1791, 1996

87. Stein CM, Pincus T, Yocum D, et al: Combination treatment of severe rheumatoid arthritis with cyclosporine and methotrexate for forty-eight weeks: an open-label extension study. The Methotrexate-Cyclosporine Combination Study Group. Arthritis Rheum 40:1843, 1997

88. Tilley BC, Alarcon GS, Heyse SP, et al: Minocycline in rheumatoid arthritis: a 48-week, double-blind, placebo-controlled trial. MIRA Trial Group. Ann Intern Med 122:81, 1995

89. Moreland LW, Pratt PW, Mayes MD, et al: Double-blind, placebo-controlled multicenter trial using chimeric monoclonal anti-CD4 antibody, cM-T412, in rheumatoid arthritis patients receiving concomitant methotrexate. Arthritis Rheum 38:1581, 1995

90. Kremer JM, Lawrence DA, Petrillo GF, et al: Effects of high-dose fish oil on rheumatoid arthritis after stopping nonsteroidal antiinflammatory drugs: clinical and immune correlates. Arthritis Rheum 38:1107, 1995

91. Arnett FC, Edworthy SM, Bloch DA, et al: The American Rheumatism Association 1987 revised criteria for the classification of rheumatoid arthritis. Arthritis Rheum 31:315, 1988

Acknowledgments

Figure 1   Provided by David Boyle, University of California, San Diego, School of Medicine, La Jolla, California.

Figures 3 and 4   Provided by Michael Weisman, M.D., University of California, San Diego, School of Medicine, La Jolla, California.

113 Seronegative Spondyloarthropathies

Frank C. Arnett, M.D.

Definition

The spondyloarthropathies are a family of clinically, epidemiologically, and genetically related inflammatory diseases that primarily affect spinal and peripheral joints. Once considered variants of rheumatoid arthritis, the spondyloarthropathies and rheumatoid disease have been shown to have such fundamental clinical and pathogenetic differences that they are now considered distinctly separate entities [*see Table 1*]. The term seronegative refers to the uniform absence of serum IgM autoantibodies to IgG (rheumatoid factor) in patients with the spondyloarthropathies. Other distinguishing characteristics are the following:

1. The sacroiliac joints are affected (sacroiliitis); ascending spinal inflammation and bony fusion (spondylitis) often follow.
2. Peripheral joints are affected, typically in an oligoarticular and asymmetrical pattern.
3. There is inflammation of sites of ligamentous insertions into bone (entheses), referred to as enthesitis or enthesopathy, in addition to inflammation of joint synovium. Inflammation occurs both along the spine and near peripheral joints.
4. There may be inflammation of extra-articular sites, including the eye, aortic valve, gastrointestinal tract, genitourinary system, and skin.
5. Disease onset typically occurs in young adulthood.
6. There is a strong familial tendency and a striking genetic association with the histocompatibility antigen HLA-B27.
7. Certain bacteria play important pathogenetic roles.

Classification

The spondyloarthropathies include the prototype spinal arthritis, ankylosing spondylitis, reactive arthritis (formerly known as Reiter syndrome), psoriatic arthritis, enteropathic arthritis (accompanying ulcerative colitis and Crohn disease), juvenile spondyloarthropathy (or juvenile ankylosing spondylitis), and such rare disorders as acne-associated arthritis (or SAPHO [synovitis, acne, pustulosis, hyperostosis, osteitis] syndrome) and Whipple disease. The various spondyloarthropathies can usually be distinguished from one another by the pattern of joint involvement and associated features [*see Table 2*]. However, some patients have overlapping clinical manifestations that defy categorization; these patients are usually designated as having undifferentiated spondyloarthropathies. Because of such patients, the European Spondyloarthropathy Study Group (ESSG) proposed classification criteria for spondyloarthropathies that may be useful in clinical diagnosis and epidemiologic studies.[1]

Epidemiology

Estimations of prevalence rates for spondyloarthropathies using the ESSG criteria are few.[1-3] Among Germans in Berlin, the prevalence of spondyloarthropathies has been reported to be 1.9%; in Eskimos in Alaska and Siberia, rates varying from 2% to 3.4% have been reported. Spondyloarthropathies appear to be rare in African and Japanese populations. These differences among ethnic groups is explainable in large part by differences in the frequency of HLA-B27.[1]

Pathogenesis

The various spondyloarthropathies appear to be complex disorders resulting from the interplay of several genetic and environmental factors, only a few of which have been identified.

GENETIC FACTORS

Heredity plays a major role in predisposition.[4] Family studies have shown that 15% to 20% of patients with ankylosing spondylitis have one or more first-degree relatives with the same disease. In the families of some patients with ankylosing spondylitis, there are relatives with other spondyloarthropathies or other associated disorders, such as uveitis, psoriasis, and inflammatory bowel disease. Concordance for ankylosing spondylitis in monozygotic twins approaches 63% to 75%, compared with 13% to 23% in dizygotic twins. Genetic modeling in twins and families indicates that ankylosing spondylitis is associated with a multiplicative, polygenic pattern of inheritance, with 97% of the susceptibility to the disease attributed to genetics. These studies suggest that the environmental factors that contribute to development of the disease are probably ubiquitous.

The HLA-B27 allele encoded by the class I *HLA-B* locus within the major histocompatibility complex (MHC) is the one genetic factor identified thus far that is strongly associated with spondyloarthropathies. This allele is present in 90% of patients with ankylosing spondylitis and confers a relative risk for the disease of over 100, but it is found less often in patients with the other spondyloarthropathies [*see Table 2*].[5] HLA-B27 shows linkage to ankylosing spondylitis in families and appears to contribute from 16% to 50% of the genetic risk; in most cases, it appears essential for disease expression.[4] Other HLA alleles, including HLA-B60, HLA-DR1, and HLA-DR8, also appear to increase the risk of ankylosing spondylitis. In addition, different HLA alleles predispose to psoriasis and psoriatic arthritis, including HLA-B13, -B17, -Cw6, -B38, and -B39.[6] The HLA region shows genetic linkage to inflammatory bowel diseases, but specific HLA alleles show only weak associations.[7] Ongoing human genome searches have revealed additional non-HLA loci linked to ankylosing spondylitis,[4,5] some of which also may be common to Crohn disease[8,9] and psoriasis.[10]

Laboratory evidence strongly suggests that the *HLA-B27* gene itself, rather than a linked locus, directly participates in the pathogenesis of ankylosing spondylitis and reactive arthritis. Transgenic rats expressing the human *HLA-B27* and β_2-microglobulin genes spontaneously develop colitis, peripheral and spinal arthritis, enthesitis, skin and nail lesions resembling psoriasis, and genitourinary inflammation.[11] Littermates raised in a germ-free environment do not develop most of these manifestations, however. That finding emphasizes the importance of both the *HLA-B27* gene and gut bacteria, especially *Bacteroides* species, in pathogenesis and suggests that antibiotics (e.g., sulfasalazine) may be useful in the treatment of reactive arthritis and ankylos-

Table 1   Comparison between Spondyloarthropathies and Rheumatoid Arthritis

	Spondyloarthropathies	*Rheumatoid Arthritis*
Distribution	Racial (more prevalent in whites)	Worldwide
Prevalence	0.2%–1.9%	1%–2%
Etiology	Genetic and bacterial	Genetic and unknown
Positive family history	Frequent	Rare
Sex distribution	More frequently diagnosed in males	More common in females
Age at onset	Peak incidence at 20–30 yr	All ages affected; peak incidence 30–50 yr
Joint involvement	Oligoarthritis; asymmetrical; large joints; lower limbs more than upper limbs	Polyarthritis; symmetrical; small and large joints; upper and lower limbs
Sacroiliac involvement	Yes	No
Spinal involvement	Ascending; all segments with fusion	Cervical only; erosions and instability
Subcutaneous nodules	No	Yes
Aortic regurgitation	Yes	No
Ocular involvement	Uveitis, conjunctivitis	Sicca syndrome; scleritis; scleromalacia perforans
Lung involvement	Upper lobe pulmonary fibrosis	Pleural effusions; lower lobe pulmonary fibrosis; nodules; Caplan syndrome
Rheumatoid factor	No	Yes
HLA-B27	Yes	No (normal frequency)
HLA-DR4	25% (normal frequency)	60%–70%
Pathology	Synovitis and enthesopathy	Synovitis
Radiographic findings	Asymmetrical erosive arthritis and periostitis; new bone formation and ankylosis; sacroiliitis, spondylitis	Symmetrical erosive arthritis with bony destruction

ing spondylitis in humans. The mechanism by which HLA-B27 promotes disease is unknown, but the following are the prevailing hypotheses[12]: (1) HLA-B27 as a major histocompatibility complex class I molecule presents a so-called arthritogenic self-peptide or bacterial peptide to cytotoxic CD8+ T cells, which causes an autoimmune attack on various self-structures; (2) stretches of amino acid sequences common to both HLA-B27 and bacterial proteins—many of which have been found—result in a cytotoxic or humoral immune response to HLA-B27 (molecular mimicry); and (3) HLA-B27, either intracellularly or extracellularly, promotes bacterial persistence or dissemination to joints and other structures.[13,14]

ENVIRONMENTAL FACTORS

Reactive arthritis provides the strongest evidence of bacterial pathogenesis in the spondyloarthropathies. Enteric infections by *Shigella flexneri*, *Salmonella* (many species), *Yersinia enterocolitica*, *Y. pseudotuberculosis*, and *Campylobacter jejuni* have all been implicated as triggers of the disease in various epidemics and in sporadic cases, especially in HLA-B27–positive persons.[15,16] Similarly, sexually acquired infections with *Chlamydia trachomatis*[15,16] and perhaps *Ureaplasma urealyticum* may cause reactive arthritis.[17] Pulmonary infection with *C. pneumoniae* has also been implicated.[18] Patients with chronic reactive arthritis have been found to have IgA antibodies to the initiating microbe, suggesting a persistent mucosal infection.[16,19] Moreover, synovial fluid T cells have been found to proliferate when challenged with the bacterium that triggered the arthritis.[12] There is no evidence, however, that these microorganisms cause ankylosing spondylitis or other

spondyloarthropathies. Normal gut flora seem more likely to be implicated in ankylosing spondylitis, as suggested by studies of the HLA-B27 transgenic rat[11] and by a high frequency of asymptomatic foci of gut inflammation in patients with ankylosing spondylitis or reactive arthritis.[20]

Pathology

Chronic inflammation with infiltrating mononuclear cells (macrophages, T cells, and B cells) occurs in both peripheral and axial joint structures of patients with spondyloarthropathy.[12,21,22] CD4+ helper T cells and CD8+ suppressor-cytotoxic T cells appear to be equally represented. A high concentration of the inflammatory cytokine tumor necrosis factor–α (TNF-α) has been found in the dense cellular infiltrates in synovial portions of sacroiliac joints.[21] When cytokines from the joints and blood of patients with spondyloarthropathies were compared with those of patients with rheumatoid arthritis, the cytokines from patients with spondyloarthropathies showed a higher ratio of immunosuppressive cytokines, such as interleukin-4 (IL-4) and IL-10, to proinflammatory cytokines, such as TNF-α and interferon gamma. This leads to a blunted T helper type 1 (Th1) response in patients with spondyloarthropathies.[22] In fact, low levels of TNF-α in the blood of patients with reactive arthritis is predictive of a more chronic course. Inherent levels of cytokines, such as TNF-α and IL-10, are determined by genetic polymorphisms in their respective genes.[22] In ankylosing spondylitis, the observed tendency for ligamentous ossification, enthesopathy, and widespread new bone formation is associated with the finding of transform-

Table 2 Features of Seronegative Spondyloarthropathies

	Ankylosing Spondylitis	Reiter Syndrome (Reactive Arthritis)	Psoriatic Arthritis	Enteropathic Arthritis
Sex distribution	Male > female	Male > female	Female > male	Female = male
Age at onset (years)	≥ 20	≥ 20	Any age	Any age
Mode of onset	Gradual	Sudden	Gradual	Peripheral sudden Spinal gradual
Peripheral joints	Often lower limbs Asymmetrical	Usually lower limbs Asymmetrical	Upper > lower limbs Asymmetrical	Lower > upper limbs Symmetrical
Enthesopathy	+	+	+	– Peripheral + Spinal
Heel pain	Occasional	Frequent	Occasional	Infrequent
Spinal involvement	+++ (always)	+ (20%)	+ (20%)	+ (10%)
Symmetry (sacroiliitis and syndesmophytes)	+	+/–	+/–	+
Familial aggregation	++	+	++	++
HLA-B27 positive	90%	63%–75%	20% (50% with sacroiliitis)	10% (50% with sacroiliitis)
Risk for B27-positive person	2% (20% when a relative)	20% (when infected)	?	?
Urethritis	–	+	–	–
Skin involvement	–	+	+++	+
Nail involvement	–	+	+++	–
Mucous membrane involvement	–	++	–	+
Cardiac involvement	+	+	Rare	Rare
Self-limiting	–	+	–	++ Peripheral – Spinal

ing growth factor–β (TGF-β) near these sites. TGF-β is a reparative cytokine that stimulates connective tissue matrix formation.

Reactive arthritis was once considered a sterile joint disease triggered in some unknown manner by a distant infection, but more recent studies of synovial fluids and tissues affected by reactive arthritis have consistently revealed the presence of intracellular bacterial antigens from each of the known offending microorganisms.[14,23,24] Moreover, with electron microscopy and polymerase chain reaction, living but dormant *C. trachomatis* has been detected in synovial macrophages and fibroblasts even after many years of disease.[23] It is still unclear whether the enteric pathogens causing reactive arthritis are viable.[14,24] Spinal joint tissue from patients with ankylosing spondylitis is difficult to obtain. Limited studies of sacroiliac joint biopsies have not revealed bacterial antigens.[25]

Ankylosing Spondylitis

EPIDEMIOLOGY

The prevalence of ankylosing spondylitis parallels the frequency of HLA-B27 in different ethnic populations.[1,26] HLA-B27 occurs in 7% to 9% of the white population, and the disease prevalence is approximately 0.2% to 0.9%.[2,3] One study from Norway, where the HLA-B27 frequency is twice as high as it is for the white populations in the United States and the United Kingdom, found that ankylosing spondylitis occurred in 1.9% to 2.2% of men and 0.3% to 0.6% of women.[3] The disease is distinct-

ly rare in African and Japanese populations, in which HLA-B27 is found in low frequency; however, ankylosing spondylitis is common in certain Native-American groups, such as the Haida and Pima Indians, in whom the frequency of HLA-B27 is high.[26]

In randomly chosen cohorts of whites possessing HLA-B27, ankylosing spondylitis developed in approximately 2% to 6%.[3] Among HLA-B27–positive relatives of patients with ankylosing spondylitis, however, some 20% to 30% are at risk for the disease. Similar estimates are not available for other ethnic groups, but estimates may differ because molecular subtypes of HLA-B27 have been discovered, each with different distributions among various ethnic groups.[5,25,26] HLA-B*2705, followed in frequency by HLA-B*2702, is predominantly found in whites; HLA-B*2704 is found in Chinese; and HLA-B*2703 is found in Africans. Most HLA-B27 subtypes appear to predispose to ankylosing spondylitis, with the possible exceptions of HLA-B*2706, found in Indonesians and Thais, and HLA-B*2709, found in Sardinians.

Ankylosing spondylitis was once considered to be almost exclusively a disease of males, but recent studies suggest a more uniform distribution by sex (the ratio of men to women is 3:1).[1] In women, the disease may be diagnosed less frequently and later in the course of disease because physicians still consider it primarily a disorder of men. Some studies suggest that women have milder disease, with less progressive spinal involvement and more peripheral arthritis. Other studies suggest that the overall pattern of disease is similar in men and women.[27]

Onset typically occurs between 16 and 30 years of age, peaking at around 24 years; it seldom begins in patients older than 40 years. Childhood onset before 16 years of age occurs in approximately 10% to 20% of cases in the United States and Europe but is more common (54%) in developing countries, suggesting earlier exposure to the environmental triggers.[28]

DIAGNOSIS

The modified New York criteria[1] are currently used to classify ankylosing spondylitis. A patient should have one or more of the following clinical criteria:

1. Low back pain of at least 3 months' duration that is alleviated by exercise and not relieved by rest.
2. Restricted lumbar spinal motion.
3. Decreased chest expansion relative to normal values for age and sex.

In addition, the patient must have definitive radiographic evidence of sacroiliitis (i.e., bilateral grade II to IV or unilateral grade III or IV) [see Figure 1].

A simpler approach in diagnosis is to accept symptomatic sacroiliitis as an adequate definition. Sacroiliitis, as defined radiographically, should be definitive (grade III or IV changes) and bilateral [see Figure 1]. In addition, the patient should have no other diseases that could cause sacroiliitis (i.e., reactive arthritis, psoriasis, or inflammatory bowel disease).

Clinical Presentation

Low back pain and stiffness are the usual presenting symptoms of ankylosing spondylitis. Because back pain is such a common complaint in the general population and its causes myriad, certain characteristics that specifically suggest inflammatory back pain have been formulated:

1. Onset in a person younger than 40 years.
2. Insidious rather than abrupt onset.
3. Persistence of back symptoms for 3 months or longer.
4. Worsening of back pain or stiffness with inactivity.
5. Subsiding of back pain or stiffness with exercise.

Some patients describe buttock pain that often alternates from one side to the other and sometimes radiates down the posterior leg, which is indicative of sacroiliac joint disease. Other patients present with a peripheral arthritis, typically monoarticular or oligoarticular, that affects lower extremity joints, often the knee. Careful questioning about subtle musculoskeletal symptoms in such patients is often fruitful. Fatigue can be a major symptom in patients with ankylosing spondylitis and has been found to correlate with level of disease activity, functional ability, global well-being, and mental health status.[29] Elicitation of a history of uveitis or the existence of family members with features of spondyloarthropathies also strongly suggests the disease. Radiologic evidence of sacroiliitis in any of these clinical presentations, however, is essential in confirming a diagnosis of ankylosing spondylitis [see Radiographic Features, below]. In patients whose sacroiliac radiographs are normal, the presence of HLA-B27 is highly suggestive but not definitive evidence of the disease. Follow-up studies of patients in whom the diagnosis was strongly suspected because of the clinical picture and HLA-B27 positivity showed that sacroiliac joint abnormalities eventually evolve, but the evolution may occur over as many as 10 years.

Patients with juvenile-onset ankylosing spondylitis typically present with peripheral oligoarthritis, often with enthesopathy and infrequently with spinal symptoms.[28] Such patients may be misdiagnosed as having juvenile rheumatoid arthritis [see Juve-

nile Spondyloarthropathy, *below*]. Spinal involvement usually appears later in young adulthood.

Physical Examination

Examination of the back may be relatively normal early in the course of the disease. Sacroiliac joints are usually painful when palpated or stressed. When the disease advances into the lumbar spine, the normal lordotic curvature may be lost, and paravertebral muscle spasm is prominent. Forward bending, or flexion, may be restricted, as measured by the Schober test. In this measurement, two points are drawn with the patient standing erect, one at the L5–S1 region and the other 10 cm above this region. With normal flexion, the distance between these two points increases by 4 to 6 cm, but when the lumbar spine becomes fused, there may be little or no increase in distance between the two points. Lateral lumbar bending and extension are also typically restricted.

Thoracic spine involvement causes an exaggerated dorsal kyphosis; with costovertebral joint fusion, chest expansion, as measured circumferentially at the fourth intercostal space from full expiration to inspiration, is reduced to 2.5 cm or less. When the disease ascends into the neck and causes fusion, cervical lordosis is lost and a fixed flexion deformity may occur. Spinal fusion often results in the patient being severely stooped forward with neck immobile and flexed; the patient has difficulty looking straight ahead.

Peripheral arthritis, especially of hips, shoulders, and knees, occurs in approximately 30% of patients with ankylosing spondylitis and further increases disability. Peripheral enthesopathic features may include Achilles tendinitis, plantar fasciitis, or costochondritis.[30]

Laboratory Findings

The HLA-B27 histocompatibility antigen is present in more than 90% of cases. HLA-B27 testing of individual patients, however, is infrequently indicated; it is done only in atypical cases, when the clinical suspicion is high but the most definitive finding—radiographic evidence of sacroiliitis—is not present. HLA-B27–positive and HLA-B27–negative patients have similar patterns and severity of arthritis, but HLA-B27–negative patients are older at disease onset, have a negative family history of spondylitis, and infrequently experience uveitis or cardiac complications.[1,26] HLA-B27 is found less commonly (50%) in patients with ankylosing spondylitis who are of African ancestry.

Elevation of the erythrocyte sedimentation rate (ESR) occurs in many patients, but it may be normal despite severe disease. Serum IgA levels are often elevated.[19] Some patients have a mild normocytic normochromic anemia because of chronic inflammation, and the platelet count may be high.

Radiographic Features

Bilateral sacroiliitis is the most specific finding that supports a diagnosis of ankylosing spondylitis, and meticulous interpretation of the radiographs is imperative. A grading system that assesses each sacroiliac joint for juxta-articular bony sclerosis, blurring or erosion of joint margins, and bony fusion has been formulated and tested [see Figure 1]. Grade 0 is normal; grade I is suspicious but not definitive; grade II shows sclerosis on both sides of a joint and is even more suspicious when bilateral but should be interpreted with great caution; and grades III and IV are definitive. Another radiographically defined entity, osteitis condensans ilii, may be misinterpreted as sacroiliitis, and vice

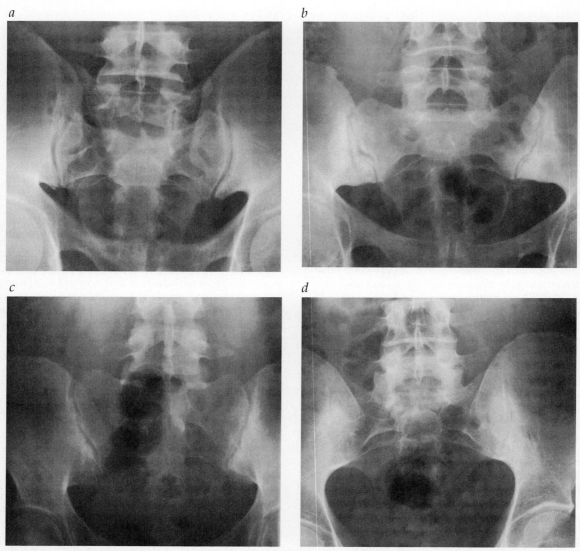

Figure 1   (*a*) **Radiograph of normal sacroiliac joints showing clearly defined joint margins and no sclerosis (grade 0). (*b*) Sclerosis on both margins of each sacroiliac joint but no joint erosions (grade II). (*c*) Sclerosis and erosions of both sacroiliac joints (grade III). (*d*) Complete bony fusion of both sacroiliac joints (grade IV).**

versa. Patients with osteitis condensans ilii have sclerosis on the iliac side of both sacroiliac joints; the condition occurs in women who have borne children. Although quantitative radionuclide scans, computed tomography, and magnetic resonance imaging have been suggested as superior diagnostic methods, well-performed plain radiographs of the sacroiliac joints (Ferguson view or oblique view) are usually adequate.

An early spinal change seen on radiographs is squaring of the normally concave anterior side of vertebral bodies [*see Figure 2*]. This phenomenon is caused by inflammation and bony erosion at the site of insertion (enthesitis) of the outer fibers of the annulus fibrosus. Later changes are ossification of ligaments, which are seen on radiographs as syndesmophytes bridging adjacent vertebral bodies [*see Figure 3*], producing the classic bamboo-spine appearance [*see Figure 4*]. Zygoapophyseal joints become fused into solid bone. Finally, diffuse osteoporosis may occur, making the spine susceptible to fracture. Bony fusion across joint spaces of affected peripheral joints in ankylosing spondylitis may be the immost distinctive change seen on radiographs.

Similar spinal changes are seen in primary ankylosing spondylitis and in the spondylitis associated with inflammatory bowel disease. In spondylitis associated with reactive arthritis and psoriatic arthritis, the sacroiliitis and syndesmophytes tend to be asymmetrical.[31] Another disease that may mimic ankylosing spondylitis is diffuse idiopathic skeletal hyperostosis (DISH).[32] DISH occurs in middle-aged and older people, especially men; it is characterized by large, flowing syndesmophytes that restrict spinal motion; sacroiliitis is not found, however, and there is no association with HLA-B27.

Extra-articular Manifestations

A number of extraskeletal features may complicate the course of ankylosing spondylitis and contribute to morbidity and mortality.

Ocular involvement   Acute anterior uveitis, usually occurring episodically and affecting one eye at a time, occurs in 25% of patients. Acute pain, redness, and photophobia are the usual

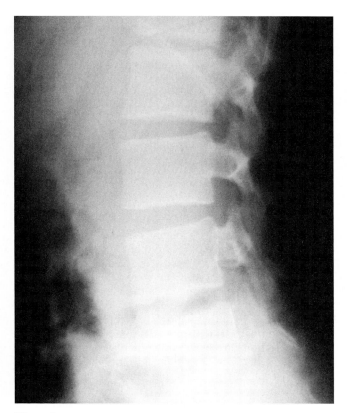

Figure 2 **Loss of the normal anterior concavity of vertebral bodies, resulting in so-called squaring in early ankylosing spondylitis.**

symptoms, and prompt referral to an ophthalmologist for treatment is essential. Uveitis does not correlate with arthritis activity or severity and shows a strong association with HLA-B27, even in patients without spondyloarthropathies.[33]

Cardiovascular disease A fibrosing cardiovascular lesion occurs in 2% to 10% of patients with ankylosing spondylitis. The lesion causes the aortic valve and proximal root to thicken, and it often extends into the conducting system, causing aortic regurgitation, atrioventricular block, or both. The lesion probably occurs with a similar frequency in patients with reactive arthritis.[34] In rare instances, mitral regurgitation may also occur. One study emphasized a high prevalence of underlying spondyloarthropathy, often undiagnosed, in men requiring cardiac pacemakers for bradyarrhythmias.[34] In addition, this study revealed the strong association of the clinical combination of lone aortic regurgitation and heart block with HLA-B27, with or without apparent arthritis. Typically appearing after many years of spondyloarthropathy, fulminant cardiac disease has been described even very early in disease. Echocardiography may detect cardiac abnormalities in some patients without clinical signs.[35] No treatment is known to prevent progression of spondylitic heart disease; most patients require permanent cardiac pacemakers, aortic valve replacement, or both.

Pulmonary disease Despite restriction of chest wall motion by joint fusion, respiratory function is preserved in most patients with ankylosing spondylitis, owing to good diaphragmatic function. Severe kyphotic deformity, however, may compromise breathing. Approximately 1% of patients with ankylosing spondylitis, usually severe, also have fibrosis in the upper lung

fields that mimics tuberculosis.[36] Cavitation may occur and may be complicated by *Aspergillus* infection. Cough, dyspnea, and even hemoptysis are typical symptoms. Currently available treatment is unsatisfactory.

Renal disease Kidney function is usually normal. The appearance of proteinuria with or without a nephrotic syndrome usually indicates complicating amyloidosis or IgA nephropathy. Secondary amyloidosis occurs in approximately 7% of patients and can be diagnosed with abdominal fat-pad or rectal biopsy.[37] There is no established treatment, but low-dose colchicine is worth trying.

IgA nephropathy is being increasingly recognized. It correlates with high serum IgA levels. Renal function may become impaired, but episodes are usually self-limited.[19]

Neurologic disease A major cause of morbidity and mortality in patients with ankylosing spondylitis is spinal fracture, with cord compression occurring even with seemingly minor trauma.[1] A rigid and osteoporotic cervical spine is most susceptible to fracture, usually at the C6 or C7 level. A high degree of suspicion for fracture is always warranted in patients with localized spinal pain, even when plain x-rays fail to reveal an acute abnormality; additional imaging with CT is often necessary.

A cauda equina syndrome occurs in rare instances, usually because of arachnoiditis around sacral nerves that leads to progressive leg weakness, paresthesias, and sphincter dysfunction.[38]

Retroperitoneal fibrosis Fibrosis in the retroperitoneum has recently been suggested as being another extra-articular feature of ankylosing spondylitis.[39]

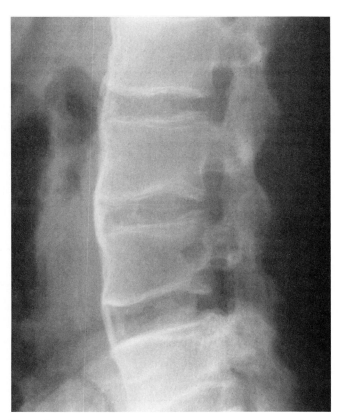

Figure 3 **Progression of ankylosing spondylitis is demonstrated by ossification of the anterior fibers of the annulus fibrosus (syndesmophytes).**

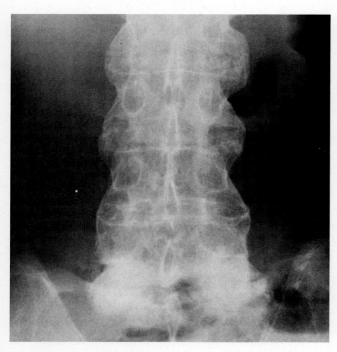

Figure 4 **Patients with severe ankylosing spondylitis may develop the classic bamboo spine, as shown in this radiograph.**

TREATMENT AND PROGNOSIS

Early diagnosis and treatment of ankylosing spondylitis appear to improve functional outcome, but it is not clear whether any drug modifies the disease pathology. Objectives of treatment are pain relief, reduction of inflammation, and maintenance of good posture and spinal function.[40]

Nonsteroidal anti-inflammatory drugs (NSAIDs) relieve inflammatory symptoms of pain and stiffness and allow patients to engage in an appropriate exercise program [*Table 3*]. Certain NSAIDs are more often effective than others as treatment for spondyloarthropathies. Indomethacin, taken at a dosage of 25 to 50 mg three times daily or as a sustained-release preparation of 75 mg every 12 hours, is often the most effective NSAID. Possible side effects are headaches, dizziness, depression, and hallucinations, which occur less often with another indoleacetic acid, tolmetin, taken at a dosage of 400 to 600 mg three times daily. Piroxicam, 20 mg daily, or diclofenac, 75 mg twice daily, may be effective in some patients. There is no evidence that any NSAIDs alter disease progression.

GI intolerance of any of the NSAIDs may present as nausea, gastric discomfort, diarrhea, or, more seriously, gut hemorrhage or perforation. Concomitant use of a gastroprotective agent, such as misoprostol or a proton pump inhibitor, may significantly reduce GI toxicity in patients treated with NSAIDs. Cyclooxygenase-2 (COX-2) inhibitors may reduce GI toxicity; their efficacy is similar to some other NSAIDs.[41] All of these drugs may decrease renal tubular capacity to secrete potassium and can cause an abrupt reduction in renal function when used in patients with renal disease or with renal hypoperfusion resulting from ineffective circulatory volume. Thus, because patients with ankylosing spondylitis will probably take NSAIDs for many years, the attending physician must diligently monitor for renal and GI tract damage.

In a recent 6-month randomized, controlled clinical trial, the bisphosphonate pamidromate, given monthly by intravenous infusion, was shown to be effective in improving symptoms and function in patients with ankylosing spondylitis whose disease was refractory to treatment with NSAIDs.[42]

Low-dose corticosteroids (e.g., prednisone, 5 to 10 mg daily) may be necessary to quell inflammation in some patients with

Table 3 Treatment for Spondyloarthropathies

Drug	Dose	Efficacy Rating	Comments
Indomethacin	50 mg t.i.d. or 75 mg SR, q. 12 hr	Effective for symptoms	Side effects: headaches, changes in mentation, peptic ulcers, GI toxicity, intolerance, renal insufficiency
Tolmetin	600 mg t.i.d.	Effective for symptoms	Side effects: peptic ulcers, GI toxicity, renal insufficiency
Celecoxib*	200 mg q.d., bi.d.	Effective for symptoms	Side effects: less GI toxicity than other NSAIDs; potential renal impairment
Rofecoxib*	25 mg q.d., bi.d.	Effective for symptoms	Side effects: less GI toxicity than other NSAIDs; potential renal impairment
Sulfasalazine*	1–3 g daily in two divided doses	Long-term efficacy; lowers acute-phase reactants	Side effects: headache, GI intolerance
Methotrexate*	7.5–20 mg weekly	Effective for skin and arthritis in psoriatic arthritis; effectiveness in other diseases unproved	Side effects: GI intolerance, hepatotoxicity, marrow suppression, pulmonary disease
Doxycycline*	100 mg bi.d.	Effective in preventing relapse and in long-term treatment of reactive arthritis only	Side effects: GI intolerance, photosensitivity
Infliximab*	5 mg/kg I.V. every 6–8 wk after loading	Highly effective and immediate response; improved inflammation in joints by MRI; long-term effects unknown	Side effects: allergic reactions; increased susceptibility to infection, especially tuberculosis
Etanercept*	25 mg subcutaneous injections twice a week	Same as infliximab	Injection-site reactions, increased risk of infections

*Potentially disease-modifying agents.
GI—gastrointestinal   MRI—magnetic resonance imaging   NSAIDs—nonsteroidal anti-inflammatory drugs   SR—slow release

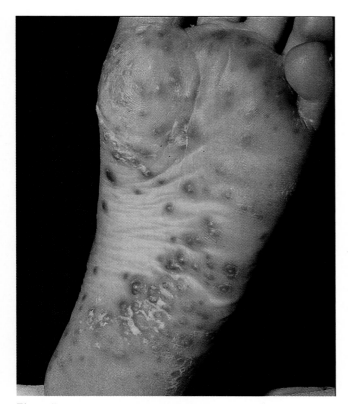

Figure 5 Typical keratoderma blennorrhagica rash of reactive arthritis on the sole of the foot.

highly active disease, but they should be used sparingly because they promote osteoporosis. Injection of repository corticosteroids into affected peripheral joints also may be useful. Injection into the sacroiliac joint, guided by either CT or MRI, may offer relief.

Sulfasalazine, 2 to 3 g daily in two divided doses, has been shown in several placebo-controlled trials to be an effective long-term treatment for ankylosing spondylitis as well as for other spondyloarthropathies.[1,40] The drug moiety responsible for its efficacy has been proved to be sulfapyridine rather than salicylate; however, it is not clear whether the efficacy results from antimicrobial or other properties of the drug.[43] Because sulfasalazine has been shown to lower acute phase reactants, such as the ESR and C-reactive protein level, it may modify disease progression; however, this desirable effect has yet to be proved.

Other long-acting agents used to treat rheumatoid arthritis, including gold salts, penicillamine, and hydroxychloroquine, are not effective in ankylosing spondylitis. Methotrexate therapy, which is highly effective for rheumatoid arthritis, requires further study in ankylosing spondylitis and other spondyloarthropathies; however, it is clearly effective in psoriatic arthritis.[6] Administration of radiation therapy to the spine was once used successfully but is no longer recommended because of the risk of subsequent malignancy.

The TNF antagonists etanercept and infliximab have recently been approved for the treatment of rheumatoid arthritis and Crohn disease.[44] An increasing number of controlled and open-label studies of the use of these agents in each of the spondyloarthropathies have shown dramatic and rapid improvement in symptoms as well as significantly reduced inflammatory changes in spine and peripheral joints, as evidenced on MRI. Long-

term efficacy and modification of disease progression and outcome have yet to be determined.[45-47]

All patients with ankylosing spondylitis should be informed of potential spinal deformities and how to prevent them. Good posture should be emphasized. A firm mattress and minimal pillow support are recommended. An exercise program of spinal extension and peripheral joint range-of-motion exercises, along with hydrotherapy, should be prescribed. Swimming is a very effective means of achieving exercise goals.[1]

Some patients who experience hip involvement—a major cause of disability—greatly benefit from total hip replacement. Wedge osteotomy for severe spinal kyphosis is available only at a few medical centers. Treatment of spinal fractures is controversial. Pregnancy does not appear to be significantly affected by ankylosing spondylitis.

Prognosis for individual patients is often difficult to ascertain.[48] Worse outcomes have been associated primarily with hip joint involvement and, to a lesser extent, early age at onset. The course of the disease in its first 10 years appears to predict its future course and functional outcome. Despite long-standing and severe disease, ankylosing spondylitis often does not affect a patient's ability to work. Mortality from the disease is infrequent but may result from cardiac or neurologic complications or amyloidosis.

Reactive Arthritis

Reactive arthritis was originally defined as the triad of nongonococcal urethritis, conjunctivitis, and arthritis. It is now recognized that most patients present with arthritis alone and have no clinical evidence of urethritis or conjunctivitis.[16,23,24] The concept of reactive arthritis arose from observations that the disease followed certain enteric infections (epidemic or postenteric form) and sexually acquired infections (endemic or postvenereal form) [*see* Pathogenesis, Environmental Factors, *above*] but was seemingly sterile when cultured for bacteria. It has been found that

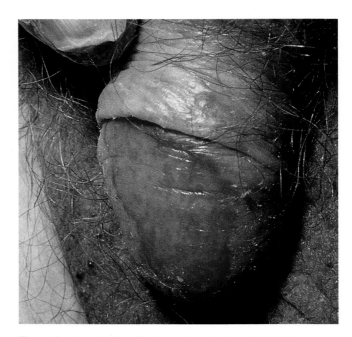

Figure 6 Superficial penile ulceration of circinate balanitis in an uncircumcised patient with reactive arthritis. Also note dystrophic fingernail.

bacterial antigens, if not viable microorganisms, are present in the joints of affected patients[15,16,26] [see Pathology, above]. Similar to ankylosing spondylitis, reactive arthritis may be complicated by sacroiliitis, spondylitis, uveitis, and the cardiac lesions. It is also strongly associated with HLA-B27 [see Table 2].

EPIDEMIOLOGY

Reactive arthritis probably has a worldwide distribution, but most epidemiologic and clinical studies have come from Europe and the United States.[16,17] The prevalence of the disease is difficult to ascertain because it changes over time, depending on sexual behavior and prevalence of enteric pathogens in different populations.[49] It was estimated that from 1950 to 1980 in Rochester, Minnesota, the incidence of reactive arthritis in men younger than 50 years was 0.035%; however, 10- to 20-fold higher rates were reported in homosexual men and in certain Native Americans in whom the frequency of HLA-B27 was high (30% to 40%) and who had endemic exposure to enteric or venereal pathogens.[15]

Reactive arthritis, probably the postvenereal form, is the most common cause of inflammatory arthritis in young men. The disease is recognized in women far less frequently and for unclear reasons, because the ratio of affected men to affected women after epidemics of gastroenteritis is typically 1:1 and, overall, approaches 1% to 2% of persons infected with any of the triggering pathogens.[15,16,26]

HLA-B27 is found in 63% to 75% of patients with both forms of reactive arthritis and confers a relative risk of approximately 37. Of persons with HLA-B27 who are infected with one of the causative bacteria, reactive arthritis develops in approximately 20%.

DIAGNOSIS

Clinical Presentation

Reactive arthritis typically develops 10 to 30 days after an episode of gastroenteritis or sexual exposure to a venereal pathogen; however, many patients deny any such antecedent events. Episodes of urethritis or conjunctivitis may have been mild and transient or not perceived at all. Thus, recognition of the pattern of musculoskeletal involvement, as well as several other mucocutaneous manifestations, are important in establishing the correct diagnosis.

The arthritis usually is oligoarticular and asymmetrical and predominantly affects lower-extremity joints, most often the knees, ankles, and feet. Diffuse painful swelling of entire digits (sausaging or dactylitis) occurs frequently. Pain in the heels from Achilles tendinitis or plantar fasciitis, or both, reflects the most common sites of enthesitis; however, enthesopathic pain at other sites is also frequent.[30] Low back pain is a complaint of 60% of patients, and 20% ultimately experience radiographically detectable sacroiliitis. An ascending spondylitis ensues in approximately 10% to 12% of patients.

One or more of the mucocutaneous features can be found on examination in more than 50% of patients, usually early in the disease. Keratoderma blennorrhagica is a papulosquamous skin rash that usually begins on the soles or palms as painless and nonpruritic excrescences resembling mollusk shells [see Figure 5]. With time, these lesions evolve into scaling plaques that may coalesce into a more generalized exfoliative dermatitis. Keratoderma blennorrhagica is clinically and histopathologically the same as the disorder pustular psoriasis. A similar scaling rash on the glans penis in circumcised men is termed circinate balanitis. Moist shallow ulcers characterize balanitis in uncircumcised men who may be unaware of the lesions unless the foreskin is re-

tracted [see Figure 6]. Similar painless oral ulcers may be found on the tongue or palate. Nails may become hyperkeratotic, thickened, and deformed, but the characteristic nail pitting of psoriasis is usually absent [see Figure 6]. It is important to search for all of these lesions; they are frequently asymptomatic but very definitive and can establish a diagnosis.

Some patients experience low-grade or high fever at disease onset; malaise—or even prostration—and significant weight loss may ensue. Acute anterior uveitis occurs in approximately 20% of patients with reactive arthritis and is more often bilateral than in ankylosing spondylitis. Cardiac bradyarrhythmia, aortic regurgitation, or both may also occur during the acute disease phase or may appear later in patients whose illness follows a chronic course.[34] Patients with reactive arthritis who are HLA-B27 positive are more likely to experience sacroiliitis and spondylitis, as well as uveitis, the cardiac lesion, or both, and to experience a prolonged disease course.

Reactive arthritis has been frequently described in patients with HIV infection; the joint and skin disease may be more severe than usual in such persons.[15,16,26] This association is now believed to result from sexually acquired enteric and venereal pathogens common to both diseases.

Laboratory Evaluation

Tests of patients with reactive arthritis usually show a modest leukocytosis, thrombocytosis, and anemia, along with elevation of the ESR, reflecting systemic inflammation. Examination of the synovial fluid reveals inflammatory changes of poor mucin clot and leukocytosis, but in contrast to septic arthritis, the glucose level is not low and bacterial cultures are negative. PCR analysis of synovial fluid or tissue biopsies has been used successfully to detect specific bacterial DNA or RNA in research laboratories; PCR kits should become clinically available soon.[50] Cultures or molecular probes for *C. trachomatis* should be obtained in patients with venereal exposure, genitourinary symptoms, or both.[51] At the same time, tests for concomitant gonorrhea, syphilis, and HIV should be performed. In patients with preceding GI symptoms, stool cultures for the triggering organisms are usually negative by the time joint symptoms appear. Serologic tests for *Salmonella* and other enteric pathogens are usually unreliable but may be useful in some cases.

Radiographic Features

X-rays are of no diagnostic value early in the disease; however, MRI may show inflammatory changes of enthesitis and arthritis. After several months of persistent joint symptoms, enthesopathic symptoms, or both, radiographs may show the distinctive changes of periostitis and bony ankylosis. Patients with chronic heel pain may show a fluffy periosteal reaction or spur formation at the Achilles or plantar tendon insertions.[30] Similar radiographic changes may be seen along metatarsal or phalangeal bones of the feet; bony fusion across joints may be visible. Sacroiliitis, when present, is more often unilateral than bilateral, and large asymmetrical syndesmophytes may be seen in the lumbar spine.[31]

TREATMENT AND PROGNOSIS

Reactive arthritis runs a self-limited course in most patients, lasting 4 to 12 months, although annoying residual musculoskeletal symptoms may persist for years.[52] From 15% to 30% of patients suffer permanent disability.[40] Relapses are not uncommon, and it is unclear whether they result from repeat infection or other endogenous mechanisms. The same NSAIDs used to treat ankylosing spondylitis [see Ankylosing Spondylitis, Treatment and Prognosis, above] [see Table 3] are usually effective in quieting inflammatory joint symptoms. Some patients with highly active disease, however, may require short courses of low-dose systemic corticosteroids or repository corticosteroid injections into joints.

Early treatment of genitourinary infections with appropriate antibiotics (tetracycline or erythromycin) has been shown to reduce the likelihood of subsequent reactive arthritis; however, even early antibiotic use in patients with gastroenteritis does not appear to prevent reactive arthritis.[15,40] A blinded, placebo-controlled trial of the use of tetracycline for the treatment of reactive arthritis demonstrated that the duration of disease was shortened only in patients who had *Chlamydia*-induced disease.[38] Ciprofloxacin has not been shown to shorten the course of chronic reactive arthritis.[40] Controlled studies have shown that sulfasalazine, used in dosages similar to those used in the treatment of ankylosing spondylitis, is effective in all the spondyloarthropathies.[40] Whether any of these antibiotic approaches change the natural history of the disease remains to be proved. Patients with spondyloarthropathy that persists despite treatment with NSAIDs and antibiotics may be benefited by use of immunosuppressive drugs such as methotrexate or azathioprine. An increasing number of studies are documenting immediate and dramatic benefit from the use of TNF-α antagonists (e.g., infliximab and etanercept) in such patients.[45] Physical therapy is important in maintaining joint motion and preventing disability.

Psoriatic Arthritis

EPIDEMIOLOGY

The prevalence of cutaneous psoriasis is estimated at 2% in most white populations and appears to be lower in populations who are of African or Asian ancestry. An inflammatory arthropathy attributable to psoriasis appears in 5% to 7% of patients with the skin disease, especially in those whose nails are affected.[6] Psoriasis is highly familial, and there is strong evidence that it is a complex genetic disease associated with several HLA alleles and other non–HLA-linked loci[53] [see Pathogenesis, above]. Genomic studies now strongly suggest major but yet unidentified loci for psoriasis susceptibility near HLA-C in the MHC region and on chromosome 17.[10] HLA-B27 is only weakly associated with psoriasis and peripheral psoriatic arthritis, but it occurs in 50% of persons who have psoriatic spondylitis. Potential environmental triggers are streptococcal infection and physical trauma. Psoriatic arthritis occurs slightly more commonly in females than in males. Psoriasis frequently first appears in childhood; psoriatic arthritis typically appears in early or middle adulthood, although there are many exceptions. The arthritis may appear before the psoriasis in as many as 40% of children and 15% of adults. Although the incidence of psoriasis and psoriatic arthritis in HIV-positive persons is similar to that in uninfected persons, severe exacerbation of both skin disease and joint disease has been observed in patients with HIV, especially as the number of CD4$^+$ T cells declines.

DIAGNOSIS

Clinical Presentation

In general, there is little relation between joint and skin severity. In fact, psoriatic skin lesions may be found only after careful scrutiny of scalp, umbilicus, or gluteal regions, and nail pitting or other changes may be the only clues supporting a diagnosis of psoriatic arthritis. Several clinical patterns of joint involvement, often overlapping, have been described:

1. Asymmetrical oligoarthritis of both small and large joints is the most common form of psoriatic arthritis. The finding of involved distal interphalangeal joints and sausage-shaped toes or fingers are highly suggestive signs. A disparity is often noted between clinical appearance and subjective symptoms; overtly involved joints may be largely asymptomatic, unlike the concordance usually found in rheumatoid arthritis.
2. Symmetrical polyarthritis may resemble rheumatoid arthritis, although the rheumatoid factor test should be negative. Uncertainty about classification is reasonable because psoriasis and rheumatoid arthritis are both relatively common diseases and are expected to occur together by chance.
3. Arthritis mutilans is the most destructive form of psoriatic arthritis; it occurs in approximately 5% of patients with psoriatic arthritis. Striking bone resorption and telescoping of fingers (opera-glass hand) are characteristic. Affected patients often have concomitant spinal involvement.
4. Psoriatic spondylitis occurs in approximately 20% of patients with psoriatic arthritis, often with unilateral sacroiliitis and large asymmetrical syndesmophytes similar to the pattern seen in patients with reactive arthritis.
5. Dominant or exclusively distal interphalangeal joint involvement with psoriatic nail changes may occur.

Laboratory Findings

An elevated ESR, anemia, and hyperuricemia may be found. Rheumatoid factor and antinuclear antibody tests are negative. Synovial fluid shows nonspecific inflammatory changes.

Radiographic Features

A characteristic change is whittling of the distal ends of phalanges, giving the joints a so-called pencil-in-cup appearance, which is radiographically distinctive for psoriatic arthritis. Periostitis—which results in whiskering around joints—bony erosions, and joint fusion in the absence of osteopenia also are common and diagnostically useful findings.

TREATMENT AND PROGNOSIS

NSAIDs similar to those used for ankylosing spondylitis [see Ankylosing Spondylitis, Treatment and Prognosis, above] [see Table 3] are the mainstay of arthritis therapy in most patients but have no effect on the skin disease, which may require separate dermatologic approaches. Sulfasalazine, methotrexate, or cyclosporine may be beneficial for both skin and joint disease in NSAID-resistant or severe, progressive disease,[6] and preliminary studies suggest that TNF-α antagonists (etanercept and infliximab) may be useful for both the arthritis and skin disease.[45] Gold, penicillamine, and hydroxychloroquine are not useful agents.

Psoriatic arthritis usually runs a more benign course than rheumatoid arthritis. Most patients with psoriatic arthritis maintain reasonable function, often despite extensive deformities.

Enteropathic Arthritis

Two major clinical patterns of arthritis associated with inflammatory bowel diseases are peripheral arthritis and spondylitis.

PERIPHERAL ARTHRITIS

Approximately 20% of patients with Crohn disease or ulcerative colitis experience an acute peripheral arthritis.[20] Symmetrical swelling, with large effusions, of knees, ankles, or wrists is the most common articular pattern. The pathogenesis of the arthritis is unknown, but the disease occurs during periods of active inflammation of the gut and may be the first sign of a bowel flare-up. HLA-B27 is not increased in frequency.

Recently, two genetic loci that predispose to Crohn disease have been found. One, termed *NOD2,* is located on chromosome 16 and may regulate bacterial processing by macrophages. The other is a tight cluster of cytokine genes located on chromosome 5.[8,9] Extraskeletal and extraintestinal manifestations may occur simultaneously and include fever, acute anterior uveitis, painful oral ulcers, erythema nodosum (in Crohn disease), and pyoderma gangrenosum (in ulcerative colitis). Treatment of the arthritis should be aimed at controlling the inflammatory bowel disease. The arthritis seldom results in deformities.

SPONDYLITIS

Sacroiliitis develops in about 10% of patients with inflammatory bowel disease, which may progress to total spinal ankylosis clinically and is radiographically indistinguishable from ankylosing spondylitis.[20] There is no correlation of the spondylitis with activity of the bowel disease. HLA-B27 is found in approximately 50% of such patients. Therapy is largely the same as for ankylosing spondylitis [*see* Ankylosing Spondylitis, Treatment and Prognosis, *above*]. Despite the bowel disease, NSAIDs are usually well tolerated.

Undifferentiated Spondyloarthropathies

Inevitably, the presentations of many patients do not conform to the typical presentations described above, and the symptoms and signs defy specific disease classification.[1,54] Examples are a patient with unilateral sacroiliitis, a sausage digit, and uveitis; a patient with typical reactive arthritis who experiences psoriatic arthritis; and a patient with typical ankylosing spondylitis who years later experiences Crohn disease. Such patients are often designated as having undifferentiated spondyloarthropathies. The European Spondyloarthropathy Study Group criteria[1] now make classification of patients with spondyloarthropathies more definitive. There remains, however, a large number of patients with formes frustes that do not fulfill the new criteria but probably fall within the spectrum of spondyloarthropathies. Such entities, which are strongly associated with HLA-B27, are chronic inflammatory back and chest pain syndromes (in which radiographs are normal), chronic dactylitis, chronic plantar fasciitis or Achilles tendinitis, pustular psoriasis (keratoderma blennorrhagica), circinate balanitis, acute anterior uveitis, and spondylitic heart disease without evidence of arthritis. In patients suspected of having a limited form of spondyloarthropathy, typing for HLA-B27 may prove clinically useful in supporting such a diagnosis.[1]

Juvenile Spondyloarthropathy

Until recently, the term juvenile rheumatoid arthritis was used, inappropriately, to describe all forms of chronic childhood arthritis. The use of careful clinical evaluation, autoantibody testing, and HLA typing has revealed a heterogeneous group of diseases in which only a small proportion of affected children truly have rheumatoid arthritis.

Juvenile spondyloarthropathy typically begins in late childhood or adolescence, most often in boys, with lower extremity oligoarthropathy and enthesopathy.[28] Spinal symptoms are rare initially but often appear years later. Bony ankylosis of the tarsal bones has been described in some of these patients. Acute anterior uveitis is not uncommon. Such patients are seronegative for rheumatoid factor and antinuclear antibodies but are positive for HLA-B27. Less often, a patient may present with chronic polyarthritis with prominent cervical spine fusion rather than lower spine involvement.

Subsets of juvenile arthritis include the following[55]:

1. Oligoarthritis appearing in early childhood, more often in girls; it is associated with antinuclear antibodies, a high risk of chronic iridocyclitis and blindness, and HLA-DR5, HLA-DR8, or HLA-DR6, as well as HLA-DP2, but not HLA-B27.
2. Polyarthritis appearing in early childhood, more often in girls who are seronegative for rheumatoid factor and antinuclear antibodies; it is associated with HLA-DR8 and HLA-DP3 but not HLA-B27.
3. Polyarthritis associated with rheumatoid factor and HLA-DR4 (but not HLA-B27), which probably represents true juvenile rheumatoid arthritis.
4. Still disease, characterized by high spiking fever, evanescent rash, hepatosplenomegaly, lymphadenopathy, and polyarthritis in patients who are seronegative and HLA-B27 negative.

Miscellaneous Arthropathies

ACNE-ASSOCIATED ARTHRITIS

A rare inflammatory oligoarthritis may occur in patients with severe forms of acne, including acne conglobata, acne fulminans, hidradenitis suppurativa, and dissecting cellulitis of the scalp.[56] Such patients experience fever and inflamed joints; symptoms resemble those of septic arthritis, but the joints are sterile by culture. Sacroiliitis has been described in some patients.

SAPHO is an acronym for a syndrome including synovitis, severe acne, palmoplantar pustulosis, hyperostosis, and osteitis and may be a form of spondyloarthritis.[57,58] These arthritides may represent forms of reactive arthritis but are usually HLA-B27 negative. Antibiotic therapy is usually of little or no benefit, but some patients respond to NSAIDs or low-dose corticosteroids. Surgical excision of the affected skin, when possible, has been reported to resolve the arthritis.

WHIPPLE DISEASE

Whipple disease is a rare multisystem disorder that usually affects men (the ratio of affected men to women is 9:1). Patients may present with arthralgias or transient episodes of additive, symmetrical polyarthritis that is nondeforming. Sacroiliitis has been reported in rare instances, and the frequency of HLA-B27 may be increased in patients with Whipple disease. Patients usually have GI symptoms, including diarrhea, steatorrhea, and profound weight loss. Other clues to diagnosis are skin hyperpigmentation, serositis (pleural effusions), lymphadenopathy, uveitis, nervous system disease (ocular palsies or encephalopathy), leukocytosis, and thrombocytosis. The diagnosis traditionally has been based on small bowel biopsies showing deposits on periodic acid–Schiff staining or electron microscopic demonstration of rodlike bacillary organisms in intestinal macrophages. The causative organism has been identified by RNA sequence analysis and recently cultured as a gram-positive actinomycete named *Tropheryma whippelii*.[59] Diagnosis can be made on the basis of results from PCR analysis of DNA from affected tissues or blood samples. Long-term treatment with tetracycline usually results in complete remission.

References

1. Khan MA: Upate on spondyloarthropathies. Ann Intern Med 136:896, 2002

2. Lawrence RC, Helmick CG, Arnett FC, et al: Estimates of the prevalence of arthritis and selected musculoskeletal disorders in the United States. Arthritis Rheum 41:778, 1998

3. Braun J, Bollow M, Remlinger G, et al: Prevalence of spondyloarthropathies in HLA-B27 positive and negative blood donors. Arthritis Rheum 41:58, 1998

4. Wordsworth P: Genes in the spondyloarthropathies. Rheum Dis Clin North Am 24:845, 1998

5. Reveille JD, Ball EJ, Khan MA: HLA-B27 and genetic predisposing factors in spondyloarthropathies. Curr Opin Rheumatol 13:265, 2001

6. Gladman DD: Psoriatic arthritis. Rheum Dis Clin North Am 24:829, 1998

7. Hampe J, Shaw SH, Saiz R, et al: Linkage of inflammatory bowel disease to human chromosome 6p. Am J Hum Genet 65:1647, 1999

8. Hugot JP, Chamaillard M, Zouali H, et al: Association of *NOD2* leucine-rich repeat variants with susceptibility to Crohn's disease. Nature 411:599, 2001

9. Rioux JD, Daly MJ, Silverberg MS, et al: Genetic variation in the 5q31 cytokine gene cluster confers susceptibility to Crohn's disease. Nat Genet 29:223, 2001

10. Höhler T, Märker-Hermann E: Psoriatic arthritis: clinical aspects, genetics and the role of T cells. Curr Opin Rheumatol 13:273, 2001

11. Taurog JD, Maika SD, Satumtira N, et al: Inflammatory disease in HLA-B27 transgenic rats. Immunol Rev 169:209, 1999

12. Märker-Hermann E, Höhler T: Pathogenesis of human leukocyte antigen B27-positive arthritis: information from clinical materials. Rheum Dis Clin North Am 24:865, 1998

13. Virtala M, Kirkveskari J, Granfors K: HLA-B27 modulates the survival of *Salmonella enteritidis* in transfected L cells, possibly by impaired nitric oxide production. Infect Immun 65:4236, 1997

14. Gaston JH, Cox C, Granfors K: Clinical and experimental evidence for persistent *Yersinia* infection in reactive arthritis. Arthritis Rheum 42:2239, 1999

15. Amor B: Reiter's syndrome: diagnosis and clinical features. Rheum Dis Clin North Am 24:677, 1998

16. Keat A: Reactive arthritis. Adv Exp Med Biol 455:201, 1999

17. Vittecoqoq O, Schaeverbeke T, Favre S, et al: Molecular diagnosis of *Ureaplasma urealyticum* in an immunocompetent patient with destructive reactive polyarthritis. Arthritis Rheum 40:2084, 1997

18. Hannu T, Puolakkainen M, Leirisalo-Repo M: *Chlamydia pneumoniae* as a triggering infection in reactive arthritis. Rheumatology 38:411, 1999

19. Montenegro V, Monteiro RC: Elevation of serum IgA in spondyloarthropathies and IgA nephropathy and its pathogenic role. Curr Opin Rheumatol 11:265, 1999

20. De Keyser F, Elewaut D, DeVos M, et al: Bowel inflammation and the spondyloarthropathies. Rheum Dis Clin North Am 24:785, 1998

21. Braun J, Bollow M, Neure L, et al: Use of immunohistologic and in situ hybridization techniques in the examination of sacroiliac joint biopsy specimens from patients with ankylosing spondylitis. Arthritis Rheum 38:499, 1995

22. Rudwaleit M, Höhler T: Cytokine gene polymorphisms relevant for the spondyloarthropathies. Curr Opin Rheumatol 13:250, 2001

23. Gerard HC, Branigan PJ, Schumacher HR, et al: Synovial *Chlamydia trachomatis* in patients with reactive arthritis/Reiter's syndrome are viable but show aberrant gene expression. J Rheumatol 25:734, 1998

24. Nikkari S, Rantakokko K, Ekman P, et al: *Salmonella*-triggered reactive arthritis. Arthritis Rheum 42:84, 1999

25. Braun J, Tuszewski M, Ehlers S, et al: Nested polymerase chain reaction strategy simultaneously targeting DNA sequences of multiple bacterial species in inflammatory joint diseases: examination of sacroiliac and knee joint biopsies of patients with spondyloarthropathies and other arthritides. J Rheumatol 24:1101, 1997

26. Lau CS, Burgos-Vargas R, Louthrenoo W, et al: Features of spondyloarthritis around the world. Rheum Dis Clin North Am 24:753, 1998

27. Gran JT, Ostensen M: Spondyloarthritides in females. Baillieres Clin Rheumatol 12:695, 1998

28. Burgos-Vargas R, Pacheco-Tena C, Vazquez-Mellado J: Juvenile-onset spondyloarthropathies. Rheum Dis Clin North Am 23:569, 1997

29. van Tubergen A, Coenen J, Landewe R, et al: Assessment of fatigue in patients with ankylosing spondylitis: a psychometric analysis. Arthritis Rheum 47:8, 2002

30. Francois RJ, Braun J, Khan MA: Entheses and enthesitis: a histopathologic review and relevance to spondyloarthropathies. Curr Opin Rheumatol 13: 255, 2001

31. Helliwell PS, Hickling P, Wright V: Do the radiological changes of classic ankylosing spondylitis differ from the changes found in the spondylitis associated with inflammatory bowel disease, psoriasis, and reactive arthritis? Ann Rheum Dis 57:135, 1998

32. Resnick D, Shapiro RF, Wiesner KB, et al: Diffuse idiopathic skeletal hyperostosis (ankylosing hyperostosis of Forestier and Rotes-Querol). Semin Arthritis Rheum 7:153, 1978

33. Banares A, Hernandez-Garcia C, Fernandez-Gutierrez B, et al: Eye involvement in the spondyloarthropathies. Rheum Dis Clin North Am 24:771, 1998

34. Bergfeldt L: HLA-B27–associated cardiac disease. Ann Intern Med 127:621, 1997

35. Roldan CA, Chavez J, Wiest PW, et al: Aortic root disease and valve disease associated with ankylosing spondylitis. J Am Coll Cardiol 32:1397, 1998

36. Casserly IP, Fenlon HM, Breatnach E, et al: Lung findings on high-resolution computed tomography in idiopathic ankylosing spondylitis: correlation with clinical findings, pulmonary function testing and plain radiography. Br J Rheumatol 36:677, 1997

37. Gratacos J, Orellana C, Sanmarti R, et al: Secondary amyloidosis in ankylosing spondylitis: a systematic survey of 137 patients using abdominal fat aspiration. J Rheumatol 24:912, 1997

38. Charlesworth CH, Savy LE, Stevens J, et al: MRI demonstration of arachnoiditis in cauda equina syndrome of ankylosing spondylitis. Neuroradiology 38:462, 1996

39. LeBlanc CM, Inman RD, Dent P, et al: Retroperitoneal fibrosis: an extraarticular manifestation of ankylosing spondylitis. Arthritis Rheum 47:210, 2002

40. Leirisalo-Repo M: Prognosis, course of disease, and treatment of the spondyloarthropathies. Rheum Dis Clin North Am 24:737, 1998

41. Dougados M, Behier JM, Jolcine I, et al: Efficacy of celecoxib, a cyclooxygenase 2–specific inhibitor, in the treatment of ankylosing spondylitis: a six-week controlled study with comparison against placebo and against a conventional non-steroidal anti-inflammatory drug. Arthritis Rheum 44: 180, 2001

42. Maksymowych WP, Jhangri GS, Fitzgerald AA, et al: A six-month randomized, controlled, double-blind, dose-response comparison of intravenous pamidronate (60 mg versus 10 mg) in the treatment of nonsteroidal antiinflammatory drug-refractory ankylosing spondylitis. Arthritis Rheum 46:766, 2002

43. Taggart A, Gardiner P, McEvoy F, et al: Which is the active moiety of sulfasalazine in ankylosing spondylitis? A randomized, controlled study. Arthritis Rheum 39:1400, 1996

44. Moreland LW, Baumgartner SW, Schiff MH, et al: Treatment of rheumatoid arthritis with a recombinant human tumor necrosis factor receptor (p75) Fc fusion protein. N Engl J Med 337:141, 1997

45. Braun J, de Keyser F, Brandt J, et al: New treatment options in spondyloarthropathies: increasing evidence for significant efficacy of anti-tumor necrosis factor therapy. Curr Opin Rheumatol 13:245, 2001

46. Gorman JD, Sack KE, Davis JC Jr: Treatment of ankylosing spondylitis by inhibition of tumor necrosis factor alpha. N Engl J Med 346:1349, 2002

47. Braun J, Brandt J, Listing J, et al: Treatment of active ankylosing spondylitis with infliximab: a randomised controlled multicentre trial. Lancet 359:1187, 2002

48. Kerr HE, Sturrock RD: Clinical aspects, outcome assessment, disease course, and extra-articular features of spondyloarthropathies. Curr Opin Rheumatol 11:235, 1999

49. Iliopoulos A, Karras D, Ioakimidis D, et al: Change in the epidemiology of Reiter's syndrome (reactive arthritis) in the post-AIDS era? An analysis of cases appearing in the Greek army. J Rheumatol 22:252, 1995

50. Li F, Schumacher HR, Kieber-Emmons T, et al: Molecular detection of bacterial DNA in venereal-associated arthritis. Arthritis Rheum 39:950, 1996

51. Sieper J, Rudwaleit M, Braun J, et al: Diagnosing reactive arthritis: role of clinical setting in the value of serologic and microbiologic assays. Arthritis Rheum 46:319, 2002

52. Thomson GD, DeRubeis DA, Hodge MA, et al: Post-*Salmonella* reactive arthritis: late clinical sequelae in a point source cohort. Am J Med 98:13, 1995

53. Gladman DD, Farewell VT: The role of HLA antigens as indicators of disease progression in psoriatic arthritis. Arthritis Rheum 38:845, 1995

54. Olivier I, Salvarani C, Cantini F, et al: Ankylosing spondylitis and undifferentiated spondyloarthropathies: a clinical review and description of a disease subset with older age at onset. Curr Opin Rheumatol 13:280, 2001

55. Grom AA, Giannini EH, Glass DN: Juvenile rheumatoid arthritis and the trimolecular complex (HLA, T cell receptor, and antigen): difference from rheumatoid arthritis. Arthritis Rheum 37:601, 1994

56. Olafsson S, Khan MA: Musculoskeletal features of acne, hidradenitis suppurativa, and dissecting cellulitis of the scalp. Rheum Dis Clin North Am 18:215, 1992

57. Winchester R: Psoriatic arthritis and the spectrum of syndromes related to the SAPHO (synovitis, acne, pustulosis, hyperostosis, and osteitis) syndrome. Curr Opin Rheumatol 11:251, 1999

58. Hayem G, Bouchaud-Chabot A, Banali K, et al: SAPHO syndrome: a long-term follow up study of 120 cases. Semin Arthritis Rheum 29:159, 1999

59. Raoult D, Birg ML, La Scola B, et al: Cultivation of the bacillus of Whipple's disease. N Engl J Med 342:620, 2000

Review

Spondyloarthropathies. Yu DYT, Ed. Rheum Dis Clin North Am 24:663, 1998

114 Systemic Lupus Erythematosus

Michael D. Lockshin, M.D.

Disease Definition and Subclassification

Lupus is a chronic autoimmune illness characterized by autoantibodies directed at nuclear antigens and causing a variety of clinical and laboratory abnormalities, including rash, arthritis, leukopenia and thrombocytopenia, alopecia, fever, nephritis, and neurologic disease. Most or all of the symptoms of acute lupus are attributable to immunologic attack on the affected organs. Many complications of long-term disease are attributable both to the disease and to its treatment.[1]

The term lupus applies to several variants of the illness [*see Table 1*], of which systemic lupus erythematosus (SLE) is the most serious and most common. SLE is the prototype of a systemic autoimmune illness, involving multiple organ systems in pathogenically similar ways. Characteristically, patients with SLE progress through periods of active inflammation (flare) and periods of quiescence (remission), both of which may occur spontaneously. The reasons for the varying course are unknown. Intense sun exposure, drug reactions, and infections are circumstances that are known to induce flare.

SLE may occur as an overlap syndrome that shares features with other autoimmune illnesses, such as mixed or undifferentiated connective tissue disease, dermatomyositis, Sjögren syndrome, rheumatoid arthritis, and scleroderma. Organ-specific autoimmune diseases, such as thyroiditis, autoimmune hemolytic anemia, and idiopathic thrombocytopenia, frequently accompany and may be part of SLE.

Lupus may also appear as a skin disease only. Discoid lupus occurs as a destructive, scarring rash, unaccompanied by systemic symptoms or autoantibodies.[2] Subacute cutaneous lupus comprises a characteristic persistent, polycyclic rash; relatively minor visceral symptoms; and strongly positive blood tests.

Drugs such as procainamide and some anticonvulsants induce a lupuslike syndrome, which is called drug-induced lupus.[3] Uncommonly, persons (often relatives of lupus patients) have positive blood tests for lupus but are clinically well. In the absence of symptoms, such persons are not considered to have lupus.

Approximately one third of lupus patients have antiphospholipid antibody, which induces blood clots and fetal death. The presence of this antibody, in the absence of clinical lupus, is referred to as primary antiphospholipid antibody syndrome.[4]

Neonatal lupus is a syndrome consisting of rash, thrombocytopenia, and congenital heart block occurring in infants born of mothers who carry antibody to the SS-A (Ro) and SS-B (La) antigens.[5] It does not evolve into SLE.

Epidemiology and Genetics

SLE is primarily a disease of young women, but the female predominance of SLE has not been explained. Women between 15 and 45 years of age are the most commonly affected; the female-to-male ratio in this age group is between 6:1 and 9:1. African Americans are four times as likely to develop lupus as are whites.[6] The disease incidence in Asians, Hispanics, and Native Americans falls between that of blacks and whites [*see Figure 1*]. No cogent explanation offered to date suggests why African Americans are more frequently affected; racial differ-ences in SLE incidence persist when socioeconomic differences have been controlled. SLE severity in men is similar to that in women. Overall survival is lower in African Americans.[7]

The familial aspects of lupus are striking: approximately 10% of persons with lupus have family members with lupus or other autoimmune disease. Susceptibility to lupus is higher in persons with specific genetic deficiencies [*see* Other Genetic Susceptibilities, *below*].

Pathophysiology and Pathogenesis

AUTOANTIBODIES

Circulating antibodies to a broad list of autoantigens characterize SLE. Antinuclear antibodies, usually defined by immunofluorescence, are present in almost all lupus patients; tests for antinuclear antibody constitute a screening test (sensitive, but not specific) for the illness. Autoantibodies to nuclear constituents—primarily to double-stranded (native) DNA but also to single-stranded (denatured) DNA, histones, ribonuclear proteins, and other nuclear antigens, such as the Smith (Sm) antigen—are likely pathogenic. For example, these autoantibodies cause glomerulonephritis by inciting inflammation when deposited as complement-fixing immune complexes on glomerular basement membranes or by binding directly to the glomerular basement membrane.[8] Both animal models and clinical observations suggest that autoantibodies in the presence of complement mediate lupus-associated glomerulonephritis, hemolysis, and thrombocytopenia. Antibodies to phospholipid-binding proteins (beta$_2$-glycoprotein I, prothrombin, and others) mediate thrombosis and fetal loss. Lupus rash and arthritis are less clearly linked to autoantibodies, but immune reactants and inflammation are demonstrable in relevant biopsy specimens, primarily at the basement membrane.[9] Among lupus manifestations, neurologic lupus is least clearly caused by anti-DNA or other autoantibody; however, anti–ribosomal P antibody may define mood disorders in neurologic lupus,[10] and antibody to a glutamate receptor may mediate cognitive dysfunction.[11]

ABNORMAL INNATE AND ADAPTIVE IMMUNITY

Genetic defects of immune complex processing are unusually frequent in lupus patients, suggesting that SLE arises because of incomplete or improper disposal of exogenous material.[12] Such defects include abnormalities in complement (deficiencies of C1q, C2, or C4), Fc receptor, apoptotic pathways, and phagocytic cells.[13] Defective clearance of immune complexes may result in their persistence in large quantities,[14] and autoantibodies may be a protective mechanism to neutralize them. Other theories of pathogenesis argue that genetic predispositions that promote T helper type 2 cell (Th2) responses or cytokine dysregulation are the underlying defects leading to the development of SLE.

In animal models, several immune defects that may cause SLE have been identified. These include abnormalities in genes affecting overall immunoreactivity (apoptosis [*Fas, Fas* ligand, *Bcl-2*]), B cell activation (*FcγRIIB, SHP-1, CD22, CD19, PD-1, Lyn,*

Table 1   Characteristic Features That Distinguish Lupus from Lupuslike Diseases

| Organ System | Lupus | | | | RA | Sjögren Syndrome |
	SLE	Discoid	Drug-Induced	Neonatal		
Skin	Specific rashes, alopecia, mucosal ulcers, periungual telangiectasia	Specific rash, alopecia, mucosal ulcers	Rash	Rash	Subcutaneous nodules	Dry eyes, dry mouth
Joints	Symmetrical nondestructive arthritis	—	Symmetrical nondestructive arthritis	—	Symmetrical destructive arthritis	Symmetrical destructive arthritis
Renal	Glomerulonephritis, renal failure	—	—	—	Amyloidosis (late)	Tubular dysfunction
CNS	Seizures, psychosis, cognitive dysfunction, stroke, myelopathy, neuropathy	—	—	—	Peripheral neuropathy	Peripheral and cranial neuropathy
Cardiac	—	—	—	Heart block	—	—
Blood ANA	Strong positive, any pattern	May be positive	Strong positive	Positive	May be positive	Positive
Complement	Low with renal disease or hemolytic anemia	Normal	Normal	Normal or low	Commonly high	Low or high
Diagnostic autoantibodies	Anti-dsDNA, anti-Sm	—	Antihistone	Anti–SS-A, anti–SS-B	Anti-IgG (rheumatoid factor)	Anti–SS-A, anti–SS-B
Other autoantibodies	Anti–SS-A (Ro), anti–SS-B (La), anti-RNP, anti-IgG, anti-ssDNA	Anti-ssDNA	Antihistone	Anti-RNP	—	Anti-IgG
Other abnormalities	Leukopenia, thrombocytopenia, hemolysis	—	Leukopenia	Thrombocytopenia, hemolysis	Leukocytosis, thrombocytosis	Hyperglobulinemia

ANA—antinuclear antibody   CNS—central nervous system   CPK—creatinine phosphokinase   dsDNA—double-stranded DNA   LLD—lupuslike disease   MCTD—mixed connective tissue disorder   PAPS— primary antiphospholipid antibody syndrome   RA—rheumatoid arthritis   RNP—ribonucleoprotein   ssDNA—single-stranded DNA   SLE—systemic lupus erythematosus   UCTD—undifferentiated connective tissue disease

(continued)

Blys-1), T cell activation (*TGF-β, TGF-βR, PD-1*), cell proliferation (*p21, Fli-1*), and cytokines (*IFN-γ, IL-4, IL-10, TNF-α*); and genes affecting autoantigen clearance (*C1q, C4, SAP, DNAse-1*).[15,16]

OTHER GENETIC SUSCEPTIBILITIES

Twin and family studies of SLE make it abundantly clear that the illness is highly heritable. HLA types DR3 and DR4 predominate in SLE patients.[17] Specific susceptibility loci on chromosomes 1, 4, and 7 (among others) have been identified.[18] Persons with genetic deficiencies of complement appear to be more susceptible to the development of lupus.[19] Specific FcIII gamma receptor alleles increase the severity of lupus nephritis, particularly in whites.[20] The genetics of lupus are extremely complex, however, and no single genetic trait is unequivocally linked to susceptibility to the illness. Several national registries are currently attempting to definitively describe the genetics of lupus.

INFECTIONS

Although an infectious trigger of SLE has long been suspected, no single infection has been found. Universal exposure of children with SLE to Epstein-Barr virus has been noted (at an age when 50% exposure is the norm), suggesting a possible link of this virus to disease.[21]

ESTROGEN

Some investigators attribute the female predominance of SLE and its occurrence in childbearing years to the upregulating effect of estrogen on the immune system, a phenomenon demonstrable largely in vitro. However, this argument applies to autoimmunity in general, not specifically to lupus, and it fails to explain why other autoimmune diseases have much less striking female-to-male ratios. Furthermore, postmenopausal estrogen replacement and oral contraceptive use do not significantly alter SLE incidence or severity, nor does pregnancy; minor differences in incidence or susceptibility have on occasion

been reported.[22-24] Alternative explanations for a high female-male ratio include an estrogen-sensitive threshold mechanism[25] or sex differences of exposure to exogenous agents (although none has been convincingly suggested).[26]

COMPLICATIONS OF CHRONIC ILLNESS

Most current information on SLE pathogenesis focuses on upregulation or downregulation of components of the immune response, genetic controls of immunity, and potential etiologic agents. However, the long-term damage of chronic disease, from tissue injury or treatment, is as important to patients as

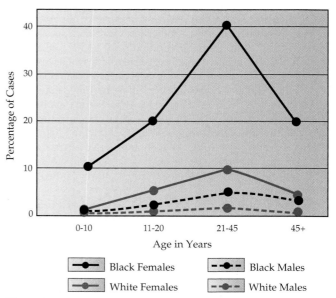

Figure 1   **Age, sex, and race distribution of the incidence of SLE.[6]**

Table 1 *(continued)*

MCTD	UCTD	PAPS	Scleroderma	LLD	Dermatomyositis
Sclerodactyly	—	Livedo reticularis	Scleroderma, periungual telangiectasia	—	Specific rash, periungual telangiectasia
Symmetrical nondestructive arthritis	Symmetrical nondestructive arthritis	—	Transient, symmetrical, early arthritis	Symmetrical nondestructive arthritis	—
—	—	Thrombotic microangiopathy	Angiotensin-driven renal crisis	—	—
—	—	Stroke, myelopathy	Hypertensive crisis	—	Myopathy
—	—	—	—	—	—
Positive, speckled Normal	May be positive Normal	May be positive Normal	Positive, speckled, nucleolar, centromere Normal	May be positive Normal	Positive Normal
Anti-RNP	—	Anticardiolipin, lupus anticoagulant	Anti–Scl-70, anticentromere (topoisomerase I)	—	Anti–Jo-1
—	—	Anti–β$_2$-glycoprotein I	—	—	—
—	—	Thrombocytopenia	High renin during crisis	—	High CPK and aldolase

acute inflammatory disease. Some elements of damage are clearly attributable to therapy: osteoporosis, osteonecrosis, cataracts, and tendon ruptures are all associated with long-term corticosteroid therapy. Other elements of damage result directly from the inflammatory and immunologic aspects of the illness, which lead to tissue necrosis and scarring: progressive renal failure, destructive joint disease, and brain infarcts. Many of these complications are more severe in patients of minority races or lower social classes.[27] Still other elements of chronicity bear an uncertain relationship to disease and treatment: accelerated atherosclerosis[28] and cognitive dysfunction and psychosocial dysfunction.

Diagnosis

The American College of Rheumatology (ACR) has defined criteria for the classification of SLE [*see Table 2*].[29] Although the ACR criteria are useful for ensuring uniformity of patients reported in medical journals, the criteria are often mistakenly used as diagnostic criteria. For individual patients, the criteria have high false negative and false positive rates.[30] For instance, a patient with biopsy-proven lupus nephritis, positive antinuclear antibody, and anti-Sm antibody as her only manifestations does not fulfill ACR criteria, whereas a patient with rheumatoid arthritis who has a positive antinuclear antibody, low positive anti-DNA antibody, and leukopenia (e.g., from Felty syndrome) does fulfill ACR criteria. As a rule, characteristic disease of one organ system (kidney, joints, skin) plus a high titer anti-dsDNA or Sm antibody suffices to make the clinical diagnosis.

In clinical practice, diagnosis of SLE is based on a combination of autoantibody assays, clinical manifestations, and laboratory studies of affected organ systems. The clinical manifestations of lupus are protean. Patients with lupus activity or damage may be asymptomatic or may present with findings that reflect the specific organ systems involved [*see Table 3*].

Symptoms and signs accumulate over time in patients with SLE [*see Table 4*].[31] At any given time, and especially at the onset of illness, most often only a few manifestations are present. Arthritis, malaise, cytopenias, and rashes are the most prominent early findings. Nephritis (with renal failure), arthritis, osteoporosis and osteonecrosis (corticosteroid complications), neurologic disease, accelerated atherosclerosis, and cardiac valvular disease dominate the late course. With disease activity and with its treatment, the risk of opportunistic infection is high. For conceptual purposes, it is easiest to consider disease activity and manifestations separately for each affected organ system.

SYSTEMIC SIGNS AND SYMPTOMS

Malaise, arthralgia, myalgias, fever (usually low grade), and weight loss are common manifestations of active SLE. Occasional patients will have high temperatures (> 40° C [104° F]).

Table 2 American College of Rheumatology Criteria for the Classification of SLE*

Malar rash
Discoid rash
Photosensitivity
Oral ulcers
Arthritis
Serositis (pleuritis or pericarditis)
Renal disorder (proteinuria > 0.5 g/day or cellular casts)
Neurologic disorder (seizures or psychosis)
Hematologic disorder (hemolytic anemia, leukopenia, lymphopenia, or thrombocytopenia)
Immunologic disorder (anti-DNA, anti-Sm, or antiphospholipid antibodies [anticardiolipin, lupus anticoagulant, or biologic false positive test for syphilis])
Antinuclear antibody

Note: these are not diagnostic criteria.
*Four criteria are required to include a patient in an SLE cohort of a research study.

Table 3   Physical Examination Abnormalities in Acute and Chronic SLE *

| Organ | Acute Disease | | Chronic Disease | |
	Common	Uncommon	Common	Uncommon
General	Fever, weight loss	Asthenia	Cachexia	
Skin	Malar rash, rash elsewhere, alopecia	Periungual telangiectasia, vasculitis	Malar rash, rash elsewhere, alopecia, striae, atrophy, pigment change	Periungual telangiectasia, skin ulcers
Nodes	Lymphadenopathy	—	—	—
Breasts	—	—	—	—
Eyes	—	Retinal hemorrhages, exudates	Hypertensive changes	Retinal hemorrhages, exudates
Ears	—	Rash in ear canal, decreased hearing	—	Scarring in ear canal, decreased hearing
Nose	—	Septal ulceration	—	Septal perforation
Throat	—	Mucosal ulcer (hard palate)	—	Mucosal scarring (hard palate)
Chest	—	Rales, pleural rub, effusion	—	Rales, effusion
Heart and vessels	Raynaud phenomenon	Pericardial rub, enlargement	Raynaud phenomenon, valve disease	Enlargement, valve insufficiency, arrhythmia
Abdomen	—	Hepatomegaly, splenomegaly	—	Hepatomegaly, splenomegaly, ascites
Muscles	Weakness, tenderness	—	Weakness, atrophy, tendon rupture	—
Bones	—	—	Fracture (vertebrae, hip), osteonecrosis	—
Joints	Synovitis, restricted motion	—	Synovitis, deformity, restricted motion	Jaccoud deformities
Neuromotor	—	Stroke, mononeuritis multiplex, seizure	—	Stroke, mononeuritis multiplex, seizure
Neurosensory	—	Peripheral neuropathy, mononeuritis multiplex	—	Peripheral neuropathy, mononeuritis multiplex
Cognitive	Depression	Psychosis, dementia	Depression	Psychosis, dementia

*This table is not comprehensive; it does not include rare abnormalities.

Even with very high fever, shaking chills are unusual; when present, they suggest infection. Like the organ-specific manifestations of lupus, the systemic symptoms vary considerably during the day and over weeks. In approximately one third of lupus patients, sun exposure, usually intense, will induce systemic flare. Sun exposure that is mild or of short duration does not harm most patients.

SKIN AND MUCOSAL INVOLVEMENT

Up to half of lupus patients manifest some degree of alopecia. Typically this takes the form of broken frontal hairs and diffuse thinning, which recovers when health is regained. Severe alopecia may occur. Discoid rashes cause focal patches of hair loss.

Most patients develop a rash at some point during their illness. The well-known butterfly rash, on both cheeks and across the bridge of the nose [see Figure 2], occurs in only a minority of patients, but most rashes involve the face in some manner. Commonly the tip of the chin, the upper lip, the eyebrows, and the hairline are also involved. The rash may consist of erythema only or may be papular and scaly or deeply pigmented (discoid rash). Discoid rashes, which may scar, are hyperpigmented at the circumference and often depigmented centrally [see Figure 3]. Patients with discoid rashes may have either discoid or systemic lupus. Other types of rashes occur only in systemic lupus.

Diagnostic inflammatory rashes are somewhat raised, scaly, and relatively uniform in appearance across the lesion; they may ulcerate; and they have sharp borders. Less diagnostic rashes occur on the extensor surfaces of the upper arms, the blush area of the neck and shoulders, and the extensor surfaces of the elbows and fingers. These are usually erythematous macular rashes. The erythematous rashes evolve over days to weeks and often leave hyperpigmentation as they recede; they may appear more prominent with fever or pregnancy. Vasculitic rashes (usually small, ulcerating papules) occur on the extensor tips of the elbows; painful, erythematous vascular lesions occur at the distal fingers and palms (lupus pernio). A polycyclic, persistent rash, primarily on the trunk, and specifically associated with anti–SS-A antibody, is known as subacute cutaneous lupus [see Figure 4]. A painful subcutaneous lesion that is deeply indurated and tender and may ulcerate is called lupus profundus.

Some patients have only erythema in distributions typical of lupus rashes. Unlike the other rashes, erythematous rashes are not by themselves diagnostic of lupus, but they add to the overall diagnostic information. Lupus rashes are often confused with rosacea (although rosacea is more oily and more papular), polymorphous light eruptions, and allergic reactions.

Chronic nasal ulcers and recurring painless mouth ulcers [see Figure 5] (particularly on the hard palate, but also on the

Table 4 Frequencies of Various Manifestations of SLE by Disease Stage[31]

Manifestation	Early Disease (%)	Late Disease (%)
Arthritis	46–53	83–95
Rash	9–11	81–88
Fever	3–5	77
Mucosal ulcers	—	7–23
Alopecia	—	37–45
Serositis	5	63
Pulmonary inflammation	—	9
Liver function test abnormalities	1	—
Vasculitis	—	21–27
Myositis	—	5
Osteoporosis	—	High
Osteonecrosis		7–24
Leukopenia	41–66	41–66
Thrombocytopenia	2	19–45
Anemia	2	57–73
CNS abnormalities	3	55–59
Nephritis	6	31–53
Renal failure	< 1	20

gums and buccal mucosa) are characteristic of more severe disease. Mucosal ulcers are irritating rather than severely painful. Periungual telangiectasias and small, ulcerating, vasculitic ulcers on the elbows also occur in more severe disease. A particular type of palmar and digital pulp erythema, known as lupus pernio, is a form of vasculitis. Rarely, subcutaneous inflammation leads to lupus profundus, consisting of local fat necrosis and painful nodules.

LYMPH NODE INVOLVEMENT

Lymphadenopathy is common in active disease. It is modest in extent and generalized (often noted on computed tomography scans of the abdomen or chest). It resolves rapidly in patients started on corticosteroid therapy for other manifestations of SLE.

CARDIOPULMONARY INVOLVEMENT

SLE is associated with a range of cardiovascular disorders [*see Table 5*]. These usually cause symptoms or abnormal phys-ical findings; it is unnecessary to test asymptomatic patients for cardiovascular disease.

Pleuropericarditis is frequently symptomatic but is not usually life-threatening. It causes pain on breathing, as well as elevation of the diaphragm that is evident on physical examination or x-ray. Atelectasis at the bases of the lungs is audible as fine crackling rales or is visible on x-ray as horizontal lines (plate atelectasis). Pulmonary function tests may reflect reduced diffusion capacity, reduced lung volumes, and reduced lung elasticity.

Pleural effusions also occur, but they are not usually large. On thoracentesis, LE cells (polymorphonuclear leukocytes with ingested nuclear debris appearing as a homogeneous round inclusion) may be found on a Wright stain of the fluid buffy coat.

A minority of patients develop respiratory insufficiency from pulmonary fibrosis. A rare manifestation is so-called lupus lung. This consists of inflammatory lung disease or pulmonary hemorrhage, either of which is life threatening.[32] Pulmonary hypertension is uncommon but serious when it occurs, which is most often in patients with intense Raynaud phenomenon, recurrent pulmonary emboli, or pulmonary fibrosis.

Echocardiography demonstrates valvular heart disease in up to 30% of patients with long-standing SLE.[33] Libman-Sacks lesions occur primarily on the mitral valve but also occur on the aortic valve and, rarely, on the pulmonic or tricuspid valves. Symptomatic valve disease may be more common in patients with antiphospholipid antibody. Pericardial effusions or thickening occur during active disease but are uncommon otherwise. Small pericardial effusions, which may be symptomatic or asymptomatic, occur often in patients with systemically active lupus. Life-threatening large effusions are uncommon.

Accelerated atherosclerosis is a risk of long-standing lupus,[34,35] leading to myocardial infarction and other vascular occlusive manifestations before the age of 40. Myocardial infarction may also be caused by coronary vasculitis, but this is less common. It is important to consider atherosclerosis, together with vasculitis and thrombosis (from antiphospholipid antibody), in patients with long-standing lupus who present with complaints of vascular insufficiency.

Diffuse nonischemic myocarditis may also occur. Newborns suffering the neonatal SLE syndrome may have complete congenital heart block and may die of congestive heart failure.

a

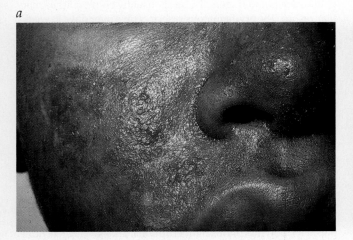

b

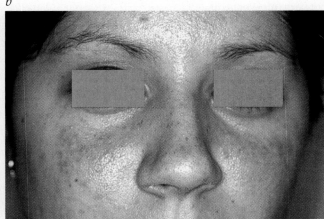

Figure 2 Most lupus rashes involve the face (*a*). The butterfly rash of lupus, on both cheeks and across the bridge of the nose (*b*), occurs in only a minority of patients.

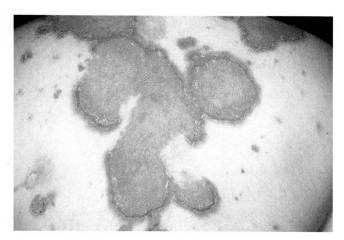

Figure 3 Discoid lupus rashes are hyperpigmented at the circumference and often depigmented centrally.

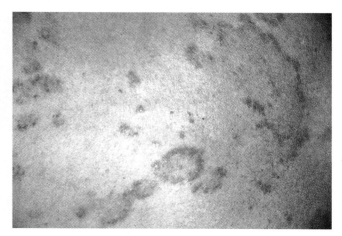

Figure 4 The rash of subacute cutaneous lupus is polycyclic and persistent.

MUSCULOSKELETAL INVOLVEMENT

The arthritis of SLE is typically painful, transient, and symmetrical, involving the wrists, small joints of the hands, elbows, knees, and ankles. Swelling and redness are modest. Less often, SLE arthritis will present as asymmetrical oligoarthritis or intensely inflamed, sustained polyarthritis resembling that of rheumatoid arthritis. Although deformity may occur as a result of ligamentous laxity (reversible subluxations, Jaccoud arthropathy),[36] rheumatoid-like joint destruction is uncommon.

Inflammatory myositis occurs primarily in patients with overlap features with scleroderma or dermatomyositis. It presents as proximal myopathy; serum levels of muscle enzymes are modestly elevated; and results of electromyography, magnetic resonance imaging, and muscle biopsy, if done, are similar to those seen in dermatomyositis. However, abnormal enzyme levels associated with proximal muscle tenderness or weakness are sufficient for diagnosis in a patient with established SLE.

Lupus does not involve bone directly. However, bone involvement can occur secondary to organ system failure (e.g., renal failure), severe illness (e.g., osteoporosis from inactivity or catabolic state), or treatment (e.g., corticosteroid-induced osteoporosis or avascular necrosis).

Osteoporosis presents as atraumatic fractures of vertebrae or long bones. Its occurrence is a severe threat to SLE patients, even premenopausal women, because of the frequent use of corticosteroids for treatment and because of inactivity attendant upon polyarthritis and systemic illness.

Avascular necrosis (osteonecrosis) most often occurs in patients who have had a severe flare treated with high-intensity corticosteroid therapy, but this complication can develop in patients who have never received corticosteroid treatment. Marked cushingoid features during steroid treatment and Raynaud phenomenon may be predictors of its occurrence.[37] The femoral head is the most commonly involved site, but shoulders, ankles, wrists, metacarpals, and shafts of long bones are also vulnerable.[38] Typically, affected areas become painful at the initial occurrence of infarction and again years later when the necrotic bone collapses. The most typical presentation of osteonecrosis is sudden hip pain 2 or 3 years after a major flare of lupus. Some patients receiving infusions of high-dose intravenous methylprednisolone complain of intense pain at preexisting osteonecrotic sites during and shortly after the infusion. Reducing the corticosteroid dose at the time of occurrence of pain has no effect on the course of the complication.

GASTROINTESTINAL AND HEPATIC INVOLVEMENT

Esophageal dysfunction is rare in SLE; it occurs primarily in patients with severe Raynaud phenomenon or in patients with scleroderma overlap disease. Gastroduodenal ulcer may occur as a result of treatment but is not directly linked to SLE. Ischemia of the small and large intestines may result from systemic vasculitis; it presents as abdominal angina, pneumatosis intestinalis, infarction or perforation, or pseudo-obstruction. Intestinal ischemia is a rare complication, occurring only in the most severely ill patients.[39]

Diverticulitis often develops in patients with long-standing SLE, especially after prolonged treatment with corticosteroids. The symptoms of diverticulitis are easily masked by corticosteroid therapy. Consequently, diverticular perforation or ab-

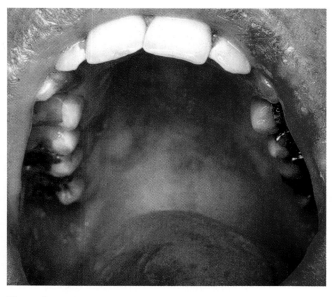

Figure 5 Painless mouth ulcers, most often found on the hard palate but also found on the gums and buccal mucosa, are characteristic of more severe lupus.

Table 5 Cardiovascular Manifestations of SLE

Pleuropericarditis
Libman-Sacks endocarditis
Valve insufficiency
Valve stenosis
Ischemic cardiomyopathy
   Accelerated atherosclerosis
   Antiphospholipid antibody syndrome
   Hypertensive heart disease
   Vasculitis
Hypertensive heart disease
Pulmonary hypertension
Peripheral arterial insufficiency
   Vasculitis
   Atherosclerosis
   Antiphospholipid antibody syndrome
Peripheral venous thrombosis
Raynaud phenomenon
Complete congenital heart block in newborns with neonatal
   lupus erythematosus

scess is frequently misdiagnosed, especially in young SLE patients.

Chemical hepatitis may follow use of nonsteroidal anti-inflammatory drugs (lupus patients appear to be unusually susceptible to this side effect) or other drugs, such as azathioprine.[40] Occasional patients suffer concomitant autoimmune hepatitis or primary biliary cirrhosis. In the absence of other causes, abnormalities of liver enzyme levels because of SLE are uncommon.

HEMATOLOGIC INVOLVEMENT

Leukopenia is such a regular feature of SLE that its absence, in untreated disease, should raise suspicion that the diagnosis is incorrect or that infection or tissue necrosis is present. Usually, lymphocyte counts show greater reductions than do granulocyte counts: a leukocyte count in the range of $3.5/mm^3$, with 10% lymphocytes, is usual. Leukopenia of this degree seldom places patients at serious risk of infection. There is usually no need to administer granulocyte-macrophage colony-stimulating factor (GM-CSF). Although GM-CSF is effective in severe leukopenia, there are anecdotal reports that administration of this agent may induce lupus flare.

Thrombocytopenia in SLE is usually low-grade, with platelet counts greater than $50,000/mm^3$. Severe thrombocytopenia may occur, however; idiopathic thrombocytopenic purpura (ITP) may be an initial presentation of SLE.

SLE may result in anemia of chronic disease and anemia from autoimmune hemolysis. The anemia of chronic disease in SLE patients responds to administration of recombinant erythropoietin.

NEUROLOGIC INVOLVEMENT

Neurologic signs and symptoms represent one of the most serious and least understood aspects of SLE. The primary neurologic manifestations of SLE consist of generalized and focal (usually vascular) brain disease, myelopathy, and peripheral neuropathy. Secondary neurologic events can also occur; these include seizures from hypertension or hemorrhage, delirium from drugs or uremia, brain or spinal cord abscess, and stroke from atheroma or embolus. Attribution of a specific neurologic symptom to active lupus (which is treatable with immunosuppression), as opposed to a complication of lupus or its treat-

ment (which is treatable by ameliorating the offending problem) requires deep investigation and good clinical judgment. Confusion about diagnostic criteria for neurologic lupus led the ACR to publish nomenclature and case-definition criteria for these syndromes.[41]

General Brain Disease

Patients with SLE frequently complain of progressive cognitive dysfunction, such as confusion, forgetfulness, and so-called foggy thinking.[42,43] Retrospective and cross-sectional studies document a high frequency of poor performance on tests of cognitive function, particularly in the executive, short-term memory, and verbal processing spheres.[44,45] It is not known whether this deficit results from immunologic attack on the brain (by antineuronal or other autoantibodies) or diffuse vascular disease. Cognitive dysfunction may respond to corticosteroid therapy. It seldom progresses to advanced dementia.

Headaches are common in SLE. A special form of migraine called lupus headache has been described, but whether it exists as a definable entity remains a matter of debate.

Focal Brain Disease

Seizures, strokes, cranial neuropathies (including blindness), and cerebellar dysfunction may occur in SLE. These events are assumed to result from vascular occlusion, but they may occur in patients with no known thrombotic diathesis, embolization, atherosclerosis, or vasculitis. Stroke is one of the most common presentations of the antiphospholipid antibody syndrome. Seizures are most common in severely active, febrile, multisystem disease. In this circumstance, they generally do not persist after the disease is brought under control.[46]

Myelopathy

Transverse myelitis occurs in two patterns: (1) abrupt onset, with progression in hours from the first symptom, often heralded by a burning, dysesthetic pain in the legs; and (2) slower progression, in a stuttering fashion, worsening over days. Unless treated immediately and aggressively, both forms may progress to advanced paraparesis or paraplegia. Although few direct data exist to support these hypotheses, it is likely that the first form represents vascular occlusion with spinal cord ischemia and the second form represents inflammatory disease. It is mandatory to exclude a space-occupying mass in all such patients.

A slowly progressive and intermittent myelopathy, very much resembling multiple sclerosis (so-called MS-like or lupoid sclerosis), develops in some lupus patients. There is no definitive way to exclude concomitant MS in these patients except by the association of the myelopathy with SLE and by its failure to progress in the way MS usually does. In this form of lupus myelopathy, cerebrospinal fluid examinations do not reveal oligoclonal bands, and MRI studies are atypical for MS.

Peripheral Neuropathy

Stocking-and-glove neuropathy is a slowly progressive lesion that tends to occur in patients with continuing, active disease. Its pathogenesis is unclear; it may result from direct immune attack on peripheral nerves or from vasculitic occlusion of the vasa nervorum. Abrupt loss of motor and sensory function, such as sudden occurrence of footdrop or wristdrop, is diagnosed as mononeuritis multiplex. This is a very serious manifestation indicating vasculitis of the vasa nervora; it implies systemic vasculitis, as well.

RENAL INVOLVEMENT

Approximately half of lupus patients develop lupus nephritis, and approximately 10% overall will progress to dialysis or transplantation. Lupus nephritis presents as proteinuria, celluria, hypertension, or rising serum creatinine, all of variable degree. In its early stages, lupus nephritis is painless and asymptomatic. In more advanced stages, edema, anemia, symptomatic hypertension, and symptomatic uremia occur. Patients with inflammatory forms of nephritis are usually hypocomplementemic; most have high levels of anti-DNA or anti-Sm antibody. Signs or symptoms of disease active in other organ systems need not accompany lupus nephritis.

The World Health Organization (WHO) has created a standard classification of lupus nephritis (now under consideration for revision) that identifies five biopsy-proven types of disease [see Table 6]. Amendments to this classification include the addition of activity and chronicity indices, which delineate acute necrosis, inflammatory infiltrate, crescent formation, scarring, and tubular atrophy to provide further prognostic information.[9] The WHO classification is a light microscopic classification. Additional information is obtainable from electron microscopy, which demonstrates immune complex deposits in subepithelial spaces in membranous lupus nephritis and in subendothelial spaces in proliferative lupus nephritis, as well as in mesangial locations. Characteristic tubuloreticular structures, thought to be RNA degradation products, also appear. Immunofluorescence studies demonstrate IgG, IgM, and C3 deposits in the same distributions. Vascular inflammation or endothelial proliferation is also seen.

Although lupus nephritis may present as anuria, acute hypertension, or fluid retention, most often it is first noted by an abnormal urinalysis. If left untreated, lupus nephritis progresses to renal insufficiency over months to years. Biopsy is necessary primarily when the result will change treatment. Urinalysis and blood chemistry results correlate only roughly with biopsy findings [see Table 7].

SPECIAL PRESENTATIONS

Neonatal Lupus Syndrome

Approximately 25% of infants born to mothers with anti–SS-A or anti–SS-B antibody will develop a photosensitive rash or thrombocytopenia, both of which are transient. A very small portion of these infants will develop, in utero, complete congenital heart block. Both the cardiac and the skin manifestations constitute the neonatal lupus syndrome. Either can be present independently. The syndrome appears to result from transplacental passage of maternal antibody, and it subsides when the antibody disappears. However, the heart block persists and may be lethal.

Antiphospholipid Antibody Syndrome

Between one third and one half of lupus patients have anticardiolipin antibody, lupus anticoagulant, or both. When the IgG or IgM isotypes are present in high titer, patients are susceptible to recurrent thromboembolic disease, thrombocytopenia, livedo reticularis, and cardiac valvular disease. Women are susceptible to recurrent pregnancy loss. These symptoms, combined with positive blood tests, constitute the antiphospholipid antibody syndrome (APS).[47] In the absence of lupus, the disorder is termed the primary antiphospholipid antibody syndrome (PAPS). When lupus or another rheumatic disease is present, the syndrome is designated secondary APS. Current research suggests that the true antigen for the syndrome is the phospholipid binding protein, beta2 glycoprotein I, rather than negatively charged phospholipids themselves. In some patients, antibody to an alternative phospholipid binding protein, such as prothrombin, induces the same syndrome. It is not known what induces clotting events in individual patients. The sites of thrombosis are not inflammatory and are best treated by anticoagulation rather than by immunosuppression.

LABORATORY TESTS

Tests of a variety of body fluids may be abnormal in patients with SLE [see Table 8]. Not all tests are abnormal in all patients. If lupus is suspected, an antinuclear antibody test, a complete blood count, and a urinalysis should be performed; if the results of these tests are all normal, SLE is excluded. However, because lupuslike illnesses are also usually suspected, it is often efficient also to obtain at first visit the following tests: erythrocyte sedimentation rate or C-reactive protein level; assays for antibodies against double-stranded DNA (dsDNA), Sm, RNP, SS-A, and SS-B; partial thromboplastin time (or other screening test for lupus anticoagulant) and cardiolipin antibodies; and a chemistry profile that includes liver function tests and serum creatinine level.

The antinuclear antibody (ANA) assay is a screening test for lupus. The ANA assay is almost always positive in high titer (>

Table 6 World Health Organization (WHO) Classification of Renal Biopsies

WHO Type	Name	Description	Clinical Presentation
I	Normal	Normal	Normal urinalysis, normal function
II	Mesangial	Infiltrating cells and proliferation of mesangium	Mild proteinuria, celluria; normal function
IIIa	Focal and segmental proliferative	Infiltrating cells and immune complex deposits in portions of the glomerulus and in < 50% of glomeruli	Variable proteinuria, celluria, normal function
IIIb	Diffuse proliferative	Infiltrating cells and moderate immune complex deposits in entire glomeruli and in > 50% of glomeruli	Variable proteinuria; celluria; often severe, decreasing function
IV*	Diffuse proliferative	Infiltrating cells and marked immune complex deposits in entire glomeruli and in > 50% of glomeruli	Moderate to marked proteinuria; celluria; often severe, decreasing function
V*	Membranous	Marked immune complex deposits without inflammatory cells	Marked proteinuria, slowly decreasing function

*Some patients have combined IV and V (membranoproliferative disease).

Table 7   Likely Renal Biopsy Findings According to
Urinalysis and Serum Creatinine Results

Urinalysis		Creatinine Level	Most Likely Pathology
Protein	Cells		
None	None	Normal	Normal or mesangial
Little	WBCs	Normal	Mesangial, focal proliferative
Moderate	WBCs, RBCs	Normal	Mesangial, focal or diffuse proliferative
Moderate	WBCs, RBCs, casts	Normal or elevated	Focal or diffuse proliferative
Severe	WBCs, RBCs, casts	Normal or elevated	Diffuse proliferative, membranoproliferative
Severe	Few	Normal or elevated	Membranous
Moderate	WBCs	Normal or elevated	Interstitial (tubular) disease (in patients with acidosis or electrolyte abnormalities)

1:80) in untreated patients with active disease, but a positive result does not by itself confirm a diagnosis of lupus. Only the anti-dsDNA antibody and anti-Sm antibodies, when present in high titer, are diagnostic of lupus. Anti-dsDNA antibody and complement levels are rough guides to disease activity, but many patients remain well for long periods of time with severely abnormal tests. Hypocomplementemia reflects proliferative lupus nephritis but not other aspects of SLE, including membranous lupus nephritis. The erythrocyte sedimentation rate remains elevated in many otherwise well SLE patients, as does the C-reactive protein level.

Brain Imaging Studies

Evaluation of neurologic involvement in SLE is complex. MRI scans, usually with contrast, are indicated for any clinical suspicion of central nervous system disease, such as seizures, cognitive dysfunction, new severe headache, chorea, or stroke symptoms. CT scans are far less definitive, except in stroke. Cerebral angiography or magnetic resonance angiography (MRA) is rarely helpful.

CT and MRI scans of the brain frequently demonstrate atrophy and infarcts (the latter including hyperintense areas in the white matter). These lesions correlate poorly with neurologic disease other than stroke syndromes.[13] Fluorodeoxyglucose positron emission tomography (PET), magnetic resonance spectrography (MRS), and single-photon emission computed tomography (SPECT) are frequently abnormal even in asymptomatic patients and correlate poorly with all but the most severe neuropsychiatric disease.[48] Interpretation of abnormal studies in asymptomatic patients is uncertain.[49,50]

Vascular Evaluation

Vascular evaluation is indicated when there is clinical suspicion of medium-size vascular occlusion. Ultrasound, Doppler studies, angiography, and MRA can demonstrate thromboembolic disease from antiphospholipid antibody or atherosclerosis. The small vessel vasculitis that occurs in SLE is usually beyond the resolution of these technologies.

Renal Evaluation

All lupus patients should have urinalyses performed, preferably at each clinic visit, because renal disease may appear de novo at any time. All patients with any abnormality on urinalysis or with an abnormal blood urea nitrogen (BUN) or serum creatinine level should have monitoring of 24-hour urine protein and creatinine clearance no less often than every 6 months. It is important to consider the results of renal testing in context:

a serum creatinine of 1.2 mg/dl may be within the laboratory range of normal, but in a 110 lb young woman, a level that high is very likely abnormal. Falling creatinine clearance always demands evaluation, even when the patient is clinically well.

Kidney biopsy   The primary indication to perform a kidney biopsy is to help the physician make a treatment decision. Although abnormal biopsies may be found in asymptomatic patients with normal urinalyses, it is not clear whether treatment of such patients improves outcome. The well patient with normal urinalysis results and normal renal function generally does not need a kidney biopsy, even if anti-DNA antibody is high and complement is low. The very ill patient with multisystem disease, including abnormal urinalysis results and abnormal renal function, likely will be treated aggressively anyway and does not need a kidney biopsy. The patient with mild systemic disease, mild urinary abnormalities, or both generally should undergo biopsy, because the decision for conservative or aggressive treatment may depend on the result. Occasionally, a biopsy is done to document end-stage, untreatable disease and thereby permit withdrawal of therapy. However, renal ultrasonography can usually provide the same information.

Cardiac Evaluation

Cardiac monitoring with echocardiography or stress tests is unnecessary on a routine basis. Because of the high frequency of accelerated atherosclerosis, however, any occurrence of dyspnea, dyspepsia, or shoulder or arm pain merits consideration of ischemic cardiac disease.

Differential Diagnosis

The differential diagnosis of lupus involves two linked questions: does the patient have a rheumatic disease, and if so, which one?

NONRHEUMATIC ILLNESSES THAT MIMIC SLE

The syndrome of fever, cytopenia, rash, and adenopathy suggests many infections, including HIV, cytomegalovirus, mononucleosis, and bacterial endocarditis. Acute polyarthritis, rash, and cytopenias can result from many viral infections, such as hepatitis, parvovirus, rubella, and others. These syndromes resolve spontaneously within several weeks. This syndrome also suggests hematologic malignancies, primarily the lymphomas, leukemias, and myelodysplastic syndromes. Although the presence of antinuclear antibody is common in many of these illnesses, the presence of anti-DNA or anti-Sm

Table 8 Commonly Abnormal Tests on Body Fluids in SLE

Test	Abnormality	Interpretation
CBC	Normochromic anemia, leukopenia (WBC ~3,000 , thrombocytopenia)	Active SLE
ESR and CRP	Elevated	Active SLE
Urinalysis	Proteinuria, hematuria, leukocyturia, cylindruria	Active lupus nephritis
Coombs and reticulocyte count	Positive, high	Hemolytic anemia
APTT, dRVVT	High	If confirmed with mixing test, lupus anticoagulant
Antinuclear antibody	Strongly positive	Positive in almost all patients during active disease; not specific for lupus
Anti-dsDNA antibody	Strongly positive	Positive in two thirds to three quarters of patients during active disease, diagnostic of lupus
Anti-Sm antibody	Positive	Positive in one quarter to one third of patients; diagnostic of lupus
Anti-SS-A, anti-SS-B, and anti-RNP antibodies	Positive	Positive in one third of patients; nonspecific
Anticardiolipin antibody	Positive	Antiphospholipid antibody syndrome
Complement C3, C4, and CH50	Low	Lupus nephritis likely; also hemolytic anemia and cryoglobulinemia
Cryoglobulin	Present	Active SLE
BUN and serum creatinine	Elevated	Severe lupus nephritis, drug toxicity
Liver function tests	Elevated	Drug toxicity (rarely, active SLE)
CSF protein and cells	Elevated	Present in a minority of patients with CNS SLE
Synovial fluid	WBC 5,000–10,000, normal glucose level	Lupus arthritis
Pleural fluid, pericardial fluid	WBC 5,000–10,000, normal glucose level, low complement, LE cells present	Lupus serositis

APTT—activated partial thromboplastin time   BUN—blood urea nitrogen   CBC—complete blood count   CNS—central nervous system   CRP—C-reactive protein   CSF—cerebrospinal fluid   dRVVT—dilute Russell viper venom time   ESR—erythrocyte sedimentation rate   WBC—white blood cells

antibodies is not; also uncommon are the specific rashes of lupus; nephritis; and vascular manifestations such as periungual telangiectasia and vasculitic papules. Photosensitivity and frontal alopecia are also characteristics of lupus that do not occur in these other illnesses.

Non-SLE causes of nephritis include poststreptococcal glomerulonephritis, Goodpasture disease, genetic nephropathies, and toxemia. The rash of rosacea is commonly mistaken for that of lupus. ITP or autoimmune hemolytic anemia may occur as isolated illnesses or as part of the multisystemic involvement of lupus. In these circumstances, full clinical and serologic evaluation for lupus will place the findings in proper context.

RHEUMATIC ILLNESSES THAT RESEMBLE SLE

Lupus may resemble a variety of other rheumatic diseases [*see Table 1*]. These include rheumatoid arthritis and Sjögren syndrome [*see Chapter 112*], as well as scleroderma [*see Chapter 115*]. The polyarthritic presentation of lupus is very similar to that of rheumatoid arthritis, Lyme disease, and other rheumatic illnesses. Early scleroderma often presents with bilateral hand edema that is mistaken for polyarthritis.

Dermatomyositis [*see Chapter 116*] peaks in three age groups: 5 to 10 years of age, late teens and early 20s, and older than 45 years. The rash of dermatomyositis is similar to that of lupus, but the former tends to involve the eyes differently: in dermatomyositis, telangiectasia causes the so-called heliotrope appearance of the eyelids; lupus rashes involve the eyebrows, but the malar rash stops abruptly at the orbits. Also, the rash in dermatomyositis commonly spares the ear canals, whereas the ear canals are commonly involved in lupus. Periungual telangiectasia is more dramatic in dermatomyositis than in lupus; it also occurs in scleroderma. Rash over the small joints of the hands suggests dermatomyositis; rash between the joints suggests lupus.

Compared with SLE, rheumatoid arthritis occurs in older persons (40 to 60 years of age) and has less of a female predominance (2:1 to 3:1). Although morning stiffness, fatigue, and weight loss are common in patients with rheumatoid arthritis, specific visceral multisystem disease is not. Leukocytosis rather than leukopenia is characteristic of rheumatoid arthritis. Renal disease is very rare, and when it does occur, it is attributable to tubular disease or amyloidosis rather than to glomerulonephritis. High fever does not occur in rheumatoid arthritis. From 10% to 20% of patients with rheumatoid arthritis have antinuclear antibodies; a small percentage have low-titer anti-DNA antibodies, and a minority have anti–SS-A and anti–SS-B antibodies. Complement levels are usually elevated. Rheumatoid factor is present in 80% of patients with rheumatoid arthritis, compared with its presence in 25% of lupus patients.

OVERLAP DISEASE

Some patients have symptoms suggestive of lupus (most commonly, arthritis, pleuritic pain, and cytopenia) but lack the specific diagnostic criteria for lupus (e.g., butterfly rash, glomerulonephritis, and high-titer anti-DNA or anti-Sm antibody). Other patients have lupuslike symptoms together with findings suggestive of rheumatoid arthritis, dermatomyositis, or scleroderma. Patients with no definable serology and a nondescript clinical picture are defined as having undifferentiated connective tissue disease (UCTD). Still other patients have inflammatory myositis, Raynaud phenomenon, and sclerodactyly together with very high titer antibodies to the ribonucleoprotein antigen (U1 RNP) and no anti-DNA or anti-Sm antibody. This set of findings is defined as mixed connective tissue disease (MCTD).

The differentiation of SLE from UCTD, MCTD, and Sjögren syndrome depends on the extent and pattern of different organ involvement (glomerulonephritis is rare in all those disorders except lupus) and on the accompanying serologic abnormalities. High-titer anti-DNA antibody or anti-Sm antibody generally indicates lupus; high-titer anti-RNP antibody with no other positive antibodies indicates MCTD; anti–SS-A and anti–SS-B antibodies are consistent with Sjögren syndrome but occur in lupus and rheumatoid arthritis, as well. Occasionally, patients have characteristic rheumatoid destructive arthritis, subcutaneous nodules, and high-titer rheumatoid factor and anti-DNA antibody. These patients, as well as those with other overlap features, should be treated as if they have both diseases.

The prognosis in patients with UCTD tends to be more benign than that in patients with SLE. Patients with MCTD do not develop glomerulonephritis, but the long-term prognosis for patients with this disorder is worsened by the eventual development of pulmonary hypertension.

Treatment

ACUTE DISEASE

Management recommendations for the acute symptoms of lupus depend on the severity and organ systems involved. Non–life-threatening manifestations, such as minor arthritis, arthralgia, malaise, myalgias, serositis, and low-grade fever can often be controlled with full doses of nonsteroidal anti-inflammatory drugs (NSAIDs). There is no specific preference among the NSAIDs, but lupus patients are unusually susceptible to hepatic and renal toxicities, which must be monitored. Also, in rare cases, lupus patients have developed abrupt high fever and meningitis after taking ibuprofen and similar drugs. Patients who do not respond to NSAIDs usually do respond to low doses (5 to 10 mg/day) of prednisone. As a rule, patients with inflammatory rashes, as well as patients anticipated to be on treatment for months or longer, should receive antimalarial therapy with hydroxychloroquine, 200 mg twice daily. Over a course of 3 months or more, hydroxychloroquine reduces arthralgia, myalgia, rash, fatigue, malaise and similar symptoms.[51] Patients expected to take corticosteroids for more than a few weeks should strongly consider bone-protective measures (see Osteoporosis, below). Such patients should also consider the addition of a lipid-lowering agent, such as a statin, to the regimen. Facial rashes, especially erythematous lesions with edema or telangiectasia, may respond to topical therapy with corticosteroid creams.

Alopecia may recover spontaneously, but it is not otherwise easily amenable to therapy. Wigs and falls or hair extenders are useful. Skillful use of makeup can cover most pigment changes caused by discoid lupus.

Low-dose corticosteroid therapy may be appropriate for modest thrombocytopenia or anemia. Leukopenia does not usually require treatment. High-dose corticosteroid therapy (60 mg of prednisone daily) is used for patients with severe systemic symptoms, renal disease, or other visceral disease that is potentially life threatening. Treatment should be initiated in split doses during the day, maintained for 4 to 6 weeks, and then tapered; too early reduction of dose usually results in recurrence of disease activity. If longer-term use of corticosteroids is anticipated, if vasculitis or life-threatening disease is present, or if corticosteroid toxicity is unacceptable, it is generally advisable to add immunosuppressive therapy. Immunosuppressive agents used for lupus include cyclophosphamide administered orally or intravenously, azathioprine, mycophenolate mofetil, and others. A standard regimen for active lupus nephritis includes a high-dose corticosteroid and intravenous cyclophosphamide. The cyclophosphamide is given in a dose of 1 g/m^2 monthly for 6 months and then every 3 months for 2 years.

Acute cerebral symptoms (other than stroke) are usually treated with high-dose corticosteroids. Hallucinations and other psychotic symptoms respond to antipsychotic medications such as haloperidol, which is often administered in conjunction with corticosteroids. Because psychosis may also result from the use of a high-dose of a corticosteroid alone, withdrawal of corticosteroids may be necessary in some cases. The distinction between so-called steroid psychosis and lupus psychosis is quite difficult. No single set of criteria distinguishes between the two; evidence of ongoing active lupus in other organ systems is an indication to treat the patient for lupus psychosis.

Many new therapies are being investigated. These are largely biologic therapies and include the use of drugs directed against receptors of immune-activating cells or recognition cells and the use of modulators of immune response, such as CD154, CTLA-4, and anti-C5b. Removal of antibody by passing patient plasma over an absorptive column is also being studied. Attempts at hormonal manipulation, as with dehydroepiandrosterone (DHEA), have had only modest success.

No single test informs the physician whether treatment for acute SLE is successful or not. Instead, it is necessary to monitor the entire clinical picture, including symptoms and results of physical examination, routine laboratory tests, and immune function studies.

INDICES OF DISEASE SEVERITY

Flare

Increase of inflammation in any SLE-affected organ system is known as flare. In a subpopulation of SLE patients, flare is a continuous, not a dichotomous, variable. In a given patient, it may occur in different organ systems at different rates and intensities; for instance, rash may become severe while nephritis remains stable. As a result, several different schemas for measuring flare exist. They differ in giving different weights to individual measures of disease activity (for instance, does new nephritis count more or less than new rash?) and whether serologic measures (antinuclear antibody titer, anti-DNA antibody, complement) do or do not count in the determination. The available indices—SLE Disease Activity Index (SLEDAI), Systemic Lupus Activity Measure (SLAM), and British Isles Lupus Assessment Group [BILAG])[52] generally agree in identifying flare in populations of patients but often disagree in specifics. There is poor consensus about distinguishing between day-to-day variation of disease activity and a definite flare. Several components of the indices (e.g., quantitation of rash or of arthritis) are sufficiently subjective that investigators in clinical trials must undergo standardization training before they can validate their scores on individual patients.

Flare in Pregnancy

Proteinuria, thrombocytopenia, and other pregnancy events that occur in the absence of lupus invalidate most scoring systems for pregnant patients. A specific instrument, the SLE Pregnancy Disease Activity Index (SLEPDAI), has been devised for use in pregnant patients.[53]

Damage

Recurring inflammation and vascular occlusion induces irreversible scarring and such permanent deficits as stroke, cataract, skin thinning, osteoporosis, osteonecrosis, and renal failure. It is common practice, therefore, to score SLE patients according to their activity (flare) indices and their damage indices. The most widely used damage index is the Systemic Lupus International Collaborating Clinics (SLICC).[54]

SLE DURING PREGNANCY

Pregnancy in patients with SLE, once thought to be contraindicated, is now a routine event. The complications of pregnancy in these patients are related to three major issues: abnormal renal function, the presence of antiphospholipid antibody, and the presence of anti–SS-A and anti–SS-B antibody. It remains debatable whether lupus is exacerbated by pregnancy, but consensus now exists that pregnant SLE patients do not need prophylactic increases of corticosteroid therapy; rather, they should be treated in the same manner as patients who are not pregnant, except that drugs with fetal toxicity should not be given.

Renal disease, particularly renal insufficiency, strongly predisposes to toxemia of pregnancy. Hypertension, reduced creatinine clearance, and active SLE all threaten the viability of the fetus. Conversely, women who enter pregnancy with no renal disease and no hypertension usually do well. Recurrent pregnancy loss, particularly in the second trimester, is one of the prime clinical manifestations of the antiphospholipid antibody syndrome; for antiphospholipid antibody–positive patients, the peripartum period is one of high risk for thromboembolic disease. Women who have antibody to the SS-A or SS-B antigen are at risk of delivering children with the neonatal lupus syndrome.

CHRONIC DISEASE AND COMPLICATIONS

The major treatment issue for long-term lupus patients is the prevention or management of damage to the arteries, kidneys, bones, and brain rather than the control of immune response and inflammation. The physician must anticipate chronic effects of both the disease and its therapy.

During treatment with high-dose corticosteroids, with or without immunosuppressive agents, avoidance of infections is a primary concern. Herpes zoster, tuberculosis, and a variety of bacterial infections are the primary threats. *Pneumocystis carinii* infection is seen relatively infrequently; most rheumatologists do not routinely suggest prophylaxis against this organism. Complications of long-term corticosteroid therapy include osteoporosis (see below) and cataracts, cutaneous striae, cuta-

neous hemorrhage, diabetes, and oral and vaginal candidiasis. In patients with long-standing disease, these complications produce as much morbidity as the disease itself.

Antiphospholipid Antibody Syndrome

Treatment of antiphospholipid antibody syndrome is anticoagulation to an international normalized ratio (INR) of 3.0. Warfarin and low-dose aspirin are used to prevent thrombotic manifestations of the syndrome; heparin or low-molecular-weight heparin are used in pregnant patients.[55] Recent data suggest that the addition of statin drugs, to downregulate endothelial activation, may also be of benefit.[56]

Atherosclerosis

Early-onset, severe atherosclerosis is a common problem in patients with long-standing SLE. Atherosclerosis most commonly presents as coronary and cerebral artery occlusion; peripheral vascular occlusion also occurs. The cause is unknown, but chronic inflammation, corticosteroid therapy, uncontrolled hypertension, diabetes, smoking, and other factors have been implicated. Most specialists in this area recommend early and vigorous treatment of known risk factors in all lupus patients. The atherosclerosis of lupus is managed in the same manner as atherosclerosis in other situations, except that vascular interventions in patients with antiphospholipid antibody syndrome are hazardous.

Osteonecrosis

Although the mechanism of osteonecrosis is not clearly known, many authorities believe that a steroid-induced increase in the volume of lipocytes increases pressure in the bone marrow, cutting off blood flow to the vulnerable areas. Consequently, if osteonecrosis is recognized before the joint has collapsed (usually by bone scan or MRI), trephining the bone to reduce intraosseous pressure (so-called core decompression) has been recommended. However, the validity of this theory and the efficacy of the treatment remain unproved. Usually, joint replacement is eventually required.[57]

Osteoporosis

Osteoporosis follows long-term corticosteroid therapy with sufficient frequency that all patients receiving such therapy should receive prophylaxis for this complication. High-dose oral calcium (i.e., 1,500 mg daily), vitamin D, and a bisphosphonate drug are the primary preventive measures; estrogen replacement may be considered in postmenopausal women who do not have antiphospholipid antibody. Weight-bearing exercise should be encouraged. Other prophylactic measures, including calcitonin and parathyroid hormone, may be appropriate. Because lupus patients are photosensitive, increased sun exposure to prevent osteoporosis is unwise. Bisphosphonates should not be used in women anticipating pregnancy.

Cardiac Disease

Inflammatory cardiomyopathy responds to corticosteroids; ischemic cardiomyopathy does not. Valvular insufficiencies and thromboemboli are late complications of lupus cardiac disease. Bacterial endocarditis rarely complicates this abnormality. Valvulitis generally does not respond to treatment, although a recent paper does state that acute valvulitis will respond to corticosteroid therapy.[58] Small numbers of patients require valve replacement, usually of the aortic or mitral valve. The mechanism of valvulopathy in SLE is unknown, as are methods of prevention.

PALLIATIVE CARE

A common mistake in the treatment of SLE is to assume that a given complaint reflects ongoing inflammatory disease, rather than irreversible damage, and that it can be controlled with anti-inflammatory and immunosuppressive therapy rather than palliation. Examples of such symptoms include seizures, dementia, and other neurologic syndromes associated with brain infarcts; cutaneous ulcers caused by long-standing vascular insufficiency; embolic phenomena from atherosclerosis; respiratory insufficiency from pulmonary fibrosis or pulmonary hypertension; arthritis from osteonecrosis, erosive rheumatoid-like arthritis, or tendinosis; and progressive renal insufficiency from arteriolonephrosclerosis, interstitial fibrosis, or glomerulosclerosis.

Dementia

Chronic neurologic disease, often in the form of dementia, is a long-term sequela of SLE. It may result from stroke (atherosclerotic, hypertensive, or thrombotic associated with antiphospholipid antibody), autoantibody attack on specific brain targets, small vessel occlusive disease, drugs, and other causes. Occasionally, patients are severely disabled. No effective prophylaxis is known.

Renal Failure

Patients with renal disease often need angiotensin-converting enzyme inhibitors for proteinuria, antihypertensives for hypertension, erythropoietin for anemia, and diuretics for edema. Renal failure in lupus occurs in two modes. In the first, acute inflammatory nephritis is characterized by distinctly abnormal urinalyses and clinically and serologically evident disease activity. Patients with this type of renal picture have rapidly rising serum creatinine levels and enter renal failure early after diagnosis. If treated aggressively, with high-dose corticosteroids and immunosuppressive drugs, renal failure will be reversible in approximately one third of these patients.[59] In the second mode of renal failure, which occurs only occasionally, patients will have renal failure from drug toxicity—usually NSAIDs—or acute tubular necrosis. Other manifestations of SLE are modified in uremia: rash is less prominent; and fever, cachexia, mucosal ulcers, and cytopenias are more prominent.

Most lupus patients, however, enter renal failure slowly after many years of disease. Characteristically, at the time renal failure first appears, the patient has little systemic illness and has had months to years of modest renal insufficiency (with creatinine clearance at 10 to 30 ml/min and serum creatinine below 3.5 mg/dl), slowly rising serum creatinine levels, relatively noninflammatory urinary sediments, and progressive anemia. Then, over a few months, the patient develops hypertension and fluid retention with or without cardiac failure. Abdominal pain is frequently present. Ultrasound shows small, fibrotic kidneys or thin, scarred renal cortices. Renal failure is only transiently reversible in such patients. Aggressive immunosuppressive therapy is not helpful at this stage; on the contrary, it may hasten renal deterioration and will complicate initiation of dialysis.

Less commonly, renal failure is caused by antiphospholipid antibody-associated thrombotic microangiopathy. In these cases, the presentation comprises modest proteinuria with bland urine sediment and slowly rising serum creatinine, often with moderate hypertension. Lupus vasculitis involving the kidneys tends to be abrupt in onset, with severely abnormal urinalyses, severe hypertension, and rapidly progressive renal failure. This complication is treated with high-dose corticosteroids and immunosuppression. However, full recovery is uncommon.

Lupus patients, particularly those who enter renal failure slowly, tolerate dialysis and renal transplantation well. However, preexisting cardiac, cerebral, and osteoarticular damage may be limiting factors. Patients who enter renal failure acutely often have other active systemic disease, with seizures and cytopenias being the most common. The common belief that lupus becomes inactive in renal failure is likely not true. Rather, in the majority of patients who enter dialysis, the lupus was already inactive systemically and remains so; probably, the renal failure results not from continuing disease but from progressive scarring. In the minority of patients who enter renal failure during an acute systemic flare, usually early in the course of the illness, active systemic disease tends to continue, and it represents a relative contraindication to renal transplantation. Patients on dialysis who have active SLE usually have high anti-DNA antibody levels and low complement levels. They respond to corticosteroid therapy, usually at lower doses than patients who are not on dialysis.

Prognosis

Prognosis in SLE has four elements: immediate prognosis for life, immediate prognosis for individual organ systems, and long-term prognosis for organ systems and for life.

During the early phases of lupus, complete reversal of almost all manifestations (i.e., rash, arthritis, fever, cytopenias, and nephritis) with aggressive therapy is expected. Exceptions include the scarring discoid rash, brain or spinal cord infarcts, and severe nephritis or nephrosis. In rare cases (< 5% of cases), patients have such severe disease that despite treatment, they rapidly progress to death within the first 2 years of illness. Because most newly diagnosed patients respond to therapy, 5-year survival is 80% to 90%, 10-year survival is 70% to 90%, and 20-year survival is nearly 70%.[6] Determinants of survival are age, renal disease, and race, with African Americans having lower overall survival than whites.[60]

One organ system (e.g., kidneys or platelets) may fail to respond completely to treatment but not directly threaten the patient's life. Such patients may be monitored without intervention. A patient may develop chronic renal insufficiency (e.g., serum creatinine, 3.0 mg/dl) or have persistent thrombocytopenia (platelet count, 30,000/mm^3) and be considered to be in remission and in no need of treatment.

Long-term prognosis is a function of organ damage from either SLE or its treatment. Pulmonary fibrosis and pulmonary hypertension respond poorly to therapy, although experimental protocols, such as infusion of prostacyclin, may be useful for pulmonary hypertension. Patients with cardiopulmonary failure who have no other system disease limitations are candidates for heart and lung transplantation. Lupus patients with renal failure are candidates for dialysis and for renal transplantation.

References

1. Zonana-Nacach A, Barr SG, Magder LS, et al: Damage in systemic lupus erythematosus and its association with corticosteroids. Arthritis Rheum 43:1801, 2000

2. Sontheimer RD: Systemic lupus erythematosus and the skin. Systemic Lupus Erythematosus, 3rd ed. Lahita RG, Ed. Academic Press, San Diego, 1999, p 631

3. Mongey A-B, Hess EV: Drug and environmental lupus: clinical manifestations and differences. Systemic Lupus Erythematosus, 3rd ed. Lahita RG, Ed. Academic Press, San Diego, 1999, p 929

4. Lockshin MD: Antiphospholipid syndrome. Kelley's Textbook of Rheumatology. Ruddy S, Harris ED Jr, Sledge C, Eds.WB Saunders, Philadelphia, 2001, p 1145

5. Buyon JP: Neonatal lupus syndromes. Systemic Lupus Erythematosus, 3rd ed. Lahita RG, Ed. Academic Press, San Diego, 1999, p 337

6. Gladman DD, Hochberg MC: Epidemiology of systemic lupus erythematosus. Systemic Lupus Erythematosus, 3rd ed. Lahita RG, Ed. Academic Press, San Diego, 1999, p 537

7. Karlson EW, Daltroy LH, Lew RA, et al: The relationship of socioeconomic status, race, and modifiable risk factors to outcomes in patients with systemic lupus erythematosus. Arthritis Rheum 40:47, 1997

8. Hahn BH: Antibodies to DNA. N Engl J Med 338:1359, 1998

9. Balow JE, Boumpas DT, Austin HA III: Systemic lupus erythematosus and the kidney. Systemic Lupus Erythematosus, 3rd ed. Lahita RG, Ed. Academic Press, San Diego, 1999, p 657

10. Bonfa E, Golombek SJ, Kaufman LD, et al: Association between lupus psychosis and anti–ribosomal P protein antibodies. N Engl J Med 317:265, 1987

11. DeGiorgio LA, Konstantinov KN, Lee SC, et al: Novel mechanism for brain injury in SLE: a subset of lupus anti-DNA antibodies cross-reacts with the NR2 glutamate receptor. Nature Med 7:1189, 2001

12. Walport MJ: Lupus, DNAse, and defective disposal of cellular debris. Nat Genet 25:135, 2000

13. Blanco P, Palucka AK, Gill M, et al: Induction of dendritic cell differentiation by IFN-alpha in systemic lupus erythematosus. Science 294:1540, 2001

14. Davies KA, Robson MG, Peters AM, et al: Defective Fc-dependent processing of immune complexes in patients with systemic lupus erythematosus. Arthritis Rheum 46:1028, 2002

15. Marrack P, Kappler J, Kotzin BL: Autoimmune disease: why and where it occurs. Nat Med 7:899, 2001

16. Davidson A, Diamond B: Autoimmune diseases. N Engl J Med 345:340, 2001

17. Reveille JD: Major histocompatibility complex class II and non–major histocompatibility complex genes in the pathogenesis of systemic erythematosus. Systemic Lupus Erythematosus, 3rd ed. Lahita RG, Ed. Academic Press, San Diego, 1999, p 67

18. Harley JB, Moser KL, Gaffney PM, et al: The genetics of human systemic lupus erythematosus. Curr Opin Immunol 10:690, 1998

19. Cook L, Agnello V: Complement deficiency and systemic lupus erythematosus. Systemic Lupus Erythematosus, 3rd ed. Lahita RG, Ed. Academic Press, San Diego, 1999, p 105

20. Zuniga R, Ng J, Peterson MG, et al: Low binding alleles of Fc gamma receptor types IIa and IIIa are inherited independently and are associated with systemic lupus erythematosus in Hispanic patients. Arthritis Rheum 44:361, 2001

21. James JA, Kaufman KM, Farris AD, et al: An increased prevalence of Epstein-Barr virus infection in young patients suggests a possible etiology for systemic lupus erythematosus. J Clin Invest 100:3019, 1997

22. Petri M, Robinson C: Review: oral contraceptives and systemic lupus erythematosus. Arthritis Rheum 40:797, 1997

23. Lockshin MD, Sammaritano LR, Schwartzman S: Lupus pregnancy. Systemic Lupus Erythematosus, 3rd ed. Lahita RG, Ed. Academic Press, San Diego, 1999, p 507

24. Ruiz-Irastorza G, Lima F, Alves J, et al: Increased rate of lupus flare during pregnancy and the puerperium: a prospective study of 78 pregnancies. Br J Rheumatol 35:133, 1996

25. Bynoe MS, Grimaldi CM, Diamond B: Estrogen up-regulates Bcl-2 and blocks tolerance induction of naive B cells. Proc Natl Acad Sci USA 97:2703, 2000

26. Cooper GS, Dooley MA, Treadwell EL, et al: Hormonal, environmental, and infectious risk factors for developing systemic lupus erythematosus. Arthritis Rheum 41:1714, 1998

27. Systemic lupus erythematosus in three ethnic groups: IX. Differences in damage accrual. LUMINA Study Group. Arthritis Rheum 44:2797, 2001

28. Salmon JE, Roman MJ: Accelerated atherosclerosis in systemic lupus erythematosus: implications for patient management. Curr Opin Rheumatol 13:341, 2001

29. Hochberg MC: Updating the American College of Rheumatology revised criteria for the classification of systemic lupus erythematosus (letter). Arthritis Rheum 40:1725, 1997

30. Lockshin MD, Sammaritano LR, Schwartzman S: Brief report: validation of the Sapporo Criteria for antiphospholipid antibody syndrome. Arthritis Rheum 43:440, 2000

31. Lahita RG: The clinical presentation of systemic lupus erythematosus. Systemic Lupus Erythematosus, 3rd ed. Lahita RG, Ed. Academic Press, San Diego, 1999, p 325

32. Lawrence EC: Systemic lupus erythematosus and the lung. Systemic Lupus Erythematosus, 3rd ed. Lahita RG, Ed. Academic Press, San Diego, 1999, p 719

33. Roldan CA, Shively BK, Crawford MH: Echocardiographic study of valvular heart disease associated with lupus erythematosus. N Engl J Med 335:1424, 1996

34. Lockshin MD, Salmon JE, Roman MJ: Atherosclerosis and lupus: a work in progress (editorial). Arthritis Rheum 44:2215, 2001

35. Roman MJ, Salmon JE, Sobel R, et al: Prevalence and relation to risk factors of carotid atherosclerosis and left ventricular hypertrophy in systemic lupus erythematosus and antiphospholipid antibody syndrome. Am J Cardiol 87:663, 2001

36. Bywaters EGL: Jaccoud's syndrome: a sequel to the joint involvement of systemic lupus erythematosus. Clin Rheum Dis 1:125, 1975

37. Mont MA, Glueck CJ, Pacheco IH, et al: Risk factors for osteonecrosis in systemic lupus erythematosus. J Rheumatol 24:645, 1997

38. Nagasawa K, Tsukamoto H, Tada Y, et al: Imaging study on the mode of development and changes in avascular necrosis of the femoral head in systemic lupus erythematosus: long-term observations. Br J Rheumatol 33:343, 1994

39. Toy LS, Mayer L: Nonhepatic gastrointestinal manifestations of systemic lupus erythematosus. Systemic Lupus Erythematosus, 3rd ed. Lahita RG, Ed. Academic Press, San Diego, 1999, p 733

40. Mackay IR: Hepatic disease and systemic lupus erythematosus: coincidence or convergence. Systemic Lupus Erythematosus, 3rd ed. Lahita RG, Ed. Academic Press, San Diego, 1999, p 747

41. The American College of Rheumatology Nomenclature and Case Definitions for Neuropsychiatric Lupus Syndromes. ACR Ad Hoc Committee on Neuropsychiatric Lupus Nomenclature. Arthritis Rheum 42:599, 1999

42. Hanly JG: Evaluation of patients with CNS involvement in SLE. Baillière's Clin Rheumatol 12:415, 1998

43. Harrison MJ, Gershengorn J: Despite low rate of global impairment in SLE patients, cognitive performance is less than expected (abstract). Arthritis Rheum 44:s197, 2001

44. Kozora E, Thompson LL, West SG, et al: Analysis of cognitive and psychological deficits in systemic lupus erythematosus patients without overt central nervous system disease. Arthritis Rheum 39:2035, 1996

45. Sanna G, Piga M, Terryberry JW, et al: Central nervous system involvement in systemic lupus erythematosus: cerebral imaging and serological profile in patients with and without overt neuropsychiatric manifestations. Lupus 9:573, 2000

46. Gladman DD, Urowitz MB, Slonim D, et al: Evaluation of predictive factors for neurocognitive dysfunction in patients with inactive systemic lupus erythematosus. J Rheumatol 27:2367, 2000

47. Wilson WA, Gharavi AE, Koike T, et al: International consensus statement on preliminary classification criteria for definite antiphospholipid syndrome: report of an international workshop. Arthritis Rheum 42:1309, 1999

48. Kozora E, West SG, Kotzin BL, et al: Magnetic resonance imaging abnormalities and cognitive deficits in systemic lupus erythematosus patients without overt central nervous system disease. Arthritis Rheum 41:41, 1998

49. Sibbitt WL Jr, Sibbitt RR, Brooks W: Neuroimaging in neuropsychiatric systemic lupus erythematosus. Arthritis Rheum 42:2026, 1999

50. West SG, Emlen W, Wener MH, et al: Neuropsychiatric lupus erythematosus: a ten-year prospective study on the value of diagnostic tests. Am J Med 99:153, 1995

51. A randomized study of the effect of withdrawing hydroxychloroquine sulfate in systemic lupus erythematosus. Canadian Hydroxychloroquine Study Group. N Engl J Med 324:150, 1991

52. Liang MH, Socher SA, Roberts WN, et al: Measurement of systemic lupus erythematosus activity in clinical research. Arthritis Rheum 31:817, 1988

53. Buyon JP, Kalunian KC, Ramsey-Goldman R, et al: Assessing disease activity in SLE patients during pregnancy. Lupus 8:677, 1999

54. Gladman DD, Goldsmith CH, Urowitz MB, et al: The Systemic Lupus International Collaborating Clinics/American College of Rheumatology (SLICC/ACR) Damage Index for systemic lupus erythematosus international comparison. J Rheumatol 27:373, 2000

55. Khamashta MA, Cuadrado MJ, Mujic F, et al: The management of thrombosis in the antiphospholipid-antibody syndrome. N Engl J Med 332:993, 1995

56. Meroni PL, Raschi E, Testoni C, et al: Statins prevent endothelial activation induced by antiphospholipid (anti-beta$_2$-glycoprotein I) antibodies: effect on the proadhesive and proinflammatory phenotype. Arthritis Rheum 44:2862, 2001

57. Mont MA, Fairbank AC, Petri M, et al: Core decompression for osteonecrosis of the femoral head in systemic lupus erythematosus. Clin Orthop 334:91, 1997

58. Nesher G, Ilany J, Rosenmann D, et al: Valvular dysfunction in antiphospholipid syndrome: prevalence, clinical features and treatment. Semin Arthritis Rheum 27:27, 1997

59. Kimberly RP, Lockshin MD, Sherman RL, et al: Reversible "end-stage" lupus nephritis: analysis of patients able to discontinue dialysis. Am J Med 74:361, 1983

60. Trends in deaths from systemic lupus erythematosus—United States, 1979–1998. MMWR Morb Mortal Wkly Rep 51(17):371, 2002

Acknowledgment

Figure 2b © 2002 Hospital for Special Surgery. http://www.Rheumatology.HSS.edu . All rights reserved. Used by permission.

115 Scleroderma and Related Diseases

George Moxley, M.D.

Scleroderma

DEFINITION AND CLASSIFICATION

Scleroderma, or systemic sclerosis, is a rare, slowly progressive rheumatic disease characterized by deposition of fibrous connective tissue in the skin and other tissues. It is often accompanied by vascular lesions, especially in the skin, lungs, and kidneys. No cure is known.

Scleroderma may be either systemic or localized. The systemic illness is either diffuse or limited. The limited form of systemic scleroderma, or CREST (calcinosis, Raynaud phenomenon, esophageal involvement, sclerodactyly, and telangiectasias), involves internal organs less often than diffuse scleroderma. Systemic scleroderma can be fatal; except when pulmonary hypertension is present, the limited form has a better prognosis than the diffuse form [*see Table 1*].

Localized scleroderma is confined to the skin, subcutaneous tissue, and muscle and is not accompanied by the Raynaud phenomenon, acrosclerosis, or visceral involvement. There are two forms of localized scleroderma: morphea, which presents as variable-sized plaques of skin induration, and linear scleroderma, which presents as bands of skin induration on the face or a single extremity. Linear scleroderma may be associated with muscle atrophy and involvement of the underlying bone. It usually afflicts children or young adults and may lead to significant growth impairment of the involved part. In morphea, the lesions may persist for months or years, after which improvement may occur [*see Table 1*]. Although there is a possibility of disfigurement, localized scleroderma is not a severe illness and is generally compatible with a normal life span.

EPIDEMIOLOGY

The Raynaud phenomenon is associated with scleroderma [*see* Diagnosis, Clinical Manifestations, *below*]. Primary Raynaud phenomenon (Raynaud phenomenon without underlying illness) is quite common, with up to 30% of young women having episodes.[1] A meta-analysis showed that the transition rate to a defined inflammatory rheumatic disease (e.g., scleroderma or lupus) is 3.2 per 100 patient-years of observation; the eventual development of an inflammatory rheumatic disease occurred in 12.6% of individuals. The best predictor of the development of inflammatory disease is an abnormal nailfold capillary pattern, which has a predictive value of 47%; a positive antinuclear antibody test has a predictive value of 30%.[2] Racial, genetic, and environmental factors have been proposed to influence scleroderma risk and disease pattern.[3] The overall global incidence of scleroderma is approximately 17 per one million population a year, with higher rates for women than for men. African Americans typically experience diffuse scleroderma more often than do other ethnic groups; whites are more often diagnosed with the CREST variant.[4] The prevalence in the United States is approximately 24 per 100,000 population[5]—fourfold to ninefold the prevalence in other countries. Mortality factors include diffuse disease, older age at onset, and internal organ involvement, particularly pulmonary and renal involvement. Some investigators have suggested that scleroderma is associated with various environmental exposures.[6] For example, workers exposed to polyvinylchloride may experience the Raynaud phenomenon and scleroderma-like skin thickening.[6] However, no substance has yet been convincingly linked with scleroderma.[7] Silicone breast implants have not been found to be associated with scleroderma.[6]

ETIOLOGY

The etiology of scleroderma is largely unknown. The disease shows familial aggregation consistent with a genetic component, and family history is the strongest risk factor.[8] Although the absolute risk of scleroderma among relatives is only about 1%, this risk represents a striking 11- to 158-fold increase over the risk in unrelated individuals.[9] One etiologic factor may be a fibrillin defect. Fibrillin is a macromolecule that is a component of elastic fibers; it is defective in Marfan syndrome. In an animal model (the tight-skin mouse, *tsk1*), a scleroderma-like condition is caused by an insertion into the fibrillin gene that apparently encodes a latent binding region for the transforming growth factor–beta (TGF-β) cytokine. One proposed explanation is that the abnormal fibrillin binds an increased number of fibroblast growth factors influencing nearby fibroblasts. The current knowledge extends to Oklahoma Choctaw scleroderma patients, who likely have a scleroderma-related genetic defect in the fibrillin chromosomal region either within or near the gene and probably inherited from a common ancestor.[9] However, other genes or environmental exposures are no doubt also involved.[9]

PATHOPHYSIOLOGY AND PATHOGENESIS

The common pathologic features of tissues with scleroderma involvement are progressive fibrosis, vascular abnormalities, and inflammation. Fibrosis involves an accumulation of excessive collagen and other extracellular matrix constituents, such as glycosaminoglycans and fibronectin. The vascular abnormalities are intimal hyperplasia with collagen deposition and adventitial fibrosis, capillary dropout, dilatation, tortuosity, and fibrotic atherosclerosis. The inflammatory changes may include cellular infiltration. These pathologic characteristics are believed to be the result of three or more interacting components: autoimmunity, an endothelial abnormality, and a skin fibroblast lesion. An alternative explanation is that these characteristics are the result of a disease process akin to graft versus host disease (GVHD).

Immune Cell and Cytokine Abnormalities

Activated thymus-derived lymphocytes predominate among the cells that infiltrate involved tissues; activated inflammatory

Table 1 Classification of Scleroderma

Form	Syndrome
Scleroderma (systemic sclerosis)	Diffuse skin involvement
	Limited skin involvement (CREST syndrome)
	Overlapping features of mixed connective tissue disease
Localized scleroderma	Morphea: single or multiple plaques or generalized lesions
	Linear scleroderma

CREST—calcinosis, Raynaud phenomenon, esophageal motility dysfunction, sclerodactyly, and telangiectasia

cells are also present. Such immune and inflammatory cells release a plethora of cytokines and soluble mediators. Of particular note are cytokines influencing fibroblast function: interleukin-1 (IL-1), IL-4, IL-6, IL-8, RANTES (regulated upon activation, normal T cell expressed and secreted), tumor necrosis factor (TNF), and TGF-β. TNF and interferon gamma are antifibrotic,[10] but the action of TGF-β results in a pattern of tissue damage similar to the pattern seen in scleroderma. TGF-β stimulates fibroblasts and vascular smooth muscle cells to make collagen, and it stimulates endothelial cells to make endothelin-1, which, in turn, causes vasoconstriction and collagen production. B cells are also activated in patients with scleroderma, but these cells do not appear to play a primary role. Although there are autoantibodies relatively specific for scleroderma, they do not appear to result in tissue damage.

Fibroblast Abnormalities

As with lymphocytes and macrophages showing activation in scleroderma, fibroblasts are also metabolically activated.[11] Such activated cells overproduce collagen, other extracellular matrix molecules, and cellular adhesion molecules.[12] The reasons why collagen gene expression is increased and sustained have not been fully explained. One possible explanation is that the presence of cytokines such as IL-4 and TGF-β strongly foster collagen production.[10] Although activated macrophages may produce TGF-β initially, TGF-β may trigger its own production from target fibroblasts. Thus, the sustained, progressive fibrosis seen in scleroderma may be the result of a process in which macrophages give rise to TGF-β, which then activates fibroblasts to secrete collagen and other matrix molecules while also inducing its own production from fibroblasts.[10]

Vascular Abnormalities

Vessels in involved tissues show disrupted pattern and function, characterized by altered endothelial permeability, adhesion of platelets and leukocytes to endothelium, and the presence of inflammatory cells.[13] Endothelial cells express increased numbers of adhesion molecules necessary for inflammatory cell adhesion and extravasation. Capillaries become obliterated but are not replaced; involved tissues may become ischemic and then reperfused. The Raynaud phenomenon [see Diagnosis, Clinical Manifestations, below] is a hallmark vascular lesion that likely represents an exaggerated response of a stiff vessel wall to a typical environmental exposure. Microscopic analysis of the nailfolds of patients with scleroderma and Raynaud phenomenon reveals capillary disappearance and dilatation. Normal vascular flow involves interactions between neural signals, circulating hormones, and mediators released from the vessel itself and from circulating cells. Neural signals are largely sympathetic and mediated through norepinephrine binding to vasoconstrictive alpha-adrenergic receptors or to vasodilating beta-adrenergic receptors. In scleroderma, small arteries develop concentric intimal fibrosis and thus become narrow; this narrowing in turn greatly increases the vascular reactivity to alpha$_2$-adrenergic agents.

Chimerism and Microchimerism

Chimerism denotes a state in which a person has cells derived from two or more other people. Many patients who undergo allogeneic marrow transplantation develop GVHD—a scleroderma-like illness characterized by progressive skin induration with ulceration, with possible involvement of the gas-

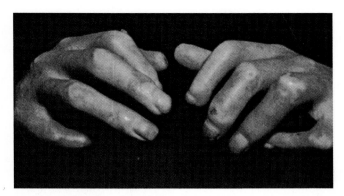

Figure 1 Severe involvement of the hands in a patient with long-standing scleroderma includes flexion contractures of the fingers related to fibrosis of the skin and of subcutaneous tissues. Increased pigmentation has occurred, and melanin loss (vitiligo) is evident in some areas. The distal aspects of the terminal phalanges in some fingers have undergone resorption or shortening. This process, termed autoamputation, usually occurs without ulceration of the terminal digit; the mechanism is unknown.

trointestinal tract, lungs, skeletal muscle, and salivary and lacrimal glands. GVHD occurs when engrafted cells react to the patient's native cells. Microchimerism, or low-level chimerism, may occur in association with pregnancy. Women who have given birth may have circulating fetal cells for many years, and maternal cells may persist in adult sons. It has therefore been suggested that scleroderma represents a sort of GVHD in which remaining foreign cells (persisting fetal cells or transfused cells) attack native body constituents.[14,15] Indeed, male DNA has been found more frequently and in higher concentrations in the circulation of women with scleroderma who have had a previous male delivery than in women without scleroderma who have also had a male delivery. In addition, microchimerism has been found in the skin of mothers with scleroderma but not in the skin of healthy mothers. However, cause and effect are not yet established,[9] and this pathogenetic explanation does not fully account for why scleroderma pa-

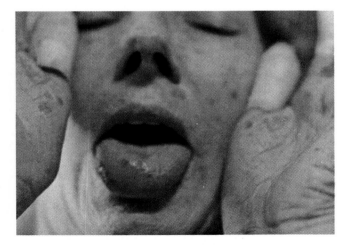

Figure 2 Telangiectasias appear on the hands, face, and tongue in a patient with the CREST (calcinosis, Raynaud phenomenon, esophageal involvement, sclerodactyly, and telangiectasias) variant of scleroderma. Thumbs are bandaged because of chronic ulcerations associated with the Raynaud phenomenon.

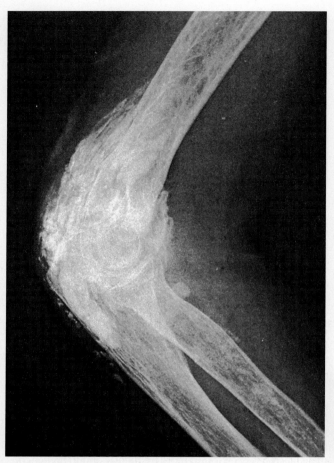

Figure 3 **In scleroderma, extensive calcinosis (hydroxyapatite crystal deposition) may be found in connective tissues and around joints. If extensive, calcinosis is usually associated with at least partial loss of joint motion.**

tients have the Raynaud phenomenon and renal disease, whereas those with chronic GVHD do not.

DIAGNOSIS

Clinical Manifestations

Skin The first signs of scleroderma in the skin are swelling and thickening of the fingers and hands, with or without involvement of the face; later in the illness, other areas of skin may become thickened. Involvement of the trunk and arms proximal to the elbows is associated with visceral involvement and a poorer prognosis. The skin continues to thicken during the first 2 to 3 years after the onset of disease; then the thickening ceases and may recede, giving the impression that the skin is softening. In subsequent years, skin atrophy occurs, with concomitant loss of hair, sebaceous glands, and sweat glands, as well as a loss of pliability. In addition, the skin becomes hidebound—tightly drawn and bound to underlying structures. Skin involvement is often most prominent in the hands and fingers (sclerodactyly); frequently, the face is also affected. A tightening of the facial skin results in decreased skin lines, a pursed appearance, and a diminution in the oral aperture. The tightness in the skin may limit mobility, especially in the fingers. Flexion contractures may also develop in the fingers [*see Figure 1*]. Several other skin abnormalities may accompany these changes. Telangiectasias

occur frequently and may be numerous [*see Figure 2*]. They are often most prominent on the face, hands, and oral mucosa. Calcinosis—the deposition of hydroxyapatite crystals in subcutaneous areas—may be limited or widespread and is usually located around joint capsules [*see Figure 3*]. Skin ulceration over calcific deposits may lead to drainage of a white material with a consistency resembling toothpaste. A diffuse increase in melanotic pigmentation may extend over the entire skin surface; areas of hypopigmentation are also commonly seen.

The Raynaud phenomenon is an episodic manifestation of numbness or pain accompanied by a two- or three-phase color change in the digits; these changes are triggered by cold temperatures or emotional stress and are relieved by warming the involved part. In severe cases, however, the relation to ambient temperature is sometimes less obvious. The episode typically begins with pallor, followed by cyanosis, and finally by redness caused by reactive hyperemia [*see Figure 4*]. Prolonged ischemia may lead to painful digits, ulceration, and even gangrene. Almost all patients (95%) with diffuse or limited scleroderma experience the Raynaud phenomenon. The Raynaud phenomenon is also seen in patients with other disorders, including other autoimmune diseases such as systemic lupus erythematosus (SLE), polymyositis, and several forms of vasculitis; in patients who are receiving certain drugs, such as

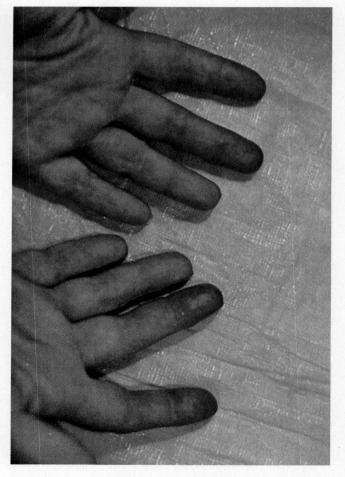

Figure 4 **Vascular pathology usually manifests itself as the Raynaud phenomenon in patients with scleroderma. The cyanotic phase of the Raynaud phenomenon often involves the distal two thirds of the second and third fingers of both hands.**

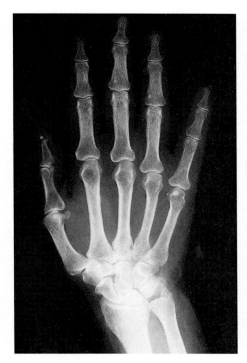
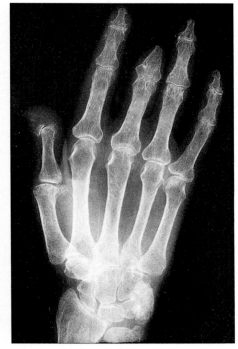

Figure 5 Over an 8-year period, radiographs taken of the hand of a patient with scleroderma demonstrate a progressive, terminal resorption of the digits. The earlier film (left) shows a loss of the spherical terminal portion of the distal phalanx of the thumb and a small, dense calcific deposit at the terminal aspect of the thumb. After an 8-year period, dramatic changes can be seen (right). An almost complete loss of the terminal phalanx of the thumb and a partial loss of the distal phalanges of the remaining fingers are observed. In addition, the entire distal phalanx of the third finger is lost along with part of the middle phalanx. Loss of the middle phalanx is less common than loss of the distal phalanges. A generalized osteopenia is present in the later stage, which is probably related to osteoporosis of disuse, and a calcific deposit has formed in the ulnar aspect of the wrist. The apparent narrowing of interphalangeal joint spaces may be associated with flexion contractures of the fingers, which are caused by the fibrous thickening of the connective tissues of the hand.

bleomycin, ergot derivatives, beta blockers, and methysergide; and after occupational exposure to vinyl chloride, cold temperatures, and vibrating tools.

In scleroderma, the Raynaud phenomenon is a manifestation of vasculopathy involving small arteries and capillaries; it occurs not only in the extremities but also in some involved viscera, such as the lungs and kidneys. Patients with scleroderma and the Raynaud phenomenon have characteristic capillary changes on nailfold microscopy. Nailfold microscopy consists of observation of the capillary structure of the periungual tissues with a handheld magnifying lens, such as that used in a standard ophthalmoscope. Patients with underlying scleroderma may exhibit loss of some capillaries and dilatation of capillaries in other nailfold areas. Such changes often occur in association with internal organ involvement and may be used to predict the development of diffuse scleroderma when visceral involvement is not clinically apparent.

Musculoskeletal system A mild, usually symmetrical, inflammatory arthritis can occur in scleroderma. Juxta-articular bone erosions occur frequently, especially in the distal interphalangeal joints, but the degree of destruction is usually less than that seen in rheumatoid arthritis. Flexion contractures of the fingers often develop and are most likely related to fibrosis of the tendons and joint capsules. Crepitus and friction rubs, detected by palpation or auscultation over tendons and bursas, are char-

acteristic findings related to fibrotic changes of underlying tissues. Another skeletal complication is acral osteolysis, which is the resorption of the terminal phalanges and surrounding soft tissue with consequent shortening of the digits [*see Figure 5*]. It may occur without infection or ulceration.

Patients with scleroderma may manifest one or more of a variety of muscle disorders.[16] Some scleroderma patients experience fatigue without objective evidence of muscle damage (i.e., normal creatine kinase [CK] levels, normal electromyographic [EMG] findings, and normal results on magnetic resonance imaging studies). Other patients have a simple myopathy with only minimal CK elevations, myopathic EMG findings, and fascial thickening or fibrosis on MRI. Yet others experience an inflammatory myositis manifested by substantial weakness with significant CK elevations, myopathic EMG changes, mononuclear cell infiltrates as evident in muscle biopsies, and brightness of muscle as shown on T_2-weighted MRI images.

GI tract Almost every part of the GI tract may be involved in scleroderma.[17] Sjögren syndrome, which causes dry eyes and dry mouth, occurs in about one third of patients with scleroderma. Esophageal hypomotility, which is demonstrated by cinefluoroscopic examination and manometric studies, occurs in more than 90% of patients with scleroderma, many of whom are asymptomatic [*see Figure 6*]. The absence of normal peristaltic waves in the lower two thirds of the esophagus may cause dysphagia; incompetence of the gastroesophageal sphincter leads to reflux esophagitis and sometimes may result in esophageal stricture. Barrett esophagus, esophageal carcinoma, and candidal esophagitis may ensue. Similarly, hypomotility of the stomach, small intestine, colon, and anorectal area may occur, possibly causing gastroparesis, pseudo-obstruction, colonic impaction, or impaired anorectal function. Telangiectasias may be present in the gastric mucosa and the mucosa of the small intestine and colon. Gas may dissect into the intestinal wall (pneumatosis intestinalis) and leak into the peritoneal cavity, simulating a perforated viscus. Characteristic wide-mouthed diverticula of the colon may develop; these are pathognomonic of scleroderma. The early lesions of the GI tract may be caused by autonomic nerve dysfunction; autonomic nerve dysfunction may in time lead to smooth muscle atrophy and irreversible muscle fibrosis of the gut. Primary biliary cirrhosis and drug-induced hepatitis may also be associated with scleroderma.

Lungs Pulmonary involvement represents an important cause of scleroderma-related morbidity and mortality[18,19]; scleroderma-related lung disease is the most frequent cause of death. Although scleroderma-related findings may range from associated malignancy and silicosis to calcinosis and hemorrhage, the most common findings are pulmonary vascular disease and interstitial inflammation and fibrosis. Isolated pulmonary hypertension is typically found in the CREST syndrome (prevalence for severe disease is about 10% in the limited cutaneous subset); interstitial pulmonary fibrosis may be found in both limited and diffuse scleroderma (at postmortem examination, the frequency is about 75%). Isolated pulmonary hypertension usually results in cough, dyspnea, and syncope; it has a severe prognostic outlook (5-year survival < 10%). Pulmonary hypertension is defined by a resting mean pulmonary arterial pressure greater than 25 mm Hg or an exercise-induced mean pulmonary arterial pressure greater than 30 mm Hg; in addition, pulmonary hypertension is often associated with abnormal diffusing capacity for carbon monoxide. Interstitial fibrosis is typically accompanied by dyspnea and cough; the 5-year survival is about 45%. Although chest roentgenograms may show linear and reticular abnormalities, high-resolution CT scanning is favored for the detection of early disease; on CT scans, alveolitis appears as patchy areas with a ground-glass appearance. Interstitial fibrosis appears to result from inflammatory alveolitis: the release of various cytokines and chemokines in the course of the inflammatory process results in fibroblast activation and extracellular matrix remodeling.

Heart Clinically evident scleroderma-related heart disease carries an adverse prognosis.[20] The myocardium is involved in approximately 20% to 25% of clinical cases of systemic scleroderma. Scleroderma-associated myocardial disease is typically characterized by patchy areas of myocardial fibrosis replacing normal muscle; this may cause hypertrophy and diminished cardiac output, particularly with exercise. Scleroderma-related myocardial fibrosis differs from myocardial fibrosis found with atherosclerotic coronary artery disease. It lacks hemosiderin deposits, and unlike fibrosis stemming from a myocardial infarction caused by a coronary artery lesion, it does not conform to a single coronary artery's distribution. Myocardial infarctions may develop in patients with scleroderma who have normal findings on coronary artery catheterization. Myocarditis may also occur in patients with scleroderma-associated inflammatory myositis. The patchy myocardial fibrosis and conduction system involvement may re-

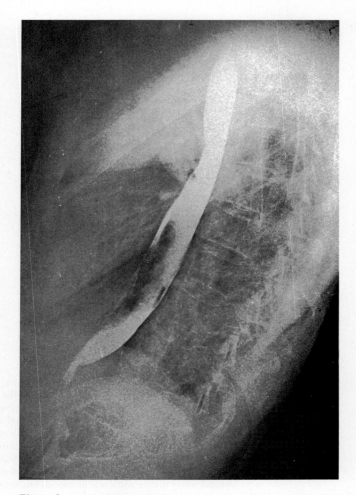

Figure 6 Hypomotility of the esophagus in scleroderma, which is demonstrated by the lack of peristaltic waves in the barium column, is frequently an asymptomatic finding, but it may be associated with dysphagia and incompetence of the gastric sphincter, which results in reflux esophagitis.

sult in various arrhythmias as well as sudden death. Pericardial disease is common at autopsy, but clinically evident pericardial manifestations occur in 5% to 16% of cases. Such pericardial disease may cause acute pericarditis, arrhythmias, pericardial effusions, or sudden death. In limited cutaneous scleroderma, apart from a similar frequency of cardiac arrhythmias and conduction defects, heart involvement is generally less frequent and less severe than in diffuse scleroderma.

Kidneys Chronic mild proteinuria and mild hypertension are common effects of scleroderma but typically do not result in significant renal dysfunction. The most significant disease process associated with scleroderma is renal crisis,[21] which consists of the rapid development of malignant hypertension, hyperreninemia, microangiopathic hemolytic anemia, and oliguric renal failure. Renal crisis typically occurs in the scleroderma that is characterized by rapidly progressive diffuse skin disease. A case-control study suggested that renal crisis was associated with antecedent high-dose corticosteroid therapy.[22] Renal crisis was formerly the most common cause of death in scleroderma, but aggressive treatment with angiotensin-converting enzyme (ACE) inhibitors early in the course of disease has greatly improved outcome.

Table 2 Antinuclear Antibodies in Scleroderma

Immunofluorescent Pattern of Antinuclear Antibody Staining	Antigens	Clinical Pattern	Approximate Frequency (%)	Specificity
Nucleolar	Nuclear ribonucleoproteins (nRNPs)	Diffuse or limited scleroderma	50	Moderate
	RNA polymerases I, II, and III	Diffuse scleroderma	23	High
	Nuclear proteins PM-1 (PM-Scl) and Ku	Scleroderma-polymyositis overlap	< 5	High, for scleroderma and polymyositis
Centromeric (large speckles)*	Centromere proteins (CENP-A, CENP-B, and CENP-C)	Usually in limited scleroderma (CREST syndrome)	50 (of patients with CREST syndrome)	High
Diffuse (fine speckles)	Topoisomerase I (Scl-70)	Diffuse scleroderma	20–33	High
Homogeneous	Histones (mainly H1 and H3)	Localized scleroderma	50	Moderate

*Requires a human epithelial carcinoma cell line (HEp-2).

Other organ systems Although scleroderma rarely involves the central nervous system, peripheral neuropathy may occur. The most frequent form is unilateral or bilateral trigeminal neuropathy of one or more of the three trigeminal branches; this neuropathy presents as progressive numbness and pain. Trigeminal neuralgia is often associated with myositis, high titers of antibodies to ribonucleoprotein, and other features of mixed connective tissue disease. Nerve entrapment with fibrous tissue and vascular lesions has been postulated, but the mechanism is unknown. Widespread autonomic nervous system dysfunction underlies the propensity for the Raynaud phenomenon and intestinal involvement. Hematopoietic consequences of scleroderma are uncommon.

Laboratory Findings

Positive test results for antinuclear antibodies are found in more than 85% of patients with scleroderma[23] [see Table 2]. Antibodies to certain nuclear antigens are specific for scleroderma,[24] and each type of antibody is associated with a particular clinical pattern of disease. The specific antibodies are directed toward topoisomerase I (Scl-70), centromere proteins, RNA polymerases, fibrillarin (U3 small nucleolar ribonucleoprotein), and the proteins of the 90 to 100 kd nucleolus organizer regions [see Table 2]. Antibodies to Scl-70 and to RNA polymerases (usually RNA polymerase III) are seen in patients with systemic scleroderma. In a meta-analysis, anti–Scl-70 antibodies had a positive predictive value of 70% for diffuse cutaneous scleroderma.[25] Anticentromere antibodies are associated with limited scleroderma (the CREST syndrome); the meta-analysis indicated a positive predictive value of 88% for limited cutaneous scleroderma.[25] Antibodies to nuclear ribonucleoprotein (nRNP) are associated with diffuse and limited scleroderma. Antibodies to PM-1 and Ku are infrequent. The presence of these antibodies is usually associated with overlapping clinical features of polymyositis and scleroderma. About 50% of patients with localized scleroderma have antibodies to histones [see Table 2].

MANAGEMENT

Management of scleroderma[26] is often a severe challenge, but it includes several potentially lifesaving interventions.

Renal Crisis

Renal crisis is a serious scleroderma-related manifestation that is manageable with appropriate therapy. A clinician will typically instruct patients with early diffuse scleroderma about daily blood pressure monitoring and will initiate antihypertensive therapy when the patient's blood pressure exceeds 130/80 mm Hg. Renal crisis is recognized by diminished renal function with new-onset hypertension (even of modest degree), microscopic hematuria, and proteinuria. Treatment of this medical emergency with the rapidly acting ACE inhibitor captopril and other potent antihypertensive drugs appears to arrest the deterioration in renal function. Even in patients who initially require dialysis, ACE inhibitors may restore renal function enough to make dialysis unnecessary.[27] However, this therapy has been shown to be more beneficial when initiated before serum creatinine levels have exceeded 3 mg/dl. In some patients, renal failure progresses despite good control of blood pressure, necessitating dialysis and possibly renal transplantation.

Pulmonary Involvement

Pulmonary involvement can usually be detected through measurements of forced vital capacity, carbon monoxide diffusing capacity, and exercise arterial blood gas levels. Patients with abnormalities may then be evaluated with bronchoalveolar lavage, where available, and high-resolution CT to detect lower respiratory inflammation. In patients with early fibrosing alveolitis, progression of pulmonary fibrosis may be halted by long-term therapy with oral cyclophosphamide and low-dose prednisone (< 10 mg/day), but this measure is not yet supported by a randomized, controlled trial.[18,28,29] Cyclophosphamide therapy is a powerful immunosuppressive medication; its use is sometimes associated with adverse events such as bacterial infections, herpes zoster, varicella-zoster virus infection, interstitial cystitis, and malignancies such as bladder transitional cell carcinoma.

Pulmonary hypertension is a serious manifestation of scleroderma that may be detected by serial echocardiographic examinations (semiannual or annual). Pulmonary hypertension was poorly controlled by therapy with vasodilators or other agents, but prostaglandins and their analogues are now used. A randomized, controlled trial of continuous prostacyclin infusion showed improved exercise capacity and cardiopulmonary function,[30] but this therapy is generally regarded as a measure for severe pulmonary hypertension that will require lung transplantation.

Cutaneous Involvement

Most patients with the Raynaud phenomenon may be managed with such measures as avoidance of cold exposure and smoking cessation. Instructions to wear warm clothing, gloves, and a hat when exposed to a cold environment may be sufficient. In addition, patients should avoid vasoconstrictive agents (e.g., decongestants, caffeine, amphetamines, beta blockers, and ergot alkaloids). For persons with attacks of the Raynaud phenomenon so frequent or so severe as to interfere with daily activities or to put them at risk for skin necrosis, pharmacologic therapy may be employed. Low-dose aspirin (81 mg daily) is recommended.[26] The calcium channel blocking agents promote vasodilatation and generally reduce the frequency and severity of the Raynaud phenomenon.[31] Although nifedipine in daily doses of 30 to 60 mg has been effective for most patients, approximately one third do not respond, and some patients experience adverse effects. In double-blind, placebo-controlled trials, other calcium channel blockers have also shown efficacy for the Raynaud phenomenon; these agents include amlodipine, 5 to 10 mg daily, and felodipine, 5 to 10 mg daily. Ischemic digital ulcerations may be difficult to treat and may progress to gangrene of the fingertips. Iloprost, an analogue of prostaglandin I_2, has been examined as an agent for severe Raynaud phenomenon in scleroderma. A randomized, double-blind study of iloprost infusion was effective for the short-term palliation of severe Raynaud phenomenon.[32] However, similar trials have found no difference between oral iloprost and placebo.[33] Sympathectomy should be reserved for severe ischemic crises.

GI Tract Involvement

Because gastroesophageal reflux is nearly universal in scleroderma, clinicians typically will instruct scleroderma patients to elevate the head of the bed and will administer H_2 receptor antagonists or proton pump inhibitors. Esophageal motility may be enhanced by use of metoclopramide. Esophageal dilatation may be required if strictures are present. Patients with diminished gastric emptying may be instructed regarding the frequent taking of small meals and may be given prokinetic medications such as metoclopramide. Small bowel motility may manifest as pain, distention, and vomiting; most episodes can be managed by increasing dietary fiber and avoiding medications that affect motility (e.g., opiates). Octreotide is used for severe small bowel dysmotility. For small bowel bacterial overgrowth with malabsorption, empirical antibiotic therapy with ciprofloxacin, metronidazole, doxycycline, or erythromycin is recommended.

Potential Disease-Modifying Therapies

Potential disease-modifying therapies have also been examined in scleroderma.[34] Penicillamine is no longer recommended because of associated toxicity and minimal efficacy. A double-blind, randomized, controlled clinical trial showed no improvement in skin thickening, mortality, or incidence of renal crisis.[35] Initial reports show that subcutaneous recombinant relaxin infusion may improve scleroderma.[36] A 24-week randomized, placebo-controlled, double-blind trial with methotrexate showed a modest favorable response, chiefly in skin manifestations,[37] but a second trial failed to replicate the findings.[38] Stem cell transplants are reserved as an experimental procedure for rapidly progressive severe scleroderma.[38] Thus, a truly effective disease-modifying therapy is not yet available.

CLINICAL COURSE

In the CREST syndrome, skin involvement is relatively limited, usually affecting only the hands and face; the prognosis for patients with this syndrome is generally favorable unless viscera are involved. However, even the limited CREST variant tends to be unremitting and slowly progressive. Many patients experience an indolent course with little change over several years, although the progression may be more rapid. Diffuse scleroderma is highly variable in its course and manifestations; therefore, its rate of progression is difficult to predict. With the exception of some of the sclerodermatous changes in mixed connective tissue disease, diffuse scleroderma rarely remits completely. Involvement of the viscera, such as the heart, lungs, or, particularly, the kidneys, indicates a poor prognosis. Two other features of scleroderma also indicate a poor outcome: (1) active inflammation, as manifested by an elevated erythrocyte sedimentation rate, and (2) evidence of cardiopulmonary disease, renal disease, or both within 1 year after diagnosis.[39] The life-threatening complications of scleroderma—severe skin involvement, pulmonary fibrosis, and renal crisis—usually occur within the first 2 to 5 years after the onset of disease. After this interval, the disease tends to run an indolent course.[40] The 5-year survival for patients with diffuse scleroderma is approximately 50%.

Eosinophilic Fasciitis

Eosinophilic fasciitis can superficially resemble scleroderma. It is characterized by pain, swelling, and tenderness of the extremities, after which induration of the skin and subcutaneous tissues occurs. Joint motion may be limited, but the Raynaud phenomenon, sclerodactyly, and other manifestations of scleroderma are not seen. Laboratory test abnormalities include peripheral blood eosinophilia, which may be marked; elevation of the erythrocyte sedimentation rate; and hyperglobulinemia. Antinuclear antibody and rheumatoid factor test results are negative. Biopsy specimens of involved areas have shown inflammation and thickening of the fascia deep to the subcutaneous tissues. The skin appears normal, but the underlying deep fascia is infiltrated with lymphocytes, plasma cells, histiocytes, and sometimes eosinophils. Eosinophilic fasciitis seems to be either self-limited or responsive to low doses of glucocorticoids. Its etiology remains unknown, but several cases have been reported after strenuous muscle exertion.

Eosinophilia-Myalgia Syndrome

In 1989, a previously unrecognized syndrome associated with ingestion of contaminated L-tryptophan appeared.[41] The eosinophilia-myalgia syndrome is characterized by peripheral eosinophilia, severe and incapacitating myalgias, and fatigue of several weeks' duration. Dyspnea and cough may also be present. Skin involvement consists of variable rashes, edema, and scleroderma-like changes, usually without the visceral manifestations of scleroderma. Interstitial pulmonary infiltrates, hypoxia, pulmonary hypertension, and hypersensitivity pneumonitis may occur. Polyneuropathy has been described in a pattern of mononeuritis multiplex. Neurocognitive disorders, such as memory disturbances and difficulty in concentration, have been reported. Most patients continue to manifest symptoms from 2 to 4 years after onset but have no new signs of inflammation.

References

1. Wigley FM, Flavahan NA: Raynaud's phenomenon. Rheum Dis Clin North Am 22:765, 1996
2. Spencer-Green G: Outcomes in primary Raynaud phenomenon: a meta-analysis of the frequency, rates, and predictors of transition to secondary diseases. Arch Intern Med 158:595, 1998

3. Mayes MD: Epidemiology of systemic sclerosis and related diseases. Curr Opin Rheumatol 9:557, 1997

4. Michet C: Update in the epidemiology of the rheumatic diseases. Curr Opin Rheumatol 10:129, 1998

5. Tan FK, Stivers DN, Foster MW, et al: Association of microsatellite markers near the fibrillin 1 gene on human chromosome 15q with scleroderma in a native American population. Arthritis Rheum 41:1729, 1998

6. Janowsky EC, Kupper LL, Hulka BS: Meta-analyses of the relation between silicone breast implants and the risk of connective-tissue diseases. N Engl J Med 16:342, 2000

7. Steen VD: Occupational scleroderma. Curr Opin Rheumatol 11:490, 1999

8. Arnett FC, Cho M, Chatterjee S, et al: Familial occurrence frequencies and relative risks for systemic sclerosis (scleroderma) in three United States cohorts. Arthritis Rheum 44:1359, 2001

9. Tan FK, Arnett FC: Genetic factors in the etiology of systemic sclerosis and Raynaud phenomenon. Curr Opin Rheumatol 12:511, 2000

10. Widom RL: Regulation of matrix biosynthesis and degradation in systemic sclerosis. Curr Opin Rheumatol 12:534, 2000

11. Jimenez SA, Hitraya E, Varga J: Pathogenesis of scleroderma. Collagen. Rheum Dis Clin North Am 22:647, 1996

12. Sato S: Abnormalities of adhesion molecules and chemokines in scleroderma. Curr Opin Rheumatol 11:503, 1999

13. LeRoy EC: Systemic sclerosis: a vascular perspective. Rheum Dis Clin North Am 22:675, 1996

14. Artlett CM, Cox LA, Jimenez SA: Detection of cellular microchimerism of male or female origin in systemic sclerosis patients by polymerase chain reaction analysis of HLA-Cw antigens. Arthritis Rheum 43:1062, 2000

15. Evans PC, Lambert N, Maloney S, et al: Long-term fetal microchimerism in peripheral blood mononuclear cell subsets in healthy women and women with scleroderma. Blood 93:2033, 1999

16. Olsen NJ, King LEJ, Park JH: Muscle abnormalities in scleroderma. Rheum Dis Clin North Am 22:783, 1996

17. Sjögren RW: Gastrointestinal features of scleroderma. Curr Opin Rheumatol 8:569, 1996

18. Bolster MB, Silver RM: Assessment and management of scleroderma lung disease. Curr Opin Rheumatol 11:508, 1999

19. Silver RM: Scleroderma: clinical problems—the lungs. Rheum Dis Clin North Am 22:825, 1996

20. Deswal A, Follansbee WP: Cardiac involvement in scleroderma. Rheum Dis Clin North Am 22:841, 1996

21. Steen VD: Scleroderma renal crisis. Rheum Dis Clin North Am 22:861, 1996

22. Steen VD, Medsger TA Jr: Case-control study of corticosteroids and other drugs that either precipitate or protect from the development of scleroderma renal crisis. Arthritis Rheum 41:1613, 1998

23. Okano Y: Antinuclear antibody in systemic sclerosis (scleroderma). Rheum Dis Clin North Am 22:709, 1996

24. Harvey GR, McHugh NJ: Serologic abnormalities in systemic sclerosis. Curr Opin Rheumatol 11:495, 1999

25. Spencer-Green G, Alter D, Welch HG: Test performance in systemic sclerosis: anti-centromere and anti–Scl-70 antibodies. Am J Med 103:242, 1997

26. Sule SD, Wigley FM: Update on management of scleroderma. Bull Rheum Dis 49:1, 2000

27. Steen VD, Medsger TA Jr: Long-term outcomes of scleroderma renal crisis. Ann Intern Med 133:600, 2000

28. Akesson A: Cyclophosphamide therapy for scleroderma. Curr Opin Rheumatol 10:579, 1998

29. White B, Moore WC, Wigley FM, et al: Cyclophosphamide is associated with pulmonary function and survival benefit in patients with scleroderma and alveolitis. Ann Intern Med 132:947, 2000

30. Badesch DB, Tapson VF, McGoon MD, et al: Continuous intravenous epoprostenol for pulmonary hypertension due to the scleroderma spectrum of disease: a randomized, controlled trial. Ann Intern Med 132:425, 2000

31. Sturgill MG, Seibold JR: Rational use of calcium-channel antagonists in Raynaud's phenomenon. Curr Opin Rheumatol 10:584, 1998

32. Wigley FM, Wise RA, Seibold JR, et al: Intravenous iloprost infusion in patients with Raynaud phenomenon secondary to systemic sclerosis: a multicenter, placebo-controlled, double-blind study. Ann Intern Med 120:199, 1994

33. Wigley FM, Korn JH, Csuka ME, et al: Oral iloprost treatment in patients with Raynaud's phenomenon secondary to systemic sclerosis: a multicenter, placebo-controlled, double-blind study. Arthritis Rheum 41:670, 1998

34. JE: Treatment of systemic sclerosis. Rheum Dis Clin North Am 22:893, 1996

35. Clements PJ, Furst DE, Wong WK, et al: High-dose versus low-dose d-penicillamine in early diffuse systemic sclerosis: analysis of a two-year, double-blind, randomized, controlled clinical trial. Arthritis Rheum 42:1194, 1999

36. Seibold JR, Korn JH, Simms R, et al: Recombinant human relaxin in the treatment of scleroderma: a randomized, double-blind, placebo-controlled trial. Ann Intern Med 132:871, 2000

37. van den Hoogen FH, Boerbooms AM, Swaak AJ, et al: Comparison of methotrexate with placebo in the treatment of systemic sclerosis: a 24 week randomized double-blind trial, followed by a 24 week observational trial. Br J Rheumatol 35:364, 1996

38. Pope JE, Bellamy N, Seibold JR, et al: A randomized, controlled trial of methotrexate versus placebo in early diffuse scleroderma. Arthritis Rheum 44:1351, 2001

39. Bulpitt KJ, Clements PJ, Lachenbruch PA, et al: Early undifferentiated connective tissue disease: III. Outcome and prognostic indicators in early scleroderma (systemic sclerosis). Ann Intern Med 118:602, 1993

40. Clements PJ: Measuring disease activity and severity in scleroderma [editorial]. Curr Opin Rheumatol 7:517, 1995

41. Varga J, Kahari VM: Eosinophilia-myalgia syndrome, eosinophilic fasciitis, and related fibrosing disorders. Curr Opin Rheumatol 9:562, 1997

116 Idiopathic Inflammatory Myopathies

Nancy J. Olsen, M.D., and Beth L. Brogan, M.D.

Idiopathic inflammatory myopathies, which include polymyositis and dermatomyositis, primarily affect skeletal muscle. The common features of these diseases are weakness of and inflammatory changes in skeletal muscle. In general, the idiopathic inflammatory myopathies are serious disorders that respond variably to therapy. Polymyositis and dermatomyositis may be linked with other rheumatic diseases, notably scleroderma, and with malignancies. Prognosis varies according to the specific syndrome that is expressed.

Classification

Classification of these heterogeneous muscle disorders into subtypes is useful for determining diagnostic and therapeutic approaches.[1,2] Categories are defined on the basis of clinical and histologic features rather than on laboratory or radiologic tests [*see Table 1*].

DERMATOMYOSITIS

Patients with dermatomyositis usually show symmetrical proximal muscle weakness in all extremities, accompanied by a characteristic skin rash. Neck and back muscles may also be weak. Areas of skin most commonly affected by the rash include extensor surfaces of the hands and knees. Subtypes of dermatomyositis include the juvenile form [*see* Juvenile Myositis, *below*]. Another recognized subtype is amyopathic dermatomyositis.[3-5] Patients with this disorder have the characteristic rash but do not have demonstrable muscle abnormalities. One study of such patients has shown that sensitive magnetic resonance imaging techniques can reveal changes after exercise that indicate a metabolic abnormality.[6]

POLYMYOSITIS

Patients with polymyositis have symmetrical proximal muscle weakness similar to that experienced in dermatomyositis, but the rash is absent. Onset of polymyositis may be more difficult to determine, in part because no rash is available as an indicator of possible inflammation. Muscle weakness and atrophy may be more profound than that usually seen in patients with dermatomyositis. However, no formal studies of long-term outcome have been carried out that prove this assertion.

JUVENILE MYOSITIS

Children ranging in age from younger than 5 years through the teen years may be affected by juvenile myositis. Most children have a skin rash, and vasculitis and soft tissue calcifications are much more common in children than in adults.[7] Although residual dermatologic changes, muscle fibrosis, and calcification may occur, the long-term outlook is generally favorable.[8]

MYOSITIS WITH MALIGNANCY

Most, but not all, cases of malignancy-associated myositis are accompanied by the typical rash of dermatomyositis. A recent study showed that patients with dermatomyositis had a relative risk of malignancy of 6.2. For patients with polymyositis or inclusion body myositis, the risk was lower but still significant.[9-11] The incidence of underlying malignancy increases with age[12] and decreases with increasing time from diagnosis.[9] Onset of the myositis may precede or follow discovery of the malignancy. Adults with dermatomyositis should be screened for occult malignancies in the first 2 years after onset of disease.

MYOSITIS WITH OTHER RHEUMATIC DISEASES

Inflammatory myositis may occur with another established rheumatic disease, most commonly scleroderma. Other conditions that can occur with myositis include rheumatoid arthritis, systemic lupus erythematosus (SLE), and Sjögren syndrome. Recent reports have linked scleromyxedema to dermatomyositis[13] and have linked inclusion body myositis to subacute cutaneous lupus.[14,15] Many patients with these overlap conditions have a relatively mild form of muscle inflammation that responds well to treatment. However, a small subset of patients, especially those with coexistent scleroderma, may have a severe and very debilitating muscle weakness that is resistant to therapy.[16]

INCLUSION BODY MYOSITIS

The pattern and severity of muscle weakness in inclusion body myositis (IBM) differs from the pattern of severity seen in the other idiopathic inflammatory myopathies. In addition to the presence of proximal weakness, distal muscles may be involved; and in some cases, muscle abnormalities are asymmetrical. Unlike most of the other muscle disorders discussed in this chapter, IBM afflicts more men than women, with approximately two thirds of affected persons being men. Response to treatment is generally poor.

Epidemiology

PREVALENCE AND INCIDENCE

The estimated prevalence of idiopathic inflammatory myopathies is approximately one case per 100,000 individuals.

Table 1 Classification of Myositis Syndromes

Clinicopathologic Category	Characteristics
Dermatomyositis	Proximal weakness, skin rash; amyopathic variant with rash only
Polymyositis	Proximal weakness without rash
Juvenile myositis	Myositis in childhood, usually with a rash
Myositis with malignancy	Myositis with associated underlying neoplastic disease
Myositis with another connective tissue disease	Coexistent syndrome, usually scleroderma, rheumatoid arthritis, or systemic lupus erythematosus
Inclusion body myositis	Severe weakness with characteristic inclusions on muscle biopsy

This prevalence makes these disorders about 1,000 times less common than rheumatoid arthritis. The rarer syndromes, such as IBM, may constitute 20% or less of all cases. In one study, the annual incidence of idiopathic inflammatory myopathies was 5.5 cases per million population.[17] Incidence rates, however, may be increasing, possibly because of improved methods of detection.

ETHNIC, RACIAL, AND GENDER GROUP DIFFERENCES

No ethnic clustering of the idiopathic inflammatory myopathies has been reported. It has been suggested that incidence rates in North America are increasing faster in African Americans than in whites.[17] In adults, polymyositis is more common than dermatomyositis, whereas in children and young adults, dermatomyositis is the predominant form. It has been suggested that incidence rates are higher in regions that have greater amounts of sun exposure.[18] Polymyositis and dermatomyositis show a female-to-male ratio of approximately 2:1. Risk of underlying malignancy increases significantly after 40 years of age.[12] Malignancies in children are rare but have been reported. The diagnosis of inclusion body myositis is rarely made in persons younger than 50 years.

Etiology and Pathogenesis

The etiology of inflammatory muscle disease remains unknown. The most widely accepted hypotheses suggest multiple factors. One possible scenario is that an initial insult—for example, a virus or another infectious agent or an environmental toxin—leads to muscle damage in a genetically susceptible host. This process in turn triggers an immune response, subsequently causing chronic muscle inflammation.[19]

INFECTIOUS AGENTS

A role for viruses in the etiology of idiopathic inflammatory myopathies has been suggested by seasonal and geographic clustering of new cases. Furthermore, infection with HIV or hepatitis C virus has been associated with the development of myopathy.[20] Most studies looking for evidence of viral genomic material in muscle tissue have failed to find such evidence.[21] Immunoreactivity for hepatitis C in involved muscle tissues has been reported in a single case.[20] Viruses may mediate tissue damage, which may in turn lead to immunologic responses that target or damage muscle tissues.[22] The relative rarity of the myositis syndromes would suggest that if a common infectious agent were involved, coexistent factors would also be required. These factors could include host-specific genetic loci that control the immune response or other noninfectious factors such as drugs or environmental toxins.[18]

NONINFECTIOUS FACTORS

Lipid-lowering agents such as clofibrate and the statin group of drugs have been associated with elevated levels of serum muscle enzymes and with muscle weakness in a small number of patients. However, most patients are asymptomatic. The list of drugs reported to be associated with development of myopathy is very long. For this reason, concomitant medications should be examined closely in any patient with unexplained muscle weakness.[23] Both HIV infection and drugs used in its treatment, such as zidovudine (AZT), have been implicated in the development of myopathy. It is possible that as yet undefined environmental toxins play a role.

GENETIC FACTORS

Familial clustering of inflammatory myositis syndromes occurs, but the great majority of cases are sporadic. Sporadic cases have been linked to HLA-DRB1*0301, whereas familial cases have shown increased prevalence of HLA-DQA1 (DQA1*0501). A form of hereditary IBM has been described in several ethnic groups. Chromosomal links with this disorder have been identified, but candidate genes are as yet undefined.[24] Many of the reported studies of genetic links in inflammatory myopathies have grouped several types of syndromes together. It is probable that future studies that perform separate analyses of the various distinct clinical syndromes will show stronger associations with genetic markers.

AUTOIMMUNE FACTORS

The presence of cellular infiltrates in muscle tissues is a defining feature of inflammatory muscle diseases [see Figure 1]. Light microscopic examination of these infiltrates reveals different patterns of infiltration. In tissues from patients with dermatomyositis, the lymphocytes are generally located around blood vessels and at the periphery of the muscle bundles. Invasion of muscle fibers by mononuclear cells is rarely observed, and there is a relative paucity of necrotic muscle fibers. Complement-mediated capillary damage is also more commonly observed in biopsy samples from dermatomyositis patients, especially those patients with an underlying malignancy. Some studies suggest that dermatomyositis patients with capillary damage who do not have a malignancy have a more acute syndrome that responds better to immunosuppressive treatment. In polymyositis, muscle fibers may be invaded by the mononuclear infiltrates, and focal areas of muscle destruction are seen. Tissues from patients with IBM usually show some degree of inflammation accompanied by intracellular rimmed vacuoles.[25]

Two groups have identified chimeric cells of maternal origin in the peripheral blood and inflammatory lesions of children with myositis. These findings support the hypothesis that

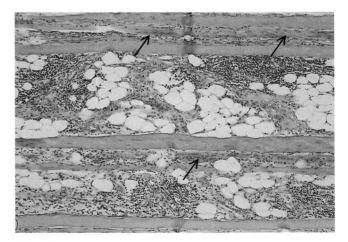

Figure 1   Extensive pathologic changes can be seen in involved muscle in myositis. These changes include a decrease in the number of striated muscle fibers and a loss of cross-striations in the remaining fibers. Some fibers demonstrate increased numbers of rounded nuclei and basophilic staining (arrows), which suggests attempted regeneration. There is also intense infiltration of the muscle by mononuclear inflammatory cells, predominantly lymphocytes and plasma cells.

childhood myositis is a manifestation of a graft-versus-host reaction.[26,27]

Differences between polymyositis and dermatomyositis are revealed by immunophenotyping of the cellular infiltrates.[28] Mononuclear cell infiltrates in polymyositis and probably in IBM tissues are predominantly of the CD8[+] cytotoxic T cell phenotype. The CD8[+] T cells in polymyositis show evidence of clonal expansion, which is most likely driven by muscle-specific antigens.[29] Activated CD8[+] T cells probably mediate cytotoxic, immune-mediated, and antigen-specific muscle cell destruction. In dermatomyositis, T cells, predominantly of the CD4[+] helper-inducer phenotype, are present along with B cells; restricted clonality is not seen.[29] These differences in histology support the hypothesis that polymyositis and dermatomyositis are distinct disorders with different etiologies.

Diagnosis

Major diagnostic criteria that were proposed by Bohan and Peter in 1975[1,2] remain useful for defining most of the myositis syndromes. However, IBM, which was not recognized at the time these criteria were written, differs somewhat from polymyositis and dermatomyositis. Although sophisticated diagnostic tests, including autoantibody profiles and imaging techniques, are now available, findings obtained through a careful history and physical examination remain indispensable for both making the initial diagnosis and evaluating responses to treatment.

CLINICAL FEATURES

Muscle Weakness

In polymyositis and dermatomyositis, the weakness is predominantly proximal. Distal strength is usually preserved. In IBM, the weakness may be asymmetrical, and diminished distal strength is commonly seen. Muscle strength can be tested in the office or at the bedside and estimated on a semiquantitative scale from 1 to 5. Devices for quantitative assessment of muscle strength, some of which can be used at the bedside, are also available.

Characteristic Skin Rash

The rash of dermatomyositis is a deep-red erythematous eruption, with or without mild scaling and atrophy. It occurs on the face, neck, upper chest, and extensor surfaces of joints such as elbows and those of the hands. Periorbital edema may appear, as may heliotrope erythema, which is characterized by a violet or lilac color, especially of the eyelids. Occasionally, the rash is more widespread or takes different forms [see Figure 2]. Erythema and telangiectasia also occur in periungual areas. In adults, vasculitis is usually confined to the skin and takes the form of urticaria, subcutaneous nodules, periungual infarcts, or digital ulcerations. Cutaneous vasculitis has been associated with underlying malignant disease.

Pulmonary Involvement

Pulmonary involvement occurs in nearly 50% of patients who have myositis, with pneumonia being the most common pulmonary abnormality. Aspiration pneumonia, which is often recurrent, is prevalent in patients who have pharyngeal muscle weakness. Ineffective coughing caused by ventilatory muscle weakness also occurs but is far less common than swallowing

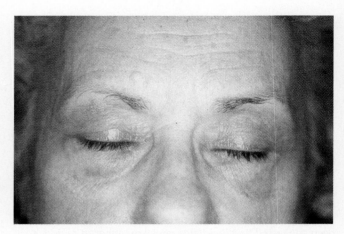

Figure 2 **Skin eruption in a patient with dermatomyositis consists of a deep-red, erythematous, papular rash over the nasal and forehead areas and a lilac-colored, or heliotrope, erythema of the upper eyelid and orbital area.**

problems. In general, the patient with recurrent aspiration pneumonia has a poor prognosis; it indicates marked dysfunction of many muscle groups. Bacterial pneumonia caused by aspiration is a major cause of death in elderly patients.[12] Opportunistic infections may occur in patients undergoing immunosuppressive drug therapy. In addition, some of these drugs, most notably methotrexate, can be associated with the development of pneumonitis, which is usually reversible but is potentially fatal.

Interstitial lung disease (ILD) occurs in up to 30% of myositis patients and in approximately 60% of patients who have antibodies directed against aminoacyl-transfer RNA (tRNA) synthetases. The advent and application of newer, sensitive diagnostic techniques such as high-resolution computed tomography may lead to an increase in the detection of pulmonary abnormalities. The most common presentation is with progressive shortness of breath, which may be accompanied by a nonproductive cough. On physical examination, basilar crepitant rales are usually detected. Progression may be slow, and symptoms may occur in patients with established disease; or onset may be rapid and may occur at the same time as the muscle weakness.[30] Hypoxemia and respiratory alkalosis may be present. In some patients, these abnormalities are detected only after exercise. High-resolution CT scanning is useful for detection of interstitial fibrosis that might not be appreciated on routine chest radiography. Pulmonary function tests may reveal reduced lung volume and diminished diffusion capacity. One of three forms of histology of ILD is usually found: interstitial pneumonia, diffuse alveolar damage, or bronchiolitis obliterans with or without organizing pneumonia. ILD occurs with or without skin involvement. There is no correlation between the development of ILD and the severity of muscle involvement, and ILD may precede or follow the onset of muscle weakness. ILD is associated with a high mortality. Treatment with cyclophosphamide or azathioprine has been reported to be beneficial in some patients.[30] A small number of patients with acute pneumonitis may respond to corticosteroid treatment alone.

Cardiac Abnormalities

Clinically significant involvement of heart muscle is unusual and is probably associated with a poor prognosis. Cardiac abnormalities may take many forms, ranging from rhythm or conduction disturbances to myocardial inflammation or fibrosis. Cardiac muscle abnormalities may be detected by radionuclide scanning studies. However, many histologic and electrical abnormalities are not clinically significant.[31] Therefore, evaluation beyond routine diagnostic studies is rarely indicated.

Calcinosis

Soft tissue calcification is seen most commonly in children. Deposits may be deep along fascial planes or in superficial dermal areas, sometimes with ulceration through the skin. Treatments have been based on largely anecdotal reports; no systematic studies have been carried out.[32] Agents that have been found to be of use in some cases include probenecid, diltiazem, and warfarin. Some patients show spontaneous regression of calcinosis without specific treatment.

Vascular Abnormalities

Raynaud phenomenon is most commonly observed in patients whose myositis is associated with another rheumatic disease (e.g., scleroderma). Clinically significant vasculitis is unusual in adults, although dermatomyositis patients may show vascular changes on histologic examination.

LABORATORY TESTS

Muscle Biopsy

Histologic confirmation of muscle inflammation is required in many, but not all, cases of inflammatory muscle disease. Patients with the characteristic skin rash of dermatomyositis and with elevated serum muscle enzyme levels may be treated without a muscle biopsy, because these two indicators can be used to follow the course of disease. In the absence of a skin rash or elevations in muscle enzyme levels, diagnosis is more difficult; in most patients, a biopsy is needed to confirm the presence of muscle inflammation. Two types of biopsy approaches are used: open surgical and closed needle. The closed-needle approach offers the advantages of decreased morbidity and of lower cost because an operating room is not required. Tissue samples obtained with the closed-needle approach can provide sufficient diagnostic information for interpretation by the muscle pathologist. However, the quality of the specimen obtained is dependent on the skill and experience of the operator. In the absence of such a resource or in special cases in which it is desirable to obtain extra tissue, the open surgical approach is preferable. Imaging studies such as MRI or CT can be used to determine the optimal site for biopsy.

All biopsy specimens require immediate handling by an experienced surgical team working closely with the pathology laboratory to ensure optimal results. Light microscopic analysis is sufficiently informative for most purposes. Because the treatment of polymyositis and that of dermatomyositis are the same, immunophenotyping of cellular infiltrates to distinguish between these two disorders is not indicated for routine diagnostic specimens. Electron microscopy may be required to demonstrate the inclusion bodies that define IBM. Examination of the biopsy specimen by a specialist in neuromuscular pathology may be helpful, because many pathologists do not see these diseases on a regular basis.

Muscle Enzymes

Most patients with inflammatory myopathy have increased muscle enzyme levels at some point during the course of active myositis.[33] The presence of intracellular muscle enzymes in the serum most likely reflects damage to muscle cell membranes. The most commonly used muscle enzyme measurement is the creatine kinase (CK) level. The CK level may rise to many times normal. The MB isozyme of CK may be elevated because of the presence of this isoform in regenerating skeletal muscle. Measurement of CK may be confounded by the presence of naturally occurring inhibitors of this enzyme. Furthermore, racial and gender variations exist for normal levels of CK, with black males generally showing the highest values.[34] Aldolase is another muscle enzyme that may be measured in the serum and may have less variability. However, aldolase is present in tissues other than muscle, and therefore, it is not specific for muscle damage. MRI studies have shown that active muscle inflammation may exist in patients with persistently normal CK serum levels.[35] Reasons for this discordance are not known, but the findings suggest that treatment strategies should be focused on the clinical status of the patient rather than on the muscle enzyme levels.[36]

Autoantibodies

Autoantibodies to nuclear and cytoplasmic antigens are found in as many as 90% of patients with an inflammatory myopathy. These antibodies are often useful in differentiating inflammatory myopathies from diseases that are not autoimmune disorders. Some of these autoantibodies are nonspecific and are seen in several autoimmune disorders. Other autoantibodies are relatively specific for the inflammatory myositis syndromes in general or for specific diagnostic categories. About 25% of patients with inflammatory myositis test positive for antinuclear antibody; in patients with overlapping rheumatic disease syndromes, the percentage is higher. The antinuclear antibody test is generally not helpful in establishing a diagnosis of myositis or one of its subsets. Autoantibodies that are in large part directed against cytoplasmic ribonucleoproteins have been designated as myositis-specific autoantibodies (MSA). Approximately 30% of patients with myositis have one or more of these autoantibodies. They are thus relatively specific but not sensitive to the presence of myositis, and as such, these autoantibodies cannot be used to screen for the presence of disease.

Three groups of patients can be defined by the MSA specificities. These subgroups differ in clinical presentation and prognosis.[37] The first group is defined by the presence of antibodies directed against aminoacyl-tRNA synthetases. The presentation in the first group is generally characterized by an acute onset of muscle disease, with a high incidence of associated interstitial lung disease. Patients in this group may also have arthritis and a hyperkeratotic rash on the hands, known as mechanic's hands. A majority of patients in this group test positive for HLA-DR3. Responses to treatment are variable, and mortality is significant. The second group includes patients with antibodies to the signal recognition particle (SRP). This protein complex facilitates translocation of newly synthesized polypeptides across the endoplasmic reticulum. Patients with anti-SRP have an abrupt onset of muscle weakness and may have associated involvement of cardiac muscle. The majority of patients in this group are African-American women. Responses to treatment are not good, and the prognosis is poor. In one series, the 5-year mortality for anti-SRP patients was 75%. A third group is identified by antibodies to Mi-2, which is a nuclear protein with unknown function. The majority of these patients have the dermatomyositis clinical syndrome with the so-called shawl-sign pattern of rash on the trunk and with cuticular overgrowth. Responses to treatment are generally good, and mortality is lower than that in the other groups. Most of these clinical associations, which were originally described in North American patients, have been confirmed in a large group of European patients.[38] Preliminary reports suggest that antibodies to a novel 155 kd protein may also be useful in identifying patients with amyopathic dermatomyositis.[39]

Electromyography

In most patients, electromyography reveals low-amplitude, polyphasic motor unit potentials, indicating a lack of synchronous contracture in muscle fibers within motor units. This finding correlates with the usually inhomogeneous distribution of muscle degeneration shown by histopathologic examination. Fibrillations and insertional irritability are evidence of membrane abnormalities. These findings are characteristic of, but not specific for, myositis.

IMAGING AND SPECTROSCOPY TECHNIQUES

Conventional radiographs have little value in evaluating skeletal muscle. However, other techniques, including ultrasonography, CT, and MRI, can enhance diagnostic approaches to many myopathies.[40] Of these modalities, MRI has been the most useful in the evaluation and longitudinal management of inflammatory muscle syndromes. However, it may not be the method of choice in all circumstances, and in some of these cases, the alternative modalities of ultrasonography and CT can provide helpful information. Advantages of these three techniques are that they are noninvasive and offer the possibility of examining a volume of muscle larger than that which can be obtained by biopsy. In patients for whom biopsy may be a difficult or traumatic experience, such as young children, imaging may provide sufficient information to proceed with treatment.

Magnetic Resonance Imaging

MRI is a very accurate method for muscle imaging that has been very useful in the diagnosis and management of patients with inflammatory muscle diseases of many kinds. Full assessment requires both T_1- and T_2-weighted images. The T_1 image

is most useful for outlining muscle anatomy because it detects changes in muscle mass caused by atrophy or fat infiltration. Inflammation is readily detected on the T_2-weighted image, where the abnormal areas appear as brightness against the usually dark background of normal muscle [see Figure 3]. Studies using MRI have clearly demonstrated the patchy nature of the muscle inflammation, perhaps explaining why some patients with significant weakness have normal biopsy results. In dermatomyositis, inflammation in the thigh muscles is seen in predominantly anterior muscle compartments, and muscle mass is generally preserved. In patients with polymyositis and inclusion body myositis, extensive fat infiltration and muscle atrophy, which can include all muscle groups, are more likely to be seen. Longitudinal MRI studies can be used to document the effectiveness of immunosuppressive therapy. Patients may be studied in the usual body coil, which allows for visualization of both legs.[41] Other studies have utilized a knee coil positioned over the anterior quadriceps, which provides a greater level of detail.[35] As in all MRI studies, patients must be very carefully questioned for the presence of any indwelling metals before being placed in the magnet.

Ultrasonography

Ultrasonography is a readily available and relatively inexpensive technique that has been used to examine a wide variety of muscle disorders.[42,43] Inflammation within muscle tissues appears on ultrasonography as areas of decreased echogenicity. In addition, blood-flow changes can be measured with related techniques such as color Doppler imaging. Ultrasonography may be useful in guiding the choice of site for needle or open muscle biopsy.

Computed Tomography

CT is not useful for the detection of inflammatory muscle changes. However, areas of atrophy or fat infiltration cause decreased muscle density, which is easily detected by CT. Soft tissue calcifications such as those seen in juvenile dermatomyositis are best visualized with CT. Sometimes, these calcifications are in deep areas that cannot be readily appreciated on physical examination.

a

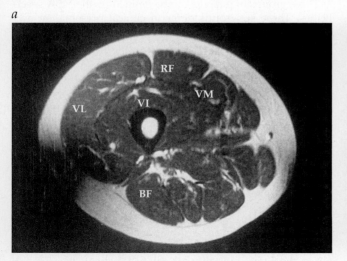

b

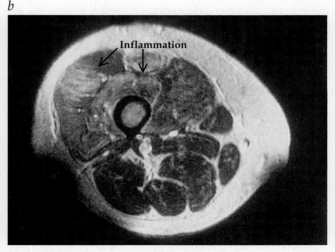

Figure 3 Magnetic resonance images of thigh muscles in a patient with dermatomyositis. The T_1-weighted image (*a*) shows uniform density in all muscle groups, identified as VL, vastus lateralis; VI, vastus intermedius; VM, vastus medialis; RF, rectus femoris; and BF, biceps femoris. The T_2-weighted image (*b*) illustrates inflammation in muscles of the quadriceps group, shown as areas of brightness or increased signal intensity.[35]

Magnetic Resonance Spectroscopy

Spectroscopy is primarily a research tool. However, studies have shown the utility of this noninvasive approach for evaluating muscle function, and applications in the clinic may become available in the near future.[35,44] In patients with dermatomyositis, loss of high-energy phosphate compounds needed for efficient muscle contraction has been documented with P-31 magnetic resonance spectroscopy.[44] Longitudinal studies have documented that correction of these metabolic abnormalities may lag behind improvement in muscle inflammation.

EVALUATION FOR UNDERLYING MALIGNANCY

Patients with dermatomyositis and polymyositis are at increased risk for an underlying malignancy. The magnitude of this risk is difficult to determine and varies greatly between reports. One study in a population-based cohort estimated the relative risk of cancer as 1.8 in males and 1.7 in females.[45] A more recent study from Scotland has indicated that the relative risk may be as high as 7.7 in patients with dermatomyositis, with a greater risk in females than in males.[46] In general, the risk is greater in patients with dermatomyositis than in patients with polymyositis and in all patients who are older than 40 years. There is general agreement that routine screening for malignancies should include chest radiography, mammography (in women), examination of stool for occult blood, complete gynecologic examination, and assessment for prostate-specific antigen (in men). Abnormalities seen on these screening tests may suggest the need for additional studies such as endoscopy, colonoscopy, and tissue biopsy. The most difficult malignancies to detect are those arising in the ovary. Uterine transvaginal ultrasonography or CT of the pelvis should be done in women older than 40 years, but some occult ovarian malignancies escape detection even with these tests. Some investigators advocate lower gastrointestinal studies to detect colon cancer in patients older than 65 years.[12] Other, more extensive screening tests for occult malignancies are generally not recommended.

Differential Diagnosis

Diagnosis of dermatomyositis is aided by the presence of the characteristic rash. However, because the rash has features of SLE, this diagnosis may be confused with SLE, especially when the antinuclear antibody test is positive. Patients with polymyositis may be difficult to distinguish from patients with other myopathic disorders [*see Table 2*]. These other disorders include metabolic myopathies, endocrine dysfunction, drug-induced disorders, infections, and miscellaneous syndromes such as sarcoidosis. Some types of dystrophies should also be considered in patients who have muscle weakness and elevated muscle enzyme levels. Myalgia syndromes, such as polymyalgia rheumatica, in which stiffness is a predominant complaint, may confuse the diagnosis in some patients. Fibromyalgia, which is associated with a primary symptom of fatigue rather than muscle weakness, is characterized by the presence of discrete tender points that are not usually present in myositis patients.

Treatment

Guidelines for treatment of the idiopathic inflammatory myopathies are not well established for several reasons. The diseases are uncommon, making it difficult to accumulate suffi-

Table 2 Differential Diagnosis of Inflammatory Myositis

Cause	Effect
Metabolic myopathies	Myophosphorylase deficiency (McArdle disease) Myoadenylate deaminase deficiency Carnitine palmitoyltransferase deficiency Glycogen storage disease Periodic paralysis Hypokalemia, hypomagnesemia
Endocrine disorders	Cushing syndrome Thyroid dysfunction
Drug-induced disorders	Ethanol toxicity Penicillamine toxicity Lipid-lowering drug (statin) toxicity Zidovudine toxicity
Infections	Viral: HIV, coxsackievirus, adenovirus, influenza virus, echovirus
Other rheumatic disorders	Systemic lupus erythematosus (rash) Polymyalgia rheumatica
Miscellaneous disorders	Sarcoidosis, eosinophilia

cient numbers of patients to carry out randomized, controlled trials. In addition, some forms of these diseases have a slow, prolonged course, requiring long periods of observation. Finally, there is as yet no uniformly accepted classification scheme for these disorders; thus, comparisons of therapies administered to different groups of patients at different times and places may not be valid. As examples, in the past, polymyositis and dermatomyositis have been included in the same category, and IBM may not have been recognized. It is now clear that different forms of these diseases vary in prognosis and in response to therapy.

DRUG THERAPY

A table showing drugs for the treatment of inflammatory muscle diseases is provided [*see Table 3*].

Glucocorticoids

Corticosteroids are the mainstay of initial therapy. Most patients with documented muscle inflammation should be started on these drugs at relatively high levels (1 mg/kg/day), given in divided doses. A standard approach has been to maintain this dosage for up to 3 months or until clinical improvement occurs. After this initial period of high-dose therapy, the dose can be consolidated into a single morning dose and then tapered, with the total daily dose being reduced by 20% to 25% each month and a maintenance dose of 5 to 10 mg daily being achieved in about 6 to 8 months. The addition of second-line drugs to the prednisone regimen is now recommended within 3 months after initiation of treatment. Older patients with comorbid conditions such as diabetes and osteoporosis are especially at risk from side effects of steroids. Side effects may include a cushingoid appearance, compression fractures, avascular necrosis, cataracts, and infections. One study has suggested that the side effects of corticosteroid therapy contribute significantly to the morbidity of polymyositis and dermatomyositis.[47] For these reasons, any patient with severe muscle weakness,

Table 3   Drugs for the Treatment of Inflammatory Muscle Diseases

Drug	Dose	Efficacy Rating	Comments
Prednisone	5–60 mg/day	Highly effective for initial treatment	Side effect: cushingoid syndrome Avoid prolonged use at high doses; taper to 10 mg/day or less
Methotrexate	15–25 mg/wk	Effective, steroid-sparing	Side effects: liver abnormalities, pneumonitis Supplement with folate
Azathioprine	100–150 mg/day	Effective, steroid-sparing	Side effect: bone marrow suppression Can be combined with methotrexate
Hydroxychloroquine	200 mg b.i.d.	Effective for skin manifestations	Side effect: retinal toxicity Can be combined with other agents
Cyclophosphamide	100–150 mg daily or as intravenous pulses every 6 wk	Possibly effective for lung involvement	Side effects: bone marrow suppression, hemorrhagic cystitis
Cyclosporine	3 mg/kg/day	Use after other immunosuppressants	Side effects: hypertension, renal dysfunction
Intravenous immunoglobulin	1 g/kg/day, 2 consecutive days monthly	Use in patients in whom other regimens have failed	High cost and limited supply

limited functional status, or underlying conditions that make steroids a high risk (e.g., diabetes mellitus or osteoporosis) should be started on second-line immunosuppressive drugs at the outset.

Methotrexate and Azathioprine

The most commonly used second-line agents for the treatment of inflammatory myopathy are methotrexate and azathioprine. Methotrexate may be given orally or subcutaneously at an initial dosage of 7.5 to 10 mg weekly and then increased gradually to 25 mg weekly. As the dosage of methotrexate is increased, the dosage of prednisone is usually tapered. In general, methotrexate is well tolerated by patients with inflammatory myopathy, but there have been reports of toxicities similar to those seen in patients with rheumatoid arthritis who have taken methotrexate. Regular monitoring of liver function is necessary. Measurement of enzymes other than aminotransferases is required to prevent interference by the ongoing muscle inflammation. γ-Glutamyltranspeptidase is a liver-specific alternative. Methotrexate may be useful in the treatment of interstitial lung disease associated with myositis, but because this drug may in rare cases cause pulmonary toxicity, it is relatively contraindicated in patients with significant lung problems.

Azathioprine has been shown to be effective in patients with myositis in a prospective, controlled, double-blind trial, but treatment for at least 6 months may be required for improvement to occur. Azathioprine therapy should be initiated at a dosage of 50 to 100 mg/day, and the dosage should be increased gradually to a maximum of 150 to 200 mg/day. Side effects include bone marrow suppression and development of infections and, possibly, malignancies. Azathioprine and methotrexate have similar efficacy in these disorders, and the choice of which to use may depend on tolerability or comorbid conditions. Patients with myositis in whom therapy with glucocorticoids and either methotrexate or azathioprine has failed may respond to a combination of methotrexate and azathioprine.[48,49]

Other Immunosuppressive Agents

Cyclophosphamide has been given both as intravenous pulse therapy and by daily oral administration. Some data suggest that it may be useful in adults with the antisynthetase syndrome and in children with vasculitis-related complications of dermatomyositis. Cyclophosphamide may be useful in the treatment of the complication of interstitial lung disease.[30] Other drugs that may be of value in patients in whom other therapies have failed include cyclosporine, FK506 (tacrolimus), chlorambucil, and mycophenolate mofetil.[50-52] The adenine analogue fludarabine has also shown some benefit in one study of refractory patients.[53]

Intravenous Immune Globulin

Intravenous immune globulin appears to benefit some patients with either polymyositis or dermatomyositis. A controlled trial of immune globulin in dermatomyositis patients demonstrated efficacy when given at a dosage of 1 g/kg/day for 2 days, repeated monthly for 3 months.[54] The combination of intravenous immune globulin and cyclosporine may be of value.[55] One controlled study suggested that intravenous immune globulin may be of benefit in IBM,[56] but studies by another group failed to show clinical improvements.[57] Treatment with intravenous immune globulin is limited by the restricted supply and very high cost and should be reserved for severe cases not responding to other therapies.

SKIN PROTECTION

The rash of dermatomyositis is usually photosensitive. Therefore, attention to protection from the sun is very important, and patients should be advised to avoid sun exposure as much as possible. Sunscreen preparations, sun-protective clothing, and tinting of windows are often effective. Some dermatologists recommend use of β-carotene, 25 to 30 mg, taken twice daily initially and then increasing to no more than five times a day. Antimalarials may be of benefit, and one report suggests the use of topical tacrolimus.[58]

PHYSICAL THERAPY

Physical therapy plays an important role in the rehabilitation of patients with myositis. During the phase of active inflammatory disease, passive range-of-motion exercises are necessary to prevent contractures. Once the inflammatory component of the disease is controlled, active resistive exercises are useful in regaining muscle strength.

References

1. Bohan A, Peter JB: Polymyositis and dermatomyositis (pt I). N Engl J Med 292:344, 1975

2. Bohan A, Peter JB: Polymyositis and dermatomyositis (pt II). N Engl J Med 292:403, 1975

3. Euwer RL, Sontheimer RD: Amyopathic dermatomyositis (dermatomyositis sine myositis). J Am Acad Dermatol 24:959, 1991

4. el-Azhara RA, Pakza SY: Amyopathic dermatomyositis: retrospective review of 37 cases. J Am Acad Dermatol 46:560, 2002

5. Caproni M, Cardinali C, Parodi A, et al: Amyopathic dermatomyositis: a review by the Italian Group of Immunodermatology. Arch Dermatol 138:114, 2002

6. Park JH, Olsen NJ, King LE, et al: MRI and P-31 magnetic resonance spectroscopy detect and quantify muscle dysfunction in the amyopathic and myopathic variants of dermatomyositis. Arthritis Rheum 38:68, 1995

7. Pachman LM, Hayford JR, Chung A, et al: Juvenile dermatomyositis at diagnosis: clinical characteristics of 79 children. J Rheumatol 25:1198, 1998

8. Collison CH, Sinal SH, Jorizzo JL, et al: Juvenile dermatomyositis and polymyositis: a follow-up study of long-term sequelae. South Med J 91:17, 1998

9. Buchbinder R, Forbes A, Hall S, et al: Incidence of malignant disease in biopsy-proven inflammatory myopathy: a population-based cohort study. Ann Intern Med 134:1087, 2001

10. Sparsa A, Liozon E, Herrmann F, et al: Routine vs extensive malignancy search for adult dermatomyositis and polymyositis: a study of 40 patients. Arch Dermatol 138:969, 2002

11. Hill CL, Zhang Y, Sigurgeirsson B, et al: Frequency of specific cancer types in dermatomyositis and polymyositis: a population-based study. Lancet 357:96, 2002

12. Marie I, Hatron PY, Levesque H, et al: Influence of age on characteristics of polymyositis and dermatomyositis in adults. Medicine (Baltimore) 78:139, 1999

13. Launay D, Hatron PY, Delaporte E, et al: Scleromyxedema (lichen myxedematosus) associated with dermatomyositis. Br J Dermatol 144:359, 2001

14. Wenzel J, Uerlich M, Gerdsen R, et al: Association of inclusion body myositis with subacute cutaneous lupus erythematosus. Rheumatol Int 21:75, 2001

15. Lindvall B, Bengtsson A, Ernerudh J, et al: Subclinical myositis is common in primary Sjögren's syndrome and is not related to muscle pain. J Rheumatol 29:717, 2002

16. Olsen NJ, King LE Jr, Park JH: Muscle abnormalities in scleroderma. Rheum Dis Clin North Am 22:783, 1996

17. Oddis CV, Conte CG, Steen VD, et al: Incidence of polymyositis-dermatomyositis: a 20-year study of hospital diagnosed cases in Allegheny County, PA 1963-1982. J Rheumatol 17:1329, 1990

18. Reed AM: Myositis in children. Curr Opin Rheumatol 13:428, 2001

19. Englund P, Nennesmo I, Klareskog L, et al: Interleukin-1alpha expression in capillaries and major histocompatibility complex class I expression in type II muscle fibers from polymyositis and dermatomyositis patients: important pathogenic features independent of inflammatory cell clusters in muscle tissue. Arthritis Rheum 46:1044, 2002

20. Kase S, Shiota G, Fujii Y, et al: Inclusion body myositis associated with hepatitis C virus infection. Liver 21:357, 2001

21. Pachman LM, Litt DL, Rowley AH, et al: Lack of detection of enteroviral RNA or bacterial DNA in magnetic resonance imaging–directed muscle biopsies from twenty children with active untreated juvenile dermatomyositis. Arthritis Rheum 38:1513, 1995

22. Ytterberg SR: Infectious agents associated with myopathies. Curr Opin Rheumatol 8:507, 1996

23. Pascuzzi RM: Drugs and toxins associated with myopathies. Curr Opin Rheumatol 10:511, 1998

24. Dalakas MC: Molecular immunology and genetics of inflammatory muscle diseases. Arch Neurol 55:1509, 1998

25. Vogel H: Inclusion body myositis: a review. Adv Anat Pathol 5:164, 1998

26. Reed AM, Picornell YJ, Harwood A, et al: Chimerism in children with juvenile dermatomyositis. 357:887, 2002

27. Artlett CM, Ramos R, Jiminez SA, et al: Chimeric cells of maternal origin in juvenile idiopathic inflammatory myopathies. Childhood Myositis Heterogeneity Collaborative Group. Lancet 356:2155, 2000

28. Engel AG, Arahata K: Mononuclear cells in myopathies: quantitation of functionally distinct subsets, recognition of antigen-specific cell-mediated cytotoxicity in some diseases, and implications for the pathogenesis of the different inflammatory myopathies. Hum Pathol 17:704, 1986

29. Mantegazza R, Andreetta F, Bernasconi P, et al: Analysis of T cell receptor repertoire of muscle-infiltrating T lymphocytes in polymyositis: restricted Vα/β rearrangements

30. may indicate antigen-driven selection. J Clin Invest 91:2880, 1993

30. Schwarz MI: The lung in polymyositis. Clin Chest Med 19:701, 1998

31. Gonzalez-Lopez L, Gamez-Nava JI, Sanchez L, et al: Cardiac manifestations in dermato-polymyositis. Clin Exp Rheumatol 14:373, 1996

32. Spiera R, Kagen L: Extramuscular manifestations in idiopathic inflammatory myopathies. Curr Opin Rheumatol 10:556, 1998

33. Hochberg MC, Feldman D, Stevens MB: Adult onset polymyositis/dermatomyositis: an analysis of clinical and laboratory features and survival in 76 patients with a review of the literature. Semin Arthritis Rheum 15:168, 1986

34. Worrall JG, Phongsathorn V, Hooper RL, et al: Racial variation in serum creatinine kinase unrelated to lean body mass. Br J Rheumatol 29:371, 1990

35. Park JH, Vital T, Ryder N, et al: MR imaging and P-31 MR spectroscopy provide unique quantitative data for longitudinal management of patients with dermatomyositis. Arthritis Rheum 37:736, 1994

36. Dalakas MC: Polymyositis, dermatomyositis, and inclusion-body myositis. N Engl J Med 325:1487, 1991

37. Love LA, Leff RL, Fraser DD, et al: A new approach to the classification of idiopathic inflammatory myopathy: myositis-specific autoantibodies define useful homogeneous patient groups. Medicine (Baltimore) 70:360, 1991

38. Brouwer R, Hengstman GJ, Vree Egberts W, et al: Autoantibody profiles in the sera of European patients with myositis. Ann Rheum Dis 60:116, 2001

39. Sontheimer RD: Would a new name hasten the acceptance of amyopathic dermatomyositis (dermatomyositis sine myositis) as a distinctive subset within the idiopathic inflammatory dermatomyopathies spectrum of clinical illness? J Am Acad Dermatol 46:626, 2002

40. Olsen NJ, Park J: Skeletal muscle imaging for the evaluation of myopathies. Diseases of Skeletal Muscle. Wortmann R, Ed. Lippincott, Williams & Wilkins, New York, 1999, p 293

41. Fraser DD, Frank JA, Dalakas M, et al: Magnetic resonance imaging in the idiopathic inflammatory myopathies. J Rheumatol 18:1693, 1991

42. Reimers CD, Fleckenstein JL, Witt TN, et al: Muscular ultrasound in idiopathic inflammatory myopathies of adults. J Neurol Sci 116:82, 1993

43. Fleckenstein JL, Reimers CD: Inflammatory myopathies: radiologic evaluation. Radiol Clin North Am 34:427, 1996

44. Newman ED, Kurland RJ: P31 magnetic resonance spectroscopy in polymyositis and dermatomyositis: altered energy utilization during exercise. Arthritis Rheum 35:199, 1992

45. Sigurgeirsson B, Lindelof B, Edhag O, et al: Risk of cancer in patients with dermatomyositis or polymyositis. N Engl J Med 326:363, 1992

46. Stockton D, Doherty VR, Brewster DH: Risk of cancer in patients with dermatomyositis or polymyositis, and follow-up implications: a Scottish population-based cohort study. Br J Cancer 85:41, 2001

47. Clarke AE, Bloch DA, Medsger TA, et al: A longitudinal study of functional disability in a national cohort of patients with polymyositis/dermatomyositis. Arthritis Rheum 38:1218, 1995

48. Joffe MM, Love, LA, Leff RL, et al: Drug therapy of the idiopathic inflammatory myopathies: predictors of response to prednisone, azathioprine, and methotrexate and a comparison of their efficacy. Am J Med 94:379, 1993

49. Villalba ML, Hicks JE, Thornton B, et al: A combination of oral methotrexate and azathioprine is more effective than high dose intravenous MTX with leucovorin rescue in treatment-resistant myositis. Arthritis Rheum 38:S307, 1995

50. Vencovsky J, Jarosova K, Machacek S: Cyclosporine A versus methotrexate in the treatment of polymyositis and dermatomyositis. Scand J Rheumatol 29:95, 2000

51. Chaudhry V, Cornblath DR, Griffin JW, et al: Mycophenolate mofetil: a safe and promising immunosuppressant in neuromuscular diseases. Neurology 56:94, 2001

52. Mowzoon N, Sussman A, Bradley WG: Mycophenolate (CellCept) treatment of myasthenia gravis, chronic inflammatory polyneuropathy and inclusion body myositis. J Neurol Sci 185:119, 2001

53. Adams EM, Pucino F, Yarboro C, et al: A pilot study: use of fludarabine for refractory dermatomyositis and polymyositis, and examination of endpoint measures. J Rheumatol 26:352, 1999

54. Dalakas MC, Illa I, Dambrosia JM, et al: A controlled trial of high-dose intravenous immune globulin infusions as treatment for dermatomyositis. N Engl J Med 329:1993, 1993

55. Danieli MG, Malcangi G, Palmieri C, et al: Cyclosporin A and intravenous immunoglobulin treatment in polymyositis/dermatomyositis. Ann Rheum Dis 61:37, 2002

56. Walter MC, Lochmuller H, Toepfer M, et al: High-dose immunoglobulin therapy in sporadic inclusion body myositis: a double-blind, placebo-controlled study. J Neurol 247:22, 2000

57. Dalakas MC, Koffman B, Fujii M, et al: A controlled study of intravenous immunoglobulin combined with prednisone in the treatment of IBM. Neurology 56:323, 2001

58. Jorizzo JL: Dermatomyositis: practical aspects. Arch Dermatol 138:114, 2002

117 Systemic Vasculitis Syndromes

Brian F. Mandell, M.D., Ph.D.

The diagnosis of a primary vasculitic syndrome is dependent on documentation of vasculitis and the exclusion of diseases that can cause secondary vasculitis. The diagnosis of a specific primary vasculitic disorder depends on the pattern of organ involvement, the pathology, and the size of affected blood vessels.

The major determinants of prognosis and therapy include the type of vasculitis, the severity of critical organ involvement, the rate of disease progression, and the etiology if identifiable. The inflammatory process is often associated with nonspecific symptoms and laboratory abnormalities (elevated erythrocyte sedimentation rate, anemia, and fevers) that do not distinguish vasculitic diseases from other inflammatory, infectious, or neoplastic diseases. The toxic nature of the therapies for systemic vasculitis dictates the need for an accurate diagnosis.

Approach to the Patient with Suspected Vasculitis

EVALUATION

The physician should not be reluctant to pursue invasive testing in the diagnostic evaluation of patients with a multisystem disease, but biopsy of clinically uninvolved tissue and obtaining less specific tests should be eschewed. An approach directed toward ruling in a specific form of vasculitis and ruling out reasonable specific alternatives should be pursued.

The first step in the diagnosis of vasculitis is to perform a detailed patient history and physical examination to document specific organ involvement. Special attention should be paid to the skin, eyes, ears, upper airway, joints, kidneys, lymph nodes, peripheral nerves, and large vessels. A few selected laboratory tests [see Table 1] should be included in the initial evaluation. Specialized studies, including serologies, should be selectively obtained only after a differential diagnosis is completed. If the urine dipstick test indicates blood or protein, a physician should immediately examine a fresh urine sediment. Urine that has been sitting for several hours before analysis is not useful for identification of cellular casts, which rapidly degenerate ex vivo. Red blood cell casts are highly suggestive of glomerulonephritis, but white cell casts may also be seen. Glomerulonephritis is usually asymptomatic. On the basis of the pattern of organ involvement, a differential diagnosis that includes the appropriate types of systemic vasculitis and other disorders can be generated.

CLASSIFICATION

Several classification schemes have been proposed for organizing the systemic vasculitic disorders into a consistent paradigm. These classifications are useful in distinguishing the clinical disorders that have distinct differences in prognosis and response to treatment.[1] No scheme is universally accepted. They all reiterate the characteristics of fulminant or classic disease, placing an emphasis on specificity of diagnosis. If a classification scheme is strictly adhered to, the newly ill patient without fully expressed disease is frequently left without a definitive diagnosis. Nonetheless, classification systems provide useful constructs for communication and the design of research protocols [see Figure 1]. The most widely used classification schemes are based on the caliber of affected blood vessels, the pattern of organ involvement, and the presence or absence of granulomas, significant immune complex deposition, and eosinophilic infiltrates. Some authors have proposed a diagnostic role for the presence or absence of specific serum antineutrophil cytoplasmic antibodies (ANCAs), particularly antibodies to proteinase 3 and myeloperoxidase. At present, the appropriate role of these tests is to support a rationally developed clinical diagnosis, not to define one. In patients who do not fit neatly into a well-defined diagnostic category, these serologic tests should not supplant an attempt to obtain a tissue diagnosis. The presence of ANCA is not equivalent to the diagnosis of vasculitis.

When the dominant symptoms and findings (i.e., neuropathy and cutaneous vasculitis) do not suggest a single specific vasculitic disorder, targeted physical examination and serologic testing may be helpful. Most valuable is biopsy confirmation of the specific disorder. The value of indiscriminate testing for antinuclear antibodies, ANCA, rheumatoid factor, and angiotensin-converting enzyme is arguable. Infection with hepatitis B or C is associated with a broad range of vasculitic syndromes, and these infections must be routinely excluded.[2]

TREATMENT

The systemic vasculitides are potentially life threatening and require potent anti-inflammatory and immunosuppressive therapy. Diagnoses should be made with as much certainty as possible. However, questions regarding alternative diagnoses or coexistent diseases may linger. Hence, even after therapy is initiated, physicians should maintain a high degree of vigilance to detect unrelated medical problems, complications of therapy, or both. The signs and symptoms of infection may transiently resolve with steroid therapy.[3] With the initiation of potent immunosuppressive therapy, there is a prolonged window of increased susceptibility to opportunistic infection. The greatest risks occur in patients with marked neutropenia or those on high doses of corticosteroids. Physicians must be particularly wary about attributing new problems to so-called flares in the underlying disease without first excluding a new or recrudescent infection. Varicella-zoster may present with fever and pain before appearance of the vesicles. *Pneumocystis carinii*, cytomegalovirus, systemic fungal infections, and reactivation of mycobacterial disease are observed more frequently than in the normal host. Immunosuppression from steroids and other medications is frequently associated with mucosal candidiasis, less commonly associated with molluscum contagiosum, and rarely associated with Kaposi sarcoma.

Methotrexate, azathioprine, and cyclophosphamide may cause leukopenia and, less often, other cytopenias. Methotrexate must be used with caution, if at all, in patients with a depressed glomerular filtration rate (GFR).

Small Vessel Vasculitis

Vasculitis that affects capillaries and venules is the most common form of vasculitis and almost invariably involves the skin. It can occur at any age and affects men and women with equal frequency.

ETIOLOGY

Small vessel vasculitis can occur as an idiopathic disorder or secondary to drug allergy, bacterial endocarditis, and viral infections such as those caused by hepatitis B or C, disseminated *Neisseria*, and rickettsiae; can be part of a defined systemic autoimmune disorder such as Sjögren syndrome, systemic lupus erythematosus (SLE), or rheumatoid arthritis; or can occur in association with hematologic, lymphoid, and solid-organ malignancies [*see Figure 2*].

DIAGNOSIS

Clinical Manifestations

Cutaneous involvement can occur in many of the primary or secondary vasculitic syndromes. Large, medium-sized, or small vessel occlusion can cause livedo, Raynaud phenomenon, or necrosis. Purpura is the most common manifestation of small vessel vasculitis. Small vessel vasculitis is frequently associated with immune complex deposition. Vasculitis primarily involving the postcapillary venules has also been termed hypersensitivity vasculitis.[4] Small vessel vasculitis can also occur in systemic vasculitis that primarily affects larger vessels (e.g., Wegener granulomatosis and microscopic polyangiitis). Primary small vessel vasculitis may be limited to the skin or may be associated with visceral involvement, including alveolar hemorrhage, intestinal ischemia or hemorrhage, and glomerulonephritis.

Purpura tends to occur in recurrent crops of lesions of similar age, and is more pronounced in gravity-dependent areas [*see Figure 3*]. When purpura is not primarily in gravity-dependent areas, cold agglutinin disease, cryoglobulinemia (which may be associated with an infection such as hepatitis C or with lymphoma), embolism, and infiltrative diseases should be excluded. Cutaneous vasculitis of any etiology may be associated with striking dependent edema.

In a case series of cutaneous small vessel vasculitis,[4] almost 100% of patients younger than 20 years had disease limited to the skin, whereas approximately 40% of the 172 patients older

Table 1 Selected Laboratory Tests for Patients with Multisystem Disease and Possible Vasculitis

Test	Comments
Platelet count	Thrombocytosis may parallel the acute-phase response Thrombocytopenia is not expected in primary vasculitic syndromes; consider SLE, marrow infiltration, hairy-cell leukemia, TTP, DIC, hypersplenism, APLS, HIV, scleroderma renal crisis, and heparin-induced thrombocytopenia
White blood cell count	Leukopenia is not expected in primary vasculitis; consider SLE, leukemia, hypersplenism, sepsis, myelodysplasia, and HIV Eosinophilia is common in Churg-Strauss syndrome; it may occur in WG, rheumatoid arthritis, or normotensive scleroderma renal crisis
Erythrocyte sedimentation rate	Relatively low ESR is seen in DIC, liver failure, and hyperviscosity; ESR is frequently low in HSP, may be low in Takayasu arteritis, and is normal in ≤ 20% of giant cell arteritis
Transaminases	ALT or AST is elevated in liver disease, myositis, rhabdomyolysis, hemolysis, or myocardial necrosis
Anti–glomerular basement membrane	Useful for evaluation of alveolar hemorrhage, with or without glomerulonephritis; also useful for evaluation of normocomplementemic glomerulonephritis
Antinuclear antibody	Order when there is clinical suspicion of SLE, not as a general screening test for sick patients
Antineutrophil cytoplasmic antibody	Order when there is clinical suspicion of WG or MPA
Drug screen	Order for unexplained CNS symptoms, myocardial ischemia, vascular spasm, panic attacks with systemic features, or tachycardia; urine screen should be done
Blood cultures	Useful for any patient with febrile, multisystem, or wasting illness; pulmonary infiltrates; or focal ischemia/infarction. Cultures are easy to obtain
APLA/PTT/RVVT	Order for unexplained venous or arterial thrombosis or thrombocytopenia
Purified protein derivative (± anergy)	Use in any patient who may require steroid therapy or who has unexplained sterile pyuria or hematuria, granulomatous inflammation, chronic meningitis, or possible exposure to tuberculosis
Examination of fresh urinary sediment	Perform in all patients with an unexplained febrile or multisystem illness
Hepatitis serologies	Order for abnormal transaminases or elevated hepatic alkaline phosphatase; portal hypertension; PAN or MPA syndrome; or unexplained cryoglobulinemia, polyarthritis, or cutaneous vasculitis
Complement C3, C4	Not a screening test for vasculitis; useful in the differential diagnosis of glomerulonephritis; low in cryoglobulinemia; may be low in endocarditis; usually normal in PAN, MPA, HSP, WG; may be low in viral hepatitis–related glomerulonephritis or vasculitis
Aldolase	Aldolase has no organ specificity; it has similar organ distribution as lactic dehydrogenase

ALT—alanine aminotransferase APLA—antiphospholipid antibody APLS—antiphospholipid antibody syndrome AST—aspartate aminotransferase DIC—disseminated intravascular coagulation ESR—erythrocyte sedimentation rate HSP—Henoch-Schönlein purpura MPA—microscopic polyangiitis PAN—polyarteritis nodosa PTT—partial thromboplastin time RVVT—Russell viper venom test SLE—systemic lupus erythematosus TTP—thrombotic thombocytopenic purpura WG—Wegener granulomatosis

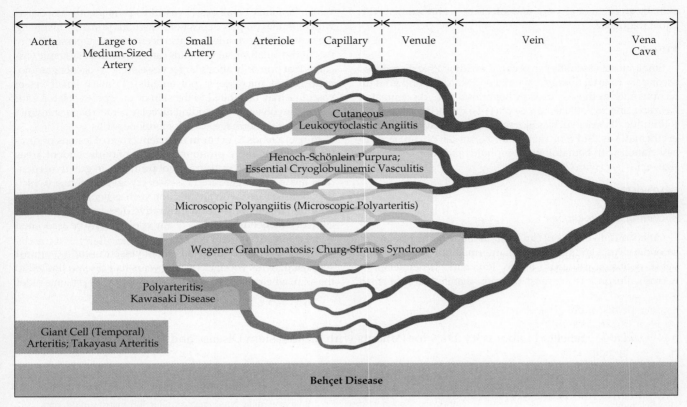

Figure 1   **Classification of the systemic vasculitis syndrome.**[1]

than 20 years had an associated or underlying systemic disorder. Seventeen adults had a systemic necrotizing vasculitis, four had malignancy, four had a bacterial infection causing the vasculitis, 11 had cryoglobulinemia, and 59 had Henoch-Schönlein purpura. The possibility of infection with hepatitis C virus, likely the most common cause of mixed cryoglobulinemia,[2] was not investigated.

Laboratory Tests

Biopsy is useful in excluding causes of nonvasculitic purpura such as amyloidosis, leukemia cutis, Kaposi sarcoma, T cell lymphomas, and cholesterol or myxomatous emboli. Tissue immunofluorescent staining is useful to support the diagnosis of Henoch-Schönlein purpura or SLE. The cells infiltrating and perhaps destroying the vessel wall may be neutrophils or lymphocytes, depending on the etiology. The pathology in most cases of small vessel vasculitis is leukocytoclastic angiitis.

CLINICAL SUBSETS

Henoch-Schönlein Purpura

Henoch-Schönlein purpura is a small vessel vasculitic syndrome in which cutaneous features are usually striking and visceral involvement is common. Henoch-Schönlein purpura, which occurs less commonly in adults than in children,[5] is usually associated with vascular and renal deposition of IgA-containing immune complexes. Common manifestations of Henoch-Schönlein purpura include purpura, urticaria, abdominal pain, gastrointestinal bleeding or intussusception (mostly in children); arthralgias or arthritis; and glomerulonephritis. Visceral symptoms may precede the skin lesions. Henoch-Schönlein purpura may

be precipitated by medications or streptococcal or viral infections. It is usually a self-limited disorder, but the associated glomerulonephritis may, in rare instances (most often in adults), progress to renal failure.

Urticarial Vasculitis

Urticarial vasculitis represents a peculiar subset of small vessel vasculitis.[6] The clinical presentation is that of wheals or serpentine papules, sometimes with surrounding or geographically separate angioedema. Individual lesions are slow to resolve, often lasting for several days. There is frequently a burning,

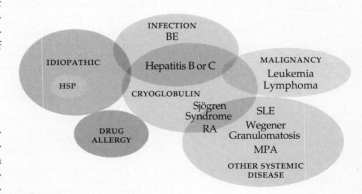

Figure 2   **A Venn diagram illustrates the relations between the causes of small vessel (hypersensitivity) vasculitis. (BE—bacterial endocarditis; HSP—Henoch-Schönlein purpura; MPA—microscopic polyangiitis; RA—rheumatoid arthritis; SLE—systemic lupus erythematosus.)**

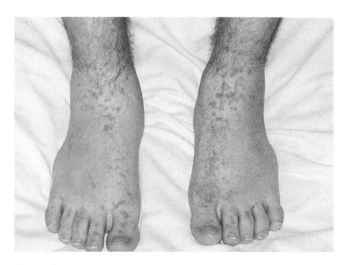

Figure 3 **Palpable purpura of the distal extremities is a common presentation of small vessel vasculitis.**

dysesthetic discomfort from the lesions. Like purpura, the lesions of urticarial vasculitis are frequently located in gravity-dependent areas and often heal with skin hyperpigmentation or an ecchymotic area. Most cases are idiopathic, although there may be an association with an underlying systemic autoimmune disorder such as SLE, IgM paraproteinemia, or a viral infection. In rare cases, urticarial vasculitis has been associated with hypocomplementemia and interstitial pulmonary disease.

TREATMENT

Therapy for cutaneous vasculitis is first directed at eliminating any underlying precipitant. Infectious etiologies should be sought out and treated. Potential offending drugs should be withdrawn. Association with myelodysplasia and myeloproliferative disease should be considered, especially if there are any hematologic abnormalities. If no precipitants are apparent, low-risk therapy can be attempted with nonsteroidal anti-inflammatory drugs, colchicine, pentoxifylline, dapsone, or short-term low-dose corticosteroids. Long-term corticosteroid therapy should be eschewed if at all possible. Compressive support stockings or panty hose may be useful to limit the significant edema that often accompanies cutaneous vasculitis.

Visceral involvement with organ dysfunction may necessitate a more aggressive approach than that used in limited cutaneous vasculitis. Moderate-dose corticosteroids are generally effective. In the setting of complications from chronic corticosteroid use or the setting of severe visceral involvement, methotrexate, azathioprine, cyclophosphamide, or other immunosuppressive agents may be required. When treating chronic, refractory small vessel disease that is not organ or life threatening, one must pay close attention to the risk-to-benefit ratio of selected therapies.

Wegener Granulomatosis

Wegener granulomatosis (WG) is a relatively uncommon, potentially lethal disease that is characterized by necrotizing granulomatous inflammation and vasculitis of small and medium-sized vessels.[7,8] Males and females of all ages can be affected.

Clinical Manifestations

In Wegener granulomatosis, multiple organs are often involved, with a predilection for the upper and lower respiratory tracts, eyes, and kidneys.

Upper respiratory tract involvement Upper airway disease may be striking but is often attributed for months or even years to routine sinus disease until other manifestations of WG are recognized. Even after the diagnosis is made and immunosuppressive treatment is provided, sinus disease may be recalcitrant to therapy. This resistance may be caused in part by superinfection of damaged tissue by *Staphylococcus aureus*. Anatomic damage can include septal perforations and saddle-nose deformities. Laryngotracheal involvement may result in subglottic stenosis. Ear involvement is common, particularly otitis media that may produce conductive hearing loss. Orbital pseudotumors may cause proptosis with intractable pain and loss of vision; these inflammatory and fibrous masses may be refractory to anti-inflammatory therapy, immunosuppressive therapy, and even radiation therapy. Conjunctivitis, uveitis, and retinal disease alone or in combination commonly occur.

Lower respiratory tract involvement Lung involvement may be absent at the onset of disease or present dramatically as diffuse alveolar hemorrhage. One third of pulmonary lesions noted on imaging studies [*see Figure 4*] are asymptomatic (CT scanning is more sensitive than radiography). Nodules often undergo necrosis leading to cavity formation. Bronchospasm is not characteristic of WG. If airway obstruction is suspected, bronchoscopy should be considered to exclude endobronchial or subglottic stenoses. It is frequently necessary to rule out infectious causes of the pulmonary infiltrates, and bronchoscopy is useful in this regard. However, tissue obtained from transbronchial biopsy is usually insufficient to make the pathologic diagnosis of WG.

Open lung biopsy often provides the optimal opportunity to demonstrate the typical pathologic findings of WG and to exclude malignancies and atypical infections. Typical open lung biopsies[9] contain areas of necrosis, frequently in a broad pattern; giant cells in the parenchymal tissue; and vasculitis. Not all histopathologic components may be present in the same section. Because these findings may also occur in chronic mycobacterial or fungal infections, special stains and cultures for these agents are essential.

Glomerulonephritis Glomerulonephritis is a common cause of morbidity and mortality in WG. Its presence or absence defines the generalized or limited forms of the disease. Glomerulonephritis may be relatively indolent or aggressive, often taking the latter course. It may be clinically and pathologically indistinguishable from idiopathic rapidly progressive crescentic glomerulonephritis. The evolution from subclinical to dialysis-dependent renal disease may occur over several weeks. Glomerulonephritis may be present at the outset of the disease, or it may develop only after the patient has been ill with an apparently limited form of the disease. The importance of frequent microscopic urinalyses in the initial and follow-up evaluation of patients with WG cannot be overemphasized. Especially in elderly or debilitated patients, valuable information may be obtained by occasional 24-hour urine collections, which

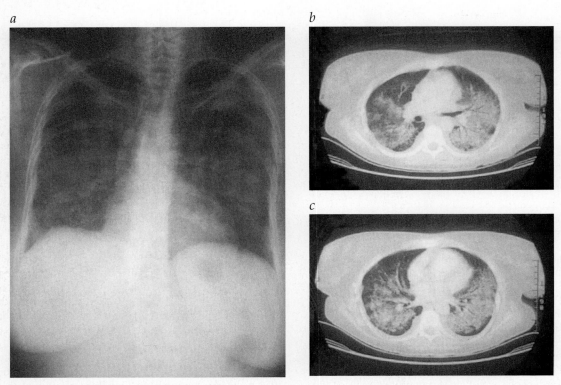

Figure 4 **The nodular infiltrates of the lung in Wegener granulomatosis are shown less extensively in a standard radiograph (*a*) than in computed tomographic scans (*b* and *c*).**

can establish a more accurate estimate of the GFR than that provided by the serum creatinine measurement. Renal biopsy may reveal focal and segmental glomerulonephritis with variable glomerular proliferative changes, crescent formation, and necrosis, in the absence of significant immune complex deposition. Although supportive of the diagnosis of WG, these findings are not diagnostic of the disease.

Additional clinical manifestations Musculoskeletal involvement occurs in over half of patients with WG. Symptoms may include migratory, additive, or fixed distribution of arthralgias or arthritis. Rheumatoid factor is frequently present in patients with WG, and it may cause diagnostic confusion with rheumatoid arthritis when joint symptoms are significant. The joint disease of WG only rarely produces bone erosions. Neurologic signs and symptoms occur in fewer than 50% of patients, peripheral neuropathy in fewer than 20%, and involvement of the central nervous system in fewer than 10%. Oculomotor defects may occur because of impingement by a retro-orbital mass. Gastrointestinal ischemia and ulcerations are infrequent but may be confused with inflammatory bowel disease, especially because the latter can be associated with ANCA (usually perinuclear ANCA, or p-ANCA) positivity. Cutaneous involvement has been reported in up to 50% of patients who have WG with purpura, panniculitis, or ulcerations. The activity of the skin disease generally parallels systemic disease activity.

Laboratory Tests

Unexplained inflammation of the respiratory tract or eye, or the presence of glomerulonephritis is consistent with the diagnosis of WG. The probability of WG is increased when multiple organ involvement is present, upper airway disease is destruc-

tive, and pulmonary nodules (especially with cavities) are demonstrated by radiography. Any combination of organ involvement is possible, but most patients exhibit upper airway involvement at the time of diagnosis.

If the entire clinical picture is compatible with WG and alternative diagnoses have been appropriately ruled out, the finding of circulating cytoplasmic ANCA, or c-ANCA, with anti–proteinase 3 specificity is sufficient to make the provisional diagnosis and initiate therapy. Approximately 20% of patients with WG may have p-ANCA with antimyeloperoxidase specificity. If there are any atypical features or special concerns regarding the initiation of immunosuppressive therapy or if the patient does not respond appropriately to therapy, tissue documentation of the diagnosis is mandatory. The presence of ANCA is not equivalent to the presence of vasculitis; ANCAs can be found in other diseases. The ANCA level is also not a reliable means to follow disease activity.[10,11] Because WG generally requires glucocorticoid plus cytotoxic drug therapy, it should be distinguished from other inflammatory disorders, including other vasculitic syndromes [*see Table 2*], which may be effectively treated with a less toxic regimen.

TREATMENT

Initial treatment of generalized WG virtually always requires dual-drug immunosuppressive therapy. Corticosteroids may produce symptomatic improvement in the upper airway, lungs, skin, and musculoskeletal system, but tapering usually results in a flare in the disease. Acutely serious disease, particularly progressing renal disease, is treated initially with corticosteroids and daily cyclophosphamide with subsequent tapering of the corticosteroids. There are some strong relative contraindications to the use of cyclophosphamide, including bladder dysfunction and leukopenia. In milder or limited WG, weekly methotrexate

Table 2   Clinical Features of Vasculitis

Disorder	Common Target Organs	Special Pathologic Features	Special Laboratory Studies	Comments
Microscopic polyangiitis	Nerve, glomerulus, lung (small vessels), GI tract	No giant cells, vasculitis, proliferative GN (no or rare immune deposits*)	p-ANCA (antimyeloperoxidase)	Rule out hepatitis B and C
Polyarteritis nodosa	Nerve, GI tract	Arteritis of medium muscular arteries, no giant cells, no GN	No ANCA	No small vessel involvement; rule out hepatitis B and C
Wegener granulomatosis	Upper airway, eye, lung (small vessels), glomerulus, nerve, musculoskeletal system	Giant cells, geographic necrosis, mild eosinophilia, vasculitis, proliferative GN (no or rare immune deposits)	c-ANCA (anti-PR3)	Chronic sinus or ear disease
Churg-Strauss syndrome	Nerve, lung infiltrates, heart, skin	Giant cells, eosinophilia, vasculitis, proliferative GN (no or rare immune deposits)	Eosinophilia ± ANCAs	Positive atopic history

*Presence of immune deposits suggests possible hepatitis B or C infection.
ANCA—antineutrophil cytoplasmic antibody   c-ANCA—cytoplasmic ANCA   GN—glomerulonephritis   p-ANCA—perinuclear ANCA   PR3—proteinase 3

(0.20 to 0.30 mg/kg, adjusted for renal function) with folic acid or leucovorin may be substituted for the cyclophosphamide.[12] Patients treated with methotrexate or cyclophosphamide must be continuously monitored for flares in disease, opportunistic infections, and side effects. Side effects include cytopenias and drug-induced pneumonitis. Methotrexate may cause hepatitis and, on rare occasions, cirrhosis. It should be avoided in the setting of significant renal insufficiency. Cyclophosphamide can cause cystitis and bladder cancer. Some authors have suggested using trimethoprim-sulfamethoxazole as adjunctive therapy for the treatment of WG and for prevention of bacterial infections that may promote flares of upper airway disease. This proposition remains controversial. Administration of trimethoprim-sulfamethoxazole three times weekly is useful, however, in protecting patients against *P. carinii* pneumonia while they are receiving intensive immunosuppression therapy. Local nasal and sinus toilet and otolaryngoscopic evaluations are a routine part of the care of patients with upper airway disease.

Churg-Strauss Syndrome

Churg-Strauss syndrome (CSS), or allergic granulomatosis angiitis, is a rare syndrome that affects small to medium-sized arteries and veins.

DIAGNOSIS

Clinical Manifestations

CSS displays clinical similarities to WG in terms of organ involvement and pathology, especially in patients with upper or lower airway disease or glomerulonephritis. CSS differs most strikingly from WG in that the former occurs in patients with a history of atopy, asthma, or allergic rhinitis, which is often ongoing. In the prevasculitic atopy phase, as well as during the systemic phase of the illness, eosinophilia is characteristic and often of striking degree ($\geq$ 1,000 eosinophils/mm^3). When eosinophilia is present in WG, it is usually more modest ($\leq$ 500 eosinophils/mm^3).

Systemic features of CSS include some combination of pulmonary infiltrates, cardiomyopathy, coronary arteritis, pericarditis, polyneuropathy (symmetrical or mononeuritis multiplex), ischemic bowel disease, eosinophilic gastroenteritis, ocular inflammation, nasal perforations, glomerulonephritis, cutaneous nodules, and purpura.[13,14]

The patchy pulmonary infiltrates of CSS are often transient and may be associated with alveolar hemorrhage. Pulmonary nodules are uncommon and rarely cavitate. Pleural effusions are common and often contain abundant eosinophils. Clinical distinction from hypersensitivity pneumonitis, allergic aspergillosis, and pulmonary lymphoma is at times difficult. Several cases of CSS have been reported after introduction of zafirlukast therapy and weaning of patients with chronic bronchial asthma off corticosteroids.

Cardiac disease can be severe and is a leading cause of mortality. Valvular heart disease is not as striking or as common as in the idiopathic hypereosinophilic syndrome. Neurologic involvement occurs in more than 60% of patients, may be severe, and is generally attributable to arteritis. Cutaneous purpura, urticaria, polymorphous erythematous eruptions, and nodules occur. Gastrointestinal involvement resulting from ischemic vasculitis, eosinophilic gastroenteritis, or both may cause pain, cramping, and diarrhea.

Laboratory Tests

Histopathology typically exhibits extravascular granulomatous inflammation, with a prominent eosinophilic infiltrate and vasculitis. Vasculitis in a given tissue section may be granulomatous or nongranulomatous. Granulomas can be found in tissue at areas separate from the demonstrable vasculitis. Eosinophilic infiltrates are more striking than in WG. Neither abundant eosinophils, granulomas, or giant cells are found in classic polyarteritis nodosa (PAN) or microscopic polyangiitis (MPA). The pathology of the nodules is not by itself sufficient to make a diagnosis of CSS, because similar pathology can be seen in lymphoma and sarcoidosis. Glomerulonephritis is not as common or severe as in WG, but when present, it is usually focal and segmental and indistinguishable from other forms of so-called pauci-immune (without significant tissue deposition of immune complexes) glomerulonephritis.

TREATMENT

CSS is generally a corticosteroid-responsive disease. Some patients are able to be withdrawn from steroids. However, bronchial asthma and sinus disease may require ongoing therapy, even if the vasculitic component of the disease has remitted. Patients with severe or refractory visceral organ involvement are empirically treated with additional agents such as cyclophosphamide, methotrexate, or azathioprine.

Polyarteritis Nodosa and Microscopic Polyangiitis

CLASSIFICATION

Attempts to separate PAN and MPA, two forms of necrotizing small to medium-sized vessel arteritis, have not been universally accepted. A recent international consensus conference proposed that the diagnosis of these disorders be based on the absence of granulomatous inflammation in both and the lack of involvement of arterioles, capillaries, venules, and glomerular capillaries in PAN. Older studies of patients with PAN did not uniformly make this distinction. Even more important, patients with viral hepatitis B or C were not excluded from older studies. The recognition of viral hepatitis is crucially important because chronic hepatitis B or C[15] can elicit a secondary vasculitic syndrome indistinguishable from PAN or MPA in presentation but distinct in response to therapy.[16] MPA involves vessels ranging in size from capillaries and venules to medium-sized arteries [see Figure 1].[17]

DIAGNOSIS

Clinical Manifestations

Glomerulonephritis, particularly rapidly progressive glomerulonephritis, and alveolar hemorrhage are common in MPA and absent, by definition, in classic PAN.

PAN affects the medium-sized muscular arteries and, like MPA, is associated with peripheral neuropathy and bowel ischemia.[18-20] Azotemia and hypertension in PAN may occur because of arteritis of the renal arteries but not because of glomerulonephritis. Microaneurysm formation in medium-sized arteries may be striking, and they may rupture.

Constitutional symptoms such as fever, asthenia, and myalgias are common in both PAN and MPA. Elevated acute-phase reactants, thrombocytosis, leukocytosis, and the anemia of inflammatory disease are common, although they are not uniformly present.

When the clinical syndrome of PAN or MPA is suspected, bacterial infection (e.g., endocarditis) and viral infection (e.g., hepatitis B and C) must be excluded. The association with hepatitis B or C infection may not dramatically alter the presentation of the PAN or MPA syndrome, except that membranous glomerulonephritis, cryoglobulinemia, immune complex–associated glomerulonephritis, hepatic failure, and thrombocytopenia are more likely to occur with viral hepatitis–associated vasculitis.

Antiphospholipid antibody syndrome (APLS) can mimic PAN by presenting as mesenteric ischemia or renal insufficiency caused by thrombotic occlusion of mesenteric and renal vessels.[21] Features of APLS and PAN include livedo reticularis [see Figure 5]. Glomerulonephritis cryoglobulinemia, immune complex–associated glomerulonephritis, and peripheral neuropathy are not expected in APLS unless the patient also has SLE. Thrombocytopenia can occur with APLS but is not expected in PAN. Cholesterol embolization[22] should also be considered as a cause of livedo, renal insufficiency, and constitutional symptoms.

Laboratory Tests

The diagnosis of MPA and PAN should ideally be based on histopathologic demonstration of arteritis and the clinical pattern of disease. The presence of serum p-ANCA with antimyeloperoxidase specificity (in 60% of MPA patients) supports the clinical diagnosis of MPA, but p-ANCA is not specific for this disease. ANCAs are not characteristic of PAN. The renal biopsy tissue in MPA, as in WG and CSS, does not contain exten-

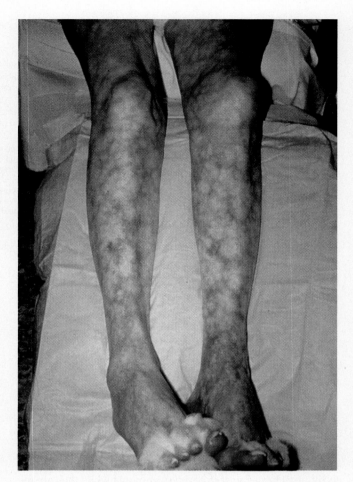

Figure 5 Livedo reticularis is characterized by reddish-blue mottling of the extremities caused by occlusion of the deep dermal arterioles.

sive immune complexes by immunofluorescent staining and electron microscopy—so-called pauci-immune glomerulonephritis. Lung biopsy in the setting of pulmonary infiltrates or hemorrhage reveals capillaritis, a histopathologic pattern that can also be seen in WG, SLE, and anti–glomerular basement membrane disease. Biopsy is most useful to rule out alternative pulmonary diagnoses; open lung and thoracoscopic techniques have a higher yield for demonstrating vasculitis than transbronchial biopsy. Classic PAN does not cause glomerulonephritis or pulmonary parenchymal disease.

Demonstrating arteritis in PAN may be difficult, especially in the setting of dominant constitutional symptoms and the absence of easily accessible, disease-affected tissue. Initial biopsy efforts should be directed toward tissue that is abnormal by symptoms or objective testing. Sural nerve biopsy has become a popular option when attempting to diagnose an arteritis that is affecting medium-sized muscular vessels. The sural nerve is an accessible pure sensory nerve, and its vasa nervorum contains small as well as medium-sized muscular arteries. Nerve conduction studies can identify a diseased ischemic nerve before the appearance of clinical symptoms.[23] Multiple reports have emphasized the low diagnostic yield from the biopsy of asymptomatic and electrically normal nerve. Even nerves with abnormal conduction study results reportedly showed no diagnostic pathology 46% of the time.[24] There is notable morbidity associated with this procedure; 13 of 60 patients experienced wound infections or delayed healing, and three patients suffered from new pain in the distribution of the biopsied sural nerve.[24] Biopsy of clinically uninvolved tissue (i.e., asymptomatic muscle) has a diagnostic yield of less than 30%.

Abdominal angiography is frequently utilized in the evaluation of patients who may have medium-sized vessel arteritis when biopsy has been unrewarding or is not an option. Arteries affected by polyarteritis nodosa and other disorders of medium-sized muscular arteries may develop microaneurysms or stenoses that can be visualized by angiography. When angiography is used in an effort to diagnose systemic necrotizing vasculitis, in the absence of pathologic evidence of the disease, several caveats must be noted. Angiography has limited spatial resolution; smaller vessels are not well seen. Patients with primarily smaller vessel disease will not likely have a diagnostic angiogram. In one study, only four of 30 patients with MPA, a disease that affects both small and medium-sized arteries, had diagnostic angiograms.[17] Different investigators have reported aneurysms in 60% to 90% of patients with PAN. Aneurysms take time to develop and may not be present early in the course of the illness. In addition to being associated with aneurysms, arteritis may also be associated with stenoses, which may be longer and smoother than typical atherosclerotic lesions or occlusion. To maximize the yield from the procedure, angiography should include the celiac, renal, and mesenteric vessels. Lack of clinical involvement of an organ (i.e., no intestinal ischemia) does not exclude the possibility of finding abnormal vessels on angiography. It has been suggested that the visualization of aneurysms in PAN denotes more severe disease; it is unclear whether their presence may alternatively relate to the actual duration of the illness. Aneurysms may resolve with successful treatment of primary or viral hepatitis–associated disease. The presence of visceral microaneurysms is not diagnostic of PAN. They have also been anecdotally described in patients with WG and MPA, likely representing medium-sized muscular artery involvement in these diseases. Microaneurysms also occur in nonvasculitic disorders. Isolated case reports have described aneurysms in patients with atrial myxoma, bacterial endocarditis, peritoneal carcinomatosis, and severe arterial hypertension and after methamphetamine abuse. Inadequate data are available to assess the sensitivity and specificity or the predictive value of abdominal angiography in the diagnosis of necrotizing arteritis. As is the case when interpreting a biopsy result of suspected vasculitis, imaging studies must be considered in the light of the entire clinical profile. Angiography is generally avoided in the setting of progressive or significant renal insufficiency.

TREATMENT

Treatment of both PAN and MPA is empirical.[25] Corticosteroids in high doses remain the initial mainstay of therapy for both disorders. Corticosteroids alone may be sufficient therapy in patients who do not have critical organ involvement, defined as renal insufficiency, gastrointestinal ischemia, cardiomyopathy, or dense peripheral neuropathy. Therapy with corticosteroids alone may fail more frequently in MPA than in PAN, given the tendency for frequent relapses in MPA.[17] Patients with markers of severe disease are usually treated with glucocorticoids and an additional immunosuppressive agent such as cyclophosphamide. Although this approach is common practice, the indications for initial combination therapy have not been adequately studied.

When active hepatitis B or C infection is present, a relatively short course of steroids should be considered on the basis of disease severity, in conjunction with antiviral therapy.

Kawasaki Disease

Kawasaki disease (KD) was first described in 1967 as mucocutaneous lymph node syndrome.[26] It typically affects infants and young children, causing dominant cutaneous manifestations, but it can on rare occasions affect adults.

DIAGNOSIS

The presence of characteristic clinical features has permitted the establishment of diagnostic criteria [see Table 3]. Vasculitis may involve vessels ranging in size from venules to the aorta. Prominent inflammation is noted in the larger coronary arteries, which results in aneurysm formation in approximately 25% of untreated patients. The immediate and delayed life-threatening cardiac complications of the disease, coupled with its unique therapy (aspirin and intravenous γ-globulin), mandates prompt clinical diagnosis.

High spiking fevers may persist for 1 to 2 weeks if untreated. Rapid defervescence is usually observed with initiation of appropriate therapy. Nonexudative conjunctivitis often appears with the fever. Aseptic (lymphocytic) meningitis is common. Oral involvement includes erythema, dryness and fissuring of the lips, nonexudative pharyngitis, and tongue erythema with very prominent papillae. Mucosal ulcerations are not characteristic of this illness. Distal limb swelling may appear days after the fever, with erythema and tenderness that are not limited to the joints. Desquamation, often in sheets, may begin days to a few weeks after the onset of fever. When desquamation occurs early in KD, it may appear concurrently with a truncal rash and eye and lip changes, and it may mimic a drug reaction or Stevens-Johnson syndrome. The rash is usually diffuse and polymorphous, with urticarial, morbilliform, annular, or plaque components, but it is not vesicular. Adenopathy, which is present in 75% of patients, is most apparent in the cervical region.

The morbidity and mortality (< 3%) of KD is overwhelmingly associated with the development of inflammatory coronary artery aneurysms, most of which are asymptomatic at the time of formation. Aneurysms may be detected by echocardiography. Thrombosis can occur in the aneurysms, resulting in direct or embolic coronary artery occlusion. Coronary events may occur weeks or even many years after the febrile illness. A baseline echocardiogram should be obtained at the time of the acute illness and repeated 2 and 6 weeks later. Early recognition of the disease and

---

Table 3 Diagnostic Criteria for Kawasaki Disease

Persistent fever (> 5 days)

plus

Four of the following five conditions:

Nonpurulent bilateral conjunctivitis

Oral mucosal involvement

  Erythematous pharynx
  Red or fissured lips
  Strawberry tongue

Soft tissue abnormalities of hands and feet

  Edema/erythema
  Desquamation

Polymorphous, nonvesicular rash

Cervical adenopathy

treatment with intravenous immunoglobulin and aspirin have significantly decreased the frequency of aneurysm formation and thrombotic coronary events.

TREATMENT

Treatment should be initiated with intravenous immunoglobulin (2 g/kg as a single dose) and aspirin (80 to 100 mg/kg/day, every 6 hours) as soon as the disease is seriously suspected.[27] Aspirin is more effective than corticosteroids in preventing aneurysms. Corticosteroid therapy is usually unnecessary, and some authors feel that it is relatively contraindicated. Fever, conjunctivitis, and rash tend to respond within several days to the institution of aspirin and intravenous immunoglobulin.

Large Vessel Arteritis

Temporal, or giant cell, arteritis (GCA) of the elderly and Takayasu arteritis (TA) are the most common inflammatory diseases of the aorta and its major branches. Similar vascular targeting may occur in Behçet disease, Cogan syndrome, and sarcoidosis. It is uncertain whether TA and GCA are distinct disorders or are the same disorder with modified expression in different age groups.

TEMPORAL OR GIANT CELL ARTERITIS

GCA generally affects individuals older than 50 years.[28,29] It is associated in many patients with the syndrome of polymyalgia rheumatica (PMR). PMR is characterized by proximal muscle pain, with nocturnal and early morning worsening. There may be a subjective sense of weakness, without true weakness on examination or elevation of serum muscle enzyme levels.

GCA is variably associated with fever, scalp tenderness, headache, masticatory muscle claudication, peripheral vascular disease, inflammatory aortic aneurysms, and retinal ischemic syndromes. Oligoarticular arthritis, often in the upper extremity, and acute carpal tunnel syndrome can occur. The ischemic symptoms and signs may be clinically indistinguishable from those occurring in arteriosclerotic obliterative disease.

Examination for symmetrical four-extremity blood pressure readings, abdominal aneurysms, and bruits must be part of the routine follow-up visits of patients with GCA. Pathologic findings of GCA can occur in superficial temporal arteries of patients with PMR, even without any symptoms of GCA. However routine biopsy of the superficial temporal arteries in patients with PMR, without any other symptoms of GCA, is not warranted.

Acute-phase reactants are elevated in more than 80% of patients. Definitive diagnosis of GCA is generally made by biopsy of the superficial temporal artery. Pathology in GCA usually reveals chronic mononuclear cell infiltrates, destruction of the internal elastic lamina, and giant cells. The presence of giant cells is not requisite to make the diagnosis. The presence of characteristic clinical features such as new headache and jaw claudication, especially with concurrent PMR, may allow for a presumptive diagnosis in the absence of a biopsy or even when the superficial temporal artery biopsy is negative. However, because other conditions can mimic GCA, including atherosclerosis, an attempt to diagnose GCA by biopsy is warranted in most patients.[30] Corticosteroid therapy will not rapidly affect the biopsy results and should not be withheld from a patient strongly suspected of having GCA who is awaiting biopsy.

TAKAYASU ARTERITIS

Takayasu arteritis (pulseless disease) is a chronic inflammatory disease affecting the aorta and its major branches.[31] Usually di-

agnosed in younger, predominantly female patients of reproductive age, TA can also occur in young children and older patients of either sex. TA is more commonly associated with stenoses and aneurysms of the aorta and aortic branch vessel than is GCA.

The presenting clinical syndrome may include a prolonged flulike illness, including a polymyalgia rheumatica pattern of muscle pain. Other patients present with symptoms of limb, cerebral, or cardiac ischemia. The characteristic features of the disease reflect the ischemia produced by the inflammatory stenoses of the aorta and its major branches. Renal ischemia can elicit high renin hypertension. Predominant sites of stenosis are the aortic arch vessels, particularly the subclavian artery. Arm claudication and the presence of bruits are common. Superficial artery pain and tenderness (e.g., carotidynia) may be found on examination but is not diagnostic of TA. Severe central hypertension caused by renal artery stenosis may not be recognized because of coexistent arm artery stenosis; thus, four-extremity blood pressure readings must be evaluated initially and monitored on a frequent basis. Occasionally, stenoses exist in all major vessels of the extremities, and cuff monitoring may be an unreliable measure of central aortic pressures. Stroke is not uncommon and is often related to undetected central hypertension. It is extremely difficult to assess the activity of TA; the presence or absence of constitutional features or elevated acute-phase reactants are poor measures of disease activity. This impression is supported by vessel histopathology obtained during reconstructive surgery. Over 40% of vascular specimens from patients thought to be in remission revealed active inflammation.

Diagnosis of TA is usually made by arteriographic demonstration of stenotic lesions; aneurysms are less commonly observed. The entire arch, as well as the abdominal aorta and renal vessels, should be evaluated. It is of paramount importance that central arterial pressure be obtained at the time of angiography and compared with simultaneously obtained arm and leg cuff pressures. The role of vascular magnetic resonance imaging in the evaluation and follow-up of these patients is currently under investigation.[32] This technique may indicate changes in vessel wall thickness and edema as well as changes in lumen size. Pathologic documentation is difficult to obtain in TA, but the histopathology, usually obtained at the time of bypass surgery, is similar to that for GCA.

TREATMENT OF GCA AND TA

Corticosteroids are the initial treatment for both TA and GCA. GCA is generally very steroid responsive, although the most appropriate initial dose remains controversial. Initial daily doses of between 20 mg and 1 mg/kg have been advocated, with tapering over 8 to 12 months. Some patients with GCA require several years of therapy. Measurement of acute-phase reactants provides an imperfect index of disease activity and should not be the sole guide for adjustment of steroid dosing. If significant steroid side effects occur or if patients experience relapses during tapering, a second-line agent such as methotrexate is often added on an empirical basis to the corticosteroid therapy. However, the value of adjunctive steroid-sparing agents in GCA is currently unproved. Vascular reconstructive surgery, angioplasty, and stent placement are adjunctive therapeutic options in some patients. The frequent involvement of the subclavian vessels in TA must be taken into consideration when choosing the graft implantation site for coronary bypass procedures. High-dose corticosteroid therapy, especially in the elderly, has potentially dangerous side effects. Special attention must be paid to prevention of opportunistic infections, osteoporosis, glaucoma, hyperglycemia, and hyperlipidemia.

References

1. Jennette C, Falk RJ, Andrassy K, et al: Nomenclature of systemic vasculitides: proposal of an international consensus conference. Arthritis Rheum 37:187, 1994

2. Agnello V, Romain PL: Mixed cryoglobulinemia secondary to hepatitis C virus infection. Rheum Dis Clin North Am 22:1, 1996

3. Lawrence EC, Mills J: Bacterial endocarditis mimicking vasculitis with steroid-induced remission. West J Med 124:333, 1976

4. Blanco R, Martinez-Taboada VM, Rodriguez-Valverde V, et al: Cutaneous vasculitis in children and adults: associated disease and etiologic factors in 303 patients. Medicine (Baltimore) 77:403, 1998

5. Szer IS: Henoch-Schönlein purpura: when and how to treat. J Rheumatol 23:1661, 1996

6. O'Donnell B, Black AK: Urticarial vasculitis. Int Angiol 14:166, 1995

7. Hoffman GS, Kerr GS, Leavitt RY, et al: Wegener's granulomatosis: an analysis of 158 patients. Ann Intern Med 116:488, 1992

8. Duna G, Galperin C, Hoffman GS: Wegener's granulomatosis. Rheum Dis Clin North Am 21:949, 1995

9. Travis WD, Hoffman GS, Leavitt RY, et al: Surgical pathology of the lung in Wegener's granulomatosis. Am J Surg 15:315, 1991

10. Hoffman GS: Classification of the systemic vasculitides: antineutrophil cytoplasmic antibodies, consensus and controversy. Clin Exp Rheumatol 16:111, 1998

11. Hoffman GS, Specks U: Antineutrophil cytoplasmic antibodies: diagnostic value in systemic vasculitis. Arthritis Rheum 41:1521, 1998

12. Sneller MC, Hoffman GS, Talar-Williams C, et al: An analysis of 42 Wegener's granulomatosis patients treated with methotrexate and prednisone. Arthritis Rheum 38:608, 1995

13. Guillevin L, Cohen P, Gayraud M, et al: Churg-Strauss syndrome: clinical study and long-term follow up of 96 patients. Medicine (Baltimore) 78:26, 1999

14. Reid AJC, Harrison BDW, Watts RA, et al: Churg-Strauss syndrome in a district hospital. Q J Med 91:219, 1998

15. Hadziyannis SJ: The spectrum of extrahepatic manifestations in hepatitis C virus infection. J Viral Hepat 4:9, 1997

16. Guillevin L, Lhote F, Cohen P, et al: Polyarteritis nodosa related to hepatitis B virus: a prospective study with long-term observation of 41 patients. Medicine (Baltimore) 74:238, 1995

17. Guillevin L, Durand-Gasselin B, Cevallos R, et al: Microscopic polyangiitis—clinical and laboratory findings in 85 patients. Arthritis Rheum 42:421, 1999

18. Travers RL, Allison DJ, Brettle RP, et al: Polyarteritis nodosa: a clinical and angiographic analysis of 17 cases. Semin Arthritis Rheum 8:184, 1979

19. Lhote F, Cohen P, Guillevin L: Polyarteritis nodosa, microscopic polyangiitis and Churg-Strauss syndrome. Rheum Dis Clin North Am 21:911, 1995

20. Mandell BF, Hoffman GS: Differentiating the vasculitides. Rheum Dis Clin North Am 20:409, 1994

21. Triplett DA: Protean clinical presentation of antiphospholipid-protein antibodies. Thromb Haemost 74:329, 1995

22. Om A, Ellahham S, DiScascio G: Cholesterol embolism: an underdiagnosed clinical entity. Am Heart J 124:1321, 1992

23. Wees SJ, Sunwoo IN, Oh SJ: Sural nerve biopsy in systemic necrotizing vasculitis. Am J Med 71:525, 1981

24. Rappaport WD, Valente J, Hunter GC, et al: Clinical utilization and complications of sural nerve biopsy. Am J Surg 166:252, 1993

25. Guillevin L, Lhote F: Treatment of polyarteritis nodosa and microscopic polyangiitis. Arthritis Rheum 41:2100, 1998

26. Schulman ST, Inocencio JD, Hirsch R, et al: Kawasaki disease. Pediatr Clin North Am 21:1013, 1995

27. Leung DY, Schlievert PM, Meissner HC: The immunopathogenesis and management of Kawasaki syndrome. Arthritis Rheum 41:1538, 1998

28. Evans JM, Hunder GG: Polyangiitis rheumatica and giant cell arteritis. Clin Geriatr Med 14:455, 1998

29. Hunder GG: Giant cell arteritis and polymyalgia rheumatica. Med Clin North Am 81:195, 1997

30. Ponge T, Barrier JH, Grolleau JY, et al: The efficacy of selective unilateral temporal artery biopsy versus bilateral biopsies for diagnosis of giant cell arteritis. J Rheumatol 15:997, 1988

31. Kerr GS, Hallahan CW, Giordano J, et al: Takayasu's arteritis. Ann Intern Med 120:919, 1994

32. Flamm SD, White RD, Hoffman GS: The clinical application of "edema-weighted" magnetic resonance imaging in assessment of Takayasu's arteritis. Int J Cardiol 66(suppl 1):S151, 1998

Acknowledgment

Figures 1 and 2   Seward Hung

118 Crystal-Induced Joint Disease

Christopher Wise, M.D.

The presence of precipitated crystals in the synovium or synovial fluid can be associated with an inflammatory response that usually manifests itself as an acute arthritis, but a variety of less common clinical features may be present. The identification of monosodium urate (MSU) crystals in the synovial fluid of patients with acute gout in 1961 by McCarty and Hollander represented the initial recognition of arthritis associated with articular crystal deposition.[1] This development was followed in 1962 by the recognition of so-called pseudogout, which is associated with calcium pyrophosphate dihydrate (CPPD) crystals.[2] Since then, a great deal has been learned about these two common types of arthritis. Other calcium-containing crystals may precipitate in or around joints and can be associated with an inflammatory reaction or degenerative process. Lipid crystals have also been described in synovial fluid but do not appear to be phlogistic. The typical characteristics of crystal-induced synovitis include a rapid-onset, self-limited arthritis, and findings of synovial fluid leukocytosis associated with phagocytosis of crystals. Definitive diagnosis of crystal-induced arthritis requires identification of crystals in synovial fluid or tissue.

Gout

DEFINITION AND CLASSIFICATION

Gout is defined as an arthritis associated with the presence of MSU crystals in synovial fluid or tissue. The development of gout tends to be associated with chronically increased levels of serum uric acid. However, a substantial minority of patients with acute gout will have normal uric acid levels, and hyperuricemia does not always lead to the development of gout.[3,4] Gout is often classified as primary or secondary [see Table 1]. Gout associated with an inborn error in metabolism or decreased renal excretion without other renal disease is referred to as primary gout, whereas gout associated with an acquired disease or use of a drug is called secondary gout. In both primary and secondary gout, chronic hyperuricemia may be the result of overproduction of uric acid caused by increased purine intake, synthesis, or breakdown or may be the result of decreased renal excretion of urate.

EPIDEMIOLOGY

Gout is predominantly a disease of middle-aged men, but there is a gradually increasing prevalence in both men and women in older age groups. The annual incidence of gout in men in most studies is in the range of one to three per 1,000 but is much lower in women.[5] In the Framingham Study, for example, the 2-year incidence of gout was 3.2 per 1,000 men versus 0.5 per 1,000 women.[6] The overall prevalence of self-reported gout in the general population is 0.7% to 1.4% in men and 0.5% to 0.6% in women. However, in people older than 65 years, prevalence increases to 4.4% to 5.2% in men and 1.8% to 2.0% in women.[7] In male populations, the prevalence of gout reaches impressive levels by the fifth decade. In a study of male medical students, the prevalence of gout reached 5.8% in whites and 10.9% in African Americans surveyed for a mean of 28 years after graduation.[8] In patients with the onset of gout after 60 years of age, prevalence in men and prevalence in women are almost equal, and in those with onset after 80 years of age, prevalence is greater in women.[9,10]

The incidence and prevalence of gout are parallel to the incidence and prevalence of hyperuricemia in the general population. Serum urate levels increase by 1 to 2 mg/dl in males at the time of puberty, but females exhibit little change in urate levels until after menopause, when concentrations approach those seen in males.[11] Most patients with elevated serum uric acid levels do not have gout, but hyperuricemia is clearly associated with an increased risk of gout.[12] For example, in persons with serum urate levels greater than 10 mg/dl, the annual incidence of gout is 70 per 1,000 and the 5-year prevalence is 30%, whereas in persons with levels less than 7 mg/dl, annual incidence is only 0.9 per 1,000 and the 5-year prevalence is 0.6%. Additional factors that correlate strongly with serum urate levels and the prevalence of gout in the general population include serum creatinine levels, body weight, height, blood pressure, and alcohol intake.

PATHOGENESIS AND ETIOLOGY

Hyperuricemia

The plasma concentration of uric acid is maintained at a relatively constant level in humans because of a balance between production and excretion. Uric acid is synthesized as an end product of dietary purines or the breakdown of purines from nucleic acids during cell turnover. A very small amount of uric acid is passively eliminated through the gastrointestinal tract.

Table 1 Classification of Hyperuricemia and Gout

Primary Hyperuricemia and Gout with No Associated Condition	Secondary Hyperuricemia and Gout with Identifiable Associated Condition
Uric acid undersecretion (80%–90%) Idiopathic Urate overproduction (10%–20%) Idiopathic HGPRT deficiency PRPP synthetase overactivity	Uric acid undersecretion Renal insufficiency (any cause) Polycystic kidney disease Lead nephropathy Drugs Diuretics Salicylates (low dose) Pyrazinamide Ethambutol Niacin Cyclosporine Didanosine Urate overproduction Myeloproliferative diseases Lymphoproliferative diseases Hemolytic anemias Polycythemia vera Other malignancies Psoriasis Glycogen storage disease Dual mechanism Obesity Ethanol consumption Hypoxemia and tissue hypoperfusion

HGPRT—hypoxanthine-guanine phosphoribosyltransferase
PRPP—phosphoribosylpyrophosphate

Almost all plasma uric acid is filtered at the glomerulus, and 80% is reabsorbed in the proximal tubule. Some of this plasma uric acid is subsequently secreted back into the lumen, with a small amount of distal reabsorption.[3,11]

Hyperuricemia can result from decreased renal excretion or increased production of uric acid. In 80% to 90% of patients with primary gout, hyperuricemia is caused by renal underexcretion of uric acid, even though renal function is otherwise normal. The defect in renal excretion of uric acid in patients with primary gout may be attributed to reduced filtration, enhanced reabsorption, or decreased secretion, but it is unclear which of these mechanisms is most important. Patients with secondary gout related to renal disease are hyperuricemic because of a decreased filtered load of uric acid, although decreased tubular secretion may play a role in some patients. The hyperuricemia associated with diuretic therapy results from volume depletion, which leads to a decreased filtered load as well as enhanced tubular reabsorption.[13] A renal mechanism is the cause of hyperuricemia associated with most other drugs as well. Low-dose aspirin can cause significant changes in renal handling of urate within a week after therapy is started, particularly in elderly patients.[14] Cyclosporine therapy has been found to be associated with hyperuricemia and gout in renal and cardiac transplantation patients. Hyperuricemia and gout appear to be the result of a combined effect of cyclosporine on renal blood flow and tubular function.[15,16]

Overproduction of uric acid, caused by increased purine synthesis, is seen in about only 10% to 20% of patients with primary gout. In addition, four specific heritable defects of purine synthesis have been identified: phosphoribosylpyrophosphate (PRPP) synthetase overactivity, glucose-6-phosphatase deficiency, and fructose-1-phosphate aldolase deficiency. The best-known heritable defect is hypoxanthine-guanine phosphoribosyltransferase (HGPRT) deficiency. Complete deficiency of this enzyme is associated with the Lesch-Nyhan syndrome in children, and a partial deficiency has been associated with early-onset gout and nephrolithiasis. Most diseases causing secondary hyperuricemia from uric acid overproduction are associated with increased nucleic acid turnover. These diseases include multiple myeloma, polycythemia, pernicious anemia, hemoglobinopathies, thalassemia, other hemolytic anemias, other myeloproliferative and lymphoproliferative disorders, and other neoplasms. In addition, some critically ill patients may experience hyperuricemia resulting from accelerated breakdown of adenosine triphosphate (ATP).

Gout has been recognized as a familial disorder since the time of Sir Alfred Garrod, with about 40% of patients reporting a family history of gout in most series.[11] The mechanisms for this association are still not understood, but most available data suggest that serum uric acid levels are controlled by multiple genes.[17]

Uric Acid Precipitation and Crystal-Induced Inflammation

Uric acid dissociates almost completely to the urate anion form at a pH of 7.4. At concentrations greater than 6.5 to 7.0 mg/dl, urate precipitates in the form of MSU crystals. Local conditions in tissues responsible for crystal precipitation and deposition include lower temperature (as is found in peripheral joints), lower pH level in extracellular fluid, and reduced urate binding to plasma proteins. Other local factors that contribute to precipitation and deposition of crystals are trauma and rapid increases in local urate concentration as a result of mobilization of water from peripheral tissues (as occurs when edematous feet are elevated during sleep).[18]

The factors responsible for the inflammatory response to crystals are not completely understood.[11] The phlogistic properties of crystals seem to be linked to their ability to bind immunoglobulins and other proteins, particularly complement and lipoproteins. These complexes bind to surface receptors on multiple cell types, leading to activation and release of proinflammatory cytokines, chemotactic factors, and other mediators. An influx of phagocytic cells—particularly neutrophils—follows. Crystals are engulfed, and subsequent disruption of lysosomes releases arachidonate metabolites, collagenases, and oxygen radicals. Several factors have been postulated to contribute to the self-termination of attacks. These factors include digestion of crystals by myeloperoxidase, increased heat and blood flow leading to dissolution and removal of crystals from the joint, and alteration of the crystal properties and bound proteins by the inflammatory process itself.

CLINICAL STAGES

Acute Gouty Arthritis

Acute gouty arthritis is usually characterized by a sudden and dramatic onset of pain and swelling, usually in a single joint. This condition occurs most often in lower extremity joints and evolves within hours to marked swelling, warmth, and tenderness. The process often extends beyond the confines of the joint and may mimic cellulitis. The pain of gout is often severe enough to make even the light pressure of bedclothes intolerable, and weight bearing is usually very difficult. Even without treatment, attacks of gout usually subside within a few days, although some attacks may last a few weeks. Early in the course of gout, affected joints usually return to normal after attacks.

The initial attack of gout is monoarticular in 85% to 90% of patients. At least half of initial attacks occur in the first metatarsophalangeal joints (a condition known as podagra), but other joints of the foot may be involved simultaneously or in subsequent attacks. Other lower extremity joints, including the ankles and knees, are often affected; in more advanced gout, attacks may occur in upper extremity joints, such as the elbow, wrist, and small joints of the fingers. In older women in particular, involvement of the small joints of the fingers (previously affected by osteoarthritis) is more commonly seen earlier in the course of the disease.[19,20] Acute episodes may also involve the bursae, particularly in the olecranon or prepatellar areas. Polyarticular gout occurs as the initial manifestation in about 10% to 15% of patients and may be associated with fever.[21]

Almost all synovial fluid aspirated early in an acute attack contains typical needlelike crystals, which are negatively birefringent and may be extracellular or within polymorphonuclear leukocytes [see Figure 1]. The leukocyte count in most gouty synovial fluid rises to a range of 10,000 to 60,000/mm³ but may be much higher in some patients.

Intercritical Gout

After the initial attack of gout subsides, the clinical course of gout may follow one of several patterns. A minority of patients never have another attack of gout, and some may not have another attack for several years. Most patients, however, have recurrent attacks over the ensuing years. In a study done before the use of hypouricemic agents, 78% of patients had a second attack within 2 years and 93% had a second attack within 10 years.[22] In many patients, symptom-free intervals between attacks become progressively shorter as episodes of

a 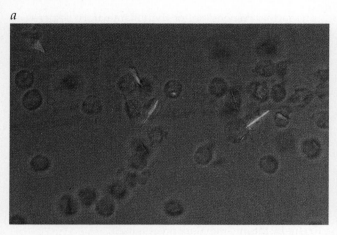   *b*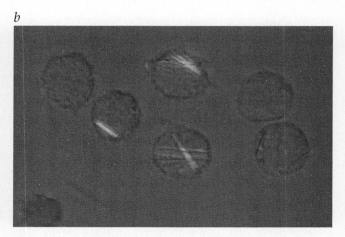

Figure 1   Gout can be diagnosed by demonstration of negatively birefringent monosodium urate crystals in synovial fluid examined by polarized-light microscopy, either free (*a*) or within polymorphonuclear leukocytes (*b*).

acute arthritis increase in frequency. In chronic disease, soft tissue swelling and joint effusions persist for longer periods after each attack. Finally, after 10 to 20 years, chronic tophaceous gout becomes apparent in patients who continue to have recurrent gouty attacks.

Chronic Tophaceous Gout

Persistent hyperuricemia with increasingly frequent attacks of gout eventually leads to a wider distribution of joint involvement and chronic joint destruction resulting from deposition of massive amounts of urate in and around joints [*see Figure 2a*]. Without therapy to lower serum uric acid levels, the average interval from the first gouty attack to the development of chronic arthritis or tophi is about 12 years.[23] After 20 years, 75% of patients have tophi, and patients with the highest urate levels are at highest risk. In elderly patients, particularly women, tophi may appear earlier in the course of the disease, sometimes in patients without a history of gouty attacks.[20] Subcutaneous tophi begin to appear in periarticular and bursal tissues, especially around the knees and elbows, along tendons of the

hands and feet, and around the interphalangeal and metacarpophalangeal joints of the hands. Tophaceous deposits are usually firm and movable, and the overlying skin may be normal or thin and reddened. When close to the surface, deposits exhibit a characteristic chalky, cream-colored or yellowish appearance. Tophi have also been described in areas not associated with joints, such as the pinna of the ear [*see Figure 2b*], and in unusual visceral locations, such as the myocardium, pericardium, aortic valves, and extradural spinal regions.

Destruction of the articular cartilage and subchondral bone eventually occurs in patients with chronic articular involvement [*see Figure 3*]. Erosive bony lesions may be seen on x-rays as well-defined punched-out lesions in periarticular bone, often associated with overhanging edges of bone.[24] These erosions are usually 5 mm or more in diameter and larger than those seen in rheumatoid arthritis. Bone mineralization appears to be generally normal in chronic tophaceous gout, and periarticular osteopenia, which is seen in rheumatoid arthritis, is usually not present. The distribution of destructive joint disease in gout is often asymmetrical and patchy.

a 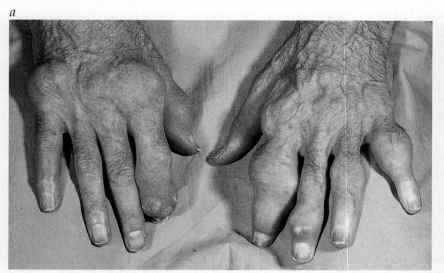   *b*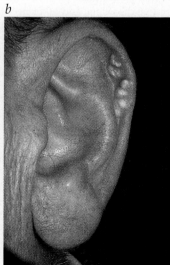

Figure 2   Tophaceous gout, demonstrating chronic swelling in and around the joints of the hand caused by bone destruction and tophaceous deposits in the hands (*a*). Tophi may also be found in extra-articular areas, such as the pinna of the ear (*b*).

Chronic Inflammation   Articular Cartilage
in Subchondral Bone   Urate Deposit

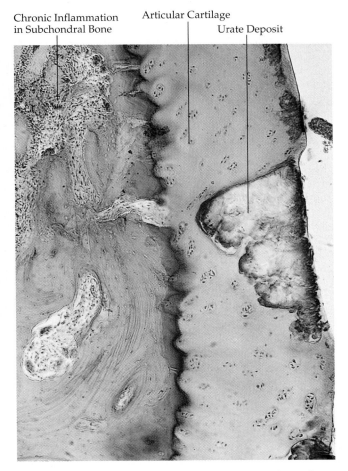

Figure 3   **Microscopic appearance of sodium urate deposits causing a defect in articular cartilage and chronic inflammation in the subchondral bone.**

Associated Conditions

A number of chronic illnesses may be associated with gout and hyperuricemia, either in primary or secondary form. The best-known association is with renal disease, which frequently occurs in patients with gout.[25,26] Most of the renal disease in patients with gout is believed to be the result of nephrosclerosis related to hypertension. However, a direct pathogenetic role for uric acid in the development of renal disease and hypertension is still possible.[27] In addition, the presence of intrarenal urate deposits associated with an inflammatory reaction in some patients suggests that urate causes some of the renal disease seen in patients with chronic tophaceous gout.[28]

Renal stones occur in 10% to 25% of patients with gout.[29] Most stones in patients with gout are composed of uric acid. However, some are composed of calcium oxalate and other constituents, and hyperuricemia is believed to contribute to the formation of these stones as well.[30] An acute urate nephropathy associated with the tumor lysis syndrome has been described in patients with leukemia or lymphoma undergoing chemotherapy.[31] This condition is associated with acute oliguria and an elevated urinary urate-to-creatinine ratio (> 1.0) and is usually treated prophylactically with allopurinol and vigorous hydration. An association of gout with renal disease and chronic lead intoxication has been noted in some populations (saturnine gout).[32] In the United States, this association has most often been attributed to illicit whiskey produced in lead-lined stills but has also been attributed to occupational lead exposure.

Gout has long been associated with an increased incidence of obesity, diabetes mellitus, hyperlipidemia, and atherosclerotic cardiovascular disease. The association with diabetes has been variable in studies, and in lipid disorders, the association is primarily with hypertriglyceridemia, which may in turn be linked to alcohol intake.[33] In addition, a correlation has been found between hyperuricemia and the insulin-resistance syndrome, possibly associated with body-fat distribution and triglyceride levels.[34,35] The association of gout and hyperuricemia with cardiovascular disease appears to be related to the link between these metabolic disorders and hypertension, and hyperuricemia is not considered to be an independent risk factor for premature atherosclerosis.[36,37]

Alcohol consumption has long been associated with the precipitation of gouty attacks in susceptible patients. In addition, chronic heavy alcohol consumption promotes hyperuricemia by interfering with renal excretion and increasing production of urate; some alcoholic beverages, particularly beer, serve as a source of dietary purine.[11] Patients with gout have an increased prevalence of hypothyroidism, and urate levels have been shown to decrease with the institution of thyroid replacement therapy, probably through a renal mechanism.[38]

DIAGNOSIS

A diagnosis of gout can be made with certainty only by confirmation of the presence of monosodium urate crystals in synovial fluid or tissue. Elements of the patient's history, physical examination, and laboratory studies can be very helpful in diagnosing gout.[39] A typical presentation of podagra in a middle-aged man with known hyperuricemia may be sufficient for an initial tentative diagnosis of gout, particularly if there is a good response to colchicine. Nodular deposits on the olecranon processes, dorsal aspects of the fingers, or finger pads should be sought, particularly in patients with a history of joint problems. Patients with gout may have a normal serum urate level at the time of an attack. With most patients, however, a review of old records reveals a history of chronic hyperuricemia. Radiographs are seldom useful during an acute attack, unless previous attacks have occurred in the area examined and unless, after years of disease, well-defined erosions in or around joints, with characteristic overhanging edges, can be seen.

The detection of needle-shaped, negatively birefringent urate crystals in synovial fluid examined under polarized light microscopy is the definitive diagnostic finding for gout. Although this test is best done on fluid obtained during an acute attack, aspiration of synovial fluid from previously affected joints or aspiration of a subcutaneous nodule suspected of being a tophus may be helpful.[40,41] The synovial fluid should be examined by someone experienced in crystal identification because an inexperienced person may not recognize the presence of crystals.[42]

Alternative diagnoses should be considered in all patients suspected of having gout. Acute arthritis can be caused by infection, other crystal-induced arthropathies, or other diseases. A Gram stain and culture of the synovial fluid and radiographs may be needed in some patients to rule out these disorders. Gout can be accompanied by fever, particularly during polyarticular attacks, and should be considered in patients with suspected acute bacterial arthritis with negative cultures.[21] In addition, gout and infection can coexist in the same joints, making therapeutic decisions difficult in individual cases. Thus, synovial fluid cultures are essential in any patient who is suspected of having gout and who has fever or purulent-appearing synovial fluid. Pseudogout [see Pseudogout (Calcium Pyrophosphate Dihydrate Deposition Disease), below] may cause an acute monoarthritis or oligoarthritis similar to gout. Radiographs in such patients may show chondrocalcinosis, and CPPD crystals in the synovial fluid are usually easily distinguishable from urate crystals. However, some patients may have both gout and pseudogout in the same joint.

TREATMENT

The goals of therapy for patients with gout include termination of the acute attack, prevention of further attacks during the intercritical period, assessment for associated and contributing factors, and consideration of long-term therapy for hyperuricemia [see Table 2].[43,44] Each aspect of therapy should be considered separately, and there should be no confusion between efforts to suppress inflammation in acute attacks and efforts to lower serum urate levels, decrease the frequency of attacks, and prevent complications in the future.

Acute Gout

Treatment of acute gout should be initiated as early in the attack as possible. Agents available for terminating the acute attack include colchicine, nonsteroidal anti-inflammatory drugs (NSAIDs), adrenocorticotropic hormone (ACTH), and corticosteroids. Each agent has a toxicity profile, with advantages and disadvantages applicable to individual circumstances. The patient's overall health and coexistent medical problems, particularly renal disease and gastrointestinal disease, often dictate the choice among these approaches. Corticosteroids and ACTH have been used more often in recent years in patients with multiple comorbid conditions because of the relatively low toxicity profile of these agents.

Colchicine has been used for centuries to treat acute attacks of gout. Given in oral dosages of 0.6 to 1.2 mg initially, followed by 0.6 mg every 2 hours, colchicine begins relieving most attacks of gout within 12 to 24 hours. However, most patients experience nausea, vomiting, abdominal cramps, and diarrhea with these dosages. Colchicine should be given more cautiously in elderly patients and should be avoided in patients with renal or hepatic insufficiency and patients already on long-term colchicine therapy.[45] Intravenous colchicine has been used for acute attacks, but recognition of the potential for bone marrow suppression and other systemic toxicities has resulted in guidelines for restricting dosage and even in a lack of availability in some countries.[46]

NSAIDs are useful in most patients with acute gout and remain the agents of choice for young, healthy patients without comorbid diseases. Indomethacin has been the most widely used agent over the years and usually begins to provide relief within hours after the initial oral dose. Most NSAIDs are comparable in efficacy, although studies comparing NSAIDs in acute gout are few. The use of all NSAIDs is limited by the risks of gastric ulceration and gastritis, acute renal failure, fluid re-

Table 2 Management of Gout

Treatment Phase	Procedure	Comments
Therapy for acute attack	Administer nonsteroidal anti-inflammatory drugs (NSAIDs) (indomethacin and others)	Ideal for healthy patients without gastrointestinal or renal disease Use with caution for limited periods and in lower doses in patients with comorbid conditions and in elderly patients
	Administer corticosteroids or corticotropin (intra-articular, oral, parenteral)	Preferable in elderly patients and those with comorbid conditions Use with caution in diabetic patients
	Administer oral colchicine	Useful two or three times a day for milder attacks; higher doses are usually not tolerated Use with caution in elderly patients and those with hepatic disease Intravenous preparation is rarely used
Interval follow-up and evaluation	Administer prophylaxis against recurrent attacks (oral colchicine or NSAID)	Use in low doses, with caution, in patients with renal disease
	Determine the presence of secondary or contributing causes	Identify underlying renal disease, concomitant drug use, dietary problems, or other diseases
	Determine the presence of associated conditions	Identify obesity, hypertension, hyperlipidemia, diabetes, or alcohol use
	Identify patient as an overproducer or underexcretor (24 hr urine collection for urate)	Underexcretor: < 700 mg/24 hr Overproducer: > 700 mg/24 hr Marked overproducer: > 1,000 mg/24 hr
	Review indications for long-term hypouricemic therapy	Tophaceous gout Erosive joint disease Frequent attacks (?over 2–3/yr) Marked hyperuricemia and ?hyperuricosuria Renal stones and persistent hyperuricemia
Therapy for chronic hyperuricemia	Administer allopurinol	Use in overproducers and underexcretors Adjust dosage for renal insufficiency Use with caution in patients with rashes and in those who display hypersensitivity
	Administer uricosuric drugs (probenecid and sulfinpyrazone)	Use in underexcretors with normal renal function Contraindicated for patients with a history of renal stones

tention, interference with antihypertensive therapy, and, in older patients, problems with mentation. Aspirin is usually avoided because of its dose-related and variable effect on urate excretion. Newly developed NSAIDs with a high specificity for cyclooxygenase-2 are now available for the treatment of rheumatoid arthritis and osteoarthritis. These agents should be much less toxic in general and appear to have very low potential for gastrointestinal toxicity and inhibition of platelet function in clinical studies. These cyclooxygenase-2–specific NSAIDs should be useful in treating acute gout, and possibly in long-term prophylaxis, in patients at risk for gastrointestinal toxicity from the currently available NSAIDs.[47]

Corticosteroids have become more widely used in the treatment of acute gout in recent years.[48] Intra-articular steroids after arthrocentesis are extremely useful in providing relief, particularly in large effusions, in which the initial aspiration of fluid results in rapid relief of pain and tightness in the affected joint. The dosage of the steroid triamcinolone depends on the size of the joint, ranging from 5 to 10 mg for small joints of the hands or feet to 40 to 60 mg for larger joints, such as the knee. Systemic corticosteroids may also be useful in patients for whom colchicine or NSAIDs are inadvisable and in patients with polyarticular attacks. Tapered doses of oral prednisone (starting at 40 to 60 mg daily) and single intramuscular injections of ACTH (40 units) or triamcinolone (40 to 60 mg) have all been shown to be as effective as NSAIDs in treating acute gout. In most studies of systemic steroids for acute gout, only a small proportion of patients have required repeated therapy for rebound attacks in the first several days after therapy.

Interval Follow-up and Evaluation

Patients remain at increased risk for another attack of gout for several weeks after resolution of the initial attack; prophylaxis with small doses of colchicine or NSAIDs should be used for most patients. Colchicine (0.6 mg one or two times a day) prevents attacks in over 80% of patients. Prophylaxis should be continued for 1 to 2 months after an acute attack, for several months in patients with a history of frequent attacks, and when urate-lowering drugs are initiated.[49] The dose of colchicine should be reduced or the duration of therapy shortened in patients with reduced renal function because bone marrow suppression and myoneuropathy have been reported in patients on long-term low-dose colchicine therapy with a creatinine clearance of less than 50 ml/min.[50]

After an acute attack of gout, a patient can be monitored for recurrent attacks and assessed for potential underlying causes of hyperuricemia. A 24-hour urine collection to measure urate excretion helps classify the patient as an overproducer or underexcretor of urate to identify the optimal drug treatment for lowering serum urate levels, if indicated.[1] If urate excretion exceeds 700 mg a day, allopurinol is the most appropriate agent for lowering urate levels, by decreasing urate production; with lower excretion levels, a uricosuric drug may be useful.

During this period, a review of the patient's overall health may reveal important coexistent diseases, medications, and habits that could contribute to hyperuricemia. In particular, alcohol consumption should be discussed as an important factor in hyperuricemia and precipitation of attacks. A review of the patient's diet may reveal heavy consumption of purine-rich foods, such as organ meats, seafood, or various legumes or other vegetables. Dietary restriction may be a useful adjunct for some patients, although the purine content of the diet usually

contributes only about 1.0 mg/dl to the serum urate concentration.[43] In addition, the intercritical period is an excellent time to assess for obesity, hyperlipidemia, and hypertension, which so often accompany gout and are important correctable risk factors for premature cardiovascular mortality.

Chronic Hyperuricemia

In general, patients with asymptomatic hyperuricemia should not be treated with hypouricemic agents. However, patients with persistent marked hyperuricemia (levels > 10 mg/dl) or hyperuricosuria (> 1,000 mg/24 hr) should be followed carefully for manifestations of gout or renal stones. Drug therapy to lower urate levels should be considered for patients who have had crystal-proven gout with recurrent attacks and persistent hyperuricemia despite efforts to identify and correct contributing factors. Most patients who have had more than two or three attacks and those with tophi or radiographic evidence of joint damage should be treated with hypouricemic therapy if they are willing to comply with a long-term regimen. Reduction of serum urate levels well into the normal range (i.e., < 6.0 mg/dl) eventually leads to prevention of further attacks and resorption of tophi.[43] Low-dose colchicine or NSAIDs should be used to prevent attacks that can occur for several months after hypouricemic therapy is started.[51]

Agents that increase renal excretion of urate (uricosuric drugs) can be used in patients with normal renal function and no history of nephrolithiasis who have a 24-hour excretion of urate less than 700 mg/day. Probenecid (1 to 2 g/day) is the most commonly used agent in this class, although sulfinpyrazone (up to 400 to 800 mg/day) can be used as well. Both agents are of limited use in patients with decreased renal function and carry a risk of precipitating renal stones. High urine volume and alkalinization with bicarbonate intake decrease this risk. Up to 25% of patients are not well controlled on uricosuric drug therapy. Benzbromarone is a uricosuric agent that has been available in Europe for over 20 years but is not available in the United States. Recent studies have shown that this agent may be useful in lowering uric acid levels in some patients with renal disease.[52]

Allopurinol, the only available inhibitor of xanthine oxidase, reduces serum urate levels in almost all compliant patients and may be used in overproducers or underexcretors. A daily dose of 300 mg is standard in patients with normal renal function, although some patients may require as much as 600 mg to achieve optimal serum urate levels. The dose should be reduced to 200 mg in patients with glomerular filtration rates (GFRs) less than 60 ml/min and to 100 mg in those with a GFR less than 30 ml/min. The dose of some other drugs, particularly azathioprine, must be reduced in patients on allopurinol because allopurinol inhibits metabolism. In approximately 2% of patients taking allopurinol, a hypersensitivity rash develops that progresses to a severe exfoliative dermatitis in a small number of these patients.[53] This disorder is more likely to occur in patients taking ampicillin or in those with renal insufficiency. Severe rashes may be accompanied by a syndrome of vasculitis, hepatitis, and interstitial renal disease, with a mortality risk of 20% reported in some series. Because of this risk, allopurinol should be discontinued in any patient who experiences a rash. Allopurinol may be reinstituted in such patients if the rash is mild. In addition, regimens of oral or parenteral desensitization have been successful in some patients but should be used with caution.

Pseudogout (Calcium Pyrophosphate Dihydrate Deposition Disease)

DEFINITION AND CLASSIFICATION

CPPD crystals may be found in deposits in and around joints and are characterized by calcification of articular cartilage, menisci, synovium, and other periarticular tissues. McCarty and colleagues first described CPPD crystals in synovial fluids from patients with goutlike attacks in 1962.[2] They used the term pseudogout for this new arthropathy, which is characterized by intra-articular calcifications (chondrocalcinosis), crystals in the synovial fluid, and acute arthropathy. Since then, other clinical presentations and a variety of disease processes have been associated with CPPD crystals. Thus, the term CPPD deposition disease has been used more often to include the various clinical presentations as part of the same general clinical syndrome.

EPIDEMIOLOGY

CPPD deposition disease is generally a disease of the elderly; the average age of patients is approximately 70 years.[54] The prevalence of articular chondrocalcinosis is very low in people younger than 40 years but increases with age and is quite common in older populations. When multiple radiologic studies are obtained, the documented prevalence in the general population is 10% to 15% in those 65 to 75 years of age and over 40% in people older than 80 years.[55,56] CPPD deposition occurs in males and females in differing distribution in different studies, but there does not seem to be a major gender predominance. An increased prevalence of CPPD deposition in certain diseases and familial groups has been reported.

PATHOGENESIS AND ETIOLOGY

The metabolic basis for CPPD formation and deposition is less well understood than that for urate crystals. CPPD crystal formation occurs almost exclusively in the articular and periarticular tissue, most often near the surface of chondrocytes.[54,57] Crystal formation is enhanced by elevated levels of either calcium or pyrophosphate (PP_i) within local tissues or local factors in the cartilage matrix that promote crystal formation. An abnormal substrate of matrix collagen and proteoglycan, as well as variations in mineral content, may promote crystal deposition. Local elevations of PP_i levels appear to be related to overactivity of a cell surface enzyme (ectoenzyme) known as nucleoside triphosphate pyrophosphohydrolase (NTPPH), which catalyzes the extracellular hydrolysis of ATP. In addition, some of the excess PP_i production may take place intracellularly through NTPPH or as a by-product of cellular proteoglycan and protein synthesis. Other factors that may contribute to excess PP_i and crystal formation include decreased activity of pyrophosphatase, degenerating cellular debris, abnormal matrix collagen, and even the local influence of growth factors (transforming growth factor and insulinlike growth factor). The mechanisms by which CPPD crystals induce inflammation are believed to be similar to those observed in gout.

CLINICAL VARIANTS

Most joints with radiographically observed chondrocalcinosis are asymptomatic, although subtle articular symptoms are more common in asymptomatic patients with chondrocalcinosis than in patients without these findings.[58] Clinically symptomatic CPPD deposition disease may take any of several forms that tend to present in acute or chronic fashion, mimicking other arthropathies.

Acute Pseudogout

Acute pseudogout is slightly more common in males than in females. Attacks of this form of CPPD deposition disease are usually acute, increase in intensity over 12 to 36 hours, and last for a few days to a few weeks. Most acute attacks of pseudogout are less intense than attacks of gout. The most commonly involved joint is the knee (seen in over half of patients), followed by the wrist and ankle. In rare cases, attacks in the first metatarsophalangeal joint may be seen.[54] Affected joints previously involved are more likely to be involved in subsequent attacks. Attacks may occur in clusters over short periods, and polyarticular attacks occur in a few patients. A moderate synovial fluid leukocytosis is common, and marked elevations mimicking a septic joint may be seen in some patients. Mild fever and leukocytosis have been described, but not as frequently as in gout.[59] Between attacks, the joint is usually asymptomatic unless there is coexistent osteoarthritis. As in gout, attacks of pseudogout seem to be precipitated in some patients by stressful events, such as surgery, trauma, and acute medical illness. The intra-articular injection of hyaluronate for the symptomatic treatment of osteoarthritis has also been reported to trigger attacks of acute pseudogout.[60]

Chronic Rheumatoid-like Arthritis

About 5% to 10% of patients with CPPD deposition disease experience a polyarticular process resembling rheumatoid arthritis that is indolent, symmetrical, and inflamed. Chronic swelling, morning stiffness, and predominant wrist and knee involvement are seen in this group of patients. Because of the relatively high frequency of incidental chondrocalcinosis and positive rheumatoid factors in elderly persons, differentiating CPPD deposition from rheumatoid arthritis can be difficult. A history of acute exacerbations in these patients may help suggest CPPD deposition, whereas the presence of subcutaneous nodules and very high titer rheumatoid factors favor a diagnosis of rheumatoid arthritis.

Osteoarthritis and CPPD Deposition

About half of patients with CPPD deposition have a chronic degenerative arthritis involving multiple joints, usually in a symmetrical pattern. Women predominate in this group of patients.[54] The knees are most commonly involved, followed by the wrist, metacarpophalangeal joints, hips, spine, and shoulders. CPPD-associated osteoarthritis may be differentiated from typical osteoarthritis by the presence of changes in atypical joints, such as the wrists, elbows, and shoulders. Some patients in this group may not have chondrocalcinosis, but CPPD crystals may be found in the synovial fluid of most of those patients without radiographic findings. In addition, radiographic features of predominantly patellofemoral involvement and femoral cortical erosions in the knee are suggestive of CPPD deposition.[61]

Conditions Associated with CPPD Deposition Disease

Most cases of CPPD deposition disease are sporadic. However, a number of kindreds with familial forms of disease and associations with metabolic diseases have been reported. Most of the familial forms have shown an autosomal dominant transmission but have displayed a variety of clinical presentations.[62] Associations with several endocrine and metabolic conditions have been reported, many of which probably represent

Table 3 **Conditions Associated with Calcium Pyrophosphate Dihydrate Deposition Disease***

Definite association	Possible or doubtful association
Hemochromatosis	Gout
Hyperparathyroidism	Familial hypocalciuric
Hypophosphatasia	hypocalcemia
Hypomagnesemia	Acromegaly
	X-linked hypophosphatemic
Probable association	rickets
Hypothyroidism	Neuropathic joints
	Amyloidosis
	Trauma

See references 53 and 62.
*As pseudogout or radiographic chondrocalcinosis.

no more than a chance occurrence of common age-related conditions [see Table 3]. Definite associations exist between CPPD deposition disease and hemochromatosis, hyperparathyroidism, hypophosphatasia, and hypomagnesemia. A distinct form of arthritis associated with hemochromatosis was first reported in 1964.[63] This arthropathy is similar to osteoarthritis and rheumatoid arthritis and may be the initial presenting feature in some patients. The most frequently involved joints are the metacarpophalangeal joints (primarily the second and third), wrists, and hips; radiologic changes consisting of hook-like osteophytes at the metacarpal heads are a characteristic finding. CPPD deposition has been described in 20% to 30% of patients with primary hyperparathyroidism, more often in older patients. Attacks of acute pseudogout after parathyroidectomy have been described and are often the first manifestation of CPPD deposition in these patients.[64]

DIAGNOSIS

Synovial fluid aspiration and examination for crystals are essential to the diagnosis. The synovial fluid in pseudogout is usually inflammatory but may be hemorrhagic. A leukocyte count of about 10,000 to 20,000 cells/mm³ is the rule, but in the small joints, such as the wrist, very high counts may be seen. Synovial fluid should be examined first under regular microscopy because CPPD crystals give a weakly positive birefringence under polarized microscopy and can be easily missed. The crystals are rhomboid or rod-shaped and may be intracellular or extracellular [see Figure 4]. Because of their weak birefringence, CPPD crystals may be missed on initial examination, so it is essential that someone experienced in crystal identification examine the fluid.

Radiographic studies of affected joints often reveal chondrocalcinosis of the articular cartilage. The fibrocartilage of the menisci in the knees [see Figure 5a] or of the triangular ligament at the radioulnar joint at the wrist [see Figure 5b] may have punctate or linear calcifications; and similar changes may be seen in the symphysis pubis, shoulder, hip, and intervertebral disks. Linear calcification of the hyaline cartilage in these joints may be seen as well. Other features may include narrowing and sclerosis of the radiocarpal and patellofemoral joints, femoral cortical erosions above the knee, and extra-articular calcifications involving tendons or ligaments.

TREATMENT

Management of the patient with pseudogout is similar to management of the patient with acute gout, with the main goal of therapy being control of the acute inflammatory reaction.[44] Rest of the inflamed joint (or joints) and administration of NSAIDs or intra-articular corticosteroid preparations are the mainstay of therapy. Aspiration of the joint is sufficient to significantly relieve pain and discomfort in some patients. Colchicine is effective in patients with acute pseudogout but should be used cautiously in older patients. At lower doses of 0.6 mg one or two times a day, colchicine can be helpful in preventing further attacks.[65] In some patients, intramuscular or subcutaneous ACTH (40 units) or intramuscular triamcinolone (60 mg) can control the acute inflammatory reaction.[66] For those with chronic pain and inflammation, physiotherapy, analgesics, and NSAIDs are alternatives for management. An evaluation of the patient for underlying metabolic abnormalities, particularly hemochromatosis and hyperparathyroidism, should be considered. However, successful treatment of these associated conditions has not been shown to alter the radiographic or clinical course of CPPD deposition disease.

Other Forms of Crystal-Associated Arthritis

BASIC CALCIUM PHOSPHATE DEPOSITION

A group of apatitelike (basic calcium phosphate) crystals has been identified in pathologic synovial fluids and articular and periarticular tissues in a variety of musculoskeletal disorders. These crystals may be found in 30% to 60% of synovial fluids from patients with osteoarthritis and may contribute to the low-grade inflammatory process of typical osteoarthritis.[67] A severe destructive arthropathy of the shoulder and knee, known as the Milwaukee shoulder-knee syndrome, that affects predominantly older women has been described.[68] This process is associated with rotator cuff degeneration and rupture, joint instability, and periarticular calcification. The synovial fluid may be serosanguineous and contains few cells, and hydroxyapatite crystals may appear as clumps or may look like intracellular shiny coins, but they are not birefringent under polarized-light microscopy. The treatment of this condition is difficult, but joint aspiration and intra-articular corticosteroid injections have been helpful in some patients.

Basic calcium phosphate crystals are also associated with acute calcific periarthritis that may affect the shoulder or other joint areas in periarticular structures. In patients with this condi-

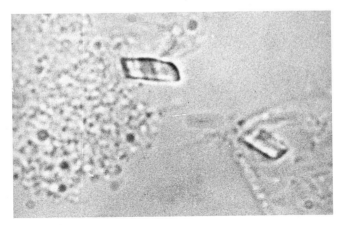

Figure 4 **Calcium pyrophosphate dihydrate crystals typical of pseudogout are rhomboid and demonstrate a weakly positive birefringence under polarized light.**

a

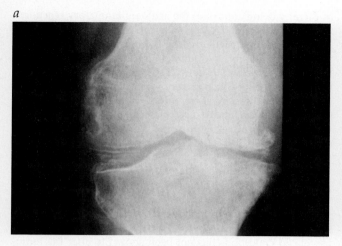

b

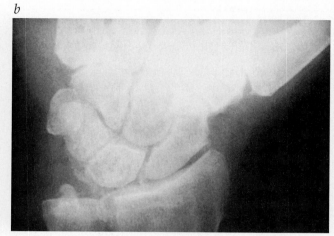

Figure 5 **Typical radiographs of chondrocalcinosis seen in CPPD deposition disease, with evidence of intra-articular calcification in the meniscus and hyaline cartilage of the knee (*a*) and the triangular cartilage of the wrist (*b*).**

tion, periarticular calcific deposits may be found in the shoulder; near the lateral trochanter of the hip; around the wrists, fingers, or knees; or in the ankle and foot. These deposits may be well defined radiographically at the beginning of attacks but often disappear over several weeks. NSAIDs and local corticosteroid injections are usually useful in the treatment of this condition.

OTHER CRYSTALS FOUND IN SYNOVIAL FLUID

A variety of other crystals in synovial fluid have been described. Cholesterol crystals may be seen in some chronic effusions and are most often associated with chronic rheumatoid bursal effusions.[69] Other lipid crystals have been seen after joint trauma, and another type of lipid crystal, which resembles a Maltese cross, has been described and may be responsible for an acute inflammatory reaction in rare cases.[70] In addition, calcium oxalate crystals have been found in the synovial fluid of patients with end-stage renal disease.[71] The pathogenetic significance of each of these types of crystals is uncertain, and therefore, they most probably represent incidental secondary phenomena.

References

1. McCarty DJ, Hollander JL: Identification of urate crystals in gouty synovial fluids. Ann Intern Med 54:452, 1961

2. McCarty DJ, Kohn NN, Faires JS: The significance of calcium phosphate crystals in the synovial fluid of arthritis patients: the `pseudogout syndrome': I. Clinical aspects. Ann Intern Med 56:711, 1962

3. Wyngaarden JB, Kelley WN: Gout and Hyperuricemia. Grune & Stratton, New York, 1976

4. Boss GR, Seegmiller JE: Hyperuricemia and gout: classification, complications and management. N Engl J Med 300:1459, 1979

5. Roubenoff R: Gout and hyperuricemia. Rheum Dis Clin North Am 16:539, 1990

6. Abbott RD, Brand FN, Kannel WB, et al: Gout and coronary artery disease: the Framingham Study. J Clin Epidemiol 41:237, 1988

7. Lawrence RC, Helmick CG, Arnett FC, et al: Estimates of the prevalence of arthritis and selected musculoskeletal diseases in the United States. Arthritis Rheum 41:778, 1998

8. Hochberg MC, Thomas J, Thomas DJ, et al: Racial differences in the incidence of gout. Arthritis Rheum 38:628, 1995

9. MacFarlane DG, Dieppe PA: Diuretic-induced gout in elderly women. Br J Rheumatol 24:155, 1985

10. Ter Borg EJ, Rasker JJ: Gout in the elderly: a separate entity? Ann Rheum Dis 46:72, 1987

11. Wortmann RL: Gout and hyperuricemia. Textbook of Rheumatology, 6th ed. Ruddy S, Harris ED, Sledge CB, Eds, WB Saunders Co, Philadelphia (in press)

12. Campion EW, Glynn RJ, DeLabry LO: Asymptomatic hyperuricemia: risks and consequences in the Normative Aging Study. Am J Med 82:421, 1987

13. Scott JT, Higgens CS: Diuretic induced gout: a multifactorial condition. Ann Rheum Dis 51:259, 1992

14. Caspi D, Lubart E, Graff E, et al: The effect of mini-dose aspirin on renal function and uric acid handling in elderly patients. Arthritis Rheum 43:103, 2000

15. Lin HY, Rocher LL, McQuillan MA, et al: Cyclosporine-induced hyperuricemia and gout. N Engl J Med 321:287, 1989

16. Burack DA, Griffith BP, Thompson ME, et al: Hyperuricemia and gout among heart transplant recipients receiving cyclosporine. Am J Med 92:141, 1992

17. Morton NE: Genetics of hyperuricemia in families with gout. Am J Med Genet 4:103, 1979

18. Simkin PA: The pathogenesis of podagra. Ann Intern Med 86:230, 1977

19. Fam AG, Stein J, Rubenstein J: Gouty arthritis in nodal osteoarthritis. J Rheumatol 23:684, 1996

20. Agudelo CA, Wise CM: Crystal-associated arthritis. Clin Geriatr Med 14:495, 1998

21. Hadler NM, Franck WA, Bress NM, et al: Acute polyarticular gout. Am J Med 56:715, 1974

22. Gutman AB: Gout. Textbook of Medicine. Beeson PB, McDermott W, Eds. WB Saunders Co, Philadelphia, 1963, p 1255

23. Gutman AB: The past four decades of progress in the knowledge of gout with an assessment of the present status. Arthritis Rheum 16:431, 1973

24. Barthelemy CR, Nakayama DA, Carrera GF, et al: Gouty arthritis: a prospective radiographic evaluation of sixty patients. Skeletal Radiol 11:1, 1984

25. Yü T-F, Berger L: Renal disease in primary gout: a study of 253 gout patients with proteinuria. Semin Arthritis Rheum 4:293, 1975

26. Yü T-F, Berger L: Impaired renal function in gout: its association with hypertensive vascular disease and intrinsic renal disease. Am J Med 72:95, 1982

27. Johnson RJ, Kivlighn SD, Kim YG, et al: Reappraisal of the pathogenesis and consequences of hyperuricemia in hypertension, cardiovascular disease, and renal disease [editorial] . Am J Kidney Dis 33:225, 1999

28. Tarng D-C, Lin H-Y, Shyong M-L, et al: Renal function in gout patients. Am J Nephrol 15:31, 1995

29. Fessel WM: Renal outcomes of gout and hyperuricemia. Am J Med 67:74, 1979

30. Pak CYC, Barilla DE, Holt K, et al: Effect of oral purine load and allopurinol on the crystallization of calcium salts in urine of patients with hyperuricosuric calcium urolithiasis. Am J Med 65:593, 1978

31. Cohen LF, Balow JE, Magrath IT, et al: Acute tumor lysis syndrome: a review of 37 patients with Burkitt's lymphoma. Am J Med 68:486, 1980

32. Reynolds PP, Knapp MJ, Baraf HSB, et al: Moonshine and lead: relationship to the pathogenesis of hyperuricemia in gout. Arthritis Rheum 26:1057, 1983

33. Takahashi S, Yamamoto T, Moriwaki Y, et al: Impaired lipoprotein metabolism in patients with primary gout: influence of alcohol intake and body weight. Br J Rheumatol 33:731, 1994

34. Vuorinen-Markkola H, Yki-Järvinen H: Hyperuricemia and insulin resistance. J Clin Endocrinol Metab 78:25, 1994

35. Cigolini M, Targher G, Tonoli M, et al: Hyperuricemia: relationships to body fat distribution and other components of the insulin resistance syndrome in 38-year-old healthy men and women. Int J Obes 19:92, 1995

36. Myers AR, Epstein FH, Dodge HJ, et al: The relationship of serum uric acid to risk factors in coronary heart disease. Am J Med 45:520, 1968

37. Culleton BF, Larson MG, Kannel WB, et al: Serum uric acid and risk for cardiovascular disease and death: the Framingham Heart Study. Ann Intern Med 131:7, 1999

38. Erickson AR, Enzenauer RJ, Nordstrom DM, et al: The prevalence of hypothyroidism in gout. Am J Med 97:231, 1994

39. Wallace SL, Robinson H, Masi AT, et al: Preliminary criteria for the classification of acute arthritis of primary gout. Arthritis Rheum 20:895, 1977

40. Agudelo CA, Weinberger A, Schumacher HR, et al: Definitive diagnosis of gout by identification of urate crystals in asymptomatic metatarsophalangeal joints. Arthritis Rheum 22:559, 1979

41. Pascual E, Batlle E, Martinez A, et al: Synovial fluid analysis for diagnosis of intercritical gout. Ann Intern Med 131:756, 1999

42. Pascual E: Gout update: from lab to the clinic and back. Curr Opin Rheumatol 12:213, 2000

43. Emmerson BT: The management of gout. N Engl J Med 334:445, 1996

44. Agudelo CA, Wise CM: Crystal deposition diseases. Treatment of the Rheumatic Diseases, 2nd ed. Weisman MH, Weinblatt ME, Louie J, Eds. WB Saunders Co, Philadelphia (in press)

45. Roberts WN, Liang MH, Stern SH: Colchicine in acute gout: reassessment of risks and benefits. JAMA 257:1920, 1987

46. Wallace SL, Singer JZ: Systemic toxicity associated with the intravenous administration of colchicine: guidelines for use (review). J Rheumatol 15:495, 1988

47. Crofford LJ, Lipsky PE, Brooks P, et al: Current comment: basic biology and clinical application of specific cyclooxygenase-2 inhibitors. Arthritis Rheum 43:4, 2000

48. Fam AG: Current therapy of acute microcrystalline arthritis and the role of corticosteroids. J Clin Rheumatol 3:35, 1997

49. Yü T-F: The efficacy of colchicine prophylaxis in articular gout: a reappraisal after 20 years. Semin Arthritis Rheum 12:256, 1982

50. Wallace SL, Singer JZ, Duncan GJ, et al: Renal function predicts colchicine toxicity: guidelines for the prophylactic use of colchicine in gout. J Rheumatol 18:264, 1991

51. Bull PW, Scott JT: Intermittent control of hyperuricemia in the treatment of gout. J Rheumatol 16:1246, 1989

52. Perez-Ruiz F, Calabozo M, Fernandez-Lopez MJ, et al: Treatment of chronic gout in patients with renal function impairment: an open, randomized, actively controlled study. J Clin Rheumatol 5:49, 1999

53. Ryan LM, McCarty DJ: Calcium pyrophosphate crystal deposition disease, pseudogout, and articular chondrocalcinosis. Arthritis and Allied Conditions, 13th ed. Koopman WJ, Ed. Williams & Wilkins, Baltimore, 1997, p 2103

54. Hande KR, Noone RM, Stone WJ: Severe allopurinol toxicity: description and guidelines for prevention in patients with renal insufficiency. Am J Med 76:47, 1984

55. Wilkins E, Dieppe P, Maddison P, et al: Osteoarthritis and articular chondrocalcinosis in the elderly. Ann Rheum Dis 42:280, 1983

56. Doherty M, Dieppe P: Crystal deposition disease in the elderly. Clin Rheum Dis 12:97, 1986

57. Reginato J: Calcium pyrophosphate and hydroxyapatite. Textbook of Rheumatology, 6th ed. Ruddy S, Harris ED, Sledge CB, Eds. WB Saunders Co, Philadelphia (in press)

58. Ellman MH, Levin B: Chondrocalcinosis in elderly persons. Arthritis Rheum 18:43, 1975

59. Bong D, Bennett R: Pseudogout mimicking systemic disease. JAMA 246:1438, 1981

60. Fam AG: What is new about crystals other than monosodium urate? Curr Opin Rheumatol 12:228, 2000

61. Resnick D, Williams G, Weisman MH, et al: Rheumatoid arthritis and pseudorheumatoid arthritis in calcium pyrophosphate dihydrate crystal deposition disease. Radiology 140:615, 1981

62. Jones AC, Chuck AJ, Arie EA, et al: Diseases associated with calcium pyrophosphate deposition disease. Semin Arthritis Rheum 22:188, 1992

63. Schumacher HR Jr: Hemochromatosis and arthritis. Arthritis Rheum 7:41, 1964

64. Rynes RI, Merzig EG: Calcium pyrophosphate crystal deposition disease and hyperparathyroidism: a controlled, prospective study. J Rheumatol 5:460, 1978

65. Alvarellos A, Spilberg I: Colchicine prophylaxis in pseudogout. J Rheumatol 13:804, 1986

66. Roane DW, Harris MD, Carpenter MT, et al: Prospective use of intramuscular triamcinolone acetonide in pseudogout. J Rheumatol 24:1168, 1997

67. Ryan LM, Cheung HS: The role of crystals in osteoarthritis. Rheum Dis Clin North Am 25:257, 1999

68. Halverson PB, Carrera GF, McCarty DJ: Milwaukee shoulder syndrome: fifteen additional cases and a description of contributing factors. Arch Intern Med 150:677, 1990

69. Wise CM, White RE, Agudelo CA: Synovial fluid lipid abnormalities in various disease states: review and classification. Semin Arthritis Rheum 16:222, 1987

70. Trostle DC, Schumacher HR Jr, Medsger TA Jr, et al: Lipid microspherule-associated acute monoarticular arthritis. Arthritis Rheum 29:1166, 1986

71. Hoffman GS, Schumacher HR, Paul H, et al: Calcium oxalate microcrystalline-associated arthritis in end-stage renal disease. Ann Intern Med 97:36, 1982

Christopher Wise, M.D.

Definition

Osteoarthritis is a common form of arthritis characterized by degeneration of articular cartilage and reactive changes in surrounding bone and periarticular tissue. The disease process results in pain and dysfunction of affected joints and is a major cause of disability in the general population. Osteoarthritis is also frequently referred to as degenerative joint disease; other terms that have been used include osteoarthrosis, hypertrophic arthritis, and atrophic arthritis.

Classification

PRIMARY OSTEOARTHRITIS

Patients without a specific inflammatory or metabolic condition known to be associated with arthritis and without a history of specific injury or trauma are considered to have primary osteoarthritis. However, a number of underlying processes are considered to be important in patients with primary osteoarthritis [see Etiologic Factors, Risk Factors, below]. In most patients, involvement is limited to one or a small number of joints or joint areas. In some patients, however, multiple joint areas are involved, and these patients are considered to have a separate variant called primary generalized osteoarthritis. Another variant, termed erosive osteoarthritis, is characterized by polyarticular involvement of the small joints of the hand and tends to occur more often in middle-aged and elderly women.

SECONDARY OSTEOARTHRITIS

Secondary osteoarthritis has been associated with several conditions that cause damage to articular cartilage through a variety of mechanisms, including mechanical, inflammatory, and metabolic processes [see Table 1]. Acute trauma, particularly intra-articular fractures and meniscal tears, can result in articular instability or incongruity and lead to osteoarthritis years after an injury.

The role of chronic trauma from certain occupational or avocational activities is not as well established as the role of acute trauma in the development of secondary osteoarthritis. Neurologic disorders that result in the loss of sensory nerve function may be associated with a particularly destructive type of degenerative arthritis (i.e., neuropathic arthritis and Charcot joint) in which cartilage and bone fragmentation are seen with relatively little pain.

Many types of inflammatory arthritis can cause destruction of articular cartilage. The best example of cartilage damage is seen in chronic rheumatoid arthritis, but similar cartilage damage can be seen in prior infectious arthritis, psoriatic arthritis, Reiter syndrome, and ankylosing spondylitis.

Congenital and developmental diseases that cause joint incongruity may result in osteoarthritis. This condition is best recognized in epiphyseal dysplasia, Perthes disease, and other processes affecting the femoral head and hip and has also been associated with generalized joint hypermobility, as seen in Ehlers-Danlos syndrome.

Primary bone disorders that affect the mechanics and articular surfaces of nearby joints may also lead to degenerative cartilage changes, particularly around major joints such as the shoulder, hip, and knee. Several metabolic and endocrine disorders have been associated directly or indirectly with the development of osteoarthritis, often with atypical patterns or in unusual locations. In most of these conditions, cartilage damage is associated with the accumulation, in articular cartilage, of a particular substance associated with the metabolic condition (e.g., uric acid or iron). In hemochromatosis, the mechanism of joint damage may also be related to an association with calcium pyrophosphate crystal deposition. In acromegaly, overgrowth of articular cartilage and subsequent mechanical problems appear to be important in the pathogenesis of the disease.

Epidemiology

Osteoarthritis is the most common type of arthritis, and it is one of the most common causes of disability and dependence in the United States.[1,2] Estimating the prevalence of osteoarthritis in the general population is difficult because of the high prevalence of asymptomatic radiographic changes of osteoarthritis and differences in case definition. The prevalence of radiographic changes of osteoarthritis in the population in general, regardless of symptoms, is roughly 30% for the hands, 21% for the feet, and 3% for the knees and hips. In persons older than 65 years, changes are seen in the knee in 33% and in the hands in almost 100%. Fortunately, most patients with radiographic changes found in population-based surveys have few symptoms or functional limitations. The overall prevalence of symptomatic osteoarthritis is equal in men and women 30 to 60 years of age (approximately 6% have affected knees and 4% have affected hips). For adults older than 60 years, however, the prevalence of symptomatic osteoarthritis (all joints) increases to 17% in men and 30% in women.[1,2]

Men and women tend be affected equally by osteoarthritis in middle age, but women are affected much more often after the age of 55, particularly in the interphalangeal joints of the fingers. Osteoarthritis is seen in all population groups, although there are certain geographic and ethnic differences in prevalence. For example, osteoarthritis of the hip is least common in Japanese, Saudi Arabian, Chinese, and African populations, and knee involvement is most common in African-American women.

Risk Factors

A number of risk factors are believed to contribute to the development of primary osteoarthritis, including age, obesity, bone density, hormonal status, nutritional factors, joint dysplasia, trauma, occupational factors, and hereditary factors.[2,3]

Age is the factor most strongly associated with radiographic and clinically significant osteoarthritis, with an exponential increase seen in more severely involved joints. The cellular or biomechanical changes in articular cartilage that occur with aging are not necessarily those seen in osteoarthritis. However, it has been speculated that these changes may facilitate the development of disease.

Obesity is clearly associated with osteoarthritis of the knee. The increased load carried by obese patients and the alterations in gait and posture that redistribute the load contribute to cartilage damage. A study in young men suggested that each increase

Table 1 Causes of Secondary Osteoarthritis

Trauma
  Acute injury
  Chronic occupational overuse
  Sports overuse
  Neuropathic arthropathy (Charcot joint)

Inflammatory arthritis
  Rheumatoid arthritis
  Infectious arthritis
  Psoriatic arthritis
  Reiter syndrome
  Ankylosing spondylitis

Dysplastic and hereditary conditions
  Congenital hip dysplasia
  Epiphyseal dysplasia
  Chondrodysplasias
  Perthes disease
  Kashin-Bek disease
  Joint hypermobility

Bone disorders
  Osteonecrosis (avascular necrosis)
  Osteochondritis
  Paget disease of bone

Metabolic and endocrine disorders
  Crystal deposition disease (gout, calcium pyrophosphate
    deposition, basic calcium phosphate)
  Hemochromatosis
  Ochronosis
  Wilson disease
  Bleeding disorders
  Acromegaly

in weight of 8 kg results in a 70% increase in the risk of symptomatic arthritis of the knee in later years.[4] Another study suggested that this association is particularly high in patients with varus malalignment of the knee, highlighting the importance of mechanical factors.[5] The relation of obesity to osteoarthritis in other weight-bearing joints is not as clear-cut and may not be much of a factor at all for hip involvement.

An association between increased bone density and osteoarthritis has been noted in several studies.[6] Women with osteoporosis and hip fractures have a decreased risk of osteoarthritis, and those affected by osteoarthritis have significantly increased bone density. This negative association suggests that soft subchondral bone absorbs impact and protects articular cartilage better than dense bone. Paradoxically, however, estrogen deficiency may contribute to the increased prevalence of osteoarthritis in women who have recently entered menopause.[2] In addition, a study showing that patients with low dietary vitamin D intake have more rapid progression of disease suggests that strong subchondral bone may be particularly important in preventing progression of osteoarthritis once it is established.[7]

Chronic repetitive impact loading is known to cause rapid degenerative changes in articular cartilage in laboratory animals. This mechanism probably accounts for the high frequency of osteoarthritis in certain occupational and athletic settings. In particular, occupational activities that require frequent knee bending increase the risk of knee involvement, and frequent lifting appears to be a risk factor for hip involvement.[8,9] Long-term weight-bearing sports activity is associated with an increased risk of developing radiographic evidence of osteoarthritis. In patients without a history of injury, clinical symptoms do not always correlate with radiographic changes, and radiographic changes do not often progress significantly.[10,11] A history of specific joint injury, usually related to sports and recreational activities, is an important risk factor for knee and hip disease.[12]

Decreased strength and proprioception have occurred in patients with osteoarthritis. Studies have found decreased strength in patients with radiographic changes and no pain, as well as decreased proprioception in unaffected knees of patients with unilateral disease.[13,14] Thus, subtle abnormalities in strength and proprioception may be risk factors for osteoarthritis.

Many patients with osteoarthritis have a positive family history, and multiple genetic factors may be responsible in various forms of osteoarthritis.[15] Primary generalized osteoarthritis with finger joint involvement and familial forms of crystal deposition disease are among the best recognized forms of arthritis with familial associations. In addition, studies have emphasized the importance of hereditary factors in osteoarthritis of the hip.[16,17] Metabolic abnormalities related to the hereditary component of osteoarthritis have been found in a number of studies. These abnormalities include associations between variations of collagen genes in familial osteoarthritis and lumbar disk disease and an abnormal vitamin D receptor gene in early osteoarthritis of the knee.[18-20] In addition to the known heritable and acquired joint dysplasias that cause secondary osteoarthritis, subclinical degrees of dysplasia may be a factor in patients with primary osteoarthritis, particularly in the hip.[21]

Physiology and Pathophysiology

NORMAL ARTICULAR CARTILAGE

Articular cartilage is specialized connective tissue that covers the weight-bearing surfaces of diarthrodial joints. It is composed of sparsely scattered cells (chondrocytes) within an extracellular matrix composed of collagen, proteoglycans, and water, with a very small component of calcium salt.[22]

Most of the collagen in cartilage is type II collagen, arranged in thick bundles parallel to the surface of the cartilage in outer portions and more perpendicular in deeper layers. This arrangement of collagen serves as a limiting membrane, distributes compressive forces, and tethers the uncalcified cartilage to the more basilar calcified cartilage and subchondral bone.

The proteoglycan component of the matrix is composed predominantly of a large molecule called aggrecan, which consists of a large core protein with covalently attached side chains of glycosaminoglycans (GAGs), most of which are chondroitin sulfate and keratan sulfate. A link protein connects aggrecan to hyaluronic acid, a long, unbranched polysaccharide molecule that can bind several hundred aggrecan molecules. This aggregate forms a very large molecule with a molecular weight of 100 million daltons or more. The molecule has a high fixed negative charge, which allows the retention of large amounts of water.

The collagen matrix and hydrophilic proteoglycan component form a resilient tissue that holds water under pressure and is capable of dissipating much of the force of weight bearing, protecting soft tissues and subchondral bone.

In normal cartilage, the turnover rate of collagen is relatively slow, whereas proteoglycan turnover is rapid. The normal turnover of these matrix components is mediated by the chondrocytes, which synthesize the components and the proteolytic enzymes responsible for their breakdown. Chondrocytes are, in

a

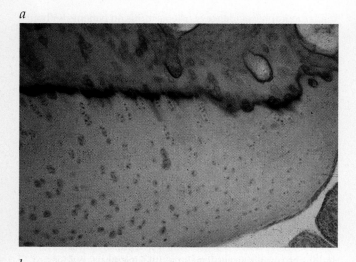

b

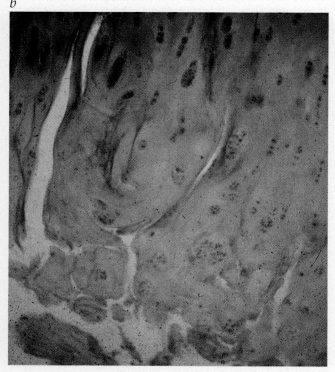

Figure 1   Microscopic appearance of normal articular cartilage (*a*) and osteoarthritic (*b*) articular cartilage. In normal cartilage, the cartilage surface is smooth and chondrocytes are regularly arranged, mostly as single cells; the background proteoglycan staining is homogeneous; and the subchondral bony plate is intact. In osteoarthritis, there is splitting fissuring of the surface, proliferation and clustering of the chondrocytes, and decreased and irregular staining of the background proteoglycan.

turn, influenced by a number of factors, including polypeptide growth factors and cytokines, structural and physical stimuli, and even the components of the matrix itself.

CHANGES IN OSTEOARTHRITIC CARTILAGE

Pathologic findings suggest that articular cartilage is the site of the primary abnormality in osteoarthritis. There is a loss of homogeneity, and disruption and fragmentation of the surface occur. Uneven staining for proteoglycans is seen in the matrix, and the

deeper layers of cartilage are invaded by capillaries from the calcified cartilage. Chondrocytes, which exist as isolated cells in normal cartilage, begin to proliferate and are found in large clusters and clones, and osteophytes are formed, which are covered by irregular hyaline and fibrocartilage [*see Figure 1*].

In early osteoarthritis, the water content of diseased cartilage increases and the cartilage swells, and the collagen fibers are usually smaller and not as tightly organized. The proteoglycan content of cartilage decreases markedly as disease progresses, with shortening of the glycosaminoglycan chains and impaired molecular aggregation.

Osteoarthritic cartilage is characterized by an increase in anabolic and catabolic activity. In early stages, the synthesis of collagen, proteoglycans, and hyaluronate is increased and chondrocytes tend to replicate. At the same time, synthesis of degradative enzymes such as collagenase, stromelysin, gelatinase, and hyaluronidase is increased, while some of the substances that inhibit cartilage destruction are themselves destroyed or inhibited. In later stages, the anabolic activities of the chondrocytes become insufficient to keep up with the degradative process. The final result is a matrix that is less structurally sound and less well organized on a macromolecular basis to withstand the forces required of articular cartilage.

Biochemical and metabolic changes in cartilage considered to be potential etiologic factors in osteoarthritis include abnormalities in collagen structure, crystal deposition, inflammatory mediators, and chondrocyte metabolism. The discovery of a familial form of osteoarthritis associated with a specific genetic defect in collagen has led to speculation that similar abnormalities in collagen or other structural components of cartilage may have etiologic importance. In addition, the association of deposition of hemosiderin, copper, or various crystals with secondary forms of osteoarthritis suggests that substances that alter matrix composition can be responsible for degenerative changes.

The relation of calcium-containing crystals to osteoarthritis is complex.[23] Both calcium pyrophosphate dihydrate and basic calcium phosphate crystals have been associated with osteoarthritic cartilage. In vitro measurement of the by-products of cartilage breakdown suggests that these crystals magnify the degenerative process by stimulation of mitogenesis in fibroblasts and secretion of proteases by cells that ingest the crystals.

The reasons for the increased anabolic and catabolic activities of chondrocytes in osteoarthritis are not well understood.[22] Chondrocytes are influenced by a number of humoral, mechanical, synovial, and cartilage matrix mediators. In particular, prostaglandins, nitric oxide, interleukin-1 (IL-1), transforming growth factor–β, estrogen, and insulinlike growth factor–1 (IGF-1) have a variety of stimulatory and inhibitory effects that may be pathogenetically important. Whether the observed abnormalities in these factors are etiologic or merely represent the response of the chondrocyte to other injury is not yet known.

The pain that patients experience in osteoarthritis may result from irritation of soft tissue structures surrounding bone, and a recent magnetic resonance study suggests that edema of subchondral bone may play an important role as well.[24]

Diagnosis

Characteristic radiographic features are usually considered essential for diagnosis but should be corroborated by the presence of compatible symptoms. Laboratory studies are useful in the evaluation of patients with osteoarthritis only in that they help to exclude other diagnoses. Thus, the erythrocyte sedimentation rate (ESR), rheumatoid factor, and routine hematologic and biochemical parameters should be normal in patients with osteoarthritis unless the osteoarthritis is attributable to comorbid conditions. Synovial fluid from involved joints is noninflammatory, with leukocyte counts being under 2,000 cells/mm³ in most patients. The presence of birefringent calcium pyrophosphate dihydrate crystals is diagnostic of a separate process that frequently overlaps with typical osteoarthritis. Basic calcium phosphate crystals, which are not birefringent, may be seen frequently in typical osteoarthritis if assessed with special stains.

Even though some patients experience multiple joint involvement, specific joints should be considered individually so that no important nonarticular or superimposed process that might be causing problems is overlooked.

CLINICAL MANIFESTATIONS

General

Typical symptoms of osteoarthritis include pain, stiffness, swelling, deformity, and loss of function. Pain is usually chronic and localized to the involved joint or joints or referred to nearby areas. Pain may be mild or moderate early in the disease but tends to worsen gradually over many years. Most of the pain is made worse with activity and improves with rest. Morning stiffness is not as prolonged as in patients with inflammatory diseases; morning stiffness in patients with osteoarthritis usually lasts less than an hour. Many patients complain of stiffening, or so-called gelling, during the day, particularly after sitting for extended periods of time. Swelling tends to be mild or moderate and is often related to bony enlargement rather than soft tissue edema. Deformity and loss of function are later manifestations, occurring after many years of disease.

Physical findings in osteoarthritis include crepitus, pain on motion, bony enlargement, and periarticular tenderness. Synovial effusions may be present, particularly in the knee. Erythema and warmth are unusual and should suggest the presence of coexistent crystal-induced inflammation or other conditions. In more advanced disease, limited range of motion, deformity, and instability may become more prominent findings.

Specific Joint Involvement and Complications

Osteoarthritis has a characteristic pattern of involvement in most patients. Joints frequently involved include the distal and proximal interphalangeal as well as the first carpometacarpal joints in the hands, the cervical and lumbar spines, the hips, the knees, and, less commonly, the small joints of the feet or the acromioclavicular joint. The wrists, metacarpophalangeal joints, elbows, shoulders, and ankles are usually not affected unless there is a history of injury to the specific joint, occupational overuse, or underlying condition that might be a cause of secondary osteoarthritis.

Hands The most commonly affected joints in the hands are the distal and proximal interphalangeal joints, resulting in bony enlargement of these joints referred to as Heberden and Bouchard nodes, respectively [see Figures 2 and 3]. The progressive enlargement of these joints occurs slowly over many years, is frequently familial, and occurs most often in middle-aged or elderly women. Individual joints may go through inflammatory phases with redness and increased swelling and pain, most of which eventually subsides to a bony enlargement. Small gelatinous cysts may develop over the dorsal aspect of the distal interphalangeal

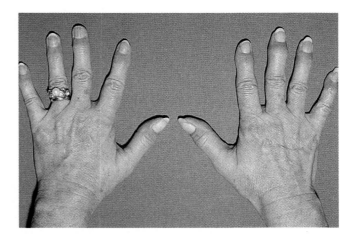

Figure 2 The hands of a patient with typical primary osteoarthritis showing bony enlargement of multiple distal interphalangeal joints (Heberden nodes), mostly on the right, and early bony enlargement of the proximal interphalangeal joints (Bouchard nodes) on the left.

joints and either persist or resolve spontaneously. Many patients with Heberden and Bouchard nodes have very little pain most of the time and may not seek medical attention. The carpometacarpal joint of the thumb is another frequently involved joint, either by itself or along with the more distal joints, that causes pain, bony enlargement, and limited motion.

Knees Osteoarthritis frequently affects the knees and may be a cause of significant disability. Most patients present with pain that is worse with activity and improves with rest; they report difficulty getting out of chairs or going up steps. Osteoarthritic knees will almost always have crepitus, limited motion, and pain on motion, and effusions may or may not be present. In more advanced disease, bony enlargement, instability, and varus angulation may be present. Many patients have involvement of the patellofemoral

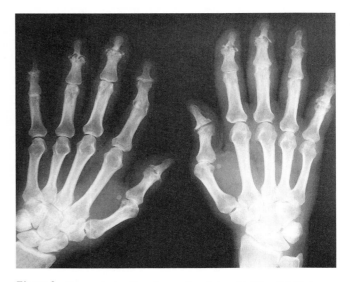

Figure 3 Severe destructive changes involving all of the distal interphalangeal joints and some of the proximal interphalangeal joints are characteristic of erosive osteoarthritis. Osteophytes are present at the margins of involved joints. Sharply demarcated bone erosions are seen in several distal interphalangeal joints, and bony fusion is seen in the proximal interphalangeal joint of the left second digit.

compartment, but isolated disease in this area should suggest the presence of calcium pyrophosphate deposition disease.

Hips   Osteoarthritis of the hips is another common cause of significant pain and disability [*see Figure 4*]. Most patients experience a progressive disabling pain usually in the upper thigh or inguinal region, sometimes radiating to the knee. Pain is worse with ambulation and may cause the patient to limp. Patients may also complain of difficulty with activities such as tying shoes, and limited hip motion is found on examination.

Spine   Osteoarthritis of the cervical and lumbar spine is referred to as spondylosis. The intervertebral disk spaces or the posterior spinal facet joints may be affected and cause chronic back or neck pain that is worse with activity and better with rest. Disk degeneration may be complicated by protrusion of the nucleus pulposus, causing nerve root compression with radicular pain or muscle weakness. In patients with extensive degenerative changes with fibrosis and osteophytes, stenosis of the spinal canal can occur, resulting in chronic cord compression in the cervical spine or compression of the cauda equina in the lumbar region. Lumbar spinal stenosis, causing chronic radicular leg pain that is worse with activity and better with rest (neurogenic claudication), is a common complication in elderly patients. A variant of spinal osteoarthritis occurring in the thoracic spine, known as diffuse idiopathic skeletal hyperostosis (DISH), is characterized by extensive bridging osteophytes and may cause loss of motion but little pain.

Radiologic Features

Typical radiographic findings in osteoarthritis include joint space narrowing, subchondral bone sclerosis, subchondral cysts, and osteophytes (bony spurs) [*see Figure 4*]. Joint space narrowing, resulting from loss of cartilage, is often asymmetrical and may be the only finding early in the disease process. In weight-bearing joints such as the knees, narrowing may be seen only in a standing view and may be missed in a film obtained with the patient in the recumbent position. In more chronic disease, the hypertrophic features of subchondral sclerosis and osteophyte formation become more prominent, and subluxations or fusion of the joint may become apparent in more severely affected joints. In the small interphalangeal joints of the fingers, central erosions may be seen within the joint space, which should be easily distinguishable from the periarticular erosions of rheumatoid arthritis.

Differential Diagnosis

Because of the high frequency of incidental radiographic changes in the general population, it is important not to attribute all musculoskeletal pain to osteoarthritis, even in patients with radiographic abnormalities. Alternative diagnoses should be made or coexistent conditions suspected in patients who are considered to be at low risk for osteoarthritis (e.g., younger patients) or in those who present with atypical pain patterns or problems in atypical joints. Patients with a relatively sudden onset of pain or with severe pain early in their presentation most often have something other than osteoarthritis. Problems in the wrists, elbows, shoulders, or ankles should raise concerns about other types of arthritis or secondary types of osteoarthritis.

Crystal-induced arthritis should always be considered in patients with acute pain, particularly if swelling and erythema are

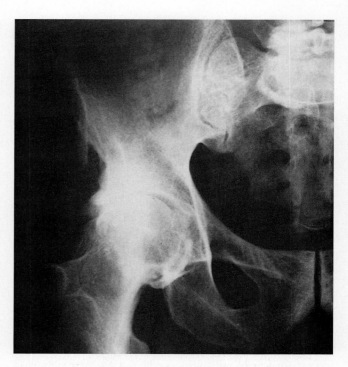

Figure 4   **The hip is a common site of involvement in osteoarthritis. Joint space narrowing is most prominent at the superior and lateral aspects of the joint. Increased bony density (sclerosis) is seen in the subchondral bone on both sides of the joint, along with early subchondral cysts and osteophytes (bony spurs) over the superior and inferior aspects of the acetabulum.**

prominent. Calcium pyrophosphate deposition disease is common in the knees and hips and often coexists with osteoarthritis. Other joints frequently involved are the wrists and shoulders. The diagnosis is dependent on the radiographic detection of chondrocalcinosis or the finding of crystals in synovial fluid. Gout usually affects foot and ankle joints in early disease and is not often confused with osteoarthritis, but involvement of the knees is common in later disease. In addition, elderly women with Heberden and Bouchard nodes in the hands may have superimposed attacks in these joints as an initial manifestation of gout. Thus, examination of fluid from these joints for urate crystals may be essential in differentiating gout from an inflammatory flare of erosive osteoarthritis.

Rheumatoid arthritis can usually be distinguished from osteoarthritis on the basis of a different pattern of joint disease, more prominent morning stiffness, and soft tissue swelling and warmth on physical examination. In some patients, the patterns of joint disease may overlap, particularly in the proximal interphalangeal joints, hips, and knees. Thus, in some patients, the presence of an elevated ESR, a high-titer rheumatoid factor, or periarticular erosive changes may be the only way to distinguish these two common conditions.

Polymyalgia rheumatica is a disease of elderly patients and is often seen in patients with underlying osteoarthritis. Patients typically have a change in the pattern of pain, more localized to the shoulder and hip girdles, with few peripheral joint symptoms. Morning stiffness is a prominent feature, and a diagnosis is usually more likely if the ESR is markedly elevated. However, because modest elevations of ESR are seen in many normal elderly individuals, the differentiation of this condition from osteoarthritis is often difficult. In some patients, a rapid response of symptoms to a low dose of corticosteroid is helpful in making a diagnosis.

Ankylosing spondylitis is usually a disease that first manifests in young adults and should not be confused with spinal osteoarthritis. However, some patients have only mild levels of pain and may not seek attention until later years. In such patients, the radiographic changes in the cervical and lumbar spine in the two conditions should make differentiation between them relatively easy.

Psoriatic arthritis, when present in a classic distribution in the distal interphalangeal joints of the fingers, may mimic Heberden nodes. Psoriatic arthritis usually occurs in younger patients and is more common in males, but differentiation between psoriatic arthritis and Heberden nodes may still be difficult. In patients, a careful search for psoriatic skin lesions and nail changes is essential. On physical examination, the swelling of involved joints is usually greater in the soft tissues, with less bony enlargement. Radiographic changes will usually show more erosive changes and fewer osteophytic changes than in typical osteoarthritis.

Disorders of bone near joints can be confused with osteoarthritis. Osteonecrosis of the hip, knee, or shoulder may cause pain and restricted motion without significant signs of inflammation. Radiographs may be normal initially, and follow-up films or magnetic resonance imaging may be necessary to differentiate this condition from osteoarthritis. Paget disease or osteoporotic fractures may cause pain in the back and hip girdle that is often similar to that of osteoarthritis, although the pain is often more severe and acute in patients with fractures.

Nonarticular pain syndromes involving tendons, bursae, peripheral nerves, and internal joint structures may cause pain similar to that of osteoarthritis. Examples include de Quervain tenosynovitis or carpal tunnel syndrome in the hand, trochanteric bursitis or meralgia paresthetica in the hip, anserine bursitis or meniscal tears in the knee, and plantar fasciitis and interdigital neuromas in the feet. A knowledge of nonarticular pain syndromes and the characteristic patterns of symptoms and physical findings in each is essential to diagnosing and differentiating these syndromes from osteoarthritis in the same area.

Management

There is no cure for osteoarthritis and no therapy known to prevent or retard the degenerative biologic process in articular cartilage. Thus, the goal of treatment is to limit or reverse the disabling effects of the condition.[25-27] Therapy for osteoarthritis is focused primarily on relieving symptoms and improving function. Treatment decisions should be based on the severity and distribution of joint involvement, considered in the setting of the patient's other medical problems that might affect the safety and effectiveness of any chosen therapy.

NONPHARMACOLOGIC MEASURES

Nonpharmacologic measures that have the potential to improve outcomes in osteoarthritis include patient education, physical and occupational therapy assessment and interventions, exercise, weight loss, and dietary vitamin C and D supplementation.[3,28] Exercise, in particular, should be a part of the therapeutic regimen in every patient. Quadriceps weakness contributes significantly to disability in patients with osteoarthritis of the knee, and exercises designed to strengthen quadriceps have potential to lessen pain and disability.[29] In addition, aerobic exercise, such as a

walking program, can improve function and reduce pain.[30,31] However, compliance with exercise programs is often low, and regular supervised follow-up may be helpful.

The role of obesity as an etiologic factor in osteoarthritis of the knee is well established, and some data suggest that weight loss may reduce the risk of development of symptoms in patients predisposed to osteoarthritis. Even though few prospective studies have been done, patients with osteoarthritis of the knees and hips should be encouraged to lose weight if they are above ideal body weight. In addition, epidemiologic studies have suggested a role for adequate dietary vitamin C and D intake in reducing the risk of progression of established osteoarthritis.[7,32] In some patients, measures designed to alter the biomechanical forces on diseased joints should be considered, including patellar taping, wedged insoles, bracing, canes, and crutches.

PHARMACOLOGIC THERAPY

The primary goal of drug therapy in osteoarthritis is to relieve pain. In some patients, simple analgesics may be as effective as nonsteroidal anti-inflammatory drugs (NSAIDs).[33] For this reason, acetaminophen in doses up to 3,000 to 4,000 mg daily should be prescribed initially in most patients. Doses should be limited in patients with exposure to other potentially hepatotoxic substances. In particular, patients who need acetaminophen regularly should be advised to limit alcohol ingestion and be warned about the increased risk of acetaminophen hepatotoxicity in heavy drinkers. Opioids are generally avoided in osteoarthritis but may be useful in selected patients. However, these agents should be used with caution in elderly patients.[34] Tramadol, a centrally acting analgesic with dual mechanisms, may give relief comparable to that achieved with acetaminophen and codeine. Topical capsaicin may be useful in some patients with involvement of the knees and hands in particular.

NSAIDs are useful in osteoarthritis mostly for their analgesic effects, although anti-inflammatory effects may have some clinical significance. Unfortunately, NSAIDs are associated with an increased risk of gastric ulcers and bleeding, particularly in patients with a history of gastrointestinal disease, those on concomitant steroids or anticoagulants, and those older than 65 years. Strategies to reduce this toxicity include the use of lower doses of NSAIDs or concomitant use of misoprostol, histamine$_2$ receptor antagonist, and proton pump inhibitors. The recently available cyclooxygenase-2 (COX-2)–specific NSAIDs celecoxib and rofecoxib have been shown to provide greater reduction of endoscopic gastritis and ulcers and serious gastrointestinal complications than the previously available nonselective cyclooxygenase inhibitors.[35,36] Intra-articular corticosteroid injections may be useful in treating selected joints, particularly during exacerbations characterized by increased pain and effusion. Some animal and in vitro studies have suggested that steroids have a detrimental effect on articular cartilage, but there are few clinical data to support this concern in patients with osteoarthritis. Nevertheless, intra-articular steroids should be used no more frequently than every 3 to 4 months in an individual joint in most patients.

Intra-articular hyaluronic acid derivatives (Hyalgan and Synvisc) have been used in osteoarthritis of the knees in Europe for many years and have recently been approved for use in Canada and the United States.[37] Depending on the product studied, a series of three to five weekly injections has been shown to be superior to placebo and comparable to oral anti-inflammatory drugs in relieving pain. The mechanism of action of these compounds is not well understood, but an anti-inflammatory effect, short-term lubrication, and stimulation of hyaluronate production by synovial cells have all been observed as potential explanations for efficacy.

SURGERY

In patients with badly damaged knees and hips, total joint replacement is an effective option. Almost all patients experience significant pain relief, and some have improved range of motion. Loosening and infection are potential late complications in prosthetic joints but are uncommon. Some patients with osteoarthritis of the knees may be helped by arthroscopic debridement, particularly when mechanical symptoms suggesting internal derangement are present. Realignment of a degenerative knee to allow redistribution of forces is sometimes attempted by a high tibial wedge osteotomy, particularly in younger patients with valgus deformities. In recent years, biologic approaches to the surgical treatment of osteoarthritis have been explored, either in the form of local enhancement of bone marrow progenitor cells or by various forms of cartilage transplantation.[25,38]

POTENTIAL THERAPIES

Therapies with potential to prevent or retard the progression of articular cartilage breakdown have received a great deal of attention in recent years.[39] Agents considered to have so-called chondroprotective potential include tetracyclines, protease inhibitors, glycosaminoglycan compounds, growth factors, and cytokine inhibitors. Oral glucosamine and chondroitin sulfate have been promoted as health food supplements to improve cartilage, but most of the clinical studies with these agents have demonstrated only modest pain relief compared with placebo, and studies to assess the effect on cartilage are ongoing.[40,41]

Tetracyclines have been shown to reduce the severity of experimental osteoarthritis in animals, probably by inhibiting metalloprotease activity, and are being studied in early human trials. Other approaches to disease modification being investigated in animal models include other agents that inhibit metalloproteases or nitric oxide synthase inhibitors.

Biologic therapies designed to augment growth factors or inhibit cytokines have also been investigated in animal models of osteoarthritis, including attempts to introduce intra-articular IL-1 receptor antagonist through the use of gene therapy.

Prognosis

Osteoarthritis is a slowly progressive condition with a variable prognosis.[2] Radiographically, most joints will usually either remain stable or gradually worsen over a 5- to 15-year period. In most patients, symptoms evolve over many years and may spontaneously remit for long periods of time without explanation. Progression in osteoarthritis of the hand is particularly hard to measure, because pain levels frequently improve after involved joints become fused. Disease may progress more rapidly in the hips and knees of older women with osteopenic bone. However, in general, predicting prognosis in osteoarthritis is difficult.

References

1. Lawrence RC, Helmick CG, Arnett FC, et al: Estimates of the prevalence of arthritis and selected musculoskeletal disorders in the United States. Arthritis Rheum 41:778, 1998

2. Felson DT, Lawrence RC, Dieppe PA, et al: Osteoarthritis: new insights. I: the disease and its risk factors. Ann Intern Med 133:635, 2000

3. Felson DT, Zhang Y: An update on the epidemiology of knee and hip osteoarthritis with a view to prevention. Arthritis Rheum 41:1343, 1998

4. Gelber AC, Hochberg MC, Mead LA, et al: Body mass index in young men and the risk of subsequent knee and hip osteoarthritis. Am J Med 107:542, 1999

5. Sharma L, Lou C, Cahue S, et al: The mechanism of the effect of obesity in knee osteoarthritis: the mediating role of malalignment. Arthritis Rheum 43:568, 2000

6. Antoniades L, MacGregor A, Matson M, et al: A cotwin control study of the relationship between hip osteoarthritis and bone mineral density. Arthritis Rheum 43:1450, 2000

7. McAlindon TE, Felson DT, Zhang Y, et al: Relation of dietary intake and serum levels of vitamin D to progression of osteoarthritis of the knee among participants in the Framingham Study. Ann Intern Med 125:353, 1996

8. McAlindon TE, Wilson PFW, Aliabadi P, et al: Level of physical activity and the risk of radiographic and symptomatic knee osteoarthritis in the elderly: the Framingham study. Am J Med 106:151, 1999

9. Coggon D, Croft P, Kellingray S, et al: Occupational physical activities and osteoarthritis of the knee. Arthritis Rheum 43:1443, 2000

10. Spector TD, Harris PA, Hart DJ, et al: Risk of osteoarthritis associated with long-term weight bearing sports: a radiologic survey of the hips and knees in female ex-athletes and population controls. Arthritis Rheum 39:988, 1996

11. Lane NE, Oehlert JW, Bloch DA, et al: The relationship of running to osteoarthritis of the knee and hip and bone mineral density of the lumbar spine: a 9 year longitudinal study. J Rheumatol 25:334, 1998

12. Gelber A, Hochberg M, Mead L, et al: Joint injury in young adults and risk for subsequent knee and hip osteoarthritis. Ann Intern Med 133:321, 2000

13. Slemenda C, Brandt KD, Heilman DK, et al: Quadriceps weakness and osteoarthritis of the knee. Ann Intern Med 127:97, 1997

14. Sharma L, Pai YC, Holtkamp K, et al: Is knee joint proprioception worse in the arthritic knee versus the unaffected knee in unilateral knee osteoarthritis? Arthritis Rheum 40:1518, 1997

15. Holderbaum D, Haqqi TM, Moskowitz RW: Genetics and osteoarthritis: exposing the iceberg. Arthritis Rheum 42:397, 1999

16. Lanyon P, Muir K, Doherty S, et al: Assessment of a genetic contribution to osteoarthritis of the hip: sibling study. BMJ 321:1179, 2000

17. MacGregor AJ, Antoniades L, Matson M, et al: The genetic contribution to radiographic hip osteoarthritis in women: results of a classic twin study. Arthritis Rheum 43:2410, 2000

18. Knowlton RG, Katzenstein PL, Moskowitz RW, et al: Genetic linkage of polymorphism to type II procollagen gene (COL 2A1) to primary osteoarthritis associated with mild chondrodysplasia. N Engl J Med 322:526, 1990

19. Keen RW, Hart DJ, Lanchbury JS, et al: Association of early osteoarthritis of the knee with a Taq I polymorphism of the vitamin D receptor gene. Arthritis Rheum 40:1444, 1997

20. Paassilta P, Lohiniva J, Goring H, et al: Identification of a novel common genetic risk factor for lumbar disc disease. JAMA 285:1843, 2001

21. Lane NE, Lin P, Christiansen L, et al: Association of mild acetabular dysplasia with an increased risk of incident osteoarthritis in elderly white women: the study of osteoporotic fractures. Arthritis Rheum 43:400, 2000

22. Goldring MB: The role of the chondrocyte in osteoarthritis. Arthritis Rheum 43:1916, 2000

23. Ryan LM, Cheung HS: The role of crystals in osteoarthritis. Rheum Dis Clin North Am 25:257, 1999

24. Felson DT, Chaisson CE, Hill CL, et al: The association of bone marrow lesions with pain in knee osteoarthritis. Ann Intern Med 134:594, 2001

25. Felson DT, Lawrence RC, Hochberg MC, et al: Osteoarthritis: new insights: II. Treatment approaches. Ann Intern Med 133:726, 2000

26. Recommendations for the medical management of osteoarthritis of the hip and knee. American College of Rheumatology Subcommittee on Osteoarthritis Guidelines. Arthritis Rheum 43:1905, 2000

27. Pendelton A, Arden N, Dougados M, et al: EULAR recommendations for the management of knee osteoarthritis: report of a task force of the Standing Committee for the International Clinical Studies Including Therapeutic Trials (ESCIST). Ann Rheum Dis 59:936, 2000

28. Puett DW, Griffin MR: Published trials of nonmedicinal and noninvasive therapies for hip and knee osteoarthritis. Ann Intern Med 121:133, 1994

29. Deyle GD, Henderson NE, Matekel RL, et al: Effectiveness of manual physical therapy and exercise in osteoarthritis of the knee: a randomized, controlled study. Ann Intern Med 132:173, 2000

30. Ettinger WH Jr, Burns R, Messier SP, et al: A randomized trial comparing aerobic exercise and resistance exercise with a health education program in older adults with knee osteoarthritis: the fitness arthritis and seniors trial (FAST). JAMA 277:25, 1997

31. Van Baar ME, Assendelft WJJ, Dekker J, et al: Effectiveness of exercise therapy in patients with osteoarthritis of the hip or knee: a systematic review of randomized clinical trials. Arthritis Rheum 42:1361, 1999

32. McAlindon T, Jacques P, Zhang Y, et al: Do antioxidant micronutrients protect against the development and progression of knee osteoarthritis? Arthritis Rheum 39:648, 1996

33. Bradley JD, Brandt KD, Katz BP, et al: Comparison of an anti-inflammatory dose of ibuprofen, an analgesic dose of ibuprofen, and acetaminophen in the treatment of patients with osteoarthritis of the knee. N Engl J Med 325:87, 1991

34. Peleso PM: Opioid therapy for osteoarthritis of the hip and knee: use it or lose it? (editorial) J Rheumatol 28:6, 2001

35. Feldman M, McMahon AT: Do cyclooxygenase-2 inhibitors provide benefits similar to those of traditional nonsteroidal anti-inflammatory drugs, with less gastrointestinal toxicity? Ann Intern Med 132:134, 2000

36. Crofford LJ, Lipsky PE, Brooks P, et al: Basic biology and clinical application of specific cyclooxygenase-2 inhibitors. Arthritis Rheum 43:4, 2000

37. Brandt K, Smith G, Simon L: Intraarticular injection of hyaluronan as treatment for

knee osteoarthritis: what is the evidence? (review) Arthritis Rheum 43:1192, 2000

38. Buckwalter JA, Mankin HJ: Articular cartilage repair and transplantation. Arthritis Rheum 41:1331, 1998

39. Dieppe PA: The management of osteoarthritis in the third millennium. Scand J Rheumatol 29:279, 2000

40. McAlindon TE, LaValley MP, Bulin JP, et al: Glucosamine and chondroitin for treatment of osteoarthritis: a systematic quality assessment and meta-analysis. JAMA 283: 1469, 2000

41. Reginster JY, Deroisy R, Rovati CL, et al: Long-term effects of glucosamine sulphate on osteoarthritis progression: a randomised, placebo-controlled clinical trial. Lancet 357: 251, 2001

Acknowledgment

Figure 1   Courtesy of Richard Hard, M.D.

120 Back Pain and Common Musculoskeletal Problems

Christopher Wise, M.D.

A large proportion of the musculoskeletal problems for which patients seek medical attention are related to periarticular structures and do not represent a true articular process or a more generalized systemic illness.[1] Knowledge of the common nonarticular regional rheumatic disorders is important because of their high prevalence in primary care practice, the dependence on clinical findings for diagnosis, and the high cost that can result from unnecessary laboratory evaluations. The ability to recognize important patterns of pain and physical signs is essential to making a correct diagnosis; in most cases, radiographic and laboratory studies are not needed. Diagnostic studies should be utilized judiciously and must be interpreted in the light of existing clinical findings and prestudy suspicion for specific diagnoses.

Most regional rheumatic disorders respond to local measures, such as application of heat or cold, splinting, and injection of glucocorticoids. Nonsteroidal anti-inflammatory drugs (NSAIDs) or mild analgesic medications are often helpful therapeutic adjuncts. Referral for surgical intervention may be indicated for patients with certain conditions. For example, in cases of cervical or lumbar disk disease or spinal stenosis with definite nerve entrapment or spinal cord compression, well-timed decompression may be necessary to restore function or prevent further functional impairment. Arthroscopic intervention is sometimes useful to better define and treat refractory knee and shoulder pain syndromes. Surgical release is indicated for entrapment neuropathies when there is evidence of motor dysfunction. Surgical consultation may be useful for a variety of other syndromes when the response to conservative measures proves to be less than optimal. Physical therapy and occupational therapy are useful for many patients—particularly those patients who have persistent back and shoulder pain—though these therapies may constitute an important part of the treatment of almost any refractory regional pain syndrome.

Common regional rheumatic disorders include various types of bursitis, tendinitis, tenosynovitis, myofascial pain, and entrapment neuropathies. Bursitis results from mechanical or inflammatory changes of one of the many bursae in the body. Bursae are synovia-lined sacs around the joints that serve to minimize friction between tendons, ligaments, and bony structures. Tendinitis usually results from trauma or overuse of tissues near sites where tendons attach to bone or at the musculotendinous junction. Myofascial pain originates at sites within muscle groups and surrounding fascial tissues that become tender and painful as a result of localized injury or overuse. Entrapment neuropathies occur at sites where peripheral nerves are compressed as they traverse periarticular areas that allow relatively little room for free movement of the affected nerves.

Neck Pain

Neck pain may result from degenerative changes in the cervical disks and zygoapophyseal (facet) joints or from a variety of muscular, ligamentous, and tendinous conditions. In whiplash injuries occurring after rapid acceleration or deceleration and hyperextension of the head in motor vehicle accidents, a number of structures may be injured.[2] Recovery from whiplash injuries is often incomplete, and a combination of physical and psychosocial factors may contribute to prolongation of pain.[3] Judicious use of analgesics, muscle relaxants, and physiotherapy are useful in some patients. Injection of the facet joints with glucocorticoids appears to have no efficacy.[4] In some patients with chronic neck pain after whiplash injury, the zygoapophyseal joints may be the source of pain, and local nerve block with an anesthetic or ablation often brings relief.[5]

The term cervical sprain denotes transient neck pain associated with muscle tenderness and spasm. Cervical sprain usually responds to heat, rest, and, occasionally, immobilization and traction. Manual therapy or exercises may provide relief in some patients.[6] In cervical disk herniation, nerve root impingement results in pain, paresthesia, and sometimes muscle weakness in the distribution of the affected nerve (usually at the C5 to C7 level). In such patients, radiographic documentation and surgical decompression are sometimes needed if symptoms do not improve with rest or traction or if significant neurologic deficit is present.[7] In some patients with long-standing cervical spondylosis, cervical stenosis may cause chronic compression of the spinal cord (most often at the C3 to C5 level). Surgical decompression is indicated in patients with evolving myelopathy.

Back Pain

Low back pain is the most common musculoskeletal complaint requiring medical attention; it is the fifth most common reason for all physician visits.[8,9] Over half of the general population will seek medical attention for back pain at some point in their lives. An increased risk of back pain is associated with male sex, smoking, frequent lifting of children or heavy objects, poor general health and conditioning, and certain occupational and sports activities.[10] In most patients, the cause of pain cannot be determined with any degree of certainty and is usually attributed to muscular or ligamentous strain, facet joint arthritis, or disk pressure on the annulus fibrosus, vertebral end plate, or nerve roots.

ACUTE BACK PAIN

Diagnosis

For patients with acute back pain, the initial history should be used to identify those who are at increased risk for serious underlying conditions, such as fracture, infection, tumor, or major neurologic deficit[8] [*see Table 1*]. The presence of such indicators in patients with acute back pain may indicate the need for radiographic and laboratory studies earlier than in patients without such indicators. The initial physical examination should include evaluation for areas of localized bony tenderness and assessment of flexion and straight leg raising. Because acute low back pain will improve within a month in over 90% of patients, further evaluation is usually unnecessary. Plain radiographs should be reserved for patients at high risk for more serious underlying conditions [*see Table 1*], because abnormal findings on plain films are common and do not correlate with back pain.

Treatment

A number of therapeutic interventions are available for acute back pain, but data supporting efficacy are minimal for most ther-

Table 1 Indications That Acute Back Pain May Involve Underlying Conditions

Patient demographics	Age > 70 yr History of cancer Glucocorticoid or immunosuppressive drug therapy Alcohol or I.V. drug abuse
Historical features	Weight loss Fever Pain increased by rest
Neurologic symptoms	Bowel or bladder dysfunction Saddle block anesthesia Progressive motor weakness

apies.[11] Strict bed rest should be kept to a minimum (no more than 2 to 4 days), and the continuation of normal activities within the limits permitted by pain will lead to a more rapid recovery than will either enforced rest or a back-mobilizing exercise program, even in patients with sciatica.[12-14] Mild analgesics and NSAIDs may be useful for early symptom control; muscle relaxants and opiates should be used sparingly. Spinal manipulation or specific exercise programs may be effective in acute back pain, but most controlled studies suggest little to no advantage of any particular regimen compared to other measures.[15-17] Patient education about the natural history of back pain may result in fewer demands for further diagnostic tests and physician visits and should improve patient satisfaction. However, a study of a preventive "back school" educational program in the workplace did not find any reduction in the frequency or severity of episodes of back pain.[18]

CHRONIC BACK PAIN

Diagnosis

Patients whose pain persists after 4 to 6 weeks of conservative treatment measures should be reassessed. Plain radiography and basic laboratory studies (e.g., complete blood count, sedimentation rate, chemistry profile, and urinalysis) should be considered to screen for systemic illnesses. A herniated lumbar disk should be considered in patients with symptoms of radiculopathy, as suggested by pain radiating down the leg with symptoms reproduced by straight leg raising. Magnetic resonance imaging may be necessary to confirm a herniated disk, but findings should be interpreted with caution because many asymptomatic persons have disk abnormalities.[19] Electromyography may be useful in differentiating lumbar radiculopathy from other causes of radicular leg pain. Most lumbar disk herniations producing sciatica occur at the L4-L5 and L5-S1 levels. Surgical intervention is indicated in patients with persistent sciatica and clear-cut evidence of a herniated disk on MRI or myelogram–computed tomographic scanning.[20]

Treatment

Patients with chronic back pain should undergo physical therapy with local modalities, an exercise program, and an education program emphasizing proper ergonomics for lifting and other activities. Light normal activity and a regular walking program should be encouraged. Judicious use of analgesics, NSAIDs, and tricyclic antidepressants may help the patient function more fully and may improve outcome.[21] In some patients with chronic low back pain that worsens with prolonged standing and extension, the source of pain may be lumbar facet joint disease. Flexion exercises and NSAIDs

may be useful, but facet joint injections with glucocorticoids do not appear to be effective.[22] Recent controlled studies have suggested that therapeutic massage or low-impact aerobic exercise provides more benefit than other strategies (e.g., acupuncture, standard physical therapy, or machine-based strengthening exercises).[23,24]

Lumbar Stenosis

Lumbar spinal stenosis, usually a result of extensive degenerative disk disease and osteophytes, should be suspected in elderly patients with chronic back pain associated with sciatica.[25] Patients typically complain of pain, numbness, and weakness in the buttocks that extends to one or both legs. Symptoms are usually brought on by standing or walking and improve when the patient assumes a flexed position or lies down (i.e., neurogenic claudication or pseudoclaudication). The diagnosis may be confirmed by MRI or myelogram–CT scanning.[26] Although conservative measures may be helpful in some patients, surgical decompression by multilevel laminectomy and fusion should be considered in patients with progressive functional deterioration.[27,28]

Shoulder Pain

Shoulder pain is one of the most common musculoskeletal problems seen in the outpatient setting.[29] Most shoulder pain results from conditions of the periarticular structures of the joint; true arthritis of the glenohumeral joint is uncommon [*see Figure 1*]. The initial evaluation of shoulder pain should include consideration of pain that may be referred from the neck, thorax, or abdomen. The examination should assess active and passive range of flexion, abduction, and internal and external rotation of the shoulder, along with forward elevation. In addition, areas of localized tenderness may help differentiate the various potential causes of shoulder pain. Plain radiographs are seldom diagnostic but are indicated in patients with a history of trauma or refractory pain or when true glenohumeral joint disease is suspected. For patients who respond poorly to conservative therapy, a variety of specialized tests (e.g., arthrography, arthroscopy, and MRI) are available for further definition of lesions that may require surgery.

ROTATOR CUFF TENDINITIS (IMPINGEMENT SYNDROME)

Rotator cuff tendinitis, or impingement syndrome, is often associated with bursitis of the overlying subacromial bursa and is the cause of most nontraumatic cases of shoulder pain. Rotator cuff tendinitis results from inflammation, degeneration, and attrition of the rotator cuff by mechanical impingement on the acromion, coracoacromial ligament, and sometimes the acromioclavicular joint.

Rotator cuff tendinitis presents most commonly in patients 35 to 60 years of age, but younger patients may be affected as a result of athletic activities involving overhand throwing. Patients report an insidious pain that may be diffuse over the lateral deltoid or more localized to the anterior acromial region. Pain worsens with reaching and may be accompanied by a catch as the patient brings the arm into an overhead position. Rotator cuff pain is often particularly bothersome at night and interferes with sleep. On examination, pain may limit movement and may be reproduced by resistance of active movement. The so-called impingement sign is elicited by forced forward elevation of the arm with the scapula stabilized from behind. A coexistent rotator cuff tear may be suspected if the patient cannot hold the arm in a horizontal position against gravity.

The goal of therapy for rotator cuff tendinitis is to relieve pain and maintain or restore range of motion. Treatment should begin with rest and a progressive program of stretching and

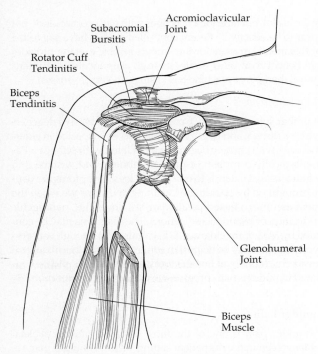

Figure 1 **Tendinitis of the rotator cuff and subacromial bursitis cause pain that is felt over the lateral aspect of the shoulder, whereas bicipital tendinitis, acromioclavicular joint disease, and glenohumeral joint disease cause anterior shoulder pain.**

strengthening exercises, facilitated by an NSAID. Injection of glucocorticoids and local anesthetic into the subacromial space or glenohumeral joint may result in dramatic relief of symptoms and may allow a more rapid, full recovery.[30,31] Avoidance of repetitive overhead activities of the arms is necessary during recovery, and job modification may be needed to prevent recurrence. In refractory cases, surgical division of the coracoacromial ligament or acromioplasty may be indicated.

CALCIFIC TENDINITIS

Calcific tendinitis is the cause of pain in a subset of patients with apparent rotator cuff disease. In most cases, a more chronic tendinitis is implicated, with associated deposition of calcium in the rotator cuff; calcification in the subacromial space is apparent radiographically. Patients usually have a more acutely painful condition, similar to that seen in crystal-induced arthritis. NSAIDs and local glucocorticoid injections are usually helpful, and surgery is indicated in selected cases. Ultrasound therapy has been shown to provide short-term improvement in symptoms and radiographic calcification when compared to placebo.[32]

BICIPITAL TENDINITIS

Bicipital tendinitis occurs in the region of the anterior shoulder, where the long head of the biceps tendon passes through the bicipital groove of the humerus and through the joint to insert over the glenoid cavity. Diagnosis is based on the localization of tenderness anteriorly, though this condition may coexist with rotator cuff tendinitis. Rupture of the tendon may occur occasionally, particularly in older patients, and often presents as a bulge in the biceps muscle. Treatment with local measures and range-of-motion exercises is effective, as in rotator cuff disease, and surgical repair of a ruptured tendon is indicated only in younger patients with acute rupture.

FROZEN SHOULDER (ADHESIVE CAPSULITIS)

Frozen shoulder, or adhesive capsulitis, is characterized by progressive pain and global loss of motion in the shoulder. This condition is usually seen in patients with an underlying rotator cuff tendinitis or bicipital tendinitis but has also been associated with stroke, myocardial infarction, cervical radiculopathy, and pulmonary disease. The pathophysiology of frozen shoulder is unclear, and controversy exists as to how significantly capsular inflammation or fibrosis really contributes to the loss of motion that is characteristic of the condition. Treatment is directed toward pain relief and restoration of function, often with a combination of exercises, local heat, ultrasonography, NSAIDs or mild analgesic medications, and periodic glucocorticoid injections. Maximal rehabilitation of a frozen shoulder often requires 1 to 2 years. Surgical procedures, capsular distention with saline injection, and closed manipulation have reportedly been useful in individual cases. Suprascapular nerve blockade has been shown to improve pain but does not improve function or range of motion in patients with frozen shoulder.[33]

MYOFASCIAL SHOULDER PAIN SYNDROME

Myofascial shoulder pain syndromes are characterized by pain over the trapezius or medial or lateral scapular borders posteriorly, with the finding of reproducible trigger points. These poorly characterized syndromes usually respond to local injection with glucocorticoids and an anesthetic, though local modalities may be needed in more chronic cases.

Chest Wall Pain

Musculoskeletal chest wall pain syndromes account for about 10% to 15% of cases in which adults are seen for chest pain in the emergency room setting, and they account for about 15% to 20% of patients who have had chest pain but whose coronary angiograms are negative.[34] The diagnosis of musculoskeletal chest wall pain requires the finding of consistent areas of tenderness that reproduce the patient's pain. In rare cases, chest pain may result from Tietze syndrome—a benign, painful, nonsuppurative localized swelling of the costosternal, sternoclavicular, or costochondral joints, most often involving the area of the second and third ribs. In most cases, only one area is involved. Young adults are more commonly affected.

More often, patients with musculoskeletal chest wall syndromes have a more diffuse pain syndrome, termed costochondritis or costosternal syndrome, the specific etiology of which is not well understood. Areas of tenderness are not accompanied by heat, erythema, or swelling; multiple areas of tenderness are found, usually in the upper costochondral or costosternal junctions. A number of less common chest wall syndromes have been described, each defined by the area of tenderness (e.g., xiphoidalgia, sternalis syndrome, and slipping rib syndrome). Musculoskeletal chest wall syndromes are usually self-limited and respond to analgesics, local heat, stretching exercises, and local glucocorticoid injection.

Elbow Pain

The most common nonarticular syndromes of the elbow include epicondylitis, olecranon bursitis, and ulnar nerve entrapment.

EPICONDYLITIS

Epicondylitis is caused by an inflammation at the origin of the tendons and muscles serving the forearm; it is usually caused by overuse or by repetitive activity.

Patients typically complain of elbow and forearm pain with activity. When the extensor muscles are involved (i.e., tennis elbow), tenderness is maximal over the lateral epicondyle and aggravated by extension of the wrist against resistance. A similar, less common process may affect the flexor muscles originating at the medial epicondyle (i.e., golfer's elbow).

Epicondylitis usually responds to rest, local heat or ice, NSAIDs, and forearm support to reduce tension at the epicondyle. Local infiltration of glucocorticoids and lidocaine often results in more rapid improvement than other measures in the first month or two but does not appear to affect the outcome over 6 to 12 months.[35,36]

OLECRANON BURSITIS

Olecranon bursitis presents as a discrete swelling with palpable fluid over the tip of the elbow. Traumatic bursitis is characterized by minimal heat or surrounding erythema. The fluid aspirated is noninflammatory and often contains multiple red cells. Infectious bursitis—usually caused by gram-positive skin organisms—is accompanied by heat, erythema, and induration. When infection is suspected, prompt aspiration and culture of the fluid are mandatory. Antibiotics should be started empirically, and the bursa should be reaspirated frequently until the fluid no longer reaccumulates and cultures are negative.[37] Olecranon bursitis may also be part of rheumatoid arthritis or gout, usually in a patient in whom a diagnosis has already been made. On occasion, an initial diagnosis of gout is made by examination of bursal fluid for urate crystals.

ULNAR NERVE ENTRAPMENT

Ulnar nerve entrapment is caused by compression of the ulnar nerve as it passes through the ulnar groove at the elbow[38] [see Chapter 181]. Patients typically complain of pain and numbness that radiates from the elbow to the little finger and the medial side of the hand. An increase in paresthesia with elbow flexion is helpful in making the diagnosis, but nerve conduction studies are often needed to confirm the diagnosis. Conservative therapy with a loose cast may help limit elbow flexion and improve symptoms in some patients; surgical decompression is indicated in patients with disabling pain or weakness.

Hand and Wrist Pain

Painful conditions of the tendons and tendon sheaths of the hand and wrist are often related to repetitive or unaccustomed activities. The resultant edema, inflammation, and fibrosis of the structures interfere with the normal function of the tendon as it moves within the sheath.

DE QUERVAIN TENOSYNOVITIS AND FLEXOR TENOSYNOVITIS

De Quervain tenosynovitis affects the abductor pollicis longus and extensor pollicis brevis. Typical symptoms are pain over the radial aspect of the wrist during activities and tenderness that is usually found over the affected tendons proximal to the level of the carpometacarpal joint of the thumb. Pain is reproduced by stretching the tendons with the thumb inside a closed fist (i.e., the Finkelstein maneuver). Flexor tenosynovitis, or trigger finger, is caused by involvement of the flexor tendons of the digits, usually at the level of the metacarpophalangeal joint. Patients complain of locking of the affected digit in a flexed position, often with a sudden painful release on extension. Treatment of de Quervain tenosynovitis and flexor tenosynovitis may require rest, local heat, immobilization with a splint, or local infiltration with glucocorticoids. Surgical release is rarely required.

CARPAL TUNNEL SYNDROME

Carpal tunnel syndrome is caused by compression of the median nerve at the wrist as it courses with the flexor tendons[38] [see Figure 2 and Chapter 181]. Entrapment is usually associated with flexor tenosynovitis related to overuse or trauma. In addition, an association has been observed with medical conditions such as diabetes mellitus, rheumatoid arthritis, pregnancy, and hypothyroidism, as well as with rare conditions, such as amyloidosis, acromegaly, and localized infection. Carpal tunnel syndrome is relatively common in the general population. A recent study found that 14% of the general population have symptoms suggestive of carpal tunnel syndrome; such symptoms were confirmed by clinical examination and electophysiologic studies in 2% to 3% of the patients studied.[39] In addition, 18% of asymptomatic people were found to have electrophysiologic evidence of median nerve entrapment. Carpal tunnel

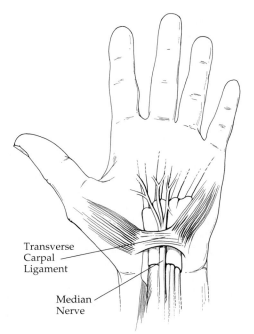

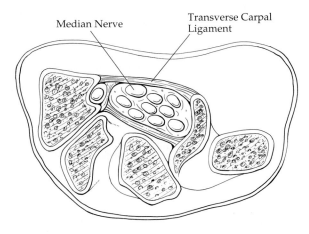

Figure 2 **Carpal tunnel syndrome involves the entrapment of the median nerve in the canal that encloses the nerve and several flexor tendons and that is formed by bones of the wrist and the transverse carpal ligament. Traumatic thickening of the flexor tendon sheaths can compress the median nerve.**

syndrome is more common in persons with occupations that require repetitive wrist movements, awkward wrist positions, or the use of vibrating tools or great force. Patients report numbness, tingling, and pain over the palmar radial aspect of the hand; these symptoms are often worse at night or after use. Reproduction of paresthesia with maximal wrist flexion (i.e., the Phalen test) or tapping over the volar aspect of the wrist (i.e., the Tinel sign) are often considered to be helpful clinical findings. However, a recent review of published studies suggests that the pattern of pain and findings of decreased sensation and weakness of thumb abduction are the most reliable diagnostic findings.[40] Because of the uncertainties in the reliability of diagnostic findings, electrodiagnostic testing is usually necessary to confirm a diagnosis, particularly when surgical intervention is considered.

Conservative treatment measures include use of NSAIDs and placement of a wrist splint in a neutral position. Local injection of glucocorticoids affords short-term relief in most patients, but long-term improvement is less predictable.[41] Surgical decompression by sectioning of the volar carpal ligament results in excellent outcome in 67% to 80% of patients; it is indicated in patients whose conditions respond poorly to conservative therapy, patients with chronic or recurrent symptoms, or patients with weakness or atrophy of the thenar muscles. In a recent study, patients with poor upper extremity function, patients who used alcohol, or patients with worse mental health status were less likely to have good results from surgical therapy.[42]

DUPUYTREN CONTRACTURE

Dupuytren contracture is a fibrosing condition of the palmar and digital fascia that results in thickening and puckering of the palmar skin with subcutaneous nodules and often in flexion contracture of the underlying digit. Dupuytren contracture may be associated with other fibrosing syndromes, with an autosomal dominant inheritance pattern, and possibly with liver disease, epilepsy, and alcoholism. Although spontaneous improvement may be seen, surgical intervention to improve function may be useful in individual cases.

STIFF-HAND SYNDROME

The stiff-hand syndrome, resembling scleroderma, is characterized by thickening of the skin and subcutaneous tissues and generalized limitation of hand and wrist motion. This condition is seen almost exclusively in young patients with long-standing insulin-dependent diabetes mellitus.[43]

Hip Girdle Pain

Pain around the hip girdle is a common complaint in clinical practice. Patients with pain resulting from diseases of the hip joint usually describe pain in the anterior thigh or inguinal region that worsens with weight bearing. More commonly, patients with a chief complaint of hip pain have a problem in one of the nonarticular structures of the hip girdle, usually located posteriorly or laterally [see Table 2]. A multitude of bursae have been described in the hip girdle region. Pain in the upper buttock in and around the gluteal muscles is often referred to as myofascial hip pain or gluteal bursitis. Pain in this area is often difficult to differentiate from referred lumbar pain. Local therapy with heat, stretching, or glucocorticoid injection is usually helpful, but many patients require long-term therapy.

Table 2 Differential Diagnosis of Hip Girdle Pain

Clinical Syndrome	Location of Pain	Diagnostic Features and Comments
Acetabular joint pain	Anterior hip (inguinal)	Worse with weight bearing Radiographic confirmation
Ileopectineal bursitis	Anterior hip (inguinal)	Pain with extension Normal radiograph ? Ultrasound or CT scanning
Meralgia paresthetica	Anterior hip (midthigh)	Numbness and tingling Normal hip movement
Trochanteric bursitis	Lateral hip, posterior hip, or both	Normal hip movement Point tenderness Relief with glucocorticoid injection
Myofascial pain	Posterior hip	Localized tenderness Relief with glucocorticoid injection ? Mimics lumbar disease
Gluteal bursitis	Posterior hip	Localized tenderness Relief with glucocorticoid injection ? Mimics lumbar disease
Ischiogluteal bursitis	Posterior hip	Normal hip movement Point tenderness

TROCHANTERIC BURSITIS (GREATER TROCHANTERIC PAIN SYNDROME)

Trochanteric bursitis is probably the most common cause of hip girdle pain, although a recent study using MRI suggests that most patients with this pain syndrome may have tendinitis or a partial tear of the gluteus medius tendon.[44] Patients typically complain of pain over the lateral aspect of the hip girdle, sometimes radiating down the thigh, that is worse at night when they lie on the affected side. Pain is sometimes present when the patient arises from a chair, but it tends to improve with ambulation. Point tenderness over the lateral or posterior aspect of the greater trochanter is usually diagnostic, though some patients with referred lumbar facet or disk disease may have a similar presentation. Patients with more severe pain may have a positive Trendelenburg sign on physical examination. Local heat and NSAIDs may be helpful, and a local glucocorticoid injection is curative in most patients. In refractory cases, repeated injections, physical therapy, and, in rare instances, surgical excision of the bursa may be indicated.

ISCHIOGLUTEAL BURSITIS

Ischiogluteal bursitis results from an irritation of the bursa in the area of the attachments of the hamstring and gluteal muscles at the ischial tuberosity. The condition may be brought on by prolonged sitting or by pressure in the area and usually responds to local heat, stretching, or glucocorticoid injection.

ILIOPECTINEAL BURSITIS

Iliopectineal bursitis, which is caused by irritation of the bursa between the iliopsoas muscle and the inguinal ligament, is an uncommon cause of inguinal pain and may mimic true hip joint disease. The diagnosis is suggested by the presence of inguinal pain that is aggravated by extension of the hip (in a patient whose hip x-ray is normal). Confirmation by ultrasonography or CT scanning may be required. Treatment is usually with local measures or, in rare cases, by means of surgical excision.

MERALGIA PARESTHETICA

Meralgia paresthetica is characterized by intermittent paresthesia, hypoesthesia, or hyperesthesia over the upper anterolateral thigh. The syndrome is caused by an entrapment of the lateral femoral cutaneous nerve at the level of the anterosuperior iliac spine where the nerve passes through the lateral end of the inguinal ligament. Causes include local trauma, rapid weight gain, and the wearing of constrictive garments around the hips. Useful therapies include avoidance of pressure in the area, weight loss, and local infiltration of glucocorticoids at the level of nerve exit.

Knee and Lower Leg Pain

Clinically, it can be difficult to differentiate articular from nonarticular knee pain. Most patients with articular knee pain have a relatively diffuse pain that is not well localized to one area of the knee. Physical examination shows loss of motion, crepitus (in osteoarthritis), warmth (in inflammatory arthritis), or the presence of effusion. If knee pain is localized or if the knee has full range of motion without warmth, crepitus, or effusion, one of the following nonarticular syndromes should be considered: infrapatellar tendinitis, Osgood-Schlatter disease, prepatellar bursitis, anserine bursitis, anterior knee pain syndromes, and restless legs syndrome.

INFRAPATELLAR TENDINITIS

Infrapatellar tendinitis, or jumper's knee, causes anterior knee pain below the patella and is often related to athletic activities. Tenderness is localized to the infrapatellar tendon, with no associated swelling, and conservative measures almost always result in resolution of symptoms.

OSGOOD-SCHLATTER DISEASE

Osgood-Schlatter disease is characterized by pain and swelling over the tibial tubercle at the tendon insertion point. This condition is seen predominantly in adolescent males and is thought to represent a traumatic avulsion injury. Symptoms usually resolve with temporary immobilization and slow resumption of activities.

PREPATELLAR BURSITIS

Prepatellar bursitis, or housemaid's knee, causes pain and swelling in the anterior knee superficial to the patella and infrapatellar tendon. An area of localized fluid collection is usually detectable; aspiration is often needed for diagnosis. As in olecranon bursitis of the elbow, prepatellar bursitis may be associated with trauma, localized bacterial infection, and, less commonly, gout, rheumatoid arthritis, and atypical infections. The differentiation between trauma and infection is particularly important for initiation of appropriate therapy.

ANSERINE BURSITIS

Anserine bursitis, which is caused by irritation of the bursa near the attachment of the sartorius and hamstring muscles at the medial tibial condyle, is a common cause of medial knee pain. Patients with this condition complain of pain at night or when climbing stairs, and an area of localized tenderness can be found on examination. Coexistent osteoarthritis of the knee joint is present in many patients, and relief with local heat or injection of glucocorticoids and anesthetic may be helpful both diagnostically and therapeutically.

ANTERIOR KNEE PAIN SYNDROMES

Anterior knee (patellofemoral) pain syndromes usually manifest themselves as pain and crepitus associated with activities that require knee flexion under load conditions (e.g., stair climbing).[45] Physical findings that help with diagnosis include (1) reproduction of pain with pressure over the patella during knee motion and (2) tenderness over the medial surface of the patella. The cause of most anterior knee pain syndromes is uncertain, but the pain may be related to misalignment of the quadriceps with lateral patellar subluxation, patella alta, hypermobility, or findings of chondromalacia of the patella on arthroscopic evaluation. Local measures and an exercise program that emphasizes isometric quadriceps strengthening is helpful in most patients. Some patients require arthroscopic intervention to diagnose and correct articular irregularities or patellar misalignment.

RESTLESS LEGS SYNDROME

Restless legs syndrome is characterized by unpleasant, deep-seated paresthesia in both legs that usually occurrs during rest and that is relieved by movement.[46] Most patients with this syndrome have associated disturbance of sleep, and many have abnormal periodic leg movements during sleep [see Chapter 187]. Although idiopathic in most patients, restless legs syndrome has been associated with iron deficiency, uremia, pregnancy, diabetes, and polyneuropathies. Patients with severe symptoms may respond to levodopa-carbidopa. However, some patients may require treatment with bromocriptine, carbamazepine, clonidine, benzodiazepines, or opioids.

Ankle and Foot Pain

Nonarticular foot and ankle pain is best approached with a consideration of the region affected: the forefoot, midfoot, or hindfoot [see Figure 3].

FOREFOOT PAIN

Hallux valgus is the leading cause of forefoot pain. It is a common deformity that causes pain because of direct pressure over the first metatarsophalangeal joint resulting from footwear or because of pressure over the lateral toe joints caused by crowding of the toes. In the lateral toes, hammer toe (i.e., plantar flexion of the proximal interphalangeal joint), claw toe (i.e., plantar flexion of the proximal and distal interphalangeal joints), or mallet toe (i.e., isolated flexion contracture of the distal interphalangeal joint) may be associated with a dorsiflexion contracture of the metatarsophalangeal joint. Initial treatment of these problems should begin with adequate footwear that allows ample width for the metatarsal heads, individualized orthoses, and surgical correction (reserved for patients with persistent pain). Morton neuroma is an entrapment neuropathy of the interdigital nerve, with or without an associated plantar neuroma, that is most commonly seen between the third and fourth metatarsal heads. Patients report pain and paresthesia radiating into the affected toes; tenderness between the metatarsal heads that reproduces the described symptoms will also be found. Orthoses to decrease pressure in the area, local glucocorticoid injection, or surgical excision of the neuroma may be needed to relieve symptoms.

MIDFOOT PAIN

Midfoot pain is usually the result of deformities of the arch of the foot or arthritic changes of the midfoot joints. Patients with a cavus foot deformity, peripheral neuropathies, or previous liga-

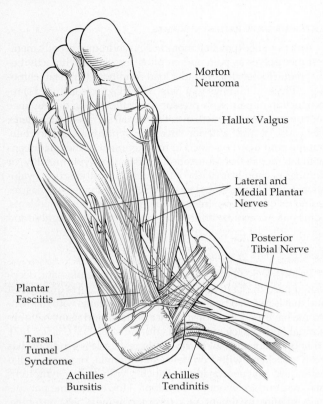

Figure 3   In the anterior foot, hallux valgus may cause diffuse pain, whereas Morton neuroma is usually localized. Tarsal tunnel syndrome causes paresthesias over the medial and plantar aspect. Plantar fasciitis and Achilles tendinitis are common causes of posterior foot pain.

mentous injuries from sprains may be predisposed to excessive stresses on the midfoot and early osteoarthritic changes. Tarsal tunnel syndrome is caused by entrapment of the posterior tibial nerve under the flexor retinaculum on the medial side of the ankle. Symptoms of pain and paresthesia over the plantar and distal foot and toes are usually present, and the Tinel sign may be positive. Tarsal tunnel syndrome is much less common and more difficult to diagnose than carpal tunnel syndrome in the wrist. Treatment consists of splinting and NSAIDs. Local glucocorticoid injection and surgical decompression are not as predictably successful as in carpal tunnel syndrome.

HINDFOOT PAIN

Plantar fasciitis is one of the most common causes of hindfoot pain. Patients report pain over the plantar aspect of the heel and midfoot that worsens with walking. Localized tenderness along the plantar fascia or at the insertion of the calcaneus is helpful in diagnosis. Plantar fasciitis is associated with obesity, pes planus, and activities that stress the plantar fascia and may also be seen in systemic arthropathies such as ankylosing spondylitis and Reiter syndrome. Although radiographic spurs in the affected area are common, they may also be seen in asymptomatic persons and are therefore not diagnostic. Orthoses, heel cord stretching exercises, NSAIDs, and local glucocorticoid injection may be helpful, whereas surgery is seldom indicated. Posterior heel pain is usually caused by Achilles tendinitis or by bursitis of the bursae that lie superficial or deep to the insertion of the Achilles tendon at the calcaneus. Although usually associated with overactivity, Achilles tendinitis may also be part of ankylosing spondylitis and Reiter syndrome. NSAIDs and orthoses designed to reduce stress

on the tendon (e.g., heel lifts) are usually helpful. In most cases, glucocorticoid injections in the Achilles tendon area should be avoided because of the risk of tendon rupture.

Fibromyalgia

Fibromyalgia is a chronic musculoskeletal pain syndrome associated with widespread pain and localized areas of deep muscle tenderness.[47] Patients typically complain of severe chronic pain, usually with stiffness that is most pronounced in the axial skeleton, shoulders, and hips, but the distal extremities are sometimes painful as well. Most patients complain of fatigue, which may be overwhelming, and nearly all patients report nonrefreshing sleep. A variety of other symptoms may be present, including headache, irritable bowel syndrome, paresthesia, swelling, and depression or anxiety. Physical examination of the joints and muscles in patients with fibromyalgia is normal except for the presence of multiple localized areas of tenderness in periarticular areas, most commonly in specific anatomic areas [*see Figure 4*]. The diagnosis of fibromyalgia is based on the history of widespread chronic pain and the findings of tender points at a majority of these typical areas. Laboratory studies such as an erythrocyte sedimentation rate, muscle enzymes, thyroid profile, antinuclear antibodies, rheumatoid factor, or radiographs of specific areas are appropriate in the initial evaluation of patients to exclude other potential causes of widespread pain and fatigue.

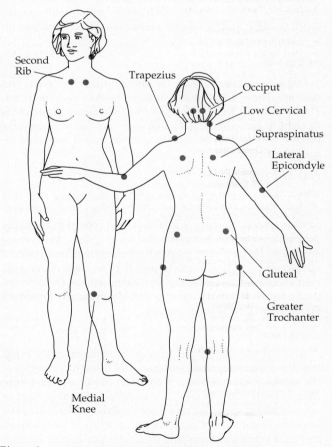

Figure 4   Patients with fibromyalgia exhibit many specific, widespread tender points that are revealed by deep palpation.

The pathogenesis of fibromyalgia is uncertain and probably complex. Most studies of patients with fibromyalgia have shown an increased incidence of previous depression or other psychological disorders, although a majority of patients are not clinically depressed at the time of diagnosis. Other abnormalities observed include disturbance of stage 4 sleep, decreased skeletal muscle high-energy phosphates, abnormalities in the concentration of substance P in the cerebrospinal fluid, subtle decreases in growth hormone, and other changes in hypothalamic-pituitary function.[48] The relationship of these changes to the etiology and pathogenesis of this syndrome is unclear.

Therapy for fibromyalgia is usually only partially effective. Low-dose tricyclic antidepressants (e.g., amitriptyline, 10 to 50 mg at bedtime) and most other antidepressants have been shown to lead to improvement in symptoms when compared to placebo.[49] Other agents that improve the quality of sleep may be effective as well. NSAIDs are less effective in general but may be useful in certain patients. Cardiovascular-fitness training and aerobic-exercise programs have been shown to be effective in many patients, and strategies that involve training patients in techniques of internal control ("mind-body therapy") may be useful as well.[50] Most patients with fibromyalgia continue to have symptoms for years. The disease course is characterized by temporary improvements and relapses; complete remission occurs in a few patients.

References

1. Sheon RP, Moskowitz RW, Goldberg VM: Soft Tissue Rheumatic Pain: Recognition, Management, Prevention, 3rd ed. Lea & Febiger, Philadelphia, 1996

2. Eck JC, Hodges SD, Humphreys SC: Whiplash: a review of a commonly misunderstood injury. Am J Med 110:651, 2001

3. Cassidy JD, Carroll LJ, Cote P, et al: Effect of eliminating compensation for pain and suffering on the outcome of insurance claims for whiplash injury. N Engl J Med 342:1179, 2000

4. Barnsley L, Lord SM, Wallis BJ, et al: Lack of effect of intraarticular corticosteroids for chronic pain in the cervical zygapophyseal joints. N Engl J Med 330:1047, 1994

5. Lord SM, Barnsley L, Wallis BJ, et al: Percutaneous radio frequency neurotomy for chronic cervical zygoapophyseal-joint pain. N Engl J Med 335:1721, 1996

6. Hoving JL, Koes BW, de Vet HC, et al: Manual therapy, physical therapy, or continued care by a general practitioner for patients with neck pain: a randomized, controlled trial. Ann Intern Med 136:713, 2002

7. Swezey RL: Conservative treatment of cervical radiculopathy. J Clin Rheumatol 5:65, 1999

8. Deyo RA, Weinstein JN: Low back pain. N Engl J Med 344:363, 2001

9. Andersson GB: Epidemiological features of chronic low-back pain. Lancet 354:581, 1999

10. Lee P, Helewa A, Goldsmith CH, et al: Low back pain: prevalence and risk factors in an industrial setting. J Rheumatol 28:346, 2001

11. Von Korff M, Moore JC: Stepped care for back pain: activating approaches for primary care. Ann Intern Med 134:911, 2001

12. Deyo RA, Diehl AK, Rosenthal M: How many days of bed rest for acute low back pain? A randomized clinical trial. N Engl J Med 315:1064, 1986

13. Malmivaara A, Hakkinen U, Aro T, et al: The treatment of acute low back pain: bed rest, exercises, or ordinary activity? N Engl J Med 332:351, 1995

14. Vroomen PC, de Krom MC, Wilmink JT, et al: Lack of effectiveness of bed rest for sciatica. N Engl J Med 340:418, 1999

15. Andersson GBJ, Lucente T, Davis AM, et al: A comparison of osteopathic spinal manipulation with standard care for patients with low back pain. N Engl J Med 341:1426, 1999

16. Cherkin DC, Deyo RA, Battie M, et al: A comparison of physical therapy, chiropractic manipulation, and provision of an educational booklet for the treatment of patients with low back pain. N Engl J Med 339:1021, 1998

17. Moffett JK, Torgerson D, Bell-Syer S, et al: Randomised controlled trial of exercise for low back pain: clinical outcomes, costs, and preferences. BMJ 319:279, 1999

18. Daltroy LH, Iverson JD, Larson MG, et al: A controlled trial of an educational program to prevent low back injuries. N Engl J Med 337:322, 1997

19. Jensen MC, Brant-Zawadzki MN, Obuchowski N, et al: Magnetic resonance imaging of the lumbar spine in people without back pain. N Engl J Med 331:69, 1994

20. Deen HG: Diagnosis and management of lumbar disk disease. Mayo Clin Proc 71:283, 1996

21. Salerno SM, Browning R, Jackson JL: The effect of antidepressant treatment on chronic back pain: a meta-analysis. Arch Intern Med 162:19, 2002

22. Carette S, Marcoux S, Truchon R, et al: A controlled trial of corticosteroid injections into facet joints for chronic low back pain. N Engl J Med 325:1002, 1991

23. Mannion AF, Muntener M, Taimela S, et al: Comparison of three active therapies for chronic low back pain: results of a randomized clinical trial with one-year follow-up. Rheumatology (Oxford) 40:772, 2001

24. Cherkin DC, Eisenberg D, Sherman KJ, et al: Randomized trial comparing traditional Chinese medical acupuncture, therapeutic massage, and self-care education for chronic low back pain. Arch Intern Med 161:1081, 2001

25. Arbit E, Pannullo S: Lumbar stenosis: a clinical review. Clin Orthop 384:137, 2001

26. Saint-Louis LA: Lumbar spinal stenosis assessment with computed tomography, magnetic resonance imaging, and myelography. Clin Orthop 384:122, 2001

27. Simotas AC: Nonoperative treatment for lumbar spinal stenosis. Clin Orthop 384:153, 2001

28. Amundsen T, Weber H, Nordal HJ, et al: Lumbar spinal stenosis: conservative or surgical management? A prospective 10-year study. Spine 25:1424, 2000

29. Steinfeld R, Valente RM, Stuart MJ: A commonsense approach to shoulder problems. Mayo Clin Proc 74:785, 1999

30. Green S, Buchbinder R, Glazier R, et al: Systematic review of randomised controlled trials of interventions for painful shoulder: selection criteria, outcome assessment, and efficacy. BMJ 316:354, 1998

31. van der Windt DA, Koes BW, Deville W, et al: Effectiveness of corticosteroid injections versus physiotherapy for treatment of painful stiff shoulder in primary care: randomised trial. BMJ 317:1292, 1998

32. Ebenbichler GR, Erdogmus CB, Resch KL, et al: Ultrasound therapy for calcific tendinitis of the shoulder. N Engl J Med 340:1533, 1999

33. Dahan TH, Fortin L, Pelletier M, et al: Double blind randomized clinical trial examining the efficacy of bupivacaine suprascapular nerve blocks in frozen shoulder. J Rheumatol 27:1464, 2000

34. Wise CM: Chest wall syndromes. Curr Opin Rheumatol 6:197, 1994

35. Hay EM, Paterson SM, Lewis M, et al: Pragmatic randomised controlled trial of local corticosteroid injection and naproxen for treatment of lateral epicondylitis of elbow in primary care. BMF 319:964, 1999

36. Smidt N, van der Windt DA, Assendelft WJ, et al: Corticosteroid injections, physiotherapy, or a wait-and-see policy for lateral epicondylitis: a randomised controlled trial. Lancet 359:657, 2002

37. Laupland KB, Davies HD: Olecranon septic bursitis managed in an ambulatory setting. The Calgary Home Parenteral Therapy Program Study Group. Clin Invest Med 24:171, 2001

38. Dawson D: Entrapment neuropathies of the upper extremities. N Engl J Med 329:2013, 1993

39. Atroshi I, Gummesson C, Johnsson R, et al: Prevalence of carpal tunnel syndrome in a general population. JAMA 282:153, 1999

40. D'Arcy CA, McGee S: The rational clinical examination: does this patient have carpal tunnel syndrome? JAMA 283:3110, 2000

41. O'Gardaigh D, Merry P: Corticosteroid injection for the treatment of carpal tunnel syndrome. Ann Rheum Dis 59:918, 2000

42. Katz JN, Losina E, Amick BC 3rd, et al: Predictors of outcomes of carpal tunnel release. Arthritis Rheum 44:1184, 2001

43. Kapoor A, Sibbitt W: Contractures in diabetes mellitus: the syndrome of limited joint mobility. Semin Arthritis Rheum 18:168, 1989

44. Bird PA, Oakley SP, Shnier R, et al: Prospective evaluation of magnetic resonance imaging and physical examination findings in patients with greater trochanteric pain syndrome. Arthritis Rheum 44:2138, 2001

45. Bernstein J: Patellar disorders. J Clin Rheumatol 5:90, 1999

46. O'Keeffe ST: Restless legs syndrome: a review. Arch Intern Med 156:243, 1996

47. Goldenberg DL: Fibromyalgia syndrome a decade later: what have we learned? Arch Intern Med 159:777, 1999

48. Crofford LJ, Clauw DJ: Fibromyalgia: where are we a decade after the American College of Rheumatology classification criteria were developed? Arthritis Rheum 46:1136, 2002

49. O'Malley PG, Balden E, Tomkins G, et al: Treatment of fibromyalgia with antidepressants: a meta-analysis. J Gen Intern Med 15:659, 2000

50. Hadhazy VA, Ezzo J, Creamer P, et al: Mind-body therapies for the treatment of fibromyalgia: a systematic review. J Rheumatol 27:2911, 2000

Acknowledgments

Figures 1 and 3   Susan E. Brust, C.M.I.

Figure 2   Lynn O'Kelley.